D1737517

OCULAR
INFECTION
&IMMUNITY

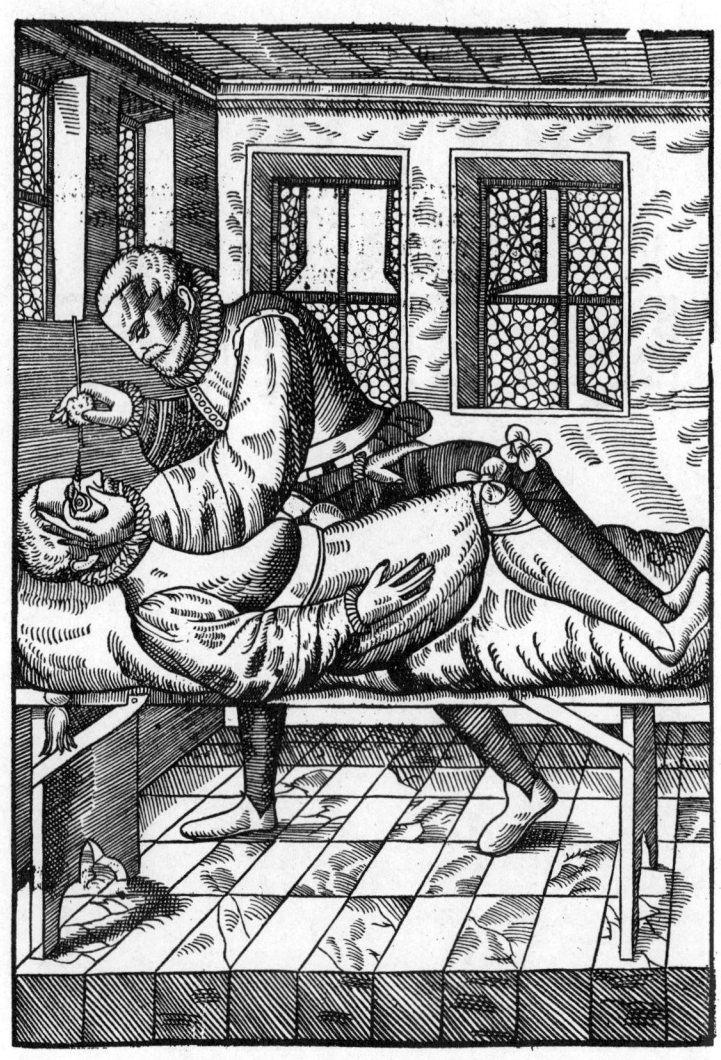

"The application of medicinal agents to the eye" is illustrated in this wood-cut, originally published in the 16th century text *Ophthalmodouleia,* by Georg Bartisch, which was one of the first large handbooks on ophthalmology to be published in Europe. Our knowledge of disease has progressed remarkably in the four centuries since Bartisch attributed a variety of maladies of the eye to witches, gnomes, and magical spells. Research, much of it in the past four decades, has brought the understanding of many ophthalmic diseases down to the molecular level. *Ocular Infection & Immunity* documents that progress in one focused, but far-reaching, discipline within ophthalmology: the study of infectious and inflammatory diseases.

OCULAR
INFECTION
& IMMUNITY

Jay S. Pepose, MD, PhD

Bernard Becker Professor of Ophthalmology,
Director, Corneal and External Diseases,
Department of Ophthalmology and Visual Sciences,
Washington University School of Medicine,
St. Louis, Missouri

Gary N. Holland, MD

Professor of Ophthalmology,
UCLA School of Medicine;
Director, UCLA Ocular Inflammatory Disease Center,
Jules Stein Eye Institute;
Chief, Ophthalmology Section,
Department of Veterans Affairs Medical Center, West Los Angeles,
Los Angeles, California

Kirk R. Wilhelmus, MD

Professor of Ophthalmology,
Department of Ophthalmology,
Baylor College of Medicine,
Houston, Texas

with 916 illustrations

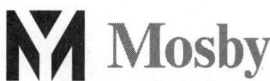 Mosby

St. Louis Baltimore Boston Carlsbad Chicago Naples New York Philadelphia Portland
London Madrid Mexico City Singapore Sydney Tokyo Toronto Wiesbaden

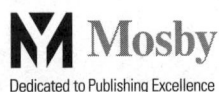
Mosby
Dedicated to Publishing Excellence

A Times Mirror
Company

Publisher: Anne S. Patterson
Senior Editor: Laurel Craven
Developmental Editor: Dana Battaglia, Kim Cox
Project Manager: Dana Peick
Production Supervisor: Cindy Deichmann
Manufacturing Manager: Betty Richmond
Editing, Design, and Production: Progressive Publishing Alternatives

Printed in the United States of America
Composition by Progressive Information Technologies
Printing/binding by Maple-Vail Book Manufacturing Group

Mosby–Year Book, Inc.
11830 Westline Industrial Drive, St. Louis, Missouri 63146

Library of Congress Cataloging-in-Publication Data

Ocular infection and immunity / [edited by] Jay S. Pepose, Gary N.
   Holland, Kirk R. Wilhelmus.
      p.   cm.
   Includes bibliographical references and index.
   ISBN 0-8016-6757-7
   1. Eye—Immunology.   2. Eye—Infections.   I. Pepose, Jay S.
II. Holland, Gary N.   III. Wilhelmus, Kirk R.
   [DNLM: 1. Eye Infections—immunology. 2. Inflammation—
immunology.   WW 160 021 1995]
   RE68.027   1995
   617.7′1—dc20
   DNLM/DLC
   for Library of Congress   95-32959
                                                              CIP

94 95 96 97 98   /   9 8 7 6 5 4 3 2 1

Contributors

MARK B. ABELSON, MD
Senior Clinical Scientist,
Department of Ophthalmology/Immunology,
Harvard Medical School,
Eye Research Institute,
Boston, Massachusetts

LEVENT AKDUMAN, MD
Clinical Fellow, Retina Service,
Department of Ophthalmology and Visual Sciences,
Washington University School of Medicine,
St. Louis, Missouri

EDUARDO C. ALFONSO, MD
Associate Professor,
Bascom Palmer Eye Institute,
University of Miami School of Medicine,
Miami, Florida

HASSAN ALIZADEH, PhD
Department of Ophthalmology,
University of Texas Southwestern Medical Center at Dallas,
Dallas, Texas

KOKI AOKI, MD, DMSc
Aoki Eye Clinic,
Sapporo, Japan

ANTHONY C. ARNOLD, MD
Chief, Neuro-Ophthalmology Division;
Director, UCLA Optic Neuropathy Center,
Jules Stein Eye Institute,
Los Angeles, California

ISAAC ASHKENAZI, MD
Department of Ophthalmology,
Goldschlager Eye Institute,
Chaim Sheba Medical Center,
Sackler School of Medicine,
Tel-Aviv University,
Tel-Aviv, Israel

SALLY S. ATHERTON, PhD
Professor,
Department of Cellular and Structural Biology,
University of Texas Health Science Center at San Antonio,
San Antonio, Texas

ANNETTE S. BACON, MA, FRCOphth
Consultant Ophthalmologist,
Royal Berkshire Hospital,
Reading, England

PAUL R. BADENOCH, PhD
Senior Hospital Scientist,
Department of Ophthalmology,
Flinders Medical Centre,
Bedford Park, South Australia, Australia

EDWARD BARON, MD
Assistant Clinical Professor,
State University of New York,
Health Sciences Center at Brooklyn,
Downstate Medical Center,
Brooklyn, New York

ROY W. BECK, MD, PhD
Director,
Jaeb Center for Health Research,
Tampa, Florida

RUBENS BELFORT, JR., MD, PhD
Professor and Chairman,
Department of Ophthalmology,
Escola Paulista de Medicina,
Hospital São Paulo,
São Paulo, Brazil

CONSTANCE A. BENSON, MD
Associate Professor of Medicine/Infectious Diseases,
Rush Medical College;
Associate Attending Physician,
Department of Medicine,
Rush-Presbyterian-St. Luke's Medical Center,
Chicago, Illinois

ETIENNE BLOCH-MICHEL, MD
Director, Ocular Immunopathology Unit
Centre Hospitalier et Universitaire Bicêtre
Paris, France;
Head, Department of Ophthalmology,
Institute Gustave Roussy,
Villesure, France

R. WAYNE BOWMAN, MD
Associate Professor,
Department of Ophthalmology,
University of Texas Southwestern Medical Center at Dallas,
Dallas, Texas

JILL M. BRODY, MD
Assistant Professor of Ophthalmology,
Southern Illinois University School of Medicine,
Springfield, Illinois

DAVID M. BROWN, MD
Vitreoretinal Consultants,
Houston, Texas

ROGER J. BUCKLEY, MA, FRCS, FRCOphth
Honorary Clinical Teacher,
Institute of Ophthalmology,
University of London;
Consultant Ophthalmologist and Director,
Contact Lens Department,
Moorfields Eye Hospital,
London, England

JOHN D. BULLOCK, MD
Professor and Chairman,
Department of Ophthalmology;
Professor of Surgery (Plastic);
Past Associate Professor of Microbiology and Immunology,
Wright State University School of Medicine,
Dayton, Ohio

CARL B. CAMRAS, MD
Professor and Vice-Chairman,
Department of Ophthalmology;
Director of the Glaucoma Service,
University of Nebraska Medical Center,
Omaha, Nebraska

DAVID M. CHACKO, MD, PhD
Assistant Professor,
Department of Ophthalmology;
Director of the Retina Service;
Director of the Residency Program,
University of Nebraska Medical Center,
Omaha, Nebraska

CHI-CHAO CHAN, MD
Chief, Section of Immunopathology,
Laboratory of Immunology,
National Eye Institute;
Ophthalmologist,
Clinical Center,
National Institutes of Health,
Bethesda, Maryland

JOHN W. CHANDLER, MD
Professor and Head,
Department of Ophthalmology and Visual Sciences;
Professor of Biochemistry,
University of Illinois at Chicago,
College of Medicine,
Chicago, Illinois

DOUGLAS J. COSTER, MBBS, FRACS, FRCS, FRACOphth
Professor and Chairman,
Department of Ophthalmology,
Flinders Medical Centre,
Bedford Park, South Australia, Australia

SCOTT W. COUSINS, MD
Assistant Professor,
Departments of Ophthalmology, Microbiology, and
  Immunology,
Bascom Palmer Eye Institute,
University of Miami School of Medicine,
Miami, Florida

WILLIAM W. CULBERTSON, MD
Professor of Ophthalmology,
Bascom Palmer Eye Institute,
University of Miami School of Medicine,
Miami, Florida

TROY E. DANIELS, DDS, MS
Professor,
Department of Stomatology,
School of Dentistry;
Department of Pathology,
School of Medicine,
University of California, San Francisco,
San Francisco, California

RAYMOND J. DATTWYLER, MD
Associate Professor of Medicine,
Department of Medicine,
State University of New York at Stony Brook,
Stony Brook, New York

PAUL T. DAVIDSON, MD
Clinical Professor of Medicine,
School of Medicine,
University of Southern California;
Director of Tuberculosis Control,
Los Angeles County Department of Health Services,
Public Health Programs and Services,
Los Angeles, California

JANET L. DAVIS, MD
Associate Professor of Ophthalmology,
Department of Ophthalmology,
Bascom Palmer Eye Institute,
University of Miami School of Medicine,
Miami, Florida

CHANDLER R. DAWSON, MD
Director,
Francis I. Proctor Foundation;
Professor of Ophthalmology,
University of California, San Francisco,
San Francisco, California

RICHARD D. DIX, PhD
Associate Professor,
Departments of Ophthalmology, Microbiology,
    Immunology, and Neurology,
Bascom Palmer Eye Institute,
University of Miami School of Medicine,
Miami, Florida

EDMUND C. DUNKEL, PhD
Assistant Professor,
Department of Ophthalmology;
Associate Scientist,
Schepens Eye Research Institute,
Harvard Medical School,
Boston, Massachusetts

JAMES P. DUNN, MD
Assistant Professor of Ophthalmology,
The Wilmer Ophthalmological Institute,
The Johns Hopkins Hospital,
Baltimore, Maryland

DAVID L. EASTY, MD
Professor of Ophthalmology;
Head, Department of Ophthalmology,
University of Bristol,
Bristol Eye Hospital;
Honorary Consultant,
Bristol Healthcare Trust,
Bristol, England

JOHN E. EDWARDS, JR., MD
Chief, Division of Infectious Diseases,
Harbor/UCLA Medical Center,
UCLA School of Medicine,
Torrance, California

JOSEPH J. ESPOSITO, PhD
Chief,
Poxvirus Section,
National Center for Infectious Diseases;
Director,
World Health Organization Collaborating Center for
    Smallpox and Other Poxvirus Infections,
Atlanta, Georgia

SANDY T. FELDMAN, MD
Assistant Professor in Residence;
Director, Refractive Surgical Service,
Department of Ophthalmology,
University of California, San Diego,
La Jolla, California

THOMAS A. FERGUSON, PhD
Assistant Professor,
Department of Ophthalmology and Visual Sciences,
Washington University School of Medicine,
St. Louis, Missouri

**LINDA A. FICKER, BSc (Hons), MBBS, FRCS,
    FRCOphth**
Director, Corneal Service,
Moorfields Eye Hospital,
Institute of Ophthalmology,
London, England

THOMAS D. FITZSIMMONS, MD
Assistant Instructor,
Department of Ophthalmology,
University of Texas Southwestern Medical Center,
Dallas, Texas

ROBERT Y. FOOS, MD
Professor of Pathology Emeritus,
Jules Stein Eye Institute,
University of California, Los Angeles
Los Angeles, California

RICHARD K. FORSTER, MD
Professor of Ophthalmology,
Bascom Palmer Eye Institute,
University of Miami School of Medicine,
Miami, Florida

C. STEPHEN FOSTER, MD, FACS
Professor of Ophthalmology,
Department of Ophthalmology;
Director, Immunology Service,
Massachusetts Eye and Ear Infirmary,
Harvard Medical School,
Boston, Massachusetts

GARY N. FOULKS, MD
Professor of Ophthalmology,
Duke University;
Director, Corneal Service,
Duke University Eye Center,
Durham, North Carolina

RUDOLPH M. FRANKLIN, MD
Director of Research,
Bob Hope Eye Research Center,
St. Joseph Hospital,
Houston, Texas

WILLIAM R. FREEMAN, MD
Department of Ophthalmology,
School of Medicine,
University of California, San Diego,
La Jolla, California

MITCHELL D. FRIEDLAENDER, MD
Director, Cornea and Refractive Surgery,
Scripps Clinic and Research Foundation;
Adjunct Member,
Scripps Research Institute,
La Jolla, California

ALAN H. FRIEDMAN, MD
Clinical Professor of Ophthalmology and Pathology,
Department of Ophthalmology and Pathology,
Mount Sinai School of Medicine,
New York, New York

J. DONALD M. GASS, MD
Professor of Ophthalmology,
Bascom Palmer Eye Institute,
University of Miami School of Medicine,
Miami, Florida

CHRISTINE GENOVESE, PhD
Associate Research Scientist,
Department of Ophthalmology,
Allegheny Singer Research Institute,
Pittsburgh, Pennsylvania

MICHELLE A. GEORGE, BS
Assistant Director, Ocular Allergy Laboratory,
Department of Immunology,
Eye Research Institute,
Boston, Massachusetts

IGAL GERY, PhD
Head, Section on Experimental Immunology,
Laboratory of Immunology,
National Eye Institute,
National Institutes of Health,
Bethesda, Maryland

BEN J. GLASGOW, MD
Assistant Professor,
Department of Ophthalmology and Pathology,
UCLA School of Medicine,
Jules Stein Eye Institute,
Los Angeles, California

ROBERT A. GOLDBERG, MD
Associate Professor of Ophthalmology,
UCLA School of Medicine;
Chief, Division of Orbital and Ophthalmic Plastic Surgery;
Director, Orbital Disease Center,
Jules Stein Eye Institute,
Los Angeles, California

LYNN K. GORDON, MD, PhD
Assistant Clinical Professor,
Department of Ophthalmology,
UCLA School of Medicine;
Associate Chief, Ophthalmology Section,
Department of Veterans Affairs Medical Center, West Los Angeles,
Los Angeles, California

Y. JEROLD GORDON, MD
Professor of Ophthalmology;
Director of Education,
Department of Ophthalmology,
University of Pittsburgh School of Medicine;
Chief, Cornea Service,
Health Center Ophthalmology,
University of Pittsburgh Medical Center,
Pittsburgh, Pennsylvania

ELIZABETH M. GRAHAM, FRCP, FRCOphth
Consultant in Medical Ophthalmology,
St. Thomas' Hospital,
National Hospital for Neurology and Neurosurgery,
London, England

ROBERT HAIMOVICI, MD
Assistant Professor of Ophthalmology,
Boston University School of Medicine,
Boston, Massachusetts

MARGARET R. HAMMERSCHLAG, MD
Professor of Pediatrics and Medicine,
Department of Pediatrics,
SUNY Health Science Center at Brooklyn,
Brooklyn, New York

DAVID R. HARDTEN, MD
Clinical Assistant Professor,
Department of Ophthalmology,
University of Minnesota;
Attending Surgeon,
Phillips Eye Institute,
Minneapolis, Minnesota;
Attending Surgeon,
St. Paul Ramsey Medical Center,
St. Paul, Minnesota

BARTON F. HAYNES, MD
Frederic M. Hanes Professor of Medicine;
Chief, Division of Rheumatology and Immunology,
Department of Medicine,
Duke University Medical Center,
Durham, North Carolina

LINDA D. HAZLETT, PhD
Professor,
Departments of Anatomy/Cell Biology and
  Immunology/Microbiology,
Wayne State University School of Medicine,
Detroit, Michigan

CRAIG J. HELM, MD
Department of Ophthalmology,
Portsmouth Naval Medical Center,
Portsmouth, Virginia

ROBERT L. HENDRICKS, PhD
Professor,
Department of Ophthalmology and Visual Sciences,
University of Illinois at Chicago;
Lions of Illinois Eye Research Institute,
Chicago, Illinois

WILLIAM G. HODGE, MD
Assistant Professor of Ophthalmology,
Ottawa Health Science Center,
University of Ottawa Eye Institute,
Ottawa General Hospital,
Ottawa, Ontario, Canada

EDWARD J. HOLLAND, MD
Associate Professor,
Director, Cornea and External Disease Service,
Department of Ophthalmology,
University of Minnesota,
Minneapolis, Minnesota

GARY N. HOLLAND, MD
Professor of Ophthalmology,
UCLA School of Medicine;
Director, UCLA Ocular Inflammatory Disease Center,
Jules Stein Eye Institute;
Chief, Ophthalmology Section,
Department of Veterans Affairs Medical Center,
  West Los Angeles,
Los Angeles, California

PHILIP L. HOOPER, MD
Assistant Professor,
Department of Ophthalmology,
University of Western Ontario,
London, Ontario, Canada

EDWARD L. HOWES, JR., MD
Professor of Pathology and Ophthalmology,
University of California, San Francisco;
Chief of Pathology,
San Francisco General Hospital,
San Francisco, California

ANDREW J.W. HUANG, MD, MPH
Assistant Professor,
Department of Ophthalmology,
Bascom Palmer Eye Institute,
University of Miami School of Medicine,
Miami, Florida

NAUSHAD HUSSEIN, MD
Adjunct Professor,
Department of Ophthalmology,
McGill University,
Quebec, Ontario, Canada

DAVID G. HWANG, MD
Assistant Professor;
Co-Director, Cornea and Refractive Surgery Service,
Department of Ophthalmology,
University of California, San Francisco School
  of Medicine,
San Francisco, California

ROBERT A. HYNDIUK, MD
Professor of Ophthalmology,
Medical College of Wisconsin,
The Eye Institute,
Milwaukee Regional Medical Center Campus,
Milwaukee, Wisconsin

NICHOLAS T. ILIFF, MD
Associate Professor of Ophthalmology and Plastic Surgery,
Department of Ophthalmology;
Director, Oculoplastic Surgery Division,
The Wilmer Ophthalmological Institute,
Johns Hopkins University School of Medicine,
Baltimore, Maryland

HAJIME INOMATA, MD, PhD
Professor and Chairman,
Department of Ophthalmology;
Faculty of Medicine,
Kyushu University,
Fukuoka, Japan

ALEXANDER R. IRVINE, MD
Professor,
Department of Ophthalmology,
University of California, San Francisco,
San Francisco, California

DOUGLAS A. JABS, MD
Professor of Ophthalmology,
Professor of Medicine,
Johns Hopkins University School of Medicine,
Wilmer Ophthalmological Institute,
Baltimore, Maryland

LEE M. JAMPOL, MD
Louis Feinberg Professor of Ophthalmology,
Chairman of Ophthalmology,
Northwestern University Medical School,
Northwestern Memorial Hospital,
Chicago, Illinois

JAMES V. JESTER, PhD
Professor of Ophthalmology,
University of Texas Southwestern Medical Center at Dallas,
Dallas, Texas

DAN B. JONES, MD
Sid W. Richardson Professor and Margaret Root Brown
    Chairman of Ophthalmology,
Department of Ophthalmology,
Cullen Eye Institute,
Baylor College of Medicine,
Houston, Texas

M. COLIN JORDAN, MD
Professor of Medicine and Microbiology;
Director, Division of Infectious Diseases,
University of Minnesota Hospital,
Minneapolis, Minnesota

JACK J. KANSKI, MD, MS, FRCS, FRCOphth
Consultant Ophthalmic Surgeon,
Prince Charles Eye Unit,
King Edward VII Hospital,
Windsor, England

HENRY J. KAPLAN, MD
Professor and Chairman,
Department of Ophthalmology and Visual Sciences,
Washington University Medical Center,
St. Louis, Missouri

ROBERT H. KENNEDY, MPH, PhD
Associate Professor of Ophthalmology,
Department of Ophthalmology,
University of Texas Southwestern Medical Center
    at Dallas,
Dallas, Texas

JOHN S. KENNERDELL, MD
Professor of Ophthalmology,
Medical College of Pennsylvania,
Philadelphia, Pennsylvania;
Chairman,
Department of Ophthalmology,
Allegheny General Hospital,
Pittsburgh, Pennsylvania

PAUL R. KINCHINGTON, PhD
Assistant Professor,
Department of Ophthalmology;
Department of Molecular Genetics and Biochemistry,
Eye and Ear Institute,
University of Pittsburgh,
Pittsburgh, Pennsylvania

GORDON K. KLINTWORTH, MD, PhD
Professor of Pathology;
Joseph A. C. Wadsworth Research Professor of
    Ophthalmology,
Duke University Medical Center,
Durham, North Carolina

DIANE J. KRAUS, MD
Assistant Clinical Instructor,
Columbia Presbyterian Medical Center,
New York, New York

ELLEN KRAUS-MACKIW, MD
Professor of Ophthalmology;
Director of Orthoptics, Pleoptics and Motility,
Disorders of the Eye,
Ruprecht-Karl University,
Heidelberg, Germany

HOWARD R. KRAUSS, MD
Assistant Clinical Professor,
Department of Ophthalmology,
UCLA School of Medicine,
Jules Stein Eye Institute,
Los Angeles, California;
Director,
Southern California Neuro-Ophthalmology and Orbital
    Surgical Associates,
Santa Monica, California

BRUCE R. KSANDER, PhD
Assistant Professor,
Department of Ophthalmology,
Harvard Medical School;
Associate Scientist,
Schepens Eye Research Institute,
Boston, Massachusetts

NAOKI KUMAGAI, MD, PhD
Department of Ophthalmology,
Yokohama City University School of Medicine,
Yokohama, Japan

SHERIDAN LAM, MD
Assistant Professor of Clinical Ophthalmology,
Department of Ophthalmology and Visual Sciences,
University of Illinois at Chicago,
Chicago, Illinois

JONATHAN H. LASS, MD
Chairman, Department of Ophthalmology,
Case Western Reserve;
Director University Hospitals of Cleveland,
Cleveland, Ohio

STEVEN F. LEE, MD
Department of Ophthalmology,
Washington University School of Medicine,
St. Louis, Missouri

PHUC LEHOANG, MD, PhD
Professor of Ophthalmology,
University of Paris;
Chairman,
Department of Ophthalmology,
Hôpital Pitié-Salpêtrière,
Paris, France

DAVID A. LEIB, PhD
Assistant Professor of Ophthalmology and Molecular
    Microbiology,
Department of Ophthalmology and Visual Sciences,
Washington University,
St. Louis, Missouri

HILEL LEWIS, MD
Chairman,
Division of Ophthalmology,
The Cleveland Clinic Foundation,
Cleveland, Ohio

THOMAS J. LIESEGANG, MD
Professor of Ophthalmology;
Chairman, Department of Ophthalmology,
Mayo Clinic Jacksonville,
Jacksonville, Florida

ROBERT P. LISAK, MD
Professor and Chairman of Neurology;
Professor of Immunology and Microbiology,
Wayne State University School of Medicine;
Neurologist-in-Chief,
Detroit Medical Center;
Chief of Neurology,
Harper Hospital,
Detroit, Michigan

CAREEN YEN LOWDER, MD, PhD
Professional Staff Surgeon,
Division of Ophthalmology,
The Cleveland Clinic Foundation,
Cleveland, Ohio

GREGG T. LUEDER, MD
Assistant Professor of Ophthalmology and Visual Sciences
    and Pediatrics,
St. Louis Children's Hospital,
Washington University School of Medicine,
St. Louis, Missouri

SHEILA A. LUKEHART, PhD
Research Professor,
Department of Medicine Division of Infectious Diseases,
University of Washington,
Harborview Medical Center,
Seattle, Washington

SID MANDELBAUM, MD
Associate Clinical Professor of Ophthalmology and Visual
    Sciences,
Albert Einstein College of Medicine,
Long Island Jewish Medical Center,
Manhattan Eye, Ear, and Throat Hospital,
New York, New York

MARK J. MANNIS, MD, FACS
Professor of Ophthalmology;
Director, Cornea and External Disease,
Department of Ophthalmology,
University of California, Davis,
Sacramento, California

TODD P. MARGOLIS, MD, PhD
Associate Professor,
Department of Ophthalmology;
Research Ophthalmologist,
Francis I. Proctor Foundation,
University of California, San Francisco School of Medicine,
San Francisco, California

ALICE Y. MATOBA, MD
Chief, Ophthalmology Service,
Department of Veterans Affairs Medical Center;
Associate Professor of Ophthalmology,
Baylor College of Medicine,
Houston, Texas

REX M. McCALLUM, MD
Assistant Professor of Medicine,
Department of Medicine,
Duke University Medical Center,
Durham, North Carolina

PETER J. McCLUSKEY, MB, BS, FRACOphth, FRACS
Doctor,
Laboratory of Ocular Immunology,
School of Pathology,
University of New South Wales,
Sydney, Australia

JAMES P. McCULLEY, MD
The David Bruton, Jr. Chair in Ophthalmology;
Professor and Chairman,
Department of Ophthalmology,
University of Texas Southwestern Medical Center at Dallas,
Dallas, Texas

JAN M. McDONNELL, MD
Associate Professor,
Departments of Ophthalmology and Pathology,
University of Southern California School of Medicine,
Los Angeles, California

ROGER F. MEYER, MD
Professor of Ophthalmology,
University of Michigan Medical School,
Ann Arbor, Michigan

NEIL R. MILLER, MD
Professor of Ophthalmology, Neurology, and Neurosurgery;
Frank B. Walsh Professor of Neuro-Ophthalmology,
Johns Hopkins University School of Medicine,
Baltimore, Maryland

MANABU MOCHIZUKI, MD
Professor and Chairman,
Department of Ophthalmology,
Kurume University School of Medicine,
Kurume, Japan

BARTLY J. MONDINO, MD
Wasserman Professor of Ophthalmology;
Chairman, Department of Ophthalmology;
Director, Jules Stein Eye Institute,
UCLA School of Medicine,
Los Angeles, California

PAUL C. MONTGOMERY, PhD
Professor and Chairman,
Department of Immunology and Microbiology,
Wayne State University Medical School,
Detroit, Michigan

RAMANA S. MOORTHY, MD
Midwest Eye Institute,
Indianapolis, Indiana

TIMOTHY G. MURRAY, MD
Assistant Professor,
Department of Ophthalmology,
Bascom Palmer Eye Institute,
University of Miami School of Medicine,
Miami, Florida

J. DANIEL NELSON, MD, FACS
Associate Professor,
Department of Ophthalmology,
University of Minnesota Medical School;
Chief, Ophthalmology,
Ramsey Clinic and St. Paul-Ramsey Medical Center,
St. Paul, Minnesota

JERRY Y. NIEDERKORN, PhD
Professor of Ophthalmology and Molecular Microbiology,
Department of Ophthalmology,
University of Texas Southwestern Medical Center at Dallas,
Dallas, Texas

ROBERT B. NUSSENBLATT, MD
Scientific Director and Head,
Laboratory of Immunology;
National Eye Institute,
National Institutes of Health,
Bethesda, Maryland

THOMAS B. NUTMAN, MD
Head, Helminth Immunology Section,
Laboratory of Parasitic Diseases,
National Institute of Allergy and Infectious Diseases,
Bethesda, Maryland

TERRENCE P. O'BRIEN, MD
Assistant Professor of Ophthalmology,
Department of Ophthalmology,
The Wilmer Ophthalmological Institute,
Johns Hopkins University School of Medicine,
Baltimore, Maryland

G. RICHARD O'CONNOR, MD
Professor of Ophthalmology Emeritus;
Director Emeritus,
Francis I. Proctor Foundation,
University of California, San Francisco,
San Francisco, California

DENIS M. O'DAY, MD
George W. Hale Professor;
Chairman, Department of Ophthalmology and Visual
    Sciences,
Vanderbilt University Medical Center,
Nashville, Tennessee

SHIGEAKI OHNO, MD, DMSc
Department of Ophthalmology,
Yokohama City University School of Medicine,
Yokohama, Japan

E. MITCHEL OPREMCAK, MD
Associate Professor,
Department of Ophthalmology,
Ohio State University College of Medicine,
Ohio State University Hospital,
Columbus, Ohio

MICHAEL S. OSATO, PhD
Research Assistant,
Veterans Administration Medical Center,
Houston, Texas

†H. BRUCE OSTLER, MD
Professor of Ophthalmology Emeritus,
Department of Ophthalmology;
Research Ophthalmologist,
Francis I. Proctor Foundation,
University of California, San Francisco,
San Francisco, California

† Deceased.

DAVID W. PARKE II, MD
President, Dean A. McGee Eye Institute;
Dean A. McGee Professor and Chairman,
Department of Ophthalmology,
University of Oklahoma,
Oklahoma City, Oklahoma

DEBORAH PAVAN-LANGSTON, MD
Associate Professor of Ophthalmology,
Harvard Medical School;
Surgeon in Ophthalmology;
Director, Clinical Virology,
Massachusetts Eye and Ear Infirmary;
Adjunct Senior Scientist,
Schepens Eye Research Institute,
Boston, Massachusetts

JAY S. PEPOSE, MD, PhD
Bernard Becker Professor of Ophthalmology,
Director, Corneal and External Diseases,
Department of Ophthalmology and Visual Sciences,
Washington University School of Medicine,
St. Louis, Missouri

THOMAS H. PETTIT, MD
Professor of Ophthalmology Emeritus,
UCLA School of Medicine,
Jules Stein Eye Institute,
Los Angeles, California

ROSS E. PETTY, MD, PhD
Professor of Pediatrics,
University of British Columbia;
Head, Division of Rheumatology,
British Columbia's Children's Hospital
Vancouver, British Columbia, Canada

STEPHEN C. PFLUGFELDER, MD
Associate Professor,
Department of Ophthalmology,
Bascom Palmer Eye Institute,
University of Miami School of Medicine,
Miami, Florida

ADOLPH POSNER, MD
Professor Emeritus,
Department of Ophthalmology,
Albert Einstein College of Medicine,
Bronx, New York

ERIC P. PURDY, MD
Assistant Clinical Professor of Ophthalmology,
Department of Ophthalmology,
Wright State University School of Medicine,
Dayton, Ohio

THOMAS C. QUINN, MD
Professor of Medicine and International Health,
Johns Hopkins University School of Medicine;
Senior Investigator,
National Institute of Allergy and Infectious Diseases,
Bethesda, Maryland

MICHAEL B. RAIZMAN, MD
Director, Cornea and Anterior Segment Service,
Department of Ophthalmology,
Tufts University School of Medicine,
New England Eye Center,
Boston, Massachusetts

NARSING A. RAO, MD
Professor,
Department of Ophthalmology and Pathology,
Doheny Eye Institute,
University of Southern California,
Los Angeles, California

PETER A. RAPOZA, MD, FACS
Assistant Professor,
Director, Cornea and External Disease Service,
Department of Ophthalmology,
University of Wisconsin,
Madison, Wisconsin

JACQUELINE L. REISS, MD
Fellow,
Division of Immunology and Allergy,
Department of Medicine,
Washington University School of Medicine,
St. Louis, Missouri

JACK S. REMINGTON, MD
Professor of Medicine,
Department of Medicine, Division of Infectious Diseases,
Standford University Medical Center,
Stanford, California;
Marcus A. Krupp Research Chair,
Department of Immunology and Infectious Diseases,
Palo Alto Medical Foundation,
Palo Alto, California

LELAND S. RICKMAN, MD
Assistant Clinical Professor of Medicine,
University of California, San Diego School of Medicine;
Medical Director,
Epidemiology Unit,
University of California, San Diego Medical Center,
San Diego, California

JOSEPH F. RIZZO III, MD
Assistant Professor of Ophthalmology,
Harvard Medical School;
Neuro-Ophthalmologist,
Massachusetts Eye and Ear Infirmary,
Boston, Massachusetts

FRANÇOIS G. ROBERGE, MD, FRCSC
National Eye Institute,
National Institutes of Health,
Bethesda, Maryland

JEFFREY B. ROBIN, MD
Head, Department of Refractive Surgery,
Cleveland Clinic Foundation,
Cleveland, Ohio

STEVEN B. ROBIN, MD
Assistant Professor,
Department of Ophthalmology,
University of Minnesota Medical School,
Minneapolis, Minnesota;
Staff Ophthalmologist,
Ramsey Clinic,
St. Paul, Minnesota

ROBERT H. ROSA, JR., MD
Fellow,
Bascom Palmer Eye Institute,
University of Miami School of Medicine,
Miami, Florida

JAMES T. ROSENBAUM, MD
Professor of Medicine, Ophthalmology, and Cell Biology;
Assistant Dean for Research;
Head, Uveitis Clinic;
Director, Inflammation Research,
Oregon Health Sciences University,
Casey Eye Institute,
Portland, Oregon

BARRY T. ROUSE, DVM, PhD
Distinguished Professor of Microbiology,
Department of Microbiology,
College of Veterinary Medicine,
University of Tennessee,
Knoxville, Tennessee

STEPHEN J. RYAN, MD
Senior Vice President for Medical Affairs,
University of Southern California;
President, Doheny Eye Institute;
Dean, University of Southern California School of
    Medicine,
Los Angeles, California

FRED SANFILIPPO, MD, PhD
Baxley Professor and Chairman,
Department of Pathology,
Johns Hopkins University School of Medicine;
Pathologist-in-Chief,
The Johns Hopkins Hospital,
Baltimore, Maryland

JULIUS SCHACHTER, PhD
Professor of Laboratory Medicine, Epidemiology,
University of California, San Francisco,
San Francisco, California

ABRAHAM SCHLOSSMAN, MD
Adjunct Associate Clinic Professor,
Department of Ophthalmology,
Mount Sinai School of Medicine;
Attending Surgeon Emeritus,
Department of Ophthalmology,
Manhattan Eye, Ear, and Throat Hospital,
New York, New York

IVAN R. SCHWAB, MD, FACS
Professor of Ophthalmology,
Department of Ophthalmology,
University of California, Davis,
Sacramento, California

DAVID V. SEAL, MD, FRCOphth, FRCPath
Consultant in Ocular Infectious Diseases,
Tennent Institute of Ophthalmology,
Western Infirmary,
Glasgow, Scotland, United Kingdom

ANTONIO G. SECCHI, MD
Professor of Ophthalmology,
Institute of Ophthalmology,
University of Padova School of Medicine,
Padova, Italy

ROBERT C. SERGOTT, MD
Co-Director, Neuro-Ophthalmology;
Attending Neuro-Ophthalmologist;
Attending Surgeon,
Wills Eye Hospital;
Attending Neuro-Ophthalmologist,
Lankenau Hospital,
Wynnewood, Pennsylvania

ROBERT P. SHAVER, MD
Professor,
Department of Ophthalmology,
University of Oklahoma,
College of Medicine,
Oklahoma City, Oklahoma

PATRICK A. SIBONY, MD
Associate Professor of Ophthalmology,
Department of Ophthalmology,
State University of New York at Stony Brook,
Stony Brook, New York

ARTHUR M. SILVERSTEIN, PhD
Professor Emeritus of Ophthalmic Immunology,
  History of Medicine,
Johns Hopkins University School of Medicine,
Baltimore, Maryland

RONALD E. SMITH, MD
Professor and Chairman,
Department of Ophthalmology,
Doheny Eye Institute,
University of Southern California School of Medicine,
Los Angeles, California

GILBERT SMOLIN, MD
Clinical Professor,
University of California, San Francisco;
Research Ophthalmologist,
Francis I. Proctor Foundation,
San Francisco, California

MILES R. STANFORD, MD
Senior Lecturer,
Department of Ophthalmology,
St. Thomas' Hospital,
London, England

RICHARD S. STEPHENS, MD
Associate Professor,
Division of Public Health, Biology, and Epidemiology,
Program in Infectious Diseases,
School of Public Health,
University of California at Berkeley,
Berkeley, California

E. RICHARD STIEHM, MD
Professor of Pediatrics;
Chief, Division of Allergy/Immunology,
UCLA School of Medicine;
Attending Pediatrician,
UCLA Medical Center,
Los Angeles, California

J. WAYNE STREILEIN, MD
President and DeWalt & Marie Ankeny Director of
  Research,
Schepens Eye Research Institute;
Professor and Vice-Chair for Research,
Department of Ophthalmology and Dermatology,
Harvard Medical School,
Boston, Massachusetts

P. MICHAEL STUART, PhD
Assistant Professor,
Department of Ophthalmology and Visual Sciences;
Department of Molecular Microbiology,
Washington University Medical Center,
St. Louis, Missouri

KHALID F. TABBARA, MD
Professor and Chairman,
Department of Ophthalmology,
King Saud University, College of Medicine,
Riyadh, Saudi Arabia

KAZUO TAJIMA, MD
Chief, Division of Epidemiology,
Aichi Cancer Center,
Research Institute,
Nagoya, Japan

QIZHI TANG
Graduate Student,
Department of Microbiology and Immunology,
University of Illinois at Chicago,
Chicago, Illinois

HUGH R. TAYLOR, MD, FRACS
Ringland Anderson Professor;
Head of Ophthalmology,
University of Melbourne;
Director of Eye Services,
Royal Victorian Eye and Ear Hospital,
Melbourne, Victoria, Australia

HOWARD TESSLER, MD
Professor of Ophthalmology;
Director of Uveitis Service,
University of Illinois,
Chicago, Illinois

†FREDERICK H. THEODORE, MD
Clinical Professor of Ophthalmology Emeritus,
Mount Sinai School of Medicine;
Associate Clinical Professor of Ophthalmology,
New York University College of Medicine,
New York, New York

PHILLIPS THYGESON, MD
Professor Emeritus,
Department of Ophthalmology,
Francis I. Proctor Foundation,
University of California, San Francisco,
San Francisco, California

---

† Deceased

ADNAN TUFAIL, FRCOphth
Visiting Assistant Professor of Ophthalmology,
Department of Ophthalmology,
UCLA School of Medicine,
Jules Stein Eye Institute,
Los Angeles, California

ANNA TYUTYUNIKOV
Associate Research Scientist,
Department of Ophthalmology,
Allegheny General Hospital,
Pittsburgh, Pennsylvania

NICHOLAS J. VOLPE, MD
Assistant Professor of Ophthalmology and Neurology,
Departments of Ophthalmology and Neurology,
University of Pennsylvania,
Scheie Eye Institute,
Philadelphia, Pennsylvania

DENIS WAKEFIELD, MD
Professor of Pathology,
Department of Immunopathology,
Prince Henry Hospital,
University of New South Wales;
Director of Immunology,
Eastern Area Health Services,
Sydney, New South Wales, Australia

J. CLIFFORD WALDREP, PhD
Assistant Professor,
Department of Molecular Physiology and Biophysics,
Baylor College of Medicine,
Houston, Texas

JACK R. WALL, MD, PhD
Professor of Ophthalmology and Medicine,
Medical College of Pennsylvania,
Hahnemann University,
Philadelphia, Pennsylvania;
Endocrinologist,
Allegheny General Hospital,
Pittsburgh, Pennsylvania

TOSHIKI WATANABE, MD, PhD
Associate Professor,
Department of Pathology,
Institute of Medical Science,
University of Tokyo,
Tokyo, Japan

H. JAMES WEDNER, MD
Chief of Clinical Allergy and Immunology,
Division of Allergy and Immunology,
Department of Medicine,
Washington University School of Medicine;
Associate Physician,
Barnes Hospital,
St. Louis, Missouri

THOMAS A. WEINGEIST, MD, PhD
Professor and Head,
Department of Ophthalmology;
Director, Vitreoretinal Service,
University of Iowa College of Medicine,
Iowa City, Iowa

JOHN P. WHITCHER, MD
Professor of Clinical Ophthalmology,
Department of Ophthalmology,
Francis I. Proctor Foundation,
University of California, San Francisco,
San Francisco, California

SCOTT M. WHITCUP, MD
Clinical Director,
National Eye Institute,
National Institutes of Health,
Bethesda, Maryland

KIRK R. WILHELMUS, MD
Professor of Ophthalmology,
Department of Ophthalmology,
Baylor College of Medicine,
Houston, Texas

NANCY WILLIAMS, MD
Assistant Professor,
Division of Ophthalmology,
Howard University Hospital,
Washington, D.C.

DAVID J. WILSON, MD
Associate Professor;
Director, Christensen Eye Pathology Laboratory,
Department of Ophthalmology,
Oregon Health Sciences University,
Portland, Oregon

FRED M. WILSON II, MD
Professor of Ophthalmology,
Department of Ophthalmology,
Indiana University School of Medicine,
Indianapolis, Indiana

LOUIS A. WILSON, MD
Professor of Ophthalmology;
Adjunct Professor of Microbiology,
Department of Ophthalmology,
Emory University School of Medicine,
Georgia State University,
Atlanta, Georgia

STEVEN E. WILSON, MD
Associate Professor,
Cleveland Clinic Foundation,
Division of Ophthalmology,
Cleveland, Ohio

JOHN R. WITTPENN, MD
Assistant Professor,
Department of Ophthalmology;
Director, Cornea and Anterior Segment,
State University of New York at Stony Brook,
Stony Brook, New York

T. RODMAN WOOD, MD
Cottage Grove, Oregon

PETER WRIGHT, MD, FRCS, FRCOphth
Retired,
Moorfields Eye Hospital and Institute of Ophthalmology,
London, England

KAZUNARI YAMAGUCHI, MD, PhD
Associate Professor,
Kumamoto University School of Medicine,
Kumamoto, Japan

LOWELL YOUNG, MD
Clinical Professor of Medicine,
University of California, San Francisco;
Director,
Kuzell Institute for Arthritis and Infectious Diseases;
Chief of Infectious Diseases,
California Pacific Medical Center,
San Francisco, California

KAMAL A. ZAKKA, MD
Assistant Clinical Professor Ophthalmology,
UCLA School of Medicine,
Los Angeles, California

To SG for your patience; DHP, MIP, SFP, and MAP for your potential; HJK for your support; and JGS for your example.

JSP

Among the many outstanding teachers with whom I have trained, two in particular stimulated my interest in uveitis and ophthalmic infectious diseases. I am pleased to offer this dedication to Drs. G. Richard O'Connor and Thomas H. Pettit, in recognition of their contributions to ophthalmology and their devotion to teaching. My decision to undertake this project was undoubtedly encouraged by their continuing influence.

Additional thanks go to my family, friends, and colleagues for their tremendous support during the preparation of this book.

GNH

For the additive effects of my clinical mentors: DBJ, DJC, and BRJ. And for synergy—C.

KRW

Foreword

In the 17th century, Descartes and Newton devised concepts to explain natural phenomena of the universe. This analytical viewpoint was subsequently applied to medicine. Germ theory and hypersensitivity mechanisms were among the many discoveries that relied on observation and experiment.

New diseases and interventions are still evolving, and acute powers of insight continue to be needed. However, clinical description is inadequate by itself to advance knowledge in the visual sciences. Diagnosis and management are becoming more reliant on the recognition of the molecular nature of eye diseases. As 19th century researchers laid the groundwork for the modern development of ocular microbiology and immunology, so today's biotechnology will shape the eye care standards of the future.

This book is organized by the disease processes that cause the major infectious and inflammatory disorders of the eye. More than a catalogue of clinical findings, the contributors present the pathogenesis, and, when known, the molecular processes that underlie these conditions and how they are applicable to clinical practice. The book provides the reader with a compendium of information, combining what is clinically important today with what are the new insights that will be important in the future. Ophthalmologists in practice and in training will find details regarding the diagnosis and management of all forms of ocular inflammation and infections. The textbook should also be a valuable and comprehensive resource to other eye care providers, as well as other physicians and scientists. By bringing together various basic and clinical science disciplines, the editors have provided a framework for a greater understanding of ocular inflammatory and infectious diseases.

Robert B. Nussenblatt, M.D.
Bethesda, Maryland

Preface

Infection and inflammation are among the leading causes of ocular morbidity and blindness. In the developing world, trachoma and onchocerciasis continue to blind millions of individuals, as they have done for thousands of years. In industrialized societies, infectious endophthalmitis, bacterial keratitis, and uveitis syndromes are among the most difficult problems that confront ophthalmologists. There are astonishing new technical and conceptual advances that have been applied to the study of these problems. In fact, few disciplines have undergone more dynamic change in recent years than the fields of infectious disease and immunology; advances in molecular biology, genetics, and pharmacology offer better understanding and management for these disorders and improved diagnosis and prognosis for patients. At the same time, however, there are new ophthalmic problems to tackle, such as the acute retinal necrosis syndrome, the ocular manifestations of AIDS, and iatrogenic disorders that include graft-versus-host disease. The abundance of new information in these disciplines poses a particular challenge to those who deal with diseases of the eye. We organized *Ocular Infection & Immunity* to help meet that challenge.

The book evolved over a four-year period. Looking back, it had its genesis in the unlikeliest of places: a German rathskellar during an international symposium on infectious diseases of the eye; the banks of the Amazon River during a Brazilian meeting on prevention of blindness; even Disneyland, during an annual meeting of the American Academy of Ophthalmology. During professional meetings at these and other colorful locations, informal discussions with colleagues from around the world continually highlighted the burgeoning interest in infectious and inflammatory diseases, yet emphasized the lack of a comprehensive reference source for the myriad problems that they can cause throughout the visual system. We recognized the need for an ophthalmological textbook on infectious and inflammatory diseases that was not constrained by the artificial limitations of our subspecialty, since it is impossible to understand these ophthalmic diseases if they are separated from their systemic counterparts. The book we envisioned would include a comprehensive review of all aspects of a disease, yet would retain the focus on the special ophthalmic features provided by a traditional ophthalmological text.

With the enthusiasm generated by these discussions, we committed ourselves to a book featuring:

- coverage of all infectious and inflammatory diseases that affect the visual system;
- a review of the basic concepts of microbiology and immunology critical for understanding these diseases;
- discussion of all aspects of a given disease, including the microbiology of its causal organism, the immunological mechanisms involved in its pathogenesis, its nonocular features, and *all* of its ophthalmic manifestations, regardless of the tissues involved;
- emphasis on disease mechanisms rather than clinical practice alone; and finally,
- the collaboration of ophthalmologists and specialists from a variety of other disciplines, thereby avoiding the insular nature and limited scope that characterizes many ophthalmological textbooks. In doing so, the textbook would be of value to ophthalmologists and nonophthalmologists alike.

We believe that *Ocular Infection & Immunity* is unique. Ophthalmological textbooks usually concentrate on one region of the eye, or on one visual system; hence there are retina and cornea books, and references dealing with neuro-ophthalmology and glaucoma. Our text is not anatomically oriented in that traditional sense. The book begins with a two-chapter Introduction that describes the history of infectious and inflammatory diseases of the eye, and how the current state of knowledge about these disciplines was achieved. The next two sections are devoted to the latest scientific knowledge about disease mechanisms and the unique anatomic and physiological features of the eye; this background can be applied to understanding the clinical aspects of disease. A brief third section, dealing with immunodeficiency disorders, illustrates the interface between clinical immunology and the study of infectious diseases. The remainder of the book is organized by clinically recognized diseases whenever possible. Chapters are divided into those dealing with inflammatory disease of uncertain cause and those known to be the result of infection. To facilitate easy reference, chapters are further grouped by the part of the eye that is most often affected.

We asked all contributors to emphasize manifestations and mechanisms of disease in their chapters. We believe strongly that a thorough understanding of the pathophysiology of disease will contribute to its appropriate clinical management, whether or not specific drugs, surgical techniques, or diagnostic tests change over time. *Ocular Infection & Immunity* is not a detailed review of practical treatment for disease; nevertheless, by providing an understanding of disease and by discussing the principles and goals of therapy, the book will be a valuable addition to the libraries of practitioners of clinical ophthalmology.

The greatest strength of this book is the group of over 200 contributors, residing across five continents, who joined together to complete this ambitious project. We are proud to have enlisted the help of renowned experts in the fields of internal medicine, pediatrics, rheumatology, immunology, microbiology, infectious diseases, pathology, and a variety of subspecialties in ophthalmology. Our contributing group is a diverse mix of laboratory and clinical scientists. Most chapters are co-authored by two or more individuals from different disciplines, backgrounds, or experiences. Long-distance collaboration was sometimes an obstacle for our co-authors, but the result has been a thorough review of each subject from various perspectives that extends beyond the frame of reference available to most ophthalmologists. We are truly indebted to these fine contributors for their enormous efforts on behalf of this book.

We would like to acknowledge specifically two individuals who passed away shortly after contributing to the textbook. H. Bruce Ostler, M.D., co-author of the chapter on Hansen disease, was Professor of Ophthalmology Emeritus at the University of California, San Francisco School of Medicine, where he was also a member of the Francis I. Proctor Foundation for Research in Ophthalmology for many years. He was a highly respected and well-liked clinician and teacher who trained a generation of external ocular disease specialists. Frederick H. Theodore, M.D. provided a special perspective to the chapter on Theodore superior limbic keratoconjunctivitis, the disease that he originally described and that now bears his name. He was Clinical Professor of Ophthalmology Emeritus at Mt. Sinai School of Medicine in New York City and Associate Clinical Professor of Ophthalmology at New York University College of Medicine. Dr. Theodore, whose career spanned more than half a century, was an internationally recognized and respected expert on a variety of subjects ranging from ocular allergies to anterior segment surgery. Our textbook was strengthened by the input from these two distinguished authorities in the field of ophthalmology.

It will not be a surprise to anyone who has edited a textbook that this project was longer, harder—and at times more frustrating—than we had originally anticipated. But now, reflecting on the finished product, we feel that we have achieved our basic goal; in a single text we have provided material that will allow ophthalmologists and other eye-care professionals to expand their understanding of disease beyond the eye, while providing nonophthalmologists with insight into the special features of infectious and inflammatory diseases found in ocular structures. It is our sincere hope that we have provided our intended audience with a useful and interesting reference that will meet their clinical and scientific needs.

Jay S. Pepose, M.D., Ph.D.
Gary N. Holland, M.D.
Kirk R. Wilhelmus, M.D.

Contents

OCULAR
INFECTION
&IMMUNITY

Ocular Infection & Immunity

This color insert contains selected figures found throughout *Ocular Infection & Immunity*. Included are clinical photographs for which color reproduction helps identify features of disease. Figure numbers identify the location of each illustration in the text, where it will have a more detailed legend. (For example, Fig. 26-3 indicates that the same figure can be found as the third black and white figure in Chapter 26.) Figures appear in sequential order on the first seven pages. On the eighth page of this insert the color illustrations for Table 81-2, "The Differential Diagnosis of Cytomegalovirus Retinitis," can be found.

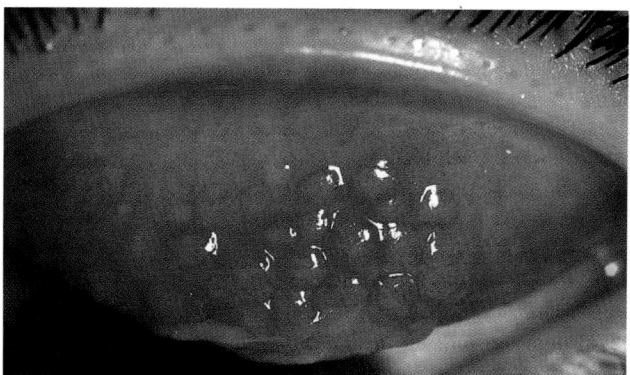

Fig. 26-3 Giant papillary conjunctivitis.

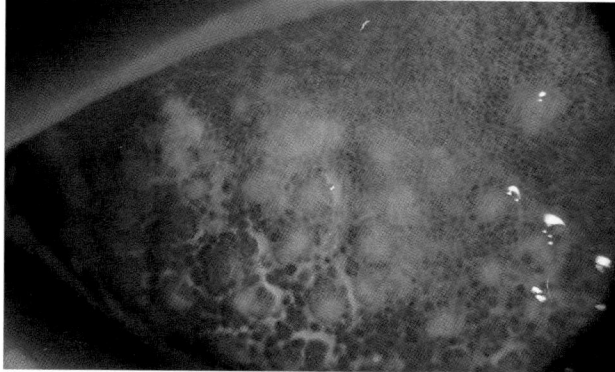

Fig. 26-5 Fluorescein staining of giant papillae.

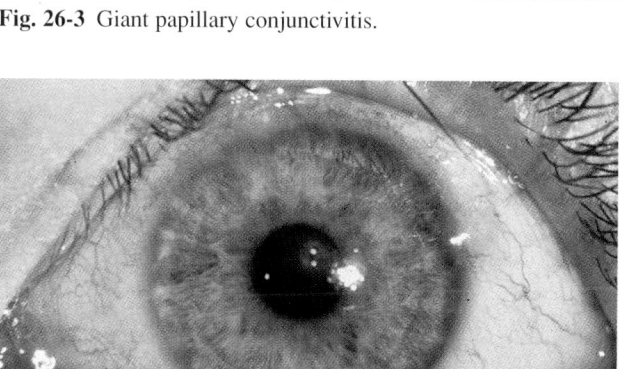

Fig. 27-4 Horner-Trantas dots.

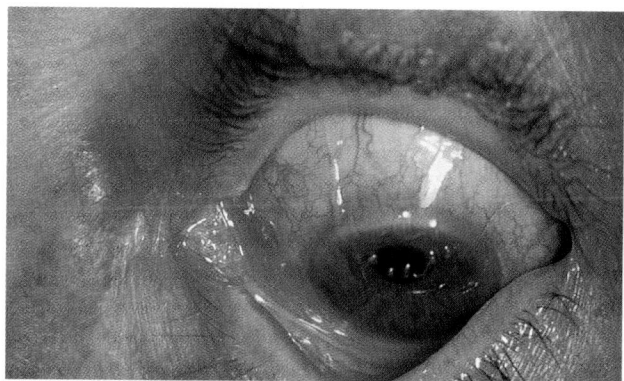

Fig. 30-6 Theodore superficial limbic keratoconjunctivitis.

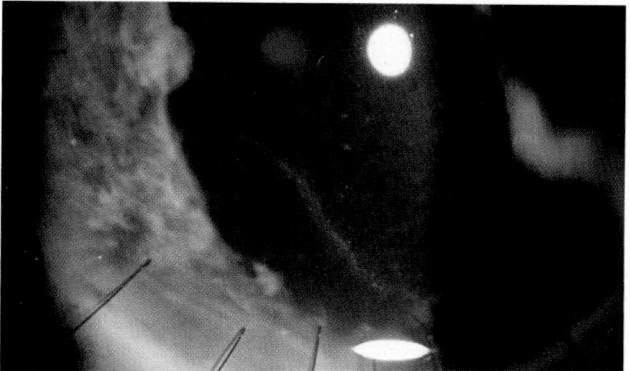

Fig. 35-4 Corneal allograft rejection (Khodadoust line).

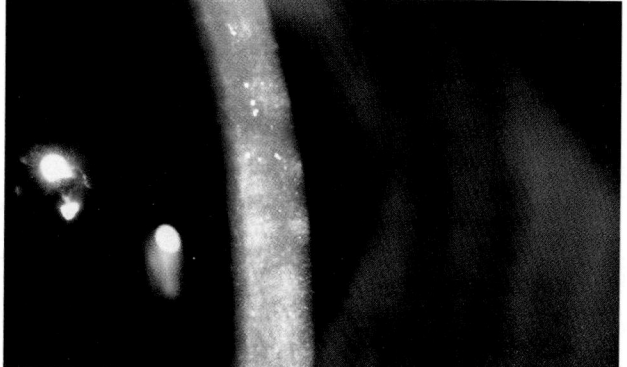

Fig. 35-5 Corneal allograft rejection (subepithelial infiltrates).

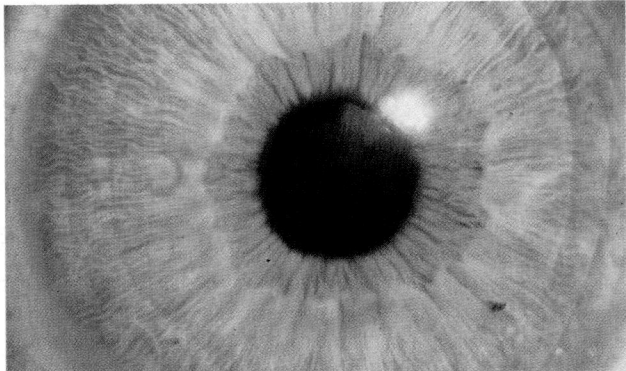

Fig. 41-1A Right eye of a patient with heterochromia caused by Fuchs uveitis syndrome in the left eye (Fig. 41-1B).

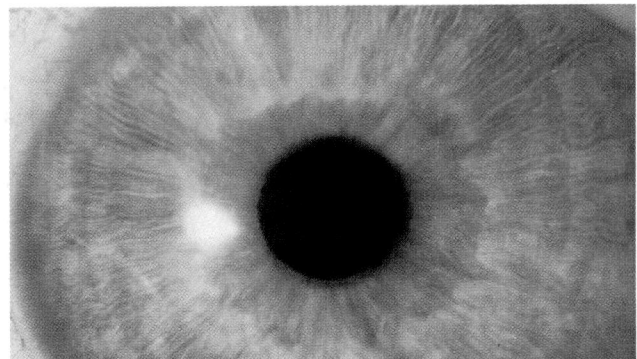

Fig. 41-1B Fuchs uveitis syndrome.

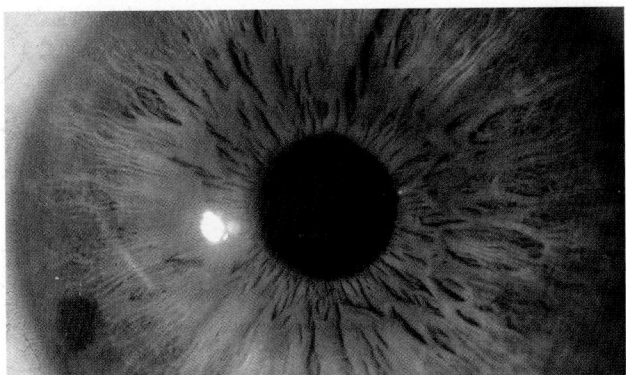

Fig. 41-2A Right eye of a patient with heterochromia caused by Fuchs uveitis syndrome in the left eye (Fig. 41-2B).

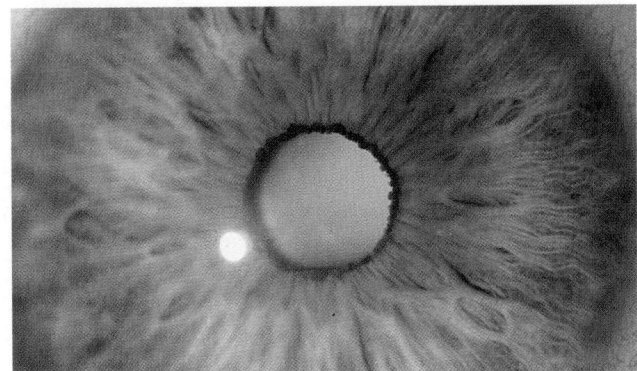

Fig. 41-2B Fuchs uveitis syndrome.

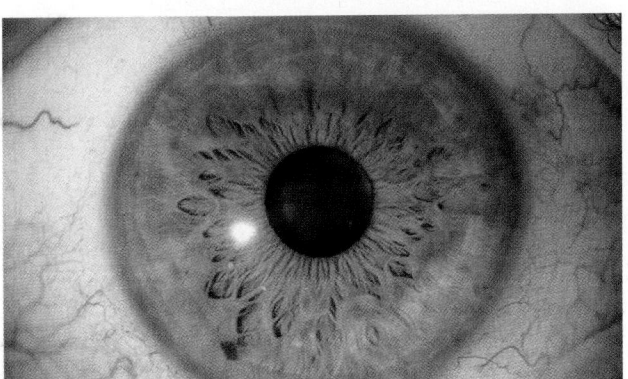

Fig. 41-3A Right eye of a patient with subtle heterochromia caused by Fuchs uveitis syndrome in the left eye (Fig. 41-3B).

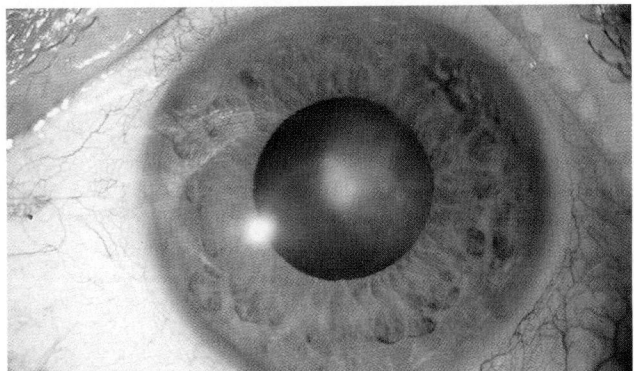

Fig. 41-3B Fuchs uveitis syndrome.

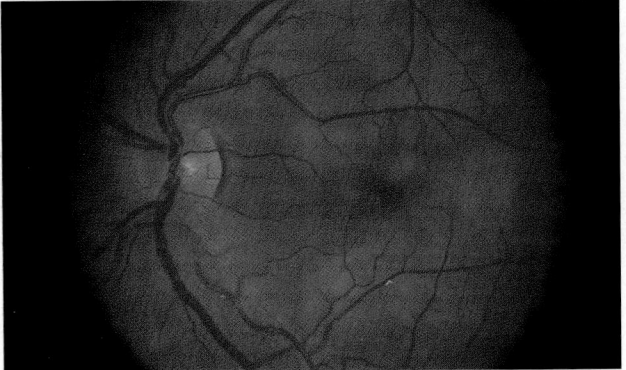

Fig. 46-2A Acute posterior multifocal placoid pigment epitheliopathy (APMPPE), acute stage.
(Note: Fig. 46-1 is located on the next page.)

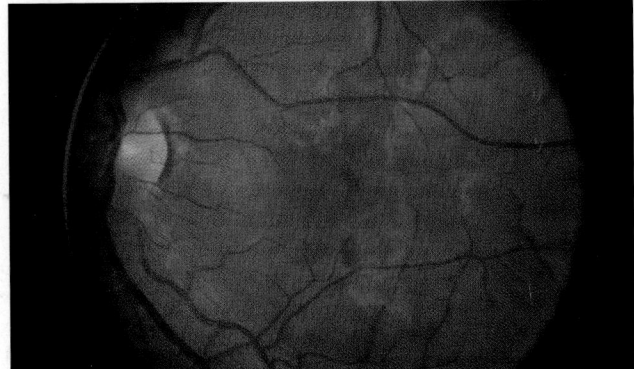

Fig. 46-2B APMPPE (same eye as Fig. 46-2A, several weeks later).

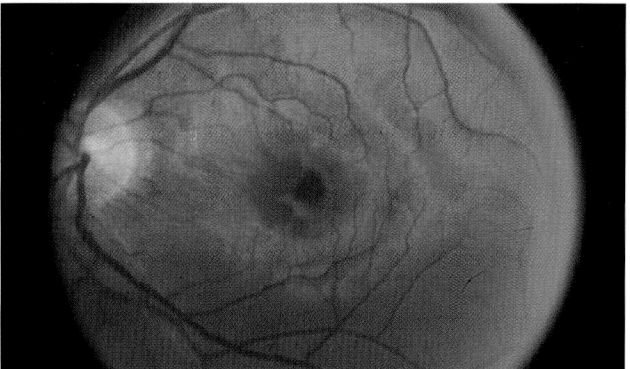

Fig. 46-1 Acute macular neuroretinopathy.

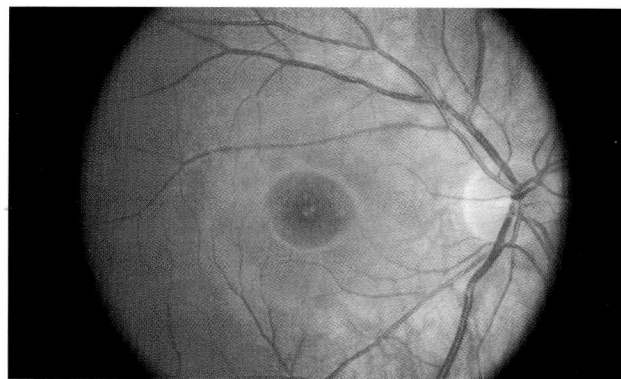

Fig. 46-3 Acute retinal pigment epitheliitis.
(Note: Figs. 46-2A and 46-2B are located on the previous page.)

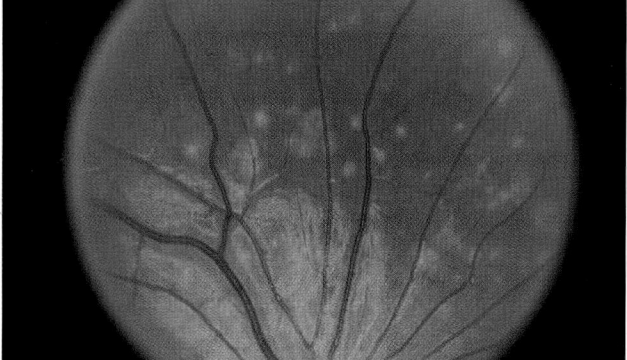

Fig. 46-8 Multiple evanescent white dot syndrome (MEWDS).

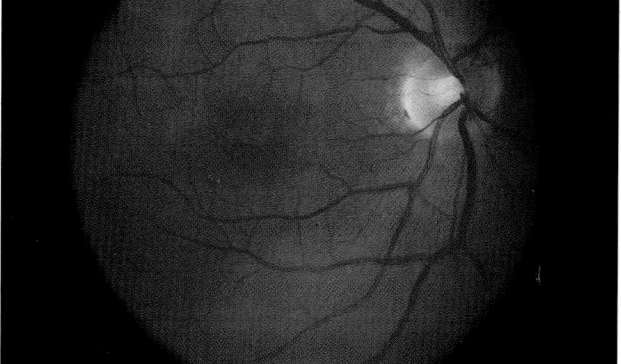

Fig. 46-9 Granular macula in a patient with MEWDS.

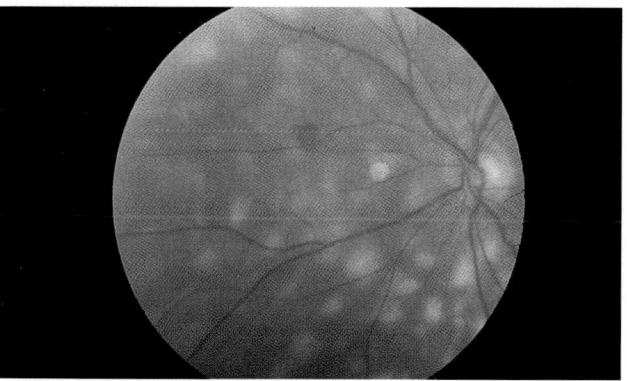

Fig. 47-1 Birdshot retinochoroidopathy.

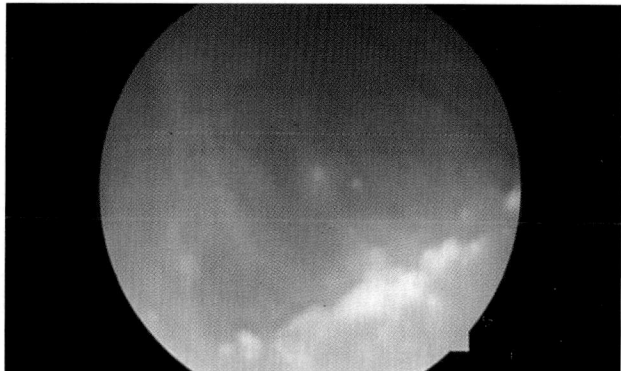

Fig. 55-1 Peripheral infiltrates in a patient with intermediate uveitis.

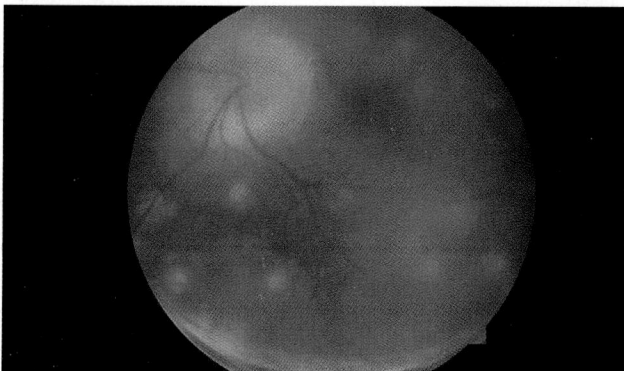

Fig. 57-1 Sympathetic ophthalmia with Dalen-Fuchs nodules.

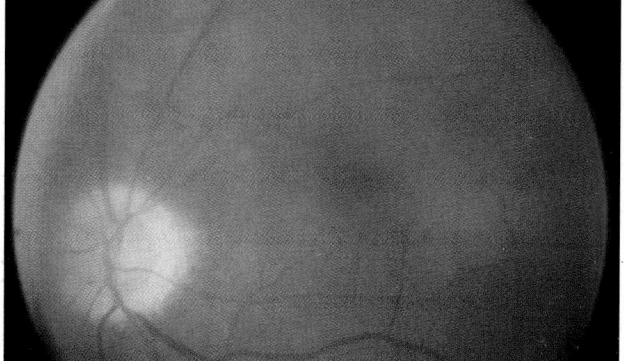

Fig. 58-2 "Sunset-glow" fundus in a patient with Vogt-Koyanagi- Harada syndrome.

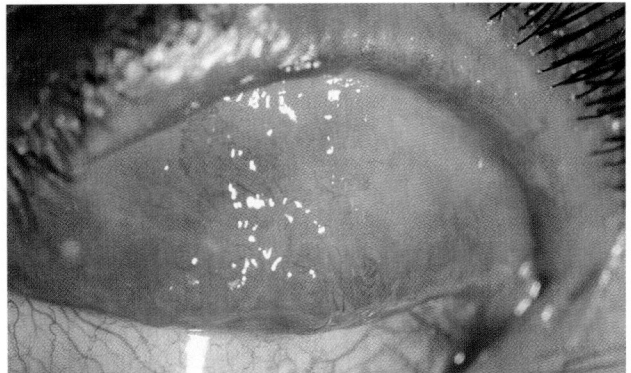

Fig. 59-5 Subconjunctival nodules in a patient with sarcoidosis.

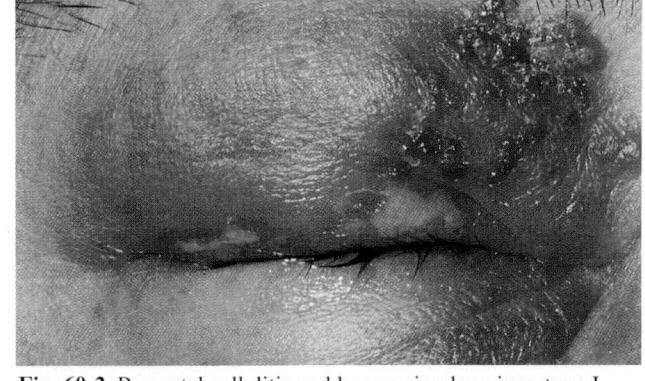

Fig. 60-2 Preseptal cellulitis and herpes simplex virus, type I blepharoconjunctivitis.

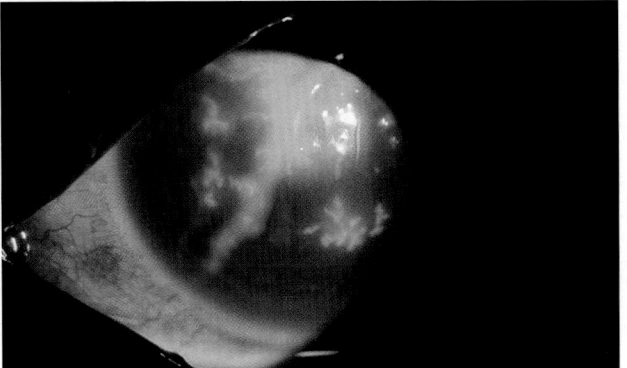

Fig. 71-1 Herpes simplex virus, type II dendriform keratitis with subepithelial infiltrates.

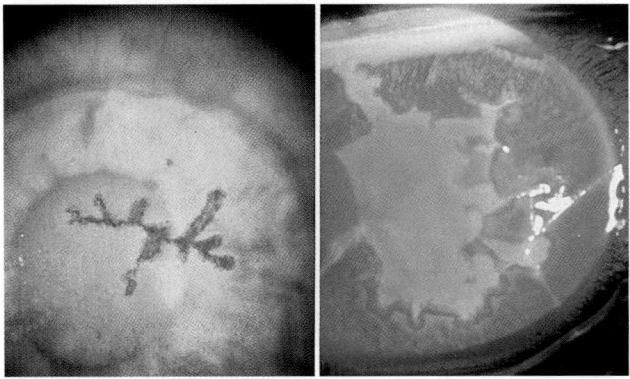

Fig. 71-8 Rose bengal staining of herpetic dendrites *(left)* and fluorescein staining of herpetic geographic ulcer *(right)*.

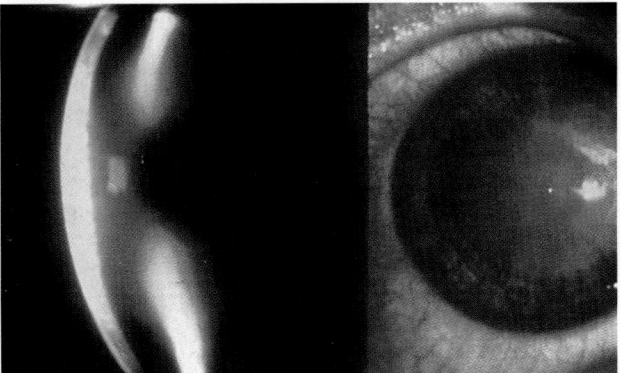

Fig. 71-9 Herpes simplex virus disciform keratitis.

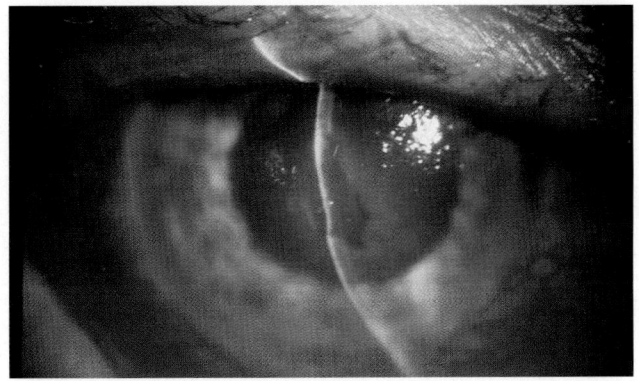

Fig. 71-22 Metaherpetic corneal ulcer.

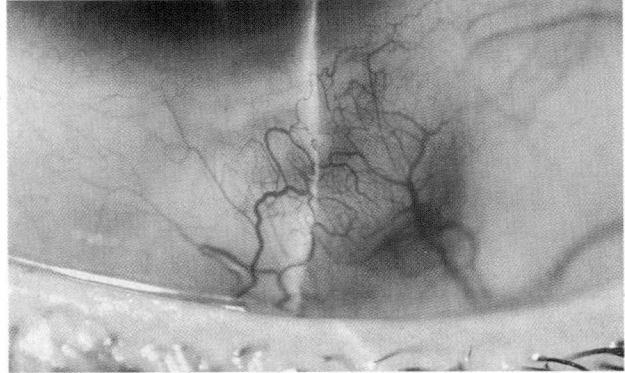

Fig. 72-4A Nodular scleritis associated with varicella-zoster virus.

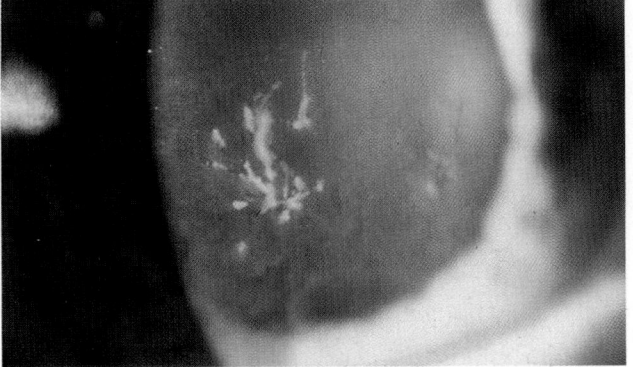

Fig. 72-4B Acute varicella-zoster virus dendriform keratitis.

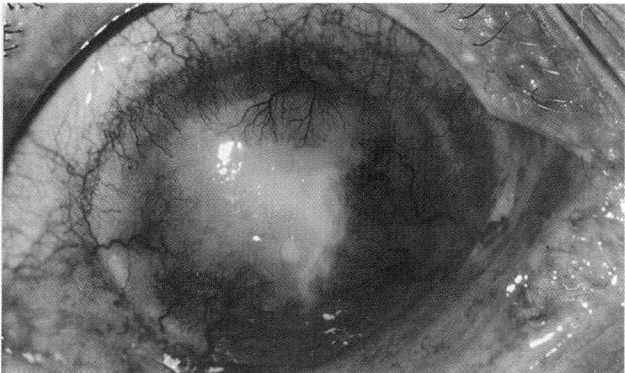

Fig. 72-5A Varicella-zoster virus limbal vasculitis and peripheral ulcerative keratitis.

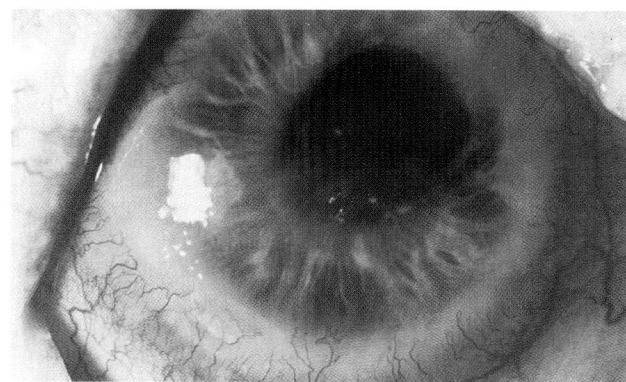

Fig. 72-5B Varicella-zoster virus limbal vasculitis and peripheral ulcerative keratitis.

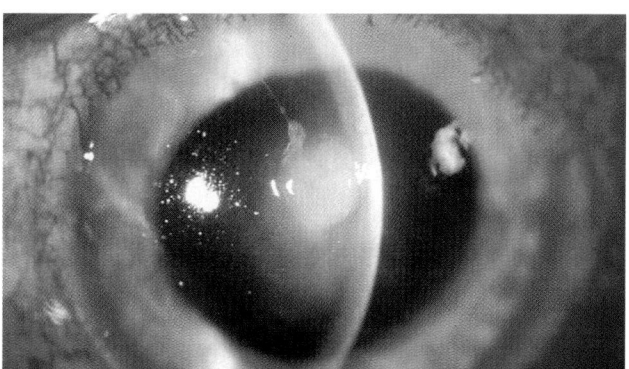

Fig. 74-5A *Staphylococcus aureus* keratitis.

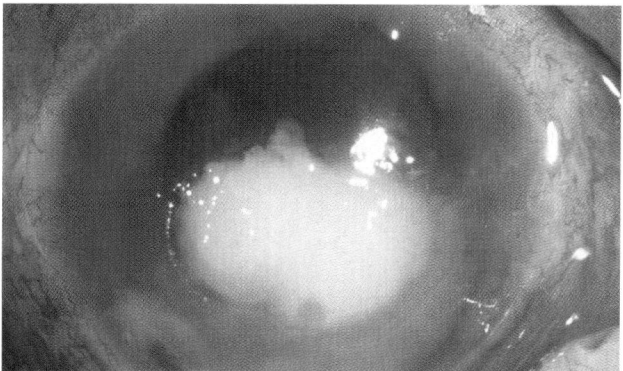

Fig. 74-5B *Streptococcus pneumoniae* keratitis.

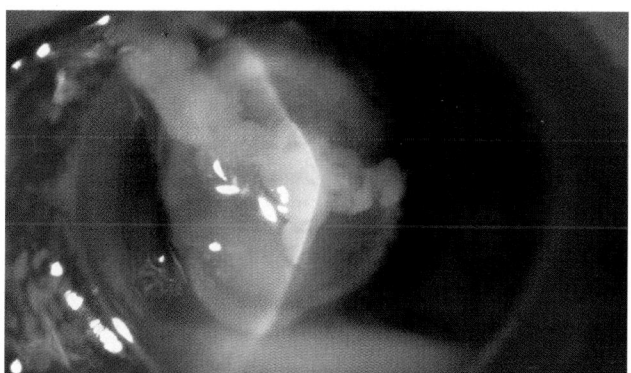

Fig. 74-13 *Pseudomonas aeruginosa* keratitis.

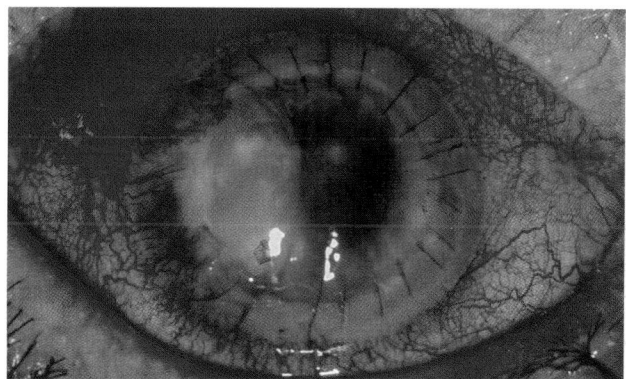

Fig. 75-3 Nontuberculous mycobacterial keratitis.

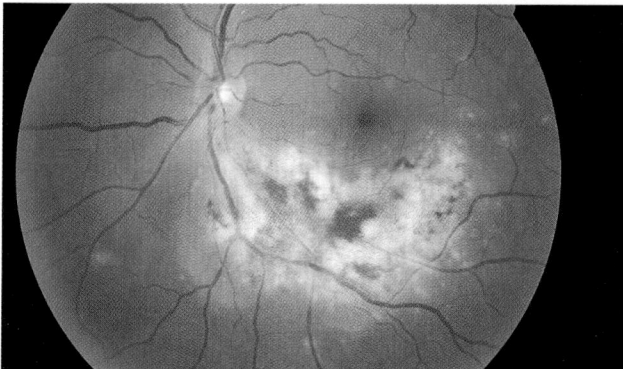

Fig. 81-1 Fulminant/edematous variant of cytomegalovirus (CMV) retinitis.

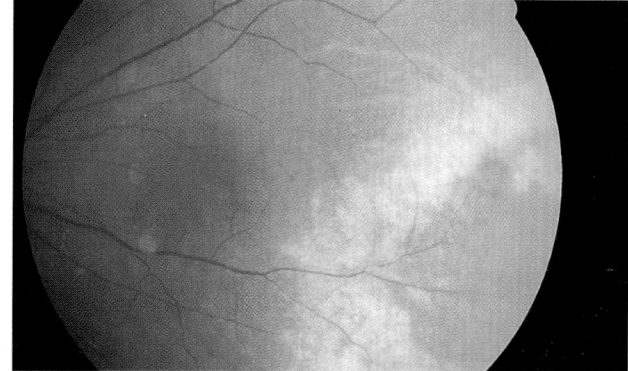

Fig. 81-2 Indolent/granular variant of CMV retinitis.

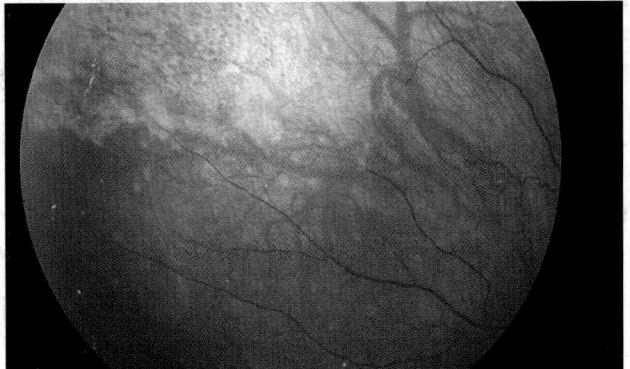

Fig. 81-3 CMV retinitis with satellite lesions.

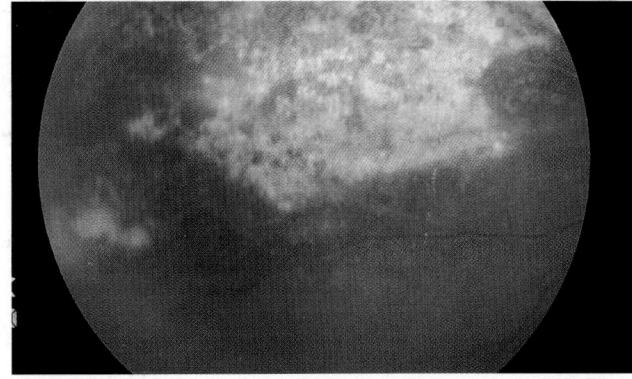

Fig. 81-17 Inactive, treated CMV retinitis with central scarring.

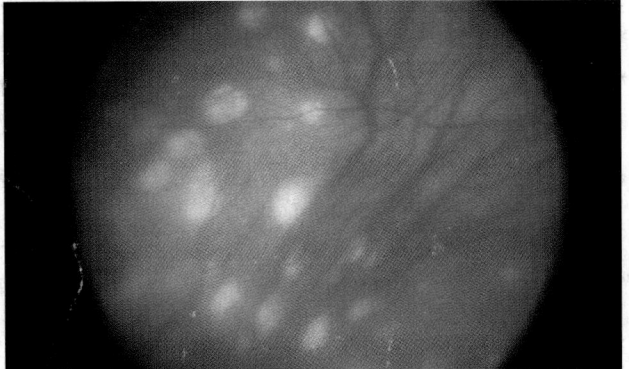

Fig. 84-1B Multifocal choroiditis and panuveitis syndrome.

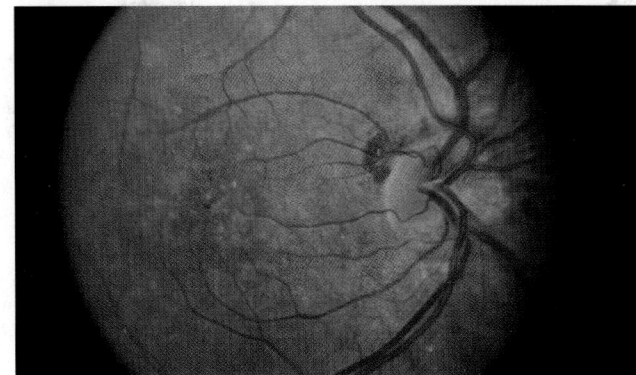

Fig. 84-2A Rubella retinopathy.

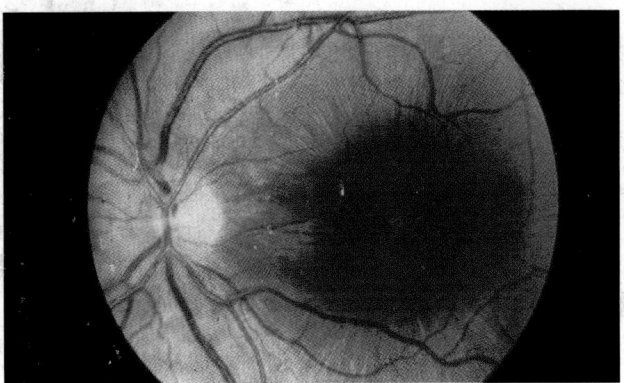

Fig. 84-4 Measles retinopathy.

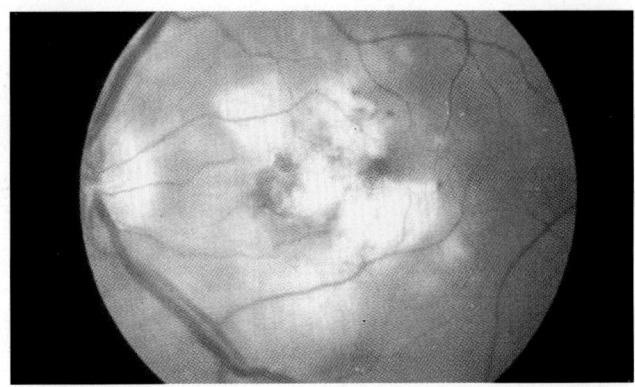

Fig. 84-5A Subacute sclerosing panencephalitis retinopathy.

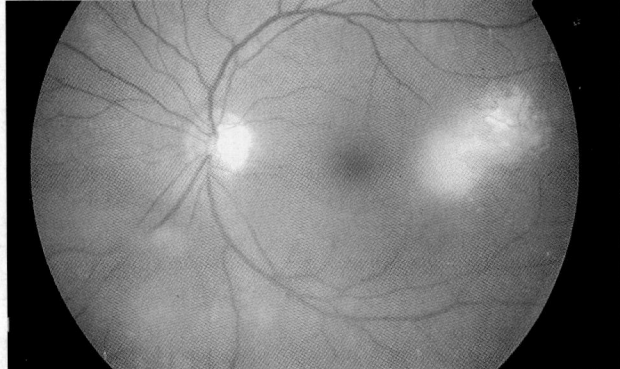

Fig. 85-10A Toxoplasmic retinochoroiditis.
(Note: Fig. 85-7 is located on the next page.)

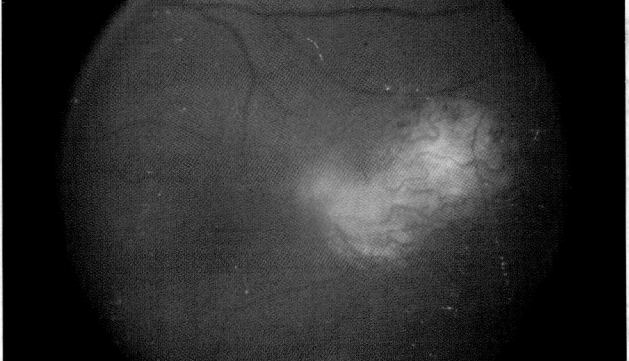

Fig. 85-10B Recurrent toxoplasmic retinochoroiditis (same eye as Fig. 85-10A).

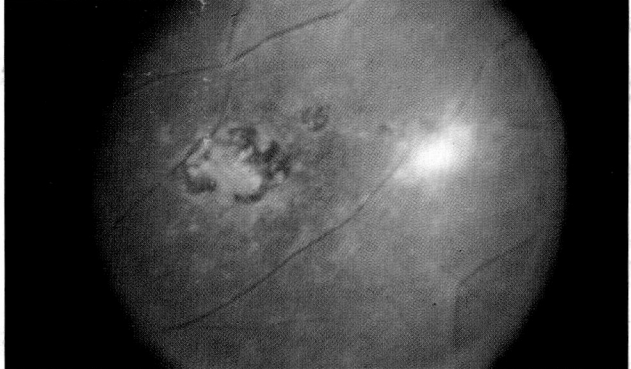

Fig. 85-7 Recurrent toxoplasmic retinochoroiditis.

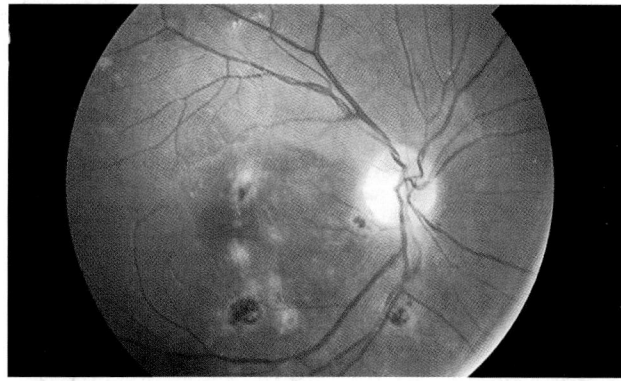

Fig. 85-12 Punctate outer retinal toxoplasmosis.
(Note: Figs. 85-10A and 85-10B are located on the previous page.)

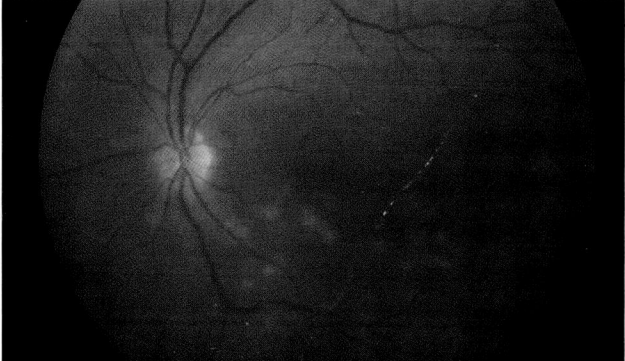

Fig. 88-1 Diffuse unilateral subacute neuroretinitis (DUSN).

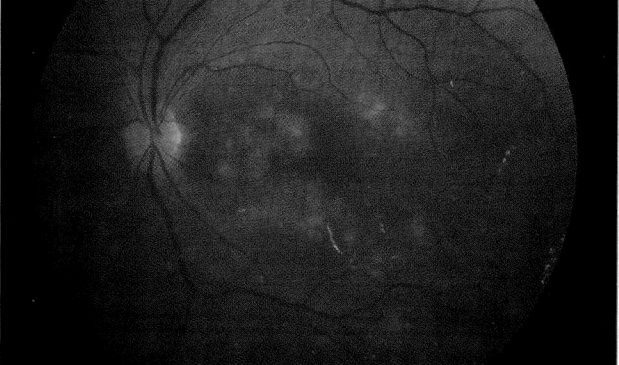

Fig. 88-2 DUSN (later photograph of the same eye shown in Fig. 88-1).

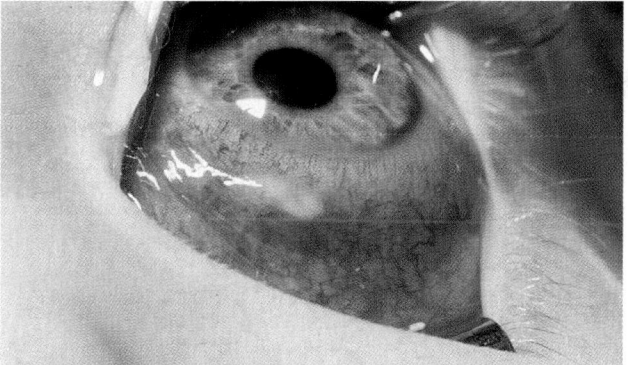

Fig. 99-4 Cat-scratch disease conjunctivitis.

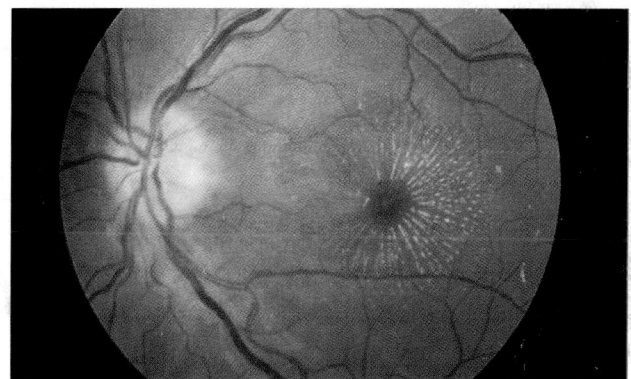

Fig. 99-5 Cat-scratch disease neuroretinitis.

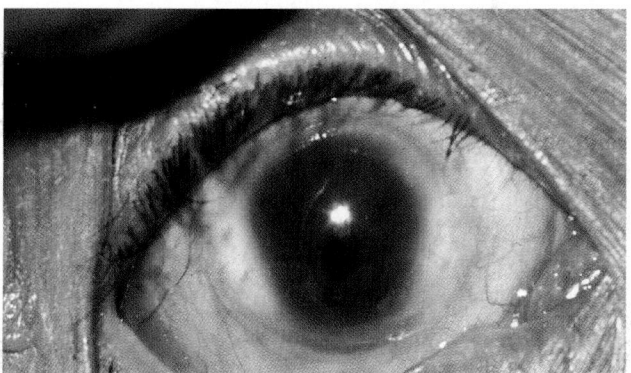

Fig. 107-8 Onchocercal keratitis.

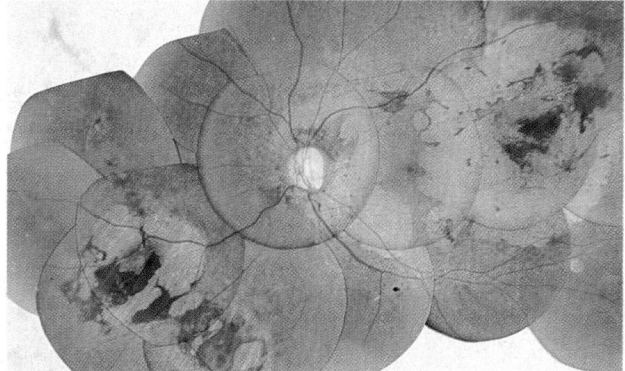

Fig. 107-10 Onchocercal chorioretinopathy.

The Differential Diagnosis of Cytomegalovirus Retinitis

Shown below are clinical photographs found in Table 81-2, which illustrates various disorders in the differential diagnosis of cytomegalovirus retinitis.

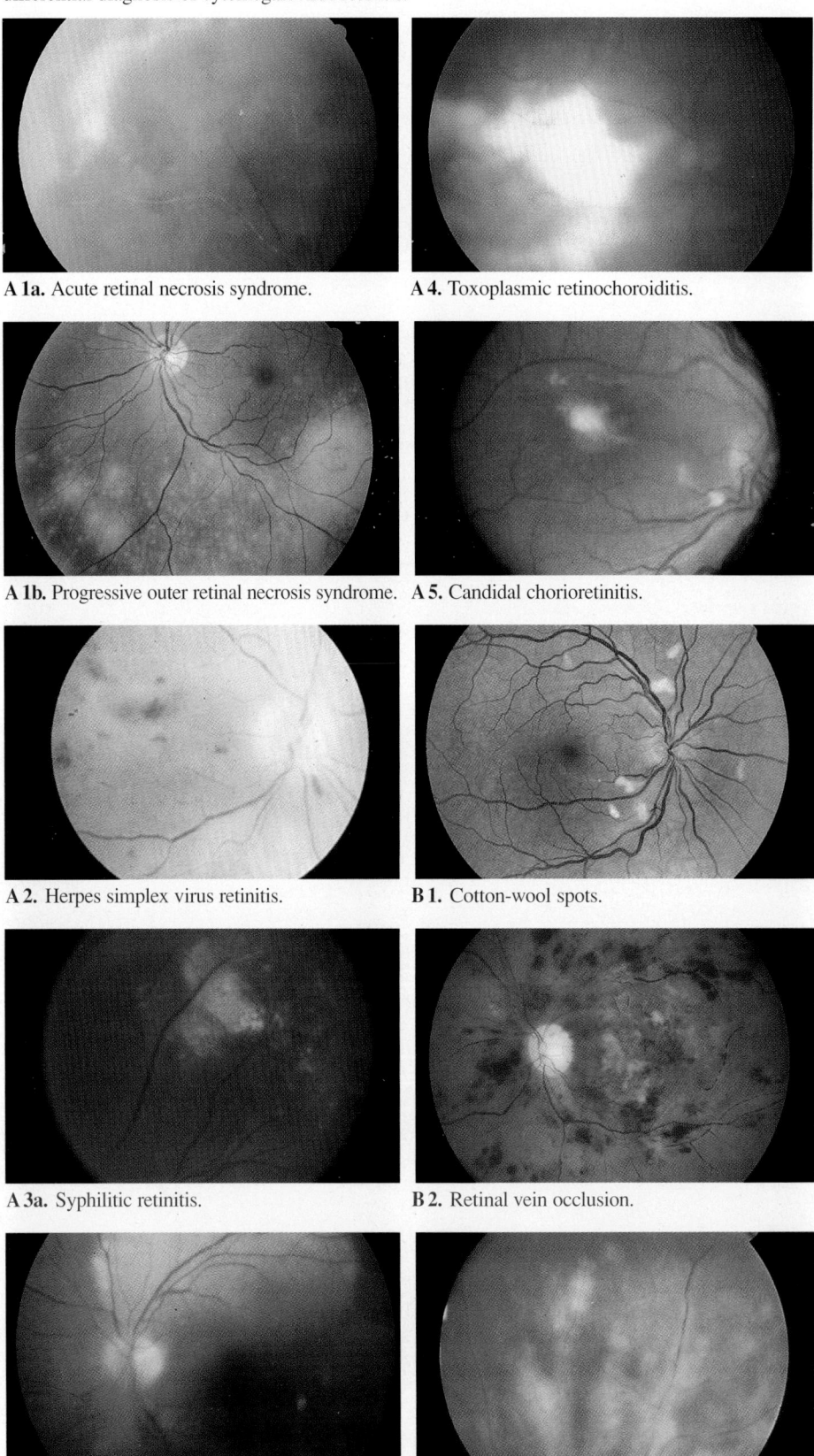

A 1a. Acute retinal necrosis syndrome.

A 4. Toxoplasmic retinochoroiditis.

A 1b. Progressive outer retinal necrosis syndrome.

A 5. Candidal chorioretinitis.

A 2. Herpes simplex virus retinitis.

B 1. Cotton-wool spots.

A 3a. Syphilitic retinitis.

B 2. Retinal vein occlusion.

A 3b. Subretinal placoid lesion caused by syphilis.

C 1. Intraocular lymphoma.

INTRODUCTION

HISTORICAL PERSPECTIVES

1 Historical Milestones in Ocular Immunology

ARTHUR M. SILVERSTEIN

The field of immunology is of special interest to sociologists of science, since during its 110 years it has affected the course of so many biological and medical disciplines and spawned so many new specialties and subspecialties. The clinical field of ophthalmology was one of the earliest influenced by the young and dynamic specialty of immunology at the start of this century. Ophthalmologists very quickly seized upon the concepts and techniques of the early immunologists, and ocular immunology slowly developed as a subdiscipline within the larger field of ophthalmology. Equally interesting is the fact that while many other clinical fields of medicine attempted transiently to integrate the turn-of-century immunological excitement into their clinical and research programs, ophthalmology is perhaps unique in having maintained that interest uninterruptedly up to the present day. This was the case even during the half-century or so when mainstream immunology abandoned its biomedical concerns in favor of more parochial immunochemical approaches.[1] Throughout this century, ophthalmology continued to adapt the newer theories and practices of immunology to its own purposes, and occasionally immunologists utilized the special characteristics of the eye to design experiments to answer nonophthalmic questions. The interaction between these two disciplines accelerated when the immunobiological revolution got fully under way in the early 1960s. Since these latest developments have been so fully recorded in numerous texts and monographs,[2] a detailed history of more recent events in the field will not be attempted. Only those modern advances that provide endpoints to earlier research trails or that illustrate the continued borrowing by ophthalmic researchers of newer findings in immunology will be sketched briefly.

THE BIRTH OF IMMUNOLOGY

Immunology was born as a laboratory and clinical science in 1880 at the hands of Louis Pasteur.[3] His demonstrations of the ability to attenuate pathogens and utilize them for preventive vaccination in the case of chicken cholera, anthrax, rabies, and other diseases excited the interest of the world, and assured that many prominent scientists would follow closely the developments in this field. These successes were further enhanced by the discovery by Behring, Kitasato, and Wernicke in 1890-92 that circulating antibodies can neutralize the toxins of diphtheria and tetanus, and that such antitoxins can even be administered passively to cure patients already showing the early symptoms of these diseases.[4] These two approaches seemed for a time to hold the promise of preventing or curing all of the infectious diseases whose etiologic agents were being discovered with great rapidity. No wonder that by the end of the 19th century, the doctrines of this as yet unnamed discipline were proving so popular and attracting the attention of the academic community in all of the medical specialties.

Ophthalmology was influenced by three components of the developing research program of the new field of immunology,[5] and applied them in turn to the explanation of its own clinical disease problems. The first of these was the "doctrine" of *cytotoxic antibodies*. At the outset, the immune response had been viewed as an evolutionary development for the protection of the individual from harmful disease agents. Ilya Metchnikoff with his phagocytic theory of immunity[6] had emphasized, and Paul Ehrlich with his side-chain theory of antibody formation[7] had implied, the Darwinian nature of these developments; and was not evolution directed toward improvement of the species? So long as the immune response appeared to be limited to mechanisms aimed at the destruction of pathogenic organisms and the neutralization of their deadly toxins, this view seemed appropriate. But in the late 1890s, antibody formation was found to be a more general phenomenon, and antibodies against such bland proteins as albumins were observed. In 1899, Jules Bordet showed[8] that antibodies might even be formed against erythrocytes, which they destroy (hemolyse) with the help of the nonspecifically-acting serum factor complement. Pandora's box had been opened, and investigators everywhere asked themselves why other tissues and

3

organs might not also stimulate an immune response that might account for the tissue destruction seen in so many diseases of unknown etiology and pathogenesis. Very quickly, suspensions or extracts of almost every available tissue and organ were injected into animals to search for specific cytotoxic antibodies, and theories were advanced to link the pathogenesis of many different diseases to this mechanism.[9]

The second relevant component of the immunological research program was the concept of *autoimmunity*. After Jules Bordet reported the finding of destructive anti-erythrocyte antibodies, Ehrlich and Julius Morgenroth wasted no time in testing whether an animal could form antibodies against *its own* erythrocytes.[10] This they never observed, causing Ehrlich to advance the dictum of *Horror Autotoxicus*,[11] which held that even if autoantibodies could be demonstrated, internal regulatory mechanisms would operate to prevent self-destructive consequences. So great was Ehrlich's prestige that his concept was accepted as law, and even the demonstrations of autocytotoxic antispermatozoa in animals by Metalnikoff[12] and of autoantibodies that cause paroxysmal cold hemoglobinuria in man by Donath and Landsteiner[13] failed to shake this belief. As a result, progress in autoimmune disease research was retarded for over 50 years.[14] Only the ophthalmologists worked consistently on this problem during this period, in the context of sympathetic ophthalmia and phacoanaphylaxis.

The third important component of the immunological research program that influenced ophthalmology was that of *anaphylaxis* and related disease mechanisms. In 1902, Paul Portier and Charles Richet reported that animals could be sensitized by a first exposure to antigen, such that a second challenge with the same antigen would lead to shock-like symptoms and even death.[15] Shortly thereafter, Maurice Arthus demonstrated that bland antigens injected repeatedly into the skin could cause local necrotizing lesions, a dermal antigen-antibody interaction thenceforth known as the Arthus phenomenon.[16] Finally, in 1906, Clemens von Pirquet and Bela Schick showed that the pathogenesis of human serum sickness involves an antibody response in the host to the injection of large quantities of foreign protein antigens.[17] Anaphylaxis the word and anaphylaxis the concept became so popular that they penetrated into all branches of medicine, and not least into ophthalmological concepts of disease. This spread of interest in anaphylaxis was accelerated when it became apparent that the human torments hayfever and asthma were also due to similar mechanisms.[18]

We shall now see how the field of ophthalmology was influenced by these three concepts. I shall discuss them in terms of their influence on the major trends in ocular immunopathology, and show how they affected the concepts of pathogenesis in a number of clinically important ophthalmic diseases.

AUTOIMMUNE DISEASES OF THE EYE

Phacoanaphylaxis

A new chapter in the history of immunology was opened up by Paul Uhlenhuth when he reported in 1903 that the antigens of the lens of the eye are organ-specific.[19] This was the first intimation that unique antigens might exist within a single organ and, further, that they might be shared among widely divergent species. It was then shown by Kraus and coworkers,[20] and by Andrejew and Uhlenhuth[21] that these lens (*phaco-*) antigens could mediate both active and passive anaphylaxis in test animals. Uhlenhuth and Haendel soon showed that a guinea pig could be rendered sensitive to *its own* lens protein and sent into anaphylactic shock with the proteins from any other lens.[22] These investigators drew no conclusions from their work that might be applied to clinical problems, although the ophthalmologist Paul Römer had earlier speculated that senile cataract formation might be mediated by autocytotoxic antibodies specific for the lens.[23] It was only when F.F. Krusius demonstrated in 1910 that rupture of the lens capsule in a *normal* guinea pig would both sensitize the animal and serve also as the disease-producing challenge[24] that the true implications of this system for ocular disease became apparent.

In a comprehensive review of the subject in 1912, Römer and Gebb considered the broader implications of these findings in a most interesting way. In a section of the review "on the question of the formation of autoanaphylactic antibodies by means of lens proteins," they asked whether autologous lens is *really* foreign in the guinea pig, or "whether the 'law of immunity research,' which Ehrlich has popularly termed horror autotoxicus, does not rather apply to the lens." Here, as early as 1912, was a foretaste of the later concept of the *sequestered antigen*. If the body *cannot* respond to self, then all such antigens able to stimulate an immune response *must* be foreign, i.e., normally sequestered somehow from contact with the host's immune system. But as true followers of Ehrlich, they finally came to the conclusion that lens is indeed self, that it does stimulate an immune response, and that "We are rather convinced that the regulatory mechanism of the organism can and will refuse to serve under special conditions. And the investigation of these situations will further promote our understanding of pathological states."[25]

Interest in lens-induced immunogenic disease continued, and important contributions were made over the years. The clinical condition was named *endophthalmitis phacoanaphylactica* by Verhoeff and Lemoine in 1922, and these investigators also reported positive skin test responses in patients with this disease.[26] Further investigation of antilens responses in patients with cataract was pursued in extensive investigations by Burky and Woods.[27] Perhaps the most significant contributions to our understanding of this autoimmune process were made in a series of reports by Marak and coworkers.[28] They produced a disease in rats histopathologically similar to that seen in the human, and were able to transfer the disease adoptively using immune serum; there seems to be little evidence that T cell mechanisms contribute significantly to the pathogenesis of "phacoantigenic uveitis."

Our story of the immunology of the lens would not be complete without mention of its application to the problem of evolution. It had been proposed as early as 1904 that the cross-reactions of the serum protein antigens of different species might be employed to measure interspecies relationships. From the 1960s on, this approach was elegantly pursued by Halbert and Manski,[29] using lens antigens from many different species, and a battery of antilens antisera. Given the evolutionary conservation of these structures, cross-reactions were detectable across the entire vertebrate spectrum, and the results proved to be fascinating.

Sympathetic Ophthalmia

Ophthalmologists were not long in responding to the doctrine of cytotoxic antibodies. Santucci suggested in 1906 that sympathetic ophthalmia might be caused by the formation of cytotoxic antibodies, following the resorption of damaged ocular tissue in the first eye. These putative antibodies would then attack the hitherto normal contralateral eye[30]. He presented experiments showing that injection of emulsified ocular tissue into rabbits and guinea pigs would cause endophthalmitis. No sooner had this thesis begun to attract attention than a counterclaim for priority appeared from the pen of S. Golowin in Russia, who stated that he had advanced this idea in 1904, in a Russian journal apparently unread in the West.[31] Golowin claimed that the iris and ciliary body were the seat of attack in the sympathizing eye, and so named these antibodies "cyclotoxins."

Then the famous Prague ophthalmologist Elschnig entered the fray. Elschnig quickly became the leading advocate of an autoimmune pathogenesis of sympathetic ophthalmia,[32] with the collaboration of the prominent immunologist Weil. They proposed that the resorption of antigen in the damaged eye led to a "hypersensitivity" that also involved the second eye. Thenceforth, the mildest disturbance in the sensitized second eye might lead to inflammation and blindness. As the result of numerous animal experiments, Elschnig identified uveal pigment as the offending antigen.

Students of sympathetic ophthalmia continued thereafter to concentrate on a pathogenesis based upon an autoimmune response to uveal pigment. The foremost American supporter of this thesis was ophthalmologist Alan Woods at Johns Hopkins, who published extensively on this subject starting as early as 1916.[33] Woods later employed uveal pigment as antigen in an intracutaneous test for sensitization in patients with sympathetic ophthalmia, and reported positive

results.[34] Woods' colleague Jonas Friedenwald demonstrated that the histopathology of the uveal pigment skin test was "consistent with an allergic reaction," thus reinforcing the concept.[35] Woods was so convinced that he understood the mechanism of the disease that he felt free to inject uveal pigment preparations into patients in a therapeutic attempt to "desensitize" them, and in fact reported favorable results.[36] It is now difficult to say what other contaminants may have been present in the crude preparations of uveal pigment then employed, but the results proved quite variable, and an etiology for sympathetic ophthalmia based upon uveal pigment slowly fell out of favor.

The absence of a satisfactory animal model of the disease was one of the chief obstacles to progress in understanding the etiology and pathogenesis of sympathetic ophthalmia. Progress was slow, until the Freund's adjuvant was introduced in 1942, a technique that advanced the cause of so many autoimmune disease models. In two landmark papers in 1949 and 1953,[37] Collins reported on the production of uveoretinitis in guinea pigs induced by uveal extracts injected in adjuvant. These observations (along with others in autoimmune hemolytic anemias, orchitis, thyroiditis, and encephalomyelitis) helped to ensure the modern revival of interest in autoimmune diseases.[38]

Some years later, Wacker and Lipton showed that retinal extracts are much more efficient in producing autoimmune disease than uveal extracts,[39] initiating a broad search for the organ-specific antigens involved. Three such antigens were found initially by this group, localized by immunofluorescent analysis to the outer segments of the retina.[40] Then, simultaneously, two different laboratories isolated and identified a soluble retinal antigen (S-antigen) able to induce autoimmune disease in animals.[41] A number of other organ-specific antigens have been implicated since then, including an interphotoreceptor retinoid-binding protein (IRBP)[42] and even the visual pigment rhodopsin itself.[43] By varying the dosage and sensitizing regimen, it has been possible to alter the previously-observed chronic inflammatory picture to that of a granulomatous form more typical of human sympathetic ophthalmia.[44] It is of some interest that experimental autoimmune uveoretinitis induced by S-antigen and IRBP is accompanied by inflammation of the pineal gland, which shares antigens in common with the retina.[45] All of the most recent data on the mechanisms of host response in this experimental model attest to its autoimmune pathogenesis and to its close relationship with human sympathetic ophthalmia.[46]

Sjögren Syndrome

Sjögren syndrome is a later addition to the list of autoimmune diseases of the eye, and is a product of the recent general interest in this area. It was first described clinically in 1933,[47] and autoantibodies were only described in 1958.[48]

It is a disease characterized by an autoimmune attack on the lacrimal and salivary glands, involving a chronic inflammatory destruction of acinar cells and ductular epithelium.[49] This results in the vexing problem of dry eyes and a dry mouth. The history, clinical aspects, and pathophysiology of this disease have been reviewed extensively by Liotet and coworkers.[50] Recent experiments appear to confirm the existence of lacrimal gland-specific antigens, able to induce autoimmune dacryoadenitis in the rat without cross-reacting involvement of the salivary gland.[51] A similar approach has shown that an experimental autoimmune disease specific only for the rat Harderian gland may also be elicited using the appropriate organ-specific antigen.[52] In these animal models of Sjögren's syndrome, T cell-mediated immunity appears to be the dominant mechanism involved.[53] The relationship between these animal models and the human disease is presently unclear, given the high degree of organ specificity of the experimental systems. They may, however, be related to a group of apparently chronic inflammatory conditions of the lacrimal gland that bear the nonspecific diagnosis "chronic dacryoadenitis".[54]

IMMUNOGENIC KERATITIS

Corneal Arthus Reactions

The first observation of an immunopathologic involvement of the cornea was by Wessely, who showed that the injection of antigen intrastromally in the central cornea of a sensitized rabbit would produce an opaque ring of interstitial keratitis.[55] This finding attracted much attention, especially on the part of Aurel von Szily, who devoted an entire book[56] to the study of this phenomenon. In a model collaboration between immunopathologists and ophthalmologists, Germuth, Maumenee, and coworkers,[57] employing modern technics such as immunofluorescent histochemical staining, proved that the Wessely ring was in fact a true intracorneal Arthus reaction, i.e., an immune complex deposit with local fixation of complement and the release of pharmacologic agents that attract polymorphonuclear leukocytes to the site. Waksman and Bullington, in a similar collaboration, had earlier demonstrated an equivalent Arthus reaction within the uveal tract.[58] These studies helped to focus attention on the possible contributions of hypersensitivity reactions and immune complex disease as possible contributors to ocular pathology.

Tuberculosis

Yet another approach to the problem of immunogenic interstitial keratitis stemmed from Robert Koch's tuberculin test, and from developments in the field of delayed hypersensitivity (later to be called cellular immunology), in which this test played so important a role. During the early period, when many new approaches to the diagnosis of tuberculosis were developed, Calmette proposed his "ophthalmoreaction,"[59] in which tuberculin dropped on the eye of a sensitized individual would lead to a more-or-less severe conjunctivitis. While this test proved to be too dangerous, it did stimulate experiments using other ocular tissues, including the cornea. It was quickly found that intracorneal injection of tuberculin into sensitized guinea pigs would yield an interstitial keratitis, whereas intracorneal injection of antigen into an anaphylactically sensitive animal would usually not lead to corneal inflammation. A different mechanism seemed to be involved, one that could operate even within the normally avascular cornea. Indeed, this difference was long used as one of the principal criteria to differentiate these two phenomena.

The hypersensitivity that accompanies tuberculosis may also be expressed by the spontaneous development of phlyctenular keratoconjunctivitis. This disease is seen most frequently at the margin between cornea and conjunctiva, and presents as an inflammatory infiltrate or nodule composed of epithelioid cells surrounded by lymphocytes, resembling a small tubercle. Descriptions of such nodules appear in the 2nd century in the writings of Paul of Aegina and of Ali ben Isa, and more recently in the 18th century treatise on ocular diseases of St. Yves.[60] The condition was produced experimentally by ophthalmologists Weekers and Riehm in the tuberculin-sensitive rabbit, following instillation of tuberculin in the conjunctiva.[61] Its association with tuberculosis has been repeatedly confirmed epidemiologically,[62] but it may also result from hypersensitivity reactions to other infectious agents and allergens.[63]

Herpesvirus Keratitis

Herpesvirus destruction of the corneal epithelium (and of the retina in intraocular infections) appears most often to be the result of direct viral cytopathogenicity, but the corneal stromal pathology associated with this virus seems to be based upon immunological (hypersensitivity) mechanisms.[64] Most investigators have favored a T cell-mediated pathogenesis,[65] although immune complex disease has also been suggested.[66]

CORNEAL TRANSPLANTATION

The attempt to transplant the cornea to restore sight has a long history,[67] but it was only around the turn of this century that technical improvements in trephines and sutures permitted the ophthalmic surgeon to begin to realize consistent success in this venture, employing what we now call allogeneic tissue. When, as frequently happened, a graft would fail, it was usually attributed to some unknown physiological factor. Despite the fact that the immunologic "laws of transplantation" were well worked out by tumor transplanters early in this century,[68] the information appears to have been unknown outside that field. It remained for Peter

Medawar to clarify the immunologic basis of allograft rejection in his elegant series of studies in the 1940s,[69] and these immediately caught the attention of transplant surgeons everywhere.

Maumenee was chiefly responsible for bringing these immunological findings to the attention of ophthalmologists, and for bringing to the attention of the transplant immunologists the special characteristics of the cornea that allow keratoplasty to succeed so often while most other tissue and organ grafts fail.[70] Again, the important mechanism responsible for the occasional graft rejection was shown to be the cellular immune response mediated by effector lymphocytes, and the high success rate of allokeratoplasty was shown to reside in an immunological privilege of the cornea, involving both the afferent and efferent limbs of the immune response, due to the avascularity and lack of lymphatic drainage in the cornea.[71] This view is supported by the observation that increased vascularization of the graft predisposes to rejection; the privilege resides mainly in the absence of visiting lymphocytes.

IMMUNOGENIC UVEITIS

It had been demonstrated from the start that the eye shares in the general hypersensitivity of the immunized or infected host,[72] and that such sensitization can be induced also by intraocular administration of antigen. But it remained for Sattler[73] to show in 1909 that bland antigen introduced into the vitreous of the rabbit eye would cause in addition a *local ocular hypersensitivity,* an observation extended by the elegant studies of the Seegals.[74] Such a sensitized eye will respond for many months thereafter with an acute anterior uveitis when specific antigen is introduced intravenously or even by feeding. Here was a possible animal model of human recurrent nongranulomatous anterior uveitis that stimulated later workers to investigate its pathogenesis.

One of the results of such studies was the finding that the tissues of the eye can support the local formation of antibody, much like a regional lymph node. This understanding emerged initially from studies of equine periodic ophthalmia, an ocular infection due to leptospira. It was shown by Goldmann and Witmer that so efficient is the eye in producing specific antibody that the high serum titers of antileptospiral antibodies found in these infected horses could have originated *solely* from local formation in that organ.[75] It was suggested later that the inflammatory response accompanying intraocular antibody formation might be the primary pathogenetic contributor to recurrent anterior uveitis, due to the persistence of specific memory cells within the uveal tract of the sensitized eye.[76] In line with developments in the general immunopathology of inflammation, it has been shown that lymphokines play an active role in the mediation of uveal inflammatory responses.[77]

Intraocular Infections and the Focal Reaction

With the finding that systemic hypersensitivity accompanies tuberculosis[78] and many other infectious diseases, many investigators wondered whether such immunologic components might not contribute to the pathogenesis of such granulomatous diseases of the eye as tuberculosis, syphilis, toxoplasmosis, and others. This notion received support from the old observation that quiescent tubercles in the eye (and elsewhere) may be reactivated during attempts to desensitize tuberculosis patients with tuberculin, the so-called focal reaction. For many years, ophthalmologists searched for the trigger of attacks of uveitis (i.e., a source of inciting antigen) at distant sites of infection, including the teeth and appendix. The possible role of hypersensitivities in these infectious uveoretinopathies was first advanced by the foremost exponent of this thesis Alan Woods,[79] who sought to prevent these flare-ups by a program of desensitization with the putative allergens involved.

Anterior Chamber Privilege

The extensive studies of H.S.N. Greene on the transplantation of tumors and endocrine tissues into the anterior chamber of the eye[80] had implied that this site might enjoy a degree of immunological privilege, although this privilege appears not to be absolute.[81] The basis of this phenomenon has been examined in detail in the immunology laboratories of Streilein and his collaborators, who suggest that an anterior chamber-associated immune deviation (ACAID) results from the induction of suppressor T cells when antigens are presented to the immune system by this route.[82]

This peculiarity of the anterior chamber has led to several curious experimental findings. In addition to the survival of otherwise immunogenic tumors in the anterior chamber,[83] infection of the mouse eye with herpesvirus results in T cell-mediated prevention of ipsilateral retinal destruction, while destruction of the contralateral retina proceeds unchecked.[84]

Ocular Immunopathology and Systemic Disease

Recent developments in immunogenetics, have led to increasing collaboration between ophthalmologists and internists, endocrinologists, geneticists, and immunologists. A significant group of systemic diseases known or suspected to involve immunopathogenetic mechanisms have been shown to manifest ocular complications, most usually uveitis or uveoretinitis. Among those with demonstrable genetic predispositions are: ankylosing spondylitis, associated with HLA-B27; Behçet syndrome, associated with HLA-B5; and Vogt-Koyanagi-Harada disease, associated with HLA-DRw54. Even sympathetic ophthalmia has been associated with HLA-DR4 and HLA-DRw53 among Japanese, although apparently not among caucasians.[85] Ocular complications in other systemic diseases where HLA association has not yet been demonstrated include lupus erythematosis, periarteritis nodosa, sarcoidosis, myasthenia gravis, and Grave's disease. The presence in the vitreous of type II collagen has also interested rheumatologists seeking to explain the ocular involvement in this group of diseases. The clinical and pathogenetic factors involved in the ocular components of these systemic diseases are reviewed in detail by Faure and colleagues.[86]

ALLERGIC CONJUNCTIVITIS

We have already seen that the conjunctiva may become inflamed by instillation of tuberculin in the sensitized individual. With the finding that hayfever and asthma are also immunologic ("anaphylactic") reactions, it became apparent that immunogenic conjunctivitis was a more general phenomenon, and ophthalmic clinicians became more interested in its pathogenesis and treatment.[87] This stimulated research on the possible immunopathogenesis of such diseases as vernal catarrh, a seasonal papillary conjunctivitis most often associated with pollen allergy.[88]

Perhaps the most interesting development along these lines was the suggestion that a chronic immune response to the antigens of *Chlamydia trachomatis* might account for the primary lesions seen in trachoma[89] and in other follicular conjunctivitides. Trachoma is characterized by the exuberant development of germinal centers beneath the conjunctival epithelium, leading Barrie Jones to liken the conjunctival sac to a lymph node cut open, where antigenic stimuli enter through an overlying epithelium.[90] Recent studies have implicated the chlamydial heat-shock protein as the stimulus for conjunctival hypersensitivity responses in this disease.[91]

Contact Allergy

Due to the widespread use of ophthalmic medications, and especially of cosmetics, contact allergy has become an increasingly important problem in industrialized societies. While the conjunctiva may be involved in the process, it is more often as a secondary complication of an allergic reaction of the skin of the eyelids. The mechanisms involved, and the many agents that may elicit this disease, are reviewed in detail by Theodore and Schlossman.[63]

INSTITUTIONALIZATION OF THE SUBDISCIPLINE

It is always difficult to assign an exact date to the formal establishment of a scientific discipline. In the case of ocular immunology/immunopathology, the components of a specific research program (involving sympathetic ophthalmia, lens-induced disease, "anaphylactic" keratitis and conjunctivitis, etc.) had already been identified by 1912, and an interacting community of clinical and laboratory researchers had formed. The first special monograph devoted to ocular immunopathology appeared in 1914,[56] and other texts and

monographs followed.[92] Departments of ophthalmology throughout the world added immunological research laboratories to their facilities.[93] These ocular immunology units soon began to hire basic science faculty members, a trend that accelerated after the Second World War with the expansion of interest in all biomedical specialties. The establishment of the National Eye Institute at the U.S. National Institutes of Health in Bethesda, Maryland in 1968 testifies to the growing scientific and political strength of ophthalmic and vision research, from the fruits of which research in ocular immunology also benefited immeasurably.

One of the hallmarks of disciplinary institutionalization is the development of first informal and then formal networks of individuals with common scientific interests. In the mid-1940s, ophthalmologists Phillips Thygeson, James Allen, and Fred Theodore organized an informal group to discuss epidemic keratitis and other problems in ocular microbiology. Immunological discussions quickly entered, and in 1966 Thygeson formalized the meeting at the Proctor Foundation in San Francisco as the Ocular Immunology and Microbiology Group. This Group served as the model for the Section on Ocular Immunology and Microbiology, when the Association for Research in Vision and Ophthalmology (ARVO) was reorganized into disciplinary sections in 1968.[94] Both the Group and the ARVO Section continue to meet annually, and the latter has grown from a few dozen persons at the start to a current membership of over 400. Whereas the earlier investigators were almost all clinicians with a bent for research, more than 50% of the current members are basic scientists with formal training in such fields as immunology, molecular biology, bacteriology, and virology.

Another prerequisite for the formation of a new discipline is the definition of its scope. A significant step in this direction was the organization in the late 1950s of a series of Macy Foundation meetings by Alan Woods and A.E. Maumenee. Prominent basic immunologists were invited to interact with clinicians in highly productive exchanges.[95] A similar set of meetings, involving ophthalmic scientists and a broad spectrum of basic immunologists, was assembled in a series of workshops sponsored by the National Eye Institute.[96] Immunology had been identified by the Eye Institute as one of the principal research areas for future exploitation, and these meetings were designed to define the current status of the field and to identify new and fruitful approaches.

Perhaps the most significant organizational development in this field was the founding in 1974 of a series of quadrennial International Symposia on the Immunology and Immunopathology of the Eye by W. Böke of Germany, R. Campinchi and E. Bloch-Michel of France, and M. Luntz of South Africa. Five such symposia have been held, whose sessions and resulting publications[97] have consolidated this specialized community of scientists, recorded the progress in the field, and stimulated new interest and activity by promoting the exchange of information with other scientific disciplines.

NOTES AND REFERENCES

1. A major transition in immunology, from an interest in biomedical problems (infectious diseases and the general pathology of inflammation) to chemical approaches, occurred about the time of the First World War. The reasons for and implications of this gestalt shift are discussed in Silverstein AM: The dynamics of conceptual change in twentieth century immunology, *Cell Immunol* 132:515, 1991.
2. Böke W: *Immunpathologie des auges,* Karger, Basel, 1968; Rahi AHS, Garner A: *Immunopathology of the eye,* Blackwell, Oxford, 1976; Faure J-P et al: *Immunopathologie de l'oeil,* Masson, Paris, 1988.
3. Pasteur L: *C R Acad Sci* 90:239, 952, 1880.
4. Behring E, Kitasato S: *Dtsch Med Wochenschr* 16:1113, 1890; Behring E, Wernicke E: *Z Hyg* 12:10, 45, 1892.
5. The six principal components of the early immunological research program are discussed by Silverstein, note 1. These were: preventive immunization, cellular (phagocytic) immunity, serotherapy, cytotoxic antibodies, serodiagnosis, and anaphylaxis and related phenomena.
6. Metchnikoff E: *L'immunité dans les maladies infectieuses,* Masson, Paris, 1901.
7. Ehrlich P: *Klin Jahrb* 6:299, 1897; *Proc R Soc London Ser B* 66:424, 1900.
8. Bordet J: *Ann Inst Pasteur* 12:688, 1899.
9. See, e.g., *Ann Inst Pasteur* 14: 1900.
10. Ehrlich P, Morgenroth J: *Berl Klin Wochenschr* 28:251, 1901.
11. Erhlich P: *Verh. 73 Ges Dtsch Naturforsch Aerzte,* 1901. Reprinted in *The collected papers of Paul Ehrlich,* Vol. 2, Pergamon, New York, 1957, p. 298.
12. Metalnikoff S: *Ann Inst Pasteur* 14:577, 1900.
13. Donath J, Landsteiner K: *Münch Med Wochenschr* 51:1590, 1904.
14. The background to this hiatus is discussed in Silverstein AM: *A history of immunology,* Academic Press, New York, 1989, pp. 160-189.
15. Portier P, Richet C: *C R Soc Biol* 54:170, 1902.
16. Arthus M: *C R Soc Biol* 55:817, 1903.
17. von Pirquet C, Schick B: *Die Serumkrankheit,* Deuticke, Vienna, 1906.
18. Wolff-Eisner A: *Das Heufieber,* Munich, 1906; Meltzer S: *J. Am Med Assoc* 55:1021, 1910.
19. Uhlenhuth P: In *Festschrift zum 60 Geburtstag von Robert Koch,* Fischer, Jena, 1903, pp. 49-74.
20. Kraus R, Doerr R, Sohma M: *Wien Klin Wochenschr* 21:1084, 1908.
21. Andrejew P, Uhlenhuth P: *Arb Kaiserl Gesundheitsamte* 30:450, 1908.
22. Uhlenhuth P, Haendel W: *Z. Immunitätsforsch* 4:761, 1910.
23. Römer P, Gebb H: *von Graefes Arch Ophthalmol* 60:175, 1905.
24. Krusius FF: *Arch Augenheilk* 67:6, 1910.
25. Römer P, Gebb H: *von Graefes Arch Ophthalmol* 81:367, 387, 1912.
26. Verhoeff FH, Lemoine AN: *Acta Int Cong Ophthalmol Washington* 1:234, 1922; *Am J Ophthalmol* 5:737, 1922.
27. Burky EL, Woods AC: *Arch Ophthalmol* 6:548, 1931; Burky EL: *Arch Ophthalmol* 12:536, 1934.
28. Marak GE et al: *Exp Eye Res* 19:311, 1974; Marak GE, Font RL, Alepa FP: *Mod Probl Ophthalmol* 16:75, 1976; *idem, Ophthalmic Res* 9:162, 1977.
29. Halbert SP, Manski W, Auerbach T: In *The structure of the eye,* Smelser GK, ed.: Academic Press, New York, 1961; Halbert SP, Manski W: *Prog Allergy* 7:107, 1963; Manski W, Halbert SP: *Invest Ophthalmol* 4:539, 1966.
30. Santucci S: *Riv Ital Ottal Roma* 2:213, 1906.
31. Golowin S: *Klin Monatsbl Augenheilk* 47:150, 1909. Golowin S: *Russky Vratch,* No. 22: May 29, 1904.
32. Elschnig A: *von Graefes Arch Ophthalmol* 75:459, 1910; 76:509, 1910; 78:549, 1911; 79:428, 1911.
33. Woods AC: *Arch Ophthalmol* 45:557, 1916; 46:8, 503, 1917; 47:161, 1918.
34. Woods AC: *Trans Ophthalmol Soc UK* 45 (part 1):208, 1925.
35. Friedenwald JS: *Am J Ophthalmol* 17:1008, 1934.

36. Woods AC: *Allergy and immunity in ophthalmology,* Johns Hopkins Press, Baltimore, 1933, pp. 76-77.
37. Collins RC: *Am J Ophthalmol* 32:1687, 1949; 36:150, 1953.
38. The almost 50 year hiatus in interest in autoimmune diseases is discussed in *A history of immunology,* note 14, pp. 160-189.
39. Wacker WB, Lipton MM: *Nature* 206:253, 1965; *J Immunol* 101:151, 1968.
40. Kalsow CM, Wacker WB: *Int Arch Allergy Appl Immunol* 44:11, 1973; 48:287, 1975.
41. Wacker WB et al: *J Immunol* 119:1949, 1977; Dorey C, Faure J-P: *Ann Immunol (Inst Pasteur)* 128:229, 1977.
42. Gery I, Mochizuki M, Nussenblatt RB: *Prog Retinal Res* 5:75, 1986.
43. Marak GE et al: *Ophthalmic Res* 12:165, 1980; Meyers-Elliot RH et al: *Clin Immunol Immunopathol* 27:81, 1983.
44. Rao NA, Wacker WB, Marak GE: *Arch Opthalmol* 97:1954, 1979.
45. Kalsow CM, Wacker WB: *Invest Ophthalmol Vis Sci* 17:774, 1978; Broekhuyse RM, Winkens HJ, Kuhlmann ED: *Curr Eye Res* 5:231, 1986; Gery I et al: *Invest Ophthalmol Vis Sci* 27:1296, 1986.
46. The most recent comprehensive review of progress in this field may be found in *Immunopathologie de l'oeil,* note 2, pp. 241-281.
47. Sjögren H: *Acta Ophthalmol Suppl* 2:1, 1933.
48. Jones BR: *Lancet* ii:773, 1958.
49. Talal N: In *The autoimmune diseases,* Rose NR, Mackay IR, eds.: Academic Press, New York, 1985, pp. 145-159.
50. Liotet S et al: *L'oeil sec,* Masson, Paris, 1987.
51. Mizejewski GJ: *Experientia* 34:1093, 1978; Liu SH, Prendergast RA, Silverstein AM: *Invest Ophthalmol Vis Sci* 28:270, 1987.
52. Pisarev MA, Altschuler N, Davison TA: *Endocrinology* 83:903, 1968; Liu SH et al: *Invest Ophthalmol Vis Sci* 28:276, 1987.
53. Jabs DA, Prendergast RA: *Invest Ophthalmol Vis Sci* 29:1437, 1988.
54. Spencer WH: *Ophthalmic pathology,* 3 vols., Saunders, Philadelphia, 1985.
55. Wessely K: *Münch Med Wochenschr* 58:1713, 1911.
56. von Szily A: *Die anaphylaxie in der augenheilkunde,* Ferdinand Enke, Stuttgart, 1914.
57. Germuth FG et al: *Am J Ophthalmol* 46:282, 1959; *J Exp Med* 115:919, 1962.
58. Waksman BH, Bullington SJ: *J Immunol* 76, 441, 1956.
59. Calmette LCA: *C R Acad Sci* 144:1324, 1907.
60. St. Yves C: *Nouveau traité des maladies des yeux,* Le Mercier, Paris, 1722.
61. Weekers L: *Arch d'Ophtalmol* 23:577, 1909; Riehm W: *Arch Augenheilk* 105:55, 1931.
62. Woods AC: *Arch Ophthalmol* 53:321, 1924; Soresby AP: *Brit J Ophthalmol* 26:159, 189, 1942.
63. Theodore FH, Schlossman A: *Ocular allergy,* Williams & Wilkins, Baltimore, 1958, pp. 281-298.
64. Metcalf JF, Kaufman HE: *Am J Ophthalmol* 82:827, 1976.
65. Sery TW, Nagy RM, Nazario H: *Ophthalmic Res* 4:137, 1972; Metcalf JF, Hamilton DF, Reichert DW: *Infect Immunity* 26:1164, 1979; Russell RG: *Invest Ophthalmol Vis Sci* 25:938, 1984.
66. Asbell P, Franklin R: *Invest Ophthalmol Vis Sci* 20 (Suppl.):228, 1981.
67. See e.g., Leigh AG: *Corneal transplantation,* Blackwell, Oxford, 1966, pp. 1-5.
68. *A history of immunology,* note 14, pp. 275-295.
69. Medawar PB: *J Anat* 78:176, 1944; 79:157, 1945; *Harvey Lect* 52:144, 1956-57.
70. Maumenee AE: *Ann NY Acad Sci* 59:453, 1955; see also Paufique L, Sourdille GF, Offret G: *Les greffes de la cornée (Kératoplasties),* Masson, Paris, 1948.
71. Billingham RE, Boswell T: *Proc Roy Soc London (Biol)* 141:392, 1953; Khodadoust AA, Silverstein AM: *Invest Ophthalmol* 11:137, 1972.
72. Nicolle M, Abt G: *Ann Inst Pasteur* 22:132, 1908.
73. Sattler CH: *Arch Augenheilk* 64:390, 1909.
74. Seegal D, Seegal BH: *Proc Soc Exp Biol Med* 27:390, 1930; *J Exp Med* 54:265, 1931.
75. Goldmann H, Witmer RH: *Ophthalmologica, Basel* 127:323, 1954; Witmer RH: *Am J Ophthalmol* 37:243, 1953; *Arch Ophthalmol* 53:811, 1955.
76. Silverstein AM: In *Immunopathology of uveitis,* Maumenee AE, Silverstein AM eds.: Williams & Wilkins, Baltimore, 1964, pp. 83-110.

77. Chandler JW, Heise ER, Weiser RS: *Invest Ophthalmol* 12:400, 1973; Liu SH, Prendergast RA, Silverstein AM: *Invest Ophthalmol Vis Sci* 24:361, 1983.

78. Rich AR: *The pathogenesis of tuberculosis,* 2nd ed., Charles C. Thomas, Springfield, Illinois, 1951.

79. Woods AC: *Endogenous inflammations of the uveal tract,* Williams & Wilkins, Baltimore, 1961.

80. Greene HSN: *Cancer Res* 2:669, 1942; 7:491, 1947. A more extensive discussion of this phenomenon will be found in Woodruff MFA: *The transplantation of tissues and organs,* Chas. C. Thomas, Springfield, Illinois, 1960.

81. Raju S, Grogan JB: *Transplantation* 7:475, 1969; Franklin RM, Prendergast RA: *J Immunol* 104:463, 1970; Niederkorn JY: *Adv Immunol* 48:191, 1990.

82. Kaplan HJ, Streilein JW: *J Immunol* 118:809, 1977; 120:689, 1978; Streilein JW, Niederkorn JY: *J Immunol* 134:603, 1984.

83. Niederkorn JY, Streilein JW, Shadduck JA: *Invest Ophthalmol Vis Sci* 20:355, 1980.

84. Whittum JA et al: *Curr Eye Res* 2:691, 1983; Whittum-Hudson JA, Farazdaghi M, Prendergast RA: *Invest Ophthalmol Vis Sci* 26:1524, 1985.

85. Ohno S et al: In *Modern trends in immunology and immunopathology of the eye,* Secchi AG, Fregona IA, eds.: Masson, Milano, 1989, p. 452.

86. *Immunopathologie de l'oeil,* note 2, pp. 291-330.

87. Lagrange H, Delthil S: *Les Conjonctivites de Nature Anaphylactique,* Doin, Paris, 1932. Advances in the field up to 1958 are summarized in *Ocular allergy,* note 63; the more recent work relating allergic conjunctivitis to IgE-mediated mechanisms is reviewed by Allansmith MR: *The eye and immunology,* Mosby, St. Louis, 1982.

88. Oguchi M: *Acta Soc Ophthalmol Jap* 58, 735, 1954; Allansmith MR, Frick OL: *J Allergy* 34:535, 1963.

89. Dhermy P et al: *Rev Int Trachome* 44, 295, 1968.

90. Jones BR: cited in Duke-Elder S, *System of ophthalmology,* vol. 8, 1965, Kimpton, London, pp. 4-5; see also Silverstein AM, Prendergast RA: In *Morphological and functional aspects of immunity,* Lindahl-Kiessling K et al., eds., Plenum, New York, 1971, p. 583.

91. Morrison RP et al: *J Exp Med* 170:1271, 1989.

92. See, e.g., *Allergy and immunity in ophthalmology,* note 36; Woods AC: *Endogenous uveitis,* Williams & Wilkins, Baltimore, 1956; Campinchi R et al: *L'uvéite, phénomènes immunologiques et allergiques,* Masson, Paris, 1970; Friedlaender MH: *Allergy and immunology of the eye,* Harper & Row, New York, 1979; D'Ermo F: *Allergia ed immunologia oculare,* Masson, Milano, 1983; Secchi AG: *Immunologia ed immunopatologia oculare,* Masson, Milano, 1984; Smolin G, O'Connor GR: *Ocular immunology,* 2nd ed., Little Brown, Boston, 1986.

93. I count at least five such laboratories in Germany and one in Prague prior to the First World War. Between the Wars, there were added two in the United States, one at Johns Hopkins University and one at Columbia University. After World War II, an additional six ocular immunology laboratories were opened in the United States, and others in at least 12 other countries throughout the world.

94. Henkind P: History of the Association for Research in Vision and Ophthalmology, *Invest Ophthalmol Vis Sci* 17 (Suppl.):2, 1978.

95. The published proceedings of these Macy Foundation Conferences are: Maumenee AE, ed.: *Uveitis, survey ophthalmol* 4 (part 2):212, 1959; Maumenee AE, ed.: *Toxoplasmosis,* Williams & Wilkins, Baltimore, 1962; *Immunopathology of uveitis,* note 76. Another significant contribution was contained in the proceedings of a Ciba Conference, Porter R, Knight J, eds.: *Corneal graft failure,* Elsevier, Amsterdam, 1973.

96. The National Eye Institute's series of workshops on *Immunology of the eye* are: Steinberg GM, Gery I, Nussenblatt RB, eds.: *I. Immunogenetics and transplantation immunity,* Information Retrieval, Washington, 1980-81; Helmsen RJ et al, eds.: *II. Autoimmune phenomena and ocular disorders,* Information Retrieval, Washington, D. C., 1981; Suran A, Gery I, Nussenblatt RB, eds.: *III. Immunological aspects of ocular diseases,* Information Retrieval, Washington, D. C., 1981.

97. Strassbourg, 1974, Böke W, Luntz MH, eds.: *Ocular immune responses,* Karger, Basel, 1976; San Francisco, 1978, Silverstein AM, O'Connor GR, eds.: *Immunology and immunopathology of the eye,* Masson, New York, 1979; Seattle, 1982, O'Connor GR, Chandler JW, eds.: *Advances in immunology and immunopathology of the eye,* Masson, New York, 1985; Padova, 1986, Secchi AG, Fregona IA, eds.: *Modern trends in immunology and immunopathology of the eye,* Masson, Milano, 1989; Tokyo, 1990, Usui M, Ohno S, Aoki K, eds.: *Ocular immunology today,* Excerpta Medica, Amsterdam, 1990; Bethesda, 1994, Nussenblatt, RB, Whitcup, SM, Caspi, RR, Gery, I, eds. *Advances in ocular immunology,* Elsevier, Amsterdam, 1994.

2 Historical Milestones in Ocular Microbiology

KHALID F. TABBARA, ROBERT A. HYNDIUK

The scientific and applied aspects of microbiology and ophthalmology are closely related. The field of ocular infectious diseases has evolved over the past centuries from the work and observations of great men and women (Table 2-1).[3,4,6,29]

Infectious diseases of the eye have long been recognized as causes of blindness. Formerly, diseases such as smallpox, syphilis, gonorrhea, tuberculosis, and trachoma were regarded as supernatural phenomena, sent by God to punish the sinful. Early records of epidemic diseases appear in the Bible, Quran, Talmud, books of other theologians and traditional healers, and moralizing poems.

From antiquity through the Renaissance, most observations pertinent to ocular microbiology were limited to clinical findings of eye inflammation and to the effects of chemical compounds on the infected eye. Microbial diseases were first observed with the development of optics in seventeenth-century Europe. Antony van Leeuwenhoek[9] (1632-1723), a Dutch draper, developed a 150X biconvex lens held in a metal frame to inspect the weave of fine cloth. After examining *animalcules*—spherical, cigarette-shaped, or spiral creatures, some of which showed rapid motion (Fig. 2-1)—he notified the Royal Society of London and the French Academy of Sciences.[9] These original observations led to the theory of "contagium animatum" and the scientific discipline of microbiology.[8]

TRANSMISSIBILITY OF OCULAR INFECTIONS

Charles St. Yves[22,39] (1667-1736), a French ophthalmologist, described a male patient with gonorrhea who contracted purulent conjunctivitis, apparently from washing his eyes with his own urine. This link between sexually transmitted diseases and the eye was furthered when he delineated the clinical manifestations of neonatal conjunctivitis.[39] Samuel Quelmalz[21] (1696-1758) noted the similarities between purulent discharge in the birth canal and neonatal conjunctivitis. Joseph Pieringer[21] (1800-1879) also sug-

gested the transmissibility of gonorrheal conjunctivitis and reproduced the disease in normal individuals by inoculating the conjunctiva with pus from conjunctival secretions. These original observations regarding communicable eye disease laid the foundations for the scientific discipline of ocular microbiology in the nineteenth century.[21]

Louis Pasteur (1822-1895) was a French chemist who disproved the doctrine of spontaneous generation by showing that fermentation and putrefaction are caused by microorganisms.[48] Joseph Lister[4] (1827-1912) applied this germ theory to surgery and introduced aseptic techniques with great success. Karl Credé[29] (1819-1892), an obstetrician in Liepzig, introduced the topical use of silver nitrate in 1881 for the prevention of neonatal conjunctivitis. Lucien Howe (1848-1928), who studied neonatal conjunctivitis in Egypt, campaigned for legislation in the United States promoting Credé prophylaxis.[8]

Further refinements in microbiologic techniques by Robert Koch[25] (1843-1910) led to the development of culture media. After observing that single colonies grow on slices of potato, he developed media containing gelatin or agar to grow pure cultures. In determining the cause of tuberculosis, Koch[26] summarized his evidence of a causative relationship between microorganisms and a specific disease: 1) the organism must always be found with a given disease, 2) the organism must be isolated in pure culture, 3) inoculation of the pure culture must produce the disease, and 4) the organism must be isolated again from the infected animal. Koch and others[26] applied these postulates to identify specific microorganisms as causes of different diseases.

MICROORGANISMS AND THE EYE

While in Egypt studying cholera, Koch[25] discovered a slender bacillus in the exudate of patients with conjunctivitis. This organism, later studied by John Weeks[52,53] (1853-1949), came to be known as the Koch-Weeks bacillus *(Hemophilus aegyptius)*.[24] Other ocular infections that are caused by specific microorganisms include gonococcal neo-

TABLE 2-1 MILESTONES OF OCULAR MICROBIOLOGY

Year	Author	Observation
400 BC	Hippocrates	Clinical observations of herpetic infections.
14	Celsus	Roughness of eyelids in trachoma.[11]
132	Galen	Described the "flow of seed" (gonorrhea).[29]
1546	Fracastoro	Introduced the concept of contagious diseases and coined the term *syphilis*.[16]
1680	van Leeuwenhoek	Microscopic observations of bacteria.[9]
1722	St. Yves	Described a man who washed his eyes with his urine and who developed purulent conjunctivitis by transmitting gonorrhea to his eyes.[22,39]
1798	Jenner	Used cowpox inoculation to prevent smallpox.[4]
1823	Werneck	Transmitted trachoma with follicular material to two volunteers.[22]
1867	Lister	Introduced the antiseptic principles in surgery.[4]
1872	Hebra	Described impetigo herpetiformis.[6]
1876	Koch	Described the cause of anthrax: *Bacillus anthracis*.[3]
1879	Neisser	Described diplococcus in urethral and conjunctival exudates.[34]
1879	Leber	Recognized and grew *Aspergillus glaucus* from corneal ulcer and reproduced the disease in rabbits.[27]
1880	Koch	Determined the cause of tuberculosis.[26]
1880	Leistikow	Cultured the gonococcus.[28]
1881	Pasteur	Developed vaccine for cholera and anthrax.[48]
1881	Koch	Developed culture media with gelatin for growth of bacteria following observation of single colonies of organisms on slices of potato.[3]
1881	Credé	Recommended the use of silver nitrate in eyes of newborn babies to prevent ophthalmia neonatorum.[29]
1882	Ehrlich	Stained the tubercle bacillus.[3]
1882	Loeffler	Grew diplococci from eyes of a patient with purulent conjunctivitis.
1883	Koch	Described slender bacillus in ocular exudates of Egyptian children with conjunctivitis.[25]
1884	Duhring	Described generalized herpes.[4]
1884	Koch	Described postulates for the determination of infectious etiology.[26]
1884	Gram	Developed staining methods for bacteria.[4]
1886	Weeks	Described acute epidemic mucopurulent conjunctivitis.[52]
1886	Weeks	Cultured Koch-Weeks bacillus (*Haemophilus aegyptius*).[53]
1889	Fuchs	Described epidemic superficial punctate keratitis (epidemic keratoconjunctivitis).[25]
1890	Pringle	Distinguished between herpes catarrhalis and herpes zoster; the former was divided into two types: herpes facialis and herpes genitalis.
1896	Morax	Subacute conjunctivitis involving angles of lids; transmitted disease to human; treated the disease with zinc sulfate.[32]
1896	Gifford	Described acute bacterial conjunctivitis caused by pneumococcus.[18]
1897	Axenfeld	Cultured the organism from angular blepharoconjunctivitis described by Morax [Morax-Axenfeld diplobacillus *(Moraxella lacunata)*].[2,49]
1899	Petit	Isolated diplobacillus from a case of serpiginous keratitis [(diplobacillus of Petit (*Moraxella liquefaciens*)].[37]
1907	Halberstaedter and von Prowazek	Described inclusion bodies from exudates of children with trachoma in Java and found the inclusion bodies infectious.[20]
1908	Ehrlich	Introduced modern chemotherapy of infectious diseases as selective toxicity.[3]
1912	Nicolle, Blaisot, and Cuénod	Transmitted trachoma to monkeys and chimpanzees with bacteria-free filtrates of scrapings and reproduced the disease.[36]
1913	Grüter	Inoculation of herpes virus in the rabbit cornea from human corneal scrapings.
1915	Lindner	Described the cause of inclusion blennorrhea and differentiated the condition from trachoma.[44]
1924	von Szily	Developed animal model of herpetic retinitis in the contralateral eye following inoculation in the anterior chamber.
1928	Griffith	Described pneumococcal types: virulent and avirulent.[19]
1929	Fleming	Discovered penicillin.[15]
1930	Fuchs	Described epidemic keratoconjunctivitis.[17]

TABLE 2-1 MILESTONES OF OCULAR MICROBIOLOGY cont'd

Year	Author	Observation
1930	Wilson	Described inclusion bodies in the conjunctiva of Egyptian children during the incubation period of trachoma.[45]
1930	Thygeson	Described the incubation period and course of inclusion blennorrhea and defined the life cycle of the inclusion bodies.[45]
1934	Thygeson	Attempted to culture the agent of trachoma in the chorioallantoic membrane of eggs.[44]
1935	Domagk	Inhibited bacteria with sulphanilamide.[10]
1935	Thygeson and Proctor	Reproduced trachoma in a volunteer with bacteria-free filtrates of conjunctival scrapings of American Indian children.[47]
1937	Rice	Observed the staining of the inclusion bodies with Lugol iodine (defining the carbohydrate matrix of the inclusion body).[44]
1938	Thygeson	Confirmed the findings of Rice.[42]
1940	Leo	Cured trachoma with sulphanilamide.[45]
1940	Woods	Introduced paraaminobenzoic acid and described the mechanism of action of sulphanilamides.[4]
1944	Avery and associates	Transformed avirulent pneumococcus mutants into virulent strains by bacterial DNA extracts.[1]
1950	Thygeson	Described the entity "superficial punctate keratitis."[43]
1952	Wilder	Identified toxoplasma in eyes of patients misdiagnosed as tuberculous uveitis.[55]
1955	Jawetz, Kimura, Nicholas, and associates	Isolated the etiologic agent of shipyard conjunctivitis: adenovirus type 8.[23]
1957	T'ang, Chang, Huang, and Wang	Isolated the etiologic agent of trachoma in the egg yolk with streptomycin *(Chlamydia trachomatis)*.[41]
1962	Kaufman	Confirmed the efficacy of IDU in the treatment of herpetic keratitis.
1971	O'Connor	Studied the pathogenesis of toxoplasmic retinochoroiditis.[40]
1972	Jones	Reported first case of *Acanthamoeba keratitis*.[40]
1973	Cohen and associates	Discovered DNA replication machinery and synthetic capacity of *Escherichia coli* by construction of biologically functional bacterial plasmids in vitro.[5]
1975	Dawson	Observed herpes virion in the stroma of patients with herpetic keratitis.[40]
1980	Moseley and associates	Introduced first practical application of recombinant DNA technology in the field of infectious diseases.[31]
1982	Burgdorfer	Described a spirochete in the tick *Ixodes dammini*, the cause of Lyme disease *(Borrelia burgdorferi)*.
1982	Culbertson and associates	Confirmed the herpetic etiology of acute retinal necrosis syndrome.[7]
1985	Wear	Identified bacterial cause of Parinaud oculoglandular syndrome.[50,51]
1988	Saiki and associates	Discovered primer-directed enzymatic amplification of DNA with a thermostable DNA polymerase (from thermophilic bacillus *Thermus aquaticus*).[34]

natal conjunctivitis caused by *Neisseria gonorrhoeae* [discovered by Albert Neisser[34] (1855-1916)] and fungal keratitis caused by *Aspergillus* sp. [discovered by Theodor Leber[27] (1840-1917)].

Victor Morax[32] (1866-1935), while at the Pasteur Institute in Paris in 1896, isolated a gram-negative diplobacillus from a case of conjunctivitis. Theodore Axenfeld (1867-1930) also conducted studies in ocular bacteriology and independently discovered this organism, subsequently referred to as the Morax-Axenfeld diplobacillus *(Moraxella lacunata)*.[49] Axenfeld[2] authored the first book on ocular bacteriology in 1907; this book was translated into English by MacNab in 1930.

Paul Petit[33,37] (1875-1950), the son-in-law of Morax,[33] studied ocular bacteriology and in 1899 described another keratitis-causing diplobacillus that later was classified as

Moraxella liquefaciens, Harold Gifford[18] (1858-1929) confirmed the findings that *Moraxella* sp. was a cause of blepharoconjunctivitis and keratitis. As microorganisms were established as causes of ocular disease, the concept of saprophytes was developed, and Gifford was among the first to evaluate the normal ocular flora.

Some eye diseases were plainly transmissible, although the filterable agent was difficult to identify. The clinical findings of epidemic conjunctivitis, for example, were first clearly delineated by Ernst Fuchs[17] (1851-1930), but it was not until 1955 that adenovirus was found to be the causal agent.[23] Eye disease caused by herpes simplex virus was also recognized as a major problem. W. Grüter[40] successfully transmitted herpes simplex virus keratitis from a patient to a rabbit in 1913. In 1924 Adolph von Szily[49] (1848-1920) described an animal model of herpetic eye disease by inject-

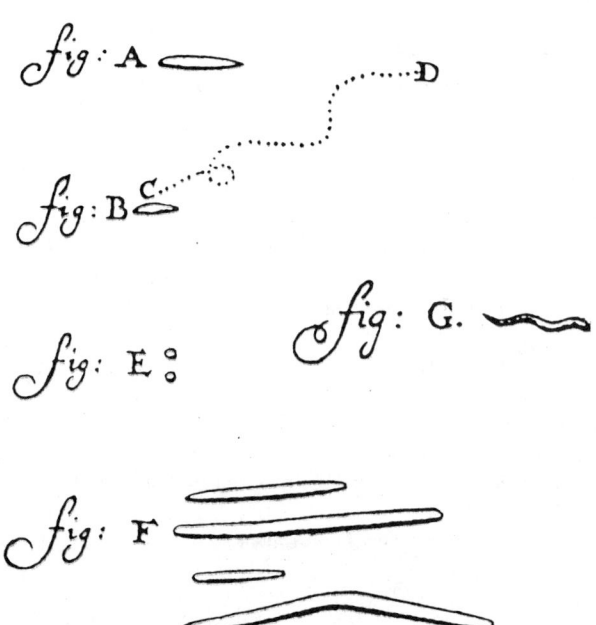

Fig. 2-1. Schematic drawing of bacteria by van Leeuwenhoek.

ing infected tissue into the anterior chamber of mice and noting contralateral retinitis.

The identification of *Chlamydia* sp. also proved elusive, even though trachoma had been recognized since antiquity. Trachoma was first transmitted to human volunteers by Wilhelm Werneck[22] in 1823, but the infectious agent remained unknown. In a joint expedition to Java in 1907, Ludwig Halberstaedter[20] and Stanislas von Prowazek[20] observed intraepithelial bodies in the conjunctival scrapings of children with active trachoma, and they successfully reproduced the disease in the eye of orangutans by using conjunctival scrapings containing these inclusion bodies.[14] In 1912 at the Pasteur Institute in Tunisia, Charles Nicolle and associates[36] transmitted trachoma to a chimpanzee by using filtration. Francis Proctor,[44] a Boston ophthalmologist who retired in Santa Fe, met Phillips Thygeson[45] in America in 1930. Financing Thygeson's experimental work on trachoma,[46] Proctor helped set up a trachoma research laboratory at a boarding school for Indian children at Fort Apache, Arizona. In 1935 Thygeson,[47] Proctor,[47] and Polk Richards of the Indian Health Service used filtered conjunctival scrapings (acquired from American Indian children) that contained elementary bodies to reproduce the disease in a volunteer, Clarence Brown. These studies supported the concept of an epithelial parasite,[42] and the agent was cultured in 1957.[41]

ANTIMICROBIAL THERAPY

In 1929 Alexander Fleming[15] (1881-1955) reported on the antibacterial action of cultures produced by a fungus. Working in London, Fleming noted that *Staphylococcus* sp. colonies underwent lysis around a fungal contaminant. This mold, *Penicillium* sp., was evidently diffusing a bacterioly-

tic substance into the surrounding medium. Furthermore, the broth in which the fungus had been growing possessed marked inhibitory effects to many types of pathogenic bacteria. Ernest Chain and Howard Florey first successfully used purified penicillin in the treatment of patients in 1942. Gerhard Domagk[10] discovered the sulfanomides in 1935 and found them to be effective against a variety of microorganisms.

The use of these new antibacterial agents revolutionized the control of many infectious eye diseases, including trachoma, purulent conjunctivitis, and suppurative keratitis. Antibiotic eyedrops and ointments were developed, and antimicrobial susceptibility testing led to the increased use of the microbiology laboratory by ophthalmologists. One of the first prospective clinical trials in ophthalmology evaluated the effects of sulfanilamide on trachoma in American Indians; Frederick Loe[44] recorded an 80% cure rate for treated patients.

PATHOGENESIS OF INFECTIOUS EYE DISEASE

Advances in molecular biology, immunology, and biochemistry are contributing to our understanding of microbial eye disease. New technologies, such as genetic engineering, are leading to a new understanding of the relationship between man and his parasites. Diseases currently thought to reflect immunologic derangement or autoimmunity may prove to be infectious in origin. The development of antiviral agents has also stimulated studies on the mechanisms of viral eye disease.

Ocular microbiology remains an applied science, but new technology is leading to research in all stages of microbial adherence and invasion. Knowledge of pathogenesis will present opportunities for the prevention of ocular infectious disease.

REFERENCES

1. Avery OT, MacLoed CM, McCarty M: Studies on the chemical nature of the substance including transformation of pneumococcal types: induction of transformation by a deoxyribonucleic acid fraction isolated from pneumococcus type III, *J Exp Med* 79:137, 1944.
2. Axenfeld T: *The bacteriology of the eye,* New York, 1908, William and Co (translated by Angus MacNab).
3. Brock TD: *Milestones in microbiology,* Englewood Cliffs, 1961, Prentice-Hall.
4. Bulloch W: *The history of bacteriology,* London, 1938, Oxford University Press.
5. Cohen SN et al.: Construction of biologically functional bacterial plasmids in vitro, *Proc Natl Acad Sci USA* 70:3240, 1973.
6. Collard P: *The development of microbiology,* New York, 1976, Cambridge University Press.
7. Culbertson WW et al.: The acute retinal necrosis syndrome. Part II. Histology and etiology, *Ophthalmology* 89:1317, 1982.
8. Derby GS: Lucien Howe: 1848-1928, *Arch Ophthalmol* 1:241, 1929.
9. Dobell C: *Antony van Leeuwenhoek and his little animals,* New York, 1938, Russell and Russell Publishers (reprinted by Dover Publications in 1960).
10. Domagk G: Ein Beitrag zur Chemotherapie der bakteriellen Infektionen, *Deutsch Med Wschr* 61:250, 1935.

11. Duke-Elder S: *System of ophthalmology: diseases of the outer eye,* 8(1), St Louis, 1965, CV Mosby.
12. Duke-Elder S, Perkins ES: *System of ophthalmology: diseases of the uveal tract,* vol 9, St Louis, 1977, Mosby.
13. Ehrlich P: Aus dem verein fur innere Medicin zu Berlin, *Deutsch Med Wschr* 8:269, 1882.
14. Finzi NS: Ludvig Halberstaedter, *Br J Radiol* 22:347, 1949.
15. Fleming A: On the antibacterial action of cultures of a penicillium: with special reference to their use in the isolation of *B. influenzae, Br J Exp* 10:226, 1929.
16. Fracastoro G: *De contagione, Contagiosis Morbis et eorum Curatione,* New York, 1930, G P Putnam and Sons (translated by Wilmer C. Wright.)
17. Fuchs E: Keratitis punctata superficialis, *Wien Klin Wschr* 2:837, 1889.
18. Gifford H: Pneumococcus of Fraenkel as a frequent cause of acute catarrhal conjunctivitis, *Graefes Arch Clin Exp Ophthalmol* 25:314, 1896.
19. Griffith F: The significance of pneumococcal types, *J Hyg* 27:113, 1928.
20. Halberstaedter L, von Prowazek S: Zur Aetiologie des Trachoms, *Deutsch Med Wschr* 33:1285, 1907.
21. Hirschberg J: Charles St. Yves, S.T. Quelmalz, W. Werneck, J. Pieringer, *Graefe-Saemisch Handbuch der Gesamten Augenheilkunde* 14(1):9, 203, 561, 577, 1911.
22. Janku J: Pathogenesa a pathologicka anatomie tak nazvaneho virozeneho kolobomu zlute skvrny oku normalne velikem a microphtalmickem nalezem parasito v. sitnici, *Gas Lek Ces* 62:1021, 1923.
23. Jawetz E et al.: New type of APC virus from epidemic keratoconjunctivitis, *Science* 122:1190, 1955.
24. Knapp A: John Elmer Weeks, *Arch Ophthalmol* 41:752, 1949.
25. Koch R: Thätigkeit der deutschen Cholerakomission in Aegypten und Ostindien, *Wein Med Wschr* 52:1548, 1883.
26. Koch R: Die Atiologie der Tuberkulose, *Mittheilungen aus dem Kaiserlichen Gesundheitsamte* 2:1-88, 1884.
27. Leber T: Keratomykosis aspergillina als Ursache von Hypopyonkeratitis, *Graefes Arch Clin Exp Ophthalmol* 25:285, 1879.
28. Leistikow L: Ueber Bacterien bei den venerischen Krankheiten, *Charité-Annalen* 7:750, 1880.
29. Locatcher-Khorazo D, Seegal BC: *Microbiology of the eye,* St Louis, 1963, CV Mosby.
30. Marquardt M: *Paul Ehrlich,* New York, 1951, Henry Schuman.
31. Morax V: Note sur un diplobacille pathogène pour la conjonctivite humaine, *Ann Inst Pasteur* 10:337, 1896.
32. Morax V, Petit PJ: *Le trachome,* Paris, 1929 (edited by Jean Morax).
33. Moseley SL et al.: Detection of enterotoxigenic *Escherichia coli* by DNA colony hybridization, *J Infect Dis* 142:892, 1980.
34. Neisser A: Ueber eine der Gonorrhoe eigentümliche Micrococcusform, *Zbl Med Wiss* 17:497, 1879.
35. Nicolle C, Manceaux L: Sur une infection à corps de leishman: ou organisms voisin due gondi, *C R Acad Sci* 147:763, 1907.
36. Nicolle C, Blaisot L, Cuénod A: Le magot animal réactif du trachome: filtrabilité du virus; pouvoir infectant des larmes, *C R Acad Sci* 155:241, 1912.
37. Petit PJ: Sur une forme particulière d'infection cornéenne à type serpigineux, *Ann Oculist* 121:166, 1899.
38. Saiki RK et al.: Primer-directed enzymatic amplification of DNA with a thermostable DNA polymerase, *Science* 239:487, 1988.
39. Shastid TH: Charles Saint-Yves, *Am Encycl Dict Ophthalmol* 15:11496, 1919.
40. Tabbara KF, Hyndiuk RA: *Infections of the eye,* Boston, 1986, Little Brown.
41. T'ang F et al.: Studies of the etiology of trachoma with special reference to isolation of the virus in chick embryo, *Chin Med J* 75:429, 1957.
42. Thygeson P: The matrix of the epithelial cell inclusion of trachoma, *Am J Pathol* 14:455, 1938.
43. Thygeson P: Superficial punctate keratitis, *J Am Med Assoc* 144:1544, 1950.
44. Thygeson P: Personal communication, October 31, 1992.
45. Thygeson P: Personal communication, May 11, 1994.
46. Thygeson P, Huges SS: A link with our past, an oral history. In *Ophthalmology oral history series,* San Francisco, 1987, Foundation of the American Academy of Ophthalmology.
47. Thygeson P, Proctor FI: The filtrability of trachoma virus, *Arch Ophthalmol* 13:1018, 1935.
48. Vallery-Radot R: *The life of Pasteur,* New York, 1926, Doubleday-Doran and Co (reprinted by Dover Publications in 1960).
49. von Szily A: Theodor Axenfeld, *Klin Monatsbl Augenheilk* 85:1, 1930.
50. Wear DJ et al.: Cat scratch disease: a bacterial infection, *Science* 221:1403, 1983.
51. Wear DJ et al.: Cat scratch disease bacilli in the conjunctiva of patients with Parinaud's oculoglandular syndrome, *Ophthalmology* 92:1282, 1985.
52. Weeks JE: The bacillus of acute conjunctival catarrh, or "pink eye", *Arch Ophthalmol* 15:441, 1886.
53. Weeks JE: *A treatise on diseases of the eye,* 255, Philadelphia, 1910, Lea and Febiger.
54. Wolf A, Cowen D, Paige BH: Toxoplasmosis: occurence in infants as an encephalomyelitis, verification by transmission to animals, *Science* 89:226, 1939.

OCULAR
IMMUNOLOGY

3 Regional Immunology of the Eye

J. WAYNE STREILEIN

The need for immune protection against a broad range of pathogenic agents exists for all tissues of the body, including the eye. Clinical and experimental evidence indicates, however, that the expression of immunity in the eye is dissimilar to the expression of immunity in many other tissues. For example, the clinical success of orthotopic transplants of solid organs, such as the kidney, heart, and liver, has been regarded as such a premier achievement in our time that the Nobel Prize in Physiology and Medicine was awarded to one of the pioneering surgeons.

UNIQUE IMMUNITY IN THE EYE

Clinical and Experimental Evidence

Orthotopic transplantation of allogenic corneas, has been practiced by ophthalmologists since the turn of the century, and the success rate is extraordinarily high. Considering that immune rejection is the last major barrier to successful transplantation of other solid organs, it is remarkable that immune rejection of corneas transplanted into nonvascularized recipient beds occurs so infrequently and that immune reactions are often readily controllable after clinical corneal transplantation. The implication is either (1) that the cornea, as a solid tissue, fails to express transplantation antigens in immunogenic form, or (2) that the orthotopic ocular bed in which corneal grafts are placed interferes with the ability of the immune system to bring destructive immune effectors to the site. Both implications appear to be correct and verify that immunity in the eye—with respect to corneal allografts —is atypical. Another example of impaired expression of immunity in the eye is the clinical observation that conventional pathogens, such as the herpes simplex virus type I (HSV-1), can establish recurrent, and even persistent, productive infections in the eye rarely found elsewhere in the body of otherwise immunologically competent individuals. Perhaps related to this example is the fact that opportunistic pathogens often preferentially infect the eye, rather than many other tissues of the body in immunocompromised individuals.

These clinical observations concerning the unusual nature of ocular immunity have their counterparts in the laboratory. Suspensions of immunogenic tumor cells, which would be promptly destroyed when implanted at conventional body sites, can quickly gain a foothold when implanted into the anterior chamber or vitreous cavity of the mouse eye.[31,52] Similarly, allogenic corneas placed orthotopically in the eyes of normal adult mice,[57] rats,[10] and other laboratory species can enjoy prolonged or even indefinite survival, even though comparable grafts of skin, kidney, or heart are routinely rejected. Along the same lines, injections of certain strains of HSV-1 into the anterior chamber of the mouse eye are often not contained locally; these infections can then set the stage for the development of acute retinal necrosis.[79]

Lest the impression be given from these illustrations that the immune system is "unable" to express itself in the eye, alternative illustrations indicate that immune responses can be mediated within the eye, often to the detriment of the visual axis. Perhaps the most dramatic example of this point is the development of sympathetic ophthalmia in a patient who has sustained penetrating trauma to one eye. There are good indications that the pathogenesis of sympathetic ophthalmia involves the activation of cell-mediated immunity directed at ocular autoantigens, and that the inflammation within the eye is an autoimmune process. Another demonstration that the immune system can, under suitable conditions, express itself in the eye is the phenomenon of stromal keratitis secondary to infection of the cornea with HSV-1. Experimental evidence strongly supports the view that the pathologic process leading to corneal clouding, scarring, and blindness in this disorder is not the direct result of virally directed cytopathology, but is mediated by T lymphocytes directing their destructive attack against HSV-1 antigens present within one or more layers of the infected cornea.[28] As a consequence, the noninfected cells and the organized extracellular matrix of the corneal stroma suffer inadvertently from an immune process carried out in their midst.

Ocular Immune Privilege

Many investigators believe that the unique aspects of immunity displayed in the eye are related to the experimentally defined phenomenon of immune privilege.[4] Foreign tissues placed in the anterior chamber of eyes of "normal" animals might survive for unexpectedly long or even indefinite periods of time.[33] Inasmuch as similar tissues implanted subcutaneously would be summarily rejected, the concept emerged that the anterior chamber is an immune-privileged site. Other privileged sites in the body include the brain, certain endocrine organs (adrenal cortex, testis, ovary), the liver, the matrix of the hair shaft, the maternal-fetal interface, and the hamster cheek pouch.[4] It was once believed that all of these tissue sites lacked lymphatic drainage routes, purporting the theory that this lack of lymphatic pathways to lymph nodes served to sequester antigenic materials in privileged sites, preventing their recognition by cells of the immune system. Although it is now known that all of these tissues actually have access to lymphatic vessels and drainage pathways to lymph nodes, the specific anatomic arrangements of lymphatic connections to the eye are unusual. This architectural feature may contribute to the privileged status, but not because antigens are sequestered in the privileged site and unavailable to the immune apparatus. Recent evidence confirms that privilege results in part from an active systemic process that stringently regulates both the quality and the quantity of immunity directed at antigens in privileged sites, including the eye.

There are microanatomic features of the eye that are special and partially account for the unusual immunity observed in this organ. As it rests within the orbit, the eye consists of two very different compartments: (1) the ocular surface (including the cornea and conjunctiva) and adnexal structures; and (2) the intraocular space (anterior chamber), vitreous cavity, subretinal space, and intraocular tissues. The ocular surface covered by conjunctiva is part of the mucosal immune system.[1,9,76] Induction and expression of immunity at this surface resembles that found at other mucosal surfaces —tracheobronchial, gastrointestinal, and genitourethral tracts. In contrast to the ocular surface, the intraocular compartments are neither integral parts of the mucosal immune system, nor relatives of the other major regional system, the skin-associated lymphoid tissues.[60] Instead, the tissues and fluid-filled spaces within the eye comprise a unique, perhaps self-contained and integrated, set of interacting molecules and cells that communicate with the rest of the body in highly distinctive ways. In this sense the eye possesses its own "regional sphere of immunologic influence," comparable in effect if not magnitude to the regional influence that is enforced along mucosal surfaces, or that pervades the integument.[61] An important feature of the ocular sphere of influence is that passage of biologic information (blood-borne molecules and cells) from the blood into the eye is meager, largely because of the existence of blood-ocular barriers.[16] These barriers are comprised of specialized endothelial cells that line the surfaces of intraocular vessels. Passage of contents of the blood via these cells is highly regulated and discriminatory. Another important feature of the ocular sphere of influence is that the escape of biologic information (molecules and cells) from the eye into the rest of the body is also tightly regulated. The vast majority of aqueous humor leaves the eye via the trabecular meshwork, entering directly into the venous circulation.[7] Except under special circumstances, movement into the lymphatics of intraocular cells and molecules that can drain the internal eye is sharply curtailed. When the uveoscleral pathway is rendered patent, the opportunity for direct communication between the internal eye and draining cervical lymph nodes exists.[7,15] These anatomic features undoubtedly play a role in creating immune privilege and in making ocular immune responses unique.

Ocular Immunity and Incident Light

Because the eye is specialized for the entrapment of light and for the faithful transmission of images of the outside world to the brain, it could be theorized that light itself might contribute to the unique features of ocular immunity. Experiments by Ferguson, Kaplan,[20] and Hayashi made this point in a dramatic fashion. These investigators discovered that the nature of systemic immune responses to antigens placed in the anterior chamber of the eye is dictated by whether or not the eye has been maintained in complete darkness. Injection of antigen-bearing splenocytes into light-adapted mouse eyes generates an unusual systemic immune response termed anterior chamber-associated immune deviation (ACAID).[49,59,75] By contrast, injection of similarly antigenic cells into the anterior chamber of dark-adapted eyes evokes a conventional systemic immune response. Although it was anticipated that the ability of visible light to promote ACAID induction would be affected by photoreceptors in the posterior pole of the eye, Ferguson and associates found that the phenomenon is dependent upon the interaction of light with the anterior segment of the eye. Another possible dimension to the effects of light on the ocular immune system derives from the realizations that ultraviolet B light (1) can have deleterious effects on the eye, (2) has been identified as a risk factor in the development of certain types of cataracts, and (3) may also play a role in the multifactorial pathogenesis of the age-related macular degeneration.[8,74,86a] In the skin, UVB light modifies cutaneous immune responses, in part by causing the intracutaneous production of tumor necrosis factor alpha that modifies the antigen-presenting capabilities of epidermal Langerhans' cells and dermal dendritic cells.[62] Although no direct evidence exists, it is conceivable that UVB radiation may also modify intraocular immune responses.

CONCEPT OF REGIONAL SPECIALIZATION IN IMMUNE RESPONSES

Theoretic Considerations

The range of disease-causing pathogens is extremely diverse. Each pathogen, moreover, has adapted successfully to its host by exploiting one or more aspects of the host's vulnerability. Consequently the immune system must adapt its functional repertoire to successfully meet the threat of an invading pathogen; irrespective of route, mode of entry, or mechanism of pathologic insult. This capacity of the immune system to meet **any** pathogen is embodied in a startlingly distinct array of specific immune effector modalities: (1) several different isotypes of antibodies, each with a defined range of effector functions, and (2) multiple subpopulations of functionally distinct T lymphocytes. In the aggregate, these effector modalities guard against exogenous and endogenous pathogens of importance. The diversity of these effectors implies that no single immune effector modality can suffice to protect against all pathogens. As a result, if an effector modality critical to the protection against a particular pathogen fails, the host is rendered vulnerable to that pathogen, even though the rest of the immune armamentarium is in place. This principle has important ramifications with regard to ocular immune responses and the vulnerability of the eye to certain pathogens.

Many immune effectors eliminate pathogens by enlisting nonspecific inflammatory mechanisms where the pathogen resides. For example, T cells of the delayed hypersensitivity type (T_{DH}) provoke the destruction of intracellular pathogens, such as the tubercle bacillus, by recruiting macrophages to the site and activating the cells such that their intracellular hydrolytic enzymes prove lethal to the microbial organism. Similarly, complement-fixing antibodies promote the elimination of bacteria by opsonizing the organism's surface, thus rendering it susceptible to phagocytosis and destruction by reticuloendothelial cells. In these examples the interaction between antigen-specific immune effectors and nonspecific plasma proteins and bone marrow-derived cells leads inevitably to a local inflammatory response that is lacking in specificity. Consequently, release of enzymes and mediators by activated inflammatory cells has the potential to injure ''innocent bystander'' cells and structures in the immediate vicinity. This potential is a threat to organs such as the eye, in which physiologic functions demand that a precise visual axis is maintained.

The concept of regional immunity[61] is based on the following considerations: (1) distinct organs and tissues are represented by a unique range of pathogens to which each is especially vulnerable, and (2) distinct organs and tissues display differential vulnerability to the injurious side effects of immune-mediated protection. Therefore the generic immune responses are subject to tissue-directed modifications that qualitatively and quantitatively mold them by promoting the generation of a selected subset of immune mediators that are consistent with, and not deleterious to, the physiologic function of the tissue (region) in question.

Features of Regional Immune Responses

Each organ or tissue possesses anatomic and physiologic features that fashion immune responses expressed in that tissue to its special requirements. These features include the following: (1) parenchymal cells that release cytokines and mediators creating a unique, local microenvironment, (2) tissue-restricted antigen-presenting cells, (3) antigen-specific, tissue-tropic lymphocytes, and (4) access via lymph and blood vasculature to an organized lymphoid tissue (lymph node, spleen) that collects immunologic information from the tissue. The tissue-specific microenvironment plays a major role in molding the manner in which local antigens are detected, recognized, and eliminated by specific immune effectors (see box).

Tissue-Restricted Antigen-Presenting Cells. During the primary immune response to an exogenous antigen, the first encounter with unprimed antigen-specific lymphocytes takes place within organized, peripheral lymphoid tissues (such as lymph nodes and spleen), rather than at the portal of antigen entry into the body. Because antigens are usually introduced to the body via the skin or mucosal surfaces, a mechanism exists to ensure that antigens are brought to draining lymphoid tissues to be recognized. In the case of particulate antigens, such as bacteria, the particles may be carried via lymph flow, or they may be phagocytosed by local tissue macrophages migrating via the lymph to the draining lymph node. In the case of soluble antigens or membrane fragments of antigenic cells, specialized bone marrow-derived cells (dendritic cells)[58] function in the local tissue as the antigen bearers. Dendritic cells constitutively

---

COMPONENTS OF THE EYE'S REGIONAL SPHERE OF IMMUNOLOGIC INFLUENCE

- Bone marrow-derived dendritic cells and macrophages located in iris, ciliary body, retina, and choriocapillaris
- Eye-seeking lymphocytes (speculative)
- Specialized filtration apparatus at trabecular meshwork for egress of intraocular fluids; uveoscleral pathway as minor route of fluid escape
- Blood-ocular barrier that limits access of blood-borne cells and molecules to internal compartments of eye
- Spleen—the primary recipient of eye-derived antigenic signals
- Aqueous humor and vitreous cavity—unique intraocular microenvironment containing immunosuppressive cytokines, neuropeptides, and mediators

express class I and class II molecules encoded by the major histocompatibility complex (MHC) and endocytose, thereby sampling their immediate microenvironment. These cells are uniquely designed to pick up, process, and even present foreign antigens on their surface. Dendritic cells can express numerous, different cell adhesion molecules (intercellular adhesion molecule-1—ICAM-1, LFA-3, B7) that promote their ability to bind nonspecifically to T lymphocytes. These cells can also secrete cytokines, such as interleukin-1, that can signal T cells via surface receptors. The high mobility of dendritic cells ensures that the antigenic information they pick up in peripheral nonlymphoid tissues is brought to the deep cortex of the draining lymph node, where a high density of potentially reactive T and B lymphocytes exists. Thus the stage is set for initial sensitization of antigen-specific lymphocytes, leading to the "induction" of a systemic state of specific immunity.

There is also evidence that tissue-restricted, bone marrow-derived dendritic cells and macrophages can function as antigen-presenting cells during the "expression" of T cell-dependent immunity. The ability of the cells to function in this manner is under the influence of two different forces. Prior to the elicitation of an immune effector response in a peripheral tissue, the functional properties of the resident antigen-presenting cells are dictated by their microenvironment, which is chiefly created by the parenchymal cells of the tissue in question. In this "resting" state, tissue-restricted APC are well equipped to activate primed effector T cells.[66] Once immune T cells have recognized antigen in this manner, the responding cells begin to elaborate a battery of lymphokines (IL-2, gamma-interferon—γ-IFN, and so on), with the potential to change dramatically the local tissue microenvironment. In turn the functional properties of the indigenous antigen-presenting cells may be modified by the novel T cell-derived cytokines elaborated at the site. Because the functional properties of tissue-restricted antigen-presenting cells are relatively plastic, their abilities to process and present antigens to T lymphocytes are heavily influenced by factors in their local environment.

Tissue-Tropic Lymphocytes. Whereas some lymphocytes are short-lived and make a single pass through the circulation before their terminal escape into the extravascular space, a large fraction of lymphocytes in the peripheral blood are long lived, and capable of recirculating throughout the vascular tree. These cells regularly exit from the blood and pass into peripheral tissues. Usually they find their way into distal lymphatic channels and are carried via lymph flow back to the circulation where the migratory process is renewed. The passage of blood-borne lymphocytes through endothelial cells into peripheral tissues is a highly regulated process.[12] At one end of the spectrum of regulation, a relatively passive mechanism (diapedesis) allows small numbers of circulating cells to trickle through fenestrations between the endothelial cells that line capillaries and

postcapillary venules of the microvasculature. When an inflammatory reaction is underway, cell adhesion molecules and their co-ligands are reciprocally induced and expressed on endothelial cells and circulating leukocytes. The resultant adhesive interactions between these cells lead to the enhanced passage of blood-borne cells into the inflamed site. At the other end of the spectrum of regulation of lymphocyte migration, highly specialized postcapillary venules (PCV) exist in organized lymphoid tissues.[42] The endothelial cells of these PCVs express unique surface ligands for which subpopulations of recirculating lymphocytes display specific co-ligands. Because of the interactions of these receptor-ligands, bulk flow of subpopulations of lymphocytes is directed into particular regions of lymphoid organs, such as the deep cortex of lymph nodes.

Within this context, ligand or receptor systems have now been described that can direct certain populations of lymphocytes into specialized, nonlymphoid tissues and organs, such as skin.[6] Lymphocytes can display the property of *tissue-tropism* such that as they recirculate throughout the body some cells preferentially migrate into one particular type of tissue (the skin), and others preferentially migrate to another tissue (the mucosal surfaces). The conjunctival surfaces of the eye appear to be integrated into the mucosally directed set of specialized recirculating lymphocytes,[22] but it remains to be determined whether other tissues of the body, such as the internal components of the eye, also possess their own set of tissue-tropic lymphocytes.

Tissue-Serving Vascular Networks. For the immune system to detect and protect against pathogens that invade a particular organ or tissue, avenues of communication between the immune system and the organ or tissue must be available. On the one hand, when an antigen is introduced into the body at a particular site, the antigenic information must be carried to a draining lymphoid organ; because only at that site can unprimed, antigen-specific lymphocytes be activated. This pathway represents the *afferent* arm of the so-called immune reflex arc, and for most tissues of the body, lymphatic channels appear to serve this function. As a consequence, the antigen-specific immune effector modalities produced following antigen-driven lymphocyte activation in lymph nodes and spleen are delivered into circulation throughout the body. On the other hand, when an antigen is reintroduced into an organ or tissue, blood-borne specific immune effectors must be mobilized and focused at the antigen-containing site. This process (1) depends upon properties expressed by the blood microvasculature of the tissue in question, (2) represents the *efferent* arm of the immune reflex arc, and (3) is the mechanism by which offending pathogens are eliminated.

Concerning the afferent limb, integrity of a lymphatic drainage route from a peripheral tissue to a lymph node is important in the induction of immunity. When a skin allograft is placed in an orthotopic site, the lymph node that drains that site undergoes a swelling response in the next several days. This response represents the accumulation, activation, and proliferation of antigen-specific T and B lymphocytes recruited in response to antigenic signals derived from the graft. Eventually the graft is rejected as specific effectors are released from the node into the general circulation. If the lymph node is surgically excised prior to placement of the allograft into the site, however, rejection does not ensue.[56] This outcome reveals that an avenue from the graft to the lymph node is absolutely essential in the induction of allograft immunity. In fact it was this observation that led Medawar and his colleagues[45] to propose that the "absence" of a demonstrable lymphatic drainage pathway for the anterior chamber was responsible for the privileged status of this site.

Concerning the efferent limb, the nature of the microvasculature within peripheral tissues dictates whether immune effectors can or will gain access to a location of relevant antigenic material. For most tissues of the body the microvasculature is fenestrated, meaning that molecules and cells from the blood can slowly but continuously escape into the perivascular connective tissue space. Included in this "silent" passage are sensitized lymphocytes and antibody molecules. When these effectors encounter their relevant antigen in the extravascular space, they secrete lymphokines and activate mediators, triggering an inflammatory response built in large measure because of the remarkable changes occurring in the microvasculature.[12] Endothelial cells respond by up-regulating those cell adhesion molecules that promote leukocyte binding and egress into the perivascular space. Cytoskeletal changes within the endothelial cells increase the effective pore size of the lumenal surface, thereby enhancing the passage of larger molecular weight plasma proteins into the tissues. The extent to which the immune system responds to and eliminates pathogens invading somatic tissues depends critically on its ability (1) to enlist the help of the local microvessels in bringing blood-borne host defense mechanisms to the site, and (2) to recruit these nonspecific inflammatory molecules and cells into the pathogen-specific destructive process. Certain tissues of the body, especially the internal compartments of the eye, are served by a restrictive microvasculature—the so-called blood-tissue barriers. As a consequence, the ability of the immune system to eliminate pathogens at these sites is partially restricted. In the eye this restriction accounts in part for immune privilege and for the vulnerability of the eye to certain pathogens.

Draining Lymphoid Organs. Peripheral lymphoid organs, such as lymph nodes, spleen, tonsils, appendix, and Peyer's patches, are designed anatomically and functionally to receive antigenic signals and to transduce them into antigen-specific immune effector modalities, including sensitized T cells and antibodies. The common anatomic features that account for this ability include the following: (1) follicles and germinal centers in which B lymphocytes proliferate and differentiate into antibody-producing plasma cells and memory B cells, and (2) parafollicular regions that entrap lymph-borne, antigen-bearing, dendritic cells and macrophages. The parafollicular regions are also served by specialized postcapillary venules that deliver large numbers of blood-borne T and B lymphocytes into the perivascular space. This remarkable confluence of tissue-derived antigenic signals and antigen-recognizing lymphocytes in a "suitable" microenvironment allows for antigen-specific lymphocyte activation and differentiation. Eventually effector and memory T and B lymphocytes are produced, and these progeny are disseminated into the vascular tree.

The word "suitable" is carefully chosen as a modifier of microenvironment in the previous paragraph. While the microenvironments found in organized lymphoid tissues generally permit antigen-driven activation of specific lymphocytes, the microenvironments of the different lymphoid organs are not all identical. For example, immune responses generated in lymph nodes that drain the skin tend to be dominated by cell-mediated immunity and by IgG antibodies that fix complement.[60] Immune responses generated in gut-associated lymphoid organs are dominated by IgA antibodies,[1,9,76] with little participation of delayed hypersensitivity.[43] In part, the pattern difference of immune effectors generated in these two distinct sets of lymphoid tissues is predicated upon the existence of recirculating tissue-tropic lymphocytes preferentially entering one or the other set of nodes. In addition, it is likely that the microenvironments within these different lymphoid organs possess special features that can drive lymphocyte activation and differentiation into unique pathways. In this context it is important to point out that the spleen represents yet a third, distinctly different microenvironment within the immune system. Antigens first encountered by lymphocytes within the spleen evoke a systemic immune response that is enriched for humoral immune responses, yet deficient in one or more components of cell-mediated immunity.[54,55] Perhaps as a consequence, the spleen appears to have a special role in the generation of regulatory lymphocytes suppressing one or more aspects of immune expression.[17,72]

Tissue-Restricted Microenvironments. In a theoretic sense, if the immune response invoked by pathogens in a particular organ or tissue is to be molded to suit the needs and requirements of that tissue, the cells that confer the differentiated function of that organ or tissue must provide the relevant information. Accordingly, the parenchymal cells of individual organs and tissues create unique local microenvironments through the factors (cytokines, mediators) they secrete locally. It is presumed that the primary function of factors elaborated by parenchymal cells is to establish intercellular communication as a means of integrating the differentiated functions of the tissue. The factors themselves are usually not tissue-restricted in their effects, however, because receptors for these factors may be expressed on other tissues, including cells in the blood. Thus if parenchymal cells of the eye continuously secrete TGF-β, cells of non-ocular origin possessing TGF-β receptors and entering the eye will come under the influence of the ocular parenchymal cells. In this manner the functional programs of migrating leukocytes entering a particular tissue or organ are suscepti-ble to modification if the cells display surface receptors for factors in the local microenvironment.

The uniqueness of the microenvironments created in the eye (as well as the central nervous system) is reinforced by the highly restrictive blood-brain and blood-ocular barriers. As discussed in the following section, the cytokines, neuro-peptides, and other factors present within the aqueous humor, vitreous body, and other internal compartments of the eye markedly influence the manner in which the immune system recognizes and responds to antigens that gain access to these sites.

Regional Specialization of Immunity in the Skin and at Mucosal Surfaces

The two major epithelial surfaces of the body (integu-ment and mucosal surfaces) that confront the environment encounter vastly different spectra of pathogenic organisms. To meet these challenges, the skin has developed a special-ized set of anatomic strategies that provide a primary, physi-cochemical barrier to ward off invasion by microorga-nisms.[33] By contrast, mucosal surfaces have developed a different set of strategies in which chemical rather than physical barriers play the more important role in preventing microbial invasion.[1,9,76] Because mucosal surfaces must allow molecules from the environment to enter into the body, these surfaces were forced to bring organized lymph-oid tissues into direct physical contact with the epithelial surface (such as tonsils and Peyer's patches). The differ-ences in potential pathogens and in barrier strategies adopted by the mucosal and integumentary surfaces led inevitably to differences in the manner in which these epithelial surfaces interact with and derive protection from the systemic im-mune apparatus.

MALT—Mucosa Associated Lymphoid Tissues. The mucosal tissues integrated into MALT include the linings of the gastrointestinal tract, the respiratory tract, the urethro-genital tract, and the conjunctiva and ocular adnexal glands. Immunity at these surfaces is dominated by IgA antibodies, rather than by other immunoglobulin isotypes. In addition, T cell-mediated immunity is accomplished primarily by CD4$^+$ cells that recruit eosinophils to carry out destruction of para-sites, rather than by T cells that mediate conventional de-layed hypersensitivity. These statements refer to immunity dependent upon T cells with alpha or beta chain receptors for antigen. Recent evidence implicates T cells with gamma or delta receptors in gut immunity.[2] The experimental evi-dence, however, is incomplete, not yet integrated into a theoretic construct, and beyond the scope of this discussion.

When mucosal immunity is initiated by exposure to an exogenous antigen at a particular mucosal site, that site, as well as other mucosal sites, eventually acquires the capacity to mediate immune protection against that antigen. For ex-ample, if exposure of an animal to an antigen by the oral routes leads to the generation of specific IgA antibodies, these antibodies are found within the secretions of the glands and secretory epithelium of the gut. Moreover, similar anti-gen-specific IgA antibodies can be found in external secre-tions at unrelated mucosal surfaces, such as the urethra and the conjunctiva. The capacity of the mucosal immune sys-tem to distribute immune effectors specific for antigens first encountered through mucosal surfaces is invested in unique populations of recirculating IgA-producing B and T cells. Homing receptors expressed on these blood-borne cells allow the cells to recognize co-ligands (addressins) that are uniquely displayed on endothelial cells of the microvascula-ture serving mucosal surfaces.[29] This process ensures that all mucosal surfaces benefit from the immunity elicited by an antigen invading one particular mucosal surface.

Examination of the systemic immunity elicited by anti-gens first experienced via mucosal surfaces reveals an inter-esting and informative spectrum of changes. Antigen-speci-fic IgA antibodies are present in mucosal fluids and usually in the blood. The blood, however, frequently contains only low titers of IgG antibodies directed at the same antigen. Moreover, T cells that mediate antigen-specific delayed hy-persensitivity (DH) are not found in the spleen or other lymphoid organs of animals immunized orally by that anti-gen. In fact, when animals immunized to an antigen via a mucosal surface are exposed subcutaneously to the same antigen in highly immunogenic form (usually in conjunction with an adjuvant), T_{DH} cells and IgG antibodies fail to ap-pear. These findings indicate that mucosal immunity is a highly specialized form of immune response in which cer-tain effector modalities are produced, whereas others are **not** elicited, but are actively suppressed.[43] The concept that re-gional specialization in immune responsiveness is accom-plished by selective down-regulation of one or more compo-nents of the immune arsenal is particularly important in explaining the unique features of immunity within the eye.

SALT—Skin Associated Lymphoid Tissues. Immune re-sponses to antigens first encountered within the skin differ remarkably from those described for mucosal surfaces. Cu-taneous immunity is dominated by T cells that mediate DH and by IgG antibodies, especially those that fix comple-ment.[60] Accordingly, intense inflammation routinely ac-companies immune elimination of antigens and pathogens from the skin. IgA antibodies are not usually observed in the blood or in mucosal secretions. As is the case with the mu-cosal immune response, immunity elicited by an initial encounter with antigen in the skin is systemically disseminated. Consequently, in an individual previously sensitized via the skin, antigen-specific DH can be elicited at virtually any cutaneous site of the body.

Induction of cutaneous immunity follows a strict set of rules. Specialized antigen-presenting cells normally reside in the epidermis (Langerhans' cells) and dermis (dermal dendritic cells). These cells capture antigens that penetrate the cutaneous barrier, carry the antigens to draining lymph nodes, and activate antigen-specific T and B cells. Sensitized T cells generated in this manner display homing receptors that restrict their subsequent migration either to lymph nodes that drain skin or to activated endothelial cells in the microvessels of inflamed skin. Once within the dermis and epidermis, these T cells can recognize their antigen of interest on indigenous dendritic cells and Langerhans' cells and thereby trigger the inflammatory response characteristic of delayed hypersensitivity.

THE EYE'S REGIONAL SPHERE OF IMMUNOLOGIC INFLUENCE

In the remainder of this chapter the algorithm deduced from MALT and SALT will be applied to the components of the ocular immune system, particularly in regard to the internal compartments of the eye. Because of anatomic considerations, the immune system interacts with the eye in two separate patterns: (1) the conjunctival surface and adnexal structures, and (2) the internal compartment of the eye. The conjunctival surface is integrated into MALT and shares many if not all of the features described for the mucosal immune system. Because the eye bears considerable structural and physiologic similarities to the brain, a consideration of the ocular immune system resembles a discussion of the specialized manner in which the immune system interacts with the brain (see box).[69]

Components of the Ocular Immune System

Eye-Restricted Antigen-Presenting Cells. In other organs and tissues of the body, professional antigen-presenting cells (APC) are represented by a distinct population of bone marrow-derived cells termed dendritic cells. This population of cells is usually complemented by tissue macrophages, which also process and present antigens to lymphocytes. Tissue-restricted APC can be readily recognized in vivo and in vitro by the dendritic shape they assume. Other critical features include: constitutive expression of class II MHC molecules (which play a central role in presenting antigenic peptide fragments to CD4$^+$ T cells), and CD45 (a marker molecule that identifies cells solely of hematopoietic origin). With the aid of these and other surface markers, several laboratories defined the intraocular distribution of dendritic cells and macrophages.[35,44,85] In the anterior segment of the eye the central cornea is virtually devoid of either dendritic

---

SPECIALIZED FEATURES OF THE OCULAR SPHERE OF IMMUNOLOGIC INFLUENCE

- Immune privilege
- Selective deficiency of T cells mediating delayed hypersensitivity
- Selective deficiency of B cells secreting complement-fixing antibodies
- Activation of cytotoxic T and B cells secreting other immunoglobulin isotypes
- Activation of regulatory T cells suppressing induction and expression of delayed hypersensitivity, as well as IgG2a-secreting B cells

---

cells (Langerhans' cells) or macrophages, except at the limbus.[70] Thus unless perturbed by inflammation, there are few if any cells in the cornea considered professional APC. By contrast, both dendritic cells and macrophages are present in the iris, trabecular meshwork, and ciliary body. McMenamin and associates[44] demonstrated that dendritic cells occupy the tissue plane between the two epithelial cell layers of the ciliary epithelium; in addition, dendritic cells adopt a position immediately beneath the single layer of iris epithelium. These investigators also found that macrophages punctuate the stroma supporting the ciliary processes and the iris. Flugel and associates[21] determined that class II MHC$^+$ cells with dendritic features are not present in the direct outflow pathway of the trabecular meshwork. Cells of this type are concentrated, however, "around" the outflow path and are particularly well represented in the ciliary muscle, along the so-called uveoscleral pathway.[21] The latter investigators detected very small numbers of rounded cells with features of macrophages directly in the aqueous outflow path of the trabecular meshwork. In the posterior compartment of the eye, typical dendritic cells were found by McMenamin and associates[44] near the ora serrata and among the neural layers of the retina. Although the choroid plexus lies immediately outside the barrier created by the retinal pigment epithelium, it may be considered part of the ocular immune system. In that regard, macrophages and dendritic cells are readily demonstrable in the connective tissues surrounding the choriocapillaris. Based on these findings, it might be expected that functional antigen presentation exists in many of the internal structures of the eye.

Experiments to examine this issue resulted in an unexpected set of findings. Williamson and associates[85] prepared single cell suspensions from murine iris and ciliary body (I/CB). Included in these suspensions were dendritic cells and macrophages. Yet when the suspensions were used as antigen-presenting cells for alloreactive T cells, no T cell activation was detected. In part, failure of the I/CB cell suspension to stimulate T cells can be ascribed to the ability of the epithelial cells (which were also present in the suspensions) to secrete immunosuppressive factors. When Streilein and Bradley[64] used flow cytometry to prepare a relatively pure population of bone marrow-derived cells from I/CB, however, the cells still failed to function in antigen presentation to T cells. Similarly, cells harvested from I/CB of eyes treated with subinflammatory doses of gamma-interferon (which increased the number and surface expression of class II MHC+ cells) were also unable to activate T cells.[65] These results imply that bone marrow-derived dendritic cells and macrophages within the anterior segment are incapable of functioning as conventional antigen-presenting cells. These results closely resemble those reported by Caspi and associates,[11] who examined the APC potential of cells in the posterior compartment. Suspensions of murine Muller cells failed to activate S antigen-specific T cell lines. Moreover, treatment of Muller cells with gamma-interferon (which up-regulates expression of class II MHC molecules) also failed to confer T cell-activating properties on them. The general conclusion from this line of investigation is that despite the existence of bone marrow-derived cells in the internal tissues of the anterior and posterior segments of the eye, these tissues are deficient in professional antigen-presenting cells, leaving the internal eye deficient in this critical immune function.

Recent studies by Wilbanks and associates[80,81,84] revealed that although the dendritic cells and macrophages of the iris and ciliary body lack conventional APC activity, these cells are not functionally silent. Injection of antigen into the anterior chamber (AC) of the eye elicits anterior chamber associated immune deviation (ACAID).[49,59,75] Wilbanks and associates produced evidence to suggest that the initial steps in ACAID induction actually begin within the eye. Using circumstantial evidence, these workers proposed that dendritic cells or macrophages of the I/CB function as specialized ocular APC, picking up intraocular antigens and migrating across the trabecular meshwork into the venous circulation. Wilbanks and associates obtained ACAID-inducing cells from two sources: (1) murine eyes into which soluble antigen has been introduced 24 hours previously, and (2) the blood of animals that received AC injections of antigen 48 hours previously. Moreover, bone marrow-derived cells obtained from normal I/CB possess ACAID-inducing properties if the cells are pulsed with antigen in vitro and are then injected intravenously into naive syngeneic recipients.

Thus the eye does appear to contain tissue-restricted antigen-presenting cells. The functional properties of these cells, however, differ sharply from APC obtained from other tissues such as skin. The inability of antigen-bearing ocular APC to activate delayed hypersensitivity T cells in vivo or to stimulate alloreactive T cells in vitro, may mean that these cells are nonfunctional. Their ability to induce regulatory splenic T cells that suppress delayed hypersensitivity in an antigen-specific manner suggests, however, that intraocular dendritic cells or macrophages function as "alternative" antigen-presenting cells that address unique populations of functionally distinct T cells found in ACAID.

Eye-Seeking Lymphocytes. Under resting conditions, the rate at which leukocytes in general, and lymphocytes in particular, penetrate across the blood-ocular barriers to enter into the internal compartments of the eye is extremely slow. When the eye is inflamed, however, marked changes in the endothelial cells of the ocular microvasculature promote the migration of blood-borne cells into the eye.[78] As in other tissues experiencing inflammation, peripheral blood leukocytes bind to cell adhesion molecules expressed on activated, ocular, vascular endothelial cells and then pass across the vessel wall. The cell adhesion molecules and ligands that promote the entry of inflammatory cells into the eye are similar to those expressed during inflammation in other organs. But they do not represent addressins and homing receptors that could selectively promote the migration of subpopulations of putative eye-seeking cells. No evidence suggests the existence of such cells. This issue, however, has been virtually unexplored experimentally, and therefore the lack of evidence should not be construed to mean that eye-seeking lymphocytes do not exist. The presence of blood-ocular and blood-brain barriers suggests either that lymphocytes are incapable of entering these organs (in the absence of inflammation), or that special mechanisms are required to promote this traffic.

Vascular Networks of the Eye. Virtually every organ and tissue of the body possesses a vascular blood supply. Exceptions include the cornea, the lens, and mature cartilage. The microvessels of the blood stream are usually associated with a second microvasculature containing lymph and representing the means by which lymph is carried to draining lymph nodes and back to the blood. These two vascular systems represent the only modes by which the immune system can communicate with, and provide protection for, somatic tissues. In this regard, the manners in which different organs are connected anatomically with the blood and lymph vascular systems are not identical. The vascular connections to the eye are particularly distinct. The internal compartments of the eye are served by a blood vasculature in which the endothelium erects a significant barrier to the passage of molecules and cells from the blood into the eye.[16] This barrier plays an important role in preventing, or at least severely restricting, blood-borne immune effector cells and molecules from penetrating the eye.[5,19] In part, immune privilege may result from the relative inability of immune effectors to reach foreign grafts placed experimentally within the eye. This vascular barrier not only limits the accessibility of immune effector cells and molecules into the eye, but it ensures that other plasma proteins are also poorly represented within the eye. For example, the complement components are present in very low concentration in aqueous humor,[47] as is alpha-2 macroglobulin. This fact is of interest because these molecules can play critical roles in amplifying or suppressing immunogenic inflammation. Their poor representation in ocular fluids may mean that the eye is unable to benefit from their abilities to regulate intraocular inflammation. The blood-ocular barrier, however, is certainly not complete. Investigators were able to induce autoimmunity directed at retina-specific antigens, and when susceptible strains of mice and rats are so immunized, uveoretinitis can be initiated and sustained. This result indicates that the blood-retina barrier can be breached under pathologic circumstances. In uveoretinitis the barrier is clearly broken, and plasma proteins can be readily detected in aqueous humor.[23,48]

Accessibility of intraocular fluids to local lymphatic vessels is greatly restricted and regulated. The bulk of aqueous humor crosses the trabecular meshwork and enters the blood vasculature directly.[7] Under resting conditions, less than 10% of aqueous humor can be traced to lymphatic vessels in the head and neck. This fact has a marked influence on the immunologic fate of antigens injected into or arising within the eye. Compared to nonocular tissues, the speed with which an antigen placed in the anterior chamber reaches draining cervical lymph nodes is noticeably reduced. Wilbanks and Streilein[82] demonstrated that greater than 99% of soluble protein antigen injected into the anterior chamber of murine eyes escapes into the blood within 24 hours. A small but potentially significant fraction of injected antigen actually remains within the eye for extended periods of time; trace amounts were detected 4 weeks postinoculation. These findings mean that under normal circumstances, the vast majority of antigens and antigen-bearing cells placed within the eye can impact the immune system only by passing directly into the blood stream. As a consequence the spleen, rather than draining lymph nodes, provides the primary focus for the initial immune response to intraocular antigens. Experimental verification of this interpretation comes from the repeated observation that splenectomy prior to intraocular administration of antigen prevents the induction of ACAID.[34,67,84] Thus the anatomic arrangement by which intraocular fluids normally drain from the eye proves to be a critical factor in dictating the nature of the immune response generated by ocular antigens.

Lymphoid Organs Receiving Eye-Derived Antigenic Signals. The previous section describes the microvascular features of the eye and indicates that these features dictate that the spleen, rather than regional lymph nodes, is the primary recipient of antigens escaping from the eye. It has long been appreciated that splenic responses to antigenic stimuli are different from lymph node responses. Generally speaking, immune responses emanating from the spleen are enriched for antibodies and deficient in cell-mediated effectors. When soluble antigens are used, the spleen-derived antibodies produced are usually of the noncomplement-fixing isotypes,

which means that elimination of antigen occurs without the aid of complement activation. Moreover, immune responses initiated within the spleen are dominated by regulatory T cells, some that suppress the induction of immunity, and others that suppress the expression of T cell-mediated, as well as antibody-mediated immunity. A satisfactory explanation for the special features of spleen-dominated immune responses has yet to be formulated.

It is relevant to this discussion that experimental evidence gathered in mice and rats implicates the spleen in the development of ACAID. Injection of soluble antigens and implantation of cellular allografts into the anterior chamber of the eye of mice with previously extirpated spleens fail to induce ACAID.[34,67,84] Instead, these animals develop conventional immunity, including antigen-specific delayed hypersensitivity. It appears that antigenic signals from the eye delivered into the blood vasculature ensure that these signals are carried primarily to the spleen, rather than to other peripheral lymphoid organs. As a consequence the features of the resulting systemic immune response bear the imprint of splenic immunity (enhanced humoral, but impaired cell-mediated immunity).

A recent study examines the systemic immune consequences when the flow of aqueous humor from the anterior chamber is deflected toward the uveoscleral pathway, rather than through the trabecular meshwork. Eichhorn and associates[18] used topical application of prostaglandin F2-alpha (PGF2α) to open the uveoscleral pathway in cynomolgus monkey eyes. When the therapeutic effect was maximal, the soluble antigen ovalbumin (OVA) was injected into the anterior chamber of the treated eye. Seven days later these monkeys were immunized with OVA in adjuvant. When they were subsequently skin challenged with OVA, they displayed vigorous OVA-specific delayed hypersensitivity. By contrast, control monkeys not treated with PGF2α that received AC injections of OVA displayed ACAID—they failed to mount cutaneous-delayed hypersensitivity responses. Bill[7] demonstrated that ocular fluids exiting via the uveoscleral pathway drain to cervical lymph nodes. Therefore, Eichhorn and others proposed that ACAID is avoided in PGF2α-treated monkeys because the antigen injected intracamerally drained primarily to cervical nodes, rather than to the spleen. These results dramatically emphasize the differences in immune effector responses elicited when different lymphoid organs receive antigenic signals. Moreover, the results imply that if fluid drainage from the eye is abnormal (directed to lymphatics, rather than the blood vasculature), antigens escaping from the eye are more likely to induce immunity of the delayed hypersensitivity type, rather than the less damaging immunity found in ACAID.

Intraocular Microenvironment. The internal components of the eye are immersed in highly distinctive intraocular fluids (aqueous humor, vitreous body). The concentration of plasma proteins and molecules in these fluids is extremely low. More important, these fluids contain cytokines, neuropeptides, and other molecules and factors that influence the growth and physiologic function of intraocular cells. Aqueous humor was subjected recently to intense study by ocular immunologists.[32] When tested in vitro, aqueous humor was found to be profoundly immunosuppressive. Normal aqueous humor (from murine, porcine, rabbit, rat, and human eyes) inhibits antigen-, mitogen-, and growth factor-dependent T cell proliferation and lymphokine production in vitro. When effector cells of delayed hypersensitivity are mixed with aqueous humor and injected subcutaneously in vivo, the anticipated, delayed, inflammatory response fails to materialize. Nonetheless, aqueous humor is not universally toxic to T lymphocytes. Fully functional cytotoxic T cells exposed to aqueous humor retain their ability to lyse their target cells. T cells are not the only type of lymphoreticular cell susceptible to aqueous humor. Exposure of conventional antigen-presenting cells (peritoneal exudate cells, peripheral blood monocytes) to aqueous humor was reported by Wilbanks and associates[81] to rob mice of their ability to acquire delayed hypersensitivity when the cells were injected into naive mice. This aspect of aqueous humor modification of APC function may form the basis of induction of ACAID in mice. Cousins and associates[14] reported that aqueous humor suppresses the expression of delayed hypersensitivity in vivo. When T cells that mediate delayed hypersensitivity are mixed with antigen and injected intracutaneously or subconjunctivally, a delayed hypersensitivity reaction ensues. If the injected cells are first mixed with aqueous humor, however, the injection elicits little or no local inflammatory response. These experimental results are the in vivo counterparts of the previously mentioned in vitro experiments, demonstrating the ability of aqueous humor to suppress effector T cell function. Aqueous humor also acts directly on macrophages, suppressing their ability to produce nitric oxide when stimulated with bacterial lipopolysaccharide and gamma-interferon (Andrew Taylor, personal communication). Aqueous humor undoubtedly has important influences on other cells, but this evidence is sufficient to indicate that this fluid is a powerful inhibitor of immunogenic inflammation—at the T cell level, at the antigen-presenting cell level, and at the level of effector macrophages.

Investigators have begun to sort out the factors in aqueous humor that may be responsible for its immunosuppressive properties. Several laboratories have now identified transforming growth factor beta (TGF-β) as a major immunosuppressive cytokine in aqueous humor.[13,23,30] Many of the inhibitory properties of aqueous humor that affect T cell and macrophage function can be ascribed to this cytokine. Of equal importance is the demonstration by Wilbanks, Mammolenti and Streilein[81] that TGF-β **alone** can confer ACAID-inducing properties on peritoneal exudate cells, implying that this capability of aqueous humor can also be ascribed to its content of TGF-β. In addition, other neuro-

peptides and cytokines are present constitutively in aqueous humor: alpha-melanocyte stimulating hormone (α-MSH), vasoactive intestinal peptide (VIP) (Andrew Taylor,[73] personal communication), and calcitonin gene-related protein.[77] Whereas TGF-β is a profound inhibitor of both T cell proliferation and secretion of gamma-interferon, α-MSH only prevents T cells from producing gamma-interferon, not from proliferating in response to antigen. It is too early to be certain of the contribution of each of these factors to the immunosuppressive properties of the anterior chamber and whether synergistic interactions prevail. Moreover, the identification of inhibitory factors is still incomplete. On the horizon, however, is the prospect that the intense current study of this ocular fluid will yield a consensus view of the extent and mechanisms of its immunosuppressive properties.

TGF-β is secreted by ciliary epithelial cells,[27,36,81] and mRNA for this cytokine was detected in both epithelial and stromal cells of several ocular tissues.[53] TGF-β was found in the supernatants of cultured iris and ciliary body cells, and its presence accounts for the ability of these supernatants to confer ACAID-inducing properties on peritoneal exudate cells.[81] It is clear, however, that supernatants of cultured I/CB cells contain other immunosuppressive factors. It may be that the neuropeptides, such as α-MSH and VIP, may actually be released from termini of axons that reach the internal compartments of the eye. Eventually it will be determined that many different cells contribute to the microenvironment of the eye and provide this environment with factors that can modify the antigen-presenting potential of indigenous APC and suppress the expression of immunogenic inflammation.

POTENTIAL CLINICAL RELEVANCE OF AN OCULAR SPHERE OF IMMUNOLOGIC INFLUENCE

The ability of the eye to influence, both qualitatively and quantitatively, the systemic immune response to antigens that gain access to or arise within the eye is important to the maintenance of the visual axis, and therefore for the preservation of vision. In general, immune responses to ocular antigens appear to be selectively deficient in those effector modalities that mediate protection by recruiting intense nonspecific inflammation. In the phenomenon of ACAID, as defined experimentally, administration of antigen via the anterior chamber of the eye not only fails to activate T cells that mediate delayed hypersensitivity; suppressor T cells that inhibit the subsequent activation and expression of delayed hypersensitivity to the original antigen are also generated. Similarly, antigen injected into the eyes of mice elicits humoral immunity selectively deficient in IgG2a antibodies —the isotype of murine antibodies that is proficient at activating complement. Because complement activation leads to intense inflammation, the lack of these antibodies combined with the lack of delayed hypersensitivity leaves animals treated in this manner deficient in their ability to mobilize molecules and cells that produce immunogenic inflammation.

Fortunately the induction of ACAID by intraocular antigen does not produce a global immune deficiency. The spleens and cervical lymph nodes of recipients of ocular injections of antigens contain activated CD4[+] and CD8[+] T cells,[3] as well as antibody-producing B cells. As a consequence, a systemic immune response to intraocular antigens is mounted that includes primed cytotoxic T cells and humoral immunity enriched for (in mice) IgG1 antibodies.[46] For many pathogens, this subset of immune effectors suffices for providing the host and the eye with protection. Not all pathogens, however, submit so readily to the immune effectors found in animals with ACAID. The herpes simplex virus may be one example (see box). Inoculation of HSV-1 (KOS strain) into the AC of BALB/c mouse eyes evokes an intense, anterior segment inflammation that is locally destructive, but apparently self-limited.[79] As the acute response within the anterior segment fades, virus is cleared and the posterior compartment of the eye is spared. Within a few days, however, the virus reemerges in the posterior compartment of the contralateral eye, and an acute retinal necrosis suddenly erupts in that eye. This occurrence reflects the inability of the immune response elicited by virus in the first eye to induce the types of immune effectors that can limit virus spread via neural connections from the injected eye to the brain and beyond.[63]

Experimentally produced intraocular tumors are another example of the inability of immunity induced by intraocular antigens to evoke complete protection. Injection of weakly histoincompatible P815 tumor cells into the AC of eyes of BALB/c mice leads to the induction of antigen-specific ACAID in recipients[68]; but as a consequence, the animals develop concomitant immunity.[51] That is, they are able to resist subsequent challenges with P815 cells, whether the tumor cells are injected subcutaneously or into the anterior chamber of the contralateral eye. These findings imply that distant metastases derived from an original intraocular tumor are not likely to develop. The precise effectors responsible for concomitant immunity in this situation have not been identified, but candidates include the primed precursor cytotoxic T cells present in spleen and lymph nodes of injected mice,[38] as well as antibodies in the blood that

react with P815 cells.[25] Despite the presence of concomitant immunity in these mice, the tumors formed at the original intraocular injection site grow progressively and eventually kill their hosts. Thus the systemic immune response to antigenic intraocular tumors can eliminate the tumor at all sites, except the site of its origination. It is presumed that elimination of tumor at the initial site requires T cells of the delayed hypersensitivity type,[39,40] which is precisely the functional set of T cells that is deficient in ACAID.

The foregoing information gives the impression that the selective deficiencies associated with ACAID are deleterious for the eye. This condition may not always, or even often, be the case. Consider the devastating form of ocular infection with HSV-1 that is termed stromal keratitis. There is convincing evidence from many laboratories that the inflammation that may lead to corneal blindness in this disease is the result of an immune response to viral antigens, rather than a direct toxic effect of the virus itself.[28] In fact, evidence strongly suggests that keratitis is produced by delayed hypersensitivity responses to viral antigens within the stroma. In human beings stromal keratitis is an "uncommon" clinical outcome (approximately 20%) of infection of the ocular surface with HSV-1, suggesting that delayed hypersensitivity to viral antigens is not the usual consequence of ocular surface infection with HSV-1. In support of this view, it was confirmed that intraocular injection of HSV-1 in most strains of mice elicits virus-specific ACAID (absence of virus-specific delayed hypersensitivity).[63] In addition, Ksander and Hendricks[37] proved that induction of ACAID by intracameral injection of HSV antigens prevents mice with corneal HSV infections from developing stromal keratitis. Moreover, MacLeish and associates[41] reported that the incidence of stromal keratitis following zosteriform spread of HSV-1 to the anterior segment of the eye is directly related to whether the animals possess virus-specific delayed hypersensitivity at the time virus reaches the eye. If virus infection of the anterior segment occurs under circumstances that delay the onset of virus-specific DH, then infection of the cornea fails to result in stromal keratitis. If virus infection precociously activates systemic-delayed hypersensitivity, however; then as virus reaches and infects the cornea, intense immunogenic inflammation is evoked—producing stromal keratitis. Because eradication of virus from the anterior segment of the eye occurs in these animals whether delayed hypersensitivity exists or not, this example suggests that the selective immune deficiency of ACAID is actually beneficial to the eye.

POTENTIAL OF TURNING OCULAR REGIONAL IMMUNITY TO THE EYE'S ADVANTAGE

It can be (and has been) argued that immune privilege and ACAID are expressions of an evolutionarily designed strategy to provide the eye with immune protection commensurate with the preservation of vision.[59,71] Because immuno-

---

RESULTS OF THE PRESENCE OF AN OCULAR SPHERE OF IMMUNOLOGIC INFLUENCE

- Survival of orthotopic corneal allografts
- Avoidance of HSV-1-dependent stromal keratitis
- HSV-1-dependent acute retinal necrosis
- Progressive growth of intraocular tumors
- Protection against metastases from intraocular tumors
- Avoidance of autoimmune and toxic uveoretinitis

genic inflammation is deleterious to the visual axis, the eye and the immune system have reached a compromise in which the latter provides **some** of the immune effector modalities at its discretion. As the example of stromal keratitis described previously suggests, an immune response that is transiently deficient in delayed hypersensitivity can spare the cornea a blinding inflammation, while at the same time promoting the elimination of virus from the eye. There are other examples of situations in which ocular injury and loss of vision occur through immunologic means: sympathetic ophthalmia and other forms of autoimmune uveoretinitis, phthisis in association with immune elimination of intraocular tumors, and rejection of orthotopic corneal allografts. In each of these examples, delayed hypersensitivity directed at antigenic material of the eye has a deleterious effect. In a sense, these illustrations represent failure of immune privilege and lack of ACAID induction.

To emphasize this point, Hara and associates[25] recently used experimental induction of ACAID with soluble retina-specific antigens to prevent autoimmune uveitis in mice; a similar strategy was used previously by Mizuno and associates[46] in rats. These studies validate the concept that the unique immune responses evoked by intraocular presentation of antigens can be used to prevent immune-mediated ocular injury and disease. Wilbanks and associates[81] demonstrated that the phenomenon of ACAID can be created in mice by in vitro techniques that do not even require an ocular injection of antigen. These investigators found that in vitro incubation of so-called professional antigen-presenting cells (obtained from peritoneal cavity or blood) with antigen in the presence of transforming growth factor beta confers upon the cells ACAID-inducing properties. Mice that receive intravenous injections of in vitro-modified cells acquire ACAID and are then incapable of developing delayed hypersensitivity to the antigen in the original incubation medium. To demonstrate the usefulness of this approach, Hara and associates[26] incubated peritoneal exudate cells with interphotoreceptor retinal-binding protein (IRBP—a retinal autoantigen) in the presence of TGF-β. The cells were then injected intravenously into B10.A mice that were subsequently immunized with IRBP in adjuvant. Unlike untreated mice, recipients of TGF-β-treated cells failed to develop uveitis.

These results indicate the power of immune privilege and the ACAID phenomenon to alter the course of immune responses to ocular antigens. It is hoped that it will be possible to develop innovative approaches based on these strategies to prevent or ameliorate immunogenic inflammation in the eye, and thereby prevent blindness caused by inappropriate intraocular expression of immunity.

REFERENCES

1. Alley CD, Mestecky J: The mucosal immune system. In Bird G, Calvert JE, editors: *B lymphocytes in human disease,* 222-254, Oxford, Great Britain, 1988, Oxford University Press.

2. Bandeira A, Itohara S, Bonneville M, et al.: Extrathymic origin of intestinal intraepithelial lymphocytes bearing T cell antigen receptor $\gamma\delta$, *Proc Natl Acad Sci USA* 88:43-47, 1991.

3. Bando Y, Ksander BR, Streilein JW: Characterization of specific T helper cell activity in mice bearing alloantigenic tumors in the anterior chamber of the eye, *Eur J Immunol* 21:1923-1932, 1991.

4. Barker CF, Billingham RE: Immunologically privileged sites, *Adv Immunol* 25:1-54, 1977.

5. Bengtsson E: Studies on the mechanism of the breakdown of the blood-aqueous barrier in the rabbit eye, *Acta Ophthalmol* S130:3-33, 1977.

6. Berg EL, Yoshino T, Rott LS, et al.: The cutaneous lymphocyte antigen is a skin lymphocyte homing receptor for the vascular lectin endothelial cell-leukocyte adhesion molecule-1, *J Exp Med* 174:1461-1466, 1991.

7. Bill A: The role of ciliary blood flow and ultrafiltration in aqueous humor formation, *Exp Eye Res* 16:287-299, 1973.

8. Blumenkranz MS, Russell SR, Robey MG, et al.: Risk factors in age-related maculopathy complicated by choroidal neovascularization, *Ophthalmology* 93:552-558, 1986.

9. Brandtzaeg P: Overview of the mucosal immune system, *Curr Top Microbiol Immunol* 146:13-25, 1989.

10. Callanan D, Peeler J, Niederkorn JY: Characteristics of rejection of orthotopic corneal allografts in the rat, *Transplantation* 45:437-443, 1988.

11. Caspi RR, Roberge FG, Nussenblatt RB: Organ-resident, nonlymphoid cells suppress proliferation of autoimmune T helper lymphocytes, *Science* 237:1029-1031, 1987.

12. Chin H-T, Falanga V, Streilein JW, Sackstein R: Specific lymphocyte-endothelial cell interactions regulate migration into lymph nodes, Peyer's patches, and skin, *Reg Immunol* 1:78-83, 1993.

13. Cousins S, McCabe M, Danielpour R, Streilein JW: Identification of transforming growth factor-beta as an immunosuppressive factor in aqueous humor, *Invest Ophthalmol Vis Sci* 32:2201-2211, 1991.

14. Cousins S, Trattler W, Streilein JW: Immune privilege and suppression of immunogenic inflammation in the anterior chamber of the eye, *Curr Eye Res* 10:287-297, 1991.

15. Crawford K, Kaufman PL, True-Gabelt B: Effect of topical PGF$_{2\alpha}$ on aqueous humor dynamics in cynomolgus monkeys, *Curr Eye Res* 6:1035-1044, 1987.

16. Davson H: *Physiology of the ocular and cerebrospinal fluids,* 195-201, London, 1956, J and A Churchill.

17. Dorf ME, Kuchroo VK, Steele JK, O'Hara RM: Understanding suppressor cells: where have we gone wrong? *Intern Rev Immunol* 3:375-392, 1988.

18. Eichhorn M, Horneber M, Streilein JW, Lutjen-Drecoll E: Anterior chamber associated immune deviation elicited via primate eyes, *Invest Ophthalmol Vis Sci* 34:2926-2930, 1993.

19. Feilder AR, Rahi AHS: Immunoglobulins of normal aqueous humor, *Trans Ophthalmol Soc U K* 99:120-125, 1979.

20. Ferguson TA, Hayashi JD, Kaplan HJ: Regulation of the systemic immune response by visible light and the eye, *FASEB J* 2:3017-3021, 1988.

21. Flugel C, Kinne RW, Streilein JW, Lutjen-Drecoll E: Distinctive distribution of bone marrow derived cells in the anterior segment of human eyes, *Curr Eye Res* 11:1173-1184, 1992.

22. Franklin RM, Remus LE: Conjunctival-associated lymphoid tissue: evidence for a role in the secretory immune system, *Invest Ophthalmol Vis Sci* 25:181-187, 1984.

23. Ghose T: Immunoglobulins in aqueous humor and iris from patient with endogenous uveitis patients with cataract, *Br J Ophthalmol* 57:897-903, 1973.

24. Granstein R, Stszewski R, Knisely T, et al.: Aqueous humor contains transforming growth factor-β and a small (<3500 daltons) inhibitor of thymocyte proliferation, *J Immunol* 144:3021-3027, 1990.

25. Hara Y, Caspi RR, Wiggert B, et al.: Suppression of experimental autoimmune uveitis in mice by induction of anterior chamber associated immune deviation with interphotoreceptor retinoid binding protein, *J Immunol* 148:1685-1692, 1992.

26. Hara Y, Caspi RR, Wiggert B, et al.: Analysis of an in vitro-generated signal that induces systemic immune deviation similar to that elicited by antigen injected into the anterior chamber of the eye, *J Immunol* 149:1531-1538, 1992.

27. Helbig H, Gurley RC, Palestine AG, et al.: Dual effect of ciliary body cells on T lymphocyte proliferation, *Eur J Immunol* 20:2457-2463, 1990.

28. Hendricks RL, Tumpey TM: Contribution of virus and immune factors to herpes simplex virus type I-induced corneal pathology, *Invest Ophthalmol Vis Sci* 31:1929-1939, 1990.

29. Holzmann B, McIntyre BW, Weissman IL: Identification of a murine Peyer's patch-specific lymphocyte homing receptor as an integrin molecule with an α chain homologous to human VLA-4α, *Cell* 56:37-46, 1989.

30. Jampel HD, Roche N, Stark WJ, Roberts AB: Transforming growth factor-β in human aqueous humor, *Curr Eye Res* 9:963-969, 1990.

31. Jiang LQ, Streilein JW: Immune privilege extended to allogeneic tumor cells in the vitreous cavity, *Invest Ophthalmol Vis Sci* 32:224-228, 1991.

32. Kaiser C, Ksander B, Streilein JW: Inhibition of lymphocyte proliferation by aqueous humor, *Reg Immunol* 2:42-49, 1989.

33. Kaplan HJ, Stevens TR: A reconsideration of immunologic privilege within the anterior chamber of the eye, *Transplantation* 19:302-309, 1974.

34. Kaplan HJ, Streilein JW: Do immunologically privileged sites require a functioning spleen? *Nature* 251:553-554, 1974.

35. Knisely TL, Bleicher PA, Vibbard CA, Granstein RD: Morphologic and ultrastructural examination of I-A$^+$cells in the murine iris, *Invest Ophthalmol Vis Sci* 32:2423-2431, 1991.

36. Knisely TL, Bleicher PA, Vibbard CA, Granstein RD: Production of latent transforming growth factor-beta and other inhibitory factors by cultured murine iris and ciliary body cells, *Curr Eye Res* 10:761-771, 1991.

37. Ksander BR, Hendricks RL: Cell-mediated immune tolerance to HSV-1 antigen associated with reduced susceptibility to HSV-1 corneal lesions, *Invest Ophthalmol Vis Sci* 28:1986-1993, 1987.

38. Ksander BR, Streilein JW: Analysis of cytotoxic T cell responses to intracameral allogeneic tumors. I. Quantitative and qualitative analysis of cytotoxic precursor and effector cells, *Invest Ophthalmol Vis Sci* 30:323-329, 1989.

39. Ksander BR, Streilein JW: Immune privilege to MHC disparate tumor grafts in the anterior chamber of the eye. I. Quantitative analysis of intraocular tumor growth and the corresponding delayed hypersensitivity response, *Transplantation* 47:661-667, 1989.

40. Luckenbach MW, Streilein JW, Niederkorn JY: Histopathologic analysis of intraocular allogeneic tumors in mice, *Invest Ophthalmol Vis Sci* 26:1368-1376, 1985.

41. MacLeish W, Rubsamen P, Atherton SS, Streilein JW: Immunobiology of Langerhans cells on the ocular surface. II. Role of central corneal Langerhans cells in stromal keratitis following experimental HSV-1 infection in mice, *Reg Immunol* 2:236-243, 1989.

42. Marchesi VT, Gowans JL: The migration of lymphocytes through the endothelium of venules in lymph nodes: an electron microscopic study, *Proc R Soc Lon [Biol]* 159:283-298, 1964.

43. Mattingly J, Waksman B: Immunologic suppression after oral administration of antigen: specific suppressor cells formed in rat Peyers' patches after oral administration of sheep erythrocytes, *J Immunol* 121:1878, 1978.

44. McMenamin PG, Holthouse I, Holt PG: Class II major histocompatibility complex (Ia) antigen-bearing dendritic cells within the iris and ciliary body of the rat eye: distribution, phenotype and relation to retinal microglia, *Immunology* 77:385-393, 1992.

45. Medawar P: Immunity to homologous grafted skin. III. The fate of skin homografts transplanted to the brain, to subcutaneous tissue, and to the anterior chamber of the eye, *Br J Exp Pathol* 29:58-69, 1948.

46. Mizuno K, Clark AF, Streilein JW: Ocular injection of retinal S antigen: suppression of autoimmune uveitis, *Invest Ophthalmol Vis Sci* 30:772-774, 1989.

47. Mondino BJ, Phinney R: The complement system in ocular allergy, *Int Ophthalmol Clin* 28:329-331, 1988.

48. Murray PI, Hoekzema R, Luyendijk L, et al.: Analysis of aqueous humor immunoglobulin G in uveitis by enzyme-linked immunosorbent assay, isoelectric focusing, and immunoblotting, *Invest Ophthalmol Vis Sci* 31:2129-2135, 1990.

49. Niederkorn JY: Immune privilege and immune regulation in the eye, *Adv Immunol* 48:191-226, 1990.

50. Niederkorn JY, Streilein JW: Analysis of antibody production induced by allogeneic tumor cells inoculated into the anterior chamber of the eye, *Transplantation* 33:573-577, 1982.

51. Niederkorn JY, Streilein JW: Intracamerally-induced concomitant immunity: mice harboring progressively growing intraocular tumors are immune to spontaneous metastases and secondary tumor challenge, *J Immunol* 131:2587-2594, 1983.

52. Niederkorn JY, Streilein JW, Shadduck JA: Deviant responses to allogeneic tumors injected intracamerally and subcutaneously in mice, *Invest Ophthalmol Vis Sci* 20:355-363, 1980.

53. Pasquale LR, Dorman-Pease ME, Lutty GA, et al.: Immunolocalization of TGF-β1, TGF-β2, and TGF-β3 in the anterior segment of the human eye, *Invest Ophthalmol Vis Sci* 34:23-30, 1993.

54. Prehn RT: Biological problems of grafting: the immunity-inhibiting role of the spleen and the effect of dosage and route of antigen administration in a homograft reaction, *Les Congres et Colloques de l'Universite de Liege* 12:163, 1959.

55. Romball CG, Weigle WO: Splenic role in the regulation of immune responses, *Cell Immunol* 34:376, 1977.

56. Sainte-Marie G, Sin YM: The lymph node: structures and possible function during the immune response, *Rev Can Biol* 27:191-207, 1968.

57. Sonoda Y, Streilein JW: Orthotopic corneal transplantation in mice: evidence that the immunogenetic rules of rejection do not apply, *Transplantation* 54:694-703, 1992.

58. Steinman RM, Van Voorhis WC, Spalding DM: Dendritic cells. In Weir DM, Herzenberg LA, Blackwell C, Herzenberg LA, editors: *Handbook of experimental immunology,* ed 4, 49, Oxford, 1986, Blackwell Scientific.

59. Streilein JW: Immune regulation and the eye: a dangerous compromise, *FASEB J* 1:199-208, 1987.

60. Streilein JW: Skin associated lymphoid tissues (SALT): the next generation. In Bos J, editor: *The skin immune system (SIS),* 26-48, 1990, CRC Press.

61. Streilein JW: Regional immunology. In *Encyclopedia of human biology,* 391-440, San Diego, CA, 1991, Academic Press.

62. Streilein JW: Sunlight and SALT: if UVB is the trigger, and TNFα is its mediator, what is the message? *J Invest Dermatol* 100:47S-52S, 1993.

63. Streilein JW, Atherton S, Vann VA: Critical role for ACAID in the distinctive pattern of retinitis that follows anterior chamber inoculation of HSV-1, *Curr Eye Res* 6:127-132, 1987.

64. Streilein JW, Bradley D: Analysis of immunosuppressive properties of iris and ciliary body cells and their secretory products, *Invest Ophthalmol Vis Sci* 32:2700-2710, 1991.

65. Streilein JW, Cousins S, Bradley D: Effect of intraocular gamma interferon on immunoregulatory properties of iris and ciliary body cells, *Invest Ophthalmol Vis Sci* 33:2304-2315, 1992.

66. Streilein JW, Grammer SF, Yoshikawa T, et al.: Functional dichotomy between Langerhans cells that present antigen to naive and to memory/effector T lymphocytes, *Immunol Reviews* 117:159-184, 1990.

67. Streilein JW, Niederkorn JY: Induction of anterior chamber-associated immune deviation requires an intact, functional spleen, *J Exp Med* 153:1058-1067, 1981.

68. Streilein JW, Niederkorn JY, Shadduck JA: Systemic immune unresponsiveness induced in adult mice by anterior chamber presentation of minor histocompatibility antigens, *J Exp Med* 152:1121-1125, 1980.

69. Streilein JW, Taylor AW: Immunologic principles within the nervous system: concerning the existence of a neurosensory immune system (NIS). In RW Keane, WF Hickey, editors: *Immunology of the nervous system,* NY, Oxford University Press, 1995.

70. Streilein JW, Toews GB, Bergstresser PR: Corneal allografts fail to express Ia antigens, *Nature* 282:326-327, 1979.

71. Streilein JW, Wilbanks GA, Cousins SW: Immunoregulatory mechanisms of the eye, *J Neuroimmunol* 39:185-200, 1992.

72. Sy M-S, Miller SD, Kowach HW, Claman HM: A splenic requirement for generation of suppressor T cells, *J Immunol* 119:2095-2102, 1977.

73. Taylor A, Streilein JW, Cousins S: Identification of alpha-melanocyte stimulating hormone as a potential immunosuppressive factor in aqueous humor, *Curr Eye Res* 11:1199-1206, 1992.

74. Taylor HR: The biological effects of UVB on the eye, *Photochem Photobiol* 50:489-492, 1989.

75. Thompsett E, Abi-Hanna D, Wakefield D: Immunological privilege in the eye: a review, *Curr Eye Res* 9:1141-1151, 1990.

76. Tomasi TB: The discovery of secretory IgA and the mucosal immune system, *Immunol Today* 13:416-418, 1992.

77. Wahlestedt C, Beding B, Ekman R, et al.: Calcitonin gene-related peptide in the eye: release by sensory nerve stimulation and effects associated with neurogenic inflammation, *Regulatory Peptides* 16:107-115, 1986.

78. Whitcup SM, Wakefield D, Li Q, et al.: Endothelial leukocyte adhesion molecule-1 in endotoxin-induced uveitis, *Invest Ophthalmol Vis Sci* 33:2626-2630, 1992.

79. Whittum JA, McCulley JP, Niederkorn JY, Streilein JW: Ocular disease induced in mice by anterior chamber inoculation of herpes simplex virus, *Invest Ophthalmol Vis Sci* 25:1065-1073, 1984.

80. Wilbanks GA, Mammolenti MM, Streilein JW: Studies on the induction of anterior chamber associated immune deviation (ACAID). II. Eye-derived cells participate in generating blood borne signals that induce ACAID, *J Immunol* 146:3018-3024, 1991.

81. Wilbanks GA, Mammolenti MM, Streilein JW: Studies on the induction of anterior chamber associated immune deviation (ACAID). III. Induction of ACAID depends upon intraocular transforming growth factor-β, *Eur J Immunol* 22:165-173, 1992.

82. Wilbanks GA, Streilein JW: The differing patterns of antigen release and local retention following anterior chamber and intravenous inoculation of soluble antigen: evidence that the eye acts as an antigen depot, *Reg Immunol* 2:390-398, 1989.

83. Wilbanks GA, Streilein JW: Distinctive humoral responses following anterior chamber and intravenous administration of soluble antigen: evidence for active suppression of IgG$_{2a}$-secreting B-cells, *Immunology* 71:566-572, 1990.

84. Wilbanks GA, Streilein JW: Studies on the induction of anterior chamber associated immune deviation (ACAID). I. Evidence that an antigen-specific, ACAID-inducing, signal exists in the peripheral blood, *J Immunol* 146:2610-2617, 1991.

85. Williamson JSP, Bradley D, Streilein JW: Immunoregulatory properties of bone marrow-derived cells in the iris and ciliary body, *Immunology* 67:96-102, 1989.

86. Young RW: Solar radiation in age-related macular degeneration, *Surv Ophthalmol* 32:252-269, 1988.

4 Humoral Immunity and the Eye

J. CLIFFORD WALDREP, BARTLY J. MONDINO

The eye is an extremely complex organ system that is functionally dependent on the transmission of light images through different cell and tissue layers and liquid media to the neurosensory retina. This visual axis possesses little tolerance for prolonged aberration or distortions within any of its conducting elements. Immune responses to invading pathogens or foreign immunogens are accompanied by a variable degree of inflammation with its many associated components: swelling, plasma protein extravasation, leukocyte infiltration, and tissue damage. Any of these sequelae can cause aberration or distortion of the visual axis. The offending element(s) must be quickly and efficiently eliminated with minimal damage to the visual axis.

With such strict requirements, there is an underlying need for a functional immune system with both cellular and humoral arms to maintain homeostasis. It has been demonstrated, however, that certain cellular aspects of the eye's immune system are unique in that intraocular presentation of some immunogens results in a selective impairment or suppression of delayed type of hypersensitivity (anterior chamber associated immune deviation).[110] In view of this ocular phenomenon, the humoral arm of immunity assumes an elevated degree of importance for the preservation of clarity within the visual axis. This chapter is limited to a discussion of the relationship between the eye and the humoral immune system; namely the immunoglobulins (IgG and subclasses, IgA and subclasses, IgM, IgD, and IgE) and antibodies (Ab), with an overview of interactions with the complement (C') system.

IMMUNOGLOBULINS AND THE EYE

The eye is a complex organ system comprised of multiple cell and tissue layers and fluid-filled chambers that will be designated as intraocular "compartments." The compartments of the eye possess unique anatomic structures, barriers, or both, as well as biochemical properties that serve important functions in regulation of accessibility, retention, and loss of soluble immune effectors. Compartments within

the eye also serve to limit or localize certain immunologic reactions.

Tears

IgA is the predominant immunoglobulin in external secretions, including the tears.[4] It is normally present in tears as secretory IgA, which consists of two IgA molecules coupled to a polypeptide J chain and secretory component. Both IgA in dimer form and chains are synthesized and complexed in plasma cells beneath the epithelial cells of the secretory surface. Estimates of the total number of plasma cells of the external eye reveal that the lacrimal gland has the most plasma cells followed by the conjunctiva and then the accessory lacrimal glands.[4,21] Secretory component is found in the epithelial cells of the acini, ducts, and tubules of the lacrimal gland[4,21] and possibly in the conjunctival epithelium.[33] IgA synthesized locally by plasma cells binds by means of its J chain to secretory component on the surface of epithelial cells before being secreted. The secretory component is thought to protect IgA from enzymatic degradation by proteolytic enzymes. In addition, serum IgA may be transferred to and contribute to secretory IgA in tears. With inflammation of the external eye, serum immunoglobulins increase in the tears probably because of leakage from conjunctival vessels that are dilated and more permeable. In this circumstance, IgG may achieve a higher level than IgA.

Ocular challenge with antigen may result in an increase in tears of specific IgA, synthesized locally by increased numbers of plasma cells.[77] Lymphoblasts with IgA-producing potential may migrate to the conjunctiva from gut- or bronchus-associated lymphoid tissue, which may be the principal source of migrating lymphoblasts to the conjunctiva. This cellular migration is antigen independent but may be increased by locally presented antigen in the eye. Circulating IgA produced at another mucosal site after immunization at that site may be another source of IgA in tears.

In rats immunized repeatedly with dinitrophenylated type III pneumococcal vaccine by the intravenous, subcutaneous, gastrointestinal, or ocular-topical routes, it was found that the gastrointestinal route was the most effective at eliciting and maintaining IgA antibody responses in tears.[77] On the other hand, following prolonged topical-ocular immunization, there were markedly diminished IgA response frequencies and antibody levels in tears. The data suggest that repeated central gastrointestinal mucosal stimulation maintained a local IgA response in tears, whereas continued topical antigen stimulation did not.

Secretory IgA is known to have antibody specificity for bacterial antigens, viruses, toxins, and dietary macromolecules.[88] Secretory IgA may act by inhibiting bacterial adherence to mucosal surfaces, thereby decreasing colonization by pathogenic organisms and allowing unbound bacteria to be swept away in the tears. Precoating *Shigella* with secretory IgA prevented keratoconjunctivitis in guinea pigs.[91]

Patients with low levels or absence of all the major serum immunoglobulins have conjunctivitis or keratoconjunctivitis associated with bacterial infection.[34] Patients who have at least one immunoglobulin class in normal concentration in the serum show no ocular inflammatory disease. Absence of only IgA, the major tear immunoglobulin, does not predispose the eye to keratoconjunctivitis. IgM alone or attached to secretory component may compensate.

Certain bacteria such as *Streptococcus sanguis, Neisseria gonorrhoeae* and *Neisseria meningitidis* elaborate IgA proteases.[88] When IgA is attached to antigen, it does not become resistant to IgA protease. Cleavage of IgA by these proteases creates isolated Fab monomers with a greatly reduced capacity as functioning antibodies. The role of IgA proteases in human ocular infections remains to be determined.

Conjunctiva and Sclera

The vessels within the conjunctiva are fenestrated and subsequently the stromal tissues are readily stained for IgG and IgA by immunohistochemistry. There is a corneo-scleral transition zone of varied GAG composition, but with free diffusional exchange between the corneal and the conjunctival stroma. The conjunctival epithelium is negative.

The sclera is a relatively avascular, highly porous structure. Consequently there is little restricted diffusion of plasma proteins throughout. Through immunohistochemical staining techniques, large amounts of IgG are detected, but lesser quantities of IgA are visible. Biochemical analysis of human eyes has detected 93 μg IgG/gram of tissue and 13 μg IgA/gram of tissue.[7] Ig that have passed out of the fenestrations into the CB/P and CC leave the eye via direct diffusion through the sclera.[14] Since IgM is excluded by the fenestrations in the CB/P and CC, this exclusion may explain the lack of detectable IgM in the sclera.

Cornea

In the quiescent eye, the avascular cornea is devoid of Ig-producing plasma cells; there is normally no Ig produced locally.[5-8] Ig is largely confined to the cornea stromal tissues.[3,5-8] The major source of corneal stromal Ig is thought to be via diffusion from the fenestrated limbal vessels.[3,5-8,47] IgG (molecular weight 160,000) is the predominant Ig in the cornea, followed by IgA.[3,5-8,60,109] Corneal concentrations of IgG, but not IgA, correlate with serum values.[6] Little or no IgM has been detected in the central cornea and limited amounts are found at the periphery.[3,5-8,60,109] The pentameric 900,000 (900K)-dalton IgM molecule is believed to be too large to diffuse into the stroma.[3,5-8,109] Thus factors that control the rate of Ig diffusion into and out of the stroma play important roles in regulating the spectrum of corneal Ig present. Factors that regulate the rate of diffusion within the cornea include the following: plasma Ig concentration, catabolic rates of degradation, and molecular diffusion coefficients.[107] It is extremely important to note that plasma Ig pools are in a dynamic state of equilibrium and are constantly changing partly as a result of past and present exposure to various immunogens. There is a continuous cycle of synthesis and degradation. By direct analogy, the Ig species within the cornea are also in a state of flux. Changes in the plasma Ig profile over time are mirrored by changes in the Ig spectrum with minor differences as a result of the time lag required for diffusion into the cornea stroma.[117,118]

Interactions between IgG and stromal tissue components, such as the anionic glycosaminoglycans (GAG) or proteoglycans (PG), also regulate tissue distributions of Ig in different intraocular tissues, including the cornea.[115,116,119] This regulation is suggested by the differential distribution of positively charged, cationic IgG and negatively charged, anionic serum albumin.[5-7] Cationic IgG is distributed throughout the central and peripheral cornea stroma, in contrast, anionic serum albumin is concentrated at the periphery and limited in the central cornea.[5-7] In the cornea stroma, anionic PG and GAG may function as fixed, anionic tissue components that indirectly regulate the distribution of soluble plasma proteins through electrostatic interactions.[4-6] The PG and GAG serve many important physiologic functions within the cornea: regulation of collagen fiber organization, pH, and swelling properties.[10,16,25,28,46,62] There is a concentration or anionic charge gradient formed by varied distribution of anionically charged, sulfated GAG and PG species from the central cornea to the limbus.[16] The electrostatic gradient within the corneal stroma may thus indirectly regulate the diffusion of certain cationically charged IgG into and out of the central and peripheral cornea.[116]

Other related parameters also regulate the egress of Ig from the circulation and its ultimate localization within the cornea. The hydration state of the cornea can affect the rate of diffusion within the stroma.[3,116] Fluid dynamics controlling the liquid flow of aqueous humor through the endothelium may alter the Ig of the cornea by "wash out" or accelerated diffusion.[3] There is a marked absence of IgG in the central and peripheral regions of many edematous corneas.[116] In contrast, acute inflammation causes alteration in the normal regulatory systems and induces the rapid influx of plasma proteins into the cornea stroma. The IgG spectrum of an acutely inflamed cornea is virtually identical to that of plasma.

The IgG subclass distribution within the cornea has been studied on a limited basis. The spectrum of cornea IgG1 to IgG4 subclasses analyzed by chromatofocusing of eye bank tissues is similar to that of the normal plasma distribution.[117] The concentration followed the plasma pattern of IgG1 > IgG2 > IgG3 > IgG4 with a similar hierarchy of electrophoretic mobility. IgG1 contained the most cationic species and IgG4 was the most anionically charged.[117] Individual profile differences were noted among individuals, most notably with IgG1 and IgG2.[117] The diversity of biologic activities attributed to the IgG subclasses within the cornea (and other parts of the eye) warrants further investigation.

The discovery that the peripheral cornea has more IgM than the central cornea may have immunologic implications. After primary exposure to an antigen, there is an early IgM response that declines rapidly.[94] The IgM antibodies bind complement and agglutinate particulate antigens, such as erythrocytes and bacteria, more effectively than other immunoglobulins do. Because IgM is the most effective agglutinant and cytolytic immunoglobulin, the higher concentration of this immunoglobulin may afford the peripheral cornea more protection initially against an invading pathogen to which it is directed. IgG, however, the most abundant immunoglobulin in the serum and the predominant immunoglobulin in the cornea, is probably the most important in microbial defense and reaches higher levels than other immunoglobulins in serum after primary and secondary exposure to antigens. Patients with rheumatoid arthritis have IgM antibody (rheumatoid factor) directed against IgG. Immune complexes of IgG and rheumatoid factor may be important in the immunopathogenesis of rheumatoid arthritis.[94] Predictably, the peripheral cornea has more rheumatoid factor than the central cornea.

Iris

The profile of iridial Ig differs from that of the cornea. Little or no IgG, IgA, and IgM (or albumin) is normally detectable in the iris stroma.[5-8] There is normally an apparent blood-iris barrier; however, in patients with iritis, IgG, IgA, and IgM forming cells have been detected.[38] Although the iris capillaries are nonfenestrated, the iris stroma is open to the flow of aqueous humor (containing IgG and IgA).[5] The iris is surrounded by Ig-containing fluids and tissues (at the ciliary body), however no Ig is detected. The continual drainage of aqueous humor (AH) may preclude the concentration of proteins around the iris. Another possible reason for the apparent lack of Ig may be the lack of sulfated GAG in the iris stroma.[12] In contrast to the cornea (and other intraocular tissues), which are richly distributed with sulfated PG and GAG, there may be little or no fixed tissue anionic

charge sites in the iris to attract and bind cationically charged Ig.

Ciliary Body

The stroma of the ciliary body processes (CB/P) contains moderate amounts of IgG detected experimentally by immunohistochemical and immunologic techniques.[5,7] Lesser concentrations of IgA have been reported.[5,7] The vasculature of the CB/P is highly fenestrated, allowing free egress of circulating molecules of varied size ranges.[83,84] Cationically charged IgG immunoglobulins rapidly traverse the fenestrations and deposit within the anionic sites of the CB/P.[115,119] Once bound within the stoma, there is a strong interaction lasting for several days.[115,119] This electrostatic mechanism is an important regulatory factor that serves to localize cationically charged Ig species within the uveal tract. Intracellular IgG and IgA have been observed in the nonpigmented ciliary epithelium, suggesting that these cells may play a role in Ig transport.[85]

Aqueous Humor and Vitreous Humor

The blood-aqueous barrier (BAB) formed by the zonula occludens of the nonpigmented ciliary epithelium and the nonfenestrated endothelium and collagen sheath of the iris stromal vessels normally limits the passage of plasma-derived proteins and cells into the aqueous humor. The AH normally contains detectable levels of IgG and specific antibodies (Abs).[23] Reported IgG levels for cataract patients average from 30 to 70 ug/mL.[7,81] The electrophoretic spectrum of the predominant IgG in the AH is between pI 6.85 to 8.45.[81] All four of the IgG subclasses have been detected partially reflecting the serum distribution profile with IgG1 at the highest percentage (56%), followed by IgG2 (29%), IgG3 (6%), and IgG4 (9%).[81] The electrophoretic mobility of IgG1 in the AH is the broadest, containing both cationic and anionic species.[117] IgG2 is similar in its spectrum to IgG3 and somewhat more anionic with IgG4, the most anionically charged subclass.[117] The IgG subclass spectrum within the AH varies from patient to patient, perhaps reflecting differences in past immunogenic exposures. Three discrete cationic IgG bands of pI 8.4 to 8.5, however, are commonly noted in both the AH and the serum.[81] The significance of these IgG species remains to be determined. During intraocular disease states, such as uveitis, there is BAB breakdown and the levels of IgG increase markedly, averaging 600 to 700 ug/mL.[38,81] There is also a corresponding increase in the levels of IgA (80 ug/mL) and IgM (45 ug/mL) in the AH.[38] These changes likely reflect the influx of plasma Ig because the relative proportions of IgG, IgA, and IgM are similar. Experimental studies in rabbits (which have much higher protein levels in the AH than humans) have demonstrated that the IgG electrophoretic profile of secondary AH formed following paracentesis is virtually indistinguishable from that of serum.[118] There is a preferential influx of some cationically charged IgG antibody species following paracentesis. After some inflammatory insults, there is a partial reestablishment of the BAB, however, there may be continued localized production of some Abs.

Analysis of the vitreal Ig has been limited. A blood-vitreal barrier restricts the passage of plasma-derived proteins and cells into the vitreous (V), where they may become trapped in the collagen-hyaluronate matrix. Subsequently the concentration of IgG in the vitreous is normally low. During inflammation, however, there is a rapid influx of plasma proteins into the V compartment. A vitreal IgG concentration of 34 ug/mL has been reported.[121] In eyes with rhegmatogenous retinal detachments, differential concentration ratios were obtained for IgG and IgM and IgA and IgM for the vitreous, subretinal fluid, and plasma, suggesting that there is unidirectional fluid movement across the retinal break.[96] Because the ratios are significantly greater than that serum, selective diffusion is suggested.[96] Analysis of vitreal IgG subclasses isolated from eye bank tissues by chromato-focusing demonstrates that there is an increased concentration of cationic IgG1 in some samples perhaps related to the high levels of anionic GAG hyaluronate. In rabbits immunized to protein antigens, little or no IgG Ab is detected within the V until day 15 after immunization, with both cationic and anionic species detected.[118] Few changes were noted in V antibody species at days 15 and 30 after immunization with the V compartment apparently reaching equilibrium with the plasma compartment. The half-life of Abs within the V compartment is unknown.

Retina

The blood-retinal barrier is formed by the zonula occludens of the retinal pigment epithelium (RPE) and the zonula occludens of the nonfenestrated endothelium of the retinal vasculature. This barrier restricts the access of plasma proteins to the retinal tissues. Subsequently the predominant Ig species are contained within the retinal vessels. Inflammation or injury results in exudation and accumulation of plasma Ig. Abs to Herpes simplex virus (HSV) and Varicella zoster virus (VZV) have been detected in subretinal fluids of acute retinal necrosis (ARN) patients.

Choroid. The choroidal tissues contain moderate amounts of IgG and IgA, which probably originate from the fenestrated capillaries within the CB/P and the choriocapillaris (CC).[83,86,119] The fenestrations of the CC are selectively permeable; cationically charged, circulating IgG Ab molecules readily traverse these barriers and deposit within the associated anionic sites of Bruchs membrane.[87,119] These anionic sites are comprised largely of the GAG chondroitin sulfate and heparan sulfate in basal lamina of the CC endothelium and the RPE.[87,93] The distribution of these anionic sites extends into pericapillary subendothelial basal lamina of the CB.[83] These anionic sites may indirectly affect the distribution of cationic IgG through electrostatic interactions by

mediating the selective uptake and retention of specific Abs.[119] Experiments have demonstrated that circulating IgG Abs of pI greater than 9.0 can actively displace the resident IgG bound within these anionic sites.[119] This relationship may serve an important regulatory function in the uvea, affecting Abs that fall within the latter extreme of the pI 5.5 to 9.5 natural range.[48] Such highly cationic molecules are normally restricted to IgG1 and IgG3 subclasses. Both of these subclasses have the potential for immunologic protection or damage to the eye via activation of the C′ cascade.

IMMUNOGLOBULIN FEATURES AFFECTING THE EYE: PLASMA AND TISSUE IMMUNOGLOBULIN CONCENTRATIONS

Much of the intraocular IgG (also IgA and IgM) is derived from the plasma, therefore the plasma IgG profile determines the repertoire generally available to the eye (exclusive of local synthesis). The normal plasma distribution and concentration of the IgG subclasses varies somewhat with 60.3 to 71.5% G1 [mean 6.6 to 8.0 g/L], 19.4 to 31.0% G2 [mean 2.2 to 3.2 g/L], 5.0 to 8.4% G3 [mean 0.58 to 0.94 g/L], and 0.7 to 4.2% G4 [mean 0.08 to 0.46 g/L].[35] Limited analysis of ocular tissues and fluids demonstrates that the average relative distribution and concentration of the IgG subclasses are similar to that of plasma.[117] On an individual basis, there is variation related, in part, to past immunogenic exposure. Other variables that influence the IgG subclass response include the following: genetic background, sex, age, and perhaps subclinical disease.[35]

The normal plasma distribution and concentration of the IgA subclasses are also variable with 75 to 93% IgA1 [mean 1.81 g/L] and 7 to 25% IgA2 [mean 0.22 g/L].[61] Monomeric forms are predominant in the plasma. Concentrations of IgA subclasses (chiefly dimeric forms) are higher in the secretory compartment and independent of the plasma.[61] Similar regulatory variables (IgG) also probably affect IgA subclass production, although the effects of immune responsiveness are less characterized.

The normal plasma IgM concentration is 0.47 to 1.47 g/L and exists predominantly in the pentameric form (19s); monomeric (7s) forms also are found in low concentrations. The 900K-dalton molecular weight of IgM limits its accessibility to the intraocular compartments.

The normal plasma concentration of IgD is approximately 0.2% [0.03 g/L] of the total Ig. Its functions are largely unknown, especially in the eye. IgD is believed to serve as a B-lymphocyte surface receptor involved in cell differentiation. Plasma IgE represents only 0.004% [0.0006 g/L] of the total Ig in circulation. IgE binds to tissue mast cells with high affinity. Its role in ocular hypersensitivity will be covered elsewhere.

Data indicate that normally there is a lag between the appearance of plasma IgG antibodies in some of the intraocular compartments.[118] Inflammation alters this temporal relationship. These factors are likely similar for IgA. It is important to note that different immunogens preferentially induce IgG or IgA subclass antibody responses. Furthermore, these subclasses have differential functional and biologic activities.

Electrophoretic Mobility

Electrostatic interactions between Ig and oppositely charged anionic intraocular tissue components (GAG and PG), regulate, in part, the accessibility, retention, and clearance of circulating IgG Abs.[115,119] In this regard, the IgG subclasses are quite varied with respect to their electrophoretic mobilities. The pI range for human IgG is 5.2 to 9.5.[100,116] IgG1 contains the widest range of electrophoretic mobilities, from pI 6.5 to 9.5; IgG3 is the most highly restricted in the cationic range with its pI range of 8.2 to 9.0; IgG2 is intermediate at pI 6.3 to 8.3; and IgG4 is the most anionic at 5.8 to 6.1.[48] The cationic species of IgG 1, 2, and 3 are predominant within the intraocular compartments.[117] Thus relationships determined by electrostatic interactions are potentially important for the eye because the IgG Ab responses to certain bacterial and viral infections are predominantly in the cationic IgG1 and IgG3 subclasses. Furthermore, for some immunogens, there is an inverse charge relationship that regulates the electrophoretic nature of the Ab response (anionic epitopes elicit cationic Ab responses).[98,101] Also, the electrophoretic mobility of antibodies to different immunogens is genetically determined such that the Ab response of inbred stains of mice to the same immunogen is different; C57 Black/6 mice produce more highly cationic Abs than Balb/c strain of mice.[31,106] In man, the response of an individual to a particular immunogen is also genetically regulated.[78] Thus there is a natural occurrence of cationic IgG Abs that possesses binding potential for different parts of the eye to mediate immune clearance or in situ immune complex formation and uveitis.

The electrophoretic mobility of other Ig is not as well characterized. The pI values reported are 4.5 to 6.5 for human IgA and 5.0 to 8.0 for human IgM.[100] Because IgA is much less cationic than IgG, the role of electrostatic interactions with intraocular components is less apparent. Although IgM is more highly cationic than IgA, its molecular diffusion coefficient (of pentameric form) normally excludes its entry into the intraocular tissues.

Phases of Synthesis and Catabolism

Plasma levels of the Ig classes and subclasses (which have been extensively studied compared to the tissues) depend on the net sum of synthesis (determined by the number of plasma cells forming a particular class or subclass) minus the catabolic rate. The rate of exchange between the intravascular and extravascular spaces as determined by the molecular diffusion coefficient also regulates plasma levels.[107]

IgG has a high diffusion coefficient and readily penetrates the extravascular spaces; in contrast, IgM has a low diffusion coefficient and is found predominantly in the plasma.[107] This relationship is extremely important for the intraocular compartments.

The synthesis of each Ig class or subclass is independently regulated. There are increasing reports of IgG and IgA class and subclass deficiencies that may or may not be associated with clinical immunodeficiency. Following most infections, the first or primary antibody class is IgM; IgG predominates in the secondary Ab response and persists after the infection has resolved providing protection against reinfection.[105] The route of infection or site of immunization regulates, in part, magnitude and the class or subclass response. The rate of IgG Ab subclass responses is dependent on multiple variables, including the age of the donor and the time elapsed after exposure to the antigen.[44] The rate of synthesis for IgG1 is 25.4 mg/kg/day and for IgG3 is 3.4 mg/kg/day.[107] IgG2 and IgG4 have not been studied. The intravascular percentages for the IgG subclasses are 51% for IgG1, 53% for IgG2, 64% for IgG3, and 54% for IgG4.[79] Therefore at any given point in time there is a range of 36 to 49% of the total IgG in the extravascular tissues.

The Ab response is highly dependent on the type of eliciting immunogen (such as bacterial, viral, or parasitic). The Ab response of adults to bacterial protein immunogens is principally IgG1 with minor IgG3 and IgG4 responses; the response to polysaccharide epitopes is predominantly IgG2.[44,92] Since bacteria are complex immunogens with different chemical types of epitopes, the Ab response is a heterogeneous mixture reactive against various immunodominant epitopes.[44] The IgG Ab subclass response to common ocular viral pathogens, such as herpes simplex virus, cytomegalovirus, and varicella zoster virus, is IgG1 and IgG3.[13,57,105] The Ab response is highly restricted with IgG3 appearing first, followed by IgG1. The IgG4 subclass has been associated with allergic conditions because of its apparent cytophilicity for basophils.[102] IgG4 is functionally monovalent and is therefore nonprecipitating.[113]

The catabolic rate for IgG accelerates as the plasma level increases, thus serving an autoregulatory function.[56] Catabolism of IgA and M are unaffected by plasma levels and the catabolic rates for IgD and IgE decrease as the plasma levels increase.[56] The half-life for each Ig class (regulated by the heavy chain constant region) is varied at 22.5 days for IgG, 5.8 days for IgA, 5.1 days for IgM, 2.8 days for IgD, and 2.5 days for IgE.[56] The half-lives of the IgG subclasses are varied with IgG3 at 7 days with 21 days for IgG1, 2, and 4.[56] The liver is the predominant site of catabolism from the circulation.[36] The catabolic rate for the various intraocular tissues is unknown.

In the plasma, IgA1 constitutes 75 to 93% of the total IgA, but it only constitutes 52 to 70% in the secretions.[61] Most of the monomeric plasma IgA is produced by plasma cells in the bone marrow in contrast to polymeric IgA, which is produced in the secretory glands and tissues.[61] The two compartments are independent of each other. IgA subclass Ab responses have, however, been infrequently studied. In general, IgA1 plasma Abs prevail in response to most bacterial and viral immunogens.[61] Plasma IgA2 Abs are prevalent in responses to carbohydrate epitopes.[44] IgA responses to environmental antigens have been implicated in immune complex (IC) diseases.[99]

Metabolic studies have demonstrated that the biosynthetic rate for plasma IgA is 18.5 to 30 mg/kg/day (24 mg/kg/day for IgA1, 4.3 mg/kg/day for IgA2).[61] The average half-life of IgA1 is 5.9 days and IgA2 is 4.5 days.[61] The fractional catabolic rate in the plasma pool is 24% for IgA1 and 34% for IgA2. Approximately 55% of the total IgA is in the intravascular compartment.[61]

Primary and Secondary Responses: Isotype Switching

Following initial exposure to a typical protein immunogen, is a complex series of cellular events involving cellular interactions within the peripheral lymphoid tissues occurs between dendritic macrophages (or other accessory cells), T-helper cells, and B cells. After clonal expansion, B cells differentiate into Ab-secreting plasma cells. There is a time lag over which no primary Ab can be detected. In the next phase the IgM Ab titer rises logarithmically, reaching a plateau phase in which the titer stabilizes. The IgM produced in the periphery, however, does not generally gain access to the inside of the eye, except at the limbus. IgG typically becomes detectable in the plasma and then at varied rates within the intraocular tissues. Inflammatory insults to the eye can rapidly alter the intraocular IgG concentrations. A decline phase normally follows, in which the Ab is cleared or catabolized. Upon secondary exposure to the immunogen, the secondary Ab response is predominantly IgG. Then a shorter lag phase occurs with an extended plateau and decline phase. The IgG Ab has a higher titer with greater affinity. During differentiation, committed B cells switch from IgM production to IgG and IgA subclasses. This isotype switching is regulated by T cells. Each of the parameters in this generalized scheme may depend on multiple variables, such as immunogenic epitopes, dosage, route of exposure, and genetic regulation.

Biologic Activities—Complement fixation, Fc Binding

Antibody molecules are bifunctional molecules: The amino-terminal portion of molecule mediates immunogen epitope-binding interactions and neutralization; the carboxy terminal portion mediates binding of the molecule to host tissues, cells, or other soluble effector systems, such as C1q.[11] The cell receptor-binding activities of the human Ig have been studied predominantly in vitro with isolated cell types. Binding activities have been described for the Fc receptors on mononuclear phagocytes (termed FcRI and FcRII).[50,95] FcRI has a high affinity for monomeric IgG1 and IgG3, whereas FcRII avidly binds IC of IgG1 and IgG3.[95] IgG4 and IgG2 are the least active. FcRIII are predominantly involved in mediation of lysis during antibody-dependent cytotoxicity.[95] FcRI binding activity is regulated by the Cg3 domain of the IgG molecule.[95] IgG1, IgG3, and IgG4 to neutrophil Fc receptors mediated through Cg2 and Cg3 domains; IgG1 through IgG4 bind lymphocyte and platelet Fc receptors.[95] Neutrophil Fc-binding activity has also been reported for both IgA1 and IgA2.[107] IgG-binding via Fc receptors has been reported in the eye for the corneal epithelium,[120] ciliary epithelium,[85,104] RPE,[26,29] and vitreal hyalocytes.[41] Binding via these receptors presumably plays a role in immune clearance.

An additional activity of some Ig molecules following epitope binding is C' fixation. Interaction with C1q of the classical pathway with fixation and activation is most efficient with IgM; the activity is variable with the IgG subclasses with IgG3 > IgG1 > IgG2 and IgG4 negative.[95] IgA, IgD, and IgE are negative. With the IgG subclass molecules, C' fixation is a function determined by the Cg2 domain (which also controls catabolic rate).[95] In certain intraocular compartments, interactions between the classical C' pathway and IgG3 and IgG1 antibodies are important because many of the antiviral Abs are within these subclasses.[13,57,105]

ANTIBODIES AND THE EYE

Antigen-antibody Interactions: Affinity, Avidity, and Biologic Significance

The binding process between the epitope and the Ab combining site is determined by the hypervariable regions of the V domain and results in hydrogen, electrostatic, and hydrophobic bonding, and Van der Waals forces. An optimal fit between the epitope and the combining site results in the formation of these attractive forces and yields a high affinity binding association. Multivalent binding or avidity describes the functional affinity of antibody binding to multiple epitopes, such as a bacterium. Affinity and avidity affect the physiologic and pathologic properties of antibodies.[108] As described earlier, affinity maturation occurs during the later stages of a humoral immune response. Such high affinity Abs more efficiently bind with immunogenic epitopes, promoting a variety of biologic activities including the following: C' fixation, immune elimination, and bacterial or viral neutralization.[95] High-affinity immune complexes are more rapidly removed from the circulation without the induction of immunopathology. Conversely, low-affinity immune complexes have been implicated in tissue deposition and in the induction of type III immune-mediated tissue injury. There may be a genetic predisposition promoting the enhanced production of low-affinity Abs.[95] An alternative hypothesis has suggested that molecular mimicry plays a role in the induction of certain autoimmune diseases, particularly uveoretinitis. The induction of low-affinity Abs through such a mechanism might promote immune complex deposition in situ.

Passive Acquisition and Local Synthesis

Each Ig class or subclass is a complex, heterogeneous group of molecules that is best visualized by the characteristic electrophoretic migration pattern.[116] It is also important to note that the spectrum of molecules is dynamic. There is continual change with simultaneous synthesis and degradation. Multiple factors play a role in regulating these processes. Most immune responses are polyclonal with the induction of multiple B-cell clones specifically reactive against distinct epitopes. Some immunogens induce oligoclonal or monoclonal responses. These have been implicated in certain disease states.

The Goldmann-Witmer Quotient (Q) has been utilized to estimate intraocular Ab production.[40] Q is calculated as follows:

$$Q = ([\text{Specific IgG Ab AH}]/[\text{Total IgG AH}])/$$
$$([\text{Specific IgG Ab plasma}]/[\text{Total IgG plasma}])$$

A value of Q = 1.0 assumes that the Abs in the AH originate from the plasma by diffusion (Q < 1.0 is indicative of active peripheral synthesis). If Q > 1.0, then intraocular Ab production is indicated. Q has been used to confirm clinical diagnoses in some cases of clinical uveitis. The validity of Q, however, has been recently questioned because there are many factors that can alter the actual values.[81,112] The IgG : albumin relative concentration ratio (RCR) has been calculated as an alternative index describing the quotient between AH or plasma IgG : albumin ratios.[81,112] Both Q and RCR are subject to the variables of selective transfer through the BAB, decreased catabolism, and polyclonal Ab production with the potential to give rise to erroneous values.[81,112] Other variables that affect both methods must include the time interval between the immune response and the sampling interval as there are marked time-dependent changes in the Ab spectrum.[118] Another variable is the presence of oligoclonal IgG.[81] Such pathologic IgG, predominantly of the IgG1 subclass, have been reported for 57% of Fuchs uveitis syndrome patients, perhaps as a result of dysregulation of B-cell clones in the eye.[81,114]

In experimental uveitis, intravitreal injection of protein antigens, such as ovalbumin or serum albumin, results in localized production of specific IgG, IgA, and IgM Abs.[43,103,112] The ocular tissues retain immunologic memory similar to organized lymphoid tissues.[103] Only a fraction of the total IgG in primary (7%) and secondary (18%) experimental uveitis is specific for the injected immunogen demonstrating the phenomenon of polyclonal activation within the eye.[43,103,112] Polyclonal activation may play a role in other forms of uveitis, most notably in autoimmune Ab production.[114] It has been postulated that there is a natural occurrence of Abs to retinal autoantigens.[114] Uncharacterized events that trigger expansion of these autoreactive clones either peripherally or within the eye may result in intraocular disease. Thus both actively and passively acquired Abs serve important functions in the eye, not only mediating immunologic protection, but also potentially causing damage via immune complex deposition.

Ocular Antibody Responses to Bacteria

Staphylococcus aureus occupies a dominant position in bacterial diseases of the eye. In addition to causing direct infections of the external eye and endophthalmitis, it is responsible for hypersensitivity diseases of the lids and cornea.[30,63] The complex relationship between the host humoral immune response to *S. aureus* has been explored in rabbit serum, tears, and the cornea.[67,70] Antibody levels to ribitol teichoic acid (RTA, the major antigenic determinant of *S. aureus*) were measured using an ELISA. After intradermal, subconjunctival, and topical application of staphylococcal antigens, an IgG antibody response to RTA was found in serum and tears and an IgA antibody response to RTA was found in tears but not serum.[70] More importantly, corneal antibody levels were measured and correlated with levels in serum and tears after immunizing rabbits using these same routes.[67] IgG titers were found consistently in corneas after intradermal, subconjunctival, and topical immunization. After intradermal immunization, IgG titers in corneas were higher than tears but lower than serum, which was presumably the source of IgG antibodies for the cornea. After subconjunctival immunization or topical immunization, IgG titers in corneas were higher than tears and generally higher than serum, suggesting that the ocular tissues were a local source of IgG. On the other hand, IgA titers were found in tears but not in serum and were found only occasionally in corneas, suggesting that IgG responses to staphylococcal antigens may be more important than IgA responses in the cornea. The results of this study suggest that corneal antibodies to RTA may be influenced by exposure to staphylococcal antigens not only in the external eye but also at sites remote from the eye. These studies measured corneal antibody levels to a bacterial antigen that may have relevance in the immunopathogenesis of hypersensitivity lesions of the cornea. Preston and associates[90a] measured corneal antibody levels to *Pseudomonas* after intracorneal infection and drew similar conclusions about the corneal antibody response.

Antibody titers to RTA were measured in the corneas of rabbits that developed hypersensitivity lesions of the cornea resembling human phlyctenules and catarrhal infiltrates.[65] Corneal lesions developed in rabbits that had the highest corneal IgG and IgA antibody titers with IgG titers being higher than IgA titers. This study showed that tissue exposure to antigen plus topical application of antigen may result in a higher corneal antibody level than either route alone. This study also correlated the corneal antibody response to an antigen with the development of corneal hypersensitivity lesions that might be related to this antigen.

Staphylococcal endophthalmitis is the most common cause of postoperative infectious endophthalmitis.[30,88] Little is known about the ocular immune response to bacterial endophthalmitis in general and S. aureus or Staphylococcus epidermidis endophthalmitis in particular. S. aureus endophalmitis was not associated with delayed hypersensitivity to the organism.[30] IgG and IgA antibody titers to RTA were measured by ELISA in serum, tears, aqueous, and vitreous after intravitreal injection of viable S. aureus. The initial IgG antibody response to S. aureus endophthalmitis was detected in serum where the levels were higher than tears, aqueous, and vitreous until day 14. The finding of serum antibody to RTA on day 3 supports the theory that antigen processing and antibody formation initially occur at extraocular sites after leakage of the antigen from the vitreous.[103] The sensitivity of the ELISA assay probably enhances the ability to detect serum antibody at this early time. A serum antibody response measured by agglutinin titers was seen as early as 4 days after the intraocular injection of typhoid vaccine before specific antibody was detected intraocularly.[100a]

Possible sources of aqueous antibody levels of RTA include leakage from serum, diffusion from vitreous, or local production by plasma cells in the ciliary body and iris. Leakage of serum IgG antibody into the aqueous after disruption of the blood-aqueous barrier by inflammation was supported by the finding that aqueous IgG antibody levels rose and fell with serum and were always less than those in serum. Serum was not a source of aqueous IgA antibody because IgA antibody was never detected in serum. Anterior segment production of IgG and IgA may occur from plasma cells found in the iris and ciliary body.

Vitreous antibody levels to RTA could originate from serum leakage or intraocular production by choroidal plasma cells. Serum IgG may contribute to vitreous IgG antibody levels after disruption of the blood-retina barrier caused by inflammation. Serum could not be the only source of IgG antibody in vitreous because vitreous antibody levels rose when serum levels were falling. Serum could not be a source of vitreous IgA antibody because IgA was not detected in serum, suggesting that vitreous IgA is produced in the eye. Choroidal plasma cells may produce IgG and IgA antibody and contribute to vitreous antibody levels. Intraocular production of IgG antibody could also explain the rising vitreous antibody levels when serum IgG levels were falling. Vitreous IgG antibody levels reached greater levels than vitreous IgA antibody levels. Shimada and Silverstein[103] also found that antigen-specific intraocular IgG antibody pro-

duction comprised more than 90% of all Ig classes present after the intravitreal injection of antigen. This fact may be important from the standpoint of host defense because IgG is a better opsonin for bacterial phagocytosis than IgA.

The host immune response to S. epidermidis endophthalmitis also was studied.[89] S. epidermidis endophthalmitis was not associated with a delayed hypersensitivity response to this organism and a much weaker antibody response in serum, aqueous, and vitreous than that associated with S. aureus. The inability of a low inoculum of S. epidermidis to elicit a strong antibody and cell-mediated immune response may help explain delayed-onset pseudophakic endophthalmitis associated with this organism. This weekly pathogenic organism may proliferate in the vitreous or within the capsular bag of the lens without eliciting a strong antibody or cell-mediated immune response to it.

IMMUNE COMPLEXES AND THE EYE

Deposition and Immunopathogenesis

Immune complexes (IC) result from the complex interaction of antigen-antibody binding. After formation, the cells of the reticuloendothelial system (RES) or other phagocytic cells within the eye remove and degrade the IC. When there is a persistence of IC caused by an overload of the normal clearance mechanisms, immunologically mediated tissue injury (type III) attributable to tissue deposition most often results. IC induce a variety of pathologic processes resulting from activation of the C' cascade with numerous consequences: elaboration of C' anaphylatoxins, leukocyte chemotaxis, release of vasoactive amines from mast cells or basophils, increased vascular permeability, platelet aggregation or microthrombus formation, release of PMN lysosomal enzymes, and tissue damage. All of these pathologic consequences are highly detrimental to the visual axis.

IC deposition is believed to occur via two basic mechanisms: 1) after vascular permeability changes in blood vessel walls caused by endothelial cell retraction or 2) after localized or in situ formation. IC deposition within the tissue and its pathologic consequences have been termed an Arthus reaction. The C' cascade (classical or alternative) and leukocytes are essential components. There are a number of variables that partially determine the consequences after IC formation. Larger IC are removed more efficiently than smaller complexes. This property may be the result of a genetic predisposition regulating the production of low affinity IC.[95] The size of the IC is determined by the epitope valence and the Ab titer and affinity. The immunogen chemical composition seems less critical since proteins, carbohydrates, and drugs have been reported in IC diseases, however, the class or subclass of the Ab is paramount. Both IgM, IgG (C' fixing subclasses), and IgA have been implicated, with precipitating and nonprecipitating Abs asso-

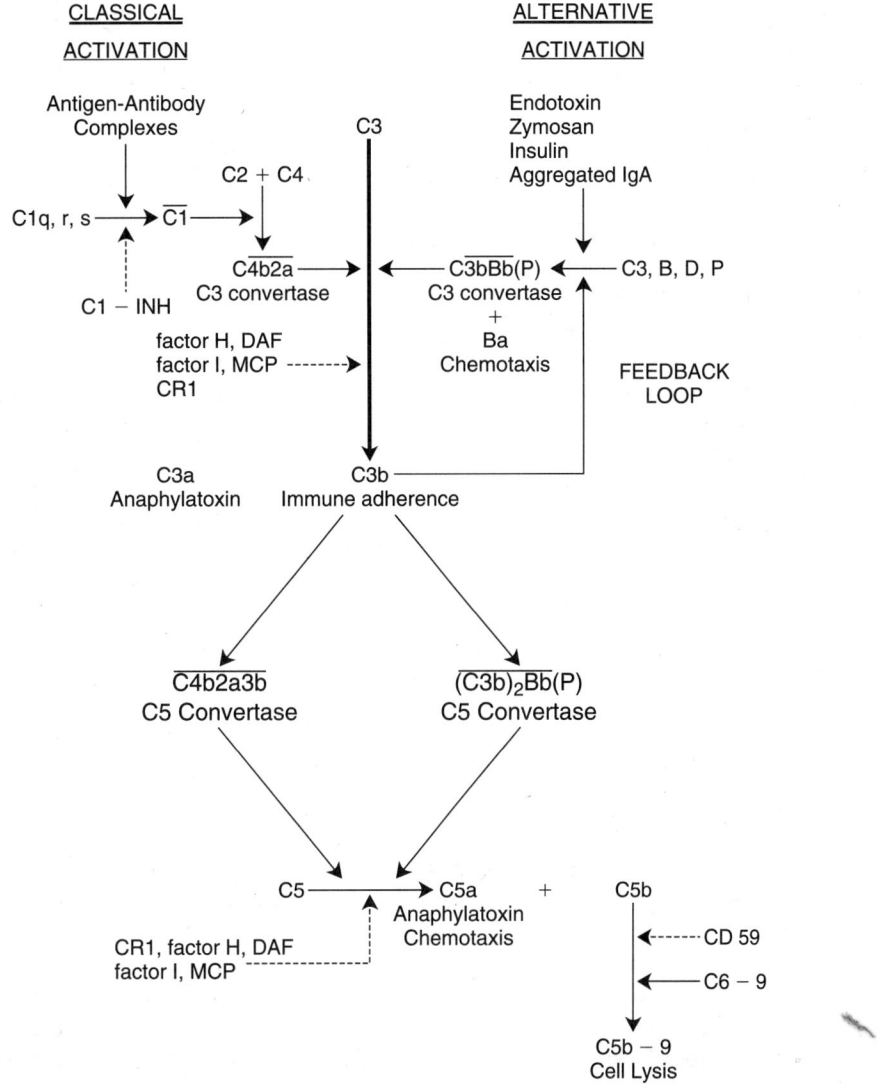

Fig. 4-2.   Diagram of classical and alternative pathways of complement activation. A bar above a complement component indicates an active enzyme. B indicates factor B, D indicates factor D, P indicates properdin, DAF represents decay accelerating factor, C1-INH represents C1 inhibitor, MCP represents membrane cofactor protein, CD59 represents membrane attack complex inhibiting protein, Factor I represents C3b inactivator, Factor H represents β-1H, CR1 represents complement receptor 1. C3 represents the pivotal component that is acted upon by both the classical and the alternative activating pathways.

either forms in solution or becomes covalently attached to the surface of the target particle. The bound C3 convertase becomes classical C5 convertase by proteolytic activation of C3 to C3a (anaphylatoxin) and binding C3b (C4b2a3b). This reaction is the most abundant of the classical pathway. C5 convertase cleaves C5a (anaphylatoxin) from the α chain of C5, with C5b becoming membrane bound and initiating the events leading to the formation of the membrane attack complex. Once C5b is bound, C6 and C7 attach to form a stable complex (C5b67) that interacts with C8 (C5b678). This unit begins cell membrane disruption and causes C9 polymerization to form transmembrane channels and ultimately cell lysis. The alternative pathway is initiated on cer-

tain "activator" surfaces by hydrolysis of the C3 internal thioester. The C3b interacts with factor B (via factor D cleaving Ba small fragments) and forms the alternative C3 convertase (C3bBb), which is bound "protected" to the activator surface away from factor I and H inhibitors. Through a C3b-dependent positive feedback mechanism, the alternative C3 convertase cleaves more C3 to generate more C3b that interacts with more B and D, thus amplifying the alternative C3 convertase, which is stabilized by properidin (C3nbPBb; n > 1). This stabilized complex forms the alternative C5 convertase that cleaves C5 to initiate the membrane attack complex, which is then identical with the classical pathway. Key regulatory components include the following: C1 esterase inhibitor, factor I, which binds free C3b; factor H, which accelerates the destructive action of factor I on C3b, anaphylatoxin inactivator (C3a, C4a, C5a); and S protein, which modulates the activity of the membrane attack complex.

The biologic consequences of C' activation are multiple. Generation of a C3b macromolecular coating on target particles is the major function.[95] Once formed, C3b coatings (and to a lesser extent C4b) facilitate the following: 1) opsonization and adherence of bacteria, viruses, and neutrophils to mononuclear phagocyte (MNP); 2) ingestion of certain bacteria by polymorphonuclear neutrophil (PMN) and MNP; and 3) augmentation of IgG-induced phagocytosis and antibody-dependent cell-mediated cytotoxicity (ADCC) cytotoxicity.[95] A C2 kinin fragment induces increased vascular permeability and smooth muscle contraction. Formation of the anaphylatoxins C3a, C4a, and C5a (plus C5a des Arg) induces a variety of consequences. C3a and C4a mediate most effects via histamine release from mast cells and basophils causing smooth muscle contraction and enhanced vascular permeability. C3a also suppresses local Ab responses. In addition to these properties, C5a and C5a des Arg induce PMN margination, chemotaxis, aggregation, release of oxygen metabolites, leukotrienes, and slow-reacting substance of anaphylaxis (SRS-A). C5a also enhances local antibody responses. The C5-9 membrane attack complex is responsible for lysis of bacteria, viral-infected or other foreign cell types. This cascade of events induces inflammation (by several different redundant systems) and ultimately leads to localization and removal of the infective agent. It is important for the maintenance of homeostasis within the eye, however, its many functions are only partially characterized.

The complement system is a fundamental element of our normal host defense against infection.[80] The fate of patients with genetic deficiencies of specific complement components underscores the importance of this system: C3 deficiency is associated with frequent, severe bacterial infections; deficiencies of C6, C7, and C8 are associated with a striking susceptibility to *Neisseria* infections; C5 deficiency or dysfunction is associated with pyogenic infections.

External Compartments (Tears, Cornea, and Sclera)

Tears. The alternative pathway of complement is present in normal tears and may play a role in the defense mechanisms of the ocular surface.[122] An intact classical pathway has been reported to be present in tears.[122] Another report indicated that tears from normal subjects contain little or no C4, C3, or C1; whereas tears from some patients with inflammation of the anterior segment had higher levels of C4.[18] In another study, absent or low activities of C1, C4, and C3 were found in normal tears, but C5 was detected in tear samples from four to seven normal subjects.[76] The minimal activities of

C1, C4, and C3 may result from low concentrations of these complement proteins in normal tears or the presence of an anticomplementary factor that interferes with hemolytic assays (as suggested by Kijlstra and Veerhuis).[54] Nevertheless, elevated hemolytic levels of C1, C3, C4, and C5 were found in tears from patients with corneal ulcers.[76] The source of elevated complement levels in tears from patients with inflamed eyes may be hyperemic conjunctival vessels with increased permeability.

In summary, it is probable that normal tears contain negligible levels of classical and perhaps even alternative pathway components of complement. Inflammation of the external eye, however, results in elevated levels of complement components so that both the classical and alternative pathways of complement may be operative in tears and may be included in the host defense against invading pathogens. Although the human cornea contains hemolytic complement, which may play a role in bacterial keratitis, elevated levels of complement in tears from eyes with corneal ulcers may contribute to host defense of the cornea against invading pathogens.

Cornea. The distribution of C' components in the eye has been identified for several different intraocular compartments. The cornea has been the most extensively studied using several different techniques. Hemolytic assays demonstrated that corneal C' was functional.[66,69] The first component of the classical pathway, C1, exists in the plasma as a trimolecular complex, C1q-C1r-C1s of 647K daltons. Its large size, therefore, is believed to limit its accessibility into the central corneal stroma (by diffusion from the limbal vessels). The ratio of C1 in the peripheral-to-central cornea is 5:1, whereas it is approximately 1.2:1 for the other C' components.[66] It is of interest to note that C1q (at 400K daltons) is highly cationic, although it is normally complexed together with the more anionic C1r and C1s by a calcium-dependent bond (perhaps neutralizing the charge of C1q). The finding of more C1 in the peripheral than central cornea may be important in peripheral inflammation and ulcers of the cornea.[63] C1 is a recognition unit of the classical pathway. Therefore antigen-antibody complexes, whether formed in the cornea or whether derived from the tears, aqueous humor, or limbal vessels, may activate C' more effectively in the peripheral than in the central cornea. The presence of any C1 in the central cornea may be explained by the fact that corneal fibroblasts, at least in tissue culture, have the ability to produce C1.[64] All of the other C' components C2, C3, C4, C5, C6, C7 (except C8 and C9) have been detected in the normal C.[69] Concentrations detected generally range from 3.2% (C1) to 27.8% (C2) of plasma values. Molecular weight may be a factor in determining the concentration of complement components in the cornea, because C1, the largest complement component with a molecular weight of 647,000, had the lowest activity in corneas relative to sera; whereas C2 and C7, with lower molecular weights of approximately 120,000, had the highest activities in corneas relative to sera. Components of the alternate pathway, properidin and factor B, have also been identified in the cornea.[72] Immunologic or chemical injuries to the cornea generate C'-derived anaphylatoxins C3a, C4a, and C5a.[75a]

In addition to these inflammatory mediators, regulatory proteins of the C' cascade—factor H (beta-1H), factor I (C3b inactivator), and C1 inhibitor—are also found in the normal cornea.[75] C1 inhibitor and C3b inactivator showed activities in corneas that were nearly as high as activities in sera. The lower molecular weights of complement inhibitors (approximately 100,000) relative to other complement components may account for their higher levels in normal cornea. These lower weights may tip the balance in favor of inhibition of complement activation in the noninflamed cornea, especially in the case of classical pathway activation of complement. As mentioned previously, C1 has the lowest concentration of all complement components in the cornea, with much less in the central than in the peripheral cornea.[66] The relative proportions of C1 and C1 inhibitor in the cornea (especially in the central cornea) may favor inhibition rather than activation of the classical pathway. These findings may be disadvantageous in initiating host defense mechanisms requiring complement activation but may be advantageous in inhibiting destructive autoimmune processes requiring complement activation.

Decay-accelerating factor (DAF) is a membrane regulatory protein that protects blood cells from autologous complement activation on their surfaces. DAF has been found in tears and on corneal and conjunctival epithelia, corneal endothelium, trabecular meshwork, and lacrimal gland acinar cells and adjacent lumens.[55] Since DAF activity is important in protecting blood cells from autologous complement attack, DAF in the tears, on the ocular surface, and within the eye may control deleterious complement activation. Two other membrane-bound complement regulatory proteins have been found in the eye: membrane cofactor protein and membrane attack complex inhibiting protein.[15] Both of these proteins were identified on the corneal epithelium and stroma. Thus the cornea would appear to contain the necessary soluble effectors that serve not only important protective functions but play a role in tissue damage as well.

The source of C' components in the corneal stroma is believed to be primarily the plasma by diffusion from the limbal vessels rather than local synthesis. Tissue culture studies have, however, demonstrated that corneal fibroblasts possess the ability to produce C1 but not C2, C3, C4, C5, C6, C7; but there is no evidence to suggest that this observation occurs in vivo.[64] Experimental studies have utilized cobra venom factor (CVF) to deplete systemic C' levels to study the relationship between the plasma and the cornea.[90] Low-to-absent corneal complement levels were present 2 days after the initial injection of cobra venom factor and persisted

for 6 days. Corneal complement depletion and restoration lagged behind serum. Moreover, the rate of complement depletion and restoration was greater for serum than cornea. This model could be used to study the influence of complement on traumatic and immunologic injuries to the cornea. Using systemic decomplementation with cobra venom factor, Cleveland and associates[20] suggested that complement may be important in corneal defense against *Pseudomonas aeruginosa.* Their experiments showed that decomplemented mice had corneal ulcers that were more severe than those of mice with normal complement levels and that decomplemented mice were unable to clear *Pseudomonas* ocular infection—unlike mice with normal complement levels.

Sclera. In the avascular sclera, the distribution of C' components is not as well characterized. Functional levels of C1, C2, C3, C4, C5, and C6 have been detected.[17] Factor B of the alternate pathway has also been detected by radial immunodiffusion.[17] Molecular weight is an important regulatory factor that apparently determines scleral C' levels. The percentages of the lower molecular C' components detected were increased relative to the serum values as compared to those with higher molecular weights. Factor B, however, was the exception to this trend. In tissue culture studies, human scleral fibroblasts produce hemolytically active C1.[45] This activity is upregulated by the addition of exogenous gamma interferon; C2 and C4 synthesis is also induced. C3, C5, C6, and C7 were not detectable. The posterior sclera has more complement than the anterior sclera except for C1.

Internal Compartments (Aqueous Humor, Vitreous, Uvea)

As with the cornea, the distribution of C' components in the AH has been extensively studied. Analysis of "normal" AH obtained from eyes without previous surgeries demonstrated that the most prevalent component is C4; C1, C3, and C5 have also been detected.[18,71] The normal levels of these components are less than those of plasma. The AH, however, contains much less C' than the cornea on a weight basis. Molecular weight is apparently not as significant a determining factor for accessibility because AH levels of C1 (647K daltons) and C3 (185K daltons) were comparable.[71] In eyes that had sustained previous injury or surgical procedures, higher C' levels were detected as a result of altered vascular permeability. Inflamed eyes had the highest C' levels. In eyes with anterior uveitis, C' fragments were also detected.[68] The pivotal component of both C' pathways, C3a was universally noted in a limited number of patients. Factor B and C3c were detected in some patients, as was Bb; suggesting activation of the alternate pathway. Similar analysis of AH for eyes with experimental endotoxin-induced anterior uveitis demonstrated the presence of chemotactically active C5a.[97]

In the other intraocular compartments there have been

few studies reporting the normal distribution of C' components or fragments. In a study of patients with retinal detachments or vitreal hemorrhages without vitritis, there were levels of C3a and C4a comparable to plasma, but with less protein; in vitritis C3a and C4a, levels were elevated 6 to 7 times higher.[73,74] C5a could not be measured accurately because of its lability. A study of proliferative vitreoretinopathy demonstrated C3, C3d, C4, and C1q-IgG.[42] The sources of the C' fragments could be activation of vitreal C' or leakage after breakdown of blood-vitreal barriers. By immunohistochemical methods, C3 has been detected within the normal stromal tissues of the choroid, CB/P, and Bruchs membrane. C3 was not detected within the retinal tissues except within the vascular lumen. The compartmental distribution in inflamed eyes was not studied, however, it is likely that C' components would accompany the influx of plasma proteins.

Low levels of C1 inhibitor and C3b inactivator may be present in aqueous humor.[75] DAF has been measured in aqueous humor and vitreous humor and has been identified in ciliary body and iris.[55] Membrane attack complex inhibiting protein has been identified in ciliary body, iris, choroid, and retina.[12] Membrane cofactor protein has been found in the retina.[12]

The role of the complement system in host defense against bacterial endophthalmitis has been studied. Guinea pigs received intravitreal injections of bacteria, and comparisons were made between bacterial counts from the vitreous of control guinea pigs and experimental guinea pigs that underwent systemic decomplementation with cobra venom factor. Decomplemented guinea pigs showed impaired host defense to endophthalmitis caused by *Pseudomonas aeruginosa*,[2] *Staphylococcus aureus*[30,39] and *Staphylococcus epidermidis*.[39,89] This defense was restored as C' levels approached normal. Complement depletion experiments also were used to underscore the importance of complement in experimental allergic uveitis.[59]

Complement Receptors: Roles Within the Eye

Activation of the C' cascade liberates several different receptor ligands on leukocytes. These ligands may either be soluble, inducing chemotaxis, or insoluble, surface bound functioning as an opsonin. Different C' receptors have been the most widely characterized, being detected on a variety of immune cells, including B-cell subsets, monocytes, and PMN. C3a and C5a receptors for chemotaxis have been identified on PMN, eosinophils, basophils, and mast cells; C3b receptors have also been identified. These have been designated as CR1 (C3b receptor, 250K daltons) and CR3 [receptor for inactivated C3b (C3bi), 260K daltons and member of the leukocyte integrin LFA-1 family]. Complement receptor one (CR1) receptors mediate phagocytosis by most MNP and PMN of C3b opsonized IC, particles, or microbes.[22,80,95] CR3 recognizes C3bi requiring high divalent cation concentrations.[22,80,95] Its principle role is in phagocytosis of infectious microbes. Other C' receptors, namely CR2 (C3dg receptor, B-cells) and CR4 (PMN, platelets) functions are poorly characterized. It is most probable that each of these C' receptors serves analogous functions on lymphocytes, MNP, and leukocytes that migrate into the eye form the periphery.

In contrast to studies on isolated lymphocytes, MNP, and leukocytes, analysis of C3 receptors on resident ocular cells has been very limited. Freshly isolated monkey RPE cells express functional CR1 receptors capable of binding C3b opsonized, IgM-coated erythrocytes.[29] The phagocytic activity via these receptors was not reported. Similar studies of isolated human RPE or uveal tissues failed to demonstrate the C3b receptor.[26] Similarly, C3b receptors were not detected on RPE isolated from Royal College of Surgeons (RCS) rats.[27] In the posterior uvea, C3b receptors were noted on the capillary endothelium and diffusely in the CP.[58] Approximately 30% of vitreal hyalocytes possess C3b receptors.[41] It seems highly probable that species differences as well as receptor lability on eye bank tissues may account for these discrepancies.

The quiescent eye selectively derives its spectral array of antibodies from the plasma. Normally, little or no localized synthesis occurs. Many different diffusion barriers, layers, and chambers have developed within the eye to regulate the Abs spectrum within the intraocular microenvironments. Each compartment is normally in a state of equilibrium with the plasma. Since the plasma antibody spectrum is in a dynamic state of flux, the intraocular compartments follow (but with a time lag). Various types of barriers selectively regulating the entry and exit of Abs inflammatory episodes markedly alter this delicate balance. C' serves as an important effector system in the eye that is responsive to both antigen-antibody interactions as well as nonimmunologic activators.

REFERENCES

1. Agoda LYC, Gauthier VJ, Mannik M: Antibody localization in the glomerular basement membrane may precede in situ immune deposit formation in rat glomeruli, *J Immunol* 134:880, 1985.
2. Aizuss DH, Mondino BJ, Sumner HL, Dethlefs BA: The complement system and host defense against *Pseudomonas* endophthalmitis, *Invest Ophthalmol Vis Sci* 26:1262-1266, 1985.
3. Allansmith M, deRamus A, Maurice D: The dynamics of IgG in the cornea, *Invest Ophthalmol Vis Sci* 18:947, 1979.
4. Allansmith M, Kajiyama G, Abelson M, Simon M: Plasma cell content of main and accessory lacrimal glands in conjunctiva, *Am J Ophthalmol* 82:819, 1976.
5. Allansmith M, Newman L, Whitney C: The distribution of immunoglobulin in the rabbit eye, *Arch Ophthalmol* 86:60, 1971.
6. Allansmith MR, McClellan BH: Immunoglobulins in the human cornea, *Am J Ophthalmol* 80:123, 1975.
7. Allansmith MR, Whitney CR, McClellan BH, Newman LP: Immunoglobulins in the human eye: location, type, and amount, *Arch Ophthalmol* 89:36, 1973.
8. Allansmith MR: *The eye and immunology*, St Louis, 1982, Mosby-Year Book.

9. Andrews BS, McIntosh J, Petts V, Penny R: Circulating immune complexes in retinal vasculitis, *Clin Exp Immunol* 29:23, 1977.

10. Anseth A: Studies on corneal polysaccharides.' V. Changes in corneal glycosamino glycans in transient stromal edema, *Exp Eye Res* 8:297, 1969.

11. Augener W, Grey HM, Cooper NR, Muller-Eberhard HJ: The reaction of monomeric and aggregated immunoglobulins with C1, *Immunochem* 8:1011, 1971.

12. Baba H: Histochemical and polarization optical investigation for glycosaminoglycans in exfoliation syndrome, *Graefes Arch Clin Exp Ophthalmol* 221:106, 1983.

13. Beck OE: Distribution of virus antibody among human IgG subclasses, *Clin Exp Immunol* 43:626, 1981.

14. Bill A: Capillary permeability to and extravascular dynamics of myoglobin, albumin, and gamma globulin in the uvea, *Acta Physiol Scand* 73:204, 1968.

15. Bora NS, Gobleman CL, Atkinson JP et al.: Differential expression of the complement regulatory proteins in the human eye, *Invest Ophthalmol Vis Sci* 34:3579, 1993.

16. Borcherding MS, Blacik LJ, Sittig RA et al.: Proteoglycans and collagen fiber organization in human cornea scleral tissue, *Exp Eye Res* 21:59, 1975.

17. Brawman-Mintzer O, Mondino BJ, Mayer FJ: The complement system in sclera, *Invest Ophthalmol Vis Sci* 29:1756, 1988.

18. Chandler J, Leder R, Kaufman H, Caldwell J: Quantitative determinations of complement components and immunoglobulins in tears and aqueous humor, *Invest Ophthalmol Vis Sci* 13:151, 1974.

19. Char DH, Stein P, Masi R, Christensen M: Immune complexes in uveitis, *Am J Ophthalmol* 87:678, 1979.

20. Cleveland RP, Hazlett LD, Leon MA, Berk RS: Role of complement in murine corneal infection caused by *Pseudomonas aeruginosa*, *Invest Ophthalmol Vis Sci* 24:237-242, 1983.

21. Cohen E, Allansmith M: Fixation techniques for secretory component in human lacrimal gland and conjunctiva, *Am J Ophthalmol* 91:789, 1981.

22. Cooper NR: The complement system. In Stites DP, Stobo JD, Fudenberg HH, Wells JV, editors: *Basic and clinical immunology,* Los Altos, 1984, Lange.

23. Dernouchamps JP: The proteins of the aqueous humor, *Doc Ophthalmol* 53:193, 1982.

24. Dernouchamps JP, Vaerman JP, Michiels J, Masson PL: Immune complexes in the aqueous humor and serum, *Am J Ophthalmol* 84:24, 1977.

25. Donn A: Cornea and sclera, *Arch Ophthalmol* 75:261, 1966.

26. Dutt K, Waldrep JC, Kaplan HJ et al.: In vitro phenotypic and functional characterization of human pigment epithelial cell lines, *Curr Eye Res* 8:435, 1989.

27. Eckert CD, Hafeman DB: Search for Fc and C3b receptors on black-eyed RCS rat RPE cells, *Curr Eye Res* 5:911, 1986.

28. Elliott GF, Goodfellow JM, Woolgar AE: Swelling studies of bovine corneal stroma without bounding membranes, *J Physiol* 298:453, 1980.

29. Elner VM, Schaffner T, Taylor K, Glagov S: Immunophagocytic properties of retinal pigment epithelium cells, *Science* 211:74, 1981.

30. Engstrom RE, Mondino BJ, Glasgow BJ et al.: Immune response to *Staphylococcus aureus* endophthalmitis in a rabbit model, *Invest Ophthalmol Vis Sci* 32:1523-1533, 1991.

31. Fahey JL, Barth W, Ovary Z: Differences in the electrophoretic mobility of antibody from inbred strains of mice, *J Immunol* 94:819, 1965.

32. Fernando AN: Immunological studies with I[131]labeled antigen in experimental uveitis, *Arch Ophthalmol* 63:515, 1960.

33. Franklin R, Prendergast R, Silverstein A: Secretory immune system of rabbit ocular adnexa, *Invest Ophthalmol Vis Sci* 18:1093, 1979.

34. Franklin R, Winkelstein J, Seto D: Conjunctivitis and keratoconjunctivitis associated with primary immunodeficiency diseases, *Am J Ophthalmol* 84:563, 1977.

35. French M: Serum IgG subclasses in normal adults. In Shakib F, editor: *Basic and clinical aspects of IgG subclasses,* Basel, 1986, Karger.

36. Fukumoto T, Brandon MR: Importance of the liver in immunoglobulin catabolism, *Res Vet Sci* 32:62, 1982.

37. Gallo GR, Caulin-Glaser T, Lamm ME: Charge of circulating immune complexes as a factor in glomerular basement membrane localization in mice, *J Clin Invest* 67:1305, 1981.

38. Ghose T, Quigley JH, Landrigan PL, Asif A: Immunoglobulins in aqueous humor and iris from patients with endogenous uveitis and patients with cataract, *Br J Ophthalmol* 57:897, 1973.

39. Giese MJ, Mondino BJ, Glasgow B et al.: The complement system and host defense against staphylococcal endophthalmitis, *Invest Ophthalmol Vis Sci*, 35:1026, 1994.

40. Goldmann H, Witmer R: Antikorper in kammerwasser, *Ophthamologica* 127:323, 1954.

41. Grabner G, Boltz G, Forster O: Macrophage-like properties of human hyalocytes, *Invest Ophthalmol Vis Sci* 19:333, 1980.

42. Grisanti S, Wiedemann P, Weller M et al.: The significance of complement in proliferative vitreoretinopathy, *Invest Ophthalmol Vis Sci* 32:2711, 1991.

43. Hall JM, Pribnow JF: Specificity of antibody formation after intravitreal immunization with bovine gamma globulin and ovalbumin. II. Non-specific enhancement of the secondary response, *Cell Immunol* 11:64, 1974.

44. Hammarstrom L, Smith CIE: IgG subclasses in bacterial infections. In Shakib F, editor: *Basic and clinical aspects of IgG subclasses,* Basel, Switzerland 1986, Karger.

45. Harrison SA, Mondino BJ, Mayer FJ: Sceral fibroblasts: human leukocyte antigen expression and complement production, *Invest Ophthalmol Vis Sci* 31:2412, 1990.

46. Hedbys BO: The role of polysaccharides in corneal swelling, *Exp Eye Res* 1:81, 1961.

47. Henkind P, Hansen RJ, Szalay J: Ocular circulation. In Duane TD, Jaeger EA, editors: *Biomedical foundations of ophthalmology,* vol 2, Philadelphia, 1983, Harper and Row.

48. Howard A, Virella G: The separation of pooled human IgG into fractions by isoelectric focusing, and their electrophoretic and immunological properties, *Protides Biol Fluids* 17:449, 1969.

49. Howes EL, McKay DG: Circulating immune complexes: effects on ocular vascular permeability in the rabbit, *Arch Ophthalmol* 93:365, 1975.

50. Huber H, Fudenberg HH: Receptor sites of human monocytes for IgG, *Int Arch Allergy* 34:18, 1968.

51. Hylkema HA, Broersma L, Kijlstra A: In vivo and in vitro deposition of immunoglobulin aggregates in the mouse eye, *Curr Eye Res* 7:593, 1988.

52. Hylkema HA, Rathman WM, Kijlstra A: Deposition of immune complexes in the mouse eye, *Exp Eye Res* 37:257, 1983.

53. Kasp-Gronchowska, Graham E, Sanders MD et al.: Autoimmunity and circulating immune complexes in retinal vasculitis, *Trans Ophthalmol Soc UK* 101:342, 1981.

54. Kijlstra A, Veerhuis R: The effect of an anticomplementary factor on normal human tears, *Am J Ophthalmol* 92:24, 1981.

55. Lass JH, Walter EI, Burris TE et al.: Expression of two molecular forms of the complement decay-accelerating factor in the eye and lacrimal gland, *Invest Ophthalmol Vis Sci* 31:1136-1148, 1990.

56. Lee SI, Heiner DC, Wara D: Development of serum IgG subclasses levels in children. In Shakib F, editor: *Basic and clinical aspects of IgG subclasses,* Basel, Switzerland, 1986, Karger.

57. Linde GA, Hammarstrom L, Pesson MAA et al.: Virus specific antibody activity of different subclasses of immunoglobulin G and A in cytomegalovirus infection, *Infect Immun* 42:237, 1983.

58. Lowder CY, Char DH: Immune complexes in ocular disease, *Int Ophthalmol Clin* 25:143, 1985.

59. Marak GE, Wacker WB, Rao N et al.: Effects of complement depletion on experimental allergic uveitis, *Ophthalmic Res* 11:97, 1979.

60. Matthews AG: Immunohistochemical investigation of the distribution of immunoglobulins G, A, and M within the anterior uvea of the normal equine eye, *Equine Vet J* 21:438, 1989.

61. Mestecky J, Russell MW: IgA subclasses. In Shakib F, editor: *Basic and clinical aspects of IgG subclasses,* Basel, 1986, Karger.

62. Mishima S, Hedbys BO: Physiology of the cornea, *Int Ophthalmol Clin* 8:527, 1968.

63. Mondino BJ: Inflammatory diseases of the peripheral cornea, *Ophthalmology* 95:463-472, 1988.

64. Mondino BJ: Studies of complement in corneal tissue. In O'Connor GR, Chandler JW, editors: *Advances in immunology and immunopathology of the eye,* Chicago, 1985, Masson.

65. Mondino BJ, Adamu SA, Pitchekian-Halabi H: Antibody studies in a rabbit model of corneal phlyctenulosis and catarrhal infiltrates related to *Staphylococcus aureus, Invest Ophthalmol Vis Sci* 32:1854-1863, 1991.

66. Mondino BJ, Brady KJ: Distribution of hemolytic complement in the normal cornea, *Arch Ophthalmol* 99:1430, 1981.

67. Mondino BJ, Brawman-Mintzer O, Adamu SA: Corneal antibody levels to ribitol teichoic acid in rabbits immunized with staphylococcal antigens using various routes, *Invest Ophthalmol Vis Sci* 28:1553-1558, 1987.

68. Mondino BJ, Glovsky MM, Ghekiere L: Activated complement in inflamed aqueous humor, *Invest Ophthalmol Vis Sci* 25:871, 1984.

69. Mondino BJ, Hoffman DB: Hemolytic complement activity in normal human donor corneas, *Arch Ophthalmol* 98:2041, 1980.

70. Mondino BJ, Laheji AK, Adamu SA: Ocular immunity to *Staphylococcus aureus, Invest Ophthalmol Vis Sci* 28:560-564, 1987.

71. Mondino BJ, Rao H: Hemolytic complement activity in aqueous humor, *Arch Ophthalmol* 101:465, 1983.

72. Mondino BJ, Ratajczak HV, Goldberg DB et al.: Alternate and classical pathway components of complement in the normal cornea, *Arch Ophthalmol* 98:346, 1980.

73. Mondino BJ, Sidikaro Y, Mayer FJ, Sumner HL: Inflammatory mediators in the vitreous humor of AIDS patients with retinitis, *Invest Ophthalmol Vis Sci* 31:798-804, 1990.

74. Mondino BJ, Sidikaro Y, Sumner H: Anaphylatoxin levels in human vitreous humor, *Invest Ophthalmol Vis Sci* 29:1195, 1988.

75. Mondino BJ, Sumner H: Complement inhibitors in normal cornea and aqueous humor, *Invest Ophthalmol Vis Sci* 25:483, 1984.

75a. Mondino BJ, Sumner H: Generation of complement-derived anaphylatoxins in normal human donor corneas, *Invest Ophthalmol Vis Sci* 31:1945-1949, 1990.

76. Mondino BJ, Zaidman G: Hemolytic complement in tears, *Ophthalmic Res* 15:208, 1983.

77. Montgomery P, Rockey J, Majumdar A et al.: Parameters influencing the expression of IgA antibodies in tears, *Invest Ophthalmol Vis Sci* 25:369, 1984.

78. Morell A, Skvaril F, Steinberg AG et al.: Correlation between the concentrations of the four subclasses of IgG and Gm allotypes in normal sera, *J Immunol* 108:195, 1972.

79. Morell A, Terry WD, Waldmann TA: Metabolic properties of IgG subclasses in man, *J Clin Invest* 49:673, 1970.

80. Muller-Eberhard HJ: Complement: chemistry and pathways. In Gallin JI, Goldstein IM, Snyderman R, editors: *Inflammation—basic principles and clinical correlates,* New York, 1988, Raven Press.

81. Murray PI, Hoekzema R, Luyendijk L et al.: Analysis of aqueous humor immunoglobulin G by enzyme-linked immunosorbent assay, isoelectric focusing, and immunoblotting, *Invest Ophthalmol Vis Sci* 31:2129, 1990.

82. Pack WL, Olson RJ: Antigen uptake and immune complex retention in collagenous ocular tissues in vitro, *J Ocular Therapy Surg* 2:95, 1984.

83. Peress NS, Tompkins DC: Pericapillary permeability of the ciliary processes: Role of molecular charge, *Invest Ophthalmol Vis Sci* 23:168, 1982.

84. Peress NS: Immune complex deposition in the ciliary process of rabbits with acute and chronic serum sickness, *Exp Eye Res* 30:371, 1980.

85. Peress NS, Perillo E: Immunoglobulin G receptor mediated phagocytosis by the pigment epithelium of the ciliary processes, *Invest Ophthalmol Vis Sci* 32:78, 1991.

86. Pino RM, Essner E: Permeability of rat choriocapillaris to heme proteins: restriction of tracers by fenestrated endothelium, *J Histochem Cytochem* 29:281, 1981.

87. Pino RM, Essner E, Pino LC: Localization and chemical composition of anionic sites in Bruch's membrane of the rat, *J Histochem Cytochem* 30:245, 1982.

88. Plaut A: Microbial IgA proteases, *New Eng J Med* 298:1459, 1978.

89. Pleyer U, Mondino BJ, Adamu SA et al.: Immune response to *Staphylococcus epidermidis* induced endophthalmitis in a rabbit model, *Invest Ophthalmol Vis Sci* 33:2650-2663, 1992.

90. Pleyer U, Mondino BJ, Sumner HL: The effect of systemic decomplementation with cobra venom factor on corneal complement levels in guinea pigs, *Invest Ophthalmol Vis Sci* 33:2212, 1992.

90a. Preston MJ, Kernacki KA, Berk JM, et al.: Kinetics of serum, tear, and corneal antibody responses in resistant and susceptible mice intracorneally infected with *Pseudomonas aeruginosa, Infect and Immun* 60:885-891, 1992.

91. Reed W, Cushing A: Role of immunoglobulins in protection against Shigella-induced keratoconjunctivitis, *Infect Immun* 11:1265, 1975.

92. Rijkers GT, Mosier DE: Pneumococcal polysaccharides induce antibody formation by human B lymphocytes in vitro, *J Immunol* 135:1, 1985.

93. Robey PG, Newsome DA: Biosynthesis of proteoglycans present in primate Bruch's membrane, *Inv Ophthalmol Vis Sci* 24:898, 1983.

94. Roitt I: *Essential immunology,* ed 4, Boston, 1982, Blackwell Scientific Publication.

95. Roitt I, Brostoff J, Male D: *Immunology,* St Louis, 1985, Mosby-Year Book.

96. Rose GE, Billington BM, Chignell AH: Immunoglobulins in paired specimens of vitreous and subretinal fluids from patients with rhegmatogenous detachment, *Br J Ophthalmol* 74:160, 1990.

97. Rosenbaum JT, Wong K, Perez HD et al.: Characterization of endotoxin induced C5-derived chemotactic activity in aqueous humor, *Invest Ophthalmol Vis Sci* 10:1184, 1984.

98. Rude E, Moses E, Sela M: Role of the net electrical charge of the complete antigen in determining the chemical nature of anti-p-azobenzenearsonate antibodies, *Biochem* 7:2971, 1968.

99. Russell MW, Mestecky J, Julian BA, Galla JH: IgA-associated renal diseases: Antibodies to environmental antigens in sera and deposition of immunoglobulins and antigens in glomeruli, *J Clin Immunol* 6:74, 1986.

100. Schibechi A, Wade AW, Depew WT, Szewczuk MR: Analysis of serum antibody repertoires by isoelectric focusing and capillary blotting onto nitrocellulose paper, *J Immunol Meth* 89:201, 1986.

100a. Seegal BC, Seegal D: Local organ hypersensitiveness: VII. Demonstration of agglutinins in tissues of the rabbit eye following immunization with Eb. typhi vaccine, *Proc Soc Exp Biol Med* 31:437-441, 1934.

101. Sela M, Moses E: Dependence of the chemical nature of antibodies on the net electrical charge of antigens, *Biochem* 55:445, 1966.

102. Shakib F: The IgG4 subclass. In Shakib F, editor: *Basic and clinical aspects of IgG subclasses,* Basel, 1986, Karger.

103. Shimada K, Silverstein AM: Local antibody formation within the eye: a study of immunoglobulin class and antibody specificity, *Invest Ophthalmol Vis Sci* 14:573, 1975.

104. Siegelman J, Peress NS: Fc receptor mediated binding and ingestion of immunoglobulin G-coated erythrocytes by the epithelium of the posterior ciliary processes: an in vitro study, *Exp Eye Res* 47:361, 1988.

105. Skvaril F: IgG subclasses in viral infections. In Shakib F, editor: *Basic and clinical aspects of IgG subclasses,* Basel, 1986, Karger.

106. Slack JH: Strain-dependent IgG subclass response patterns, *J Immunol* 139:3734, 1987.

107. Spiegelberg HL: Biological activities of immunoglobulins of different classes and subclasses, *Adv Immunol* 22:259, 1974.

108. Steward MW: The biological significance of antibody affinity, *Immunol Today* 7:134, 1981.

109. Stock EL, Aronson SB: Corneal immune globulin distribution, *Arch Ophthalmol* 84:355, 1970.

110. Streilein JW: Immune regulation and the eye: a dangerous compromise, *FASEB J* 1:199, 1987.

111. Suzuki Y, Maruyama Y, Arakawa M, Oite T: Preservation of fixed anionic sites in the GBM in the acute proteinuric phase of cationic antigen-mediated in situ immune complex glomerulonephritis in the rat, *Histochem* 81:243, 1984.

112. Van der Voet JCM, Liem A, Otto AJ, Kijlstra A: Intraocular antibody synthesis during experimental uveitis, *Invest Ophthalmol Vis Sci* 30:316, 1989.

113. van der Zee JS, van Swieten P, Aalberse RC: Serologic aspects of IgG4 antibodies. II. IgG4 antibodies form small, nonprecipitating immune complexes due to functional monovalency, *J Immunol* 137:3566, 1986.

114. Waldrep JC, Donoso LA: Auxiliary production of antibodies to intraocular antigens in experimental autoimmune uveoretintis, *Curr Eye Res* 9:241, 1990.
115. Waldrep JC, Kaplan HJ, Warbington M: In situ immune complex formation in the uvea. Potential role for cationic antibody, *Invest Ophthalmol Vis Sci* 28:1191, 1987.
116. Waldrep JC, Noe RL, Stulting RD: Analysis of human corneal IgG by isoelectric focusing, *Invest Ophthalmol Vis Sci* 29:1538, 1988.
117. Waldrep JC, Schulte JR: Characterization of human IgG subclasses within intraocular compartments, *Reg Immunol* 2:22, 1989.
118. Waldrep JC, Wood JD: Kinetic analysis of antibody localization within the eye, *Invest Ophthalmol Vis Sci* 31:302, 1990.

119. Waldrep JC: Uveal IgG distribution: Regulation by electrostatic interactions, *Curr Eye Res* 6:897, 1987.
120. Wang HM, Jeng JE, Kaplan HJ: Fc receptors in corneal epithelium, *Curr Eye Res* 8:123, 1989.
121. Weller M, Clausen R, Bresgen M et al.: Immunoglobulin G, complement factor C3, and lymphocytes in proliferative intraocular disorders, *Int Ophthalmol* 14:277, 1990.
122. Yamamoto G, Allansmith M: Complement in tears from normal humans, *Am J Ophthalmol* 88:758, 1979.

5 Chemical Mediators of Ocular Inflammation

SCOTT W. COUSINS, BARRY T. ROUSE

Inflammation is the process by which white blood cells and fluids accumulate within a tissue.[213] At the macroscopic level, inflammation is a tissue reaction triggered by various stimuli (trauma, infection, or immunity) that results in the classic "cardinal" clinical signs (pain, redness, swelling, warmth, and loss of function). Specific physiologic responses mediate the clinical findings: redness and heat are caused by vasodilation and cellular metabolism; swelling is a result of extravascular fluid, fibrin deposition, and cellular accumulation; and pain is attributable to stimulation of nerve endings.

At the microscopic level, inflammation is infiltration by neutrophils, monocytes and lymphocytes, fibrin deposition, and extracellular edema. Each of the pathophysiologic responses is regulated by complex interactions between soluble mediators and cellular effectors, resulting in enhanced binding to adjacent surfaces, transmigration through matrices, release of cytoplasmic granules and vacuoles, activation or deactivation of genes, upregulation or downregulation of synthesis of specific cellular enzymes and products, as well as other changes in cellular metabolism.[77,78,188,213]

Knowledge of the identity and function of the cellular and soluble participants is a critical issue in understanding inflammation. Leukocytes are the most important cells, but platelets, vascular endothelium, and parenchymal cells of the local tissue (epithelium, fibroblasts, and other specialized cell types) also participate. Important soluble mediators include free radicals, vasoactive amines, lipid mediators, cytokines, plasma-derived factors, and other molecules.

CELLULAR EFFECTORS OF INFLAMMATION

Tissue infiltration with blood-borne leukocytes is one of the principal components of inflammation. Although the triggering stimuli of inflammation may initially interact with local parenchymal cells within tissues (such as vascular endothelium), most of the inflammatory process is mediated through the products generated and secreted by infiltrating leukocytes recruited into the site. Much general information for the three leukocyte subsets (granulocytes, lymphocytes, and monocytes) has been detailed in several reviews.[78,109] All three families of leukocytes participate in ocular inflammation.

Leukocytes and Inflammation

Granulocytic Leukocytes. Granulocytes represent a family of three bone marrow-derived cell types (neutrophils, eosinophils, and basophils) that have prominent cytoplasmic granules and participate as effector cells in inflammation. All three types mature within bone marrow and are released into the circulation.[18]

Neutrophils. Neutrophils, also called polymorphonuclear leukocytes (PMNs), are the most abundant granulocytes in the blood.[18] They are efficient phagocytes and readily invade tissues and degrade ingested material. They act as important effector cells through the release of granule products and cytokines. Through specific receptors (such as F_c, anaphylatoxin, or complement receptors), PMNs can be recruited and triggered by immune mechanisms. Via poorly characterized receptors and their ligands, PMNs are recruited and activated at sites of injury by nonimmune mechanisms, such as the formyl peptides.

In experimental models and clinical examples of active bacterial infections of the conjunctiva, sclera, cornea, and vitreous, PMNs dominate the infiltrate.[86] This fact is also true in many models of active viral infections of the cornea (herpes simplex virus keratitis)[153] and retina (herpes simplex virus retinitis).[44] PMNs are the principal cell type in lipopolysaccharide-induced[45] and cytokine-induced inflammation.

PMN infiltration can be triggered by immunologic mechanisms, particularly by immune complex formation. PMNs are numerous in animal models for keratitis[80] or uveitis resulting from immune complex activation (or Arthus reactions).[12,165] Similarly, in animal models (especially in mice and rats), neutrophil infiltrates often predominate in the early phases of acute T cell-mediated lesions.[48,65] During acute T cell-mediated delayed hypersensitivity reactions in the anterior chamber, cornea, or conjunctiva, PMNs often predominate; although monocytes and other granulocyte populations become prominent in subacute lesions.[47,99] In experimental allergic uveoretinitis induced by S antigen (a T cell-mediated autoimmune disorder), PMNs are prominent in the retinal infiltrate.[54] Many forms of lens-associated uveitis are characterized by a predominance of PMNs. Thus PMNs often dominate in ocular inflammation regardless of the cause, making histologic detection of PMNs an unreliable immunodiagnostic tool.[65]

Eosinophils. Eosinophils are similar to PMNs in that they contain abundant cytoplasmic granules and lysosomes.[82] Eosinophils, however, differ in the biochemical nature of the granules (which are more basic and bind acidic dyes) and in the way they respond to certain triggering stimuli. Eosinophils have receptors for and become activated to many mediators, of which interleukin-5 (IL-5) is especially important. Eosinophil granule products, such as major basic protein or ribonucleases, are ideal for destroying parasites, and eosinophils accumulate at sites of parasitic infection. Eosinophils are numerous in skin infiltrates during the late phase allergic response and atopic lesions, and in lung infiltrates during asthma. T cell production of IL-5 within the infiltrated site is probably an important regulator of eosinophil function locally, although many of the specific mechanisms for regulation of eosinophil recruitment, activation, or function remain unknown.[216]

Eosinophils are abundant in the conjunctiva and tears in many forms of atopic conjunctivitis, especially vernal and allergic conjunctivitis.[7] Eosinophils are not major effectors for intraocular inflammation, except during helminthic infections of the eye, such as toxocariasis.[86]

Basophils and Mast Cells. Basophils are the blood-borne equivalent of the tissue-bound mast cell.[101,135] Mast cells exist in two major subtypes, connective tissue and mucosal types. Connective tissue mast cells contain high histamine and heparin levels and release prostaglandin D_2 as a lipid metabolite. Mucosal mast cells require T cell cytokines for granule formation, contain low histamine levels, and make chiefly leukotrienes. The granule type and functional activity can be altered by the tissue location, but the regulation of these important differences is not well understood.

Basophils and mast cells differ from other granulocytes in several important ways. The granule contents are different and mast cells express high-affinity F_c receptors for IgE. Mast cells act as the major effector cells in IgE-mediated, immune-triggered, inflammatory reactions, especially allergy or immediate hypersensitivity. Mast cells may also participate in the induction of cell-mediated immunity, as inhibitors of mast cell degranulation or granule function prevent the early-triggering phase of delayed hypersensitivity in animal models.[14]

The normal human conjunctiva contains significant numbers of mast cells localized in the substantia propria but not in the epithelium.[8] In certain atopic and allergic disease states, such as vernal conjunctivitis, not only do the number of mast cells increase in the substantia propria, but the epithelium also becomes densely infiltrated.[8] In careful anatomic studies performed in rats, the sclera, choroid, and anterior uvea also contain significant densities of connective tissue type of mast cells, whereas the cornea has none. Histamine, one of the major mediators derived from mast cell degranulation, is responsible for many of the effects of basophil- and mast cell-mediated inflammation.

Monocytes and Macrophages. The monocyte (the circulating cell) and the macrophage (the tissue-infiltrating equivalent) are important effectors in all forms of inflammation.[4] Monocytes are relatively large cells (12 to 20 μ in suspension, but up to 40 μ in tissues) and traffic through many normal sites. Most normal tissues contain macrophages, and in many tissues these have been given tissue-specific names (for example, Kupffer cells in the liver and alveolar macrophages in the lungs).

Macrophages serve three primary functions: (1) as antigen-presenting cells for T lymphocytes, (2) as inflammatory effector cells, and (3) as regulators in other processes, such as fibrosis. In vitro studies indicate that ''quiescent'' monocytes can be activated through various signals into efficient antigen-presenting cells and, upon additional activation signals, into effector cells. Exposure to various bacterial toxins (such as lipopolysaccharide), phagocytosis of antibody-coated or complement-coated pathogens, or exposure to mediators released during inflammation (interleukin-1 or interferon gamma), are effective activation stimuli. Only upon full activation are macrophages most efficient at synthesis and release of inflammatory mediators and killing and degradation of phagocytosed pathogens.[134] At some sites of inflammation, a macrophage can undergo a morphologic change both in size and in histologic features into an *epithelioid cell*.[182] Epithelioid cells can fuse into multinucleated *giant cells*.[182]

Macrophages are extremely important effector cells in ocular inflammation, particularly in immune-triggered events. They are often detectable in acute ocular infections, even if other cell types such as PMNs are more numerous.[55]

Dendritic Cells and Langerhans Cells. Dendritic cells are terminally differentiated, bone marrow-derived, circulating, antigen-presenting cells distinct from the macrophage-monocyte lineage. They comprise approximately 0.1 to 1% of blood mononuclear cells.[17,192] They are large (15 to 20 μm) cells, that upon infiltration into tissue sites, form cytoplasmic veils that extend 2 to 3 times the diameter of the cell. Together with macrophages and B cells, dendritic cells play an important role in processing and presentation of antigens to T cells.[205,212] Dendritic cells may be the most potent antigen-presenting cells for generating primary T cell-dependent immune responses, and they are capable of initiating the activation of quiescent lymphocytes.[192]

Dendritic cells form a system of antigen-presenting cells found in many nonlymphoid and lymphoid organs. These sites are interconnected by defined migration pathways, and in each site, dendritic cells share features of structure and function. Epidermal Langerhans cells are the best-characterized nonlymphoid dendritic cells. Langerhans cells represent about 3 to 8% of cells in most human epithelia, including the skin and mucosa (counting conjunctiva and peripheral cornea).[76] They are identified on the basis of many dendrites, an electron dense cytoplasm, and Birbeck granules. At most sites, resident Langerhans cells are not efficient antigen-presenting cells; however, after exposure to specific growth factors they become activated. As a result Langerhans cells lose their granules, transform into the appearance of typical dendritic cells, and acquire antigen-presenting capacity. Langerhans cells can leave the skin and move via the afferent lymph to draining lymphoid organs.[185] Langerhans cells are important components of the immune system and their elimination from skin before antigen challenge inhibits the induction of the contact hypersensitivity response. Langerhans cells are important in antigen presentation, control of lymphoid cell traffic, differentiation of T cells, and induction of delayed hypersensitivity.[76]

The limbus and conjunctiva are richly invested with Langerhans cells, and these cells contribute to the normal immunoreactivity of the extraocular surface. They are absent from the midcornea and central cornea, a finding that partially explains the success of corneal allografting.[152] Many kinds of irritation to the cornea can result in centripetal migration of peripheral Langerhans cells, altering the immunobiology of this tissue.[152] For example, induction of Langerhans cell migration into the central corneal before herpes simplex virus corneal infection results in accelerated and enhanced delayed hypersensitivity response to viral antigen challenge and increased severity of corneal inflammation.[131] The type of corneal inflammation induced by different virus strains may reflect their capacity to induce the migration of Langerhans cells into the cornea.

The uvea is richly invested with non-Langerhans type of dendritic cells. The iris and ciliary body of mice contain a dense network of dendritic cells, many adjacent to nerve endings.[110] Dendritic cells have been observed to intercalate between the pigmented and nonpigmented epithelium of the ciliary body and are abundant in the choroid.[132,133] The role of these cells in antigen presentation within the eye remains poorly characterized, but recent experiments indicate that many of these cells can recirculate to the spleen, where they induce antigen-specific suppressor T cells.[219]

Lymphocytes. Lymphocytes are small (10 to 20 u) cells with large dense nuclei and are derived from stem cell precursors within the bone marrow.[160] Unlike other leukocytes, lymphocytes require subsequent maturation in peripheral lymphoid organs. Originally characterized and differentiated based on a series of ingenious but esoteric laboratory tests, lymphocytes can now be subdivided based on detection of specific cell surface proteins. These surface "markers" are related to functional and molecular activity of individual subsets. Three broad categories of lymphocytes have been determined: (1) B cells, (2) T cells, and (3) non-T, non-B lymphocytes. T cells can be further divided into CD4 positive and CD8 positive subsets, and CD4 positive T cells have recently been divided into two functional T helper types (Th1 and Th2).[144] The non-T, non-B lymphocytes, often called "null" cells, include natural killer cells and other granule-containing lymphocytes.

T Cells. In ocular infectious diseases, especially viral infections, T cells are crucially important in providing protection against spread of infection, in regulating the severity of the inflammatory response to infection, and in assisting the eventual clearance of the infectious agent.[180] In animal models of herpes simplex virus stromal keratitis, a specific subset of T helper cells (Th1 subset) appears to regulate the immune-mediated, inflammatory component of this disorder.[153] In experimental cytomegaloviral retinitis, depletion of T cells allows efficient infection of the retina and retinal pigment epithelium, and both CD4+ and CD8+ T cell subsets appear to participate.[16] In herpes simplex virus retinitis in mice, both T cells and natural killer cells contribute.[198]

B Cells. B cells predominate in other ocular inflammatory disorders. In Fuchs uveitis syndrome the anterior uveal tract is infiltrated with B cells and plasma cells. Other forms of nonviral uveitis are also mediated by B cells.

Regulation of Leukocytic Infiltration

The generation of a tissue inflammatory response requires that leukocytes be recruited from their normal location in the blood to sites of injury. Such recruitment occurs rapidly and is a tightly controlled process. It involves multiple *cell adhesion molecules* on leukocytes and on endothelial cells in postcapillary venules and other microvessels adjacent to the inflammatory site. The process is complex and dynamic with various possible outcomes depending on the nature of the inflammatory stimuli, the tissue or organ involved, and the duration of the reaction. Acute reactions involving bacteria are typically dominated by PMNs. Eosinophils may be more prominent in parasite-mediated inflammatory responses, and viral lesions often have a predominance of mononuclear leukocytes. Inversely, PMNs are almost never found in lymph nodes except for certain specific diseases (for example, cat-scratch fever). Most of the current information on adhesion events associated with inflammation concerns PMNs and lymphocytes, and the topic has been the subject of several succinct reviews.[36,156,157,226]

For leukocytes to escape from blood vessels, an essential adhesion with vascular endothelial cells must occur. Neutrophil recruitment has been best characterized and serves as the model for other leukocytes. Molecules on the two cell types belonging to at least three sets of cell adhesion molecule families are involved: (1) the selectins, (2) the integrins, and (3) molecules in the immunoglobulin (Ig) superfamily.[226] The primary interactive events are mediated largely by members of the selectin family and occur within minutes of injury. The ligands for selectin molecules are as yet poorly characterized oligosaccharides found in the cell membranes of target cells.[191] The initial phase involves neutrophil rolling, a process by which cells bind loosely but reversibly to endothelial cells. Nonactivated PMNs express L-selectin, which mediates a weak bond to endothelial cells. Upon exposure to activating factors such as thrombin, histamine, leukotrienes, and other agonists, these cells express at least two selectins (E and P) by which they can bind to PMNs and help stabilize the interaction.[226] Subsequently, additional adhesion molecules mediate a firmer interaction between PMNs and endothelial cells. Thus the activated endothelial cells are induced to express biologically active molecules at their cell membranes. One such molecule, platelet-activating factor, probably subserves at least two functions; it may mediate attachment to PMNs by binding to a G protein-linked cell surface receptor and may serve to activate PMNs to express at least two adhesion molecules of the β integrin family, LFA-I and MAC-I. Other stimuli to PMNs, such as various cytokines and bacterial products, also cause functional upregulation of β integrins.[11] As integrins are expressed, the L-selectins are shed and PMNs bind firmly to endothelial cells via at least two intercellular adhesion molecules of the Ig superfamily (ICAM 1 and 2).[157] Both ICAM molecules are upregulated on activated endothelial cells. A summary of the principal molecules involved in PMN adhesion to endothelial cells is presented in Fig. 5-1.

Another outcome of endothelial cell activation is the production and secretion of interleukin-8, a powerful chemoattractant and activating factor for PMNs.[121] Activating and binding by platelet-activating factor and IL-8 are perhaps the most potent stimulants for β integrin upregulation and serve to enhance transmigration to the adjacent inflammatory site.

Although little is known about the various molecules involved in monocyte adhesion and migration, considerable information is available with regard to adhesion behavior and migration of lymphocytes, a process called *homing*.[184,190] Lymphocytes are normally migratory cells that pass from the circulation into various tissues from which they subsequently depart and pass by way of lymphatics to reenter the circulation. Homing involves the variable interaction of multiple adhesion molecules between lymphocytes and target cells. These include the receptor-counterreceptors for PMNs as well as additional adhesion molecules. Memory cells, which express higher levels of certain adhesion molecules than do naive cells, are the only types of lymphocytes that migrate into tissues. Naive lymphocytes migrate to lymphoid tissues, where they may meet their cognate antigen; but inflammation changes the rules and breaks down homing patterns. Thus at inflammatory sites, the volume of lymphocyte migration is far greater, and selection is much less precise. Migration of activated and memory cells, however, exceeds that of naive cells. Activated T cells express higher levels of the integrins LFA-I and MAC-I that mediate the necessary adhesion to endothelial cells.[184]

The specificity and activational status of inflammatory lymphocytes varies markedly according to the site, the inflammatory stimulus, and the stage of inflammation. For example, during stromal keratitis, the Th1 subset of CD4+ T cells predominates over both Th2 subset of CD4+ T cells or CD8+ T cells.[153] The molecular reasons for such preferential accumulation have not been elucidated. Following the transendothelial migration of lymphocytes, other activational events can occur if T cells recognize antigen at the inflammatory site.

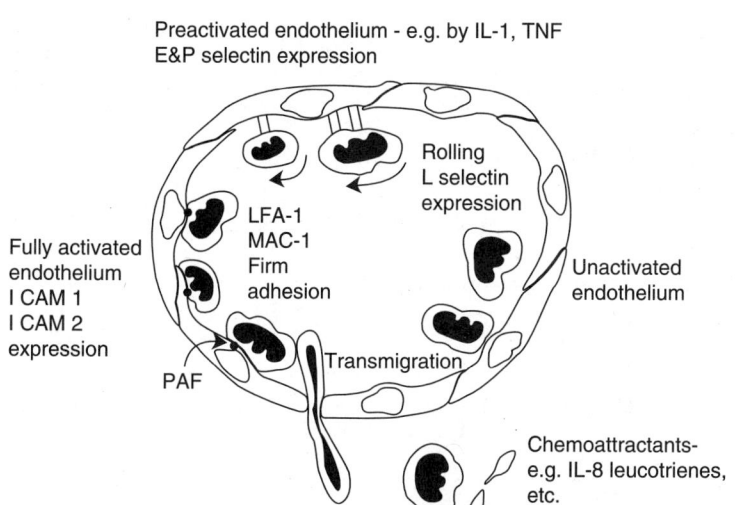

Fig. 5-1. Schematic representation of the events important to cellular adhesion, emigration, and infiltration.

Leukocyte Traffic in the Eye and the Blood-Ocular Barrier. The anterior chamber and retina possess a barrier for cells and macromolecules.[50] The normal blood-ocular barrier allows regulated and selective transmigration of blood-borne leukocytes. The uveal tract is richly invested with certain leukocyte subsets, especially macrophages, dendritic cells, and mast cells.[132,133] Since cell transmigration is an active, directed process, the vascular endothelium of the uvea must constitutively express cell adhesion molecules for these leukocytes. The ability of leukocytes to enter the retina through the normal retinal vasculature is limited; transmigration of leukocytes through the retinal vessels is an early sign of inflammation.[87]

Both physiologically and functionally, the blood-ocular barrier to movement of plasma-derived macromolecules is quite different when compared with the barrier to the movement of leukocytes. Plasma-derived proteins and intravascularly administered diagnostic dyes are excluded from some of the ocular compartments by tight junctions.[50] In the retinal circulation, the blood-ocular barrier exists at the level of tight junctions between adjacent endothelial cells and the absence of fenestrations.[167] In contrast, the vessels of the uveal tract are highly permeable to macromolecules. The tight junctions between the nonpigmented ciliary epithelium and retinal pigmented epithelium provide a more exclusive barrier, preventing extravascular macromolecules from permeating directly through the uvea into the aqueous humor or retina.[87,167] Macromolecules, however, can sieve through the iris stroma to the anterior iris surface, where they can enter into the anterior chamber.[227] During inflammation, blood-ocular barriers to leukocyte transmigration and to protein leakage are altered.[87] The factors responsible for these changes are related but not identical, and selective regulation of the barrier for cells can occur independently of that for macromolecules.[87]

Cellular Enzymes and Free Radicals

The inflammatory response is generally a protective one that results in microbial killing, removal of debris, and clearance of antigenic material. Although extracellular biochemical processes may mediate some of these protective properties, the most efficient and effective protective event is phagocytosis by PMNs and macrophages.[223] Phagocytosis is a selective, receptor-mediated process. The two most important receptors are the Ig F_c receptor and the complement receptors. Pathogens complexed with Ig or activated complement components are specifically bound to the cell surface by membrane-expressed F_c or complement (C) receptors and are effectively ingested. Other receptors may also mediate attachment to phagocytes.[223]

The actual process of particle ingestion is an energy-requiring process that is modulated by several biochemical events within the cells. Concomitant processes during ingestion include membrane synthesis, lysosomal enzyme synthesis, generation of metabolic products of oxygen and nitrogen, and the migration of various granules toward the phagosome. Ultimately, several granules fuse with the phagosomes. If this fusion occurs prior to complete invagination, granule contents spill outside of the phagocyte.

Phagocytes destroy microorganisms by antimicrobial polypeptides that reside within cytoplasmic granules, by reactive oxygen radicals generated from oxygen during the respiratory burst, and by reactive nitrogen radicals. Although these mechanisms are primarily designed to destroy pathogens, released contents may contribute to inflammation and tissue damage.[91] In addition to spillage, which may be more characteristic of PMNs, leukocytes can release or secrete intracellular contents to the extracellular environment. PMNs can also be detonated to secrete, particularly under conditions in which phagocytosis is "difficult" ("frustrated" phagocytosis).[91] Thus the antimicrobial mechanisms of leukocytes produce inflammation and bystander damage to tissues.

Granulocyte Products. A large number of antimicrobial polypeptides are present in the many types of granules found in human PMNs (see Box). PMNs also contain numerous other molecules not directly involved in antimicrobial defense. These include hydrolytic enzymes, elastase, adhesins, receptors, myeloperoxidase, gelatinase, vitamin B_{12} binding protein, cytochrome b_{558}, and several others. Granule contents remain inert and membrane bound when the granules are intact but become active and soluble when granules fuse to the phagocytic vesicles or plasma membrane. The principal antimicrobial polypeptides found in human PMNs granules are bacteriocidal permeability-increasing factors, defensins, lysozyme, lactoferrin, serine proteases, and metalloproteinases.[118]

Exactly how the various granulocyte products enhance inflammation is not clear. The original idea was that the

---

ANTIMICROBIAL POLYPEPTIDES OF NEUTROPHILS

Primary Granules
Myeloperoxidase
Defensins
Cathepsin G
Azurocin
Bactericidal permeability-increasing factor
Hydrolases
Secondary Granules
Lysozyme
Lactoferrin
Vitamin B_{12}-binding protein
Adhesion receptors
Chemoattractant receptors
Gelatinase
Cytochrome b_{2558}

release of proteases and other enzymes directly degraded the extracellular matrix of inflamed sites, thereby enabling the recruitment of additional leukocytes, damaging the integrity of microvessels, and injuring the parenchymal cells.[92] Recent evidence suggests that hypochlorous acid derived from toxic oxygen by-products must interact with proteases and protease inhibitors in a complex fashion to enhance the tissue-destructive effects of PMNs granule products.[214]

The role of PMN-derived proteases in ocular inflammation remains unclear. Collagenases are believed to contribute to corneal injury and liquefaction during bacterial keratitis and scleritis, especially in *Pseudomonas* infections.[112] Collagenases also contribute to peripheral corneal melting syndromes secondary to rheumatoid arthritis[187] and other rheumatic diseases.

Toxic Oxygen Products. Phagocytes exposed to a wide variety of stimuli undergo changes in oxidase utilization and oxygen consumption, generating reactive products that are damaging and destructive to microorganisms. The principal oxidase involved in the reactions is membrane-associated nicotinamide adenine dinucleotide phosphate (NADPH) oxidase, but others include NADH oxidase, xanthine oxidase, and aldehyde oxidase.[151] NADPH oxidase catalyses the transfer of electrons from NADPH (or nicotinamide adenine dinucleotide (NADH)) to oxygen or hydrogen peroxide to form intermediates such as the reactive oxygen radical, superoxide anion. Two electrons can be transferred to molecular oxygen, a process that normally occurs in the peroxisomes.

$$O_2 + e^- = \cdot O_2^-$$

Alternatively, the transfer of a single electron to oxygen forms superoxide anion, an unstable radical that can either dismutase spontaneously (one of the molecules gains an electron and the other loses one), or the reaction can be catalyzed by the enzyme superoxide dismutase to form hydrogen peroxide and oxygen.[108]

$$\cdot O_2^- + \cdot O_2^- + 2H^+ = O_2 + H_2O_2$$

This process results in hydrogen peroxide (H_2O_2), a molecule that has feeble microbicidal activity. H_2O_2 can be catalyzed by enzymes such as catalase and glutathione peroxidase to take up two more electrons to form water. This process is summarized in Fig. 5-2.

Hydrogen peroxide is involved in two processes with marked microbicidal potential. First, one electron can be added to form hydroxyl anion along with the highly reactive hydroxyl radical.[220] Second, H_2O_2 may be catalyzed by myeloperoxidase, an abundant protein found in PMNs, to react with halide or the pseudohalide (thiocyanate) substrates to form extremely toxic products that are highly damaging to bacteria[108] and tissues. These include hypohalous acids, halogens, chloramines, and hydroxyl radicals (with main methods of toxicity involving halogenation and oxidation). Halogenation replaces hydrogen atoms in crucial locations with halides, resulting in loss of molecular function. With iodine as the halide, iodination of tyrosines is the most likely mechanism. Possibly the most damaging oxidation products are hydroxyl radicals.[220] These radicals interact with several potential targets giving effects such as lipid peroxidation of the lipid bilayers, loss of energization, and cellular stores of adenosine triphosphate (ATP) caused by loss of the inner membrane of the mitochondria and the appearance of single-strand breaks in DNA.[70]

Oxygen-free radicals are likely mediators in many forms of ocular inflammation. Toxic oxygen radicals are involved in retinal injury during experimental autoimmune uveoretinitis.[166] The generation of toxic oxygen intermediates is associated with PMN and monocyte infiltration in experimental uveitis. Various methods for detecting lipid peroxidation

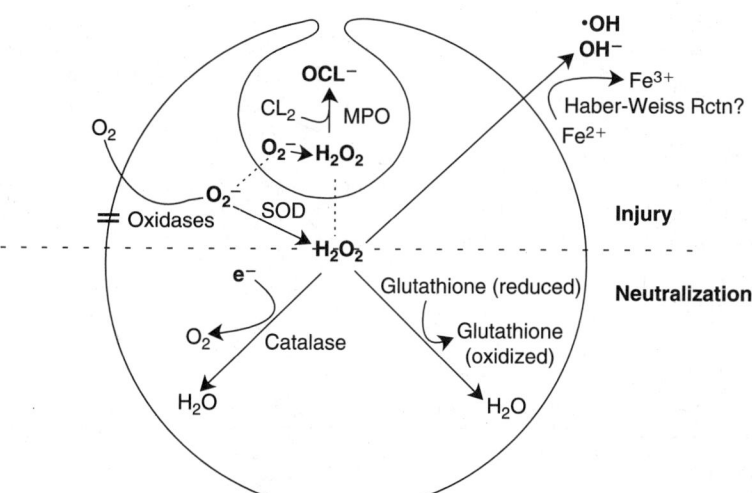

Fig. 5-2. Overview of the essential intracellular and extracellular pathways in oxygen radical generation and neutralization. SOD = superoxide dismutase, OCL^- = hypochlorous acid, MPO = myeloperoxidase.

products indicated that peroxidation of photoreceptor membranes, especially the depletion of polyunsaturated fatty acid docosahexaenoic acid 22 : 6, occurs simultaneously with the onset of free radical formation and electrophysiologic loss of photoreceptor function. The peroxidation products are chemotactic for PMNs, thereby providing a mechanism for amplifying the cycle of inflammatory tissue destruction. Some argue that free radical damage is less important in the anterior segment because of diminished content of polyunsaturated lipids and increased concentration of natural antioxidants and free radical scavengers.

Protection studies with various agents that inhibit the formation of toxic oxygen metabolites, such as catalase (an antioxidant enzyme), dimethylsulfoxide (a free radical scavenger), superoxide dismutase (an antioxidant enzyme), aminicotinamide (an NADPH inhibitor), vitamin E (a free radical scavenger), and desferoxamine (an iron chelation), indicate a role for toxic oxygen moieties in autoimmune[166] and lens-associated[123] uveitis. It remains to be seen if similar events occur in chronic uveitis models, especially when macrophage infiltrates predominate.

Toxic Nitrogen Products. Another important pathway of nonspecific defense involves toxic products of nitrogen. This pathway was first observed in patients with a deficiency of the respiratory burst enzymes. As such, their PMNs and macrophages were unable to generate reactive oxygen intermediates, but were still able to mount effective antimicrobial function via a toxic nitrogen product, nitric oxide (NO).[217] How NO functions to kill microorganisms is not known with certainty. Likely possibilities include interaction with the Fe-S groups of aconitase (an enzyme important for the control of DNA synthesis and RNA production) or complex I and complex II of the mitochondrial electron transport system.[62,217] NO may also interact with O_2 to form the toxic hydroxyl radical as well as NO_2.[19]

The formation of NO is dependent upon the enzyme nitric oxide synthase that is located in the cytosol and is NADPH-dependent.[126] NO is formed from the terminal guanidino-nitrogen atoms of L-arginine. Two forms of nitric oxide synthase are known: constitutive and inducible. Many cells produce basal levels of NO, which is secondary to the calcium-dependent, constitutive form of the enzyme. Activation induces enhanced production of NO in certain cells, especially macrophages. This enhanced production appears to be secondary to the induced synthesis of a second, calcium-independent form of NO synthase.[126] Cytokines may play an important role in the modulation of NO production in the inducible system. Both IFN-γ and TNF-α induce NO,[149,151] but both cytokines additionally require a second stimulus, such as lipopolysaccharide, to cause maximal NO production. If both cytokines are used in combination, second stimuli are not required and the combination is synergistic.[149,151] In addition, other cytokines can inhibit NO synthesis, including a macrophage deactivation factor and TGF β.[59]

The contribution of reactive nitrogen radicals to ocular inflammation remains to be investigated thoroughly. Preliminary evidence for a role for macrophage-derived NO in ocular inflammation has been suggested for a model of lens-associated uveitis[221] in herpes simplex virus stromal keratitis and for endotoxin-induced uveitis.

Lymphocyte and Macrophage Secretory Products. Leukocytes contribute to inflammation by releasing their contents into tissues during phagocytosis. Macrophages function normally as secretory cells, and upon activation, secrete even more products, including many soluble mediators (Table 5-1).[91] A partial list of macrophage secretory products is presented in Table 5-1. Although the extracellular release of granule products is probably unintentional in the case of PMNs, certain lymphocytes (such as cytotoxic T cells and the large granular lymphocytes of the ''null cell'' series) also contain cytoplasmic granules that are designed for extracellular release.[21] These granule products include a number of specialized molecules and enzymes capable of killing tumor and host cells. For example, perforin, a molecule similar to the complement membrane attack complex, causes pore formation and cell lysis.[163] The exact role that these other leukocyte products play in inflammation is uncertain, and almost nothing is known about the function of these molecules in ocular inflammation.

TABLE 5-1 SECRETORY PRODUCTS OF MACROPHAGES

Constitutive	Induced
Proteins	
Apolipoprotein E	Acid hydrolases
Alpha$_2$-macroglobulin	Angiogenesis factors
Complement (C_{1q}, C_2, C_4)	Arginase
Factor H, Factor I	Interferon-β
Lipoprotein lipase	Tumor necrosis factor-α
Lysozyme	Collagenase
	Colony-stimulating factors
	Elastase
	Factor B
	Interleukins (IL-1 and IL-6)
	Macrophage-derived growth factor
	Plasminogen activator
	Chemokines
Lipids	
	Leukotriene C_4
	Platelet-activating factor
	Prostaglandins E_2, F_2
	6-Keto-prostaglandin F
Others	
Thymidine	Hydrogen peroxide
	Superoxide anion
	Hydroxyl radical

SOLUBLE MEDIATORS OF INFLAMMATION

Inflammatory responses involve the passage of fluids and cells from nearby blood vessels. Certain molecules found in plasma, released by leukocytes, produced by inflamed tissues, or generated by microorganisms may produce the cardinal manifestations of inflammation. Molecules generated within the host that induce inflammation are termed inflammatory mediators, and several categories of molecules qualify as mediators. Most mediators act on target cells via receptor-mediated processes, and some act in enzymatic cascades that interact in a complex fashion.[150]

In evaluating the role of a specific mediator in inflammation, three types of experimental studies, "injection, detection, and protection," are required to confirm its contribution. Direct tissue injection ("injection") of a mediator proves that a mediator can, at the very least, induce some component of inflammation, such as a cellular infiltrate or vascular leakage. Transgenic mice, genetically engineered to inappropriately synthesize a specific factor within the eye, have become an elegant method to replace injection studies for some cytokines. Measurement of mediator concentration during inflammation ("detection"), especially in association with temporal changes in severity, is good evidence of an association of a mediator with the inflammatory response. Finally, demonstration that inflammation is diminished by pharmacologic inhibitors, natural antagonists, or neutralizing antibodies ("protection") provides evidence of participation of a specific mediator in a particular model of inflammation. Unfortunately, this trio of studies has not been performed in the eye for many important mediators. Furthermore, this approach does not address the complex interactions between multiple mediators. Nevertheless, the three-way approach permits speculation about how the principal groups of soluble inflammatory mediators may participate in ocular inflammation.

Vasoactive Amines

Histamine and serotonin are small preformed molecules released early during inflammatory responses that cause smooth muscle contraction and strongly influence vascular permeability. Both amines subserve other functions in addition to those that are inflammatory. For example, serotonin also functions as a neurotransmitter.

Histamine is present in the granules of mast cells and basophils and is actively secreted following exposure of cells to a wide range of secretagogues.[69,218] One pathway for degranulation is antigen crosslinking of IgE bound to mast cell IgE receptors, but during most acute inflammatory responses this pathway is not involved. Many inflammatory stimuli can induce histamine release.[218] Histamine acts by binding to one of at least three known types of receptors present differentially on target cells.[32,69] In addition to direct proinflammatory effects, histamine also causes inflammation by stimulating cytokine production and receptor expression.[69]

Platelets provide the principal source of serotonin. Platelets release serotonin from granules following activation or aggregation.[215] Platelet plasma membranes are highly activatable and respond rapidly to a wide variety of injuries and inflammatory stimuli. Platelets also act as a source of other inflammatory mediators, such as platelet-activating factors and thromboxanes, the latter causing platelet aggregation and further activation.[215] Serotonin is also released by mast cells. Mast cell-derived products, especially serotonin, have been postulated to contribute to the initiation of delayed hypersensitivity by producing transient altered vascular permeability that mediates the later onset of cellular infiltration.[14]

Vasoactive amines are important mediators for certain types of ocular inflammation, especially allergic reactions of the ocular surface. When topically applied, histamine induces hyperemia (vascular leakage of the conjunctiva) in rabbits[88] and symptoms of allergy in humans.[2] Moreover, elevated tear histamine has been detected in vernal conjunctivitis in association with degranulated mast cells of the conjunctiva.[3] Mast cell stabilizers, such as cromolyn and lodoxamide, are effective in reducing symptoms in vernal conjunctivitis and other related disorders.[75]

The contribution of histamine to intraocular inflammation remains equivocal. Histamine can be detected in normal aqueous humor,[2] but increased levels with inflammation have not been documented. Upon injection of high doses into the anterior chamber or vitreous cavity, histamine causes breakdown of the blood-eye barrier.[13] Treatment with antihistamines protects against breakdown of the blood-eye barrier in immune complex (IC)-mediated uveitis[155] but has less effect in lipopolysaccharide-induced uveitis, diminishing vascular leakage but not cellular infiltrates.[45,100]

Serotonin occurs as a normal constituent of aqueous humor[127] and could play a role in uveitis. Cyproheptadine, a serotonin (and H_1) receptor antagonist, and methysergide are partially efficacious in diminishing vascular leakage associated with lipopolysaccharide-uveitis.[45,100] These antagonists are less efficacious in preventing cellular infiltration. In several studies, a combination of antihistamines and serotonin antagonists had an additive effect.[45,100]

Plasma-Derived Proteins

Complement Factors. Components and fragments of the complement cascade, accounting for approximately 5% of blood proteins, are important endogenous mediators of inflammatory responses. The complement system can be activated directly by foreign stimuli and undergoes self-amplification, giving rise to a rapid and substantial role during inflammation.[145,169]

Many stimuli associated with inflammatory responses can initiate complement activation pathways. Immune complexes activate complement via the classical pathway; microorganisms, their products, or injured cell surfaces generally activate complement via the alternative pathway. Both activation pathways generate products that contribute to the inflammatory process.

Complement serves three basic functions during inflammation: (1) coating antigenic or pathogenic surfaces by C3b to enhance phagocytosis; (2) causing lysis of cell membranes through pore formation by membrane attack complexes; and (3) recruiting of PMNs and inducing of inflammation through generation of small polypeptides called anaphylatoxins (C3a, C4a, and C5a). The anaphylatoxins, so named because they cause anaphylaxis upon systemic administration into animals, are the principal complement-derived mediators. Their effects include chemotaxis and changes in cell adhesiveness mediated principally by C5a, and release of preformed and newly synthesized mediators from mast cells and platelets, mediated by all three anaphylatoxins.[35,145] The latter effects include those caused by vasoactive amines, arachidonic acid metabolites, and platelet-activating factors.[186] The proinflammatory complement mediator, C5a, also stimulates oxidative metabolism, production and release of toxic oxygen radicals from leukocytes, and extracellular discharge of leukocyte granule contents.

Complement is an important inflammatory mediator in the eye. Injection of C5a into the conjunctiva, cornea, or vitreous induces infiltration by PMNs and monocytes.[20] Intact components of the complement cascade occur in most ocular tissues, including conjunctiva, sclera, and cornea.[142] As such, C3a and C4a (but not C5a) could be generated within normal corneas after triggering complement activation with either the alternative or classical pathways. C3a and C4a are present in the aqueous humor or vitreous fluid of patients with a variety of bacterial or viral causes of intraocular inflammation.[141,143] C5a has also been detected in the aqueous humor of rabbit eyes with lipopolysaccharide-induced vascular leakage but, paradoxically, without evident cellular infiltrate.[176]

Protection studies can be performed by inhibiting the complement cascade with systemic administration of the cobra venom factor that depletes C3.[109] This technique of complement inactivation was employed to demonstrate that complement plays an important role in many different experimental models of immune-triggered inflammation, including corneal inflammation,[209] lens-associated uveitis,[124] and intraocular Arthus reaction to autoantigens.[125] Studies are needed to determine the source of production of complement components (derived from blood versus produced locally in the eye by fibroblasts or macrophages), to determine the regulation of the breakdown of anaphylatoxins within ocular tissues, and to assess the contribution of complement to human immunogenic inflammation and other disorders.[42]

Kinin-Forming System. Kinins are low-molecular-weight polypeptides derived from precursors, called kininogens, in plasma and tissue fluids. They mediate numerous inflammatory effects including vasodilation, pain, constriction of smooth muscle, increased vascular permeability, and stimulation of arachidonic acid metabolism.[164] The proinflammatory action of kinins appears to result from an active nonapeptide moiety, binding to one of at least two receptors.[168] Although no known physiologic antagonists of kinins have been identified, their activity is curtailed by enzymatic degradation by kininogenases and kininases found in tissue fluids as well as in PMNs.[183]

The generation of kinins proceeds in multiple steps typical of cascade reactions, and more than one pathway exists. In one pathway, the inflammatory trigger activates the Hageman factor. This activation, in turn, converts inactivate proenzymes (prekallikrein) into active forms (kallikrein). Substrates for the kallikrein enzymes are kininogens that are converted into kinins. The best known kinin product of the Hageman factor-dependent pathway is bradykinin. A second kinin, lysbradykinin, is derived from tissue kininogens. These are enzymatically degraded into kinins by tissue kallikreins, which are generated from prekallikrein precursors probably by tissue or cellular proteases.[168] Four cascade systems (kinin, fibrinolytic, clotting, and complement) all interact via the Hageman factor, a plasma protein activatable by numerous stimuli. These include negatively charged surfaces (urate crystals), collagen, trypsin, plasmin, kallikrein, clotting, factor XI, and lipopolysaccharide.

The role of ocular kinin activation has not been thoroughly investigated. Conjunctiva and intraocular tissues contain kallikrein and its precursors, so activation of the kininogens within the eye is possible.[116] Injection of high concentrations of bradykinin into the vitreous apparently induces blood-eye barrier breakdown and miosis.[41] These effects appeared to be mediated indirectly through the neurogenic release of a neuropeptide, substance P.[37] Bradykinins and related peptides might serve a physiologic role in regulating aqueous humor production, intraocular pressure, and ocular blood flow.[117] Both bradykinin and substance P are related to a family of structurally similar peptides, called tachykinins, which are naturally occurring, neurally derived homologous proteins present in ocular nerves.[181]

Fibrin. Fibrin deposition has long been considered a clinical sign of delayed hypersensitivity. Fibrin deposits in skin lesions of delayed hypersensitivity give the skin a ''hardened'' or indurated feeling upon palpation, and extracellular fibrin deposits are visible by histologic examination.[24,65] Fibrin is released from its circulating zymogen precursor, fibrinogen, upon cleavage by thrombin, also a zymogen.[170] Polymerization of smaller units gives rise to the characteristic fibrin plugs or clots. Fibrin dissolution is mediated by plasmin and activated from its zymogen precursor, plasminogen, by plasminogen activators. In experimental animals, measurements of fibrin deposition reveal that quantitative increases in fibrin deposition are associated with T cell-mediated delayed hypersensitivity, but substantial deposits also occur in other forms of inflammation.[24,65] Inhibition of fibrin deposition lessens the severity of delayed hypersensitivity. Prevention of clot formation with heparin or other anticlotting agents diminishes experimental delayed hypersensitivity reactions.[105]

The role of fibrin deposits in the eye during uveitis is unknown. Intraocular fibrin deposition has been studied in the context of trauma and intraocular scarring diseases, such as proliferative vitreoretinopathy. In these disorders, fibrin clot formation provides a scaffold for aberrant intraocular growth of retinal pigment epithelium and other scar tissue cells.[122] Recombinant plasminogen activator (tPA), an enzyme that activates plasminogen into plasmin, effectively dissolve clots caused by postoperative inflammation after vitrectomy[102] or cataract surgery.[107] Fibrin deposition presumably contributes to synechiae formation in uveitis. Although fibrin clots are prominent clinical signs in acute uveitis, clots fail to form in chronic cases, presumably because high aqueous humor levels of natural plasminogen activators and plasmin are present.

Other Plasma Components. The contribution of other plasma components to inflammation and lymphocyte activation has received little investigation. In vitro studies reveal that serum and plasma contain numerous bioactive substances that enhance lymphocyte and macrophage activation, including cell attachment factors and cytokines. For example, platelet-derived growth factor (PDGF) in serum alters the pattern of T cell activation and cytokine synthesis.[51] The contribution of other active agents in plasma has not been as well defined, including the role of arginine (as a substrate for macrophage nitric oxide synthase), transferrin or iron (crucial for proliferation and free radical production), steroid hormones, and proteases. An increasing number of cytokines are known to be released in an inactive precursor form that requires an extracellular activation step. Plasma-derived proteases might be one source of enzymes for activation; conversely, plasma might be a source of protease inhibitors that prevents cell surface-associated proteases from activating the zymogens.[52]

An intact blood-ocular barrier excludes serum proteins from the normal eye. Studies of the impact of serum proteins in uveitis are lacking, primarily as a result of the lack of models for chronic inflammation. Secondary aqueous humor containing high serum protein content stimulates lymphocyte and macrophage activation in vitro,[200] however. This serum effect may result from the addition of stimulating factors (perhaps PDGF), plus the loss of inhibitory factors from aqueous humor caused by the protease inhibitor alpha$_2$-macroglobulin, which binds and neutralizes some of the natural immunosuppressive factors in aqueous humor. Conversely, lymphocytes incubated in serum-free assays tend to be more sensitive to immunomodulation by suppressor factors in aqueous humor than those incubated in the presence of serum. A therapeutic strategy targeting restoration of the blood-eye barrier might enable better immuno-suppressive control of the cellular activation with other agents.

Lipid Mediators — Eicosanoids and Platelet-Activating Factors

Two groups of lipid molecules synthesized by stimulated cells act as powerful mediators and regulators of inflammatory responses: arachidonic acid metabolites (the eicosanoids) and acetylated triglycerides, usually called platelet-activating factors (PAF). Both groups of molecules are rapidly generated from the same lysophospholipid precursors by the enzymatic action of cellular phospholipases such as phospholipase A$_2$.

Eicosanoids. Eicosanoids are biologic mediators of many physiologic functions, including the inflammatory responses. All eicosanoids are derived from arachidonic acid that is liberated from membrane phospholipids by phospholipase A (activated by various agonists). Arachidonic acid is oxidized by two major pathways to generate the various mediators: the cyclooxygenase pathway derivatives (prostaglandins, thromboxanes, and prostacyclins) and the 5-lipoxygenase pathway derivatives (hydroxyeicosatetraenoic acid, lipoxins, and leukotrienes). Fig. 5-3 illustrates these pathways, and Table 5-2 lists the principal functions of these metabolites.

The cyclooxygenase-derived mediators are evanescent compounds induced by a variety of stimuli, including other inflammatory mediators (PAF and some cytokines). They act in the immediate environment of their release to mediate many proinflammatory activities, often interacting with other mediators to modulate particular functions.[162] More-

TABLE 5-2   ACTIVITIES OF SOME EICOSANOIDS OF OCULAR IMPORTANCE

Molecule	Effect
Cyclooxygenase Derivatives	
Prostaglandin E$_2$	Increased blood flow
	Activation of pain receptors
	Release of histamine and serotonin
	Pyrogenic
	Increased vascular permeability
	T cell inhibition
	Suppression of LTB$_4$ synthesis by PMN or macrophages
Prostaglandin I$_2$	Vasodilatation
Thromboxane B$_2$	Vasoconstriction
Lipoxygenase Derivatives	
Leukotriene B$_4$	Leukocyte adhesion
	Chemotaxis and diapedesis
	Lysozomal enzyme release
Lipoxins	Superoxide anion production

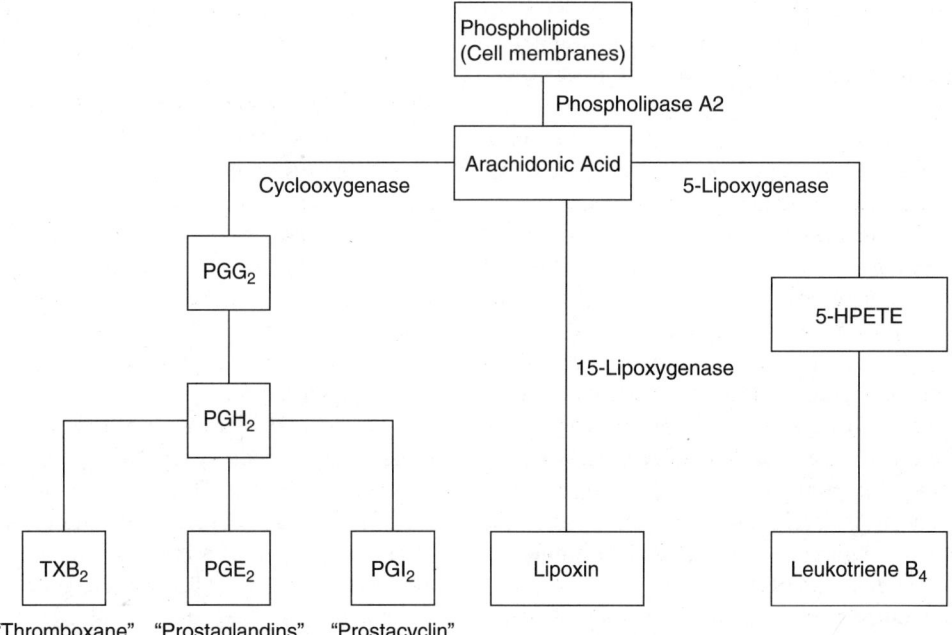

Fig. 5-3.   Schematic overview of the major eicosanoid pathways.

over, some compounds are taken up by cells and are further metabolized into active mediators.

The other major pathway of arachidonic acid metabolism is via the 5-lipoxygenase pathway, an enzyme found mainly in granulocytes and mast cells. Lipoxygenase derivatives have been also detected in the brain and retina. The products of this pathway are numerous and some are extremely potent mediators of the inflammatory response.[119] One of the best characterized is leukotriene B_4 (LTB$_4$), a potent chemotactic factor that also causes lysosomal enzyme release and reactive oxygen radical production by granulocytes. Some leukotrienes may have 1000-fold the activity of histamine on vascular permeability. Another lipoxygenase product, lipoxin, is a potent stimulator of superoxide anion.

Prostaglandins and other eicosanoids play a major role in regulating ocular processes beyond participating as mediators of inflammation.[31] Interest in the role of prostaglandins in ocular inflammation began with the discovery of "irin," an inflammatory substance extracted from rabbit irises.[9] Subsequently, irin was found to contain prostaglandins E and F.[10] Even though some of the eicosanoids are probably crucial to ocular inflammation, much of the extensive literature is difficult to interpret. Differential responsiveness among species, variability in experimental conditions, unknown purity of reagents in early studies, and degradation within ocular tissues influence interpretation of experimental data. Even the active inflammatory mediator in irin is in dispute, as some have postulated that nonprostaglandin contaminants of the early preparations, such as neuropeptides, were active components.[194]

Prostaglandins clearly regulate vascular permeability in the eye, but their role in mediating cellular infiltration is uncertain. Topical, intracameral, or intravitreal administration of various prostaglandins indicate that many cyclooxygenase derivatives induce vasodilation and breakdown of the blood-eye barriers.[161,222] The ability of prostaglandin injections to induce acute cellular inflammation is equivocal,[66,206] however. Although prostaglandins can be detected in the aqueous humor during uveitis,[27] after trauma,[30] and following ocular surgery,[38] it is likely that eicosanoids have a complex relationship to inflammation. Inhibitors of cyclooxygenase to prevent prostaglandin production afford only incomplete protection,[25] and a blockade of prostaglandin production is associated with only partial inhibition of cellular infiltration.[45,114]

In contrast, leukotrienes contribute directly to inflammatory infiltration. Injection of leukotriene B_4 into rabbit eyes causes PMN infiltration,[26] and this mediator is present in aqueous humor of animals[28] and patients[158] with uveitis. Although specific inhibitors of leukotriene synthesis are not widely available, one experimental inhibitor, BWA4C, inhibits cellular infiltrates but not vascular permeability in experimental uveitis.[28] The proinflammatory role of other eicosanoids, especially various prostacyclins or thromboxanes, remains to be investigated.

The eicosanoids have been postulated to contribute to various other sequela of inflammation. Much interest has been generated concerning the role of prostaglandins in miosis of the pupil during inflammation, although most prostaglandins have minimal or no significant miotic activity on nonhuman, primate, or human eyes.[136] Some eicosanoids have been hypothesized to cause corneal neovascularization.[195] Prostaglandins may be the cause of macular edema in association with anterior segment surgery or inflammation.[137-139] Posterior diffusion of one or more of the eicosanoids through the vitreous is presumed to alter capillary permeability of the perifoveal capillary network, leading to the characteristic pattern of intraretinal fluid accumulation and cyst formation. Clinical trials in humans have indicated that topical treatment with cyclooxygenase inhibitors diminish the onset of mild cystoid macular edema after cataract surgery[137,139] and might be efficacious in the treatment of severe, persistent macular edema.[104]

Platelet-Activating Factors. Platelet-activating factors (PAF) are potent agonists for most inflammatory cells and function by binding to one or more protein-associated receptors on target cells.[162] Some of the widespread effects of PAF associated with inflammatory responses are depicted in Table 5-3. Several species of PAFs can be produced by individual cells and their physiologic effects on target cells may differ. Multiple PAFs seem to orchestrate many aspects of the inflammatory response and interact with numerous eicosanoids.[162]

PAFs are associated with ocular inflammation.[178] Contradictory evidence has been generated in relation to the ability of PAF to directly induce inflammation. One study indicated that PAF might cause retinal vascular constriction and inflammation after intravenous administration in rabbits,[34] but another study failed to confirm these findings.[178] Detection of PAF in fluids or tissues of eyes with inflammation has not been reported, reflecting the rapid uptake and clearance of PAF from tissues.

Other lines of evidence indicate that PAF is an important cofactor in ocular inflammation. Both the anterior segment and retina can synthesize PAF and express receptors for PAF.[173] Significant levels of PAF were detected in media conditioned by iris and ciliary body explants obtained from rabbit eyes with lipopolysaccharide-induced uveitis, but the source of the PAF (leukocytes, nonpigmented epithelium of the ciliary body or endothelium) was not determined.[173]

Protection studies with PAF receptor inhibitors diminish the severity of the leakage after procedures that break the blood-eye barrier by trauma in the absence of inflammation.[179] In uveitis models caused by immune complex-mediated inflammation or intravitreal IL-1 injection, both vascular permeability and cell infiltration were diminished by administration of PAF inhibitors.[177] The interpretation of these studies depends upon the specificity of the activity of the inhibitors. Since PAF is suspected to initiate the production of various eicosanoids, it may participate as a regulator or initiator of other mediators. The complex nature of its interaction with prostaglandins and other mediators needs better characterization.

Cytokines

Cytokines are polypeptide mediators synthesized and released by cells at the site of inflammation to act on neighboring cells (paracrine action) or on the synthesizing cell itself (autocrine action). In other cases, some cytokines are

TABLE 5-3 SOME EFFECTS OF PLATELET-ACTIVATING FACTORS ON CELLS OF THE INFLAMMATORY RESPONSE (MODIFIED FROM PINCKARD AND ASSOCIATES[162])

Cell	Activities
Vascular endothelial cell	Calcium uptake
	Neutrophil adherence
	Plasminogen activator release
Neutrophil	Chemotaxis
	Chemokinesis
	Aggregation
	Enhanced adherence
	Lysosomal enzyme release
	Leukotriene synthesis
	HETE production
	Superoxide anion production
	Calcium uptake
	Phosphatidylinositol turnover
Vascular smooth-muscle cell	Prostaglandin synthesis
	Calcium efflux
	Phosphatidylinositol turnover
Monocyte-macrophage	Chemotaxis
	Aggregation
	Superoxide anion production
	Differentiation
	Calcium uptake
	Prostaglandin and thromboxane
Production	Increased spreading
	IL-I production
	TNF production
Eosinophil	Chemotaxis
	Leukotriene production
	Superoxide anion production
Platelet	Secretion
	Aggregation
	Calcium uptake
	Phosphatidylinositol turnover
	Thromboxane synthesis
	Myosin phosphorylation

released into the blood to act on a distant site (hormonal action). Many cytokines contribute to inflammation, such as uveitis,[53] but the precise role of individual molecules during a specific inflammatory response is difficult to determine. Most studies focus on the isolated activity of a particular cytokine, discussed in terms of one of the "cardinal triads" of studies (injection, detection, or protection). The function of a specific cytokine must be interpreted in the context of the inflammatory milieu in which many factors act simultaneously. Cytokines usually have pleiotropic activities that overlap and counteract depending upon the target. Consequently, cytokine interactions might be combinatorial (two factors combining for greater effect than the sum of their individual activities), synergistic (two factors enabling a new activity not manifest by either alone), or antagonistic. In addition, for some cytokines, an immunoregulatory role may be more important than its direct action on parenchymal tissues as mediators of inflammation. The function of various cytokines might change during the course of an inflammatory response. Some cytokines appear to have paradoxic, bifunctional activities—stimulatory in one context but inhibitory in another setting.

Interleukin 1 (IL-1). Interleukin 1, which is present in two forms, IL-1α and IL-1β (each of approximately 17 kD), is one of the major cytokines that participates in inflammatory responses.[60] Many cell types produce IL-1, but macrophages are probably the principal source.[58] Numerous stimuli induce cells to produce IL-1, including signals, such as lipopolysaccharide, complement fragments, and other cytokines, particularly TNF.[140] IL-1 acts on a broad spectrum of target cells and induces them to express numerous proinflammatory effects. IL-1 is also an important regulator of the immune response. The effects of IL-1 are mediated via binding to high-affinity receptors on target cells.[61]

Of the numerous proinflammatory effects of IL-1, the production and release of prostaglandins from parenchymal cells, such as fibroblasts and endothelial cells, appear crucial.[64,228] IL-1 also causes the secretion of tissue-damaging proteases from phagocytes, procoagulants, and plasminogen activator from macrophages.[140] It stimulates the release of other cytokines such as TNF-α and IL-6,[64] and IL-1 is responsible for increased expression of molecules such as the adhesins that play a role during cell migration to inflammatory sites. Overproduction of IL-1 can be a major contributory factor in disseminated intravascular coagulation and chronic inflammation.[63] Physiologic IL-1 receptor antagonists are produced by inflammatory cells, resulting in a natural downregulation of the effects of IL-1.[130] The use of such receptor antagonists and their synthetic derivatives has been considered as therapy for controlling inflammation.[57]

IL-1 is difficult to measure because several biologic forms are released.[56] IL-1 lacks the classical signal peptide sequence necessary for conventional secretory pathways, implying that IL-1 (particularly IL-1α) might function as a cell surface-retained signal or be secreted in a unique fashion. This cell-associated form would not be released into the extracellular environment even though it was very bioactive. In addition, a latent form of soluble IL-1 (IL-1 propeptide) has been recognized that might be measured as active in some assays, but not fully functioning and contributing to the inflammatory process.[56] Furthermore, IL-1 avidly binds to plasma α_2-macroglobulin, a plasma-derived protease inhibitor and natural scavenger of cytokines. Yet, bound IL-1 remains in bioactive form, so that IL-1 bound to α_2-macroglobulin can be delivered into the site by leakage of plasma and be protected from clearance by other proteases.[33] This form of IL-1 is detectable by bioassay but not by ELISA.

The natural antagonists to IL-1, including soluble receptors, can interfere with certain bioassays for this cytokine. Therefore, detection studies for IL-1 and probably for all cytokines, should be carefully scrutinized for these types of confounding variables.

Direct injection of IL-1 into the eye produces altered vascular permeability and acute cellular infiltration of the uvea and retina with PMNs, and later with monocytes.[113,175] The inflammatory response resolves within several days. Intracorneal injection of IL-1β caused induction of IL-8 in corneal explants, indicating that some of the ocular effects of IL-1 are likely to be indirect, via the induction of other signals.[67] In addition, IL-1 is a potent stimulator of ocular prostaglandin and PAF activation.[113] Protection from the inflammatory effects of IL-1 has been attempted with several modalities. Intravitreal injection with neutralizing antibodies can block the effects of IL-1 up to 6 hours after cytokine injection, suggesting that the early inflammatory effects of IL-1 are the consequence of direct actions of the cytokine.[128] Similarly, protection from the infiltration and protein leakage can be demonstrated with intravitreal injection of the IL-1 receptor antagonist or soluble IL-1 receptors only when the eye is pretreated and not if the antagonists are injected after onset of inflammation.[172] The antagonist had little effect, however, upon lipopolysaccharide-induced uveitis indicating that other cytokines in addition to IL-1 are contributing to inflammation in this model. Finally, some of the inflammatory effects of intravitreally injected IL-1 can be blocked by pharmacologic inhibitors of PAFs and prostaglandins.[177] The detection of IL-1 during uveitis has not been documented.

Tumor Necrosis Factor (TNF-α or TNF-β). TNF exists in two homologous forms (TNF-α or TNF-β), each of approximately 17 kD.[5] First recognized as a factor capable of inducing tumor cell death and ischemic necrosis of whole tumors, the tumor necrosis factor's main function is mediating acute inflammation. When present in high concentrations in blood, it is associated with the accompanying effects of wasting disease (cachexia) and bone resorption.[22] TNF-β was formerly called cachectin. TNF-α is mainly produced by macrophages, whereas T cells generate TNF-β, a related molecule with high homology and nearly identical activity.[11]

TNF-α has a broad range of activities and alters the function of multiple-target cells.[22] The profile of its effects closely resembles IL-1 and may in part be mediated by IL-1. Thus TNF-α induces IL-1 from inflammatory cells. TNF-α is a major mediator of cell adhesion and chemotaxis and largely contributes to the regulation of cell migration during inflammation. Other prominent effects include the triggering of lipid mediators of inflammation, induction of reactive oxygen radicals, and the production and release of proinflammatory enzymes from cells.[23] The effects of TNF-α are mediated via binding of the cytokine to one of at least two receptors that have been identified and cloned.[199] As with

IL-1, natural inhibitors for TNF-α have been recognized that may downregulate the effects of TNF-α. TNF-α injection into tissue sites induces acute inflammation, vascular injury, and fibrin deposition.[1] Since vascular plugging, fibrin deposition, and ischemic necrosis are features of delayed hypersensitivity reactions, TNF-α is probably one of the major mediators of this response. TNF-α has also been shown to be a major mediator in the Shwartzman reaction.[1]

Intravitreal injections of microgram amounts of TNF-α result in protein leakage and mononuclear cell infiltration, but various features suggest that TNF-α works indirectly through the stimulation of other chemical mediators. First, the onset of TNF-α-induced infiltration is slightly delayed (24 to 48 hours) and longer lasting compared to that induced by injections of other cytokines, consisting of greater density of monocytes and less neutrophils.[72,174] Second, intracorneal injection of TNF-α induces IL-8 production by stomal keratocytes.[67] Pharmacologic blockade of the effects of intravitreal TNF-α has been attempted with cyclooxygenase inhibitors or PAF antagonists. Treatment with both antagonists was most effective, resulting in decreased vascular permeability without profound effect on cell infiltrate. TNF-α induces inflammation indirectly via the activation of lipid mediators.[73] TNF-α has a complex, synergistic interrelationship with other mediators of ocular inflammation, especially IL-1 and lipopolysaccharide.

Although detection of TNF-α in ocular fluids has been difficult, it has been detected by cytoplasmic immunostaining within infiltrating lymphocytes obtained from vitrectomy specimens in eyes with AIDS-associated retinitis.[97] A preliminary report indicates that aqueous TNF levels are elevated in lipopolysaccharide-induced uveitis.[53]

Interleukin 6 (IL-6). Interleukin 6 is another cytokine that regulates the function of multiple-cell types including those involved in inflammatory responses. IL-6, ranging in size between 21 to 30 kD, is an important regulator of T and B cell function and stimulates growth and differentiation of hemopoietic cells.[208] IL-6 is probably a principal mediator of acute phase protein production by hepatocytes.[79] Because the large number of acute phase proteins limit tissue damage and facilitate healing, the hepatic effects of IL-6 may be important in limiting the extent of inflammation.[23] Multiple-cell types produce IL-6, but only in response to appropriate stimulation. Included among the stimulants are the inflammatory cytokines Il1 and TNF. Rather than acting alone in mediating many of its effects, IL-6 may interact synergistically with IL-1 and perhaps TNF.[64,111] Evidence for synergy has been obtained mainly for effects on T cell proliferation and acute phase protein production. Increasing evidence suggests that IL-6 overproduction may be associated with certain chronic inflammatory responses such as psoriasis, rheumatoid arthritis, and glomerulonephritis.[93]

Intravitreal injection of IL-6 produces altered vascular permeability and severe uveal and retinal infiltration with PMNs.[95,96] Repeated injections of IL-6 result in desensitization and unresponsiveness.[94] Aqueous humor levels of IL-6 are correlated with the clinical inflammation in lipopolysaccharide-induced uveitis. Elevated aqueous humor IL-6 levels have been detected in many forms of human uveitis, especially Fuchs uveitis syndrome.[96,146,147] IL-6 is an important mediator in other intraocular diseases, such as proliferative vitreoretinopathy.[120]

Interleukin 8 (IL-8) and the Chemokines. IL-8 is the best-characterized member of a larger family of polypeptide mediators called the chemokines.[225] All members of this family (IL-8, monocyte chemotactic protein-2, and many others) have a similar molecular size (8-10 kD), structure, and function.[225] IL-8 is primarily a potent chemotactic factor for PMNs[40] and, to a lesser extent, other granulocytes and lymphocytes.

The chemokines resist degradation in conditions typical of inflammatory responses, such as low pH and activated proteolytic enzymes. IL-8 is produced by several cell types, including lymphocytes, macrophages, fibroblasts, epithelial cells, and vascular endothelial cells.[171] IL-8 production by vascular endothelium may regulate migration of PMNs from blood vessels into tissues. Most cells produce IL-8 in response to exogenous signals, especially to the cytokines IL-1 and TNF-α[171] or even some bacterial products. Thus IL-8 is indirectly regulated through the action of other cytokines produced earlier in the inflammatory response.

The ocular effects of IL-8 have not been well characterized. Intravitreal injection of IL-8 produces a mild infiltration of PMNs and vascular permeability, becoming maximal within 24 hours.[71] A preliminary report indicates that IL-8 is present in the vitreous of patients with uveitis. IL-8 synthesis can be induced in corneal fibroblasts after treatment with IL-1 or TNF.[67]

Interferon Gamma (IFN-γ). Interferon-γ is a 15 kD polypeptide that is primarily produced by antigen-stimulated T cells or natural killer cells.[148] This factor functions during immune-mediated inflammatory lesions and exerts numerous activities on cells. At high concentrations, it is an inflammatory mediator inducing the recruitment of PMNs and monocytes if injected into the skin. At lower concentrations, IFN-γ is an immunomodulator without direct inflammatory activities, including the ability to induce cell activation, the secretion of proinflammatory mediators from cells,[29] the up-regulation of cell adhesion molecules, and an increased susceptibility to other cytokines. IFN-γ is a potent activator of macrophage effector cell function,[134] and paracrine feedback of this molecule from T cells to macrophages may be a T cell strategy for amplifying inflammation.

When high concentrations are injected into the vitreous, IFN-γ induces a significant inflammatory infiltrate within the uvea, aqueous humor, and vitreous that consists of PMNs and monocytes.[115] Transgenic mice, which inappropriately synthesize IFN-γ in the eye, develop spontaneous ocular inflammation. Systemic injection of this agent,[89] or intracameral injection of low concentration of IFN-γ,[47] induces noninflammatory, physiologic changes in the eye, including upregulation of class II molecules on intraocular cells and recruitment of additional leukocytes (probably macrophages) into the iris. IFN-γ also induces prostaglandin synthesis when added to cultures of nonpigmented epithelium and occurs in ciliary body explants if cultured after anterior chamber injection with IFN-γ.[197]

Little information exists about levels of IFN-γ in ocular fluids during experimental or clinical uveitis. As expected, normal ocular fluids or vitreous from eyes with hemorrhage or retinal detachment contain no IFN-γ.[98,141] Some eyes of patients with infectious retinitis, including those with AIDS, have significant vitreous levels,[141] however. Additionally, IFN-γ-producing T cells have been identified infiltrating the cornea during experimental herpes simplex virus keratitis[204] and in the retina during experimental autoimmune uveoretinitis.[39] Protection from the effects of IFN-γ with neutralizing antibodies may suppress autoimmune retinitis.[15]

Transforming Growth Factor Beta (TGF-β). TGF-β is a 25-kD polypeptide cytokine with numerous, often seemingly contradictory biologic activities.[189] As the name suggests, TGF-β was initially defined by its ability to transform the phenotype of nonneoplastic cells in culture. TGF-β, however, was subsequently found to mediate other additional functions, including effects on cells involved in inflammation and the immune response. At least five related TGF-β homologous molecules have been identified, but TGF-β 1, 2, and 3 are most important in mammals.[129] The biology of TGF-β is somewhat unique, in that it is secreted as a biologically inactive precursor (latent TGF-β) that must be activated extracellularly into the bioactive "mature" TGF-β molecule. Measurement of TGF-β must differentiate between "latent" inactive and "mature" bioactive TGF-β. TGF-β_2 is the predominate isoform produced by neuroectoderm, including production by the nonpigmented epithelium of the ciliary body.[90] Little differences in biologic activity between TGF-β isoforms have been found, but better characterization of the specific receptors and their expression will probably lead to future discovery of differential bioactivities.

Perhaps no other cytokine better demonstrates the paradox of bifunctionality and need for "interpretation in context" than does TGF-β. Some early work suggested that TGF-β might be an important inflammatory mediator.[211] When injected into inflamed joints, TGF-β can exacerbate arthritis.[6] TGF-β's immunosuppressive and antiinflammatory activities have been the focus of more recent studies.[106] In vitro, TGF-β acts as a potent inhibitor of both T and B cell activation.[150] This cytokine is immunosuppressive, and it inhibits cytokine production and lymphocyte proliferation by various culture systems for lymphocytes.[68] TGF-β prevents macrophage activation and is a potent inhibitor of

macrophage function.[203] Treatment of macrophages with TGF-β alters the antigen-presenting cell function of these cells.[219] Systemic administration of TGF-β is profoundly immunosuppressive and diminishes inflammatory reactions dependent upon immune-triggered delayed hypersensitivity.[196] The ultimate biologic role of TGF-β may be to downregulate inflammatory responses that involve T cells as immune effector cells.

TGF-β may have an important role in a reparative healing response to inflammation. TGF-β causes chemotaxis of fibroblasts and induces PDGF and basic fibroblast growth factor gene activation in monocytes and fibroblasts.[210] TGF-β stimulates collagen and fibronectin synthesis in fibroblasts. Consequently, TGF-β stimulates both angiogenesis and fibrosis and thereby contributes to tissue repair and wound healing.

Direct injection of TGF-β into the vitreous has minimal effect, unless combined with other attachment factors such as fibronectin.[43] In this case, fibrosis and retinal detachment occurs without significant inflammation. When microgram quantities are injected intravitreally (adjacent to the retina during vitrectomy), TGF-β functions as a biologic glue to induce fibrotic or gliotic proliferation and closure of retinal holes.[81] High (nanogram) concentrations of both latent and active TGF-β_2 are present within normal aqueous humor[46,85,103] and the vitreous.[224] Immunostaining reveals the presence of the protein in the normal uveal tract.[159] Decreased levels of bioactive TGF-β are present in secondary and inflamed aqueous humor.[200] Thus rather than acting as a mediator of inflammation, TGF-β may serve an important protective role in maintaining immune privilege of the normal eye.

Other Cytokines and Growth Factors. Other cytokines important to the immune system, such as IL-2, IL-3, IL-4, IL-5, IL-12, and the colony-stimulating factors may also contribute to ocular inflammation. IL-2-expressing T cells can be found in vitreous specimens of eyes with chronic uveitis[98] and in the cornea during herpetic keratitis.[153] Even less is known about the role of the other interleukins.

Colony-stimulating factors may be released by macrophages at sites of ocular inflammation. Transgenic mice that overexpress granulocyte-CSF or monocyte-CSF develop severe infiltration of both eyes with monocytes, a process that might be regulated by the GM-CSF induction of other cytokines (IL-1-α, TNF, and bFGF).[49]

Neuropeptides

Neuropeptides represent a wide range of small polypeptide mediators that were originally associated with neurons and were initially believed to function solely as neurotransmitters.[193,206] It is now recognized that neuropeptides are produced by many different cells, including mast cells, keratinocytes, macrophages, and lymphocytes.[83] Although some neuropeptides are released upon neural stimulation, nonneural cells release neuropeptides as paracrine mediators either constitutively or in response to inflammatory stimuli. Consequently, neuropeptides can modify cell responses to other stimuli and cytokines. Because the functions of neuropeptides are diverse, a simple categorization is difficult to achieve.

Most neuropeptides were formerly considered to be mediators of local inflammation, and analogies were made to actions of the vasoactive amines.[74] More recent studies have implicated neuropeptides in more subtle and complex regulation of neuroimmune interactions.[84,154] Table 5-4 lists the important neuropeptides and their potential role in inflammation. A simplistic generalization is that substance P is probably proinflammatory and immunostimulatory, whereas vasoactive intestinal peptide (VIP) and alpha-melanocyte-stimulating hormone (α-MSH) tend to be immunosuppressive.

Abundant neuropeptides exist within the normal eye.[193,206] Picomolar concentrations of α-MSH,[201] calcitonin gene-related peptide (CGRP),[207] substance P, and nanomolar amounts of VIP[202] are present in aqueous humor from normal mice, rabbits, or humans. Using immunohistochemical staining, most neuropeptides appear to be associated with uveal nerve fibers or in the retinal neurons. Other sources of neuropeptides, such as the ciliary body epithelium and mast cells, cannot be ruled out, however. The contribution of neuropeptides to the physiology of the normal eye is unknown, although regulation of pupil constriction and ocular blood flow are suspected functions.[193] Certain of the neuropeptides might assist in the regulation of ocular immune privilege.

It remains to be seen how various neuropeptides contribute to ocular inflammation. Studies based on intracameral injection are difficult to interpret because injections of nonphysiologic quantities of neuropeptide are required to induce an effect. Nevertheless, intraocular injections of micromolar quantities of substance P, α-MSH, VIP, and others may induce breakdown of the blood-aqueous barrier, but not cellular infiltration.[193] Detection of neuropeptides in inflamed fluids has been difficult, because blood-derived proteases generally degrade neuropeptides.

TABLE 5-4   IMMUNOREGULATORY FUNCTIONS OF NEUROPEPTIDES IN THE EYE

Neuropeptide	Location in Eye	In vitro or Systemic Inflammatory Effect	Ocular Inflammatory Effect

Substance P	Nerves of anterior segment
	Retina
	Aqueous humor (10 pM)
		Proinflammatory
		  Chemotactic for macrophage and PMN
		  Enhance H_2O_2 by PMN
		  Enhance T helper/inhib T suppressor activation
		  Induces mast cell degranulation
			Breakdown of blood-eye barrier (massive dose)

Enkephalins	Retina	Immunosuppressive Inhibits T cell proliferation	None

Vasoactive intestinal peptide	Retina
	Nerves in anterior choroid and ciliary process
	Aqueous humor (10 nM)
		Immunosuppressive
		  Modulates lymphocyte homing
		  Inhibits T cell proliferation and IFN-γ production
			Breakdown of blood-eye barrier (massive dose)

Calcitonin gene-related peptide	Aqueous humor (15–20 pM, increase to 40–45 pM after neural stim)
	Nerves of anterior uvea
		Antiinflammatory
		  Inhibits oxygen-free radical production
		  Inhibits IFN-γ by T cells
			Unknown

Alpha-MSH	Aqueous humor (10–30 pM)	Immunosuppressive
		  Inhibits systemic effects of IL-1 and TNF
		  Local application inhibits contact hypersensitivity of skin
		  Inhibits PMN migration
		  Inhibits IFN-γ by T cells
			Breakdown of blood-eye barrier (massive dose)

Somatostatin	Uncertain	Antiinflammatory
		  Inhibits T cell proliferation
		  Inhibits mast cell degranulation
			Unknown

REFERENCES

1. Abbas AK, Lichtman AH, Pober JS: *Molecular and cellular immunology,* Philadelphia, 1991, WB Saunders.
2. Abelson MB, Allansmith MR: Histamine and the eye. In Silverestein AR, O'Connor GR, editors: *Immunology and immunopathology of the eye,* New York, 1979, Mason.
3. Abelson MB, Baird BS, Allansmith MR: Tear histamine levels in vernal conjunctivitis and ocular inflammation, *Ophthalmology* 87:812-814, 1980.
4. Adams DO, Hamilton TA: Macrophages as destructive cells in host defense. In Gallin JI, Goldstein IM, Snyderman R, editors: *Inflammation: basic principles and clinical correlates,* 637-662, New York, 1992, Raven Press.
5. Aggarwal BB: Tumor necrosis factor. In Aggarwal BB, Gutterman JU, editors: *Human cytokines,* 270-299, Boston, 1991, Blackwell Scientific.
6. Alkin JB, Manthey CL, Hand AR, et al.: Rapid onset of synovial inflammation and hyperplasia induced by transforming growth factor-β, *J Exp Med* 171:231-247, 1990.
7. Allansmith MR, Baird RS, Henriquez AS, Bloch KJ: Sequence of mast cell changes in ocular anaphylaxis, *Immunology* 49:281-287, 1983.
8. Allansmith MR, Greiner JV, Baird RS: Number of inflammatory cells in the normal conjunctiva, *Am J Ophthalmol* 86:250-259, 1978.
9. Ambache N: Irin, a smooth-muscle contracting substance present in rabbit iris, *J Physiol* 129:65P-66P, 1955.
10. Ambache N, Kavanagh L, Whiting J: Some differences in uveal reaction between cats and rabbits, *J Physiol* 182:110-130, 1966.
11. Arai KI, Lee F, Miyajima A, et al.: Cytokines: coordinators of immune and inflammatory responses, *Annu Rev Biochem* 59:783-836, 1990.
12. Aronson SB, McMaster PRB: Passive transfer of experimental allergic uveitis, *Arch Ophthalmol* 91:60-65, 1971.
13. Ashton N, Cunha-Vaz JG: Effect of histamine on the permeability of ocular vessels, *Arch Ophthalmol* 73:211-216, 1973.
14. Askenase PW, van Loveren M: Delayed-type hypersensitivity: activation of mast cells by antigen-specific T cell factors initiate a cascade of cellular interactions, *Immunol Today* 4:259-263, 1984.
15. Atalla LR, Yoser S, Rao NA: In vivo treatment of experimental uveoretinitis with monoclonal antibody to gamma-interferon. In Usui M, Ohno S, Aoki K, editors: *Ocular immunology today,* 65-68, Amsterdam, 1990, Elsevier Science.
16. Atherton SS, Newel CK, Kanter MY, Cousins SW: T cell depletion increases susceptibility to murine cytomegalovirus retinitis, *Invest Ophthalmol Vis Sci* 33:3353-3360, 1992.
17. Austyn JM: The basis for the immunoregulatory role of macrophages and other accessory cells, *Immunology* 62:161-169, 1987.
18. Bainton DF: Developmental biology of neutrophils and eosinophils. In Gallin JI, Goldstein IM, Snyderman R, editors: *Inflammation: basic principles and clinical correlates,* 303-324, New York, 1992, Raven Press.
19. Beckman JS, Beckman TW, Chen J, et al.: Apparent hydroxyl radical production by peroxynitrite: implications for endothelial injury form nitric oxide and superoxide, *Proc Natl Acad Sci USA* 87:1620-1624, 1990.
20. Ben-Zvi A, Rodrigues MM, Gery I, Schiffman E: Induction of ocular inflammation by synthetic mediators, *Arch Ophthalmol* 99:1436-1444, 1981.
21. Berke G: Functions and mechanism of lysis induced by cytotoxic T lymphocytes and natural killer cells. In Paul WE, editor: *Fundamental immunology,* New York, 1989, Raven Press.
22. Beutler B, Cerami A: Cachectin: more than a tumor necrosis factor, *N Engl J Med* 316:379-385, 1987.
23. Beutler B, Cerami A: The biology of cachectin/TNF—a primary mediator of the host response, *Annu Rev Immunol* 7:625-655, 1989.
24. Bevilacqua MP, Gimbrone MA: Inducible endothelial functions in inflammation and coagulation, *Semin Thromb Hemost* 13:425-433, 1987.
25. Bhatacherjee P: Release of prostaglandin-like substances by Shigella endotoxin and its inhibition by nonsteroidal anti-inflammatory compounds, *Br J Pharmacol* 54:489-494, 1975.
26. Bhattacherjee P: The role of arachidonate metabolites in ocular inflammation. In Bito LZ, Stjernschantz J, editors: *The ocular effects of prostaglandins and other eicosanoids,* 211-227, New York, 1989, Adam R Liss.
27. Bhattachejee P, Eakins EA: Lipoxygenase products: mediation of inflammatory responses and inhibition of their function. In Charkin LW, Belly DM, editors: *Leukotrienes: chemistry and biology,* 195-214, London, 1985, Academic Press.
28. Bhattacherjee P, Hammond B, Salmon JA, Eakins KE: Effect of lipoxygenase products on leukocyte accumulation in the rabbit eye: advances in prostaglandin, *Thromboxane Leukotriene Res* 9:325-330, 1982.
29. Billiau A: Gamma-interferon: the match that lights the fire, *Immunol Today* 9:37-40, 1988.
30. Bito LZ: Species differences in the response of the eye to irritation and trauma: a hypothesis of divergence in ocular defense mechanisms and the choice of experimental animals for eye research, *Exp Eye Res* 39:807-829, 1984.
31. Bito LZ, Stjernschantz J: *The ocular effects of prostaglandins and other eicosanoids,* New York, 1989, Adam R Liss.
32. Black JW, Duncan WA, Durant CJ, et al.: Definitions and antagonism of histamine H2-receptors, *Nature* 236:385-390, 1972.
33. Borth W, Scheer B, Urbansky A, et al.: Binding of IL-1β to α-macroglobulins and release by thioredoxin, *J Immunol* 145:3747-3754, 1990.
34. Braquet P, Vidal RF, Braquet M, et al.: Involvement of leukotrienes and PAF-acether in the increased microvascular permeability of the rabbit retina, *Agents Actions* 15:82-85, 1984.
35. Brown EJ: Complement receptors and phagocytosis, *Curr Opin Immunol* 3:76-82, 1991.
36. Butcher EC: Leukocyte-endothelial cells recognition: three (or more) steps to specificity and diversity, *Am J Pathol* 67:1033-1036, 1991.
37. Bynke G, Hakanson R, Horig J, Leander S: Bradykinin contracts the pupillary sphincter and evokes ocular inflammation through release of neuronal substance P, *Eur J Pharmacol* 91:469-475, 1983.
38. Camras CB, Miranda OC: The putative role of prostaglandins in surgical miosis. In Bito LZ, Stjernschantz J, editors: *The ocular effects of prostaglandins and other eicosanoids,* 197-210, New York, 1989, Adam R Liss.
39. Charteris DG, Lightman SL: Interferon-gamma production in vivo in EAU, *Immunology* 75:463-467, 1992.
40. Colditz I, Zwahlen R, Dewald B, Baggiolini M: In vivo inflammatory activity of neutrophilactivating factor, a novel chemotactic peptide derived from human monocytes, *Am J Pathol* 134:755-760, 1989.
41. Cole DF, Unger WG: Action of bradykinin on intraocular pressure and pupillary diameter, *Ophthalmic Res* 6:308-314, 1974.
42. Colten HR: Tissue-specific regulation of inflammation, *J Appl Physiol* 72:1-7, 1992.
43. Connor TB, Roberts AB, Sporn MB, et al.: Correlation of fibrosis and transforming growth factor-β type 2 levels in the eye, *J Clin Invest* 83:1661-1669, 1989.
44. Cousins SW, Gonzalez A, Atherton SS: Herpes simplex retinitis in the mouse: clinicopathologic correlations, *Invest Ophthalmol Vis Sci* 30:1485-1494, 1989.
45. Cousins SW, Guss RB, Howes EL, Rosenbaum JT: Endotoxin-induced uveitis in the rat: observations on altered vascular permeability, clinical findings and histology, *Exp Eye Res* 39:665-676, 1984.
46. Cousins SW, McCabe MM, Danielpoor D, Streilein JW: Identification of transforming growth factor-β as an immunosuppressive factor in aqueous humor, *Invest Ophthalmol Vis Sci* 32:2201-2211, 1991.
47. Cousins SW, Trattler WB, Streilein JW: Immune privilege and suppression of immunogenic inflammation in the anterior chamber, *Curr Eye Res* 10:287-297, 1991.
48. Crowle AJ: Delayed hypersensitivity in the mouse, *Adv Immunol* 20:197-264, 1975.
49. Cuthbertson RA, Lang RA, Coghlan JP: Macrophage products IL-1 alpha, TNF-alpha and bFGF mediate multiple cytopathic effects in the developing eyes of GM-CSF transgenic mice, *Exp Eye Res* 51:335-344, 1990.
50. Davson H: *Physiology of the eye,* ed 5, New York, 1990, Pergamon Press.

51. Daynes R, Dowel T, Araneo BA: Platelet-derived growth factor is a potent response modifier of T cells, *J Exp Med* 174:1323-1333, 1991.
52. Daynes RA, Araneo BA: Natural regulators of T-cell lymphokine production in vivo, *J Immunother* 12:174-179, 1992.
53. De Vos AF, Hoekzema R, Kijlstra A: Cytokines and uveitis: a review, *Curr Eye Res* 11:581-597, 1992.
54. DeKozak Y, Sakai J, Thillaye B, Faure JP: S-antigen-induced experimental autoimmune uveoretinitis in rats, *Curr Eye Res* 6:327-334, 1981.
55. Dijkstra CD, Dopp EA, Huitinga I, Damoiseaux JGMC: Macrophages in experimental autoimmune diseases in the rat: a review, *Curr Eye Res* 11(supp):75-79, 1992.
56. Dinarello CA: Elisa kits based on monoclonal antibodies do not measure total IL-1β synthesis, *J Immunol Methods* 148:255-259, 1992.
57. Dinarello CA, Thompson RC: Blocking IL-1: interleukin receptor antagonist in vivo and in vitro, *Immunol Today* 12:404-410, 1991.
58. Dinarello CA, Wolff SM: The role of interleukin-1 in disease, *N Engl J Med* 328:106-113, 1993.
59. Ding A, Nathan CF, Graycar J, et al.: Macrophage deactivation factor and transforming growth factors — β 1, β 2 and β 3 inhibit induction of macrophage nitrogen oxide synthesis by IFN-γ, *J Immunol* 145:940-944, 1990.
60. Dower SK: Interleukin-1. In Aggarwal BB, Gutterman JU, editors: *Human cytokines,* 46-80, Boston, 1991, Blackwell Scientific.
61. Dower SK, Kronheim SR, March CJ, et al.: Detection and characterization of high affinity plasma membrane receptors for human interleukin 1, *J Exp Med* 162:501-515, 1985.
62. Drapier JC, Hibbs JBJ: Murine cytotoxic activated macrophages inhibit aconitase in tumor cells: inhibition involved the iron-sulfur prosthetic group and is reversible, *J Clin Invest* 78:790-797, 1986.
63. Dunn CJ: Cytokines as mediators of chronic inflammatory disease. In Kimball ES, editor: *Cytokines and inflammation,* London, 1991, CRC Press.
64. Durum SK, Oppenheim JJ: Macrophage derived mediators: interleukin 1, tumor necrosis factor, interleukin 6, interferon and related cytokines. In Paul WE, editor: *Fundamental immunology,* New York, 1989, Raven Press.
65. Dvorak HF, Galli SJ, Dvorak AM: Cellular and vascular manifestations of cell-mediated immunity, *Hum Pathol* 17:122-137, 1986.
66. Eakins KE: Prostaglandin and non-prostaglandin mediated breakdown of the blood-aqueous barrier, *Exp Eye Res* 25:483-498, 1977.
67. Elner VM, Strieter RM, Pavilack MA, et al.: Human corneal interleukin-8 IL-1 and TNF-induced gene expression and secretion, *Am J Pathol* 139:977-988, 1991.
68. Espevik T, Figari IS, Shalaly MR, et al.: Inhibition of cytokine production by cyclosporin A and TGF-β, *J Exp Med* 166:571-579, 1987.
69. Falus A, Meretey K: Histamine: an early messenger in inflammatory and immune reactions, *Immunol Today* 13:154-156, 1992.
70. Farber JL, Kyle ME, Coleman JB: Mechanisms of cell injury by activated oxygen species, *Lab Invest* 62:670-679, 1990.
71. Ferrick MR, Thurau SR, Oppenheim MH, et al.: Ocular inflammation stimulated by intravitreal interleukin-8 and interleukin-1, *Invest Ophthalmol Vis Sci* 32:1534-1539, 1991.
72. Fleisher LN, Ferrel JB, McGahan MC: Ocular inflammatory effects of intravitreal injection of tumor necrosis factor-α and endotoxin, *Inflammation* 14:325-335, 1990.
73. Fleisher LN, Ferrel JB, Smith MG, McGahan MC: Lipid mediators of TNF-α induced uveitis, *Invest Ophthalmol Vis Sci* 32:2393-2399, 1991.
74. Foreman JC: Peptides and neurogenic inflammation, *Br Med Bull* 43:386-400, 1987.
75. Foster CS, Duncan BA: Randomized clinical trial of topically administered cromolyn sodium for vernal keratoconjunctivitis, *Am J Ophthalmol* 90:175-181, 1980.
76. Friedman PS: The immunobiology of the Langerhans cell, *Immunol Today* 2:124-127, 1981.
77. Gallin JI: Overview. In Gallin JI, Goldstein IM, Snyderman R, editors: *Inflammation: basic principles and clinical correlates,* 1-4, New York, 1992, Raven Press.
78. Gallin JI, Goldstein IM, Snyderman R, editors: *Inflammation: basic principles and clinical correlates,* ed 2, New York, 1992, Raven Press.
79. Gauldie J, Baumann H: Cytokines and acute phase protein expression. In Kimball ES, editor: *Cytokines and inflammation,* London, 1991, CRS Press.
80. Germuth FG, Maumenee AE, Senterfit LB, Pollack AD: Immunohistologic studies on antigen-antibody reactions in the avascular cornea. I. Reaction in rabbits sensitized to foreign proteins, *J Exp Med* 115:99-925, 1962.
81. Glaser BM, Michels RG, Kupperman BD, et al.: Transforming growth factor-beta 2 for the treatment of full-thickness macular holes: a prospective randomized study, *Ophthalmology* 99:1162-1172, 1992.
82. Gleich GJ, Adolphson CR, Leiferman KM: Eosinophils. In Gallin JI, Goldstein IM, Snyderman R, editors: *Inflammation: basic principles and clinical correlates,* 663-700, New York, 1992, Raven Press.
83. Goetzl EJ, Adelman DC, Sreedharan SP: Neuroimmunology, *Adv Immunol* 48:161-191, 1991.
84. Goetzl EJ, Spector NH: *Neuroimmune networks: physiology and diseases,* New York, 1989, Alan R Liss.
85. Granstein R, Staszlaski R, Knisely TL, et al.: Aqueous humor contains transforming growth factor-β and a small (< 3500 dalton) inhibitor of thymocyte proliferation, *J Immunol* 144:3021-3026, 1990.
86. Green WR: Uveal tract. In Spencer WH, editor: *Ocular pathology: an atlas and textbook,* 1792-2013, Philadelphia, 1986, WB Saunders.
87. Greenwood J: The blood-retinal barrier in experimental autoimmune uveoretinitis (EAU): a review, *Curr Eye Res* 11(supp):25-32, 1992.
88. Hagedorn WG, Maas ER: The effect of histamine on the rabbit cornea, *Am J Ophthalmol* 42:89-97, 1956.
89. Hamel CP, Detrick B, Hooks JJ: Evaluation of Ia expression in rat ocular tissues following inoculation with interferon-γ, *Exp Eye Res* 50:173-182, 1990.
90. Helbig H, Kittredge KL, Coca-Prados M, et al.: Mammalian ciliary-body epithelial cells in culture produce transforming growth factor-β, *Graefes Arch Clin Exp Ophthalmol* 229:84-91, 1991.
91. Henson PM: Phagocytic cells degranulation and secretion. In Gallin JI, Goldstein M, Snyderman R, editors: *Inflammation: basic principles and clinical correlates,* 363-390, New York, 1988, Raven Press.
92. Henson PM, John RB: Tissue injury in inflammation: oxidants, proteases and cationic proteins, *J Clin Invest* 79:669-693, 1987.
93. Hirano T, Matsuda T, Turner M, et al.: Excessive production of interleukin 6/B cell stimulatory factor-2 in rheumatoid arthritis, *Eur J Immunol* 18:1797-1801, 1988.
94. Hoekzema R, Murray PI, Kijlstra A: Cytokines and intraocular inflammation, *Curr Eye Res* 9(supp):207-211, 1990.
95. Hoekzema R, Murray PI, Van Haren MAC, et al.: Analysis of interleukin-6 in endotoxin-induced uveitis, *Invest Ophthalmol Vis Sci* 32:88-95, 1991.
96. Hoekzema R, Verhagen C, Van Haren M, Kijlstra A: Endotoxin-induced uveitis in the rat, *Invest Ophthalmol Vis Sci* 33:532-539, 1992.
97. Hofman F, Hinton DR: Tumor necrosis factor-α in the retina in acquired immune deficiency syndrome, *Invest Ophthalmol Vis Sci* 33:1829-1835, 1992.
98. Hooks JJ, Chan CC, Detrick B: Identification of the lymphokines interferon-γ and interleukin-2 in inflammatory eye disease, *Invest Ophthalmol Vis Sci* 29:1444-1451, 1988.
99. Howes EL: Cellular hypersensitivity in the cornea, *Arch Ophthalmol* 83:475-488, 1970.
100. Howes EL, McKay DG: Comparison of the ocular effects of circulating endotoxin and immune complexes, *J Immunol* 114:734-737, 1975.
101. Huntley JF: Mast cells and basophils: a review of their heterogeneity and function, *J Comp Pathol* 107:349-372, 1992.
102. Jaffe GJ, Abrams GW, Williams GA, Han DP: Tissue plasminogen activator for postvitrectomy fibrin formation, *Ophthalmology* 97:184-189, 1990.
103. Jampel H, Roche N, Stark WJ, Roberts AB: Transforming growth factor-β in aqueous humor, *Curr Eye Res* 10:963-970, 1991.
104. Jampol LM: Pharmacologic therapy of aphakic and pseudophakic cystoid macula edema: 1985 update, *Ophthalmology* 92:807-810, 1985.
105. Kakakios AM, Ryan J, Geczy CL: Effect of locally administered heparins on delayed-type hypersensitivity reactions, *Int Arch Appl Immunol* 93:300-307, 1990.

106. Kehrl JH, Taylor A, Kim S-J, Fauci AS: Transforming growth factor-β is a negative regulator of human lymphocytes, *Ann NY Acad Sci* 628:345-353, 1991.

107. Kimura M, Eguchi S, Araie M, et al.: Anticoagulant and fibrinolytic therapies for anterior chamber fibrin following cataract surgery in the rabbit eye, *Acta Soc Opthalmol Jap* 96:1240-1247, 1992.

108. Klebanoff SJ: Phagocytic cells: products of oxygen metabolism. In Gallin GI, Goldstein IM, Snyderman R, editors: *Inflammation: basic principles and clinical correlates*, New York, 1988, Raven Press.

109. Klein J: *Immunology*, Boston, 1990, Blackwell Scientific.

110. Knisely TL, Anderson TM, Sherwood ME, et al.: Morphologic and ultrastructural examination of I-A+ cells in the murine iris, *Invest Ophthalmol Vis Sci* 32:2432-2440, 1991.

111. Kovacs EJ: Fibrogenic cytokine: the role of immune mediators in the development of scar tissue, *Immunol Today* 12:17-23, 1991.

112. Kreger AS, Gray LL: Purification of *Pseudomonas aeruginosa* proteins and microscopic characterization of pseudomonal protein-induced rabbit corneal damage, *Infect Immun* 19:630-638, 1978.

113. Kulkarni P, Mancino M: Studies on intraocular inflammation produced by intravitreal human interleukins in the rabbit, *Exp Eye Res* 56:275-279, 1993.

114. Kulkarni PS, Bhattacherjee P, Eakins KE, Srinivasan BD: Anti-inflammatory effects of betamethasone phosphate, dexamethasone phosphate and indomethacin on rabbit ocular inflammation induced by bovine serum albumin, *Curr Eye Res* 1:43-49, 1981.

115. Kusuda M, Gaspari AA, Chan CC, et al.: Expression of Ia antigen by ocular tissues of mice treated with interferon-γ, *Invest Ophthalmol Vis Sci* 30:764-768, 1989.

116. Kuznetsova TP, Chesnokova NB, Paskhina TS: Activity of tissue and plasma kallikrein and level of their precursors in eye tissue structures and media of healthy rabbits, *Vap Medit Khim* 37:79-82, 1991.

117. Laliberte M-F, Laliberte F, Alhenc-Gelas F, Chevillard C: Immunochemistry of angiotensin I-converting enzyme in rat eye structures involved in aqueous humor regulation, *Lab Invest* 59:263-270, 1988.

118. Lehrer RI, Ganz T: Antimicrobial polypeptides of human neutrophils, *Blood* 76:2169-2181, 1990.

119. Lewis RA, Austin KF: Leukotrienes. In Gallin JI, Goldstein M, Snyderman R, editors: *Inflammation: basic principles and clinical correlates*, 121-128, New York, 1992, Raven Press.

120. Limb A, Little BC, Meager A, et al.: Cytokines in proliferative vitreoretinopathy, *Eye* 5:686-693, 1991.

121. Lorant DE, Patel KD, McIntrye TM, et al.: Coexpression of GMP-140 and PAF by endothelium stimulated by histamine or thrombin: a juxtacrine system for adhesion and activation of neutrophils, *J Cell Biol* 115:223-234, 1991.

122. Mansour AM, Chess J, Henkind P: Fibrinogen-induced vitreous membranes, *Ophthalmic Res* 19:164-169, 1987.

123. Marak GE: Phacoanaphylactic endophthalmitis, *Surv Ophthalmol* 36:325-329, 1992.

124. Marak GE, Font RL, Alepa FP, Ward PA: Effects of C3 inactivator factor on the development of experimental lens-induced granulomatous endophthalmitis, *Ophthalmic Res* 9:416-420, 1977.

125. Marak GE, Wacker WB, Rao NA, et al.: Effects of complement depletion on experimental allergic uveitis, *Ophthalmic Res* 11:97-107, 1979.

126. Marletta MA: Nitric oxide: biosynthesis and biological significance, *Trends Biochem Sci* 14:488-492, 1989.

127. Martin XD, Brennan MC, Lichter PR: Serotonin in aqueous humor, *Ophthalmology* 95:1221-1226, 1988.

128. Martiney JA, Litwak M, Berman JW, et al.: Pathophysiologic effect of interleukin-1β in the rabbit retina, *Am J Pathol* 137:1411-1423, 1990.

129. Massague J, Chiefetz S, Laiho M, et al.: Transforming growth factor-β, *Cancer Surv* 12:81-103, 1992.

130. Mazzei GJ, Shaw AR: Purification and characterization of a 26 Kd competitive inhibitor of interleukin 1, *Eur J Immunol* 20:683, 1990.

131. McLeish W, Rubsamen P, Atherton SS, Streilein JW: Immunobiology of Langerhans cells on the ocular surface. II. Role of central corneal Langerhans cells in stromal keratitis following HSV-1 infection in mice, *Reg Immunol* 2:236-243, 1989.

132. McMenamin PG, Holthouse I: Immunohistochemical characterization of dendritic cells and macrophages in the aqueous outflow pathways of the rat eye, *Exp Eye Res* 55:315-324, 1992.

133. McMenamin PG, Holthouse I, Holt PG: Class II major histocompatibility complex (Ia) antigen bearing dendritic cells within iris and ciliary body of the rat eye: distribution, *Immunology* 77:385-393, 1992.

134. Meltzer MS, Nacy CA: Delayed-type hypersensitivity and induction of activated, cytotoxic macrophages. In Paul WE, editor: *Fundamental immunology*, New York, 1989, Raven Press.

135. Metcalfe DD, Costa JJ, Burd PR: Mast cells and eosinophils. In Gallin JI, Goldstein IM, Snyderman R, editors: *Inflammation: basic principles and clinical correlates*, 709-725, New York, 1992, Raven Press.

136. Miranda OC, Bito LZ: Putative and demonstrated miotic effects of prostaglandins in mammals. In Gallin JI, Goldstein IM, Snyderman R, editors: *Inflammation, basic principles and clinical correlates*, 171-195, New York, 1988, Raven Press.

137. Mishima H, Masuda K, Miyake K: The putative role of prostaglandins on cystoid macula edema. In Bito LZ, Stjernschantz J, editors: *The ocular effects of prostaglandins and other eicosanoids*, 251-264, New York, 1989, Adam R Liss.

138. Miyake K: Indomethacin in the treatment of postoperative cystoid macula edema, *Surv Ophthalmol* 28:554-568, 1984.

139. Miyake K, Shirasowa E, Hikita M: Hypothesis on the role of prostaglandins in the pathogenesis of epinephrine maculopathy and aphakic cystoid macula edema. In Bito LZ, Stjernschantz J, editors: *The ocular effects of prostaglandins and other eicosanoids*, 265-276, New York, 1989, Adam R Liss.

140. Mizel SB: The interleukins, *FASEB J* 3:2379-2388, 1989.

141. Mondino BJ, Sidaharo Y, Meyer IJ, Sumner HJ: Inflammatory mediators in the vitreous humor of AIDS patients, *Invest Ophthalmol Vis Sci* 31:798-804, 1990.

142. Mondino BJ, Sumner HL: Generation of complement-derived anaphylatoxins in normal human donor corneas, *Invest Ophthalmol Vis Sci* 31:1945-1949, 1990.

143. Mondino BJ, Sidiharo Y, Sumner H: Anaphylatoxin levels in human vitreous humor, *Invest Ophthalmol Vis Sci* 29:1195-1198, 1988.

144. Mosmann T, Coffman RC: TH1 and TH2 cells: different patterns of lymphockine secretion lead to different functional properties, *Annu Rev Immunol* 7:145-173, 1989.

145. Muller-Eberhard HJ: Molecular organization and function of the complement system, *Annu Rev Biochem* 57:321-347, 1988.

146. Murray PI, Hoekzema R, Van Haren MA, et al.: Aqueous humor analysis of Fuch's heterochromic cyclitis, *Curr Eye Res* 5:686-693, 1991.

147. Murray PI, Hoekzema R, Van Haren MAC, et al.: Aqueous humor interleukin-6 levels in uveitis, *Invest Ophthalmol Vis Sci* 31:917-920, 1990.

148. Nathan C: Interferon-γ. In Gallin JI, Goldstein IM, Snyderman R, editors: *Inflammation: basic principles and clinical correlates*, New York, 1992, Raven Press.

149. Nathan C: Nitric oxide as a secretory product of mammalian cells, *FASEB J* 6:3051-3064, 1992.

150. Nathan C, Sporn M: Cytokines in context, *J Cell Biol* 5:981-986, 1991.

151. Nathan CF, Stuehr DJ: Does endothelium derived nitric oxide have a role in cytokine-induced hypotension? *J Nat Cancer Inst* 82:726-728, 1990.

152. Niederkorn JY: Immune privilege and immune regulation in the eye, *Adv Immunol* 48:191-226, 1991.

153. Niemialtowski MG, Rouse BT: Predominance of Th1 cells in ocular tissues during herpetic stromal keratitis, *J Immunol* 149:3035-3039, 1992.

154. Nio DA, Moylan RN, Roche JK: Modulation of T lymphocyte function by neuropeptides: evidence for their role as local immunoregulatory elements, *J Immunol* 150:5281-5288, 1993.

155. Okada M, Shimada K: The effects of various pharmacologic agents on the allergic inflammation of the eye, *Invest Ophthalmol Vis Sci* 19:176-183, 1980.

156. Osborn L: Leukocyte adhesion to endothelium in inflammation, *Cell* 62:3-6, 1990.

157. Pardi R, Inverardi L, Bender JR: Regulatory mechanisms in leukocyte adhesion: flexible receptors for sophisticated travelers, *Immunol Today* 13:224-230, 1992.

158. Parker JA, Goetzel ED, Friedlaender MH: Leukotrienes in the aqueous humor of patients with uveitis, *Arch Ophthalmol* 104:722-724, 1986.

159. Pasquale LR, Dorma-Pease ME, Lutty GA, et al.: Immunolocalization of TGF-β1, β2, β3 in the anterior segment of the human eye, *Invest Ophthalmol Vis Sci* 34:22-30, 1993.

160. Paul WE: Development and function of lymphocytes. In Gallin JI, Goldstein IM, Snyderman R, editors: *Inflammation: basic principles and clinical correlates,* 775-790, New York, 1992, Raven Press.

161. Peyman GA, Bennet TO, Vilchik J: Effects of intravitreal prostaglandins in retinal vasculature, *Arch Ophthalmol* 7:279-288, 1975.

162. Pinckard RN, Ludwig J, McManus LM: Platelet activating factors. In Gallin JI, Goldstein M, Snyderman R, editors: *Inflammation: basic principles and clinical correlates,* 139-168, New York, 1988, Raven Press.

163. Podack ER: Perforin: structure, function and regulation, *Curr Top Microbiol* 178:175-184, 1992.

164. Proud D, Kaplan AP: Kinin formation: mechanisms and role in inflammatory disorders, *Annu Rev Immunol* 6:49-83, 1988.

165. Rahi AHS, Tripathi RC: Anatomy of the reverse passive Arthus reaction in the cornea: a preliminary communication, *Mod Prob Ophthalmol* 16:165-170, 1976.

166. Rao NA: Role of oxygen free radicals in retinal damage associated with experimental uveitis, *Trans Am Ophthalmol Soc* 89:797-850, 1990.

167. Raviola G: The structural basis of the blood-ocular barrier, *Exp Eye Res* 23:27-63, 1977.

168. Regoli D, Barake S: Pharmacology of bradykinin and related kinins, *Pharmacol Rev* 31:1980.

169. Reid KB: Activation and control of the complement system, *Essays Biochem* 22:27-68, 1986.

170. Robbins KC: Fibrinolytic therapy: biochemical mechanisms, *Semin Thromb Hemost* 17:1-6, 1991.

171. Rolfe MW, Kunkel SL, Standiford TJ, et al.: Pulmonary fibroblast expression of interleukin-8: a model for alveolar macrophage-derived cytokine networking, *Am J Respir Cell Mol Biol* 5:493-501, 1991.

172. Rosenbaum JT, Boney RS: Use of interleukin-1 receptor to inhibit ocular inflammation, *Curr Eye Res* 10:1137-1139, 1991.

173. Rosenbaum JT, Boney RS, Samples JR, Valone FH: Synthesis of PAF by ocular tissues from inflamed eye, *Arch Ophthalmol* 109:410-413, 1991.

174. Rosenbaum JT, Howes EL, Samples JR: Ocular inflammatory effects of intravitreally-injected tumor necrosis factor, *Am J Pathol* 133:47-53, 1988.

175. Rosenbaum JT, Samples JR, Hefeneider SH, Howes EL: Ocular inflammatory effects of intravitreal IL-1, *Arch Ophthalmol* 105:1117-1120, 1987.

176. Rosenbaum JT, Wong K, Perez HD, et al.: Characterization of endotoxin-induced C5-derived chemotactic activity in aqueous humor, *Invest Ophthalmol Vis Sci* 25:1184-1191, 1984.

177. Rubin RM, Rosenbaum JT: A platelet activating factor antagonist inhibits interleukin-1 induced inflammation, *Biochem Biophys Res Commun* 154:429-436, 1988.

178. Rubin RM, Rosenbaum JT: The role of platelet-activating factor in ocular inflammation. In Handley DA, Saunders RN, Houlihan WJ, Tomesch JC, editors: *Platelet activating factor in endotoxin and immune diseases,* 189-205, New York, 1990, Marcel Dekker.

179. Rubin RM, Samples JR, Rosenbaum JT: Prostaglandin-independent inhibition of ocular vascular permeability by a platelet-activating factor antagonist, *Arch Ophthalmol* 106:1116-1120, 1988.

180. Scott P, Kaufman SHE: The role of T-cell subsets and cytokines in the regulation of infection, *Immunol Today* 12:346-348, 1991.

181. Shaw C, Foy WL, Johnston CF, Buchanan KD: Identification and characterization of multiple tachykinin immunoreactivities in bovine retina: evidence for the presence of a putative oxidative system for substance P, *J Neurochem* 53:1547-1554, 1989.

182. Sheffield EA: The granulomatous inflammatory response, *J Pathol* 160:1-2, 1990.

183. Sheikh IA, Kaplan AP: Studies of the digestion of bradykinin, lys-bradykinin, and des-Arg9-bradykinin by angiotensin converting enzyme, *Biochem Pharmacol* 35:1951-1956, 1986.

184. Shimizu Y, Newman W, Tanaka Y, Shaw S: Lymphocyte interactions with endothelial cells, *Immunol Today* 13:106-112, 1992.

185. Silberberg-Sinakin L, Thjorberke RL, Baer RL, et al.: Antigen-bearing Langerhans cells in skin, dermal lymphatics and in lymph nodes, *Cell Immunol* 25:137-145.

186. Sims PJ, Wiedmer T: The response of human platelets to activated components of the complement system, *Immunol Today* 12:338-342, 1991.

187. Smolin G, Thoft RA: *The cornea: scientific foundations and clinical practice,* ed 3, Boston, 1994, Little, Brown and Company.

188. Snyderman R: Injury and tissue destruction in the rheumatic diseases. In Wyngaarden JB, Smith LH, Bennett Jr JC, editors: *Cecil's textbook of medicine,* 1898-1906, Philadelphia, 1992, WB Saunders.

189. Sporn MB, Roberts AB, Wakefield LM, Assoian RK: Transforming growth factor-β: biological function and chemical structure, *Science* 233:532-534, 1986.

190. Springer TA: Adhesion receptors of the immune system, *Nature* 346:425-434, 1990.

191. Springer TA, Lasky LA: Cell adhesion: sticky sugars for selectins, *Nature* 349:196-197, 1991.

192. Steinman RM: The dendritic cell system and its role in immunogenicity, *Annu Rev Immunol* 9:271-305, 1991.

193. Stjernschantz J: Autocoids and neuropeptides. In Sears ML, editor: *Pharmacology of the eye,* 311-365, London, 1984, Springer Verlag.

194. Stjernschantz J, Bito LZ: The ocular effects of eicosanoids and other autocoids: historical background and the need for a broader perspective. In Bito LZ, Stjernschantz J, editors: *The ocular effects of prostaglandins and other eicosanoids,* 1-13, New York, 1989, Adam R Liss.

195. Stjernschantz J, Nilson SFE, Astin M: Vasodynamic and angiogenic effects of eicosanoids in the eye. In Bito LZ, Stjernschantz J, editors: *The ocular effects of prostaglandins and other eicosanoids,* 155-170, New York, 1989, Adam R Liss.

196. Strassman G, Bertolini DR, Eidelman O: Inhibition of immune reactions in vivo by liposome encapsulated TGF-type β1, *Clin Exp Immunol* 86:53-56, 1991.

197. Streilein JW, Cousins SW, Bradley D: Effect of intraocular γ-interferon on the immunoregulatory properties of iris and ciliary body cells, *Invest Ophthalmol Vis Sci* 33:2304-2315, 1992.

198. Tamesis RR, Foster CS: Natural killing of HSV-1 infected and non-infected target cells in Igh-1 disparate mice. In Usui M, Ohno S, Aoki K, editors: *Ocular immunology today,* 157-160, Amsterdam, 1990, Elsevier Science.

199. Tartaglia LA, Goeddel DV: Two TNF receptors, *Immunol Today* 13:151-153, 1992.

200. Taylor AW, Streielin JW, Cousins SW: Alpha$_2$-macroglobulin may neutralize ocular immune privilege, *FASEB J* (supp):1042, 1992.

201. Taylor AW, Streilein JW, Cousins SW: Identification of alpha melanocyte stimulating hormone as a possible immunoregulatory factor in aqueous humor, *Curr Eye Res* 12:1199-1206, 1992.

202. Taylor AW, Streilein JW, Cousins SW: Neuropeptides in aqueous humor may regulate T-lymphocytes within the eye, *Invest Ophthalmol Vis Sci* 33(supp):1283, 1993.

203. Tsunawaki S, Sporn M, Ding A, Nathan C: Deactivation of macrophages by transforming growth factor-β, *Nature* 334:260-263, 1988.

204. Tumpey TM, Finnegan A, Hendricks RL: Lymphokine-secreting cells in HSV-1 infected mouse corneas, *Invest Ophthalmol Vis Sci* 33(supp):786, 1992.

205. Unanue ER, Allen PM: The immunoregulatory role of macrophages and other accessory cells, *Science* 236:551-554, 1987.

206. Unger WG: Mediation of the ocular response to injury and irritation: peptides versus prostaglandins. In Bito LZ, Stjernschantz J, editors: *The ocular effects of prostaglandins and other eicosanoids,* 293-328, New York, 1989, Adam R Liss.

207. Unger WG, Terenghi G, Ghatei MA, et al.: Calcitonin gene-related polypeptide as a mediator of the neurogenic ocular injury response, *J Ocul Pharmacol* 1:189-199, 1985.

208. Van Snick J: Interleukin-6: an overview, *Annu Rev Immunol* 8:253-278, 1990.

209. Verhagen C, Breebaart AC, Kijlstra A: The effects of complement depletion on corneal inflammation in rats, *Invest Ophthalmol Vis Sci* 33:273-279, 1992.

210. Wahl SM: Transforming growth factor beta (TGF-beta) in inflammation: a cause and a cure, *J Clin Immunol* 12:61-74, 1992.

211. Wahl SM, McCartney-Francis N, Mergenhagen SE: Inflammatory and immunomodulatory role of TGF-β, *Immunol Today* 10:258-261, 1989.

212. Weaver CT, Unanue ER: The costimulatory function of antigen-presenting cells, *Immunol Today* 11:49-53, 1990.

213. Weisman G: Inflammation: historical perspective. In Gallin JI, Goldstein IM, Snyderman R, editors: *Inflammation: basic principles and clinical correlates,* 5-9, New York, 1992, Raven Press.

214. Weiss SS: Tissue destruction by neutrophils, *N Engl J Med* 320:365-376, 1989.

215. Weksler BB: Platelets in inflammation. In Gallin JI, Goldstein M, Snyderman R, editors: *Inflammation: basic principles and clinical correlates,* 543-557, New York, 1988, Raven Press.

216. Weller PF: Immunobiology of eosinophils, *N Engl J Med* 324:1110-1118, 1991.

217. Wharton M, Granger DL, Durack DT: Mitochondrial iron loss from leukemia cells injured by macrophages: a possible mechanism for electron transport chain defects, *J Immunol* 141:1311-1317, 1988.

218. White MV, Kaliner MA: Histamine. In Gallin JI, Goldstein M, Snyderman R, editors: *Inflammation: basic principles and clinical correlates,* 169-193, New York, 1988, Raven Press.

219. Wilbanks GA, Streilein JW: Fluids from immune privileged sites endow macrophages with the capacity to induce antigen-specific immune deviation via a mechanism involving transforming growth factor-β, *Eur J Immunol* 22:1031-1036, 1992.

220. Winterbourn CC, Sutton HC: Hydroxyl radical production from hydrogen peroxide and enzymatically generated paraquat radicals: catalytic requirements and oxygen dependence, *Arch Biochem* 235:116-126, 1984.

221. Winton A, Eshbaugh C, Roth E, Cousins SW: Intraocular macrophage activation and lens-associated uveitis, *Invest Ophthalmol Vis Sci* 34(supp):1482, 1993.

222. Wong KL, Howes EL: Intraocular injection of prostaglandins modifies responsiveness to circulating endotoxin, *Arch Ophthalmol* 101:275-279, 1983.

223. Wright SD: Receptors for complement and the biology of phagocytosis. In Gallin JI, Goldstein IM, Snyderman R, editors: *Inflammation: basic principles and clinical correlates,* 477-496, New York, 1992, Raven Press.

224. Yoshitushi T, Shichi H: Immunosuppressive factors in procine vitreous body, *Curr Eye Res* 10:1141-1144, 1991.

225. Zacharae COC: Interleukin-8. In Aggarwal BB, Gutterman JU, editors: *Human cytokines,* Boston, 1991, Blackwell Scientific.

226. Zimmerman GA, Prescott SM, McIntyre TM: Endothelial cell interactions with granulocytes: tethering and signaling molecules, *Immunol Today* 13:93-100, 1992.

227. Zirm M: Proteins in aqueous humor, *Adv Ophthalmol* 40:100-172, 1980.

228. Zucali JR, Dinarello CA, Oblon DJ, et al.: Interleukin 1 stimulates fibroblasts to produce granulocyte-macrophage colony-stimulating activity and prostaglandin E2, *J Clin Invest* 77:1857-1863, 1986.

6 Cellular Immunity and the Eye

ROBERT L. HENDRICKS, QIZHI TANG

Cellular immunology originated with the observations of Elie Metchnikoff that mobile phagocytic cells, which he referred to collectively as phagocytes, eliminate foreign material from the body through phagocytosis. The cellular immunity theory of Metchnikoff was in direct conflict with the humoral theory of immunity of Robert Koch, Emil von Behring, and associates. These investigators confirmed that bacteria and toxins can be neutralized by immune serum in the absence of cells. Thus was spawned one of the great debates of immunology regarding the relative importance of cellular versus humoral factors in immunity.

Although the phagocytic cells described by Metchnikoff were clearly mobilized by an infection, their activity was not antigen specific (did not constitute an acquired response to a specific antigen that is associated with immunity). Moreover, the distinction between cell-mediated and humoral immunity became somewhat clouded when it was discovered that the antibodies that mediated humoral immunity were produced by lymphocytes, and that antibody binding to foreign material (opsonization) greatly increased the phagocytic activity of macrophages and neutrophils. It wasn't until the early 1960s that studies by J.F.A.P. Miller in London,[66a] Waksman and Yankowic in Boston,[35a] and Robert A. Good[4a,50a,121a] in Minnesota confirmed that the thymus, then considered a vestigial organ, actually played a central role in immunologic processes. Their studies plainly established that a distinct subpopulation of lymphocytes used the thymus as a site of maturation.

These thymus-dependent lymphocytes (T lymphocytes) did not produce antibodies, but were soon shown to be responsible for the delayed type of hypersensitivity (DTH) reaction that was described earlier by Robert Koch, and shown by Karl Landsteiner and Merrill Chase to be transferable with cells but not serum. Thus the concept of cell-mediated versus humoral immunity reemerged with T lymphocytes as the central characters in the former and B lymphocytes as the central characters in the latter.

T Lymphocyte Subpopulations and Functions

Major Histocompatibility Complex Restriction. T cell recognition of foreign antigens bound to self major histocompatibility complex (MHC) molecules is called MHC restriction. This concept arose in the early 1970s from experiments by Kindred and Shreffler,[53] and Katz, Hamaoka, and Benacerraf[52] demonstrating that the interaction between T cells and B cells requires the interacting cells to share the same MHC molecules. Similar MHC restriction was later shown for the interaction between T cells and antigen-presenting cells in lymphoproliferative responses,[91] as well as the interaction of cytotoxic T lymphocytes (CTL) and their target cells.[100,126] T helper cells that help antibody responses and proliferate in lymphoproliferative assays were found to recognize foreign antigens in the context of MHC class II, whereas CTL recognized foreign antigen in the context of MHC class I.

T Cell Receptor. In 1896 Paul Ehrlich introduced the *side-chain* theory of antibody production. According to this theory, antibodies originated as side-chains on the surface membrane of cells, where they served as antigen receptors. He further proposed that upon interaction with antigen, these receptors were released from the surface of the cells and were ultimately overproduced by those cells, leading to the appearance of antibodies in the serum. Indeed, Ehrlich's theory was found to be largely correct in that antibody molecules represent the antigen-specific receptor on B lymphocytes. The fact that T lymphocytes also react to antigens with a high degree of specificity led to the prediction of a similar antigen-specific T cell receptor (TCR). Because TCRs are not secreted like antibodies, however, the nature of the TCR remained elusive until the early 1980s. During the brief period from 1982 through 1984 the TCR was identified, isolated, and sequenced; and several TCR genes were cloned.* Although the TCR bears structural similarities to

---

*References 2, 15, 41, 93, 103, 125.

71

the immunoglobulin receptor on B cells, the two receptors are functionally quite dissimilar. For instance, (1) immunoglobulins are secreted, whereas TCRs are not; (2) immunoglobulins generally recognize the nascent form of an antigen, whereas TCRs require processing of the antigen prior to recognition; and (3) immunoglobulins recognize antigens in soluble form, whereas TCRs recognize antigens bound to MHC molecules on the surface of antigen-presenting cells (APC).

Two theories have been offered to explain the MHC restriction of antigen recognition by the TCR. One theory postulated a single polymorphic T cell receptor recognizing "altered self" determinants resulting from the physical interaction of an antigenic fragment with self MHC. The second theory proposed two polymorphic receptors, one recognizing MHC and the other recognizing antigen. These two receptors could be present on individual molecules that become associated on the T cell membrane, or they could represent separate sites on the same molecule.

T Cell Subpopulations. *CD4 and CD8.* Functional studies revealed heterogeneity within the T cell population. Thus functional T cell subpopulations were defined based on their capacity to (1) mediate DTH responses, (2) provide helper function for the differentiation and antibody production of B lymphocytes, and (3) mediate cytolysis of target cells expressing specific foreign antigens. These functional studies converged with the phenotypic work of Cantor and Bois,[13] who generated antisera specific for three antigens (Lyt-1, Lyt-2, and Lyt-3) that were expressed on T lymphocytes but not on B lymphocytes.[13] Moreover, it was determined that Lyt-2 and Lyt-3 were expressed on CTL but not on T helper cells. The molecules recognized by anti-Lyt-2 and anti-Lyt-3 antibodies represent the alpha and beta chains, respectively, of the T cell marker that has now been given the cluster of differentiation (CD) designation CD8. Monoclonal antibodies have subsequently been developed that recognize a monomeric CD4 T cell marker. Most mature T cells express the phenotype CD4$^+$ CD8$^-$, or CD4$^-$CD8$^+$. The CD4$^+$ T lymphocytes are often referred to as T helper (Th) cells because they contain the cells that provide helper function for antibody responses. CD4 cells also regulate the activity of T effector cells, such as CTL, and are responsible for most DTH responses. More importantly, the CD4 and CD8 markers define T lymphocyte subpopulations that recognize foreign antigens in the context of MHC Class II and MHC Class I antigens, respectively.

Th1 and Th2 Subpopulations of CD4 T Cells. For the most part, T lymphocytes mediate their immunologic functions through the elaboration of soluble mediators. These mediators, usually glycoproteins are referred to either as lymphokines if they are exclusively the product of lymphocytes, or by the generic term cytokines. A plethora of functionally defined cytokines were described during the early and middle 1970s. Through the use of monoclonal anticytokine antibodies and molecular biologic techniques, the genes

encoding a variety of cytokines have now been cloned and large quantities of cytokines have been produced in recombinant form. It is now clear that many of the functional characteristics that were previously ascribed to different cytokines are actually mediated by the same pleotropic cytokine molecule. When a cytokine that is involved in immune regulation is purified, molecularly cloned, and expressed, it can be given an interleukin (IL) designation by the International Union of Immunological Societies Nomenclature Committee. The total array of cytokines is very large and growing, and only those cytokines that perform a key function in cell-mediated immune responses will be discussed in this chapter (Table 6-1).

Mosmann and associates[14,68] have defined Th1 and Th2 subpopulations of mouse CD4$^+$ T cells based on the array of cytokines produced by individual T cell clones. Th1 clones are defined by the production of IL-2 and interferon gamma (IFN-γ), whereas Th2 cells produce IL-4, IL-5, IL-6, and IL-10, (Table 6-1). The different patterns of cytokine production expressed by Th1 and Th2 clones are associated with different functional characteristics of the cells. For instance, IFN-γ is responsible for at least part of the induration at sites of DTH reactions.[32] Accordingly, Th1 clones are capable of mediating DTH, whereas Th2 clones are not.[14,69] Conversely, IL-4 and IL-5 are involved in B cell differentiation and antibody production, and Th2 cells are thought to be primarily involved in regulating antibody responses. Moreover, IL-4 induces an isotype switch in B cells favoring production of IgE. IL-4 also induces the expression of IgE Fcϵ receptors on B cells,[45] and in conjunction with IL-3 induces mast cell proliferation. IL-5 induces the proliferation of eosinophils.[96] Thus Th2 cells would be expected to be a key part of immediate hypersensitivity reactions. In agreement with this theory, Maggi and associates[62] recently described the accumulation of Th2-like helper T cells in the conjunctiva of patients with vernal conjunctivitis.

Not only do Th1 cells and Th2 cells appear to subserve different functions, but they may also be capable of cross-regulating each other's activities. For instance, the Th1 product IFN-γ can inhibit the proliferation of Th2 clones, but not Th1 clones, in vitro.[28,34] IFN-γ also inhibits the effects of IL-4 on B cells.[87,106] In contrast, the Th2 product IL-4 can serve as an autocrine growth factor for Th2 clones in the presence of IL-1,[37] but is much less effective in inducing the proliferation of Th1 clones. In addition, the Th2 product IL-10 can inhibit IFN-γ and IL-2 production by Th1 clones.[29,30,102] This functional cross-regulation of Th1 and Th2 cells may be reflected in the reciprocal relationship between the DTH and antibody response in vivo. A strong antibody response is often associated with weak DTH and vice versa. Preferential activation of Th1 or Th2 cells may simultaneously upregulate one response while downregulating the other. This reciprocal regulation may lead to a more efficient response to a particular infection. For example, Th1 cells mediate DTH, and the Th1 products IFN-γ and IL-2 are

TABLE 6-1 CHARACTERISTICS OF SELECTED CYTOKINES

Cytokine	Molecular Weight	Major Cell Source	Major Functions
IL-1α/β	17.5 kd	Macrophages, epithelial cells, keratinocytes, B cells, PMNs	Endogenous pyrogen, cofactor for thymocyte proliferation, PMN activation, induces growth factor responsiveness in Th2 clones, fibroblast activation and proliferation, induces adhesion molecule expression
IL-2	15-20 kd	T cells (except Th2 and some CD8)	Growth factor for T, B, and NK cells
IL-4	15-19 kd	Th2 cells, mast cells	B cell isotype switching to IgG1 and IgE, growth factor for T and B cells
IL-5	43 kd homodimer	Th2 cells, mast cells	B cell growth factor, enhances IgA synthesis by LPS-stimulated B cells, eosiniphil growth and differentiation factors
IL-6	21-28 kd	Macrophages, T cells, fibroblasts	B cell differentiation, hepatocyte stimulation (acute phase protein synthesis), thymocyte and plasmacytoma/hybridoma growth factor
IL-7	25 kd	Bone marrow and thymic stromal cells	Growth and differentiation of immature B and T cells, induces CTL and LAK activity
NAP-1/IL-8	8-10 kd	Macrophages, T cells, PMN, fibroblasts, endothelial cells, keratinocytes	Stimulatory and chemotactic for PMN, chemotactic for T cells, stimulates mast cells, angiogenic
IL-10	19 kd	Th2 cells, some B cells, activated monocytes, EBV-transformed cell lines, mast cells	Inhibits antigen presentation by macrophage by downregulating MHC class II, inhibits IFN-γ, IL-2, and other cytokines by Th1 cells, inhibits TNF-α, IL-1, and IL-6 release by macrophage, growth and differentiation factor for B cells, maintains viability and, in synergy with IL-3 and IL-4 growth of mast cells
IL-12	35, 40 kd heterodimer	B cells, macrophages, EBV-transformed B cell lines	Induces proliferation and differentiation of T and NK cells, induces IFN-γ production by T and NK cells, activates LAK cells
IFN-γ	20-24	Th1 and CD8 T cells, NK cells	Induces MHC expression, inhibits virus replication, B cell isotype switch to IgG2a, inhibits proliferation of Th2 cells and B cells in response to IL-4, activates macrophage
TNF-α	15-25 kd multimers	Macrophages, keratinocytes, T cells	Cachexia, macrophages and PMN activation and chemotaxis, cytotoxic for virus-infected cells, fever induction, induces adhesion molecule expression, in synergy with IFN-γ induces IL-8 production by keratinocytes, induces proliferation of fibroblasts, B cells, and thymocytes, LC migration, induces production of extracellular matrix, induces MHC class I, angiogenic
LT/TNF-β	15-25 kd multimers	Th1 and CD8 T cells	Cytotoxic for virus-infected and some tumor cells, induces production of extracellular matrix, induces MHC class I expression, B cell differentiation and proliferation, angiogenic
GM-CSF	22 kd	T cells, keratinocytes	Hemopoietic growth factor, activation of PMN and LC
MIP-1α/β	8-10 kd	Activated T cells, B cells and macrophages	Chemotactic for and activates PMN in vivo, differentially chemotactic for lymphocyte subpopulations in vitro, induces fever
TGF-β	12.5 kd homodimer	Platelets, activated macrophages and T cells	Proinflammatory: chemotactic for PMN, T cells, and monocytes, upregulates β1 integrins, induces CD16 expression on monocytes, induces proinflammatory cytokines Antiinflammatory: inhibits T cell proliferation and IL-1 receptor expression, functional maturation of CTL, NK and LAK cells, O_2^- radical production by macrophage
IL-1ra	17-25 kd	Many of the cells that produce IL-1	Inhibits IL-1 functions by competitively binding to the IL-1 receptor

Abbreviations: IL, interleukin; PMN, polymorphonuclear leukocyte; Th1/2, T helper type 1/2; CD, cluster of differentiation; NK, natural killer cell; LPS, lipopolysaccharide; CTL, cytotoxic T lymphocyte; LAK, lymphokine-activated killer cell; NAP, neutrophil activating protein; EBV, Epstein-Barr virus; IFN, interferon; TNF, tumor necrosis factor; LC, Langerhans cell; LT, lymphotoxin; GM-CSF, granulocyte/macrophage colony stimulating factor; MIP, macrophage inflammatory protein; TGF, transforming growth factor; IL-1ra, IL-1 receptor antagonist.

involved in the proliferation and differentiation of CTL precursors.[26,104] These responses appear to control infections by intracellular parasites such as viruses. In contrast, the capacity of Th2 cells to regulate antibody responses would favor their involvement in reactions to infections by free-living organisms such as bacteria. Not only do the Th1 and Th2 cytokine patterns seem to be stable phenotypes in mouse T cell clones, it is apparent that these T cell subpopulations have their origin in normal T cells in vivo. This fact is illustrated by the contrasting roles of Th1 and Th2 cells in certain infectious diseases.

Naive and Memory T Cell Subpopulations. The capacity of the immune system to respond more quickly to antigens that have previously been encountered is referred to as immunologic memory. It is now obvious that naive T cells (those that have not yet been stimulated by antigen) are phenotypically and functionally distinguishable from memory T cells (T cells that have been stimulated by antigen). Naive and memory T cells are most readily identified by antibodies specific for different isoforms of the leukocyte common antigen (CD45). CD45 is expressed on all nucleated hematopoietic cells. The molecular weight of CD45 ranges from 180 to 220 kd because of alternative splicing of its exons encoding the extracytoplasmic domain. The CD45 gene is composed of 34 exons. Among them, exons 4, 5, and 6 (also called exons A, B, and C, respectively) are alternatively spliced. The splicing pattern of CD45 is differentially regulated in various cell types and is developmentally regulated during T cell maturation. Moreover, naive T cells and activated or memory T cells express different isoforms of CD45, that is, naive T cells express CD45RO, whereas activated and memory T cells express CD45RA. This expression not only provides a convenient cell surface marker to study different subpopulations of T cells, it also reflects a change of cell status, during and after activation, that may be functionally important.

Memory T cells also express higher levels of a variety of adhesion molecules including the following: CD2, CD11a/CD18 (LFA-1), CD44 (Pgp-1), CD58 (LFA-3), CD54 (ICAM-1) and very late antigens 4, 5, and 6 (VLA-4, -5, -6). These adhesion molecules perform an important function in T cell activation and in the homing patterns of T cells and other inflammatory cells, and will be discussed in that context in the subsequent sections of this chapter dealing with the afferent and efferent limbs of the T cell response.

The enhanced expression of these adhesion molecules is probably responsible, at least in part, for the accelerated response of memory T cells to antigens upon secondary exposure. Moreover, CD45, CD4, and CD8 molecules form a stable complex with the TCR in memory, but not naive T cells. Because these molecules appear to augment T cell responsiveness under suboptimal stimulatory conditions, a stable complex of these accessory molecules with the TCR may enhance the responsiveness of memory T cells upon reexposure to antigen.

αβ TCR⁺ and γδ TCR⁺ T Cell Subpopulations. Most T cells in the lymphoid organs and circulation of adult animals express heterodimeric TCR consisting of an α and a β chain. A second subpopulation of T cells has now been identified,[12] however, that expresses a heterodimeric TCR consisting of a γ and a δ chain. Most $\gamma\delta$ TCR⁺ cells exhibit the double-negative (CD4⁻ CD8⁻) phenotype. Although $\gamma\delta$ T cells represent a minor subpopulation in the lymphoid organs, they are the major lymphocyte subset in the epithelium of nonlymphoid organs such as the skin, intestines, vagina, and uterus. Epidermal $\gamma\delta$ T cells have a dendritic morphology, embody the Thy-1 and CD3 surface antigens, but do not display either the CD4 or CD8 T cell antigens.[5,40] $\gamma\delta$ T cells represent about 60% of T cells in the intestinal epithelia. These cells are unique among $\gamma\delta$ cells in that they express the CD8 molecule. Unlike $\alpha\beta$ T cells that exhibit a heterodimeric form of CD8 consisting of an α and β chain, however, $\gamma\delta$ T cells in the intestinal epithelium bear a CD8α homodimer. $\gamma\delta$ T cells represent about half of the lymphocyte population associated with mucosal epithelia or organs such as the tongue, vagina, and uterus.[49] These cells exhibit CD3 but do not show CD4 or CD8 and only half express Thy-1.

The function of $\gamma\delta$ cells is still not clear. $\gamma\delta$ cell lines and clones have been described that preferentially lyse tumor cells,[94] virus-infected cells,[51] and natural killer (NK)-sensitive targets.[18] Like their $\alpha\beta$ T cell counterparts, $\gamma\delta$ cells can be activated by signals that result from cross-linking of the TCR-CD3 complex. Activation results in proliferation and cytokine production. The nature of the ligand that is recognized by $\gamma\delta$ T cells is not apparent. The lack of CD4 and CD8 on the vast majority of $\gamma\delta$ cells has prompted studies to determine if antigen recognition by these cells is MHC restricted. The results to date suggest that some $\gamma\delta$ cells display MHC-restricted antigen recognition, whereas many do not.[50,51,55] Many $\gamma\delta$ clones are restricted by the virtually nonpolymorphic MHC class Ib (Qa and TL) molecules.[10,118] A surprisingly large proportion of $\gamma\delta$ T cells recognize mycobacterial antigens, particularly mycobacterial heat shock protein 65 (HSP65), which is essentially identical to the mammalian homologue.[50] This observation has led to the hypothesis that highly conserved antigens such as HSP might serve as the major ligand for $\gamma\delta$ T cells. Some interesting corollaries to this hypothesis include the following: (1) the participation of HSP-reactive $\gamma\delta$ T cells that are activated during bacterial infections in autoimmune reactions to autologous HSP; (2) the prolongation of inflammatory responses caused by the reaction of $\gamma\delta$ T cells to HSP in inflamed tissue following the elimination of the inciting foreign antigen; and, conversely, (3) the participation of HSP-reactive $\gamma\delta$ cells in the resolution of inflammatory responses by eliminating activated macrophages that express HSP65 on their surface. None of these possibilities have been confirmed. The developmental relationship between $\alpha\beta$ TCR⁺ and $\gamma\delta$ TCR⁺ T cells is not obvious. Ontogenetically, $\gamma\delta$ TCR⁺ cells precede $\alpha\beta$ TCR⁺ cells, representing the majority of thymocytes in the fetal thymus until day 17 or 18 of gestation. $\alpha\beta$ TCR$^+$ cells then appear and become the predominant subpopulation thereafter. The mechanisms that regulate TCR gene expression are only beginning to be understood. A recent study[80] determined that mice that are homozygous for a disrupted TCRα gene lack $\alpha\beta$ TCR$^+$ cells, but their $\gamma\delta$ TCR$^+$ T cells developed in normal numbers. It appears, therefore, that regulation of $\gamma\delta$ TCR expression is independent of the presence of $\alpha\beta$ TCR$^+$ cells.

Maturation and Selection of T Cells in the Thymus. T lymphocytes originate from pluripotent stem cells within the bone marrow. The T cell precursors (pre-T cells) become committed to the T lymphocytic pathway of differentiation prior to emergence from the bone marrow. These pre-T cells then leave the bone marrow and migrate via the circulation to the thymus. It is within the microenvironment of the thymus that they acquire the characteristics of mature T lymphocytes.

Pre-T cells enter the thymus cortex as CD4$^-$, CD8$^-$ lymphoblasts. These cells then rearrange and express their TCR genes (description follows) and differentiate into CD4$^+$, CD8$^+$ double-positive cells, which may represent an intermediate stage in the differentiation to CD4$^+$ or CD8$^+$ single-positive cells expressing a low density of the TCR-CD3 complex. The maturing thymocytes undergo a somewhat paradoxical double-selection process in which cells with TCR that can recognize self MHC are both positively and negatively selected.

The MHC-restricted manner in which the TCR recognizes foreign antigens necessitates a positive selection for cells with TCR that can recognize a combination of self MHC plus antigenic peptide. Although the mechanism of this positive selection is not obvious, it seems to result from an interaction of the maturing thymocyte with MHC antigens on thymic epithelial cells. A successful interaction between the TCR and MHC permits further thymocyte maturation and avoids programmed cell death, which appears to be the fate of most thymocytes. Conversely, the export of functionally mature T cells capable of reacting to self MHC alone could lead to autoimmune disease. Cells with TCR that are reactive to self-MHC determinants are present among immature thymocytes. It appears, however, that most of these cells are eliminated within the thymus through a negative selection process. In this process, too strong a reaction between TCR and MHC antigens on bone marrow-derived macrophage or dendritic thymic APC leads to programmed cell death. The net result of these two selection processes is an MHC-restricted but self-tolerant T cell repertoire. Mature thymocytes leave the thymus and migrate via the lymphatics or circulation to the secondary lymphoid organs. Emigration of mature T cells from the thymus occurs at the relatively low rate of 1 to 2 million cells per day.

Export of Naive T Cells to the Secondary Lymphoid Organs. The secondary lymphoid organs (including lymph nodes, spleen, and Peyers patches) have developed special-ized means of recruiting T cells, particularly naive T cells, from the circulation.[81] Selective recruitment is accomplished via distinctive postcapillary venules. The first step in the extravasation of T cells into the secondary lymphoid organs involves binding of the circulating lymphocyte to the endothelium of postcapillary venules. The lymph nodes and Peyers patches have evolved specialized venules that are called high endothelial venules (HEV) as a result of the cuboid morphology of the endothelial cells that line the lumen of these vessels. These HEV are highly efficient at trapping and recruiting lymphocytes. The spleen lacks HEV, but has specialized endothelial cells lining the sinuses of the white pulp that contribute to lymphocyte recruitment.[7] Diapedesis of naive T cells into secondary lymphoid organs is a multiple step process that is mediated by adhesion molecules (Table 6-2). The first step in the binding of naive T cells to the HEV endothelium of peripheral lymph nodes results from the interaction of the lymphocyte selectin (L-selectin, mouse Mel-14, or its human homologue—LAM-1) homing receptor to sialyated oligosaccharide determinants on the peripheral lymph node vascular addressin (PNAd). Expression of PNAd on lymph node HEV and of L-selectin on naive T cells is constitutive. The interaction between these two homing receptors retards the flow of the T cell, enabling it to attach to the endothelial surface of the HEV. The second step in the interaction between naive T cells and HEV involves the binding of the $\beta 2$ integrin, LFA-1 (CD11a-CD18) to a counter receptor on the HEV. The known ligands for LFA-1 include the intercellular adhesion molecules -1, -2, and -3 (ICAM-1, -2, -3). Antibodies to ICAM-1 do not block extravasation of naive T cells into lymph nodes. The possible involvement of ICAM-2 and ICAM-3 has not been tested. A different combination of homing receptor and vascular addressin regulates extravasation into Peyers patches. Thus antibodies to L-selectin or to PNAd effectively inhibit extravasation of naive T cells into peripheral lymph nodes, but not into Peyers patches. Conversely, a monoclonal antibody, MECA-367, specific for a vascular addressin on Peyers patches HEV blocks extravasation of T cells into Peyers patches but not into lymph nodes. The nature of the homing receptor on T cells that binds to the Peyers patches vascular addressin is not known.

Afferent Limb of the Cellular Immune Response

The afferent limb of cellular immunity is the process by which the invasion of foreign antigen leads to activation of T lymphocytes that are specifically reactive to that antigen. It can be further divided into a cognitive phase and an activation phase. In the cognitive phase, foreign antigens are transported from a site of administration to a regional secondary lymphoid tissue and are presented to T lymphocytes. T cells recognize, via TCR, antigenic fragments in conjunction with MHC molecules on the surface of APC. This highly specific interaction, in conjunction with other co-

TABLE 6-2 CHARACTERISTICS OF ADHESION MOLECULES THAT APPEAR TO PLAY AN IMPORTANT ROLE IN IMMUNE/INFLAMMATORY RESPONSES

Leukocyte Receptor				Counter Receptor				
Molecule	Family	Induction	Distribution	Molecule	Family	Induction	Distribution	Function
L-selectin, Mel-14, LAM-1, LECCAM-1	Selectin	Constitutive	Resting lymphs, PMN, monocytes	MECA-79, sgp50, sgp90, glyCAM-1	CHO	Constitutive	HEV	L-selectin-lymph homing to LN
sLeX-related structure	CHO	Constitutive	PMN	E-selectin, ELAM-1, LECCAM-2	Selectin	IL-1, TNF, LPS	Endothelial cells	Initial interaction (rolling) of PMN on vascular endothelium
				P-selectin, CD62, PADGEM, GMP-140	Selectin	Thrombin, Histamine, H_2O_2	Endothelial cells, platelets	
LFA-1, CD11a/CD18	$\beta2$-Integrin	IL-2, IFN-γ, IL-8, PAF, TCR cross-linking (avidity change)	Lymphs (T, B, NK), PMN, monocytes, Mϕ	ICAM-1, CD54	Ig	IL-1,TNF, IFN-γ	Endothelial, epithelial, dendritic B, T, NK, monocyte	T cell-APC/target interaction
				ICAM-2	Ig	Constitutive	Endothelial cells	Extravasation, Migration T cell signal transduction
Mac-1, CD11b/CD18	$\beta2$-Integrin	PAF IFN-γ IL-8	Ly1+ B, CD8 (subpopulation), NK, PMN, monocyte, Mϕ	ICAM-1, CD54, several ECM proteins, C3bI				
VLA-4, $\alpha4$, $\beta1$, CD49d/CD29	$\beta1$-Integrin	TCR cross-linking (avidity change)	B, T, monocyte, LC	VCAM-1	Ig	IL-4 IL-1 TNF	Endothelial cells	Extravasation T cell activation?

Abbreviations: LAM, leukocyte adhesion molecule; LECCAM, lectin-epidermal growth factor-complement related cell adhesion molecules; PMN, polymorphonuclear leukocytes; sgp, sulfated glycoprotein; CAM, cell adhesion molecule; CHO, carbohydrate; HEV, high endothelial venule; LN, lymph node; sLeX, sialyated Lewis-X blood group antigen; ELAM, endothelial leukocyte adhesion molecule; PADGEM, platelet activation dependent granule external membrane; GMP, granule membrane protein; PAF, platelet-activating factor; TCR, T cell receptor; ICAM, intercellular adhesion molecule; ECM, extracellular matrix; VLA, very late activation; VCAM, vascular cell adhesion molecule.

stimulatory signals provided by APC or the microenvironment, triggers the activation phase, which involves a cascade of changes of cellular biochemical status within the T cell. Activation of T cells is marked by proliferation, functional maturation, and differentiation. T helper lymphocytes are essential in initiating the immune response. They become activated by interacting with antigen-bearing APC and produce cytokines, which in turn help to activate B cells and cytotoxic T cells.

Transport of Antigen to the Lymphoid Organs. The first line of protection against microbial invasion is a physical barrier: the epidermal layer of the skin and the epithelium of internal organs. This shield not only provides mechanical protection, it also represents the frontier of immune surveillance. Langerhans cells (LC) are an important part of this surveillance system in the skin. These bone marrow-derived cells have dendritic morphology and display receptors for the Fc portion of IgG and IgE, as well as complement receptors. LC also constitutively express MHC class II antigen. Although LC are considered nonphagocytic, they can take up antigens by means of pinocytosis and possibly receptor-mediated endocytosis when the antigens are complexed with complement or antibodies. The latter may be especially important in secondary immune responses. Moreover, recent evidence suggests that immature LC are capable of phagocytosis.[47] Circumstantial in vivo and in vitro evidence implies that, upon exposure to antigens, LC undergo functional maturation and gain the ability to present antigens to CD4 T cells. Changes include increase in size, increased MHC class II expression, and possibly production of co-stimulatory factors. Cytokines, such as IL-1 and GM-CSF that are secreted by keratinocytes, induce the maturation process in vitro and have been proposed to carry out a similar function in vivo. Coincident with functional maturation, LC (with antigens) migrate from the epithelium to draining lymph nodes via the afferent lymphatic channels. A recent report proposed a role for TNF-α in the induction of LC migration to draining lymph nodes.[19] After entering the lymph node, LC home to the cortical and paracortical regions, where T cell activation occurs. Antigens are presented to T cells by interdigitating dendritic cells (IDC). It is still controversial whether LC deliver antigens to IDC, or alternatively, that they transform into IDC and present antigen themselves.

Antigen Processing and Presentation. In contrast to B cell receptors, which recognize native protein antigens, TCRs recognize processed antigenic peptides. Early evidence of this difference came from a study by Gell and Benacerraf[35] in 1959. They observed that DTH, which was known at that time to be mediated by mononuclear cells, could be provoked by both native and denatured protein, whereas antibody mediated anaphylaxis could only be elicited by native protein. The significance of this phenomenon remained unexplained until the 1970s, however, when the role of macrophages in generating immune responses was investigated

extensively. Through the combined efforts of many laboratories, it became apparent that, to activate helper T cells, APC must take up antigens, pass them through intracellular compartments, and express them on the cell surface as antigenic peptides bound to MHC molecules. This process is now referred to as antigen processing. Generally speaking, antigen processing is defined as partial degradation of protein to oligopeptides. When antigens are in the form of small peptides or simple proteins, antigen processing can be just unfolding of the secondary structure or processing may not be required at all.

To activate T cells, processed antigens must be bound to MHC on the surface of APC. MHC antigens were initially discovered as transplantation antigens in the 1940s. Using outbred strains of mice, Snell and associates found that a tumor arising spontaneously in one mouse was usually rejected when transplanted to another mouse. In some cases, however, the tumor did grow. To map the genetic loci responsible for this phenomenon, they undertook extensive breeding studies that led to the development of inbred strains of mice and the Nobel Prize-winning discovery of MHC molecules. Tumors arising from one member of an inbred strain were accepted by another member of the same strain, but readily rejected by members of other inbred strains. It was thus concluded that the antigens responsible for tumor rejection were not tumor-associated, but were antigens present in normal tissues. This interpretation was further supported by skin and other tissue transplantation studies between inbred strains. Genetic analysis revealed a single locus was responsible for most of the rejection phenomena. Through experiments using sera obtained from mice undergoing transplant rejection, the antigens responsible for the rejection were identified on the cell surface of the transplanted tumor as well as on normal donor tissue. These transplant antigens were referred to as antigen II by Snell's group, and the genetic region was called histocompatibility-2 or simply H-2. Because the H-2 region contained several different yet closely linked genes that were largely responsible for transplant rejection, this region was more generally referred to as the major histocompatibility complex. The human MHC is referred to as the human leukocyte antigen (HLA) genes.

It was not until 20 years later that the MHC region was found to play an important role in regulating physiologic immune responses. Benacerraf and associates mapped genes that control the immune responsiveness to certain synthetic peptides to the MHC in inbred mice and guinea pigs. The genes were therefore called immune response (Ir) genes. The central role of Ir genes in immune responses was further elucidated in the 1970s by the same group. They found that T cells can recognize antigenic peptides only when they are noncovalently bound to MHC molecules.[52]

There are two types of MHC molecules, class I and class II. Both are membrane glycoproteins composed of one alpha

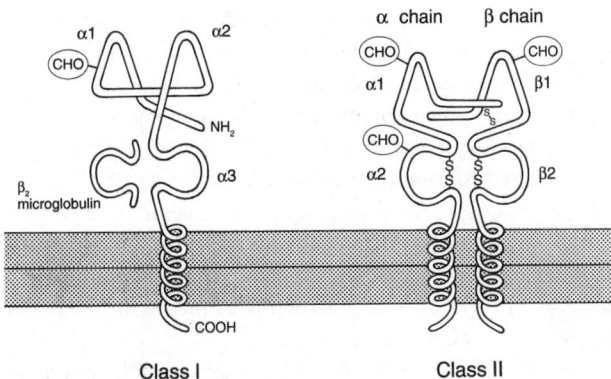

Fig. 6-1. Structural characteristics of major histocompatibility complex (MHC) class I and class II molecules.

chain and one beta chain (Fig. 6-1). The class I alpha chain is about 47 kd in mice and 44 kd in humans. The extracellular portion has three domains, namely, α1, α2, and α3. The α1 and α2 domains, which form the peptide-binding region, are polymorphic; whereas the α3 domain is monomorphic. The β chain of class I is also called β2 microglobin. It is monomorphic and associates with the α chain noncovalently. It is about 12 kd in both humans and mice. The α chain (32 to 34 kd) and the β chain (29 to 32 kd) of class II molecules are of similar size. Both are polymorphic, and each has two extracellular domains. The peptide-binding region is formed between the α1 and β1 domains.

The murine MHC is located on chromosome 17, whereas its human homolog is on the short arm of chromosome 6.

The organization of both loci is shown in Fig. 6-2. Murine class I genes are also called H-2 genes. Two major alleles that encode the α chain of class I molecules are H-2K and H-2D. The gene for the β chain of class I molecules (β2 microglobin) is located on chromosome 2. The I region, located between the K and D loci, codes for murine class II genes. It is further divided into I-A and I-E regions. Both contain genes encoding their own α and β chains. HLA-A, B, and C are genes for human class I α chains. HLA-DP, DQ, and DR are human class II genes. Each locus contains genes for both α and β chains. All the alleles are co-dominantly expressed.

Class II Restricted Responses. As noted earlier, APC present exogenously derived antigen to CD4 T cells in conjunction with MHC class II molecules. The current model for the processing and presentation of antigens in the context of MHC class II is shown in Fig. 6-3, *B*. There are several requisite properties that allow a cell to function as an APC. First, the cell must be able to endocytose antigens and process them to peptides. Virtually all cells are capable of endocytosis by means of phagocytosis, pinocytosis, or receptor-mediated endocytosis. This process is sensitive to fixation by chemicals such as formaldehyde. The internalized antigens are then gradually degraded while being transported from endocytic vesicles (endosomes) to lysosomes. During their intracellular passage, endosomes become acidified. This change of pH along with activation of acid pH-dependent proteases leads to denaturation and initial fragmentation of the internalized antigen. If peptide fragments are

Human HLA complex Chromosome #6

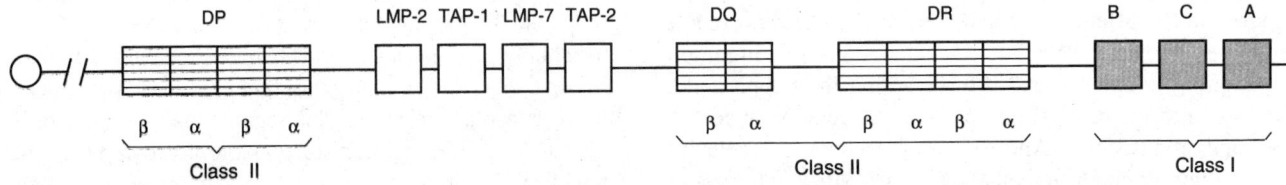

Mouse H-2 complex Chromosome #17

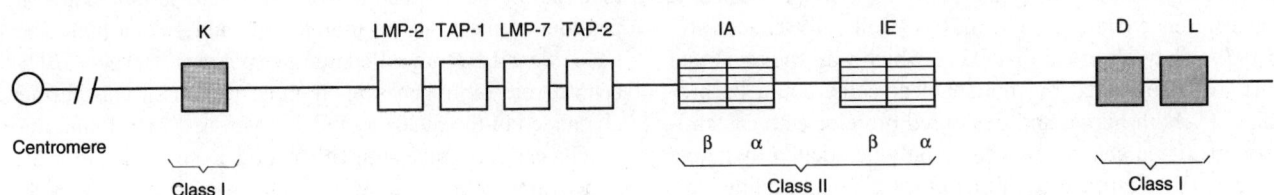

Fig. 6-2. Organization of the human and murine MHC gene loci. LMP, low molecular mass polypeptide; TAP, transporter associated with antigen processing.

not protected from degradation by binding to class II molecules in the late endosomal compartment, they will eventually be transported to lysosomes and completely degraded. This degradation pathway is almost universal to all cell types. It is sensitive to the protease inhibitor leupeptin as well as reagents, such as chloroquine and ammonia, that elevate intracellular pH.

The second requirement for an APC is expression of class II antigen. Macrophages, B cells, lymphoid dendritic cells, and epidermal LC all express class II antigens constitutively. They are considered to be professional APC. Class II expression can be induced by cytokines in a variety of cell types. Epithelial, glial, mesenchymal, and vesicular endothelial cells can express class II upon cytokine induction and present antigen in vitro. The physiologic significance of antigen presentation by nonprofessional APC in vivo is not clear. It is conceivable that immune responses are first initiated by interaction of professional APC with CD4 T cells. Activated CD4 T cells then secrete IFN-γ at sites of antigen entry and induce class II expression on nonprofessional APC, which, in turn, activate more T cells locally. One potential problem in this hypothetical amplification mecha-

nism, however, is that expression of class II alone is not sufficient to enable a cell to activate most T cells. Professional APC provide T cells with some co-stimulatory signals in addition to MHC-peptide complex. As will be discussed in more detail later, MHC-peptide interaction with the TCR —without co-stimulatory factors—may result in T cell anergy.

To interact with processed peptides, class II molecules within APC must be sorted to the endolysosome compartment before being transported to the cell surface. This fact was demonstrated in several laboratories in the late 1980s. Regulation of class II expression is primarily at the transcription level. Transcription of α and β chain mRNA is coordinately regulated. The mRNA for both chains of class II molecules is translated by endoplasmic reticulum (ER)-bound ribosomes and transported into the lumen of the ER cotranslationally.

Soon after entering the ER, α and β chains, together with γ chain, associate with each other noncovalently to form a trimeric complex. The γ chain of class II molecules is also called invariant chain (li) because of its lack of polymorphism. Its gene is not linked to the MHC locus in humans or

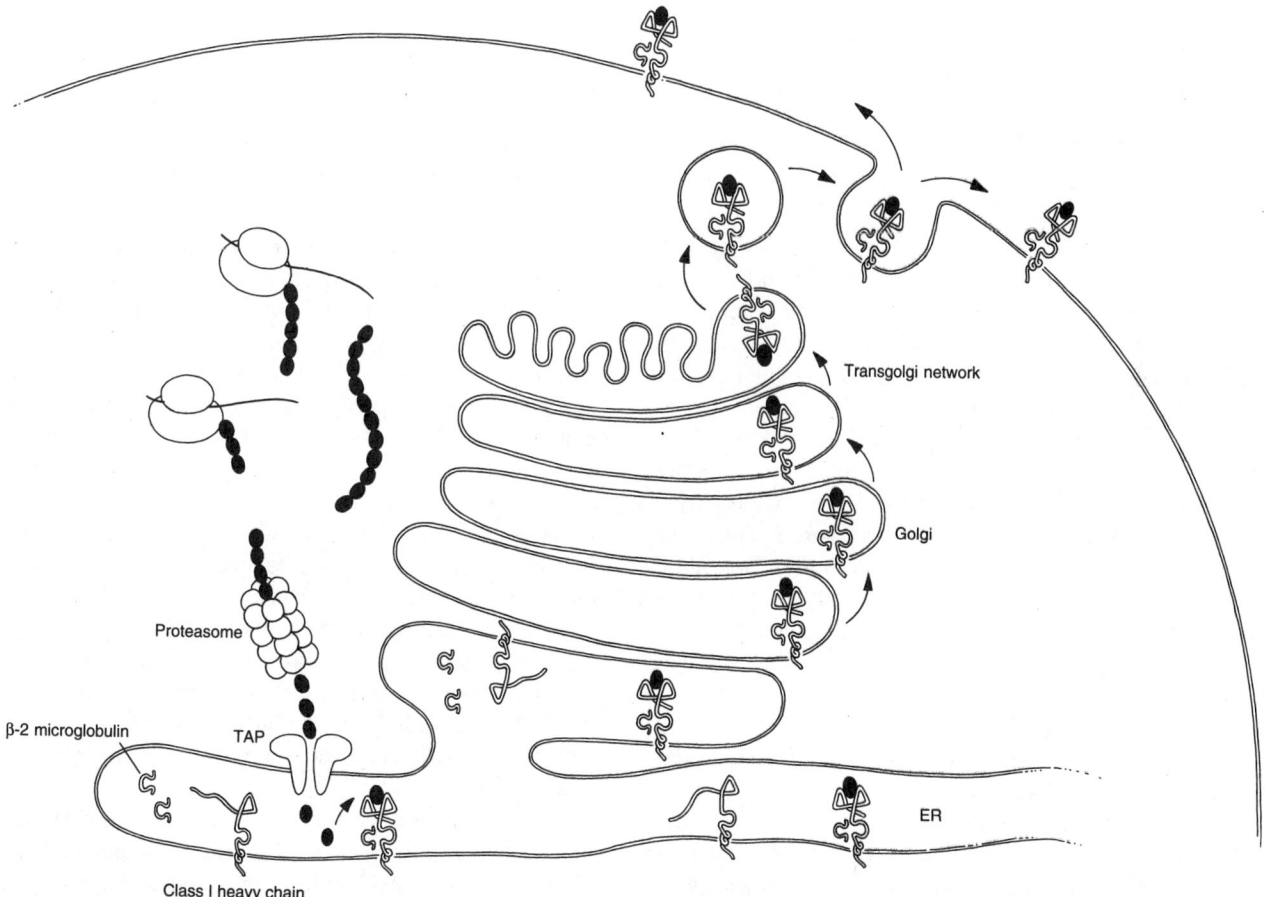

Fig. 6-3. **A,** current model for the processing of endogenous antigens for presentation by MHC class I.

Continued

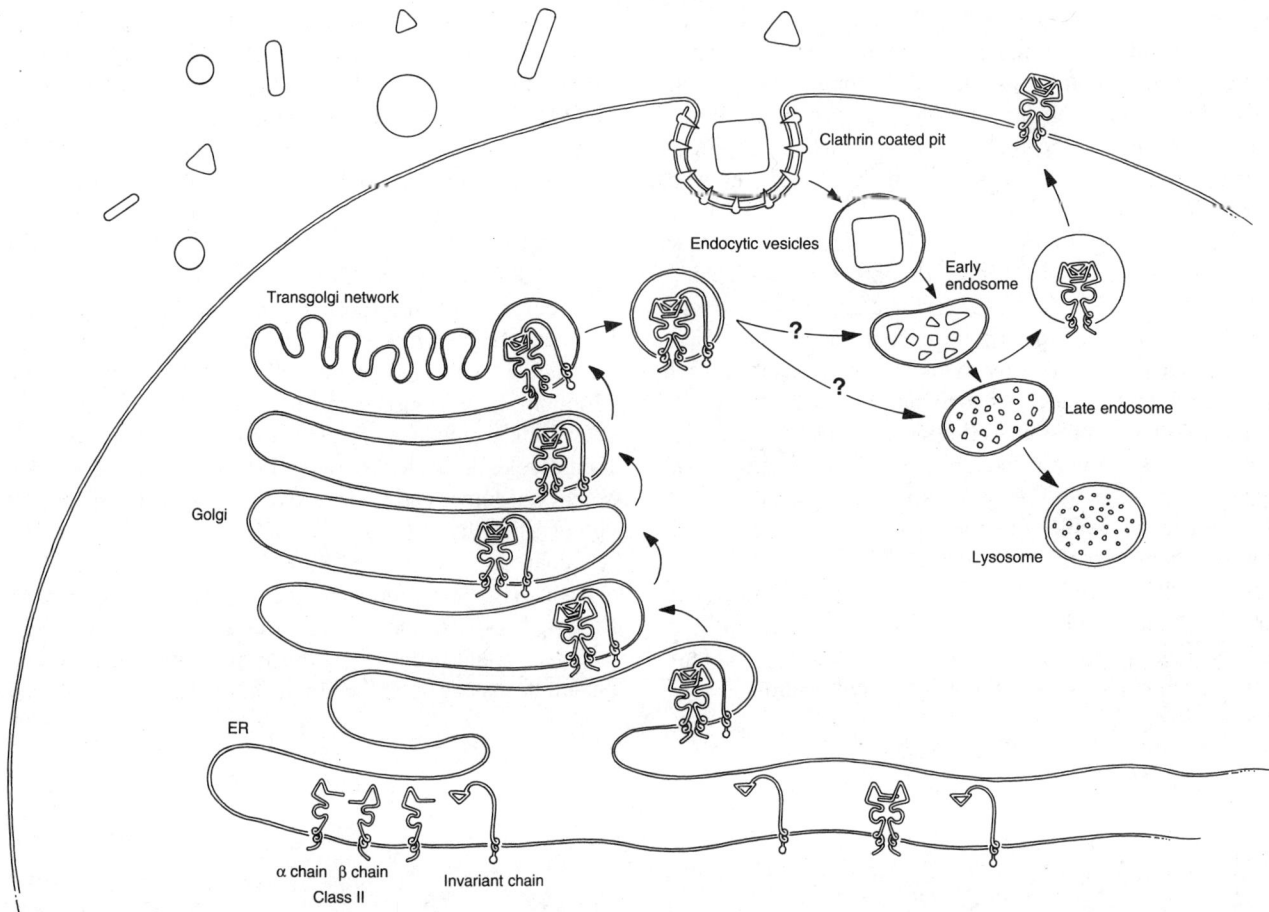

Fig. 6-3, cont'd. **B,** current model for the processing of exogenous antigens for presentation by MHC class II (see text for details).

mice. Its expression, however, is regulated coordinately with that of α and β chains. It has a molecular weight of 31 kd. Like α and β chains, it is also a transmembrane protein. The trimeric complex of class II molecules is transported from the ER to the Golgi apparatus, following the cellular default transportation for cytoplasmic proteins. From the trans-Golgi network, however, transport of class II diverges from the default pathway and is redirected to the endolysosomal compartment. Invariant chain is responsible for this divergence. Its cytoplasmic domain contains a sorting signal for the endolysosomal compartment. In addition to providing this sorting signal, invariant chain is thought to shield the peptide-binding groove with its axoplasmic domain, so that no peptide can bind before class II reaches the endolysosomal compartment, where class II meets endocytosed antigens.

After arriving at the endolysosome, invariant chain is degraded and released from the α and β chains to expose the peptide-binding site. This model explains the preferential presentation of exogenously acquired processed antigens over endogenously produced antigens in the context of MHC class II. The precise compartment where class II molecules meet peptides still remains to be determined. It is

likely to occur after the late endosome and before the lysosome. Following assembly, class II peptide complexes are transported to the cytoplasmic membrane via an undefined route.

Several biochemical characteristics of class II binding peptides have been identified. They usually contain 13 to 17 amino acid residues. About 2000 different peptides bind to the same class II molecules. No common structural motif can be found among them, however. Despite the promiscuousness of peptide MHC interaction, the antigenicity of a particular peptide still can be predicted from its primary amino acid sequence. Mutational analysis has shown that all antigenic peptides have some amino acid residues that point downward, contacting the class II molecule, while others point away from the peptide-binding groove of the MHC making contact with the TCR. Thus peptides bound to class II may not be antigenic if they fail to express residues that contact the TCR.

Loading of peptides onto class II molecules in endolysosomes occurs at low pH. The resulting weak interaction is stabilized when the pH increases to the physiologic level of the cell cytoplasm. The binding of peptides to class II does not occur completely at random. Experiments in mice have shown that some peptides can bind to different I-A gene products (for example, I-A^d and I-A^k), but fail to bind to I-E encoded by any I-E gene. Because of co-dominant expression of both haplotypes and random association of α and β chains encoded by different alleles, however, most individuals express 10 to 20 different class II molecules on a cell surface. With binding potential of thousands of different peptides per molecule, this expression provides ample binding opportunities for antigenic peptides. Nonetheless, some antigens are presented more effectively by certain class II molecules. Accordingly, those antigens are more immunogenic in animals that express the class II molecule, which is likely the basis for the aforementioned Ir gene regulation of immune responsiveness.

Class I Restricted Responses. Class I restricted antigen presentation was decidedly shown for the first time by Zinkernagel and Doherty[126] in 1974. They confirmed that CD8 T cells from the spleen of virally infected mice can only lyse infected fibroblasts that express homologous H-2 antigens.

Distinct from the class II pathway, class I antigens present peptides that are synthesized within the cell. Early evidence of two different pathways came from studies by Morrison and associates[67] in 1986. Their experiments revealed that class I-restricted CTL lysed target cells infected with live viruses, whereas class II-restricted T cells responded to APC infected with both live and UV-inactivated viruses. Feeding APC with purified viral proteins sensitized them for class II-restricted recognition. Additionally, inhibition of protein synthesis after live viral infection abrogated the class I-restricted lysis but not the class II-restricted response. The fact that presentation of viral antigens by class I molecules is sensitive to inhibitors of protein synthesis suggests that class I presents endogenously produced antigens. Because purified viral antigens and UV-inactivated viruses were internalized into the cell via an endocytic route, the resulting processed viral peptides were presented by class II molecules. The fact that the class I-restricted response is unaffected by chloroquine treatment further supports the contention that the processing pathway leading to class I presentation is distinct from the pathway leading to class II presentation. In the early 1980s, when studying influenza virus-reactive CTL clones, Townsend and associates[114] found some of the clones were specific for viral nuclear protein (NA) instead of the membrane protein hemagglutinin (HA). This result was completely unexpected, because NA is synthesized in the cytoplasm of the cell and does not have a signal peptide for exporting to ER. Therefore NA is not expressed on the cell surface. Their observation was further supported by transfection experiments. Transfection of cells with a gene encoding a truncated form of HA lacking the signal peptide sequence rendered them sensitive to lysis by HA-specific CTL clones. HA proteins in the transfectants were produced in the cytoplasm and rapidly degraded, so the intact molecule never gained entry into the secretory path-

way. These experiments clearly demonstrated that class I is capable of presenting cytosolic antigens. More importantly, the results also implied that there must be machinery in the cytoplasm (that processes cytosolic protein into peptides) and an active transporter (that pumps antigens from the cytoplasm into a secretory pathway to reach the extracellular domain of class I molecules). Inhibition of class I-restricted presentation by brefeldin A, which blocks transport of membrane proteins from the ER to the Golgi, further infers that peptides enter the secretory pathway in a pre-Golgi compartment, presumably the ER.

The current model of processing and transport of endogenous antigens for presentation by class I molecules is shown in Fig. 6-3, *A*. Proteins presented by class I molecules are synthesized by cytosolic-free ribosomes. It has been proposed that proteasomes, particularly those designated low molecular mass polypeptide (LMP) complexes then degrade the protein into peptides. The 580-kd LMP is composed of 16 polypeptides, each of molecular weight 15 to 30 kd. Genes for two subunits, LMP1 and LMP2, are MHC linked. The LMP complex is closely related to proteasomes in antigenic and biochemical properties. Proteasomes are 1500-kd cytoplasmic multicatalytic proteinase complexes. They are present in most cells tested and are evolutionarily conserved. They may mediate ubiquitin-dependent proteolysis in the cytoplasm, which plays an important role in antigen processing for class I presentation. It has been postulated that LMP degrades proteins into peptides in a "breadslicer" model (cut at different sites simultaneously to produce multiple peptides). By changing the binding frame, proteasomes may generate overlapping sets of peptides of the same antigen.

Peptides generated by LMP complexes are then transferred to ER transporters. It has been proposed that LMP complexes may contact transporters directly and deliver peptides themselves. The putative transporters are transmembrane proteins in the ER and belong to the family of ATP-dependent transport proteins. Genes for the transporter, TAP1 and TAP2 (transporters associated with antigen processing), have been cloned in mice, humans, and other species. Both genes are mapped to the class II region of the MHC locus (see Fig. 6-2). Apparently, TAP1 and TAP2 associate with each other and form heterodimers in the ER membrane. The mechanism by which TAP function to transport peptides is still unknown. The fact that class I presentation in TAP mutants is reduced by more than 95% suggests that most of the peptides presented by class I are transported from the cytoplasm by TAP, and few ER peptides or peptides directed into ER by signal sequence are presented by class I.

After entering the lumen of the ER, peptides bind to class I. Peptide binding is required for proper folding of the α chain, association of α and β chains, and expression of class I on the cell surface. Presumably, peptide-binding induces conformational changes in the α chain, thus increasing thermostability of the complex.

Several unique characteristics have been attributed to class I presentation. Unlike class II, class I has strict size restrictions for peptides. Peptides bound to class I usually have 9 ± 1 residues, and for a given class I molecule, peptide bonds usually have conserved amino acid residues at both ends. This observation implies that peptides may be anchored to the class I molecule at both ends, whereas residues in the middle reach out to contact the TCR. The reason for the size restriction of class I presentation is still not certain. Theoretically, every step in the pathway described previously may contribute to the selection of peptides that are homogenous in size. The possibility that peptides are trimmed to nanomers after binding to class I has also been proposed. Another characteristic of class I presentation is that it is sensitive to protein synthesis inhibitors like cycloheximide. This fact implies that ordinarily only newly synthesized peptides are presented by class I molecules. Peptides may be rapidly degraded into single amino acids, unless they are protected by binding to class I.

Comparison of Class I and Class II Pathways of Antigen Presentation. Despite several differences, the two pathways of antigen presentation (class I and class II) do have some common features. Neither class I nor class II discriminate self and nonself peptides, that is both can bind and present foreign antigens as well as self proteins. The rule that class I presents endogenous antigens, whereas class II presents exogenously acquired antigens is not absolute. Presentation of exogenous antigen by class I, as well as presentation of endogenous antigen by class II, although unusual, has been demonstrated under certain experimental conditions.

Recognition of MHC-Peptide Complex by T Cells. Recognition of the MHC-peptide complex by TCR initiates an elaborate intracellular signal transduction pathway within the T cell. It is mediated by many different membrane molecules on the surfaces of T cells and their ligands on APCs (or target cells). Molecules like TCR and MHC-peptide complex determine the specificity of T cell activation. CD3 molecules associate with the TCR and are part of the TCR complex. Other molecules involved in the interaction are not antigen specific and can be grouped into two categories. Molecules that transduce signals across the T cell membrane are referred to as stimulatory molecules. Molecules that serve to strengthen the binding of T cells to APC (or target cells) are called adhesion molecules. These designations are not absolute, however, because many molecules carry out both functions.

TCR. As stated earlier, T cells can be divided into two subpopulations based on their expressions of $\alpha\beta$ or $\gamma\delta$ TCR. Chains for both types of TCR are transmembrane glycoproteins that belong to the Ig superfamily. TCR protein structure (Fig. 6-4, *A*) as well as gene organization (Fig. 6-4, *B*)

and expression resemble those of immunoglobulins. Each TCR locus consists of multiple genes for variable (V), joining (J), and constant (C) regions. β and δ chains have additional gene segments for diversity (D) region. The δ locus is unique in that the entire locus resides within the α locus, on chromosome 14 in both humans and mice. The β chain locus is on chromosome 7 in humans and on chromosome 6 in mice, whereas the γ chain locus is on chromosome 7 in humans and chromosome 13 in mice.

Shortly after arriving at the thymus, thymocytes start to rearrange TCR genes such that one coding gene for each region (V, J, D, C) is randomly selected and joined together, whereas intervening nonselected gene segments are permanently deleted from the genome. Rearrangement of $\gamma\delta$ genes precedes that of $\alpha\beta$ genes.

The mechanism of rearrangement is believed to be similar to that of immunoglobulins. Details of the process are not yet fully characterized. For both TCR and Ig, gene rearrangement is mediated by a lymphoid-specific recombinase complex, which recognizes recombination signal sequences (RSS) that flank all recombinant-competent gene segments. After binding to RSS, the recombinase brings two joining gene segments close to each other, presumably excising the intervening sequence and ligating the two segments. Two recombination-activating genes, RAG1 and RAG2, are expressed exclusively in developing lymphocytes. Transfec-

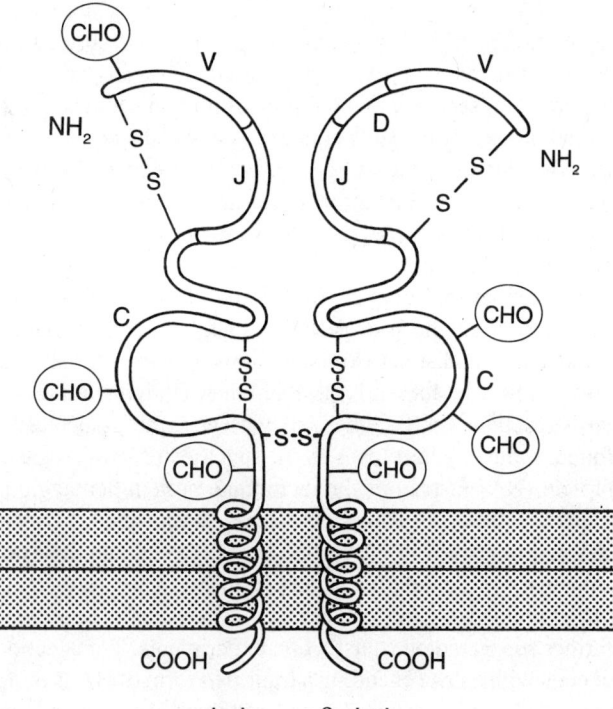

Fig. 6-4. T cell receptor (TCR): **A,** structure showing the variable (V), joining (J), diversity (D), and constant (C) regions of the $\alpha\beta$ TCR.

A.

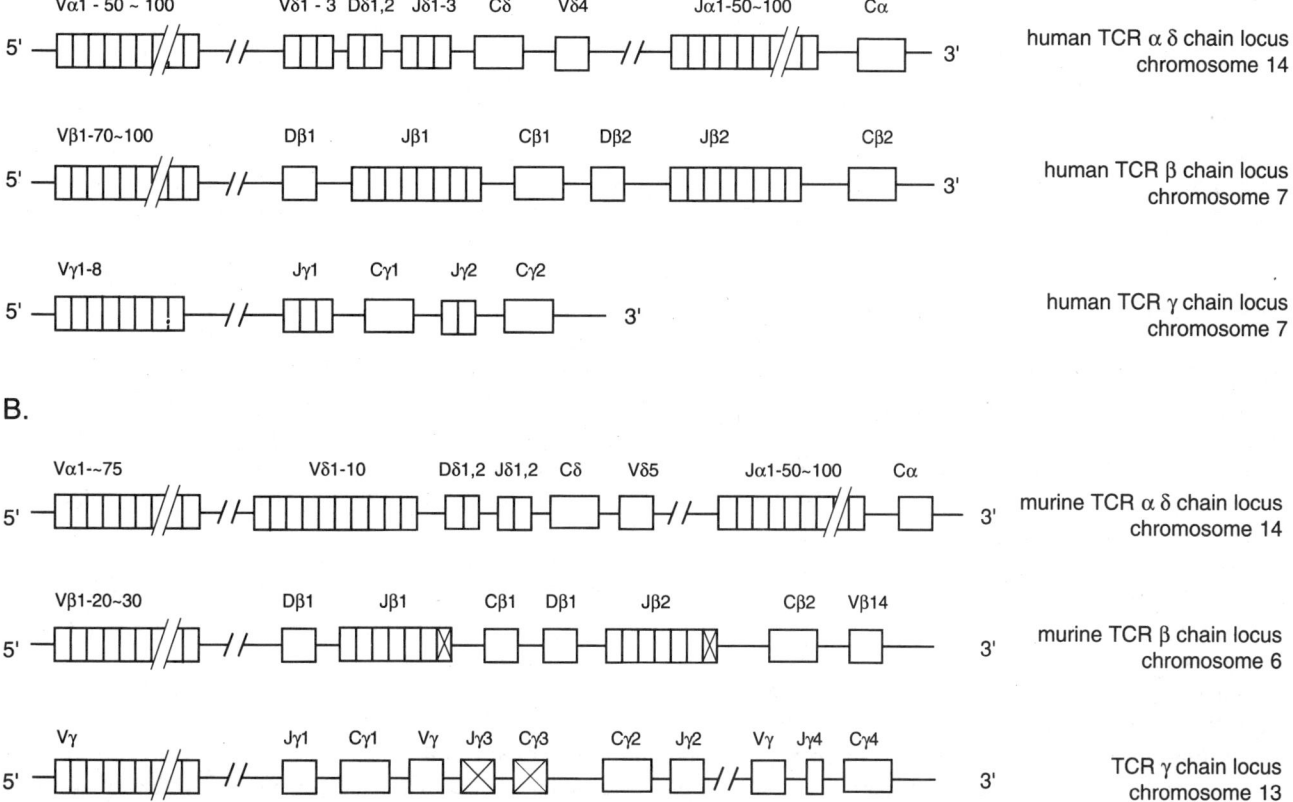

Fig. 6-4, cont'd.   **B**, gene organization. Note that the TCRδ gene lies within the TCR α locus. The approximate number of gene segments is given where the precise number is not known. An X indicates a pseudogene.

tion of both genes into fibroblasts induces recombination at RSS sites in the transfectant. It has been speculated that both RAG gene products may either upregulate recombinase activity in lymphocytes or, alternatively, participate directly in the recombination process.[75]

Rearrangement of the TCR genes occurs on only one of the two alleles. When successful rearrangement of one allele is completed, rearrangement of the second allele is suppressed. This phenomenon is referred to as allelic exclusion. Because of the mechanism of allelic exclusion, every individual T cell expresses only one type of TCR on its surface. Allelic exclusion can also be accomplished artificially in transgenic animals. When DNA encoding rearranged TCR genes are introduced into embryonic cells, TCR gene rearrangement in the cellular genome is suppressed. Thus animals developed from such embryos express only or predominantly the transgenic TCR on their T cells.

Specificities of the unselected immature T cell repertoire have been estimated to range from 10^{10} to 10^{15}. Mechanisms that contribute to generating the diversity include the following: (1) multiple V, D, and J gene segments in the germline; (2) random recombination of V, D, and J segments; (3) N-segment diversity (the joining sites of different gene segments may not be precise, and more nucleotides may be added between the two joining segments); (4) random assortment of α and β or γ and δ TCR chains. There is no evidence that somatic mutation contributes to TCR diversity, as it does in immunoglobulins.

Two TCR chains are held together by a disulfide bond between the constant regions of the extracellular domain. Variable regions are on the distal end of the extracellular domain. Variable regions of α and γ chains are encoded by V and J genes. Those for β and δ chains are encoded by V, D, and J genes. Variable regions of both pairing TCR chains act together to recognize antigens in association with MHC molecules on the surface of APC. Transmembrane domains of all TCR have one unusual positively charged lysine residue in each. The positive charge may help to bring TCR and CD3 chains into close proximity on the cell membrane, because the later have negatively charged aspartic acid residues in their transmembrane domains. Cytoplasmic domains of different TCR chains have no more than 12 amino acid residues, too short to function as signal transducers. TCR antigen recognition is coupled to cell activation by noncovalent association of TCR with molecules, such as CD3 and p59[fyn], that activate the intracellular signal transduction pathway.

CD3. CD3 refers to a group of five nonpolymorphic transmembrane proteins that are expressed on all mature T cells. These five polypeptides are called γ, δ, ε, ζ, and η chains, with molecular weights of 16 to 28 kd. The γ, δ, and ε chains are expressed as monomers. They share a high degree of sequence homology and are all members of the Ig superfamily. It has been proposed that their genes all arose from the same ancestral gene through gene duplication. On the other hand, ζ chains are expressed as a homodimer on 90% of T cells, or as ζ and η heterodimers on the other 10% of T cells. The ζ and η chains are homologous to each other, but both are unrelated to γ, δ, and ε chains. All five chains of CD3 associate closely with the TCR. They are often referred to as part of the integrated TCR-CD3 complex. All CD3 chains are nonpolymorphic and therefore do not participate in the antigen recognition process. They are involved in the regulation of TCR expression and T cell signal transduction.

Expression of CD3 and TCR chains is mutually dependent. In humans with CD3 mutations, the density of the TCR-CD3 complex is reduced to 10% to 50% of the normal level. Moreover, in TCR α chain knockout transgenic mice, essentially no independent CD3 expression is found. The regulation of expression occurs at a posttranslational level. Preassembly of the complete seven-chain complex, either αβγδεζζ or αβγδεζη, is required for surface expression of the complex. Incomplete complexes are rapidly degraded within the cell. CD3 chains have cytoplasmic domains of sufficient size to transduce signal. None of them, however, share sequence homology with any known signal-transducing proteins. Cross-linking of each CD3 chain with monoclonal antibodies produces nonspecific activation of T cells. Target sites for tyrosine protein kinase and an ATP-binding sequence have been found in the cytoplasmic domain of ζ chain. Cytoplasmic domains of γ, δ, and ε chains all contain target sites for serine phosphorylation. Phosphorylation of γ, δ, and ε chains on serine residues and phosphorylation of ζ chain on tyrosine residues have been demonstrated during T cell activation. It has been reported recently that cytoplasmic tails of ζ and ε chains can activate T cells independently of each other and of other components of the receptor complex.[48,58,122]

A src-like tyrosine kinase p59[fyn] associates noncovalently with ε and ζ chains of CD3. The src family includes a group of cytoplasmic nonreceptor tyrosine kinases, which mediate signal transduction and cause cell transformation when hyperactive. p59[fyn] has been implicated in T cell signal transduction. Overexpression of p59[fyn] in thymocytes led to hyperresponsiveness when the cells were stimulated with anti-TCR antibody, while expression of a mutant form of p59[fyn] abolished the proliferative response.[17] p59[fyn] knockout mice exhibited defective signal transduction in immature thymocytes, but apparently had normal signal transduction in peripheral T cells.[3,109]

Molecules Associated with TCR. CD4 and CD8. CD4 is a 55-kd monomeric transmembrane glycoprotein. CD8 is expressed on the cell membrane as a disulfide-linked homodimer of two 34-kd α chains, or as a heterodimer of α and β chains, or even as a multimeric complex. Both CD4 and CD8 molecules belong to the Ig gene superfamily. Expression of CD4 and CD8 on mature T cells is mutually exclusive. About 65% of peripheral T cells express CD4, whereas the other 35% express CD8.

CD4 binds to the monomorphic domain of class II MHC molecules and is important in class II-restricted responses. On the other hand, CD8, the functional analog of CD4, interacts with the monomorphic region of class I MHC molecules and plays a key role in class I-restricted responses. Binding of CD4/CD8 molecules to MHC is thought to be important in initial adhesion and avidity of the interaction between T cells and APC-target cells. It is still not clear whether CD4/CD8 molecules and TCR bind to the same MHC-peptide complex, though this theory is a common assumption. This assumption is supported by the observation that during T cell activation, CD4 molecules become closely associated with TCR-CD3 complex at the site of cell-cell contact. For this reason, CD4 and CD8 are also referred to as coreceptors of the TCR-CD3 complex.

In addition to the role in adhesion, CD4 and CD8 also participate in signal transduction in T cells. The intracellular domains of CD4 and CD8 have special sequences that bind to another src family tyrosine kinase, p56[lck] (which is expressed at high levels in T cells) and together with p59[fyn] phosphorylates phospholipase C (PLC)γ1, and CD3ζ and η chains at tyrosine residues during T cell activation.[58,71,76,123] Tyrosine phosphorylation is the earliest change detected in T cells during activation, followed by phosphotidyl inositol 4,5-bisphosphate (PIP2) breakdown. PLC resides in the inner leaf of the plasma membrane. Upon phosphorylation and activation, it cleaves PIP2 into inositol 1,4,5-triphosphate (IP3) and diacylglycerol (DAG), which in turn induce Ca^{2+} influx and protein kinase C (PKC) activation, respectively. The activity of p56[lck] is regulated by phosphorylation at tyrosine residues. Tyrosine residue 394 is weakly stimulatory when phosphorylated, whereas tyrosine residue 505 is inhibitory when phosphorylated. During T cell activation, when CD4 and CD8 become physically associated with the TCR, tyrosine kinase activity of p56[lck] is delivered to the TCR complex at the same time. Through this process the coreceptors augment the signal transmitted through the TCR-CD3 complex. It has been estimated that, with the coreceptors, 30- to 300-fold less ligand density is needed to activate T cells.

CD45. CD45 was formerly called leukocyte common antigen. Its pattern of expression was discussed in the section on naive and memory T cell population earlier in this chapter. A ligand for CD45 has been identified as CD22 on B cells. Several lines of evidence support the importance of CD45 in T cell function. First, CD45 knockout mice do not have T cells in the periphery. Second, cross-linking of CD45 with antibodies can either co-stimulate or inhibit T cell activation, depending on the CD45 epitope that is recognized by the antibody. Third, CD45-deficient cell lines show a profound defect in cellular proliferation and signal transduction through the TCR. Finally, the cytoplasmic domain of CD45 displays a high degree of homology with tyrosine phosphatase isolated from placenta, and purified CD45 has tyrosine phosphatase activity. CD45 is responsible for more than 90% of membrane bond tyrosine phosphatase activity in T cells. When cross-linked to CD4 or CD8, CD45 can dephosphorylate p56^{lck}. A plausible model proposes that CD45 modulates p56^{lck} activity when it becomes incorporated into the TCR-CD3 co-receptor complex during antigen recognition. Definitive elucidation, however, awaits further experimental support.

CD28. CD28 is a homodimeric transmembrane protein expressed on approximately 80% of human peripheral T lymphocytes. The molecular weight of the CD28 monomer is 44 kd. Constitutive expression of CD28 is upregulated during T cell activation. Recently a transmembrane protein on T lymphocytes called CTLA-4 (cytotoxic T lymphocyte associated antigen 4) shares a high degree of homology with CD28. Unlike CD28, CTLA-4 is a monomeric protein of 44 kd, and it is only expressed on activated T cells. Both CD28 and CTLA-4 belong to the Ig gene superfamily, and more importantly, they bind to the same ligand called B7-BB1, which is expressed on all professional antigen-presenting cells.

Cross-linking of CD28 with antibody can stimulate T cells to proliferate. Anti-CD28 antibody can also augment the T cell proliferation induced by a suboptimal dose of anti-CD2, anti-CD3, anti-TCR, and phytohemagglutinin (PHA). More importantly, the T cell response induced by Phorbol 12-Myristate 13-Acetate (PMA) in conjunction with anti-CD28 antibody is resistant to the immunosuppressive drug Cyclosporin A. Thus signal transduction through CD28 is biochemically distinct from that via the TCR-CD3 complex, which is sensitive to Cyclosporin A. In addition to inducing T cell proliferation, signaling through CD28 also potently activates T cell effector functions, such as lymphokine production and cytotoxicity.[33] The mechanism of this functional activation is twofold. Early in the response (less than 1 hour after stimulation), upregulation of lymphokine production is mainly caused by lymphokine mRNA stabilization. Later, an increase in transcription becomes prominent.

It has long been appreciated that T cell activation requires a second co-stimulatory signal in addition to the signal provided by TCR and MHC-peptide complex engagement. In fact, the TCR signal alone appears to cause T cells to enter a state of long-term unresponsiveness to the antigen, referred to as clonal anergy. This state of anergy persists even when the T cells are properly stimulated at later times.[70] Recent studies indicated that the interaction between CD28 and B7-BB1 provides the requisite co-stimulatory signal. Fixed APCs are deprived of their co-stimulatory ability and induce clonal anergy. Addition of anti-CD28 antibody to fixed APCs can correct the defect and stimulate T cells to proliferate. Moreover, pretreatment of animals with the fusion protein CTLA4Ig, which binds to B7-BB1 and blocks its interaction with CD28, suppresses the immune response to transplanted tissue, thus prolonging survival of the transplant. In contrast to conventional immunosuppressive drugs like Cyclosporin A, the suppressed immune response induced by CTLA4Ig is specific for the transplant.[57,59] This finding emphasizes the vital role of CD28 in T cell activation in vivo.

CD11a-CD18 (LFA-1). Leukocyte function-associated antigen-1 (LFA-1) is a heterodimeric, transmembrane protein composed of noncovalently linked CD11a and CD18 molecules. LFA-1 is expressed on a variety of cell types, including polymorphonuclear leukocytes, lymphocytes, and monocytes. Its ligands are ICAM-1, ICAM-2, and ICAM-3.

The primary function of LFA-1 is adhesion. Anti-LFA-1 antibodies block T cell activation in vitro, presumably by preventing adherence of T cells to APC or target cells. LFA-1, however, does not mediate adhesion of resting T cells. Prior activation of T cells with PMA, anti-CD3, anti-CD2, or antigen is required. PMA induces phosphorylation of the CD18 chain of LFA-1. It has been suggested that phosphorylation causes a conformational change in LFA-1, resulting in increased affinity for its ligands.

T Cell Signal Transduction and T Cell Activation. A hallmark of T cell activation is the requirement for cell-cell contact and multivalent stimulation. Fig. 6-5 summarizes the current model of this process. While interacting with antigen on an APC or target cell, the TCR-CD3 complex, CD4 or CD8 coreceptors, and CD45 are brought into close proximity. This action allows CD45 to activate p59^{fyn} and p56^{lck} by dephosphorylation. These tyrosine kinases then phosphorylate CD3ζ chain, PLCγ1, and other cellular substrates. Activated PLC cleaves PIP2 into IP3 and DAG. IP3 opens the calcium channel and increases the intracellular Ca^{2+} concentration. Ca^{2+} binds to calmodulin and activates calcineurin. Calcineurin, a Ca^{2+}-dependent phosphotase, in turn activates IL-2 gene transcription through an unknown mechanism (presumably by inducing nuclear translocation of transcription factors). The two widely used immunosuppressants, Cyclosporin A and FK506, both act on calcineurin to block T cell activation.[16,31,60] DAG activates protein kinase C, which can also activate IL-2 gene transcription. This PLC-initiated signaling cascade is a major pathway in T cell activation, but it is not the only one. CD3ζ chain and CD28 have a distinct signaling mechanism of their own. A suc-

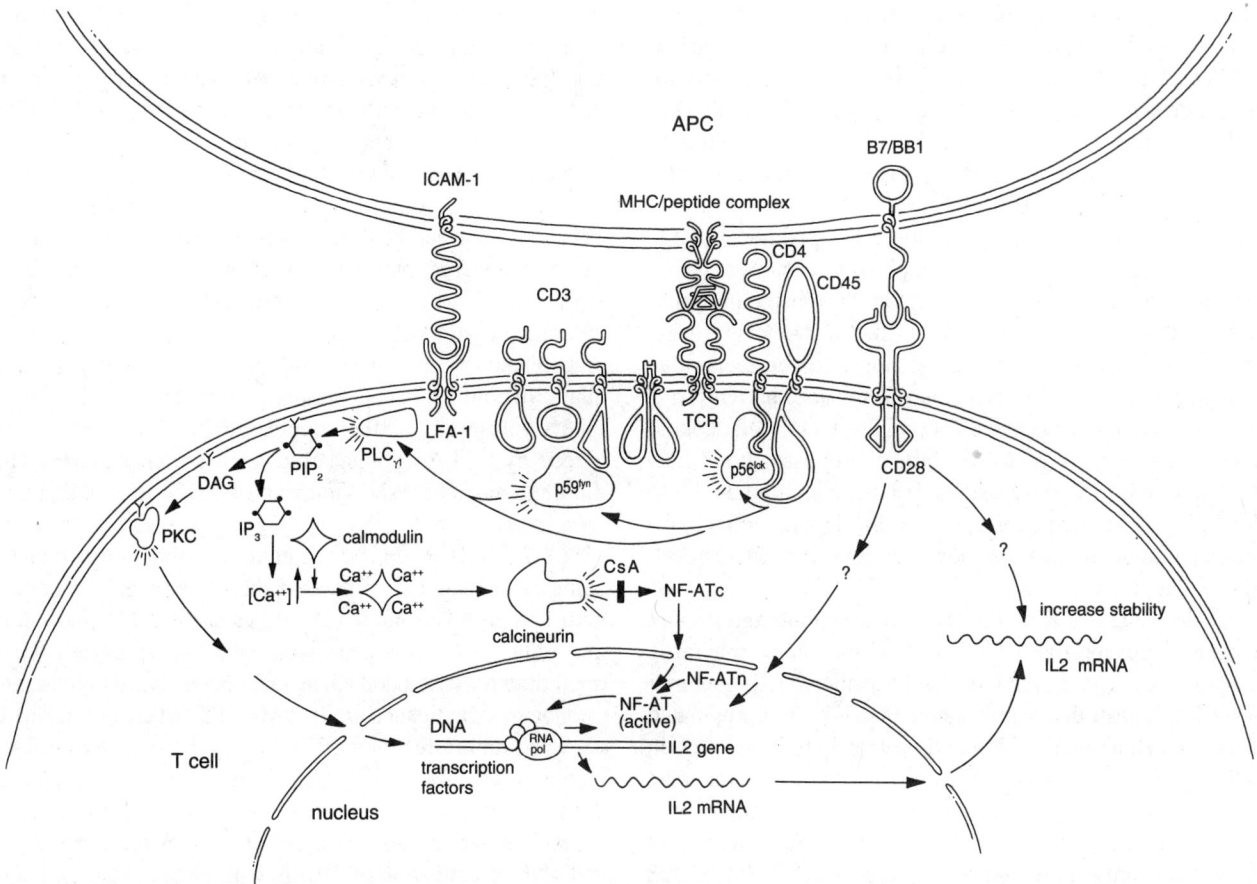

Fig. 6-5. Signal transduction pathways during T cell activation (see text for details). DAG: Diacylglycerol; PKC: Protein Kinase C; CsA: cyclosporin A; NF-AT: nuclear factor of activated T cells; NF-ATc: cytoplasmic subunit of NF-AT; NF-ATn: nuclear subunit of NF-AT.

cessful interaction between T cell and APC leads to induction of IL-2 synthesis and IL-2 receptor expression. IL-2 binds to IL-2 receptor and induces T cell proliferation in an autocrine or paracrine fashion, which leads to expansion of T cells of the selected antigen specificity.

Efferent Limb of the Cellular Immune Response

Cellular Trafficking. *Adhesion Molecules.* The effector function of B lymphocytes is exerted through the production of relatively stable soluble mediators (immunoglobulins) in copious amounts. Thus B cells can participate in immune responses from a distance. In contrast, T lymphocytes exert their effector functions through the elaboration of minute amounts of soluble mediators (cytokines) that are short lived in vivo and through direct cognate interaction with target cells. For this reason, infiltrating sites of infection or antigen deposition is an essential component of the effector function of T lymphocytes. In recent years a great deal of information has emerged about the mechanisms that control cellular trafficking of T lymphocytes and other inflammatory cells, particularly neutrophils and macrophages. It is now obvious that trafficking patterns are controlled, at least in part,

through the regulated expression of adhesion molecules on inflammatory cells and vascular endothelium. The expression of these adhesion molecules is controlled by cytokines, some of which also serve as chemotactic factors that direct the migration of inflammatory cells into sites of antigen deposition.

Extravasation of inflammatory cells at sites of inflammation appears to involve the sequential, transient expression or activity of adhesion molecules on circulating inflammatory cells and vascular endothelium, prompting the term "adhesion cascade". The variable composition of the inflammatory infiltrate that is induced by different infectious agents, or even by the same infectious agent at different anatomic sites, implies that the extravasation of different leukocyte populations may be differentially regulated. This differential regulation is now beginning to be understood at the molecular level. In all cases, extravasation is initiated by binding of the inflammatory cell to endothelial cells lining the lumen of postcapillary venules at the inflammatory site. The fascinating story of the mechanism of this interaction is now rapidly unfolding.

Naive T cells are constantly in search of antigen. Antigens that are deposited in cutaneous and mucosal tissues are picked up by the lymphatics or by local APCs and carried to the draining lymph nodes. Thus naive T cells can enhance their chances of encountering antigen by traveling from lymph node to lymph node. Once a T cell is activated by antigen, however, its goal is to migrate as rapidly as possible to the site of antigen deposition. The phenotypic changes that occur in lymphocytes following activation reflect the changing objective of the T cell. As previously mentioned, L-selectin plays a significant part in the homing of naive T cells to lymph nodes. T cell activation downregulates L-selectin expression and upregulates the expression and affinity of integrins. The loss of L-selectins from activated T cells discourages these now unnecessary excursions through lymph nodes. Moreover, the enhanced expression of integrins favors an interaction of activated T cells with vascular endothelium at inflammatory sites and ultimately their reactivation through interaction with APCs within those sites. Extravasation of T cells at inflammatory sites requires an initial binding or "tethering" of the T cell to the vascular endothelium. It has recently been demonstrated that under the sheer forces created by the flow conditions within the venules, the interaction of selectins with their ligands is of prime importance.[105]

The three members of the selectin family include the following: (1) E-selectins, endothelial leukocyte adhesion molecule-1 (ELAM-1); (2) the P-selectins (also called CD62) granule membrane protein-140 (GMP-140) and platelet activation dependent granule external membrane (PADGEM); and (3) the L-selectins, also referred to as Mel-14–LAM-1, LECCAM-1, gp90[Mel-14], Leu 8, TQ1, and Ly22.

The L-selectins perform an important function in the initial binding or tethering of neutrophils to vascular endothelium at inflammatory sites but appear to be of lesser importance for T cell tethering, particularly of activated or memory T cells, which often do not express L-selectin. L-selectins are constitutively expressed on neutrophils, thus enabling resting neutrophils to bind to the carbohydrate ligand of L-selectin on activated vascular endothelium. E-selectins are also involved in the initial binding of neutrophils and at least a subpopulation[8,101] of memory T cells to activated vascular endothelium at inflammatory sites.

E-selectins are not normally expressed on vascular endothelium, but their expression is rapidly induced upon exposure of vascular endothelium to a variety of inflammatory mediators including IL-1β tumor necrosis factor (TNF)-α, TNF-β, and LPS. E-selectin expression is transient and no longer detectable 48 hours after stimulation of endothelial cells. A member of a class of sialyated and fucosylated structures related to the sialyated Lewis-X blood group antigen (SLex) has been identified as an E-selectin ligand. P-selectin expression is also inducible on vascular endothelium. Unlike E-selectins, P-selectin expression does not require de novo protein synthesis. P-selectins are stored in the secretory α granules of platelets and Weibel-Palade bodies of

vascular endothelial cells and redistribute to the cell surface within minutes of exposure of the endothelial cells to thrombin, histamine, phorbol esters, and hydrogen peroxide. P-selectins are clearly involved in the initial binding of neutrophils to vascular endothelium, but their involvement in T cell binding has not been confirmed. The interaction of selectins with their ligand retards the flow of neutrophils and causes them to roll along the surface of the vascular endothelium. This rolling phenomenon has not been determined for T cells.

Following the initial tethering, the second step in the extravasation of inflammatory cells involves the firm binding of the inflammatory cell to the vascular endothelium that is mediated by an interaction between two families of inducible adhesion molecules (the integrins and certain members of the Ig superfamily). The integrins are heterodimeric cell surface molecules consisting of a noncovalently linked α and β chain. Three distinct subfamilies of integrins (β1, β2, and β3) have been identified based on the presence of a common β chain. Three members of the β2 integrin family that share a common β chain (CD18) include LFA-1 (CD11a-CD18), Mac-1 (CD11b-CD18), and p150, 95 (CD11c-CD18). LFA-1 is constitutively expressed on neutrophils and T cells, and expression is transiently increased following activation of both cells. Activation also causes a transient conformational change in LFA-1, resulting in greater affinity for its ligand. Mac-1 is constitutively expressed on neutrophils but not T cells, and its expression is transiently increased following neutrophil activation. Mac-1 is also expressed on a subset of activated CD8 T cells.[66] LFA-1 and Mac-1 share a common ligand—intercellular adhesion molecule 1 (ICAM-1), an Ig superfamily member. ICAM-1 is expressed at low levels on normal vascular endothelium, but its expression is upregulated by exposure of the vascular endothelium to IL-1, TNF, and IFN-γ.[107] ICAM-1 has five Ig-like domains. The N-terminal domain of ICAM-1 binds to LFA-1, whereas the third domain binds to Mac-1.[21,108]

The current paradigm for neutrophil extravasation is as follows: Interaction of selectins with their carbohydrate ligands slows the progress of the neutrophil and causes it to roll along the surface of the vascular endothelium. Cytokines and other factors produced at the site of inflammation activate the vascular endothelium, upregulating expression of ICAM-1 and ELAM-1, and also activating the neutrophil once it has come in contact with the endothelium. Neutrophil activation results in upregulation of LFA-1 and Mac-1 and simultaneous release of L-selectins. Mac-1 and LFA-1 provide firm attachment to the vascular endothelium via an interaction with ICAM-1, and in the case of LFA-1, ICAM-2 as well. In response to a chemotactic gradient, the neutrophil then passes through the endothelial junctions and migrates through the vascular basement membrane and into the tissue. Recent evidence suggests that transendothelial migration of neutrophils may be mediated largely by Mac-1, which has a broad range of ligand specificities including not only ICAM-1 but also a variety of extracellular matrix proteins that are present in the vascular basement membrane and in the surrounding tissue.[113] The importance of β2 integrins for neutrophil extravasation is illustrated by an experiment in nature. The disease leukocyte adhesion deficiency (LAD) is characterized by a genetic deficiency in the production of the β2 chain CD18. These patients suffer frequent life-threatening infections caused by the inability of their neutrophils to infiltrate sites of infection.

Activated T cells utilize an additional set of adhesion molecules for extravasation. Expression of the β1 integrin VLA-4 is upregulated on the surface of activated T cells. The counter receptor for VLA-4 on activated vascular endothelium is a member of the Ig superfamily VCAM-1. Although memory T cells use both LFA-1 and VLA-4 for binding to activated vascular endothelium, the fact that LAD patient T cells are capable of extravasating into inflammatory sites implies that the LFA-1-ICAM interaction is not required for their extravasation. This interpretation is in agreement with the results of antibody-blocking studies. Antibodies to VLA-4 or VCAM-1 are much more effective in blocking the binding of memory T cells to activated vascular endothelium than are antibodies to ELAM-1, LFA-1, or ICAM-1,* and the blocking effect of these latter antibodies in combination with antibody to VCAM-1 is additive.[36,82,88,101]

Cytokines. The composition of the inflammatory infiltrate appears to be determined by at least two factors: (1) the combination of adhesion molecules expressed on the inflammatory cells and on the activated vascular endothelium; and (2) the nature of the chemotactic stimulant that attracts the inflammatory cells. The expression of adhesion molecules on the vascular endothelium is regulated by cytokines and lipid mediators that are produced at the site of inflammation. Many of these same molecules enhance the expression and affinity of integrins on the surface of neutrophils and T cells. The expression on vascular endothelium of the selectin ELAM-1 and the Ig superfamily molecules ICAM-1 and VCAM-1 is regulated by unique but overlapping groups of activators (see Table 6-2). The relative importance of ICAM-1–β2 integrin interaction for neutrophil extravasation and of the VCAM-1–VLA-4 interaction for T cell extravasation infers that differential expression of these two molecules might influence the composition of the inflammatory infiltrate. Thus upregulation of ICAM-1 but not VCAM-1 by IFN-γ might favor a neutrophilic infiltrate. In contrast, upregulation of VCAM-1 and downregulation of ICAM-1 and ELAM-1 by IL-4 would seem to favor a T cell infiltrate. It must be noted, however, that the regulatory ef-

*References 25, 36, 38, 82, 88, 101.

fects of these cytokines was established with cultures of vascular endothelial cells in vitro, and a similar in vivo regulatory role has not yet been established. Other mediators released at sites of inflammation that can induce adhesion molecule expression on vascular endothelium include thrombin, histamine, and oxygen radicals.

The extravasation and directed migration of leukocytes into inflammatory sites is mediated largely by chemotactic factors. It is suggested that the interaction of leukocytes with vascular endothelium at inflammatory sites induces phenotypic changes in the leukocytes that may enhance their capacity to migrate through the extracellular matrix of tissues. This activation-dependent phenotypic change seems to reflect the activity of cytokines and lipid mediators that are produced by vascular endothelium as well as other cells at sites of antigen deposition. Platelet-activating factor (PAF) is a potent lipid mediator of inflammation. PAF is expressed on the membrane of vascular endothelial cells when exposed to thrombin and histamine, but very little PAF is secreted. This membrane-associated PAF can activate bound leukocytes[84] and enhancing the expression and affinity of integrins, thus facilitating their transendothelial migration.

A new class of low-molecular weight cytokines has been described that belongs to the platelet factor 4 (PF4) superfamily.[97] This superfamily is defined by the conservation of a four-cysteine motif and other predicted structural similarities. The members of this group of chemokines can be divided, based on the position of the first two cysteines in the conserved motif. One branch of the PF4 superfamily (C-X-C) is characterized by the separation of the first two cysteines in the primary structure, by an intervening amino acid. In another branch (C-C), the first two cysteines are directly adjacent.

IL-8, also known as neutrophil attractant-activation protein-1 (NAP-1), is the most thoroughly studied member of the C-X-C branch of the PF4 superfamily. IL-8 is produced by macrophages, vascular endothelial cells, and other cells such as keratinocytes and fibroblasts. IL-8 is a strong chemoattractant for neutrophils, lymphocytes, and basophils, and induces the accumulation of neutrophils in rabbit skin when administered in vivo.[85] In vitro studies suggest that IL-8 may enhance neutrophil emigration in two ways. Mast cells, present in the perivascular space, have receptors for IL-8.[92] When activated by IL-8, mast cells release stored mediators including histamine and TNF-α. These mediators upregulate the expression of P-selectins and E-selectins on vascular endothelium. Thus IL-8 may indirectly enhance the selectin-mediated initial interaction between neutrophils and the vascular endothelium. In addition, vascular endothelial cells produce IL-8 when stimulated with TNF-α, IL1-β, or LPS.[111] IL-8 activates neutrophils, causing the release of L-selectin and enhanced expression of integrins. This phenotypic change would inhibit the initial interaction of neutrophils with vascular endothelium, but may favor the transendothelial migration of neutrophils that are already attached to the vascular endothelium. It has been suggested that IL-8 that is bound to the membrane of vascular endothelial cells may stimulate neutrophil release of L-selectin after their attachment to vascular endothelium, thus favoring neutrophil extravasation. In contrast, serum IL-8 (secreted by vascular endothelial cells) may stimulate neutrophils to release L-selectin before their attachment to vascular endothelium, thus discouraging extravasation.[61] Recent evidence also proposes that IL-8 is angiogenic, causing ingrowth of blood vessels into the cornea.[54]

Several members of the C-C branch of the PF4 superfamily have been described. Those of human origin are referred to as the RANTES-SIS cytokine family. The best defined members of this family include the macrophage inflammatory protein 1 (MIP-1), monocyte chemotactic protein-1 (MCP-1), and RANTES. Murine MIP-1 causes swelling and neutrophilic infiltration in vivo and is mildly chemotactic for neutrophils in vitro.[97] MIP-1 consists of two related proteins designated MIP-1α and MIP-1β. Recent studies with recombinant human MIP-1α and MIP-1β imply that these molecules attract distinct subpopulations of lymphocytes in vitro. MIP-1β attracts naive CD4$^+$ cells, whereas MIP-1α attracts killer T cells and B lymphocytes.[97] MCP-1 is produced by T cells, monocytes, endothelial cells, and fibroblasts when stimulated with IL-1, TNF, or LPS.[97] MCP-1 has potent monocyte chemotactic activity, but is not chemotactic for neutrophils. MCP-1 induces a monocytic infiltration into rat ears that begins 6 hours after injection and is maximal after 16 hours. RANTES is primarily produced by T lymphocytes. In vitro studies demonstrated that RANTES is chemotactic for monocytes and a subpopulation of T lymphocytes, but not for neutrophils. RANTES selectively attracts memory CD4 T lymphocytes. Based on these in vivo and in vitro studies, the composition of an inflammatory infiltrate may be regulated, at least in part, by the array of cytokines and lipid mediators produced by vascular endothelial cells and other cells in the perivascular space.

Antigen Presentation at Inflammatory Sites. *Professional Antigen-Presenting Cells.* ''Professional APC'' are present in most, if not all tissues of the body. These professional APC express high levels of MHC class I and class II antigens and are capable of processing and presenting foreign antigenic peptides to T lymphocytes in an immunogenic form. The presence of these professional APC in non-lymphoid tissue probably reflects, in part, a need for restimulation of memory T cells through TCR ligation and delivery of accessory signals by APC at sites of immunologic reactions. This requirement for restimulation is probably attributable to the short duration of cytokine mRNA expression following the removal of the T cell activating signal.[99]

Langerhans cells are professional APC that are present in epidermal and mucosal surfaces. LC are the only corneal cells that constitutively express MHC class II antigens. LC are normally absent from the central cornea.[90] Any of a variety of irritations to the central cornea, however, [including herpes simplex virus (HSV) infection] can result in the centripetal migration of LC that reside in large numbers in the peripheral corneal and contiguous conjunctival epithelia.[43,78] The mechanism that normally excludes LC from the central cornea is not apparent. Niederkorn and associates[74] have confirmed, however, that injection of IL-1β into the central corneal epithelium can induce LC migration. Because corneal epithelial cells produce IL-1, this induction may represent a physiologic mechanism that regulates LC migration into injured corneas. Moreover, when injected intradermally, TNF-α induces the migration of LC from the skin to the draining lymph nodes. Thus both TNF-α and IL-1 can directly or indirectly induce LC migration.

Evidence suggesting the capacity of LC to participate in the afferent limb of the immune response through the uptake and processing of antigens encountered in the epidermis and through transport of the processed antigens to the T cell regions of the regional lymph nodes was described earlier in this chapter. A role of LC in the efferent limb of the immune response in the cornea has also been suggested.[43]

Although resident APC such as LC may be important early in an inflammatory process, as the inflammation progresses, other professional APC (including macrophages and B lymphocytes) infiltrate the inflammatory site. In humans, both B cells and macrophages constitutively express MHC class II antigens. Most mouse macrophages do not constitutively display MHC class II antigens, but their expression is rapidly induced by a variety of cytokines (including IFN-γ and IL-4) that may be present at sites of inflammation. When activated, both macrophages and B cells can take up and process antigen, present the antigenic peptides in a binary complex with MHC class II, and provide the adhesive interactions and co-stimulatory signals that are necessary for efficient T cell activation. Because of their phagocytic capability, macrophages are probably most effective at processing particulate antigens, such as whole bacteria. B cells are likely more effective at processing soluble antigens, which are internalized in endocytic vesicles. The endocytic process is most effective when mediated through surface receptors on B cells (viz, Fc or complement receptor-mediated binding of immune complexes, or specific binding of antigen to the immunoglobulin receptors on antigen-reactive B cells).

Presentation by Tissue Cells at Inflammatory Sites. Although constitutive expression of MHC class II antigens is restricted to a few bone marrow-derived professional APC, many other cells (including fibroblasts, keratinocytes, keratocytes, epithelial cells, and vascular and corneal endothelial cells) can be induced to express MHC class II antigens when exposed to IFN-γ. Indeed, these cells are often found to express MHC class II antigens at sites of inflammation. The role they play in antigen presentation to T cells at inflammatory sites is not entirely clear, however. In vitro studies infer that these cells vary in their capacity to serve as APC. Although they can all process and present immunogenic peptides complexed with MHC class II antigens, they differ in their capacity to provide the co-stimulatory signals that are variably required by T cells at different stages of activation. Thus under certain circumstances, MHC class II positive fibroblasts and keratinocytes can present antigens in a stimulatory manner to antigen-specific T cell lines. These cells, however, are incapable of stimulating resting T cells reactive to the same antigen.[116] This reflects differences in the co-stimulatory requirements of activated versus resting T cells. Most T cells use IL-2 as an autocrine or paracrine growth factor, and failure of fibroblasts to stimulate resting T cells has been associated with inadequate induction of IL-2 production. In fact, presentation of antigens to resting T cells in the absence of the necessary co-stimulatory signals can actually lead to a state of clonal anergy.

Cytokines. Cytokines plainly perform a key function in the body's defense against invasion by infectious and noninfectious agents. Once the invading material is eliminated, cytokines regulate the processes that lead to tissue repair and return to homeostasis. Unfortunately, the defensive mechanisms that are mediated by cytokines can be unnecessary (induced by antigenic material remaining after elimination of an infectious agent), destructive (septic shock resulting from the overproduction of TNF-α and IL-1), or misdirected against self components (autoimmune inflammatory diseases such as rheumatoid arthritis and uveitis). In addition, the tissue repair process itself can lead to loss of organ function (the loss of corneal clarity caused by scar tissue deposited following corneal inflammation).

This section will review the available information implicating specific cytokines in protective or immunopathologic responses. It must be noted, however, that no single cytokine can mediate a protective or pathologic response. It emerges from the previous sections of this chapter that a variety of cytokines are involved in the activation, trafficking, and effector functions of T cells. Nonetheless, recent studies imply that in certain infectious diseases, specific cytokines are essential in determining if the net result of infection is protection, susceptibility, or immunopathology.

Role in Protective Immunity. The susceptibility to infection displayed by immunologically compromised humans and animals underscores the essential role of the immune system in eradicating disease. The exact nature of the immunologic mechanisms that provide resistance to infectious diseases remains largely undefined, however. Defining the essential protective mechanisms is rendered difficult by the duplicity and functional diversity of the mechanisms that are evoked by most infectious agents. For instance, many cytokines have overlapping functions, and any one cytokine can

mediate a variety of functions. These functions may be protective or detrimental depending on when the cytokine is produced, how much is produced, in what tissue it is produced, and how it interacts with other present cytokines. Nonetheless, distinct cytokine patterns have recently been shown to be associated with protective immune responses to certain infectious agents.

For instance, resistance of mice to certain intracellular parasites such as *Listeria, Leishmania* species, and mycobacteria is genetically determined and closely associated with IFN-γ production. Thus treatment of normally resistant mice with antibodies to IFN-γ or disruption of their gene for IFN-γ or IFN-γ receptor renders them susceptible to the parasites.[20,42,44] Conversely, susceptibility to these parasites is associated with production of IL-4, which is functionally antagonistic to IFN-γ. Recently the cytokine mRNA profiles of lesions from patients with the resistant tuberculoid form and the susceptible lepromatous form of leprosy were analyzed using PCR technology.[124] A clear bias toward IL-2 and IFN-γ mRNA production (characteristic of Th1 cells) was observed in tuberculoid lesions, whereas IL-4, IL-5, and IL-10 mRNA (characteristic of Th2 cells) predominated in lepromatous lesions.

The reciprocal role of Th1 and Th2 cytokines is a common factor in several parasitic infections. These observations have important implications for vaccine development. Epitopes that specifically, or at least preferentially, activate Th1 cells would engender protective cell-mediated immune responses, whereas those epitopes that activate Th2 cells would favor antibody production and inhibit the more protective cell-mediated immune responses. The results of some studies seem to support the feasibility of developing subunit vaccines that favor Th1 cell activation. Thus *Listeria* major-reactive Th1 and Th2 clones were identified that responded to different L. major-derived peptides.[98] In addition, infection of mice with Schistosoma mansoni generated predominantly T cells that produced the Th2 pattern of cytokines when stimulated with antigen or mitogens in vitro.

In contrast, vaccination with attenuated larval stages generated T cells that produced the Th1 pattern of cytokines when stimulated in vitro.[77] Again in this model, the Th1 cytokine pattern was associated with protection, whereas the Th2 cytokine pattern was not. A recent study by Reiner and colleagues,[86] however, demonstrated a common, restricted TCR repertoire among L. major-reactive CD4 cells of both Th1 and Th2 type, and from resistant and susceptible mice. The results of that study suggested that antigen-independent factors may influence the expansion of Th1 or Th2 clones and the associated pattern of susceptibility to leishmaniasis. Better characterization of the epitopes recognized by Th1 and Th2 clones may help to resolve this issue.

TNF-α also plays an essential protective role in certain bacterial and parasitic infections. Thus pretreatment with

TNF-α enables mice to survive a lethal dose and more rapidly clear a sublethal dose of Listeria monocytogenes.[39] Conversely, antibody to TNF-α can render lethal a normally sublethal Listeria infection.[72] Similar studies determined an essential role for TNF-α in protection against salmonellosis[73] and legionellosis.[9]

Role in Immunopathology. When an immune response causes an unacceptable level of tissue destruction, the response is considered to be immunopathologic. It should be noted that tissues may vary with regard to the degree of tissue destruction they can tolerate. Thus a response that is "protective" in one tissue may be "immunopathologic" in another. This condition is particularly true in the eye, where the requirement for clarity necessitates careful control of inflammatory responses in the tissues comprising the visual axis. Like protective immune responses, immunopathologic responses are largely mediated by cytokines produced by the milieu of inflammatory cells that are present in the inflamed tissue. An initially protective immune response may become immunopathologic as a result of the failure of regulatory systems to reestablish homeostasis. The involvement of cytokines in this type of situation can be difficult to evaluate for two reasons: (1) the role of any given cytokine may change from protective to immunopathologic during the course of the response, and (2) failure of the immune system to eliminate the inducing agent may result in tissue destruction by the agent itself. Establishing a role for specific cytokines in immunopathologic reactions can be most readily accomplished in systems in which the inducing agent itself does not cause tissue destruction. Examples of these types of situations would include autoimmune diseases, graft-versus-host disease (GVHD) and transplantation rejection reactions, and responses to infections that are normally self-limiting but can induce immunologically mediated tissue destruction. In these instances failure of the immune system to eliminate the inducing agent is a favorable, or at least acceptable, outcome.

A role for TNF-α and IL-1 in the pathology associated with GVHD was established in studies in which the activity of these cytokines was neutralized by in vivo treatment with antibodies or, in the case of IL-1, with a recombinant IL-1 receptor antagonist (IL-1ra). IL-1ra is a newly defined member of the IL-1 family[4,64] that binds with high affinity to the 80-kDa IL-1 receptor on T cells and fibroblasts,[22] and with lower affinity to the 67-kDa IL-1 receptor on B cells and neutrophils.[23] IL-1ra lacks agonist activity but blocks binding and signal transduction by IL-1. Treatment of mice with antibodies to TNF-α or with IL-1ra virtually eliminated the severe skin and intestinal lesions and reduced the mortality associated with GVHD.[65,83]

TNF-α has also been implicated in the rejection of transplanted solid tissues. Elevation of serum levels of TNF-α was observed during the course of acute renal allograft reactions[63] and after liver and heart transplantations.[117] Moreover, anti-TNF-α antibody treatment enhances cardiac allograft survival in rats,[46] and when combined with anti-IFN-γ, enhances skin graft survival in monkeys.[110]

A number of cytokines have been implicated in the pathogenesis of rheumatoid arthritis. Synovial fluid of rheumatoid arthritis patients contains elevated levels of TGF-β, TNF-α, IL-6, and IL-1. TGF-β is a family of at least five homodimeric polypeptides that share 70% to 80% amino acid sequence homology and many biologic functions. TGF-β1, TGF-β2, and TGF-β3 are found in mammalian tissues. The mature TGF-β molecule is secreted in an inactive or latent form because of its noncovalent association with the 75-kd glycosylated latency-associated protein (LAP), which is covalently linked to a 135-kd-binding protein.[89,121] Latent TGF-β is activated by proteases, such as plasmin and cathepsin, and by transient exposure to acidic conditions. TGF-β is perhaps the most potent chemoattractant for monocytes with activity in the femtomolar concentrations.[120] TGF-β is also chemotactic for neutrophils[11,27] and T cells.[1] In addition to being chemotactic, TGF-β may enhance inflammatory cell migration through tissues by its capacity to upregulate their expression of the β2 integrins, VLA-3 and VLA-5 (which bind to laminin, collagen, and fibronectin), and by its capacity to induce monocyte production of type IV collagenases. This latter function would facilitate the movement of inflammatory cells through the collagen matrix of the vascular basement membrane and of tissues. This function may be of particular importance in avascular tissues such as the cornea, where cells extravasating from limbal vessels early in an inflammatory response must negotiate several millimeters of collagenous tissue enroute to the central cornea. TGF-β also induces the rapid expression of CD16 (FcqRIII) on monocytes[79] (thus increasing their phagocytic function) and reportedly induces the differentiation of naive CD4 T lymphocytes to the memory phenotype and their production of IL-2.[56,112] TGF-β also enhances levels of mRNA for several inflammatory cytokines including IL-1, TNF, PDGF, basic fibroblast growth factor (bFGF), and IL-6 in monocytes. TGF-β is produced rapidly and in large amounts by platelets at sites of immunologic challenge and injury[6] and is also produced by activated monocytes and T lymphocytes. Thus TGF-β possesses strong proinflammatory activity and is likely involved in the early stages of a variety of inflammatory responses, including rheumatoid arthritis. This conclusion is supported by the fact that local administration of TGF-β exacerbates synovial inflammation and tissue destruction,[119] and antibodies to TGF-β inhibit these reactions.

Interestingly, TGF-β is also a potent immunosuppressive agent. TGF-β inhibits (1) T cell proliferation and IL-1 receptor expression,[24] (2) the development of CTL, NK, and LAK activity, and (3) reactive oxygen intermediate metabolism by macrophages.[115] Susceptibility to these immunosuppressive effects of TGF-β depends on the level of activation of the cell, however. Activated T cells upregulate TGF-β receptor expression and are thus exquisitely sensitive to the antiproliferative effects of TGF-β. While proliferation of activated T cells is inhibited by TGF-β, their cytokine production is not. Moreover, it appears that a subpopulation of CD8 cells is much less sensitive to the antiproliferative effects of TGF-β than CD4 cells. These TGF-β-resistant CD8 cells produce IL-4, IL-5, and IL-10 and suppress the proliferation and activity of Th1 CD4 cells.[95] Conversely, activation of monocytes by IFN-γ, LPS, or TGF-β results in downregulation of TGF-β receptor expression. Thus high concentrations of TGF-β at inflammatory sites would seem to favor activation but limit proliferation of T cells and may have little effect on monocytes because of modulation of their TGF-β receptors during activation.

Immune Defenses of the Eye

The immune-inflammatory system is a highly sophisticated army that is charged with protecting the body against foreign invasion. This army has sentinels, such as LC, that first detect the foreign invader and carry information to the nearest camp (lymph node, spleen and so on). Neutrophils are relatively unsophisticated advanced troops, charged with delaying the advance of the foreign invasion until more sophisticated lymphoid cells can enter the foray. Lymphocytes can remember an enemy from a previous encounter and organizing an accelerated response to future invasions. Among the lymphocytes, B cells are the artillery. They can attack the enemy from great distances through the elaboration of antibody molecules. T cells are the foot soldiers who engage the enemy at short range through cognate interactions and through the elaboration of mediators that, for the most part, function regionally. The story of these sophisticated foot soldiers is now rapidly unfolding. New information about the mechanisms by which T cells are (1) activated, (2) transported to the site of invasion, (3) rendered capable of orchestrating the destruction of the foreign material, and (4) disengaged from battle is emerging at a furious pace. The foregoing was a brief excerpt from that story. As the tale unfolds, the lessons that are learned will undoubtedly lead to improved modalities for controlling the invasion of foreign organisms as well as the occasional aberrant attack of the immune system on self components.

REFERENCES

1. Adams DH, Hathaway M, Shaw J, et al.: Transforming growth factor-beta induces human T lymphocyte migration in vitro, *J Immunol* 147:609-612, 1991.
2. Allison JP, McIntyre BW, Bloch D: Tumor-specific antigen of murine T-lymphoma defined with monoclonal antibodies, *J Immunol* 129:2293, 1982.
3. Appleby MW, Gross JA, Cooke MP, et al.: Defective T cell receptor signaling in mice lacking the thymic isoform of p59fyn, *Cell* 70:751-763, 1992.
4. Arend WP, Joslin FG, Thompson RC, Hannum CH: An IL-1 inhibitor from human monocytes: production and characterization of biologic properties, *J Immunol* 143:1851-1858, 1989.
4a. Arnason BG, Jankovic BD, Waksman BH, Wennersten C: Role of the thymus in immune reactions in rats. II. Suppressive effect of thymectomy at birth on reactions of delayed (cellular) hypersensitivity and the circulating small lymphocyte, *J Exp Med* 116:177-186, 1962
5. Asarnow DM, Kuziel WA, Bonyhadi M, et al.: Limited diversity of gamma delta antigen receptor genes of thy-1+ dendritic epidermal cells, *Cell* 55:837, 1988.
6. Assoian RK, Komonya A, Meyers CA, et al.: Transforming growth factor-β in human platelets, *J Biol Chem* 258:7155-7160, 1983.
7. Berg EL, Picker LJ, Robinson MK, et al.: Vascular addressins: tissue selective endothelial cell adhesion molecules for lymphocyte homing. In Cochrane C, Gimbrone MAJ, editors: *Cellular and molecular mechanisms of inflammation,* San Diego, 1991, Academic Press.
8. Bevilacqua MP, Stengelin S, Gimbrone MA Jr, Seed B: Endothelial leukocyte adhesion molecule 1: an inducible receptor for neutrophils related to complement regulatory proteins and lectins, *Science* 243:1160, 1989.
9. Blanchard DK, Djeu JY, Klein TW, et al.: Protective effects of tumor necrosis factor in experimental Legionella pneumophilia infections of mice via activation of PMN function, *J Leukoc Biol* 43:429-435, 1988.
10. Bonneville M, Ito K, Krecko EG, et al.: Recognition of a self major histocompatibility complex TL region product by âë T cell receptors, *Proc Natl Acad Sci USA* 86:5928, 1989.
11. Brandes ME, Mai UEH, Ohura K, Wahl SM: Human neutrophils express type 1 TGF-b receptors and chemotax to TGF-b, *J Immunol* 147:1600-1606, 1991.
12. Brenner MB, McLean J, Dialynas D, et al.: Identification of a putative second T cell receptor, *Nature* 322:145-149, 1986.
13. Cantor H, Boyse EA: Functional subclasses of T lymphocytes bearing different Ly antigens. II. Cooperation between subclasses of Ly+ cells in the generation of killer activity, *J Exp Med* 141:1390, 1975.
14. Cher DJ, Mosmann TR: Two types of murine helper T cell clone. II. Delayed-type hypersensitivity is mediated by t-h-1 clones, *J Immunol* 138:3688-3694, 1987.
15. Chien Y-H, Becker DM, Lindsten T, et al.: A third type of murine T-cell receptor gene, *Nature* 312:31-35, 1984.
16. Clipstone NA, Crabtree GR: Identification of calcineurin as a key signaling enzyme in T lymphocyte activation, *Nature* 357:695-697, 1992.
17. Cooke MP, Abraham KM, Forbush KA, Perlmutter RM: Regulation of T cell receptor signaling by a src family protein-tyrosine kinase (p59fyn), *Cell* 65:281-291, 1991.
18. Cron RQ, Gajewski TF, Sharrow SO, et al.: Phenotypic and functional analysis of murine CD3+, CD4−, CD8-TCR-γ δ expressing peripheral T cells, *J Immunol* 142:3754, 1989.
19. Cumberbatch M, Kimber I: Dermal tumour necrosis factor-à induces dendritic cell migration to draining lymph nodes, and possibly provides one stimulus for Langerhans' cell migration, *Immunology* 75:257-263, 1992.
20. Dalton DK, Pitts-Meek S, Keshav S, et al: Multiple defects of immune cell function in mice with disrupted interferon-δ genes, *Science* 259:1739-1742, 1993.
21. Diamond MS, Staunton DE, De Fougerolles AR, et al.: ICAM-1 (CD54): a counter receptor for Mac-1 (CD11b/CD18), *J Cell Biol* 111:3129-3139, 1990.
22. Dripps DJ, Brandhuber BJ, Thompson RC, Eisenberg SP: Interleukin-1 (IL-1) receptor antagonist binds to the 80-kDa IL-1 receptor but does not initiate IL-1 signal transduction, *J Biol Chem* 266:10331-10336, 1991.
23. Dripps DJ, Verderber E, Ng RK, et al.: Interleukin-1 receptor antagonist binds to the type II interleukin-1 receptor on B cells and neutrophils, *J Biol Chem* 266:20311-20315, 1991.
24. Dubois CM, Ruscetti FW, Palaszynski EW, et al.: Transforming growth factor β is a potent inhibitor of interleukin 1 (IL-1) receptor expression: proposed mechanism of inhibition of IL-1 action, *J Exp Med* 172:737-744, 1990.

25. Dustin ML, Springer TA: Lymphocyte function-associated antigen-1 (LFA-1) interaction with intercellular adhesion molecule-1 (ICAM-1) is one of at least three mechanisms for lymphocyte adhesion to cultured endothelial cells, *J Cell Biol* 107:321-331, 1988.

26. Erard F, Corthesy P, Nabholtz M, et al.: Interleukin 2 is both necessary and sufficient for the growth and differentiation of lectin-stimulated cytolytic T lymphocyte precursors, *J Immunol* 134:1644-1652, 1985.

27. Fava RA, Olsen NJ, Postlethwaite AE, et al.: Transforming growth factor á1 (TGF-á1) induced neutrophil recruitment to synovial tissues: implications for TGF-á-driven synovial inflammation and hyperplasia, *J Exp Med* 173:1121-1132, 1991.

28. Fernandez-Botran R, Sanders VM, Mosmann TR, Vitetta ES: Lymphokine-mediated regulation of the proliferative response of clones of T helper 1 and T helper 2 cells, *J Exp Med* 168:543-558, 1988.

29. Fiorentino DF, Bond MW, Mosmann TR: Two types of mouse T helper cell. IV. Th2 clones secrete a factor that inhibits cytokine production by Th1 clones, *J Exp Med* 170:2081-2095, 1989.

30. Fiorentino DF, Zlotnik A, Vieira P, et al.: Il-10 acts on the antigen-presenting cell to inhibit cytokine production by Th1 cells, *J Immunol* 146:3444-3451, 1991.

31. Flanagan WM, Corthesy B, Bram RJ, Crabtree GR: Nuclear association of a T cell transcription factor blocked by FK-506 and cyclosporin A, *Nature* 352:803-807, 1991.

32. Fong TAT, Mosmann TR: The role of IFN-ç in delayed-type hypersensitivity mediated by Th1 clones, *J Immunol* 143:2887-2893, 1989.

33. Fraser JD, Irving BA, Crabtree GR, Weiss A: Regulation of interleukin-2 gene enhancer activity by the T cell accessory molecule CD28, *Science* 251:313-316, 1991.

34. Gajewski TF, Joyce J, Fitch FW: Antiproliferative effect of INF-ç in immune regulation. III. Differential selection of TH1 and TH2 murine helper T lymphocyte clones using recombinant IL-2 and recombinant INF-ç, *J Immunol* 143:15-22, 1989.

35. Gell PGH, Benacerraf B: Studies on Hypersensitivity. II. Delayed hypersensitivity to denatured proteins in guinea pigs, *Immunology* 2:64-70, 1959.

35a. Good RA, Dalmasso AP, Martinez C, et al.: The role of the thymus in development of immunologic capacity in rabbits and mice, *J Exp Med* 116:773-795, 1962.

36. Graber N, Gopal TV, Wilson D, et al.: T cells bind to cytokine-activated endothelial cells via a novel, inducible sialogylycoprotein and endothelial leukocyte adhesion molecule-1, *J Immunol* 145:819-830, 1990.

37. Greenbaum LA, Horowitz JB, Woods A, et al.: Autocrine growth of CD4+ T cells: differential effects of IL-1 on helper and inflammatory T cells, *J Immunol* 140:1555-1560, 1988.

38. Haskard DO, Cavender DE, Beatty P, et al.: T lymphocyte adhesion to endothelial cells: mechanisms demonstrated by anti-LFA-1 monoclonal antibodies, *J Immunol* 137:2901-2906, 1986.

39. Havell EA: Evidence that tumor necrosis factor has an important role in antibacterial resistance, *J Immunol* 143:2894-2899, 1989.

40. Havran WL, Grell S, Durve H, et al.: Limited diversity of T-cell receptor â-chain expression of murine Thy-1+ dendritic epidermal cells revealed by Vâ3-specific monoclonal antibody, *Proc Natl Acad Sci USA* 86:4185, 1989.

41. Hedrick SM, Cohen DI, Nielsen EA, Davis MM: Isolation of cDNA clones encoding T-cell specific membrane-associated proteins, *Nature* 308:149, 1984.

42. Heinzel FP, Sadick MD, Holaday BJ, et al.: Reciprocal expression of interferon gamma or interleukin 4 during the resolution or progression of murine leishmaniasis, *J Exp Med* 169:59-72, 1989.

43. Hendricks RL, Janowicz M, Tumpey TM: Critical role of corneal Langerhans cells in the CD4- but not CD8-mediated immunopathology in herpes simplex virus-1-infected mouse corneas, *J Immunol* 148:2522-2529, 1992.

44. Huang S, Hendricks W, Althage A, et al: Immune response in mice that lack the interferon-γ receptor, *Science* 259:1742-1745, 1993.

45. Hudak SA, Gollnick SO, Conrad DH, Kehry MR: Murine B cell stimulatory factor 1 (interleukin 4) increases expression of the Fc receptor for IgE on mouse B cells, *Proc Natl Acad Sci USA* 84:4606-4610, 1987.

46. Imagawa DK, Millis JM, Olthoff KM, et al.: The role for tumor necrosis factor in allograft rejection. II. Evidence that antibody therapy against tumor necrosis factor-alpha and lymphotoxin enhances cardiac allograft survival in rats, *Transplantation* 50:189-193, 1990.

47. Inaba K, Inaba M, Naito M, Steinman RM: Dendritic cell progenitors phagocytose particulates, including Bacillus-Guerin organisms, and sensitize mice to mycobacterial antigens in vivo, *J Exp Med* 178:479-488, 1993.

48. Irving BA, Weiss A: The cytoplasmic domain of the T cell receptor zeta chain is sufficient to couple to receptor-associated signal transduction pathways, *Cell* 64:891-901, 1991.

49. Itohara S, Farr AG, Lafaille JJ, et al: Homing of a âë thymocyte subset with homogeneous T-cell receptors to mucosal epithelia, *Nature* 343:754, 1990.

50. Janis EM, Kaufmann SHE, Schwartz RH, Pardoll DM: Activation of âë T cells in the primary immune response to mycobacterium tuberculosis, *Science* 244:713, 1989.

50a. Jankovic BD, Waksman BH, Arnason BG: Role of the thymus in immune reactions in rats. I. The immunologic response to bovine serum albumin (antibody formation, Arthus reactivity, and delayed hypersensitivity) in rats thymectomized or splenectomized at various times after birth, *J Exp Med* 116:159-176, 1962.

51. Johnson RM, Lancki DW, Sperling AI, et al: A murine CD4-, CD8- T cell receptor-gammaë T lymphocyte clone specific for herpes simplex virus glycoprotein I, *J Immunol* 148:983-988, 1992.

52. Katz DH, Hamaoka T, Benacerraf B: Cell interactions between histocompatible T and B lymphocytes. II. Failure of physiologic cooperative interactions between T and B lymphocytes from allogeneic donor strains in humoral response to hapten-protein conjugates, *J Exp Med* 137:1405-1418, 1973.

53. Kindred B, Shreffler DC: H-2 dependence of cooperation between T and B cells in vivo, *J Immunol* 109:940-943, 1972.

54. Koch AE, Polverini PJ, Kunkel SL, et al.: Interleukin-8 as a macrophage-derived mediator of angiogenesis, *Science* 258:1798-1804, 1992.

55. Kozbor D, Trinchieri G, Monos DS, et al.: Human TCR-gamma+/delta+, CD8+ T lymphocytes recognize tetanus toxoid in an MHC-restricted fashion, *J Exp Med* 169:1847, 1989.

56. Lee HM, Rich S: Co-stimulation of T cell proliferation by transforming growth factor-β 1, *J Immunol* 147:1127-1133, 1991.

57. Lenschow DJ, Zeng Y, Thistlethwaite JR, et al.: Long-term survival of xenogeneic pancreatic islet grafts induced by CTLA4Ig, *Science* 257:789-792, 1992.

58. Letourneur F, Klausner RD: Activation of T cells by a tyrosine kinase activation domain in the cytoplasmic tail of CD3 epsilon, *Science* 255:79-82, 1992.

59. Linsley PS, Wallace PM, Johnson J, et al.: Immunosuppression in vivo by a soluble form of the CTLA-4 T cell activation molecule, *Science* 257:792-794, 1992.

60. Liu J, Farmer JDJ, Lane WS, et al.: Calcineurin is a common target of cyclophilin-cyclosporin A and FKBP-FK506 complexes, *Cell* 66:807-815, 1991.

61. Lloyd AR, Oppenheim JJ: Poly's lament: the neglected role of the polymorphonuclear neutrophil in the afferent limb of the immune response, *Immunol Today* 13:169-172, 1992.

62. Maggi E, Biswas P, Del Prete G, et al.: Accumulation of Th-2-like helper T cells in the conjunctiva of patients with vernal conjunctivitis, *J Immunol* 146:1169, 1991.

63. Maury C, Teppo A: Raised serum levels of cachectin/tumor necrosis factor- α in renal allograft rejection, *J Exp Med* 166:1132-1137, 1987.

64. Mazzei GJ, Seckinger PL, Dayer J-M, Shaw AR: Purification and characterization of a 26-kDa competitive inhibitor of interleukin 1, *Eur J Immunol* 20:683-689, 1990.

65. McCarthy PL Jr, Abhyankar S, Neben S, et al.: Inhibition of interleukin-1 by an interleukin-1 receptor antagonist prevents graft-versus-host disease, *Blood* 78:1915-1918, 1991.

66. McFarland HI, Nahill SR, Maciaszek ZW, Welsh RM: CD11b (Mac-1): a marker for CD8+ cytotoxic T cell activation and memory in virus infection, *J Immunol* 149:1326-1333, 1992.

66a. Miller JF: Immunological function of the thymus, *Lancet* 2:748, 1961.

67. Morrison LA, Lukacher AE, Braciale VL, et al.: Differences in antigen presentation to MHC class I- and class II-restricted influenza virus-specific cytolytic T lymphocyte clones, *J Exp Med* 163:903-921, 1986.

68. Mosmann TR, Cherwinski H, Bond MW, et al.: Two types of murine helper T cell clones. I. Definition according to profiles of lymphokine activities and secreted proteins, *J Immunol* 136:2348-2357, 1986.

69. Mosmann TR, Coffmann RL: Heterogeneity of cytokine secretion patterns and functions of helper T cells, *Adv Immunol* 46:111, 1989.

70. Mueller DL, Jenkins MK, Schwartz RH: Clonal expansion versus functional clonal inactivation: costimulatory signalling pathway determines the outcome of T cell antigen receptor occupancy, *Annu Rev Immunol* 7:445-480, 1989.

71. Mustelin T, Coggeshall KM, Isakov N, Altman A: T cell receptor-mediated activation of phospholipase C requires tyrosine phosphorylation, *Science* 247:1584-1587, 1990.

72. Nakane A, Minagawa T, Kato K: Endogenous tumor necrosis factor (cachectin) is essential to host resistance against Listeria monocytogenes infection, *Infect Immun* 56:2563-2569, 1988.

73. Nakano Y, Onozuka K, Terada Y, et al.: Protective effect of recombinant tumor necrosis factor-α in murine salmonellosis, *J Immunol* 144:1935-1941, 1990.

74. Niederkorn JY, Peeler JS, Mellon J: Phagocytosis of particulate antigens by corneal epithelial cells stimulates interleukin-1 secretion and migration of Langerhans cells into the central cornea, *Reg Immunol* 2:83-90, 1989.

75. Oettinger MA, Schatz DG, Gorka C, Baltimore D: RAG-1 and RAG-2: adjacent genes that synergistcaly activate V(D)J recombination, *Science* 248:1517-1523, 1990.

76. Park DJ, Rho HW, Rhee SG: CD3 stimulation causes phosphorylation of phospholipase C-γ 1 on serine and tyrosine residues in a human T-cell line, *Proc Natl Sci USA* 88:5453-5456, 1991.

77. Pearce E, Caspar P, Grzych J-M, et al.: Downregulation of Th1 cytokine production accompanies induction of Th2 responses by a parasitic helminth: Schistosoma mansoni, *J Exp Med* 173:159-166, 1991.

78. Pepose JS: The relationship of corneal langerhans cells to herpes simplex antigens during dendritic keratitis, *Curr Eye Res* 8:851-858, 1989.

79. Phillips JH, Chang C, Lanier LL: Platelet-induced expression of FcgammaRIII (CD16) on human monocytes, *Eur J Immunol* 21:895-899, 1991.

80. Philpott KL, Viney JL, Kay G, et al.: Lymphoid development in mice congenitally lacking T cell receptor àá-expressing cells, *Science* 256:1448-1452, 1992.

81. Picker LJ, Butcher EC: Physiological and molecular mechanisms of lymphocyte homing, *Annu Rev Immunol* 10:561-591, 1992.

82. Picker LJ, Kishimoto TK, Smith CW, et al.: ELAM-1 is an adhesion molecule for skin-homing T cells, *Nature* 349:796-799, 1991.

83. Piguet PF, Grau GE, Allet B, Vassalli P: Tumor necrosis factor/cachectin is an effector of skin and gut lesions of the acute phase of graft-vs-host disease, *J Exp Med* 166:1280-1289, 1987.

84. Pober JS, Cotran RS: The role of endothelial cells in inflammation, *Transplantation* 50:537-544, 1990.

85. Rampart M, Van Damme J, Zonnekeyn L, Herman AG: Granulocyte chemotactic protein/interleukin-8 induces plasma leakage and neutrophil accumulation in rabbit skin, *Am J Pathol* 135:21-25, 1989.

86. Reiner SL, Wang Z-E, Hatam F, et al.: TH1 and TH2 cell antigen receptors in experimental leishmaniasis, *Science* 259:1457-1460, 1993.

87. Reynolds DS, Boom WH, Abbas AK: Inhibition of B lymphocyte activation by interferon-gamma, *J Immunol* 139:767, 1987.

88. Rice GE, Munro JM, Bevilacqua LP: Inducible cell adhesion molecule 110(INCAM-110) is an endothelial cell receptor for lymphocytes: a CD11/CD18-independent adhesion mechanism, *JEM* 171:1369-1374, 1990.

89. Roberts AB, Sporn MB: The transforming growth factor betas, *Handbk Exp Pharm* 95:419-458, 1990.

90. Rodrigues MM, Rowden G, Hackett J, Bakos I: Langerhans cells in the normal conjunctiva and peripheral cornea of selected species, *Invest Ophthalmol Vis Sci* 21:759-765, 1981.

91. Rosenthal AS, Shevach EM: Function of macrophages in antigen recognition by guinea pig T lymphocytes. I. Requirement for histocompatible macrophages and lymphocytes, *J Exp Med* 138:1194, 1973.

92. Rot A: Endothelial cell binding of NAP-1/IL-8: role in neutrophil emigration, *Immunol Today* 13:291-294, 1992.

93. Saito H, Kranz DM, Takagaki Y, et al.: A third rearranged and expressed gene in a clone of cytotoxic T lymphocytes, *Nature* 312:36-40, 1984.

94. Saito T, Pardoll DM, Fowlkes BJ, Ohno H: A murine thymocyte clone expressing gamma delta T cell receptor mediates natural killer-like cytolytic function and Th1-like lymphokine production, *Cell Immunol* 131:284, 1990.

95. Salgame P, Abrams JS, Clayberger C, et al.: Differing lymphokine profiles of functional subsets of human CD4 and CD8 T cell clones, *Science* 254:279-282, 1991.

96. Sanderson CJ, O'Garra A, Warren DJ, Klaus GG: Eosinophil differentiation factor also has B-cell growth factor activity: proposed name interleukin 4, *Proc Natl Acad Sci USA* 83:437-440, 1986.

97. Schall TJ: Biology of the RANTES/SIS cytokine family, *Cytokine* 3:165-183, 1991.

98. Scott P, Natovitz P, Coffman RL, et al.: Immunoregulation of cutaneous leishmaniasis: T cell lines that transfer protective immunity or exacerbation belong to different T helper subsets and respond to distinct parasite antigens, *J Exp Med* 168:1675-1684, 1988.

99. Shaw G, Kamen R: A conserved AU sequence from the 3′ untranslated region of GM-CSF mRNA mediates selective mRNA degradation, *Cell* 46:659-667, 1986.

100. Shearer GM: Cell-mediated cytotoxicity to trinitrophenyl-modified syngeneic lymphocytes, *Eur J Immunol* 4:527-533, 1974.

101. Shimizu Y, Shaw S, Graber N, et al.: Activation-independent binding of human memory T cells to adhesion molecule ELAM-1, *Nature* 349:799-802, 1991.

102. Silva JS, Morrissey PJ, Grabstein KH, et al.: Interleukin 10 and interferon gamma regulation of experimental trypanosoma cruzi infection, *J Exp Med* 175:169-174, 1992.

103. Sim GK, Yague J, Nelson J, et al.: Primary structure of human T-cell receptor a-chain, *Nature* 312:771-775, 1984.

104. Simon MM, Landolfo S, Diamantstein T, Hochgeschwender U: Antigen- and lectin-sensitized murine cytolytic T lymphocyte precursors require both interleukin 2 and endogenously produced immune (gamma) interferon for their growth and differentiation into effector cells, *Curr Top Microbiol Immunol* 126:173-185, 1986.

105. Smith CW, Kishimoto TK, Abbass O, et al.: Chemotactic factors regulate lectin adhesion molecule 1 (LECAM-1)-dependent neutrophil adhesion to cytokine-stimulated endothelial cells in vitro, *J Clin Invest* 87:609-618, 1991.

106. Snapper CM, Paul WE: Interferon-gamma and B cell stimulatory factor-1 reciprocally regulate Ig isotype production, *Science* 236:944-947, 1987.

107. Springer TA: Adhesion receptors of the immune system, *Nature* 346:425-434, 1990.

108. Staunton DE, Dustin ML, Erickson HP, Springer TA: The arrangement of the immunoglobulin-like domains of ICAM-1 and the binding sites for LFA-1 and rhinoviruses, *Cell* 61:243-254, 1990.

109. Stein PL, Lee H, Rich S, Soriano P: pp59fyn mutant mice display differential signaling in thymocytes and peripheral T cells, *Cell* 70:741-750, 1992.

110. Stevens HPJD, van der Kwast TH, van der Meide PH, et al.: Synergistic immunosuppressive effects of monoclonal antibodies specific for interferon-γ and tumor necrosis factor-α, *Transplantation* 50:856-861, 1990.

111. Strieter RM, Kunkel SL, Showell HJ, et al.: Endothelial cell gene expression of a neutrophil chemotactic factor by TNF-à, LPS, and IL-1á, *Science* 243:1467-1469, 1989.

112. Swain SL, Huston G, Tonkonogy S, Weinberg A: Transforming growth factor-β and IL-4 cause helper T cell precursors to develop into distinct effector helper cells that differ in lymphokine secretion pattern and cell surface phenotype, *J Immunol* 147:2991-3000, 1991.

113. Thompson HL, Matsushima K: Human polymorphonuclear leucocytes stimulated by tumour necrosis factor-α show increased adherence to extracellular matrix proteins which is mediated via the CD11b/18 complex, *Clin Exp Immunol* 90:280-285, 1992.

114. Townsend AR, McMicheal AJ, Carater NP, et al.: Cytotoxic T cell recognition of the influenza nucleoprotein and hemagglutinin expressed in transfected mouse L cells, *Cell* 39:13-35, 1984.

115. Tsunawaki S, Sporn M, Ding A, Nathan C: Deactivation of macrophages by transforming growth factor-β, *Nature* 334:260-262, 1988.

116. Umetsu DT, Katzen D, Jabara HJ, Geha RS: Antigen presentation by human dermal fibroblasts: activation of resting T lymphocytes, *J Immunol* 136:440, 1986.

117. Vassalli P: The pathophysiology of tumor necrosis factors, *Annu Rev Immunol* 10:411-452, 1992.

118. Vidovic D, Roglic M, McKune K, et al.: Qa-1 restricted recognition of foreign antigen by a âë T cell hybridoma, *Nature* 340:646, 1989.

119. Wahl SM, Allen JB, Brandes ME: Cytokine modulation of bacterial cell wall-induced arthritis. In *Progress in inflammation research and therapy,* 29-34, Basel, 1991, Burkhauser Verlag.

120. Wahl SM, Hunt DA, Wakefield LM, et al.: Transforming growth factor-β (TGF-β) induces monocyte chemotaxis and growth factor production, *Proc Natl Acad Sci USA* 8488:5788-5792, 1987.

121. Wakefield LM, Smith DM, Flanders KC, Sporn MB: Latent transforming growth factor-β from human platelets: a high molecular weight complex containing precursor sequences, *J Biol Chem* 263:764-766, 1988.

121a. Waksman BH, Arnason BG, Jankovic BD: Role of the thymus in immune reactions in rats. III. Changes in the lymphoid organs of thymectomized rats, *J Exp Med* 116:187-206, 1962.

122. Wegener AM, Letourneur F, Hoeveler A, et al.: The T cell receptor/CD3 complex is composed of at least two autonomous transduction modules, *Cell* 68:83-95, 1992.

123. Weiss A, Koretzky G, Schatzman RC, Kadlecek T: Functional activation of the T cell receptor induces tyrosine phosphorylation of phospholipase C-1, *Proc Natl Acad Sci USA* 88:5484-5488, 1991.

124. Yamamura M, Uyemura K, Deans RJ, et al.: Defining protective responses to pathogens: Cytokine profiles in leprosy lesions, *Science* 254:277-279, 1991.

125. Yanagi Y, Yoshikai Y, Leggett K, et al.: A human T cell-specific cDNA clone encodes a protein having extensive homology to immunoglobulin chains, *Nature* 308:145-149, 1984.

126. Zinkernagel RM, Doherty PC: Immunological surveillance against altered self components by sensitized T lymphocytes in lymphocytic choriomeningitis, *Nature* 251:547-548, 1974.

7 Anterior Chamber Associated Immune Deviation (ACAID)

JERRY Y. NIEDERKORN, THOMAS A. FERGUSON

The unique immunologic attributes of the anterior chamber of the eye were recognized over a century ago when researchers observed that tumor xenografts survived in this ocular compartment longer than they did at other sites.[2] In the 1940s, Greene and Lund[16] reported that human tumors grew in the anterior chambers of experimental animals and metastasized to distant organs. Subsequent investigators used the anterior chamber of the rabbit as an effective, albeit cumbersome, tool for propagating a variety of human and animal tumors.

IMMUNOLOGIC PRIVILEGE OF THE ANTERIOR CHAMBER

Until the mid-1970s, the immunologic privilege of the anterior chamber was a well recognized but poorly understood immunologic anomaly. The most widely accepted explanation for the anterior chamber's immunologic privilege was that this ocular compartment lacked identifiable lymphatic drainage pathways. The absence of lymphatic drainage to regional lymph nodes was believed to sequester antigens (for example, histocompatibility antigens) and thus produce afferent blockade of the systemic immune apparatus.[2] In the past 15 years, however, experimental findings from several laboratories have clearly indicated that the immunologic privilege in the anterior chamber is the product of a complex array of both local and systemic immunoregulatory processes.[42,51,52]

ANTERIOR CHAMBER ASSOCIATED IMMUNE DEVIATION (ACAID)

The theory that alloantigens placed into the anterior chamber were sequestered from the systemic apparatus was independently disproved by several scientists.[13,23,24,25,44] Kaplan and Streilein[23,24,25] provided the first compelling evidence that antigens delivered into the anterior chamber not only escaped from the eye but also subverted the systemic cell-mediated alloimmune apparatus in an antigen-specific manner. By transplanting semiallogeneic (F_1) cells into the anterior chamber of allogeneic parental strain rats, these researchers demonstrated that the alloantigenic cells were perceived by the host's immunologic apparatus. Hosts primed via the anterior chamber produced hemagglutinating antibodies against the donor alloantigens and, more importantly, displayed an impaired capacity to reject skin allografts from the donor strain used for the anterior chamber priming. The same hosts, however, rejected third-party skin allografts in a normal fashion, thereby confirming the antigen specificity of this phenomenon. The antigen-specific impairment of extraocular orthotopic skin allografts indicated that antigens presented into the anterior chamber were not sequestered in this compartment, but were processed in a manner that would promote the survival of allografts residing in the anterior chamber. Since inoculation of allogeneic lymphoid cells normally sensitizes the host and accelerates rejection of orthotopic skin allografts, the deviant immune response produced by anterior chamber inoculation of semiallogeneic lymphocytes was termed "lymphocyte-induced immune deviation" to connote the aberrant nature of this phenomenon.[24]

Studies in mice confirmed and characterized the dynamic nature of the aberrant cell-mediated immune responses produced by anterior chamber priming. The first studies to examine the immunologic privilege in the anterior chamber of the mouse used tumor allografts to deliver minor histocompatibility antigens into the eye.[35,47] DBA-2 mastocytoma cells (P815) underwent swift rejection following subcutaneous inoculation in BALB-c mice caused by the recognition of minor histocompatibility antigens expressed on the allogeneic tumor cells. Transplantation of P815 cells into the anterior chamber (AC) of BALB-c mice resulted, however, in progressively growing intraocular tumors. The unrestricted growth of the intraocular tumors was accompanied by an equally impressive antigen-specific suppression of cell-mediated alloimmunity.[28,42,52] BALB-c hosts bearing intraocular DBA-2 tumors were unable to reject extraocular DBA-2 skin allografts, yet were perfectly capable of rejecting third-party skin allografts.[42,52] Thus anterior chamber priming resulted in immunologic privilege that extended beyond the boundaries of the eye and was manifested systemically. The profound impairment of skin and tumor allograft rejection suggested that the anterior chamber priming paralyzed all aspects of the host's alloimmune response. This theory, however, was proved incorrect. Further investigations involving this same model revealed the surprising finding that although skin and tumor allograft rejection was inhibited, cytotoxic T lymphocyte (CTL) and humoral antibody responses were specifically activated in response to anterior chamber priming.[28,39] This puzzling spectrum of alloimmune responses elicited by anterior chamber presentation of antigen was termed "anterior chamber associated immune deviation" (ACAID) to connote the dynamic nature of this phenomenon and the participation of the anterior chamber in its induction.[50] Later studies revealed that anterior chamber priming with tumor allografts resulted in active inhibition of the delayed type of hypersensitivity (DTH) to the donor's histocompatibility antigens.[28,51] To date, the primary detectable immunologic lesion induced by anterior chamber presentation of alloantigen appears to be antigen-specific downregulation of DTH reactivity.[37,47,48] Thus the hallmarks of ACAID include (1) progressive growth of intraocular tumor allografts, (2) normal serum antibody production, (3) normal systemic CTL responses, (4) inhibition of orthotopic skin allograft rejection, and (5) antigen-specific inhibition of systemic DTH to the donor strain minor histocompatibility antigens (Table 7-1).

Several researchers have confirmed the basic principles of ACAID in mice using a variety of antigens.[37,47,48] Wetzig, Foster, and Greene[56] and Waldrep and Kaplan[54] showed that AC inoculation of hapten-derivatized lymphoid cells induced suppressed DTH responses. These studies also revealed that a T-suppressor system was responsible for the inhibition of DTH. Subsequent studies have shown that ACAID can be induced by a constellation of antigens including (1) herpes simplex virus (HSV),[58,59] (2) melanoma-associated antigens,[35] (3) soluble proteinaceous antigens,[31] (4) retinal S antigen,[32,33] and (5) hapten-derivatized cells.[54,56]

Although the list of antigens that induce ACAID is impressive, numerous antigens do **not** induce ACAID, but pro-

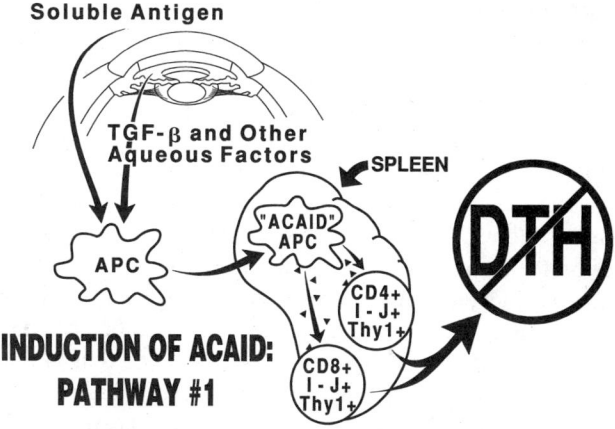

Fig. 7-1. Hypothetic pathway for the induction of ACAID to antigens introduced into the anterior chamber. Soluble factors (for example, TGF-β) in the aqueous humor render local antigen-presenting cells (APC) tolerogenic. The putative "tolerogenic" APC migrate via the blood vasculature to the spleen, where they present antigen in a manner that culminates in T-suppressor cells that inhibit DTH responses systemically.

voke strong DTH responses following anterior chamber presentation. These include (1) highly immunogenic, syngeneic, ultraviolet, irradiation-induced regressor tumors[24]; (2) large, simian, virus-40 T antigens (Niederkorn[28a] and associates, unpublished results); (3) HSV-1 in C57BL-6 hosts[26]; (4) purified protein derivative (PPD) of *Mycobacterium tuberculosis* antigens (Ferguson and associates, unpublished results); (5) mutagenized clone of P815 mastocytoma[38]; (6) Ia+ allogeneic lymphoid cells and; (7) Ia+ tumor allografts.[4] The reason some antigens produce persistent suppression of DTH responses following anterior chamber presentation, whereas other antigens induce prompt DTH responses remains unclear. Unraveling this dichotomy will undoubtedly shed light on the inductive mechanisms of ACAID.

INDUCTIVE SIGNALS OF ACAID

Recent findings propose that the anterior chamber contains a unique population of antigen-presenting cells (APC) that preferentially direct antigen-specific immune responses toward a suppressed state.[60,61,63] Cells isolated from the iris, choroid, and ciliary body of the mouse eye inhibit proliferative responses of lymphocytes in vitro.[7,8,17,28,64] Moreover, the inhibition was mediated by soluble factors secreted by the resident ocular cells.* Presumably, the soluble immunosuppressive mediator secreted by the iris and ciliary body cells accumulates in the aqueous and creates an immunosuppressive environment that favors aberrant antigen processing and the eventual development of ACAID (Fig. 7-1).

TABLE 7-1   HALLMARKS OF ACAID

Antigen Administration	Cellular Responses			Antibody Responses
	CTL	DTH	T$_s$	
Extraocular	+++	+++	−	+++
Anterior chamber (eusplenic host)	+++	−	+	+++
Anterior chamber (splenectomized host)	+++	+++	−	−

*References 7, 8, 15, 17, 18, 21, 28, 64.

This hypothesis was tested by Wilbanks and associates,[60,61,63] who determined that resident iris and ciliary body cells pulsed with soluble antigens and injected intravenously into normal mice produce suppression of DTH identical to that which occurs in ACAID. Moreover, similar suppression was produced by incubating normal peritoneal macrophages in aqueous humor during antigen pulsing.[60,63] This phenomenon, however, appears to be restricted to soluble protein antigens. For example, attempts to reproduce this form of suppression using viruses, hapten-derivatized spleen cells, or antigenic tumor cells have failed.[10a] Unlike soluble antigens, particulate antigens elicit a T cell reaction in the anterior chamber that produces a soluble, serum-borne molecule that homes to the spleen and induces suppressor T cells.[10]

Numerous studies have demonstrated the antiproliferative characteristics of aqueous humor.* Considerable interest has focused on transforming growth factor-β (TGF-β) as a molecule likely responsible for the immunomodulatory effects of aqueous humor.[8,17,28,61] Significant quantities of TGF-β can readily be identified in normal aqueous humor,[8,15,18,21] and iris and ciliary body cells can produce this cytokine.[64] Although TGF-β exercises pleiotropic effects, it is noteworthy that it inhibits a variety of immunologic responses, including DTH.[30] Thus the presence of TGF-β and other inhibitory molecules in the aqueous humor and the strategic location of suppressorogenic APC in the iris and ciliary body create an environment that not only favors the induction of DTH suppressor cells, but also nonspecifically inhibits the expression of DTH effector cells in oculi.

Although the participation of the eye in the induction of ACAID is axiomatic, this requirement is only temporary because removal of the antigen-injected eye 7 days after anterior chamber priming does not prevent the development of ACAID.[40,49] The antigenic signal that emanates from the eye is perceived in the spleen, where a suppressor cell system is activated. The second signal of ACAID originates in the spleen, within approximately 7 days.[40,49] Removal of the spleen, either before or shortly after anterior chamber priming, prevents the induction of ACAID and results in the development of positive DTH responses to the intraocular antigens.[22,50] The concomitant requirement of an intact eye and a functional spleen led to the proposition of a camerosplenic axis for the induction of ACAID.[22,50] Presumably, the first signal of ACAID is generated by unique, antigen-presenting cells in the anterior chamber. These cells either migrate to the spleen or induce T cells that have entered the eye to release a blood-borne, antigen-specific signal. This signal is transduced in the spleen, where suppressor cells are activated and then disseminated systemically.

---

*References 8, 17, 28, 61, 62, 63.

THE NATURE OF ACAID SUPPRESSOR CELLS

The major characteristic of ACAID is the consistent development of T suppressor cells that inhibit the induction and expression of systemic DTH responses. Wetzig, Foster, and Greene[56] were the first to show the presence of antigen-specific suppressor cells in AC-primed mice. Using azobenzenearsonate-derivatized spleen cells, these investigators determined that AC priming induced antigen-specific, T suppressor cells that lacked the azobenzenearsonate cross-reactive idiotype and functioned at the efferent mode of the immune response. Waldrep and Kaplan[54,55] employed trinitrophenol (TNP)-derivatized spleen cells as antigen and showed that AC priming evoked two distinct suppressor cell systems. The first suppressor cell apparatus was antigen-specific and cyclophosphamide-sensitive, and it acted at the efferent phase of the DTH response. The second suppressor cell population was antigen-nonspecific and cyclophosphamide-insensitive. It acted at the efferent mode and was regulated by a third population of spleen cells that displayed contrasuppressor activity. Ferguson and Kaplan[11] employed two novel monoclonal antibodies specific for T suppressor inducer (T_{si}) and T suppressor effector (T_{se}) factors to characterize the suppressor cells in TNP-induced ACAID. To induce ACAID to TNP-coupled cells, the AC inoculum needed to contain two distinct cell populations: one was CD5+ and I-J+, and the other population was CD5+, which also expressed the surface phenotype of T_{si} (14-30+). Further analysis of the first cell population revealed that the cells expressed the CD4+ phenotype. The ability of these cells to induce ACAID was abolished by treatment with either cycloheximide or cytochalasin-B, thereby indicating that protein synthesis was necessary for the induction of DTH suppression.[10] Cell proliferation was not required for the induction of suppressor cells, however, because treatment with 2000 cGy of gamma-irradiation did not prevent the induction of ACAID.[10] Although the two cell populations needed to be introduced into the AC to induce ACAID, they did not need to physically interact or reside in the same intraocular milieu because they could be inoculated into separate eyes and still induce suppression of DTH. These TNP-coupled cells elaborated a soluble T_{si} factor that was antigen-specific, genetically restricted, and reactive with a monoclonal antibody that specifically identifies T_{si}. The putative soluble T_{si} factor was elaborated by the hapten-coupled T_{si} cells in the AC prior to entering the bloodstream. The blood-borne T_{si} factor induced the formation of TNP-specific suppressor cells in the spleen. Recent studies suggest that this "ACAID-inducing factor" is a soluble form of the T cell receptor-bearing determinants identical to the T cell receptor α-chain (Ferguson and associates, unpublished findings). Passive transfer of the blood-borne T_{si} factor to naive hosts results in characteristic ACAID suppressor spleen cells; however, suppression is not induced in splenectomized recipients. Thus the T_{si} factors necessary for the induction of TNP-ACAID arise within the AC, but are transported to the spleen where they elicit the generation of two phenotypically and functionally distinct suppressor cells that can adoptively transfer ACAID (Fig. 7-2). One population of splenic suppressor cells is CD5$^+$ and I-J$^+$, and the other is CD8$^+$, which expresses a surface determinant (14-12$^+$) characteristic of T_{se} cells.[10,11]

Anterior chamber priming with either herpes simplex virus (HSV) or minor histocompatibility antigens also results in the appearance of T suppressor cells that inhibit antigen-specific DTH responses.[51,59] In the case of minor histocompatibility antigens, the ACAID suppressor T cells are antigen-specific, I-J$^+$, CD8$^+$, cyclophosphamide-resistant, and they act at the efferent phase.[51] A second, less common suppressor cell population also occurs in response to AC priming with minor histocompatibility antigens. This suppressor cell population is also I-J$^+$, cyclophosphamide-resistant, but it expresses the CD4 surface phenotype instead of the CD8 antigen.[16]

The absence of lymphatic drainage of the AC requires that antigens introduced into this compartment depart by venous routes. Thus it has been proposed that presentation of antigens into the AC is merely a complicated intravenous (I.V.) injection. It was recognized over a quarter of a century ago that I.V. injection of antigen produced an "immune deviation" in which DTH was selectively inhibited.[1] Thus some researchers have submitted that ACAID is simply another form of the intravenous immune deviation. The ability of aqueous humor, however, to render normal macrophages

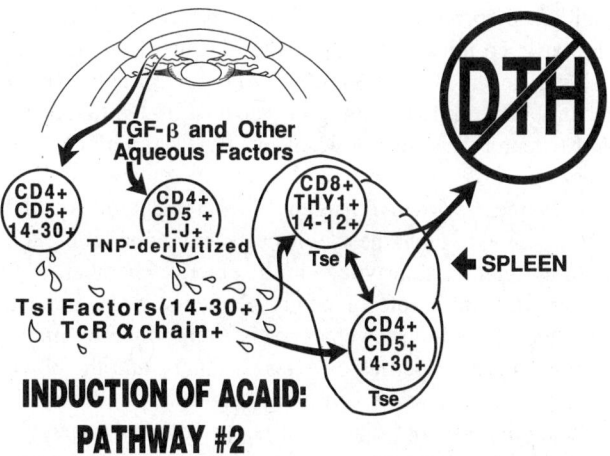

INDUCTION OF ACAID: PATHWAY #2

Fig. 7-2. Hypothetic pathway for the induction of ACAID to hapten-derivatized syngeneic cells introduced into the anterior chamber. Soluble factors (for example, TGF-β) in the aqueous humor provoke TNP-derivatized CD4$^+$, CD5$^+$, TNP-derivatized T cells, and CD4$^+$, CD5$^+$, I-J$^+$, 14-30$^+$ T cells to elaborate the T-suppressor inducer (T_{si}) factor that enters the bloodstream and the spleen, where it activates two populations to T-suppressor effector (T_{se}) cells that inhibit systemic DTH responses.

tolerogenic implies that factors present in the intraocular milieu exert profound tolerizing properties not found in the bloodstream. Moreover, the suppressor cells induced by AC inoculation differ from those induced by I.V. injection in several fundamental ways. Using bovine-serum albumin as an antigen, Wilbanks and Streilein[62] compared the suppressor cells induced by I.V. injection with those produced in ACAID. They found that I.V.-induced suppressor cells acted only at the afferent phase, whereas ACAID suppressor cells functioned effectively at the efferent mode.[62] Moreover, the afferent suppressor cells induced by I.V. injection of bovine-serum albumin were CD8$^+$, whereas ACAID suppressor cells were CD4$^+$. Although the spleen is required for the induction of ACAID, there is no apparent splenic requirement for the induction of I.V.-induced immune deviation.[53] Thus the weight of evidence indicates that the suppression induced by AC priming is distinctly different from that induced by I.V. injection.

MODULATION AND ABROGATION OF ACAID

The unique form of DTH suppression that occurs in ACAID requires the active participation of an intact eye and a functional spleen.[40,49,50] Removal of the eye 3 to 5 days after intracameral inoculation of either HSV-1[49] or P815[40] antigens prevents the development of ACAID. Based on the previous studies by Streilein and associates,[24,40,49] it could be concluded that antigen must reside within the anterior chamber for a finite period of time either to ensure processing by the tolerogenic antigen-processing cells of the iris and ciliary body,[60,63,64] to provide adequate exposure to the immunomodulatory properties of the aqueous humor or to allow the activation of Tsi cells.*

Early experiments in the rat model of ACAID clearly revealed the need for a camero-splenic axis.[24,50] Splenectomy prior to anterior chamber priming with semiallogeneic lymphoid cells prevented the suppression of skin allograft rejection in the lymphocyte-induced immune deviation model.[24] Subsequent studies in mouse models of ACAID confirmed the requirement of an intact spleen and demonstrated that the spleen needed to remain in the anterior chamber-primed host for at least 6 days for ACAID to be successfully induced and expressed systemically.[50] In the P815 tumor allograft model of ACAID, splenectomy produces three remarkable effects indicating the abolition of ACAID. First and most obvious is the ablation of immunologic privilege in the anterior chamber. P815 tumor allografts do not grow progressively in the eyes of splenectomized BALB-c hosts, but instead undergo an ischemic necrotizing form of immune-mediated rejection that histopathologically resembles an exaggerated DTH response.[50]

---

*References 7, 8, 12a, 15, 17, 18, 21, 34, 61-64.

The second striking indicator that splenectomy abolishes ACAID is the accelerated rejection of donor-specific orthotopic skin allografts. Instead of surviving indefinitely as they do in ACAID, orthotopic DBA-2 skin allografts undergo swift rejection in splenectomized BALB-c hosts primed intracamerally with P815 mastocytoma cells. Skin allografts undergo second-set rejection indicative of allospecific priming. The third and most obvious confirmation that splenectomy abrogates ACAID is the full development of systemic DTH responses in splenectomized hosts that have been primed intracamerally.

Similar studies in the TNP-ACAID model revealed the splenic requirement for the induction of suppressed DTH responses to hapten-derivatized cells introduced into the anterior chamber.[10] Following anterior chamber inoculation, TNP-derivatized lymphoid cells elaborate a T_{si} factor that enters the bloodstream and induces the maturation of DTH suppressor cell populations in the spleen. Premature removal of the spleen prevents the blood-borne factor from activating the splenic suppressor cell system and thus circumvents ACAID.

Other manipulations can produce more subtle perturbations in the induction and expression of ACAID. Studies that analyzed the underlying suppressor cell system of ACAID revealed that in vivo treatment with α-I-J monoclonal antibodies prevented ACAID and allowed the AC primed hosts to mount positive DTH responses to anterior chamber antigens.[51]

The successful induction and execution of DTH involves a constellation of cytokines and the participation of second-level effector cells, including granulocytes and macrophages. The obligatory participation of various cytokines and accessory cells has led some investigators to suspect that ACAID might be the consequence of perturbations in one or more cytokine pathways. Murine lymphoma allografts that constitutively secrete interleukin-2 (IL-2) consistently fail to induce ACAID and consequently, undergo immunologic rejection in the anterior chamber.[36] A similar circumvention of ACAID was produced through the systemic administration of recombinant IL-2 in hosts primed in the anterior chamber with lymphoma allografts that did not produce IL-2 and that normally induced ACAID. The IL-2-treated hosts mounted positive DTH responses, whereas the sham-treated hosts displayed ACAID.[36] Further studies indicated that a similar effect could be produced through the systemic administration of IL-1, which presumably promoted the elaboration of endogenous IL-2 in hosts primed in the anterior chamber with tumor allografts.[3]

In recent years it has become clear that immune responses are modulated by at least two distinct T helper cell subsets that cross-regulate each other.[34] Mosmann and associates[34] have identified and defined the Th_1 and Th_2 subsets based on their characteristic cytokine patterns and functional attributes. Th_1 cells represent classical DTH T cells and secrete IL-2, interferon-γ (IFN-γ), and lymphotoxin. By contrast, Th_2 cells produce IL-4, IL-5, IL-6, and IL-10. In vivo administration of Th_2 cytokines (for example, IL-10) inhibits Th_1 responses, whereas administration of Th_1 cytokines (for example, IFN-γ) interferes with Th_2-mediated responses and disease processes.[34] Thus some researchers have considered the in vivo administration of Th_1 and Th_2 cytokines as a method for modulating ACAID. The notion that ACAID might result in preferential induction of one of these subsets of Th cells is suggested by the recent results by Ferguson and colleagues.* Using Th clones, it was shown that only Th_2 type of clones would produce the characteristic, antigen-specific suppression of DTH following injection into the anterior chamber. This induction was restricted to AC injection because inoculation of identical numbers of cells at other sites (intravenous or subcutaneous) did not produce ACAID. The cytokine profile of the Th_2 cells seemed crucial to the system. It was further explained that inclusion of Th_2 cytokines with antigen and a Th_1 clone produced antigen-specific suppression of DTH. Interestingly, suppression in this system was always antigen-specific and conformed to the specificity of the injected clone and not the cytokine-producing cell. Thus downregulation of Th_1 (DTH-mediating) T cells by Th_2 cytokines as demonstrated in other systems also extends to ACAID. It appears that the response is not related to the dose or form of the antigen, as seen in other systems, but it is significantly influenced by the microenvironment of the eye. The eye clearly possesses a mechanism that preferentially activates Th_2 over Th_1 cells.

Other studies have determined a role for several cytokines in the induction of ACAID.[10b] Antibodies to tumor necrosis factor alpha (TNF-α), when co-injected with TNP-conjugated spleen cells, prevent the induction of ACAID. Similarly, co-injection of antibodies against IL-4 and IL-10 also prevents the induction of ACAID. Interestingly, when a cocktail of neutralizing antibodies against IL-1α, IL-1β, and IL-1 receptor was used; or when anti-IL-2 was administered, suppression of DTH was not blocked. Thus a defined series of cytokines is involved in the development of ACAID, thereby implying that these molecules are important in regulating immunologic privilege in the anterior chamber.

The obligatory role of ocular elements in the immune privilege of the anterior chamber is exemplified by immunosuppressive properties of aqueous humor and the downregulatory characteristics of antigen-presenting cells of the iris and ciliary body.† The visual, light-perceiving elements of the eye also contribute to the immunologic privilege in the anterior chamber. By comparing the responses of mice maintained in the dark with those maintained in the light, Ferguson and associates[9,12] established that visible light di-

---

*References 7, 8, 10a, 15, 17, 18, 21, 28, 64.
†References 17, 18, 28, 61, 62, 64.

rectly influences the induction of ACAID. Animals maintained in the dark for even brief periods of time failed to develop ACAID. Moreover, only 1 to 2 lux of illumination of light were needed to permit the development of ACAID. Interestingly, neither the retina nor the pineal gland (the two major light-absorbing organs) was necessary for this effect. Although the precise target cell involved in the light-dependent phase of ACAID remains a mystery, it appears that expression of immunologic privilege in the anterior chamber is more complicated than previously recognized and involves multiple cell populations and regulatory processes found no where else in the body.

WHAT IS THE MEANING OF ACAID?

The eye is an anatomic and embryologic extension of the brain and like the brain, possesses very limited regenerative capacities. Before images can be focused and even perceived by the neural elements of the retina, they must pass through a clear and properly contoured cornea. Thus maintaining corneal clarity is a critical prerequisite for normal vision. The hygroscopic nature of the corneal stroma necessitates a healthy and vibrant pumping mechanism to maintain corneal deturgescence and clarity. This important function is performed by the single-cell-layered corneal endothelium that is unable to undergo mitosis. Thus the only thing standing between normal vision and blindness is a single cell layer with essentially no regenerative capacity. Accordingly, immunologic responses in the anterior segment of the eye must be closely regulated to prevent unwitting immune-mediated injury to such tissues. In the case of the corneal endothelium, at least two adaptations reduce the risk of immune-mediated injury: (1) avoidance of CTL-mediated cytolysis, and (2) inhibition of DTH responses in the anterior chamber. Like neurons of the brain,[6,20] corneal endothelial cells express little or no class I MHC antigens[14,29,43,59] and therefore, should be resistant to lysis by virus-specific CTL. Neurons of the brain avoid CTL recognition and lysis by their failure to present viral peptides complexed by MHC glycoproteins.[20] By expressing little or no class I MHC antigens, virally infected corneal endothelial cells would avoid lysis by class I-restricted CTL. The obvious risk of this strategy is the persistence of virus in the cornea. Alternate immunologic effectors such as interferon-γ, however, might be invoked to eliminate infectious virus without inflicting irreparable damage to the endothelium. The raison d'etre of ACAID is the avoidance of "innocent bystander" damage to ocular tissues by exuberant DTH responses to ocular antigens. Since the corneal endothelium lines a large portion of the anterior chamber, it is in a strategic location to benefit from the effects of ACAID. It is particularly noteworthy that some intraocular regressor tumors do not induce ACAID. They elicit vigorous, systemic DTH responses and become infiltrated with lymphocytes that can produce classical DTH lesions following local adoptive transfer to extraocular sites,

but they are "silenced" within the eye.[5] Thus even if systemic DTH responses are activated, the **expression** of DTH is inhibited within the anterior chamber.[5]

The inhibitory effects of aqueous humor on both antigen-specific and antigen-nonspecific immune responses is well recognized. Moreover, the aqueous humor also exercises neutralizing effects on toxic oxygen radicals elaborated by polymorphonuclear leukocytes.[45] Although inflammatory responses can occur within the anterior chamber, the eye possesses redundant strategies for restricting injurious immune-mediated responses.

The posterior regions of the eye may also benefit from ACAID and the ancillary downregulatory systems of the eye. Although the retina is a relatively large tissue, the point of maximum visual acuity is represented by the fovea. This structure lies within the macula, and the focusing of light in this region provides sharp and detailed vision necessary for the survival of many organisms. The fovea comprises only a few hundred microns of the total retinal surface, but plays a crucial role in the visual process. Thus protecting this critical tissue from immune-mediated injury, even at the risk of invasion by pathogens, is of paramount importance. A DTH reaction on or near this region would inflict irreparable damage on the fovea and other elements of the retina that are crucial for normal vision. Therefore, expression of ACAID in the posterior regions of the eye would have enormous benefit. Studies by Mizuno and associates[31] indicate that anterior chamber priming with retinal S antigen induces ACAID and results in significant mitigation of S antigen-induced uveitis in mice.

It is clear that although we have learned a great deal about the relationship between the eye and the immune apparatus, much still remains to be uncovered. It is likely that applying the principles learned in the study of immunologic privilege and ACAID will help in the design of rational treatments for a variety of ocular diseases and refinement of corneal transplantation.[46] It is even feasible to consider applying the basic tenets of ACAID for promoting the acceptance of retinal transplants.[19]

REFERENCES

1. Asherson GL, Stone SH: Selective and specific inhibition of 24 hr skin reactions in the guinea pig. I. Immune deviation: description of the phenomenon and the effect of splenectomy, *Immunology* 9:205-217, 1965.
2. Barker CF, Billingham RE: Immunologically privileged sites, *Adv Immunol* 25:1-54, 1977.
3. Benson JL, Niederkorn JY: Interleukin-1 abrogates anterior chamber-associated immune deviation, *Invest Ophthalmol Vis Sci* 31:2123-2128, 1990.
4. Benson JL, Niederkorn JY: The presence of donor-derived class II-positive cells abolishes immune privilege in the anterior chamber of the eye, *Transplantation* 51:834-838, 1991.
5. Benson JL, Niederkorn JY: In situ suppression of delayed-type hypersensitivity: another mechanism for sustaining the immune privilege of the anterior chamber, *Immunology* 74:153-159, 1991.

6. Berah M, Hors J, Dausset J: A study of HL-A antigens in human organs, *Transplantation* 9:185-192, 1970.

7. Cousins SW, Trattler WB, Streilein JW: Immune privilege and suppression of immunogenic inflammation in the anterior chamber of the eye, *Curr Eye Res* 10:287-297, 1991.

8. Cousins SW et al.: Identification of transforming growth factor-β as an immunosuppressive factor in aqueous humor, *Invest Ophthalmol Vis Sci* 32:2201-2211, 1991.

9. Ferguson TA, Hayashi JD, Kaplan HJ: Regulation of the systemic immune response by visible light and the eye, *FASEB J* 2:3017-3021, 1988.

10. Ferguson TA, Hayashi JD, Kaplan HJ: The immune response and the eye. III. Anterior chamber-associated immune deviation can be adoptively transferred by serum, *J Immunol* 143:821-826, 1989.

10a. Ferguson TA, Herndon JM: The immune response and the eye. V. The ACAID inducing signal is dependent on the nature of the antigen, *Invest Ophthal Vis Sci* 35:3085, 1994.

10b. Ferguson TA, Herndon JM, Dube P: The immune response and the eye. IV. A role for tumor necrosis factor in anterior chamber associated immune deviation, *Invest Ophthal Vis Sci* 35:2643, 1994.

11. Ferguson TA, Kaplan HJ: The immune response and the eye. I. The effects of monoclonal antibodies to T suppressor factors in anterior chamber-associated immune deviation (ACAID), *J Immunol* 139:346-351, 1987.

12. Ferguson TA et al.: The wavelength of light governing intraocular immune reactions, *Invest Ophthalmol Vis Sci* 33:1788-1795, 1992.

12a. Ferguson TA, Waldrep JC, Kaplan HJ: The immune response and the eye. II. The nature of T-suppressor cell induction in anterior chamber associated immune deviation (ACAID), *J Immunol* 139:352, 1987.

13. Franklin RM, Prendergast RA: Primary rejection of skin allografts in the anterior chamber of the rabbit eye, *J Immunol* 104:463-469, 1970.

14. Fujikawa LS et al.: Expression of HLA-A/B/C and -DR locus antigens on epithelial, stromal, and endothelial cells of the human cornea, *Cornea* 1:213-222, 1982.

15. Granstein RD et al.: Aqueous humor contains transforming growth factor-β and a small (< 3500 daltons) inhibitor of thymocyte proliferation, *J Immunol* 144:3021-3027, 1990.

16. Greene HSN, Lund PK: The heterologous transplantation of human cancers, *Cancer Res* 4:352-363, 1944.

17. Helbig H et al.: Dual effect of ciliary body cells on T lymphocyte proliferation, *Eur J Immunol* 20:2457-2463, 1990.

18. Hooper P et al.: Inhibition of lymphocyte proliferation by resident ocular cells, *Curr Eye Res* 10:363-372, 1991.

19. Jiang LQ, Streilein JW: Immunity and immune privilege elicited by autoantigens expressed on syngeneic neonatal neural retina grafts, *Curr Eye Res* 11:697-709, 1992.

20. Joly E, Mucke L, Oldstone MBA: Viral persistence in neurons explained by lack of major histocompatibility class I expression, *Science* 253:1283-1285, 1991.

21. Kaiser CJ, Ksander BR, Streilein JW: Inhibition of lymphocyte proliferation by aqueous humor, *Reg Immunol* 2:42-49, 1989.

22. Kaplan HJ, Streilein JW: Do immunologically privileged sites require a functioning spleen? *Nature* (London) 251:553-554, 1974.

23. Kaplan HJ, Streilein JW: Immune response to immunization via the anterior chamber of the eye. I. F$_1$ lymphocyte-induced immune deviation, *J Immunol* 118:809-814, 1977.

24. Kaplan HJ, Streilein JW: Immune response to immunization via the anterior chamber of the eye. II. An analysis of F$_1$ lymphocyte induced immune deviation, *J Immunol* 120:689-693, 1978.

25. Kaplan HJ, Streilein JW, Stevens TR: Transplantation immunology of the anterior chamber of the eye. II. Immune response to allogeneic cells, *J Immunol* 115:805-810, 1975.

26. Kielty D, Cousins SW, Atherton SS: HSV-1 retinitis and delayed hypersensitivity in DBA/2 and C57BL/6 mice, *Invest Ophthalmol Vis Sci* 28:1994-1999, 1987.

27. Knisely TL et al.: Destructive and nondestructive patterns of immune rejection of syngeneic intraocular tumors, *J Immunol* 138:4515-4523, 1987.

28. Knisely TL et al.: Production of latent transforming growthfactor-β and other inhibitory factors by cultured murine iris and ciliary body cells, *Curr Eye Res* 10:761-771, 1991.

28a. Ma D et al.: Capacity of simian virus 40 T antigen to induce self tolerance but not immunological privilege in the anterior chamber of the eye, *Transplantation* 57:718-725, 1994.

29. Mayer DJ et al.: Localization of HLA-A,B,C and HLA-DR antigens in the human cornea: practical significance for grafting technique and HLA typing, *Transplant Proc* 15:126-129, 1983.

30. Meade R et al.: Transforming growth factor-beta inhibits murine immediate and delayed type hypersensitivity, *J Immunol* 149:521-528, 1992.

31. Mizuno K, Clark AF, Streilein JW: Anterior chamber associated immune deviation induced by soluble antigens, *Invest Ophthalmol Vis Sci* 30:1112-1119, 1989.

32. Mizuno K, Clark AF, Streilein JW: Ocular injection of retinal S antigen: suppression of autoimmune uveitis, *Invest Ophthalmol Vis Sci* 30:182-184, 1989.

33. Mizuno K et al.: Histopathologic analysis of experimental autoimmune uveitis attenuated by intracameral injection of S-antigen, *Curr Eye Res* 8:113-121, 1989.

34. Mosmann TR, Coffman RL: Two types of mouse helper T-cell clones, *Immunol Today* 8:223-227, 1987.

35. Niederkorn JY: Suppressed cellular immunity in mice harboring intraocular melanomas, *Invest Ophthalmol Vis Sci* 25:447-454, 1984.

36. Niederkorn JY: Exogenous recombinant interleukin-2 abrogates anterior-chamber-associated immune deviation, *Transplantation* 43:523-528, 1987.

37. Niederkorn JY: Immune privilege and immune regulation in the eye, *Adv Immunol* 48:191-226, 1990.

38. Niederkorn JY, Meunier PC: Spontaneous immune rejection of intraocular tumors in mice, *Invest Ophthalmol Vis Sci* 26:877-884, 1985.

39. Niederkorn JY, Streilein JW: Analysis of antibody production induced by allogeneic tumor cells inoculated into the anterior chamber of the eye, *Transplantation* 33:573-577, 1982.

40. Niederkorn JY, Streilein JW: Induction of anterior chamber-associated immune deviation (ACAID) by allogeneic intraocular tumors does not require splenic metastases, *J Immunol* 128:2470-2474, 1982.

41. Niederkorn JY, Streilein JW: Alloantigens placed into the anterior chamber of the eye induce specific suppression of delayed type hypersensitivity but normal cytotoxic T lymphocyte responses, *J Immunol* 131:2670-2674, 1983.

42. Niederkorn JY, Streilein JW, Shadduck JA: Deviant immune responses to allogeneic tumors injected intracamerally and subcutaneously in mice, *Invest Ophthalmol Vis Sci* 20:355-363, 1980.

43. Pepose JS et al.: Detection of HLA class I and II antigens in rejected human corneal allografts, *Ophthalmology* 92:1480-1484, 1985.

44. Raju S, Grogan JB: Allograft implants in the anterior chamber of the eye of the rabbit, *Transplantation* 7:475-483, 1969.

45. Rao et al.: Superoxide dismutase in ocular structures, *Invest Ophthalmol Vis Sci* 26:1778-1781, 1985.

46. She S-C, Steahly LP, Moticka EJ: Intracameral injection of allogeneic lymphocytes enhances corneal graft survival, *Invest Ophthalmol Vis Sci* 31:1950-1956, 1990.

47. Streilein JW: Immune regulation and the eye: a dangerous compromise, *FASEB J* 1:199-208, 1987.

48. Streilein JW: Anterior chamber associated immune deviation: the privilege of immunity in the eye, *Sur Ophthalmol* 35:67-73, 1990.

49. Streilein JW, Atherton SS, Vann V: A critical role for ACAID in the distinctive pattern of retinitis that follows anterior chamber inoculation of HSV-1, *Curr Eye Res* 6:127-131, 1987.

50. Streilein JW, Niederkorn JY: Induction of anterior chamber-associated immune deviation requires an intact, functional spleen, *J Exp Med* 153:1058-1067, 1981.

51. Streilein JW, Niederkorn JY: Characterization of the suppressor cell(s) responsible for anterior chamber-associated immune deviation (ACAID) induced in BALB/c mice by P815 cells, *J Immunol* 20:603-622, 1984.

52. Streilein JW, Niederkorn JY, Shadduck JA: Systemic immune unresponsiveness induced in adult mice by anterior chamber presentation of minor histocompatibility antigens, *J Exp Med* 152:1121-1125, 1980.

53. Sy M-S et al.: Splenic requirement for the generation of suppressor T cells, *J Immunol* 119:2095-2099, 1977.

54. Waldrep JC, Kaplan HJ: Anterior chamber associated immune deviation induced by TNP-splenocytes (TNP-ACAID). I. Systemic tolerance mediated by suppressor T-cell, *Invest Ophthalmol Vis Sci* 24:1086-1092, 1983.

55. Waldrep JC, Kaplan HJ: Cyclophosphamide-sensitive contrasuppression in TNP-anterior chamber associated immune deviation (TNP-ACAID), *J Immunol* 131:2746-2750, 1983.

56. Wetzig RP, Foster CS, Greene MI: Ocular immune responses. I. Priming of A/J mice in the anterior chamber with azobenzenearsonate-derivatized cells induces second-order-like suppressor T cells, *J Immunol* 128:1753-1757, 1982.

57. Whitsett CF, Stulting D: The distribution of HLA antigens on human corneal tissue, *Invest Ophthalmol Vis Sci* 25:519-524, 1984.

58. Whittum JA et al.: Intracameral inoculation of herpes simplex virus type 1 induces anterior chamber associated immune deviation, *Curr Eye Res* 2:691-697, 1983.

59. Whittum JA et al.: The role of suppressor T cells in herpes simplex-induced immune deviation, *J Virol* 51:556-558, 1984.

60. Wilbanks GA, Mammolenti M, Streilein JW: Studies on the induction of anterior chamber-associated immune deviation (ACAID). II. Eye-derived cells participate in generating blood borne signals that induce ACAID, *J Immunol* 146:3018-3024, 1991.

61. Wilbanks GA, Mammolenti M, Streilein JW: Studies on the induction of anterior chamber-associated immune deviation (ACAID). III. Induction of ACAID depends upon intraocular transforming growth factor-beta, *Eur J Immunol* 22:65-73, 1992.

62. Wilbanks GA, Streilein JW: Characterization of suppressor cells in anterior chamber-associated immune deviation (ACAID) induced by soluble antigen: evidence for two functionally and phenotypically distinct T-suppressor cell populations, *Immunology* 71:383-389, 1990.

63. Wilbanks GA, Streilein JW: Studies on the induction of anterior chamber-associated immune deviation (ACAID). I. Evidence that an antigen-specific, ACAID-inducing, cell-associated signal exists in the peripheral blood, *J Immunol* 146:2610-2617, 1991.

64. Williamson JSP, Bradley D, Streilein JW: Immunoregulatory properties of bone marrow derived cells in the iris and ciliary body, *Immunology* 67:96-102, 1989.

8 Ocular Surface Immunology

JOHN W. CHANDLER

The ocular surface, which consists of the cornea, the conjunctiva, and the limbus, is the site of frequent inflammatory and immunologic reactions.[11,14] The biologic requirements for the maintenance of an optically normal cornea give the sequence of pathophysiologic responses major importance. Whereas scarring and disorganization of the extracellular matrix at the site of a labial herpetic lesion may be inconsequential, the same response in the cornea may lead to a marked visual loss. Unlike most other epithelial surfaces (skin and mucous membranes), the convergence of the cornea and conjunctiva at the limbus separates two vastly different tissues. The arrangement of the corneal extracellular matrix (with its lack of blood vessels or lymphatics) is very dissimilar from that of the adjacent limbus and conjunctiva. At the same time, the corneal epithelial stem cells originate at the limbus,[5,29] and immunoglobulins diffuse from the limbus into the cornea.[19] IgG is the predominant immunoglobulin in the cornea, followed by IgA. Only small amounts of IgM are located in corneal tissue, and those are restricted to the periphery. The resultant distribution of immunoglobulins may underlie a number of peripheral corneal diseases [such as the limbal corneal guttering seen in rheumatoid arthritis, in which immune complexes of IgG and rheumatoid factors (IgM) are localized at the peripheral cornea]. The corneal epithelium contains Fc receptors.[56] The role of antibodies, complement, and complement regulatory proteins in the immunology of the ocular surface is the subject of Chapter 4.

The near constant exposure of the ocular surface to potentially antigenic materials including microbes and toxic substances from the environment (chemicals, environmental pollutants), continually places the ocular surface at risk for immunopathophysiologic events. It also makes the ocular surface a potential site for antigen presentation and the initiation of systemic immune responses. Likewise, the immunologic components of the ocular surface may become involved in a systemic immunologic response and lead to untoward sequelae involving the conjunctiva, the cornea, or both. A noteworthy clinical example is ocular cicatricial pemphigoid, in which the conjunctiva becomes infiltrated with T cells, macrophages, B cells, plasma cells, and dendritic cells; which leads to subepithelial fibrosis, scarring, symblepharon, and keratinization.[42]

The ocular surface is an ideal location to study immunologic responses. It can be easily examined with high magnification in the living animal. The properties of the normal cornea allow studies of such immunologic sequelae as the following: (1) angiogenesis, (2) epithelial and stromal wound healing (including scar formation), (3) dissolution of extracellular matrix (which leads to corneal perforation), and (4) biologic changes in immune cell populations such as lymphocytes, mast cells, and dendritic epithelial Langerhans cells. This chapter describes the current understanding of control mechanisms in the ocular surface and correlates them with the involved cell populations, cytokines, and adhesion molecules. Conceptually, it may be useful to consider the anatomic sites of the conjunctiva, the limbus, and the cornea in terms of a cytokine-adhesion molecular network. This approach has been helpful in epidermal immunopathology for understanding normal control mechanisms as well as for depicting the pathogenesis of diseases involving the skin.[27,57]

Cytokines are proteins of low-molecular weights that are produced and released by diverse immune and non-immune cells.[18,26,44,45] They control a mixture of biologic responses including cell growth, differentiation, immunity, inflammation, wound repair, production of cytokines, production of extracellular matrix receptors and adhesion molecules, and other functions by both different and identical cell types. Cytokines are capable of potent effects. Therefore it is vital that a variety of control mechanisms exist including downregulation of cytokine production, cytokine inhibitors, differential effects of the same cytokine on different cell populations (perhaps caused by differences in receptor densities), and cytokine inactivators to destroy cytokines once they are released. A more extensive discussion of cytokine networks is provided in Chapter 5.

Adhesion molecules are involved in the important function of bringing leukocytes and other cell types in close contact so that biologic events can occur.[1,9,28] For example, leukocytes need to adhere to vascular endothelial cells before they can migrate from the blood vessels into injured tissue. Adhesion molecules are expressed by most cell types and specific recognition leads to cell-cell contact. These molecules also play a role in the maturation of leukocytes in lymphoid organs, the ''homing'' of leukocytes to specific tissues, the attachment of leukocytes to extracellular matrix, and the cell interactions involving T cells, B cells, and monocytes.[42,51]

The complete elucidation of cytokines and adhesion molecules in the ocular surface remains to be accomplished, especially in the normal state. This chapter looks at the cell types, cytokines, and adhesion molecules that are likely operative in the ocular surface and unifies these observations through an ocular surface cytokine network. Future studies will lead to further modifications of these concepts, delineate the normal state, and provide the essential data for therapeutic advances in the management of ocular surface diseases.

COMPONENTS OF THE OCULAR SURFACE

Anatomic Considerations

The ocular surface is composed of the conjunctiva, the limbus, and the cornea. The palpebral and bulbar portions of the conjunctiva (as well as the caruncle) have localized areas of unique cell populations including: goblet cells, mast cells, and accessory lacrimal glands.[54] The lacrimal gland and its contribution of tearfilm components via the lacrimal ducts are important as well.

The conjunctival epithelium and the underlying tissue (with its blood vessels and lymphatics) are similar to the epidermal-dermal junction in the skin.[4,53] The limbus is a unique anatomic area where the corneal epithelial stem cells reside while blood vessels and lymphatic channels, common in the conjunctiva, terminate prior to entry into the normal cornea.[2,8,13,47] The limbus is approximately 1.0 mm wide and its central edge begins where the Bowman layer terminates. There is a striking concentration of mast cells in the substantia propia of the limbus in conjunction with the blood vessels and lymphatics.[47] The role of most cells in allergic ocular diseases is discussed in detail in Chapters 25, 27, and 29. The normal quantity and chemical composition of the tearfilm, the normal contours and apposition of eyelid margins during blinks and sleep, the precorneal mucus layer, and an intact ocular surface epithelial layer are essential for a normal cornea and conjunctiva. If these are absent or compromised, a diversity of pathophysiologic processes may

occur that lead to visually significant corneal changes. Even in the presence of all of these ocular surface features, however, a variety of stimuli from pollens to microbes may initiate clinically evident ocular surface inflammatory or immune responses. In some diseases and nutritional conditions, major alterations in cell populations within the ocular surface may occur.

The limbal and conjunctival lymphatics drain to the preauricular and submandibular lymph nodes. Thus ocular surface Langerhans cells can easily initiate immune responses following an encounter with antigen on the conjunctiva and limbus. The blood vessels that supply the palpebral conjunctiva also supply eyelids, and those that supply the bulbar conjunctiva are frequently branches from the ophthalmic artery. The venous drainage has a similar pattern. The characteristics of the capillaries in the conjunctiva are similar to those of the skin. The conjunctival epithelium is two to five cell layers thick and the basal layer rests on a thin basement membrane that is not crossed by lymphatics or blood vessels. At the limbus, the relationships between the epithelium and stroma of the conjunctiva and cornea are formed by the radially oriented palisades of Vogt.[8,13] At this site, there is the transition of conjunctival to corneal epithelium along with the concentration of corneal epithelial stem cells.[10] The capillaries and lymphatics extend only to the edge of the Bowman layer, which demarcates the edge of the corneal epithelium under normal conditions. Angiographic data suggest that the endothelial cell junctions of the limbal capillaries are not very permeable.[13] At the limbus, the lymphatic channels extend into the palisades of Vogt and are in subepithelial and deeper stromal locations.[2,47] Similar relative locations appear in the palpebral and bulbar conjunctiva.

The microvascular endothelial cells from the human limbus have been isolated and grown in tissue culture.[21] These endothelial cells have been partially characterized and resemble human dermal microvascular endothelial cells.[36] Among the shared characteristics are the following: (1) factor VIII-related antigen (von Willebrand factor), (2) class I MHC antigen expression, (3) induced expression of class II MHC antigen by interferon gamma (IFN-τ), and (4) production of interleukin-1 alpha (IL-1α). These common characteristics suggest that the limbal microvascular endothelium has functional characteristics similar to its dermal counterpart that support the concept of an analogous site for a cytokine network.

Cell Types of the Ocular Surface

With the exception of dendritic Langerhans cells, no immune cells exist in the normal ocular surface at birth.[33] In early life, collections of lymphocytes can be identified in the conjunctiva. They have an overlying specialized lymphoepithelium and are part of the mucosal-associated lymphoid tissue found in the gut and respiratory system.[12] The ocular

TABLE 8-1   IMMUNOLOGIC AND INFLAMMATORY CELLS IN THE NORMAL OCULAR SURFACE

	Conjunctiva		Cornea	
Cell Type	**Epithelium**	**Substantia Propria**	**Epithelium**	**Stroma**
Dendritic cells	+	+	+ (periphery)	–
Lymphocytes				
T cells	+	+	Few	Few
α-β	+	+	?	?
τ-δ	+	–	?	?
T-helper	+	+	Few	Few
T-suppressor	+	+	Few	Few
B cells	–	+	Rare	Rare
Plasma cells	–	+	–	–
Polymorphonuclear leukocytes	+	+	–	–
Mast Cells	–	+	–	–
Basophils	–	–	–	–
Eosinophils	–	–	–	–

surface component is conjunctival-associated lymphoid tissue. Its specific role in ocular surface immune responses remains speculative.[20] In addition to dendritic Langerhans cells, the ocular surface (especially the conjunctiva) has populations of immune-inflammatory cells throughout life despite a normal clinical appearance of the external eye.[6,23,48,52] This fact suggests that there are control mechanisms that ordinarily downregulate immunologic and inflammatory responses.

Table 8-1 lists the cell types that are normal components of the healthy ocular surface by their locations. It is important to recognize the following: (1) epithelial cells may, under specific conditions, produce or release IL-1 and other cytokines and, (2) epithelial cells play a crucial role in the initiation of ocular surface responses.[24] For example, following the phagocytosis of killed *Staphylococcus aureus* or latex beads, corneal epithelial cells secrete increased quantities of IL-1 that directly or indirectly induce the migration of dendritic Langerhans cells into the central portion of the cornea.[10] Along with the epithelial cells; dendritic cells, polymorphonuclear leukocytes, and T cells are adjacent to the conjunctival surface; and dendritic cells and the epithelium are poised at the surface of the cornea. Similarly, polymorphonuclear leukocytes also reside in the substantia propria of the conjunctiva along with B cells, plasma cells, and mast cells. The normal adult cornea also has low numbers of B cells, and CD4- and CD8-positive T cells.[44,54] The addition of other cell types is secondary to perturbations of the ocular surface. Adhesion molecules and cytokines are the most likely mechanisms for the trafficking of immunologic and inflammatory cells into and away from the ocular surface.* These mechanisms could account for such clinically

recognizable conditions as papillary or follicular responses, migration of inflammatory cells or blood vessels into the cornea, or the dissolution of corneal or scleral tissue. For example, failed corneal transplants, as well as inflamed corneal tissue removed at the time of transplantation, express a variety of adhesion molecules that are absent in normal corneas except for the minimal expression of ICAM-1 (including ICAM-1, VCAM-1, E-selection, LFA, PECAM-1, and HLA-DR).[7,34]

The conjunctiva has anatomic relationships that are similar to those in other mucous membranes and the skin. The relationship of the epithelium to the substantia propria along the location of the capillary network and the lymphatic channels gives a typical anatomic milieu for the operation of adhesion molecules and cytokine networks. The cornea, however, is anatomically different. It can be viewed as an epithelium and thick basement membrane, and as a Bowman layer. It can also be regarded with an epidermis or dermis type of relationship, but only at the border of the terminus of the Bowman layer, circumferentially at the limbus. This unusual anatomic relationship creates a paradox. It helps protect the visually important central cornea from immune responses but also deprives the central cornea of rapid inflammatory and immune responses in the early phases of microbial keratitis.

The limbus is unique because it has a mixture of anatomic and cellular features that distinguish it from either the cornea or the conjunctiva. Biologically, the limbus is of major importance because of the concentration of corneal epithelial stem cells.[5,29] The cytokeratins expressed by the stem cells are unique to this anatomic region.[29] Unlike conjunctival epithelium, limbal and corneal epithelial layers are devoid of goblet cells. The substantia propria of the limbus has capillaries, lymphatics, sensory nerve endings, and mast cells that are similar to the conjunctiva.[2,8,13,47] These terminate, how-

*References 1, 9, 18, 26, 28, 42, 44, 45, 51.

ever, at the edge of the Bowman layer in the normal situation and are not present within or beneath the corneal epithelium. Dendritic Langerhans cells are normally located within the epithelium in all components of the ocular surface except the central corneal epithelium.[33] Their cell bodies are in a suprabasilar location. Dendritic Langerhans cells are of bone marrow origin and their homing in epithelia is not yet un-derstood. The cell surface glycoprotein Sialyl Lewis,[x] however, is a ligand for endothelial-leukocyte adhesion molecules (ELAM-1). Epidermal dendritic Langerhans cells that bear human leukocyte antigens DR[+] and CD1a[+] also are Siayl Lewis[x+].[37,38] These observations suggest that dendritic Langerhans cells may home within epithelia by this mechanism.[38] In the ocular surface, dendritic Langerhans cells

TABLE 8-2 CYTOKINES OPERATIVE IN THE OCULAR SURFACE

Cytokine	Produced By	Stimulant	Target	Action
IL-1	Monocytes, macrophages, corneal epithelium, conjunctival epithelium	Exog. agents, infectious agent products, IFN, TNF-α, IL-2, IL-3, IL-1, products of lipoxygenase, pathways of arachidonic acid pathway	T cells B cells Epithelial cells Fibroblasts	IL-2 and IL-2r production proliferation, IL-6, IL-8, TNF-α, production development activation, A6 proliferation, type IV collagen production Proliferation, collagenase production
IL-2	Activated T cells	IL-1	T cell subsets B cells, NK Macrophages	Activation, proliferation IL-1 production proliferation, phagocytosis
IL-3	T cells, NK, keratinocytes	Ag activation, may involve IgE, parasitic infections	Mast cells, macrophages, PMN, eosinophils, basophil	Growth stimulation
IL-4	T cells, mast cells	Ag activation	B cells Macrophages Fibroblasts	Induces proliferation, expression class II MHC, Ab "switching" factor Induces class I and II MHC expression, granuloma formation Induces proliferation
IL-6	T cells, B cells, monocytes, macrophages, epithelium, vascular endothelium, mast cells	Endotoxin, cytokines (esp. IL-1 and TNF)	B cells	Growth, Ab production
IL-8	Monocytes, macrophages Keratinocytes, fibroblasts (skin and cornea) vascular endothelium	IL-1 TNF α basophils	PMN T cells chemotaxis Vascular endothelium	Chemotaxis Chemotaxis Histamine release, angiogenesis
IL-10	T cells, keratinocytes	Ag activation	T cells, macrophages	Inhibits cytokine synthesis
TNF-α	Monocytes, macrophages, T cells, B cells	Endotoxin, infectious agent products	Leukocytes Fibroblasts Vascular endothelium	MHC expression, T cell activation, IL-1 and IL-6 synthesis Cell growth, collagenase release Angiogenesis, upregulation of ICAM, ELAM, MHC
TNF-β	T cells, B cells	Antigen activation	Cytolytic T cells, helper-killer T cells, NK	Mediates apoptotic target cell death
TGF-β	VIrtually all cells	Inflammation	Fibroblasts Epithelia Immune cells	Produce ECM, collagen, fibronectin, enhance or prohibit proliferation or differentiation, downregulations growth and differentiation, locally promoted inflammation by induction of IL-1

have another unusual feature. Those residing within conjunctival and limbal epithelia are mature, whereas those within the normal peripheral corneal epithelium are immature.[55] The dichotomy can be viewed to have teleologic importance as it may protect the cornea from inflammatory responses. The pressure of increased amounts of IL-1, or possibly downstream cytokines, or other factors; however, may stimulate the centripetal migration of mature dendritic Langerhans from the limbal region.

Cytokines

Primarily following activation, a wide variety of cell types produce diverse, low-molecular-weight proteins that are involved in inflammation, immunity, cell growth, apoptic death, differentiation, and wound repair. These proteins have been designated as cytokines.[26,28,45] Most of their effects are at their site of production. Activity is achieved with picogram to nanogram amounts of a particular cytokine. Typically, activated cells produce a cytokine for only a few days; however, some chronic inflammatory diseases are associated with prolonged cytokine production. The nomenclature of cytokines remains diverse. Some are referred to as interleukins; others are classified as interferons or growth factors, and some have more than one designation. A discussion of all known cytokines and their actions is beyond the scope of this chapter and this area of immunobiology is rapidly advancing. Further information is provided in Chapter 5.

Table 8-2 lists cytokines that have been studied in the skin, mucus membranes, and ocular surface, or are important in the immunobiologic responses of the ocular surface. In many instances, the investigators looked at a possible relationship with a single cytokine. Following a perturbation of the ocular surface, there appears to be simultaneous, interacting production and function of multiple cytokines in a dynamic fashion. Therefore such observations may not completely capture the symphonic operation of the cytokine network. Nevertheless, the studies of cytokines provide us with new clues about the immunopathogenesis of ocular surface inflammation. For example, stimulation of corneal epithelial cells to produce enhanced amounts of IL-1 leads to migration of limbal dendritic Langerhans cells into the central cornea.[10] Likewise, infection of human corneal stromal fibroblasts with herpes simplex virus leads to the synthesis of IL-8 mRNA and release of IL-8, which may account for polymorphonuclear leukocyte infiltration in herpetic keratitis. Conversely, corneal epithelial cells did not produce IL-8 protein or mRNA under the same conditions.[30]

Cells in the normal ocular surface (Table 8-3) are active, crucial components of the cytokine networks. These cells can initiate a wide variety of processes when they release cytokines following disparate perturbations. Their cytokines can influence the surrounding cells and also attract other cell types to the area by controlling the expression of adhesion

TABLE 8-3 CELL POPULATIONS OF THE NORMAL OCULAR SURFACE AND CYTOKINES PRODUCED BY THESE CELLS

Cell Type	Cytokines
Epithelial cells	
Conjunctival	IL-1, IL-6, IL-10
Corneal	IL-1, IL-6, IL-10
Langerhans cells	IL-1
Fibroblasts	IL-1, IL-3, IL-6, IL-8, IFN-τ
Corneal stromal keratocytes	IL-1, IL-3, IL-6, IL-8, IFN-τ
Vascular endothelium	IL-6, IL-8
Neurons	Substance P
Mast cells	IL-4, IL-6

molecules on different cells. The models for cytokine networks in the skin are prototypes for what probably occurs in the ocular surface.[4,15,53] The anatomic relationships have many similarities and the differences in the relationships of the limbus and cornea are still likely to operate in an analogous manner.

The condition known as Mooren ulcer is a poorly understood, possibly autoimmune disorder that has recently been related to hepatitis C virus as well as to a corneal antigen.[3,31,40,44] The condition leads to perilimbal corneal dissolution, which may proceed circumferentially, as well as centrally onto the cornea. The histologic picture is dominated by plasma cells and lymphocytes in the adjacent conjunctiva. In the melting corneal stroma, polymorphonuclear leukocytes predominate with smaller numbers of plasma cells and lymphocytes. In some cases, resection of the limbal conjunctiva leads to healing. It seems reasonable to conclude that the limbal and corneal relationship is similar to the more standard epithelial-dermal relationship in the described skin cytokine networks.

Many investigators have found various cytokines in the ocular surface, whereas others have studied their putative functions by either topical application or injection in association with a particular ocular surface challenge or perturbation. For example, following the seminal discovery of IL-1 by Gery and associates, IL-1 production by corneal and conjunctival epithelia was confirmed.[18,24] Other researchers have shown that corneal angiogenesis can be induced in association with applications of IL-2 and IL-8.[32,58] It seems reasonable to assume that these may be direct effects. It must be kept in mind, however, that the exogenous addition of one cytokine may upregulate as well as downregulate one or more other cytokines, and that the observed outcome is an indirect effect of the putative cytokine. Since these chemical compounds work in picogram or nonogram amounts and are rapidly formed, the large added amount may precipitate responses that do not occur with physiologic levels. This area needs much more investigation before definitive conclusions can be made that correlate with pathogenetic mechanisms.

It is also important to consider other mechanisms that control ocular surface inflammation along with cytokines. All three layers of the cornea, both within cells and in the extracellular matrix, contain α-1 proteinase inhibitor, which is a major inhibitor polymorphonuclear leukocyte elastase.[25] As such, it protects the cornea from proteolytic degradation in association with inflammation. Synthesis of α-1 proteinase inhibitor by corneal epithelial cells has been demonstrated.[39] It can also be detected in tears and aqueous humor. Conversely, production and release of IL-l alpha by corneal cells may play a central role in mediating collagenase expression, which is important in diseases leading to corneal thinning or melting, as well as remodeling of corneal wounds.[59]

Adhesion Molecules

Another important group of biologic elements involved in the functioning of immunologic and inflammatory responses of the ocular surface are adhesion molecules.[12-14,35,36] Potentially, they could play crucial roles in two situations. The first circumstance is lymphocyte trafficking and recirculation in the ocular surface. This condition probably occurs through the conjunctival-associated lymphoid tissue (CALT), as part of the secondary lymphoid organs of the mucosal-associated lymphoid tissues (including Peyers patches).[15] This system allows lymphocytes to continuously home to mucosal sites and move out of the circulation by specific receptor-ligand binding in postcapillary, high-endothelial venules. This action is followed by emigration into CALT and into lymphatics so that an eventual reentering of the blood stream takes place via the thoracic duct. This function has not yet been elucidated.

In the second situation, the recirculating lymphocytes recognize antigen that is presented by dendritic cells either in secondary lymphoid tissues such as CALT[28] or within the ocular surface cells. The dendritic cells were epithelial Langerhans cells that migrated to the secondary lymphoid tissue and possibly the regional lymph nodes. During their migration, the cells enhanced MHC class II antigens and intercellular adhesion molecule-1 expression (ICAM-1).[51] This expression of ICAM-1 enhances lymphocyte-dendritic cell adhesion via the receptor-ligand binding of ICAM-1 with lymphocyte function-associated antigen-1 (LFA-1) expressed by virtually all T cells, B cells, and monocytes-macrophages.[16,52] This occurrence is an antigen-specific event, however, it also activates these cells to release a variety of cytokines, such as IL-1, IL-4, IFN-τ, and TNF-α.[10-12] These cytokines, in turn, lead to ICAM-1 expression by vascular endothelial cells, epithelial cells, fibroblasts, and even corneal endothelial cells, as well as the production of the cyto-

kine repertoire of these cells.[53-56] Thus the presentation of antigen sets off a cascade of events that lead to an ocular surface inflammatory response.

The sequence of immunologic events leading to the debilitating, clinically-evident condition of ocular cicatricial pemphigoid (OCP) is an example. Conjunctival biopsies demonstrate the deposition of immunoglobulins and complement components in the epithelial basement membrane zone and on epithelial cells that also exhibit metaplasia. The substantia propria contains increased numbers of mast cells, dendritic cells and macrophages, T and B lymphocytes, and plasma cells along with fibrosis. The mast cells produce IL-4, which induces fibroblast proliferation. The profiles of heat shock proteins (HSP) have also been studied. Expression on conjunctival epithelium from OCP patients is lower than normal tissue. In contrast, some members of the HSP family (HSP 90 and HSP 27) are greatly increased on cells in the substantia propria, as well as on conjunctival vessels in OCP.[57] Undoubtedly, cytokines and adhesion molecules are important, but other molecules may be vital as well.

It is essential to recognize that the initial localization of immune cells is an example of an effective immune surveillance system, and that the adhesion molecules involved in that system are unique and separate from those that are operative once antigens are effectively presented in secondary lymphoid tissue. The anatomic specifications of the involved blood vessels for an immune surveillance system are restricted to postcapillary high-endothelial venules (HEV) and the lymphocyte-HEV receptor-ligand pairs appear to be unique for secondary lymphoid tissue as compared to peripheral lymph nodes.[15,58] The HEV have a thicker endothelial lining than other capillaries, and the individual endothelial cells are cuboidal or columnar rather than flattened. While the receptor-ligand pairs are less well identified, CD44 is found on a variety of cells, both immune and nonimmune, and may bind to so-called vascular addressins on HEV as the first step in the normal recirculation of lymphocytes through ocular surface CALT.

There may be additional trafficking mechanisms for immune surveillance as well. The author's laboratory has found a small but consistent conjunctival population of widely dispersed τ-α as well as CD4$^+$ and CD8$^+$ T lymphocytes in normal murine strains. The preferential homing of τ-δ T cells to epidermal and mucus membrane cells is now well recognized but its full implications are not yet elucidated. A recent observation that τ-δ T cells demonstrate preferential adherence to fibroblasts, including an enhanced adherence to fibroblasts pretreated with interferon-τ, provides new concepts that need to be investigated.[59]

CONCLUSION

The adhesion molecules provide an ideal mechanism for bringing various immune and inflammatory cells in contact with one another and with nonimmune cells. The intimately related expression of cytokine cascades by the various cells helps restrict the locations and intensity of immune and inflammatory responses in the ocular surface. Although not all of the puzzle pieces have been completely elucidated, the overall picture is consistent with that of other sites and can be applied to the typical relationships in the conjunctiva, as well as to the unique sites of the limbus and cornea. The challenges are still significant. The missing pieces must be found and the normal state completely elucidated. The adhesion molecule and cytokine networks for specific clinical conditions need to be determined. Once these goals are achieved, new specific therapies based on cytokine networks need to be conceptually determined and tested. In the interim, most ocular surface inflammation will be treated by corticosteroids, nonsteroidal antiinflammatory drugs, or both.

REFERENCES

1. Akira S, Hirano T, Taga T, Kishimoto T: Biology of multifunctional cytokines: IL-6 and related molecules (IL-1 and TNF), *FASEB J* 4:2860-2867, 1990.
2. Albelda SM, Buck CA: Integrins and other cell adhesion molecules, *FASEB J* 4:2868-2880, 1990.
3. Allansmith MR, Greiner JV, Baird RS: Number of inflammatory cells in the normal conjunctiva, *Am J Ophthalmol* 86:250-259, 1978.
4. Allansmith MR, McClennon B: Immunoglobulins in the human cornea, *Am J Ophthalmol* 80:125-132, 1975.
5. Barker JNWN, Mitra RS, Griffiths CEM, et al.: Keratinocytes as initiators of inflammation, *Lancet* 337:211-214, 1991.
6. Berra A, Dutt JE, Nouri M, Foster CS: Heat shock protein expression in human conjunctiva, *Invest Ophthalmol Vis Sci* 35:352-357, 1994.
7. Bienenstock J, Befus AD: Mucosal immunity, *Immunology* 41:249-270, 1980.
8. Bos JD, Kapsenberg ML: The skin immune system: its cellular constituents and their interactions, *Immunol Today* 7:235-240, 1986.
9. Brown SI: Mooren's ulcer: histopathology and proteolytic enzymes of adjacent conjunctiva, *Br J Ophthalmol* 59:670-674, 1975.
10. Brown SI, Mondino BJ, Robin BS: Autoimmune phenomenon in Mooren's ulcer, *Am J Ophthalmol* 82:835-840, 1976.
11. Chandler JS, Cummings M, Gillette TE: Presence of Langerhans cells in the central corneas of normal human infants, *Invest Ophthalmol Vis Sci* 26:113-116, 1985.
12. Chandler JW, Axelrod AJ: Conjunctiva-associated lymphoid tissue: a probable component of the mucosa-associated lymphoid tissue. In O'Connor GR, editor: *Immunologic diseases of the mucous membranes: pathology, diagnosis and treatment,* 63-70, New York, 1980, Masson.
13. Chandler JW, Gillette TE: Immunologic defense mechanisms of the ocular surface, *Ophthalmology* 90:585-991, 1983.
14. Chandler JW, Heise ER, Weiser RS: Induction of delayed-type sensitivity-like reactions in the eye by the injection of lymphokines, *Invest Ophthalmol Vis Sci* 12:400-409, 1973.
15. Cooper KD: Immunoregulation in the skin. In vanVloten WA, Willemze R, Lange-Vejlsgaard G, Thomsen K, editors: *Cutaneous lymphoma: current problems dermatology,* Basel, 1990, Karger.
16. Cumberbatch M, Peters SW, Gould SJ, Kimber I: Intercellular adhesion molecule-1 (ICAM-1) expression by lymph node dendritic cells: comparison with epidermal Langerhans cells, *Immunol Lett* 32:105-110, 1992.
17. Detmar M, Tenorio S, Hettmannspeerger U, et al.: Cytokine regulation of proliferation and ICAM-1 expression of human dermal microvascular endothelial cells in vitro, *J Invest Dermatol* 98:147-153, 1992.
18. Dustin ML, Singer KH, Tuck DT, Springer TA: Adhesion of T lymphoblasts to epidermal keratinocytes is regulated by interferon τ and is mediated by intercellular adhesion molecule 1 (ICAM-1), *J Exp Med* 167:1323-1340, 1988.
19. Ebato B, Friend J, Thoft RA: Comparison of limbal and peripheral human corneal epithelium in tissue culture, *Invest Ophthalmol Vis Sci* 29:1533-1537, 1988.
20. Epstein RJ, Hendricks RL, Stulting RD: Interleukin-2 induces corneal neovascularization in A/J mice, *Cornea* 9:318-323, 1990.
21. Garcia-Gonzalez E, Swerlick RA, Lawley TJ: Cell adhesion molecules, *Am J Dermatopathol* 12:188-192, 1990.
22. Gery I, Gershon RK, Waksman BH: Potentiation of the T-lymphocyte response to mitogens. I. The responding cells, *J Exp Med* 136:128-142, 1972.
23. Gillette TE, Chandler JW, Greiner JV: Langerhans cells of the ocular surface, *Ophthalmology* 89:700-711, 1982.
24. Goldberg MF, Bron AJ: Limbal palisades of Vogt, *Trans Am Ophthalmol Soc* 80:155-169, 1982.
25. Goldberg MF, Ferguson TA, Pepose JS: Detection of cellular adhesion molecules in inflamed human corneas, *Ophthalmology* 101:161-168, 1994.
26. Grabner G, Luger TA, Smolin G, Oppenheim JJ: Corneal epithelial cell-derived thymocyte-activating factor (CETAF), *Invest Ophthalmol Vis Sci* 23:757-763, 1982.
27. Hynes RO: Integrins: a family of cell surface receptors, *Cell* 48:549-554, 1987.
28. Iwamoto T, Smelser GK: Electron microscope studies on the mast cells and blood and lymphatic capillaries of the human corneal limbus, *Invest Ophthalmol Vis Sci* 4:815-834, 1965.
29. Koch AE, Polverini PJ, Kunkel SL, et al.: Interleukin-8 as a macrophage-derived mediator of angiogenesis, *Science* 258:1798-1801, 1992.
30. Lawrenson JG, Ruskell GL: The structure of corpuscular nerve endings in the limbal conjunctiva of the human eye, *J Anat* 177:75-84, 1991.
31. Luger TA, Schwarz T: Evidence for an epidermal cytokine network, *J Invest Dermatol* 95:1005-1045, 1990.
32. Marlin SD, Springer TA: Purified intercellular adhesion molecule-1 (ICAM-1) is a ligand for lymphocyte function-associated antigen 1 (LFA-1), *Cell* 51:813-819, 1987.
33. Marreu F, Boisjoly HM, Wagner E, et al.: Long-term culture and characterization of human limbal microvascular endothelial cells, *Exp Eye Res* 51:645-650, 1990.
34. Mizel SB: The interleukins, *FASEB J* 3:2379-2388, 1989.
35. Nickoloff BJ: The cytokine network in psoriasis, *Arch Dermatol* 127:871-884, 1991.
36. Niederkorn JV, Peeler JS, Mellon J: Phagocytosis of particulate antigens by corneal epithelial cells stimulates interleukin-1 secretion and migration of Langerhans cells into the central cornea, *Reg Immunology* 2:83-90, 1989.
37. Oakes JE, Monteiro CA, Cubitt CL, Lausch RN: Induction of interleukin-8 gene expression is associated with herpes simplex virus infection of human corneal keratinocytes but not human corneal epithelial cells, *J Virol* 67:4777-4784, 1993.
38. Pavilack MA, Elner VM, Elner SG, et al.: Differential expression of human corneal and perilimbal ICAM-1 by inflammatory cytokines, *Invest Ophthalmol Vis Sci* 33:564-573, 1992.
39. Philips M, Nudelman E, Gaeta FCA, et al.: ELAM-1 mediates cell adhesion by recognition of a carbohydrate ligand, *Science* 250:1130-1132, 1990.
40. Piela-Smith TH, Broketa G, Hand A, Korn JH: Regulation of ICAM-1 expression and function in human dermal fibroblasts by IL-4, *J Immunol* 148:1375-1381, 1992.
41. Sacks E, Rutgers J, Jakobiec FA, et al.: A comparison of conjunctival and monocular dendritic cells utilizing new nonoclonal antibodies, *Ophthalmology* 93:1089-1097, 1986.
42. Sacks EH, et al.: Immunophenotypic analysis of the inflammatory infiltrate in ocular cicatricial pemphigoid: further evidence for a T cell-mediated event, *Ophthalmology* 96:236-243, 1989.
43. Sacks EH, Wieczorek R, Jakobiec FA, Knowles DM: Lymphocytic subpopulations in the normal human conjunctiva: a monoclonal antibody study, *Ophthalmology* 93:1276-1283, 1986.
44. Scheiffarth OF et al.: T lymphocytes of the normal human cornea, *Br J Ophthalmol* 71:384-386, 1987.
45. Schermer A, Galvin S, Sun T-T: Differentiation-related expression of a major 64K corneal keratin in vivo and in culture suggests limbal location of corneal epithelial stem cells, *J Cell Biol* 103:49-62, 1986.
46. Seto SK, Gillette TE, Chandler JW: HLA-DR+/T6− Langerhans cells in the human cornea, *Invest Ophthalmol Vis Sci* 28:1719-1722, 1987.

47. Soukiasian SH, Rice B, Foster CS, Lee SJ: The T cell receptor in normal and inflamed human conjunctiva, *Invest Opthalmol Vis Sci* 33:453-459, 1992.
48. Stoolman LM: Adhesion molecules controlling lymphocyte migration, *Cell* 56:907-910, 1989.
49. Swerlick RA, Lawley TJ: Role of microvascular endothelial cells in inflammation, *J Invest Dermatol* 100:1115-1155, 1993.
50. Tabata N, Aiba S, Nakagawa S, et al.: Sialyl Lewis^{X} expression on human Langerhans cells, *J Invest Dermatol* 101:175-179, 1993.
51. Townsend WM: The limbal palisades of Vogt, *Trans Am Ophthalmol Soc* 89:721-756, 1991.
52. Twining SS, Everse SJ, Wilson PM, et al.: Localization and quantification of α-1-proteinase inhibitor in the human cornea, *Curr Eye Res* 8:389-393, 1989.
53. Twining SS, Fukuchi T, Yue BJYT, et al.: Corneal systhesis of α1-proteinase inhibitor (α1-antitrypsin), *Invest Ophthalmol Vis Sci* 35:458-462, 1994.
54. Vantrappen L et al.: Lymphocytes and Langerhans cells in the normal human cornea, *Invest Ophthalmol Vis Sci* 26:220-225, 1985.
55. Walz G, Aruffo A, Kolanus W, et al.: Recognition by ELAM-1 of the Sialyl-Le determinant on myeloid and tumor cells, *Science* 250:1132-1135, 1990.
56. Wang HM, Jeng JE, Kaplan HJ: Fc receptors in corneal epithelium, *Can Eye Res* 8:123, 1989.
57. Wawryk SO, Novotny JR, Wicks IP, et al.: The role of the LFA-1/ICAM-1 interaction in human leukocyte homing and adhesion, *Immunol Rev* 108:135-161, 1989.
58. Wei Z-G, Wu R-L, Lavker RM, Sun T-T: In vitro growth and differentiation of rabbit bulbar, fornix and conjunctival epithelium, *Invest Ophthalmol Vis Sci* 34:1814-1828, 1993.
59. West JA, Strissel KJ, Girard MT, Fini ME: Endogenously produced interleukin 1-α mediates collagenase synthesis by corneal fibroblasts, *Invest Ophthalmol Vis Sci* 35(suppl):1457, 1994.
60. Whitcup SM, Nussenblatt RB, Price FW, Chan C-C: Expression of cell adhesion molecules in corneal graft failure, *Cornea* 12:475-480, 1993.
61. White B, Korn JH, Piela-Smith TH: Preferential adherence of human τ/a, CD8+, and memory T cells to fibroblasts, *J Immunol* 152:4912-4918, 1994.
62. Wilson SE, Lee WM, Murakami C, et al.: Mooren's corneal ulcers and hepatitis C virus, *N Engl J Med* 329:62, 1993.
63. Wood TD, Kaufman HE: Mooren's ulcer, *Am J Ophthalmol* 71:417-422, 1971.
64. Yednock TA, Rosen SD: Lymphocyte homing, *Adv Immunol* 44:313-378, 1989.

9 Postinflammatory Neovascularization

GORDON K. KLINTWORTH

Blood vessels form within the ocular tissues in numerous pathologic states.[298] The cornea and surfaces of the retina and iris are particularly vulnerable to clinically significant angiogenesis.[95] Important causes of retinal neovascularization encompass diabetes mellitus, retinopathy of prematurity, retinal branch vein occlusion, and sickle cell disease. The common denominator in most cases of retinal neovascularization is impaired retinal circulation. Potent stimuli of vascular proliferation on the anterior surface of the iris (rubeosis iridis) include long-standing retinal detachment, retinoblastoma, and anterior uveitis.

Inflammation includes vascular responses (hyperemia, increased vascular permeability, and adherence of leukocytes to the vascular endothelium) as well as the migration of leukocytes from the circulation into the extravascular compartment. Vascular dilatation, increased vascular permeability, and edema account for three of the cardinal signs of inflammation: rubor (redness), tumor (swelling), and calor (heat). The inflammatory reaction involves numerous concurrent interacting mediators (complement, kinin system, clotting and fibrinolytic cascades, vasoactive amines, mediators derived from leukocytes, cyokines, growth factors, metabolites of arachidonic acid, platelet-activating factor, reactive oxygen metabolites, neuropeptides, endothelial-derived mediators) as well as polymorphonuclear leukocytes (PMNs), lymphocytes, monocytes, eosinophils, basophils, mast cells, and platelets with the relative proportion of the components varying with the nature of the inflammation-evoking stimulus.

The inflammatory response embraces all traditional clinical and morphologic events plus the relevant concealed molecular events that lead to the tissue reaction known as inflammation. Although wound healing has commonly been regarded as a postinflammatory event, it is more reasonably considered part of the inflammatory response (from which it cannot usually be separated). According to conventional concepts, inflammatory angiogenesis is part of wound healing (as in granulation tissue); but as corneal studies have shown, neovascularization can occur within days of injury—before wound healing begins—and not after inflammation has subsided.

INFLAMMATORY ANGIOGENESIS

The evidence for inflammatory neovascularization is strongest for the cornea. In a wide variety of natural and experimental situations [including corneal injuries produced by chemicals, antigens, and metabolic disorders[89-91,141] (Figs. 9-1 and 9-2)], capillaries invade the normally avascular cornea after leukocytes. Inflammatory factors are probably involved in at least some cases of intraocular and retinal angiogenesis (for example, posterior segment inflammatory disease involving the retinal vasculature[112], sarcoidosis,[59] Behçet's syndrome,[132] Eales disease,[6] and toxoplasmosis[97]). Most cases of subretinal neovascularization, which is a feature of age-related macular degeneration, have inflammatory components and a perivascular leukocytic infiltrate within the choroid. Moreover, inflammation is an element in one experimental model of iris neovascularization.[261]

Inflammatory angiogenesis has been extensively studied in the cornea and in the granulation tissue of wound healing. Sequential morphologic observations on heterotopic corneal grafts (from various sources and after diverse forms of pretreatment) in the hamster cheek pouch (Fig. 9-3) led to the hypothesis that corneal neovascularization is a manifestation of inflammation and that leukocytes might play an important pathogenetic role. Reviews of numerous experimental models of corneal vascularization revealed that an inflammatory reaction occurs in association with angiogenesis and the degree of angiogenesis is often proportional to the vigor of the inflammatory reaction.[141] Many studies emphasize the association of corneal vascularization with the inflammatory response[141] and most facets of corneal neovascularization are identical to inflammatory angiogenesis in other tissues. Further support for the hypotheses that corneal vascularization is a component of inflammation and that leukocytes

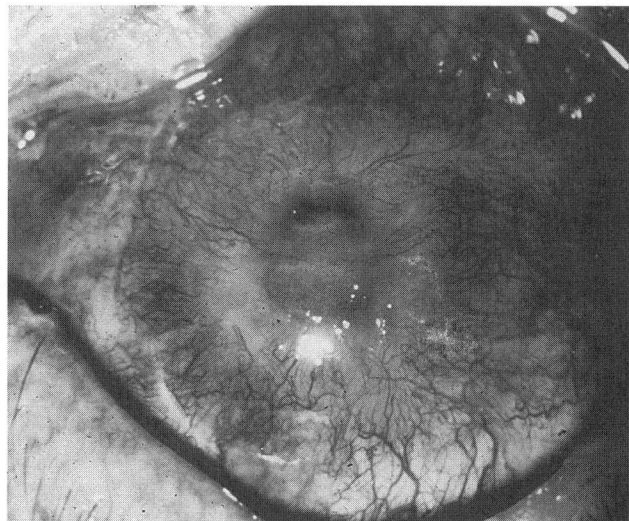

Fig. 9-1. Clinical photograph of markedly vascularized human cornea.

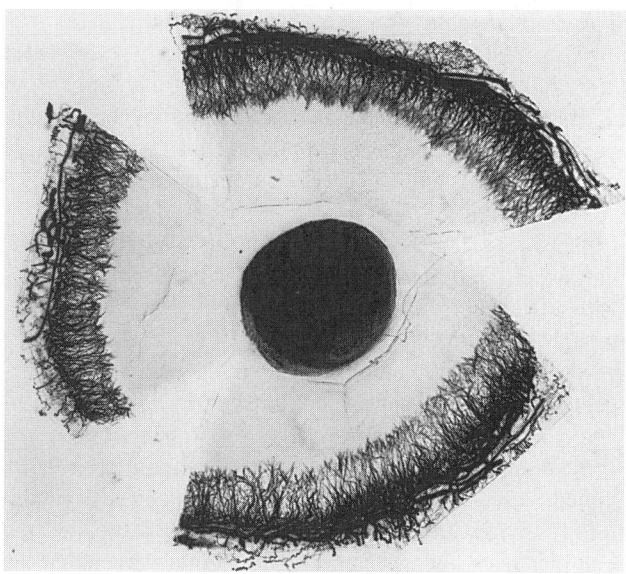

Fig. 9-2.   Flat preparation of rat cornea after perfusion with India Ink showing corneal blood vessels. (Reproduced with permission from Culton M, Chandler DB, Proia AD, Hickingbotham D, Klintworth GK: The effect of oxygen on corneal neovascularization, *Invest Ophthalmol Vis Sci* 31:1277-1281, 1990).

play a cardinal role in the angiogenesis stems from experiments that suppress angiogenesis in which the leukocytic infiltration into the cornea is markedly diminished. Corneal neovascularization is suppressed by corticosteroids, nonsteroidal antiinflammatory drugs, and irradiation. Different corticosteroids inhibit corneal angiogenesis in various clinical and experimental circumstances.[141] The timing of the drug administration affects the degree of angiogenesis, with most angiogenic suppression occurring with treatment prior to, or immediately after, corneal injury rather than after the onset of the lesion.[141]

Inhibitors of Inflammatory Angiogenesis

Aside from their effect on corneal angiogenesis, corticosteroids suppress angiogenesis around a freeze injury to the cerebral cortex[14] and in the granulation tissue of healing gastric ulcers.[118] Such suppression of angiogenesis by corticosteroids presumably relates, at least in part, to the antiinflammatory action that results from the binding of the steroid to a cytoplasmic receptor, followed by the translocation of this complex to the nucleus where the synthesis of lipocortin is induced. This "second messenger" protein prevents the activation of phospholipase-A_2. This repression interferes with the hydrolysis of phospholipids to nonesterified fatty acids, the liberation of arachidonic acid from cell membranes, and the synthesis of the entire cascade of eicosanoids [prostaglandins (PGs), leukotrienes, HETEs and other metabolites of arachidonic acid] by the cyclooxygenase and lipooxygenase pathways.[75] Corticosteroids inhibit the migration of leukocytes toward sites of injury,[43,90,207,221] inhibit the dilation and increased permeability of blood vessels to PMLs,[28] cause a marked reduction in the macrophage population of some lesions,[14] destroy lymphocytes,[44] and diminish other participants of the inflammatory response.

Corticosteroids stabilize lysosomal membranes[289] and hence inhibit the release of hydrolytic enzymes from PMLs, diminish the increased vascular permeability that accompanies inflammation,[267] and inhibit the production of several cytokines, including IL-1 and TNF.[19,20,260] Moreover, systemic corticosteroids induce monocytopenia.[151] Corticosteroids even inhibit prostacyclin synthesis by vascular endothelial cells.[135] Hydrocortisone has a slight inhibitory effect on DNA synthesis and cell growth of certain vascular endothelial cells.[14]

Medroxyprogesterone decreases substantially the PML

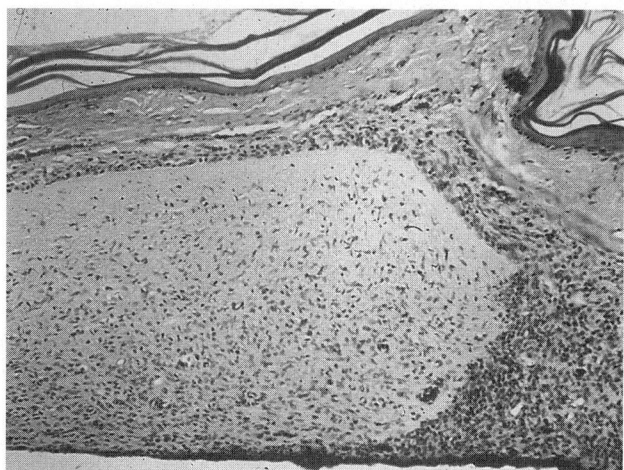

Fig. 9-3.   Tissue section of corneal graft in hamster cheek pouch illustrating blood vessels and numerous inflammatory leukocytes within corneal stroma. Masson trichrome stain.

and vascular infiltration into sensitized rabbit corneas with experimental herpes simplex virus keratitis.[146] It decreases corneal neovascularization following thermal burns[207] or PGE₁ induction.[43] This angiostatic steroid inhibits plasminogen activator—an enzyme implicated in angiogenesis—in endothelial cells.[5] Glucocorticoids even reduce plasminogen activator activity.[293]

Nonsteroidal antiinflammatory agents that retard corneal neovascularization include inhibitors of fatty acid cyclooxygenase (flurbiprofen, indomethacin, and Ketorolac).[141] Although not eliminating the ability of PGs to trigger blood vessel proliferation, indomethacin seems to confine the perpetuation of angiogenesis and its extent.[15] Inhibitors of lipooxygenase have not suppressed experimentally induced corneal angiogenesis. For reasons that remain to be determined, certain dual cyclooxygenase-lipooxygenase inhibitors (BW 755C and BW A540C) do not reduce—even at high doses[120]—new vessel formation in the cornea that can be induced by silver-potassium nitrate cautery in the rat. Another dual inhibitor (SK&F 86002) represses corneal neovascularization in a dose-dependent fashion,[119] but it inhibits its IL-1 production by monocytes and reduces the PMN infiltrate in certain situations—possibly by inhibiting leukotriene B.[119]

Corneal angiogenesis is severely suppressed by total body irradiation[65,90,103,232,255] and total lymphoid irradiation.[266] It is less severely suppressed by head irradiation[103] and by total body irradiation followed by bone marrow transplantation.[103] Although corneal vascularization follows irradiation of the head, the amount is less than in nonirradiated animals,[103,256] presumably because the blood vessels that invade the cornea in those cases are formed only from endothelial cell migration rather than in the usual manner by migration and mitosis. Antineutrophil serum enhances the leukopenic effect of total body irradiation.[255] In quantitative studies of corneal vascularization in inbred mice following chemical cautery, the degree of angiogenic suppression produced by total body irradiation is significantly less if a total marrow transplant is performed immediately after the irradiation. This evidence supports the belief that bone marrow-derived elements are involved in corneal angiogenesis in that model.[103] Corneal angiogenesis is diminished in leukopenic rabbits following total body irradiation with eyes shielded.[66] In rats, a single dose of irradiation severely inhibits angiogenesis if delivered prior to wounding in the Selye pouch.[281]

For poorly understood reasons, heparin combined with cortisone enhances the antiangiogenic effect of cortisone on posttraumatic,[200] alkali-induced,[262] and PGE₁-induced[43] corneal vascularization. These two compounds inhibit the growth of new capillary blood vessels in the chick embryo and in the rabbit cornea following tumor implantation.[79] Cycloamyloses, which act as carriers for hydrophobic molecules such as certain corticosteroids, adsorb to endothelial cells and have an even stronger synergism with corticoste-

roids against angiogenesis induced on the CAM.[81] Even corticosteroids that lack glucocorticoid or mineralocorticoid activity inhibit angiogenesis in the CAM in the presence of heparin or heparin fragments.[50] They also inhibit endotoxin-induced corneal inflammatory neovascularization. Whereas corticosteroids retards corneal neovascularization, cortisone alone does not inhibit tumor angiogenesis except in the presence of heparin.[79]

Inflammatory Corneal Angiogenesis

The closely related processes of inflammation and angiogenesis are claimed to be independent of each other,[77] but this hypothesis lacks convincing supporting evidence. Moreover, inflammatory angiogenesis is seldom an isolated phenomenon, which suggests that an angiogenic factor that stimulates only vascular endothelium may not exist. Aside from vascular endothelial activation, other cells react during new vessel formation.[141] When blood vessels invade tissues (such as the avascular cornea) in different experimental models, several cell types that do not normally reside in a tissue, such as leukocytes (PMLs, monocytes, lymphocytes) and mast cells, invade the tissue.[141] Even lymphatic vessels and Langerhans cells invade the cornea during neovascularization.[141]

In all circumstances that have been thoroughly studied to date, corneal angiogenesis has been part of the inflammatory reaction.[141] Even when corneal neovascularization is induced experimentally by nutritional deficiencies, such as ascorbic acid, vitamin A deficiency, or complete starvation, it is not a direct consequence of the deficiency state but a complication of it. The duration of the prevascular latent period is directly related to the time that it takes for the initial leukocytic infiltration to begin.[89] In different experimental models, new vessels only grow into the cornea in areas in which leukocytes are present.[89] The extent and nature of the inciting agent as well as the degree of inflammation influence the amount and duration of corneal neovascularization. Despite their differences, all experimental models of corneal neovascularization display three phases: an early prevascular phase in which leukocytes infiltrate the cornea, a second phase in which leukocytes and blood vessels occur together, and a later phase in which corneal blood vessels persist in the absence of leukocytes.[89] Numerous experiments indicate that the initial event that triggers blood vessels to invade tissue occurs early in the inflammatory response and the vascularization involves a complex cascade of concurrent and overlapping events that are extremely difficult to dissect.

NONINFLAMMATORY ANGIOGENESIS

New blood vessels form in several physiologic and apparently noninflammatory pathologic circumstances in which cell replication is pronounced. These include embryonic development and the growth of solid neoplasms. Also, a circulatory system evolved during the evolution to metazoa. Angiogenesis in all of these situations is preceded by an increased cellularity and, in all likelihood, tissue hypoxia. Vast quantities of cells in close proximity to each other compete for oxygen and existing nutrients, and certain metabolites accumulate, which alters the cellular milieu. Presumably, the cells then liberate some factor(s) that are capable of inducing directional vascular growth. In pathologic states that prominently feature new vessel formation, such as proliferative diabetic retinopathy and the retinopathy of prematurity, ample evidence exists for an antecedent tissue hypoxia. The possibility of an angiogenic substance being liberated by nonperfused or ischemic retina was originally proposed by Michaelson[177] in 1948. The identity of the hypoxia-inducing angiogenic factor remains unknown; but lactate, a product of anerobic metabolism, stimulates macrophages to secrete angiogenic factors.[134]

The increased cellularity in the granulation tissue of healing wounds and in the vascularizing corneal tissue which is caused by the inflammatory cell infiltrate brings up the question of whether inflammatory angiogenesis is triggered by tissue hypoxia involving a similar basic mechanism as noninflammatory angiogenesis. Because the normal corneal stroma is relatively acellular, could an increased cellularity contribute to the invasion of the cornea by blood vessels?

The difference between inflammatory and noninflammatory angiogenesis is not clear and common pathways are probably involved in both varieties of neovascularization. Although tumor and inflammatory angiogenesis may be different, they have many similarities and the distinction remains to be clarified; particularly since an inflammatory reaction usually surrounds all solid tumors—especially those that are malignant. For instance, whereas angiogenesis that is induced by tumors may be noninflammatory in type, inflammatory pathways may contribute to the new blood vessels found in solid neoplasms. Moreover, their new vessels manifest an increased permeability which, as discussed later, can lead to angiogenesis.

Noninflammatory Corneal Angiogenesis

The question of whether there is a noninflammatory form of corneal angiogenesis remains open. Tissue hypoxia may contribute to contact lens-induced neovascularization, which may involve the inflammatory response. Corneal angiogenesis that is induced with extended wear contact lenses is suppressed with the antiinflammatory agent flurbiprofen (a cyclooxygenase inhibitor).[60] Extended hydrogel contact lens wear causes deep stromal vascularization that is associated with leukocytes.[162] To date, a convincing model of noninflammatory corneal neovascularization has not been found. Alleged noninflammatory models have either lacked adequate documentation or, on closer scrutiny, have turned out not to be valid. When angiogenesis is induced in the absence of an associated inflammatory response (1) microscopic evaluations need to be performed prior to and during

the early neovascularization after the angiogenic stimulation and (2) noncellular constituents of the inflammatory response need to be ruled out. The corneas of certain strains of mice [nude mice (nu/nu), hairless mice (hr/hr), DBA, and corn-1] vascularize spontaneously. Although all of these strains of mice have not yet been fully studied, our research has found blood vessels in nude and hairless mice to be preceded by an inflammatory response.[148]

STAGES OF INFLAMMATORY ANGIOGENESIS

The invasion of tissues by capillaries depends on the migration of endothelial cells as well as on their ability to replicate and become aligned in an orderly manner. As in noninflammatory angiogenesis, blood vessels form in several discrete but overlapping phases (Fig. 9-4).

Early Events

Latent Period Between Injury and Onset of Angiogenesis. Following injury, a remarkably similar sequence of events occurs before neovascularization in different experimental models. Vasodilation, increased vascular permeability, and edema conspicuously precede corneal and other forms of inflammatory angiogenesis. Surrounding blood

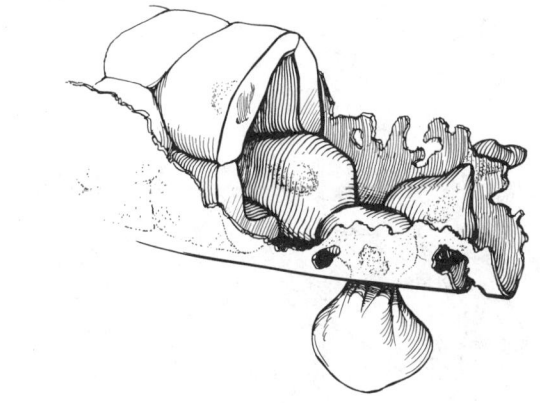

A

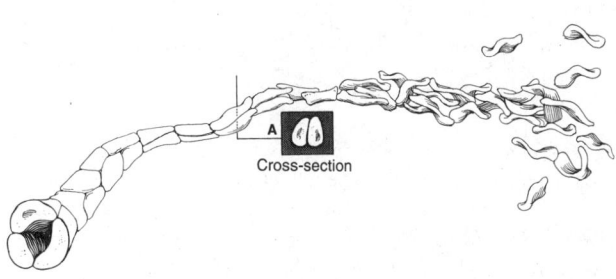

B

Fig. 9-4. Schematic depiction of early events in angiogenesis. **A,** Early stage of angiogenesis depicting degradation of vascular endothelial basal lamina and the migration of endothelial cells through the defects in the basal lamina. **B,** Conceptional view of possible new vessel formation at tip of vascular sprout which lacks a lumen. Individual endothelial cells may lose contact with each other and migrate independently into the tissue.

Continued

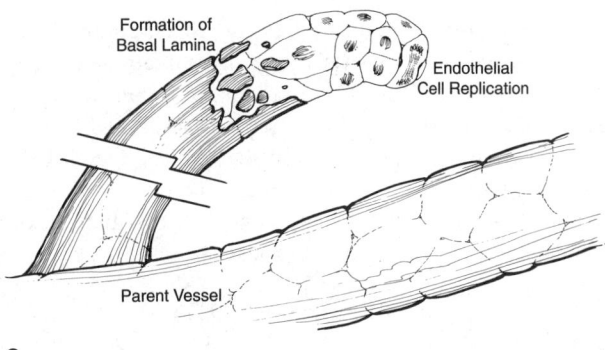

C

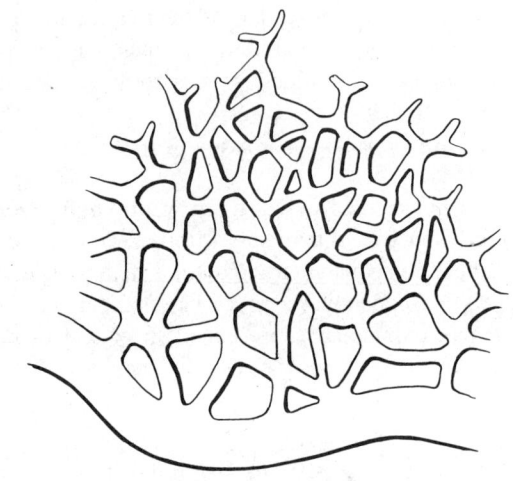

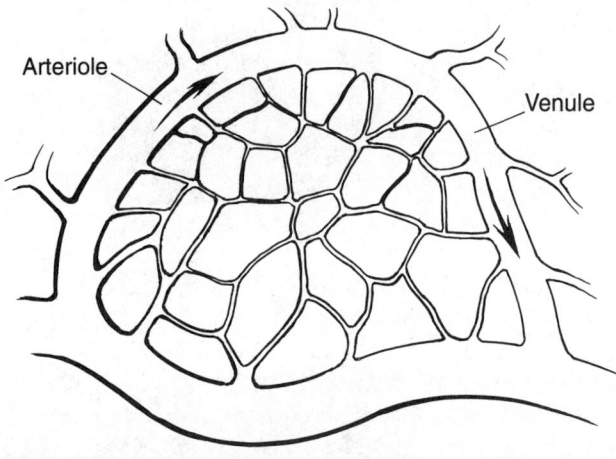

D

Fig. 9-4, cont'd. **C,** At the tip of vascular sprouts the basal lamina is defective and the endothelial cells undergo cell replication. **D,** After the individual new capillaries unite to form a capillary network (Top), some vessels differentiate into arterioles or venules while other capillaries become obliterated (Bottom).

vessels dilate within minutes of injury, and for a few hours leukocytes and platelets become conspicuous within the dilated vascular channels. PMLs migrate from the microvasculature into the adjacent tissue. The onset of these events, the nature of the cellular infiltrate, and the length of time that

precedes the neovascularization following injury varies with the experimental model.

The latent period between the initial angiogenic-provoking event and the appearance of new vessels varies considerably in different situations. In some settings, the vascular endothelial cells begin to migrate and proliferate within 24 hours; under other circumstances, the onset of neovascularization takes days or weeks. At least in the cornea, angiogenesis is delayed when the leukocytic infiltrate is retarded; whereas injuries that provoke a rapid and extensive invasion by leukocytes elicit an early and enhanced neovascularization.

Increased Vascular Permeability and Edema. Like inflammatory edema elsewhere, the edema within the corneal stroma that antecedes and accompanies the growth of blood vessels into the cornea is caused by an increased vascular permeability, rather than by a functionally impaired corneal endothelium. Stromal edema facilitates the growth of blood vessels into the cornea by separating the normally compact collagen fibers and thereby providing capillaries with space into which they can grow in planes of diminished resistance.[47]

The increased vascular permeability of inflammation occurs primarily between endothelial cells of postcapillary venules. It is mediated by numerous factors and can be counteracted by several autacoids (such as epinephrine, vasopressin, and cortisone) and drugs (such as $\beta 2$ receptor agonists, antihistaminics, glucocorticoids, and xanthines).[267]

Newly formed blood vessels within different tissues lack firm intercellular junctional complexes and are permeable to many molecules of variable size.[242] During the increased vascular permeability that accompanies inflammation and neovascularization, fibrinogen, fibronectin, and other plasma constituents enter the extracellular space. The edema continues while the invading new vessels remain permeable, and this situation persists until the newly formed vascular endothelial cells become united and develop a basal lamina with supporting cells.

Following extravasation of fibrinogen, the A and B fibrinopeptides become cleaved and produce fibrin monomers that polymerize and form cross-linked fibrin as tissue procoagulants interact with plasma-clotting factors.[64] For several reasons fibrin and products of its degradation are suspected of being important in angiogenesis: (1) fibrin deposition consistently precedes new-vessel growth in solid tumors and healing wounds,[64] (2) the invasion of tissue by blood vessels is enhanced by antifibrinolysins,[259] (3) fibrin degradation products induce angiogenesis in the CAM,[271] (4) when implanted subcutaneously, fibrin gels around tumors progressively vascularize[61-63,223] and induce an angiogenic response in the absence of tumor cells and platelets,[64] (5) vascular endothelial cells form a confluent monolayer on fibrin gels, but invade it following treatment with 4β-phorbol 12-myristate 13-acetate (PMA) in the absence of plasminogen or fibrinolytic inhibitors,[185] (6) fibrinogen is chemotactic for vascular endothelium,[57] (7) fibrinogen fragment E is not angiogenic in the CAM until cleaved with thrombin,[273] and (8) other lines of evidence support a role for the fibrinolytic system in angiogenesis.[296] The addition of plasminogen to a type 1 collagen gel matrix increases the length of endothelial cell tubes in culture, and inhibitors of plasmin suppress the enhancing effect of plasminogen.[296]

Endothelial Cell Activation with Retraction and Decreased Cell Junctions. As evidenced by DNA synthesis, the endothelium of the pericorneal vasculature can respond within 21 hours of corneal cauterization.[36,176] By 24 hours, these vascular endothelial cells and pericytes manifest morphologic features of activation (prominent nucleoli, abundant polyribosomes, plumper cells, and more prominent cytoplasmic organelles). The initial direct evidence of new vessel formation appears as enlargement of the nuclei and nucleoli of the vascular endothelium and the incorporation of H[3]-thymidine within the nuclei of these same cells.

Degradation of Endothelial Cell Basal Lamina. Because migrating and dividing endothelial cells penetrate through their basal lamina as well as through the surrounding connective tissue, proteases (such as plasminogen activator and collagenase) are suspected of contributing to new vessel formation. As new vessels form, the basal lamina surrounding the vascular endothelium becomes degraded, presumably by proteolytic enzymes derived from one or more potential sources (the growing vascular endothelium, PMLs, mononuclear phagocytes, mast cells, other tissue cells, microorganisms), which allows the endothelial cells to migrate into the extracellular matrix. Certain stimulators of angiogenesis, including phorbol esters[190] and basic fibroblast growth factor (bFGF), induce the synthesis and secretion of proteases by vascular endothelial cells.[114,115,186,192] Plasminogen activator has been implicated in localized extracellular proteolysis and in neovascularization.[18,105] Blood vessels grow into the cornea following the instillation of plasminogen activator and this reaction is accompanied by a leukocytic infiltration. Moreover, the reaction is diminished if the urokinase is inactivated by heat or an inhibitor.[18] Although the angiogenic activity of plasminogen activator may reflect proteolysis, this enzyme shares amino acid sequences with epidermal growth factor (EGF). Thrombin potentiates the FGF-stimulated growth response of cultured vascular endothelial cells.[108] Angiogenesis is induced by agents that stimulate plasminogen activators and suppressed by inhibitors of plasminogen activators.[293]

In the presence of fibrinolytic proteases, such as plasminogen, vascular endothelial cells may not invade a fibrin matrix.[185] Depending on their site of origin, cultured endothelial cells may or may not synthesize plasminogen activator and latent collagenase.

Vascular Sprouting

Endothelial Cell Migration and Replication. The assembly of new vessels depends on the simultaneously occurring, but independent, migration and mitoses of endothelial cells.

Vascular sprouting is not dependent on endothelial cell division in the silver nitrate cauterization model of corneal vascularization.[254] The tips of the growing new vessels extend toward the vascularized area, whereas mitoses occur in the more proximal cells on the capillary buds.[294,295] Migrating vascular endothelial cells form provisional lumens before they undergo cell division. The first buds appear shortly before vascular endothelial cells undergo cell division.[34] Following x-irradiation, injuries can still evoke endothelial cell migration and vascular sprouting despite the absence of cell division.[103,256]

Normal vascular endothelium has a turnover time of 2 months or longer. With certain injuries, morphologic alterations and the H[3]-thymidine incorporation occur within 24 hours.[36] Because the combined duration of the S and G_2 phases of the cell cycle in most cell types lasts about 10 to 12 hours, the first mitotic figures within endothelial cells should appear within 36 hours of injury, and indeed this occurs.

Pericytes also contribute to new vessel formation. They manifest prominent nucleoli and abundant polyribosomes and become labeled with H[3]-thymidine following injuries that elicit blood vessels.[36,176]

Vascular Sprouting, Lumen Formation, and Establishment of Anastomoses. In numerous situations vascular sprouts arise largely from postcapillary venules and preexisting capillaries and not from small arteries or arterioles. Because interstitial fluid normally drains into the venous side of the microcirculation, this may reflect a tendency of an angiogenic substance(s) to drain with the extracellular fluid. It is noteworthy, however, that in inflammatory angiogenesis, leukocytes emigrate predominantly from the postcapillary venules.[194] New blood vessels emerge and extend toward the site of the injury. In the cornea this occurs within 33 hours of injury by silver nitrate cauterization. A maze of proliferating channels set in a sea of inflammatory cells extend into the cornea. After blind vascular channels form, the newly created capillaries become linked to each other and establish a circulation.

Vascular Maturation

Formation of Basal Lamina Around Newly Formed Vessels. The endothelium of new-forming vessels lacks a continuous basal lamina and one or more layers of pericytes until the vessels secrete components of the extracellular matrix.[83] Laminin has been noted throughout the newly formed vessels, as well as in individual cells at the migrating, proliferating tips.[83] In contrast, type IV collagen correlates with lumen formation and is not detected at the vessel tips.

Phase of Capillary Regression and Vascular Maturation. As demonstrated experimentally, a persistent stimulus is required for the maintenance of newly formed blood vessels. For example, blood vessels grow into the cornea following the implantation of tumor cells, but they regress following tumor removal. Within a week of chemical cauterization, the vascular lattice simplifies as many newly formed channels apparently resorb, while other vessels enlarge and extend as loops to and from the site of injury. Except for theopaqueness caused by the vascularity, the cornea regains its clarity after the edema and inflammatory infiltrate resolve. Fluorescein angiography combined with transmission electron microscopy has disclosed that the surviving vessels that receive blood directly acquire attributes of arterioles, whereas draining vessels develop features of venules.[35] The vasculature about a healed corneal lesion becomes inconspicuous without blood flow (''ghost vessels''), but may become apparent again when vasodilation is induced—as with acute inflammation provoked by an additional new injury.

ANGIOGENIC FACTORS

The precise trigger of angiogenesis remains unknown, but diffusible factors probably initiate directional capillary growth in many normal and diseased tissues. Studies in a wide variety of biologic systems suggest that angiogenesis can arise by several mechanisms via different pathways. A century ago, Loeb[157] postulated that some trophic chemical might be responsible for vascularization in general, and soon thereafter Wiesner claimed that injured cells might liberate substances capable of stimulating cell proliferation. In 1907 Goldman[106] suggested that neoplasms produce an angiogenic agent, when he noted that neovascularization could be traced to regions in which the tumor had not yet advanced, and he stressed that ''the impetus which gives rise to the proliferation of blood vessels emanates from the invading cell.'' In 1968, using hamster cheek pouch chambers, Greenblatt and Shubik[113] provided convincing evidence that tumors produce a diffusible angiogenic factor. Since then, largely as a result of studies by Folkman and associates,* an increasing body of evidence has accumulated which supports the long-suspected view that locally generated factor(s) trigger angiogenesis. When a localized abnormality provokes neovascularization, the new blood vessels usually emerge from vessels nearest to the lesion. Newly formed capillaries extend toward and into vascularizing transplanted tissue in hamster cheek pouches, the chick chorioallantoic membrane (CAM), and other systems.[100,140,282,283] As first pointed out by Campbell and Michaelson[37] more than four decades ago, a localized injury elicits angiogenesis only if it is situated within a critical distance of the closest microvasculature. This fact suggests that a factor produced within the lesion diffuses centripetally—as its concentration diminishes—until it becomes ineffective beyond a critical distance from the point of injury. In the cornea, newly formed capillaries often extend into the tissue within an isosceles triangle having its base at the corneal periphery.[37]

Numerous oncogenes and growth factors influence the growth of many cell types, including the vascular endothelium.[127,187,250] Some growth factors stimulate protein phosphorylation.[27] Biologically active substances that influence

*References 11, 50, 76-81, 100, 128, 129, 268.

TABLE 9-1 SUBSTANCES IMPLICATED IN ANGIOGENESIS

Heprarin-binding Growth Factor

Heparin-binding growth factor-1
  (Acidic fibroblast growth factor, aFGF)[125,156,264,271]
Heparin-binding growth factor-2
  (Basic fibroblast growth factor, bFGF)*
Macrophage-derived growth factor (MDGF)
  (Probably identical to bFGF)[101,168]

Other Growth Factors

Angiogenin[26, 188, 290]
Endothelial cell-stimulating factor (ESAF)[141]
Epidermal growth factor (EGF)†
Human angiogenic factor (HAF)[92]
Platelet-derived endothelial cell growth factor (ENDO-GF, PD-ECGF)[130,137]
Platelet-derived growth factor (PDGF)[53,299]
Transforming growth factor α (TGF-α)[247]
Transforming growth factor TGF-β (TGF-β)‡
Vascular permeability factor (VPF)
  (Also called vascular endothelial growth factor, VEGF)§

Cytokines

Interleukin 1 (IL-1)[17,58,121,147]
Interleukin 1β (IL-1β)[56]
Interleukin 2 (IL-2)[70,117]
Interleukin 6 (IL-6)[193]
Interleukin 8 (IL-8)[102,142]
Angiotropin[124]
Tumor necrosis factor α (TNFα)[225,236,237,238,266]

Other Compounds

ATP[141]
Bradykinin[141]
Eicosanoids[15,155,215,300,302]
Fibrin[61-64,259,272]
Heparin|
Histamine[141,166,270]
Nicotinamide and a nicotinamide-containing complex[145]
Proteases[141]
Serotonin[141]

*References 30, 31, 33, 55, 73, 84, 88, 107, 192, 201, 218, 239, 300.
†References 38, 54, 99, 107,110, 170, 247, 277.
‡References 74, 86, 133, 219, 220, 284, 291.
§References 49, 131, 136, 152, 180, 191, 205, 249, 269, 276.
|References 2, 11, 14, 76, 79, 80, 85, 166, 174, 175, 215, 216.

the gene expression, migration, mitotic activity or other functions of vascular endothelial cells have been identified in normal plasma or serum, as well as in numerous normal and pathologic tissues† (Table 9-1) (Fig. 9-5). Some angiogenic factors activate enzymes like procollagenase.[288] Almost none of these putative angiogenic factors act solely and

†References 52a, 68, 93, 98, 141, 154, 160, 161, 196, 199, 209, 212, 234, 245.

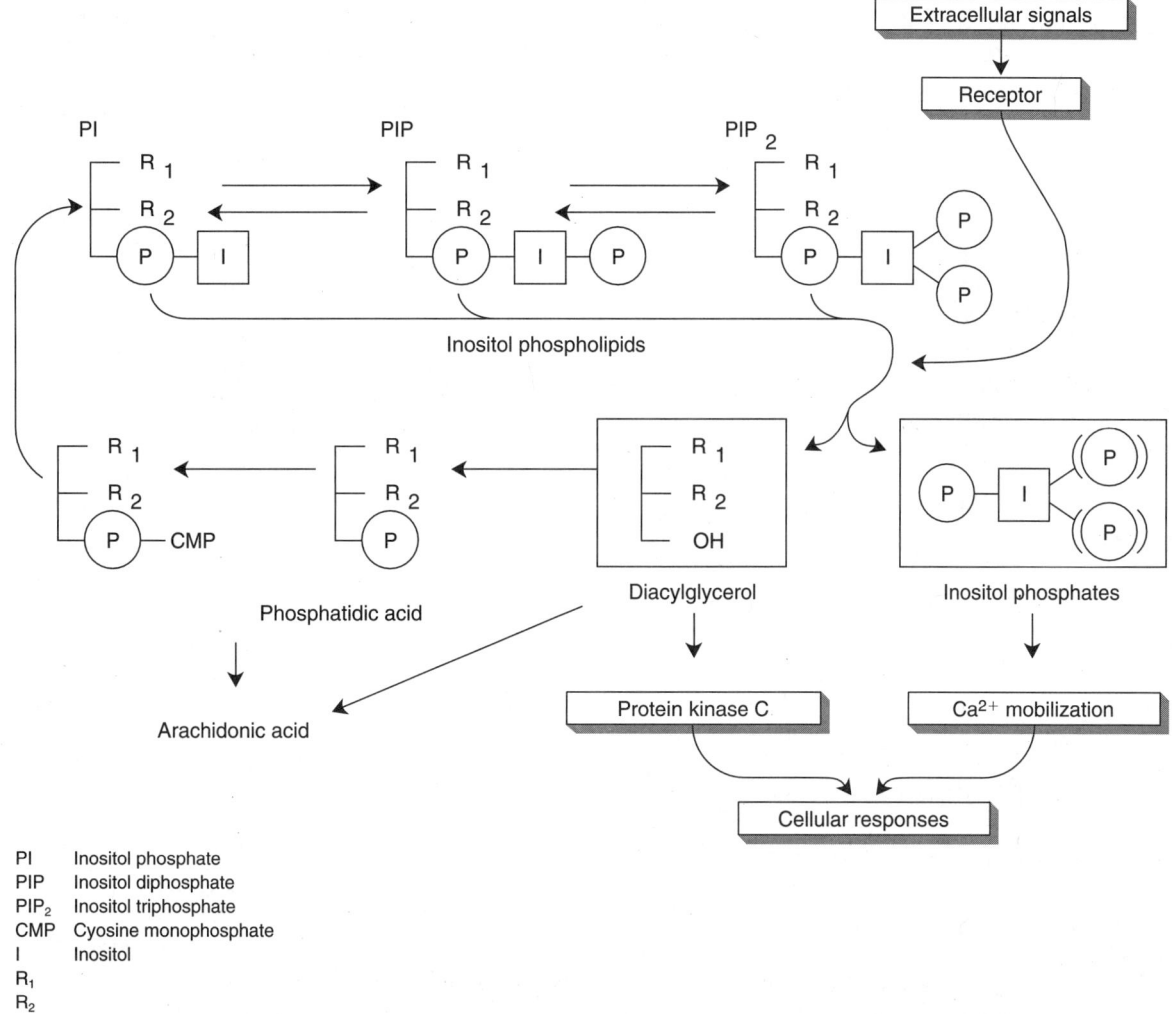

PI   Inositol phosphate
PIP   Inositol diphosphate
PIP$_2$ Inositol triphosphate
CMP   Cyosine monophosphate
I   Inositol
R$_1$
R$_2$

Fig. 9-5. Diagram depicting some of the presumed interactions between putative angiogenic factors and the vascular endothelium relationship between certain cells and the vascular endothelium. (Reproduced with permission from Klintworth GK: *Corneal angiogenesis: a comprehensive critical review,* New York, 1991, Springer Verlag).

specifically on vascular endothelium. Some factors, such as inteferon lymphotoxin and transforming growth factor β, inhibit certain endothelial cell functions.[32,195,279] Other aspects of wound healing may also be inhibited.[265]

ASSAYS FOR ANGIOGENESIS

A major difficulty in isolating angiogenic factors stems from the lack of a specific, sensitive assay system. Various viable and nonviable, normal and neoplastic cells and tissues, as well as specific substances, have been introduced into the cornea in an attempt to assay angiogenic activity. Reasons for using the cornea have included the misconceptions that the inflammation can be detected clinically and that the cornea is an immune-privileged site where the rejection of implanted materials is delayed.[303] Many materials elicit angiogenesis within the cornea, but the intracorneal instillation of most extraneous substances elicits a nonspecific, but variable, inflammatory reaction—especially when

foreign antigens are involved. Indeed, tissue surrounding an inoculum is usually infiltrated with leukocytes for at least several hours, regardless of the nature of the introduced material.

The study of Ryu and Albert[232] illustrates the difficulty of infering angiogenic activity to corneal implants. They found that the implantation of both viable and nonviable tumor cells into the cornea produces not only neovascularization, but also a nonspecific localized keratitis. They failed, however, to detect a significant difference between the corneas containing live or dead tumors. Moreover, in immunodeficient rabbits, the implanted tumors induced a negligible inflammatory cell infiltrate and negligible vascularization. Ryu and Albert[232] found that the vascular invasion of the cornea following tumor implantation was not modified by denaturation of the transplanted tumor by boiling or formalin fixation, both of which might be expected to inactivate a tumor angiogenic factor or to prevent its synthesis.

POTENTIAL SOURCES OF ANGIOGENIC FACTORS IN INFLAMMATION

Within the complex cellular and humoral events of the inflammatory response, many potential sources for molecules involved in the initiation and potentiation of angiogenesis exist: the denatured tissue, the injurious agent, local tissue cells, hematogenously derived cells, vascular cells, as well as plasma and other body fluids (Figs. 9-6 and 9-7).

Cellular Components of Inflammation

Much evidence supports the notion that leukocytes produce factors that stimulate directional vascular growth and several factors stimulate neutrophils or induce the release of the contents of their granules.[138,139,141,278] The events that precede and accompany inflammatory angiogenesis in diverse experimental models are essentially similar, and in almost all thoroughly studied models of corneal neovascularization, leukocytes have invaded the cornea before blood vessels.[141] Even though new vessels can apparently form in their absence, leukocytes augment the process.

As pointed out years ago by Carrel,[39,40] leukocytes and their extracts contain substances capable of stimulating the proliferation of cells. Several cell types are implicated in inflammatory angiogenesis (Table 9-2) and the relative importance of each cell type varies with the inducer of vascularization.

Polymorphonuclear Leukocytes (PMNs). PMLs, common companions of newly formed blood vessels in many tissues, enter the cornea prior to angiogenesis.[48,89] Interleukin-1 plays a role in the neutrophil emigration from blood vessels induced by some stimuli, such as endotoxin.[51] A direct relationship between the PMN infiltrate and the neovascular response has been noted in the rabbit cornea following thermal cautery.[240] Peripheral corneal burns elicit both a PMN infiltrate and neovascularization, whereas central burns evoke neither response.[240] Extracts of PMLs are weakly mitotic for endothelial cells.[233] Corticosteroids, as well as nonsteroidal antiinflammatory drugs (flurbiprofen and indomethacin), that suppress angiogenesis in the cornea inhibit the PML migration following corneal injury.[221]

A vast body of information emphasizes extracellular proteases in the regulation of mitogenesis in many cell types.[241] Proteases may (1) convert progrowth factors to active moieties, (2) act directly on cell surfaces thus causing transmembrane signals that lead to the stimulation of mitosis, and (3) by inducing the secretion of other proteases in a multicascade of proteolytic events. PLMs may promote angiogenesis via collagenase and other proteases[155] or by prostaglandins (PGs—especially PGE₁).[155]

Even if PMLs contribute to inflammatory angiogenesis, in some way this cell type is frequently present within pathologic tissue in the absence of associated neovascularization. For example, blood vessels do not grow into necrotic or

TABLE 9-2 CELLS IMPLICATED IN ANGIOGENESIS AND POSSIBLE MEDIATORS

Cellular Component	Possible Mediator
Lymphocyte	Cytokines
	Prostaglandins
Macrophage	Angiotropin
	(bFGF)MDGF
	Cytokines
	IL-I
	TNFα
	TNFβ
	HAF
	Prostaglandins
	Proteases
Mast cell	ATP
	Heparin
	Histamine (possibly via increased vascular permeability)
	Prostaglandins
	Proteases
	Serotonin (possibly via increased vascular permeability)
Platelet	ATP
	TGFα
	TGFβ[122]
	PD-ECGF
	PDGF
	Prostaglandins
	Serotonin (possibly via increased vascular permeability)
Polymorphonuclear leucocyte	Collagenase
	Other proteases
	Prostaglandins

suppurative tissue containing excessive PMNs, presumably because of the unfavorable tissue acidity and overabundance of extracellular proteolytic enzymes. Moreover, some investigators have been unable to induce angiogenesis by injecting PMLs into the cornea.[45,189,213] Besides, even if PMLs are not essential for the initiation of inflammatory angiogenesis, as in the cornea, the current consensus is that they play a facilitatory role.

Lymphocytes. Lymphocytes are known to interact with vascular endothelial cells.[211] An association between vascular proliferation and lymphoid cells has been recognized for decades[159,204,257] and much evidence implicates activated lymphocytes in angiogenesis in several tissues.[141] The intradermal transfer of immunocompetent lymphocytes induces endothelial cell proliferation.[258] The intracorneal implantation of homologous, but not autologous, adult lymph nodes[78] and allogeneic lymphocytes[71] induces corneal angiogenesis in the rabbit. Neovascularization has been induced in the

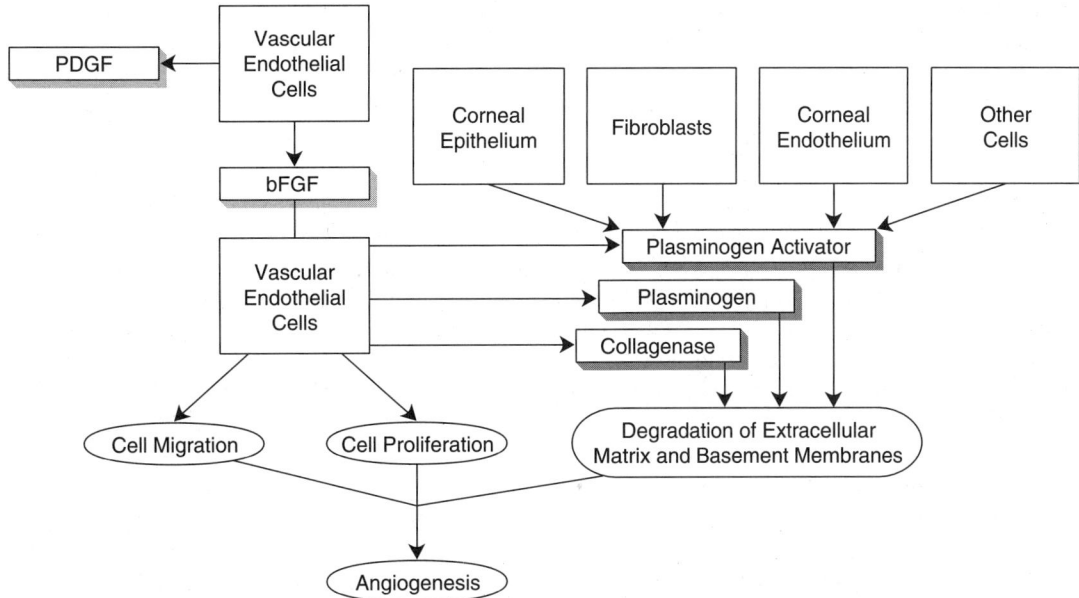

Fig. 9-6. Diagram of some factors contributing to inflammatory angiogenesis. (Modified from Klintworth GK: *Corneal angiogenesis: a comprehensive critical review,* New York, 1991, Springer Verlag).

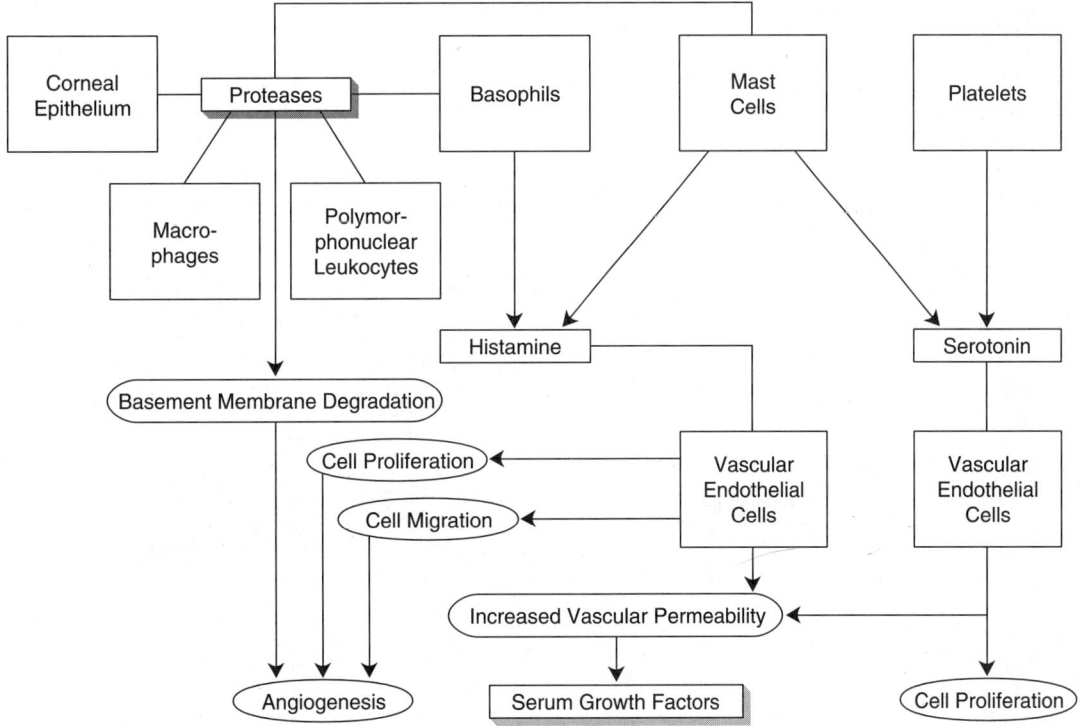

Fig. 9-7. Diagram depicting relationship between certain cells and the vascular endothelium. (Reproduced with permission from Klintworth GK: *Corneal angiogenesis: a comprehensive critical review,* New York, 1991, Springer Verlag).

mouse with corneal implants of whole lymph node fragments[197] and concanavalin A (con A)-stimulated allogeneic lymphocytes.[72] Moreover, lipopolysaccharide as well as con A-stimulated lymphocytes evoke vascular endothelial proliferation.[16]

Following stimulation by mitogens, lymphocytes secrete biologically active substances, including some implicated in angiogenesis: PGs[15,82] and cytokines.[9] Activated T cells may mediate new vessel formation by activating resident macrophages and by producing a proliferation-inducing endothelial cell lymphokine.[287] Interferon γ (IFNγ)—produced by activated T cells—may contribute to the induction of angiogenesis by increasing the release of superoxide by endothelial cells.[169]

Nevertheless, the belief that lymphocytes induce inflammatory angiogenesis remains controversial, as some investigators were unable to elicit new blood vessels by implanting normal and activated lymphocytes into corneas.[213]

Macrophages. Several observations suggest that activated macrophages play a role in angiogenesis: (1) endothelial proliferation occurs at the height of the delayed sensitivity reaction in the skin of guinea pigs, (2) macrophages may be the only inflammatory cells at a wound site capable of initiating new vessel formation, (3) intracorneal injections of activated macrophages, or conditioned medium derived from them, produce angiogenesis in a high percentage of animals, (4) stimulated macrophages produce a potent growth factor (macrophage-derived growth factor), (5) lactate has been found to cause macrophages to secrete angiogenic factors (6) the angiogenic activity of macrophage-conditioned media is enhanced following exposure of cultured macrophages to endotoxin, latex particles, viable microorganisms, or phorbol myristate acetate.[101,134,141,189,213]

Macrophages, however, are probably not essential for new vessel growth in nonimmunologic acute inflammation. Monocytes obtained from the citrated blood buffy coat of healthy adult human donors fail to stimulate angiogenesis in the rat cornea, whereas monocytes activated with con A or endotoxin are potently angiogenic.[143] Antigenically stimulated macrophages secrete increased amounts of mitogens,[104] but hypoxic macrophages do not.[134]

Macrophages could induce angiogenesis in several ways (Fig. 9-8). Activated macrophages produce several cytokines implicated in angiogenesis: IL-1,[181] FGF,[181] TNFα,[111] TNFβ,[7,87,150,208,220] MDGF,[101,149,168] angiotropin,[124] and human angiogenic factor (HAF)—a 67-kDa protein with a pI of 5.0 that does not have a marked affinity to heparin.[92] Macrophages release proteases,[198,217] which may contribute to new vessel formation because of their capability to induce mitogenesis and degrade the extracellular matrix.

Platelets. During the early hours of the inflammatory response, platelets are prominent in the dilated stagnant blood vessels, and they have been noted in the pericorneal vasculature prior to corneal angiogenesis.[176] These cellular elements aggregate and degranulate thus releasing numerous biologically active substances that stimulate DNA synthesis and migration in vascular endothelium.[46,137,158,285,286] These compounds, which may play a role in angiogenesis, include PGs, platelet-derived growth factor (PDGF), TGF-α, TGF-β, adenosine triphosphate (ATP), 5-hydroxytryptamine (serotonin), and platelet-derived endothelial growth factor (PD-ECGF, ENDO-GP). PAF is angiogenic

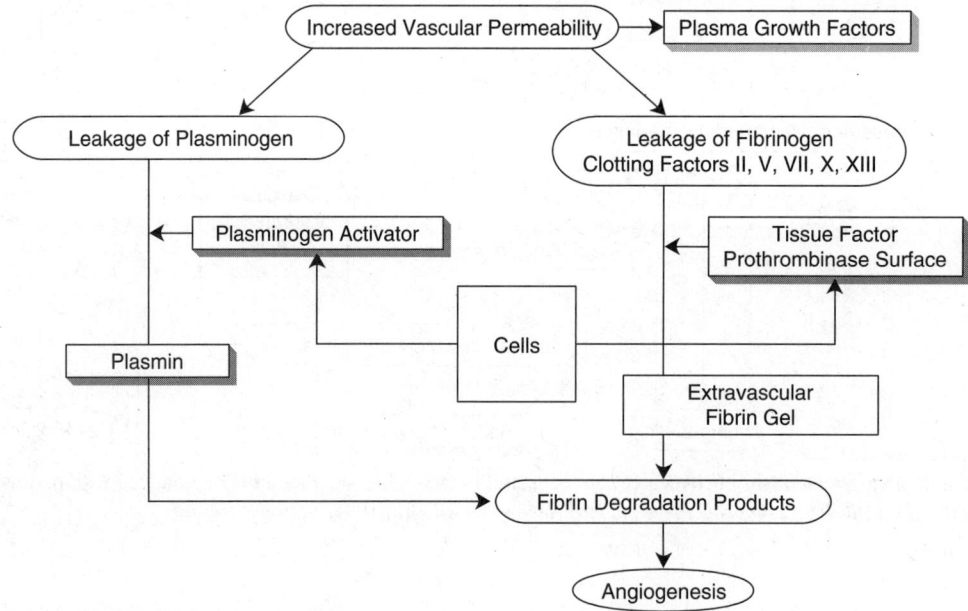

Fig. 9-8. Diagram depicting some effects of macrophages on vascular endothelial cells. (Reproduced with permission from Klintworth GK: *Corneal angiogenesis: a comprehensive critical review,* New York, 1991, Springer Verlag).

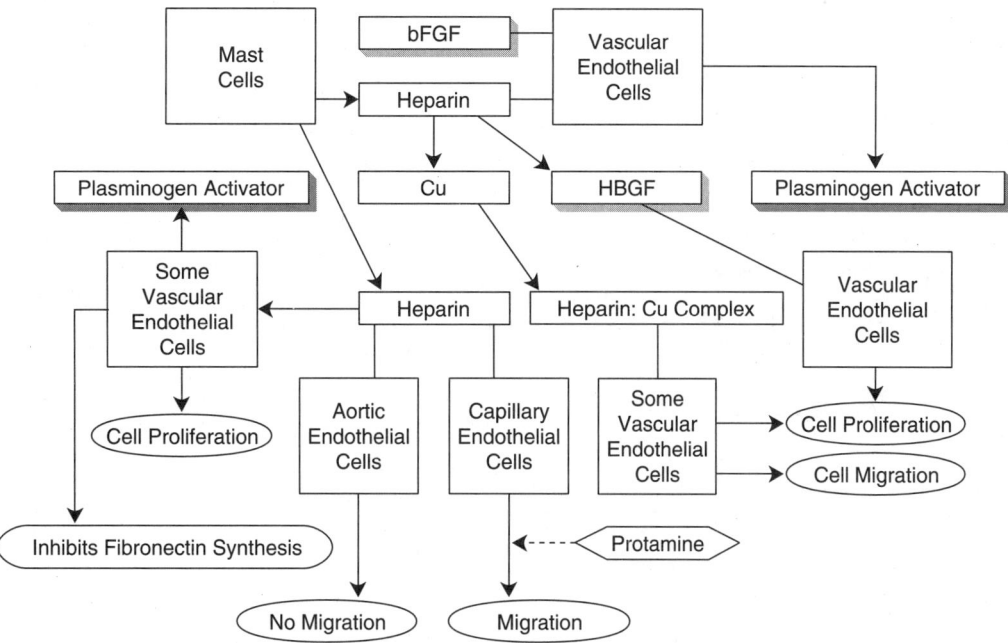

Fig. 9-9. Diagram depicting relationship between mast cells, heparin, and the vascular endothelium. (Reproduced with permission from Klintworth GK: *Corneal angiogenesis: a comprehensive critical review,* New York, 1991, Springer Verlag).

after tissue infiltration by fibrin and PMNs in some implants.*

Some components of the inflammatory reaction probably counteract the angiogenic stimulation of other factors, and the relative proportions of proangiogenic and antiangiogenic factors probably influence—not only the extent of the neovascularization—but the duration of the reaction. For example, IFNα and IFNβ inhibit the migration of vascular endothelial cells, and platelet factor-4 inhibits angiogenesis —in different systems. The latter inhibition is abrogated by heparin (for which it has a high affinity). Moreover, transforming growth factor β (TGFβ) either stimulates or inhibits cell growth, depending on the cell type and other growth factors present.[141,165]

Mast Cells. Mast cells have been implicated in angiogenesis (Fig. 9-9),[141,166,202,227,228] but they are not prominent in some situations with inflammatory angiogenesis and are not essential for new vessel formation (which can be elicited in mast cell-deficient mice).[10] Although heparin does not promote endothelial cell proliferation in certain systems,[11,42,268] it enhances the growth of some vascular endothelial cells. Heparin even potentiates the proliferative effect of aFGF on endothelial cells in culture[274] and protects some growth factors, such as FGF, from inactivation.[109] Relevant to the potential role of mast cells in angiogenesis is the avid binding of heparin to a family of growth factors with putative angiogenic activity (heparin-binding growth factor) (see Table

9-1). Mast cells not only release heparin but also heparin proteoglycans and other proteins and proteoglycans.[251] Heparin enhances the binding of endothelial cell growth factors to surface receptors on these vascular cells.[246]

Heparin and several nonanticoagulant fragments of it inhibit new-vessel growth induced by tumor in the CAM and cornea in the presence of cortisone or hydrocortisone,[79,81] or on the CAM by other corticosteroids.[50,128] Heparin with and without hydrocortisone slightly inhibits DNA synthesis and cell growth by murine cerebral endothelial cells.[14]

Humoral Aspects of Inflammation

Many biologically active substances, including eicosanoids, biogenic amines, plasminogen activator, and numerous cytokines, are liberated within the injured tissue during the inflammatory response. Furthermore, as a consequence of the increased vascular permeability of acute inflammation, constituents of plasma—such as fibrinogen, fibronectin, and a wide variety of growth factors (including mesodermal growth factor, insulin, PDGF, EGF, and FGFs) that are capable of enhancing the proliferation of vascular endothelium and other cell types—gain access to tissues (Fig. 9-10).

Biogenic Amines (Histamine, Bradykinin, and Acetylcholine). Histamine, a potent component of the inflammatory response and a constituent of mast cell granules, has long been suspected of being angiogenic. This biogenic amine is mitogenic to human microvascular and umbilical vein endothelial cells in culture.[37,141,166] Histamine may enhance angiogenesis through the resultant increased

---

*References 3, 8, 53, 130, 137, 141, 219, 226, 252, 200.

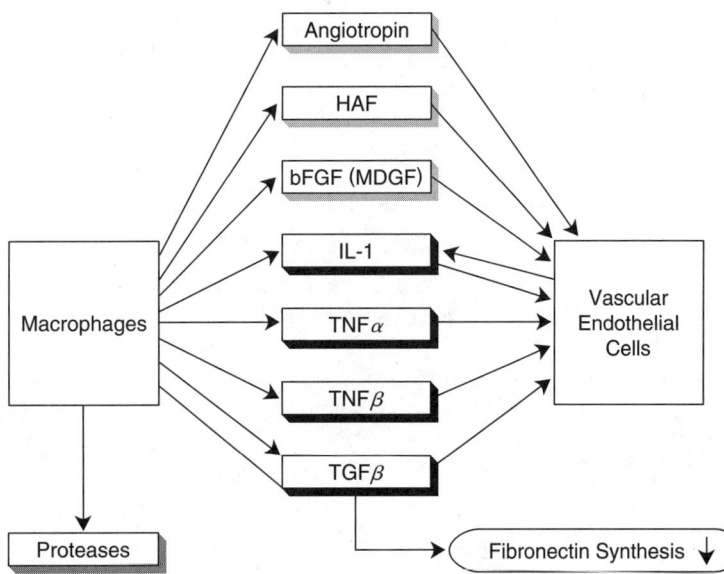

Fig. 9-10. Diagram depicting influence of increased vascular permeability on angiogenesis. (Reproduced with permission from Klintworth GK: *Corneal angiogenesis: a comprehensive critical review,* New York, 1991, Springer Verlag).

vascular permeability that it causes in the inflammatory response.

Eicosanoids. Soon after tissue injury, cellular phospholipids become degraded by phospholipases to liberate nonesterified fatty acids, including arachidonic acid. The latter is metabolized further both by the cyclooxygenase pathway to prostaglandins (PG), thromboxanes, and prostacyclin and by lipoxygenase pathways to produce hydroxyeicosatetraenoic acids (HETEs) and leukotrienes. Angiogenic activity has been attributed to PGs and notably PGE_1.[15,155,216,302] The theory that PGs participate in the cascade of events leading to angiogenesis finds support in several observations: (1) the intracorneal instillation of certain PGs (especially PGE_1) induces angiogenesis,[15,301] (2) an elevated PG concentration has been noted in the aqueous humor during corneal angiogenesis secondary to experimentally produced anterior uveal ischemia[178] and (3) corneal neovascularization is suppressed by inhibitors of PG synthesis.[141]

Most cells, including PMNs, activated lymphocytes,[15] macrophages,[126] and aggregated platelets,[252] synthesize PGs. The high content of leukocyte phospholipase provides inflamed tissue with an ample source of arachidonic acid for PG production.

Even if PGs contribute to angiogenesis, this effect may be mediated by leukocytes. These cellular elements not only synthesize PGs and chemotactic leukotrienes,[12,13] but PMLs are attracted chemotactically to metabolites of arachidonic acid.[1,123,144] Also, corneas that become markedly vascularized following implants that sequester PGE_1 are infiltrated by PMLs.[15] Corticosteroids and nonsteroidal antiinflammatory drugs that block PG synthesis suppress the leukocytic infiltrate, partly because certain PGs are chemotactic for PMLs.[1,123,144]

Another potential role of PGs in inflammatory angiogenesis involves their ability to mobilize copper ions, which

have been implicated in neovascularization.[2,171,216] Indeed, some investigators consider these ions necessary to induce new vessel formation in vivo and endothelial cell migration in vitro.[173,215] Prior to the onset of angiogenesis which follows the implantation of intracorneal pellets containing PGE_1, the corneal copper level increases and the tissue synthesizes several enzymes (including the copper-dependent benzylamine oxidase).[301] Moreover, a dietary deficiency of copper prevents PGE_1-induced corneal angiogenesis.[302] Several copper-containing molecules trigger angiogenesis and this property is lost when the copper is removed.[214,215] How copper is involved in angiogenesis remains unclear, but copper ions stimulate collagenase production by PMLs in a dose-dependent manner.[155]

The induction of newly formed capillaries by PGE_1 or bFGF is enhanced by the intracorneal instillation of gangliosides. An elevated ganglioside content has been found within the cornea prior to PGE_1-induced neovascularization.[300]

Leukotrienes and other metabolites of arachidonic acid may play a role in angiogenesis. HETEs (hydroxyeicosatetraenoic acids) and leukotriene D_4 (LTD_4) induce endothelial cell migration[174] and leukotriene C_4 (LTC_4) promotes endothelial cell growth in culture.[179] PMLs possess specific membrane receptors for leukotriene B_4 (LTB_4), which is a potent chemoattractant for PMNs;[25] however, the implantation of pellets with LTB_4 in the rabbit induces a marked leukocytic infiltration—but apparently without neovascularization.[222] In addition, 12-HETE is chemokinetic and chemotactic for PMLs.[25]

Vascular Endothelium

A potential source of the initiator of inflammatory angiogenesis is the endothelium of the microvasculature from which the new vessels arise.[248] Even sprouting endothelial cells may modulate themselves in an autocrine fashion by producing relevant factors. Following activation by a wide variety of inflammatory mediators, the vascular endothelium produces many biologically active proteins including tissue factor, fibronectin,[172] von Willebrand factor, inhibitors of fibrinolysis,[229] endothelial-leukocyte adhesion molecule 1 (ELAM-1), intercellular adhesion molecule 1 (ICAM-1) and 2 (ICAM-2), and vascular cell adhesion molecule 1 (VCAM-1). Integrins are involved in endothelial cell migration, proliferation, and new vessel formation[69] and numerous integrin subunits have been identified in vascular endothelial cells.

Adhesion molecules are involved in causing the adherence of PMLs, lymphocytes, or monocytes to the vascular endothelium.[2,22–24,210] bFGF and TGFβ upregulate the biosynthesis of certain integrins, including some that bind endothelial cells to matrix components involved in angiogenesis by vascular endothelium.[69] IL-1β and TNFα induce human vascular endothelial cells to synthesize and secrete a chemoattractant, which may contribute to the accumulation of monocytes at sites of inflammation.[224] Like mast cells, the vascular endothelium itself produces a biologically active heparinlike species.[41] The endothelium also self-regulates procoagulant events.[263] The changes in the endothelial cells include active participation in the increased microvascular permeability[230,231] and their loss following cytolysis.[275] During the inflammatory response, the vascular endothelium can be injured passively by microorganisms or leukocytes or actively to specific mediators such as bradykinin, cytokines (including IL-1), or thrombin.[229] Plasminogen binds to cultured endothelial cells and becomes a substrate for conversion to plasmin by tissue plasminogen activator.[116]

The activated endothelial cells of the microvasculature synthesize metalloproteinases and plasminogen activator. These proteases may digest the basal lamina that normally surround the microvasculature as well as the adjacent extracellular matrix during the endothelial migratory aspect of angiogenesis.[116,153] Endothelial cells not only express the bFGF gene, but produce bFGF in culture. FGF stimulates capillary endothelial cells to produce a urokinase type of plasminogen activator.[186] Vascular endothelial cells migrating from the edges of a wounded confluent monolayer of cells in culture produce an increased amount of plasminogen activator.[206] Bovine aortic endothelial cells secrete a platelet-derived protein growth factor.[141] Vascular endothelial cells synthesize several growth factors including bFGF, TGFβ, insulinlike growth factor 1, PDGF-AA, and PDGF-BB.[4,235]

Tissue Constituents

A variety of cell types other than leukocytes are suspected of producing angiogenic factors in various tissues;[141] but if normal tissue cells produce an angiogenic factor, they clearly do not liberate significant quantities of it until the cells are stimulated to liberate the factor. Within the cornea, the epithelium is a prime suspect for producing an angiogenic factor. Because blood vessels can grow into corneas devoid of an epithelium,[96,297] however, this cell layer is not essential for corneal neovascularization. Nevertheless, several observations suggest that a reactive epithelium may contribute to an angiogenic response: (1) corneal epithelial injury frequently coexists with an underlying stromal neovascularization, (2) heat stable homogenates of freshly excised or cultured normal corneal epithelial cells induce angiogenesis when infused into the cornea of rabbits[65-67], (3) corneal epithelial cells and medium from cultures of them stimulate the growth of cultured vascular endothelium in a dose-dependent manner[66], (4) the vascular endothelium in thermally injured skin has a higher labeling index beneath foci of incomplete reepithelialization compared to nonepithelialized injured sites[253], (5) an extract from skin epidermis incites angiogenesis in the hamster cheek pouch.[292]

Because the corneal epithelium synthesizes PGs and plasminogen activator,[141] mechanisms involved in inflammation may account for some observations that implicate these cells in angiogenesis. Moreover, corneas perfused with an epithelial homogenate induce a dense leukocytic infiltrate (mononuclear leukocytes and PMLs) within the corneal stroma.[66] If an angiogenic factor arises in damaged tissue from local constituents, it could be anticipated that a particular injury would consistently provoke vascularization; but similarly treated corneal tissue that is implanted into hamster cheek pouches does not evoke angiogenesis reproducibly.[140]

Extracellular Matrix

The extracellular matrix influences gene expression and may play a cardinal role in the formation of new blood vessels by binding to specific receptors on the cell surface of vascular endothelial cells. A functional relationship between the vascular endothelium, extracellular matrix, and certain growth factors seems to exist.[163] Capillary endothelial cells proliferate in response to certain putative angiogenic factors, such as EGF, only if they are plated on fibronectin or on native collagen.[170] Collagenous components of the extracellular matrix influence the ability of endothelial cells to form capillarylike tubular structures.[164,182-184,186] The proliferative capability and biosynthetic activity of microvascular endothelial cells in culture is also influenced by components of the matrix.[129,243,244] The proliferation of vascular endothelial cells is significantly greater on laminin than on either plasma fibronectin, interstitial collagen types I and III, or basement membrane collagen type IV.[83]

Fibronectin or fragments of it are chemotactic for endothelial cells[29] and blood monocytes.[203] Some cells, such as monocytes, bear membrane receptors for surface-bound fibronectin[21] and these may stimulate macrophages to generate products, such as MDGF, plasminogen activator, and elastase.[140,167] Fibronectin enhances endothelial cell migration in cell culture and heparin enhances this effect.[280] Moreover, fibronectin antiserum blocks the migration of the endothelial cells and neutralization of the antiserum restores the mobilization.[280]

Products of Injurious Agents. Some noxious agents, such as bacteria, may possess angiogenic activity and induce inflammatory angiogenesis by themselves. A bacterial product of *Bartonella bacilliformis* stimulates vascular proliferation as well as an increased production of tissue plasminogen activity in vascular endothelial cells in vitro. The organism also stimulates the formation of new blood vessels in subcutaneous wounds.[94]

PROGNOSIS

Inhibition of Angiogenesis

Corneal and other forms of inflammatory angiogenesis are inhibited by corticosteroids, non-steroidal antiinflammatory drugs and irradiation. Numerous other inhibitors of angiogenesis have been, and continue to be, developed. These include angiostatic steroids, thrombospondin, angioinhibins, thalidomide and related analogues.[25a,52,213a]

Future Developments

A vast body of information has been accumulated about the various cellular and humoral elements within the inflammatory response that participate in inflammatory angiogenesis, but a considerable hiatus remains in our knowledge about the relative importance of these components. Innocent bystanders have not all been definitely distinguished from active participants in angiogenesis. Some involved elements may initiate, or be components of, relevant cascades that culminate in neovascularization. We hope future studies on inflammatory angiogenesis will lead to a clearer understanding of the factors and their relative contributions that are involved in different pathologic states.

REFERENCES

1. Adams SS, Burrows CA, Skeldon N, Yates DB: Inhibition of prostaglandin synthesis and leukocyte migration by flurbiprofen, *Curr Med Res Opin* 5:11-16, 1977.
2. Alessandri G, Raju K, Gullino PM: Mobilization of capillary endothelium in vitro induced by effectors of angiogenesis in vivo, *Cancer Res* 43:1790-1797, 1983.
3. Andrade SP, Vieira LBGB, Bakhle YS, Piper PJ: Effects of platelet activating factor (PAF) and other vasoconstrictors on a model of angiogenesis in the mouse, *Int J Exp Pathol* 73:503-513, 1992.
4. Antonelli-Orlidge A, Saunders KB, Smith SF, D'Amore PA: An activated form of transforming growth factor β is produced by cocultures of endothelial cells and pericytes, *Proc Natl Acad Sci USA* 86:4544-4548, 1989.
5. Ashino-Fuse H, Takano Y, Oikawa T et al.: Medroxyprogesterone acetate, an anti-cancer and anti-angiogenic steroid, inhibits the plasminogen activator in bovine endothelial cells, *Int J Cancer* 44:859-864, 1989.
6. Ashton N: Pathogenesis and aetiology of Eales's disease. In *XIX Congress of Ophthalmology*, 828-840, New Delhi, 1962, YKC Pandit, Bombay.
7. Assoian RK, Fleurdelys BE, Stevenson HC et al.: Expression and secretion of type transforming growth factor by activated human macrophages, *Proc Natl Acad Sci USA* 84:6020-6024, 1987.
8. Assoian RK, Komoriya A, Meyers CA et al.: Transforming growth factor-β in human platelets, *J Biol Chem* 258:7155-7160, 1983.
9. Auerbach R: Angiogenesis-inducing factors: a review. In Pick E, Landy M, editors: *Lymphokines: a forum for immunoregulatory cell products,* vol 4, 69-88, New York, 1981, Academic Press.
10. Auerbach R: Discussion of Fraser RA, Simpson JG: Role of mast cells in experimental tumour angiogenesis. In Nugent J, O'Connor M, editors: *Development of the vascular system,* 120-131, Ciba Foundation Symposium 100, London, 1983, Pitman Books.
11. Azizkhan RG, Azizkhan JC, Zetter BR, Folkman J: Mast cell heparin stimulates migration of capillary endothelial cells in vitro, *J Exp Med* 152:931-944, 1980.
12. Bazan HEP, Birkle DL, Beuerman RW, Bazan NG: Cryogenic lesion alters the metabolism of arachidonic acid in rabbit cornea layers, *Invest Ophthalmol Vis Sci* 26:474-480, 1985.
13. Bazan HEP, Birkle DL, Beuerman RW, Bazan NG: Inflammation induced stimulation of the synthesis of prostaglandins and lipoxygenase reaction products in rabbit cornea, *Curr Eye Res* 4:175-179, 1985.
14. Beck DW, Olson JJ, Linhardt RJ: Effect of heparin, heparin fragments, and corticosteroids on cerebral endothelial cell growth in vitro and in vivo, *J Neuropathol Exp Neurol* 45:503-512, 1986.
15. BenEzra D: Neovasculogenic ability of prostaglandins, growth factors, and synthetic chemoattractants, *Am J Ophthalmol* 86:455-461, 1978.
16. BenEzra D, Gery I: Stimulation of keratocyte metabolism by products of lymphoid cells, *Invest Ophthalmol Vis Sci* 18:317-320, 1979.
17. BenEzra D, Hemo I, Maftzir G: In vivo angiogenic activity of interleukins, *Arch Ophthalmol* 108:573-576, 1990.
18. Berman M, Winthrop S, Ausprunk D et al.: Plasminogen activator (urokinase) causes vascularization of the cornea, *Invest Ophthalmol Vis Sci* 22:191-199, 1982.
19. Besedovsky H, del Rey A, Sorkin E, Dinarello CA: Immunoregulatory feedback between interleukin-1 and glucocorticoid hormones, *Science* 233:652-654, 1986.
20. Beutler B, Krochin N, Milsark IW et al.: Control of cachectin (tumor necrosis factor) synthesis: mechanisms of endotoxin resistance, *Science* 232:977-980, 1986.
21. Bevilacqua MP, Amrani D, Mosesson MW, Bianco C: Receptors for cold-insoluble globulin (plasma fibronectin) on human monocytes, *J Exp Med* 153:42-60, 1981.
22. Bevilacqua MP, Pober JS, Wheeler ME et al.: Interleukin-I acts on cultured human vascular endothelium to increase the adhesion of polymorphonuclear leukocytes, monocytes and related leukocyte cell lines, *J Clin Invest* 76:2003-2011, 1985.
23. Bevilacqua MP, Pober JS, Wheeler ME et al.: Interleukin-I activation of vascular endothelium: effects on procoagulant activity and leukocyte adhesion, *Am J Pathol* 121:394-403, 1985.
24. Bevilacqua MP, Stengelin S, Gimbrone MA Jr, Seed B: Endothelial leukocyte adhesion molecule 1: an inducible receptor for neutrophils related to complement regulatory proteins and lectins, *Science* 243:1160-1165, 1989.
25. Bhattacherjee P, Eakins KE: Lipoxygenase products: mediation of inflammatory responses and inhibition of their formation. In Charkin LW, Belley DM, editors: *Leukotrienes chemistry and biology,* 195-214, London, 1984, Academic Press.
25a. Bicknell R: Vascular targeting and the inhibition of angiogenesis. *Ann Oncol* 5(suppl 4):s45-s50, 1994.
26. Bicknell R, Vallee BL: Angiogenin activates endothelial cell phospholipase C, *Proc Natl Acad Sci USA* 85:5961-5965, 1988.
27. Blackshear PJ, Witters LA, Girard PR et al.: Growth factor-stimulated protein phosphorylation in 3T3-L1 cells, *J Biol Chem* 260:13304-13315, 1985.
28. Boggs DR, Athens JW, Cartwright GE, Wintrobe MM: The effects of adrenal glucocorticosteroids upon the cellular composition of inflammatory exudates, *Am J Pathol* 44:763-773, 1964.
29. Bowersox JC, Sorgente N: Chemotaxis of aortic endothelial cells in response to fibronectin, *Cancer Res* 42:2547-2551, 1982.

30. Broadley KN, Aquino AM, Hicks B et al.: The diabetic rat as an impaired wound healing: stimulatory effects of transforming growth factor beta and basic fibroblast factor, *Biotechnol Ther* 1:55-68, 1989.

31. Broadley KN, Aquino AM, Woodward SC et al.: Monospecific antibodies implicate basic fibroblast growth factor in normal wound repair, *Lab Invest* 6:571-575, 1989.

32. Brouty-Boye D, Zetter BR: Inhibition of cell motility by interferon, *Science* 208:516-518, 1980.

33. Buckley-Sturrock A, Woodward SC, Senior RM et al.: Differential stimulation of collagenase and chemotactic activity in fibroblasts derived from rat wound repair tissue and human skin by growth factors, *J Cell Physiol* 138:70-78, 1989.

34. Burger PC, Chandler DB, Klintworth GK: Corneal neovascularization as studied by scanning electron microscopy of vascular casts, *Lab Invest* 48:169-180, 1983.

35. Burger PC, Chandler DB, Klintworth GK: Experimental corneal neovascularization: biomicroscopic, angiographic, and morphologic correlation, *Cornea* 4:35-41, 1985.

36. Burger PC, Klintworth GK: Autoradiographic study of corneal neovascularization induced by chemical cautery, *Lab Invest* 45:328-335, 1981.

37. Campbell FW, Michaelson IC: Blood vessel formation in the cornea, *Br J Ophthalmol* 33:248-255, 1949.

38. Carpenter G, Cohen S: Epidermal growth factors, *Annu Rev Biochem* 48:193-216, 1979.

39. Carrel A: Growth-promoting function of leucocytes, *J Exp Med* 36:385-391, 1922.

40. Carrel A, Ebeling H-H: Trephones embryonnaires, *C R Soc Biol* 89:1142-1144, 1923.

41. Castellot JJ Jr, Addonizio ML, Rosenberg RD, Karnovsky MJ: Cultured endothelial cells produce a heparin-like inhibitor of smooth muscle cell growth, *J Cell Biol* 90:372-379, 1981.

42. Castellot JJ Jr, Kambe AM, Dobson DE, Spiegelman BM: Heparin potentiation of 3T3-adipocyte stimulated angiogenesis: mechanisms of action on endothelial cells, *J Cell Physiol* 127:323-329, 1986.

43. Chang C-T, Chen Y-L, Lee S-H et al.: The inhibition of prostaglandin E$_1$-induced corneal neovascularization by steroid eye drops, *J Formos Med Assoc* 88:707-711, 1989.

44. Claman HN: Corticosteroids and lymphoid cells, *New Eng J Med* 287:388-397, 1972.

45. Clark RA, Stone RD, Leung DYK et al.: Role of macrophages in wound healing, *Surg Forum* 27:16-18, 1976.

46. Clemmons DR, Isley WL, Brown MT: Dialyzable factor in human serum of platelet origin stimulates endothelial cell replication and growth, *Proc Natl Acad Sci USA* 80:1641-1645, 1983.

47. Cogan DG: Vascularization of the cornea: its experimental induction by small lesions and a new theory of its pathogenesis, *Arch Ophthalmol* 41:406-416, 1949.

48. Collin HB: Limbal vascular response prior to corneal vascularization, *Exp Eye Res* 16:443-455, 1973.

49. Connolly DT, Heuvelman DM, Nelson R et al.: Tumor vascular permeability factor stimulates endothelial cell growth and angiogenesis, *J Clin Invest* 84:1470-1478, 1989.

50. Crum R, Szabo S, Folkman J: A new class of corticosteroids inhibits angiogenesis in the presence of heparin or a heparin fragment, *Science* 230:1375-1378, 1985.

51. Cybulsky MI, Colditz IG, Movat HZ: The role of interleukin-I in neutrophil leukocyte emigration induced by endotoxin, *Am J Pathol* 124:367-372, 1986.

52. D'Amato RJ, Loughnan MS, Flynn E, Folkman J: Thalidomide is an inhibitor of angiogenesis. *Proc Natl Acad Sci USA* 91:4082-4085, 1994.

52a. D'Amore PA, Glaser BM, Brunson SK, Fenselau AH: Angiogenic activity from bovine retina: partial purification and characterization, *Proc Natl Acad Sci USA* 78:3068-3072, 1981

53. D'Amore PA, Shepro D: Stimulation of growth and calcium influx in cultured, bovine, aortic endothelial cells by platelets and vasoactive substances, *J Cell Physiol* 92:177-184, 1977.

54. Davidson J, Buckley A, Woodward S et al.: Mechanisms of accelerated wound repair using epidermal growth factor and basic fibroblast growth factor. In Barbul A, Pineo E, Caldwell M, Hunt TK, editors: *Growth factors and other aspects of wound healing: biological and clinical implications,* 63-75, New York, 1988, Alan R Liss.

55. Daviet I, Herbert JM, Maffrand JP: Involvement of protein kinase C in the mitogenic and chemotaxis effects of basic fibroblast growth factor on bovine cerebral cortex capillary endothelial cells, *FEBS Lett* 259:315-317, 1990.

56. Day S, DuPlessie M, Klintworth GK: In vivo quantification of corneal angiogenesis induced by recombinant interleukin-1 beta, *Invest Ophthalmol Vis Sci* 34(suppl):998, 1993.

57. Dejana E, Languino LR, Polentarutti N et al.: Interaction between fibrinogen and cultured endothelial cells: induction of migration and specific binding, *J Clin Invest* 75:11-18, 1985.

58. Dinarello CA: Interleukin-1 and its biologically related cytokines, *Adv Immunol* 44:153-205, 1989.

59. Doxanas MT, Kelley JS, Prout TE: Sarcoidosis with neovascularization of the optic nerve head, *Am J Ophthalmol* 103:1143-1149, 1985.

60. Duffin RM, Weissman BA, Glasser DB, Pettit TH: Flurbiprofen in the treatment of corneal neovascularization induced by contact lenses, *Am J Ophthalmol* 93:607-614, 1982.

61. Dvorak HF: Tumors—wounds that do not heal similarities between tumor stroma generation and wounding healing, *New Eng J Med* 315:1650-1659, 1986.

62. Dvorak HF, Dvorak AM, Manseau EJ et al.: Fibrin-gel investment associated with line 1 and line 10 solid tumor growth, angiogenesis, and fibroplasia in guinea pigs: role of cellular immunity, myofibroblasts, microvascular damage, and infarction in line 1 tumor regression, *J Natl Cancer Inst* 62:1459-1472, 1979.

63. Dvorak HF, Form DM, Manseau EJ, Smith BD: Pathogenesis of desmoplasia. I. Immunofluorescence identification and localization of some structural proteins of line 1 and line 10 guinea pig tumors and of healing wounds, *J Natl Cancer Instit* 73:1195-1205, 1984.

64. Dvorak HF, Harvey VS, Estrella P et al.: Fibrin containing gels induce angiogenesis: implications for tumor stroma generation and wound healing, *Lab Invest* 57:673-686, 1987.

65. Eliason JA: Leukocytes and experimental corneal vascularization, *Invest Ophthalmol Vis Sci* 17:1087-1095, 1978.

66. Eliason JA: Angiogenic activity of the corneal epithelium, *Exp Eye Res* 41:721-732, 1985.

67. Eliason JA, Maurice DM: Angiogenesis by the corneal epithelium, *Invest Ophthalmol Vis Sci* 17(suppl):141, 1978.

68. Elstow SF, Schor AM, Weiss JB: Bovine retinal angiogenesis factor is a small molecule (molecular mass < 600), *Invest Ophthalmol Vis Sci* 26:74-79, 1985.

69. Enenstein J, Waleh NS, Kramer RH: Basic FGF and TGF-β differentially modulate integrin expression of human microvascular endothelial cells, *Exp Cell Res* 203:499-503, 1992.

70. Epstein RJ, Hendricks RL, Stulting RD: Interleukin-2 induces corneal neovascularization in A/J mice, *Cornea* 9:318-323, 1990.

71. Epstein RJ, Hughes WF: Lymphocyte-induced corneal neovascularization: a morphologic assessment, *Invest Ophthalmol Vis Sci* 21:87-94, 1981.

72. Epstein RJ, Stulting RD: Corneal neovascularization induced by stimulated lymphocytes in inbred mice, *Invest Ophthalmol Vis Sci* 28:1505-1513, 1987.

73. Esch P, Baird A, Ling N et al.: Primary structure of bovine pituitary basic fibroblast growth factor (FGF) and comparison with the amino-terminal sequence of bovine brain acidic FGF, *Proc Natl Acad Sci USA* 82:6507-6511, 1985.

74. Fiegel VD, Knighton DR: Transforming growth factor-β (TGFβ) causes indirect angiogenesis by recruiting monocytes, *Fed Proc* 2:A1601, 1988.

75. Flower RJ, Blackwell GJ: Anti-inflammatory steroids induce biosynthesis of a phospholipase A$_2$ inhibitors which prevents prostaglandin generation, *Nature* 278:456-459, 1979.

76. Folkman J: Angiogenesis: initiation and control, *Ann NY Acad Sci* 401:212-227, 1982.

77. Folkman J, Brem H: Angiogenesis and inflammation. In Gallin JI, Goldstein M, Snyderman R, editors: *Inflammation: basic principles and clinical correlates,* ed 2, 821-839, New York, 1992, Raven Press.

78. Folkman J, Cotran R: Relation of capillary proliferation to tumour growth, *Int Rev Exp Pathol* 16:207-248, 1976.

79. Folkman J, Langer R, Linhardt RJ et al.: Angiogenesis inhibition and tumor regression caused by heparin or a heparin fragment in the presence of cortisone, *Science* 221:719-725, 1983.

80. Folkman J, Taylor S, Spillberg C: The role of heparin in angiogenesis. In *Development of the vascular system,* Ciba Foundation Symposium 100, London, 1983, Pitman Rooks.

81. Folkman J, Weisz PB, Joullie MM et al.: Control of angiogenesis with synthetic heparin substitutes, *Science* 243:1490-1493, 1989.

82. Form DM, Auerbach R: PGE_2 and angiogenesis, *Proc Soc Exp Biol* 172:214-218, 1983.

83. Form DM, Pratt BM, Madri JA: Endothelial cell proliferation during angiogenesis: in vitro modulation by basement membrane components, *Lab Invest* 55:521-530, 1986.

84. Fox GM: The role of growth factors in tissue repair. III. Fibroblast growth factor. In Clark RAF, Henson PM, editors: *The molecular and cellular biology of wound repair,* New York, 1988, Plenum.

85. Fraser RA, Ellis M, Stalker AL: Experimental angiogenesis in the chorioallantoic membrane. In Lewis DH, editor: *Current advances in basic and clinical microcirculatory research,* 25-26, Basel, Switzerland, 1979, Karger.

86. Frater-Schröder M, Müller G, Birchmeier W, Böhlen R: Transforming growth factor-β inhibits endothelial cell proliferation, *Biochem Biophys Res Commun* 137:295-302, 1986.

87. Frater-Schröder M, Risau W, Hallmann R et al.: Tumor necrosis factor type α, a potent inhibitor of endothelial cell growth in vitro, is angiogenic in vivo, *Proc Natl Acad Sci USA* 84:5277-5281, 1987.

88. Freisel R, Burgess WH, Mehlman T, Maciag T: The characterization of the receptor for endothelial cell growth by covalent ligand attachment, *J Biol Chem* 261:7581-7584, 1986.

89. Fromer CH, Klintworth GK: An evaluation of the role of leukocytes in the pathogenesis of experimentally induced corneal vascularization. I. Comparison of experimental models of corneal vascularization, *Am J Pathol* 79:537-554, 1975.

90. Fromer CH, Klintworth GK: An evaluation of the role of leukocytes in the pathogenesis of experimentally induced corneal vascularization. II. Studies on the effect of leukocyte elimination on corneal vascularization, *Am J Pathol* 81:531-544, 1975.

91. Fromer CH, Klintworth GK: An evaluation of the role of leukocytes in the pathogenesis of experimentally induced corneal vascularization. III. Studies related to the vasoproliferative capability of polymorphonuclear leukocytes and lymphocytes, *Am J Pathol* 82:157-167, 1976.

92. Frühbeis B, Zwadlo G, Brocker E-B et al.: Immunolocalization of an angiogenic factor (HAF) in normal, inflammatory and tumor tissues, *Int J Cancer* 42:207-212, 1988.

93. Gamble JR, Harlan JH, Klebanoff SJ, Vadas MA: Stimulation of the adherence of neutrophils to umbilical vein endothelium by human recombinant tumor necrosis factor, *Proc Natl Acad Sci USA* 82:8667-8671, 1985.

94. Garcia FU, Wojta J, Broadley KN et al.: Bartonella bacilliformis stimulates endothelial cells in vitro and is angiogenic in vivo, *Am J Pathol* 136:1125-1135, 1990.

95. Garner A: Ocular angiogenesis, *Int Rev Exp Pathol* 28:249-306, 1986.

96. Gasset AR, Dohlman CH: The tensile strength of corneal wounds, *Arch Ophthalmol* 79:595-602, 1968.

97. Gaynon MW, Boldrey EE, Strahlman ER, Fine SL: Retinal neovascularization and ocular toxoplasmosis, *Am J Ophthalmol* 98:585-589, 1968.

98. Gerritsen ME, Bloor CM: Endothelial cell gene expression in response to injury, *FASEB J* 7:523-532, 1993.

99. Gill GN, Bertics PJ, Santon JB: Epidermal growth factor and its receptor, *Mol Cell Endocrinol* 53:169-186, 1987.

100. Gimbrone MA Jr, Cotran RS, Leapman SB, Folkman J: Tumor growth and neovascularization: an experimental model using the rabbit cornea, *J Natl Cancer Inst* 52:413-427, 1974.

101. Gimbrone MA Jr, Martin BM, Baldwin WM et al.: Stimulation of vascular cell growth by macrophage products. In Nossel HL, Vogel HJ, editors: *Pathobiology of the endothelial cell,* 3-17, New York, 1982, Academic Press.

102. Gimbrone MA Jr, Orbin MS, Brock AF et al.: Endothelial interleukin-8: a novel inhibitor of leukocyte-endothelial interactions, *Science* 246:1601-1603, 1989.

103. Glatt HJ, Klintworth GK: Corneal vascularization in irradiated inbred mice reconstituted with bone marrow, *Invest Ophthalmol Vis Sci* 25(suppl):67, 1984.

104. Glenn KC, Ross R: Human monocyte-derived growth factor(s) for mesenchymal cells: activation of secretion by endotoxin and concanavalin A, *Cell* 25:603-615, 1981.

105. Goldfarb RH: Proteases in tumor invasion and metastasis. In Liotta LA, Hart LR, editors: *Tumor cell invasion and metastasis,* 375-390, The Hague, 1982, Martinus Nijhoff.

106. Goldman E: The growth of malignant disease in man and the lower animals, with special reference to the vascular system, *Proc R Soc Med* 1(Surgical section):1-13, 1907.

107. Gospodarowicz D, Bialecki H, Thakral TK: The angiogenic activity of the fibroblast and epidermal growth factor, *Exp Eye Res* 28:501-514, 1979.

108. Gospodarowicz D, Brown KD, Birdwell CR, Zetter BR: Control of proliferation of human vascular endothelial cells: characterization of the response of human umbilical vein endothelial cells to fibroblast growth factor, epidermal growth factor, and thrombin, *J Cell Biol* 77:774-778, 1978.

109. Gospodarowicz D, Cheng J: Heparin protects basic and acidic FGF from inactivation, *J Cell Physiol* 128:475-484, 1986.

110. Gospodarowicz D, Mescher AL, Birdwell CR: Stimulation of corneal endothelial cell proliferation in vitro by fibroblast and epidermal growth factors, *Exp Eye Res* 25:75-89, 1977.

111. Gospodarowicz D, Neufeld G, Schweigerer L: Molecular and biological characterization of fibroblast growth factor, an angiogenic factor which also controls the proliferation and differentiation of mesoderm and neuroectoderm derived cells, *Cell Diff* 19:1-17, 1986.

112. Graham EM, Stanford MR, Shilling JS, Sanders MD: Neovascularisation associated with posterior uveitis, *Br J Ophthalmol* 71:826-833, 1987.

113. Greenblatt M, Shubik P: Tumor angiogenesis: transfilter diffusion studies in the hamster by transparent chamber techniques, *J Natl Cancer Inst* 41:111-124, 1968.

114. Gross JL, Moscatelli D, Jaffe EA, Rifkin DB: Plasminogen activator and collagenase produced by cultured capillary endothelial cells, *J Cell Biol* 95:974-981, 1982.

115. Gross JL, Moscatelli D, Rifkin DB: Increased capillary endothelial cell protease activity in response to angiogenic stimuli in vitro, *Proc Natl Acad Sci USA* 80:2623-2627, 1983.

116. Hajjar KA, Harpel PC, Jaffe EA, Nachman RL: Binding of plasminogen to cultured human endothelial cells, *J Biol Chem* 261:11656-11662, 1986.

117. Hall WK, Sydenstricker VP, Hock CW, Bowles LL: Protein deprivation as a cause of vascularization of the cornea in the rat, *J Nutr* 32:509-524, 1946.

118. Hase S, Nakazawa S, Tsukamoto Y, Segawa K: Effects of prednisolone and human epidermal growth factor on angiogenesis in granulation tissue of gastric ulcer induced by acetic acid, *Digestion* 42:135-142, 1989.

119. Haynes WL, Hirakata A, Proia AD: Inhibition of corneal neovascularization in the rat by SK&F 86002, a dual inhibitor of arachidonic acid metabolism, *Exp Eye Res* 55:189-191, 1992.

120. Haynes WL, Proia AD, Klintworth GK: Effect of inhibitors of arachidonic acid metabolism on corneal neovascularization in the rat, *Invest Ophthalmol Vis Sci* 30:1588-1593, 1989.

121. Hemo I, BenEzra D, Maftzir G, Birkenfeld V: Angiogenesis and interleukins. In BenEzra D, Ryan SJ, Glaser DM, Murphy RP, editors: *Ocular circulation and neovascularization,* Dordrecht, 1987, Martinus Nijhoff/Dr. W Junk.

122. Hermark RL, Twardzik DR, Schwartz SM: Inhibition of endothelial regeneration by type-β transforming growth factor from platelets, *Science* 233:1078-1080, 1986.

123. Higgs GA, McCall E, Youlten LJF: A chemotactic role for prostaglandins released from polymorphonuclear leukocytes during phagocytosis, *Br J Pharmacol* 53:539-546, 1975.

124. Hockel M, Sasse J, Wissler JH: Purified monocyte-derived angiogenic substance (angiotropin) stimulates migration, phenotypic changes, and "tube formation" but not proliferation of capillary endothelial cells in vitro, *J Cell Physiol* 133:1-13, 1987.

125. Huang SS, Huang JS: Association of bovine brain-derived growth factor receptor with protein tyrosine kinase activity, *J Biol Chem* 261:9568-9571, 1986.

126. Humes JL, Bonney RJ, Pelus J et al.: Macrophages synthesize and release prostaglandins in response to inflammatory stimuli, *Nature* 269:149-150, 1977.

127. Hunter T: Oncogenes and growth control, *Trends Biochem Sci* 10:275, 1985.

128. Ingber DE, Madri JA, Folkman J: A possible mechanism for inhibition of angiostatic corticosteroids: induction of capillary basement membrane dissolution, *Endocrinology* 119:1768-1775, 1986.

129. Ingber DE, Madri JA, Folkman J: Endothelial growth factors and extracellular matrix regulate DNA synthesis through modulation of cell and nuclear expansion, *In Vitro Cell Dev Biol* 23:387-394, 1987.

130. Ishikawa F, Miyazono K, Hellman U et al.: Identification of angiogenic activity and the cloning and expression of platelet-derived endothelial cell growth factor, *Nature* 338:557-562, 1989.

131. Jaye M, Howk R, Burgess W et al.: Human endothelial cell growth factor: cloning, nucleotide sequence, and chromosome localization, *Science* 233:541-545, 1986.

132. Jebejian R, Kalfayan B: Le syndrome oculo-buccogénital, *Ann Ocul* 179:481-491, 1946.

133. Jennings JC, Mohan S, Linkhart TA, Widstrom R: Quantitation of beta 1 and beta 2 TGF in bone matrix extracts and bone cell conditioned medium using unique biological and radioreceptor assays, *Endocrinology* 122(suppl):A1222, 1988.

134. Jensen JA, Hunt TK, Scheuenstuhl H, Banda MJ: Effect of lactate, pyruvate, and pH on secretion of angiogenesis and mitogenesis factors by macrophages, *Lab Invest* 54:574-578, 1986.

135. Jorgensen KA, Stoffersen E: Hydrocortisone inhibits platelet prostaglandin and endothelial prostacyclin production, *Pharmacol Res Commun* 13:579-586, 1981.

136. Keck PJ, Hauser SD, Krivi G et al.: Vascular permeability factor, an endothelial cell mitogen related to PDGF, *Science* 246:1309-1312, 1989.

137. King GL, Buchwald S: Characterization and partial purification of an endothelial cell growth factor from human platelets, *J Clin Invest* 73:392-396, 1984.

138. Klebanoff SJ, Vadas MA, Harlan JM et al.: Stimulation of neutrophils by tumor necrosis factor, *J Immunol* 136:4220-4225, 1986.

139. Klempner MS, Dinarello CA, Gallin JI: Human leukocyte pyrogen induces release of specific granule contents from human neutrophils, *J Clin Invest* 61:1330-1336, 1978.

140. Klintworth GK: The hamster cheek pouch: an experimental model of corneal vascularization, *Am J Pathol* 73:691-710, 1973.

141. Klintworth GK: *Corneal angiogenesis: a comprehensive critical review,* 1-135, New York, 1991, Springer-Verlag.

142. Koch AE, Polverini PJ, Kunkel SL et al.: Interleukin-8 as a macrophage-derived mediator of antiogenesis, *Science* 258:1798-1801, 1992.

143. Koch AE, Polverini J, Leibovich SJ: Induction of neovascularization by activated human monocytes, *J Leuko Biol* 39:233-238, 1986.

144. Kulkarni PS, Bhattacherjee P, Eakins KE, Srinivasan BD: Anti-inflammatory effects of betamethasone phosphate, dexamethasone phosphate and indomethacin on rabbit ocular inflammation induced by bovine serum albumin, *Curr Eye Res* 1:43-47, 1981.

145. Kull FC Jr, Brent DA, Parikh I, Cuatrecacas P: Chemical identification of a tumor-derived angiogenic factor, *Science* 236:843-845, 1987.

146. Lass JH, Berman MB, Campbell RC et al.: Treatment of experimental herpetic interstitial keratitis with medroxyprogesterone, *Arch Ophthalmol* 98:520-527, 1980.

147. Le J, Vilcek J: Tumor necrosis factor and interleukin 1: cytokines with multiple overlapping biological activities, *Lab Invest* 56:234-248, 1987.

148. Lee HW-H, Klintworth GK: An evaluation of spontaneously developing corneal angiogenesis in nude (nu/nu) and hairless (hr/hr) mice, *Invest Ophthalmol Vis Sci* 33(suppl):777, 1992.

149. Leibovich SJ, Polverini PJ: Partial purification of macrophage derived growth factor (MDGF) and macrophage-derived angiogenic activity (MDAA) by gel filtration high-pressure liquid chromatography, *Br J Rheumatol* 24(suppl 1):197-202, 1985.

150. Leibovich SJ, Polverini PJ, Shepard HM et al.: Macrophage-induced angiogenesis is mediated by tumor necrosis factor-α, *Nature* 329:630-632, 1987.

151. Leibovich SJ, Ross R: The role of the macrophage in wound repair: a study with hydrocortisone and antimacrophage serum, *Am J Pathol* 78:71-100, 1975.

152. Leung DW, Cachianes G, Kuang W-J et al.: Vascular endothelial growth factor is a secreted angiogenic mitogen, *Science* 246:1306-1309, 1989.

153. Levin EG, Loskutoff DJ: Cultured bovine endothelial cells produce both urokinase and tissue-type plasminogen activators, *J Cell Biol* 94:631-636, 1982.

154. Libby P, Ordovas JM, Auger KR et al.: Endotoxin and tumor necrosis factor induce interleukin-1 gene expression in adult human vascular endothelial cells, *Am J Pathol* 24:179-185, 1986.

155. Lin MT, Chen YL, Lue CM: The involvement of collagenase from polymorphonuclear leucocyte (PMN) in PGE_1 induced corneal neovascularization, *Fed Proc* 2:A1715, 1988.

156. Lobb RR, Alderman EM, Fett JW: Induction of angiogenesis by bovine brain derived class 1 heparin-binding growth factor, *Biochemistry* 24:4969-4973, 1985.

157. Loeb J: Ueber die Entwicklung von Fischembryonen ohne Kreislauf, *Arch Gesammte Physiol Bonn* 54:525-531, 1893.

158. Maca RD, Fry GL, Hoak JC, Loh PT: The effects of intact platelets on cultured human endothelial cells, *Thromb Res* 11:715-727, 1977.

159. Mach KW, Wilgram GF: Characteristic histopathology of cutaneous lymphoplasia (lymphocytoma), *Arch Dermatol* 94:26-32, 1966.

160. Maciag T: Molecular and cellular mechanisms of angiogencsis. In Devita Jr VT, Hellman S, Rosenberg SA, editors: *Important advances in oncology,* 85-98, Philadelphia, 1990, Lippincott.

161. Maciag T, Kadish J, Wilkins L et al.: Organizational behavior of human umbilical vein endothelial cells, *J Cell Biol* 94:511-520, 1982.

162. Madigan MC, Penfold PL, Holden BA, Billson FA: Ultrastructural features of contact lens-induced deep corneal neovascularization and associated stromal leukocytes, *Cornea* 9:144-151, 1990.

163. Madri JA, Pratt BM, Tucker AM: Phenotypic modulation of endothelial cells by transforming growth factor-β depends on the composition and organization of the extracellular matrix, *J Cell Biol* 106:1375-1384, 1988.

164. Madri JA, Williams SK: Capillary endothelial cell cultures: phenotypic modulation by matrix components, *J Cell Biol* 97:153-165, 1983.

165. Maione TE, Gray GS, Petro J et al.: Inhibition of angiogenesis by recombinant human platelet factor-4 and related peptides, *Science* 247:77-79, 1990.

166. Marks RM, Roche WR, Czerniecki M et al.: Mast cell granules cause proliferation of human microvascular endothelial cells, *Lab Invest* 55:289-294, 1986.

167. Martin BM, Gimbrone MA Jr, Majeau GR et al.: Stimulation of human monocyte- and macrophage-derived growth factor (MDGF) production by plasma fibronectin, *Am J Pathol* 111:367-373, 1983.

168. Martin BM, Gimbrone MA Jr, Unanue ER, Cotran RS: Stimulation of nonlymphoid mesenchymal cell proliferation by a macrophage derived growth factor, *J Immunol* 126:1510-1515, 1981.

169. Matsubara T, Ziff M: Increased superoxide anion release from human endothelial cells in response to cytokines, *J Immunol* 137:3295-3298, 1986.

170. McAuslan BR, Bender V, Riley W, Moss BA: New functions of epidermal growth factor: stimulation of capillary endothelial cell migration and matrix dependent proliferation, *Cell Biol Int Rep* 9:175-182, 1985.

171. McAuslan BR, Gole GA: Cellular and molecular mechanisms in angiogenesis, *Trans Ophthalmol Soc UK* 100:354-358, 1980.

172. McAuslan BR, Hannah GN, Reilly W, Stewart FHC: Variant endothelial cells: fibronectin as a transducer of signals for migration and neovascularization, *J Cell Physiol* 104:177-186, 1980.

173. McAuslan BR, Reilly W: Endothelial cell phagokinesis in response to specific metal ions, *Exp Cell Res* 130:147-157, 1980.

174. McAuslan BR, Reilly W, Hannan GN: Inducers of neovascularization: criteria for definition of a putative direct acting angiogenic factor. In Courtice FC, Garlick DG, Perry MA, editors: *Progress in microcirculation research II,* Proceedings of Second Australia and New Zealand Symposium on the Microcirculation, Sydney, New South Wales, 1983.

175. McAuslan BR, Reilly WG, Hannan GN, Gole GA: Angiogenic factors and their assay: activity of formyl methionyl leucyl phenylalanine, adenosine diphosphate, heparin, copper, and bovine endothelium stimulating factor, *Microvasc Res* 26:323-338, 1983.

176. McCracken JS, Burger PC, Klintworth GK: Morphologic observations on experimental corneal vascularization in the rat, *Lab Invest* 41:519-530, 1979.

177. Michaelson IC: The mode of development of the vascular system of the retina with some observations on its significance for certain retinal diseases, *Trans Ophthalmol Soc UK* 68:137-180, 1948.

178. Miki H, Yamane A, Tokura T, Sano T: Corneal neovascularization after anterior uveal ischemia by occlusion of both long ciliary arteries in rabbit's eye, *Proc Int Soc Eye Res* 4:17, 1986.

179. Modat G, Muller A, Mary A et al.: Differential effects of leukotrienes B4 and C4 on bovine aortic endothelial cell proliferation in vitro, *Prostaglandins* 33:531-538, 1987.

180. Monacci WT, Merrill MJ, Oldfield EH: Expression of vascular permeability factor, vascular endothelial growth factor in normal rat tissue, *Cell Physiol* 33:C995-C1002, 1993.

181. Montesano R, Mossaz A, Ryser J-E et al.: Leukocyte interleukins induce cultured endothelial cells to produce a highly organized, glycosaminoglycan-rich pericellular matrix, *J Cell Biol* 99:1706-1715, 1984.

182. Montesano R, Orci L: Tumor-promoting phorbol esters induce angiogenesis in vitro, *Cell* 42:469-477, 1985.

183. Montesano R, Orci L: Phorbol esters induce angiogenesis in vitro from large-vessel endothelial cells, *J Cell Physiol* 130:284-291, 1987.

184. Montesano R, Orci L, Vassalli P: In vitro rapid organization of endothelial cells into capillary-like networks is promoted by collagen matrices, *J Cell Biol* 97:1648-1652, 1983.

185. Montesano R, Pepper MS, Vassalli JD, Orci L: Phorbol ester induces cultured endothelial cells to invade a fibrin matrix in the presence of fibrinolytic inhibitors, *J Cell Physiol* 132:509-516, 1987.

186. Montesano R, Vassalli JD, Baird A et al.: Basic fibroblast growth factor induces angiogenesis in vitro, *Proc Natl Acad Sci USA* 83:7297-7301, 1986.

187. Moolenaar WH, Tertoolen LGJ, de Laat SW: Na +/H + exchange and cytoplasmic pH in the action of growth factors in human fibroblasts, *Nature* 304:645-648, 1983.

188. Moore F, Riordan JF: Angiogenin activates phospholipase C and elicits a rapid incorporation of fatty acid into cholesterol esters in vascular smooth muscle cells, *Biochemistry* 29:228-233, 1990.

189. Moore JW, Sholley MM: Comparison of the neovascular effects of stimulated macrophages and neutrophils in autologous rabbit corneas, *Am J Pathol* 120:87-98, 1985.

190. Morris PB, Hida T, Blackshear PJ et al.: Tumor-promoting phorbol esters induce angiogenesis in vivo, *Am J Physiol* 254 (Cell Physiol):C318-322, 1988.

191. Moscat J, Moreno F, Herrero C et al.: Endothelial cell growth factor and ionophore A23187 stimulation of production of inositol phosphates in porcine aortic endothelial cells, *Proc Natl Acad Sci USA* 85:659-663, 1988.

192. Moscatelli D, Presta M, Rifkin DB: Purification of a factor from human placenta that stimulates capillary endothelial cell protein production, DNA synthesis and migration, *Proc Natl Acad Sci USA* 83:2091-2095, 1986.

193. Motro B, Itin A, Sachs L, Keshet E: Pattern of interleukin 6 gene expression in vivo suggests a role for this cytokine in angiogenesis, *Proc Natl Acad Sci USA* 87:3092-3096, 1990.

194. Movat HZ: *The inflammatory reaction,* 1-365, Amsterdam, 1985, Elsevier Biochemical.

195. Muller G, Behrens J, Nussbaumer U et al.: Inhibitory action of transforming growth factor β on endothelial cells, *Proc Natl Acad Sci USA* 84:5600-5604, 1987.

196. Mullins DE, Rifkin DB: Stimulation of motility in cultured bovine capillary endothelial cells by angiogenic preparations, *J Cell Physiol* 119:247-254, 1984.

197. Muthukkaruppan VR, Auerbach R: Angiogenesis in the mouse cornea, *Science* 205:1416-1418, 1979.

198. Nathan CF: Secretory products of macrophages, *J Clin Invest* 79:319-326, 1987.

199. Nawroth P, Bank I, Handley D et al.: Tumor necrosis factor/cachectin interacts with endothelial cell receptors to induce release of interleukin-1, *J Exp Med* 163:1363-1375, 1986.

200. Nikolic L, Friend J, Taylor S, Thoft RA: Inhibition of vascularization in rabbit corneas by heparin: cortisone pellets, *Invest Ophthalmol Vis Sci* 27:449-456, 1986.

201. Noji S, Matsuo T, Koyama E et al.: Expression pattern of acidic and basic fibroblast growth factor genes in adult rat eyes, *Biochem Biophys Res Commun* 168:343-349, 1990.

202. Norrby K, Jakobsson A, Sorbo J: Mast-cell secretion and angiogenesis, a quantitative study in rats and mice, *Virchows Arch B Cell Pathol* 57:251-256, 1989.

203. Norris DA, Clark RAF, Swigart LM et al.: Fibronectin fragments are chemotactic for human peripheral blood monocytes, *J Immunol* 129:1612-1618, 1982.

204. Oehlschlaegel G, Stollmann K, Schropl F: Ungewohnliche Hamangiomatose der Haut bei Plasmocytose, *Hautarzt* 19:210-215, 1968.

205. Pepper MS, Ferrara N, Orci L, Montesano R: Potent synergism between vascular endothelial growth factor and basic fibroblast growth factor in the induction of angiogenesis in vitro, *Biochem Biophys Res Commun* 189:824-831, 1992.

206. Pepper MS, Vassalli JD, Montesano R, Orci L: Urokinase-type plasminogen activator is induced in migrating capillary endothelial cells, *J Cell Biol* 105:2535-2541, 1987.

207. Phillips K, Arffa R, Cintron C et al.: Effects of prednisolone and medroxyprogesterone on corneal wound healing, ulceration, and neovascularization, *Arch Ophthalmol* 101:640-643, 1983.

208. Plunkett ML, Hailey JA: Methods in laboratory investigation: an in vivo quantitative angiogenesis model using tumor cells entrapped in alginate, *Lab Invest* 62:510-517, 1990.

209. Pober JS, Bevilacqua MP, Mendick DL et al.: Two-distinct monokines, interleukin-I and tumor necrosis factor, each independently induce biosynthesis and transient expression of the same antigen on the surface of cultured human vascular endothelial cells, *J Immunol* 136:1680-1687, 1986.

210. Pober JS, Cotran RS: Cytokines and endothelial cell biology, *Physiol Rev* 70:427-451, 1990.

211. Pober JS, Gimbrone MA Jr, Collins T et al.: Interactions of T lymphocytes with human vascular endothelial cells: role of endothelial cells surface antigens, *Immunobiology* 168:483-494, 1984.

212. Pober JS, Gimbrone MA Jr, Cotran RS et al.: Ia expression by vascular endothelium is inducible by activated T cells and by human γ interferon, *J Exp Med* 157:1339-1353, 1983.

213. Polverini PJ: Macrophage-induced angiogenesis: a review. In Sorg C, editor: *Macrophage-derived regulatory factors,* vol. 1. *Cytokines* 1:54-73, 1989.

213a. Proia AD, Hirakata A, McInnes JS et al.: The effect of angiostatic steroids and β-cyclodextrin tetradecasulfate on corneal neovascularization in the rat. *Exp Eye Res* 57:693-698, 1993.

214. Raju KS: Isolation and characterization of copper-binding sites of human ceruloplasmin, *Mol Cell Biochem* 56:81-88, 1983.

215. Raju KS, Alessandri G, Ziche M, Gullino PM: Ceruloplasmin, copper ions, and angiogenesis, *J Natl Cancer Inst* 69:1183-1188, 1982.

216. Raju KS, Alessandri G, Ziche M, Gullino PM: Characterization of a chemoattractant for endothelium induced by angiogenesis effectors, *Cancer Res* 44:1579-1584, 1984.

217. Reiko T, Werb Z: Secretory products of macrophages and their physiologic functions, *Am J Physiol* 246:C1-C9, 1984.

218. Reilly TM, Taylor DS, Herblin WF et al.: Monoclonal antibodies against basic fibroblast growth factor which inhibit its biological activity in vitro and in vivo, *Biochem Biophys Res Commun* 164:736-743, 1989.

219. Roberts AB, Sporn MB: Regulation of endothelial cell growth, architecture, and matrix synthesis by TGF-β, *Am J Respir Dis* 140:1126-1128, 1989.

220. Roberts AB, Sporn MB, Assoian RK et al.: Transforming growth factor type β: rapid induction of fibrosis and angiogenesis in vivo and stimulation of collagen formation in vitro, *Proc Natl Acad Sci USA* 83:4167-4171, 1986.

221. Robin JB, Regis-Pacheco LF, Kash RL, Schanzlin DJ: The histopathology of corneal neovascularization: inhibitor effects, *Arch Ophthalmol* 103:284-287, 1985.

222. Rochels R: Tierexperientelle Untersuchungen zur Rolle von EntzUndungsmediatoren bei der Hornhautneovaskurisation, *Docum Ophthalmol* 57:215-262, 1984.

223. Rohr S, Toti F, Brisson C et al.: Quantitative image analysis of angiogenesis in rats implanted with a fibrin gel chamber, *Nouv Rev Fr Hematol* 34:287-294, 1992.

224. Rollins BJ, Yoshimura T, Leonard EJ, Pober JS: Cytokine-activated human endothelial cells synthesize and secrete a monocyte chemoattractant, MCP-1/JE, *Am J Pathol* 136:1229-1233, 1990.

225. Rosenbaum JT, Howes EL Jr, Rubin RM, Samples JR: Ocular inflammatory effects of intravitreally-injected tumor necrosis factor, *Am J Pathol* 133:47-53, 1988.

226. Ross R: The pathogenesis of atherosclerosis—an update, *New Eng J Med* 314:488-500, 1986.

227. Ryan TJ: Factors influencing the growth of vascular endothelium in the skin, *Br J Dermatol* 82(suppl 15) 99, 1970.

228. Ryan TJ: Factors influencing growth of vascular endothelium in the skin. In Jarrett A, editor: *The physiology and pathophysiology of the skin,* vol 2. *The Nerves and Blood Vessels,* London, 1973, Academic Press.

229. Ryan US: The endothelial surface and responses to injury, *Fed Proc* 45:101-108, 1986.

230. Ryan US, Ryan JW: Endothelial cells and inflammation. In Ward PA, editor: *Clinics in Laboratory Medicine,* 577-599, Philadelphia, 1983, Saunders.

231. Ryan US, Ryan JW: Inflammatory mediators, contraction and endothelial cells. In Courtice FC, Garlick DG, Perry MA, editors: *Progress in microcirculation research.* II. 424-438, Sydney, Australia, Committee in Postgraduate Medical Education, University of New South Wales, 1984.

232. Ryu S, Albert DM: Evaluation of tumor angiogenesis factor with the rabbit cornea model, *Invest Ophthalmol Vis Sci* 18:831-841, 1979.

233. Saba HL, Hartmann RC, Saba SR: Effect of polymorphonuclear leukocytes on endothelial cell growth, *Thromb Res* 12:397-407, 1978.

234. Saksela O, Moscatelli D, Rifkin DB: The opposing effects of basic fibroblast growth factor and transforming growth factor beta on the regulation of plasminogen activator activity in capillary endothelial cells, *J Cell Biol* 105:957-963, 1987.

235. Sato N, Beitz JG, Kato J et al.: Plate-derived growth factor indirectly stimulates angiogenesis in vitro, *Am J Pathol* 142:1119-1130, 1993.

236. Sato N, Fukuda K, Nariuchi H, Sagara N: Tumor necrosis factor inhibiting angiogenesis in vitro, *J Natl Cancer Inst* 79:1383-1391, 1987.

237. Sato N, Goto T, Haranaka K et al.: Actions of tumor necrosis factor on cultured vascular endothelial cells: morphologic modulation, growth inhibition, and cytotoxicity, *J Natl Cancer Inst* 76:1113-1121, 1986.

238. Sato N, Sawasaki Y, Haranaka K et al.: Growth inhibitory and cytotoxic action of rabbit tumor necrosis factor against bovine capillary endothelial cells in vitro, *Proc Jpn Acad* 61(B):471-474, 1985.

239. Sato Y, Rifkin DB: Autocrine activities of basic fibroblast growth factor: regulation of endothelial cell movement, plasminogen activator synthesis, and DNA synthesis, *J Cell Biol* 107:1199-1205, 1988.

240. Schanzlin DJ, Cyr RJ, Friedlaender MH: The histopathology of corneal neovascularization, *Arch Ophthalmol* 101:472-474, 1983.

241. Scher W: Biology of disease: the role of extracellular proteases in cell proliferation and differentiation, *Lab Invest* 57:607-633, 1987.

242. Schoefl GI: Studies on inflammation. III. Growing capillaries: their structure and permeability, *Virchows Arch Pathol Anat* 337:97-141, 1963.

243. Schor AM, Schor SL, Allen TD: Effects of culture conditions on the proliferation, morphology and migration of bovine aortic endothelial cells, *J Cell Sci* 62:267-285, 1983.

244. Schor AM, Schor SL, Kumar S: Importance of a collagen substratum for stimulation of capillary endothelial cell proliferation by tumour angiogenesis factor, *Int J Cancer* 24:225-234, 1979.

245. Schor AM, Schor SL, Weiss JB et al.: Stimulation by a low molecular weight angiogenic factor of capillary endothelial cells in culture, *Br J Cancer* 41:790-799, 1980.

246. Schreiber AB, Kenney J, Kowalski WJ et al.: Interaction of endothelial cell growth factor with heparin: characterization by receptor and antibody recognition, *Proc Natl Acad Sci USA* 82:6138-6142, 1985.

247. Schreiber AB, Winkler ME, Derynck R: Transforming growth factors: a more potent angiogenic mediator than epidermal growth factor, *Science* 232:1250-1253, 1986.

248. Schweigerer L, Neufeld G, Friedman J et al.: Capillary endothelial cells express basic fibroblast growth factor, a mitogen that promotes their own growth, *Nature* 325:257-259, 1987.

249. Senger DR, Connolly DT, van De Water L et al.: Purification and NH$_2$-terminal amino acid sequence of guinea pig tumor secreted vascular permeability factor, *Cancer Res* 50:1774-1778, 1990.

250. Senior RM, Huang SS, Griffin GL, Huang JS: Brain-derived growth factor is a chemoattractant for fibroblasts and astroglial cells, *Biochem Biophys Res Commun* 141:67-72, 1986.

251. Serafin WE, Katz HR, Austen KF, Stevens RL: Complexes of heparin proteoglycans, chondroitin sulfate E proteoglycans, and [^{3}H] diisopropyl fluorophosphate-binding proteins are exocytosed from activated mouse bone marrow-derived mast cells, *J Biol Chem* 261:15017-15021, 1986.

252. Shio H, Ramwell P: Effect of prostaglandin E$_2$ and aspirin on the secondary aggregation of human platelets, *Nature New Biol* 236:45-46, 1972.

253. Sholley MM, Cavallo T, Cotran RS: Endothelial proliferation in inflammation: I. Autoradiographic studies following thermal injury to the skin of normal rats, *Am J Pathol* 89:277-290, 1977.

254. Sholley MM, Ferguson GP, Seibel HR et al.: Mechanisms of neovascularization: vascular sprouting can occur without proliferation of endothelial cells, *Lab Invest* 51:624-634, 1984.

255. Sholley MM, Gimbrone MA Jr, Cotran RS: The effects of leukocyte depletion on corneal neovascularization, *Lab Invest* 38:32-40, 1978.

256. Sholley MM, Wilson JD, Montour JL, Ruffolo JJ Jr: Radiation response of corneal neovascularization, *Invest Ophthalmol Vis Sci* 19(suppl):254, 1980.

257. Sidky YA, Auerbach R: Lymphocyte-induced angiogenesis: a quantitative and sensitive assay of the graft-versus-host reaction, *J Exp Med* 141:1084-1100, 1975.

258. Sidky YA, Auerbach R: Lymphocyte-induced angiogenesis in tumor-bearing mice, *Science* 192:1237-1238, 1976.

259. Smith RS, Smith LA: Effects of BP961 on corneal wound healing, *Invest Ophthalmol Vis Sci* 19(suppl):254, 1980.

260. Snyder DS, Unanue ER: Corticosteroids inhibit murine macrophage la expression and interleukin 1 production, *J Immunol* 129:1803-1805, 1982.

261. Stefansson E, Landers MB III, Wolbarsht ML, Klintworth GK: Neovascularization of the iris: an experimental model in cats, *Invest Ophthalmol Vis Sci* 25:361-364, 1984.

262. Stein MB, Asbell PA, Kamenar T et al: Inhibition of corneal neovascularization by combination heparin-steroid therapy, *Invest Ophthalmol Vis Sci* 28(suppl):231, 1987.

263. Stern DM, Bank I, Nawroth PP et al.: Self-regulation of procoagulant events on the endothelial cell surface, *J Exp Med* 162:1223-1235, 1985.

264. Stokes CL, Rupnick MA, Williams SK, Lauffenburger DA: Chemotaxis of human microvessel endothelial cells in response to acidic fibroblast growth factor, *Lab Invest* 63:657-668, 1990.

265. Stout AJ, Gresser I, Thompson WD: Inhibition of wound healing in mice by local interferon α/β injection, *Int J Exp Pathol* 74:79-85, 1993.
266. Suvarnamani C, Halperin EC, Proia AD, Klintworth GK: The effect of total lymphoid irradiation on corneal vascularization in the rat following chemical cautery, *Radiat Res* 117:259-272, 1989.
267. Svensjo E, Grega GJ: Evidence for endothelial cell-mediated regulation of macromolecular permeability by postcapillary venules, *Fed Proc* 45:89-95, 1986.
268. Taylor S, Folkman J: Protamine is an inhibitor of angiogenesis, *Nature* 297:307-312, 1982.
269. Terman BI, Dougher-Vermazen M, Carrion ME et al.: Identification of the KDR tyrosine kinase as a receptor for vascular endothelial cell growth factor, *Biochem Biophys Res Commun* 187:1579-1586, 1992.
270. Thompson WD, Brown FI: Quantitation of histamine-induced angiogenesis in the chick chorioallantoic membrane: mode of action of histamine is indirect, *Int J Microcirc Clin Exp* 6:343-357, 1987.
271. Thompson WD, Campbell R, Evans AT: Fibrin degradation and angiogenesis: quantitative analysis of the angiogenic response in the chick chorioallantoic membrane, *J Pathol* 145:27-37, 1985.
272. Thompson JA, Haudenschild CC, Anderson KD et al.: Heparin-binding growth factor 1 induces the formation of organoid neovascular structures in vivo, *Proc Natl Acad Sci USA* 86:7928-7932, 1989.
273. Thompson WD, Smith EB, Stirk CM et al.: Angiogenic activity of fibrin degradation products is located in fibrin fragment E, *J Pathol* 168:47-53, 1992.
274. Thornton SC, Mueller SN, Levine EM: Human endothelial cells: use of heparin in cloning and long-term serial cultivation, *Science* 222:623-625, 1983.
275. Till GO, Johnson KJ, Kunkel R, Ward PA: Intravascular activation of complement and acute lung injury: dependency on neutrophils and toxic oxygen metabolites, *J Clin Invest* 69:1126-1135, 1982.
276. Tishcer E, Gospodarowicz D, Mitchell R et al.: Vascular endothelial growth factor: a new member of the platelet-derived growth factor gene family, *Biochem Biophys Res Commun* 165:1198-1206, 1989.
277. Todderud G, Carpenter G: Epidermal growth factor: the receptor and its function, *Biofactors* 2:11-15, 1989.
278. Tsujimoto M, Yokota S, Vilcek J, Weissmann G: Tumor necrosis factor provokes superoxide anion generation from neutrophils, *Biochem Biophys Res Commun* 137:1094-1100, 1986.
279. Tsuruoka N, Sugiyama M, Tawaragi Y et al.: Inhibition of in vitro angiogenesis by lymphotoxin and interferon-γ, *Biochem Biophys Res Commun* 155:429-436, 1988.
280. Ungari S, Katari RS, Alessandri G, Guillino PM: Cooperation between fibronectin and heparin in the mobilization of capillary endothelium, *Invasion Metastasis* 5:193-205, 1985.
281. Van den Brenk HAS, Sharpington C, Orton C, Stone M: Effects of x-irradiation on growth and function of the repair blastema (granulation tissue). II. Measurement of angiogenesis in the Selye pouch in the rat, *Int J Radiat Biol* 25:277-289, 1974.
282. Vu MT, Burger PC, Klintworth GK: Angiogenic activity in injured rat corneas as assayed on the chick chorioallantoic membrane, *Lab Invest* 53:311-319, 1985.
283. Vu MT, Smith CF, Burger PC, Klintworth GK: Methods in laboratory investigation: an evaluation of methods to quantitate the chick chorioallantoic membrane assay in angiogenesis, *Lab Invest* 53:499-508, 1985.
284. Wahl SM, Hunt DA, Wakefield LM et al.: Transforming growth factor type β induces monocyte chemotaxis and growth factor production, *Proc Natl Acad Sci USA* 84:5788-5792, 1987.
285. Wall RT, Harker LA, Quadracci LJ, Striker GE: Factors influencing endothelial cell proliferation in vitro, *J Cell Physiol* 96:203-213, 1978.
286. Wall RT, Harker LA, Striker GE: Human endothelial cell migration: stimulation by a released platelet factor, *Lab Invest* 39:523-529, 1978.
287. Watt SL, Auerbach R: A mitogenic factor for endothelial cells obtained from mouse secondary mixed leukocyte cultures, *J Immunol* 136:197-202, 1986.
288. Weiss JB, Hill CR, Davis RJ et al.: Activation of procollagenase by a low molecular weight angiogenesis factor, *Biosci Rep* 3:171-177, 1983.
289. Weissmann G: The role of lysosomes in inflammation and disease, *Ann Rev Med* 18:97-112, 1967.
290. Weremonicz S, Fox EA, Morton CC, Valle BL: Localization of the human angiogenin gene to chromosome band 14q11, proximal to the T cell receptor α/δ locus, *Am J Hum Genet* 47:973-981, 1990.
291. Wiseman DM, Polverini PJ, Kamp DW, Leibovich SJ: Transforming growth factor β (TGF-β) is a chemoattractant for monocytes and induces their expression of angiogenic activity, *J Cell Biol* 105:163a, 1987.
292. Wolf JE, Harrison RG: Demonstration and characterization of an epidermal angiogenic factor, *J Invest Dermatol* 61:130-141, 1973.
293. Wolff JEA, Guerin C, Laterra J et al.: Dexamethasone reduces vascular density and plasminogen activator activity in 9L rat brain tumors, *Brain Res* 604:79-85, 1993.
294. Yamagami I: Electron microscopic study of the cornea. I. The mechanisms of experimental new vessel formation, *Acta Soc Ophthalmol Jpn* 73:1222-1242, 1969.
295. Yamagami I: Electron microscopic study of the cornea. I. The mechanism of experimental new vessel formation, *Jpn J Ophthalmol* 14:41, 1970.
296. Yasunaga C, Nakashima Y, Sueishi K: A role of fibrinolytic activity in angiogenesis: quantitative assay using in vitro method, *Lab Invest* 61:698-704, 1989.
297. Zauberman H, Refojo MF: Keratoplasty with glued-on lenses for alkali burns: an experimental study, *Arch Ophthalmol* 89:46-48, 1973.
298. Zetter BR: Angiogenesis: state of the art, *Chest* 93(suppl):159, 1988.
299. Zetter BR, Antoniades HN: Stimulation of human vascular endothelial cell growth by a platelet-derived growth factor and thrombin, *J Supramol Struct* 11:361-370, 1979.
300. Ziche M, Alessandri G, Gullino PM: Gangliosides promote the angiogenic response, *Lab Invest* 61:629-634, 1989.
301. Ziche M, Banchelli G, Caderni G et al.: Copper-dependent amine oxidases in angiogenesis induced by prostaglandin E$_1$ (PGE$_1$), *Microvasc Res* 34:133-136, 1987.
302. Ziche M, Jones J, Gullino PM: Role of prostaglandin E$_1$ and copper in angiogenesis, *J Natl Cancer Inst* 69:475-482, 1982.
303. Ziche M, Morbidelli L, Alessandri G, Gullino PM: Angiogenesis can be stimulated or repressed in vivo by a change in GM3 : GD3 ganglioside ratio, *Lab Invest* 67:711-715, 1992.

10 Lacrimal Gland Immunology

RUDOLPH M. FRANKLIN, PAUL C. MONTGOMERY

The lacrimal gland provides substances that are essential for function at the ocular surface. Although the lipid and the mucus content of the tear film each plays an important role in maintaining a healthy ocular surface, the lacrimal gland contributes a number of biologically active molecules to the tear film, each with a unique protective role. For instance, lysozyme is present in human tears at a concentration of 1 mg/ml and exerts its bacteriolytic action by disrupting cell walls.[36] The acinar cells of the lacrimal gland are the source of the lysozyme production. Likewise, lactoferrin is produced by the acinar cells of the lacrimal gland[18] and exerts a bacteriocidal action by chelating metals that are essential for the growth of microorganisms.

IMMUNITY AT THE OCULAR SURFACE

Acquired immunity at the ocular surface is provided primarily by an immune system common to mucosal tissues. A distinct feature of the mucosal or secretory immune system is a general predominance of immunoglobulin A (IgA) in mucosal secretions. The high ratio of IgA to other immunoglobulins (Igs) in tears is unlike that of serum, in which immunoglobulin G (IgG) predominates. Initial studies of human tears showed an average level of 0.07 mg/ml of IgA, with only a trace of IgG.[9] Further studies confirmed an even higher concentration of IgA in tears, 0.5 mg/ml, with very low levels of IgG.[36] The IgA is produced locally, predominantly in lacrimal glands, and is actively transported into tears.[46,55] Low levels of IgG and occasionally other Igs are present in tears and may represent transudation.

Mucosal Immune System

Secretory IgA (S-IgA) differs from its serum counterpart in several distinct ways. S-IgA is usually a dimer of IgA molecules (when examined in tears), and it has two additional polypeptides, the J chain and the secretory component.[37] The J chain is covalently linked to the heavy (H) chains of the IgA dimer, and the secretory component (SC) is linked to the dimer through interactions with both the J chain and the IgA heavy chains. Fig. 10-1 diagrams the structural features of the S-IgA molecule.

Mucosal tissues typically show plasma cells that produce polymeric IgA (pIgA), which consists of the IgA dimer linked by the J chain with the adjacent epithelium-producing SC. Fig. 10-2 presents the biosynthetic events that lead to the production of the S-IgA molecule. SC, which functions as part of the receptor for the transepithelial transport of polymeric immunoglobulin (poly Ig receptor),[52] is acquired from lacrimal gland epithelial cells during the transport of pIgA into tears.[18] Additional features of this system involve regulatory T cells and specialized cell traffic patterns that localize the IgA-producing plasma cells within tissues at mucosal sites. Studies with human, rat, rabbit, and mouse lacrimal glands show features typical of this system.

The origin of the mucosal IgA plasma cells has been a subject of intense investigation. It has become clear that the precursor cells—IgA-committed B cells—arrive at the mucosal destinations through the circulation.[12] These IgA-committed B cells arise from specialized lymphoid tissues associated with certain mucosal surfaces. For instance, specialized collections of lymphoid tissue located along the ileum, gut, or gastrointestinal-associated lymphoid tissue (GALT), contain lymphoid follicles known as Peyer patches. The Peyer patches transfer gut luminal antigens through specialized surface M (microfold or membranous) cells.[44] Once within the lymphoid portion of the Peyer patches, antigen initiates a series of cellular interactions involving macrophages, T cells, and B cells that leads to antigen-reactive B cells committed to IgA synthesis. These IgA-committed B cells then traffic throughout the body and localize specifically within mucosal tissues. Fig. 10-3 summarizes the major features of the mucosal immune network as they relate to GALT. A similar mechanism has been demonstrated for bronchial tissue, wherein inhaled antigens can initiate a commitment to specific IgA production.[5] In the rabbit a conjunctival-associated lymphoid tissue (CALT) shares certain histologic characteristics with the gastrointes-

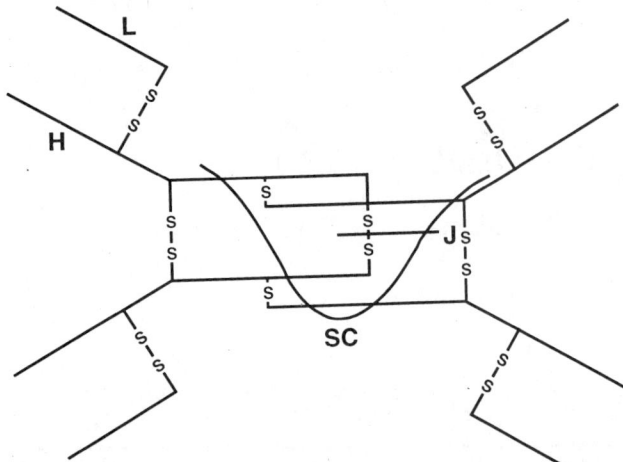

Fig. 10-1. Diagrammatic representation of the S-IgA molecule. IgA monomers, each containing two heavy (α) and two light (k or λ) chains, are linked covalently through the J chain. Secretory component *(SC)* interacts with the polymeric IgA molecule through association with J chain and the $C\alpha$ domains of the heavy chains of each monomeric unit.

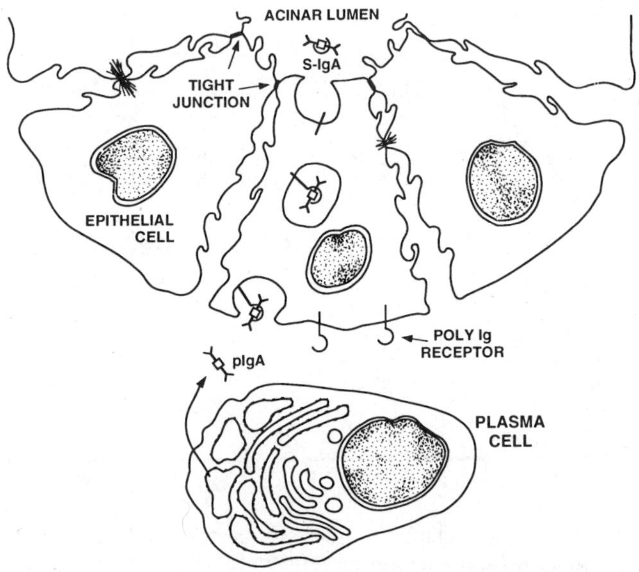

tinal and bronchial lymphoid tissues. It has been speculated that antigen triggers cells in CALT to subsequently seed lacrimal glands and other mucosal tissues.[20] To date, the relationship of CALT to the other well-defined components of the mucosal network has not been established.

Mucosal Immune Function

Defense at mucosal surfaces is predominantly mediated by S-IgA antibodies. IgA functions at three levels: in mucosal secretions, within epithelial cells, and extracellularly within the lamina propria.* IgA-mediated bacterial defense occurs mainly in mucosal secretions and functions by agglutination, direct killing, prevention of epithelial attachment or invasion, inactivation of bacterial enzymes or toxins, and possibly by opsonization or cell-mediated killing mechanisms.[7,34,35,58] IgA-mediated protection against viruses mainly involves neutralization, which occurs both in secretions and within epithelial cells.† For both bacteria and viruses, IgA antibodies can interact with antigenic components that cross the epithelium or are produced in mucosal tissues; and the resulting immune complexes can be actively transported back into the luminal contents and out of the body.[26,32] In this later case complexes of at least 925 kDa can be transported.[26]

With respect to the ocular compartment, little information is available regarding the function of S-IgA. In one study, however (involving tear IgA from rabbits previously immunized with herpes simplex virus), type 1 did inhibit the

---

*References 7, 17, 32, 34, 35, 58.
†References 7, 31, 32, 34, 35, 58.

Fig. 10-2. Schematic representation of S-IgA biosynthesis in the lacrimal gland. Polymeric IgA (pIgA) is synthesized in plasma cells located adjacent to the acinar epithelial cells. pIgA interacts with the poly Ig receptor on the surface of the acinar epithelial cell, is internalized and transported to the apical surface, and is released into the glandular lumen. Prior to release of the S-IgA molecule, the poly Ig receptor is cleaved, leaving behind the cytoplasmic domain. The remainder of the poly Ig receptor remains associated with the S-IgA molecule and is designated secretory component *(SC)*. (Redrawn from Franklin RM, Kenyon KR, Tomasi TB: Immunohistologic studies of human lacrimal gland: localization of immunoglobulins, secretory component and lactoferrin, *J Immunol* 110:984, 1973).

attachment of the virus to cultured cells.[30] Although the in vivo protective capacity of S-IgA in the eye remains to be documented, the in vitro findings suggest a potential role for S-IgA in the blocking of viral attachment to host tissue.

Relationship of the Lacrimal Gland to the Mucosal Network

Although it is general knowledge that the lacrimal gland contains the components that are characteristic of other tissues of the mucosal immune system, documentation of a functional interrelationship is a more recent finding. With respect to antibody expression, IgA antibodies in tears possess specificity for ingested microbes.[21] In addition, after human volunteers ingested heat-killed *Streptococcus mutans,* S-IgA antibodies were found in their tears and saliva, but no serum IgA antibodies were detected.[38] Following a second oral immunization, a marked increase in S-IgA antibodies was noted for the tears and saliva, with no serum response. Using a murine cell transfer system, it was subsequently shown that IgA-committed cells from gastrointestinal lymphoid tissue seeded the lacrimal gland as well as other mucosal sites.[39,59] Based on these observations, it was

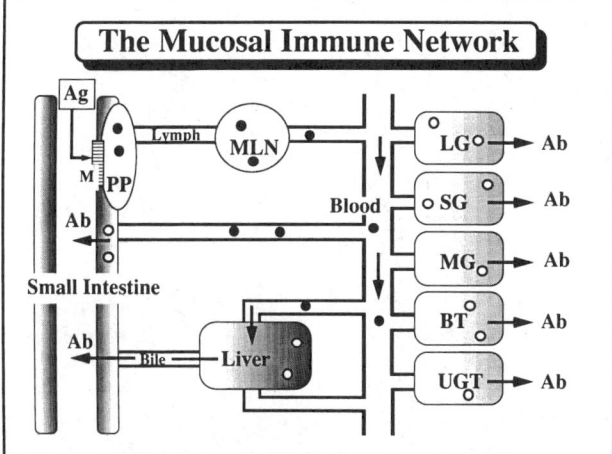

The Mucosal Immune Network

Fig. 10-3. Diagrammatic representation of the major features of the mucosal immune network as they relate to GALT. Intestinal antigens *(Ag)* are taken up by microfold *(M)* cells overlying Peyer patches *(PP)* and are delivered to lymphoid cells in the PP. T cells and IgA-committed B cells (●) migrate to the mesenteric lymph nodes *(MLN)*, enter the circulation, and traffic to the lacrimal *(LG)*, salivary *(SG)*, and mammary *(MG)* glands as well as to the lamina propria of the small intestine, the bronchial *(BT)*, the urogenital *(UGT)* tracts, and the liver. B lymphocytes that lodge in mucosal tissues differentiate into IgA-secreting plasma cells *(O)*, producing pIgA, which is transported into external secretions as S-IgA antibody *(Ab)*. In some species the liver directly transports significant quantities of pIgA from the circulation into bile. (From Montgomery PC, O'Sullivan NL, Martin LB, Skandera CA, Peppard JV, Pockley AG: *Regulation of lacrimal gland immunoresponses.* In Sullivan DA, editor: *The lacrimal gland, tear film and dry eye syndromes. Basic science and clinical relevance,* New York, 1994, Plenum).

concluded that the lacrimal gland was a functional component of the mucosal immune network.

GLANDULAR STRUCTURE AND CELLULAR COMPOSITION

Tissue Organization

The lacrimal gland in the human is located in the anterior, superolateral portion of the orbit with a number of ducts emptying into the superotemporal conjunctival cul-de-sac. A variable number of much smaller accessory lacrimal glands are located in the upper conjunctiva, where they empty directly through the conjunctival epithelium. The lower conjunctiva contains only a few small clusters of accessory lacrimal glands. Many animal species also possess lacrimal glands, and glands from such animals demonstrate a variable location either within the orbit or over the external orbital rim.

The lacrimal gland is composed of acini connected by ductules, which form the collecting ducts. The interconnected acini form lobules and numerous lobules form the lobes of each gland. As illustrated in Fig. 10-4, plasma cells and lymphocytes are located in the connective tissue between the numerous acini, lobules, and ducts.[24]

Each acinus consists of an epithelium with flattened myoepithelial cells interspersed between the secretory epithelial cells along the basal surface.[24,50] The secretory epithelial cells show an abundance of granules, although occasional cells may show considerably fewer of these secretory granules (Fig. 10-5). It is likely that the epithelial cells vary in their secretory state, depending on the degree of stimulation. The various ducts of the gland are lined with a pseudostratified epithelium of between one and four layers. These ductule epithelial cells, as well as the secretory epithelial cells of the acini, display apical zonula occludens.[50]

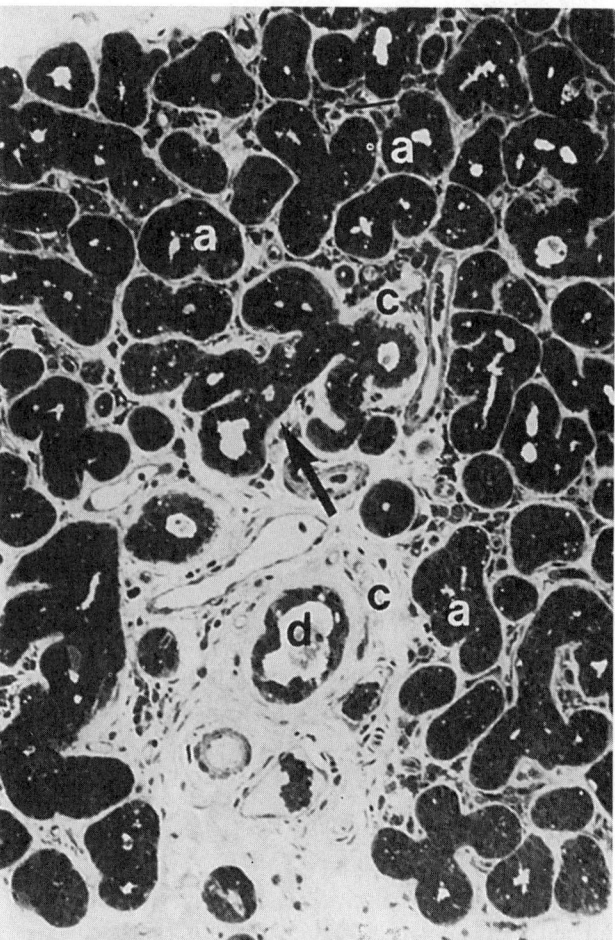

Fig. 10-4. Photomicrograph of normal human lacrimal gland that shows a lobule consisting of acini *(a)*, intralobular connective tissue *(c)*, and an intralobular duct *(d)*. The arrow shows a transition zone between the acinus and the duct (Methylene blue-azure II stain, ×184). (From Iwamoto T, Jakobiec FA: A comparative ultrasound study of the lacrimal gland and its epithelial tumors, *Human Path* 13:236, 1982).

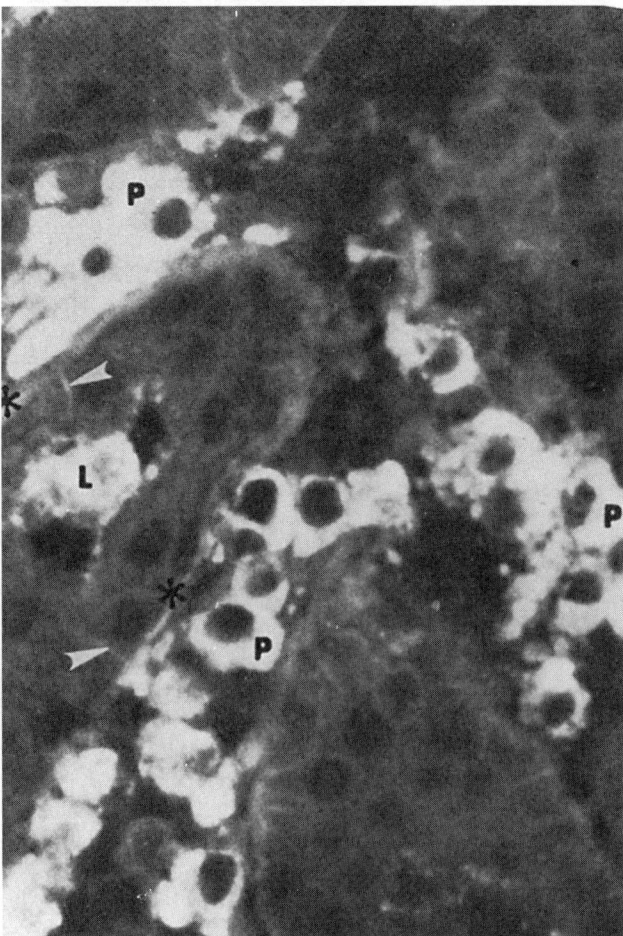

Fig. 10-5. Electron micrograph of an acinus that consists of a central lumen *(L)* and a layer of secretory epithelial cells *(SE)* that contain large secretory granules *(g)* in the apical and middle portions of the cell. Flattened cisternae of rough-surfaced endoplasmic reticulum *(re)* are located in the basal portion of the cytoplasm. A discontinuous layer of myoepithelial cells *(ME)* surrounds the acinar periphery. Other features include apical junctional complexes *(arrows)*, microvilli *(mv)*, lipid droplets *(l)*, and the multilaminar basement membrane *(bm)* (×6,300). *Inset,* higher-power electron micrograph of the junctional complex shown in the main figure: zonula occludens *(o)*, zonula adherens *(a)*, and desmosomes *(d)* (×38,000). (From Iwamoto T, Jakobiec FA: A comparative ultrasound study of the normal lacrimal gland and its epithelial tumors, *Human Path* 13:236, 1982).

Fig. 10-6. Photomicrograph showing the acinar organization of the human lacrimal gland. IgA staining is seen within the clustered plasma cells *(P)*, along the epithelial basement membrane (*), in intracellular spaces *(arrowheads)*, and within the acinar lumen *(L)*. (Fluorescein-conjugated anti-IgA serum and Evans blue staining ×475). (From Franklin RM, Kenyon KR, Tomasi TB: Immunohistologic studies of human lacrimal gland: localization of immunoglobulins, secretory component and lactoferrin, *J Immunol* 110:984, 1973).

Cells in the Lacrimal Gland

The predominant cell type in lacrimal glands is the acinar epithelial cell, which is a relatively large (greater than 15 micrometers) secretory cell. The next most common cell type is the ductal epithelial cell, and even fewer myoepithelial cells are seen both in sections and in dissociated gland preparations. The acinar and ductal epithelial cells contain SC, which appears controlled (at least in part) by hormonal mechanisms.[54] In addition, the acinar cells contain lactoferrin and lysozyme. The acinar epithelial cells may represent a source for the various cytokines that are responsible for local proliferation and possible differentiation of lymphoid cells within the lacrimal gland.

As shown in Fig. 10-6, plasma cells are a major lymphoid population present in lacrimal glands. These cells are commonly of the IgA isotype.[18] Variable percentages of IgG and IgM cells have been found in different animal species as well as in humans; and occasionally, IgE has been identified within human plasma cells of lacrimal glands. These plasma cells are scattered throughout the interstitium of the gland, not only adjacent to the acinar structures, but in some instances adjacent to ducts and ductules. B cells of the major isotypes have been identified in mouse and rat lacrimal glands, as well as T cells with helper and suppressor phenotypes[33,41] (although the functional capabilities of these T cell subpopulations have yet to be elucidated).

Macrophages have been confirmed within rat lacrimal glands; and human glands contain only occasional neutrophils, but no other polymorphonuclear leukocytes. Mast cells have rarely been found in human lacrimal glands, and no basophils are present.

ORIGIN OF IMMUNOCOMPETENT CELLS

Antibody Expression in Tears

As noted previously, antigen administration by the gastrointestinal route has elicited tear IgA antibody responses in both humans and animals. In addition, topical application of antigen to the conjunctiva in certain animal models induces tear IgA antibody responses. In the rat model, in which direct comparisons of the gastrointestinal and conjunctival routes have been made using a nonreplicating particulate antigen, the conjunctival route consistently elicits higher levels of tear IgA antibodies.[40,45] Although the mechanism by which topical antigen application elicits a tear IgA antibody response is not known, the placement of antigen at the surface of the conjunctiva (as opposed to subconjunctival injection) is critical. Although it is tempting to speculate that cells traffic from the conjunctiva (or CALT) to the lacrimal gland (perhaps via a draining lymph node), no hard evidence currently supports this hypothesis.

Lymphocyte Traffic to Lacrimal Glands

The murine model has been particularly useful in detailing lymphocyte traffic patterns in vivo. Using adoptive cell transfer, lymphocytes from GALT have been shown to selectively seed the lamina propria of gastrointestinal, bronchial, and urogenital tissues as well as glandular sites such as mammary (lactating animals), salivary, and lacrimal glands (Fig. 10-3).[39,59] As has been the case for other mucosal tissues, the traffic of B lymphocytes to lacrimal glands has been studied more extensively than T cells. With respect to B cells, the IgA-committed cells from Peyer patches pass through the mesenteric lymph node, enter the thoracic duct lymph, reach the blood, and selectively populate mucosal sites, including lacrimal glands. After lodging in mucosal tissues, these B lymphocytes differentiate into IgA-secreting plasma cells. T lymphocytes are also known to traffic but, thus far, there has been little information to suggest that distinct T cell subsets exhibit a specific migratory tropism for glandular mucosal tissues.

Mechanisms That Control Lymphocyte Lodging in Lacrimal Glands

It is now well documented that lymphocyte traffic to organized lymphoid tissue is mediated by an organ-specific recognition system that involves lymphocyte-high endothelial venule (HEV) interactions.[4,8,47,51,53] Generally, these interactions involve lymphocyte homing receptors, which recognize vascular addressins on HEVs or other specialized endothelial cells. As noted earlier, lymphocytes traffic to glandular mucosal tissues, such as lacrimal glands; but the precise mechanisms responsible for their preferential accumulation, lodging, or retention of specific lymphoid populations are not well defined. Such control mechanisms could exist at two possible levels: at the blood vessel wall or within the stroma of the lacrimal tissue itself. While there is presently no reason to rule out some type of control at the level of exit from the vasculature, such a mechanism would most likely involve interaction with endothelial cells. Because there are no HEVs in lacrimal glands, and, thus far, no documented "selective" interaction with glandular endothelium, it appears that lymphocyte entry into lacrimal glands (and perhaps other glandular tissues) may be random.[33] In fact, based on accumulating data, it now appears that selective retention of circulating lymphocytes occurs within the lacrimal tissue microenvironment. Early studies proposed that retention of B cells, in particular those committed to IgA production, resulted from a direct interaction with T cells located in lacrimal tissue.[19] Although such interactions may contribute to B cell localization, the mechanism accounting for T cell retention was not addressed. More recently, a direct interaction of circulating lymphocytes with acinar epithelial cells found in the lacrimal gland has been established.[42] Further, this selective lymphocyte-acinar epithelial cell interaction extends to at least one other type of glandular tissue—salivary glands—although the pattern of interaction varies within salivary gland types. With respect to lacrimal glands, both B cells and T cells participate in this interaction. Current studies have centered on classifying the lymphocyte-lacrimal acinar epithelial cell interaction within the context of defined families of adhesion molecules. It appears that lymphocyte homing receptors, which mediate HEV binding, may be involved in binding to lacrimal tissue; although it is not yet clear if the lymph node homing receptor, Peyer patch homing receptor, or a distinct receptor is directly involved. Whereas the involvement of integrins or cartilage-link protein adhesion molecule families has not been ruled out, carbohydrate inhibition patterns are similar to those noted for HEV binding and are suggestive of a selectin interaction.[43] At present there is no definitive information regarding the nature of the acinar epithelial cell ligand or counter receptor.

IMMUNE REGULATION

Immune Potentiators

A variety of compounds have been employed to modulate immune responses in both humans and animal models. Nonspecific immune potentiators, or adjuvants, have been widely used to enhance antibody responses in vivo. Classical adjuvants are generally not host-derived, although subsequent sections will discuss host products that can exert regulatory adjuvant-like effects. Whereas the specific mechanisms responsible for response enhancement vary for each adjuvant and are often not well defined, they are thought to function by one or a combination of mechanisms. These include increasing the influx of inflammatory cells, promotion of antigen presentation, and increasing antigen uptake. With respect to mucosal adjuvants, cholera toxin has been studied in great detail.[29] Enhanced mucosal responses appear to depend on the binding of the B subunit of cholera toxin to the GM_1 ganglioside (which is displayed on the luminal surface of enterocytes) as well as on the toxin's modulatory effects on B cells, T cells, and antigen-presenting cells.[14] The toxin can function when it is delivered with antigen or as a carrier when conjugated to antigen. Presently, cholera toxin does not enhance lacrimal gland-mediated IgA antibody responses to antigen administered by the gastrointestinal route. The potential use of antigens conjugated to cholera toxin or its B subunit, administered by the gastrointestinal or conjunctival route, has yet to be fully investigated, however. Other mucosal adjuvants, such as avridine and muramyl tripeptide, have been administered with antigen by the conjunctival route.[45] Thus far, no enhancement of lacrimal gland-mediated IgA antibody responses has been noted.

Cytokines

Cellular growth and differentiation factors, collectively termed cytokines, clearly exert a variety of important regulatory effects on cells that participate in immune responses.[1,16] These factors are produced by many cell types, with those being produced by lymphoid cells classified as interleukins. The genes for many of the interleukins have been cloned and recombinant molecules are available in quantities that allow a detailed functional assessment. Certain cytokines, transforming growth factor-β (TGF-β), interleukin-5 (IL-5), and interleukin-6 (IL-6), augment in vitro IgA responses in murine B cell cultures and are thought to exert important regulatory influences on mucosal IgA responses.* TGF-β is believed to increase IgA synthesis by inducing B cells to switch to IgA production[10]; whereas IL-5 and IL-6 apparently induce IgA^+ B cells to terminally differentiate into IgA-producing plasma cells.[2,3] With respect to lacrimal glands, IL-5 and IL-6 specifically enhance IgA production in a rat in vitro lacrimal gland tissue fragment culture system.[48] Further, IL-5 and IL-6, in combination with antigen, enhance specific tear IgA antibody responses following topical administration to rat conjunctiva.[49] Presently, little is known regarding the mechanism of this enhancement and the regulatory role, as well as the therapeutic potential, of these interleukins (and other cytokines) needs to be fully explored.

Hormonal Regulation

Neuroendocrine products are involved in immune regulation. Recently, hormones and neural agonists have been

shown to exert significant modulatory influences on the mucosal system.[54] The effects of these molecules on lacrimal gland immunoregulation have been well documented in animal models.[56] In experimental animals sexual dimorphism and aging affect SC and IgA production.[57] Androgens increase SC biosynthesis in lacrimal gland acinar cell cultures, enhance the production of IgA in lacrimal tissue, and enhance IgA production in vivo. Evidence suggests that the effect on SC production involves hormonal association with specific receptors on lacrimal acinar cells and subsequent promotion of SC mRNA transcription and translation.[27] The mechanisms that control IgA biosynthesis remain unknown, although increased SC production appears to account for enhanced expression of IgA in tears. It is interesting to note that the effects on SC and IgA synthesis may be unique to lacrimal tissues. With respect to humans, gender differences have been noted, but the direct influence of androgens on SC and IgA production has yet to be documented.

Idiotypic Networks

It is now clear that the immune system encompasses a balanced network of lymphocyte clones that express antigen-specific receptors. Another class of molecules that is directly involved in immune regulation is antiidiotypic antibodies.[6,13,23] In general, antiidiotypic antibodies recognize determinants located in the variable regions of antigen-specific receptors on both B cells and T cells, as well as on antibodies. Although a number of antiidiotypic antibody subclasses have been defined, operationally and functionally, two major subclasses will be considered here: (1) antiidiotypic antibodies that recognize framework epitopes (Ab2α) and (2) antiidiotypic antibodies that recognize binding site epitopes in the antibody variable region (Ab2β). Fig. 10-7 provides a simplified schematic of the idiotype concepts relevant to the current discussion. Ab2α generally mark families of antibody molecules within inbred species and exert regulatory influences on the immune system. Ab2β carry the internal image of the antigen-reactive site of Ab1 and, under the appropriate conditions, are able to induce Ab3, which can interact with the original antigenic stimulus. The later subclass of antiidiotypic antibodies (Ab2β) has been of interest because it has the potential to be useful for vaccine purposes. With respect to the mucosal system, recent data indicate that mucosally targeted vaccination with antiidiotypic antibodies elicits protective salivary[25] and gastrointestinal responses.[28] Although recent unpublished evidence proposes that Ab2β (combining site-specific, internal image) applied topically to the conjunctiva can induce antigen-specific tear IgA responses comparable to those obtained with antigen, these data require confirmation. Finally, with respect to regulation, no information is currently available regarding the capacity of antiidiotypic antibodies to exert regulatory influences on the B and T cell compartments of the lacrimal gland.

---

*References 2, 3, 10, 11, 15, 22.

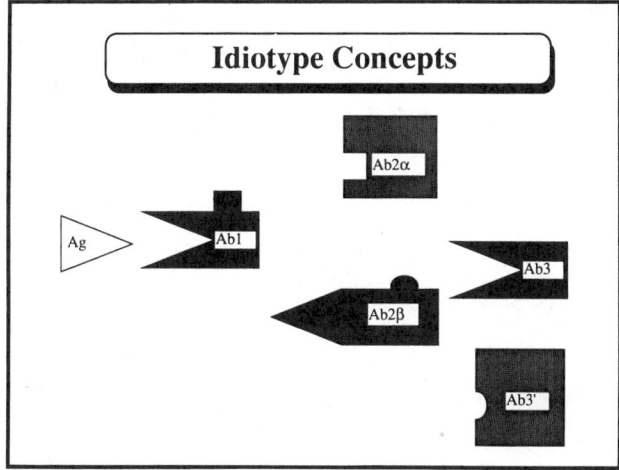

Fig. 10-7. Antigen *(Ag)* elicits antibody 1 *(Ab1).* Ab1 elicits Ab2α, which interacts with framework epitopes and Ab2β, which interacts with combining site epitopes. Ab2β elicits Ab3 and Ab3' in a similar fashion. Ab3 has the capacity to interact with the original antigenic stimulus. (From Montgomery PC, O'Sullivan NL, Martin LB, Skandera CA, Peppard JV, Pockley AG: *Regulation of lacrimal gland immune responses.* In Sullivan DA, editor: *The lacrimal gland, tear film and dry eye syndromes. Basic science and clinical relevance,* New York, 1994, Plenum).

Regulation of Immune Responses

The lacrimal gland is a functional effector site in the mucosal immune network. It is linked to the mucosal network through the emigration of B lymphocytes and T lymphocytes. B cell populations committed to IgA synthesis arrive from mucosal inductive sites and differentiate into IgA-producing plasma cells. T cell traffic to lacrimal glands also occurs, but the precise subset involvement remains to be defined. Lymphocyte retention in lacrimal gland tissue appears to be regulated by specific interactions with acinar epithelial cells. Recent research suggests that the regulation of immune responses in lacrimal tissues, like other compartments of the immune system, is subject to a variety of factors including: immune potentiators, cytokines, hormones, and idiotypic networks. Further investigation is required to determine the precise influence of these regulatory processes on the appearance of antibodies in tears and effector cells within lacrimal glands.

REFERENCES

1. Arai K, Lee F, Miyajima A, et al.: Cytokines: coordinators of immune and inflammatory responses, *Annu Rev Biochem* 59:783-836, 1990.
2. Beagley KW, Eldridge JH, Kiyuno H, et al.: Recombinant murine IL-5 induces high rate IgA synthesis in cycling IgA-positive Peyer's patch B cells, *J Immunol* 141:2035-2042, 1988.
3. Beagley KW, Eldridge JH, Lee F, et al.: Interleukins and IgA synthesis: human and murine interleukin 6 induce high rate IgA secretion in IgA-committed B cells, *J Exp Med* 169:2133-2148, 1989.
4. Bevilacqua MP: Endothelial-leukocyte adhesion molecules, *Annu Rev Immunol* 11:767-804, 1993.
5. Bienenstock J, Johnston N, Perey DYE: Bronchial lymphoid tissue. I. morphologic characteristics, *Lab Invest* 28:686-698, 1973.
6. Burdette E, Schwartz RS: Idiotypes and idiotypic networks, *N Engl J Med* 317:219-224, 1987.
7. Childers NK, Bruce MG, McGhee JR: Molecular mechanisms of immunoglobulin: a defense, *Annu Rev Microbiol* 43:503-536, 1989.
8. Chin YH, Sackstein R, Cai JP: Lymphocyte homing receptors and preferential migration pathways, *Proc Soc Exp Biol Med* 196:374-380, 1991.
9. Chodirker WB, Tomasi TB: Gammaglobulins: quantitative relationships in human serum and nonvascular fluids, *Science* 142:1080-1081, 1963.
10. Coffman RL, Lebman DA, Shrader B: Transforming growth factor β specifically enhances IgA production by lipopolysaccharide-stimulated murine B lymphocytes, *J Exp Med* 170:1039-1044, 1989.
11. Coffman RL, Shrader B, Carty J, et al.: A mouse T cell product that preferentially enhances IgA production. I. Biologic characterization, *J Immunol* 139:3685-3690, 1987.
12. Craig SW, Cebra JJ: Peyer's patches: an enriched source of precursors for IgA-producing immunocytes in the rabbit, *J Exp Med* 134:188-196, 1974.
13. Davie JM, Seiden MV, Greenspan NS, et al.: Structural correlates of idiotypes, *Annu Rev Immunol* 4:147-165, 1986.
14. Dertzbaugh MT, Elson CO: Cholera toxin as a mucosal adjuvant. In Spriggs DR, Koff WC, editors: *Topics in vaccine adjuvant research,* 119-131, Boca Raton, 1990, CRC Press.
15. Ehrhardt RO, Strober W, Harriman GR: Effect of transforming growth factor (TGF)-β1 on IgA isotype production, *J Immunol* 148:3830-3836, 1992.
16. Finkelman FD, Holmes J, Katona IM, et al.: Lymphokine control of *in vivo* immunoglobulin selection, *Annu Rev Immunol* 8:303-333, 1990.
17. Franklin RM: The ocular secretory immune system: a review, *Curr Eye Res* 8:599-606, 1989.
18. Franklin RM, Kenyon KR, Tomasi TB: Immunohistologic studies of human lacrimal gland: localization of immunoglobulins, secretory component and lactoferrin, *J Immunol* 110:984-992, 1973.
19. Franklin RM, McGee DW, Shepard KF: Lacrimal gland-directed B cell responses, *J Immunol* 135:95-99, 1985.
20. Franklin RM, Remus LE: Conjunctival-associated lymphoid tissue: evidence for a role in the secretory immune system, *Invest Ophthalmol Vis Sci* 25:181-187, 1984.
21. Gregory RL, Allansmith MR: Naturally occurring IgA antibodies to ocular microorganisms in tears saliva and colostrum: evidence for a common mucosal immune system and local immune response, *Exp Eye Res* 43:739-749, 1986.
22. Harriman GR, Kuminoto DY, Elliot JF, et al.: The role of IL-5 in IgA B cell differentiation, *J Immunol* 140:3033-3039, 1988.
23. Hiernaux JR: Idiotypic vaccines and infectious diseases, *Infect Immun* 56:1407-1413, 1988.
24. Iwamoto T, Jakobiec FA: A comparative ultrasound study of the normal lacrimal gland and its epithelial tumors, *Hum Pathol* 13:236-262, 1982.
25. Jackson S, Mestecky J, Childers NK, Michalek SM: Liposomes containing antiidiotypic antibodies: an oral vaccine to induce protective secretory immune responses specific for pathogens of mucosal surfaces, *Infect Immunity* 58:1932-1936, 1990.
26. Kaetzel CS, Robinson JK, Chintalacharuyu KR, et al.: The polymeric immunoglobulin receptor (secretory component) mediates transport of immune complexes across epithelial cells: a local defense function for IgA, *Proc Natl Acad Sci USA* 88:8796-8800, 1991.
27. Kelleher RS, Hann LE, Edwards JA, Sullivan DA: Endocrine, neural and immune control of secretory component output by lacrimal gland acinar cells, *J Immunol* 146:3405-3412, 1991.
28. Lucas GP, Cambiaso CL, Vaerman JP: Protection of rat intestine against cholera toxin challenge by monoclonal antiidiotypic antibody immunization via external and parenteral routes, *Infect Immun* 59:3651-3658, 1991.
29. Lycke N, Holmgren J: Strong adjuvant properties of cholera toxin on gut mucosal immune responses to orally presented antigens, *Immunology* 59:301-308, 1986.
30. Malaty R, Gebhardt BM, Franklin RM: HSV-specific IgA from tears blocks virus attachment to the cell membrane, *Curr Eye Res* 7:313-320, 1988.

31. Mazanec MB, Kaetzel CS, Lamm ME, et al.: Intracellular neutralization of virus by immunoglobulin A antibodies, *Proc Natl Acad Sci USA* 89:6901-6905, 1992.

32. Mazanec MB, Kaetzel CS, Nedrud JG, Lamm ME: New thoughts on the role of immunoglobulin A in mucosal immunity, *Mucosal Immunol Update* 1:1-15, 1993.

33. McGee DW, Franklin RM: Lymphocyte migration into the lacrimal gland is random, *Cell Immunol* 86:75-82, 1984.

34. McGhee JR, Mestecky J: In defense of mucosal surfaces: development of novel vaccines for IgA responses protective at the portals of entry of microbial pathogens, *Infect Dis Clin North Am* 4:315-341, 1990.

35. McGhee JR, Mestecky J, Dertzbaugh MT, et al.: The mucosal immune system: from fundamental concepts to vaccine development, *Vaccine* 10:75-88, 1992.

36. McGill J, Liakos GM, Goulding NJ, Seal DV: Normal tear protein profiles and age-related changes, *Br J Ophthalmol* 68:316-320, 1984.

37. Mestecky J, McGhee JR: Immunoglobulin A (IgA): molecular and cellular interactions involved in IgA biosynthesis and immune responses, *Adv Immunol* 40:153-245, 1987.

38. Mestecky J, McGhee JR, Arnold RR, et al.: Selective induction of an immune response in human external secretions by ingestion of bacterial antigen, *J Clin Invest* 6:731-737, 1978.

39. Montgomery PC, Ayyildiz A, Lemaitre-Coelho IM, et al.: Induction and expression of antibodies in secretions: the ocular immune system, *Ann NY Acad Sci* 409:428-439, 1983.

40. Montgomery PC, Majumdar AS, Skandera CA, Rockey JH: The effect of immunization route and sequence of stimulation on the induction of IgA antibodies in tears, *Curr Eye Res* 3:861-865, 1984.

41. Montgomery PC, Peppard JV, Skandera CA: Isolation and characterization of mononuclear cell populations from lacrimal glands. In Secchi AG, Fregona IA, editors: *Modern trends in immunology and immunopathology of the eye*, 339-343, Milan, 1989, Masson.

42. O'Sullivan NL, Montgomery PC: Selective interactions of lymphocyte with neonatal and adult lacrimal gland tissues, *Invest Ophthalmol Vis Sci* 31:1615-1622, 1990.

43. O'Sullivan NL, Raja R, Montgomery PC: Lymphocyte adhesive interaction with lacrimal gland acinar epithelium involves carbohydrate recognition. In Sullivan DA, editor: *The lacrimal gland, tear film and dry eye syndromes: basic science and clinical relevance*, New York, 1994, Plenum.

44. Owen RL, Jones AL: Epithelial cell specialization within human Peyer's patches: an ultrastructural study of intestinal lymphoid follicles, *Gastroenterology* 66:189-203, 1974.

45. Peppard JV, Mann RV, Montgomery PC: Antibody production in rats following ocular-topical or gastrointestinal immunization: kinetics of local and systemic antibody production, *Curr Eye Res* 7:471-481, 1988.

46. Peppard JV, Montgomery PC: Studies on the origin and composition of IgA in rat tears, *Immunology* 62:193-198, 1987.

47. Picker LJ, Butcher EC: Physiological and molecular mechanisms of lymphocyte homing, *Annu Rev Immunol* 10:561-591, 1992.

48. Pockley AG, Montgomery PC: The effects of interleukins 5 and 6 on immunoglobulin production in rat lacrimal glands, *Reg Immunol* 3:242-246, 1991.

49. Pockley AG, Montgomery PC: In vivo adjuvant effects of interleukins 5 and 6 on rat tear IgA antibody responses, *Immunology* 73:19-23, 1991.

50. Shabo AL, Kenyon KR, Franklin RM: Electron microscopic localization of a blood-tear barrier to tracer protein in the primate lacrimal gland, *Lab Invest* 28:185-193, 1973.

51. Shimizu Y, Newman W, Tanaka Y, Shaw S: Lymphocyte interactions with endothelial cells, *Immunol Today* 13:106-112, 1992.

52. Solari R, Kraehenbuhl JP: The biosynthesis of secretory component and its role in the transepithelial transport of IgA dimer, *Immunol Today* 6:17-20, 1985.

53. Stoolman LM: Adhesion molecules controlling lymphocyte migration, *Cell* 56:907-910, 1989.

54. Sullivan DA: Hormonal influence on the secretory immune system of the eye. In Frier S, editor: *The neuroendocrine-immune network,* Boca Raton, 1990, CRC Press.

55. Sullivan DA, Allansmith MR: Source of IgA in tears of rats, *Immunology* 53:791-799, 1984.

56. Sullivan DA, Allansmith MR: Hormonal influence on the secretory immune system of the eye: androgen modulation of IgA levels in tears or rats, *J Immunol* 134:2978-2982, 1985.

57. Sullivan DA, Allansmith MR: The effect of aging on the secretory immune system of the eye, *Immunology* 63:403-410, 1988.

58. Underdown BJ, Schiff JM: Immunoglobulin A: strategic defense initiative at the mucosal surface, *Annu Rev Immunol* 4:389-417, 1986.

59. Weisz-Carrington P, Roux ME, McWilliams M, et al.: Organ and isotope distribution of plasma cells producing specific antibody after oral immunization: evidence for a generalized secretory immune system, *J Immunol* 123:1705-1708, 1979.

11 Immunologic Basis of Uveitis

IGAL GERY, ROBERT B. NUSSENBLATT

Inflammatory diseases of the eye are commonly seen by the ophthalmologist. Fifty years ago most intraocular inflammatory diseases were thought to originate from an infectious agent—usually tuberculosis or syphilis.[89] Over the years the growing understanding of the complex ocular immune response has invalidated the aforementioned causes for intraocular inflammatory conditions. The role of the immune system in ocular inflammatory disorders—some caused by infectious agents, and others caused by putative autoimmune mechanisms—is clear but somewhat ill-defined.

This chapter summarizes the involvement of the immune system in uveitis in man and in animals. The latter studies have added remarkably to the knowledge of both the immunopathogenic processes that produce uveitis and the new approaches for their modulation.

IMMUNE SYSTEM IN HUMAN UVEITIS

Types of Hypersensitivity Responses

The immune response in humans has classically been divided into four major hypersensitivity responses. The type I response is mediated by IgE and is the main mechanism by which classic ocular allergy is mediated. The type II response is mediated by cytotoxic antibodies—antibodies that upon adhering specifically to a cell, either activate the complement cascade and puncture the cell membrane or consort with other cells to kill the target cell. It is assumed that some of the alterations to mucous membranes and the ocular surface in ocular pemphigoid are the result of this mechanism. The type III hypersensitivity is mediated via immune complex formation. Once thought to be the major cause of injury in ocular inflammatory diseases, this mechanism may be important in a more limited number of disorders including lens-induced uveitis, certain types of anterior uveitis, and perhaps the ocular manifestations of systemic collagen vascular disorders. The type IV hypersensitivity reaction is cell-mediated, meaning that T cells dominate the induction of the immune response. This mechanism has been intoned

for many disorders, including sarcoidosis and Behçet's syndrome.

It is clear that the pathogenic immune response is not necessarily relegated to only one type of hypersensitivity reaction, enabling histologic evidence of several mechanisms to be present. It is also certain, however, that a dominant mechanism can frequently be discerned, underscoring the importance of one mechanism over another. Such observations have practical implications, as therapies will become increasingly more specific, and the need to identify the dominant disease-causing mechanism will become even greater.

Tests to Evaluate the Immune System in Uveitis

Antibody Studies. Perhaps the most common tests determined the presence of antibodies that were directed against a specific organism or autoantigen. Several blood tests that demonstrate the role of the immune system in eye disease are used in the clinic. Possibly the best accepted is that of the toxoplasmosis titer. There has been an unconfirmed observation that antibodies to the early activation antigens of the Epstein-Barr virus have been associated with multifocal choroiditis.[211]

Autoimmunity is an accepted possible mechanism for a number of the diseases in man, including many diseases of the eye. Elevated levels of antibodies to bovine S-antigen (S-Ag) were found in patients with uveitis,[64,83] but later studies could not differentiate between uveitis patients and the controls in their levels of antibodies against retinal antigens.[58,72,98] Kasp and associates[111] reported that antibodies to S-Ag in sera of patients with retinal vasculitis exhibit lower affinity than those in control subjects.

The presence of autoantibodies against ocular antigens was shown by immunostaining techniques. Chan and associates[28] confirmed that sera of patients with the Vogt-Koyanagi-Harada (VKH) syndrome contain large amounts of antibodies that selectively bind to the outer portions of the

141

retina. Other disorders, such as Behçet's syndrome, also reveal a specific staining pattern.[28] It is of note that Behçet patients also produce an antibody that adheres to the lip of guinea pigs.[118,145] Research proposes that this antibody may not be as specific to Behçet's syndrome as initially thought, but may also be seen in other ocular inflammatory conditions.[70]

The presence of autoantibodies against nonocular antigens plays an important diagnostic role in some diseases. A classic finding would be a child with juvenile rheumatoid arthritis who does not have circulating rheumatoid factor, but who does have circulating antinuclear antibodies (ANA).[25] Similarly, the evaluation of a patient with the ocular manifestations of Wegener granulomatosis requires the search for antineutrophil cytoplasmic antibody located in the cytoplasm (cANCA).[214]

The interpretation, however, of the presence of circulating antibodies to organisms or antigens relevant to eye disease is difficult at best. Clearly, sensitization does not necessarily indicate participation in the disease process. Indeed, it could suggest even an epiphenomenon that occurred as a result of another process altogether. In an attempt to identify immune responses that may be particularly relevant to the eye, however, much work has centered on evaluating ocular fluids for the presence of antibody. The quotient used by Desmonts and associates[54] has become a standard way to evaluate the importance of antibodies in the eye. The underlying hypothesis is that if an infectious process is centered in the eye, for example, toxoplasmosis, then the relative amount of specific antibody in the eye will be higher than in the systemic circulation when compared to the total amount of immunoglobulin. This concept has been applied to putative viral infections in the eye as well. Employing this quotient, Kaplan and associates[107] submitted that several ocular inflammatory disorders are caused by the measles and zoster virus.

Immune Complexes. The mechanism of immune reactivity was implicated as one of the most important modes by which injury to ocular tissue occurred. The presence of circulating immune complexes has been reported in a number of diseases, including Behçet's syndrome,[126,165] and has been detected in the eye.[50,165] Other work suggests, however, that immune complexes may not play a pathogenic role and that, in fact, their presence in the blood of retinal vasculitis patients improves their visual outcome,[64,203] perhaps because of a certain protective value these complexes may have.

Cellular Immunity. The role of cell-mediated immune reactions in the pathogenesis of uveitis has been indicated mainly by four lines of indirect evidence:

1. Immunohistochemical examination has indicated that T cells accumulate in inflammatory sites of uveitic eyes.[30] Moreover, analysis of the lymphocyte subpopulations in eyes with sympathetic ophthalmia (SO) showed that, similar to the observation in rat eyes with experimental autoimmune uveoretinitis (EAU),[29] CD4 cells (the helper-inducer subset) were present in high proportions in Dalen-Fuchs nodules at the early phase of the disease, whereas CD8 lymphocytes (the suppressor-cytotoxic subset) were more numerous at the later phase.[30]

2. Cytokines that are specifically produced by T lymphocytes, such as interferon-gamma (IFN-γ) or interleukin (IL) -2, were found in inflammatory sites.[74,100]

3. The animal disease, EAU, that serves as a model for certain uveitic conditions in man, is mediated by T cells.

4. Patients with uveitis often exhibit increased activity of T lymphocytes that recognize uveitogenic antigens.[52,58,159] The recognition, routinely determined by the proliferative response of peripheral blood lymphocytes in vitro, is considered the equivalent of the in vivo anamnestic response. The increased activity, as compared to control groups, has been determined both by the higher proliferative response of whole lymphocyte cultures and by the elevated frequency of responsive cells.[53,168] The antigens used in these assays induce EAU in experimental animals, including primates,[69,160] and mainly include S-Ag and interphotoreceptor retinoid-binding protein (IRBP). Proliferative responses were also observed with uveitogenic peptides that were derived from the sequence of S-Ag or IRBP.[51,52] Of particular interest is the high percentage of patients with birdshot retinochoroidopathy that shows enhanced response to S-Ag.[162] Combined with the strong HLA association, this lymphocyte response makes this disease a prime candidate for an autoimmune entity.

Other Tests. As knowledge of the immune system increases, new assays become available to further analyze the immunologic changes that accompany the development of uveitis. Thus patients with uveitis differ from controls by several parameters including the level of soluble IL-2 receptor in the blood[6] and the increased expression of "activation markers" on T lymphocytes.[56]

Relationship Between HLA and Disease

The major histocompatibility complex (MHC), a group of genes located on chromosome 6 in humans, is a major factor controlling each individual's immune response. Therefore an attempt to demonstrate possible correlations between the MHC and disease entities was a logical approach.[209] Research of this kind (focusing on the eye) revealed that ocular disease is strongly associated with the MHC as well.

Significant levels of association were reported (1) between HLA-B27 and anterior uveitis among Caucasians,[11,158] (2) between DR-53 and VKH syndrome among Japanese,[166] and (3) between HLA-B51 and Behçet's patients from Japan and the Middle East (but not from Northern Europe).[27,148,149,167] Other associations were shown between VKH in Japan and class II antigens HLA-DR4, DRw53, and Dw15, and class I antigen HLA-Bw54.[166] The associations between VKH and antigens HLA-DR4 and DRw53 were also observed in the United States[42] and, in addition, Davis and associates[42] noted a close similarity between VKH and SO in their association with specific HLA antigens. S. Ohno's group reported that the frequency of HLA-DQw1 is significantly low among patients with Behçet's syndrome.[148]

The association of HLA and certain ethnic groups emphasizes the important role the genetic background of the patient plays in determining the immune response. Birdshot retinochoroidopathy is such an example. This disorder is associated with HLA-A29[4,162] and is found almost exclusively in Caucasians, particularly those of North European origin. The relative risk of this disorder is 80 to 100, indicating that a Caucasian who bears HLA-A29 has an 80 to 100 times greater chance of developing birdshot retinochoroidopathy than someone not bearing this antigen. Research has shown that two forms of the HLA-A29 antigen exist, and that one subgroup (that of HLA-A29.2 subtype) was associated with this disorder[207]; therefore the structural differences could explain the association between this antigen and this disease. Investigation has also shown, however, that the distribution of these subgroups is not equal in the general population and that patients with this entity can bear either subtype of HLA-A29.[55]

Expression of MHC Antigens and Adhesion Molecules in Uveitis

MHC class II gene products are normally expressed only on lymphoid cells that are involved in antigen presentation.[212] Under pathologic conditions, however, these molecules are also expressed by tissue resident cells,[212] presumably because of the effect of IFN-γ.[100] Expression of class II molecules on ocular resident cells was observed in uveitic conditions,[31,157] suggesting that these cells could present antigens to lymphocytes.[31,172]

Adhesion molecules play a pivotal role in both immune responses[202] and inflammatory processes.[169] Studies by Whitcup and associates revealed the increased expression of two adhesion molecules (LFA-1 and ICAM-1) in eyes with uveitis,[222] thus indicating that these proteins are involved in ocular inflammation. Moreover, interfering with these molecules inhibits uveitis in experimental animals and may offer a new approach for treatment of uveitis in man.

Immunosuppression of Uveitic Conditions

The immunosuppressive agents most readily available to the clinician are those that are the most nonspecific in their actions. Both corticosteroids and cytotoxic agents will have effects that go beyond the immune response, but the major therapeutic influence on an inflammatory condition is on the inflammatory cells involved in the disease. Indeed, the fact that these agents have a beneficial therapeutic effect on the group of diseases usually called "endogenous" uveitis is by itself evidence of the important role that the immune system plays in these diseases.

Compounds with selective effect toward immune cells were successfully applied for treatment of uveitis. The search for such compounds benefited from the availability of animal models for the human conditions; new drugs are routinely tested in animals prior to being applied for the human condition. The first of these selective drugs was cyclosporine.[163] This medication's effect is limited to those cells containing cyclophilin, a cytoplasmic-binding protein for the agent.[194] Though several cells have this binding protein, the practical clinical influence of cyclosporine is on T cells.[196] Cyclosporine has been used for the treatment of many human ocular inflammatory conditions, with numerous beneficial results, especially with Behçet's syndrome.[5,140,163]

The preceding findings can be considered more a beginning than an end. The relative success of cyclosporine points more to the fact that a standard has been established against which new medications can be effectively evaluated. It is in this context that FK506 was evaluated in the animal model, was found to be effective,[114] and is now being used in human studies.[153] Newer medications continue to be developed and evaluated.

Attempts at immunosuppression without the use of pharmacologic agents are being studied as well. Feeding of uveitogenic antigens has been extensively evaluated in the experimental uveitis model and has been found to effectively suppress disease. Following the success in a small pilot study, a randomized, masked clinical trial is now ongoing.

Autoimmune Processes in the Human Eye: Hypothetic Initiating Mechanisms

Although the concept of autoimmune-driven ocular disease is generally well accepted, little is known about the mechanisms that trigger the immunopathogenic process. Autoimmune disease may be caused by "forbidden clones" of lymphocytes,[87] which could initiate uveitic conditions. Supporting evidence for this notion has been provided by Ichikawa and associates,[104] who showed that spontaneous uveoretinitis may develop in nude mice that have been reconstituted with embryonic rat thymi. Moreover, the disease could be adoptively transferred to naive nude mice by CD4 lymphocytes.[104] The involvement of other mechanisms has been indicated by other animal models that are induced by immunization with ocular antigens. One such mechanism is tissue damage produced by mechanical injury (as in SO), or as consequence to infection (for example, toxoplasmosis). Although attempts to induce an experimental model for SO by injuring one eye have all failed, damage to the retina, by cryopexy, enhances EAU induction in rats.[43] In addition to compromising the blood-retina barrier[43] and exposing tissue antigens to the immune system, it is conceivable that tissue damage provokes modifications of autologous nonimmunogenic antigens, thus rendering them "foreign" and immunogenic. These notions are in accord with the finding that immune responses against retinal antigens often develop in patients with retinitis pigmentosa[13,156] or retinal detachment.[12]

The most common cause for tissue damage in the eye is microbial infection. In addition to causing damage, however, infectious agents may initiate autoimmunity through other effects. One such effect is the microbial *adjuvant* activity. Experimental autoimmune diseases are routinely induced by injecting uveitogenic antigens in emulsion with complete Freund adjuvant (CFA). The pivotal component of CFA, the mycobacterium, is a powerful stimulant for the immune system and triggers a massive production of cytokines.[155,226] At least one of the cytokines, IL-2, can initiate autoimmunity by stimulating *anergic* lymphocyte clones.[88] Another bacterial adjuvant, endotoxin, is also a potent inducer of cytokines[37] that interferes with tolerance induction.[171]

The mitogenic effect of certain microorganisms has been attributed to their *superantigenic* components. Superantigens are mitogenic to large subpopulations of lymphocytes[36] and are thought to trigger autoimmune processes.[36] Superantigens were found to stimulate immunopathogenicity,[173a] but their administration can also produce anergy[112] and even to inhibit the development of autoimmune diseases.[116,173a,186]

Another possible mechanism whereby microorganisms can initiate ocular autoimmunity is by the homology between the sequence of their proteins and the sequence of uveitogenic determinants of ocular antigens. Such sequence homology, or "mimicry," was found to exist between S-Ag and several microbial antigens.[200,201] Injection of the microbial molecules was found to induce uveitis in rats.[200,201] Although the mimicking peptides were active at exceedingly high doses, these observations suggest that mimicry may be one mechanism by which autoimmunity against ocular antigens is initiated.

UVEITIS IN EXPERIMENTAL ANIMALS

As mentioned previously, the notion that the majority of noninfectious uveitis in man is immune-mediated is supported by the fact that similar uveitic diseases can be induced in experimental animals by manipulation of their immune systems. These animal models for the human conditions have been used in studies aimed at learning about the pathogenesis of uveitis, as well as about procedures and agents that can modulate the inflammatory eye diseases.[19,68,78]

For the sake of simplicity, the experimental diseases are grouped here according to the procedure used for their induction. The relationship between the animal model and the human disease is indicated by their similar anatomic location, type of inflammation, or known cause.

Immunogenic Uveitis (Albumin-Induced Uveitis)

Immunogenic uveitis is an experimental disease that is induced by injecting a foreign antigen (usually albumin) into the vitreous of animals that have been hyperimmunized against that antigen.[101,131] The pathogenic mechanism of this disease is assumed to be identical to the one that mediates the Arthus skin response, that is, type III hypersensitivity or immune complex-mediated process. There is no known similar entity in humans but the pathogenic mechanism of this experimental disease resembles that of lens-induced endophthalmitis (see chapter 40).

Bacterial Product-Induced Uveitis

Uveitis in man is often associated with systemic disorders including Reiter syndrome, ankylosing spondylitis, juvenile rheumatoid arthritis, inflammatory bowel disease, and sarcoidosis.[181] Little is known about the pathogenic mechanisms of these diverse diseases, but bacterial infection has been proposed as a potential cause.[158,183] In support of this theory, it has been shown that inflammatory processes can be induced in the eyes of experimental animals by injection of bacteria or bacterial products. Several bacterial products have been used to induce uveitis in animals and the diseases are designated according to the injected product (for example, *endotoxin-induced uveitis (EIU)*). To unify these diseases, an integrating term has been proposed, *bacterial product-induced uveitis (BPIU)*.

BPIU: Induction Procedures. Whole bacteria were used in a few experiments to induce this disease, but two bacterial components have been used in the majority of studies: (1) muramyl dipeptide (MDP), a component of gram-positive bacteria[122,219] and (2) endotoxin, the lipopolysaccharide (LPS) component of gram-negative bacteria.[94,183] The bacteria and bacterial products induced uveitis either when they were injected into the eyeball, or systemically, by several different routes—intravenously, intraperitoneally, or subcutaneously. The experimental disease can be induced in several animals including rabbits,[122,123,182] rats of different inbred strains,[183] and mice [at least one strain (C_3H/HeN)].[109,208]

BPIU: Pathologic Changes. The clinical and histologic changes in the eyes of animals with BPIU are described in detail in several of the references at the end of this chapter.[39,99,122,183,219] In rabbits and rats the inflammatory changes localize mainly in the anterior segment and consist of inflammatory cell accumulation, as well as proteinaceous exudate. In addition, cellular infiltration may also be seen in these animals in the vitreous and choroid.[39,122] In the mouse, on the other hand, the inflammation is localized mainly in the posterior vitreous that surrounds the optic disc, and milder infiltration is seen in the anterior chamber.[109]

BPIU: Pathogenic Mechanisms. Inflammatory processes are mediated and regulated by complex circuits of cytokines.[3,218] Because bacterial products, such as LPS or MDP, are powerful inducers of cytokines,[37,57,217] it has been proposed that BPIU is mediated by locally produced cytokines.[99,184] This theory is in line with the following observations:

1. Bacterial products are localized in the eye—even when administered systemically.[102]
2. Several cytokines, such as IL-1, IL-6, IL-8, or tumor necrosis factor alpha (TNF-a), produce acute inflammatory reactions when injected into the eye.[9,71,99,123,184]
3. A correlation was found between the development of uveitis and the presence of IL-6 in the aqueous humor of rats that had been injected with LPS.[99]
4. Prior to the onset of uveitis, ocular resident cells express surface molecules that are induced by proinflammatory cytokines. These molecules include class II MHC gene products that are induced by IFN-γ[100,117] and adhesion molecules, such as ELAM-1 and ICAM-1,[221] that are expressed under the influence of IL-1 and TNF-α.[169]
5. Treatment of rats either with chlorpromazine (which inhibits the production and release of TNF-α[108]) or with antibodies against ICAM-1 significantly suppresses the development of EIU.[223] On the other hand, the involvement of cytokines, such as TNF or IL-1, in the pathogenesis of BPIU has been questioned in view of data showing that procedures that neutralize the systemic activities of these cytokines did not inhibit and even exacerbate the ocular inflammation of EIU.[109,182] These paradoxical observations are not understood, but they imply that the inflammatory processes within the eyeball differ from those in other tissues.

Other studies have shown the participation of inflammatory mediators, such as prostaglandin E2, thromboxane B2, leukotriene B4, substance P,[94] and phospholipase A2.[33] Accordingly, the inflammatory process can be inhibited by antiinflammatory agents, such as corticosteroids[10,117] or phospholipase A2 inhibitors.[33]

Lens-Induced Uveitis

Endophthalmitis phacoanaphylactica, or lens-induced uveitis, may develop following rupture of the lens capsule and is attributed to an autoimmune response against the lens proteins, the crystallins. This theory is in accord with the finding that a similar disease can be induced in animals by immunization against lens proteins and subsequent disruption of the lens capsule. The animal disease was introduced by Burky[18] and has been further developed by Marak and his associates,[136,137] who have produced two disease models in the rat—*experimental lens-induced granulomatous endophthalmitis* (ELGE) and *Arthus type of panophthalmitis* (AP). In both models the lens is punctured after hyperimmunization, with the difference being the antigen—allogeneic or syngeneic lens proteins are used in ELGE, whereas xenogeneic proteins are employed in AP.

Pathologic Changes in Lens-Induced Uveitis. The ocular inflammation in ELGE is less severe than in AP and more closely resembles the human disease. It is of interest that granulomata develop at later stages of both animal diseases.[136,137,170]

The Pathogenesis of Lens-Induced Uveitis. Marak's group proved that the inflammation in both the AP and ELGE models is a type III, Arthus-like reaction that is mediated by antigen-antibody complexes and the complement cascade.[134,135,138] This theory was further corroborated by other studies.[79,170]

The granulomatous nature of the lens-induced uveitis is of interest because granuloma formation is usually the result of cellular immune responses.[174] Yet granulomata are often seen in eyes at sites of damaged membranes.[97] It is conceivable, therefore, that the granulomata in ELGE and AP are formed in response to the damaged lens capsule.

Experimental Autoimmune Uveitic Diseases

As mentioned earlier, the theory that autoimmune processes play a pathogenic role in certain uveitic conditions is in accord with the observation that inflammatory diseases may be induced in animals by immunization with ocular-specific antigens. These diseases are designated and divided according to the affected ocular tissues.

Experimental Autoimmune Anterior Uveitis (EAAU). In a recent series of elegant studies, Broekhuyse and associates[15,16,17] described a new experimental autoimmune disease that affects mainly the anterior segment. The disease, EAAU, supports the theory that autoimmune processes may be involved in the pathogenesis of anterior uveitis in man. This disease has also been termed *experimental melanin-protein-induced uveitis (EMIU),*[33a] or *experimental allergic ivitis (EAI).*[106a]

Induction of EAAU. The molecule that induces EAAU has not been defined except for its association with melanin granules. EAAU-inducing preparations have been isolated from several bovine ocular tissues including the retinal pigment epithelium (RPE), the iris and choroid, and the skin.[16,17] Uveitogenic preparations were also isolated from tissues of other species, including humans.[16] EAAU is readily induced in Lewis rats by immunization with the antigen emulsified in CFA, or Hunter adjuvant, along with pertussis toxin.[17] Disease was induced with the melanin-associated protein at a dose as low as 1μg/rat.[15]

EAAU: Pathologic Features. Clinical changes in EAAU include hyperemia and lesions in the iris, pupil constriction, and flare and cells in the aqueous.[17] The histopathologic changes are characterized by infiltration of the ciliary body and iris with mononuclear (MNL) and polymorphonuclear (PMN) leukocytes, and exudate of protein and cells in the anterior and posterior chambers[17] (Fig. 11-1). In severe cases, mild choroiditis also develops.[15] Significantly, essentially no involvement of the retina is observed in eyes with EAAU, in contrast to the heavy involvement of the retina in rats with retinal antigen-induced EAU.

EAAU: Pathogenic Mechanisms. Like EAU, EAAU is mediated by T cells, as evidenced by the findings that the disease can be adoptively transferred by sensitized CD4 lymphocytes,[15] but not by hyperimmune serum,[15] and is inhibited by cyclosporine.[17]

Of particular interest is the relationship between the localization of the uveitogenic antigen and the inflammatory lesions in rats with EAAU. It is of note that the affected tissues in the albino Lewis rat contain no pigment. On the other hand, rats immunized with RPE or choroidal preparations develop minimal or no inflammation in these tissues.[16,17] The latter observation was hypothetically attributed by Broekhuyse and associates[16] to low expression of MHC class II antigens on cells of these tissues. These facts support the theory that the localization of inflammation is determined to a large extent by the expression of adhesion molecules, in particular on endothelial cells (unpublished data).

Experimental Autoimmune Posterior Uveitis (EAPU). Broekhuyse and associates[14] described an experimental disease in rats that is sufficiently different from other autoimmune uveitic diseases. The disease, EAPU, is induced in Lewis rats by immunization with PEP-65, a protein isolated from the RPE. EAPU is characterized by granulomatous lesions, along one or both sides of Bruch's membrane, that resemble Dalen-Fuchs nodules and by vitreous cell infiltration. EAPU also differs from the typical EAU, induced by S-Ag or IRBP, by its chronicity and lack of pineal involvement. Yet as discussed in the following section, the inflammatory changes of EAU may vary remarkably when uveitic challenges of different intensities are used. More investigation is needed, therefore, to further define the uniqueness of EAPU.

Experimental Autoimmune Uveoretinitis (EAU). EAU has been the animal disease model used in the great majority of studies that investigated pathogenic autoimmune processes in the eye. As mentioned earlier, the assumption that autoimmunity plays an important role in the pathogenesis of certain uveitic conditions in man is supported by the findings that (1) a large portion of these patients exhibit immune responses against retinal-specific antigens, and (2) immunization with these antigens produces uveitic changes in animals that resemble those seen in human diseases. The following text summarizes information on these antigens and the diseases they induce in animals.

Uveitogenic Antigens of the Retina. Extensive studies in the last two decades have identified three major retinal antigens with uveitogenic capacity—S-Ag, IRBP, rhodopsin, and recoverin. These proteins selectively localize in the retina and the other vision-associated organ, the pineal gland. An additional retinal protein, phosducin, has been reported to be uveitogenic.[63]

S-Antigen (S-Ag). S-Ag is a highly conserved protein that is found in photoreceptor cells in the eyes of a very wide range of species including invertebrates such as starfish, scallop, or Drosophila.[129,147] S-Ag has been identified as the "48K" retinal protein or "arrestin"—a molecule that is believed to have a pivotal regulatory role in vision—by competing with transducin for photoexcited and phosphorylated rhodopsin.[173,197] The biophysical and immunologic properties of S-Ag have been thoroughly reviewed,[79,197] so this chapter will focus on studies in which the submolecular components of this protein have been analyzed. T lymphocytes recognize proteins in the form of peptides that are associated with MHC molecules[195] and thus, much research has been done to identify the peptide determinants of S-Ag that are uveitogenic in animals and those that are recognized by lymphocytes from patients with uveitis. In early studies, L. Donoso and his associates[60] found that two peptides, derived from S-Ag sequences and designated "M" and "N," are uveitogenic in Lewis rats and other animals.[199] Both peptides, however, were uveitogenic only at doses much higher (on a molar basis) than those of whole S-Ag and do not play any significant role in the EAU-inducing activity of this protein. Later studies, on the other hand, have identified

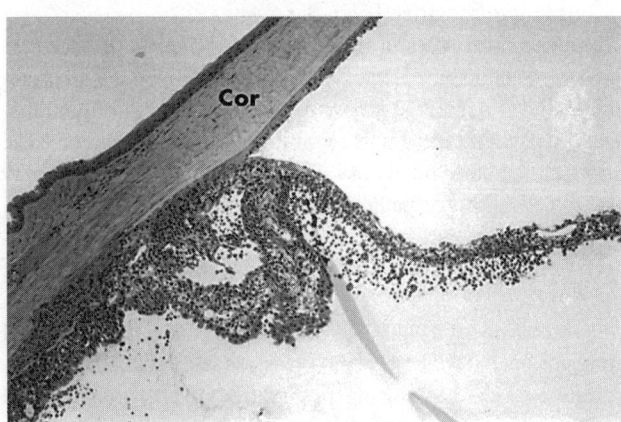

Fig. 11-1. Histopathologic changes in a Lewis rat eye with EAAU. The eye was obtained 15 days after immunization with 50 μg bovine melanin[14] in Hunter adjuvant, along with 10^{10} *B. pertussis* bacteria. The changes mainly include infiltration with inflammatory cells in the iris, ciliary body, and trabecular meshwork. In addition, inflammatory cells are adhered to the corneal endothelium. Cor, cornea (Hematoxylin and eosin ×100). By courtesy of Dr. C.-C. Chan.

two other sequences of S-Ag (333-352 and 352-364) that were uveitogenic in Lewis rats at submicrogram doses and are believed to be the major uveitogenic determinants in this rat strain.[85,144] The two latter peptides are also recognized by lymphocytes of rats that were immunized against whole S-Ag and can be defined, therefore, as "immunodominant."[8,77]

S-Ag peptides were also found to be stimulatory for lymphocytes both from patients with uveitis[51,52] and those following laser photocoagulation.[216] Significantly, most patients responded to more than one peptide and often the responses to peptides were higher than those against the whole S-Ag protein.[51,52]

Interphotoreceptor Retinoid-Binding Protein (IRBP). IRBP, a glycoprotein of approximately 140 KDa, is the major soluble protein of the interphotoreceptor matrix of vertebrate retinas and is assumed to function in the transport of retinoids between the neural retina and the RPE.[26] IRBP is highly uveitogenic in Lewis rats,[80] monkeys,[97] rabbits,[67] and mice,[23] but, unlike S-Ag, is poorly uveitogenic in guinea pigs.[215] Similar to S-Ag, IRBP is also found in the pineal glands of vertebrates,[180] and animals that have been immunized with IRBP usually develop pinealitis as well.[23,80,97]

Several determinants have been identified in the IRBP sequence that show uveitogenic capacity in Lewis rats. Donoso and associates[61] investigated the human IRBP molecule by testing 120 overlapping peptides, corresponding to the entire 1262 amino acid sequence of the protein. Five of the peptides were uveitogenic, with one of these—at sequence 521-540—being active at doses as low as 0.1 μg/rat. A second group used another approach, that is, testing peptides that were selected from the bovine IRBP sequence for their high amphipathicity.[188,189] Of the ten selected peptides, three were uveitogenic in Lewis rats: 1091-1115,[121] 1158-1180,[188] and 1169-1191.[189] Two of these peptides, 1158-1180 and 1169-1191, were also found to be uveitogenic in primates.[190] Of particular interest is peptide 1169-1191. This peptide is uveitogenic in Lewis rats at the exceedingly low dose of 0.01 nmol/rat,[189] which is only approximately five-fold higher than the minimal uveitogenic dose of whole IRBP[73] and is much smaller than the uveitogenic doses of the other IRBP-derived peptides.[132,188] This potency of peptide 1169-1191 is assumed to be related to the fact that it is an immunodominant determinant of IRBP in Lewis rats. The immunodominance of peptides is thought to be determined in part by their high affinity toward the MHC molecules on antigen-presenting cells (APC).[8,132] In line with this assumption, peptide 1169-1191 exhibits a strong affinity, as indicated by its capacity to stimulate sensitized lymphocytes at concentrations much lower than those needed for other IRBP-derived peptides.[132]

Testing truncated forms of peptide 1169-1191 revealed that the immunodominance and other activities of this determinant reside within the nonamer 1182-1190, with the smallest form to exhibit the maximum potency of the peptide being 1179-1191.[120] The IRBP molecule exhibits a fourfold repeat structure with partial homology in the amino acid sequence of the four repeats.[26,119] Two of the repeats of 1179-1191, peptides 271-283 and 880-892, were also found to be uveitogenic.[119]

Rhodopsin. Rhodopsin, a glycoprotein with a molecular weight of ~40 KDa that plays a crucial role in vision, is present in large amounts in the retina and meets all criteria for being an organ-specific antigen. Yet rhodopsin is poorly uveitogenic in animals and its capacity to induce EAU had been in doubt for some time.[78] Its uveitogenicity has been clearly established only in recent years, when highly purified rhodopsin became available. Rhodopsin induces EAU in Lewis rats when injected at the relatively high doses of 50 to 100 mg/rat[192]; these doses are higher by two orders of magnitude than the minimal uveitogenic doses of S-Ag or IRBP.[73] Schalken and associates[193] later confirmed that rhodopsin is also uveitogenic in primates and produces severe chorioretinitis with concomitant anterior uveitis. These scientists also proved that rhodopsin is more pathogenic than opsin, both in the Lewis rat[192] and in monkeys.[193] Adamus, Moticka, and their associates[1] identified several peptide determinants of rhodopsin that are uveitogenic in Lewis rats.

Recoverin. This ~23 KDa calcium-binding protein was recently found to be highly uveitogenic in rats, producing severe EAU as well as pinealitis at doses as low as 10 μg per rat.[77a] This observation is of interest since recoverin was also identified as the target for the putative pathogenic autoimmune process of cancer-associated retinopathy.[208a]

EAU: Pathologic Changes. Analysis of the inflammatory changes in eyes of animals with EAU has revealed that the pattern of disease is affected by the animal species, as well as by the strength of the uveitogenic challenge.

The variability among species is well depicted by comparing the changes characteristic for IRBP-induced EAU in rats and primates. In Lewis rats the disease is acute, usually developing 8 to 12 days postimmunization (p.i.) and subsiding within 5 to 10 days thereafter.[80] In primates, on the other hand, the earliest signs of IRBP-induced EAU were detected 3 weeks p.i. and the inflammatory process continued for at least 6 months.[97] The two species also differ by the typical histopathologic changes in the affected eyes. In the Lewis rat the inflammation localizes mainly in the anterior segment and the retina, with minimal involvement of the choroid[80] (Fig. 11-2). In contrast, in primates the choroid is the tissue most affected[97] (Fig. 11-3), whereas the retina is involved to a lesser degree and minimal or no inflammation is found in the anterior segment.[97] In addition, the inflammation in the Lewis rat is of the "acute" type, with many PMN leukocytes,[80] whereas in primates the inflammation is "chronic," with many granulomata.[97]

The effect of the potency of the uveitogenic challenge was clearly demonstrated in mice that had been injected with

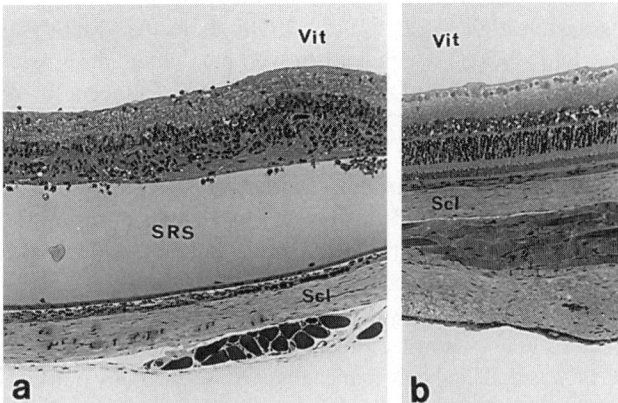

Fig. 11-2. IRBP-induced EAU in the Lewis rat. **A,** Histopathologic changes in the posterior segment of an eye obtained 16 days after immunization with 30 μg bovine IRBP in CFA, along with 10^{10} B. pertussis bacteria.[79] The retina is severely detached and infiltrated with inflammatory cells. The photoreceptor cell layer is virtually destroyed. Fibrinous exudate with some inflammatory cells is present in the subretinal space (SRS). The choroid is only minimally infiltrated. **B,** A control normal eye. Vit, vitreous; Scl, sclera (Hematoxylin and eosin ×150).

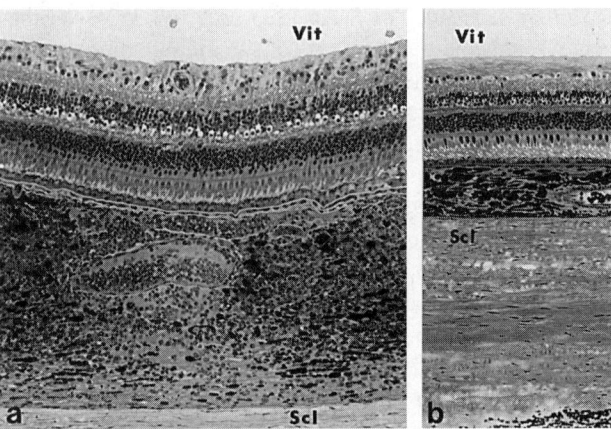

Fig. 11-3. IRBP-induced EAU in a monkey eye. **A,** Histopathologic changes in the posterior segment of an eye of a cynomolgus monkey that has been immunized with bovine IRBP (Monkey #M683 in reference 97). The main changes are seen in the choroid, which is remarkably thickened and heavily infiltrated with inflammatory cells (mainly MNLs). The section also shows an engorged vein in the choroid. The retina is much less involved, with mild edema and slight inflammatory infiltration, mainly in the ganglion cell layer. A few cells are also seen in the vitreous. **B,** A section of a control normal monkey eye. Vit, vitreous; Scl, sclera (Hematoxylin and eosin ×150).

different amounts of IRBP and pertussis toxin.[32] Animals that had been challenged with high doses of both agents developed an acute disease, with an early onset and short duration; whereas lower doses of IRBP or the toxin induced a chronic form of EAU, with a late onset and extended duration. Moreover, the potency of the challenge also affected the type of histopathologic changes: mice injected with high doses of IRBP and pertussis toxin developed changes similar to those regularly seen in rats with IRBP-induced EAU, that is, extensive serous retinal detachment and diffuse photoreceptor cell damage. On the other hand, immunization with lower doses produced focal photoreceptor damage, retinal vasculitis, choroidal thickening, and mild uveitis.[32] It is noteworthy that these recent observations with mice closely resemble the finding of Rao and associates[175] that different patterns of EAU develop in guinea pigs that have been immunized with different doses of S-Ag. In Lewis rats, reducing the dose of S-Ag or IRBP delays the onset of disease and reduces its severity,[73] but does not modify the acute type of inflammation. Granulomatous inflammation can be induced in Lewis rats, however, by using molecules that are weakly uveitogenic, such as IRBP peptide 1158-1180.[188]

EAU: Pathogenic Mechanisms. Studies in the last decade have defined EAU to be a T cell-mediated (type IV) immunopathogenic process.[19,78] As in the following discussion, this is a highly complex process, involving numerous cells and their products.

Possible Roles of Antibodies. Antibodies against ocular antigens probably do not play any direct pathogenic role in EAU.[78] de Kozak and associates[44] determined, however, that IgE antibodies could be involved in the early phase of the process by activating mast cells. In addition, Kasp and associates[110] presented data suggesting that circulating immune complexes play regulatory and pathogenic roles in EAU.

Mast Cells in EAU. Several lines of evidence indicate that mast cells play an important role in the EAU process:

1. A good correlation was found between the susceptibility of rat inbred strains to EAU and the number of mast cells in the animals' choroid,[150] iris, and ciliary body.[127]
2. The number of choroidal mast cells increases in rat eyes 5 to 6 days after immunization with S-antigen.[44]
3. A massive mast cell degranulation develops 1 or 2 days prior to the onset of EAU.
4. EAU development can be attenuated by drugs that affect mast cells.[45]

Lymphocytes in EAU. The pivotal role of T lymphocytes in the pathogenesis of EAU is well established. This has been shown indirectly by the reduced capacity to develop EAU in animals in which the T cell population was depleted or suppressed.[161,187] Direct evidence for the T cell function has been provided by the finding that these lymphocytes can adoptively transfer EAU into naive recipients. The adoptive transfer of disease can be achieved with either donor-supplied lymphocytes that have been sensitized with uveitogenic antigens,[141,151] or cell line lymphocytes that have been sensitized against uveitogenic antigens.[22,103] The cell lines consist of relatively homogenous populations and thus, they could be used to collect information concerning the lymphocytes that induce EAU. These cells express on their surface the CD4 molecule and the marker for the helper-inducer subset, and they exhibit high levels of MHC restriction in their interaction with APC.[22,103] In addition, uveitogenic cell lines selectively express certain T cell receptor (TCR) gene products: all S-Ag specific uveitogenic cell lines express the Vβ8.2 gene product, whereas nonuveitogenic lines usually do not.[65,86] Lymphocyte lines specific toward IRBP, on the other hand, express the Vβ8.3 gene product as well.[66] The relationship between the expression of these TCR components and the immunopathogenicity of lymphocytes is not clear, but it is of note that Vβ8.2 is also selectively expressed by lymphocytes capable of inducing another disease—experimental allergic encephalomyelitis (EAE).[92] Moreover, in a recent study, Egwuagu and associates[66a,133] found that lymphocytes that express Vβ8.2 accumulate in rat eyes with S-Ag-induced EAU in proportions much higher than in the peripheral blood of these animals; whereas lymphocytes that express both Vβ8.2 and Vβ8.3 selectively accumulate in eyes with IRBP-induced EAU.

Cytokines and Adhesion Molecules in EAU. Researchers have underscored the complexity of the type IV immune response and have identified some of its major participants. This process is reviewed in more detail in this volume by R. Hendricks (Chapter 6). The process is initiated by CD4 T lymphocytes that exert their effect by releasing several cell products—cytokines—that affect various other cells, some of which add to the cascade by releasing their own cytokines. The cytokines that play major roles in the process include IFN-γ, TNF-α, IL-1, IL-2, IL-6, and IL-8. These cytokines recruit inflammatory cells and stimulate them, as well as tissue resident cells, to express (on their surface) adhesion molecules that promote the interaction between the different cells of the inflammatory process. Of particular importance are the adhesion molecules that facilitate the interaction between leukocytes and endothelial cells, in particular LFA-1, VLA-4, and Mac-1 on the lymphoid cells and their counter ligands—ICAM-1, ICAM-2, VCAM-1, and ELAM-1 on the endothelial cells.[169]

The participation of cytokines in EAU has not been completely analyzed yet, but data accumulating so far have documented the increased expression of IL-2, IL-4 lymphotoxin, and IFN-γ.[34,35] It is noteworthy that antibodies against IFN-γ were found to exacerbate the disease,[20] despite the presumed local effect of IFN-γ of augmenting the expression of MHC antigens.[90,124,125] Information also becomes available concerning adhesion molecules in the EAU process: increased expression of ICAM-1, LFA-1, and Mac-1 has been observed in eyes that are developing EAU.[224] Moreover, the expression of ICAM-1 was found to precede by a few days the earliest detectable inflammatory process, and treatment with antibodies effectively inhibited the development of disease in experimental animals.[224]

Expression of MHC Antigens in EAU. The MHC antigens play a major role in the immune system by enabling the interaction between T lymphocytes and their target antigenic peptides.[195] MHC class I antigens are found on virtually all nucleated cells, whereas the class II antigens are normally expressed only on "professional" APC of hematopoietic lineage. Class II antigens are expressed, however, on nonhematopoietic cells following certain stimuli, in particular exposure to IFN-γ.[212] Class II antigens were detected on many ocular cells in animals that were injected with IFN-γ,[90,124,125] or in those that were developing EAU.[75] Little is known, however, about the function of these cells. It has been speculated that cells of RPE or vascular endothelium may actually present autologous peptides to T lymphocytes and thus, may be active participants in the immunopathogenic process of EAU.[75,172] This assumption has been challenged, however, by later studies showing that these cells function poorly as APC (as compared to professional APC) and may even be inhibitory to lymphocytes.[93] Moreover, a theory has been put forward suggesting that class II-expressing resident cells play a regulatory role by inhibiting the disease that induces T lymphocytes.[20,21,93]

EAU: The Hypothetic Early Immunopathogenic Events. Whereas the inflammatory process of EAU is quite well understood, little is known about the initial immunologic reaction that actually triggers this response. It has been hypothesized that the immunopathogenic process is initiated by a few sensitized lymphocytes that randomly circulate through the eye and interact there with "professional" APC that process the retinal antigens and present uveitogenic peptides in combination with class II MHC antigen. Hickey and associates[95] provided data to propose that such a process initiates EAE, and the presence of professional APC in the eye was shown by McMenamin and associates.[142] Following stimulation, the T lymphocytes trigger the cascade of events of EAU by releasing cytokines (mentioned earlier). A major component of the pathogenic process is the invasion of recruited inflammatory cells into ocular tissues. This process critically depends on the interaction between complementary adhesion molecules on the inflammatory cells and the vascular endothelium, as well as on structural changes in the endothelium. Studies by McMenamin and associates[143] and by L. E. Casper-Velu (personal communication) determined that the endothelium of retinal venules undergoes profound changes, in particular a significant increase in thickness. The venules with thickened endothelium resemble the characteristic high-endothelium venules of lymph nodes[143] and probably serve as the entry site for the recruited inflammatory cells. Indeed, Casper-Velu and associates[18a] noted the attachment of lymphocytes to the thickened endothelium and Greenwood and associates[82a] observed the actual penetration of lymphocytes through these endothelial cells in rat eyes that were developing EAU.

Several investigators examined the blood-retina barrier

(BRB) in rats with EAU. A breakdown of BRB was clearly seen in eyes at advanced inflammatory stages,[130] but, unlike the observation in EAE,[41,106] no increased BRB permeability was detected prior to lymphocytic infiltration.[130]

Immunosuppression of EAU. As mentioned previously, EAU has been extensively used in studies aimed at testing drugs and other agents for their capacity to inhibit or modulate immune-mediated inflammatory eye diseases. Using agents of known mode of action has also provided information on the pathogenic mechanisms of EAU and, by implication, of related diseases in humans.[20]

Antiinflammatory and Immunosuppressive Drugs. Like other immune-mediated inflammatory conditions, EAU is inhibited by antiinflammatory agents such as corticosteroids,[152] antioxidants,[47,176] or cytotoxic compounds like cyclophosphamide.[152,206] EAU has been particularly useful for testing drugs with selectivity toward T lymphocytes, for example, cyclosporine,[152,161] FK-506,[114] and rapamycin.[179] Significantly, these drugs inhibit both the afferent and efferent limbs of the immune response[114] and can be used for treatment of animals even when given at postimmunization intervals.[114,161] EAU has also been used to show the effect of the chimeric toxin IL-2-PE40 that selectively affects activated T cells.[178] EAU has been employed to test the activity of experimental compounds such as mycophenolate mofetil,[81] linomide,[198] or the synergism between drugs of different modes of action.[139]

Antibodies Against Cellular Components. EAU can be inhibited by treatment with antibodies against a variety of components of cells that participate in the immunopathogenic process of this disease. Active antibodies in this system include those against CD4,[2] class II MHC antigen,[177,220] IL-2 receptor,[96] TCR,[154] and adhesion molecules ICAM-1 and LFA-1.[224] The inhibitory activity of these antibodies could be attributed to masking essential molecules or eliminating cells that express these molecules.

Manipulation of the Idiotypic Network. Immune responses against idiotypes on antibodies or T cell receptors are a natural regulatory mechanism of the immune response.[105,185] This immunoregulatory system has been used by deKozak and her colleagues[46] to achieve suppression of EAU in rats and guinea pigs by immunization with a monoclonal antibody (mAb) against an epitope of S-antigen. The suppression could be adoptively transferred by lymphocytes that are assumed to be specific against the idiotype.[48] Yet the mechanism of suppression is not completely understood and could be attributed at least in part to the sequence homology between the S-antigen peptide that is the target for the mAb and the cytokine TNF-α.[49]

Immunization against idiotypes on TCR has been applied for inhibition of several experimental autoimmune diseases.[38,128] The procedure, termed *vaccination,* consists of immunization against the specific immunopathogenic lymphocytes at subpathogenic numbers or in inactive forms.[38]

Vaccination against a uveitogenic cell line was found by Beraud and associates[7] to partially inhibit EAU that was induced by the same line.

Another approach for vaccination[213] consists of immunization against peptide determinants that are derived from the sequence of the Vβ8.2 component of TCR, which is selectively used by most lymphocytes that produce EAE.[92] As mentioned earlier, most uveitogenic cell lines also express the Vβ8.2 molecule, but a trial in which the procedure of Vandenbark and associates[213] was used yielded equivocal results, thus casting doubt as to the usefulness of this procedure for inhibition of EAU.[113]

Antigen-Specific Immunosuppression. Selective unresponsiveness, or "tolerance," toward immunopathogenic antigens is the most desirable approach for immunosuppression of autoimmune diseases and has been successfully used for inhibition of EAU. This disease can be suppressed (1) by exposing naive animals to the antigens that are in *tolerogenic* form (in aqueous solution),[191] or that are attached to chemically-modified splenocytes,[62] or (2) by administering the antigens via tolerogenic routes (the alimentary canal)[84,164,210] or the anterior chamber.[91] The uveitogenic antigens used in these studies have included S-Ag, IRBP, or peptides that were derived from their sequence.[84,210]

The mechanisms involved in induction of unresponsiveness by the various procedures are not completely clear. Because immunologically mature animals are used in all procedures cited previously, it is assumed that extrathymic mechanisms are involved, namely, clonal anergy and activation of suppressor cells. The participation of both anergy and suppressor cells has been shown in animals that were rendered unresponsive by feeding,[84] and antigens that were injected into the anterior chamber provoke the well-analyzed phenomenon of *anterior chamber-associated immune deviation* (ACAID).[205] A cytokine, TGF-β, plays a major role in both the feeding[146] and ACAID[205] procedures.

Natural Immunosuppressive Mechanisms. Accumulating data show that the eye is protected from destructive immune-mediated inflammation by naturally occurring mechanisms. These mechanisms have been best analyzed in the anterior segment, where immunosuppressive substances have been detected[40,82,205] and the tolerance-inducing ACAID phenomenon is triggered by immunogens.[205] In addition, several resident ocular cells have been found to be inhibitory toward lymphocytes and are believed to exert immunosuppression effects in vivo as well. These cells include Muller cells,[21] ciliary body epithelial cells,[93] iris-ciliary body parenchymal cells,[204] corneal fibroblasts,[59] and corneal endothelial cells.[115]

Immunogenetics of EAU. Rats. Rats of different inbred strains were found to profoundly differ in their susceptibility to EAU induction.[73,127,150,206] It is noteworthy that a good correlation was observed between the susceptibility of rat strains to EAU that was induced by S-antigen or IRBP, as well as between the susceptibility to these diseases and to another experimental disease, experimental allergic encephalomyelitis.[73] The susceptibility to EAU is assumed to be affected by the MHC gene products, but other factors also play a role, as shown by the low susceptibility of the Fischer (F344) rats that share the RT1[l] gene with the highly susceptible Lewis or CAR strains.[73] Other factors include the number of mast cells in ocular tissue[127,150] or the hormonal balance, in particular of the hypothalamic-pituitary-adrenal axis.[76]

Mice. The relationship between susceptibility to EAU and the genetic makeup has been thoroughly studied by R. Caspi and her colleagues[23,24] in the mouse. Using a large number of haplotypes, these investigators showed that IRBP-induced EAU develops particularly well in strains of the H-2^k haplotype and to lesser degrees in the H-2^r, H-2,^{b} and H-2^d haplotypes. In addition, the susceptibility was mapped to the I-A subregion of the H-2^k, and the I-E^k gene product was found to have an ameliorating effect on the disease. Testing strains with the same H-2 on different backgrounds has shown, however, that the final expression of EAU in susceptible haplotypes is largely determined by background, non-MHC genes. Thus the strains that showed the highest susceptibility were those with the B10 background; lower levels of susceptibility were observed in strains with the A or LP backgrounds. Caspi and associates[24] have speculated that the level of permissiveness of the genetic background is a complex balance of factors such as hormonal interplay, mast cell numbers, and responses to lymphokines.

CONCLUDING REMARKS

Although there is compelling evidence to support the theory regarding the involvement of immune mechanisms in uveitis, several issues remain to be further addressed. These issues include the following:

1. The role of microbial factors in initiating uveitis should be further analyzed in both animals and humans, mainly with regard to their capacity to trigger cytokine production and to initiate autoimmunity.
2. The accumulating data concerning the putative involvement of autoimmunity in uveitis in humans meets and even exceeds the four ''postulates'' put forward by Witebsky[225] to indicate the autoimmune nature of human diseases. Yet additional pieces of information are still needed to ascertain this theory. In particular, more investigation is needed with regard to (1) the ocular antigens and their peptide determinants that are the actual target for the putative pathogenic autoimmune processes and (2) the characteristics of the disease-inducing lymphocytes, mainly concerning their clonality and selective usage, if any, of TCR gene products.
3. The factors and mechanisms that regulate the inflammatory process in the eye are not fully known. In particular, useful information is to be yielded by studies that analyze the recruitment of inflammatory cells and the interaction between these cells and vascular endothelium.
4. Despite recent advances in immunosuppression, the available modalities for the treatment of uveitis are inadequate. It can be predicted that new modalities, in addition to new immunosuppressive compounds, will be developed by using antibodies or antagonists to cytokines and adhesion molecules that are pivotal for the immune-mediated inflammatory process. In addition, regulation of pathogenic immune responses may be achieved by newly introduced procedures that may induce antigen-specific unresponsiveness or selective elimination of pathogenic lymphocyte clones.

REFERENCES

1. Adamus G et al.: Induction of experimental autoimmune uveitis with rhodopsin synthetic peptides in Lewis rats, *Curr Eye Res* 11:657-677, 1992.
2. Ando K et al.: The influence of H-2 genes and the effect of T cell depletion on experimental autoimmune uveoretinitis (EAU), *Invest Ophthalmol Vis Sci* 34(suppl):1480, 1993.
3. Arai K et al.: Cytokines: coordinators of immune and inflammatory responses, *Annu Rev Biochem* 59:783-836, 1990.
4. Baarsma GS, Priem HA, Kijlstra A: Association of birdshot retinochoroidopathy and HLA-A29 antigen, *Curr Eye Res* 9(suppl):63-68, 1990.
5. BenEzra D et al.: Ciclosporin (CyA) versus conventional therapy in Behçet's disease: preliminary observations of a masked study. In Schindler R, editor: *Ciclosporin in autoimmune diseases,* Berlin, 1985, Springer-Verlag.
6. BenEzra D et al.: Serum levels of interleukin-2 receptor in ocular Behçet's disease. *Am J Ophthalmol* 115:26-30, 1993.
7. Beraud E et al.: Control of experimental autoimmune uveoretinitis by low dose T-cell vaccination, *Cell Immunol* 140:112-122, 1992.
8. Berzofsky JA: Immunodominance in T lymphocyte recognition, *Immunol Lett* 18:83-92, 1988.
9. Bhattacherjee P, Henderson B: Inflammatory responses to intraocularly injected interleukin-1, *Curr Eye Res* 6:929-934, 1987.
10. Bhattacherjee P, Williams RN, Eakins KE: A comparison of the ocular anti-inflammatory activity of steroidal and nonsteroidal compounds in the rat, *Invest Ophthalmol Vis Sci* 24:1143-1146, 1983.
11. Brewerton DA et al.: Acute anterior uveitis and HLA-A27, *Lancet* ii:994-996, 1973.
12. Brinkman CJJ, Broekhuyse RM: Cell-mediated immunity after retinal detachment as determined by lymphocyte stimulation, *Am J Ophthalmol* 86:260-265, 1978.
13. Brinkman CJJ, Pinckers AJLG, Broekhuyse RM: Immune reactivity to different retinal antigens in patients suffering from retinitis pigmentosa, *Invest Ophthalmol Vis Sci* 19:743-750, 1980.
14. Broekhuyse RM, Kuhlmann ED, Winkens HJ: Experimental autoimmune posterior uveitis accompanied by epitheloid cell accumulations (EAPU): a new type of experimental ocular disease induced by immunization with PEP-65, a pigment epithelial polypeptide preparation, *Exp Eye Res* 55:819-829, 1992.
15. Broekhuyse RM, Kuhlmann ED, Winkens HJ: Experimental autoimmune anterior uveitis (EAAU). II. Dose-dependent induction and adoptive transfer using a melanin-bound antigen of the retinal pigment epithelium, *Exp Eye Res* 55:401-411, 1992.

16. Broekhuyse RM, Kuhlmann ED, Winkens HJ: Experimental autoimmune anterior uveitis (EAAU). III. Induction by immunization with purified uveal and skin melanins, *Exp Eye Res,* 56:575-583, 1993.

17. Broekhuyse RM et al.: Experimental autoimmune anterior uveitis (EAAU), a new form of experimental uveitis. I. Induction by a detergent-insoluble intrinsic protein fraction of the retinal pigment epithelium, *Exp Eye Res* 52:465-474, 1991.

18. Burky EL: Experimental endophthalmitis phaco-anaphylactica in rabbits, *Arch Ophthalmol* 12:536-546, 1934.

18a. Casper-Velu LE et al.: Ultrastructural changes of retinal vascular endothelial cells at the onset of experimental autoimmune uveitis. In Dernouchamps JP and associates, editors: *Recent advances in uveitis,* Amsterdam, 1993, Kugler Publications.

19. Caspi RR: Basic mechanisms in immune-mediated uveitic disease. In Lightman S, editor: *Immunology of Eye Diseases,* 61-86, Dordrecht, 1989, Kluwer Academic.

20. Caspi RR, Nussenblatt RB: Natural and therapeutic control of ocular autoimmunity—rodent and man. In Coutinho A, Kazatchkine M, editors: *Autoimmunity,* New York, 1994, Wiley-Liss.

21. Caspi RR, Roberge FG, Nussenblatt RB: Organ-resident, nonlymphoid cells suppress proliferation of autoimmune T-helper lymphocytes, *Science* 237:1029-1032, 1987.

22. Caspi RR et al.: T cell lines mediating experimental autoimmune uveoretinitis (EAU) in the rat, *J Immunol* 136:928-933, 1986.

23. Caspi RR et al.: A new model of autoimmune disease: experimental autoimmune uveoretinitis induced in mice with two different retinal antigens, *J Immunol* 140:1490-1495, 1988.

24. Caspi RR et al.: Genetic control of susceptibility to experimental autoimmune uveoretinitis in the mouse model, *J Immunol* 148:2384-2389, 1992.

25. Cassidy JT et al.: A study of classification criteria for a diagnosis of juvenile rheumatoid arthritis, *Arthritis Rheum* 29:274-281, 1986.

26. Chader GJ: Interphotoreceptor retinoid-binding protein (IRBP): A model protein for molecular biologic and clinically relevant studies, *Invest Ophthalmol Vis Sci* 30:7-22, 1989.

27. Chajek-Shaul T et al.: HLA-B51 may serve as an immunogenetic marker for a subgroup of patients with Behçet's syndrome, *Am J Med* 83:666-672, 1987.

28. Chan CC et al.: Anti-retinal autoantibodies in Vogt-Koyanagi-Harada's syndrome, Behçet's disease, and sympathetic ophthalmia, *Ophthalmology* 92:1025-1028, 1985.

29. Chan CC et al.: T-lymphocyte subsets in experimental autoimmune uveitis, *Clin Immunol Immunopathol* 35:103-110, 1985.

30. Chan CC et al.: Sympathetic ophthalmia, *Ophthamology* 93:690-695, 1986.

31. Chan CC et al.: HLA-DR antigens on retinal pigment epithelial cells from patients with uveitis, *Arch Ophthalmol* 104:725-729, 1986.

32. Chan CC et al.: Pathology of experimental autoimmune uveoretinitis in mice, *J Autoimmun* 3:247-255, 1990.

33. Chan CC et al.: Effects of antiflammins on endotoxin-induced uveitis in rats, *Arch Ophthalmol* 109:278-281, 1991.

33a. Chan CC et al.: Experimental melanin-protein-induced uveitis in the Lewis rat. Immunopathologic processes. *Ophthalmology* 101:1275-1280, 1994.

34. Charteris DG, Lightman SL: Interferon gamma (IFN-γ) production in vivo in experimental autoimmune uveoretinitis, *Immunology* 75:463, 1992.

35. Charteris DG, Lightman SL: In vivo lymphokine production in experimental autoimmune uveoretinitis, *Immunology* 78:387-392, 1993.

36. Chatila T, Geha RS: Superantigens, *Curr Opin Immunol* 4:74-78, 1992.

37. Chen TY et al.: Lipopolysaccharide receptors and signal transduction pathways in mononuclear phagocytes, *Curr Top Microbiol Immunol* 181:169-188, 1992.

38. Cohen IR: Regulation of autoimmune disease physiologic and therapeutic, *Immunol Rev* 94:6-21, 1986.

39. Cousins SW et al.: Endotoxin-induced uveitis in the rat: observations on altered vascular permeability, clinical findings and histology, *Exp Eye Res* 39:665-676, 1984.

40. Cousins S et al.: Identification of transforming growth factor-beta as an immunosuppressive factor in aqueous humor, *Invest Ophthalmol Vis Sci* 32:2201-2211, 1991.

41. Daniel PM, Lam DKC, Pratt OE: Relation between the increase in the diffusional permeability of the blood central-nervous system barrier and other changes during the development of experimental allergic encephalomyelitis in the Lewis rat, *J Neurol Sci* 60:367-376, 1983.

42. Davis JL et al.: HLA associations and ancestry in Vogt-Koyanagi-Harada disease and sympathetic ophthamia, *Ophthalmology* 97:1137-1142, 1990.

43. de Bara R et al.: Cryopexy enhances experimental autoimmune uveoretinitis (EAU) in rats, *Invest Ophthalmol Vis Sci* 30:2165-2173, 1989.

44. de Kozak Y et al.: Evidence for immediate hypersensitivity phenomena in experimental autoimmune uveoretinitis, *Eur J Immunol* 11:612-617, 1981.

45. de Kozak Y et al.: Pharmacological modulation of IgE-dependent mast cell degranulation in experimental autoimmune uveoretinitis, *Jpn J Ophthalmol* 27:598-608, 1983.

46. de Kozak Y et al.: Prevention of experimental autoimmune uveoretinitis by active immunization with autoantigen-specific monoclonal antibodies, *Eur J Immunol* 17:541-547, 1987.

47. de Kozak Y et al.: Effect of antioxidant enzymes on experimental uveitis in rats, *Ophthalmic Res* 21:230-234, 1989.

48. de Kozak Y et al.: Modulation of experimental autoimmune uveoretinitis by adoptive transfer of cells from rats immunized with anti-S-antigen monoclonal antibody, *Reg Immunol* 2:311-320, 1989.

49. de Kozak Y et al.: Humoral immune response against the S-antigen/TNF common epitope in rat EAU suppressed by the monoclonal antibody S2D2, *Curr Eye Res* 11(suppl):119-127, 1992.

50. Dernouchamps JP et al.: Immune complexes in the aqueous humor and serum, *Am J Ophthalmol* 84:24-31, 1977.

51. de Smet MD et al.: Cellular immune responses to fragments of S-antigen in patients with uveitis. In Usui M, Ohno S, Aoki K, editors: *Ocular immunology today,* 285-288, Amsterdam, 1990, Excerpta Medica.

52. de Smet MD et al.: Cellular immune responses of patients with uveitis to retinal antigens and their fragments, *Am J Ophthalmol* 110:135-142, 1990.

53. de Smet MD et al.: Determination of the precursor frequency of response to S-Ag in uveitis patients and controls, *Invest Ophthalmol Vis Sci* 33(suppl):930, 1992.

54. Desmonts G: Definitive serological diagnosis of ocular toxoplasmosis, *Arch Ophthalmol* 76:839-853, 1986.

55. de Waal LP et al.: HLA-A29 subtypes and birdshot chorioretinopathy, *Immunogenetics* 35:51-53, 1992.

56. Dick AD et al.: Immunocytochemical analysis of blood lymphocytes in uveitis, *Eye* 6:643-647, 1992.

57. Dinarello CA: Interleukin 1, *Rev Infect Dis* 6:59-95, 1984.

58. Doekes G et al.: Humoral and cellular immune responsiveness to human S-antigen in uveitis, *Curr Eye Res* 6:909-919, 1987.

59. Donnelly J, Xi MS, Rockey J: Inhibition of mixed lymphocyte responses by human corneal fibroblasts, *Invest Ophthalmol Vis Sci* 30(suppl):440, 1989.

60. Donoso LA et al.: S-antigen: characterization of a pathogenic epitope which mediates experimental autoimmune uveitis and pinealitis in Lewis rats, *Curr Eye Res* 6:1151-1159, 1987.

61. Donoso LA et al.: Human interstitial retinoid-binding protein: a potent uveitopathogenic agent for the induction of experimental autoimmune uveitis, *J Immunol* 143:79-83, 1989.

62. Dua HS, Gregerson DS, Donoso LA: Inhibition of experimental autoimmune uveitis by retinal photoreceptor antigens coupled to spleen cells, *Cell Immunol* 139:292-305, 1992.

63. Dua HS et al.: Induction of experimental autoimmune uveitis by the retinal photoreceptor cell protein, phosducin, *Curr Eye Res* 11(suppl):107-111, 1992.

64. Dumonde DC et al.: Anti-retinal autoimmunity and circulating immune complexes in patients with retinal vasculitis, *Lancet* ii:787-792, 1982.

65. Egwuagu CE et al.: T cell receptor β-chain usage in experimental autoimmune uveoretinitis, *J Autoimmun* 4:315-324, 1992.

66. Egwuagu CE et al.: Predominant usage of Vβ8.3 T cell receptor in a T cell line that induces experimental autoimmune uveoretinitis (EAU), *Clin Immunol Immunopathol* 65:152-160, 1992.

66a. Egwuagu CE et al.: Evidence for selective accumulation of Vβ8$^+$ T lymphocytes in experimental autoimmune uveoretinitis induced with two different retinal antigens. *J Immunol* 151:1627-1636, 1993.

67. Eisenfeld AJ, Bunt-Milam AH, Saari JC: Uveoretinitis in rabbits following immunization with interphotoreceptor retinoid-binding protein, *Exp Eye Res* 44:425-438, 1987.

68. Faure JP: Autoimmunity and the retina, *Curr Top Eye Res* 2:215-302, 1980.

69. Faure JP et al.: Uveo-rétinite experimentale induite par l'antigène S rétinien chez le singe: induction, histopathologie, *J Fr Ophtalmol* 4:465-472, 1981.

70. Fenton RM et al.: The use of indirect immunofluorescence testing and guinea pig lip mucosa for the evaluation of Behçet's and non-Behçet's uveitis, *Invest Ophthalmol Vis Sci* 33(suppl):942, 1992.

71. Ferrick MR et al.: Ocular inflammation stimulated by intravitreal interleukin-8 and interleukin-1, *Invest Ophthalmol Vis Sci* 32:1534-1539, 1991.

72. Forrester JV, Scott DI, Hercus KM: Naturally occurring antibodies to bovine and human retinal S antigen: a comparison between uveitis patients and healthy volunteers, *Br J Ophthalmol* 73:155-159, 1989.

73. Fox GM et al.: Experimental autoimmune uveoretinitis (EAU) induced by retinal interphotoreceptor retinoid-binding protein (IRBP): differences between EAU induced by IRBP and by S-antigen, *Clin Immunol Immunopathol* 43:256-264, 1987.

74. Franks WA et al.: Cytokines in human intraocular inflammation, *Curr Eye Res* 11(suppl):187-191, 1992.

75. Fujikawa LS et al.: Retinal vascular endothelium expresses fibronectin and class II histocompatibility complex antigens in experimental autoimmune uveitis, *Cell Immunol* 98:139-150, 1987.

76. Fujino Y et al.: The role of steroid hormone in the regulation of EAU, *Invest Ophthalmol Vis Sci* 32(suppl):932, 1991.

77. Gammon G et al.: The choice of T-cell epitopes utilized on a protein antigen depends on multiple factors distant from, as well as at the determinant site, *Immunol Rev* 98:53-73, 1987.

77a. Gery I, Chanaud NP, Anglade E: Recoverin is highly uveitogenic in Lewis rats. *Invest Ophthalmol Vis Sci* 35:3342-3345, 1994.

78. Gery I, Mochizuki M, Nussenblatt RB: Retinal specific antigens and immunopathogenic processes they provoke, *Prog Retinal Res* 5:75-109, 1986.

79. Gery I, Nussenblatt R, BenEzra D: Dissociation between humoral and cellular immune responses to lens antigens, *Invest Ophthalmol Vis Sci* 20:32-39, 1981.

80. Gery I et al.: Uveoretinitis and pinealitis induced by immunization with interphotoreceptor retinoid-binding protein, *Invest Ophthalmol Vis Sci* 27:1296-1300, 1986.

81. Gery I et al.: Inhibition of experimental autoimmune uveoretinitis (EAU) by mycophenolate mofetil (MM), *Invest Ophthalmol Vis Sci* 34(suppl):1480, 1993.

82. Granstein RD et al.: Aqueous humor contains transforming growth factor-β and a small (<3500 dalton) inhibitor of thymocyte proliferation, *J Immunol* 144:3021-3027, 1990.

82a. Greenwood J et al.: The blood-retinal barrier in experimental autoimmune uveoretinitis. Leukocyte interactions and functional damage. *Lab Invest* 70:39-52, 1994.

83. Gregerson DS, Abrahams IW, Thirkill CE: Serum antibody levels of uveitis patients to bovine retinal antigens, *Invest Ophthalmol Vis Sci* 21:669-680, 1981.

84. Gregerson DS, Obritsch WF, Donoso LA: Oral tolerance in experimental autoimmune uveoretinitis. Distinct mechanisms of resistance are induced by low dose vs high dose feeding protocols. *J Immunol* 151:5751-5761, 1993.

85. Gregerson DS et al.: Identification of a potent new pathogenic site in human retinal S-antigen which induces experimental autoimmune uveoretinitis in LEW rats, *Cell Immunol* 128:209-219, 1990.

86. Gregerson DS et al.: Conserved T cell receptor V gene usage by uveitogenic T cells, *Clin Immunol Immunopathol* 58:154-161, 1991.

87. Gutierrez JC et al.: Insights into autoimmunity: from classical models to current perspectives, *Immunol Rev* 118:73-101, 1990.

88. Gutierrez-Ramos JC, Moreno de Alboran I, Martinez-AC: In vivo administration of interleukin-2 turns on anergic self-reactive T cells and leads to autoimmune disease, *Eur J Immunol* 22:2867-2872, 1992.

89. Guyton JS, Woods AC: Etiology of uveitis: a clinical study of 562 cases, *Arch Ophthalmol* 26:983-1018, 1941.

90. Hamel CP, Detrick B, Hooks JJ: Evaluation of Ia expression in rat ocular tissues following inoculation with interferon gamma, *Exp Eye Res* 50:173-182, 1990.

91. Hara Y et al.: Suppression of experimental autoimmune uveitis in mice by induction of anterior chamber-associated immune deviation with interphotoreceptor retinoid-binding protein, *J Immunol* 148:1685-1692, 1992.

92. Heber-Katz E, Acha-Orbea H: The V-region disease hypothesis: evidence from autoimmune encephalomyelitis, *Immunol Today* 10:164-169, 1989.

93. Helbig H et al.: Dual effect of ciliary body cells on T lymphocyte proliferation, *Eur J Immunol* 20:2457-2463, 1990.

94. Herbort CP, Okumura A, Mochizuki M: Endotoxin-induced uveits in the rat: a study of the role of inflammation mediators, *Graefe's Arch Clin Exp Ophthalmol* 226:553-558, 1988.

95. Hickey WF, Hsu BL, Kimura H: T-lymphocyte entry into the central nervous system, *J Neurosci Res* 28:254-260, 1991.

96. Higuchi M et al.: Combined anti-interleukin-2 receptor and low dose cyclosporin therapy in experimental autoimmune uveoretinitis, *J Autoimmun* 4:113-124, 1991.

97. Hirose S et al.: Uveitis induced in primates by interphotoreceptor retinoid-binding protein, *Arch Ophthalmol* 104:1698-1702, 1986.

98. Hoekzema R et al.: Serum antibody response to human and bovine IRBP in uveitis, *Curr Eye Res* 9:1177-1183, 1990.

99. Hoekzema R et al.: Endotoxin-induced uveitis in the rat: the significance of intraocular interleukin-6, *Invest Ophthalmol Vis Sci* 33:532-539, 1992.

100. Hooks JJ, Chan CC, Detrick B: Identification of the lymphokines, interferon-γ and interleukin-2, in inflammatory eye diseases, *Invest Ophthalmol Vis Sci* 29:1444-1451, 1988.

101. Howes EL Jr, Char DH, Christensen M: Aqueous immune complexes in immunogenic uveitis, *Invest Ophthalmol Vis Sci* 23:715-718, 1982.

102. Howes EL Jr et al.: Ocular localization of circulating bacterial lipopolysaccharide, *Exp Eye Res* 38:379-389, 1984.

103. Hu LH et al.: Rat T-cell lines specific to a nonimmunodominant determinant of a retinal protein (IRBP) produce uveoretinitis and pinealitis, *Cell Immunol* 122:251-261, 1989.

104. Ichikawa T et al.: Spontaneous development of autoimmune uveoretinitis in nude mice following reconstitution with embryonic rat thymus, *Clin Exp Immunol* 86:112-117, 1991.

105. Jerne NK: Idiotypic networks and other preconceived ideas, *Immunol Rev* 79:5-24, 1984.

106. Juhler M: Pathophysiological aspects of acute experimental allergic encephalomyelitis, *Acta Neurol Scand Suppl* 78:1-21, 1988.

106a. Kaplan AD et al.: Experimental allergic ivitis, a new model of autoimmune uveitis. *Invest Ophthalmol Vis Sci* 34 (Suppl): 1480, 1993.

107. Kaplan HJ et al.: Viral antibodies in the aqueous humor in idiopathic uveitis. In Saari KM, editor: *Uveitis update,* 214-219, Amsterdam, 1984, Excerpta Medica.

108. Kasner L et al.: The effect of chlorpromazine on endotoxin-induced uveitis in the Lewis rat, *Curr Eye Res* 11:843-848, 1992.

109. Kasner L et al.: The paradoxical effect of tumor necrosis factor alpha (TNF-α) in endotoxin-induced uveitis, *Invest Ophthalmol Vis Sci,* 1993 (in press).

110. Kasp E et al.: Circulating immune complexes may play a regulatory and pathogenic role in experimental autoimmune uveoretinitis, *Clin Exp Immunol* 88:307-312, 1992.

111. Kasp E et al.: Antibody affinity to retinal S-antigen in patients with retinal vasculitis, *Am J Ophthalmol* 113:697-701, 1992.

112. Kawabe Y, Ochi A: Selective anergy of Vβ8+, CD4+ T-cells in staphylococcus enterotoxin B-primed mice, *J Exp Med* 172:1065-1070, 1990.

113. Kawano YI et al.: Trials of vaccination against experimental autoimmune uveoretinitis with a T-cell receptor peptide, *Curr Eye Res* 10:789-795, 1991.

114. Kawashima H, Mochizuki M: Effects of a new immunosuppressive agent, FK506, on the efferent limb of the immune response, *Exp Eye Res* 51:565-572, 1990.

115. Kawashima H et al.: Inhibitory effects of corneal endothelial cells on autoimmune T cells in vitro, *Invest Ophthalmol Vis Sci* 33(suppl):986, 1992.
116. Kim C, Siminovitch KA, Ochi A: Reduction of lupus nephritis in MRL/lpr mice by a bacterial superantigen treatment, *J Exp Med* 174:1431-1437, 1991.
117. Kim MK et al.: Expression of class II antigen in endotoxin induced uveitis, *Curr Eye Res* 5:869-876, 1986.
118. Klok AM et al.: Antibodies against ocular and oral antigens in Behçet's disease associated with uveitis, *Curr Eye Res* 8:957-962, 1989.
119. Kotake S et al.: Repeated determinants within the retinal interphotoreceptor retinoid-binding protein (IRBP): immunological properties of the repeats of an immunodominant determinant, *Cell Immunol* 126:331-342, 1990.
120. Kotake S et al.: Analysis of the pivotal residues of the immunodominant and highly uveitogenic determinant of interphotoreceptor retinoid-binding protein, *J Immunol* 146:2995-3001, 1991.
121. Kotake S et al.: Unusual immunologic properties of the uveitogenic interphotoreceptor retinoid-binding protein-derived peptide R23, *Invest Ophthalmol Vis Sci* 32:2058-2064, 1991.
122. Kufoy EA et al.: Modulation of the blood-aqueous barrier by gram-positive and gram-negative bacterial cell wall components in the rat and rabbit, *Exp Eye Res* 50:189-195, 1990.
123. Kulkarni PS, Mancino M: Studies on intraocular inflammation produced by intravitreal human interleukins in rabbits, *Exp Eye Res* 56:275-279, 1993.
124. Kusuda M et al.: Expression of Ia antigen by ocular tissues of mice treated with interferon gamma, *Invest Ophthalmol Vis Sci* 30:764-768, 1989.
125. Lee SF, Pepose JS: Cellular immune response to Ia induction by intraocular gamma-interferon, *Ophthalmic Res* 22:310-317, 1990.
126. Levinsky RJ, Lehner T: Circulating soluble immune complexes in recurrent oral ulceration and Behcet's syndrome, *Clin Exp Immunol* 32:193-198, 1978.
127. Li Q et al.: Association between mast cells and the development of experimental autoimmune uveitis in different rat strains, *Clin Immunol Immunopathol* 65:294-299, 1992.
128. Lider O et al.: Anti-idiotypic network induced by T-cell vaccination against experimental autoimmune encephalomyelitis, *Science* 239:181-183, 1988.
129. Lieb WE et al.: Identification of an S-antigen-like molecule in Drosophila melanogaster: an immunohistochemical study, *Exp Eye Res* 53:171-178, 1991.
130. Lightman S, Greenwood J: Effect of lymphocytic infiltration on the blood-retinal barrier in experimental autoimmune uveoretinitis, *Clin Exp Immunol* 88:473-477, 1992.
131. Lightman S, Palestine AG, Nussenblatt RB: Immunohistopathology of experimental immunogenic uveitis induced by a non-ocular antigen, *Curr Eye Res* 5:857-862, 1986.
132. Lipham WJ et al.: Immunological features of synthetic peptides derived from the retinal protein IRBP: differences between immunodominant and nondominant peptides, *Curr Eye Res* 9:95-98, 1990.
133. Mahdi RM et al.: Selective accumulation of Vβ8+ T lymphocytes in EAU, *Invest Ophthalmol Vis Sci* 34(suppl):1144, 1993.
134. Marak GE Jr: Phacoanaphylactic endophthalmitis, *Surv Ophthalmol* 36:325-339, 1992.
135. Marak GE Jr, Font RL, Alepa FP: Experimental lens-induced granulomatous endophthalmitis: passive transfer with serum, *Ophthalmic Res* 8:117-120, 1976.
136. Marak GE Jr, Font RL, Alepa FP: Arthus-type panophthalmitis in rats sensitized to heterologous lens protein, *Ophthalmic Res* 9:162-170, 1977.
137. Marak GE Jr et al.: Experimental lens-induced granulomatous endophthalmitis: preliminary histopathologic observations, *Exp Eye Res* 19:311-316, 1974.
138. Marak GE Jr et al.: Effects of C3 inactivator factor on the development of experimental lens-induced granulomatous endophthalmitis, *Ophthalmic Res* 9:416, 1977.
139. Martin DF et al.: Synergistic effect of rapamycin and cyclosporine A on the inhibition of experimental autoimmune uveoretinitis, *Invest Ophthalmol Vis Sci* 34(suppl):1476, 1993.
140. Masuda K et al.: Double masked trial of cyclosporine versus colchicine and long term open study of cyclosporine in Behçet's disease, *Lancet* i:1093-1096, 1989.
141. McAllister CG et al.: Uveitogenic potential of lymphocytes sensitized to interphotoreceptor retinoid-binding protein, *J Immunol* 138:1416-1420, 1987.
142. McMenamin PG, Holthouse I, Holt PG: Class II major histocompatibility complex (Ia) antigen-bearing dendritic cells within the iris and cilliary body of the rat eye: distribution, phenotype and relation to retinal microglia, *Immunology* 77:385-393, 1992.
143. McMenamin PG et al.: Ultrastructural pathology of experimental autoimmune uveitis: quantitative evidence of activation and possible high endothelial venule-like changes in retinal vascular endothelium, *Lab Invest* 67:42-45, 1992.
144. Merryman CF et al.: Characterization of a new, potent immunopathogenic epitope in S-antigen which elicits T cells expressing Vβ8 and Vα2-like genes, *J Immunol* 146:75-80, 1991.
145. Michaelson JB, Chisari FV, Kansu T: Antibodies to oral mucosa in patients with ocular Behçet's disease, *Ophthalmology* 92:1277-1281, 1985.
146. Miller A et al.: Suppressor T-cells generated by oral tolerization to myelin basic protein suppress both in vitro and in vivo immune responses by the release of TGF-β following antigenic specific triggering, *Proc Natl Acad Sci USA* 89:421-425, 1992.
147. Mirshahi M et al.: Retinal S-antigen epitopes in vertebrate and invertebrate photoreceptors, *Invest Ophthalmol Vis Sci* 26:1016-1021, 1985.
148. Mizuki N et al.: Association of HLA-B51 and lack of association of class II alleles with Behçet's disease, *Tissue Antigens* 40:22-30, 1992.
149. Mizuki N et al.: Human leukocyte antigen serologic and DNA typing of Behçet's disease and its primary association with B51, *Invest Ophthalmol Vis Sci* 33:3332-3340, 1992.
150. Mochizuki M et al.: An association between susceptibility to experimental autoimmune uveitis and choroidal mast cell numbers, *J Immunol* 133:1699-1701, 1984.
151. Mochizuki M et al.: Adoptive transfer of experimental autoimmune uveoretinitis in rats: immunopathogenic mechanisms and histologic features, *Invest Ophthalmol Vis Sci* 26:1-9, 1985.
152. Mochizuki M et al.: Effects of cyclosporine and other immunosuppressive drugs on experimental autoimmune uveoretinitis in rats, *Invest Ophthalmol Vis Sci* 26:226-232, 1985.
153. Mochizuki M et al.: Preclinical and clinical study of FK506 in uveitis, *Curr Eye Res* 11(suppl):87-95, 1992.
154. Montes C et al.: Treatment of murine experimental autoimmune uveoretinitis with T cell receptor (TCR) V-β specific antibody, *Invest Ophthalmol Vis Sci* 33(suppl):934, 1992.
155. Munk ME et al.: Target cell lysis and IL-2 secretion by γ/δ T lymphocytes after activation by bacteria, *J Immunol* 145:2434-2439, 1990.
156. Newsome DA, Nussenblatt RB: Retinal S-antigen reactivity in patients with retinitis pigmentosa and Usher's syndrome, *Retina* 4:195-199, 1984.
157. Ni M et al.: Iris inflammatory cells, fibronectin, fibrinogen and immunoglobulin in various ocular diseases, *Arch Ophthalmol* 106:392-395, 1988.
158. Nussenblatt RB, Palestine AG: Uveitis. In *Fundamentals and clinical practice*, Chicago, 1989, Year Book Medical.
159. Nussenblatt RB et al.: Cellular immune responsiveness of uveitis patients to retinal S-antigen, *Am J Ophthalmol* 89:173-179, 1980.
160. Nussenblatt RB et al.: S-antigen uveitis in primates: a new model for human disease, *Arch Ophthalmol* 99:1090-1092, 1981.
161. Nussenblatt RB et al.: Cyclosporin A: inhibition of experimental autoimmune uveitis in Lewis rats, *J Clin Invest* 67:1228-1231, 1981.
162. Nussenblatt RB et al.: Birdshot retinochoroidopathy associated with HLA-A29 antigen and immune responsiveness to retinal S-antigen, *Am J Ophthalmol* 94:147-158, 1982.
163. Nussenblatt RB et al.: Cyclosporin A therapy of intraocular inflammatory disease, *Lancet* ii:235-238, 1983.
164. Nussenblatt RB et al.: Inhibition of S-antigen induced experimental autoimmune uveoretinitis by oral induction of tolerance with S-antigen, *J Immunol* 144:1689-1695, 1990.

165. O'Connor GR: Factors related to the initiation and recurrences of uveitis: XL Edward Jackson memorial lecture, *Am J Ophthalmol* 96:577-599, 1983.

166. Ohno S: Immunological aspects of Behcet's and Vogt-Koyanagi-Harada's diseases, *Trans Ophthalmol Soc UK* 101:335-341, 1981.

167. Ohno S et al.: HLA-Bw51 and Behcet's disease, *JAMA* 240:529, 1978.

168. Opremcak EM et al.: Enumeration of autoreactive helper T-lymphocytes in uveitis, *Invest Ophthalmol Vis Sci* 32:2561-2567, 1991.

169. Osborn L: Leukocyte adhesion to endothelium in inflammation, *Cell* 62:3-6, 1990.

170. Palestine AG et al.: The failure of cyclosporin to inhibit granulomatous inflammation in acute Arthus-like panophthalmitis, *Immunol Lett* 9:235-237, 1985.

171. Parks DE, Walker SM, Weigle WO: Bacterial lipopolysaccharide (endotoxin) interferes with the induction of tolerance and primes thymus-derived lymphocytes, *J Immunol* 126:938-942, 1981.

172. Percopo CM et al.: Cytokine-mediator activation of a neuronal retinal resident cell provokes antigen presentation, *J Immunol* 145:4101-4107, 1990.

173. Pfister C et al.: Retinal S-antigen identified as the 48K protein regulating light dependent phosphodiesterase in rods, *Science* 228:891-893, 1985.

173a. Racke MK et al.: Superantigen modulation of experimental allergic encephalomyelitis. Activation of anergy determines outcome. *J Immunol* 152:2051-2059, 1994.

174. Ragheb S, Boros DL: Characterization of granuloma T-lymphocyte function from *Schistosoma mansoni*—infected mice, *J Immunol* 142:3239-3246, 1989.

175. Rao NA, Wacker WB, Marak GE Jr: Experimental allergic uveitis: clinicopathologic features associated with varying doses of S-antigen, *Arch Ophthalmol* 97:1954-1958, 1979.

176. Rao NA et al.: Role of oxygen radicals in experimental allergic uveitis, *Invest Ophthalmol Vis Sci* 28:886-892, 1987.

177. Rao NA et al.: Suppression of experimental uveitis in rats by anti-I-A antibodies, *Invest Ophthalmol Vis Sci* 30:2348-2355, 1989.

178. Roberge FG et al.: Selective immunosuppression of activated T-cells with the chimeric toxin IL-2-PE40: inhibition of experimental autoimmune uveoretinitis, *J Immunol* 143:3498-3502, 1989.

179. Roberge FG et al.: Treatment of autoimmune uveoretinitis in the rat with rapamycin, an inhibitor of lymphocyte growth factor signal transduction, *Curr Eye Res* 12:197-203, 1993.

180. Rodrigues MM et al.: Interphotoreceptor retinoid binding protein in retinal red cells and pineal gland, *Invest Ophthalmol Vis Sci* 27:844-850, 1986.

181. Rosenbaum JT: Uveitis. An internist's view, *Arch Intern Med* 149:1173-1176, 1989.

182. Rosenbaum JT, Boney RS: Activity of an interleukin 1 receptor antagonist in rabbit models of uveitis, *Arch Ophthalmol* 110:547-549, 1992.

183. Rosenbaum JT et al.: Endotoxin-induced uveitis in rats as a model for human disease, *Nature* 286:611-613, 1980.

184. Rosenbaum JT et al.: Ocular inflammatory effects of intravitreally-injected tumor necrosis factor, *Am J Pathol* 133:47-53, 1988.

185. Rossi F, Dietrich G, Kazatchkine MD: Anti-idiotypes against autoantibodies in normal immunoglobulins: evidence for network regulation of human autoimmune responses, *Immunol Rev* 110:135-149, 1989.

186. Rott O, Wekerle H, Fleischer B: Protection from experimental allergic encephalomyelitis by application of a bacterial superantigen, *Int Immunol* 4:347-353, 1992.

187. Salinas-Carmona MC, Nussenblatt RB, Gery I: Experimental autoimmune uveitis in athymic nude rat, *Eur J Immunol* 12:480-484, 1982.

188. Sanui H et al.: Synthetic peptides derived from IRBP induce EAU and EAP in rats, *Curr Eye Res* 7:727-735, 1988.

189. Sanui H et al.: Identification of an immunodominant and highly immunopathogenic determinant in the retinal interphotoreceptor retinoid-binding protein (IRBP), *J Exp Med* 169:1947-1958, 1989.

190. Sanui H et al.: Uveitis and immune responses in primates immunized with IRBP-derived synthetic peptides, *Curr Eye Res* 9:193-199, 1990.

191. Sasamoto Y et al.: Immunomodulation of experimental autoimmune uveoretinitis by intravenous injection of uveitogenic peptides, *Invest Ophthalmol Vis Sci* 33:2641-2649, 1992.

192. Schalken JJ et al.: Experimental autoimmune uveoretinitis in rats induced by rod visual pigment: rhodopsin is more pathogenic than opsin, *Graefes Arch Clin Exp Ophthalmol* 226:255-261, 1988.

193. Schalken JJ et al.: Rhodopsin-induced experimental autoimmune uveoretinitis in monkeys, *Br J Ophthalmol* 73:168-172, 1989.

194. Schreiber SL: Chemistry and biology of the immunophilins and their immunosuppressive ligands, *Science* 251:283-287, 1991.

195. Schwartz RH: T-lymphocyte recognition of antigen in association with gene products of the major histocompatibility complex, *Annu Rev Immunol* 3:237-261, 1985.

196. Shevach EM: The effects of cyclosporine A on the immune response, *Annu Rev Immunol* 3:397-423, 1985.

197. Shinohara T et al.: S-antigen: structure, function and experimental autoimmune uveitis (EAU), *Prog Retinal Res* 8:51-66, 1988.

198. Shirkey BL et al.: Linomide, a novel immunomodulator, inhibits experimental autoimmune uveoretinitis (EAU) in mice and rats, *Invest Ophthalmol Vis Sci* 34(suppl):1475, 1993.

199. Singh VK et al.: Identification of a uveitopathogenic and lymphocyte proliferation site in bovine S-antigen, *Cell Immunol* 115:413-419, 1988.

200. Singh VK et al.: Molecular mimicry: yeast histone H3-induced experimental autoimmune uveitis, *J Immunol* 142:1512-1517, 1989.

201. Singh VK et al.: Molecular mimicry between a uveitopathogenic site of S-antigen and viral peptides: induction of experimental autoimmune uveitis in Lewis rats, *J Immunol* 144:1282-1287, 1990.

202. Springer TA: Adhesion receptors of the immune system, *Nature* 346:425-434, 1990.

203. Stanford MR et al.: A longitudinal study of clinical and immunologic findings in fifty-two patients with retinal vasculitis, *Br J Ophthalmol* 72:442-447, 1988.

204. Streilein JW, Bradley D: Analysis of immunosuppressive properties of iris and ciliary body cells and their secretory products, *Invest Ophthalmol Vis Sci* 32:2700-2710, 1991.

205. Streilein JW, Wilbanks GA, Cousins SW: Immunoregulatory mechanisms of the eye, *J Neuroimmunol* 39:185-200, 1992.

206. Suzuki I: Experimental autoimmune uveoretinitis (EAU) in rats: isolation of S-antigen, EAU susceptibility of rat strains, genetic control of EAU induction and effects of cyclophosphamide and irradiation on EAU, *Jpn J Ophthalmol* 33:13-26, 1989.

207. Tabary T et al.: Susceptibility to birdshot retinochoroidopathy is restricted to the HLA-A29.2 subtype, *Tissue Antigens* 36:177-179, 1990.

208. Tanouchi Y et al.: Endotoxin-induced uveitis in LPS-susceptible C3H/HeN mice, *Invest Ophthalmol Vis Sci* 32(suppl):792, 1991.

208a. Thirkill CE et al.: The cancer-associated retinopathy antigen is a recoverin-like protein. *Invest Ophthalmol Vis Sci* 33:2768-2772, 1992.

209. Thomson G: HLA disease associations: models for insulin dependent diabetes mellitus and the study of complex human genetic disorders, *Annu Rev Genet* 22:31-50, 1988.

210. Thurau SR et al.: Induction of oral tolerance to S-antigen induced experimental autoimmune uveitis by a uveitogenic 20 mer peptide, *J Autoimmun* 4:507-516, 1991.

211. Tiedeman JS: Epstein-Barr viral antibodies in multifocal choroiditis and panuveitis, *Am J Ophthalmol* 103:659-663, 1987.

212. Unanue ER, Allen PM: Comment on the finding of Ia expression in non-lymphoid cells, *Lab Invest* 55:123-125, 1986.

213. Vandenbark AA, Hashim G, Offner H: Immunization with a synthetic T-cell receptor V-region peptide protects against experimental autoimmune encephalomyelitis, *Nature* 341:541-544, 1989.

214. Venning MC et al.: Antibodies directed against neutrophils (C-ANCA and P-ANCA) are of distinct diagnostic value in systemic vasculitis, *Q J Med* 77:1287-1296, 1990.

215. Vistica BP et al.: IRBP from bovine retina is poorly uveitogenic in guinea pigs and is identical to A-antigen, *Curr Eye Res* 6:409-417, 1987.

216. Vrabec TR et al.: S-antigen. Identification of human T-cell lymphocyte proliferation sites, *Arch Ophthalmol* 108:1470-1473, 1990.

217. Wahl SM et al.: Macrophage activation by mycobacterial water soluble compounds and synthetic muramyl dipeptide, *J Immunol* 122:2226-2231, 1979.

218. Wakefield D, Lloyd A: The role of cytokines in the pathogenesis of inflammatory eye disease, *Cytokine* 4:1-5, 1992.
219. Waters RV, Terrell TG, Jones GH: Uveitis induction in the rabbit by muramyl dipeptides, *Infect Immun* 51:816-825, 1986.
220. Wetzig R et al.: Anti-Ia antibody diminishes ocular inflammation in experimental autoimmune uveitis, *Curr Eye Res* 7:809-818, 1988.
221. Whitcup SM et al.: Endothelial leukocyte adhesion molecule-1 in endotoxin-induced uveitis, *Invest Ophthalmol Vis Sci* 33:2626-2630, 1992.
222. Whitcup SM et al.: Expression of cell adhesion molecules in posterior uveitis, *Arch Ophthalmol* 110:662-666, 1992.
223. Whitcup SM et al.: Monoclonal antibody against C116/CD18 inhibits endotoxin-induced uveitis, *Invest Ophthalmol Vis Sci* 34:673-681, 1993.
224. Whitcup SM et al.: Monoclonal antibodies against ICAM-1 (CD54) and LFA-1 (CD11a/CD18) inhibit experimental autoimmune uveitis, *Clin Immunol Immunopathol,* 67:143-150, 1993.
225. Witebsky E et al.: Chronic thyroiditis and autoimmunization, *JAMA* 164:1439-1447, 1957.
226. Yamamura M et al.: Cytokine patterns of immunologically mediated tissue damage, *J Immunol* 149:1470-1475, 1992.

12 Immunology of Ocular Tumors

BRUCE R. KSANDER, TIMOTHY G. MURRAY

Malignant transformation of a variety of cell types within the eye can result in the formation of ocular tumors. Most immunologic studies have been directed at the two most common ocular tumors—uveal melanoma and retinoblastoma. Studies of the identification, expression, and immune response against specific and nonspecific tumor antigens expressed by these tumors are at a relatively early stage. This situation contrasts with the extensive immunologic studies conducted during the past decade of antigens expressed on nonocular tumors.

This chapter will initially review the immunologic studies of nonocular tumors to provide the background necessary for evaluating the past and present immunologic studies of ocular tumors. This chapter will provide the following: (1) a brief overview of cell-mediated and antibody-mediated immunity, (2) recent studies that characterize tumor-specific T cells, the antigens recognized by these cells, and the genes that encode tumor antigens, (3) the development of immunotherapies that manipulate and augment antitumor immunity, (4) the mechanisms used by tumor cells to escape immune recognition, and (5) the relationship between immune privilege and human spontaneous tumors. Research in these different areas has recently redefined tumor immunology and renewed hope that the immune response may be used as a therapeutic tool in the treatment of cancer. As ocular tumors provide many unique immunologic opportunities and challenges, it may be possible to apply these new concepts to the study of intraocular tumors.

HISTORICAL BACKGROUND

Early studies (1950s to 1960s) of the immune response against tumor cells were conducted using animal models in which tumors were induced by treatment with either (1) chemical carcinogens, (2) ultraviolet light, or (3) oncogenic tumor viruses. In all of these animal models the tumor cells were immunogenic, and it was relatively easy to induce a tumor-specific T cell response that was protective in vivo. By contrast, researchers in the 1970s were unable to detect T cells that were specific for human spontaneous tumors and, for this reason, it was believed that spontaneous tumors were not immunogenic and did not express antigens that were recognized by T cells. Therefore the use of animal models to study antitumor immunity was considered controversial because these tumors were highly immunogenic, and human tumors did not appear to be immunogenic.[47]

This controversy has been resolved recently with the conclusive documentation that at least some human spontaneous tumors express tumor-specific antigens that are recognized by T cells. These data demonstrate that patients generate an antitumor immune response and possess clonally expanded populations of tumor-specific T cells. Although some patients generate an antitumor immune response, there is no indication that this immune response successfully controls tumor growth. Therefore these new data raise several important questions that must be addressed: (1) If tumors express specific antigens, why is the immune response unable to eliminate tumor cells? and (2) Can the tumor-specific T cell response be manipulated to successfully control tumor growth?

ANTITUMOR IMMUNE RESPONSE

This section will describe the different types of cell-mediated and antibody-mediated immune responses that can be generated against tumors. Although these effector cells are typically studied in murine tumor models, they have also been observed and characterized in patients with spontaneous tumors.

Antigen-Specific Effector Cells

Tumor-Specific and Tumor-Associated Antigens. Two types of antigens are expressed by tumor cells that can be recognized by the immune system: tumor-specific antigens and tumor-associated antigens. Tumor-specific antigens are expressed only on tumor cells and are not found on normal nonmalignant cells. Recent studies identifying genes that encode tumor-specific antigens determined that these antigens were small peptide fragments presented on the surface of tumor cells by major histocompatibility complex (MHC) class I molecules. Proteins that contain these peptides are not required to be displayed on the tumor cell surface, because peptide fragments are derived from the proteolysis of proteins within the cytosol. Thus proteins within the cytoplasm of tumor cells can be immunogenic and induce a specific T cell response when they are broken down into peptides in the cytoplasm and transported to the cell surface by MHC class I molecules. As these antigens are small peptide fragments (approximately nine amino acids long) that rest within the "groove" of MHC class I molecules, it is not possible to generate antibodies specific for these antigens. Peptides are only recognized by antigen-specific receptors on T cells. Therefore tumor-specific antigens are associated with cell-mediated immunity and not the humoral immune response. Recent evidence suggests that ocular melanoma and retinoblastoma may express tumor antigens that are recognized by tumor-specific T cells.

By contrast, tumor-associated antigens (TAA) are found on both malignant and normal cells; however, malignant cells express greatly elevated levels of TAA. TAA that have been identified include gangliosides and proteins expressed only during differentiation of embryonic cells. These proteins must be expressed on the tumor cell surface to be recognized by the immune system. An example of a tumor-associated antigen found on ocular tumors is the GD3 ganglioside found on choroidal melanoma cells (the expression of TAA on ocular tumors is discussed later in this chapter).

Specific T Cell Responses: Cytotoxic T Cells, T_{DH} Cells, and T_H Cells. Several subpopulations of T cells are involved in the antitumor T cell response:

- T_C—cytotoxic T cells and precursors of cytotoxic T cells (pT_C)
- T_{DH}—T cells that mediate delayed hypersensitivity (DH)—a subpopulation of Th cells.
- T_H—T cells that secrete lymphokines required for activation of pT_C and the effectors of DH.

Cytotoxic T cells (T_C) are CD8+, CD4− T cells, restricted by MHC class I molecules, that specifically lyse tumor cells expressing specific antigens. Experiments using murine tumor models have demonstrated T_C are effective in eliminating tumor cells in vitro and in vivo. T_C lyse tumor cells by a complex series of events that is initiated when T_C bind target cells via the TCR/CD3 (T cell antigen receptor/cluster designation) complex, resulting in T cell stimulation. Stimulated T cells reorient cell-surface molecules and increase expression of adhesion molecules that strengthen cell-cell binding. Microtubules within the cytoplasm of T_C are also reoriented to direct vesicles containing lytic factors toward the point of contact with tumor cells. At the point of contact

with the tumor cell, T_C release lytic factors that mediate tumor-cell lysis via multiple mechanisms. T_C have the ability to recycle and repeatedly bind and lyse multiple tumor cells. The initial induction and amplification of populations of specific cytotoxic T cells occur in a series of sequential steps that begins with the clonal expansion of CD8+ pT_C (precursor cytotoxic T cells) and CD4+ T_H (T helper cells) within the draining lymph node, and culminates in the lymphokine-driven terminal differentiation of pT_C into cytolytic T cells (Fig. 12-1). There is evidence that pT_C proceed through several distinct stages of differentiation before obtaining cytolytic activity, and these separate stages are each driven by distinct lymphokines. Thus the generation of tumor-specific cytotoxic T cells and the mechanism by which they effect tumor cell lysis are complex processes.[1]

T cells that mediate delayed hypersensitivity (T_{DH}) are contained within a subpopulation of T helper cells called Th1 cells. T helper cells (T_H/T_{DH}) cells are CD4+, CD8−, MHC class II restricted T cells. Activation of T_{DH} cells by recognition of specific tumor antigens results in the release of lymphokines that recruit and activate macrophages, resulting in a local inflammatory response. Elimination of tumor cells via delayed hypersensitivity occurs mainly by cytotoxic and cytostatic factors released by macrophages. Experimental systems using murine tumor models have demonstrated that both cytotoxic T cells and T cells that mediate delayed hypersensitivity can mediate tumor rejection. The relative roles of each of these effector cells are unclear and may vary depending on the tumor cell type.

Lymphokine Driven Differentiation of Cytotoxic T cells

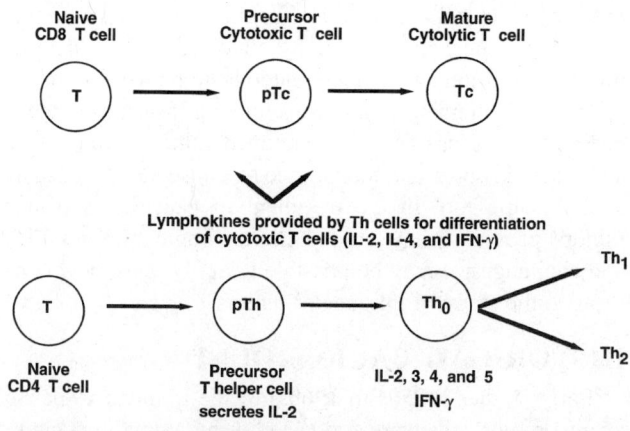

Fig. 12-1. The activation of cytolytic T cells starts with the clonal expansion of CD8+ precursor cytotoxic T cells and CD4+ precursor helper T cells. Differentiation of precursor cells is driven by lymphokines secreted by T helper cells and occurs in a series of sequential steps. The ability of cytolytic T cells to lyse tumor cells is acquired in the final stage of maturation.

Nonspecific Effector Cells

Natural Killer Cells. Natural killer (NK) cells compose approximately 5% of peripheral blood lymphocytes and express $CD56^+$, $CD2^+$, $NKH1^+$, and $CD3^-$ cell surface markers. NK cells eliminate tumor cells via two separate mechanisms: (1) the direct binding and lysing of tumor cells through the release of cytolytic factors, and (2) the indirect activation of antitumor immune responses by the secretion of IFN-γ. Although NK cells are nonspecific and lack the TCR/CD3 receptor complex, they demonstrate limited specificity and can recognize and lyse (1) virus-infected, but not uninfected, target cells, (2) a wide range of malignant, but not normal, target cells, and (3) a limited number of transformed cell lines. At present it is not known what type of receptor(s) and ligand(s) NK cells use to identify these different target cells. NK cells are activated by IFN-γ to proliferate and display increased cytolytic activity for tumor target cells. Evidence that NK cells are involved in antitumor immunity is derived from experiments that demonstrate NK-deficient beige mice are unable to eliminate some tumors that are rejected in mice with normal NK activity. In addition, accelerated tumor growth is observed when NK cells are depleted in vivo by injection of NK-specific complement-fixing antibodies.

Several laboratories have studied the relationship between the susceptibility of tumor cells to NK-mediated lysis and the expression of cell-surface MHC class I molecules.[31] These studies revealed that NK-mediated tumor cell lysis is inversely related to MHC class I expression on the surface of tumor cells. In other words, MHC class I deficient tumor cells are more susceptible to NK lysis, and tumor cells that express MHC class I are resistant to NK lysis. Because tumor cells may downregulate MHC class I expression in an effort to escape T cell-mediated immunity, NK-mediated lysis may represent an important mechanism to combat MHC class I deficient tumor cells. It is important to note, however, that not all MHC class I deficient tumor cells display increased susceptibility to NK-mediated lysis. Future studies in this area may yield important information on how NK cells identify tumor target cells. NK cells also lyse tumor cells by a distinct killing mechanism termed ADCC (antibody-dependent cell-mediated cytotoxicity) that is described later in this chapter.

Lymphokine-Activated Killer Cells. Peripheral blood lymphocytes cultured in vitro for 5 to 7 days in the presence of high concentrations of interleukin-2 (1000 units/ml) proliferate rapidly, resulting in the expansion of a heterogeneous population of cytotoxic cells termed lymphokine-activated killer (LAK) cells. LAK cells are a very heterogeneous population of lymphocytes; however, a large percentage of LAK cells is derived from the activation of NK cells. LAK cells are nonspecific cytotoxic cells that lyse a wide variety of tumor target cells from different histologic origins. Al-

though LAK cells are nonspecific effector cells, they display a limited degree of specificity for malignant target cells and fail to lyse nonmalignant cells. Some reports indicate LAK cells preferentially lyse fresh tumor cells, but fail to lyse tumor cell lines cultured in vitro for a prolonged time. Experiments using the adoptive transfer of LAK cells prevented tumor growth in murine models and resulted in considerable enthusiasm and hope that LAK cells could be used to treat human tumors.[63] Results from clinical trials using LAK cells are discussed in the section on Immunotherapeutic Treatment of Tumors.

Macrophages. Resting macrophages display almost no cytotoxic activity toward tumor cells; by contrast, activated macrophages are tumoricidal and release cytolytic and cytostatic factors. Macrophages are activated by either endotoxins or Th cell-secreted lymphokines such as IFN-γ. Activated macrophages are nonspecific cytotoxic cells that can distinguish between malignant and nonmalignant target cells, but are unable to recognize tumor cells in an antigen-specific manner. Experimental evidence suggests that macrophages are involved in antitumor immunity and eliminate some types of tumors. If macrophages are deleted by either specific antibody treatment or treatment with silica (a macrophage inhibitor), tumor growth is accelerated in some murine tumor models. In addition, stimulation of macrophages decreases tumor growth. Macrophages also participate in antibody-dependent cell-mediated cytotoxicity (ADCC) as described in the following section.

Antitumor Antibody Response

Tumor-Associated Antigens. Monoclonal antibodies specific for tumor-associated antigens (TAA) can be generated in vitro using the currently available technology. In addition, there are a few reports in the literature documenting the presence of antibodies specific for TAA in the autologous serum of some cancer patients, although the antitumor effects of these antibodies remain controversial. Although complement-fixing antibodies specific for TAA lyse tumor cells in vitro, the adoptive transfer of similar antibodies in animal tumor models has demonstrated limited tumor-inhibiting potential. This failure to reject tumors is probably due to a failure of the antibodies to gain access to the tumor cells in vivo. The high interstitial pressure found within most tumors results in poor perfusion and may prevent movement of antibodies from the blood vasculature into the tumor. An additional problem with antibodies specific for TAA is the nonspecific binding of antibodies to normal cells. Recent efforts using antitumor antibodies bound to toxins (immunotoxins), however, have led to some limited success in treating patients with B cell lymphoma.

Antibody Immunotoxins. Antibody immunotoxins consist of specific antibodies that are coupled to a toxin. In vitro studies demonstrated that A chain immunotoxins specifically killed tumor cells. Initial in vivo studies, however, were hampered by (1) instability of the toxin-antibody conjugate, (2) failure of the antibodies to gain access to the tumor, (3) nonspecific binding of the antibodies to normal cells, and (4) generation of antiimmunotoxin antibodies after repeated immunotoxin treatments. Current attempts at solving these problems should result in more effective immunotoxin treatments for cancer patients in the future.[95]

Antibody-Dependent Cell-Mediated Cytotoxicity. Macrophages and a subpopulation of NK cells (originally called K cells) express Fcγ receptors that bind antibodies specific for tumor-associated antigens. Tumor cells coated with specific antibodies are bound by macrophages or NK cells via these receptors. Binding of the Fcγ receptor on NK cells and macrophages activates a killing mechanism that lyses tumor target cells. It should be noted, however, that NK cells participating in ADCC mediate tumor destruction via a mechanism distinct from NK lysis of tumor cells. This situation was demonstrated by the observation that ADCC requires NK cells that express Fcγ receptors, whereas NK cells lacking Fcγ receptors are still able to bind and lyse tumor target cells.

TUMOR-SPECIFIC T CELL RESPONSE

Characterization and Identification of Specific T Cells in Cancer Patients

The remainder of this chapter will focus on studies of the induction and expression of tumor-specific T cells in patients with progressively growing tumors. This population of effector cells is considered by some to possess the most potential for effectively eliminating tumors. This belief is based on the following: (1) data using animal tumor models indicate specific T cells are more efficient and effective than nonspecific effectors (NK and LAK cells) at eliminating tumors, (2) specific T cells display a high degree of specificity for malignant cells and therefore can eliminate tumors with minimal damage to surrounding normal tissue, and (3) new data on the molecular basis of specific tumor antigens have provided an approach for the development of gene therapies and immunotherapies directed at manipulating specific T cells. As tumor-specific T cells in patients with metastatic cutaneous melanoma have been studied extensively, this chapter will concentrate on this group of patients. Similar studies have been conducted on a variety of other types of tumors, however. The relevance of these results to the study of the immune response to ocular melanoma will be discussed.

Tumor-Specific T Cells Within the Peripheral Blood. Originally it was difficult to detect tumor-specific T cells among peripheral blood lymphocytes (PBL) recovered from patients with recurrent and/or metastatic melanoma. In these experiments PBL were isolated and immediately tested for the ability to lyse autologous melanoma cells. Results from these experiments demonstrated that PBL were unable to lyse tumor target cells, and therefore it was concluded that ''fresh'' PBL did not contain terminally differentiated specific cytotoxic T cells. For many years these experimental results were used as evidence that patients did not possess T cells specific for antigens on autologous tumor cells. In the 1980s, however, several laboratories reported that tumor-specific cytotoxic T cells could be detected in the PBL of melanoma patients, if PBL were restimulated in vitro under specific conditions.[62] Mixtures of PBL and x-irradiated autologous tumor cells were cultured in vitro for 5 to 7 days in the presence of exogenous interleukin-2 (IL-2). Restimulated lymphocytes recovered from these cultures lysed specifically autologous tumor cells. The addition of IL-2 during restimulation in vitro was essential for detecting specific cytotoxic cells, and no cytotoxic activity could be detected in the absence of IL-2. These results suggested that PBL from melanoma patients contained precursor cytotoxic T cells that were tumor-specific, but unable to lyse tumor cells unless additional differentiation signals were provided by lymphokines such as IL-2. Restimulation of precursor cells in cultures containing IL-2 provided the necessary differentiation signal for pT_C to mature into cytotoxic T cells that lysed tumor cells. The reason(s) precursor cytotoxic cells fail to differentiate in situ in cancer patients will be discussed later in this chapter.

Investigators were able to establish and maintain bulk cultures of melanoma-specific cytotoxic T cells by continued restimulation of T cells with autologous tumor cells plus IL-2. Clones of specific T cells were isolated from these bulk cultures using limiting dilution techniques. Obtaining clones of specific T cells provided investigators with a sufficient number of lymphocytes to conduct extensive studies on these T cells.[41,71] Cloned melanoma-specific cytotoxic T cells ($CD3^+$, $CD8^+$, $CD4^-$) lysed autologous melanoma tumor cells and failed to lyse nonmalignant Epstein-Barr virus-transformed B cells or fibroblasts isolated from the same patient. Lysis of autologous tumor cells was HLA class I restricted, as demonstrated by the failure of specific T cells to lyse allogeneic melanoma cells, isolated from a series of other patients, that did not share common HLA class I loci with the original patient. Further evidence that these specific T cells were HLA class I restricted was provided by experiments in which antibodies specific for monomorphic HLA class I determinants prevented the killing of autologous tumor cells in cytotoxicity assays by precluding T cell receptors from recognizing antigens presented by class I molecules. Melanoma-specific T cells lysed autologous melanoma cells, but failed to lyse other types of malignant target cells recovered from tumors of other histologic origins that either shared HLA class I loci or were disparate at all HLA class I loci. Together, these results demonstrate that lymphocytes, recovered from the peripheral blood lymphocytes of melanoma patients and restimulated in vitro, contain tumor-specific, HLA class I restricted, cytotoxic T cells.

Frequency of Specific T Cells in the Peripheral Blood. To determine the frequency of tumor-specific T cells in cancer patients, Coulie and associates[23] used limiting dilution techniques to quantitate the number of specific precursor cytotoxic T cells among peripheral blood lymphocytes of melanoma patients. These studies determined the number of specific T cells with the potential to lyse autologous tumor cells. Their results revealed that in seven different melanoma patients the frequency of specific pT_C ranged from 1/900 to 1/33,000 (specific pT_C/peripheral lymphocytes). In comparison, the frequency of pT_C to minor alloantigens is within this range. These results demonstrate that spontaneous tumors induce the clonal expansion of a population of specific T cells, and that the size of this population is similar to that observed for other types of immunogenic antigens.

Tumor-Specific T Cells Within the Tumor Site. The detection of precursor cytotoxic T cells among peripheral blood lymphocytes of melanoma patients led to speculation on whether these cells were able to migrate from the blood vasculature and infiltrate the tumor site. As subcutaneous melanomas frequently contain infiltrating lymphocytes, techniques were developed to recover tumor-infiltrating lymphocytes by the enzymatic digestion of tumor tissue. The cells recovered were then analyzed to determine if specific T cells were present. Tumor-infiltrating lymphocytes recovered from metastatic melanomas and assayed immediately for cytotoxic activity exhibited poor lysis of autologous tumor cells and NK-sensitive target cells. In addition, tumor-infiltrating lymphocytes displayed minimal in vitro proliferative responses to autologous tumor cells and mitogenic stimulation. Thus lymphocytes within the tumor were similar to peripheral blood lymphocytes in failing to contain mature cytotoxic T cells or cells that proliferate in response to stimulation by tumor antigens.

By contrast, restimulation of tumor-infiltrating lymphocytes in IL-2-containing cultures routinely resulted in proliferation and expansion of a population of lymphocytes with significant cytotoxic activity.[40,88] Characterization of restimulated tumor-infiltrating lymphocytes from different patients indicated that some patients possessed highly specific cytotoxic T cells that lysed autologous tumor cells in an HLA class I restricted manner. Although most tumors contained infiltrating lymphocytes that could be expanded in cultures containing IL-2, not all tumors possessed lymphocytes with specific cytotoxic activity.

Three patterns of cytotoxic activity were reported: (1) highly specific killing of only autologous tumor cells, (2) mixed specificity, in which autologous tumor cells are lysed more efficiently than allogeneic tumor target cells, and (3) nonspecific lysis of both autologous and allogeneic melanoma cells. Further investigation revealed that these patterns of cytotoxic activity coincided with the infiltration of (1) specific precursor cytotoxic T cells, (2) a mixture of specific T cells and nonspecific NK/LAK cells, and (3) only nonspecific NK/LAK cells. The frequency of melanoma patients that possess highly specific T cells among tumor-infiltrating lymphocytes is unclear at the present time. It is difficult to determine if the failure to detect specific T cells is due to either the absence of specific T cells or whether specific T cells are present, but the culture conditions fail to provide the necessary differentiation signals to detect these cells.

T Cell Receptors Used by Melanoma-Specific T Cells. The expression of tumor-specific antigens on melanoma cells could drive the accumulation of tumor-specific T cells within the tumor site. Moreover, melanoma cells expressing a limited number of tumor antigens could result in the accumulation of an oligoclonal population of T cells that express a limited number of T cell receptor (TCR) specificities. By contrast, if the number of tumor antigens is very large, or there is no selective pressure for the accumulation of specific T cells within the tumor, then tumor-infiltrating lymphocytes will display a great diversity of T cell receptor specificities.

To distinguish between these two possibilities several laboratories have examined the T cell receptor α and β chain genes used by tumor-infiltrating lymphocytes to determine if they display a polyclonal or oligoclonal pattern.[79,86,96] Polymerase chain reaction (PCR) amplification techniques were used to recover and analyze RNA for T cell receptor $V\alpha$ and $V\beta$ genes among fresh and cultured tumor-infiltrating lymphocytes and peripheral blood lymphocytes. Although the results are still controversial, several different laboratories have reported the preferential use of a limited number of T cell receptor $V\alpha$ and $V\beta$ genes among tumor-infiltrating lymphocytes, compared with peripheral blood lymphocytes from normal donors. The most frequently reported genes are $V\alpha4$, $V\alpha22$, $V\beta8$, and $V\beta2$. These results suggest that cutaneous melanoma tumor cells may express a limited number of shared and/or specific tumor antigens, and that these antigens drive the preferential accumulation of specific T cells within the tumor site.

T Cells Specific for Primary and Metastatic Tumor Cells. The previous studies indicated that cutaneous melanoma-specific T cells are found in the peripheral blood and tumor-infiltrating lymphocytes of some patients. This raised several questions about the expression of tumor antigens on melanoma cells: (1) Are multiple antigens expressed on tumor cells from a single patient? (2) If there are multiple antigens, can tumor cells present only one or many antigens? and (3) Are the same antigens expressed on primary and metastatic tumors? In addition, some investigators questioned whether these melanoma antigens were the result of cultural artifacts, as these studies used melanoma cell lines cultured in vitro for a prolonged period of time.

To determine the extent of heterogeneity among melanoma tumor cells cultured from a single patient, subclones of melanoma cells were obtained and tested against a panel of cloned specific cytotoxic T cells. These studies revealed that clones of melanoma cells were resistant to lysis by some T cell clones, but could still be lysed by others.[46,100] Further studies indicated that at least three distinct tumor antigens were present on these tumor cells and that a single subpopulation of tumor cells expressed all three antigens on individual cells. These initial studies have important implications for the development of immunotherapies that use tumor-specific T cells, because they indicate that the expression of tumor antigens is heterogeneous and that a specific T cell response must be directed at several different tumor antigens to effectively eliminate all tumor cells.

Permanent melanoma tumor cell lines that are cultured in vitro for a long time are required for experiments that analyze tumor-specific T cell clones. Tumor cell lines are necessary, as prolonged culture of specific T cells requires continued restimulation with autologous tumor cells. This fact raises the possibility that tumor antigens recognized by T cells are cultural artifacts occurring as a result of prolonged culture of tumor cells in vitro. In support of this idea is the observation that culturing tumor cell lines in vitro can change the immunogenicity of tumor cells. To ensure that antigens recognized by specific T cell clones were not the result of cultural artifacts, Boon and associates[26] tested the reactivity of clones derived from a long-established melanoma cell line against a freshly collected metastatic relapse from a single patient, and found that T cell clones lysed freshly isolated metastatic tumor cells not cultured in vitro. These results demonstrate that tumor antigens recognized by specific T cell clones are expressed by tumor cells in vivo and also are found on permanent melanoma cell lines. In addition, these results demonstrate that T cells specific for a primary tumor can also recognize tumor antigens on a metastatic tumor that develops after a prolonged disease-free interval.

Tumor-Specific T Helper Cells. The differentiation of precursor cytotoxic T cells into mature cytolytic cells is mediated by lymphokine-secreting T helper cells. For this reason, the study of the T helper cell response in melanoma patients may provide important insights into why mature cytotoxic T cells are absent, and why the immune response fails to control tumor growth. Unlike the recovery and culture of CD8$^+$ specific T cells, it has been extremely difficult to detect or culture tumor-specific CD4$^+$ Th cells from melanoma patients.

This problem may stem from the fact that either (1) tumor cells possess antigens that stimulate CD8$^+$ T cells, but fail to display antigens that stimulate CD4$^+$ T helper cells, or (2) culture conditions currently used in experiments are unable to support the growth of CD4$^+$ T helper cells. Data in support of the latter were recently supplied by Cohen and associates[20] and indicated tumor-specific CD4$^+$ T helper cells restimulated with a combination of tumor cells, antigen-presenting cells, and different combinations of exogenous IL-2, IL-7, and IFN-γ resulted in the propagation of CD4$^+$ T cells from the peripheral blood of several melanoma patients. Tumors may fail to present antigens that stimulate CD4$^+$ T helper cells. Animal models of tumor rejection by specific cytotoxic T cells indicate that successful rejection of tumors requires a sustained source of lymphokine-secreting T helper cells. Therefore this area of research is likely to be critical in identifying a potential defect in the T cell response that allows immunogenic tumor cells to escape elimination.

Specific Tumor Antigens and Shared Tumor Antigens. Initial experimental results indicated that either HLA-A, HLA-B, or HLA-C class I molecules were capable of presenting melanoma tumor antigens to specific T cells. A more recent detailed analysis of the HLA class I restricting elements used by specific T cells revealed a slightly more complicated situation—there were both specific tumor antigens and shared tumor antigens recognized by T cells.[70] Specific T cells that recognize melanoma antigens presented by HLA-A1 class I molecules are tumor-specific and fail to lyse HLA-A1$^+$ normal melanocytes. By contrast, T cells that recognize melanoma antigens in the context of HLA-A2.1 class I molecules recognize a tumor antigen that is shared and found on melanoma cells and "normal" A2.1 positive melanocytes. Because T cells effectively lyse HLA-A2 positive tumor cells, but are less effective in lysing normal HLA-A2 positive melanocytes, it is likely that shared antigens are expressed at elevated levels on tumor cells.

Together these results indicate that specific T cells are HLA class I restricted, and recognition of tumor cells requires expression of (1) the relevant tumor antigen, and (2) the appropriate HLA class I molecule. There appear to be at least two types of tumor antigens presented by class I molecules: (1) antigens that are tumor-specific and not found on normal cells, or (2) antigens that are shared and found on both malignant and nonmalignant cells. The molecular difference between specific and shared melanoma antigens is discussed in the following section.

Conclusions. The results from these experiments indicate that tumor-specific CD8$^+$ T cells are clonally expanded in some patients and can be found in both the peripheral blood and the primary tumor site. In situ, these specific T cells remain in an early precursor stage of development and are unable to effect lysis of tumor cells. Although precursor T cells are inactive in situ, they can be restimulated in vitro to differentiate into mature cytotoxic T cells that display potent antitumor cytotoxic activity. These results imply that spontaneous tumors are immunogenic and induce the expansion of specific precursor T cells with the potential to eliminate autologous tumor cells; however, tumors escape immune-mediated elimination when these precursor cells fail to fully mature into cytotoxic effector cells.

Identification of Antigens Recognized by Specific T Cells

Historically, the search for tumor-specific antigens started with an effort to generate antibodies that would specifically bind tumor cells. Although this approach yielded interesting results, it was difficult to obtain antibodies that were truly specific for autologous tumor cells. Most of these antibodies recognized tumor-associated antigens—antigens found on normal cells, but present in larger quantities on tumor cells. These disappointing results led some researchers to question the existence of tumor-specific antigens. The preceding section discussed the data (obtained by cellular immunologists) identifying populations of tumor-specific T cells in some cancer patients. In spite of this evidence, the existence of tumor antigens remained controversial. In 1991, however, Boon and associates[93] identified a gene, which encoded a tumor antigen on melanoma cells, that was recognized by cytotoxic T cells (providing conclusive proof that T cells recognize specific tumor antigens). These studies provided a molecular basis for the observation that some spontaneous tumors were immunogenic, and renewed interest in the development of therapies directed at manipulating tumor-specific T cells.

Cloning Tumor Antigen Genes. The initiation of a tumor-specific CD8$^+$ T cell response requires that unique tumor antigens are presented by HLA class I molecules on the surface of tumor cells. The pathway by which endogenous antigens gain access to HLA class I molecules is discussed in detail in Chapter 6—Cellular Immunity and the Eye. Boon's approach[11] to identify tumor antigens was based on the concept that only T cell receptors could recognize the relevant tumor antigen, and therefore only specific T cells could identify these antigens. Using this rationale, he developed a unique method for identifying genes that encode tumor antigens[11] (Fig. 12-2). A cosmid library was prepared from genomic DNA isolated from a melanoma cell line that expressed an antigen recognized by a clone of tumor-specific cytotoxic T cells. Small segments of the cosmid library (40 kb) were packaged into a selectable vector system. To screen the entire genomic DNA library, 7×10^5 different cosmid vectors were prepared. A variant of the original melanoma cell line was isolated that failed to express the tumor antigen and therefore was no longer lysed by the T cell clone. It was possible to obtain this "antigen-loss-variant," because the original melanoma cell line was heterogeneous and not a cloned cell line. Specific T cells were used to identify, isolate, and subclone the antigen-loss-variant melanoma clone. Different cosmid vectors were then transfected into the antigen-loss variant and screened with the specific T cell clone for the expression of the tumor antigen. If a par-

Cloning of Tumor Antigen Genes

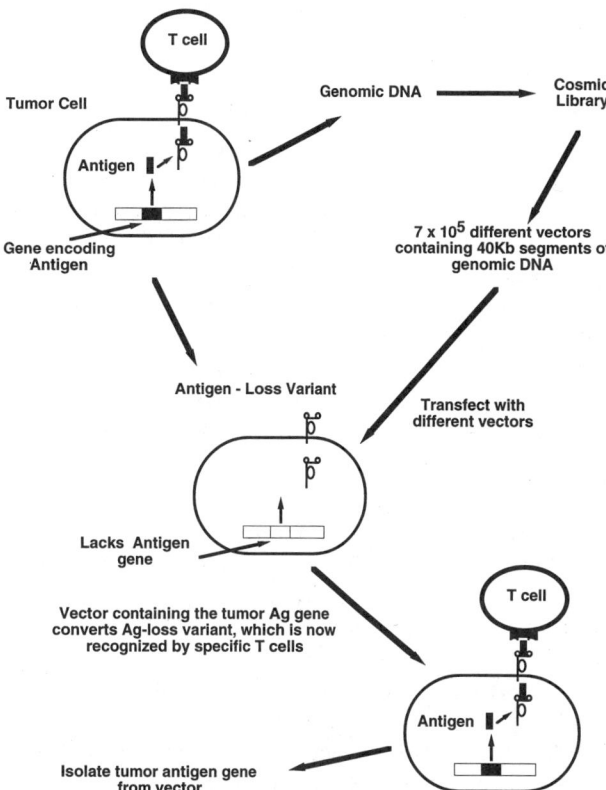

Fig. 12-2. Expression cloning was used successfully to identify genes that encode tumor-specific antigens on both mouse and human tumor cells.

ticular vector contained the gene for the relevant antigen, it would convert the antigen-loss variant into an antigen-positive cell that would be lysed by the T cell clone. The analysis of over 6000 different transfected melanoma cell lines revealed several transfectants that restored expression of the tumor antigen. Cosmid DNA was retrieved from these cells and further dissected with restriction enzymes. The analysis of these smaller fragments of DNA revealed a gene that transferred expression of the tumor antigen recognized by specific cytotoxic T cells. This procedure (called "expression cloning") was used successfully by Boon and associates[92,93] to identify tumor-specific antigens on both mouse and human tumor cells.

Genes Encoding Melanoma Antigens. Expression cloning was used to isolate a family of genes from human cutaneous melanoma cells that encode for antigens recognized by T cells. These genes, termed MAGE genes (for melanoma antigen genes), are present in all normal cells but transcriptionally active only in tumor cells.[27,90] There is a family of 11 different MAGE genes (MAGE 1-11) that are all highly homologous and found on chromosome 6. MAGE-1 expression was analyzed by PCR amplification of MAGE-1 mRNA and revealed the MAGE-1 gene was expressed in (1) several different melanoma cell lines, (2) fresh melanoma tumor tissue, and (3) both primary and metastatic tumors. MAGE-1 mRNA was not detected in lymphocyte clones, muscle cells, skin fibroblasts, or kidney cells. The MAGE-1 gene was found transcriptionally active in 37% of all melanoma cell lines tested, 33% of small cell lung carcinomas, and 17% of breast tumors. By contrast, MAGE-1 mRNA was not detected in colon carcinoma, renal cell carcinoma, or leukemic cells. It is interesting to note that the testes is the only normal tissue in which MAGE-1 mRNA was detected. The significance of this finding is unclear and currently under investigation. The MAGE-1 gene codes for a nanomer peptide that binds to HLA-A1 class I and is recognized by specific cytotoxic T cells. HLA-A1 positive nonmalignant cells, with a transcriptionally silent MAGE-1 gene, do not express the relevant antigen and are not lysed by MAGE-1 specific T cells. If these cells are transfected with a plasmid that contains a transcriptionally active MAGE-1 gene, however, this transfers sensitivity to MAGE-1 specific T cells and leads to cell lysis.

Techniques Used to Identify Tumor Antigens. The first successful isolation of a tumor antigen gene was accomplished using the expression cloning technique described previously; however, as this technique is very labor intensive, laboratories have attempted to use other techniques to identify tumor antigens. Recently tumor antigens were identified by using acid elution techniques to extract peptides from denatured cell-surface HLA class I molecules, that were then analyzed by HPLC (high-performance liquid chromatography) fractionation for peptides that stimulate T cell clones. Identification of a specific antigenic peptide sequence would allow further studies directed at isolating the relevant gene. This technique has been used successfully to identify immunogenic peptides from virus-infected cells and is currently being employed in several laboratories in an attempt to identify tumor-specific antigens.[81,82] Another technique currently being employed to identify tumor antigens uses the fact that binding of immunogenic peptides to HLA class I molecules requires critical anchor residues within the peptide sequence. As these anchor residues are required for peptides to bind HLA class I, it is possible to analyze known peptide sequences and predict if they possess a potential HLA class I binding motif. Because many mutant oncogenes have already been sequenced, it is possible to screen these different sequences for peptides with a potential HLA class I binding motif. This method recently identified an immunogenic peptide fragment from a mutant p53 gene.[101] Thus currently there are three different methods to identify tumor antigens: (1) expression cloning, (2) acid elution of HLA class I peptides, and (3) screening mutant oncogene sequences for HLA class I peptide-binding motifs. Which of these techniques is the most effective at identifying tumor antigens remains to be determined.

Types of Tumor Antigens Identified. Using the techniques described previously, four categories of tumor antigens have been identified on human tumors that are recognized by specific T cells: (1) oncogene proteins, (2) tumor-suppressor gene products, (3) tumor virus gene products, and (4) MAGE-type tumor genes (Table 12-1). An example of antigens derived from oncogene products is the proto-oncogene p210$^{BCR-ABL}$, which is found in chronic myelogenous leukemia. This gene is a fusion (of the ABL and BCR genes) that occurs during malignant transformation. The p210$^{BCR-ABL}$ gene codes for a protein with tyrosine kinase activity that is expressed only in malignant cells. Studies by Cheever and associates[18] indicate that the gene product encodes for unique peptides that are presented by HLA class I molecules and recognized by specific T cells. Another example of antigens derived from oncogenes is the p21 ras oncogene. Point mutations that occur in the p21 ras oncogene are found in several different types of tumors and give rise to immunogenic peptides that bind either HLA-DQ7, DP3, or DR2. These peptides are recognized by a CD4$^+$ T cell clone restricted by HLA-DR2. The function of these CD4$^+$ T cells remains to be determined.[30,36] These results demonstrate that tumor antigens derived from oncogenes encode peptides that also bind HLA class II molecules and are recognized by HLA class II restricted CD4$^+$ T cells.

Tumor suppressor genes (sometimes called antioncogenes) are a family of genes in which the gene product normally prevents uncontrolled proliferation and therefore "suppresses" tumor development. In normal cells these genes are active and functional; however, if mutations occur that alter and prevent the tumor suppressor gene product from functioning normally, malignant transformation can occur. The classic example of a tumor suppressor gene is the retinoblastoma (Rb) gene, which was the first tumor suppressor gene identified. p53 is also a tumor suppressor gene that is mutated and/or overexpressed in a variety of human tumors. Recent studies indicate that peptides derived from mutant p53 bind HLA-A2.1 and are immunogenic.[39] In these

TABLE 12-1 TYPES OF SPECIFIC TUMOR ANTIGENS

Tumor Antigen	Example	Responding T Cells
Oncogene proteins	Mutated p21 ras	CD4$^+$ T cells
	p210 ABL and BCR genes	CD8$^+$ T cells
Tumor suppressor gene products	Mutated p53	CD8$^+$ T cells
Tumor virus gene products	Human papilloma virus	CD8$^+$ T cells
Silent genes activated during transformation	MAGE	CD8$^+$ T cells

experiments specific CD8$^+$ cytotoxic T cells were obtained from peripheral blood lymphocytes that were restimulated in vitro with mutant p53 peptides "loaded" into antigen-presenting cells (antigen-presenting cells incubated with mutant p53 peptides that bind class I on the cell surface). As the retinoblastoma gene is a tumor suppressor gene functioning in a manner similar to p53, retinoblastoma tumors may also yield peptides presented by HLA class I molecules on the surface of retinoblastoma cells.

Immunogenic peptides have also been identified from tumor virus gene products such as (1) human papilloma virus gene products associated with cervical carcinoma, and (2) Epstein-Barr virus gene products associated with Hodgkin disease. The final category of tumor antigens contains the MAGE genes isolated from human cutaneous melanoma. These genes are present in normal cells, but are transcriptionally active only in tumor cells. These tumor antigens are different from those described previously, simply because the normal function of these "silent" genes remains unknown. **Proposed Mechanisms by Which Tumor Antigens Are Formed.** From their studies Boon and associates[91] have hypothesized that tumor antigens can be formed by three dif-

ferent mechanisms during malignant transformation of cells: (1) point mutations that allow new peptides to bind HLA class I, (2) point mutations that alter peptides that already bind HLA class I, or (3) activation of a gene that is normally silent and not transcribed in nonmalignant cells. The first two proposed mechanisms use mutational events induced by either chemical carcinogens or UV exposure. Not all peptide fragments are able to bind HLA class I molecules, and therefore some peptides are not presented on the cell surface. A point mutation may occur, however, enabling the peptide to bind HLA class I molecules. These altered peptide fragments are expressed on the cell surface and can now be recognized by T cells (Fig. 12-3, *A*). On the other hand, point mutations may also alter peptides that already bind HLA class I and are presented on the cell surface. The host is normally tolerant to these endogenous peptides, and therefore they are not immunogenic. A point mutation that alters these peptides may expose a new and/or novel epitope that becomes immunogenic and is recognized as foreign on tumor cells (Fig. 12-3, *B*). The final proposed mechanism occurs when normally silent genes are activated. A gene that is normally silent in nonmalignant cells is not transcribed

Proposed Mechanisms by which Tumor Antigens are Formed

A. Point mutations that allow new peptides to bind Class I

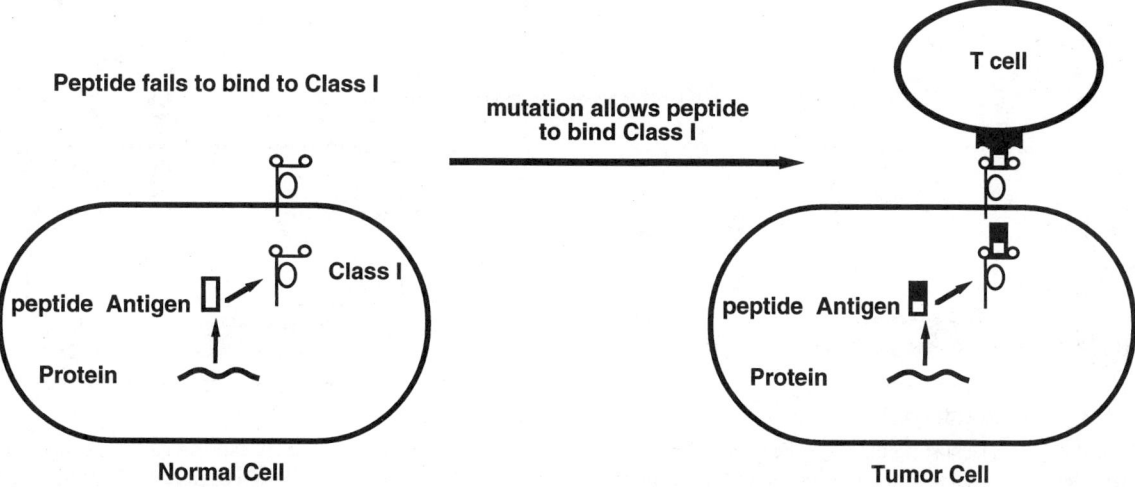

Fig. 12-3. The hypothetical mechanisms for the formation of specific antigens on tumor cells that are recognized by T cells. **A,** Point mutations allow new peptides to bind HLA class I molecules and this allows these new antigens to be expressed on the tumor cell surface.

Continued

Proposed Mechanisms by which Tumor Antigens are Formed

B. Mutations that expose new epitopes on peptides that already bind to Class I

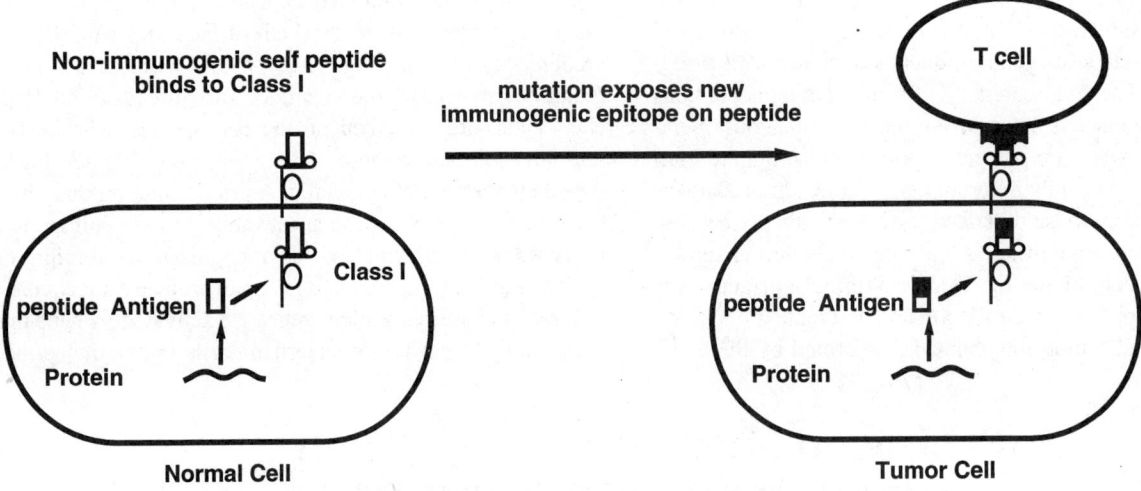

C. Activation of a gene normally silent and not transcribed in non-malignant cells

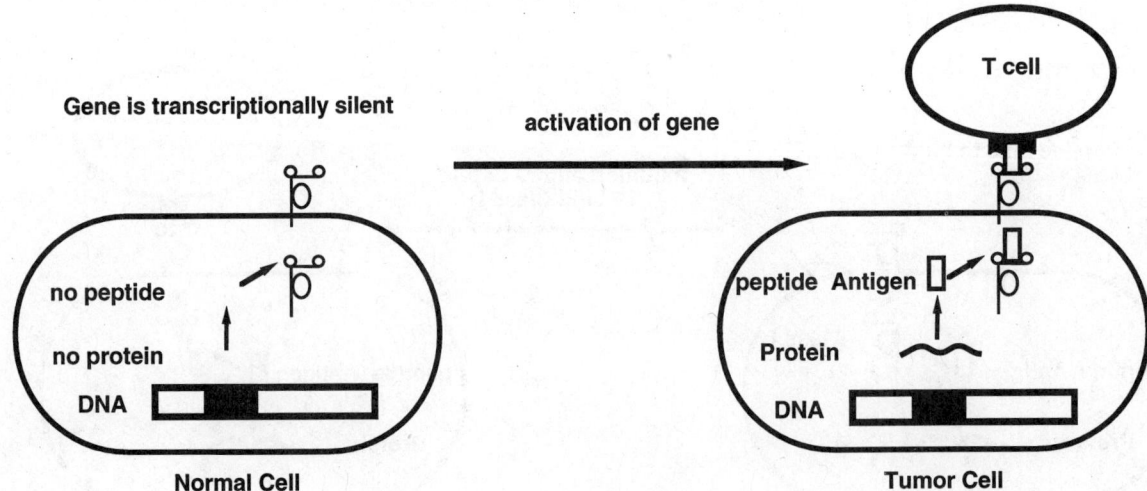

Fig. 12-3, cont'd.   B, The host is normally tolerant to "self" peptides that bind class I molecules and are expressed on the surface of normal cells. Mutations that expose new immunogenic epitopes on these peptides form novel antigens that are recognized by specific T cells. **C,** Normal cells possess genes that are transcriptionally silent, and therefore no peptide antigens are derived from proteins encoded by these genes. Malignant transformation may activate these genes, resulting in the expression of new immunogenic peptides on the tumor cell surface.

and therefore does not provide any endogenous peptides that can be presented by HLA class I. As the gene is not active in normal cells, there is no reason for the host to be tolerant to proteins encoded by this gene. If the gene is activated during malignant transformation, however, new immunogenic peptides are now presented on the cell surface by HLA class I molecules that can be recognized by specific T cells (Fig. 12-3, *C*).

Determining which of these mechanisms occurs most frequently in different types of tumors is important for the development of immunotherapeutic treatments. There are an unlimited number of possible antigens that could result from point mutations. Each individual tumor would therefore express unique antigens not found on similar types of tumors from other patients. Immunotherapies generating immune responses to these antigens would require that each individual tumor be isolated and the antigens identified. By contrast, antigens resulting from the activation of a silent normal gene are likely to be conserved and more homogeneous. Moreover, as the probability is high that the same gene will be present and activated in tumors of common histologic origins, it is likely all tumors of a certain type would share common antigens. If this were the case, patients that share the same HLA class I haplotype would express the same tumor antigens. Thus immunotherapies could be developed for specific types of tumors that would be effective among all patients sharing HLA class I loci.

In conclusion, a variety of techniques are currently used to identify and isolate genes that encode different tumor antigens. These initial studies have provided valuable evidence that spontaneous tumors are immunogenic. As these studies continue, it is likely many additional novel tumor antigens will be identified. Moreover, this research will probably become the basis for experiments that will determine (1) the molecular mechanism by which tumor cells fail to induce a successful immune response, and (2) the development of methods that manipulate the antitumor immune response.

MECHANISMS USED BY TUMOR CELLS TO ESCAPE IMMUNE RECOGNITION AND ELIMINATION

The identification of genes that encode tumor antigens resolved the long-debated issue of whether tumor cells express antigens recognized by specific T cells. An obvious question resulting from this research is: If tumors are immunogenic, why is the immune response unable to eliminate these cells? The following section describes several methods used by tumor cells to avoid and escape the immune system. In general, tumor cells block either the induction of immunity (afferent phase of the immune response) or the expression of immunity (efferent phase of the immune response). Blocking the afferent arm of immunity prevents the immune system from recognizing and detecting malignant cells. This

block can be accomplished by altering normal routes of antigen processing, antigen presentation, or the delivery of co-stimulatory signals to T cells. By contrast, once the immune system detects and responds to tumor antigens, tumors may block the efferent phase of immunity by creating a local immunosuppressive environment around the tumor site that downregulates effector cells infiltrating the tumor.

Defects in Antigen Presentation

Tumor cells present antigenic peptide fragments via cell-surface HLA class I molecules to specific CD8[+] T cells. These antigenic peptides are derived from proteins in the cell cytosol that are unfolded and cleaved by proteolytic enzymes (proteasomes). In the absence of cell-surface HLA class I molecules, antigenic peptides remain trapped in the cell cytosol and are unable to access the cell surface. Thus T cells are unable to recognize antigens on tumor cells deficient in cell-surface HLA class I molecules (Fig. 12-4). The downregulation of class I expression has been reported in many different types of tumors and may be achieved by

Defects in Antigen Presentation

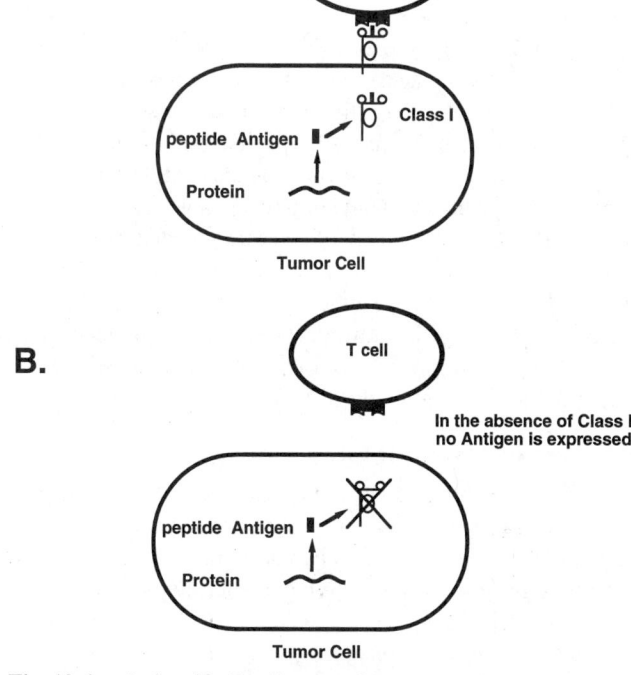

Fig. 12-4. **A,** Specific T cells recognize tumor antigens expressed on the cell surface by HLA class I molecules. **B,** In the absence of class I molecules, antigenic peptides are not expressed on the cell surface and T cells are unable to recognize the tumor cell.

either (1) the loss of class I α chain alleles, or (2) the loss of B_2-microglobulin (B_2-M).[35] The binding of B_2-microglobulin to class I α chain occurs in the endoplasmic reticulum and is required for proper folding of the α chains, and stabilizing the class I plus peptide complex. It is also involved in transporting class I molecules to the cell surface. In the absence of B_2-M, class I is not expressed on the cell surface. It has been reported that complete loss of class I α chains requires multiple mutations in the coding regions of these structural genes. By contrast, only two cumulative mutations in B_2-M are sufficient to induce the complete loss of cell-surface MHC class I molecules. For this reason, tumor cells may favor the loss of B_2-M as a mechanism to downregulate expression of class I and escape immune recognition.

Defects in Antigen Processing

Proteasomes form complexes with LMP (low molecular mass polypeptide) and are responsible for degrading proteins into peptide fragments in the cell cytosol. LMP-proteasome complexes may also deliver peptide fragments directly to transporter molecules encoded by TAP1 and TAP2 genes (transporters associated with antigen processing) that transport peptide fragments from the cytosol into the endoplasmic reticulum. For this reason LMP and TAP gene products are essential for proper processing of peptide fragments made available to class I molecules in the endoplasmic reticulum. Defects in proteasomes, LMP, or transporter molecules could either prevent proteolytic cleavage of proteins, or prevent transport of cleaved peptides from the cytosol into the endoplasmic reticulum. These defects would block antigen processing by preventing endogenous peptide fragments from gaining access to class I molecules in the endoplasmic reticulum. Recently Restifo and associates[75] reported that several human small-cell lung carcinoma cell lines were unable to present endogenous peptide fragments. This was associated with low or undetectable levels of LMP and TAP mRNA. Treatment of these tumor cells with IFN-γ increased the expression of TAP and LMP mRNA and restored the ability of these tumor cells to present peptide antigens via the class I pathway. These results indicate that tumor cells with altered TAP or LMP genes may escape immune recognition by blocking antigen processing.

Defects in Co-stimulator Signals

Effective stimulation of tumor-specific CD8$^+$ T cells requires at least two signals from antigen-presenting cells: (1) a peptide fragment presented by class I molecules, and (2) a second signal provided by soluble factors and/or co-stimulatory molecules. The second signal may be provided by either cytokines, adhesion molecules (ICAM-1, LFA-3, VLA-4), and/or the B7 co-stimulatory molecule. Recent evidence suggests that the B7 co-stimulatory molecule may play a pivotal role in stimulating naive T cells.[43,74] The receptor for B7 is CD28 and is found on 50% of CD8$^+$ T cells. B7 is expressed on antigen-presenting cells, but the cell-surface expression of B7 is highly regulated. High levels of B7 are found on antigen-presenting cells within the lymphoid tissues (activated B cells and splenic dendritic cells), and low levels are found on antigen-presenting cells outside the lymphoid tissues (peripheral monocytes and epidermal Langerhans cells). Stimulation of naive T cells is initiated when antigen-presenting cells endocytose antigenic material in the periphery and migrate to the draining lymph node where they present peptide fragments to specific T cells. Recent data suggest that antigen-presenting cells in the periphery upregulate B7 expression during their migration from the peripheral tissues to lymphoid organs.[54] It is not until after antigen-presenting cells express B7 that they are competent to stimulate specific T cells within the lymphoid tissues. Thus the expression of B7 appears to be critical in initiating a T cell response.

As mentioned previously, secondary stimulatory signals can also be provided by either cytokines or various adhesion molecules. These secondary signals are, however, fundamentally different from the co-stimulatory signals provided by B7. Antibodies specific for cytokines or adhesion molecules can block the delivery of these stimulatory signals and prevent T cell stimulation. The addition of cytokines and adhesion molecules to subsequent cultures (secondary stimulation), however, leads to successful T cell activation. By contrast, if anti-CD28 antibodies (Fab fragments only) are used to block the delivery of B7 co-stimulatory signals, T cell stimulation is prevented, and secondary stimulation is also blocked. Thus stimulating T cells in the absence of B7 co-stimulatory signals results in T cell anergy[83] (Fig. 12-5).

Tumor antigens can be presented to specific T cells via two routes: (1) directly by tumor cells themselves, and (2) by host antigen-presenting cells that migrate into a tumor site and reprocess tumor antigens. Tumor cells that express class I molecules can present endogenous tumor antigens directly to T cells; however, in the absence of a second co-stimulator signal provided by B7, this may be a tolerizing event. Tumor-specific precursor T cells that migrate into the tumor site can bind tumor cells expressing class I plus the relevant antigenic peptide fragment. Because tumor cells fail to express B7, however, these T cells fail to receive a second co-stimulatory signal, resulting in anergic T cells unable to differentiate and respond to further stimulatory signals. For this reason, it may be a selective advantage for tumor cells to express antigenic peptides, as long as they do not also express co-stimulatory B7 molecules. In an attempt to correct this block in stimulation of T cells, recent gene therapy experiments have been directed at transfecting tumor cells with vectors that contain cDNA for B7. Tumor cells, manipulated so that they express B7, effectively stimulate T cells in vitro and in vivo. These experiments are discussed in detail in the section Gene Therapy.

Immunosuppressive Tumor Microenvironment

There is mounting evidence that tumor cells secrete immunosuppressive factors such as TGF-β. These factors may create a suppressive environment around the site of tumor growth that alters the function of lymphocytes and antigen-presenting cells infiltrating the tumor. This suppressive environment may act directly on infiltrating lymphocytes, preventing them from terminally differentiating and mediating antitumor effector functions. In addition, antigen-presenting cells that infiltrate the tumor site and are exposed to suppressive factors may be unable to reprocess and present tumor antigens effectively. An example of this latter situation follows.

It is generally believed that endogenous antigens are only presented by class I molecules, and exogenous antigens are only reprocessed and presented by class II molecules on host antigen-presenting cells. Thus endogenous tumor antigens could be presented by class I molecules on tumor cells, or

Defects in Co-stimulation

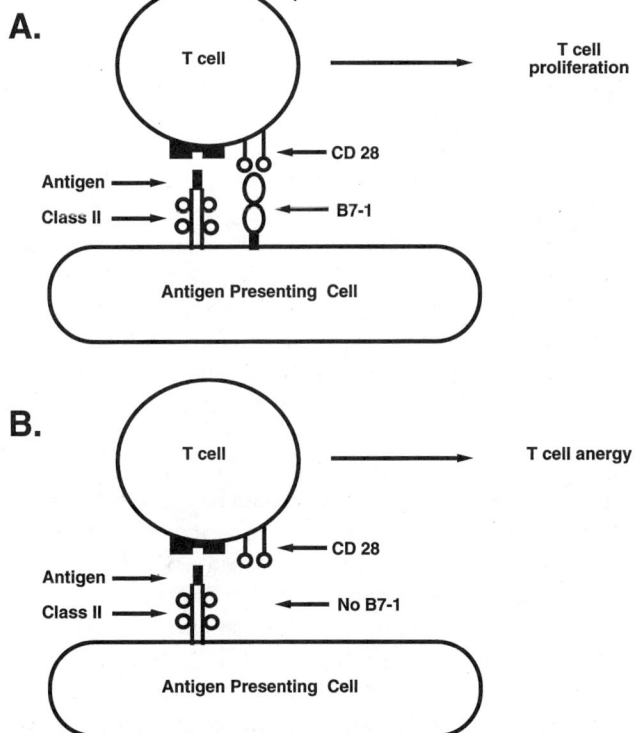

Fig. 12-5. A, Successful stimulation of T cells by professional antigen-presenting cells requires two signals, the antigenic peptide presented by HLA molecules and a second co-stimulatory signal provided by B7-1. **B,** In the absence of the second co-stimulatory signal, specific T cells are anergic and unable to respond to secondary stimulation.

Immunosuppressive Tumor Microenvironment

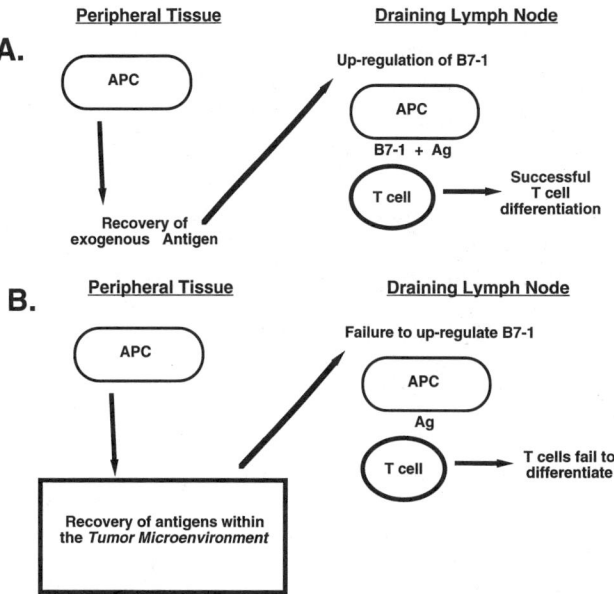

Fig. 12-6. A, Antigen-presenting cells migrate through peripheral tissues, recovering exogenous antigens that are transported to the draining lymph node. In the peripheral tissues, antigen-presenting cells fail to express the B7-2 co-stimulatory molecule; however, within the draining lymph node, B7-1 expression is upregulated. It is believed that the expression of B7-1 is required to successfully stimulate specific T cells. **B,** Antigen-presenting cells that migrate into the site of tumor growth are exposed to the local tumor microenvironment that contains factors secreted by tumor cells. If these factors prevent the subsequent upregulation of B7-1 on antigen-presenting cells, then the tumor antigens carried by these antigen-presenting cells will not induce T cell differentiation.

reprocessed and presented by class II molecules on host antigen-presenting cells. Under these circumstances class I restricted tumor antigens could only be presented by tumor cells and would not be presented by host antigen-presenting cells. This is an important difference considering that host antigen-presenting cells provide the necessary co-stimulatory signals to T cells. Preliminary evidence from Pardoll, however, indicates that tumor antigens may be reprocessed by host antigen-presenting cells and presented via the class I pathway, although it is unclear at this time how these exogenous antigens gain access to the class I pathway. These data indicate that host antigen-presenting cells that migrate into the tumor site process tumor antigens and present them via class I molecules to CD8[+] T cells in the draining lymph nodes. As host antigen-presenting cells have the potential to upregulate B7, this should lead to successful stimulation of specific T cells. In fact, this may be the mechanism that initiates the clonal expansion of specific CD8$^+$ precursor cytotoxic T cells found in the peripheral blood of cancer patients. It is also possible, however, that antigen-presenting cells that migrate into the tumor microenvironment and are exposed to immunosuppressive factors, are unable to upregulate B7 when they migrate to the draining lymph node. Thus antigen-presenting cells that migrate through the tumor site may be unable to properly stimulate T cells in the draining lymph node (Fig. 12-6). This view presents another possible mechanism by which tumor cells may escape immune recognition. Experiments that examine the functional properties of antigen-presenting cells recovered from within the tumor site should provide important information on the ability of these cells to properly stimulate tumor-specific T cells.

RELATIONSHIP BETWEEN IMMUNE PRIVILEGE AND HUMAN SPONTANEOUS TUMORS

A significant amount of research has been conducted on the immune response to immunogenic tumors growing within the anterior chamber of mouse eyes. The basis for this research is the observation that the anterior chamber is an immune-privileged site in which immunogenic tumor cells grow progressively and escape immune-mediated elimination. Although this model has been accepted as a valuable tool in dissecting the mechanisms by which immune privilege is established and maintained within the eye, its usefulness as a model for human ocular tumors has remained controversial. The reason for this is apparent in the obvious differences between this murine model and human ocular tumors (histologic origin of the tumor cells, the anatomic site and pattern of tumor growth, and so on). There is mounting evidence, however, that this model may provide insights into the mechanism(s) by which ocular and nonocular tumors evade T cell-mediated immune destruction. Moreover, these studies may suggest methods by which the immune response can be manipulated to successfully treat human spontaneous tumors.

The observation that human spontaneous tumors are immunogenic and induce a tumor-specific T cell response in some patients presents an immunologic paradox: Immunogenic tumor cells that grow progressively within an immunocompetent patient are capable of generating a T cell response to antigens presented on the surface of tumor cells. In 1977 Spitalny and North[80] were the first investigators to suggest a relationship between immune privilege and tumor growth. They proposed that tumors escape immune-mediated elimination by establishing a local microenvironment conveying immune privilege to the developing tumor. An immune-privileged site is defined as an anatomic site in which immunogenic cells or tissue survives for an extended time in an immunocompetent host. Spontaneous tumors develop in a variety of anatomic sites that are, for the most part, considered nonprivileged (in that allogenic grafts placed at

these sites are rapidly rejected). It was proposed that as spontaneous tumors form they convert the tumor site into an immune-privileged site, possibly by the secretion of local immunosuppressive factors. Since this hypothesis was originally proposed, many studies have reported that the local microenvironment plays an important role in establishing and maintaining immune privilege within the eye, brain, testis, and at the maternal-fetal junction. It still remains to be proved, however, whether suppressive factors alone can "create" an immune-privileged site. Two types of experimental evidence suggest that tumors can establish immune privilege locally. First, alloantigenic cells injected into the tumor microenvironment survive and are not eliminated. Second, if immunogenic tumor cells are injected into an already established immune-privileged site, tumors form and induce a T cell response similar to that induced by spontaneous human tumors.

To determine whether tumor sites establish a local immune-privileged environment, it is necessary to demonstrate that immunogenic tissue or cells survive within the tumor. Spitalny and North demonstrated that mice were incapable of eliminating an inoculation of *Listeria* injected into a progressively growing tumor in the right hind footpad. By contrast, mice easily eliminated the same inoculation of *Listeria* injected into the tumor-free left hind footpad. The authors speculated that the failure to eliminate *Listeria* from the tumor site resulted from the secretion of factors by the tumor that suppress the function of *Listeria*-specific T cells and macrophages.

A more elaborate series of experiments was performed by Perdrizet and associates[72] in 1990 demonstrating that immunogenic cells within the tumor microenvironment fail to induce an effective immune response. By contrast, if the same antigen is presented by cells on a normal skin graft, an effective immune response eliminates the graft. These investigators provided further evidence that the failure of the immune response to eliminate immunogenic tumor cells was not due to (1) the lack of a strong rejection antigen, (2) release of tumor antigens that caused the host to become unresponsive, or (3) rapid proliferation of tumor cells that outstrips the capacity of the immune system to respond. They postulated that factors secreted by the tumor cells prevented the induction of an effective local immune response. These experiments demonstrate that immunogenic cells within the tumor microenvironment induce a systemic immune response, but this response fails to successfully eliminate tumor cells. By definition, the extended survival of immunogenic tumor cells within the tumor microenvironment indicates that the tumor environment is acting as an immune-privileged site.

Additional circumstantial evidence that tumors form immune-privileged sites was obtained from experiments examining the immune response induced against immunogenic tumor cells injected into an already established immune-privilege site. The immune response induced against these tumors is remarkably similar to the response observed among patients with spontaneous human tumors. When minor histoincompatible P815 tumor cells are inoculated into the anterior chamber of the eye, they grow progressively and escape immune-mediated elimination, despite the fact that they induce the clonal expansion of tumor-specific precursor cytotoxic T cells. Precursor cells migrate systemically and infiltrate the tumor-containing eye, but they fail to terminally differentiate into cytolytic T cells that eliminate tumor cells.[5,6,51,52] Thus immunogenic tumor cells escape elimination by cytotoxic T cells within the immunologically privileged anterior chamber because precursor T cells fail to terminally differentiate into cytolytic T cells. The failure of precursor cells to differentiate locally coincides with (1) a lack of memory T helper cells that secrete lymphokines required to initiate precursor differentiation, and/or (2) suppression of precursor differentiation by the local microenvironment within the anterior chamber. In general, this type of immune response is very similar to the immune response observed among patients with metastatic cutaneous melanoma. These patients possess high frequencies of tumor-specific precursor cytotoxic T cells in their peripheral blood. These precursor cells infiltrate into the tumor site, but there is no evidence that they terminally differentiate into cytolytic T cells. Moreover, it is difficult to demonstrate that these patients possess tumor-specific CD4+ T helper cells. Together, these results indicate that spontaneous immunogenic tumors induce a specific, but unique, spectrum of T cell responses similar to immune responses induced within immune-privileged sites.

If tumors do establish an immune privilege-like microenvironment to escape immune elimination, it is likely that tumors accomplish this by the local secretion of immunosuppressive factors. The study of immune-privileged sites may provide some insights into the factors secreted by these tumors. One factor present within all immune-privileged sites (eye, brain, testis, and the maternal-fetal junction) is TGF-β_2. It is interesting to note that recent reports indicate that some human metastatic cutaneous melanomas secrete TGF-β_2.

IMMUNOTHERAPEUTIC TREATMENT OF TUMORS

Since the early 1950s it was believed that tumors might be eliminated by activation of a tumor-specific immune response. Among the different types of immune effector cells, the T cell response is particularly well suited for eliminating tumor cells, as T cells are specifically designed to distinguish between autologous and foreign antigens, responding only to cells expressing foreign antigens. Moreover, it seemed intuitive that during malignant transformation, cells might express new or altered antigens that would be recognized as foreign by the immune system. In spite of the logic

behind this argument, early attempts at immune-mediated elimination of tumors were generally disappointing. Early tumor immunotherapies typically involved treating patients with a mixture of nonspecific adjuvants and/or tumor cell lysates. As it is now known that tumor antigens are small peptide fragments presented on the cell surface by HLA class I molecules, it is not surprising that these early attempts at immunizing patients to tumor cell lysates failed to control tumor growth or induce specific T cells.

In the late 1980s a new generation of immunotherapies was developed that used different lymphokines with T cell growth and stimulatory properties. These new therapies became possible only after the development of molecular biologic techniques that allowed the isolation, purification, and cloning of lymphokine genes. This development made available large quantities of highly purified recombinant lymphokines that were tested for their ability to stimulate antitumor immunity. One of the first lymphokines used was interleukin-2 (IL-2), which was shown to stimulate antitumor immunity and control tumor growth in several different animal models. In general, these new immunotherapies have demonstrated limited success in clinical trials. Recent studies in mice using novel forms of gene therapy to manipulate the antitumor immune response have renewed the hope that a successful immunotherapy can be developed. The following section will discuss the immunotherapies currently in clinical trials and the recent advances in the use of gene therapy to treat cancer. This segment will be followed by studies that have attempted to eliminate ocular tumors in mice by immune-mediated mechanisms, and a discussion of the potential of treating ocular tumor patients with immunotherapeutic techniques.

Interleukin-2 Treatment

The rationale behind this treatment was based on the observation that high doses of IL-2 activated LAK cells in vitro. LAK cells are nonspecific cytotoxic cells that lyse a broad range of malignant tumor cells, but fail to lyse normal cells. Experiments conducted in animal models indicated that high doses of IL-2 injected intravenously activated LAK cells in situ that effectively controlled metastatic tumor growth. In general, the protocol used to treat metastatic cancer patients with IL-2 includes intravenous bolus injections of recombinant IL-2 every 8 hours at a concentration of 100,000 units/kg for 5 days, followed by 7 to 10 days of rest, followed by 5 more days of treatment. Metastatic cutaneous melanoma patients demonstrated a response rate of approximately 24% (including both partial and complete responses).[77] Most patients receiving high-dose IL-2 treatment display toxic side effects related to an IL-2-induced vascular leak syndrome manifested by hypotension, tachycardia, and oliguria. Treatment-related deaths caused by myocardial infarction have been reported. High doses of IL-2 are required, as the half-life of IL-2 in serum is extremely short, and an effective concentration in situ is only achieved with large IL-2 doses. In an effort to reduce the concentration of IL-2 required to initiate a response, LAK cells were isolated via hemopheresis, stimulated in vitro, and administered along with IL-2. A variety of other cytokines (IL-4, IL-6, IL-7, GM-CSF, TNF, IFN-α, and IL-12) are currently in various stages of phase I/II clinical trials to determine their efficacy and toxicity in cancer patients when injected intravenously.

LAK Plus Interleukin-2 Treatment

To increase the effectiveness of IL-2 treatments and minimize the related morbidity, autologous LAK cells were injected with a lower dose of IL-2.[77] Patients received 5 days of intravenous IL-2 injections followed by 5 days of leukapheresis to obtain peripheral blood lymphocytes. LAK cells were obtained by culturing peripheral blood lymphocytes for 4 to 5 days in vitro with 1000 units/ml of IL-2. LAK cells were reinfused into the patient along with IL-2 over the next 5 days. Patients typically received a cumulative dose of 5 to 10×10^{10} LAK cells. Although there was a slight increase in the effectiveness of this treatment (compared with IL-2 alone), and prolonged remissions were reported in some patients, the overall effectiveness of this treatment was disappointing. In an effort to further increase effectiveness, the next type of immunotherapy used tumor-specific T cells instead of nonspecific LAK cells. This decision was based on studies using mice that indicated tumor-specific T cells were 50 to 100 times more effective than nonspecific LAK cells in eliminating tumors.

Tumor-Infiltrating Lymphocytes Plus Interleukin-2 Treatment

Tumor-Infiltrating Lymphocytes (TIL) Plus Interleukin-2 treatment was based on the observation that lymphocytes extracted from freshly resected tumors can be expanded in vitro with IL-2 and often demonstrate specific lysis of autologous tumor cells. This treatment protocol required resection of tumors weighing between 10 and 30 grams and enzymatic digestion of tumor tissue to obtain TIL, that were then cultured for 4 to 8 weeks in IL-2. Restimulated TIL were reinfused into patients in 1 to 7 injections over 2 days, with the total number of cells injected ranging from 3 to 75 $\times$ 10^{10}. IL-2 was injected along with TIL, as in the treatments described previously. Although an early initial response rate of 60% was reported among metastatic cutaneous melanoma patients, more extensive clinical trials have yielded more limited success. The effectiveness of this treatment appears to be limited by the failure of in vitro stimulated TIL to recirculate and infiltrate into the tumor site. Thus although a large number of TIL are infused into the patient, very few gain access to the tumor site.

Gene Therapy

To increase the immunogenicity of tumor cells and generate a more effective immune response, several laboratories have recently demonstrated that different types of tumor cells transfected with one of several different cytokine genes can induce varying degrees of protective immunity in mice. In these experiments tumor cells were transfected with a selectable vector (retroviral and episomal vectors have both been used) containing cDNA for a specific cytokine gene. Transfected tumor cells are selected for the constitutive secretion of high levels of the appropriate cytokine, expanded in vitro, and then reinoculated into mice to induce an effective immune response. Prior to re-inoculation, transfected tumor cells were first x-irradiated to prevent continued proliferation of tumor cells; however, this did not prevent continued secretion of the cytokine, which continued for up to 2 weeks. Using this protocol, several laboratories observed that transfection of tumor cells with either TNF-α, IL-4, or GM-CSF prevented tumor growth by a non-T cell-mediated mechanism.[21,84,85] By contrast, tumor cells that secreted either IFN-γ, IL-2, IL-4, or IL-7 prevented tumor growth by a T cell-mediated mechanism.[22,37,38,76] Conflicting results have been reported using IL-4 transfected renal carcinoma cells (T cell-mediated rejection) and IL-4 transfected plasmacytoma cells (non-T cell-mediated) and may reflect differences in the immunogenicity of these two types of tumor cells. Not all cytokines induced a protective response, as demonstrated by the accelerated tumor growth observed after transfection of tumor cells with genes that encode for either TGF-β, IL-3, IL-5, or IL-6.[9] Together these data indicate that transfection of tumor cells with several different cytokine genes can induce protective immunity.

The data from several laboratories suggest that immunization with IL-2-secreting tumor cells protects mice by activating specific cytotoxic T cells. Although the exact mechanism by which IL-2-secreting tumor cells induce cytotoxic T cells is uncertain, transfected tumor cells may directly stimulate precursor T cells that bind tumor cells (Fig. 12-7). Immunogenic "untransfected" tumor cells induce the clonal expansion of specific CD8$^+$ precursor cytotoxic T cells, but are poor inducers of CD4$^+$ T helper cells that provide the lymphokines required to properly activate precursor cells into cytolytic T cells. Therefore in the absence of lymphokine-secreting T helper cells, precursor T cells fail to differentiate and remain in the precursor state. Precursor cells that infiltrate the tumor site and bind IL-2-secreting tumor cells are stimulated to differentiate and mature into cytolytic T cells. The most important aspect of the immune response induced against transfected tumor cells is that specific cytolytic T cells lyse untransfected parental tumor cells. In other words, transfected tumor cells activate cytolytic T cells that recirculate and lyse untransfected tumor cells at distant sites. Therefore cancer patients immunized with transfected tumor cells would induce an immune response that eliminates metastatic tumors occurring at a variety of sites.

These experiments are an attempt to transform tumor cells into antigen-presenting cells that will stimulate T cells. Therefore the most effective approach should be to transfect tumor cells with genes that encode for cytokines and co-stimulatory molecules normally displayed by antigen-presenting cells. As mentioned previously, the complete activation of specific CD8+ T cells by antigen-presenting cells requires presentation of antigenic peptides by cell-surface MHC class I molecules plus a second signal provided by either (1) soluble factors, and/or (2) co-stimulatory B7 molecules. Thus the B7 gene is a strong candidate for these transfection experiments, because B7 is expressed only on antigen-presenting cells and is believed to provide a powerful co-stimulatory signal to T cells. The following experiments indicate that transfecting tumor cells with B7 induces a potent and protective immune response. For this reason it is important to review the background of B7,[32,42,55,56,57] as transfection of tumor cells with B7 appears effective at inducing specific T cells and is likely to be involved in future treatment of human tumors by gene therapy. B7 is a 45- to 55-kDa B cell activation antigen first described as BB-1. The binding of B7 by CD28 receptors on T cells stimulates IL-2 production and T cell proliferation by upregulating IL-2 gene transcription and stabilizing IL-2 mRNA. The signal provided by triggering CD28 on T cells appears to be distinct from the signaling pathway used by the Tcr/CD3 complex and involves activation of a unique DNA-binding protein that increases IL-2 mRNA synthesis by binding to an enhancer region of the IL-2 gene. The interaction of B7 and CD28 appears to be distinct from the stimulatory signals provided by adhesion molecules in that triggering specific T cells in the absence of B7 results in T cell anergy.

Two sets of experiments conducted recently indicate tumor cells that express B7 induce a very effective antitumor

IL-2 cDNA Transfected Tumor Cells Activate Cytotoxic T Cells

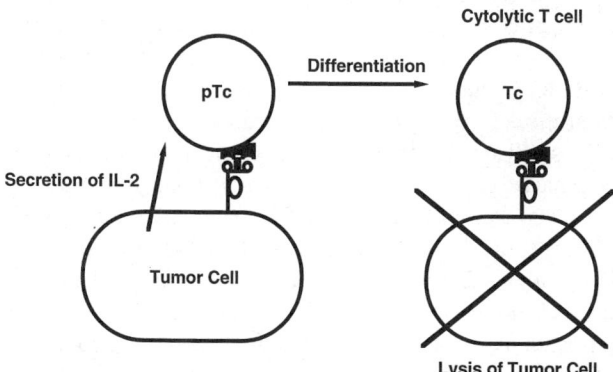

Fig. 12-7. Tumor cells transfected with vectors containing IL-2 cDNA constitutively secrete IL-2. When precursor cytotoxic T cells bind and recognize specific tumor antigens, these cells are exposed to the IL-2 secreted by the tumor cell. Precursor cytotoxic T cells responding to specific antigens in the presence of IL-2 are induced to differentiate into mature cytolytic T cells that can now lyse untransfected tumor cells.

Tumor Cells That Express B7-1 Co-stimulatory Signals Activate Cytotoxic T Cells

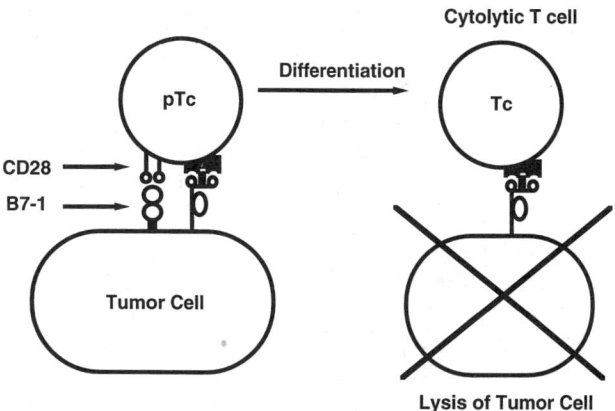

Fig. 12-8. Tumor cells transfected with vectors containing B7-1 cDNA constitutively express B7-1 on the surface of the tumor cell. When precursor cytotoxic T cells bind tumor cells that express specific tumor antigens, the CD28 receptor on the precursor cell recognizes B7-1, resulting in proliferation and differentiation into mature cytolytic T cells that can now lyse tumor cells that do not express B7-1.

T cell response. First, UV-induced melanomas that express B7 were rejected when inoculated into syngeneic mice.[89] Tumor rejection was mediated by CD8+ T cells, as demonstrated by the growth of B7+ tumors in either nude mice, or CD8+ T cell-depleted mice. By contrast, CD4+ T cells were not required and B7+ tumors were rejected from mice depleted of CD4+ T cells. Most importantly, mice that rejected B7+ tumors were protected from a second tumor challenge of B7 negative melanoma cells. These data suggest that the expression of B7 on tumor cells renders them capable of directly stimulating CD8+ T cells in the absence of CD4+ T helper cells. A second series of experiments reported by Chen and associates[17] demonstrated that rejection of B7+ tumors coincided with the activation of specific cytotoxic T cells. In addition, they demonstrated that "established" tumors were eliminated following treatment with B7+ tumor cells. The proposed mechanism for the activation of specific T cells by B7+ transfected tumor cells is illustrated in Fig. 12-8.

IMMUNOTHERAPY OF OCULAR TUMORS

Immunotherapeutic Treatment of Ocular Tumors in Animal Models

Niederkorn and associates[7,65,68] first demonstrated that lymphokine treatment can prevent formation of ocular tumors in the anterior chamber of mouse eyes. Their data indicate that either systemic delivery of lymphokines or injection of lymphokine-secreting tumor cells into the anterior chamber can induce protective immunity to intraocular tumors. Systemic delivery of either IL-2 or IL-1 by an osmotic pump placed in a subcutaneous pocket in the mid-dorsal region of the mouse prior to anterior chamber inoculation of tumor cells resulted in the induction of tumor-specific delayed hypersensitivity and abrogation of anterior chamber associated immune deviation (ACAID). In another series of experiments they demonstrated that tumor cells that secrete either IL-2 or IL-1 failed to form progressively growing tumors when inoculated into the anterior chamber of the eye. Tumor rejection coincided with the induction of specific delayed hypersensitivity in these mice. Together, these experiments demonstrate that exogenous lymphokines can induce a protective tumor-specific T cell response that prevents the formation of tumors within the anterior chamber.

In a related series of experiments Ruitenberg and associates[78] observed complete regression in three of five cows with ocular squamous cell carcinoma treated with intralesional injections of recombinant IL-2. Bovine ocular squamous cell carcinoma is a spontaneously forming tumor that occurs in a high frequency of cows in some countries. Interleukin-2 was injected into the tumor site daily for 5 consecutive days, followed by 2 days of rest, and then the cycle was repeated. No IL-2-associated toxicity was observed using this treatment protocol. Tumor regression was accompanied by infiltration of lymphocytes into the tumor-containing eye. Tumor-infiltrating lymphocytes possessed cytotoxic activity and lysed autologous carcinoma cells in vitro; however, the phenotype and specificity of these infiltrating cells remains to be determined. The dose of IL-2 used to treat these animals was surprisingly low, only 2500 units per injection. This dose is considerably lower than the dose typically administered intravenously in other animal models. The direct injection of lymphokines into the tumor site may have several advantages as compared with intravenous injection lymphokines. Lower doses should be required to achieve a clinical effect because of the direct delivery of lymphokines into the tumor site. In addition, the injection of lymphokines into the tumor site may preferentially activate specific T cells, as it is believed a high number of tumor-specific T cells are present within the tumor site. The direct intralesional injection of lymphokines has been reported to be more effective in controlling tumor growth in several other animal models.

Miki and associates[61] demonstrated that terminally differentiated, tumor-specific cytotoxic T cells injected directly into an intraocular tumor are capable of eliminating the tumor completely. In these experiments antigen-specific pTc (obtained from the spleen or draining lymph nodes) were restimulated in vitro to obtain fully functional tumor-specific CD8+ cytolytic T cells that were injected directly into eyes containing anterior chamber tumors. Cytolytic T cells completely eliminated tumors in 100% of the mice when injected within 3 days of tumor formation. Rejection of

tumors did not require the participation of the recipient's T cells, because intraocular injection of T cells also eliminated ocular tumors from immunoincompetent SCID (severe combined immunodeficiency) mice. By determining the frequency of tumor-specific cytotoxic T cells in the effector cell inocula, it was estimated that it is possible to cure intraocular tumors when the ratio of cytotoxic T cells to tumor cells is less than 1 : 50, and the total tumor burden at the time T cells are injected is less than 80,000 viable tumor cells. These experiments indicate that direct intraocular injection of cytolytic T cells can mediate rejection of tumors within the anterior chamber.

Sight-Destroying Versus Sight-Preserving Tumor Rejection

The ultimate goal of the immunotherapeutic treatment of ocular tumors is to generate a local immune response that completely eliminates all tumor cells from the eye and preserves normal ocular tissues. This condition requires that the immune response eliminate ''only'' malignant cells and leave the surrounding normal nonmalignant cells intact. The experiments of Niederkorn and associates suggest that this will require the induction of a highly regulated cellular immune response that activates cytolytic T cells in the absence of an inflammatory delayed hypersensitivity response. Luckenbach and associates[58] first described histologically two types of immune-mediated ocular tumor rejection in different mouse strains: (1) sight-destroying rejection, and (2) sight-preserving rejection. Sight-destroying tumor rejection resulted in complete destruction of normal ocular tissue during rejection of ocular tumor cells from the anterior chamber. In these mice, tumor rejection was accompanied by a massive mononuclear cell infiltrate and a vigorous local inflammatory response that eventually subsided, and was replaced by fibrovascular scarring. This type of tumor rejection results in atrophy of the eye (phthisis) and complete loss of vision. By contrast, sight-preserving tumor rejection is accompanied by significantly less mononuclear cell infiltration and virtually no local inflammatory response. Complete rejection of ocular tumors results in no contraction scarring and preserves the basic anatomic structures of the eye.

These distinct patterns of tumor rejection suggest that two separate effector mechanisms may mediate tumor rejection. Delayed hypersensitivity (DH) involves activation of tumor-specific T cells that release lymphokines (such as IFN-γ) and subsequently activate a nonspecific host response. DH therefore can result in a high burden of ''innocent bystander'' destruction of normal tissue. By contrast, sight-preserving tumor rejection is suggestive of a more specific T cell response. Tumor-specific cytotoxic T cells have exquisite specificity for tumor cells and therefore can distinguish between normal and malignant cells. Thus Niederkorn and associates[8,66,67] have hypothesized that sight-destroying tumor rejection results from nonspecific destruction of normal ocular tissue during elimination of tumor cells by CD4$^+$ T cells that mediate delayed hypersensitivity. Sight-preserving tumor rejection is mediated by specific cytotoxic T cells that lyse malignant, but not normal, cells. Recent experiments from this laboratory support this hypothesis.

Several new animal models that spontaneously develop intraocular tumors should prove valuable tools for studying the induction and development of the immune response to ocular tumors. Two different lines of mice were created by the insertion of a transgene that allows tissue-specific expression of a selected gene. A murine model of retinoblastoma was created using a transgene that drives bilateral retinal tumor development in 100% of transgenic mice.[99] This model uses a retinal-specific promoter sequence to direct the expression of SV40 large T antigen to neural crest tissues, resulting in the spontaneous development of intraocular tumors. The most important feature of this animal model is that the ocular tumors are histopathologically and clinically identical to human retinoblastoma. A second line of transgenic mice was created that express a transgene containing the tyrosinase promoter and the SV40 early region transforming sequences.[59] These mice develop rapidly growing primary ocular tumors that consist of a mixture of choroidal melanomas and retinal pigment epithelial carcinomas. It was recently shown that these mice are tolerant to the immunogenic T antigen expressed on the tumor cells.

Potential New Treatments for Patients with Ocular Tumors

A new and more effective therapy is needed for both ocular melanoma and retinoblastoma patients. Ocular melanoma patients have a limited number of therapeutic choices that include either enucleation or scleral plaque radiotherapy. Although either of these treatments can control primary tumor growth, neither is able to control metastatic tumor spread, which occurs in an estimated 50% of patients. Moreover, vision is not preserved among patients receiving enucleation, and complications limit vision in a significant number of patients within 5 years of radiation therapy.[12] The therapeutic choices for retinoblastoma patients are also limited to either laser and/or cryotherapy, external beam radiotherapy, or enucleation. Although these treatments can control tumor growth, none is completely successful in preserving vision, and complications limit vision in many treated eyes. This fact is significant in that a large number of retinoblastoma patients have bilateral tumors and therefore a serious risk of complete blindness. The ultimate goal for treating retinoblastoma or ocular melanoma would be to eliminate the primary tumor, preserve normal vision, and control metastatic tumor spread. Recent advances in tumor immunology may provide the necessary information to develop novel immunotherapies to achieve this goal.

Several novel immunotherapies, described in the preced-

ing section, have recently been developed in an effort to treat nonocular tumors. Although the rationale for these immunotherapies is experimentally sound, the initial clinical trials have yielded only limited success and demonstrated that these treatments are labor intensive and have significant side effects. Current efforts to solve these problems should result in more effective immunotherapies in the future. There are several compelling reasons why these therapies may be highly successful in treating patients with ocular tumors. Ocular tumors are usually detected early, when the tumor is relatively small. This circumstance allows initiation of treatment early in the development of the disease, which is important because immunotherapies are thought to provide the greatest benefit when the tumor burden is low. In addition, most ocular melanomas are slow-growing tumors, allowing more therapy time. Tumors also grow within a contained space, and surgical techniques are available for the delivery of intra-tumor injections of cytokines and/or lymphocytes. Finally, ocular melanoma patients experience a long disease-free interval prior to the development of secondary metastases. This interval allows initiation of treatment prior to formation of clinically detectable metastatic tumors, when the tumor burden is extremely small. By contrast, immunotherapy of nonocular tumors has been conducted on patients at an advanced stage of metastatic disease, during a time when the total tumor burden is large. For these reasons, it is believed that immunotherapies may be highly successful in treating patients with intraocular tumors.

Immunotherapies may be used to successfully control growth of primary ocular tumors and/or prevent the metastatic spread of tumor cells from the eye. Potential treatments for primary ocular tumor include the following: (1) local intratumor injection of lymphokines, (2) local intratumor injection of lymphokines plus either LAK cells or specific T cells, and (3) use of gene therapy to immunize patients with genetically altered tumor cells. Treatments that use nonspecific LAK cells would not require tumor tissue obtained from the patient, as peripheral blood lymphocytes are stimulated in vitro with IL-2 only. By contrast, treatments that use tumor-specific T cells would require tumor cells obtained from the patient. For treatment of primary ocular melanoma, tumor cells would have to be obtained by fine needle biopsies. If a case of bilateral retinoblastoma required enucleation of one eye, the tissue could be used to initiate immunotherapy for the remaining eye. Future treatments to prevent the metastatic spread of ocular melanoma could include systemic treatment with tumor-specific T cells or gene therapy to immunize the patient against tumor antigens. Both of these therapies are designed to eliminate micrometastases. Systemic treatment with specific T cells is a form of adoptive immunotherapy in which the patient's T cells are restimulated and activated in vitro and then injected intravenously back into the patient. The theory behind this approach is that specific T cells would recirculate, identify, and eliminate micrometastases of ocular melanoma cells. A second approach uses gene therapy to immunize patients to specific tumor antigens that would provide long-term protection from the development of metastases. Ocular tumor cells recovered from an enucleated eye could be transfected with vectors containing cDNA for lymphokine and/or co-stimulatory molecules. If these altered tumor cells are immunogenic in situ, it may be possible to immunize patients with these tumor cells to induce an immune response that prevents development of secondary tumors. Although there is evidence that primary ocular melanomas are immunogenic, it is unknown if metastatic tumors display the same, or different, tumor antigens. Thus it will be important to determine if an immune response induced against antigens on primary tumor cells is also able to recognize antigens on metastatic tumor cells. Studies of cutaneous melanoma indicates that at least some primary and secondary tumors express similar tumor antigens and, in the case of MAGE-1 antigens, metastatic tumors express elevated levels of this antigen.

IMMUNE RESPONSE TO HUMAN OCULAR TUMORS

Uveal Melanoma

Background. Malignant transformation of melanocytes in the iris, ciliary body, or choroid of the eye can lead to the development of uveal melanoma; however, the most common site of tumor formation within the eye is the choroid. Although ocular and cutaneous melanoma are both derived from melanocytes, the pathobiology of ocular melanoma is unique. Cutaneous melanoma can be separated histologically into discrete sequential stages: nevus, dysplastic nevus, radial growth phase, vertical growth phase, and metastases. The vertical growth phase is a histologic phenotype typically associated with tumors that acquire competence for metastatic tumor spread. When metastases develop, they can occur at a variety of sites, typically within 5 years after treatment of the primary tumor. By contrast, ocular melanomas do not progress through discrete sequential stages. Two histologic patterns of growth are typically observed, nodular and diffuse, with the majority of patients displaying the characteristic mushroom-shaped nodular form. The less-common diffuse tumors are associated with a more malignant phenotype. Melanoma cells can disseminate from the tumor-containing eye and develop into secondary tumors, but it is unclear when or how tumor cells are dispersed from the eye. Tobal and associates[87] recently conducted experiments using reverse transcription polymerase chain reaction amplification of tyrosinase gene mRNA to detect circulating melanocytes. This technique is highly sensitive and can detect as few as 10 circulating melanocytes in 5 ml of peripheral blood. Using this technique, these investigators detected tyrosinase mRNA among the peripheral blood cells of two patients with metastatic disease. The blood samples were obtained after the appearance of the metastases. Interestingly, they also detected a positive signal in a patient 9 months prior to the development of clinically detectable metastases. Three patients that remained disease-free and control blood samples displayed negative results. This technique may prove an extremely valuable tool in determining the time and mechanism of tumor cell dispersal from the eye.

A significant number of ocular melanoma patients have a prolonged disease-free interval between the time primary tumors are removed and the development of metastases. The literature reports several dramatic cases in which more than 40 years passed before secondary tumors developed. Metastases occur most frequently in the liver; and in contrast to their prolonged delay in initial development, once secondary tumors are clinically detectable, they progress at an accelerated pace, resulting in a median survival time of only 2 to 6 months.[73] Initial attempts at treating a small number of these patients with nonspecific immunotherapies (IL-2 or IFN-γ) have been unsuccessful.* These initial attempts at therapy were conducted in patients after metastases were already established. The lack of response is not surprising, as these hepatic metastases are also highly resistant to conventional forms of chemotherapy—only 4% to 5% of patients demonstrate a detectable response. The only reported form of therapy with any success has been hepatic arterial chemoembolization of cisplatin, which increased the median survival time to 11 months in 33 patients.[60]

The unique pathobiology of ocular melanomas may be related to the unique functional properties of ocular melanocytes. The fact that ocular melanocytes are different from melanocytes at other anatomic sites may not be readily apparent, as all melanocytes are derived from stem cells that migrate from the neural crest during embryogenesis. These stem cells establish populations of melanocytes in the skin, hair, and eyes; however, melanocytes residing in the iris, ciliary body, and choroid of the eye are all functionally and morphologically distinct.[10] These cells are melanogenically dormant during adult life and are actively involved in pigment synthesis only during gestation. Moreover, the melanin synthesized by these cells is retained within the cytoplasm in large, numerous melanosomes that are not transferred to other cells. By contrast, melanocytes within the skin are continuously synthesizing small melanosomes that are then transferred to keratinocytes. The unique metabolic properties of ocular melanocytes may be important in the unusual growth pattern of tumors that results from the malignant transformation of these cells.

Expression of Cell-Surface Molecules. Another way in which ocular and cutaneous melanomas are different is in

---

*M. Lotze, NCI, personal communication.

the expression of cell-surface molecules recognized by monoclonal antibodies.[13,45,64,94] Generally speaking, melanoma-associated antigens, found frequently on cutaneous melanomas, are absent from ocular melanomas or are present on a significantly fewer number of tumors. Several different groups of investigators have used various panels of monoclonal antibodies, which were raised against cutaneous melanomas, to determine if these antibodies recognize similar cell-surface molecules on ocular melanomas. ICAM-1, S100 (α and β), and the melanoma-associated antigens identified by antibodies Muc 18 and Muc 54 are all frequently found on cutaneous melanomas, but are absent from ocular tumors. Similarly, the majority of cutaneous melanomas ($> 90\%$) express the ganglioside GD3; by contrast, less than 50% of ocular melanomas are found to react with anti-GD3 antibodies. Thus the majority of cell-surface molecules routinely found on cutaneous tumors are not found on ocular melanomas. Because these studies all used monoclonal antibodies raised against cutaneous melanomas, it is unclear whether the reverse is true and ocular melanomas express membrane-bound molecules not found on skin melanomas. To address this question, Donoso and associates[28] developed a monoclonal antibody to ocular melanoma cells that identified a 40- to 50-KDa protein; however, this protein was also expressed on a large number of skin tumors. Similar results were obtained by Damato and associates.[24] Additional studies will be required to determine if ocular melanomas express unique cell-surface antigens.

T Cell Response. Experiments conducted by Char and associates[14] in the early 1970s provided the first evidence that patients with ocular melanoma mount an immune response against their tumors. In these experiments patients with ocular melanoma were tested for the development of delayed hypersensitivity against a soluble melanoma extract using a skin test. A significant DH response was observed in 90% of ocular melanoma patients; however, a number of false-positive responses were observed among normal donors (21%). The nonspecific DH response observed in these skin tests probably resulted from the tumor cell extracts used in the assay. Nonspecific DH responses were observed frequently in studies that used skin tests to detect DH to tumor antigens. The poor specificity of the melanoma DH assay prevented its use in the clinical diagnosis of ocular melanoma. These results, however, were the first to suggest that ocular melanomas are immunogenic and can induce a T cell response in patients. More recent studies have begun to identify and characterize the function of ocular-melanoma specific T cells. Nitta and associates[69] used reverse transcriptase polymerase chain reaction techniques to examine T cell receptor Vα chain gene transcription among lymphocytes infiltrating uveal melanomas. Their surprising results indicate that tumors from seven out of eight patients contained lymphocytes expressing the Vα7 gene. These results suggest that an oligoclonal population of T cells may be present in a high frequency of ocular melanoma patients. This condition is characteristic of specific T cells that are responding to melanoma antigen(s). It also suggests that a high frequency of uveal melanomas may be infiltrated by tumor-specific T cells, as a common T cell receptor gene was found in $> 80\%$ of the specimens examined.

Ksander and associates[50] also reported evidence that tumor-specific T cells infiltrate into ocular melanomas. In these experiments cell suspensions were prepared enzymatically from a choroidal melanoma and cultured in vitro in an effort to generate a melanoma cell line and obtain tumor-infiltrating lymphocytes. Even though a histologic study of the tumor failed to reveal "significant" infiltrating bone marrow-derived cells, lymphocytes were readily generated in cultures to which interleukin-2 was added. A phenotypic analysis of the cultured lymphocytes indicated that T cells, natural killer cells, and lymphokine activated killer cells were present. Moreover, functional studies of the cultured lymphocytes revealed NK activity, LAK activity, and, most important, tumor antigen-specific cytotoxic T cell activity. These results indicate that ocular melanomas can express unique tumor-specific antigens, and that the immune system of a patient bearing such an ocular tumor can perceive these tumor antigens, because antigen-specific precursor cytotoxic T cells were already present in the tumor-containing eye at the time of enucleation.

Evidence that T cells specific for tumor-associated antigens were present among the peripheral blood lymphocytes of ocular melanoma patients was provided by Mitchell and associates.[44] Peripheral blood lymphocytes were restimulated in vitro for several days in the presence of interleukin-2 and allogeneic ocular melanoma stimulator cells. Following restimulation, cytotoxic T cells were recovered from these cultures that displayed restricted specificity for melanoma target cells. Together these results suggest that tumor antigens expressed on melanoma cells within the eye are detected by the immune system, resulting in the expansion of a population of antigen-specific T cells. These T cells recirculate and can infiltrate the tumor site within the eye. These results also imply that tumor antigens must escape from the eye. Two routes of escape are possible: (1) by antigen-present cells that migrate into the eye, phagocytose tumor cells, and then migrate to the draining lymph node, or (2) by tumor cells that are shed from the eye through the blood vasculature and are deposited in the spleen.

Tumor-Infiltrating Lymphocytes. Studies of lymphocytic infiltration of cutaneous melanomas indicate that tumor infiltration by lymphocytes is associated with a better prognosis and increased survival. For this reason several studies have examined the lymphocytic infiltration of ocular melanomas to determine if the presence of lymphocytes within the tumor site also coincides with a better prognosis. Microscopic analysis of lymphocytic infiltration of ocular melanomas revealed few tumors (approximately 12%) displayed "heavy" infiltration of lymphocytes. Surprisingly, the presence of lymphocytes within ocular tumors coincided with a "poor" survival as compared to tumors displaying little or no infiltration.[53]

A second study examined the infiltration of T and B cells using immunohistochemical staining and microscopic examination of formalin-fixed, paraffin-embedded tissue. Among patients with heavy lymphocytic infiltration, T cells were more prominent than B cells. Once again, T cell infiltration coincided with a poorer survival.[98] Flow cytometric analysis of freshly frozen tumor cell suspensions allowed analysis of T cell subsets among tumor-infiltrating lymphocytes.[29] These studies demonstrated that CD8+ T cells were more prevalent than CD4+ T cells or B cells. The percentage of CD8+ T cells was elevated within the tumor site as compared with the percentage of CD8+ T cells within the peripheral blood, suggesting a preferential accumulation of CD8+ T cells within the tumor site. Although the correlation between lymphocyte infiltration and increased survival among patients with cutaneous melanoma has never been particularly strong, it is still surprising that increased infiltration corresponds with decreased survival among ocular melanoma patients.

Experiments conducted by Ksander and associates suggest that tumor-infiltrating T cells present within the eye are not active in situ and only become effective cytotoxic T cells after restimulation in vitro. This theory would explain the lack of correlation between lymphocytic infiltration and a better prognosis; however, this would not explain the correlation with decreased survival. Whelchel and associates[98] suggest that heavy lymphocytic infiltration may be associated with more aggressive ocular tumors that seed tumor cells from the eye. Thus these tumors would induce a more potent immune response; but because the specific T cell response is not effective, this immune response is unable to provide any protection, resulting in a decreased survival among these patients. It should be noted, however, that if these lymphocytes were "activated" by immunotherapeutic techniques, it might be possible to control the growth of these aggressive ocular tumors.

Retinoblastoma

Background. Although retinoblastoma is a relatively rare ocular tumor, occurring in approximately 1 in 14,000 live births, it is the third most frequent intraocular tumor and is one of the most frequent childhood malignancies (along with leukemia and neuroblastoma). Malignant transformation of retinal precursor cells results in bilateral or unilateral tumors, which are typically detected by the age of three and rarely occur after the age of seven. Tumors may arise within any layer of the sensory retina, and tumor growth is usually not focal or cohesive with tumor cells disseminating throughout the eye. The genetic analysis of families with a positive history of retinoblastoma resulted in Knudson's

1971 two-hit hypothesis in which he predicted that at least two mutational events at the retinoblastoma gene locus were required for malignant transformation. Patients that inherit a predisposition for the formation of tumors (first mutational event) require an additional mutation at the retinoblastoma gene for tumors to develop. Because retinal precursor cells undergo terminal differentiation during the first few years of life and the retinoblastoma gene regulates terminal differentiation, patients with a germline mutation in this gene lack the regulatory mechanism to override transformation. This circumstance explains the fact that 80% of patients with a positive family history develop bilateral, multifocal tumors at an early age. By contrast, the majority of patients with retinoblastoma tumors lack germline mutations and have two somatic mutational events that occur within the retina. Typically these characteristics result in unilateral, unifocal tumors that occur later in development and present at a more advanced age.

During the past decade the molecular biology of the retinoblastoma susceptibility gene has been studied extensively.[97] The retinoblastoma gene was the first tumor-suppressor gene to be identified in which malignant transformation corresponds with mutations, resulting in the loss of the retinoblastoma gene product. The most recent experimental evidence* suggests that the normal function of the retinoblastoma gene is to control cellular proliferation by downregulating the transcription of genes expressed as cells progress from the quiescent G_o phase to G_1 and S phase. The retinoblastoma gene product is thought to be active in an unphosphorylated state in cells in G_o; phosphorylation and inactivation of retinoblastoma occurs as cells progress from G_1 to S phase. It is believed that the active retinoblastoma gene product binds and inactivates cellular transcription factors (E2F) involved in upregulating the transcription of genes required for cellular proliferation. In other words, the active form of the retinoblastoma protein functions as a negative sink for transcription factors and blocks them from continually activating genes that initiate cellular proliferation. In the absence of a functional retinoblastoma gene, it is thought that cellular transcription factors are released from this negative control, resulting in sustained and continued proliferation and malignant transformation.

Although the molecular biology of retinoblastoma has been studied extensively over the past decade, experiments that examine the induction and expression of tumor-specific T cell responses in retinoblastoma patients have not been conducted. This lack of information occurs despite the fact that circumstantial evidence indicates retinoblastomas may be highly immunogenic.[33] The rate of spontaneous regression of retinoblastoma tumors has been reported to be as high as 1.0%—a surprisingly high frequency when com-

---

*References 2, 3, 4, 16, 19, 25.

pared with the spontaneous regression of other malignant diseases, which is estimated at 0.01%. The mechanism of retinoblastoma regression is unknown; however, several theories have been proposed. Regression may result from ischemic necrosis when tumor cells outgrow the stromal blood supply. Although local areas of necrosis are commonly seen, it seems unlikely that this mechanism could account for complete termination of all tumor growth, as at least some tumor cells should have access to the choroidal blood vasculature.

An alternative mechanism proposed by Gallie and associates[34] suggests that the spontaneous regression of retinoblastoma does not result from the termination of tumor growth, but is a benign retinoma (hyperplastic nodule of differentiated cells). Whether a retinoma or retinoblastoma develops is dependent on the stage of differentiation of the retinoblast when the final mutation of the retinoblastoma gene occurs. If the final mutation occurs in an immature retinoblast, it would result in the formation of a retinoblastoma. If the mutation occurs in a partially differentiated cell prior to terminal differentiation, it would result in the formation of a retinoma. Finally, it has also been proposed that the spontaneous regression of retinoblastoma is the result of an immune-mediated tumor rejection. Although there is no direct evidence supporting the immune-mediated rejection of these tumors, a local inflammatory response has been reported to accompany spontaneous regression of retinoblastomas. If regression is immune-mediated, it is possible that tumor-specific antigens recognized by T cells may participate in preventing tumor growth.

An interesting and unusual aspect of the spontaneous regression of retinoblastoma is that two distinct types of ocular pathology coincide with tumor regression: (1) regression accompanied by phthisis and blindness (sight-destroying tumor rejection), and (2) regression with useful vision (sight-preserving tumor rejection). It is believed that sight-destroying tumor rejection (phthisis) coincides with the appearance of a vigorous inflammatory response characterized by proliferation of capillary vascular channels and infiltration of macrophages and lymphocytes. As the acute inflammatory response subsides, it is replaced by fibrovascular scarring and destruction of the normal ocular architecture. These two patterns of spontaneous regression are similar to the patterns of intraocular tumor rejection observed in the murine model of immune-mediated tumor rejection described earlier.

Retinoblastoma-Associated Antigens Recognized by Antibodies. Char and associates[15] identified retinoblastoma-associated antigens by developing monoclonal antibodies against the Y-79 retinoblastoma cell line. The antibodies obtained bound Y-79 tumor cells, other retinoblastoma cell lines, and fresh retinoblastoma tumor tissue. Fab antibody fragments also bound retinoblastoma cells, indicating that binding was not due to nonspecific Fc binding. These antibodies were specific for retinoblastoma cells and did not bind neuroblastoma, glioma, melanoma, normal fibroblasts, or extracts from normal retinas. These results indicate retinoblastoma cells express tumor-associated antigens that can be recognized by specific antibodies. The nature of the antigen(s) is unknown and, in addition, it is not known if serum from retinoblastoma patients contains antibodies specific for these antigens.

T Cell Response to Retinoblastoma. Data from Ksander and associates[48] support the hypothesis that retinoblastomas are immunogenic tumors and patients possess specific T cells that recognize antigens presented by HLA class I molecules. In these experiments, tumors were examined for the presence of tumor-specific infiltrating lymphocytes. Tumor tissue was treated with collagenase to obtain single-cell suspensions cultured with or without recombinant interleukin-2. After 13 days in culture, the cells were examined by flow cytometry for the presence of T cells. Cultures containing interleukin-2 possessed a population of $CD45^+$, $CD8^+$, and $CD4^-$ T lymphocytes that were absent from identical cultures lacking interleukin-2. Activated infiltrating lymphocytes were tested for their ability to lyse a panel of retinoblastoma target cells. The lymphocytes demonstrated specific cytotoxicity toward autologous tumor cells, failing to lyse two different retinoblastoma target cells from other patients. These results indicate that retinoblastomas are immunogenic tumors infiltrated by specific T cells that can be recovered and activated in vitro with interleukin-2 to kill specifically the patient's own tumor cells. Thus it may be possible to eliminate retinoblastomas if specific T cells, present within the tumor, were properly activated in situ.

As mentioned earlier, a transgenic mouse strain was created recently that spontaneously develops retinoblastoma within 2 months after birth. An analysis of these tumors indicates that they are similar to human retinoblastoma histologically, ultrastructurally, and by immunohistochemical staining. Transgenic retinoblastoma cells, but not other tissues, express Tag mRNA that is highly immunogenic and can induce a specific T cell response in which $CD8^+$ T cells recognize peptide fragments of Tag presented by MHC class I molecules. Previous investigations of the T cell response to Tag indicate that the magnitude of the T cell response depends in part on the phenotype of the class I MHC molecules expressed on the cell surface; a vigorous, moderate, or no response occurs when Tag is presented by K^b, D^d, or K^d class I molecules, respectively. Because the phenotype of class I molecule is important in determining the response of T cells, retinoblastoma cells from transgenic mice were examined for the expression of class I molecules.[49] Flow cytometry and allospecific cytotoxic T cells were used to evaluate quantitatively the expression of class I on tumor cells. Surprisingly, all retinoblastoma cells from $H-2^{b/d}$ transgenic mice failed to express detectable levels of K^b and only one mouse out of eight expressed D^d. By contrast, low levels of K^d were observed on tumor cells from all mice tested. Thus the highest class I expression occurred for K^d, which fails to induce Tag specific T cell responses. Class I K^b, which can induce vigorous Tag immunity, was not expressed on tumor cells. These results indicate that the expression of MHC class I on retinoblastoma tumor cells from transgenic mice is inversely related to their ability to induce Tag-specific T cell responses. These results imply that retinoblastoma cells induce a Tag-specific immune response that selectively eliminates tumor cells that express class I molecules. Under these conditions class I deficient mutant retinoblastoma cells develop and form classical ocular tumors.

Additional experiments were performed to determine if retinoblastoma transgenic mice possessed Tag-specific T cells. Spleen cells from retinoblastoma transgenic mice were primed for a Tag-specific cytotoxic T cell response and cytotoxic T cells were obtained when spleen cells were restimulated in vitro with x-irradiated Tag-positive fibroblasts. These cytotoxic T cells lysed Tag-positive, but not Tag-negative fibroblast target cells, indicating the T cells were specific for Tag. Tumor cells from retinoblastoma transgenic mice that possessed Tag mRNA, however, were not lysed by these cytotoxic T cells. The failure to lyse retinoblastoma tumor target cells coincided with the downregulation of cell-surface class I molecules. T cells specific for Tag presented by class I K^b were unable to lyse tumor cells for $H-2K^b$ mice, because these tumor cells failed to express K^b class I on the tumor cell surface. Retinoblastoma cells treated with IFN-γ upregulated class I expression and were now lysed by T cells from transgenic mice. These results suggest that transgenic mice generate tumor-specific T cells that eliminate tumor cells from the eye; however, it is suspected that tumor cells are eliminated slowly, allowing for the development of class I deficient mutant retinoblastoma cells. These cells escape immune-mediated elimination because the T cells are unable to detect their presence. This transgenic model will allow a detailed study of the mechanism(s) used by tumor cells to escape immune detection.

PROGNOSIS

In the past five years there have been many important advances in the study of the immune response to tumors: (1) tumor-specific antigens have been identified and the genes that encode these antigens cloned, (2) tumor-specific T cell subpopulations have been characterized, (3) lymphokines and co-stimulatory molecules have been identified that activate tumor-specific T cells, (4) new clues have been obtained on the molecular basis for defects in the immune response that allow immunogenic tumor cells to escape elimination, and finally (5) new immunotherapeutic techniques have been developed that manipulate tumor-specific T cells. Although this new information has yet to be applied to the immunologic study of ocular tumors, it is likely that future research may furnish the necessary information to develop a novel immunotherapy that successfully controls intraocular tumor growth.

REFERENCES

1. Bach FH, Geller R, Nelson P et al.: A minimal signal stepwise activation analysis of functional maturation of T lymphocytes, Immunol Rev 111:35, 1989.
2. Bagchi S, Weinmann R, Raychaudhuri P: The retinoblastoma protein copurifies with E2F-I, and E1A-regulated inhibitor of the transcription factor E2F, Cell 65:1063, 1991.
3. Bandara LR, Adamczewski JP, Hunt T, La Thangue NB: Cyclin A and the retinoblastoma gene product form complex with a common transcription factor, Nature 352:249, 1991.
4. Bandara LR, La Thangue NB: Adenovirus E1a prevents the retinoblastoma gene product from complexing with a cellular transcription factor, Nature 351:494, 1991.
5. Bando Y, Ksander BR, Streilein JW: Characterization of specific T helper cell activity in mice bearing alloantigenic tumors in the anterior chamber of the eye, Eur J Immunol 21:1923-1931, 1991.
6. Bando Y, Ksander BR, Streilein JW: Incomplete activation of lymphokine-producing T cells by alloantigenic intraocular tumours in anterior chamber-associated immune deviation, Immunology 78:266-272, 1993.
7. Benson JL, Niederkorn JY: Interleukin-1 abrogates anterior chamber-associated immune deviation, Invest Ophthalmol Vis Sci 31:2123-2128, 1990.
8. Benson JL, Niederkorn JY: In situ suppression of delayed-type hypersensitivity: another mechanism for sustaining the immune privilege of the anterior chamber, Immunology 74:153-159, 1991.
9. Blankenstein T, Rowley DA, Schreiber H: Cytokines and cancer: experimental systems, Curr Opin Immunol 3:694-698, 1991.
10. Boissy RE: The melanocyte—its structure, function, and subpopulations in skin, eyes, and hair, Dermatol Clin 6:161, 1988.
11. Boon T: Toward a genetic analysis of tumor rejection antigens, Adv Cancer Res 58:177-210, 1992.
12. Bosworth JL, Packer S, Rotman M et al.: Choroidal melanoma: I-125 plaque therapy, Radiology 169:249, 1988.
13. Carrel S, Schreyer M, Gross N, Zografos L: Surface antigenic profile of uveal melanoma lesions analyzed with a panel of monoclonal antibodies directed against cutaneous melanoma, Anticancer Res 10:81, 1990.
14. Char DH, Hollinshead A, Cogan DG et al.: Cutaneous delayed hypersensitivity reactions to soluble melanoma antigen in patients with ocular melanoma, N Engl J Med 291:274, 1974.
15. Char DH, Wood IS, Huhta K et al.: Retinoblastoma: tissue culture lines and monoclonal antibody studies, Invest Ophthalmol Vis Sci 25:30-40, 1984.
16. Chellappan SP, Hiebert S, Mudryj M et al.: The E2F transcription factor is a cellular target for the RB protein, Cell 65:1053, 1991.
17. Chen L, Ashe S, Brady WA et al.: Costimulation of antitumor immunity by the B7 counterreceptor for the T lymphocyte molecules CD28 and CTLA-4, Cell 71:1093-1102, 1992.
18. Chen W, Peace D, Rovira D et al.: T cell immunity to the joining region of p210bcr-abl protein, Proc Natl Acad Sci USA 89:1468-1472, 1992.
19. Chittenden T, Livingston DM, Kaelin WG: The T/E1A binding domain of the retinoblastoma product can interact selectively with a sequence-specific DNA-binding protein, Cell 65:1073, 1991.
20. Cohen PA, Kim H, Fowler DH et al.: Use of interleukin-7, interleukin-2, and interferon-gamma to propagate CD4+ T cells in culture with maintained antigen specificity, J Immunother 14:242-252, 1993.
21. Colombo MP, Lombardi L, Stoppacciaro A et al.: Granulocyte colony-stimulating factor (G-CSF) gene transduction in murine adenocarcinoma drives neutrophil-mediated tumor inhibition in vivo: neutrophils discriminate between G-CSF-producing and G-CSF-nonproducing tumor cells, J Immunol 149:113-119, 1992.
22. Connor J, Bannerji R, Saito S et al.: Regression of bladder tumor in mice treated with interleukin 2 gene modified tumor cells, J Exp Med 177:1127-1134, 1993.
23. Coulie PG, Somville M, Lehmann F et al.: Precursor frequency analysis of human cytolytic T lymphocytes directed against autologous melanoma cells, Int J Cancer 50:289-297, 1992.
24. Damato BE, Campbell AM, McGuire BJ, Lee WR: Monoclonal antibodies to human primary uveal melanomas demonstrate tumor heterogeneity, Invest Ophthalmol Vis Sci 27:1362, 1986.

25. DeFeo-Jones D, Huang PS, Jones RE et al.: Cloning of cDNAs for cellular proteins that bind to the retinoblastoma gene product, *Nature* 352:251, 1991.

26. Degiovanni G, Hainaut P, Lahaye T et al.: Antigens recognized on a melanoma cell line by autologous cytolytic T lymphocytes are also expressed on freshly collected tumor cells, *Eur J Immunol* 20:1865-1868, 1990.

27. de Smet C, Lurquin C, Van der Bruggen P et al.: Sequence and expression pattern of the human *MAGE2* gene, *Immunogenetics* 39:121-129, 1994.

28. Donoso LA, Shields A, Augsburger JJ et al.: Antigenic and cellular heterogeneity of primary uveal malignant melanomas, *Arch Ophthalmol* 104:106, 1986.

29. Durie FH, Campbell AM, Lee WR, Damato BE: Analysis of lymphocytic infiltration of uveal melanoma, *Invest Ophthalmol Vis Sci* 31:2106-2110, 1990.

30. Fossum B, Gedde-Dahl III T, Hansen T et al.: Overlapping epitopes encompassing a point mutation (12 Gly → Arg) in p21 ras can be recognized by HLA-DR, -DP and -DQ restricted T cells, *Eur J Immunol* 23:2687-2691, 1993.

31. Franksson L, George E, Powis S et al.: Tumorigenicity conferred to lymphoma mutant by major histocompatibility complex-encoded transporter gene, *J Exp Med* 177:201-205, 1993.

32. Fraser JD, Irving BA, Crabtree GR, Weiss A: Regulation of IL-2 gene enhancer activity by the T cell accessory molecule CD28, *Science* 251:313, 1991.

33. Gallie BL, Dupont B, Whitsett C et al.: *HLA and malignancy,* New York, 1977, Alan R. Liss.

34. Gallie BL, Ellsworth RM, Abramson DH, Phillips RA: Retinoma: spontaneous regression of retinoblastoma or benign manifestation of the mutation, *Br J Cancer* 45:513, 1982.

35. Garrido F, Cabrera T, Concha A et al.: Natural history of HLA expression during tumour development, *Immunol Today* 14:491-499, 1993.

36. Gedde-Dahl III T, Fossum B, Eriksen JA et al.: T cell clones specific for p21 ras-derived peptides: characterization of their fine specificity and HLA restriction, *Eur J Immunol* 23:754-760, 1993.

37. Golumbek PT, Lazenby AJ, Levitsky HI et al.: Treatment of established renal cancer by tumor cells engineered to secrete interleukin-4, *Science* 254:713-716, 1991.

38. Hock H, Dorsch M, Kunzendorf U et al.: Mechanisms of rejection induced by tumor cell-targeted gene transfer of interleukin 2, interleukin 4, interleukin 7, tumor necrosis factor, or interferon, *Proc Natl Acad Sci USA* 90:2774-2778, 1993.

39. Houbiers JGA, Nijman HW, Van der Burg SH et al.: *In vitro* induction of human cytotoxic T lymphocyte responses against peptides of mutant and wild-type p53, *Eur J Immunol* 23:2072-2077, 1993.

40. Itoh K, Platsoucas CD, Balch CM: Autologous tumor-specific cytotoxic T lymphocytes in the infiltrate of human metastatic melanomas. Activation by interleukin 2 and autologous tumor cells, and involvement of the T cell receptor, *J Exp Med* 168:1419, 1988.

41. Itoh K, Salmeron MA, Morita T et al.: Distribution of autologous tumor-specific cytotoxic T lymphocytes in human metastatic melanoma, *Int J Cancer* 52:52-59, 1992.

42. Jenkins MK, Taylor PS, Norton SD, Urdhl KB: CD28 delivers a costimulatory signal involved in antigen-specific IL-2 production by human T cells, *J Immunol* 147:2461-2466, 1991.

43. June CH, Ledbetter JA, Linsley PS, Thompson CB: Role of the CD28 receptor in T-cell activation, *Immunol Today* 11:211-216, 1990.

44. Kan-Mitchell J, Liggett PE, Harel W et al.: Lymphocytes cytotoxic to uveal and skin melanoma cells from peripheral blood of ocular melanoma patients, *Cancer Immunol Immunother* 33(5):333-340, 1991.

45. Kan-Mitchell J, Liggett PE, Taylor CR et al.: Differential S100b expression in choroidal and skin melanomas: quantitation by the polymerase chain reaction, *Invest Ophthalmol Vis Sci* 34:3366-3375, 1993.

46. Knuth A, Wolfel T, Klehmann E et al.: Cytolytic T-cell clones against an autologous human melanoma: specificity study and definition of three antigens by immunoselection, *Proc Natl Acad Sci USA* 86:2804-2808, 1989.

47. Kripke ML: Immunoregulation of carcinogenesis: past, present, and future, *JNCI* 80:722-727, 1988.

48. Ksander BR, Geer DC, Murray TG: Studies of tumor-infiltrating-lymphocytes from human retinoblastoma, *Proc Am Assoc Cancer Res* 34:488, 1993.

49. Ksander BR, Geer DC, O'Brien JM et al.: Retinoblastoma specific T cells fail to eliminate intraocular tumors, *Invest Ophthalmol Vis Sci* 34(suppl):974, 1993.

50. Ksander BR, Rubsamen PE, Olsen KR et al.: Studies of tumor-infiltrating lymphocytes from a human choroidal melanoma, *Invest Ophthalmol Vis Sci* 32:3198-3208, 1991.

51. Ksander BR, Streilein JW: Recovery of activated cytotoxic T cells from minor H incompatible tumor graft rejection sites, *J Immunol* 143:426-431, 1989.

52. Ksander BR, Streilein JW: Failure of infiltrating precursor cytotoxic T cells to acquire direct cytotoxic function in immunologically privileged sites, *J Immunol* 145:2057-2063, 1990.

53. Lang JR, Davidorf FH, Baba N: The prognostic significance of lymphocytic infiltration in malignant melanoma of the choroid, *Cancer* 40:2388-2394, 1977.

54. Larsen CP, Ritchie SC, Pearson TC et al.: Functional expression of the costimulatory molecule, B7/BB1, on murine dendritic cell populations, *J Exp Med* 176:1215-1220, 1992.

55. Lindsten T, June CH, Ledbetter JA et al.: Regulation of lymphokine mRNA stability by a surface-mediated T cell activation pathway, *Science* 244:339, 1989.

56. Linsley PS, Brady W, Grosmaire L et al.: Binding of the B cell activation antigen B7 to CD28 costimulates T cell proliferation and interleukin 2 mRNA accumulation, *J Exp Med* 173:721-730, 1991.

57. Linsley PS, Greene JL, Tan P et al.: Coexpression and functional cooperation of CTLA-4 and CD28 on activated T lymphocytes, *J Exp Med* 176:1595-1604, 1992.

58. Luckenbach MW, Streilein JW, Niederkorn JY: Histopathologic analysis of intraocular allogeneic tumors in mice, *Invest Ophthalmol Vis Sci* 26:1368-1376, 1985.

59. Ma D, Comerford S, Bellingham D et al.: Capacity of simian virus 40 T antigen to induce self-tolerance but not immunologic privilege in the anterior chamber of the eye, *Transplantation* 57:718-725, 1994.

60. Mavligit GM, Charnsangavej C, Carrasco CH et al.: Regression of ocular melanoma metastatic to the liver after hepatic arterial chemoembolization with cisplatin and polyvinyl sponge, *JAMA* 260:974, 1988.

61. Miki S, Ksander BR, Streilein JW: Complete elimination ('cure') of progressively growing intraocular tumors by local injection of tumor-specific CD8 + T lymphocytes, *Invest Ophthalmol Vis Sci* 34:3622-3634, 1993.

62. Mukherji B, Guha A, Chakraborty NG et al.: Clonal analysis of cytotoxic and regulatory T cell responses against human melanoma, *J Exp Med* 169:1961, 1989.

63. Mule JJ, Shu S, Schwarz SL, Rosenberg SA: Adoptive immunotherapy of established pulmonary metastases with LAK cells and recombinant interleukin-2, *Science* 225:1487-1489, 1984.

64. Natagli PG, Bigotti A, Nicotra MR et al.: Analysis of the antigenic profile of uveal melanoma lesions with anti-cutaneous melanoma-associated antigen and anti-HLA monoclonal antibodies, *Cancer Res* 49:1269, 1989.

65. Niederkorn JY: Exogenous recombinant interleukin-2 abrogates anterior-chamber-associated immune deviation, *Transplantation* 43:523-528, 1987.

66. Niederkorn JY: The immunopathology of intraocular tumour rejection, *Eye* 5:186-192, 1991.

67. Niederkorn JY, Knisely TL: Immunological analysis of a destructive pattern of intraocular tumor resolution, *Curr Eye Res* 7:515-526, 1988.

68. Niederkorn JY, Streilein JW: Lymphoma allografts abrogate immune privilege within the anterior chamber of the eye, *Invest Ophthalmol Vis Sci* 27:1235-1243, 1986.

69. Nitta T, Oksenberg JR, Rao NA, Steinman L: Predominant expression of T cell receptor Va7 in tumor-infiltrating-lymphocytes of uveal melanoma, *Science* 249:672, 1990.

70. O'Neil BH, Kawakami Y, Restifo NP et al.: Detection of shared MHC-restricted human melanoma antigens after vaccinia virus-mediated transduction of genes coding for HLA, *J Immunol* 151:1410-1418, 1993.

71. Pandolfino M-C, Viret C, Gervois N et al.: Specificity, T cell receptor diversity and activation requirements of CD4$^+$ and CD8$^+$ clones derived from human melanoma-infiltrating lymphocytes, *Eur J Immunol* 22:1795-1802, 1992.

72. Perdrizet GA, Ross SR, Strauss HJ et al.: Animals bearing malignant grafts reject normal grafts that express through·gene transfer the same antigen, *J Exp Med* 171:1205-1220, 1990.

73. Rajpal S, Moore R, Karakousis CP: Śurvival in metastatic ocular melanoma, *Cancer* 52:334, 1983.

74. Razi-Wolf Z, Freeman GJ, Galvin F et al.: Expression and function of the murine B7 antigen, the major costimulatory molecule expressed by peritoneal exudate cells, *Proc Natl Acad Sci USA* 89:4210-4214, 1992.

75. Restifo NP, Esquivel F, Kawakami Y et al.: Identification of human cancers deficient in antigen processing, *J Exp Med* 177:265-272, 1993.

76. Restifo NP, Spiess PJ, Karp SE et al.: A nonimmunogenic sarcoma transduced with the cDNA for interferon gamma elicits CD8$^+$ T cells against the wild-type tumor: correlation with antigen presentation capability, *J Exp Med* 175:1423-1431, 1992.

77. Rosenberg SA, Lotze MT, Yang JC et al.: Prospective randomized trial of high-dose interleukin-2 alone or in conjunction with lymphokine-activated killer cells for the treatment of patients with advanced cancer, *JNCI* 85:622-632, 1993.

78. Rutten VP, De Jong WA, Klein WR et al.: Immunotherapy of bovine ocular squamous cell carcinoma: isolation, culture and characterization of lymphocytes present in the tumor, *Anticancer Res* 11:1259-1264, 1991.

79. Sensi M, Salvi S, Castelli C et al.: T cell receptor (TCR) structure of autologous melanoma-reactive cytotoxic T lymphocyte (CTL) clones: tumor-infiltrating lymphocytes overexpress in vivo the TCR b chain sequence used by an HLA-A2-restricted and melanocyte-lineage-specific CTL clone, *J Exp Med* 178:1231-1246, 1993.

80. Spitalny GL, North RJ: Subversion of host defense mechanisms by malignant tumors: an established tumor as a privileged site for bacterial growth, *J Exp Med* 145:1264, 1977.

81. Storkus WJ, Zeh III HJ, Maeurer MJ et al.: Identification of human melanoma peptides recognized by class I restricted tumor infiltrating T lymphocytes, *J Immunol* 151:3719-3727, 1993.

82. Storkus WJ, Zeh III HJ, Salter RD, Lotze MT: Identification of T-cell epitopes: rapid isolation of class I-presented peptides from viable cells by mild acid elution, *J Immunother* 14:94-103, 1993.

83. Tan P, Anasetti C, Hansen JA et al.: Induction of alloantigen-specific hyporesponsiveness in human T lymphocytes by blocking interaction of CD28 with its natural ligand B7/BB1, *J Exp Med* 177:165-173, 1993.

84. Teng MN, Park BH, Koeppen HK et al.: Long term inhibition of tumor growth by TNF in the absence of cachexia or T cell immunity, *Proc Natl Acad Sci USA* 88:3535-3539, 1991.

85. Tepper RI, Coffman RL, Leder P: An eosinophil-dependent mechanism for the antitumor effect of interleukin-4, *Science* 257:548-551, 1992.

86. Thor Straten P, Scholler J, Hou-Jensen K, Zeuthen J: Preferential usage of T-cell receptor ab variable regions among tumor-infiltrating lymphocytes in primary human malignant melanomas, *Int J Cancer* 56:78-86, 1994.

87. Tobal K, Sherman LS, Foss AJE, Lightman SL: Detection of melanocytes from uveal melanoma in peripheral blood using the polymerase chain reaction, *Invest Ophthalmol Vis Sci* 34:2622-2625, 1993.

88. Topalian SL, Solomon D, Rosenberg SA: Tumor-specific cytolysis by lymphocytes infiltrating human melanomas, *J Immunol* 142:3714, 1989.

89. Townsend SE, Allison JP: Tumor rejection after direct costimulation of CD8$^+$ T cells by B7-transfected melanoma cells, *Science* 259:368-370, 1993.

90. Traversari C, Van der Bruggen P, Luescher IF et al.: A nonapeptide encoded by human gene MAGE-1 is recognized on HLA-A1 by cytolytic T lymphocytes directed against tumor antigen MZ2-E, *J Exp Med* 176:1453-1457, 1992.

91. Traversari C, Van der Bruggen P, Van den Eynde B et al.: Transfection and expression of a gene coding for a human melanoma antigen recognized by autologous cytolytic T lymphocytes, *Immunogenetics* 35:145-152, 1992.

92. Van den Eynde B, Lethe B, Van Pel A et al.: The gene coding for a major tumor rejection antigen of tumor P815 is identical to the normal gene of syngeneic DBA/2 mice, *J Exp Med* 173:1373-1384, 1991.

93. Van der Bruggen P, Traversari C, Chomez P et al.: A gene encoding an antigen recognized by cytolytic T lymphocytes on a human melanoma, *Science* 254:1643-1647, 1991.

94. Van der Pol JP, Jager MJ, De Wolff-Rouendaal D et al.: Heterogeneous expression of melanoma-associated antigens in uveal melanomas, *Curr Eye Res* 6:757, 1987.

95. Vitetta ES, Thorpe PE, Uhr JW: Immunotoxins: magic bullets or misguided missiles? *Immunol Today* 14:252-259, 1993.

96. Weidmann E, Elder EM, Trucco M et al.: Usage of T-cell receptor Vb chain genes in fresh and cultured tumor-infiltrating lymphocytes from human melanoma, *Int J Cancer* 54:383-390, 1993.

97. Weinberg RA: Tumor suppressor genes, *Science* 254:1138-1146, 1991.

98. Whelchel JC, Farah SE, McLean IW, Burnier MN: Immunohistochemistry of infiltrating lymphocytes in uveal malignant melanoma, *Invest Ophthalmol Vis Sci* 34:2603-2606, 1993.

99. Windle JJ, Albert DM, O'Brien JM et al.: Retinoblastoma in transgenic mice, *Nature* 343:665-669, 1990.

100. Wolfel T, Klehmann E, Muller C et al.: Lysis of human melanoma cells by autologous cytolytic T cell clones, *J Exp Med* 170:797, 1989.

101. Yanuck M, Carbone DP, Pendleton CD et al.: A mutant *p53* tumor suppressor protein is a target for peptide-induced CD8$^+$ cytotoxic T-cells, *Cancer Res* 53:3257-3261, 1993.

OCULAR MICROBIOLOGY

13 Natural Defense Mechanisms of the Ocular Surface

MARK J. MANNIS, GILBERT SMOLIN

The surface of the eye is uniquely modified to subserve the function of vision. This part of the integument is armed with mechanical and immunologic functions that equip it for defense against a hostile environment and provide it with the mechanisms for both normal and pathologic immune responses. The defense mechanisms of the eye are both native and acquired, generalized and specific.[2,3,21] These defenses work together to effectively protect the eye from injury and infection.

ANATOMIC DEFENSES

The bony orbital rim of the eye protects the globe from injury by large objects. The most generalized and purely mechanical protectors of the ocular surface are the eyelids. The cilia function as accurate sensors, and lid closure reflexes serve as effective barriers to foreign material. The sweeping action of the lids cleans the ocular surface by virtue of its excursion over the entire exposed surface of the eye as well as its augmentation of the lacrimal pump mechanism. The lid contributes to the stability of the tear film by providing the lipid component from the meibomian glands.

The tear film bears both general and specific defense mechanisms. The flushing action of the tears, with the aid of the lids, sweeps debris, microbes, and potential allergens from the ocular surface and protects the corneal epithelium from desiccation and mechanical trauma.[28] The neutral pH of the tear film (7.14-7.82) may contribute to the neutralization of noxious or toxic substances introduced onto the ocular surface. The mucin layer of the tear film, aside from its primary function as a surface active agent, functions as a network to entrap foreign material and carry it into the conjunctival cul-de-sac.[1] Within the mucin network is an oxygen radical-producing system with antibacterial properties.[42] The metabolic activity of the corneal surface, which is responsible for maintaining epithelial integrity, is also supported in part by substrates carried in the tear film. The tear film is rich in substances such as lysozyme, lactoferrin, and other antimicrobial agents that defend against potentially pathogenic organisms. The tear film also carries a variety of specific immunoglobulins.

The tightly adherent, nonkeratinized, squamous epithelium of the conjunctiva and cornea is a strong barrier against pathogenic microbial invasion or penetration of antigenic material (Fig. 13-1). The complex and richly cellular conjunctiva provides both native and specific immune defenses by virtue of the accessory lacrimal glands, goblet cells, and a panoply of humoral and cellular immune components brought to the site by the conjunctival vasculature. Even the indigenous aerobic and anaerobic ocular flora of the skin of the lids and of the mucosal ocular surface serve a protective function by minimizing the opportunity for pathogenic organisms to colonize.[20,26] Acquired very early in life, the normal flora consists largely of aerobic *Staphylococcus epidermidis* and diphtheroid species.[37,39,40,41,48] The most common anaerobe is *Propionibacterium acnes.*[38] This confluence of mechanisms allows for protection of an otherwise delicate and exposed ocular surface. Anatomic or functional disruption of this defense complex by local anatomic changes or immunosuppression leaves the eye prey to disease.

VASCULAR DEFENSES

The rich blood supply to the eye can be thought of as a major conduit of immune defense. The eyelids, conjunctiva, extraocular muscles, and lacrimal glands are supplied by the superior and inferior medial palpebral arteries, the lacrimal artery, and the muscular branches of the ophthalmic artery.[54] Although the cornea is avascular, its immune defense system depends largely on components supplied by the adjacent vessels as well as on its poor recognition of antigens. Vascularization of the cornea (in the context of inflammatory disease caused by pathogenic invasion) alters the corneal response to immunologic stimuli.[27]

The ocular inflammatory response is characterized by vascular dilation followed by the exudation of serum and blood elements—macrophages, polymorphonuclear leukocytes, lymphocytes, C-reactive protein, and immunoglobulins—

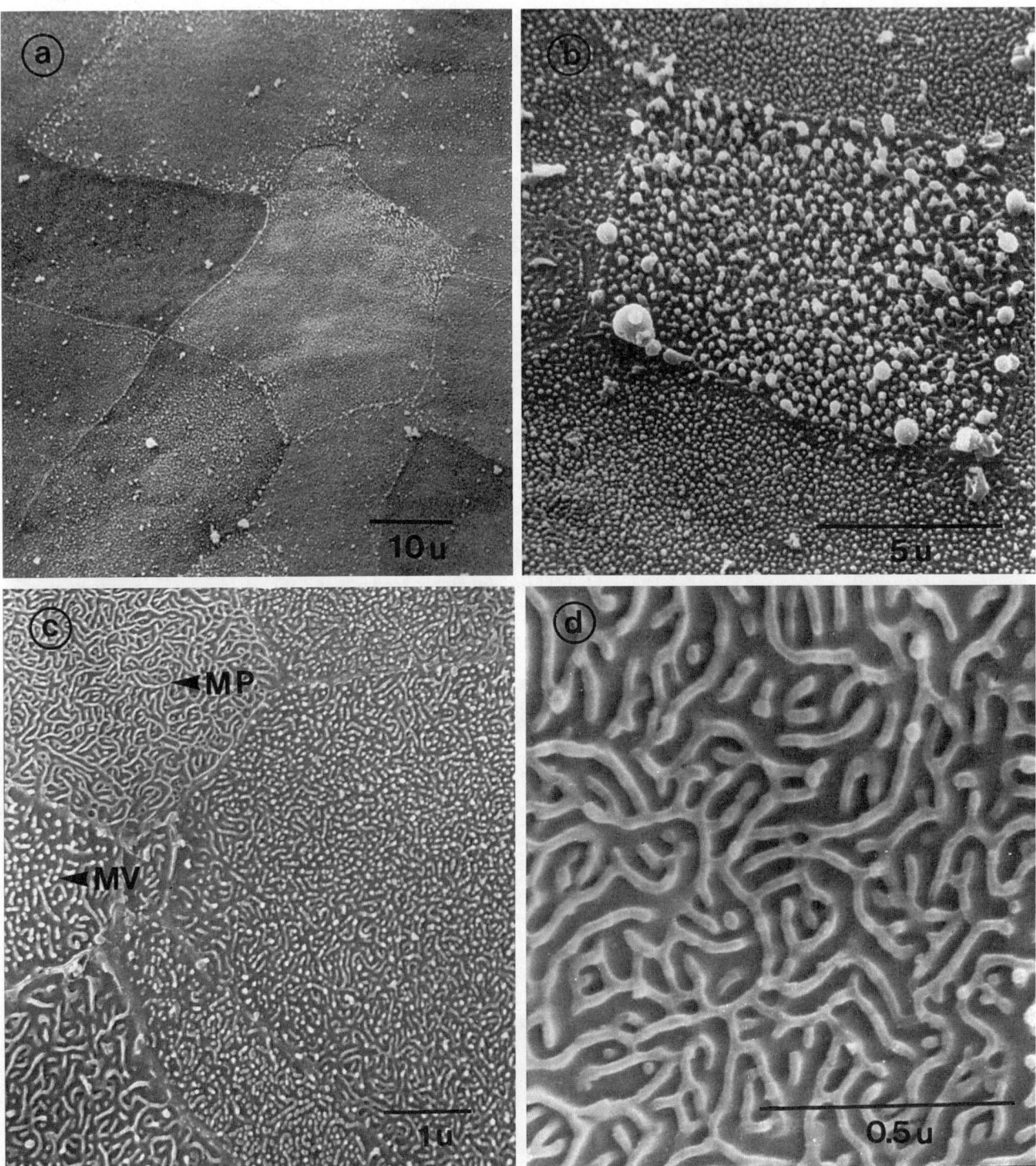

Fig. 13-1. Scanning electron micrographs of normal corneal epithelium. **A,** Polygonal mosaic of surface epithelial cells. **B,** Higher power showing microvilli that are longer on some cells. **C,** Microvilli (MV) and microplicae (MP) on adjacent epithelial cells. **D,** Interlacing microplicae with occasional stubby microvilli of an older cell. (Reprinted from Pfister RR: The effects of chemical injury in the ocular surface, *Ophthalmology* 90:601-609, 1983.)

into the extravascular spaces. In addition, the cornea and conjunctiva can produce prostaglandins, thromboxanes, and leukotrienes C, D, and E.[34,46]

The bulbar conjunctiva contains lymphatics that are divided into two networks. One network is superficial and is located just under the vascular capillaries. The second is deep and consists of the larger vessels in the fibrous layer of the conjunctiva. The bulbar lymphatics begin as a series of arcades at the limbus, and the interconnecting plexuses drain toward the palpebral commissures, joining the lymphatics of the lids. The lymphatic drainage to the palpebral conjunctiva is also divided naturally into pretarsal and posttarsal plexuses that are interconnected by cross-channels. The pretarsal channels serve the skin, and the posttarsal plexus serves the conjunctiva and tarsal glands. The lateral lymphatics drain into the preauricular and parotid lymph nodes, and the medial lymphatics drain into the submandibular lymph nodes. The avascular cornea is devoid of lymphatics, unless the cornea becomes vascularized, at which time there is an ingrowth of lymphatic channels.[15,45]

DEFENSES OF THE TEAR FILM

The human tear film serves many purposes. Ranging in thickness from 7 to 10 μm, the tear volume in a relatively unstimulated state ranges between 6 and 8 μl, with production in the resting state at approximately 1.2 μl/minute. The trilayered tear film consists of a lipid layer variably 800 to 2000 Å thick, depending on the state of closure of the lids. The largest portion of the tear film is the aqueous layer, approximately 7 μm thick. Finally, the mucin layer forms a thin blanket over the surface epithelial microvilli and is approximately 0.02 to 0.05 μm thick.

Table 13-1 lists the primary components of the tear film. Other components include enzymes of energy-producing metabolism such as lactate dehydrogenase and lysosomal enzymes as well as amylase, peroxidase, plasminogen activator, and collagenase. Cholesterol, glucose, lactate, urea, catecholamines, histamine, and prostaglandins[50] are also on the list. The tear film is rife with immunoactive substances, both general and specific. These include lactoferrin, tear-specific albumin, lysozyme, beta-lysin, and secretory IgA.[8,30] Other immune components that can be found in the tear film include properdin, properdin factor B, complement, interferon, prostaglandins, leukotrienes, ceruloplasmin, and prealbumin.[8,10]

Lactoferrin

Lactoferrin represents one of the main proteins in human tears with a mean concentration of 2 ng/ml.[32] It is synthesized and secreted by the lacrimal gland. Considered a mainstay in the nonspecific defense against a variety of bacteria, lactoferrin was thought to function by virtue of its iron-binding capacity.[6,7] More recent studies indicate that it

TABLE 13-1 COMPONENTS OF THE TEAR FILM[50]

Electrolytes	Concentration in mmol/l
Na$^+$	120-170
K$^+$	6-26
Ca^{++}	0.5-1.1
Mg^{++}	0.3-0.6
Cl$^-$	118-138
HCO$_3^-$	26

Antiproteases	mg%
Alpha$_1$-antitrypsin	1.5
Alpha$_1$-antichymotrypsin	1.4
Inter-alpha-trypsin inhibitor	0.5
Alpha$_2$-macroglobulin	3

Antimicrobial Factors	Function
Lysozyme	Bacterial cell wall lysis
Lactoferrin	Binds iron used in microbial metabolism
β-lysin	Ruptures bacterial cell membrane
Immunoglobulin A	Interferes with bacterial adherence
Immunoglobulin G	Promotes phagocytosis and complement fixation
Immunoglobulin E	Activates mast cells
Complement	Causes bacterial cell lysis

has a direct effect on certain bacterial strains and that its action may be the result of interaction with specific antibodies. It helps regulate the production of granulocyte-derived and macrophage-derived colony-stimulating factors. Lactoferrin prevents the formation of biologically active complement fragments C3a and C5a by inhibiting the formation of the classical C3 convertase of the complement system.[31] In this fashion, it may prevent complement activation and thus decrease inflammation.

Lysozyme

Lysozyme accounts for up to 30% of the protein content of the tears.[8,43] It is active against selected gram-positive bacteria and enhances bacteriolysis by secretory IgA in the presence of complement.

β-lysin

β-lysin is another tear component with antimicrobial action that functions by causing lysis of bacterial cell membranes.

Immunoglobulins

Secretory IgA is found in much higher concentration in the tears than in the serum. It prevents the adherence of bacteria to the mucosal surface and modulates the normal flora, allowing saprophytic growth that prevents colonization by potential pathogens.[24] Secretory IgA also agglutinates bacteria and can neutralize viruses and toxins.[47] The antibacterial activity of secretory IgA may be enhanced by the mucin layer of the tear film, which concentrates immunoglobulins at the mucosal surface.[19]

Serum IgG can neutralize viruses and toxins, cause bacteriolysis, enhance opsonization, and form complement-binding immune complexes that result in immune adherence, neutrophil chemotaxis, and release of anaphylatoxins. IgG concentration increases in the tear film during episodes of acute inflammation that are caused principally by an increase in vascular permeability and the resulting outpouring of IgG into the tears.[4] Although present in the cornea, IgG probably plays a limited role in corneal inflammatory reactions.

IMMUNE DEFENSES OF THE CONJUNCTIVA AND CORNEA

Conjunctival Defenses

The conjunctival mucosa contains a wide variety of immunoactive components. Mast cells are present in the submucosal tissue and, in response to an allergen or to injury, release histamines, platelet-activating factor, leukotrienes, and heparin. This release causes vascular dilation and increased permeability. The resulting transudate has antimicrobial properties.[3]

The tissue-associated immune defense system is histologically distinct lymphoid tissue, referred to as the conjunctiva-associated lymphoid tissue (CALT). CALT sites consist of multiple lymphoid nodules packed with multiple small and medium-size lymphocytes.[13,14,18,19] Lymphocytes are also packed into the adjacent lymphatics. The CALT sites are the loci of antigen-processing in the conjunctiva. The mucosal tissue also contains plasma cells that synthesize immunoglobulins, chiefly IgA.

The conjunctiva may also be populated by a variety of T cells (helper cells, suppressor cells) and natural killer cells in cases of neoplasm or virus infection.[9] Macrophages are also present, particularly near the vascular limbus (where they can trap immune complexes and initiate further immune activity). Immunoglobulins are in rich supply in the conjunctiva. IgG, IgA, and IgM emanate from the vascular supply, from abundant plasma cells, and from the tear film.[5] IgE may be present on the mast cell surfaces in the conjunctiva.

Corneal Defenses

Immune mechanisms available in the avascular cornea are limited. IgG is present in half the concentration of serum levels, and IgA is at only one fifth of serum levels. Their distribution over the cornea is uniform. IgM is less common and is rarely found in the central cornea.[5] The stroma is the

site of immunoglobulin concentration. In the presence of damage, the corneal epithelium may release a thymocyte-activating factor (CETAF) that attracts polymorphonuclear leukocytes, lymphocytes, and fibroblasts and may stimulate prostaglandin release.[25]

Corneal Antigens

Class I antigens can be found regularly in cell cultures derived from human corneal epithelium, stroma, or endothelium by the cytotoxic-plating inhibition test or by using monoclonal antibodies in an indirect immunofluorescence assay. Class II antigens are not expressed.[52] With sensitive immunoperoxidase techniques, Class I antigens are also noted in human corneal epithelium, stroma, and endothelium of fresh donor buttons.[49] The corneal epithelium has the most antigen; the periphery has more than the center. Basic fibroblast growth factor, epidermal growth factor receptor, transforming growth factor β-1, and interleukin 1-alpha have been found in corneal epithelial cells and stromal fibroblasts.[53]

Class II antigens are found on cells that are scattered throughout the central and peripheral epithelium and the stroma.[49] The cells in the stroma with Class II antigens (HLA-DR positive) appear dendritic. The region of HLA-DR positivity in the stroma begins at a distance of 3.5 to 4.0 mm from the center.[12,39] The HLA-DR positive cells (Langerhans cells) are present in the periphery of the corneal epithelium (Fig. 13-2). Langerhans cells function in the processing of antigen that is presented via the epithelial surface and stroma, and carry histocompability antigens needed to stimulate T and B lymphocytes.[14] Present primarily in the vascular limbus and peripheral corneal epithelium, Langerhans cells may be found in small numbers near the center of the cornea.[51]

Centripetal migration occurs with a central inflammatory stimulus (Fig. 13-3). Along with the CALT system, Langerhans cells stimulate helper T and B cells. T and B lymphocytes in the regional lymph nodes migrate via the blood stream to the ocular adnexa. Activated T cells occupy sub-

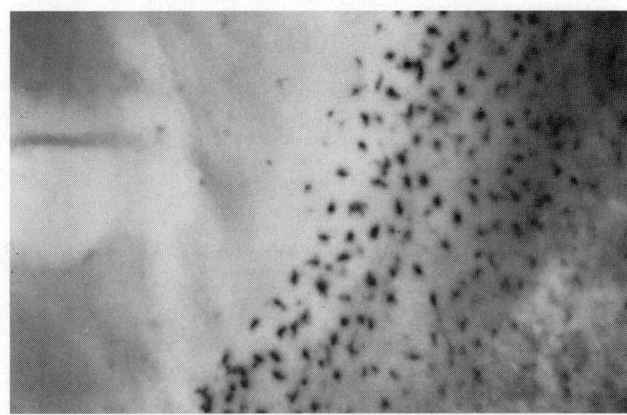

Fig. 13-2. Langerhans cells at the corneal limbus (ADPase stain).

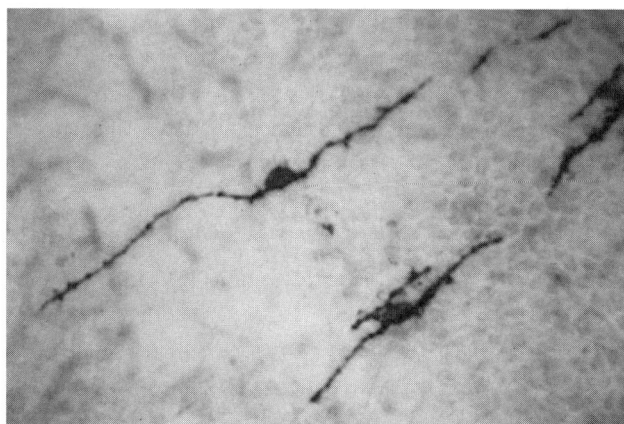

Fig. 13-3. Langerhans cells streaming into the cornea after stimulation (ADPase stain).

mucosal sites in the conjunctiva, whereas B cells concentrate in the lacrimal glands and produce a variety of immunoglobulins, particularly IgA. B cells appear in the corneal endothelium during primary immunogenic uveitis, and Class II antigens have been reported in the human corneal endothelium after incubation with interferon.[17] Epikeratophakia lenticules express Class I antigens but no Class II antigens.

LEUKOCYTE DEFENSES

The central role of the polymorphonuclear leukocyte in immune defense is based on its ability to ingest and kill microorganisms. The bactericidal activity of the neutrophils functions through at least two antimicrobial mechanisms. The oxygen-dependent killing pathway is based on the post-phagocytic intracellular production of potent oxidants such as hydrogen peroxide, hydroxyl radical, hypochlorous acid, and chloramines.[33] The oxygen-independent killing pathway is based on the presence of intracellular antimicrobial proteins that are contained in cytoplasmic granules and released into the phagocytic granules. Among these antimicrobial proteins are cathepsin G, cationic antimicrobial peptide, bactericidal-increasing factor, permeability-increasing factor, lysozyme, and defensins.[23,35,44]

The defensins—variably cationic, arginine-rich, nonglycolsylated peptides that are composed of 30 to 35 amino acids—form a major component of the oxygen-independent killing pathway of the neutrophil in mammals.[36] Defense peptides with parallel activity have been demonstrated in a variety of animal groups, including the magainins in frogs,[55] the mellitins in bees,[11] and the cecropins in moths.[29,31] In each case, the peptides possess broad-spectrum antimicrobial activity and function as part of the native defense system.

Three principal defensins (HNP-1, 2, and 3) are present in the neutrophils of humans; similar proteins are found in the neutrophils and macrophages of guinea pigs, rabbits, and rats.[22] Purified mammalian defensins have a remarkably broad spectrum of antimicrobial activity in vitro, killing a wide variety of gram-positive and gram-negative bacteria as well as selected fungi and enveloped viruses. Their efficacy against virulent ocular pathogens, including *Pseudomonas aeruginosa,* streptococcal species, *Staphylococcus aureus,* and *Candida albicans* has been demonstrated in vitro.[16] Defensins probably play a role in the intracellular antimicrobial defenses of the ocular surface. Their role outside the cell is yet to be determined.

REFERENCES

1. Adams AD: The morphology of human conjunctival mucus, *Arch Ophthalmol* 97:730, 1979.
2. Allansmith MR: *The eye and immunology,* St Louis, 1982, Mosby.
3. Allansmith MR: Defense of the ocular surface, *Ophthalmol Clin* 12(6):93, 1979.
4. Allansmith MR, McClelland B: Immunoglobulins in the human cornea, *Am J Ophthalmol* 80:123, 1975.
5. Allansmith MR, O'Connor GR: Immunoglobulins: structure, function and relation to the eye, *Surv Ophthalmol* 14:367, 1970.
6. Arnold RR, Cole MF, McGhee JR: A bacterial effect for human lactoferrin, *Science* 197:263, 1977.
7. Arnold RR, Russell JE, Champion WJ et al.: Bactericidal activity of human lactoferrin: differentiation from the stasis of iron deprivation, *Infect Immun* 35:792, 1982.
8. Berta A: *Enzymology of the tears,* Boca Raton, 1992, CRC Press.
9. Bhan AK, Fujikawa L, Foster CS: T-cell subsets and Langerhans cells in normal and diseased conjunctiva, *Am J Ophthalmol* 94:205, 1982.
10. Bluestone R: Lacrimal immunoglobulins and complement quantified by counter-immunoelectrophoresis, *Br J Ophthalmol* 59:279, 1975.
11. Boman HG, Hultmark D: Cell-free immunity in insects, *Annu Rev Microbiol* 41:103, 1987.
12. Catry L, van den Oord J, Foets B, Missotten L: Morphologic and immunophenotypic heterogeneity and corneal dendritic cells, *Graefes Arch Clin Ophthalmol* 229:182, 1991.
13. Chandler JW, Axelrod AJ: Conjunctiva-associated lymphoid tissue. In O'Connor GR, editor: *Immunologic diseases of the mucous membranes,* New York, 1980, Masson.
14. Chandler JW, Gillette TE: Immunologic defense mechanisms of the ocular surface, *Ophthalmology* 90:585, 1983.
15. Collin HB: Lymphatic draining of I[131]-albumin from the vascularized cornea, *Invest Ophthalmol* 9:146, 1970.
16. Cullor JS, Mannis MJ, Murphy CJM et al.: In vitro antimicrobial activity of defensins against ocular pathogens, *Arch Ophthalmol* 108:864, 1990.
17. Foets BJ, van den Oord J, Billiau A et al.: Heterogeneous induction of MHC class II antigens on corneal endothelium by interferon, *Invest Ophthalmol Vis Sci* 32:341, 1991.
18. Franklin RM, Remus LE: Conjunctival-associated lymphoid tissue: evidence for a role in the secretory immune system, *Invest Ophthalmol Vis Sci* 25:181, 1984.
19. Franklin RM, Rice CD: Autoimmune diseases of the conjunctiva. In O'Connor GR, editor: *Immunologic diseases of the mucous membrane,* New York, 1980, Masson.
20. Frederickson AB: Behavior of mixed culture of microorganisms, *Annu Rev Microbiol* 31:63, 1969.
21. Friedlaender MH: Immunology of ocular infections. In *Allergy and immunology of the eye,* Philadelphia, 1979, Harper & Row.
22. Ganz T, Selsted ME, Szklarek D et al.: Defensins: natural peptide antibiotics of human neutrophils, *J Clin Invest* 76:1435, 1985.
23. Ganz T, Lehrer RI: Defensins, *Curr Opin Immunol,* 6:584, 1994.
24. Gibbons RJ: Bacterial adherence to the mucosal surfaces and its inhibition by secretory antibodies, *Adv Exp Med Biol* 45:315, 1974.
25. Grabner G et al.: Corneal epithelial cell-derived thymocyte-activating factor, *Invest Ophthalmol Vis Sci* 23:757, 1982.
26. Halbert SP, Swick LS, Sonn C: Characteristics of antibiotic-producing strains of ocular bacterial flora, *J Immunol* 70:400, 1953.
27. Henley WL, Okas S, Leopold IH: Clinical experiments in cellular immunity in eye disease, *Invest Ophthalmol* 12:520, 1973.

28. Holly FJ, Lemp MA: Tear physiology and dry eyes, *Surv Ophthalmol* 22:69, 1977.
29. Hultmark D, Steiner H, Rasmuson T, Boman HG: Insect immunity: purification and properties of three inducible bactericidal proteins from the hemolymph of immunized pupae of *Hyalophora cecropia, Eur J Biochem* 1106:7, 1980.
30. Janssen PT, Van Bijsterveld OP: Origin and biosynthesis of human tear fluid proteins, *Invest Ophthalmol Vis Sci* 24:623, 1983.
31. Kijlstra A, Jerissen SHM: Modulation of classical C_3 convertase of complement by tear lactoferrin, *Immunology* 47:263, 1982.
32. Kijlstra A, Jeuissen SHM, Koning KM: Lactoferrin levels in normal human tears, *Br J Ophthalmol* 67:199, 1983.
33. Klebanoff SJ: Phagocytic cells: products of oxygen metabolism. In Gallin JI, Goldstein IM, Snyderman R, editors: *Inflammation: basic principles and clinical correlates,* ed 2, New York, 1992, Raven Press.
34. Kulkarni PS, Srinivasan BD: Synthesis of slow reacting substance-like activity in rabbit conjunctiva and anterior uvea, *Invest Ophthalmol Vis Sci* 24:1079, 1983.
35. Lehrer RI, Ganz T: Antimicrobial polypeptides of human neutrophils, *Blood* 76:2181, 1990.
36. Lehrer RI, Ganz T, Selsted ME: Defensins: endogenous antibiotic peptides of animal cells, *Cell* 64:230, 1991.
37. Locatcher-Khorazo D, Seegal BC: The bacterial flora of the healthy eye. In Locatcher-Khorazo D, Seegal B, editors: *Microbiology of the eye,* St Louis, 1972, CV Mosby.
38. McNatt J, Allen SD, Wilson LA, Dowell VR Jr: Anaerobic flora of the normal human conjunctival sac, *Arch Ophthalmol* 96:1448, 1978.
39. Mayer DJ et al.: Localization of HLA-A,B,C and HLA-DR antigens in the human cornea, *Transplant Proc* 15:126, 1983.
40. Okumoto M: Normal flora in the defense of the conjunctiva against infection. In O'Connor GR, editor: *Immunologic disease of the mucous membranes; pathology, diagnosis, and treatment,* New York, 1980, Masson.
41. Perkins RE, Kundsin RB, Pratt MV et al.: Bacteriology of normal and infected conjunctiva, *J Clin Microbiol* 1:147, 1975.
42. Proctor P, Kirkpatrick D, McGinness JA: A superoxide-producing system in the conjunctival mucous thread, *Invest Ophthalmol Vis Sci* 16:762, 1977.
43. Rotkis WM: Lysozyme: its significance in external ocular disease. In O'Connor GR, editor: *Immunologic diseases of the mucous membranes: pathology, diagnosis, and treatment,* New York, 1980, Masson.
44. Selsted ME, Harwig SSL, Ganz T et al.: Primary structures of human defensins: three antimicrobial peptides from blood neutrophils, *J Clin Invest* 76:1436, 1985.
45. Smolin G, Hyndiuk RA: Lymphatic drainage from vascularized rabbit cornea, *Am J Ophthalmol* 72:147, 1971.
46. Taylor L, Menconi M, Leibowitz MH, Polgar P: The effect of ascorbate, hydroperoxidases, and bradykinin on prostaglandin production by corneal and lens cells, *Invest Ophthalmol Vis Sci* 23:387, 1982.
47. Tomasi TB: *The immune system of secretion,* Englewood Cliffs, 1976, Prentice-Hall.
48. Torrey JC, Reese MK: Initial aerobic flora of newborn infants; selective tolerance of the upper respiratory tract for bacteria, *Am J Dis Child* 69:208, 1945.
49. Treseler PA, Foulks GN, Sanfilippo F: The expression of HLA antigens by cells in the human cornea, *Am J Ophthalmol* 98:763, 1984.
50. Van Haeringen NJ: Clinical biochemistry of tears, *Surv Ophthalmol* 26:96, 1981.
51. Vantrappen L, Geboes K, Missotten L et al.: Lymphocytes and Langerhans' cells in the normal human cornea, *Invest Ophthalmol Vis Sci* 26:220, 1985.
52. Whitsett CF, Stulting RD: The distribution of HLA antigens on human corneal tissue, *Invest Ophthalmol Vis Sci* 25:519, 1984.
53. Wilson SE, Schultz GS, Chegini N et al.: Epidermal growth factor, transforming growth factor alpha, transforming growth factor beta, acidic fibroblast growth factor, basic fibroblast growth factor, and interleukin-1 proteins in the cornea, *Exp Eye Res* 59:63, 1994.
54. Wolff E: *Anatomy of the eye and orbit,* Philadelphia, 1961, Saunders.
55. Zasloff M: Antibiotic peptides as mediators of innate immunity, *Curr Opin Immunol* 4:3, 1992.

14 Normal Ocular Flora

MICHAEL S. OSATO

The concept that microbes can establish resident communities on and within the human body without inducing overt infection has been known since the early days of microscopy.[61] Microorganisms indigenous to man are a selection of microbic species from the environment.

The normal flora is a heterogenous collection of bacteria. Regulatory processes that control the normal flora derive from the host and from the microbiota. These processes include paraimmunologic effects (natural immunity, natural resistance, anatomic barrier function, nutrient competition, metabolic end-product inhibition, and bacteriocin production) and specific immunologic phenomena.[12] These interactions reduce the opportunity for microbes with greater pathogenic potential to become established. Because colonization of the ocular surface is inevitable, it is advantageous that colonization be by commensals.[62] Under normal circumstances, the resident indigenous microbial community induces minimal activation of the host's inflammatory and immune responses.

The exact microbial population depends upon the anatomic site and the age of the host. In most instances, the microbial composition is independent of geography or climate,[42] although fungi may be more prevalent in tropical regions. Most members of the microbial community are specialized bacteria that form complex biochemical and physiologic interactions to optimally use the available nutrients in an otherwise hostile environment. Often, these bacteria possess structures to facilitate attachment to body surfaces.[16,58,63] Selective adherence, once achieved, is difficult to disrupt and can protect microorganisms from the mechanical defenses of the external eye.

INDIGENOUS MICROBIOTA OF THE EXTERNAL EYE

The normal flora of the eyelids and conjunctiva principally consists of aerobic bacteria.[5,37,41,56] *Staphylococcus epidermidis*, *Staphylococcus aureus*, and diphtheroids (alone or in combination) can be isolated from the conjunctivae of normal healthy individuals (Table 14-1). When appropriate culture conditions and media are used, other important components of the indigenous ocular flora can be identified: *Propionibacterium acnes*,[34,44,46,56] *Malassezia furfur (Pityrosporum ovale)*,[26,54] and *Candida* species.[2,3] Other anaerobes and filamentous fungi can be recovered from the external ocular surfaces, but their numbers and recovery rates vary from one study population to another.*

Age Differences

The eye harbors bacteria at birth and throughout life. *S. aureus*, *S. epidermidis*, streptococci, and *Escherichia coli* are transferred from mother to child following delivery through the vaginal canal.[42] Neonatal acquisition of the indigenous ocular flora also occurs via transfer from skin as determined by culturing of the face, nose, and hands. The flora undergoes minimal change during the first two decades of life; streptococci and pneumococci are more prevalent during those years. With increasing age, there is a trend toward the recovery of more gram-negative bacteria, but *S. epidermidis*, *S. aureus*, and diphtheroids remain the predominant bacteria on the conjunctivae and the eyelids (Table 14-1).[42]

Geographic Differences

The relative stability of the eye's microbial community is evident by the studies of individuals from widely separated geographic regions (Table 14-2).[13,36,42,67] Although viridans streptococci and *Streptococcus pneumoniae* are detected in a small proportion of certain populations, *S. epidermidis*, *S. aureus*, and diphtheroids are the predominant flora of the conjunctiva—regardless of location.[42] The isolation of streptococci may reflect the increased proportion of children and adolescents in these study populations.

---

*References 2, 3, 34, 44, 46, 56.

TABLE 14-1 BACTERIA RECOVERED FROM NORMAL CONJUNCTIVA AT DIFFERENT AGES

Bacteria	Age (Years)					
	0-5	6-14	15-29	30-49	50-69	70+
Staphylococcus epidermidis	41%	39%	43%	39%	42%	45%
Staphylococcus aureus	25%	24%	24%	21%	25%	23%
Streptococcus haemolyticus	<1%	<1%	3%	<1%	2%	<1%
Viridans streptococci	8%	4%	2%	3%	4%	1%
Streptococcus pneumoniae	13%	2%	2%	3%	2%	1%
Diphtheroids	25%	24%	28%	38%	42%	45%
No growth	20%	23%	20%	20%	14%	12%

From Locatcher-Khorazo D, Guitierrez E: Ocular flora of 1,024 children (1–10 years old), 1,786 young adults (20-25), and 7,461 patients awaiting ocular surgery with no known infection. 1952-1968. In Locatcher-Khorazo D, Seegal BC, editors: *Microbiology of the eye.* St. Louis, 1972, CV Mosby.

Variations in Location

The resident microbiota of the external ocular surfaces are not distributed evenly across the ocular surface, but inhabit restricted domains. The conjunctival surface provides a broad expanse for colonization. The mechanical flushing action of tears, coupled with the activities of its natural antimicrobial components, restrict implantation to microbes that possess adhesive mechanisms and are resistant to the effects of the tear-film components. Anaerobic components of the ocular surface flora are localized to the crypts of the inferior fornix, the sebaceous glands, the meibomian glands, and the hair follicles where the lowered oxidation-reduction potential favors growth of microaerophilic, facultative, and obligate anaerobes.

Normal Parasites

Bacteria and yeasts are part of the indigenous microbiota of the external ocular surfaces. Viruses and amebae are not.

TABLE 14-2 GLOBAL COMPARISON OF THE CONJUNCTIVAL MICROBIAL FLORA OF NORMAL EYES

Bacteria	Percent of Positive Cultures			
	USA	China	Germany	England
Staphylococcus epidermidis	37%	10%	65%	22%
Staphylococcus aureus	40%	10%	11%	8%
Corynebacterium species	3%	3%	83%	57%
Streptococcus pneumoniae	<1%	10%	5%	2%
Moraxella species	<1%	17%	0%	0%

Soudakoff PS: Bacteriologic examination of the conjunctiva. A survey on 3,000 patients. *Am J Ophthalmol,* 38:374-376, 1954.

The intracellular habitat of viruses, in which the host cell's replicative and maintenance mechanisms are diverted to viral propagation, reflects a parasitic (rather than a commensalistic) association. *Acanthamoeba* spp. are not encountered on the external ocular surfaces, except perhaps in contact lens wearers where the flora may reflect contaminated contact lens paraphernalia rather than normal ocular microbiota.

The role of the acarian parasites, *Demodex folliculorum* and *Demodex brevis,* in the stability of the indigenous microbiota of the eyelids is uncertain. They are commonly detected on the lid margins of normal healthy individuals and become more prevalent with advancing age. Infestation rates vary from approximately 20% in teenagers to nearly 100% in the elderly. Though closely related, the two species occupy entirely different habitats. *D. folliculorum* is found in hair follicles above the level of the sebaceous glands, and *D. brevis* occurs in sebaceous and meibomian glands and ducts of the deeper villus hairs. They consume gland cells and can cause plugging of the meibomian and sebaceous gland ducts.[72]

Demodex infestation may be associated with the spread of indigenous bacteria over the lid margins. The life cycle of *Demodex* involves random meanderings of the protonymphs and adult mites across the eyelid margins with frequent entry into hair follicles, sebaceous glands, and meibomian glands. Bacteria, attached to the mites, are deposited at various sites on the lids, which has led to speculation that they may be responsible for inciting local infection. The role of *Demodex,* however, in the pathogenesis of blepharitis is still undetermined.[72]

SELECTIVE INFLUENCES ON THE NORMAL OCULAR FLORA

Anatomic Barriers

The eyelids serve as an anatomic and mechanical barrier to bacterial colonization.[47] The blinking reflex protects against inadvertent deposition of airborne microbes on the ocular surfaces. The cilia sweep particulate matter from the air before reaching the eyelid surface or the conjunctiva. Each time the eyelids close, they mechanically sweep tear fluid, mucus, and suspended bacteria toward the lacrimal puncta. The blinking response then pumps bacteria into the lacrimal sac for subsequent drainage to the nose.

Microbial Adherence

Microbial attachment is initiated by a molecular interaction between bacterial surface glycoprotein adhesins (invasins) and protein receptors (integrins) on the epithelial cell surface. Adherence to cells of the ocular surface is a crucial step in the initiation of infection because it protects bacteria from mechanical washout. The teichoic acid fraction of the *S. aureus* cell wall functions as an adhesin to nonocular epithelial mucosal cells and may also be important in their adherence to epithelial cells of the conjunctiva and the lids.[4,6,30,35,43] Adherence of gram-negative bacteria such as *Pseudomonas* sp., *Neisseria* sp., *Moraxella* sp., and *Haemophilus* sp. can occur by pili (fimbriae).[16,58,63]

Slime[51] production can also prevent dislodgement by the flushing action of tears, and this biofilm enhances the survival of adherent microbes over the planktonic community. There are a number of other microbial surface components that facilitate microbial adherence to tissue. These microbial surface components recognizing adhesive matrix molecules (MSCRAMMs) distinguish varied cell surface ligands as collagen, laminin, fibronectin, fibrinogen, vitronectin, heparan sulfate, thrombospondin, and elastin.[55] Adherence of microbes to the ocular surface by multiple mechanisms resists washout by the mechanical action of tear flow.

The conjunctival tissue of the eye is unique among mucosal membranes in its ability to transdifferentiate by a process of environmental modulation when placed over the cornea.[78] The process is both reversible and incomplete. Conjunctival epithelial stem cells may reside in the fornix and impart unique characteristics to the conjunctival tissue that may play an important role in the temporal expression of surface receptors. These characteristics may explain the predilection of certain bacteria to colonize the conjunctiva of infants and adolescents but not adults. Furthermore, the organisms that colonize the ocular surface are limited to a select few bacteria. The predilection of these species for the conjunctival surface may be explained, to some extent, by the differential ability of these organisms to adhere to different types of epithelial cells.

Bacteriocins

Bacteriocins are bacterial proteins that are lethal to closely related bacteria (Table 14-3). Bacteria that produce a specific bacteriocin are resistant to its antagonistic action but are susceptible to bacteriocins produced by other bacteria. Bacteriocins may give some bacteria a competitive advantage over others that are trying to exist in the same ecologic niche. An important example is the colicins —bacteriocins produced by strains of *E. coli* and related

TABLE 14-3 BACTERIOCIN PRODUCERS

Gram-Positive Bacteria	Gram-Negative Bacteria
Bacillus	*Bacteroides*
Clostridium	*Brucella*
Corynebaterium	*Cardiobacterium*
Lactobacillus	*Caulobacter*
Lactococcus	*Citrobacter*
Leuconostoc	*Enterobacter*
Listeria	*Escherichia*
Micrococcus	*Halobacterium*
Mycobacterium	*Klebsiella*
Pediococcus	*Neisseria*
Propionibacterium	*Pasteurella*
Sarcina	*Proteus*
Staphylococcus	*Pseudomonas*
Streptococcus	*Salmonella*
	Serratia
	Vibrio

From Barefoot SF, Harmon KM, Grinstead DA, Nettles CG: Bacteriocins, molecular biology. In Lederberg J, editor: *Encyclopedia of microbiology,* vol 1, New York, 1992, Academic Press.

members of the Enterobacteriaceae family in the gastrointestinal tract.

Bacteriocins are widespread throughout the prokaryotic world and demonstrate diverse chemical and physical properties (Table 14-4). Most bacteriocin genes are encoded on plasmids, but some chromosomally encoded bacteriocins have been identified (microcin H47, lactacin B, helveticin, plantaricin, nisin, and lactastrepcin). The bacteriocins nisin, subtilin, pep 5, and epidermidin compose a distinct subset of bacteriocins called lantibiotics. This subset contains unusual amino acids including didehydroalanine and didehydrobutyrine and is distinguished by unique structural characteristics such as intramolecular rings between the thioester amino acids lanthionine and 3-methyllanthionine.[8]

The indigenous microbiota of the eyelid and conjunctiva encompass a narrow spectrum of microorganisms. Of the bacterial microflora, staphylococci, corynebacteria, and propionibacteria are all known bacteriocin producers. Their ability to synthesize and secrete toxins that are detrimental to the growth of other closely related bacteria could afford these bacteria the necessary competitive advantage to survive in this microenvironment. The production and secretion of bacteriocins is an energy-demanding process, however. In a microenvironment that is sufficient in the necessary growth nutrients (including electrolytes and amino acids), the modest population densities attained by the indigenous bacteria may be a reflection of the constant demands of energy diversion to bacteriocin production.

Microbial Metabolic End Products

Inhibitory products that resemble bacteriocin activity include excreted metabolites such as lactic and acetic acids.

TABLE 14-4 MECHANISM OF ACTION OF SELECTED BACTERIOCINS

Mechanism	Example
Membrane pore formation	Colicin A, B, E1, 1a, 1b, K, L, V
Functions as a DNAse	Colicin E2, E7
Functions as an RNAse	Colicin E3, E5 Cloacin DF13
Protein synthesis inhibitor	Colicin D Microcin A15, C17, 15m Lactocin LP27
Peptidoglycan synthesis inhibitor	Colicin M
Causes cell lysis	Colicin N
Blocks DNA replication	Microcin B17
Cationic detergent	Nisin Subtilin Pep 5 Epidermidin
Terminates DNA, RNA, and protein syntheses	Diplococcin Lactostrepcins
Causes ATP and ion efflux and disrupts cell membrane	Microcin D15, D140, E492 Lactocin L27 Pediocin AcH
Inhibits RNA synthesis	Microcin 15m
Undetermined mechanisms	Caseicin 80 Colicin E4 Helveticin Lactacin B, F Microcin H47 Pediocin PA1, A Plantaricin

From Barefoot SF, Harmon KM, Grinstead DA, Nettles CG: Bacteriocins, molecular biology. In Lederberg J, editor: *Encyclopedia of microbiology,* vol 1, New York, 1992, Academic Press.

Lactic acid produced by *Lactobacillus acidophilus* inhibits the putrefactive activity of clostridia in mixed cultures.[74] Similarly, acetic and formic acids from culture filtrates of *Bifidobacterium bifidus (A. bifidus)* inhibit the growth of *E. coli* and enterococci.[75] Other metabolic end products such as pyocyanin, hyaluronidase, and hydrogen peroxide possess potent antibacterial and tissue-destructive activities that can affect the bacterial composition of the community by altering the surrounding microenvironment.

Eyelid Lipids

Lipids of the human meibomian glands are composed of sterol esters (30% of total lipid), wax esters (35%), diesters (8%), triglycerides (5%), free sterols (2%), free fatty acids (2%), and phospholipids (15%).[49] The presence of unsaturated branched-chain fatty acids in the lipid fraction ac-

counts for the low melting point of 35°C.[53] These lipids maintain the optical properties of the tear film, retard the evaporative rate of the tear film when the eye is exposed to the ambient environment, prevent tear overflow onto the skin adjacent to the globe, and provide lubrication to the lid-ocular interface. Free fatty acids possess surfactant properties that assist spread of the hydrophobic wax esters and sterol esters over the tear film.[49]

Unsaturated fatty acids of the skin are bactericidal for hemolytic streptococci, pneumococci, and *Corynebacterium diphtheriae;*[11] and long-chain fatty acids (linolenic acid) can inhibit the growth of dermatophytic fungi.[48] The indigenous bacterial lid flora are relatively resistant to acids and can contribute to the degradation of lipids, thus releasing free fatty acids[17,18] into the surrounding environment. The lowered pH may prove advantageous to members of the resident community by inhibiting colonization by other organisms less able to tolerate acidic environments. Lipases of *S. aureus,* in addition, inhibit granulocyte function and thereby escape cellular destruction by cells of the inflammatory response.[60]

Soluble Tear-Film Components

The tear film contains numerous proteins,* electrolytes,[59] amino acids,[59] vitamins,[59] and metabolic intermediates.[59] The various proteins, of which more that 60 have been identified, include those known to possess antimicrobial activity, as well as proteins whose biologic functions in the tear-film have not yet been clearly elucidated. While some tear-film components have direct antimicrobial effects, other components express their antibacterial action indirectly by subverting microbial access to essential nutrients.

Lysozyme. Lysozyme comprises 20% to 40% of the total protein content of tears.[9,71] It is active against many grampositive bacteria[22] and catalyzes the hydrolysis of the β-1-4 glycosidic linkages of the polysaccharide backbone of mureins to yield disaccharides of N-acetyl-D-glucosamine and N-acetylmuramic acid. Gram-negative bacteria are not susceptible to the action of lysozyme because of the presence of a protective lipopolysaccharide sheath overlying the murein backbone. Although Fleming[22] initially reported lysozyme to be active against gram-negative bacteria, corroboration of this finding was not forthcoming until 1955. Lysozyme greatly accelerates the lysis of gram-negative bacteria in the presence of specific antiserum and complement. These accessory components affect bacteriolysis by altering the protective lipopolysaccharide coat, thus facilitating access of the murein backbone to the action of lysozyme.

Micrococci and gram-negative bacteria are isolated infrequently from the conjunctival sacs of normal healthy individuals. Their susceptibility to the effects of lysozyme and the accessory components in the tear film restrict their habitats to areas distant from these lytic components. Staphylococci are resistant to lysozyme and are commonly isolated from the normal conjunctival surfaces of man. Similarly, corynebacteria and the closely related propionibacteria are not affected by the action of lysozyme because of their cell-wall composition (meso-diaminopimelic acid and arabinogalactan) and lipid content (short-chain mycolic acids and dihydrogenated menaquinones).[14] The genus *Corynebacterium* is most closely related to the mycobacteria and *Nocardia,* two genera noted for their resistance to antimicrobial eradication.

Lysozyme production decreases in the aged. These decreased levels may predispose the conjunctival surfaces of the elderly to colonization with bacterial species not commonly found on the conjunctivae of younger eyes. Demographic data tend to support this hypothesis (Table 14-5).

Lactoferrin and Other Metal-Chelating Proteins. Lactoferrin was first isolated from bovine milk and subsequently identified in human tears. It binds reversibly to two atoms of iron and copper and has an affinity for IgA, IgG, and albumin. Lactoferrin has both bacteriostatic and bactericidal properties and may interact with specific antibody and complement.[10,25,39] Other metal-chelating proteins identified in normal human tears include transferrin and ceruloplasmin, which afford protection by binding metal cofactors necessary to enzyme function.[59]

The binding of iron to lactoferrin can interfere with bacterial iron uptake and decrease the virulence of several bacteria, including *Pseudomonas* spp., and render them more susceptible to other enzymes and lysozyme.[59] Meningococci are a prime example of the detrimental effect of iron limitation. Meningococci express many surface-accessible proteins that specifically bind iron-containing proteins such as lactoferrin and transferrin. These proteins represent the principal mechanism of iron acquisition by the organism.[64,65] When adequate levels of transferrin are present in serum, infection in experimental animals progresses. Resolution of infection occurs in concert with the disappearance of plasma transferrin iron.[32]

β-Lysin. β-Lysin is a bactericidal protein found in human tears.[73] It has a molecular weight of between 5000 to 7500 daltons and is heat-labile at 100°C. β-Lysin acts directly on the bacterial cytoplasmic membrane but functions optimally when combined with lysozyme for a synergistic action.[23,24] β-Lysin derives from platelets, but since these cells are absent in human tears it is probably actively secreted or filtered into the tear film.

Complement. Complement is a series of proteins that, when activated, initiates a cascade of reactions that ultimately results in the lysis of bacteria. There are two distinct but interrelated complement pathways, and the components of each are found in the normal tear film.[38,80] Release of pharmacologically active by-products of the activated complement cascade occurs by specific complement-mediated cleavage. These cleavage products promote immune adherence and cause neutrophil chemotaxis. The classical path-

TABLE 14-5 INCIDENCE OF MICROBIAL RECOVERY FROM CONJUNCTIVAE AND EYELIDS OF NORMAL EYES

Microorganism	Average Percent Positive					
	1-18 Years Conj.	Eyelid	20-35 Years Conj.	Eyelid	40-90 Years Conj.	Eyelid
Staphylococcus epidermidis	65%	72%	70%	70%	69%	72%
Staphylococcus aureus	37%	39%	36%	38%	38%	39%
Diphtheroids	22%	22%	35%	38%	28%	36%
Viridans streptococci	1.6%	1.6%	0.5%	0.6%	3.0%	3.0%
Streptococcus pneumoniae	7.0%	7.0%	1.8%	0.9%	0.6%	0.7%
Escherichia coli	0.2%	0.3%	1.5%	0.9%	1.7%	2.3%
Klebsiella pneumoniae	1.8%	1.8%	1.7%	0.8%	0.7%	1.2%
Klebsiella ozaenae	0%	0%	0%	0%	0.4%	0.4%
Proteus vulgaris	0.2%	0.2%	0.2%	0.2%	1.8%	2.5%
Morganella morganii	0.2%	0.2%	0.2%	0.4%	1.8%	1.7%
Proteus mirabilis	0.2%	0.2%	0.3%	0.6%	1.6%	1.6%
Providencia ruttgeri	0%	0%	0%	0%	0.7%	0.7%
Moraxella catarrhalis	2.0%	0.9%	0.7%	0.9%	0.7%	0.7%
Neisseria sicca	0.7%	1.5%	1.1%	1.6%	0.7%	0.8%
Neisseria flava	0%	0%	0.4%	0.6%	0.8%	0.8%

From Locatcher-Khorazo D, Guitierrez E: Ocular flora of 1,024 children (1-10 years old), 1,786 young adults (20-35), and 7,461 patients awaiting ocular surgery with no known infection. 1952-1968. In Locatcher-Khorazo D, Seegal BC, editors: *Microbiology of the eye,* St. Louis, 1972, CV Mosby.

way requires fixed antibody on the bacterial cell for activation to occur, whereas the alternative pathway can be activated by bacterial products such as lipopolyssacharides. The end results of the activation schemes are identical: killing pathogenic microbes that initiated the cascade.

Immunoglobulins. Immunoglobulins are present in tears under normal conditions.* Secretory immunoglobulin A is the predominant immunoglobulin and comprises about 17% of the total protein content of tears. Secretory IgA consists of two 7S monomers joined by a nonimmunoglobulin glycoprotein, the J chain, and a secretory component. This is unlike serum IgA, which consists of only one 7S monomer. The IgA monomers are produced by plasma cells that are located in interstitial tissues of the main and accessory lacrimal glands and the substantia propria of the conjunctiva. The role of IgA in host protection is in the prevention of bacterial adherence to epithelial cells by entrapping microorganisms in mucous. IgA may also have direct antimicrobial activity against bacteria, but this is still unclear. IgA can activate the alternative complement pathway and may, in combination with other tear components such as lysozyme, induce bacteriolysis. IgA can also neutralize both extracellular toxins and viruses.

IgG is present, but in somewhat lower concentrations. It exerts its action through the activation of the classical complement cascade, which results in enhanced phagocytosis and lysis of pathogenic microorganisms.

The role of IgE in the defense against infections is not known. It can facilitate eradication of pathogenic organisms by indirect means. IgE that is bound to the surface of mast cells can bind antigen and trigger a chain of events that lead to the release of vasoactive amines. These substances cause vasodilatation of the conjunctival vessels with leakage of various serum components into the conjunctival sac. The net result of these phenomena is the removal of organisms by the flushing action of the tears.

IgM and IgD are rarely detected in normal tears.[59] Under certain pathologic conditions, elevated levels of these and other immunoglobulin classes are found. This probably results from increased serum transudation from the engorged vasculature. No known tear-film regulatory role has been identified for either of these immunoglobulin classes.

Cellular Tear-Film Components

Large numbers of dead or dying desquamated cells of the conjunctiva, cornea, and eyelid are present in the normal tear film.[50] Viable epithelial cells, possess limited phagocytic potential and can engulf bacteria and small particles. The cellular fraction of tears contains approximately 5×10^5 cells/cm^2 and a substantial population of functioning lymphocytes (700/cm^2) and polymorphonuclear leukocytes (50/

cm^2)[50,59] that contribute to the microbial scavenging apparatus. These cells can recognize implantation of pathogenic organisms and initiate nonimmunologic and specific immunologic phenomena to eradicate invading organisms. The importance of these leukocytes in controlling the normal flora is uncertain.

ALTERATIONS OF THE INDIGENOUS MICROBIAL POPULATION

The indigenous microbiota of the skin, mucous membranes, and gut[1,76] are characterized by their stability. On the eye, short-term changes in physical and chemical parameters such as lowered oxygen tensions during sleep, exposure to cold or heat, or immersion in water during swimming do not result in significant alterations in the composition of the indigenous microbial population. Sterilization of the ocular surface by intensive antibiotic treatment (total antimicrobial modulation) and subsequent repopulation of the ocular surface with a less virulent or completely nonpathogenic bacterial population is possible but unlikely.[27,28] Selective antimicrobial modulation—the elimination of the pathogenic aerobic microorganisms with minimal disturbance of the normal anaerobic bacterial flora—may be more efficacious but is highly dependent upon homeostatic mechanisms. These mechanisms favor the establishment of a select microbial population in which the biochemical and physical interactions of the previous unaltered state are extant. Should an organism provide fully for these strict requirements, implantation may occur with displacement of the original strain.

Antibiotic Effects

Changes in the composition of the indigenous microbiota can occur following application of antiseptics or antibiotics to the eyelids or into the conjunctival cul-de-sac. Although all antibiotics induce changes in the composition of the indigenous microbiota of the external eye, it is the narrow-spectrum antibiotics that are the most detrimental. The predominantly gram-positive nature of the indigenous microbial population (>95%) enhances its susceptibility to agents such as erythromycin, first-generation penicillins and cephalosporins, vancomycin, clindamycin, rifampin, and trimethoprim-sulfamethoxazole. Aminoglycosides, second-generation and third-generation penicillins and cephalosporins, chloramphenicol, and tetracyclines have greater anti-gram-negative effects.

Parenterally administered antibiotics can also alter the composition of the indigenous microbiota. Following systemic dosing, tear-film levels can be achieved with ampicillin, chloramphenicol, cephalothin, cephaloridine, and cephalexin.[40] Ocular penetration is rapid for penicillin, methicillin, neomycin, vancomycin, gentamicin, colistin, polymyxin, erythromycin, cefoxitin, and cefamandole[40] following parenteral administration. Even at subtherapeutic

---

*References 15, 25, 39, 45, 62.

levels, antibiotics can exert selective pressures to effect qualitative, as well as quantitative, changes in the indigenous microbial population.

Disruption of the normal microbiota can allow implantation of other microorganisms. Yeast superinfection and recolonization with antibiotic-resistant pathogens following prolonged use of antibiotics are typical examples. The protection afforded by the normal indigenous microbiota is compromised and exposes the external ocular surfaces to overgrowth or recolonization by other microbes present in the indigenous microbial population. Further therapeutic options may be affected by the implantation of these more pathogenic microorganisms. Recovery of the natural microbial composition occurs slowly and normal levels are not reached until all local conditions are reestablished and the selective influence of the antibiotic, disinfectant, or antiseptic wanes.

Effects of Contact Lens Wear

Prolonged contact lens use has been associated with changes in the indigenous conjunctival flora. Whereas short-term ($<$ 7 days) contact lens use produces no variation in the normal resident conjunctival flora,[19,21] significant changes occur after two months of extended wear (removed every 7 days for cleaning).[20] These changes include an increase in the occurrence of potentially pathogenic eye strains, an increase in the number of negative cultures, and a decrease in the incidence of eyes harboring only normal conjunctival flora. These data reflect the selective pressures, both physical and biochemical, that accompany application of a contact lens to the ocular surface. Physiologic changes include a reduced blink rate, stagnation of tears under the lens, reduced oxygenation of tissues, a switch from aerobic to more anaerobic metabolic activity of the tissue with increased lactic acid production, and selective adhesion of bacteria to the contact lens itself. Furthermore, contact lens disinfectants select for microorganisms resistant to their effects, thereby heightening the probability of recovering more pathogenic strains from the ocular surface.

INFECTION OF THE OCULAR SURFACE BY THE NORMAL FLORA

Infection occurs when microbes overwhelm host defense mechanisms. Many of the manifestations of bacterial infection of the ocular surface undoubtedly involve constituents and products of the microorganisms that are known collectively as virulence factors. Bacteria avoid the clearance mechanisms of the tear film by secreting IgA protease that cleaves the proline-rich hinge region of the IgA or by inhibiting phagocytosis or chemotaxis of neutrophils, thereby permitting attachment and colonization. Exotoxins, primarily exoenzymes such as elastase and alkaline phosphatase, degrade proteoglycans, types III and IV collagens, and gelatins; hyaluronidase can digest glycosaminoglycan ground substance; and phospholipases can destroy cellular membranes. Bacterial endotoxin, the lipopolysaccharide of the outer membrane of gram-negative bacteria, can activate various inflammatory reactions. Stimulated macrophages produce peptides and lipids that attract other inflammatory cells and activate the alternate complement pathway to induce leukocyte chemotaxis and the release of lysosomal enzymes.

Some conditions such as, Bruton hypogammaglobulinemia,[31] Sjögren syndrome, and xerophthalmia predispose to infection by changes in the composition of the tear film. Lack of IgA in Bruton disease, decreased activity of antibacterial enzymes in Sjögren syndrome, and an abnormal tear mucus in xerophthalmia reduce the innate resistance of the ocular surface to bacterial infection.

The nutrient load of the tear film, though much diluted, provides all the necessary constituents required to support bacterial growth. Microbial overgrowth on the exposed ocular surface is a rare occurrence because of the efficacy of the ocular defense mechanisms. After death, bacterial proliferation, including gram-negative bacilli, of the conjunctival flora validates the powerful nature of the paraimmunologic and immunologic defense mechanisms of the ocular surface.[57,69]

REFERENCES

1. Abrams GD, Bishop JA: Effect of the normal microbial flora on the resistance of the small intestine to infection, *J Bacteriol* 92:1604-1608, 1966.
2. Ainley R, Smith B: Fungal flora of the conjunctival sac in healthy and diseased eyes, *Br J Ophthalmol* 49:505-515, 1965.
3. Albus A, Arbeit RD, Lee JC: Virulence of *Staphylococcus aureus* mutants altered in type 5 capsule production, *Infect Immun* 59:1008-1014, 1991.
4. Allansmith MR, Ostler HB, Butterworth M: Concomitance of bacteria in various areas of the eye, *Arch Ophthalmol* 82:37-42, 1969.
5. Ando N, Takatori K: Fungal flora of the conjunctival sac, *Am J Ophthalmol* 94:67-74, 1982.
6. Baddour LM, Smalley DL, Hill MM, Christensen GD: Proposed virulence factors among coagulase-negative staphylococci from two healthy populations, *Can J Microbiol* 34:901-905, 1988.
7. Barefoot SF, Harmon KM, Grinstead DA, Nettles CG: Bacteriocins, molecular biology. In Lederberg J, editor: *Encyclopedia of microbiology,* vol 1, 191-202, New York, 1992, Academic Press.
8. Barlati S, Marchina E, Quaranta CA et al.: Analysis of fibronectin, plasminogen activators and plasminogen in tear fluid as markers of corneal damage and repair, *Exp Eye Res* 51:1-9, 1990.
9. Bonavida B, Sapse AT: Human tear lysozyme. II. Quantitative determination with standard Schirmer strips, *Am J Ophthalmol* 66:70-76, 1968.
10. Broekhuyse RM: Tear lactoferrin: a bacteriostatic and complexing protein, *Invest Ophthalmol Vis Sci* 13:550-554, 1974.
11. Burtenshaw JML: The mechanism of self-disinfection of the human skin and its appendages, *J Hyg* 42:184-210, 1942.
12. Chandler JW, Gillette TE: Immunologic defense mechanisms of the ocular surface, *Ophthalmology* 90:585-591, 1983.
13. Chang HL: Bacterial flora of the normal conjunctiva, *Chin Med J* 75:233-235, 1957.
14. Coyle MB, Lipsky BA: Coryneform bacteria in infectious diseases: clinical and laboratory aspects, *Clin Microbiol Rev* 3:227-246, 1990.
15. Coyle PK, Sibony PA, Johnson C: Electrophoresis combined with immunologic identification of human tear proteins, *Invest Ophthalmol Vis Sci* 30:1872-1878, 1989.

16. Davis SD, Kushmaryov YM, Hyndiuk RA: Role of pili in virulence of *Pseudomonas aeruginosa* for the corneal epithelium. Presented at the Ocular Microbiology and Immunology Group Meeting, Chicago, 1983.

17. Dougherty JM, McCulley JP: Analysis of the free fatty acid component of meibomian secretions in chronic blepharitis, *Invest Ophthalmol Vis Sci* 27:52-56, 1986.

18. Dougherty JM, McCulley JP: Bacterial lipases and chronic blepharitis, *Invest Ophthalmol Vis Sci* 27:486-491, 1986.

19. Elander TR, Goldberg MA, Salinger CL et al.: Microbial changes in the ocular environment with contact lens wear, *CLAO J* 18:53-55, 1992.

20. Fleiszig SM, Efron N: Conjunctival flora in extended wear of rigid gas permeable contact lenses, *Optom Vis Sci* 69:354-357, 1992.

21. Fleiszig SM, Efron N: Microbial flora in eyes of current and former contact lens wearers, *J Clin Microbiol* 30:1156-1161, 1992.

22. Fleming A, Allison VD: Observations on a bacteriolytic substance ("lysozyme") found in secretions and tissues, *Br J Exp Pat* 3:252-262, 1922.

23. Ford LC, DeLange RJ, Petty RW: Identification of a nonlysozymal bactericidal factor (beta lysin) in human tears and aqueous humor, *Am J Ophthalmol* 81:30-33, 1976.

24. Friedland BR, Anderson DR, Forster RK: Non-lysozyme antibacterial factors in human tears, *Am J Ophthalmol* 74:52-59, 1972.

25. Ganchon AM, Verrelle P, Betail G, Dastugue B: Immunological and electrophoretic studies of human tear proteins, *Exp Eye Res* 29:539-553, 1979.

26. Gots JS, Thygeson P, Waisman M: Observations on *Pityrosporum ovale* in seborrheic blepharitis and conjunctivitis, *Am J Ophthalmol* 30:1485-1494, 1947.

27. Guiot HFL, van Furth R: Partial antibiotic decontamination, *Br Med J* 1:800-802, 1977.

28. Guiot HFL, van der Meer J, van Furth R: Selective antimicrobial modulation of human microbial flora: infection prevention in patients with decreased host defense mechanisms by selective elimination of potentially pathogenic bacteria, *J Infect Dis* 143:644-654, 1981.

29. Halbert SP: Inhibitory properties of the ocular flora. In Locatcher-Khorazo D, Seegal BC, editors: *Microbiology of the eye,* 24-40, St Louis, 1972, CV Mosby.

30. Hancock IC: Encapsulation of coagulase-negative staphylococci, *Int J Med Microbiol* 272:11-18, 1989.

31. Hansel TT, O'Neill DP, Yee ML et al.: Infective conjunctivitis and corneal scarring in three brothers with sex linked hypogammaglobulinemia (Bruton's disease), *Br J Ophthalmol* 72:118-120, 1990.

32. Holbein BE: Iron-controlled infection with *Neisseria meningitidis* in mice, *Infect Immun* 29:886-891, 1980.

33. Hsu C, Wiseman GM: Antibacterial substances from staphylococci, *Can J Microbiol* 13:947-955, 1967.

34. Johnson AP, Karcioglu ZA, Johnson MK: In vivo demonstration of the adherence of *Staphylococcus aureus* to rabbit corneal epithelial cells, *Invest Ophthalmol Vis Sci* 25(suppl):1394, 1984.

35. Johnson AP, Wool BM, Johnson MK: Adherence of *Staphylococcus aureus* to rabbit corneal epithelial cells, *Arch Ophthalmol* 102:1229-1231, 1984.

36. Jones DB, Robinson NM: Anaerobic ocular infections, *Trans Am Acad Ophthalmol Otolaryngol* 83:309-331, 1977.

37. Khorazo D, Thompson R: The bacterial flora of the normal conjunctiva, *Am J Ophthalmol* 18:1114-1116, 1935.

38. Kijlstra A, Veerhuis R: The effect of an anticomplementary factor on normal human tears, *Am J Ophthalmol* 92:24-27, 1981.

39. Kuizenga A, van Haeringen NJ, Kijlstra A: SDS-Minigel electrophoresis of human tears. Effect of sample treatment on protein patterns, *Invest Ophthalmol Vis Sci* 32:381-386, 1991.

40. Leopold IH: Antiinfective agents. In Sears ML, editor: *Handbook of experimental pharmacology: pharmacology of the eye,* vol 69, 385-457, New York, 1984, Springer-Verlag.

41. Locatcher-Khorazo D, Guitierrez E: Ocular flora of 1,024 children (1-10 years old), 1,786 young adults (20-35), and 7,461 patients awaiting ocular surgery with no known infection. In Locatcher-Khorazo, Seegal, editors: *Microbiology of the eye,* 14, New York, 1972, CV Mosby.

42. Locatcher-Khorazo D, Seegal BC: The bacterial flora of the healthy eye. In Locatcher-Khorazo D, Seegal BC, editors: *Microbiology of the eye,* St Louis 1972, CV Mosby.

43. Matoba AY, Hamill RJ, Osato MS: The effects of fibronectin on the adherence of bacteria to corneal epithelium, *Cornea* 10:87-89, 1991.

44. Matsuura H: Anaerobes in the bacterial flora of the conjunctival sac, *Jpn J Ophthalmol* 15:116-124, 1971.

45. McClellan BH, Whitney CR, Newman LP, Allansmith MR: Immunoglobulins in tears, *Am J Ophthalmol* 76:89-101, 1973.

46. McNatt J, Stephen D, Allen MD et al.: Anaerobic flora of the normal human conjunctival sac, *Arch Ophthalmol* 96:1448-1450, 1978.

47. Nassif KF: Ocular surface defense mechanisms. In Tabbara KF, Hyndiuk RA, editors: *Infections of the eye,* 37-44, Boston, 1986, Little Brown.

48. Nathanson RB: The fungistatic action of oleic, linoleic, and linolenic acids on *Trichophyton rubrum in vitro, J Invest Dermatol* 35:261-263, 1960.

49. Nicolaides N, Kaitaranta JK, Rawdah TN et al.: Meibomian gland studies: comparison of steer and human lipids, *Invest Ophthalmol Vis Sci* 20:522-536, 1981.

50. Norn MS: The conjunctival fluid: its height, volume, density of cells, and flow, *Acta Ophthalmol* 44:212-222, 1966.

51. Obana Y, Nishino T: Studies on the biologic activity of slime isolated from staphylococci, *Kansenshogaku Zasshi* 63:991-996, 1989.

52. Ohashi Y, Motokura M, Kinoshita Y et al.: Presence of epidermal growth factor in human tears, *Invest Ophthalmol Vis Sci* 30:1879-1882, 1989.

53. Osgood JK, Dougherty JM, McCulley: The role of wax and sterol esters of meibomian secretions in chronic blepharitis, *Invest Ophthalmol Vis Sci* 30:1958-1961, 1989.

54. Parunovic A, Halde C: *Pityrosporum obiculare:* its possible role in seborrheic blepharitis, *Am J Ophthalmol* 63:815-820, 1967.

55. Patti JM, Allen BL, McGavin MJ, Hook M: MSCRAMMs mediated adherence of microorganisms to host tissues, *Clin Infect Dis* (in press).

56. Perkins RE, Kundsin BB, Pratt MV et al.: Bacteriology of normal and infected conjunctiva, *J Clin Microbiol* 2:147-149, 1975.

57. Polack FM, Locatcher-Khorazo D, Gutierrez E: Bacteriologic study of "donor" eyes: evaluation of antibacterial treatments prior to corneal grafting, *Arch Ophthalmol* 78:219-225, 1967.

58. Punsalang AP, Sawyer WD: Role of pili in the virulence of *N. gonorrhoeae, Infect Immun* 8:255-263, 1973.

59. Records RE: The tearfilm. In Tasman W, Jaeger EA, editors: *Biomedical foundations of ophthalmology,* vol 2, 1-22, Philadelphia, 1985, JB Lippincott.

60. Rollof J, Braconier JH, Soderstrom C, Nilsson-Ehle P: Interference of *Staphylococcus aureus* lipases with human granulocyte function, *Eur J Clin Microbiol Infect Dis* 7:505-510, 1988.

61. Rosebury T: *Microorganisms indigenous to man,* New York, 1962, McGraw-Hill Book.

62. Sapse AT, Bonavida B, Stone W Jr, Sercarz EE: Proteins in human tears, *Arch Ophthalmol* 81:815-819, 1969.

63. Sato H, Okinaga K, Saito H: Role of pili in the pathogenesis of *Pseudomonas aeruginosa* burn infection, *Microbiol Immunol* 32:131-139, 1988.

64. Schryvers AB, Morris LJ: Identification and characterization of the human lactoferrin-binding protein from *Neisseria meningitidis, Infect Immun* 56:1144-1149, 1988.

65. Schryvers AB, Morris LJ: Identification and characterization of the transferrin receptor from *Neisseria meningitidis, Mol Microbiol* 2:281-288, 1988.

66. Selinger DS, Selinger RC, Reed WP: Resistance to infection of the external eye: the role of tears, *Surv Ophthalmol* 24:33-38, 1979.

67. Smith CH: Bacteriology of the healthy conjunctiva, *Br J Ophthalmol* 38:719-726, 1954.

68. Soudakoff PS: Bacteriologic examination of the conjunctiva: a survey on 3,000 patients, *Am J Ophthalmol* 38:374-376, 1954.

69. Sperling S, Sorensen IG: Decontamination of cadaver corneas, *Acta Ophthalmol* 59:126-133, 1981.

70. Stanifer RM, Andrews JS, Kretzer FL: Tear film. In Anderson RA, editor: *Biochemistry of the eye,* 1983, American Academy of Ophthalmology, San Francisco.

71. Stuchell RN, Farris RL, Mandel ID: Basal and reflex human tear analysis. II. Chemical analysis: lactoferrin and lysozyme, *Ophthalmology* 88:858-862, 1981.

72. Tabbara KF: Other parasitic infections. In Tabbara KF, Hyndiuk RA, editors: *Infections of the eye,* 679-695, Boston, 1986, Little Brown.

73. Thompson R, Callardo E: The antibacterial action of tears on staphylococci, *Am J Ophthalmol* 24:635-640, 1941.

74. Torrey JC, Kahn MC: The inhibition of putrefactive spore-bearing anaerobes by *Bacterium acidophilus, J Infect Dis* 33:482-497, 1923.

75. Upton MF: The effect of filtrates of certain intestinal microbes upon bacterial growth, *J Bacteriol* 17:315-327, 1929.

76. van der Waaij D, Berghuis JM: Determination of the colonization resistance of the digestive tract of individual mice, *J Hyg* 72:379-387, 1974.

77. van Setten G-B, Viinikka L, Tervo T et al.: Epidermal growth factor is a constant component of normal human tear fluid, *Graefes Arch Clin Exp Ophthalmol* 227:184-187, 1989.

78. Wei ZG, Wu RL, Lavker RM, Sun TT: In vitro growth and differentiation of rabbit bulbar, fornix, and palpebral conjunctival epithelia: implications on conjunctival epithelial transdifferentiation and stem cells, *Invest Ophthalmol Vis Sci* 34:1814-1828, 1993.

79. Weiber H, Andersson C, Murne A et al.: β-Microseminoprotein is not a prostate-specific protein: its identification in mucous, glands and secretions, *Am J Pathol* 137:593-603, 1990.

80. Yamamoto GK, Allansmith MR: Complement in tears from normal humans, *Am J Ophthalmol* 88:758-763, 1979.

81. Yen MT, Pflugfelder SC, Crouse CA, Atherton SS: Cytoskeletal antigen expression in ocular mucosa-associated lymphoid tissue, *Invest Ophthalmol Vis Sci* 33:3235-3241, 1992.

15 Pathogenesis of Ocular Infection

TERRENCE P. O'BRIEN, LINDA D. HAZLETT

The pathogenesis of ocular infectious disease is determined by the intrinsic virulence of the microorganism, the nature of the host response, and the anatomical features of the site of infection.[2] The unique anatomical structure of the cornea with its clarity, avascularity, and specialized microenvironment (Fig. 15-1) predisposes to potential alteration and destruction by invading microorganisms, microbial virulence factors, and host responses. Understanding the mechanisms of attachment and invasion during viral, bacterial, fungal, and parasitic eye infections is fundamental to the design of therapeutic strategies to eliminate the organism, to control nonsuppurative and suppurative inflammation, to minimize the action of virulence factors, to prevent permanent structural alterations, and ultimately to preserve vision.

MOLECULAR ASPECTS OF MICROBIAL ADHERENCE AND PATHOGENICITY

Microbes colonize body sites by engaging adhesins at their surface with receptors on host cells. The binding site of many adhesins often requires a particular receptor. For example, certain adhesins can discriminate between sialic acid linked to the 3- or 6-position of galactose; others require sialic acid to be acetylated; and yet another requires it to be N-glycosylated.[9]

Besides adherence, microbial adhesins also contribute to the ensuing interaction. Microbial invasion may be initiated either through virulence factors or by secondary effector molecules. Host defense mechanisms may be upregulated or downregulated. The more complex the adhesin, the greater are the possibilities. Adhesins may even be toxins.[4] Thus receptor recognition is merely the first step in the pathogenesis of infection directed by microbial adhesin molecules.[46]

Considerable knowledge exists on the structure and sequence of adhesins. Many bacteria display several adhesins on fimbriae (pili) and nonfimbrial structures. These adhesive proteins often recognize carbohydrates on eukaryotic cells, although protein-protein interactions also occur. Some bacteria have been grouped according to their ability to recognize several common monoamine sugars (such as galactose, mannose, or sialic acids) on eukaryotic glycoproteins and glycolipids.[53,58] Studies employing such glycoconjugates have determined the critical structural requirements for many adhesins. The domains of many adhesin molecules that mediate receptor recognition, however, remain to be characterized. Similarly, although much is known about the arrangement of carbohydrates preferred as receptors, more information is needed about the molecules with which the receptors associate. As functional domains of adhesins are elucidated, relationships will become apparent between microbial adhesins and other biologic effector molecules involved in intercellular systems.[46]

PATHOGENESIS OF VIRAL OCULAR INFECTION: HERPES SIMPLEX VIRUS

Herpetic viral infection of the cornea is a leading nontraumatic cause of blindness.[74] Acute infection of the corneal surface is a manifestation of virus-induced cytolysis. The stroma may also be involved, particularly as a result of recurring infections associated with reactivation from latency.[77] Stromal inflammation involves an immunopathologic process that often leads to corneal scarring, neovascularization, permanent endothelial dysfunction, and vision impairment.[54] Herpes simplex virus also causes dermatitis, blepharitis, conjunctivitis, iridocyclitis, and retinitis.

Viral Adherence

Identification of a cell-surface molecule as a virus receptor (or of multiple cell-surface molecules as alternate receptors) needs to fulfill at least two criteria. First, presence of the receptor should be a prerequisite for binding of the virus to a cell and for subsequent infection. Its absence should prevent specific binding of the virus to the cell and allow the cell to be resistant to infection. Second, the virus must interact physically with the cell-surface molecule(s).[95]

Genetic evidence using cell mutants defective in various aspects of glycosaminoglycan synthesis[26] has shown that

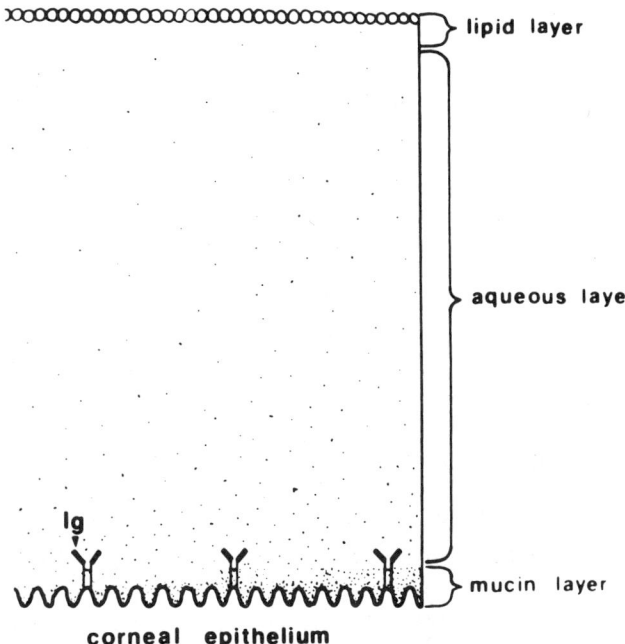

Fig. 15-1. The ocular surface. The tear film, the microvilli of epithelial cells, and associated antibody (Ig) form a physicochemical barrier to microbial invasion.

cell-surface heparan sulfate, but not other glycosaminoglycans or growth factors, fulfills these criteria as a receptor for herpes simplex virus (HSV).[95] Additionally the level of N-sulfation of heparan sulfate significantly influences the amount of virus that binds to and infects cells. Support for heparan sulfate as a receptor for HSV also is provided from experiments involving removal of heparan sulfate from human cells by enzymatic treatment. This reduces the ability of the cells to bind virus and renders the cells partially resistant to HSV infection.

Characterization of the virion glycoprotein that mediates binding of HSV to cells supports the conclusion that heparan sulfate is the receptor. Two of the virion glycoproteins (gB and gC) have heparin-binding activity (heparin is related closely in structure to heparan sulfate[44]), and gC is principally responsible for the binding of virions to cells. The latter is based on the finding that gC-negative virions are impaired in ability to bind to cells, whereas absence of any of the other glycoproteins required for HSV infectivity (gB, gD, and gH) blocks penetration of virus into cells but not binding of virus to cells.[14,21,64,65,91] Passive transfer of monoclonal antibodies specific for defined epitopes on gD of HSV-1 protects mice against development of persistent necrotizing stromal keratitis,[60] indicating that gD can serve as a target for effective antibody therapy in the mouse. Possibly, carbohydrates could be an important determinant in specificity of the HSV ligand (antireceptor), as binding of HSV can be inhibited by pretreatment of cells with wheat-germ agglutinin, which binds to N-acetylglucosa-

mine and sialic acid residues.[109,113] Higher sulfated fractions of heparan sulfate or heparin also inhibit HSV binding to cells, whereas chondroitin or dermatan sulfate inhibit poorly.[67]

Cell-surface heparan sulfate is required for the binding of both serotypes of HSV (HSV-1 and HSV-2) to cells.[112] Because the HSV-1 and HSV-2 forms of gC and gB differ in amino-acid sequence,[13,24,103,104] it is possible that there are serotype-specific differences in the structural features of heparan sulfate required for virus binding.

Viral Penetration

After binding of HSV to a cell, virus penetration into the cells can occur by fusion of the virion envelope with the cell's plasma membrane.[30,73] Events required for viral penetration are not known, but depend on the activities of at least three HSV glycoproteins designated gB, gD, and gH.[14,21] Whether there is a single path for viral binding and entry into cells or multiple pathways is not known. High-efficiency infection of most cultured adherent cells with HSV, however, appears to rely on the presence of cell-surface heparan sulfate, as heparin inhibits infection by HSV of many cell types and species, and absence of cell-surface heparan sulfate renders human, monkey, and rodent cells resistant to HSV infection.[112]

Host Response

Most of the understanding of ocular pathogenesis mechanisms of herpetic stromal keratitis comes from studies using rabbit and mouse models.[69,79] The rabbit is useful for the histopathology and study of the effects of treatment. In the rabbit the disease usually takes the necrotizing form and polymorphonuclear neutrophils (PMNs) predominate. The severity of the disease is markedly suppressed if neutrophils are depleted or complement activity is inhibited.[70] Consequently, the pathologic mechanisms may be a combination of direct viral damage with immune complex-mediated immunopathology.[86] Resolution of this immunologic issue in the rabbit has proved difficult.

It is the mouse model that provides a better understanding of the role of immune responses in tissue damage. Mice are experimentally infected with certain strains of HSV and develop keratitis. Wounding of the cornea before infection is usually required, however, and only some mouse strains (BALB/c and A/J) are susceptible.[102] Stromal keratitis in the mouse is a model of disciform nonnecrotizing keratitis in which the inflammation may be dominated (after an initial stage) by lymphocytes and other mononuclear cells, depending on the virus strain.[43] The mouse model may also not be ideal to simulate human stromal disease, as the latter usually results from repeated recurrent infections, whereas in the mouse it is usually a progressive disease. Spontaneous recurrences from latent infections do not occur experimentally. When they are induced experimentally, mice do not express clinical disease.[77]

Leukocytes. Stromal keratitis is T cell-mediated, but the mechanisms remain controversial. In effect, either the lesion primarily represents a CD8 +-mediated response with in vivo cytotoxicity playing a principal part,[40] or the lesion represents a CD4 +-mediated one.[42,75] In the latter, CD4 + cells are assumed to release various cytokines, including destructive ones such as tumor necrosis factor, or may themselves mediate cytotoxicity. Langerhans cells, normally resident at the periphery of the cornea, migrate centripetally after HSV-1 infection.[63] These cells play a critical role in activation of HSV-reactive CD4 + T cells in mouse cornea.[41] Direct cytotoxicity of virally infected corneal cells is another mechanism by which CD4 + cells might participate in HSV immune-mediated pathogenesis. This type of cellular immunity predominates in human HSV infections. Moreover, keratocytes readily express MHC class II molecules upon stimulation by interferon (IFN)-gamma and can present HSV antigens to autologous CD4 + cells. Both IFN-gamma and IL-2 appear to be important elements in the T cell response to HSV-1 antigen.[43]

PATHOGENESIS OF BACTERIAL OCULAR INFECTION: *PSEUDOMONAS AERUGINOSA*

Bacterial infections of the eye are an important public health problem. The intrinsic virulence of an organism relates to its ability to invade tissue, resist host defense mechanisms, and produce tissue damage.[76b] With few exceptions, exogenous penetration of bacteria into the cornea requires a defect in the surface epithelium. A few species of bacteria, such as *Neisseria gonorrhoeae, N. meningitidis, Corynebacterium diptheriae,* and *Shigella* spp., may directly penetrate corneal epithelium to initiate stromal suppuration. In general, disruption of the normal ocular surface predisposes the eye to microbial adherence, invasion, and infectivity. Bacterial keratitis, in particular, is a common, sight-threatening disease.

Pseudomonas corneal infections often result from contact lens wear and can lead to a highly destructive process resulting in vision loss.[59] Bacterial adherence to soft contact lenses appears to be an active process, as killed or altered bacteria do not adhere as well.[52] Both new and used lenses bind bacteria, although adherence to worn lenses can be associated with large focal deposits.[12] More hydrophobic bacteria putatively adhere in greater numbers than bacteria that are more hydrophilic.

Treatment of *Pseudomonas* infections is difficult, despite the availability of potent antibacterial agents. Extensive, irreparable corneal damage often occurs because of rapid onset, delay in diagnosis, production of proteases, and relative resistance to many common antibiotics.[1] Sustaining adequate concentrations of antibiotics may be problematic, and the tendency for infection to recur after apparent remission

makes *P. aeruginosa* one of the most serious causes of bacterial keratitis.[5]

Bacterial Adherence

P. aeruginosa has many virulence factors that contribute to pathogenesis. Cell-associated structures such as pili[22,110] and flagella[47,48] and extracellular products such as alkaline protease,[76] elastase,[76] exoenzyme S,[4] exotoxin A,[50] endotoxin,[20] slime polysaccharide,[18] phospholipase C,[76] and leukocidin[76] are associated with virulence, invasiveness, and colonization. Unlike gram-positive bacteria such as *Staphylococcus aureus* that adhere to host tissues via fibronectin and collagen,[82,105] *P. aeruginosa* attaches to cell surfaces devoid of fibronectin.[111]

Adhesin Receptors. Colonization of host tissue by *P. aeruginosa* depends on its ability to bind to the host epithelial cell surface either by direct molecular interactions, through hydrophobic bonds, or by interactions attributable to surface charge (Fig. 15-2).

Bacteria adhere to injured tissue areas,[34,84] to exposed corneal stroma,[34,100] or to immature nonwounded cornea.[11,31,97] Studies have implicated several carbohydrates, sialic acid,[31,84,85] N-acetylmannosamine,[34] mannose,[98] galactose,[51] N-acetylglucosamine,[108] and L-fucose,[23] as host receptors for *P. aeruginosa*. Glycosphingolipids (gangliotriosylceramide and gangliotetraosylceramide) also bind *Pseudomonas* organisms with GalNAcβ1-4Gal as the minimal binding unit.[58] In rabbit corneal epithelium grown in cell culture, *Pseudomonas* spp. binds to nonsialylated neutral glycolipids but not to the gangliosides.[80] In the adult mouse, both protease-sensitive and lipase-sensitive epithelial receptors have been identified,[36,96] whereas in the nonwounded epithelium of the immature mouse only protease-sensitive receptors are present.[90] The corneal epithelial receptors for

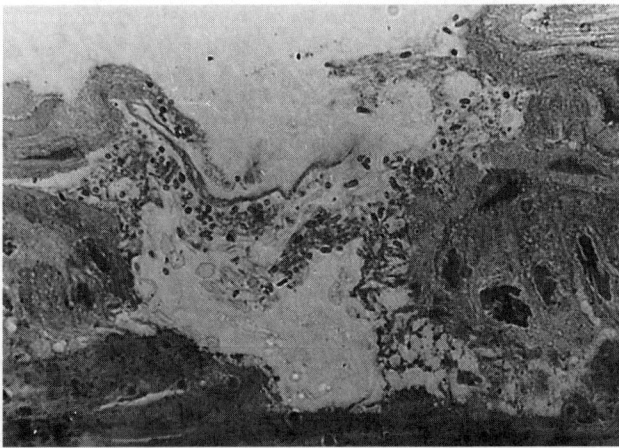

Fig. 15-2. Wounded mouse corneal epithelium illustrating *Pseudomonas aeruginosa* binding to epithelial cells and exposed stroma ($\times$600).

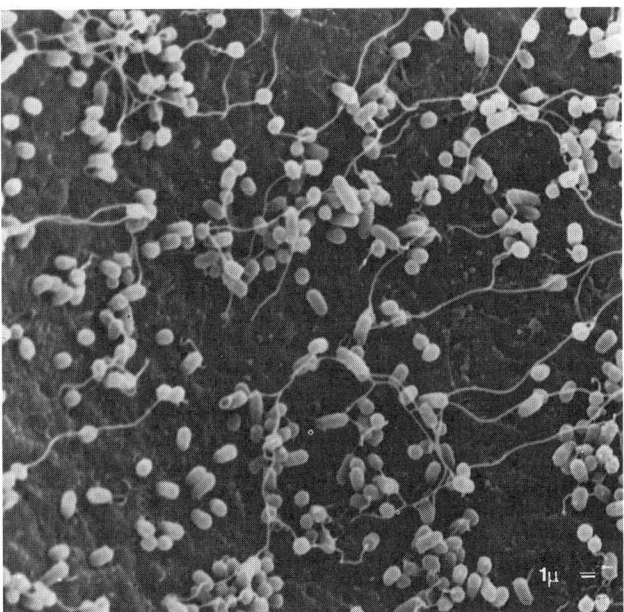

Fig. 15-3.   Scanning electron micrograph showing *P. aeruginosa* bound to exposed human corneal stroma (×6000, bar = μm).

Pseudomonas spp. are glycoproteins,[37,87] and a similar interaction presumably occurs when bacteria bind directly to the stroma (Fig. 15-3).

Pili. Pili (fimbriae) are thin (4 to 10 nm in diameter) protein filaments found on the surfaces of many types of bacteria. Most strains of *P. aeruginosa* have from 2 to 12 chromosomally encoded, retractile polar pili that promote infection by various pilus-specific bacteriophages. Research on pseudomonal pili has focused on two strains, strain K (PAK) and strain O (PAO), with pilins of similar molecular weights[29] and amino acid composition.[92,93,94] The *N*-terminus of each pilin subunit consists of a methylated phenylalanine[81] that is associated with a highly conserved, hydrophobic region of about 30 amino-acid residues. The central region of pilin is hypervariable, and the C-terminal region is semi-conserved, containing two half-cysteine residues (129 and 144) linked through a disulfide bridge in the native protein.[61]

In ocular[66] and nonocular in vitro studies, purified pili successfully compete for binding with whole bacteria by saturating available binding sites on the host cell surface. Pilus-specific monoclonal antibody has allowed identification of five major pilus-binding human epithelial glycoproteins by immunoblotting.[23] Similarly, monoclonal antibodies specific for *Pseudomonas* pili and a peptide, PAK 128-144(OX) conjugated to alkaline phosphatase, allowed identification of host corneal receptor molecules.[87,88] Three corneal epithelial proteins of similar migratory patterns on SDS-gels (molecular weights: 38, 42 to 45, and 66 kD) from immature and adult mice, and a fourth protein (57 kD) in the adult, bind purified pili. In lectin-binding assays, these cor-

neal epithelial proteins are glycoproteins containing sialic acid, *N*-acetylglucosamine, galactose β(1,3) *N*-acetylgalactosamine, mannose, and L-fucose.

Characterization of these receptor proteins[87,88] indicates that carbohydrates are necessary for receptor activity. In competitive inhibition experiments, sialic acid was the only amino sugar able to completely inhibit pilus binding to mouse corneal epithelial proteins, indicating that in the mouse, it is an important constituent of the pilus receptor. Other studies show that *Pseudomonas* pili adhere to human, rat, and rabbit corneal epithelial glycoproteins[37] (Fig. 15-4).

Pili can be used to protect against *P. aeruginosa* corneal infection.[66] Pili have considerable antigenic variation between strains,[62] however, and bacteria possess an array of other virulence factors including nonpilus adhesins.[90] Increased efforts should be directed toward study of these nonpilus adhesins, in light of the fact that many clinical isolates of *P. aeruginosa* are purportedly nonpiliated.[5]

Flagella. Flagella are subcellular filamentous organelles (16 to 18 nm in diameter) that originate in the cell membrane and extend 15 to 20 μm from its surface. They are responsible for bacterial motility, which establishes the organism and allows it to disseminate in the host.[25] The most prominent extracellular portion of a flagellum is the helical fila-

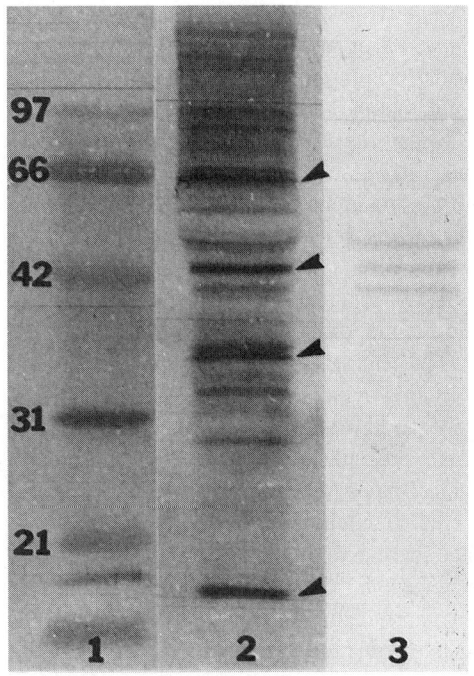

Fig. 15-4.   Immunoblot of human corneal epithelial proteins reacted with bacterial pili and a specific antipili monoclonal antibody. Lanes: 1, nitrocellulose blot of low-molecular-weight markers in kD; 2, *P. aeruginosa* pili with antipili monoclonal antibody (*arrowheads* indicate strongly reactive proteins); 3, control (antipili antibody alone).

ment, usually composed of self-assembling subunits of a single protein, flagellin.

Flagella contain immunospecific proteins that may be the basis for a vaccine, because their large surface exposure and availability make them highly susceptible to antibody binding. Antigenicity without phase variation resides in two basic types, a and b. In *P. aeruginosa,* the flagellins of the antigenic homologous type b are 53 kD and found on 50% to 60% of *P. aeruginosa* isolates,[2] whereas the heterologous type of flagellin ranges from 45 to 52 kD. The latter contains a common subtype, a0, and one or more additional subtypes. More than 95% of *P. aeruginosa* clinical isolates are flagellated.[3]

Most research examining flagellum as a virulence factor in *P. aeruginosa* infection and/or as a vaccine candidate has focused on the burned-mouse model.[48,71] Considerable loss of virulence was seen in flagella-deficient mutants.[71] Active or passive immunization with flagella protects mice against burn wound infection.[25] Similarly, active or passive systemic, as well as topical immunization with flagella or topical antiflagellar antibody homologous to the infecting strain of bacteria, protects mice against *P. aeruginosa* corneal infection.[89] Protection may occur by inhibiting flagella motility or by competitively inhibiting bacterial binding to the cornea.

Host Response

Once *Pseudomonas* organisms infect the cornea, complex tissue reactions occur: inflammation, angiogenesis, cellular and humoral immune responses, and degradation of stromal matrix. Various host factors are resolved in producing ocular damage during infection.

Cytokines. During inflammation, leukocyte adhesion to vascular endothelium is enhanced by interleukin-1 (IL-1) and tumor necrosis factor (TNF), products of T cells and macrophages.[19] IL-1 is a potent intercellular mediator of inflammatory and immune reactions and a potent chemotactic for neutrophils. TNF causes leukopenia, stimulates immunocompetent cells, and induces release of IL-1 and interleukin-6 (IL-6) from macrophages and other cells.[27] *Pseudomonas* organisms induce the release of TNF-α and IL-1 in human mononuclear cells. Bacterial exotoxin A downregulates TNF, IL-1, and lymphotoxin by inhibiting the cell's ability to produce these cytokines.[99]

Leukocytes. The host inflammatory response to *Pseudomonas* spp. has been studied in mice designated as susceptible or resistant. The former fail to restore corneal clarity, and the latter are capable of doing so within 1 month after ocular challenge.[7] Initially, the number of corneal leukocytes is significantly greater in resistant animals. The peak cellular response also is greater in resistant mice who have a shorter duration of inflammatory cells and bacteria in cornea. Susceptible mice are hyporesponsive cellularly[38] and in their ability to produce antibody.[8]

The importance of the host neutrophil response in *Pseudomonas* infections is highlighted by studies showing that if neutrophils are experimentally depleted, many resistant animals die of *Pseudomonas* septicemia within 48 hours.[32] In aged mice, neutrophil deficiencies in phagocytosis have been described[35] that may provide a clue to the age-related susceptibility of animals that are naturally resistant as young adults. In other studies, preimmunization of rats with phenol-killed organisms results in massive corneal stromal degradation caused by neutrophils in the absence of viable bacteria. Naive, unimmunized rats show little stromal damage during the first 18 h, despite the presence of bacteria throughout the cornea. Thus immune recognition is involved in the host corneal response to *Pseudomonas* spp. and appears required for efficient phagocytosis, but not for neutrophil recruitment.[106]

Complement. Complement component C3 also is important in host resistance in experimental *P. aeruginosa* ocular disease. Resistant mice, experimentally depleted of C3 by cobra venom and corneally infected with *Pseudomonas,* respond with delayed leukocyte mobility, bacterial persistence in cornea, and subsequent vision loss.[15]

Corneal Enzymes. Some studies suggest that at 48 h after the onset of ocular infection, host lysosomal enzymes and oxidative substances produced by neutrophils, keratocytes, and epithelial cells may be more important than the damage caused by *Pseudomonas* spp.[101] Two eukaryotic gelatinase species have been characterized: type IV collagenase (72 kD) and type V collagenase (90 to 100 kD).[45] Corneal epithelial cells produce predominantly the 92-kD form of progelatinase, whereas stromal fibroblasts synthesize mostly the 72 kD progelatinase.[28] The latter is cleaved by pseudomonal elastase to produce active forms of the gelatinase.[56,68] Although controlled expression or activation of gelatinases might facilitate homeostatic processes, overexpression or inappropriate activation of these enzymes, as in bacterial infections, could have detrimental tissue-degrading effects.

Bacterial Toxins and Enzymes

P. aeruginosa produces many toxic substances able to cause necrotic central corneal ulceration. Toxin A inhibits protein synthesis like diphtheria toxin by catalyzing the transfer of the adenosine 5'-diphosphate ribose (ADPR) portion of nicotinamide adenine dinucleotide to mammalian elongation factor EF-2.[50] Exoenzyme S is another ADP-ribosyl transferase whose host cell targets are the p21 product of H ras and K ras[17] and the 10-nm filament, vimentin.[16] The toxin may be an adhesin[4] and may also contribute to dissemination of the organism.

Two bacterial proteases, elastase and alkaline protease, cause necrosis of the cornea when injected intrastromally.[49,78] Injection of purified elastase intrastromally also results in severe corneal damage. Inhibition of elastase activity with 2-mercaptoacetyl-L-phenylalanine-L-leucine[10] prevents corneal dissolution. The proteases contribute to pathogenesis by degrading basement membrane,[39] laminin, proteoglycans, extracellular matrix,[107] and collagen.[6] They interfere with host defense systems by degrading complement, immunoglobulins, interferon, interleukin-1, interleukin-2, and tumor necrosis factor.[55] These actions result in decreased neutrophil chemotaxis, T cell function, and NK cell function.[55] Mutants produce infections that are less severe and do not persist in the eye as long as the parent strain. Use of alkaline protease-deficient mutants[49] suggests that this enzyme is required to establish corneal infections. More recent antibody/substrate specificity studies show that bacterial heat-labile phospholipase C is produced in mouse ocular infections,[83] implicating it as a potential virulence factor. Bacterial lipopolysaccharide (LPS) also elicits extensive PMN infiltration into the cornea,[33,57] with subsequent corneal opacification.

Attempts to understand the mechanisms of host defense against bacterial infection show that vaccination with monoclonal antibodies against specific outer membrane proteins[72] of the organism confers partial protection against keratitis. Active immunization with lipopolysaccharide mediates restoration of corneal clarity.[57] Active immunization with elastase or passive immunization with antielastase antibody does not allow mice to recover from corneal infection, but does reduce its severity.[57]

PATHOGENESIS OF FUNGAL OCULAR INFECTION

Fungi are ubiquitous, opportunistic agents of ocular infection.[76b] Fungi rarely infect the normal eye with intact surface epithelium. In a compromised or immunosuppressed cornea, however, virtually any fungal species is capable of producing infection.[52a,52b,52d,52e,77a] Fungal keratitis is more prevalent in warmer climates. There is often a marked seasonal variation in the incidence of fungal keratitis, especially those caused by filamentous fungi. Environmental factors may account for this seasonal variation. In India the incidence of fungal keratitis is greatest in the autumn during harvesting,[82a] whereas in Florida the incidence is highest between November and March during the cool, dry, and windy season.[63a]

Corneal infection with yeast is more commonly encountered in cooler climates, as compared with filamentous fungi, and there is considerably less seasonal variation. Risk factors for candidal keratitis include protracted epithelial ulceration, topical corticosteroid therapy, keratoplasty treated with topical corticosteroids, and therapeutic soft contact lens wear. In patients with local ocular surface abnormalities (such as dry eyes, exposure keratopathy, and previous herpes simplex keratitis) or those with systemic immunosuppression, infection with Candida is more common.

The septate filamentous fungi are the most common causes of fungal keratitis, with a variable geographic distribution. *Fusarium solani* is the most common etiologic organism, which has been isolated in up to 65% of the cases.[21a,52c] *Aspergillus,*[94b] *Curvularia, Paecilomyces, Phialophora, Blastomyces, Sporothrix, Exophiala, Pseudallescheria,* and many other fungi can cause keratitis. Nonseptate filamentous fungi such as Mucoraceae rarely are responsible. The most common predisposing factor to fungal keratitis with filamentous organisms is corneal injury, usually by tree branches or vegetative material. Fungi can contaminate contact lenses and contact lens solutions.[23a,95a,112a] Unlike bacteria, fungal organisms surprisingly infrequently cause keratitis in association with contact lens wear.[112a] Filamentous fungi are more frequently associated with keratitis in extended cosmetic or aphakic soft contact lens wearers, whereas yeasts are more likely to cause keratitis in individuals using therapeutic or bandage soft contact lenses.

Over the past few decades an increased number of fungal infections of the eye have been reported, caused in part by increased clinical awareness and improved laboratory techniques, but perhaps more significantly reflecting the widespread use of antibiotics, immunosuppression, chemotherapy, and ocular prosthetic devices. While the number of cases of oculomycoses has increased, the number of antifungal agents available for therapy is few compared with the number of fungal pathogens capable of infecting the eye. Successful medical treatment of fungal keratitis and endophthalmitis depends not only on the spectrum of antifungal activity of the particular drug, but is also largely influenced by the pharmacokinetic properties of the agent (i.e., its ability to achieve therapeutic concentrations in the cornea and/or vitreous).

Compared with bacterial infections, there are relatively few studies on the pathogenesis of oculomycoses, and a complete understanding of appropriate therapy is still lacking. The pathogenic mechanisms of fungi include direct physical damage by adherence, followed by invasion, growth of fungal elements, damage resulting from the host response, and damage directly produced by fungal toxins and enzymes.

Fungal Adherence

As *Candida albicans* and related species are the leading cause of disseminated fungal infection in the immunocompromised host, the diabetic, the neonate, and the postoperative patient, a considerable body of evidence has accumulated regarding the adherence and receptor relationships of *Candida* spp.[14a,48a] The cell wall of *C. albicans* is composed primarily of the polysaccharides mannan, glycan, and chitin. The major chemical components in the cell wall layers of *C. albicans* have been determined by experiments using various extractants, chemical stains, conjugated antibodies, and conjugated lectins.[14b,82b,105c] The outer fibrillar layer of the cell wall of both yeast and filamentous cells is composed of mannan or mannoprotein. The outer layer has also been described as a mucous coat or capsule[83b] and is sloughed off during infection.[85c]

The prevailing data strongly indicate that the ligand-receptors of *C. albicans* are mannoproteins. These components are located at the cell surface, where they are associated with the outer, fibrillar-floccular layers. Adhesion-ligand interactions have been divided into three categories: (1) protein-protein interactions (e.g., the integrin analogue, iC3b receptor or CR3-like protein, and the fibronectin receptor); (2) lectinlike interactions, including mannoproteins recognizing fucose or N-acetylglucosamine; and (3) incompletely defined interactions such as those involving secretory aspartyl proteinase and Factor 6. The following list summarizes the major adhesins of *C. albicans* and other fungi.

Integrin Analogues. Candidal proteins exhibiting antigenic and functional similarities to human complement receptors 3 and 4 (CR3 and CR4) are known as integrin analogues.[17a] The mammalian integrins are expressed as transmembrane proteins on a wide variety of mammalian cells, including epithelium and leukocytes.[49b] The participation of integrin analogues and epithelial adhesion in *Candida albicans* has been confirmed by identifying a specific protein; by blocking its activity with specific inhibitors including monoclonal antibodies, ligands, and peptides; and by defining the epithelial ligand itself. Additional evidence for integrin analogues as virulence factors derives from their role in the inhibition of phagocytosis.[30c]

Fibronectin Receptor. The binding of fibronectin by *C. albicans* and other species has been demonstrated.[97a] Radiolabeled yeast cells were deposited in fibronectin-coated wells. Through counting the radioactivity in washes of the wells, it was determined that approximately 30% to 40% of *C. albicans* cells adhered in a calcium-dependent fashion. The participation of a fibronectin receptor has also been studied in relation to *Candida albicans* adherence to endothelium.

Adhesive Mannoproteins. The interaction of mannoproteins of *C. albicans* with fucose-containing moieties on epithelial cells has undergone much investigation and provides an explanation for the correlation of candidal carriage and blood group O.[9a] Hosts having blood group O express the H-antigen, a glycoside containing D-galactose, N-acetyl-D-glycocyamine, N-acetyl-D-galactosamine, and alpha-1,2-fucose moiety on their buccal and vaginal epithelial cells. A crude mannoprotein preparation from budding yeast inhibited adhesion of *C. albicans* to epithelial cells in a strain specific fashion.[68a] The interaction of lectinlike mannoproteins on *C. albicans* and fucosalated antigens on buckle or vaginal epithelial cells has been proposed as an explanation for the predilection of nonsecretors and hosts with blood group O for oral or vaginal candidiasis.[105b]

Secretory Aspartyl Proteinase. The role of extracellular (secretory) aspartyl proteinase in epithelial adhesion has not been completely determined, despite purification of the pro-

teinase, the sequencing of the related genes, and several studies indicating decreased virulence in proteinase-deficient strains.[8a,30a,49a] Evidence implicating a role for aspartyl proteinase includes the demonstration of the proteinase on both blastospores and invading germ tubes of *C. albicans* and *C. tropicalis,* but not *C. parapsilosis,* by immunoperoxidase staining of oral mucosa during experimental infection.[8a] In addition, pepstatin, an inhibitor of aspartyl proteinase, prevented the formation of cavitations surrounding blastospores already adherent to murine epidermal corneocytes but did not block candidal adhesion or invasion.[85a]

Factor 6. A second type of incompletely defined interaction is represented by Factor 6, an epitope in the outer chain of candidal mannoprotein that is composed of the terminal side chains of mannoresidues, bound via beta-linkage to the inner branch structures. A mutant lacking Factor 6 was derived from a *Candida albicans* strain and displayed reduced adhesion to human squamous cell oral carcinoma cell line.[70b] Several Factor 6-deficient mutants have been isolated more recently with an agglutinating monoclonal antibody against antigen 6. These mutants have shown reduced adhesion to exfoliated buccal epithelial cells.[70c]

Endothelial Adhesins. The adherence of *Candida* to endothelium has also been studied. There are several important differences between epithelial and endothelial adhesion. In contrast to epithelial adhesion, which typically occurs at the point of initial contact of the blastospore with the host, endothelial adhesion is a late consequence of the organisms having invaded the submucosal vessels or having been inoculated via an intravascular catheter. In addition, epithelial adhesion is predominantly a calcium-independent process, whereas endothelial adhesion is largely calcium-dependent except for the integrin analogue. Interference with epithelial adhesion could conceivably interrupt or decrease candidal colonization, thereby reducing the risk of fungemia. Inhibition of endothelial adhesion, however, would prevent the formation of metastatic abscesses in tissue, but not necessarily blood stream invasion. Thus adhesion in *Candida albicans* is not only a species-specific event but is also tissue-specific.

Fibrinogen Receptor. Little is known about the molecular basis of adherence of filamentous fungal organisms to host tissues. Various proteins or glycoproteins have been proposed as ligands for the pathogenic filamentous fungi at the host cell surface. Fibrinogen is a dimeric glycoprotein having a molecular mass of 340 kDa. It comprises two sets of three nonidentical polypeptide chains (2 alpha [A], 2 beta [B], and 2 gamma chains) held together by numerous disulfide bonds.[23b] The native molecule presents a polydomanial structure with two identical globular domains at the extremities of the molecule, the D domains, and a central globular domain, the E domain, linked by interdomanial super-coiled alpha helioses. A variety of techniques, including immunofluorescence, electron microscopy, and binding assays using radio-labeled ligands, have been used to demonstrate the binding of human fibrinogen to conidia, the infectious airborne form of *Aspergillus fumigatus*.[8b] The interaction appears to be specific and mediated by the outer D domains.[2a] Flow cytometry studies using fluorescein isthiocyanate-conjugated fibrinogen confirm that binding of human fibrinogen to the conidia of *Aspergillus fumigatus* was dose-dependent and specific.[19b] Binding was inhibited by unlabeled fibrinogen and by basement membrane lamina. Moreover, the expression of fibrinogen receptors at the surfaces of conidia seems to be related to the maturation of the conidia. Binding sites appear to be located in the D domains of the fibrinogen molecule. Conidia strongly adhered to human fibrinogen and to laminin but not to fibronectin. Adhesion to fibrinogen substrates was specific since it was inhibited by soluble fibrinogen and by specific antibodies and seemed to be mediated by the D domains of the molecule. Study of the adhesion of numerous strains or clinical isolates of *Aspergillus* to various mammalian fibrinogens did not reveal any particular affinity of strains for some animal species.

Fungal Penetration

Histopathologic observations of corneal fungal infections demonstrate that invasion of the mycelia of filamentous fungi usually occurs parallel to the corneal lamellae but may by perpendicular with more virulent organisms.[74a] In either case, the result of invasion is disruption of the normal orderly arrangement of collagen fibers within the stroma. Yeast forms of *C. albicans,* particularly those strains with surface mannoprotein adhesions, are also capable of penetrating into the cornea to establish infection.[74b] In addition, increased virulence of some strains of *C. albicans* has been particularly associated with the ability to produce hyphae. This increased virulence is presumably based on the greater potential adherence of hyphal forms and on the assumption that hyphae penetrate tissues more readily. Within tissues, hyphal and pseudohyphal mannoproteins have also been shown to inhibit the attachment of neutrophils, thereby allowing the fungal pathogen to escape phagocytosis. In vaginal candidiasis electron microscopic studies have shown that hyphal forms of *Candida albicans* directly invade host epithelial cells.[83c] Direct invasion of leukocytes by yeast has also been documented and some strains of *Candida* are able to germinate after ingestion by neutrophils.[19a]

Filamentous fungal organisms may penetrate Descemet membrane with hyphae.[51a] The ability of filamentous fungi organisms to penetrate Descemet membrane may account for the recurrence of mycotic keratitis in corneal grafts and its initial presentation as posterior stromal keratitis in certain cases. It is also known that *Fusarium* spp. elaborate extracellular proteases that may be responsible for their pathogenicity.[25a] These enzymes may assist fungal pathogens in intrastromal penetration.

Host Response

Once fungal organisms infect the cornea, complex tissue reactions also occur, including inflammation, cellular and humoral immune responses, and degradation of stromal matrix. Although incompletely studied, various host factors appear to be involved in producing ocular damage during infection.

Cytokines. During inflammation, the cascade of events as previously described following bacterial infection with *Pseudomonas* may result in elaboration of several potent mediators of inflammatory and immune reactions as well as chemotactic factors. The precise cytokines elaborated during fungal keratitis have not been elucidated.

Leukocytes. Infiltration of the cornea with host leukocytes plays an important role in fungal keratitis. Extensive migration of polymorphonuclear neutrophils, plasma cells, and rare eosinophils around fungal hyphae are characteristically observed histopathologically. Acute inflammatory cells are also present in areas of stromal destruction where hyphae are not present.[28a] The size of fungal hyphae may preclude ingestion by polymorphonuclear neutrophils. The mechanisms by which neutrophils attempt to destroy fungal hyphae may contribute to destruction of the surrounding stromal tissue with consequent extracellular release of lysosomal enzymes and oxygen metabolites.[21b] Certain strains of yeast forms differing in surface mannoprotein expression may vary in susceptibility to ingestion and in killing by neutrophils.

Fungal Toxins and Enzymes

Microbial toxins are broadly divided into those substances that are spontaneously liberated by actively multiplying organisms (exotoxins) and those associated with cell walls that are released only after cell death and autolysis (endotoxins). A variety of endotoxins and exotoxins have been implicated in causing destruction during fungal eye infections.

Mycotoxins are low-molecular-weight fungal products that may be toxic to higher organisms. Only a few studies have investigated the role of fungal enzymes and toxins as contributing factors in corneal infections.

Early experimental studies using extracts of filamentous fungi showed that corneal damage could be induced in animal models. It was postulated that proteolytic enzymes within the extract were presumably causing the corneal damage. Further studies assessing the role of fungal proteases utilized a clinical isolate of *Aspergillus flavus*.[112b] A strain of *A. flavus* isolated from a severe case of keratitis was grown with a variety of substrates as nitrogen sources, under conditions that would be expected to de-repress the production of extracellular proteases. When grown on minimal medium with milk protein as a nitrogen source, the fungus appeared to produce primarily a metalloprotease, which has a zinc cofactor. When grown with insoluble collagen or elastin as a nitrogen source, a serine protease and cysteine protease as well as the metalloprotease were produced. The strain was further noted to grow with collagen, but not elastin, as a sole source of carbon as well as nitrogen. Since these enzymes had no activity against elastin, it was suggested that it was possibly the collagenolytic activity that was responsible for the pathogenicity of the particular *Aspergillus* isolate. Although elastase activity was not present in the *A. flavus* ocular isolate studied, clinical isolates of *A. flavus* that produce serine proteases with activity against elastin have been demonstrated in infective lung tissues.[85b]

Other predominant types of mycotoxins include aflatoxins, trichothecenes, and zearalenones. A few strains of *Aspergillus* produce aflatoxins and ochratoxins.[14c] Aflatoxins have carcinogenic potential and have been implicated as a cause of hepatocellular carcinoma. The specific role of aflatoxin in corneal infection produced by *Aspergillus* is not known. *Fusarium* and *Acremonium* organisms produce trichothene toxins, which elicit an inflammatory response even at low doses and may cause destruction of many cell types at higher concentrations.[109a] *Penicillium, Aspergillus,* and *Glicladium* organisms may produce gliotoxins that have been characterized as epipolythiodioxopiperzines. These gliotoxins have antibacterial, antiviral, antitumor, and antiphagocytic effects and may suppress immune function. A variety of clinical isolates of candidal species have been demonstrated to produce a gliotoxinlike metabolite.[94b]

A variety of proteolytic enzymes have been characterized from yeast and fungal species. Some neutral and carboxyl proteases having keratinolytic and collagenolytic activity have been demonstrated.[30c] Yeast strains have also been demonstrated to produce phospholipases, which assist in tissue invasion. Canditotoxin, a high-molecular-weight toxin, may be cytotoxic and modulate the immune response. Canditotoxin may be lethal in mice.

Although fungal corneal infections represent a major cause of corneal blindness in the developing tropical world, the precise mechanisms of fungal organism corneal pathogenicity remain incompletely understood. Further investigations into fungal organism adherence, penetration, cytokine release, host immune responses, and enzyme/toxin elaboration are essential to advance therapeutic strategies and minimize corneal destruction in fungal eye infections.

PATHOGENESIS OF PARASITIC OCULAR INFECTION: *ACANTHAMOEBA*

Parasitic infections of the eye are a leading cause of blindness in many parts of the world and have been increasing in frequency in developed nations. Factors related to the increasing incidence of parasitic infections include the frequency of international travel, increased immigration from endemic areas, spread of debilitating disease, including the acquired immunodeficiency syndrome, and the increased use of prosthetic devices, including contact lenses with in-

adequate hygienic practice. *Acanthamoeba* organisms are small, free-living protozoa that are widely distributed in nature. *Acanthamoeba* species have been found in soil, fresh water, sewage, sludge, brackish water, sea water, swimming pools, hot tubs, bottled water, tap water, water baths, condensate in air-conditioning units, trough water, soft contact lenses, contact lens cases and solutions, tissue cultures, and air.[55a,94a,108a]

Epidemiologic studies have established contact lens wear as the most significant risk factor in the United States.[99a] Trauma is the second most significant factor. Poor lens hygiene is frequently encountered with an association with tap water rinsing. *Acanthamoeba* organisms may be recovered from contact lens cases in approximately 10% of asymptomatic users.[59b] The prevalence of *Acanthamoeba* appears to peak during warmer weather. *Acanthamoeba* can be isolated from the nasopharynx of some asymptomatic adults and children.[85d] Demonstration of humoral immunity to *Acanthamoeba* appears to be common in the general population.[19c] Despite frequent and constant exposure to *Acanthamoeba*, clinical ocular infections rarely result. Opportunistic circumstances, such as a break in the corneal epithelium to facilitate entry of organism and/or repeated exposure or inoculation into an immunoprivileged site, such as the cornea, may be required to establish infection. Co-infection with bacteria (especially gram-negative rods), fungi, or viruses may also be additional factors required to establish *Acanthamoeba* infection.[52f] Some species appear to be more pathogenic than others, but the specific factors that determine virulence have not been completely identified.

Amoebic Adherence

Early efforts to produce consistently reliable animal models analogous to human acanthamoebic keratitis were unsuccessful, despite a variety of strategies in immunocompetent and immunosuppressed animals of several species. The corneas of mice and rats inoculated with various *Acanthamoeba* species returned to normal shortly after injection. In early studies acanthamoebic keratitis could be produced in rats only if the parasites were co-injected with *Corynebacterium xerosis*.[3a] The precise role of corynebacteria in the pathogenesis of acanthamoebic keratitis in rats remains incompletely understood. Keratitis of short clinical duration could be induced in rats by intrastromal inoculation of *Acanthamoeba polyphaga*.[59a] From these experimental observations, it was concluded that *Acanthamoeba* was less infective for the rat cornea than human cornea. A series of in vitro studies examined the ability of *Acanthamoeba castellanii* to adhere, invade, and damage normal, intact corneas of several mammalian and one avian species.[76a] *A. castellanii* trophozoites and cysts were incubated with corneas and examined by scanning electron microscopy. Results disclosed that parasites not only failed to produce cytopathic effects but did not even bind to the corneal epithelium of mice, rats, cotton rats, horses, guinea pigs, cows, chickens, dogs, or rabbits. However, parasites were observed to adhere, invade, and produce severe damage in human, pig, and chinese hamster corneas. Additional experiments quantified the binding of *A. castellanii* to the corneas of selected susceptible and nonsusceptible species. In vitro binding assays determined that scant binding of parasites to mouse, rat, and rabbit occurred. In contrast, extensive binding was observed on chinese hamster, pig, and human corneas. The results of these investigations indicate that *A. castellanii* exercises rigid host specificity at the host cell surface.

Scanning and transmission electron microscopic study of human corneal buttons exposed to trophozoites and cysts of *A. castellanii* disclosed limited regions of attachment of trophozoites to the epithelium.[107a] There were, however, extensive regions of attachment ot trophozoites to each other observed. Attachment regions were characterized as plaque-like maculae of an incomplete desmosome junction.

Adhesins. The cell surface of *A. castellanii* is a highly specialized region that is not active in the active transport of solutes but is involved directly in the uptake of nutrients by endocytosis, membrane fusion events and cell motility.[56a,107b] The plasma membrane turns over as much as 50 times per hour. The plasma membrane consists of carbohydrate, protein, and lipophosphoglycan in equal proportions. Glycoproteins have also been detected in the plasma membrane of *Acanthamoeba* species.[79b] Bacterial binding to the cell surface of *A. castellanii* has been demonstrated to involve carbohydrate-containing heterogenous receptors.[83a] Pathogenicity is associated with alterations in lectin-induced agglutination, with pathogenic strains exhibiting less sensitivity to the lectin and possessing fewer lectin-binding sites exposed at the cell surface. Electron-dense amorphous material in association with ferritin-labeled concanavalin-A was found in contact regions of the agglutinated avirulent amoebas on electron photomicrographs.[101a] Electron-dense, calcium-dependent deposits against the plasma membrane of trophozoites have also been observed in arrangements similar to the desmosome-like structures previously observed.[97b]

Adhesin Receptors. In vitro studies assessing corneal pathogenicity disclosed that rabbit and human corneal epithelial cells in culture induced excystment of amoeba to the active trophozoite form.[59c] Total destruction of corneal epithelial cell monolayers was observed for both a human corneal and environmental isolate of *Acanthamoeba,* which were dependent on incubation time and amoebic concentration. Using a human epithelial sheet culture system[76] with morphologically intact epithelial sheets having preserved intracellular junctions, acanthamoebic adherence was observed to increase with time and to decrease with rinsing.

The precise role of intact corneal epithelium for pathogenesis of acanthamoebic keratitis has been a source of controversy. In one in vitro system,[79a] damage to the epithelium was a prerequisite for penetration; however, using human corneas exposed to a high concentration of amoeba, abrading the corneal epithelium did not significantly alter amoebic penetration.[105d]

In patients with trauma as an antecedent risk factor for subsequent development of acanthamoebic keratitis, it is reasonable to presume that the trophozoite gained access to the stroma through a physical gap in the corneal epithelium. *Acanthamoeba* species have been observed to elevate and infiltrate between individual epithelial cells of cultured corneal tissue.[72a]

Amoebic Penetration

After initial invasion of corneal epithelium by *Acanthamoeba,* a sequence involving four successive stages of infection has been proposed based on histopathologic examination of human cases.[30c] The first stage (initial infection) involves amoebic invasion of the superficial stromal lamellae without significant inflammatory response. The second stage (keratocyte depletion) is manifested by a reduced keratocyte population of the anterior stroma. Some replacement with scar tissue formation has occasionally been observed. The loss of keratocytes appears to be independent of the inflammatory reaction. The third stage (inflammatory response) is associated with an acute inflammatory cell infiltration.[105a] The precise stimulus to leukocyte infiltration is uncertain but perhaps is a direct response to the parasite.[67a] A relative absence of lymphocytes and plasma cells has been noted. The fourth stage (stromal necrosis) results in a reduced thickness of the stroma in association with acute inflammatory cell infiltration and stromal cell loss. The stromal keratolysis may be comparable to the nuetrophil-mediated collagenolysis described in experimental corneal alkali burns.[52g] The presence of stromal necrosis in the absence of a significant leukocytic response suggests possible additional factors, such as collagenolytic enzymes secreted by the trophozoites.[38a]

Other factors potentially correlating with in vitro invasiveness and in vivo pathogenicity include the degree of plasminogen activator activity in acanthamoebic strains.[70a] Electron microscopic studies have confirmed the occurrence of bacterial endosymbionts in *Acanthamoeba* species isolated from corneal, environmental, and contact lens specimens.[28b] There was no difference between the number of endosymbiont strains originating from clinical and environmental amoebic isolates, suggesting that the presence alone of these principally gram-negative bacteria does not enhance amoebic infectivity. Gram-negative rods and cocci were found in both clinical and environmental isolates from different geological areas, demonstrating their widespread occurrence in nature. These recent findings suggest that endosymbiosis occurs commonly among members of the family *Acanthamoeba* and that the endosymbionts comprise a diverse taxonomic assemblage.

Host Response

Complement. It has been demonstrated that both *Acanthamoeba* species and *Naegleria fowleri* can activate complement via the alternate pathway.[27a] It has been postulated that the activation of complement via the alternative pathway is an important host defense against these amoebae due to generation of opsonic factors that promote binding and damage by neutrophils.[27b]

Antibodies. Antibodies against pathogenic *Acanthamoeba* have been demonstrated in human serum. The antibodies are of the IgM and IgG isotypes and are capable of neutralizing cytopathogenic effects of *Acanthamoeba*. Antibodies in human serum also promote killing of *Acanthamoeba* by cytokine-activated human neutrophils.[27c] The high prevalence of humoral antibody and the occurrence of clinical acanthamoebic keratitis suggest the inadequacy of humoral factors alone for protection. Thus expression of immunity against *Acanthamoeba* species most likely requires collaboration between cellular components and humoral factors.

Leukocytes. Phagocytic cells play an important role in host immunity to *Acanthamoeba*. Studies have demonstrated that *Acanthamoeba* can be killed by neutrophils. The role of cell-mediated immunity and resistance against *Acanthamoeba* is still unclear. The production of lymphokines by activated T-cells may directly damage or inhibit the growth of amoeba. Lymphokines may activate macrophages in antibody-dependent cellular cytotoxicity against *Acanthamoeba*.[27d] The possibility that amoebae are immunosuppressive exists, yet the precise mechanisms of chronic infection remain to be clearly defined.

REFERENCES

1. Allan JD, Moellering Jr RC: Management of infections caused by gram-negative bacilli: the role of antimicrobial combination, *Rev Infect Dis* 7:S559-S571, 1985.
2. Allison JS et al.: Electrophoretic separation and molecular weight characterization of *Pseudomonas aeruginosa* H-antigen flagellin, *Infect Immun* 49:770-774, 1985.
2a. Annaix V, Bouchara JP, Larcher G et al.: Specific binding of human fibrinogen fragment D to *Aspergillus fumigatus* conidia, *Infect Immun* 60:1747-1755, 1992.
3. Ansorg RA et al.: Differentiation of the major flagellar antigens of *Pseudomonas aeruginosa* by the slide coagglutination technique, *J Clin Microbiol* 20:84-88, 1984.
3a. Badenoch RP, Johnson AM, Christy PE et al.: Pathogenicity of *Acanthamoeba* and a corynebacterium in the rat cornea, *Arch Ophthalmol* 108:107, 1990.
4. Baker NR: *Pseudomonas aeruginosa* exoenzyme S is an adhesin, *Infect Immun* 59:2859-2863, 1991.
5. Baum J, Panjwani NJ: Adherence of *Pseudomonas* to soft contact lenses and cornea: mechanisms and prophylaxis. In Cavanaugh HD, editor: *The cornea: transactions of the World Congress on the cornea III*, New York, 1988, Raven Press.
6. Bejarano PA et al.: Degradation of basement membranes by *Pseudomonas aeruginosa* elastase, *Infect Immun* 57:3783-3787, 1989.
7. Berk RS, Beisel K, Hazlett LD: Genetic studies on the murine corneal response to *P. aeruginosa*, *Proc Soc Exp Biol Med* 172:488-491, 1983.
8. Berk RS et al.: Antibody hyporesponsiveness in resistant BALB/cJ mice intracorneally infected with *Pseudomonas aeruginosa*, *Reg Immunol* 3:186-192, 1991.
8a. Borg M, Ruchel R: Expression of extracellular acid proteinase by proteolytic *Candida* spp. during experimental infection of oral mucosa, *Infect Immun* 56:626-631, 1988.
8b. Bouchara JP, Bouali A, Tronchin G et al.: Binding of fibrinogen to the pathogenic *Aspergillus* species, *J Med Vet Mycol* 26:327-334, 1988.
9. Brandley BK, Schnaar RJ: Cell surface carbohydrates in cell recognition and responce, *J Leuk Biol* 40:97-111, 1986.
9a. Buford MA, Weber JC, Willoughby AM: Oral carriage of *Candida albicans*, ABO blood group and secretor status in healthy subjects, *J Med Vet Mycol* 26:49-56, 1988.
10. Burns FR, Gray RP, Paterson CA: Inhibition of alkali-induced corneal ulceration and perforation by a thiol peptide, *Invest Ophthalmol Vis Sci* 31:107-114, 1990.
11. Burns RP, Rhodes Jr DH: *Pseudomonas* eye infection as a cause of death in premature infants, *Arch Ophthalmol* 65:517-525, 1960.
12. Butrus SI, Klotz SA: Contact lens surface deposits increase the adhesion of *Pseudomonas aeruginosa*, *Curr Eye Res* 9:717-724, 1990.
13. Bzik DJ et al.: The nucleotide sequence of the gB glycoprotein gene of HSV-2 and comparison with the corresponding gene of HSV-1, *Virology* 155:322-333, 1986.
14. Cai W, Gu B, Person S: Role of glycoprotein B of herpes simplex virus type 1 in viral entry and cell fusion, *J Virol* 62:2596-2604, 1988.
14a. Calderone RA, Braun PC: Adherence and receptor relationships of *Candida albicans*, *Microbiol Rev* 55:1-20, 1991.
14b. Cassone A, Mattia E, Boldrini L: Agglutination of blastospores of *Candida albicans* by concanavalin-A and its relationship with the distribution of mannan polymers and the ultrastructure of the cell wall, *J Gen Microbiol* 105:263-273, 1978.
14c. Christensen CM: *Molds, mushrooms, and mycotoxins*, 59-113, Minneapolis, 1975, University of Minnesota Press.
15. Cleveland RP et al.: The role of complement in *Pseudomonas* ocular infections, *Invest Ophthalmol Vis Sci* 24:237-242, 1983.
16. Coburn J et al.: Exoenzyme S of *Pseudomonas aeruginosa* ADP-ribosylates the intermediate filament protein vimentin, *Infect Immun* 57:996-998, 1989.
17. Coburn J et al.: Several GTP-binding proteins including p21c-H-ras, are preferred substrates of *Pseudomonas aeruginosa* exoenzyme S, *J Biol Chem* 264:9004-9008, 1989.
17a. Corbi AL, Kishimoto TK, Miller LJ et al.: The human leukocyte adhesion glycoprotein Mac-1 (complement receptor type III, CD11b) α subunit, *J Biol Chem* 263:12403-12411, 1988.
18. Costerton JW: *Pseudomonas aeruginosa* in nature and diseases. In Sabath LD, editor: *Pseudomonas aeruginosa: the organisms, the disease it causes, and their treatment*, Bern, 1980, Hans Huber.
19. Cotran RS: New roles for the endothelium in inflammation and immunity, *Am J Pathol* 129:407-413, 1987.
19a. Coulot P, Bouchara JP, Reiner G et al.: Specific interaction of *Aspergillus fumigatus* with fibrinogen and its role in cell adhesion, *Infect Immun* 62:2169-2177, 1994.
19b. Cryz SJ et al.: Role of lipopolysaccharide in virulence of *Pseudomonas aeruginosa*, *Infect Immun* 44:508-513, 1984.
19c. Cursons RTM, Brown TJ, Keys EA: Immunity to pathogenic free-living amoeba, *Lancet* 1:877, 1977.
20. Cutler JE: Putitive virulence factors of *Candida albicans*, *Annu Rev Microbiol* 45:187, 1991.
21. Desai PJ, Schaffer A, Minson AC: Excretion of non-infectious virus particles lacking glycoprotein H by a temperature sensitive mutant of herpes simplex virus type I: evidence that gH is essential for virus infectivity, *J Gen Virol* 69:1147-1156, 1988.
21a. DeVoe AG, Silva-Hunter M: Fungal infections of the eye. In Locatcher-Khorazo D, Seegal BC, editors: *Microbiology of the eye*, 208, St Louis, 1972, Mosby.
21b. Diamond RD, Krzesicki R, Wellington J: Damage to pseudohyphal forms of *Candida albicans* by neutrophils in the absence of serum in vitro, *J Clin Invest* 61:349, 1978.
22. Doig P et al.: Role of pili in the adhesion of *Pseudomonas aeruginosa* to human respiratory epithelial cells, *Infect Immun* 56:1641-1646, 1988.

23. Doig P et al.: Human buccal epithelial cell receptors of *Pseudomonas aeruginosa:* identification of glycoproteins with pilus binding activity, *Can J Microbiol* 35:1141-1145, 1989.

23a. Donzis PB et al.: Microbial contamination of contact lens care systems, *Am J Ophthalmol* 104:325, 1987.

23b. Doolittle RF: Fibrinogen and fibrin, *Annu Rev Biochem* 53:195-229, 1984.

24. Dowbenko DJ, Lasky LA: Extensive homology between the herpes simplex virus type 2 glycoprotein F gene and the herpes simplex virus type I glycoprotein C gene, *J Virol* 52:154-163, 1984.

25. Drake D, Montie TC: Flagella, motility and invasive virulence of *Pseudomonas aeruginosa, J Gen Microbiol* 134:43-52, 1988.

25a. Dudley MA, Chick EW: Corneal lesions produced by an extract of *Fusarium moniliforme, Arch Ophthalmol* 72:346, 1964.

26. Esko JD et al.: Animal cell mutants defective in glycosaminoglycan biosynthesis, *Proc Natl Acad Sci USA* 82:3197-3201, 1985.

27. Fajardo LF: The complexity of endothelial cells: a review, *Am J Clin Pathol* 92:241-250, 1989.

27a. Ferrante A, Rowan-Kelly B: Activation of the alternative pathway of complement by *Acanthamoeba culbertsoni, Clin Exp Immunol* 54:477, 1983.

27b. Ferrante A, Mocatta TJ: Human neutrophils require activation by mononuclear leukocyte condition medium to kill pathogenic free-living amoeba, *Clin Exp Immunol* 56:559, 1984.

27c. Ferrante A, Abell TJ: Condition medium from stimulated mononuclear leukocytes augments human neutrophil-mediated killing of a virulent *Acanthamoeba* spp., *Infect Immun* 51:607, 1986.

27d. Ferrante A: Free-living amoeba: pathogenicity and immunity, *Parasite Immunol* 13:31-47, 1991.

28. Fini ME, Girard MT: Expression of collagenolytic/gelatinolytic metalloproteinases by normal cornea, *Invest Ophthalmol Vis Sci* 32:2997-3001, 1991.

28a. Fons A et al.: Histopathology of experimental *Aspergillus fumigatus* keratitis, *Mycopathologia* 101:129, 1988.

28b. Fritsche TR, Gautom RK, Seyedirashti S et al.: Occurrence of bacterial endosymbionts in *Acanthamoeba* spp.: isolated from corneal and environmental specimens and contact lenses, *J Clin Microbiol* 31:1122-1126, 1993.

29. Frost LS, Paranchych W: Composition and molecular weight of pili purified from *Pseudomonas aeruginosa* K, *J Bacteriol* 131:259-269, 1977.

30. Fuller AO, Spear PG: Anti-glycoprotein D antibodies that permit adsorption but block infection by herpes simplex virus I prevent virion cell fusion at the cell surface, *Proc Natl Acad Sci USA* 84:5454-5458, 1987.

30a. Ganesan K, Banerjee A, Datta A: Molecular cloning of the secretory acid proteinase gene from *Candida albicans* and its use as a species-specific probe, *Infect Immun* 59:2972-2977, 1991.

30b. Garner A: Pathogenesis of *Acanthamoeba* keratitis: hypothesis based on a histological analysis of 30 cases, *Br J Ophthalmol* 77:366-370, 1993.

30c. Ghannoum MA, Abu-Elteen KH: Pathogenicity determinants of *Candida, Mycoses* 33:265, 1990.

30d. Gilmore BJ, Retsinas EM, Lorenz JS et al.: An iC3b receptor on *Candida albicans:* structure, function, and correlates for pathogenicity, *J Infect Dis* 157:38-46, 1988.

31. Hazlett LD, Moon MM, Berk R: In vivo identification of sialic acid as the ocular receptor for *Pseudomonas aeruginosa, Infect Immun* 51:687-689, 1986.

32. Hazlett LD, Rosen D, Berk RS: Experimental *Pseudomonas* eye infection in cyclophosphamide-treated mice, *Invest Ophthalmol Vis Sci* 16:649-652, 1977.

33. Hazlett LD et al.: Murine corneal response to heat-inactivated *Pseudomonas aeruginosa, Ophthalmic Res* 10:73-81, 1978.

34. Hazlett LD et al.: Evidence for N-acetylmannosamine as an ocular receptor for *P. aeruginosa* adherence to scarified cornea, *Invest Ophthalmol Vis Sci* 28:1978-1985, 1987.

35. Hazlett LD et al.: Aging alters the phagocytic capability of inflammatory cells induced into cornea, *Curr Eye Res* 9:124-138, 1990.

36. Hazlett LD et al.: Proteinase K decreases *Pseudomonas aeruginosa* adhesion to wounded cornea, *Exp Eye Res* 55:579-588, 1992.

37. Hazlett LD et al.: *Pseudomonas aeruginosa* pili mediate binding to human corneal epithelial glycoproteins, *10th Intl Congress Eye Res,* Stresa, Italy, 1992.

38. Hazlett LD, Zucker M, Berk RS: Distribution and kinetics of the inflammatory cell response to ocular challenge with *P. aeruginosa* in susceptible vs. resistant mice, *Ophthalmic Res* 24:32-39, 1992.

38a. He Y, Niederkorn JY, McCulley JP et al.: In vivo and in vitro collagenolytic *Acanthamoeba castellanii, Invest Ophthalmol Vis Sci* 31:2235-2240, 1990.

39. Heck LW, Morihara K, Abrahamson DR: Degradation of soluble laminin and depletion of tissue-associated basement laminin by *Pseudomonas aeruginosa* elastase and alkaline protease, *Infect Immun* 54:149-153, 1986.

40. Hendricks RL, Epstein RJ, Tumpey T: The effects of cellular immune tolerance to HSV-I antigens on the immunopathology of HSV-I keratitis, *Invest Ophthalmol Vis Sci* 30:105-115, 1989.

41. Hendricks RL, Janowicz M, Tumpey TM: Critical role of corneal Langerhans cells in the CD4 − but not CD8 mediated immunopathology in herpes simplex virus-I infected mouse corneas, *J Immunol* 148:2522-2529, 1992.

42. Hendricks RL, Tumpey T: Contribution of virus and immune factors to herpes simplex type I virus induced corneal pathology, *Invest Ophthalmol Vis Sci* 31:1929-1939, 1990.

43. Hendricks RL, Tumpey TM, Finnegan AL: IFN-γ and IL-2 are protective in the skin but pathologic in the corneas of HSV-1 infected mice, *J Immunol* 149:3023-3028, 1992.

44. Herold BC et al.: Glycoprotein C of herpes simplex virus type I plays a principal role in the adsorption of virus to cells and in infectivity, *J Virol* 65:1090-1098, 1991.

45. Hibbs MS et al.: Gelatinase (type IV collagenase) immunolocalization in cells and tissues: use of an antiserum to rabbit bone gelatinase that identifies high and low Mr forms, *J Cell Sci* 92:487-495, 1989.

46. Hoepelman AIM, Tuomanen EI: Consequences of microbial attachment: directing host cell functions with adhesins, *Infect Immun* 60:1729-1733, 1992.

47. Holder IA, Naglich JG: Experimental studies of the pathogenesis of infections due to *Pseudomonas aeruginosa* infection, *J Trauma* 26:118-122, 1986.

48. Holder IA, Wheeler R, Montie TC: Flagellar preparations from *Pseudomonas aeruginosa:* animal protection studies, *Infect Immun* 35:276-280, 1982.

48a. Hostetter MK: Adhesins and ligands involved in the interaction of *Candida albicans* spp.: with epithelial and endothelial surfaces, *Clin Microbiol Rev* 7:29-42, 1994.

49. Howe TR, Iglewski BH: Isolation and characterization of alkaline protease-deficient mutants of *Pseudomonas aeruginosa* in vitro and in vivo, *Infect Immun* 3:1058-1063, 1984.

49a. Hube B, Turner CJ, Odds FC et al.: Sequence of the *Candida albicans* gene and coding the secretory aspartate proteinase, *J Med Vet Mycol* 29:129-132, 1991.

49b. Hynes RO: Integrins: versatility, modulation, and signaling in cell adhesion, *Cell* 69:11-25, 1992.

50. Iglewski BH, Liu PV, Kabat D: Mechanism of action of *Pseudomonas aeruginosa* exotoxin A: adenosine diphosphate-ribosylation of mammalian elongation factor 2 in vitro and in vivo, *Infect Immun* 15:138-144, 1977.

51. Iida T, Kotoh M, Matsuo Y: Physical and chemical factors affecting the adherence of *Pseudomonas aeruginosa* to a rabbit corneal cell line (SIRC) cells, *Hiroshima J Med Sci* 34:201-207, 1985.

51a. Ishida N, Brown AC, Rao GN et al.: Recurrent *Fusarium* keratomycosis: a light and electron microscopic study. *Ann Ophthalmol* 16:354-366, 1984.

52. John T et al.: Adherence of viable and nonviable bacteria to soft contact lenses, *Cornea* 8:21-33, 1989.

52a. Jones BR: Principles and the management of oculomycosis, *Trans Am Acad Ophthalmol Otolaryngol* 79:15, 1975.

52b. Jones BR, Richards AB, Morgan G: Direct functional infections of the eye in Britain, *Trans Ophthalmol Soc UK* 89:727, 1969.

52c. Jones DB, Forster RK, Rebell G: *Fusarium solani* keratitis treated with natamycin (pimaricin): eighteen consecutive cases, *Arch Ophthalmol* 88:147, 1972.

52d. Jones DB: Pathogenesis of bacterial and fungal keratitis, *Trans Ophthalmol Soc UK* 98:367-371, 1978.

52e. Jones DB: Diagnosis and management of fungal keratitis. In Tasman W, Jaeger E, editors: *Duane's clinical ophthalmology,* vol 4, chapter 21, 1-22, Philadelphia, 1986, Lippincott.

52f. Jones DB: *Acanthamoeba*—the ultimate opportunist? *Am J Ophthalmol* 102:527, 1986.

52g. Kao WWY, Ebert J, Kao CWC et al.: Development of monoclonal antibodies recognizing collagenase from rabbit PMN: the presence of this enzyme in ulcerating corneas, *Curr Eye Res* 5:801-815, 1986.

53. Karlsson KA: Animal glycosphingolipids as membrane attachment sites for bacteria, *Annu Rev Biochem* 58:309-350, 1989.

54. Kaufman HE: Herpetic keratitis, *Invest Ophthalmol Vis Sci* 17:941-957, 1978.

55. Kharazami A: Mechanisms involved in the evasion of the host defense by *Pseudomonas aeruginosa, Immunol Lett* 30:201-205, 1991.

55a. Kingston D, Warhurst DC: Isolation of amoeba from the air, *J Med Microbiol* 2:27, 1969.

56. Kirschner SE, Twining SS: The effect of *Pseudomonas aeruginosa* exoproducts on corneal proteases, *Invest Ophthalmol Vis Sci* 31(suppl):487, 1990.

56a. Korn ED, Wright PL: Macromolecular composition of an amoeba plasma membrane, *J Biol Chem* 246:439-447, 1973.

57. Kreger AS et al.: Immunization against experimental *Pseudomonas aeruginosa* and *Serratia marcescens* keratitis vaccination with lipopolysaccharide endotoxin and proteases, *Invest Ophthalmol Vis Sci* 27:932-939, 1986.

58. Krivan HC, Roberts DD, Ginsburg V: Many pulmonary pathogenic bacteria bind specifically to the carbohydrate sequence GalNacβ1-4Gal found in some glycolipids, *Proc Natl Acad Sci USA* 85:6157-6161, 1988.

59. Laibson PR: Annual review: cornea and sclera, *Arch Ophthalmol* 88:553-574, 1972.

59a. Larkin DFP, Easty DL: Experimental *Acanthamoeba* keratitis. I. Preliminary findings, *Br J Ophthalmol* 74:551, 1990.

59b. Larkin DF, Kilvington S, Easty DL: Contamination of contact lens storage cases by *Acanthamoeba* and bacteria, *Br J Ophthalmol* 74:133, 1990.

59c. Larkin DFP, Berry M, Easty DL: In vitro corneal pathogenicity of *Acanthamoeba, Eye* 5:560-568, 1991.

60. Lausch RN et al.: Prevention of herpes keratitis by monoclonal antibodies specific for discontinuous and continuous epitopes on glycoprotein D, *Invest Ophthalmol Vis Sci* 32:2735-2740, 1991.

61. Lee KK et al.: Immunological studies of the disulfide bridge region of *Pseudomonas aeruginosa* PAK and PAO pilins, using anti-PAK pilus and antipeptide antibodies, *Infect Immun* 57:502-526, 1989.

62. Lee KK et al.: Mapping the surface regions of *Pseudomonas aeruginosa* PAK pilin: the importance of the C-terminal region of adherence to human buccal epithelial cells, *Mol Biol* 3:1493-1499, 1989.

63. Lewkowisz-Moss SJ et al.: Quantitative studies on Langerhans cells in mouse corneal epithelium following infection with herpes simplex virus, *Exp Eye Res* 45:127-140, 1987.

63a. Liesegang TJ, Forster RF: Spectrum of microbial keratitis in South Florida, *Am J Ophthalmol* 90:38, 1980.

64. Ligas MW, Johnson DC: A herpes simplex virus mutant in which glycoprotein D sequences are replaced by β-galactosidase sequences binds to but is unable to penetrate into cells, *J Virol* 62:1486-1494, 1988.

65. Little SP et al.: A virion-associated glycoprotein essential for infectivity of herpes simplex virus type I, *Virology* 115:149-160, 1991.

66. Liu X, Hazlett LD, Berk RS: Systemic and topical protection studies using pseudomonas flagella or pili, *Invest Ophthalmol Vis Sci* 31:449, 1990.

67. Lycke et al.: Binding of herpes simplex virus to cellular heparan sulfate an initial step in the adsorption process, *J Gen Virol* 72:1131-1137, 1991.

67a. Mathers W, Stevens G, Rodrigues M et al.: Immunopathology and electron microscopy of *Acanthamoeba* keratitis, *Am J Ophthalmol* 103:626,635, 1987.

68. Matsumoto K, Shams NBK, Hanninen LA, Kenyon KR: Proteolytic activation of corneal matrix metalloproteinase by *Pseudomonas aeruginosa* elastase, *Curr Eye Res* 11:1105-1110, 1992.

68a. McCourtie J, Douglas LJ: Extracellular polymer of *Candida albicans*: isolation, analysis, and role in adhesion, *J Gen Microbiol* 131:495-503, 1985.

69. Metcalf JF, Kaufman HE: Herpetic stromal keratitis: evidence for cell-mediated immunopathogenesis, *Am J Ophthalmol* 82:827-837, 1976.

70. Meyers-Elliot RH, Chitjian PA: Immunopathogenesis of corneal inflammation in herpes simplex virus stromal keratitis: role of the polymorphonuclear leucocyte, *Invest Ophthalmol Vis Sci* 20:784-798, 1981.

70a. Mitra MM, Taylor WM, Alizadeh H et al.: Level of plasminogen activator activity correlates with pathogenicity in *Acanthamoeba, Invest Ophthalmol Vis Sci* 36(suppl):862, 1995.

70b. Miyakawa Y, Kagaya K, Kuribayashi T et al.: Isolation and chemical and biological characterization of antigenic mutanants of *Candida albicans* serotype-A, *Yeast* 5:S225-229, 1989.

70c. Miyakawa Y, Kuribayashi T, Kagaya K et al.: Role of specific determinants in mannan of *Candida albicans* serotype-A and adherence to human buccal epithelial cells, *Infect Immun* 60:2493-2499, 1992.

71. Montie TC et al.: Motility, virulence, and protection with a flagella vaccine against *Pseudomonas aeruginosa* infection, *Antibiot Chemother* 39:233-248, 1987.

72. Moon MM et al.: associates: Monoclonal antibodies provide protection against ocular *Pseudomonas aeruginosa* infection, *Infect Immun* 29:1277-1284, 1988.

72a. Moore MB, Ubelaker JE, Martin JH et al.: In vitro penetration of human corneal epithelium by *Acanthamoeba castellanii:* A transmission and scanning electron microscopy study, *Cornea* 10:291-298, 1991.

73. Morgan C, Rose HM, Mednis B: Electron microscopy of herpes simplex virus I. Entry, *J Virol* 2:507-516, 1968.

74. The National Advisory Eye Council: External ocular infections and inflammatory diseases: herpes simplex. *In Vision research. A national plan 1987 evaluation and update,* 1987, United States Department of Health and Human Services, Public Health Service, National Institute of Health Publ. No 87-2755.

74a. Naumann G, Green WR, Zimmerman LE: Mycotic keratitis: the histopathologic study of 73 cases, *Am J Ophthalmol* 64:668, 1967.

74b. Nelson RD et al.: *Candida* mannan: chemistry, suppression of cell-mediated immunity and possible mechanism of action, *Clin Microbiol Rev* 4:1, 1991.

75. Newell CK et al.: Herpes simplex virus-induced stromal keratitis: role of T-lymphocyte subsets in immunopathogenesis, *J Virol* 63:769-775, 1989.

76. Nicas TI, Iglewski BH: Toxins and virulence factors of *Pseudomonas aeruginosa.* In Sokatch JR, editor: *The bacteria,* vol X, *The biology of Pseudomonas,* New York, 1986, Academic Press.

76a. Niederkorn JY, Ubelaker JE, McCulley JP et al.: Susceptibility of corneas from various animal species to in vitro binding and invasion by *Acanthamoeba castellanii, Invest Ophthalmol Vis Sci* 33:104-112, 1992.

76b. O'Brien TP, Green WR: Fungus infections of the eye and periocular tissues. In Garner A, Klintworth GK, editors: *Pathobiology of ocular diseases: A dynamic approach,* 229-333, New York, 1994, Marcel Dekker.

77. O'Brien WJ: Herpesvirus. In Rapp F, editor: *Herpetic eye diseases in animals as models for therapeutic studies of acute and latent herpesvirus infections,* New York, 1984, Liss.

77a. O'Day et al.: Influence of corticosteroid on experimentally induced keratomycosis, *Arch Ophthalmol* 109:1601, 1991.

78. Ohman DE, Burns RP, Iglewski BH: Corneal infection in mice with toxin A and elastase mutants of *Pseudomonas aeruginosa, J Infect Dis* 142:547-555, 1980.

79. Opremcak EM et al.: Histology and immunohistology of the Igh-I restricted herpes simplex keratitis in BALB/c congenic mice, *Invest Ophthalmol Vis Sci* 31:305-312, 1990.

79a. Osato MS, Pyron M, Elizondo M et al.: Adherence and penetration of human corneal epithelium by *Acanthamoeba, Invest Ophthalmol Vis Sci* 31(suppl):420, 1990.

79b. Paatero GIL, Gahmberg CG: Detection of glycoproteins in the *Acanthamoeba* plasma membrane, *Exp Cell Res* 179:253-262, 1988.

80. Panjwani N et al.: Binding of *Pseudomonas aeruginosa* to glycosphingolipids of rabbit corneal epithelium, *Infect Immun* 58:114-118, 1990.

81. Paranchych W: Molecular studies on N-methylphenylalanine pili. In Iglewski BH, Clark VL, editors: *The bacteria, vol. XI: molecular basis of bacterial pathogenesis,* New York, 1990, Academic Press.

82. Patti JM, Allen BL, McGavin MJ, Höök M: MSCRAMM-mediated adherence of microorganisms to host tissues, *Ann Rev Microbiol* 48:585-617, 1994.

82a. Poria VC et al.: Study of mycotic keratitis, *Indian J Ophthalmol* 33:229, 1985.

82b. Poulain D, Hopwood V, Vernes A: Antigenic variability of *Candida albicans, Crit Rev Microbiol,* 12:223-270, 1985.

83. Preston M et al.: Kinetics of serum, tear and corneal antibody responses in resistant and susceptible mice intracorneally infected with *Pseudomonas aeruginosa, Infect Immun* 60:885-891, 1992.

83a. Preston TM, King CA: Binding sites for bacterial flagella at the surface of soil amoeba, *J Gen Microbiol* 130:1449-1458, 1984.

83b. Pugh D, Cawson RA: The surface layer of *Candida albicans, Microbios* 23:19-23, 1979.

83c. Ragasingham KC, Challacombe SJ, Tovey D: Ultrastructure and possible processes involved in the invasion of host epithelial cells by *Candida albicans* and vaginal candidosis, *Cytobios* 60:11, 1989.

84. Ramphal R, Mcniece MT, Polack FM: Adherence of *Pseudomonas aeruginosa* to the injured cornea: a step in the pathogenesis of corneal infections, *Ann Ophthalmol* 13:421-425, 1981.

85. Ramphal R, Pyle M: Evidence for mucins and sialic acid as receptors for *Pseudomonas aeruginosa* in the lower respiratory tract, *Infect Immun* 41:339-344, 1983.

85a. Ray TL, Payne CD: Scanning electron microscopy of epidermal adherence and cavitation in murine candidiasis: a role for candida acid proteinase, *Infect Immun* 56:1942-1946, 1988.

85b. Reichard U et al.: Purification and characterization of an extracellular serine protease from *Aspergillus fumigatus* and its detection in tissue, *J Med Microbiol* 33:243, 1990.

85c. Reiss E, DeRepentigny L, Kuykendall RJ et al.: Monoclonal antibodies against *Candida tropicalis* mannan: antigen detection by enzyme immunoassay and immunofluorescence, *J Clin Microbiol* 24:796-802, 1986.

85d. Rivera F et al.: Pathogenic and free-living protozoa cultured from the nasopharyngeal and oral regions of dental patients, *Environ Res* 33:428, 1984.

86. Rouse BT: The herpesviruses. In Roizman B, Lopez C, editors: *Immunopathology of herpesvirus infection,* New York, 1985, Plenum.

86a. Ruchel R, DeBernardis F, Ray TL et al.: Candida acid protenases (CAP), *J Med Vet Mycol* 30(suppl)1:123-132, 1992.

87. Rudner XL et al.: Corneal epithelial glycoproteins exhibit *Pseudomonas aeruginosa* pilus binding activity, *Invest Ophthalmol Vis Sci* 33:2185-2193, 1992.

88. Rudner XL et al.: *Pseudomonas aeruginosa* pili interact differently with glycosylated proteins of immature cornea, *Invest Ophthalmol Vis Sci* 33(suppl):844, 1992.

89. Rudner XL, Hazlett LD, Berk RS: Systemic and topical protection studies using *Pseudomonas aeruginosa* flagella in an ocular model of infection, *Curr Eye Res* 11:727-738, 1992.

90. Saiman L, Ishimoto K, Lory S, Prince A: The effect of piliation and exoproduct expression on the adherence of *Pseudomonas aeruginosa* to receptor monolayers, *J Infect Dis* 161:541-548, 1990.

91. Sarmiento M, Haffey M, Spear PG: Membrane proteins specified by herpes simplex viruses. III. Role of glycoprotein VP7(B2) in virion infectivity, *J Virol* 29:1149-1158, 1979.

92. Sastry PA et al.: Amino acid sequence of pilin isolated from *Pseudomonas aeruginosa* PAK, *FEBS Lett* 151:253-256, 1983.

93. Sastry PA et al.: Studies on the primary structure and antigenic determinants of pilin isolated from *Pseudomonas aeruginosa* K, *J Biochem Cell Biol* 63:284-291, 1985.

94. Sastry PA et al.: Comparative studies of the amino acid and nucleotide sequences of pilin derived from *Pseudomonas aeruginosa* PAK and PAO, *J Bacteriol* 164:557-577, 1985.

94a. Sawyer TK, Visvesvara GS, Harle B: Pathogenic amoebas from brackish and ocean sediments with a description of *Acanthamoeba hatchetti, Science* 196:1324, 1977.

94b. Searl SS, Udell IJ, Sadun A et al.: *Aspergillus* keratitis with intraocular invasion, *Ophthalmology* 88:1244, 1981.

94c. Shah DT, Larsen B: Clinical isolates of yeasts produce a glicotoxin-like substance, *Mycopathologia* 116:203, 1991.

95. Shieh M-T et al.: Cell surface receptor for herpes simplex virus are heparan sulfate proteoglycans, *J Cell Biol* 116:1273-1281, 1992.

95a. Simmons RB et al.: Morphology and ultrastructure of fungi in extended-wear soft contact lenses, *J Clin Microbiol* 24:21, 1986.

96. Singh A, Hazlett LD, Berk RS: Characterization of *Pseudomonas aeruginosa* adherence to mouse corneas in organ culture, *Infect Immun* 58:1301-1307, 1990.

97. Singh A, Hazlett LD, Berk RS: Characterization of *Pseudomonas aeruginosa* adherence to unwounded cornea, *Invest Ophthalmol Vis Sci* 32:2096-2104, 1991.

97a. Skerl KG, Calderone RA, Segal E et al.: In vitro binding of *Candida albicans* yeast cells to human fibronectin, *Can J Microbiol* 30:221-227, 1984.

97b. Soboto A, Przelecka A: Developmental changes in the localization of calcium binding sites in *Acanthamoeba castellanii, Histochem J* 71:135-144, 1981

98. Spurr-Michaud SJ, Barza M, Gipson IK: An organ culture system for study of adherence of *Pseudomonas aeruginosa* to normal and wounded corneas, *Invest Ophthalmol Vis Sci* 29:379-386, 1988.

99. Staugas REM et al.: Induction of tumor necrosis factor (TNF) and interleukin-1 (IL-1) by *Pseudomonas aeruginosa* and exotoxin A-induced supression of lymphoproliferation and TNF, lymphotoxin, gamma interferon, and IL-1 production in human leukocytes, *Infect Immun* 60:3162-3168, 1992.

99a. Stehr-Green JK, Bailey TM, Visvesvara GS: The epidemiology of *Acanthamoeba* keratitis in the United States, *Am J Ophthalmol* 107:331, 1989.

100. Stern GA, Weitzenkorn D, Valenti J: Adherence of *Pseudomonas aeruginosa* to the mouse cornea: epithelial v. stromal adherence, *Arch Ophthalmol* 100:1956-1958, 1982.

101. Steuhl KP et al.: Effect of immunization on corneal infection by *Pseudomonas aeruginosa, Invest Ophthalmol Vis Sci* 28:1559-1568, 1987.

101a. Stevens AR, Kaufman AE: Concanavalin-A-induced agglutination of *Acanthamoeba, Nature* 252:43-45, 1974.

102. Stulting RD, Kindler JC, Nahmias AJ: Patterns of herpes simplex keratitis in inbred mice, *Invest Ophthalmol Vis Sci* 26:1360-1367, 1985.

103. Stuve et al.: Structure and expression of the herpes simplex virus type 2 glycoprotein gB gene, *J Virol* 61:326-335, 1987.

104. Swain MA, Peet RW, Galloway DA: Characterization of the gene encoding herpes simplex virus type 2 glycoprotein C and comparison with the type I counterpart, *J Virol* 53:561-569, 1985.

105. Switalski LM et al.: Collagen receptor of *Staphylococcus aureus*. In Hook M, Switalski L, editors: *Microbial adhesion and invasion,* New York, 1992, Springer-Verlag.

105a. Theodore FH, Jakobiec FA, Juechter KB et al.: The diagnostic value of a ring infiltrate in *Acanthamoeba* keratitis, *Ophthalmology* 92:1471-1479, 1985.

105b. Thom SM, Blackwell CC, MacCallum CJ et al.: Non-secretion of blood group antigens and susceptibility to infection by *Candida* species, *FEMS Microbiol Immunol* 1:401-405, 1989.

105c. Tronchin G, Poulain D, Herbaut J, Biguet J: Cytochemical and ultrastructural studies of *Candida albicans*. II. Evidence for a cell wall coat using concanavalin-A, *J Ultrastruct Res* 75:50-59, 1981.

105d. Tschumper RC, Sloan LM, Rosenblatt JE et al.: A human in vitro model for *Acanthamoeba* keratitis, *Invest Ophthalmol Vis Sci* 31:419, 1990.

106. Twining SS, Lohr KM, Moulder JE: The immune system in experimental keratitis: model and early effects, *Invest Ophthalmol Vis Sci* 27:507-515, 1986.

107. Twining SS, Davis SD, Hyndiuk RA: Relationship between proteases and descemetocele formation in experimental *Pseudomonas* keratitis, *Curr Eye Res* 5:503-510, 1986.

107a. Ubelaker, Moore MB, Martin JH et al.: In vitro intracellular adherence of *Acanthamoeba castellanii:* a scanning and transmission electron microscopy study, *Cornea* 10:299-304, 1991.

107b. Victoria EJ, Korn ED: Enzymes of phospholipid metabolism in the plasma membrane of *Acanthamoeba castellanii*, *J Lipid Res* 16:54-60, 1975.

108. Vishwanath S, Ramphal R: Tracheobronchial mucin receptor for *Pseudomonas aeruginosa:* predominance of amino sugars in binding sites, *Infect Immun* 48:331-335, 1985.

108a. Warhurst DC: Pathogenic free-living amoebae, *Parasitol Today* 1:24, 1985.

108b. Wilhelmus KR et al.: Fungal keratitis in contact lens wearers, *Am J Ophthalmol* 106:708, 1988.

109. Wittels M, Spear PG: Penetration of cells by herpes simplex virus does not require a low pH-dependent endocytic pathway, *Virus Res* 18:271-290, 1991.

109a. Wogan GN: Mycotoxins, *Annu Rev Pharmacol Toxicol* 15:437, 1975.

110. Woods DE et al.: Role of pili in adherence of *P. aeruginosa* to mammalian buccal epithelial cells, *Infect Immun* 29:1146-1151, 1980.

111. Woods DE et al.: Role of fibronectin in the prevention of adherence of *Pseudomonas aeruginosa* to buccal cells, *J Infect Dis* 143:784-790, 1981.

112. WuDunn D, Spear PG: Initial interaction of herpes simplex virus with cells is binding to heparan sulfate, *J Virol* 63:52-58, 1989.

112a. Yamaguchi T et al.: Fungus growth on soft contact lenses with different water contents, *CLAO J* 10:166, 1984.

112b. Zhu WS, Wojdyla K, Donlon K et al.: Extracellular proteases of *Aspergillus flavus*: fungal keratitis, proteases and pathogenesis, *Diagn Microbiol Infect Dis* 13:491-497, 1990.

113. Ziegler RJ, Pozos RS: Effects of lectins on peripheral infection by herpes simplex virus of rat sensory neurons in culture, *Infect Immun* 34:588-595, 1981.

16 Biomaterials and Ocular Infection

LOUIS A. WILSON

Microbial colonization of indwelling and implanted biomedical devices can lead to serious, often lethal infection.[11] Polymers, silicones, and metals used for the fabrication of devices such as cerebrospinal fluid shunts, vascular and urinary catheters, percutaneous sutures, synthetic vascular grafts, joint prostheses, artificial hearts, cardiac valves, and pacemakers have all been implicated.* The infecting organisms may be introduced percutaneously, intraoperatively, or via a transient episode of bacteremia that is associated with minor surgical procedures. The indwelling or implanted material is subsequently colonized by microorganisms that elaborate a protective matrix, shielding the organisms from host defense mechanisms and standard concentrations of circulating antimicrobial drugs. Within this matrix, the organisms are sessile, yet viable. They can reproduce and are shed as free-floating planktonic cells that can cause persistent localized infection or that can disseminate to give rise to distant foci of infection.

Bacteria, both gram-positive and gram-negative, are the predominant pathogens. *Staphylococcus epidermidis* is the most frequent agent that causes infection related to the use of intravenous catheters, orthopedic devices, synthetic vascular grafts, prosthetic heart valves, central nervous system shunts, and peritoneal dialysis catheters.[68] Alpha-hemolytic streptococci selectively adhere to tooth surfaces, are primary colonizers of dental plaque, and are a major cause of subacute bacterial endocarditis.[37] Gram-negative bacteria, particularly strains of *Escherichia coli,* more commonly colonize urinary catheters and may result in uroepithelial cell infection.[123,127] *Candida* spp. can colonize catheters and cause intermittent fungemia with distant metastases.[60,111,112]

MICROORGANISMS THAT CAUSE BIOMEDICAL DEVICE-ASSOCIATED INFECTION

The etiopathic agents of biomaterial-related infections are, for the most part, resident microbiota in a specific area of the body and thus represent a constant reservoir of oppor-

tunistic pathogens. For example, strains of *E. coli,* other gram-negative bacteria, enterococci, and some *Candida* species are resident to the lower digestive tract and conveniently available to contaminate and colonize urinary catheters. A biomedical device creates a pathway of extraluminal access to the lower urinary tract which leads to infection of uroepithelial cells by the colonizing organisms. The longer the device remains indwelling, the greater the chance of infection. Similarly, a transcutaneous vascular catheter can be readily colonized by microbial residents of the skin, leading to hematogenous dissemination of one or more organisms.

Staphylococcus epidermidis, an organism routinely found on the skin, is a frequent cause of infection that is associated with biomedical devices.[68,112] *Staphylococcus aureus* may also adhere to vascular catheters that are coated with host-derived fibronectin.[126] *Pseudomonas aeruginosa* and *Candida parapsilosis* have also been reported in cases of vascular catheter-related sepsis.[112] Organisms adherent to infected catheters may disseminate to, and colonize, other previously implanted devices. Microbiota introduced intraoperatively may also adhere to and subsequently colonize the implanted material. Transient bacteremia associated with minor surgical procedures (such as dental extractions) may likewise lead to colonization of prosthetic devices. This risk forms the rationale for the prophylactic use of antibiotics prior to and following such procedures.

MECHANISMS OF INFECTION ASSOCIATED WITH BIOMATERIALS

On a mucosal surface such as the conjunctiva, colonizing organisms initially form a weak or reversible attachment called "association" (Fig. 16-1A). This is facilitated—or prevented—by factors including comparative electrostatic surface charges, the hydrophobicity or hydrophilicity of the pathogen and host cell surface, and the presence or absence of a carbohydrate-rich extrinsic mucosal cell surface coat (that is, host-cell glycocalyx). If the microorganism is not repelled following association, a relatively stable, irreversible attachment of the microbial cell to the host cell occurs

---

*References 8, 9, 40, 43, 44, 55, 61, 70, 123.

215

Colonization of Conjunctival Surface (mucosa) by Bacteria

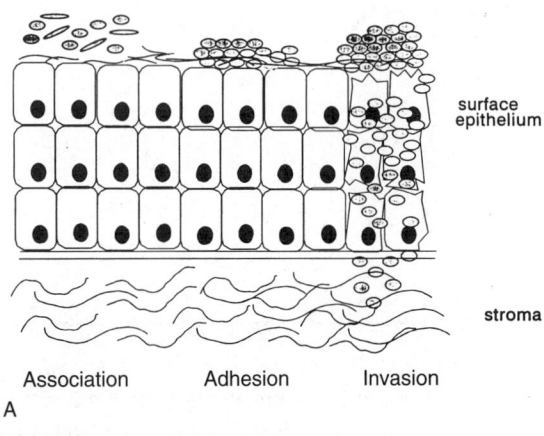

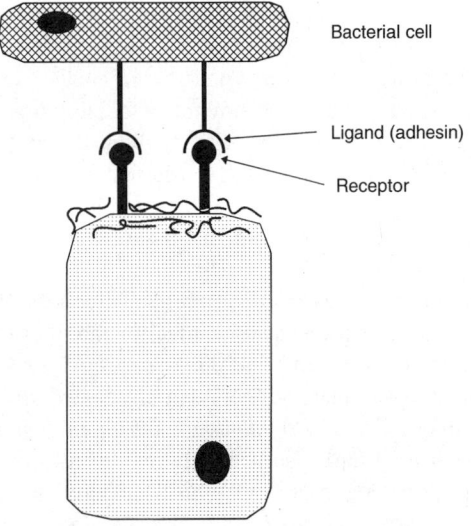

Fig. 16-1. **A,** Schematic representation of bacterial colonization of conjunctival mucosal surface: Invasion is suggestive of a more virulent organism causing hyperacute bacterial conjunctivitis. **B,** Schematic representation of a bacterial cell that has overcome electrostatic repulsion attaching via ligand-receptor couplings to a conjunctival epithelial cell.

—an event termed *adhesion* or *adherence.* This is often facilitated by complementary structures or molecules present on the surface of both the microbial and host cell. Fimbriae are fine, hairlike structures on some bacterial cells (for example, *E. coli*) that display *adhesins* to a host cell surface. A *ligand* is a microbial surface molecule that performs as an adhesin, exhibiting specific binding properties to a complementary substrate molecule on the surface of a host cell called a *receptor* (Fig. 16-1B). Following adhesion to a mucosal surface, the pathogen may initiate noninvasive clinical infection by surface growth or by elaboration of toxins. It may penetrate the mucosal barrier (''invasion'') to establish

growth within epithelial cells or subjacent stroma (Fig. 16-1A). In either instance, microbial attachment is critically important as an initial event in the infection of mucosal surfaces.

Other examples of human disease caused by fimbriae-host cell attachment are bacterial dysentery and gonorrhea. It is likely that some forms of invasive bacterial conjunctivitis follow the same series of events. For instance, in bovine keratoconjunctivitis caused by *Moraxella bovis,* fimbrial attachment is followed by production of a cytotoxic pitting agent that facilitates invasion of ocular surface epithelium. Similarly, microbial keratitis may occur in the absence of known predisposing injury or environmental factors.[56,110]

Nonproteinaceous, nonfimbrial adhesins are best represented by the teichoic and lipoteichoic acid molecules on *S. aureus* and streptococcal cells, respectively, that serve as ligands and facilitate attachment to epithelial cell receptor sites.[4]

Certain bacteria, notably strains of *S. epidermidis* and *P. aeruginosa,* also secrete an extracellular polymeric substance (glycocalyx) that functions as a nonspecific adhesin that mediates attachment of these bacteria to animate and inanimate surfaces. The substrate adsorbs these substances which then encases the microbial cells and glues them onto the surface (Fig. 16-2). The increasing mass of the bacterial glycocalyx is an anionic, polysaccharide matrix that can be stained with polyanion-specific stains such as ruthenium red[69] (Fig. 16-3). Within this matrix, attached sessile organisms metabolize and reproduce occasionally, releasing free-floating planktonic cells into what is most often a fluid environment (Fig. 16-2). As imbedded microcolonies increase in size, they become confluent and give rise to a mucilaginous slime, frequently referred to as a microbial *biofilm.*

This nonspecific adherence to an inanimate surface with subsequent biofilm formation is a basic survival mechanism for environmental organisms—particularly those in an aquatic setting.[23] It is also the mechanism with which some

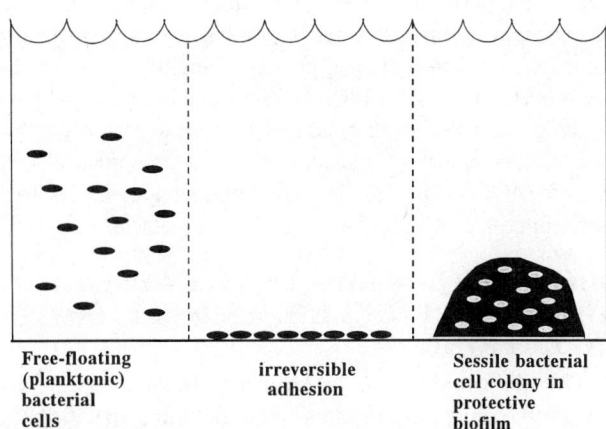

Fig. 16-2. Planktonic bacterial cells forming irreversible adherence to an inanimate surface. Sessile bacteria secrete and reproduce in a protective matrix-biofilm.

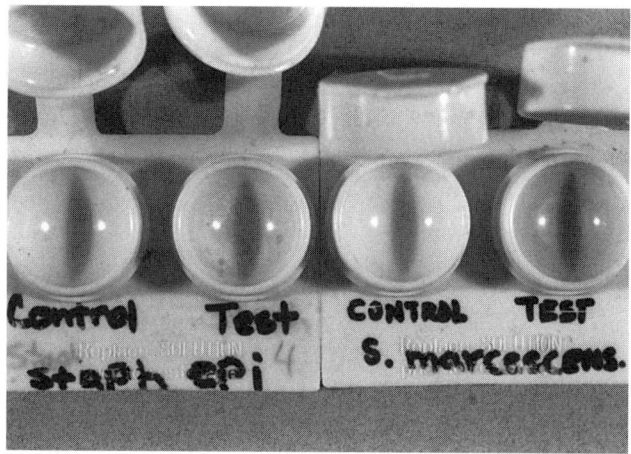

Fig. 16-3. Polyethylene contact lens case with adherent microbial films stained with ruthenium red *(S. epidermidis, S. marcescens).*

strains of *S. epidermidis* and *P. aeruginosa* colonize indwelling and implanted medical devices.[17,31,53] The presence of host fibronectin on some of these devices provides for a more specific ligand-receptor mechanism of attachment for some strains of coagulase-negative staphylococci and *S. aureus.*[126]

In summary, several factors explain the mechanisms of infection that are associated with biomedical devices:

1. Intraoperative contamination of the device at the time of surgical implantation or extraluminal migration of organisms along a transcutaneous canula or indwelling urinary catheter permit opportunistic pathogens access across the protective barriers.

2. The microbial production of mucoid exopolymeric substances enhances the stickiness of the colonizing organisms while protecting them from host defense mechanisms and circulating antimicrobial agents.

3. The presence of plasma proteins on the surface of the biopolymer, particularly fibronectin, selectively promotes staphylococcal and probably *Candida* species attachment to its surface.[14,126]

BIOMATERIALS IN OPHTHALMOLOGY

Contact lens plastics and their storage cases are the most frequently used class of biopolymers in ophthalmic practice —with monofilament suture materials a close second. Silicone encircling bands, sponges, and segmental plates are biomaterials commonly used in retinal detachment repair. Silicone plugs are marketed in the United States for closure of the lacrimal puncta in cases of keratoconjunctivitis sicca. Polymethylmethacrylate (PMMA), hydrogel, and silicone polymers are widely employed in the fabrication of intraocular lenses for use during cataract surgery. In many instances, monofilament polypropylene is the biopolymer that constitutes the haptic of the prosthetic intraocular lens. Poly-

methylmethacrylate, aluminum oxide ceramics, and poly-tetrafluoroethylene (Teflon) are used in the fabrication of keratoprosthetic devices that restore vision in patients with corneal blindness who are not amendable to standard penetrating keratoplasty.[66,108]

All of these biomaterials are subject to nonspecific microbial colonization in much the same manner as those materials used to fabricate catheters and nonophthalmic prosthetic devices. Ophthalmologists are now recognizing the importance of colonization and how it relates to various ocular infections.

Contact Lenses

Contact lenses and their storage cases are frequently used polymers in ophthalmic practice. During a five-year period (1987-1992), the number of Americans wearing these devices increased from slightly over 18 million to 24 million.[13,51] The vast majority of these people wore soft contact lenses designed for daily (DWSCL) or extended wear (EWSCL) or both, and an increasing percentage of new fits or refits are with disposable soft lenses (DSCL).[13] Rigid gas-permeable contact lenses (RGP) are composed mostly of variable percentages of silicone polymer and PMMA with or without fluoro or styrene polymers. These have almost completely replaced the older hard contact lenses (HCL) that were fabricated entirely from PMMA.

Ocular infection associated with contact lens wear is not a recent phenomenon. A 1966 nationwide survey reported severe keratitis that resulted in diminished or lost vision among HCL wearers.[28] Two additional cases of HCL-related pseudomonal keratitis were described in 1971, and in both instances the same organism was isolated from the contact lens case.[41] Following the availability of hydrogel contact lenses during the 1970s, instances of microbial keratitis were principally caused by gram-negative bacteria and contamination of the contact lens case and or lens solution(s).[22,50,63] Lens case contamination, chiefly by gram-negative bacteria, was noted in over one third of soft lens wearers, suggesting inadequate DWSCL disinfection as a major contributing factor.[106] Cases of pseudomonal keratitis were linked to the use of saline soaking solutions prepared from distilled water and sodium chloride tablets.[135]

A fairly extensive literature review of ulcerative keratitis in 1987 noted that up to 34% of all cases were associated with contact lens wear: the predominant lens type was hydrogel (DWSCL and EWSCL), and *P. aeruginosa* was a major etiopathic agent.[129] The same report graphically depicted a notable increase in the institutional incidence at selected American referral centers and an increase in the number of published reports since the advent of hydrogel contact lenses. Subsequent studies have calculated the relative risk of contact lens-associated microbial keratitis for DWSCL, EWSCL, and rigid lens wearers and noted a significant increase in risk for EWSCL wearers compared to DWSCL or rigid lens wearers. Also, a comparison was made of the annualized rate of ulcerative keratitis among users of these devices.[107,113] Disposable soft contact lenses are now known to predispose to ulcerative keratitis.[13,73]

All contact lens wearers are at risk of corneal infection. Extended overnight wear is the most important risk factor among soft contact lens wearers.

Microorganisms. *Bacteria.* Gram-negative bacteria in general and *P. aeruginosa* in particular predominate as causes of corneal infection associated with contact lens wear.* *Serratia marcescens,* a gram-negative enteric bacillus, is also an important cause.[3,22,87,100] Of the gram-positive bacteria, *Staphylococcus* spp. are most commonly encountered.[114]

Protozoa (Acanthamoeba). *Acanthamoeba* spp. are small free-living amoebae with a life cycle that is characterized by a trophozoite stage and a cyst stage.[72] They are commonly isolated from human surroundings including swimming ponds and pools, drinking water, sand from sand boxes, and dust from various habitat locations.[82] Although still a relatively uncommon cause of corneal disease, acanthamoebic keratitis has been increasingly recognized as a sight-threatening corneal infection that may be difficult to diagnosis and recalcitrant to medical management. Although corneal infection by *Acanthamoeba* spp. is not limited to contact lens wear, a fairly extensive survey in the United States noted 85% of cases were contact lens wearers.[121] In Europe, the percentage of patients diagnosed as having acanthamoebic keratitis has also been linked to contact lens wear, ranging between 76% and 100% of all cases.[20] In addition to DWSCL and EWSCL use, RGP lens and DSCL wear have also been associated with instances of acanthamoebic keratitis.[49,62]

Fungi. Fungal infection of the cornea that is related to contact lens wear is uncommon. All lens types have been associated with mycotic keratitis, but soft lenses for aphakia and therapeutic extended wear are most frequently implicated.[120,128,134] Soft lenses for cosmetic and aphakic extended wear are more often associated with filamentous fungal pathogens (hyphomycetes), whereas yeast fungi are more frequently implicated with therapeutic soft lens wear.[128] Fungal spores adhere to the surface of a continuously worn soft lens and, supported by tear film nutrients, germinate, sending hyphae into the matrix of the soft lens (Fig. 16-4*A*). Chitinous hyphae projecting through the posterior surface may then penetrate the corneal epithelium, thus giving rise to fungal keratitis[118] (Fig. 16-4*B*).

Microbial Adhesion and Biofilm Formation. Given suitable conditions (for example, bullous keratopathy) just about any organism can cause microbial keratitis. Nevertheless, in most patients who do not wear contact lenses, there is generally some form of antecedent trauma that breeches the protective epithelial layer. The causative agent may either be

---

*References 3, 10, 16, 19, 32, 38, 87, 98, 100, 129.

inoculated by the instrument of trauma (for example, mascara brush) or be an environmental opportunist. In either case, specific or nonspecific microbial adherence to corneal epithelium or stroma occurs, cell reproduction ensues, and infection begins.

In contact lens wearers with ulcerative keratitis, a history of trauma is usually absent. A spontaneous irritation or foreign-body sensation ordinarily escalates to persistent pain, photophobia, redness, and decreased vision. The rapidity of onset of symptoms and the clinical findings depend, in large measure, on the mechanisms of pathogenicity that characterize the agent (that is, virulence, invasiveness, toxigenicity, and pathogenicity).

The microbial production of a sticky, mucoid, exopolymeric biofilm is one of the more important components of the pathogenesis of biopolymer-associated infection. This biofilm permits establishment and persistence of a microbial colony on the plastic surface of the contact lens or its soaking case (Fig. 16-3). Additional prerequisites are minimal nutritional requirements and environmental universality.

Contact lens-related polymers (rigid and hydrogel lenses, contact lens cases, and plastic containers for care system fluids) may be nonspecifically colonized by bacteria, protozoa, and some fungi. Whereas initial microbial attachment is dependent on hydrophobic interactions and electrostatic attraction, bacterial colonization of the polymer surface is associated with an extracellular polysaccharide matrix, or slime, that protects the microbial cells from the action of many chemical biocides. The subsequent release of free-swimming, planktonic cells from the adherent biofilm permits a similar attachment to, and colonization of, the contact lens soaking in the contaminated solution. Substantial glycocalyx formation may occur on the lens surface, particularly if the contact lens soaks in the contaminated case fluid for prolonged periods of time. When placed on the eye, the contact lens acts as a mechanical vector bringing opportunistic pathogens into contact with the corneal surface.

P. aeruginosa. Perhaps no single agent is as efficacious in meeting these requirements as is *P. aeruginosa*. It is well-adapted for growth in an aquatic environment because it can fix nitrogen and metabolize dissolved carbon dioxide. *Pseudomonas* spp. can grow in distilled water and is an almost universal inhabitant of inanimate, moist environments such as sinks and bathtubs and is present in some tap and bottled water.[34] Cultures of swimming pools and whirlpools have shown that *P. aeruginosa* is frequently present in low numbers despite proper chlorination.[52,64] The success of *Pseudomonas* spp. in colonizing and proliferating in such diverse environments is a function not only of its minimal nutritional needs but, perhaps more importantly, of its ability to exist and grow as a mobile, swimming, planktonic cell and as a sessile member of an adherent microcolony encased within an anionic polysaccharide matrix. It is this secreted slime that initially facilitates nonspecific attachment and

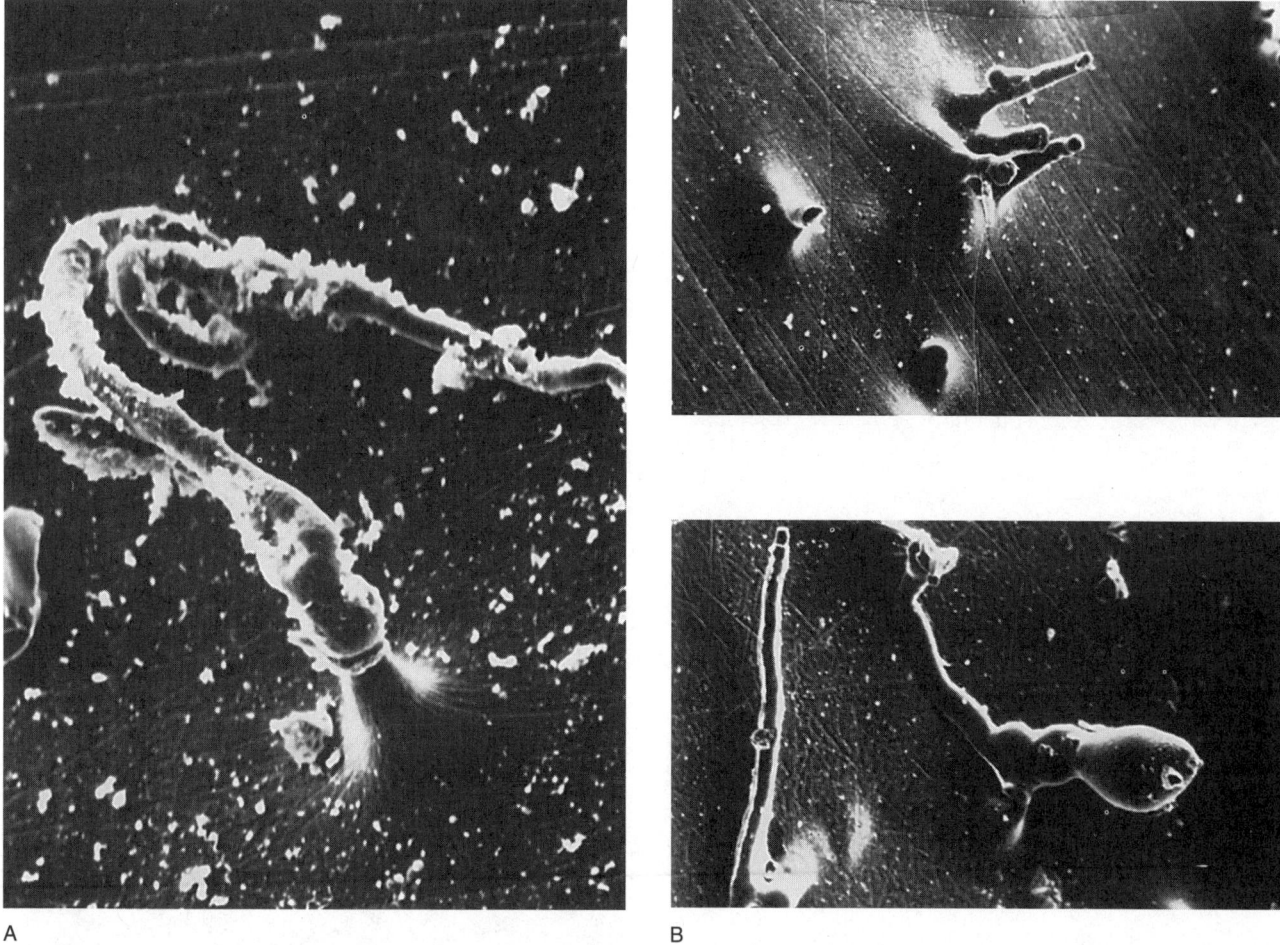

A   B

Fig. 16-4. **A,** Attached spore of *Curvularia lunata* germinating; hyphae penetrating surface of a 55% water hydrogel contact lens. **B,** Hyphae of *C. lunata* having penetrated the surface of a 55% water soft contact lens now emerged from the opposite surface.

then protects the sessile, adherent pseudomonads from potentially lethal chemicals such as chlorine (hypochlorous acid) in a swimming pool environment.

A contact lens case can be reasonably compared to a whirlpool or swimming pool environment. Most of the planktonic pseudomonal cells inoculated into a case with a contact lens disinfecting solution will die, but some may nonspecifically adhere to the plastic case wall and, within a biofilm, be protected from the disinfectant. As with a swimming pool, the addition of fresh disinfectant may clear the solution of planktonic bacterial cells but, with time, the biofilm gives release to additional planktonic cells that may survive and replicate in the presence of a weakened disinfectant (Figs. 16-5*A,* 16-5*B*).

Pseudomonas spp. can adhere to new and protein-coated soft contact lenses and, in greater numbers, to RGP contact lenses.[84-86] Thus a contact lens soaking in a contaminated environment may have bacteria attached to its surface and transfer bacterial cells to the corneal surface when the lens is placed on the eye (Fig.16-5*B*).

This sequence of events caused by *P. aeruginosa* as the prototype bacterial corneal infection in contact lens wear is strongly suggested by the following observations:

1. *P. aeruginosa* is a ubiquitous organism.
2. *P. aeruginosa* is the most common isolate in contact lens-associated microbial keratitis.[129]
3. *P. aeruginosa* is a frequent isolate from contaminated care systems.[30,74]
4. Isolates of *P. aeruginosa* from corneal ulcers and the contaminated saline solutions of a given patient are often identical.[75,135]
5. *P. aeruginosa* adheres to, and subsequently elaborates a biofilm glycocalyx on the surface of polyethylene and polyvinylchloride, both of which are plastics used in fabricating contact lens cases.[5,131]
6. *P. aeruginosa* adheres to new and used contact lens polymers, both soft and rigid[84-86] (Figs. 16-6*A,* 16-6*B*).
7. Within the biofilm glycocalyx, the sessile pseudo-

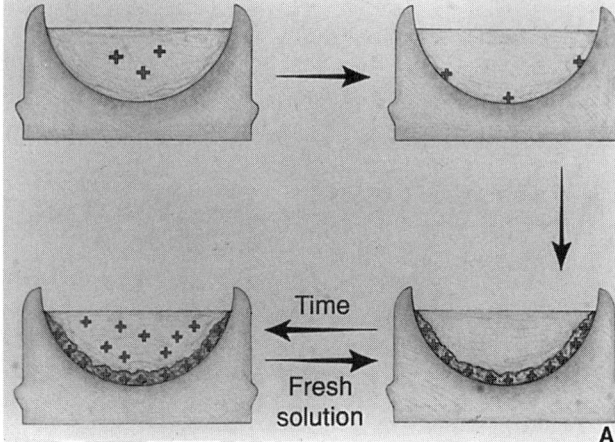

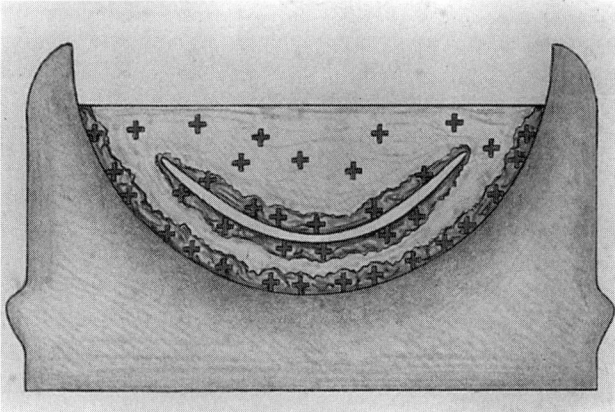

Fig. 16-5. **A,** A bacterial inoculum in a contact lens case survives to adhere to the contact lens case surface. A biofilm is produced, protecting the sessile cells from the disinfecting fluids. Over a period of time, planktonic cells emerge from the biofilm and survive in a weak disinfecting solution. **B,** A contact lens soaking in such a system may have adherent bacteria with biofilm formation on its surface.

monads are protected from the action of some disinfectants and surfactants.[5,54] Some contact lens disinfecting-soaking solutions, even when used in accordance with the manufacturer's recommendations, fail to eliminate *P. aeruginosa* cells within a biofilm adherent to the contact lens case surface.[131]

***Serratia* spp.** *Serratia marcescens* is a nonfastidious, enteric, aerobic, gram-negative rod with chromogenic and nonchromogenic features. It has been reported in 5% to 10% of gram-negative corneal ulcers and as a contaminant in the care systems of patients with contact lens-related *Serratia* keratitis.[74,100] *S. marcescens* is encountered as a contaminant in not only the contact lens case solution but also within the dispensing bottle of disinfectant-soaking solutions recommended for PMMA and RGP contact lenses.[1,39,99] The disin-

fectants are benzalkonium chloride and chlorhexidine gluconate—the former used frequently as a preservative in topical ophthalmic medications. Survival of *S. marcescens* in benzalkonium chloride contributes to epidemic septic arthritis, and prolonged survival in 2% chlorhexidine has been attributed to formation of a *Serratia* spp. biofilm on the internal surface of the plastic container.[71,94] Of nine patients with ulcerative keratitis (all wearing RGP contact lenses and all using a chlorhexidine-preserved soaking-conditioning solution[91]) eight had *Serratia* spp. isolated from their contact lens cases and seven had it isolated from their dispensing bottle. *S. marcescens* contamination was identified in the chlorhexidine-preserved bottle of the soaking-conditioning solution in 63% of patients, and 36% became contaminated within 7 days of being opened and used for lens care.[90]

Adaptation of *Serratia* spp. in the presence of chlorhexidine is attributed to alterations of the outer bacterial cell membrane and increased adherence to polyethylene.[39] Poly-

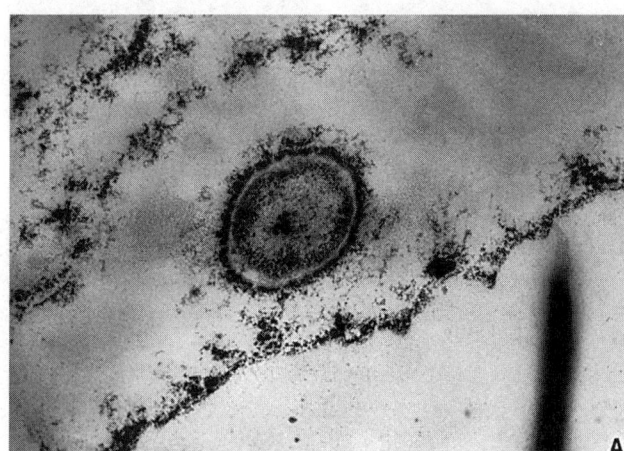

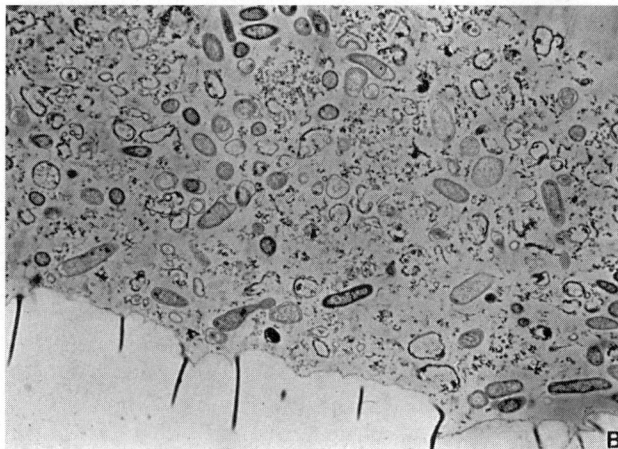

Fig. 16-6. **A,** Transmission electron photomicrograph of a single *P. aeruginosa* cell attaching to the surface of an unused soft contact lens via nonspecific adhesion (glycocalyx). **B,** Transmission electron photomicrograph of sessile *Pseudomonas* cells encased in a biofilm attached to the surface of a new soft contact lens.

ethylene is a polymer used in the manufacture of both plastic bottles and contact lens cases. Contamination in the dispensing bottle of a contact lens soaking-conditioning solution exposes contact case fluids and the contact lens to high densities of *S. marcescens,* which may in turn adhere to and form biofilms on their respective surfaces.

Staphylococcus spp. Both *S. aureus* and *S. epidermidis* have been isolated from contact lens cases, and both have been reported to cause contact lens-associated keratitis.[30,114,129] *S. epidermidis* is part of the resident, aerobic microbiota of the normal outer eye and is readily available to adhere to and colonize contact lens and lens case polymers.[67] Biofilm production by some strains constitutes a virulence factor in infections associated with nonophthalmic biomaterials.[17,31] Biofilm-producing strains of *S. epidermidis* and other microorganisms may adhere to polyethylene contact lens case surfaces and be resistant to disinfectant action in the same manner as *P. aeruginosa.*[131]

The nonspecific adherence of coagulase-positive *S. aureus* to contact lens or case plastic has not been directly investigated, but adherence to nonophthalmic plastics has been noted and is facilitated in the presence of fibronectin.[126]

Acanthamoeba. Given the prevalence of *Acanthamoeba* spp. in the human environment, it is not surprising that there are reported cases of acanthamoebic keratitis unrelated to contact lens wear.[115] Nonetheless, contact lens wear is the principal risk factor in its occurrence.[121] Initially, the disease was most common among DWSCL users who soaked their contact lenses in unpreserved, home-prepared saline solution without adequate heat disinfection.[88,121]

Acanthamoebic keratitis in lens wearers is frequently associated with the presence of this parasite as a contaminant of the lens care system, along with synchronous bacterial contamination, chiefly by gram-negative organisms.[29,65,88] A synergy exists between amoebae and bacterial contaminants in that the bacteria support amebic growth.[12]

While home-prepared saline for soaking and storing contact lenses is rarely suggested today, contact lens wear persists as a significant risk factor in the development of acanthamoebic keratitis. This causal relationship may be summarized by the following observations:

1. *Acanthamoeba* spp. are ubiquitous in the environment and may readily gain access to a contact lens care system, particularly with frequent use of nonsterile water as a rinsing solution.
2. Established bacterial biofilms in contact lens cases are generally resistant to the recommended 4 to 6 hours of soaking in most chemical and one hydrogen peroxide disinfection system available for use with hydrogel lenses.[131] Rigid gas-permeable contact lenses, soaking in conditioning solutions preserved with chlorhexidine, are frequently contaminated while "in use" with *S. marcescens* and/or other bacteria.[65,90,91,99] Once introduced into the contaminated case-care system, *Acanthamoeba* spp. uses these bacterial contaminants as a nutritional substrate for growth.
3. *Acanthamoeba* spp. cysts and trophozoites exhibit firm, nonspecific adherence to the surface of hydrogel contact lenses. Trophozoites also bind to the protein coating on used RGP lenses. When transferred onto the ocular surface, both amebic forms can give rise to experimental keratitis.[48,58,89]
4. *Acanthamoeba* organisms exhibit specific adhesion to corneal epithelium and may gain access to the corneal stroma by penetrating the epithelial layer.[89,92,95]

Fungi. While the indigenous aerobic bacterial flora of the outer eye is composed mainly of staphylococci and diphtheroids, a normal fungal flora is probably nonexistent. Most likely, fungi isolated from the healthy outer eye are caused by random seeding from the environment.[133] These transient fungal propagules may alight on the surface of a hydrogel lens while it is being worn. Normally, they would be removed by surface cleaning of the contact lens on removal from the eye, prior to the soaking-disinfecting process. Noncompliance with lens hygiene or wearing the lens for a prolonged period of time, however, may permit adherence and subsequent penetration of the lens matrix (Figs. 16-4*A*, 16-4*B*). Continued wear of a hydrogel lens supporting fungal growth may lead to ocular irritation or, more seriously, a fungal corneal ulcer[120,128,134] (Fig. 16-7).

Although filamentous fungi are occasionally isolated from the lens care system, there are no data available that show nonspecific adherence to contact lens case plastic via biofilm formation or a synergistic relationship to *Acantha-*

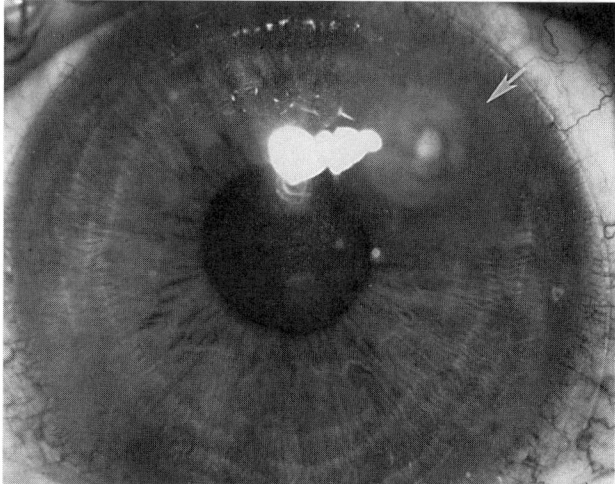

Fig. 16-7. Fungal thallus (*Fusarium* spp.) growing within the matrix of a 71% water extended wear soft contact lens on the patient's eye. Ocular irritation but no corneal ulcer was present.

moeba spp. in contact lens care fluids. *Candida albicans* (a dimorphic yeast fungus) adheres, within a biofilm, to polyethylene contact lens case plastic and is more resistant to the action of contact lens disinfectants than bacteria.[131]

Opportunities for Prevention. Not all instances of contact lens-associated microbial keratitis can be attributed to contaminated care systems. There are sufficient data linking the two events, however, as to make it imperative that the person fitting and dispensing these devices understand fully the mechanics of contamination and the relative merits of various contact lens cleaning and disinfecting regimens.

Cleaning the contact lens on removal from the eye — prior to placement in a soaking-disinfecting solution — is necessary, not only for the removal of tear protein deposits, but to debulk the lens of any attached microorganisms. A contact lens cleaner containing isopropyl alcohol in combination with surfactants may kill adherent microbial cells including those of *Acanthamoeba* spp.[104]

Sterile, commercial, preserved, or preservative-free saline solutions should not be used as soaking solutions without thermal disinfection. Thermal disinfection is efficacious in killing microorganisms including *Acanthamoeba* spp. within the case, but in today's convenience-oriented climate it is not considered user friendly and is recommended infrequently in lens care.

Home-prepared saline is prone to bacterial and protozoal contamination and should not be used in contact lens care.[106,121,135] Chemical-disinfecting solutions vary considerably in their microbicidal efficacy. Thimerosal-chlorhexidine and thimerosal-alkyl triethanol ammonium chloride are effective biocides within the recommended storage times against both bacteria and some fungi.[103,105] Thimerosal hypersensitivity among contact lens wearers has restricted their use in the United States, however. Chlorhexidine-based solutions for soft contact lens disinfection appear effective against microbial films and lens cases — especially when combined with air-drying the lens case when not in use.[131] When used as a preservative for RGP contact lens soaking and conditioning solutions, however, chlorhexidine appears less than effective — allowing dangerous levels of bacterial cells (especially *S. marcescens*) to populate, not only the fluid within the lens case, but also the fluid within the plastic dispensing bottle.[39,90,99] Chemical disinfectants for soft lenses such as polyquaternium-1 and polyaminopropyl biguanide are less effective against established biofilms within contact lens cases and their use should be in combination with hand washing, adequate lens cleaning, daily replacement of lens case solutions, and air drying of the plastic lens case when not in use. Because planktonic bacterial cells are generally susceptible to these later biocides, the attention to hand washing, lens cleaning, and air drying the case when not in use should result in diminished microbial inocula, microbial attachment, and subsequent biofilm formation.

Hydrogen peroxide (H_2O_2) soft lens disinfecting solutions are microbicidal when used in excess of 10 minutes for most bacteria and at least 60 minutes for some filamentous fungi.[102,103,131] Systems wherein the H_2O_2 is neutralized almost instantaneously by platinum catalytic discs are considerably less effective and may permit microbial contamination about the catalytic discs with subsequent microbial colonization (Figs. 16-8*A, B, C, D*). Dichloroisocyanurate dihydrate-effervescent base tablets are available for soft lens disinfection in Europe. Added to saline, approximately 3 to 5 ppm of available chlorine equivalent is released. In laboratory studies, these tablets were not effective against *S. marcescens* or *Candida parapsilosis*.[105]

Because of its role in therapeutically recalcitrant keratitis, *Acanthamoeba* spp. susceptibility to various contact lens disinfectants has been extensively investigated. These studies, however, do not address the "real-life" situation of synchronous bacterial contamination that most likely precedes *Acanthamoeba* spp. contamination in the contact lens case.[29] Nonetheless, some lens care guidelines are inferred. In one study, chlorhexidine and nondisc neutralized 3% H_2O_2 were quite effective in eliminating both trophozoite and cyst stages of two species of *Acanthamoeba,* but polyquaternium-1 and polyaminopropyl biguanide were not amebicidal within 8 hours.[117] Another study confirmed these results, but 4 hours of 3% H_2O_2 exposure was required to eliminate the cysts of the same two species of *Acanthamoeba.*[25]

On the basis of published studies and aside from thermal disinfection, overnight soaking of soft lenses in 3% H_2O_2 (longer than 4 hours) with morning neutralization using thiosulfate solution, catalase solution, or catalase tablets is perhaps the safest way to ensure killing of bacteria, *Acanthamoeba* spp., and fungi. In the United States, however, polyquaternium-1 and polyaminopropyl biguanide are en-

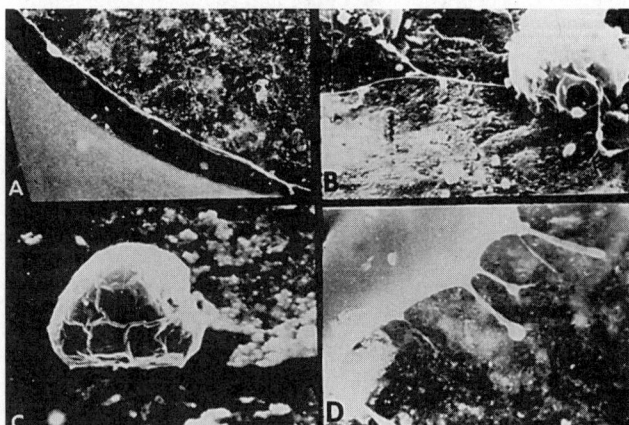

Fig. 16-8. **A,** Platinum-coated neutralizing disc in one-step H_2O_2 soft contact lens disinfecting system with an observed surface biofilm on transmission electron microscopy ($\times$ 4000). **B,** Enlargement illustrating *Acanthamoeba* spp. cyst on the disc surface covered with *P. aeruginosa* cells. **C,** *Acanthamoeba* cyst on the surface of the platinum neutralizing disc. **D,** Trophozoite stage of *Acanthamoeba* on the neutralizing disc surface after the addition of saline.

dorsed by more contact lens fitters—presumably because of perceived simplicity in use and greater wearer compliance. If these disinfectants are recommended, it is essential that good lens care instruction with regard to hand washing, lens cleaning, and following the manufacturer's guidelines for disinfection time be given the wearer. Simple reinforcement of lens care instructions can significantly reduce, but not eliminate, in-use care system microbial contamination.[132] Since microbial contamination and biofilm formation within the contact lens case environment are not entirely preventable with many of today's care systems, the case itself should be periodically cleaned, thermally disinfected, or replaced.

Ophthalmic Sutures

Previous studies have shown that synthetic materials such as polyester (Dacron) and Teflon, when used as suture materials or as vascular grafts, may be variably colonized by adherent bacteria and may give rise to infection.[18,47] Many of these materials are multifilament, considerably larger in diameter than ophthalmic sutures, and have a porosity that facilitates bacterial adherence. Polyamide monofilament (Ethilon), polypropylene monofilament (Prolene), and polyester fiber monofilament (Mersilene) are biopolymers used extensively in ophthalmic surgery as suture materials. Postoperative wound infections are not infrequently initiated in the vicinity of such suture lines, particularly when the sutures remain exposed.

Microbial Adhesion. Nonspecific microbial attachment by electrostatic forces and polymer hydrophobicity probably influences bacterial adherence to monofilament suture materials. Colonization of the exposed suture via adhesive biofilm formation can result in a microbial reservoir and a pathway for extension into the depth of the wound[21] (Fig. 16-9). This sequence is the likely series of events that leads to infectious crystalline keratopathy following penetrating keratoplasty (Figs. 16-10, 16-11).

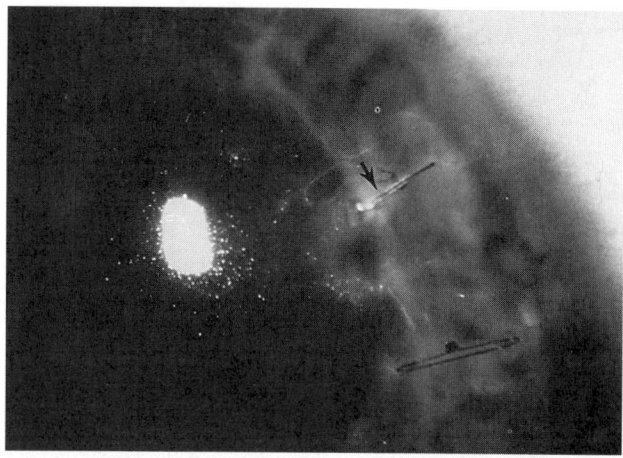

Fig. 16-10.   Exposed strand of 10-0 nylon following keratoplasty. Note the biofilm forming along the length of exposed suture.

The relative adherence of some bacterial strains to Ethilon and Prolene suture materials was evaluated quantitatively by measuring the attachment of radiolabeled cells to a given surface area of the two suture polymers.[2] All test organisms adhered to both Prolene and Ethilon in significant density, but enterococci and *S. aureus* attached in greater numbers than *S. marcescens* and *P. aeruginosa* (Figs. 16-12, 16-13*A, B*). The greater attachment of gram-positive bacteria to these polymers may result from facilitation of adherence by cell-wall adhesins that normally mediate adherence to host-cell receptors. This is consistent with the frequency of gram-positive isolates in cases of infectious crystalline keratopathy.[76,97] These organisms can secrete an intrastromal glycocalyx, an attribute which renders them relatively impervious to standard antimicrobial concentrations.[97]

Opportunities for Prevention.   An excellent motive for burying monofilament sutures and knots is to avoid microbial colonization of the suture with the potential risk of infection adjacent to or within the suture track. Cases

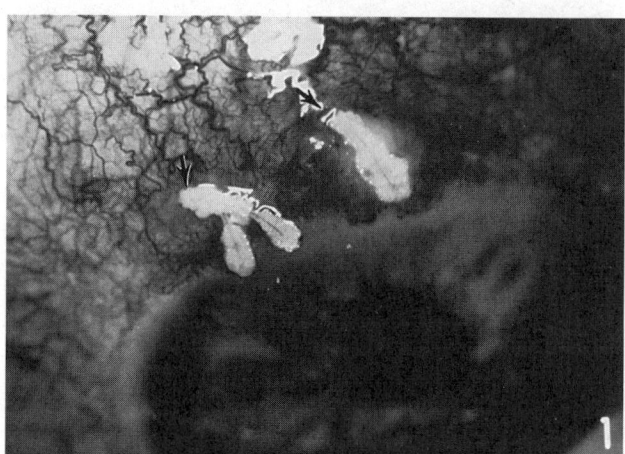

Fig. 16-9.   Colonization of exposed 10-0 nylon sutures by biofilm-colony of *Moraxella catarrhalis*. (Courtesy Dr. D. Harris.)

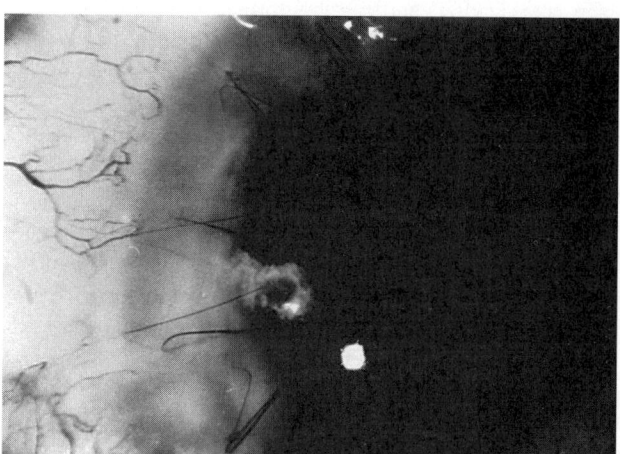

Fig. 16-11.   Infectious crystalline keratopathy within the stroma of a corneal graft and along the exposed loop of a running 10-0 nylon suture. (Courtesy Dr. G. O. Waring III.)

Adherence of Bacteria to Sutures

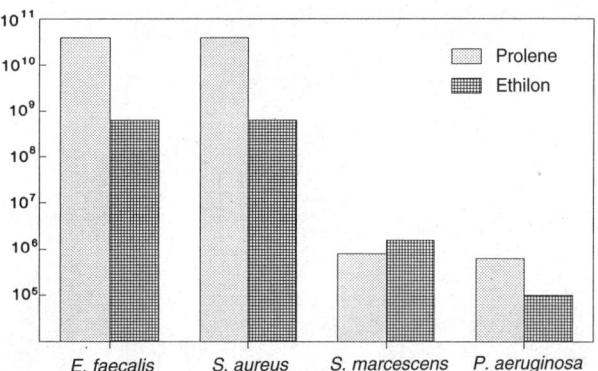

Fig. 16-12. Quantitative attachment of two gram-positive and two gram-negative bacterial species to monofilament Ethilon and Prolene sutures after 12 hours exposure to washed and labeled cells in sterile buffered saline. The number of tests per bacterium and suture were five; the standard deviation was not statistically significant.

of delayed-onset endophthalmitis following penetrating keratoplasty have been reported in association with exposed monofilament sutures.[21]

Punctal Occluders

Punctal plugs are marketed for the management of dry eye syndromes. The silicone rubber plug is fabricated in variable lengths and diameters and requires insertion with a rod developed for that purpose. Previous models were 1.6 to 2.8 mm in length, difficult to insert and remove, and designed with a dome that protruded above the punctal orifice. A central core extends within the plug and facilitates placement with the insertion rod. The dome and central core are exposed to the periocular environment and to resident and transient microbiota. These devices are left in situ for considerable periods of time and, as with other biopolymer materials, are subject to nonspecific microbial attachment, surface colonization, and biofilm formation. Whereas newer designs have a flatter dome, the older models had an exposed dome that caused corneal abrasion on adduction and depression of the globe.

Microbial Adhesion. After a variable period of time, a bacterial biofilm may be observed adherent to the exposed dome and within the core of the plug (Figs. 16-14*A, B*). A host-protein coating on the surface of a silicone elastomer polymer is not necessary for slime-producing strains of coagulase-negative staphylococci to nonspecifically adhere to its surface.[93] Following removal of silicone plugs with observed surface slime, cultures have yielded exuberant growth of staphylococci (Fig. 16-14*B*). In one instance, a patient with mycotic keratitis caused by *Curvularia lunata* was observed to have a dematiaceous fungus colonizing the core of the silicone plug; on removal, *C. lunata* was isolated from the plug (Fig. 16-15).

Qualitatively, the adherence of a biofilm-producing strain of *P. aeruginosa* to silicone plugs was evaluated.[2] The plugs were exposed for 45 minutes to an 18-hour culture of *P. aeruginosa* in tryptic soy broth, followed by fixation. Bacteria readily adhered to the silicone rubber plug with apparent elaboration of a protective glycocalyx (Figs. 16-16*A, B, C*). **Opportunities for Prevention.** Once colonized, silicone rubber plugs can act as a reservoir of opportunistic pathogens encased in a biofilm, thus representing a threat of ocular infection. In managing patients with a dry eye, the safest route is to effect temporary canalicular occlusion with collagen or gelatin rods—followed, if successful, by a electrothermal closure of the punctal opening and/or canaliculi.

Biopolymers in Vitreoretinal Surgery

Bacterial infection of the episclera and sclera following retinal buckling procedures with either solid or sponge silicone polymer explants has been reported over the past several decades.[83,130] In one large series, the incidence was 0.6%

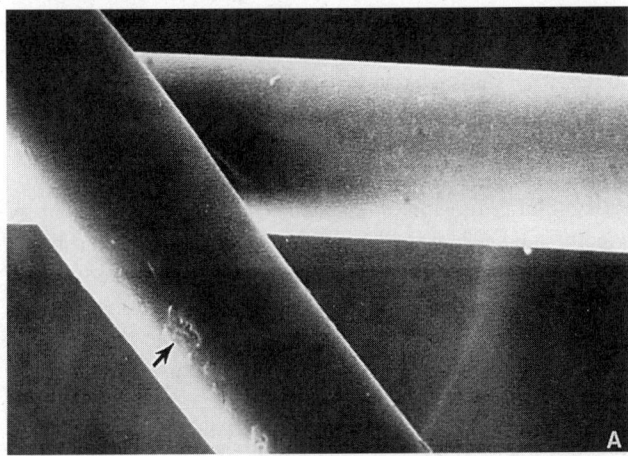

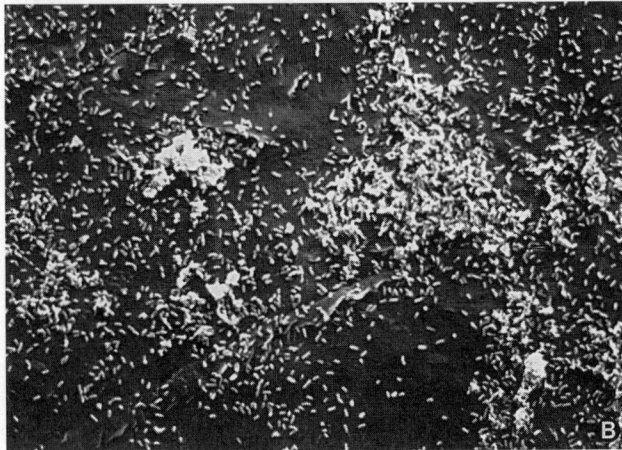

Fig. 16-13. **A,** Transmission electron photomicrograph of a monofilament Ethilon suture with foci of adherent *S. marcescens* cells. **B,** Enlargement of the area of attached bacterial cells showing biofilm formation.

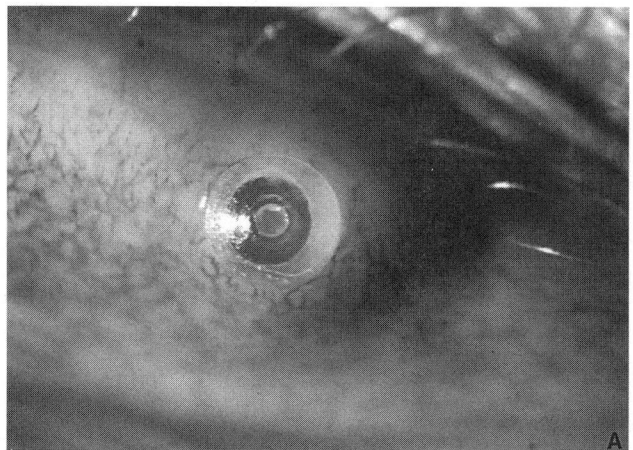

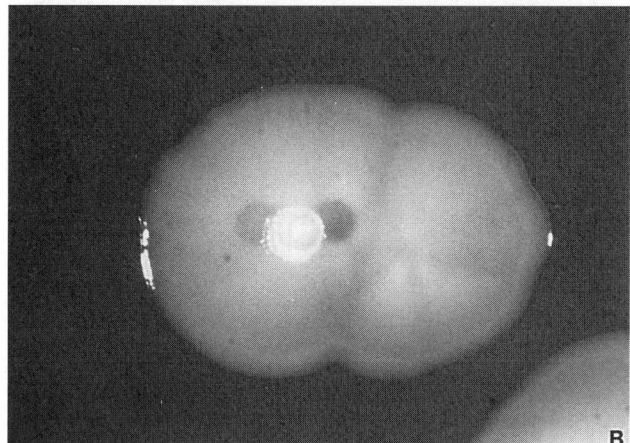

Fig. 16-14.   A, Silicone punctal plug with biofilm-matrix within the central core. **B,** Growth of *S. epidermidis* from punctal plug on chocolate agar at 37°C, 5% CO_2 for 24 hours.

over a 14-year period,[35] and in others the rate was between 3% and 5%.[45,46] The time from surgery to the onset of clinical symptoms depends on the virulence of the infecting agent and has ranged from 2 days to 13 years.[35] Removal of the explant and encircling band, if present, may be necessary because of severe pain, recalcitrance to antibiotic therapy, and scleral necrosis with impending perforation (Fig. 16-17).

S. aureus and *S. epidermidis* are the most frequent isolates from cultures of removed buckles and explants.[35] Gram-negative bacteria including *P. aeruginosa, Proteus* spp. and *Moraxella catarrhalis* have also been reported as etiopathic agents associated with infected buckles and explants.[15,46] Bacteria contaminate the operative field at the time of surgery.[77,78] *S. epidermidis* is the aerobic organism most frequently cultured from the operative field and from removed silicone explants.[46]

Microbial Adhesion. As with implantable biomaterials elsewhere in the body, microorganisms can attach to the inanimate surface of a silicone, rubber, or sponge explant or

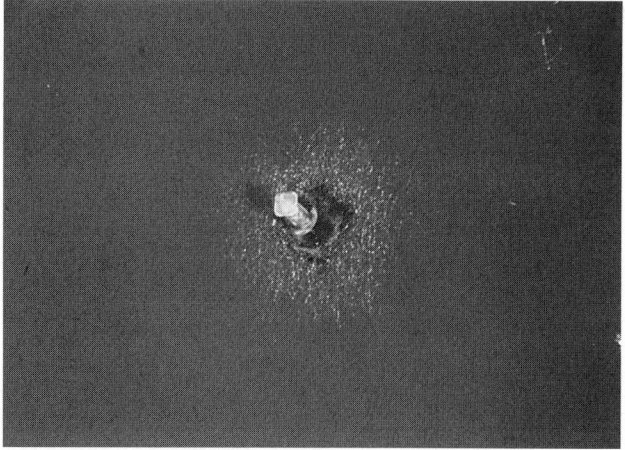

Fig. 16-15.   *Curvularia lunata* mycelium growing from a removed punctal plug on chocolate agar, 25°C at 24 hours.

encircling band and elaborate a protective carbohydrate or polypeptide matrix. Depending on the organism, adherent microbes give rise to early postoperative signs of infection or remain silent for weeks to months before eliciting signs of inflammation. If the operative field is not free of resident or transient bacteria at the time of surgery, then microbial cell attachment to the silicone elements can occur.

The operative field is not necessarily sterile. Because resident microflora are chiefly coagulase-negative staphylococci, many explanted elements yield *S. epidermidis* on culture. Overlying conjunctival dehiscence may expose an explant or encircling band to microbial colonization with resident or transient microorganisms (Fig. 16-18). Standard antimicrobial therapy may be somewhat less than effective because the dosages of the antimicrobial drug used may be below the concentration required for the elimination of bacteria growing in a glycocalyx-protected biofilm.[6] Addition-

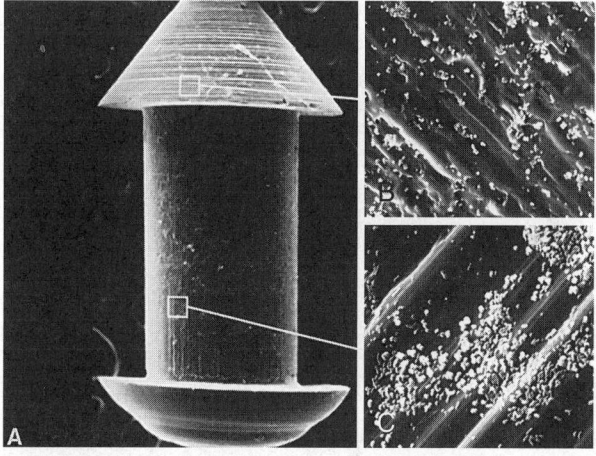

Fig. 16-16.   A, Foci of *P. aeruginosa* cells adhering to silicone punctal plug. **B,** Adherent *P. aeruginosa* cells on the stem of the punctal plug. **C,** *Pseudomonas aeruginosa* adherent to the inserted end of the punctal plug with biofilm formation.

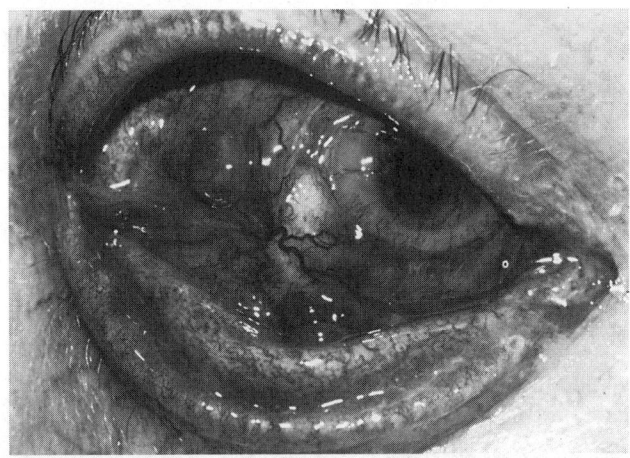

Fig. 16-17. Infected encircling silicone buckle following retinal detachment surgery: nontuberculous mycobacteria were isolated on culture. (Courtesy Dr. P. Sternberg.)

ally, the extracellular slime substance is inhibitory to human neutrophil bactericidal activity.[96]

The occurrence of biofilm formation on silicone explants used during retinal detachment surgery is probably dependent on the ability of staphylococci (as *Pseudomonas* spp., *Moraxella* spp., or other bacteria) to elaborate a protective slime layer.[17,31] Microbial attachment and subsequent biofilm formation to both silicone rubber and sponge explant polymer has been evaluated qualitatively by exposing the polymer to bacteria for several hours.[2] Representative pieces of each polymer show bacterial adherence and biofilm formation. Bacteria adhere in greater numbers to the sponge polymer when compared to the silicone rubber (Figs. 16-19*A, B*).

Opportunities for Prevention. Improved surgical techniques and avoidance of scleral dissection and/or diathermy shorten the time required for retinal detachment surgery and

lessen the chance for postoperative infection. The problem has not been eliminated, however. The retinal surgeon should have an understanding of the periocular microbiota, microbial attachment, and biofilm formation on explant or encircling band polymers. The surgeon must also be aware of the possible need for biomaterial removal if a resultant infection cannot be eliminated medically. Strategies for prevention include meticulous attention to preoperative prepping to diminish intraoperative contamination of the operative field. Preoperative soaking of the silicone sponge polymer in an antibiotic solution has been suggested as useful in minimizing the risk of postoperative infection associated with microbial colonization of the explant.[7]

Intraocular Lenses

Many of the polymers used in manufacturing intraocular lenses (IOLs) are essentially the same as those previously mentioned, that is, hydrogel polymers, polypropylene monofilament, and silicone elastomers. Bacteria can adhere to the PMMA optical zone of the IOL, but greater adherence

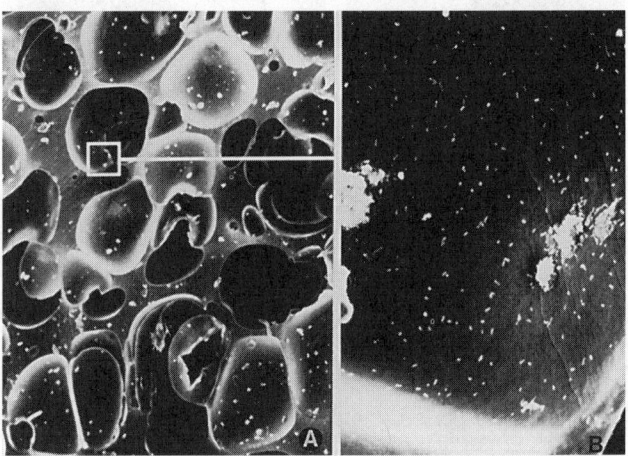

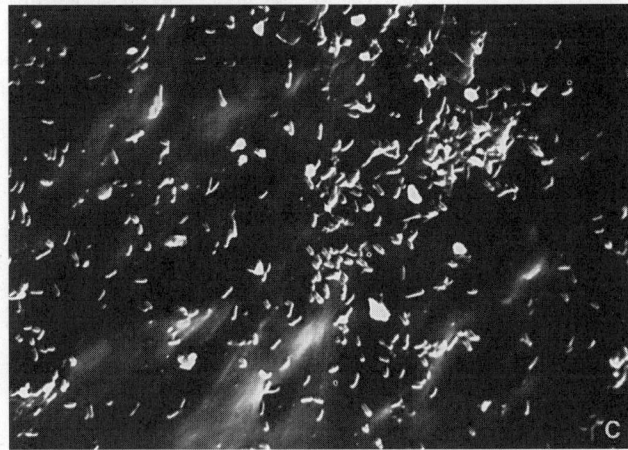

Fig. 16-19. **A,** Adherence of *Pseudomonas* bacteria to silicone sponge explant polymer. **B,** With enlargement. **C,** Adherence of *P. aeruginosa* cells to silicone explant rubber polymer.

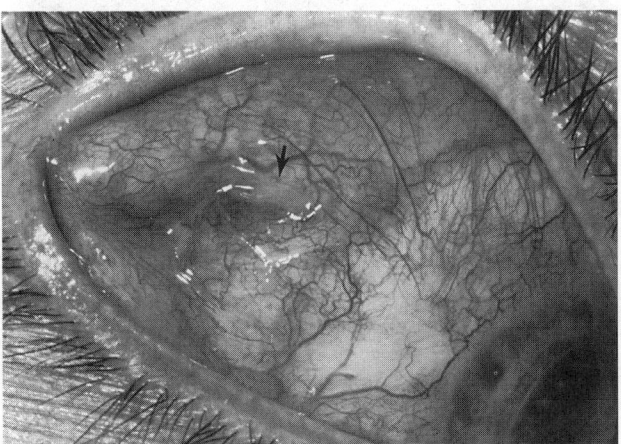

Fig. 16-18. Dehiscence of the conjunctiva overlying a silicone plate after retinal detachment surgery. Cultures of the creamy biofilm yielded *S. epidermidis*.

appears to be to polypropylene haptics when they are present.[27,42,109,124] At least one study suggests a greater risk of postoperative endophthalmitis when an IOL with polypropylene haptics is implanted when compared with an all-PMMA IOL.[81]

Whereas streptococci, gram-negative rods, and fungi occasionally cause postoperative endophthalmitis, the predominant pathogens are staphylococci, especially *S. epidermidis*.[119] Because staphylococci constitute the main aerobic periocular microflora, they can be compared to infection related to colonization of polymers used in percutaneous sutures or vascular catheters. As previously described, there is nonspecific adhesion to the smooth polymer surface, followed by glycocalyx formation and sustained growth in a protective biofilm. Following wound closure during cataract surgery, conjunctival and aqueous humor cultures often yield microbial growth, mostly *S. epidermidis*.[26,116] *S. epidermidis* can then be postulated to adhere to the IOL either on insertion or as a contaminant of anterior chamber fluid following IOL implantation. Subsequent development of intraocular infection depends on irreversible attachment to the IOL optical zone, haptic, or both, with subsequent biofilm formation and later release of infecting bacterial cells into the aqueous or vitreous.

Bacterial attachment to the implanted IOL results in chronic intraocular inflammation. In one report, bacteria were present on IOLs that were removed because of chronic inflammation.[24] Whereas the authors of that report observed at least one explanted IOL with adherent bacteria and an extracellular matrix suggestive of biofilm, other explanted IOLs were observed to have adherent bacterial cells without biofilm formation. In another case of delayed-onset endophthalmitis, the explanted IOL revealed heavy *S. epidermidis* colonization of the IOL haptic.[57]

Propionibacterium acnes is a gram-positive, anaerobe that constitutes the majority of anaerobic microflora of the healthy human eye.[79] It has been described as a cause of delayed-onset, chronic postoperative endophthalmitis.[80] Although it is likely that *P. acnes* gains access to the posterior chamber, capsular bag, or vitreous humor during surgery, the role of the IOL polymer(s) as a mechanical vector is less than clear, and no attachment phenomena or biofilm formation for this bacterium has been reported. In such situations, *P. acnes* endophthalmitis that is chronic and recurs after antimicrobial therapy may require IOL removal.[122]

Having presented microbial attachment and biofilm formation as potential mechanisms for endophthalmitis caused by *S. epidermidis,* and possibly other bacteria, it is necessary to consider some contradictions. *S. epidermidis* is normal periocular microbiota and apparently gains access to anterior chamber fluids in a large percentage of patients during cataract removal.[24,26] Endophthalmitis is uncommon, however. Whereas slime production by attached *S. epidermidis* cells constitutes a virulence factor, nonslime-producing strains

also adhere firmly to the surface of PMMA and polypropylene IOL polymers.[42] In addition, some cases of postoperative endophthalmitis caused by *S. epidermidis* can be managed without removal of the IOL.[101] Furthermore, *S. epidermidis* has been cultured from the aqueous and vitreous of patients with endophthalmitis following cataract extraction without IOL implantation.[36,125]

It thus appears that the bacteria can gain entry to aqueous and/or vitreous humors at surgery, independent of IOL implantation. If an IOL is implanted, resident bacteria like *S. epidermidis* may adhere to the IOL, particularly if it is not rinsed (electrostatic attraction) or if it touches the conjunctiva (especially if coated with adhesive viscoelastic substances). It is also possible that bacteria contaminating the anterior chamber fluid may adhere to the IOL. In either case, subsequent release of planktonic bacteria may access the aqueous and/or vitreous compartment. If a biofilm matrix is secreted onto the surface of the IOL, haptic, or optical zone, microorganisms are protected from host phagocytic cells and antibiotics (Fig. 16-20*A, B*). Single-dose, intravitreal

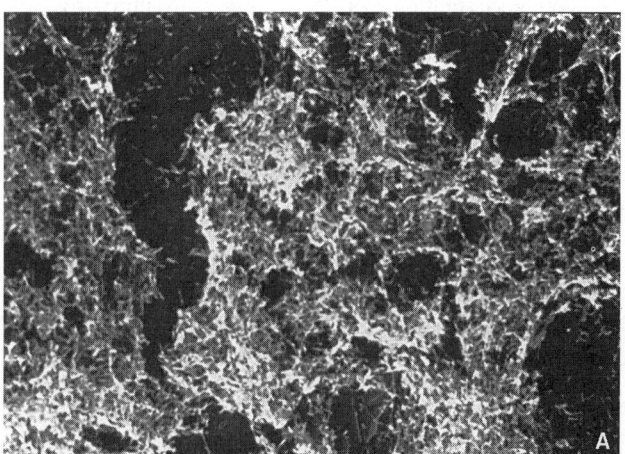

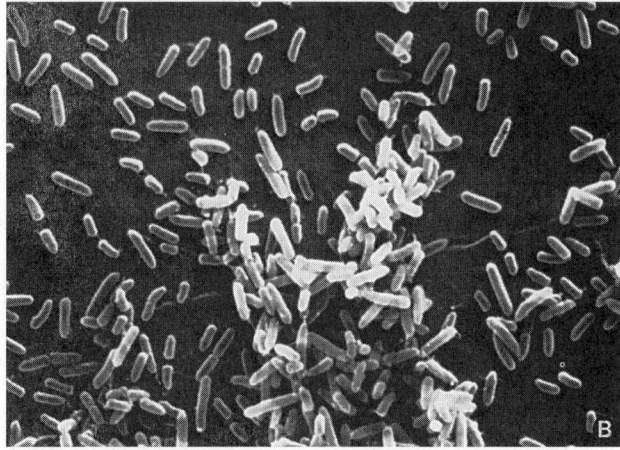

Fig. 16-20.   A, *Pseudomonas aeruginosa* biofilm is adherent to the Prolene haptic of a new, unused IOL. **B,** *Pseudomonas* cells attach to the PMMA optic of the same IOL.

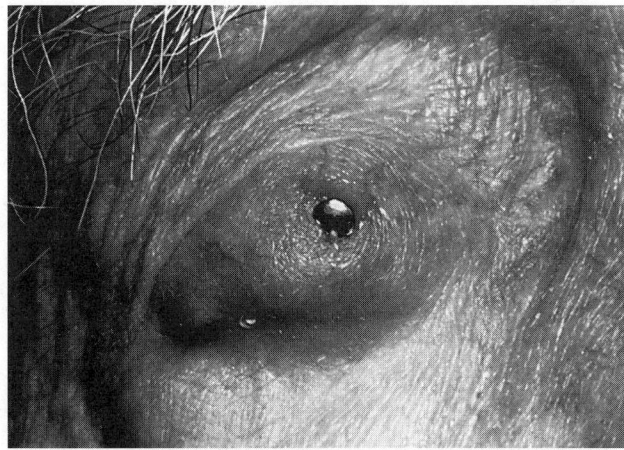

Fig. 16-21. Protruding PMMA cylinder of a keratoprosthesis with creamy biofilm at its edges. There is surrounding edema and hyperemia of the cutaneous and subcutaneous tissues. Cultures yielded *Candida albicans*.

antibiotics may or may not penetrate the biofilm to eliminate the infecting agent. If not, recurrent infection is likely to develop, necessitating repeated injections of intravitreal antimicrobics and/or explantation of the IOL.

Keratoprostheses

Although infection can occur with its use, there are no data on microbial adherence to the component parts of a keratoprosthesis. As staphylococci can attach to PMMA, there is no reason to suspect that *S. epidermidis* or *S. aureus* would not adhere to other keratoprosthesis materials such as ceramic or fluoroethylene polymers.[66,108] Once attached, any biofilm produced would make it difficult to eradicate colonizing organisms (Fig. 16-21). Compounding the potential for infection is the exterior or interior nature of the device. No matter how well-protected by cuffs of host or donor-derived tissues, the exteriorized optical column is exposed constantly to resident and transient microflora—any or all of which represent opportunistic pathogens.

Orbital Implants

Infection has been reported in association with silicone, supramid, and teflon alloplastic biomaterials used in the treatment of orbital wall and floor fractures.[59] Employed to prevent herniation of orbital tissue and possible enophthalmos, they frequently are exposed to the paranasal sinuses and to colonization by nasal pharyngeal microflora. Orbital infection, however, is an infrequent complication.

PREVENTION OF MICROBIAL ADHESION TO OPHTHALMIC BIOMATERIALS

As with biomaterials used elsewhere in the body, microorganisms can nonspecifically adhere to ophthalmic biopolymers and are often embedded in a thick extracellular matrix of polysaccharides or glycoproteins called slime, glycocalyx, or biofilm. Prevention of ophthalmic biopolymer-related infections is much preferred over treatment. This requires an awareness of the common etiopathogens as well as their sources and the mechanism-colonizing polymer surfaces. With this information, strategies for prevention can be developed.

Careful instruction in contact lens cleaning, selection of effective disinfectant solutions, and air drying the contact lens case are useful strategies, as is periodic thermal disinfection or replacement of the lens case itself. Certainly inexpensive, disposable contact lens cases should be as available as disposable soft contact lenses.

Monofilament sutures should be buried to avoid microbial colonization, and if silicone punctal plugs are inserted, they should be observed frequently for biofilm formation. Meticulous preoperative prepping with occlusive draping minimizes microbial contamination of the operative field with periocular microbial flora. This might lessen the chance for (1) bacterial attachment to silicone polymer materials in retinal detachment surgery or (2) anterior chamber fluid contamination during cataract surgery.

Finally, it would be very useful, in a prophylactic sense, if industry could provide a nontoxic coating or additive to ophthalmic biomaterials that would decrease or inhibit microbial attachment to the polymer surface. This appears to have been partly achieved, via coating silicone or polyurethane catheters with salicylic acid.[33] This technology needs to be explored for possible ophthalmic use.

REFERENCES

1. Ahearn DG, Penley CA, Wilson LA: Growth and survival of *Serratia marcescens* in hard contact lens wetting solutions, *CLAO J* 10:172-174, 1984.
2. Ahearn DG, Wilson LA: Unpublished data.
3. Alfonso E, Mandelbaum S, Fox MJ et al.: Ulcerative keratitis associated with contact lens wear, *Am J Ophthalmol* 101:429-433, 1986.
4. Aly R, Levit S: Adherence of *Staphylococcus aureus* to squamous epithelium: role of fibronectin and teichoic acid, *Rev Infect Dis* 9(suppl 4):S341-S350, 1987.
5. Anderson RL, Holland BW, Carr JK et al.: Effect of disinfectants on pseudomonads colonized on the interior surface of PVC pipes, *Am J Public Health* 80:17-21, 1990.
6. Anwar H, Dasgupta MK, Costerton JW: Testing the susceptibility of bacteria in biofilms to antibacterial agents, *Antimicrob Agents Chemother* 34:2043-2046, 1990.
7. Arribas NP, Olk RJ, Schertzer M: Preoperative antibiotic soaking of silicone sponges: does it make a difference? *Ophthalmology* 91:1684-1689, 1984.
8. Baddour LM, Christensen GD, Simpson WA: Microbial adherence. In Mandell GL, Douglas RG, Bennett JE, editors: *Principles and practice of infectious disease,* ed 3, 9-25, New York, 1990, John Wiley and Sons.
9. Bandyk DF: Diagnosis and treatment of biomaterial-associated vascular infections, *Infect Dis Clin N Am* 6:719-729, 1992.
10. Baum J, Barza M: *Pseudomonas* keratitis and extended-wear soft contact lenses, *Arch Ophthalmol* 108:663-664, 1990 (editorial).
11. Bisno AL, Waldvogel F, editors: *Infections associated with indwelling medical devices,* Washington DC, 1989, American Society for Microbiology.
12. Bottone EJ, Madayag RM, Qureshi MN: *Acanthamoeba* keratitis: synergy between amebic and bacterial co-contaminants in contact lens care systems as a prelude to infection, *J Clin Microbiol* 30:2447-2450, 1992.

13. Buehler PO, Schein OD, Stamler JF et al.: The increased risk of ulcerative keratitis among disposable soft contact lens users, *Arch Ophthalmol* 110:1555-1558, 1992.

14. Calderone RA, Scheld WM: Role of fibronectin in the pathogenesis of candidal infections, *Rev Infect Dis* 9(suppl 4):S400-S403, 1987.

15. Callanan D, Rubsamen PE: Moraxella infection of a scleral buckle, *Am J Ophthalmol* 114:637-638, 1992 (letter).

16. Chalupa E, Swarbrick HA, Holden BA et al.: Severe corneal infections associated with contact lens wear, *Ophthalmology* 94:17-22, 1987.

17. Christensen GD, Simpson WA, Bisno AL: Adherence of slime-producing strains of *Staphylococcus epidermidis* to smooth surfaces, *Infect Immun* 37:318-326, 1982.

18. Chu CC, Williams DF: Effects of physical configuration and chemical structure of suture materials on bacterial adhesion: a possible link to wound infection, *Am J Surg* 147:197-204, 1984.

19. Cohen EJ, Laibson PR, Arentsen JJ: Corneal ulcers associated with cosmetic extended-wear soft contact lenses, *Ophthalmology* 94:109-114, 1987.

20. Colin J, Malet F, Robinet A et al.: The epidemiology of *Acanthamoeba* keratitis in Europe, *Contactologia* 12E:54-56, 1990.

21. Confino J, Brown SI: Bacterial endophthalmitis associated with exposed monofilament sutures following corneal transplantation, *Am J Ophthalmol* 99:111-113, 1985.

22. Cooper RL, Constable IJ: Infective keratitis in soft contact lens wearers, *Br J Ophthalmol* 61:250-254, 1977.

23. Costerton JW, Marrie TJ, Cheng KJ: Phenomena of bacterial adhesion. In Savage DC, Fletcher M, editors: *Bacterial adhesion, mechanisms and physiological significance,* New York, 1985, Plenum Publishing.

24. Cusumano A, Busin M, Spitznas M: Is chronic intraocular inflammation after lens implantation of bacterial origin? *Ophthalmology* 98:1703-1710, 1991.

25. Davies DJG, Anthony Y, Meakin BJ et al.: Evaluation of the antiacanthamoebal activity of five contact lens disinfectants, *Int Contact Lens Clin* 17:14-20, 1990.

26. Dickey JB, Thompson KD, Jay WM: Anterior chamber aspirate cultures after uncomplicated cataract surgery, *Am J Ophthalmol* 112:278-282, 1991.

27. Dilly PN, Sellors PJ: Bacterial adhesion to intraocular lenses, *J Cataract Refract Surg* 15:317-320, 1989.

28. Dixon JM, Young CA Jr, Baldone JA et al.: Complications associated with the wearing of contact lenses, *JAMA* 195:901-903, 1966.

29. Donzis PB, Mondino BJ, Weissman BA et al.: Microbial analysis of contact lens care systems contaminated with *Acanthamoeba, Am J Ophthalmol* 108:53-56, 1989.

30. Donzis PB, Mondino BJ, Weissman BA et al.: Microbial contamination of contact lens care systems, *Am J Ophthalmol* 104:325-333, 1987.

31. Drewry DT, Galbraith L, Wilkinson BJ et al.: Staphylococcal slime: a cautionary tale, *J Clin Microbiol* 28:1292-1296, 1990.

32. Ehrlich M, Weissman BA, Mondino BJ: *Pseudomonas* corneal ulcer after use of extended-wear rigid gas-permeable contact lens, *Cornea* 8:225-226, 1989.

33. Farber BF, Wolff AG: The use of nonsteroidal anti-inflammatory drugs to prevent adherence of *Staphylococcus epidermidis* to medical polymers, *J Infect Dis* 166:861-865, 1992.

34. Favero MS, Carson LA, Bond WW et al.: *Pseudomonas aeruginosa:* growth in distilled water from hospitals, *Science* 173:836-838, 1971.

35. Folk JC, Cutkomp J, Koontz FP: Bacterial scleral abscesses after retinal buckling operations: pathogenesis, management, and laboratory investigations, *Ophthalmology* 94:1148-1154, 1987.

36. Forster RK, Zachary IG, Cottingham AJ Jr et al.: Further observations on the diagnosis, cause, and treatment of endophthalmitis, *Am J Ophthalmol* 81:52-56, 1976.

37. Frandsen EV, Pedrazzoli V, Kilian M: Ecology of viridans streptococci in the oral cavity and pharynx, *Oral Microbiol Immunol* 6:129-133, 1991.

38. Galentine PG, Cohen EJ, Laibson PR et al.: Corneal ulcers associated with contact lens wear, *Arch Ophthalmol* 102:891-894, 1984.

39. Gandhi PA, Sawant AD, Wilson LA et al.: Adaptation and growth of *Serratia marcescens* in contact lens disinfectant solutions containing chlorhexidine gluconate, *Appl Environ Microbiol* 59:183-188, 1993.

40. George R, Leibrock L, Epstein M: Long-term analysis of cerebrospinal fluid shunt infections: a 25-year experience, *J Neurosurg* 51:804-811, 1979.

41. Golden B, Fingerman LH, Allen HF: *Pseudomonas* corneal ulcers in contact lens wearers: epidemiology and treatment, *Arch Ophthalmol* 85:543-547, 1971.

42. Griffiths PG, Elliot TSJ, McTaggart L: Adherence of *Staphylococcus epidermidis* to intraocular lenses, *Br J Ophthalmol* 73:402-406, 1989.

43. Gristina AG, Dobbins JJ, Giammara B et al.: Biomaterial-centered sepsis and the total artificial heart: microbial adhesion vs. tissue integration, *JAMA* 259:870-874, 1988.

44. Gristina AG, Price JL, Hobgood CD et al.: Bacterial colonization of percutaneous sutures, *Surgery* 98:12-19, 1985.

45. Hadden OB: Infection after retinal detachment surgery, *Aust NZ J Ophthalmol* 14:69-73, 1986.

46. Hahn YS, Lincoff A, Lincoff H: Infection after sponge implantation for scleral buckling, *Am J Ophthalmol* 87:180-185, 1979.

47. Harris JM, Martin LF: An in vitro study of the properties influencing *Staphylococcus epidermidis* adhesion to prosthetic vascular graft materials, *Ann Surg* 206:612-620, 1987.

48. He YuGuang, McCulley JP, Alizadeh H et al.: A pig model of *Acanthamoeba* keratitis: transmission via contaminated contact lenses, *Invest Ophthalmol Vis Sci* 33:126-133, 1992.

49. Heidemann DG, Verdier DD, Dunn SP et al.: *Acanthamoeba* keratitis associated with disposable contact lenses, *Am J Ophthalmol* 110:630-634, 1990.

50. Herbst RW: *Herellea* corneal ulcer associated with the use of soft contact lenses, *Br J Ophthalmol* 56:848-850, 1972.

51. Herman CL: An FDA survey of contact lens wearers, *Contact Lens Spectrum* 2:89-92, 1987.

52. Hoadley AW, Ajello G, Masterson N: Preliminary studies of fluorescent pseudomonads capable of growth at 41°C in swimming pool waters, *Appl Environ Microbiol* 29:527-531, 1975.

53. Hoyle BD, Williams LJ, Costerton JW: Production of mucoid exopolysaccharide during development of *Pseudomonas aeruginosa* biofilms, *Infect Immun* 61:777-780, 1993.

54. Hoyle BD, Jass J, Costerton JW: The biofilm glycocalyx as a resistance factor, *J Antimicrob Chemother* 26:1-5, 1990.

55. Inman RD, Gallegos KV, Brause BD et al.: Clinical and microbial features of prosthetic joint infection, *Am J Med* 77:47-53, 1984.

56. Jackman SH, Rosenbusch RF: In vitro adherence of *Moraxella bovis* to intact corneal epithelium, *Curr Eye Res* 3:1107-1112, 1984.

57. Jansen B, Hartmann C, Schumacher-Perdreau F et al.: Late onset endophthalmitis associated with intraocular lens: a case of molecularly proved *S. epidermidis* aetiology, *Br J Ophthalmol* 75:440-441, 1991.

58. John T, Desai D, Sahm D: Adherence of *Acanthamoeba castellanii* cysts and trophozoites to extended wear soft contact lenses, *Rev Infect Dis* 13(suppl 5):S419-S420, 1991.

59. Jordan DR, St Onge P, Anderson RL et al.: Complications associated with alloplastic implants used in orbital fracture repair, *Ophthalmology* 99:1600-1608, 1992.

60. Kennedy MJ, Rogers AL, Yancey RJ Jr: Environmental alteration and phenotypic regulation of *Candida albicans* adhesion to plastic, *Infect Immun* 57:3876-3881, 1989.

61. Kluge RM: Infections of prosthetic cardiac valves and arterial grafts, *Heart Lung* 11:146-151, 1982.

62. Koenig SB, Solomon JM, Hyndiuk RA et al.: *Acanthamoeba* keratitis associated with gas-permeable contact lens wear, *Am J Ophthalmol* 103:832, 1987.

63. Krachmer JH, Purcell JJ Jr: Bacterial corneal ulcers in cosmetic soft contact lens wearers, *Arch Ophthalmol* 96:57-61, 1978.

64. Kush BJ, Hoadley AW: A preliminary survey of the association of *Pseudomonas aeruginosa* with commercial whirlpool bath waters, *Am J Public Health* 70:279-281, 1980.

65. Larkin DF, Kilvington S, Easty DL: Contamination of contact lens storage cases by *Acanthamoeba* and bacteria, *Br J Ophthalmol* 74:133-135, 1990.

66. Legeais JM, Rossi C, Renard G et al.: A new fluorocarbon for keratoprosthesis, *Cornea* 11:538-545, 1992.

67. Locatcher-Khorazo D, Gutierrez EH: The bacterial flora of the healthy eye. In Locatcher-Khorazo D, Seegal BC, editors: *Microbiology of the eye,* 13-73, St Louis, 1972, CV Mosby.

68. Lowy FD, Hammer SM: *Staphylococcus epidermidis* infections, *Ann Intern Med* 99:834-839, 1983.

69. Luft JH: Ruthenium red and violet. I. Chemistry, purification, methods of use for electron microscopy and mechanism of action, *Anat Rec* 171:347-368, 1971.

70. Marrie TJ, Costerton JW: Morphology of bacterial attachment to cardiac pacemaker leads and power packs, *J Clin Microbiol* 19:911-914, 1984.

71. Marrie TJ, Costerton JW: Prolonged survival of *Serratia marcescens* in chlorhexidine, *Appl Environ Microbiol* 42:1093-1102, 1981.

72. Martinez AJ: *Free-living amebas: natural history, prevention, diagnosis, pathology and treatment of disease*, 33-34, Boca Raton, 1985, CDC Press.

73. Matthews TD, Frazer DG, Minassian DC et al.: Risks of keratitis and patterns of use with disposable contact lenses, *Arch Ophthalmol* 110:1559-1562, 1992.

74. Mayo MS, Schlitzer RL, Ward MA et al.: Association of *Pseudomonas* and *Serratia* corneal ulcers with use of contaminated solutions, *J Clin Microbiol* 25:1398-1400, 1987.

75. Mayo MS, Cook WL, Schlitzer RL et al.: Antibiograms, serotypes, and plasmid profiles of *Pseudomonas aeruginosa* associated with corneal ulcers and contact lens wear, *J Clin Microbiol* 24:372-376, 1986.

76. McDonnell PJ, Kwitko S, McDonnell JM et al.: Characterization of infectious crystalline keratitis caused by a human isolate of *Streptococcus mitis*, *Arch Ophthalmol* 109:1147-1151, 1991.

77. McMeel JW, Wapner JM: Infections and retina surgery. I. Bacteriologic contamination during scleral buckling surgery, *Arch Ophthalmol* 74:42-44, 1965.

78. McMeel JW: Infections and retina surgery. II. Incidence and significance of positive wound site cultures, *Arch Ophthalmol* 74:45-47, 1965.

79. McNatt J, Allen SD, Wilson LA et al.: Anaerobic flora of the normal human conjunctival sac, *Arch Ophthalmol* 96:1448-1450, 1978.

80. Meisler DM, Palestine AG, Vastine DW et al.: Chronic *Propionibacterium* endophthalmitis after extracapsular cataract extraction and intraocular lens implantation, *Am J Ophthalmol* 102:733-739, 1986.

81. Menikoff JA, Speaker MG, Marmor M et al.: A case-control study of risk factors for postoperative endophthalmitis, *Ophthalmology* 98:1761-1768, 1991.

82. Mergeryan H: The prevalence of *Acanthamoeba* in the human environment, *Rev Infect Dis* 13(suppl 5):S390-S391, 1991.

83. Michels RG, Wilkinson CP, Rice TA: *Retinal detachment,* 1032, St Louis, 1990, CV Mosby.

84. Miller MJ, Wilson LA, Ahearn DG: Effects of protein, mucin and human tears on adherence of *Pseudomonas aeruginosa* to hydrophilic contact lenses, *J Clin Microbiol* 26:513-517, 1988.

85. Miller MJ, Ahearn DG: Adherence of *Pseudomonas aeruginosa* to hydrophilic contact lenses and other substrata, *J Clin Microbiol* 25:1392-1397, 1987.

86. Miller MJ, Wilson LA, Ahearn DG: Adherence of *Pseudomonas aeruginosa* to rigid gas-permeable contact lenses, *Arch Ophthalmol* 109:1447-1448, 1991.

87. Mondino BJ, Weissman BA, Farb MD: Corneal ulcers associated with daily-wear and extended-wear contact lenses, *Am J Ophthalmol* 102:58-65, 1986.

88. Moore MB, McCulley JP, Newton C et al.: *Acanthamoeba* keratitis: a growing problem in soft and hard contact lens wearers, *Ophthalmology* 94:1654-1661, 1987.

89. Moore MB, Ubelaker J, Silvany R et al.: Scanning electron microscopy of *Acanthamoeba castellanii*: adherence to surfaces of new and used contact lenses and to human corneal button epithelium, *Rev Infect Dis* 13(suppl 5):S423, 1991.

90. Morgan JF: Personal communication, 1993.

91. Morgan JF: Clinical approach to the care of rigid gas permeable lenses. Paper presented at the annual meeting of the Contact Lens Society of Ophthalmologists, New Orleans, January 20, 1993.

92. Morton LD, McLaughlin GL, Whiteley HE: Adherence characteristics of three strains of *Acanthamoeba*, *Rev Infect Dis* 13(suppl 5):S424, 1991.

93. Muller E, Takeda S, Goldmann DA et al.: Blood proteins do not promote adherence of coagulase-negative staphylococci to biomaterials, *Infect Immun* 59:3323-3326, 1991.

94. Nakashima AK, Highsmith AK, Martone WJ: Survival of *Serratia marcescens* in benzalkonium chloride and in multiple-dose medication vials: relationship to epidemic septic arthritis, *J Clin Microbiol* 25:1019-1021, 1987.

95. Niederkorn JY, Ubelaker JE, McCulley JP et al.: Susceptibility of corneas from various animal species to in vitro binding and invasion by *Acanthamoeba castellani*, *Invest Ophthalmol Vis Sci* 33:104-112, 1992.

96. Noble MA, Reid PE, Park CM et al.: Inhibition of human neutrophil bacteriocidal activity by extracellular substance from slime-producing *Staphylococcus epidermidis*, *Diagn Microbiol Infect Dis* 4:335-339, 1986.

97. Ormerod LD, Ruoff KL, Meisler DM et al.: Infectious crystalline keratopathy: role of nutritionally variant streptococci and other bacterial factors, *Ophthalmology* 98:159-169, 1991.

98. Ormerod LD, Smith RE: Contact lens-associated microbial keratitis, *Arch Ophthalmol* 104:79-83, 1986.

99. Parment P-A, Rönnerstam R, Walder M: Persistence of *Serratia marcescens*, *Serratia liquefaciens* and *E coli* in solutions for contact lenses, *Acta Ophthalmol* 64:456-462, 1986.

100. Parment PA, Rönnerstam RA: Soft contact lens keratitis associated with *Serratia marcescens*, *Acta Ophthalmol* 59:560-565, 1981.

101. Pavan PR, Brinser JH: Exogenous bacterial endophthalmitis treated without systemic antibiotics, *Am J Ophthalmol* 104:121-126, 1987.

102. Penley CA, Llabres C, Wilson LA et al.: Efficacy of hydrogen peroxide disinfection systems for soft contact lenses contaminated with fungi, *CLAO J* 11:65-68, 1985.

103. Penley CA, Ahearn DG, Schlitzer RL et al.: Laboratory evaluation of chemical disinfection of soft contact lenses. II. Fungi as challenge organisms, *Contact Intraocul Lens Med J* 7:196-204, 1981.

104. Penley CA, Willis SW, Sickler SG: Comparative antimicrobial efficacy of soft and rigid gas permeable contact lens solutions against *Acanthamoeba*, *CLAO J* 15:257-260, 1989.

105. Penley CA, Schlitzer RL, Ahearn DG et al.: Laboratory evaluation of chemical disinfection of soft contact lenses, *Contact Intraocul Lens Med J* 7:101-110, 1981.

106. Pitts RE, Krachmer JH: Evaluation of soft contact lens disinfection in the home environment, *Arch Ophthalmol* 97:470-472, 1979.

107. Poggio EC, Glynn RJ, Schein OD et al.: The incidence of ulcerative keratitis among users of daily-wear and extended-wear soft contact lenses, *N Engl J Med* 321:779-783, 1989.

108. Polack FM, Heimke G: Ceramic keratoprostheses, *Ophthalmology* 87:693-698, 1980.

109. Raskin EM, Speaker MG, McCormick SA et al.: Influence of haptic materials on the adherence of staphylococci to intraocular lenses, *Arch Ophthalmol* 111:250-253, 1993.

110. Rogers DG, Cheville NF, Pugh GW Jr: Pathogenesis of corneal lesions caused by *Moraxella bovis* in gnotobiotic calves, *Vet Pathol* 24:287-295, 1987.

111. Rotrosen D, Calderone RA, Edwards JE Jr: Adherence of *Candida* species to host tissues and plastic surfaces, *Rev Infect Dis* 8:73-85, 1986.

112. Salzman MB, Isenberg HD, Rubin LG: Use of disinfectants to reduce microbial contamination of vascular catheters, *J Clin Microbiol* 31:475-479, 1993.

113. Schein OD, Glynn RJ, Poggio EC et al.: The relative risk of ulcerative keratitis among users of daily-wear and extended-wear soft contact lenses: a case-control study, *N Engl J Med* 321:773-778, 1989.

114. Schein OD, Ormerod LD, Barraquer E et al.: Microbiology of contact lens-related keratitis, *Cornea* 8:281-285, 1989.

115. Sharma S, Srinivasan M, George C: *Acanthamoeba* keratitis in non-contact lens wearers, *Arch Ophthalmol* 108:676-678, 1990.

116. Sherwood DR, Rich WJ, Jacob JS et al.: Bacterial contamination of intraocular and extraocular fluids during extracapsular cataract extraction, *Eye* 3:308-312, 1989.

117. Silvany RE, Dougherty JM, McCulley JP et al.: The effect of currently available contact lens disinfection systems on *Acanthamoeba castellanii* and *Acanthamoeba polyphaga*, *Ophthalmology* 97:286-290, 1990.

118. Simmons RB, Buffington JR, Ward M: Morphology and ultrastructure of fungi in extended-wear soft contact lenses, *J Clin Microbiol* 24:21-25, 1986.
119. Speaker MG, Milch FA, Shah MK: Role of external bacterial flora in the pathogenesis of acute postoperative endophthalmitis, *Ophthalmology* 98:639-649, 1991.
120. Starr MB: *Paecilomyces lilacinus* keratitis: two case reports in extended-wear contact lens wearers, *CLAO J* 13:95-101, 1987.
121. Stehr-Green JK, Bailey TM, Visvesvara GS: The epidemiology of *Acanthamoeba* keratitis in the United States, *Am J Ophthalmol* 107:331-336, 1989.
122. Stern GA, Engel HM, Driebe WT Jr: Recurrent postoperative endophthalmitis, *Cornea* 9:102-107, 1990.
123. Sugarman B: Adherence of bacteria to urinary catheters, *Urol Res* 10:37-40, 1982.
124. Vafidis GC, Marsh RJ, Stacey AR: Bacterial contamination of intra-ocular lens surgery, *Br J Ophthalmol* 68:520-523, 1984.
125. Valenton MJ, Brubaker RF, Allen HF: *Staphylococcus epidermidis (albus)* endophthalmitis: report of two cases after cataract extraction, *Arch Ophthalmol* 89:94-96, 1973.
126. Vaudoux P, Pittet D, Haeberli A et al.: Fibronectin is more active than fibrin or fibrinogen in promoting *Staphylococcus aureus* adherence to inserted intravenous catheters, *J Infect Dis* 167:633-641, 1993.
127. Virkola R, Westerlund B, Holthofer H et al.: Binding characteristics of *Escherichia coli* adhesins in human urinary bladder, *Infect Immun* 56:2615-2622, 1988.
128. Wilhelmus K, Robinson NM, Font RA: Fungal keratitis in contact lens wearers, *Am J Ophthalmol* 106:708-714, 1988.
129. Wilhelmus KR: Review of clinical experience with microbial keratitis associated with contact lenses, *CLAO J* 13:211-214, 1987.
130. Williams GA, Aaberg TM: Retina. In Ryan SJ, Glaser BM, Michaels RG, editors: *Surgical retina,* vol 3, 139-140, St Louis, 1989, CV Mosby.
131. Wilson LA, Sawant AD, Ahearn DG: Comparative efficacies of soft contact lens disinfectant solutions against microbial films in lens cases, *Arch Ophthalmol* 109:1155-1157, 1991.
132. Wilson LA, Sawant AD, Simmons RB: Microbial contamination of contact lens storage cases and solutions, *Am J Ophthalmol* 110:193-198, 1990.
133. Wilson LA, Ahearn DG, Jones DB et al.: Fungi from the normal outer eye, *Am J Ophthalmol* 67:52-56, 1969.
134. Wilson LA, Ahearn DG: Association of fungi with extended-wear soft contact lenses, *Am J Ophthalmol* 101:434-436, 1986.
135. Wilson LA, Schlitzer RL, Ahearn DG: *Pseudomonas* corneal ulcers associated with soft contact lens wear, *Am J Ophthalmol* 92:546-554, 1981.

17 Inflammatory Responses to Ocular Infection

SCOTT W. COUSINS, BARRY T. ROUSE

Inflammation is the process by which white blood cells and fluid accumulate within a tissue. At the macroscopic level, inflammation is manifest by the "cardinal" clinical signs: pain, redness, swelling, warmth, and loss of function. Inflammation is ultimately determined at the cellular level via complex interactions between tissue sites, effector leukocytes, and soluble mediators. Three major concepts pertain to (1) how inflammation is initiated, (2) how it injures tissues, and (3) how it is terminated.

Inflammation can be triggered independently by one of at least three initiating mechanisms: infection (tissue colonization and replication of a microorganism), immune response, and injury.[102] Microbial-induced inflammation has a dual pathogenesis. In some cases the intrinsic properties of the microorganism can directly trigger inflammation, whereas in other cases the immune response to the microorganism acts as the trigger.

Infections do not always initiate inflammation; some ocular parasitic infections develop inflammation only when the parasite dies.[19] Other examples of ocular infection without inflammation include crystalline keratopathy,[73] latent herpetic infection of the trigeminal ganglion,[90] latent Epstein-Barr viral infection of the lacrimal gland, and *Propionibacterium acnes* growth in the lens capsule.[67] Conversely, significant tissue inflammation can occur in the absence of immunity, such as experimental herpes simplex virus retinitis in athymic mice[11] and cytomegaloviral retinitis in AIDS.[76]

The instruments of tissue injury during inflammation are complex. In spite of an extensive literature on the soluble mediators and cellular effectors of inflammation, how these two factors actually damage the eye remains unclear. Even less is known of the reparative response following injury. To understand infectious eye disease it is important to consider how inflammation is regulated and ultimately terminated.

TRIGGERING MECHANISMS FOR MICROBIALLY INDUCED INFLAMMATION

Intrinsic Properties of Microorganisms That Trigger Inflammation

Bacterial Lipopolysaccharide (LPS). Bacterial lipopolysaccharide (endotoxin), an intrinsic component of most gram-negative bacterial cell walls, consists of three components: lipid A, polysaccharide, and a protein core.[69] Of these, lipid A is responsible for most of the inflammatory effects of LPS. Lipid A-associated proteins enhance the biologic potency of lipid A itself, and these proteins vary depending on the source of LPS or the way it is prepared.

LPS is an important cause of morbidity during infections with gram-negative bacteria. It is the major cause of shock, fever, and other pathophysiologic responses to bacterial sepsis.[71] The pleiotropic effects of LPS include activation of monocytes and polymorphonuclear leukocytes (PMN), leading to upregulation of genes for various cytokines (IL-1, IL-6, TNF), degranulation, activation of complement via the alternative pathway, and direct influence on vascular endothelium. The cellular effects of LPS are the result of interactions with specific cell receptors such as CD 18-CR3, a specific LPS scavenger receptor on macrophages and lymphocytes. A circulating LPS binding protein has been identified. Binding by the LPS-binding protein complex with the CD 14 molecule on the macrophage surface results in activation.[107] Because of its devastating physiologic properties during septicemia, LPS is a target of novel therapeutic strategies (neutralizing antibodies and soluble CD 14 molecules).[65]

Systemic Administration

Intravenous exposure to LPS triggers ocular inflammation in animals, and this effect occurs at lower doses of LPS than those that cause apparent systemic effects. In rabbits, plasma protein leakage through uveal vessels and loosening of the tight junctions between the nonpigmented epithelia of the ciliary body cause a breakdown of the blood ocular barrier.[29,51] Rats and mice develop an acute cellular infiltrate in the iris and ciliary body within 24 hours.[27,35,84] The precise mechanism of LPS-induced ocular effects after systemic administration is unknown. One possibility is that LPS circulates and binds to the vascular endothelium (or other sites) within the anterior uvea, producing a localized physiologic change. Alternatively, LPS might cause leukocytes to preferentially adhere to the anterior uveal vascular endothelium.

Rapid accumulation and degranulation of platelets are among the first histologic changes in LPS uveitis, probably mediated by eicosanoids, platelet-activating factor (PAF), and vasoactive amines.[51-53] The subsequent intraocular generation of several mediators, especially LTB_4, thromboxane B_2, PGE_2, and IL-6, correlates with the subsequent development of the cellular infiltrate and vascular leakage.[46,47] Humans are intermittently exposed to low doses of endotoxin that are released from the gut, particularly during episodes of diarrhea and dysentery; and exposure to LPS is thought to play a role in dysentery-related uveitis, arthritis, and Reiter syndrome.[82] Ocular inflammation, however, was not observed when eye exams were performed during systemic LPS administration, even though significant effects were noted in other organ systems.[48]

Local Administration

Direct injection of LPS into various ocular sites can initiate a severe localized inflammatory response. Intravitreal injection of LPS triggers a dose-dependent infiltration of the uveal tract, retina, and vitreous with PMNs and monocytes.[54] Injection of LPS into the central cornea results in the development of a "ring infiltrate" caused by the infiltration of PMNs circumferentially from the limbus.[68]

Repeated exposure to LPS causes a paradoxical phenomenon. LPS desensitization (or tolerance) occurs after repeated exposure to low systemic doses of LPS.[29] Rabbits with LPS tolerance are resistant to the uveitis induced by subsequent intraocular LPS injections.[54] This desensitization response may include resistance to certain cytokines and might be the basis for the reported utility of "fever therapy" as a treatment for uveitis in the presteroid era.[89]

Other Bacterial Cell-Wall Components. The bacterial cell wall is complex, with numerous polysaccharide and protein structures.[101] Some of these components have been implicated in experimental models of arthritis and uveitis.

The classical model that is dependent on bacterial cell wall-associated products is adjuvant disease in rats. Immunization with Freund adjuvant produces polyarthritis, cutaneous inflammation, and uveitis that closely resemble the clinical features of Reiter syndrome and, to a lesser extent, rheumatoid arthritis.[99] Early work indicated that inflammation might be directed against muramyl dipeptide, a cell-wall component of *Mycobacterium tuberculosis* present in the adjuvant.[75] Other studies, however, have focused on the pathogenic role of other bacterial proteins.[98]

Another arthritis and uveitis model identified inflammation that was directed against bacterial cell walls. Upon intraperitoneal injection of bacterial cells walls or muramyl dipeptide, rats and rabbits developed arthritis,[97] and in some cases, ocular inflammation.[100] Repeated intravenous injection of muramyl dipeptide induced chronic anterior uveitis that is associated with the breakdown of the blood-eye barrier and cellular infiltrate.[64,74] The mechanism of this model is unclear, but "antigen trapping" of bacterial cell debris within the hyperpermeable uveal tract has been postulated to occur and might be relevant to uveitis associated with bacterial dysentery, gingivitis, and other nonocular infections.[36,83]

Exotoxins and Other Secretory Products of Bacteria. Various bacteria secrete products such as exotoxins.[41,101] Many of these products are enzymes and, although not directly inflammatory, cause tissue damage which subsequently results in inflammation. Examples include collagenases, hemolysins (such as streptolysin O that can kill neutrophils by causing cytoplasmic and extracellular release of their granules),[17] and phospholipases (such as *Shiga* toxins that kill cells and cause necrosis by disrupting cell membranes).[96] The metabolic byproducts of bacterial physiology also result in nonspecific tissue alterations (such as tissue pH changes) that predispose to inflammation.

Some bacteria secrete small formyl-peptide molecules that are related to the tripeptide, N-formyl-methionyl-leucyl-phenylalanine (FMLP). These formyl peptides are potent triggering stimuli for inflammation. FMLP interacts with specific receptors on leukocytes, resulting in their recruitment into the site.[23] FMLP activates neutrophils, causes degranulation, and stimulates chemotaxis. Injection of FMLP into the cornea, conjunctiva, or vitreous produces infiltration with neutrophils and monocytes. This ocular inflammation can be prevented by pretreatment with corticosteroids, cyclooxygenase inhibitors, and competitive inhibitors of FMLP.[13]

Bacteria release some products that are immunosuppressive. For example, some bacterial proteases—especially those derived from *Pseudomonas* species—can degrade various immunoregulatory cytokines, which inhibit lymphocyte activation and proliferation.[63] A specialized family of exotoxins, called superantigens, are potent triggers of lymphocyte activation.

Viral Properties That Trigger Inflammation. Viruses trigger inflammation in a variety of ways. These include the effects of direct cell destruction, the release of viral products, and the induction of inflammatory molecules such as various cytokines in infected cells. Added to these direct effects are interactions between viral products and host immunity.[20,56,79]

Bacterial and Viral Superantigens. Superantigens are proteins that can activate T cells in the absence of preexisting immunity.[66] They do so by simultaneously binding specific sites on the T cell antigen receptor with the MHC class II molecule on the antigen-presenting cell. Several bacterial exotoxins are superantigens, primarily those produced by staphylococci, streptococci, and mycoplasma. Some viral proteins are superantigens.[2] Superantigens contribute to toxic shock syndrome by activating the patient's T cells, thereby releasing high levels of cytokines such as TNF and IL-6, which results in shock.[66] Although the role of superantigens in ocular disease remains unexplored, superantigen-mediated T cell activation might contribute to inflammation in several ocular infections, such as endophthalmitis.

Immune Responses Against Infection as Triggers of Inflammation

Immune responses directed against infectious agents may act as major triggers of inflammation.

Antibody-Mediated Inflammation. Antibody-antigen interactions are important triggers of inflammation. Two different processes should be distinguished: deposition of preformed circulating complexes and the local formation of immune complexes within the eye (Chapter 4). In situ formation of immune complexes can occur when high concentrations of antigen and antibody accumulate within tissues. The resultant tissue-restricted immune complex formation and complement activation cause a severe inflammatory reaction, known as an Arthus reaction.[32,39] Such a reaction can occur in the vitreous[8,78] and cornea[40] under many different experimental conditions. It is possible for antibody-induced phagocytosis or complement-mediated lysis of microorganisms or infected cells to occur in the absence of overt inflammation.

The ocular deposition of circulating immune complexes is probably not a common triggering device for inflammation in man,[72] even though some animal models that produce intravascular soluble immune-complex overload (serum sickness) can induce inflammatory effects.[105] Circulating immune complexes have been reported in the blood of uveitis patients.[6] Widespread ocular deposition of circulating immune complexes is usually avoided in man, however, because immune complexes are efficiently taken up by erythrocytes. Red blood cells have high-affinity receptors for IC-C3b, which permit subsequent sequestration and destruction of immune complexes in the spleen and liver.[86] Many of the early studies that analyzed the role of circulating immune complexes in ocular inflammation did not differentiate between soluble and erythrocyte-associated immune complexes, dislodged at the time of phlebotomy.

Lymphocyte-Mediated Inflammation. Two fundamentally different forms of lymphocyte-mediated inflammation are recognized. Cytotoxic lymphocytes, representing three functional categories of effector lymphocytes (CD8 cytotoxic T lymphocytes [CTLs], natural killer cells, and lymphokine-activated killer cells), can recognize infected host cells and kill the cells through lysis or apoptosis. This form of immunity occurs in the absence of severe inflammation and thereby rids the host of the invading pathogen with minimal tissue destruction.[60] CTLs control the spread of virus and allow the clearance of virus after infection. In contrast, CD4 T lymphocytes are designed to trigger severe inflammation that results in bystander tissue damage as a tradeoff for killing the pathogen. Initial antigen recognition and activation of CD4 T cells occur in lymph nodes, followed by release into the venous circulation via lymphatics. After transmigration into the site, antigen-specific delayed hypersensitivity T cells must recognize antigen within the tissue, become activated, and release proinflammatory cytokines locally.[60]

T cells require very specific homing signals (via cell-adhesion molecules on the vascular endothelium) to be recruited into a tissue site. How these homing molecules are upregulated in the absence of other inflammatory stimuli is unknown. That is, how can the T cell be directed to go to the site before the site is inflamed and expresses the appropriate cell-adhesion molecules? The nonimmunologic inflammation triggered by many bacterial toxins often contributes to the ultimate recruitment and functional activation of delayed-hypersensitivity T cells during infections.[36] Additionally, the mechanism by which the relatively low concentration of cytokines released by a few antigen-specific T cells is amplified into a signal that initiates a severe inflammatory response is not understood.[26] T cells mediate their effect indirectly by the recruitment and activation of inflammatory effector cells (especially macrophages and neutrophils). The complexity of animal models of infectious uveitis make it difficult to clearly distinguish the contribution of antigen-specific delayed hypersensitivity from other triggering stimuli.

Important differences exist in the immunoregulatory control of T cell activation at these different sites, primarily within different ocular compartments. In particular, the conjunctiva is probably more susceptible to delayed hypersensitivity reactions than is the uveal tract because of the physiologic differences between the two sites. The natural production of immunosuppressive cytokines (such as TGF-β or neuropeptides) within the iris and ciliary body provide a relative degree of protection from intraocular delayed hypersensitivity reactions.

Combined Antibody- and Cell-Mediated Mechanisms. Interaction between antibodies and effector cells can trigger inflammation in different ways. First, the ability of an effector cell to recognize the F_c portion of an antibody bound to a pathogenic target can produce a localized inflammatory response that is similar to that of the cytotoxic lymphocyte. This mechanism, often called antibody-directed cell-mediated cytotoxicity (ADCC), might help to rid the host of virally infected cells in the absence of widespread nonspecific inflammation.[60] Receptors on the macrophages recognize the F_c portion of lg molecules bound to infected target cells. Second, mast cell degranulation via surface-bound IgE is considered another form of combination cell-antibody triggered inflammation. Finally, the opsinization of pathogens and the subsequent phagocytosis, especially by macrophages and neutrophils, can lead to the activation of the phagocytic cell. For instance, after phagocytosis, the macrophage is often changed from a quiescent monocyte into an effector cell by undergoing an oxidative burst and synthesizing a wide range of mediators in an effort to destroy the ingested substance or pathogen. Immune complexes can also initiate granulomatous reactions and produce many of the histologic features that are associated with chronic inflammation.[85]

Molecular Mimicry and Autoimmunity

Autoimmunity may play an important role in the pathogenesis of inflammatory ocular diseases. One mechanism whereby autoimmunity to self-antigens in the eye or central nervous system might be triggered by infection is through molecular mimicry, the immunologic cross-reaction between epitopes of an unrelated foreign antigen and self-epitopes with similar structures. Theoretically, these epitopes would be similar enough to stimulate an immune response but different enough to cause a breakdown of immunologic tolerance.

At least two related processes might be relevant to the eye. Foreign antigens (such as those present within yeast, viruses, or bacteria) may induce the formation of antibodies or the activation of effector lymphocytes, which, in turn, react with homologous epitopes of a self-antigen. For example, yeast histone shares significant homology with retinal S antigen, and the immunization of rats against the yeast antigen results in bilateral retinitis similar to experimental autoimmune uveoretinitis.[88]

Other possibilities for molecular mimicry are immune responses against stress or heat-shock proteins (HSPs). HSPs are cellular proteins that are not highly expressed in normal cells unless they are induced by a stress response such as cellular injury. Inflammation that is directed against bacteria often results in immune responses against bacterial heat-shock protein.[98] Because many antigenic determinants on the bacterial HSP are conserved among human HSP, cross-reactivity is possible. For instance, evidence has implicated immune responses against mycobacterial HSP 65 as a source of autoreactive T cells in an animal model for ar-

thritis and uveitis following immunization with Freund adjuvant.[98]

Amplification of Triggering Stimuli Into Sustained Inflammation

How a triggering stimulus becomes amplified into overt inflammation remains a mystery. Simply demonstrating that a particular stimulus can initiate inflammation does not indicate how the initiating stimulus accomplishes this process. Four possibilities are postulated.

First, many of the triggering stimuli are part of self-amplifying cascades. Complement activation and fibrin formation are two such examples.

Second, the temporal activation of cytokine and mediator genes usually results in a pattern of proinflammatory mediator synthesis and release as part of a "program." That is, genes for many proinflammatory mediators are activated in coordinated fashion to the same stimulus.[92] Furthermore, proinflammatory mediators tend to be synthesized and released early after activation, whereas some downregulatory signals are not activated until later.

Third, it is possible that temporal differences in the activity between the intrinsic stimuli of pathogens (immediate) versus the immune-mediated trigger to pathogens (delayed by several days) contribute to a dual mechanism for maintaining inflammation.

Fourth, nonantigen-specific "polyclonal" activation of lymphocytes might enhance a low level, antigen-specific triggering stimulus.[4,12] For example, the concept of trans-stimulation has been suggested for T cells, in which a small but highly efficient number of activated antigen-specific T cells create a microenvironment in which many nonantigen-specific T cells become activated at a lower "efficiency." These nonspecific T cells might be induced to proliferate for a few cycles or release some proinflammatory cytokines, even though they would eventually die off from a lack of antigen.

The various components of the ocular inflammatory response are represented in Fig. 17-1. This illustration forms a guide to understanding the rationale for present and future treatment modalities (Table 17-1).

INJURY AND HEALING AFTER OCULAR INFLAMMATION

Ocular Injury Caused by Inflammation

Injury is the direct consequence of inflammation. Physical or physiologic alterations allow fluid and cells to enter the tissue. A conceptual overview of the processes by which the products of inflammation mediate injury is depicted in Fig. 17-2.

Free-radical injury is the only well-characterized biochemical mediator of cellular injury in the eye. Oxygen-free

Evolution of acute inflammation in the eye

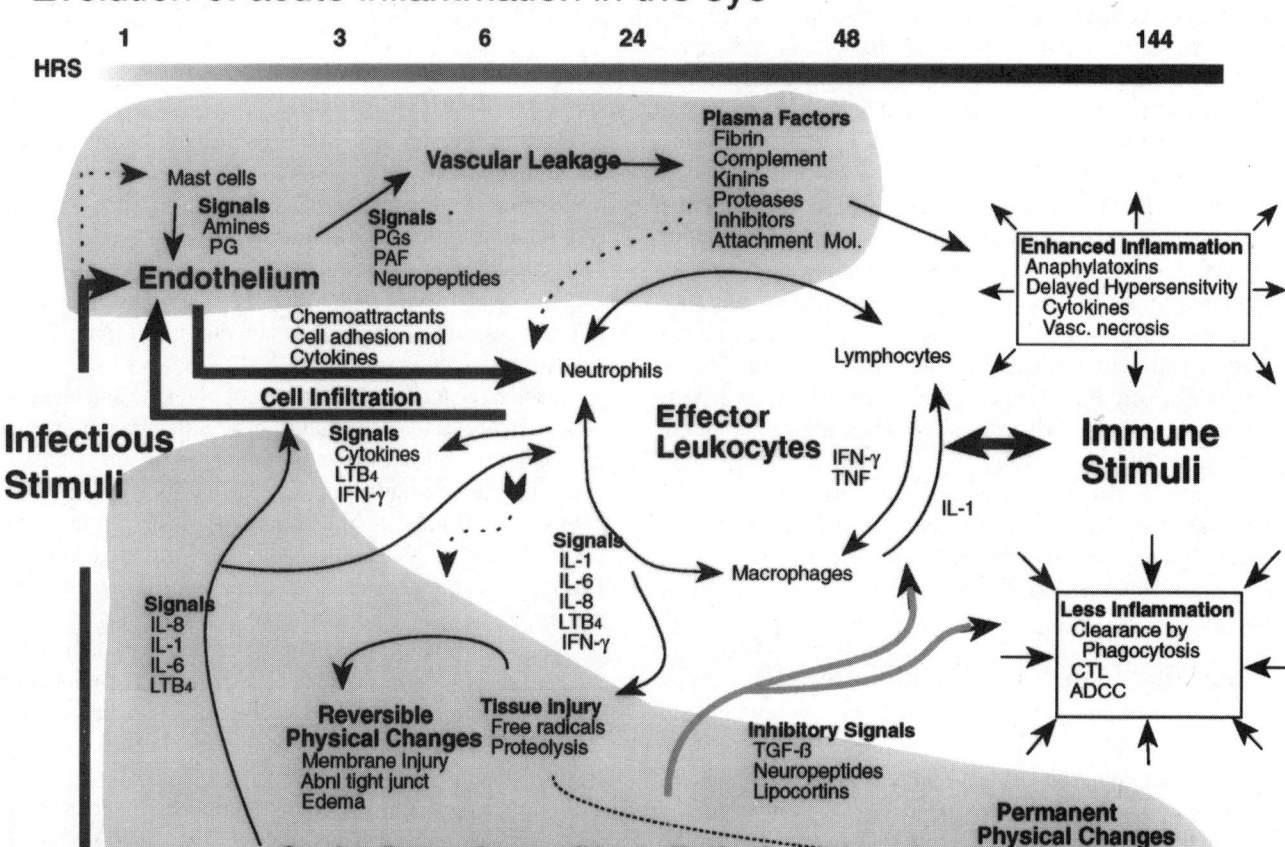

Fig. 17-1. Diagrammatic representation of the complex interrelationships within the eye during evolution of acute inflammation.

radicals produce lipid peroxidation, resulting in loss of membrane function. Intact cell membranes are particularly important for neurons and secretory epithelia, which depend on membrane ionic pumps for normal function. Free radicals also lead to denaturation of proteins, thus disrupting cell-surface receptors and adhesion molecules. Mutations in DNA can be caused by free-radical interference with protein synthesis. Nitrogen-free radicals block energy generation by the respiratory metabolism in mitochondria and inhibit enzymes important in RNA synthesis. Free-radical injury has been convincingly demonstrated as a mediator of retinal injury during experimental uveitis.[80] The role of free-radical injury in the anterior segment may be less important as a result of the presence of high concentrations of antioxidants and low levels of target lipids in cell membranes.

Two other inflammation-induced forms of localized cell injury can occur. Lysis refers to cell death caused by pore formation in the plasma membrane, leading to swelling and loss of cytoplasmic contents and nuclei.[16] Complement and cytotoxic lymphocytes are the major mediators of lytic activity. Lysis is the usual device for the immune destruction of virally infected cells and tumor cells. Apoptosis refers to

the cellular process of "programmed cell death."[22] Every cell has the intrinsic capacity for self destruction via the activation of a specialized program of "death proteins," essentially deoxyribonucleases and other degradatory enzymes. Apoptosis is the mediator of physiologic cell death caused by aging or developmental remodeling of tissue. Apoptosis, however, can be initiated by the products of leukocytes as well. Certain T cells, especially CTL cells, release granule products that can activate apoptosis. It is likely that exposure of cells to the "correct" combination of soluble cytokines and mediators during an inflammatory response can activate apoptosis. For example, the combination of nitric oxide and TNF can result in the death of some cell lines. The role of apoptosis as a biochemical mediator of cell injury in uveitis has not been well characterized.

Vascular endothelial injury is important in some forms of inflammation. Disrupted tight junctions between capillary endothelia are a primary cause of fluid leakage. The subsequent accumulation of extracellular protein macromolecules alters the osmotic pressure gradient, leading to extracellular edema. In the eye, disruption of tight junctions between ad-

TABLE 17-1   THERAPEUTIC CONSIDERATIONS FOR CONTROLLING INFLAMMATION

Strategy	Mechanism	Example
Prevent vascular leakage/restore blood-ocular barrier	Block action of vasoactive amines	Histamine receptor blocker/serotonin antagonist
	Prevent PG or PAF synthesis	Cyclooxygenase inhibitors/PAF inhibitors
	Prevent certain neuropeptide release	Substance P inhibitor
Prevention of cell infiltration	Block cell adhesion molecule binding site	RGD peptides Cell-adhesion blocking antibodies
Prevent activation of lipid mediators	Phospholipase inhibitors	Glucosteroids Lipocortins
	Leukotriene inhibitors PAF inhibitors	
Interruption of cytokine action	Bind up/neutralize cytokine	Neutralizing antibodies Soluble receptors
	Cytokine receptor blockade	Blocking antibody Receptor antagonists
Imunomodulation with exogenous compounds	Immunosuppressive drugs	Cyclosporine Local delivery of antimetabolites
	Immunosuppressive cytokines	Transforming growth factor-β Certain interleukins Neuropeptides
	Immunotoxins	Antibody-toxin conjugates Cytokine-toxin conjugates
Paracrine immunomodulation	Induce production of immunosuppressive factors by host tissue	Retinoids to induce transforming growth factor-β Steroids to induce lipocortins
Prevention of tissue injury from free radicals	Antioxidant enzymes Free-radical scavengers	Superoxide dismutase/catalase Vitamins E,C

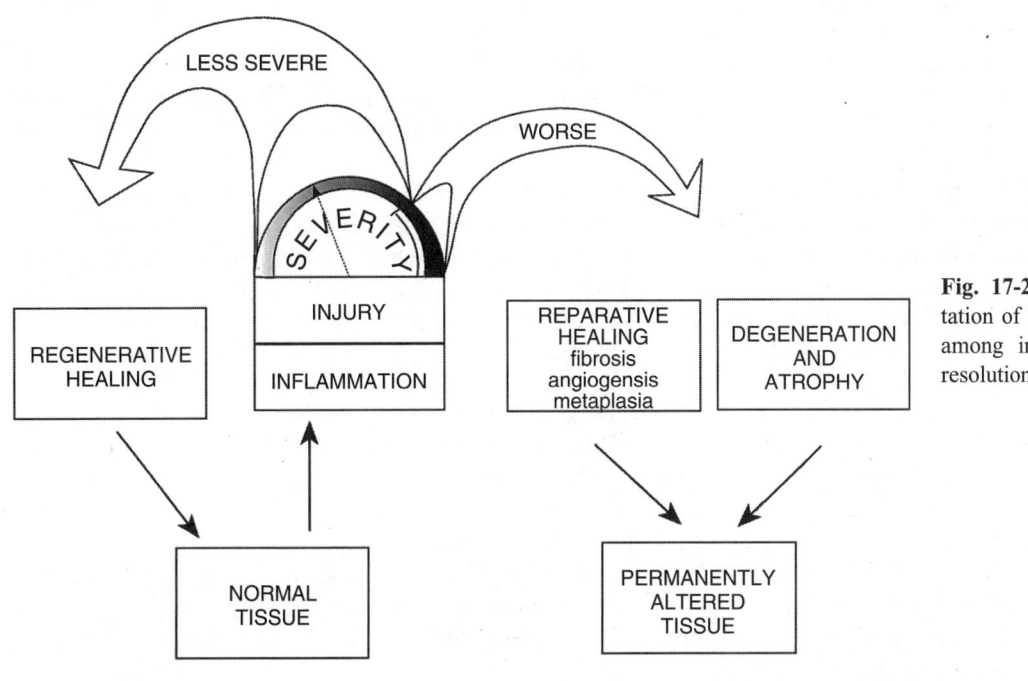

Fig. 17-2. Diagrammatic representation of the conceptual relationships among inflammation, tissue injury, resolution, and permanent damage.

jacent nonpigmented epithelial cells or retinal pigmented epithelial cells produces edema.[43,53]

Another form of vascular injury leads to capillary occlusion and ischemia. The resulting hypoxia and metabolic derangement cause ischemic necrosis of the tissue subserved by the capillary bed.[15,33] Necrosis indicates that the pattern of injury is widespread, resulting in devitalization of major blocks of the tissue. Presumably, capillary endothelial cells are induced to alter their surface and synthesize thrombin and platelet-activating factors, leading to intravascular clotting and scattered vascular plugging. Capillary blood flow is interrupted, causing hypoxia, accumulation of cellular metabolic byproducts, and depletion of crucial nutrients. Evidence of thrombosis and occlusion of larger vessels is usually absent, however. Reperfusion can paradoxically worsen the injury via enhanced production of oxygen radicals and other mechanisms.[38] Ischemic necrosis contributes to severe ocular inflammation following ocular delayed hypersensitivity responses (principally tumor rejection),[61] and immune-complex deposition can also produce ischemic necrosis. At nonocular sites, exposure to certain cytokines, particularly TNF, can mimic the pattern of ischemic necrosis.[1]

Finally, proteolytic digestion of extracellular matrix and cell surface receptors has been classically considered as a major contributor to inflammatory injury, but it may be less important than previously thought. Theoretically, leukocyte-derived enzymes might reshape the extracellular matrix and injure basement membranes. The interstitial matrix acts as a major storage site for sequestered cytokines and growth factors,[45] which, upon proteolytic disruption of the matrix, would become activated and released. Experiments designed to evaluate the contribution of this device in nonocular tissues have indicated that serum-derived protease inhibitors and other regulatory mechanisms tend to prevent significant injury from proteolytic enzymes.[103]

Healing from Injury Caused by Inflammation

In the eye, structure and function are closely interdependent. Structural changes that are induced by healing from inflammation can be extremely disruptive to vision. Many similarities exist between the mechanisms of inflammation and those of wound healing. Indeed, many of the cytokines and factors that are generated within a healing wound are the same as those found during inflammation, and both lymphocytes and macrophages are crucial in normal wound healing.[25,50,62]

Regenerative healing is the most desirable outcome in the eye. Injured cell membranes are rapidly regenerated if the insult is removed and normal cell physiology is returned. Even the retinal photoreceptor outer segment can repair itself if the cell body is alive.[80] Vascular endothelium regenerates, and tight junctions between adjacent cells become reestablished. Edema fluid is pumped out by restoration of osmotic and oncotic gradients. External ocular tissues (chiefly the conjunctival and corneal epithelia) have excellent regenerative powers, but the corneal stroma is less resilient. Intraocular tissues can only regenerate to a limited extent.

At some point during the inflammatory response, the sum total of "inflammatory factors" overloads the "threshold tolerance," and permanent tissue injury follows (Fig. 17-2). Degeneration or atrophy refers to the condition when a tissue has been depopulated of normal parenchymal cells. The capacity of ischemic necrosis to cause degeneration and atrophy is self-evident. Even apoptosis or lysis, which are relatively benign when localized to a few cells, can seriously destroy the function of the eye if widespread. For example, retinal photoreceptor degeneration is a major source of vision loss in chronic posterior uveitis, even in eyes without clinical evidence of severe, acute retinal inflammation.[80]

Reparative healing refers to a vigorous attempt of the tissue to repair itself by one or more of three physiologic processes including fibrosis, angiogenesis, and metaplasia. The conjunctiva can tolerate substantial fibrosis and scarring without major loss of function, but adhesions can occur.[90] Corneal and intraocular structures have minimal tolerance for reparative healing. Corneal vascularization, retinal neovascularization, and cyclitic membrane formation are examples of intraocular reparative responses that result in permanent tissue alterations, often threatening the function of the eye.

RESOLUTION AND THE REGULATION OF THE OCULAR INFLAMMATORY RESPONSE

Inflammation is usually described as acute or chronic—according to its temporal course. Acute inflammation usually proceeds in a stereotypical way to resolution within days or weeks. Characterized at first by neutrophils, the inflammatory infiltrate eventually transforms into a mononuclear cell pattern.[50] If the inflammatory reaction represents the response to infection, then nonimmune triggering devices are largely responsible for initiating the response. Immune mechanisms participate 5 to 7 days later. Severe changes in vascular permeability are present, with fibrin deposition a prominent feature. Upon resolution, normal anatomic and physiologic properties of the eye can return without apparent tissue alteration.

Chronic inflammation is inflammation that fails to resolve spontaneously, usually after more than 2 weeks. Histologically, chronic inflammatory responses show wide variation. In the *nongranulomatous* form, lymphocytes and monocytes predominate[25] (Fig. 17-3). Although numerous T lymphocytes appear to be activated, less than 1% (perhaps as

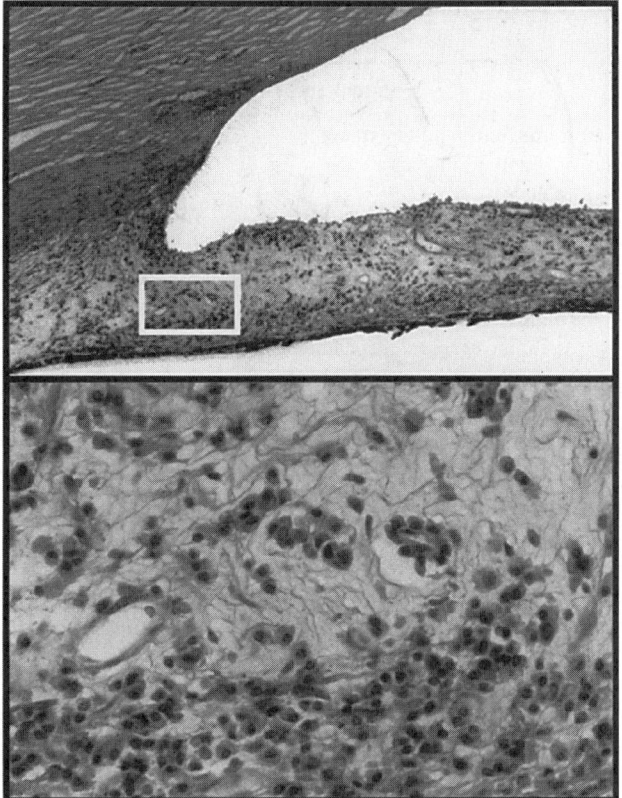

Fig. 17-3. *Top,* Photomicrograph of an eye with chronic non-granulomatous inflammation. *Bottom,* High-power view *(inset)* demonstrating that the infiltrate is mostly plasma cells and mononuclear leukocytes.

few as 0.01%) of the T cells are antigen-specific, indicating that either the T cells are nonspecifically activated or they have become activated to other antigens within the site (such as autoantigens).[59] Vascular permeability is often abnormal, but fibrin deposits are less prominent.

Some chronic responses become intensely infiltrated by macrophages, epithelioid cells, and giant cells and are referred to as *granulomatous* reactions[3,87] (Fig. 17-4). Eliciting agents include paraffin oil (in adjuvants), mycobacterial waxes, talc, and other foreign bodies. Mycobacterial, fungal, and certain anaerobic infections are associated with granulomatous inflammation. In these infections, the typical histologic pattern probably occurs because the intracellular pathogens survive and persist within macrophages, in association with a vigorous delayed hypersensitivity T-cell reaction to pathogen-related antigens. Evidence from experimental granulomata indicates that T cell-derived cytokines, interferon-γ and TNF, are probably crucial mediators.[10] In some cases, local immune-complex formation has been associated with granulomatous inflammation.[85] Chronic inflammation results in numerous anatomic and functional sequelae.

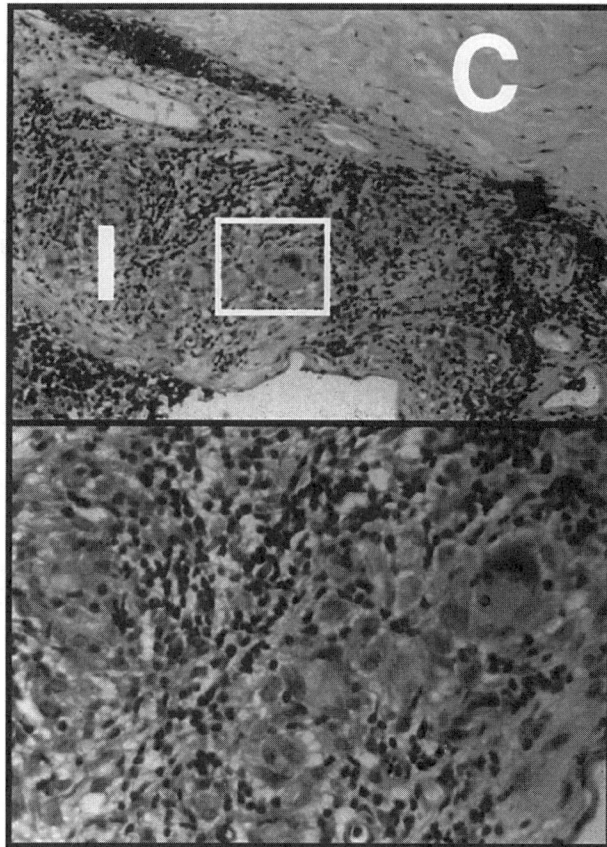

Fig. 17-4. *Top,* An eye with chronic granulomatous inflammation with the iris, **I**, adherent to the cornea, **C**, *Bottom,* High-power view *(inset)* revealing epithelioid cells and a granuloma surrounded by lymphocytes.

Regulatory Mechanisms of the Inflammatory Response

The difference between acute and chronic inflammation is the absence of spontaneous resolution of the latter. Resolution indicates that the inflammatory process can be regulated at the site.[24] Cessation of inflammation requires termination of cellular infiltration, necessitating the down-regulation of cell-adhesion molecules on endothelium and the disappearance of chemoattractants. The local synthesis and release of leukocyte mediators cease. Finally, the production of soluble factors by parenchymal cells within the tissue itself must return to normal. A number of speculations are suggested in Table 17-2 as potential mechanisms that determine whether inflammation resolves or becomes chronic.

Role of Pathogen. The most commonly cited mechanism leading to resolution is the removal of the triggering stimulus. Injection of labeled antigen into the conjunctiva or anterior chamber demonstrates that 99% of the antigen is cleared in a few hours.[104] Antigen deposited into the vitreous persists for much longer.[34] In animal models of immunogenic

TABLE 17-2   COMPARISON OF FACTORS LEADING TO RESOLUTION VERSUS CHRONIC INFLAMMATION

Resolution	Chronicity
Stimulus/antigen clearance Immune clearance by phagocytosis Degradation by enzymes	**Stimulus/antigen persistence** Intracellular infection Latency Sequestration Molecular mimicry and/or sensitization to autoantigens
Restoration of blood-eye barrier Exclusion of serum proteases, fibrin, and attachment factors	**Permanent loss of blood-eye barrier** Anatomic changes in endothelial cells or other intercellular tight junctions due to injury
Restoration of normal physiologic microenvironment Production of suppressive cytokines and neuropeptides by parenchymal tissues	**Loss of normal physiologic cell/tissue relationships** Persistent production of proinflammatory cytokines by parenchymal cells (endothelium, fibroblasts, ciliary body, or retinal pigment epithelia)
Downregulation of cell-adhesion molecules Termination of stimulatory cytokines	**Long-lived induction of cell-adhesion molecules and chemoattractants** Neovascularization and granulation tissue Tissue injury (peroxidation products) Lymphoid conversion (transformation)
Regenerative healing Repair injury and return to normal status	**Degeneration, atrophy, or reparative healing** Granulation tissue Neovascularization Vitreous gel liquefaction

inflammation, the inflammatory course is usually correlated with the clearance of antigen, and such clearance is quickly followed by resolution.[34]

In contrast, persistent infection can produce chronicity. Infectious agents have evolved several ingenious devices to escape elimination, such as sequestration, encystation, or glycocalyx (biofilm) formation.[77] Certain organisms produce inhibitory substances, thereby preventing elimination by the inflammatory response. For example, *Pseudomonas* is believed to elaborate molecules that are immunosuppressive. Some intracellular bacteria, such as mycobacteria, have substances that prevent fusion of the phagosome with the lysosome, thereby impeding the macrophage from killing the bacterium. Certain microorganisms might induce autoimmunity by molecular mimicry.

Role of Ocular Microenvironment. The immunoregulatory interactions of specific tissue sites with the immune and inflammatory responses can alter the pattern of inflammation. Each tissue site, especially various sites within the eye, is a different microenvironment that contributes certain attributes to the underlying inflammatory reaction. For example, the anterior chamber demonstrates immune privilege—defined as the survival of tissue grafts or tumors within the eye—when a similar graft is rejected elsewhere.[30] Although the mechanism of privilege is complex, the downregulation

of immune effectors by immunosuppressive cytokines within the eye is one physiologic component.

The anterior uveal tissue and aqueous humor contain large quantities of immunosuppressive factors such as TGF-β[14,28] and certain neuropeptides (α-MSH[94] or VIP[95]). Upon exposure to these factors or to fluids containing a cocktail of these factors (such as aqueous humor), macrophages are partially prevented from becoming activated and T lymphocytes are blocked from proliferation and cytokine synthesis. In turn, the physiologic inhibition of these inflammatory effector cells renders the anterior chamber less responsive to certain immune-mediated triggers of inflammation.[31] Delayed hypersensitivity immune responses are downmodulated, and the eye is protected from immunogenic inflammation. Certain stimuli (primarily nonspecific, non-immune-triggered inflammation[31]) may antagonize the effects of these immunosuppressive factors, thereby abrogating immune privilege and rendering the anterior chamber susceptible to delayed hypersensitivity. Thus environmental insults, such as trauma, infection, and surgery, may temporarily deplete the anterior chamber of immune privilege. Perhaps if ocular parenchymal cells could synthesize and release more immunosuppressive cytokines, the suppressor factors might function in paracrine fashion to downregulate the inflammatory response. The ability to manipulate local tissues to produce immunosuppressive factors ("paracrine immunosuppression") might be a novel approach to treating ocular inflammation.

Antiinflammatory Proteins. Local ocular production of the lipocortins and/or the antiflammins may be another instrument for local paracrine immunoregulation in the eye. Lipocortins are a family of proteins induced after treatment of certain cells with glucocorticosteroids, and they inhibit phospholipase A_2 from releasing arachidonic acid from cell membrane lipids.[42] Lipocortin induction is a potential physiologic device by which corticosteroids inhibit prostaglandin and leukotriene synthesis. Antiflammins are smaller peptides with sequence homology and functional similarity to the lipocortins.[21] The modulatory role of these proteins in ocular inflammation is unknown, but the antiinflammatory potential of local lipocortin or antiflammin production within the eye is very attractive.

Plasmin

Downregulatory cascades are used by the eye to terminate inflammation. Although altered vascular permeability and fibrin deposition are important components of conjunctival and intraocular inflammation, the plasmin cascade (which produces the clot-dissolving enzyme plasmin) is simultaneously activated and leads to the eventual dissolution of the clot. Plasminogen activators are present in normal aqueous humor, presumably produced locally by cells within the eye.

Cytokines

The mediators of inflammation generated within the inflamed site are sometimes immunosuppressive, which demonstrates the complexity of their interactions and paradoxic bifunctional behavior. Although PGE_2, nitric oxide, and other metabolites produced by macrophages or neutrophils during inflammation cause tissue injury, these compounds can also inhibit the activation of T cells or macrophages in vitro.[5,57] Proinflammatory cytokines (such as IFN-γ) can contribute to downregulation of inflammation and, paradoxically, IFN-γ can be immunosuppressive when administered in some sites. Even though local treatment of the anterior chamber with low doses of IFN-γ overrides certain aspects of immune privilege and renders the anterior chamber more susceptible to delayed hypersensitivity responses, it simultaneously causes the ciliary body to produce more PGE_2.[91] Accordingly, a proinflammatory stimulus is partially balanced by a (perhaps) less effective immunosuppressive one.

Additional T cell-derived cytokines can downregulate other T cells. IFN-γ can downregulate the activation of certain T cell subsets (especially the Th2 subset), resulting in a preponderance of Th1 type of T cells within the lesion and the exacerbation of delayed hypersensitivity.[70] Conversely, IL-4 or IL-10 production by Th2 subset can downregulate cytokine production by the Th1 subset, producing the inverse outcome.[70] Thus complex regulation of inflammation and immunity is occurring within the inflamed site, but these interactions might provide clues for novel therapeutic approaches.

Lymphocytes

Several authors have suggested the concept of the "eye as a lymph node,"[58] but the capacity of ocular tissue to undergo physiologic transformation into "lymphoid" tissue has not been established. Lymph follicles, or even granulomata, are highly organized structures that are tightly regulated and do not occur spontaneously in tissues without stimulus and direction.

In many respects, some chronically inflamed eyes resemble lymph follicles or granulomata. Intraocular T cell activation, B cell activation, and antibody formation occur in uveitis, supporting the "lymphoid" nature of the inflamed eye. Several parenchymal cell types, such as Mueller cells and retinal pigment epithelium, may present antigens to T cells under some conditions.[81] If the concept of the chronically inflamed eye as a "lymphoid structure" is true, this conversion indicates a transformation into a proinflammatory tissue that might sustain inflammation.

Role of Blood-Eye Barrier. Restoration of the intact blood-eye barrier is suspected by clinicians to be another mechanism for downregulating inflammation. Flare, a clinical sign of increased protein caused by altered vascular permeability, is one of the important clinical signs of inflammation.[49] The persistence of plasma-derived factors within ocular tissues indicates that the eye has not returned to normal. For example, the extremely large blood-borne protease inhibitor α_2-macroglobulin is essentially excluded from aqueous humor by the normal blood-eye barrier.[108] High concentrations of α_2-macroglobulin, however, occur in the aqueous humor of eyes with breakdown of the blood-eye barrier in the absence of inflammation.[93] α_2-Macroglobulin not only transports bioactive IL-1 into the eye (thereby promoting inflammation),[18] but α_2-macroglobulin also binds to and neutralizes locally produced TGF-β (thereby preventing local paracrine immunosuppression).[55] Thus the presence of persistent, altered permeability and flare possibly indicates that the microenvironment is tilted toward a proinflammatory status, perhaps causing the eye to be at greater risk for recurrent inflammation.[7,9] The contribution of altered vascular permeability to recurrent ocular inflammation occurs in an experimental model for immune-complex-associated uveitis.[37]

Interplay Between Healing and Persistence of Inflammation

The reparative response to inflammation can lead to anatomic and physiologic alterations that contribute to chronicity. New blood vessel growth is both a sequela and a cause of chronic inflammation.

Keratitis. New vessel growth in the cornea is often the result of chronic inflammation, particularly in the case of stromal vessels that grow in response to infection (interstitial keratitis).[90] Vascularized corneas are prone to inflammatory events, mainly allograft rejection after corneal transplantation. New vessels are permeable, allow plasma proteins to leak into the tissue, and express higher levels of cell-adhesion molecules.

Uveitis. Pars plana neovascularization, in association with a reparative "granulation response," is occasionally the sequelae of chronic inflammation in intermediate uveitis.[72] An organized "snowbank" (consisting of fibrous tissue, blood vessels, and granulomatous inflammation) sustains chronic inflammation and causes permanent alteration of the blood-ocular barrier. Perhaps the snowbank is analogous to pannus in chronic experimental arthritis, in which the inflammatory reaction becomes unresponsive to immunomodulation even though T cells initiated the response.

Vitreitis. The importance of physiologic and anatomic changes in the vitreous gel during inflammation remains controversial. During inflammation the vitreous gel often becomes infiltrated with leukocytes that are centered in the anterior uvea or retina. The gel can retain antigen, provide extracellular matrix molecules for sustaining lymphocyte activation, sequester and store proinflammatory mediators, and prevent the permeation of topical drugs throughout the eye. Surgical removal of the vitreous has been advocated as a therapeutic procedure. Conversely, the intact gel might provide a relative barrier to cellular transmigration and activation, because it contains high levels of the inhibitory cytokine TGF-β.[106] Recurrent bouts of vitreous inflammation produce liquefaction of the hyaluronic acid gel, the consequences of which are unclear.

Sequelae of Ocular Inflammation. The physiologic consequences of the chronic exposure to inflammatory mediators on the important secretory and neural elements within the eye has not been characterized.

Chronic exposure of the uveal tract to inflammatory mediators is unknown. Cultured ciliary body epithelia respond to cytokines and mediators by altering functional activity, suggesting an "activated metabolism" and transdifferentiation.[44] Abnormal expression of cell surface markers and ICAM can also be induced. The clinical consequences of these experimental observations is uncertain, but if the ciliary body epithelia became "transdifferentiated" in vivo, inappropriate local production of inflammatory mediators, hypotony, cyclitic membrane formation, and other complications would follow.

The physiologic effects of chronic exposure to cytokines and other mediators on distant, uninflamed tissue must also be considered. For example, macular edema is one of the most important causes of visual loss in anterior uveitis. Inflammatory mediators released in the anterior segment presumably diffuse through the vitreous to act on the retina, leading to leakage and intraretinal fluid accumulation in the macula.

REFERENCES

1. Abbas AK, Lichtman AH, Pober JS: *Molecular and cellular immunology,* Philadelphia, 1991, WB Saunders.
2. Acha-Orbea H, Palmer E: Mls-a retrovirus exploits the immune system, *Immunol Today* 12:356-361, 1991.
3. Adams DO: The granulomatous response, *Am J Pathol* 84:164-191, 1976.
4. Akbar AN, Salmon M, Ianossy G: The synergy between naive and memory T cells during activation, *Immunol Today* 12:184-188, 1991.
5. Al-Ramadi BK, Miesler JJ, Huang D, Eisenstein TK: Immunosuppression induced by nitric oxide and its inhibition by interleukin-4, *Eur J Immunol* 22:2249-2254, 1992.
6. Andrews BS, Pelts V, McIntosh J: Circulating immune complexes in acute uveitis, *Arthritis Rheum* 20:106-110, 1976.
7. Aronson SB, Elliot JH: *Ocular inflammation,* St Louis, 1972, CV Mosby.
8. Aronson SB, McMaster PRB: Passive transfer of experimental allergic uveitis, *Arch Ophthalmol* 91:60-65, 1971.
9. Aronson SB, Moore TB, O'Day DM: The effect of structural alterations on anterior ocular inflammation, *Am J Ophthalmol* 70:886-893, 1970.
10. Asano M, Nakane A, Minagawa T: Endogenous gamma interferon is essential in granuloma formation induced by glycolipid-containing mycolic acid in mice, *Infect Immun* 61:2872-2878, 1993.
11. Atherton SS, Altman NH, Streilein JW: Histopathologic study of herpes virus-induced retinitis in athymic BALB/c mice: evidence for an immunopathogenic process, *Curr Eye Res* 8:1179-1186, 1989.
12. Augustin AA, Julius MH, Cosenza H: Antigen-specific stimulation and trans-stimulation of T cells in long term culture, *Eur J Immunol* 9:665-670, 1979.
13. Ben-Zvi A, Rodrigues MM, IG Schiffman E: Induction of ocular inflammation by synthetic mediators, *Arch Ophthalmol* 99:1436-1444, 1981.
14. Benson JL, Niederkom JY: In situ suppression of delayed-type hypersensitivity: another mechanism for sustaining the immune privilege of the anterior chamber, *Immunology* 74:153-159, 1991.
15. Bevilacqua MP, Gimbrone MA: Inducible endothelial functions in inflammation and coagulation, *Semin Thromb Hemost* 13:425-433, 1987.
16. Bhakdi S, Tranum-Jensen J: Complement lysis: a hole is a hole, *Immunol Today* 12:318-320, 1991.
17. Bohack GA, Fast DJ, Nelson RD, Schlevert PM: Staphylococcal and streptococcal pyrogenic toxins involved in toxic shock syndrome and related illnesses, *Crit Rev Microbiol* 17:251-272, 1990.
18. Borth W, Scheer B, Urbansky A et al.: Binding of IL-1β to α-macroglobulins and release by thioredoxin, *J Immunol* 145:3747-3754, 1990.
19. Byers B, Kimura SJ: Uveitis after death of a larva in the vitreous, *Am J Ophthalmol* 77:63-66, 1974.
20. Carrasco L: *Mechanism of viral toxicity in mammalian cells,* Boca Raton, 1987, CRC Press.
21. Chan C-C, Ming N, Miele L et al.: Antiflammins: inhibition of endotoxin-induced uveitis in Lewis rats. In Usui M, Ohno S, Aoki K, editors: *Ocular immunology today,* 467-470, Amsterdam, 1990, Elsevier Science.
22. Cohen JJ: Apoptosis, *Immunol Today* 14:126-130, 1993.
23. Colditz I, Zwahlen R, Dewald B, Baggiolini M: In vivo inflammatory activity of neutrophilactivating factor, a novel chemotactic peptide derived from human monocytes, *Am J Pathol* 134:755-760, 1989.
24. Colten HR: Tissue-specific regulation of inflammation, *J Appl Physiol* 72:1-7, 1992.
25. Cotran RS, Kumar V, Robbins SL: *Robbins pathological basis of disease,* ed 4, Philadelphia, 1985, WB Saunders.
26. Cousins SW: T cell activation in different intraocular compartments. In *Modern developments in ophthalmology,* 23:150-155, 1992.
27. Cousins SW, Guss RB, Howes EL, Rosenbaum JT: Endotoxin-induced uveitis in the rat: observations on altered vascular permeability, clinical findings and histology, *Exp Eye Res* 39:665-676, 1984.
28. Cousins SW, McCabe MM, Danielpoor D, Streielin JW: Identification of transforming growth factor-β as an immunosuppressive factor in aqueous humor, *Invest Ophthalmol Vis Sci* 32:2201-2211, 1991.

29. Cousins SW, Rosenbaum JT, Guss RB, Egbert PR: Ocular albumin fluorometric quantitation of endotoxin-induced vascular permeability, *Infect Immun* 36:730-736, 1982.

30. Cousins SW, Streilein JW: Immune privilege and its regulation by immunosuppressive growth factors in aqueous humor. In Usui M, Ohno S, Aoki K, editors: *Ocular immunology today,* 81-84, Amsterdam, 1990, Elsevier Science.

31. Cousins SW, Trattler WB, Streilein JW: Immune privilege and suppression of immunogenic inflammation in the anterior chamber, *Curr Eye Res* 10:287-297, 1991.

32. Crawford JP, Movat HZ, Ranadive N, Hay JB: Pathways to inflammation induced by immune complexes, *Fed Proc* 41:2583-2587, 1982.

33. Dvorak HF, Galli SJ, Dvorak AM: Cellular and vascular manifestations of cell-mediated immunity, *Hum Pathol* 17:122-137, 1986.

34. Fernando AN: Immunological studies with I[131] labeled antigen in experimental uveitis, *Arch Ophthalmol* 63:515-539, 1960.

35. Forrester JV, Worgul BV, Merriam GR: Endotoxin-induced uveitis in the rat, *Graefes Arch Clin Exp Ophthalmol* 213:221-233, 1980.

36. Fox A: Role of bacterial debris in inflammation of the joint and eye, *APMIS* 98:957-968, 1990.

37. Gamble CN, Aronson SB, Brescia FS: Experimental uveitis. II. The pathogenesis of recurrent immunologic (Auer) uveitis, *Arch Ophthalmol* 84:331-341, 1970.

38. Garcia JH, Anderson ML: Physiology of cerebral ischemia, *Crit Rev Neurobiol* 4:303-324, 1989.

39. Gell PGH, Hinde IT: Observations and histology of the Arthus reaction and its relation to other known types of skin hypersensitivity, *Int Arch Appl Immunol* 5:23-54, 1954.

40. Germuth FG, Maumenee AE, Senterfit LB, Pollack AD: Immunohistologic studies on antigen-antibody reactions in the avascular cornea. I. Reaction in rabbits sensitized to foreign proteins, *J Exp Med* 115:99-925, 1962.

41. Gill DM: Toxins. In Gorbich SL, Bartlett JG, Blacklo NR, editors: *Infectious disease,* 17-22, Philadelphia, 1992, WB Saunders.

42. Goulding NJ, Guyre PM: Regulation of inflammation by lipocortins, *Immunol Today* 13:295-297, 1992.

43. Greenwood J: The blood-retinal barrier in experimental autoimmune uveoretinitis (EAU): a review, *Curr Eye Res* 11(supp):25-32, 1992.

44. Helbig H, Kittredge KL, Coca-Prados M et al.: Mammalian ciliary-body epithelial cells in culture produce transforming growth factor-β, *Graefes Arch Clin Exp Ophthalmol* 229:84-91, 1991.

45. Henson PM, John RB: Tissue injury in inflammation: oxidants, proteases and cationic proteins, *J Clin Invest* 79:669-693, 1987.

46. Herbort CP, Okumura A, Mochizaki M: Endotoxin-induced uveitis in the rat: a study of the role of inflammatory mediators, *Graefes Arch Clin Exp Ophthalmol* 226:553-558, 1988.

47. Herbort CP, Okumura A, Mochizaki M: Immunopharmacologic analysis of endotoxin-induced uveitis in the rat, *Exp Eye Res* 48:693-705, 1989.

48. Herman DC, Suffredini AF, Parillo JE, Plaestine AG: Ocular permeability after systemic administration of endotoxin in humans, *Curr Eye Res* 10:121-126, 1991.

49. Hogan MJ, Kimura SJ, Thygeson P: Signs and symptoms of uveitis. I. Anterior uveitis, *Am J Ophthalmol* 47:155-170, 1959.

50. Howes EL: Basic principles. In Spencer WH, editor: *Ocular pathology: an atlas and textbook,* 1986, Philadelphia, WB Saunders.

51. Howes EL, Aronson SB, McKay DG: Ocular vascular permeability-effect of systemic administration of bacterial endotoxin, *Arch Ophthalmol* 84:360-367, 1970.

52. Howes EL, McKay DG: Comparison of the ocular effects of circulating endotoxin and immune complexes, *J Immunol* 114:734-737, 1975.

53. Howes EL, McKay DG, Aronson SB: An ultrastructural study of the ciliary processes in the rabbit following systemic administration of bacterial endotoxin, *Lab Invest* 3:217-228, 1971.

54. Howes EL, Rosenbaum JT: LPS tolerance inhibits eye inflammation. II. Preliminary study on the mechanism, *Arch Ophthalmol* 103:261-265, 1985.

55. James K: Interactions between cytokines and alpha 2-macroglobulin, *Immunol Today* 11:63-66, 1990.

56. Joiner KA: Virulence factors. In Gorbich SL, Bartlett JG, Blacklo NR, editors: *Infectious disease,* 23-29, Philadelphia, 1992, WB Saunders.

57. Jordan ML, Simmons RL: A reevaluation of the role of prostaglandin E2 as an immunoregulator, *Transplant Proc* 19:3388-3390, 1987.

58. Kaplan HJ: Immunologic insights into the eye and uveitis. In Krause-Maciw E, O'Connor GR, editors: *Uveitis: pathophysiology and therapy,* Thieme Medical Publishers, New York, 1983.

59. Kaufman SHE, Vath U, Thole JER et al.: Enumeration of T cell reactive with *Mycobacterium tuberculosis* organisms and specific recombinant mycobacterial 64-kD protein, *Eur J Immunol* 17:351-359, 1987.

60. Klein J: *Immunology,* Boston, 1990, Blackwell Scientific.

61. Knisely TL, Lukenbach MW, Fischer BJ, Niederkorn JY: Destructive and nondestructive patterns of immune rejection of syngeneic ocular tumors, *J Immunol* 138:4515-4522, 1987.

62. Kovacs EJ: Fibrogenic cytokine: the role of immune mediators in the development of scar tissue, *Immunol Today* 12:17-23, 1991.

63. Kreger AS, Gray LL: Purification of *Pseudomonas aeruginosa* proteins and microscopic characterization of pseudomonal protein-induced rabbit corneal damage, *Infect Immun* 19:630-638, 1978.

64. Li T, Fox K, Fox A, Pakalnis V: Recurrent anterior uveitis induced by multiple systemic injections of muramyl dipeptide, *Exp Eye Res* 57:79-87, 1993.

65. Lynn WA, Golenbock DT: Lipopolysaccharide antagonists, *Immunol Today* 13:271-275, 1992.

66. Marrack P, Kappler J: The staphylococcal enterotoxins and their relatives, *Science* 248:707-711, 1990.

67. Meisler DM, Mandelbaum S: *Propionibacterium*-associated endophthalmitis after extracapsular cataract extraction, *Ophthalmology* 96:54-60, 1988.

68. Mondino BJ, Rabin BS, Kessler E et al.: Corneal rings with gram-negative bacteria, *Arch Ophthalmol* 95:2222-2227, 1977.

69. Morrison DC, Ulevitch RJ: The effects of bacterial endotoxins on host mediation systems, *Am J Pathol* 93:525-617, 1978.

70. Mosmann T, Coffman RC: TH1 and TH2 cells: different patterns of lymphockine secretion lead to different functional properties, *Annu Rev Immunol* 7:145-173, 1989.

71. Nathanson C, Eichenholz PW, Dann RL: Endotoxin and TNF challenges in dogs simulate the cardiovascular profile of human septic shock, *J Exp Med* 169:823-832, 1989.

72. Nussenblatt RB, Palestine AG: *Uveitis: fundamentals and clinical practice,* 2nd ed, St. Louis, Mosby Year Book, 1995.

73. Ormerod LD, Ruoff KL, Wasson PJ et al.: Infectious crystalline keratopathy: role of nutritionally variant streptococci and other bacterial factors, *Ophthalmology* 98:159-169, 1991.

74. Parks C, Pakalnis A, Kufoy EA et al.: Modulation of the blood-aqueous barrier by gram-positive and gram-negative cell wall components in the rat and rabbit, *Exp Eye Res* 50:189-195, 1990.

75. Pearson CM, Chang YH: Adjuvant disease: pathology and immune reactivity, *Ann Rheum Dis* 38(suppl):102-110, 1979.

76. Pepose JS, Holland GN, Nestor MS et al.: Acquired immunodeficiency syndrome: pathogenic mechanisms, *Ophthalmology* 92:75-84, 1985.

77. Pincus SH, Rosa PA, Spangrude GJ, Heineman JA: The interplay of microbes and their hosts, *Immunol Today* 13:471-473, 1992.

78. Rahi AHS, Tripathi RC: Anatomy of the reverse passive Arthus reaction in the cornea: a preliminary communication, *Mod Prob Ophthalmol* 16:155-170, 1976.

79. Ramsay AJ, Ruby J, Ramshaw IA: A case for cytokines as effector molecules in the resolution of virus infection, *Immunol Today* 14:155-157, 1993.

80. Rao NA: Role of oxygen free radicals in retinal damage associated with experimental uveitis, *Trans Am Ophthalmol Soc* 89:797-850, 1990.

81. Roberge FG, Caspi RR, Chan CC, Nussenblatt RB: Inhibition of T lymphocyte proliferation by retinal glial Muller cells: reversal of inhibition by glucocorticoids, *J Autoimmunity* 4:307-314, 1991.

82. Rosenbaum JT: Why HLA-B27: an analysis of two animal models, *Ann Intern Med* 21:261-263, 1981.

83. Rosenbaum JT, Cousins SW: Uveitis and arthritis: experimental models and clinical correlates, *Semin Arthritis Rheum* 11:383-389, 1982.

84. Rosenbaum JT, McDevitt HO, Guss RB, Egbert PR: Endotoxin-induced uveitis in rats as a model for human disease, *Nature* 286:611-613, 1980.

85. Scherzer H, Ward PA: Lung injury produced by immune complexes of varying composition, *J Immunol* 121:947-952, 1978.

86. Schifferli JA, Ng YC, Peters DK: The role of complement and its receptor in the elimination of immune complex, *New Engl J Med* 315:482-495, 1986.

87. Sheffield EA: The granulomatous inflammatory response, *J Pathol* 160:1-2, 1990.

88. Singh VK, Yamaki K, Donoso LA, Shinohara T: Yeast histone H3-induced experimental autoimmune uveitis, *J Immunol* 142:1512-1517, 1989.

89. Skrzpypczak KE: Typhoid endotoxin in the treatment of uveitis and other ocular inflammations, *Am J Ophthalmol* 64:937-946, 1969.

90. Smolin G, Thoft RA: *The cornea: scientific foundations and clinical practice*, ed 2, Boston, 1987, Little, Brown.

91. Streilein JW, Cousins SW, Bradley D: Effect of intraocular gamma-interferon on the immunoregulatory properties of iris and ciliary body cells, *Invest Ophthalmol Vis Sci* 33:2304-2315, 1992.

92. Taniguchi T: Regulation of cytokine gene expression, *Annu Rev Immunol* 6:439-464, 1988.

93. Taylor AW, Streilein JW, Cousins SW: Alpha$_2$-macroglobulin may neutralize ocular immune privilege, *FASEB J* (suppl):1042, 1992.

94. Taylor AW, Streilein JW, Cousins SW: Identification of alpha melanocyte stimulating hormone as a possible immunoregulatory factor in aqueous humor, *Curr Eye Res* 12:1199-1206, 1992.

95. Taylor AW, Streilein JW, Cousins SW: Neuropeptides in aqueous humor may regulate T-lymphocytes within the eye, *Invest Ophthalmol Vis Sci* 33(suppl):1283, 1993.

96. Tesh VL, O'Brien AD: The pathogenic mechanism of shiga toxin and the shiga-like toxins, *Mol Microbiol* 5:1817-1822, 1991.

97. van der Broek M: Streptococcal cell wall-induced polyarthritis in the rat, *APMIS* 97:861-897, 1989.

98. van Eden W: Heat-shock proteins as immunogenic bacterial antigens with the potential to induce and promote autoimmunity, *Immunol Rev* 121:5-28, 1991.

99. Waksman BH, Bullington SJ: Studies of other lesions induced in rats by injection of mycobacterial adjuvant. II. Lesions of the eye, *Arch Ophthalmol* 64:751-762, 1960.

100. Waters RV, TG T, Jones GH: Uveitis induction in the rabbit by muramyl dipeptide, *Infect Immun* 51:816-825, 1986.

101. Weinstein L, Swartz MN: Pathogenic properties of microorganisms. In Sodeman WA, Sodeman TM, editors: *Sodeman's patholophysiologic mechanisms of disease*, 523-539, Philadelphia, 1985, WB Saunders.

102. Weisman G: Inflammation: Historical perspective. In Gallin JI, Goldstein IM, Snyderman R, editors: *Inflammation: basic principles and clinical correlates*, 5-9, New York, 1992, Raven Press.

103. Weiss SS: Tissue destruction by neutrophils, *New Engl J Med* 320:365-376, 1989.

104. Wilbanks GA, Streilein JW: The differing patterns of antigen release and local retention following anterior chamber and intravenous inoculation of soluble antigen: the eye is an antigen depot, *Reg Immunol* 2:390-389, 1989.

105. Wong VG, Anderson RR, McMaster PRB: Endogenous immune uveitis, *Arch Ophthalmol* 85:93-102, 1971.

106. Yoshitushi T, Shichi H: Immunosuppressive factors in procine vitreous body, *Curr Eye Res* 10:1141-1144, 1991.

107. Ziegler-Heitbrock HWL, Ulevitch RJ: CD14: cell surface receptor and differentiation marker, *Immunol Today* 14:121-125, 1993.

108. Zirm M: Proteins in aqueous humor, *Adv Ophthalmol* 40:100-172, 1980.

18 Structural Consequences of Ocular Infection

DAVID J. WILSON, EDWARD L. HOWES JR.

The residual effects of ocular infections depend on the tissue(s) involved, the amount of disruption of normal tissue integrity, and the subsequent restoration attempts. The disruption of normal tissues is, in turn, dependent on the quantity and nature of the infectious agent and the accompanying inflammatory response. The degree of acute tissue disturbance affects the extent of regeneration and repair. In certain circumstances, such as in cicatricial diseases of the conjunctiva and chronic low-grade intraocular inflammatory processes, reparation efforts appear to be the primary clinical problem.

The eye is profoundly affected by minor alterations in structure. This characteristic originates from the need for optical transparency and critical alignment of intraocular structures. Ocular tissues must be maintained in the proper position by a protective outer layer and a stable intraocular pressure. Outside of trauma, infectious diseases most threaten the structure of the eye.

Structural alterations are caused by the infectious agent and by the host response to the infection. Viruses are capable of direct cell infection and destruction. Cytomegalovirus and herpes simplex virus cause cytopathic cell injury, which involves the proliferation of these agents within the cells and eventually leads to the death of the host cell. Bacterial exotoxins may also directly cause cell death. The classic example of this bacterial injury is that caused by the alpha toxin (a lecithinase) of *Clostridia perfringens*. The structural damage ensuing from direct cell injury can be profound (Fig. 18-1).

Infectious agents generally result in direct alterations in the extracellular matrix of ocular tissues. Bacteria, fungi, and parasites produce various enzymes that help them spread through tissue. Parasitic organisms that migrate through ocular tissues leave a path of tissue destruction (Fig. 18-2).

Despite the importance of the direct effects of the infectious agents in producing the structural alterations associated with ocular infections, most damage is indirect and dependent on the inflammatory response to the infection. This response not only reflects the virulence of the infectious agent but also the immunologic status and inflammatory capabilities of the host. With some acute infections, inflammation may either be diminished or enhanced, depending on preexistent immunity or development of an immune response during the infection. With indolent and chronic infections, the immune response often perpetuates inflammation through immunopathologic mechanisms that involve acute hypersensitivity, antibody-directed injury, immune-complex formation, and/or cell-mediated hypersensitivity. Each of these devices may have different effects on tissue disruption, perpetuation of inflammation, and subsequent repair mechanisms. Postinflammatory changes vary, depending on the nature of the inflammatory response.

During inflammation, the interaction between the tissue extracellular matrix and various growth factors as well as cytokines determines tissue repair or disease progression.[14] Within an infected tissue the spatial and temporal expression of growth factors and cytokines may vary along with the expression of integrins, fibronectins, proteoglycans, and different types of collagen.[14]

In the eye and the central nervous system, astrocytic and fibroblast proliferation plus associated gliosis and fibrosis are important mechanisms of repair. At the same time, epithelial cells regenerate, and their proliferation (whether it be epidermis, corneal epithelium, or pigmented and nonpigmented epithelia within the eye) adds to the complexity of the response. These interactions between connective tissues and epithelia are only partially understood.

The postinfectious, structural changes that occur depend on the type of inflammation. The principal patterns of ocular inflammation include chronic edema, necrotizing inflammation, acute and suppurative inflammation, mononuclear inflammation, and chronic inflammation with scarring. Structural changes may also result from therapeutic interventions.

EDEMA

Edema is a widespread component of the inflammatory response that accompanies infection. It is generally the con-

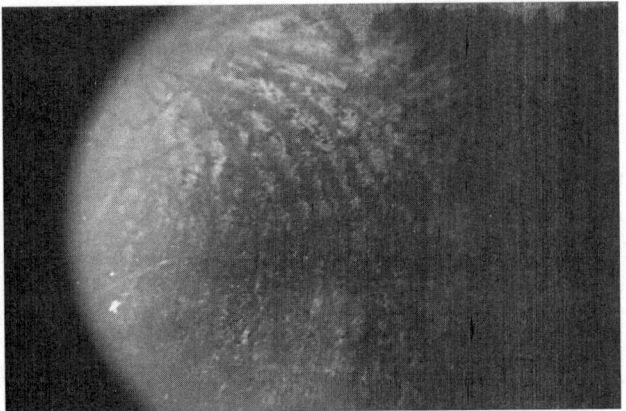

A

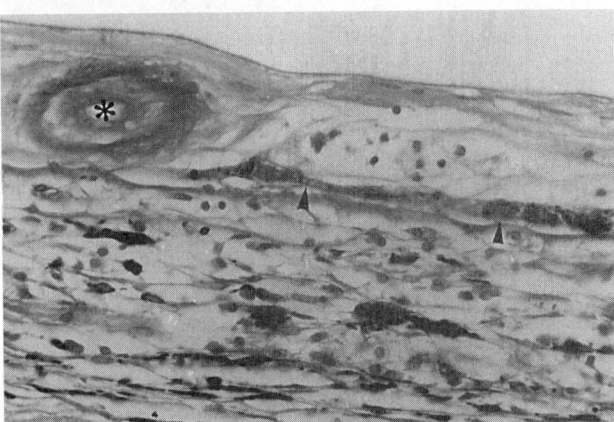

B

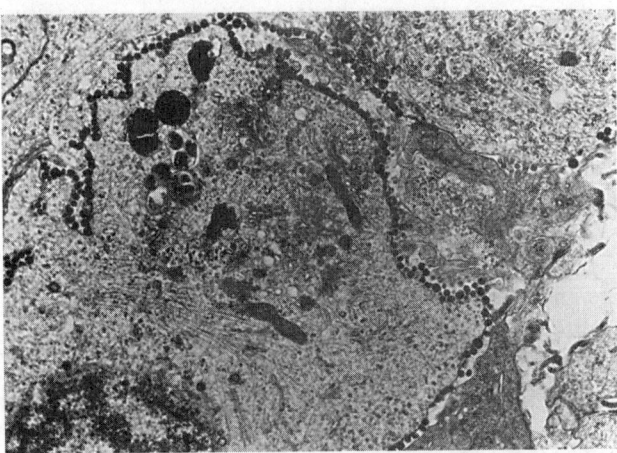

C

Fig. 18-1. Untreated CMV retinitis. **A,** The retina is markedly thinned and the retinal vessels are atrophic. There is RPE hyperplasia and the choroidal vessels are prominent. **B,** The retina has been reduced to a thin gliotic scar, and none of the normal retinal layers are identifiable. An acellular retinal vessel is present *(asterisk).* The RPE *(arrowheads)* is intact and slightly hyperplastic. There is a mild chronic inflammatory infiltrate in the choroid. **C,** Viral particles *(arrowheads)* on the surface of a photoreceptor cell in a patient with CMV retinitis. Same patient as illustrated in Figure 18-15.

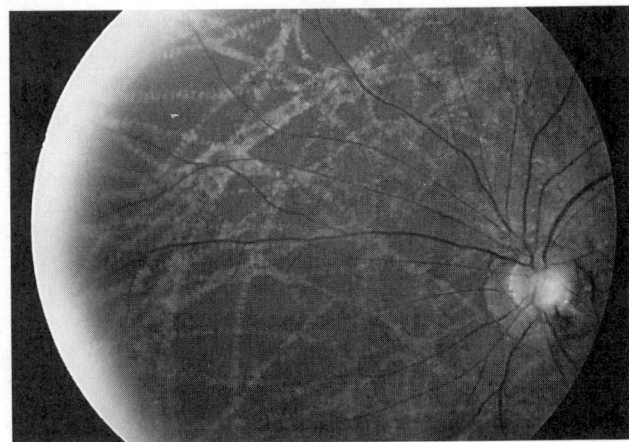

Fig. 18-2. Ophthalmomyiasis. Subretinal tracts produced by a migrating fly larva.

sequence of increased vascular permeability in reply to various vasoactive amines, neuropeptides, and prostaglandins[28] and may develop chronicity from vascular endothelial injury.[15,18] Edema in the eye becomes visually significant when it affects the cornea or the macula.

Corneal edema may be acute and transient, as in the edema accompanying herpes simplex epithelial keratitis (Fig. 18-3). Corneal edema may also become chronic, as in herpes simplex stromal keratitis or postinflammatory corneal endothelial damage. Corneal endothelial injury from acute infections is probably attributable to the presence of acute inflammatory cells in proximity to the corneal endothelium (Fig. 18-4). If this damage is severe enough, the endothelium will cease maintenance of normal corneal dehydration, and the corneal edema will become permanent.

Macular edema may occur when retinal infections take place in the vicinity of the macula or as a result of traction on the macula by inflammatory membranes (Fig. 18-5).

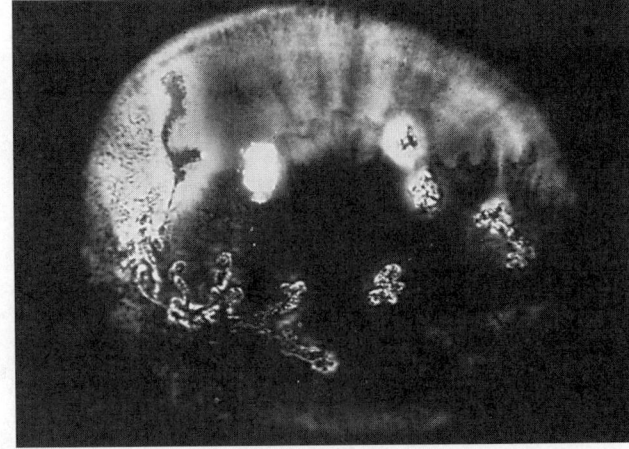

Fig. 18-3. Corneal edema at margins of dendrite secondary to epithelial herpes simplex virus infection.

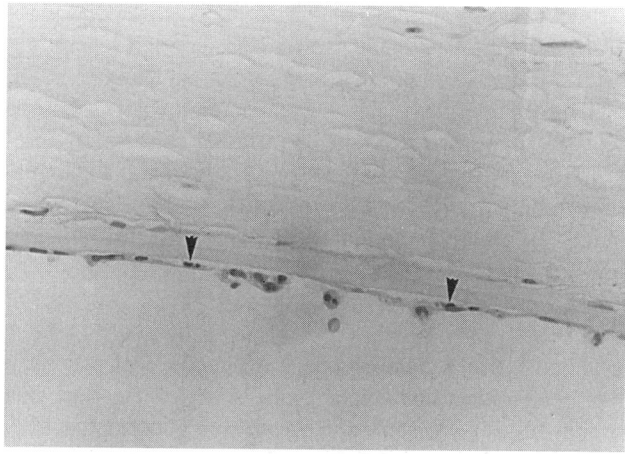

Fig. 18-4. Neutrophils present along the corneal endothelium. There are neutrophils present between the endothelium and Descemet's membrane *(arrowheads)* as well as along the anterior chamber surface of the endothelial cells.

CHANGES CAUSED BY INFLAMMATION

Necrotizing Inflammation

Cell and tissue destruction produces necrotizing inflammation. The direct cytopathic effect of cytomegalovirus and other viruses on the retina produces extensive necrosis. The end result of necrotizing retinitis is atrophy and gliosis. Often, only a thin glial membrane remains (Fig. 18-4). In acute toxoplasmic chorioretinitis, necrosis of the retina occurs which may, in part, be on an immunopathologic basis. In these conditions not only may the retina become atrophic and gliotic, but focal chorioretinal scarring can take place with proliferation of retinal pigment epithelium (Fig. 18-5).

Infectious agents may also engender injury by causing ischemia. Ischemia may be produced at the capillary level, as is characteristic of AIDS retinopathy (Fig. 18-6).[16,23] Ischemia may also be generated by the occlusion of larger vessels, as is typical of the occlusive vasculitis of ophthalmic zoster[21] or the vascular invasion of nonseptate, filamentous fungi during orbital mucormycosis (Fig. 18-7).[22]

Suppurative Inflammation

Suppurative inflammation is most apt to arise during acute bacterial keratitis, endophthalmitis, or orbital cellulitis. Abscess formation or ulceration with accompanying tissue destruction may also ensue. Although the infectious agents may directly affect the tissues,[20] many of the changes are secondary to the effects of leukocytes (particularly polymorphonuclear leukocytes). These cells produce various oxidants, proteases, and cationic proteins at the site of inflammation.[15] The exact role and the interaction of these different elements in the tissue injury produced by infection has not

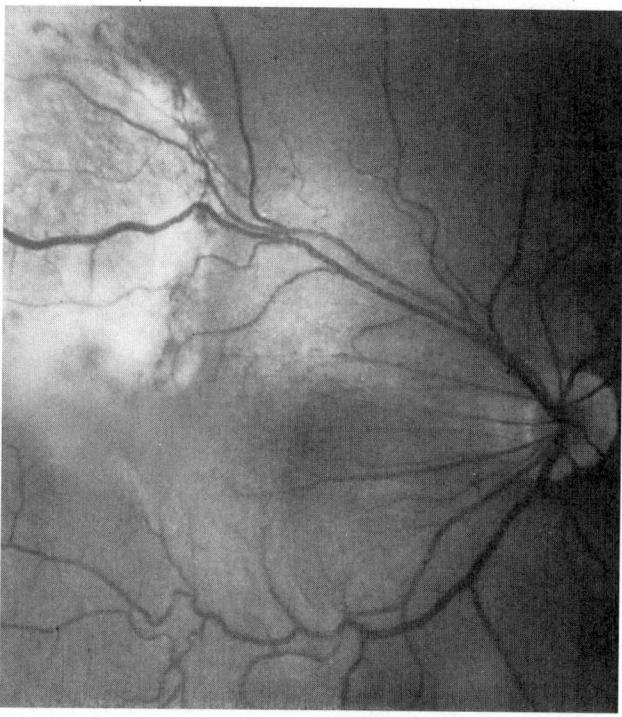

Fig. 18-5. Traction by a preretinal membrane resulting in distortion of the macula and macular edema in a patient with toxoplasmosis.

been fully clarified. Leukocytes exposed to microorganisms create abundant reactive oxygen species that, in addition to being microbicidal, damage ocular tissues.[15,17] Lysosomes contain very potent proteases that degrade collagen, basement membrane, elastic tissue, and fibrin and may also contribute to the tissue damage that accompanies infections.[18] Leukocytes also produce cationic proteins that can produce tissue injury as well as increase vascular permeability.[15]

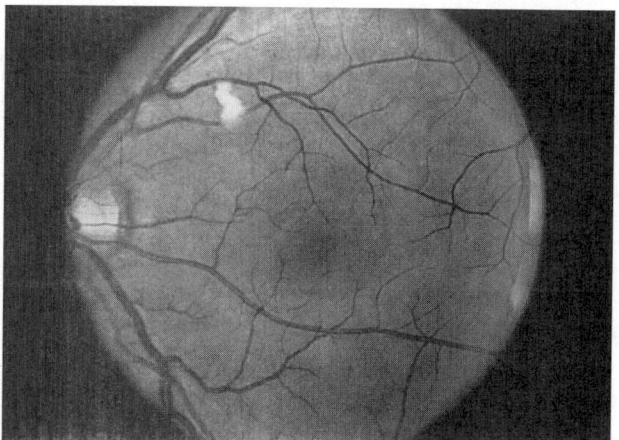

Fig. 18-6. AIDS retinopathy. Cotton wool spot is present superotemporal to the optic disc in a patient with AIDS.

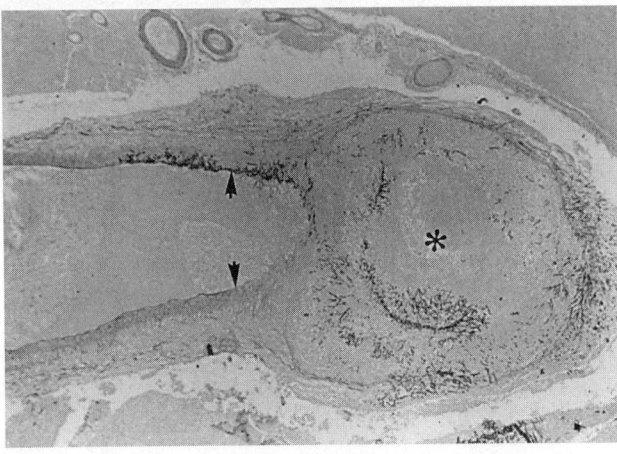

A

B

Fig. 18-7. Aspergillosis. Production of a mycotic aneurysm by vascular invasion of a medium-sized artery by *Aspergillus fumigatus* in a heart transplant patient. Vessel wall, *arrowheads.* Aneurysm, *asterisk* (**A,** Hematoxylin and eosin, **B,** Gomori methenamine silver).

If tissue injury is sufficient, a repair response is initiated that brings on fibroblastic proliferation and collagen deposition. This scarring may cause structural damage by rendering transparent ocular tissue opaque or by distorting the normal position of intraocular tissues. Reparative responses may be further complicated by intraocular hemorrhage and the byproducts of the clotting and fibrinolysis cascades.

Chronic Inflammation

Viruses, intracellular bacteria and parasites, immunologic responses, partially treated acute inflammations, and nonspecific low-grade inflammatory stimulation of unknown cause may undergo this form of inflammation. Within the eye this type of inflammation may have particu-

larly devastating results including subtle vascular and fibrovascular membranes, anterior and posterior syncheae, rubeosis iridis, and vitreous and retinal membranes. Cell-cell interactions, changes in extracellular matrix, and the release of cell products such as growth factors and cytokines are of major consequence in this subtle inflammation.[14] Early granuloma formation (for example in sarcoidosis) is an additional aspect of this inflammatory pattern.

SCARRING

Conjunctival inflammations, scarring and contractions of the lids, keloids and hypertrophic scars of the skin, and orbital fibrosis are some of the scarring patterns that may occur around the eye. Inflammatory masses may develop and lead to diagnostic confusion. Scarring of the conjunctiva arises after a variety of ocular infections. Trachoma results in progressive corneal injury caused by exposure and is a major cause of blindness in many parts of the world (Fig. 18-8).[3,8]

Corneal scarring is characteristic of most corneal infections. The main consequence of corneal stromal scarring is the loss of normal corneal clarity. The collagen laid down in the area of scarring lacks the regular lamellar arrangement of normal corneal collagen. Subepithelial and stromal scarring is a feature of many types of viral keratitis (Fig. 18-9). Salzmann modular degeneration and other forms of subepithelial fibrosis can follow several causes of corneal injury. Another important variety of corneal scarring is the formation of retrocorneal membranes. Retrocorneal membranes are typical of infections that result in corneal perforation, endothelial damage, and a pronounced inflammatory infiltrate in the anterior chamber (Fig. 18-10).[6]

Cyclitic membranes frequently form after severe intraoc-

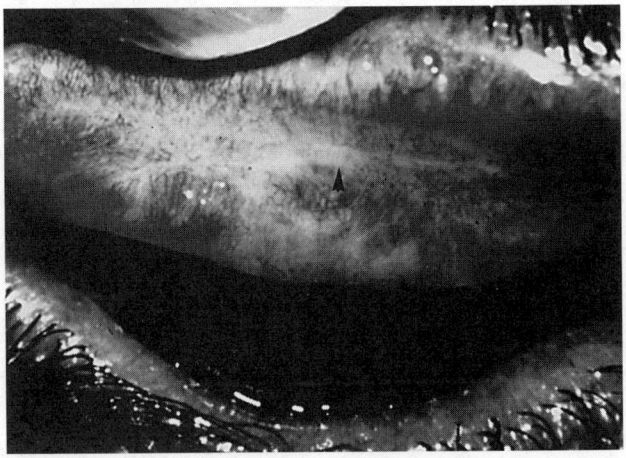

Fig. 18-8. Scarring of the palpebral conjunctiva of the eyelids caused by conjunctival infection with *Chlamydia trachomatis.* Arlt's line *(arrowhead).*

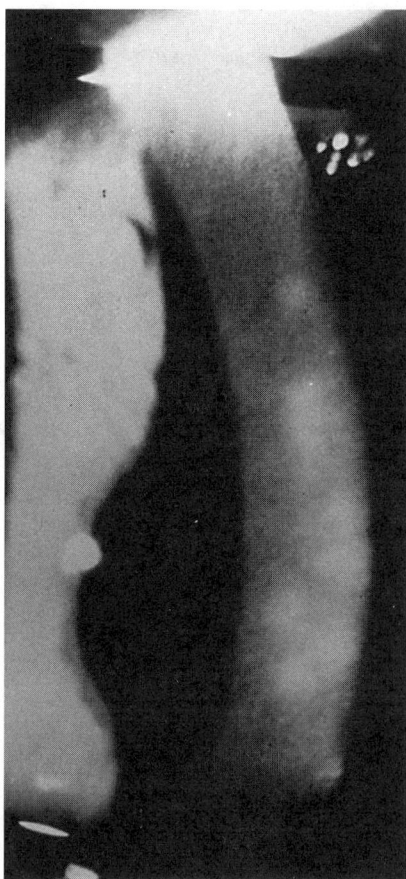

Fig. 18-9. Subepithelial scarring following viral keratitis.

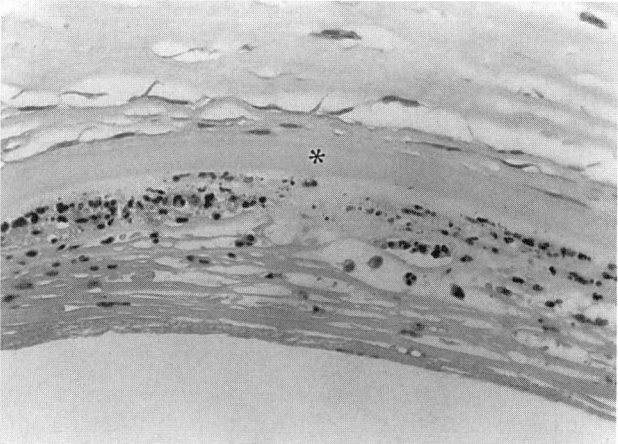

Fig. 18-10. Retrocorneal membrane after bacterial keratitis. There are numerous neutrophils remaining within the forming membrane. Descemet's membrane *(asterisk)* is devoid of endothelial cells.

ULCERATION, THINNING, AND PERFORATION

Loss of the extracellular matrix is a common consequence of infections of the cornea and sclera, and certain patterns of structural change may follow acute and chronic inflammations. When there is only partial-thickness ulceration of the cornea or sclera, healing will result in thinning. If these structures are thinned to the degree that they can no longer tolerate the intraocular pressure, a staphyloma may develop (Fig. 18-13). Thinning and/or staphyloma are clinically important when they conclude in an irregular refractive surface.

Perforation may occur acutely as an outcome of full thickness destruction of the cornea or the sclera, or sub-

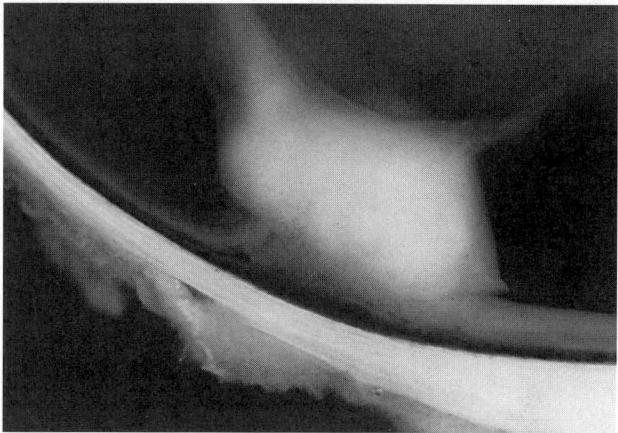

Fig. 18-11. Vitreous membrane extending from the surface of a site of fungal infection of the retina and choroid. Traction by membranes such as these can produce traction retinal detachments as well as traction-induced macular edema.

ular infections, such as bacterial endophthalmitis, and are fibroglial proliferations. These membranes may lead to loss of vision by producing a media opacity, but more importantly by causing progressive traction on the peripheral retina and the ciliary epithelium. Ciliary body detachment and/ or ciliary epithelial involvement with the cyclitic membrane may conclude in progressive hypotony and phthisis bulbi.

Preretinal membranes may also form as a result of intraocular infections. These membranes often span the vitreous cavity and connect one site of infection with others (Fig. 18-11). Many of the cell types present in these membranes contain intracellular actin filaments that enable these cells to exert traction on the tissue to which they are anchored.[13]

Chorioretinal scarring is the consequence of some infections, most notably histoplasmosis, and may produce persistent fibrovascular tissue.[19] This subretinal fibrovascular tissue may initiate structural damage by the production of recurrent hemorrhages (Fig. 18-12). Epidemiologic evidence suggests that this type of scarring may follow viral infections of the retina as well.[9,29]

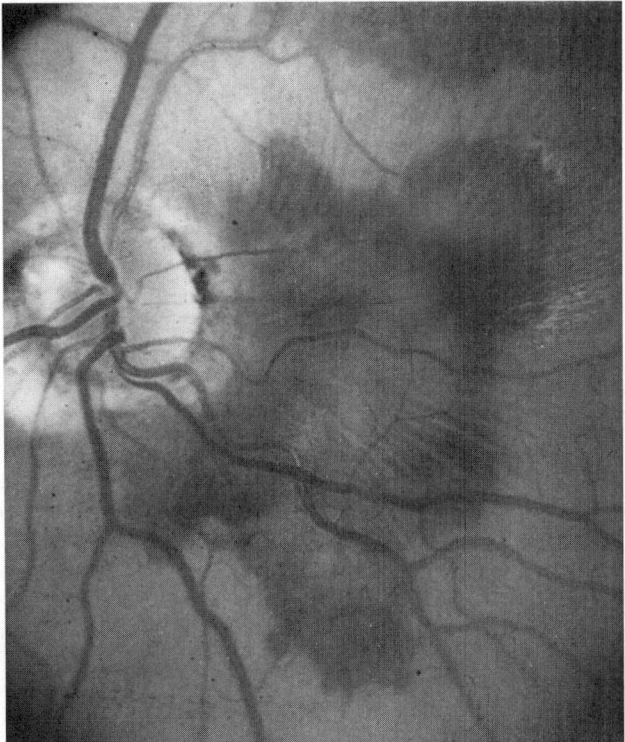

Fig. 18-12. Fibrovascular scar and subretinal hemorrhage in the macula and justapapillary retina of a patient with ocular histoplasmosis.

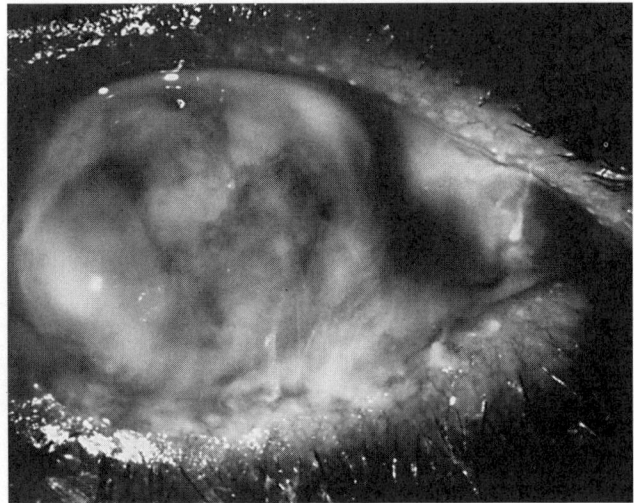

A

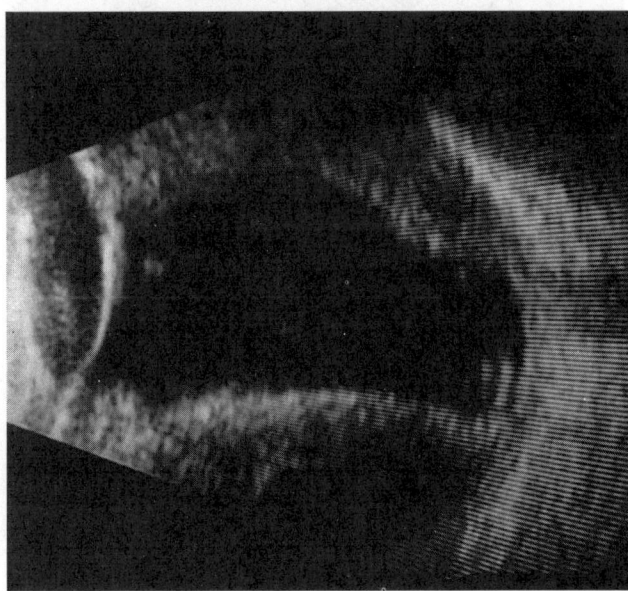

B

Fig. 18-14. Gram negative bacterial keratitis after varicella-zoster keratitis. **A,** Descemetocoele from suppurative bacterial keratitis. **B,** Ultrasound revealed serous choroidal detachments. Despite intensive topical therapy, the patient developed a corneal perforation and expulsive choroidal hemorrhage, requiring enucleation.

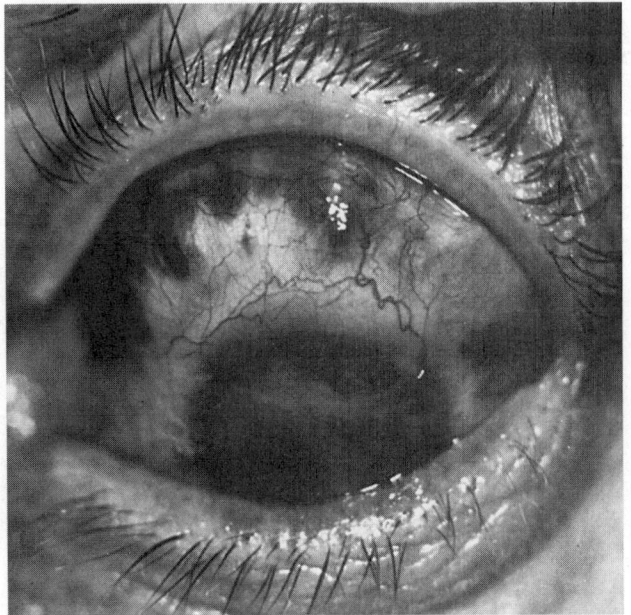

Fig. 18-13. Limbal staphyloma. There is marked thinning of the limbus with prominent protrusion of the uvea.

acutely because of progressive thinning in an area of earlier infection. If untreated, perforations may lead to total loss of the globe caused by progressive intraocular infection or choroidal effusion eventually followed by expulsive hemorrhage (Fig. 18-14).

Thinning and perforation of the retina are sequelae of viral infections of the retina. Retinal detachments are a frequent complication of CMV retinitis and the acute retinal necrosis syndrome. In both of these infections the retinal

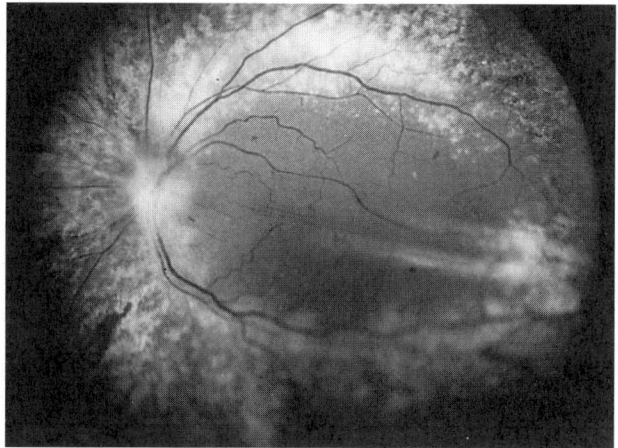

Fig. 18-15.   Retinal detachment secondary to CMV retinitis.

tears tend to form in areas where the retina has been thinned by viral infection (Fig. 18-15).[10,11,26]

STRUCTURAL CHANGES RELATED TO THERAPY

Structural changes may arise from therapeutic intervention. The employment of intraocular antibiotics and antifungal agents may have significant structural effects on the retina (Fig. 18-16).* The use of topical or systemic corticosteroids may aggravate thinning of the cornea and/or sclera.[1,12,24] In some circumstances, therapeutic intervention may lead to unusual structural patterns such as infectious crystalline keratopathy after penetrating keratoplasty and topical corticosteroids.

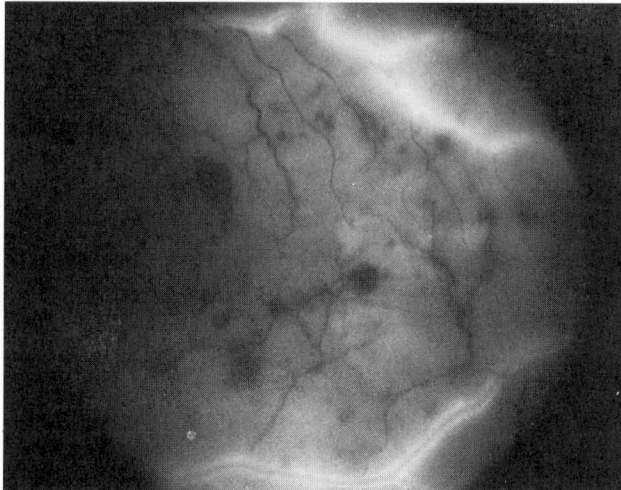

Fig. 18-16.   Fluorescein angiogram showing characteristic macular hypoperfusion in a patient who was treated with intravitreal gentamicin for bacterial endophthalmitis.

*References 2, 4, 5, 7, 25, 27.

REFERENCES

1. Aquavella JV, Gasset AR, Dohlman CH: Corticosteroids in corneal wound healing, *Am J Ophthalmol* 58:621-626, 1964.
2. Axelrod AJ, Peyman GA, Apple DJ: Toxicity of intravitreal injection of amphotericin B, *Am J Ophthalmol* 76:578-583, 1973.
3. Badhir G, Wilson RP, Maxwell-Lyons F: The histopathology of trachoma, *Bull Egyptian Ophthalmol Soc* 46:97-129, 1953.
4. Baldinger J et al.: Retinal toxicity of amphotericin B in vitrectomized and non-vitrectomized eyes, *Br J Ophthalmol* 70:657-661, 1986.
5. Balian JV: Accidental intraocular tobramycin injection: a case report, *Ophthalmic Surg* 14:353-354, 1983.
6. Brown SI, Kitano S: Pathogenesis of the retrocorneal membrane, *Arch Ophthalmol* 75:518-525, 1966.
7. Campochiaro PA, Conway BP: Aminoglycoside toxicity—a survey of retinal specialists, *Arch Ophthalmol* 109:946-950, 1991.
8. Dawson CR et al.: Severe endemic trachoma in Tunisia, *Br J Ophthalmol* 60:245-252, 1976.
9. Dreyer RF, Gass JDM: Multifocal choroiditis and panuveitis, *Arch Ophthalmol* 102:1176-1184, 1984.
10. Dugel PU et al.: Repair of retinal detachment caused by cytomegalovirus retinitis in patients with the acquired immunodeficiency syndrome, *Am J Ophthalmol* 112:235-242, 1991.
11. Duker JS, Blumenkranz MS: Diagnosis and management of the acute retinal necrosis syndrome, *Surv Ophthalmol* 35:327-343, 1991.
12. Fraunfelder FT: *Drug-induced ocular side effects and drug interactions,* ed 3, 327, Philadelphia, 1989.
13. Glaser BM, Cardin A, Biscoe B: Proliferative vitreoretinopathy: the mechanism of development of retinal traction, *Ophthalmology* 94:327-332, 1987.
14. Haralson MA: Extracellular matrix and growth factors: an integrated interplay controlling tissue repair and progression to disease, *Lab Invest* 69:369-372, 1993.
15. Henson PM, Johnston RB Jr: Tissue injury in inflammation, *J Clin Invest* 79:669-674, 1987.
16. Holland GN, Pepose JS, Pettit TH et al.: Acquired immune deficiency syndrome: ocular manifestations, *Ophthalmology* 90:859-873, 1983.
17. Jesaitis AJ, Quinn MT, Mukherjee G et al.: Death by oxygen: radical views, *New Biologist* 3:651-655, 1991.
18. Madri JA: Inflammation and healing. In Kissane JM, editor: *Anderson's pathology,* 67-110, St Louis, 1990, CV Mosby.
19. Meredith TA et al.: Ocular histoplasmosis: clinicopathologic correlation of 3 cases, *Surv Ophthalmol* 22:189-205, 1977.
20. Morrison DC, Ryan JL: Endotoxins and disease mechanisms, *Annu Rev Med* 38:417-432, 1987.
21. Naumann GOH, Gass JDM, Font RL: Histopathology of herpes zoster ophthalmicus, *Am J Ophthalmol* 65:533-541, 1968.
22. Parfrey NA: Improved diagnosis and prognosis of mucormycosis: a clinicopathologic study of 33 cases, *Medicine* 65:113-123, 1986.
23. Pepose JS, Holland GN, Nestor MS et al.: Acquired immune deficiency syndrome: pathogenic mechanism of ocular disease, *Ophthalmology* 92:160-166, 1985.
24. Petroutsos G et al.: Corticosteroids and corneal epithelial wound healing, *Br J Ophthalmol* 66:705-708, 1982.
25. Peyman GA et al.: Intraocular injection of gentamicin: toxic effects and clearance, *Arch Ophthalmol* 92:42-47, 1974.
26. Sidikaro Y, Silver L, Holland GN, Kreiger AE: Rhegmatogenous retinal detachments in patients with AIDS and necrotizing retinal infections, *Ophthalmology* 98:129-135, 1991.
27. Souri EN, Green WR: Intravitreal amphotericin B toxicity, *Am J Ophthalmol* 78:78-81, 1974.
28. VanArsdel PP Jr: Acute inflammatory reaction. In Roitt IM, Delves PJ, editors: *Encyclopedia of immunology,* 15-16, San Diego, 1992, Academic Press.
29. Watzke RC, Packer AJ et al.: Punctate inner choroidopathy, *Am J Ophthalmol* 98:572-584, 1984.

19 Transmission of Infection in Ophthalmic Practice

WILLIAM G. HODGE, JOHN P. WHITCHER, DENIS M. O'DAY

The transmission of infection in an ophthalmic practice is an important public health issue. Some communicable pathogens, including adenovirus and enterovirus, are frequently encountered as causes of ocular disease. Other infectious agents, such as the human immunodeficiency virus and hepatitis B virus, are potentially communicable in the ophthalmologist's office and can produce severe systemic complications. Ophthalmologists must prevent microbial transmission among patients and eye-care personnel.

TRANSMISSION OF INFECTIOUS DISEASE

The causal pathway of an infectious process involves an agent that initiates an infection via a specific mode of transmission to a susceptible host. Each of these components exists in a communicable infection.

Infectious Agents

The term *pathogenicity* describes an organism's disease-causing potential. For example, adenovirus has high local pathogenicity, whereas *Staphylococcus epidermidis* has very low pathogenicity for the healthy eye. Many factors are involved in an organism's pathogenic potential. Depending on the microbe—various mechanisms of adherence, the production of enzymes and exotoxins, or the presence of endotoxin can be responsible. Antibiotic resistance, which can be chromosomal-mediated or plasmid-mediated, is another important component. An organism's *virulence* is a relative concept and has different meanings depending on the context. From a public health point of view, virulence refers to the agent's potential for causing morbidity, mortality, and high rates of communicability. Clinically, virulence pertains to the severity of the disease produced. An example of a highly virulent ophthalmic pathogen, regardless of the context, is *Neisseria gonorrhoeae*. The *invasiveness* of the organism alludes to its ability to penetrate and spread through the tissue involved. Gonococci are invasive ophthalmic pathogens that can penetrate intact corneal epithelium.

The number of organisms necessary to produce an infection is known as the *infective dose*. The utility of this term is limited by the route of transmission and host susceptibility. The physical characteristics of the organism can strongly influence the incidence of disease. Adenovirus can survive in a desiccated state for extended periods of time—a crucial factor in its high pathogenicity. The *antigenic variation* of an organism can change with time, and as a result *antigenic drifts* are a principal reason for the cyclical, highly contagious nature of influenza virus epidemics.[30]

With some infections, it is important to differentiate between the reservoir and the source of the agent to carry out control measures. The organism is normally found in the reservoir, whereas the organism is immediately transmitted from the source. In a patient with unmanageable blepharitis who is a "chronic staph carrier," the reservoir and source may be the same (for example, the patient's own nares).

Transmission

After pathogenicity of the organism, transmission is the second component in the causal pathway of infection. Generally, contact, common vehicle, air, and vector are the recognized routes of transmission. The *contact* route, as the name implies, involves contact between the source and the host. Direct contact is associated with person-to-person touch and is a mode of transmission familiar to ophthalmologists. Indirect contact (also called passive transfer) involves the presence of an inanimate object, such as a tonometer head or fomite, in the transmission process. Droplet spread is another contact transmission that is possible when organisms are larger than 5 μm in diameter. Streptococcal infections can be transmitted in this way. *Common-vehicle* spread is a term that describes transmission when an inanimate vehicle transmits an agent to multiple hosts. In *airborne transmission* the agent is transported by droplet or dust particles in the air to the host. Infection with *Mycobacterium tuberculosis* is the most commonly cited example of airborne transmission. *Vectorborne* transmission involves insects or other intermediate hosts.[9]

Host

The host's defense mechanisms are the final consideration in the infectious pathway. Nonspecific barrier mechanisms include the protective effects of the lids and corneal epithelium. Only a few known bacterial species can invade an intact corneal epithelium—*Neisseria gonorrhoeae, Neisseria meningitidis, Listeria monocytogenes, Corynebacterium diphtheriae,* and *Haemophilus* sp.[4] The tears provide protection by the physical action of washing away organisms as well as by the presence of antibacterial components such as lactoferrin, lysozyme, and immunoglobulins A and G. Conjunctival lymphoid tissue provides another source of host protection.

STERILIZATION AND DISINFECTION

Adherence to the principles of microbial eradication prevents infectious outbreaks in ophthalmic practice. Sterilization is the destruction of all contaminating organisms. This destruction is the ultimate goal for surgical instruments, but such strict criteria are unrealistic and impractical for much office equipment. Many methods of sterilization are available, including heat, gases, chemical, irradiation, and filtration. Heat and gas are the most common and practical[13] processes for ophthalmic use.

Heat sterilization, the oldest and most widely used practice, is the method of choice for sterilizing surgical instruments. Moist heat is superior to dry heat because it kills organisms at a faster rate, requires less exposure time, and penetrates many materials. By saturating steam under high pressure, the temperature of the steam can be raised well above 100°C (Boyle's law). The autoclave is the most common means of heat sterilization. Although standardized cycle times, temperatures, and pressures are available, the exact conditions required for sterilization of instruments vary. Because bacterial endospores are relatively heat resistant, they should indicate the completeness of the process. Thus weekly biologic sterility testing with spores of *Bacillus stearothermophilus* is recommended by the Centers for Disease Control and Prevention (CDC) and the Joint Commission on Accreditation of Hospitals (JCAH). Viruses are particularly vulnerable to heat sterilization. Most are inactivated at 60°C within 20 minutes, though more rigorous conditions are necessary for small nonenveloped RNA viruses.[50]

"Flash" sterilization is a method of autoclaving unwrapped materials using steam at 132°C for 3 minutes. Instruments contaminated during surgery are often flashed, but the Association for the Advancement of Medical Instrumentation (AAMI) has recommended that it be restricted to unplanned or emergency situations. Although flash sterilization failure is rare compared to standard autoclaving, serious nosocomial infections have been reported from flash failure including infections from *Pseudomonas aeruginosa.*

The second most common method of sterilization is with the gas ethylene oxide. In general, the use of ethylene oxide is restricted to those cases in which heat sterilization is not possible. Typically, this includes electronic equipment and items made of plastic, rubber, cotton, wool, or silk. The microbicidal activity of gas depends on the alkylation of nucleic acids. Because spores of *B. subtilis* are relatively resistant, this organism is the indicator of choice for gas sterilization. A few of the disadvantages of using ethylene oxide include marbling of some plastics and fogging of instruments with transparent surfaces. Furthermore, the Occupational Safety and Health Administration (OSHA) has declared that exposure to ethylene oxide presents a carcinogenic, mutagenic, and neurologic hazard; and strict time-regulated permissible exposures have been outlined.[22]

Disinfection refers to the elimination of all vegetative microorganisms (but not bacterial or fungal spores) from inanimate objects. Disinfection is the goal in the office setting. Spaulding[84] has described an approach to disinfection by chemicals that is based on the level of their germicidal action—high, intermediate, and low (Table 19-1), and on the type of instrumentation used—critical, semicritical, and noncritical (Table 19-2). The highest level is critical and applies to agents introduced into a sterile body area. Instruments that come into direct contact with the ocular surface (tonometer heads, ophthalmodynemometer, scleral depressors) are considered to be semicritical and require high-level disinfection with agents such as glutaraldehyde, hydrogen peroxide, ethyl alcohol, or chlorine. Noncritical instruments, which only have potential contact with skin, just need to be disinfected with low-level disinfectants.

An antiseptic is a substance that is applied to skin or other vital tissue to prevent the growth or action of a microorganism. A germicide destroys microbes on either inanimate objects or vital tissue. Cleaning refers to the removal of

TABLE 19-1   RECOMMENDATIONS FOR LEVELS OF DISINFECTION BASED ON MICROORGANISM

	Level of Disinfection		
	High	**Intermediate**	**Low**
Bacteria			
Vegetative	+	+	+
TB	+	+	−
Spores	+	+/−	+/−
Fungi	+	+	+/−
Viruses			
Lipid & medium-size	+	+	+
Nonlipid & small	+	+/−	−

Modified from Spaulding EH: Chemical disinfection of medical and surgical materials. In Lawrence CA, Block SS, editors: *Disinfection, Sterilization, and Preservation,* Philadelphia, 1968, Lea and Febiger.

TABLE 19-2 GUIDELINES FOR CLEANING, DISINFECTING, AND STERILIZING MEDICAL EQUIPMENT

Classification	Definition	Example	Minimum Level of Disinfection	Methods
Critical	An object introduced into a sterile body area	Surgical equipment	Sterilization	Heat Ethylene oxide
Semicritical	Mucous membrane contact	Tonometer head	High-level chemical disinfectant	Glutaraldehyde Hydrogen peroxide Ethyl alcohol Chlorine
Noncritical	Skin contact	Table top	Low-level chemical disinfectant	Many

Modified from Spaulding EH: Chemical disinfection of medical and surgical materials. In Lawrence CA, Block SS, editors: *Disinfection, Sterilization, and Preservation,* Philadelphia, 1968, Lea and Febiger.

foreign organic material from objects, and decontamination is the removal of pathogenic microorganisms from inanimate objects so that they are safe to handle.[13]

CONTROL OF COMMUNICABLE OCULAR PATHOGENS

Some common and clinically important ocular and systemic pathogens are potentially transmissible in an ophthalmic practice.

Adenovirus

Of the more than 65 outbreaks of epidemic keratoconjunctivitis that have been reported in the literature, at least half have resulted from nosocomial spread in medical settings such as eye clinics and hospitals.[36] Adenoviral conjunctivitis is the most significant communicable ocular infection.

Conjunctivitis that is attributable to adenovirus was initially reported in Austria in 1889 and was named keratitis punctata superficialis.[2] The first report of an adenoviral epidemic took place in Bombay in 1901,[43] but it was exclusively a community outbreak. In 1936 the earliest nosocomial epidemic was reported in California.[45] Although the infectious nature of this disease had been suspected for years, the first identified serotype was isolated in 1955 by Jawetz, Kimura, and Nicholas.[48]

The adenoviruses are a group of nonenveloped double-stranded DNA viruses that belong to the family Adenoviridae.[70a] There are 42 human serotypes, with 5 more awaiting official classification. For adenoviral infection to occur, the virus must first attach to and penetrate the target cell. A complicated sequence of viral mRNA synthesis and DNA replication takes place at the expense of the host cell. During the viral replicative cycle, host DNA and mRNA synthesis are severely curtailed.[39a,57a]

Although the molecular mechanisms are not clear, one of the important physical characteristics of the virus is its ability to survive for extended periods in unfavorable environments. Adenovirus-19 can maintain its infectivity on dried tonometer tips for up to 11 days and in ophthalmic solutions for 20 days.[42] The type of material and its surface characteristics may be important in promoting prolonged adenoviral recovery. Adenovirus-19 can be recovered in a desiccated state for up to 8 days on paper and up to 10 days on cloth, metal, and plastic. The amount of virus that is recoverable from nonporous surfaces is significantly greater than that recoverable from porous surfaces. Desiccated virus on a nonporous plastic surface remains viable for more than one month![69] These studies clearly demonstrate the robust nature of the virus and the potential significance of fomite spread.

Transmission. The incidence of nosocomial adenoviral conjunctivitis is difficult to determine. Varied viral strains have different pathogenicity, virulence, and infective dose. Moreover, these characteristics may change with geographic region and with the extent of patient crowding. Case series incidences are prone to several biases including patient underreporting of ''trivial'' or subclinical infection. Disease misclassification biases may be the result of clinical diagnostic error or diverse methods of laboratory diagnostic criteria. Reported attack rates have ranged from as low as 0.8%[90] to as high as 49%.[21]

Numerous potential sources of adenoviral nosocomial infection have been identified including the hands of caregivers[46,81,86] and tonometer tips.[55,74,91] Other sources are ophthalmoscopes,[56] slit-lamps,[31] phoropters,[52] trial contact lenses,[15] ophthalmic wash solutions,[44,85] topical anesthetic solutions,[86] foreign-body removal instruments,[20,85,86] and towels.[52]

Control Measures. Measures to control the spread of adenoviral ocular infection are important. Specific antiviral therapy (including trifluridine, dexamethasone,[89] and topical interferon)[78] is not available. Some general measures to control and prevent potential outbreaks include using unit doses of ophthalmic solutions, avoiding the use of cloth towels, encouraging patient segregation, quarantining infected staff, postponing elective procedures, and educating patients and staff.

The two most important measures for controlling adenoviral infection are staff handwashing and proper use of disinfectants. Handwashing decreases the number of viral particles available for infection. Germicides are more effective when applied to surfaces void of organic material.[82] Handwashing is the principal means of controlling an outbreak,[20,78] but handwashing alone is not a panacea. Most ethanol-based and proviodine-based hand washes are unpredictable and inconsistent in their ability to inactivate adenovirus.[32] Handwashing inactivated virus in only 50% of hands that were contaminated with adenovirus-infected tears.[49] Gloves should be used to examine patients during adenoviral outbreaks.[26,49]

Chemical disinfection is often used to prevent nosocomial adenoviral infections. One recent study systematically analyzed the effectiveness of different disinfectants.[82] Chlorine-containing disinfectants can eradicate adenovirus from a metallic surface within 1 minute, but only at relatively high concentrations (free chlorine = 1000 ppm). Unfortunately, many commercial disinfectants have free chlorine concentrations between 25 and 500 ppm. Iodine 1% is not effective in eradicating the virus, but 70% ethanol is effective. Glutaraldehyde 2% has broad viricidal activity and is often used as an endoscope disinfectant. Quaternary ammonium compounds are useless against adenovirus when used alone but can be effective when combined with other substances. Another poorly performing yet widely available commercial disinfectant is the class of phenolics.

Enterovirus

The enteroviruses are a group of nonenveloped DNA viruses that present clinical findings similar to those seen in adenoviral infections. These include an acute follicular conjunctivitis and a palpable preauricular node. Because of the often dramatic subconjunctival hemorrhages associated with this infection, the infection is often referred to as "acute hemorrhagic conjunctivitis." The first reported outbreak occurred in 1969 in Ghana during the Apollo space mission and has been referred to as "Apollo conjunctivitis."

The physical characteristics of the enteroviruses are similar to the adenoviruses, but in vitro studies clearly demonstrate that enteroviruses are much less pathogenic. Undoubtedly an important reason is the inability of this virus to survive in a desiccated state.[42] Whereas desiccated adenovirus can be recovered from tonometer heads for days or weeks, enterovirus-70 levels are decreased 4 log units 4 hours after drying, and virus is not recoverable after 6 hours. In a moistened state (for example, ophthalmic solutions), however, enterovirus can be recovered at the same titer as adenovirus for up to 3 weeks.

Transmission. Perhaps because of the the reduced pathogenicity of these viruses compared to adenoviruses, only a few outbreaks of enteroviral conjunctivitis have been reported.[5,6,47,93] There is some evidence that droplet spread is an important method of transmission[93] and that heat and humidity are important conditions promoting outbreaks.[5,6] Fewer data are available for attack rates for nosocomial enterovirus infections than for adenovirus, making valid estimates of the incidence virtually impossible.

Control Measures. The general measures described previously for nosocomial adenoviral control apply to these viruses as well. In terms of the choice of specific disinfectants, using coxsackievirus B3 as the prototype, the spectrum of efficacy is similar to that of adenovirus with some exceptions (Table 19-3).[82] Ethanol solutions did not reduce viral recovery as they did with adenovirus. Moreover, the quaternary ammonium compounds and their derivatives were less effective against enterovirus compared to adenovirus.

Herpes Simplex Virus

Clinical descriptions of herpes infections date back to the time of Hippocrates.[92] The word "herpes" is derived from the Greek word meaning "to creep." The infectious nature of herpes simplex lesions was first demonstrated in 1919 by Lowenstein, who produced corneal epithelial dendrites in rabbits with material derived from human herpes simplex virus keratitis and labialis.[58]

Herpes simplex virus (HSV) is an enveloped double-stranded DNA virus. The overall diameter is between 150 and 200 nm. HSV-1, the serotype responsible for ocular and labial herpes, is differentiated from HSV-2 (its genital counterpart) by several biologic and biochemical characteristics. These include pock size on chick embryo chorioallantoic membranes, the ability to form plaques in chick embryo cultures, the formation of giant cells in cell culture, sensitivity to heparin, and DNA base composition.[39,62,67,70]

Transmission. Herpes simplex has a worldwide distribution, and the human is the only known natural host.[12] The prevalence of HSV antibodies is heavily dependent on socioeconomic status, but the overall risk of acquiring infection is between 60% to 80%.[19,68] For HSV-1 the prevalence rate rises most rapidly in childhood. Approximately 10% of adults shed HSV-1 at any given time.[24,29] Whereas there have been laboratory and nonocular nosocomial outbreaks, nosocomial epidemics of ocular disease have not been reported.[17,37,41,47]

Direct contact with infected secretions is the principal mode of distribution. During contact transmission, the development of disease depends on the dose and strain of virus. The age of the exposed individual may also play a role as, in general, resistance to infection changes with age.[51]

Several factors may account for the lack of nosocomial epidemics despite this identification of the tonometer as a

TABLE 19-3 DISINFECTANT EFFICACY OF VARIOUS FORMULATIONS AGAINST ADENOVIRUS AND ENTEROVIRUS

Disinfectant	Concentration (%) and Approx. PH	Reduction of Virus Titer by >99.9%	
		Adenovirus*	Enterovirus†
Hypochlorite	0.01 (8.0)	−	−
	0.10 (9.4)	−	−
	0.50 (11.0)	+	+
	1.00 (11.4)	+	+
Organo-chlorine	0.01 (7.0)	−	−
	0.10 (8.0)	−	−
	0.30 (8.0)	+	+
	0.50 (8.0)	+	+
Povidine-iodine	10.00 (3.0) (1% iodine)	−	−
Ethanol	70.00 (4.0)	+	−
Glutaraldehyde	2.00 (7.0)	+	+
Quaternary ammonium	0.04 (6.0)	−	−
Quaternary ammonium with HCl	0.04 (1.0) 7.00	+	+
Quaternary ammonium with EtOH	0.04 (5.0) 70.00	+	−
Chlorhexidine	0.08 (5.0)	−	−
Chlorhexidine with ethanol	0.50 (4.5) 70.00	+	−
Phenolics		−	−

Modified from Sattar SA, Springthorpe US, Karim Y, and associates: Chemical disinfection of non-porous inanimate surfaces experimentally contaminated with four human pathogenic viruses, *Epidemiol Infect* 102(3):493-505, 1989.
*c-Adenovirus-5 used as prototype adenovirus
†b-Coxsackievirus B3 used as prototype enterovirus

possible mode of dispersion. First, HSV is an enveloped virus and these viruses are more sensitive to disinfectants than their nonenveloped counterparts. Second, dried surfaces harbor herpes viruses for only a short period of time. For example, whereas herpes simplex virus persists for up to 8 hours on a moist toxometer tip, it can be recovered for less than 2 hours on dried tips.[87] Third, because most adults already have anti-HSV antibodies, the critical transmissibility coefficient needed to begin and sustain an epidemic is unlikely to be attained.[3] Nonetheless, the possibility of individual transmission in an ophthalmologist's office should always be a consideration.

Control Measures. HSV-1 ocular infection is one of the few viral diseases for which effective chemotherapeutic intervention is available. Asymptomatic viral shedding can periodically occur, however.

Because HSV-1 has a lipid envelope, it is more vulnerable to disinfection than adenovirus and enterovirus. Following the wiping of tonometer tips with 70% isopropyl alcohol, HSV can no longer be recovered.[87] In general, lower concentrations of chlorine disinfectants reduce the recovery of enveloped viruses compared to their nonenveloped counterparts.[82]

Human Immunodeficiency Virus

The acquired immunodeficiency syndrome first appeared in North America in a small series of homosexual men with *Pneumocystis carinii* pneumonia in Los Angeles in 1981.[23a] Since that time this disease has become one of the most important epidemics of this century. The human immunodeficiency virus (HIV-1) has been isolated from the tears of as many as two thirds of patients with AIDS[1] and from conjunctival, corneal, and retinal tissue and from intraocular fluids. Whereas there are no reported cases of AIDS attributable to transmission in ophthalmic practice, germicides should be used to destroy the viability of this virus in eye-care and other settings.[25,61,75]

Control Measures. HIV is a retrovirus that employs the enzyme reverse transcriptase to produce its own DNA. Studying the potency of different disinfectants against this virus is complicated and results must be interpreted cautiously. The delicate cell lines used to assay the virus in tissue culture are very sensitive to the toxicity of most disinfectants. Thus the inhibitory activity of a disinfectant may only reflect its tissue culture toxicity. Sufficient follow-up of cell cultures is also important because the eclipse and growth period of the virus can be as long as 7 days. Lastly, obtaining final viral concentrations in the cell culture assays that resemble those in vivo is often very difficult on both a theoretical and practical level.[7]

For high-water content trial contact lenses, chemical treatment with a surfactant cleaner containing a chlorhexidine-containing agent and a hydrogen peroxide disinfectant is recommended.[27] There is controversy as to whether heat disinfection is adequate.[64] Instrumentation disinfection has been studied with various chemicals (Table 19-4). Benzalkonium chloride 2%, 1% Triton X, and 1% sodium hypochlorite can all inactivate high concentrations of the virus completely.[7] Benzalkonium chloride, however, requires as much as 5 minutes of contact time to completely inactivate the virus, whereas the other two require only one minute. In contrast, 100% ethanol inactivates only small concentrations of HIV.

Hepatitis B Virus

The first recorded cases of serum hepatitis occurred after the administration of the smallpox vaccine in 1833.[59] In the first half of the 20th century, the importance of percutaneous transmission of this virus became evident.[11,60,63] Only in the

TABLE 19-4 HIV INACTIVATION BY VARIOUS DISINFECTANTS

Disinfectant	Incubation Time	Complete Inactivation
Benzalkonium chloride (2%)	15 s	−
	30 s	−
	1 min	−
	5 min	+
Triton-X 100 (1%)	15 s	−
	30 s	+/−
	1 min	+
	5 min	+
Sodium hypochlorite (1%)	15 s	−
	30 s	+/−
	1 min	+
	5 min	+
Ethanol (100%)	30 s	−
	1 min	−
	5 min	−
	10 min	−

Modified from Aranda-Anzaldo A, Viza D, Busnel RG: Chemical inactivation of human immunodeficiency virus in vitro, *J Virol Methods* 37:71-82, 1992.

middle of this century was the antigenic and biologic complexity of this virus unraveled.[14] In 1968 Bayer and associates[8] used the electron microscope to identify the hepatitis B surface antigen. Today this virus is one of the world's most important and prevalent infectious diseases, with carrier rates exceeding 10% in some areas. Approximately 170 million people are infected worldwide.

HBV is a small DNA virus with unique antigenic and ultrastructural features.[79,80] The DNA is very small, circular, and partly single-stranded. The complete virion (hepatitis B surface antigen) has a diameter of just over 40 nm with a surrounding lipid envelope 7 nm in width and an electron dense internal core (Hepatitis B core antigen).[28] Hepatitis B antigen (HB_sAg) is released from the core by detergent treatment and is found as a soluble antigen in serum. At least five antigenic specificities can be found on hepatitis B antigen particles. This virus has a striking propensity for liver parenchymal cells and the unusual ability to cause persistent infection (the carrier state).

Transmission. Blood and blood products are the best documented sources of hepatitis B transmission. HBsAg has also been isolated from virtually every human fluid including tears.[85a] Hepatitis B transmission can occur through fomite contact of skin breaks or mucous membranes with household articles (such as toothbrushes and toys) and hospital equipment (including endoscopes and respirators).[76] Oral transmission has been verified, but in these cases invasion is via breaks in the oral mucous membranes as opposed to the gastrointestinal tract.[23] Although frank epidemics are rare, hepatitis B is clearly an infection that can be easily transmitted in the ophthalmologist's office. Health-care personnel (such as ophthalmologists) are at a higher risk of acquiring the infection than the general public.[57,66]

Control Measures. Immunization of all health-care personnel is strongly recommended. General measures of control for this virus parallel control measures for other infectious agents and include segregation of patients known to be infected, routine handwashing, patient education, and consistent case reporting. For sterilization of instruments, heat is the method of choice when plausible. Boiling in water for 10 minutes, autoclaving at 121°C and 15 psi for 15 minutes, or dry heat at 160°C for 2 hours will inactivate all hepatitis B viral particles. Gas sterilization with ethylene oxide is also effective. Chemical disinfectants presumed to be effective include sodium hypochlorite 0.5% to 1.0% (free chlorine— 5000 to 10,000 ppm) for 30 minutes, 40% aqueous formalin or 16% aqueous formaldehyde for 12 hours, or 1% sodium dodecyl sulfate for an indeterminate contact time.[80]

Bacterial Causes of Epithelial Parasitism

The number of potential bacterial pathogens transmissible in the ophthalmologist's office is, like viruses, extensive. Some genera can invade intact corneal epithelium and cause corneal ulcers in previously healthy corneas. Many others can adhere to sites of epithelial trauma and lead to suppurative keratitis.

Neisseria gonorrhoeae. The gonococcus causes one of the oldest human infectious diseases. References to it can be found in ancient Chinese writings and the Old Testament. This organism generates epithelial parasitism but is best known for its ability to produce hyperacute adult and neonatal conjunctivitis. The vast majority of cases are transmitted sexually or perinatally. Fortunately, nosocomial spread of this organism is rare because of its fastidious nature. It does not tolerate drying, and any commercial disinfectant can be used on office surfaces or instruments after examining a patient infected with these bacteria.[73] Different povidine-iodine concentrations are effective against gonococcus; complete sterilization occurs with 5%, 1%, and 0.1% solutions.[10]

Neisseria meningitidis. Despite being a close relative to gonococcus, the pathogenic nature of this bacteria wasn't described until 1805 by Vieusseaux.[88] The mode of transmission of this organism is much less understood than that of gonococcus. The main route appears to be via respiratory droplet spread, but precise data concerning this or other mechanisms do not exist. Moreover, an elucidation of the means for preventing infection with this bacteria is hampered by the facts that its epidemic nature is very sporadic, certain populations have different susceptibilities, and nonsymptomatic carrier states are not uncommon.[38]

Neisseria meningitidis resembles gonococcus in that it is a very fastidious organism. Routine use of germicides and segregation of patients afflicted with this organism should suffice in halting any office transmission. Ocular infection with *N. meningitidis* demands mandatory infectious disease consultation and notification of regional public health personnel. Case series of meningococcal meningitis have been reported in which the portal of entry was felt to be an ocular infection.[33]

Haemophilus species. *Haemophilis aegyptius* is a small, pleomorphic, gram-negative coccobacillus (Koch-Weeks bacillus) that is so similar morphologically and biochemically to *H. influenza* that some investigators feel that the two organisms should be classified together.[53,54] *Haemophilus* spp. is capable of epithelial parasitism and is a frequent cause of acute conjunctivitis in warm climates. *H. aegyptius* is responsible for the oculosystemic disease Brazilian purpuric fever,[16] which is characterized by purulent conjunctivitis, fever, a purpuric rash, and septic shock.

Because many *Haemophilus* species are present in the flora of the upper respiratory tract, airborne transmission is considered the usual method of spread. These organisms are very fastidious, requiring hemin and nicotinamide adenine dinucleotide for growth on blood agar and preferring moderate levels of carbon dioxide. Office transmission can be easily prevented with routine antiseptic and disinfectant techniques.

Listeria monocytogenes. This gram-positive, nonspore-forming aerobic rod is motile at room temperature and produces a ring of hemolysis on blood agar. It was first isolated as a mammalian pathogen in 1926[83] and from a human in 1929.[71] *Listeria* sp. is a peculiar organism because it is ubiquitous in nature[77] and extremely invasive through both eye and skin,[40] yet the attack rate for both eye and systemic infections is extremely low (approximately 2 to 3 cases per million per year). Clearly the immune system is important in keeping this organism in check.[18] The usual source and mode of transmission is not known.

Corynebacterium diphtheriae. The first outbreak of diphtheria occurred in the 1700s, but because of public health measures, it has been reduced to a medical curiosity.[34] The pathophysiology of corneal infection is thought to involve lid pressure, exotoxins, and thrombosis of limbal capillaries.[35] *Corynebacterium diphtheriae* is very sensitive to desiccation, and fastidious growth requirements make transmission prevention fairly routine.

Pseudomonas aeruginosa. This gram-negative aerobic rod has minimal nutritional requirements and can tolerate a wide variety of physical conditions. This organism is one of the most important nosocomial pathogens.

Pseudomonas sp. has been found in hospitals and clinics, in medicines and contact lens solutions, in sinks, and even in disinfectants.[65] As many as one million CFU/ml could be isolated from a "sterile" eye wash.[72] In corneal infections associated with contact lens wear, the lens case is a source of the pathogen.

Because *Pseudomonas* sp. can survive in a variety of physical environments, preventing its transmission in the office setting requires a multifactorial approach. Trial contact lens disinfection with heat or chemicals is critical. In the office, no medication dispenser should be used for a prolonged period of time. Preservative-free solutions should be discarded after 1 day of use, and preserved solutions should not be used longer than 2 weeks.[27] High-chlorine-concentration disinfectants are advisable for periodic use on office equipment. One of the few environmental conditions inhibitory to *Pseudomonas* sp. survival is desiccation.

REFERENCES

1. Ablashi DV, Sturzenegger S, Hunter EA et al.: Presence of HTLV-III in tears and cells from the eyes of AIDS patients, *J Exp Pathol* 3(4):693-703, 1987.
2. Adler H: Keratitis subepithelialis, *Zentralbl Prakt Augenheilkd* 13:289-294, 1889.
3. Anderson RM, May: *The basic model: statics in: infectious diseases of humans,* Oxford, 1992, Oxford University Press.
4. Antonios S, Tabbara KF: Bacterial conjunctivitis. In Tabbara KF, Hyundiuk RA, editors: *Infections of the eye,* Boston, 1986, Little, Brown.
5. Aoki K, Kawana R, Matsumoto I et al.: An epidemic of acute hemorrhagic conjunctivitis in the city of Sao Paulo, *Jpn J Ophthalmol* 31(4):532-537, 1987.
6. Aoki K, Sawada H, Ishikawa H et al.: An outbreak of acute hemorrhagic conjunctivitis due to Coxsackievirus type A24 variant in Japan, *Jpn J Ophthalmol* 32(1):1-5, 1988.

7. Aranda-Anzaldo A, Viza D, Busnel RG: Chemical inactivation of human immunodeficiency virus in vitro, *J Virol Methods* 37:71-82, 1992.
8. Bayer ME, Blumberg BS, Werner B: Particles associated with Australia antigen in the sera of patients with leukemia, Down's syndrome and hepatitis, *Nature* 218:1057-1059, 1968.
9. Benenson AS, editor: *Control of communicable diseases in man,* ed 13, Washington, 1980, APHA.
10. Benevento WJ, Murray P, Reed CA et al.: The sensitivity of *Neiseria gonorrheae, Chlamydia trachomatis,* and herpes simplex type II to disinfection with proviodine-iodine, *Am J Ophthalmol* 109(3):329-333, 1990.
11. Bigger JW, Dubi SD: Jaundice in syphilitics under treatment, *Lancet* 1:457-461, 1943.
12. Black FL: Infectious diseases in primitive societies, *Science* 187:515-519, 1975.
13. Block SS: Definition of terms. In Block SS, editor: *Disinfection, sterilization, and preservation,* ed 4, Philadelphia, 1991, Lea and Febiger.
14. Blumberg BS, Alter HJ, Visnich S: A "new" antigen in leukemia sera, *JAMA* 191:541, 1965.
15. Braley AE: Epidemic keratoconjunctivitis, *Trans Am Acad Ophthalmol Otolaryngol* 48:153-174, 1944.
16. Brazilian Purpuric Fever Study Group: Brazilian purpuric fever: epidemic purpura fulminans associated with antecedent purulent conjunctivitis, *Lancet* 2:757-761, 1987.
17. Buchman TG, Roizman B, Adams G et al.: Restriction endonuclease fingerprinting of herpes simplex virus DNA: a novel epidemiologic tool applied to a nosocomial outbreak, *J Infect Dis* 138:488, 1978.
18. Buchner LH, Schneierson SS: Clinical and laboratory aspects of *Listeria monocytogens* infections with a report of ten cases, *Am J Med* 45:904-909, 1968.
19. Buddingh GJ, Schrum DI, Lanier JC et al.: Studies on the natural history of herpes simplex infection, *Pediatrics* 11:595-601, 1953.
20. Buehler JW, Finton RJ, Goodman RA et al.: Epidemic keratoconjunctivitis: report of an outbreak in an ophthalmology practice and recommendations for prevention, *Infect Control* 5:390-394, 1984.
21. Buffington J, Chapman LE, Stobierski MG et al.: Epidemic keratoconjunctivitis in a chronic care facility: risk factors and measures for control, *J Am Geriat Soc* 41(11):1177-1181, 1993.
22. Caputo RA, Odlaug TE: Sterilization with ethylene oxide and other gases. In Block SS, editor: *Disinfection, sterilization, and preservation,* ed 4 Philadelphia, 1991, Lea and Febiger.
23. Centers for Disease Control: *Hepatitis Surveillance Report No 41,* September 1977.
23a. Centers for Disease Control: Pneumocystis pneumonia-Los Angeles, *MMWR* 30:250, 1981.
24. Centifanto YM, Drylie DM, Deardourff SL et al.: Herpes type II in the male genitourinary tract, *Science* 178:318-322, 1972.
25. Chermann JC, Barre-Sinoussi F, Henin Y et al.: HIV inactivation by a spermicide containing benzalkonium chloride, *AIDS-Forsch* 2:85-86, 1987.
26. Clarke SKR, Dean Hart JC, Barnard DL: The disinfection of instruments and hands during outbreaks of epidemic keratoconjunctivitis, *Trans Ophthalmol Soc UK* 92:613-618, 1972.
27. Cohen EJ: Is your office safe? Yes, *Cornea* 9(Suppl):S41-S43, 1990.
28. Dane DS, Cameron CH, Briggs M: Virus-like particles in serum of patients with Australia antigen associated hepatitis, *Lancet* 2:695-698, 1970.
29. Douglas RG Jr, Couch RB: A prospective study of chronic herpes simplex virus infection and recurrent herpes labialis in humans, *J Immunol* 104:289, 1970.
30. Dowdle WR, Coleman MT, Gregg MB: Natural history of influenza type A in the United States: 1957-1972, *Prog Med Virol* 17:91-96, 1974.
31. Adenovirus keratoconjunctivitis, *Br J Ophthalmol* 61:73-75, 1977 (editorial).
32. Eggers HJ: Experiments on antiviral activity of hand disinfectants: some theoretical and practical considerations, *Int J Med Microbiol* 273(1):36-51, 1990.
33. Ellis M, Weindling AM, Davidson DC et al.: Neonatal meningococcal conjunctivitis associated with meningococcal meningitis, *Arch Dis Child* 67:1219-1220, 1992.
34. English PC: Diphtheria and theories of infectious disease: centennial appreciation of the critical role of diphtheria in the history of medicine, *Pediatrics* 76:1-9, 1985.
35. Fedukowicz HB, Stenson S: *External infections of the eye,* Norwalk, 1985, Appleton-Century-Crofts.
36. Ford E, Nelson KE, Warren D: Epidemiology of epidemic keratoconjunctivitis, *Epidemiol Rev* 9:244-261, 1987.
37. Francis DP, Herrmann KL, MacMahon JR et al.: Nosocomial and maternally acquired herpesvirus hominis infections, *Am J Dis Child* 129:889-893, 1975.
38. Gauld JR, Nitz RE, Hunter DH et al.: Epidemiology of meningococcal meningitis at Ford Ord, *Am J Epidemiol* 82:56-72, 1965.
39. Gentry GA, Randal CC: The physical and chemical properties of the herpesviruses. In Kaplan AS, editor: *The herpesviruses,* New York, 1973, Academic Press.
39a. Ginsberg HS: Adenoviruses. In Davis BD, Dulbecco R, Eisen HN et al.: *Microbiology,* Hagerstown, 1980, Harper & Row.
40. Gray ML, Killinger AH: Listeria monocytogenes and listeric infections, *Bacteriol Rev* 30:309-315, 1966.
41. Hale BD, Rendtorff RC, Walker LC et al.: Epidemic herpetic stomatitis in an orphanage nursery, *JAMA* 183:1068-1073, 1963.
42. Hara J, Okamoto S, Minekawa Y et al.: Survival and disinfection of adenovirus type 19 and enterovirus 70 in ophthalmic practice, *Jpn J Ophthalmol* 34:421-427, 1990.
43. Herbert H: Superficial punctate keratitis associated with an encapsulated bacillus, *Ophthalmol Res* 20:339-345, 1901.
44. Hierholzer JC, Sprague JB: Five-year analysis of adenovirus 8 antibody levels in an industrial community following an outbreak of keratoconjunctivitis, *Am J Epidemiol* 110:132-140, 1979.
45. Hobson LC: Acute epidemic superficial punctate keratitis, *Am J Ophthalmol* 21:1153-1155, 1938.
46. Holmes WJ: Epidemic infectious conjunctivitis, *Hawaii Med J* 1:11-12, 1941.
47. Ishii K, Uchida Y, Miyamura K et al.: *Acute hemorrhagic conjunctivitis,* 1989, University of Tokyo Press.
48. Jawetz E, Kimura S, Nicholas AN et al.: New type of APC virus from epidemic keratoconjunctivitis, *Science* 122:1190-1191, 1955.
49. Jernigan JA, Lowry BS, Hayden FG et al.: Adenovirus type 8 epidemic keratoconjunctivitis in an eye clinic: risk factors and control, *J Infect Dis* 167:1307-1313, 1993.
50. Joslyn L: Sterilization by heat. In Block SS, editor: *Disinfection, sterilization, and preservation,* ed 4, Philadelphia, 1991, Lea and Febiger.
51. Kaye SB, Shimeld C, Grinfeld E et al.: Non-traumatic acquisition of herpes simplex virus infection through the eye, *Br J Ophthalmol* 76(7):412-418, 1992.
52. Keenlyside RA, Hierholzer JC, D'Angelo LJ: Keratoconjunctivitis associated with adenovirus type 37: an extended outbreak in an ophthalmologist's office, *J Infect Dis* 147:191-198, 1983.
53. Kilian M: A taxonomic study of the genus *Haemophilus* with the proposal of a few species, *J Gen Microbiol* 93:9-62, 1976.
54. Kilian M: *Haemophilus.* In Lennette EH, Ballows A, Hausler WJ Jr, Shadomy HJ, editors: *Manual of clinical microbiology,* ed 4, Washington, 1985, American Society for Microbiology.
55. Kjer P, Mordhorst CH: Studies of an epidemic of keratoconjunctivitis caused by adenovirus type 8. II. Clinical and epidemiological aspects, *Acta Ophthalmol* 39:984-992, 1961.
56. Leopold IH: Characteristics of hospital epidemics of epidemic keratoconjunctivitis, *Am J Ophthalmol* 43(4 II):93-97, 1957.
57. Lewis TL, Alter HJ, Chalmers TC: A comparison of the frequency of hepatitis B antigen and antibody in hospital and non-hospital personnel, *New Eng J Med* 289:647-650, 1973.
57a. Londberg-Holm K, Philipson L: Early events of virus cell interactions in an adenovirus system, *J Virol* 4:323-338, 1969.
58. Lowenstein A: Aetiologische untersuchungen uber den fieberhaften Herpes, *Munch Med Wochenschr* 66:768, 1919.
59. Lurman A: Eine icterus epidemic, *Berl Klin Wochenscher* 22:20, 1855.
60. MacCallum FO: Transmission of arsenotherapy jaundice by blood: failure with feces and nasopharyngeal washings, *Lancet* 1:342-345, 1945.
61. Malkovsky M, Newell A, Dalgleish AG: Inactivation of HIV by nonoxynol-9, *Lancet* 1:645, 1988.

62. Marks-Hellman S, Ho M: Use of biological characteristics to type herpes-virus hominis types 1 and 2 in diagnostic laboratories, *J Clin Microbiol* 3:277, 1976.
63. McNatty AS: *Great Britain Ministry Health Report of Chief Medical Officer, Annual Report,* London, 1937.
64. Moo KB: Necessity and methods of HTLV-III inactivation in contact lens practice, *J Am Optom Assoc* 58:180-186, 1987.
65. Morrison AJ, Wenzel RP: Epidemiology of infections due to *Pseudomonas aeruginosa, Rev Infect Dis* 6(suppl):627-642, 1984.
66. Mosley JW, Edwards VM, Casey BS: Hepatitis virus infection in dentists, *New Eng J Med* 293:730-734, 1975.
67. Nahmias AJ, Josey WE: Epidemiology of herpes simplex viruses 1 and 2. In Kaplan AS, editor: *Viral infections of humans: epidemiology and control,* ed 2, New York, 1982, Plenum.
68. Nahmias AJ, Josey WE, Naib AM et al.: Antibodies to herpesvirus hominis types 1 and 2 in humans. I. Patients with genital herpes infections, *Am J Epidemiol* 91:539-545, 1970.
69. Nauheim RC, Romanowski EG, Araullo-Cruz T et al.: Prolonged recoverability of desiccated adenovirus type 19 from various surfaces, *Ophthalmology* 97:1450-1453, 1990.
70. Nordlund JJ, Anderson C, Hsiung GD: The use of temperature sensitive and selective cell culture systems for differentiation of herpes simplex virus types 1 and 2 in a clinical laboratory, *Proc Soc Exp Biol Med* 155:118, 1977.
70a. Norrby E, Bartha A, Boulanger P et al.: Adenoviridae, *Intervirology* 7:117-125, 1976.
71. Nyfeldt A: Etiologiede la mononucleose infectieuse, *Compt Rend Soc Biol* 101:590-594, 1929.
72. Paszko-Kolva C, Yamamoto H, Shahamat M et al.: Isolation of amoeba and *Pseudomonas* and *Legionella* species from eyewash stations, *Appl Environ Microbiol* 57:163-167, 1991.
73. Pedersen AHB, Bonin P: Screening females for asymptomatic gonorrhea infection, *Northwest Med* 70:255-261, 1971.
74. Pellitteri OJ, Fried JJ: Epidemic keratoconjunctivitis: report of a small office outbreak, *Am J Ophthalmol* 33:1596-1599, 1950.
75. Polsky B, Baron PA, Gold JWM et al.: In vitro inactivation of HIV-1 by contraceptive sponge containing nonoxynol-9, *Lancet* 2:1456, 1988.
76. Prince AM, Hargrove RI, Szmuness W: Immunologic distinction between infectious and serum hepatitis, *New Eng J Med* 282:987-990, 1970.
77. *Proceedings of the Third International Symposium on Listeriosis,* Bilthaven, Netherlands, 1966.
78. Reilly S, Dhillon BJ, Nkanza KM et al.: Adenovirus type 8 keratoconjunctivitis—an outbreak and its treatment with topical human fibroblast interferon, *J Hyg* 96:557-575, 1986.

79. Robinson WS: Genetic variation among hepatitis B and related viruses, *Ann NY Acad Sci* 354:371-378, 1980.
80. Robinson WS, Marion PL, Feitleson M et al.: The hepadna virus group: hepatitis B and related viruses. In Szmuness W, Alter HJ, Maynard JE, editors: *Viral hepatitis,* Philadelphia, 1982, Franklin Institute Press.
81. Sanders M, Gulliver FD, Forchheimer LL et al.: Epidemic keratoconjunctivitis: clinical and experimental study of an outbreak in New York City: further observations on the specific relationship between a virus and the disease, *JAMA* 121:25-255, 1943.
82. Sattar SA, Springthorpe US, Karim Y et al.: Chemical disinfection of non-porous inanimate surfaces experimentally contaminated with four human pathogenic viruses, *Epidemiol Infect* 102:493-505, 1989.
83. Seeliger HPR, Jones D: Genus *Listeria.* In Sneath PHA, Mair NS, Sharpe ME, Holt JG, editors: *Bergey's manual of systematic bacteriology,* volume 2 Baltimore, 1986, Williams and Wilkins. pp 1235-1245.
84. Spaulding EH: Chemical disinfection of medical and surgical materials. In Block SS, editors: *Disinfection, sterilization, and preservation,* ed 4 Philadelphia, 1991, Lea and Febiger.
85. Sprague JB, Hierholzer JC, Currier RW II et al.: Epidemic keratoconjunctivitis: a severe industrial outbreak due to adenovirus type 8, *New Eng J Med* 289:1341-1346, 1973.
85a. Su CS, Bowden S, Fong LP, Taylor HR: Detection of hepatitis B virus DNA in tears by polymerase chain reaction, *Arch Ophthalmol* 112:621-625, 1994.
86. Thygeson P: The epidemiology of epidemic keratoconjunctivitis, *Trans Am Ophthalmol Soc* 46:366-385, 1948.
87. Ventura LM, Dix RD: Viability of herpes simplex virus type 1 on the applanation tonometer, *Am J Ophthalmol* 103:48-52, 1987.
88. Vieusseaux M: Memoire sur le maladie qui a regne a Geneve au printempts de 1805, *J Med Chir Pharmacol* 11:163, 1805.
89. Ward JB, Siojo LG, Waller SG: A prospective masked clinical trial of trifluridine, dexamethasone, and artificial tears in the treatment of epidemic keratoconjunctivitis, *Cornea* 12:216-221, 1993.
90. Warren D, Nelson KE, Farrar JA et al.: A large outbreak of epidemic keratoconjunctivitis: problems in controlling nosocomial spread, *J Infect Dis* 160:938-943, 1989.
91. Wegman DH, Guinee VF, Milliani SJ: Epidemic keratoconjunctivitis, *Am J Public Health* 60:1230-1237, 1970.
92. Wildy P: History and classification. In Kaplan AS, editor: *The herpesviruses,* New York, 1973, Academic Press.
93. Yin-Murphy M, Goh KT, Phoon MC et al.: A recent epidemic of acute hemorrhagic conjunctivitis, *Am J Ophthalmol* 116:212-217, 1993.

IMMUNO-
DEFICIENCIES

20 Opportunistic Infections

CONSTANCE A. BENSON, FRED M. WILSON II, LOWELL YOUNG

One of the first observations suggesting a relationship between susceptibility to infection and ineffective immune response was recorded by James Ewing in 1940 in a document stating "In the material gathered in New York where the disease is very common, tuberculosis follows Hodgkin's disease like a shadow."[34] Ruskin and Remington[104] first coined the term "compromised host" in an article about *Pneumocystis carinii* pneumonia published in 1967. The term "immunocompromised host" was adopted by consensus during a 1980 international symposium on "Infections in the Immunocompromised Host."[2] It is only in the last two decades that major advances in the treatment of neoplastic, inflammatory, and immunodeficiency disorders (Table 20-1) have resulted in prolonged survival of patient populations with less-than-effective immune function. One outcome of this success has been the emergence of infections caused by opportunistic pathogens as a conspicuous threat to the quality of life and duration of survival for such patients (Table 20-2). A rational, directed approach to clinical recognition, diagnosis, treatment, and prevention requires not only knowledge of the microbial pathogens that cause infection in immunocompromised patients but also an understanding of the defects in host defense and the patterns of infection associated with the underlying disease processes.

The term "opportunistic" is conventionally defined in a medical context as "capable of adapting to a tissue or host other than the normal one."[40] This definition implies that opportunistic infections occur in abnormal hosts. A number of elements impair the natural ability of a host to defend against infection, thus rendering that host abnormal. These factors include damage to or interruption of mucosal or skin surface barriers, defective or insufficient numbers of phagocytic cells, cellular or humoral immune dysfunction, alterations in normal microbial flora, and abnormalities induced by medical procedures or equipment. An "immunocompromised" host specifically refers to one with impaired immune function. Even in the presence of host or tissue compromise, the ability of microorganisms to cause disease is determined by a variety of virulence factors, such as those that facilitate attachment, adherence, or penetration of anatomic barriers, the elaboration of toxins, or the presence of capsules or cell-wall products that allow the organism to evade host defenses.

Opportunistic infections of the eye are a clinically important group of diseases caused by microorganisms that are normally commensal or saprophytic, weakly virulent, or rarely cause infection except in those individuals with impaired host defenses (Table 20-3). Many of these organisms can cause clinically important disease, but they rarely generate serious ocular infections or disseminated or life-threatening systemic infections in either immunocompetent patients or patients with anatomically intact ocular structures. Examples of these organisms are *Pseudomonas aeruginosa,* *Candida* spp., cytomegalovirus (CMV), and *Toxoplasma gondii.* Other opportunistic organisms, such as *Pneumocystis carinii,* virtually never cause disease unless the host is impaired. True pathogens, in contrast, are those that regularly cause significant disease—even in immunologically intact individuals—unless previous infection or immunization has rendered the host immune. Examples of true ocular pathogens are adenovirus, *Chlamydia trachomatis, Neisseria gonorrhoeae,* and *Streptococcus pneumoniae* among others. This chapter provides an overview of important opportunistic infections of the eye and the pathogens that cause them in patients with compromised immune function.

PROTOZOA

Pneumocystis carinii

P. carinii is at present classified as a protozoan, although analysis of ribosomal RNA suggests that it shares many biologic properties with fungi.[32] Cysts of *P. carinii* are large (5 to 8 microns), thick-walled organisms that contain up to eight sporozoites. The cysts can be detected in tissue

TABLE 20-1 DEFECTS OF IMMUNE FUNCTION AND ASSOCIATED SELECTED PRIMARY AND ACQUIRED IMMUNODEFICIENCY DISORDERS

Immune Defect	Immunodeficiency Disorder	Immune Defect	Immunodeficiency Disorder
B-Lymphocyte Defects		**Combined B- and T-Lymphocyte Defects**	
Primary	X-linked agammaglobulinemia		
	Common variable immunodeficiency	Primary	Severe combined immunodeficiency
	Selective IgA deficiency		Wiskott-Aldrich syndrome
Acquired	Acquired immunodeficiency syndrome		Ataxia telangiectasia
	Splenectomy	Acquired	Acquired immunodeficiency syndrome
	Multiple myeloma		Lymphoreticular malignancies (Non-Hodgkin/Hodgkin lymphomas, leukemias)
	Waldenstrom macroglobulinemia		Bone marrow transplantation
	Non-Hodgkin/Hodgkin lymphoma		Solid organ transplantation
T-Lymphocyte Defects		**Phagocytic Cell Defects**	
Primary	Purine nucleoside phosphorylase deficiency	Primary	Chronic granulomatous disease
	Chronic mucocutaneous candidiasis		Chediak-Higashi syndrome
	DiGeorge anomaly		Leukocyte adhesion defect
			Cyclic neutropenia
Acquired	Acquired immunodeficiency syndrome	Acquired	Drug-induced neutropenia
	Lymphoreticular malignancies (Non-Hodgkin/Hodgkin lymphomas, leukemias)		Immune-mediated neutropenia
			Infiltrative disease of the bone marrow
	Cytotoxic chemotherapy		Corticosteroid therapy
	Corticosteroid therapy	**Complement Deficiencies**	
	Cyclosporine therapy	Primary	C1, C4, C2, C3, C5 terminal complement deficiencies
			Factor 1 deficiency
		Acquired	Severe liver disease

by silver stains that stain the cyst wall. Sporozoites are released from mature cysts and in turn develop into trophozoites. Trophozoites may be numerous in infected tissue, are usually found in clusters of small, pleomorphic organisms of 1 to 4 microns in diameter, and are detected using Giemsa or similar stains that stain the nucleus red and the cytoplasm blue.[119] *Pneumocystis carinii* is worldwide in its distribution, although its natural environment is unknown; it has only been detected in animal or human hosts. It is likely that genetically distinct organisms infect different animal species or humans.[117] Organisms are probably acquired as lung saprophytes in early childhood through inhalation of aerosolized or airborne organisms.[57] As most children and adults have antibodies to *P. carinii* in the absence of clinically apparent disease, it is likely that normal immune surveillance is sufficient to control infection.[95]

Disease in Compromised Hosts. The major risk associated with development of disease caused by *P. carinii* is a defect in cell-mediated immune function, either as a consequence of specific neoplastic or immunologic disease or of corticosteroid or cytotoxic chemotherapy. Studies in animal models using polyclonal or monoclonal antibodies as passive immunoprophylaxis showed that these agents could decrease organism load, thereby suggesting a role for humoral immunity as well.[45,102] Neoplastic or immunodeficiency disorders that create a risk for *P. carinii* disease include acute lymphocytic leukemia, rhabdomyosarcoma and its associated therapy in children,[59] bone marrow transplantation,[85,86] primary severe combined immunodeficiency syndrome,[72] solid organ transplantation requiring broad spectrum immunosuppression for prevention of rejection,[23,49] and human immunodeficiency virus (HIV) infection with advanced immunosuppression, as reflected by a CD4+ T-lymphocyte count of less than 200 cells/μl.[80,97] Among chemotherapeutic modalities, high-dose corticosteroid therapy is most frequently associated with the development of *P. carinii* disease; the greatest risk is incurred during periods when corticosteroid doses are being tapered or when other cytotoxic

TABLE 20-2 COMMON PATHOGENS CAUSING INFECTION IN PATIENTS WITH SELECTED DEFECTS IN IMMUNE FUNCTION

Defects	Common Pathogens Causing Infection
B-Lymphocyte Defects	Encapsulated bacteria (*Streptococcus pneumoniae, Haemophilus* spp., *Neisseria* spp., *Escherichia coli, Klebsiella* spp., and others) *Giardia lamblia* Enteroviruses
T-Lymphocyte Defects	*Listeria monocytogenes* Fungi (*Candida* spp., *Histoplasma capsulatum, Blastomyces dermatitidis, Cryptococcus neoformans, Coccidioides immitis, Sporothrix schenckii, Trichosporon begelii,* and others) Mycobacteria Protozoa (*Pneumocystis carinii, Toxoplasma gondii,* Cryptosporidia, Microsporidia) *Salmonella* spp. Viruses (cytomeglovirus, varicella-zoster virus, herpes simplex virus, among others)
Combined B- and T-Lymphocyte Defects	Same as B- and T-lymphocyte defects above
Phagocytic Cell Defects	*Staphylococcus aureus* Other *staphylococcus species* *Capnocytophaga* spp. *Enterobacteriaceae* *Candida* spp. *Aspergillus* spp. *Nocardia* spp.
Complement Deficiencies	*Neisseria* spp. *S. pneumoniae*

chemotherapeutic agents are added to high-dose corticosteroid regimens.[13,58,108,109] It has been suggested that the relationship with corticosteroid withdrawal may relate to recovery of the ability of the immune system to respond to infection with an inflammatory reaction.[108] Other cytotoxic chemotherapeutic agents that have been associated with development of *P. carinii* disease include cytarabine, methotrexate, fluorouracil, bleomycin, cyclosporine, L-asparaginase, dactinomycin, desferoxamine, colloidal gold, and busulfan.[15] These agents have in common the ability to impair CD4+ T-lymphocyte number and function.

The mechanism by which disease occurs in the immunosuppressed host is thought to be reactivation of latent infection. Because *P. carinii* cannot be reproducibly cultivated in vitro, the precise stimuli for reactivation and whether or not reinfection occurs remain unknown. The most common presentation of *P. carinii* disease is a pneumonitis syndrome characterized by fever, nonproductive cough, dyspnea, hypoxemia, and interstitial infiltration on chest radiograph. Extrapulmonary pneumocystosis remains uncommon, occurring in up to 1% to 3% of patients with *P. carinii* pneumonia.[110] It has been reported primarily among persons with AIDS, particularly those who have had a prior episode of *P. carinii* pneumonia and have received either no or only aerosolized pentamidine prophylaxis.[110] *P. carinii* organisms spread outside the lung to ocular structures through hematogenous dissemination. Organisms are found localized to the choroidal layer of the eye with minimal surrounding inflammatory reaction.

Diagnosis of *P. carinii* disease is based on the demonstration of cysts or trophozoites in tissue. A number of stains can be used to detect organisms. These stains include toluidine blue-O and methenamine silver, which stain only the cyst wall; Giemsa and Diff-Quik, which stain intracystic bodies and trophozoites; and monoclonal antibody immunofluorescence stains.[67]

TABLE 20-3 OPPORTUNISTIC PATHOGENS AND THEIR ASSOCIATED OCULAR DISEASES

Ocular Opportunistic Pathogens	Ocular Disease
Staphylococcus epidermidis	Blepharokeratoconjunctivitis Corneal ulcers Endophthalmitis
Pseudomonas aeruginosa and other gram-negative bacilli	Corneal ulcers Endophthalmitis
Mycobacterium leprae	Hansen disease (leprosy)
Mycobacterium tuberculosis and atypical mycobacteria	Corneal ulcers Endophthalmitis
Propionibacteria acnes	Chronic endophthalmitis
Candida spp. and other fungi	Chronic blepharitis or conjunctivitis Corneal ulcers Endogenous endophthalmitis
Fusarium spp. and other soil saprophytes	Corneal ulcers
Herpes simplex virus, varicella-zoster virus	Blepharitis Keratitis Conjunctivitis Scleritis Uveitis Retinitis
Acanthamoeba spp.	Chronic keratitis
Toxoplasma gondii	Retinochoroiditis
Pneumocystis carinii	Choroidopathy
Microsporidia	Chronic keratoconjunctivitis

Toxoplasma gondii

Toxoplasma gondii is a protozoan species ubiquitous in the environment. It exists in three forms: the oocyst (production of which is unique to the feline intestinal mucosa), the tissue cyst, and the tachyzoite; the latter is the form that invades host cells — where it actively proliferates, causing cell lysis.[81] The cat serves as the categorical host, with humans as a fortuitous intermediate host.[81] Cats ingest either oocysts from soil or tissue cysts from contaminated meat. Following ingestion, cysts break down and organisms invade feline intestinal epithelial cells, where they undergo asexual schizogony and sexual gametogony, producing oocysts that are shed in feces.[81] Under appropriate conditions, sporulation occurs. Breakdown of tissue cysts by contact with digestive enzymes leads to release of trophozoites that can then invade tissue or host cells and disseminate.[81] Once inside the host cell, tachyzoites replicate within a cytoplasmic vacuole; and as replication continues, the host cell is either destroyed or incorporated into tissue cysts. Tissue cysts are of variable size and may contain up to 3000 organisms.[81]

Serosurveys suggest that anywhere from 15% to 68% of humans in the United States are infected with *T. gondii,* with overall seropositivity rates largely a function of geographic location and socioeconomic, cultural, and dietary practices.[81] Transmission to humans can occur through ingestion of tissue cysts present in poorly cooked meat products, inadvertent ingestion of oocysts from soil or material contaminated by cat feces, transplacental transmission during gestation, autoinoculation, organ transplantation, or transfusion of contaminated blood products.[81,90,100,106]

Disease in Compromised Hosts. Persons with intact immune function rarely experience clinically overt disease following acute infection with *T. gondii.* Those who do often experience a benign, self-limited illness that resolves without specific treatment. Once infection occurs, organisms remain latent unless there is a defect in cell-mediated immunity that allows reactivation by as yet unknown mechanisms. *T. gondii* organisms have a predilection for the central nervous system, and skeletal and cardiac muscle — the precise reason for which is unknown. Ocular localization may occur as a consequence of contiguous spread from other infected central nervous system sites or by lymphohematogenous dissemination. The cellular location of latent organisms is thought to be tissue mononuclear phagocytes.

Excluding congenital infection, those at increased risk of disease caused by *T. gondii* are (1) those with hematopoietic or lymphoproliferative malignancies, (2) those receiving cytotoxic chemotherapy for hematopoietic or solid organ malignancies, (3) those receiving immunosuppressive therapy or corticosteroids for prevention of transplant rejection or treatment of other diseases, and (4) those with AIDS.* Each

---

*References 48, 62, 91, 105, 129.

of these disorders has the same defects of cell-mediated immunity including, but not limited to, abnormalities of monocyte or macrophage number or function, decreased CD4⁺ T-lymphocyte number or function, or dysregulation of mononuclear phagocyte cytokine production. It is unclear why only a small proportion of *T. gondii*-seropositive patients at risk actually develop toxoplasmosis when they become immunocompromised. Host genetic predisposition or virulence factors associated with infecting strains of the organism both may contribute to the susceptibility to disease.[76]

Microsporidia

Microsporidia are obligate intracellular pathogens. They are prevalent in the environment in a variety of wild and domestic animals; the latter are thought to be the likeliest sources for human infection.[14] Microsporidia are transmitted to humans through fecal-oral, transplacental, or transovarial routes or through direct inoculation.[14,98] Only five of the many microsporidia genera infect humans. They include *Nosema, Entercytozoon, Encephalitozoon, Pleistophora,* and *Septada* species. *Enterocytozoon, Encephalitozoon,* and *Septada* species are the species most commonly implicated in human disease. They are spore-forming protozoa; spores contain a central tubule that, following ingestion by the host, is ejected from the spore to penetrate and infect the target host cell cytoplasm. Replication continues, resulting in maturation of new spores that multiply, ultimately infecting new cells or passing into the environment, where they may viably persist for several months.[118]

Disease in Compromised Hosts. Although sporadic cases of disease caused by various microsporidia have been reported in humans who had no apparent immune dysfunction, the majority of cases have occurred in immunocompromised hosts, predominantly those with AIDS. Several of the cases occurring in nonimmunosuppressed patients had in common apparent acquisition of infection following exposure in tropical locations.[4,9,98] Ocular disease most frequently arises as a consequence of direct inoculation of organisms onto ocular surfaces. As many species cannot be reliably cultivated in vitro, it has been difficult to characterize the precise immune defect that predisposes to development of microsporidiosis; however, among persons with AIDS, those with very low CD4⁺ T-lymphocyte counts (usually < 100 cells/μl) appear to be at highest risk for disease.

Diagnosis is based on clinical presentations coupled with the demonstration of organisms by light or electron-microscopic examination of tissue specimens. Although isolation of microsporidia from clinical specimens is not generally possible in routine clinical laboratory settings, organisms can be cultivated from corneal and conjunctival tissue in research or reference laboratory settings.[29] Detection of organisms in tissue specimens can also be accomplished using electron or light microscopy. A chromotrope-based modified trichrome stain or a chitin-specific stain has been used for identifying microsporidia in stool or urine specimens of infected patients, but these techniques require expert laboratory personnel, are not widely available, and may not be applicable to ocular tissue.[122]

Acanthamoeba species

Acanthamoeba spp. are small, free-living amoebae that are ubiquitous in nature, especially in freshwater sources. They have been implicated as unusual causes of encephalitis, sinusitis, pneumonitis, and skin lesions in immunocompromised hosts, and often severe and destructive keratitis in immunocompetent hosts. The organisms exist as either tachyzoites or tissue cysts in human tissue and are probably acquired by inhalation, penetration of the nasal epithelium, or by autoinoculation of mucosal surfaces. Organisms have been recovered from nasopharyngeal swabs of otherwise healthy volunteers.[120]

Disease in Compromised Hosts. Of the reported cases of systemic disease, the majority have occurred in (1) individuals with underlying malignancies undergoing cytotoxic chemotherapy, (2) individuals receiving high-dose corticosteroids, (3) renal transplant recipients, and (4) patients with AIDS.[39,51,79] Primary sites of infection are most likely the sinuses, lung, or skin. Infection of these sites may be followed by hematogenous dissemination to the central nervous system or other organs. Infection of the corneal surface generally occurs through direct inoculation, whereas other ocular structures, although rarely involved, may be infected by hematogenous dissemination or contiguous spread from other central nervous system or sinus sites.[111a]

In the immunocompromised patient, disseminated *Acanthamoeba* sp. infection most often results in a granulomatous amoebic encephalitis that is rapidly progressive and ultimately lethal in the majority of cases. Disease limited to the skin has been reported in four patients with AIDS.[111a] The primary ocular manifestation of *Acanthamoeba* sp. disease in humans is keratitis, a disease entity most often seen in the normal host and rarely seen in those who are immunocompromised, except in the context of more widespread or disseminated disease.

VIRUSES

Cytomegalovirus

Cytomegalovirus is a double-stranded DNA virus of the herpesviridae family that, like its counterparts, is widespread in nature. Human CMV is species-specific and capable of latently infecting human host cells with periodic reactivation—particularly in those patients who are immunosuppressed. The host cells thought to most frequently harbor latent viruses are circulating or tissue mononuclear phagocytes, although other cells may also be infected.[101]

Seroepidemiologic studies show a bimodal pattern of CMV infection in humans with peaks in early childhood and in young adulthood.[54] From 40% to 70% of the adult population in the United States is seropositive for CMV, although the proportion infected varies with age and demographic characteristics.[54] Transmission occurs through direct contact with virus-infected body fluids (urine, saliva, sexually transmitted fluids), through blood-product transfusion, organ transplantation, and transplacental and perinatal passage.

Disease in Compromised Hosts. Most infections in immunocompromised hosts are thought to occur as a consequence of reactivation of latent virus, although primary infection following transplantation of latently infected donor tissue into seronegative recipients accounts for a substantial number of cases among organ or bone marrow transplant recipients. Specific triggers of reactivation are unknown. With the exception of congenital or perinatal CMV syndromes, the most frequent conditions associated with an increased risk of developing end-organ disease caused by CMV are those accompanied by defects in cell-mediated immunity, more specifically, those defects affecting CD4+ T-lymphocyte, CD8+ suppressor T-lymphocyte, cytotoxic T-lymphocyte, or natural killer cell number or function. Disorders include bone marrow transplantation, solid organ transplantation, lymphoreticular malignancies, conditions requiring prolonged therapy with high doses of corticosteroids, and AIDS.

CMV end-organ disease manifestations differ according to the patient population (and possibly the immunologic defect) in question. For example, in those with bone marrow or solid organ transplants, CMV pneumonitis is the single most common end-organ disease syndrome, characteristically occurring 30 to 90 days posttransplantation. CMV retinitis occurs most often in those with AIDS, developing in up to 40% of HIV-infected patients, and is distinctly less common in other immunocompromised patient populations.[41,54] CMV retinitis is most frequently a late opportunistic infection in patients with AIDS, occurring in those with advanced immunosuppression as reflected by a CD4+ T-lymphocyte count of less than 50 cells/μl.[41]

The eye is usually infected through hematogenous dissemination of virus, although it is unclear why there appears to be a predilection for retinal tissue, particularly in individuals with AIDS. In patients with HIV disease, the presence of HIV retinopathy may create a locus of decreased resistance that allows the virus to invade ocular structures more readily; however, there does not appear to be any clear-cut relationship between HIV retinopathy, cotton wool spots, and the eventual occurrence of CMV retinitis in patients with AIDS.[38]

CMV disease in the immunosuppressed host can result in one or more syndromes including interstitial pneumonitis, gastrointestinal tract ulceration, hepatitis, papillary stenosis with sclerosing cholangitis, pancreatitis, adrenalitis, encephalitis, myelopathy, and disseminated multiorgan disease. The characteristic ocular manifestation of active CMV infection is retinitis.

The diagnosis of CMV retinitis is a clinical one. The presence of IgG antibody is nearly universal but only indicates prior infection; shedding of CMV in the urine and blood can be seen in the absence of end-organ disease and cannot be used as a reliable indicator of active disease.

Varicella-Zoster Virus

Similar to CMV, varicella-zoster virus (VZV) is a double-stranded DNA virus member of the herpesviridae family capable of causing latent infection and reactivation disease. Primary infection with VZV causes the common childhood infection varicella (chicken pox), and reactivation disease generally causes zoster (shingles). In the previously infected individual, the virus is thought to travel along efferent pathways of nerves to the dorsal root ganglion, where it survives in a latent state until triggered to reactivate; at that point replicating virions travel along the nerve to reach distal portions of the dermatome supplied by a given nerve root. The clinical manifestations of disease caused by VZV are manifest in the cutaneous surface supplied by that nerve root.[82,115]

Most individuals acquire VZV in childhood; more than 90% are seropositive with demonstrable IgG antibody by the time they reach adulthood.[83,84,115] The virus is transmitted by aerosol droplet, direct contact with infected secretions, or (rarely) by transplacental or transplanted tissue routes.

Disease in Compromised Hosts. Infections caused by VZV occur in normal and immunocompromised hosts alike. As with the majority of the opportunistic infections discussed in this chapter, individuals with defects of cell-mediated immunity, particularly defects of VZV-specific T-lymphocyte proliferative responses and CD4+ and CD8+ cytotoxic T-lymphocyte function, are at increased risk for disease: disseminated varicella (if not previously infected) or recurrent or disseminated zoster caused by reactivation of virus (in those who have been previously infected).[3] Ocular disease can occur in either setting. Conditions that predispose to VZV infection as a consequence of their associated abnormalities of cell-mediated immune function include lymphoreticular malignancies such as lymphoma and leukemia, solid organ or bone marrow transplantation, high-dose corticosteroid or cytotoxic chemotherapy administration, and AIDS. Among recipients of organ or bone marrow transplants, clinical infection related to VZV occurs in the late posttransplantation period, after day 90 to 180. Among patients with AIDS, disease caused by VZV can occur early, before advanced immunosuppression intervenes, or it can occur in individuals with very low CD4+ T-lymphocyte counts, suggesting that functional as well as quantitative defects in cell-mediated immunity are important in the pathogenesis of infection caused by VZV in this patient population.

Compared to disease in the immunocompetent individual, dermatomal zoster ophthalmicus in immunosuppressed patients may be more complicated, often associated with prolonged vesiculopustular cutaneous lesions, severe neuralgia, keratitis, and anterior uveitis.[20,31,78] Spread outside a single dermatome, widespread dissemination, intracranial cerebral angiitis, thrombotic vasculopathy, or other neurologic sequelae are not uncommon complications.[53,115]

Herpes Simplex Virus

There are two distinct herpes simplex viruses (HSV), type 1 and type 2. They share similar morphologic and biologic properties and can both cause similar clinical syndromes; although in general, HSV-1 is more likely to be associated with orolabial, oropharyngeal, ocular, and central nervous system infections, whereas HSV-2 is more likely to be associated with genital infections.[21,22] Both viruses are prevalent worldwide. Seroepidemiologic surveys demonstrate that antibodies to HSV-1 are detectable early in childhood and their prevalence rises with age such that 30% to 100% of adults, depending on geographic and socioeconomic characteristics of the population studied, are seropositive.[126] For HSV-2, seropositivity rates begin to rise with the onset of sexual activity and reach 3% to 70% by adulthood, again depending on the characteristics of the population under investigation.[21,22,126] Both HSV-1 and HSV-2 induce latency and reactivate, although HSV-1 is more likely to recur in orolabial locations and HSV-2 in genital locations.[21,22,126] Recurrent HSV keratitis is less common.[16]

HSV is most often transmitted by direct contact with infected secretions, usually through skin or mucosal surfaces. Ocular infection generally occurs through direct inoculation of virus onto epithelial or corneal surfaces. Transmission may be partly dependent on the viral inoculum present at the time of contact; those lesions with the highest virus load are lesions of recent onset (for cutaneous lesions, the vesicular or ulcerative stages within the first 24 to 96 hours of onset) in persons with true primary infection.[21,22,126] Asymptomatic shedding of virus in oral secretions or from the genital tract in the absence of skin lesions does occur and has been associated with transmission, but the virus load is low in such instances and the efficiency of transmission arguably less.[12,83]

Disease in Compromised Hosts. HSV-1 and HSV-2 often cause disease in immunocompetent hosts and, as such, are not clearly opportunistic pathogens. Characteristics of disease in those with compromised immune function, however, may substantially differ from those in the immunocompetent host. Abnormalities of cell-mediated immune function may be associated with more aggressive or atypical localized disease, and failure to locally contain viral replication results in subsequent viremia and hematogenous dissemination to other sites. Appropriate CD4+ T-lymphocyte, natural killer cell, and cytotoxic T-lymphocyte function and adequate interferon production appear necessary to prevent unabated local viral replication; in the absence of these defenses, response to antiviral therapy may be diminished, delayed, or absent. Acyclovir-resistant strains of virus have been recovered primarily from those individuals with underlying abnormalities of immune function.[5]

Those who appear to be at particular risk of severe, chronic, or progressive disease caused by HSV are solid organ or bone marrow transplant recipients (particularly in the immediate posttransplant period when immunosuppressive regimens are maximal); patients with lymphoreticular malignancies; those with AIDS; and those at extremes of age (particularly neonates), when cell-mediated immunity is immature or waning.[21,22,126]

Once epithelial cells are infected, ongoing viral replication causes cell lysis with release of cytokines that induce a localized inflammatory reaction resulting in the characteristic clinically recognized lesions. In the immunosuppressed host, viremia and hematogenous dissemination of HSV to other organs may occur, whereas those with competent cell-mediated immunity, primarily natural killer cell and sensitized virus-specific cytotoxic T-lymphocyte responses, contain local infection and heal.[22,75,126] Following primary infection, latency is induced through travel of HSV along sensory nerve pathways to sensory neural ganglia, where viral DNA and RNA can be localized.[6,22,82,114] Whereas the precise mechanisms for reactivation remain to be determined, a variety of physical and immunologic stimuli, acting at central or peripheral sites, appear to trigger viral reactivation; these stimuli vary from person to person.[82]

Prevention of infection is best afforded by avoiding contact with infected secretions. Patients with active cutaneous lesions should be instructed to avoid activity that might transfer infected secretions from the lesions to the eye. Barrier protection such as latex gloves and careful handwashing for medical personnel or anyone coming in personal or household contact with infected lesions should be recommended. For individuals with frequently recurrent lesions, chronic suppression with oral acyclovir may reduce the frequency and duration of episodes and, thereby, also reduce the risk of transmission, although this strategy has been evaluated primarily for genital tract HSV disease.[64]

FUNGI

Candida species

Candida spp. are fungi that exist predominately as unicellular yeasts—small, oval cells that reproduce by budding and that can produce pseudohyphae or hyphae in clinical specimens.[33] Candida albicans is the most common pathogen responsible for invasive or disseminated candidal infections in immunocompromised patients. Other Candida spp. responsible for similar clinical syndromes in these patient populations include C. tropicalis, C. krusei, C. glabrata (or Torulopsis glabrata), C. lusitaniae, and C. parapsilosis. Increasingly recognized invasive disease caused by C. krusei, C. lusitaniae, and C. tropicalis has been linked to their relative or frank resistance to amphotericin B and the azoles, resulting in a higher likelihood of fatal disease in those who are immunosuppressed.[11,37,66,99,128] The adherence characteristics of Candida spp. organisms probably play a major role in their virulence.[103]

Candida albicans and other Candida spp. can be found in soil, foods, and hospital environmental surfaces; C. albicans are also common commensal organisms that can be found on the skin and in the upper respiratory, gastrointestinal, and genital tracts of humans. Infection generally results from natural or iatrogenic breakdown of epithelial or mucosal barriers or hematogenous spread in individuals who have abnormal immune function. Once Candida spp. traverse epithelial or mucosal surfaces or gains access to the bloodstream, host defense mechanisms are complex. Neutrophils, monocytes, and eosinophils phagocytose and kill Candida spp. Complement and possibly antibody appear necessary for adequate opsonization of organisms to facilitate phagocytosis.[42,111] Cell-mediated immunity also plays a role in host defense against Candida spp. infections with CD4+ T-lymphocytes and natural killer cells as the operant components. With such a complex array of immune mechanisms involved in host defense against these organisms, deficiencies in any one can be associated with increased risk of severe or invasive candidiasis.

Disease in Compromised Hosts. Ocular disease can result from either direct inoculation, particularly during or following eye surgery, or by hematogenous dissemination. Factors that may predispose to candidal disease include neutropenia or neutrophil dysfunction; interruption of epithelial or mucosal surface integrity, as might be engendered by intravascular catheterization; surgical or traumatic injury or cytotoxic chemotherapy-induced mucosal ulceration; suppression of normal gut bacterial flora allowing Candida spp. overgrowth; primary or acquired immunoglobulin or complement deficiency states; or a reduction in CD4+ T-lymphocyte number or function. Patient populations at risk include those with congenital defects of neutrophil number or function; patients undergoing cytotoxic chemotherapy or receiving corticosteroid therapy in the presence of other risk factors that allow access of fungi to the blood stream; those with chronic indwelling vascular access devices; parenteral drug users; patients receiving broad-spectrum antibacterial therapy for prolonged periods, particularly those who have indwelling catheters or who have undergone surgical procedures; those receiving parenteral hyperalimentation; patients with congenital or acquired immunoglobulin deficiencies; and patients with AIDS.

Cryptococcus neoformans

Cryptococcus neoformans is an encapsulated yeast, 4 to 6 μm in diameter, that, like *Candida* spp., reproduces by budding. There are four different serotypes of *C. neoformans*, A, B, C, and D, based on capsular polysaccharide antigen determination; A and D are most commonly associated with clinical disease.[26] The organism is worldwide in its distribution. Infection is thought to be acquired by inhalation of aerosolized organisms from contaminated soil. Concentrations of organisms are highest in soil contaminated by bird excreta, particularly pigeon droppings, although pigeons are not infected and contact with pigeons or their excreta cannot be implicated in many cases of cryptococcosis.[26] Cases of cryptococcosis have also occurred in laboratory workers cutaneously inoculated with organisms and following corneal transplantation in which the donor had cryptococcosis.[10,46]

Disease in Compromised Hosts. Although cryptococcal infections can occur in immunologically intact persons, disease caused by these fungi is more likely to occur in the immunosuppressed host. As with the majority of opportunistic infections discussed thus far, cell-mediated immune function is critical for protection from invasive infection caused by *C. neoformans*. Those individuals who have primary or acquired defects of cell-mediated immunity are at greatest risk for disease caused by cryptococci; they include patients receiving corticosteroid therapy, those with lymphoreticular malignancies, solid organ transplant recipients —including those who have undergone renal, liver, heart, or heart-lung transplants (although in many instances the predisposition may be related to high doses of corticosteroids used in the immunosuppressive regimens following transplantation), and patients with AIDS.

In the normal host, clearance of cryptococci consists of an initial neutrophil phagocytic response followed by intracellular killing; this phenomena may be inhibited to some degree by the large polysaccharide capsule surrounding cryptococci.[28] Organisms not ingested by neutrophils may be engulfed and killed by activated macrophages, antibody-dependent cytotoxic T-lymphocytes, and natural killer cells.[52,74,88,123] Anticryptococcal antibodies may enhance the ability of natural killer cells.[52,74,88,123] The major virulence factor contributing to impaired killing is the polysaccharide capsule, a glucuronoxylomannan structure. Cryptococcal polysaccharide appears to inhibit phagocytosis and impair leukocyte migration.[68] Although high concentrations of capsular polysaccharide activate the alternative complement pathway, anticryptococcal antibody and complement do not damage the organism.[27,68,69] The latter do appear necessary, however, as opsonic and chemotactic factors in the intact host immune response to infection. Thus abnormalities of immune function that interfere with this complex array of host immune responses to cryptococci can increase the predilection for serious cryptococcal infection.

Cryptococcus neoformans can cause a variety of clinical syndromes in the immunocompromised patient including meningitis, prostatitis, pneumonia, skin and soft tissue abscesses, bone infection, myocarditis, and disseminated multiorgan disease. The organism has a predilection for the central nervous system in humans that is likely related to the relative absence of antibody, complement activity, or other soluble anticryptococcal factors in the cerebrospinal fluid and the presence of substances that enhance local cryptococcal proliferation.[60,70] The most common clinical syndrome associated with *C. neoformans* then is meningoencephalitis. Ocular abnormalities seen in the course of cryptococcal meningitis include papilledema, extraocular muscle paresis, nystagmus, and optic atrophy.[92] *C. neoformans* is an uncommon cause of endophthalmitis, which is clinically indistinguishable from other fungal causes of endophthalmitis. Intraocular cryptococcal disease is usually seen in the setting of disseminated or multiorgan cryptococcal infection.

The diagnosis of cryptococcal infection is based on recovery of the organism in culture from infected tissue sites or from blood. Ancillary studies may be helpful in cases where tissue is unavailable or cultures are negative; the most useful of these is cryptococcal antigen detection, usually performed by latex agglutination and present in infected cerebrospinal fluid or serum. The height of the antigen titer has some prognostic significance when present in the face of meningeal infection, although similar associations have not been made with ocular or other organ-invasive disease.[107]

Aspergillus species

The two most common *Aspergillus* species associated with human disease are *A. fumigatus* and *A. flavus*. *Aspergillus* spp. are molds that grow well or persist in a wide variety of environments including soil, decaying vegetation, and hospital air supply sources or filters.[7] They are worldwide in their distribution. Hyphae are 2 to 4 μm in diameter, septate, and branched.[7] Sporulation does not occur in tissue; spores or conidia are found in environmental sources and are 2 to 3 μm in diameter, which is sufficiently small to reach human alveoli following inhalation. Human infection occurs through inhalation of aerosolized or airborne spores. As spores can be carried in hospital air supplies, contamination of wounds or inoculation through traumatic interruption of skin or other surfaces may serve as a source of infection, particularly among immunosuppressed patients.[7]

Disease in Compromised Hosts. Phagocytic cells, including neutrophils, monocytes, and macrophages, are necessary to the host defense against *Aspergillus* spp. Oxidative killing within phagocytic cells is thought to play a central role.[121] Those at greatest risk for invasive *Aspergillus* spp. infections are individuals with intrinsic defects of phagocyte number or function, such as those with chronic granulomatous disease and those with acquired neutropenia, as seen in the setting of lymphoreticular malignancies with bone marrow infiltration, cytotoxic chemotherapy, or other drug-induced immunosuppressive states. Prolonged neutropenia appears to be a particular risk.[25] *Aspergillus* spp. infection is an uncommon cause of pulmonary disease in patients with AIDS; it usually occurs in patients with HIV-associated or drug-induced neutropenia or advanced stages of immunosuppression in which multiple concomitant opportunistic infections are present.[24] Rarely, invasive aspergillosis has resulted, in an otherwise normal host, from direct trauma to a mucosal or cutaneous surface with inoculation of spores into the wound or caused by inoculation of organisms into the bloodstream through injection drug use.[65]

Disease syndromes caused by *Aspergillus* spp. in immunocompromised patients include pneumonitis with pulmonary infarction, sinusitis with vascular invasion, invasive pseudomembranous tracheobronchitis, and disseminated disease. *Aspergillus* spp. are rare causes of fungal endophthalmitis; in most reported instances, this entity has occurred as a consequence of contiguous spread from infected sinuses or hematogenous dissemination in immunosuppressed patients or injection drug users.[30,87,89]

Because *Aspergillus* spp. are frequently recovered in culture as commensal organisms from a variety of sites and surfaces within the hospital environment and are frequent contaminants of culture media, the presence of a few colonies growing in cultures does not conclusively indicate that *Aspergillus* spp. organisms are the cause of the clinical syndrome in question. Histopathologic confirmation of septate branching hyphae invading involved tissues is often necessary. Positive blood cultures and serologic tests may provide ancillary evidence of systemic infection, but the yield from these studies is usually low—even, and sometimes especially, in those with profound immunosuppression.

Other Fungi

A number of other fungal pathogens cause clinically significant disease in immunosuppressed patients, but their relative importance as causes of ocular infection remains small. The most prevalent of these fungi is *Histoplasma capsulatum,* which causes disease in both immunocompetent and immunosuppressed individuals. This pathogen has a geographic distribution corresponding to the central United States and the Caribbean; most cases occur in persons who have been exposed to the pathogen in these geographic locations. The organism is found in soil contaminated by bird or bat excreta and is acquired by humans through inhalation of infectious aerosols. In the immunocompromised host, *H. capsulatum* causes a disseminated multiorgan disease only

rarely involving ocular structures. Patients with AIDS appear to be at highest risk for this entity, although sporadic cases occur among patients with lymphoreticular malignancies, those treated with corticosteroids, and those who have undergone solid organ or bone marrow transplantation and are receiving immunosuppressive therapy.[125] The immune defect common to these individuals is an abnormality of cell-mediated immune function. The diagnosis of histoplasmosis is based on culture of the organism from clinical specimens. A radioimmunoassay that detects *Histoplasma* sp. polysaccharide antigen in body fluids can be used as presumptive evidence of infection and as a monitor of the effects of therapy.[124]

Other fungi that cause disease in immunosuppressed patients and may occasionally cause disease of ocular structures include *Coccidioides immitis, Blastomyces dermatitidis, Penicillium marneffei, Sporothrix schenckii, Fusarium* spp. and others.

BACTERIA

Bacterial pathogens tend to be virulent and often cause clinically significant ocular infections in both immunocompetent and immunosuppressed patients. This section will concentrate only on those bacterial organisms that are conventionally categorized as opportunistic pathogens.

Listeria monocytogenes

Listeria monocytogenes is an aerobic, gram-positive bacillus. It is occasionally pleomorphic in appearance in Gram stains of clinical specimens. The presence of pleomorphic rods in pairs in microscopic specimens may result in their misinterpretation as gram-positive cocci or, if overdecolorized, with pleomorphic gram-negative rods.[1] The organisms may also be incorrectly reported as diphtheroids or laboratory contaminants.[43]

Listeria monocytogenes is ubiquitous and can be recovered from soil, water, and a wide variety of animals, fish, and insects. A small proportion of humans may be asymptomatically infected with or be fecal carriers of *L. monocytogenes.*[1] The route of transmission or portal of entry of *L. monocytogenes* infection is not always evident. Transmission to humans occurs (1) through ingestion of contaminated cow's milk, cheese, other dairy products or meat; (2) through direct inoculation from contact with infected animals or in the laboratory; or (3) through transplacental transmission. In many instances, however, no documented exposure or route of acquisition can be elicited.[1]

Disease in Compromised Hosts. Although infections caused by *L. monocytogenes* do occur in immunologically intact individuals, up to one half of all human infections occur in those who are immunosuppressed.[19,43] Immunocompromised hosts in whom *L. monocytogenes* infections are seen most often include those at extremes of age (neonates or the elderly); pregnant women (particularly in the third trimester); those receiving high-dose or long-term corticosteroid therapy; solid organ transplant recipients, particularly renal transplant recipients; and those with lymphoreticular malignancies, most frequently non-Hodgkin lymphoma. This organism is an uncommon cause of disease among patients with AIDS, although the infection rate is higher in this patient population than for those of similar ages who are not HIV-infected.[19,43]

Mononuclear phagocytes and T-lymphocytes seem to be of primary importance in the host immune response to this organism. Ingestion and killing of the organism requires activation of mononuclear phagocytes by T-lymphocyte-dependent mechanisms and opsonization of the organism by immunoglobulin and complement-mediated mechanisms, although it is likely that other host responses also play a role.[1,63,77] Those who have global or isolated defects in one or more of these host responses seem to be at greatest risk for infections with *L. monocytogenes*.

The most common clinical syndromes caused by *L. monocytogenes* are disseminated, bacteremic infections or meningoencephalitis. The latter often results from a previous bacteremic infection. Other localized infectious processes, such as endocarditis, brain abscess, osteomyelitis, or lymphadenitis, are also generally the consequence of prior bacteremic seeding of these sites. Local skin or ocular infections can result from direct inoculation, although ocular disease also appears more likely to be a focal manifestation of systemic infection. When ocular infection occurs through direct inoculation, the most frequent clinical manifestation is a purulent conjunctivitis. Other ocular syndromes reported include acute anterior uveitis and endophthalmitis.[44] The clinical signs and symptoms are usually indistinguishable from other bacterial causes of conjunctivitis, uveitis, or endophthalmitis.

Recovery of organisms in culture from ocular structures, including purulent material from the conjunctiva or vitreous, provides confirmation of the diagnosis. Enrichment techniques, such as cold enrichment or the use of selective media, may be necessary.[43] Serologic assays are not routinely available. Positive cultures from blood, cerebrospinal fluid, or other normally sterile sites are useful ancillary studies.

Nocardia species

Similar to *Listeria monocytogenes, Nocardia* spp. cause infections in immunocompetent and immunocompromised hosts alike. *Nocardia asteroides* is the most prevalent species that causes disease in humans; *N. brasiliensis* and *N. caviae* are occasional causes of disease, more often in immunosuppressed individuals.[73] These bacteria are soil saprophytes. Branching, filamentous, weakly gram-positive and irregularly stained rods, which fragment into bacillary

and coccobacillary pieces, are recognized in clinical specimens and in smears made from primary culture.[73] Many, but not all, species are acid-fast in tissue or primary colonies; a modified Ziehl-Neelsen stain, which uses sulfuric acid rather than acid alcohol for decolorization, is best able to demonstrate this characteristic in tissue specimens.

The organisms are usually introduced by inhalation.[73] Hematogenous dissemination to other sites from the respiratory tract is the most common mode of spread. Person-to-person transmission is unlikely, although rare clusters or hospital outbreaks suggest this mode is possible.[113] Ocular infections occur both as a consequence of bloodstream invasion or, more frequently, following traumatic inoculation of ocular structures.[17,71]

Disease in Immunosuppressed Hosts. The host mechanisms responsible for containment of nocardiosis include initial neutrophil chemotaxis and recruitment followed by phagocytosis and killing of organisms by activated mononuclear phagocytes and cytotoxic T-lymphocytes.[35,36]

Disease caused by *Nocardia* spp. is most often seen in patients with defects of neutrophil function or cell-mediated immunity. The patient populations at greatest risk are those with chronic granulomatous disease, lymphoreticular malignancies, solid organ or bone marrow transplant recipients, patients on long-term corticosteroids, those with AIDS, and those with dysgammaglobulinemia or other leukocyte defects.

Based on its usual route of acquisition, pneumonia is the most common presentation and is often accompanied by bacteremia and central nervous system invasion, where a localized suppurative mass or brain abscess develops, resulting in a "lung-brain syndrome." Localized keratoconjunctivitis and endophthalmitis are the most frequent ocular manifestations of infection. The clinical presentation of these infections is similar to that seen with other bacterial pathogens, although a more subacute or chronic infection with intermittent exacerbations and remissions may be seen.

A Gram stain or modified acid-fast stain of purulent material obtained from infected sites will provide a presumptive diagnosis. Culture is the definitive diagnostic technique, but the laboratory must be alerted to the possibility of *Nocardia* spp. because the normally small colonies may be obscured by rapidly growing bacteria present in clinical specimens, and well-formed identifiable colonies may take 2 to 4 weeks for sufficient growth.[73]

Mycobacteria

Mycobacteria are not numerically important causes of ocular infection; their role is only briefly described here. As noted with the other bacteria in this section, disease caused by mycobacteria can occur in both normal and immunosuppressed individuals, although because they are obligate intracellular pathogens, immunocompromised persons are at increased risk for active mycobacterial infection and disseminated disease. Most mycobacteria are aerobic, slowly growing, acid-fast bacilli that produce colonies on media after 3 to 6 weeks of growth.[47] *Mycobacterium tuberculosis, M. avium* complex, and *M. kansasii* are probably the most prevalent human pathogens. *M. tuberculosis* is transmitted by respiratory droplet inhalation from person-to-person, whereas *M. avium* complex organisms are present in a number of environmental sources including water, soil, foods, and a variety of animal species.[47,56] Infection with the latter is acquired either by inhalation or ingestion of organisms; saprophytic infection or colonization of both the respiratory tract and the gastrointestinal tract in the absence of clinical disease states has been suggested by a number of epidemiologic studies.[18,50] Person-to-person transmission has not been described. *M. kansasii* is also probably acquired by a respiratory route based on the fact that pulmonary disease is the most frequent clinical manifestation of infection with this organism.

Disease in Compromised Hosts. Intact cell-mediated immunity is necessary for an appropriate host response to mycobacteria. CD4[+] T-lymphocytes appear to be necessary because the deficiency of these cells in patients with AIDS is the most consistent marker of risk for disseminated infection; most patients with AIDS who develop *M. avium* complex disease or disseminated tuberculosis do so only after a decline in CD4[+] T-lymphocyte count to below 50 cells/μl. Other cell fractions necessary for the normal immune response to these organisms include natural killer cells, cytotoxic T-lymphocytes, and activated mononuclear phagocytes.[8,61,93] Production and release of a number of cytokines by these cells may contribute to the host response; unregulated production of some, such as tumor necrosis factor, may contribute to the symptoms associated with systemic disease.[8,61,93]

The diagnosis of mycobacterial infections is dependent on demonstrating the organisms in tissue, by using appropriate stains (acid-fast, flurochrome stains) and by growing them in culture followed by species identification. A positive acid-fast smear is presumptive evidence of mycobacterial infection but does not distinguish among the many species, nor is it indicative of the presence of viable organisms. In the present milieu of rising rates of tuberculosis (particularly drug-resistant tuberculosis) in some urban areas, a positive acid-fast smear should be considered indicative of *M. tuberculosis* infection until proved otherwise. The use of radiometric detection methods for culture and nucleic acid probe assays for species identification can substantially reduce the time required for a positive culture. Demonstration of a granulomatous inflammatory reaction in histopathologic specimens is characteristic of mycobacterial infection, although those with profound immuno-

suppression may be incapable of producing well-formed granulomata.

CONCLUSION

Isolated aberration of any segment of host defense, including phagocytic dysfunction, complement deficiency, abnormalities of humoral immunity, or breakdown of anatomic barriers, may be sufficient to allow development of an opportunistic infection. Nevertheless, the majority of opportunistic pathogens causing serious disease, as discussed in this chapter, have their occurrence predominantly in the setting of disorders of phagocytosis or cell-mediated immunodeficiency states. For the immunocompetent host, these opportunistic pathogens lack specific virulence factors that allow them to adhere to and invade host tissue or to evade normal host defenses; or the pathogens are normally present in sufficiently low inocula that normal immune surveillance mechanisms keep them in check. Development of a clinically apparent opportunistic infection requires a breakdown of host immune or natural barrier defenses. For example, breakdown in natural barrier defenses alone may allow development of an opportunistic infection in an otherwise normal host, as can occur with the fungemia that results from an infected indwelling catheter or a contaminated needle used for injection drug use. In addition, debilitating diseases, including malignancies, diabetes mellitus, burns, and malnutrition, may increase the risk of both ocular and systemic infections.

With regard to immune and natural defenses, there are a number of factors unique to the ocular surface that must be considered. The corneal epithelium and eyelids serve as physical barriers, and some components of tears, including tear lysozyme and lactoferrin, serve an antimicrobial function. The normal flushing action of the tears with blinking is also an important protection. Traditionally, it is believed that only a few bacteria can penetrate corneal epithelium; they include *Neisseria gonorrhoeae, Neisseria meningitidis, Corynebacterium diphtheriae, Listeria* sp., and *Hemophilus influenza,* biotype 3 (previously known as *H. aegyptius* or the Koch-Weeks bacillus). It should be noted that there is little experimental evidence of the ability of these bacteria to penetrate corneal epithelium; it has been inferred clinically from the development of invasive corneal disease in the absence of known preexisting structural abnormalities of the eye.

A number of factors can breach the protective barriers of the ocular surface including blunt or sharp trauma, tear deficiencies, trichiasis, and contact lens use. Contact lenses are believed to increase the risk of corneal infections (1) by microscopic trauma to the corneal epithelium, (2) by reducing the availability of oxygen to the cornea, (3) by affecting the flushing action of tears, and (4) by serving as a vehicle for carrying infectious agents to the eye. Topical anesthetic abuse increases the risk of corneal infection by its toxic effect on the epithelium and by reducing the stimulus for protective reflex blinking.[127] Patching may pose a risk to the ocular surface by increasing its temperature and altering the flushing action of normal eyelid function.[94] Topical corticosteroid use is believed to have increased the rates of fungal, certain bacterial, and viral infections of the cornea since they were first introduced in the 1950s.[116] Large inocula of infectious agents may also overwhelm the immune and natural protections against ocular surface infections.

When considering opportunistic pathogens, the tissue involved must also be taken into account. *Streptococcus pyogenes,* for example, regularly causes a purulent or membraneous conjunctivitis, even in immunologically normal hosts that have no physical abnormalities of the ocular surface; however, unlike *Streptococcus pneumoniae,* which is traditionally considered to be a true corneal pathogen, conjunctival infection with *Streptococcus pyogenes* rarely spreads to involve a normal cornea.

The incidence, clinical manifestations, and severity of opportunistic infections and the degree to which different pathogens cause disease also vary according to the type and degree of immunosuppression. To illustrate, *P. carinii* and serious varicella-zoster virus infections in children with acute lymphocytic leukemia are common, but in one study, their incidence varied substantially according to the level of immunosuppression induced by chemotherapy maintenance regimens. They ranged from 5% and 10%, respectively, for children receiving methotrexate alone to 43% and 29%, respectively, for children receiving four chemotherapeutic agents plus mediastinal radiation.[58] Also, the clinical manifestations of disease caused by the same pathogen differ according to the underlying host defect. Again using *P. carinii* as an example, pneumonia caused by this pathogen often has a more acute and explosive presentation in bone marrow transplant recipients but a more insidious presentation in many patients with AIDS. Many pathogens considered to be opportunistic are ones that latently infect large segments of the population and only cause serious disease when acquired immunodeficiency intervenes. For instance, from 40% to 70% of the general population is latently infected with CMV,[54] as measured by IgG antibody levels, yet serious end-organ disease is seen almost exclusively in those with serious impairment of cell-mediated immune function.

Opportunistic ocular infections have become progressively more common in recent years, usually as part of a systemic illness. Knowledge of predisposing factors and clinical recognition of disease syndromes will improve our diagnostic capabilities and, as understanding of the immunopathogenesis of disease caused by these pathogens expands, improvement in our ability to treat and prevent serious infection more effectively will follow.

REFERENCES

1. Armstrong D: *Listeria monocytogenes.* In Mandell GL, Douglas RG Jr, Bennett JE, editors: *Principles and practice of infectious disease,* ed 3, 1587-1593, New York, 1990, Churchill Livingstone.
2. Armstrong D: History of opportunistic infection in the immunocompromised host, *Clin Infect Dis* 17(suppl 2):S318-S321, 1993.
3. Arvin AM: Cell-mediated immunity to varicella-zoster virus, *J Infect Dis* 166(suppl 1):S35-S41, 1992.
4. Ashton N, Wirasinha PA: Encephalitozoonosis (nosematosis) of the cornea, *Br J Ophthalmol* 57:669-674, 1973.
5. Balfour HH, Benson C, Braun J et al.: Management of acyclovir-resistant herpes simplex and varicella-zoster virus infections, *J Acquir Immune Defic Syndr* 7:254-260, 1994.
6. Baringer JR, Swoveland P: Recovery of herpes-simplex virus from human trigeminal ganglions, *N Engl J Med* 288:648-650, 1973.
7. Bennett JE: *Aspergillus* species. In Mandell GL, Douglas RG Jr, Bennett JE, editors: *Principles and practice of infectious disease,* 1958-1962, ed 3, New York, 1990, Churchill Livingstone.
8. Benson CA, Ellner JJ: *Mycobacterium avium* complex infection and AIDS: advances in theory and practice, *Clin Infect Dis* 17:7-20, 1993.
9. Bergquist NR, Stintzing G, Smedman L et al.: Diagnosis of encephalitozoonosis in man by serological tests, *Br Med J* 288:902, 1984.
10. Beyt Jr BE, Waltman SR: Cryptococcal endophthalmitis after corneal transplantation, *New Eng J Med* 298:825-826, 1978.
11. Blinkhorn RJ, Adelstein D, Spagnuolo PJ: Emergence of a new opportunistic pathogen: *candida lisitianiae, J Clin Microbiol* 27:236-240, 1989.
12. Brock BV, Selke S, Benedetti J et al.: Frequency of asymptomatic shedding of herpes simplex virus in women with genital herpes, *JAMA* 263:418-420, 1990.
13. Browne MJ, Hubbard SM, Longo DL et al.: Excess prevalence of *Pneumocystis carinii* pneumonia in patients treated for lymphoma with combination chemotherapy, *Ann Intern Med* 104:338-344, 1986.
14. Bryan RT: *Microsporidia.* In Mandell GL, Douglas RG Jr, Bennett JE, editors: *Principles and practice of infectious disease,* ed 3, 2130-2134, New York, 1990, Churchill Livingstone.
15. Burke BA, Good RA: *Pneumocystis carinii* infection, *Medicine* 52:23-51, 1973.
16. Carroll JM, Martola EL, Laibson PR et al.: The recurrence of herpetic keratitis following idoxuridine therapy, *Am J Ophthalmol* 63:103-107, 1967.
17. Chen CJ: *Nocardia asteroides* endophthalmitis, *Ophthalmic Surg* 14:502-505, 1983.
18. Chin DP, Hopewell PC, Yajko DM et al.: *Mycobacterium avium* complex in the respiratory or gastrointestinal tract and the risk of *M. avium* complex bacteremia in patients with human immunodeficiency virus infection, *J Infect Dis* 169:289-295, 1994.
19. Ciesielski CA, Hightower AW, Parsons SK et al.: Listeriosis in the United States: 1980-1982, *Arch Intern Med* 148:1416-1419, 1988.
20. Cole EL, Meisler DM, Clabrese LH et al.: Herpes zoster ophthalmicus and acquired immune deficiency syndrome, *Arch Ophthalmol* 102:1027-1029, 1984.
21. Corey L, Adams HG, Brown ZA et al.: Genital herpes simplex virus infections: clinical manifestations, course, and complications, *Ann Intern Med* 98:958-972, 1983.
22. Corey L, Spear PG: Infections with herpes simplex viruses, *N Engl J Med* 14:686-691, 749-757, 1986.
23. Cryzan S, Paradis IL, Zeevi A et al.: Unexpectedly high incidence of *Pneumocystis carinii* infection after lung-heart transplantation. Implications for lung defense and allograft survival, *Am Rev Respir Dis* 137:1268-1274, 1988.
24. Denning DW, Follansbee SE, Scolaro M et al.: Pulmonary aspergillosis in the acquired immunodeficiency syndrome, *N Engl J Med* 324:654-662, 1991.
25. Denning DW, Stevens DA: Antifungal and surgical treatment of invasive aspergillosis: review of 2,121 published cases, *Rev Infect Dis* 12:1147-1201, 1990.

26. Diamond RD: *Cryptococcus neoformans.* In Mandell GL, Bennett JE, Dolin R, editors: *Principles and practice of infectious disease,* ed 4, 2331-2340, New York, 1995, Churchill Livingstone.
27. Diamond RD, Erickson NF III: Chemotaxis of human neutrophils and monocytes induced by *Cryptococcus neoformans, Infect Immun* 38:380-382, 1982.
28. Diamond RD, Root RK, Bennett JE: Factors influencing killing of *Cryptococcus neoformns* by human leukocytes in vitro, *J Infect Dis* 125:367-376, 1972.
29. Didier ES, Didier PJ, Friedberg DN et al.: Isolation and characterization of a new human microsporidian, *Encephalitozoon hellem* (n sp), from three AIDS patients with keratoconjunctivitis, *J Infect Dis* 163:617-621, 1991.
30. Doft BH, Clarkson JG, Febell G et al.: Endogenous *Aspergillus* endophthalmitis in drug abusers, *Arch Ophthalmol* 98:859, 1980.
31. Dunn JP, Holland GN: Human immunodeficiency virus and opportunistic ocular infections, *Infect Dis Clin North Am* 6:909-923, 1992.
32. Edman JC, Kovacs JA, Masur H et al.: Ribosomal RNA sequence shows *Pneumocystis carinii* to be a member of the fungi, *Nature* 334:519-522, 1988.
33. Edwards JE, Jr: *Candida* species. In Mandell GL, Bennett JE, Dolin R, editors: *Principles and practice of infectious disease,* ed 4, 2289-2306, New York, 1995, Churchill Livingstone.
34. Ewing J: *Neoplastic diseases: a treatise on tumors,* Philadelphia, 1940, WB Saunders.
35. Filice GA, Niewoehner DE: Contribution of neutrophils and cell-mediated immunity to control *Nocardia asteroides* in man. In Ortiz-Ortiz L, Bojalil LF, Yakoleff V, editors: *Biological, biochemical, and biomedical aspects of actinomycetes,* Orlando, Fla, Academic Press.
36. Filice GA, Niewoehner DE: Contribution of neutrophils and cell-mediated immunity to control of *Nocardia asteroides* in murine lungs, *J Infect Dis* 156:113-121, 1987.
37. Fisher MA, Shen S-H, Haddad J et al.: Comparison of in vivo activity of fluconazole with that of amphotericin B against *Candida tropicalis, Candida glabrata,* and *Candida krusei, Antimicrob Agents Chemother* 33:1443-1446, 1989.
38. Freeman WR, Chen A, Henderly DE et al.: Prevalence and significance of acquired immunodeficiency syndrome-related retinal microvasculopathy, *Am J Ophthalmol* 107:229-235, 1989.
39. Friedland LR, Raphael SA, Deutsch ES et al.: Disseminated *Acanthamoeba* infection in a child with symptomatic human immunodeficiency virus infection, *Pediatr Infect Dis J* 11:404-407, 1992.
40. Friel JP, editor: *Dorland's illustrated medical dictionary,* ed 25, Philadelphia, 1974, WB Saunders.
41. Gallant JE, Moore RD, Richman DD et al.: Incidence and natural history of cytomegalovirus disease in patients with advanced human immunodeficiency virus disease treated with zidovudine. The Zidovudine Epidemiology Study Group, *J Infect Dis* 166:1223-1227, 1992.
42. Gelfand JA, Jurley DL, Fauci AS et al.: Role of complement in host defense against experimental disseminated candidiasis, *J Infect Dis* 138:9-16, 1978.
43. Gellin BG, Broome CV: Listeriosis, *JAMA* 261:1313-1320, 1989.
44. Goodner EK, Okumoto MA: Intraocular listeriosis, *Am J Ophthalmol* 64:682, 1967.
45. Gigliotti F, Hughes WT: Passive immunoprophylaxis with specific monoclonal antibody confers partial protection against *Pneumocystis carinii* pneumonitis in animal models, *J Clin Invest* 81:1666, 1988.
46. Glaser JB, Garden A: Inoculation of cryptococcosis without transmission of the acquired immunodeficiency syndrome, *N Engl J Med* 313:266, 1985.
47. Haas DW, DesPrez RM: *Mycobacterium tuberculosis.* In Mandell GL, Bennett JE, Dolin R, editors: *Principles and practice of infectious diseases,* ed 4, 2213-2243, New York, 1995, Churchill Livingstone.
48. Hakes TB, Armstrong D: Toxoplasmosis: problems in diagnosis and treatment, *Cancer* 140:330-342, 1983.
49. Hardy AM, Wajszczuk CP, Suffredini AF et al.: *Pneumocystis carinii* pneumonia in renal-transplant recipients treated with cyclosporine and steroids, *J Infect Dis* 149:143-147, 1984.
50. Havlik JA Jr, Metchock B, Thompson SE III et al.: A prospective evaluation of *Mycobacterium avium* complex colonization of the respiratory and gastrointestinal tracts of persons with human immunodeficiency virus infection, *J Infect Dis* 168:1045-1048, 1993.
51. Helton J, Loveless M, White CR Jr: Cutaneous *Acanthamoeba* infection associated with leukocytoclastic vasculitis in an AIDS patient, *Am J Dermatopathol* 15:146-149, 1993.
52. Hidore MR, Murphy JW: Correlation of natural killer cell activity and clearance of *Cryptococcus neoformans* from mice after adoptive transfer of splenic nylon wool-nonadherent cells, *Infect Immun* 51:547-555, 1986.
53. Hilt DC, Buchholz D, Krumholz A et al.: Herpes zoster ophthalmicus and delayed contralateral hemiparesis caused by cerebral angiitis: diagnosis and management approaches, *Ann Neurol* 14:543-553, 1983.
54. Ho M: Cytomegalovirus. In Mandell GL, Bennett JE, Dolin R, editors: *Principles and practice of infectious disease,* ed 4, 1351-1364, New York, 1995, Churchill Livingstone.
55. Holland GN: Ocular toxoplasmosis in the immunocompromised host, *Int Ophthalmol* 13:399-402, 1989.
56. Horsburgh CR Jr, Selik RM: The epidemiology of disseminated nontuberculous mycobacterial infection in the acquired immunodeficiency syndrome (AIDS), *Am Rev Respir Dis* 139:4-7, 1989.
57. Hughes WT: Natural mode of acquisition for de novo infection with *Pneumocystis carinii, J Infect Dis* 145:842-848, 1982.
58. Hughes WT, Feldman S, Aur RJA et al.: Intensity of immunosuppressive therapy and the incidence of *Pneumocystis carinii* pneumonitis, *Cancer* 36:2004-2009, 1975.
59. Hughes WT, Kuhn S, Chaudhary S et al.: Successful chemoprophylaxis for *Pneumocystis carinii* pneumonitis, *N Engl J Med* 297:1419-1426, 1977.
60. Igel JH, Bolande RP: Humoral defense mechanisms in cryptococcosis: substances in normal human serum, saliva and cerebrospinal fluid affecting the growth of *Cryptococcus neoformans, J Infect Dis* 116:75-83, 1966.
61. Inderlied CB, Kemper CA, Bermudez LEM: The *Mycobacterium avium* complex, *Clin Microbiol Rev* 6:266-310, 1993.
62. Israelski DM, Remington JS: Toxoplasmosis in patients with cancer, *Clin Infect Dis* 17(suppl 2):S423-S435, 1993.
63. Isselutz TB, Lee SHS, Bortolussi R: Immune response to *Listeria monocytogenes.* In Rose NR, Friedman H, Fahey JL, editors: *Manual of clinical laboratory immunology,* ed 4, 402-407, Washington, DC, 1992, American Society for Microbiology.
64. Kaplowitz LG, Baker D, Gelb L et al.: Prolonged continuous acyclovir treatment of normal adults with frequently recurring genital herpes simplex virus infection, *JAMA* 265:747-751, 1991.
65. Karam GH, Griffin FM Jr: Invasive pulmonary aspergillosis in nonimmunocompromised, nonneutropenic hosts, *Rev Infect Dis* 8:357-363, 1986.
66. Komshian SV, Uwaydah AK, Sobel JD et al.: Fungemia cause by *Candida* species and *Torulopsis glabrata* in the hospitalized patient: frequency, characteristics, and evaluation of factors influencing outcome, *Rev Infect Dis* 11:379-390, 1989.
67. Kovacs JA: Diagnosis, treatment, and prevention of *Pneumocystis carinii* pneumonia in HIV-infected patients, *AIDS Updates* 6:1-13, 1993.
68. Kozel TR, Hermerath CA: Binding of cryptococcal polysaccharide to *Cryptococcus neoformans, Infect Immun* 43:879-886, 1984.
69. Kozel TR, Pfrommer GST: Activation of the complement system by *Cryptococcus neoformans* leads to binding of iC3b to the yeast, *Infect Immun* 52:1-5, 1986.
70. Kwon-Chung KJ, Rhodes JC: Encapsulation and melanin formation as indicators of virulence in *Cryptococcus neoformans, Infect Immun* 51:218-223, 1986.
71. Lass JH, Thoft RA, Bellows AR et al.: Exogenous *Nocardia asteroides* endophthalmitis associated with malignant glaucoma, *Ann Ophthalmol* 13:317-321, 1981.
72. Leggiadro RJ, Winkelstein JA, Hughes WT: Prevalence of *Pneumocystis carinii* pneumonitis in severe combined immunodeficiency, *J Pediatr* 99:96-98, 1981.
73. Lerner PI: *Nocardia* species. In Mandell GL, Bennett JE, Dolin R, editors: *Principles and practice of infectious disease,* ed 4, 2273-2280, New York, 1995, Churchill Livingstone.

74. Lipscomb MR, Alvarellos T, Toews GB et al.: Role of natural killer cells in resistance to *Cryptococcus neoformans* infections in mice, *Am J Pathol* 128:354-361, 1987.

75. Lopez C: Resistance to herpes simplex virus-type 1 (HSV-1), *Curr Top Microbiol Immunol* 92:15, 1981.

76. Luft BJ, Remington JS: Toxoplasmic encephalitis in AIDS, *Clin Infect Dis* 15:211-222, 1992.

77. MacGowan AP, Peterson PK, Keane W et al.: Human peritoneal macrophage phagocytic, killing, and chemiluminescent responses to opsonized *Listeria monocytogenes, Infect Immun* 40:440, 1983.

78. Mader TH, Stulting RD: Viral keratitis, *Inf Dis Clin North Am* 6:831-849, 1992.

79. Martinez AJ: Is *Acanthamoeba* encephalitis an opportunistic infection? *Neurology* 30:567-574, 1980.

80. Masur H, Ognibene FP, Yarchoan R et al.: CD4 counts as predictors of opportunistic pneumonias in human immunodeficiency virus (HIV) infection, *Ann Intern Med* 111:223, 1989.

81. McCabe RE, Remington JS: *Toxoplasma gondii.* In Mandell GL, Douglas RG Jr, Bennett JE, editors: *Principles and practice of infectious disease,* ed 3, 2090-2103, New York, 1990, Churchill Livingstone.

82. Meier JL, Straus SE: Comparative biology of latent varicella-zoster virus and herpes simplex virus infections, *J Infect Dis* 166(suppl 1):S13-S23, 1992.

83. Mertz GJ, Coombs RW, Ashley R et al.: Transmission of genital herpes in couples with one symptomatic and one asymptomatic partner: a prospective study, *J Infect Dis* 157:1169-1177, 1988.

84. Meunch R, Nassim C, Niku S et al.: Seroepidemiology of varicella, *J Infect Dis* 153:153-155, 1986.

85. Meyers JD, Flournoy N, Thomas ED: Nonbacterial pneumonia after allogeneic marrow transplantation: a review of ten years' experience, *Rev Infect Dis* 4:1119-1132, 1982.

86. Meyers JD, Pifer LL, Sale GE et al.: The value of *Pneumocystis carinii* antibody and antigen detection for diagnosis of *Pneumocystis carinii* pneumonia after marrow transplantation, *Am Rev Respir Dis* 120:1283-1287, 1979.

87. Michelson JB, Freedman SD, Boyden DG: *Aspergillus* endophthalmitis in a drug abuser, *Ann Ophthalmol* 14:1051, 1982.

88. Nabavi N, Murphy JW: Antibody-dependent natural killer cell-mediated growth inhibition of *Cryptococcus neoformans, Infect Immun* 51:556-562, 1986.

89. Naidoff MA, Green WR: Endogenous *Aspergillus* endophthalmitis occurring after kidney transplant, *Am J Ophthalmol* 79:502, 1975.

90. Neu HC: Toxoplasmosis transmitted at autopsy, *JAMA* 202:284, 1967.

91. Nicholson DH, Wolchok EB: Ocular toxoplasmosis in an adult receiving long-term corticosteroid therapy, *Arch Ophthalmol* 94:248-254, 1976.

92. Okun E, Butler WT: Ophthalmologic complications of cryptococcal meningitis, *Arch Ophthalmol* 71:52, 1964.

93. Orme IM, Andersen P, Boom WH: T cell response to *Mycobacterium tuberculosis, J Infect Dis* 167:1481-1497, 1993.

94. Ostler HB, Okumoto M, Wilkey C: The changing pattern of the etiology of central bacterial corneal (hypopyon) ulcer, *Trans Pac Coast Oto-Ophthalmol Soc* 57:235, 1976.

95. Peglow SL, Smulian AG, Linke MJ et al.: Serologic responses to *Pneumocystis carinii* antigens in health and disease, *J Infect Dis* 161:296, 1990.

96. Pflugfelder SC, Flynn HW: Infectious endophthalmitis, *Inf Dis Clin North Am* 6:859-873, 1992.

97. Phair J, Munoz A, Detels R et al.: The risk of *Pneumocystis carinii* pneumonia among men infected with human immunodeficiency virus type 1, *N Engl J Med* 322:161, 1990.

98. Pinnolis M, Egbert PR, Font RL et al.: Nosematosis of the cornea, *Arch Ophthalmol* 99:1044-1047, 1981.

99. Powderly WG, Kobayashi GS, Herzig GP et al.: Amphotericin B-resistant yeast infection in severely immunocompromised patients, *Am J Med* 84:826-832, 1988.

100. Remington JS, Desmonts G: Toxoplasmosis. In Remington JS, Klein JO, editors: *Infectious diseases of the fetus and newborn infant,* 143, Philadelphia, 1983, WB Saunders.

101. Rinaldo CR, Black PH, Hirsch MS: Interaction of cytomegalovirus with leukocytes from patients with mononucleosis due to cytomegalovirus, *J Infect Dis* 136:667-678, 1977.

102. Roths JB, Sigman CL: Single and combined humoral and cell-mediated immunotherapy of *Pneumocystis carinii* pneumonia in immunodeficient scid mice, *Infect Immunol* 61:1641, 1993.

103. Rotrosen D, Calderone RA, Edwards JE Jr: Adherence of *Candida* species to host tissues and plastic surfaces, *Rev Infect Dis* 8:73-85, 1986.

104. Ruskin J, Remington JS: The compromised host and infection. I. Pneumocystis carinii pneumonia, *JAMA* 202:1070-1074, 1967.

105. Ruskin J, Remington JS: Toxoplasmosis in the compromised host, *Ann Intern Med* 84:193-199, 1976.

106. Ryning FW, McLeod R, Maddox JC et al.: Probable transmission of *Toxoplasma gondii* by organ transplantation, *Ann Intern Med* 90:47-49, 1979.

107. Saag MS, Powderly WG, Cloud GA et al.: Comparison of amphotericin B with fluconazole in the treatment of acute AIDS-associated cryptococcal meningitis, *New Eng J Med* 326:83-89, 1992.

108. Sepkowitz KA: *Pneumocystis carinii* pneumonia in patients without AIDS, *Clin Infect Dis* 17(suppl 2):S416-S422, 1993.

109. Sepkowitz KA, Brown AE, Telzak EE et al.: *Pneumocystis carinii* pneumonia among patients without AIDS at.a cancer hospital, *JAMA* 267:832-837, 1992.

110. Sha BE, Benson CA, Deutsch T et al.: *Pneumocystis carinii* choroiditis in patients with AIDS: clinical features, response to therapy, and outcome, *J Acquir Immune Defic Syndr* 5:1051-1058, 1992.

111. Solomkin JS, Mills EL, Giebink GS et al.: Phagocytosis of *Candida albicans* by human leukocytes: opsonic requirements, *J Infect Dis* 137:30-37, 1978.

111a. Stehr-Green JK, Bailey TM, Brandt FH et al.: *Acanthamoeba* keratitis in soft contact wearers: a case-control study, *JAMA* 258:57-60, 1987.

112. Slater CA, Sickel JZ, Visvesvara GS et al.: Brief report: successful treatment of disseminated acanthamoeba infection in an immunocompromised patient, *New Eng J Med* 331:85-87, 1994.

113. Stevens DA, Pier AC, Beaman BL et al.: Laboratory evaluation of an outbreak of nocardiosis in immunocompromised hosts, *Am J Med* 71:928-934, 1981.

114. Stevens JG, Wagner EK, Dovi-Rao GB et al.: RNA complementary to a herpesvirus and gene in RNA in prominent in latently infected neurons, *Science* 236:1056, 1987.

115. Straus SE, Ostrove JM, Inchauspe G et al.: Varicella-zoster virus infections: biology, natural history, treatment, and prevention, *Ann Intern Med* 108:221-237, 1988.

116. Thygeson P: The immunology and immunopathology of corneal infection, *Trans Pac Coast Oto-Ophthalmol Soc* 57:357, 1976.

117. Wakefield AE, Pixley FJ, Banerji S et al.: Amplification of mitochondrial ribosomal RNA sequences from *Pneumocystis carinii* DNA of rat and human origin, *Mol Biochem Parasitol* 43:69, 1990.

118. Waller T: Sensitivity of *Encephalitozoon çuniculi* to various temperatures, disinfectants and drugs, *Lab Anim* 13:227-230, 1979.

119. Walzer PD: *Pneumocystis carinii.* In Mandell GL, Bennett JE, Dolin R, editors: *Principles and practice of infectious diseases,* ed 4, 2475-2487, New York, 1995, Churchill Livingstone.

120. Wang SS, Feldman HA: Isolation of *Hartmanella* species from human throats, *New Eng J Med* 277:1174-1179, 1967.

121. Washburn RG, Gallin JI, Bennett JE: Oxidative killing of *Aspergillus* proceeds by parallel myeloperoxidase-dependent and myeloperoxidase-independent pathways, *Infect Immun* 55:2088-2092, 1987.

122. Weber R, Bryan RT, Owen RL et al.: Improved light-microscopical detection of microsporidia spores in stool and duodenal aspirates, *N Engl J Med* 326:161-166, 1992.

123. Weinberg PB, Becker S, Granger DL et al.: Growth inhibition of *Cryptococcus neoformans* by human alveolar macrophages, *Am Rev Respir Dis* 136:1242-1247, 1987.

124. Wheat LJ, Kohler RB, Lewari RP: Diagnosis of disseminated histoplasmosis by detection of *Histoplasma capsulatum* antigen in serum and urine specimens, *N Engl J Med* 314:83-88, 1986.
125. Wheat LJ, Connolly-Stringfield PA, Baker RL et al.: Disseminated histoplasmosis in the acquired immunodeficiency syndrome: clinical findings, diagnosis and treatment, and review of literature, *Medicine* 69:361-374, 1990.
126. Whitley RJ: Herpes simplex viruses. In Fields BN, Knipe DM, editors: *Virology,* ed 2, 1843-1888, New York, 1990, Raven Press.
127. Wilson FM II: Adverse external ocular effects of topical ophthalmic medications, *Surv Ophthalmol* 24:57, 1979.
128. Wingard JR, Merz WG, Rinaldi MG et al.: Increase in *Candida krusei* infection among patients with bone marrow transplantation and neutropenia treated prophylactically with fluconazole, *N Engl J Med* 325:1274-1277, 1991.
129. Wreghitt TG, Hakim M, Cory-Pearce R et al.: The impact of donor-transmitted CMV and *Toxoplasma gondii* disease in cardiac transplantation, *Trans Proc* 18:1375-1376, 1986.

21 Ocular Disease and Immunodeficiency Disorders

E. RICHARD STIEHM, MITCHELL H. FRIEDLAENDER

Primary immunodeficiency syndromes are inherited defects of the immune system that are associated with undue susceptibility to infection. These conditions may result in protean ocular manifestations.[1a] Afflicted patients, principally infants and children, have defects in one or more components of their immune system: the B lymphocytes, the T lymphocytes, the phagocytic cells, or the complement system. Primary immunodeficiency is classified into five categories: (1) antibody (B cell) immunodeficiencies, (2) cellular (T cell) immunodeficiencies, (3) combined B cell and T cell immunodeficiencies, (4) disorders of phagocytic function, and (5) complement abnormalities.

Antibody (B cell) deficiencies account for one half of the primary immunodeficiency diseases. The remaining half are attributed to (in descending order of frequency) combined B cell and T cell disorders (20%), phagocytic disorders (18%), T cell disorders (10%), and complement disorders (2%).[50] Because of the interaction of T cells with other components of the immune system, overlap exists in several syndromes.

In 1992 the World Health Organization (WHO) identified 45 distinct primary immunodeficiency syndromes (Table 21-1).[56a] Several other congenital or hereditary diseases (Down syndrome, congenital asplenia, Bloom syndrome) also have consistent immunologic defects (Table 21-2).[56a]

The overall incidence of primary immunodeficiency is 1:10,000 (excluding selective IgA deficiency), so in the United States there may be 400 new victims born annually. About two thirds of the patients are male,[16] reflecting the numerous X-linked disorders. Selective IgA deficiency is the most common primary immunodeficiency, with a reported incidence ranging from 1:40 to 1:1,000.[13] Severe primary immunodeficiencies such as X-linked agammaglobulinemia, severe combined immunodeficiency (SCID), and chronic granulomatous disease occur with an incidence of about 1:100,000 live births.

B CELL (ANTIBODY) IMMUNODEFICIENCIES

Patients with antibody deficiency have recurrent respiratory infection and/or severe infection with encapsulated organisms, such as *Streptococcus pneumoniae*. In addition to having a deficiency of circulating immune globulins and antibodies, these patients lack secretory antibodies that enable bacteria, viruses, and parasites to attach more easily to mucosal surfaces.[24] Frequent gastrointestinal and respiratory tract infections occur. The ocular surface may also be at increased risk for infection. Lack of antibody can limit the action of nonspecific immune defense mechanisms, such as complement activation by immune complexes or phagocytosis of antibody-coated organisms.

Patients with *X-linked agammaglobulinemia* have repeated bouts of infection and sepsis. Keratoconjunctivitis has been reported in a few of these patients,[24] but in most cases the eyes are unaffected.[12,25] In one family, three brothers with X-linked agammaglobulinemia had recurrent purulent conjunctivitis caused by *Haemophilus influenzae* and two of them developed corneal scarring.[31] They all had no detectable IgA in their tears, although tear lysozyme levels were normal. Eczema is common in this condition[21] and may affect the eyelids; and benign lymphoid infiltration of the vitreous (which is resistant to corticosteroids and cytotoxic agents) may cause visual impairment.[35]

Selective IgA deficiency (IgA < 10 mg/dl) is the most common primary immunodeficiency, occurring in 1 of 400 individuals.[1,13] Ocular infection in IgA deficiency is rare, despite the fact that IgA is the main immunoglobulin in tears and the conjunctiva.[1,22] Ocular disease is more common when other immunoglobulin classes are also deficient.[24] Hemorrhagic retinitis was described in one case of IgA deficiency, but may actually have been the result of systemic lupus erythematosus.[28]

It is not feasible to provide serum IgA to an IgA-deficient patient. There is minimal IgA in immunoglobulin prepara-

TABLE 21-1 1992 WHO CLASSIFICATION OF PRIMARY AND SECONDARY IMMUNODEFICIENCIES

Groups	Inheritance*	Groups	Inheritance†
A. Predominantly antibody deficiencies		b) Autosomal recessive (CGD)	AR
1. X-linked agammaglobulinemia	XL	1. p 22 phox†	
2. Ig deficiency with increased IgM ("Hyper-IgM syndrome")	Various: XL, AR, unknown	2. p 47 phox	
3. Ig heavy chain gene deletions	AR	3. p 67 phox	AR
4. κ chain deficiency	AR	20. Leukocyte adhesion defect [deficiency of beta chain (CD18) of LFA-1, Mac 1, p150,95]	
5. Selective deficiency of IgG subclasses (with or without IgA deficiency)	Unknown	21. Neutrophil G6PD deficiency	XL
6. Common variable immunodeficiency (CVID)	Various: AR, AD, or unknown	22. Myeloperoxidase deficiency	AR
7. IgA deficiency	Various: AR, unknown	23. Secondary granule deficiency	AR
8. Transient hypogammaglobulinemia of infancy	Unknown	E. Complement deficiencies Deficiency	Inheritance
B. Combined immunodeficiencies		24. C1q	AR
9. Severe combined immunodeficiency (SCID):		25. C1r	AR
a) X-linked	XL	26. C4	AR
b) Autosomal recessive	AR	27. C2	AR
10. Adenosine deaminase (ADA) deficiency	AR	28. C3	AR
11. Purine nucleoside phosphorylase (PNP) deficiency	AR	29. C5	AR
12. MHC class II deficiency	AR	30. C6	AR
13. Reticular dysgenesis	AR	31. C7	AR
14. CD3 γ or CD3 ε deficiency	AR	32. C8α	AR
15. CD8 deficiency	AR	33. C8γ	
C. Other well-defined immunodeficiency syndromes		34. C8β	AR
16. Wiskott-Aldrich syndrome	XL	35. C9	AR
17. Ataxia-telangiectasia	AR	36. C1 inhibitor	AD
18. DiGeorge anomaly	Unknown	37. Factor I	AR
D. Defects of phagocytic function		38. Factor II	AR
19. Chronic granulomatous disease (CGD)		39. Factor D	?AR or XL
a) X-linked CGD (deficiency of 91 kD binding chain of cytochrome b)	XL	40. Properdin	XL
		F. Other primary immunodeficiency diseases	
		41. Primary CD4 deficiency	
		42. Primary CD7 deficiency	
		43. IL-2 deficiency	
		44. Multiple cytokine deficiency	
		45. Signal transduction deficiency	

From WHO Scientific Group. Primary immunodeficiency diseases, *Immunodeficiency Reviews* 3:195-236, 1992.
*XL—X-linked, AR—autosomal recessive, AD—autosomal dominant
†Phagocyte oxidase

tions and its half life (7 days) is too rapid to maintain therapeutic levels. Patients with IgA deficiency may also develop anti-IgA antibodies and anaphylactic response to treatment with immunoglobulins specifically the IgA component.[14] The IgA present in secretions (such as tears) is locally produced and does not come from the circulating IgA. Secretory IgA is usually in a dimer form and contains two serum IgA molecules plus a secretory piece and a joining chain.

Patients with hypogammaglobulinemia and *IgG subclass*

deficiency may have ophthalmic abnormalities. Franklin and associates[24] reported nonfollicular, nonpurulent conjunctivitis in eight patients with severe hypogammaglobulinemia including three with X-linked agammaglobulinemia, four with common variable ("acquired") immunodeficiency, and one with a combined immunodeficiency. *Haemophilus influenzae* was isolated from five patients, two of whom were also infected by *Staphylococcus aureus; Staphylococcus epidermidis* was isolated from another patient.

TABLE 21-2   CONGENITAL OR HEREDITARY DISEASES ASSOCIATED WITH IMMUNODEFICIENCY

Chromosome abnormalities
  Bloom syndrome
  Fanconi anemia
  Down syndrome
  Abnormal condensation of heterochromatin in chromosomes 1, 9, and 16

Multiple-organ system abnormalities
  Partial albinism
  Chediak-Higashi syndrome
  Cartilage hair hypoplasia
  Agenesis of the corpus callosum

Hereditary metabolic defects
  Transcobalamin 2 deficiency
  Acrodermatitis enteropathica
  Type I orotic aciduria
  Biotin dependent carboxylase deficiency

Hypercatabolism of Ig
  Familial hypercatabolism of Ig
  Intestinal lymphangiectasia

Other
  Hyper IgE syndrome
  Chronic mucocutaneous candidiasis
  Hypo- or aspenia
  EBV-associated immunodeficiency (X-linked lymphoproliferative syndrome)

From WHO Scientific Group. Primary immunodeficiency diseases, *Immunodeficiency Reviews* 3:195-236, 1992.

Among approximately 500 cases of hypogammaglobulinemia in the United Kingdom, one patient had acute unilateral uveitis[38] and another had an acute annular detachment of the choroid and retina with panuveitis. These findings may have been incidental and cannot be attributed specifically to the immunodeficiency.

Multiple chalazia and hordeola, marginal corneal infiltrates, and vascularization of the limbus have been reported in patients with IgG4 deficiency.[34] Other cases, however, have reported no ocular findings.[4]

Little information is available about ophthalmic involvement with other selective antibody disorders. *Selective IgM deficiency* results in systemic sepsis, severe eczema, verrucae vulgaris, and recurrent bacterial infections of the skin.[21] Periorbital cellulitis has been reported with this condition.[13] Patients with *immunodeficiency with hyper-IgM* develop severe verrucae vulgaris,[21] which can involve the eyelids. One patient with hypogammaglobulinemia, a 10-year-old girl, had diplopia caused by Brown superior oblique tendon syndrome.[7]

COMBINED IMMUNODEFICIENCIES

These disorders have defects of both antibody and cellular immunity and range from life-threatening illness to prolonged survival with minimal morbidity. Several immunologic syndromes (Wiskott-Aldrich syndrome, ataxia-telangiectasia) have combined defects and fit into this category.

Severe combined immunodeficiency syndrome (SCID) is a multifactorial disorder with potentially fatal, profound defects in both cellular and humoral immunity. SCID actually includes a spectrum of syndromes with various enzymatic defects, modes of inheritance, and levels of cellular differentiation (Table 21-1). Inheritance may be X-linked, autosomal recessive, autosomal dominant, or sporadic. Because of the severe lack of immunocompetence, infants with SCID are at risk for overwhelming infection by all types of pathogens: viruses (Fig. 21-1), bacteria, fungi, and protozoa. Sufferers often succumb to infection during the first year of life, although bone marrow transplantation can reconstitute a majority of these patients.

These patients are particularly susceptible to normally mild viral respiratory pathogens such as parainfluenza, adenovirus, and respiratory syncytial virus.[22] Reports of fatal, disseminated adenoviral infection in these children have not mentioned the cornea or conjunctiva as sites of the disease.

Perhaps because of the rapidly fatal nature of SCID, reports of opportunistic eye infections are rare. Cytomegalovirus (CMV) retinopathy has been reported in a child with SCID.[8] The patient was treated by bone marrow transplantation. Severe disseminated CMV infections occur frequently in patients who undergo transplantation, and therefore the relationship between the retinal infection and the immunologic defects of SCID is uncertain. Conjunctivitis was reported by Franklin and associates[24] in a child with SCID.

Nezelof syndrome refers to an illness with a severe cell-mediated immune defect and an embryonic thymus, but with normal circulating immunoglobulins; it is a variant of SCID. There has been some inconsistency in the use of this term, and therefore it is difficult to compare reports of its manifes-

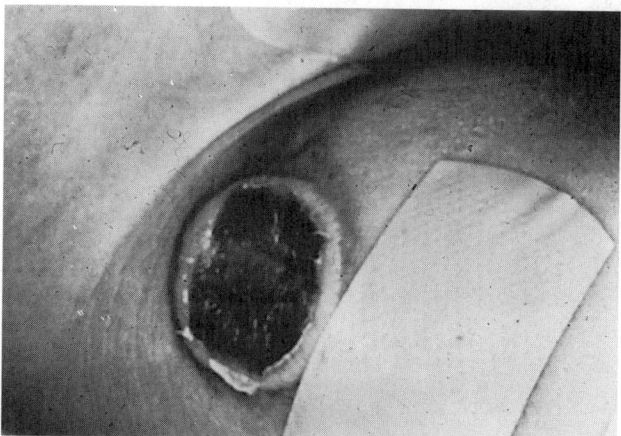

Fig. 21-1.   Disseminated vaccinia in a child with severe combined immunodeficiency syndrome.

tations. Among five patients with Nezelof syndrome, *Staphylococcus aureus* blepharitis was identified in one and *Pseudomonas aeruginosa* blepharoconjunctivitis in another (Fig. 21-2).[26] The other patients were without apparent ophthalmic disease.

Bare lymphocyte syndrome is a rare autosomal recessive combined immunodeficiency syndrome that is associated with absent HLA antigens on the lymphocyte surfaces. Candidal retinitis has been reported in a patient with this disorder, but the patient had other, well-established risk factors for disseminated candidiasis including indwelling catheters and systemic use of broad-spectrum antibiotics.[17] The infection cleared with appropriate antifungal therapy.

Wiskott-Aldrich syndrome is a combined X-linked congenital immunodeficiency disease that is characterized by eczema, thrombocytopenia, and increased susceptibility to infection. Immunologically it is characterized by deficiency of antibody responses to polysaccharide antigens and a partial T cell immunodeficiency. Serum IgM levels and isoagglutinin titers are characteristically reduced, and serum IgG, IgA, and IgE levels are usually elevated. Patients have recurrent bronchitis, gastroenteritis, pyoderma, and otitis. Infection is caused most frequently by pyogenic bacteria, but patients also are susceptible to a variety of fungi, viruses, and protozoa. Kaposi varicelliform eruption, a disseminated form of cutaneous herpes simplex virus infection, may occur.

Patients are thrombocytopenic at birth, and bleeding complications are severe and lifelong. Infections become apparent by 6 months of age, and susceptibility to infection and secondary malignancies increases with age. Death generally occurs in the first decade of life because of bleeding or infection. Bone marrow transplantation has cured many of these patients.

Several ophthalmic disorders are associated with Wiskott-Aldrich syndrome.[11,45] Patients may develop ocular

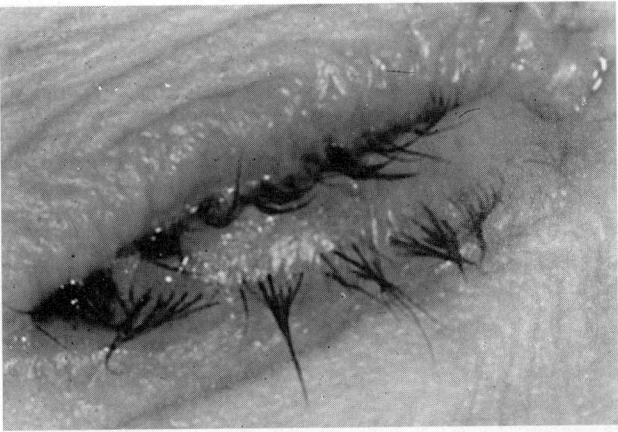

Fig. 21-2. Patient with Nezelof syndrome and severe bilateral blepharoconjunctivitis from which *Pseudomonas aeruginosa* and *Serratia marcescens* were cultured.

surface disease including eczema on the eyelids, blepharoconjunctivitis and pannus formation associated with molluscum contagiosum lesions, and recurrent, sometimes bilateral, herpes simplex virus keratitis. In many reported cases, the specific pathogens that are responsible for conjunctivitis are not mentioned. Marginal infiltrates and episcleritis also have been reported; these findings have been attributed to an altered immune response to infectious agents. Papilledema and oculomotor disorders have been attributed to intracranial lesions. Hemorrhage may occur both intraocularly and on the ocular surface.

In a review of reported cases, Podos and associates[45] found that ophthalmic disease (excluding eczema of the eyelids) has been mentioned in 18 of 80 Wiskott-Aldrich syndrome cases. Fifteen patients had infections and five had bleeding of the conjunctiva, periorbital tissues, retina, or into the vitreous. Excision of molluscum contagiosum lesions by expression and curettage must be performed with caution in these patients because of the increased risk of hemorrhage.

Ataxia-telangiectasia (A-T) is a rare, autosomal recessive disorder that is characterized by progressive neurologic degeneration, cerebellar ataxia, vascular changes of the conjunctiva and skin, recurrent respiratory infections, and malignancies (especially lymphomas). Patients have alterations in both humoral and cellular immune functions, and a markedly decreased IgA level is frequently present. The disease is progressive, with gradual loss of immunologic and neurologic function. Patients may become mentally retarded. They usually die of their disease before age 20.

Conjunctival vascular changes and eye movement disorders constitute the ophthalmic manifestations of A-T.[3,30,32] Dilated venules and irregular vascular segments in the horizontal exposure area give the eye an injected appearance. They appear in most patients between the ages of 2 and 7. These vascular changes have no functional significance. Similar vascular changes occur on the nose, ears, and extremities. Ocular telangiectasias are seen in virtually all cases.[58]

A-T patients have a variety of eye movement disorders including (1) nystagmus—an increased delay time for initiation of voluntary horizontal and vertical saccades, (2) hypometria of voluntary saccades—an abnormality in the initiation of the fast component of involuntary saccades (induced by optokinetic or vestibular stimuli), with deviation of the eyes in the direction of the slow component (rather than in the direction of the fast component as in normal subjects), and (3) decreased slow component velocity of optokinetic nystagmus.[3] Patients may have head thrusts when making horizontal refixations that are identical to those in patients with congenital oculomotor apraxia,[18] in an attempt to redirect the eyes for fixation on objects of interest. A combination of ocular motor apraxia, cerebellar oculomotor abnormalities, and periodic alternating nystagmus should strongly suggest a diagnosis of ataxia telangiectasia.[49]

Visual acuity, pupillary responses, and funduscopic examination are normal. Recently the gene for ataxia-telangiectasia was mapped to chromosome 11q23.[59] In one family congenital cataracts accompanied ataxia and microcephaly.

Autopsy examinations have revealed severe abnormalities of the thymus in patients with ataxia-telangiectasia. A unifying mechanism to explain the broad spectrum of abnormalities in the syndrome has not been determined, but a defect in DNA repair is suspected. Not all of the clinical manifestations can be explained on the basis of the associated immunodeficiency.

T CELL IMMUNODEFICIENCIES

Chronic mucocutaneous candidiasis (CMC) is a cellular immune defect that is associated with a specific T lymphocyte defect against *Candida* species. Patients with CMC have severe skin and mucous membrane infections including ulcerative candidal blepharitis and candidal keratoconjunctivitis.[23] Keratopathy with photophobia may be the first symptom of disease. Findings may include fine punctate erosions of the upper cornea, superficial pannus, and superficial stromal infiltration with scarring. Easty[22] believes that these findings are the result of bacterial, rather than fungal, infections, but organisms are rarely identified. The cellular defect does not, however, result in candidemia or systemic candidiasis because antibody and phagocytic functions are intact. CMC patients, therefore, do not develop endogenous candidal chorioretinitis or endophthalmitis.

CMC may occur as an isolated disorder, or it may be a component of several different syndromes. In 1962 Gass[29] reported that keratoconjunctivitis was a frequent initial finding in young children with multiple endocrine deficiencies, autoimmune disease, and candidiasis—a disorder that is usually associated with idiopathic hypoparathyroidism and adrenal insufficiency. Organisms were isolated from the conjunctiva in only one of these cases; it was suggested that the conjunctival disease was an immunologic reaction to a fungal antigen. More recently Wagman and associates[54] reported a series of sixteen patients with CMC, four of whom had keratitis, anterior stromal vascularization, and scarring. A report of two siblings with CMC mentioned the additional findings of eyelash and eyebrow loss in both patients and small diffuse keratic precipitates in one.[52] Wong and Kirkpatrick[57] reported clinical improvement in one patient with CMC following treatment with allogeneic lymphocytes and administration of transfer factor and amphotericin B.

CMC is also part of a syndrome that includes keratitis, ichthyosis, and deafness *(KID syndrome).*[33] The precise immunologic defect has not been identified, and evidence of candidiasis has been found in approximately 20% of cases. Corneal vascularization apparently occurs in most patients with KID syndrome, and loss of eyelashes and eyebrows is common.

Cowan and associates[20] described *multiple carboxylase*

deficiency in a family with mucocutaneous candidiasis. Three siblings had defects in lymphocyte function and antibody production that the authors attributed to a defect in biotin metabolism.[20] Clinical findings included central nervous system dysfunction and severe mucocutaneous candidiasis with blepharoconjunctivitis and corneal ulceration. Although candidal infections are usually associated with defects in cellular immunity, antibody defects (as occurred in these patients) may play a role in their development as well.[23]

PHAGOCYTIC DEFICIENCIES

Neutrophils, monocytes, and eosinophils comprise the nonspecific phagocytic system and provide immunologic defense against pyogenic bacteria such as *Staphylococcus aureus* and fungi, and *Aspergillus* species. To accomplish this role, phagocytes must be capable of several sequential functions including chemotaxis, adhesion, opsonization, ingestion, and intracellular microbial lysis. Defects in one or more of these functions may result in chronic or recurrent infections that are refractory to antibiotic therapy. Targets of infection include skin, mucous membranes, lungs, bone, lymph nodes, and components of the reticuloendothelial system.

Disorders of phagocytic function can occur in combination with other immune defects. Wheeland and associates[55] described a father and son with chronic purulent blepharitis and secondary corneal ulceration who had abnormal neutrophil function and cellular immunodeficiency. This disorder did not fit other well-established syndromes.

Chronic granulomatous disease (CGD) is an inherited disorder that is characterized biochemically by the inability of phagocytes to use molecular oxygen for the generation of reactive oxygen intermediates such as hydrogen peroxide, hydroxyl radical, and superoxide anion. This incapacity makes patients susceptible to recurrent life-threatening infections despite normal T cell and antibody functions.[27] In the majority of families CGD is transmitted as an X-linked recessive trait, although both autosomal recessive and autosomal dominant inheritance with variable penetration have been reported.[27,51] The genetic heterogeneity of the disease reflects different point mutations in the complex oxidative metabolic pathways of the neutrophil. Female carriers of the X-linked form of the disease can be identified by various tests. Recently the abnormal gene in X-linked CGD was identified.[47] The diagnosis is usually made by a nitroblue tetrazolium (NBT) test; the activated granulocytes from these patients are unable to reduce the colorless NBT dye to blue.

CGD is characterized by recurrent and chronic infections that involve the lungs, lymph nodes, skin and soft tissues, liver, gastrointestinal tract, bone, and brain. The pathogens that are involved most frequently in the disease are *Staphylococcus aureus, Aspergillus* species, *Chromobacterium violaceum, Pseudomonas cepacia,* and *Nocardia* species, which survive intracellularly and cause granulomata which can be observed microscopically. Most of the pathogens are catalase-positive microorganisms. Catalase-positive microbes destroy the hydrogen peroxide they generate. CGD phagocytes are defective in hydrogen peroxide generation and are thus deprived of an alternative source of hydrogen peroxide by which their microbial function could be maintained. Infections with catalase-negative microbes, such as *Streptococcus pneumoniae,* are rare in CGD.

The ocular signs of CGD fall into two groups: recurrent blepharokeratoconjunctivitis and chorioretinal lesions.[15,39,44] The focal, pigmented chorioretinal lesions appear to be a consistent finding in CGD. They usually are perivascular and peripapillary in distribution and can progress to large areas of chorioretinal atrophy.[39,44] Macular lesions and decreased acuity have not been reported, but visual field defects may occur that correspond to the location of chorioretinal scars.[44] Histopathologic studies of the chorioretinal lesions revealed almost total atrophy of choroid and retina and irregular proliferation of retinal pigment epithelium at the scar margin. No inflammatory cells, microorganisms, or pigmented lipid histiocytes were observed in these lesions, and microbial cultures from fresh autopsy eyes were negative.

Chronic blepharoconjunctivitis and marginal or punctate keratitis have been reported in patients with CGD, frequently accompanied by both pannus formation and perilimbal infiltrates.[39,46] These findings represent an immune reaction to staphylococcal antigens or toxins, rather than a direct invasion of the cornea by organisms. Because it is caused by catalase-positive bacterium, staphylococcal blepharitis is often a chronic condition in patients with CGD and requires regular lid hygiene and the selective use of topical antibiotics and corticosteroids to prevent corneal neovascularization and scarring.[44]

Chédiak-Higashi syndrome (CHS) is a rare autosomal recessive disorder, usually found in the offspring of consanguineous parents, that is characterized by partial oculocutaneous albinism, increased susceptibility to both viral and bacterial infections, anemia, leukopenia, thrombocytopenia, cutaneous ulcers, and peripheral and central neurologic changes including cerebral atrophy.[6] CHS often leads to death in early childhood from infections or, less commonly, from hemorrhage. Neutrophil abnormalities that are associated with CHS include neutropenia, reduced-marrow neutrophil reserves, and reduced-neutrophil chemotaxis. Abnormal granules in neutrophils and eosinophils can be seen on routine peripheral blood smears and also are present in other granule-containing cells such as hepatocytes, renal tubular cells, melanocytes, Schwann cells, and thyroid cells.[56] Natural killer function is also generally reduced.

Children that survive early childhood may be later afflicted with an "accelerated phase" of the disease that is characterized by lymphohistiocytic infiltration of the liver, spleen, nerves, and other tissues. Neoplastic transformation of these cells may occur. In addition to antimicrobial chemotherapy for infections, antineoplastic drugs and corticosteroids have been used to treat this accelerated phase.

Oculocutaneous albinism may be a predominant feature of CHS; an ultrastructural defect of melanosomes distinguishes this condition from true forms of albinism. Giant abnormal melanosomes, believed to be the result of fusion of smaller abnormal organelles, have been reported. Hair color ranges from blond to light brown but most frequently has been reported as silver or gray.[6,37] The iris is translucent with variable color. The amount of pigment in the uveal tract is variable and may be within normal limits. Histologic examination of the eyes also has revealed decreased pigmentation of the retinal pigment epithelium, ciliary body, and choroid. The abnormal granules have been observed in monocytes and polymorphonuclear leukocytes that are present in the corneal limbus, iris, and choroid.*

COMPLEMENT DEFICIENCIES

The complement system consists of approximately 20 serum proteins that are critical mediators of opsoninization, inflammation, and augmentation of antigen-antibody reactions. Sequential activation of the complement proteins (complement cascade) is caused by either antibody-antigen interaction (via the "classic" pathway that involves C1, C4, and C2) or by a variety of stimulants such as lipopolysaccharide, aggregated immunoglobulin, cobra venom, thrombin, or proteases (via the "alternate" pathway). These elements activate C3 directly, bypassing C1, C4, and C2.

Specific complement components, fragments, and complexes of more than one complement protein serve different functions. C3b, for example, promotes immune adherence, phagocytosis, lymphokine production, and antibody-dependent cell-mediated cytotoxicity. C1, C4, and C1,2,3,4 complexes aid in the neutralization of viruses to which antibodies have attached. The completed complement cascade leads to lysis of viruses, *Mycoplasma,* protozoa, and spirochetes by creating holes in membranes, capsules, or envelopes.

Deficiencies have been reported for each of the proteins that comprise the complement system (Table 21-1). Persons with complement disorders are susceptible to specific infectious agents that are related to the position of the deficient component(s) in the sequential cascade. For example, C2-deficient patients generally do not have problems with recurrent infections unless other components, acting later in the cascade, are deficient as well. In contrast, a deficiency of C3, which plays an integral role in both the classic and alternate pathways, results in repeated infections. Deficiencies of the later-acting components (C6, C7, or C8) have been

---

*References 5, 6, 10, 36, 48, 53.

linked with serious and sometimes fatal infections with *Neisseria meningitidis* and *Neisseria gonorrhea*.

Although complement has been found in tears,[42] cornea,[40] aqueous humor,[41] and sclera[9]; ocular infections are not prominent features of complement disorders.[22] Patients will be at risk, however, for ocular infections with the same pathogens that are seen in nonocular sites. Experimental evidence in animal models shows that the complement system may protect the eye against corneal infection[19] and endophthalmitis[2] that are caused by *Pseudomonas aeruginosa* (an organism whose endotoxin activates the alternate pathway).

Complement levels are increased in the vitreous of inflamed eyes.[43] Patients with complement deficiencies who develop intraocular infections for some other reason may therefore have more severe disease than their immunocompetent counterparts.

SECONDARY IMMUNODEFICIENCIES

In addition to the primary immunodeficiencies, there are a large number of illnesses that lead to transient or permanent immunodeficiency. These include such illnesses as malnutrition, specific vitamin and mineral deficiencies, immunosuppressive therapy, leukemia and lymphoma, protein-losing states, metabolic states (diabetes, uremia), genetic disorders (Down syndrome, Bloom syndrome), and infection including HIV. In general these are more common than primary immunodeficiencies, and most of them involve transient or permanent depression of the T cell (cellular immune system).[48]

REFERENCES

1. Addison DJ, Rahi AH: Immunoglobulin A (IgA) deficiency and eye disease, *Trans Ophthalmol Soc UK* 101:9, 1981.
2. Aizuss DH et al.: The complement system and host defense against *Pseudomonas* endophthalmitis, *Invest Ophthalmol Vis Sci* 26:1262, 1985.
3. Baloh RW et al.: Eye movements in ataxia-telangiectasia, *Neurology* 28:1099, 1978.
4. Beck CS, Heiner DC: Selective immunoglobulin IgG4 deficiency and recurrent infections of the respiratory tract, *Am Rev Respir Dis* 124:94, 1981.
5. Bedoya V, Grimley PM, Duque O: Chédiak-Higashi syndrome, *Arch Pathol* 88:340, 1969.
6. BenEzra D et al.: Chédiak-Higashi syndrome: ocular findings, *J Pediatr Ophthalmol* 17:68, 1980.
7. Binkley K et al.: Acquired Brown's syndrome associated with hypogammaglobulinemia, *J Rheumatol* 18:139-141, 1991.
8. Boone WB et al.: Acquired CMV chorioretinitis in severe combined immunodeficiency, *Clin Immunol Immunopathol* 9:129, 1978.
9. Brawman-Mintzer O, Mondino BJ, Mayer F: The complement system in sclera, *Invest Ophthalmol Vis Sci* 29:1756, 1988.
10. Bregeat P, Dhermy P, Hamard H: Manifestations oculaires du syndrome de Chédiak-Higashi, *Arch Ophthalmol (Paris)* 26:661, 1966.
11. Brunova B: Ocni projevy u Wiskottova-Aldrichova syndromu, *Cesk Oftalmol* 29:298, 1973.
12. Bruton OC: Agammaglobulinemia, *Pediatrics* 9:722, 1952.
13. Buckley RH: Immunodeficiency diseases, *JAMA* 258:2841, 1987.
14. Burks AW, Sampson HA, Buckley RH: Anaphylactic reactions following gamma globulin administration in patients with hypogammaglobulinemia: detection of IgE antibodies to IgA, *N Engl J Med* 314:560, 1986.
15. Carson MJ et al.: Thirteen boys with progressive septic granulomatosis, *Pediatrics* 35:405, 1965.
16. Chandra RK: Diagnosis. In Chandra RK, editor: *Primary and secondary immunodeficiency disorders,* 24, New York, 1983, Churchill Livingstone.
17. Chess J et al.: *Candida* retinitis in bare lymphocyte syndrome, *Ophthalmology* 93:696, 1986.
18. Churchyard A, Stell R, Mastaglia FL: Ataxia telangiectasia presenting as an extrapyramidal movement disorder and ocular motor apraxia without overt telangiectasia, *Clin Exp Neurol* 28:90-96, 1991.
19. Cleveland RP et al.: Role of complement in murine corneal infection caused by *Pseudomonas aeruginosa, Invest Ophthalmol Vis Sci* 24:237, 1983.
20. Cowan MJ et al.: Multiple biotin-dependent carboxylase deficiencies associated with defects in T-cell and B-cell immunity, *Lancet* 1:115, 1979.
21. Dwyer JM: Cutaneous manifestations of immunogenetic deficiency disorders, *Birth Defects* 17:93, 1981.
22. Easty DL: Infection in the compromised eye, *Trans Ophthalmol Soc UK* 105:61, 1986.
23. Edwards JE Jr et al.: Severe candidal infections: clinical perspective, immune defense mechanisms, and current concepts of therapy, *Ann Intern Med* 89:91, 1978.
24. Franklin RM, Winkelstein JA, Seto DS: Conjunctivitis and keratoconjunctivitis associated with primary immunodeficiency diseases, *Am J Ophthalmol* 84:563, 1977.
25. Frenkel M, Russe HP: Retinal telangiectasis associated with hypogammaglobulinemia, *Am J Ophthalmol* 63:215, 1967.
26. Friedlaender MH et al.: Ocular microbial flora in immunodeficient patients, *Arch Ophthalmol* 98:1211, 1980.
27. Gallin JI et al.: Recent advances in chronic granulomatous disease, *Ann Intern Med* 99:657, 1983.
28. Gallo M et al.: Lupus-like connective tissue disease with severe hemorrhagic retinitis in a patient with total IgA deficiency, *Z Rheumatol* 42:362, 1983.
29. Gass DGM: The syndrome of keratoconjunctivitis, superficial moniliasis, idiopathic hypoparathyroidism and Addison's disease, *Am J Ophthalmol* 54:660, 1962.
30. Greenwald MJ, Weiss A: Ocular manifestations of the neurocutaneous syndromes, *Pediatr Dermatol* 2:98, 1984.
31. Hansel TT et al.: Infective conjunctivitis and corneal scarring in three brothers with sex-linked hypogammaglobulinemia (Bruton's disease), *Br J Ophthalmol* 74:118-120, 1990.
32. Harley RD, Baird HW, Cravaen EM: Ataxia-telangiectasia: report of seven cases, *Arch Ophthalmol* 77:582, 1977.
33. Harms M et al.: KID syndrome and chronic mucocutaneous candidiasis: case report and review of the literature, *Pediatr Dermatol* 2:1, 1984.
33a. Holland GN, Pepose JS, Dinning WJ: Ophthalmic disorders associated with selected primary and acquired immunodeficiency diseases. In Tasman W, Jaeger EA, editors: *Duane's clinical ophthalmology,* 1-20, Philadelphia, 1989, JB Lippincott.
34. Insler MS, Gordon RA: Absolute IgG4 deficiency and recurrent bacterial blepharokeratoconjunctivitis, *Am J Ophthalmol* 98:243, 1984.
35. Johns KJ et al.: Cellular infiltration of the vitreous in a patient with X-linked immunodeficiency with increased IgM, *Am J Ophthalmol* 113:183-186, 1992.
36. Johnson DL et al.: Histopathology of eyes in Chédiak-Higashi syndrome, *Arch Ophthalmol* 75:84, 1966.
37. Kinnear PE, Jay B, Witkip CP: Albinism, *Surv Ophthalmol* 30:75, 1985.
38. Lever AM et al.: Chronic *Campylobacter* colitis and uveitis in patient with hypogammagloblinaemia, *Br Med J* 288:531, 1984.
39. Martyn LJ et al.: Chorioretinal lesions in familial chronic granulomatous disease of childhood, *Am J Ophthalmol* 73:403, 1972.
40. Mondino BJ, Brady KJ: Distribution of hemolytic complement in the normal cornea, *Arch Ophthalmol* 99:1430, 1981.

41. Mondino BJ, Rao H: Complement levels in normal and inflamed aqueous humor, *Invest Ophthalmol Vis Sci* 24:380, 1983.

42. Mondino BJ, Sidikaro Y, Sumner H: Anaphylatoxin levels in human vitreous humor, *Invest Ophthalmol Vis Sci* 29:1195, 1988.

43. Mondino BJ, Zaidman GW: Hemolytic complement in tears, *Ophthalmic Res* 15:208, 1983.

44. Palestine AG et al.: Ocular findings in patients with neutrophil dysfunction, *Am J Ophthalmol* 95:598, 1983.

45. Podos SM et al.: Ophthalmic manifestations of the Wiskott-Aldrich syndrome, *Arch Ophthalmol* 82:322, 1969.

46. Rodriguez MM et al.: Histopathology of ocular changes in chronic granulomatous disease, *Am J Ophthalmol* 96:810, 1983.

47. Royer-Pokora B et al.: Cloning the gene for an inherited human disorder—chronic granulomatous disease—on the basis of its chromosomal location, *Nature* 322:32-38, 1986.

47a. Shearer WT, Anderson DC: The secondary immunodeficiencies. In Stiehm ER, editor: *Immunologic disorders in infants and children,* ed 3, 400-438, Philadelphia, 1989, WB Saunders.

48. Spencer WH, Hogan MJ: Ocular manifestations of Chédiak-Higashi syndrome, *Am J Ophthalmol* 50:1197, 1960.

49. Stell R et al.: Ataxia telangiectasia: a reappraisal of the ocular motor features and their value in the diagnosis of atypical cases, *Mov Disord* 4:320-329, 1989.

50. Stiehm ER et al.: Infectious complications of the primary immunodeficiencies, *Clin Immunol Immunopathol* 40:69, 1986.

51. Tauber AI et al.: Chronic granulomatous disease: the syndrome of phagocyte oxidase deficiencies, *Medicine* 62:286, 1983.

52. Traboulsi EI et al.: Ocular findings in the candidiasis-endocrinopathy syndrome, *Am J Ophthalmol* 99:486, 1985.

53. Valenzuela R, Morningstar WA: The ocular pigmentary disturbance of human Chédiak-Higashi syndrome: a comparative light- and electron-microscopic study and review of the literature, *Am J Clin Pathol* 75:591, 1981.

54. Wagman RD et al.: Keratitis associated with the multiple endocrine deficiency autoimmune disease, and candidiasis syndrome, *Am J Ophthalmol* 103:569, 1987.

55. Wheeland RG et al.: Chronic blepharitis and pyoderma of the scalp: an immune deficiency state in a father and son with hypercupremia and decreased intracellular killing, *Pediatr Dermatol* 1:134, 1983.

56. White CJ, Gallin JI: Phagocyte defects, *Clin Immunol Immunopathol* 40:50, 1986.

56a. WHO Scientific Group: Primary immunodeficiency diseases, *Immunodefic Rev* 3:195-236, 1992.

57. Wong VG, Kirkpatrick CH: Immunologic reconstitution in a patient with keratoconjunctivitis, superficial candidiasis and hypoparathyroidism: the role of immunocompetent lymphocyte transfusion and transfer factor, *Trans Am Ophthalmol Soc* 71:254, 1973.

58. Woods CG, Taylor AM: Ataxia telangiectasia in the British Isles: the clinical and laboratory features of 70 affected individuals, *Q J Med* 82:169-179, 1992.

59. Ziv Y et al.: Ataxia telangiectasia: linkage analysis in highly inbred Arab and Druze families and differentiation from an ataxia-microcephaly-cataract syndrome, *Hum Genet* 88:619-626, 1992.

22 Acquired Immunodeficiency Syndrome

DOUGLAS A. JABS, THOMAS C. QUINN

The acquired immunodeficiency syndrome (AIDS) was first recognized in the United States in 1981. Since then AIDS has become a global pandemic with more than 750,000 cases officially reported to the World Health Organization (WHO) from 173 countries. Because of under-reporting in many areas, the WHO estimates that over 2.5 million cases of AIDS have occurred worldwide along with one million deaths since 1981.[268] In 1984 the human immunodeficiency virus type 1 (HIV-1) was identified as the casual agent of AIDS. Since then immunologic, virologic, and epidemiologic studies have clearly demonstrated that AIDS represents only one part of the clinical spectrum of HIV infection. From natural history studies of HIV-infected individuals, the median time from HIV exposure to the development of AIDS is approximately 11 years, demonstrating the prolonged and progressive nature of HIV infection.[155]

With the advent of serologic tests for HIV, it became possible to identify HIV-infected people before the development of AIDS, thereby providing opportunities for antiviral therapy and prophylaxis against opportunistic infections in an effort to prolong the lives of infected individuals. In addition, early identification of infected individuals provided the opportunity for education and counseling in an effort to prevent further transmission. Despite these and other efforts to control the AIDS epidemic, the WHO now estimates that approximately 14 million individuals are infected with HIV worldwide, and that by the year 2000 nearly 40 million will be infected.[267] These HIV-infected individuals represent the human reservoir from which further transmission may occur, eventually resulting in further escalation in AIDS cases and fatalities. Consequently, it is likely that AIDS will continue to have a profound medical, social, and cultural impact on our global society into the next decade.

EPIDEMIOLOGY

Within a relatively short period, HIV infection spread rapidly to all areas of the world, predominantly by three routes of transmission: (1) sexual transmission, which can be homosexual, bisexual, or heterosexual; (2) parenteral transmission, including transfusion of infected blood products or injection with blood-contaminated needles or syringes; and (3) perinatal transmission, which may occur *in utero,* during delivery, or postnatally. In developing countries where nearly 70% of all HIV-infected individuals reside, heterosexual transmission continues to be the major mode of spread, a trend that is becoming increasingly common in developed countries as well. In sub-Saharan Africa there are nearly 8 million HIV-infected individuals and in the Americas over 2.5 million.[267] The area with the most recent explosive growth of HIV infection is Southeast Asia where over 1.5 million cases became infected during a 3-year period in the early 1990s.

In some urban centers of sub-Saharan Africa, Western Europe and the Americas, AIDS has already become the leading cause of death for both men and women, aged 15 to 49 years.[46,229,259] It has also been estimated that the HIV pandemic may have already resulted in the death of nearly 750,000 children worldwide, and by the year 2000, ten million children under 15 years of age may be orphaned because of the premature death of an HIV-infected mother or father from AIDS.[28] Overall, infant and child mortality rates will increase as much as 30% greater than previously projected as a direct consequence of perinatal HIV infection. Pediatric AIDS is now threatening much of the progress that has been made in child survival in developing countries during the past 20 years.

Although the vast majority of HIV-infected individuals reside in developing countries, the United States has officially reported the highest number of AIDS cases worldwide, with over 315,000 cases and nearly 200,000 fatalities as of June 1993.[27] During the 1980s HIV infection emerged as one of the leading causes of death among young men and women in the United States.[229,259] In 1991 HIV infection was ranked as the second leading cause of death among men aged 25 to 44 years and the fifth leading cause of death among women in this age group. Although deaths from all causes in this age group comprised only 7% of total U.S. deaths in 1991, they impose a disproportionately high impact on society because of the loss of productive years of life and the loss of parents from families with young children. The impact of HIV infection on death patterns is even greater in many large cities than in the total U.S. population. For example, if a person was aged 25 to 44 years in 1990, HIV was the leading cause of death among men in 64 (37%) of 172 cities with populations of at least 100,000 and among women in 9 (5%) of such cities.[259] The high death rates from HIV infection were also higher for blacks and Hispanics than for other racial/ethnic groups, consistent with reported rates and the incidence of AIDS. Differences in risk among racial/ethnic groups may reflect social, economic, behavioral, or other factors rather than race/ethnicity directly.

It is also likely that the impact of HIV infection on U.S. mortality patterns is even greater than that described previously. These data were based on the underlying cause of death recorded on death certificates; however, previous studies suggest that persons aged 25 to 44 years, whose cause of death is designated as HIV, represent 65% to 85% of HIV-related deaths among men and 55% to 80% of those among women.[16,215]

Risk Groups

Initially an epidemic among homosexual men, HIV infection rapidly spread to intravenous (IV) drug users and to heterosexuals similar to patterns seen in other areas of the world. This trend of increasing AIDS cases among heterosexuals is more evident when comparing the proportional increases by risk group in 1992 compared to 1991. In 1992 47,095 cases of AIDS were reported to Centers for Disease Control and Prevention (CDC), an increase of 3.5% over the previous year (Fig. 22-1).[258] Most of these cases (52%) were attributable to transmission of HIV among homosexual/bisexual men. When compared to the previous year, however, there was a slight decline (1.1%) in the number of AIDS cases among homosexual/bisexual men. In contrast, there

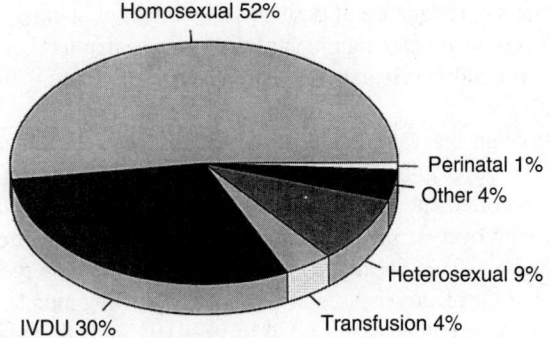

Fig. 22-1 Proportion of AIDS cases in 1992 by risk factor. From Centers for Disease Control and Prevention. HIV/AIDS Surveillance Report 5:1-20, 1993.

CONDITIONS INCLUDED IN THE 1993 AIDS SURVEILLANCE CASE DEFINITION

- Candidiasis of bronchi, trachea, or lungs
- Candidiasis, esophageal
- Cervical cancer, invasive*
- Coccidioidomycosis, disseminated or extrapulmonary
- Cryptococcosis, extrapulmonary
- Cryptosporidiosis, chronic intestinal (>1 month's duration)
- Cytomegalovirus disease (other than liver, spleen, or nodes)
- Cytomegalovirus retinitis (with loss of vision)
- Encephalopathy, HIV-related
- Herpes simplex virus: chronic ulcer(s) (>1 month's duration); or bronchitis, pneumonitis, or esophagitis
- Histoplasmosis, disseminated or extrapulmonary
- Isosporiasis, chronic intestinal (>1 month's duration)
- Kaposi sarcoma
- Lymphoma, Burkitt (or equivalent term)
- Lymphoma, immunoblastic (or equivalent term)
- Lymphoma, primary, of brain
- *Mycobacterium avium* complex or *M. kansasii,* disseminated or extrapulmonary
- *Mycobacterium tuberculosis,* any site (pulmonary* or extrapulmonary)
- *Mycobacterium,* other species or unidentified species, disseminated or extrapulmonary
- *Pneumocystis carinii* pneumonia
- Pneumonia, recurrent*
- Progressive multifocal leukoencephalopathy
- *Salmonella* sp. septicemia, recurrent
- Toxoplasmosis of brain
- Wasting syndrome caused by HIV infection

From Centers for Disease Control. 1993 revised classification system for HIV infection and expanded surveillance case definition for AIDS among adolescents and adults, *MMWR* 41(R-17), 1992 (with permission).
* Added in the 1993 expansion of the AIDS Surveillance Case Definition.

---

was a larger proportionate increase in reported cases among women (9.8%) than among men (2.5%). For women, rates were higher for blacks and Hispanics (31.3 and 14.6 per 100,000, respectively) than for non-Hispanic whites (1.8 per 100,000). The number of cases attributable to IV drug use increased slightly, representing nearly one fourth of reported cases. Heterosexual contact accounted for the largest proportional increase (17.1%) in reported cases. The proportionate increase in cases attributable to heterosexual contact was greater for men (26.3%) than for women (11.5%). Women accounted for most persons infected through heterosexual contact (59.4%). The second largest proportionate increase was in perinatal transmission (13.4%).

In 1992 the number of AIDS cases among women infected through heterosexual contact actually exceeded those infected through intravenous drug use for the first time. The pattern varied by region; IV drug use was the predominant mode of transmission among women in the Northeast, whereas heterosexual transmission equaled or surpassed IV drug use among women in the South, the Midwest, the West and the U.S. territories. Among those cases attributed to heterosexual transmission, most (56.8%) involved sex with an infected drug user.

These data reflect the evolving nature of the HIV epidemic in the United States, which is a composite of multiple epidemics in different regions and among different population subgroups. The rate of increase of AIDS cases among women and others with heterosexual contact along with an accompanying decrease in AIDS cases among homosexual men illustrates the increasing importance of heterosexual spread of HIV.

Case Definitions for AIDS

One of the hallmarks of progressive immunodeficiency among HIV-infected individuals is a steady decline in the absolute number of CD4+ T-lymphocytes (see Pathogenesis section).[176] Multiple studies have shown that as the CD4+ T-lymphocyte count declines, the risk for developing a broad spectrum of illnesses, including those meeting the 1987 AIDS-defining criteria, increases.[21,56,157,188] Monitoring CD4+ T-lymphocyte counts is therefore a part of the recommended standard of care for persons with HIV infection and the CD4+ T-lymphocyte counts are used to guide clinical decisions regarding the use of antiretroviral therapy and prophylaxis against *Pneumocystis carinii* pneumonia (PCP).[64,91,262]

In 1993 the CDC revised its classification of HIV infection and expanded the AIDS surveillance definition to include those individuals with severe immunosuppression (defined as a CD4+ T-lymphocyte count of less than 200 cells/μl without a diagnosis of an opportunistic infection in an HIV-infected person).[23] The immediate effect of this expanded AIDS surveillance definition was that many persons with severe immunosuppression who had not developed an AIDS indicator condition would now be reported to the CDC.

As of January 1993 the CDC classification schema for HIV infection stages all patients along two axes: the presence of HIV-related symptoms or diseases and the level of CD4+ T-lymphocytes.[23] Each axis is subdivided into three categories, resulting in a three by three matrix for nine categories, as outlined in Table 22-1. Patients are classified as having AIDS when they either have category "C" AIDS-indicator diseases or category "3" level of immunodeficiency (CD4+ T-lymphocyte count < 200 cells/μl). The AIDS-indicator diseases are listed in the box entitled Conditions Included in the 1993 AIDS Surveillance Case Definition.

The CDC estimated that as of January 1992, 115,000 to 170,000 U.S. residents or 10% of the estimated number of HIV-infected individuals would have a severe immunosuppression as defined by depressed CD4+ T-lymphocyte counts less than 200 cells/μl.[202] Only about 50,000 of these persons were receiving medical care for HIV-related conditions and were known to have a CD4+ T-lymphocyte count less than 200 cells/μl. Although the number of persons with severe immunosuppression was estimated to be 130,000 to 205,000 by January 1995, the actual number is more in the lower half of this range than the upper half. The expanded HIV surveillance definition that includes severe immunosuppression resulted in an increase of approximately 50% of the number of persons reported during 1993 and an increase of less than 20% in 1994 compared with the number of persons who would have been reported had the definition not been changed.[202] Projections of future AIDS cases incorpo-

TABLE 22-1 1993 REVISED CLASSIFICATION SYSTEM FOR HIV INFECTION AND EXPANDED AIDS SURVEILLANCE CASE DEFINITION FOR ADOLESCENTS AND ADULTS*

CD4+ T-lymphocyte Categories	(A) Asymptomatic, Acute (Primary) HIV or PGL†	(B) Symptomatic, not (A) or (C) Conditions	(C) AIDS-Indicator Conditions‡
(1) ≥ 500/μl	A1	B1	C1
(2) 200-499/μl	A2	B2	C2
(3) < 200/μl§	**A3**	**B3**	C3

From Centers for Disease Control. 1993 revised classification system for HIV infection and expanded surveillance case definition for AIDS among adolescents and adults, *MMWR* 41(R-17), 1992 (with permission).
* The bolded cells illustrate the expanded AIDS surveillance case definition. Persons with AIDS-indicator conditions (Category C) as well as those with CD4+ T-lymphocyte counts < 200/μl (Categories A3 or B3) will be reportable as AIDS cases in the United States and Territories, effective January 1, 1993.
† PGL = persistent generalized lymphadenopathy. Clinical Category A includes acute (primary) infection.
‡ See box Conditions Included in the 1993 AIDS Surveillance Case Definition.
§ AIDS-indicator; T-lymphocyte count.

rating this new definition demonstrate that the number of U.S. residents with HIV-related morbidity is likely to increase.

CLINICAL FEATURES

Approximately 3 to 6 weeks after initial exposure to HIV infection, 50% to 70% of patients with primary HIV infection develop an acute nonspecific viral syndrome (Fig. 22-2).[255] This acute syndrome resolves spontaneously and patients may remain free of symptoms for 10 years or longer.

Opportunistic Infections

As the CD4+ T-lymphocyte count declines below 200 cells/μl, clinical deterioration becomes more progressive, witnessed by the appearance of multiple opportunistic infections.

***Pneumocystic carinii* Pneumonia.** In the United States PCP is still the initial life-threatening opportunistic infection, occurring in 50% to 60% of persons with AIDS.[100,132,177] The usual presentation is the combination of a nonproductive cough, dyspnea and fever that often evolves slowly over a period of several days or weeks. Chest X-ray usually shows bilateral and interstitial infiltrates, although 10% to 15% of X-rays are normal, requiring additional diagnostic tests such as gallium scan, blood gases to detect hypoxia, or pulmonary function tests to detect abnormal diffusing capacity. Diagnosis is usually established with induced sputum or bronchoalveolar lavage (BAL) from fiber optic bronchoscopy.

Multiple studies have now proved the efficacy of PCP prophylaxis, which should be provided to any HIV-infected individual with a CD4+ T-lymphocyte count less than 200 cells/μl (primary prophylaxis) and to any patient with a history of PCP (secondary prophylaxis).[25] Comparative trials recently showed trimethoprim-sulfamethoxasole (TMP-SMX) to be superior to aerosolized pentamidine for preventing recurrent PCP.[19,98,222] Unfortunately, 30% to 50% of patients with HIV may experience side effects to TMP-SMX, the most common being rash, fever, or abdominal pain. Most patients can be treated despite mild reactions, or they can be treated with reduced doses; the lowest dose regimen with established efficacy is one double-strength tablet three times per week. Most physicians prefer one double-strength tablet per day as compliance may be easier and this dose may be superior in preventing infections caused by other microbes such as *Streptococcus pneumoniae*, *Haemophilus influenza*, *Listeria* sp., *Nocardia* sp., *Legionella* sp., *Salmonella* sp. When alternative treatment is necessary, the major options are dapsone or aerosolized pentamidine; occasional patients may be treated with Fansidar (sulfadoxine and pyrimethamine).[165]

Other Opportunistic Infections. Other opportunistic infections that are frequently observed in individuals with CD4+ T-lymphocyte counts less than 200 cells/μl include toxoplasmic encephalitis, candidal esophagitis, disseminated *Mycobacterium avium* complex and *M. tuberculosis* infections, cryptococcal meningitis, and disseminated cytomegalovirus (CMV) infection. Most opportunistic infections are rare until the CD4+ T-lymphocyte count is less than 200 cells/μl and most occur when the average CD4+ T-lymphocyte count is between 50 to 100 cells/μl. Mucocutaneous candidiasis, shingles, oral hairy leukoplakia, salmonellosis, tuberculosis, and pneumococcal pneumonia tend to occur at higher CD4+ T-lymphocyte levels.

Neoplasms

Prior to the AIDS epidemic Kaposi sarcoma was a rare tumor occurring in specific populations, particularly elderly men of Mediterranean origin. Other affected populations included African children and renal transplant recipients.[99,217] In 1981 a sudden and dramatic increase in an aggressive form of Kaposi sarcoma among young homosexual men was observed as one of the manifestations of AIDS. AIDS-associated Kaposi sarcoma was distinguished from classic forms of Kaposi sarcoma by its epidemiologic features and its more aggressive course, particularly visceral involvement. Early in the AIDS epidemic Kaposi sarcoma was seen almost exclusively in homosexual and bisexual men. Whereas this risk group for AIDS still represents the vast majority of patients with AIDS and Kaposi sarcoma, cases have been described in other risk groups, including heterosexual women.[217] Epidemiologic studies have suggested a decrease in the frequency of Kaposi sarcoma among HIV-infected patients in the late 1980s.[101]

Kaposi sarcoma generally presents with multiple red to violaceous macules, papules, and/or nodules. Classic Kaposi sarcoma lesions are cutaneous and involve the lower extremity. In patients with AIDS and Kaposi sarcoma, lesions tend to occur on the upper trunk, head, and neck. Visceral involvement, including the lymph nodes, gastrointestinal tract, and lungs is much more common in patients with AIDS. The characteristic histopathologic findings on biopsy

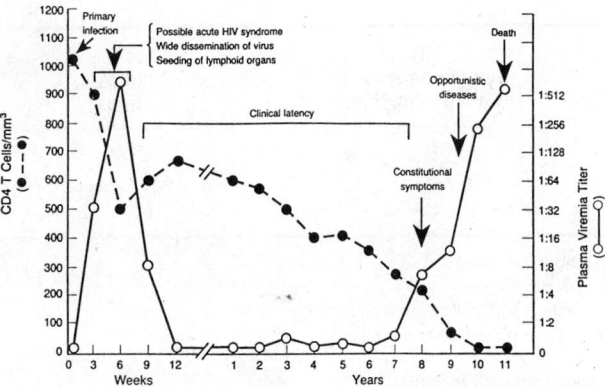

Fig. 22-2 Clinical course of HIV infection. From Pantaleo GP et al.: The immunopathogenesis of human immunodeficiency virus infection, *N Engl J Med* 328:327-335, 1993 (with permission).

TABLE 22-2 OCULAR MANIFESTATIONS OF AIDS

Lesion	Frequency
Microangiopathy	
Conjunctival microangiopathy	75%
HIV retinopathy	50-67%
Opportunistic ocular infections	
Anterior segment	
Microsporidial keratoconjunctivitis	<1%
Zoster ophthalmicus	4%
Posterior segment	
Cytomegalovirus retinitis	20-25%
Varicella zoster virus retinitis	<1%
Acute retinal necrosis syndrome	
Progressive outer retinal necrosis syndrome	
Toxoplasmic retinochoroiditis	1-2%
Choroidal pneumocystosis	<1%
Ocular neoplasms	
Eyelid Kaposi sarcoma	1-2%
Conjunctival Kaposi sarcoma	1-2%
Orbital lymphoma	<1%
Neuroophthalmic lesions	10%

include bands of spindle cells and vascular structures embedded in collagen and reticular fibers.

Ophthalmic Disease

Since 1982, when Holland and associates[111] reported eye changes in patients with AIDS, it has become clear that ocular manifestations are seen in the majority of patients with AIDS. Multiple series have reported an abnormal eye exam in 52% to 100% of patients with AIDS.* Usually, the ocular manifestations of HIV infection are classified into four areas: (1) a noninfectious microangiopathy, most often seen in the retina and often referred to as "HIV retinopathy"; (2) opportunistic ocular infections; (3) ocular adnexal involvement by those neoplasms seen in patients with AIDS; and (4) neuroophthalmic lesions.

The microangiopathy is the most frequent ocular manifestation, and CMV retinitis is the most frequent opportunistic ocular infection.† Although CMV retinitis was a rare disease prior to the AIDS epidemic, it has now become a major public health problem and appears to be the most common intraocular infection now seen in major urban medical centers. The various ocular manifestations seen in patients with AIDS are outlined in Table 22-2.

HIV Retinopathy. HIV retinopathy is the most frequent form of ocular involvement seen in patients with AIDS. Clinically, HIV retinopathy is manifested most often by cotton-wool spots (Fig. 22-3), but also occasionally by intraretinal hemorrhages.

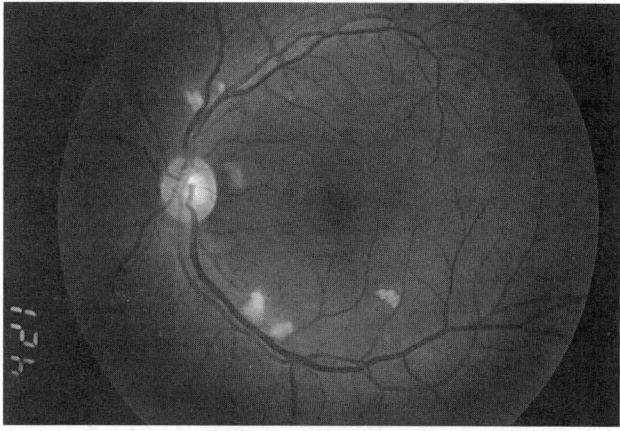

A

B

Fig. 22-3 HIV retinopathy (cotton-wool spots).

Cotton-wool spots have been reported in 28% to 92% of patients with AIDS, with most series reporting a frequency of greater than 50%. In the largest reported series of patients with AIDS, retinopathy was present in approximately two thirds of these patients.[123] Cotton-wool spots are sometimes referred to as microinfarcts of the nerve fiber layer of the retina, although they are not true areas of coagulative necrosis. The pathogenesis of cotton-wool spots is one in which ischemia disrupts axonal transport, resulting in swelling of the axons in the nerve-fiber layer, thus producing the characteristic white, opaque patches.

Intraretinal hemorrhages are considerably less frequent than cotton-wool spots, but have been reported in 0% to 54% of patients with AIDS, with most series reporting their presence in less than 20% of patients.*

Perivascular sheathing without infectious retinitis has also been reported, but it is uncommon in the United States.[181,194] Most often, perivascular sheathing is seen in association with CMV retinitis or other opportunistic ocular infections. Perivascular sheathing has been reported to occur

*References 74, 76, 112, 121, 123, 181, 185, 194, 211, 227, 228.
†References 76, 110, 112, 121, 123, 134, 136, 180, 181, 185, 194, 211, 228.

*References 74, 76, 112, 123, 181, 185, 194, 211, 227, 228.

in 15% of African patients with AIDS and 60% of African patients with AIDS-related complex (ARC, a fairly nonspecific term used for patients with HIV disease in categories B1, B2 of the current CDC classification system), but less than 1% of U.S. patients with AIDS or ARC.[134] Reasons for the reported difference in the frequency of perivascular sheathing between patients in Africa and the United States are unclear.

Fluorescein angiographic and histologic studies have suggested that microangiopathy may be present in an even greater percentage of patients than seen clinically. The fluorescein angiographic study by Newsome and associates[181] found microangiopathic changes, including microaneurysms and telangiectatic vessels, in all 12 patients studied. The autopsy series reported by Pepose and associates[194] found ocular involvement in 94% of patients studied and some evidence of retinal microangiopathy in 89%. Histologic findings related to this microangiopathy have included a loss of pericytes, microaneurysm formation, thickened vascular walls with deposition of amorphous material and luminal narrowing, swelling of endothelial cells, and thickening of the vascular basement membrane. This vascular damage results in the formation of cotton-wool spots. Many of the clinical and histologic features of microangiopathy are similar to those seen with diabetic retinopathy.

HIV retinopathy is associated with the level of immunodeficiency. In the study reported by Jabs and associates[123] in 1989, retinopathy was present in 66% of patients with AIDS, 40% of patients with ARC, 1% of patients with asymptomatic HIV infection, and 0% of non-HIV infected homosexual men. Similarly, Freeman and associates[74] reported that HIV retinopathy was associated with a lower CD4+ T-lymphocyte count.

Opportunistic Infections. Multiple opportunistic ocular infections have been reported in patients with AIDS. Over a dozen infectious agents have been reported to cause retinal disease. Most retinal infections occur infrequently; those reported most frequently are identified in Table 22-2.

CMV Retinitis. CMV retinitis is the most common intraocular infection in patients with AIDS. Estimates of the cumulative frequency of CMV retinitis in patients with AIDS have varied from 6% to 45%.* Although earlier data suggested that approximately 20% to 25% of patients with AIDS will develop CMV retinitis at some time during the course of their disease, more recent data suggest that with the use of prophylaxis against PCP, the frequency is closer to 40%.[117]

CMV retinitis is a relatively late-stage event in HIV infection. It is generally associated with CD4+ T-lymphocyte counts less than 50 cells/μl.[81,117,196] Cross-sectional analyses of patients with CMV retinitis have revealed mean and median CD4+ T-lymphocyte counts on the order of 20 to 30 cells/μl.[108,117,145,249] Occasionally, patients with higher CD4+ T-lymphocyte counts have been reported, but only rarely will a patient have a CD4+ count greater than 100 cells/μl.[108]

The epidemiologic study by Pertel and associates[196] reported that 42% of patients with CD4+ T-lymphocyte counts less than 50 cells/μl would develop CMV retinitis over 27 months of follow-up. The level of immunodeficiency was clearly associated with the risk of developing CMV retinitis (with a relative risk of 4.62 for a CD4+ T-lymphocyte count less than 50 cells/μl, and a relative risk of 2.47 for a CD4+ T-lymphocyte count of 50 to 100 cells/μl compared to those patients with a CD4+ T-lymphocyte count greater than 100 cells/μl). In this study, no patient developed CMV retinitis without first having a CD4+ T-lymphocyte count less than 50 cells/μl.

In the study by Gallant and associates,[81] of patients with a CD4+ T-lymphocyte count less than 100 cells/μl, 10% developed CMV retinitis within 1 year. No difference could be detected between patients with a CD4+ T-lymphocyte count less than 50 cells/μl and those with CD4+ T-lymphocyte counts between 50 and 100 cells/μl. Cross-sectional studies have occasionally reported patients with CD4+ T-lymphocyte counts greater than 100 cells/μl and a high count of 323 cells/μl, but these cases are unusual.[108] Hence, the level of immunodeficiency is a risk factor for the development of CMV retinitis, with the highest rate seen in patients with CD4+ T-lymphocytes less than 50 cells/μl. Only an occasional patient with CMV retinitis will have a CD4+ T-lymphocyte greater than 100 cells/μl.

Further immunosuppression, such as corticosteroid therapy, appears to further increase the risk of CMV retinitis.[179] Although CMV retinitis is common in patients with AIDS, it is (relatively speaking) uncommon with immunosuppression, such as after organ transplantation. Studies of renal transplant patients have suggested that CMV retinitis occurs in approximately 1% to 2% of patients after renal transplantation, and studies of bone marrow transplantation have suggested that it occurs in less than 1% of patients. Reasons for the difference in frequency between transplant patients and patients with AIDS are not known. Cytomegalovirus is ubiquitous herpes family virus, and approximately 50% of the general population have antibodies to CMV, suggesting previous exposure. Nearly 100% of homosexual men will have antibodies to CMV, suggesting a greater exposure among this group than in the population at large.[36,250] In the immunologically normal host, CMV exists in a harmless, latent state. When immunodeficiency or immunosuppression is present, CMV can reactivate, spread hematogenously to the retina, invade retinal cells, and establish a productive infection. At least part of the explanation for the greater frequency of CMV retinitis in patients with AIDS may be the greater baseline exposure to CMV and the more profound and sustained level of immunodeficiency seen in patients with AIDS, when compared to patients who are immunosuppressed pharmacologically.

---

*References 76, 112, 117, 122, 123, 185, 194, 211.

In addition, HIV and CMV have been demonstrated to transactivate each other in vitro.[45] Hence, cells co-infected with HIV and CMV may provide higher yields of both viruses than cells infected with either virus alone. This transactivation may also contribute to the greater frequency of CMV retinitis in patients with AIDS.

The diagnosis of CMV retinitis can usually be made reliably on ophthalmoscopy by an experienced observer.[13] CMV retinitis may be asymptomatic, particularly if the lesion is small or peripheral, or minimally symptomatic. The most frequent symptoms are floaters or a vague sense of blurred vision. More posteriorly located lesions will produce a scotoma or loss of vision. The study reported by Kuppermann and associates[145] suggested that 54% of patients with CMV retinitis were asymptomatic, and that there may be significant underdiagnosis of CMV retinitis.

Clinically, the most characteristic feature of CMV retinitis is a yellowish-white area of retinal necrosis with a granular border extending into the surrounding retina (Fig. 22-4). Hemorrhages may or may not be present. Lesions that have extensive necrosis and hemorrhage are sometimes termed "fulminant," whereas those without hemorrhage are sometime described as "granular" or "indolent."[113]

Untreated CMV retinitis is a progressive and blinding disorder.[122] Areas of retina previously infected with CMV show total destruction of the retinal architecture and replacement by a thin gliotic scar. As the lesion spreads, the central area will become scarred and atrophic, whereas the borders will remain active and edematous. The progression of the borders has been termed "a brush-fire" lesion. Ultrastructural studies show that active CMV retinitis replication occurs at the border of the lesion.[193,195] The end stage of this process is a totally destroyed retina, often with retinal detachment, and resulting in total loss of vision.

As of April 1994, two drugs have been approved for the treatment of CMV retinitis in patients with AIDS: ganciclovir and foscarnet. Ganciclovir is a nucleoside analog, whereas foscarnet is a pyrophosphate analog. Both drugs suppress viral replication, and multiple series have documented the efficacy of each drug in arresting the progression of CMV retinitis.* As with other opportunistic infections, discontinuation of therapy results in relapse. With CMV retinitis, relapse occurs promptly (with most patients relapsing within 3 weeks).[127] Hence, long-term suppressive (maintenance) therapy is required. Despite the use of long-term suppressive therapy, relapse occurs; it is now estimated that, given enough time, nearly all patients with CMV retinitis will relapse while on chronic maintenance therapy. As such, the efficacy of an anti-CMV agent can be measured by its ability to prolong the time to relapse. In a randomized controlled trial, Palestine and associates[187] demonstrated that foscarnet prolonged the time to relapse over observation alone in patients with small peripheral CMV retinitis lesions. Similarly, the relative efficacy of two drugs can be compared by measuring their relative times to relapse. In the Foscarnet-Ganciclovir CMV Retinitis Trial,[249] foscarnet and ganciclovir were equivalent in prolonging the time to relapse; hence, they are considered to have equal efficacy in controlling CMV retinitis. In this study, however, foscarnet was associated with a longer survival, a result that could not be fully explained by differential use of antiretroviral therapy in the study, and may be due, in part, to an anti-HIV effect of foscarnet. CMV resistant to anti-CMV drugs has been reported[49,59] and appears to be associated with prolonged treatment with an anti-CMV agent.

Because currently approved therapies for initial or "induction" treatment are available only as intravenous formulations, local, intraocular therapy has been investigated. Intravitreous therapy with either foscarnet or ganciclovir appears to be effective in controlling the disease, but necessitates weekly intravitreous injections for maintenance.[18,31,102,260] More recently, an intraocular sustained-release device has been developed and used investigationally to deliver ganciclovir.[6,216,241] This device releases ganciclovir at a steady rate for several months and also appears to suppress retinitis. The development of contralateral ocular and/or visceral disease in patients treated with local therapy may represent a limitation to this form of therapy. Furthermore, the comparative efficacy of local therapy awaits the results of controlled clinical trials.

Retinal detachments represent a serious problem in patients with CMV retinitis. Case series suggest that 18% to 25% of patients with CMV retinitis will develop retinal detachments.† One retrospective study suggested that the cumulative incidence of retinal detachments at 1 year would be 50%.[126] Retinal detachments were described as a consequence of CMV retinitis prior to the use of anti-CMV agents.[15,173] Early in the AIDS epidemic, it was suggested that antiviral therapy of CMV retinitis might increase the

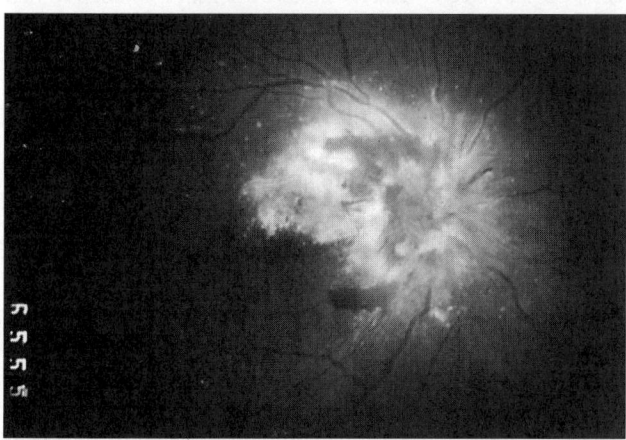

Fig. 22-4 Cytomegalovirus retinitis in a patient with AIDS.

*References 7, 17, 35, 92, 103, 114, 116, 122, 126-129, 151, 183, 186, 187, 249, 263.

†References 52, 77, 78, 126, 184, 208, 236.

rate of retinal detachment by causing premature involution of the retinal scar.[77] Subsequently it has become clear that the rate of retinal detachments is actually greater in patients not treated for CMV retinitis than in those treated.[126] Detachments appear to occur most often in those patients with large lesions extending into the periphery, particularly out to the ora serrata.[77,78,126] Multiple series have reported the efficacy of vitrectomy with silicone oil for the treatment of CMV retinitis-associated retinal detachments.* Local, delimiting laser photocoagulation may have some benefit in treating small peripheral retinal detachments.[184] Whereas the detachment will generally "break through" the laser barrier over time, such laser therapy may retard the development of "macula-off" retinal detachments.

Cytomegalovirus retinitis is discussed in greater detail in Chapter 81.

Ocular Toxoplasmosis. In the United States infection of the eye by *Toxoplasma gondii* occurs in approximately 1% to 2% of patients with AIDS.[123,228] Series from France, where the baseline seroprevalence of antibodies to *T. gondii* is higher, suggest a somewhat greater frequency of ocular toxoplasmosis in patients with AIDS there.[32] In patients with AIDS, ocular toxoplasmic lesions may show the classic focal necrotizing retinitis or may be atypical (Fig. 22-5).[12,109,189,264] They may present as a diffuse necrotizing retinitis,[189] which may be bilateral or multifocal.[12] In the series reported by Holland and associates,[109] the majority of lesions appeared to represent acquired ocular infection. In series reported by Cochereau-Massin and associates[32] from France, approximately 12% of the cases represented acquired toxoplasmosis, as evidenced by a positive IgM antibody to toxoplasmosis, whereas the remaining cases represented reactivation of latent *T. gondii* infection. The apparent discrepancy between the clinical appearance of the ocular disease most often representing acquired ocular infection and the serologic studies most often suggesting reactivation of previously acquired infection may be resolved by the presence of parasitemia in patients with AIDS and toxoplasmosis. Because of the profound immunodeficiency seen in patients with AIDS, parasitemia can be detected in those with central nervous system toxoplasmosis.[257] As such, reactivation of any toxoplasmic infection could result in dissemination of the infection to the retina and an acquired ocular lesion. Toxoplasmic infection in patients with AIDS is generally associated with CD4+ T-lymphocyte counts less than 100 cells/μl.

Ocular toxoplasmosis generally responds to treatment with standard drugs: pyrimethamine, sulfadiazine, and/or clindamycin.[32,109] Long-term maintenance therapy is generally required to prevent relapse of the disease.[109] Corticosteroid treatment, often given to immunologically normal hosts

*References 52, 77, 78, 126, 208, 236.

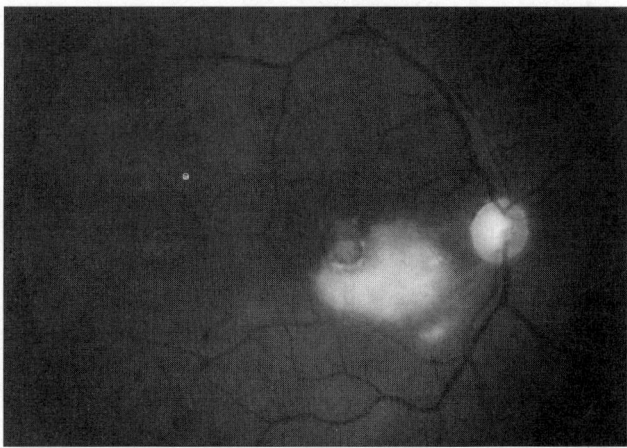

Fig. 22-5   Toxoplasmic retinochoroiditis in a patient with AIDS.

with ocular toxoplasmosis, is not needed in patients with AIDS and ocular toxoplasmosis, as the infection responds to antibiotics alone.

Toxoplasmosis is discussed in greater detail in Chapter 85.

Varicella-Zoster Virus Retinitis. Overall, varicella-zoster virus (VZV) retinitis (Fig. 22-6) occurs in less than 1% of patients with HIV infection.[123] Clinically, VZV retinitis may occur in two different forms. The first is the acute retinal necrosis (ARN) syndrome.[125,230] This form is generally associated with a peripheral necrotizing retinitis, often with multiple scalloped or "thumb print" lesions, which then coalesce. The lesions have little retinal hemorrhage and respond to treatment with intravenous acyclovir.[14] In patients with HIV infection, long-term suppressive therapy with acyclovir is required.[130] In the series by Sellitti and colleagues,[230] 17% of immunocompromised patients with zoster ophthalmicus subsequently developed ARN syndrome. The second form of VZV retinitis is progressive outer retinal necrosis (PORN) syndrome.[71,164] This latter form of VZV retinitis is associated with profound immunodeficiency, generally with CD4+ T-lymphocyte counts less than 50 cells/μl. In PORN syndrome, there are multiple deep retinal yellowish lesions with extensive posterior pole involvement. These lesions rapidly coalesce and result in retinal destruction. The response to treatment with intravenous acyclovir is poor. In patients with HIV infection, the ARN syndrome variant may occur at any level of CD4+ T-lymphocyte count, whereas the PORN syndrome variant is, as noted previously, associated with very low CD4+ T-lymphocyte counts.

Varicella-zoster virus retinitis is discussed in greater detail in Chapter 82.

Fungal Retinitis. Candidal chorioretinitis or endophthalmitis has been reported in patients with AIDS, but occurs in much less than 1% of patients with AIDS.[123] Although oral or esophageal candidiasis is common in patients with HIV

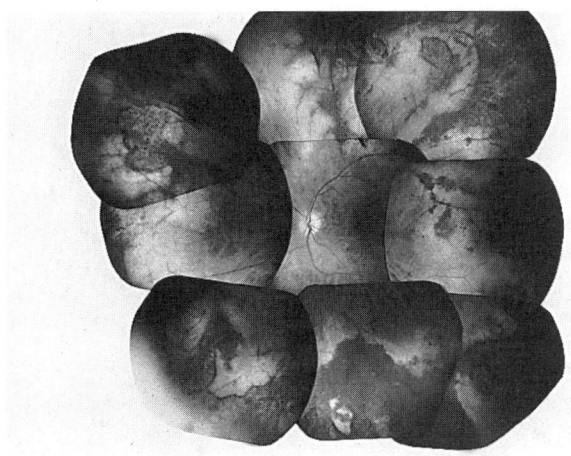

Fig. 22-6   Varicella zoster virus retinitis in a patient with AIDS.

infection, disseminated or visceral infection with *Candida* sp. is uncommon. Disseminated bilateral chorioretinitis caused by *Histoplasma capsulatum* has also been reported.[160] Cryptococcal infection of the choroid and occasionally the retina have been reported in patients with cryptococcal meningitis.[123,134,175,194]

Bacterial Infections. The most common bacterial infection in patients with HIV is syphilis, which can occur at any stage of HIV infection. Ocular syphilis can cause either uveitis or neuroophthalmic lesions.[8,20,191,248] Syphilis in the HIV-infected patient can be treated with appropriate antibiotics (e.g. penicillin) but will often require higher doses and/or more prolonged therapy. Autopsy studies have demonstrated infection of the choroid with *Mycobacterium avium* complex (MAC).[123,175,194] In patients with AIDS, infection with MAC is generally associated with low CD4+ T-lymphocyte counts (less than 100 cells/μl). MAC infection is also associated with a bacteremia, which is presumably the mechanism by which the choroid is involved. MAC infection of the choroid is generally clinically silent.

An unusual bacterial retinitis has been reported in two patients with AIDS, both of whom responded to therapy with tetracycline.[44]

Choroidal Pneumocystosis. Choroidal pneumocystosis (Fig. 22-7) was first described by Rao and associates[207] in 1989. This disorder is a form of extrapulmonary pneumocystosis. *Pneumocystis carinii* has traditionally been considered a protozoan parasite, but there is recent evidence that it might be classified as a fungus.[55,120,270] It has ribosomal RNA sequences that share greater homology with some fungi than with protozoa. Also, it has a soluble translation factor unique to fungal protein synthesis.

The disease is characterized by multiple yellow-white subretinal plaques, 300 to 3000 μ in diameter, that are scattered throughout the posterior pole (Fig. 22-7). As many as several dozen lesions may be seen, but unilateral and unifocal disease has been reported.[72] Lesions are not observed

anterior to the equator. Untreated lesions enlarge slowly at a rate of 750 μ/month.[111,231] As lesions enlarge, they sometimes acquire irregular, multilobular shapes; such enlargement suggests that organisms spread by invasion of choroidal vascular spaces.[111] Eventually, lesions can coalesce, resulting in large geographic patches. On fluorescein angiography, there is early hypofluorescence of lesions with late staining.[75,231] Vitreous cells are not seen with choroidal pneumocystosis, presumably because infection does not extend into the retina. Serous detachment of the retina overlying choroidal lesions has been reported,[72] and there may be retinal pigment epithelium alterations overlying some lesions.[207,242] At autopsy, lesions have been found to be collections of *P. carinii* organisms surrounded by a "frothy" material.[111,207] There are almost no inflammatory cells in lesions.

Many patients with choroidal pneumocystosis also have concurrent CMV retinitis. There is a known association between infections caused by *P. carinii* and CMV in other organs of immunocompromised patients; they have been found to occur together at rates higher than would be predicted from chance alone, based on their individual frequencies.[111] Whether such a relationship exists for the eye is not known. Because *P. carinii* and CMV infect different layers of the eye, their association may only be coincidental because of the high prevalence of CMV retinitis in patients with AIDS.

Patients with choroidal pneumocystosis are frequently asymptomatic or have only mild visual symptoms, even when lesions are under the fovea.[143] Some patients may complain of "intermittent blurring" of vision and may display subtle changes on visual field testing,[231] but even with lesions directly below the foveal avascular zone, objective visual acuity measurements can be as good as 20/25.[143]

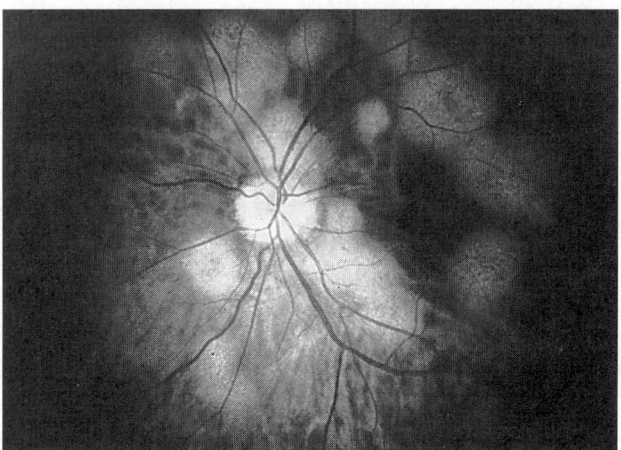

Fig. 22-7   Choroidal pneumocystosis in a patient with AIDS. From Rao NA et al.: A clinical, histopathologic, and electron microscopic study of *Pneumocystis carinii* choroiditis, *Am J Ophthalmol* 107:218-228, 1989 (with permission).

The most important implication of choroidal pneumocystosis is the fact that it can be an early sign of disseminated, life-threatening *P. carinii* infection. Each of the initial patients described by Rao and associates[207] was also found at autopsy to have *P. carinii* infections of multiple organs.[207] Average survival after diagnosis of choroidal pneumocystosis is reported to be 4 months.[231]

Choroidal pneumocystosis is most often seen in patients treated with aerosolized pentamidine as PCP prophylaxis.[50,75,231] In the aggregate series reported by Shami and associates[231] 86% of the 21 patients with choroidal pneumocystosis had aerosolized pentamidine as their form of prophylaxis. Because aerosolized pentamidine does not have systemic absorption, but does effectively prevent the development of *P. carinii* pneumonia, these patients were able to develop extrapulmonary replication of the organisms, including replication in the eye.

This disorder occurs in less than 1% of patients with AIDS and responds therapeutically to systemically administered anti-*P. carinii* therapy,[231] such as intravenous TMP-SMX or intravenous pentamidine. With the demonstration that oral TMP-SMX is superior to aerosolized pentamidine for PCP prophylaxis,[19,98,222] and the subsequent widespread use of oral TMP-SMX as the first-line prophylactic agent, the frequency of choroidal pneumocystosis appears to be declining.

Zoster Ophthalmicus. Zoster ophthalmicus has been reported to occur in approximately 4% of patients with AIDS and 3% of patients with ARC.[123] Ocular complications are common in patients with zoster ophthalmicus and HIV infection; they include scleritis, iridocyclitis, sixth cranial nerve palsies, and retinitis.[34,135,220,230] In HIV-infected patients zoster ophthalmicus can cause a widespread necrotizing and destructive cutaneous lesion with damage to the eyelids. Long-term problems attributed to exposure may result. Although zoster ophthalmicus responds to acyclovir therapy, long-term suppressive therapy may be required.

Other Ocular Infections. Bacterial and fungal corneal ulcers have been reported in patients with AIDS.[190,221] They are relatively infrequent and often occur as a consequence of damage to ocular structures from other problems (e.g. zoster ophthalmicus or radiation therapy for ocular Kaposi sarcoma).

Microsporidial keratoconjunctivitis is a chronic debilitating infection of the corneal and conjunctival epithelium; it is described in more detail in Chapter 79 of this textbook.[79,158]

Ocular Neoplasms. Ocular involvement by Kaposi sarcoma has been reported in 2% of patients with AIDS.[123] Of patients with AIDS and Kaposi sarcoma, 15% to 22% will develop ocular involvement of either the eyelids or conjunctiva.[51,123,235] Conjunctival Kaposi sarcoma (Fig. 22-8) may not require therapy, as the lesions grow slowly and do not invade the eye. Treatment is directed only to those lesions that compromise vision. Conversely, eyelid involvement by

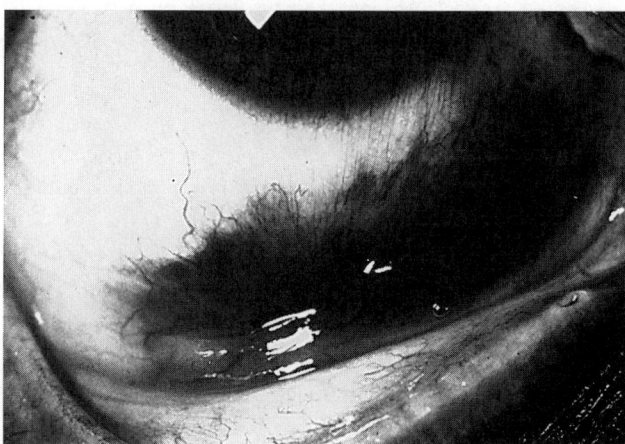

Fig. 22-8 Conjunctiva Kaposi sarcoma in a patient with AIDS. From Jabs DA et al.: Ocular manifestations of acquired immune deficiency syndrome, *Ophthalmology* 96:1092-1099, 1989 (with permission).

Kaposi sarcoma often requires therapy when the lesions become sufficiently large to obscure vision either by eyelid edema or tumor. Local excision, cryotherapy, radiation therapy, and systemic chemotherapy have all been associated with a good response in some patients.[53,86,235]

In patients with HIV infection, high-grade lymphoma is an AIDS-defining indicator disease.[21] There are case reports of orbital involvement by lymphoma, but orbital lymphoma appears to occur in much less than 1% of patients with AIDS.[80,123]

Neuroophthalmic Lesions. Neuroophthalmic lesions may occur in patients with AIDS, either caused by opportunistic central nervous system infections or HIV infection of the central nervous system.* The most common cause of neuroophthalmic lesions is cryptococcal meningitis, which accounts for approximately 50% of neuroophthalmic lesions.[123] Of patients with AIDS and cryptococcal meningitis, one third will have a neuroophthalmic lesion on careful ophthalmologic examination.[123] These lesions include cranial nerve palsies (particularly sixth nerve palsies), papilledema (Fig. 22-9), optic neuropathy, and hemianopsia.[33,124,137] Profound vision loss can result from optic nerve involvement in *Cryptococcus neoformans* infection,[33,137] but this complication fortunately appears to be uncommon.[137]

Other causes of neuroophthalmic lesions include zoster ophthalmicus, viral encephalitis, and central nervous system lymphoma.[166]

In addition, subtle ocular motility defects in patients with AIDS can be detected using eye movement recordings. These defects include slowed saccades, fixational instability, and abnormal pursuit.[41,182] They appear to be directly

---

*References 41, 97, 123, 166, 182, 238, 265.

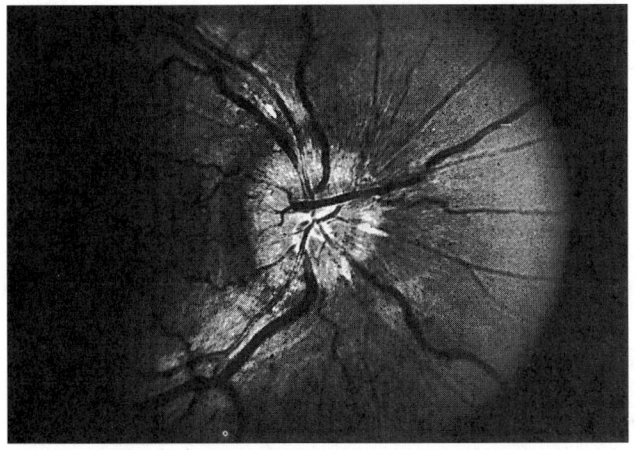 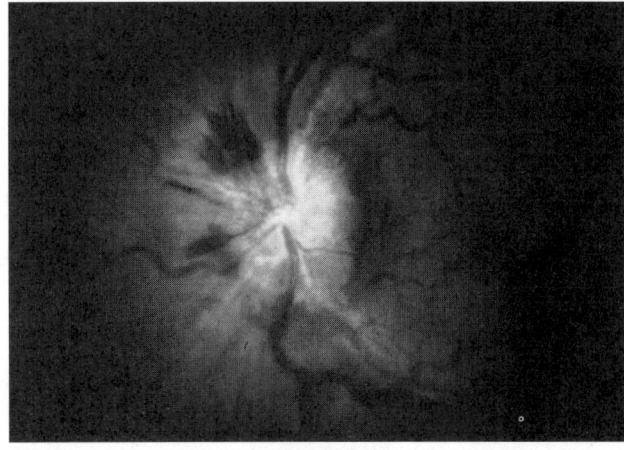

A
B

Fig. 22-9 Papilledema in a patient with cryptococcal meningitis and AIDS. From Jabs DA et al.: Ocular manifestations of acquired immune deficiency syndrome, *Ophthalmology* 96:1092-1099, 1989 (with permission).

related to HIV infection of the central nervous system and may correlate with the AIDS dementia complex.

PATHOGENESIS

Although the vast majority of HIV-infected individuals are without symptoms, HIV has the ability to cause an insidious and progressive deterioration of the host's immune function, leading to profound immunosuppression. Central to the immunopathogenesis of HIV is its interaction with the CD4 molecule in the helper/inducer subset of T-lymphocytes.[139,169] As CD4+ T-lymphocytes play a key role in the induction of most immunologic responses, HIV-induced damage of the CD4+ T-lymphocyte population results in the abrogation of a wide range of immune functions, ultimately leading to extreme immunosuppression manifested by opportunistic infections and neoplasms pathognomonic for AIDS.

Life Cycle of HIV

Following entry of HIV into the blood system of an exposed individual, HIV binds with high affinity to the CD4 molecule via its envelope (env) glycoprotein gp120.[43,139,169] HIV then enters the CD4+ T-lymphocyte by direct fusion of the HIV env with the host T-lymphocyte membrane.[9,161] A recent study now suggests that CD26, another human protein of CD4+ T-lymphocyte, may be required for complete entry into the cytoplasm of the CD4+ T-lymphocyte (unpublished data; Hovanessian and associates). Following entry into the cell, the viral particles are converted into an enzymatically active nucleoprotein complex.[261] After the virion-associated reverse transcriptase transcribes the RNA genome into unintegrated double-stranded DNA, the virally-encoded endonuclease (integrase) enables the viral DNA to integrate into the host cell's chromosomal DNA.[206] In HIV infection a substantial amount of HIV DNA is in an

unintegrated form potentially contributing to the cytopathogenicity observed in HIV infection.[233]

Once the HIV proviral DNA is integrated into the host cell's chromosomal DNA, viral replication may enter a restrictive, latent phase, depending on the state of activation of the infected cell.[107] In an activated cell, host-cell signals initiate transcription of viral DNA into genomic RNA and messenger RNA (mRNA). The mRNA are spliced and translated into viral proteins that subsequently undergo posttranslational modifications including cleavage and glycosylation. The virion RNA and core proteins associate with viral envelope env proteins that are located at the cell membrane, and the mature virion forms by budding from the cell surface.

HIV is an extremely complex virus with genes that may facilitate either high levels of virus production and cell death, restricted chronic virus replication, or latent infection.[214] Viral regulatory proteins influence the levels of viral RNA transcription, splicing of mRNA, and packaging of mature virions. The HIV regulatory genes can interact with each other in a regulatory network that may switch from one pathway to another, depending on cellular factors.[159] Interaction between cellular factors and the HIV genome is thought to play a major role in the maintenance of the long and variable asymptomatic phase of the infected individual and the subsequent progressive immunologic deterioration.

Course of HIV Infection

The period of acute HIV illness is associated with high levels of viremia as documented by either p24 antigenemia or plasma virus culture.[29,42] HIV is widely disseminated during this early stage of infection, suggesting that the subsequent course of HIV infection may be influenced by this early seeding of the virus, particularly to lymphoid organs.[62,188,214] There is a highly HIV-specific immunologic response initiated during this stage that is effective in decreasing the level of viremia.[2] This immunity is apparently inadequate to suppress viral replication completely, however, because HIV expression persists in lymph nodes and peripheral blood CD4+ T-lymphocytes, even though plasma viremia is difficult to detect and mRNA is virtually undetectable in peripheral blood mononuclear cells. As the acute syndrome resolves, levels of CD4+ T-lymphocytes may rebound to 80% to 90% of their original level.[62] Nevertheless, many patients equilibrate to a CD4+ T-lymphocyte level that is moderately or even markedly depressed. The majority of patients then enter a period of clinical latency that may last for 10 years or longer, during which time very few cells in the peripheral blood (1 in 1000 to 1 in 10,000) are infected with HIV.[224,226] Although patients are generally free of symptoms during this period, immune deterioration progresses, manifested by the gradual attrition of circulating CD4+ T-lymphocytes.[63]

It has now been documented that during the clearance of HIV from peripheral blood during the acute primary infection, HIV is trapped within lymph nodes that paradoxically may contribute to further immune deterioration.[73,245,266] When HIV becomes trapped in the follicular dendritic cells within germinal centers of lymph nodes, additional CD4+ T-lymphocytes become vulnerable to HIV infection as they migrate to the lymph node in response to antigenic challenge.[62] In the microenvironment of the lymph node, cytokines are released and a general state of immune activation ensures.[216] Activated CD4+ T-lymphocytes are highly susceptible to HIV infection,[68,168] and cytokines are able to induce HIV replication in latently infected cells.[197,212] The combination of immune activation and cytokine production, in concert with a large pool of susceptible CD4+ T-lymphocytes, may result in the propagation of HIV infection within the lymphoid tissue.

Electron microscopy (EM) analysis of lymph nodes excised from an individual during the early stage of infection reveals large amounts of virus, coated with antibody attached extracellularly to processes of the follicular dendritic cells.[73] EM studies also show that the architecture of the lymph node and the follicular dendritic cell network are relatively intact at this stage. Later in the course of disease, when the numbers of circulating CD4+ T-lymphocytes have declined significantly, plasma viremia once again becomes detectable.[62] EM studies of lymph nodes from late-stage patients show a marked disruption of the architecture of the germinal center and necrosis of the follicular dendritic cell processes. The loss of virus-trapping function likely results in the decreased virus burden in the lymph node as virus increases in the bloodstream. This decreased ability of the follicular dendritic cell network to trap virus, along with accelerated virus replication seen in the late stages of HIV disease, probably explains the increase in plasma viremia seen at this stage.[188] Moreover, the loss of the lymph node's

crucial antigen-trapping and antigen-presenting functions likely compounds the severe immunosuppression that results from the loss of functional CD4+ T-lymphocytes. Investigators conclude from these studies that the term "latency" should be used with caution in the context of HIV disease because HIV is actively replicating in the lymphoid tissues, even when little or no virus is evident in peripheral blood.[62,188] It is highly unlikely that a true state of microbiologic latency exists at any time during HIV infection.

Activation Factors

Within the lymph node, the HIV-infected T-lymphocyte is exposed to a number of activating factors that may directly or indirectly induce further HIV replication. Agents shown to upregulate the expression of HIV in cells in vitro include antigens and mitogens; genes from heterologous viruses including CMV, herpes simplex virus, human herpes virus type 6, and human T-lymphtrophic virus type 1; mycoplasma; and other co-infecting microbes.[85,156,205,212] Some of these agents have been shown to induce HIV expression in the host cell by activating DNA-binding proteins such as NF-kB.[178,212] Such proteins initiate viral expression through interactions with specific sequences within the HIV long terminal repeat (LTR).[237,257]

A wide variety of endogenous cytokines (soluble factors responsible for normal immune homeostasis) may also be induced, which then act on HIV replication. In vitro studies with latently or chronically infected promonocytic or key lymphocytic cell lines have shown that a number of cytokines directly influence HIV replication.[54,67,70,199] Tissue necrosis factor-α appears to upregulate HIV expression by inducing transcription factors that bind to the NF-kB binding region of HIV LTR, resulting in new HIV transcription and virion formation.[213,237,257] This effect can be blocked by use of anti-tumor necrosis factor (TNF)-α antibodies. Other cytokines such as interleukin (IL)-6 and granulocyte-monocyte colony-stimulating factor (GM-CSF) also induce HIV expression, predominantly through posttranscriptional mechanisms.[198] It has been observed, however, that various cytokines can act synergistically in the induction of HIV expression, and when IL-6 and GM-CSF act in concert with TNF-α, transcriptional upregulation involving activation of NF-kB occurs.[213]

B-lymphocyte abnormalities have also been seen in HIV-infected individuals and are manifested by polyclonal activation and spontaneous production of immunoglobulin.[3,4] Interestingly, B-lymphocytes from HIV-infected individuals may secrete high levels of TNF-α and IL-6, which can further upregulate HIV expression.[133] Activated B-lymphocytes from an HIV-infected patient, when cultured with autologous T-lymphocytes, appear to up-regulate HIV expression.[210] These findings suggest a mechanism for HIV expression in the lymph node during clinical latency. Fauci and associates[63] postulated that B-lymphocytes in the germinal center of HIV-infected individuals are in an activated state and secrete high levels of TNF-α and IL-6.[62,188] These cytokines are likely contributors to the induction of virus replication in infected CD4+ T-lymphocytes, both in the paracortical areas of the lymph node and in the germinal center itself, where CD4+ T-lymphocytes may have infiltrated.

CD4+ T-Lymphocyte Depletion

As described earlier, the hallmark of HIV infection is a steady, progressive decline in the number of CD4+ T-lymphocytes, the target cell for HIV.* Although several mechanisms by which HIV destroys CD4+ T-lymphocytes have been postulated, the exact mechanisms are not known at present. One possible cell-killing mechanism may be the formation of microholes in the cell membrane that are the result of intense virus budding.[153] Another direct mechanism of cell-killing involves (1) the accumulation of unintegrated viral DNA in the cell cytoplasm and (2) accumulation of high levels of heterodisperse RNAs containing repetitive sequences that do not contain long open reading frames.[141,192] It has also been suggested that the binding of HIV env proteins to intracellular CD4 molecules may result in cell death.[118] In support of this hypothesis, there have been several reports that correlate expression of the env gene with cytopathic effect on CD4+ T-lymphocytes.[65,243]

Several indirect mechanisms of CD4+ T-lymphocyte destruction have also been implicated in the pathogenesis of HIV infection. The dramatic depletion of CD4+ T-lymphocytes that occurs in AIDS patients may be the consequence of HIV infection of CD4+ T-lymphocyte precursors, which secrete factors that can stimulate the propagation of the entire lymphoid cell pool.[61] It has been shown that bone marrow progenitor cells and thymic precursor cells can be infected with HIV in vitro.[69,225] Another potential mechanism of depletion involves the generation of multinucleated giant cells in vitro that result from the high affinity binding of gp120 CD4 molecules on neighboring uninfected CD4+ T-lymphocytes.[243,269] It is thought that these syncytia die soon after formation and contribute to the indirect cytopathic effects of HIV infection. Autoimmune phenomena play a role in the pathogenesis of HIV infection. It is hypothesized that the binding of soluble gp120 to CD4 receptors on uninfected T-lymphocytes may render these cells susceptible to immune clearance.[138]

The premature induction of apoptosis has also been proposed as a mechanism of CD4+ T-lymphocyte loss during HIV infection.[62] Apoptosis, a form of programmed cell death, is a common physiologic process first described in the context of clonal deletion of autoreactive T-lymphocytes in the human thymus.[167,239] In HIV-infected individuals it has

been hypothesized that gp120 alone or bound to anti-gp120 antibodies cross-link CD4 receptors; this occurrence may result in a negative signal to the CD4+ T-lymphocyte.[5,93] Apoptosis may then be triggered by subsequent antigenic stimulation of the T-lymphocyte receptor.[93] Apoptosis has been demonstrated in vitro in acute HIV infection of lymphoid blastoid cells or activated peripheral blood mononuclear cells.[152,253] It should be noted, however, that the data reported so far are inconsistent with apoptosis being a selective mechanism for CD4+ T-lymphocyte depletion, and that both CD4+ and CD8+ T-lymphocytes in asymptomatic HIV-infected individuals have been reported to undergo apoptosis spontaneously in vitro.[90,174]

Precise mechanisms responsible for the functional defects and depletion of CD4+ T-lymphocytes leading to the immune deterioration of HIV disease are complex and not well understood. Further understanding of these complex interactions of HIV with the human immune system are critical for the design of effective vaccine and therapeutics in the ultimate control of HIV disease.

In addition to depletion of CD4+ T-lymphocytes, functional abnormalities of viable and normal-appearing CD4+ T-lymphocytes have been noted at all stages of HIV infection. CD4+ T-lymphocytes are defective in their ability to induce B-lymphocytes to secrete immunoglobulin and to respond to alloantigens.[95,149] Although lymphocytes from patients with AIDS respond normally to mitogens, they were shown defective in their ability to recognize and proliferate in response to soluble antigens.[87,150,234] Abnormal T-lymphocyte responses to soluble antigens were observed early in the course of the infection, prior to a significant decline in the number of CD4+ T-lymphocytes.[119,150] Defective T-lymphocyte cloning efficiency is another measure of functional impairment of CD4+ T-lymphocytes in HIV infection.[162] Suppression of in vitro lymphocyte activation has been shown to occur upon normal T-lymphocytes exposure to sera from AIDS patients.[40] The inhibitory activity of AIDS sera occurred even when added several hours after phytohemagglutinin stimulation of normal T-lymphocytes and could be diluted out with normal sera. It is thought that the inhibitory factor or factors cause a decline in IL-2r expression.[47]

There are several potential mechanisms to explain how HIV can cause a functional impairment of antigen-responsive CD4+ T-lymphocytes in the absence of cell infection. HIV or its products may interfere with CD4-mediated monocyte-T-lymphocyte interaction.[214] Interaction of CD4 molecules on the surface of CD4+ T-lymphocytes with MHC class II molecules on the surface of monocytes is required for antigen-specific responses.[48,83] Because HIV gp120-CD4 interactions occur with a very high affinity, the binding of HIV or free gp120 may prevent the MHC class II molecule from binding to CD4 and thus block the antigen-specific response. Although it has recently been shown that the bind-

---

*References 21, 56, 89, 157, 163, 176, 188, 254.

ing site on the CD4 molecule for MHC class II is distinct from that of gp120, CD4 MHC class II binding may require a more extensive area of contact that can be inhibited by CD4-gp120 binding.[30,148] It is also possible that infection with HIV may also downregulate other cellular genes including CD3, CD4, and CD8 levels, as well as IL-2 and IL-2r.[246,271] Downregulation of IL-2 or IL-2r gene expression may contribute to the functional deficits for antigen-specific responses that require IL-2 for amplification.[214]

Abnormalities of Monocytes and Macrophages

Monocytes and macrophages are also susceptible to HIV infection. Infection may occur through phagocytosis of HIV particles or through attachment to the CD4 receptor present on the surface of monocyte/macrophages.[39,247] HIV infection of these cells appears persistent and does not result in significant cell death or syncytial formation that occurs after infection of CD4+ T-lymphocytes.[105,154,218] In HIV-infected macrophages, virus particles are often located within cytoplasmic vacuoles.[82] Some investigators have even reported that certain isolates of HIV display specific tropisms for monocyte/macrophages or CD4+ T-lymphocytes. HIV isolated from lung and brain macrophages of infected individuals was shown to infect macrophages more readily than T-lymphocytes compared with a standard tissue culture strain of HIV (HTLV-IIIb) that prefers T-lymphocyte infection.[82,144]

The role of circulating monocytes in HIV infection is presently unknown. Although it has been reported by polymerase chain reaction (PCR) analysis that the level of infection in circulating monocytes is nearly equal to that in CD4+ T-lymphocytes,[170] several investigators have found very few HIV-infected monocytes in the peripheral blood of HIV-infected individuals.[203,244] Nevertheless, the function of monocyte/macrophages in HIV-infected individuals is abnormal. There is reduced monocyte chemotaxis,[240] monocyte-dependent T-lymphocytes proliferation,[201] Fc receptor function,[10] and C3 receptor-mediated clearance.[11] Thus the detection of HIV in macrophages from the lung and brain along with recent data that show monocyte/macrophages are readily infected with HIV following differentiation suggest that the tissue-specific macrophages may be a significant target for HIV in vivo.[84] The sequestration of the virus within monocyte/macrophages in these infected cells may function as a reservoir for infection in the body similar to other lentivirus systems.[84] The relative lack of extracellular budding virus in these cells may help explain why the HIV-specific immune response is unsuccessful in eliminating HIV. In addition, the infected monocyte/macrophage may be responsible for transporting HIV to the lung or brain, resulting in neuropsychiatric problems.

Microvasculopathy

Three hypotheses have been proposed for the pathogenesis of HIV retinopathy: (1) immune complex disease, (2) HIV infection of the retinal vascular endothelium, and (3) hemorheologic abnormalities. HIV retinopathy is related to HIV disease itself and not to any opportunistic ocular infection.[146,194] The first hypothesis suggested for the pathogenesis of HIV retinopathy was that of circulating immune complexes. Circulating immune complexes can be detected in the majority of patients with AIDS and ARC.[94] Pepose and associates[194] have demonstrated immunoglobulin deposition within arterial walls, a finding that supports this hypothesis. Furthermore, AIDS is characterized by polyclonal B-lymphocyte activation and hypergammaglobulinemia, which are immunologic abnormalities associated with microangiopathy in autoimmune disorders such as systemic lupus erythematosus.[149,223]

Although immune complex deposition disease remains a possibility for the pathogenesis of HIV retinopathy, HIV infection of the retinal vascular endothelial cells is an alternative explanation. Pomerantz and associates[200] were able to culture HIV from the retina of patients with AIDS and have localized HIV proteins to the retinal vascular endothelium using immunohistochemical techniques. Other authors[228] have reported electron micrographic evidence of HIV infection of the retina. Furthermore, HIV is known to infect the central nervous system.[106,140,232] Hence, HIV retinopathy could be a direct consequence of HIV infection of the vascular endothelial cells, in which the virus damages the vascular endothelium and produces arteriolar occlusion. Alternatively, HIV infection of the vascular endothelial cells could lead to anti-HIV antibodies binding to the retinal vascular endothelium and result in vascular occlusion.

In addition to the microangiopathy seen in the retina, abnormalities of blood vessels have been reported in the conjunctiva, including vascular occlusion and telangiectatic vessels.[251] Engstrom and associates[57] reported that systemic hemorheologic abnormalities, as evidenced by an elevated zeta sedimentation rate, were correlated with the ocular microangiopathy, particularly the anterior segment findings. Hence, abnormalities of blood flow, due to HIV infection, could also be a contributing factor in HIV retinopathy.

Whereas each of these hypotheses could explain the abnormalities seen, the complete pathogenesis of disease remains unknown at this time. It is also possible that a combination of factors may produce HIV retinopathy. Fortunately, although HIV retinopathy is common in patients with AIDS, it is generally visually asymptomatic. Usually the lesions come and go without clinical visual symptoms. More recently, subtle abnormalities of color vision and contrast sensitivity have been reported in patients with HIV infection.[204] The pathogenesis of these abnormalities is not clear, but two hypotheses exist: the first is that they are due to HIV infection of the retina and/or optic nerve; and the second is that they represent cumulative damage from the microvasculopathy. Histologic morphometric studies have suggested a loss of nerve fibers in the optic nerve supporting the concept of subtle damage to the retina and optic nerve.[252] These histologic changes cannot distinguish between a direct effect of HIV infection and a cumulative damage from a microangiopathy, however.

Kaposi Sarcoma

The cause of Kaposi sarcoma remains unknown. Although the cell of origin has been debated, the current hypothesis maintains it is a multipotential cell of mesenchymal origin[217] and the cause is multifactorial. HIV infection alone is not sufficient, as Kaposi sarcoma occurs in other populations, and the HIV gene has not been detected in the lesions of KS. The occurrence of Kaposi sarcoma with variable CD4+ T-lymphocyte counts suggests that immunodeficiency alone is not the primary cause; however, the occurrence of Kaposi sarcoma in renal transplant patients and the much greater incidence in patients with AIDS suggests that immune dysfunction is an important contributing factor. Infectious agents have been proposed as contributing factors, including CMV, human papilloma virus (HPV)-16, and an as yet unidentified transmissible agent.[88,217] CMV has been of particular interest because of the demonstration of elevated antibody levels in the sera of patients with Kaposi sarcoma and the presence of CMV antigens and CMV-DNA sequences within the tumor itself.[88] None of the hypotheses concerning causation have been widely accepted, however.

In the 1980s it became possible to culture Kaposi sarcoma cells and produce Kaposi sarcoma cell lines. These cell lines expressed cytokines and demonstrated autocrine and paracrine growth effects and angiogenic activity. Multiple cytokines have been demonstrated to have a growth-promoting activity for Kaposi sarcoma cells, including IL-1, fibroblast growth factor, IL-6, the HIV transactivating (Tat) protein and, to a lesser degree, TNF-α, transforming growth factor-β, and IL-4. The effect of these cytokines on tumor cell growth suggests a role for the immune system in the propagation of this tumor and potential avenues for therapy.

THERAPY

This section deals with the therapy of HIV disease in general. The treatment of specific opportunistic infections are discussed in other chapters of this textbook that deal with those specific disorders.

With evidence of ongoing HIV replication during the entire course of an HIV-infected individual's disease, one of the primary objectives of the clinician is to prevent or slow further virus replication through antiviral therapy. In 1987 antiretroviral therapy with the nucleoside analog zidovudine (ZDV) was found effective for delaying the onset of opportunistic infections and prolonging survival in patients with AIDS and advanced HIV disease.[64] In 1990 the benefit of ZDV in individuals who were asymptomatic with CD4+ T-lymphocyte counts less than 500 cells/μl was demon-

strated.[262] Although the latter study demonstrated a significant delay in progression to AIDS or advanced HIV disease, the study did not demonstrate a difference in mortality within two years of use of ZDV. Further follow-up of these patients is ongoing. This study also showed that the group treated with the lower dose of ZDV (500 mg/day) experienced significantly less toxicity than the higher-dose group. Retrospective studies also support the beneficial effects of ZDV on the survival of patients. Analysis of the multicenter AIDS cohort study data suggests that the early initiation of ZDV may prolong survival.[91] The mortality rate was significantly reduced in patients who received ZDV before the development of an AIDS diagnosis. This effect was in addition to the beneficial effect of prophylaxis for PCP.

Preliminary results from the Concorde trial were published in 1993 and generated a controversy regarding early therapy.[1] This study recruited 1749 asymptomatic HIV individuals who were randomized to one gram daily of ZDV or matching placebo. The CD4+ T-lymphocyte counts in those receiving ZDV rose to significantly higher levels than those on placebo. Although this study showed a beneficial effect of ZDV on the progression of the disease at 1-year follow-up, there was no significant difference in clinical progression of HIV disease or in survival at 3 years of follow-up. The subsequent Australian-European study suggested that ZDV was beneficial in the prevention of minor symptoms of HIV, and delayed the decline of CD4+ T-lymphocytes to less than 350 cells/μl.[38] The latter study did not demonstrate a benefit of ZDV in delay of progression to AIDS or severe HIV symptoms, however, and did not report survival data.

As a result of these studies, a National Institutes of Health (NIH) panel recently provided recommendations regarding antiretroviral therapy (see box). Zidovudine remains the initial drug of choice when starting therapy, but the availability of other antiretroviral agents has provided patients with other options should they develop intolerance to ZDV or experience further clinical deterioration. Although reasons for a lack of response to ZDV may be complex, it appears that resistance to ZDV may develop over time.[209] Intolerance to ZDV because of anemia, neutropenia, nausea, insomnia, headaches, and/or fatigue may also necessitate a change in therapy. Didanosine (ddI) and zalcitabine (ddC) are available options for individuals who cannot tolerate ZDV or have failed to respond to it.[37,131,172] Their toxicity profile is different from ZDV, and their major adverse effects are peripheral neuropathy and pancreatitis.

Other Management Considerations

In addition to assessing immune function via CD4+ T-lymphocyte testing and initiating antiretroviral treatment and PCP prophylaxis, many other issues in the clinical management of individuals with HIV infection are of primary importance (see the box.) These issues include the detection and treatment of other infections such as tuberculosis and syphilis (which may occur very early in the natural history of HIV disease), oral care, eye care, the provision of preventive measures including immunizations, the evaluation and management of patients' psychologic and emotional needs, and the prevention of further transmission of HIV infection. A detailed medical history is crucial and should emphasize the review of HIV test results, previous infections including opportunistic infections, and sexual and substance use history. A comprehensive physical examination, with attention to eye and oral examination, neurologic examination, careful skin and lymph node assessment, as well as HIV-associated signs and symptoms such as weight loss and diarrhea, allows the provider to define the stage of HIV infection and determine the appropriate course of management and treatment in the individual patient. Testing for CD4+ T-lymphocyte counts should be performed every 6 months, and if abnormal, repeated prior to institution of antiretroviral therapy or PCP prophylaxis. Each patient should have a PPD with an

---

RECOMMENDATIONS FOR EARLY HIV INFECTION EVALUATION AND CARE

Review of HIV serology with counseling

Detailed medical history including substance abuse and sexual history

Comprehensive physical examination

Baseline lab studies: CBC with differential, chemistry panel, CD4+ T-lymphocyte count, VDRL, hepatitis and toxoplasmosis serology, PPD with anergy panel

Vaccinations: influenza, pneumococcal, hepatitis B, tetanus, mumps, rubella and measles vaccines when indicated

Antiretroviral therapy and prophylaxis against *Pneumocystis carinii* pneumonia if indicated according to symptoms and CD4+ T-lymphocyte count

---

NIAID CONSENSUS RECOMMENDATIONS FOR THE TREATMENT OF HIV-INFECTED PATIENTS, JUNE 1993

1. For patients without symptoms whose CD4+ T-lymphocyte counts are above or equal to 500 cells/μl, antiviral therapy should not be given, and clinical and immunologic monitoring should occur every 6 months.
2. For patients without symptoms with CD4+ T-lymphocyte counts between 200 to 500 cells/μl, the physician may either initiate antiretroviral therapy or continue observation and monitoring for clinical laboratory evidence of deterioration, at which point antiretroviral therapy should be initiated.
3. For patients with CD4+ T-lymphocyte counts between 200 and 500 cells/μl who present with symptoms related to HIV disease, antiretroviral therapy should be started.
4. Zidovudine (ZDV) should be used as first-line therapy in patients who have received prior antiretroviral therapy. The recommended dose is 600 mg per day in divided doses.
5. Combination therapy using ZDV and didanosine (ddI) or zalcitabine (ddC) may be considered, although clinical trials have not conclusively demonstrated clinical benefit to date.
6. For patients whose CD4+ T-lymphocyte counts decline below 300 cells/μl while on ZDV, ZDV can be continued or switched to ddI. Strongest data supporting a change to ddI were in patients who had already been on ZDV for 4 months or longer (median duration 13 months).
7. For patients who are intolerant to ZDV or experience progression of disease despite ZDV therapy, patients should be switched to ddI or ddC monotherapy.

---

anergy panel including *Candida albicans,* tetanus toxoid, and mumps. If PPD positive, INH prophylaxis should be instituted.[22,24,26] Serologic tests for syphilis, hepatitis B, and hepatitis C should be obtained, and if negative for hepatitis B, the patient should be vaccinated with the hepatitis B vaccine.

Toxoplasmosis serology (IgG) is also advocated to assist in the later diagnosis of toxoplasmic encephalitis. Seroprevalence rates in the United States range from 10% to 40%, and most patients with this complication have a positive serologic test. Use of the serologic test as a screening test when patients are asymptomatic is somewhat arbitrary, but some have argued that it is more likely to be positive in the early stages of disease when the humoral response is more effective. It is probable that the prophylaxis for PCP may also be effective in preventing toxoplasmosis. Other immunizations that should be considered include influenza, pneumococcal, tetanus, rubella, and measles vaccines. For guidelines regarding effective treatments, suppression of disease, and potential prophylaxis against secondary infections, the reader is referred to a more general text on HIV disease.

REFERENCES

1. Aboulker P et al.: Preliminary analysis of the Concorde trial, *Lancet* 341(8849):889-890, 1993 (letter to editor).
2. Albert J et al.: Rapid development of isolate-specific neutralizing antibodies after primary HIV-1 infection and consequent emergency of virus variants which resist neutralization by autologous sera, *AIDS* 4:107-112, 1990.
3. Amadori A, Chieco-Binachi L: B-cell activation and HIV-1 infection: deeds and misdeeds, *Immunol Today* 11:374-379, 1990.
4. Amadori A et al.: HIV-1-specific B cell activation: a major constituent of spontaneous B cell activation during HIV-1 infection, *J Immunol* 143:2146-2152, 1989.
5. Ameisen JC, Capron A: Cell dysfunction and depletion in AIDS: the programmed cell death hypothesis, *Immunol Today* 7:115-119, 1986.

6. Anand R et al.: Control of cytomegalovirus retinitis using sustained release of intraocular ganciclovir, *Arch Ophthalmol* 111:223-227, 1993.

7. Aweeka F, Gambertoglio J, Mills J et al.: Pharmacokinetics of intermittently administered intravenous foscarnet in the treatment of acquired immunodeficiency syndrome patients with serious cytomegalovirus retinitis, *Antimicrob Agents Chemother* 33:742-745, 1989.

8. Becerra LI, Ksiazek SM, Savino PT et al.: Syphilitic uveitis in human immunodeficiency virus-infected and noninfected patients, *Ophthalmology* 96:1727-1730, 1989.

9. Bedinger P et al.: Internalization of the human immunodeficiency virus does not require the cytoplasmic domain of CD4, *Nature* 334:162-165, 1988.

10. Bender BS et al.: Defective reticuloendothelial system Fc-receptor function in patients with acquired immunodeficiency syndrome, *J Infect Dis* 152:409-412, 1985.

11. Bender BS et al.: Demonstration of defective C3-receptor-mediated clearance by the reticuloendothelial system in patients with acquired immunodeficiency syndrome, *J Clin Invest* 79:715-720, 1987.

12. Berger BB et al.: Miliary toxoplasmic retinitis in acquired immunodeficiency syndrome, *Arch Ophthalmol* 111:373-376, 1993.

13. Bloom JN, Palestine AG: The diagnosis of cytomegalovirus retinitis, *Ann Intern Med* 109:963-969, 1988.

14. Blumenkranz MS, Culbertson WW, Clarkson JG et al.: Treatment of the acute retinal necrosis syndrome with intravenous acyclovir, *Ophthalmology* 93:296-300, 1986.

15. Broughton WL, Cupples HP, Parver LM: Bilateral retinal detachment following cytomegalovirus retinitis, *Arch Ophthalmol* 96:618-619, 1978.

16. Buehler JW, Berkelman RL, Stehr-Green JK: The completeness of AIDS surveillance, *J Acquir Immune Defic Syndr* 5:257-264, 1992.

17. Buhles WC et al.: Ganciclovir treatment of life- or sight-threatening cytomegalovirus infection: experience in 314 immunocompromised patients, *Infect Dis Clin North Am* 10(3):S495-S506, 1988.

18. Cantrill HL, Henry K, Melroe NH et al.: Treatment of cytomegalovirus retinitis with the intravitreal ganciclovir: long-term results, *Ophthalmology* 96:367-374, 1989.

19. Carr A et al.: Trimethoprim-sulfamethoxazole appears more effective than aerosolized pentamidine as secondary prophylaxis against *Pneumocystis carinii* pneumonia in patients with AIDS, *AIDS* 6:165-171, 1992.

20. Carter JB, Hamill RJ, Matoba AY: Bilateral syphilitic optic neuritis in a patient with a positive test for HIV, *Arch Ophthalmol* 105:1485-1486, 1987.

21. Centers for Disease Control: Revision of the CDC surveillance case definition for acquired immunodeficiency syndrome, *MMWR CDC Surveill Summ* 36(suppl 1S):1S-5S, 1987.

22. Centers for Disease Control: Purified protein derivative (PPD)-tuberculin anergy and HIV infection: guidelines for anergy testing and management of anergic persons at risk of tuberculosis, *MMWR* 37:600-608, 1988.

23. Centers for Disease Control: Guidelines for prophylaxis against *Pneumocystis carinii* pneumonia for adults and adolescents infected with human immunodeficiency virus, *MMWR* 41(RR-4):1-11, 1992.

24. Centers for Disease Control: National action plan to combat multidrug-resistant tuberculosis; meeting the challenge of multidrug-resistant tuberculosis: summary of a conference; management of persons exposed to multi-drug resistant tuberculosis, *MMWR* 41(RR-11):1-71, 1992.

25. Centers for Disease Control: 1993 revised classification system for HIV infection and expanded surveillance case definition for AIDS among adolescents and adults, *MMWR CDC Surveill Summ* 41(No. RR-17), 1992.

26. Centers for Disease Control: Treatment of tuberculosis: recommendations of the Advisory Council for the elimination of tuberculosis, *MMWR,* 1993.

27. Centers for Disease Control and Prevention: *HIV/AIDS Surveillance Report* 5(3):1-20, 1993.

28. Chin J: Current and future dimensions of the HIV epidemic, *Lancet* 336:221-224, 1990.

29. Clark SJ et al.: High titers of cytopathic virus in plasma of patients with symptomatic primary HIV-1 infection, *N Engl J Med* 324:954-960, 1991.

30. Clayton LK et al.: Identification of human CD4 residues affecting class II MHC versus HIV-1 gp120 binding, *Nature* 339:548-551, 1989.

31. Cochereau-Massin I et al.: Efficacy and tolerance of intravitreal ganciclovir in cytomegalovirus retinitis in acquired immune deficiency syndrome, *Ophthalmology* 98:1348-1355, 1991.

32. Cochereau-Massin I et al.: Ocular toxoplasmosis in human immunodeficiency virus-infected patients, *Am J Ophthalmol* 114:130-135, 1992.

33. Cohen DB, Glasgow BJ: Bilateral optic nerve cryptococcosis in sudden blindness in patients with acquired immune deficiency syndrome, *Ophthalmology* 100:1689-1694, 1993.

34. Cole EL, Meisler DM, Calabrese LH et al.: Herpes zoster ophthalmicus and acquired immune deficiency syndrome, *Arch Ophthalmol* 102:1027-1029, 1984.

35. Collaborative DHPG Treatment Study Group: Treatment of serious cytomegalovirus infections with 9-(1,3-dihydroxy-2-propoxymethyl) guanine in patients with AIDS and other immunodeficiencies, *N Engl J Med* 314:801-805, 1986.

36. Collier AC, Meyers JD, Corey L et al.: Cytomegalovirus infection in homosexual men, *Am J Med* 82:593-601, 1987.

37. Cooley TP et al.: Treatment of AIDS in AIDS-related complex with 2′, 3′ dideoxyinosine given once daily, *Rev Infect Dis* 12(suppl 5):S552-S560, 1990.

38. Cooper DA et al.: Zidovudine in persons with asymptomatic HIV infection and CD4$^+$ cell counts greater than 400 per cubic millimeter, *N Engl J Med* 329(5):297-303, 1993.

39. Crowe S, Mills J, McGrath MS: Quantitative immunocytofluorographic analysis of CD4 surface antigen expression and HIV infection of human peripheral blood monocyte/macrophages, *AIDS Res Hum Retroviruses* 3:135-145, 1987.

40. Cunningham-Rundles S, Michelis MA, Masur H: Serum suppression of lymphocyte activation in vitro is acquired immunodeficiency disease, *J Clin Immunol* 3:156-165, 1983.

41. Currie J, Benson E, Ramsden B et al.: Eye movement abnormalities as a predictor of the acquired immunodeficiency syndrome dementia complex, *Arch Neurol* 45:949-953, 1988.

42. Daar ES et al.: Transient high levels of viremia in patients with primary human immunodeficiency virus type 1 infection, *N Engl J Med* 324:961-964, 1991.

43. Dalgleish AG et al.: The CD4 (T4) antigen is an essential component of the receptor of the AIDS retrovirus, *Nature* 312:763-767, 1984.

44. Davis JL, Nussenblatt RB, Bachman DM et al.: Endogenous bacterial retinitis in AIDS, *Am J Ophthalmol* 107:613-623, 1989.

45. Davis MG et al.: Immediate-early gene region of human cytomegalovirus trans-activates the promoter of human immunodeficiency virus, *Proc Natl Acad Sci USA* 84:8642-8646, 1987.

46. DeCock KM et al.: AIDS—the leading cause of adult death in the West African city of Abidjan, Ivory Coast, *Science* 249:793-796, 1990.

47. Donnelly RP, La Via MF, Tsang KY: Humoral-mediated suppression of interleukin 2-dependent target cell proliferation in acquired immune deficiency syndrome (AIDS): interference with normal IL-2 receptor expression, *Clin Exp Immunol* 68:488-499, 1987.

48. Doyle C, Strominger JL: Interaction between CD4 and class II MHC molecules mediates cell adhesion, *Nature* 330:256-259, 1987.

49. Drew WL et al.: Prevalence of resistance in patients receiving ganciclovir for serious cytomegalovirus infection, *J Infect Dis* 163:716-719, 1991.

50. Dugel PU, Rao NA, Forster DJ et al.: *Pneumocystis carinii* choroiditis after long-term aerosolized pentamidine therapy, *Am J Ophthalmol* 110:113-117, 1990.

51. Dugel PU et al.: Ocular adnexal Kaposi's sarcoma in acquired immunodeficiency syndrome, *Am J Ophthalmol* 110:500-503, 1990.

52. Dugel PU et al.: Repair of retinal detachment caused by cytomegalovirus retinitis in patients with the acquired immunodeficiency syndrome, *Am J Ophthalmol* 112:235-242, 1991.

53. Dugel PU et al.: Treatment of ocular adnexal Kaposi's sarcoma in acquired immune deficiency syndrome, *Ophthalmology* 99:1127-1132, 1992.

54. Duh EJ et al.: Tumor necrosis factor-alpha activates human immunodeficiency virus-1 through induction of nuclear factor binding to the NF-KB sites in the long terminal repeat, *Proc Natl Acad Sci USA* 86:5974-5978, 1989.

55. Edman JC et al.: Ribosomal RNA sequence shows *Pneumocystis carinii* to be a member of the Fungi, *Nature* 334:519-522, 1988.

56. Embretson J et al.: Massive covert infection of helper T lymphocytes and macrophages by HIV during the incubation period of AIDS, *Nature* 362:359-362, 1993.

57. Engstrom RE et al.: Hemorhelogic abnormalities in patients with human immunodeficiency virus-infection and ophthalmic microvasculopathy, *Am J Ophthalmol* 153-161, 1990.

58. Ensoli B et al.: AIDS-Kaposi's sarcoma-derived cells express cytokines with autocrine and paracrine growth effects, *Science* 243:223-226, 1989.

59. Erice A, Chou S, Biron KK et al.: Progressive disease due to ganciclovir-resistant cytomegalovirus in immunocompromised patients, *N Engl J Med* 320:291-293, 1989.

60. Farrell PL, Heinemann MH, Roberts CW et al.: Response of human immunodeficiency virus-associated uveitis to zidovudine, *Am J Ophthalmol* 106:7-10, 1988.

61. Fauci AS: AIDS: immunopathogenic mechanisms and research strategies, *Clin Res* 35:503-510, 1987.

62. Fauci AS: Immunopathogenesis of HIV infection, *J Acquir Immune Defic Syndr* 6:655-662, 1993.

63. Fauci AS et al.: NIH conference: immunopathogenic mechanisms in human immunodeficiency virus (HIV) infection, *Ann Intern Med* 114:678-693, 1991.

64. Fischl MA et al.: The safety and efficacy of zidovudine (AZT) in the treatment of subjects with mildly symptomatic human immunodeficiency virus type 1 (HIV) infection: a double-blind, placebo-controlled trial, *Ann Intern Med* 112:727-737, 1990.

65. Fisher AG et al.: Infectious mutants of HTLV-III with changes in the 3' region and markedly reduced cytopathic effects, *Science* 233:655-659, 1986.

66. Flores-Aguilar M et al.: Pathophysiology and treatment of clinically resistant cytomegalovirus retinitis, *Ophthalmology* 100:1022-1031, 1993.

67. Folks T et al.: Characterization of a continuous T-cell line susceptible to the cytopathic effects of the acquired immunodeficiency syndrome (AIDS)-associated retrovirus, *Proc Natl Acad Sci USA* 82:4539-4543, 1985.

68. Folks T et al.: Susceptibility of normal human lymphocytes to infection with HTLV-III/LAV, *J Immunol* 136:4049-4053, 1986.

69. Folks TM et al.: Infection and replication of HIV-1 in purified progenitor cells of normal human bone marrow, *Science* 242:919-922, 1988.

70. Folks TM et al.: Tumor necrosis factor-alpha induces the expression of the human immunodeficiency virus from a chronically infected T cell clone, *Proc Natl Acad Sci USA* 86:2365-2368, 1989.

71. Forster DJ et al.: Rapidly progressive outer retinal necrosis in the acquired immunodeficiency syndrome, *Am J Ophthalmol* 110:341-348, 1990.

72. Foster RE et al.: Presumed *Pneumocystis carinii* choroiditis: unifocal presentatin, regression with intravenous pentamidine, and choroiditis recurrence, *Ophthalmology* 98:1360, 1991.

73. Fox CH et al.: Lymphoid germinal centers are reservoirs of human immunodeficiency virus type 1 RNA, *J Infect Dis* 164:1051-1057, 1991.

74. Freeman WR, Chen A, Henderly DE et al.: Prevalence and significance of acquired immunodeficiency syndrome-related retinal microvasculopathy, *Am J Ophthalmol* 107:229-335, 1989.

75. Freeman WR, Gross JG, Labelle J et al.: *Pneumocystis carinii* choroidopathy: a new clinical entity, *Arch Ophthalmol* 107:863-867, 1989.

76. Freeman WR, Lerner CW, Mines JA et al.: A prospective study of the ophthalmologic findings in the acquired immune deficiency syndrome, *Am J Ophthalmol* 97:133-142, 1984.

77. Freeman WR et al.: Prevalence, pathophysiology, and treatment of rhegmatogenous retinal detachment in treated cytomegalovirus retinitis, *Am J Ophthalmol* 103:527-536, 1987.

78. Freeman WR et al.: Surgical repair of rhegmatogenous retinal detachment in immunosuppressed patients with cytomegalovirus retinitis, *Ophthalmology* 99:466-474, 1992.

79. Friedberg DN, Stenson SM, Orenstein JM et al.: Microsporidial keratoconjunctivitis in acquired immunodeficiency syndrome, *Arch Ophthalmol* 108:504-508, 1990.

80. Fujikawa LS, Schwartz LK, Rosenbaum EH et al.: Acquired immune deficiency syndrome associated with Burkitt's lymphoma presenting with ocular findings, *Ophthalmology* 90(suppl):50, 1983 (abstract).

81. Gallant JE et al.: Incidence and natural history of cytomegalovirus disease in patients with advanced human immunodeficiency virus disease treated with zidovudine, *J Infect Dis* 166:1223-1227, 1992.

82. Gartner S et al.: The role of mononuclear phagocytes in HTLV-III/LAV infection, *Science* 233:215-219, 1986.

83. Gay D et al.: Functional interaction between human T-cell protein CD4 and the major histocompatibility complex HLA-DR antigen, *Nature* 328:626-629, 1987.

84. Gendelman HE et al.: Slow, persistent replication of lentiviruses: role of tissue macrophages and macrophage precursors in bone marrow, *Proc Natl Acad Sci USA* 82:7086-7090, 1985.

85. Gendelman HE et al.: Trans-activation of the human immunodeficiency virus long terminal repeat sequence by DNA viruses, *Proc Natl Acad Sci USA* 83:9759-9763, 1986.

86. Ghabrial R et al.: Radiation therapy of acquired immunodeficiency syndrome-related Kaposi's sarcoma of the eyelids and conjunctiva, *Arch Ophthalmol* 110:1423-1426, 1992.

87. Giorgi JV et al.: Early effects of HIV on CD4 lymphocytes in vivo, *J Immunol* 138:3725-3730, 1987.

88. Giraldo G, Beth E, Huang E: Kaposi's sarcoma and its relationship to cytomegalovirus. III. CMV, DNA and CMV early antigens in Kaposi's sarcoma, *Int J Cancer* 26:23-29, 1980.

89. Goedert JJ et al.: A prospective study of human immunodeficiency virus type 1 infection and the development of AIDS in subjects with hemophilia, *N Engl J Med* 321:141-148, 1989.

90. Gougeon ML et al.: Evidence for an engagement process towards apoptosis in lymphocytes of HIV-infected patients, *CR Acad Sci III* 312:529-537, 1991.

91. Graham NMH et al.: Effect of zidovudine and *Pneumocystis carinii* pneumonia prophylaxis on progression of HIV-1 infection to AIDS, *Lancet* 338:265-269, 1991.

92. Gross JG, Bozzette SA, Mathews WC et al.: Longitudinal study of cytomegalovirus retinitis in acquired immune deficiency syndrome, *Ophthalmology* 97:681-686, 1990.

93. Groux H et al.: Activation-induced death by apoptosis in CD4+ T cells from human immunodeficiency virus-infected asymptomatic individuals, *J Exp Med* 175:331-340, 1992.

94. Gupta S, Licorish K: Circulating immune complexes in AIDS, *N Engl J Med* 310:1530-1531, 1984.

95. Gupta S, Safai B: Deficient autologous mixed lymphocyte reaction in Kaposi's sarcoma associated with deficiency of Leu-3+ responder T cells, *J Clin Invest* 71:296-300, 1983.

96. Guyer DR, Jabs DA, Brant AM et al.: Regression of cytomegalovirus retinitis with zidovudine: a clinicopathologic correlation, *Arch Ophthalmol* 107:868-874, 1989.

97. Hamed LM, Schatz NJ, Galetta SL: Brainstem ocular motility defects in AIDS, *Am J Ophthalmol* 106:437-442, 1988.

98. Hardy WD et al.: A controlled trial of trimethoprimsulfamethoxazole or aerosolized pentamidine for secondary prophylaxis of *Pneumocystis carinii* pneumonia in patients with the acquired immunodeficiency syndrome, *N Engl J Med* 327:1842-1848, 1992.

99. Harwood AR et al.: Kaposi's sarcoma in recipients of renal transplants, *Am J Med* 67:759-765, 1979.

100. Haverkos HW et al.: Assessment of therapy for *Pneumocystis carinii* pneumonia: PCP therapy project group, *Am J Med* 76:508, 1984.

101. Haverkos HW et al.: The changing incidence of Kaposi's sarcoma among patients with AIDS, *J Am Acad Dermatol* 22:6(Pt 2)1250-1253, 1990.

102. Heinemann MH: Long-term intravitreal ganciclovir therapy for cytomegalovirus retinopathy, *Arch Ophthalmol* 107:1767-1772, 1989.

103. Henderly DE, Freeman WR, Causey DM et al.: Cytomegalovirus retinitis and response to therapy with ganciclovir, *Ophthalmology* 94:425-434, 1987.

104. Henderly DE, Freeman WR, Smith RE et al.: Cytomegalovirus retinitis as the initial manifestation of the acquired immune deficiency syndrome, *Am J Ophthalmol* 103:316-320, 1987.

105. Ho DD, Rota TR, Hirsch MS: Infection of monocyte/macrophages by human T lymphotropic virus type III, *J Clin Invest* 77:1712-1715, 1986.

106. Ho DD, Rota TR, Schooley RT et al.: Isolation of HTLV-III from cerebrospinal fluid and neural tissues of patients with neurologic syndromes related to the acquired immunodeficiency syndrome, *N Engl J Med* 313:1493-1497, 1985.

107. Ho DD et al.: Pathogenesis of infection with human immunodeficiency virus, *N Engl J Med* 317:278-286, 1987.

108. Hoechster H et al.: Toxicity of combined ganciclovir and zidovudine for cytomegalovirus disease associated with AIDS, *Ann Intern Med* 113:111-117, 1990.

109. Holland GN, Engstrom RE, Glasgow BJ et al.: Ocular toxoplasmosis in patients with the acquired immunodeficiency syndrome, *Am J Ophthalmol* 106:653-667, 1988.

110. Holland GN, Gottlieb MS, Yee RD et al.: Ocular disorders associated with a new severe acquired cellular immunodeficiency syndrome, *Am J Ophthalmol* 93:393-402, 1982.

111. Holland GN, McArthur LJ, Foos RY: Choroidal pneumocystosis, *Arch Ophthalmol* 109:1454, 1991.

112. Holland GN, Pepose JS, Pettit JH et al.: Acquired immune deficiency syndrome: ocular manifestations, *Ophthalmology* 90:859-873, 1983.

113. Holland GN, Shuler JD: Progression rates of cytomegalovirus retinopathy in ganciclovir-treated and untreated patients, *Arch Ophthalmol* 110:1435-1442, 1992.

114. Holland GN, Sidikaro Y, Kreiger AE et al.: Treatment of cytomegalovirus retinopathy with ganciclovir, *Ophthalmology* 94:815-823, 1987.

115. Holland GN, Sison RF, Jatulis DE et al.: Survival of patients with acquired immune deficiency syndrome after development of cytomegalovirus retinopathy, *Ophthalmology* 97:204-211, 1990.

116. Holland GN et al.: A controlled retrospective study of ganciclovir treatment for cytomegalovirus retinopathy: use of a standardized system for the assessment of disease outcome, *Arch Ophthalmol* 107:1759-1766, 1989.

117. Hoover DR et al.: Clinical manifestations of AIDS in the era of *Pneumocystis* prophylaxis, *N Engl J Med* 329:1922-1926, 1993.

118. Hoxie JA et al.: Alterations in T4 (CD4) proteins and mRNA synthesis in cells infected with HIV, *Science* 234:1123-1227, 1986.

119. Hoy JF, Lewis DE, Miller GG: Functional versus phenotypic analysis of T cells in subjects seropositive for the human immunodeficiency virus: a prospective study of in vitro responses to *Cryptococcus neoformans*, *J Infect Dis* 158:1071-1078, 1988.

120. Hughes WT: *Pneumocystis carinii*: taxing taxonomy, *Eur J Epidemiol* 5:265-269, 1989.

121. Humphry RC, Parkin JM, Marsh RJ: The ophthalmological features of AIDS and AIDS related disorders, *Trans Am Ophthalmol Soc* 105:505-509, 1986.

122. Jabs DA, Enger C, Bartlett JG: Cytomegalovirus retinitis and acquired immunodeficiency syndrome, *Arch Ophthalmol* 107:75-80, 1989.

123. Jabs DA, Green WR, Fox R et al.: Ocular manifestations of acquired immune deficiency syndrome, *Ophthalmology* 96:1092-1099, 1989.

124. Jabs DA, Newman C, de Bustros S et al.: Treatment of cytomegalovirus retinitis with ganciclovir, *Ophthalmology* 94:824-830, 1987.

125. Jabs DA, Schachat AP, Liss R et al.: Presumed varicella zoster retinitis in immunocompromised patients, *Retina* 7:9-13, 1987.

126. Jabs DA et al.: Retinal detachments in patients with cytomegalovirus retinitis, *Arch Ophthalmol* 109:794-799, 1991.

127. Jacobson MA, O'Donnell JJ, Brodie HR et al.: Randomized prospective trial of ganciclovir maintenance therapy for cytomegalovirus retinitis, *J Med Virol* 25:339-349, 1988.

128. Jacobson MA, O'Donnell JJ, Mills J: Foscarnet treatment of cytomegalovirus retinitis in patients with the acquired immunodeficiency syndrome, *Antimicrob Agents Chemother* 736-741, 1989.

129. Jacobson MA, O'Donnell JJ, Porteous D et al.: Retinal and gastrointestinal disease due to cytomegalovirus in patients with the acquired immune deficiency syndrome: prevalence, natural history, and response to ganciclovir therapy, *QJM* 67:473-486, 1988.

130. Johnston WH et al.: Recurrence of presumed varicella-zoster virus retinopathy in patients with acquired immunodeficiency syndrome, *Am J Ophthalmol* 116:42-50, 1993.

131. Kahn JO et al.: A controlled trial comparing continued zidovudine with didanosine in human immunodeficiency virus infection, *N Engl J Med* 327:581-587, 1992.

132. Kales CP et al.: Early predictors of in-hospital mortality for *Pneumocystis carinii* pneumonia in acquired immunodeficiency syndrome, *Arch Intern Med* 147:1413-1417, 1987.

133. Kehrl JH et al.: Lymphokine production by B cells from normal and HIV-infected individuals, *Ann NY Acad Sci* 651:220-227, 1992.

134. Kestelyn P, Lepage P, Perre PVD: Perivasculitis of the retinal vessels as an important sign in children with AIDS-related complex, *Am J Ophthalmol* 100:614-615, 1985.

135. Kestelyn P, Stevens AM, Bakkers E et al.: Severe herpes zoster ophthalmicus in young African adults: a marker for HTLV-III seropositivity, *Br J Ophthalmol* 71:806-809, 1987.

136. Kestelyn P, Van de Perre P, Rouvroy D et al.: A prospective study of the ophthalmologic findings in the acquired immune deficiency syndrome in Africa, *Am J Ophthalmol* 100:230-238, 1985.

137. Kestelyn P et al.: Ophthalmic manifestations of infections with *Cryptococcus neoformans* in patients with the acquired immunodeficiency syndrome, *Am J Ophthalmol* 116:721-727, 1993.

138. Klatzmann D, Gluckman JC: HIV infection: facts and hypotheses, *Immunol Today* 7:291-296, 1986.

139. Klatzmann D et al.: T-lymphocyte T4 molecule behaves as the receptor for human retrovirus LAV, *Nature* 312:767-768, 1984.

140. Koenig S, Gendelman HE, Orenstein JM et al.: Detection of AIDS virus in macrophages in brain tissue from AIDS patients with encephalopathy, *Science* 233:1089-1093, 1986.

141. Koga Y et al.: High levels of heterodisperse RNAs accumulate in T cells infected with human immunodeficiency virus and in normal thymocytes, *Proc Natl Acad Sci USA* 85:4521-4525, 1988.

142. Kohn SR: Molluscum contagiosum in patients with acquired immune deficiency syndrome, *Arch Ophthalmol* 105:458, 1987.

143. Koser MW, Jampol LM, MacDonell K: Treatment of *Pneumocystis carinii* choroidopathy, *Arch Ophthalmol* 108:1214, 1990.

144. Koyanagi Y et al.: Dual infection of the central nervous system by AIDS viruses with distinct cellular tropisms, *Science* 236:819-822, 1987.

145. Kuppermann BD et al.: Correlation between CD4+ counts and prevalence of cytomegalovirus retinitis and human immunodeficiency virus-related noninfectious retinal vasculopathy in patients with acquired immunodeficiency syndrome, *Am J Ophthalmol* 115:575-582, 1993.

146. Kwok S, O'Donnell JJ, Wood IS: Retinal cotton-wood spots in a patient with *Pneumocystis carinii* infection, *N Engl J Med* 307:185, 1982.

147. LaHoang P, Girard B, Robinet TM et al.: Foscarnet in the treatment of cytomegalovirus retinitis in acquired immune deficiency syndrome, *Ophthalmology* 96:864-865, 1989.

148. Lamarre D et al.: The MHC-binding and gp120-binding functions of CD4 are separable, *Science* 245:745-746, 1989.

149. Lane HC, Masur H, Edgar LC et al.: Abnormalities of B-cell activation and immunoregulation in patients with the acquired immunodeficiency syndrome, *N Engl J Med* 309:453-458, 1983.

150. Lane HC et al.: Qualitative analysis of immune function in patients with the acquired immunodeficiency syndrome: evidence for a selective defect in soluble antigen recognition, *N Engl J Med* 313:79-84, 1985.

151. Laskin OL, Cederberg DM, Mills J et al.: Ganciclovir for the treatment and suppression of serious infections caused by cytomegalovirus, *Am J Med* 83:201, 1987.

152. Laurent-Crawford AG et al.: The cytopathic effect of HIV is associated with apoptosis, *Virology* 185:825-839, 1991.

153. Leonard R et al.: Cytopathic effect of human immunodeficiency virus in T4 cells is linked to the last stage of virus infection, *Proc Natl Acad Sci USA* 85:3570-3574, 1988.

154. Levy JA et al.: AIDS-associated retroviruses (ARV) can productively infect other cells besides human T helper cells, *Virology* 147:441-448, 1985.

155. Lifson AR, Rutherford GW, Jaffe HW: The natural history of human immunodeficiency virus infection, *J Infect Dis* 158:1360-1367, 1988.

156. Lo SC et al.: Enhancement of HIV-1 cytocidal effects in CD4+ lymphocytes by the AIDS-associated mycoplasma, *Science* 251:1074-1076, 1991.

157. Longini IMJ et al.: The dynamics of CD4+ T-lymphocyte decline in HIV-infected individuals; a Markov modeling approach, *J Acquir Immune Defic Syndr* 4:1141-1147, 1991.

158. Lowder CY, Meisler DM, McMahon JT et al.: Microsporidia infection of the cornea in a man seropositive for human immunodeficiency virus, *Am J Ophthalmol* 109:242-244, 1990.

159. Luciw PA et al.: Molecular cloning of AIDS-associated retrovirus, *Nature* 312:760-763, 1984.

160. Macher A, Rodriguex MM, Kaplan W et al.: Disseminated bilateral chorioretinitis due to *Histoplasma capsulatum* in a patient with the acquired immunodeficiency syndrome, *Ophthalmology* 92:1159-1164, 1985.

161. Maddon PI et al.: HIV infection does not require endocytosis of its receptor, CD4, *Cell* 54:865-874, 1988.

162. Margolick JB et al.: Clonal analysis of T lymphocytes in the acquired immunodeficiency syndrome: evidence for an abnormality affecting individual helper and suppressor T cells, *J Clin Invest* 76:709-715, 1985.

163. Margolick JB et al.: Changes in T-lymphocyte subsets in intravenous drug users with HIV-1 infection, *JAMA* 267:631-636, 1992.

164. Margolis TP et al.: Varicella-zoster virus retinitis in patients with the acquired immunodeficiency syndrome, *Am J Ophthalmol* 112:119-131, 1991.

165. Martin MA et al.: A comparison of the effectiveness of three regimens in the prevention of *Pneumocystis carinii* pneumonia in human immunodeficiency virus infected patients, *Arch Intern Med* 152:523-528, 1992.

166. McArthur J: Neurologic manifestations of AIDS, *Medicine* 66:407-437, 1987.

167. McConkey D et al.: Ca++-dependent killing of immature thymocytes by stimulation via CD3/RCR complex, *J Immunol* 143:1801-1806, 1989.

168. McDougal JS et al.: Cellular tropism of the human retrovirus HTLV-III/LAV 1. Role of T cell activation and expression of the T4 antigen, *J Immunol* 135:3151-3162, 1985.

169. McDougal JS et al.: Binding of HTLV-III/LAV to T4+ T cells by a complex of the 110K viral protein and the T4 molecule, *Science* 231:382-385, 1986.

170. McElrath MJ, Steinman RM, Cohn ZA: Latent HIV-1 infection in enriched populations of blood monocytes and T cells from seropositive patients, *J Clin Invest* 87:27-30, 1991.

171. McLeish WM, Pulido JS, Holland S et al.: The ocular manifestations of syphilis in the human immunodeficiency virus type 1-infected host, *Ophthalmology* 97:196-203, 1990.

172. Meng TC et al.: Combination therapy with zidovudine and dideoxycytidine in patients with advanced human immunodeficiency virus infection: a phase I/II study, *Ann Intern Med* 116:13-20, 1992.

173. Meredith TA, Aaberg TM, Reeser FH: Rhegmatogenous retinal detachment complicating cytomegalovirus retinitis, *Am J Ophthalmol* 87:793-796, 1979.

174. Meyaard L et al.: Programmed death of T cells in HIV-1 infection, *Science* 257:217-219, 1992.

175. Morinelli EN et al.: Infectious multifocal choroiditis in patients with acquired immunodeficiency syndrome, *Ophthalmology* 100:1014-1021, 1993.

176. Munoz A et al.: Acquired immunodeficiency syndrome (AIDS)-free time after human immunodeficiency virus type 1 (HIV-1) seroconversion in homosexual men, *Am J Epidemiol* 130:530-539, 1989.

177. Murray JF et al.: NHLBI workshop summary: pulmonary complications of the acquired immunodeficiency syndrome, *Am Rev Resp Dis* 135:504-508, 1987.

178. Nabel G, Baltimore D: An inducible transcription factor activates expression of human immunodeficiency virus in T cells, *Nature* 326:711-713, 1987.

179. Nelson MR et al.: Treatment with corticosteroids—a risk factor for the development of clinical cytomegalovirus disease in AIDS, *AIDS* 7:375-378, 1993.

180. Newman NM, Mandel MR, Gullett J et al.: Clinical and histologic findings in opportunistic infections, *Arch Ophthalmol* 101:396-401, 1983.

181. Newsome DA, Green WR, Miller ED et al.: Microvascular aspects of acquired immune deficiency syndrome retinopathy, *Am J Ophthalmol* 98:590-601, 1984.

182. Nguyen N, Rimmer S, Katz B: Slowed saccades in the acquired immunodeficiency syndrome, *Am J Ophthalmol* 107:356-360, 1989.

183. Orellana J, Teich SA, Friedman AH et al.: Combined short- and long-term therapy for the treatment of cytomegalovirus retinitis using ganciclovir (BW B759U), *Ophthalmology* 94:831-838, 1987.

184. Orellana J et al.: Treatment of retinal detachments in patients with the acquired immune deficiency syndrome, *Ophthalmology* 98:939-943, 1991.

185. Palestine AG, Rodrigues MM, Macher AM et al.: Ophthalmic involvement in acquired immunodeficiency syndrome, *Ophthalmology* 91:1092-1099, 1984.

186. Palestine AG, Stevens G, Lane HC et al.: Treatment of cytomegalovirus retinitis with dihydroxy propoxymethyl guanine, *Am J Ophthalmol* 101:95-101, 1986.

187. Palestine AG et al.: A randomized, controlled trial of foscarnet in the treatment of cytomegalovirus retinitis in patients with AIDS, *Ann Intern Med* 115:665-673, 1991.

188. Pantaleo GP, Graziosi C, Fauci AS: The immunopathogenesis of human immunodeficiency virus infection, *N Engl J Med* 328:327-335, 1993.

189. Parke DW, Font RL: Diffuse toxoplasmic retinochoroiditis in a patient with AIDS, *Arch Ophthalmol* 104:571-575, 1986.

190. Parrish CM, O'Day DM, Hoyle TC: Spontaneous corneal ulcer as an ocular manifestation of AIDS, *Am J Ophthalmol* 104:302-303, 1987.

191. Passo MS, Rosenbaum JT: Ocular syphilis in patients with human immunodeficiency virus infection, *Am J Ophthalmol* 106:1-5, 1988.

192. Pauza CD, Galindo JE, Richman DD: Reinfection results in accumulation of unintegrated viral DNA in cytopathic and persistent human immunodeficiency virus type 1 infection of CEM cells, *J Exp Med* 172:1035-1042, 1990.

193. Pepose JS, Hilborne LH, Cancilla PA et al.: Concurrent herpes simplex and cytomegalovirus retinitis and encephalitis in the acquired immune deficiency syndrome (AIDS), *Ophthalmology* 91:1669-1677, 1984.

194. Pepose JS, Holland GN, Nestor MS et al.: Acquired immune deficiency syndrome: pathogenic mechanisms of ocular disease, *Ophthalmology* 92:472-484, 1985.

195. Pepose JS, Newman C, Bach MC et al.: Pathologic features of cytomegalovirus retinopathy after a treatment with the antiviral agent ganciclovir, *Ophthalmology* 94:414-424, 1987.

196. Pertel P et al.: Risk of developing cytomegalovirus retinitis in persons infected with the human immunodeficiency virus, *J Acquir Immune Defic Syndr* 5:1069-1974, 1992.

197. Poli G, Fauci AS: The effect of cytokines and pharmacologic agents on chronic HIV infection, *AIDS Res Hum Retroviruses* 8:191-197, 1992.

198. Poli G et al.: Interleukin 6 induces human immunodeficiency virus expression in monocytic cells alone and in synergy with tumor necrosis factor alpha by transcriptional and post-transcriptional mechanisms, *J Exp Med* 172:151-158, 1990.

199. Poli G et al.: Tumor necrosis factor alpha functions in an autocrine manner in the induction of human immunodeficiency virus expression, *Proc Natl Acad Sci USA* 87:782-785, 1990.

200. Pomerantz RJ, Kuritzkes R, Monte M et al.: Infection of the retina by human immunodeficiency virus type I, *N Engl J Med* 317:1643-1647, 1987.

201. Prince HE et al.: Defective monocyte function in acquired immune deficiency syndrome (AIDS): evidence from a monocyte-dependent T-cell proliferative system, *J Clin Immunol* 5:21-25, 1985.

202. Projections of the number of persons diagnosed with AIDS and the number of immunosuppressed HIV-infected persons—United States, 1992-1994, *MMWR* 41(No. RR-18):1-29, 1992.

203. Psallidopoulos MC et al.: Integrated proviral human immunodeficiency virus type 1 is present in CD4+ peripheral blood lymphocytes in healthy seropositive individuals, *J Virol* 63:4626-4632, 1989.

204. Quiceno JI et al.: Visual dysfunction without retinitis in patients with acquired immunodeficiency syndrome, *Am J Ophthalmol* 113:8-13, 1992.
205. Quinnan GV Jr et al.: Herpesvirus infections in the acquired immune deficiency syndrome, *JAMA* 252:72-77, 1984.
206. Rabson AB: The molecular biology of HIV infection. In Levy JA, editor: *AIDS: pathogenesis and treatment,* 231-256, New York, 1988, Marcel Dekker.
207. Rao NA, Zimmerman PL, Boyer D et al.: A clinical, histopathologic, and electron microscopic study of *Pneumocystis carinii* choroiditis, *Am J Ophthalmol* 107:218-228, 1989.
208. Regillo CD et al.: Repair of retinitis-related retinal detachments with silicone oil in patients with acquired immunodeficiency syndrome, *Am J Ophthalmol* 113:21-27, 1992.
209. Richman DD et al.: Effect of stage of disease and drug dose on zidovudine susceptibilities of isolates of human immunodeficiency virus, *J Acquir Immune Defic Syndr* 3:743-746, 1990.
210. Rieckmann P et al.: Activated B lymphocytes from human immunodeficiency virus-infected individuals induce virus expression in infected T cells and a promonocytic cell line, U1, *J Exp Med* 173:1-5, 1991.
211. Rosenberg PR, Uliss AE, Friedland GH et al.: Acquired immunodeficiency syndrome: ocular manifestations in ambulatory patients, *Ophthalmology* 90:874-878, 1983.
212. Rosenberg ZF, Fauci AS: Induction of expression of HIV in latently or chronically infected cells, *AIDS Res Hum Retroviruses* 5:1-4, 1989.
213. Rosenberg ZF, Fauci AS: Immunopathogenic mechanisms of HIV infection: cytokine induction of HIV expression, *Immunol Today* 11:176-180, 1990.
214. Rosenberg ZF, Fauci AS: Immunopathogenesis of HIV infection. In Quinn TC, editor: *Sexually transmitted diseases,* 165-200, New York, 1992, Raven Press.
215. Rosenblum L et al.: Completeness of AIDS case reporting, 1988: a multisite collaborative surveillance project, *Am J Public Health* 82:1,495-499, 1992.
216. Rouse RV, Ledbetter JA, Weissman IL: Mouse lymph node germinal centers contain a selected subset of T cells with the helper phenotype, *J Immunol* 128:2243-2246, 1982.
217. Safai B, Dias BM: Kaposi's sarcoma and cloacogenic carcinoma associated with AIDS. In Broder S, Merigan TC Jr, Bolognesi D, editors: *Textbook of AIDS medicine,* 401-414, Baltimore, 1994, Williams and Wilkins.
218. Salahuddin SZ et al.: Human T lymphotrophic virus type III infection of human alveolar macrophages, *Blood* 68:281-284, 1986.
219. Sanborn GE et al.: Sustained-release ganciclovir therapy for treatment of cytomegalovirus retinitis: use of an intravitreal device, *Arch Ophthalmol* 110:188-195, 1992.
220. Sandor EV, Millman A, Croxson S et al.: Herpes zoster ophthalmicus in patients at risk for the acquired immune deficiency syndrome (AIDS), *Am J Ophthalmol* 101:153-155, 1986.
221. Santos C, Parker J, Dawson C et al.: Bilateral fungal corneal ulcers in a patient with AIDS-related complex, *Am J Ophthalmol* 102:118-119, 1986.
222. Schneider MME et al.: A controlled trial of aerosolized pentamidine or trimethoprim-sulfamethoxazole as primary prophylaxis against *Pneumocystis carinii* pneumonia in patients with human immunodeficiency virus infection, *N Engl J Med* 327:1836-1841, 1992.
223. Schnittman SM, Lane HC, Higgins SE et al.: Direct polyclonal activation of human B lymphocytes by the acquired immune deficiency syndrome virus, *Science* 233:1084-1086, 1986.
224. Schnittman SM et al.: The reservoir for HIV-1 in human peripheral blood is a T cell that maintains expression of CD4, *Science* 245:305-308, 1989.
225. Schnittman SM et al.: Evidence for susceptibility of intrathymic T-cell precursors and their progeny carrying T-cell antigen receptor phenotypes TCR alpha beta + and TCR gamma delta + to human immunodeficiency virus infection: a mechanisms for CD4+ (T4) lymphocyte depletion, *Proc Natl Acad Sci USA* 87:7727-7731, 1990.
226. Schnittman SM et al.: Increasing viral burden in CD4+ T cells from patients with human immunodeficiency virus (HIV) infection reflects rapidly progressive immunosuppression and clinical disease, *Ann Intern Med* 113:438-443, 1990.
227. Schuman JS, Friedman AH: Retinal manifestations of the acquired immune deficiency syndrome (AIDS): cytomegalovirus, candida albicans, toxoplasmosis, and *Pneumocystis carinii, Trans Ophthalmol Soc UK* 103:177-190, 1983.
228. Schuman JS, Orellana J, Friedman AH et al.: Acquired immunodeficiency syndrome (AIDS), *Surv Ophthalmol* 31:384-410, 1987.
229. Selik RM, Chu SY, Buehler JW: HIV infection as leading cause of death among young adults in U.S. cities and states, *JAMA* 269:2991-2994, 1993.
230. Sellitti TP et al.: Association of herpes zoster ophthalmicus with acquired immunodeficiency syndrome and acute retinal necrosis, *Am J Ophthalmol* 116:297-301, 1993.
231. Shami MJ et al.: A multicenter study of *Pneumocystis* choroidopathy, *Am J Ophthalmol* 112:15-22, 1991.
232. Shaw GM, Harper ME, Hahn BH et al.: HTLV-III infection in brains of children and adults with AIDS encephalopathy, *Science* 227:177-182, 1985.
233. Shaw GM et al.: Molecular characterization of human T-cell leukemia (lymphotropic) virus type III in the acquired immune deficiency syndrome, *Science* 226:1165-1171, 1984.
234. Shearer GM et al.: A model for the selective loss of major histocompatibility complex self-restricted T cell immune responses during the development of acquired immune deficiency syndrome (AIDS), *J Immunol* 137:2514-2521, 1986.
235. Shuler JD et al.: Kaposi sarcoma of the conjunctiva and eyelids associated with the acquired immunodeficiency syndrome, *Arch Ophthalmol* 197:858-862, 1989.
236. Sidikaro Y et al.: Rhegmatogenous retinal detachments in patients with AIDS and necrotizing retinal infections, *Ophthalmology* 98:129-135, 1991.
237. Siekevitz M et al.: Activation of the HIV-1 LTR by T cell mitogens and the trans-activator protein of HTLV-I, *Science* 238:1575-1587, 1987.
238. Slavin ML, Mallin JE, Jacob HS: Isolated homonymous hemianopsia in the acquired immunodeficiency syndrome, *Am J Ophthalmol* 108:198-200, 1989.
239. Smith CA et al.: Antibodies to CD4/TCR complex induce death by apoptosis in immature T cells in thymic culture, *Nature* 337, 181-184, 1989.
240. Smith PD et al.: Monocyte function in the acquired immune deficiency syndrome: defective chemotaxis, *J Clin Invest* 74:2121-2128, 1984.
241. Smith TJ et al.: Intravitreal sustained-release ganciclovir, *Arch Ophthalmol* 110:255-258, 1992.
242. Sneed SR et al.: *Pneumocystis carinii* choroiditis in patients receiving inhaled pentamidine, *N Engl J Med* 322:936, 1990.
243. Sodroski J et al.: Role of the HTLV-III/LAV envelope in syncytium formation and cytopathicity, *Nature* 332:470-474, 1986.
244. Spear GT et al.: Analysis of lymphocytes, monocytes, and neutrophils from human immunodeficiency virus (HIV)-infected persons for HIV DNA, *J Infect Dis* 162:1239-1244, 1990.
245. Spiegel H et al.: Follicular dendritic cells are a major reservoir for human immunodeficiency virus type 1 in lymphoid tissues facilitating infection of CD4+ T-helper cells, *Am J Pathol* 140:15-22, 1992.
246. Stevenson M, Zhang XH, Volsky DJ: Downregulation of cell surface molecules during noncytopathic infection of T cells with human immunodeficiency virus, *J Virol* 61:3741-3748, 1987.
247. Stewart SJ, Fujimoto J, Levy R: Human T lymphocytes and monocytes bear the same Leu- 3(T4) antigen, *J Immunol* 136:3773-3778, 1986.
248. Stoumbos VD, Klein ML: Syphilitic retinitis in a patients with acquired immunodeficiency syndrome-related complex, *Am J Ophthalmol* 103:103-104, 1987.
249. Studies of Ocular Complications of AIDS Research Group, in collaboration with the AIDS Clinical Trials Group: Mortality in patients with the acquired immunodeficiency syndrome treated with either foscarnet or ganciclovir for cytomegalovirus retinitis, *N Engl J Med* 326:213-220, 1992.
250. Tange M, Klein EB, Kornfield H et al.: Cytomegalovirus isolation from healthy homosexual man, *JAMA* 252:1908-1910, 1984.
251. Teich SA: Conjunctival vascular changes in AIDS and AIDS-related complex, *Am J Ophthalmol* 103:332-333, 1987.

252. Tenhula WN et al.: Morphometric comparisons of optic nerve axon loss in acquired immunodeficiency syndrome, *Am J Ophthalmol* 113:14-20, 1992.
253. Terai C et al.: Apoptosis as a mechanism of cell death in culture T lymphoblasts acutely infected with HIV-1, *J Clin Invest* 87:1710-1715, 1991.
254. The Italian Seroconversion Study: Disease progression and early predictors of AIDS in HIV-seroconverted injecting drug users, *AIDS* 6:421-426, 1992.
255. Tindall B, Cooper DA: Primary HIV infection: host responses and intervention strategies, *AIDS* 5:1-14, 1991.
256. Tirard DV et al.: Diagnosis of toxoplasmosis in patients with AIDS by isolation of parasite from the blood, *N Engl J Med* 324:634, 1991.
257. Tong-Starksen SE, Luciw PA, Peterlin BM: Human immunodeficiency virus long terminal repeat responds to T-cell activation signals, *Proc Natl Acad Sci USA* 84:6845-6849, 1987.
258. Update: Acquired Immunodeficiency Syndrome—United States, 1992, *MMWR* 42(28):547, July 1993.
259. Update: Mortality attributable to HIV infection/AIDs among persons aged 25-44 years—United States, 1990 and 1991, *MMWR* 42(25):481-485, July 1993.
260. Ussery FM, Gibson SR, Conklin RH et al.: Intravitreal ganciclovir in the treatment of AIDS-associated cytomegalovirus retinitis, *Ophthalmology* 95:640-648, 1988.
261. Varmus H: Retroviruses, *Science* 240:1427-1435, 1988.
262. Volberding PA et al.: Zidovudine in asymptomatic human immunodeficiency virus infection: a controlled trial in persons with fewer than 500 CD4-positive cells per cubic millimeter, *N Engl J Med* 322:941-949, 1990.
263. Walmsley SL, Chew E, Read SE et al.: Treatment of cytomegalovirus retinitis with trisodium phosophonoformate hexahydrate (foscarnet), *J Infect Dis* 157:569-572, 1988.
264. Wiess A, Margo CE, Ledford DK et al.: Toxoplasmic retinochoroiditis as an initial manifestation of the acquired immune deficiency syndrome, *Am J Ophthalmol* 103:248-249, 1987.
265. Winward KE, Hamed LM, Glaser JS: The spectrum of optic nerve disease in human immunodeficiency virus infection, *Am J Ophthalmol* 107:373-380, 1989.
266. Wood GS: The immunohistology of lymph nodes in HIV infection: a review, *Prog AIDS Pathol* 2:25-32, 1990.
267. World Health Organization: AIDS—Global Data: the current global situation of the HIV/AIDS pandemic, *Wkly Epidemiol Rec* 68:9-11, January 1993.
268. World Health Organization: AIDS—Global Data: the current global situation of the HIV/AIDS pandemic, *Wkly Epidemiol Rec* 68:193-195, July 1993.
269. Yoffe B et al.: Fusion as a mediator of cytolysis in mixtures of uninfected CD4+ lymphocytes and cells infected by human immunodeficiency virus, *Proc Natl Acad Sci USA* 84:1429-1433, 1987.
270. Ypma-Wong MF, Fonzi WA, Sypherd PS: Fundus-specific translation elongation factor 3 gene present in *Pneumocystis carinii*, *Infect Immun* 60:4140-4145, 1992.
271. Yuille MAR, Hugunin M, John P et al.: HIV-1 infection abolishes CD4 biosynthesis but not CD4 mRNA, *J Acquir Immune Defic Syndr* 1:131-137, 1988.

IMMUNE-MEDIATED OCULAR DISEASES

23 Sjögren Syndrome

STEPHEN C. PFLUGFELDER, JOHN P. WHITCHER, TROY E. DANIELS

Sjögren syndrome or sicca syndrome describes the clinical conditions characterized by a combination of aqueous tear deficiency (also referred to as keratoconjunctivitis sicca) and dry mouth.

HISTORICAL BACKGROUND

Published case reports of patients with the combination of keratoconjunctivitis sicca (KCS) and dry mouth can be found in the literature as far back as 1888[122]; however, this syndrome is named after the Swedish ophthalmologist, Henrik Sjögren,[123] who authored a comprehensive monograph combining the clinical and pathologic findings of this condition into a single entity in 1933.

EPIDEMIOLOGY

A recent epidemiologic study performed in Sweden reported that the prevalence of Sjögren syndrome is approximately 0.4%.[82] A strong gender predilection exists for Sjögren syndrome, because 95% of the patients are women. Three clinical subsets of Sjögren syndrome are recognized: (1) patients who have systemic immune dysfunction but no defined connective tissue disease, (2) patients who lack evidence of systemic immune dysfunction or a defined connective tissue disease, and (3) patients who have a defined connective tissue disease (most commonly rheumatoid arthritis). The first two subsets are referred to as primary Sjögren syndrome, whereas the latter group is termed secondary Sjögren syndrome.[24] In all cases progressive lymphocytic infiltration of the lacrimal and salivary glands is accompanied by secretory dysfunction of these glands, resulting in severe (and occasionally disabling) ocular and oral dryness.

DIAGNOSIS

Sjögren syndrome is classically defined as the presence of at least two components of a clinical triad consisting of dry mouth, dry eyes, and autoimmune disease (usually rheumatoid arthritis).[46] Although a diagnosis of Sjögren syn-

drome is often considered in the differential diagnosis of patients complaining of dry mouth and dry eyes, these symptoms are highly subjective and are not specific for this disorder.[24,25] In 1986 there was an attempt to establish well-defined objective criteria for the diagnosis and classification of Sjögren syndrome. At the First International Seminar on Sjögren syndrome held in Copenhagen, four different sets of diagnostic criteria for Sjögren syndrome were presented.[142] All but one set of criteria required patient symptoms of dry mouth and/or dry eyes, and all proposed criteria included diagnostic tests to identify and grade the severity of the ocular and oral components. Serum autoantibody tests to screen for systemic immune dysfunction were also included in the California set of diagnostic criteria.

The most comprehensive diagnostic criteria for Sjögren syndrome are those proposed by Fox and associates[46] (see box): (1) clinical confirmation of KCS defined by an abnormally low Schirmer test and the presence of rose bengal or fluorescein staining, (2) objective evidence of decreased salivary gland flow, (3) proof of lymphocytic infiltration of the labial salivary glands, exhibited by a biopsy specimen containing at least four glandular lobules with an average of at least two foci of fifty or more lymphocytes per 4 mm^2 of tissue, and (4) verification of a systemic autoimmune process as manifested by the presence of serum autoantibodies [either antinuclear antibody, rheumatoid factor, or Sjögren syndrome-specific antibodies such as anti-Ro (SS-A) or anti-La (SS-B)]. Following Fox's criteria, a diagnosis of "definite Sjögren syndrome" can be made only when all four criteria are met. A diagnosis of "possible Sjögren syndrome" is made when only three of the four criteria are met. Although these criteria are admittedly much more stringent than those previously accepted, their use probably increases the likelihood of identifying patients with a similar cause for their sicca symptoms.

When considering the diagnosis of Sjögren syndrome in a patient with sicca symptoms, a complete history and physical examination are of utmost importance. Sjögren syn-

---

PROPOSED CRITERIA FOR THE DIAGNOSIS OF SJÖGREN SYNDROME[46]

1. Keratoconjunctivitis
   a. Decreased tear flow, using Schirmer test
   b. Rose bengal and/or fluorescein dye staining in characteristic pattern
2. Xerostomia
   a. Symptomatic xerostomia
   b. Decreased parotid flow rate
3. Lymphocytic infiltrate on labial salivary gland biopsy (focus score of at least 2 per 4 mm2)
4. Laboratory evidence of a systemic autoimmune disease
   a. Positive antinuclear antibody (titer $\geq$ 1 : 160), or
   b. Positive rheumatoid factor (titer $\geq$ 1 : 160), or
   c. Positive SS-A or SS-B antibody

---

drome is a multisystem disorder that may have a varied and complex clinical presentation and can often be diagnosed only by taking a careful history and asking pertinent questions. The diagnosis may then be confirmed by a series of tests to identify the oral, ocular, and systemic components of the disease.

DIAGNOSIS OF OCULAR COMPONENT

Diagnosis of the ocular component of Sjögren syndrome is usually made by (1) biomicroscopic examination of the ocular surface for signs of aqueous tear deficiency, (2) tests to quantitate aqueous tear production, and in some cases (3) cytologic evaluation of the conjunctival epithelium.

Slit Lamp Examination

Inspection of the Tear Meniscus. Normal tear production should result in a continuous, full, slightly concave tear meniscus, approximately 0.5 mm in width, between the eyelid margin and the inferior bulbar conjunctiva where the eyelid touches the globe. In subjects with aqueous tear deficiency, the meniscus is often reduced or absent and may contain debris or mucus.

Fluorescein Staining. Touching a dry fluorescein strip to the inferior bulbar conjunctiva (1) indicates the wetness of the ocular surface, (2) stains the tear film, allowing the tear meniscus to be more easily appreciated, and (3) provides useful information regarding the integrity of the ocular surface epithelium. Fluorescein stains a diseased epithelium that has increased permeability to fluorescein caused by disrupted intercellular junctions, as well as connective tissue in areas of denuded or absent epithelium.[33] In patients with KCS, punctate or blotchy corneal (and occasionally conjunctival) epithelial staining is often seen in the interpalpebral exposure zone, and the staining is typically most intense in the inferior cornea.

Rose Bengal Staining. Experimental evidence suggests that rose bengal dye stains epithelial cells lacking a protective mucin coating.[34] Mild to severe rose bengal staining of the corneal and conjunctival epithelia is normally observed in Sjögren syndrome and may result from pathologic alterations of the ocular surface epithelia (discussion follows). The staining pattern may vary from fine punctate staining of the conjunctiva in the interpalpebral area in mild clinical cases to coarse blotchy staining of the bulbar conjunctiva and inferior cornea in moderate clinical cases. In severe clinical cases there is usually diffuse corneal staining and also confluent staining of the bulbar conjunctiva in a "wedge-shaped" pattern within the interpalpebral area. Corneal filaments, which are frequently observed in Sjögren syndrome, also stain brilliantly with rose bengal.[124] A grading scale for quantitating rose bengal staining on the ocular surface has been proposed by van Bijsterveld.[139] Rose bengal is one of the most specific ocular diagnostic tests for Sjögren syndrome and should be used as a key clinical parameter in diagnosing and grading the severity of KCS in patients with Sjögren syndrome and in documenting the progression of this clinical disease.[106]

Tear Film Breakup Time (TBUT). The TBUT is measured after fluorescein has been instilled into the eye and before the lids and/or the tear film are manipulated.[74] To determine TBUT, the patient is instructed to blink and then hold the lids open as long as possible. The eye is then examined with the biomicroscope and blue light illumination, and a measurement is made of the time in seconds it takes for the first "dark spot" to appear in the precorneal tear film after blinking. In normal individuals the TBUT is usually 10 seconds or greater.[75] In patients with KCS the TBUT may be a few seconds or less. A TBUT of 10 seconds or less implies an unstable tear film; however, this may result from lipid, aqueous, and/or mucin[75] tear deficiencies[103a] and therefore is not specific for Sjögren syndrome.

Ocular Diagnostic Procedures

Schirmer Test. The Schirmer test is the most commonly employed, objective, clinical test used to quantify aqueous tear production. To perform a Schirmer test, a standardized strip of filter paper is placed over the temporal lower lid margin into the tear film to act as a wick to absorb tears by capillary action. The amount of wetting of the strip is measured in millimeters after 5 minutes. A strip placed against an unanesthetized normal eye (Schirmer I test) usually stimulates reflex tearing. As such, the Schirmer test measures both basal and reflex tearing. Approximately 70% of normal subjects without ocular irritation will have a Schirmer I value of 10 mm or more in 5 minutes,[139] although significant variability has been noted with repeated testing of the same eye.[14] Because of the variation in Schirmer I values, there is no uniform consensus regarding the normal lower limit of Schirmer test values. Schirmer I values in the range from 5 to 10 mm of strip wetting are suggestive of a mild aqueous tear deficiency, and readings between 10 to 15 mm must be carefully correlated with clinical findings and other tests before a diagnosis of aqueous tear deficiency can be made. Patients with severe aqueous tear deficiency, such as that characteristically found in Sjögren syndrome, almost uniformly have a Schirmer I test result of 5 mm or less in at least one eye. A Schirmer test may also be performed after instillation of topical anesthetic (basic secretion test). This test predominantly measures basal tear production, and values below 7 to 9 mm are frequently observed, even in normal individuals.[73] The Schirmer I test gives the most useful and reproducible information regarding aqueous tear production.[14] Nasal stimulation during a Schirmer I test to measure reflex tearing is a more specific diagnostic test for Sjögren syndrome than a Schirmer I test alone, because Sjögren syndrome patients lose their ability to reflex tear early in the course of the disease.[134]

Fluorescein Dilution Test. Evaluation of the clearance of fluorescein dye instilled into the preocular tear film is a clinically useful parameter for quantitating aqueous tear production.[93,151] Tear fluorescein concentrations can be accurately quantitated by a fluorophotometer,[93] however, this instrument is expensive and not readily available. A less accurate, but more practical, method of quantitating tear fluorescein concentration is by visually inspecting fluorescein staining of Schirmer test strips placed into the tear lake at various times after instillation of fluorescein.[97] In patients with normal tear production and drainage, fluorescein cannot be detected in the tear film 20 minutes after instillation of 5 μl of a 1% fluorescein solution into the inferior conjunctival cul-de-sac (unpublished data).[103a] In Sjögren syndrome patients, a marked delay in fluorescein clearance is the result of reduced aqueous tear production, and fluorescein is often detected on the filter paper strip 30 minutes after instillation.[97]

Tear Lysozyme and Lactoferrin Tests. Both lysozyme and lactoferrin are antimicrobial proteins produced by lacrimal gland secretory acini and secreted into the tears. Patients with aqueous tear deficiency have reduced concentrations of both of these tear proteins. Lacrimal gland secretory function can be evaluated by quantitatively measuring the concentration of these proteins in the tears. Tear specimens for lysozyme determination may be collected on filter paper strips and placed on agar media that has been inoculated with a suspension of *Micrococcus lysodeikticus.* A zone of inhibition indicates the presence of lysozyme. The concentration of tear lysozyme can also be quantitated by measuring the rate at which a standardized suspension of *M. lysodeikticus* is lysed, producing a decrease in the optical density of the suspension.[111] Tear lactoferrin can be measured using a commercially available immunoassay (Lactoplate®, MacKeen Consultants, Bethesda, Md.). Studies comparing the lactoferrin assay with rose bengal staining in the diagnosis of KCS indicate that both tests have a specificity of 90% or greater.[57]

Tear Osmolarity Determination. Tear fluid has an osmolarity of 302 ± 6.3 mOsm/L in normal individuals.[53] Gilbard[54] reported that in patients with KCS, the tear film osmolarity increases to between 330 and 340 mOsm/L because of reduced tear flow and increased tear evaporation. Gilbard suggested that tear osmolarity determination may be superior to Schirmer testing, TBUT, and rose bengal staining for diagnosing KCS. Lucca and associates[81] noted that in patients with a known diagnosis of Sjögren syndrome, an elevated tear osmolarity has a 90% sensitivity and a 95% specificity. Unfortunately, the high cost and limited availability of the microosmolmeter required to measure tear osmolarity has limited the clinical utility of this technique.

Conjunctival Impression Cytology. Impression cytology is a simple and noninvasive technique to evaluate pathologic changes of the ocular surface epithelium. Superficial epithelial cells are obtained by placing nitrocellulose acetate filter papers against the conjunctiva. One study evaluated conjunctival impression cytology obtained from four groups of subjects: Sjögren syndrome, aqueous tear deficiency without Sjögren syndrome, seborrheic blepharitis, and normal controls. The following features were observed with a significantly greater frequency in cytology specimens from the eyes of Sjögren syndrome patients than cytology specimens from the eyes of the other groups: squamous metaplasia (enlarged cytoplasmic/nuclear ratio) of the temporal and inferior bulbar conjunctiva, extensive goblet cell loss of the temporal bulbar conjunctiva, mucous aggregates on the conjunctival epithelia, and inflammatory cells in the inferior tarsal conjunctiva.[98] Aguilar[3] has also documented moderate to severe conjunctival epithelial squamous metaplasia in 94% of conjunctival impression cytology specimens taken from patients with clinical and laboratory evidence of Sjögren syndrome.

Conjunctival Scrapings. Giemsa-stained conjunctival scrapings from patients with Sjögren syndrome also show characteristic cytologic changes of goblet cell loss, metaplastic epithelial cells, and occasional keratinized cells. Cellular debris plus mucus strands and filaments may also be observed.

Oral Diagnostic Tests

All of the current diagnostic criteria for Sjögren syndrome include a salivary component. Although the salivary component of Sjögren syndrome was originally described as "xerostomia,"[11] neither symptoms nor signs of dry mouth are useful as diagnostic criteria for Sjögren syndrome. Symptoms of dry mouth are subjective, are common to many conditions,[25] and correlate poorly with changes in salivary flow rate.[38] For these reasons, labial salivary gland biopsy is recommended for diagnosing the oral component

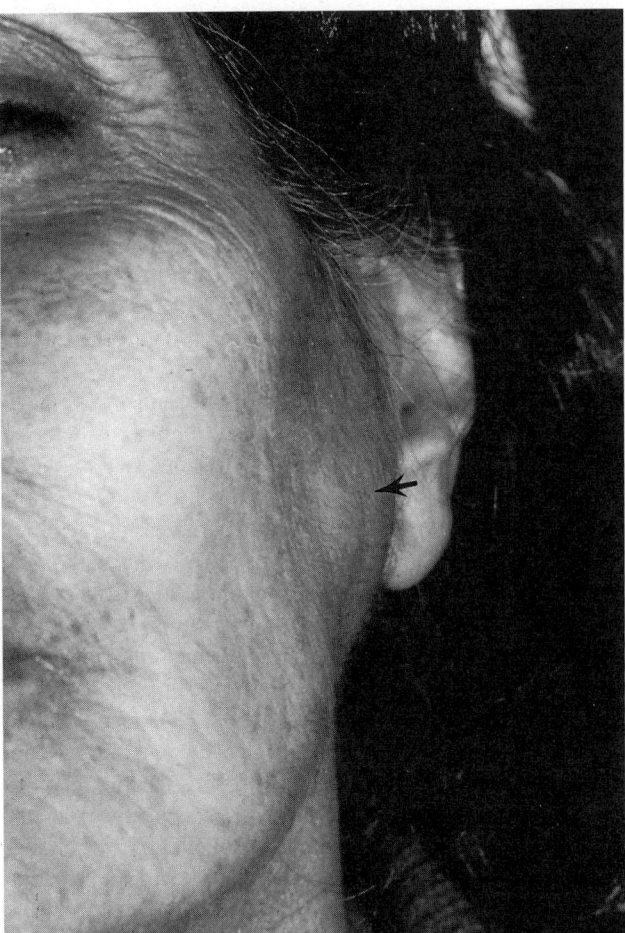

Fig. 23-1. Parotid gland enlargement *(arrow)* in 68-year-old Sjögren syndrome patient.

of Sjögren syndrome. Also, this diagnostic tool is the most disease-specific means to confirm or rule out the salivary component of Sjögren syndrome.* As outlined in the following discussion, the characteristic appearance of minor salivary glands in Sjögren syndrome is focal lymphocytic infiltration. After nonspecific chronic sialadenitis has been ruled out, the amount of focal infiltration is usually assessed with a focus score to provide a diagnostic threshold and severity assessment. Foci containing 50 or more lymphocytes are counted, and focus scores greater than 1 focus/ 4 mm² support the diagnosis of the salivary component of Sjögren syndrome. A horizontal incision through the lower labial mucosa yielding five to ten minor glands separated from their surrounding connective tissue will provide an adequate specimen for diagnosis and severity assessment. Labial salivary gland morbidity is minimal when the glands are dissected free of neural and muscular tissues under direct visualization.[20]

---

*References 7, 20, 22, 46, 121, 147.

Biopsy of the parotid gland is not indicated for routine diagnostic evaluation. Even though the procedure has little morbidity when current surgical techniques are used,[85] assessment of parotid tissue does not yield better diagnostic accuracy than minor gland biopsy and, in some cases, gives false negative results.[147] In cases of persistent parotid enlargement, biopsy of the affected gland should be considered (Fig. 23-1). Although these cases usually reveal a benign lymphoepithelial lesion, a high index of suspicion of malignant lymphoma should be maintained in this patient population.[65] Persistently enlarged glands with continually increasing size should be followed closely, and changes in the nature of the enlarged region (from a soft, diffuse swelling to a hard, nodular density) may indicate malignant transformation. The appearance of a serum monoclonal gamma globulin spike in a patient with persistent gland enlargement should prompt major gland biopsy. Immunophenotyping of biopsy tissue may be helpful in distinguishing benign from malignant lesions.[42]

DIAGNOSIS—SYSTEMIC TESTS

Patients with dry mouth and dry eyes should be evaluated for the presence of serum autoantibodies that are commonly detected in Sjögren syndrome [antinuclear antibodies, rheumatoid factor (RF), and anti-Ro (SS-A) and anti-La (SS-B)], because autoantibody positivity greatly supports a diagnosis of Sjögren syndrome. A recent case-control study investigating immunologic dysfunction in patients with aqueous tear deficiency stated that the presence of serum autoantibodies correlated with the severity of aqueous tear deficiency.[97] Antinuclear antibodies (ANA) were the most frequently detected autoantibodies in aqueous tear-deficient patients and were observed in 80% of patients with severe aqueous tear deficiency.[97] Positive RF and SS-A were detected in 65% and 30%, respectively, of severe aqueous tear deficiency patients. In patients diagnosed with Sjögren syndrome using the criteria proposed by Fox and associates[46] at the Bascom Palmer Eye Institute over the past decade, the prevalence of serum autoantibodies was: ANA 63%, RF 76%, SS-A 67%, and SS-B 47%. The difference in reported prevalence of autoantibodies in Sjögren syndrome patients probably reflects differences in diagnostic criteria, sensitivity of detection techniques, and the antigen substrate used.

CLINICAL FEATURES

Sjögren syndrome occurs most commonly in postmenopausal women[76,84]; however, the average age of patients with primary Sjögren syndrome who were diagnosed by the Cornea/External Disease service of the Bascom Palmer Eye Institute from 1984 to 1994 is 43—with the age of onset ranging from 22 to 70. Sjögren syndrome symptoms may have an acute or insidious onset. Patients usually have predominantly oral or ocular complaints, although a careful history will usually reveal that the patient is experiencing both oral and ocular sicca symptoms. Occasionally patients will experience simultaneous onset of moderate to severe oral and ocular complaints.

Ocular

Individuals with the ocular manifestations of Sjögren syndrome generally report severe and occasionally disabling eye irritation, especially while reading. The majority of patients complain of a foreign body sensation that is usually most pronounced in the late afternoon or evening. The foreign body sensation is exacerbated by moving the eyes from side to side with the eyelids closed and by locating in dry environments such as airplanes. Ocular foreign body sensation worsens as the day progresses. This symptom is helpful in differentiating the symptoms from those produced by meibomian gland dysfunction, a condition that typically causes the greatest ocular irritation on awaking in the morning. When questioned about their ability to tear even with marked mechanical, chemical, or psychologic stimulation, most Sjögren syndrome patients will reveal that they cannot produce tears. Patients with Sjögren syndrome often complain of excessive mucous secretion. The lids may be stuck together on awaking in the morning, but more commonly, strands of mucus collect in the fornices, irritating the patient to the point that he constantly pulls them from the eye. Sjögren syndrome patients also frequently complain of burning, itching, redness, photophobia, and intermittent blurring of vision. The external ocular manifestations of Sjögren syndrome are occasionally misdiagnosed and treated as bacterial conjunctivitis. Table 23-1 summarizes the ocular symptoms of patients with KCS that is caused by Sjögren syndrome.

Individuals with KCS attributable to Sjögren syndrome exhibit a number of characteristic clinical ocular signs. One of the most obvious signs that can be appreciated on routine slit lamp examination is the absence or dimunition of the

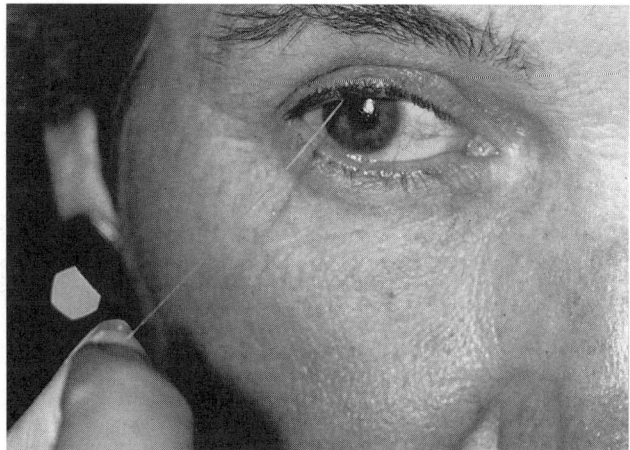

Fig. 23-2. Tenacious mucous strand being pulled from an eye of a Sjögren syndrome patient.

inferior tear meniscus. The tear meniscus should be examined prior to instillation of drops into the conjunctival sac and may be more easily visualized by staining the preocular tear film with a dry fluorescein strip. Patients with KCS also frequently have long strands of rubbery tenacious mucus in the inferior fornix and the superior cul-de-sac. These strands can be readily appreciated by everting the upper lid. The abnormal mucus appears to be polymerized into long filaments that can frequently be teased out to several centimeters in length (Fig. 23-2). In some cases there is also hyperemia of the conjunctiva, and both the inferior forniceal and the tarsal conjunctiva may appear edematous, infiltrated, and thrown into folds. With intense infiltration there may be a follicular reaction of the conjunctiva (Fig. 23-3).

The most clinically evident ocular surface changes in Sjögren syndrome involve the cornea and the bulbar conjunctiva in the interpalpebral (or exposure) zone. The precorneal tear film looks viscous and may contain mucous

TABLE 23-1 OCULAR SYMPTOMS OF KERATOCONJUNCTIVITIS SICCA IN 50 PATIENTS WITH SJÖGREN SYNDROME

Symptoms	Percent
Foreign body sensation	68
Excessive secretion	66
Burning	62
Redness	62
Photophobia	58
Blurred vision	56
Itching	52
Pain	52
Inability to tear	44

Whitcher JP: Clinical diagnosis of the dry eye, *Int Ophthalmol Clin* 27:7-24, 1987.

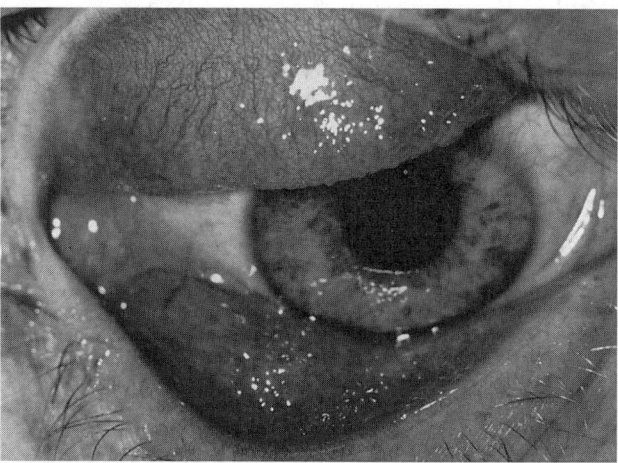

Fig. 23-3. Follicular reaction on inferior and superior tarsal conjunctiva.

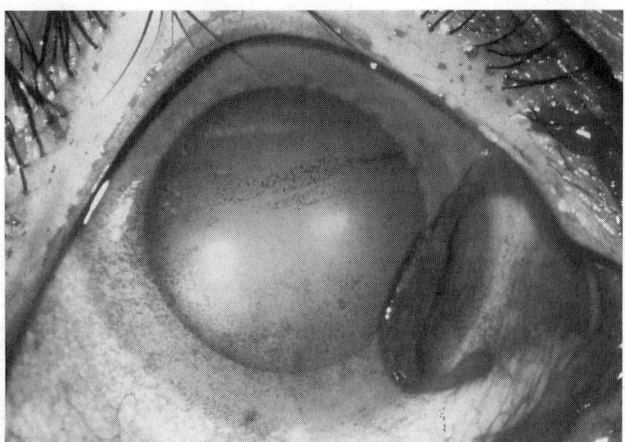

Fig. 23-4. Ocular surface mucous strands and characteristic exposure zone corneal and conjunctival rose bengal staining.

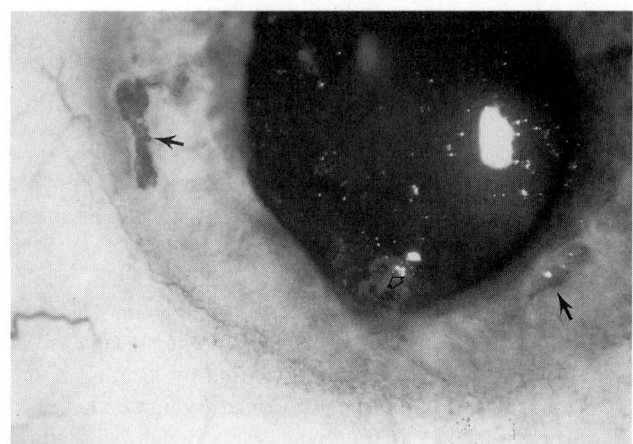

Fig. 23-5. Corneal filaments *(arrows)* are readily stained with rose bengal dye in a case of Sjögren syndrome.

strands and particulate debris (Fig. 23-4). With fluorescein staining, the tear film appears to be very thin and breaks up rapidly after blinking. Small, round, grayish depressions in the corneal epithelium (punctate epithelial erosions or PEE) are frequently observed with the biomicroscope. PEE are more easily visualized after staining with fluorescein or rose bengal dyes. The density of the PEE is usually greatest on the inferior cornea, where occasionally they become confluent (Fig. 23-4). In severe cases, diffuse corneal PEE may be noted. In addition to punctate staining, blotchy corneal epithelial fluorescein staining (presumably the result of altered epithelial fluorescein permeability) is also frequently observed. One of the most striking clinical findings in patients with KCS is the presence of corneal filaments. Filaments can occur singly but are usually numerous. Filaments are usually located on the inferior rather than than the superior cornea, and they stain brilliantly with rose bengal dye (Fig. 23-5). Occasionally, mucus adheres to the cornea in a cobweblike pattern that may markedly decrease vision (Fig. 23-6).

Pathologic changes of the conjunctiva in Sjögren syndrome are most easily appreciated by rose bengal dye staining. Typically, "wedge-shaped" staining of the bulbar conjunctiva in the exposure zone is observed with the base of the wedge adjacent to the limbus. In mild cases, punctate rose bengal staining is usually noted on the nasal bulbar conjunctiva. In moderate or severe cases, punctate, patchy, or confluent rose bengal staining may be observed on both the nasal and temporal exposure zone bulbar conjunctiva in addition to the cornea (Fig. 23-4). Rose bengal staining of the bulbar conjunctiva can be seen with greater contrast by using the green filter on the slit lamp for illumination.

Other corneal manifestations of Sjögren syndrome may occasionally be observed. Punctate epithelial keratitis and subepithelial infiltrates resembling the lesions in adenovirus ocular infection are occasionally seen. The most severe and sight-threatening corneal complication associated with this condition is corneal ulceration. Sterile corneal ulcers in primary Sjögren syndrome normally have the following characteristics: they are circular or oval, they measure less than 3 mm in diameter, they are located in the central or paracentral cornea (Fig. 23-7), and they resemble paracentral sterile corneal ulcers associated with rheumatoid arthritis.[68] Occasionally, the corneal stroma in the area of ulceration may rapidly thin and perforate. Sjögren syndrome is a significant risk factor for microbial keratitis.[90] These microbial ulcers may result from increased susceptibility of the ocular surface to infection caused by reduced tear concentrations of antimicrobial tear proteins as well as alterations in the protective tear coating and surface epithelium. Corneal ulcers in Sjögren syndrome are most often caused by *Staphylococcus* sp. and *Streptococcus* species.[94,100] Sterile or infectious corneal ulceration in Sjögren syndrome can occasionally recur, develop bilaterally, and progress to blindness or enucleation.[94,100]

Oral

The principal oral symptom of Sjögren syndrome is continuous oral dryness with a broad range of severity. Not all patients complain of dryness; specifically, many describe difficulty in swallowing food, problems in wearing complete dentures, changes in their sense of taste, increase in the incidence of dental caries, chronic burning symptoms from the oral mucosa, intolerance to acidic or spicy foods, or the inability to eat dry food or to speak continuously for more than a few minutes.[19] Chronic symptoms of dry mouth may be caused by a variety of other conditions. The oral symptoms of Sjögren syndrome usually have an insidious onset and progress gradually. Dysphagia in Sjögren syndrome results from alteration of oral swallowing patterns by a prolongation of the oral phase of swallowing with and without water.[13] Nutrition may be compromised and sleep may be

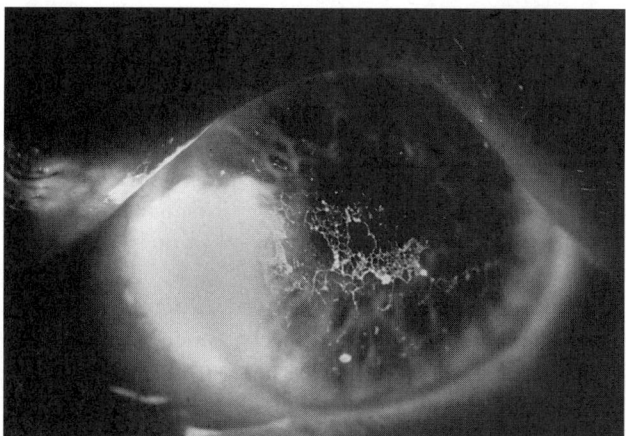

Fig. 23-6. Cobweblike coating of corneal surface with mucus in severe Sjögren syndrome.

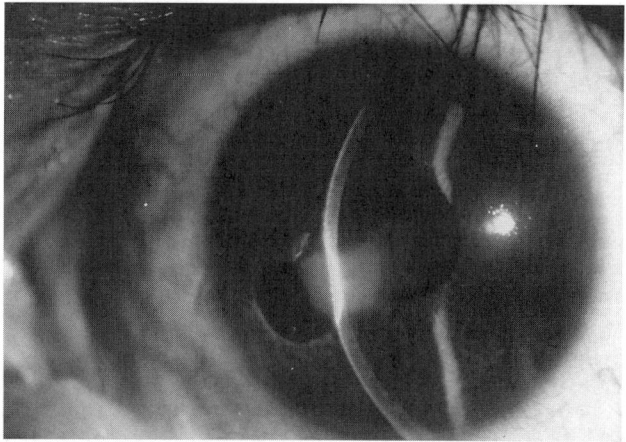

Fig. 23-7. Characteristic paracentral corneal ulceration in Sjögren syndrome patient.

disturbed by nocturia caused by an increased fluid intake. Impaired clearance of esophageal acid and chronic esophagitis resulting from a lack of salivary buffering may leave patients more susceptible to gastroesophageal reflux disease.[70]

The intraoral signs, like the symptoms, have a wide range of severity and are generally nonspecific, appearing also in chronic xerostomia of other causes. These signs include dry, sticky, oral mucosal surfaces; primary or recurrent dental caries at the necks or incisal edges of the teeth; absence of pooled saliva in the mouth floor; expression of cloudy or no saliva from the major salivary gland ducts; and patchy or generalized oral mucosal erythema with dorsal tongue papillary atrophy and angular cheilitis. The oral mucosal sign of papillary atrophy—erythema and fissuring on the dorsal tongue (with or without erythema in other oral mucosal sites)—is usually caused by overgrowth of the common, normally harmless yeast *Candida albicans*. This presentation is termed chronic erythematous candidiasis and develops in about one third of patients with Sjögren syndrome as a result of their salivary hypofunction and other unknown factors.[60] This pathogen usually causes burning mucosal symptoms and intolerance to acidic and spicy foods in affected patients.

Although dental caries is one of the most troubling sequelae of Sjögren syndrome, little attention has been given to it. One study of 65 patients with Sjögren syndrome found cervical or incisal dental caries at the time of initial diagnosis in 63% of the patients with primary Sjögren syndrome and 45% of the patients with secondary Sjögren syndrome who had remaining teeth.[19] Their mean stimulated parotid flow rates were reduced by 82% and 45%, respectively, as compared with patients who had a connective tissue disease alone.

About one third of Sjögren syndrome patients develop salivary gland enlargement during the course of the disease

(Fig. 23-1). Major salivary glands in Sjögren syndrome may develop firm, diffuse, nontender or slightly tender enlargement, usually bilaterally. In early or mild cases, there may be slight induration of the glands without enlargement. Patients with more severe gland dysfunction and inflammation are more likely to have enlargement than patients with mild disease.[20] Submandibular glands may be affected before parotids,[20] but this may not be observed unless these glands are specifically examined by palpation. Some patients report that their salivary gland enlargement occurs in episodes lasting for many weeks or months, whereas other patients have chronic enlargement with little or no fluctuation in size. A cream-colored exudate may be apparent at the orifice of the major salivary gland ducts, but smear preparations of the exudate usually reveal mostly lymphocytes, with few polymorphonuclear leukocytes. Superimposed acute bacterial sialadenitis occurs uncommonly, and unless the patient has symptoms and signs of acute sialadenitis, treatment with antibiotics is not indicated.

Systemic

Patients with Sjögren syndrome may develop, in addition to the exocrine gland manifestations, involvement of numerous other organ systems (see box). In patients with Sjögren syndrome and a defined connective tissue disorder (classified as secondary Sjögren syndrome), the systemic involvement is often typical of their connective tissue disease. Features of these diseases will not be reviewed here. Patients with primary Sjögren syndrome often have systemic complaints and occasionally develop serious and potentially fatal systemic complications. Unfortunately, few epidemiologic studies have been performed to establish the relative risk of systemic symptoms and nonexocrine gland organ involvement.

One of the most common complaints of patients with Sjögren syndrome is severe and occasionally disabling fa-

AUTOIMMUNE DISORDERS ASSOCIATED WITH SJÖGREN SYNDROME

Rheumatoid arthritis
Systemic lupus erythematosus
Scleroderma
Polymyositis
Polyarteritis nodosa
Hashimoto thyroiditis
Chronic hepatobiliary cirrhosis
Lymphocytic interstitial pneumonitis
Thrombocytopenic purpura
Hypergamma globulinemia
Waldenstrom macroglobulinemia
Raynaud phenomenon
Progressive systemic sclerosis
Dermatomyositis
Interstitial nephritis

tigue. Other common systemic symptoms include dry skin, hair loss, pruritis, scaling of the skin, and a decreased capacity for sweating. The skin is commonly thin and smooth and may have an almost transparent quality. Vaginal dryness is also a prevalent problem. The patient may develop frequent urinary tract infections and burning pain on urination. Dyspareunia may be a severe intractable complication.

Sjögren syndrome patients may occasionally experience numerous other symptoms including low grade fever, myalgia, and aching joints. These symptoms are often unaccompanied by objective clinical findings of connective disease, and this makes the evaluation of the symptoms frustrating for the clinician and the patient.

Signs and symptoms of gastrointestinal and hepatobiliary disease may develop in Sjögren syndrome and can occasionally result in weight loss and malnutrition. Poor appetite, loss of smell and taste sensation, difficulty swallowing, nausea, chronic indigestion, inability to tolerate certain foods, and abdominal pain are the most common gastrointestinal complaints. These symptoms may result from involvement of the stomach, small bowel, or pancreas. Decreased volume and acid content of gastric secretions has been reported in Sjögren syndrome. Atrophic gastritis has been observed endoscopically, and biopsy of the stomach mucosa may show CD4 T cell infiltration.[69] Small intestine involvement in Sjögren syndrome includes primary malabsorption syndrome and adult celiac disease. Acute pancreatitis or subclinical pancreatic deficiency may develop as a result of lymphocytic infiltration and fibrosis of the pancreas.[132] An association between primary Sjögren syndrome and liver disease has been recognized for many years.[17] The liver disease in Sjögren syndrome may manifest as abnormal biochemical tests, chronic active hepatitis, or primary biliary or crytogenic cirrhosis. The prevalence of Sjögren syndrome in patients with primary biliary cirrhosis is between 69% and 81%; and because of this association, patients with Sjögren syndrome should have liver function tests to screen for liver involvement.[17]

Respiratory symptoms may also develop that are secondary to inflammatory cell infiltration of the bronchi and parenchyma of the lungs. Sjögren syndrome patients with pulmonary involvement may have a chronic, dry, nonproductive cough and a decreased vital capacity with shortness of breath.[18]

Renal involvement in Sjögren syndrome may be overt or latent and consists primarily of interstitial disease caused by lymphocytic infiltration, tubular atrophy, and fibrosis. Clinical manifestations of renal pathologic findings in Sjögren syndrome include hyposthenuria, renal tubular acidosis, and (rarely) Fanconi syndrome (characterized by glucosuria, aminoaciduria, phosphaturia, and uricosuria). Glomerulonephritis has been reported in a small number of cases of Sjögren syndrome.[66]

Vasculitic complications of Sjögren syndrome may affect numerous organs. A variety of vasculitic skin lesions have been described in Sjögren syndrome including the following (in decreasing frequency of occurrence): purpura, urticaria-like lesions, petechia, digital ulcers, erythema multiforme, erythema perstans, erythema nodosum, erythema macules, and subcutaneous nodules.[107]

Peripheral and central nervous system vasculitis may develop in Sjögren syndrome. Several forms of peripheral neuropathy have been described.[4] These varied forms are attributable to vasculitis of small blood vessels in the epineurium and vasa nervosum. The most common peripheral nervous system manifestation of primary Sjögren syndrome is distal symmetrical sensory polyneuropathy, which affects the lower extremity more frequently than the upper extremity. Motor nerve dysfunction is less prevalent. Cranial nerve palsies may also develop. Trigeminal sensory neuropathy is the most common cranial neuropathy in Sjögren syndrome. Facial nerve palsies, neurosensory hearing loss, and peripheral vestibular dysfunction are less frequently observed.

Central nervous system manifestations of Sjögren syndrome include focal deficits (such as hemiparesis and hemisensory defects), seizure disorders, movement disorders, aseptic meningitis, and dementia. Involvement of the spinal cord may manifest as paraparesis and neurogenic bladder.[5]

Sjögren syndrome patients have an increased risk of developing lymphoproliferative disorders. The spectrum of lymphoproliferation in Sjögren syndrome ranges from benign lymphocytic infiltration of the salivary and lacrimal glands to low-grade monoclonal B lymphoproliferation to high-grade lethal nonHodgkin's lymphoma. Kassan and associates[65] estimated that patients with Sjögren syndrome have a 43.8%-fold greater risk of developing a salivary lymphoma than normal individuals. Biopsies of clinically enlarged parotid salivary glands from Sjögren syndrome show *myoepithelial sialadenitis* (MESA), also termed benign lymphoepithelial lesions.[15,23] Monoclonal B cell proliferations have been demonstrated by immunohistochemical and immunogenetic techniques in glands with MESA.[35,116] In a small percentage of Sjögren syndrome patients, extension of lymphoproliferation to extraglandular sites such as the lung, kidney, lymph nodes, skin, gastrointestinal tract, and bone marrow may develop. When extraglandular lymphoproliferation develops, diagnosis of malignant lymphoma may be clinically and histologically difficult. These extraglandular lymphoproliferations are most often non-Hodgkin B cell (IgM-kappa) lymphomas.[15] In some Sjögren syndrome patients who developed malignant lymphoma following MESA, malignant transformation has been associated with karyotypic alteration and has resulted in abnormal high-level expression of proto-oncogenes.[47] An increased frequency of chromosomal translocation (t14:18) in lymphomas arising in Sjögren syndrome patients has recently been reported.[47] This translocation results in opposition of the BCL-2 proto-oncogene to the immunoglobulin heavy chain gene, which leads to high-level expression of the BCL-2 gene. Increased expression of the BCL-2 protein may interfere with preprogrammed cell death (apoptosis) and thus increase the chance of malignant transformation. Thus development of malignant lymphoma in Sjögren syndrome may represent a multistep transition from benign exocrine gland lymphoproliferation to non-Hodgkin B cell lymphoma.

PATHOLOGY

Lacrimal Gland

The human lacrimal gland consists of tubuloacinar structures composed of morphologically and immunohistochemically distinct epithelial cell components.[150] The lacrimal gland also contains an immunoarchitecture that reflects its

role as a component of the secretory immune system.[145] Lymphoid follicles that contain central B cells and peripheral CD4 T cells resembling lymph node germinal centers are typically found in the center of lacrimal gland lobules (Fig. 23-8). Numerous lymphocytes consisting predominantly of IgA-secreting plasma cells and CD8 T lymphocytes reside in the interstitium of the normal lacrimal gland and surround the secretory acini.

A lymphoproliferation develops in the lacrimal glands of Sjögren syndrome patients (Fig. 23-9) in much the same way it develops in the salivary glands. Early in the course of the disease, single or multiple foci of lymphocytes are noted in lacrimal gland lobules, with more foci located in the center than in the periphery of lacrimal gland lobules (Fig. 23-10).[99] As the disease progresses, the lymphoproliferation surrounds epithelial ducts and islands and eventually replaces secretory acini (Fig. 23-11). In advanced cases of Sjögren syndrome, the majority of lacrimal gland lobules may be filled with mononuclear inflammatory cells (Fig. 23-12).

The lymphoproliferation in the Sjögren syndrome lacrimal gland consists predominantly of B and CD4 T lymphocytes (Fig. 23-13 A and B).[95] Immunoglobulin gene rearrangements on Southern hybridization[95] and the predominance of one immunoglobulin light chain in the majority of lobules in Sjögren syndrome lacrimal gland biopsies[99] suggest that the B lymphoproliferation in Sjögren syndrome lacrimal glands may be clonal. The B lymphoproliferation typically contains large B cells that express CD23 (blast-2 antigen) and ICAM-1 centrally, and smaller B cells in the periphery.[99] Less than 5% of cells within the lymphoproliferation in Sjögren syndrome lacrimal glands express plasma cell-associated differentiation antigens.

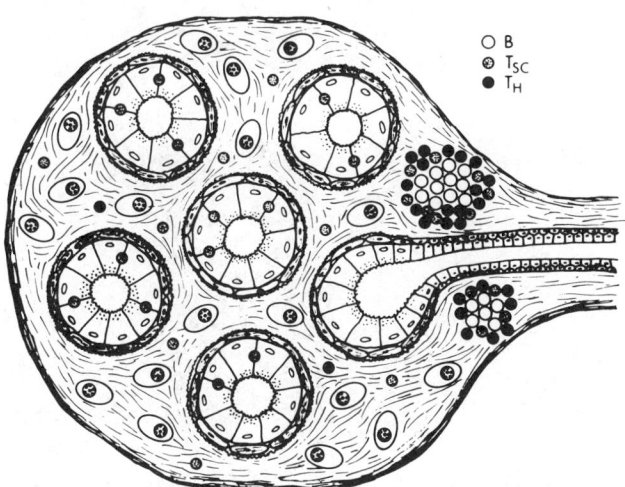

Fig. 23-8. Diagram of immunoarchitecture of the normal lacrimal gland showing location of B lymphocytes within lymphoid follicles that are most often located adjacent to intralobular ducts (B = B cells, Tsc = suppressor/cytotoxic T cells, T_H = helper T cells). (Published courtesy of *Ophthalmology* 97:1599-1605.)

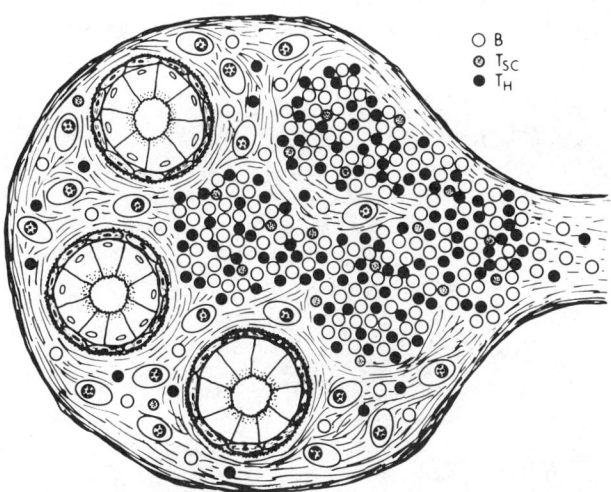

Fig. 23-9. Lymphoproliferation in the lacrimal glands of Sjögren syndrome replaces secretory acini and consists predominantly of B and helper T cells (B = B cells, Tsc = suppressor/cytotoxic T cells, T_H = helper T cells).

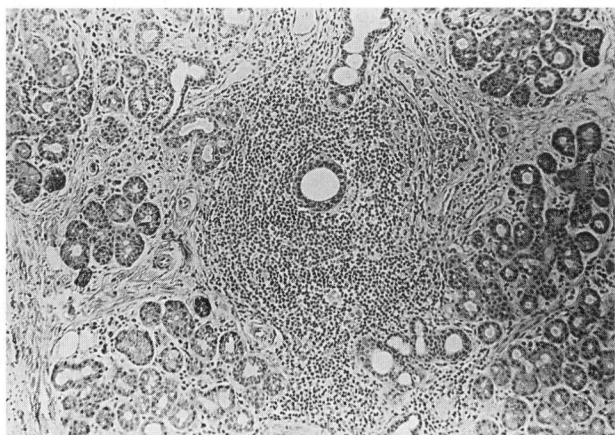

Fig. 23-10. Central focus of lymphoproliferation in lacrimal gland biopsy of Sjögren syndrome patient.

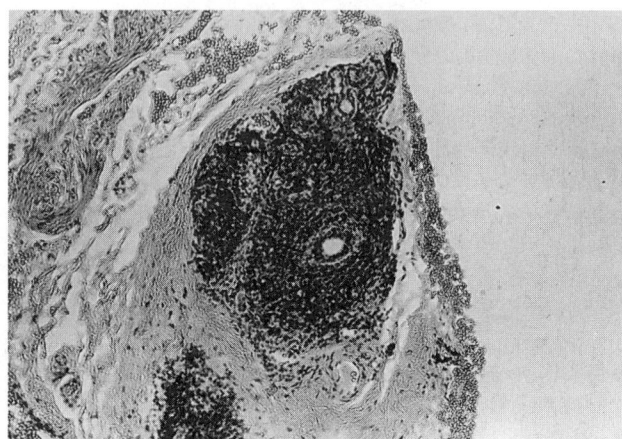

Fig. 23-12. Lacrimal gland lobule in lacrimal gland biopsy of Sjögren syndrome patient almost entirely filled with lymphocytes.

In the normal lacrimal gland, CD4 cells are found predominantly in lymphoid follicles in the center of lobules, and CD8 lymphocytes are the prevailing T cell population in the interstitium.[95,145] CD4 cells are more commonly observed in the lymphoproliferation in Sjögren syndrome lacrimal glands than CD8 cells, which results in a significant increase in the CD4-CD8 ratio compared to normal lacrimal glands (0.3 in normal glands compared to 3.0 in Sjögren syndrome LGs).[99]

The epithelial pathologic features in Sjögren syndrome lacrimal glands consist of dysfunction and loss of secretory acinar epithelia, retention and proliferation of ductal epithelia, and formation of epithelial islands.[99] The tubuloacinar structures in Sjögren syndrome lacrimal gland lobules often show abnormal morphology. Total loss of secretory acini was observed in 45% of lacrimal gland lobules and epithelia islands were noted in 26% of lobules.[99] Although these epithelial islands have previously been referred to in the literature as epimyoepithelial islands,[36] they do not stain with muscle-specific actin antibodies that show strong immuno-

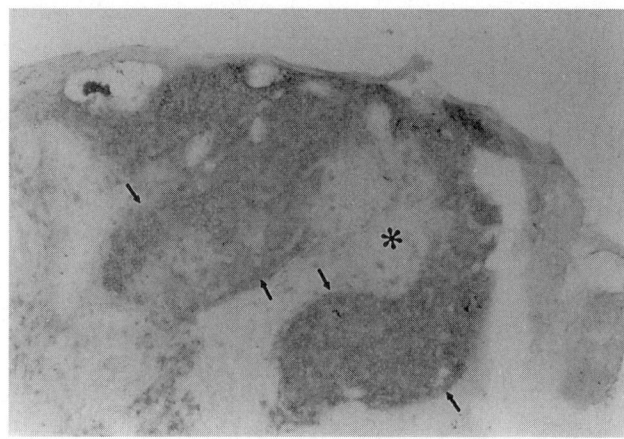

A

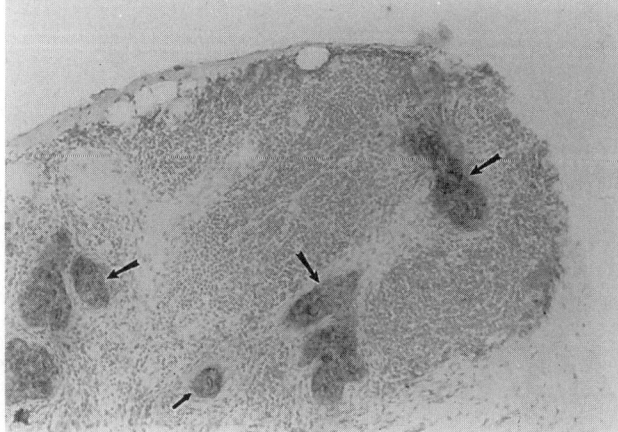

B

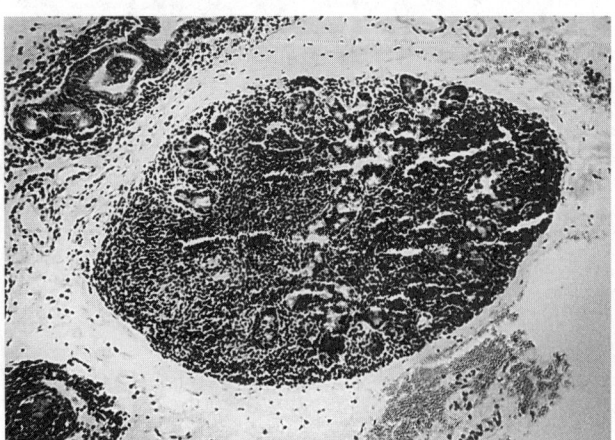

Fig. 23-11. Extensive lymphoproliferation surrounding residual ducts in lacrimal gland biopsy of Sjögren syndrome patient.

Fig. 23-13. **A,** B lymphoproliferation *(arrows)* surrounding epithelial island *(asterisk)* (100× original magnification). **B,** Epithelial island *(arrows)* in Sjögren syndrome lacrimal gland biopsy stained with cytokeratin-specific antibody (100× original magnification).

reactivity with the myoepithelia that surround the tubulo-acinar structures in normal lacrimal glands.[99]

There are several possible causes for the lacrimal gland epithelial and immune pathology of Sjögren syndrome. These include altered immunoregulation and CD4-derived, cytokine-driven B lymphoproliferation. A second possibility is that lacrimal gland acini can be destroyed by direct T cell cytotoxicity or inflammatory cytokines that are produced by activated T cells. Third, there is increasing evidence that an abnormal, persistent, type 1 EBV infection in the lacrimal glands of Sjögren syndrome patients may directly contribute to glandular destruction.

The theory that direct T cell cytotoxicity may be responsible for acinar epithelial destruction is supported by the Tsubota and associates[135] report, which states that the expression of perforin, a protein released from cytoplasmic granules of cytotoxic lymphocytes that punches holes in the cell membrane of target cells, is upregulated in Sjögren syndrome lacrimal glands. T cell cytokines may also create adverse conditions for acinar survival in the Sjögren syndrome lacrimal gland.

Epstein-Barr virus (EBV) has been implicated as a risk factor for Sjögren syndrome, based on the following: a number of case reports of primary Sjögren syndrome immediately following infectious mononucleosis,[52,103,144] detection of elevated EBV serology in Sjögren syndrome patients,[97,149] and detection of EBV genomes in a significantly greater percentage of peripheral blood lymphocytes, salivary and lacrimal gland biopsies, and tear specimens of Sjögren syndrome patients than normal controls.[101,102] Because EBV is capable of persistent infection in normal lacrimal and salivary glands, some investigators consider EBV to be too ubiquitous a virus to be involved in the pathogenesis of the exocrine glandular pathologic features of Sjögren syndrome. There are differences in the cellular sites, the extent of EBV infection, the pattern of antigen expression, and the strain of infecting virus in Sjögren syndrome lacrimal gland biopsies compared to those obtained from normal controls.[102] By in situ hybridization, EBV was found in intraductal epithelia in a small percentage of lobules in 21% of normal human lacrimal glands. In contrast, EBV was detected in mononuclear cells in areas of B lymphoproliferation as well as in the majority of residual epithelia in 86% of Sjögren syndrome LGs. EBV genomic sequences were amplified from 36% of normal and 88% of Sjögren syndrome lacrimal gland biopsies by PCR. Only EBV nuclear antigen 2 (EBNA-2), deleted, type 2 EBV sequences were amplified from normal lacrimal glands. In contrast, only type 1 (but not EBNA-2, deleted, EBV sequences) was amplified from Sjögren syndrome lacrimal gland biopsies. No EBV antigens were observed in normal lacrimal glands by immunohistochemical staining. In contrast, EBNA-2 and LMP (two EBV antigens associated with B cell transformation) were noted in areas of B lymphoproliferation, and lytic cycle antigens were observed in residual epithelia in Sjögren syndrome lacrimal gland biopsies.

A difference in EBV EBER1 expression was noted in lacrimal gland biopsies of Sjögren syndrome patients compared to normal control lacrimal gland biopsies.[103a] EBERs are small (166bp), abundantly expressed mRNAs (approximately 10^7 copies per cell) in cells with active latent EBV infection. Because of their high copy number, they make excellent targets for in situ hybridization. EBERs exist in vivo as ribonuclear protein particles complexed to the cellular antigen, La (also termed SS-B). EBERs were rarely seen in acinar epithelia (<0.1% of cells) in normal lacrimal glands. In contrast, EBER expression was observed in a significantly greater percentage of acinar epithelia (10% to 62%) in 80% of Sjögren syndrome lacrimal glands, and was also recognized in lymphocytes in areas of B lymphoproliferation in two thirds of Sjögren syndrome lacrimal glands. The detection of EBERs in the acinar epithelia of Sjögren syndrome lacrimal glands suggests that EBV infection may play a role in lacrimal gland acinar epithelial dysfunction and destruction in Sjögren syndrome. Serum antibodies to La antigen (SS-B) were detected in 47% of Sjögren syndrome patients followed in one clinic (unpublished data).[99] These antibodies could be directed to EBER-expressing acinar epithelia in Sjögren syndrome lacrimal glands or alternatively, they could result from sensitization to cellular La antigens that are released from dead or degenerating acinar epithelia.

Ocular Surface

Characteristic corneal and conjunctival epithelial pathologic changes are noted in Sjögren syndrome. Corneal changes include punctate and diffuse fluorescein staining, punctate rose bengal staining that is usually greatest in the inferior cornea, filamentary keratitis, adherent mucous strands, central and peripheral sterile corneal ulceration, and microbial keratitis. Thinning of the corneal epithelia has been noted in some histologic sections,[122] and a smaller than normal diameter and a persistence of nuclei have been observed in superficial corneal epithelial cells by specular microscopy.[78,137]

Impression cytology has greatly contributed to the knowledge regarding the conjunctival pathologic changes in Sjögren syndrome. Superficial conjunctival epithelia (in impression cytology taken from eyes of Sjögren syndrome patients) show enlarged cytoplasmic-nuclear ratios (Fig. 23-14), mild keratinization, reduced density or total loss of goblet cells, and adherent mucous aggregates.[3,98] These changes are more pronounced in the exposure zone of the conjunctiva. Acanthosis was seen in bulbar conjunctival biopsies of Sjögren syndrome patients (Fig. 23-15). Mild to severe punctate rose bengal staining of the conjunctival epithelium, particularly in the exposure zone, may be observed as it was in the corneal epithelium. Rose bengal staining of

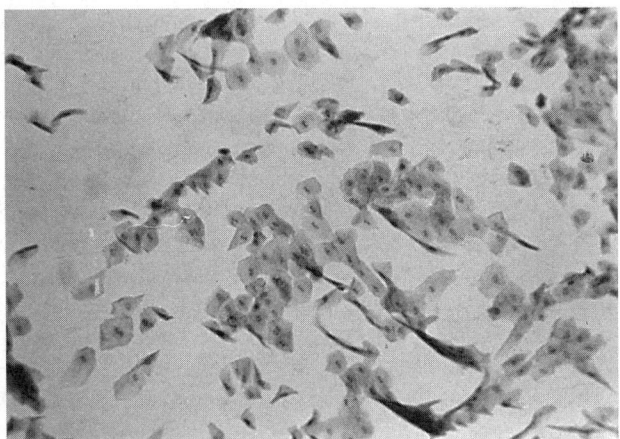

Fig. 23-14. Impression cytology from temporal bulbar conjunctiva of primary Sjögren syndrome patient showing enlarged cytoplasmic-nuclear ratio of epithelia and loss of goblet cells (also termed squamous metaplasia, 100× original magnification).

ocular surface epithelia may be caused by the lack of a protective mucin coating (that normally prevents intracellular penetration of rose bengal dye) on stained epithelial cells.[34] This theory for the mechanism of ocular surface epithelial rose bengal staining is supported by decreased epithelial mucin expression in a significantly lower percentage of bulbar conjunctival epithelia in Sjögren syndrome patients compared to normal eyes.[103a]

The pathogenesis of the ocular surface epithelial changes in Sjögren syndrome has not yet been established. It is possible that these changes result from one or more of the following: mechanical trauma related to decreased aqueous and mucin tear layers, osmotic cellular damage caused by increased tear osmolarity,[55] lack of tear-borne growth factors essential for growth and differentiation of ocular surface epithelia, and conjunctival inflammation. Immunopathologic changes occur in the conjunctival epithelia of Sjögren syndrome patients. These changes include T cell infiltration[98,108] and aberrant conjunctival epithelial expression of interleukin-6 (IL-6) plus HLA Class II antigens and ICAM-1 (two inflammatory cell membrane proteins that are typically induced by exposure to interferon gamma).[63] Similar immunopathologic changes are observed in epidermis in psoriasis plaques, and IL-6 has been implicated as an autocrine growth factor that stimulates epithelial hyperproliferation in psoriasis. IL-6 may contribute to the conjunctival epithelial pathologic features in Sjögren syndrome.

Salivary Gland

A common feature of all organs affected by Sjögren syndrome is a potentially progressive lymphocytic infiltration. These infiltrates presumably cause the functional changes in affected organs and the diverse clinical features of this disorder. Two types of pathologic appearance must be considered in the salivary component of Sjögren syndrome: the benign lymphoepithelial lesion (occurring primarily in the parotid glands) and focal lymphocytic sialadenitis (occurring in the other major and minor salivary glands).

The benign lymphoepithelial lesion apparently represents both proliferation of intraparotid lymphoid tissue and infiltration of lymphocytes into the gland. These proliferating cells replace the glandular epithelium and cause clinical enlargement of the gland. The proliferating lymphocytes are associated with hyperplasia and metaplasia of salivary ductal epithelia, forming the epimyoepithelial islands that characterize the lesion. The normal lobular architecture of the gland is maintained. Lymphoid follicles with germinal centers may or may not be present. Plasma cells and polymorphonuclear leukocytes are usually not a significant component of this infiltration. Batsakis[9] described the pathologic

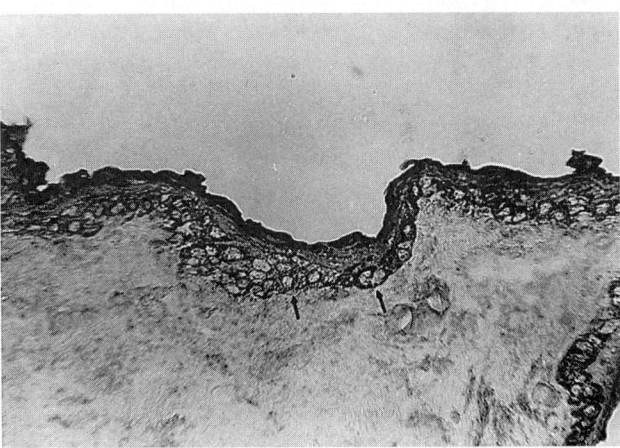

A

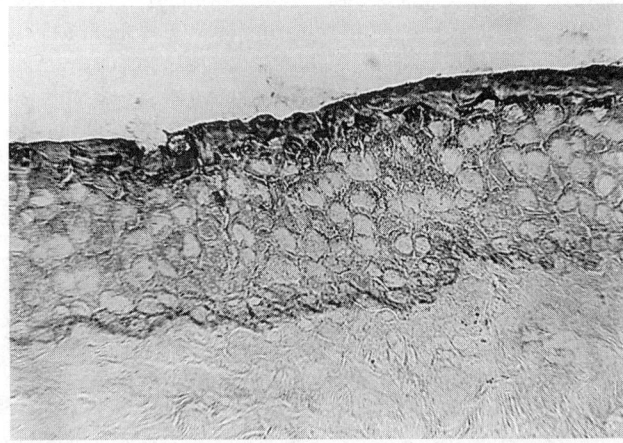

B

Fig. 23-15. **A,** Biopsy of normal temporal bulbar conjunctiva stained with cytokeratin-specific antibodies showing approximately four epithelial cell layers *(arrows)* (400× original magnification). **B,** Biopsy of temporal bulbar conjunctiva in Sjögren syndrome patient stained with cytokeratin-specific antibodies showing acanthosis (400× original magnification).

appearance of the benign lymphoepithelial lesion as a "distinctive, yet not pathognomonic, sialadenopathy."

Microscopic examination of enlarged parotid or submandibular glands from patients with Sjögren syndrome **usually** reveals the benign lymphoepithelial lesion. Only 40% of 22 major salivary gland specimens from Sjögren syndrome patients, 10 of whom had enlarged salivary glands at the time of biopsy, revealed benign lymphoepithelial lesions.[11] The benign lymphoepithelial lesion may also occur in patients who do not have Sjögren syndrome or other systemic disease. Furthermore, these lesions do not always remain benign and may be associated with (or transform into) lymphomas in patients with or without Sjögren syndrome.[23] There is evidence suggesting that benign lymphoepithelial lesions in patients with Sjögren syndrome may in some cases represent clonal expansion of populations of infiltrating T or B lymphocytes.[35,48] This expansion may signify a step in the uncommon progression of Sjögren syndrome to lymphoma.

The characteristic histopathologic feature of minor salivary glands in Sjögren syndrome is focal lymphocytic sialadenitis.[20,21,23] This feature consists of a primary lymphocytic infiltrate in otherwise normal-appearing glands and is characterized by (1) focal aggregates of 50 or more (usually many more) lymphocytes adjacent to normal-appearing acini, and (2) consistent presence of these foci in all or most of the glands in the specimen. Plasma cells are often seen interstitially, but seldom in the lymphocytic foci. Lymphoid germinal centers are often found within large infiltrates, but the epimyoepithelial islands characteristic of the benign lymphoepithelial lesion in major salivary glands occur uncommonly in minor glands.

The microscopic differential diagnosis in minor glands includes mild-to-moderately severe nonspecific chronic sialadenitis. Nonspecific chronic sialadenitis is characterized by (1) diffuse atrophy of glandular epithelium in lobules or entire glands, usually with duct dilation and interstitial fibrosis; and (2) infiltration by lymphocytes or plasma cells in scattered, interstitial, or focal patterns.[21,23] Nonspecific chronic sialadenitis is found in specimens from people who have no history of Sjögren syndrome or other connective tissue disease. This disease increases in frequency with age and appears in women at an earlier age than in men.[119]

PATHOGENESIS

Immunopathology

The primary immunopathologic process in Sjögren syndrome is infiltration of affected organs by lymphocytes. It is a dynamic process in which metabolically active cells affect the surrounding tissue and participate in their own proliferation. This process may signal generalized or regional changes in lymphocyte regulation. Early studies of lymphocytes in salivary glands from patients with Sjögren syndrome detected immunoglobulin synthesis[129] and found that the proportion of T lymphocytes in infiltrates was greater in the specimens with more and larger infiltrates.[130]

Later studies with monoclonal antibodies and more sensitive labeling systems allowed phenotypic identification of the infiltrating cells. Labial salivary glands from patients with primary Sjögren syndrome contained more than three times as many T helper cells (CD4+) as T suppressor cells (CD8+), and this pattern was generally unrelated to the proportion of these cells in the peripheral blood.[41] More than 75% of the infiltrating cells were T lymphocytes (mainly T helper type); only 5% to 20% were B lymphocytes; and about 50% of the cells expressed lymphocyte activation markers, compared with only 15% in the peripheral blood.[2]

An immunocytochemical study of benign lymphoepithelial lesions suggested that there is a characteristic and consistent distribution of inflammatory cells that resembles the distribution in reactive lymph nodes.[6] Natural killer cell activity by peripheral blood mononuclear cells is significantly reduced in patients with Sjögren syndrome,[43,87,97] but those cells have been observed in the germinal centers of benign lymphoepithelial lesions.[6]

A large number of immunologic mediators have been described in salivary glands from patients with Sjögren syndrome. Little is known, however, about the role of cytokines and growth factors in normal regulation of salivary gland differentiation or function, making it difficult to ascribe immunopathologic actions to any of the factors found in glands affected by Sjögren syndrome. The cytokines probably contribute to the inflammatory destruction of tissue and may also stimulate the intense B cell hyperactivity seen in affected patients.

Epithelial cells in minor salivary glands from Sjögren syndrome patients express the class II major histocompatibility complex antigen HLA-DR, whereas glands from normal subjects do not.[80] Subsequently, class I major histocompatibility complex antigens, as well as HLA-DP and DQ antigens, have been detected in salivary glands from Sjögren syndrome patients.[64,112] The extent of HLA-DR expression has been correlated with the number of inflammatory cells within the gland,[126] but not with gland function.[59] The class II antigen expression by glandular epithelium does not appear to be a specific autoimmune mechanism, because it was also seen in glands with traumatically induced nonspecific sialadenitis.[126] These results suggest that HLA class II antigen expression is the result of inflammatory cell infiltration and not an event initiating this autoimmune process.

Viral Pathogenesis of Salivary Gland Disease

Viruses have long been suspected of playing a role in the initiation or perpetuation of autoimmune diseases, especially Sjögren syndrome. A number of viruses have been found in the salivary glands or their secretions including EBV,[148] cytomegalovirus, mumps virus, several enteroviruses, and human immunodeficiency virus.[120] Of these viruses, EBV has been the most investigated as a causal agent; perhaps because there have been several reports of the development of Sjögren syndrome following acute EBV infection.[52,103,144]

Previous studies that evaluated parotid and minor salivary gland biopsies from Sjögren syndrome patients for EBV infection contain conflicting results. Using polymerase chain reaction (PCR), Saito and associates[113] amplified EBV genomic sequences in 78% of Sjögren syndrome salivary gland biopsies compared to only 13% of biopsies from normal controls. Mariette and associates[83] amplified EBV DNA by PCR in 86% of minor salivary gland biopsies from primary Sjögren syndrome patients, 60% in secondary Sjögren syndrome patients, and 29% of normal controls. Also using PCR, Deacon and associates[26] reported that 90% of Sjögren syndrome minor salivary gland biopsies and 70% of normal salivary gland biopsies harbored EBV DNA. Mariette and associates[83] detected EBV DNA in ductal epithelia and lymphocytes in 50% of primary Sjögren syndrome biopsies and only 8% of controls by in situ hybridization with probes reactive with the Bam HI W region of the EBV genome. In contrast, Venables and associates[140] found EBV in 17% of primary Sjögren syndrome, 33% of secondary Sjögren syndrome, and 71% of normal controls using in situ DNA hybridization.

Salivary gland biopsies from normal controls and Sjögren syndrome patients have also been evaluated for EBV antigens. Fox and associates[45] reported ductal epithelial staining with anti-EA-D antibodies in 8/14, with gp350/220-specific antibodies in 2/14 salivary gland biopsies from Sjögren syndrome patients, and 0/10 control glands. In contrast, Venables and associates[140] found anti-EA-D staining of ductal epithelia in 30% of primary Sjögren syndrome, 66% of secondary Sjögren syndrome, and 86% of controls; and anti-membrane antigen staining in 17% of primary Sjögren syndrome, 20% of secondary Sjögren syndrome, and 66% of controls. Deacon and associates[26] described a lack of specific immunoreactivity of salivary gland biopsies from primary and secondary Sjögren syndrome patients and normal controls with monoclonal antibodies specific for EBV latent (EBNA 2,LMP) or lytic (EA-D,EA-R,VCA) infection antigens.

There are several possible explanations for the differences in the type of EBV infection observed in salivary glands compared to that seen in lacrimal glands (described previously) in Sjögren syndrome. First, the immunoarchitecture phenotype of resident lymphocytes and the inflammatory response of the minor salivary gland are not equivalent to the lacrimal gland. In Sjögren syndrome patients undergoing simultaneous LG and minor salivary gland biopsies for diagnosis of Sjögren syndrome, greater inflammation is noted in the lacrimal gland than in the salivary gland.[115] Second, in most of the previous evaluations of Sjögren syndrome salivary gland biopsies for EBV infection,

EBV antigens and DNA were detected primarily in ductal epithelia; and an EBV-associated B lymphoproliferation surrounding infected ducts was not noted. Furthermore, the lymphocytic infiltration in published photomicrographs of Sjögren syndrome salivary glands generally appears to be less severe than that typically observed in Sjögren syndrome LG biopsies. A recent study by Tsubota and associates[136] using quantitative PCR suggests that the amount of EBV DNA in the LG is ten times that in the salivary gland when both tissues were obtained from the same Sjögren syndrome patient.[136]

The description of a Sjögren syndromelike condition in HIV-infected patients has offered the possibility that a retrovirus is involved in the pathogenesis of Sjögren syndrome. Recent reports, however, describe significant differences between the salivary lesions found in this HIV-associated salivary gland disease and those in Sjögren syndrome.[62,118] It is likely that sicca syndrome in patients with HIV infection is a distinct syndrome associated with a CD8 lymphocytosis and a different HLA type (HLA-DR5) than primary Sjögren syndrome (discussion follows). Another retroviral link is advanced by the presence of antibodies to HIV-1 group-specific protein p24 in 57% of sera from Sjögren syndrome patients and in 5% of normal sera,[140] and by the presence of retroviral particles in minor salivary glands from Sjögren syndrome patients that were distinct from, but antigenically related to, HIV.[51] These data suggest the presence of an agent that can stimulate production of retrovirus-associated antibody, but not of a retroviral cause of Sjögren syndrome.

A pathogenesis for Sjögren syndrome involving an immunologic response to the presence of viral antigens in a genetically susceptible host, possibly modified by environmental factors, has not been proved. But this remains an intriguing possibility.

Immunogenetics

In addition to female gender, the other significant risk factor for Sjögren syndrome is HLA type. The first HLA antigen reported to be a risk factor for Sjögren syndrome was HLA-DR3 (Dw3) in 1977.[16] In 1979 Moutsopoulos and associates[89] verified that there were differences in the frequencies of certain HLA types in patients with primary Sjögren syndrome compared to those with secondary Sjögren syndrome. Primary Sjögren syndrome patients had a significantly increased frequency of HLA B8 and DR3, and secondary Sjögren syndrome patients had an increased frequency of DR4. Since that time, a number of studies have been performed confirming and extending the knowledge regarding the immunogenetic risk factors for Sjögren syndrome. The HLA-B8, DR3, DRw52a, DQW2.1 haplotype, and (less often) HLA-DR2 have been found at significantly increased frequencies in Caucasians of Western European descent with primary Sjögren syndrome. In Caucasians with secondary Sjögren syndrome, those with rheumatoid arthritis have an increased frequency of HLA-DR4, whereas Sjö-gren syndrome patients with systemic lupus erythematosus often have DR2 or DR3 genes. Thus far the DRw52a antigen that is encoded by the DR β3 gene is the best candidate as the primary genetic marker for Sjögren syndrome.[109]

HLA type is also strongly correlated with the production of SS-A (Ro) and SS-B (La) autoantibodies in Sjögren syndrome patients. In fact, the presence of these autoantibodies is more strongly correlated with HLA type than clinical manifestations of the disease. Combined Ro and La positivity occurs most commonly in patients with primary Sjögren syndrome, and these patients usually have the HLA B8 haplotype. The highest relative risk for anti-Ro and anti-La positivity or anti-Ro positivity alone is conferred by the DQw1.2/DW2.1 heterozygous state.[109]

The relationship of HLA type with the pathogenesis of Sjögren syndrome has not been established. HLA class I and II antigens are involved in presentation of foreign antigens to T lymphocytes. Furthermore, the magnitude of an individual's immune response to foreign microorganisms has been correlated with HLA type. Because viruses have been implicated in the pathogenesis of the lacrimal and salivary gland pathologic features of Sjögren syndrome, it is possible that the HLA types associated with Sjögren syndrome result in an aberrant immune response to an infecting virus. As mentioned previously in this chapter, EBV has been consistently detected in a significantly greater percentage of blood mononuclear cells, lacrimal and salivary gland biopsies, and tear specimens of primary Sjögren syndrome patients. Genotype analysis indicates that the abnormal persistent EBV infection in blood mononuclear cells and in the lacrimal glands of Sjögren syndrome patients is caused by type 1 EBV strains.[102] Recently Misko and associates[86] reported that EBV-specific cytotoxic lymphocytes isolated from individuals with the HLA B8 haplotype have an inherent inability to lyse target EBV-infected B lymphocytes. This inability was not caused by a defective T cell function and probably represents an inability of effective EBV antigen presentation to HLA class I restricted CTLs by the class I restricted HLA B8 antigen. These data suggest that Sjögren syndrome patients may develop an abnormal persistent EBV infection if they are infected by certain type I EBV strains to which their cellular immune system cannot respond.

THERAPY

Ocular Component

Current treatment of ocular irritation associated with Sjögren syndrome is largely directed to providing symptomatic relief.[27,49] Current treatment strategies are aimed at lubricating the ocular surface and conserving endogenously produced tears. Topically applied lubricating drops and ointments continue to be the mainstay of therapy for the ocular component of Sjögren syndrome. Although these agents often provide temporary symptomatic relief, they do not appear to reverse the ocular surface cellular pathologic features.[91] Commercially available lubricant drops are aqueous solutions containing polymers to increase their retention time or their adherence to the ocular surface.[77] In some cases they also contain buffers and electrolytes. Unfortunately, there are no true therapeutic tear replacements with biologic activity at the present time. Some patients with severe ocular irritation find they must instill lubricant drops several times per hour to keep their symptoms tolerable. This frequency of instillation combined with reduced tear clearance as a result of aqueous tear deficiency (and in some cases punctal occlusion) makes Sjögren syndrome patients particularly susceptible to ocular surface epithelial toxicity from preservatives in lubricant solutions or ointments, particularly benzalkonium chloride.[61,96] The advent of preservative-free lubricants in the past decade represents a major advance by allowing patients to use these preparations as frequently as they desire without experiencing ocular surface epithelial toxicity.[1] It is currently recommended that preservative-free lubricants be considered for treatment of patients who feel they must instill these medications greater than four times per day to relieve their symptoms. Lubricant ointments are particularly useful for instillation before going to bed because they have a longer contact time than drops and will coat the ocular surface during sleep (when aqueous tear production is normally decreased). Severe Sjögren syndrome patients may also use lubricant ointments during the day, but most patients are bothered by the blurred vision and sticky sensation experienced after instillation of ointments.

One sustained-release lubricant preparation has been marketed (Lacrisert®, Merck Sharpe and Dohme).[27] It consists of hydroxypropyl cellulose rods that slowly dissolve into the tear film after being placed onto the ocular surface. These sustained-release lubricants have theoretical advantages over lubricant drops and ointments; however, because they slowly dissolve over a 6- to 12-hour period, they are often not well tolerated by patients with severe aqueous tear deficiency, who lack a sufficient tear volume to hydrate and dissolve the polymer. Additionally, the polymer tends to increase tear viscosity and blur vision. These sustained-released preparations are occasionally well tolerated by patients with mild to moderate aqueous tear deficiency.

Topical aqueous solutions containing the glycosaminoglycans hyaluronic acid and chondroitin sulfate have been evaluated for the treatment of keratoconjunctivitis sicca because of their increased viscosity and prolongation of tear breakup times following topical instillation. Two retrospective, noncontrolled studies reported that artificial tear preparations containing sodium hyaluronate improved symptoms and ocular surface signs of dry eye patients.[28,104] In contrast, a prospective, controlled study reported that a topically applied solution consisting of hyaluronic acid, chondroitin sulfate, and polyvinyl alcohol was no better than a commercial artificial tear containing polyvinyl alcohol and preserved with benzalkonium chloride.[79] Similarly, an unpreserved artificial tear substitute containing 0.1% sodium hyaluronate was verified to have clinical efficacy equal to a preparation containing polyvinyl alcohol and chlorbutanol.[91]

Patients who remain symptomatic on maximal lubricant therapy may benefit from therapies aimed at conserving their reduced volume of innately produced aqueous tears. A humidified environment is recommended to reduce tear evaporation. Room humidification is particularly beneficial in dry climates and high altitudes. Tear evaporation can also be inhibited by placement of side shields on eyeglasses. Covering the eye at night may also reduce tear evaporation. This may be accomplished by wearing swim goggles or taping a plastic shield or plastic wrap over the eyelids.

Punctal occlusion is one of the most useful and practical treatments for conserving tears. This technique may increase tear volume, and the retention of aqueous tears may also increase the concentration of biologically active constituents in the tears. Although there have been no controlled studies evaluating the effectiveness of punctal occlusion, clinical series have reported an improvement in symptoms and decreased ocular surface signs following this treatment.[29,138,146] It is recommended that temporary punctal occlusion with collagen, plastic plugs, or chromic suture be performed prior to permanent punctal occlusion to determine whether patients will experience bothersome epiphora following punctal occlusion. These side effects are unlikely in most severe Sjögren syndrome patients, who often have very low aqueous tear production.

Permanent punctal occlusion is most commonly performed with a disposable thermocautery[72] in the examination room after application of topical anesthesia and/or infiltration of the lid with local anesthetic. Punctal occlusion can also be performed with the argon laser,[8] but the results of this technique are variable. One advantage to the laser technique is that it can surround the puncta, causing stenosis, but not permanent closure. Therefore the amount of stenosis can be titrated based on the patient's tear function.

At the present, there are no therapeutic agents (termed secretogouges) marketed in the United States that stimulate the lacrimal gland to produce tears. Bromhexine is a mucolytic agent currently marketed in many foreign countries that stimulates aqueous tear production and increases tear film stability in patients with Sjögren syndrome. Unfortunately, no decrease in ocular surface rose bengal staining or subjective improvement in ocular irritation was noted in clinical trials of Bromhexine.[50,105] Topical application of another secretogouge, 3-isobutyl-1-methylxanthine (IBMX), was reported to increase tear production, lower tear osmolarity, and decrease ocular surface rose bengal staining in an open-label clinical trial on patients with aqueous tear deficiency; however, this study did not specify whether these patients had Sjögren syndrome.[56]

Over the past decade, cyclosporin A (CSA), a potent suppressor of T cell function, has been evaluated for treatment of Sjögren syndrome. Drosos and associates[31] announced the results of a double-masked trial of oral CSA for the treatment of primary Sjögren syndrome. Subjects in this trial were treated with either oral CSA (5 mg/kg/day) or a placebo for 6 months. The majority of subjects receiving oral CSA noted improvement in their dry mouth symptoms; however, only 20% noted improvement of their ocular irritation. Furthermore, no difference in aqueous tera production by Schirmer testing was noted between the CSA-treated group and the control group.

More recently, topical CSA has been reported to stimulate aqueous tear production in dogs with spontaneous keratoconjunctivitis sicca,—a disease that may be a canine correlate of human Sjögren syndrome.[67] Stimulation of aqueous tear production was noted 3 to 60 days after initiation of topical CSA. The mechanism of increased tear production in these animals has not been established; however, CSA has been reported to be a lacrimal gland secretogouge both in vitro and in vivo.[67] A recent pilot trial of 1% CSA ophthalmic ointment for treatment of keratoconjunctivitis sicca demonstrated that patients receiving CSA described significantly less foreign body sensation and a greater number of hours of symptom control per day compared to subjects treated with a placebo. Patients treated with CSA also had less ocular surface rose bengal staining than controls, but no difference in Schirmer test values or tear breakup times were noted.[71] A prospective, masked trial of 1% CSA ointment for treatment of the ocular manifestations of Sjögren syndrome was recently completed; however, the results have not yet been published. Topical 2% CSA solution was recently reported to successfully treat paracentral corneal ulcers in patients with rheumatoid arthritis and secondary Sjögren syndrome.[68]

Both glucocorticoids and androgenic corticosteroids have shown beneficial therapeutic effects for the ocular manifestations of Sjögren syndrome. Tabbara and Frayha[128] recorded that the majority of patients treated with alternate day oral prednisone (40 mg) showed improved aqueous tear production defined as the following: 5 mm or greater increase in Schirmer test strip wetting (71% of subjects), decreased rose bengal staining (86% of subjects), and elevated tear lysozyme levels (64% of subjects).[128] It has been hypothesized that the low incidence of Sjögren syndrome in males may be a result of protection from disease by androgenic hormones such as testosterone.[127] Bizzarro and associates[10] evaluated the therapeutic effects of testosterone undecanoate (TU) in three patients with primary Sjögren syndrome (fulfilling the diagnostic criteria of Fox and associates[46] presented in box on page 314). The patients were initially treated with placebo for 60 days, followed by TU (120 mg/day) for 60 days. Compared to placebo therapy, all of the TU-treated subjects showed a significant improvement in Schirmer test values and a reduction in ocular surface rose bengal staining. Treatment of two different murine models of Sjögren syndrome (NZB/NZW F1 and MRL/Mp-1pr/1pr mice) with systemic androgen hormone therapy decreases the number and size of lacrimal gland lymphocytic foci, reduces the extent of lymphocytic infiltration, and ameliorates the immune-associated effects on lacrimal gland acinar and ductal epithelia.[114,141] Additionally, tear volumes increased significantly in NZB/NZW F1 mice treated with testosterone.[141] In summary, these studies suggest that systemically administered corticosteroids or androgen hormones may suppress the immune-mediated lacrimal gland disease of Sjögren syndrome and may improve lacrimal gland secretory function.

Clinical trials have also been performed evaluating the efficacy of therapies that may directly influence the ocular surface disease of Sjögren syndrome. In 1985 Tseng and associates[133] reported the results of a nonrandomized clinical trial of tretinoin (all transretinoic acid) ointment for the treatment of various dry-eye conditions. This study included one group of patients with KCS associated with Sjögren syndrome.[133] All of these subjects recounted an improvement in their clinical symptoms and a reduction in ocular surface rose bengal staining and squamous metaplasia. Subsequently, a multicenter, placebo-controlled, double-masked study evaluating the efficacy of tretinoin for KCS was performed.[125] This trial failed to find a beneficial therapeutic effect of tretinoin; however, the selection criteria for entry into this study did not require documentation that the patients had aqueous tear deficiency, nor did this study indicate the percentage of patients with KCS associated with Sjögren syndrome.[125] It appears that additional clinical trials are needed to determine if topical retinoids have a role in the therapy of ocular Sjögren syndrome. Fox and associates[44] reported that compared to placebo, artificial tears made with autologous sera (1 : 3 dilution with normal saline) resulted in a significant improvement in symptoms of ocular irritation and a decrease in ocular surface rose bengal staining. Additional studies evaluating artificial tears containing autologous sera have not been performed.

Oral Component

Although Sjögren syndrome is not curable, it is certainly manageable to the extent of both significantly reducing a patient's symptoms and preventing irreversible damage to the teeth and eyes. Managing the oral component of Sjögren syndrome includes the following: (1) treating and preventing dental caries, (2) reducing oral mucosal symptoms by treating and retreating oral candidiasis, (3) stimulating remaining salivary glands to produce more saliva, and (4) selectively using saliva substitutes.

Dental Caries. The dental caries associated with Sjögren syndrome and with other causes of chronic salivary hypofunction are called root caries because they attack the teeth near the gingiva and at the margins of dental restorations, above or below the gum. Because patients with severe salivary hypofunction may not be able to wear a complete lower denture, preventing caries and preserving the dentition is an especially important aspect of treatment for all patients with Sjögren syndrome who have remaining teeth. Although much remains unknown about this form of dental caries, frequent fluoride applications and plaque control have been established as greatly reducing the frequency of caries in patients with postradiation caries.[30] These measures seem to be of similar benefit for patients with Sjögren syndrome.

Methods of preventing new and recurrent dental caries in patients with Sjögren syndrome need to be individualized by the dentist according to their dentition and the severity of their salivary hypofunction. Caries prevention for patients with chronic salivary hypofunction usually includes the following: (1) regular use of a fluoride-containing dentifrice supplemented by daily topical fluoride application; (2) avoidance of all sugar-containing foods or beverages between meals; (3) careful daily removal of plaque deposits from the teeth; and (4) regular dental supervision and care. Fluoride tablets and fluoridated water supplies, which help prevent tooth decay in developing teeth of children, are of no help to adults.

Oral Candidiasis. Antifungal drugs applied topically in the mouth (usually for several months) can eliminate chronic erythematous candidiasis, allowing the oral mucosa to return to normal.[60] Effective treatment is important because it eliminates painful mucosal symptoms and intolerance to acidic or spicy foods for most patients, even though the oral dryness continues. Because the secretory hypofunction of Sjögren syndrome is chronic, however, fungal overgrowth commonly recurs. Therefore each case must be followed for reappearance of the mucosal symptoms or signs and retreated as necessary. Systemic antifungal drugs such as ketoconazole may be ineffective in patients with severe salivary hypofunction.

Many topical antifungal drugs are available, but the oral forms are usually not effective for treating chronic erythematous candidiasis. Liquid preparations (for example, nystatin oral suspension) cannot be kept in the mouth for a sufficient amount of time to be effective; other oral preparations have low drug concentrations (for example, clotrimazole oral troche); and all oral preparations contain sufficient quantities of sugar to significantly increase the risk of dental decay when used chronically. The most generally effective treatment is for patients to dissolve nystatin vaginal tablets orally for 20 to 30 minutes, beginning at two or three per day. Most patients find these unflavored tablets acceptable for the long treatment regimens that are often necessary. Patients with very dry mouths usually require periodic sips of water to help the tablets dissolve within 30 minutes. The effects of treatment are monitored by noting improvement in oral symptoms and resolution of the oral mucosal lesions.

To permit the drug access to all mucosal sites, patients must remove their dentures while antifungal tablets are dissolving. The dentures themselves also need to be treated to eliminate the yeast. To avoid damaging the dentures, the method and frequency of denture disinfection should be decided in consultation with the patient's dentist.

Stimulation of Salivary Flow. Patients with residual salivary gland function may benefit from stimulating their salivary flow with either local or systemic methods. For patients with mild salivary hypofunction, salivary stimulation with sugarless candies or chewing gum is often effective. Even sugarless products, however, may contain carbohydrates that have cariogenic potential in the presence of reduced salivary function.[12] Limitations to these approaches are that the duration of action for the stimulation is short and that a patient must constantly have something in the mouth.

Systemic sialogogues, such as the mucolytic agent bromhexine, have been assessed for salivary and lacrimal effects in several studies with Sjögren syndrome patients. An objective increase in salivary flow has not been demonstrated with bromhexine.[39] Anetholetrithione showed significant effects on saliva output in one study of Sjögren syndrome patients with mild-to-moderate secretory dysfunction.[32] A later study in Sjögren syndrome patients with more severe hypofunction failed to find a significant response to the agent, however.[117]

A series of controlled clinical trials with systemic administered pilocarpine has verified the efficacy of pilocarpine HCl as a systemic secretogogue.[37,40,58] A 5-mg dose increases salivary flow significantly for several hours, as compared with placebo, and may be given three times daily.[40,58] Side effects are common, especially sweating, flushing, and increased urination. There are no serious side effects (such as significant cardiovascular or other systemic alterations), however, during up to 5 months of active drug treatment.[40] At present, pilocarpine is the most effective systemic sialogogue available for persons with reduced, but residual, salivary gland function.

Saliva Substitutes. Several saliva substitutes that contain some of the constituents of normal saliva are available without prescription. Most of these are water-based and remain in the mouth only a short time. In controlled studies, these were found to be more effective than distilled water for relieving general symptoms of xerostomia, and more effective than a glycerine mouth rinse for relieving oral discomfort at night. Recently mucopolysaccharide-containing[110] and gel-based preparations have been introduced that may remain in the mouth longer. For patients with severe xerostomia, use of these preparations may be helpful, especially at night and for those wearing complete dentures. Patients with mild or even moderately severe xerostomia, however, may find frequent sips of water as effective. Oral lubricants containing lemon flavor and citric acid have been suggested to stimulate salivary flow; but for those patients with remaining natural teeth, the acid can damage dental enamel.

REFERENCES

1. Adams J, Wilcox MJ, Trousdale MD et al.: Morphologic and physiologic effects of artificial tear formulations on corneal epithelial derived cells, *Cornea* 11:234-241, 1992.
2. Adamson TC, Fox RI, Frisman DM et al.: Immunohistologic analysis of lymphoid infiltrates in primary Sjögren's syndrome using monoclonal antibodies, *J Immunol* 130:203-208, 1983.
3. Aguilar AJ, Fonseca L, Croxatto JO: Sjögren syndrome: a comparative study of impression cytology of the conjunctiva and the buccal mucosa, and salivary gland biopsy, *Cornea* 10(3):203-206, 1991.
4. Alexander EL: Neuromuscular complications of Sjögren syndrome. In Talal N, Moutsopoulos HM, Kassan S, editors: *Sjögren's syndrome, clinical and immunological aspects,* 61-82, Berlin, 1987, Springer Verlag.
5. Alexander EL: Central nervous system disease in Sjögren's syndrome: new insights into immunopathogenesis, *Rheum Dis Clin N Am* 18:637-672, 1992.
6. Andrade RE, Hagen KA, Manivel JC: Distribution and immunophenotype of the inflammatory cell population in the benign lymphoepithelial lesion (Mikulicz disease), *Hum Pathol* 19:932-941, 1988.
7. Atkinson JC, Travis WD, Slocum L et al.: Serum anti-Sjögren's syndrome-B/La and IgA rheumatoid factor are markers of salivary gland disease activity in primary Sjögren's syndrome, *Arthritis Rheum* 35:1368-1372, 1992.
8. Awan KJ: Laser punctoplasty for the treatment of punctal stenosis, *Am J Ophthalmol* 100:341-342, 1985.
9. Batsakis JG: Lymphoepithelial lesion and Sjögren's syndrome, *Ann Otol Rhinol Laryngol* 96:354-355, 1987.
10. Bizzarro A, Valentini G, DiMartino G et al.: Influence of testosterone therapy on clinical and immunologic features of autoimmune disease associated with Klinefelter's syndrome, *J Clin Endocrinol Metab* 64:32-35, 1987.
11. Bloch KJ, Buchanan WW, Wohl MJ et al.: Sjögren's syndrome: a clinical, pathological and serological study of sixty-two cases, *Medicine* 44:187-231, 1965.
12. Bowen WH, Young DA, Pearson SK: The effects of sucralose on coronal and root-surface caries, *J Dent Res* 69:1485-1487, 1990.
13. Caruso AJ, Sonies BC, Atkinson JC et al.: Objective measures of swallowing in patients with primary Sjögren's syndrome, *Dysphagia* 4:101-105, 1989.
14. Clinch TE et al.: Schirmer's test: a closer look, *Arch Ophthalmol* 101:1383-1386, 1983.
15. Chin SS, Sheibani K, Fishleder A et al.: Monocytoid B-cell lymphoma in patients with Sjögren's syndrome: a clinical pathologic study of 13 patients, *Hum Pathol* 22:422-430, 1991.
16. Chused TM, Kassan SS, Opelz G et al.: Sjögren's syndrome associated with HLA-Dw3, *New Eng J Med* 296:895-897, 1977.
17. Constantopoulos SH, Tsianos EB, Moutsopoulos HM: Pulmonary and gastrointestinal manifestations of Sjögren's syndrome, *Rheum Dis Clin North Am* 18:617-635, 1992.
18. Constantopoulos SH, Moutsopoulos HM: The respiratory system in Sjögren's syndrome. In Talal N, Moutsopoulos HM, Kassan S, editors: *Sjögren syndrome: clinical and immunological aspects,* 83-88, Berlin, 1987, Springer Verlag.
19. Daniels TE, Silverman S, Michalski JP et al.: The oral component of Sjögren's syndrome, *Oral Surg Oral Med Oral Pathol* 39:875-885, 1975.
20. Daniels TE: Labial salivary gland biopsy in Sjögren's syndrome: assessment as a diagnostic criterion in 362 suspected cases, *Arthritis Rheum* 27:147-156, 1984.
21. Daniels TE: Salivary histopathology in diagnosis of Sjögren's syndrome, *Scand J Rheumatol Suppl* 61:36-43, 1986.
22. Daniels TE: Clinical assessment and diagnosis of immunologically mediated salivary gland disease in Sjögren's syndrome, *J Autoimmun* 2:529-541, 1989.
23. Daniels TE: Benign lymphoepithelial lesion and Sjögren's syndrome. In Ellis GL, AuClair PL, Gnepp DR, editors: *Surgical pathology of the salivary glands,* 83-106, Philadelphia, 1991, WB Saunders.
24. Daniels TE, Talal N: Diagnosis and differential diagnosis of Sjögren syndrome. In Talal N, Moutsopoulos HM, Kassan S, editors: *Sjögren's syndrome: clinical and immunological aspects,* 193-199, Berlin, 1987, Springer Verlag.

25. Dawes C: Physiological factors affecting salivary flow rate, oral sugar clearance, and the sensation of dry mouth in man, *J Dent Res* 66:648-653, 1987.

26. Deacon EM, Matthews JB, Potts AJ et al.: Detection of Epstein-Barr virus antigens and DNA in major and minor salivary glands using immunocytochemistry and polymerase chain reaction: possible relationship with Sjögren's syndrome, *J Pathol* 163:351, 1991.

27. DeLuise VP: Management of dry eyes, vol 3, module 3, *Focal Point,* San Francisco, 1985, American Academy of Ophthalmology.

28. DeLuise VP, Peterson WS: The use of topical Healon tears in the management of refractory dry-eye syndrome, *Ann Ophthalmol* 16:823-824, 1984.

29. Dohlman CH: Punctal occlusion in keratoconjunctivitis sicca, *Ophthalmology* 85:1277-1281, 1978.

30. Dreizen S, Brown LR, Daly TE et al.: Prevention of xerostomia-related dental caries in irradiated cancer patients, *J Dent Res* 56:99-104, 1977.

31. Drosos AA, Skopouli FN, Galanopoulou K et al.: Cyclosporin A therapy in patients with primary Sjögren's syndrome: results at one year, *Scand J Rheumatol* 61(suppl):246-249, 1986.

32. Epstein JB, Decoteau WE, Wilkinson A: Effect of sialor in treatment of xerostomia in Sjögren's syndrome, *Oral Surg Oral Med Oral Pathol* 56:495-499, 1983.

33. Feenstra RPG, Tseng SCG: Comparison of fluorescein and rose bengal staining, *Ophthalmology* 99:605-617, 1992.

34. Feenstra RPG, Tseng SCG: What is actually stained by rose bengal, *Arch Ophthalmol* 110:984-993, 1992.

35. Fishleder A, Tubbs R, Hesse B et al.: Uniform detection of immunoglobulin-gene rearrangement in benign lymphoepithelial lesions, *New Eng J Med* 316:1118-1121, 1987.

36. Font RL, Yannoff M, Zimmerman LE: Benign lymphoepithelial lesion of the lacrimal gland and its relationship to Sjögren's syndrome, *Am J Clin Pathol* 48:365-376, 1967.

37. Fox PC, van der Ven PF, Baum BJ et al.: Pilocarpine for the treatment of xerostomia associated with salivary gland dysfunction, *Oral Surg Oral Med Oral Pathol* 61:243-248, 1986.

38. Fox PC, Busch KA, Baum BJ: Subjective reports of xerostomia and objective measures of salivary gland performance, *J Am Dent Assoc* 115:581-584, 1987.

39. Fox PC: Systemic therapy of salivary gland hypofunction, *J Dent Res* 66:689-692, 1987.

40. Fox PC, Atkinson JC, Macynski AA et al.: Pilocarpine treatment of salivary gland hypofunction and dry mouth (xerostomia), *Arch Intern Med* 151:1149-1152, 1991.

41. Fox RI, Carstens SA, Fong S et al.: Use of monoclonal antibodies to analyze peripheral blood and salivary gland lymphocyte subsets in Sjögren's syndrome, *Arthritis Rheum* 25:419-426, 1982.

42. Fox RI, Howell FV, Bone RC et al.: Primary Sjögren's syndrome: clinical and immunopathologic features, *Semin Arthritis Rheum* 14:77-105, 1984.

43. Fox RI, Hugli TE, Lanier LL et al.: Salivary gland lymphocytes in primary Sjögren's syndrome lack lymphocyte subsets defined by Leu-7 and Leu-11 antigens, *J Immunol* 135:207-214, 1985.

44. Fox RI, Cheng R, Michelson JB et al.: Beneficial affects of artificial tears made with autologous serum in patients with keratoconjunctivitis sicca, *Arthritis Rheum* 27:459, 1984.

45. Fox RI, Pearson G, Vaughan JH: Detection of Epstein-Barr virus-associated antigens and DNA in salivary gland biopsies from patients with Sjögren's syndrome, *J Immunol* 137:3162-3168, 1986.

46. Fox RI, Robinson CA, Curd JG et al.: Sjögren's syndrome: proposed criteria for classification, *Arthritis Rheum* 29:577-585, 1986.

47. Fox RI, Hang HI: Pathogenesis of Sjögren's Syndrome, *Rheum Dis Clin North Am* 18:517-538, 1992.

48. Freimark B, Fantozzi R, Bone R et al.: Detection of clonally expanded salivary gland lymphocytes in Sjögren's syndrome, *Arthritis Rheum* 32:859-869, 1989.

49. Friedlaender MH: Ocular manifestations of Sjögren's syndrome: keratoconjunctivitis sicca, *Rheum Dis Clin North Am* 18:591-608, 1992.

50. Frost-Larsen K, Isager H, Manthorpe R: Sjögren's syndrome treated with bromhexine: a randomized clinical study, *Br Med J* 1:1579-1581, 1978.

51. Garry RF, Fermin CD, Hart DJ et al.: Detection of human intracisternal A-type retroviral particle antigenically related to HIV, *Science* 250:1127-1129, 1990.

52. Gaston JSH, Rowe M, Bacon P: Sjögren's syndrome after infection by Epstein-Barr virus, *J Rheumatol* 17:558, 1990.

53. Gilbard JP, Farris L, Santamaria J: Osmolarity of tear microvolumes in keratoconjunctivitis sicca, *Arch Ophthalmol* 96:677-681, 1978.

54. Gilbard JP: Tear film osmolarity and keratoconjunctivitis sicca, *CLAO J* 11:243-250, 1985.

55. Gilbard JP, Farris RL: Tear osmolarity and ocular surface disease in keratoconjunctivitis sicca, *Arch Ophthalmol* 97:1642, 1979.

56. Gilbard JP, Rossi SR, Heyda KG, Dartt DA: Stimulation of tear secretion and treatment of dry-eye disease with 3-isobutyl-1-methylxanthine, *Arch Ophthalmol* 109:672-676, 1991.

57. Goren MB, Goren SB: Diagnostic tests in patients with symptoms of keratoconjunctivitis sicca, *Am J Ophthalmol* 106:570-574, 1988.

58. Greenspan D, Daniels TE: Effectiveness of pilocarpine in postradiation xerostomia, *Cancer* 59:1123-1125, 1987.

59. Hedfors E, Lindahl G: Variation of MHC class I and II antigen expression in relation to lymphocytic infiltrates and interferon-gamma positive cells, *J Rheumatol* 17:743-750, 1990.

60. Hernandez YL, Daniels TE: Oral candidiasis in Sjögren's syndrome: prevalence, clinical correlations and treatment, *Oral Surg Oral Med Oral Pathol* 68:324-329, 1989.

61. Ichijima H, Petrol WM, Jester JV, Cavanaugh HD: Confocal microscopic studies of living rabbit cornea treated with benzalkonium chloride, *Cornea* 11:221-225, 1992.

62. Itescu S, Brancato LJ, Winchester R: A sicca syndrome in HIV infection: association with HLA-DR5 and CD8 lymphocytosis, *Lancet* ii:466-468, 1989.

63. Jones DT, Monroy D, Ji Z et al.: Sjögren's syndrome: cytokine and Epstein-Barr viral gene expression within the conjunctival epithelium. *Invest Ophthalmol Vis Sci* 35:3493-3504, 1994.

64. Jonsson R, Klareskog L, Bäckman K et al.: Expression of HLA-D-locus (DP, DQ, DR)-coded antigens, β2-microglobulin, and the interleukin 2 receptor in Sjögren's syndrome, *Clin Immunol Immunopathol* 45:235-243, 1987.

65. Kassan S, Thomas T, Moutsopolous H: Increased risk of lymphoma in sicca syndrome, *Ann Intern Med* 89:888-892, 1978.

66. Kassan S: Sjögren syndrome. In Talal N, Moutsopoulos HM, Kassan S, editors: *Sjögren syndrome. Clinical and immunological aspects,* 96-101, Berlin, 1987, Springer Verlag.

67. Kazwan RL, Salisbury MA, Ward DA: Spontaneous canine keratoconjunctivitis sicca: a useful model for human keratoconjunctivitis sicca: treatment with cyclosporine eye drops, *Arch Ophthalmol* 106:484-487, 1988.

68. Kervick GN, Pflugfelder SC, Haimovici R et al.: Paracentral rheumatoid corneal ulceration: clinical features and cyclosporin therapy, *Ophthalmology* 99:80-88, 1992.

69. Kilpi A, Bergroth V, Konttinen YT et al.: Lymphocyte infiltrations of the gastric mucosa in Sjögren's syndrome, *Arthritis Rheum* 26:1196-1200, 1983.

70. Korsten MA, Rosman AS, Fishbein S et al.: Chronic xerostomia increases esophageal acid exposure and is associated with esophageal injury, *Am J Med* 90:701, 1991.

71. Laibovitz RA, Solch S, Andriano K et al.: Pilot trial of Cyclosporine 1% ophthalmic ointment in the treatment of keratoconjunctivitis sicca, *Cornea* 12:215-323, 1993.

72. Lamberts DW: Punctal occlusion, *Int Ophthalmol Clin* 27:44-47, 1987.

73. Lamberts DW, Foster CS, Perry HD: Schirmer test after topical anesthesia and tear meniscus height in normal eyes, *Arch Ophthalmol* 97:1082-1085, 1979.

74. Lemp M, Hamill JR: Factors affecting tear break-up in normal eyes, *Arch Ophthalmol* 89:103-105, 1973.

75. Lemp MA, Dohlman CH, Kuwabara T et al.: Dry eye secondary to mucus deficiency, *Trans Am Acad Ophthalmol Otolaryngol* 75:1223-1227, 1971.

76. Lemp MA: General measures in management of the dry eye, *Int Ophthalmol Clin* 27:36-43, 1987.

77. Lemp MA: Artificial tear solutions, *Int Ophthalmol Clin* 13:221-230, 1973.

78. Lemp MA, Gold JB, Wong S et al.: An in vitro study of cornea surface morphologic features in patients with keratoconjunctivitis sicca, *Am J Ophthalmol* 98:426-428, 1984.

79. Limberg MB, McCaa C, Kissling GE, Kufman HE: Topical application of hyaluronic acid and chondroitin sulfate in the treatment of dry eyes, *Am J Ophthalmol* 103:194-197, 1987.

80. Lindahl G, Hedfors E, Klareskog L et al.: Epithelial HLA-DR expression and T lymphocyte subsets in salivary glands in Sjögren's syndrome, *Clin Exp Immunol* 61:475-482, 1985.

81. Lucca JA, Nunez JN, Farris RL: A comparison of diagnostic tests for keratoconjunctivitis sicca: lactoplate, Schirmer, and tear osmolarity, *CLAO J* 16(2):109-112, 1990.

82. Manthorpe R, Axell T, Hansen B et al.: Prevalence of primary Sjögren's syndrome in patients with multiple sclerosis, *Clin Exp Rheumatol* 9:326 1991 (abstract).

83. Mariette X, Golzan J, Clerc D et al.: Detection of Epstein-Barr virus DNA by in situ hybridization and polymerase chain reaction in salivary gland biopsy specimens from patients with Sjögren's syndrome, *Am J Med* 90:286-294, 1991.

84. Manthorpe R, Frost-Larsen K, Isager H, Prause JU: Sjögren's syndrome: a review with emphasis on immunologic features, *Allergy* 36:139-153, 1981.

85. Marx RE, Hartman KS, Rethman KV: A prospective study comparing incisional labial vs incisional parotid biopsies in the detection and confirmation of sarcoidosis, Sjögren's disease, sialosis and lymphoma, *J Rheumatol* 15:621-629, 1988.

86. Misko IS, Schmidt C, Honeyman M et al.: Failure of Epstein-Barr virus-specific cytotoxic T lymphocytes to lyse B cells transformed with the B95-8 strain is mapped to an epitope that associates with the HLA B8 antigen, *Clin Exp Immunol* 87:65-71, 1992.

87. Miyasaka N, Seaman W, Bakshi A et al.: Natural killing activity in Sjögren's syndrome, *Arthritis Rheum* 26:954-960, 1983.

88. Morgan DG, Niederman JC, Miller G et al.: Site of Epstein-Barr virus replication in the oropharynx, *Lancet* ii:1154-1157, 1979.

89. Moutsopolous HM, Mann DL, Johnson AH, Chused TM: Genetic differences between primary and secondary sicca syndrome, *New Eng J Med* 301:761-763, 1979.

90. Musch DC, Sugar A, Meyer RF: Demographic and predisposing factors in corneal ulceration, *Arch Ophthalmol* 101:1545-1548, 1983.

91. Nelson JD, Farris RL: Sodium hyaluronate and polyvinyl alcohol artificial tear preparations. A comparison in patients with keratoconjunctivitis sicca, *Arch Ophthalmol* 106:484-487, 1988.

92. Norn MS: Lacrimal apparatus tests, *Acta Ophthalmol* 43:557-566, 1965.

93. Occhipinti JR, Mosier MA, LaMotte J, Monji GT: Fluorophotometric measurement of human tear turnover rate, *Curr Eye Res* 10:995-1000, 1988.

94. Ormerod DL, Fong LP, Foster CS: Corneal infections in mucosal scarring disorders and Sjögren syndrome, *Am J Ophthalmol* 105:512-518, 1988.

95. Pepose JS, Akata RF, Pflugfelder SC, Voight W: Mononuclear cell phenotypes and immunoglobulin gene rearrangements in lacrimal gland biopsies from patients with Sjögren syndrome, *Ophthalmology* 97:1599-1605, 1990.

96. Pfister RR, Burstein N: The effects of ophthalmic drugs, vehicles, and preservatives on corneal epithelium: a scanning electron microscopic study, *Invest Ophthalmol* 15:246-259, 1976.

97. Pflugfelder SC, Tseng SCG, Pepose JS et al.: Chronic Epstein-Barr viral infection and immunologic dysfunction in patients with aqueous tear deficiency, *Ophthalmology* 97:313-323, 1990.

98. Pflugfelder SC, Huang AJW, Feuer W et al.: Conjunctival cytologic features of primary Sjögren syndrome, *Ophthalmology* 97:985-991, 1990.

99. Pflugfelder SC: Lacrimal gland epithelial and immunopathology of Sjögren syndrome. In Homma M, editor: *Proceedings of the IV international Sjögren syndrome symposium*, Amsterdam, 1994, Kugler.

100. Pflugfelder SC, Wilhelmus KR, Osato MS et al.: The autoimmune nature of aqueous tear deficiency, *Ophthalmology* 93:1513-1517, 1986.

101. Pflugfelder SC, Crouse C, Pereira I, Atherton SS: Amplification of Epstein-Barr virus genomic sequences in blood cells, lacrimal glands, and tears from primary Sjögren syndrome patients, *Ophthalmology* 97:976-984, 1990.

102. Pflugfelder SC, Crouse CA, Monroy D et al.: Epstein-Barr virus and the lacrimal gland pathology of Sjögren syndrome, *Am J Pathol* 143:49-64, 1993.

103. Pflugfelder SC, Roussel TJ, Culbertson WW: Primary Sjögren syndrome after infectious mononucleosis, *JAMA* 257:1049-1050, 1987 (letter).

103a. Pflugfelder SC et al.: manuscript in publication.

104. Pollack FM, McNiece MT: The treatment of dry eyes with Na hyaluronate (Healon®), *Cornea* 1:133-136, 1982.

105. Prause JU, Frost-Larsen K, Hoj L et al.: Lacrimal and salivary secretion in Sjögren syndrome: the effect of systemic treatment with bromhexine, *Acta Ophthalmol* 62:489-497, 1984.

106. Prause JU et al.: Rose Bengal score: a possible key parameter when evaluating disease level and progression in primary Sjögren's syndrome, *J Autoimmun* 2(4):501-507, 1989.

107. Provost TT, Watson R: Cutaneous manifestations of Sjögren syndrome, *Rheum Dis Clin North Am* 18:609-620, 1992.

108. Raphael M, Bellefgih S, Piette J Ch et al.: Conjunctival biopsy in Sjögren's syndrome: correlations between histologic and immunohistochemical features, *Histopathology* 13:191-202, 1988.

109. Reveille JD, Arnett FC: The immunogenetics of Sjögren's syndrome, *Rheum Dis Clin North Am* 18:609-620, 1992.

110. Rhodus NL, Schuh M: Effectiveness of three artificial salivas as assessed by mucoprotective relativity, *J Dent Res* 70:407, 1991 (abstract 1133).

111. Ronen D et al.: A spectrophotometric method for quantitative determination of lysozyme in human tears: description and evaluation of the methods and screening of 60 healthy subjects, *Invest Ophthalmol* 14:479-484, 1975.

112. Rowe D, Griffiths M, Stewart J et al.: HLA class I and II, interleukin 2, and the interleukin 2 receptor expression on labial biopsy specimens from patients with Sjögren's syndrome, *Ann Rheum Dis* 46:580, 1987.

113. Saito I, Servenius B, Compton T, Fox RI: Detection of Epstein-Barr virus DNA by polymerase chain reaction in blood and tissue biopsies from patients with Sjögren's syndrome, *J Exp Med* 169:2191-2198, 1989.

114. Saito EH, Ariga H, Sullivan DA: Impact of androgen therapy in Sjögren syndrome: hormonal influence on lymphocyte populations and IA expression in lacrimal glands of MRL/Mp-1pr/1pr mice, *Invest Ophthalmol* 33:2537-2545, 1992.

115. Sarada K: Histopathological studies of the lacrimal gland in Sjögren's syndrome. II. Correlation with histologic findings in labial salivary glands, *Folia Ophthalmologica Japonica* 32:2457-2470, 1981.

116. Schmid U, Helbron D, Lennert K: Development of malignant lymphoma in myoepithelial sialadenitis (Sjögren's syndrome), *Virchows Arch [A]* 395:11-43, 1982.

117. Schiødt M, Oxholm P, Jacobsen A: Treatment of xerostomia in patients with primary Sjögren's syndrome with sulfarlem, *Scand J Rheumatol Suppl* 61:250-252, 1986.

118. Schiødt M, Greenspan D, Daniels TE et al.: Parotid gland enlargement and xerostomia associated with labial sialadenitis in HIV-infected patients, *J Autoimmunity* 2:415-425, 1989.

119. Scott J: Qualitative and quantitative observations on the histology of human labial salivary glands obtained postmortem, *J Biol Buccale* 8:187-200, 1980.

120. Scully C: Viruses and salivary gland disease: are there associations? *Oral Surg Oral Med Oral Pathol* 66:179-183, 1988.

121. Shah F, Rapini RP, Arnett FC et al.: Association of labial salivary gland histopathology with clinical and serological features of connective tissue diseases, *Arthritis Rheum* 33:1682-1687, 1990.

122. Sjögren H, Bloch KJ: Keratoconjunctivitis sicca and the Sjögren's syndrome, *Surv Opthalmol* 16(3):145-159, 1971.

123. Sjögren HS: Zur kenntnis der keratoconjunctivitis sicca (Keratitis folliformis bei hypofunktion der tranendrusen), *Acta Ophthalmol (kobenhavn)* 11:1-151, 1933.

124. Shearn MA: Sjögren's syndrome. In Smith LH, editor: *Major problems in medicine*, vol 2, Philadelphia, 1971, WB Saunders.

125. Soong HK, Martin NF, Wagoner MB et al.: Topical retinoid therapy for squamous metaplasia of various ocular surface disorders, *Ophthalmology* 95:1442-1446, 1998.

126. Speight PM, Cruchley A, Williams DM: Epithelial HLA-DR expression in labial salivary glands in Sjögren's syndrome and non-specific sialadenitis, *J Oral Pathol Med* 18:178-183, 1989.

127. Sullivan DA: Hormonal influence on the secretory immune system of the eye. In Freier S, editor. *The Neuroendocrine-Immune Network*, 199-238, Boca Raton, 1990, CRC Press.

128. Tabbara KF, Frayha RA: Alternate-day steroid therapy for patients with primary Sjögren's syndrome, *Ann Ophthalmol* 358-361, 1983.

128a. Talal N: Renal disease in Sjögren syndrome. In Talal N, Moutsopoulos HM, Kassan S, editors: *Sjögren syndrome: clinical and immunological aspects,* 96-101, Berlin, 1987, Springer Verlag.

129. Talal N, Asofsky R, Lightbody P: Immunoglobulin synthesis by salivary gland lymphoid cells in Sjögren's syndrome, *J Clin Invest* 49:49-54, 1970.

130. Talal N, Sylvester RA, Daniels TE et al.: T and B lymphocytes in peripheral blood and tissue lesions in Sjögren's syndrome, *J Clin Invest* 53:180-189, 1974.

131. Talal N, Dauphinée MJ, Dang H et al.: Detection of serum antibodies to retroviral proteins in patients with primary Sjögren's syndrome (autoimmune exocrinopathy), *Arthritis Rheum* 33:774-781, 1990.

132. Trevino H, Tsianos EB, Schenker S: Gastrointestinal and hepatobiliary features. In Talal N, Moutsopoulos HM, Kassan S, editors: *Sjögren's syndrome: clinical and immunological aspects,* 89-95, Berlin, 1987, Springer Verlag.

133. Tseng SCG, Maumenn AE, Stark WJ et al.: Topical retinoid treatment for various dry-eye disorders, *Ophthalmology* 92:717-727, 1985.

134. Tsubota K: The importance of the schirmer test with nasal stimulation, *Am J Ophthalmol* 111:106-108, 1991.

135. Tsubota K, Terauchi K, Shimuta M et al.: Detection of granulozyme A and perforin expression in lacrimal gland of Sjögren's syndrome, *Invest Ophthalmol Vis Sci* 34:823, 1993 (ARVO abstracts).

136. Tsubota K, Fujishima H, Toda I et al.: Increased level of Epstein-Barr virus DNA in lacrimal and salivary glands of patients with Sjögren's syndrome, *Invest Ophthalmol Vis Sci* 32:807, 1991 (ARVO abstracts).

137. Tsubota K, Yamada M, Naoi S: Specular microscopic observation of human corneal epithelial abnormalities, *Ophthalmology* 98:184-191, 1991.

138. Tuberville AW, Frederick WR, Wood P: Punctal occlusion in tear deficiency syndromes, *Ophthalmology* 89:1170-1172, 1982.

139. van Bijsterveld OP: Diagnostic tests in sicca syndrome, *Arch Ophthalmol* 82:10-14, 1969.

140. Venables PJW, Teo CG, Baboonian C et al.: Persistence of Epstein-Barr virus in salivary gland biopsies from healthy individuals and patients with Sjögren syndrome, *Clin Exp Immunol* 75:359-364, 1989.

141. Vendramini ACLM, Soo C, Sullivan DA: Testosterone-induced suppression of autoimmune disease in lacrimal tissue of a mouse model (NZB/NZW F1) of Sjögren's syndrome, *Invest Ophthalmol Vis Sci* 32:3002-3006, 1991.

142. Vitali C, Bombardieri S: Diagnostic criteris for Sjögren syndrome: the state of the art, *Clin Exp Rheumatol* 8(suppl 5):13-16, 1990.

143. Whitcher JP: Clinical diagnosis of the dry eye, *Int Ophthalmol Clin* 27:7-24, 1987.

144. Whittingham S, McNeilage J, Mackay IR: Primary Sjögren's syndrome after infectious mononucleosis, *Ann Intern Med* 102:490-493, 1987.

145. Wieczorek R, Jakobiec FA, Sachs EH, Knowles DM: The immunoarchitecture of the normal human lacrimal gland: relevancy for understanding pathologic conditions, *Ophthalmology* 95:100-109, 1988.

146. Willis RM, Folberg R, Kratchmer JH, Holland EJ: The treatment of aqueous-deficient dry eye with removal punctal plugs: a clinical and impression-cytologic study, *Ophthalmology* 84:514-518, 1987.

147. Wise CM, Agudelo CA, Semble EL et al.: Comparison of parotid and minor salivary gland biopsy specimens in the diagnosis of Sjögren's syndrome, *Arthritis Rheum* 31:662-666, 1988.

148. Wolf H, Haus M, Wilmes E: Persistence of Epstein-Barr virus in the parotid gland, *J Virol* 51:795-798, 1984.

149. Yamaoka K, Miyasaka N, Yamamoto K: Possible involvement of Epstein-Barr virus in polyclonal B cell activation in Sjögren's syndrome, *Arthritis Rheum* 31:1014-1021, 1988.

150. Yen M, Pflugfelder SC, Crouse CA, Atherton SS: Immunohistochemical evaluation of cytoskeletal antigen expression in human ocular mucosal associated lymphoid tissue, *Invest Ophthalmol Vis Sci* 33:3235-3241, 1992.

151. Zappia RJ, Milder B: Lacrimal drainage function, *Am J Ophthalmol* 74:16-62, 1972.

24 Meibomian Gland Dysfunction and Rosacea

R. WAYNE BOWMAN, JAMES P. McCULLEY, JAMES V. JESTER

Rosacea is a chronic oculodermal disorder, primarily affecting the sebaceous glands of the face and the meibomian glands of the eyelids. Some patients develop meibomian gland dysfunction (ocular rosacea) as part of the cutaneous syndrome, and others have changes limited to the eyelid margins. Chronic blepharitis is occasionally associated with other anterior segment changes including conjunctivitis, episcleritis, marginal keratitis, and corneal neovascularization.[15,113]

Blepharitis is an inflammation of the eyelids and other ocular structures with important long-term implications. Maintaining a healthy patient-physician relationship in the management of this chronic disorder can be a time-consuming and challenging task. Ongoing assessment of the complex interaction that exists between the lids and the ocular surface is required to determine the optimal treatment that will delay or prevent serious sequelae.

HISTORICAL BACKGROUND

Many of the facial features of rosacea have been recognized for centuries. In 1387 Chaucer described an individual with the cutaneous characteristics of rosacea, and in 1480 Ghirlandaio painted a grandfather with obvious rhinophyma.[90] Ophthalmologists, however, have been slow to associate blepharitis with other skin changes. In the 1940s Thygeson[106] emphasized the importance of *Staphylococcus aureus* as a cause of lid disease, sometimes in conjunction with seborrheic blepharitis. It later became evident that *S. aureus* was not the sole organism involved in acute blepharitis, and coagulase-negative staphylococci were found to be more common.[23] More importantly, seborrheic blepharitis, alone or in combination with meibomitis, became widely accepted as an entity with a spectrum of clinical manifestations. In 1864 Arlt had first described the association between conjunctivitis and keratitis in patients with rosacea. Blepharitis was subsequently identified as the principal ophthalmic manifestation of rosacea. Recent work has detailed the clinical findings in the spectrum of meibomian gland

dysfunction.[72,73] Whether alone or in association with rosacea, meibomian gland dysfunction is now recognized as a common cause of chronic lid disease.

EPIDEMIOLOGY

Eyelid disease is an important part of ophthalmic practice. Meibomian gland dysfunction is the most common cause of blepharitis,[45,69] and up to 20% to 40% of patients undergoing routine eye examinations show evidence of meibomian gland dysfunction.[43] Blepharitis is also an important reason for patient visits in general medicine. Two British studies showed that ophthalmic problems account for 2% to 6% of outpatient visits to a general practitioner or acute-care facility[27,74] and that blepharitis or conjunctivitis is diagnosed in 70% of these patients. Meibomian gland dysfunction and rosacea may be even more common than generally appreciated. Three fourths of patients referred to a rheumatology clinic with a preliminary diagnosis of cutaneous lupus erythematosus were found to have rosacea.[9]

Patients affected with rosacea are usually between 40 and 60 years old. Blepharitis can occur during acne vulgaris, but rosacea and meibomian gland dysfunction are uncommon in children.[28] Age-related changes may contribute to the increased occurrence of meibomian gland dysfunction in older individuals.[46] There are no definite gender or ethnic differences. Clinical features may be more easily seen in fair-skinned people from northern Europe, but rosacea occurs in blacks[16,91] and other populations.

Epidemiologic studies pertaining to blepharitis are limited by uncertainties in the type of lid margin disease. A clinical classification scheme has been proposed that categorizes the principal forms of blepharitis.[71] By combining the proportion of patients with seborrheic blepharitis and meibomitis, the spectrum of changes involved in meibomian gland dysfunction accounts for a majority of patients with blepharitis. Clinical signs of meibomian gland dysfunction are present in three fourths of patients with lid margin inflammation. About one fourth of patients with rosacea and meibomian gland dysfunction present with eye problems only, one fourth develop eye and skin changes together, and one half have skin lesions first. Over one half of patients with a chalazion have the skin changes of rosacea.[60]

Conjunctivitis is often an associated finding. Corneal involvement is relatively uncommon, although an incidence of 5% or higher has been reported. Keratitis and corneal neovascularization may be more common in patients with severe disease.

CLINICAL FEATURES

Many of the findings of meibomian gland dysfunction and rosacea (see box) are subtle and easily overlooked. The most frequent ocular symptoms are foreign-body sensation, discomfort, and burning.[47] There is some overlap with age-related changes in lid thickness, vascularity, and keratinization.[46]

The lid is often thickened, and the posterior lid margin is rounded, thereby interfering with normal apposition of the lid to the globe. Vascularization of the lid margin can extend around the meibomian orifices. Hyperkeratinization at the orifices and irregularity of the lid margin may also develop. The meibomian gland orifices may appear to open in mucosal tissue because of the anteroplacement of the mucocutaneous junction or, more commonly, the retroplacement of the mucocutaneous junction with keratinization and posterior movement of the orifices. One manifestation of keratinization or epithelialization of the orifices is capping.[54] Pouting, dilatation, and reduction in the number of meibomian gland orifices may be observed. The meibomian gland secretions are normally clear, but in meibomian gland dysfunction they may vary from a cloudy, fluid secretion to a

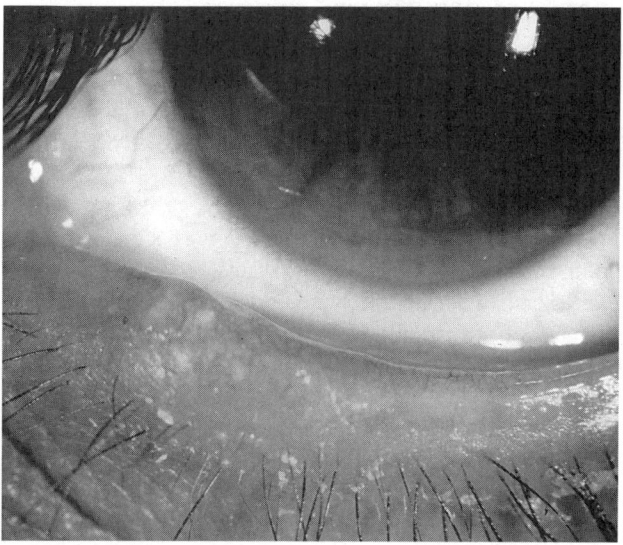

Fig. 24-1. Inflammatory nodule of the eyelid margin.

semisolid plug or toothpastelike strand. Frequently, this material is not true meibum but consists of keratinized epithelial cells.[40]

Meibomitis can be either localized or generalized. Localized meibomitis presents as a posterior (internal) hordeolum, chalazion, or spotty meibomitis secondary to anterior blepharitis. Generalized meibomitis includes meibomian seborrhea and can be associated with keratoconjunctivitis.

Localized Meibomitis: Hordeolum and Chalazion

A posterior hordeolum is an inflammatory or infectious process involving an individual meibomian gland.[22] Typically, the onset is abrupt and painful. The initial inflammatory signs may be localized around the orifice of the involved meibomian gland. The entire lid may become erythematous and edematous. Rarely, a posterior hordeolum may progress to orbital cellulitis or result in cavernous sinus thrombosis.[33,110] A yellowish nodule may be apparent through the tarsal conjunctiva and may spontaneously rupture to drain posteriorly through the tarsal conjunctiva. Secretions from within the involved gland are often either nonexpressible or purulent. As the inflammation resolves, a sterile nodule may remain.

A chalazion is a noninfectious, localized inflammatory process involving an individual meibomian gland. Although it may arise from a posterior hordeolum (Fig. 24-1), it more commonly develops de novo. For unknown reasons, a lipogranulomatous reaction develops, presumably to extravasated meibomian secretions. The course is more indolent and produce fewer symptoms (such as pain and inflammation) than a posterior hordeolum. Chalazia may rarely be suppurative, but more commonly, they slowly increase in size, then shrink a variable amount. Many completely re-

---

OCULAR SIGNS OF ROSACEA

Common
  Meibomitis
  Lid margin telangiectasia
  Conjunctival hyperemia
  Papillary conjunctivitis
  Foam, mucin particles, and excess oil in tear film
  Reduced tear-film breakup time and volume
  Punctate corneal epithelial granularity and erosions
  Episcleritis
  Hordeolum
  Chalazion
Less Common
  Entropion
  Marginal corneal infiltration
  Corneal neovascularization
Rare
  Corneal perforation
  Scleritis
  Iritis

sorb. Spontaneous drainage usually develops posteriorly but can occur anteriorly through the eyelid skin. Cosmetic complaints are common. An upper lid chalazion may induce substantial corneal astigmatism. Some patients develop recurrent chalazia.

Generalized Meibomitis

There is a spectrum of posterior lid margin disease. Meibomian gland dysfunction represents the minimally inflamed end, and generalized meibomitis indicates diffuse lid margin inflammation. Confusion in terminology has resulted in different authors using these terms in different ways.

The term *meibomian seborrhea* was coined in 1922,[20] and this condition has been included as a subset of seborrheic blepharitis.[54] But meibomian seborrhea is not seborrheic meibomitis because there is no inflammation. Meibomian seborrhea characteristically has excessive meibomian secretions with little or no inflammation.[108] There is a buildup of excess secretions with the meibomian glands that can be easily expressed. The expressed secretions are relatively normal, as they are liquid and fairly clear. Solidification is uncommon unless there is inflammation within the meibomian ducts. It has been assumed, but not established, that meibomian seborrhea is the result of overproduction of secretions by the meibomian glands. Ductule stasis with a slow secretory rate could also result in an apparent excess of secretions, but the rapid reaccumulation of excessive secretions after therapeutic expression makes overproduction more likely.[12]

Patients with abnormal meibomian gland secretions often have moderate-to-marked burning that is most pronounced in the morning. Clinical signs of meibomian seborrhea include easily expressed meibomian secretions, a foamy tear meniscus, and minimal inflammation (usually consisting of bulbar conjunctival infection).[71,108] Anterior seborrheic blepharitis may be present. Dermatologic evaluation has revealed generalized sebaceous gland dysfunction.[70,71] It has not been established whether or not excessive (but normal) meibomian secretions are capable of producing disease. The presence of foam in the tear meniscus and on the outer lid margin suggests that the excessive fatty acid soaps and abnormal secretions contain biochemical abnormalities responsible for the clinical signs.[80] Free fatty acids are irritating to the skin; and although they have not been shown irritating to the lid and ocular surface, this is likely.[31,55,87]

Meibomitis is produced by inflammation surrounding the meibomian gland orifices. Stagnation and solidification of the meibomian gland secretions produce dilatation of the acini and ductules of the meibomian glands. This dilatation can be demonstrated by transilluminating the eyelids with a fiberoptic light source and by using special infrared photographic techniques.[49,105] A prominent feature of primary meibomitis is the formation of semisolid or solid plugs that

contribute to stagnation and buildup of secretions within the glands. Pressure on the tarsus may express these plugs and the underlying secretions. The stagnant secretions are white or yellow—not as a result of inflammatory cells—but rather because of their viscosity; just as candle wax is relatively clear when liquid and opaque when solid.

The diagnosis of secondary meibomitis is made in the context of concomitant anterior lid margin blepharitis such as staphylococcal blepharitis or seborrheic blepharitis. Secondary meibomian gland involvement tends to be patchy with clusters of glands involved. The lid tissue surrounding the affected glands is inflamed, and there is stagnation of secretions with dilatation of the glands and their ductules. Other ocular findings are identical to those found in primary meibomitis, and severity correlates to the extent of secondary meibomian gland involvement. Staphylococcal growth on the lid margins probably contributes to the inflammatory signs,[107] but rarely do bacteria invade the meibomian glands to the extent that a suppurative meibomitis develops. In the rare case with a meibomian gland abscess, however, *S. aureus* is usually the cause.[65] In secondary meibomitis, staphylococci may be contributory, not as a direct infection, but in relation to enzymatic activity on meibomian lipids.

Ocular Surface Changes

Full-blown meibomian gland blockage, dilatation, and inflammation will produce inflammation of the ocular surface. The tarsus becomes thickened, and the meibomian glands may pout above the lid surface. About one third of patients with rosacea have diminished tear production,[59] and pH changes may occur.[1,14] A loss of the normal lipid layer of the precorneal tear film leads to a rapid tear breakup time that produces dry spots in the interpalpebral fissure zone. The tear-film abnormalities account for the frequent complaints of blurred vision, tearing, and burning that occur during meibomian gland dysfunction.

Conjunctival injection is common. Blepharoconjunctivitis usually displays more inflammation inferiorly. A follicular reaction can be occasionally seen in the inferior fornix, but papillary conjunctivitis is more typical. Contact lens wearers with meibomian gland dysfunction are prone to develop giant papillary conjunctivitis,[68] and episcleritis sometimes occurs.[11]

The corneal changes probably result from a combination of factors. Tear-film instability, manifested by a rapid tear breakup time, leads to inconsistent ocular surface wetting. The resultant superficial punctate epitheliopathy often occurs in the inferior one third and interpalpebral fissure areas of the cornea, and is best demonstrated with rose-bengal staining. Other factors that may contribute to epithelial keratopathy include the irregular lid margin and tarsal conjunctival surface, inflammatory mediators, abnormal meibomian lipids, and keratin in the meibomian secretions.

The corneal changes can be diffuse and may lead to ul-

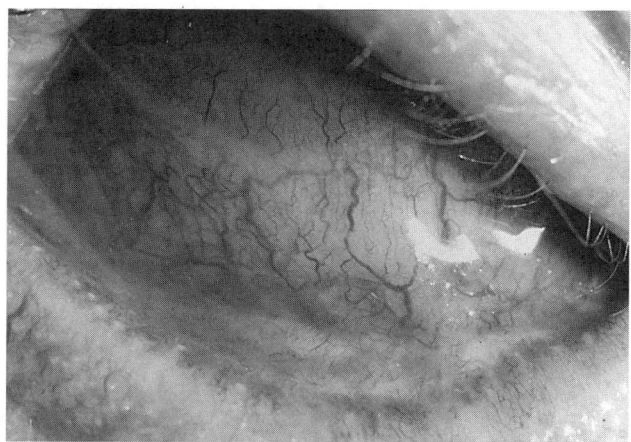

Fig. 24-2. Meibomian gland dysfunction with chronic blepharo-conjunctivitis and corneal neovascularization associated with rosacea.

ceration, peripheral infiltration, and neovascularization.[32] Visual acuity can be decreased because of ocular surface irregularity or scarring (Fig. 24-2). Anterior membrane changes indistinguishable from map-dot-fingerprint dystrophy may be present. Phlyctenular keratoconjunctivitis may develop at the limbus and can progress centrally with repeated attacks; iritis also has been reported.[113] Ulcerative keratitis can rarely progress to corneal perforation.[32]

Dermatitis

Clinical recognition of rosacea may require dermatologic consultation. Ocular signs may develop before cutaneous changes,[11] but abnormalities in the facial skin can be found in many patients. Flushing is generally the earliest manifestation and involves the cheeks, forehead, nose, chin, neck, and upper chest. Telangiectasias develop and result in chronic erythema in the same areas as the flushing. Whereas most patients show no further progression of their disease, others develop papules and pustules.[88] With long-term involvement, hypertrophy of the nasal sebaceous glands and connective tissue and subcutaneous lymphedema can produce rhinophyma.[22]

PATHOGENESIS

The eyelid margins are a transition zone between the skin and the conjunctival mucous membrane. Besides mechanically protecting the eye, the eyelids create a continuous tear film with an anterior lipid layer made of meibomian gland oils.[18] The spreading behavior of the meibomian lipids is important for tear-film integrity.[51,52] Meibomian gland lipids reduce tear-film evaporation[67] and retard nocturnal drying.[4,14] By stabilizing the tear film through a lowering of its surface tension, meibomian lipids prevent tears from spilling over the lid margin. Meibomian gland secretions also seal the ocular surface from contamination by sebum.

TABLE 24-1 CLINICOPATHOLOGIC CORRELATES OF ROSACEA DERMATITIS AND BLEPHAROCONJUNCTIVITIS

Clinical Features	Pathologic Findings
Facial erythema and telangiectasia	Perivascular infiltration with lymphocytes, monocytes, and plasma cells
Papulopustular dermatitis	Disruption of superficial dermal collagen with elastosis
Rhinophyma	Sebaceous gland hypertrophy with follicular dilatation and increased connective tissue
Meibomian gland inspissation	Keratinization of orifice with lymphocytic infiltration around dilated meibomian glands
Conjunctivitis	Vascular dilatation with subepithelial infiltration by lymphocytes and epithelioid cells

The meibomian glands open just anterior to the mucocutaneous junction. This position is essential for proper delivery of meibomian gland lipid to the precorneal tear film. The meibomian glands are visible through the conjunctiva within the tarsal plate and are more easily seen in younger patients.[12] Acinar lobules are yellow, grapelike clusters on either side of the main duct of these tubuloacinar glands.[101] The duct openings normally are flush with the surface of the lid margin. The inner cuffs of the meibomian gland orifice and duct are partially composed of keratinized squamous epithelium.[50] Keratinization of the meibomian ductules may play an important role in the pathogenesis of meibomitis.[48,49] Keratin proteins are present in the meibomian secretion of experimental animals.[81] Histopathologic examinations (Table 24-1) of patients with meibomian gland dysfunction have shown abnormalities of meibomian gland keratinization (involving the ductules) similar to those in sebaceous glands of patients with rosacea.[37]

Bacterial Lipases

The role of bacteria in meibomian disease is more complex than previously thought. Bacteria such as staphylococci play a direct role in posterior (internal) hordeolum, a lesion analogous to an acneiform infection of the eyelid. Bacteria may also play an important part in chronic meibomian gland disease. Patients with blepharitis have more bacteria colonizing their eyelid margin and skin.[34]

Some bacteria present on the lid margin possess enzymes

capable of altering meibomian gland secretions. For example, lipases break down lipids into free fatty acids that can destabilize the tear film. Production of these enzymes by bacteria on the eyelid margin could alter the meibomian gland secretions near the gland orifices. This theory is consistent with the observation that expression of material from deeper within the meibomian gland will normalize the tear film's breakup time. S. aureus, coagulase-negative staphylococci, lipophilic corynebacteria, and Propionibacterium acnes—the most commonly isolated bacteria from the eyelid margin—exhibit lipolytic enzyme activity.[25] S. aureus produces cholesteryl esterase, fatty wax esterase, and triglyceride lipase. P. acnes possesses fatty wax esterase and triglyceride lipase but lacks cholesteryl esterase. Lipolytic enzyme production by coagulase-negative staphylococci is variable, but the production of fatty wax esterase correlates with meibomian gland dysfunction. In addition, cholesteryl esterase production by coagulase-negative staphylococci correlates with the presence of not only meibomian gland dysfunction but mixed seborrheic and staphylococcal blepharitis as well. Differences in lipase production by coagulase-negative staphylococci could account for some of the clinical variability in blepharitis patients.[25] Coagulase-negative staphylococcal strains capable of hydrolyzing cholesteryl oleate are present in greater amounts on the lids of patients with meibomian gland dysfunction.

Altered Lipid Composition

Meibomian gland secretions of normal subjects are of two types: those with very low levels of both cholesterol esters and esterified unsaturated fatty acids (the normal cholesterol absent, NCA, group) and those with high levels of cholesterol esters and esterified unsaturated fatty acids (the normal cholesterol present, NCP, group). Only when cholesterol esters are present do wax and sterol esters containing unsaturated fatty acids accumulate. It is known that meibomian gland fatty alcohols can be formed from the corresponding fatty acids.[56] In meibomian gland dysfunction the ratio of unsaturated C18 fatty acids to cholesterol in the wax and sterol esters is significantly different from the NCP group.[98] Additionally, patients with meibomian gland dysfunction possess an alcohol not present in patients with other conditions. The presence and hydrolysis of cholesterol esters of meibomian secretions may contribute to the proliferation of staphylococci.[100] Even in the two normal subgroups, the normal cholesterol present (NCP) subgroup contained twice the number of coagulase-negative staphylococci showing cholesterol ester lipase activity. This increase may be from a change in bacterial growth rate caused by the presence of cholesterol esters.[39]

Abnormalities in meibomian gland secretions may be the primary cause of meibomian gland dysfunction. Obstruction of the meibomian gland, rather than inflammation, may be the primary disorder as inflammatory cells are absent in many biopsy specimens obtained from patients with meibomian gland dysfunction.[37] Although earlier reports of pooled meibomian gland secretions failed to confirm any alterations of meibomian lipids during meibomian gland dysfunction,[19,54,78] these studies involved small numbers of patients and used relatively insensitive techniques. With more extensive chromatography, differences in minor fatty acids suggest that an altered lipid composition contributes to the disease process.[24]

Biochemical abnormalities of meibomian secretion could result from several different mechanisms. There may be a basic defect in lipid secretion, or there may be secondary changes that arise from intrinsic abnormalities of the ductules of the meibomian glands. Exogenous alteration of secretions (caused by the action of bacterial enzymes) may also occur at the lid surface. Lipid abnormalities could also result from aberrant peroxisomal function or from an abnormal interaction of peroxisomes with endoplasmic reticulum.[99]

Fatty waxes and cholesterol esters make up 60% of meibomian gland secretions.[79] Triglycerides constitute less than 5% of meibomian lipids but are also an important component.[78] Patients with meibomian gland dysfunction show a shift in the fatty wax-sterol ester fraction, with significantly lower amounts of fatty wax esters and higher levels of sterol esters. This shift may raise the melting point of meibomian secretions as sterol esters have higher melting points than wax esters. Even small changes in lipid composition can have large effects on the physical properties of lipid secretions. Animal studies have demonstrated that triglycerides containing (n-10) fatty acids have melting points at least 15°C higher than either the (n-9) or the (n-11) isomers.[38] A higher percentage of saturated fatty acids and alcohols would result in a higher melting point and a more viscous meibomian secretion. Increased viscosity and a higher melting point could then lead to glandular blockage, secretion stagnation, and lid margin changes. No comparable alterations in meibomian gland secretion have been detected in patients with other types of blepharitis. The types of triglycerides and the presence of unsaturated fatty acids may also be important. As analyses become more complete and precise, it is possible that a specific lipid profile will prove to be typical of meibomian gland dysfunction.

Sebaceous Gland Dysfunction

The pathogenesis of rosacea remains an enigma. Many hypotheses have been proposed including bacterial infection, climatic exposure, psychosomatic alterations, and an abnormality of vasodilatation.[15] Cultures of the skin surface and skin biopsies of patients with rosacea have not shown a consistent bacteriologic cause.[64] Skin surface swabs typically grow coagulase-negative staphylococci and S. aureus. Skin biopsies are sterile nearly half the time and yield normal flora in the remainder. Analyses of bacterial enzymes similar to studies performed on patients with meibomian gland dysfunction have not been done, although bacterial lipases may play a role in diffuse sebaceous gland disease. Antibiotics seem to have a beneficial effect on the symptoms of rosacea patients.[65]

A role for climatic exposure has been proposed because of the observation that two thirds of rosacea patients have a flare-up of disease activity during the spring.[102] An equal number of rosacea patients, however, report exacerbation of symptoms during cold weather as do with hot weather. Other patients have ascribed seasonal fluctuations to sun and wind exposure.[90,106,113]

A variety of gastrointestinal disorders (including alkaline gastric secretions, achlorhydria, and jejunal mucosal atrophy) have been linked to patients with rosacea. None of these conditions, however, can be consistently linked with rosacea.[90,106]

Biopsies of rosaceous skin show hypertrophy and plugging of sebaceous glands. Implicating rosacea as a diffuse sebaceous gland disease agrees with finding meibomian gland dysfunction in many patients with rosacea. Ductule and lipid abnormalities are often present in early rosaceous dermal lesions. Although sebaceous gland hypertrophy is not always seen in early rosacea,[66] these changes may take time to develop. Significant lipid differences have not yet been demonstrated between patients with rosacea and normal controls, but these studies have only examined total fatty acid composition.[84] More detailed analyses of the exact composition of skin lipid in the presence of rosacea may uncover differences similar to those found in meibomian gland dysfunction.

Hyperemia and Inflammation

Hyperemia is a common feature of both rosacea and meibomitis, but the cause of dilated blood vessels of the face and along the lid margins is not readily apparent. The presence of rhinophyma in some carcinoid patients suggests an abnormality in the release of endogenous substances,[103] but the levels of specific metabolites are normal in rosacea patients.[92] Ethanol-induced flushing and the inhibition by naloxone pretreatment suggest either an abnormally high level of endorphins or an increased sensitivity to endorphins.[8] An abnormality in neurotransmitter release or sensitivity, however, has not been proved. More likely, vascular dilatation is secondary to an altered connective-tissue framework in the dermis. This alteration in the skin of rosacea patients apparently makes them susceptible to solar damage; greater elastotic degeneration occurs in patients with rosacea—even when compared with people who have greater sun exposure.

Inflammation is an occasional component of meibomian gland dysfunction and of the cutaneous changes of rosacea. Biopsy findings obtained from patients with rosacea suggest a hypersensitivity reaction.[66] The upper dermis exhibits prominent vascular dilatation with perivascular infiltration composed of histiocytes, lymphocytes, and (occasionally) plasma cells. In papular rosacea, granulomatous inflammation with multinucleated giant cells may be present. Most lymphocytes found in rosacea lesions are helper-inducer (CD4) T cells.[93] The conjunctiva in ocular rosacea is also infiltrated by inflammatory cells, (mainly CD4 cells), and the response resembles a cell-mediated hypersensitivity reaction.[42] Immunoglobulin and complement deposition have also been reported,[63] although immunoglobulin deposition might passively occur from chronic vasodilatation. Rosacea patients have a higher incidence of autoimmune disorders,[63] and circulating antinuclear antibody of IgM type is occasionally detected.

Lymphocytes sometimes surround degenerating *Demodex* spp. mites. *Demodex* spp. infestation can trigger an immune response,[93,96] and *Demodex* spp. mites can be pathogenic when present in extremely large numbers. *Demodex folliculorum* has been implicated in the pathogenesis of rosacea and blepharitis, but many investigators dispute its importance.[6,89] *Demodex* spp. do feed on sebum, and treatments effective against *Demodex* spp. have resulted in improvement of rosacea.[42]

DIFFERENTIAL DIAGNOSIS

Various causes of lid margin inflammation must be evaluated by a careful examination of the lids, lashes, conjunctiva, and face. Physical examination may reveal clues to the particular type of blepharitis. Many causes of dermatoblepharitis have distinctive findings such as herpes simplex blepharitis, molluscum contagiosum, lice infestation, and atopic dermatitis. Medication toxicity can be a component of chronic blepharoconjunctivitis, especially as patients with meibomian gland dysfunction may have seen multiple physicians and tried several topical agents. Distinguishing meibomian gland dysfunction from staphylococcal blepharitis is important. Laboratory studies are usually not indicated in patients with rosacea, but lid margin cultures may assist in the diagnosis of staphylococcal blepharoconjunctivitis.

Blepharitis may contribute to tear-film instability. Dry eye syndrome may coexist with meibomian gland dysfunction and rosacea.[36,59] Careful attention should be paid to the tear meniscus, tear breakup time, and ocular surface staining pattern with rose bengal. Schirmer testing should be considered. Speculations that primary Sjögren syndrome[83] may be caused by a dysfunctional immune reaction at the ocular surface suggests that a similar phenomenon could contribute to obstruction and inflammation of the meibomian gland ductules.

The clinical diagnosis of rosacea can be difficult. The presence of facial telangiectasis or papules does not confirm the diagnosis. Rosacea can be indistinguishable from acne vulgaris in young patients, except for the presence of comedos in the latter. Telangiectasia increases with aging, sun exposure, corticosteroid use, and alcohol ingestion. Flushing may occur in alcohol abuse and in carcinoid syndrome. Cutaneous changes similar to rosacea can occur with corticosteroid use,[61] alcohol misuse,[41] and phototherapy.[75] Medical conditions that may simulate rosacea include lupus erythematosus, sarcoidosis,[26] syphilis, tuberculosis, nontuberculous mycobacterial infection,[76] sporotrichosis,[21] disseminated histoplasmosis,[111] angiosarcoma,[82] lymphoma,[97] and nasal septal carcinoma.[58] Basal cell carcinoma can mimic rhinophyma.[53]

Malignancy must be considered in patients with persistent or recurrent unilateral eyelid inflammation.[17] Sebaceous gland carcinoma is a rare tumor, representing only 1% of all eyelid malignancies; but a high degree of suspicion and early diagnosis are essential.[10] The earliest possible diagnosis is important, as the 4-year survival rate decreases from 87% to 57% if symptoms have been present longer than 6 months prior to treatment.[85,86] All patients with chronic blepharoconjunctivitis or recurrent chalazion should undergo biopsy if malignancy is suspected. Frozen sections stained with oil red O can demonstrate sebaceous material within tumor cells.[86]

THERAPY

The management of meibomian gland dysfunction is directed at the forms of lid margin inflammation present and the associated conditions such as tear-film disturbances, exposure, and medication toxicity. A dermatologist is consulted to aid in managing the skin disease. Educating patients about the goals of therapy helps them to maintain a realistic attitude about the management plan. Helping affected patients to achieve an understanding of the natural history of their condition can alleviate part of the frustration that both the physician and patient experience.

Eyelid Hygiene

Eyelid cleansing should be a part of the treatment regimen. Warm compresses help to dilate local blood vessels and unplug the meibomian lipids of the involved glands. The melting points of many meibomian secretions are near body temperature, but secretions insulated within inspissated meibomian ducts can solidify.[104] Moist compresses serve to liquify these secretions and aid in spontaneous draining. Local packs may be efficiently done by placing two washcloths in a basin of heated water and alternating their use every 10 minutes.

Lid scrubs are often performed with commercially prepared pads and solutions. Traditional methods using a facecloth and diluted baby shampoo or cleansing solution may be more cost effective. Local lid hygiene should be performed vigorously, especially in the morning when symptoms are usually the worst, to remove the previous night's buildup of debris and oils.

Management of Hordeolum and Chalazion

A posterior hordeolum usually responds to conservative treatment but may require incision and drainage when chronic. If a posterior hordeolum progresses to a chalazion, then curettage should also be performed. Many chalazia resolve spontaneously. If a chalazion is persistent or chronically inflamed, if it induces symptomatic visual blurring from astigmatism, or if it creates a cosmetic defect, then the chalazion should be incised and curetted. Any protruding granulation tissue can be shaved off flush with the lid surface. Lid massage following warm compresses may be beneficial in preventing recurrences. The amount of lid pressure required to express meibomian secretions can be determined using the slit-lamp biomicroscope, and then demonstrated to the patient.

Topical Ophthalmic Agents

Although short-term antibacterial therapy may be beneficial in suppressing bacterial overgrowth and in reducing bacterial enzymes on the eyelid margin, topical ophthalmic antibiotics are generally reserved for an infected hordeolum. An ointment is preferred for application onto the lid margin. Given the usual spectrum of bacteria that may infect a meibomian gland, bacitracin (with or without polymyxin B) and erythromycin ointments are among the suggested choices. Long-term topical antibiotics are rarely required, except in children who excessively rub their eyes or manipulate nasal secretions. With the prolonged use of antibiotics, it is advisable to rotate agents to minimize the emergence of resistant strains.

Topical corticosteroids have no primary use in the treatment of meibomian gland dysfunction, unless inflammation of the lid margin or ocular surface is present. Steroids are not appropriate for chronic use. Although topical corticosteroids may yield short-term improvement, patient expectations can be difficult to maintain with chronic use or without risking unacceptable side effects. The more severe inflammatory processes such as keratitis and episcleritis may require the judicious use of topical corticosteroids.

Many rosacea patients require artificial tears to control the dry eye that occasionally coexists with lid margin disease.[36,59] Preservative-free eyedrops are ideal for rosacea patients. Certain preservatives such as benzalkonium chloride that can destabilize the tear film should be avoided. Decreased tear function makes these patients more susceptible to the toxic effects of topical medications that may produce corneal epithelial erosions and ulceration.

Topical Dermatologic Agents

The cutaneous treatment of rosacea is best directed by a dermatologist. A variety of topical agents are available including metronidazole, clindamycin, hexachlorocyclohexane, and corticosteroids. Metronidazole may work by inhibiting oxidative tissue injury[3] and is marketed as a 0.75% gel. Although it is effective for inflammatory lesions and erythema,[5,62,95] metronidazole can be irritating if it contacts the eyes.

Ketoconazole shampoo is beneficial in treating seborrhea of the scalp. A topical 2% solution results in apparent improvement to the eyelid margins,[77] but few patients have been evaluated in comparative clinical trials. The dermatologic ointment can be irritating to the eye.

Oral Agents

Systemic agents may be required to control meibomian gland dysfunction when local measures fail to control symptoms or when associated keratoconjunctivitis or recurrent chalazia occur. Oral antibiotics such as tetracycline and its derivatives are an important component of the treatment of ocular rosacea.[7,47,94] The initial dosage of tetracycline is 250 mg orally, four times per day, taken with water on an empty stomach. The action of tetracycline depends not on its antibacterial effect alone but also on the stabilization of meibomian lipids through inhibiting bacterial enzymes such as lipase.[13,29,109,112] In pregnant women or women of child-bearing age local measures are best used, but if oral antibiotics are indicated then erythromycin should be substituted for tetracycline. Tetracycline should also be avoided with children under 13 years of age. Although more expensive, doxycycline may be useful for patients unable to tolerate tetracycline. Tetracycline has been reported to improve symptoms faster than doxycyline.[30] Patients on tetracycline should protect themselves from ultraviolet light exposure and be alert to diarrhea as *Clostridium difficile* colitis is a rare complication. Once control has been achieved, the minimal maintenance dosage should be determined. At that point, patient education is key, because patients need to understand that the problem has been controlled—but not cured. An understanding of the natural history of chronic blepharitis and rosacea will help the patient appreciate that treatment may need to be continued indefinitely.

Isotretinoin has been used for severe rosacea.[44] Unfortunately, oral retinoids may cause blepharitis and conjunctivitis.[35,44] Symptoms caused by oral isotretinoin are related to decreased meibomian gland function[57] and increased tear evaporation and tear osmolality. Other agents effective in controlling the cutaneous disease include low-dose spironolactone in some male patients.[2]

Surgical Management

Corneal thinning may require a conjunctival flap or a tectonic corneal graft. An impending or small perforation can be treated with tissue adhesive. Corneal transplantation may be required for a larger perforation. Corneal vascular-

ization, recurrent inflammation, and dry eye increase the postoperative complication rate.

REFERENCES

1. Abelson MB, Sadun AA, Udell IF, West JH: Alkaline tear pH in ocular rosacea, *Am J Ophthalmol* 90:866-869, 1980.
2. Aizawa H, Miimura M: Oral spironolactone therapy in male patients with rosacea, *J Dermatol* 19:293-297, 1992.
3. Akamatsu H, Oguchi M, Nishijima S et al.: The inhibition of free radical generation by human neutrophils through the synergistic effects of metronidazole with palmitoleic acid: a possible mechanism of action of metronidazole in rosacea and acne, *Arch Dermatol Res* 282:449-454, 1990.
4. Andrews JS: The meibomian secretion, *Int Ophthalmol Clin* 13:23-28, 1973.
5. Aronson IK, Rumsfeld JA, West DP et al.: Evaluation of topical metronidazole gel in acne rosacea, *Drug Intel Clin Pharmacol* 221:346-351, 1987.
6. Ayres S, Ayres S: Demodectic eruptions (demodicidosis) in the human, *Arch Dermatol* 83:816-827, 1961.
7. Bartholomew RS, Reid BJ, MacDonald M, Galloway NR: Oxytetracycline in the treatment of ocular rosacea: a double-blind trial, *Br J Ophthalmol* 66:386, 1982.
8. Bernstein JE, Soltani K: Alcohol-induced rosacea flushing blocked by naloxone, *Br J Dermatol* 107:59-62, 1982.
9. Black AA, McCauliffe DP, Sontheimer RD: Prevalence of acne rosacea in a rheumatic skin disease subspecialty, *Lupus* 1:229-237, 1992.
10. Boniuk M, Zimmerman LE: Sebaceous carcinoma of the eyelid, eyebrow, caruncle, and orbit, *Int Ophthalmol Clin* 12:225, 1972.
11. Borrie P: Rosacea with special reference to its ocular manifestations, *Br J Ophthalmol* 656:458, 1953.
12. Bron AJ, Benjamin L, Snibson GR: Meibomian gland disease: classification and grading of lid changes, *Eye* 5:395-411, 1991.
13. Brown SI, Shahinian L: Diagnosis and treatment of ocular rosacea, *Ophthalmology* 85:779, 1978.
14. Browning DJ: Tear studies in ocular rosacea, *Am J Ophthalmol* 99:530-533, 1985.
15. Browning DJ, Proia AD: Ocular rosacea, *Surv Ophthalmol* 31:145-158, 1986.
16. Browning DJ, Rosenwasser G, Lugo M: Ocular rosacea in blacks, *Am J Ophthalmol* 101:441-444, 1986.
17. Brownstein B, Codere F, Jackson WB: Masquerade syndrome, *Ophthalmology* 87:259, 1980.
18. Chew CK, Hykin PG, Jansweijer C et al.: The casual level of meibomian lipids in humans, *Curr Eye Res* 12:255-259, 1993.
19. Cory CC, Hinks W, Burton JL, Shuster S: Meibomian gland secretions in the red eyes of rosacea, *Br J Dermatol* 88:25, 1973.
20. Cowper HW: Meibomian seborrhea, *Am J Ophthalmol* 5:25-30, 1922.
21. Day TW, Gibson GH, Guin JD: Rosacea-like sporotrichosis, *Cutis* 33:549-552, 1984.
22. Donshik PC, Hoss DM, Ehlers WH: Inflammatory and papulosquamous disorders of the skin and eye, *Dermatol Clin* 10:533-547, 1992.
23. Dougherty JM, McCulley JP: Comparative bacteriology of chronic blepharitis, *Br J Ophthalmol* 68:524, 1984.
24. Dougherty JM, McCulley JP: Analysis of the free fatty acid component of meibomian secretions in chronic blepharitis, *Invest Ophthalmol Vis Sci* 27:52-56, 1986.
25. Dougherty JM, McCulley JP: Bacterial lipases and chronic blepharitis, *Invest Ophthalmol Vis Sci* 27:486-491, 1986.
26. Drolet B, Paller AS: Childhood rosacea, *Pediatr Dermatol* 9:22-26, 1992.
27. Edwards RS: Ophthalmic emergencies in a district general hospital casualty department, *Br J Ophthalmol* 71:938, 1987.
28. Erzurum SA, Feder RS, Greenwald MJ: Acne rosacea with keratitis in childhood, *Arch Ophthalmol* 111:228-230, 1993.
29. Freinkel RK, Strauss JS, Yip SY, Pochi PE: Effect of tetracycline on the composition of sebum in acne vulgaris, *N Engl J Med* 373:850, 1965.

30. Frucht-Pery J, Sagi E, Hemo I, Ever-Hadani P: Efficacy of doxycycline and tetracycline in ocular rosacea, *Am J Ophthalmol* 116:88-92, 1993.

31. Fulton JE Jr: Lipases: their questionable role in acne vulgaris, *Int J Dermatol* 15:732, 1976.

32. Goldsmith AJB: The ocular manifestations of rosacea, *Br J Dermatol* 3:446-451, 1953.

33. Gozberk R: Sur un cas de septicemia à staphylocoques consécutive à une meibomite suppurée, *Ann Oculist* 175:159, 1938.

34. Groden LR, Murphy B: Lid flora in blepharitis, *Cornea* 10:50-53, 1991.

35. Gross EG, Helfgott MA: Retinoids and the eye, *Dermatol Clin* 10:521-531, 1992.

36. Gudmundsen KJ, O'Donnell BF, Powell FC: Schirmer testing for dry eyes in patients with rosacea, *J Am Acad Dermatol* 26:211-214, 1992.

37. Gutgessell VJ, Stern GA, Hood CI: Histopathology of meibomian gland dysfunction, *Am J Ophthalmol* 94:383-387, 1982.

38. Hagemann JW, Tallent WH, Barve JA et al.: Polymorphism in single-acid triglycerides of positional and geometric isomers of octadecenoic acid, *J Am Oil Chem Soc* 52:204-207, 1975.

39. Hayami M, Okabe A, Kariyama R et al.: Lipid composition of *Staphylococcus aureus* and its derived L-forms, *Microbiol Immunol* 23:435-442, 1979.

40. Henriquez AS, Korb DR: Meibomian glands and contact lens wear, *Br J Ophthalmol* 65:108-111, 1981.

41. Higgens EM, du Vivier AW: Cutaneous disease and alcohol misuse, *Br Med Bull* 50:85-98, 1994.

42. Hoang-Xuan T, Rodriguez A, Zaltas MM et al.: Ocular rosacea: a histologic and immunopathologic study, *Ophthalmology* 97:1468-1475, 1990.

43. Hom MM, Martinson JR, Knapp LL, Paugh JR: Prevalence of meibomian gland dysfunction, *Optom Vis Sci* 67:710-712, 1990.

44. Hoting E, Paul E, Plewig G: Treatment of rosacea with isotretinoin, *Int J Dermatol* 25:660-663, 1986.

45. Huber-Spitzy V, Baumgartner I, Bohler-Sommeregger K, Grabner G: Blepharitis—a diagnostic and therapeutic challenge: a report on 407 consecutive cases, *Graefes Arch Clin Exp Ophthalmol* 229:224-227, 1991.

46. Hykin PG, Bron AJ: Age-related morphological changes in lid margin and meibomian gland anatomy, *Cornea* 11:334-342, 1992.

47. Jenkins MNS, Brown SI, Lempert SL et al.: Ocular rosacea, *Am J Ophthalmol* 88:618-622, 1979.

48. Jester JV, Nicolaides N, Kiss-Polvolgyi I, Smith RE: Meibomian gland dysfunction. II. The role of keratinization in a rabbit model of meibomian gland dysfunction, *Invest Ophthalmol Vis Sci* 30:936-945, 1989.

49. Jester JV, Nicolaides N, Smith RE: Meibomian gland dysfunction. I. Keratin protein expression in normal human and rabbit meibomian glands, *Invest Ophthalmol Vis Sci* 30:927-935, 1989.

50. Jester JV, Rife L, Nii D et al.: In vivo biomicroscopy and photography of meibomian glands in a rabbit model of meibomian gland dysfunction, *Invest Ophthalmol Vis Sci* 22:660-667, 1982.

51. Kaercher T, Honig D, Mobius D: Brewster angle microscopy: a new method of visualizing the spreading of Meibomian lipids, *Int Ophthalmol* 17:341-348, 1993-94.

52. Kaercher T, Mobius D, Welt R: Biophysical characteristics of the Meibomian lipid layer under in vitro conditions, *Int Ophthalmol* 16:167-176, 1992.

53. Keefe M, Wakeel RA, McBride DI: Basal cell carcinoma mimicking rhinophyma: case report and literature review, *Arch Dermatol* 124:1077-1079, 1988.

54. Keith CG: Seborrheic blepharo-kerato-conjunctivitis, *Trans Ophthalmol Soc UK* 87:85, 1967.

55. Kellum RE: Acne vulgaris: studies in pathogenesis: relative irritancy of free fatty acids from C2 to C16, *Arch Dermatol* 97:722, 1968.

56. Kolattukudy PE, Rogers L: Acyl-coA reductase and acyl-coA: fatty alcohol acyltransferase in the microsomal preparation from the bovine meibomian gland, *J Lipid Res* 27:404, 1986.

57. Kremer I, Gaton DD, David M et al.: Toxic effect of systemic retinoids on meibomian glands, *Ophthalmic Res* 26:124-128, 1994.

58. Law TH, Jackson IT, Muller SA: Nasal septal carcinoma masquerading as acne rosacea, *J Dermatol Surg Oncol* 13:1021-1024, 1987.

59. Lemp MA, Mahmood MA, Weiler HH: Association of rosacea and keratoconjunctivitis sicca, *Arch Ophthalmol* 102:556-557, 1984.

60. Lempert SL, Jenkins MS, Brown SI: Chalazia and rosacea, *Arch Ophthalmol* 97:1652, 1979.

61. Litt JZ: Steroid-induced rosacea, *Am Fam Physician* 48:67-71, 1993.

62. Lowe NJ, Henerson T, Millikan LE et al.: Topical metronidazole for severe and recalcitrant rosacea: a prospective open trial, *Cutis* 43:283-286, 1989.

63. Manna V, Marks R, Holt P: Involvement of immune mechanisms in the pathogenesis of rosacea, *Br J Dermatol* 107:203, 1982.

64. Marks R: Concepts in the pathogenesis of rosacea, *Br J Dermatol* 80:170-177, 1968.

65. Marks R: Comparative effectiveness of tetracycline and ampicillin in rosacea, *Lancet* 2:1049-1052, 1971.

66. Marks R, Harcourt-Webster JN: Histopathology of rosacea, *Arch Dermatol* 100:682-691, 1969.

67. Mathers WD: Ocular evaporation in meibomian gland dysfunction and dry eye, *Ophthalmology* 10:347-351, 1993.

68. Mathers WD, Billborough M: Meibomian gland dysfunction and giant papillary conjunctivitis, *Am J Ophthalmol* 114:188-192, 1992.

69. Mathers WD, Shields WJ, Sachdev MS et al.: Meibomian gland dysfunction in chronic blepharitis, *Cornea* 10:277-285, 1991.

70. McCulley JP, Dougherty JM: Blepharitis associated with acne rosacea and seborrheic dermatitis, *Int Ophthalmol Clin* 25:159, 1985.

71. McCulley JP, Dougherty JM, Deneau DG: Classification of chronic blepharitis, *Ophthalmology* 89:1173-1180, 1982.

72. McCulley JP, Sciallis GF: Meibomian keratoconjunctivitis, *Am J Ophthalmol* 84:788, 1977.

73. McCulley JP, Sciallis GF: Meibomian keratoconjunctivitis: oculodermal correlates, *Contact Intraocul Lens Med J* 9:130, 1983.

74. McDonnell PJ: How do general practitioners manage eye disease in the community? *Br J Ophthalmol* 72:733, 1988.

75. McFadden JP, Powles AV, Walker M: Rosacea induced by PUVA therapy, *Br J Dermatol* 121:413, 1989.

76. Nedorost ST, Elewski B, Tomfort JW, Camisa C: Rosacea-like lesions due to familial *Mycobacterium avium-intracellulare* infection, *Int J Dermatol* 30:491-497, 1991.

77. Nelson ME, Midgley G, Blatchford NR: Ketoconazole in the treatment of blepharitis, *Eye* 4:151-159, 1990.

78. Nicolaides N, Kaitaranta JK, Rowdan TN: Meibomian gland studies: comparison of steer and human lipids, *Invest Ophthalmol Vis Sci* 20:522, 1981.

79. Nicolaides N, Ruth EC: Unusual fatty acids in the lipids of steer and human meibomian gland excreta, *Curr Eye Res* 2:93-98, 1983.

80. Norn MS: Foam at outer palpebral canthus, *Acta Ophthalmol* 41:531, 1963.

81. Ong BL, Hodson SA, Wigham T et al.: Evidence for keratin proteins in normal and abnormal human meibomian gluids, *Curr Eye Res* 10:1213-1219, 1991.

82. Panizzon R, Schneider BV, Schnyder UW: Rosacea-like angiosarcoma of the face, *Dermatologica* 181:252-254, 1990.

83. Pflugfelder SC, Huang AJ, Feuer W et al.: Conjunctival cytologic features of primary Sjögren's syndrome, *Ophthalmology* 97:985-991, 1990.

84. Pye RJ, Meyrick G, Burton JL: Skin surface lipid composition in rosacea, *Br J Dermatol* 94:161-164, 1976.

85. Rao NA, McLean IW, Zimerman LE: Sebaceous carcinoma of the eyelids and caruncle: correlation of clinicopathologic features with prognosis. In Jakobiec FA, editor: *Ocular and adnexal tumors*, 461, Birmingham, 1978, Aesculapius.

86. Raskin EM, Speaker MG, Laibson PR: Blepharitis, *Infect Dis Clin North Am* 6:777-787, 1992.

87. Ray T, Kellum RE: Acne vulgaris: studies in pathogenesis: free fatty acid irritancy in patients with and without acne, *J Invest Dermatol* 57:6, 1971.

88. Rebora A: Rosacea, *J Invest Dermatol* 88:56-60, 1987.

89. Robinson TWE: *Demodex folliculorum* and rosacea, *Arch Dermatol* 92:542-544, 1965.

90. Rolleston JD: A note on the early history of rosacea, *Proc R Soc Med* 26:327-329, 1932.

91. Rosen T, Stone MS: Acne rosacea in blacks, *J Am Acad Dermatol* 17:70-73, 1987.

92. Rowell NR, Summerscales JW: Urinary excretion of 5-hydroxyindole-acetic acid in rosacea, *J Invest Dermatol* 36:405-406, 1961.

93. Rufli T, Buchner SA: T-cell subsets in acne rosacea lesions and the possible role of *Demodex folliculorum, Dermatologica* 169:1-5, 1984.

94. Salamon SM: Tetracyclines in ophthalmology, *Surv Ophthalmol* 29:265-275, 1985.

95. Schmadel LK, McEvoy GK: Topical metronidazole: a new therapy for rosacea, *Clin Pharm* 9:94-101, 1990.

96. Shelley WB, Shelley ED, Burmeister V: Unilateral demodectic rosacea, *J Am Acad Dermatol* 20:915-917, 1989.

97. Sherertz EF, Westwick TJ, Flowers FP: Sarcoidal reaction to lymphoma presenting as granulomatous rosacea, *Arch Dermatol* 122:1303-1305, 1986.

98. Shine WE, McCulley JP: The role of cholesterol in chronic blepharitis, *Invest Ophthalmol Vis Sci* 32:2272-2280, 1991.

99. Shine WE, McCulley JP: Role of wax ester fatty alcohols in chronic blepharitis, *Invest Ophthalmol Vis Sci* 34:3515-3521, 1993.

100. Shine WE, Silvany R, McCulley JP: Relation of cholesterol-stimulated *Staphylococcus aureus* growth to chronic blepharitis, *Invest Ophthalmol Vis Sci* 34:2291-2296.

101. Sirigu P, Shen RL, Pinto da Silva P: Human meibomian glands: the ultrastructure of acinar cells as viewed by thin section and freeze-fracture transmission electron microscopies, *Invest Ophthalmol Vis Sci* 33:2284-2292, 1992.

102. Sobye P: Aetiology and pathogenesis of rosacea, *Acta Dermatol* 30:137-158, 1950.

103. Starr PAJ, MacDonald A: Oculocutaneous aspects of rosacea, *Proc R Soc Med* 62:9-11, 1969.

104. Stevens AJ: The meibomian secretions, *Int Ophthalmol Clin* 13:23, 1973.

105. Tapie R: Etude biomicroscopique des glandes de meibomius, *Ann Ocul* 210:637, 1977.

106. Thygeson P: Etiology and treatment of blepharitis: a study on military personnel, *Arch Ophthalmol* 36:445, 1946.

107. Thygeson P: Complications of staphylococcic blepharitis, *Am J Ophthalmol* 68:446, 1969.

108. Thygeson P, Kimura SJ: Chronic conjunctivitis, *Trans Am Acad Ophthalmol Otolaryngol* 67:494, 1963.

109. Vavrecka M, Petrasek R, Poledne R: The effect of tetracycline antibiotics on fat metabolism, *Prog Biochem Pharmacol* 3:468, 1967.

110. Vittadini A: Un caso letde di sellicemia stafilococcia consecutiva ad orizaiols meibomians, *Boll Ocul* 12:683, 1933.

111. Wasserteil V, Jimenez-Acost FJ, Kerdel FA: Disseminated histoplasmosis presenting as a rosacea-like eruption in a patient with the acquired immunodeficiency syndrome, *Int J Dermatol* 29:649-651, 1990.

112. Weaber K, Freedman R, Eudy WW: Tetracycline inhibition of a lipase from *Corynebacterium acnes, Appl Microbiol* 21:639, 1971.

113. Wise G: Ocular rosacea, *Am J Ophthalmol* 26:591-609, 1943.

25 Allergic Conjunctivitis

JACQUELINE REISS, MARK B. ABELSON, MICHELLE A. GEORGE,
H. JAMES WEDNER

Ocular allergy encompasses a variety of diseases. Classically these have been divided into five categories: allergic conjunctivitis (often referred to as hay fever conjunctivitis or seasonal conjunctivitis), atopic keratoconjunctivitis, vernal keratoconjunctivitis, giant papillary conjunctivitis, and contact conjunctivitis. These diseases are all IgE-mediated or type I immediate hypersensitivity reactions, with the exception of contact conjunctivitis, which is a type IV or cell-mediated hypersensitivity reaction. The most common ocular allergy is allergic conjunctivitis. This disease is very often associated with allergic rhinitis, and when they appear together the term often used is allergic rhinoconjunctivitis. This chapter will review the pathogenesis, clinical presentation, and treatment of allergic rhinoconjunctivitis.

Allergic rhinoconjunctivitis is a type I or immediate hypersensitivity reaction[31] to a specific allergen or allergens in a sensitized individual. The process begins with allergen (antigen) mixing with tears, permeating the conjunctiva, and coming into contact with mast cells surrounding the conjunctival vessels. The allergen then attaches to IgE antibodies bound to the mast cell surface via the high affinity $Fc\epsilon$ receptor (CD64). IgE cross-linking then occurs, leading to degranulation of the mast cells and release of soluble mediators. It is the degranulation and release of the mast cell products that produces the symptoms and signs of allergic disease, including ocular allergy. Although the symptoms of allergic conjunctivitis are disconcerting, the disease rarely leads to altered vision.

In contrast to allergic conjunctivitis, vernal conjunctivitis and atopic conjunctivitis have more serious sequelae, possessing both inflammatory and cytotoxic components that can lead to impaired vision or blindness. Giant papillary conjunctivitis occurs primarily in contact lens wearers, but can be induced by other types of palpebral conjunctival trauma such as exposed sutures and/or prostheses, suggesting that both immune and mechanical elements contribute to its etiology. Contact conjunctivitis is generally associated with specific drugs, for instance neomycin and/or the pre-servative thimerosal, and shares many similar characteristics of its dermatologic counterpart.

A number of groups have investigated the role of IgE, specific and nonspecific, in allergic conjunctivitis. Several of these studies have detected elevated levels of total tear IgE as well as pollen-specific tear IgE levels.[52,70] In contrast, Ballow and associates[24] reported the absence of detectable specific IgE antibody levels in a group of their patients with the clinical features of seasonal allergic conjunctivitis. Instead, these authors noticed an elevation in tear antigen-specific IgG levels. Both IgG_1 and IgG_4 antibodies specific to ragweed and rye grass pollen antigens were detected in tears. IgG_1 has a high binding affinity for C1q and therefore can activate the classical complement cascade. The function of IgG_4 is more controversial. It has been suggested that IgG_4 can mediate immediate type hypersensitivity reactions. Additionally, IgG_4 can serve as a blocking antibody.

EPIDEMIOLOGY

Allergic diseases in general and allergic rhinoconjunctivitis in particular are among the most common health problems in the United States. For example, a survey of 7945 patients in suburban Cook County revealed that allergies were the second most common medical complaint (dental problems were the most common). The prevalence rate in this population was 9.4%. Other estimates of the incidence of allergic diseases suggest that over 18% of the population (> 40 million) have allergic rhinitis and/or allergic conjunctivitis, 10% have allergic cutaneous disorders, and 4.4% have bronchial asthma.[77] Other studies have suggested that these may be underestimates, particularly the incidence of bronchial asthma. It is of interest with respect to the topic of allergic conjunctivitis, that in a study of 5000 children undergoing immunotherapy, ocular signs and symptoms were the only manifestation of allergic disease in 32%.[96]

The majority of allergy sufferers develop their disease in childhood. A portion of these allergic children will lose their allergic sensitivity during puberty; however, the percentage is 50% or less, and a portion of children who lose allergic reactivity will regain their disease later in life. Of the pediatric population, there is a strong male preponderance. A second group of patients will develop allergies later in life. The peak incidence is very broad—usually between 18 and 35 years. For this group of patients, an equal number of males and females are affected. There is a third group of patients who develops asthma later in life. Currently, workers in the field are debating whether this represents an allergic disease.

There is a strong familial component to allergic disease. This is true for the atopic state as a whole and for individual allergic manifestations, including conjunctivitis. For example, it has been shown that a child with one atopic parent has about a fourfold increase in their chance of developing any allergic disease, and the presence of two affected parents increases the chance of developing allergies to tenfold greater than the normal population. The exact mode of inheritance is not well understood. A gene has been demonstrated that appears to be linked to the development of bronchial asthma; however, how this gene affects individuals has not yet been determined. In addition, several groups have failed to confirm this initial report. It should be pointed out that the genetics of allergies is complicated by the fact that the inheritance involves first the predisposition to make the class switch to IgE production and second the genetic ability to make IgE to a specific allergen. The former is believed to be at the level of the B cell, whereas the latter is related to T cell reactivity.

Both seasonal and perennial allergens can trigger an allergic immune response. Seasonal allergens include tree pollens (early spring), grasses (May-July), weed (ragweed) pollen (Aug-Oct), and outdoor molds such as *Cladosporium, Alternaria, Epicoccum,* and *Basidiospores,* although mold aerospora varies widely throughout the United States. The perennial allergens are house dust mites (*Dermatophagoides farinea* and *D. pteronyssinus*), indoor molds [largely *Aspergillus* (*A. flavis* and *A. fumigatus*), and *Penicillium* spp.] and animal danders (most often cat and dog). Although indoor molds and dust are usually considered perennial allergens, they may have a strong seasonal component, particularly in temperate climates. The seasonal form of allergic conjunctivitis, especially that caused by pollen, is more prevalent than the perennial form.[53] This is of interest, as the most common allergy is to dust mite—a perennial allergen. This fact suggests that certain allergens may be better able to penetrate the conjunctiva.

PATHOGENESIS

Allergen challenges in most tissues, including the eye, reveal both an early-phase response (0 to 60 min) and a late-phase response (4 to 24 hr). In the ocular early phase, conjunctival scrapings and tear cytology from patients stimulated with specific allergen reveal increased numbers of neutrophils and eosinophils. The presence of eosinophils is enough to make a diagnosis of allergic conjunctivitis, although the absence of eosinophils does not rule out this diagnosis.[11] In severe allergic responses, eosinophils infiltrate the conjunctiva within 1 to 6 hours after challenge. Both eosinophils and neutrophils return to baseline levels by 24 hours.[93] The increase in eosinophils and neutrophils is the result, in part, of the appearance of CD54 (noted in the following section). Clinically, the early phase is associated with conjunctival edema and hyperemia, palpebral edema, and mild mucous discharge.

Several authors have described varying types of ocular late phases. These late phases range from biphasic to multiphasic to sustained.[75] A human provocation study using rye grass-sensitive patients, who were challenged with increasing doses of rye grass allergen, demonstrated the presence of neutrophils at 20 minutes, eosinophils at 6 hours, and neutrophils, lymphocytes, and eosinophils at 12 to 24 hours after challenge. Interestingly, the clinical features of the late-phase response were only witnessed at the highest dose of allergen (320,000 BU/ml) tested.[32] (Note: BU or biologic unit is a method of measuring allergen concentration common in Europe. In the United States, most allergens are measured in weight to volume [w/v] or protein nitrogen unit [PNU]. Currently, allergy unit [AU] is used for dust mite and biologic allergy unit [BAU] is used for cat allergy.) The clinical features associated with the late phase response were induration of the lid margin and, occasionally, erythema of the lid and conjunctiva.[75]

Mast Cells

Quiescent mucosal mast cells have been identified and described in the normal conjunctiva of rats[16] and humans.[17] Of the approximately 50 million mast cells reportedly found in the ocular and adnexal tissues of the human eye,[12] the majority are located in the substantia propria of the normal conjunctiva. In disease states, they are found in other areas.[14,15,17,56]

There are two morphologically and functionally distinct types of human mast cells. The morphologic distinction is based on the mast cell's neutral protease composition. Mast cells that contain tryptase, chymase, and a cathepsin G-like protein in their granules (MCtc mast cells) are located in connective tissues. The second type of mast cell, MCt, has granules that contain only tryptase. The MCt cells are located in the lung and on mucosal surfaces. The two cells can be distinguished morphologically using high resolution electron microscopy. The MCt cells have a scroll pattern in their granules, whereas MCtc cells have a lattice pattern. Frequently, mast cells are found at portals of entry and interfaces between the internal and external environment. The conjunctiva is one example of this interface.[84] Human studies have identified the MCtc as the predominant mast cell in the normal palpebral conjunctiva. These cells are usually found beneath the basement membrane, near blood vessels.

Patients with vernal conjunctivitis, allergic conjunctivitis, and giant papillary conjunctivitis show an increased number of mucosal mast cells (MCt) in the inflamed conjunctiva.[67] This is in contrast to the nose, where an increase in serosal mast cells (MCtc) has been seen in atopic patients.

Each mast cell contains granules filled with inflammatory mediators. Preformed mediators include histamine, tryptase, chymase, cathepsin G-like protein, carboxypeptidase, and the matrix proteins—heparin and chondroitin sulfate. These preformed substances are released upon degranulation.

Just prior to degranulation, the allergen cross-links IgE molecules on the surfaces of mast cells and basophils. Activation of the mast cell occurs and calcium ions pour into the mast cells. Microtubule formation occurs and leads to the movement of the granules. The granules fuse with the plasma membrane and release the preformed mediators. Additionally, phospholipase A2 is activated and releases arachidonic acid from plasma membrane-bound phospholipid. The free arachidonic acid then can be metabolized by lipoxygenase and cyclooxygenase enzymes to form mediators. Some of the newly formed mediators from the arachidonic acid pathway include leukotriene B4 (LTB4), LTC4, LTE4, prostaglandin D2 (PGD2), and platelet activating factor (PAF). Recent studies have demonstrated that cytokines (largely IL-3, IL-4 and IL-5) are produced by activated mast cells and play a prominent role in the allergic response. In contrast to the lipid mediators, cytokine products require a significantly longer time before they are secreted because of the need for gene activation and subsequent protein production.

Mast Cell Mediators

Histamine. Histamine is a preformed, biogenic amine stored by both mast cells and basophils. Histamine acts directly on smooth muscle and blood vessels. There are three identified types of histamine receptors designated H1, H2, and H3. The major locations for H1 receptors are on bronchial and gastrointestinal smooth muscle and in the brain. H_2 receptors are located in gastric mucosa, uterus, brain, and blood vessel walls. H_3 receptors are located in the brain and bronchial smooth muscle. Of these three types of histamine receptors, only H1[84] and H2[9] exist on the ocular surface. Selective H1 receptor activation results in itching, whereas selective H2 receptor activation causes mainly redness. Abelson and associates[3] produced both ocular itching and conjunctival redness by topically applying histamine to the human eye. Maximal histamine release in response to conjunctival challenge with allergen has been correlated with peak itching response.[26] Although the principal roles of each receptor subtype have been elucidated, the level of discretion between these receptor populations is still being determined. Histamine has been identified in both normal human tears and in the tears of allergic subjects after antigen challenge. Allergic patients, however, were found to have significantly greater levels of histamine in their tears than the controls.[80] In the past there was a problem quantitating levels of histamine secondary to both histaminase and histamine methyltransferase that degrade histamine to imidazoleacetic acid (IAA) and methylhistamine, respectively. More recent methods for assaying histamine or IAA have circumvented these problems.

Animal studies with presensitized guinea pigs demonstrated that histamine release was maximal after 10 minutes and returned to baseline 1 hour after challenge. In addition, a late phase was noted in 2 of the animals 4 to 8 hours after antigen challenge. Histamine may also act as a stimulant for the release of prostacyclin (PGI1).[65] Animal models of ocular anaphylaxis demonstrate 70% to 100% mast cell degranulation.[2]

Tryptase. Tryptase is a preformed endoprotease stored in both subtypes of mast cells. It is specific for mast cells and, therefore, is an identifiable marker for mast cell-mediated diseases. Provocation studies have identified elevated tear levels of tryptase in subjects with active ocular allergies. In addition, elevated levels of tryptase have been found in tears of patients after rubbing of the eyes and provocation with compound 48/80, which nonspecifically releases mediators from mast cells (but not basophils).[43] In addition to the eye, tryptase has been found in other biologic fluids such as serum,[86] bronchial lavage fluid,[98] nasal lavage secretions,[48] and skin.[85] Tryptase also has the ability to degrade neuropeptides such as vasoactive intestinal peptide (VIP), peptide histidine-methionine (PHM), and calcitonin gene-related peptide (CGRP). Of these, VIP is a prominent bronchodilator. It is postulated that in asthma, tryptase may increase bronchomotor tone and bronchial hyperresponsiveness[91] by destroying VIP. Whether a similar mechanism is present in the eye has not been evaluated.

Chymase. Chymase is a preformed stored serine endoprotease found in the MCtc subset of mast cells. It is inhibited by plasma proteinase inhibitors.[82] Chymase release has not yet been demonstrated in the eye, although release might be anticipated because the majority of the conjunctival mast cells are of the MCtc phenotype.

Platelet Activating Factor. Platelet activating factor (PAF, acetylglycerolether (s,n)-phosphoryl-choline) is a unique phospholipid derived from membrane phospholipids following the action of phospholipase A2. Both the ether linkage of the long chain fatty acid and the acetyl group at the 2 position are critical for PAF action. PAF is released from the majority of bone marrow-derived inflammatory cells including macrophages, eosinophils, neutrophils, basophils, monocytes, and mast cells. PAF is among the most potent mast cell mediators. PAF has several systemic actions including aggregating platelets, increasing vascular permeability, chemotaxis and degradation of eosinophils and neutrophils, bronchoconstriction, increased bronchial responsiveness, and hypotension.

Histologically, PAF has been found to be chemotactic for neutrophils and eosinophils in the conjunctiva of both rabbits and humans.[60] PAF has been studied in the external eyes of humans and rabbits by dose challenge method. Hyperemia and chemosis developed upon PAF exposure. Intravenous injection of PAF in rabbits resulted in marked retinal ischemia and microvascular leakage.[39]

Arachidonic Acid Metabolites

Prostaglandins and Thromboxanes. During an allergic response, phospholipase A_2 is rapidly activated. The cell membrane contains phospholipids that are metabolized by phospholipase A_2, resulting in the release of arachidonic acid from the 2 position. Once removed, the arachidonic acid serves as a substrate for either cyclooxygenase or lipoxygenase.

The cyclooxygenase pathway produces prostacyclins, prostaglandins (PG), and thromboxanes (TX) (Fig. 25-1). The primary prostaglandins include PGD_2, PGE_2, and $PGF_{2\alpha}$ isomers. PGD_2 and $PGF_{2\alpha}$ have similar pharmacologic actions including bronchoconstriction, peripheral vasodilation, coronary and pulmonary vasoconstriction, inhibition of platelet aggregation, neutrophil chemoattraction, and augmentation of basophil histamine release. PGE_2 has relaxant effects on human airways and produces vasodilation and erythema. PGI_2 has been shown to inhibit macrophage spreading and surface adherence. Thromboxane A_2 (TXA_2) actions include vasoconstriction, platelets aggregation, and bronchoconstriction. Recent evidence suggests a role for TXA_2 in bronchial asthma. The role of TXA_2 in ocular allergies is not clear.

PGD_2 is the major prostaglandin produced by mast cells and is generated after activation via the IgE receptor or when mast cells are incubated with Ca^{++} ionophores. Conjunctival studies have identified PGD_2 generation in tear fluid.[80] Topical application of PGD_2 to human eyes induces characteristic changes similar to allergic conjunctivitis such as redness, chemosis, mucous discharge, and eosinophil infiltration.[10] PGE_2 and PGD_2 act synergistically with PGB_2 to enhance vascular permeability, edema formation, and neutrophil infiltration.[10] Prostaglandins are believed to induced

a state of hyperalgesia by increasing pain receptor sensitivity to stimuli.[47]

Leukotrienes. Leukotrienes are products of arachidonic acid metabolism by the 5-lipoxygenase pathway. The initial product 5-hydroperoxyeicosatetraenoic acid (5-HPETE, LTA_4) can be converted to 5-hydroxy HETE, 5,12-d1-hydroxy HETE (LTB_4), or the sulfidopeptide leukotrienes LTC_4, LTD_4, and LTE_4. LTC_4, LTD_4, and LTE_4 have been identified in tears after allergen challenge.[27] Systemically, the leukotrienes have many actions.

LTB_4 is produced predominantly by eosinophils and basophils but also by neutrophils, macrophages, and monocytes. Ocular tissue produces LTB_4[73], and it acts as a potent neutrophil chemotactic agent and has platelet-aggregating activity in vitro. In humans a subcutaneous injection of LTB_4 causes a wheal and flare response followed 2 to 3 hours later by a tender indurated lesion consisting of a dermal infiltrate of mainly neutrophils.[88] Topical application of LTB_4 to hamster conjunctivae did not demonstrate a change in conjunctival vascular permeability.[102] In guinea pigs[89] and rats,[94] however, LTB_4 did cause eosinophil and neutrophil chemotaxis. LTB_4 and PGD_2 together can produce mast cell degranulation.

LTC_4, LTD_4, and LTE_4 are potent bronchoconstrictors in animals[63] and man.[64] LTD_4 additionally causes smooth muscle contraction and increases vascular permeability. LTC_4 and LTD_4 have myocardial depressant properties.[41] LTE_4 has several systemic effects that include causing vasodilation and potentiating increased vascular permeability produced by histamine and bradykinin. There is controversy as to the amount of LTC_4 in tears of atopic versus control subjects. More importantly, Weston and associates[99] reported that instillation of LTC_4 in the eyes of New Zealand albino rabbits produced no effect.[99] This finding suggests that leukotrienes have little role in ocular allergies.

HPETE and HETE. Hydroperoxyeicosatetraenoic acid (HPETE) and hydroxyeicosatetraenoic acid (HETE) are products of the arachidonic acid lipoxygenase pathway. Their role in ocular allergy is, as of yet, undefined. HETE and HETE2 levels have been identified in the tears of vernal

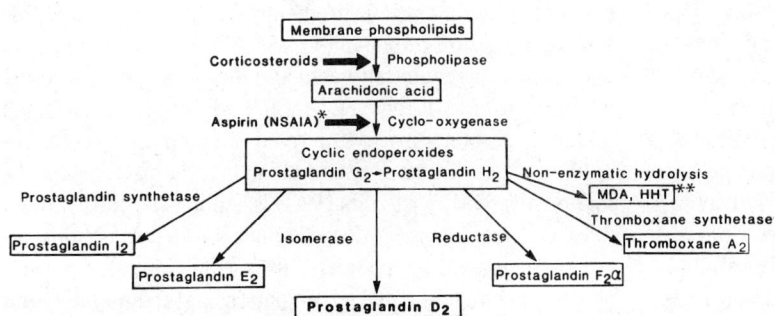

Fig. 25-1. Cyclooxygenase arm of arachidonic acid cascade. Enzymes and sites of activity of representative therapeutic agents are specified.

*nonsteroidal anti-inflammatory agents
**Malondialdehyde and heptadecatrienoic acid

conjunctivitis, pemphigoid, and rosacea patients,[1] suggesting a role in ocular inflammation is likely.

Interleukins

IL-3 is produced by immunologically stimulated lymphocytes. In long-term culture of splenic lymphocytes, the addition of IL-3 produced cells resembling mast cells and basophils.[66] An exact role in mast cell proliferation has not been identified. IL-3 stimulates the growth of precursors of the hematopoietic cell lines. Some of these known cells include macrophages, red blood cells, and granulocytes.

One study from Italy used PHA-stimulated T cells from patients with vernal conjunctivitis. These authors found that large numbers of conjunctival T cell clones produced IL-4. Almost all of these cells provided helper function for IgE synthesis in allogeneic normal B cells. It was also noted that none of these cells produced interferon γ.[76]

Eosinophils and Neutrophils

Conjunctival scrapings[34] and tear cytology[33] reveal increased eosinophils and neutrophils after ocular stimulation with allergen. As noted previously, the presence of eosinophils alone can make the diagnosis of allergic conjunctivitis. The absence of eosinophils does not necessarily rule out allergic conjunctivitis, as eosinophils are often in the deep layers of the conjunctiva and may be absent in the more superficial layers.

Eosinophil Chemotactic Factor and Eosinophil-Derived Enzymes

Eosinophil chemotactic factor (ECF) is released from T cells, mast cells, and basophils. It is a potent chemotactant for eosinophil migration into the conjunctiva. The eosinophil-derived enzymes include histaminase, which inactivates histamine, and phospholipase, which inactivates platelet activating factor.[13] The eosinophil contains a number of granule proteins that are toxic to mast cells. These include eosinophil-derived major basic protein (MBP), eosinophil-derived major cationic protein (MCP), and eosinophil-derived neurotoxin (EDN). MBP is an arginine-rich protein with a pI of 10.9 making it the most basic protein known. This basic protein is the main toxic element in the eosinophil granule. MCP is nearly as basic as MBP, with a pI of 10.8. MCP shares significant homology with the third toxic protein EDN. Both EDN and MCP are members of the ribonuclease multigene family. A final cationic protein found in eosinophil granules is eosinophil-derived peroxidase (EPO). This is a heme protein related to, but distinct from, myeloperoxidase. EPO is toxic to cells and this toxicity is markedly enhanced by H_2O_2 and halide ions.[72]

Eosinophil Granule Major Basic Protein. Eosinophil granule major basic protein is the primary mediator released by eosinophils. This protein accounts for 50% of the eosinophil granule-derived protein.[19] MBP can elicit mast cell de-granulation.[95] MBP activates basophils and mast cells for noncytotoxic histamine release.[95] MBP deposition has been confirmed by immunofluorescence studies in the conjunctiva from patients with vernal conjunctivitis and giant papillary conjunctivitis.[95]

Complement

The complement system consists of two major divisions: the classical pathway and the alternative pathway. Antigen-antibody complexes (IgG or IgM) activate the classical pathway via C1. Thereafter, sequential activation of C4, C2, C3, C5, C6, C7, C8, and C9 occur. The alternative pathway is initiated by IgA, endotoxin, and zymosan. This course is entered at the C3 level and continues on as in the classical pathway. Normal human corneas have demonstrated C1q, C3, C4, C5, properdin, and factor B.[79] A recent review by Fearon[55] contains a more complete review of complement.

C3 tear levels are higher in patients with allergic conjunctivitis. By using transferrin as a marker, C3 has been shown to be locally produced by conjunctival tissues in giant papillary conjunctivitis and vernal conjunctivitis.[23]

Because complement activation occurs with inflammation, several regulatory proteins protect "self" from attack. These proteins, membrane cofactor protein (MCP, CD46), decay accelerating factor (DAF, CD55), and membrane attack complex inhibitory protein (CD59), exist in the human eye, thereby protecting tissue from destruction by the complement-activating system.[35]

Adhesion Molecules

Intercellular adhesion molecules are membrane-bound proteins that allow cells to interact with one another. Cells can modulate their interactions with other cells by increasing or decreasing the amount or avidity of these adhesion molecules. There are several groups of adhesion molecules. One of these groups, the integrins, is a member of the immunoglobulin supergene family that includes CD54 (intracellular adhesion molecule-1 or ICAM-1). CD54 is normally expressed on endothelium, but can be induced on other tissues by cytokines. Ciprandi and associates[51] studied CD54 expression on conjunctival epithelium in allergic patients. Their study demonstrated no CD54 expression at baseline; however, antigen stimulation resulted in CD54 expression on epithelial cells. Because CD54 may actually have a central role in allergic inflammation and may be a sensitive marker of inflammatory changes,[51] these findings are significant for ocular allergy.

CLINICAL FEATURES

The hallmark of allergic conjunctivitis is itching. Patients also may complain of tearing, burning, redness, and pressure behind the eyes and ears. The timing and duration of these symptoms depend largely on the allergen, whether perennial or seasonal. Hence some patients may have relief or exacerbations during particular seasons and exposures. In addition, different climates can exacerbate symptoms. Dry, warm climates tend to worsen symptoms, whereas cooler, wet climates tend to ameliorate symptoms by removing pollen and mold spores from the air.

The ocular exam may reveal minimal findings. Conjunctival hyperemia, chemosis (even if only visible by slit lamp exam), lid and/or periorbital swelling typify the reaction. Often the conjunctiva appears milky or pale pink as a result of edema and dilatation of the conjunctival vessels. In the acute setting, patients may exhibit a clear to white discharge. In the chronic setting, however, a mucopurulent, thick, or stringy exudate is more common. Also frequently present are "allergic shiners" (the hyperpigmented periorbital coloring is thought to be secondary to impaired venous return in the skin and subcutaneous tissue)[59] and Dennie line (prominent folds on the lower eyelid).

Clinical Approach

The first step to an accurate diagnosis is obtaining a careful history with special emphasis on the patient's environment and potential triggers. Additionally important is the patient's personal or family history of atopy, that is, allergies, asthma, or eczema.

The physical examination should focus on the conjunctiva, cornea, limbus, and eyelids. Findings suggestive of allergic conjunctivitis include early age at onset, bilateral conjunctivitis, marked itching, recurrence of symptoms, mild eyelid edema, edema of the conjunctiva, and hypertrophy of the small papillae on the upper tarsal conjunctiva. Corneal involvement is rare in acute allergic conjunctivitis, other than the occasional dellen adjacent to an area of extensive chemosis.

The presence of purulent discharge, follicles, cobbles, or keratitis is inconsistent with a sole diagnosis of allergic conjunctivitis.

DIFFERENTIAL DIAGNOSIS

Allergic conjunctivitis can be particularly difficult to differentiate from dry eye syndrome. Both conditions may produce mild conjunctival vasodilation and a burning sensation with intermittent exacerbations. Ocular allergic symptoms rarely include a foreign body sensation, although this symptom is commonly reported in dry eye. Dry eye patients may be more prone to allergic conjunctivitis as a result of inadequacies in the tear film compromising the ability of tears to dilute and wash allergens from the conjunctival surface. Blepharitis, inspissation of the meibomian glands, and inflammation of the lid margin may be associated with staphylococcal infections and/or seborrhea. Symptoms and signs usually associated with blepharitis include irritation and burning, lid erythema, conjunctival injection, a frothy tear film, lid scurf and collarettes, and scaly or flaky lid margins.[87] The diagnostic tools available for the detection of dry eye, such as rose bengal staining, tear meniscus height, Schirmer test, and tear breakup time evaluation, should be

used during the exam to properly diagnose these conditions.

The infectious types of conjunctivitis are not seasonal and tend to be worse upon awakening. Matting of the eyelashes and lids in the morning is a common complaint. The ocular discharge can range from serous to purulent. Organisms include *Neisseria gonorrhoeae* (associated with a hyperacute conjunctivitis), *Neisseria meningitidis*, *Streptococcus pneumoniae*, *Haemophilus influenzae*, *Staphylococcus* species, *Moraxella*, *Chlamydia*, and viruses. Basophilic intracytoplasmic inclusion bodies in epithelial cells from scrapings of the conjunctiva are indicative of chlamydial infection. In contrast, allergic conjunctivitis is usually seasonal, tends to have a stringy or ropy discharge, and is culture negative.

Vernal keratoconjunctivitis is a condition seen more commonly in young men ages 8 to 20 that manifests as severe itching, a burning sensation, and a tenacious, ropy mucous discharge. Examination reveals giant papillae and cobblestone papillae on the upper eyelid. The cornea may be involved and shield ulcers are not uncommon.

Atopic keratoconjunctivitis can be present at various stages of life and can have serious ocular sequelae. Clinical signs and symptoms include chronic exudative conjunctivitis with severe itching and burning. Examination reveals thickened eyelid margins, corneal changes (including pannus, keratitis, ulceration), and chronically red eyes. Keratoconus, subcapsular and polar cataracts, and susceptibility to staphylococcus and herpetic ocular infections are also associated. These patients often concurrently manifest atopic dermatitis, particularly of the eyelids and ocular adnexa.

Giant papillary conjunctivitis is most frequently seen in people who wear contact lenses or have ocular prostheses. An exposed suture can also cause the disease. Eversion of the upper lid will reveal giant follicles often in apposition to the offending lens, prosthesis, or suture. Symptoms include redness, burning, itching, and mucous discharge.

Contact allergic conjunctivitis is characterized by erythema, chemosis, and induration and edema of the lids in the acute phase. This reaction is a type IV, cell-mediated, hypersensitivity. In chronic cases, findings include crusting and lichenification. Affected areas are those exposed to the noxious substance. Sensitization to components of cosmetics or ophthalmic preparations is the common etiologic pathway. Examples include topical neomycin, atropine, and preservatives. Epithelial defects, corneal opacities, and keratitis are complications that may occur in extreme cases.

LABORATORY INVESTIGATIONS

If the diagnosis is uncertain, several tests can be performed: conjunctival scrapings for eosinophils, tear levels of specific IgE, allergy skin testing to aeroallergens, and ocular challenge with allergens.[6]

In allergic conjunctivitis, the prevalence of eosinophils in conjunctival scrapings ranges from 20% to 80%. Abelson and associates[7] found approximately 45% of their patients with hay fever conjunctivitis had eosinophils in their conjunctival scrapings. This difference in percentages is thought to be secondary to the level and depth of the biopsy or scrapings. Eosinophils may be located more deeply in the conjunctiva than the level of the scraping; thus a negative scraping for eosinophils may not rule out the diagnosis of allergic conjunctivitis. Tear levels of IgE can be measured by radioallergosorbent testing (RAST).[42]

Skin tests can be helpful in confirming a diagnosis of a specific suspected allergy. The tests are performed by epicutaneous (prick) and, if necessary, intradermal methods. The usual allergens tested include tree, grass and weed pollens, mites, and animal danders. The specific antigens endemic to different geographic areas vary, and therefore testing may differ slightly across the country. In addition to the allergens, both a positive control (histamine and/or codeine phosphate) and a negative control (saline) are placed. The IgE-mediated reaction in the skin is a dermal response characterized by a wheal and flare reaction. The immediate reaction is dependent on mast cell degranulation after antigen (allergen) exposure. The advantages of this form of testing are simplicity, low cost, and high sensitivity. The disadvantages of skin testing are possibility of an adverse reaction, inability to perform test with certain skin conditions or medications, and need for an experienced tester.

The radioallergosorbent test (RAST) is one of a number of in vitro methods that measure the specific IgE level against a specific allergen. The allergen is covalently bound to a cellulose disc. Test antibody (IgE) is added and binds to the allergen. The unbound antibody is washed away. Then radiolabeled anti-IgE is added next. The unbound radiolabeled antibody is washed away. The radioactivity of the disc is counted on a gamma counter. Because the RAST is less sensitive and more expensive than skin testing, RAST or other in vitro methods should be used only when skin testing cannot be performed, that is, severe skin rash such as atopic eczema, dermatographism or antihistamines that cannot be stopped.

Elevated tryptase tear levels can be detected by sensitive immunoassays[97] and have been demonstrated in allergic conjunctivitis.[43] Because tryptase is released from mast cells, it is seen only in the early-phase reaction. Potentially, a tryptase level is useful in monitoring the effectiveness of treatment with mast cell stabilizing drugs. The ability to measure tryptase tear levels is now commercially available.

In the United States ocular allergen challenges are used mostly for experimental data to quantitate mediators after antigen challenge. European countries, in contrast, continue to perform ocular allergen challenges for diagnosis. Ocular challenges can be useful clinically in identifying a specific allergen and clarifying the particular eye disease. A positive challenge is one in which itching results within 3 to 5 minutes and conjunctival hyperemia occurs at 20 minutes and

lasts 1 to 1½ hours. If the test is initially negative, doses are increased until 312.5 AU/dose is achieved.[42] Ocular allergens challenges are not recommended. Skin testing is as reliable and is significantly safer.

THERAPY

Treatment of allergic conjunctivitis, like all allergic diseases, is centered around three steps: environmental control, pharmacologic therapy, and immunotherapy. The first step in successful treatment is eliminating the allergen from the patient's environment. This elimination, however, is not always possible, especially if the patient is allergic to outdoor allergens. Several airborne indoor allergens can be controlled. Dust mite avoidance measures emphasize the bedroom. In the bedroom, allergen-proof encasings for the mattress, pillow, and boxspring are effective. Additionally, washing the bedding in hot water (130° F) once a week, reducing the humidity indoors to below 50%, and removing the carpeting from the bedroom or using specialized chemicals such as benzylbenzoate (Acarasan[R]) or 3% tannic acid (available commercially as Allergy Control Solution[R]) that eliminate dust mites from the carpeting or denature the mite allergens are all effective measures to reduce mite load.

Mold is a difficult problem, as spores are not visible. For those areas of the house that are mildewed or demonstrate mold, cleansing with fungicides is reasonable. Additionally, patients should be told to avoid wet basements and keep the humidity low.

Animals are best eliminated from the environment. If the animals are not eliminated, then they should at least be kept out of the bedroom. Keeping the animals out of the bedroom decreases a significant exposure, but may not be effective. Allergen, particularly cat Fel d1 (which is sticky), can be carried into the bedroom. Additionally, the animal, cat or dog, can be washed once a month to decrease its dander load.[61]

Pharmacotherapy

Depending on the severity of the disease and symptoms, several treatment plans can be formulated. For mild symptoms, cold compresses and sterile saline irrigations are useful to help relieve the itching. This is effective presumably by washing allergen away from the eye. For more severe disease, pharmacologic agents are necessary.

Antihistamines. Antihistamines are available in either systemic or topical forms (Fig. 25-2). Systemic antihistamines may relieve ocular symptoms; however, in many instances, the response will be only partial. In the past, oral antihistamines were only available in sedating forms. More recently, three nonsedating oral antihistamines have become available. A comparative study with two nonsedating antihistamines, astemizole (Hismanal) and terfenadine (Seldane), found them to equally control pollen-induced rhinoconjunctivitis.[69]

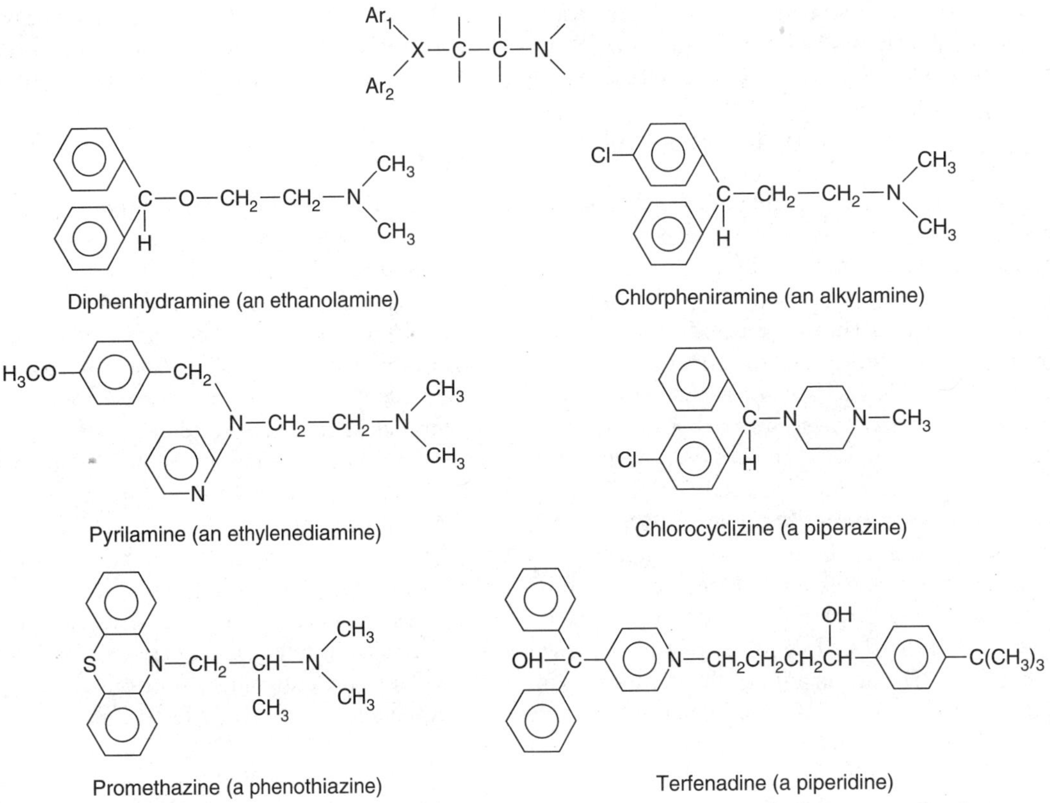

Fig. 25-2. Molecular structures of some common antihistamines. The basic structure is represented at the top.

Antihistamines exert their ocular effect by competitively and reversibly blocking the histamine receptors located primarily in the conjunctiva and the lids. Neither H1 nor H2 blockers have an effect on the release of endogenous histamine itself. There are reports of rare occurrences of cardiac arrhythmias in association with the use of certain nonsedating antihistamines, particularly when they are combined with erythromycin, its analogs or ketoconazole.

Topical H1 antihistamines are usually combined with vasoconstrictors. These preparations act synergistically to alleviate the itching, redness, and swelling.[4,8] The H1 antihistamine inhibits the ocular itching, whereas the alpha adrenergic agent maximizes the alleviation of conjunctival redness (Fig. 25-3). Sensitization and rebound congestion can occur with prolonged use of any decongestant and lead to conjunctivitis medicamentosa. Examples of common combination antihistamine-vasoconstrictor include various preparations of naphazoline-pheniramine maleate. The National Academy of Sciences—National Research Council, however, has classified this drug combination as "possibly" effective for treatment of allergic ocular conditions. Currently, the only antihistamine-vasoconstrictor preparation approved by the FDA for treatment of allergic conjunctivitis is 0.05% antazoline phosphate/0.5% naphazoline hydrochloride (Vasocon-A).

Levocabastine (Levsin®), a new cyclohexylpiperidine derivative, is a very potent and highly specific H1 antihistamine with a rapid onset of action and relatively long duration of action. A number of studies have examined this topical antihistaminic in patients with allergic conjunctivitis (Fig. 25-4). Levocabastine has been shown to be an effective therapeutic agent when compared with placebo in alleviating the majority of the symptoms and signs of conjunctivitis. It has been shown to be 15,000 times more potent than chlorpheniramine in the rat model of 40/80-induced mortality.[9] When compared to cromolyn sodium, this drug was as effective or superior.[20,100] Levocabastine has recently been approved for use by the FDA and is available as a 0.05% topical solution. A recent double-blind parallel group study in patients with allergic conjunctivitis compared topical levocabastine with oral terfenadine. The study found better improvement in symptoms (especially ocular itching) with levocabastine.[21]

H2 antihistamines have been tried on an experimental level. Studies have been done with cimetidine and pyrilamine. Leon and associates[74] found an added effective benefit with both agents, but no benefit with either singly.[74] Currently there is not an available topical H2 antihistamine.

Mast Cell Stabilizing Agents. Several therapeutic agents have been developed that appear to act by decreasing or eliminating the release of mast cell mediators. Their exact mechanism is not known, however.

Cromolyn. The first of this class, disodium cromoglycate or cromolyn sodium, is effective in a variety of allergic

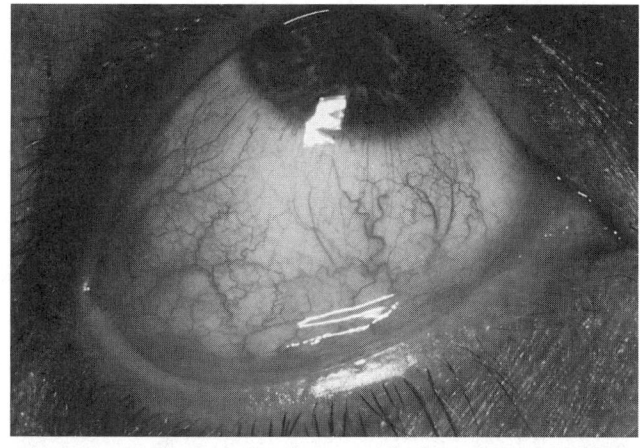

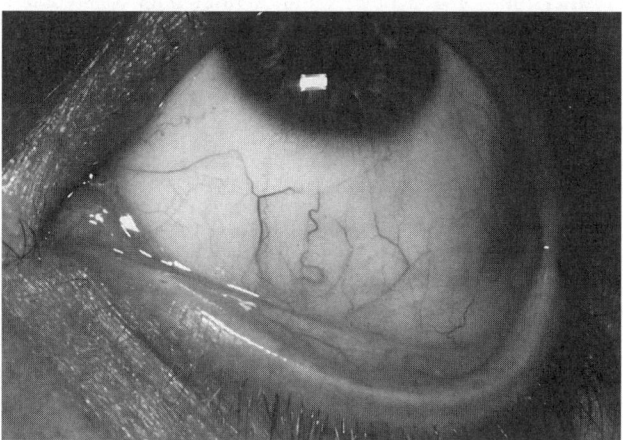

Fig. 25-3. Allergic conjunctivitis. **A,** Right eye treated with placebo. **B,** Left eye of same individual treated with a naphazoline/pheniramine combination product. (Note: Photographs taken at same point in time.)

are burning and stinging, which have been attributed to the preservative. Recently 4% cromolyn (Opticrom) was withdrawn from the United States market as a result of manufacturing problems. It is available in Europe, however. A new formulation of 4% cromolyn sodium (Crolom) has been approved and is now available.

Nedocromil. Nedocromil sodium (Tilade) also inhibits mast cell mediator release and blocks activation and mediator release from eosinophils, neutrophils, macrophages, monocytes, and platelets. As with cromolyn, the exact mode of action is not known. In allergic asthma, nedocromil sodium appears to have a slightly broader activity range than cromolyn sodium. In a guinea pig model of allergic conjunctivitis, nedocromil sodium was found to be as effective as cromolyn sodium.[45] Nedocromil sodium 2%, administered BID in a double-blind placebo-controlled study of allergic conjunctivitis patients during ragweed season, was shown to decrease pruritus, injection and severity of dis-

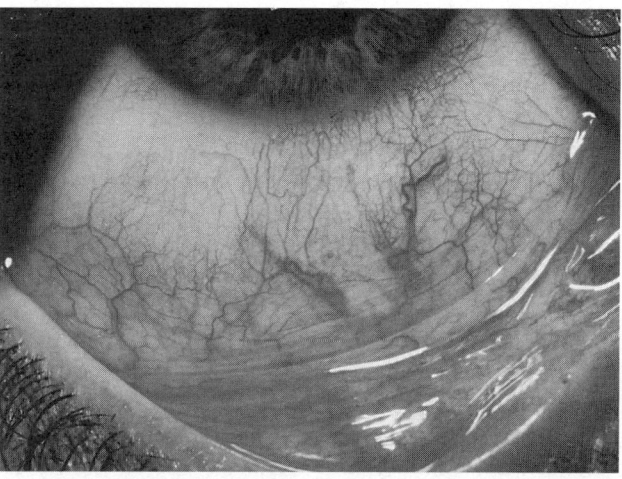

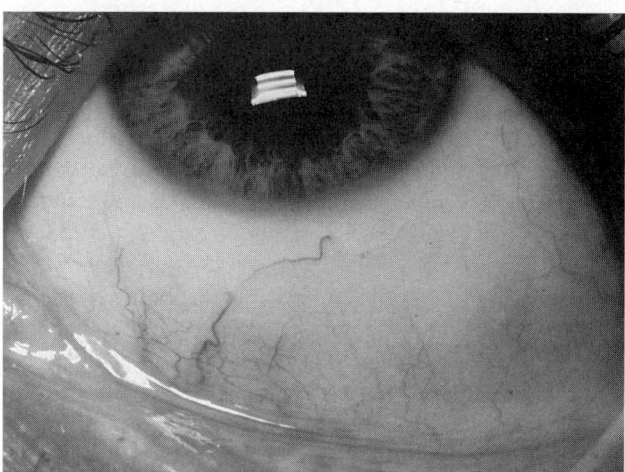

Fig. 25-4. Allergic conjunctivitis. **A,** Right eye treated with placebo. **B,** Left eye of same individual treated with 0.05% levocabastine. (Note: Photographs taken at same point in time.)

states including allergic conjunctivitis. Studies have suggested that cromolyn may also inhibit the activation of neutrophils, eosinophils, and monocytes, as well as stabilize the mast cell; however, this may be a secondary effect. Cromolyn may also inhibit the release of substance P and other neuropeptides from sensory nerve endings.[58] Studies performed with 2% and 4% cromolyn in saline (Opticrom) have shown this agent to be effective in relieving symptoms and signs of allergic conjunctivitis.[18] One study performed in ragweed-sensitive patients demonstrated a reduction in symptom scores and improvement in patient symptoms with use of cromolyn.[62] There have been no reports of a well-designed placebo-controlled study showing efficacy of cromolyn in treating allergic conjunctivitis. Furthermore, cromolyn was not effective in the allergen challenge model of acute allergic conjunctivitis in contrast to antihistamine-vasoconstrictors, corticosteroids, NSAIDS, and anti-IgE compounds. Cromolyn sodium is not active orally because of extremely poor absorption. Side effects of cromolyn therapy ease.[30] At this time, topical nedocromil is not available in the United States.

Lodoxamide. Lodoxamide (Alomide), a third mast cell stabilizing agent, has recently been approved for use in the United States for the treatment of vernal conjunctivitis. It is also being studied in atopic and giant papillary conjunctivitis. Caldwell and associates[44] compared lodoxamide 0.1% with cromolyn sodium 4% in 120 patients with vernal conjunctivitis using a double-blind parallel design. This group found a greater and earlier improvement with lodoxamide.[44] Lodoxamide was more effective than cromolyn sodium in controlling pruritus, epiphora, and foreign body sensation in patients with vernal conjunctivitis. A fourth drug in this class, ketotifen (Zatiden[R]) is effective orally but is not yet approved in the United States.

Corticosteroids. Corticosteroids have a variety of actions that play a role in suppressing allergic diseases. The effect of corticosteroids may relate to the classical pathway of steroid action in which the steroid molecule interacts with an intracellular steroid-binding protein and migrates into the nucleus. There it interacts with steroid-responsive elements in the genome to increase or decrease transcription and translation with a concomitant increase or decrease in protein synthesis. Other actions are not consistent with this mechanism; however, the exact biochemical pathway is not known. An example of the former mechanism is the inhibition of phospholipase A2 caused by the action of corticosteroids on intracellular transcortin. The inhibition of phospholipase A2 prevents the release of arachidonic acids from membrane phospholipids and, as a result, the synthesis of newly formed mediators of allergic inflammation. These include prostaglandins, LTC, LTD and LTE (SRS-A), HPETEs and HETEs. An example of the latter mechanism is the increase in the availability of beta-adrenergic receptors that are downregulated during ongoing allergic reactions. Topical corticosteroids also reduce the number of mast cells within the mucosa. The mechanism for this effect is not well understood.

In both clinical and experimental situations, corticosteroids profoundly suppress the late-phase allergic reaction. In contrast, most studies have demonstrated that this class of drugs only slightly suppresses the immediate response. These studies were being taken to suggest a limited effect of corticosteroids on the mast cell. Other studies, however, have shown that corticosteroids may be as effective as other agents that can alter the immediate response. For example, studies in the rat have shown that dexamethasone pretreatment resulted in a 40% decrease in Evans Blue dye extravasation compared with 44% reduction with pyrilamine (an H1 antihistaminic) applied three times daily, 10% reduction with pyrilamine applied once daily, and 55% with disodium cromoglycate.[46] Studies by several groups have evaluated the effect of corticosteroids on human mast cells. In vitro,

dexamethasone does not inhibit the release of mediators from airway, skin, or intestinal mast cells. In contrast, topical corticosteroid treatment partially inhibited mediator release in the nose in vivo.[83]

Topical corticosteroids are very effective in the treatment of allergic conjunctivitis. In all but the worst cases, however, the serious side effects of this class of drug outweigh their benefits. Some of these side effects include elevated intraocular pressure in steroid responders, cataractogenesis, potential exacerbation of herpes simplex virus keratitis (which may be more common in atopic individuals), delayed wound healing, and secondary bacterial and fungal infections. Topical corticosteroids should be reserved for those situations in which other forms of therapy are not effective. In general, the least potent steroid for the shortest possible time should be the rule. On the other hand, a brief burst of a potent steroid, such as dexamethasone or 1% prednisolone acetate, may be more effective than a prolonged course with a less potent formulation. Trials with prednisolone 0.12% given twice or three times a day have proved effective with few complications.[10] Systemic corticosteroids should be avoided in allergic rhinoconjunctivitis.

Nonsteroidal Antiinflammatory Drugs (NSAIDs). NSAIDs are a large class of chemically diverse drugs (aspirin, indomethacin, ibuprofen, and so on) that exert potent antiinflammatory, antipyretic, and analgesic properties. These drugs all inhibit arachidonic acid cyclooxygenase and thus inhibit the formation of prostacyclins, thromboxanes, and prostaglandins. Because of their antiinflammatory activity they are often useful alternatives to corticosteroids. In many allergic diseases, however, the large number of untoward pseudoallergic reactions associated with NSAIDs has tempered the use of this class of drug. For example, 5% to 10% of asthmatic patients have been reported to have "aspirin sensitive asthma" and there is marked cross-reactivity among all of the NSAIDs. Another group of patients will develop urticarial and rhinoconjunctivitis associated with aspirin or other NSAIDs.

Nonetheless, a number of groups have examined the role of NSAIDs in the treatment of allergic conjunctivitis. Abelson and associates[5] found aspirin to be beneficial in controlling vernal keratoconjunctivitis in three patients with uncontrolled disease. These patients demonstrated improvement in conjunctival and episcleral disease; however, other oral NSAIDs have not been shown to be beneficial.[90]

Ketorolac. Ketorolac tromethamine 0.5% (Acular) is a NSAID that inhibits prostaglandin synthetase and has been shown to be effective when administered four times daily. Ketorolac relieves the symptoms, conjunctival inflammation, ocular itching, swollen eyes, tearing, and conjunctival injection of patients with acute allergic conjunctivitis.[22,92] Significant decreases from baseline were noted in ketorolac-treated eyes, with a 0.5 and 1.55 grade decrease at the mid-week visit and a 0.95 and 1.80 grade decrease at the final visit for conjunctival inflammation and itching, respectively. Ketorolac was also shown to be superior to placebo for both conjunctival inflammation and itching at the final visit.[92] The safety of ocular NSAIDs in aspirin-sensitive patients of either type, as described previously, has not been demonstrated.[90]

Flurbiprofen. In a study examining the efficacy of 0.03% flurbiprofen topical ophthalmic solution (Ocufen) with its vehicle in subjects with allergic conjunctivitis induced by topical antigen challenge, flurbiprofen was found to be significantly superior to vehicle control at reducing conjunctival, ciliary and episcleral hyperemia and ocular itching.[28] Thus blocking the cyclooxygenase pathway while allowing a concomitant increase in leukotriene synthesis does not appear to exacerbate the signs and symptoms of allergic conjunctivitis.[28]

Suprofen. Suprofen (Profenal) is a topical NSAID that has been shown to be effective in treating the signs and symptoms of giant papillary conjunctivitis. The study was a randomized, double-masked study that compared the suprofen 1.0% solution to the suprofen vehicle solution (placebo). Subjects treated with suprofen had a greater reduction in ocular signs and symptoms than placebo. Especially notable were reductions in papillae and mucous strands in the suprofen group.[101]

Oral Flurbiprofen. Flurbiprofen (Ansaid[R]) is a new oral NSAID that may be beneficial in some patients with allergic rhinoconjunctivitis. Brooks and Karl,[40] in a blinded clinical trial, demonstrated transient improvements in allergic symptoms when flurbiprofen was used as an adjuvant to oral antihistamines. The improvements in symptoms consisted of less nasal congestion, nasal running, and sneezing. Flurbiprofen had some nasal effects, but it had little effect on the eye symptoms in these patients.[40] Although studies have demonstrated improvement in eye symptoms, this drug has not yet been approved for allergic eye disease.[40]

Oral Deflazocort. Deflazocort, an oral derivative of prednisolone, has calcium and glucose sparing effects. It has been demonstrated to have significant reductions in the late phase reactions and CD54 expression on conjunctival epithelium.[50]

Cyclosporin A. Cyclosporin A is an immunosuppressive agent that inhibits activated T cells. It has been used as a 2% solution diluted in various oils in the treatment of refractory vernal keratoconjunctivitis, and studies have demonstrated an improvement.[25,29]

Lipoxygenase Inhibitors. Lipoxygenase inhibitors are currently being investigated and may have a role in the treatment of ocular allergy at a future date. REV 5901 has been demonstrated to be the most potent lipoxygenase inhibitor in reducing lens protein-induced ocular inflammation in rabbits.[49] MK-571 is a selective and potent leukotriene D_4 receptor antagonist. It has been demonstrated in vitro to competitively inhibit binding of [^{3}H] leukotriene D_4 in guinea pig (IC_{50} value 0.9 nM) and human (IC_{50} value 8.5 nM) lung homogenates. MK-571 has been shown to block leukotriene D_4-induced bronchoconstriction in several animal models and is presently being evaluated in asthmatics with or without bronchial provocation.[57] MK-886 is selective for the 5-lipoxygenase pathway and has potent in vitro and in vivo effects. Future clinical studies of MK-886 will help define the role of leukotrienes in pathologic processes. This information can be compared with results obtained with MK-571 and help delineate the importance of leukotrienes other than leukotriene D_4.[57]

Immunotherapy

Immunotherapy is the third arm of the treatment plan of patients with allergic diseases that also includes environmental control and pharmacotherapy. Immunotherapy should be considered when allergic conjunctivitis symptoms are severe and are not controlled by environmental modifications and appropriate topical and oral medications.

Immunotherapy was first introduced into clinical practice by Noon and Freeman in 1911[79a]. It is only in the last 25 years, however, that carefully controlled studies have truly demonstrated the efficacy of this therapeutic modality. The mechanism by which immunotherapy specifically alters the immune response is not known. Early studies suggested that an increase in specific IgG and later, IgG$_4$, antibodies might serve a "blocking function" that would prevent the allergen from reaching IgE bound to mast cells. Although this mechanism may be effective, particularly in immunotherapy for stinging insect venoms, in general, there is little correlation between the increase in IgG levels and the clinical efficacy. Indeed, in many instances challenge studies have shown a significant decrease in allergic sensitivity prior to the rise in specific IgG levels.

Inhibition of IgE has also been suggested as a major effect of immunotherapy. A large number of studies have demonstrated that IgE levels rise and then fall during the course of immunotherapy. Most importantly, there is a blunting of the postseasonal rise in specific IgE in patients with seasonal allergies. Nonetheless, like the increase in IgG levels, the decrease in specific IgE occurs well after the change in allergic sensitivity, strongly suggesting that changes in IgE level cannot account for the therapeutic efficacy of immunotherapy.

For these reasons, recent interest has focused on the T cell and its role in allergic sensitivity. Although the experimental data are sketchy, it has been demonstrated, for example, that immunotherapy results in an increase in specific CD8$^+$ T cells. In addition, evidence now exists of a shift in helper T cells (CD4$^+$) from the Th2 cell secreting cytokines that stimulate the production of IgE to the Th1 cell that stimulates γ interferon, a known inhibitor of IgE biosynthesis.

Finally, a number of histamine-releasing factors synthesized and excreted by T cells, monocytes, or platelets have been identified. It has been demonstrated that immunotherapy can decrease the production of these histamine-releasing factors and this, too, may be one of the modes of action of immunotherapy. In addition, a histamine release inhibitory factor has also been described. Changes in this factor, associated with immunotherapy, have not yet been demonstrated, but an elevation in this factor might be associated with specific immunotherapy. For a review of the immunology of allergy immunotherapy see the review by Bousquet and Michel.[38]

Despite the lack of understanding of the underlying immunologic basis for immunotherapy, its efficacy in rhinoconjunctivitis has clearly been demonstrated. This has been shown for seasonal allergens, including grasses and ragweed pollen, and for a mold, *Cladosporium*.[36,37,54,68,71] Finally, it should be pointed out that interesting studies on the use of oral immunotherapy with birch pollen have demonstrated the efficacy of this therapeutic modality in the treatment of rhinoconjunctivitis in children.[78]

Immunotherapy is based on the demonstration of specific IgE. This should always be done by the use of epicutaneous and intradermal allergy skin testing. Skin testing is preferred to in vitro (RAST, and so on) techniques. Skin testing is more sensitive, gives immediate results, and is significantly cheaper than in vitro procedures. It is recommended that in vitro procedures be limited to those instances in which skin testing cannot be performed. This includes patients who have significant skin disease, who are dermatographic, or who have been on agents known to inhibit skin test reactivity. These include H1 type antihistaminics, particularly of the long-acting variety [astemizole (Hismanal) may inhibit skin test reactivity for up to 14 weeks], tricyclic antidepressants that have a significant H1 antihistaminic potential, and high-dose corticosteroids. Once the specific allergens have been determined, then immunotherapy is performed using small and increasing doses of the allergens.[81]

REFERENCES

1. Abelson MB: Lipoxygenase products in ocular inflammation, *Invest Ophthalmol Vis Sci* 24(suppl):42, 1983.
2. Abelson MB: *Immunology and immunopathology of the eye,* 1985, New York, Masson Publishing.
3. Abelson MB, Allansmith MR: Histamine and the eye. In Silverstein AM, O'Connor GR, editors: *Immunology and immunopathology of the eye,* 1979, Masson Publishing.
4. Abelson MB, Allansmith MR, Friedlander MH: Effects of topically applied ocular decongestant and antihistamine, *Am J Ophthalmol* 90:254, 1980.
5. Abelson MB, Butrus SI, Weston JH: Aspirin therapy in vernal conjunctivitis, *Am J Ophthalmol* 95:502-505, 1983.
6. Abelson MB, Chamber WA, Smith LM: Conjunctival allergen challenge: a clinical approach to studying allergic conjunctivitis, *Arch Ophthalmol* 108:84-88, 1990.
7. Abelson MB, Madiwale N, Weston JH: Conjunctival eosinophils in allergic ocular disease, *Arch Ophthalmol* 101:555-556, 1983.
8. Abelson MB, Paradis A, George MA et al.: The effects of Vasacon-A in the allergen challenge model of acute conjunctivitis, *Arch Ophthalmol* 108:520, 1990.
9. Abelson MB, Rombaut N, Vanden Bussche G: Levocabastine: evaluation in human ocular histamine and 48/80 models, *Allergol Immunologia Clin* 2:3(281), 1987.
10. Abelson MB, Schaeffer K: Conjunctivitis of allergic origin: immunologic mechanisms and current approaches to therapy, *Surv Ophthalmol* 38(suppl):115-132, 1993.
11. Abelson MB, Udell IJ, Weston JH: Conjunctival eosinophils in compound 48/80 rabbit model, *Arch Ophthalmol* 101:631-633, 1983.
12. Abelson MB, Weston JH: Antihistamines. In Lamberts DW, Potter DE, editors: *Clinical ophthalmic pharmacology,* 1987, Boston, Little, Brown.
13. Allansmith MR: *Immunology of the eye. The eye and immunology,* St Louis, 1982, Mosby.
14. Allansmith MR, Baird RS: Percentage of degranulated mast cells in vernal conjunctivitis and giant papillary conjunctivitis associated with contact lens wearers, *Am J Ophthalmol* 91:71, 1981.
15. Allansmith MR, Baird RS, Greiner JV et al.: Late-phase reactions in ocular prophylaxis in the rat, *J Allergy Clin Immunol* 73:49, 1984.
16. Allansmith MR, Baird RS, Kashima K et al.: Mast cells in ocular tissues of normal rats and rats infected with *Nippostringylus brasiliensis, Invest Ophthalmol Vis Sci* 18:863, 1979.
17. Allansmith MR, Greiner JV, Baird RS: Number of inflammatory cells in the normal conjunctiva, *Am J Ophthalmol* 86:250, 1978.
18. Allansmith MR, Ross RN: Ocular allergy and mast cell stabilizers, *Surv Ophthalmol* 30:229-244, 1986.
19. Archer GT, Hirsch JG: Isolation of granules from eosinophil leukocytes and study of their enzyme content, *J Exp Med* 140:313, 1974.
20. Azevedo M, Castel-Branco MG, Oliveira JF et al.: Double-blind comparison of levocabastine eye drops with sodium cromoglycate and placebo in the treatment of seasonal allergic conjunctivitis, *Clin Exp Allergy* 21:689-694, 1991.
21. Bahmer FA, Ruprecht KW: Safety and efficacy of topical Levocabastine compared with oral terferadine, *Ann Allergy* 72:429-434, 1994.
22. Ballas Z, Blumenthal M, Tinkelman DG et al.: Clinical evaluation of ketorolac tromethamine 0.5% ophthalmic solution for the treatment of seasonal allergic conjunctivitis, *Surv Ophthalmol* 38(suppl):141-148, 1993.
23. Ballow M, Donshik PC, Mendelson L: Complement proteins C3 anaphylatoxin in the tears of patients with conjunctivitis, *J Allergy Clin Immunol* 76:473-476, 1985.
24. Ballow M, Mendelson L, Donshik P et al.: Pollen specific IgG antibodies in the tears of patients with allergic-like conjunctivitis, *J Allergy Clin Immunol* 73:376-380, 1984.
25. Benezra D, Pe'er J, Brodsky M, Cohen E: Cyclosporin eye drops for the treatment of severe vernal keratoconjunctivitis, *Am J Ophthalmol* 101:272-278, 1986.
26. Berdy GJ, Levine RB, Bateman ST: Identification of histaminase activity in human tears with conjunctival antigen challenge, *Invest Ophthalmol Vis Sci* (suppl):65, 1990.
27. Bisgaard H, Ford-Hutchinson AW, Charleson A et al.: Production of leukotrienes in human skin and conjunctival mucosa after specific allergen challenge, *Allergy* 40:417, 1985.
28. Bishop K, Abelson MB, Cheetham J et al.: Evaluation of flurbiprofen in the treatment of antigen-induced allergic conjunctivitis, *Invest Ophthalmol Vis Sci* 31:487, 1990.
29. Bleik JH, Tabbora KF: Topical cyclosporin in vernal keratoconjunctivitis, *Ophthalmology* 98:1679-1684, 1992.
30. Blumenthal M, Casale T, Dockhorn R et al.: Efficacy and safety of nedocromil sodium ophthalmic solution in treatment of seasonal allergic conjunctivitis, *Am J Ophthalmol* 113:56-63, 1992.
31. Bonini S, Bonini S: IgE and non-IgE mechanisms in ocular allergy, *Ann Allergy* 71:296-299, 1993.
32. Bonini S, Bonini S, Berruto A et al.: Conjunctival provocation test as a model for the study of allergy and inflammation in humans, *Int Arch Allergy Appl Immunol* 88:144-148, 1989.
33. Bonini ST, Bonini SE, Todini V et al.: Persistent inflammatory changes in the conjunctival late reaction of humans, *Invest Ophthalmol Vis Sci* 29(suppl):230, 1988.

34. Bonini ST, Bonini SE, Vecchione A et al.: Inflammatory changes in conjunctival scrapings after allergen provocation in humans, *J Allergy Clin Immunol* 82:462, 1988.

35. Bora NS, Golbleman CL, Atkinson JP et al.: Differential expression of the complement regulatory proteins in the human eye, *Invest Ophthalmol Vis Sci* 34:3579-3584, 1993.

36. Bousquet J, Hejjaoui A, Soussana M, Michel F-B: Double-blind, placebo-controlled immunotherapy with mixed grass-pollen allergoids, *J Allergy Clin Immunol* 85:490-497, 1990.

37. Bousquet J, Maasch H, Hejjaoui A et al.: Double-blind placebo controlled immunotherapy with mixed grass pollen allergoids. III. Comparison with an unfractionated allergoid, a fractionated allergoid and a standardized orchard grass pollen in rhinitis, conjunctivitis, and asthma, *J Allergy Clin Immunol* 84:546-556, 1989.

38. Bousquet J, Michel FB: Advances in specific immunotherapy, *Clin Exp Allergy* 22:889-896, 1992.

39. Braquet P, Vidal RF, Braquet M et al.: Involvement of leukotrienes and PAF-acether in the increased microvascular permeability of the rabbit retina, *Agents Actions* 15:82, 1984.

40. Brooks CD, Karl KJ: Hay fever treatment with combined antihistamines and cyclooxygenase-inhibiting drugs, *J Allergy Clin Immunol* 81:1110-1117, 1988.

41. Burke JA, Levi R, Corey EJ: Cariovascular effects of pure synthetic leuktotrienes C and D, *Fed Proc* 40:1015, 1981.

42. Butrus SI, Abelson MB: Laboratory evaluation of ocular allergy, *Int Ophthalmol Clin* 28(4):324-328, 1988.

43. Butrus SI, Ochsner KI, Abelson MB, Schwartz LB: The level of tryptase in human tears: an indicator of activation of conjunctival mast cells, *Ophthalmology* 97:1678-1683, 1990.

44. Caldwell DR, Verin P, Hartwich-Young R et al.: Efficacy and safety of lodoxamide 0.1% vs cromolyn sodium 4% in patients with vernal keratoconjunctivitis, *Am J Ophthalmol* 113:632-637, 1992.

45. Calonge M, Herreras JM, Juberias JR et al.: Efficacy of 2% nedocromil sodium compared to 2% sodium cromoglycate in a model of allergic conjunctivitis in the guinea pig, *Invest Ophthalmol Vis Sci* 34:844, 1993.

46. Calonge MC, Pastor JC, Herreras JM, Gonzalez JL: Pharmacologic modulation of vascular permeability in ocular allergy in the rat, *Invest Opthalmol Vis Sci* 31:176-180, 1990.

47. Capetola RJ, Rosenthale ME, Dubinsky B, McGuire JL: Peripheral analgesics, *Clin Pharmacol* 23:545-556, 1983.

48. Castells M, Schwartz LB: Tryptase levels in nasal-lavage fluid as an indicatory of the immediate allergic response, *J Allergy Clin Immunol* 82:348-355, 1988.

49. Chiou LY, Chiou GCY: Ocular anti-inflammatory action of a lipoxygenase in the rabbit, *J Ocul Pharmacol* 1:383-390, 1985.

50. Ciprandi G, Buscaglia S, Pesce G et al.: Allergic subjects express intercellular adhesion molecule-1 (ICAM-1 or CD54) on epithelial cells of conjunctiva after allergen challenge, *J Allergy Clin Immunol* 91:783-792, 1993.

51. Ciprandi G, Buscaglia S, Pesce GP et al.: Deflazacort protects against late-phase but not early-phase reactions induced by the allergen specific conjunctival provocation test, *Allergy* 48:421-430, 1993.

52. Dart JKG, Buckley RJ, Monnickenda M, Prasad J: Perennial allergic conjunctivitis: definition, clinical characteristics, and prevalence, *Trans Ophthalmol Soc UK* 105:513-520, 1986.

53. Donshik PC: Allergic conjunctivitis, *Int Ophthamol Clin* 28:294-302, 1988.

54. Dreborg S, Agrell B, Foucard T et al.: A double-blind, multicenter immunotherapy trial in children, using a purified and standardized *Cladosporium herbarum* preparation. I. Clinical results, *Allergy* 41:131-140, 1986.

55. Fearon DT: Complement, *J Allergy Clin Immunol* 71:520-529, 1983.

56. Ferreira SH: Prostaglandins, aspirin-like drugs and analgesia, *Nature New Biol* 240:200-203, 1972.

57. Ford-Hutchinson AW: Regulation of the production and action of leukotrienes by MK-571 and MK-886, *Advances in Prostaglandin, Thromboxane and Leukotriene Research* 20:9-16, 1990.

58. Foreman JC: Substance P and calcitonin gene-regulated peptide: effects on mast cells and in human skin, *Int Arch Allergy Appl Immunol* 82:366, 1987.

59. Friedlander MH: Conjunctivitis of allergic origin: clinical presentation and differential diagnosis, *Surv Ophthalmol* 38(suppl):105-114, 1993.

60. George MA, Smith LM, Berdy GJ et al.: Platelet activating factor induced inflammation following topical ocular challenge, *Invest Ophthalmol Vis Sci* 31(suppl):63, 1990.

61. Glinert R, Wilson P, Wedner HJ: Fel D1 is markedly reduced following sequential washing of cats, *J Allergy Clin Immunol* 85:327, 1990.

62. Greenbaum J, Cockcroft D, Hargreave FE, Dolovich J: Sodium cromoglycate in ragweed-allergic conjunctivitis, *J Allergy Clin Immunol* 59:437-439, 1977.

63. Hansson G, Bjorck T, Dahlen SE et al.: Specific allergen induces contraction of bronchi and formation of leukotrienes C_4, D_4 and E_4 in human asthmatic lung, *Adv Prostaglandin Thromboxane Leukot Res* 12:153-159, 1983.

64. Hedqvist P, Dahlen SE, Gustafsson L et al.: Biologic profile of leukotrienes C4 and D4, *Acta Physiol Scand* 110:331-333, 1980.

65. Helleboid L, Khatami M, Wei Z-G, Rockey JH: Histamine and prostacyclin: primary and secondary release in allergic conjunctivitis, *Invest Ophthalmol Vis Sci* 32:2281-2289, 1991.

66. Ihle JN, Pipersack L, Rebar L: Regulation of T cell differentiation in vitro induction of 20 α-hydroxysteroid dehydrogenase in splenic lymphocytes is mediated by a unique lymphokine, *J Immunol* 126:2184, 1981.

67. Irani AMA, Butrus SI, Tabbora KF, Schwartz LB: Human conjunctival mast cells: distribution of MCt and MCtc in vernal conjunctivitis and giant papillary conjunctivitis, *J Allergy Clin Immunol* 86:34-40, 1990.

68. Juniper EF, Roberts RS, Kennedy P et al.: Polyethylene glycol-modified ragweed pollen extract in rhinoconjunctivitis, *J Allergy Clin Immunol* 75:578-585, 1985.

69. Juniper ER, White J, Dolovich J: Efficacy of continuous treatment with astemizole and terfenadine in ragweed pollen-induced rhinoconjunctivitis, *J Allergy Clin Immunol* 82:670-675, 1988.

70. Kari O, Salo OP, Bjorksten F, Blackman A: Allergic conjunctivitis total and specific IgE in the tear fluid, *Acta Ophthalmol* 63:97-99, 1985.

71. Karlsson R, Agrell B, Dreborg S et al.: A double-blind, multicenter immunotherapy trial in children, using a purified and standardized *Cladosporium herbarum* preparation. II. *In vitro* results, *Allergy* 41:141-150, 1986.

72. Kay AB: Eosinophils as effector cells in immunity and allergic disorders. In Korenblat P, Wedner HJ, editors: *Allergy, theory and practice,* ed 2, Philadelphia, 1992, WB Saunders.

73. Kulkarni PS, Srinivasan BD, Kaufman P: Comparison of cyclooxygenase and lipoxygenase pathways in rabbit and monkey ocular tissues, *Invest Ophthalmol Vis Sci* 26(suppl):191, 1985.

74. Leon J, Charap A, Duzman E et al.: Efficacy of cimetidine/pyrilamine eyedrops. A dose response study with histamine challenge, *Ophthalmology* 93:120-123, 1986.

75. Leonardi A, Secchi AG, Briggs R, Allansmith MR: Conjunctival mast cells and the allergic late phase reaction, *Ophthalmic Res* 24:234-242, 1992.

76. Maggi E, Biswas P, Del Prete G et al.: Accumulation of Th-2-like helper T cells in the conjunctiva of patients with vernal conjunctivitis, *J Immunol* 146:1169-1174, 1991.

77. Meltzer EO: Evaluating rhinitis: clinical rhinomanometric, and cytologic assessment, *J Allergy Clin Immunol* 82:900-908, 1988.

78. Moller C, Dreborg S, Lanner A, Bjorksten B: Oral immunotherapy of children with rhinoconjunctivitis due to birch pollen allergy, *Allergy* 41:271-279, 1986.

79. Mondino BJ, Ratajczak HV, Goldberg DB et al.: Alternate and classical pathway components of complement in normal cornea, *Arch Ophthalmol* 98:346-349, 1980.

79a. Noon L: Prophylactic inoculation against hayfever, *Lancet* 1:1572, 1911.

80. Proud D, Sweet J, Stein P et al.: Inflammatory mediatory release on conjunctival provocation of allergic subjects with allergen, *J Allergy Clin Immunol* 85:896-905, 1990.

81. Sale S: Immunotherapy. In Korenblat P, Wedner HJ, editors: *Allergy: theory and practice,* ed 2, 279-294, Philadelphia, 1992, WB Saunders.

82. Schechter NM, Choi JK, Slavin DA et al.: Identification of a chymotrypsin-like proteinase in human mast cells, *J Immunol* 137:962, 1986.

83. Schleimer RP: Effects of glucocorticosteroids on inflammatory cells relevant to their therapeutic applications in asthma, *Am Rev Respir Dis* 141:S59-S69, 1990.

84. Schwartz L, Huff T: Biology of mast cells and basophils. In Korenblat P, Wedner HJ, editors: *Allergy: principles and practice,* 135-168, St Louis, 1993, Mosby.

85. Schwartz LB, Atkins PC, Bradford TR et al.: Release of tryptase together with histamine during the immediate cutaneous response to allergen, *J Allergy Clin Immunol* 141:821-826, 1988.

86. Schwartz LB, Metcalfe DD, Miller JS et al.: Tryptase levels as an indicator of mast-cell activation in systemic anaphylaxis and mastocytosis, *N Engl J Med* 316:1622-1626, 1987.

87. Smolin B, Okumoto M: Staphylococcal blepharitis, *Arch Ophthalmol* 95:812-816, 1983.

88. Soter NA, Lewis RA, Corey EJ, Austen KF: Local effects of synthetic leukotrienes (LTC_4, LTD_4, LTE_4, and LTB_4) in human skin, *J Invest Dermatol* 80:115, 1983.

89. Spada CS, Woodward DF, Hawley SB et al.: Leukotrienes cause eosinophil migration into conjunctival tissue, *Prostaglandins* 31:795, 1986.

90. Stock EL, Pendleton RB: Pharmacological treatment of ocular allergic diseases, *Int Ophthalmol Clin* 33:52, 1993.

91. Tam EK, Caughey GH: Degradation of airway neuropeptides by human lung tryptase, *Am J Respir Cel Mol Biol* 3:27, 1990.

92. Tinkelman D, Rupp G, Kaufman H et al.: Double-masked, paired-comparison clinical study of ketorolac tromethamine 0.5% ophthalmic solution compared with placebo eyedrops in the treatment of seasonal allergic conjunctivitis, *Surv Ophthalmol* 38(suppl):133-140, 1993.

93. Trocme SD, Bonini ST, Bakey NP et al.: Late-phase reaction in topically induced ocular anaphylaxis in the rat, *Curr Eye Res* 7:437-443, 1988.

94. Trocme SD, Gilbert CM, Allansmith ML et al.: Characteristics of the cellular response of the rat conjunctiva to topically applied leukotriene B4, *Ophthalmic Res* 21:297, 1989.

95. Trocme SD, Kephart GM, Allansmith MR et al.: Conjunctival deposition of eosinophil granule major basic protein in vernal keratoconjunctivitis and contact lens-associated giant papillary conjunctivitis, *Am J Ophthalmol* 108:57, 1989.

96. Wallace W IV: Diseases of the conjunctiva. In Bartlett JD, Jaanus SD, editors: *Clinical ocular pharmacology,* 533, Boston, 1984, Butterworths.

97. Wenzel SE, Fowler AA, Schwartz LB: Activation of pulmonary mast cells by bronchoalveolar allergen challenge: in vivo release of histamine and tryptase in atopic subjects with and without asthma, *Am Rev Res Dis* 137:1002-1008, 1988.

98. Wenzel S, Irani AA, Sander JM et al.: Immunoassay of tryptase from human mast cells, *J Immunol Methods* 80:139-142, 1986.

99. Weston JH, Abelson MB: Leukotriene C4 in rabbit and human eye, *Invest Ophthalmol Vis Sci* 26(suppl):191, 1985.

100. Wihl JA, Rudblad S, Kjellen H, Blychert LA: Levocabastine eyedrops vs. sodium cromoglycate in seasonal allergic conjunctivitis, *Clin Exp Allergy* 21:37-38, 1991.

101. Wood TS, Stewart RH, Bowman RW et al.: Suprofen treatment of contact lens-associated giant papillary conjunctivitis, *Ophthalmology* 95:822-826, 1988.

102. Woodward DF, Ledgard SE: Comparison of leukotrienes as conjunctival microvascular permeability factors, *Ophthalmic Res* 17:318, 1985.

26 Giant Papillary Conjunctivitis

ROGER J. BUCKLEY, ANNETTE S. BACON

HISTORY AND EPIDEMIOLOGY

In 1950 MacIvor[44] gave the first description of the syndrome now recognized as giant papillary conjunctivitis (GPC) or contact lens associated papillary conjunctivitis (CLAPC). Although in the 1950s people did not wear contact lenses, McIvor found that 8 out of 100 patients fitted with plastic ocular prostheses developed a contact allergy, and some of those so afflicted also showed positive skin patch results to the plastics used. The problem was resolved by removing buried implants in two patients and substituting glass for plastic in the other six. The condition as it relates to contact lens wearers was first depicted (in clinical and histologic detail) by Spring[65] in 1974: 78 of 176 soft lens wearers managed by him became symptomatic between 3 and 33 months after starting to use lenses. Spring is generally credited with the first description of GPC in modern times.

GPC was so named by Allansmith and associates[1a] in 1977 in a classic paper that established that the syndrome can affect wearers of both hard and soft contact lenses. The authors reported increased numbers of mast cells, eosinophils, and basophils in the conjunctiva, as well as large quantities of neutrophils, lymphocytes, and plasma cells.[1,2] They concluded from these histologic findings that the cause of GPC was immunologic. The condition was compared with vernal keratoconjunctivitis (VKC) by Allansmith[1,3] and has even been termed ''secondary vernal'',[45] although the clinical course is usually less severe and does not threaten eyesight.

In 1979 Srinivasan[66] described similar clinical manifestations and identical histologic findings in patients with cosmetic shells. Later Sugar[68] recognized that protruding corneal nylon sutures could induce a similar conjunctival reaction, and this was confirmed by others using nylon sutures of a larger diameter.[74]

GPC affects a significant percentage of most reported populations at risk[1,16,32]; for example, it is thought to affect 1% to 5% of soft-lens wearers in the United States,[1a] and probably closer to 1% of the rigid-lens wearers (although the prevalence in the United Kingdom soft-lens wearers has been estimated at 10%).[16]

Hart,[33] in a retrospective study, showed that GPC was induced a mean 31.4 months after the start of lens wear; although Allansmith estimated that GPC took 10 months to develop in soft-lens wearers and 8.5 years in rigid-lens wearers.[1a]

PATHOGENESIS

Mechanical and Deposit Theories

GPC has traditionally been associated with the wearing of contact lenses and ocular prostheses, and more recently with protruding corneal sutures and other elevations (such as an extruded scleral buckle[59] and corneal deposits).[22] Several authors[23,24] proposed that the foreign body mechanically traumatizes the upper lid with each blink (the frequency of which, in this condition, is likely to exceed the normal rate of around 20,000 per day).

Deposits on the surface of the contact lens have been implicated in causing trauma: Fowler[25] showed that deposits covered 90% of the surface of a lens worn by a GPC patient and only 5% of one worn by an asymptomatic individual. Soft contact lenses, in particular, accumulate deposits that cannot be removed even by professional cleaning;[27] these deposits include mucus, cellular debris, and bacteria.[28] Bucci[15] performed a controlled comparison between disposable lenses and soft contact lenses (SCL) in GPC[15] and found that the former was more comfortable (although the handling of the latter was better). Mackie and Wright[45] reported that after cleaning lenses with deproteinating agents, symptoms might disappear for two months. Digesting proteinaceous deposits with enzymes such as papain may increase lens tolerance.[40] There is some evidence that deposits on lathe-cut contact lenses may be more resistant to cleaning than deposits on moulded or spun-cast lenses.[26] The oxygen permeability of the materials from which rigid gas permeable (RGP) lenses are made also appears to influence the incidence of GPC.[21]

Meibomitis and meibomian gland dropout have recently been associated with GPC by two groups.[46,47] It is possible that meibomian dysfunction with consequent tear film instability and dryness may compound mechanical trauma caused by the lens on the conjunctiva, although Heidemann and associates[34] have found no link between tear breakup time and GPC. Alternatively, the atopic state itself may explain the occurrence of meibomitis and GPC together. There is evidence that patients with GPC may have reduced levels of tear lactoferrin.[8] Such lower levels of lactoferrin may allow the deposition of larger numbers of bacteria and their products on the lenses,[62] and may predispose to infection— particularly by staphylococci.[45,67] A course of tetracycline was reported to alleviate the symptoms of GPC in three of Mackie's[45] cases.

Type I Hypersensitivity

Type I hypersensitivity may play a part in the pathogenesis of GPC. Some authors have shown a strong association between atopy and GPC.[11] It occurs more in March than in February,[64] with a marked seasonal variation.[11] Other authors, including Allansmith, have doubted a connection with atopy.

Mast cells may be demonstrated in the epithelium in GPC, as in other forms of allergic conjunctivitis. A large proportion of the mast cells seen histologically in GPC are in a degranulated state;[5] Henriquez[35] found 30% of mast cells degranulated in GPC and as many as 80% in VKC. Raised levels of free IgE in the tears[16,19] also indicate the ingredients of classic Type I hypersensitivity, with mast cell degranulation occurring as a result of surface IgE cross-linkage in GPC. The fact that the cellular infiltrate also includes basophils, eosinophils, and neutrophils[1,3] is consistent; because these are attracted by inflammatory mediators released by the degranulation of the mast cell, with that cell's subsequent secretion of proinflammatory cytokines. The vasoactive and chemical mediators released by mast cells include histamine, serotonin, leukotrienes, prostaglandins, tryptase, chymase, carboxypeptidase, cathepsin G, PAF and eosinophil and neutrophil chemotactic factors.[17]

Irani[36] found that mast cells [of the normal MC_{TC} (T cell-independent) type] had migrated into the epithelium in three of six GPC patients, their position indicating the heightened activity of the tissue. Her finding that there were subepithelial MC_T type cells in VKC only, could indicate that in VKC (but perhaps not in GPC) T cell influence is dominant.

Delayed Type Hypersensitivity

Ballow[9] considers that in GPC there is a delayed type of hypersensitivity to deposits on the contact lens. Metz[51a] has recently shown that a marked infiltrate of CD4+ lympho-

cytes is seen in both GPC and VKC, and that these cells bear the characteristics of memory T cells (CD45Ro+). They are HLA-DR positive, suggesting that they are activated. An increase in macrophage numbers also indicates the occurrence of active antigen presentation.

Contribution of Other Cells

Although macroscopic eosinophil collections[51] (such as those represented by Trantas's dots in VKC) are rarely seen in GPC, eosinophils are found in increased numbers in the conjunctival stroma in GPC.[1,2] Basic tear proteins will adhere to contact lenses.[62] Trocme[70] found deposition of eosinophil major basic protein (MBP) in conjunctival biopsies from both GPC and VKC patients, but he detected MBP on contact lenses only in atopic subjects.[71] Rigal[58] discovered fewer eosinophils in GPC than in VKC, and Udell[73] found MBP only in the tears in VKC, but not in GPC.

Numerous neutrophils were counted by Allansmith[2] in biopsies from GPC patients. Tear LTC4 production is increased in GPC, confirming the activity of neutrophils in the condition; tear LTC4 production may initially be reduced if disposable contact lenses (DCL) are used (although after a month of DCL, there is little difference).[1] Neutrophil Chemotactic Factor (NCF) has been detected at 15 times the normal level in tears of GPC patients,[20] where it is probably being released by injured conjunctival cells.[24] NCF indicates a link between trauma and GPC. CL wearers who did not have GPC had only three times the normal level of NCF. The findings of neutrophilia and active neutrophil attraction both support the theory that simple physical trauma plays a part early in the pathogenesis of GPC.

The characteristic thick and stringy mucus of GPC is produced both by the goblet cells (which are of normal density but occupy an abnormally large surface area[4]) and by nongoblet epithelium.[30]

Conjunctival Immunohistochemistry in GPC

The bulbar and tarsal conjunctivae of nine untreated patients with GPC were biopsied during an exacerbation of disease. Using a method of glycolmethacrylate resin embedding,[14] it was possible to perform immunohistochemical stains of the tissue on 1.5- to 2-micron thick sections, allowing accurate cell counts. Four of the patients were atopic on tear and serum IgE testing. The results of subepithelial cell counts are shown in Fig. 26-1. For comparison, counts are shown with those of 16 nonatopic normal biopsies and of 14 patients with vernal keratoconjunctivitis (13 out of 14 of whom were atopic in this UK population).

There is evidently a contribution to the inflammatory process from several cell types. Both Type I and Type IV hypersensitivity are implicated from the raised numbers of mast cells and of CD4+ T cells. The infiltrate has similarities to that of VKC, though with a more pronounced neutro-

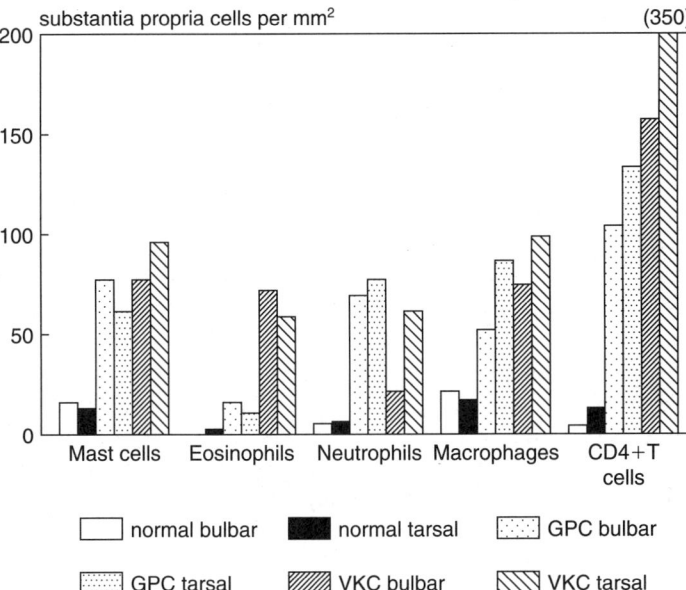

Fig. 26-1. The cellular infiltrates of GPC and VKC contrasted with normal controls.

philia and fewer CD4[+] T cells. The infiltrate of eosinophils, a striking feature of VKC, is much less significant in GPC. This is consistent with the lack of corneal involvement in GPC as compared with the acute and chronic erosive keratopathy that may characterize severe vernal disease.

Adhesion Molecules

Vascular-endothelial adhesion molecules may be instrumental in GPC, as in other forms of allergic conjunctivitis, in the cellular infiltration of the tissues. The immunoglobulin-like molecules InterCellular Adhesion Molecule-1 (ICAM-1) and Vascular Cell Adhesion Molecule-1 (VCAM-1), as well as E-selectin and others, are expressed on the vascular endothelium after induction by a variety of cytokines (IL-1, IL-4, TNFa, and IFgamma) or are upregulated from their basal level of expression (ICAM-1). They grip the circulating leukocytes bearing their ligands (receptors) during margination in the vessels and then aid extravasation through the vessel wall. Directed travel along chemical gradients of inflammatory mediators may be less important than these cell-bound attractants.[61]

Fig. 26-2 demonstrates the levels of adhesion molecule expression (figures expressed represent the percentage of vessels in the tissue staining for the molecule). There is high expression of ICAM-1 and E-selectin in GPC, the ligands for which are expressed on neutrophils, macrophages, and lymphocytes. VCAM-1, however, is expressed on a smaller proportion of the vessels in GPC than VKC (tarsal tissue), consistent with the observed lower eosinophil and lymphocyte counts in GPC.

Immunoglobulins

In an animal model of GPC,[9] cynomolgus monkeys were made to wear (1) used CLs from GPC patients, (2) used CLs from normals, or (3) new CLs. GPC was reproduced only in monkeys with previously worn CLs. The tears showed raised IgA, IgG, and IgE levels, and plasma cells, lymphocytes, and mast cells were found in the conjunctival stroma.

In normal subjects, immunoglobulin levels in the tears are higher in HCL wearers (although still within normal limits) than in SCL wearers,[69] possibly because corneal sen-

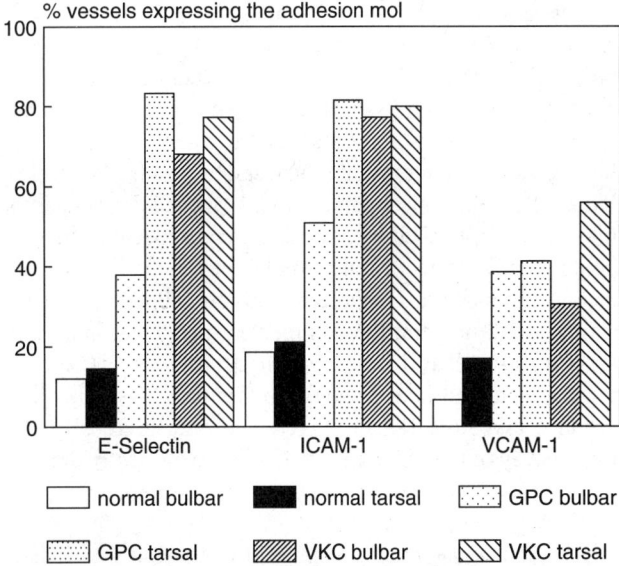

Fig. 26-2. Cell-vascular adhesion molecules expressed in GPC, VKC, and normal controls.

sitivity is reduced to a greater extent with HCLs than with SCLs. The evidence is very varied, however: normal levels have been found in GPC by some,[31,42] and raised levels by others. Raised IgE, IgM, and IgG have been reported by Donshik[19] and raised tear IgE in GPC and VKC reported by Barishak.[10] Meisler[49] found plasma cells of all five types in the substantia propria in a prosthesis wearer. The ratio of IgM to IgA was used as an index of immune inflammatory stress by Jones and Sack[38] and was highest with high water content hydrogel lenses. Richard[57] found a statistically significant difference in deposits of IgM (but not of other immunoglobulins, lysozyme, or lactoferrin) on the contact lenses of patients with GPC versus controls.

Predictably, with the heightened humoral and cellular immunologic activity, various complement products are found in the tears.[6] Of these complement products, C3a and C5a (anaphylatoxins) may contribute to mast cell activation.

Other Theories

Van Aalst and van Bijsterveld postulate that in GPC, antidromic stimulation of unmyelinated (C) nerve fibers results in mast cell degranulation,[72a] so that a larger than expected area of disease process involvement may be produced by direct stimulation; this may explain the mechanism of suture GPC. Cromoglycate can prevent reflex stimulation of primary afferent nerve endings initiated by capsaicin,[18] a compound that releases and depletes neuropeptides. Yano[76] found that Substance P (which is released from peripheral sensory nerve endings) caused mast cell degranulation in mice, with secondary granulocyte infiltration, tissue swelling, and increased vascular permeability.

A Unifying Theory

Severe focal GPC has been caused by corneal deposits[22] alone in a nonatopic patient and by an elevated filtering bleb.[34] Examples such as these indicate that there may not be a specific antigen on the plastic of the contact lens, prosthesis, or suture, but simply mechanical trauma. A weal and flare reaction is the most obvious sign of mast cell degranulation after mechanical stimulation. Mast cell degranulation may be accomplished by several different mechanisms, including antidromic neural stimulation. Human skin mast cells degranulate in response to substance P, VIP, somatostatin, morphine, and the complement anaphylatoxins C5a and C3a, as well as to cross-linkage of surface IgE (explaining the weal and flare response to trauma). Mast cells also produce and store IL4.[14,56,60] IL4 may induce T cell help, particularly of the Th2 type, and therefore indirectly dictates an "allergic" profile of cytokine elaboration, including IL4 and IL5.

The somewhat smaller degree of eosinophil infiltrate in GPC as compared with VKC[58] may be related to the degree and type of T cell help and the atopic phenotype. Eosinophils require the influence of the Th2-type CD4[+] T cell that produces IL5 (as well as IL4 and other cytokines). In the nonatopic individual, Th1 and Th2 cells exert some inhibitory influence on each other; but in the atopic patient (and in VKC), there may be runaway positive feedback of Th2 cells, with a resulting magnification of one pattern of cytokine production, activating and attracting eosinophils. Those GPC patients who are atopic are, of course, subject to the same influences.

In those who are nonatopic, degranulation of the mast cell by means other than the cross-linkage of specific surface IgE may be the first step on the same path. Prolonged mechanical stimulation in the lens or prosthesis wearer will lead to chronic mast cell degranulation, as described by Allansmith.[5] If mast cells are still the first step in the inflammatory process, it is not surprising that the cellular infiltrate (and therefore the clinical picture) becomes very similar to the allergic conjunctivitis of hayfever—or worse, VKC—once T cells and eosinophils are involved.

CLINICAL FEATURES

GPC is characterized by severe itching of the affected eye, especially on lens removal, and by a stringy mucous discharge. There may be excessive movement of the lens during blinking, as the lens is carried on a tide of mucus. Most important for the patient is the resulting loss of lens tolerance. The loss of daily wear time may progress to the point at which the lens cannot be worn at all.

The clinician sees papillae on the tarsal conjunctiva, particularly of the upper lid; this is the most striking feature of the disease. These papillae may be true giant papillae (> 1.0 mm diameter, Fig. 26-3) or "macropapillae" (0.3-1.0 mm diameter, Fig. 26-4). Macropapillary conjunctivitis (MPC) is a developmental stage of GPC or a milder variant, with similar clinical manifestations and histopathologic findings.[16] When the disease is active, there is obvious tissue edema, hyperaemia, and cellular infiltration; and the epithelium at the tips of the papillae may be eroded, so that it stains with

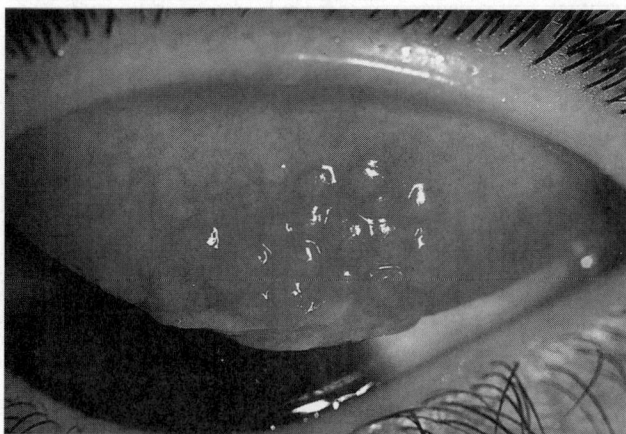

Fig. 26-3. Giant papillae (diameter > 1 mm) in the upper tarsal conjunctiva in GPC. (Figure also in color insert.)

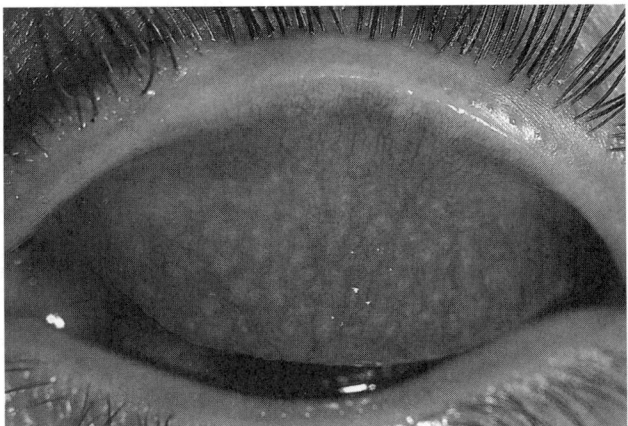

Fig. 26-4. Macropapillae (diameter 0.3-1.0 mm) in the upper tarsal conjunctiva in MPC (a developmental stage of GPC or a milder variant).

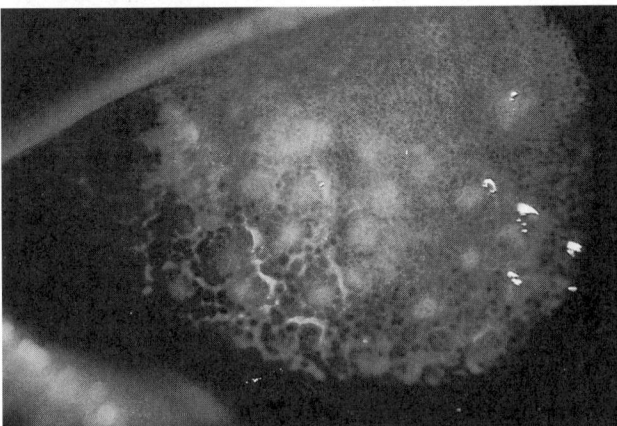

Fig. 26-5. Fluorescein staining of the tips of giant papillae in a case of suture GPC. The sutures were of 10/0 monofilament nylon in a peripheral corneal cataract section; some had loosened and two had broken, so that the material had eroded through the epithelium. (Figure also in color insert.)

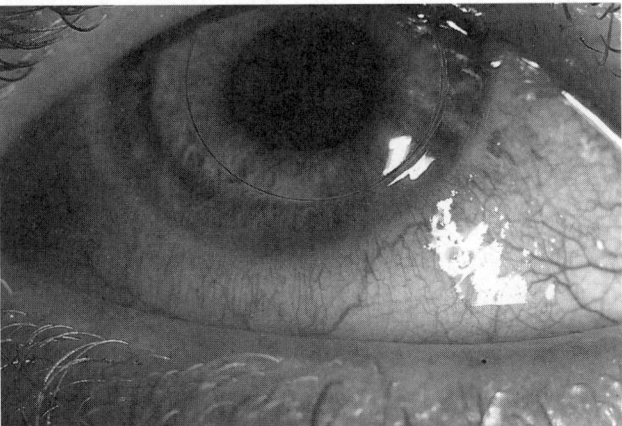

Fig. 26-6. Limbal edema and hyperemia in GPC. The patient wore GP corneal lenses for keratoconus, and continued to do so despite severe symptoms, as his vision with glasses was very poor.

fluorescein (Fig. 26-5). The abnormal mass of the upper lid sometimes leads to ptosis.[45,52] Limbal involvement, such as in VKC,[51] is uncommon (Fig. 26-6). There is no corneal involvement.

In many contact lens wearers, asymptomatic giant papillary tarsal conjunctival hypertrophy is seen at regular routine examinations. Active management of the condition at this stage may prevent its development to a symptomatic phase.

The differential diagnosis of GPC includes atopic keratoconjunctivitis and vernal keratoconjunctivitis, both conditions presenting itching symptoms, excessive mucus production, and the appearance of abnormally large or irregular papillae on the tarsal surfaces—although the presence of keratopathy distinguishes these from GPC. Bacterial conjunctivitis may occasionally resemble GPC, but the exudate is purulent rather than white and stringy. The follicles of a chlamydial, adenoviral, or primary herpetic conjunctivitis may occasionally be mistaken for giant papillae. The history of exposure to a foreign body (such as a contact lens, prosthesis, or suture) usually gives a clear pointer to the diagnosis.

THERAPY

The principles of the conventional management of GPC are as follows:

1. Reduction of deposits on the foreign surface that is in contact with the conjunctiva.
2. Reduced exposure of the conjunctiva to the foreign surface.
3. Optimization of contact lens or prosthesis fit and type.
4. Drug therapy.

Reduction of Deposits

Contact lenses should be cleaned with a surfactant cleaner after each period of wear (usually once daily); afterwards, they should be rinsed (preferably with sterile unpreserved saline) and then placed in the disinfection system (cold chemical or pasteurization). In addition, protein deposits (if judged problematic by the practitioner) should be removed by the use of enzyme solution (made up from tablets) at a frequency to be determined by the practitioner.[40] Since the availability of disposable contact lenses, it has been held by some that frequent replacement of the surface causing the problem is a legitimate management of GPC (and indeed this may work in some patients). Effective cleaning of both disposable and reusable lenses may, however, produce similar results.

Prostheses should be cleaned daily (or more often if necessary) with a simple household detergent such as soap or baby shampoo (unscented); then thoroughly rinsed in sterile saline, cool, recently boiled water or rising main tap water; then stored dry (or if desired replaced in the socket). Some wearers use contact lens cleaning solutions.

It is always necessary to ask contact lens or prosthesis wearers for exact details of their maintenance routine; nothing can be taken for granted. Experience suggests that an improvement in device hygiene can be advised for more than half of all patients. Lustine[43] found that the continued use of aging lenses and suboptimal lens care were the most important common factors in 47 patients with GPC. These patients obtained resolution of symptoms in 79% of their cases by improved cleaning, replacement of lenses, and the use of sodium cromoglycate. Infrequent lens change, with the older lens affecting patients unilaterally, was also reported recently by Palmisano.[55]

Reduced Exposure

The symptoms of GPC are usually dose-dependent, reducing with lesser exposure of the conjunctival surface to the foreign surface. Most contact lens wearers can reduce their daily wear time; for example, myopes can often be persuaded to remove their lenses and to substitute glasses on arrival home from work. Those who wear their lenses only socially or for sports can be encouraged to minimize the wear time on each occasion. Sometimes one lens can be worn for the first half of the day, and the other for the remainder. A reduced wear schedule may be adequate (in conjunction with scrupulously maintained lens hygiene) to control the symptoms of GPC.

Prosthesis wearers are in a less fortunate position in terms of reduced wear time, as an empty socket is always a cosmetic disaster; but they can be prevailed upon to remove the device at night. Ocularists (prosthetists) often instruct their clients to wear their cosmetic shells or artificial eyes continuously to maintain the elasticity of the adnexal tissues, but this is rarely necessary.

The ultimate reduction in wear is cessation. It was formerly believed that GPC would always regress if the offending foreign body was removed, although this is not always the case[54] in more advanced disease.

Optimization of Device Fit and Type

A lens that fits poorly is more likely to cause or to perpetuate GPC. Attention should always be paid to the profile of the lens, particularly its edge. Lenses with excessive edge lift are traumatic to the upper tarsal surface. Large diameter lenses, with their correspondingly large surface area, are more apt than smaller lenses to cause the condition.[48]

It is the practice of many contact lens practitioners to refit their soft lens GPC patients in RGP lenses. This practice is logical for two reasons: GP materials deposit less than most soft materials, and they are smaller in diameter.

The prosthesis wearer may be helped by switching to another type or material: for example, there are a few patients who develop GPC when wearing standard PMMA prostheses, who can be rendered asymptomatic by provision of glass prostheses. However, glass prostheses can also cause GPC, and their surfaces degrade more quickly.

Drug Therapy

Topical sodium cromogycate (cromolyn 4%), a mast cell stabilizing drug, is an effective treatment for mild to moderate cases of giant papillary conjunctivitis.[41,48,50] Cromolyn allowed 14 of 20 intolerant patients to wear their contact lenses.[41] Cromolyn inhibits activation of neutrophils, eosinophils, and monocytes.[18,39] There is a newer drug, nedocromil sodium,[6] that also reduces itching and mucus production. Nedocromil prevents inflammatory mediator release[30] and activation of the same cells.[53] Lodoxamide is another mast cell stabilizing agent, 2500 times more potent than cromolyn in vitro,[37] that may also be as effective as cromolyn in vivo and has the advantage of a faster onset.[73] Nonsteroidal antiinflammatory agents, such as suprofen, have shown some benefit in GPC[75]; and the search for further mast cell stabilizing agents has produced promising candidates, such as N-acetyl aspartyl glutamic acid.

Topical corticosteroid preparations are effective, but contraindicated, in GPC, because the complications (glaucoma, cataract, infection enhancement) that they may cause are unacceptable in the context of a nonsight-threatening disease. The same does not apply in prosthesis GPC, in which there is no eye present to be harmed in this way; in such cases, topical steroid preparations may be given if necessary.

PROGNOSIS

The usual outcome of the disease process is resolution, with flattening of the papillae, subepithelial fibrosis, and cessation of the symptoms. Contact lens wear may once again be possible, but at this stage many patients will have given up the use of contact lenses or reduced their dependency on them, and consequently will not wish to resume full time lens wear. Only a few cases become autonomous and remain chronically active.

It is therefore possible to inform patients with GPC of the likelihood their condition will resolve, and without visual loss. Keratoconjunctivitis sicca, conjunctival cicatrisation, tarsal marginal entropion, and other sequelae of chronic conjunctival inflammation are not seen in GPC.

REFERENCES

1. Abbasoglu O: *Effect of disposable contact lenses on tear film LTC4 in giant papillary conjunctivitis.* Unpublished data presented at the 23rd Congress of the European Contact Lens Society of Ophthalmologists, Amsterdam, May 1993.
1a. Allansmith MR, Korb DR, Greiner JV et al.: Giant papillary conjunctivitis in contact lens wearers, *Am J Ophthalmol* 83:697-708, 1977.
2. Allansmith MR, Korb DR, Greiner JV: Giant papillary conjunctivitis induced by hard or soft contact lens wear: quantitative histology, *Ophthalmology* 85:766-778, 1978.

3. Allansmith MR, Baird RS, Greiner JV: Vernal conjunctivitis and contact lens-associated giant papillary conjunctivitis compared and contrasted, *Am J Ophthalmol* 87:544-555, 1979.

4. Allansmith MR, Baird RS, Greiner JV: Density of goblet cells in vernal conjunctivitis and contact lens-associated giant papillary conjunctivitis, *Arch Ophthalmol* 99:884-885, 1981.

5. Allansmith MR, Baird RS: Percentage of degranulated mast cells in vernal conjunctivitis and giant papillary conjunctivitis associated with contact lens wear, *Am J Ophthalmol* 91:71-75, 1981.

6. Bailey CS, Buckley RJ: Nedocromil sodium in contact lens-associated papillary conjunctivitis, *Eye* 9(suppl)7:29-33, 1993.

7. Ballow M, Donshik PC, Mendelson L: Complement proteins and C3 anaphylatoxin in the tears of patients with conjunctivitis, *J Allergy Clin Immunol* 76:473-476, 1985.

8. Ballow M, Donshik PC, Rapacz P, Samartino L: Tear lactoferrin levels in patients with external inflammatory ocular disease, *Invest Ophthalmol Vis Sci* 28:543-545, 1987.

9. Ballow M, Donshik PC, Rapacz P et al.: Immune responses in monkeys to lenses from patients with contact lens induced giant papillary conjunctivitis, *CLAO J* 15:64-70, 1989.

10. Barishak Y, Zavaro A, Samra Z, Sompolinsky D: An immunologic study of papillary conjunctivitis due to contact lenses, *Curr Eye Res* 3:1161-1168, 1984.

11. Begley CG, Riggle A, Tuel JA: Association of giant papillary conjunctivitis with seasonal allergies, *Optom Vis Sci* 67:192-195, 1990.

12. Ben-Sasson SZ, LeGros G, Conrad DH et al.: *Proc Natl Acad Sci USA* 87:1421-1425, 1990.

13. Bradding P, Feather IH, Howarth PH et al.: Interleukin 4 is localized to and released by human mast cells, *J Exp Med* 176:1381-1386, 1992.

14. Britten KM, Howarth PH, Roche WR: Immunohistochemistry on resin sections: a comparison of resin embedding techniques for small mucosal biopsies, *Biotech Histochem,* 1993 (in press).

15. Bucci FA, Lopatynsky MO, Jenkins PL et al.: Comparison of the clinical performance of the Acuvue disposable contact lens and CSI lens in patients with giant papillary conjunctivitis, *Am J Ophthalmol* 115:454-459, 1993.

16. Buckley RJ: Pathology and treatment of giant papillary conjunctivitis. II. The British perspective, *Clin Ther* 9:451-457, 1987.

17. Church MK, Caulfield JP: Mast cell and basophil functions. In Holgate ST, Church MK, editors: *Allergy,* 1993, London and New York, Gower Medical Publishing.

18. Dixon JM, Jackson DM, Richards IM: The action of sodium cromoglycate on 'C' fibre endings in the dog lung, *Br J Pharmacol* 70:11-13, 1980.

19. Donshik PC, Ballow M: Tear immunoglobulins in giant papillary conjunctivitis induced by contact lenses, *Am J Ophthalmol* 96:460-466, 1983.

20. Donshik P, Downes RT, Gotasky K, Elgebaly SA: The detection of neutrophil chemotactic factors in tear fluids of contact lens wearers with active giant papillary conjunctivitis, *Invest Ophthalmol Vis Sci* 29(suppl):230, 1988.

21. Douglas JP, Lowder CY, Lazouik R, Meisler DM: Giant papillary conjunctivitis associated with rigid gas permeable contact lenses, *CLAO J* 14:143-147, 1988.

22. Dunn JP Jr, Weissman BA, Mondino BJ, Arnold AC: Giant papillary conjunctivitis associated with elevated corneal deposits, *Cornea* 9:357-358, 1990.

23. Ehrlers WH, Fishman JB, Donshik PC et al.: Neutrophil chemotactic factors derived from conjunctival epithelial cells: preliminary biochemical characterisation, *CLAO J* 17:65-68, 1991.

24. Elgebaly SA, Donshik PC, Rahhal F, Williams W: Neutrophil chemotactic factors in the tears of giant papillary conjunctivitis patients, *Invest Ophthalmol Vis Sci* 32:208-213, 1991.

25. Fowler SA, Korb DR, Finnemore VM, Allansmith MR: Surface deposits on worn hard contact lenses, *Arch Ophthalmol* 102:757-759, 1984.

26. Fowler SA, Gaertner KL: Scanning electron microscopy of deposits remaining in soft contact lens polishing marks after cleaning, *CLAO J* 16:214-218, 1990.

27. Fowler SA, Allansmith MR: Evolution of soft contact lens coatings, *Arch Ophthalmol* 98:95-99, 1980.

28. Fowler SA, Greiner JV, Allansmith MR: Attachment of bacteria to soft contact lenses, *Arch Ophthalmol* 97:659-660, 1979.

29. Gonzalez JP, Brogden RN: Nedocromil sodium: a preliminary review of its pharmacodynamic and pharmaocokinetic properties, and therapeutic efficacy in the treatment of reversible obstructive airways disease, *Drugs* 34:560-577, 1987.

30. Greiner JV, Kenyon KR, Henriquez AS et al.: Mucus secretory vesicles in conjunctival epithelial cells of wearers of contact lenses, *Arch Ophthalmol* 98:1843-1846, 1980.

31. van Haeringen NJ: Clinical biochemistry of tears, *Surv Ophthalmol* 26:84-96, 1981.

32. Hamano H, Kitano J, Mitsunaga S et al.: Adverse effects of lens wear in a large Japanese population, *CLAO J* 11:141-147, 1985.

33. Hart DE, Scholnik JA, Bernstein S et al.: Contact lens induced giant papillary conjunctivitis: a retrospective study, *J Am Optom Assoc* 60:195-204, 1989.

34. Heidemann DG, Dunn SP, Siegal MJ: Unusual causes of giant papillary conjunctivitis, *Cornea* 12:78-80, 1993.

35. Henriquez AS, Kenyon KR, Allansmith MR: Mast cell ultrastructure: comparison in contact-lens associated giant papillary conjunctivitis and vernal conjunctivitis, *Arch Ophthalmol* 99:1266-1272, 1981.

36. Irani A-M A, Butrus SI, Tabbara KF, Schwartz LB: Human conjunctival mast cells: distribution of MC_T and MC_{TC} in vernal conjunctivitis and giant papillary conjunctivitis, *J Allergy Clin Immunol* 86:34-39, 1990.

37. Johnson HG, Van Hout CA, Wright JB: Inhibition of allergic reactions by cromoglycate and by a new anti-allergy drug, U-42,585E: I Activity in rats, *Int Arch Allergy Appl Immunol* 56:416-423, 1978.

38. Jones B, Sack R: Immunoglobulin deposition on soft contact lenses: relationship to hydrogel structure and mode of use and giant papillary conjunctivitis, *CLAO J* 16:43-48, 1990.

39. Kay AB, Walsh GM, Moqbel R et al.: Disodium cromoglycate inhibits activation of human inflammatory cells in vitro, *J Allergy Clin Immunol* 80:573-577, 1987.

40. Korb DR, Greiner JV, Finnemore VM, Allansmith MR: Treatment of contact lenses with papain: increase in wearing time in keratoconic patients with papillary conjunctivitis, *Arch Ophthalmol* 101:48-50, 1983.

41. Kruger CJ, Ehrlers WH, Luistro AE, Donshik PC: Treatment of giant papillary conjunctivitis with cromolyn sodium, *CLAO J* 18:46-48, 1992.

42. Little JM, Certifanto YM, Kaufman HE: Immunoglobulins in human tears, *Am J Ophthalmol* 68:898-905, 1969.

43. Lustine T, Bouchard CS, Cavanagh HD: Continued contact lens wear in patients with giant papillary conjunctivitis, *CLAO J* 17:104-107, 1991.

44. MacIvor J: Contact allergy to plastic artificial eyes: preliminary report, *Can Med Assoc J* 62:164, 1950.

45. Mackie IA, Wright P: Giant papillary conjunctivitis (secondary vernal) in association with contact lens wear, *Trans Ophthalmol Soc UK* 98:3-9, 1978.

46. Martin NF, Rubinfeld RS, Malley JD, Manzitti V: Giant papillary conjunctivitis and meibomian gland dysfunction blepharitis, *CLAO J* 18:165-169, 1992.

47. Mathers WD, Billborough M: Meibomian gland function and giant papillary conjunctivitis, *Am J Ophthalmol* 114:188-192, 1992.

48. Matter M, Rahi AHS, Buckley RJ: Sodium cromoglycate in the treatment of contact lens-associated giant papillary conjunctivitis, *Proc VII Congress Europ Soc Ophthalmol, Helsinki* 383-384, 1985.

49. Meisler DM, Krachmer JH, Goeken JA: An immunopathologic study of giant papillary conjunctivitis associated with an ocular prosthesis, *Am J Ophthalmol* 92:368-371, 1981.

50. Meisler DM, Berzins UJ, Krachmer JH, Stock EL: Cromolyn treatment of giant papillary conjunctivitis, *Arch Ophthalmol* 100:1608-1610, 1982.

51. Meisler DM, Zaret CR, Stock EL: Trantas dots and limbal inflammation associated with soft contact lens wear, eosinophil degranulation, with the deposition of MBP occurs in both VKC and GPC, *Am J Ophthalmol* 89:66-69, 1980.

51a. Metz D: *T cells in chronic atopic conjunctivitis,* PhD thesis submitted to University of London, 1993.

52. Molinari JF: Transient ptosis secondary to giant papillary conjunctivitis in a hydrogel lens patient, *J Am Optom Assoc* 54:1007-1009, 1983.

53. Moqbel R, Cromwell O, Walsh GM et al.: Effects of nedocromil sodium (Tilade) on the activation of human eosinophils and neutrophils and the release of histamine from mast cells, *Allergy* 43:268-276, 1988.

54. Neuhann T: Papillomatous hyperplastic conjunctivitis caused by contact lenses, *Klin Monatsbl Augenheilkd* 182:46-50, 1983.

55. Palmisano PC, Ehrlers WH, Donshik PC: Causative factors in unilateral giant papillary conjunctivitis, *CLAO J* 19:103-107, 1993.

56. Piccinni M-P, Macchia D, Parronichi P et al.: Human bone marrow non-B, non-T cells produce interleukin 4 in response to cross linkage of Fc epsilon and Fc gamma receptors, *Proc Natl Acad Sci USA* 88:8656-9660, 1991.

57. Richard NR, Anderson JA, Tasevska ZG, Binder PS: Evaluation of tear protein deposits on contact lenses from patients with and without giant papillary conjunctivitis, *CLAO J* 18:143-147, 1992.

58. Rigal K, Harrer S, Rubey F: Differential diagnosis and therapy of gigantopapillary conjunctivitis, *Klin Monatsbl Augenheilkd* 186:377-379, 1985.

59. Robin JB, Regis-Pacheco LF, May WN et al.: Giant papillary conjunctivitis associated with an extruded scleral buckle, *Arch Ophthalmol* 105:619, 1987.

60. Romagnani S: Induction of TH1 and TH2 responses: a key role for the "natural" immune response? *Immunol Today* 13:379-381, 1992.

61. Rot A: Endothelial binding of NAP-1/1L8: role in neutrophil emigration, *Immunol Today* 13:291-294, 1992.

62. Sach RA, Jones B, Antignani A et al.: Specificity and biologic activity of the protein deposited on the hydrogel surface: relationship of polymer structure to biofilm formation, *Invest Ophthalmol Vis Sci* 28:842, 1987.

63. Skrypuch OW, Willis NR: Giant papillary conjunctivitis from an exposed prolene suture, *Can J Ophthalmol* 21:189-192, 1986.

64. Soni PS, Hathcoat G: Complications reported with hydrogel extended wear contact lenses, *Am J Optom Physiol Opt* 65:545-551, 1988.

65. Spring TF: Reaction to hydrophilic contact lenses, *Med J Aust* 1:449, 1974.

66. Srinivasan BD, Jakobeic FA, De Voe AG: Giant papillary conjunctivitis with ocular prosthesis, *Arch Ophthalmol* 97:892-895, 1979.

67. Stenson S: Focal giant papillary conjunctivitis from retained contact lenses, *Ann Ophthalmol* 14:881-885, 1982.

68. Sugar A, Meyer RF: Giant papillary conjunctivitis after keratoplasty, *Am J Ophthalmol* 91:239-242, 1981.

69. Temel A, Kazokoglu H, Taga Y, Orkan AL: The effect of contact lens wear on tear immunoglobulins, *CLAO J* 17:69-71, 1991.

70. Trocme SD, Kephart GM, Allansmith MR et al.: Conjunctival deposition of eosinophil major basic protein in vernal keratoconjunctivitis and contact lens-associated giant papillary conjunctivitis, *Am J Ophthalmol* 108:57-63, 1989.

71. Trocme SD, Kephart GM, Bourne WM et al.: Eosinophil granular major basic protein in contact lenses of patients with giant papillary conjunctivitis, *CLAO J* 16:219-222, 1990.

72. Udell IJ, Gleich GJ, Allansmith MR et al.: Eosinophil granule major basic protein and Charcot-Leyden crystal protein in human tears, *Am J Ophthalmol* 92:824, 1981.

72a. van Aalst, van Bijsterveld: The Axon Reflex in GPC. Unpublished data presented at 23rd Congress of the European Contact Lens Society of Ophthalmologists, Amsterdam, 1993.

72b. van Bijsterveld OP, Aalders-Deenstra V: Clinical evaluation of N-acetylaspartyl glutamic acid eyedrops in subacute and chronic atopic conjunctivitis, *Klin Monatsbl Augenheilkd* 188:625-627, 1986.

73. Verstappen AA, Rosenthal AL, McDonald TO: Alomide versus sodium cromoglycate in patients with vernal, atopic or giant papillary conjunctivitis, *Arq Bras Ophtalm* 52:4, 1989.

74. Wille H, Molgaard IL: Giant papillary conjunctivitis in connection with corneoscleral supramid (nylon) suture knots, *Acta Ophthalmol (Copenh)* 62:75-83, 1984.

75. Wood TJ, Stewart RH, Bowman RW et al.: Suprofen treatment of contact lens-associated giant papillary conjunctivitis, *Ophthalmology* 95:822-826, 1988.

76. Yano H, Wershil BK, Arizono N, Galli SJ: Substance P-induced augmentation of cutaneous vascular permeability and granulocyte infiltration in mice is mast cell dependent, *J Clin Invest* 84:1276-1286, 1989.

27 Vernal Conjunctivitis

JILL M. BRODY, C. STEPHEN FOSTER

Vernal conjunctivitis, or more accurately, vernal kerato-conjunctivitis (VKC), is a bilateral, chronic, external ocular inflammatory disease of unknown cause that is related to atopy and has environmental and racial predilections. Atopic individuals develop reactions to ubiquitous environmental antigens. The major atopies include eczema, asthma, and urticaria. VKC primarily affects children and young adults and is most common in the spring, hence the name "vernal." The afflicted patients suffer from a collection of external symptoms, most prominently itching, tearing, photophobia, and mucus discharge. The disease is usually "self-limiting," but the morbidity of it can be severely disabling. The current treatment modalities of proven efficacy include topical adrenocorticosteroids and mast cell stabilizers.

EPIDEMIOLOGY

VKC is an episodic, bilateral, inflammatory condition of the conjunctiva that is most frequently seen in children and young adults; it is rarely seen in individuals who are under 3 years of age or over 30.[13] About 60% of VKC patients are between the ages of 11 and 20 years, 17% are between 21 and 30, and 6% are older than 30.[31] Males with VKC outnumber females by a ratio of 2 or 3 to 1 until puberty, when the number of females afflicted with VKC increases gradually until the ratio approaches 1:1 by age 20. Episodes typically occur over a 2- to 10-year period, and the underlying condition often resolves around puberty. VKC has a seasonal nature; although in a few unfortunate patients, the disease is perennial and evolves into the cicatrizing condition of adult allergic keratoconjunctivitis (AKC). VKC is associated with keratoconus, atopy, and atopic cataract.

VKC occurs worldwide and affects all races; but it has an increased incidence in hot, dry environments such as West Africa, the Mediterranean, the Balkans, and parts of India and Central and South America. VKC may represent as much as 3% of serious ophthalmic disease in some regions,[5] whereas in Northern Europe and North America the incidence is approximately 1 in 5000 cases of eye disease.[22] The increased incidence in warmer climates is thought to be secondary to relatively high levels of pollution by pollens and other allergens. Seasonal changes or symptom-free intervals are less common in the tropics, as is regression of the disease.

HISTORICAL BACKGROUND

A chronology of the early descriptions of VKC is shown in Fig. 27-1. The early authors highlighted the conjunctival changes in VKC. Arlt reported the first series of young patients with perilimbal swelling in 1846.[31] Nine years later, Desmarres published a detailed description of limbal VKC, and in 1871 von Graefe described a case with both limbal changes and the classical cobblestone papillary response of the upper tarsal conjunctiva. The parallels between VKC and the allergic diseases, asthma and hay fever, were drawn in 1886 by Berkart and Gradle, respectively.[7,31]

Saemisch enlightened the ophthalmic world on two major aspects of VKC. In 1872 he highlighted the seasonal nature of the disease with the name "fruhjahrkatarrh" (spring or vernal catarrh). In 1876, when Saemisch published a lengthy review of the literature (along with his substantial series of 182 VKC patients), he commented on the rare involvement of the cornea.[7] Similarly, Axenfeld noted corneal manifestations of VKC in his 1907 review,[7] but like Saemisch, he considered them to be of trivial importance. Trantas[34] expounded on the corneal involvement in VKC in his treatise of 1910; he detailed a wider range of keratopathies, including corneal plaques and punctate superficial epitheliopathy. Trantas[33,34] described peculiar, limbal, white concretions ("point blancs") in 1899; however, in 1910 he acknowledged the earlier contributions of Horner in describing what are now known as Horner-Trantas dots.[7]

Gabrielides published a more detailed account of the vernal plaque in 1909. In Herbert's 1903 work on vernal plaque, he noted eosinophils in the involved tissues and the peripheral blood.[7,31] Pascheff's histologic examination of the epi-

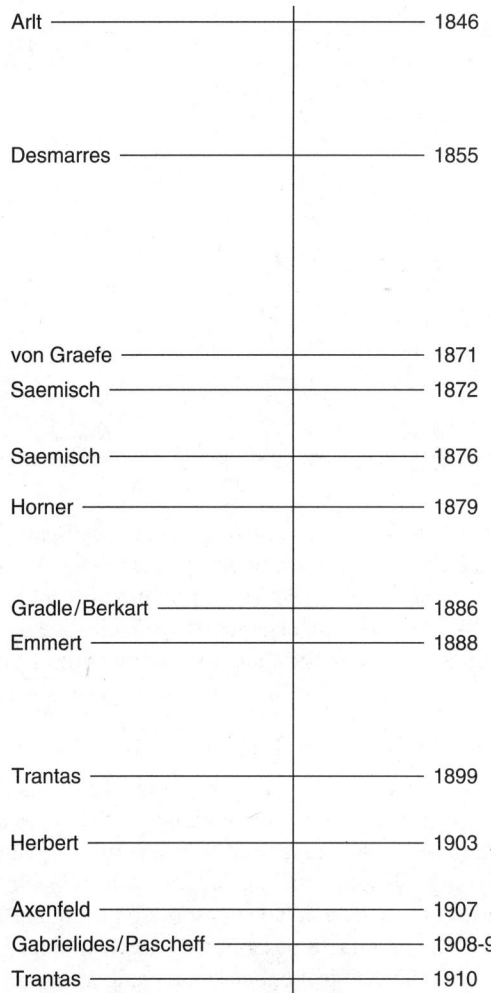

Arlt	1846
Desmarres	1855
von Graefe	1871
Saemisch	1872
Saemisch	1876
Horner	1879
Gradle/Berkart	1886
Emmert	1888
Trantas	1899
Herbert	1903
Axenfeld	1907
Gabrielides/Pascheff	1908-9
Trantas	1910

Fig. 27-1. Major contributors to the description of vernal kerato-conjunctivitis.

thelium of the tarsal conjunctiva in VKC revealed a substantial number of mast cells.[7]

PATHOGENESIS

VKC probably involves more than one immune mechanism. Direct and indirect evidence supports the hypothesis that a Gell and Coombs type 1 hypersensitivity reaction (an immediate, IgE-dependent, allergic response) underlies many of the symptoms suffered by patients with VKC.[4,15] Careful questioning of patients reveals a concomitant atopy or a family history of atopy. The elevated histamine levels in the tears, the histopathologic findings of many degranulated mast cells in the substantia propria and conjunctival epithelium, and the response to cromolyn sodium all point to an IgE mast cell-mediated process.[7,16] There has been a report of low histaminase activity in tears of patients with VKC; and histaminase deficiency or dysfunction may play a role in the pathogenesis.[5a] Although it is rare to identify a specific causal agent evoking the exuberant inflammatory response

of VKC, carefully performed scratch and intradermal skin testing often discloses sensitivity to several ubiquitous environmental allergens; sensitivity to house dust mites is especially prominent among these patients.[6a]

The type 1 hypersensitivity reaction cannot account for all of the histopathologic findings in VKC, however. Histopathologic and immunopathologic characteristics of the affected conjunctiva have led[3,6] to the conclusion that VKC is a combination of type 1 (immediate) and type 4 (delayed or cell-mediated) hypersensitivity reactions. Histopathologic studies of the conjunctival papillae reveal large collections of mononuclear cells, fibroblasts, and newly secreted collagen in addition to cells typically associated with allergic reactions (mast cells and eosinophils). Immunohistochemical studies show that the mononuclear cells are rich in helper (CD4) T cells (particularly TH2, the interleukin-4-secreting cells), and that the cytokines being produced by the inflammatory cells are, among other things, inducing elevated expression of Class II HLA glycoproteins on epithelium of the conjunctiva and on stromal cells.[6]

CLINICAL FEATURES

The classic hallmark of this bilateral disease is the giant papillae, usually on the upper tarsal conjunctiva (Fig. 27-2), but sometimes on the conjunctiva of the corneoscleral limbus (Fig. 27-3). The most prominent symptom, itching, is persistent. It is commonly the presenting symptom. Often the itching intensifies toward the evening, after a full day of exposure to exacerbating conditions and allergens such as dust, dander, bright lights, wind, sweat, and rubbing of the eyes. Other symptoms include ocular irritation and foreign body sensation, photophobia, burning, excessive tearing, and mucus discharge. Variation in the symptomatology is a prominent feature in the early course of VKC; as the disease progresses, the symptoms can intensify and, in some cases, become perennial. Emmert's 1888 description classified the

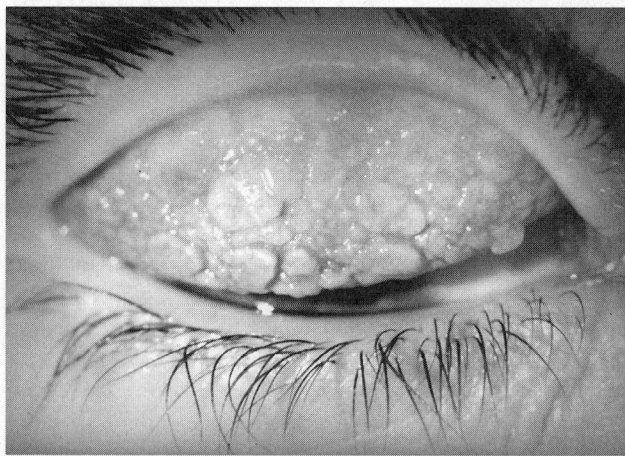

Fig. 27-2. Cobblestone pattern of giant papillae in vernal kerato-conjunctivitis.

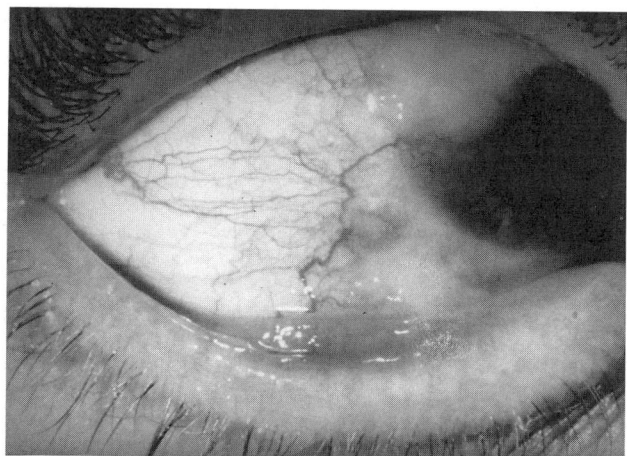

Fig. 27-3.   Limbal vernal keratoconjunctivitis.

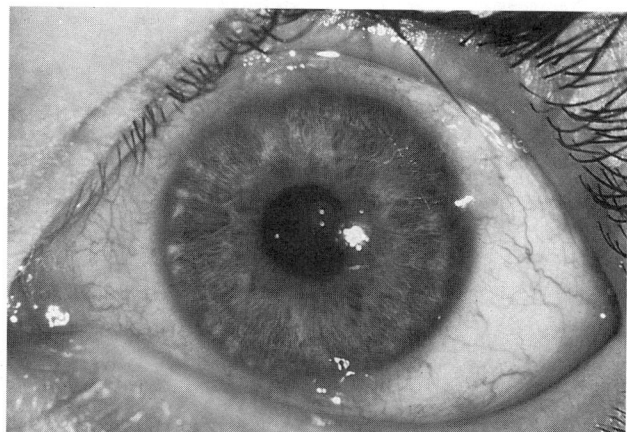

Fig. 27-4.   Horner-Trantas dots. (Figure also in color insert.)

disease as palpebral, limbal, or mixed[31]; but individual cases seldom fall neatly into one of these categories, and it is more useful to think of VKC in terms of the severity of symptoms. The disease can be described, however, by addressing the clinical changes in each ocular tissue affected.

Conjunctiva

VKC has its main influence on the bulbar and palpebral conjunctiva. The upper palpebral conjunctiva is classically involved with a cobblestone papillary reaction that may be confluent. These polygonal, flat-topped, giant papillae of the superior tarsal conjunctiva can be seen on simple external examination. The finding of giant papillae is not, however, pathognomonic. Slit lamp examination (Fig. 27-2) reveals papillae 1 mm to 8 mm in diameter that usually abut one another. Each has a central core of blood vessels (in contrast to follicles, which have blood vessels coursing over their top surfaces). Fluorescein stains their apices. Lying between these giant papillae and covering their surfaces (giving them a dull appearance) is a ropey, lardacious discharge that often forms a tenacious pseudomembrane (Maxwell-Lyons sign).[18,31] A follicular response is never seen in conjunctiva affected by VKC.

Limbal manifestations of VKC most often occur in people of color. Gelatinous limbal nodules or elevations appear in the area of the corneoscleral limbus (Fig. 27-3). Although the limbal conjunctiva can be involved 360 degrees, these papillae usually appear along the superior half of the limbus. Small, white excrescences (Horner-Trantas dots), composed of inflammatory cells rich in eosinophils, can be found at the apices of these papillae (Fig. 27-4). Thickening, broadening, and opacification of the limbal conjunctiva can also be detected.[7]

Cornea

The degree of corneal involvement in VKC is a good indicator of the severity of the disease. Beigelman[5] reported

that up to 50% of patients with palpebral VKC have corneal manifestations. In a study of 120 patients with VKC, Dart[14] found that corneal complications occurred almost exclusively in patients with palpebral or mixed palpebral and limbal VKC.

A superficial epithelial keratitis, consisting of punctate, dull gray opacities in the upper half of the cornea, is the most frequent corneal finding. Often described as a flour dusting overlying the cornea (Fig. 27-5), these points can break down, uniting to form a macroerosion. The margins of this shallow-based erosion are raised and can form a collection of compacted layers of cellular debris and mucus, known as a vernal plaque (Fig. 27-6). These plaques, also called "shield ulcers," are usually found only in the very young patients; most often, they are located superiorly and are transversely oval. They inhibit normal reepithelialization; and therefore the area of the erosion heals slowly, often resulting in a permanent, gray, oval, subepithelial opacity. These corneal plaques seldom vascularize, unless the corneal inflammation has become chronic.[31] These ulcers,

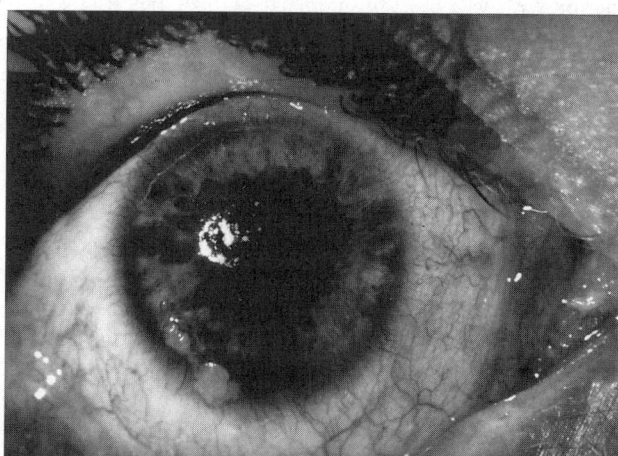

Fig. 27-5.   Superficial epithelial keratitis of vernal keratoconjunctivitis.

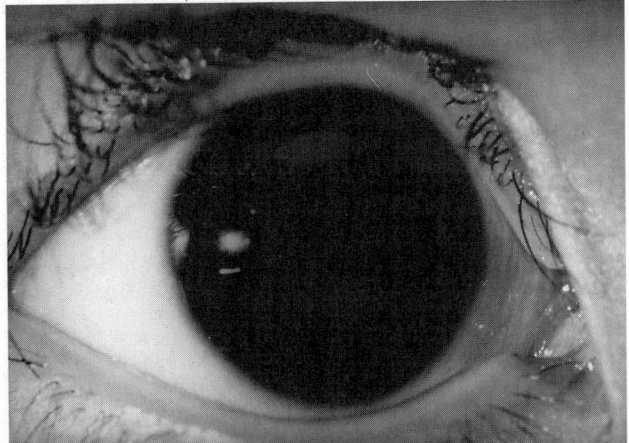

Fig. 27-6. Vernal plaque or shield ulcer.

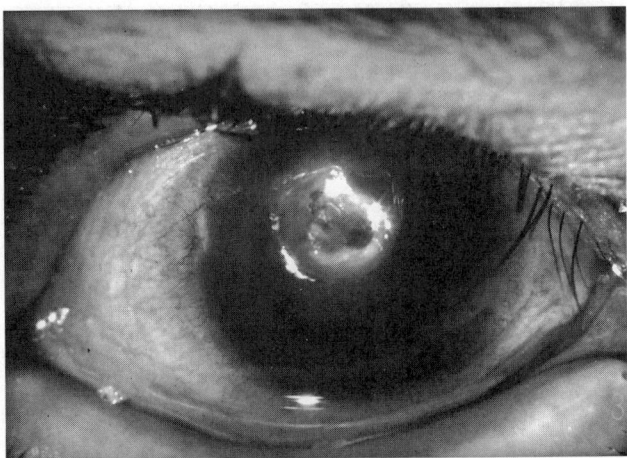

Fig. 27-7. Secondary microbial infection of a shield ulcer.

however, present the risk of secondary microbial infection with permanent corneal consequences (Fig. 27-7).

Stromal keratitis may also occur in VKC. The degenerative change most often observed in the cornea is pseudogerontoxon, which resembles arcus senilis.[31] This arc-shaped opacification of the superficial stroma appears in the peripheral cornea, which has an intervening clear zone separating it from the limbus. In some cases this focal, yellow-gray opacity ulcerates, causing a peripheral furrowing. Subsequent steepening of the cornea in the area of the furrow causes myopic astigmatism. The pseudogerontoxon is associated with new vessel growth into the corneal periphery, which waxes and wanes depending on the limbal inflammatory activity. Likewise, the occasional formation of a superior pannus is usually a consequence of these limbal changes.[31]

Other ulcerations have been noted in the literature; Shuler and associates[30] reported inferior corneal ulcerations associated with palpebral VKC. Corneal ectasias (keratoconus, keratoglobus, pellucid marginal degeneration, and superior marginal corneal thinning) have also been described in association with VKC.[11,27] In summary, corneal alterations such as astigmatism, keratoconus, keratoglobus, marginal corneal degeneration, or pseudogerontoxon can result from VKC; but, except in the rare cases in which the disease is unrelenting and evolves into AKC, blinding complications such as severe corneal scarring or pannus formation are unusual.

External

Examination of the eyelids may reveal signs of VKC. Ptosis, believed to be secondary to the weight of the vernal papillary hypertrophy, is common. Dennie line, an extra fold in the lower lid skin, may be seen as well.

DIFFERENTIAL DIAGNOSIS

The differential diagnosis of VKC includes most of the conditions resulting in an allergic response of the conjunctiva. The classic textbook case of severe VKC, with signs of

papillary cobblestone reaction, shield ulcer, Horner-Trantas dots, and ocular allergic symptoms, is unmistakable. Less severe cases of VKC, however, are more difficult to discern. Some laboratory tests that are helpful in diagnosis are discussed later in this chapter.

Because it requires aggressive treatment, the most important contender in the differential diagnosis of VKC is AKC, which can be easily confused early in the disease process.[17] Epidemiologically, AKC affects patients from their teens to mid-life; it is almost always perennial, and has a longer disease course than VKC. Externally, the lids of AKC patients show the signs of chronic blepharitis and eczema. Unlike VKC, AKC causes conjunctival scarring, subepithelial fibrosis, and foreshortening of the lower fornix (cicatrization). Other signs and symptoms help to differentiate the two conditions: AKC principally affects the lower palpebral conjunctiva, causing small papillae; neovascularization of the cornea is usually deeper in AKC; the discharge of AKC is watery, whereas the discharge of VKC is viscous; Horner-Trantas dots are rarely found in AKC; and conjunctival scrapings seldom contain eosinophilic granules.

Hay fever conjunctivitis, or seasonal allergic conjunctivitis (SAC), is one of the most common afflictions seen in an ophthalmology practice. Rapid onset (with conjunctival injection, chemosis, and occasionally lid edema) follows exposure to allergen. Unlike VKC patients, SAC patients often have a concomitant allergic rhinitis or sinusitis. Corneal changes are rarely observed in SAC.

Giant papillary conjunctivitis (GPC) is usually related to allergens or foreign bodies that directly contact the conjunctiva. In the past few decades, GPC has been most widely associated with contact lenses; but other irritants, such as exposed ends of unburied sutures or ocular prostheses, may also stimulate GPC. The conjunctival papillary response of the upper tarsus and the significant mucus production closely resemble the changes seen in VKC; however, a good history and careful examination will lead to the correct diagnosis. Signs and symptoms of GPC will disappear when the inciting agent is removed.

Chemical (or toxic) conjunctivitis from drug hypersensitivity also produces signs and symptoms similar to those of VKC. Agents notorious for causing drug hypersensitivity reactions in the conjunctiva are atropine, topical anesthetics, antibiotics, phenylepherine, and various drug vehicles. In chemical conjunctivitis, the papillary conjunctival response is less dramatic, and the inferior fornix is more substantially affected than in VKC.

Finally, a differential diagnosis may need to include trachoma. Trachoma causes many pathologic changes in the upper tarsal conjunctiva and superior corneolimbal area. Unlike VKC, however, it produces conjunctival scarring, a follicular conjunctivitis, and Arlt line (horizontal subepithelial fibrosis). Conjunctival scrapings from trachoma patients do not disclose eosinophils. Interestingly, VKC and trachoma can coexist in the same patient; this phenomenon is not surprising, considering the diseases' common predilection for warmer climates.[19]

PATHOLOGY

VKC is proliferative in nature, characterized by increased formation of hyalinized connective tissue. In the conjunctiva, hypertrophy produces papillae covered by hyperplastic epithelium; increased numbers of goblet cells are noted, especially along the walls of abutting papillae.[16] Each papillae has a central blood vessel tuft; the central blood vessel is surrounded by edematous tissues infiltrated extensively with plasma cells, eosinophils, mast cells, and lymphocytes.[35] Active phagocytosis by histiocytes and neutrophils can be seen. In the limbal region, both conjunctival epithelium and subepithelial fibrovascular connective tissue undergo hyperplasia and infiltration by the same kind of cells; the characteristic gelatinous nodules develop as a result.[35] The Horner-Trantas dots overlying some of the affected limbal areas are rich in eosinophils.

Eosinophilic degeneration and hyalinization of the connective tissue, along with neovascularization of the substantia propria, eventually lead to endothelial swelling and hyalinization of capillary walls, and finally to degeneration of the blood vessels.[16] The proliferating epithelium forms as many as 10 layers of edematous epithelial cells in the palpebral conjunctiva and 30 to 40 layers in the bulbar conjunctiva at the limbus. The conjunctival epithelial layers thin at the apex of the papillae, and this area may show punctate staining.[7,35]

Although the corneal manifestations of VKC have been described as "frictional," chemical toxicity from the degranulation of mast cells and eosinophils is a far more important cause of the corneal changes.[7] Mast cells, normally present in the conjunctival substantia propria, are found in the involved conjunctival epithelium and are in varying stages of degranulation.[35] Degeneration and sloughing of the corneal epithelium results in punctate keratopathy.

Immunohistochemical analysis of the conjunctiva discloses large numbers of helper T cells, with a reversal of the helper-to-suppressor (CD 4 to CD 8) ratio, and an increased number of Langerhans cells.[6] Many of the plasma cells in the involved conjunctiva in VKC are designated IgE plasma cells. Many of the activated T cells express the CD 25 (IL-2 receptor) glycoprotein on their surface membranes. Gamma interferon and other cytokines secreted by these immunologically active cells induce the expression of Class II HLA glycoprotein by epithelial cells.[26] Maggi and associates[23] discovered that the majority of T cells in the conjunctiva of VKC patients are Th2-like helper cells that produce interleukin-4 (IL-4), but not gamma interferon, and show a helper function for IgE synthesis. IL-4 is a growth factor for mast cell and B cells, and therefore the Th2-like cells may be responsible for the increased accumulation of mast cells and B cells in the conjunctiva of VKC patients.

LABORATORY INVESTIGATIONS

Classical VKC is easy to diagnose, but some cases of VKC are indistinct. Although few of the laboratory tests and examinations described in the following discussion are commonly used, they can be helpful in identifying some types of ocular allergy.

Allergy testing is indicated for patients with atopy or systemic allergy and sometimes for patients with refractory cases of VKC. In a collaborative study, Foster noted multiple sensitivities in 41 of 65 patients with VKC.[15] Such testing should measure the response of the patient to the usual allergens in his environment.

Conjunctival Cytology

Conjunctival scrapings can also aid the diagnosis of patients' ocular allergy. The normal human conjunctiva does not contain eosinophils or eosinophilic granules, and therefore the finding of either in a Giemsa-stained conjunctival scraping confirms the presence of an allergic process.[8] Similarly, electron microscopy of conjunctival biopsy specimens can identify mast cells, basophils, and eosinophils and/or eosinophilic granules.[8] Electron microscopy is preferred for the identification and counting of mast cells and their associated granules; in VKC, many mast cells have undergone extensive degranulation, making them difficult to recognize under light microscopy.[20]

The clinically useful diagnostic tests listed previously are varied and have given rise to laboratory research into the nature of the disease itself. In 1990 Irani and associates[21] examined the distribution of human tryptase-positive, chymase-negative mast cells (MC_T) and tryptase-positive, chymase-positive mast cells (MC_{TC}) in conjunctival biopsy specimens from patients with active VKC and GPC. The results were compared with findings obtained from patients with allergic conjunctivitis, from asymptomatic contact lens wearers, and from normal controls. In VKC conjunctiva, the percentages of MC_T and total mast cell concentrations in the substantia propria were dramatically higher than in conjunctiva from other patients or controls.

Tear Composition

Examination of tears can also be useful. The demonstration of eosinophils, neutrophils, or lymphocytes in tears indicates an allergic condition.[8] Elevated tear histamine levels are also occasionally detected in patients with ocular allergy, but not with the consistency found in VKC.[1] Dart[14] found higher-than-normal levels of IgE, and IgE specific to cat dander and house dust mites, in the serum and tear IgE levels in VKC patients.[14]

Tryptase levels in tears reflect the degree of mast cell involvement in ocular allergies. In 1990 Butrus and associates[9] studied tryptase levels in the unstimulated tears of controls and of patients with VKC, other ocular allergies, or nonallergic inflammation. They also measured tear tryptase amounts in tears brought on by common allergen challenge, instillation of compound 48/80, or ocular rubbing. Dramatically elevated tryptase levels were found in unstimulated tears of ocular allergy patients; and marginal elevation was seen in atopic individuals provoked with topical allergens and compound 48/80, and in controls incited with compound 48/80 and traumatic eye rubbing. Elevated tear tryptase is a harbinger of mast cell involvement in the disease process and its detection can be a useful marker for mast cell involvement in vernal and other ocular allergies.

Levels of two important tear proteins, lactoferrin and lysozyme, are reduced in keratoconjunctivitis sicca. In 1988 Rapacz and associates[25] demonstrated that tears from patients with VKC or GPC have reduced levels of lactoferrin, but normal levels of lysozyme, compared with controls. This pattern of decreased lactoferrin and normal lysozyme levels was felt to be unique to VKC and GPC; further studies may elucidate its cause.

THERAPY

Therapy of VKC can be divided into three broad categories: general, chemotherapeutic or medical, and surgical or procedural. Historically, the types of therapies for VKC have varied greatly.[7] Heavy metals, calcium therapy, acids, vitamins, and local anesthetics are a few of the local medical therapies used in the past. Surgical treatments have included cautery, electrolysis, tarsectomy, and conjunctival advancements; most were injurious to the conjunctiva and caused permanent scarring. Although current measures are more effective, the patient suffering from debilitating VKC still presents an ongoing dilemma to the ophthalmic practitioner.

First and foremost, the clinician should keep in mind the self-limiting nature of the disease and the usual good outcome of the disease. Iatrogenic disease must be avoided. Steroid drugs are so effective in controlling inflammation that the physician is sometimes tempted to underestimate the possibility of complications (cataract, glaucoma, enhancement of infections) arising from overuse. The risks and benefits of therapies must be carefully explained to the patients (or their parents), so that they may make informed decisions.

General Measures

General measures must include alteration of the VKC patient's environment. Although it is usually an unpleasant, expensive, time-consuming exercise, policing of the patient's environment and scrupulous removal of all potential allergen provocateurs is critical to the patient's long-term stability. Involvement of an expert allergist is essential, especially in refractory VKC patients. A knowledgeable, experienced specialist performs the appropriate patch, scratch, and prick tests, as well as the serum Rast tests; this professional does the environmental detective work and provides the motivation and education necessary for a successful environmental program. Obviously, the patient's family must be convinced of the long-term benefits to the whole family, as well as to the patient, before they embark on a complex program that sometimes requires removal of expensive carpeting, installation of air conditioning and air-filtering systems in the home heating system, elimination of beloved pets, etc. Nonetheless, the wisdom, importance, and prophylactic benefit of this component of the total care of the VKC patient cannot be overemphasized.

Desensitization by immunotherapy often produces disappointing results, but it can benefit severely affected patients who are strikingly sensitive to a limited number of allergens. Performing desensitization immunotherapy on a patient with ocular allergy by his allergist, however, is not easy; and some features of this treatment differ from the typical practice of desensitization immunotherapy in the patient with allergies not affecting the eyes.

Cool compresses and ice packs may provide some respite. Patients report that they are less symptomatic when their eyes are closed; similarly, occlusive therapy (patching, occlusive goggles, or a tarsorrhaphy) provides temporary relief. The symptoms recur after cessation of the occlusive therapy. Soft contact lenses have been used to protect the cornea from the irritative effect of the vegetations on the upper tarsal conjunctiva. The fitting of contact lenses in patients with VKC can be very difficult, however; and the increased susceptibility to infections in patients using topical corticosteroids make contact lenses a temporary and risky measure.

Medical Therapy

Drug therapy of VKC has evolved dramatically over the last two decades from reliance on nonspecific treatment of symptoms (for example, topical vasoconstrictors) toward treatment of their causes. The medical treatment of VKC, however, often remains moderately palliative at best; and to the novice, it may seem broad and haphazard. The challenge is to fashion a regimen that provides comfort for the patient and uses the smallest amount of topical adrenocorticosteroid possible.

Antihistamines

Beginning with systemic medications, systemic antihistamine therapy is preferred[6a] to topical ocular antihistamines used in the past, primarily because these allergic eye diseases last a long time; but also because allergic individuals sometimes become sensitized to the preservatives present in the commercially available ocular antihistamines. Terfenadine, 60 mg twice a day, and/or astemizole, 10 mg twice a day, is usually sufficient. In patients with significant *neuro-conjunctivitis* (a cycle of itch, scratch, itch), slowly escalating doses of hydroxazine (beginning with 50 mg at bedtime and slowly increasing as needed) may interrupt the vicious cycle.

Corticosteroids

Adrenocorticosteroids remain a mainstay of therapy for VKC, especially in the case of the most severely diseased patients. Experts agree that short courses (burst and taper) of topical corticosteroids are very useful in getting acute exacerbations under control and breaking the inflammatory cycle. A typical short-course strategy consists of 1% prednisolone sodium phosphate taken four times a day for two days, then taken twice daily for two more days, followed by once daily dosing for an additional three days, and subsequent discontinuation. Steroid solutions are believed to be better than suspensions, whose particles can get lodged between the papillae, causing irritation and possibly corneal abrasions. Because the complications arising from unmonitored adrenocorticosteroid use can be severe, the practice of long-term, "low-dose," maintenance therapy with topical corticosteroids is not recommended.[6a]

Mast-cell Stabilizers

In some practices,[6a] mast-cell stabilizing agents have become the mainstay of treatment of VKC. Their primary effect, stabilization of the mast cell membrane, prevents degranulation and the subsequent release of vasoactive substances responsible for the immediate hypersensitivity response. Thus these agents greatly reduce the need for topical corticosteroids. Topical cromolyn sodium, which interferes with calcium transport by cell membranes, is thought to raise the intracellular levels of cAMP (cyclic adenosine monophosphate) by inhibiting cAMP-phosphodiesterase. Every clinical study using 2% to 4% cromolyn to treat VKC has shown efficacy. Most convincing was a randomized, double-blind, placebo-controlled, multicenter study performed in the United States that demonstrated unequivocally that cromolyn sodium was safe and effective.[15] The study stratified the results in terms of the atopy status of the patients and revealed that atopic patients had a better response

to the drug than nonallergic patients. Although cromolyn sodium is ineffective against acute exacerbations (topical corticosteroids should be used initially under these circumstances to get the inflammation under control), it is invaluable[6a] as a "preventive maintenance" drug, enabling the clinician to discontinue or decrease topical steroid usage. Disodium cromoglycate in 2% to 4% ophthalmic solution is also effective, although its availability in the United States is limited at this time.

Caldwell and associates[10] conducted a double-masked, parallel-group, clinical study that compared the efficacy and safety of lodoxamide 0.1% with that of cromolyn sodium 4% ophthalmic solution in the treatment of VKC. Both drugs proved to be safe; however, lodoxamide 0.1% effected greater and earlier improvement in several primary symptoms and signs of VKC. Further studies are underway to confirm these findings and to test the usefulness of other mast-cell stabilizers (such as 2% nedocromil sodium) for the treatment of VKC.

Nonsteroidal Antiinflammatory Drugs

Nonsteroidal antiinflammatory agents commercially available and approved for ophthalmic use in the United States are the cyclooxygenase inhibitors diclofenac, suprofen, flurbiprofen, and ketorolac. Ketorolac is the first ophthalmic nonsteroidal antiinflammatory agent tried and approved for the treatment of ocular allergy. Keratolac tromethamine 0.5% ophthalmic solution has been approved by the FDA for the treatment of seasonal allergic conjunctivitis; supporting data came from two multicenter, double-masked, randomized comparative trials.[28] Flurbiprofen and suprofen are approved by the FDA for inhibition of intraoperative miosis, and diclofenac is approved for treatment of postoperative inflammation.

Supplemental Agents

Topical mucolytic agents are sometimes used to loosen or dissolve the thick, stringy discharge of VKC. Monohydrated sodium carbonate (1% to 2%) and other very dilute acid solutions have been used. Acetyl cysteine (Mucomyst) 10% solution has also been tried to control the discharge, and it has had some effect.

Topical vasoconstrictors, which temporarily reduce edema and hyperemia of the conjunctiva, may offer some relief to the VKC patient. Other medical therapies for VKC have included cyclosporine A ophthalmic solution, systemic aspirin, indomethacin, and tolmetin.[2,12,24,29,32] Randomized, double-blind, placebo-controlled studies have not been performed to support their efficacy, however.

Frank corneal epithelial defects (shield ulcers) are trophic in nature and often defy the normally successful therapeutic strategies for dealing with corneal abrasions or epithelial defects (that is, lubrication, patching, soft contact lens). The longer corneal epithelial defects persist, the greater the likelihood of stromal ulceration and permanent corneal scarring. Successful treatment of such defects therefore requires at least temporary control of the ocular inflammation with topical corticosteroids. Once this is achieved, the aforementioned treatments (lubrication, patching, soft contact lenses) can be used or the superficial plaque can be removed by keratectomy to aid in the reepithelialization.

Surgical Measures

Long-term complications from these surgical procedures include scarring, trichiasis, tear deficiency, and entropion. In the meantime, the basic underlying immunologic derangement guarantees that the process affecting the conjunctiva will recur unless definitive environmental and medical measures are taken. Nonetheless, the surgeon, frustrated by the unrelenting nature of VKC, may resort to a surgical procedure to produce a "cure." Rarely, conjunctival transposition or conjunctival autografts are employed with limited benefits. Cryotherapy of the tarsal conjunctival surface often relieves the symptoms of VKC for a while, probably by killing the inflammatory cells in the giant papillae and thereby temporarily eliminating or reducing the inflammatory mediators bathing the ocular surface; surgical removal of the large vegetative papillae has the same result. In both cases, the papillae soon recur and the symptoms resume.

Surgical removal of the vernal plaques by superficial keratectomy can be useful because it encourages the reepithelialization of the cornea in the area of the trophic shield ulcer. Radiotherapy, used extensively in the past, has unacceptable adverse effects and has fallen into disrepute.

PROGNOSIS

VKC is most often self-limiting, with a clinical course of two to ten years. The conjunctival changes do eventually resolve and leave no signs of scarring unless the conjunctiva has been abused by procedural measures or the rare case when the disease transforms into AKC.

In a 1989 study of 120 patients, Dart[14] reported that 27% lost some visual acuity as a result of VKC; and he commented that "therapeutic complications"—from steroid misuse, for example—are "common and may lead to blindness." Although the corneal changes of VKC (pannus formation, astigmatism, keratoconus, keratoglobus, marginal corneal degeneration, subepithelial scarring, or pseudogerontoxon) can be permanent, corneal sequelae rarely diminish visual acuity in a way that cannot be corrected by semirigid contact lenses or surgery.

REFERENCES

1. Abelson MB, Baird RS, Allansmith MR: Tear histamine levels in vernal conjunctivitis and other ocular inflammations, *Ophthalmology* 87:812-814, 1980.
2. Abelson MB, Butrus SI, Weston JH: Aspirin therapy in vernal conjunctivitis, *Surv Ophthalmol* 95:502-505, 1983.
3. Allansmith MA: Vernal conjunctivitis. In Duane T, editor: *Clinical ophthalmology,* Hagerstown, 1978, Harper and Row.
4. Allansmith MR, Ross RN: Ocular allergy and mast cell stabilizers, *Surv Ophthalmol* 30:229-244, 1986.
5. Beigelman MN: *Vernal conjunctivitis,* Los Angeles, 1950, University of Southern California Press.
5a. Berdy GJ et al.: Identification of histaminase activity in human tears after conjunctival antigen challenge, *Invest Ophthalmol Vis Sci* 31(suppl):65, 1990.
6. Bhan AK, Fujikawa LS, Foster CS: T-cell subsets and Langerhans cells in normal and diseased conjunctiva, *Surv Ophthalmol* 94:205-212, 1982.
6a. Brody JM, Foster CS: Unpublished data.
7. Buckley RJ: Vernal keratoconjunctivitis, *Surv Ophthalmol* 28:303-308, 1988.
8. Butrus SI, Abelson MB: Laboratory evaluation of ocular allergy, *Surv Ophthalmol* 28:324-328, 1988.
9. Butrus SI, Ochsner KI, Abelson MB, Schwartz LB: The level of tryptase in human tears: an indicator of activation of conjunctival mast cells, *Ophthalmology* 97:1678-1683, 1990.
10. Caldwell DR, Verin P, Hartwich-Young R et al.: Efficacy and safety of lodoxamide 0.1% vs cromolyn sodium 4% in patients with vernal keratoconjunctivitis, *Surv Ophthalmol* 113:632-637, 1992.
11. Cameron JA, Al-Rajhi AA, Badr IA: Corneal ectasia in vernalkeratoconjunctivitis, *Ophthalmology* 96:1615-1623, 1989.
12. Chaudhary K: Evaluation of combined systemic aspirin and cromolyn sodium in intractable vernal catarrh, *Ann Ophthalmol* 22:314-318, 1990.
13. Coutu RB: Treatment of vernal keratoconjunctivitis: a retrospective clinical case study, *Optom Vis Sci* 68:561-564, 1991.
14. Dart JKG: The epidemiology of vernal keratoconjunctivitis. In *Proceedings of the second fisions international ophthalmology workshop,* Bollington, Cheshire, England, 1989, Pennine Press.
15. Foster CS: Evaluation of topical cromolyn sodium in the treatment of vernal keratoconjunctivitis, *Ophthalmology* 95:194-201, 1988.
16. Foster CS: Vernal keratoconjunctivitis, *Perspec Ophthalmol* 4:35-38, 1980.
17. Foster CS, Calonge M: Atopic keratoconjunctivitis, *Ophthalmology* 97:992-1000, 1990.
18. Friedlaender MH: Ocular diseases with immunologic features. In Friedlaender MH, editor: *Allergy and immunology of the eye,* Hagerstown, 1979, Harper and Row.
19. Friedlaender MH, Cameron JA: Vernal keratoconjunctivitis and trachoma, *Int Ophthalmol* 12:47-51, 1988.
20. Henriquez AS, Kenyon KR, Allansmith MR: Mast cell ultrastructure: comparison in contact lens-associated giant papillary conjunctivitis and vernal conjunctivitis, *Arch Ophthalmol* 99:1266-1272, 1981.
21. Irani AA, Butrus SI, Tabbara KF, Schwartz LB: Human conjunctival mast cells: distribution of MC_T and MC_{TC} in vernal conjunctivitis and giant papillary conjunctivitis, *J Allergy Clin Immunol* 86:34-39, 1990.
22. Jones BR, Andrews BE, Henderson WG, Schofield PB: The pattern of conjunctivitis at Moorefield's during 1956, *Trans Ophthalmol Soc UK* 77:291-305, 1957.
23. Maggi E, Biswas P, Del Prete G, Parronchi P et al.: Accumulation of TH2-like helper T cells in the conjunctiva of patients with vernal conjunctivitis, *J Immunol* 146:1169-1174, 1991.
24. Meyer E, Kraus E, Zonis S: Efficacy of antiprostaglandin therapy in vernal conjunctivitis, *Br J Ophthalmol* 71:497-499, 1987.
25. Rapacz P, Tedesco J, Donshik PC, Ballow M: Tear lysozyme and lactoferrin levels in giant papillary conjunctivitis and vernal conjunctivitis, *CLAO J* 14:207-209, 1988.
26. Rice BA, Foster CS: Immunopathology of cicatricial pemphigoid affecting the conjunctiva, *Ophthalmology* 97:1476-1483, 1990.
27. Rosenthal WN, Insler MS: Vernal keratoconjunctivitis: new corneal findings in fraternal twins, *Cornea* 3:288-290, 1985.
28. Rupp G: Keratolac tromethamine: a nonsteroidal anti-inflammatory agent for ophthalmic use in the management of ocular itching associated with seasonal allergic conjunctivitis, *Allergan technical report,* Irvine, Calif., 1992, Allergan.

29. Secchi AG, Tognon S, Leonardi A: Topical use of cyclosporin in the treatment of vernal keratoconjunctivitis, *Am J Ophthalmol* 110:641-645, 1990.
30. Shuler JD, Levenson J, Mondino BJ: Inferior corneal ulcers associated with palpebral vernal conjunctivitis, *Am J Ophthalmol* 106:106-107, 1988.
31. Smolin G, O'Connor GR: Atopic diseases affecting the eye. In Smolin G, O'Connor GR, editors: *Ocular immunology,* 135-192, Philadelphia, 1981, Lea and Febiger.
32. Sybopoulos S, Gilbert D, Easty DL: Double-blind comparison of a steroid (prednisolone) and a nonsteroid (tolmetin) in vernal keratoconjunctivitis, *Cornea* 5:35-39, 1986.
33. Trantas A: Le catarrhe printanier en Turquie, *Arch Ophthalmol* 25:717-731, 1905.
34. Trantas A: Sur le catarrhe printanier, *Arch Ophthalmol* 30:503-621, 1910.
35. Yanoff M, Fine BS: *Ocular pathology: a text and atlas,* 281-282, Philadelphia, 1989, JB Lippincott.

28 Atopic Keratoconjunctivitis

THOMAS J. LIESEGANG

Atopic dermatitis is a disease that is difficult to define precisely. It is an intensely pruritic, chronic, inflammatory, cutaneous condition that usually begins in childhood and is associated with a personal or family history of one or more atopic diseases (asthma, allergic rhinitis, conjunctivitis). The skin lesions are polymorphous and include erythemato-vesiculo-bullous elements, lichenifications, and nodular lesions. Atopic dermatitis has no specific cutaneous lesion, laboratory parameter, or characteristic histology; rather, the diagnosis is made on a cluster of clinical features. Atopic dermatitis is one of the eczemas—a generic term implying exudative dermatitis. Atopic keratoconjunctivitis is a chronic manifestation of several ocular surface disorders seen in the context of atopic dermatitis.[26]

HISTORICAL BACKGROUND

Besnier was the first to characterize atopic dermatitis and his name is still used by Europeans in describing the disease (prurigo Besnier). Several other names have been applied to this disease by authors from different countries.[32] Eczema was used in the United States for a number of years, but this depicts a weeping dermatitis that is more typical of the infantile form than the adult form of atopic dermatitis. Atopy was coined by Coca and Cooke[18] to portray strange skin hypersensitivities in patients with a hereditary background of allergic disease. Major atopic conditions include hay fever, allergic asthma, perennial allergic rhinitis, and atopic dermatitis. Minor atopic diseases include food allergies, urticaria, and nonhereditary angioedema. Wise and Sulzberger[78] assigned the term *atopic dermatitis* to encompass the spectrum of diseases from infancy to adulthood as well as to recognize the frequent association with other atopic conditions.

EPIDEMIOLOGY AND RISK FACTORS

Atopic Dermatitis

Epidemiologic studies of atopic dermatitis have been difficult to evaluate because of differences in the diagnostic criteria, poor follow-up of a disease that may remit, and the retrospective nature of most studies. Atopic dermatitis is predominantly a disease of infancy and childhood, with 60% of the victims having their onset within the first year and 85% within the first five years.[61] Fewer than 2% have their onset after age 20. Current estimates are that 3% to 10% of the population may be affected at some time, and about 0.7% are affected at any one time.[62] There appears to be an increasing incidence of atopic dermatitis in recent years,[32,47,62] so the medical impact can be considerable. Increased exposure to airborne allergens (dust, mites, dander, pollen), irritants (cigarette smoke, pollution), or food allergens may contribute to this increase (see box).

The familial nature of atopic dermatitis is strong, with two out of three patients having a family history of another atopic disease.[62] The high concordance in monozygotic twins also confirms a strong genetic basis.[37,47] There are contradictory articles in the literature, but more recent studies suggest a multifactorial pattern of inheritance with probable autosomal dominance.[20] A genetically inherited bone marrow-derived cell is central to the immunopathogenesis of atopic dermatitis as explained in the following discussion. Gene linkage analysis has demonstrated a strong association between IgE reactivity and chromosome 11q.[19]

The presence of functionally abnormal, defectively controlled cells in the skin or in the respiratory mucosa probably sets the stage for environmental factors to trigger the atopic hyperresponsiveness.[31] For the skin, irritants are the most frequent environmental stimuli, whereas allergenic triggers are less frequent. Geographic, climatic, psychologic, and occupational factors control the status in genetically predisposed individuals. Epidemiologic data reflects these multifactors. It is possibly the arrival of the abnormal, bone marrow-derived cell in the skin or in the respiratory mucosa that sets the stage for environmental allergens or irritants to trigger the atopic hyperresponsiveness. Atopic dermatitis can plausibly only develop in genetically susceptible individuals after these appropriate secondary environmental exposures.

FLARE FACTORS FOR ATOPIC DERMATITIS
Irritants
Allergens (eg. mild, soy, wheat, egg, peanut)
Inhalants (eg. dust, mites, pollens, animals)
Sweating
Heat
Low humidity
Sudden changes in temperature
Rapid elevation atmospheric pressure
Contact of skin with irritating chemicals
Rough clothing (wool, acrylic)
Emotional anxiety
Scratching
High bacterial or fungal counts on the skin

Atopic dermatitis affects all races but has a higher incidence in urban areas and in cooler temperate zones, possibly related to environmental factors or psychologic stress.[32,37] This may also explain why the disease occasionally appears for the first time in adults. Correspondingly, some patients with atopic tendencies may exacerbate the condition in association with occupations involving water or chemicals (such as hair dressing or medical care work). Up to 80% of occupational dermatitis occurs in atopic individuals.[69] Even patients with resolved atopic dermatitis remain at risk for developing irritant contact dermatitis and have a hyperreactive immune response of the skin. Atopic dermatitis has been an exclusionary factor from military service because of the high risk of exacerbation during stress. Atopic dermatitis is a risk factor for asthma, and even adults with atopic dermatitis without a history of asthma have methacholine-reactive airways.[8]

Atopic Keratoconjunctivitis

Ocular disease is seen in 25% to 40% of patients with atopic dermatitis.[28,43,63] Large series, reported by a number of investigators, indicate that the disease is occasionally sight threatening.[26,28,41,73] Atopic eye disease is bilateral and symmetric in patients between the ages of 30 and 50 and has a predilection for males. These patients usually have a history of childhood eczema, although they suffered no other ocular symptoms until their late teens. The initial manifestations are always extraocular and consist of dermatitis, hay fever, or asthma.[26] The characteristics are frequently nonspecific and include itching, watering, photophobia, and a mucous discharge from the eyes. The symptoms are perennial and persistent, although they are usually worse in hot weather. The majority of patients have a family history of atopic dermatitis. The ocular inflammation may flare, independent of the skin condition. In distinction to vernal disease, atopic ocular disease frequently continues into the fifties or sixties.

PATHOGENESIS

Atopic Dermatitis

The pathogenesis of atopic dermatitis has been extensively studied but remains elusive. It involves a complex interrelationship between precipitating environmental factors and the genetic factors relating to immune response, vascular reactivity, and neuroimmune and neurocutaneous responses.[21] Many investigators have researched the disease, but bias is frequently present in their reports. The close and prolonged contact with antigens can be causative; but the exact role of environmental factors such as irritants, emotional stress, foods, *Staphylococcus aureus,* viruses, mites, molds, yeasts, and human dander has not been fully elucidated. There is no single, primary, underlying cause to explain the eczematoid, and later lichenified, changes of atopic dermatitis. The inflammation of atopic dermatitis does not fit any one of the four distinct hypersensitivity reaction patterns described by Coombs, but rather, multiple types of inflammation may be involved.

Atopic dermatitis has been transferred by bone marrow transplantation, suggesting a basic defect in the bone marrow stem cells.[3] Other immunologic changes in atopic dermatitis are compatible with an inherited immune dysregulation. Transplantation of normal bone marrow has also eliminated flexural eczema of the Wiskott-Aldrich syndrome, a T cell immunodeficiency disease.[67] The two major recognized immune aberrations in atopic dermatitis (IgE overproduction and diminished cell-mediated immunity) are probably both T cell dependent and the result of the abnormal immune response, rather than the basic disease defect.

A number of immunologic abnormalities exist in atopic dermatitis with no coherent synthesis of data available to explain them (box).[20a] Lymphocytes (predominantly CD4+ T cells), Langerhans cells, and mast cells are increased in the skin involved with atopic dermatitis. T cells and mast cells in the skin appear dysfunctional with the resultant increase in viral, fungal, and bacterial infections, anergic skin reactions, and hypersensitivity to irritants and allergens. Dysfunctional B cells result in excessive production of IgE, the formation of IgE immune complexes, and the absorption of IgE with subsequent involvement of T cell mediators, macrophage activators, and other cell mediators. These mediators are soluble molecules that are not antigen-specific, although they may be antigen-driven (as discussed in Chapter 5). Collectively, they are called cytokines, and those produced by lymphocytes are termed lymphokines. The mediators that act between leukocytes are labeled interleukins.[16] These may have overlapping functions and are produced by a variety of cell types. There is a reduction in the function and number of natural killer cells in the skin of active atopic dermatitis, independent of any steroid effect.[55]

There is controversy in the literature over the status of the

IMMUNE ABNORMALITIES IN ATOPIC DERMATITIS

IgE-mediated immediate hypersensitivity
  Increase serum IgE
  Reduced suppressors for IgE production
  Positive radioallergosorbent tests
  Positive skin tests
  Biphasic skin response after antigen challenges
Depressed cell-mediated immunity
  Defective delayed-type skin responsiveness to antigens
  Decreased lymphocyte response to mitogens and antigens
  Increased susceptibility to cutaneous viral infections
  Defective generation of cytotoxic T lymphocyte response
Impaired mononuclear, macrophage and neutrophil chemotaxis, phagocytosis and bacterial killing
Abnormal cytokine production
Increased mast cell and basophil histamine release
Increased cyclic adenosine monophosphate-specific phosphodiesterase

circulating T lymphocytes in atopic dermatitis, although recent control studies suggest normal circulating T cell and T cell subsets.[55] The T lymphocyte has a relative affinity for the epidermis and there is controversy as to whether normal circulating T lymphocytes traffic through the epidermis. Some of the features in the histology of atopic dermatitis suggest a type IV lymphocyte-mediated interaction with intracellular edema, vesiculation, and an epidermal infiltrate of macrophages and CD4 lymphocytes along with major basic protein. T cells in atopic dermatitis may have inadequate interferon gamma production combined with excessive interleukin 4 production.[13,50] This may be central to explain the immune and inflammatory defects associated with atopic dermatitis.

Interferons are a group of cytokines that interfere with superinfection of virally infected cells. Three major classes are identified. Interferon alpha is produced by leukocytes. Interferon beta is generated by epithelial cells and fibroblasts. Interferon gamma (originated by activated T cells) is a major activator of macrophages but is antagonistic to interleukin 4.[16] Interleukin 4 is produced by the T cells and influenced by both the T cells and monocytes; it appears to program normal human B cells for IgE synthesis.[35] This suggests a potential role of gamma interferon in treatment.

The dendritic Langerhans cells reside in the epidermis and have recognized immunologic function. They have a surface that encourages adhesion and a function for antigen presentation similar to that of macrophages.[23] Langerhans cells are increased in the dermis in atopic dermatitis. IgE is adherent to Langerhans cells in atopic dermatitis, although it is also seen in other conditions with elevated IgE. Macrophages and Langerhans cells can release mediators and proinflammatory cytokines (interleukin 1 and 6) following stimulation via its IgE allergic-induced reaction. A defect in monocytes and other antigen-presenting cells has been detected[23,31] that further explains some of the pharmacophysiologic abnormalities in atopic dermatitis.[31]

There is an association between elevated serum IgE and atopic dermatitis. Two signals are required for in vitro IgE synthesis: interleukin 4 and a B cell-activating signal.[42] Interferon gamma inhibits interleukin 4-induced IgE synthesis, and there appears to be decreased production of gamma interferon in atopic dermatitis. Eighty percent of all patients will have increased IgE, and there is a rough correlation between levels of serum IgE and disease activity. IgE will decline slowly as the activity becomes quiescent. Twenty percent of atopic individuals, however, will have normal IgE; and approximately 15% of the normal population have elevated IgE, so the significance remains unclear. No single laboratory test can confirm atopic dermatitis.[55] In infants, radioallergosorbent testing generally shows that IgE is almost completely directed against food stuffs (milk, fish, eggs). In older children and adults, the IgE appears directed against inhaled allergens (house dust, mites, dander, pollens). There is a relatively good correlation between prick testing and specific IgE. Delayed cutaneous testing with aeroallergens may identify allergens in some.[17] Avoidance of these allergens, however, does not necessarily result in a cure of atopic dermatitis. In some patients, an allergy can be associated with an episode of angioedema (a Type I reaction) and is then followed by an exacerbation of atopic dermatitis.

Hanifin[35] suggests that the initiation of atopic dermatitis from an immunologic viewpoint is caused by specific antigen stimulation and disturbance of genetically predisposed T lymphocytes, resulting in excessive (and perhaps spontaneous) IgE and interleukin production. Leung's hypothesis[49] is that the chronic manifestations of atopic dermatitis are the result of sustained cellular activation of T cells and macrophages. T cells control both IgE responses and the composition of inflammatory cell responses by the release of various cytokines (interleukins 2, 3, 4, 5, 6, 9, 10 and interferon gamma). These cytokines may result in an increased number of mast cells as well as the activation of neutrophils, eosinophils, and macrophages for the release of chemical mediators.[49] These reactions are physiologic and the more compelling question in atopic dermatitis deals with why these patients fail to terminate the normal chain of cellular responses to the allergen (or other triggers). The cause could be either the continuous exposure to allergens and/or a regulatory T cell defect involving the production of cytokines required to terminate the immune response.[49] Levels of T suppressor cells are decreased, supporting the latter hypothesis.

In addition to these immunocellular abnormalities in

atopic dermatitis, disordered chemical mediators are in the forefront of the clinical manifestations of the disease. Some investigators believe that the atopic dermatitis reaction begins with the release of mast cell-derived mediators in response to any number of stimuli (such as a Type I reaction).[34] Stimulated mast cells can release histamine, prostaglandins, leukotrienes, and various other inflammatory factors.[34] Both histamine-releasing factors secreted by T cells and macrophages could play a role in acute mast cell degranulation.[35] In addition to mediators, the mast cells also release chemotactic cytokines (including interleukins and interferons) that contribute to focal infiltration with inflammatory cells. The mast cells, basophils, and eosinophils may not be present in large numbers initially. Eosinophils migrate into the reactive site and disintegrate, leaving deposition of a toxic basic protein within the dermis.[34,48] Basophils and neutrophils infiltrate rapidly, and later a mononuclear leukocytic infiltrate occurs making late phase reactions appear intermixed with delayed hypersensitivity reactions.

Alternately, defects in the cyclic nucleotide regulatory system may be central to the pathogenesis of atopic dermatitis and may account for both the immune and pharmocophysiologic abnormalities. Measurements of cyclic adenosine monophosphate (cAMP) phosphodiesterase activity in mononuclear leukocytes of patients with atopic dermatitis reveal substantially elevated activity even in persons whose disease is in remission.[30] The cause and biologic relevance of elevated phosphodiesterase activity in immune cells remain uncertain, but may represent a basic gene-related defect and a marker for epidemiologic and genetic studies.[31,36]

Stimulation of atopic mononuclear leukocytes with adenylate-cyclase-active agonists also reveals a deficient cyclic-AMP response level, probably because of hydrolysis by the phosphodiesterase.[36] Further studies suggest that the increased phosphodiesterase may be the result of increased protein kinase A and decreased protein kinase C activity.[71] A close correlation exists between both phosphodiesterase activity and leukocyte histamine release,[14] and IgE production by B cells[22] and interleukin activity. The exact elucidation of the relationship between altered nucleotide metabolism and the excessive immune and inflammatory activity characteristic of atopic dermatitis may provide a key to the disease or a mechanistic clarification, probably on the basis of a permissive effect.[31] Treatment strategies may be possible because agonists or inhibitors of these compounds are available.

Overall, there are a variety of cutaneous antigens or factors that act on a dysfunctional immune system in atopic dermatitis in many different ways. Activation of T cells through antigen-presenting cells, direct chemotaxis, activation of macrophages and granulocytes, and degranulation of mast cells bearing antigen-specific IgE molecules are just some of these mechanisms.[21] A single coordinated working concept of the disease is still lacking.

Atopic Keratoconjunctivitis

The pathogenesis of atopic keratoconjunctivitis is unclear, complex; and the initiating event remains unknown. Structures of the eye in contact with the external environment are well supplied with inflammatory cells such as the following: neutrophils, lymphocytes, mast cells, macrophages, Langerhans cells, and plasma cells. Eosinophils and basophils can appear in response. Mast cells may differ between anatomic sites.[5,72] Humans have a high density of mast cells in the conjunctiva (5000 cells per mm^3), with more at the limbal area. The cornea has none. Local mediators from mast cell degranulation (such as histamine, leukotrienes, platelet-activating factor, prostaglandin E, and bradykinin) produce the symptoms of acute keratoconjunctivitis; but a secondary migration of eosinophils (with prolonged production of eosinophil-granule major basic protein) may initiate epithelial breakdown and enhance degranulation of mast cells.[29,73] The influx of lymphocytes, as a result of delayed hypersensitivity, may contribute to the development of subepithelial fibrosis. Mechanical irritation by eye rubbing may also influence the recruitment of additional cells.

Tear IgE values may be increased but not as uniformly as serum IgE.[73] Neither serum nor tear IgE distinguishes well between different atopic groups and does not reflect the severity of ocular disease. Local IgE is produced in atopic individuals with or without clinical signs of disease.[73] Although patients with atopic dermatitis have an increased number of IgE-bearing B lymphocytes in their peripheral blood, it is not clear why some atopic individuals have increased migration of these primed IgE-secreting B cells to their mucosal surface and why only some develop ocular disease.

PATHOLOGY

Histopathology of the Skin in Atopic Dermatitis

The histopathology of atopic dermatitis is that of an eczematous condition without a distinctive diagnostic feature or identifying laboratory marker. In acute lesions there is epidermal parakeratosis and hyperkeratosis with irregular acanthosis and spongiotic edema between and within the epidermal cells.[61] This condition produces the clinical appearance of the eczematoid weeping lesion. Some inflammatory mononuclear cells are observed in the epidermis, along with a mononuclear dermal infiltrate. Lymphocytes, rare monocytes, and macrophages are present around the venus plexus in the dermis with a normal number of mast cells, Langerhans cells, basophils, and eosinophils.[65]

In chronic lesions of atopic dermatitis, there is (1) hyperplasia of the epidermis with elongation of the rete ridges, (2) prominent hyperkeratosis, and (3) areas of parakeratosis. Monocytes, macrophages, and lymphocytes are present in both the perivenular and intervascular areas. Mast cells, eosinophils, and Langerhans cells increase in number in chronic lesions.[48,65,75] Sebaceous glands may appear immature or hypoplastic in the involved skin only. The presence of spongiosis in the orifices of hair follicles may be a specific histologic abnormality in atopic dermatitis.[77]

The cellular components of the skin in atopic dermatitis will be further described under pathogenesis. Immunohistochemical analysis of inflammatory infiltrates reveals that the mononuclear infiltration in the dermis consists primarily of T cells bearing CD3 and CD4 surface antigens (helper or inducer phenotype).[50,65] Most of the cells in the infiltrate are highly positive for HLA class II antigen, indicating they are "activated."[65] An increased number of Langerhans cells are an important component of this reaction. The Langerhans cells serve as antigen-presenting cells for T cells and are surface IgE positive. The chronic infiltration of eczematous skin with activated macrophages and T cells probably promotes collagen deposition and epidermal hyperplasia, with subsequent thickening and lichenification of the skin.

Histopathology of the Conjunctiva in Atopic Keratoconjunctivitis

The histopathology of atopic keratoconjunctivitis reveals the following: (1) increased conjunctival goblet cell proliferation, (2) epithelial pseudotubular formation, (3) eosinophil and mast cell invasion of the epithelium, and (4) a pronounced mononuclear, eosinophil, and mast cell infiltration of the substantia propria (often with a frank granuloma formation and perivasculitis[27]). The conjunctival epithelium shows increased numbers of T helper cells, activated T cells, dendritic cells, and macrophages. In the substantia propria there are increased T helper and T suppressor or cytotoxic cells, macrophages, activated T cells, B cells, and dendritic cells.[27] The majority of T cells express interleukin-2 receptor protein.[27]

The immunopathology of the conjunctiva in atopic keratoconjunctivitis suggests a complex immunoregulatory dysfunction at the local ocular surface. There is an abundance of activated T cells, B cells, and antigen-presenting cells (macrophages, Langerhans cells) and chemical mediators (histamine, leukotrienes, cytokines) causing chronic inflammation and scarring. The induction of class II antigen expression on conjunctival cells (epithelial, fibroblasts, and vascular endothelium) also indicates that the etiology is far more complex than just mast cell degranulation.

CLINICAL FEATURES

Atopic Dermatitis

There is no specific disease marker for atopic dermatitis and the patients frequently have subtle clinical manifestations. A set of diagnostic criteria was established by Hani-

---

DIAGNOSTIC CRITERIA FOR ATOPIC DERMATITIS

Major Features (must have 3 or more)
Pruritus
Typical morphology and distribution
Flexural lichenification or linearity in adults
Facial and extensor involvement in infants and children
Chronic or chronically relapsing course
Personal or family history of atopy
Plus Minor Features (must have 3 or more)
Xerosis
Pityriasis alba
Itch when sweating
Ichthyosis/palmer hyperlinearity/keratosis pilaris
Immediate skin-test reactivity
Elevated serum IgE
Early age of onset
Tendency toward cutaneous infection/impaired cell-mediated immunity
Nonspecific hand or foot dermatitis
Nipple eczema
Cheilitis
Keratoconus
Anterior subcapsular cataracts
Recurrent or chronic conjunctivitis
Orbital darkening and/or Dennie-Morgan infraorbital fold
Facial pallor/facial erythema
Anterior neck folds
Intolerance to wool and lipid solvents
Perifollicular accentuation
Food hypersensitivity
Course influenced by environmental/emotional factors
White dermographism/delayed blanch

---

fin[38] in 1977 but was later modified by an international conference to provide a definitional structure and guidelines for prospective dermatitis investigations (box).[39]

There is a continuum of atopic dermatitis through three phases: infantile, childhood, and adult (box). In the infantile form (2 months of age through 2 years), atopic dermatitis is typically an erythematous papulovesicular rash on the face and the extensor surfaces of the extremities. In more severe cases, generalized skin involvement with weeping lesions often is seen. Periauricular fissuring and cradle cap are common. Most cases of infantile atopic dermatitis clear up by age 2 or 3. The disease may reappear in childhood or adulthood. In childhood eczema (3 years of age through puberty), the tendency for weeping eczematoid dermatitis during infancy gradually converts to a more lichenified morphology. It is probably the pruritus, erythema, and papulation (the earliest clinical features of atopic dermatitis) that give rise to rubbing and scratching, and eventually excoriation and li-

PATTERN OF SKIN LESIONS IN ATOPIC DERMATITIS

Infantile stage (2 mo-2 yrs)
Erythematous, papulovesicular, exudative, intensely pruritic rash which may have prurigo (follicular) papules
Cheek, facial area and scalp involved first
Trunk and extensor extremities later
Childhood stage (3 yrs-10 yrs)
Lesions less exudative, drier, and more papular
Face, especially perioral, and periocular area
Moves from extensor for flexural areas of involvement
Antecubital and popliteal flexures
Hands, feet, buttocks, thighs
Young adult and adult stage
Erythematous vesicular patches or lichenified patches
Face, neck and upper trunk
Antecubital and popliteal flexures
Periocular area

chenification. Childhood atopic dermatitis is characterized by an erythematous papular rash on the flexural surfaces as well as on the face and neck. The predominant extensor involvement of infancy may persist to the pubertal years, but usually the typical flexural pattern is established by early childhood.

In the adult phase (puberty and beyond), the involvement shifts to the antecubital and popliteal flexure areas, with hand and foot dermatitis becoming significant clinical and occupational problems. Persistent inflammation of the face, sides and back of neck, axilla, shoulders, thorax, antecubital and popliteal areas is characteristic in adults. Perifollicular accentuation is seen in dark-skinned patients and can give a pebbly skin appearance. Pigmentary defects such as vitiliginous depigmentation or hyperpigmentation of scars also occur.

All patients with atopic dermatitis have dry skin, exacerbated by low humidity. The cracked and roughened skin typical of atopic dermatitis results from inadequate stratum corneum maturation of the skin caused by inflammation-induced hyperproliferation in the epidermis. Some patients have concomitant ichthyosis with keratosis pilaris and hyperlinear palms. The defective stratum corneum barrier probably allows irritants and allergens to gain access to cellular elements of the skin, thus provoking the inflammatory response. A major focus of skin treatment is in hydration. Irritants in the environment, especially chemicals and detergents, further damage the stratum corneum. Hand dermatitis is observed in 70% of patients with atopic dermatitis from these environmental irritants.[4] Patients learn to avoid occupations with frequent chemical exposure. Other recognized exacerbating factors include infection, bathing with soaps

and detergents, emotional stress, and sweating and itching (box).[24] Fewer than 10% of children have food allergens as a contributory factor in their atopic dermatitis, although the frequency may be higher in children with severe atopic dermatitis.[37,66] The most common allergy-causing foods are eggs, milk, seafood, nuts, wheat, and soy. The diagnosis of food-induced eczemas can only be made with a positive, persistent, pruritic response after exposure. Evidence is lacking for a specific food avoidance regimen in older children and adults.[37] Pet allergies are a frequently suspected, but poorly documented, cause of atopic dermatitis; however, avoidance measures are reasonable. The role of mite allergy remains unclear.[37]

Children with severe atopic dermatitis typically are asthenic with reduced linear growth.[37] Multiple factors may be involved. Cutaneous infection is a significant problem related partly to immune dysfunction and partly to excoriation of skin lesions. Ninety percent of adult patients with atopic dermatitis are colonized with *Staphylococcus aureus* rather than the usual staphylococcal flora,[52] so that weeping and crusting lesions of atopic dermatitis should be considered infected. The *S. aureus* is usually resistant to penicillin. Although the lesions are superficial, systemic antibiotics are frequently required. It is not clear if bacteria are secondary invaders or play a role in perpetuating the disease. Hyposensitization to bacteria seldom provides therapeutic benefit.

Patients with atopic dermatitis have increased susceptibility to local and generalized herpes simplex virus infections. *Kaposi varicelliform eruption (eczema herpetiform)* is the term applied to the widespread eruption most commonly seen in children. This infection is usually cutaneous but may be prolonged and spreading. Vesicular lesions may be accompanied by fever and secondary bacterial skin infections. In severe cases viral infection of the lungs, brain, and adrenal glands can occur. Eczema herpeticum may be increasing

CUTANEOUS PHYSIOLOGIC ABNORMALITIES AND RESPONSES IN ATOPIC DERMATITIS

Increased trans-epidermal water loss
Decreased water binding capacity of stratum corneum
Decreased sebum production
Altered fatty acid content of sebum
Decreased itch threshold
White dermographism
Delayed blanch to cholenergic stimuli
Paradoxical response to nicotinic acid
Reduced acral skin temperature
Rapid vasoconstriction and slow rewarming
Increased cold-pressor response
Increased piloerection

in frequency in adults and may represent a recurrent disease.[11] Recalcitrant warts and molluscum contagiosum infections are more frequent in atopic dermatitis. This may relate to the decrease in natural killer T cell activity. Immunomodulators may enhance the immune response to these viral infections.

Although the disease is capricious and marked by (often unexplained) exacerbations and remissions, the natural course indicates a general tendency toward resolution with age in approximately 40% of those afflicted.[64] The tendency for dry irritated skin persists in all patients with atopic dermatitis. Prognostic signs indicative of a less favorable course include late onset, reverse pattern (flexure surface involvement instead of extensor surface), widespread infantile dermatitis, family history of atopic dermatitis, early evidence of food allergy, and associated allergic rhinitis.[64,65]

Atopic Keratoconjunctivitis

The face may show several phases of atopic dermatitis. An acute eczematoid reaction can be seen in children and young adults (Fig. 28-1). This stage may progress into a chronic inflammation of the lids characterized by thickening of the dermis, scaling of the epidermis, exaggeration of eyelid skin folds, and variation in pigmentation. In the majority of adults, a diffuse lichenification is present with a grayish white complexion or scaling accentuated on the eyelids (Fig. 28-2). Alternatively, facial erythema may be present during active bouts of atopic dermatitis.

Eyelid thinning or tightening is sometimes evident. The eyelids have the thinnest epidermis and stratum corneum on the body but are continually exposed to allergens and irritants. This exposure results in the itching that causes rubbing and subsequent thickening, scaling, and lichenification. The lids are not usually puffy with edema. The swelling and

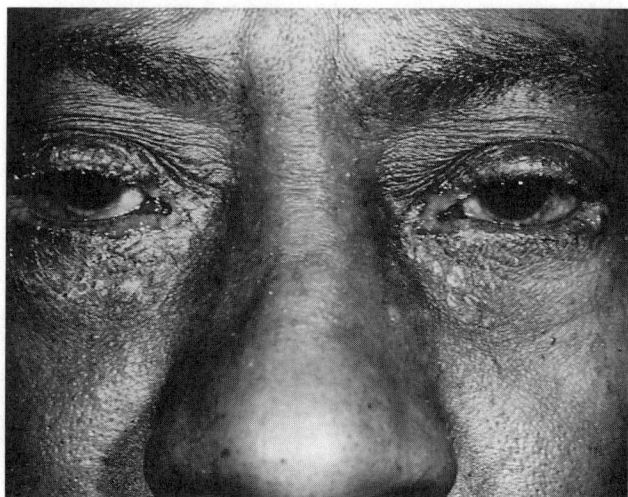

Fig. 28-2. The dry scaling grayish lichenified eyelid and periocular skin in a black adult female with chronic atopic dermatitis. There is hyperpigmentation of the periocular skin.

lichenification can proceed to ectropion and epiphora. Thickening of the lids or ptosis may occur in exacerbations. Pigmentation of the eyelids is increased in some patients, although a periocular pallor is seen in others. The eyelids may be glued shut upon awakening, with the lashes pointed and clumpy. A mucoid exudate may be seen along the lid margin. Maceration of the inner and outer canthi may occur from tearing, with associated blepharitis and meibomitis (Fig. 28-3). *Staphylococcus aureus* is isolated from the lids in up to 67% of those afflicted.[73] A Dennie-Morgan crease, which is an extra single (or occasionally a double) infraorbital eyelid fold, is caused by lower eyelid dermatitis (Fig. 28-4).[57,59]

Atopic keratoconjunctivitis is a term introduced by Hogan[41] to describe patients with chronic conjunctivitis and

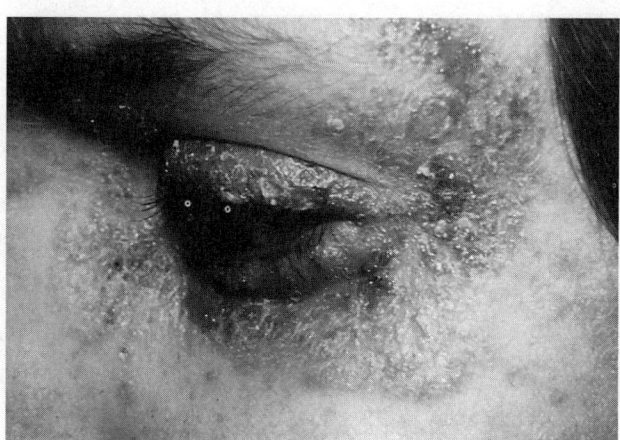

Fig. 28-1. A weeping eczematoid atopic dermatitis of the lids and periocular skin in a young adult. She has a history of childhood eczematoid dermatitis.

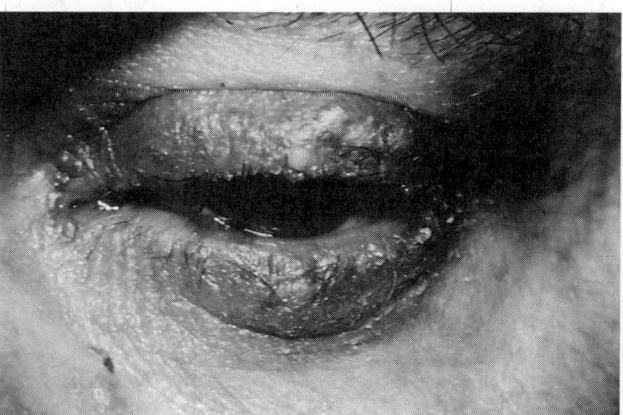

Fig. 28-3. An indurated lid with eczematoid skin changes of atopic dermatitis in a young adult. There are superimposed abscesses of the eyelid hair follicles (hordeolum) and eyelid margin blepharitis from *Staphylococcus aureus*.

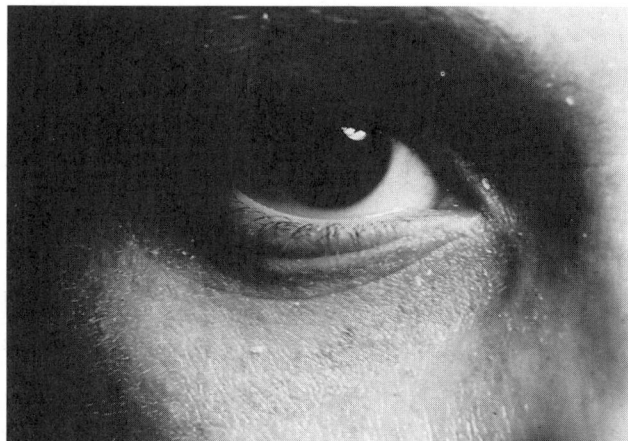

Fig. 28-4. A double infraorbital eyelid fold (Dennie-Morgan crease) in a young female caused by chronic atopic dermatitis.

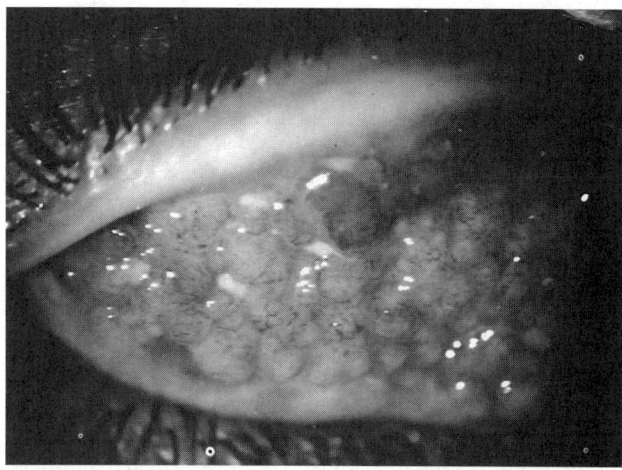

Fig. 28-6. Giant papillary conjunctival reaction with scarring and flat topped papules on the upper tarsal conjunctiva in an adult with chronic atopic keratoconjunctivitis.

progressive keratitis in the presence of atopic dermatitis. Atopic keratoconjunctivitis is a chronic manifestation of various ocular surface disorders in the context of atopic dermatitis with several possible hypersensitivity reactions involved.[26] This disease is always bilateral with symptoms of itching, burning, tearing, and variable mucoid discharge. Resultant structural changes involve the conjunctiva and cornea.

Conjunctival involvement in atopic keratoconjunctivitis is primarily in the inferior fornix and palpebral conjunctiva. The conjunctiva has an overall pale appearance; but during inflammatory exacerbations there may be chemosis, limbal hyperemia, as well as papillary hypertrophy of the superior and inferior tarsal regions (Fig. 28-5). Giant papillae (greater than 1 mm) may develop on the upper tarsal conjunctiva, although most are scarred with flat tops (Fig. 28-6). Both conjunctival and episcleral vessels can be dilated, sometimes continually. Patients become resolved to having red

eyes. Occasionally a gelatinous papillary reaction of the perilimbal conjunctiva may develop[26] (Fig. 28-7); this may be a form fruste of vernal keratoconjunctivitis. Over time, and with chronic disease, conjunctival subepithelial fibrosis leads to scarring and foreshortening, especially in the inferior fornix. Symblepharons may develop between the lower palpebral and bulbar conjunctiva. These adhesions can appear similar to symblepharon of ocular pemphigoid but are usually less extensive and less progressive. A biopsy for fluorescent antibody studies characteristic of pemphigoid may occasionally be indicated. Mucous discharge is a result of this chronic inflammatory process and resultant dry eyes are an additive insult to the surface. Tears contain major basic protein, similar to vernal conjunctivitis.[1]

Corneal complications are seen in up to 75% of cases.[12,26]

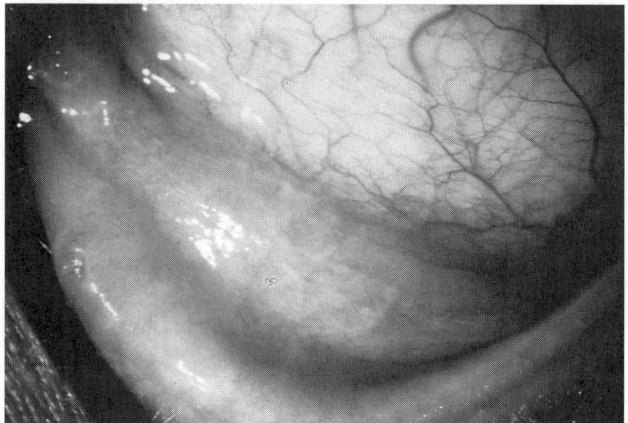

Fig. 28-5. Boggy pale conjunctiva with minimal subepithelial fibrosis and beginning inferior cul de sac foreshortening secondary to atopic conjunctivitis in an adult.

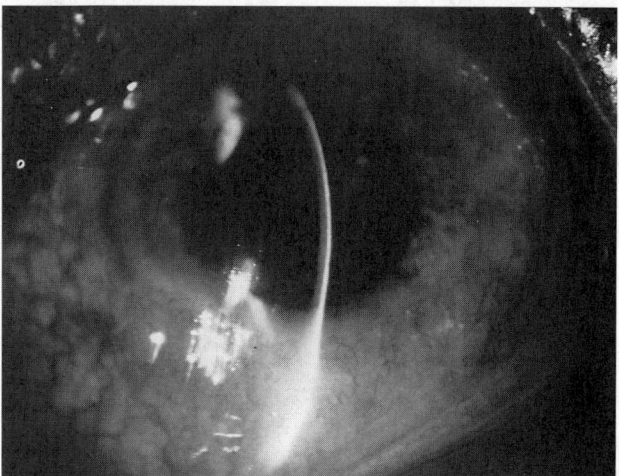

Fig. 28-7. Conjunctival and episcleral injection and phlyctenular like scar and neovascularization of the inferior cornea in an adult with chronic atopic keratoconjunctivitis.

These complications can occur along with or after repeated exacerbations of blepharoconjunctivitis. Punctate epithelial keratitis and intraepithelial microcysts are evident in almost all patients with conjunctival involvement.[43] Peripheral corneal pannus and neovascularization may be observed in up to 65% of victims, especially in the superior quadrants (Fig. 28-7).[73] These conditions are stimulated by punctate keratitis and may progress to peripheral ulcerative keratitis. Lipid deposition from leaking corneal vessels is possible. Shield-shaped anterior stromal scars may be the residual of central macroulcerations or persistent epithelial defects. These scars can progress to thinning. Microbial keratitis is a constant threat to these patients. Gelatinous hypertrophy at the limbus may be an expression of the conjunctival disease (Fig. 28-8). Keratoconus is seen in up to 16% of those afflicted, although the exact pathogenesis is not known.[15,73] Corneal astigmatism and thinning are more frequent in atopes than in the general population.[46]

Ocular herpes simplex virus is noted in about 13% to 22% of those affected.[11,26,73] The ocular herpes is frequently bilateral, and is more widespread and more difficult to treat in these patients than in non-atopic patients (Fig. 28-9).[56] Compounding insults to the cornea occur because of concomitant staphylococcal blepharitis, trichiasis, ectropion, exposure, and keratitis sicca.[26] The carriage rate of *Staphylococcus aureus* on the lids is higher in patients with atopic dermatitis than in the normal population, but this does not correspond to the production of keratopathy.[73] Corneal transplantation in highly atopic individuals is fraught with potential problems including an early, aggressive inflammatory response resulting in the accumulation of mucus and the loosening of the transplant sutures (Fig. 28-10).[54]

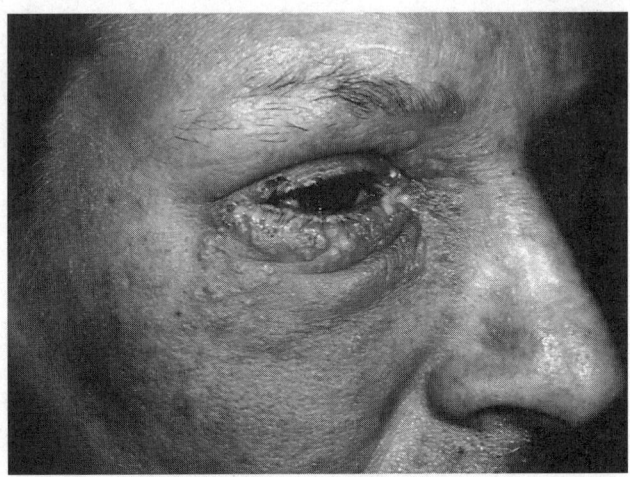

Fig. 28-9. Herpes simplex virus vesicles involving the face, eyelids, and conjunctiva in a young adult female with an underlying chronic atopic dermatitis. Patient went on to develop eczema herpeticum.

Shieldlike anterior subcapsular or posterior polar cataracts are observed in about 10% of patients, but a larger number of sufferers have some form of lens opacity (Fig. 28-11).[9] Cataracts tend to develop quickly in middle-aged atopes. Intracapsular cataract surgery may have a higher incidence of retinal detachment in patients with severe atopic dermatitis.[73] Self-inflicted ocular contusion by tapping of eyes may be the cause of retinal detachment in atopic dermatitis.[60a] Some victims have reported an increased incidence of uveitis, although the disease otherwise is restricted to the ocular surface.

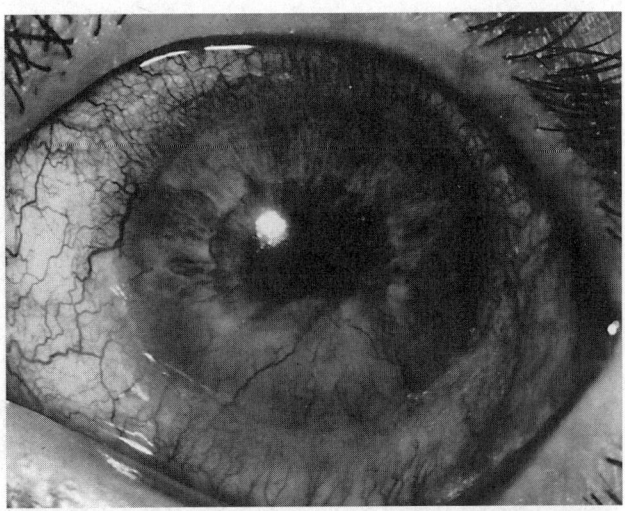

Fig. 28-8. Conjunctival and episcleral injection along with gelatinous hypertrophy of the limbal conjunctiva and a mild diffuse haze to the corneal epithelium in an adult with an exacerbation of atopic keratoconjunctivitis.

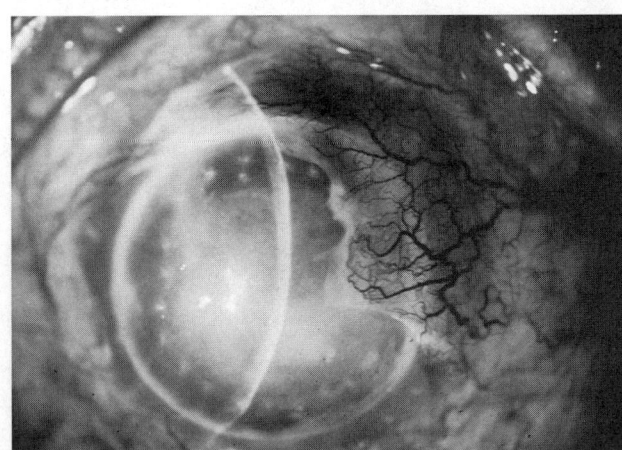

Fig. 28-10. A corneal pannus advancing toward a hazy corneal transplant performed in an older adult with severe atopic keratoconjunctivitis and recurrent herpes simplex viral stromal keratitis. The graft opacified from rejection and pannus formation.

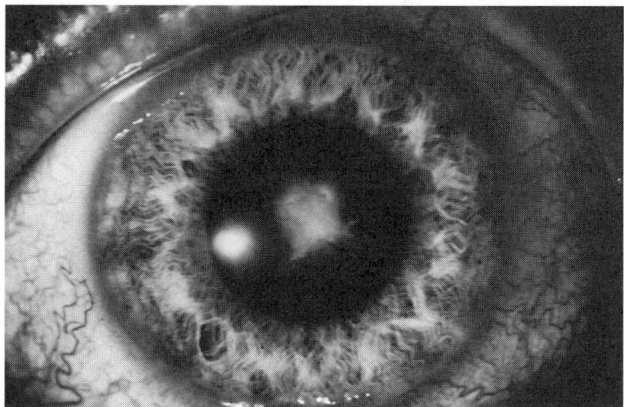

Fig. 28-11. Typical anterior subcapsular shield cataract in an adult with atopic dermatitis. These cataracts are sometimes said to have a "bear-rug" configuration.

LABORATORY INVESTIGATIONS

There are numerous cutaneous and systemic physiologic and pharmacologic abnormalities in atopic dermatitis. It remains unclear whether these are pharmacologic overreactions to antigen stimulation, or whether a basic biochemical defect in the regulation of the immune and inflammatory reactions causes these overreactions. Elevated leukocyte cyclic AMP-phosphodiesterase accounts for low intracellular cyclic AMP levels and may be at the crux of this problem.[33]

The cutaneous physiologic responses most evident in atopic dermatitis are listed in the box. White dermographism refers to the observation that streaking of the skin of a patient with atopic dermatitis produces a paradoxical blanching of the skin rather than a red line. It appears early in an exacerbation of atopic dermatitis and can be elicited even in minimally affected skin.[33] Skin blood flow is decreased in this response, which appears to be a local, and not a neural or systemic, response. A number of reactions to temperature change have been observed.[31,33] There is reduced basal skin temperature, especially over the acral areas. Skin vasculature constricts rapidly in a cold environment and dilates slowly in a warmer one. Patients have an inappropriate elevation of blood pressure when an extremity is immersed in ice water and show increased piloerection and exaggerated cutis anserina in the cold. Sweating is abnormal in atopic dermatitis and is a stimulus to itching, but the studies on sweating in the literature are contradictory.[31]

There are numerous abnormal pharmacologic responses that can be divided into cholinergic, adrenergic, and histamine groupings.[31,33] The delayed blanch to acetycholine is demonstrated in 70% of patients and occasionally only in areas of active dermatitis.[74] This reaction reflects vascular lability and defective vasoregulatory mechanisms resulting from cholinergic hyperresponsiveness.[31,33] This fact correlates with the subnormal methacholine bronchoconstriction threshold in patients with atopic dermatitis but without al-

lergic respiratory disease.[7] There are conflicting studies concerning increased cholinergic sweat responses in atopic dermatitis.[45,60] Overall, it appears that patients with atopic dermatitis have abnormal cholinergic responsiveness, but it is not clear whether these are primary defects or secondary to inflammation in cutaneous and pulmonary tissues.

The adrenergic responsiveness and the role of catecholamines in atopic dermatitis remain uncertain. Szentivanyi proposed the adrenergic blockade theory suggesting that beta-adrenergic hyporesponsiveness and alpha-adrenergic hyperresponsiveness are responsible for the vasoconstriction and mast cell histamine release of atopic dermatitis.[42] Atopic individuals may have the following: (1) blunting of epinephrine-induced hypoglycemia,[53] (2) increased vascular reactivity to intracutaneous adrenergic agonists,[44] (3) in-

---

OCULAR CHANGES WITH ATOPIC DERMATITIS

Eyelids
Eczema of the eyelids
Indurated and lichenified lid margins
Thickening of the dermis
Exaggeration of eyelid folds
Increased or decreased eyelid pigmentation
Ectropion
Ptosis
Staphylococcal blepharitis
Meibomitis
Secondary skin infections

Conjunctiva
Pale conjunctiva
Hyperemia and mucoid discharge
Papillary hypertrophy, giant papilla
Thickening of the conjunctiva, especially at the limbus
Subepithelial fibrosis and scarring
Forniceal foreshortening
Symblepharon formation
Keratinization

Cornea
Punctate epithelial keratitis
Peripheral or central ulceration
Peripheral or central corneal scarring
Pannus and deep corneal vessels
Horners spots (Trantas dots)
Keratoconus
Lipid keratopathy
Susceptibility to Staphylococcal and herpes simplex infections

Lens
Anterior shield-like subcapsular cataracts
Posterior polar cataracts

Other
Uveitis (?)
Retinal detachment (?)

creased tissue levels of norepinephrine,[70] (4) heightened alpha-adrenergic tone with increased piloerection, and (5) increased pupillary responsiveness to phenylephrine.[40]

Responses to histamine are abnormal. A flare response is absent after intradermal histamine administration.[58] There may be increased erythema to intramuscular histamine at sites of predilection of atopic dermatitis—specifically the face, neck, and the antecubital and popliteal flexures.[40] A similar flushing is seen in patients during spontaneous flares of atopic dermatitis or after allergen challenges. There are elevated numbers of mast cells, especially in areas of chronic dermatitis with increased histamine levels in both involved and uninvolved skin. The basophil numbers are normal in tissue and blood, but histamine releasability is raised in basophils from patients with atopic dermatitis.[31] A role for substance P, a neural peptide discharged by antidromic stimulation from sensory C type fibers in the skin, in the release of histamine has been suggested.[31] The release of leukotrienes and prostaglandins from mast cells may comprise other components of the atopic response.

Whatever the mechanism of its production (increased mast cells, expanded skin histamine concentration, increased leukotrienes, or additional substance P), the itch of atopic dermatitis leads to the excoriations, erosions, and lichenification of the skin. The scratching itself results in the following: (1) interleukin 1 and interleukin 3 secretion by keratinocytes, (2) subsequent T cell activation with secretion of interleukin 3 through 6, and histamine-releasing factors —all of which perpetuate the reaction.[42] The itch threshold in atopic dermatitis is low, the duration of the itch is prolonged, and nighttime scratching movements may be frequent or almost continual. The heightened cyclic AMP-phosphodiesterase activity in leukocytes from atopic individuals appears to remove an inhibitory factor and results in cellular hyperresponsiveness with raised histamine releasability.

THERAPY

Treatment of Atopic Dermatitis

Because the cause of atopic dermatitis appears to be multifactorial and there is no cure, several approaches exist for the treatment of this disease (box). Overall management includes environmental, systemic, and topical approaches to incorporating stress control, removing allergens and trigger factors, topical corticosteroids, systemic antibiotics, antihistamines, immunosuppresives, ultraviolet light, and hospitalization. Recent approaches also take into account the immunologic and chemical events taking place in the skin.[49] Pruritus is the cardinal feature, although it is not clear whether it is an initiator or a response to the skin lesion. It may relate to allergen exposure or mediator release. Potential irritants, allergens, or flare factors should be avoided. Irritants include soaps or detergents, exposure to heat and

---

> **THERAPEUTIC APPROACHES TO TREATMENT OF ATOPIC DERMATITIS**
>
> **General**
> Removal of irritant and flare factors
> Allergan avoidance
> Avoidance temperature change
> Skin hydration
> **Antiinflammatory**
> Corticosteroids
> Ultraviolet therapy
> Tar emulsion
> **Mediator-directed**
> Antihistamine
> Cromolyn and other mast cell stabilizers
> Evening primrose oil
> Phosphodiesterase inhibitors
> Leukotriene antagonists
> Platelet—activating factor antagonists
> **Immunomodulatory**
> Thymopentin
> Interferon—gamma
> IV gamma globulin
> IgE pentapeptide
> Cyclosporine
> **Control of infection**
> **Hospitalization**
> **Psychotherapy**

---

humidity, and contact with wool or acrylic. Identification of allergens may be obtained by taking a careful history and carrying out immediate skin tests for allergens in the environment. Foods or inhalants are significant trigger factors. Avoidance of the food allergens is effective, but malnutrition needs to be monitored in children. Peanut, egg, milk, fish, soy, and wheat account for almost 90% of positive food challenges. A dust-free environment may help. Hyposensitization has generally not been helpful. The dry lackluster skin of patients with atopic dermatitis can be improved with frequent tap water baths followed by immediate trapping of the water in the skin by hydrophobic agents such as mineral oil or petrolatum. Hydration and moisturization must be continually provided. Petroleum products are the best moisturizers and should be applied immediately after tepid baths.

In addition to the preventative measures, a number of specific therapeutic options are available. For acute weeping eczematous dermatitis, wet compresses of Burow's solution are recommended. Tar preparations act as antipruritics, disinfectants, and desquamating agents when used either in the bath or applied topically. Reducing the skin inflammation of erythematous papular lesions or follicular eczema is most effective with topical corticosteroids. Corticosteroids decrease capillary permeability and block influx of inflammatory cells. A mid-strength topical corticosteroid applied to the skin is usually sufficient. Topical triamcinolone 0.1% is effective in controlling flare and hydrocortisone 1% cream or ointment provides maintenance therapy. Topical corticosteroids cause thinning of the skin and striae if used chronically. Potent corticosteroids can be used when flares occur. Occasionally brief 4- to 6-day courses of systemic corticosteroids are needed with high doses over the first few days.[37] Fluorinated corticosteroids should not be applied to the face or intertriginous areas for prolonged periods. Lichenified and/or edematous skin has a reduced absorption of topical corticosteroids, and lichenified skin does not respond well to corticosteroids.

Ultraviolet radiation from a sunlamp (UV-B) or psoralen chemotherapy followed by UV-A (PUVA) may be antiinflammatory by reducing cell trafficking to the skin and reducing the capacity of antigen-presenting cells to activate the T cells. There is increased risk of accelerated photoaging and skin cancer with this therapy. Tar emulsion can be used in a bath, or topical coal tar ointment may be combined with ultraviolet light. Superficial x-ray reduces inflammation.

Administration of drugs to counteract the chemical mediators released by inflammatory cells has limited use at present but may have expanded application as the chemical responses in atopic dermatitis are better defined. Inflammatory cells contain two major enzymes (cycloxygenase and 5-lipoxygenase) that convert arachidonic acid into products (prostaglandins and leukotrienes) with a role in inflammation. Aspirin, Indocin, and others inhibit cycloxygenase and can be useful in alleviating pruritis. Systemic H1 receptor-blocking antihistamines such as hydroxyzine (Atarax) or diphenhydramine (Benadryl) are effective for both sedative and antipruritic effects, especially during the early evening hours when scratching seems excessive. Other agents include terfenadine (Seldane) and astemizole (Hismanal). Mast cell stabilizers prevent the flux of calcium across cell membranes and may also inhibit activation of neutrophils, eosinophils, and monocytes. Potentially useful agents include cromolyn, lodoxamide, and nedocromil. Topical sodium cromoglycate[45a] and topical doxepin[24a] have been effective in controlled studies. Dietary supplementation with eiocosapentenoic acid and oil of evening primrose may improve the skin by effecting prostaglandin synthesis and regulation of T lymphocytes. Use of phosphodiesterase inhibitors is an attractive hypothesis, but it has not been extensively evaluated.

Therapy directed at the immune dysfunction represents an alternative approach.[21a,49] The immunoregulators thymopentin and interferon gamma have been used.[10,51,62a,70a] Thymopentin is a synthetic pentapeptide that promotes differentiation of thymocytes and effector T cell function and may relieve the pruritis and erythema of atopic dermatitis. Interferon gamma suppresses the interleukin-4-induced IgE synthesis and, in a small, uncontrolled pilot study, appeared to reduce the severity of atopic dermatitis. Intravenous gamma globulin may also inhibit IgE synthesis. IgE pentapeptide can block the binding of intact IgE to specific cell receptors and has been applied topically.[25] Cyclosporin is a cyclic peptide with immunosuppressive effects, because it reduces IgE production and inflammation by inhibiting the transcription of proinflammatory cytokines (such as interleukin-2) by T cells.[76] It has been used systemically and topically.[76a]

Because of the increased susceptibility to cutaneous infections with bacteria, viruses, and dermatophytes, patients need to be vigilant. Frequent tap water baths aid in debridement of the extensive crusting and weeping lesions. Systemic antibiotics are frequently needed because the incidence and density of *Staphylococcus aureus* colonization is increased in patients with atopic dermatitis. It may manifest with superficial small pustules that are frequently excoriated because of intense pruritis. Staphylococcal infections in patient with atopic dermatitis are almost always penicillin-resistant and frequently erythromycin- and methicillin-resistant. Topical mupirocin may be used, but systemic cephalosporin or dicloxacillin is frequently needed for widespread infection.

Patients with widespread herpes simplex virus involvement and toxicity should be treated with systemic acyclovir. Herpes simplex virus frequently behaves differently on the skin of patients with atopic dermatitis. The availability of oral acyclovir has lead to treatment of some patients with chronic therapy as an alternative to exacerbations of severe dermatitis secondary to herpes simplex virus.

Hospitalization is frequently beneficial for recalcitrant or widespread dermatitis. Psychotherapy is useful for relieving accompanying emotional stress. Plasmapheresis may help some patients with high IgE and IgE antistaphylococcal antibodies.[6] This treatment may work by (1) removing circulating IgE or high-molecular immune complexes containing either IgE or IgG with anti-E activity or (2) depleting a chemotactic factor produced by mononuclear cells.[6]

Treatment of Atopic Blepharitis and Keratoconjunctivitis

The treatment of eyelid dermatitis has been outlined previously. Avoidance of irritants is recommended and sparing use of topical corticosteroid creams (0.5% to 1% hydrocortisone) to eyelids can help reduce edema and inflammation. Atrophy and telangiectasia are complications of steroid use. Management of coexisting blepharitis with lid scrubs should be maintained.

Atopic keratoconjunctivitis varies in severity and can be recalcitrant to treatment. Again, avoidance of irritants, allergens, and dust is advised. Systemic antihistamines may help some of the ocular symptoms of itching and watering. Preparations of antihistamines for topical ophthalmic use include alkylamines (pheniramine), ethylenediames (antazoline and pyrilamine), and levablastine. The combination of a topical antihistamine (antazoline) and a vasoconstrictor (naphazoline) is more effective than either agent used separately.[2] Mast cell stabilizers have been effective in relieving some symptoms in about two out of three patients.[43] Four percent cromolyn sodium has been most commonly used four times a day for both prophylactic and maintenance therapy.[43] This treatment reduces the need for topical steroid therapy. Lodoxamide, nedocromil, and tromethamine are other topical ophthalmic agents being evaluated. Mast cell stabilizers may have additional roles in inhibiting activation of other inflammatory cells.[72] Ocular lubricants can occasionally be soothing, although they rarely provide dramatic nor prolonged relief. A trial of a wide range of artificial tears may be appropriate. Punctal occlusion or tarsorrhaphy has not been helpful. The mucous discharge is usually not sufficient to suggest a trial of mucomyst.

Topical ophthalmic corticosteroids can be used over short periods for crisis management of the inflammatory conjunctivitis or punctate epithelial keratitis. Their long-term use is discouraged because of sensitization to preservatives, as well as the increased risk of cataracts, glaucoma, and infections.[26] Medrysone (HMS) ophthalmic solution is preferred because it has minimal ocular penetration and fewer side effects. Occasionally systemic corticosteroids are required. Patients need to be continually monitored for complications of *Staphylococcus aureus* blepharitis and the occurrence of herpes simplex viral disease of the eyelids, conjunctiva, or cornea. Topical inhibitors of cyclooxygenase (0.1% suprofen and 0.03% flurbiprofen) may have a role. Eczema herpeticum is a distinct threat and is treated with oral acyclovir and topical trifluorothymidine.[56]

The role of immunosuppressives and plasmapheresis is not well defined in ocular disease. Topical cyclosporine in castor oil has been used to treat persistent conjunctivitis in both vernal and atopic keratoconjunctivitis.[26,68] Systemic cyclosporine is a remedy for resistant cases of atopic dermatitis. Plasmapheresis may be useful therapy in rare patients with severe atopic dermatitis and in the hyper IgE syndrome.[6] Treatment of the generalized atopic dermatitis condition and (occasionally) hospitalization or psychotherapy may be necessary in selected cases of ocular disease.

Patients need to be continually monitored for infection as well as for progression of limbal hyperemia and pannus with resultant corneal vascularization, scarring, and thinning. Treatment of corneal neovascularization with laser probably would not be successful because these vessels are smaller and very numerous. A bandage contact lens may provide structural support to a thinned cornea. A vascular pannus may form under the contact lens and help avoid perforation. Small perforations can be treated with cyanoacrylate glue or a small therapeutic lamellar keratoplasty. Larger perforations may require more extensive corneal reconstructive procedures or a corneal transplant. Tarsorrhaphy may protect a new graft, but many of these patients have developed a chronic ptosis from long-term ocular protective mechanisms. Corneal transplantation runs the risk of hyper rejection or the occurrence or recurrence of herpes simplex virus. Lid reconstruction is occasionally necessary for severe ectropion.

Therapy overall is aimed at limiting the symptoms rather than the disease process. There is no simple or single cure for the disease; and sympathetic understanding, counseling, encouragement, and a multitreatment approach over time yield the best results.

REFERENCES

1. Abelson MB, Baird RD, Allansmith MR: Tear histamine levels in vernal conjunctivitis and other ocular inflammations, *Ophthalmology* 87:812-814, 1980.
2. Abelson MB, Paradis A, George MA et al.: Effects of Vasocon A in the allergen challenge model of acute allergic conjunctivitis, *Arch Ophthalmol* 108:520-524, 1990.
3. Agosti JM, Sprenger JD, Lum LG et al.: Transfer of allergen-specific IgE mediated hypersensitivity with allogeneic bone marrow transplantation, *N Engl J Med* 319:1623-1628, 1988.
4. Agrup G: Hand dermatitis and other hand dermatoses in South Sweden, *Acta Derm Venereol* 49(suppl):1, 1969.
5. Allansmith MR, Ross RN: Ocular allergy, *Clin Exp Allergy* 18:1-13, 1988.
6. Aswad MI, Tauber J, Baum J: Plasmapheresis treatment in patients with severe atopic keratoconjunctivitis, *Ophthalmology* 95:444-447, 1988.
7. Barker AF, Hanifin JM, Hirshman CA, D'Silva R: Airway hyperactivity in patients with atopic dermatitis, *Am Rev Respir Dis* 131:A41, 1985.
8. Barker AF, Hanifin JM, Hirshman CA et al.: Airway responsiveness in patients with atopic dermatitis, *J Allergy Clin Immunol* 87:780-783, 1991.
9. Beetham WP: Atopic cataracts, *Arch Ophthalmol* 24:21-37, 1940.
10. Boguniewicz M, Jaffe HS, Izer A et al.: Recombinant gamma interferon in the treatment of patients with atopic dermatitis and elevated IgE levels, *Am J Med* 88:365-370, 1990.
11. Bork K, Brauninger W: Increasing incidence of eczema herpeticum: analysis of seventy five cases, *J Am Acad Dermatol* 19:1024, 1988.
12. Braude LS, Chandler JW: Atopic corneal disease, *Int Ophthalmol Clin* 24(2):145-146, 1984.
13. Brown MA, Hanifin JM: Atopic dermatitis, *Curr Opin Immunol* 2:531-534, 1990.
14. Butler JM, Chan SC, Stevens SR, Hanifin JM: Increased leukocyte histamine release with elevated cyclic AMP-phosphodiesterase activity in atopic dermatitis, *J Allergy Clin Immunol* 71:490-497, 1983.
15. Cameron JA, Al-Rajhi A, Badr IA: Corneal ectasia in vernal keratoconjunctivitis, *Ophthalmology* 96:1615-1623, 1989.
16. Claman HN: The biology of the immune response, *JAMA* 268:2790-2796, 1992.
17. Clark RAF, Adinoff AD: Aeroallergen contact can exacerbate atopic dermatitis: patch tests as a diagnostic tool, *J Am Acad Dermatol* 21:863-869, 1989.
18. Coca AF, Cooke RA: On the classification of the phenomena of hypersensitiveness, *J Immunol* 8:163-182, 1923.
19. Cookson W, Faux JA, Hopkin J et al.: Linkage between immunoglobin-E responses underlying asthma and rhinitis and chromosome 11q, *Lancet* 1:1292-1295, 1989.
20. Cookson W, Hopkin JM: Dominant inheritance of atopic immunoglobin-E responsiveness, *Lancet* 1:86-88, 1988.
20a. Cooper KD: Atopic dermatitis: Recent trends in pathogenesis and therapy. *J Invest Dermatol* 102:128-37, 1994.
21. Cooper KD: Mechanisms of atopic dermatitis, *Immunol Sem* 46:247-276, 1989.
21a. Cooper KD: New therapeutic approaches in atopic dermatitis. *Clin Rev Allergy* 11:543-59, 1993.

22. Cooper KD, Kang K, Chan SC, Hanifin JM: Phosphodiesterase inhibition by RO 20-1724 reduces hyper-IgE synthesis by atopic dermatitis cell in vitro, *J Invest Dermatol* 84:477-482, 1985.

23. Cooper KD, Taylor RS, Hammerberg C et al.: Abnormal Langerhans cell differentiation in atopic dermatitis: increased CD36, CD16, CD1C expression in associated with increased autostimulatory capacity, *Clin Res* 38:835A, 1990.

24. Dahl MV: Flare factors and atopic dermatitis, *J Dermatol Sci* 1:311-318, 1990.

24a. Drake LA, Fallon JD, Sober A: Relief of pruritus in patients with atopic dermatitis after treatment with topical doxepin cream. The Doxepin Study Group. *J Am Acad Dermatol* 31:613-6, 1994.

25. Floyd R, Kalpaxis J, Thayer T, Rangus K: Double-blind comparison of HEPP (IgE pentapeptide) 0.5% ophthalmic solution (H) and sodium cromolyn ophthalmic solution, USP 4% (O) in patients having allergic conjunctivitis, *Invest Ophthalmol Vis Sci* 29:45, 1988 (abstract).

26. Foster CS, Calonge M: Atopic keratoconjunctivitis, *Ophthalmology* 97:992-1000, 1990.

27. Foster CS, Rice BA, Dutt JE: Immunopathology of atopic keratoconjunctivitis, *Ophthalmology* 98:1190-1196, 1991.

28. Garrity JA, Liesegang TJ: Ocular complications of atopic dermatitis, *Can J Ophthalmol* 19:19-24, 1984.

29. Gleich GJ, Frigas E, Loegering DA et al.: Cytotoxic properties of the eosinophil major basic protein, *J Immunol* 123:2925-2927, 1979.

30. Grewe SR, Chan SC, Hanifin JM: Elevated leukocyte cyclic AMP-phosphodiesterase in atopic disease: a possible mechanism for C AMP-agonist hyporesponsiveness, *J Allergy Clin Immunol* 70:452-457, 1982.

31. Hanifin JM: Pharmacophysiology of atopic dermatitis, *Clin Rev Allergy* 4:43-65, 1986.

32. Hanifin JM: Epidemiology of atopic dermatitis. Monogr, *Allergy* 21:116-131, 1987.

33. Hanifin JM: Pharmacological abnormalities in atopic dermatitis, *Allergy* 44:41-46, 1989.

34. Hanifin JM: Recognizing and managing clinical problems in atopic dermatitis, *Allergy Proc* 10(6):397-402, 1989.

35. Hanifin JM: Immunologic aspects of atopic dermatitis, *Dermatol Clin* 8:747-750, 1990.

36. Hanifin JM: Phosphodiesterase and immune dysfunction in atopic dermatitis, *J Dermatol Sci* 1:1-6, 1990.

37. Hanifin JM: Atopic dermatitis in infants and children, *Pediatr Clin North Am* 38:763-789, 1991.

38. Hanifin JM, Lobitz WC: Newer concepts of atopic dermatitis, *Arch Dermatol* 113:663-670, 1977.

39. Hanifin JM, Rajka G: Diagnostic features of atopic dermatitis, *Acta Derm Venereol Suppl* 92(S):44-47, 1980.

40. Henderson WR, Shelhammer JH, Rheingold DB et al.: Alph-adrenergic hyper-responsiveness in asthma, *N Engl J Med* 300:642-647, 1979.

41. Hogan MJ: Atopic keratoconjunctivitis, *Am J Ophthalmol* 36:937-947, 1953.

42. Horan RF, Schneider LC, Sheffer AL: Allergic skin disorders and mastocytosis, *JAMA* 268:2858-2868, 1992.

43. Jay TL: Clinical features and diagnosis of adult atopic keratoconjunctivitis and the effect of treatment with sodium cromoglycate, *Br J Ophthalmol* 65:335-340, 1981.

44. Juhlin L: Skin reactions to iontophoretically administered epinephrine and norepinephrine in atopic dermatitis, *J Invest Dermatol* 37:201-205, 1961.

45. Kaliner M: The cholenergic nervous system and immediate hypersensitivity. I. Eccrine sweat responses in allergic patients, *J Allergy Clin Immunol* 58:308-315, 1976.

45a. Kimata H, Hiratsuka: Effect of topical cromoglycate solution on atopic dermatitis: combined treatment of sodium cromoglycate solution with the oral antiallergic medication, oxatomide. *Eur J Pediatr* 153:66-71, 1994.

46. Kerr Muir MG, Woodward EG, Leonard TJK: Corneal thickness, astigmatism, and atopy, *Br J Ophthalmol* 71:207-211, 1987.

47. Larsen FS, Holm NV, Henningsen K: Atopic dermatitis: a genetic-epidemiologic study in a population-based twin sample, *J Am Acad Dermatol* 15:487-494, 1986.

48. Leiferman KM, Ackerman SJ, Sampson HA et al.: Dermal deposition of eosinophilgranule major basic protein in atopic dermatitis, *New Eng J Med* 313:282, 1985.

49. Leung DYM: Immune mechanisms in atopic dermatitis and relevance to treatment, *Allergy Proc* 12:339-346, 1991.

50. Leung DYM, Geha RS: Immunoregulatory abnormalities in atopic dermatitis, *Clin Rev Allergy* 4:67-86, 1986.

51. Leung DYM, Hirsch RL, Schneider L et al.: Thymopentin therapy reduces the chemical severity of atopic dermatitis, *J Allergy Clin Immunol* 85:927-934, 1990.

52. Leyden JE, Marples RR, Kligman AM: *Staphylococcus aureus* in the lesions of atopic dermatitis, *Br J Dermatol* 90:525-530, 1974.

53. Lockey S, Glennon J, Reed C: Comparison of some metabolic responses in normal and asthmatic subjects to epinephrine and glucagon, *J Allergy* 40:349-354, 1967.

54. Lyons CJ, Dart JKG, Aclimandos WA et al.: Sclerokeratitis following keratoplasty in atopy, *Ophthalmology* 97:729-833, 1990.

55. MacKie RM: The immunology of atopic dermatitis, *Clin Exp Allergy* 21:290-293, 1991.

56. Margolis TP, Ostler HB: Treatment of ocular disease in eczema herpeticum, *Am J Ophthalmol* 110:274-279, 1990.

57. Meenan FOC: The significance of Morgan's fold in children with atopic dermatitis, *Acta Derm Venereol Suppl* 92:42-43, 1980.

58. Moller H, Rorsman G: Studies on vascular permeability factors with sodium fluorescein. II. The effect of intracutaneously injected histamine and serum in patients with atopic dermatitis, *Acta Derm Venereol* 38:243-250, 1958.

59. Morgan DB: A suggestive sign of allergy, *Arch Dermatol Syphilol* 57:1050, 1984.

60. Murphy GM, Smith SE, Greaves MW: Autonomic function in cholinergic urticaria and atopic eczema, *Br J Dermatol* 110:581-586, 1984.

60a. Oka C, Ideta H, Nagasaki H et al.: Retinal detachment with atopic dermatitis similar to traumatic retinal detachment. *Ophthalmology* 101:1054-4, 1994.

61. Prose PH, Sedlis E: Morphologic and histochemical studies of atopic dermatitis in infants and children, *J Invest Dermatol* 34:149, 1960.

62. Rajka G: Natural history and clinical manifestations of atopic dermatitis, *Clin Rev Allergy* 4:3-26, 1986.

62a. Reinhold U, Kukel S, Brzoska J, Kreysel HW: Systemic interferon gamma treatment in severe atopic dermatitis. *J Am Acad Dermatol* 29:58-63, 1993.

63. Rich LF, Hanifin JM: Ocular complications of atopic dermatitis and other eczemas, *Int Ophthalmol Clin* 25:4-76, 1985.

64. Roth HL, Kierland RR: The natural history of atopic dermatitis, *Arch Dermatol* 89:209-214, 1964.

65. Sampson HA: Pathogenesis of eczema, *Clin Exp Allergy* 20:459-467, 1990.

66. Sampson HA, McCaskill CC: Food hypersensitivity and atopic dermatitis. Evaluation of 113 patients, *J Pediatr* 107:669-675, 1985.

67. Saurat JH: Eczema in primary immune-deficiencies, *Acta Derm Venereol* 114:125-128, 1985.

68. Secchi AG, Tognon MS, Leonardi A: Topical use of cyclosporin in the treatment of vernal keratoconjunctivitis, *Am J Ophthalmol* 110:641-645, 1990.

69. Shmunes E, Keil JE: Occupational dermatosis in South Carolina: a descriptive analysis of cost variables, *J Am Acad Dermatol* 9:861-866, 1983.

70. Solomon LM, Wentzel HE, Tulsky E: The physiological disposition of C14-norepinephrine in patient with atopic dermatitis and other dermatoses, *J Invest Dermatol* 43:193-200, 1964.

70a. Stiller MJ, Shupack JL, Kenny C et al.: A double-blind, placebo-controlled clinical trial to evaluate the safety and efficacy of thymopentin as an adjunctive treatment in atopic dermatitis. *J Am Acad Dermatol* 30:597-602, 1994.

71. Trask DM, Chan SC, Sherman SE, Hanifin JM: Altered leukocyte activity in atopic dermatitis, *J Invest Dermatol* 90:526-531, 1988.

72. Trocme SD, Raizman MB, Bartley GB: Medical therapy for ocular allergy, *Mayo Clin Proc* 67:557-565, 1992.

73. Tuft SJ, Kemeny M, Dart JKG, Buckley RJ: Clinical features of atopic keratoconjunctivitis, *Ophthalmology* 98:150-158, 1991.

74. Uehara M, Ofuji S: Abnormal vascular reactions in atopic dermatitis, *Arch Dermatol* 113:627-629, 1977.
75. Uno H, Hanifin JM: Langerhans cells in acute and chronic epidermal lesions of atopic dermatitis, observed by L-Dopa histofluorescence, glycol methyacrylate thin section, and electron microscopy, *J Invest Dermatol* 75:52-60, 1980.
76. Van Joost T, Stolz E, Heule F: Efficacy of low dose cyclosporin in severe atopic skin disease, *Arch Dermatol* 123:166-167, 1987.

76a. Van Joost T, Heule F, Korstanje M, et al.: Cyclosporin in atopic dermatitis: a multicentre placebo-controlled study. *Br J Dermatol* 130:634-40, 1994.
77. White CR Jr: Histopathology of atopic dermatitis, *Semin Dermatol* 2:34, 1983.
78. Wise E, Sulzberger MB: Editorial remarks in *Year book of dermatology and syphilogy,* 59, Chicago, 1933, Year Book Medical Publishers.

29 Kawasaki Disease

NAOKI KUMAGAI, SHIGEAKI OHNO

Kawasaki disease is a systemic inflammatory illness of childhood with prominent mucocutaneous manifestations. It was first described in Japan by Dr. Tomisaku Kawasaki in 1967[16]; he later described the disease in an English language report in 1974.[17] Kawasaki disease starts as a sudden, persistent fever followed by bilateral congestion of the bulbar conjunctivae (Fig. 29-1), reddening of the lips, a strawberry tongue (Fig. 29-2), reddening of the palms and soles, indurative cutaneous edema of the hands and feet, polymorphous exanthema (Fig. 29-3), redness and crusting at the site of BCG inoculation, and unilateral swelling of the cervical lymph nodes. During the convalescent stage, membranous desquamation begins at the fingertips (Fig. 29-4).

Although most of the reactions associated with Kawasaki disease are self-limited and reversible, coronary artery aneurysm or myocardial infarction can occur as a late manifestation. Because of its association with life-threatening coronary artery disease, Kawasaki disease is considered a refractory disease of childhood. Aneurysms can also occur in other medium-size arteries of the kidneys, spleen, and lung. Cardiac sequelae, such as dilatation or stenosis of coronary arteries, myocardial infarction, and valve lesions, occur in 16.3% of patients.[27] The mortality rate is 0.3% to 0.4%.[34]

EPIDEMIOLOGY

Kawasaki disease is now recognized as a relatively common childhood disease. It can occur in children of nearly all racial backgrounds, but has a much higher incidence and prevalence in the Japanese population.[6] In Japan about 5000 children develop Kawasaki disease every year, and the cumulative number of reported patients is above 100,000. Individuals of Japanese descent who are born in other countries also have an increased prevalence of the disease.[12]

Kawasaki disease occurs in epidemics at intervals of 3 years. In Japan the incidence of Kawasaki disease was much higher in 1979, in 1982, and in the winter of 1985 to 1986 than in the intervening years. For example, in 1982 the incidence of Kawasaki disease was as high as 194.7/100,000, which was a 2.4-fold increase over the previous year.[34] The epidemics of Kawasaki disease spread in a wavelike fashion to adjacent regions of the country over a period of months. Outbreaks may also occur when new groups of susceptible children are added to the population.

Siblings of Kawasaki disease patients have a much greater risk of developing Kawasaki disease.[7,34,35] Within 1 year after the onset of the first case in a family, the second-case rate was as much as 2.1% for siblings, whereas the overall incidence in the general population of children 0 to 4 years of age in Japan was approximately 0.19%.[7] More than half of the second familial cases developed Kawasaki disease within 10 days after the onset of the first case, suggesting a common exposure to an unknown causal agent.

CLINICAL FEATURES

Kawasaki disease induces a variety of ocular signs and symptoms (Table 29-1). Although ocular involvement does not usually lead to severe visual disturbances, it is of great diagnostic importance because ocular symptoms develop in the early stage of Kawasaki disease and are among the principal diagnostic features of the disease (as described in a following section).

Conjunctivitis

Conjunctival injection, the most common ocular manifestation, is found in about 90% of cases.[28] It is always bilateral, and the severity of injection is similar in both eyes. Injection is localized to the bulbar conjunctiva. Medium- to large-size vessels of the bulbar conjunctiva are engorged and tortuous. Patients have no or minimal ocular discharge despite the bulbar conjunctival injection. Palpebral conjunctiva shows minimal change, and no hyperemia or pseudomembrane formation is observed on the palpebral conjunctiva. Preauricular lymphadenopathy, which is often found with adenovirus infection, does not occur in Kawasaki disease.

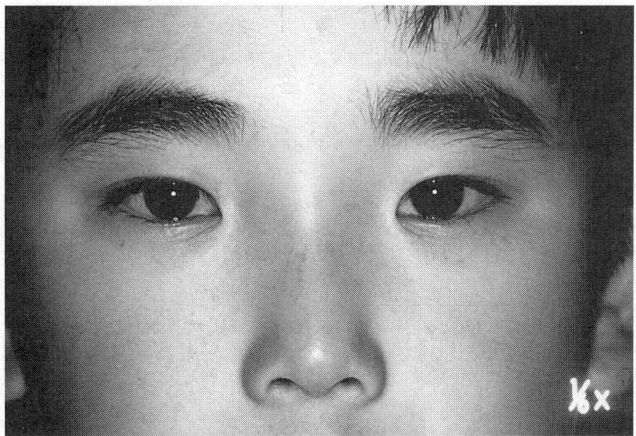

Fig. 29-1. Bilateral bulbar conjunctival injection in a boy with Kawasaki disease on the fifth day of illness.

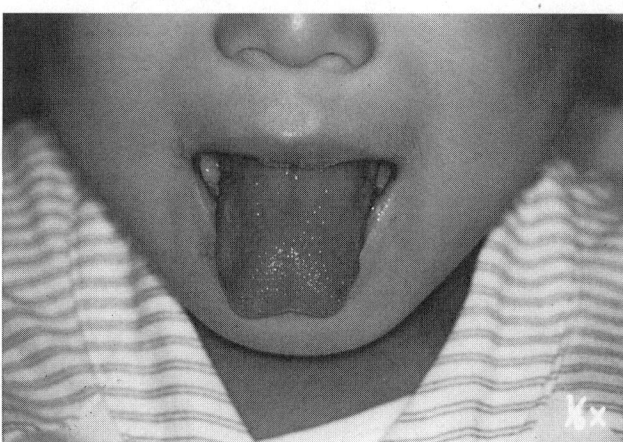

Fig. 29-2. Strawberry tongue of a boy with Kawasaki disease.

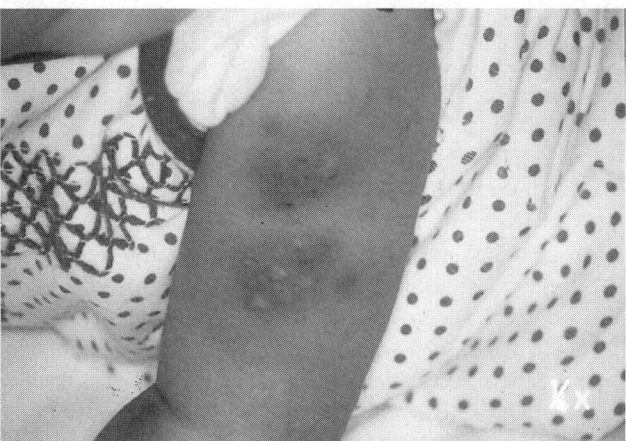

Fig. 29-3. Polymorphous exanthema of a girl with Kawasaki disease.

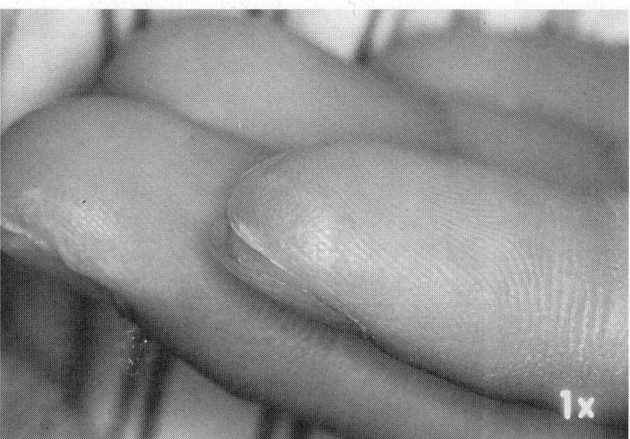

Fig. 29-4. Membranous desquamation of the fingertips of a boy with Kawasaki disease at the convalescent stage.

The conjunctival injection is severe in the acute stage of the disease and gradually decreases in intensity without local treatment. The conjunctival injection usually disappears within 2 to 4 weeks (Fig. 29-5). Sometimes unilateral or bilateral subconjunctival hemorrhage is also observed (Fig. 29-6).

Puglish and associates[29] examined the conjunctival lesion histologically and found engorgement of vessels with mild infiltration of polymorphonuclear and plasma cells in the substantia propria. IgG, IgA and C3 were demonstrated on the surface of the plasma cells by immunohistochemical studies.

Anterior Uveitis

Acute, nongranulomatous iridocyclitis is another important clinical feature of Kawasaki disease and is observed in about 80% of diseased children.[28] The frequency of iridocyclitis is highest in children 2 years of age or older (Fig. 29-7),

but there is no correlation between the severity of the iridocyclitis and patient age. Like bulbar conjunctival injection, the iridocyclitis is always bilateral, and its severity is quite similar between eyes. It is noteworthy that ciliary injection is not usually observed. Acute iridocyclitis begins a little later than the conjunctival injection, and inflammatory cells in the anterior chamber are most numerous between days 5 and 8 (Fig. 29-8). In a study of 41 patients, Burns and associates[4] found that 20 of 24 patients (83%) examined during the first week of their disease had anterior uveitis, whereas anterior uveitis was present in only seven of 17 patients (41%) examined after 1 week.[4] The difference was statistically significant, indicating that the iridocyclitis associated with Kawasaki disease is self-limited.

Like conjunctival injection, aqueous cells are markedly diminished after 2 to 3 weeks and leave no ocular complications such as posterior synechia of the iris, secondary cataract formation, or secondary glaucoma. There is a positive

TABLE 29-1 FREQUENCY OF OCCURRENCE OF OCULAR SIGNS AND SYMPTOMS IN KAWASAKI DISEASE

Ocular Signs and Symptoms	Frequency of Occurrence
Injection of bulbar conjunctiva	32/36 (89%)
Nongranulomatous iridocyclitis	28/36 (78%)
Superficial punctate keratitis	8/36 (22%)
Vitreous opacities	4/36 (12%)
Papilledema	4/36 (11%)
Subconjunctival hemorrhage	1/36 (3%)
Retinal vasculitis	0/28 (0%)
Retinochoroiditis	0/28 (0%)

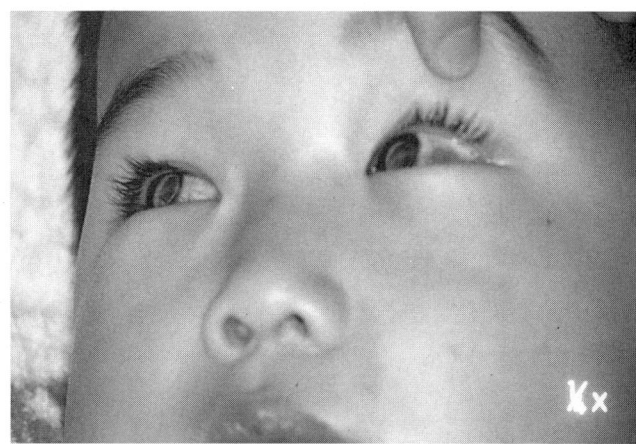

Fig. 29-6. Bilateral bulbar conjunctival injection and subconjunctival hemorrhage in the left eye of a patient with Kawasaki disease on the fifth day of illness.

correlation between the intensity of cells in the anterior chamber and the intensity and duration of conjunctival injection. In relapsing Kawasaki disease, iridocyclitis is not observed.

Keratitis

Superficial keratitis occurs in about 20% of affected children. This keratitis is localized to the area of the palpebral fissure. In a few cases, transient corneal stromal opacity can be observed. Stromal lesions resolve spontaneously without leaving visual impairments.

Posterior Segment Disease

In Kawasaki disease, the posterior segment is also involved. Vitreous opacification, papilledema, tortuous, dilated retinal vessels, retinal folds, and subretinal hemorrhage can be observed. Posterior ocular changes in Kawasaki disease usually resolve without specific treatment. Nevertheless, because sight-threatening changes such as acute retinal

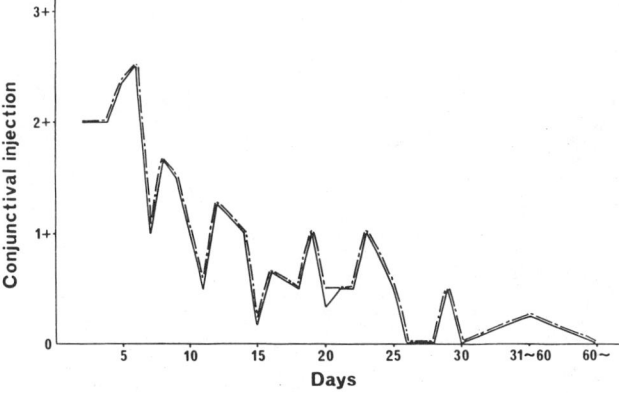

Fig. 29-5. Clinical course of 18 patients with Kawasaki disease showing the average score for conjunctival injection on each day. Solid line indicates right eye and broken line indicates left eye. (From Ohno S et al.: *Am J Ophthalmol* 93:713-717, 1982.)

necrosis or preretinal membrane formation can occur in rare cases, the ophthalmologist should look for ocular fundus diseases as well as external ocular changes. The severity of retinal vascular change does not correlate with the severity of systemic vascular involvement.

PATHOGENESIS

There are several epidemiologic features indicating that Kawasaki disease may have an infectious cause. They include the following observations:

- Kawasaki disease occurs almost exclusively in children.
- It occurs in epidemics at several-year intervals.
- Its incidence is higher in siblings of affected patients.
- Siblings develop Kawasaki disease at almost the same time.
- The epidemics of Kawasaki disease spread in a wavelike fashion.

House dust mites,[10] *Propionibacterium acnes,*[14] Epstein-Barr virus,[19] *Streptococcus sanguis,*[26] and retrovirus infection[32] are candidates for the cause of Kawasaki disease, but none has been confirmed.

Recently, however, knowledge has been accumulated to support the theory that bacterial toxins, acting as superantigens, are the real cause of Kawasaki disease. Kawasaki disease shares some immunologic and clinical features with diseases caused by superantigens, which include streptococcal and staphylococcal toxic shock syndrome, streptococcal scarlet fever, and staphylococcal scalded-skin syndrome. There is a selected expansion of T-lymphocytes expressing specific TCR regions (Vβ2 and, to a lesser extent, Vβ8) in the acute phase of Kawasaki disease.[1] The selective expansion of T-lymphocytes with specific V regions is character-

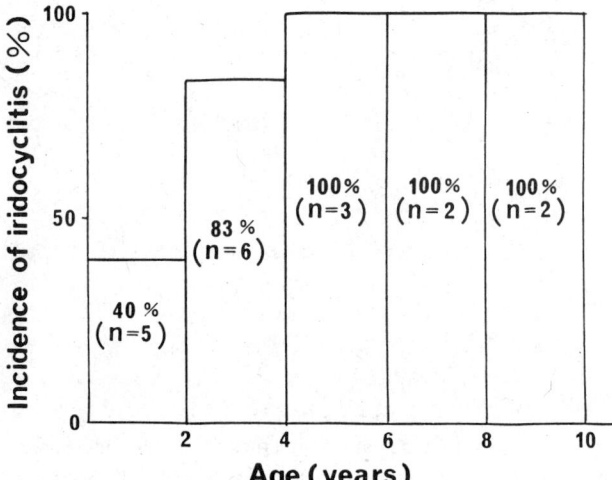

Fig. 29-7. Incidence of bilateral iridocyclitis and the age of the children at the beginning of Kawasaki disease. (From Ohno S et al.: *Am J Ophthalmol* 93:713-717, 1982.)

istic of diseases caused by antigens acting as superantigens. The selective expansion of T-lymphocytes with Vβ2 region, for example, is observed in toxic shock syndrome, a disease that is caused by a bacterial toxin acting as a superantigen.[5] In addition, Leung and associates[23] isolated toxic shock syndrome toxin-secreting *Staphylococcus aureus* and pyogenic exotoxin-secreting streptococci in 13 of 15 patients with Kawasaki disease; these toxins are known to stimulate Vβ2 T-lymphocytes. *Staphylococcus aureus* colonies isolated from patients were unusual because they produced less lipase, haemolysin, and protease than controls. *Staphylococcus aureus* colonies isolated from Kawasaki disease patients were white and could be easily mistaken for coagulase-negative staphylococci, whereas colonies of non-Kawasaki disease isolates were gold.[23]

Kawasaki disease is characterized by both immunoregulatory abnormalities and diffuse vasculopathy. The acute phase of Kawasaki disease is characterized by marked activation of the immune system leading to (1) increased levels of circulating cytokines [interleukin-1,[25] interleukin-6,[33] tumor necrosis factor-α,[8] and interferon-γ,[31]] produced by immune effector cells, (2) the induction of activation antigens on their vascular endothelium, and (3) the generation of lytic antibodies directed against vascular endothelial cells stimulated with cytokines.[21] The vascular disease is characterized histologically by endothelial necrosis, immunoglobulin deposition, and mononuclear infiltrates around small- and medium-size blood vessels. Gross and microscopic features of the vasculitis, as well as the location of the vessels involved are quite similar in Kawasaki disease and infantile periarteritis nodosa.[20] The dilatation of vessels was most vigorous on the fourth day of the illness and then gradually

decreased. The number of mast cells increased in both superficial arteriolar and venular plexus areas, and degranulation was frequent.[11]

Patients have activated T- and B-lymphocytes as well as macrophages-monocytes.[9] There is a reduced ratio of CD8+ to CD4+ T-lymphocytes.[22] Patients with active Kawasaki disease have IgM antibodies to human umbilical vein endothelial cells and human saphenous vein endothelial cells, but only after cells have been induced to express antigenic determinants by interferon-γ, as might occur in the presence of activated T-lymphocytes.[24] These antibodies resulted in killing of the endothelial cells in vitro, which might be one possible mechanism of vascular damage. Similar cell lysis did not occur with other tissues, such as fibroblasts or even human vascular smooth muscle cells. The induced antigens do not appear to be major histocompatibility complex determinants.

The severity of the aqueous cellular reaction has a positive relationship with erythrocyte sedimentation rate and serum C-reactive protein levels,[28] indicating that the severity of the iridocyclitis is a reflection of the severity of systemic acute inflammation. The panvasculitis that occurs in various organs in the acute stage of Kawasaki disease probably also causes ocular lesions such as bulbar conjunctival injection and nongranulomatous iridocyclitis.

The pathogenesis of corneal involvement is not clear, although it is assumed that limbic vasculitis, intracorneal peripheral neuritis, or changes of tear component lead to epithelial breakdown.

The immunogenetic basis of Kawasaki disease has been studied by several authors. As for the HLA class I antigens, the presence of HLA-Bw22 was reported to be correlated with Kawasaki disease in Japanese patients.[15] Another report stated that HLA-Bw51 is related to Kawasaki disease in

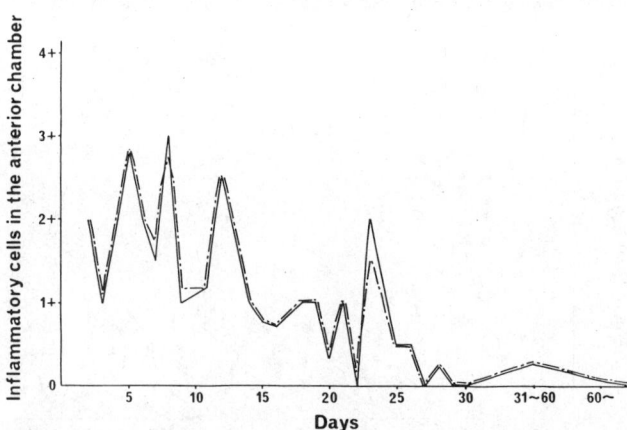

Fig. 29-8. Clinical course of nongranulomatous iridocyclitis in 18 patients with Kawasaki disease showing the average score for inflammatory cells in the anterior chamber on each day. Solid line indicates right eyes and broken line indicates left eyes. (From Ohno S et al.: *Am J Ophthalmol* 93:713-717, 1982.)

TABLE 29-2 DIAGNOSTIC GUIDELINES FOR KAWASAKI DISEASE

Kawasaki disease is a disease of unknown cause most frequently affecting infants and young children under 5 years of age. Signs and symptoms can be classified into two categories: principal signs and other significant symptoms or findings.

A. Principal Signs
  1. Fever persisting 5 days or more
  2. Changes in peripheral extremities
     Initial stage: reddening of palms and soles, indurative cutaneous edema of the hands and feet
     Convalescent stage: Membranous desquamation of the fingertips
  3. Polymorphous exanthema
  4. Bilateral conjunctival congestion
  5. Changes of lips and oral cavity
     Reddening of lips, strawberry tongue, diffuse injection of oral and pharyngeal mucosa
  6. Acute, nonpurulent cervical lymphadenopathy

At least five items of 1-6 should be satisfied for diagnosis of Kawasaki disease; however, if four principal signs are present, Kawasaki disease can be diagnosed when coronary aneurysm is recognized by two-dimensional echocardiography or coronary angiography.

B. Other Significant Symptoms or Findings
  The following symptoms and findings should be clinically considered:
  1. Cardiovascular: auscultation (heart murmur, gallop rhythm, distant heart sounds), ECG changes (prolonged PR, QT intervals, abnormal Q wave, low voltage, ST-T changes, arrhythmias), chest x-ray findings (cardiomegary), 2-dimensional echocardiographic findings (pericardial effusion, coronary aneurysms), aneurysm of peripheral arteries other than coronary (axillary), angina pectoris, or myocardial infarction
  2. Gastrointestinal tract: diarrhea, vomiting, abdominal pain, hydrops of gallbladder, paralytic ileus, mild jaundice, slight increase of serum transaminase
  3. Blood: leukocytosis with shift to the left, thrombocytosis, increased ESR, positive C-reactive protein, hypoalbuminemia, increased alpha-2-globulin, slight decrease in erythrocyte and hemoglobin levels
  4. Urine: proteinuria, increase of leukocytes in urine sediment
  5. Skin: redness and crusting at the site of BCG inoculation, small pustules, transverse furrows of the fingernails
  6. Respiratory: cough, rhinorrhea, abnormal shadow on chest x-ray film
  7. Joints: pain, swelling
  8. Neurologic: pleocytosis of mononuclear cells in CSF, convulsion, unconsciousness, facial palsy, paralysis of the extremities

(From Japan Kawasaki Disease Research Committee: *Guidelines of Kawasaki & Disease*, 4 rev ed., Tokyo, Japan Kawasaki Disease Research Comittee, 1984.)

white patients.[18] Because these data have not been confirmed by other researchers, the true relationship between class I antigens and Kawasaki disease remains unknown. Barron and associates[3] investigated HLA class II alleles in Kawasaki disease by molecular genetic typing using the polymerase chain reaction technique, which is currently the most reliable method for the study of immunogenetics. They found that the frequency of HLA-DRB3*0301 is significantly increased in Caucasian patients in Houston compared to Caucasian controls in the same city. Nevertheless, because no HLA alleles were found to be significantly associated with Kawasaki disease in Caucasian, Asian or African-American patients in Toronto, Canada, they concluded that their data failed to support a consistent role for HLA class II alleles in the pathogenesis of Kawasaki disease.

As described previously, bacterial antigens acting as superantigens may play a major role in the pathogenesis of Kawasaki disease. Because the actions of superantigens are not HLA-restricted, it is assumed that the importance of HLA associations is limited for Kawasaki disease. Further immunologic and molecular biologic studies will be needed to clarify the true nature of this disease.

LABORATORY INVESTIGATIONS

A specific diagnostic test for Kawasaki disease does not exist. Diagnosis is based on characteristic clinical signs and symptoms, which are classified as principal clinical findings and other significant symptoms and findings in the *Fourth Revised Edition of Diagnostic Guidelines for Kawasaki Disease,* published by the Japan Kawasaki Disease Research Committee in 1984 (Table 29-2).[13] Principal symptoms include fever lasting 5 days or longer, bilateral congestion of conjunctiva, changes in the mucous membranes of the oral cavity, changes in the peripheral extremities, polymorphous exanthem, and acute nonsuppurative swelling of the cervical lymph nodes. Similar diagnostic criteria have been formulated by United States Centers for Disease Control and Prevention[30] and the American Heart Association.[2]

Acute bilateral nongranulomatous iridocyclitis occurs in as many as 80% of diseased children and can be considered an important diagnostic feature, even though it is not included as a principal sign in the diagnostic criteria for Kawasaki disease.

THERAPY

The anterior uveitis associated with Kawasaki disease may be treated with topical corticosteroids, if severe, in an attempt to prevent complications. The majority of cases, however, appear to be mild and self-limited, and they resolve spontaneously—even without treatment. The prognosis for retention of normal vision is excellent.

REFERENCES

1. Abe J et al.: Selective expansion of T cells expressing T-cell receptor variable regions Vβ2 and Vβ8 in Kawasaki disease, *Proc Natl Acad Sci USA* 89:4066, 1992.
2. American Heart Association Committee on Rheumatic Fever, Endocarditis, and Kawasaki disease: Diagnostic guidelines for Kawasaki disease, *Am J Dis Child* 144:1220-1221, 1990.
3. Barron KS et al.: Major histocompatibility complex class II alleles in Kawasaki syndrome—lack of consistent correlation with disease or cardiac involvement, *J Rheumatol* 19:1790-1793, 1992.
4. Burns JC et al.: Anterior uveitis associated with Kawasaki syndrome, *Pediatr Infect Dis* 4:258-261, 1985.
5. Choi Y et al.: Selective expansion of T cells expressing Vβ2 in toxic shock syndrome, *J Exp Med* 172:981-984, 1990.
6. Cook DH et al.: Results from an international survey of Kawasaki disease in 1979-82, *Can J Cardiol* 5:389, 1989.
7. Fujita Y et al.: Kawasaki disease in families, *Pediatrics* 84:666, 1989.
8. Furukawa S et al.: Peripheral blood monocyte/macrophage and serum tumor necrosis factor in Kawasaki disease, *Clin Exp Immunol* 48:247-251, 1988.
9. Furukawa S et al.: Expression of FcϵR2/CD23 on peripheral blood macrophages/monocytes in Kawasaki disease, *Clin Immunol Immunopathol* 56:280, 1990.
10. Furusho K et al.: Possible role for mite antigen in Kawasaki disease, *Lancet* ii:194, 1981.
11. Hirose S et al.: Morphological observations on the vasculitis in the mucocutaneous lymph node syndrome, *Eur J Pediatr* 129:17, 1978.
12. Ichida F et al.: Epidemiologic aspects of Kawasaki disease in a Manhattan hospital, *Pediatrics* 84:235, 1989.
13. Japan Kawasaki Disease Research Committee: Diagnostic guidelines of Kawasaki disease, 4 rev ed, Tokyo, Japan Kawasaki Disease Research Committee, 1984.
14. Kato H et al.: Variant strains of *Propionibacterium acnes:* a clue to the aetiology of Kawasaki disease, *Lancet* 2:1383, 1983.
15. Kato S et al.: HLA antigens in Kawasaki disease, *Pediatrics* 61:252-255, 1978.
16. Kawasaki T: Acute febrile mucocutaneous syndrome with lymphoid involvement with specific desquamation of the fingers and toes in children, *Jpn J Allegol* 16:178, 1967.
17. Kawasaki T et al.: A new infantile acute febrile mucocutaneous lymph node syndrome (MLNS) prevailing in Japan, *Pediatrics* 54:271-276, 1974.
18. Kernsky A et al.: HLA antigens in mucocutaneous lymph node syndrome in New England, *Pediatrics* 67:741-743, 1981.
19. Kikuta H et al.: Kawasaki disease and an unusual primary infection with Epstein-Barr virus, *Pediatrics* 73:413, 1984.
20. Landing BM et al.: Are infantile periarteritis nodosa with coronary artery involvement and fatal mucocutaneous lymph node syndrome the same? Comparison of 20 patients from North America with patients from Hawaii and Japan, *Pediatrics* 59:651-662, 1977.
21. Leung DY: The potential role of cytokine-mediated vascular endothelial activation in the pathogenesis of Kawasaki disease, *Acta Paediatr Jpn* 33:739, 1991.
22. Leung DY et al.: Immunoregulatory abnormalities in mucocutaneous lymph node syndrome, *Clin Immunol Immunopathol* 23:100, 1982.
23. Leung DY et al.: Toxic shock syndrome toxin-secreting Staphylococcus aureus in Kawasaki syndrome, *Lancet* 342:1385, 1993.
24. Leung DY et al.: Immunoglobulin M antibodies present in the acute phase of Kawasaki syndrome lyse cultured vascular endothelial cells stimulated by gamma interferon, *J Clin Invest* 77:1428-1435, 1986.
25. Maury CP et al.: Circulating interleukin-1b in patients with Kawasaki disease, *New Eng J Med* 319, 1670-1671, 1988.
26. Nakagawa N et al.: A study of Streptococcus sanguis isolated from dental plaque of MCLS patients and their mothers, *J Dent Health* 35:435, 1985.
27. Nakamura Y et al.: Cardiac sequelae of Kawasaki disease in Japan: Statistical analysis, *Pediatrics* 88:1144, 1991.
28. Ohno S et al.: Ocular manifestations of Kawasaki's disease (mucocutaneous lymph node syndrome), *Am J Ophthalmol* 93:713-717, 1982.
29. Puglish JV et al.: Ocular features of Kawasaki's disease, *Arch Ophthalmol* 100:1101-1103, 1982.
30. Rauch A et al.: Center of Disease Control definition of Kawasaki syndrome, *Pediatr Infect Dis J* 4:702-703, 1985.
31. Rowley AH et al.: Serum interferon concentrations and retroviral serology in Kawasaki syndrome, *Pediatr Infect Dis J* 7:663-667, 1988.
32. Shulman ST, Rowley AH: Does Kawasaki disease have a retroviral aetiology? *Lancet* 2:545, 1986.
33. Ueno Y et al.: The acute phase nature of interleukin 6: studies in Kawasaki disease and other febrile illnesses, *Clin Exp Immunol* 76:337-342, 1989.
34. Yanagawa H et al.: Nationwide survey on Kawasaki disease in Japan, *Pediatrics* 80:58, 1987.
35. Yanagawa H et al.: A nationwide incidence survey of Kawasaki disease in 1985-1986 in Japan, *J Infect Dis* 158:1296, 1988.

30 Theodore Superior Limbic Keratoconjunctivitis

J. DANIEL NELSON, FREDERICK H. THEODORE

Superior limbic keratoconjunctivitis of Theodore (SLK) is a disease of unknown cause that is characterized by recurrent chronic keratoconjunctivitis involving inflammation of the superior bulbar conjunctiva, superior palpebral conjunctiva, superior limbus, and adjacent cornea. Filaments of the superior cornea and limbus are identified in one third to one half of episodes in patients with SLK. Patients who do not have filaments during one episode may have them at another.

HISTORICAL BACKGROUND

In 1953 Braley and Alexander[3] performed microbiologic studies on patients with Thygeson superficial punctate keratitis (TSPK). In some patients, filaments and superior corneal involvement were seen. Since these observations are not typical of TSPK, they may have been instances of SLK. In June 1961 Theodore[23] reported on cases of limbic keratoconjunctivitis with filaments. In August 1961 Thygeson,[31] in a paper on TSPK, noted that some of the cases with filaments and severe bulbar conjunctivitis were undiagnosed and belonged to another clinical picture. In November 1962 at the annual convention of the American Academy of Ophthalmology, Thygeson and Kimura, in a detailed and comprehensive paper on chronic conjunctivitis and keratoconjunctivitis, briefly included general observations on 17 ''unidentified'' cases (clearly SLK) that they referred to as ''chronic keratoconjunctivitis with filaments.'' Theodore (whose paper entitled ''Superior Limbic Keratoconjunctivitis'' was in press and published 2 months later in January 1963[24]) presented a detailed description, clearly defining and establishing SLK as a distinct entity. Thygeson and Kimura's paper, including Theodore's discussion, was published in July 1963.[33] Later in 1963, in his paper on filamentary keratitis, Thygeson[32] urged general acceptance of the name SLK as well as Theodore's description and delineation of this clinical entity. Over the years, Theodore and associates[25,27-30] contributed additional reports on SLK.

EPIDEMIOLOGY

SLK occurs in all adult age groups but more commonly in patients between the ages of 30 to 55 years. Women (70%) tend to be afflicted more often than men.[14] The disease is usually bilateral (70%) but can occur unilaterally. Asymmetric involvement is not unusual. About one third of patients with SLK have associated thyroid disease.* One fourth of patients have decreased Schirmer test values.[8,16,18,24,32] SLK has been reported in identical twins.[9]

PATHOGENESIS

The exact cause of SLK remains unknown. Infectious agents,[31] immunologic disease,[4] keratoconjunctivitis sicca, and mechanical trauma have been proposed as underlying causes.[17,38] Culture and electron microscopic methods have failed to demonstrate a viral cause.[18] The minimal inflammation found by light microscopy, the lack of immunoglobulin deposition, the absence of circulating antibodies and eosinophils, and the poor response to topical corticosteroids make an immunologic mechanism very unlikely.[11] Dry eye is not a probable cause as it is only found in about one quarter of patients with SLK.

Wright[38] proposed that a chronically inflamed upper lid and palpebral conjunctiva may disturb the normal maturation of the cells of the bulbar conjunctiva and could give rise to the symptoms and signs of SLK. The superior tarsal conjunctiva, however, is often only mildly inflamed; and it is difficult to determine whether the superior bulbar or the superior palpebral conjunctiva is the initial site of inflammation.[10] Ostler[17] submitted that mechanical trauma of the superior limbus and bulbar conjunctiva arises because of movement of a tightly applied upper eyelid over a lax superior bulbar conjunctiva.[17] The fact that SLK has been reported in twins suggests a genetic predisposition. Environ-

---

*References 4, 16, 18, 21, 24, 38.

mental factors, such as airborne particulate material, may be involved.[7]

Evidence that a multitude of seemingly unrelated therapies, which either remove or cause a tightening of the superior bulbar conjunctiva, reduce the symptoms and signs of SLK supports a mechanical cause. It may be that an initial insult, such as hyperthyroidism or allergy, results in transient edema and inflammation of the superior conjunctiva. This condition then leads to laxity and redundancy of the superior bulbar conjunctiva. The mechanical action of a tightly applied upper eyelid moving over and traumatizing the loose bulbar conjunctiva leads to the clinical and histologic signs of SLK.

The disease involves a chronic, prolonged course with a gradual and complete clearing. Short remissions, seen early in the course of the disease, slowly lengthen until the disease abates. Treatment of underlying thyroid disease,[14] which occurs in about one third of patients with SLK, may result in improvement of signs and symptoms of SLK.

CLINICAL FEATURES

Symptoms

Patients with SLK usually complain of irritation, foreign-body sensation, burning, photophobia, redness, and a mucoid discharge from the eye. Symptoms vary in severity with time, environment, and activity; and generally parallel clinical signs. Blepharospasm and pseudoptosis may occur. The presence of filaments is associated with marked discomfort, especially when they spontaneously tear off the epithelium.

Signs

The characteristic findings of SLK are listed in Table 30-1 and shown diagramatically in Fig. 30-1. The disease affects the superior palpebral conjunctiva, superior bulbar conjunctiva, and the superior limbus and cornea. There is a papillary reaction of the superior palpebral conjunctiva with a normal-appearing inferior palpebral conjunctiva. The su-

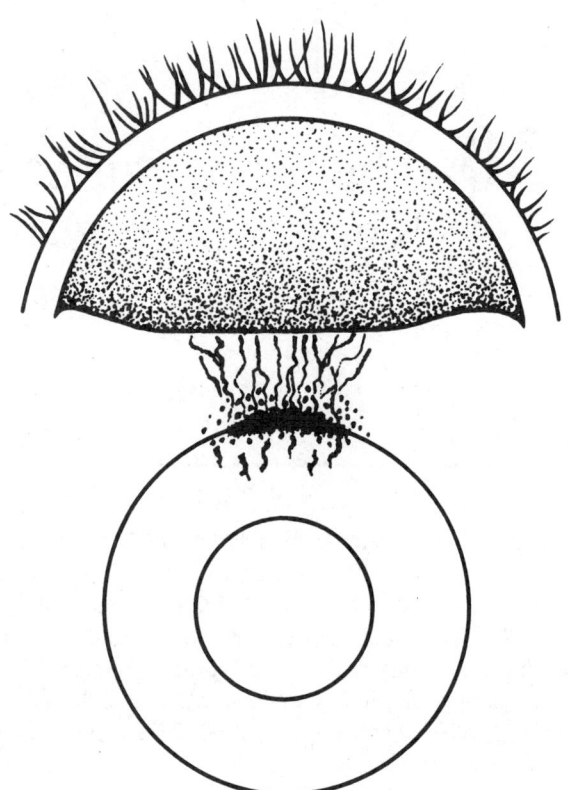

Fig. 30-1. Schematic representation of the characteristic clinical findings in SLK showing the following: (1) superior palpebral conjunctival papillae, (2) injection of the superior bulbar conjunctiva, (3) punctate rose bengal staining of the superior bulbar conjunctiva, (4) superior limbal epithelial proliferation, and (5) corneal filaments. (Modified after Theodore[25]).

perior bulbar conjunctiva is hyperemic, thickened, and lusterless. It is usually positioned in a 10-mm arc centered at the twelve o'clock superior corneoscleral limbus and directed posteriorly toward the superior rectus muscle (Figs. 30-2 and 30-3). This area typically stains with rose bengal and less so with fluorescein and alcian blue. Occasionally a

TABLE 30-1 CHARACTERISTICS OF SLK

Characteristic	Finding
Clinical course	Recurring episodes
Duration	1-10 years
Prognosis	Evenutally clears
Superior palpebral conjunctiva	Papillary reaction
Superior bulbar conjunctiva	Injection, fine punctate staining
Superior cornea	Fine punctate staining, filaments
Rose bengal staining	Superior cornea and conjunctiva

Braley AE, Alexander RC: Superficial punctate keratitis, *Arch Ophthalmol* 50:147-54, 1953.
Nelson JD: Superior limbic keratoconjunctivitis, *Eye* 3:180-189, 1989.
Theodore FH: Superior limbic keratoconjunctivitis (Theodore's SLK). In Fraunfelder, FT, Roy FH, editors: *Current ocular therapy,* Philadelphia, 1980, WB Saunders.

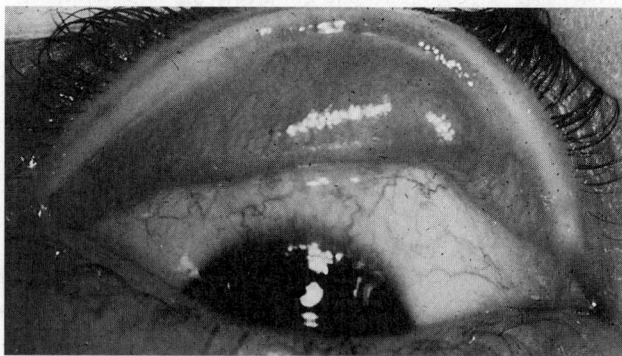

Fig. 30-2. Superior palpebral conjunctival papillae and superior limbal proliferation in a patient with Theodore SLK. (Published courtesy of *Trans Am Acad Ophthalmol Otolaryngol* 71:341-351, 1967).

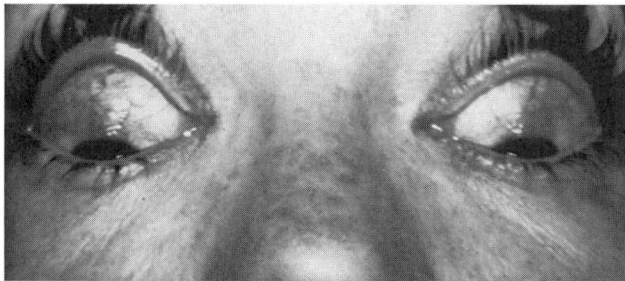

Fig. 30-3. Marked bilateral inflammation of the superior bulbar conjunctiva in a patient with Theodore SLK. (Published courtesy of *Arch Ophthalmol* 84:481-484, 1970, American Medical Association.)

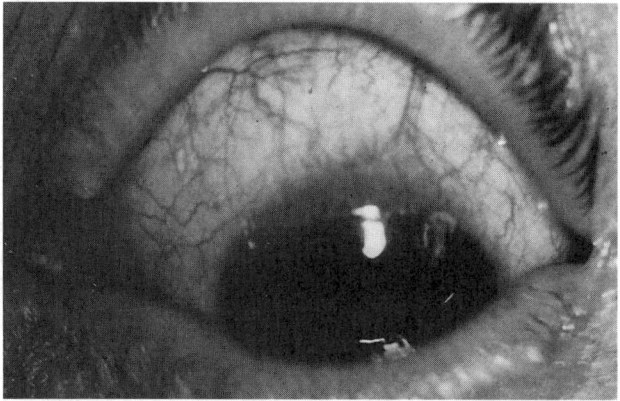

Fig. 30-4. Superior bulbar injection, limbal proliferation, and filaments in a patient with Theodore SLK.

pseudomembrane[24] or a subconjunctival hemorrhage may be seen.[37]

There are fine punctate epithelial erosions involving the superior one third of the cornea that stain with rose bengal and fluorescein. From one third to one half of the patients have multiple filaments that may be found on the superior cornea and superior limbus.[14] Acquired with-the-rule astigmatism, that disappears with resolution of SLK, has been reported.[4] Decreased aqueous tear secretion, as measured by Schirmer testing, is seen in about one quarter of SLK patients.[14] Table 30-2 summarizes the frequency of findings associated with SLK.

PATHOLOGY

Conjunctival scrapings,[30] biopsy,[2,5] and impression cytology[14] show keratinization of the superior bulbar conjunctival epithelium. Biopsy specimens also show swollen, degenerated epithelial cells with few goblet cells present (Fig. 30-4).[34] Condensed epithelial cell nuclear chromatin ("snakelike" chromatin) has been noted in some patients.[35] Conjunctival impression cytology demonstrates superior bulbar conjunctival squamous metaplasia with loss of goblet cells.[15] The conjunctival stroma shows signs of edema with dilated lymphatics but few inflammatory cells (Fig. 30-5).[10]

Transmission electron microscopy reveals extensive in-

tracellular accumulation of glycogen granules with increased (1) numbers and clumping of microfilaments, (2) presence of secondary lysosomes, (3) thickening of the epithelial cellular membranes, and (4) the presence of keratohyaline granules in the cytoplasm.[5,10] The superior palpebral conjunctiva shows infiltration of polymorphonuclear neutrophilic leukocytes, lymphocytes, and plasma cells. The epithelium is usually normal, and goblet cells are increased in numbers.[38]

DIFFERENTIAL DIAGNOSIS

Most instances of SLK are easily recognized by the presence of superior conjunctival and corneal staining, especially when filaments are present (Fig. 30-6). Other filament-associated conditions that should be considered include ptosis or lid occlusion, keratoconjunctivitis sicca (where filaments occur predominately in the lower half of the cornea), neuroparalytic keratopathy, recurrent erosions, corneal trauma, neurotrophic keratopathy, herpes simplex

TABLE 30-2 FREQUENCY OF FINDINGS IN SLK

Finding	Occurrence in SLK
Age	85% between 30-55
Gender	70% women
Bilaterality	70%
Filaments	30-50% of episodes
Decrease Schirmer's test	25%
Thyroid disease	33%

Braley AE, Alexander RC: Superficial punctate keratitis, *Arch Ophthalmol* 50:147-54, 1953.
Nelson JD: Superior limbic keratoconjunctivitis, *Eye* 3:180-189, 1989.
Theodore FH: Superior limbic keratoconjunctivitis (Theodore's SLK). In Fraunfelder, FT, Roy FH, editors: *Current ocular therapy,* Philadelphia, 1980, WB Saunders.

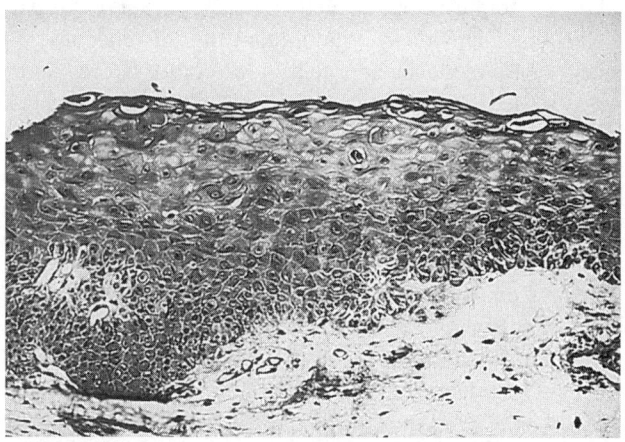

Fig. 30-5. Keratinization of the bulbar conjunctival surface, acanthosis, and mild dyskeratosis, along with neovascularization of the stroma in a patient with Theodore SLK (hematoxylin and eosin, original magnification × 180). (Published courtesy of *Arch Ophthalmol* 84:481-484, 1970.)

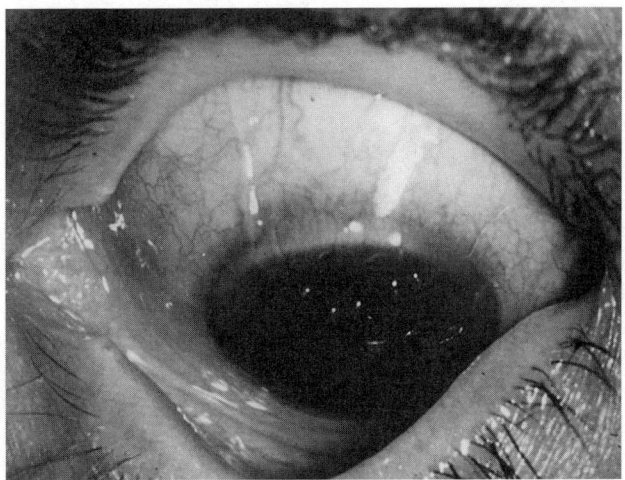

Fig. 30-6. Numerous corneal filaments in a patient with Theodore SLK. (Published courtesy of *Trans Am Acad Ophthalmol Otolaryngol* 71:341-351, 1967.) (Figure also in color insert.)

TABLE 30-3   COMPARISON OF SLK AND CONTACT LENS-INDUCED KERATOPATHY (CLK)

Finding	SLK	CLK
Filaments	Present	Absent
Corneal involvement	Superior limbus	Superior 1/2
Bulbar conjunctiva	Inflamed superiorly	Inflamed
Superior palpebral conjunctiva	Papillae	Papillae
Conjunctival scrapings	Neutrophils, lymphocytes, plasma cells	Eosinophils
Topical steroids	Minimal, if any, effect	Improves symptoms
Contact lenses	Improves symptoms	Worsens symptoms

virus keratitis, chronic bullous keratopathy, nystagmus, and keratitis medicamentosa.[1] All of these entities, except dry eye syndrome, can have filaments involving any part of the cornea.

When filaments are not present, other entities should be considered. These include trachoma, superficial punctate keratitis (Thygeson SPK), the limbal form of vernal keratoconjunctivitis, and phlyctenulosis (if the lesions occur at twelve o'clock).

The syndrome of contact lens keratopathy or keratoconjunctivitis (CLK) has been misdiagnosed as SLK or contact lens-induced SLK.[2,12,19,20] Whereas early cases of CLK may be confused with Theodore SLK, advanced cases show marked differences (Table 30-3). SLK is essentially conjunctival with definite injection superiorly. Corneal involvement is primarily at the superior limbus with filaments limited to the upper few millimeters. CLK is mainly corneal, although confluent or enlarged papillae of the superior palpebral conjunctiva may occur. Initially this disorder superficially involves the superior half of the cornea but may progress to deeper opacification with superior corneal pannus and impaired vision. Corneal filaments occur rarely, if at all. The syndrome is attributed to an allergy to lipoprotein deposits on contact lenses or to preservatives, especially thimerosal.[2,12,19,20,37] Conjunctival scrapings may show eosinophils, which are never seen in SLK, suggesting drug allergy. Stopping contact lens wear improves symptoms in these patients, and symptoms of true SLK are often improved with hydrophilic contact lenses. Improvement with topical corticosteroids, which do not help in SLK, usually occurs in CLK.

THERAPY

Although immediate amelioration usually takes place with several types of therapy, relapses of varying severity occur over a period of years. Following longer intervals between recurrences, the condition eventually clears.

Silver Nitrate

Experience of over 30 years shows that a very weak, 0.5% solution of silver nitrate applied to the superior bulbar and palpebral conjunctiva (never the cornea), as initially proposed by Theodore, is the mainstay of management for SLK. It usually gives immediate relief. When filaments are present, they almost always fall off a few minutes after this treatment. A cotton-tipped applicator, wet but not dripping, is gently touched to the entire superior palpebral conjunctiva and to the involved area of the superior bulbar conjunctiva (with the patient looking down). Irrigation with normal saline is done 2 to 3 minutes later. The cornea is never treated as deposition of silver and corneal opacification lasting for years may occur, especially if there is an absence of epithelium. Moreover, it is not necessary. Should the cornea be touched, it should be immediately irrigated.

It is very important to be sure that a proper and accurate solution concentration has been prepared by the pharmacy. Solutions should be reasonably fresh, as evaporation of standing solutions may increase their concentration. Concentrations over 1.0% should not be used. *Washings from silver nitrate sticks (75% strength) or the sticks themselves should never be used.* Topical anesthesia for silver nitrate treatment is not necessary and, on rare occasions, may cause an immediate (within 30 minutes) idiosyncratic reaction (especially with proparacaine) that may be falsely attributed to the silver nitrate.[26]

Although extremely rare, mild silver salt deposition with pigmentation of the conjunctiva may occur from repeated silver nitrate treatments given over many years for other conditions. This has not been reported for silver nitrate treatment in SLK, as the treatments are less frequent, less intense, and less extensive.

Silver nitrate treatments are often given on a weekly basis, but may be given more frequently. As improvement occurs, longer intervals between treatments suffice. As noted earlier, recurrences are not unusual. Eventually, the condition appears to clear completely, but sometimes it remains for years. The effects of silver nitrate may be related to a transient tightening or shrinkage of the superior limbal conjunctiva.

Soft Contact Lenses

Large therapeutic hydrophilic contact lenses that extend beyond the limbus are useful in reducing the signs and symptoms of SLK. Caution is advised in patients with impaired tear secretion. To treat SLK, frequent reexamination is indicated in all patients using contact lenses. Discontinuation of the lens often results in recurrence of SLK.

Other Nonsurgical Treatments

Topical or systemic antibiotics and antivirals are ineffective and should be avoided, except when secondary infection is feared. Corticosteroids are not effective, and long-term use may cause cataracts, glaucoma, and other complications.[29] Topical artificial lubricants may reduce symptoms, especially in patients with dry eyes. Topical methylcellulose, acetylcysteine,[38] vitamin A,[16] and cromolyn sodium[6] alleviate the symptoms and signs of SLK to a variable extent. Patching[13] may also offer relief, especially when a corneal erosion from torn-off filaments has occurred. In patients with a hyperactive thyroid, medical measures have proven useful, including radioactive iodine.[4,21]

Surgical Treatment

In cases where silver nitrate therapy and other therapies mentioned previously are not satisfactory, various surgical procedures have been used. Minor procedures such as diagnostic scrapings of the superior palpebral and bulbar conjunctivae can be symptomatically helpful, at least temporarily. Apparently, almost any moderate mechanical treatment of the involved bulbar conjunctiva gives good but temporary results. Thermal cautery[34] of the involved superior bulbar conjunctiva (never the cornea) is reported to give temporary relief for a number of weeks to months. Transient increased vascularity may be noted following treatment.

Surgical resection of the superior limbic conjunctiva usually is more successful for much longer periods with immediate and continued relief of symptoms.[10,18,22] First, a superior peritomy from ten o'clock to two o'clock is performed. Then an arcuate segment of conjunctiva and Tenon's capsule, measuring 5 mm in the twelve o'clock meridian is resected. Although the remaining conjunctival edge can be sutured to the sclera, it is not necessary. Recession of the involved bulbar conjunctiva has also been performed, but resection is preferred. While good long-term results do occur in many patients, when the superior bulbar conjunctiva regenerates—the disease may recur.

Procedures for treating SLK may be complicated by inflammatory reactions of varying degrees. Dry eyes not only may aggravate the symptoms of SLK but also complicate treatment. Signs and symptoms of dry eyes should be sought in advance and treated as intensively as indicated, including punctal occlusion if necessary. Severe thinning of the exposed sclera has occurred after conjunctival resection in cases of SLK with severe dryness.[36] Indications for other forms of ocular surgery should be carefully evaluated in patients with SLK. Pseudoptosis, which may be present in some cases, may lead to unneeded ptosis surgery and aggravated SLK.

REFERENCES

1. Arffa RC: *Grayson's diseases of the cornea,* ed 3, 48, St Louis, 1991, Mosby.
2. Bloomfield SE, Jakobiec FA, Theodore FH: Contact lens-induced keratopathy. A severe complication extending the spectrum of keratoconjunctivitis in contact lens wearers, *Ophthalmology* 91:290-294, 1984.
3. Braley AE, Alexander RC: Superficial punctate keratitis, *Arch Ophthalmol* 50:147-154, 1953.
4. Cher I: Clinical features of superior limbic keratoconjunctivitis in Australia, *Arch Ophthalmol* 82:580-586, 1969.
5. Collin HB et al.: Keratinization of the superior bulbar conjunctival epithelium in superior limbic keratoconjunctivitis in humans, *Acta Ophthalmol* 56:531-543, 1978.
6. Confino J, Brown SI: Treatment of superior limbic keratoconjunctivitis with topical cromolyn sodium, *Am J Ophthalmol* 19:129-131, 1987.
7. Corona R, Abraham JL: Superior limbic keratoconjunctivitis apparently related to particulate material from a ventilation system, *N Engl J Med* 320:1354, 1989 (correspondence).
8. Corwin ME: Superior limbic keratoconjunctivitis, *Am J Ophthalmol* 66:338-340, 1968.
9. Darrell RW: Superior limbic keratoconjunctivitis in identical twins, *Cornea* 11:262-263, 1992.
10. Donshik PC et al.: Conjunctival resection treatment and ultrastructural histopathology of superior limbic keratoconjunctivitis, *Am J Ophthalmol* 85:101-110, 1978.
11. Eiferman RA, Wilkins EL: Immunological aspects of superior limbic keratoconjunctivitis, *Can J Ophthalmol* 14:85-87, 1979.
12. Fuerst DJ, Sugar J, Worobec S: Superior limbic keratoconjunctivitis associated with cosmetic soft contact lens wear, *Arch Ophthalmol* 101:1214-1216, 1983.
13. Mondino BJ, Zaidman GW, Salamon SW: Use of pressure patching and soft contact lenses in superior limbic keratoconjunctivitis, *Arch Ophthalmol* 100:1932-1934, 1982.
14. Nelson JD: Superior limbic keratoconjunctivitis, *Eye* 3:180-189, 1989.
15. Nelson JD, Wright JC: Goblet cell densities in ocular surface disease, *Arch Ophthalmol* 102:1049-1051, 1984.
16. Ohasi Y et al.: Vitamin A eye drops for superior limbic keratoconjunctivitis, *Am J Ophthalmol* 105:523-527, 1988.
17. Ostler HB: Superior limbic keratoconjunctivitis. In Smolin G, Thoft RA, editors: *The cornea,* 296-298, Boston/Toronto, 1987, Little Brown.
18. Passons GA, Wood TO: Conjunctival resection for superior limbic keratoconjunctivitis, *Ophthalmology* 91:966-968, 1986.
19. Sendele DD, Kenyon KR, Mobilia EF et al.: Superior limbic keratoconjunctivitis in contact lenses wear, *Ophthalmology* 90:617-622, 1983.
20. Stenson S: Superior limbic keratoconjunctivitis associated with soft contact lens wear, *Arch Ophthalmol* 101:402-404, 1983.
21. Tenzel RR: Comments on superior limbic filamentous keratoconjunctivitis. part 2, *Arch Ophthalmol* 78:505, 1968.
22. Tenzel RR: Resistant superior limbic keratoconjunctivitis, *Arch Ophthalmol* 89:439, 1973.

23. Theodore FH: *The collected letters of the international correspondence society of ophthalmologists and otolaryngologists,* series VI, June 30, 1961.

24. Theodore FH: Superior limbic keratoconjunctivitis, *Eye Ear Nose Throat Month* 42:25-28, 1963.

25. Theodore FH: Further observations on superior limbic keratoconjunctivitis, *Trans Am Acad Ophthalmol Otolaryngol* 71:341-351, 1967.

26. Theodore FH: Idiosyncratic reactions of the cornea from proparacaine, *Eye Ear Nose Throat Month* 47:66-71, 1968.

27. Theodore FH: Superior limbic keratoconjunctivitis: further studies. In *Proceedings of the XXI international congress,* Amsterdam, 1970, Excerpta Medica.

28. Theodore FH: Superior limbic keratoconjunctivitis: a summary, *Mod Probl Ophthalmol* 9:23-26, 1971.

29. Theodore FH: Superior limbic keratoconjunctivitis (Theodore's SLK). In Fraunfelder FT, Roy FH, editors: *Current ocular therapy,* 387-388, Philadelphia, 1980, WB Saunders.

30. Theodore FH, Ferry AP: Superior limbic keratoconjunctivitis: clinical and pathologic correlations, *Arch Ophthalmol* 84:481-484, 1970.

31. Thygeson P: Further observations on superficial punctate keratitis, *Arch Ophthalmol* 66:158-167, 1961.

32. Thygeson P: Observations on filamentary keratitis transactions of AMA section on Ophthalmology 112th Annual Meeting, 1963.

33. Thygeson P, Kimura SJ: Observations on chronic conjunctivitis and chronic keratoconjunctivitis, *Trans Am Acad Ophthalmol* 67:494-517, 1963.

34. Udell IJ, Kenyon KR, Sawa M: Treatment of superior limbic keratoconjunctivitis by thermocauterization of the superior bulbar conjunctiva, *Ophthalmology* 93:162-166, 1986.

35. Wander AH, Masukawa T: Unusual appearance of condensed chromatin in conjunctival cells in superior limbic keratoconjunctivitis, *Lancet* 2:42-43, 1981.

36. Wander AH: Superior limbic keratoconjunctivitis (Theodore's SLK). In Fraunfelder FT, Roy FH, editors: *Current ocular therapy,* 457-458, Philadelphia, 1990, WB Saunders.

37. Wilson LA, McNatt J, Reitschel R: Delayed hypersensitivity to thimerosal in soft contact lens wearers, *Ophthalmology* 88:804-809, 1981.

38. Wright P: Superior limbic keratoconjunctivitis, *Trans Ophthalmol Soc UK* 92:555-560, 1972.

31 Thygeson Superficial Punctate Keratopathy

IVAN R. SCHWAB, PHILLIPS THYGESON

Thygeson superficial punctate keratopathy (TSPK) is an insidious, chronic epithelial keratitis of unknown cause, with no known association with any systemic disease. Patients usually have a long history replete with spontaneous remissions, exacerbations of intermittent foreign body sensation, but minimal, if any, conjunctival reaction.

HISTORICAL BACKGROUND

In 1889 Ernst Fuchs[6] was probably the first to use the term *keratitis punctata superficialis* or *superficial punctate keratitis (SPK)*, but he was referring to what later became known as epidemic keratoconjunctivitis. Unfortunately, the term SPK was later used to describe, indiscriminately, all manner of spotty superficial keratopathies.[20]

Thygeson[18] first reported 26 cases of true TSPK in 1950, some of which he had been following for 24 years. Thygeson first noted TSPK in Denver, where it was called miliary dendritic keratitis by Jackson and Fenoff, who had observed (but not described) the disease. Thygeson's[20a] initial impression was to differentiate TSPK from herpes simplex virus keratitis, because there was no loss of corneal sensation in TSPK. Shortly after Thygeson's initial description, Braley[2] recounted one case in which an uncharacterized virus was isolated from the cornea. The virus was passaged in embryonic mouse brain maintained in organ culture. Its original pathogenicity, when inoculated directly into rabbit cornea, was lost after serial passage. Many observers, including the authors, believe this rare isolate to be a result of a laboratory accident. Braley and Alexander[3] later expanded their original report to include nine cases with some different clinical features. They reported hyperemia of the superior bulbar conjunctiva and the association of filamentary keratitis, although most observers now believe these patients had superior limbic keratoconjunctivitis. In 1961 Thygeson[19] added 29 cases and first stated the 5 diagnostic features that would differentiate TSPK from other forms of epithelial keratitis: (1) the chronic bilateral punctate epithelial nature of the disease, (2) the long duration with remissions and exacerba-

tions, (3) the eventual healing without scars, (4) the lack of response to antibiotics, and (5) the striking symptomatic response to topical corticosteroids. A majority of these cases healed within 2 to 4 years, although some were of a much shorter duration.

Jones[9] reported 27 cases in 1963 and also recounted a faint opacification of the superficial stroma underlying the epithelial opacity. He believed this stromal change had the grey appearance of lamellar separation caused by edema, rather than the hard or dotlike appearance of cellular infiltration. Additionally, in retroillumination, this stromal change was transparent or translucent, suggesting edema. Jones[9] also emphasized that the disease should be called Thygeson superficial punctate keratitis, and that "SPK" should not be used to describe other forms of keratitis.

In 1966 Thygeson[20] added another 27 previously unreported cases and distinguished superior limbic keratoconjunctivitis from TSPK. In this work Thygeson noted that the disease usually lasted from 6 months to 4 years.

Thygeson[20] pointed out in 1966 that a viral cause of superficial punctate keratitis was strongly suggested by (1) the absence of bacteria or other microorganisms, (2) the resistance of the disease to antibacterial agents, (3) the scanty mononuclear cell exudate on conjunctival scrapings, and (4) the viral type characteristics of the epithelial lesions.

Quere,[14] in 1968, believed the disease had 3 stages: (1) the primary stage of onset lasting 1 to 2 weeks, (2) a developmental stage of up to 8 months, and (3) a stage of regression of several months to 3 years. During the stage of onset there was catarrhal inflammation, photophobia, and tearing. During the second stage (developmental phase) the signs of conjunctival inflammation disappeared entirely, leaving the epithelial lesions. During the regressive phase, the lesions became fewer in number and smaller in size until they finally vanished. Quere and associates[14] also suggested that this disease was potentially longer lasting than initially thought and proposed that the disease could be chronic, although these patients had been placed on corticosteroids.

Total duration of the disease in these patients ranged from 4 months to 30 years, with an average of 7.5 years and a median of 4 years. Tabbara and associates,[17] in their review of 45 cases, found cases to be active for as briefly as 1 month or as long as 24 years.[17]

In 1974 Lemp and associates[10] isolated varicella-zoster from the corneal epithelium of a patient with TSPK. This isolated finding may have reflected a laboratory accident or perhaps even spontaneous shedding. The role of varicella-zoster in TSPK remains unconfirmed.

EPIDEMIOLOGY

Most authors report no sex predilection, although Darrell[4] did find a mild female preponderance (25 women and 7 men). van Bijstervelt and associates,[22] in a large retrospective series of 54 cases of TSPK, found significantly more women affected than men. These latter investigators also suggested that the median age of onset was younger for women than for men.[22] Conversely, in another series Tabbara and associates[17] had 28 men and 17 women. Without sex-specific population rates or properly performed prevalence studies, these numbers mean very little.

The onset of the disease occurs most frequently during the second and third (or perhaps fourth) decades, presenting with characteristic corneal lesions and generally no conjunctival involvement. Occasional isolated reports suggest that a mild conjunctivitis may precede early attacks.[18] At diagnosis, patients have ranged in age from 2.5 years to over 70 years of age, with a mean age of 29. There is often a delay between the onset of symptoms and the diagnosis.[17]

CLINICAL FEATURES

Symptoms include photophobia, foreign body sensation, burning, tearing, and occasional blurring of vision—depending on axial location. The conjunctiva may be mildly injected but can be completely quiet. Classic clinical signs seen in the cornea include oval or round, grouped punctate intraepithelial deposits comprised of many discrete, fine, granular, white-to-grey, dotlike opacities (Figs. 31-1 and 31-2). These three-dimensional ellipsoidal or round intraepithelial opacities usually develop a raised center that breaks through the epithelial surface and may occasionally show tiny hairlike filaments that are probably mucus. The corneal lesions may have a ragged edge or, rarely, a stellate appearance. The stellate or dendriform appearance sometimes leads to an incorrect diagnosis of herpes simplex virus keratitis.

Thygeson described as few as 3, or as many as 20 lesions,[18] and other observers have described from 1 to 50 of these lesions with an average of 15 to 20.[9,19] Mild epithelial and subepithelial edema is occasionally observed with the opacities, but no infiltration is evident. The opacities are evanescent and do not necessarily remain in the same location from week to week, although they do favor the central cornea and the visual axis. Untreated individual attacks usually last 1 to 2 months and then resolve into remission—only to recur 6 to 8 weeks later. During the inactive stage, the lesions may disappear completely unless subepithelial scarring has left a "footprint".

During exacerbations, these focal opacities are elevated above the superficial epithelium and stain with fluorescein and rose bengal. During remissions, the inactive lesions appear to be flat, intraepithelial, grey dots wholly within the epithelium that do not stain with fluorescein or rose bengal.

Corneal sensation is not generally affected, although sometimes patients are found to have a mild decrease in corneal sensation. This disease is almost exclusively bilateral, with fewer than 1 patient in 20 having unilateral disease. In bilateral cases, the disease may first present in one eye and it is not uncommon to have one eye that is more symptomatic throughout the course of the disorder. Onset of

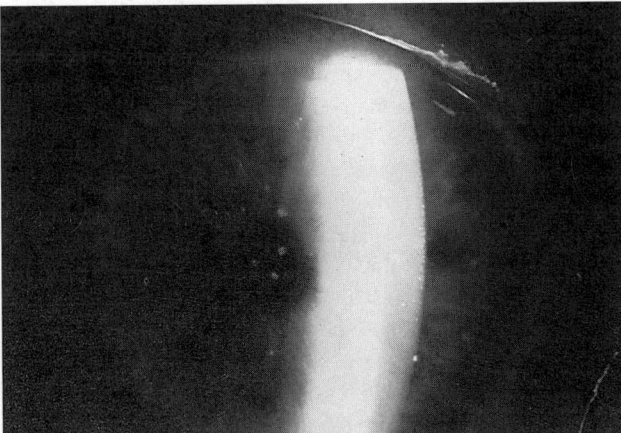

Fig. 31-1. Thygeson superficial punctate keratitis. Note the round-to-oval grouped intraepithelial opacities, each with a granular appearance.

Fig. 31-2. Thygeson superficial punctate keratitis. Note the size of the lesions and the relative clustering of the opacities to the central cornea. These are round-to-oval lesions and entirely intraepithelial.

the disease occurs most frequently in the second, third, or fourth decade of life with little or no conjunctival reaction. Although the course is chronic and may last more than two decades, signs and symptoms often resolve spontaneously in spite of, but probably not in response to, treatment. The acute symptoms are responsive to several methods of treatment.

THERAPY

Treatment generally consists of topical corticosteroids during acute exacerbations. Some evidence suggests that corticosteroids will prolong the overall course and that these medications should be used sparingly and in low dose, if at all. Tabbara and associates[17] concluded that the average course of the disease was prolonged in the patients receiving corticosteroid therapy. Thygeson's early reports included patients who were not treated with corticosteroids whose disease never exceeded 6 years. Tabbara and associates, however, reported cases with longer disease intervals that had been treated with corticosteroids. These authors concluded that corticosteroids may prolong this otherwise self-limited disease. Hence, corticosteroids should be used sparingly and in very low dose, although TSPK does respond to these drugs. Therapeutic soft contact lenses used on an extended wear basis offer an alternative treatment to be used during exacerbations, although potential complications, such as microbial keratitis, exist with this modality.[16] Rapid resolution of the epithelial lesions and immediate symptomatic relief with soft contact lenses have been reported by various authors.[5,7] Therapeutic contact lenses are not without complications, and one must weigh these potential problems against other treatment measures and against the patient's disease.

Other topical agents have been tried with little or no success. Idoxuridine (IDU), specifically, produces subepithelial scarring and is contraindicated. In an unmasked, uncontrolled study, Nesburn and associates[12] treated six eyes of four separate patients with TSPK with topical trifluridine. They reported improvement in five of six eyes but noted that the signs and symptoms disappeared more slowly than lesions treated with corticosteroids.

Interestingly, 1 patient with an 11-year history of topical corticosteroid dependence was treated successfully with trifluridine. Nesburn et al concluded that trifluridine is an effective and safe alternative to corticosteroids, noting only mild irritation and transient limbal follicle formation as side effects of the trifluridine.[12] Other investigators have not had similar experience with trifluridine. The natural history of this disease is to spontaneously wax and wane. Therefore, these unmasked observations should be critically evaluated, especially in light of the previous known problems with IDU.

Some investigators, including Darrell,[4] believe that certain patients may spontaneously develop subepithelial opacities without IDU or other medication. In the investigation of Tabbara and associates,[17] 20 (44%) of the 45 patients had subepithelial ghost opacities. Eighteen of these twenty patients had received topical idoxuridine. The remaining two were believed to have mild, transient subepithelial edema.[17] Epithelial debridement and/or chemical cauterization (previously done with iodine) of the active lesions does not help and may also produce scarring and even ulceration.

PROGNOSIS

Generally, the visual outcome in such patients with TSPK is good, although a prolonged course is a harbinger for possible complications. Visual prognosis is excellent, although inappropriate treatment with IDU can lead to subepithelial scarring. Injudicious treatment with corticosteroids can probably prolong the disease and lead to larger cumulative doses of corticosteroid therapy, thus exposing the patient to the potential treatment side effects such as cataracts or glaucoma.

One patient described by Abbott and Forster[1] had a prolonged course of TSPK (16 years) and later developed Salzmann nodular degeneration. Curiously, this patient suffered subepithelial opacities without concomitant antiviral therapy. This case raises an interesting question because Salzmann nodular degeneration is otherwise so rare in TSPK (although Salzmann nodular degeneration is known to occur in other chronic corneal diseases). Possibly, another ocular inflammatory disease contributed to the Salzmann nodular degeneration and the subepithelial opacities. Some authors believe the subepithelial opacity can be seen in patients who have not had antiviral agents,[1,4,7] although Thygeson[20a] does not.

DIFFERENTIAL DIAGNOSIS

In general, the differential diagnosis should not be difficult because the disease is so distinctive. Thygeson, however, mentioned several possible diagnoses that might prove confusing including the epithelial keratitis of staphylococcal blepharitis; pneumococcal conjunctivitis; seborrheic blepharitis; keratoconjunctivitis sicca; neurotrophic and exposure keratopathy; vernal, molluscum, verruca, occupational, and traumatic keratopathy. TSPK can be differentiated from adenoviral keratoconjunctivitis (or epidemic keratoconjunctivitis) by (1) the lack of conjunctivitis, (2) the absence of preauricular lymphadenopathy or lid swelling, and (3) the chalklike intraepithelial opacification with irregular borders as opposed to the subepithelial, larger infiltrative lesions seen in later stages of epidemic keratoconjunctivitis. Other observers have considered varicella-zoster virus, herpes simplex, recurrent erosion syndrome, rosacea, Reiter syndrome, leprosy, measles keratitis, and medicamentosa within the differential diagnosis.

PATHOGENESIS

The pathogenesis of TSPK is not understood. Conjunctival scrapings show scant mononuclear cells, and corneal scrapings reveal atypical epithelial cells with vacuolated cytoplasm, occasional neutrophils, mononuclear cells, degenerating epithelial cells, and mucus.

Bacterial cultures have shown normal conjunctival flora. Ten of the forty-five patients with TSPK in the report by Tabbara and associates[17] had their corneal epithelium removed for culture or electron microscopy. These authors noted that the epithelium did not come off readily, suggesting that the basement membrane and its hemidesmosomal attachments were intact.

Viral Studies

All viral cultures have been negative, with the exceptions of the work by Braley[2] and later Lemp,[10] who reported viral isolation from the corneal epithelium of two affected individuals. Many questions have been raised about the significance or validity of these viral isolation data. Curiously, the lesions of TSPK do resemble the viral lesions of rubeola, rubella, mumps, and adenovirus. Both TSPK and chronic adenovirus keratitis can develop grouped epithelial lesions, although in TSPK these lesions have a specific morphology of oval-shaped, grouped punctate keratitis. Subepithelial lesions are more prominent in adenovirus keratitis but can be found in TSPK. The subepithelial infiltrates in adenovirus keratitis are comprised of histiocytes and lymphocytes.[11,21]

Human papilloma virus (HPV) has been mentioned as a possible source because it is a virus capable of infecting the ocular surface while causing minimal inflammation. Corneal scrapings from two patients with TSPK were examined using polymerase chain reaction to evaluate HPV as the infective agent, but both patients were negative.*

In 1971 Wakui and associates[23] described the clinical and electron microscopy (EM) of TSPK. EM did not reveal virus particles but did show cell destruction confined to one discrete area. This finding was in contrast to the cell-to-cell spread of destruction observed in herpes simplex virus keratitis. Other investigators in more recent studies have not detected viruses by either tissue culture techniques or with EM.[14,17] Nevertheless, TSPK has several features in common with known viral infections of the cornea. For example, the intraepithelial lesions, the long duration, the exacerbations and remissions, and the mononuclear cell response suggest a persistent or reactivating latent virus or defective virion as the causative agent. Such diseases as adenovirus and measles can have similar presentations under certain circumstances. Measles and adenovirus both have been known to show similar characteristics to TSPK. Ostler[13] submitted that a slow virus may be responsible for TSPK, although there are no data to support this hypothesis.

Immunologic Studies

Quere[14,15] in 1968 and 1973 suggested an allergic cause for TSPK because some of his patients had eczema, urticaria, or asthma and because the lesions responded to corticosteroids. The lack of eosinophils in smears and the lack of other signs or symptoms of ocular allergy make this possibility less likely, however. Jones,[9] in 1963, proposed TSPK to be a dyskeratosis, although histologic and ultrastructural studies do not support this hypothesis. Physical examination and clinical history have failed to reveal any consistent associated systemic disease. van Bijstervelt[22] evaluated plasma cortisol levels in patients with TSPK and found them to be within normal limits for both sexes but significantly higher in females. This finding must be viewed with circumspection because the values were normal. In these same patients, the serum protein and protein fraction concentration were normal.

HLA-DW3 and HLA-DR3 antigens were found by Darrell[4] to be associated with an increased relative risk of developing TSPK. Other diseases associated with these antigens include gluten-sensitive enteropathy, dermatitis herpetiformes, chronic hepatitis, Addison disease, primary Sjögren syndrome, Graves syndrome, insulin-dependent diabetes mellitus, and systemic lupus erythematosus. Conceivably, TSPK may be caused by a common virus whose replication in the corneal epithelium and stroma or local immune response is influenced by the presence of HLA-DR3. Certain features of TSPK imply the contribution of an immune-mediated process. The monocytes in corneal epithelium as observed by electron microscopy, the marked effect of corticosteroids on the corneal lesions, and the chronic course of TSPK with remissions and exacerbations all suggest an immunologic component.

REFERENCES

1. Abbott RL, Forster RK: Superficial punctate keratitis of Thygeson associated with scarring and Salzmann's nodular degeneration, Am J Ophthalmol 87:296-298, 1977.
2. Braley AE: Virus diseases of the cornea, Med Rec Ann 44:102, 1950.
3. Braley AE, Alexander RC: Superficial punctate keratitis: isolation of a virus, Arch Ophthalmol 50:147-154, 1953.
4. Darrell RW: Thygeson's superficial punctate keratitis: natural history and association with HLA-DR3, Trans Am Ophthalmol Soc 74:486-516, 1981.
5. Forstot SL, Binder PS: Treatment of Thygeson's superficial punctate keratopathy with soft contact lenses, Am J Ophthalmol 88:186-189, 1979.
6. Fuchs E: Keratitis punctate superficialis, Klin Wochenschr 2:837-839, 1889.
7. Goldberg DB, Schanzlin DJ, Brown SI: Management of Thygeson's superficial punctate keratitis, Am J Ophthalmol 89:22-24, 1980.
8. Jones BR: The differential diagnosis of punctate keratitis, Trans Ophthalmol Soc UK 80:665-675, 1960.
9. Jones BR: Thygeson's superficial punctate keratitis, Trans Ophthalmol Soc UK 83:245-253, 1963.
10. Lemp MA, Chambers RW Jr, Lundy J: Viral isolate in superficial punctate keratitis, Arch Ophthalmol 91:8-10, 1974.
11. Lund E, Stefani FH: Corneal histology after epidemic keratoconjunctivitis, Arch Ophthalmol 96:2085-2088, 1978.
12. Nesburn AB, Lowe GH, Lepoff NJ, Maguen E: Effect of topical trifluridine on Thygeson's superficial punctate keratitis, Ophthalmology 91:1188-1192, 1984.
13. Ostler HB: Suspected infectious etiology. In Smolin G, Thoft RA, editors: The cornea: scientific foundations and clinical practice, ed 3, Boston, 1994, Little, Brown.

*Unpublished data.

14. Quere MA, Diallo J, Rogez JP: La kératite de Thygeson (A propos de 116 cas de kératite ponctuée superficielle), *Bull Soc Ophtalmol Fr* 68:276-280, 1968.

15. Quere MA, Delplace MP, Rossazza C et al.: Frequence et etiopathogenie de la kératite de Thygeson, *Bull Soc Ophtalmol Fr* 73:629-631, 1973.

16. Sundmacher R, Press M, Neumann-Haefelin D et al.: Keratitis superficialis punctata Thygeson, *Klin Monatsbl Augenheilkd* 170:908-916, 1977.

17. Tabbara KF, Ostler HB, Dawson C et al.: Thygeson's superficial punctate keratitis, *Ophthalmology* 88:75-77, 1981.

18. Thygeson P: Superficial punctate keratitis, *JAMA* 144:1544-1549, 1950.

19. Thygeson P: Further observations on superficial punctate keratitis, *Arch Ophthalmol* 66:34-38, 1961.

20. Thygeson P: Clinical and laboratory observations on superficial punctate keratitis, *Am J Ophthalmol* 61:1344-1349, 1966.

20a. Thygeson P: Personal communication, 1992.

21. Tullo AB, Ridgway AEA, Lucas DR, Richmond S: Histopathology of adenovirus type 8 keratitis, *Cornea* 6:234, 1987.

22. van Bijsterveld OP, Mansour KH, Dubois FJ: Thygeson's superficial punctate keratitis, *Ann Ophthalmol* 17:150-153, 1985.

23. Wakui K, Komoriya S, Hayashi E et al.: Corneal and epithelial dystrophies, *Rinsho Ganka* 25:1103-1123, 1971.

32 Ocular Cicatricial Pemphigoid

BARTLY J. MONDINO

Cicatricial pemphigoid (CP) is a chronic disease characterized by recurrent blisters or bullae. Skin and mucous membranes have the predilection for scar formation in this disease.[31] Other names for this disease are essential shrinkage of the conjunctiva, ocular pemphigus, and benign mucous membrane pemphigoid. Pemphigoid is presumed to be an autoimmune disease. Ocular involvement includes progressive conjunctival shrinkage, symblepharon, entropion with trichiasis and distichiasis, dry eye, and finally, reduced vision from corneal opacification.[32]

EPIDEMIOLOGY

Pemphigoid has no geographic or racial predilection. In a series of 108 patients,[31] the mean age at initial examination was 70 years, with a range of 43 to 88 years. Patients may develop this disease at a younger age, however. This disease of the elderly affects more women than men, with a ratio of approximately 2 : 1.[12,31,32]

PATHOGENESIS

CP is characterized by the binding of immunoglobulins (most commonly IgG) and components of both the classical and alternative complement pathways to the basement membrane zone of skin and oral mucosa.[20] Circulating antibodies to the basement membrane zone can be demonstrated occasionally.[20] CP and bullous pemphigoid antigens are distinct but have a common localization within the lamina lucida of the dermal-epidermal junction.[8] The bullous pemphigoid antigen is present on the blister roof in close association with basal cells, whereas CP antigen is present on the blister floor.

Conjunctival biopsies (Fig. 32-1) demonstrate immunoglobulins and complement that are bound to the basement membrane in most, but not all, patients with CP.* Immunoglobulin deposition on the conjunctival basement membrane

---

*References 14, 16, 17, 28, 35, 39, 45.

can be found in other diseases.[2,16,28,35] In one study, immunoreactant deposition at the basement membrane zone of the conjunctiva was found in patients with Mooren ulcer and staphylococcal keratitis.[35] A more linear deposition of immunoglobulins was found in CP, and a more granular deposition was described in the other conditions. A CP case has been reported, however, with granular IgA and C3 complement deposition along the basement membrane zone, suggesting that immune-complex deposition may provide an alternative pathogenetic mechanism to basement membrane zone autoantibody formation.[45] Another study also proposed that direct immunofluorescence is useful—but not absolutely diagnostic—for CP. This proposal was based on the fact that linear deposition of immunoglobulins was found along the conjunctival basement membrane of two of seven patients with cicatrizing conjunctivitis associated with other diseases.[28] Additionally, both bullous pemphigoid[16] and linear IgA disease[2] can cause conjunctival shrinkage associated with linear immunoreactant deposition at the conjunctival basement membrane zone.

The percentage of patients that demonstrate circulating antibodies to conjunctival basement membrane varies from 0% to 50%.[12,14,15,39] In one study the ability to detect these antibodies correlated with the degree of clinical activity.[15]

In CP, autoimmune phenomena may be directed against the conjunctival epithelium and its basement membrane. Some patients show immunoglobulins bound to the conjunctival epithelium.[16,35,39] In addition, circulating antibodies that bind to the conjunctival and corneal epithelium have been demonstrated.[35,39]

The conjunctiva of patients with CP show increased numbers of dendritic cells (which process antigen locally) and T lymphocytes located within the epithelium and substantia propria.[51] There was a greater increase in T helper than T suppressor cells in the epithelium—with the reverse found in the substantia propria. Activated interleukin 2 receptor-positive lymphocytes were found in both the epithe-

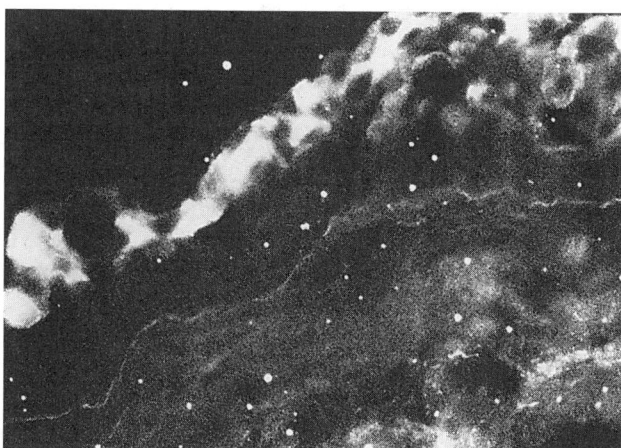

Fig. 32-1. Immunofluorescent staining of conjunctival epithelium and basement membrane zone for IgA in a patient with cicatricial pemphigoid.

lium and substantia propria. Macrophages were the next most common cells found in the substantia propria, followed by B cells and plasma cells. Another study reported similar findings, except that a reversal of the T helper-suppressor ratio was not found in the substantia propria, presumably because the patients displayed clinical activity.[48]

Approximately one half of patients with CP have elevated serum IgA levels.[35,39] Patients with CP have reduced numbers of circulating T lymphocytes as determined by E rosette formation.[38] In one study an association of CP with HLA-B12 was shown, suggesting that there is an immunogenetic susceptibility to the development of this disease.[36] In another study CP was associated with HLA-DR4.[56]

The immunopathologic mechanisms underlying CP are not known. The binding of antibody and complement to the basement membrane zone of the conjunctiva could be important in the development of conjunctival disease. Activation of the complement cascade by antibody-antigen complexes generates anaphylatoxins (C3a, C4a, and C5a) that cause vasodilation, increased vascular permeability, histamine release from mast cells, and lysosomal protease release from neutrophils and macrophages. C5a also is a potent chemotactic factor for neutrophils and macrophages. Eosinophil chemotactic factor released by mast cells attracts eosinophils to the site of the lesion. Cell-mediated immunity may also be important in the development of conjunctival disease.[48,51] The increased T lymphocytes in the conjunctival infiltrates may be responsible for an immunoregulatory defect that allows local B lymphocytes to produce autoantibodies to the basement membrane zone. They may also elaborate cytokines that promote fibroplasia. The increased dendritic cells in the conjunctiva may provide the basis for local antigen processing for B and T cell reactivity.

In contrast to CP, pemphigus is characterized by (1) the binding of immunoglobulins and complement to the inter-

cellular space of the epithelium, and (2) circulating antibodies to this location that correlate with disease severity. On the other hand, bullous pemphigoid is associated with immunoglobulins (mainly IgG) and complement that are bound to the basement membrane zone as well as circulating antibodies to this region that do not correlate consistently with disease activity.

Drug-Induced Ocular Cicatricial Pemphigoid

Topical drugs associated with conjunctival scarring include idoxuridine,[27] echothiophate iodide,[43] pilocarpine,[22] demecarium,[22] epinephrine,[26] and timolol.[9] Drug-induced conjunctival shrinkage may represent a spectrum of disease ranging from a self-limited toxic form to a progressive, immunologic form that is indistinguishable from CP.[9] Patients with drug-induced conjunctival shrinkage may show immunoglobulins bound to the conjunctival basement membrane.[27,28,43] In a histopathologic study of drug-induced CP affecting the conjunctiva, light and electron microscopy of the conjunctiva revealed findings identical to those reported for idiopathic CP.[44] The patients in four of these studies did not have extraocular involvement of mucous membranes or skin.[9,22,27,43]

There are several possible explanations for the relationship between drugs and conjunctival scarring: (1) the drug may cause conjunctival scarring that only mimics CP, because the scarring is not progressive; (2) drug use and CP may be coincidental; (3) the drug may promote or accelerate the development of CP, which can take place later anyway; (4) the drug may be a cause of CP; or (5) CP causes scarring that may obstruct collecting vessels of the outflow system and result in glaucoma that requires topical therapy. As mentioned previously, glaucoma has been associated with CP.[54]

A practical approach to the problem of drug-induced conjunctival scarring involves discontinuing the topical agents (if this can be done) and following the patient for progressive conjunctival shrinkage.[30] If the latter develops, or if the patient has skin or extraocular mucous membrane lesions, then the patient probably has CP and will require immunosuppressive therapy. If the drugs are absolutely essential to control glaucoma, then they should be continued. If progressive conjunctival shrinkage occurs, then immunosuppressive therapy may be warranted. The determination of whether these drugs simply generate scarring that mimics CP, or whether they actually cause or promote CP in a particular patient can be made only by long-term follow-up. This follow-up should take place after drug discontinuation for the development of chronic, progressive, conjunctival shrinkage (which is the hallmark of CP) or the development of extraocular lesions. Histopathologic and immunopathologic examination of conjunctival biopsies cannot distinguish between CP and drug-induced conjunctival shrinkage.

CLINICAL FEATURES

Cutaneous Involvement

The skin is involved less frequently than the mucous membranes. Skin involvement has been reported in 9% to 24% of cases.[12,29,31,32] There are two types of skin lesions in CP: (1) a recurrent, vesiculobullous, nonscarring eruption (that may involve the inguinal area and extremities) that occasionally becomes generalized (Fig. 32-2); and (2) localized, erythematous plaques (with overlying vesicles and bullae) that appear on the scalp and face (near the affected mucous membranes) and heal leaving smooth, atrophic scars.[40]

Mucous Membrane Involvement

In addition to the conjunctiva, CP may involve the following mucous membranes: nose, mouth, pharynx, larynx, esophagus, anus, vagina, and urethra. In a dermatologic study, oral lesions were found in 91% and conjunctival lesions in 66% of patients with CP.[29] In ophthalmic studies, 15% to 50% of patients showed involvement of the oral mucosa, and 100% had ocular involvement.[12,30,33] CP is associated with two types of oral lesions: (1) a desquamative gingivitis that may be patchy or diffuse, heals slowly, and may persist for years; and (2) vesicles and bullae of the oral mucosa that develop rapidly, remain intact for a few days, and then rupture.[40] Scarring and even strictures may result from mucous membrane lesions and can be fatal. Stenosis of the nasopharynx or larynx may cause obstructive sleep apnea, and esophageal strictures may result in asphyxiation and death when food is swallowed.[21] The presence of mucous membrane or skin lesions may be important in the diagnosis of CP, when a patient with conjunctival scarring is undergoing evaluation.

Ocular Involvement

Although CP may begin in one eye, both eyes are eventually involved. The initial symptoms of CP are nonspecific and include irritation, burning, and tearing.[37] Bacterial blepharoconjunctivitis frequently complicates CP and is highlighted by a mucopurulent discharge. As the disease advances, breakdown of the corneal epithelium leads to foreign body sensation, photophobia, and finally, reduced visual acuity from corneal vascularization and opacification. The hallmark of CP is fibrosis beneath the conjunctival epithelium.[7,19] Fibrosis may take the form of symblephara, which are fibrotic bands that pass between the palpebral and bulbar conjunctiva. They involve the inferior fornix first. The best way to demonstrate them early in the disease is to draw the lower eyelid down and have the patient look up (Fig. 32-3). Extensive conjunctival scarring may limit ocular motility and increase intraocular pressure when the patient looks up or down.

CP eventually results in a dry eye that may have several components. To begin with, fibrosis beneath the conjunctival epithelium may cause occlusion of the ducts of the lacrimal and accessory lacrimal glands, leading to decreased aqueous tear secretion. The reduced numbers of mucus-producing goblet cells that are found[46] may contribute to an unstable tearfilm. Moreover, conjunctival scarring causes lagophthalmos (with abnormal blinking and exposure) and entropion (with trichiasis and distichiasis). All these factors may cause a breakdown of the ocular surface epithelium.

Although conjunctival and corneal bullae have been described,[19] they are rarely observed. The blinking action of the eyelids may cause the bullae to rupture soon after their development. Breakdown of the corneal epithelium most commonly results from entropion with trichiasis (Fig. 32-4),

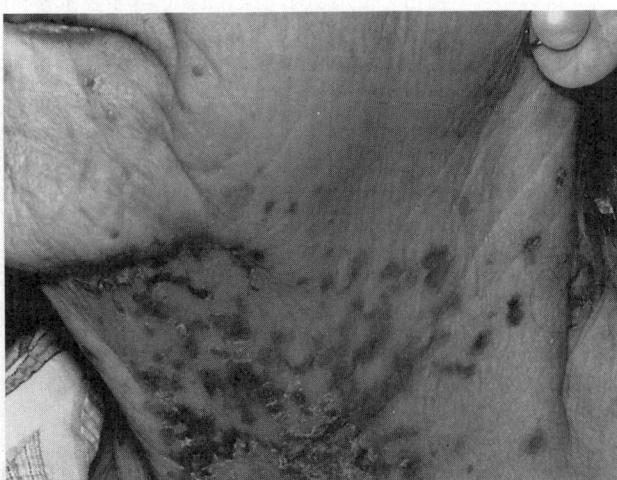

Fig. 32-2. Patient with cicatricial pemphigoid showing vesiculobullous eruption involving the neck and anterior chest. Most of the lesions have ruptured and show crusting and scaling.

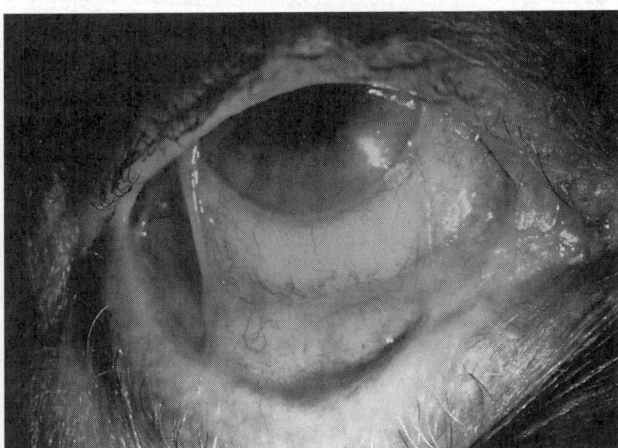

Fig. 32-3. Patient with ocular cicatricial pemphigoid shows prominent temporal symblepharon of the right eye, which is best demonstrated by drawing the lower eyelid down and having the patient look up.

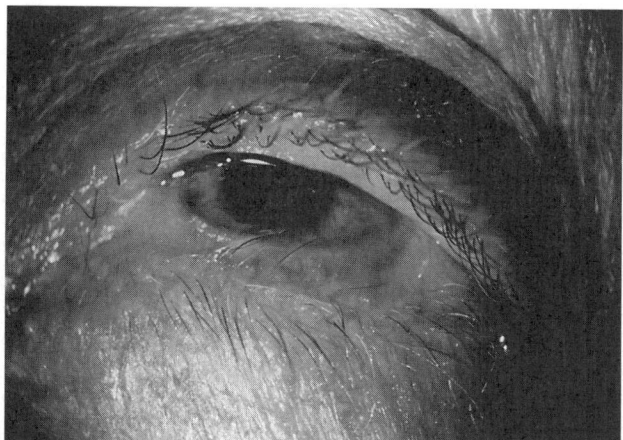

Fig. 32-4. Entropion with trichiasis of lower lid in patient with cicatricial pemphigoid.

lagophthalmos with abnormal blinking and exposure, and a diminished, unstable tearfilm. Secondary bacterial infiltrates and ulcers may be associated with the compromised corneal epithelium. Predisposing factors for the development of microbial keratitis include topical corticosteroids, bandage contact lenses, trichiasis, corneal surgery, lagophthalmos, and meibomitis.[42] Eventually, corneal neovascularization may develop in the form of a pannus or pseudopterygium (Fig. 32-5).

Giemsa stain of conjunctival scrapings from patients with CP shows neutrophils, keratinized squamous cells, and eosinophils.[41] In a study of the bacterial flora of patients with CP, potential pathogens (mainly mannitol-positive staphylococci) were recovered from the eyelids and/or conjunctiva of 81% of patients.[32] Glaucoma may be more prevalent in patients with CP and was reported in 26% of the cases in one series.[54]

Course Of Ocular Disease

CP usually runs a chronic course defined by progressive shrinkage of the conjunctiva. The end stage of this disease is characterized by absent tears, obliterated conjunctival fornices, ankyloblepharon, and a keratinized ocular surface epithelium. Episodes of acute disease activity may punctuate the chronic disease course and result in rapid shrinkage of the conjunctiva.[34] Acute disease activity may be precipitated by surgical procedures that include conjunctival biopsy, lysis of symblepharon, oculoplastic procedures on the eyelids, and cataract extraction. The acute manifestations of CP consist of localized, ulcerated, conjunctival mounds (Fig. 32-6) or diffuse, severe, conjunctival hyperemia and edema. Before concluding that acute inflammatory activity is caused by the disease process itself, it is necessary to eliminate confounding factors such as trichiasis, exposure, or bacterial blepharoconjunctivitis.

When evaluating a patient with CP, it is extremely important to determine the extent of conjunctival shrinkage that already has taken place. The most useful positions for examination and photography are the upward gaze with the lower eyelid retracted and the downward gaze with the upper eyelid retracted. The staging system of Mondino and Brown[32,33] is based on the percentage of conjunctival shrinkage. As the disease advances in stage, a patient with CP is more likely to have a dry eye, corneal vessels, trichiasis, and positive cultures of the lids and/or conjunctiva for potential pathogens.[31,32,33] On the other hand, the staging system of Foster[12] rests more heavily on the presence or absence of symblephara.

In addition to staging the extent of conjunctival shrinkage that has taken place, it is important to assess the degree of conjunctival inflammatory activity (hyperemia and edema) that is present. Both stage and inflammatory activity are important parameters to assess, but they are not necessarily

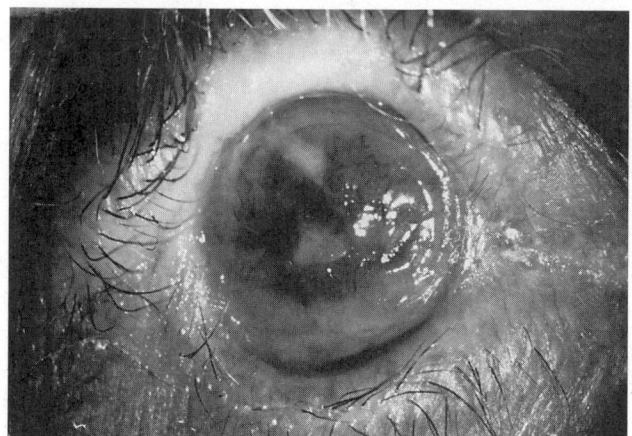

Fig. 32-5. Patient with severe shrinkage of the conjunctival fornices shows extensive vascularization and opacification of the cornea in the wake of repeated corneal epithelial breakdown and infiltrates.

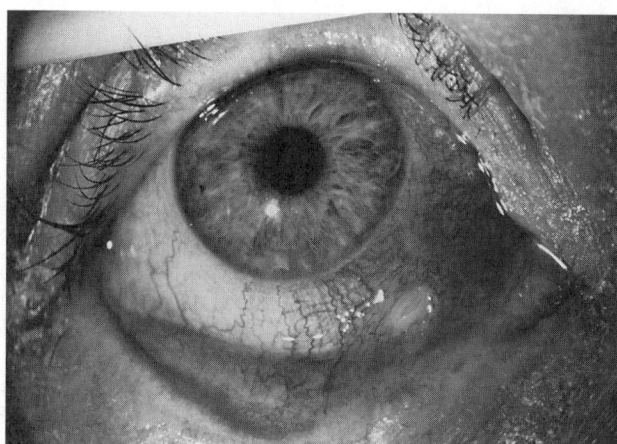

Fig. 32-6. Ulceration of inferonasal conjunctiva of right eye following conjunctival biopsy in patient with cicatricial pemphigoid.

correlated. For example, an eye at stage 4 may show no conjunctival inflammatory activity, whereas an eye at stage 1 may show severe conjunctival inflammatory activity.

Disease progression should be determined by clinical examination and comparison with previous photographs of the external eye.[32,33] Progression is defined as increased conjunctival shrinkage that may involve loss of fornix, new symblepharon formation, or enlargement of existing symblephara. Other important parameters to assess are tear volumes, keratinization of the conjunctiva, breakdown of the corneal epithelium, and corneal neovascularization.

A previous study of the natural course of CP suggested that it may be asymmetric in severity (both eyes may not be at the same stage) and progression (both eyes may not progress at the same rate).[33] Although most eyes advanced, the untreated disease had a variable course, because there were eyes in all stages that did not necessarily progress. Progression was more likely to occur over a given period of time in the later stages, that is, an eye at stage 3 was more likely to proceed than an eye at stage 1.

LABORATORY INVESTIGATIONS

CP is characterized by blisters or bullae in a subepithelial location. The separation at the margin of a blister is located within the lamina lucida between the plasma membrane of the basal cells and the electron-dense lamina densa.[29] Bullous pemphigoid also is associated with subepithelial blisters, but pemphigus is defined by blisters within the epithelium.

The conjunctival epithelium in CP (Fig. 32-7) shows squamous metaplasia with parakeratosis and keratinization.[1] Mucus-producing goblet cells are scarce or absent.[25,46] Because the mitotic rate of conjunctival epithelium from patients with CP was higher than that in controls, this disease was presumed to be associated with hyperproliferation of the

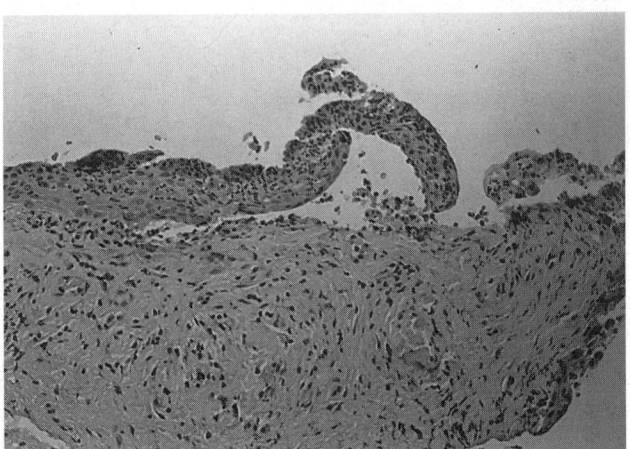

Fig. 32-8. Patient with acute inflammatory activity shows numerous neutrophils within and beneath the conjunctival epithelium and a subepithelial blister (hematoxylin and eosin, original magnification × 200).

conjunctival epithelium with a failure of conjunctival differentiation caused by the reduced goblet cell density.[55]

In the early stages of conjunctival disease, granulation tissue is found beneath the conjunctival epithelium with an infiltration of lymphocytes, plasma cells, occasional eosinophils, and relatively few neutrophils.[1,41] Later, pronounced fibrosis takes place in the conjunctival stroma and is responsible for the conjunctival shrinkage that characterizes this disease.[7,19] Hyperproliferation of conjunctival fibroblasts from patients with CP has been demonstrated in tissue culture.[49] One study described perivascular inflammatory cell infiltration in 20% of specimens and substantial mast cell participation and degranulation.[12] In addition to the chronic inflammatory cells found in this disease, patients with acute manifestations of CP (Fig. 32-8) show numerous neutrophils within and beneath the conjunctival epithelium.[34]

An electron microscopic study of conjunctival epithelium from patients with CP showed increased desmosomes and prominent tonofilaments and tonofibrils throughout the epithelial cytoplasm.[5,18] The basal lamina showed areas of discontinuity, duplication, and focal thickening. Collagen fibrils were highly disorganized, and the vascular space was reduced. Scanning electron microscopy demonstrated a homogeneous granular sheet of amorphous, mucinlike material covering extensive areas of the conjunctival surface in patients with CP, but not in controls.[13]

DIFFERENTIAL DIAGNOSIS

The clinical diagnosis of CP depends on the documentation of progressive conjunctival shrinkage. The presence of skin and extraocular mucosal lesions supports the diagnosis. Conjunctival biopsies that demonstrate immunoreactant binding to the conjunctival basement membrane zone are important to confirm the diagnosis, especially if immunosuppressive therapy is under consideration. False-positive

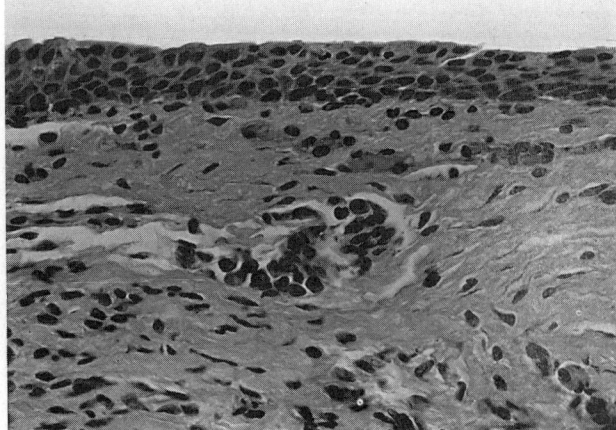

Fig. 32-7. Conjunctival biopsy from patient with cicatricial pemphigoid showing squamous metaplasia with absent goblet cells. An infiltration of mononuclear cells is seen beneath the conjunctival epithelium (hematoxylin and eosin, original magnification × 400).

and false-negative findings are possible, however, as discussed previously. Other causes of conjunctival shrinkage and symblepharon must be excluded.

Conjunctival scarring may result from radiation and severe chemical burns, especially alkali. Symblephara have also been reported with Sjögren syndrome,[23] atopic keratoconjunctivitis, and sarcoidosis[10]—but not to the extent, and not with the relentless progression, of CP. Conjunctival scarring may develop in association with scleral buckles and conjunctival carcinoma, but these conditions are usually unilateral—unlike CP. Progressive systemic sclerosis (scleroderma) may be associated with a dry eye and progressive conjunctival shrinkage.[11] Trachoma causes conjunctival scarring, but this usually begins and predominates in the superior fornix and palpebral conjunctiva.

A membranous conjunctivitis that results in conjunctival scarring may be caused by adenovirus types 8 and 19, a primary infection of herpes simplex, diphtheria, or beta-hemolytic Streptococcus spp.[6,17] The acute, self-limited nature of these infections contrasts with the chronic, progressive, conjunctival shrinkage found in CP.

Conjunctival shrinkage may be associated with systemic practolol,[24] topical epinephrine, echothiophate iodide, idoxuridine, pilocarpine, timolol, and dipivefrin.[9,22,26,27,43] Whether this drug-induced conjunctival shrinkage is self-limited or is actual CP is discussed previously.

Other bullous diseases usually do not cause much diagnostic confusion with CP. Bullous pemphigoid and pemphigus do not usually cause conjunctival scarring.[3,16] Erythema multiforme major may cause conjunctival shrinkage as a result of the acute episode, but the shrinkage is not chronically progressive as it is with CP. Patients with erythema multiforme major and their families have little difficulty recalling the acute event.

THERAPY

Lubrication is extremely important in the treatment of the dry eye associated with CP. Artificial tears without preservatives are useful if the preservatives in commercial tear preparations irritate the eyes, if allergies develop to them, or if the patient requires artificial tear installation more than 4 or 5 times each day. Punctal occlusion can be performed, but it is rarely necessary because the puncta are usually occluded by scarring.

CP may be complicated by secondary bacterial blepharoconjunctivitis. As mentioned previously, potential pathogens, especially mannitol-positive staphylococci, were recovered from the eyelids or conjunctiva of 81% of patients with this disease.[32] Therefore, cultures of the eyelids and conjunctiva should be performed at initial examination and at regular intervals. Topical antibiotic drops or ointments should be administered, depending on the results of specific antibiotic sensitivity testing. The staphylococcal blepharitis that frequently accompanies this condition may be treated at bedtime with eyelid scrubs followed by an antibiotic oint-

ment such as erythromycin or bacitracin. Oral tetracycline or doxycycline may be useful in the treatment of the meibomian dysfunction that is often found.

In the presence of sufficiently deep fornices, therapeutic soft contact lenses may be used in selected patients to protect the corneal epithelium from trichiasis and drying. Some patients with CP develop recurrent, painful, corneal, epithelial defects that require almost continuous use of a pressure patch or tarsorrhaphy. In these cases, therapeutic soft contact lenses may keep the corneal epithelium intact and the patients comfortable. Artificial tears must be used frequently to prevent dessication of the lenses. Because patients who have dry eyes and wear contact lenses are at increased risk of infection, they must be followed carefully.

Cryotherapy or electrocautery may be used to eliminate distichiasis or trichiasis. Entropion with a keratinized lid margin or trichiasis may be corrected early in the disease course by oculoplastic surgical techniques (such as mucous membrane grafts). In the advanced stages of the disease, the benefits of oculoplastic procedures (including mucous membrane grafts) may be negated by the disease itself—if the patient is not in remission. In fact, surgery on the conjunctiva (including biopsy) may entail a risk of setting off acute inflammatory activity that may lead to rapid and alarming shrinkage of the conjunctiva.[34]

If patients with CP show conjunctival inflammation or evidence of progressive conjunctival shrinkage, cataract surgery or oculoplastic surgery on the lids and conjunctiva should be deferred until the disease is controlled by systemic immunosuppressive therapy. Once disease activity is controlled and progression halted, mucous membrane grafts may be used to reconstruct or expand the fornices. Favorable results were reported for patients on systemic immunosuppression at the time of cataract surgery.[52] Bacterial endophthalmitis is a concern, however, in patients on immunosuppressive therapy who undergo intraocular surgery. On the other hand, patients who are stable and do not showconjunctival inflammation may not require systemic immunosuppression prior to surgery, but may require postoperative systemic corticosteroids if acute inflammatory activity develops. Systemic corticosteroids are useful in the treatment of the acute manifestations of CP.[34] If a conventional lid speculum and a retrobulbar injection are used at the time of cataract surgery, increased posterior pressure may result in the presence of severe conjunctival scarring. To overcome this problem, general anesthesia as well as lid sutures could be used. Another approach is to make a horizontal incision (running from the medial to the lateral canthus) in the superior and inferior fornix; this facilitates the placement of a conventional lid speculum.

Immunosuppressive Therapy

Topical therapy is ineffective in halting disease progression. Foster and associates[14] and Mondino and Brown[33] found that long-term systemic immunosuppressive therapy suppressed conjunctival inflammatory activity and inhibited progression of conjunctival shrinkage. An eye at stage 1 or stage 2 was less likely to progress, and more likely to respond, to immunosuppressive therapy than an eye at stage 3.[31,33] Not all patients responded to immunosuppressive therapy, however, and some developed complications that required tapering or even discontinuation (Figs. 32-9 and 32-10). Therefore, elderly patients with limited lifespans should not be subjected to the risk of immunosuppressive therapy unless their eyes are at stage 2 (moderate conjunctival shrinkage) and demonstrate ongoing progression of conjunctival shrinkage. Patients taking immunosuppressive agents should be monitored by an internist, oncologist, or rheumatologist who is familiar with the toxicity and side-effects of these potent drugs.

Dapsone has been used to treat CP,[50] but it should be

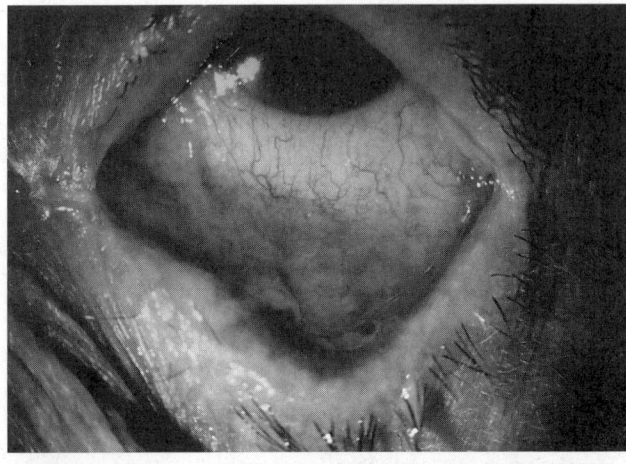

A

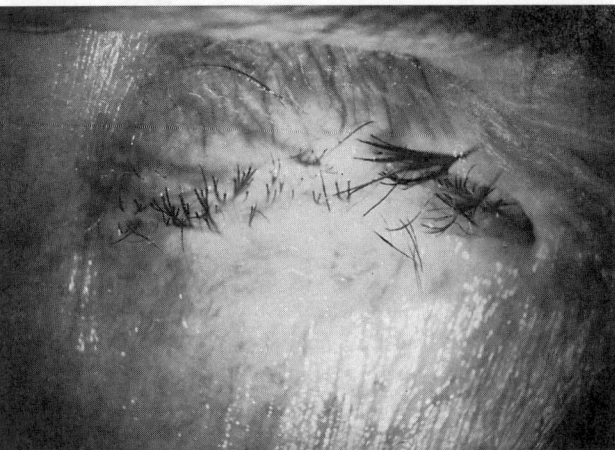

B

Fig. 32-10. Patient who underwent treatment with cyclophosphamide and prednisone. **A,** External eye prior to immunosuppressive therapy. **B,** Patient progressed to end stage of cicatricial pemphigoid despite immunosuppressive therapy.

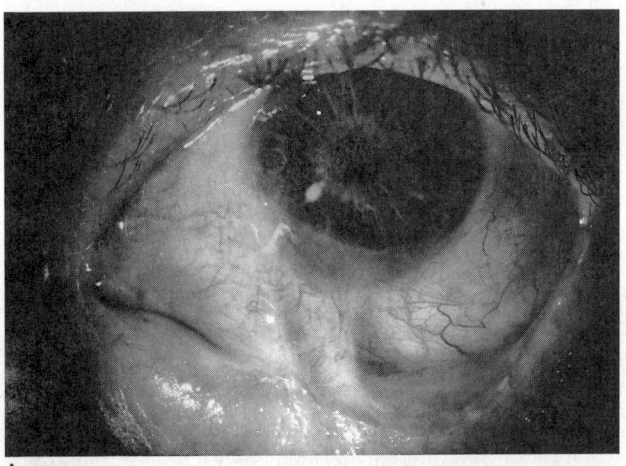

A

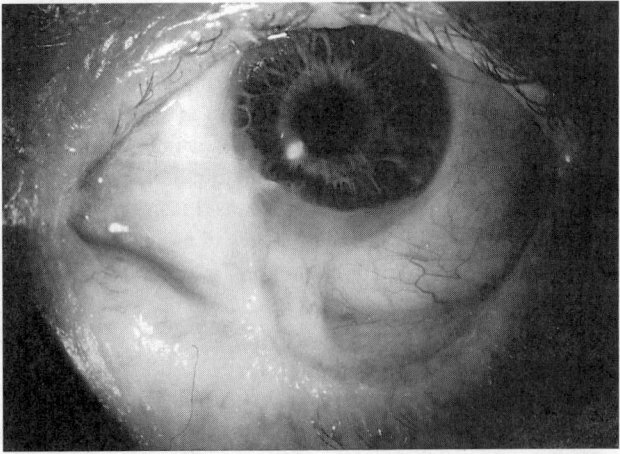

B

Fig. 32-9. Patient with cicatricial pemphigoid underwent immunosuppressive therapy with cyclophosphamide for 2 years and did not show progression of conjunctival shrinkage. **A,** External eye prior to onset of immunosuppressive therapy. **B,** External eye 2 years later with reduced hyperemia and no change in conjunctival shrinkage.

avoided in patients who have a history of sulfa allergy or glucose-6-phosphate dehydrogenase deficiency. Hemolysis may be associated with high-dose dapsone therapy. Tauber and associates[53] believe that dapsone may be the best initial therapy for patients with CP (which shows mild to modest inflammatory activity and is not rapidly progressive), whereas cyclophosphamide may be the best initial choice for highly active cases.

Keratoprosthesis

In the final stages of CP, a keratoprosthesis may be inserted to restore some sight to the patients with obliterated conjunctival fornices and a keratinized ocular surface epithelium.[47] Complications associated with the use of a keratoprosthesis include retroprosthetic membrane, extrusion, endophthalmitis, choroidal hemorrhage, and retinal detachment. Unfortunately, the long-term prognosis for these devices is dismal in this setting.

REFERENCES

1. Andersen SR, Jensen OA, Kristensen EB: Benign mucous membrane pemphigoid. III. Biopsy, *Acta Ophthalmol* 52:455-463, 1974.
2. Aultbrinker EA, Starr MB, Donnenfeld ED: Linear IgA disease—The ocular manifestations, *Ophthalmology* 95:340-343, 1988.
3. Bean SF, Holubar K, Gillett RB: Pemphigus involving the eyes, *Arch Dermatol* 111:1484-1486, 1975.
4. Bean SF, Furey N, West CE et al.: Ocular cicatricial pemphigoid (immunologic studies), *Trans Am Acad Ophthalmol Otolaryngol* 81:806-812, 1976.
5. Carroll JM, Kuwabara T: Ocular pemphigus, *Arch Ophthalmol* 80:683-695, 1968.
6. Darougar S, Quinlan MP, Gibson JA: Epidemic keratoconjunctivitis and chronic papillary conjunctivitis in London due to adenovirus type 19, *Br J Ophthalmol* 61:76-85, 1977.
7. Duke-Elder S, editor: *System of ophthalmology*, vol 8, part 1. Diseases of the outer eye, *Conjunctiva*, St Louis, 1965, CV Mosby.
8. Fine JD: Epidermolysis bullosa: variability of expression of cicatricial pemphigoid, bullous pemphigoid, and epidermolysis bullosa acquisita antigens in clinically uninvolved skin, *J Invest Dermatol* 85:47-49, 1985.
9. Fiore PM, Jacobs IH, Goldberg DB: Drug-induced pemphigoid, *Arch Ophthalmol* 105:1660-1663, 1987.
10. Flach A: Symblepharon in sarcoidosis, *Am J Ophthalmol* 85:210-214, 1978.
11. Foster CS: Non-rheumatoid acquired collagen vascular diseases. In Smolin G, Thoft RA, editors: *The cornea, scientific foundations and clinical practice*, ed 3, 385-407, Boston, 1994, Little, Brown.
12. Foster CS: Cicatricial pemphigoid, *Trans Am Ophthalmol Soc* 84:527-663, 1986.
13. Foster CS, Shaw CD, Wells PA: Scanning electron microscopy of conjunctival surfaces in patients with ocular cicatricial pemphigoid, *Am J Ophthalmol* 102:584-591, 1986.
14. Foster CS, Wilson LA, Ekins MB: Immunosuppressive therapy for progressive ocular cicatricial pemphigoid, *Ophthalmology* 89:340-353, 1982.
15. Franklin RM, Fitzmorris CT: Antibodies against conjunctival basement membrane zone, *Arch Ophthalmol* 101:1611-1613, 1983.
16. Frith PA, Venning VA, Wojnarowska F et al.: Conjunctival involvement in cicatricial and bullous pemphigoid: a clinical and immunopathological study, *Br J Ophthalmol* 73:52-56, 1989.
17. Furey N, West C, Andrews T et al.: Immunofluorescent studies of ocular cicatricial pemphigoid, *Am J Ophthalmol* 80:825-831, 1975.
18. Galbavy EJ, Foster CS: Ultrastructural characteristics of conjunctiva in cicatricial pemphigoid, *Cornea* 4:127-136, 1985.
19. Gazala JR: Ocular pemphigus, *Am J Ophthalmol* 48:355-362, 1959.
20. Griffith MR, Fukuyama K, Tuffanelli D, Silverman S: Immunofluorescent studies in mucous membrane pemphigoid, *Arch Dermatol* 109:195-199, 1974.
21. Hanson RD, Olsen KD, Rogers RS: Upper aerodigestive tract manifestations of cicatricial pemphigoid, *Ann Otol Rhinol Laryngol* 97:493-499, 1988.
22. Hirst LW, Werblin T, Novak M: Drug-induced cicatrizing conjunctivitis simulating ocular pemphigoid, *Cornea* 1:121-128, 1982.
23. Jones BR: The ocular diagnosis of benign mucous membrane pemphigoid, *Proc R Soc Med* 54:109-110, 1961.
24. Jones DB: Prospects in the management of tear-deficiency states, *Trans Am Acad Ophthalmol Otolaryngol* 83:693-700, 1977.
25. Kinoshita S, Kiorpes TC, Friend J, Thoft RA: Goblet cell density in ocular surface disease, *Arch Ophthalmol* 101:1284-1287, 1983.
26. Kristensen EB, Norn MS: Benign mucous membrane pemphigoid. I. Secretion of mucus and tears, *Acta Ophthalmol* 52:266-281, 1974.
27. Lass JH, Thoft RA, Dohlman CH: Idoxuridine-induced conjunctival cicatrization, *Arch Ophthalmol* 101:747-750, 1983.
28. Leonard JN, Hobday CM, Haffenden GP et al.: Immunofluorescent studies in ocular cicatricial pemphigoid, *Br J Dermatol* 118:209-217, 1988.
29. Lever WF: Pemphigus and pemphigoid, *J Am Acad Dermatol* 1:2-31, 1979.
30. Mondino BJ: Discussion of drug-induced cicatricial pemphigoid affecting the conjunctiva, *Ophthalmology* 93:782-783, 1986.
31. Mondino BJ: Bullous diseases of the skin and mucous membranes. In Duane T, editor: *Clinical ophthalmology*, vol 4, 1-19, Hagerstown, 1991, Harper & Row.
32. Mondino BJ, Brown SI: Ocular cicatricial pemphigoid, *Ophthalmology* 88:95-100, 1981.
33. Mondino BJ, Brown SI: Immunosuppressive therapy in ocular cicatricial pemphigoid, *Am J Ophthalmol* 96:453-459, 1983.
34. Mondino BJ, Brown SI, Lempert S, Jenkins MS: The acute manifestations of ocular cicatricial pemphigoid: diagnosis and treatment, *Ophthalmology* 86:543-555, 1979.
35. Mondino BJ, Brown SI, Rabin BS: Autoimmune phenomena of the external eye, *Ophthalmology* 85:801-817, 1978.
36. Mondino BJ, Brown SI, Rabin BS: HLA antigens in ocular cicatricial pemphigoid, *Arch Ophthalmol* 97:479, 1979.
37. Mondino BJ, Manthey R: Dermatological diseases and the peripheral cornea, *Int Ophthalmol Clin* 26(4):121-136, 1986.
38. Mondino BJ, Rao H, Brown SI: T and B lymphocyte enumerations in ocular cicatricial pemphigoid, *Am J Ophthalmol* 92:536-542, 1981.
39. Mondino BJ, Ross AN, Rabin BS, Brown SI: Autoimmune phenomena in ocular cicatricial pemphigoid, *Am J Ophthalmol* 83:443-450, 1977.
40. Moschella SL, Pillsbury DM, Hurley HJ: *Dermatology*, 466-468, Philadelphia, 1975, Saunders.
41. Norn MS, Kristensen EB: Benign mucous membrane pemphigoid. II. Cytology, *Acta Ophthalmol* 52:282-290, 1974.
42. Ormerod LD, Fong LP, Foster CS: Corneal infection in mucosal scarring disorders and Sjogren's syndrome, *Am J Ophthalmol* 105:512-518, 1988.
43. Patten JT, Cavanagh HD, Allansmith MR: Induced ocular pseudopemphigoid, *Am J Ophthalmol* 82:272-276, 1976.
44. Pouliquen Y, Patey A, Foster CS et al.: Drug-induced cicatricial pemphigoid affecting the conjunctiva, *Ophthalmology* 93:775-781, 1986.
45. Proia AD, Foulks GN, Sanfilippo FP: Ocular cicatricial pemphigoid with granular IgA and complement deposition, *Arch Ophthalmol* 103:1669-1672, 1985.
46. Ralph RA: Conjunctival goblet cell density in normal subjects and dry eye syndromes, *Invest Ophthalmol* 14:299-302, 1975.
47. Rao GN, Blatt HL, Aquavella JV: Results of keratoprosthesis, *Am J Ophthalmol* 88:190-196, 1979.
48. Rice BA, Foster CS: Immunopathology of cicatricial pemphigoid affecting the conjunctiva, *Ophthalmology* 97:1476-1483, 1990.
49. Roat MI, Sossi G, Lo C-Y, Thoft RA: Hyperproliferation of conjunctival fibroblasts from patients with cicatricial pemphigoid, *Arch Ophthalmol* 107:1064, 1989.
50. Rogers RS, Seehafer JR, Perry HO: Treatment of cicatricial (benign mucous membrane) pemphigoid with dapsone, *J Am Acad Dermatol* 6:215-223, 1982.
51. Sacks EH, Jakobiec FA, Wieczorek R et al.: Immunophenotypic analysis of the inflammatory infiltrate in ocular cicatricial pemphigoid: further evidence for a T cell-mediated disease, *Ophthalmology* 96:236-243, 1989.
52. Sainz de la Maza M, Tauber J, Foster CS: Cataract surgery in ocular cicatricial pemphigoid, *Ophthalmology* 95:481-486, 1988.
53. Tauber J, Brookline MA, Sainz de la Maza M, Foster CS: Systemic chemotherapy for ocular cicatricial pemphigoid, *Ophthalmology* 95(suppl):146, 1988.
54. Tauber J, Melamed S, Foster CS: Glaucoma in patients with ocular cicatricial pemphigoid, *Ophthalmology* 96:33-37, 1989.
55. Thoft RA, Friend J, Kinoshita S et al.: Ocular cicatricial pemphigoid associated with hyperproliferation of the conjunctival epithelium, *Am J Ophthalmol* 98:37-42, 1984.
56. Zaltas MM, Ahmed R, Foster CS: Association of HLA-DR4 with ocular cicatricial pemphigoid, *Curr Eye Res* 8(2):189-193, 1989.

33 Stevens-Johnson Syndrome

EDWARD J. HOLLAND, DAVID R. HARDTEN

Erythema multiforme major (Stevens-Johnson syndrome) was first described in 1922 as an acute blistering disorder affecting the skin and mucous membranes.[111] Stevens-Johnson syndrome can follow ingestion of an inciting medication or can occur after an infectious process. Erythema multiforme is a less serious blistering disorder of the skin and does not often involve the ocular surface. Toxic epidermal necrolysis is a rare, but acute, life-threatening syndrome that involves the mucous membranes and skin. Patients with toxic epidermal necrolysis have involvement of over 20% of the skin, with sloughing of the skin in sheets.[93] The ocular consequences of these disorders can be severe, involving pathologic changes of the eyelids, the bulbar and palpebral conjunctiva, and the cornea.

HISTORICAL BACKGROUND

The nomenclature surrounding bullous reactions of the skin with mucosal involvement has changed multiple times, and there is still no clear agreement as to terminology. Much of this confusion is because of the separate reports of different aspects of this multisystem disorder.

In 1866 Hebra[42] described a cutaneous disease with erythematous lesions of the skin and proposed the name erythema exudativum multiforme. He reported severe stomatitis and a purulent conjunctivitis associated with erythema multiforme. A generalized cutaneous eruption of the skin with round, erythematous lesions was portrayed in association with pseudomembranous conjunctivitis by Fuchs[32] in 1876 with the term *herpes iris type*.

In 1922 Stevens and Johnson[111] recorded two classic cases and renamed the disease eruptive fever with stomatitis and ophthalmia. Since that time erythema multiforme major has most commonly been referred to as the Stevens-Johnson syndrome. Erythema multiforme is now used to describe cutaneous eruption of the skin alone, without mucous membrane involvement.

Toxic epidermal necrolysis is a more extensive form of erythema multiforme in which more than 20% of the skin is involved.[20,57,58,86] This disease has been referred to as Lyell syndrome after Lyell's classic descriptions.[57,58,59] Lyell has recently suggested that the term *exanthematic necrolysis* be used rather than *toxic epidermal necrolysis*.[60] He feels that this term provides a short, clear name for this sudden outbreak of prostration and widespread skin eruption.

As more is learned about the distinct etiopathologic entities, the terminology will inevitably undergo further change. The Chan and associates[20] classification system will be used throughout this chapter.

EPIDEMIOLOGY

Incidence of Systemic Disease

Erythema multiforme, Stevens-Johnson syndrome, and toxic epidermal necrolysis are very uncommon. Chan and associates[20] reported an incidence of erythema multiforme, Stevens-Johnson syndrome, or toxic epidermal necrolysis of 4.2 per million person-years. The incidence of toxic epidermal necrolysis is only 0.5 per million person-years. Schöph and associates[105] found an overall risk of 0.93 and 1.1 per million for toxic epidermal necrolysis and Stevens-Johnson syndrome, respectively. An incidence of 1.2 to 1.3 per million per year was noted in France,[95] and an incidence of 0.6 cases per million per year was described in an Italian population.[71] Erythema multiforme may be more common in patients with the acquired immunodeficiency syndrome (AIDS).[67]

Incidence of Ocular Complications

Ocular complications from erythema multiforme major and toxic epidermal necrolysis vary with the degree of severity of the systemic disease. Ocular involvement occurs in approximately 80% of patients hospitalized with Stevens-Johnson syndrome or toxic epidermal necrolysis.[84] In more severe cases, acute ocular involvement may include keratitis; and corneal perforation can lead to endophthalmitis.[13,122] Chronic complications are conjunctival scarring, symblepharon, entropion, and dry eye syndrome. These conditions may cause late corneal damage, the most important long-term complication for survivors of toxic epidermal necrolysis and Stevens-Johnson syndrome.[4,13,122] Approximately one third of patients with ocular involvement caused by Stevens-Johnson syndrome experience permanent visual changes.[4,46,124] Because patients with AIDS may already have decreased lacrimation, they may be at increased risk for ocular complications of Stevens-Johnson syndrome and toxic epidermal necrolysis.[11,104]

HLA Association

Patients with ocular lesions of Stevens-Johnson syndrome have a significantly increased incidence of HLA-B12.[70] An increased incidence of HLA-B12 is also seen in white patients with toxic epidermal necrolysis.[96] In a subset of toxic epidermal necrolysis patients in whom the condition could be associated with sulfonamide use, there was a significant increase in the frequency of HLA-A29, B12, and DR7.[70] It is difficult to tell whether these individuals have a genetic susceptibility to toxic epidermal necrolysis, or whether the presence of these antigens in a population that survives toxic epidermal necrolysis may indicate a protective mechanism for a better systemic prognosis.

RISK FACTORS

Erythema multiforme is associated with several causal factors. Some cases are associated with systemic medications, topical medications, infections, malignancy, and collagen-vascular disease.

Medications

Drug-related cases of erythema multiforme, Stevens-Johnson syndrome, and toxic epidermal necrolysis typically arise within 3 weeks after initiation of drug therapy.[20] If the patient is reexposed to the inciting drug, a reaction may begin within hours of restarting drug therapy. Fifty to sixty percent of erythema multiforme cases are secondary to drugs.[14,116] The sulfonamides are the best-documented agents causing erythema multiforme in healthy patients and in patients with human immunodeficiency virus infection or AIDS.[22,30,53,66,72] Anticonvulsants (such as phenytoin and the barbiturates) and nonsteroidal antiinflammatory drugs (such as phenylbutazone) are also well-documented agents that cause erythema multiforme.[27,88] Other drugs associated with erythema multiforme are the penicillins and the salicylates.[27,88]

In one study, implication of drugs as causal factors was postulated in 77% of patients by the onset of the eruption 7 to 21 days after first administration of the drug, or an eruption beginning within 48 hours of drug administration when the patient had been previously exposed.[39] In this same study, though, 23% had evidence that a systemically administered drug was not causative because improvement continued to occur despite continued drug use. Onset before 24 hours or after 21 days of administration of the drug also made it unlikely that the drug caused the erythema multiforme. Although drugs have been implicated in patients as young as 2 and as old as 90, adults and children less than 5 years old are more likely to have drug-associated erythema multiforme than are patients between 20 and 64 years of age.[20]

Erythema multiforme has been described after the use of topical medications. Ophthalmic scopolamine, sulfonamide, or tropicamide may be associated with erythema multiforme.[34,37,38,61,98]

Infections

Postinfectious erythema multiforme has been reported following herpes simplex disease, mycoplasma pneumonia, *Yersinia enterocolitica* infection, measles infection, smallpox vaccination, and other infections.[77,83,106,116] Herpes virus has been implicated in several cases. The virus itself, or more likely an immunologic process directed against the virus or viral-changed host antigens, may cause the skin lesions.[17,106,112] Bacterial infections have also been noted. In Lyell's review[58] of toxic epidermal necrolysis, one fourth of the cases were associated with cutaneous staphylococcal infections, and all of these occurred in children.

PATHOGENESIS

The stimulus for the immunological events of Stevens-Johnson syndrome remains unknown.[68] Although drugs are the most frequent provocative factors, clinical features and laboratory studies do not support a type 1, immediate hypersensitivity, IgE-mediated mechanism.[64,65] Similarly, whereas infectious agents are sometimes implicated, none have been confirmed to be the ultimate cause or explanation for the pathogenesis.[64]

A profound depletion of OKT4-positive cells (helper T cells) occurs during acute Stevens-Johnson syndrome that returns to normal after patient recovery.[97] The majority of cells in the dermal infiltrate of toxic epidermal necrolysis are of the OKT4 subset.[65] It is not known whether this sequestration of T cells damages the epidermal basal cells, or whether it is a consequence of damage. Langerhans cells are also thought to play a role, and it has been postulated that they may serve as antigen-presenting cells or produce lymphokines that attract T helper-inducer cells into these sites.[93]

More recent reports have shown an increase in CD8 lymphocytes in blister fluid of patients with toxic epidermal necrolysis.[22] These cells lack the CD45RA marker and have higher levels of CD29, which suggests that they are antigen-primed cytotoxic T cells. This suggestion implies that these cells also play a role as regulators and effector cells. Interferon gamma-1b may also aid in the development of erythema multiforme. Interferon gamma occurs in response to antigenic stimuli and induces expression of intracellular adhesion molecules—that enable killer T cells to attach to epidermal cells.[75]

CLINICAL FEATURES

Erythema multiforme, Stevens-Johnson syndrome, and toxic epidermal necrolysis share many clinical features and account for the majority of severe cutaneous reactions following drug therapy. There has been much debate over the proper diagnostic criteria for these three diseases.[9,23,80,99] Chan and associates[20] used the diagnostic criteria in the box in their study of the incidence of erythema multiforme, Stevens-Johnson syndrome, and toxic epidermal necrolysis.

The clinical picture of erythema multiforme minor is variable, although the eruption typically is monomorphous in any individual patient. Individual lesions are less than 3 cm in diameter, with less than 20% of the body surface area involved. The rash of erythema multiforme minor appears suddenly and typically is found on the dorsal aspect of the hands and feet and on the extensor surfaces of forearms, legs, palms, and soles.[88] The initial lesions are erythematous annular macules and papules that undergo concentric alter-

ations and produce target, iris, and bull's-eye lesions.[1,28] Some of the lesions may coalesce, becoming vesicular or bullous. Urticarial plaques may also appear. This eruption usually lasts less than 4 weeks. If the lesions are limited only to the skin and there is minimal or no mucous membrane involvement, erythema multiforme minor is the name given to the disease process (see box).

If at least two areas of mucous membrane are involved, then Stevens-Johnson syndrome or erythema multiforme major is the term assigned. Constitutional symptoms including fever, malaise, sore throat, myalgias, arthralgias, and vomiting can occur. The inflammatory bullous eruption involves the oral pharyngeal mucosa, the lips, conjunctiva, genital surfaces, and occasionally the viscera[3,12,28] (Fig. 33-1). Less than 20% of the total body surface area is involved in Stevens-Johnson syndrome.

Toxic epidermal necrolysis is frequently preceded by constitutional symptoms such as malaise, fever, and burning irritation of the conjunctiva and skin.[88] The rash is initially more morbilliform and involves the face and extremities. The lesions later coalesce, leading to huge bullae formation, and resulting in large portions of the skin denuding (Fig. 33-2). Involvement of more than 20% of the body surface is characteristic of toxic epidermal necrolysis. A positive Nikolsky sign is present when friction applied to healthy areas of the skin causes the epidermis to wrinkle and separate. The mucosa are involved with severe erosions of the lips, oral surface, conjunctiva, and genital areas. Fever, leukocytosis, renal dysfunction, sepsis, pulmonary embolism, or gastrointestinal bleeding can occur.[90]

Initial Ocular Disease

In the Stevens-Johnson syndrome, a nonspecific conjunctivitis usually occurs concurrently with lesions on the

---

DIAGNOSTIC CRITERIA FOR BULLOUS SKIN DISEASES (ADAPTED FROM CHAN AND ASSOCIATES[20])

Erythema Multiforme (Erythema Multiforme Minor)
Target (iris) lesions (typical or atypical)
Individual lesions less than 3 centimeters in diameter
No or minimal mucous membrane involvement
Less than 20% of body area involved in reaction
Biopsy specimen compatible with erythema multiforme minor

Stevens-Johnson Syndrome (Erythema Multiforme Major)
Less than 20% of body area involved in first 48 hours
Greater than 10% body area involvement
Target (iris) lesions (typical or atypical)
Individual lesions <3 centimeters in diameter (lesions may coalesce)
Mucous membrane involvement (at least 2)
Fever
Biopsy specimen compatible with erythema multiforme major

Toxic Epidermal Necrolysis
Bullae and/or erosions over 20% of body area
Bullae develop on erythematous base
Occurs on nonsun-exposed skin
Skin peels off in >3 centimeter sheets
Mucous membrane involvement is frequent
Tender skin within 48 hours of onset of rash
Fever
Biopsy specimen compatible with toxic epidermal necrolysis

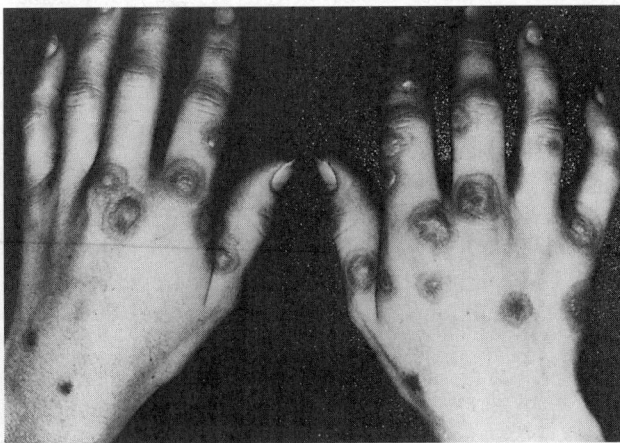

Fig. 33-1. Bull's-eye lesions of the hands in a patient with Stevens-Johnson syndrome. (Reproduced with permission from Araujo and Flowers.[3])

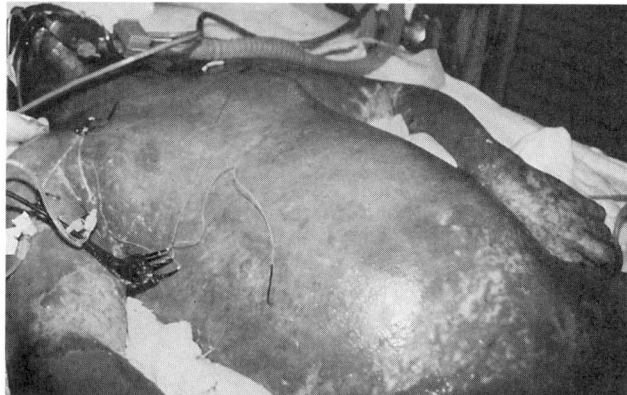

Fig. 33-2. Skin sloughing in a patient with phenytoin-induced toxic epidermal necrolysis.

skin and other mucous membranes, but the conjunctivitis may precede the skin eruption.[26,77,122] Bilateral catarrhal, purulent, or pseudomembranous conjunctivitis occurs in 15% to 75% of patients with Stevens-Johnson syndrome.[6,14,46,82] Severe anterior uveitis may occur. Corneal ulceration may be seen during the acute stage of the disease, which lasts from 2 to 4 weeks.[82] Monocular involvement is unusual.[6]

Chronic Ocular Disease

The ophthalmologist usually becomes involved in managing and following the chronic stages of Stevens-Johnson syndrome and toxic epidermal necrolysis. Cicatrization of the conjunctiva results from the inflammatory process. Symblepharon, entropion, trichiasis, corneal vascularization, keratinization, and instability of the tear film can be seen[4,26,122] (Fig. 33-3). An orbital cyst may occur when epithelial cells become trapped between adhesions of the tarsal and bulbar conjunctiva.[25] Cicatrization of the lacrimal ducts in association with destruction of the conjunctival goblet

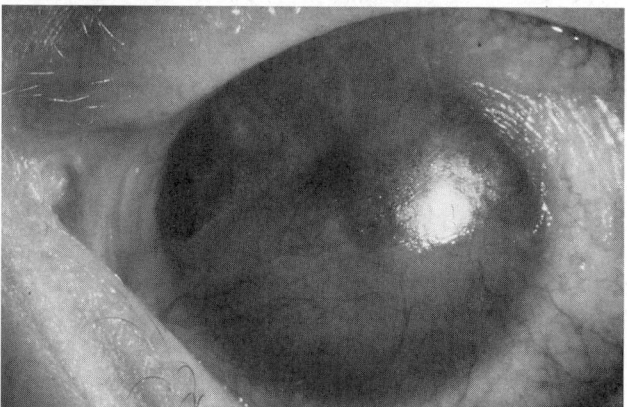

Fig. 33-3. Corneal vascularization in a patient with sulfa-induced Stevens-Johnson syndrome.

cells may lead to tear film abnormalities.[4,69,85] If there is no scarring of the lacrimal ducts, then the patients can be photophobic with considerable lacrimation. The tear film abnormality in these patients results from the absence of mucus with instability of the tear film and poor wetting of the cornea.[26] Entropion and trichiasis can result in chronic irritation of the cornea with resultant persistent epithelial defects.[110] A degenerative pannus can occur that can be easily stripped from the Bowman membrane, with the stroma remaining surprisingly unaffected for several weeks.[26] These corneal manifestations are not the result of the initial acute inflammation, but are the consequence of the goblet cell dysfunction, trichiasis, and dry eye.

Recurrent Ocular Disease

A small number of Stevens-Johnson syndrome patients develop recurrent conjunctival inflammation that is not associated with trichiasis, entropion, keratoconjunctivitis sicca, or lid margin keratinization.[31] In these patients, conjunctival inflammation lasting from 8 days to 5 weeks occurred without recurrence of the typical skin lesions of erythema multiforme. One patient had recurrent oral mucosal ulcers, but these were not concurrent with the development of episodes of conjunctivitis.

PATHOLOGY

Dermatopathology

In erythema multiforme major, separation of the epidermis and basement membrane from the dermis occurs[28,88] (Fig. 33-4). Endothelial swelling, lymphocytic-histiocytic

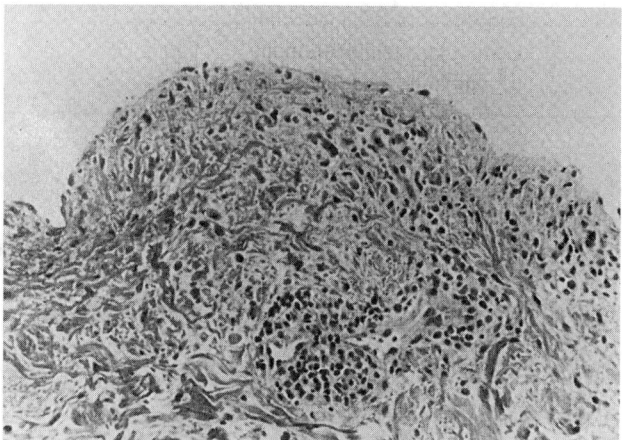

Fig. 33-4. Histopathology of the skin in erythema multiforme. Subepidermal bulla with vascularization and hyalinization of individual keratocytes, papillary edema, and a hematoxylin-mononuclear infiltrate are characteristic of erythema multiforme. (Hematoxylin-eosin stain, × 420, reproduced with permission from Raviglione and associates.[88])

perivascular infiltration, and papillary dermal edema occur. Orfanos and associates[76] described two different histologic patterns. In the first type, pure dermal damage occurs with dermal edema, intradermal bullae formation, and erythematous papular lesions. Epidermal damage characterizes the second type, resulting in bullae formation at the dermal-epidermal junction with the basal laminae at the floor of the bullae in "target lesions." Tissue eosinophilia can be seen in skin lesions of drug-induced Stevens-Johnson syndrome.[79]

Toxic epidermal necrolysis has a histopathologic picture similar to the epidermal type of erythema multiforme major.[76] Eosinophilic necrosis of the epidermis occurs with a cleavage plane above the basement membrane at the basal cell layer (Fig. 33-5). Endothelial swelling may be seen in the dermal vessels, although they do not undergo major histopathologic change. The earliest changes observed are vacuolar changes at the dermoepidermal junction, which progress to dermoepidermal separation and subepidermal blister formation.[64] The epidermis becomes dyskeratotic and then necrotic. The majority of the inflammatory cells of the dermal infiltrate are of the helper-inducer T lymphocyte subsets.[65] Deposition of immunoglobulins and/or complement that use immunofluorescent techniques is usually not evident.[64]

Ocular Histopathology

A nonspecific inflammatory response is seen in the acute phase in enucleated eyes of patients with erythema multiforme.[35,92] Widespread necrosis of arterioles and venules occurs with fibrinoid degeneration of the associated collagen.[2] During the chronic phase, the effects of cicatrization on the cornea, conjunctiva, and eyelids are most prominent (Fig. 33-6). Conjunctival biopsies in Stevens-Johnson syndrome show an absence of the mucous-producing goblet cells as a sequela to cicatrization.[26,69] Conjunctival goblet cells are decreased to 1% to 2% of normal when measured by impression cytologic techniques.[73] Nonspecific mononuclear inflammation can characterize the acute phase of Stevens-Johnson syndrome, affecting the subepithelial layers of the conjunctiva.[10] Circulating immune complexes have been found as well as immune complexes in the mucosal subepithelial tissue microvasculature.[49,102,113,123] Increased proliferation of basal epithelial cells has been demonstrated in Stevens-Johnson syndrome, and an increased percentage of proliferating conjunctival cells appears to be correlated with the severity of the disease.[121]

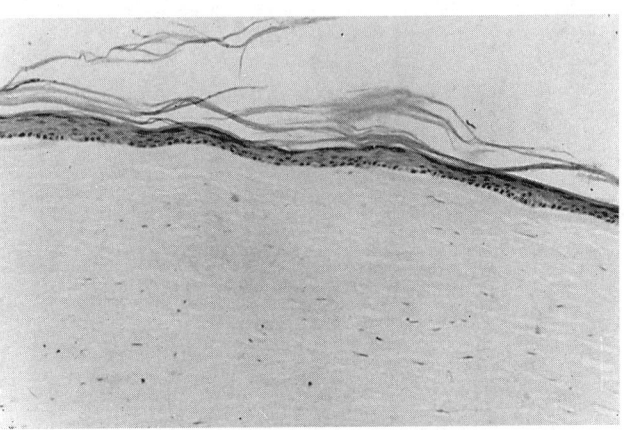

Fig. 33-6. Keratinization of the conjunctival epithelium in toxic epidermal necrolysis.

DIFFERENTIAL DIAGNOSIS

Acute Oculocutaneous Disease

The striking clinical picture of extensive erythema of the skin and epidermal sloughing is mimicked by few other diseases. Staphylococcal scalded skin syndrome can be confused with toxic epidermal necrolysis or Stevens-Johnson syndrome.[93] It is important to make this diagnosis quickly because the management and prognosis are different. Staphylococcal scalded skin syndrome most commonly occurs in children.[41,56,89,94] Clinically, these patients show more intense cutaneous tenderness and a less severe systemic toxicity. The epidermis quickly regenerates and effectively restores its barrier functions in the staphylococcal scalded skin syndrome. No mucous membrane lesions are found, and only the top layer of epidermis peels off. Cultures can be confusing because lesions of Stevens-Johnson syndrome and toxic epidermal necrolysis can be secondarily colonized. This disease occurs because of a toxin released by *Staphylococcus aureus* that results in intraepidermal damage. This disease is treated with appropriate antibiotics.

Toxic shock syndrome, Kawasaki disease, Leiner disease, and erythroderma secondary to other causes should be

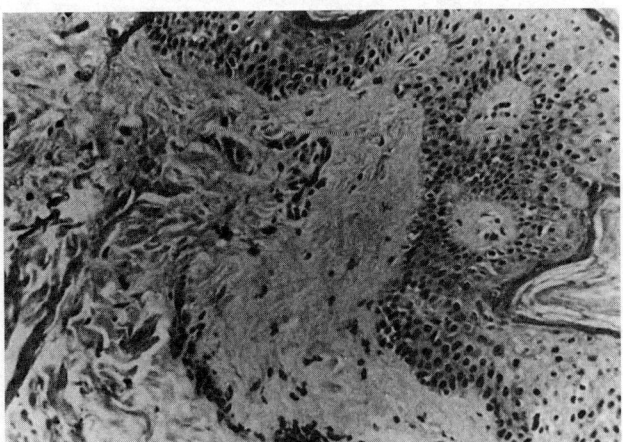

Fig. 33-5. Histopathology of the skin in toxic epidermal necrolysis. Marked epidermal necrosis, hyalinization, and cell loss with an inflammatory cell infiltrate is characteristic of toxic epidermal necrolysis. (Hematoxylin-eosin stain, ×420, reproduced with permission from Raviglione and associates.[88])

included in the differential diagnosis for toxic epidermal necrolysis and Stevens-Johnson syndrome. Contact dermatitis from thermal burns or poisonings should also be considered.[59,78]

Chronic Ocular Disease

The chronic ocular findings in Stevens-Johnson syndrome and toxic epidermal necrolysis can resemble cicatricial ocular pemphigoid. The symblepharon are rarely as pronounced in Stevens-Johnson syndrome and toxic epidermal necrolysis as they are in cicatricial ocular pemphigoid.[26] A history of the typical skin lesions of Stevens-Johnson syndrome or toxic epidermal necrolysis helps to make the diagnosis in the chronic stages. Chronic scarring of the ocular mucosae that appears clinically similar to ocular cicatricial pemphigoid can persist up to 31 years after an episode of Stevens-Johnson syndrome.[21] Biopsies of the mucosa in patients with ocular cicatricial pemphigoid show linear immune deposits along the basement membrane.

The differential diagnosis also includes chronic keratoconjunctivitis caused by bacteria, medications, allergies, chemical burns, avitaminosis A, and trachoma.[26] The history will usually provide the clues necessary to make the correct diagnosis.

THERAPY

Systemic Treatment

The management of patients with severe Stevens-Johnson syndrome and toxic epidermal necrolysis is difficult. These patients are critically ill and require specialized nursing and medical care. Careful monitoring of fluid balance, respiratory function, nutritional requirements, and wound care are crucial.[93] Patients are best managed in an intensive burn care unit.[24,29,44,78,91] Proper fluid balance management is crucial because of the loss of the stratum corneum.[29]

More than half of all deaths occurring in toxic epidermal necrolysis are secondary to sepsis, so control of infection is critical.[91] It is generally felt that antibiotics should be reserved for culture-proven sepsis, with less emphasis on wide-spectrum prophylactic antibiotic coverage.[29,44,91] Silver nitrate solution can be used as an antibacterial on the denuded skin.[78] Biological dressings such as cadaver skin, porcine skin, amniotic membrane, and iodoplex can be used to reduce pain and evaporative loss and to protect against infection.[5,24,44,48,91]

In cases of Stevens-Johnson syndrome or toxic epidermal necrolysis caused by an inciting medication, the offending drug should be discontinued.[88]

The use of systemic corticosteroids in patients with Stevens-Johnson syndrome and toxic epidermal necrolysis is still controversial.* Some studies suggest that high-dose

corticosteroids might arrest the necrolysis and benefit the patient's systemic recovery.[15,33,80,81,107] Systemic steroid dosages range from 40 mg of prednisone to 750 mg of methylprednisolone daily. In some cases, dramatic reversal of disease progression follows institution of corticosteroids.

Because evidence for beneficial effects of corticosteroids is lacking, other authors feel that the use of corticosteroids in severe cutaneous drug reactions is not recommended and does not positively affect the final outcome.* Some patients' symptoms progress despite institution of corticosteroids. The risks of using high-dose corticosteroids in patients with compromised barrier defenses are of concern. Secondary infections can be more serious when systemic corticosteroids are used. There is an increased propensity toward gastrointestinal hemorrhage.

The course of toxic epidermal necrolysis and Stevens-Johnson syndrome is variable and unpredictable, which casts doubt on uncontrolled observations on steroid use. Because of the potential complications of steroid therapy (including increased susceptibility to infection, masking of early signs of sepsis, gastrointestinal hemorrhage, impaired wound healing, and prolonged recovery), use of corticosteroid therapy for severe Stevens-Johnson syndrome and toxic epidermal necrolysis should be decided on an individualized basis. A definitive answer may never be possible because of the variable course of the disease.[80]

There has been a case report of cyclosporine therapy slowing the progression of toxic epidermal necrolysis after failure of high-dose steroid therapy.[100] This patient developed no permanent sequelae on follow-up examination. The use of cyclosporine in this disease requires further delineation. Cyclophosphamide is also useful in treating toxic epidermal necrolysis.[45] Case reports of plasma exchange therapy in patients with toxic epidermal necrolysis have been reported.[47,103]

Ocular Treatment

Good hygiene of the ocular surface should be maintained during the acute stages of Stevens-Johnson syndrome and toxic epidermal necrolysis. This includes frequent conjunctival irrigation with balanced saline solution and installation of prophylactic antibiotics to combat secondary infection.[4,26,46,82] Frequent nonpreserved, artificial tear supplements should be used to protect the integrity of the corneal epithelium. Cycloplegics should be used for the anterior uveitis that is often associated with the external inflammation in Stevens-Johnson syndrome and toxic epidermal necrolysis.

The role of topical corticosteroids is still unclear. Their use can be associated with secondary infection in these patients with an unstable ocular surface. They do tend to de-

*References 33, 36, 40, 50, 52, 58, 74, 90, 91, 99, 107, 115.

*References 40, 50, 52, 62, 74, 87, 91, 99, 115.

crease the inflammation, although symblepharon can form despite the use of topical corticosteroids.[26] Topical corticosteroids should be judiciously used to treat the inflammatory process, while observing the patient closely to detect early complications. If a keratitis does occur, careful cultures should be obtained, and vigorous antibiotic therapy should be started with fortified antibiotics.

The role of topical cyclosporine has not been studied, although one case in which systemic treatment was used suggested that it may be of use in this disease.[100]

Lamellar or penetrating keratoplasty can be used if perforation is impending or has occurred. A conjunctival flap is also a valuable option for treatment of the ocular surface disorder in the acute stage. Daily lysis of the symblepharon can be attempted, but it is usually ineffective in preventing recurrence of the symblepharon. Saran Wrap or a symblepharon ring can be used in association with a bandage soft contact lens to line the palpebral surface and prevent symblepharon formation.[101] The plastic wrap is used to line the palpebral surface by placing one edge in the fornix and draping it over the palpebral surface, eyelid margin, and skin. Mattress sutures are used to anchor the Saran Wrap in the fornix. The plastic wrap is left in place until the acute episode is over. This plastic wrap is better tolerated in children than a symblepharon ring and bandage soft contact lens.

Treatment of Chronic Ocular Disease

The treatment of the chronic stages of Stevens-Johnson syndrome and toxic epidermal necrolysis is challenging. Trichiasis can be a difficult problem. Epilation, cryotherapy, argon laser, electrolysis, or blepharotomy can be used to destroy lashes.[8,43] A rapid freeze of the eyelid margin to −20° C to −30° C, followed by a slow thaw, will irreversibly damage approximately 80% of the eyelashes.[43] The probe is placed on the conjunctiva 2 to 3 mm behind the posterior lid margin. Forty to sixty seconds of freezing is required to reach the appropriate tissue temperature. A double freeze technique is recommended with a period for thawing between the two freezing periods.

Cicatricial entropion and epidermalization of the conjunctiva can lead to mechanical trauma to the cornea. Entropion repair, possibly combined with mucous membrane grafting, should be performed to correct lid problems.[13,19,55,63] Nasolacrimal duct obstruction and canalicular obstruction or stenosis can occur. Sometimes this offsets the relatively dry eye state and may not need correction. Epiphora or dacryocystitis may be symptomatic and require dacryocystorhinostomy and silicone tube insertion.[7]

Artificial tear supplementation should be used to treat the keratoconjunctivitis sicca that develops after scarring of the conjunctiva and lacrimal ducts in Stevens-Johnson syndrome and toxic epidermal necrolysis. Nonpreserved methylcellulose lubricants should be used because of the toxicity observed with preservatives in patients with such severe dry eye states.

Topical corticosteroids control the inflammation and prevent further symblepharon formation. Mucolytics such as 10% N-acetyl-cysteine control filament formation or abnormal mucous discharge. A lateral or medial tarsorrhaphy can improve the status of the ocular surface by decreasing the surface area available for evaporation. Bandage soft contact lenses can manage persistent epithelial defect.[18] Care should be taken to watch these patients for tight lens syndrome because of their compromised ocular surface and low mucin production.[16] Microbial keratitis is a risk with bandage lenses.

Topical transretinoic acid can reverse conjunctival transdifferentiation that follows ocular surface injury.[118,119] Topical and systemic vitamin A was used to treat a child with Stevens-Johnson syndrome, with improvement in his ocular surface appearance.[108] Improvement in clinical symptoms, visual acuity, rose bengal staining, Schirmer test, or squamous metaplasia has been seen after treatment with topical retinoids.[119] Topical vitamin A in a 0.01% or 0.025 % ointment is commercially available and should be used twice daily. Blepharitis or ocular inflammation may increase after initiation of topical vitamin A and can be tapered to minimize these side effects.[109]

Keratoepithelioplasty is a procedure that is useful in the treatment of persistent epithelial dysfunction caused by toxic epidermal necrolysis and Stevens-Johnson syndrome. Keratoepithelioplasty has been described for the treatment of persistent epithelial defects in patients who lack healthy donor tissue from their other eye.[114] Lenticules of donor limbus are placed at the limbus after a superficial keratectomy (Fig. 33-7). The epithelium spreads and covers the conjunctiva and cornea.[51,114,120]

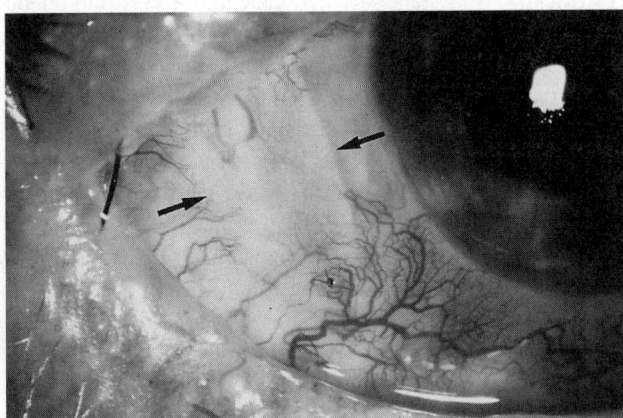

Fig. 33-7. Keratoepithelioplasty lenticules 3 months postoperatively in a patient with persistent epithelial defect following an episode of toxic epidermal necrolysis.

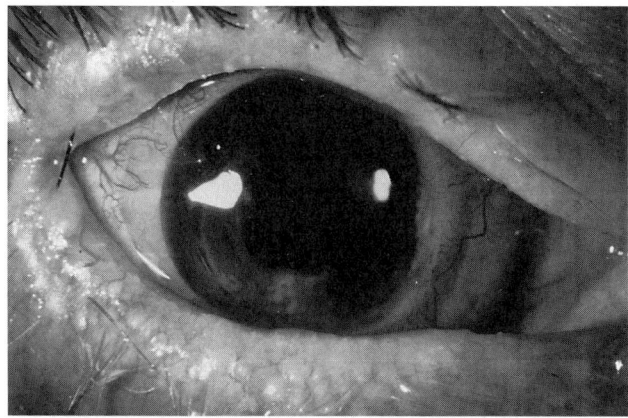

Fig. 33-8. Clear corneal transplant with regular epithelium 3 months following keratoepithelioplasty and penetrating keratoplasty in a patient with toxic epidermal necrolysis.

Once the epithelium has been stabilized, corneal transplantation can be performed to improve the vision by removing the corneal stromal scarring and providing a clear transplant (Fig 33-8). The main postoperative complications in these patients are related to epithelial toxicity from medications, trichiasis, and mucin deficiency.

A keratoprosthesis has been recommended for patients with Stevens-Johnson syndrome who have poor epithelial healing.[54] This procedure can be complicated by eyelid cellulitis, extrusions of the keratoprosthesis, aqueous leaks, retroprosthetic membranes, endophthalmitis, or progressive glaucoma.

PROGNOSIS

Erythema multiforme major (Stevens-Johnson syndrome) and toxic epidermal necrolysis are potentially fatal disease processes. The ocular complications can be one of the lasting sequela for survivors of these diseases. The outcome depends on the severity of the initial event much more than it does on the initial treatment. To minimize visual impairment, prevention of complications is paramount. Careful attention to ophthalmic examinations during the early period of the skin reaction, and recognizing the complications of trichiasis, epithelial surface disease, and secondary infection can improve the outcome.

The risk-benefit ratio of systemic steroid use should be evaluated individually for each patient because of the unclear efficacy and potential for severe systemic side effects and secondary infection. When topical corticosteroids are used, careful monitoring of the ocular surface should be performed to detect early secondary bacterial or fungal infections.

Improved management of ocular surface disease with keratoepithelioplasty, tarsorrhaphy, nonpreserved artificial lubricants, and treatment of trichiasis may improve the prognosis of this disease.

REFERENCES

1. Ackerman AB, Penneys NS, Clark WH: Erythema multiforme exudativum: distinctive pathological process, *Br J Dermatol* 84:554-566, 1971.
2. Alexander MK, Cope S: Erythema multiforme exudativum major (Stevens-Johnson syndrome), *J Pathol Bacteriol* 68:373-380, 1954.
3. Araujo OE, Flowers FP: Stevens-Johnson syndrome, *J Emerg Med* 2:129-135, 1984.
4. Arstikaitis MJ: Ocular aftermath of Stevens-Johnson syndrome: review of 33 cases, *Arch Ophthalmol* 90:376-379, 1973.
5. Artz CP, Rittenbury MS, Yarbrough DR: An appraisal of allografts and xenografts as biological dressings for wounds and burns, *Ann Surg* 175:934-938, 1972.
6. Ashby DW, Lazar T: Erythema multiforme exudativum major (Stevens-Johnson syndrome), *Lancet* 260:1091-1095, 1951.
7. Auran JD, Hornblass A, Gross WD: Stevens-Johnson syndrome with associated nasolacrimal duct obstruction treated with dacryocystorhinostomy and Crawford silicone tube insertion, *Ophthal Plast Reconstr Surg* 6:60-63, 1993.
8. Bartley GB, Lowry JC: Argon laser treatment of trichiasis, *Am J Ophthalmol* 113:71-74, 1992.
9. Bastuji-Garin S, Rzany B, Stern RS et al.: Clinical classification of cases of toxic epidermal necrolysis, Stevens-Johnson syndrome, and erythema multiforme, *Arch Dermatol* 129:92-96, 1993.
10. Bedi TR, Pinkus H: Histopathological spectrum of erythema multiforme, *Br J Dermatol* 95:243-250, 1976.
11. Belfort R Jr, deSmet M, Whitcup SM et al.: Ocular complications of Stevens-Johnson syndrome and toxic epidermal necrolysis in patients with AIDS, *Cornea* 10:536-538, 1991.
12. Benichou C, Brini A, Abensour M, Grosshans E: Lesions oculopalpebrales dans les erythè mes polymorphes graves: prevention du symblepharon, *Bull Soc Ophtalmol Fr* 88:391-396, 1988.
13. Beyer CK: The management of special problems associated with Stevens-Johnson syndrome and ocular pemphigoid, *Trans Am Acad Ophthalmol Otolaryngol* 83:701-707, 1977.
14. Bianchine JR, Macaraeg PVJ Jr, Lasagna L et al.: Drugs as etiologic factors in the Stevens-Johnson syndrome, *Am J Med* 44:390-405, 1968.
15. Björnberg A: Fifteen cases of toxic epidermal necrolysis (Lyell), *Acta Derm Venereol* 53:149-152, 1973.
16. Bouchard CS, Lemp MA: Tight lens syndrome associated with a 24 hour disposable collagen lens: a case report, *CLAO J* 17:141-142,1991.
17. Brice SL, Krzemien D, Weston WL, Huff JC: Detection of herpes simplex virus DNA in cutaneous lesions of erythema multiforme, *J Invest Dermatol* 93:183-187, 1989.
18. Brown SI, Weller CA, Akiya S: Pathogenesis of ulcers of the alkali-burned cornea, *Arch Ophthalmol* 83:205-208, 1970.
19. Callahan A: Correction of entropion from Stevens-Johnson syndrome, use of nasal septum and mucosa for severely cicatrized eyelid entropion, *Arch Ophthalmol* 94:1154-1155, 1976.
20. Chan HL, Stern RS, Arndt KA et al.: The incidence of erythema multiforme, Stevens-Johnson syndrome, and toxic epidermal necrolysis: a population-based study with particular reference to reactions caused by drugs among outpatients, *Arch Dermatol* 126:43-47, 1990.
21. Chan LS, Soong HK, Foster CS et al.: Ocular cicatricial pemphigoid occurring as a sequela of Stevens-Johnson syndrome, *JAMA* 266:1543-1546, 1991.
22. Correia O, Delgado L, Ramos JP et al.: Cutaneous T-cell recruitment in toxic epidermal necrolysis. Further evidence of CD8+ lymphocyte involvement, *Arch Dermatol* 129:466-468, 1993.
23. Crosby SS, Murray KM, Marvin JA et al.: Management of Stevens-Johnson syndrome, *Clin Pharm* 5:682-689, 1986.
24. Demling RH, Ellerbe S, Lowe NJ: Burn unit management of toxic epidermal necrolysis, *Arch Surg* 113:758-759, 1978.
25. Desai VN, Shields CL, Shields JA: Orbital cyst in a patient with Stevens-Johnson syndrome, *Cornea* 11:592-594, 1992.
26. Dohlman CH, Doughman DJ: The Stevens-Johnson syndrome, *Trans New Orleans Acad Ophthalmol* 24:236-252, 1972.

27. Dunagin WG, Millikan LE: Drug eruptions, *Med Clin North Am* 64:983-1003, 1980.
28. Elias PM, Fritsch PO: Erythema multiforme. In Fitzpatrick et al., editors: *Dermatology and general medicine,* 555-563, New York-St Louis, 1987, McGraw-Hill Book.
29. Finlay AY, Richards J, Holt PJ: Intensive therapy unit management of toxic epidermal necrolysis: practical aspects, *Clin Exp Dermatol* 7:55-60, 1982.
30. Fischel MA, Dickinson GM: Fansidar prophylaxis of pneumocystis pneumonia in the acquired immunodeficiency syndrome, *Ann Intern Med* 105:629, 1986.
31. Foster CS, Fong LP, Azar D, Kenyon KR: Episodic conjunctival inflammation after Stevens-Johnson syndrome, *Ophthalmology* 95:453-462, 1988.
32. Fuchs E: Herpes iris conjunctivae, *Klin Monatsbl Augenheilkd* 14:333-351, 1876.
33. Garabiol B, Touraine R: Syndrome de Lyell de l'adulte: éléments de prognostic et déductions thérapeutiques: étude de 27 cas, *Ann Med Interne (Paris)* 127:670-672, 1976.
34. Genvert GI, Cohen EJ, Donnenfeld ED, Blecher MH: Erythema multiforme after use of topical sulfacetamide, *Am J Ophthalmol* 99:465-468, 1985.
35. Ginandes GJ: Eruptive fever with stomatitis and ophthalmia: atypical erythema exodativum multiforme (Stevens-Johnson), *Am J Dis Child* 49:1148-1160, 1935.
36. Ginsburg CM: Stevens-Johnson syndrome in children, *Pediatr Infect Dis J* 1:155-158, 1982.
37. Gottschalk HR, Stone OJ: Stevens-Johnson syndrome from ophthalmic sulfonamide, *Arch Dermatol* 112:513-514, 1976.
38. Guill MA, Goette DK, Knight CG et al.: Erythema multiforme and urticaria, *Arch Dermatol* 115:742-743, 1979.
39. Guillaumue JC, Roujeau JC, Revuz J et al.: The culprit drugs in 87 cases of toxic epidermal necrolysis (Lyell's syndrome), *Arch Dermatol* 123:1166-1170, 1987.
40. Halebian PH, Madden MR, Finklestein JL et al.: Improved burn center survival of patients with toxic epidermal necrolysis managed without corticosteroids, *Ann Surg* 204:503-512, 1986.
41. Hawley HB, Aronson MD: Scalded-skin syndrome in adults, *New Eng J Med* 288:1130, 1973.
42. Hebra F: *On diseases of the skin, including the exanthematha,* vol 1, London, 1866, New Sydenham Society. (Translated and edited by CH Fagge).
43. Hecht SD: Cryotherapy of trichiasis with use of the retinal cryoprobe, *Ann Ophthalmol* 9:1501-1503, 1977.
44. Heimbach DM, Engrav LH, Marvin JA et al.: Toxic epidermal necrolysis: a step forward in treatment, *JAMA* 257:2171-2175, 1987.
45. Henz MC, Allen SG: Efficacy of cyclophosphamide in toxic epidermal necrolysis: clinical and pathophysiologic aspects, *J Am Acad Dermatol* 25:778-786, 1991.
46. Howard GM: The Stevens-Johnson syndrome: ocular prognosis and treatment, *Am J Ophthalmol* 55:893-900, 1963.
47. Kamanabroo D, Schmitz-Landgraf W, Czarnetzki BM: Plasmapheresis in severe drug-induced toxic epidermal necrolysis, *Arch Dermatol* 121:1548-1549, 1985.
48. Kaufman T, Shechter H, Bar-Joseph G, Hirshowitz B: Topical treatment of toxic epidermal necrolysis with iodoplex, *J Burn Care Rehabil* 12:346-348, 1991.
49. Kazmierowski JA, Wuepper KD: Erythema multiforme: immune complex vasculitis of the superficial cutaneous microvasculature, *J Invest Dermatol* 71:366, 1978.
50. Kim PS, Goldfarb IW, Gaisford JC, Slater H: Stevens-Johnson syndrome and toxic epidermal necrolysis: a pathophysiologic review with recommendations for a treatment protocol, *J Burn Care Rehabil* 4:91-100, 1983.
51. Kinoshita S, Ohashi Y, Ohji M, Manabe R: Long-term results of keratoepithelioplasty in Mooren's ulcer, *Ophthalmology* 98:438-445, 1991.
52. Kint A, Geerts ML, de Weert J: Le syndrome de Lyell, *Dermatologica* 163:433-454, 1981.
53. Kovacs JA, Masur H: *Pneumocystis carinii* pneumonia: therapy and prophylaxis, *J Infect Dis* 158:254-259, 1988.
54. Kozarsky AM, Knight SH, Waring GO III: Clinical results with a ceramic keratoprosthesis placed through the eyelid, *Ophthalmology* 94:904-911, 1987.
55. Leone CR Jr: Mucous membrane grafting for cicatricial entropion, *Ophthalmic Surg* 5(2):24-28, 1974.
56. Levine G, Norden CW: Staphylococcal scalded-skin syndrome in an adult, *New Eng J Med* 287:1339-1340, 1972.
57. Lyell A: Toxic epidermal necrolysis: an eruption resembling scalding of the skin, *Br J Dermatol* 68:355-361, 1956.
58. Lyell A: A review of toxic epidermal necrolysis in Britain, *Br J Dermatol* 79:662-671, 1967.
59. Lyell A: Toxic epidermal necrolysis (the scalded-skin syndrome): a reappraisal, *Br J Dermatol* 100:69-86, 1979.
60. Lyell A: Requiem for toxic epidermal necrolysis, *Br J Dermatol* 122:837-838, 1990.
61. Margolis DJ, Bondi EE: Toxic epidermal necrolysis associated with sulfonamides, *Int J Dermatol* 29:153, 1990.
62. Marvin JA, Heimbach DM, Engrav LH, Harnar TJ: Improved treatment of the Stevens-Johnson syndrome, *Arch Surg* 119:601-605, 1984.
63. McCord CD Jr, Chen WP: Tarsal polishing and mucous membrane grafting for cicatricial entropion, trichiasis and epidermalization, *Ophthalmic Surg* 14:1021-1025, 1983.
64. Merot Y, Saurat JH: Clues to pathogenesis of toxic epidermal necrolysis, *Int J Dermatol* 24:165-168, 1985.
65. Merot Y, Gravallese E, Guillén FJ, Murphy GF: Lymphocyte subsets and Langerhan's cells in toxic epidermal necrolysis: report of a case, *Arch Dermatol* 122:455-458, 1986.
66. Miller KD, Lobel HO, Satriale RF et al.: Severe cutaneous reactions among American travelers using pyrimethamine-sulfadoxine (Fansidar) for malaria prophylaxis, *Am J Trop Med Hyg* 35:451-458, 1986.
67. Miller L, Cohn D: High rates of recurrent pneumocystis pneumonia and toxicity in AIDS patients taking pyrimethamine-sulfadoxine, International Conference on AIDS, 5:294, 1989 (abstract number T.B.P. 317).
68. Mok CH, Stevens FRT: Stevens-Johnson syndrome, *Med J Aust* 51:591-592, 1964.
69. Mondino BJ, Brown SI: Ocular cicatricial pemphigoid, *Ophthalmology* 88:95-100, 1981.
70. Mondino BJ, Brown SI, Biglan AW: HLA antigens in Stevens-Johnson syndrome with ocular involvement, *Arch Ophthalmol* 100:1453-1454, 1982.
71. Nadli L, Locati F, Marchesi L, Cainelli T: Incidence of toxic epidermal necrolysis in Italy, *Arch Dermatol* 126:1103-1104, 1990.
72. Navin TR, Miller KD, Satriale RF, Lobel HO: Adverse reactions associated with pyrimethamine-sulfadoxine prophylaxis for pneumocystis carinii infections in AIDS, *Lancet* 1:1332, 1985.
73. Nelson JD, Wright JC: Conjunctival goblet cell densities in ocular surface disease, *Arch Ophthalmol* 102:1049-1051, 1984.
74. Nethercott JR, Choi BCK: Erythema multiforme (Stevens-Johnson syndrome)—chart review of 123 hospitalized patients, *Dermatologica* 171:383-396, 1985.
75. Nickoloff BJ: Role of interferon − γ in cutaneous trafficking of lymphocytes with emphasis on molecular and cellular adhesion events, *Arch Dermatol* 124:1835-1843, 1988.
76. Orfanos CE, Schaumburg-Lever G, Lever WF: Dermal and epidermal types of erythema multiforme: a histopathologic study of 24 cases, *Arch Dermatol* 109:682-688, 1974.
77. Ostler HB, Conant MA, Groundwater J: Lyell's disease, the Stevens-Johnson syndromes, and exfoliative dermatitis, *Trans Am Acad Ophthalmol Otolaryngol* 74:1254-1265, 1970.
78. Parsons JM: Management of toxic epidermal necrolysis, *Cutis* 36:305-311, 1985.
79. Patterson JW, Parsons JM, Blaylock WK, Mills AS: Eosinophils in skin lesions of erythema multiforme, *Arch Pathol Lab Med* 113:36-39, 1989.
80. Patterson R, Dykewicz MS, Gonzalzles A et al.: Erythema multiforme and Stevens-Johnson syndrome. Descriptive and therapeutic controversy, *Chest* 98:331-336, 1990.
81. Patterson R, Grammer LC, Greenberger PA et al.: Stevens-Johnson syndrome (SJS): effectiveness of corticosteroids in management and recurrent SJS, *Allergy Proc* 13:89-95, 1992.

82. Patz A: Ocular involvement in erythema multiforme, *Arch Ophthalmol* 43:244-256, 1950.
83. Pedrazzoli P, Rosti V, Rossi R, Cazzola M: Toxic epidermal necrolysis following Yersenia enterocolitica infection, *Int J Dermatol* 32:74, 1993.
84. Prendiville JS, Herbert AA, Greenwald MJ, Esterly NV: Management of Stevens-Johnson syndrome and toxic epidermal necrolysis in children, *J Pediatr* 115:881-887, 1989.
85. Ralph RA: Conjunctival goblet cell density in normal subjects and in dry eye syndromes, *Invest Ophthalmol* 14:299-302, 1975.
86. Rasmussen JE: Toxic epidermal necrolysis, *Med Clin North Am* 64:901-920, 1980.
87. Rasmussen JE: Erythema multiforme in children: response to treatment with systemic corticosteroids, *Br J Dermatol* 95:181-186, 1976.
88. Raviglione MC, Pablos-Mendez A, Battan R: Clinical features and management of severe dermatological reactions to drugs, *Drug Saf* 5:39-64, 1990.
89. Reid L, Weston WL, Humbert JR: Staphylococcal scalded-skin syndrome. Adult onset in a patient with deficient cell-mediated immunity, *Arch Dermatol* 109:239-241, 1974.
90. Revuz J, Penso D, Roujeau JC et al.: Toxic epidermal necrolysis: Clinical findings and prognosis factors in 87 patients, *Arch Dermatol* 123:1160-1165, 1987.
91. Revuz J, Roujeau JC, Guillaume JC et al.: Treatment of toxic epidermal necrolysis: Créteil's experience, *Arch Dermatol* 123:1156-1158, 1987.
92. Richards JM, Romaine HH: Keratoconjunctivitis sicca: a sequela to purulent erythema exudativum multiforme (Stevens-Johnson's disease), *Am J Ophthalmol* 29:1121-1125, 1946.
93. Rohrer TE, Ahmed AR: Toxic epidermal necrolysis, *Int J Dermatol* 30:457-466, 1991.
94. Rothenberg R, Renna FS, Drew TM, Feingold DS: Staphylococcal scalded skin syndrome in an adult, *Arch Dermatol* 108:408-410, 1973.
95. Roujeau JC, Guillaume JC, Fabre JP et al.: Toxic epidermal necrolysis (Lyell syndrome): incidence and drug etiology in France, 1981-1985, *Arch Dermatol* 126:37-42, 1990.
96. Roujeau JC, Huynh TN, Bracq C et al.: Genetic susceptibility to toxic epidermal necrolysis, *Arch Dermatol* 123:1171-1173, 1987.
97. Roujeau JC, Moritz S, Guillaume JC et al.: Lymphopenia and abnormal balance of T-lymphocyte subpopulations in toxic epidermal necrolysis, *Arch Dermatol Res* 277:24-27, 1985.
98. Rubin Z: Ophthalmic sulfonamide-induced Stevens-Johnson syndrome, *Arch Dermatol* 113:235-236, 1977.
99. Ruiz-Maldonado R: Acute disseminated epidermal necrosis types 1, 2, and 3: study of sixty cases, *J Am Acad Dermatol* 13:623-635, 1985.
100. Renfro L, Grant-Kels JM, Daman LA: Drug-induced toxic epidermal necrolysis treated with cyclosprine, *Int J Dermatol* 28:441-444, 1989.
101. Robin JB, Dugel R: Immunologic disorders of the cornea and conjunctiva. In Kaufman HE, Barron BA, McDonald MV, Waltman SR, editors: *The cornea*, New York, 1988, Churchill Livingstone.
102. Safai B, Good RA, Day NK: Erythema multiforme: report of two cases and speculation on immune mechanisms involved in the pathogenesis, *Clin Immunol Immunopathol* 7:379-385, 1977.
103. Sakellariou G, Koukoudis P, Karpouzas J et al.: Plasma exchange (PE) treatment in drug-induced toxic epidermal necrolysis, *Int J Artif Organs* 14:634-638, 1991.
104. Schiodt M, Greenspan D, Daniels TE et al.: Parotid gland enlargement and xerostomia associated with labial sialadenitis in HIV-infected patients, *J Autoimmun* 2:415-425, 1989.
105. Schöph E, Stühmer A, Rzany B et al.: Toxic epidermal necrolysis and Stevens-Johnson syndrome: an epidemiologic study from West Germany, *Arch Dermatol* 127:839-842, 1991.
106. Shelley WB: Herpes simplex virus as a cause of erythema multiforme, *JAMA* 201(3):71-74, 1967.
107. Simons HW: Acute life-threatening dermatologic disorders, *Med Clin North Am* 65:227-243, 1981.
108. Singer L, Brook U, Romem M, Fried D: Vitamin A in Stevens-Johnson syndrome, *Ann Ophthalmol* 21:209-210, 1989.
109. Soong HK, Martin NF, Wagoner MD et al.: Topical retinoid therapy for squamous metaplasia of various ocular surface disorders: a multicenter, placebo-controlled double-masked study, *Ophthalmology* 95:1442-1446, 1988.
110. Stark HH: Membranous conjunctivitis of over four years' duration, *Am J Ophthalmol* 1:91, 1918.
111. Stevens AM, Johnson FC: A new eruptive fever associated with stomatitis and ophthalmia, *Am J Dis Child* 24:526-533, 1922.
112. Ström J: Herpes simplex virus as a course of allergic mucocutaneous reactions (ectodormosis erosiva plurioficialis, Stevens-Johnson's syndrome, etc.) and generalized infection, *Scand J Infect Dis* 1:3-10, 1969.
113. Swinehart JM, Weston WL, Huf C, McIntosh R: Identification of circulating immune complexes in erythema multiforme, *Clin Res* 26:577A, 1978.
114. Thoft RA: Keratoepithelioplasty, *Am J Ophthalmol* 97:1-6, 1984.
115. Ting HC, Adam BA: Erythema multiforme-response to corticosteroid, *Dermatologica* 169:175-178, 1984.
116. Tonnesen MG, Soter NA: Erythema multiforme, *J Am Acad Dermatol* 1:357-364, 1979.
117. Tseng SCG, Farazdaghi M: Reversal of conjunctival transdifferentiation by topical retinoic acid, *Cornea* 7:273-279, 1988.
118. Tseng SCG, Hirst LW, Farazdaghi M, Green WR: Inhibition of conjunctival transdifferentiation by topical retinoids, *Invest Ophthalmol Vis Sci* 28:538-542, 1987.
119. Tseng SCG, Maumenee AE, Stark WJ et al.: Topical retinoid treatment for various dry eye disorders, *Ophthalmology* 92:717-727, 1985.
120. Turgeon PW, Nauheim RC, Roat MI et al.: Indications for kerato-epithelioplasty, *Arch Ophthalmol* 108:233-236, 1990.
121. Weissman SS, Char DH, Herbort CP et al.: Alteration of human conjunctival proliferation, *Arch Ophthalmol* 110:357-359, 1992.
122. Wright P, Collin JR: The ocular complications of erythema multiforme (Stevens-Johnson syndrome) and their management, *Trans Ophthalmol Soc UK* 103:338-341, 1983.
123. Wuepper KD, Watson PA, Kazmierowski JA: Immune complexes in erythema multiforme and the Stevens-Johnson syndrome, *J Invest Dermatol* 74:368-371, 1980.
124. Yetiv JZ, Bianchine JR, Owen JA: Etiologic factors of the Stevens-Johnson syndrome, *South Med J* 73:599-602, 1980.

34 Ocular Complications of Bone Marrow Transplantation

DOUGLAS JABS

Since its initial clinical success in the 1970s, bone marrow transplantation (BMT) has been used increasingly for the treatment of aplastic anemia or hematologic malignancies that have relapsed or have a poor prognosis. Bone marrow transplantation consists of the obliteration of the patient's own bone marrow using cytoreductive chemotherapy and/or irradiation. This procedure is followed by transplantation of donor marrow to reconstitute the patient's (host's) hematologic and immune functions.

BONE MARROW TRANSPLANTATION

There are three types of bone marrow transplants: (1) autologous, in which the patient's own stored marrow is transplanted; (2) syngeneic, in which marrow from an identical twin is transplanted; and (3) allogeneic, in which marrow from an HLA-matched donor, such as a sibling, is used. More recently, HLA-"mismatched" transplants (in which there is a single antigen mismatch) and transplants from unrelated donors have been performed.

Preparative, marrow-ablative regimens are standardized according to the pretransplant diagnosis. Whereas these conditioning regimens are standardized within institutions —they vary among institutions—which may account for some of the differences in the various complications. At some centers, patients with aplastic anemia are treated with cyclophosphamide (50 mg/kg intravenously for 4 days).[12] Other common regimens include cyclophosphamide and total body irradiation (TBI). Patients with acute nonlymphocytic leukemia (for example, acute myelocytic leukemia), chronic myelogenous leukemia, or many types of lymphomas are treated with busulfan (4 mg/kg daily for 4 days), followed by cyclophosphamide (50 mg/kg intravenously, daily for 4 days).[25] Patients with acute lymphocytic leukemia (or with some types of lymphoma) are treated with cyclophosphamide (50 mg/kg intravenously, daily for 4 days), followed by total body irradiation (at 3 Gy daily for 4 days) with a lung shield for the third dose.[38]

For allogeneic and syngeneic transplants, marrow is harvested from the donor using multiple aspirations from the iliac bones in a sterile operating room. The pooled, aspirated marrow is passed through stainless-steel screens of successively smaller openings to produce a single-cell suspension. No long-lasting effects occur from the removal of a small fraction of the bone marrow—a rapidly replicating tissue —from the donor. For autologous transplants, bone marrow is harvested from the patient when he is in remission. Harvested bone marrow can then be "purged" using ex vivo treatment with medications such as 4-hydroperoxy-cyclophosphamide or with monoclonal antibodies.[41] After the conditioning regimen has been completed, bone marrow is infused into the recipient through a right atrial catheter. The donor bone marrow circulates and then lodges in the marrow cavity of the host. Once the marrow has engrafted, it begins to replicate and produce hematopoietic elements.

Indications

Bone marrow transplantation for severe aplastic anemia has revolutionized the treatment of this disease. In patients with untransfused aplastic anemia, the rate of 10-year actual survival is estimated to be 82%.[1,29] For children with acute lymphoblastic leukemia in second or subsequent remission, bone marrow transplantation appears superior to chemotherapy.[22] Patients with chronic myelogenous leukemia in the initial chronic phase have a 5-year survival rate of 50% to 70% following BMT.[16,33] Finally, for patients with acute myelogenous leukemia, BMT is associated with (1) a significantly lower rate of leukemic relapse than consolidation chemotherapy, and (2) possibly an improved 5-year survival rate.[6,25] Because of the ability to engraft enzymatically normal marrow cells, bone marrow transplantation is also being used investigationally in certain genetic storage diseases. In patients with leukemia—but without an HLA-matched donor—autologous transplantation using the patient's own marrow [after ex vivo treatment with chemotherapy (purging)] has produced results similar to allogeneic transplantation.[8,41] In addition, autologous BMT has been used in lymphoma and other solid tumors in an effort to deliver very high doses of chemotherapy followed by "marrow rescue."[8]

Complications

Although bone marrow transplantation has clearly improved the prognosis for many of these disorders, significant complications occur. Complications following bone marrow transplantation are generally divided into those that occur early (within the first 6 months after BMT), and those that occur late. Immediately following transplant and prior to recovery of the donor marrow in the host, there is a period of aplasia that may be associated with either hemorrhage or infection. During this time, patients receive vigorous transfusion support, including transfusions of packed red cells and platelets. In addition, patients are treated with standardized antibiotic protocols for the first fever and for persistent or recurrent fever in an effort to minimize bacterial and/or fungal infections during aplasia. Other potential early complications include toxicity from the chemotherapy, such as oropharyngeal mucositis and bladder toxicity caused by cyclophosphamide. Graft rejection, a major problem early in the history of BMT, has become much less common in recent years as a result of more effective conditioning regimens. Early herpetic infections, such as herpes simplex virus mucositis, have been largely abolished by prophylactic acyclovir.[6,31,35,39,40] Interstitial pneumonitis, often caused by cytomegalovirus, may occur and has been associated with mortality, despite treatment in some centers. Intrahepatic veno-occlusive disease occurs in approximately 5% of patients transplanted for malignancies and is related to the toxic effects of high-dose chemotherapy and radiation. In addition to the early aplasia, patients undergoing BMT have profound abnormalities of both T and B lymphocytes following successful engraftment. Recovery usually occurs between 6 and 12 months after transplant. Late infections with viruses, such as varicella-zoster virus are common.[31,40]

Graft-versus-Host Disease

The most problematic complication of bone marrow transplantation is graft-versus-host disease (GVHD), in which the immunocompetent graft mounts an immunologically mediated attack on the now immuno-incompetent host. Graft-versus-host disease has been classified clinically into two types: acute GVHD and chronic GVHD. Acute GVHD occurs within the first 100 days after transplant, whereas chronic GVHD occurs later. The two types of GVHD have distinct clinical paradigms, but the successful use of prophylactic agents for GVHD has blurred the traditional clinical pictures and timing.

PATHOGENESIS

There are three essential requirements for the induction of GVHD. As stated by Billingham,[4] they are: "1) the graft must contain immunologically-competent cells; 2) the host must possess important transplantation isoantigens that are lacking the graft donors, so that the host appears foreign to it, and is, therefore, capable of stimulating it antigenically; 3) the host must be incapable of mounting an effective immunologic reaction against the graft, at least for sufficient time for the latter to manifest its immunologic capabilities (i.e., must have security of tenure)."[4]

In allogeneic transplants, data have implicated minor histocompatibility antigens as the inciting antigens and cytotoxic T cells as the effectors of GVHD. The occurrence of syngeneic and autologous GVHD, however, suggests that GVHD is more complex than minor histocompatibility antigen recognition. Cytotoxic T cells recognizing self class II antigens are found in animals with syngeneic GVHD, and autoreactivity in normal animals and man can be demonstrated using autologous mixed lymphocyte reactions. Hence, syngeneic and autologous GVHD appear to represent the failure of the immune system to discriminate self from nonself, resulting in the generation of autoreactive cells.[37]

CLINICAL FEATURES

Acute Graft-versus-Host Disease

The earliest clinical manifestation of acute GVHD is usually a maculopapular skin rash. On average, the rash occurs 20 days after transplant. Symptoms include pruritus or a sunburn sensation. The rash has a typical distribution that begins with the palms, soles, and ears (Fig. 34-1). The trunk, face, and extremities become involved later as the rash progresses. In severe disease, bullous lesions with desquamation of the epidermis may be seen (Fig. 34-2).[6,37]

Other organs commonly linked with acute GVHD include the liver and the gastrointestinal tract (primarily the

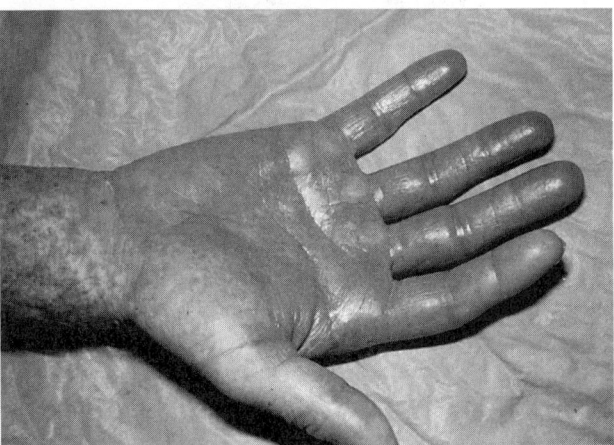

Fig. 34-1. Palm of a patient with acute graft-vs-host disease, showing intense erythema and edema. (From Vogelsang GB and associates.[37] Used with permission.)

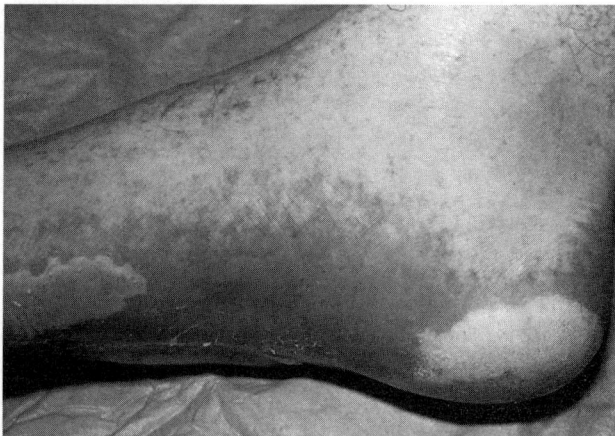

Fig. 34-2. Foot of a patient with acute graft-vs-host disease, showing erythema and blister formation on the sole with a macular rash involving the rest of the foot. (From Vogelsang GB and associates.[37] Used with permission.)

TABLE 34-1 CLINICAL STAGING OF ORGAN SYSTEM ACUTE GVHD

Organ System	Stage	Description
Skin	1	Maculopapular rash < 25% of body surface area
	2	Maculopapular rash 25-50% of surface area
	3	Generalized erythroderma (> 50% of body surface area)
	4	Generalized erythroderma with bulla formation
Liver	1	Bilirubin 2-3 mg/dl
	2	Bilirubin 3-6 mg/dl
	3	Bilirubin 6-15 mg/dl
	4	Bilirubin > 15 mg/dl
Intestinal tract	1	> 500 ml diarrhea/day
	2	> 1000 ml diarrhea/day
	3	> 1500 ml diarrhea/day
	4	severe abdominal pain with or without ileus

Modified from Thomas ED, Storb R, Clift RA and associates: Bone-marrow transplantation (second of two parts), *New Engl J Med* 1975, 202:895-902. Used with permission.

colon). Involvement of the liver by GVHD is manifested principally by an elevated bilirubin. Other liver function tests, such as transaminases, may also be abnormal. The differential diagnosis of liver GVHD includes veno-occlusive disease of the liver following transplant and viral hepatitis. A liver biopsy can establish the diagnosis of hepatic GVHD; histopathologically, hepatic GVHD is portrayed by a cholestatic picture with bile duct atypia and degeneration.[6,37]

Intestinal GVHD is characterized by diarrhea and crampy, abdominal pain. Intestinal GVHD is difficult to treat, in part because of the associated infectious complications. The distinction between infectious enteritis and intestinal GVHD may require a biopsy. Histopathologically, intestinal GVHD shows crypt cell necrosis. With increasing severity of disease, more extensive damage may occur, leading to crypt dropout. With severe intestinal GVHD, there is total loss of the intestinal epithelium.[37]

The severity of acute GVHD is classified as outlined in Tables 34-1 and 34-2.[34,35] Organ GVHD is staged according to the amount of organ involvement (Table 34-1), and the overall clinical GVHD is grouped in accordance with the severity of the overall disease process (Table 34-2). Cutaneous acute GVHD is staged in keeping with the extent of the skin disease, going from grade 1 (involvement of <25% of the body surface area) to grade 3 (generalized erythroderma), and grade 4 (bulla formation). Hepatic GVHD is staged to conform with the level of elevation of the bilirubin, whereas intestinal GVHD is staged according to the volume of diarrhea. The overall clinical stage is similarly graded on a 0 to IV scale based on the overall severity. It should be noted that stage I is cutaneous involvement only, whereas stages II and above have visceral or "systemic" involvement as well.

It is estimated that (1) half of the patients receiving an allogeneic BMT will develop some degree of acute GVHD, and (2) half of those patients will ultimately succumb to either the GVHD, its complications, it, or complications from the GVHD immunosuppressive therapy.[37]

Chronic Graft-versus-Host Disease

Chronic GVHD generally occurs 100 days or more after BMT. The clinical picture of chronic GVHD is markedly different from that of acute GVHD. Instead of an erythematous skin disease progressing to bulla formation, cutaneous association by chronic GVHD is usually characterized by either sclerodermatoid or lichenoid skin involvement.[28,31,32,37] Hepatic involvement in chronic GVHD is detected by abnormal liver function tests including elevations of alkaline phosphatase, transaminases, and bilirubin. Oral involvement may take two forms: (1) an inflammatory mu-

TABLE 34-2 OVERALL CLINICAL STAGING OF ACUTE GVHD

Clinical Stage	Stage of Organ Involvement			Decrease in Clinical Performance
	Skin	Liver	Intestinal Tract	
I	1-2	0	0	None
II	1-3	1	1	Mild
III	2-3	2-4	2-3	Marked
IV	2-4	2-4	2-4	Extreme

Modified from Thomas ED, Storb R, Clift RA and associates: Bone-marrow transplantation (second of two parts), *New Engl J Med* 1975, 202:895-902. Used with permission.

cositis that resembles oral lichen planus; and/or (2) a fibrosing sialoadenitis that resembles Sjögren syndrome and results in a dry mouth. Other manifestations include esophageal reflux, myositis, and fasciitis, resulting in contracture.[37]

Chronic GVHD develops in approximately 20% to 40% of recipients of allogeneic BMT. Chronic GVHD may occur (1) de novo (in which case there was no prior acute GVHD), (2) after a period of quiescent GVHD, or (3) after progressively evolving directly from poorly controlled acute GVHD. The most important risk factor for the development of chronic GVHD is a history of acute GVHD. The 10-year actual survival rate after the onset of chronic GVHD is approximately 40%.[37,39] Chronic GVHD with (1) a progressive presentation, (2) lichenoid changes on skin biopsy, or (3) liver involvement with an elevated serum bilirubin is predictive of an increased mortality.[39]

Ocular Graft-versus-Host Disease

Ocular complications are commonly observed in patients undergoing transplantation.[5,9,11,14,17-21] Whereas many of the early reports merely listed the different ocular complications, it later became evident that certain complications are caused directly by involvement of the conjunctiva by GVHD; and others are the result of the involvement of the lacrimal and salivary glands by GVHD. A characteristic finding of ocular association of acute GVHD is the development of conjunctivitis. Early conjunctival influence is manifested by erythema; and with more severe involvement, there is development of chemosis or a serosanguineous exudate, followed by pseudomembrane formation. The pseudomembranes consist of sloughed conjunctival epithelium. In the worst cases, pseudomembranous conjunctivitis is accompanied by sloughing of the corneal epithelium (Fig. 34-3). In this situation, only a thin rim of epithelium is left at the limbus. The process is analogous to cutaneous involvement by acute GVHD and can be staged (Table 34-3) in a manner analogous to other organ system involvement. Conjunctival involvement at stage 2 or greater occurs in 12% of patients with acute GVHD, is a marker for severe GVHD, and is

associated with a 90% mortality. In the study from Johns Hopkins, the median day of onset of conjunctival involvement was 14 days after the median onset of the patient's first manifestations of acute GVHD.[20] Median survival after the development of conjunctival involvement was 36 days.[20] This survival was similar to that for severe systemic GVHD, suggesting that conjunctival involvement at stage 2 or higher is a marker for severe systemic GVHD.[20]

Conjunctival involvement may also be seen in patients with chronic GVHD. In the study from Johns Hopkins, it occurred in 11% of patients with chronic GVHD and 2% of patients undergoing transplant.[20] In patients with chronic GVHD and conjunctival involvement, there was also severe systemic GVHD; although the survival implications were less clear than with conjunctival involvement by acute GVHD. Patients developing conjunctival involvement in association with chronic GVHD who survive, may develop a severe scarring reaction of the conjunctiva, similar to that seen with cicatricial pemphigoid (Fig. 34-4).

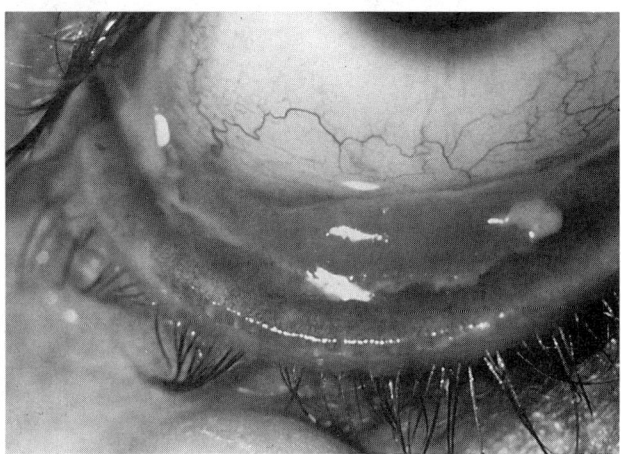

A

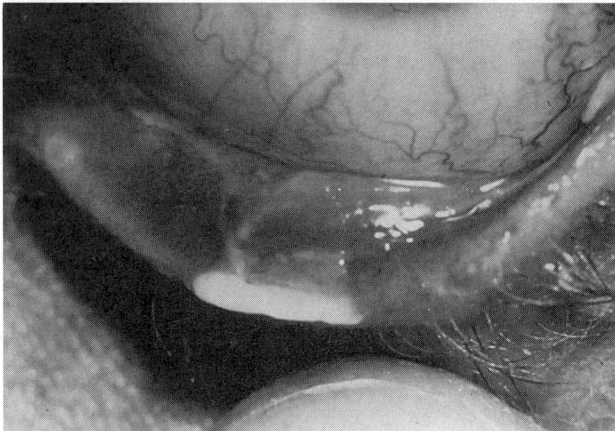

B

Fig. 34-3. Pseudomembranous conjunctivitis after bone marrow transplant. **A,** right eye and **B,** left eye, showing early changes;

Continued

TABLE 34-3 CLINICAL STAGING OF CONJUNCTIVAL GVHD

Stage	Description
1	Conjunctival hyperemia
2	Conjunctival hyperemia with chemotic response or serosanguineous exudate
3	Pseudomembranous conjunctivitis
4	Pseudomembranous conjunctivitis plus corneal epithelial slough

From Jabs DA, Wingard J, Green WR and associates: The eye in bone marrow transplantation. III. Conjunctival graft-versus-host disease, *Arch Ophthalmol* 1989, 107:1343-1348. Used with permission.

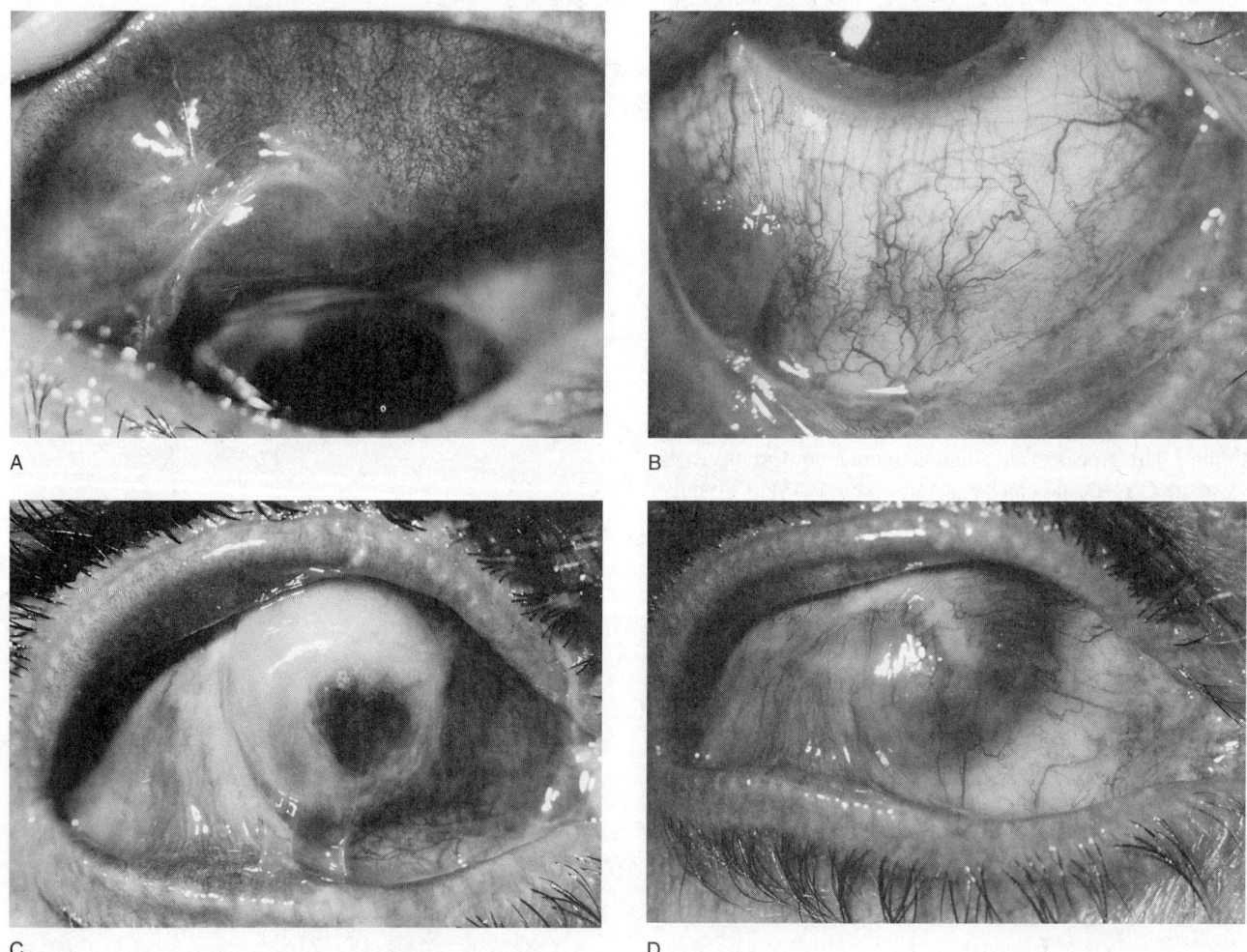

C

D

Fig. 34-3, cont'd. **C,** right eye and **D,** left eye, one month later with severe changes and Stage 4 disease. Conjunctival ulcerations are apparent along the lid margin, and only a rim of corneal epithelium remains. (From Jabs DA and associates.[20] Used with permission.)

A

B

C

D

Fig. 34-4. Conjunctival scarring after pseudomembranous conjunctivitis due to chronic graft-vs-host disease. **A** and **B,** early conjunctivitis; **C,** progressive scarring with pannus formation; **D,** end-stage process with ankyloblepharon.

The lacrimal gland also may be involved by either acute or chronic GVHD. In acute GVHD, there is often a stasis picture with large dilated ductules filled with inspissated material.[17,18] Electron microscopy can show large accumulations of granules in the apices in the secretory cells.[18] With chronic GVHD, there appears to be an inflammatory infiltrate into the lacrimal gland, resulting in lacrimal gland damage.[24] The long-term outcome of a drying trend in the early posttransplant period remains unclear. In patients with chronic GVHD who develop dry eyes, however, the probability of recovery of tear function appears low. Approximately 50% of patients with chronic GVHD will develop dry eyes and a Sjögren-like picture.[32]

PATHOLOGY

Because cutaneous involvement is almost always seen in patients with acute GVHD, and because the skin biopsy is relatively easy to perform; grading of the histologic severity of GVHD on the skin biopsy has become a widely accepted clinical tool. A standardized grading system for cutaneous involvement is outlined in Table 34-4.[13,35] Early changes are nonspecific and include basal epithelial vacuolization and the migration of lymphocytes into the epithelial layer. With more advanced disease, there are the specific findings of dyskeratotic cells in the epithelium that may progress to microvesiculation, and finally to desquamation and loss of the epidermis.[13,35] As noted previously, in acute GVHD, the pathologic finding in the liver is a cholestatic picture. In the intestine, it is one of epithelial necrosis, and with severe disease—desquamation.[35,37]

Research with a limited number of conjunctival biopsies and with autopsy data suggests that the findings in the conjunctiva of patients with conjunctival involvement by acute GVHD are similar to those in the skin (Fig. 34-5).* It appears that the cutaneous grading system for histologic changes can also be used for the conjunctiva.[18,20] In particular, pseudomembranous conjunctivitis is histologically grade 4 disease, as there is a desquamation of the conjunctival epithelium (Fig. 34-6).

The cutaneous pathologic feature of chronic GVHD is either one of a scleroderma-like skin reaction or a lichenoid skin reaction, similar to lichen planus. Because dry eyes as a consequence of lacrimal gland damage are the most common ocular complication of chronic GVHD, the pathologic feature most often identified in the conjunctiva is one of keratinization caused by a chronic dry eye picture.[18] In patients with active chronic GVHD and dry eyes, a minor salivary gland biopsy will often show a mononuclear cell inflammatory infiltrate.[24]

---

*Unpublished data.

TABLE 34-4 HISTOLOGICAL GRADING OF CUTANEOUS ACUTE GVHD

Grade	Description
1	Basal epithelial vacuolization; lymphocyte migration into epithelium
2	Dyskeratosis
3	Microvesiculation
4	Epidermal loss

Modified from Thomas ED, Storb R, Clift RA and associates: Bone-marrow transplantation (second of two parts). *N Engl J Med* 1975, 202:895-902. Used with permission.

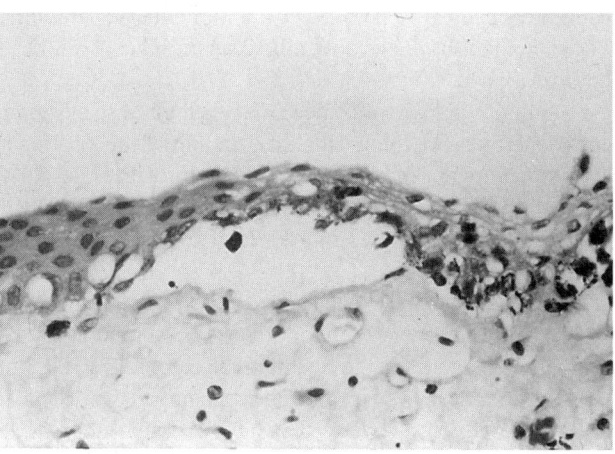

Fig. 34-5. Lymphocyte migration into the basal layer and microvesiculation of the conjunctiva with acute graft-vs-host disease (hematoxylin and eosin, X410). (From Jabs DA and associates.[18] Used with permission.)

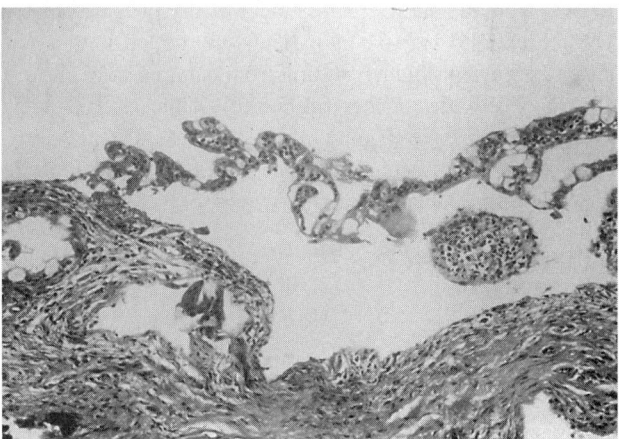

Fig. 34-6. Grade 4 conjunctival changes due to acute graft-vs-host disease, showing an inflammatory infiltrate in the substantia propria and separation of the conjunctival epithelium (hematoxylin and eosin, X130). (From Jabs DA and associates.[20] Used with permission.)

THERAPY

All patients undergoing bone marrow transplantation receive prophylaxis with medications to prevent the development of GVHD. Although early in the history of BMT, immunosuppressive drugs such as methotrexate or cyclophosphamide were used, the prophylaxis of GVHD has been revolutionized by the use of cyclosporine. Cyclosporine, when given in combination with other agents, markedly decreases the severity of acute GVHD and is now the most commonly used agent.[26] Cyclosporine is started at the time of transplantation and continued until 6 months after transplant. At that time, if there is no evidence of active GVHD, it is discontinued. Another strategy for the prophylaxis of GVHD is the purging of donor marrow of lymphocytes using mechanical separation or antithymocyte globulin. These methods have met with mixed success, but continue to be investigated.[36]

The initial therapy of acute GVHD is high-dose systemic corticosteroids. At Johns Hopkins, the initial protocol consists of 2.5 mg/kg of intravenous methylprednisolone for 4 days, followed by a tapering schedule. Refractory GVHD is treated either with increasing doses of cyclosporine or antithymocyte globulin.

The initial therapy of chronic GVHD is oral corticosteroids.[32] More recently, thalidomide has been used as an investigational agent for the treatment of chronic GVHD, but its relative efficacy is currently being compared in clinical trials to that of corticosteroids and immunosuppressive drugs.[36]

In patients who develop ocular complications of GVHD, the treatment is that of the underlying systemic disease. Topical corticosteroids have little effect on the treatment of the pseudomembranous conjunctivitis in association with GVHD.* Similarly, local antiinflammatory therapy appears to play a small role in the treatment of dry eyes associated with chronic GVHD. Many patients will be left with a persistent dry eye problem resulting from damage from chronic GVHD, even after successful control of the GVHD using immunosuppressive therapy. The liberal use of tear substitutes and punctal occlusion when necessary, contribute to the long-term management of dry eyes.

COMPLICATIONS

Cataract

Cataracts are a common complication after bone marrow transplantation. Cataracts may be attributable to a variety of causes, including the use of systemic corticosteroids and total body irradiation. Fractionated radiation has markedly reduced the incidence of cataracts. In an early study from Seattle, patients receiving single-dose total body irradiation developed cataracts with an incidence of 75% at 6 years, whereas those receiving fractionated total body irradiation had a projected incidence of only 25% at 5 years.[10,31] In a more recent study from Johns Hopkins, cataracts developed in only 10% of the group.[11] A univariate analysis suggested that chronic GVHD, steroid therapy, and total body irradiation were all risk factors for the subsequent development of cataracts. In the multivariate analysis, only chronic GVHD and steroid therapy were significantly associated. For those not receiving corticosteroids, the projected incidence of cataracts at 5 years was 5% to 8% (no TBI versus TBI); and for those receiving corticosteroids, the probability of cataracts was 23% to 26% (no TBI versus TBI). In this study, fractionated TBI was given to all patients.[11]

Ocular Infection

Bacterial infections in the eye following transplantation are uncommon in the early posttransplant period, presumably because of the aggressive use of systemic antibiotics for the first fever. In a series of nearly 400 patients from Johns Hopkins, there were no cases of bacterial endophthalmitis following BMT.[9] Fungal retinitis and/or endophthalmitis is the most common ocular infection observed in patients undergoing BMT. In a prospective series of patients undergoing BMT at Johns Hopkins and followed weekly during the early post transplant period, 4% developed fungal endophthalmitis.[17] A later retrospective series gave an estimate of 1.5%.[9] Candidal endophthalmitis was the most common cause, but aspergillus endophthalmitis was also seen.[9] Late infectious complications of BMT include viral retinitis, with either varicella-zoster virus (VZV) or with cytomegalovirus (CMV). Both CMV and VZV retinitis are uncommon, occurring in less than 0.5% of patients undergoing transplant.[9,19] Toxoplasmic retinitis may also be a late complication after BMT. Toxoplasmic retinitis after BMT occurs in less than 0.5% of BMT patients; but the clinical picture may be atypical and coexistent central nervous system toxoplasmosis may be present.[9]

Retinopathy

Leukemia patients who undergo transplantation may develop an occlusive microvasculopathy.* Prevalence estimates for retinopathy have varied from 4% to 10%.[3,9] The pathogenesis appears to be multifactorial. In a study from Johns Hopkins, only chronic GVHD was a significantly associated risk factor, with an odds ratio of 4.7.[9] Other studies have suggested that cyclosporine and/or chemotherapy and total body irradiation may contribute to the problem.[3,15,23] In the series from Johns Hopkins,[9] the lesions generally resolved without long-term sequelae. In the series of eight patients with "BMT retinopathy" from Emory[23] (where the

---

*Unpublished data.

*References 3, 5, 9, 15, 23, 30.

preparative regimen was high-dose cytarabine hydrochloride and TBI) proliferative retinopathy developed in one patient, and macular edema in four.

Other Complications

Other ocular complications have included intraretinal and vitreous hemorrhages during the early posttransplant period, associated with the aplasia immediately after BMT. These hemorrhages have generally resolved without long-term sequelae.[9] Subconjunctival hemorrhages are commonly seen during this time period as well, and also resolve without sequelae.[18] Occasionally, relapses of the leukemia may occur in the eye.[9,27] In these situations, aggressive diagnostic procedures, such as paracentesis, diagnostic vitrectomy, and/or retinal biopsy may be necessary to establish the proper diagnosis. Indeed, early relapse of leukemia may simulate fungal endophthalmitis.[9]

An optic neuropathy, presumably secondary to cyclosporine, has also been reported and occurs in approximately 2% of patients undergoing transplantation.[2,9] This optic neuropathy is characterized by bilateral optic disc edema, usually without visual loss, and resolves with discontinuation of cyclosporine.[2] Other causes of papilledema in patients undergoing BMT include meningitis, intracerebral bleed, and central nervous system leukemic relapse. Serous retinal detachments associated with disseminated intravascular coagulopathy occur in approximately 0.5% of patients undergoing transplant.[9]

REFERENCES

1. Anasetti C, Doney KC, Storb R et al.: Marrow transplantation for severe aplastic anemia: long-term outcome in fifty "untransfused" patients, *Ann Intern Med* 104:461-466, 1986.
2. Avery R, Jabs DA, Wingard JR et al.: Optic disc edema after bone marrow transplantation, *Ophthalmology* 98:1294-1301, 1991.
3. Bernauer W, Gratwohl A, Keller A et al.: Microvasculopathy in the ocular fundus after bone marrow transplantation, *Ann Intern Med* 115:925-930, 1991.
4. Billingham RE: The biology of graft-versus-host reactions, *Harvey Lec* 62:21-78, 1966-67.
5. Bray LC, Carey PJ, Proctor SJ et al.: Ocular complications of bone marrow transplantation, *Br J Ophthalmol* 75:611-614, 1991.
6. Champlin RE, Gale RP: The early complications of bone marrow transplantation, *Semin Hematol* 2:101-108, 1984.
7. Champlin RE, Ho WG, Gale RP et al.: Treatment of acute myelogenous leukemia: a prospective controlled trial of bone marrow transplantation versus consolidation chemotherapy, *Ann Intern Med* 102:285-291, 1985.
8. Cheson BD, Lacerna L, Leyland-Jones B: Autologous bone marrow transplantation: current status and future directions, *Ann Intern Med* 110:51-56, 1989.
9. Coskuncan NM, Jabs DA, Dunn JP et al.: The eye in bone marrow transplantation. VI. Retinal complications, *Arch Ophthalmol* 112:372-379, 1994.
10. Deeg HJ, Flournoy N, Sullivan KM et al.: Cataracts after total body irradiation and marrow transplantation: a sparing effect of dose fractionation, *Int J Radiat Oncol Biol Phys* 10:957-964, 1984.
11. Dunn JP, Jabs DA, Wingard J et al.: The eye in bone marrow transplantation. V. Cataracts after bone marrow transplantation, *Arch Ophthalmol* 111:1367-1373, 1993.

12. Elfenbein GJ, Mellits ED, Santos GW: Patients with aplastic anemia: engraftment and survival after allogeneic bone marrow transplantation for severe aplastic anemia, *Transplant Proc* 15:1412-1416, 1983.
13. Farmer ER: The histopathology of graft-vs-host disease, *Adv Dermatol* 1:173-188, 1986.
14. Franklin RM, Kenyon KR, Tutschka PJ et al.: Ocular manifestations of graft-vs-host disease, *Ophthalmology* 90:4-13, 1983.
15. Gloor B, Gratwohl A, Hahn H et al.: Multiple cotton wool spots following bone marrow transplantation for treatment of acute lymphatic leukaemia, *Br J Ophthalmol* 69:320-325, 1985.
16. Goldman JM, Apperley JF, Jones L et al.: Bone marrow transplantation for patients with chronic myeloid leukemia, *New Eng J Med* 314:202-207, 1986.
17. Hirst LW, Jabs DA, Tutschka PJ et al.: The eye in bone marrow transplantation. I. Clinical study, *Arch Ophthalmol* 101:580-584, 1983.
18. Jabs DA, Hirst LW, Green WR et al.: The eye in bone marrow transplantation. II. Histology, *Arch Ophthalmol* 101:585-590, 1983.
19. Jabs DA, Wingard JR, de Bustros S et al.: BW B759U for cytomegalovirus retinitis: intraocular drug penetration, *Arch Ophthalmol* 104:1436-1437, 1986.
20. Jabs DA, Wingard JR, Green WR et al.: The eye in bone marrow transplantation. III. Conjunctival graft vs host-disease, *Arch Ophthalmol* 107:1343-1348, 1989.
21. Jack MK, Jack GM, Sale GE et al.: Ocular manifestations of graft-v-host disease, *Arch Ophthalmol* 101:1080-1084, 1983.
22. Johnson FL, Thomas ED, Clark BS et al.: A comparison of marrow transplantation with chemotherapy for children with acute lymphoblastic leukemia in second or subsequent remission, *New Eng J Med* 305:846-851, 1981.
23. Lopez PF, Sternberg P, Dabbs CK et al.: Bone marrow transplant retinopathy, *Am J Ophthalmol* 112:635-646, 1991.
24. Sale GE, Shulman HM, Schubert MM et al.: Oral and ophthalmic pathology of graft versus host disease in man: predictive value of the lip biopsy, *Hum Pathol* 12:1022-1030, 1981.
25. Santos GW, Tutschka PJ, Brookmeyer R et al.: Marrow transplantation for acute nonlymphocytic leukemia after treatment with busulfan and cyclophosphamide, *New Eng J Med* 309:1347-1353, 1983.
26. Santos GW, Tutschka PJ, Brookmeyer R et al.: Cyclosporine plus methylprednisolone versus cyclophosphamide plus methylprednisolone as prophylaxis for graft vs. host disease: a randomized double-blind study in patients undergoing allogeneic marrow transplantation, *Clin Transplant* 1:21-28, 1987.
27. Schachat AP, Jabs DA, Graham ML et al.: Leukemic iris infiltration, *J Pediatr Ophthalmol Strabismus* 25:135-138, 1988.
28. Shulman HM, Sullivan KM, Weiden PL et al.: Chronic graft-versus-host syndrome in man: a long-term clinicopathologic study of 20 Seattle patients, *Am J Med* 69:204-217, 1980.
29. Storb R, Prentice RL, Buckner CD et al.: Graft-versus-host disease and survival in patients with aplastic anemia treated by marrow grafts from HLA-identical siblings, *New Eng J Med* 308:302-307, 1983.
30. Stuckenschneider BJ, Meiler WF: Ocular findings following bone marrow transplantation, *Ophthalmology* 92(suppl):152, 1992 (abstract).
31. Sullivan KM, Deeg HJ, Sanders JE et al.: Late complications after marrow transplantation, *Semin Hematol* 21:53-63, 1984.
32. Sullivan KM, Shulman HM, Storb R et al.: Chronic graft-versus-host disease in 52 patients: adverse natural course and successful treatment with combination immunosuppression, *Blood* 57:267-276, 1981.
33. Thomas ED, Clift RA, Fefer A et al.: Marrow transplantation for the treatment of chronic myelogenous leukemia, *Ann Intern Med* 104:155-163, 1986.
34. Thomas ED, Storb R, Clift RA et al.: Bone-marrow transplantation (first of two parts), *New Eng J Med* 292:832-843, 1975.
35. Thomas ED, Storb R, Clift RA et al.: Bone-marrow transplantation (second of two parts), *New Eng J Med* 202:895-902, 1975.
36. Vogelsang GB, Farmer ER, Hess AD et al.: Thalidomide for the treatment of chronic graft-versus-host disease, *New Eng J Med* 326:1055-1058, 1992.
37. Vogelsang GB, Hess AD, Santos GW et al.: Acute graft-versus-host disease: clinical characteristics in the cyclosporine era, *Medicine* 67:163-174, 1988.

38. Wingard JR, Piantadosi S, Santos GW et al.: Allogeneic bone marrow transplantation for patients with high-risk acute lymphoblastic leukemia, *J Clin Oncol* 8:820-830, 1990.

39. Wingard JR, Piantadosi S, Vogelsang GB et al.: Predictors of death from chronic graft-versus-host disease after bone marrow transplantation, *Blood* 74:1428-1435, 1989.

40. Winston DJ, Gale RP, Meyer DV et al.: Infectious complications of human bone marrow transplantation, *Medicine* 58:1-31, 1979.

41. Yeager AM, Kaizer H, Santos GW et al.: Autologous bone marrow transplantation in patients with acute nonlymphocytic leukemia, using ex vivo marrow treatment with 4-hydroperoxy-cyclophosphamide, *New Eng J Med* 315:141-147, 1985.

35 Corneal Allograft Rejection

GARY N. FOULKS, JERRY Y. NIEDERKORN, FRED SANFILIPPO

Corneal transplantation is one of the most successful transplants accomplished in humans, yet corneal allograft rejection continues to be the most common cause of corneal graft failure.[62] With over 40,000 corneal grafts performed annually in the United States, the reported incidence of allograft rejection has decreased over the past 20 years from 44% to the present range of 5% to 15%—depending on the disease being treated and the overall health of the eye.[3,31,41,91]

Although some of the improvement in graft survival certainly is the result of better surgical techniques, early recognition and aggressive therapy of allograft rejection reaction represent the most significant advances in achieving successful corneal transplantation. Local immunosuppression with topical corticosteroids has been the mainstay of therapy, but selective systemic use of corticosteroids has become an integral part of the management of severe allograft reactions. The newer immunosuppressive agents look promising, yet the limited understanding of the mechanism of action of these agents and their potential toxicities restricts their usefulness. Although much has been learned about the immunologic characteristics of the eye (in general) and allograft rejection reaction (in particular), the lack of understanding of the process of allograft rejection in the cornea limits the ability to prevent immunologically mediated corneal graft failure.

HISTORICAL BACKGROUND

A brief historic review highlights the progress achieved in understanding and preventing corneal allograft rejection. In 1948 Paufique, Sourdille, and Offret[55] viewed graft failure (''maladie du greffon'') as an opacification of the graft occurring after an interval of clarity, and they suggested host sensitivity to the donor as the cause. Maumenee[71] confirmed that sensitization of the host to the donor was the underlying basis of this graft outcome. Maumenee[72,73] also extensively characterized the clinical features of corneal allograft failure in the 1960s, emphasizing the importance of the endothelium as a target of immunologic attack. In the late 1960s

Silverstein and Khodadoust[64] demonstrated the clinical and histopathologic events of allograft rejection in experimental animals and observed that each layer of the cornea (epithelium, stroma, and endothelium) could induce host sensitization and undergo allograft rejection individually or in concert. Polack[92] extended these observations and determined experimentally the fate of the various layers of the transplanted cornea. Polack's work[92] showed that there was a rapid turnover of epithelial components, but that stromal and endothelial tissues persisted and remained subject to immunologic attack. Subsequent allograft rejection was therefore thought to be a form of delayed hypersensitivity.

Further characterization of corneal allograft survival by analysis of clinical risk factors occurred in the 1970s and 1980s through the work of Casey[6] in England, Volker-Dieben[124] in the Netherlands, Arentsen[3] in the United States, and later by Boisjoly[10] in Canada. This research confirmed the higher risk associated with vascularization of the host cornea either preoperatively or postoperatively.[84] An early clinical observation that larger diameter corneal grafts were more prone to rejection was initially explained by proximity of the graft-host junction to the limbal vasculature.[9,20] Studies by Gillete and Chandler,[42] however, suggested that (1) the presence of Langerhans cells in the peripheral cornea could also account for this finding, and (2) the occurrence of such cells in the central cornea might increase the risk of allograft rejection. The presence of preexisting inflammation in the eye also correlated with graft reaction, as did the presence of iris synechiae to the graft-host junction.[3,89] Loose sutures, whether by induction of vascularization or localized inflammation, also increase the risk of rejection.[84] Several studies documented a higher risk of rejection in younger recipients.[3,10]

Attempts to improve the success rate of corneal transplantation by applying histocompatibility strategies used in solid organ transplantation advanced understanding of the rejection process. This progression took place despite the fact that the results of HLA matching of the donor tissue and the recipient patient were found to be beneficial by some investigators,[6,9,103,124,125] but not by others.[1,21,110] Certain immunologic risk factors are reflected in serologic presensitization to histocompatibility antigens with lymphocytotoxic antibodies and with antibodies to minor transplantation antigens. These risks have correlated with reduced graft survival in some studies.[46,83,101]

CLINICAL FEATURES

The classic clinical characteristics of corneal allograft rejection are those of inflammation. Conjunctival and episcleral vascular engorgement, particularly in the circumcorneal vessels, is one of the earliest clinical signs of rejection (Fig. 35-1). The accumulation of leukocytes (predominantly lymphocytes) can appear in the epithelium (Fig. 35-2). Similar inflammatory cell infiltrates can occur in the anterior chamber, with focal aggregations on the endothelium (keratic precipitates, Fig. 35-3), and may progress to linear accumulations on the endothelium (Khodadoust line, Fig. 35-4). As these cells march across the corneal endothelium (destroying corneal endothelial cells), interstitial edema in the corneal stroma ensues, and epithelial edema subsequently occurs. Occasionally, focal greyish-white infiltrates (resembling those observed in viral epidemic keratoconjunctivitis) will appear in the subepithelial anterior stroma; such infiltrates can precede or coincide with the other features of corneal allograft rejection (Fig. 35-5).[40] Arentsen[3] and Allredge and Krachmer[2] chronicled the incidence and concurrence of these clinical features. Epithelial rejection occurs in about 10% to 14% of corneal grafts and usually precedes other more destructive rejection events. Subepithelial infiltrates are often subtle and evanescent, and therefore occur less frequently in about 2% to 15% of grafts. They can occur concurrently with epithelial or endothelial rejection lines, but they also may be an early harbinger of a more aggressive reaction and should be treated accordingly. En-

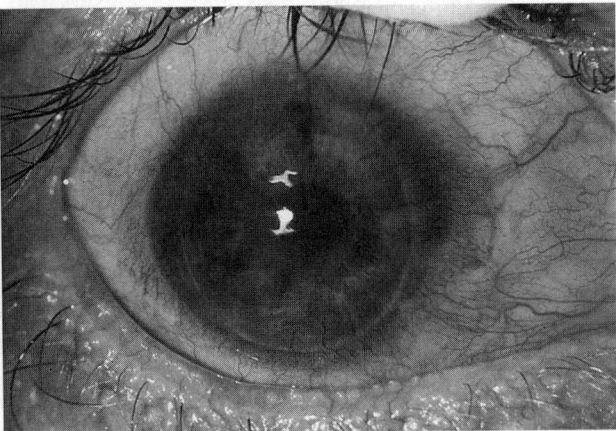

Fig. 35-1. Circumcorneal conjunctival and episcleral vascular engorgement as an early clinical sign of corneal allograft rejection.

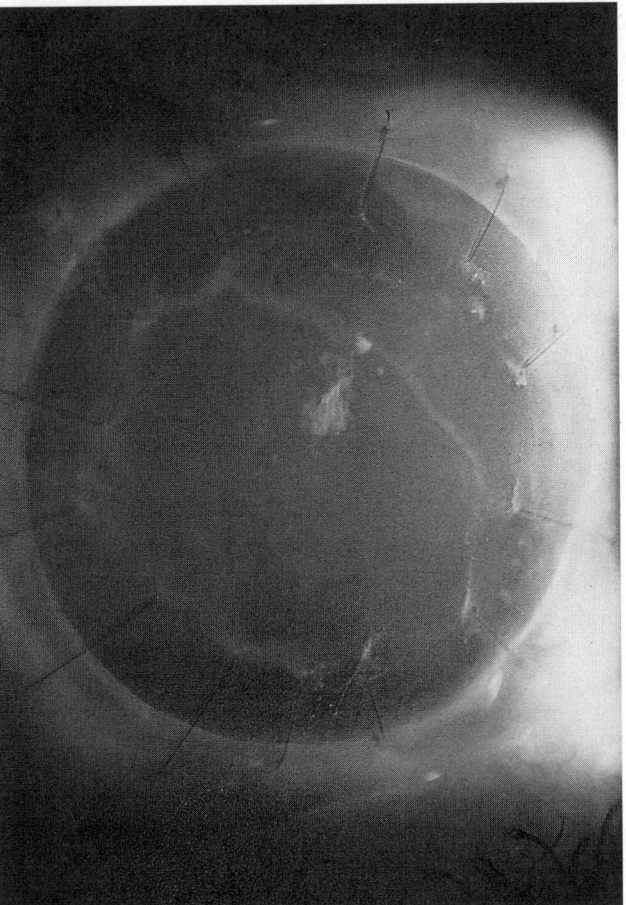

Fig. 35-2. Leukocytes infiltrating the epithelium in an epithelial rejection line as a sign of epithelial rejection.

dothelial rejection occurs in from 12% to 44% of grafts with endothelial keratic precipitates that can evolve to definable rejection lines in about 45% of episodes.[3] Inflammatory cells can infiltrate the corneal stroma directly. Symptomatically, all these signs of allograft rejection can be accompanied by the symptoms of a red eye, decreased vision, photophobia, and discomfort.

Other manifestations of corneal allograft rejection are less common, but highly important, because they pose other risks to the graft and the eye in general. Elevated intraocular pressure can occur either as a premonitory sign or during active rejection, and it probably results from edema in the trabecular meshwork tissue during the early stages of the inflammatory response.[35,93] The pressure elevation can be high enough to cause pain and, if prolonged, can damage the optic nerve.

Acute defects and erosions in the corneal epithelium can be a manifestation of allograft rejection that occurs commonly in the very young patient.[114] The epithelial defect can predispose to further corneal infiltration with inflammatory cells, secondary infection, or aggravated corneal vascular-

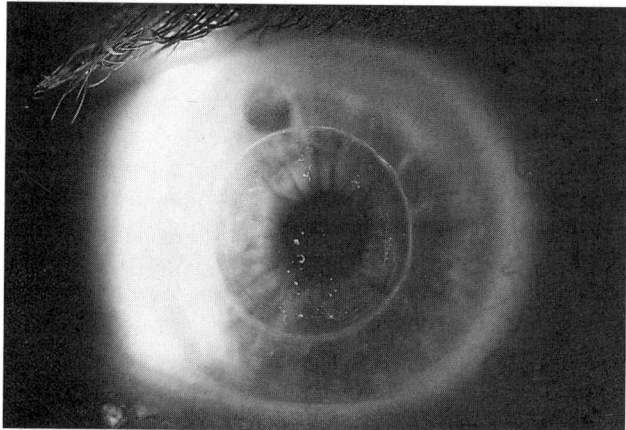

Fig. 35-3. Keratic precipitates (leukocytes) deposited on the endothelium as part of an allograft rejection reaction.

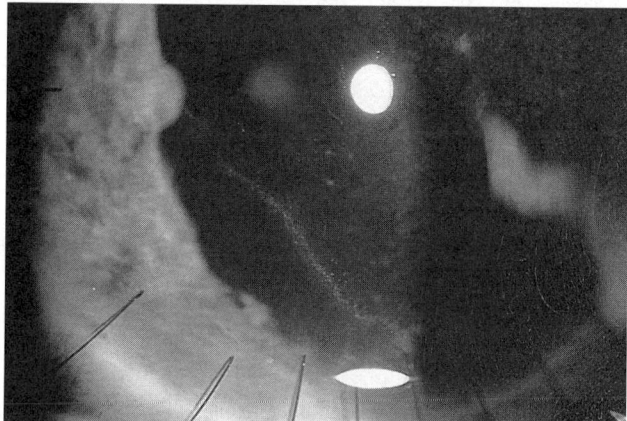

Fig. 35-4. Linear distribution of keratic precipitates (leukocytes) on the corneal endothelium as a clinical sign of endothelial rejection (Khodadoust Line). (Figure also in color insert.)

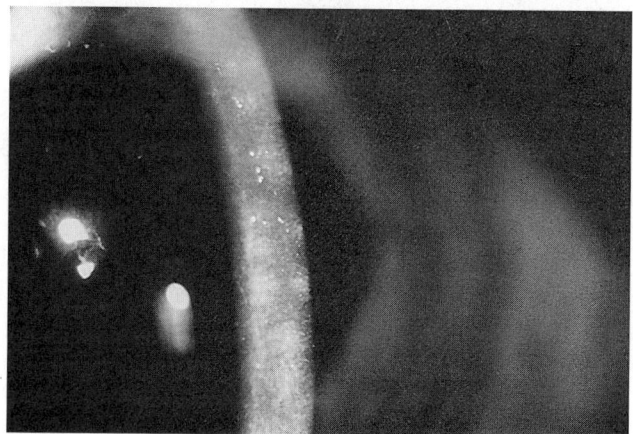

Fig. 35-5. Subepithelial infiltrates present in the anterior cornea as an early sign of corneal allograft rejection. (Figure also in color insert.)

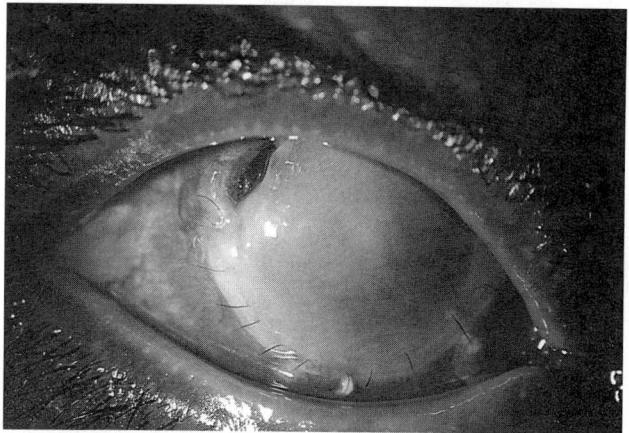

Fig. 35-6. Keratolysis of the edge of the corneal graft in a young, black patient with keratoconus occurring as part of the corneal allograft rejection.

ization. The occurrence of such an epithelial defect in the peripheral cornea, particularly in young black males receiving grafts for treatment of keratoconus, can result in lysis of the stroma with resultant corneal melting to the point of perforation (Fig. 35-6).[36] Even in the absence of epithelial defects, the allograft reaction can result in neovascularization and invade the corneal stroma.

RISK FACTORS

Avascularity of the cornea is probably the major reason that corneal transplantation is generally so successful. Indeed, numerous studies have confirmed the increased risk of rejection associated with corneal stromal vascularization, whether it be preoperative or postoperative vascularization.[34,84] The risk incurred by vascularization is probably the result of enhanced access to the tissue by both afferent and efferent arms of the immune response.[65] Blood vessels into the cornea certainly facilitate access of immune-competent cells (capable of antigen recognition) and effector cells (such as activated lymphocytes).[90] The presence of lymphatic channels in association with the new blood vessels also adds a route for enhanced immune recognition and stimulation. Likewise, iris synechiae to the graft-host junction increase the risk of rejection.[3]

Alterations of the cellular composition of the cornea can increase the risk of rejection, and certain disease states are more apt to produce such changes. Chemical burns and inflammatory disease often result in accumulation of inflammatory cells and increase the risk of rejection.[128] Langerhans cells that serve as effective antigen-presentation cells can be induced in the cornea and can facilitate rejection.[98]

Prior allograft rejection failure is well recognized as a major risk factor for subsequent rejection.[62] Recent studies suggest that such patients (who have been presensitized to major histocompatibility antigens as manifested by the presence of circulating lymphocytotoxic antibodies to class I and class II HLA antigens) may be at increased risk of both allograft rejection and immune-mediated rejection.[46,111] Similarly, sensitization to minor histocompatibility antigens is associated with increased graft rejection[77]; and multiple minor histocompatibility antigens can serve as excellent targets for allodestructive immune responses.[59a,61,98,107] Donor-recipient ABO blood group incompatibility may also be associated with increased corneal graft rejection.[21]

LABORATORY INVESTIGATIONS

Recognition of specific antigens in the donor tissue initiates the afferent arc of the immune response. The cornea has both antigenic and immunogenic specificities that are expressed in constitutive and inducible phases. The expressed antigens are structural proteins, hematopoetic cell-derived antigens, intercellular adhesion molecules, and histocompatibility antigens.[30,39,119,120,127] Recognition of the transplanted antigen by an effective antigen-presenting or antigen-processing cell (through intercellular adhesion) allows subsequent communication to specific lymphocyte subsets (Th cells). These subsets, when activated, produce cytokines that induce T lymphocytes capable of direct cellular attack on target cells. The cytokines also induce B lymphocytes (capable of elaborating antibodies directed against the recognized antigen) to produce direct damage or damage by antibody dependent cell-mediated cytolysis (ADCC). The antibodies also may recruit other immune cells or provoke additional inflammation. Whereas corneal graft damage is thought primarily to be mediated by cellular response,[13] considerable evidence exists to implicate the humoral response as well.[29,44,46,109,121]

In spite of the extraordinary success of corneal allografts, a significant number of grafts fail because of immunologic rejection. Early investigations in a rabbit model of keratoplasty revealed that all three layers of the corneal graft were vulnerable to immunologic rejection.[64] The adherence of lymphocytes to the corneal endothelium and the subsequent piecemeal necrosis of the endothelial cells suggest that cytotoxic T lymphocytes mediate corneal graft rejection. The infiltration of macrophages and the extensive necrosis that occurs in the stroma, however, indicate a possible role for delayed-type hypersensitivity (DTH). Thus simple histopathologic tools have failed to provide conclusive evidence as to the mechanism of rejection or the identity of the immune cells that mediate this process. In an effort to resolve this dilemma, investigators employed four basic strategies: (1) immunohistochemical identification of immune cells that infiltrate a rejecting human or rodent corneal allograft; (2) functional analysis of allospecific immune responses in experimental animals before, during, and after corneal allograft rejection; (3) adoptive transfer of selectively depleted lymphoid cell suspensions to immune-compromised rodents prior to corneal transplantation; and (4) selective in vivo depletion of T cell subsets prior to corneal transplantation in rodents.

The most direct approach for identifying the cellular immune elements involved in corneal graft rejection is simply to examine the rejecting corneal allografts and determine the phenotype of the infiltrating cells. This determination can be made by immunohistologic staining with monoclonal antibodies that recognize specific leukocyte populations. This approach assumes that a predominance of a specific leukocyte population in rejecting corneal allografts is conclusive evidence for cause and effect. The presence of a given leukocyte subset does not necessarily indicate if the cell population found in a rejected graft initiated rejection or simply entered the graft in response to rejection. Moreover, the immune system displays extraordinary versatility such that rigidly assigning a T cell phenotype to a specific effector function can lead to erroneous conclusions. Although CD8[+] cells are often considered classical cytotoxic T lymphocytes (CTL),[17] some CD4[+] T lymphocyte populations can express cytotoxic functions.[8,12] Likewise, some CD8[+] T lymphocyte populations can produce DTH lesions.[76,130] Examination of biopsy specimens of rejecting corneal allografts has revealed a mixed cellular infiltrate comprised of both CD4[+] and CD8[+] T lymphocytes and macrophages.[87,88] Similar findings were reported in heterotopic and orthotopic corneal allografts in rats.[57,116] Thus although in situ analyses of rejecting corneal allografts (in both humans and rodents) consistently find a mixed inflammatory infiltrate predominantly comprised of CD4[+] T lymphocytes, CD8[+] T lymphocytes, and macrophages; these analyses have not revealed the exact mechanism of rejection nor firmly established which populations mediate tissue damage.

A second, albeit less direct, approach for identifying the mechanism of corneal allograft rejection is to evaluate allospecific immune effector functions before, during, and after rejection. This strategy assumes that a sharp increase in the relevant immune effector function either precedes or coincides with corneal graft rejection. Studies using heterotopic corneal allografts in mice[86] and rats[16] indicated that allospecific CTL responses coincided with graft rejection. Interestingly, DTH responses to donor alloantigens were not detected before, during, nor after the rejection of murine heterotopic allografts.[86] Similar results were reported with a rat orthotopic corneal allograft model in which allospecific CTL responses peaked at the time of corneal allograft rejection, yet systemic allospecific DTH responses were undetectable.[16] The inability to detect systemic DTH responsiveness to donor alloantigens before, during, or after heterotopic corneal graft rejection initially suggested that DTH was not directly involved in this process.[86] However, subsequent studies revealed that under certain conditions heterotopic corneal allografts could induce strong donor-specific DTH.[77a] Indirect evidence also suggests that DTH might be involved in corneal allograft rejection. Sonoda and Streilein reported that mice that rejected their orthotopic corneal grafts also developed vigorous DTH responses to donor alloantigens, while hosts bearing longterm clear corneal allografts failed to mount DTH, even if the hosts were immunized subcutaneously with donor lymphoid cells.[108] The latter finding led to the conclusion that the success of orthotopic corneal allografts relied on the allograft's peculiar capacity to induce active suppression of systemic DTH.

Adoptive transfer of alloreactive lymphocytes to unprimed recipients is a tool used for assessing the role of specific lymphoid cell subsets in the rejection of various types of allografts.[47] Using this approach, Khodadhoust and Silverstein[66] showed that corneal allograft rejection was a cell-mediated event. Subsequent studies in mice indicated that either CD4[+] or CD8[+] T lymphocytes could initiate the rejection of heterotopic corneal allografts.[70]

Recently systemic administration of monoclonal antibodies against T specific antigens has been used effectively to inactivate CD4[+] and CD8[+] T lymphocyte populations in vivo, thereby providing further insight into the role of the respective T cell subsets in the rejection of various categories of allografts. In both mice[51] and rats,[4] in vivo administration of anti-CD4[+] monoclonal antibodies resulted in a sharp reduction in the incidence and tempo of orthotopic corneal allograft rejection. By contrast, anti-CD8[+] monoclonal antibody failed to reduce significantly the incidence of orthotopic corneal allograft rejection in either species.[4,51] These results suggest that classical CD8[+] CTL are not required for corneal allograft rejection, although it is possible that CD4[+]CD8[-] CTL-mediated direct cytolysis can occur. Alternatively, CD4[+] T lymphocytes might activate second-level antigen-nonspecific effector cells (for example, macrophages) that act as mediators of graft destruction.

In spite of almost a half century of investigation, the identity of the immune cells that mediate corneal graft rejection remains obscure, and the immunologic mechanism itself remains poorly understood. Prospective studies in rodents implicate CD4[+] T cells as crucial participants in corneal graft rejection. CD4[+] cells could act directly as cytotoxic effector cells or indirectly by activating second level effector cells. Considering the plasticity and redundancy of the immune system, it is quite possible that under different conditions, multiple pathways contribute to corneal graft rejection and that the CD4[+] T cell serves many functions in this process.

PATHOGENESIS

The interesting immunologic feature of corneal transplantation is not that the grafts fail, but that they so often survive. This feature has been ascribed to immunologic privilege of the cornea and anterior segment of the eye. Attempts to explain such privilege have included the following proposals: (1) the donor cells are replaced by host cells, (2)

the cornea is not immunogenic, or (3) there is a blockade to the normal host immunologic response in either the afferent or efferent immune pathway.

Extensive work by Khodadhoust and Silverstein[64] and Polack[92] established that although the epithelial tissue is ultimately replaced by the host, both donor stroma and endothelium persist. Furthermore, there are several elegant immunohistochemical studies demonstrating antigen expression in epithelial, stromal, and endothelial layers of the cornea.[118,119,127] Some of these studies characterizing the differential expression of the major histocompatibility antigens suggest that the immunologic benefit bestowed upon a corneal transplant is attributable to the lack of significant class II HLA antigen expression in the normal central cornea.[98] The various layers of the cornea will, however, provoke both an antigenic and immunogenic response when transplanted to a heterotopic, vascularized location.[117,120]

Lafferty and associates[68] proposed that immunologically competent passenger cells in transplanted tissue are capable of mediating an immune response by enhancing antigen processing of the donor tissue by the host. This theory may be a vital factor in cornea transplantation, because studies by Gillette and Chandler[42] have correlated the importance of the presence of dendritic class II positive Langerhans cells in the corneal immunologic response. The work of Ross and associates[98,99,100] also underscores the value of Langerhans cells in corneal allograft reaction and suggests that donor Langerhans cells are crucial to the effective antigen presentation of the donor to the host. Their work suggests that a relative blockade of the afferent arc of the immune response is in part responsible for the success of corneal transplantation.

A substantial body of evidence supports the premise that the success of corneal transplantation is the result of a relative blockade of the efferent arc of the immune response. Khodadhoust and Silverstein[65] documented the benefit incurred by the lack of vascularization and lymphatic supply, and how such benefit is lost when vascularization occurs. More recently, Sonada and Streilein[106,107] demonstrated cytokine suppression of the efferent arm of the immune response in the eye. Their work submitted that the ocular microenvironment—in communication with the splenic system—mutes or inhibits immune effector cells, resulting in protection of the graft as well as induction of anterior chamber associated immune deviation (ACAID).

The strategic positioning of the orthotopic corneal allograft over the anterior chamber may contribute to graft survival. It has been recognized for over a century that the anterior chamber of the eye provides an immunologically privileged environment for a variety of allografts.[77,113] The basis for immune privilege in the anterior chamber is believed to be the result of a dynamic immunoregulatory mechanism in which systemic cell-mediated immunity is actively downregulated.[77,113] The unique spectrum of immune responses leading to suppression of cellular immunity is termed anterior chamber associated immune deviation (ACAID).[77,113] The hallmarks of ACAID include the elicitation of normal humoral antibody and CTL responses, but a profound suppression of allospecific DTH. In addition to suppressed antigen-specific DTH, hosts accept orthotopic skin allografts prepared from the same donor strain used for the anterior chamber priming.[79] The ability of anterior chamber priming to downregulate systemic cellular alloimmune responses led She and associates[104] to consider this approach as a strategy for promoting corneal allograft survival in rats.[104] Intracameral inoculation of allogeneic lymphocytes prior to orthotopic corneal transplantation substantially reduced the incidence of rejection of corneal grafts from the same donor strain used for intracameral inoculation, but it had no effect on corneal grafts from third party strains. Thus antigen-specific downregulation of systemic cellular immune responses (that is, ACAID) promoted corneal allograft survival. Along similar lines, Sonoda and Streilein[108] reported that mice bearing clear orthotopic corneal allografts resisted systemic immunization with donor strain alloantigenic lymphocytes and failed to develop DTH. The inability to generate DTH to donor-specific alloantigens suggested that the long-term accepted corneal allografts had induced ACAID. By contrast, corneal grafts that underwent rejection presumably did not induce ACAID, because the hosts were capable of mounting DTH responses to donor alloantigens.

The results of these studies show a strong correlation between inhibition of DTH (ACAID) and corneal graft survival and suggest that corneal graft rejection is mediated primarily by DTH. However, the piecemeal lysis of corneal endothelial cells in orthotopic corneal allografts undergoing rejection is inconsistent with a DTH-mediated process. Considering the plasticity and redundancy of the immune system and the lessons learned from studies on other organ allografts, it is likely that corneal allograft rejection can occur by multiple pathways involving different effector mechanisms. It is remarkable that this seemingly simple allograft remains an immunological enigma despite so much ongoing research and despite the information obtained in the past 20 years.

As the general understanding of immune processes improves, and the specific molecular aspects of immune regulation become increasingly clear, the importance of intercellular communication becomes apparent. This is particularly true of signaling between antigen-processing cells and subsequently activated lymphocytes whose clonal expansion provides the effectors of graft destruction specific to the allograft rejection reaction.

THERAPY

The most important aspects of clinical treatment of corneal allograft reaction are early recognition and early insti-

tution of therapy. About 66% of allograft reactions in both low-risk and high-risk patients can be reversed if aggressive treatment is started early—after onset of the reaction.[36]

Once the symptoms and signs of corneal allograft rejection appear, the mainstay of therapy is glucocorticosteroids.[53,54,97] Whereas topical application is usually effective in mild reactions, the use of oral systemic therapy or pulse intravenous corticosteroids is advisable when a severe reaction is encountered. Administration of subconjunctival steroid injections is occasionally used, although such treatment is not necessary in a compliant patient capable of administering topical drop medication. A regimen found effective in a recent clinical study was that of topical prednisolone acetate (1% suspension hourly during waking hours) and dexamethasone ointment at night for mild reactions. In severe cases, pulse intravenous methylprednisolone 250 to 500 mg can be added, followed by 1 mg/kg per day oral prednisone for 5 days.[21] For significant photophobia, the patient may obtain relief with topical homatropine (5%) or scopolamine (0.25% drops twice a day).

The entire mechanism of steroid immunosuppression is not fully understood, but it is clear that corticosteroids help prevent the manifestations of both humoral and cellular aspects of the immune response. This prevention is probably accomplished by disruption of intercellular communication of lymphokines and interference with antigen expression on both lymphoid and nonlymphoid tissue. Certainly much of the effectiveness of corticosteroids stems from (1) the antiinflammatory properties of an inhibition of phospholipase-A2 and the prostaglandin cascade, (2) a decrease in fibrinous exudation and cellular tissue infiltration, (3) an inhibition of neovascularization, and (4) a restoration of excessive capillary permeability.[28] Redistribution and sequestration of T lymphocytes may explain some of the systemic immunosuppressive effects of corticosteroids,[32,33] but direct inhibition of cytokine production or function on macrophages and lymphocytes provides more direct immunosuppression.[11]

Glucocorticoids affect many cellular components of the immune system. Although B lymphocytes are relatively resistant to the in vivo immunosuppressive effects of corticosteroids, an initial increase in immunoglobulin catabolism and subsequent decrease in production of immunoglobulins occur with exposure to corticosteroids.[15] T lymphocytes are more sensitive to the effects of corticosteroids. Glucocorticoids interfere with several of the activation events and proliferative responses of T lymphocytes by inhibiting the completion of RNA synthesis and limiting gene expression; all of which results in decreased production of IL-2, IL-6, and IFN-gamma.[11] Finally, glucocorticoids can result in direct lysis of both immature and mature lymphoid cells by activating an endonuclease that cleaves chromatin and leads to apoptosis of the cells.[80]

Macrophage and monocyte function is also suppressed by glucocorticoids. There is decreased chemotaxis and phagocytosis,[96] and reduced expression of Fc and C3 receptors.[38] Glucocorticosteroids downregulate expression of class II major histocompatibility antigens in macrophages by repressing gene expression.[18] Glucocorticosteroids can prevent induction of antigen expression on nonlymphoid tissue by inhibiting both IFN-gamma and non-IFN-gamma MHC-class II-inducing mediators.[102] Steroids also inhibit macrophage production of IL-1, IL-6, and other cytokines.[11] Finally, there is evidence that corticosteroids can abolish the expression of surface molecules on subsets of Langerhans cells or destroy those cells.[40]

PREVENTION

Several strategies exist for improving corneal graft survival. The two main approaches are (1) to make the donor tissue less visible to the host immune system (afferent intervention), and (2) to suppress the effector cells of the host immune response (efferent intervention).

One extensively investigated method for improving corneal graft survival in the high-risk patient is histocompatibility antigen matching. Whereas a number of studies in England,[6] the Netherlands,[125,126] the United States,[103] and Canada[10] support the benefits of histocompatibility matching for donor and recipients in high-risk patients; a large collaborative clinical trial recently completed in the United States showed no benefit from histocompatibility matching when both high-dose steroid therapy and close postoperative follow-up were employed in treatment.[21] Interestingly, despite no demonstrable benefit of antigen matching, that same study showed an increased risk of rejection in the subgroup of patients who had serologically identifiable lymphocytotoxic antibodies to class I and class II histocompatibility antigens.[46] A further intriguing observation in this study was that ABO blood group compatibility had a positive effect on graft survival.[21] This result contrasts with most previous reports showing no benefit from ABO compatibility,[1,126] but it coincides with a smaller number of reports that do support such benefit.[50,95] Additional controlled clinical trials will be needed to validate this finding before routine ABO blood group testing can be advocated for donor-recipient allocation.

To date, clinical studies have neglected the role of minor histocompatibility antigens in provoking corneal graft rejection. Results from animal studies indicate that 30-50% of MHC matched penetrating keratoplasties will undergo immunological rejection due to the recognition of foreign multiple minor histocompatibility antigens on the corneal allograft.[59a,61,98,107] Therefore, any benefit achieved by MHC matching of donor and recipient might be offset by the significant immunogenicity produced by foreign multiple minor histocompatibility antigens that are expressed by the corneal allograft. Although MHC matching does not significantly improve graft survival in some studies, the conclusion that MHC antigens do not represent barriers to successful

corneal transplantation is untenable. Studies on penetrating keratoplasty in rats and mice have shown that corneal grafts in which the donor and recipient are matched at all minor histocompatibility loci but mismatched at the entire MHC undergo immunological rejection.[61,107] Thus, efforts to improve corneal graft survival will need to take into account both MHC antigens and multiple minor histocompatibility antigens.

Attempts to deplete the antigens in the donor tissue also have been made. Simple removal of surface epithelium at the time of keratoplasty has been advocated by some[122] to reduce rejection reaction, but this method has not been successful in a larger prospective study using survival statistical analysis.[115] The additional risks of failure of epithelial healing with persistent epithelial defect formation and subsequent vascularization of the graft also limit the utility of epithelial removal, particularly in those patients with damaged or incompetent ocular surface epithelium (for example, chemical burn, atopic dermatitis). Specific depletion of class II MHC antigen positive cells by exposinq the tissue to hyperbaric oxygen, ultraviolet light, and specific monoclonal antibodies[78,129] has been attempted in animal models with variable success. The risk posed to the viability of the donor cells by each of these treatments has limited the clinical application of such strategies. It is recognized that organ culture storage methods also can deplete cells expressing class II MHC antigens in the cornea, but such depletion alone is not enough to prevent allograft rejection.[25]

Immunosuppression continues to be an active area of investigation for the prevention of allograft reaction. Animal studies of both systemic and topical cyclosporine A (CyA) therapy have resulted in improved graft survival,[7,19] yet the correlative human studies are inconclusive.[7,52,55]

The immunophilin-specific class of drugs provides a novel avenue of immunosuppression. Beginning with cyclosporine A and expanding with FK-506, these agents have shown excellent immunosuppression in solid organ transplantation.[60,82,112] The hydrophobic drugs selectively and reversibly interfere with certain populations of immunocompetent cells—with no generalized cytotoxic effect.[37] The mechanism of action is through binding of the agent to an intracellular cytoplasmic protein (immunophilin) that has enzymic (peptidyl-prolyl isomerase) activity in regulating intracellular protein synthesis.[48,49,105] The resultant inhibition of transcription of lymphokine genes interferes with the production of IL-2 that, in turn, inhibits proliferation and function of cytotoxic T cells.[14,43] Production of IFN-gamma is also reduced in the T helper cell population.[94] Additionally, there is inhibition of expression of the high-affinity IL-2 receptor. This fact suggests that cyclosporine may be able to mitigate the initial sensitization of the graft if CyA is present prior to or concurrent with grafting.[123]

The potential risks of epithelial defect formation and aggravation of recurrent herpes simplex viral disease cloud the clinical benefit of topical CyA. The hydrophobic nature of the drug requires preparation with a lipid vehicle (such as corn oil or olive oil), and the penetration into tissue is uncertain. One recent clinical study in humans, evaluating an ointment vehicle preparation, failed to demonstrate effectiveness in preventing graft rejection in high-risk patients[22]; but a rodent study, evaluating the effectiveness of topical cyclosporine A in unilamellar liposome-encapsulated form, showed a statistically significant prolongation of corneal graft survival.[75] Although some preliminary studies with FK-506 have been promising, more data and further studies are needed.[24,56] The successful use of rapamycin and 15-desoxyspergualin to prolong survival in animal models is also provocative, but the systemic toxicities of even limited dose-combined therapy are worrisome.[56]

More specific immunomodulatory therapy may be possible with the use of monoclonal antibodies and their immunoconjugates. Treatment directed against the efferent arm of the rejection reaction has seen both animal and human application. Anti-CD4 monoclonal antibodies, which affect class II MHC-restricted (predominantly regulatory) T cells, demonstrate some effectiveness in interfering with the efferent arm of the immune response in animal studies.[26,51] Use of a combination of anti-CD4 and anti-CD8 monoclonal antibodies was shown to be more effective in one animal study in mice, but the systemic toxicity was unacceptable.[27] Anti-CD3 and CD6 monoclonal antibodies have been used successfully by intracameral injection to abort acute allograft reactions in humans.[59] Cell adhesion molecules play a critical role in a wide variety of immunological processes. The increased expression of cell adhesion molecules on inflamed corneas[42a] and corneal allografts undergoing rejection[126a] suggests that disruption of cell adhesion molecule expression and function might promote corneal allograft survival. This prediction is supported by results from animal studies in which systemic administration of monoclonal antibodies against leukocyte function antigen-1 (LFA-1) and intercellular adhesion molecule-1 (ICAM-1) greatly reduced the rejection of heterotopic and orthotopic corneal allografts in mice.[45,51a]

Another exciting possible method of prevention of allograft rejection is the induction of immune tolerance by presentation of associated donor antigen in either oral feeding or nasal mucosal application. Although the specific antigens necessary for such induction of tolerance are not presently defined for the cornea, the observation in animals that oral feeding of retinal antigens can avert or ameliorate experimental autoimmune uveoretinitis (EAU) is encouraging.[81] A similar observation that T cell-mediated EAU can be aborted by intranasal administration of retinal antigens further recommends exploration of a search for allograft tolerance.[23]

One of the most provocative, yet distant, possibilities is that of genetic manipulation of antigen expression in donor cells either by treatment in tissue culture or transfection strategies. Alteration of antigen expression can be accomplished in tissue culture by exposure of cells to nicotinamide (nonspecifically) or triplex-forming oligonucleotides (specifically), both of which will suppress HLA-DR expression[69] and ICAM-1 expression.[58] Such modification of the donor cell might prevent cell recognition and thereby elude the initial immune response. It remains to be seen, however, if such treatment of the donor would preclude the subsequent induction of expression of HLA class I and II or ICAM-1 antigens, which could at a later time serve to induce allograft rejection.

Until new immunosuppressive strategies are perfected, the best clinical approach to prevent corneal graft failure (caused by allograft rejection) is to recognize those patients at high risk of rejection and follow them closely in the postoperative period. While treating the patient with frequent topical glucocorticoid corticosteroids in the postoperative period, it is still necessary to maintain a low threshold for signs of allograft rejection and treat vigorously with additional topical or short pulse systemic corticosteroids at the early sign of an allograft rejection reaction.

REFERENCES

1. Allansmith MR, Fine M, Payne R: Histocompatibility typing and corneal transplantation, *Trans Am Acad Ophthalmol Otolarygol* 78:445-451, 1974.
2. Alldredge OC, Krachmer JH: Clinical types of corneal rejection: their manifestations, frequency, preoperative correlates, and treatment, *Arch Ophthalmol* 99:599-610, 1981.
3. Arentsen JJ: Corneal transplant allograft rejection: possible predisposing factors, *Trans Am Ophthalmol Soc* 81:361-402, 1983.
4. Ayliffe W, Alam Y, Bell EB et al.: Prolongation of rat corneal graft survival by treatment with anti-CD4 monoclonal antibody, *Br J Ophthalmol* 76:602-606, 1992.
5. Baer J, Foster CS: Control of corneal vascularization by 577 nm yellow dye laser, *Ophthalmology* 99:173-179, 1992.
6. Batchelor JR, Casey TA, West A et al.: HLA matching and corneal grafting, *Lancet* 1:551-554, 1976.
7. Belin MW, Bouchard CS, Phillips TM: Update on topical cyclosporine A: background, immunology, and pharmacology, *Cornea* 9:184-195, 1990.
8. Blanchard D, Els CV, Aubry J-P et al.: CD4 is involved in a postbinding event in the cytolytic reaction mediated by human CD4$^+$ cytotoxic T lymphocyte clones, *J Immunol* 140:1745-1752, 1988.
9. Boisjoly HM, Bernard PM, Dube I et al.: Effect of factors unrelated to tissue matching on corneal transplant endothelial rejection, *Am J Ophthalmol* 107:647-654, 1989.
10. Boisjoly HM, Roy R, Bernard PM et al.: Association between corneal allograft reactions and HLA compatibility, *Ophthalmology* 97:1689-1698, 1990.
11. Boumpas DT, Paliogianni F, Anastassiou ED, Balow JE: Glucocorticosteroid action on the immune system: molecular and cellular aspects, *Clin Exp Rheumatol* 9:413-423, 1991.
12. Braakman E, Rotteveel FTM, van Bleek G et al.: Are class II-restricted cytotoxic T lymphocytes important? *Immunol Today* 8:265-267, 1987.
13. Braude LS, Chandler JW: Corneal allograft rejection: the role of the major histocompatibility complex, *Surv Ophthalmol* 27:290-330, 1983.
14. Britton S, Palacios R: Cyclosporin A—usefulness, risks, and mechanism of action, *Immunol Rev* 65:5-10, 1982.
15. Butler WT, Rossen RD: Effects of corticosteroids on immunity in man: decreased serum IgG concentration caused by 3 or 5 days of high doses of methylprednisolone, *J Clin Invest* 52:2629-2640, 1973.

16. Callanan D, Peeler J, Niederkorn JY: Characteristics of rejection of orthotopic corneal allografts in the rat, *Transplantation* 45:437-443, 1988.

17. Cantor H, Boyse EA: Functional subclasses of T lymphocytes bearing different Ly antigens. II. Cooperation between subclasses of Ly+ cells in the generation of killer activity, *J Exp Med* 141:1390-1399, 1975.

18. Celada A, McKercher S, Maki RA: Repression of major histocompatibility complex Ia espression by glucocorticoids: the glucocorticoid receptor inhibits the DNA binding of the X box DNA binding protein, *J Exp Med* 177:691-698, 1993.

19. Chen YF, Gebhardt BM, Reidy JJ, Kaufman HE: Cyclosporine containing collagen shields suppress corneal allograft rejection, *Am J Ophthalmol* 109:132-137, 1990.

20. Cherry PMH et al.: An analysis of corneal transplantation. I. Graft clarity, *Ann Ophthalmol* 11:461-469, 1979.

21. Collaborative Corneal Transplantation Studies Research Group: Effectiveness of histocompatibility matching in high risk corneal transplantation, *Arch Ophthalmol* 110:1392-1403, 1992.

22. Collaborative evaluation of topical sandimmune sandimmune™ in high risk keratoplasty (unpublished results).

23. Dick AD, Cheng YF, McKinnon et al.: Nasal administration of retinal antigens suppresses the inflammatory response in experimental allergic uveoretinitis, *Brit Jour Ophthalmol* 77:171–175, 1993.

24. Dickey JB, Cassidy EM, Bouchard CS: Periocular FK-506 delays allograft rejection in rat penetrating keratoplasty, *Cornea* 12:204-207, 1993.

25. Doughman DJ: Prolonged donor cornea preservation in organ culture: long term clinical evaluation, *Trans Am Acad Ophthalmol Otolaryngol* 81:567-570, 1980.

26. Duguid IGM, Koulmanda M, Mandel TE: Prolongation of heterotopic human corneal graft survival in mice treated with anti-CD4 monoclonal antibody, *Transplantation Proc* 22:2107-2108, 1990.

27. Duguid IGM, Koulmanda M, Mandel TE: Effect of monoclonal antibody on corneal graft survival across major and minor histocompatibility mismatches, *Transplant Proc* 25:844, 1993.

28. Duke-Elder S, Ashton N: Action of cortisone on tissue reactions of inflammation and repair with special reference to the eye, *Br J Ophthalmol* 35:695-705, 1951.

29. Ehlers N, Olsen T, Johnsen HE: Corneal graft rejection probably mediated by antibodies, *Acta Ophthalmol* 59:119-125, 1981.

30. Elner VM et al.: Intercellular adhesion molecule-1 (ICAM) in human corneal endothelium, *Am J Pathol* 138:525-531, 1991.

31. Eye Bank Association of America annual report, 1992.

32. Fauci AS: Mechanism of corticosteroid action on lymphocyte subpopulations. I. Redistribution of circulating T and B lymphocytes to the bone marrow, *Immunology* 38:669-680, 1975.

33. Fauci AS, Dale DC, Balow JE: Glucocorticosteroidal therapy: mechanism of action and clinical considerations, *Ann Intern Med* 84:304-315, 1976.

34. Fine M, Stein M: The role of corneal vascularization in human corneal graft reactions, Corneal Graft Failure CIBA Foundation Symposium, 193-204, Amsterdam, 1973, Elsevier.

35. Foulks GN: Glaucoma associated with penetrating keratoplasty, *Ophthalmology* 94:871-874, 1987.

36. Foulks GN: Unpublished data.

37. Foxwell BMJ, Ruffel B: The mechanisms of action of cyclosporine, *Cardiol Clin* 8:107-117, 1990.

38. Fries LF, Brickman CM, Frank MM: Monocyte receptors for the Fc portion of IgG increase in number in autoimmune hemolytic anemia and other hemolytic states and are decreased by glucocorticoid therapy, *J Immunol* 131:1240-1245, 1983.

39. Fujikawa LS, Colvin RV, Bahn AK et al.: HLA-A/B/C and -DR locus antigens on epithelial, stromal, and endothelial cells of the human cornea, *Cornea* 1:213-222, 1982.

40. Furue M, Katz SI: Direct effects of glucocorticosteroids on epidermal Langerhans cells, *J Invest Dermatol* 92:342-347, 1989.

41. Gibbs DC, Batchelor JR, Werb A et al.: The influence of tissue-type compatibility on the fate of full thickness corneal grafts, *Trans Ophthalmol Soc UK* 94:101-126, 1974.

42. Gillette TE, Chandler JW, Greiner JV: Langerhans cells of the ocular surface, *Ophthalmology* 89:700-710, 1982.

42a. Goldberg MF, Ferguson TA, Pepose JS: Detection of celular adhesion molecules in inflamed human corneas. *Ophthalmology* 101:161–168, 1994.

43. Granelli-Piperno A, Andrus L, Steinman RM: Lymphokine and non-lymphokine mRNA levels in stimulated human T cells: kinetics, mitogen requirements, and effects of cyclosporin A, *J Exp Med* 163:922-930, 1986.

44. Grunnet N, Kristensen T, Kissemeyer-Nielsen F, Ehlers N: Occurrence of lymphocytotoxic lymphocytes and antibodies after corneal transplantation, *Acta Ophthalmol* 54:167-172, 1976.

45. Guymer RH, Mandel TE: Immunosuppression using a monoclonal antibody to ICAM-1 in murine allotransplantation, *Transplantation* 24:218-219, 1992.

46. Hahn AB, Foulks GN, Sanfilippo F, Enger C et al.: The role of lymphocytotoxic antibodies in high risk corneal transplant rejection, *Transplantation* (in press).

47. Hall BM: Cells mediating allograft rejection, *Transplantation* 51:1141-1151, 1991.

48. Harding MW, Handschumacher RE: Cyclophilin, a primary target molecule for cyclosporine: structural and functional implications, *Transplantation* 46:29s, 1988.

49. Harding MW, Galat A, Uehling DE et al.: A receptor for the immunosuppressant FK-506 is a cis-trans peptidyl-prolyl isomerase, *Nature* 341:758-760, 1989.

50. Havener WH: Donor cornea selection by blood type, *Arch Ophthalmol* 60:443-446, 1958.

51. He YG, Ross J, Niederkorn JY: Promotion of murine orthotopic corneal allograft survival by systemic administration of anti-CD4 monoclonal antibody, *Invest Ophthalmol Vis Sci* 32:2723-2728, 1991.

51a. He Y-G, Mellon J, Apte R, Niederkorn JY: Effect of LFA-1 and ICAM-1 antibody treatment on murine corneal allograft survival. *Invest Ophthalmol Vis Sci* 35:3218-3225, 1994.

52. Hill JC: The use of cyclosporine in high risk keratoplasty, *Am J Ophthalmol* 107:506-510, 1989.

53. Hill JC, Maske R, Watson PG: The use of a single pulse of intravenous methylprednisolone in the treatment of corneal graft rejection, *Eye* 5:420-424, 1991.

54. Hill JC, Maske R, Watson P: Corticosteroids in corneal graft rejection: oral versus single pulse therapy, *Ophthalmology* 98:329-333, 1991.

55. Hoffmann F, Wiederholt M: Local treatment of corneal transplants in the human with cyclosporine A, *Klin Monatsbl Augenheilkd* 187:92-96, 1985.

56. Holland EJ: Immunosuppression of corneal allograft rejection. In Brightbill FS, editor: *Corneal surgery: theory, technique, and tissue*, ed 2, St Louis, 1993, Mosby.

57. Holland EJ, Chan C-C, Wetzig RP et al.: Clinical and immunohistologic studies of corneal rejection in the rat penetrating keratoplasty model, *Cornea* 10:374-380, 1991.

58. Hwang DG, Tam S, Garovoy M et al.: Inhibition of HLA and ICAM-1 expression in cultured human corneal endothelial cells, *Invest Ophthalmol Vis Sci* 34:772, 1993.

59. Ippoliti G, Fronterre A: Usefulness of CD3 or CD6 anti-T monoclonal antibodies in the treatment of acute corneal graft rejection, *Transplant Proc* 21:3133-3134, 1989.

59a. Joo CK, Pepose JS, Stuart PM: T-cell mediated responses in a murine model of orthotopic corneal transplantation. *Invest Ophthalmol Vis Sci* 36:1530-1540, 1995.

60. Kahan BD et al.: Cyclosporine immunosuppression mitigates immunologic risk factors in renal transplantation, *Transplant Proc XV* 4:2469-2478, 1983.

61. Katami M, White DJG, Watson PG: An analysis of corneal graft rejection in the rat, *Transplant Proc* 21:3147-3149, 1989.

62. Khodadoust AA: The allograft rejection reaction: the leading cause of late failure of clinical corneal grafts. In Corneal Graft Failure Ciba Symposium, 151-167, Amsterdam, 1973, Elsevier.

63. Khodadoust AA, Abizadeh A: The fate of corneal regrafts after previous rejection reactions. In Silverstein AM, O'Connor GR, editors: *Immunology and immunopathology of the eye*, 167-173, New York, 1979, Masson Publishing.

64. Khodadoust AA, Silverstein AM: Transplantation and rejection of individual cell layers of the cornea, *Invest Ophthalmol Vis Sci* 8:180-195, 1969.

65. Khodadhoust AA, Silverstein AM: Studies on the nature of the privilege enjoyed by corneal allografts, *Invest Ophthalmol Vis Sci* 11:137-148, 1972.

66. Khodadoust AA, Silverstein AM: Induction of corneal allograft rejection by passive cell transfer, *Invest Ophthalmol Vis Sci* 15:89-95, 1976.

67. Krachmer JH, Alldredge OC: Subepithelial infiltrates: a probable sign of corneal transplant rejection, *Arch Ophthalmol* 96:2234-2237, 1978.

68. Lafferty KJ, Prowse SJ, Simeonovic CJ: Immunobiology of tissue transplantation: a return to the passenger leukocyte concept, *Ann Rev Immunol* 1:143-173, 1983.

69. Lui GM, Tam S, Weiss T et al.: Modulation of HLA-DR and ICAM-1 expression in human retinal pigment epithelial cells by nicotinamide and triple helix forming oligonucleotides, *Invest Ophthalmol Vis Sci* 34:870, 1993.

70. Matoba AY, Peeler JS, Niederkorn JY: T cell subsets in the immune rejection of murine heterotopic corneal allografts, *Invest Ophthalmol Vis Sci* 27:1244-1254, 1986.

71. Maumenee AE: The influence of donor-recipient sensitization on corneal grafts, *Am J Ophthalmol* 34:142-152, 1951.

72. Maumenee AE: Clinical aspects of the corneal homograft reaction, *Invest Ophthalmol Vis Sci* 1:244-252, 1962.

73. Maumenee AE: Clinical patterns of corneal graft failure, Corneal Graft Failure Ciba Symposium, 5-15, Amsterdam, 1973, Elsevier.

74. Mehri P, Becker B, Oglesby R: Corneal transplants and blood types: a clinical study, *Am J Ophthalmol* 47:48-53, 1959.

75. Milani JK, Pleyer U, Dukes A et al.: Prolongation of corneal allograft survival with liposone-encapsulated cyclosporine in the rat eye, *Ophthalmology* 100:890-896, 1993.

76. Moskophidis D, Fang L, Gossman J et al.: Virus specific delayed-type hypersensitivity (DTH): cells mediating lymphocytic choriomeningitis virus specific CTH reaction in mice, *J Immunol* 144:1926-1934, 1990.

77. Niederkorn JY: Immune privilege and immune regulation in the eye, *Adv Immunol* 48:191-226, 1990.

77a. Niederkorn JY, Mayhew E: "Subthreshold stimulation" of allospecific delayed hypersensitivity by corneal allografts. *Immunology* 80:605-610, 1993.

78. Niederkorn JY, Callanan D, Ross JR: Prevention of the induction of allospecific cytotoxic T lymphocyte and delayed type hypersensitivity responses by ultraviolet irradiation of corneal allografts, *Transplantation* 50:281-286, 1990.

79. Niederkorn JY, Streilein JW, Shadduck JA: Deviant immune responses to allogeneic tumors injected intracamerally and subcutaneously in mice, *Invest Ophthalmol Vis Sci* 20:355-363, 1981.

80. Nieto MA, Lopez-Rivas A: Glucocorticoids activate a suicide program in mature T lymphocytes. *Ann NY Acad Sci* 650:115-120, 1992.

81. Nussenblatt RB: Experimental autoimmune uveitis: mechanisms of disease and clinical therapeutic indications, *Invest Ophthalmol Vis Sci* 32:3131-3141, 1991.

82. Oyer PE et al.: Cyclosporin in cardiac transplantation, *Transplant Proc XV* 4:2552-2564, 1983.

83. Page B, Roy R, Lille S et al.: Anti-endothelial antibodies: implication in corneal allograft rejection, *Invest Ophthalmol Vis Sci* 34:1365, 1993.

84. Paque J, Poirier RH: Corneal allograft reaction and its relationship to suture site neovascularization, *Ophthalmol Surg* 8:71-74, 1977.

85. Paufique L, Sourdille P, Offret G: *Les Greffes del la Cornee,* Paris, 1948, Masson et Cie.

86. Peeler J, Niederkorn J, Matoba A: Corneal allografts induce cytotoxic T cell but not delayed hypersensitivity responses in mice, *Invest Ophthalmol Vis Sci* 26:1516-1523, 1985.

87. Pepose JS, Foos RY, Gardner KM et al.: Composition of cellular infiltrates in rejected human corneal allografts, *Graefe's Arch Ophthalmol* 222:128-133, 1985.

88. Pepose JS, Foos RY, Gardner KM et al.: Detection of HLA Class I and II antigens in rejected human corneal allografts, *Ophthalmology* 92:1480-1484, 1985.

89. Polack FM: The effect of ocular inflammation on corneal grafts, *Am J Ophthalmol* 60:259-269, 1965.

90. Polack FM: The pathologic anatomy of corneal graft rejecton, *Surv Ophthalmol* 11:391-404, 1966.

91. Polack FM: Clinical and pathological aspects of the corneal graft reaction, *Trans Am Acad Ophthalmol* 77:418-431, 1973.

92. Polack FM: *Corneal transplantation,* 22, New York, 1977, Grune and Stratton.

93. Polack FM: Glaucoma occurring with corneal graft rejection, *Am J Ophthalmol* 101:294-297, 1986.

94. Reem GH, Cook LA, Vilcek JV: Gamma interferon synthesis by human thymocytes and T lymphocytes inhibited by cyclosporine A, *Science* 221:63-65, 1983.

95. Richter S: Untersuchugen uber isoantikosper be keratoplastik, *Albrecht Graefe Arch* 168:131-135, 1965.

96. Rinehart JJ, Balcerzak SP, Sagone AL, Lobuglio AF: Effects of corticosteroids on human monocyte function, *J Clin Invest* 54:1337-1343, 1975.

97. Rinne JR, Stulting RD: Current practices in the prevention and treatment of corneal graft rejection, *Cornea* 11:326-328, 1992.

98. Ross JR, He Y-G, Pidherney M et al.: The differential effects of donor versus host Langerhans cells in the rejection of MHC-matched corneal allografts, *Transplantation* 52:857-861, 1991.

99. Ross JR, Callanan DG, Kunz H, Niederkorn JY: Evidence that the timing of class II expression determines the fate of class II disparate corneal grafts, *Transplantation* 51:532-536, 1991.

100. Ross JR, He Y-G, Niederkorn JY: Class I disparate corneal grafts enjoy afferent but not efferent blockade of the immune response, *Curr Eye Res* 10:889-892, 1991.

101. Roy R, Boisjoly HM, Wagner E, Langlois A et al.: Pretransplant and posttransplant antibodies in human corneal transplantation, *Transplantation* 54:463-467, 1992.

102. Ruers TJM, Leeuwenberg JFM, Spronken EEM et al.: The effect of steroids on the regulation of major histocompatibility complex-class II expression on non-lymphoid tissue, *Transplantation* 47:492-499, 1989.

103. Sanfilippo F, MacQueen JM, Vaughn WK, Foulks GN: Reduced graft rejection with good HLA-A and HLA-B matching in high risk corneal transplantation, *New Engl J Med* 315:29-35, 1986.

104. She S-C, Steahly LP, Moticka EJ: Intracameral injection of allogeneic lymphocytes enhances corneal graft survival, *Invest Ophthalmol Vis Sci* 31:1950-1956, 1990.

105. Siekierka JJ, Hung SHY, Poe M et al.: A cytosolic binding protein for the immunosuppressant FK-506 has peptidyl-prolyl isomerase activity but is distinct from cyclophilin, *Nature* 341:755-757, 1989.

106. Sonoda Y, Ksander B, Streilein JW: Impaired cell mediated immunity (ACAID) induced in mice that accept orthotopic corneal allografts indefinitely, *Invest Ophthalmol Vis Sci* 33:843, 1992.

107. Sonoda Y, Streilein JW: Orthotopic corneal transplantation in mice—evidence that the immunogenetic rules of rejection do not apply, *Transplantation* 54:694-704, 1992.

108. Sonoda Y, Strelein JW: Impaired cell-mediated immunity in mice bearing healthy orthotopic corneal allografts, *J Immunol* 150:1727-1734, 1993.

109. Stark WJ: Transplantation immunology of penetrating keratoplasty, *Tr Am Ophthalmol Soc* 78:1079-1095, 1980.

110. Stark WJ, Taylor HR, Datiles M et al.: Transplantation antigens and keratoplasty, *Aust NZ J Ophthalmol* 11:333-337, 1983.

111. Stark WJ et al.: Sensitization to human lymphocyte antigens by corneal transplantation, *Invest Ophthalmol Vis Sci* 12:639-642, 1973.

112. Starzl TE et al.: Report of Colorado-Pittsburgh liver transplantation studies, *Transplant Proc XV* 4:2582-2585, 1983.

113. Streilein JW: Immune regulation and the eye: a dangerous compromise, *FASEB J* 1:199-208, 1990.

114. Stulting RD: Penetrating keratoplasty in children. In Brightbill FS, editor: *Corneal surgery: theory, technique, and tissue,* ed 2, 374-385, St Louis, 1993, Mosby.

115. Stulting RD, Waring GO, Bridges WZ, Cavanagh HD: Effect of donor epithelium on corneal transplant survival, *Ophthalmology* 95:803-812, 1988.

116. Treseler PA, Foulks GN, Sanfilippo F: Immunity to class I major histocompatibility complex (MHC) antigens evoked by heterotopic corneal allografts in the rat, *Invest Ophthalmol Vis Sci* 25(suppl):299, 1984.
117. Treseler PA, Foulks GN, Sanfilippo F, Treseler CB: Allospecific cellular and humoral immunity to rat corneal transplants, *Transplantation Proc* 18:789-791, 1985.
118. Treseler PA, Foulks GN, Sanfilippo F: Expression of HLA antigens by cells in the human cornea, *Am J Ophthalmol* 98:763-772, 1984.
119. Treseler PA, Foulks GN, Sanfilippo F: Expression of ABO blood group, hematopoetic, and other cell-specific antigens by cells in the human cornea, *Cornea* 4:157-168, 1986.
120. Treseler PA, Foulks GN, Sanfilippo F: The relative immunogenicity of corneal epithelium, stroma and endothelium, *Transplantation* 41:229-234, 1986.
121. Treseler PA, Sanfilippo F: Humoral immunity to heterotopic corneal allgrafts in the rat, *Transplantation* 39:139-145, 1985.
122. Tuberville AW, Foster CS, Wood TO: The effect of donor cornea epithelium removal on the incidence of allograft rejection reactions, *Ophthalmology* 90:1351-1356, 1983.
123. Ueda H, Wayne HW, Yuk-Chun C et al.: The mechanism of synergistic interaction between anti-interleukin 2 receptor monoclonal antibody and cyclosporine therapy in rat recipients of organ allografts, *Transplantation* 50:545-550, 1990.
124. Volker-Dieben HJ, D'Amaro J, Kok-van Alphen CC: Hierarchy of prognostic factors for corneal allograft survival, *Aust NZ J Ophthalmol* 15:11-20, 1987.
125. Volker-Dieben HJ, Kok-van Alphen CC, Krut PJ: Advances and disappointments, indications and restrictions regarding HLA matched corneal grafts in high risk cases, *Doc Ophthalmol* 46:219-226, 1979.
126. Volker-Dieben HJ, Kok-van Alphen CC, Lansbergen Q, Persijn GG: The effect of prospective HLA-A and -B matching on corneal graft survival, *Acta Ophthalmol* 60:203-212, 1982.
126a. Whitcup SM, Nussenblatt RB, Price Jr FW, Chan C-C: Expression of cell adhesion molecules in corneal graft failure. *Cornea* 12:474-480, 1993.
127. Whitsett CF, Stulting RD: The distribution of HLA antigens on human corneal tissue, *Invest Ophthalmol Vis Sci* 25:519-524, 1984.
128. Williams KA, Ash JK, Coster DJ: Histocompatibility antigents and passenger cell content of normal and diseased human cornea, *Transplantation* 39:265-269, 1985.
129. Young E, Olkowski ST, Dana M et al.: Pretreatment of donor corneal endothelium with ultraviolet-B irradiation, *Transplant Proc* 21:3145-3146, 1989.
130. Zangemeister-Wittke U, Kyewski B, Schirrmacher V: Recruitment and activation of tumor-specific immune T cells in situ: CD8+ cells predominate the secondary response in sponge matrices and exert both delayed-type hypersensitivity-like and cytotoxic T lymphocyte activity, *J Immunol* 143:379-385, 1989.

36 Cogan Syndrome

REX M. McCALLUM, BARTON F. HAYNES

Cogan syndrome is an inflammatory disease that is characterized by ocular inflammation (typically interstitial keratitis) and is associated with Menière-like vestibuloauditory dysfunction.[1,47]

EPIDEMIOLOGY

Cogan syndrome, first described by Dr. David Cogan in 1945,[25] is an uncommon illness with approximately 150 cases reported in the world's literature.[11,47,65,86,99] Most reports of Cogan syndrome are individual cases or small series, although recently, larger series of Cogan syndrome cases have been reported.[47,65,99]

In addition to eye and ear inflammation, vascular inflammatory disease has been noted in approximately 10% of patients.[47,65] Previous reports have divided patients into "typical" and "atypical" subsets, based on the presence of only interstitial keratitis, conjunctivitis, or iritis (typical) versus other types of ocular inflammation (atypical).[47] Given that patients with typical ocular features can subsequently develop atypical types of ocular inflammation, these clinical subsets are less clinically useful than once thought.[1,65]

PATHOGENESIS

The pathogenesis of Cogan syndrome is unknown but is presumed to be autoimmune. Clues to the underlying mechanism are (1) the type of ocular inflammation, (2) the abnormal laboratory parameters of inflammation (erythrocyte sedimentation rate), (3) the infiltration of affected tissues with inflammatory cells (Figs. 36-1 and 36-2), and (4) the response of eye, ear, and vascular inflammation to antiinflammatory and/or immunosuppressive therapy.* Approximately one half (40% to 65%) of patients with Cogan syndrome have an antecedent upper respiratory illness.[48] This fact suggests a role for infection in disease initiation, as has been noted for other immune-mediated illnesses.[84]

Infectious Etiology

No organism has been isolated or identified at the time of acute Cogan syndrome onset, despite repeated attempts by several investigators.* Serologic studies, however, have implied an association with various infections. For example, one Cogan syndrome patient had a significant rise in serum antibodies to type 1 poliovirus during the acute phase of Cogan syndrome.[12]

Cogan-like syndromes have been associated with chlamydial infections of the eye and ear.[32] Two thirds of the patients with either acute or nonacute Cogan syndrome in the original National Institutes of Health series had evidence of elevated IgM and IgG antichlamydial antibody titers, respectively.[47] The importance of these findings remains unclear, and subsequent attempts to find direct evidence of chlamydial infection in ocular biopsy specimens (using culture[24,100] and a monoclonal antibody against chlamydial elementary body antigen[73]) were negative.[64]

A recent report has associated Cogan syndrome with Lyme disease.[42] It is interesting to note that syphilis, also caused by a spirochete, has long been recognized as a major differential diagnostic consideration in Cogan syndrome.[25,47] A report of "pseudo-Cogan syndrome" secondary to acquired syphilis has also recently been published.[88] Cogan syndrome is, by original definition, nonluetic in origin.[25] It is doubtful that Lyme disease is the cause of Cogan syndrome because several Cogan syndrome patients live in nonendemic areas of the United States where *Borrelia burgdorferi* infestation of the appropriate tick vector is low.[21]

Thus although Cogan syndrome may be initiated by an infectious agent, primary infection by a pathologic agent does not seem to be the main pathogenetic mechanism of disease. Current evidence points to an autoimmune hypersensitivity reaction.

---

*References 1, 11, 47, 48, 65, 72.

*References 23, 26, 34, 36, 47, 99.

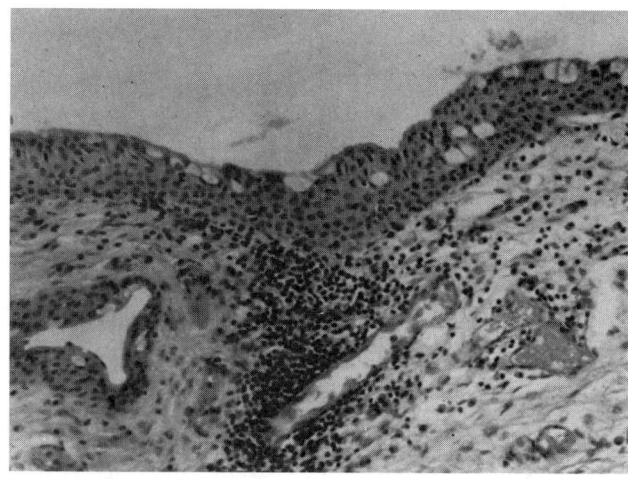

Fig. 36-1. Conjunctival biopsy from a patient with active Cogan syndrome. Note the intense inflammatory cell infiltrate beneath a normal-appearing conjunctival epithelium in this hematoxylin and eosin stained section.

Autoimmune Etiology

Support for an immune-mediated origin of Cogan syndrome is found in studies of humoral and cellular immunity. T cell anergy has been noted in some studies but not others.[99] Different research has demonstrated autoantibodies against inner ear and corneal tissue in Cogan syndrome.[2,3,4] Abnormal tests of cellular immunity have been noted using inner ear antigen[51] and pooled corneal antigen.[20]

Cogan syndrome has been suggested to be a primary vasculitis[21,79] and is associated with vasculitis in approximately 10% of patients. The majority of patients never develop signs nor symptoms of vasculitis, however, and vascular inflammation of the eye and ear is not the primary pathophysiology of the syndrome.[47,65] Rather, inflamed ocular and auditory tissues have infiltration with T and B lymphocytes in the absence of vascular damage.

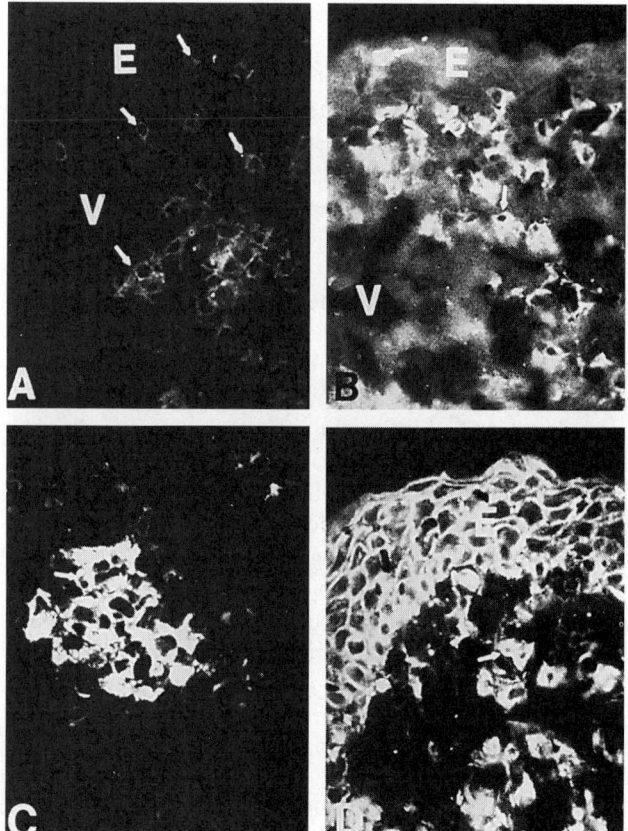

Fig. 36-2. Phenotypic characterization of conjunctival infiltrating cells and epithelial cells in Cogan syndrome using direct immunofluorescence assay on frozen tissue sections. Acetone-fixed 4-micron-thick frozen sections of conjunctiva were prepared from tissue taken during a flare of anterior uveitis and conjunctivitis. Tissue was reacted with monoclonal antibodies against CD4 or CD8 T cell antigens or with anti-MHC Class II or antitransferrin antibodies. **A,** shows CD4 + infiltrating cells, and **B,** shows CD8 + cells. **C,** shows a foci of activated T cells in the conjunctival stroma that were antitransferrin receptor +, and **D,** shows MHC Class II + stromal macrophages and MHC Class II + conjunctival epithelium (E). (Reproduced with permission from Haynes BF and associates: Pathogenesis and immunotherapy of Cogan's syndrome. In Eisenbarth GS, editor: *Immunotherapy of diabetes and selected autoimmune diseases,* Boca Raton, 1989, CRC Press.)

CLINICAL FEATURES

The average age of disease onset for patients with Cogan syndrome is 29 years (range 3 to 50 years),[47,65] although at least two patients have been reported with disease onset in the seventh decade of life.[39,80] Previous literature reviews indicate that the number of male and female patients are equal,[48,100] but a recent series show approximately twice as many women as men.[47,65,99] One half of the patients present with ocular problems, one fourth with vestibuloauditory problems, and one fourth with both (within one month of each other)[65,99] (Table 36-1).

Eye Findings

The most common presenting ocular symptoms are eye discomfort, redness, and photophobia.[65] Additional symptoms include disturbances of visual acuity, tearing, diplopia, foreign-body sensation, and visual-field deficit.[23,47,99] Ocular findings in the Duke/National Institutes of Health series patients included interstitial keratitis (72%), conjunctivitis (34%), iritis (32%), scleritis/episcleritis (20%), corneal ulceration (4%), vitreitis, choroiditis, subretinal neovascular membrane (2%), pars planitis (2%), orbital pseudotumor (2%), and cotton-wool spots (2%).[65] Ocular findings can be evanescent, and repetitive examinations may be necessary to demonstrate evidence of ocular inflammatory disease, particularly interstitial keratitis.[26,99]

Cogan described the interstitial keratitis in Cogan syndrome as "a granular type of corneal infiltrate, patchy in distribution, situated predominantly in the posterior half of the cornea. Later in the course of Cogan's syndrome the cornea can become vascularized."[26] The most common early corneal findings are "faint peripheral, anterior stromal, subepithelial corneal infiltrates, measuring 0.5 to 1.0 mm in diameter mimicking lesions seen in adenoviral or chlamydial keratitis"[23] (Fig. 36-3). These corneal lesions resolved promptly with the institution of topical or systemic glucocorticoids, although faint subepithelial scars remained in 2 of 13 patients studied.[23] Epithelial erosions may overlie the stromal infiltrates in less than 5% of Cogan syndrome patients.[99]

The late sequelae of corneal scarring and vascularization are rarely seen in Cogan syndrome if appropriate antiinflammatory therapy is undertaken early.[23] The corneal findings of Cogan syndrome described by Cogan[25,26] occur later

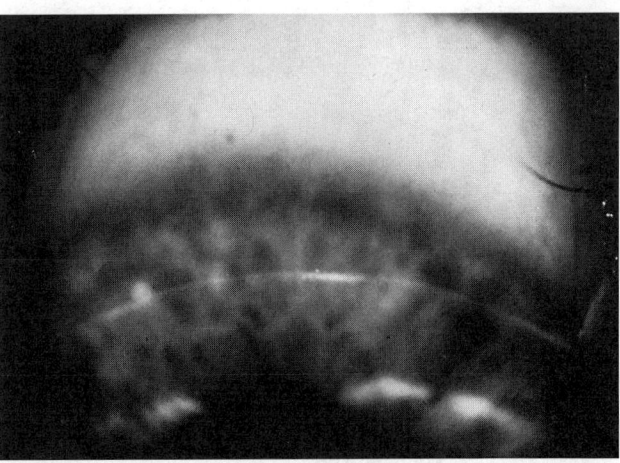

Fig. 36-3. Discrete, anterior stromal, subepithelial corneal infiltrate observed in a patient with Cogan's syndrome and early interstitial keratitis. (Reproduced with permission from Cobo LM, Haynes BF: Early corneal findings in Cogan's syndrome, *Ophthalmology* 91:903-907, 1984.)

in the course of the keratitis and may not develop with early topical corticosteroid therapy.[23] Less than 5% of steroid-treated patients demonstrate late corneal opacification.[30] In one of these patients, corneal scarring was severe enough to lead to corneal transplantation.[29]

Conjunctivitis and mild anterior uveitis, either isolated or associated with interstitial keratitis, are frequently noted in Cogan syndrome.[23,65,99] Other reported ocular manifestations include posterior uveitis, vitreitis, retinochoroiditis, papillitis, vitreous hemorrhage, conjunctival nodule, central venous occlusion, and retinal arterial disease.[47,99] The association of any ocular inflammatory disease with vestibuloauditory complaints should raise the question of Cogan syndrome.

Ear Findings

Patients frequently have the sudden onset of the Menière-like symptoms of nausea, emesis, tinnitus, downfluctuation of hearing, and severe vertigo.[47,65] Presenting vestibuloauditory symptoms are vertigo, sudden decrease in hearing, sudden nausea and vomiting, tinnitus, ataxia, and gradual decrease in hearing.[65] Vestibuloauditory features include Menière-like symptoms with hearing loss (92%), nystagmus (32%), oscillopsia (15%), Menière-like symptoms without hearing loss (4%), and hearing loss only (4%). Less than 5% had vestibuloauditory symptoms without hearing loss.[65] Vestibular symptoms are acutely incapacitating for many patients, requiring hospitalization. Examination frequently reveals nystagmus, decreased auditory acuity, and ataxia. Reduced or absent caloric responses and abnormal auditory-evoked responses have been noted.[7,51,99]

Cardiovascular Findings

Some of the systemic symptoms may be secondary to systemic necrotizing vasculitis. Inflammatory vascu-

TABLE 36-1 PRESENTING SYSTEM INVOLVEMENT IN PATIENTS WITH COGAN SYNDROME

Eye	50%
Ear	30%
Both eye and ear	15%
Neither eye nor ear	5%

lar manifestations occur in approximately 10% of patients.[11,47,65,99] Evaluation can reveal large-vessel (Takayasu-like) vasculitis, aortitis, aortitis with large-vessel vasculitis, and medium-vessel (polyarteritis nodosalike) vasculitis.[65]

Aortic insufficiency has developed in 10% of Cogan syndrome patients,[11] secondary to an inflammatory aortitis. The cardiac symptoms and signs of aortic insufficiency range from an asymptomatic murmur to exertional dyspnea and chest pain secondary to severe aortic insufficiency (with or without coronary disease).* Aortitis may develop within weeks to years after the onset of Cogan syndrome.[1,43,47,99] Associated findings may include the following: valvular fenestrations,[37,43] ostial coronary disease,[43,61] aneurysms of the valve cusps,[37,43] myocardial infarction,[29] coronary arteritis with or without myocardial infarction,[1,37] pericarditis,[61,77] aortic dilatation,[61] left ventricular hypertrophy,[99] and arrhythmias.[99] These findings have been documented at cardiac catheterization and in pathologic studies. The development of an aortic insufficiency murmur in a patient with Cogan syndrome is an indication for evaluation and strong consideration of antiinflammatory therapy.[1,47] All patients with Cogan syndrome should have periodic screening for the development of aortic insufficiency by physical examination and echocardiography.[63]

The systemic necrotizing vasculitis syndrome observed in patients with Cogan syndrome is typically a large-vessel (Takayasu-like) vasculitis syndrome (Fig. 36-4).† Medium-vessel (polyarteritis nodosalike) disease has also been reported.[31,40,65] Early accounts of systemic necrotizing vasculitis in association with Cogan syndrome were often based on clinical, rather than angiographic or pathologic, evidence or were associated with the use of foreign proteins.[48] Subsequent studies have appropriately documented the association of systemic necrotizing vasculitis with Cogan syndrome in a minority of patients.[1,47,65,99] The presenting symptoms of large-vessel vasculitis include the following: (1) abdominal pain leading to laparotomy with discovery of vasculitis in a gastric ulcer and enlarged spleen secondary to vasculitis,[1] (2) lower extremity claudication,[1] (3) new-onset femoral bruit,[64] and (4) symptoms of mesenteric insufficiency.[24] The presenting symptoms of medium-vessel vasculitis include gastrointestinal bleeding,[31] upper extremity vascular symptoms,[64] proteinuria and microscopic hematuria,[64,99] ischemic loss of limbs,[40] and neurologic complaints.[99] The diagnosis of systemic necrotizing vasculitis is made via angiography and/or review of pathologic material.‡ Systemic necrotizing vasculitis has been documented in the following sites in patients with Cogan syndrome: coronary,[1,37] gastrointestinal tract (Fig. 36-5, B),[1] subclavian,[1,24] femoral,[1] renal,[1] skin (Fig. 36-5, A),[31,40,104] testicle,[41] and muscle.[32]

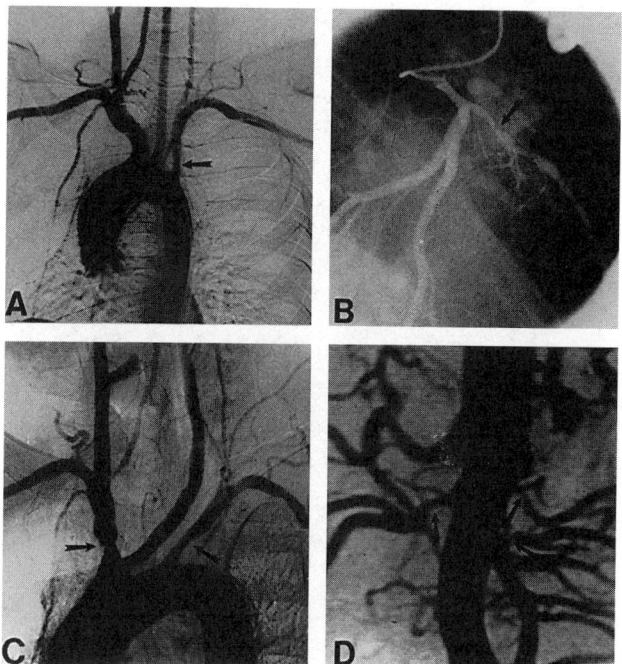

Fig. 36-4. Arteriographic demonstration of large-vessel lesions in Cogan syndrome: **A,** Stenotic lesion in the left subclavian artery *(arrow).* **B,** Stenotic lesions in the left anterior descending coronary artery *(arrows)* with poststenotic dilatation. **C,** Stenotic lesions in the right innominate artery *(left arrow)* and the left subclavian artery *(right arrow).* **D,** Multiple lesions in the single right and duplicated left renal arteries *(arrows).* (Reproduced with permission from Allen NB and associates: Use of immunosuppressive agents in the treatment of severe ocular and vascular manifestations of Cogan's syndrome, *Am J Med* 88:296-301, 1990.)

Other Findings

Systemic symptoms are common in patients with Cogan syndrome (Table 36-2). Many systemic symptoms are nonspecific, such as fever, weight loss, fatigue, headache, arthralgias, and myalgias.[11,47,65,99] Male patients may note testicular pain,[99] although this is uncommon.[47,65] Central nervous system manifestations of Cogan syndrome have included the following: meningismus, encephalitis, psychosis, seizures, localized cerebral infarction, cavernous sinus thrombosis, and trigeminal neuralgia.[11,47,99] One patient had pulmonary nodules that resolved over a period of weeks without specific therapy. Dermatologic findings of Cogan syndrome that have been described are skin nodules and nonspecific rashes.[99] Ulcers, palpable purpura, and oral ulcers have also been described.[78,99] Systemic features generally resolve with the institution of appropriate antiinflammatory therapy. One patient with Cogan syndrome had a pauciarthritis that remained active despite medium-dose glucocorticoids, methotrexate, cyclosporine, and cyclophosphamide.

Cogan syndrome has occurred in association with inflammatory bowel disease, acute sarcoidosis, hypothyroid-

---

*References 1, 9, 24, 28, 37, 43, 47, 61, 77, 99.
†References 1, 11, 21, 47, 58, 65, 99.
‡References 1, 24, 31, 47, 58, 99.

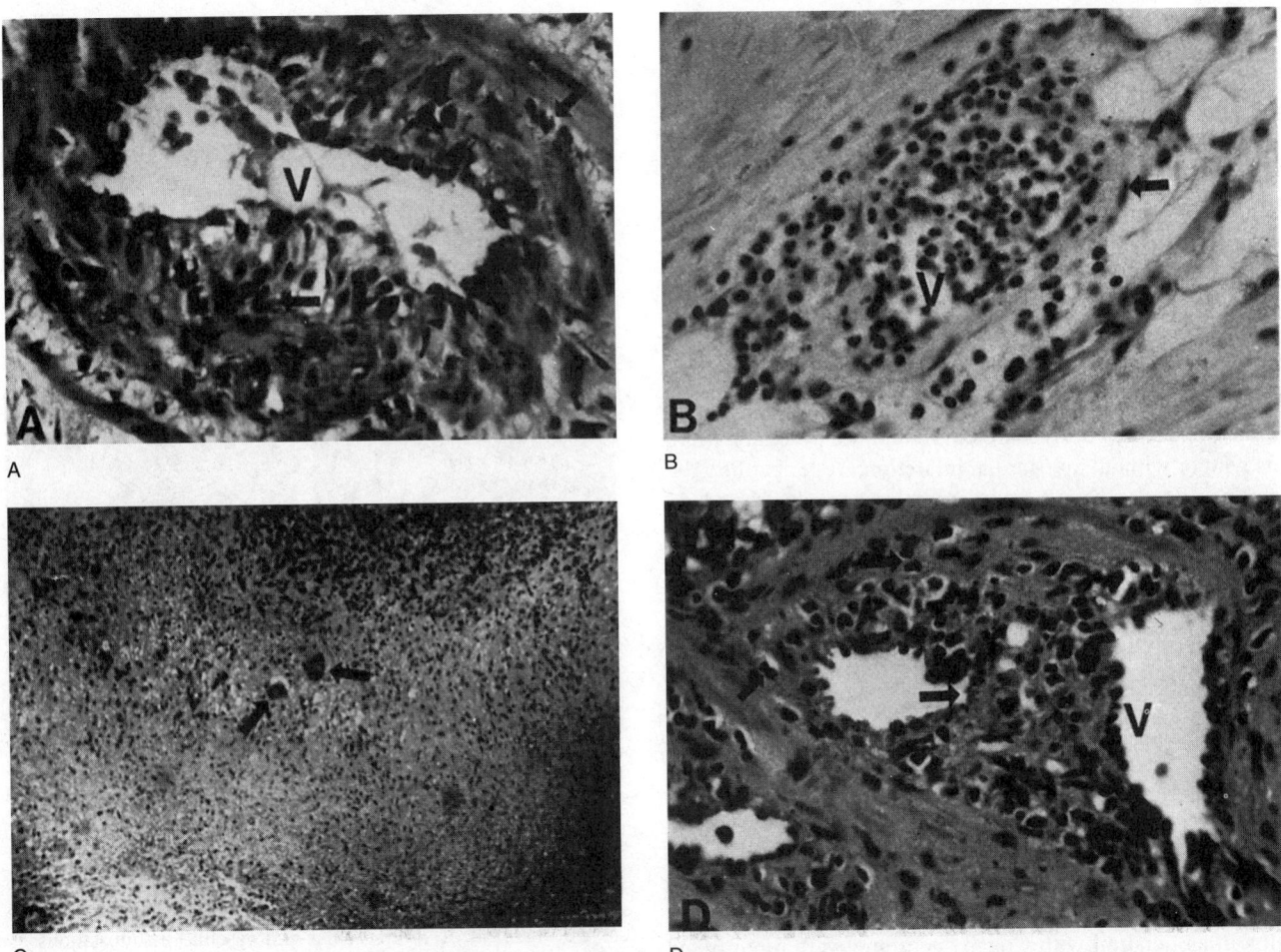

Fig. 36-5. Histology of vascular and splenic inflammation in a patient with Cogan syndrome: **A,** A medium-size blood vessel in skin dermis with inflammatory cells in and around the vessel wall *(arrows)*. V shows the vessel lumen. **B,** Inflammatory infiltrate in the lumen (V) and in and around a vessel in gastric serosa. *Arrow* points to vessel wall. **C,** Giant cells *(arrows)* in splenic granulomatous inflammatory infiltrate. **D,** A splenic muscular artery with inflammatory cells in a thrombus in the lumen and in the vessel wall *(arrows)*. All panels are hematoxylin and eosin. (Reproduced with permission from Allen NB and associates: Use of immunosuppressive agents in the treatment of severe ocular and vascular manifestations of Cogan's syndrome, *Am J Med* 88:296-301, 1990.)

ism, and interstitial nephritis leading to renal failure and dialysis.[65]

COMPLICATIONS

The natural history of Cogan syndrome is progression to deafness and corneal opacification following one or several attacks of Cogan syndrome, unless inflammatory vascular disease develops.[47] Interstitial keratitis is initially limited to inflammatory stromal edema and infiltration, but may advance to corneal vascularization and a marked opacity if the patient does not receive topical and/or systemic glucocorticoid therapy.[23,29] Eighty percent of patients progress to deafness unless treated with systemic corticosteroid or systemic corticosteroid and immunosuppressive therapy.[47,48,65] Aortic insufficiency progresses to death from congestive heart failure if not treated early and aggressively with immunosuppressive therapy and, if necessary, aortic valve replace-

ment.[1,11,24,37] Systemic necrotizing vasculitis may be fatal unless treated with systemic glucocorticoid and/or immunosuppressive therapy.*

LABORATORY INVESTIGATIONS

Blood and Cerebrospinal Fluid Testing

Hematologic laboratory parameters are frequently abnormal in patients with Cogan syndrome: 75% of patients have leukocytosis (median 13,700 with a range of 1,600 to 47,000) and 10% have a maximal (white blood cell) WBC count of >24,000/mm[3].[99] About 50% manifest neutrophilia,[99] 25%—relative lymphopenia,[99] and 17%—mild eosinophilia.[47] Monocytosis[99] and leukemoid reaction[31]

---

*References 1, 31, 40, 43, 45, 65.

TABLE 36-2   SYSTEMIC MANIFESTATIONS OF COGAN SYNDROME

Manifestations	Proportion of Cases
Fever	25%
Fatigue	20%
Weight loss	15%
Arthralgias/myalgias	15%
Arthritis	15%
Abdominal	10%
Gastrointestinal bleeding	10%
Lymphadenopathy	10%
Hepatomegaly	10%
Splenomegaly	10%
Abnormal urine sediment	10%
Abnormal chest x-ray	5%
Pleuritis	5%
Rash	5%
Cutaneous nodules	5%
Central nervous system findings	5%
Peripheral nervous system findings	<5%
Polychondritis	<5%

have been reported. Thirty-three percent of Cogan syndrome patients have anemia, and approximately 30% manifest thrombocytosis.[99] Erythrocyte sedimentation rates are > 20/hour in 75% of patients, with a median value of 40 and range of 3 to 128.[99]

Serologic studies have failed to reveal consistent abnormalities. A low-titer rheumatoid factor is present in 14% of patients, in the absence of rheumatoid arthritis.[47,99] Low-titer antinuclear antibodies occur in 17%.[99] Cryoglobulins were found in 3 of 13 (23%) patients in the original National Institutes of Health series,[47] but they were noted in transient trace in only 1 of 6 (17%) of patients in the Mayo Clinic series.[99] A false-positive VDRL was noted infrequently.[47,99] An increased frequency of HLA-B17, HLA-A9, HLA-Bw35, and HLA-Cw4 has been reported in patients with Cogan syndrome, but the significance of these studies is unclear.[20,47,52] Total hemolytic complement is diminished in 17% of patients, C_3 decreased in 21% of patients, and C_4 diminished in 17% of patients in the Mayo Clinic series.[99] Abnormalities of the serum protein electrophoresis suggesting nonspecific inflammation have been noted.[99] No monoclonal proteins have been described in association with Cogan syndrome. A positive heterophil has been reported in two patients with Cogan syndrome.[14,31] Other tests have been consistently negative or normal, including the following: Coomb test, anti-DNA, anti-smooth muscle, anti-Ro, anti-La, and hepatitis B antigen.[99]

Cerebrospinal fluid studies have been abnormal in 25% of patients studied.[99] Cerebrospinal fluid abnormalities include leukocytosis,[47,99] elevated protein, and increased γ-globulin fraction.[33]

Clinical Diagnostic Tests

Echocardiography is abnormal in Cogan syndrome patients with aortic insufficiency murmurs.[1,65,99] Echocardiographic abnormalities described in Cogan syndrome include "fluttering" of the anterior mitral leaflet,[99] Doppler evidence of regurgitant flow,[1,99] thickening of valve cusps,[57,99] paradoxical movement of the ascending aorta during systole,[1] and left ventricular enlargement.[1,57,99] No patient has had significant valvular abnormality without a clinically evident aortic insufficiency murmur. Cardiac catheterization can characterize the degree of aortic insufficiency,[1,24,61] reveal ostial coronary stenosis associated with aortitis,[24,43,61] and show any distal coronary arteritis.[1]

Radiographic studies are used to exclude a central nervous system mass lesion (for example, acoustic neuroma) and to assist in the diagnosis of systemic necrotizing vasculitis. Two patients have had meningiomas documented at sites away from the eight cranial nerves.[64] Angiography has documented changes compatible with systemic necrotizing vasculitis (Fig. 36-4).*

Audiograms are almost always abnormal in patients with Cogan syndrome[11,47,65,99]; only about 5% of patients have a normal audiogram.[65,99] Hearing loss is most pronounced at the extreme frequencies, with relative sparing of the midrange (Fig. 36-6), as is frequently noted in patients with Menière syndrome.[68] Short-increment sensitivity index testing is abnormal in all patients tested,[47,64] indicating cochlear pathology.[47] Brainstem auditory-evoked potential studies are also suggestive of cochlear disease. Caloric testing is normal in 4% of patients, absent in 70%, and abnormal but present in 26% of patients.[99] A glycerol test was positive in at least one reported patient,[47] suggesting cochlear hydrops. This test is no longer routinely performed.[80]

Ophthalmologic photography is helpful in documenting and following corneal disease and in watching the uncommon Cogan syndrome patient with posterior-segment disease.[23] Fluorescein angiography can be useful diagnostically and in following the efficacy of therapy in patients with retinal vasculitis and retinochoroiditis.[88]

Diagnostic Approach to the Patient

The care of Cogan syndrome patients requires coordination between ophthalmologists, otolaryngologists, audiologists, and internists. Cogan syndrome patients frequently have systemic symptoms and require vigilant monitoring for the development of inflammatory vascular disease.

The potential Cogan syndrome patient requires careful ophthalmologic evaluation to seek evidence of inflammatory eye disease, remembering that interstitial keratitis can be evanescent, subtle, and viral-like in appearance. Pure-tone audiograms should be performed (in Cogan syndrome these tests are usually abnormal). Short-increment sensitiv-

---

*References 1, 20, 24, 58, 65, 99.

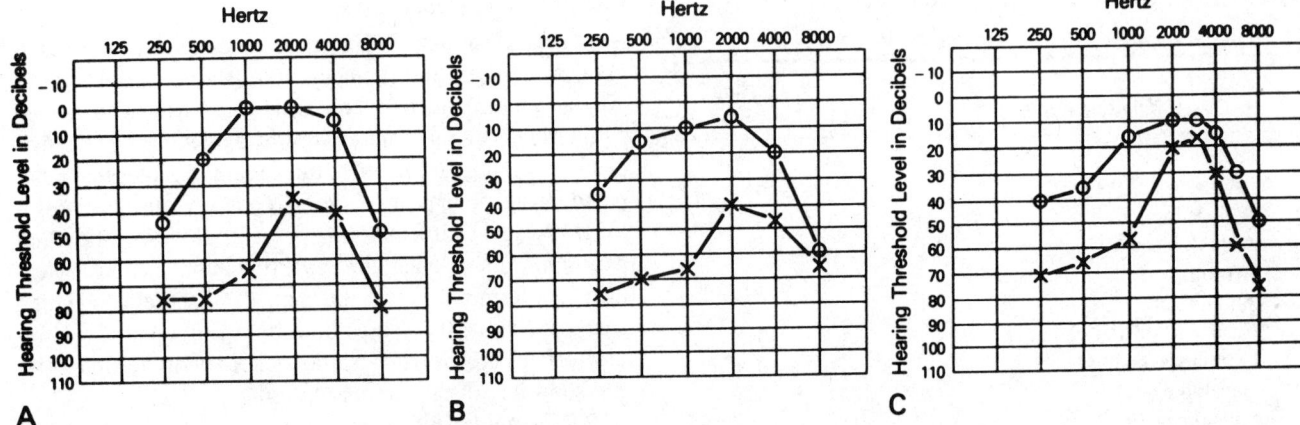

Fig. 36-6. Serial pure-tone audiogram over an 8-year period in a patient with Cogan syndrome: **A,** Audiogram 2 months after the onset of Cogan syndrome while on daily systemic corticosteroids. **B,** Five years later, the patient's corticosteroid therapy had been tapered to an alternate day regimen. **C,** Audiogram demonstrating stable hearing acuity in both ears over the total 8-year period. (O—O, right ear; X—X, left ear.) (Reproduced with permission from Haynes BF and associates: Cogan syndrome: studies in thirteen patients, long term follow-up, and review of the literature, *Medicine* 59:426-440, Williams & Wilkins, 1980.)

ity index testing should be accomplished to assess cochlear pathology, and brain imaging should be undertaken to exclude the possibility of acoustic neuroma or other brainstem lesions. An internist should evaluate the patient, paying particular attention to the vestibular and cardiovascular systems. Evidence of nystagmus and ataxia should be sought. Auscultation of the heart should seek the murmur of aortic insufficiency, and all pulses should be carefully palpated and auscultated for evidence of bruits.

Laboratory studies should include complete blood counts (with differential), serum electrolytes, creatinine, urinalysis, liver function tests, erythrocyte sedimentation rate, VDRL, and FTA-abs. Serologic tests for Lyme disease depend on the local incidence of tick infestation. Other serologic tests for arthritis, connective-tissue disease, infection, and HLA-typing are not routinely indicated or clinically helpful. 2D-echocardiography is advantageous to absolutely exclude aortic insufficiency and to establish a baseline for future follow-up studies. Cardiac catheterization is used to further characterize aortic insufficiency before consideration of aortic valve replacement and, in the patient with chest pain, to exclude coronary artery disease. Angiography and/or appropriate tissue biopsy should be performed in the patient suspected of having vasculitis.

PATHOLOGY

Eye

In an autopsy of a patient with Cogan syndrome, both eyes revealed thickened corneal epithelium, lymphocytic infiltration of the corneal stroma (greatest at the limbus), and neovascularization of the cornea with moderate hyalinization. Lymphocytes with some plasma cells also extended into the adjacent sclera, iris, ciliary body, and choroid.[40] Similar findings were noted in another report of Cogan syndrome.[59]

Two Cogan syndrome patients have received corneal transplants for corneal opacity.[29,71] Both corneas showed deep corneal stromal neovascularization, one with infiltration of lymphocytes and plasma cells[71] and the other with hypercellularity and relatively few lymphocytes.[29] In one cornea, Descemet membrane was three times normal thickness with abundant birefringent crystals and intracellular and extracellular sudanophilic material in the deep layers of the corneal stromal (Fig. 36-7).[29]

Conjunctival biopsies in patients with active interstitial keratitis have revealed plasma cell, T cell, and monocyte infiltration (Fig. 36-2, *A,B,D*).[47,64] Activated T cells have been noted in conjunctival biopsies (Fig. 36-2, *C*).[64]

Ear

An autopsy of a patient with Cogan syndrome revealed the following: (1) infiltration of the ligamentum spirale of the cochlea with lymphocytes and plasma cells, (2) slightly thickened membranous lining of the cochlea, (3) semicircular canals, utricle, saccule, and cochlear duct filled with dense acidophilic coagulum, (4) the organ of Corti had relatively few nuclei, (5) the cochlear and vestibular branches of the eighth nerve showed demyelination and atrophy, and (6) the vestibular and spiral ganglion exhibited marked satellitosis.[40]

Other reports of ear pathology revealed fibropurulent crust in the niche of the round window[99] and ruptured outer walls of the saccule of the cochlea, new bone formation in the round window membrane, hydrops of the labyrinth and cochlea, atrophy of the spiral ganglion of the cochlea, and a cyst of the stria vascularis.[105]

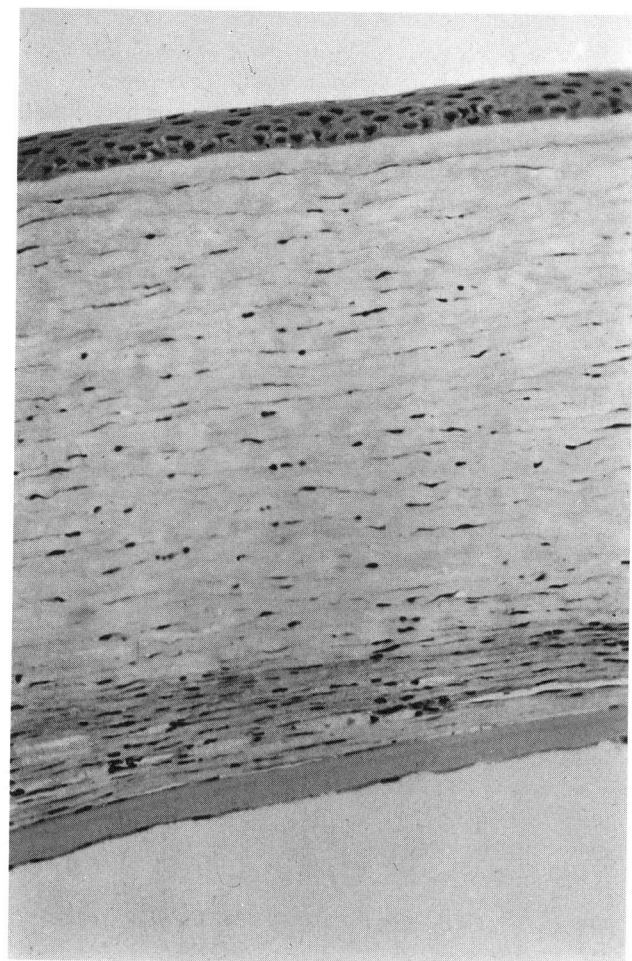

Fig. 36-7. Full-thickness section of cornea from patient with Cogan syndrome who underwent corneal transplantation secondary to corneal opacity that interfered with vision. The epithelium and Bowman membrane are normal. There is fibroplasia in the posterior stroma, thickened Descemet membrane, and mildly increased cellularity in the stroma.

Cardiovascular System

Aortic valve involvement in patients with Cogan syndrome has also been documented pathologically.[47,99] Gross descriptions of abnormalities have included deformed and fibrotic aortic valve,[99] thickened and retracted valves,[24] receded left coronary cusp with detached edge at commissure,[43] prolapsing left coronary cusp,[58] floppy and prolapsing aortic valves,[77] thinned aortic leaflets with incompetence secondary to coronary sinus dilatation,[61] and aneurysm of the aortic cusps with fenestration of the right cusp and irregularly thickened, opaque endocardium.[37] Histologic evaluation of aortic valves has revealed acute and chronic inflammation with a combination of neutrophils, lymphocytes, and histiocytes,[20,37,43,83] neovascularization,[20,44] fibrinoid necrosis,[21,38] myxomatous changes with inflammation,[21] and myxomatous changes without inflammation.[24,43] Immuno-

fluorescent staining for immunoglobulin, C_3, and fibrin was negative.[20]

Proximal and distal aortitis have been described pathologically in patients with Cogan syndrome. Ascending aortic disease has commonly been delineated[20,24,40,43,61] with only one example of pathologically documented descending and abdominal aortic disease.[28] Proximal aortic dilatation,[61,99] thickening,[43] firm and rubbery texture,[20] "curdlike" material on the intimal surface,[61] and rigidity[24] have all been described. Histologic evaluation has revealed panarteritis with diffuse-to-focal inflammatory infiltration characterized by lymphocytes, histiocytes,[24,43,61] and neutrophils.[29,44] Other features noted include fibrinoid necrosis,[39,43,61] endothelial proliferation and hypertrophy of small arteries/arterioles,[28,43] giant cells,[43] neovascularization,[43] intimal thickening,[24,43,61] media with muscle and elastic tissue replaced by connective tissue,[28,61] and thickened collagenous adventitia.[28,61] Aortic disease may extend into the proximal coronary arteries and the sinus of Valsalva.[20,28,37,43]

Inflammatory involvement of vessels beyond the aorta has been documented.[47,99] This vasculitis involves all three layers of the artery with inflammatory infiltration by lymphocytes and plasma cells.[1,40,99] Vessels with vasculitis pathologically documented in patients with Cogan syndrome include skin (Fig. 36-4, A),[79,104] extremities,[40] renal,[40] hepatic,[41] splenic (Fig. 36-4, C,D),[31,40,47] gastrointestinal tract (Fig. 36-4, B),[1,31] brain,[31] kidneys,[16,31] muscle,[83] and innominate.[25] Proximal involvement of the coronary arteries has been associated with aortitis,[24,43,61] and more distal involvement[38,41] has been described.

Other Organs

Other tissues examined from patients with Cogan syndrome have revealed nonspecific inflammation or normal findings.[99] The spleen has shown extensive necrosis with noncaseating granuloma and negative cultures in at least two patients (Fig. 36-4, C).[1,99] A third patient with similar findings yielded a "scant growth of coagulase-negative staphylococci and diphtheroids."[83] Pathologic material has been reported for lymph nodes, liver, kidney, bone marrow, testicle, gastrointestinal tract, nervous system, and synovial tissue.[47,99]

DIFFERENTIAL DIAGNOSIS

Infectious Diseases

Since Cogan's original report,[25] ocular inflammation due to syphilis and other infections should be considered in the differential diagnosis. A major consideration is congenital syphilis,[47] although several characteristics of congenital syphilis and Cogan syndrome differ.[47] Interstitial keratitis in Cogan syndrome often varies from day-to-day and from eye-to-eye; whereas in congenital syphilis it is of gradual onset, progressive, bilateral, consistent, and far more severe

---

**DIFFERENTIAL DIAGNOSIS OF
COGAN SYNDROME**

Infections
  Congenital syphilis
  Acquired syphilis
  Lyme disease
  Chlamydia
  Virus
  Tuberculous with streptomycin therapy
Vasculitis
  Polyarteritis nodosa
  Wegener granulomatosis
  Temporal arteritis
  Takayasu arteritis
Rheumatic Diseases
  Rheumatoid arthritis
  Relapsing polychondritis
  Behçet's disease
Toxins
  3-methyl-1-pentyn-3-yl acid phthalate (Whipcide)
  Cobalt
  Desferioxamine
Others
  Sarcoidosis
  Vogt-Koyanagi-Harada
  Menière's disease with eye inflammation

---

than Cogan syndrome.[47] In Cogan syndrome corneal inflammation and swelling is anterior or midstromal, whereas posterior corneal findings are generally normal. In congenital syphilis, intense, progressive, vision-threatening, generally posterior corneal swelling, and vascularization are noted early. Vestibuloauditory difficulties in Cogan syndrome are acute—with sudden hearing loss and Menière-like symptoms—whereas deafness evolves gradually, without vertigo or vestibular features, in congenital syphilis.[47] Syphilis serologies are usually positive in congenital syphilis, and the stigmata of congenital syphilis (skeletal, dental, cardiac, and so on) are present[95]; these features are absent in Cogan syndrome.[25,47] Acquired syphilis has been associated with Cogan-like features in at least two reported cases.[47,94]

Cogan syndrome has been associated with seroreactivity to Lyme borreliosis. One patient had initial improvement in hearing and interstitial keratitis with antibiotic therapy.[42] A recurrent episode of interstitial keratitis 11 months after onset was associated with recurrent seroreactivity to *Borrelia burgdorferi*.[42] In addition, interstitial keratitis,[5] ischemic optic neuropathy,[83] iritis followed by panophthalmitis,[96] bilateral choroiditis and exudative retinal detachments,[10] birdshot chorioretinopathy[98] and optic disc edema[106] have all been associated with Lyme borreliosis. Vertigo, tinnitus, Menière-like symptoms, ear pain, ear fullness, and hearing loss have been linked with Lyme disease.[56,70,87]

Chlamydial organisms have been connected with the development of keratitis and hearing loss, the latter generally of acute onset and associated with otitis media rather than Menière-like attacks.[23] One patient has been reported with *Chlamydia psittaci* (isolated from the conjunctiva) and recurrent interstitial keratitis, deafness, aortic insufficiency, aortitis, and sacroiliitis.[32]

The cause of interstitial keratitis and other ocular inflammatory diseases is rarely tuberculosis.[82] Tuberculosis keratitis is usually monocular and isolated with minimal neovascularization.[81] Tuberculosis could indirectly be associated with deafness, if treated with streptomycin (which can cause deafness and Menière-like vestibular toxicity).[101]

Many viral infections have been connected with interstitial keratitis. Mumps, varicella-zoster, and rubeola have been linked with deafness and labyrinthitis.[30,84,97] Many viruses cause labyrinthitis and conjunctivitis.[99]

Vasculitic and Rheumatic Diseases

Systemic necrotizing vasculitis associated with ocular inflammation and vestibuloauditory symptoms could be called Cogan syndrome with vasculitis. This proffers a semantics problem that is solved by the presentation of the patient. A patient diagnosed with systemic necrotizing vasculitis who develops ocular inflammation and vestibuloauditory difficulties would have systemic necrotizing vasculitis with eye and ear involvement, whereas a patient having ocular inflammation and vestibuloauditory symptoms, who is then diagnosed with systemic necrotizing vasculitis, would have Cogan syndrome associated with vasculitis. Both ocular inflammation and vestibuloauditory dysfunction have been associated with classic polyarteritis nodosa,[4,27,66,90] Wegener granulomatosis,[16,35,46,91] temporal arteritis,[18] and Takayasu arteritis.[13]

Other systemic rheumatic illnesses could manifest both ocular inflammation and vestibuloauditory dysfunction. Rheumatoid arthritis has often been associated with ocular inflammatory disease[103] but rarely with vestibuloauditory dysfunction.[2,8,93] Relapsing polychondritis is commonly linked with corneo-scleral inflammatory disease of the anterior segment and can manifest Menière-like vestibuloauditory dysfunction.[62,69] In Behçet disease ocular inflammation is a major and potentially vision-threatening feature.[74] Vestibuloauditory dysfunction has also been noted in Behçet disease and includes hearing loss, unsteadiness, vertigo, nystagmus, and abnormal caloric stimulation tests.[15,38,44] Antiinflammatory therapy and immunosuppression can lead to improvement in the vestibuloauditory and ocular inflammatory symptoms in Behçet disease.[38,74]

Vogt-Koyanagi-Harada syndrome is a cause of ocular inflammation and auditory dysfunction. Symptoms include headache, orbital pain, vertigo, stiff neck, fever, dysacousia, tinnitus, and hypersensitivity to touch of hair and skin.[76] Clinical findings include panuveitis, vitiligo, poliosis, vitiligo, aseptic meningitis, and hearing loss.[76] Interstitial keratitis has not been described with Vogt-Kayanagi-Harada, but the inflammation in other ocular anatomic sites is often severe and vision-threatening. Hearing loss occurs in 75% of Vogt-Kayanagi-Harada patients.[76]

Sarcoidosis can be associated with ocular inflammation at almost any site,[53,75] and interstitial keratitis has been described.[77] Vestibuloauditory symptoms are rare in sarcoidosis but have been noted.[49]

Toxicity

Whipcide (3-methyl-1-pentyn-3-yl acid phtalate), for the treatment of whipworm infections, has been associated with a Cogan-like syndrome, 12 hours after its administration. This syndrome is characterized by conjunctivitis, interstitial keratitis, tinnitus, and deafness—all of which resolved upon discontinuation of the drug.[50] Cobalt toxicity can manifest with decreased visual acuity, optic atrophy, and an abnormal fluorescein angiography with vestibuloauditory symptoms of decreased auditory acuity, tinnitus, and vertigo.[60,67] Desferrioxamine, when used by patients on hemodialysis, is associated with decreased visual acuity, tritan-type dyschromatopsy in the Farnsworth test, hearing loss, and tinnitus.[18] This is often asymptomatic, but vestibuloauditory symptoms can occur. Actual ocular inflammation has not been described. The hearing loss with desferrioxamine is sensorineural, and auditory-evoked potential studies are compatible with a cochlear lesion.[19]

Menière Disease

The combination of Menière disease with ocular inflammatory disease could be indistinguishable from Cogan syndrome.[47] Menière disease is not corticosteroid-responsive.[80] Given that Cogan syndrome is rare, the concurrence of two common disorders (such as conjunctivitis and otitis media) could also lead to confusion.[47,99]

THERAPY

Management of Ocular Disease

Interstitial keratitis and iritis should be treated with topical ocular corticosteroids and mydriatic for inflammation control, the prevention of synechiae, and comfort.[63] Weaker types of topical corticosteroid therapy may be sufficient to treat the interstitial keratitis. Systemic corticosteroid therapy is also effective for interstitial keratitis and iritis, but there are no clear indications for this type of treatment, except the rare patient who fails to respond to topical therapy.[47,63] Failure of interstitial keratitis to respond to topical therapy in a patient with Cogan syndrome should raise concerns about other potential causes of interstitial keratitis.

Chlamydia can cause Cogan-like syndromes,[32] and cultures for Chlamydia should be undertaken in the patient with a lack of response to topical therapy. A therapeutic trial of tetracycline should be considered.[102]

Ocular symptoms in Cogan syndrome usually respond to treatment within 3 to 7 days with concomitant improvement in signs of ocular inflammation.[99] Chronic corneal opacity occurred in at least one Cogan syndrome patient who did not receive topical corticosteroid therapy.[29] Given that corneal opacities are unusual because of the widespread use of this treatment, early topical therapy may prevent the development of these changes; however, one patient has been described with progressive late corneal opacity despite the lack of inflammation.[29] If corneal opacity interferes with visual function, it is an indication for consideration of corneal transplantation.[29] The most common indication for surgery in Cogan syndrome is likely the development of cataracts that interfere with visual acuity. Cataracts may develop prematurely in patients with Cogan syndrome secondary to corticosteroid therapy, and they may require surgery at an earlier stage secondary to associated deafness and the need to lip read and use sign language.

Other forms of anterior-segment inflammation including conjunctivitis, scleritis, and episcleritis should also be treated with a topical corticosteroid. Nonsteroidal antiinflammatory therapy, topical and/or systemic, could be considered in patients with episcleritis or scleritis.[100] The presence of nodular scleritis is an indication to consider systemic corticosteroids or other immunosuppressive therapy.[41]

Posterior-segment inflammation is unusual in Cogan syndrome, although pars planitis,[23,65] papillitis,[100] posterior scleritis,[1] vitreous hemorrhage,[99] central retinal vein occlusion,[99] and retinochoroiditis[1] have been described. Posterior-segment ocular inflammation should be treated with systemic corticosteroid therapy if it is progressive or persistent and interferes with the patient's visual function.[1,47,63] Patients who have progressive visual loss on systemic corticosteroid should be considered for other forms of systemic immunosuppression such as cyclophosphamide or cyclosporine[1,63]; such treatment has been effective.[1]

Management of Auditory Disease

The presence of compromised auditory acuity in a patient with newly diagnosed Cogan syndrome is an indication for a trial of therapy with systemic corticosteroid.[47,48,63,65] The degree of abnormality should be quantitated with an audiogram. Therapy is started with systemic corticosteroid at a dose of 1 to 2 mg/kg/day of prednisone or equivalent corticosteroid therapy.[47,63] This medicine can be started in divided doses for the first 3 to 7 days with subsequent consolidation to a single morning dose.[63] If a good response is noted subjectively and by audiogram in 10 to 14 days, then prednisone is continued for 2 to 4 weeks with subsequent institution of a corticosteroid taper.[63] An attempt should be made to taper the prednisone to an every-other-day regimen at 6 to 8 weeks, with subsequent tapering off of the drug by 3 to 4 months of treatment, provided that auditory acuity remains stable.[63] Certain patients have required continued daily corticosteroid therapy and/or have been unable to taper totally off prednisone because of recurrent episodes of decreased auditory acuity;[64] however, efforts to taper the prednisone to a dose of < 10 mg/day should continue.

Systemic corticosteroid therapy may be effective in maintaining auditory acuity in patients with Cogan syndrome. Auditory acuity was < 60 decibels in 17% of patients who received no corticosteroid therapy and in 81% patients who received systemic corticosteroid therapy.[65] If the patient does not respond to oral prednisone within 14 days, then the decision must be made to either declare the case a treatment failure and rapidly taper the patient off corticosteroid or give the patient a trial of other immunosuppressive therapy.[63] Cyclophosphamide can be used. If this path is chosen, criteria for response and length of treatment must be determined at the time therapy is instituted.[63] Criteria for response might depend, in part, on auditory acuity at the onset of immunosuppressive therapy; but it could consist of at least a 10-decibel improvement in hearing within 6 to 8 weeks of therapy that persists, despite prednisone taper. There is insufficient experience to ensure the efficacy of immunosuppressive therapy in this circumstance.

If persistently decreased auditory acuity is noted with attempted prednisone taper, then an increased dose of prednisone is indicated. On subsequent tapers of prednisone that are associated with decreased auditory acuity, a trial of other immunosuppressive therapy should be considered, unless the effective dose of prednisone is 10 mg/day or less.[63] Cyclophosphamide, methotrexate, and azathioprine have been used successfully under these circumstances.[64] Again, criteria for response and length of treatment should be determined at the time other immunosuppressive therapy is instituted. Response criteria might include stabilized or improved hearing on a lesser dose of prednisone after 3 months of additional immunosuppressive therapy. Subsequent attempts should be made to taper off of prednisone. Use of cyclophosphamide for more than one year should be approached cautiously, given fears regarding lymphoreticular neoplasm and bladder cancer.[55] There is insufficient experience to ensure the efficacy of other immunosuppressive drugs under these circumstances; however, a hearing threshold of < 60 decibels was noted in about three fourths of patients treated with corticosteroids alone and in those requiring corticosteroid plus other immunosuppressive therapy.[65] A major indication for other immunosuppressive therapy was auditory acuity that required excessive doses of corticosteroid to maintain (steroid-sparing therapy).[64,65] FK-506 is successful in the treatment of hearing loss in Cogan syndrome.[87]

Patients can develop cochlear hydrops after prolonged inflammation.[6,47] This can be associated with hearing fluctu-

ations that are not inflammation-related and are short-lived (hours to 3 to 5 days). Auditory acuity fluctuation caused by cochlear hydrops may be precipitated by the menstrual cycle in women, eating salty foods, allergies, or upper respiratory illnesses. It is impossible to absolutely distinguish such an episode from a bout of recurrent cochlear and vestibular inflammation, but the association with elevated erythrocyte sedimentation rate, recurrent ocular inflammation, and increased vestibular symptoms suggests a recurrent episode of inflammation. Downfluctuations in hearing that are thought to be caused by inflammation should be documented by audiography and treated with increased doses of corticosteroids to 0.5 to 2.0 mg/kg/day of prednisone equivalent therapy. If the fluctuation in hearing is not inflammatory, monitoring of status without therapeutic change, institution of diuretic therapy for presumed cochlear hydrops,[64,81] and time may lead to resolution of the hearing fluctuation. If no improvement in hearing is noted after 3 to 5 days, then a trial of prednisone should be considered. Two patients have undergone cochlear implants[55] because of profound hearing loss, with improvement.

Management of Cardiovascular Disease

The inflammatory vascular complications of Cogan syndrome assume two forms, aortitis and systemic necrotizing vasculitis.[11,47,65,99] The development of aortic insufficiency in a patient with Cogan syndrome implies aortitis, unless another clear cause is evident.[47,99] If infection is ruled out by blood cultures, corticosteroid therapy is indicated.[1] An echocardiogram should (1) assess the degree of regurgitate flow, (2) look for vegetations, and (3) evaluate left ventricular function.[1] If aortic insufficiency develops on corticosteroid therapy, other immunosuppressive therapy should be considered.[1] Cyclophosphamide is frequently chosen, at a dose of 2 to 3 mg/kg/day with appropriate monitoring of the patient's leukocyte count.[63] Many of these patients have come to aortic valve replacement soon after the discovery of aortic insufficiency,[11,47,99] although one patient stabilized for a period of years with aggressive medical therapy.[1] The development of angina in association with aortitis is an indication for coronary angiography, given the frequent association of coronary ostial stenosis with aortitis.[43,61]

Systemic necrotizing vasculitis in patients with Cogan syndrome has generally been large-vessel (Takayasu-like) or medium-vessel (polyarteritis nodosa-like) vasculitis.[11,47,65,99] Systemic necrotizing vasculitis must be considered with examination of pulses and careful monitoring of the patient's general status. When documented by angiography and/or tissue biopsy, systemic necrotizing vasculitis should be treated with prednisone at 1 mg/kg/day and other immunosuppressive therapy. Large-vessel vasculitis has been treated with cyclosporine at a dose of < 5 mg/kg/day,[1,63] and medium-vessel vasculitis is treated with cyclophosphamide.[45,60] After 4 to 6 weeks, the prednisone is tapered over 6 to 8 weeks to every-other-day therapy. Prednisone is subsequently stopped if clinical parameters of disease activity allow. Cyclosporine is used for one year after the systemic necrotizing vasculitis is felt stabilized or in remission.[1,63] With stabilization or remission of the systemic necrotizing vasculitis, cyclophosphamide is used for a total of one year.[1,63] In large-vessel vasculitis, a dose of prednisone < 10 mg/day is continued chronically in some patients.[92] If cyclosporine or cyclophosphamide is ineffective, the other drug should be considered.[63] Response is monitored using clinical parameters of disease activity such as sedimentation rate, active renal sediment, pulses, bruits, and repeat angiography.

The development of angina in a patient with Cogan syndrome should lead to coronary angiography.[1,40] Surgical procedures may be indicated to obtain material for diagnostic biopsy or to bypass diseased vessels with ischemic symptoms in distal structures (coronary artery bypass grafting in angina or extremity bypass in claudication).[1,58] It is important to submit any tissue available at corrective cardiac or vascular surgery for pathologic examination. Procedures for ischemic symptoms should be avoided in the face of active inflammation, if possible, because inflammation can cause technical difficulties for the surgeon[63]; however, if clinically necessary, corrective cardiac or vascular surgery should proceed regardless of whether inflammation is present or not.

PROGNOSIS

The ocular outcome of Cogan syndrome is excellent. In one series only 6% of patients with available follow-up data manifested visual acuity of worse than 20/30 in either eye, with 20/60 the worst.[66] These results compared with blindness in 5% of eyes reported in another review.[99] Severe visual loss was noted in 4% of patients in a literature review.[47] Blindness and severe visual loss were associated with ocular inflammation beyond the anterior segment.[47,99]

Progression to deafness in Cogan syndrome is frequent and occurs 25% to 50% of patients.[65,99] Loss of auditory acuity is the major debilitating sequelae in most patients with Cogan syndrome.[47,65,72,99] Vestibular symptoms and signs usually improve with time, but persistent oscillopsia was noted by 15% of patients.[66] One patient had severe and persistent vertigo for greater than 2 years after disease onset and underwent a right transmastoid labyrinthectomy for the treatment of these persistent symptoms.

Inflammatory vascular symptoms stabilize or resolve with proper therapy in most affected patients, although one patient developed a large-vessel vasculitis while being treated with cyclosporine for aortitis and later required cyclophosphamide.[65]

REFERENCES

1. Allen NB et al.: Use of immunosuppressive agents in the treatment of severe ocular and vascular manifestations of Cogan's syndrome, *Am J Med* 88:296-301, 1990.

1a. Arnold W, Gebbers J-O: Serum-antikörper gegen Kornea und innenohrgewebe beim Cogan-syndrome, *Laryng Rhinol Otol* 63:428-432, 1984.

2. Arnold GE, Ohsaki K: Two cases of sudden deafness: one from acquired syphilis; and one associated with possible collagen disease, *Ann Otol Rhinol Laryngol* 72:605-620, 1963.

3. Arnold W, Pfaltz R, Altermatt H-J: Evidence of serum antibodies against inner ear tissues in the blood of patients with certain sensorineural hearing disorders, *Acta Otolaryngol* 99:437-444, 1985.

4. Bakaar GL, Gibbs DD: Polyarteritis nodosa presenting with bilateral nerve deafness, *J R Soc Med* 71:144-147, 1978.

5. Baum J et al.: Bilateral keratitis as a manifestation of Lyme disease, *Am J Ophthalmol* 105:75-77, 1988.

6. Beckman H, Trotsky MB: Cogan's syndrome treated with oral glycerine: report of a case, *Arch Otolaryngol* 91:179-182, 1970.

7. Benitez JT: Evidence of central vestibulo-auditory dysfunction in atypical Cogan's syndrome: a case report, *Am J Otol* 11:131-134, 1990.

8. Bennett FM: Bilateral recurrent episcleritis: associated with posterior corneal changes, vestibulo-auditory symptoms and rheumatoid arthritis, *Am J Ophthalmol* 55:815-818, 1963.

9. Bernhardt O et al.: Cogan syndrome ber angiitis von humerven, aortitis, endoharditis, and glomerulonephritis, *Dtsch Med Worhensche* 101:373-377, 1967.

10. Bialasiewicz AA et al.: Bilateral diffuse choroiditis and exudative retinal detachments with evidence of Lyme disease, *Am J Ophthalmol* 105:419-420, 1988.

11. Bielory L, Conti J, Frohman L: Cogan's syndrome, *J Allergy Clin Immunol* 85:808-815, 1990.

12. Bonamour M, Gehin M: A propos du syndrome de Cogan, *Bull Soc Ophthalmol* 5-6:382-385, 1961.

13. Bonventre MV: Takayasu's disease revisited, *NY State J Med* 74:1960-1967, 1974.

14. Boyd GG: Cogan's syndrome: report of two cases with signs and symptoms suggesting periarteritis nodosa, *Arch Otolaryngol* 65:24-25, 1957.

15. Brama I, Fainaru M: Inner ear involvement in Behçet's disease, *Arch Otolaryngol* 106:215-217, 1980.

16. Bullen CL et al.: Ocular complications of Wegener's granulomatosis, *Ophthalmology* 90:279-290, 1983.

17. Carpio JK, Espinoza LR, Osterland CK: Cogan's syndrome and HLA BW17, *N Engl J Med* 295:1262-1263, 1976.

17a. Carter F, Nabarro J: Cromoglycate for Cogan's syndrome, *Lancet* 1:858, 1987.

18. Caselli RJ, Hunder GG, Whisnant JP: Neurologic disease in biopsy-proven giant cell (temporal) arteritis, *Neurology* 38:352-359, 1988.

19. Cases A et al.: Ocular and auditory toxicity in hemodialyzed patients receiving desferrioxamine, *Nephron* 56:19-23, 1990.

20. Char DH, Cogan DG, Sullivan WR: Immunologic study of nonsyphilitic interstitial keratitis with vestibuloauditory symptoms, *Am J Ophthalmol* 80:491-494, 1975.

21. Cheson BD, Bluming AZ, Alroy J: Cogan's syndrome: a systemic vasculitis, *Am J Med* 60:549-555, 1976.

22. Ciesielski CA et al.: The geographic distribution of Lyme disease in the United States, *Ann NY Acad Sci* 539:283-288, 1988.

23. Cobo LM, Haynes BF: Early corneal findings in Cogan's syndrome, *Ophthalmology* 91:903-907, 1984.

24. Cochrane AD, Tatoulis J: Cogan's syndrome with aortitis, aortic regurgitation, and aortic arch vessel stenoses, *Ann Thorac Surg* 52:1166-1167, 1991.

25. Cogan DG: Syndrome of nonsyphilitic interstitial keratitis and vestibuloauditory symptoms, *Arch Ophthalmol* 33:144-149, 1945.

26. Cogan DG: Nonsyphilitic interstitial keratitis with vestibuloauditory symptoms: report of four additional cases, *Arch Ophthalmol* 42:42-49, 1949.

27. Cogan DG: Corneoscleral lesions in periarteritis nodosa and Wegener's granulomatosis, *Trans Am Ophthalmol Soc* 53:321-344, 1955.

28. Cogan DG, Dickerson GR: Nonsyphilitic interstitial keratitis with vestibuloauditory symptoms: a case with fatal aortitis, *Arch Ophthalmol* 71:172-175, 1964.

29. Cogan DG, Kuwabara T: Late corneal opacities in the syndrome of interstitial keratitis and vestibulo-auditory symptoms, *Acta Ophthalmol* 67:182-187, 1989.

30. Crabtree JA: Herpes zoster oticus, *Layrngoscope* 78:1853-1878.

31. Crawford WJ: Cogan's syndrome associated with polyarteritis nodosa: a report of three cases, *Penn Med J,* 60:835-838, 1957.

32. Darougar S et al.: Isolation of *Chlamydia psittaci* from a patient with interstitial keratitis and uveitis associated with otological and cardiovascular lesions, *Br J Ophthalmol,* 62:709-714, 1978.

33. Djupesland G et al.: Cogan syndrome: the audiological picture, *Arch Otolaryngol* 99:218-225, 1974.

34. Donald RA, Gardner WJ: Keratitis with deafness, *Am J Ophthalmol* 33:889-892, 1950.

35. Drachman DA: Neurological complications of Wegener's granulomatosis, *Arch Neurol* 8:45-55, 1963.

36. Edstrom S, Vahlne A: Immunological findings in a case of Cogan's syndrome, *Acta Otolaryngol* 82:212-215, 1976.

37. Eisenstein B, Taubenhaus M: Nonsyphilitic interstitial keratitis and bilateral deafness (Cogan's syndrome) associated with cardiovascular disease, *N Engl J Med* 258:1074-1079, 1958.

38. Elidan J et al.: Effect of Cyclosporine A on the hearing loss in Behçet's disease, *Ann Otol Rhinol Laryngol* 100:464-468, 1991.

39. Fidler H, Jones NS: Late onset Cogan's syndrome, *J Laryngol Otol* 103:512-514, 1989.

40. Fisher ER, Hellstrom HR: Cogan's syndrome and systemic vascular disease, *Arch Pathol* 72:96-116, 1961.

41. Foster CS: Immunosuppressive therapy for external ocular inflammatory disease, *Ophthalmology* 87:140-150, 1980.

42. Fox GM, Heilskov T, Smith JL: Cogan's syndrome and seroreactivity to Lyme borreliosis, *J Clin Neuroophthalmol* 10:83-87, 1990.

43. Gelfand ML, Kantor T, Gorstein F: Cogan's syndrome with cardiovascular involvement: aortic insufficiency, *Bull NY Acad Med* 48:647-660, 1972.

44. Gemignani F et al.: Hearing and vestibular disturbances in Behçet's syndrome, *Ann Otol Rhinol Laryngol* 100:459-463, 1991.

45. Haynes BF, Allen NB, Fauci AS: Diagnostic and therapeutic approach to the patient with vasculitis, *Med Clin N Am* 70:355-368, 1986.

46. Haynes BF et al.: The ocular manifestations of Wegener's granulomatosis: fifteen years experience and review of the literature, *Am J Med* 63:131-141, 1977.

47. Haynes BF et al.: Studies in thirteen patients, long-term follow-up, and a review of the literature, *Medicine* 59:426-440, 1980.

48. Haynes BF et al.: Successful treatment of sudden hearing loss in Cogan's syndrome with corticosteroids, *Arth Rheum* 24:501-503, 1981.

49. Hedges TR, Taylor GW: Uveal and vestibuloauditory disease with sarcoid, *Arch Ophthalmol* 48:88-89, 1952.

50. Hoekenga MT: Ocular toxicity of whipcide (3-methyl-1-pentyn-3-YL acid phthalate) in humans, *J Am Med Assoc* 161:1252-1253, 1956.

51. Hughes GB et al.: Autoimmune reactivity in Cogan's syndrome: a preliminary report, *Otolaryngol Head Neck Surg* 91:24-32, 1983.

52. Kaiser-Kupfer MI et al.: The HLA antigens in Cogan's syndrome, *Am J Ophthalmol* 86:314-316, 1978.

53. Klintworth GK: Sarcoidosis. In Gold DH, Weinfeist TA, editors: *The eye in systemic disease,* Philadelphia, 1990, JB Lippincott.

54. Kohut RI et al.: Cochlear implants, *Nat Inst Health Consens Dev Conf Statement* 7(2):1-9, 1988.

55. Kovarsky J: Clinical pharmacology and toxicology of cyclophosphamide: emphasis of use in rheumatic diseases, *Sem Arthr Rheum* 12:359-372, 1983.

56. Krejcova H et al.: Otoneurological symptomatology in Lyme disease, *Adv Otorhinolaryngol* 42:210-212, 1988.

57. Kundell SP, Ochs HD: Cogan syndrome in childhood, *J Ped* 97:96-98, 1980.

58. LaRaja RD: Cogan syndrome associated with mesenteric vascular insufficiency, *Arch Surg* 111:1028-1031, 1976.

59. Leff IL: Cogan's syndrome, *NY State J Med* 67:2249-2257, 1967.

60. Licht A, Oliver M, Rachmilewitz EA: Optic atrophy following treatment with cobalt chloride in a patient with pancytopenia and hypercellular marrow, *Isr J Med Sci* 8:61-66, 1972.

61. Livingston JZ, Hutchins GM, Shapiro EP: Coronary involvement in Cogan's syndrome, *Am Heart J* 123:528-530, 1992.

62. McAdam LP et al.: Relapsing polychondritis: prospective study of 23 patients and a review of the literature, *Medicine* 55:193-215, 1976.

63. McCallum RM: Cogan's syndrome. In Fraunfelder FT, Hampton R, editors: *Current ocular therapy,* ed 4, Philadelphia, 1993, WB Saunders.

64. McCallum RM, Haynes BF: Unpublished observations.

65. McCallum RM et al.: Cogan's syndrome: clinical features and outcomes, *Arthr Rheum* 35(supp 9):S51, 1992.

66. McNeil NF, Ferke M, Reingold IM: Polyarteritis nodosa causing deafness in an adult: report of a case with special reference to concepts about the disease, *Ann Int Med* 37:1253-1267, 1952.

67. Meecham HM, Humphrey P: Industrial exposure to cobalt causing optic atrophy and nerve deafness: a case report, *J Neurol Neurosurg Psychiatry* 54:374-375, 1991.

68. Meyerhoff WL, Paparella MM, Gudbrandsson FK: Clinical evaluation of Meniese's disease, *Laryngoscope* 91:1663-1668, 1981.

69. Michet CJ et al.: Relapsing polychondritis: survival and predictive role of early disease manifestations, *Ann Int Med* 104:74-78, 1986.

70. Moscatello AL et al.: Otolaryngologic aspects of Lyme disease, *Laryngoscope* 101:592-595, 1991.

71. Negroni L, Tiberia G: La sindrome di cogan, *Riv Otoneuroophthalmol* 44:199-203, 1969.

72. Norton EWD, Cogan DG: Syndrome of nonsyphilitic interstitial keratitis and vestibuloauditory symptoms: a long-term follow-up, *Arch Ophthalmol* 61:47-49, 1959.

73. Nowinski RC et al.: Monoclonal antibodies for diagnosis of infectious diseases in humans, *Science* 219:637-644, 1983.

74. Nussenblatt RB, Palestine AG: Behçet's disease and other retinal vasculitides. In *Uveitis: fundamentals and practice,* Chicago, 1989, Mosby.

75. Nussenblatt RB, Palestine AG: Sarcoidosis. In *Uveitis: fundamentals and practice,* Chicago, 1989, Mosby.

76. Nussenblatt RB, Palestine AG: The Vogt-Kayanagi-Harada syndrome. In *Uveitis: fundamentals and practice,* Chicago, 1989, Mosby.

77. Obenauf CD et al.: Sarcoidosis and its ophthalmic manifestations, *Am J Ophthalmol* 86:648-655, 1978.

78. Ochonisky S et al.: Cogan's syndrome: an unusual etiology of urticarial vasculitis, *Dermatologica* 183:218-220, 1991.

79. Oliner L et al.: Nonsyphilitic interstitial keratitis and bilateral deafness (Cogan's syndrome) associated with essential polyangitis (periarteritis nodosa), *N Engl J Med* 248:1001-1008, 1953.

80. Paparella MM et al.: Meniere's disease and other labyrinthine diseases. In Papatella MM, Shumrick DA, Gluckman JL, Meyerhoff WL, editors: *Otolaryngology: otology and neurotology,* Philadelphia, 1991, WB Saunders.

81. Pau H: Parenchymatous (interstitial) keratitis. In *Differential diagnosis of eye diseases,* Philadelphia, 1978, WB Saunders.

82. Peiffer RL, Lewen RM, Yin H: Tuberculosis. In Gold DH, Weingeist TA, editors: *The eye in systemic disease,* Philadelphia, 1990, JB Lippincott.

83. Pinals RS: Cogan's syndrome with arthritis and aortic insufficiency, *J Rheumatol* 5:294-298, 1978.

84. Pomeroy C, Jordan MC: Mumps. In Hoeprich PD, Jordan MC, editors, *Infectious diseases: a modern treatise of infectious processes,* Philadelphia, 1990, JB Lippincott.

85. Roat MI et al.: Treatment of Cogan's syndrome with FK 506: a case report, *Transplantation Proc* 23:3347, 1991.

86. Roberts J: Cogan's syndrome. *Med J Aust,* 1:186-190, 1965.

87. Rosenhall U, Hanner P, Kaijser B: Borrelia infection and vertigo, *Acta Otolaryngol* 106:111-116, 1988.

88. Schatz H: Fluorescein angiography: basic principles and interpretation. In Ryan SJ, Schachat AP, Murphy RB, Patz A, editors: *Retina: Vol 2, Medical retina,* St Louis, 1989, Mosby.
89. Schechter SL: Lyme disease associated with optic neuropathy, *Am J Med* 81:143-145, 1986.
90. Sergent JS et al.: Vasculitis with hepatitis B antigenemia: long-term observations in nine patients, *Medicine* 55:1-18, 1976.
91. Sevel D: Necrogranulomatous keratitis: associated with Wegener's granulomatosis and rheumatoid arthritis, *Am J Ophthalmol* 63:250-255, 1967.
92. Shelhamer JH et al.: Takayasu's arteritis and its therapy, *Ann Int Med* 103:121-126, 1985.
93. Smith JL: Cogan's syndrome, *Laryngoscope* 80:121-132, 1970.
94. Smith JL: Cogan's syndrome and Lyme serology, *J Clin Neuro-ophthalmol* 10:264-265, 1990.
95. Speck WT, Toltzu P: Spirochetal diseases 12.50 syphilus. In Behaman RE, Kliegman RM, Niko WE, Vaughan VC, editors: *Nelson textbook of pediatrics,* ed 14, Philadelphia, 1992, WB Saunders.
96. Steere AC et al.: Unilateral blindness by infection with the Lyme disease spirochete, *Borrelia burgdorferi, Ann Int Med* 103:382-384, 1985.
97. Sullivan CJ, Jordan MC: Measles. In Hoeprich PD, Jordan MC, editors: *Infectious diseases: a modern treatise of infectious processes,* Philadelphia, 1990, JB Lippincott.
98. Suttorp-Schulten MSA et al.: Birdshot chorioretinopathy and Lyme borreliosis, *Am J Ophthalmol* 115:149-153, 1993.
99. Vollertsen RS et al.: Cogan's syndrome: 18 cases and a review of the literature, *Mayo Clin Proc* 61:344-361, 1986.
100. Watson PG: The diagnosis and management of scleritis, *Ophthalmology* 87:716-720, 1980.
101. Weinstein L: Antimicrobial agents. In Goodman LS, Gilman A, editors: *The pharmacologic basis of therapeutics,* ed 5, New York, 1975, McMillan Publishing.
102. Whitcher JP: Chlamydial diseases. In Smolin G, Thoft RA, editors: *The cornea: scientific foundations and clinical practice,* Boston, 1983, Little Brown.
103. Whitson WE, Krachmer JH: Adult rheumatoid arthritis. In Gold DH, Weingeist TA, editors: *The eye in systemic disease,* Philadelphia, 1990, JB Lippincott.
104. Wohlgethan JR, Stilmant MM, Smith HR: Palpable purpura and uveitis precipitated by splenectomy in an atypical case of Cogan's syndrome, *J Rheumatol* 18:1100-1103, 1991.
105. Wolff D et al.: The pathology of Cogan's syndrome causing profound deafness, *Ann Otol Rhinol Laryngol* 74:507-520, 1965.
106. Wu G et al.: Optic disc edema and Lyme disease, *Ann Ophthalmol* 18:252-255, 1986.

37 Peripheral Corneal Disorders Associated with Systemic Immune-Mediated Disease

STEVEN B. ROBIN, JEFFREY B. ROBIN, BARTLY J. MONDINO

The peripheral cornea is a vaguely defined area that marks the transition from the central and paracentral cornea across the corneal periphery and limbus to the adjoining tissues of the conjunctiva and sclera. The peripheral cornea may be the target of inflammatory reactions caused by infections and hypersensitivity reactions.[94] Noninfectious inflammations of the sclera and conjunctiva frequently spread to involve the adjacent cornea. The peripheral cornea is sometimes involved in systemic disease (Table 37-1), most commonly vasculitic disorders. Marginal corneal infiltration or ulceration may be the presenting sign of rheumatoid arthritis, polyarteritis nodosa, and Wegener granulomatosis. Other systemic conditions, particularly dermatologic diseases and merabolic disorders, commonly have manifestations in the peripheral cornea. Intrinsic disorders of the peripheral cornea include marginal degenerations and certain neoplasms.

PATHOGENESIS

The unique anatomy of the peripheral cornea is the key to understanding the various disorders that may affect it. Although clear-cut borders are delineated, the central limit of the peripheral cornea is arbitrarily considered to coincide with the flattening of the normal corneal curvature (usually 3.5 to 4.5 mm from the visual axis). The peripheral cornea is arbitrarily assigned to the junction of the gradually opacifying limbus with the conjunctiva and sclera. Compared to the central cornea, the thickness of the peripheral cornea is greater (up to 0.7 mm), near the adjoining sclera. The periphery of the cornea is best considered as a transition zone that encompasses the histologic characteristics of the cornea, conjunctiva, episclera and sclera (including the blood vessels, lymphatic channels, and corneal nerves).

The vascular supply to the limbus and peripheral cornea consists of capillary arcades that extend approximately 0.5 mm into the clear cornea.[56] These capillary arcades are derived from the anterior conjunctival and deep episcleral arteries, branches of the anterior ciliary arteries. Unlike the avascular central cornea, the limbus and peripheral cornea derive part of their nutrient supply from these blood vessels. Interruption of this vascular supply can potentially result in peripheral necrosis and ulceration. The presence of these vessels also allows for limited diffusion of small-molecular-weight molecules (for example, fluorescein and smaller immunoglobulins)[2] into the peripheral corneal stroma. Inflamed capillaries become more permeable, resulting in the movement of more or larger molecules from the circulation into the corneal periphery. Although the central cornea may be eventually involved, the peripheral cornea is invariably affected first. The presence of this vasculature may also explain the predilection of the peripheral cornea to be involved in systemic hypersensitivity disorders or autoimmune diseases.

Channels from the subconjunctival lymphatics accompany the capillaries into the peripheral cornea.[56] These drain into regional lymph nodes, providing a mechanism for the afferent arm of corneal immunologic reactions. The peripheral cornea contains a reservoir of inflammatory cells, including polymorphonuclear leukocytes, lymphocytes, plasma cells, eosinophils, and mast cells.[56] These cells and their products make the peripheral cornea susceptible to the effects of hypersensitivity and immunologic reactions and account for the operating mechanisms of several peripheral corneal disorders.

The systemic vasculitides, particularly the collagen-vascular diseases, often involve the peripheral cornea and/or adjacent sclera. Corneal changes in these conditions may result from inflammatory collagen destruction, ischemic necrosis, or tear deficiency.

Microbially Induced Corneal Ring

Noninfectious, ring-shaped infiltration of the corneal stroma (commonly known as a Wessely ring) is described most frequently in association with corneal infections caused by gram-negative bacteria,[83] particularly *Pseudomonas aeruginosa*,[10] herpes simplex virus, and varicella-zoster virus.[79] These rings are believed to result from the intracorneal interaction of antigens (from the infecting orga-

TABLE 37-1 SYSTEMIC CONDITIONS THAT MAY AFFECT THE PERIPHERAL CORNEA

Vasculitides

Rheumatoid arthritis
Sjogren syndrome
Relapsing polychondritis
Juvenile rheumatoid arthritis
Systemic lupus erythematosus
Progressive systemic sclerosis
Wegener granulomatosis
Polyarteritis nodosa
Giant-cell arteritis
Cogan syndrome

Dermatologic Conditions

Ectodermal dysplasia
Benign mucous membrane pemphigoid
Stevens-Johnson syndrome
Rosacea
Psoriasis
Ichthyosis
Acrodermatitis enteropathica
Darier disease (keratosis follicularis)

Metabolic Conditions

Chrysiasis
Argyrosis
Hyperlipidemias
Wilson hepatolenticular degeneration

nism and antibody) diffusing into the cornea from the limbal blood vessels and plasma cells.[10,79] This immune reaction then activates complement by the classical pathway, attracting inflammatory cells, and resulting in stromal infiltration. Certain gram-negative bacteria may elaborate endotoxins that activate the alternate complement pathway, resulting in a similar clinical picture.[83]

Histopathologic and immunopathologic studies have shown that antigen-antibody complexes, complement, and polymorphonuclear leukocytes are contained in corneal immune rings.[83] Herpesvirus antigens have been demonstrated in both experimental[78] and clinical[79] cases of herpetic Wessely rings. Experimental corneal immune rings have been produced by introducing an antigen into the peripheral cornea of a previously sensitized animal.

CLINICAL FEATURES

The wide variety of disorders that may involve the peripheral cornea leads to a long list of potential symptomatology. Conditions resulting in inflammatory infiltration, epithelial erosion, or ulceration usually cause photophobia, foreign body sensation, and pain. Visual acuity may be af-

fected if the inflammatory process involves the central cornea or if peripheral structural alterations are severe enough to cause astigmatism. Noninflammatory peripheral thinning disorders are frequently asymptomatic, except for visual distortion caused by altered corneal topography. Itching may be a prominent component of some ocular hypersensitivity conditions. The physician should determine whether the symptoms are acute or chronic, worse in the morning or evening, or have a seasonal variation.

A careful history of previous ocular infection, trauma, surgery, and current and previous medications is important. Contact lens tolerance and care habits should be investigated in lens wearers. The use of topical medications should be ascertained, including illicit drugs such as crack cocaine.[96] The patient should be asked about any infectious diseases, allergic symptoms, arthritis, respiratory difficulties, skin changes, headaches, difficulties with maintaining balance, mouth dryness, or severe diarrhea. Such systemic complaints may point to underlying illnesses associated with, or responsible for, the peripheral corneal disorder.

Patients with peripheral corneal disorders should have a thorough ocular examination, highlighting several areas. The presence of any blepharitis should be carefully noted. The degree and location of conjunctival hyperemia, discharge, papillary formation, or follicles are important to document. Areas of episcleritis or scleritis are best identified by examining the patient in natural light. The marginal corneal lesions should be carefully documented with descriptions, photographs, and drawings of the area of infiltration, ulceration, thinning, vascularization, pigmentation, or lipid deposition. Corneal sensation should be ascertained. The application of sodium fluorescein and rose bengal will delineate any areas of epithelial loss. Careful examination of the anterior chamber and iris should be made to determine the presence and extent of any ocular inflammation.

Special attention should be given to certain aspects of the general physical examination. The skin should be closely examined for the presence of telangiectatic blood vessels, pustules, papules, abnormal texture, eczema, scarring, and scaling. The nail beds should be examined for ridging. The scalp, hair, and teeth should be noted for abnormalities stemming from one of the ectodermal dysplasias. The face should be examined for the development of rhinophyma, pigmentary or cartilaginous abnormalities of the auricles, or palpable anomalies of the temporal arteries. Thorough examination of the joints may be indicated in symptomatic patients; limited range of motion, pain, and distortion may denote the presence of one of the collagen vascular diseases.

Rheumatoid Arthritis

Rheumatoid arthritis is the most common collagen-vascular disorder that affects the peripheral cornea. Adult rheumatoid arthritis is a chronic multisystem disorder characterized by symmetric inflammation of the peripheral joints. It affects approximately 2.5% to 3% of adults (primarily women) and has an average age of onset between 35 and 40 years.[67] Any joint may eventually be affected; however, the interphalangeal and metacarpophalangeal joints are characteristically involved. Affected patients may have a mild onset characterized by prodromal symptoms (weight loss, malaise, fatigue) followed by mild joint pain and stiffness. Alternatively, some patients have an acute onset characterized by moderate to severe pain and swelling in multiple joints accompanied by fever and chills. Periarticular involvement, manifested by tenosynovitis, tendinitis, and muscular and bone atrophy, is common. Furthermore, about 25% of rheumatoid arthritis patients will have extraarticular manifestations, including subcutaneous nodules, cardiac involvement, pulmonary disease, splenomegaly, or ocular disease.[67]

The exact cause of rheumatoid arthritis is unknown, although it is probably immunologically based. Additional factors (genetic susceptibility, environmental stimuli) may eventually become implicated in the pathogenesis of this disease.[80] Immunologic findings in adult rheumatoid arthritis include serum and synovial fluid rheumatoid factor, serum and synovial fluid immune complexes, depressed levels of synovial fluid complement, serum cryoglobulins, and antinuclear antibodies.[67]

Ocular involvement in adult rheumatoid arthritis includes keratoconjunctivitis sicca (Sjögren syndrome), scleritis, episcleritis, and a variety of corneal changes. These complications tend to occur more frequently in those patients with evidence of advanced disease, particularly subcutaneous nodules, vasculitis, and cardiac involvement.[61] Corneal damage in rheumatoid arthritis may result from an adjacent scleritis with sclerosing keratitis or from corneal stromal melting that may or may not be associated with scleritis.[18] In addition to scleritis-associated changes, the corneas of rheumatoid arthritis patients are frequently affected by keratoconjunctivitis sicca arising from an associated Sjögren syndrome.[42] Sialochemical analyses,[11] as well as lacrimal and salivary gland biopsies,[40] have demonstrated evidence of Sjögren syndrome in 24% to 31% of adult rheumatoid arthritis patients. Of the patients with sialochemical abnormalities, 80% had clinical evidence of keratoconjunctivitis sicca.[11]

Sclerokeratitis. The reported incidence of scleritis in adult rheumatoid arthritis has ranged from 0.67%[82] to 6.3%.[62] Scleritis tends to occur in patients having both severe arthritic and extraarticular disease.[61,75] Its development is a particularly ominous sign of an ongoing systemic vasculitis; untreated, most of these patients will die within 5 years.[42,112] Adult rheumatoid arthritis accounts for 10% to 30% of scleritis cases.[75,112] Additional conditions that may cause scleritis include other collagen vascular diseases, syphilis, tuberculosis, gout, Reiter disease, ophthalmic zoster, and ankylosing spondylitis. In 55% of scleritis cases, no asso-

ciated systemic diseases can be identified.[112] Corneal involvement occurs in 28% to 37% of all scleritis patients.[75] Of those scleritis patients having adult rheumatoid arthritis, the reported incidence of corneal abnormalities ranges from 46% to 69%.[71,75] The peripheral cornea is most commonly involved, usually as a direct extension of the scleral inflammatory process. Four patterns of peripheral corneal involvement in scleritis have been described: sclerosing keratitis, acute stromal keratitis, furrowing (limbal guttering), and keratolysis.[61,111,112,113]

Sclerosing keratitis is the most common corneal complication associated with scleritis.[75,112,113] It is characterized by a peripheral thickening and grayish opacification of the stroma adjacent to the site of scleral inflammation. The process will usually progress centrally, having crystalline stromal opacities behind the advancing edge. Vascular infiltration follows slowly and usually involves the superficial stroma. Late complications include scarring, vascularization, and lipid deposition.

Acute stromal keratitis manifests as superficial and/or midstromal peripheral infiltrates in association with nodular or diffuse, nonnecrotizing scleritis. These infiltrates may either develop simultaneously with or after the onset of the scleritis. They may coalesce to a diffuse peripheral opacification that may eventually become vascularized. Additionally, these opacities may result in epithelial breakdown and stromal melting. With vigorous treatment of the scleritis, however, resolution with resultant linear stromal scars is the rule.

Peripheral corneal furrowing (Fig. 37-1) is a well-recognized complication of rheumatoid scleritis.[18,75,113] It frequently begins in an area of sclerosing keratitis, but may progress circumferentially to involve the entire periphery.[61,70,75] The degree of thinning is usually severe, especially in cases associated with necrotizing scleritis. Addi-

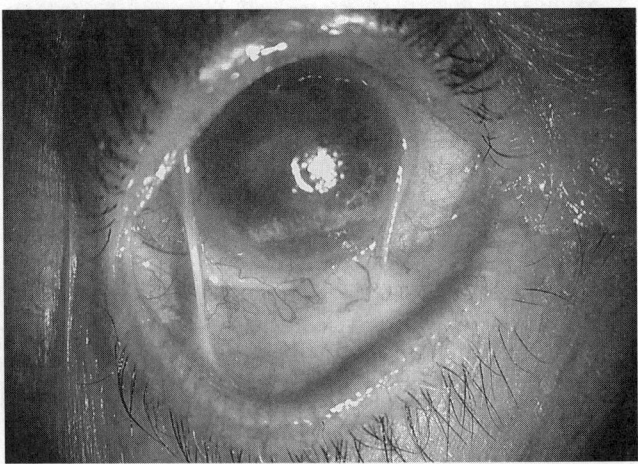

Fig. 37-1. Peripheral corneal furrow associated with rheumatoid arthritis.

tionally, peripheral furrowing is ordinarily accompanied by vascularization of, and eventual lipid deposition into, the stromal gutter. The epithelium customarily remains intact throughout the entire disease process.

Keratolysis is an acute, severe melting of clear cornea that occurs in association with marked necrotizing scleritis or scleromalacia perforans.[112,113] In this process, the entire stroma is rapidly destroyed, resulting in descemetocele formation in as little as 4 days. These corneas are especially prone to rupture following minor trauma.

Limbal Furrow. Peripheral corneal melting in the form of limbal furrowing can occur in adult rheumatoid arthritis patients without an associated scleritis.[18,32,61,97] The corneal epithelium usually remains intact, and the furrow ordinarily does not become vascularized.

Episcleritis with Corneal Changes. Peripheral corneal abnormalities may also be observed in association with episcleritis in adult rheumatoid arthritis patients.[112,113] Corneal involvement occurs in approximately 15% of rheumatoid episcleritis cases and is generally milder than the involvement associated with rheumatoid scleritis. The most frequent signs are stromal edema and infiltration occurring adjacent to the episcleral inflammation. This process usually remains in the periphery. Recurrent attacks may result in permanent stromal opacification and vascularization. Additionally, areas of peripheral stromal thinning may occur, as dellen, adjacent to elevated episcleritic nodules.

Sjögren Syndrome

Sjögren syndrome is a chronic, multisystem autoimmune disorder, characterized clinically by keratoconjunctivitis sicca and xerostomia.[99] Two forms of the disease are recognized: (1) dry eye and xerostomia alone ("primary sicca syndrome") and (2) the combination of dry eye and xerostomia in association with another connective tissue or collagen vascular disease, most commonly rheumatoid arthritis ("secondary sicca syndrome").[85]

Ocular findings in Sjögren syndrome primarily consist of those caused by aqueous tear deficiency. In addition, Sjögren syndrome patients are predisposed to develop peripheral corneal infiltrates, thinning, ulceration, and even perforation.[3,26,50,68,91] Peripheral sterile infiltrates occur in approximately 10% of patients, and they resemble the infiltrates of staphylococcal hypersensitivity. Most of the reported cases of peripheral thinning in Sjögren syndrome have been in those patients with associated rheumatoid arthritis.[22,26,50,68,91] Additionally, an association seems to exist between the perforation of these peripheral furrows and the use of topical corticosteroids.[26,68,91]

Systemic Lupus Erythematosus

Systemic lupus erythematosus is a multisystem disorder that may affect the articular, cutaneous, renal, hematologic, pulmonary, neurologic, cardiovascular, and ocular systems.

Ocular complications of lupus include scleritis, keratitis, corneal furrowing, and retinal vasculitis.[41]

The major corneal manifestation associated with systemic lupus erythematosus is a punctate epitheliopathy.[39,41] This finding may be related to disease severity. The incidence of punctate corneal staining varies between 6.5% of outpatients with controlled lupus[47] and 88% of patients with disease activity severe enough to require hospitalization.[103] Schirmer testing usually shows normal aqueous tear production.[103] Superficial keratopathy, therefore, does not appear to be related to keratoconjunctivitis sicca.

Corneal stromal involvement in systemic lupus erythematosus is rare. Bilateral deep interstitial keratitis in a band-shaped pattern has been reported.[52,92] Quiet, nonfiltrative marginal melts may occur. Marginal ulcers with vascularization and infiltration have occasionally been noted.[113]

Discoid lupus erythematosis is a related collagen vascular disorder that affects only the skin and mucous membrane.[39] Superficial punctate keratitis is the major corneal complication in discoid lupus.[29,39] Diagnosis can be made by skin biopsy, and the keratitis resolves during systemic therapy with chloroquine or quinacrine.[29,39]

Relapsing Polychondritis

Relapsing polychondritis, first described in 1923,[91] is an uncommon, multisystem disorder characterized by recurrent episodes of inflammation in cartilaginous tissues throughout the body. Systemic manifestations consist of a migratory polyarthritis, fever, and a diffuse chondritis. The latter eventually involves the external ear, and the nasal, costal, tracheal, and laryngeal cartilages. Potential systemic complications include myocardial and aortic disease, anemia, abnormal liver function tests, and airway obstruction.[117] Although relapsing polychondritis may be associated with autoimmune disorders (for example, Sjögren syndrome), the pathogenesis of the chondritis remains unknown.[30] Recent evidence[77] suggests that anticollagen antibodies may play a pathogenic role in this disease.

Ocular complications occur in approximately 60% of relapsing polychondritis patients.[30] These complications include episcleritis, scleritis, iritis, conjunctivitis, keratoconjunctivitis sicca, keratitis, exudative choroidopathy, exudative retinal detachments, optic neuritis, proptosis, and abducens nerve palsy.[3,57,72,76,95]

Episcleritis and scleritis are the most common ocular manifestations, occurring in 30% to 60% of patients.[3,30,57] Corneal disease, reported in 11% of patients, consists primarily of sclerokeratitis or marginal ulceration.

Peripheral corneal edema and stromal infiltrates have been noted in association with relapsing polychondritis, episcleritis, or scleritis.[3,12,54,63] The epithelium may remain intact over the infiltrates; corneal vascularization may occur with infiltrate resolution. Marginal ulceration or limbal furrowing have been reported, both with[57,117]—and without[7,74]—an associated scleritis. This process of marginal thinning may spread circumferentially to involve the entire periphery[117] and may become severe enough to cause perforation.[7,74] In one case of marginal furrowing[117] a normal anterior segment angiogram was noted, suggesting that neither a vasculitic nor ischemic process was responsible for the corneal changes. Peripheral corneal involvement in relapsing polychondritis usually responds well to topical and/ or systemic corticosteroids.[12,117] Resistant cases may be treated with dapsone.[73,81]

Wegener Granulomatosis

Wegener granulomatosis is an idiopathic, multisystem respiratory vasculitis. Its classic clinicopathologic triad consists of necrotizing granulomatous inflammation of the upper respiratory tract, granulomatous inflammation of the lower respiratory tract, and a focal glomerulonephritis.[48,93] In most cases, a diffuse systemic granulomatous vasculitis accompanies this triad. Presenting symptoms and signs usually involve the upper respiratory tract,[48] although some patients may have ocular abnormalities.[104] Additionally, a limited form of Wegener granulomatosis has been described.[20] It has a milder clinical course and lacks renal involvement. The systemic, pathologic, and ocular findings in both the classic and limited forms have been well reviewed.[19,93]

Reports of the incidence of ocular involvement in Wegener granulomatosis have varied from 28% to 45%.[19,105] Ophthalmic manifestations consist of secondary orbital involvement from contiguous sinus disease, as well as primary, focal, ocular disease. Focal disease includes scleritis, episcleritis, uveitis, keratitis, retinal vasculitis, conjunctivitis, and retinal detachment.[19,93,104,105]

Peripheral corneal involvement in Wegener granulomatosis usually consists of an ulcerative keratitis. This process is ordinarily bilateral, is classically associated with an adjacent scleritis, and may be the presenting sign of the disease. The keratitis customarily begins as multiple, peripheral, stromal infiltrates, similar to those seen in staphylococcal hypersensitivity. Eventually, the epithelium and uninvolved stroma overlying these infiltrates ulcerate. Progression of the ulcerative keratitis is generally circumferential; a 360° peripheral ring ulcer may result. In some cases, the ulcer may extend centrally, with an overhanging central edge similar to that seen in Mooren ulcer. Untreated, the central and peripheral ulcerations may perforate.

The histopathologic features of peripheral keratitis in Wegener granulomatosis[25,37,44] include the following: necrosis of the epithelium and superficial stroma; stromal infiltration by inflammatory cells; and, occasionally, the presence of epithelioid and giant cells surrounding the ulcer base. This necrotizing granulomatous inflammation may extend into the adjacent sclera and ciliary body. The pathogenesis of peripheral ulcerative keratitis in Wegener granulomatosis is believed to involve an occlusive vasculitis of the adjacent intrascleral blood vessels.[6,17,44]

Polyarteritis Nodosa

Polyarteritis nodosa is a chronic, idiopathic, necrotizing vasculitis that primarily affects medium- and small-sized arteries. The disease has protean manifestations and is seen most frequently in 20- to 40-year-old males.[41] Its pathogenesis, although unknown, probably involves an immune complex-mediated vasculitis.

Ocular involvement occurs in approximately 20% of polyarteritis nodosa patients and includes scleritis, choroidal vasculitis, retinal vasculitis, optic atrophy, exudative retinal detachment, papilledema, and keratitis.[41]

The keratitis in polyarteritis nodosa is usually peripheral, bilateral, ulcerative, and progressive.[25,84] It may begin with marginal stromal infiltrates, and eventually the overlying epithelium and anterior stroma ulcerate. This process generally spreads circumferentially and may also extend Mooren-like into the central cornea. Frequently, the keratitis is associated with an adjacent necrotizing scleritis.[53] Like Wegener granulomatosis, peripheral ulcerative keratitis may be the presenting sign in polyarteritis nodosa. Furthermore, as is the case with Wegener granulomatosis, topical ocular therapy of the corneoscleral manifestations is usually ineffective, and successful management is predicated upon full systemic therapy of the disease. The recommended treatment regimen for the systemic disease is a combination of systemic corticosteroids and cyclophosphamide.[35] Local measures (for example, conjunctival resection, cyanoacrylate adhesive, therapeutic soft contact lenses, and collagenase inhibitors) may slow the corneal disease process while the patient is being systemically treated.[41]

Progressive Systemic Sclerosis (Scleroderma)

Progressive systemic sclerosis is a multisystem disorder that primarily affects women. The skin, blood vessels, esophagus, joints, kidneys, heart, and lungs are the most common targets. Raynaud phenomenon is a nearly universal finding and a common presenting sign. The skin becomes thickened and hardened during the disease course. The pathogenesis of the disease is as yet unknown. Foster[41] believes that this disease involves an immunologic sensitization to skin antigens along with a subsequent proliferation of dermal fibroblasts, an overproduction of immature collagen, and a vascular ingrowth.

Ocular manifestations in progressive systemic sclerosis include keratitis, keratoconjunctivitis sicca, conjunctival shrinkage, choroidal vasculopathy, and extraocular muscle myositis.[41] The majority of corneal changes result from keratoconjunctivitis sicca. Secondary sicca (Sjögren) syndrome is noted in more than 70% of patients.[65] Occasionally, these patients may have peripheral ulcerations or furrowing unassociated with keratoconjunctivitis sicca.[27]

Giant-Cell Arteritis

The peripheral cornea may also be involved during the course of other vasculitides. Marginal corneal ulcers can be the presenting sign of cranial arteritis.[46] These corneal lesions were associated with conjunctival ulcerations and scleromalacia. Slow resolution of the corneal and conjunctival ulcerations[10] achieved with systemic corticosteroids.

Cogan Syndrome

In 1945 Cogan[24] described a vasculitic syndrome characterized by nonsyphilitic interstitial keratitis, vertigo, and deafness. An atypical form was also noted, consisting of ocular orbital inflammatory disease (not involving the cornea) and vestibuloauditory symptoms. The most common ocular findings in early, typical Cogan syndrome are bilateral, peripheral, subepithelial nummular opacities.[23] Treatment for the corneal changes consists of topical corticosteroids. Systemic corticosteroids are eventually necessary to prevent deafness.

Psoriasis

Psoriasis is a relatively common condition. Characterized by hyperproliferation of epidermal cells), psoriasis results in plaquelike, keratotic skin lesions. Arthritis is the most frequent nondermatologic manifestation. Ocular involvement occurs in about 10% of cases. The limbus and peripheral cornea may be affected by phlyctenule-like lesions, superficial and deep opacities, as well as epithelial erosions and stromal melting.[16]

Crohn Disease and Ulcerative Colitis

Crohn disease and ulcerative colitis are inflammatory disorders of the intestinal tract. Extraintestinal complications of inflammatory bowel disease are common and include arthritis, erythema nodosum, stomatitis, ankylosing spondylitis, hepatitis, cholangitis, and pyelonephritis.[101]

Ocular involvement is a well-recognized complication of both Crohn disease and ulcerative colitis. Uveitis is probably the most common ocular complication, occurring in 0.5% to 11.8% of cases.[116] Anterior uveitis may occur coincident with, or before, the intestinal symptoms.[28,116] Peripheral uveitis has been associated with the ulcerative colitis patient.[116] Other ocular manifestations in inflammatory bowel disease include conjunctivitis,[101] episcleritis, scleritis, and keratitis.[90]

Peripheral corneal involvement has been documented in Crohn disease and ulcerative colitis. Peripheral subepithelial infiltrates[33,71,90,98] and nodules[66] have been reported. These infiltrates may be associated with an adjacent scleritis or episcleritis, and they respond well to topical corticosteroids. In advanced cases, the overlying epithelium may ulcerate, resulting in sterile marginal ulcers.[33]

DIFFERENTIAL DIAGNOSIS

The peripheral cornea can be affected by several infectious and hypersensitivity disorders. Some of these are similar to central corneal inflammatory reactions. Others, including allergic reactions to bacterial toxins and airborne antigens, preferentially affect the corneal periphery. Peripheral corneal involvement has been occasionally noted in acute anaphylaxis, usually after an intravenous diagnostic test.[11,94] Corneal changes consist of bilateral peripheral stromal infiltrates separated from the limbus by a clear interval.

Microbial Keratitis

All organisms that infect the central cornea can produce peripheral corneal infections. The clinical manifestations of central or peripheral infectious keratitis are not pathognomonic for a particular organism.

Peripheral keratitis may begin as an epithelial defect and stromal infiltrate near the limbus. It may then spread along the limbus, toward the center of the cornea, or into the adjacent sclera. A ring ulcer is a circumferential ulceration just inside the limbus, and it results from the coalescence of several peripheral ulcers or from progression of a circumferential keratitis. A ring abscess is a rapidly progressive, circumferential, purulent infiltration of the cornea that is typically 1 to 2 millimeters wide and separated from the limbus by approximately 1 millimeter of clear cornea.

The most common bacteria infecting the peripheral cornea are *Staphylococcus* species, *Streptococcus pneumoniae, Pseudomonas aeruginosa, Hemophilus influenzae,* and *Moraxella* sp. *Staphylococcus aureus* and *Streptococcus pneumoniae* classically produce round or oval, gray-white, well-circumscribed corneal ulcers. Peripheral infections by *Streptococcus pneumoniae* tend to spread centrally, resulting in an "acute serpiginous ulcer." *Moraxella* species typically produces shallow, grey-white ulcers with irregular borders. Most *Moraxella* sp. peripheral corneal ulcers do not spread circumferentially or centrally.

Nearly one third of all *Pseudomonas* species corneal infections involve the peripheral cornea initially. Peripheral involvement is particularly common if certain predisposing factors, such as trauma or lagophthalmos, are present. Peripheral *Pseudomonas* sp. keratitis frequently spreads circumferentially, producing a ring ulcer or a ring abscess. These lesions may also extend into the sclera (an extremely poor prognostic sign because limbal perforation frequently results). *Pseudomonas* spp. infections of the peripheral cornea are generally more difficult to treat than their central counterparts; limbal cryotherapy may be a possible adjunct in the treatment of cases unresponsive to antibiotic therapy.

As with bacterial keratitis, nearly all of the fungi that affect the central cornea can affect the corneal periphery and limbus. Approximately 20% of fungal keratitis cases primarily involved the peripheral cornea. Peripheral ulcers sometimes respond better to medical therapy than the central or diffuse ulcers: only 43% of the former required surgical intervention as opposed to 73% of the latter. Lamellar keratectomy and inlay conjunctival flap are useful for the treatment of peripheral fungal keratitis refractory to medical therapy.

Acanthamoeba spp. keratitis may present as a peripheral corneal infiltrate and can be associated with anterior scleritis.

Chlamydial Keratitis

Chlamydial ocular infections commonly affect the limbus and peripheral cornea. Involvement consists of edema and infiltration of the limbal conjunctiva, punctate epithelial keratitis, subepithelial infiltrates, limbal follicles, extension of limbal blood vessels into the cornea forming a microscopic or gross pannus, and vascularized ulcers. The keratitis associated with Reiter syndrome preferentially involves the peripheral cornea.

Viral Keratitis

Several viruses can affect the peripheral cornea, including herpes simplex virus, varicella-zoster virus, adenovirus, vaccinia, molluscum contagiosum, and Epstein-Barr virus. Peripheral herpes simplex virus keratitis may be difficult to diagnose because of its atypical presentation. In recurrent peripheral herpetic keratitis, stromal infiltrates often follow dendrite formation; these infiltrations may be mistaken for catarrhal ulcers. Differentiation is important because the corticosteroid therapy recommended for catarrhal ulcers may exacerbate a herpetic infection. As compared to central disease, peripheral herpetic keratitis (1) usually results in more severe stromal disease, (2) is more frequently accompanied by iritis and keratitic precipitates, and (3) tends to run a more prolonged and refractory course.

Varicella-zoster virus can preferentially involve the peripheral cornea. Peripheral corneal infiltrates occurring during varicella or zoster sometimes resemble corneal phlyctenules. Peripheral stromal involvement may result in perilimbal infiltration and vascularization. Zoster peripheral infiltrative and ulcerative keratitis is associated with an adjacent scleritis.

Peripheral corneal involvement with vaccinia usually takes the form of limbal pustules. These may spread into the peripheral clear cornea and result in frank corneal ulceration. Other forms of peripheral keratitis including superficial punctate, interstitial, and disciform lesions may also occur.

Viruses that produce eyelid margin lesions, such as molluscum contagiosum and verruca vulgaris, frequently have an associated peripheral epithelial keratitis. The keratitis is believed to be toxic and begins as punctate epithelial erosions. It can progress, leading to infiltration and vascularization. The keratitis usually resolves with the removal of the eyelid lesion. Primary corneal disease caused by molluscum is relatively rare, but has been reported, as a limbal nodule, in a few patients with the acquired immune deficiency syndrome.

Systemic Infections Associated with Peripheral Keratitis

In onchocerciasis, most of the microfilariae are in the superficial third of the corneal stroma at the periphery of the nasal and temporal interpalpebral areas. A superficial punctate keratitis with fluffy, longitudinal stromal opacities develops around dead microfilariae. As a late complication, vascularization of the limbus and peripheral cornea may occur.

Other systemic infections have been associated with peripheral sterile corneal infiltration or ulceration. These include bacillary dysentery, brucellosis, mumps, influenza, infectious mononucleosis, dengue fever, and systemic hookworm infestation. The pathogenesis of these corneal changes is unclear.

Marginal Keratitis Associated with Blepharoconjunctivitis

Corneal hypersensitivity responses, often called "catarrhal" infiltrates and ulcers, probably represent the most common form of peripheral corneal disorder. Catarrhal marginal keratitis usually occurs with a concomitant blepharoconjunctivitis.[21] Severe marginal keratitis has been described in younger patients suffering from neutrophil dysfunction[89] or Wiskott-Aldrich syndrome.[51]

Catarrhal lesions typically begin as one or more, grey-white, peripheral stromal infiltrates with the long axis parallel to the limbus.[21,109] These lesions are almost always separated from the limbus by a zone of clear, uninvolved cornea. There is usually an associated conjunctival reaction with hyperemia and chemosis. Affected patients complain of pain, foreign-body sensation, and photophobia. If left untreated, the natural course of these lesions involves breakdown of the overlying epithelium and eventual ulceration. The ultimate course, however, is usually benign; healing generally occurs in 2 to 4 weeks with little, if any, vascularization. Recurrences of marginal keratitis are quite common. Microbial cultures of the involved areas are sterile, although cultures of the lid margins or conjunctiva may reveal microorganisms.

As early as 1946, Thygeson[109] observed that catarrhal infiltrates and ulcers were hypersensitivity reactions to chronic staphylococcal blepharitis or conjunctivitis. He had previously[108] noted that the ocular pathogenic effects of staphylococci were caused not only by the organism, but also by the toxins it elaborated. Chignell and associates[21] cultured staphylococci from the eyelid margins and/or conjunctiva in nearly 30% of a series of marginal keratitis patients (as opposed to an 11% culture rate in unaffected controls). Other organisms rarely implicated in cases of marginal keratitis are *Streptococcus pneumoniae, Haemophilus* sp., *Bacillus* sp., *Moraxella* sp., *Actinomycetes* sp., *Neisseria gonorrhoeae,* and *Escherichia coli.*[109]

Marginal corneal infiltrates and ulcerations are believed to be the result of deposition of antigen-antibody complexes in the peripheral cornea.[45] The antigen is probably derived from the associated local bacteria; and the antibody diffuses into the cornea from the limbal vasculature. An animal model of catarrhal infiltrates and phlyctenulosis uses staphylococcal cell-wall antigens in previously sensitized rabbits.[82] The deposition of immune complexes into the peripheral cornea activates the classical complement pathway and leads to polymorphonuclear leukocyte infiltration.[4] These inflammatory cells elaborate collagenase and other hydrolytic enzymes, resulting in epithelial denudation and stromal ulceration.

Phlyctenulosis

Phlyctenulosis is thought to be a local conjunctival and/or corneal immune response, probably cell-mediated, to an antigen to which the host has been previously sensitized. In the past, the disease was closely linked to the tuberculin antigen. Today, phlyctenulosis is much more commonly associated with *Staphylococcus aureus*.[82] Other implicated organisms include *Coccidioides immitis, Chlamydia lymphogranulomatosis, Ascaris lumbricoides, Ancylostoma duodenale, Enterobius vermicularis, Entamoeba histolytica, Hymenolopis nana,* and several viruses including adenovirus and herpes simplex virus.[1]

Phlyctenular disease is usually bilateral and may affect the conjunctiva or cornea.[9] Isolated corneal phlyctenules, without conjunctival involvement, are infrequent. The first attack usually involves the limbus, but bulbar or tarsal conjunctival lesions have been described. The typical phlyctenule is a pinkish-white limbal nodule, usually adjacent to an area of conjunctival hyperemia. It may be solitary or multiple, and it varies in size from pinpoint to several millimeters. These elevated nodules become grayish in color, ulcerate, and eventually resolve. Resolution usually involves corneal vascularization and scarring; the conjunctival side remains unscarred. The process may remain isolated at the limbus or spread centrally in what is termed a ''wandering'' fashion. The active corneal lesions usually have a small circular ulceration at the central margin with a sharply demarcated band of blood vessels covering the healed area of peripheral ulceration. These vascularized lesions are classically wedge-shaped, with the base toward the limbus, and usually affect the inferior cornea. Although stromal involvement is typically superficial, deeper involvement may occur in staphylococcal phlyctenulosis.[87] Corneal phlyctenules generally ulcerate and resolve with a vascularized scar within 10 to 15 days. Histopathologically, corneal phlyctenules are characterized by accumulations of lymphocytes, even in acute attacks, that are analogous to marginal ulcers.

Symptomatology depends on the location of the lesions. Isolated conjunctival lesions cause redness, lacrimation, and foreign-body sensation. Corneal involvement results in the classical symptom of extreme photophobia. Photophobia in acutely affected children may be so severe as to preclude ocular examination.[9]

In endemic tuberculosis areas, patients with typical phlyctenular lesions should have a tuberculin skin test and, if the skin test is positive, a chest roentgenogram. In most of the developed world, eyelid margin and conjunctival cultures are the only diagnostic tests of potential use.

Vernal and Atopic Keratoconjunctivitis

Vernal and atopic keratoconjunctivitis are recurrent, bilateral inflammations of the tarsal and limbal conjunctivae that may also involve the peripheral and paracentral cornea. Vernal eye disease occurs primarily in warm climates and usually affects children under the age of 14. The prevalence of this condition appears to be much higher in males than females, particularly in those cases having their onset prior to puberty. In most cases, the disease process lasts between 4 and 10 years.

Ocular findings are characteristic. There may be a slight ptosis (1 to 3 mm) caused by excessive thickening of the tarsal conjunctiva. Most patients have a characteristic conjunctival discharge; it is yellowish, mucoid, and occurs in a rope-strand that can be easily pulled from the cul-de-sac. There are two patterns of conjunctival involvement: palpebral and limbal. Both of these are usually noted, in some degree, in a given patient. The palpebral form primarily affects the superior tarsal conjunctiva, particularly at the superior border of the tarsal plate. The predominant finding is a papillary hypertrophy that may begin as diffuse small papillae, but usually progresses to form the large, flat-topped ''cobblestone'' papillae. The lower tarsal conjunctiva, although frequently unaffected, may show a mild papillary response.

Limbal vernal is characterized by gelatinous thickening and opacification of the superior limbus. The superior peripheral cornea may be covered by the thickened conjunctiva. Raised nodules may appear in the gelatinous conjunctiva. Frequently, whitish Horner-Trantas dots may be observed in these masses that are composed of concretions of eosinophils.

Corneal involvement may be divided into two groups: punctate keratitis and ulcerative keratitis. The punctate keratitis generally involves the superior third of the cornea, and consists of fine epithelial disruptions that stain with rose bengal. In more severe cases, patches of necrosing epithelium may be seen in the superior cornea; these stain well with fluorescein. Ulcerative keratitis has a characteristic clinical appearance. The ulcer is usually solitary, shieldlike in shape, and almost invariably in the superior cornea. It is characteristically shallow and surrounded by raised edges of dead epithelium. The course of these ulcers is usually indolent, with healing and subsequent subepithelial scarring the rule.

Terrien Marginal Corneal Degeneration

Terrien marginal degeneration is classically described as an idiopathic, ectatic, noninflammatory degeneration.[43,106,107] Some patients with corneal changes typical of Terrien's, however, have suffered concomitant recurrent bouts of ocular inflammation consisting of episcleritis or superficial scleritis.[5,15] Whether these patients provide a clue to an immunologic mechanism for the disease remains a matter of speculation.

LABORATORY INVESTIGATIONS

Laboratory investigations may reveal causative or predisposing ocular or systemic conditions. Local ocular infections may be diagnosed by staining and culturing samples from suspected tissues or discharges. Ocular scrapings may also reveal the presence of eosinophils and other inflammatory cells in local hypersensitivity conditions. Tear-film determinations should be routine adjuncts in the investigation of peripheral corneal disorders. Biopsy and histopathologic studies may be necessary in the identification of limbal mass lesions.

Laboratory studies are frequently necessary to confirm the diagnosis of systemic conditions. If collagen vascular diseases are suspected, serologic studies should include rheumatoid factor, antinuclear antibodies, and complement levels. Roentgenographic studies may be helpful in delineating the nature of arthritides, in demonstrating the pulmonary and/or upper respiratory involvement characteristic of Wegener granulomatosis, and in highlighting inflammatory bowel changes. Tissue biopsy may be necessary to confirm the diagnosis of Wegener granulomatosis, polyarteritis nodosa, temporal arteritis, and the collagen-vascular diseases.

The diagnosis of metabolic conditions that involve the peripheral cornea frequently rests on the determination of serum levels of the suspected metabolic product or carrier and/or histopathologic identification of the product in tissue biopsies. The diagnosis of blood dyscrasias involving the peripheral cornea depends on appropriate peripheral blood or bone-marrow studies.

Many systemic disorders can be associated with peripheral keratitis and thinning. A general physical examination and appropriate consultation with an internist or rheumatologist are important.

Screening laboratory testing can include the following: complete blood count, sedimentation rate, serum chemistries (including serum urea nitrogen, creatinine, and uric acid), rheumatoid factor, antinuclear antibody, antineutrophil cytoplasmic antibody, immune-complex evaluation,[13] and complement levels. A chest x-ray and PPD skin testing are usually recommended to determine whether antituberculous prophylaxis will be needed during systemic corticosteroid therapy and to detect asymptomatic pulmonary disease.

THERAPY

The primary therapy for peripheral corneal changes associated with immunologic disorders is directed at aggressively controlling the systemic vasculitis and autoimmune process with systemic corticosteroids and/or immunosuppressive agents.* Topical corticosteroids may be useful in controlling sclerosing keratitis and scleritis.[111,113] These agents should usually not be used in noninflammatory cor-

neal furrowing or keratolysis, as they may enhance the possibility of perforation.[18,31,61,113] Topical collagenase inhibitors,[100] topical cyclosporine,[64,69] therapeutic soft contact lenses, or cyanoacrylate glue may prove effective in these cases.[38,61] Similarly, conjunctival resection has been shown to halt the progression of furrowing in refractory cases, both with and without an associated scleritis.[32,36,115] Lamellar or penetrating keratoplasty may be required either acutely to prevent perforation or, after control of the scleritis, to restore visual acuity.[14,102] Although penetrating keratoplasty often provides anatomic success, the prognosis is poor for both the vision and survival of the patient after surgery.[88]

The mainstay of management for the corneal complications in Sjögren syndrome consists of ocular surface lubrication. In cases with peripheral infiltrates, a short course of topical corticosteroids is recommended. These agents should not be used in the presence of corneal thinning. Peripheral furrowing and ulcerations can usually be managed successfully with therapeutic soft contact lenses.[91] In the case of perforation, management may include therapeutic lenses, cyanoacrylate adhesive, and lamellar or penetrating keratoplasties.[55,58,91,114]

Local treatment of corneoscleral involvement in Wegener granulomatosis is generally unsuccessful. Most cases will resolve only after institution of both appropriate systemic immunosuppressive agents (particularly cyclophosphamide) that are necessary to save the patient's life and systemic corticosteroids. Impending or actual corneal perforations can be acutely managed with cyanoacrylate adhesive,[44] conjunctival flap, or lamellar and/or penetrating keratoplasty.[49,119]

Therapy for band keratopathy focuses on disodium ethylenediamine tetraacetic acid (EDTA), a chelator of calcium.[49] A cellulose sponge saturated with 0.25 M disodium edetate is placed on the band keratopathy for 3 to 5 minutes. Because of the toxicity of edetate, it should be kept away from nondiseased tissue. The dissolved portion of band is then scraped away, with the procedure repeated until clear cornea is reached. A bandage therapeutic contact lens is then placed on the eye to aid in reepithelialization and comfort.

REFERENCES

1. Al-Hussaini MK, Khalifa R, Al-Ansary ATA et al.: Phlyctenular eye disease in association with *Hymenolepis nana* in Egypt, *Br J Ophthalmol* 63:627-631, 1979.
2. Allansmith MR, McClellan BH: Immunoglobulins in the human cornea, *Am J Ophthalmol* 80:123-132, 1975.
3. Anderson B: Ocular lesions in relapsing polychondritis and other rheumatoid syndromes, The Edward Jackson Memorial Lecture, *Am J Ophthalmol* 64:35-50, 1967.
4. Aronson SB, Elliott JH, Moore TE, O'Day DM: Pathogenetic approach to therapy of peripheral corneal inflammatory disease, *Am J Ophthalmol* 70:65-90, 1970.
5. Austin P, Brown SI: Inflammatory Terrien's marginal corneal disease, *Am J Ophthalmol* 92:185-192, 1981.
6. Austin P, Green WR, Sallyer DC et al.: Peripheral corneal degeneration and occlusive vasculitis in Wegener's granulomatosis, *Am J Ophthalmol* 85:311-317, 1978.

*References 32, 40, 59, 60, 112, 113.

7. Barth WF, Berson EL: Relapsing polychondritis, rheumatoid arthritis and blindness, *Am J Ophthalmol* 85:613-614, 1978.
8. Baum JL, Bierstock SR: Peripheral corneal infiltrates following intravenous injection of diatrizoate meglumine, *Am J Ophthalmol* 85:613-614, 1978.
9. Beauchamp GR, Gillette TE, Friendly DS: Phlyctenular keratoconjunctivitis, *J Pediatr Ophthalmol Strabismus* 18:22-28, 1981.
10. Belmont JR, Ostler HB, Dawson CR, Schwat I: Noninfectious ring-shaped keratitis associated with *Pseudomonas aeruginosa*, *Am J Ophthalmol* 93:338-341, 1982.
11. Ben-Aryeh H, Nahir M, Scharf Y et al.: Sialochemistry of patients with rheumatoid arthritis, *Oral Surg* 45:63-70, 1978.
12. Bergaust B, Abrahamson AM: Relapsing polychondritis: report of a case presenting multiple ocular complications, *Acta Ophthalmol* 47:174-181, 1969.
13. Berkowitz PT, Arentsen JJ, Felberg NT, Larbin PR: Presence of circulatory immune complexes in patients with peripheral corneal diseases, *Arch Ophthalmol* 101:242-245, 1983.
14. Biglan AW, Brown SI, Cignetti FE, Linn JG: Corneal perforation in Wegener's granulomatosis treated with corneal transplantation: case report, *Ann Ophthalmol* 9:799-801, 1977.
15. Binder PS, Zavala EY, Stainer GA: Noninfectious peripheral corneal ulceration: Mooren's ulcer or Terrien's marginal degeneration? *Ann Ophthalmol* 14:425-435, 1982.
16. Boss JM, Peachey RDG, Easty DSL, Thomsitt J: Peripheral corneal melting syndrome in association with psoriasis: a report of two cases, *Br Med J* 282:609-610, 1981.
17. Brady HR, Israel MR, Lewin WH: Wegener's granulomatosis and corneoscleral ulcer, *JAMA* 193:248-249, 1965.
18. Brown SI, Grayson M: Marginal furrows: a characteristic corneal lesion of rheumatoid arthritis, *Arch Ophthalmol* 79:563-567, 1968.
19. Bullen CL, Liesegang TJ, McDonald TJ, Remee RA: Ocular complications of Wegner's granulomatosis, *Ophthalmology* 90:270-290, 1983.
20. Carrington CB, Liebow AA: Limited forms of angiitis and granulomatosis of Wegener's type, *Am J Med* 41:497-527, 1966.
21. Chignell AH, Easty DL, Chesterton JR, Thomsitt J: Marginal ulceration of the cornea, *Br J Ophthalmol* 54:433-440, 1970.
22. Chudwin DS, Daniels TE, Wara DW et al.: Spectrum of Sjögren's syndrome in children, *J Pediatr* 98:213-217, 1981.
23. Cobo LM, Haynes BF: Early corneal findings in Cogan's syndrome, *Ophthalmology* 91:903-907, 1984.
24. Cogan DG: Syndrome of nonsympathetic interstitial keratitis and vestibuloauditory symptoms, *Arch Ophthalmol* 33:144-149, 1945.
25. Cogan DG: Corneoscleral lesions in periarteritis nodosa and Wegener's granulomatosis, *Trans Am Ophthalmol Soc* 53:321-344, 1965.
26. Cohen KL: Sterile corneal perforation after cataract surgery in Sjögren's syndrome, *Br J Ophthalmol* 66:179-182, 1982.
27. Coyle EF: Scleroderma of the cornea, *Br J Ophthalmol* 40:239-241, 1956.
28. Daum F, Gould HB, Gold D et al.: Asymptomatic transient uveitis in children with inflammatory bowel disease, *Am J Dis Child* 13:170-171, 1979.
29. Doesschate JT: Corneal complications in lupus erythematosis discoides, *Ophthalmologica* 132:153-156, 1956.
30. Dolan DL, Lemmon GB, Teitlebaum FR: Relapsing polychondritis: analytical literature review and studies on pathogenesis, *Am J Med* 41:285-299, 1966.
31. Easty DL, Madden P, Jayson MIV et al.: Systemic immunosuppression in marginal keratolysis, *Trans Ophthalmol Soc UK* 98:410-417, 1978.
32. Eiferman RA, Carothers DJ, Yankeelov JA: Peripheral rheumatoid ulceration and evidence for conjunctival collagenase production, *Am J Ophthalmol* 87:703-709, 1979.
33. Ellis PP, Gentry JH: Ocular complications of ulcerative colitis, *Am J Ophthalmol* 58:779-785, 1964.
34. Ericson S, Sundmark E: Studies on the sicca syndrome in patients with rheumatoid arthritis, *Acta Rheum Scand* 16:60-80, 1970.
35. Fauci AS, Doppman IL, Wolff SM: Cyclophosphamide-induced remissions in advanced polyarteritis nodosa, *Am J Med* 64:890-894, 1978.
36. Feder RS, Krachmer JH: Conjunctival resection for the treatment of the rheumatoid corneal ulceration, *Ophthalmology* 91:111-115, 1984.
37. Ferry AP, Leopold IH: Marginal (ring) corneal ulcer as presenting manifestation of Wegener's granulomatosis, *Ophthalmology* 74:1276-1282, 1970.
38. Fogle JA, Kenyon KR, Foster CS: Tissue adhesive arrests stromal melting in the human cornea, *Am J Ophthalmol* 89:795-802, 1980.
39. Foster CS: Ocular surface manifestations of neurological and systemic disease, *Int Ophthalmol Clin* 19(2):207-242, 1979.
40. Foster CS: Immunosuppressive therapy for external ocular inflammatory disease, *Ophthalmology* 87:140-150, 1980.
41. Foster CS: Nonrheumatoid acquired collagen vascular diseases. In Smolin G, Thoft RA, editors: *The cornea: scientific foundations and clinical practice,* 264-284, Boston, 1994, Little, Brown.
42. Foster CS, Forstot SI, Wilson LA: Mortality rate in rheumatoid arthritis patients developing necrotizing scleritis or peripheral ulcerative keratitis: effects of systemic immunosuppression, *Ophthalmology* 91:1253-1263, 1984.
43. Francois J: La degenerescence marginale de la cornée, *Arch Ophthalmol (Paris)* 53:540-547, 1936.
44. Frayer WC: The histopathology of perilimbal ulceration in Wegener's granulomatosis, *Arch Ophthalmol* 64:58-64, 1960.
45. Friedlander MH: Ocular allergy and immunology, *J Allergy Clin Immunol* 63:51-60, 1979.
46. Gerstle CC, Friedman AH: Marginal corneal ulceration (limbal guttering) as a presenting sign of temporal arteritis, *Ophthalmology* 87:1173-1176, 1980.
47. Gold DH, Morris DA, Henkind P: Ocular findings in systemic lupus erythematosus, *Br J Ophthalmol* 56:800-804, 1972.
48. Goodman GC, Churg J: Wegener's granulomatosis: pathology and review of the literature, *Arch Pathol* 58:533-553, 1954.
49. Grant WM: New treatment for calcific corneal opacities, *Arch Ophthalmol* 48:681-685, 1952.
50. Gudas PP, Altman B, Nicholson DH, Green WR: Corneal perforations in Sjögren's syndrome, *Arch Ophthalmol* 90:470-472, 1973.
51. Guss RB, McCulley JP: Abnormal immune responses in the ocular presentation of Wiskott-Aldrich syndrome, *Ann Ophthalmol* 14:1058-1060, 1982.
52. Halmay O, Ludwig K: Bilateral band-shaped deep keratitis and iridocyclitis in systemic lupus erythematosis, *Br J Ophthalmol* 48:558-562, 1964.
53. Harbart F, McPherson SD: Scleral necrosis in polyarteritis nodosa, *Am J Ophthalmol* 30:727-732, 1947.
54. Harwood TR: Diffuse perichondritis, chondritis, and iritis: report of an autopsied case, *Arch Pathol* 65:81-87, 1958.
55. Hirst LW, DeJaun E: Sodium hyaluronate and tissue adhesive in treating corneal perforations, *Ophthalmology* 89:1250-1253, 1982.
56. Hogan MJ, Alvarado JA: The limbus. In *History of the human eye: an atlas and textbook,* ed 2, 112-182, Philadelphia, 1971, WB Saunders.
57. Hughes RAC, Berry CL, Seifert M, Leesof MH: Relapsing polychondritis: three cases with a clinicopathologic study and literature review, *Q J Med* 61:363-380, 1972.
58. Hyndiuk RA, Hull DS, Kinyoun JL: Free tissue patch and cyanacrylate in corneal perforations, *Ophthalmic Surg* 5:50-55, 1974.
59. Jakobiec FA, Lefkowitch J, Knowles DM: B- and T-lymphocytes in ocular disease, *Ophthalmology* 91:635-654, 1984.
60. Jampol LW, West C, Goldberg MF: Therapy of scleritis with cytotoxic agents, *Am J Ophthalmol* 86:266-271, 1978.
61. Jayson MIV, Easty DL: Ulceration of the cornea in rheumatoid arthritis, *Ann Rheum Dis* 36:428-432, 1977.
62. Jayson MIV, Jones DED: Scleritis and rheumatoid arthritis, *Ann Rheum Dis* 30:343-347, 1971.
63. Kaye RI, Sones DA: Relapsing polychondritis: clinical and pathologic features in fourteen cases, *Ann Intern Med* 60:653-664, 1964.
64. Kervick GN, Pflugfelder SC, Haimovici R et al.: Paracentral rheumatoid corneal ulceration: clinical features and cyclosporine therapy, *Ophthalmology* 99:80-88, 1992.
65. Kirkham TH: Scleroderma and Sjögren's syndrome, *Br J Ophthalmol* 53:131-133, 1969.
66. Knox DL, Snip RC, Stark WJ: The keratopathy of Crohn's disease, *Am J Ophthalmol* 90:862-865, 1980.

67. Koffler D: The immunology of rheumatoid diseases, *Clin Symp* 31(4):1-36, 1979.
68. Krachmer JH, Laibson PR: Corneal thinning and perforation in Sjögren's syndrome, *Am J Ophthalmol* 78:917-920, 1974.
69. Liegner JT, Yee RW, Wild JH: Topical cyclosporine therapy for ulcerative keratitis associated with rheumatoid arthritis, *Am J Ophthalmol* 109:610-612, 1990.
70. Lyne AJ: "Contact lens" cornea in rheumatoid arthritis, *Br J Ophthalmol* 54:410-415, 1970.
71. Macoul KL: Ocular changes in granulomatous ileocolitis, *Arch Ophthalmol* 84:95-97, 1970.
72. Magargal LE, Donoso LA, Goldberg RE et al.: Ocular manifestations of relapsing polychondritis, *Retina* 1:96-99, 1981.
73. Martin J, Roenigk HH, Lynch W, Tingwald FR: Relapsing polychondritis treated with dapsone, *Arch Dermatol* 112:1271-1274, 1976.
74. Matoba A, Plager S, Barber J, McCulley JP: Keratitis in relapsing polychondritis, *Ann Ophthalmol* 16:367-369, 1984.
75. McGavin DDM, Williamson J, Forrester JV et al.: Episcleritis and scleritis: a study of their clinical manifestations and association with rheumatoid arthritis, *Br J Ophthalmol* 60:192-226, 1976.
76. McKay DAR, Watson PG, Lyne AJ: Relapsing polychondritis and eye disease, *Br J Ophthalmol* 58:600-605, 1974.
77. Meyer O, Cyna J, Dryll A et al.: Relapsing polychondritis-pathogenic role of anti-native collagen type II antibodies, *J Rheumatol* 8:820-824, 1981.
78. Meyers RL, Pettit TH: The pathogenesis of corneal inflammation due to HSV. I. Corneal hypersensitivity in the rabbit, *J Immunol* 111:1031-1042, 1973.
79. Meyers-Elliott RL, Pettit TH, Maxwell A: Viral antigens in the immune ring of herpes simplex stromal keratitis, *Arch Ophthalmol* 98:897-904, 1980.
80. Mondino BJ: Inflammatory diseases of the peripheral cornea, *Ophthalmology* 95:463-472, 1988.
81. Mondino BJ, Brown SI, Mondzelewski JP: Peripheral corneal ulcers with herpes zoster ophthalmicus, *Am J Ophthalmol* 86:611–614, 1978.
82. Mondino BJ, Kowalski RP: Phlyctenulae and catarrhal infiltrates, *Arch Ophthalmol* 100:1968-1971, 1982.
83. Mondino BJ, Rabin BS, Kessler E et al.: Corneal rings with gram-negative bacteria, *Arch Ophthalmol* 95:2222-2225, 1977.
84. Moore JG, Sevel D: Corneoscleral ulceration in polyarteritis nodosa, *Br J Ophthalmol* 50:651-655, 1966.
85. Moutsopoulos HM, Chuset TM, Mann DL et al.: Sjögren's syndrome (sicca syndrome): current issues, *Ann Intern Med* 92:212-226, 1980.
86. Neetens A, Burvenich H: Anaphylactic marginal keratitis, *Bull Soc Belge Ophtalmol* 186:69-72, 1979.
87. Ostler HB: Corneal perforation in nontuberculous (staphylococcal) phlyctenular keratoconjunctivitis, *Am J Ophthalmol* 79:446-448, 1975.
88. Palay DA, Stulting RD, Waring GO et al.: Penetrating keratoplasty in patients with rheumatoid arthritis, *Ophthalmology* 99:622-627, 1992.
89. Palestine AG, Meyers SM, Fauci AS, Gallin JI: Ocular findings in patients with neutrophil dysfunction, *Am J Ophthalmol* 95:598-604, 1983.
90. Petrelli EA, McKinley M, Troncale FJ: Ocular manifestations of inflammatory bowel disease, *Ann Ophthalmol* 14:356-360, 1982.
91. Pfister RR, Murphy GE: Corneal ulceration and perforation associated with Sjögren's syndrome, *Arch Ophthalmol* 98:89-94, 1980.
92. Reeves JA: Keratopathy associated with systemic lupus erythematosus, *Arch Ophthalmol* 74:159-160, 1965.
93. Robin JB, Schanzlin DJ, Meisler DM et al.: Ocular involvement in the respiratory vasculitides, *Surv Ophthalmol* 30:127-140, 1985.
94. Robin JB, Schanzlin DJ, Verity SM et al.: Peripheral corneal disorders, *Surv Ophthalmol* 31:1-36, 1986.
95. Rucker CW, Ferguson RH: Ocular manifestations of relapsing polychondritis, *Trans Am Ophthalmol Soc* 62:167-172, 1964.
96. Sachs R, Zagelbaum BM, Hersh PS: Corneal complications associated with the use of crack cocaine, *Ophthalmology* 100:187-191, 1993.
97. Scharf Y, Meyer E, Nahir M, Zonis S: Marginal mottling of cornea in rheumatoid arthritis, *Ann Ophthalmol* 16:924-926, 1984.
98. Schulman MF, Sugar A: Peripheral corneal infiltrates in inflammatory bowel disease, *Ann Ophthalmol* 13:109-111, 1981.
99. Sjögren H, Bloch KJ: Keratoconjunctivitis and the Sjögren syndrome, *Surv Ophthalmol* 16:145-159, 1971.
100. Slansky HH, Dohlman CH: Collagenase and the cornea, *Surv Ophthalmol* 14:402-416, 1970.
101. Smith JN, Winship DH: Complications and extraintestinal problems in inflammatory bowel disease, *Med Clin North Am* 64:1161-1171, 1980.
102. Smith RE, Dippe DW, Miller SD: Phlyctenular keratoconjunctivitis. Results of penetrating keratoplasty in Alaskan natives, *Ophthalmic Surg* 6:62-65, 1975.
103. Spaeth GK: Corneal staining in systemic lupus erythematosus, *New Eng J Med* 276:1168-1171, 1967.
104. Spalton DJ, Graham EM, Page NGR, Sanders MD: Ocular changes in Wegener's granulomatosis, *Br J Ophthalmol* 65:553-563, 1981.
105. Straatsma BR: Ocular manifestations of Wegener's granulomatosis, *Am J Ophthalmol* 44:785-799, 1957.
106. Suveges I, Levai G, Alberth B: Pathology of Terrien's disease: histochemical and electron microscopic study, *Am J Ophthalmol* 74:1191-1200, 1972.
107. Terrien F: Dystrophic marginale symetrique des deux cornées, *Arch Ophtalmol* 20:12-14, 1900.
108. Thygeson P: Bacterial factors in chronic catarrhal Conjunctivitis. I. Role of toxin-forming staphylococci, *Arch Ophthalmol* 18:373-387, 1937.
109. Thygeson P: Marginal corneal infiltrates and ulcers, *Trans Am Acad Ophthalmol Otolaryngol* 51:198-207, 1946.
110. Tyner GS: Wegener's granulomatosis: a case report, *Am J Ophthalmol* 50:1203-1207, 1960.
111. Watson PG: Diseases of the episclera and sclera. In Duane TD, editor: *Clinical ophthalmology*, vol 4, Philadelphia, 1984, Harper & Row.
112. Watson PG, Hayreh SS: Scleritis and episcleritis, *Br J Ophthalmol* 60:163-191.
113. Watson PG, Hazelman BL: *The sclera and systemic disorders*, Philadelphia, 1976, WB Saunders.
114. Webster RG, Slansky HH, Refojo MF et al.: The use of adhesive for the closure of corneal perforations, *Arch Ophthalmol* 80:705-709, 1968.
115. Wilson FM II, Grayson M, Ellis FD: Treatment of peripheral corneal ulcers by limbal conjunctivectomy, *Br J Ophthalmol* 60:713-719, 1976.
116. Zaidman GW, Coles RS: Peripheral uveitis and ulcerative colitis, *Ann Ophthalmol* 13:73-75, 1981.
117. Zion VM, Brackup AH, Weingeist S: Relapsing polychondritis, erythema nodosum and sclerouveitis. Case report with anterior segment angiography, *Surv Ophthalmol* 19:107-110, 1974.

38 Mooren Ulcer

STEVEN B. ROBIN, JEFFREY B. ROBIN

Mooren ulcer is an idiopathic condition characterized by progressive inflammatory thinning and ectasia of the cornea. The process initially involves the peripheral cornea, but eventually spreads both circumferentially and centrally. The disease affects both sexes equally and is limited primarily to adults (although some cases of pediatric involvement have been reported).[42]

HISTORICAL BACKGROUND

Bowman, in 1849, was the first to describe chronic serpiginous ulceration of the peripheral cornea, also termed "ulcus rodens." In 1867 Mooren described similar cases and postulated that they were a distinct clinical entity.[34] The first large series of cases was reported by Nettleship in 1902.[36]

CLINICAL FEATURES

Two clinical types of Mooren ulcer have been described.[49] The first is the unilateral, limited type that occurs mostly in older patients and responds well to therapy. The second type occurs in younger patients, particularly in blacks, is usually bilateral; has a more aggressive course, and responds poorly to all forms of therapy. This second type of Mooren ulcer is frequently seen in Africa, especially in Nigeria, and affects young healthy males. Additionally, Mooren ulcer has been noted to occur in patients who have had previous chronic ocular surface disorders or previous ocular trauma.

Symptomatically, patients suffer from extreme ocular pain, and marked photophobia and lacrimation may be present. Other ocular features occasionally noted include a mild-to-moderate anterior uveitis, secondary glaucoma, and cataract.

Mooren ulceration is characterized by unilateral or bilateral painful ulceration and ectasia of the peripheral cornea. The ulceration begins as grayish infiltrations in the perilimbal cornea, usually in the interpalpebral fissures. Within a few weeks, this is followed by breakdown of the overlying epithelium and degeneration of the anterior stroma. Typi-

cally, coalescence of these areas occurs, eventually resulting in circumferential progression. As the ulcer advances, stromal infiltration precedes epithelial breakdown. Disease activity can be ascertained by following the extent of epithelial denudation with repeated fluorescein applications.

The process eventually undermines the central wall of the thinned tissue, leading to the characteristic "overhanging" central edge. If this progresses, central spread of the ulcer results. The conjunctiva, episclera, and sclera surrounding the involved areas are usually quite inflamed. Blood vessels from these tissues eventually cover the remaining stroma and Descemet membrane after destruction of the anterior lamellae. Although spontaneous perforation is uncommon, these eyes are characteristically quite vulnerable to perforation with minimal trauma.

PATHOGENESIS

The cause of Mooren ulceration is unknown.[31] No pathogenic features or predisposing systemic conditions have been noted in the unilateral cases. In the bilateral cases, however, epidemiologic studies performed on patients in Africa have demonstrated a high incidence of concomitant parasitic infestation, particularly helminthiasis.[25,28] The ulcerative process has been arrested in Nigerian patients treated for systemic helminthiasis. Although direct corneal infection has not been demonstrated in any of these cases, immunologic reactions to helminth antigens deposited in the cornea or to corneal antigens altered by helmith infestation may be pathogenic factors.[44]

Other infections have been linked to Mooren ulcer, including hepatitis C virus infection,[48] but most patients have no other disease manifestations.

The pathogenesis of Mooren ulcer seems to be immunologically based.[5,8,43] Histologically, polymorphonuclear leukocytes, lymphocytes (especially CD4 lymphocytes), and plasma cells have been found in the affected cornea,[14,32,50] as well as in conjunctiva adjacent to the ulcer. Mast cells[35] and eosinophils have also been noted. Serum elevations of IgA have been noted in some patients. Similarly, one report showed an increase in circulating serum immune complexes.[2] Immunopathologic examinations have shown tissue-fixed immunoglobulins and complement in both the adjacent conjunctiva[15,16] and in the corneal epithelial basement membrane.[20]

There is some evidence that autoimmunity to corneal and/or conjunctival tissue may play a role in the pathogenesis of Mooren ulcer. Mooren ulcer has occurred, for example, after penetrating keratoplasty.[22,33] Circulating antibodies against cornea and conjunctiva have been reported by several investigators. Cellular immune deviations, suggestive of antigenic transformation of corneal tissue, have also been reported. T-helper and/or T-inducer (CD4) cells and B cells infiltrate the peripheral cornea in excess of T-cytotoxic suppressor (CD8) cells.[27,35] Unchecked helper T cells could lead to overproduction of antibody, resulting in immune-complex deposition, complement activation, inflammatory-cell infiltration, and release of destructive enzymes.[3] Most corneal epithelial cells and keratocytes express class II antigens in Mooren ulcer.[27] Aberrant expression of HLA-DR antigens of limbal cells may promote autoimmune reactivity of the peripheral cornea during Mooren ulcer.

DIFFERENTIAL DIAGNOSIS

Differentiation of Mooren ulceration from noninflammatory peripheral ectasias (Terrien marginal degeneration and pellucid marginal degeneration) is not usually difficult. The epithelium generally remains intact in these noninflammatory ectasias. Mooren ulcer patients, additionally, have the hallmark of severe pain and ocular inflammation; these are rarely, if ever, seen in Terrien or pellucid degeneration patients. Also, the central overhanging edge of the Mooren ulcer is typically not a feature of either Terrien or pellucid marginal degenerations. Several systemic vasculitides can also cause peripheral corneal ulcerations and ectasia. Differentiation of these from early Mooren ulceration may be made on the basis of associated systemic features and laboratory tests.

LABORATORY INVESTIGATIONS

Many systemic disorders can be associated with peripheral keratitis and thinning. General physical examination and appropriate serologic tests are important to exclude a systemic vasculitis or connective-tissue disorder. Circulating anticorneal antibodies[40] and immune complexes can sometimes be found.[2] Hepatitis C antibody testing should be considered.

THERAPY

Treatment of Mooren ulcer is difficult and frequently unsatisfactory. The prime therapeutic concern in Mooren ulcer is arresting the inflammatory process and thereby preserving the structural integrity of the eye.[7] The most effective medical therapies are topical corticosteroids[37] and systemic immunosuppressive agents (corticosteroids, cyclophosphamide, methotrexate).[13,19,21,45,47] Collagenase inhibitors and heparin have been recommended but usually prove ineffective in halting disease progression. Topical and systemic Cyclosporine has been recommended in light of its ability to increase the population of suppressor T cells.[24,46,51] Plasma exchange is not usually done.[9] Systemic interferon has been suggested for hepatitis-associated Mooren ulcer.[48]

An effective treatment for cases of Mooren ulcer that are refractory to medical therapy involves excision or cryotherapy of the adjacent perilimbal conjunctiva.[1,4,10,17,41] Excision or destruction of the conjunctiva probably is effective because it removes the source of antibody and inflammatory cells that may be mediating the ulcerative reaction. Additional surgical therapies in the acute phase include lamellar keratectomy, delimiting keratotomy,[18,29,39,52] conjunctival flaps, and periosteal graft.[12] Corneal perforations must be rapidly managed by cyanoacrylate glue or surgical repair.[38]

After the inflammatory process has been medically or surgically ameliorated, lamellar or penetrating keratoplasties may be performed to restore visual acuity.[6,11,23] Ocular surface replacement has been attempted with keratoepithelioplasty.[26] A keratoprosthesis may be a surgical option for selected patients. Mooren ulcer may recur after keratoplasty.[30]

REFERENCES

1. Aviel E: Combined cryoapplications and peritomy in Mooren's ulcer, *Br J Ophthalmol* 56:48-51, 1978.
2. Berkowitz PT, Arentsen JJ, Felberg NT, Laibson PR: Presence of circulatory immune complexes in patients with peripheral corneal disease, *Arch Ophthalmol* 101:242-245, 1983.
3. Brown SI: Collagenolytic enzymes in corneal pathology, *Isr J Med Sci* 8:1537-1542, 1972.
4. Brown SI: Mooren's ulcer: treatment by conjunctival excision, *Br J Ophthalmol* 59:675-682, 1975.
5. Brown SI: What is Mooren's ulcer? *Trans Ophthalmol Soc UK* 98:390-392, 1978.
6. Brown SI, Mondino BJ: Penetrating keratoplasty in Mooren's ulcer, *Am J Ophthalmol* 89:255-258, 1980.
7. Brown SI, Mondino BJ: Therapy of Mooren's ulcer, *Am J Ophthalmol* 98:1-6, 1984.
8. Brown SI, Mondino BJ, Rabin BS: Autoimmune phenomenon in Mooren's ulcer, *Am J Ophthalmol* 82:835-840, 1968.
9. Carmichael TR, Mervitz MD, Bezwoda W, Rush PS: Plasma exchange in the treatment of Mooren's ulcer, *Ann Ophthalmol* 7:311-314, 1985.
10. Chihara E, Nishi R, Asayama K, Tsukahara I: Treatment of Mooren's ulcer by conjunctival excision, *Ophthalmologica* 179:258-264, 1979.
11. Cowden JW, Copeland RA Jr, Schneider MS: Large diameter therapeutic penetrating keratoplasties, *Refract Corneal Surg* 5:244-248, 1989.
12. Dingeldein SA, Insler MS, Barron BA, Kaufman HE: Mooren's ulcer treated with a periosteal graft, *Ann Ophthalmol* 22:56-57, 1990.
13. Easty DL, Madden P, Jayson MIV et al.: Systemic immunosuppression in marginal keratolysis, *Trans Ophthalmol Soc UK* 98:410-417, 1978.
14. Edwards WC, Reed RE: Mooren's ulcer: a pathologic case report, *Arch Ophthalmol* 80:361-364, 1968.
15. Eiferman RA, Hyndiuk R: IgE in limbal conjunctiva in Mooren's ulcer, *Can J Ophthalmol* 12:234-236, 1977.
16. Eiferman RA, Hyndiuk RA, Hensley GT: Limbal immunopathology of Mooren's ulcer, *Ann Ophthalmol* 10:1203-1206, 1978.
17. Faye M, Lam A, Borzeix A: Traitement de l'ulcère de Mooren par l'association periectomie-córticothèrapie: a propos de 6 cas, *J Fr Ophtalmol* 14:629-632, 1991.

18. Ferguson CE, Carreno OB: Mooren's ulcer and delimiting keratotomy, *South Med J* 62:1170-1174, 1969.
19. Foster CS: Systemic immunosuppressive therapy for progressive bilateral Mooren's ulcer, *Ophthalmology* 92:1436-1439, 1985.
20. Foster CS, Kenyon KR, Greiner J et al.: The immunopathology of Mooren's ulcer, *Am J Ophthalmol* 88:149-159, 1979.
21. Genvert G, Sakauye CM, Arentsen JJ: Treatment of marginal corneal ulcers with cryotherapy and conjunctival recession or resection, *Cornea* 3:256-261, 1984.
22. Gottsch JD, Liu SH, Stark WJ: Mooren's ulcer and evidence of stromal graft rejection after penetrating keratoplasty, *Am J Ophthalmol* 113:412-417, 1992.
23. Grana PC: Therapeutic keratoplasty in Mooren's ulcer, *Arch Ophthalmol* 62:414-418, 1959.
24. Hill JC, Potter P: Treatment of Mooren's ulcer with cyclosporin A: report of three cases, *Br J Ophthalmol* 71:11-15, 1987.
25. Kietzman B: Mooren's ulcer in Nigeria, *Am J Ophthalmol* 65:788-791, 1968.
26. Kinoshita S, Ohashi Y, Ohji M, Manabe R: Long-term results of keratoepithelioplasty in Mooren's ulcer, *Ophthalmology* 98:438-445, 1991.
27. Lopez JS, Price FW Jr, Whitcup SM et al.: Immunohistochemistry of Terrien's and Mooren's corneal degeneration, *Arch Ophthalmol* 109:988-992, 1991.
28. Majekodunmi AA: Ecology of Mooren's ulcer in Nigeria, *Doc Ophthalmol* 49:211-219, 1980.
29. Martin NF, Stark WJ, Maumenee AE: Treatment of Mooren's and Mooren's-like ulcer by lamellar keratectomy: report of six eyes and literature review, *Ophthalmic Surg* 18:564-569, 1987.
30. McDonnell PJ: Recurrence of Mooren's ulcer after lamellar keratoplasty, *Cornea* 8:191-194, 1989.
31. Mondino BJ, Brown SI, Rabin BS: Autoimmune phenomena of the external eye, *Ophthalmology* 85:801-817, 1978.
32. Mondino BJ, Brown SI, Rabin BS: Cellular immunity in Mooren's ulcer, *Am J Ophthalmol* 85:788-791, 1978.
33. Mondino BJ, Hofbauer JD, Foos RY: Mooren's ulcer after penetrating keratoplasty, *Am J Ophthalmol* 103:53-56, 1987.
34. Mooren A: *Ophthalmologische Beobachturges,* 107, Berlin, 1867, A Hirschwald.
35. Murray PI, Rahi AHS: Pathogenesis of Mooren's ulcer: some new concepts, *Br J Ophthalmol* 68:182-187, 1984.
36. Nettleship E: Chronic serpiginous ulcer of the cornea (Mooren's ulcer), *Trans Ophthalmol Soc UK* 22:103-115, 1902.
37. Pandey R: Topical cortisone in the treatment of Mooren's ulcer, *J All India Ophthalmol Soc* 17:114-117, 1969.
38. Parunovic A, Brkic S, Vuckovic S: Corneal perforation in Mooren's ulcer—immunological and clinical follow-up, *Graefes Arch Clin Exp Ophthalmol* 226:330-331, 1988.
39. Rycroft BW, Romantes GJ: Lamellar corneal grafts—clinical report on 62 cases, *Br J Ophthalmol* 36:337-351, 1952.
40. Schaap OL, Feltkamp TEW, Breenbaart AJ: Circulating antibodies to corneal tissue in a patient suffering from Mooren's ulcer (ulcus rodens corneae), *Clin Exp Immunol* 5:365-370, 1969.
41. Stilma JS: Conjunctival excision or lamellar scleral autograft in 38 Mooren's ulcers from Sierra Leone, *Br J Ophthalmol* 67:475-478, 1983.
42. Taylor SJ: Notes of a case of rodent ulcer of the cornea in a child, *Trans Ophthalmol Soc UK* 22:98-99, 1902.
43. Trojan HJ: Ulcus rodens (Mooren)—Aspekte der Aetiologie, des Verlaufs und der Therapie, *Klin Monatsbl Augenheilkd* 174:166-176, 1972.
44. van der Gaag R, Abdillahi H, Stilma JS, Vetter JCM: Circulating antibodies against corneal epithelium and hookworm in patients with Mooren's ulcer from Sierra Leone, *Br J Ophthalmol* 67:623-628, 1983.
45. Wakefield D, McCluskey P, Penny R: Intravenous pulse methylprednisolone therapy in severe inflammatory eye disease, *Arch Ophthalmol* 104:847-851, 1986.
46. Wakefield D, Robinson LP: Cyclosporin therapy in Mooren's ulcer, *Br J Ophthalmol* 71:415-417, 1987.
46a. Watson PG, Richardson E: Large corneal transplants in corneal destructive disease, Klin Monatsbl Augenheilkd 205:280-283, 1994.
47. Wilson FM II, Grayson M, Ellis FD: Treatment of peripheral corneal ulcers by limbal conjunctivectomy, *Br J Ophthalmol* 60:713-719, 1976.
48. Wilson SE, Lee WM, Murakami C et al.: Mooren-type hepatitis C virus-associated corneal ulceration, *Ophthalmology* 101:736-745, 1994.
49. Wood TO, Kaufman HE: Mooren's ulcer, *Am J Ophthalmol* 71:417-421, 1971.
50. Young RG, Watson PG: Light and electron microscopy of corneal melting syndrome (Mooren's ulcer), *Br J Ophthalmol* 66:341-356, 1982.
51. Zhao JC, Jin XY: Immunological analysis and treatment of Mooren's ulcer with cyclosporin A applied topically, *Cornea* 12:481-488, 1993.
52. Zu D: Mooren's ulcer treated by lamellar kcratoplasty, *Jpn J Ophthalmol* 23:257-261, 1979.

39 HLA B27-Associated Diseases

JAMES T. ROSENBAUM

Few studies have attempted to determine the incidence or prevalence of uveitis. Some of the best data can be found in a Mayo Clinic survey that recorded 15 new cases of uveitis per 100,000 patients per year in the geographic area served by that clinic.[17] Anterior uveitis was four times more common than posterior uveitis. Although the differential diagnosis of anterior uveitis includes infections, systemic diseases, and Fuchs uveitis syndrome, the most common form of anterior uveitis is that associated with the major histocompatibility complex antigen, HLA B27.

EPIDEMIOLOGY

A British study found that 52% of patients with acute anterior uveitis were HLA B27 positive.[9] HLA B27 is even more strongly associated with precisely defined subsets of anterior uveitis, especially in patients with unilateral, recurrent disease of sudden onset.[60]

In some geographic areas, such as Japan[70] or Africa,[46] HLA B27 is rare; and consequently, HLA B27-related eye disease is less common. In the United States approximately 6% of the population is HLA B27 positive. One small study found that 30% of HLA B27 positive, male blood bank donors had stigmata, such as debris on the anterior lens capsule, suggesting prior iritis.[15] A Dutch study, however, estimated that the cumulative, lifetime risk of iritis for an HLA B27 positive individual was only 1%.[44]

Often patients with HLA B27-associated anterior uveitis will have a systemic disease such as Reiter syndrome, ankylosing spondylitis, psoriatic arthritis, inflammatory bowel disease, or a juvenile form of ankylosing spondylitis or Reiter syndrome. Among individuals with HLA B27-associated joint disease (that is, Reiter syndrome or ankylosing spondylitis) the risk of iritis during a lifetime is approximately 20% to 40%.* Males are roughly three times more likely than females to develop HLA B27-associated anterior uveitis. Although children or elderly individuals can develop

HLA B27-associated anterior uveitis, the disease is especially common in adults between the ages of 20 and 40.[66,85]

Although 10% of patients with ankylosing spondylitis are HLA B27 negative[71] and as many as 40% of patients with Reiter syndrome are HLA B27 negative,[92] fewer than 5% of patients with either Reiter syndrome or ankylosing spondylitis and iritis at the Oregon Health Sciences University are HLA B27 negative.* In series of patients with uveitis, Reiter syndrome, ankylosing spondylitis, or the diagnosis of HLA B27-associated anterior uveitis normally account for a significant percentage of all patients (as shown in Table 39-1). As demonstrated in this table, series vary widely with regard to the frequency of these diagnoses. The difference reflects ethnic variation, referral bias, environmental factors, and different approaches to differential diagnosis. For example, experts vary as to whether they routinely order HLA B27 typing or how diligently they seek evidence of related joint disease.

RISK FACTORS

The majority of patients with HLA B27-associated anterior uveitis have no obvious precipitating event. Some have reported that the eye disease is seasonal, tending to occur in the fall.[66] Reiter syndrome may be triggered by a variety of infectious agents including *Salmonella, Shigella, Yersinia, Campylobacter,* and *Chlamydia* species. One study found that a specific plasmid distinguished arthritogenic isolates of *Shigella* species.[81] Following an epidemic of an arthritogenic gram-negative dysentery, such as that caused by *Shigella* species, both reactive arthritis and conjunctivitis would typically begin 1 to 4 weeks after the onset of diarrhea.[75,94] Iritis may occur during this immediate postinfectious period, or it may be delayed for several years.[68]

Patients with ankylosing spondylitis, who develop a predisposing infection, will frequently have manifestations of Reiter syndrome. Family studies suggest that first degree

---

*References 5, 26, 32, 41, 42, 59, 90.

*Unpublished data.

TABLE 39-1 FREQUENCY OF REITER SYNDROME, ANKYLOSING SPONDYLITIS, OR HLA B27-ASSOCIATED ANTERIOR UVEITIS AMONG PATIENTS WITH UVEITIS

Location of Patient Population	HLA B27-associated Iritis	Ankylosing Spondylitis	Reiter Syndrome
Oregon, USA[61]	1.7%	5.5%	7.2%
Iowa, USA[54]	ND	5.8%	5.2%
Southern California, USA[28]	3%	1.5%	1%
England[54]	ND	10.5%	17.2%
The Netherlands[65]	12.1%	5.5%***	ND
Israel*[87]	3%	3.3%	1%
Turkey[79]	0.6%	1.9%	0%
China[14]	10.8%**	22.1%	4.2%

ND = not determined.
Data expressed as the percent of patients relative to the total series.
* Includes only patients with chronic uveitis
** Includes patients with psoriatic arthropathy
*** Reiter syndrome and ankylosing spondylitis are classified together as seronegative spondyloarthropathy

relatives of patients with Reiter syndrome are more likely to develop Reiter syndrome. Similarly, first degree relatives of patients with ankylosing spondylitis are more likely to develop that syndrome.[31] A plausible explanation for this observation is that the disease has more than one genetic factor in addition to HLA B27. Obviously, environmental factors are involved in Reiter syndrome and possibly in ankylosing spondylitis as well.

CLINICAL FEATURES

Rheumatologic Disorders

Both Reiter syndrome and ankylosing spondylitis have a predilection to involve the sacroiliac joint and the spine. Accordingly, each is labeled a seronegative spondyloarthropathy. The term *seronegative* contrasts these diseases with rheumatoid arthritis, because most patients with rheumatoid arthritis have a positive serum test for rheumatoid factor.

Reiter syndrome and ankylosing spondylitis are closely related diseases (Table 39-2). Approximately 90% of patients with ankylosing spondylitis are HLA B27 positive,[10,71] whereas the association is less strong in Reiter syndrome. Roughly 60% of patients with Reiter disease possess this HLA marker.[11,29] By definition, sacroiliac involvement (Fig. 39-1) is symmetric and universal among patients with ankylosing spondylitis. In contrast, only about 60% of patients with Reiter syndrome develop sacroiliac involvement. In both diseases, other joints in addition to the vertebral column

TABLE 39-2 DISTINCTIONS BETWEEN ANKYLOSING SPONDYLITIS AND REITER SYNDROME

	Ankylosing Spondylitis	Reiter Syndrome
Sacroiliitis	Always	60%
Peripheral arthritis	Often	Often
Iritis	Common	Common
HLA B27	90%	60%
Aortic insufficiency	Rare	Rare
Occult bowel inflammation	Common	Common
Urethritis	Never	Common
Keratodermia	Never	Common
Conjunctivitis	Never	Common
Oral ulcers	Never	Common
Nail changes	Never	Common

can be involved, and the distribution is very similar. Aortic root inflammation and cardiac conduction defects rarely occur in either disease.[55]

The peripheral joint disease in either Reiter syndrome or ankylosing spondylitis is generally pauciarticular, that is, it involves a few joints. In addition it is generally asymmetric and tends to involve the joints of the lower extremities—especially large joints. When digits are involved, the entire finger or toe tends to be swollen, resulting in dactylitis (Fig. 39-2). In about 60% of patients with Reiter syndrome, the sacroiliac joints are involved, often asymmetrically. In addition to eye and joint disease, patients with Reiter syndrome also have mucosal involvement, which consists of a psoriasiform rash on the palms and soles known as keratodermia, a mild aphthous stomatitis, and a rash on the glans penis known as balanitis. The nails may also be affected, resulting

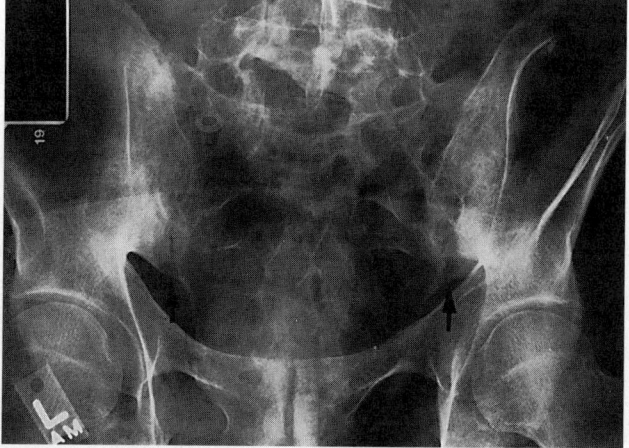

Fig. 39-1. X-ray of the pelvis. *Arrows* mark the inferior margins of the sacroiliac joints. Both joints have irregular margins and sclerosis is present superior to the arrows. These changes are consistent with sacroiliitis.

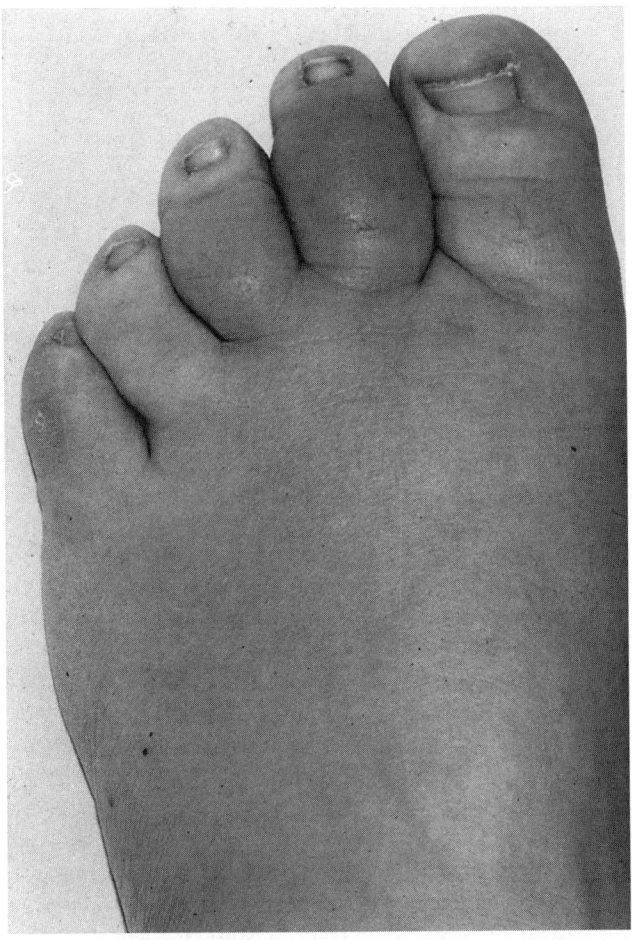

Fig. 39-2. The second and third toes are markedly swollen. This dactylitis is characteristic of seronegative spondyloarthritis.

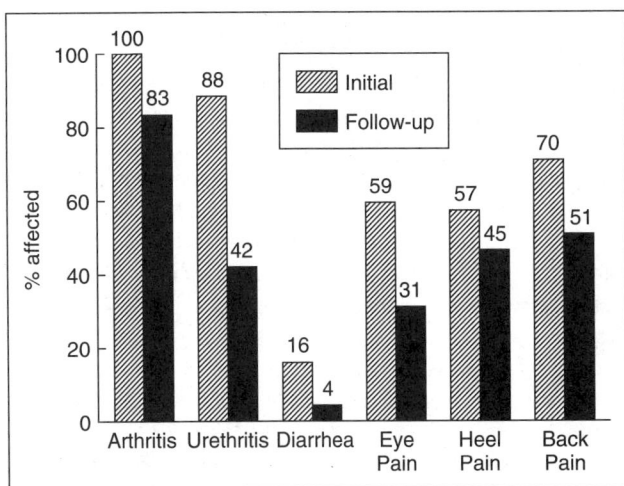

Fig. 39-3. Symptoms of Reiter syndrome as determined by a large clinical series. Data derived from Fox and associates.[22]

interphalangeal joints in association with nail disease. Other subsets of psoriatic arthritis include (1) spondyloarthritis, (2) a pauciarticular peripheral disease, (3) a symmetric peripheral disease that mimics rheumatoid arthritis, and rarely, (4) arthritis mutilans affecting a few digits. HLA B27 is especially associated with spondyloarthritis.

Ocular Disorders

Conjunctivitis in association with Reiter disease is usually bilateral and occurs at the onset of the disease. It is generally self-limited and without marked visual consequences. A keratitis has also been reported in association with Reiter syndrome.[47,50]

Whether the patient has Reiter syndrome or ankylosing spondylitis, the iritis associated with HLA B27 is similar in character and has a sudden onset.[60] A one- or two-day pro-

in oncholysis. Some patients with Reiter syndrome will have significant diarrhea. Fig. 39-3 shows the frequency of symptoms in Reiter syndrome based on the report by Fox and associates.[22]

The features of Reiter syndrome may include arthritis, dermatitis, urethritis, aphthous stomatitis, nail changes, and aortic root disease in addition to the eye disease.[22] Reiter syndrome is distinguished from ankylosing spondylitis by virtue of the mucosal involvement of the conjunctiva, mouth, gut, or urethra as well as the cutaneous involvement (Table 39-2).

The term *enthesopathy* is frequently used to describe the joint involvement of Reiter syndrome or ankylosing spondylitis as well as the closely related diseases psoriatic arthritis and the arthritis associated with inflammatory bowel disease. This term refers to the predilection of these diseases to involve tendinous insertions (Fig. 39-4).

The term *psoriatic arthritis* is used to describe joint disease in association with psoriasis. Approximately 10% of patients with psoriasis have some form of joint involvement. The most common form is primarily a disease of the distal

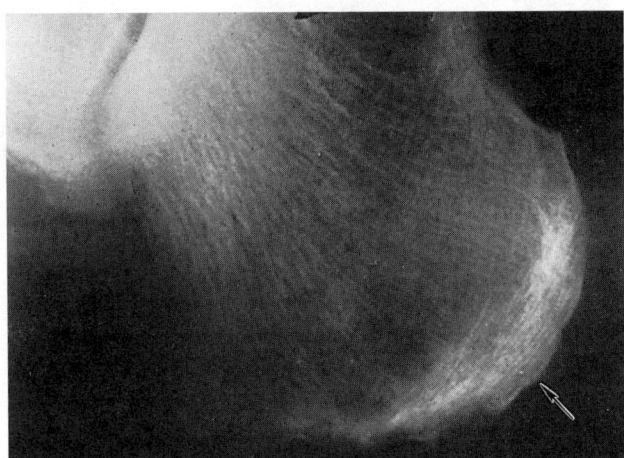

Fig. 39-4. Heel x-ray from a patient with plantar fasciitis secondary to Reiter syndrome. The irregular cortical bone margin *(arrow)* is typical of an enthesopathy.

drome of ocular discomfort and perhaps photosensitivity is generally followed by marked redness, pain, and miosis. Keratic precipitates are always nongranulomatous.[19] Typically, the intraocular pressure in the affected eye will be lower than in the contralateral eye.[19] Attacks are virtually always unilateral.[19,60] There is a marked tendency for posterior synechiae to form, and cystoid macular edema is common as well. Episodes usually subside within 6 to 8 weeks, but then tend to recur. These recurrences may involve the contralateral eye.[60] Although hypopyon is rarely associated with this form of iritis, one study from southern California found that most patients with hypopyon in association with noninfectious iritis are HLA B27 positive.[16] The clinical features of the iritis associated with HLA B27 are summarized in the box. Occasionally, patients with Reiter syndrome or ankylosing spondylitis will experience uveitis that is bilateral, chronic in duration, or posterior to the lens. Such cases are usually seen in patients with a history of multiple episodes of unilateral disease, or in patients whose past episodes of uveitis have been inadequately treated. Chorioretinal lesions are not reported.

A number of researchers have studied the likelihood of associated joint disease affecting victims of HLA B27-associated anterior uveitis. These studies are summarized in Table 39-3. The estimates of patients so affected vary from

---

CHARACTERIZATION OF HLA B27-ASSOCIATED UVEITIS

Anterior
Sudden onset
Unilateral
Brief duration (usually less than 3 months)
Recurrent, sometimes in the contralateral eye
Reduced intraocular pressure
Cystoid macular edema common
Posterior synechiae common
Fibrin or hypopyon sometimes present
Nongranulomatous
Usually male
Commonly associated with systemic joint disease

---

roughly 30% to 90%. The disease is more common in males. Patients with HLA B27-associated anterior uveitis who do not develop arthritis are likely to be either female or very young (less than 15 years of age).

Iritis as a complication of either psoriatic arthritis or inflammatory bowel disease is less common and less well characterized. Approximately 2% of patients with inflammatory bowel disease will develop iritis.[4,25] One study, however, found that 11.8% of patients with ulcerative colitis had a history of anterior uveitis that often co-existed with the presence of sacroiliitis.[93] In this series, 17.4% of patients with ulcerative colitis had sacroiliitis. Fifty-two percent of the patients with sacroiliitis had a history of anterior uveitis. Patients rarely had anterior uveitis without sacroiliitis. Although HLA B27 typing was not performed in this study (published in 1964), HLA B27 is a likely factor to account for the co-occurrence of sacroiliitis and anterior uveitis. The finding of eye involvement also correlates with other extracolonic manifestations of the disease, including dermal involvement such as pyoderma gangrenosum and mucositis. The relationship between HLA B27, iritis, and inflammatory bowel disease has not been well studied. Experience suggests that the iritis associated with ulcerative colitis is frequently unilateral and sudden in onset, but the uveitis associated with Crohn disease is much more variable (it may be bilateral, posterior to the lens, and long-standing in duration). A variety of retinal, choroidal, and optic nerve inflammatory signs have been reported to be associated with inflammatory bowel disease.[18a] A retinal vasculitis may occur as well.[72]

The relationship between B27 and iritis in association with psoriasis has not been well studied. Only 7% of patients with psoriatic arthritis reportedly developed iritis.[39,84] The subset of psoriatic arthritis characterized by sacroiliitis-spondylitis is especially at risk for iritis. Similarly, only 20% to 40% of patients with psoriatic arthritis are HLA B27 positive, with most of those falling into the spondyloarthritic subset of psoriatic arthritis.

TABLE 39-3 REPRESENTATIVE STUDIES ON THE LIKELIHOOD OF RHEUMATIC DISEASE WITH IRITIS

Author	Conclusion
Beckingsale and associates[3]	60% of patients with HLA B27-associated anterior uveitis had significant back pain
Feltkamp[20]	90% of patients with HLA B27-associated anterior uveitis had definite or possible AS
Haarr[26]	34% of patients with acute iritis had AS
Linssen and associates[43]	73% of HLA B27-positive patients with acute anterior uveitis had rheumatic disease
Pedersen[53]	33% of patients with acute anterior uveitis had rheumatic disease
Rosenbaum[60]	84% of patients with HLA B27-associated anterior uveitis had AS, RS, or incomplete RS
Russell and associates[67]	63% of patients with acute anterior uveitis had sacroiliitis by radio-nuclide scan
Saari and associates[69]	51% of HLA B27-associated anterior uveitis had rheumatic disease
Stanworth & Sharp[80]	42% of patients with nongranulomatous anterior uveitis had AS or RS
Vinje and associates[84]	35% with acute anterior uveitis had radiographic sacroiliitis

Adapted from Rosenbaum JT: Acute anterior uveitis and spondyloarthropathies, *Rheum Dis Clin North Am,* 18:143, 1992.

PATHOGENESIS

Recent findings have focused attention on the cause of HLA B27-related joint disease. HLA B27 is a class I major histocompatibility complex antigen that is present on the surface of all nucleated cells. HLA class I antigens can be identified by classic serologic typing or by newer techniques involving analysis of nucleic acid or amino acid sequences. HLA antigens are inherited and therefore immutable.

At least eight subsets of HLA B27 have now been defined.[8,30,45] The subsets differ by only a few amino acid changes. Most, if not all, of these subsets can predispose to disease including ankylosing spondylitis, Reiter syndrome, or recurrent, unilateral anterior uveitis of sudden onset. The mechanism by which HLA B27 predisposes to disease is not known, but a variety of biochemical and epidemiologic observations help to clarify the role of HLA B27 in the disease process. First, it is clear that Reiter syndrome or reactive arthritis can be triggered by infectious processes.[76] These processes include gram-negative dysenteries (as noted previously) caused by *Shigella*, *Salmonella*, *Campylobacter*, and *Yersinia* species. In addition, a variety of causes of nongonococcal urethritis, such as *Chlamydia* species, can precipitate Reiter syndrome.

A major experiment toward understanding the pathogenesis of HLA B27-related disease has been to develop transgenic rats that are HLA B27 positive.[27] Hammer and associates[27] have created lines of rats that express the human histocompatibility antigen HLA B27, along with beta-2-microglobulin (a co-factor that is necessary for cell surface organization of HLA class I molecules). Many of these rats develop a spontaneous disease that seems to be preceded by colon inflammation and diarrhea. The rats subsequently develop involvement of the spine as well as peripheral arthritis. Furthermore, the rats develop skin, nail, and penile changes that are very clinically and histologically reminiscent of the HLA B27-associated spectrum of diseases. These studies show definitively that HLA B27 itself (rather than a co-factor inherited with HLA B27) contributes to the predisposition to disease.

The normal bowel flora are critical in the development of the disease. Rats that are reared in a germ-free environment appear to escape the joint disease as well as much of the bowel inflammation.[83]

The HLA B27 gene has been sequenced, and the amino acids in HLA B27 have been identified. In addition, the crystallographic structure of class I HLA molecules has been reported.[6] Site-directed mutagenesis has been helpful in distinguishing critical amino acids in the HLA B27 molecule.[82] The function of the class I molecule is, in part, to present antigen to the T cell receptor on CD8+ suppressor-cytotoxic T-lymphocytes.

The understanding of the structure-function relationships of class I HLA molecules and the HLA B27 transgenic studies have provided exciting new insights into the pathogenesis of HLA B27-related disease, but the mechanism by which HLA B27 predisposes to disease in patients is still unclear. If the molecule is functioning as a unique antigen-presenting factor, an explanation is needed as to why a variety of infections can trigger eye and joint inflammation.

Several intriguing observations may help to explain the pathogenesis of HLA B27-related inflammation. First, biopsy studies with colonoscopy showed that many patients with either Reiter syndrome or ankylosing spondylitis have occult bowel inflammation.[49] This finding might relate to the priority that bowel inflammation plays in the pathogenesis of transgenic rat disease. In addition, it helps to relate the complications of inflammatory bowel disease to the joint manifestations of Reiter syndrome and ankylosing spondylitis. Abnormal bowel permeability has also been noted in spondyloarthritis.[78]

Second, HLA B27 may have a variety of cross-reactivities with gram-negative bacteria.[57,74] A computer data base search has shown that HLA B27 is unique among class I molecules in sharing many peptide sequences with proteins from a variety of gram-negative bacteria. Other class I molecules do not show nearly this degree of homology. Furthermore, the B27 homologies are particularly common with gram-negative bacterial products, as opposed to viruses or other peptides. Monoclonal antibodies to HLA B27 cross-react with gram-negative bacteria, and antibodies to some gram-negative bacteria cross-react with HLA B27.[95,96] The expression of HLA B27 facilitates penetration of gram-negative bacteria into cells based on transfection studies.[33] Patients with ankylosing spondylitis or HLA B27-associated iritis are more likely than controls to have bowel colonization with *Klebsiella* species.[73,89]

In addition, gram-negative products have been found within joint tissue from patients with reactive arthropathy. The bacterial cell wall of *Salmonella* species, for example, has been found in neutrophils within the joints of patients who have been infected with that agent and developed Reiter syndrome.[23] Similarly, yersinial antigens have been found in joint tissues of patients with postyersinial infection arthritis.[24] Chlamydial antigens may be present in the joints[56] of patients whose Reiter syndrome has developed after chlamydial infection. Lymphocytes from these joints show heightened reactivity against the triggering antigen.[21]

Two additional animal models may also provide insight into the pathogenesis of HLA B27-related disease. An injection of killed mycobacteria (adjuvant) or killed streptococcal cell wall[13] will provoke a reactive arthritis in rats that has many similarities to Reiter syndrome. The inciting injection can be placed into a number of tissues including the tail, foot pad, or skin. Joint disease begins approximately 10 days later. The joint inflammation resembles Reiter syndrome by virtue of its asymmetric nature as well as the tendency to form new bone (a feature that is distinctly different from the arthritis associated with rheumatoid arthritis). In addition, rats will develop tail ankylosis, a finding that resembles the vertebral column arthritis characteristic of spondyloarthritis.

Extraarticular manifestations have also been reported including uveitis, balanitis, and urethritis.[52] In adjuvant arthritis, the uveitis generally begins 1 to 3 weeks after the adjuvant injection, similar to when the arthritis begins. Eye disease occurs in only a minority of rats. It is usually unilateral and nongranulomatous, but bilateral disease, iris nodules, and mutton fat keratic precipitates do occur. Other ocular structures such as conjunctiva, cornea, and episclera are commonly involved.[86a] In adjuvant or poststreptococcal disease, the bacterial cell walls have been recovered from the joint tissue[88] and an immune response directed against the bacterial cell wall may play a prominent role in disease pathogenesis. T-lymphocyte responses to other antigens, including a heat shock protein and collagen, have also been implicated in this disease.

A second animal model that may be linked to the HLA B27-related diseases is endotoxin-induced uveitis.[37,63] An injection of endotoxin into the foot pad, subcutaneous tissue, peritoneum, or vein of many rat strains and some murine strains will provoke anterior uveitis of acute onset. The disease does differ from HLA B27-related disease in that it tends to be bilateral. It generally begins within 24 hours of the endotoxin exposure. In contrast, the human disease is characterized by a unilateral anterior uveitis that may begin 1 to 4 weeks after the endotoxemia associated with several gram-negative dysenteries. Still, the possible association between HLA B27 and a variety of gram-negative organisms makes this model of potential interest in understanding the pathogenesis of uveitis in HLA B27 positive patients.

The insights that link HLA B27 to gut pathology are summarized in the box below. Those observations that apply specifically to B27-related disease and gram-negative bacteria are summarized in the box in the next column.

Several broad theories have been espoused to explain the relationship between HLA antigens and disease in general. Most of the diseases whose likelihood is influenced by an HLA antigen are autoimmune diseases, which fits well with the knowledge that HLA antigens are markedly involved in controlling immune responses. One popular hypothesis is

---

OBSERVATIONS THAT LINK GRAM-NEGATIVE BACTERIA TO HLA B27-ASSOCIATED DISEASES

1. Infection with certain gram-negative bacteria such as *Salmonella* species triggers Reiter syndrome
2. HLA B27 transgenic rats raised in a germ-free environment develop less joint disease
3. Antigens from gram-negative bacteria are present in synovial fluid from patients with postdysenteric arthritis
4. HLA B27 has protein sequence homologies with gram-negative bacterial proteins
5. Monoclonal antibodies to certain gram-negative bacteria cross-react with HLA B27 or vice-versa
6. Endotoxin from gram-negative bacterial cell wall produces iritis in experimental animals
7. The therapeutic efficacy of sulfasalazine may depend on its action on bowel flora

---

that a particular HLA allele confers an altered immune response to a triggering antigen that directly relates to the disease. For example, a virus or an environmental antigen might trigger a heightened immune response that would result in direct tissue damage or immune complex formation. A second possibility is known as molecular mimicry. It is known, for example, that some bacterial antigens resemble tissue antigens. This finding is true for certain streptococcal antigens and certain yeast histones.[77] An immune response against one of these proteins could result in autoimmune disease by triggering an immune response against the patient. There is some evidence of autoantibodies in patients with HLA B27-associated arthritis,[23] although spondyloarthropathy is not usually considered to be an autoimmune disease in the same sense as rheumatoid arthritis or systemic lupus erythematosis. A third possibility is a reduction in immune responsiveness by virtue of a particular HLA allele. For example, the cross-reactivity between HLA B27 and a variety of gram negative bacteria may permit the alterations in gut flora because of the molecular mimicry. Eventually, the gram-negative bacterial product may escape the gut and lodge in tissue such as joint or iris. Bacterial antigens could become the focus of an immune response. Bacterial endotoxin could alter local vascular permeability and facilitate the deposition of immune complexes or the transendothelial migration of cells from the immune system.

In addition to HLA B27, other factors have been investigated as contributors to HLA B27-associated eye disease. For example, circulating immune complexes have been detected in HLA-B27 positive patients with iritis.[1] Certain immunoglobulin allotypes are especially prevalent when ankylosing spondylitis is associated with iritis.[36] Iris autoantibodies and reductions in circulating T-lymphocytes have been noted in patients with B27-associated anterior uveitis.[86]

OBSERVATIONS THAT LINK BOWEL PATHOLOGY TO HLA B27-RELATED DISEASES

1. HLA B27 transgenic rats develop bowel inflammation prior to joint disease
2. Patients with Reiter syndrome or ankylosing spondylitis have occult bowel inflammation
3. Patients with inflammatory bowel disease develop eye, oral mucous membrane, and joint disease similar to Reiter syndrome
4. Patients with Reiter syndrome or ankylosing spondylitis have increased gut permeability

Although the observation is somewhat controversial, several studies have concluded that AIDS or HIV infection is associated with worsening of Reiter syndrome or psoriatic arthritis.[34,91] This observation is a conundrum because T-lymphocytes immunodeficiency might reduce pathology in a disease mediated by CD4+ T-lymphocytes, as is true of rheumatoid arthritis. Conceivably, CD8+ T-lymphocytes play a more critical role in seronegative arthritis. The effect of AIDS on HLA B27-associated iritis is not well described.

DIFFERENTIAL DIAGNOSIS

The differential diagnosis of anterior uveitis includes the following: (1) infections with agents such as herpes simplex virus and varicella-zoster virus; (2) infectious diseases such as syphilis and leprosy; (3) syndromes confined to the eye such as Fuchs uveitis syndrome or Posner-Schlossman syndrome; (4) masquerade syndromes such as an iris melanoma or pigmentary dispersion syndrome; and (5) iritis in association with systemic diseases such as spondyloarthritis, sarcoidosis, interstitial nephritis, and allergic reactions to foreign substances such as medications.

Although many identifiable forms of anterior uveitis are specifically discussed elsewhere in this textbook, Posner-Schlossman syndrome (Chapter 43) deserves some additional explanation.[1,2] Also known as glaucomatocyclitic crisis, this eponym describes a distinct syndrome of recurrent, unilateral anterior uveitis in association with elevated intraocular pressure.[1,2] Distinctive features include marked pressure rises in association with mild inflammation; an episodic, unilateral nature; and a pupil that becomes slightly dilated after recurrent attacks. Although the disease begins suddenly, pain and redness are usually mild. Topical corticosteroids are beneficial. Episodes should resolve completely within 1 month. Despite the elevated intraocular pressure, gonioscopy shows no structural impairment of aqueous flow.

The iritis in association with HLA B27 is distinct, as noted previously. The majority of patients with an acute onset, unilateral, recurrent iritis will be HLA B27 positive. The likelihood of this diagnosis is further supported by characteristic changes such as a lower intraocular pressure, fibrin in the anterior chamber, posterior synechiae, or hypopyon. Additional supportive evidence comes from a history of chronic low back pain and/or peripheral arthritis (usually of the lower extremities in an asymmetric fashion). The low back pain can generally be distinguished from other causes of chronic low back pain (such as herniation of a disc) by virtue of its characteristics. The low back pain in association with HLA B27 generally has an insidious onset, chronic duration, stiffness in the morning, improvement with exercise, and nondermatomal distribution of pain.[12] In contrast, mechanical low back pain often begins suddenly, worsens with exercise, follows a nerve route distribution, and remits after days to weeks.

LABORATORY INVESTIGATIONS

HLA B27 typing may be useful in defining a subset of patients with anterior uveitis. As noted previously, patients who are HLA B27 positive are more likely to follow a typical clinical course. It may not be necessary to test for HLA B27 in a patient with iritis and previously diagnosed, typical Reiter syndrome or ankylosing spondylitis. Frequently, however, patients will not have a classic presentation. The joint disease may be mild and undiagnosed. In one series, two thirds of patients with spondyloarthritis and iritis did not have a diagnosis for the joint disease prior to the eye inflammation.[61] The back pain may be minimized by the patient and the physician. In this setting, HLA B27 can help to establish a diagnosis. The test, of course, must be interpreted with caution because the majority of patients who are HLA B27 positive do not develop eye disease, and the possibility is always present that the HLA antigen is a coincidence rather than a causal factor. The presence of HLA B27, however, does give prognostic information,[43] because it helps to predict complete resolution within 2 months, good vision between attacks, and the possibility of contralateral involvement with recurrence.

X-ray studies of the sacroiliac joints can also help to establish a diagnosis of spondyloarthritis, but plain radiographs of these joints are often difficult to interpret because of the oblique angulation of the joint (Fig. 39-1). A computerized tomography exam gives better definition of the joint but, of course, entails increased cost.[38] Furthermore, early in the disease process, radiographic changes may be absent, despite the presence of inflammation.[35] A clinical finding of note is reduced spinal mobility, which can be quantitated with a Schober test. In this maneuver the examiner demarcates two points (10 cm apart) along the lumbar spine. With maximal forward flexion, the distance between these points should increase to 14 cm or more if spinal mobility is normal. The physician should, of course, carefully seek a history for psoriasis, diarrhea, abdominal pain, aphthous stomatitis, penile discharge, rash, or nail changes.

THERAPY

The treatment of HLA B27-associated eye disease usually differs little from treatment for other causes of acute-onset anterior uveitis. Frequent use of topical corticosteroids and a dilating drop are indicated. In general, the prognosis is good and the frequency of medication can be rapidly adjusted as the inflammation wanes. On rare occasions, treatment will require a periocular corticosteroid injection. Brief courses of oral corticosteroids can also be used sparingly for the most severe forms of this inflammation. With resolution of inflammation, corticosteroid therapy can usually be discontinued altogether without recrudescence of disease. The eye appears normal between episodes, if there have been no complications (such as posterior synechiae formation) at the time of the acute disease.

When Reiter syndrome is triggered by a recognized infection, such as a urethritis or a dysentery, antibiotic therapy is appropriate. Some recent studies have suggested that the joint disease is reduced by prolonged therapy with antibiotics.[2,40] The role of this approach for treatment of eye disease has not been studied. Furthermore, the majority of patients with HLA B27-associated eye disease will not provide a history of a recent discrete antecedent-triggering infection.[64]

Many patients with HLA B27-associated eye disease will be receiving an oral nonsteroidal antiinflammatory drug, such as indomethacin or ibuprofen. The effects of such a medication on the eye disease have not been studied in detail. There is anecdotal experience to suggest that for some patients, chronic use of an oral nonsteroidal antiinflammatory drug might reduce the frequency or intensity of iritis episodes. Nevertheless, the long-term toxicity and expense of such treatment must be weighed with its potential benefit. Frequent toxicities from oral nonsteroidal antiinflammatory drugs include an increased risk of peptic ulcer disease. This problem is especially significant in patients who have a previous history of ulcer disease or who have other risk factors for an ulcer such as smoking, alcohol use, or aspirin use. The risk of developing an ulcer from a nonsteroidal antiinflammatory drug increases with the patient's age, duration of the medication use, and dosage of the medication. Other potential side effects from nonsteroidal antiinflammatory drugs include frequent mood alteration (such as depression) and rare renal toxicity (such as fluid retention, hypertension, hyperkalemia, or an allergic type nephritis).

Sulfasalazine has recently been used effectively to treat spondyloarthropathy as well as psoriatic arthritis and inflammatory bowel disease.[48,51,58] Two preliminary studies have suggested that sulfasalazine might be effective in the treatment of iritis.[7,18] For patients with HLA B27-associated anterior uveitis, sulfasalazine appears to reduce the frequency and intensity of recurrent attacks. Sulfasalazine might act, in part, by altering bowel flora. Based on the studies in transgenic rats, this flora may be critical to the disease pathogenesis. Again, the expense and potential risk of using this medication must be considered before beginning treatment of a disease that is episodic and often unpredictable with regard to its recurrence rate.

For patients with inflammatory bowel disease, the eye inflammation may respond to control of the bowel disease. This control can be achieved with corticosteroids by enema for proctitis or orally for more widespread disease. In addition, surgical removal of the inflamed bowel might reduce the extracolonic disease.[64,73]

REFERENCES

1. Andrews BS, McIntosh J, Petts V, Penny R: Circulating immune complexes in acute uveitis: a possible association with the histocompatibility complex locus antigen B27, *Int Arch Allergy Appl Immunol* 58:313, 1979.
2. Bardin T, Enel C, Cornelis F et al.: Antibiotic treatment of venereal disease and Reiter's syndrome in a Greenland population, *Arthritis Rheum* 35:190, 1992.
3. Beckingsale AB, Davies J, Gibson JM, Rosenthal AR: Acute anterior uveitis, ankylosing spondylitis, back pain and HLA B27, *Br J Ophthalmol* 68:741, 1984.
4. Billison FA, De Dombal FT, Watkinson G, Goligher JC: Ocular complications of ulcerative colitis, *Gut* 8:102, 1967.
5. Birkbeck MQ, Buckler WS, Mason RM, Tegner WS: Iritis as the presenting symptom in ankylosing spondylitis, *Lancet* 2:802, 1951.
6. Bjorkman PJ, Saper MA, Samourai B et al.: Structure of the human class I histocompatibility antigen-HLA-A2, *Nature* 329:506, 1987.
7. Breitbart A, Bauer H, Krastel H et al.: Sulfasalazine in recurrent anterior uveitis: a new therapeutical strategy, *Arthritis Rheum* 36(suppl):S225, 1993.
8. Breur-Viesendorp BS, Neefjes JT, Huir B et al.: Identification of new B27 subtypes, *Hum Immunol* 16:163, 1986.
9. Brewerton DA, Caffrey M, Nicholls A et al.: Acute anterior uveitis and HLA B27, *Lancet* 2:994, 1973.
10. Brewerton DA, Hart FD, Nicholls A et al.: Ankylosing spondylitis and HL-A27, *Lancet* 1:904, 1973.
11. Brewerton DA, Nicholls A, Caffrey M et al.: HL-A 27 and arthropathies associated with ulcerative colitis and psoriasis, *Lancet* 1:956, 1974.
12. Calin A, Porta J, Fries JF, Schurman DJ: Clinical history as a screening test for ankylosing spondylitis, *J Am Med Assoc* 237:2613, 1977.
13. Case JP, Sano H, Lafyatis R et al.: Transin/stromelysin expression in the synovium of rats with experimental erosive arthritis, *J Clin Invest* 84:1731, 1989.
14. Chung Y-M, Yeh T-S, Liu J-H: Endogenous uveitis in Chinese—an analysis of 240 cases in a uveitis clinic, *Jpn J Ophthalmol* 32:64, 1988.
15. Cohen LM, Mittal KK, Schmid FR et al.: Increased risk for spondylitis stigmata in apparently healthy HL-AW27 men, *Ann Intern Med* 84:1, 1976.
16. D'Alessandro LP, Forster DJ, Rao NA: Anterior uveitis and hypopyon, *Am J Ophthalmol* 112:317, 1991.
17. Darrell RW, Wagener HP, Kurland LT: Epidemiology of uveitis, incidence and prevalence in a small urban community, *Arch Ophthalmol* 68:100, 1962.
18. Dougados M, Berenbaum F, Maetzel A, Amor B: The use of sulfasalazine for the prevention of attacks of acute anterior uveitis associated with spondylarthropathy, *Arthritis Rheum* 34(suppl): 1991.
18a. Ernst BB, Lowder CY, Meisler DM, Gutman FA: Posterior segment manifestations of inflammatory bowel disease, *Ophthalmology* 98:1272-1280, 1991.
19. Feltkamp TEW: HLA B27, acute anterior uveitis, and ankylosing spondylitis, *Adv Inflamm Res* 9:211, 1985.
20. Feltkamp TEW: HLA-B27 and acute anterior uveitis, *Curr Eye Res* 9:213, 1990.
21. Ford DK, Schulzer M: Synovial lymphocyte responses to microbial antigens differentiate the arthritis of enteric reactive arthritis from the arthritis of inflammatory bowel disease, *J Rheum* 15:1239, 1988.
22. Fox R, Calin A, Gerber RC, Bigson D: The chronicity of symptoms and disability in Reiter's syndrome, *Ann Intern Med* 91:190, 1979.
23. Granfors K, Jalkanen S, Lindberg AA et al.: Salmonella lipopolysaccharide in synovial cells from patients with reactive arthritis, *Lancet* 335:685, 1990.
24. Granfors K, Jalkanen S, Von Essen R et al.: Yersinia antigens in synovial-fluid cells from patients with reactive arthritis, *N Engl J Med* 320:216, 1989.
25. Greenstein AJ, Janowitz HD, Sachar DB: The extra-intestinal complications of Crohn's disease and ulcerative colitis: a study of 700 patients, *Medicine* 55:401, 1976.
26. Haarr M: Rheumatic iridocyclitis, *Acta Ophthalmol* 38:37, 1960.
27. Hammer RE, Maika SD, Richardson JA et al.: Spontaneous inflammatory disease in transgenic rats expressing HLA-B27 and human β-2 microglobulin: an animal model of HLA-B27-associated human disorders, *Cell* 63:1099, 1990.

28. Henderley DE, Genstler AJ, Smith RE, Rao NA: Changing patterns of uveitis, *Am J Ophthalmol* 103:131, 1987.
29. Heuer DK, Gager WE, Reeser FH: Ischemic optic neuropathy associated with Crohn's disease, *J Clin Neuroophthalmol* 2:175, 1982.
30. Hill AVS, Kwiatkowski D, Greenwood BM et al.: HLA class I typing by PCR: HLA-B27 and an African B27 subtype, *Lancet* 337:640, 1991.
31. Hochberg MC, Bias WB, Arnett FC Jr: Family studies in HLA-B27 associated arthritis, *Medicine* 57:463, 1978.
32. Horvath G, Fajnor KI: Uveal changes in spondylitis ankylopoetica, *Acta Rheum Scand* 14:1, 1974.
33. Kapasi KJ, Inman RD: HLA-B27 expression modulates gram-negative bacterial invasion into transfected L cells, *J Immunol* 148:3554, 1992.
34. Kaye BR: Rheumatologic manifestations of infection with human immunodeficiency virus (HIV), *Ann Intern Med* 111:158, 1989.
35. Khan MA, van der Linden SM, Kushner I et al.: Spondylitic disease without radiologic evidence of sacroiliitis in relatives of HLA-B27 positive ankylosing spondylitis patients, *Arthritis Rheum* 28:40, 1985.
36. Kijlstra A, Linssen A, Ockhuizen T: Association of Gm allotypes with the occurrence of ankylosing spondylitis in HLA-B27-positive anterior uveitis, *Am J Ophthalmol* 98:732, 1984.
37. Kogiso M, Tanouchi Y, Mimura Y et al.: Endotoxin-induced uveitis in mice. I. Induction of uveitis and role of T lymphocytes, *Jpn J Ophthalmol* 36:281, 1992.
38. Kozin F, Carrera GF, Ryan LM et al.: Computed tomography in the diagnosis of sacroiliitis, *Arth Rheum* 24:1479, 1981.
39. Lambert JR, Wright V: Eye inflammation in psoriatic arthritis, *Ann Rheum Dis* 35:354, 1976.
40. Lauhio A, Leirisalo-Repo M, Lahdevirta J et al.: Double-blind, placebo-controlled study of three-month treatment with lymecycline in reactive arthritis, with special reference to chlamydia arthritis, *Arthritis Rheum* 34:6, 1991.
41. Lehtinen K: 76 patients with ankylosing spondylitis seen after 30 years of disease, *Scand J Rheumatol* 12:5, 1983.
42. Lenoch F, Kralik V, Bartos J: Rheumatic iritis and iridocyclitis, *Ann Rheum Dis* 18:45, 1959.
43. Linssen A, Dekker-Saeys AJ, Dijkstra PF et al.: The use of HLA-B27 as a diagnostic and prognostic aid in acute anterior uveitis (AAU) in the Netherlands, *Doc Ophthalmol* 64:217, 1986.
44. Linssen A, Rothova A, Valkenburg HA et al.: The lifetime cumulative incidence of acute anterior uveitis in a normal population and its relation to ankylosing spondylitis and histocompatibility antigen HLA-B27, *Invest Ophthalmol Vis Sci* 32:2568, 1991.
45. Maclean IL, Iqball S, Woo P et al.: HLA-B27 subtypes in the spondarthropathies, *Clin Exp Immunol* 91:214, 1993.
46. Maier G, Miller B, Freedman J, Baumgarten I: HLA antigens in acute anterior uveitis in South African blacks, *Br J Ophthalmol* 64:329, 1980.
47. Mark DB, McCulley JB: Reiter's keratitis, *Arch Ophthalmol* 100:781, 1982.
48. Medina-Rodriguez F, Jara LJ, Miranda JM et al.: Sulfasalazine treatment in Reiter's syndrome patients may not be sufficient: comment on the article by Youssef and associates, *Arthritis Rheum* 36:726, 1993.
49. Mielants H, Erick M, Veys RJ et al.: Repeat ileocolonoscopy in reactive arthritis, *J Rheumatol* 14:456, 1987.
50. Mills RP, Kalina RE: Reiter's keratitis, *Arch Ophthalmol* 87:447, 1972.
51. Nissila M, Lehtinen K, Leirisalo-Repo M et al.: Sulfasalazine in the treatment of ankylosing spondylitis, *Arthritis Rheum* 31:1111, 1988.
52. Pearson CM, Waksman BH, Sharp JT: Studies of arthritis and other lesions induced in rats by injection of mycobacterial adjuvant, *J Exp Med* 113:485, 1961.
53. Pedersen OO: Acute anterior uveitis, *Scand J Rheumatol* 32(suppl):226, 1980.
54. Perkins ES, Folk J: Uveitis in London and Iowa, *Ophthalmologica* 189:36, 1984.
54a. Posner A, Schlossman A: Syndrome of unilateral attacks of glaucoma with cyclitic symptoms, *Arch Ophthalmol* 39:517, 1948.
55. Qaiyumi S, Hassan ZU, Toone E: Seronegative spondyloarthropathies in lone aortic insufficiency, *Arch Intern Med* 145:822, 1985.
56. Rahman MU, Cheema MA, Schumacher HR, Hudson AP: Molecular evidence for the presence of chlamydia in the synovium of patients with Reiter's syndrome, *Arthritis Rheum* 35:521, 1992.
57. Raybourne RB, Bunning VK, Williams KM: Reaction of anti-HLA-B monoclonal antibodies with envelope proteins of Shigella species: evidence for molecular mimicry in the spondyloarthropathies, *J Immunol* 140:3489, 1988.
58. Rijk MCM, van Hogezand RA, van Lier HJJ, van Tongeren JHM: Sulphasalazine and prednisone compared with sulphasalazine for treating active Crohn disease, *Ann Intern Med* 114:445, 1991.
59. Romanus H: Pelvo-spondylitis ossificans in the male, *Acta Med Scand* 280(suppl):1953.
60. Rosenbaum JT: Characterization of uveitis associated with spondyloarthritis, *J Rheumatol* 16:792, 1989.
61. Rosenbaum JT: Uveitis: an internist's view, *Arch Intern Med* 149:1173, 1989.
62. Rosenbaum JT: Acute anterior uveitis and spondyloarthropathies, *Rheum Dis Clin North Am* 18:143, 1992.
63. Rosenbaum JT, McDevitt HO, Guss RB, Egbert PR: Endotoxin-induced uveitis in rats as a model for human disease, *Nature* 286:611, 1980.
64. Rosenbaum JT, Tammaro J, Robertson JE Jr: Uveitis precipitated by non-penetrating ocular trauma, *Am J Ophthalmol* 112:392, 1991.
65. Rothova A, Buitenhuis HJ, Meenken C et al.: Uveitis and systemic disease, *Br J Ophthalmol* 76:137, 1992.
66. Rothova A, van Veenedaal MS, Linssen A et al.: Clinical features of acute anterior uveitis, *Am J Ophthalmol* 103:137, 1987.
67. Russell AS, Lentle BC, Percy JS, Jackson FI: Scintigraphy of sacroiliac joints in acute anterior uveitis: a study of thirty patients, *Ann Int Med* 85:606, 1976.
68. Saari KM, Vilppula A, Lassus A et al.: Ocular inflammation in Reiter's disease after salmonella enteritis, *Am J Ophthalmol* 90:63, 1980.
69. Saari R, Lahti R, Saari KM: Frequency of rheumatic diseases in patients with acute anterior uveitis, *Scand J Rheumatol* 11:121, 1982.
70. Sasaki T, Kusalba Y, Yamamoto et al.: HLA B27 and acute anterior uveitis in the Japanese population, *Jpn J Ophthalmol* 23:374, 1979.
71. Schlosstein L, Terasaki PI, Bluestone R, Pearson CM: High association of an HL-A antigen, W27, with ankylosing spondylitis, *New Eng J Med* 288:704, 1973.
72. Schneiderman JH, Sharpe JA, Sutton DMC: Cerebral and retinal vascular complications of inflammatory bowel disease, *Ann Neurol* 5:331, 1979.
73. Schwimmbeck PL, Oldstone MB: Klebsiella pneumoniae and HLA B27-associated diseases of Reiter's syndrome and ankylosing spondylitis, *Curr Top Microbiol Immunol* 144:45, 1989.
74. Scofield RH, Warren WL, Koelsch G, Harley JB: A hypothesis for the HLA-B27 immune dysregulation in spondyloarthropathy: contributions from enteric organisms, B27 structure, peptides bound by B27, and convergent evolution, *Proc Natl Acad Sci USA* 90:9330, 1993.
75. Short CL: III. Clinical description of infectious and other types of arthritis, *New Eng J Med* 236:468, 1947.
76. Simon DG, Kaslow RA, Rosenbaum JT et al.: Reiter's syndrome following epidemic shigellosis, *J Rheumatol* 8:6, 1981.
77. Singh VJ, Yamaki K, Donoso LA, Shinohara T: Molecular mimicry. Yeast histone H3-induced experimental autoimmune uveitis, *J Immunol* 142:1512, 1989.
78. Smith MD, Gibson RA, Brooks PM: Abnormal bowel permeability in ankylosing spondylitis and rheumatoid arthritis, *J Rheumatol* 12:299, 1985.
79. Soylu M, Ersoz TR, Haciyakupoglu G, Eroglu A: Aetiological distribution of uveitis patients in Southern Turkey, *Ocul Immunol Inflamm* 1:355, 1993.
80. Stanworth A, Sharp J: Uveitis and rheumatic diseases, *Ann Rheum Dis* 15:140, 1956.
81. Stieglitz H, Fosmine S, Lipsky P: Identification of a 2-Md plasmid from Shigella flexneri associated with reactive arthritis, *Arthritis Rheum* 32:937, 1989.
82. Taurog JD, El-Zaatari AK: In vitro mutagenesis of HLA-B27, *J Clin Invest* 82:987, 1988.
83. Taurog JD, Hammer RE, Montafiez S et al.: Effect of germfree state on the inflammatory disease of HLA-B27 transgenic rats. A split result, *Arthritis Rheum* 36(suppl):546, 1993.
83a. Theodore FH: Observations on glaucomatocyclitic crises (Posner-Schlossman syndrome), *Br J Ophthalmol* 36:207, 1952.
84. Vinje O, Dale K, Moller P: Radiographic changes, HLA B27 and back pain in patients with psoriasis or acute anterior uveitis, *Scand J Rheumatol* 12:219, 1983.

85. Wakefield D, Easter J, Penny R: Clinical features of HLA B27 anterior uveitis, *Aust J Ophthalmol* 12:191, 1984.

86. Wakefield D, Easter J, Robinson P, Penny R: Immunological features of HLA-B27 anterior uveitis, *Aust J Ophthalmol* 11:15, 1983.

86a. Waksman BH, Bullington SJ: Studies of arthritis and other lesions induced in rats by injection of mycobacterial adjuvant. II. Lesions of the eye, *Arch Ophthalmol* 64:751-762, 1960.

87. Weiner A, BenEzra D: Clinical patterns and associated conditions in chronic uveiis, *Am J Ophthalmol* 112:151, 1991.

88. Wells A, Pararajasegaram G, Baldwin M et al.: Uveitis and arthritis induced by systemic injection of streptococcal cell walls, *Invest Ophthalmol Vis Sci* 27:1986.

89. White L, McCoy R, Tait B, Ebringer R: A search for gram-negative enteric micro-organisms in acute anterior uveitis: association of klebsiella with recent onset of disease, HLA-B27, and B7 CREG, *Br J Ophthalmol* 68:750, 1984.

90. Wilkinson M, Bywaters EGL: Clinical features and course of ankylosing spondylitis as seen in a follow-up of 222 hospital referred cases, *Ann Rheum Dis* 17:209, 1958.

91. Winchester R, Bernstein DH, Fischer HD et al.: The co-occurrence of Reiter's syndrome and acquired immunodeficiency, *Ann Intern Med* 106:19, 1987.

92. Woodrow JC: HL-A 27 and Reiter's syndrome, *Lancet* 2:671, 1973.

93. Wright R, Lumsden K, Luntz MH et al.: Abnormalities of the sacroiliac joints and uveitis in ulcerative colitis, *Q J Med* 34:229, 1965.

94. Young RH, McEwen EG: Bacillary dysentry as the cause of Reiter's syndrome, *J Am Med Assoc* 134:1456, 1947.

95. Yu DT, Choo SY, Schaack T: Molecular mimicry in HLA-B27-related arthritis, *Ann Intern Med* 111:581, 1989.

96. Zhang J-J, Hamachi M, Hamachi T et al.: The bacterial outer membrane protein that reacts with anti-HLA-B27 antibodies is the OMPA protein, *J Immunol* 143:2955, 1989.

40 Chronic Childhood Arthritis and Uveitis

JACK J. KANSKI, ROSS E. PETTY

An association between intraocular inflammation and chronic arthritis in children has been recognized since the early descriptions by Ohm[42] and Blegvad.[3] The association was not firmly established, however, until the publication by Vesterdal and Sury[82] in which 34 patients with arthritis and uveitis were presented, and the published information on an additional 31 patients reviewed. Since then, a number of reports have expanded and refined the clinical knowledge of this association.*

The spectrum of childhood arthritis includes both acute and chronic disorders. Limited data suggest that acute transient arthritis, presumably related to infection, accounts for the majority of childhood arthritis cases; nevertheless, chronic arthritis represents a more significant health problem.[31] This chapter focuses on uveitis that occurs with the chronic arthritides of childhood.

SYSTEMIC DISEASE

Chronic inflammatory arthritis in childhood is uncommon, but not rare. Estimates of the incidence vary widely, depending on the criteria used for diagnosis and the methods of ascertainment. An overall incidence of approximately 25 per 100,000 children per year under the age of 16 years and a prevalence of approximately 150 per 100,000 children under 16 years of age may be appropriate.

Chronic inflammatory arthritis in childhood is a heterogeneous group of disorders for which there is no universally agreed classification. The American College of Rheumatology (ACR) has defined juvenile rheumatoid arthritis (JRA) as chronic arthritis of one or more joints that has an onset prior to age 16 years.[4] The ACR further defines three subsets of JRA according to the behavior of the disease during the first 6 months after onset: oligoarticular disease, in which there is arthritis in one to four joints; polyarticular

disease, in which there is arthritis in five or more joints; and systemic disease, in which there can be any number of affected joints plus characteristic fever and, usually, other systemic features. All other rheumatic diseases are excluded from this definition. The European League Against Rheumatism (EULAR) criteria for the classification of juvenile chronic arthritis (JCA)[41] differ in two important ways: first, the term "juvenile rheumatoid arthritis" is restricted to those children who have polyarticular arthritis and rheumatoid factor (RF); second, children with the seronegative spondyloarthropathies [juvenile ankylosing spondylitis, juvenile psoriatic arthritis, Reiter syndrome, and the arthropathies of inflammatory bowel disease (all of which are excluded from the ACR definition of JRA)] are included in the EULAR definition of JCA. It is hoped that this confusion will be resolved in the near future;[57] for this chapter, the ACR terminology will be used.

Juvenile Rheumatoid Arthritis

Juvenile rheumatoid arthritis is a form of chronic arthritis that begins before the sixteenth birthday and is categorized into three types based on the behavior of the disease at onset (during the first 6 months). In all types, arthritis persists for at least 6 weeks (3 months in the EULAR classification system). The estimated annual incidences range from 9.2 per 100,000[79] to 13.9 per 100,000.[80] The prevalence estimated in a Mayo Clinic report[80] was 113.4 per 100,000 children.

Oligoarticular JRA. Pauciarticular or oligoarticular JRA accounts for at least 50% of all children with JRA. By definition, 4 or fewer joints are affected during the first 6 months of disease. It affects girls five times as often as boys and is most common in young children, with a peak age of onset at around 2 years of age (Table 40-1). Involvement of the knees and, less frequently, the ankles and wrists is characteristic. Although the cervical spine and temporomandibular joints are sometimes affected, small joints are usually spared, and systemic complications do not occur. The prog-

---

*References 6, 7, 8, 9, 10, 12, 13, 21, 22, 23, 24, 25, 26, 27, 28, 29, 30, 34, 46, 50, 59, 66, 67, 70, 71, 72, 73, 74, 75, 77, 78, 86.

TABLE 40-1 CHARACTERISTICS OF JRA BY TYPE OF ONSET

	Oligoarticular	Polyarticular	Systemic
Frequency of cases	50%	40%	10%
Number of joints involved	<5	>4	Variable
Age at onset	Early childhood	Throughout childhood	Throughout childhood
	Peak at 1–3 yr	Peak at 1–2 yr	No peak
Sex ratio (F:M)	5:1	3:1	1:1
Systemic involvement	None	Moderate	Prominent
Chronic anterior uveitis	20%	5%	Rare
Rheumatoid factor present	Rare	10%	Rare
Antinuclear antibody present	75-85%*	40-50%	10%
Prognosis	Good to excellent†	Fair to good	Poor to good

Adapted from Cassidy JT, Petty RE: *Textbook of pediatric rheumatology,* ed 3, Philadelphia, 1994, Saunders
* Especially frequent in girls with uveitis
† Visual prognosis may be guarded

nosis is variable: many children have complete resolution of their joint disease after months or years of activity; others progress to have polyarticular disease; still others have a remission followed by recurrence of oligoarticular disease after many years. The overall outlook, however, is generally favorable. About 20% of children develop chronic anterior uveitis.

Polyarticular JRA. Polyarticular JRA affects 5 or more joints during the first 6 months of disease. Arthritis often affects large and small joints symmetrically. Three times as many girls as boys are affected by polyarticular JRA, which occurs in a somewhat older age group than oligoarticular JRA. The disease course is usually chronic and the long-term functional outcome guarded. IgM RF is present in the serum of 10% of children with polyarticular JRA and is associated with the presence of subcutaneous nodules, erosions, and a poor prognosis. Chronic anterior uveitis occurs in approximately 5% of children.

Systemic Onset JRA. Children with systemic onset JRA are usually acutely ill. The disease occurs with equal frequency in boys and girls and can occur at any age. In addition to polyarthritis, children with systemic onset JRA have a characteristic quotidian fever that reaches 39° C or 40° C during the late afternoon or evening and falls to normal or below during the morning. A characteristic transient macular rash occurs in 95% of patients, hepatosplenomegaly in 75%, pericarditis in 35%, pleuritis in 20%, and abdominal pain in 10%. The early course is dominated by the systemic features; later, chronic polyarthritis predominates. Chronic anterior uveitis is extremely rare in this subgroup.

Spondyloarthropathies

The spondyloarthropathies comprise a group of disorders characterized by enthesitis and arthritis of the joints of the axial skeleton: juvenile ankylosing spondylitis, juvenile psoriatic arthritis, Reiter syndrome, and the arthropathies of inflammatory bowel disease.[52] Enthesitis, an inflammation

of the sites of attachment of ligaments, tendons, capsule, or fascia to bone, is a hallmark of these disorders. This constellation of findings has led to the delineation of a syndrome of seronegativity, enthesitis, and arthritis (SEA syndrome)[61] that identifies children with arthritis who are likely to develop a spondyloarthropathy, especially juvenile ankylosing spondylitis.[5] Features common to the spondyloarthropathies are shown in the box. Extraarticular disease serves to separate the individual members of the spondyloarthropathies. As a group, children with inflammation of the axial skeleton (lumbosacral spine and sacroiliac joints) have a high frequency of the histocompatibility antigen HLA-B27.

Juvenile Ankylosing Spondylitis. Juvenile ankylosing spondylitis is the prototype of the spondyloarthropathies. It is a chronic arthropathy that most frequently affects boys after the age of 10 years. Enthesitis (especially around the feet and knees) together with arthritis, which usually affects large and small joints of the lower extremity, characterize the clinical presentation. Although the lumbosacral spine and sacroiliac joints are ultimately affected, involvement is usually subclinical and radiographs normal during the early months or years of the disease. Rheumatoid factor and antinuclear antibodies (ANA) are not present. Recurrent attacks

---

CHARACTERISTICS OF THE SPONDYLOARTHROPATHIES[55]

Family history of spondyloarthropathies
High frequency of HLA-B27
Onset in late childhood or adolescence
More common in boys than girls
Frequent sacroiliitis
Frequent enthesitis
Absence of IgM rheumatoid factor
Absence of antinuclear antibodies

of unilateral acute anterior uveitis occur in 5% to 15% of children.[15a,65a]

Juvenile Reiter Syndrome. Reiter syndrome is uncommon in children, although a number of well-documented cases have been reported.[60] Reiter syndrome is a reactive arthritis that is frequently found to have an antecedent extraarticular bacterial infection, usually in the gastrointestinal tract *(Yersinia enterocolitica, Salmonella typhimurium, Shigella flexneri, or Campylobacter jejuni),* or in the genitourinary tract *(Chlamydia trachomatis).* The arthritis is characteristically acute in onset, is very painful, and affects a few joints. There is often an associated tenosynovitis. The Reiter syndrome triad includes arthritis, conjunctivitis, and urethritis; other systemic features include fever, rash (keratoderma blenorrhagicum), oropharyngeal mucosal changes, and balanitis. RF and ANA are not present, but close to 90% of children have HLA-B27.[58a] The course is usually brief, lasting a few days to several weeks, but it may recur and may become chronic. About 2% of patients develop acute anterior uveitis.[20a]

Arthropathies Associated with Inflammatory Bowel Disease. Both Crohn disease (regional enteritis) and ulcerative colitis may be associated with arthritis in childhood.[33] Two patterns of joint disease are recognized. The most common pattern is acute transient peripheral arthritis usually associated with active inflammation of the gut. A less common articular manifestation is sacroiliitis and lumbosacral spine disease, which resembles juvenile ankylosing spondylitis and is associated with HLA-B27. This type of arthropathy tends to be chronic and its manifestations do not necessarily reflect the activity or extent of the gut inflammation. Chronic anterior uveitis, which may be granulomatous, has been reported occasionally in children with peripheral joint disease,[64] whereas unilateral anterior uveitis of sudden onset may occur in those who are HLA-B27 positive. The characteristics of the latter form of uveitis are similar to those seen in HLA-B27 positive adults. In patients with Crohn disease, chronic anterior uveitis is more common in those with inflammation of the colon (rather than the small bowel) and in those in whom the gut disease is accompanied by arthritis.[64]

Juvenile Psoriatic Arthritis. Juvenile psoriatic arthritis has been included with the spondyloarthropathies by longstanding tradition, although it is apparent that this disorder differs significantly from other members of this group. Juvenile psoriatic arthritis can be defined as arthritis occurring with psoriasis or with three of the following criteria: dactylitis (inflammation of joints and tendon sheaths of a finger or toe resulting in a "sausage digit"), nail pitting, family history of psoriasis, or a rash that is not entirely typical of psoriasis.[76] Juvenile psoriatic arthritis usually presents as an asymmetric oligoarticular (sometimes polyarticular) arthritis that affects both large and small joints. Dactylitis is characteristic and often associated with pitting or onycholysis of the nail of the same digit. Other patterns of joint involvement (predominant distal interphalangeal joint disease, sa-

croiliitis, arthritis mutilans)[38] are very uncommon. ANA of undetermined specificity are common, but RF is absent. There is no particular HLA association, except in those children with sacroiliitis who are likely to be HLA-B27 positive. Unlike other members of the spondyloarthropathies group, the anterior uveitis that occurs in 10% to 15% of these children is usually chronic and asymptomatic.[76]

Other Arthritides in Childhood

Two other arthropathies of childhood are frequently complicated by uveitis. Their onset is usually very early in life, often before 6 months of age.

Sarcoidosis. Although sarcoidosis is uncommon in childhood,[62] it can cause chronic arthritis and uveitis. Infantile sarcoidosis consists of a syndrome that includes arthritis, a papular dermatitis, and uveitis. The arthritis is usually polyarticular and symmetric, affecting large and small joints. Affected joints are frequently described as "boggy" and are usually not acutely inflamed. RF and ANA are usually absent. The course is prolonged and may be complicated by involvement of the viscera. Although the uveitis of infantile sarcoidosis may begin as chronic iridocyclitis indistinguishable from that seen in JRA, involvement of the posterior uveal tract will clearly distinguish it from that seen with other chronic childhood arthritides.

Neonatal Onset Multisystem Inflammatory Disease. Neonatal onset multisystem inflammatory disease (NOMID) is a rare familial disorder of neonatal onset characterized by arthritis, a variable nonpruritic urticarial rash, central nervous system signs (chronic meningitis, spasticity, intellectual impairment), and ocular abnormalities (papilledema, optic atrophy, uveitis).[56] The disease is prolonged, generally unresponsive to therapy, and frequently fatal.

RISK FACTORS

The occurrence of chronic anterior uveitis in children with arthritis is influenced by age, sex, disease type, and genetic factors (Table 40-2). In general, uveitis is much

TABLE 40-2 RISK OF UVEITIS IN CHILDREN WITH JRA

Factor	Low Risk	High Risk
Sex	Male	Female
Age at onset of arthritis	>6 yr	<6 yr
Type of onset of arthritis	Systemic	Oligoarticular
Duration of arthritis	>4 yr	<4 yr
Antinuclear antibody	Absent	Present
Rheumatoid factor	Present	Absent
HLA-DR4	Present	Absent
HLA-DR5	Absent	Present

From Cassidy JT, Petty RE: *Textbook of pediatric rheumatology,* ed 3, Philadelphia, 1994, Saunders

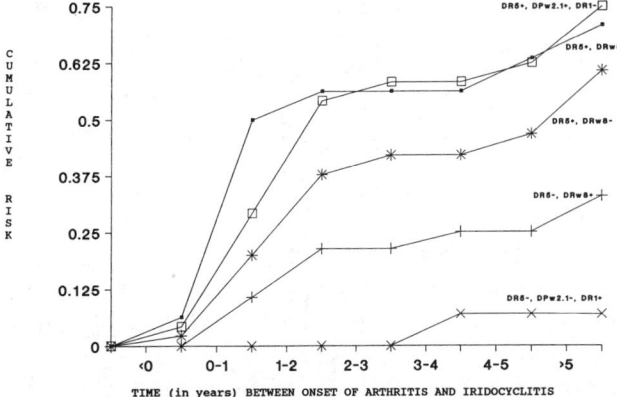

Fig. 40-1. The relationship of HLA antigens to the cumulative risk of development of chronic anterior uveitis in children with oligoarticular JRA. Children with highest risk have DR5 and DP2.1, but are DR1 negative. Those with both HLA-DR5 and DPw8 are also at very high risk. Children who lack DR5 and DRw8 are also at high risk. Children who lack DR5 and DPw2.1 and are DR1 positive have the lowest risk. (Reprinted with permission from Fiannini EH, Malagon CN, Van Kerhove C et al.: Longitudinal analysis of HLA-associated risks for iridocyclitis in juvenile rheumatoid arthritis, *J Rheumatol* 18:1394-1397, 1991)

more common in children in whom the age at onset of arthritis is below 6 years.[8] Chronic anterior uveitis occurs with greater frequency in girls than boys; the female to male ratio is approximately 5 to 1. Children with oligoarticular JRA or juvenile psoriatic arthritis are particularly at risk, and those with systemic onset JRA are at very low risk. Genetic factors undoubtedly play a role in explaining these associations but also appear to contribute to the risk of uveitis per se. Thus although HLA-DR8 is associated with oligoarticular JRA, HLA-DR5 is associated with uveitis in these children.[35] Conversely, HLA-DR1 and HLA-DR4 are negatively associated with uveitis.[35] Hoffman and associates[18] reported the association of HLA-DP 2.1 with uveitis in JRA. An analysis of the contribution of HLA antigens to the cumulative risk of children with early onset oligoarticular JRA developing chronic uveitis is shown in Fig. 40-1.[14] In children with ankylosing spondylitis, the class I antigen HLA-B27 is associated with unilateral anterior uveitis of sudden onset.

CLINICAL FEATURES

Chronic Anterior Uveitis

In JRA and juvenile psoriatic arthritis, the intraocular inflammation is bilateral in about 75% of cases.[47] In most instances both eyes are involved either simultaneously or within a few months of each other, and it is unusual for children whose uveitis is unilateral initially to develop uveitis in the second eye after more than 12 months have elapsed. The onset of uveitis is usually asymptomatic and its presence is often initially detected by routine slit lamp biomicro-

scopic examination of those at risk. Even during exacerbations with numerous (up to 4+) cells in the aqueous humor, the eye is almost invariably noninjected to external inspection. The patients usually have no symptoms, although a few older children may report slight blurring of vision and an increase in the amount of vitreous floaters.

In the vast majority of patients the intraocular inflammation is nongranulomatous, although Koeppe nodules and mutton fat keratic precipitates may rarely be present. The keratic precipitates are usually small to medium in size and located mainly in the inferior half of the corneal endothelium. In eyes with moderate to severe uveitis, cells are frequently seen in the anterior vitreous humor. During acute exacerbations of inflammation, the entire endothelium may become covered by many hundreds of minute keratic precipitates (endothelial dusting). This sign is particularly helpful when detailed slit lamp examination of the aqueous is difficult in an uncooperative child.

Acute Anterior Uveitis

The uveitis associated with juvenile spondyloarthropathies is similar to that seen in HLA-B27 positive adults. It usually has a fairly sudden, symptomatic onset and persists for 6 weeks or less. The attacks are unilateral, although either eye may be involved at different times. Treatment of acute attacks with topical corticosteroids and, if necessary, anterior sub-Tenon injections of corticosteroids is usually very effective. The long-term visual prognosis is good and vision-threatening complications are rare, although a small percentage of children subsequently develop chronic inflammation similar to that seen with JRA.

PATHOGENESIS

The cause of uveitis associated with childhood arthritis is unknown.[47] Reports of examination of ocular tissue have been infrequent and have invariably involved the study of tissue removed after years of chronic disease.[11,15,17,37,63] In these studies an intense inflammatory infiltrate consisting predominantly of lymphocytes and plasma cells was observed in the iris and ciliary body.[15,17,37,63] These nonspecific changes have contributed little to understanding pathogenesis and still less to understanding the underlying cause of the uveitis. Reports of mollicutelike organisms (cell wall deficient bacteria, classified with the mycoplasma) in ocular fluids and tissues from adults with juvenile onset arthritis and uveitis[85] have not been confirmed.

Serologic studies of children with arthritis and uveitis have yielded limited information. Antinuclear antibodies are found in almost all children with arthritis and uveitis, but they are also present in over 80% of children with oligoarticular JRA who do not have uveitis.[36] Thus the absence of ANA is of some help in predicting which child will probably not develop uveitis, but their presence does not aid in the prediction of the subsequent development of uveitis. The antigenic specificities of ANA in children with uveitis are not known. Alspaugh and Miller[1] showed that ANA in children with uveitis and JRA are not directed to DNA, Sm, RNP, Ro, or La antigens. There have been reports of the association of antihistone ANA with uveitis.[39,43,45] Rosenberg and Gilmer[58] reported that 100% of their patients with oligoarticular JRA and uveitis had antibodies that reacted with chromosomes.[58] Antibodies to a 15-kDa protein have also been associated with uveitis.[40]

Because type II collagen is restricted in its distribution to hyaline cartilage, which is present in joints and vitreous humor, immunity to this protein might contribute to both uveitis and arthritis. Furthermore, type II collagen induces arthritis, and, occasionally, uveitis in animals. In children with arthritis and uveitis, however, antibodies or cell-mediated immunity to native or denatured human or bovine collagen is not more frequent in children with uveitis than in those with arthritis alone.[51] Frequencies of antibodies to types I, III, and IV collagen, which are also present in the anterior uveal tract,[68] were similar in both groups.[51]

Immunity to ocular antigens has also been studied in children with arthritis and uveitis. Immunity to the soluble retinal antigen (S antigen) is present in approximately two thirds of such children.[54,81] Because S antigen is found in the retina, but not the anterior uveal tract, these findings may indicate that the extent of ocular involvement in JRA also includes the posterior uveal tract, despite the lack of obvious clinical findings in that portion of the eye. One ill-defined antigen from the iris reacts with antibodies from the serum of children with JRA and uveitis.[20] Whether any of these immune reactions represents a pathogenic mechanism, or whether they simply reflect an immune response to ocular tissue damaged by other mechanisms is not known.

The frequent association of uveitis with arthritis suggests either a common cause or predisposition, or an interdependent pathogenesis wherein one disorder causes changes that lead to the other. Such potential mechanisms are shown schematically in Fig. 40-2.

Animal Models

Very limited application of animal models has been made to the study of arthritis and uveitis.[49] Most animal models of uveitis affect primarily the posterior uveal tract and are therefore of limited interest. In the rat model of chronic arthritis induced by complete Freund adjuvant, uveitis occurs in approximately one third of arthritic Lewis and Lewis SsN rats.[55,83] Uveitis follows the development of arthritis by several days, persists for 10 to 14 days, and affects primarily the anterior uveal tract. Uveitis can occasionally be induced by adoptive transfer of lymphocytes from injected donors to naive recipients.[53] Intraperitoneal injection of *Mycobacterium butyricum* also induces chronic arthritis accompanied by a high frequency (80%) of anterior uveitis.[53] Arthritis in-

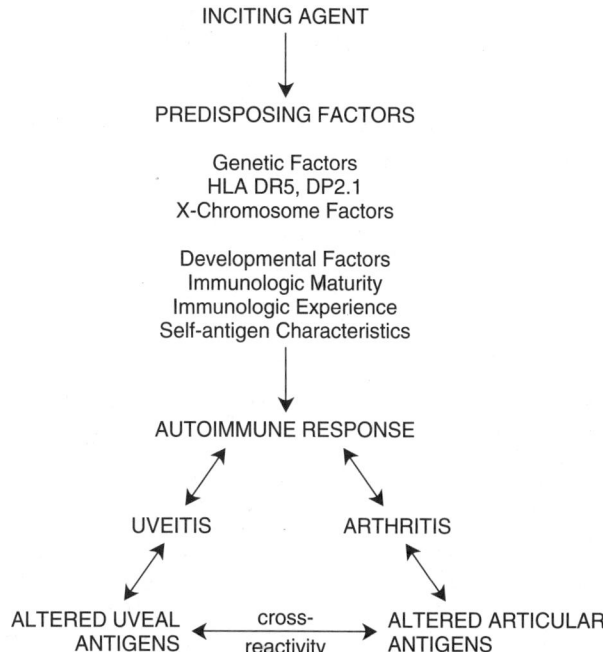

Fig. 40-2. The figure outlines some factors that could play a role in the interaction between arthritis and uveitis. An inciting agent (possibly an infectious agent), under appropriate circumstances, including genetic and developmental factors, could induce an autoimmune response resulting in uveitis and/or arthritis. Inflammation of the joint or eye could result in alteration of tissue specific antigens which, by their cross-reactivity could induce further disease, and perpetuate the process. There is little direct evidence to support or refute such a model.

duced by type II collagen is also occasionally accompanied by anterior uveitis indistinguishable from that induced by complete Freund adjuvant.[19] Uveitis and arthritis may also be induced by injection of streptococcal cell walls.[84]

THERAPY

Because most children with arthritis and uveitis are asymptomatic, it is incumbent on physicians to recognize the risk factors and to monitor the child by slit lamp biomicroscopy. Similarly, those with little or no risk of ocular complications should be identified to spare the patients and parents the inconvenience of unnecessary visits to the ophthalmologist. The recent recommendations of the Sections of Rheumatology and Ophthalmology of the American Academy of Pediatrics are shown in Table 40-3.[2] These guidelines are appropriate, if children who have had uveitis are also considered to be at high risk, because the frequency of recurrence is high. Additional risk factors may be used to refine these recommendations. For example, it is unusual for a child who does not have ANA to develop uveitis. Likewise, children with HLA-DR1 or HLA-DR4 rarely develop ocular disease.

TABLE 40-3 RISK OF UVEITIS AND SUGGESTED FREQUENCY OF SLIT LAMP EXAMINATIONS FOR CHILDREN WITH JRA AND WITHOUT KNOWN IRIDOCYCLITIS

JRA Subtype at Onset	Risk	
	Age at Onset	
	< 7 yr*	> 7 yr†
Oligoarticular		
ANA +	High‡	Medium
ANA −	Medium	Medium
Polyarticular		
ANA +	High‡	Medium
ANA −	Medium	Medium
Systemic	Low	Low

Slit lamp examination should be performed in children in the high-risk category every 3-4 mo, in the medium-risk group every 6 mo, and in the low-risk group every 12 mo. ANA indicates results of test for antinuclear antibodies

Adapted from Guidelines for ophthalmic examinations in children with juvenile rheumatoid arthritis, *Pediatrics* 92:295-296, 1993

* All patients with onset under 7 yr of age are considered at low risk 7 yr after the onset of arthritis and should have yearly ophthalmologic examinations indefinitely

† All patients with onset at age 7 yr or more are considered at low risk 4 yr after onset of arthritis and should have yearly ophthalmologic examinations indefinitely

‡ All high-risk patients are considered at medium risk 4 yr after onset of arthritis

Mydriatics

The formation of posterior synechiae can be best prevented by keeping the pupil mobile with a short-acting mydriatic such as tropicamide 1%. In mild cases the mydriatic can be instilled once at bedtime to prevent difficulties with accommodation during the day. The pupil should not be kept constantly dilated with atropine, because synechiae can still develop when the pupil is immobilized in the dilated position. In a young child unilateral atropine-induced cycloplegia may result in amblyopia.

Corticosteroids

In most patients the uveitis can be controlled by the appropriate use of potent topical corticosteroids such as dexamethasone, prednisolone, or betamethasone. The most frequent reason for failure of therapy is inadequate use of topical medication caused by fear of corticosteroid-induced complications such as cataract and secondary glaucoma. Unfortunately, fluorometholone (which has much less effect on intraocular pressure) is, at best, of minimal value in treating anterior uveitis.

Acute exacerbations of chronic inflammation usually respond well to a three-day course of hourly topical corticosteroid instillation. The frequency of administration can then be reduced to four times a day. If the inflammation is under good control with no more than 1 + cells in the aqueous humor, the rate of instillation can be gradually tapered even further over the next few months, and then stopped. Following cessation of treatment, the patient should be reexamined within a few days to ensure that the uveitis has not recurred.

Patients who are unresponsive to topical medication occasionally respond to oral corticosteroid therapy. In some cases, however, intravenous methylprednisolone in a dose of 30 mg/kg/day on 1 to 3 consecutive days with appropriate in-hospital monitoring is required to control the inflammation so the patient can revert to topical therapy. Alternatively, anterior sub-Tenon injections of a depot preparation of corticosteroid, such as methylprednisolone acetate or triamcinolone acetonide, can be used when topical medication is ineffective or compliance is poor. It is very important for all patients receiving corticosteroid medication to have regular measurements of intraocular pressure. Topical indomethacin may be a useful substitute for glucocorticoids in some patients with acute anterior uveitis,[65] and oral nonsteroidal antiinflammatory drugs may have a modest effect in chronic uveitis.[32] Nonsteroidal antiinflammatory drugs are less effective than corticosteroids, however, and most clinicians have not found these drugs useful in the management of uveitis.

Systemic Immunosuppressive Drugs

The treatment of intractable corticosteroid-resistant uveitis with systemic immunosuppressive agents is controversial. In one study seven patients with bilateral uveitis were treated with prolonged low-dosage chlorambucil.[44] Only two patients were judged to have had long-term benefit in both eyes, and one patient had a transient response in one eye. Three patients developed serious drug-induced adverse effects (varicella-zoster virus infection, ovarian failure, and bone marrow depression). A second study found that immunosuppressive therapy can be both safe and effective if carefully administered and closely supervised.[16] In six of eight patients, treatment with a variety of systemic immunosuppressive drugs (methotrexate, azathioprine, and chlorambucil) was successful in the abolition of intraocular inflammation. Cyclosporine has been successful in treatment of posterior uveitis, but its use in the management of anterior uveitis is anecdotal. Cytotoxic agents must be used with great care in children because of the risk of significant short- and long-term side effects.

COMPLICATIONS AND PROGNOSIS

Many children with chronic anterior uveitis have no residual complications.[48] In some, however, complications persist long after the inflammatory disease has ceased and may contribute to vision loss. Although variable and difficult to predict early in the disease course, there is little doubt that the visual outcome in children with arthritis complicated by uveitis is improving, probably as a result of earlier detection and more effective antiinflammatory treatment. Early reports described a poor prognosis for sight, with blindness resulting in 15% to 38% of patients.[8,10,28,74]

More recent studies record a more favorable prognosis.[6,24,35,69,86] In one long-term study[24] of 103 patients in whom uveitis was initially diagnosed prior to the development of complications, about 25% either required no treatment or responded very well to topical corticosteroids. At the other end of the spectrum were patients with very severe and prolonged inflammation that responded poorly to topical therapy; this group accounted for about 25% of cases. The vast majority required surgery for complications. The remaining 50% had moderate to severe uveitis and required topical therapy for many months, and in many cases, several years. The visual prognosis in this subgroup was fair. A similar study[86] found that the severity of vision loss was correlated with the degree of inflammation found in initial examination. Of 58 eyes that were initially normal or had only mild inflammation, cataract subsequently developed in 28%, glaucoma in 17%, and band keratopathy in 5%. Only 3% of eyes in this group had a final visual acuity of 20/200 or less. Of 31 eyes that had posterior synechiae on initial examination, cataract developed in 81%, glaucoma in 45%, and band keratopathy in 77%. In this group 58% of eyes had a final visual acuity of 20/200 or less. The results of the most recent study of 49 patients (82 affected eyes) are summarized in Table 40-4.[6] Corrected visual acuity was 20/20 to

20/40 in 85%, 20/50 to 20/100 in 5%, and 20/200 or worse in 10%.

Optimal outcome requires close cooperation between physicians who are thoroughly familiar with the uveitis that complicates childhood arthritis and with the potential risks and benefits of specific therapies.

TABLE 40-4 OCULAR COMPLICATIONS AND VISUAL ACUITY AT MOST RECENT FOLLOW-UP OF 49 PATIENTS WITH UVEITIS

	Maximum Follow-up Period			
	2-4 yr	5-9 yr	>9 yr	Total
Patients with uveitis	7	23	19	49
Eyes with uveitis	12	37	33	82
Eyes with complications	5	13	9	27
Frequency (%) of specific complications in eyes with uveitis				
Synechiae	33	19	27	24
Band keratopathy	33	13	15	17
Cataract	33	19	18	21
Glaucoma	8	11	6	12
Phthisis bulbi	0	0	3	1
Visual outcome of all eyes with uveitis (%) (corrected acuity)				
20/20–20/40	92	84	85	85
20/50–20/100	0	8	3	5
20/200 or worse	8	8	12	10

Modified from Cabral DA, Petty RE, Malleson PN and associates: Visual prognosis in children with chronic anterior uveitis and arthritis, *J Rheumatol* 21:2370-2375, 1994.

REFERENCES

1. Alspaugh M, Miller JJ III: A study of specificities of antinuclear antibodies in juvenile rheumatoid arthritis, *J Pediatr* 90:391-395, 1977.
2. American Academy of Pediatrics, Subcommittees of Rheumatology and Ophthalmology: Guidelines for ophthalmologic examinations in children with juvenile rheumatoid arthritis, *Pediatrics* 92:295-296, 1993.
3. Blegvad O: Iridocyclitis and disease of the joints in children, *Acta Ophthalmol* 19:219-236, 1941.
4. Brewer EJ, Bass J, Baum J et al.: Current proposed revision of JRA criteria, *Arthritis Rheum* 20(suppl):195-199, 1977.
5. Cabral DA, Oen KG, Petty RE: SEA syndrome revisited: a long-term follow-up of children with a syndrome of seronegative enthesopathy and arthropathy, *J Rheumatol* 19:1282-1285, 1992.
6. Cabral DA, Petty RE, Malleson PN et al.: Visual prognosis in children with chronic anterior uveitis and arthritis, *J Rheumatol* 21:2370-2375, 1994.
7. Calabro JJ, Parrino GR, Atchoo PD et al.: Chronic iridocyclitis in juvenile rheumatoid arthritis, *Arthritis Rheum* 13:406-413, 1970.
8. Cassidy JT, Sullivan DB, Petty RE: Clinical patterns of chronic iridocyclitis in children with juvenile rheumatoid arthritis, *Arthritis Rheum* 20(suppl):224-227, 1977.
9. Chylack LT Jr: The ocular manifestations of juvenile rheumatoid arthritis, *Arthritis Rheum* 20(suppl):217-223, 1977.
10. Chylack LT Jr, Bienfang DC, Bellows AR et al.: Ocular manifestations of juvenile rheumatoid arthritis, *Am J Ophthalmol* 79:1026-1033, 1975.
11. Chylack LT Jr, Dueker DK, Pihlaja DJ: Ocular manifestations of juvenile rheumatoid arthritis: pathology, fluorescein iris angiography and patient care patterns. In Miller JJ, editor: *Juvenile rheumatoid arthritis,* 149-163, Littleton, 1978, PSG Publishing.
12. Franceshetti A, Blum JD, Bamatter F: Diagnostic value of ocular symptoms in juvenile chronic polyarthritis (Still's Disease), *Trans Ophthalmol Soc UK* 71:17-26, 1951.
13. Galea P, D'Amato B, Goel KM: Ocular complications in juvenile chronic arthritis (JCA), *Scott Med J* 30:164-167, 1985.
14. Giannini EH, Malagon CN, Van Kerkhove C et al.: Longitudinal analysis of HLA associated risks for iridocyclitis in juvenile rheumatoid arthritis, *J Rheumatol* 18:1394-1397, 1991.
15. Godfrey WA, Lindsley CB, Cuppage FE: Localization of IgM in plasma cells in the iris of a patient with iridocyclitis and juvenile rheumatoid arthritis, *Arthritis Rheum* 24:1195-1198, 1981.
15a. Hafner R: Die juvenile Spondarthritis. Retrospektive Untersuchung an 71 Patienten. *Manatsschr Kinderheilkd* 135:41-46, 1987
16. Hamady RK, Baer JC, Foster CS: Immunosuppressive drugs in the management of progressive, corticosteroid-resistant uveitis associated with juvenile rheumatoid arthritis. *International Ophthalmology Clinics,* 32:241-252, 1992.
17. Hinzpeter EN, Naumann G, Bartelherman HK: Ocular histopathology in Still's disease, *Ophthalmic Res* 2:16-24, 1971.
18. Hoffman RW, Shaw S, Francis LC et al.: HLA-DP antigens in patients with pauciarticular juvenile rheumatoid arthritis, *Arthritis Rheum* 29:1057-1062, 1986.
19. Hunt DWC, Corson L, Barker HD et al.: Relationship between collagen-induced and adjuvant arthritis in the Lewis rat, *J Autoimmun* 6:691-700, 1993.
20. Hunt DWC, Petty RE, Millar F: Iris protein antibodies in serum of patients with juvenile rheumatoid arthritis and uveitis, *Int Arch Allergy Appl Immunol* 100:314-318, 1993.
20a. Iveson JMI, Nanda BS, Hancock JAH et al.: Reiter's disease in three boys. *Ann Rheum Dis* 34:364-368, 1975.
21. Jose DG, Good RA: Iridocyclitis and pauciarticular juvenile rheumatoid arthritis, *Pediatrics* 78:910-911, 1971.

22. Kanski JJ: Clinical and immunological study of anterior uveitis in juvenile chronic polyarthritis, *Trans Ophthalmol Soc UK* 96:123-130, 1976.

23. Kanski JJ: Anterior uveitis in juvenile rheumatoid arthritis, *Arch Ophthalmol* 95:1794-1797, 1977.

24. Kanski JJ: Uveitis in juvenile chronic arthritis: incidence, clinical features and prognosis, *Eye* 2:641-645, 1988.

25. Kanski JJ: Screening for uveitis in juvenile chronic arthritis, *Br J Ophthalmol* 73:225-228, 1989.

26. Kanski JJ: Juvenile arthritis and uveitis, *Surv Ophthalmol* 34:253-267, 1990.

27. Kanski JJ, Shun-Shin A: Systemic uveitis syndromes in childhood: an analysis of 340 cases, *Ophthalmology* 91:1247-1251, 1984.

28. Key SN, Kimura SJ: Iridocyclitis associated with juvenile rheumatoid arthritis, *Am J Ophthalmol* 80:425-429, 1975.

29. Kimura SJ, Hogan MJ, O'Connor GR et al.: Uveitis and joint disease: a review of 191 cases, *Trans Am Ophthalmol Soc* 64:291-305, 1966.

30. Kohoutek J, Havelka S: The results of the ophthalmic examination in rheumatoid arthritis in children: the eye in juvenile rheumatoid arthritis, *Rheumatologica* 5:47-50, 1967.

31. Kunnamo I, Kallio P, Pelkonen P: Incidence of arthritis in urban Finnish children, *Arthritis Rheum* 29:1232-1238, 1986.

32. Lindsley CB, Olson NY, Godfrey WA: Treatment of chronic childhood iridocyclitis with nonsteroidal anti-inflammatory drugs, *Am J Dis Child* 142:1289-1292, 1988.

33. Lindsley CB, Schaller JG: Arthritis associated with inflammatory bowel disease in children, *J Pediatr* 84:16-20, 1974.

34. Lipton NL, Crawford JS, Greenberg ML et al.: The risk of iridocyclitis in juvenile rheumatoid arthritis, *Can J Ophthalmol* 11:26-30, 1976.

35. Malagon C, Van Kerckhove C, Giannini EH et al.: The iridocyclitis of early onset pauciarticular juvenile rheumatoid arthritis: outcome in immunogenetically characterised patients, *J Rheumatol* 19:160-163, 1992.

36. Malleson P, Petty RE, Fung M, Candido EPM: Reactivity of antinuclear antibodies with histones and other antigens in juvenile rheumatoid arthritis, *Arthritis Rheum* 32:919-923, 1989.

37. Merriam JC, Chylack LT, Albert DM: Early onset pauciarticular juvenile rheumatoid arthritis. A histopathologic study, *Arch Ophthalmol* 101:1085-1092, 1983.

38. Moll JMH, Wright V: Psoriatic arthritis, *Semin Arthritis Rheum* 3:55-78, 1973.

39. Monestier M, Losman JA, Fasy TM et al.: Antihistone antibodies in antinuclear antibody-positive juvenile arthritis, *Arthritis Rheum* 33:1836-1841, 1990.

40. Neuteboom GH, Hertzberger-ten Cate R, de Jong J et al.: Antibodies to a 15 kD nuclear antigen in patients with juvenile chronic arthritis and uveitis, *Invest Ophthalmol Vis Sci* 33:1657-1660, 1992.

41. Nomenclature and classification of arthritis in children, European League Against Rheumatism (EULAR) Bulletin 4; Basel, 1977, National Zeitung AG.

42. Ohm J: Brandformige Hornhauttrubung bei einem neunjahrigen Madchen und ihre Behandlung mit Subconjunktivalen. Sodkaliumeinspitzungen, *Klin Montasbl Augenheilkd* 48:243-246, 1918.

43. Ostensen M, Fredriksen K, Kass E, Rekvig OP: Identification of antihistone antibodies in subsets of juvenile chronic arthritis, *Ann Rheum Dis* 48:114-117, 1989.

44. Palmer RG, Kanski JJ, Ansell BM: Chlorambucil in the treatment of intractable uveitis associated with juvenile chronic arthritis, *J Rheumatol* 12:967-970, 1985.

45. Pauls JP, Silverman E, Laxer RM, Fritzler MJ: Antibodies to histones H1 and H5 in sera of patients with juvenile rheumatoid arthritis, *Arthritis Rheum* 32:877-883, 1989.

46. Perkins ES: Patterns of uveitis in children, *Br J Ophthalmol* 50:169-185, 1966.

47. Petty RE: Current knowledge of the etiology and pathogenesis of chronic uveitis accompanying juvenile rheumatoid arthritis, *Rheum Dis Clin North Am* 13:19-36, 1987.

48. Petty RE: Ocular complications of rheumatic diseases of childhood, *Clin Orthop* 259:51-59, 1990.

49. Petty RE: Is there a useful model for the study of childhood uveitis and arthritis, *Clin Exp Rheumatol* 11(suppl 9):S7-S8, 1993.

50. Petty RE, Cassidy JT, Sullivan DB: Clinical correlates of antinuclear antibodies in juvenile rheumatoid arthritis, *J Pediatr* 83:386-389, 1973.

51. Petty RE, Hunt DWC: Immunity to ocular and collagen antigens in childhood arthritis and uveitis, *Int Arch Allergy Appl Immunol* 89:31-37, 1989.

52. Petty RE, Malleson P: Spondyloarthropathies of childhood, *Pediatr Clin North Am* 33:1079-1096, 1986.

53. Petty RE, Hunt DWC, Mathers DM et al.: Experimental arthritis and uveitis in rats associated with Mycobacterium butyricum, *J Rheumatol* 21:1491-1496, 1994.

54. Petty RE, Hunt DWC, Rollins DF et al.: Immunity to soluble retinal antigen in patients with uveitis accompanying juvenile rheumatoid arthritis, *Arthritis Rheum* 30:287-293, 1987.

55. Petty RE, Johnston W, McCormick AQ et al.: Uveitis and arthritis induced by adjuvant: clinical, immunologic and histologic characteristics, *J Rheumatol* 16:499-505, 1989.

56. Prieur AM, Griscelli C, Lampert F et al.: A chronic, infantile, neurological, cutaneous and articular (CINCA) syndrome: a specific entity analysed in 30 patients, *Scand J Rheumatol Suppl* 66:57-68, 1987.

57. Prieur AM, Petty RE: Definitions and classifications of chronic arthritis in children, *Baillieres Clin Pediatr* 1:695-702, 1993.

58. Rosenberg AM, Gilmer SM: Cell cycle specific patterns of autoantibody reactivity in juvenile rheumatoid arthritis (JRA), *J Rheumatol Suppl* 19:117, 1982.

58a. Rosenberg AM, Petty RE: Reiter's disease in children. *Am J Dis Child* 133:394-398.

59. Rosenberg AM, Oen KG: The relationship between ocular and articular disease activity in children with juvenile rheumatoid arthritis and associated uveitis, *Arthritis Rheum* 29:797-800, 1986.

60. Rosenberg AM, Petty RE: Reiter's disease in children, *Am J Dis Child* 133:394-398, 1979.

61. Rosenberg AM, Petty RE: A syndrome of seronegativity, enthesopathy and arthropathy in children, *Arthritis Rheum* 25:1041-1047, 1982.

62. Rosenberg AM, Yee EH, MacKenzie JW: Arthritis in childhood sarcoidosis, *J Rheumatol* 10:987-990, 1983.

63. Sabates R, Smith T, Apple O: Ocular histopathology in juvenile rheumatoid arthritis, *Ann Ophthalmol* 11:733-737, 1979.

64. Salmon JF, Wright JP, Murray AD: Ocular inflammation in Crohn's disease, *Ophthalmology* 98:480-484, 1991.

65. Sand B, Krogh E: Topical indomethacin, a prostaglandin inhibitor, in acute anterior uveitis: a controlled clinical trial of non-steroid versus steroid anti-inflammatory treatment, *Acta Ophthalmologica* 69:145-148, 1991.

65a. Schaller J: Ankylosing spondylitis of childhood onset, *Arthritis Rheum* 20(Suppl):398-401, 1977.

66. Schaller JG, Johnson DG, Holborow EJ et al.: The association of antinuclear antibodies with chronic iridocyclitis in juvenile rheumatoid arthritis (Still's disease), *Arthritis Rheum* 17:409-416, 1974.

67. Schaller JG, Kupfer C, Wedgwood RJ: Iridocyclitis in juvenile rheumatoid arthritis, *Pediatrics* 44:92-100, 1969.

68. Schmut O: The organization of tissues of the eye by different collagen types, *Albrecht von Graefes Arch Klin Exp Ophthalmol* 207:189-199, 1978.

69. Sherry DD, Mellins ED, Wedgwood RJ: Decreasing severity of chronic uveitis in children with pauciarticular arthritis, *Am J Dis Child* 145:1026-1028, 1991.

70. Smiley WK: The eye changes in Still's disease, *Proc R Soc Med* 51:597-600, 1957.

71. Smiley WK: The visual prognosis of Still's disease with eye involvement, *Proc R Soc Med* 53:196-199, 1960.

72. Smiley WK: Iridocyclitis in Still's disease, *Trans Ophthalmol Soc UK* 85:351-356, 1965.

73. Smiley WK: Ocular involvement in juvenile rheumatoid arthritis (Still's disease), *Proc R Soc Med (Lond)* 66:47-48, 1973.

74. Smiley WK: The eye in juvenile rheumatoid arthritis, *Trans Ophthalmol Soc UK* 94:817-829, 1974.

75. Smiley WK, May E, Bywaters EGL: Ocular presentations of Still's disease and their treatment. Iridocyclitis in Still's disease: its complications and treatment, *Ann Rheum Dis* 16:371-383, 1957.

76. Southwood TR, Petty RE, Malleson PN: Juvenile psoriatic arthritis—an analysis of 60 cases, *Arthritis Rheum* 32:1007-1013, 1989.

77. Spalter HF: The visual prognosis in juvenile rheumatoid arthritis, *Trans Am Ophthalmol Soc* 773:554-570, 1975.
78. Stewart AJ, Hill RH: Ocular manifestations in juvenile rheumatoid arthritis, *Can J Ophthalmol* 2:58-67, 1967.
79. Sullivan DB, Cassidy JT, Petty RE: Pathogenic implications of age of onset in juvenile rheumatoid arthritis, *Arthritis Rheum* 18:251-255, 1975.
80. Towner SR, Michet CJ Jr, O'Fallon WM, Nelson AM: The epidemiology of juvenile rheumatoid arthritis in Rochester, Minnesota, *Arthritis Rheum* 26:1208-1213, 1983.
81. Uusitalo RJ, Stjernschartz J, Mahlborg K et al.: Serum antibody levels to S-antigen in children with chronic uveitis, *Br J Ophthalmol* 69:212-216, 1985.

82. Vesterdal E, Sury B: Iridocyclitis and band-shaped corneal opacity in juvenile rheumatoid arthritis, *Acta Ophthalmol* 28:321-337, 1950.
83. Waksman B, Bullington S: Studies of arthritis and other lesions induced in rats by injection of mycobacterial adjuvant II, *Arch Ophthalmol* 64:751-760, 1960.
84. Wells A, Pararajesgaram G, Baldwin M et al.: Uveitis and arthritis induced by systemic injection of streptococcal cell walls, *Invest Ophthalmol Vis Sci* 27:921-925, 1986.
85. Wirostko E, Johnson L, Wirostko W: Juvenile rheumatoid arthritis inflammatory eye disease: parasitization of ocular leukocytes by Mollicute-like organisms, *J Rheumatol* 16:1446-1453, 1989.
86. Wolf MD, Lichter PR, Ragsdale CG: Prognostic factors in the uveitis of juvenile rheumatoid arthritis, *Ophthalmology* 94:1242-1248, 1987.

41 Fuchs Uveitis Syndrome

THOMAS J. LIESEGANG

When Fuchs uveitis syndrome appears in its classic (limited) form, the diagnosis is straightforward. The large spectrum of manifestations of this syndrome, however, causes the diagnosis to be frequently overlooked. Because it is a panophthalmic disease and because it may lack obvious heterochromia, the term Fuchs uveitis syndrome is preferred over Fuchs heterochromic uveitis or Fuchs heterochromic cyclitis. Recognition is essential both to eliminate unnecessary testing and to allow better prognostication for some patients in a field (uveitis) in which a precise understanding of disease is frequently lacking.

HISTORICAL BACKGROUND

In 1906 Ernst Fuchs, from the University of Vienna, produced a comprehensive summary of 38 patients with features of the condition that now bears his name.[32] Although Lawrence[60] was the first to describe some components of this specific form of indolent uveitis in 1843, and Weill[103] had described other components in 1904, Fuchs described both the clinical and pathologic features of the disease with a remarkably descriptive accuracy in an era prior to the availability of the slit lamp biomicroscope. With the recognition over the past several years that multiple portions of the eye can be involved with the inflammatory process, other features have been added to those described by Fuchs.

EPIDEMIOLOGY

The frequency with which Fuchs uveitis syndrome is identified depends on the observational skills and experience of the examiner. In 1955 Kimura[51] was one of the first to recognize the expanded spectrum of Fuchs uveitis syndrome in 23 patients. At the same time, Franceschetti[31] was expanding his recognition of its spectrum in 62 patients. In 1973 Loewenfeld and Thompson[62,63] reviewed Fuchs uveitis syndrome. Additional series in the literature have added to the recognition of a more complete spectrum of the disease.*

---

*References 21, 43, 47, 49, 61, 96.

In its strict "classic" form, as originally described by Fuchs (and as written in the major teaching texts), the disease is relatively rare (see first box). With recognition of the "expanded" spectrum of the disease, however, it is more common (see second box). In several reported series the prevalence of Fuchs uveitis syndrome has varied from 1.2% to 4.5% of patients with uveitis.[13,18,25,104] The true prevalence is probably higher because the ophthalmologist who does not see a large number of patients with uveitis fails to appreciate the atypical variants of this syndrome. It is especially difficult to recognize the disease in an individual with brown eyes because the heterochromia is less marked or is absent.

The disease has no racial or sexual predilection and can involve either eye in patients of all ages.[61] About 7.8% to 10% of patients have bilateral disease, which requires an astute clinician for recognition of the syndrome.[47] If the disease is unilateral at presentation, it usually remains a unilateral disease.

Early studies suggested a hereditary disposition.[6,95] Fuchs uveitis syndrome has been occasionally diagnosed in several members of a family, including monozygotic twins.[64] Discordance has also been reported for monozygotic twins.[50] The vast majority of large series show only a small number of cases that suggest a genetic basis for the syndrome, and it certainly is not transmitted as a simple Mendelian trait.[63]

Although several types of uveitis have been strongly linked to HLA specificities,[29] data on HLA typing in Fuchs uveitis syndrome has been either contradictory, or supportive of only a very weak association. An association with HLA-B18 has been reported in one series,[78] but refuted in other series.[24,85] A decreased frequency of both HLA-Cw3[24] and HLA-DRw53[85] has been described, although the significance is difficult to discern.[49]

Neither familial concurrence nor HLA association have a direct role in the disease, although they may play a role in the predisposition to the disease.

CLINICAL FEATURES

Fuchs uveitis syndrome is readily recognized when it appears in its "classic" clinical form. Fuchs,[32] as well as Ki-

---

CLASSIC FUCHS UVEITIS SYNDROME

Quiet external eye
Heterochromia with involved eye lighter in color
Unilateral disease (approximately 90%)
Anterior iris atrophy, especially peri-pupillary
Hyaline keratic precipitates with intervening filaments
Minimal anterior chamber cell and flare
Absence of posterior synechiae
Occasional Koeppé or Busacca nodules
Vitreous humor cells
Cataract beginning with posterior subcapsular changes
Occasional secondary glaucoma
Amsler sign (hyphema or filiform hemorrhage after sudden reduction in intraocular pressure during surgery)
Occasional chorioretinal scars
Long insidious course
Prognosis good

---

mura[52] and Franceschetti,[31] have summarized the essential features of this condition. The patient is ordinarily a young adult with heterochromia of the irides (usually lighter iris in the involved eye) and mild visual symptoms. The condition is customarily unilateral, with absence of conjunctival injection or external signs of inflammation. Specific atrophic changes within the iris lead to heterochromia (depending on the combined changes of the anterior and posterior layers of the iris). There are minimal and variable cell and flare, along with widely scattered, small, round, nonconfluent keratic precipitates with stellate precipitates in between. These keratic precipitates represent one of the most characteristic features of Fuchs uveitis syndrome. They typically have a granular appearance and are translucent or opalescent, in contrast to the more dense, white keratic precipitates seen in other forms of anterior uveitis. They are commonly found above the visual axis, in contrast to many other forms of uveitis in which keratic precipitates occur primarily in the inferior quandrant of the cornea. Vitreous humor cells and occasional vitreous veils are observed. Posterior synechiae are only present following anterior segment surgery. A complicated cataract invariably develops and glaucoma is variably present.

There are atypical variants of this "classic" presentation and, consequently, variation in the prognosis of the condition. The "expanded" spectrum of the disease is more commonly encountered than the "classic" description. This "expanded" spectrum retains the essentials of the "classic" definition but adds subtle features that help to establish the diagnosis in more patients, thereby offering them a better prognostic forecast. The descriptive features of this "classic" and "expanded" spectrum follows.

Symptoms

Patients with Fuchs uveitis syndrome usually are not treated as emergencies. They frequently are discovered during the course of a routine examination. These patients may complain of symptoms of floaters (from vitreous debris) or symptoms of cataracts. The heterochromia may not be apparent to the patient, even after being recognized by the ophthalmologist. The heterochromia is a rare prompter for the eye examination. Some patients may have external ocular perilimbal injection and, others may have signs or symptoms of recurrent hyphema or symptoms consistent with elevated intraocular pressure. Patients do not usually complain of photophobia.

The referral patient with the condition may have chronic and variable symptoms. Ophthalmologists frequently miss or dismiss this syndrome when it does not have the heterochromia they expect to see. Many victims have undergone a uveitis workup and several have undergone cataract surgery without the benefit of the correct diagnosis.

Heterochromia and the Iris Surface

The presence of heterochromia has been an overemphasized feature of Fuchs uveitis syndrome. The heterochromia can show wide variation and is an inconsistent feature of the disease. Some patients remain unaware of it; in others, the signs are very subtle; and some victims describe having the heterochromia or iris changes since youth.[47,49,61] Daylight examination is usually best for detecting subtle heterochromia. Heterochromia is usually most evident in patients with blue eyes (Fig. 41-1). Typically, the iris of the affected eye has a paler hue and is more uniform in color, having lost the scattered brown highlights that are often present on the anterior iris surface. In brown irides (in either whites,[51] blacks,[96] or Asians[43]) the heterochromia can be subtle or absent be-

---

EXPANDED SPECTRUM OF FUCHS UVEITIS SYNDROME

A panophthalmic disease
Any age group affected
Occasionally presents with red external eye
Absent or reversed heterochromia
May have heterochromia without evident iris atrophy
May have iris atrophy without evident heterochromia
Patchy atrophy of posterior pigmented layer of iris
Pupil irregular from sphincter atrophy
Frequent small peripheral anterior synechiae
Increased visibility of iris radial vessels
Fine iris rubeosis or gross rubeosis
Spontaneous or induced hyphema
Cataract develops in all patients
Prognosis variable with cataract surgery
Secondary glaucoma in up to 60%
Poor prognosis with glaucoma
Dense vitreous veils or vitreous hemorrhage
Increased incidence of central and peripheral corneal edema

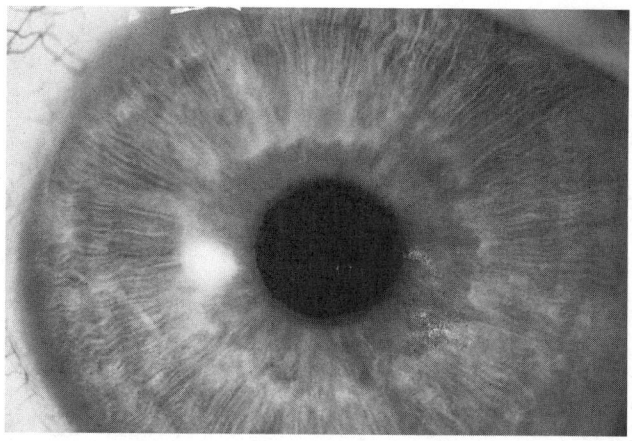 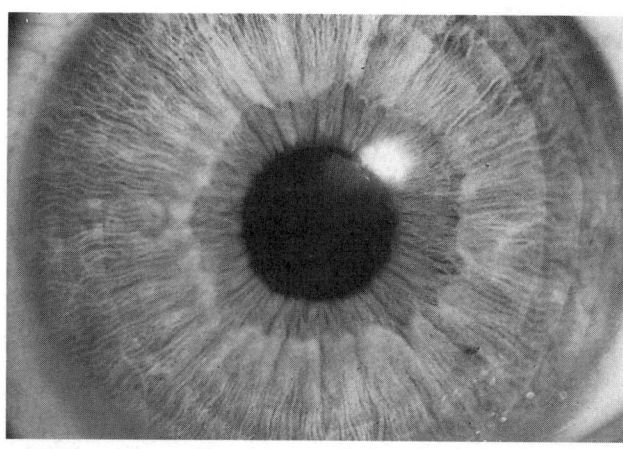

A   B

Fig. 41-1. Both eyes of a blue-eyed patient with Fuchs uveitis syndrome in the left eye. Obviously lighter left eye, **A,** has loss of anterior iris color, lack of crisp iris detail, and absence of some pupillary ruff. The patient also has fine iris rubeosis and Russell bodies on the iris surface (not evident in photo). The right eye, **B,** is normal. (Figures also in color insert.)

cause both layers of the iris (anterior and posterior) are of the same color and texture (Figs. 41-2 and 41-3).[74] In some individuals there is more atrophy of the anterior iris layer, such that the iris can appear darker in the affected eye (reversed heterochromia) from the pigmentation of the posterior iris layer. If both eyes are involved, there can be an absence of heterochromia. In some patients heterochromia never develops, although the anterior iris stroma maintains a washed-out appearance in comparison with the normal eye.[61] In each of these situations, there are other features present that establish the diagnosis.[20,28]

A variable degree of iris atrophy involves both the anterior iris stroma and the posterior pigmented layer. The anterior iris atrophy is evident as a generalized blunting, flattening, blurring, or washed-out appearance of the surface markings of the iris crypts or rugae, especially in compari-

son with the normal fellow eye at the biomicroscope or in slit lamp photographs.[47] A smooth pale iris surface with a dull stroma or loss of crisp iris detail is most evident in the pupillary zone. Anterior stromal thinning can affect the iris sphincter, causing an irregular and enlarged pupil (Figs. 41-4 and 41-5). The pupillary ruff frequently has gaps, or it may be absent. The iris demonstrates overall rarefaction with transparency and a moth-eaten appearance. Transillumination defects in the posterior pigmented layer may be evident, sometimes as patchy holes.

Iris Lesions and Anterior Chamber Reaction

Small gelatinous nodules on the iris surface (Busacca nodules) or at the pupillary margin (Koeppé nodules) are seen in a variable number of patients with Fuchs uveitis syndrome (Fig. 41-6). Although some series have rarely re-

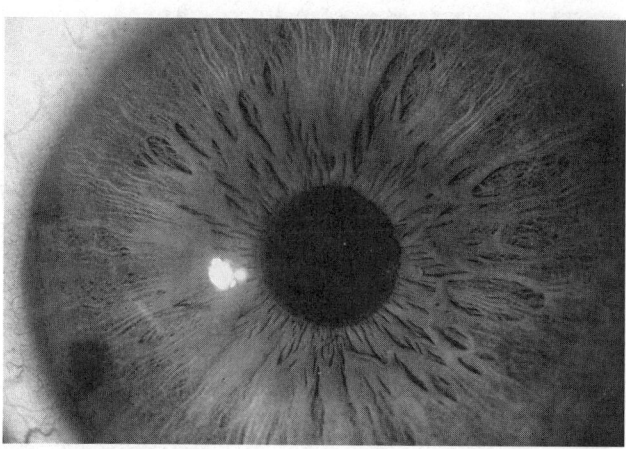 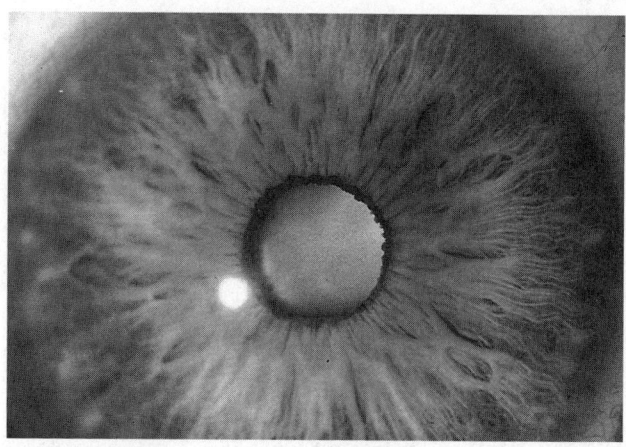

A   B

Fig. 41-2. **A, B,** Both eyes of a brown-eyed patient with Fuchs uveitis syndrome in the left eye. The patient has a lighter left iris, **B,** with disturbance of the pupillary ruff, smudgy loss of iris detail, and a maturing cataract. The right eye, **A,** is normal. (Figures also in color insert.)

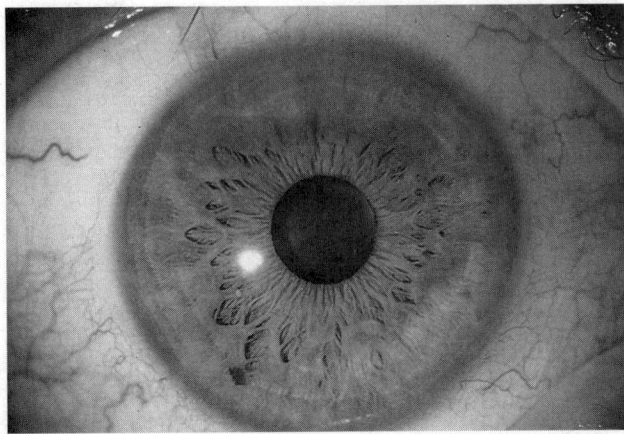

A

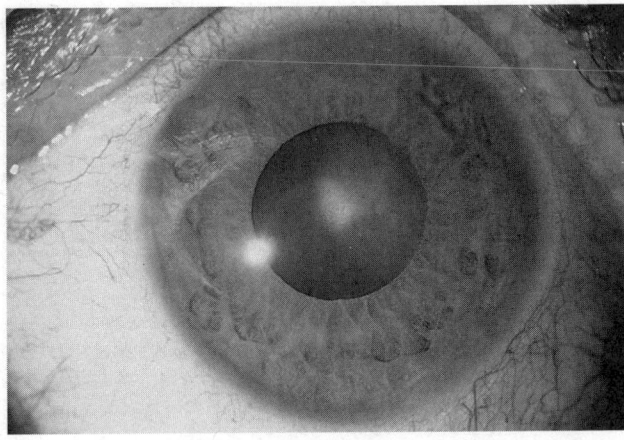

B

Fig. 41-3. **A, B,** Both eyes of a brown-eyed patient with Fuchs uveitis syndrome in the left eye. The patient has a subtle lighter left iris, **B,** with peripupillary iris atrophy, smudgy iris surface, and a posterior subcapsular cataract. The right eye, **A,** is normal. (Figures also in color insert.)

ported them,[61,74] in other large series they have been described in 20% to 30% of patients.[31,43,47,96] These nodules are more likely to be present in the early stages of the disease and may be quite small and transparent, making them easy to overlook. Other small, glistening, crystalline deposits on the surface of the iris (termed Russell bodies) probably represent plasma cells choked with immunoglobulin. They are infrequently observed.[10,58]

Posterior synechiae do not occur in Fuchs uveitis syndrome prior to a surgical intervention; their absence remains a constant and differentiating feature of this specific syndrome. Posterior synechiae rarely occur after anterior segment surgery.[47,61] The Koeppé nodules may be associated with a transient posterior synechiae, but they are evanescent and leave just a small amount of residual pigment on the anterior lens surface (Fig. 41-7).

Cells in the anterior chamber are usually present in patients with Fuchs uveitis syndrome, although they are rarely more than moderate (2+) in number and are usually asymptomatic. Prominent flare is even less common; it is rarely more than moderate (2+) in amount. The magnitude of the cell and flare can vary in individuals over time. The keratic precipitates of Fuchs uveitis syndrome are characteristic and probably pathognomonic. There are typically small, round, hyaline keratic precipitates that are nonpigmented, translucent, sharply circumscribed, and never confluent or greasy (Fig. 41-8). Fine stellate cotton-wisp filaments are almost always present between the hyaline precipitates. Although the keratic precipitates are most common in the lower triangular portion of the cornea (as in other types of uveitis), the keratic precipitates in Fuchs uveitis syndrome are frequently scattered over the entire posterior surface of the cornea, out

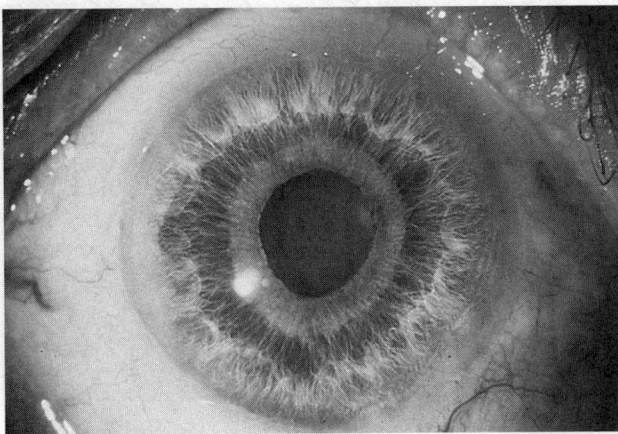

Fig. 41-4. Extensive anterior stromal iris atrophy accentuated in the peripupillary area with absence of the pupillary ruff and irregular pupil from sphincter atrophy.

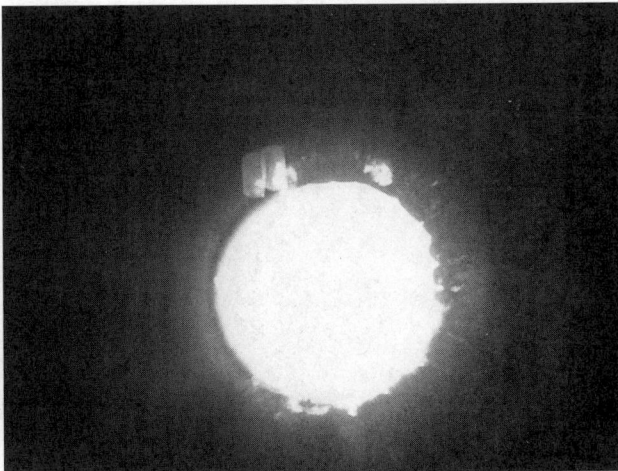

Fig. 41-5. Same patient as Fig. 41-4 with retroillumination demonstrating the gaps in the pupillary ruff, the sphincter muscle atrophy, and the patchy atrophy of the posterior pigmented layer of the iris.

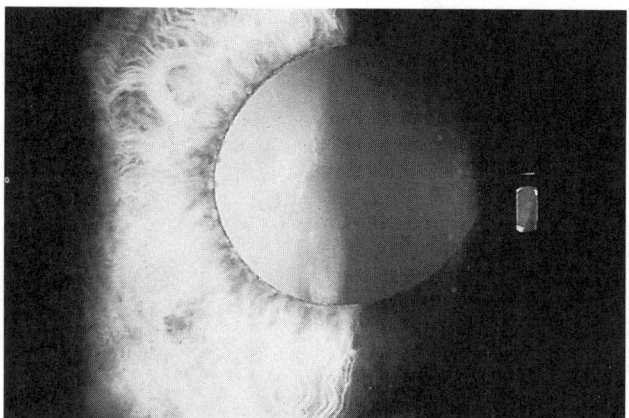

Fig. 41-6. Koeppé nodules in Fuchs uveitis syndrome. Multiple small brown Koeppé nodules at the pupillary margin. The patient has anterior iris stromal atrophy and a maturing cataract.

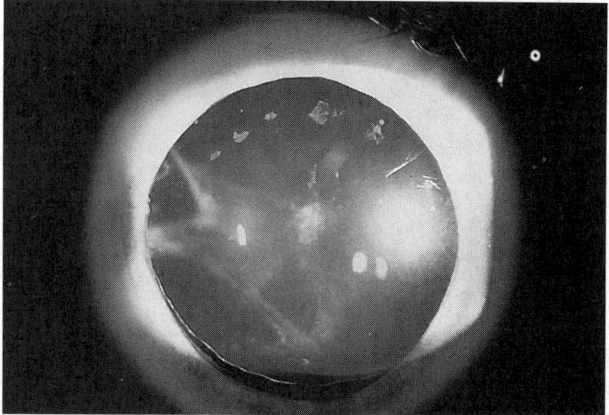

Fig. 41-7. Residual pigment debris on the anterior lens surface from previous broken anterior synechiae of Koeppé nodules. The patient has a posterior subcapsular cataract and dense veils in the anterior vitreous.

of proportion to the anterior chamber reaction. The presence of keratitic precipitates on the upper portion of the cornea may be a pathognomonic sign of Fuchs uveitis syndrome. The presence and location of the keratitic precipitates can vary dramatically with each patient visit. The cell, flare, and keratic precipitates may entirely disappear over time.[49]

Iris Vessels

With the progressive anterior iris atrophy of Fuchs uveitis syndrome, the blood vessels within the iris stroma become more visible and also straighter and narrower.[47,49,61] In addition to this increased prominence of normal radial vessels, there is the occasional development of a fine rubeosis meandering over the iris surface, the angle, and possibly the ciliary body* (Fig. 41-9). In some eyes, a gross rubeosis develops.

Fluorescein angiography of the iris in several patients with Fuchs uveitis syndrome has demonstrated an ischemic vasculopathy and infarction, along with increased permeability of the vessels in the anterior segment.† The vessels of the iris surface, limbus, or ciliary body can all be involved. New vessel fronds can be identified more dramatically with angiography. Sector iris atrophy, however, is not a feature of Fuchs uveitis syndrome.[49,84] The fragile blood vessels in the iridocorneal angle are susceptible to either spontaneous bleeding or bleeding in association with a sudden reduction of pressure in the anterior chamber. Blood-containing cysts in the ciliary body can occasionally give rise to vitreous hemorrhage.[74]

More exquisite studies with fluorophotometry have confirmed a frequent breakdown of the blood aqueous barrier in Fuchs uveitis syndrome.[45,62,63] The site of the fluorescein

*References 8, 43, 47, 61, 75, 96.
†References 8, 9, 62, 63, 77, 84, 100.

leakage (the iris or ciliary body) has not been definitively established.

Anterior Chamber Angle

An abnormal angle with peripheral anterior synechiae or rubeotic vessels is seen in about 20% to 30% of patients with Fuchs uveitis syndrome.[40,61] The rubeotic vessels are usually delicate, but occasionally, large vessels have been described in the angle. The iris atrophy contributes to an increased visualization of even normal vessels in the angle. The angle can have a dirty dullness or filmy appearance, but there is no increased pigmentation.[61]

The filiform hemorrhage observed in the chamber angle, in the peripheral iris after paracentesis, or in association with cataract surgery, glaucoma surgery, or posterior capsulot-

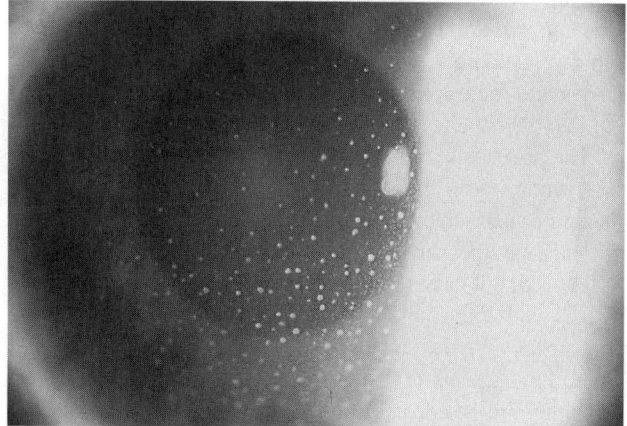

Fig. 41-8. The typical hyaline keratic precipitates of Fuchs uveitis syndrome. They have a tendency to involve the whole posterior surface of the cornea including the superior cornea. There are fine cotton-wisp filaments between the hyaline keratic precipitates.

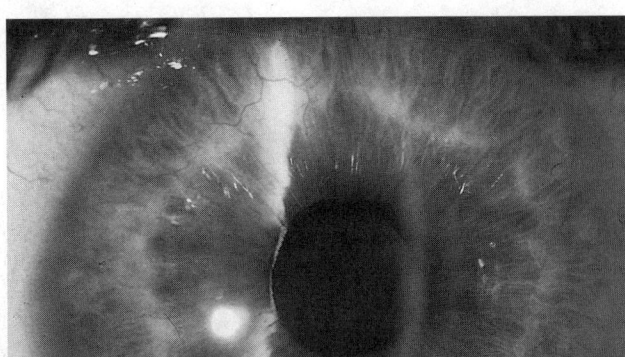

Fig. 41-9. Fuchs uveitis syndrome with rubeosis. Lighter iris with peripupillary iris atrophy and fine rubeotic vessels meandering across the iris surface.

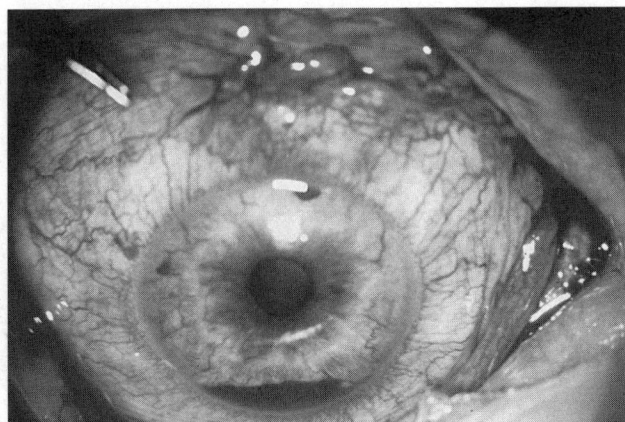

Fig. 41-10. Amsler sign in Fuchs uveitis syndrome. A hyphema and increased iris vascular congestion at the completion of a trabeculectomy.

omy* is characteristic (but not diagnostic) of Fuchs uveitis syndrome[74] (Amsler sign—Fig. 41-10). A hyphema may also occur in association with trivial trauma, gonioscopy, applanation tonometry, mydriasis; or it may occur spontaneously.[30,47,48] The occurrence of hyphema does not necessarily correlate with the clinical signs of iris neovascularization or with the presence of abnormal vessels in the iridocorneal angle.[47,61]

The anterior synechiae are usually small, nonconfluent, and irregular.[31,61] They are perhaps more frequent after intraocular surgery, although they are not concentrated at the incision site. They do not progress to broad-based synechiae, even with the presence of angle neovascularization.

Cataract

Cataracts are an invariable feature after prolonged follow-up of Fuchs uveitis syndrome. They originate as posterior subcapsular cataracts and have a tendency to mature rapidly. Cataracts may progress to shrunken hypermature lenses and the iris heterochromia may become more prominent as the cataract matures.[61]

The prognosis for cataract surgery fluctuates in the literature according to the variability and severity of the overall disease process in the individual eye. It is ironic that patients with classic Fuchs uveitis syndrome usually are more readily diagnosed, but have a milder form of the disease and probably do well with cataract surgery. Patients with more severe iris atrophy, vitreous debris, and severe glaucoma more often have a subtle heterochromia, go unrecognized as Fuchs uveitis syndrome, but have a worse prognosis with cataract surgery.

Glaucoma

Glaucoma has been described in up to 59% of patients after prolonged follow-up and is the most common cause of permanent vision loss in patients with Fuchs uveitis syndrome.[61] It is more prevalent in patients with progressive iris atrophy. The cause of the glaucoma remains obscure, although trabeculitis may be a mechanism early in the course.[75] A number of pathophysiologic mechanisms may cause the glaucoma including peripheral anterior synechiae, rubeotic vessels, trabecular sclerosis, lens-induced glaucoma, an abnormal feltlike membrane in the angle, trabecular spaces filled with plasma cells, or corticosteroid induction.* The peripheral anterior synechiae and the fine rubeotic angle vessels usually remain isolated and do not appear to be significant factors in most patients with glaucoma.

The glaucoma may be initially intermittent and may respond to corticosteroids (a trabeculitis), but gradually it becomes recalcitrant to both corticosteroids and glaucoma medications.[52,61]

Cornea

Although the cornea may appear clinically normal and the endothelial cell density has been reported as normal in most patients with Fuchs uveitis syndrome,[1,93] a number of corneal abnormalities (for example, guttata[61]) have been described. Some patients have large areas of abnormal endothelium demonstrated on specular microscopy as areas of darkness spanning several endothelial cells, intracellular blebs, and altered cellular morphology.[1,14] Some studies have documented increased endothelial cell loss after cataract surgery; there is the suggestion of decreased endothelial

---

*References 5, 34, 40, 44, 46, 67, 82.

*References 7, 8, 36, 37, 41, 48, 59, 62, 74, 75.

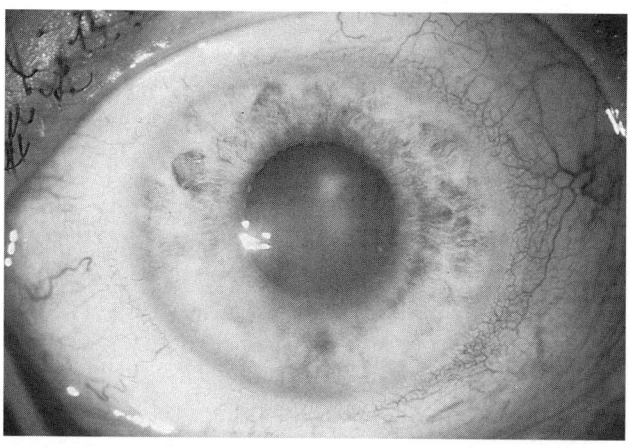
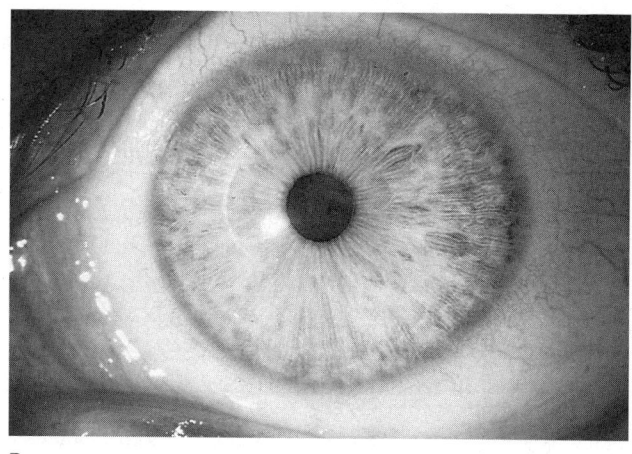

A

B

Fig. 41-11.   A, B, Both eyes of a patient with Fuchs uveitis syndrome in the right eye. There is iris atrophy, fine rubeosis, gaps in the pupillary ruff, a posterior subcapsular cataract, central corneal edema, a quiet external eye, and glaucoma in the right eye, **A.** The left eye, **B,** is normal.

tolerance to intraocular surgery in patients with Fuchs uveitis syndrome.[1] Anterior chamber fluorophotometry has confirmed an increased endothelial permeability to fluorescein.[45]

Research has verified clinically evident corneal edema after cataract surgery.[51,61] The corneal edema can be central or peripheral with the latter similar to that described by Brown and McLean[15] (Figs. 41-11 and 41-12). Peripheral corneal edema may occur prior to cataract surgery.

A cellular and humoral immune response to a major corneal stromal and/or epithelial antigen (54 Kd) has been found with a high frequency in patients with Fuchs uveitis syndrome.[56,99] This immune response may account for the inflammatory cells in the anterior chamber, the keratic precipitates, and the endothelial changes observed by specular microscopy.

Vitreous Humor and Fundus

Vitreous humor cells are present in almost all patients with Fuchs uveitis syndrome. The cells may remain dustlike or progress to heavy, stringy veils as they cling to a degenerative vitreous framework (Fig. 41-13). They can interfere

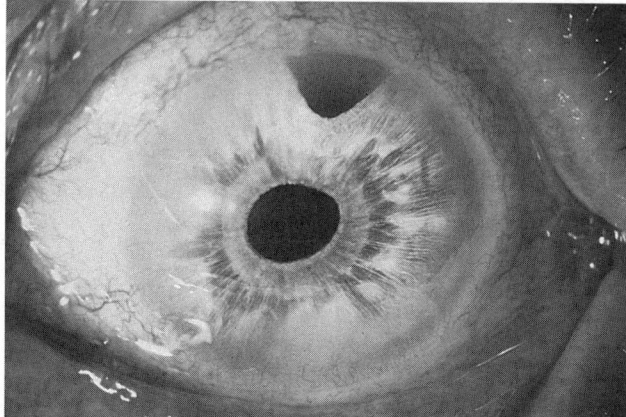

Fig. 41-12.   Peripheral corneal edema (Brown McLean syndrome) from 2 o'clock to 8 o'clock in a patient following intracapsular cataract surgery for a mature cataract in Fuchs uveitis syndrome.

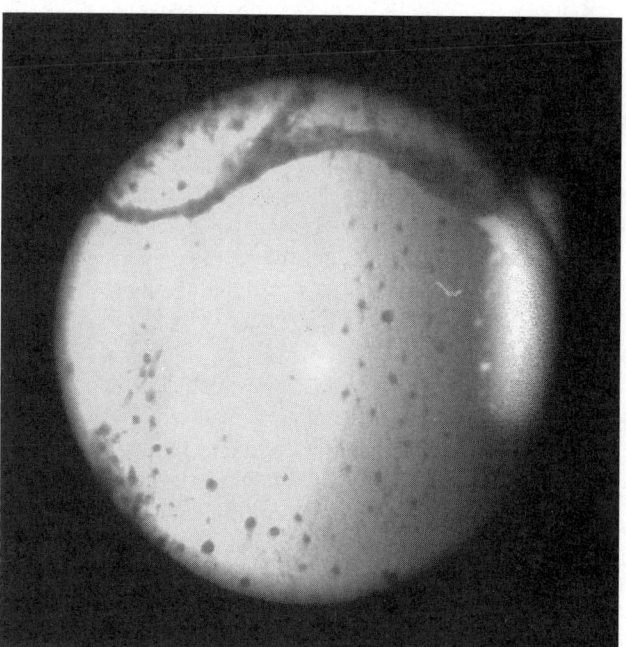

Fig. 41-13.   Retroillumination photograph demonstrated the small hyaline keratic precipitates on the back surface of the cornea and dense anterior vitreous veils in a patient with Fuchs uveitis syndrome.

with vision and/or become an annoyance. The vitreous debris can vary in density over time. With cataract surgery (especially intracapsular cataract surgery), dense vitreous veils can form, possibly related to bleeding from a ciliary body blood cyst. Vitrectomy is occasionally necessary to eliminate the heavy vitreous veils.[47,61,102]

Both Fuchs[32] and Kimura[52] recognized peripheral choroidal inflammatory scars in a few patients with Fuchs uveitis syndrome. Franceschetti[31] and Liesegang[61] also described peripheral chorioretinal scars in a small percentage of patients. These chorioretinal scars are usually small, focal, atrophic lesions with hyperpigmented borders in the peripheral choroid, and are consistent with lesions of ocular toxoplasmosis. Most patients with Fuchs develop significant cataracts, so this fundus finding is often underreported. Beginning in 1982, observers have reported the frequency of chorioretinal lesions to be much higher.[23] A discussion of the significance of these findings will follow.

PATHOLOGY

There are no distinct histopathologic or electron microscopy findings in Fuchs uveitis syndrome that permit its differentiation from other types of uveitis. Fuchs described the histopathologic examination of iris tissue in six patients, reporting (1) abnormal stromal pigmentation, (2) hyalinization and endothelial cell proliferation of blood vessel walls, and (3) the presence of plasma cells and Russell bodies.[32] Other researchers have confirmed the following: (1) atrophy of the iris stroma, (2) hyalinization of blood vessels, (3) sphincter muscle sclerosis and atrophy, (4) patchy loss and vacuolization of the iris pigment epithelium, (5) an increase in mononuclear chronic inflammatory cells within both the iris and the smaller melanosomes in the iris.[35,62,65,80]

Electron microscopy of the iris in patients with Fuchs uveitis syndrome has demonstrated endoplasmic reticulum damage with cytolysis.[65,66,105] Iris melanocytes are decreased in number with abnormal intracellular melanin granules.[65,66] Large numbers of plasma cells surround the melanocytes.

PATHOGENESIS

In addition to the possibility of a weak genetic predisposition, other theories concerning the cause of Fuchs uveitis syndrome can be listed under neurogenic, infectious, vascular, and inflammatory-immunologic categories.[49,62,63] At present there is still inadequate information to formulate a pathophysiologic mechanism that can encompass the multiple features of this condition.

Neurogenic Theory

A neurogenic cause of Fuchs uveitis syndrome was championed for a number of years. A congenital paralysis of the sympathetic system can cause heterochromia; congenital or acquired Horner syndrome was initially considered the cause of Fuchs uveitis syndrome.[11,12,81] Loewenfeld and Thompson[62,63] extensively reviewed the evidence without finding convincing proof of a sympathetic cause. "Status dysraphicus", the unilateral syndrome of dysmorphism and asymmetry, has been suggested as a cause by some,[38,39] although it is largely unsupported.[63] Isolated cases of Fuchs uveitis syndrome have been found in association with Romberg syndrome of hemifacial atrophy[33,47] and Moebius syndrome.[42] Although these diseases can all produce iris heterochromia, they are not associated with intraocular inflammation. Other large series have failed to find evidence to support a role for the sympathetic nervous system for the condition.[47,49,61]

Infectious Theory

There is an association between Fuchs uveitis syndrome and chorioretinal scars. In their descriptions of the disease, both Fuchs[32] and Kimura[52] noted the presence of peripheral choroidal inflammatory scars in a small number of patients. Peripheral choroidal lesions were noticeably absent in the large review of the disease by Loewenfeld and Thompson[62,63] and Liesegang.[61] In Brazil in 1982, De Abreu and associates[23] reported chorioretinal scars consistent with ocular toxoplasmosis in 56.5% of 23 Fuchs uveitis syndrome patients and confirmed serologic evidence of *Toxoplasma gondii* infection. A number of other investigators from Brazil,[91] France,[86,98] and the United States[3,88,96] have also reported a relationship between the presence of chorioretinal scars and the existence of antibodies against *T. gondii* in the blood or aqueous humor of patients with Fuchs uveitis syndrome. A number of these chorioretinal scars have been nondescript and not characteristic of toxoplasmic retinochoroiditis lesions.

Although the association between chorioretinal scars and Fuchs uveitis syndrome is variable and strong, the role of toxoplasmosis remains controversial. In the United States over 50% of adults are seropositive for *T. gondii* infection,[53] and the prevalence in Brazil is much higher.[89] La Hey and associates[58] have analyzed the association with ocular toxoplasmosis with a number of laboratory tests that analyze both the serum and the aqueous humor specimens. They have concluded that there is no significant link between Fuchs uveitis syndrome and *T. gondii* infection, although there appears to be an association between chorioretinal scars and Fuchs uveitis syndrome.

Saraux and associates[86] suggested that *T. gondii* infection of the retina permits sensitization to a retinal antigen that may elicit Fuchs uveitis syndrome. Others have suggested that the chorioretinal scar itself may incite a retinal antigen that leads to Fuchs uveitis syndrome.[3] Experimental models of uveitis associated with S-antigen, however, do not cause a clinical picture that resembles Fuchs uveitis syndrome.[101] It remains possible that Fuchs uveitis syndrome is a secondary phenomenon.

Vascular Theory

A vascular pathogenesis involving localized iris vessels may be at the crux of the disease. Iris fluorescein angiography demonstrates distinct peripupillary fluorescein leakage, delayed iris filling, and sectors of ischemia frequently associated with neovascularization.[8,83] A characteristic filiform hemorrhage with anterior chamber paracentesis is a hallmark of the disease.[2] Light microscopy has disclosed hyalinization and endothelial proliferation of iris vessel walls with narrowing of the vessel lumen.[35] Immune complexes have been detected in the serum and aqueous humor of some patients,[27] and these immune complexes may be causative in the localized iris vascular occlusions. La Hey and associates[57] have observed deposits of immunoglobulin and complement in the iris vessel wall of patients, although no specific immune deposits were discovered within the iris stroma of these patients. This finding suggests that the immune reactants originate from the circulation rather than from local iris processes, and that the complexes bind to activated iris vascular endothelial cells perhaps because of the action of cytokine mediators.[57]

Inflammatory Theory

The presence of inflammatory cells has been a fertile investigatory stimulus for an immune cause. Lymphocytes, plasma cells, mast cells, and eosinophils are a constant feature of the inflammatory cell infiltrate in Fuchs uveitis syndrome. Russell bodies and crystalloid immunoglobulin from a hypersecretion of plasma cells are occasionally present.[10,94]

In the peripheral blood, the B- and T-lymphocyte number and function have been reported as normal by some,[70] although others have recounted activation of B- and T-lymphocytes.[4] A depression of CD8 + T-lymphocyte activity has been described,[69] perhaps correlating with circulating immune complexes.[27] Receptors for interleukin-2, a T-lymphocyte proliferation stimulator, have been reported to be high in the peripheral blood.[4] Anterior chamber levels of interleukin-6 rose in the absence of an increase in peripheral levels.[71] Increased B-lymphocyte activity in the anterior chamber has been supported by the findings of some investigators,[35,65] although not by others.[72] Increased intraocular production of IgG has been reported in patients[72] as a possible result of the increased anterior chamber levels of interleukin-6.

High levels of serum antibodies against corneal epithelial protein (54 Kd) have been described[54,55,56,99] and may be a causative factor in the corneal features of the disease. Antibodies to iris components have not yet been identified. Although Fuchs uveitis syndrome has several features suggesting an immune basis, it is not clear whether these immune reactions are a cause or an epiphenomena. The generator of the stimulatory immune response remains unknown, and the assembly of present immunologic findings does not allow a tidy understanding.

THERAPY

The uveitis is frequently asymptomatic or mild, and can fluctuate over time. The cells, flare, and keratic precipitates do not cause intraocular destruction. In most instances, therapy is not indicated. On occasion, Fuchs uveitis syndrome can be associated with discomfort, ciliary injection, a sudden increase in floaters, or increasing keratic precipitates or cells. These symptoms may warrant topical corticosteroid therapy for a short period. In general, corticosteroid therapy should be minimal, because it is not possible to render the condition quiescent.

Vitreous debris and veils can cause a significant visual disturbance. This problem is perhaps most dramatic after intracapsular cataract surgery in which blood may be mixed with the abnormal vitreous.[102] On rare occasions, vitrectomy may be necessary to clear the vitreous humor.[47]

The frequency of glaucoma varies in different series from 6.3% to 59.0%.[49] Glaucoma developed in 59% of 54 patients in a series followed over a prolonged time period, and 66% required a glaucoma surgical procedure.[61] Most other authors have described fewer problems with glaucoma.*

The glaucoma is more difficult to control than primary open angle glaucoma. In the early stages, the elevated intraocular pressure may be intermittent and associated with increased intraocular inflammation.[76] At this stage, the elevated pressure may respond to topical corticosteroids. Topical and systemic glaucoma medications are later required, with a variable long-term effect. Argon laser trabeculoplasty is usually not successful and may be contraindicated in view of the inflammatory nature of the condition and the presence of peripheral anterior synechiae, fine vessels in the angle, or a feltlike membrane in the angle. Glaucoma filtration surgery is frequently necessary but has all the attendant risks associated with glaucoma surgery in a uveitis patient, including bleb failure.[48,61] The role of adjunctive wound modulators (5-fluorouracil, mitomycin C) with filtration surgery has not been extensively evaluated. Use of light cryotherapy prior to filtration surgery may reduce complications related to neovascularization.[74] Patients who do not respond to filtration surgery may need shunt implantation. Rare patients have required enucleation because of absolute or rubeotic glaucoma.[48,59,61,73]

Several studies address the treatment of cataracts in patients with Fuchs uveitis syndrome. In the era of intracapsular cataract extraction, variable results were reported.[61,73,102,106] Ward and Hart[102] described nine patients who had extensive complications with intracapsular cataract

---

*References 16, 22, 26, 38, 48, 62, 63, 76, 91, 96, 98.

extraction including capsule rupture, vitreous hemorrhage, vitreous loss, hyphema, and progressive glaucoma. Liesegang[61] reported 17 patients who had significant problems with intracapsular surgery including hyphema, glaucoma, pupillary membranes, and central and peripheral bullous keratopathy. Others have reported only a slight increase in complications with intracapsular cataract extraction.[73,106] Smith and O'Connor[92] retrospectively reviewed the records of 29 patients and declared both intracapsular and extracapsular cataract surgery to be without a significantly increased risk. The use of an intraocular implant in association with intracapsular cataract extraction further complicates the question with some favorable[68] and unfavorable reports.[67]

The prognosis for cataract surgery in the age of extracapsular cataract extraction and phacoemulsification with intraocular lens implantation has been provided by another series of papers.* These authors generally report favorable results. Patients with preexisting glaucoma, severe iris atrophy, abnormal iris vasculature, history of spontaneous hyphema, the presence of Busacca and Koeppe nodules, and prolonged disease represent the high-risk patients.[46,49]

Specific problems in patients after cataract surgery include new or exacerbated glaucoma, severe uveitis, hyphema, formation of synechiae, pigment deposition on the intraocular lens, vitreous opacification, and corneal decompensation.[5,44,46] There can occasionally be a severe rubeotic glaucoma resulting in enucleation. Cystoid macula edema and hypotony have been noticeably lacking.[49,61]

In view of the potential increased complication rate and the young age of many of these patients, surgery should be approached cautiously. A posterior chamber implant placed completely in the capsular bag is probably most appropriate. Patients with severe Fuchs uveitis syndrome with iris atrophy and rubeosis may wish to avoid an intraocular lens.[46] A peripheral iridectomy is probably not necessary. Preoperative control of uveitis and glaucoma is essential, perhaps with a burst of corticosteroids prior to surgery. A neodymium: YAG laser discission of the opacified posterior lens capsule will probably be needed in a higher percentage of these patients than in the general population, and it may precipitate a marked increase in intraocular pressure.[82]

SUMMARY

Fuchs uveitis syndrome is a clinically described disorder that is readily identified in its classic form, but frequently not recognized in its subtle or more expanded forms. The essential features of the disease, however, remain in all forms. The criteria for the diagnosis of Fuchs uveitis syndrome include the following: (1) absence of acute symptoms; (2) presence of characteristic small, white, round and stellate keratic precipitates; (3) minimal cell and flare in the anterior chamber; (4) diffuse iris stromal atrophy, with or without patchy loss of the iris pigment epithelium; (5) absence of posterior synechiae; and (6) presence of cells or opacities in the vitreous humor. Heterochromia and glaucoma are variable features; all eyes will develop a cataract over time.

The disease is unilateral in 90% of those afflicted and has a long and insidious course. It is more common than reported because it is frequently missed. The clinical spectrum is extremely variable and, subsequently, so is the prognosis. With prolonged follow-up, approximately 40% of the victims maintain 20/40 or better visual acuity.[61] Cataracts cause decreased vision that is potentially restorable. A large number of patients lose their vision permanently from glaucoma, and several eyes have had to be removed.[61] Not all patients tolerate cataract or glaucoma surgery well. The prognosis may differ between the classic form (with a good prognosis) and the more common variants of the syndrome (with a poorer prognosis). Patients with this condition need to be constantly monitored, especially for glaucoma and progression of iris atrophy, which may be related to the ultimate prognosis.

There is no unifying cause or known inciting factor for Fuchs uveitis syndrome that is reflected in its multiple and variable clinical features. The disease affects many different tissues in the eye. The clinical features of the disease, however, are limited to the eye and disease recognition obviates an extensive medical workup and intensive antiinflammatory treatment.

REFERENCES

1. Alanko HI, Vuorre I, Saari KM: Characteristics of corneal endothelial cells in Fuchs heterochromic cyclitis, *Acta Ophthalmologica* 64:623-631, 1986.
2. Amsler M, Verrey F: Heterochromic de Fuchs et fragilite vasculaire, *Ophthalmogica* 111:177, 1946.
3. Arffa RC, Schlaegel TF: Chorioretinal scars in Fuchs heterochromic iridocyclitis, *Arch Ophthalmol* 102:1153-1155, 1984.
4. Arocker-Mettinger E, Asenbauer T, Ulbrich S, Grabner G: Serum interleukin-2 receptor levels in uveitis, *Curr Eye Res* (suppl) 9:25-29, 1990.
5. Baarsma GS, de Vries J, Hammudoglu CD: Extracapsular cataract extraction with posterior chamber lens implantation in Fuchs heterochromic cyclitis, *Br J Ophthalmol* 75:306-308, 1991.
6. Becker J: Heterochromiglaukom bei Mutter und Tochter, *Klin Monatsbl Augenheilkd* 78:707, 1927.
7. Benedikt O, Roll P, Zirm M: The glaucoma in heterochromic cyclitis of Fuchs: gonioscopic studies and electron microscopic investigations of the trabecular meshwork, *Klin Monatsbl Augenheilkd* 173:523-533, 1978.
8. Berger BB, Tessler HH, Kottow MH: Anterior segment ischaemia in Fuchs heterochromic cyclitis, *Arch Ophthalmol* 98:499-501, 1980.
9. Bernsmeier H, Kluxen G, Friedberg D: Fluorescence angiographical findings in complicated heterochromia of Fuchs, *Ber Dtsch Ophthalmol Gesellsch* 78:49-52, 1981.
10. Bialasiewicz AA, Gierth K, Naumann GOH: Heterochromia complicata Fuchs, crystalline iridopathy, and elevation of IgG concentration in aqueous humor, *Klin Monatsbl Augenheilkd* 198:205-206, 1991.
11. Bistis J: Heterochromic und Kataractbildung, *Zentralbl Prakt Augenheilkd* 22:136-137, 1898.

---

*References 17, 19, 34, 40, 44, 46, 79, 87, 90, 97.

12. Bistis J: La paralysie du sympathique dans l'étiologic de l'héterochromie, *Arch Ophtalmol* 32:578-583, 1912.
13. Bloch-Michel E: Physiopathology of Fuchs heterochromic cyclitis, *Trans Ophthalmol Soc UK* 101:384-386, 1981.
14. Brooks AMV, Robertson IF, Grant G, Gillies WE: Progressive corneal endothelial cell changes in anterior segment disease, *Aust NZ J Ophthalmol* 15:71-78, 1987.
15. Brown SI, McLean JM: Peripheral corneal edema after cataract extraction; a new clinical entity, *Trans Am Acad Ophthalmol Otolaryngol* 79:465-469, 1969.
16. Calixto N: Fuchs heterochromic cyclitis and glaucoma, *Rev Bras Oftalmol* 37:331-358, 1978.
17. Chung YM, Yeh TS: Intraocular lens implantation following extracapsular cataract extraction in uveitis, *Ophthalmic Surg* 21:272-276, 1990.
18. Chung YM, Yeh TS, Liu JH: Endogenous uveitis in Chinese—an analysis of 240 cases in a uveitis clinic, *Jpn J Ophthalmol* 32:64-69, 1988.
19. Chung YM, Yeh TS, Din W et al.: Intraocular lens implantation in Fuchs heterochromic cyclitis, *Folia Ophthalmol Jpn* 38:1120-1125, 1987.
20. Ciarnella Cantani A, Leonardi E: Bilateral Fuchs syndrome of heterochromic cyclitis, *Clin Oculist Patol Oculare* 3:91-94, 1982.
21. Comhaire-Poutchinian Y, Berthe-Bonnet S: La cyclite hétérochromique de Fuchs, *Bull Soc Belge Ophtalmol* 230:19-25, 1989.
22. Daus W, Kraus-Mackiw E: Fuchs heterochromic cyclitis: case reports of patients treated at Heidelberg University Eye Hospital since 1978, *Klin Monatsbl Augenheilkd* 185:410-411, 1984.
23. De Abreu MT, Belfort R, Hirata PS: Fuchs heterochromic cyclitis and ocular toxoplasmosis, *Am J Ophthalmol* 93:739-744, 1982.
24. De Bruyere M, Dernouchamps J-P, Sokal G: HLA antigens in Fuchs heterochromic iridocyclitis, *Am J Ophthalmol* 102:392-393, 1986.
25. Dernouchamps JP: Fuchs heterochromic cyclitis: an IUSG study on 550 cases. In Saari KM, editor: *Uveitis update,* 129-135, Amsterdam, 1984, Elsevier.
26. Dernouchamps JP: Fuchs heterochromic cyclitis, *Acta Ophthalmol* 62(suppl 63):49, 1984.
27. Dernouchamps JP, Vaerman JP, Michiels J, Masson PL: Immune complexes in the aqueous humor and serum, *Am J Ophthalmol* 84:24-31, 1977.
28. Donoso LA, Eigerman RA, Magargal LE: Fuchs heterochromic cyclitis associated with subclavian steal syndrome, *Ann Ophthalmol* 13:1153-1155, 1981.
29. Feldkamp TEW: Ophthalmological significance of HLA associated uveitis, *Eye* 4:839-844, 1990.
30. Feldman ST, Deutsch TA: Hyphema following Honan balloon use in Fuchs heterochromic iridocyclitis, *Arch Ophthalmol* 104:967, 1986.
31. Franceschetti A: Heterochromic cyclitis (Fuchs syndrome), *Am J Ophthalmol* 39:50-58, 1955.
32. Fuchs E: Über Komplikationen der Heterochromic, *Z Augenheilkd* 15:191-212, 1906.
33. Fulmek R: Hemiatrophia progressiva faciei (Romberg syndrome) associated with heterochromia complicata (Fuchs syndrome), *Klin Monatsbl Augenheilkd* 164:615-628, 1974.
34. Gee SS, Tabbara KF: Extracapsular cataract extraction in Fuchs heterochromic iridocyclitis, *Am J Ophthalmol* 108:310-314, 1989.
35. Goldberg MF, Erozan YS, Duke JR, Frost JK: Cytopathologic and histopathologic of Fuchs heterochromic iridocyclitis, *Arch Ophthalmol* 74:604-609, 1965.
36. Hart CT: The IOP in Fuchs heterochromic cyclitis, *Trans Ophthalmol Soc UK* 91:771-775, 1971.
37. Hart CT, Ward DM: Intraocular pressure in Fuchs heterochromic uveitis, *Br J Ophthalmol* 51:739-743, 1967.
38. Hollwich F: Heterochromic cyclitis (Fuchs syndrome), *Medica ICS* 450:1030-1033, 1979.
39. Hollwich F: Fuchs heterochromia complicata, *Klin Monatsbl Augenheilkd* 192:87-96, 1988.
40. Hooper PL, Rao NA, Smith RE: Cataract extraction in uveitis patients, *Surv Ophthalmol* 35:120-144, 1990.
41. Huber A: Das Glaukom bei Komplizierten Heterochromie Fuchs, *Ophthalmologica* 142:66-115, 1961.
42. Huber A, Kraus-Machiw E: Fuchs heterochromic cyclitis in Moebius syndrome, *Klin Monatsbl Augenheilkd* 178:182-185, 1981.
43. Jain IS, Gupta A, Gangwar DN, Dhir SP: Fuchs heterochromic cyclitis: some observations on clinical picture and on cataract surgery, *Ann Ophthalmol* 15:640-642, 1983.
44. Jakeman CM, Jordan K, Keast-Butler J, Perry S: Cataract surgery with intraocular lens implantation in Fuchs heterochromic cyclitis, *Eye* 4:543-547, 1990.
45. Johnson D, Liesegang TJ, Brubaker RF: Aqueous humor dynamics in Fuchs uveitis syndrome, *Am J Ophthalmol* 95:783-787, 1983.
46. Jones NP: Extracapsular cataract surgery with and without intraocular lens implantation in Fuchs heterochromic uveitis, *Eye* 4:145-150, 1990.
47. Jones NP: Fuchs heterochromic uveitis: a reappraisal of the clinical spectrum, *Eye* 5:649-661, 1991.
48. Jones NP: Glaucoma in Fuchs heterochromic uveitis: aetiology, management and outcome, *Eye* 5:662-667, 1991.
49. Jones NP: Fuchs heterochromic uveitis: an update, *Surv Ophthalmol* 37:253-272, 1993.
50. Jones NP, Read AP: Is there a genetic basis for Fuchs heterochromic uveitis? Discordance in monozygotic twins, *Br J Ophthalmol* 76:22-24, 1992.
51. Kimura SJ: Fuchs syndrome of heterochromic cyclitis in brown-eyed patients, *Trans Am Ophthalmol Soc* 76:76-89, 1978.
52. Kimura SJ, Hogan JH, Thygeson P: Fuchs syndrome of heterochromic cyclitis, *Arch Ophthalmol* 54:179-186, 1955.
53. Krick JA, Remington JS: Current concepts in parasitology: toxoplasmosis in the adult—an overview, *N Engl J Med* 298:550-553, 1978.
54. Kruit PH, van der Gaag R, Broersma L, Kijlstra A: Autoimmunity against corneal antigens. I. Isolation of a soluble 54Kd corneal epithelium antigen, *Curr Eye Res* 5:313-320, 1986.
55. Kruit PJ: Cellular immunity against the 54 Kd corneal epithelium antigen in chronic ocular diseases. In *Corneal autoimmunity: a clinical and experimental approach,* 72-78, Amsterdame, 1987, Vrije Universiteit Uitgeverij.
56. La Hey E, Baarsma GS, Rothova A et al.: High incidence of corneal epithelium antibodies in Fuchs heterochromic cyclitis, *Br J Ophthalmol* 72:921-925, 1988.
57. La Hey E, Mooy CM, Baarsma GS et al.: Immune deposits in iris biopsy specimens from patients with Fuchs heterochromic iridocyclitis, *Am J Ophthalmol* 113:75-80, 1992.
58. La Hey E, Rothova A, Baarsma S et al.: Fuchs heterochromic iridocyclitis is not associated with ocular toxoplasmosis, *Arch Ophthalmol* 110:806-811, 1992.
59. Lerman S, Levy C: Heterochromic iritis and secondary neovascular glaucoma, *Am J Ophthalmol* 57:479-481, 1964.
60. Lawrence W: Changes in colour in the iris. In Hays I, editor: *A treatise on disease of the eye,* 411-416, Philadelphia, 1843, Lea & Blanchard.
61. Liesegang TJ: Clinical features and prognosis in Fuchs uveitis syndrome, *Arch Ophthalmol* 100:1622-1626, 1982.
62. Loewenfeld IE, Thompson S: Fuchs heterochromic cyclitis: a critical review of the literature. I. Clinical characteristics of the syndrome, *Surv Ophthalmol* 17:394-457, 1973.
63. Loewenfeld IE, Thompson S: Fuchs heterochromic cyclitis: a critical review of the literature. II. Etiology and mechanisms, *Surv Ophthalmol* 18:2-61, 1973.
64. Makley TA: Heterochromic cyclitis in identical twins, *Am J Ophthalmol* 41:768-772, 1956.
65. McCartney AC, Bull TB, Spalton DJ: Fuchs heterochromic cyclitis: an electron microscopy study, *Trans Ophthalmol Soc UK* 105:324-329, 1986.
66. Melamed S, Lahav M, Sandbank U et al.: Fuchs heterochromic iridocyclitis: an electron microscopic study of the iris, *Invest Opthalmol Vis Sci* 17:1193-1198, 1978.
67. Mills KB, Rosen ES: Intraocular lens implantation following cataract extraction in Fuchs heterochromic uveitis, *Ophthalmic Surg* 13:467-469, 1982.
68. Mooney D, O'Connor M: Intraocular lenses in Fuchs heterochromic cyclitis, *Trans Ophthalmol Soc UK* 100:510, 1980.

69. Murray PI, Dinning WJ, Rahi AHS: Contrasting relations between suppressor cell number and function in acute anterior uveitis and heterochromic cyclitis, *Acta Ophthalmologica* 62 (suppl 163):52, 1984.

70. Murray PI, Dinning WJ, Rahi AHS: T-lymphocyte subpopulations in uveitis, *Br J Ophthalmol* 68:746-749, 1984.

71. Murray PI, Hoekzema R, van Haren MAC et al.: Aqueous humor analysis in Fuchs heterochromic cyclitis, *Curr Eye Res* 9:53-57, 1990.

72. Murray PI, Mooy CM, Visser-de-Jong E et al.: Immunohistochemical analysis of iris biopsy specimens from patients with Fuchs heterochromic cyclitis, *Am J Ophthalmol* 109:394-399, 1990.

73. Norn MS: Cataract extraction in Fuchs heterochromia: follow-up of 19 cases, *Acta Ophthalmologica* 46:685-699, 1968.

74. O'Connor GR: Heterochromic iridocyclitis, *Trans Ophthalmol Soc UK* 104:219-231, 1985.

75. Perry HD, Yanoff M, Scheie HG: Rubeosis in Fuchs heterochromic iridocyclitis, *Arch Ophthalmol* 93:337-339, 1975.

76. Pietruschka G, Priesz G: Secondary glaucoma with heterochromia cyclitis according to Fuchs, *Klin Monatsbl Augenheilkd* 164:609-615, 1974.

77. Pivetti Pezzi P, Bozzoni F, DeLiso P et al.: Iris fluorescein angiography in Fuchs heterochromic iridocyclitis, *Boll Oculist* 63:879-886, 1984.

78. Pivetti Pezzi P, Catarinelli G, Paroli MP, Polisena P: Fuchs heterochromic iridocyclitis. II. Immunogenetic aspects, *Clin Oculist Patol Oculare* 11:123-127, 1990.

79. Razzak A, Al-Samarrai A: Intraocular lens implantation following cataract extraction in Fuchs heterochromic uveitis, *Ophthalmic Res* 22:134-136, 1990.

80. Redslob E, Brini A: Les lèsions histo-pathologiques dans le iris atteints de la maladie de Fuchs, *Bull Soc Fr Ophtalmol* 62:116-119, 1957.

81. Regenbogen LS, Naveh-Floman N: Glaucoma in Fuchs heterochromic cyclitis associated with congenital Horner's syndrome, *Br J Ophthalmol* 71:844-849, 1987.

82. Roussel TJ, Coster DJ: Fuchs heterochromic cyclitis and posterior capsulotomy, *Br J Ophthalmol* 69:449-451, 1985.

83. Saari M, Vuorre I, Nieminen H: Fuchs heterochromic cyclitis: a simultaneous bilateral fluorescein angiographic study of the iris, *Br J Ophthalmol* 62:715-721, 1978.

84. Saari M, Vuorre I, Nieminen H: Infra-red transillumination stereophotography of the iris in Fuchs heterochromic cyclitis, *Br J Ophthalmol* 62:110-115, 1978.

85. Saari M, Vuorre I, Tiilikainen A, Algvere P: Genetic background of Fuchs heterochromic cyclitis, *Can J Ophthalmol* 13:240-246, 1978.

86. Saraux H, Laroche L, Le Hoang P: Secondary Fuchs heterochromic cyclitis: a new approach to an old disease, *Ophthalmologica* 190:193-198, 1985.

87. Schulze F, Beck R, Tungler O: Implantations of artificial eye lenses in patients with cataracta syndermatotica, cataracta heterochromica (Fuchs) and cataracta complicata, *Folia Ophthalmol* 10:199-202, 1985.

88. Schwab IR: Fuchs heterochromic iridocyclitis, *Int Ophthalmol Clin* 30:252-256, 1990.

89. Schwab IR: The epidemiologic association of Fuchs heterochromic iridocyclitis and ocular toxoplasmosis, *Am J Ophthalmol* 111:356-362, 1991.

90. Sherwood DR, Rosenthal AR: Cataract surgery in Fuchs heterochromic iridocyclitis, *Br J Ophthalmol* 76:238-240, 1992.

91. Silva HS, Orefice F, Pinheiro SRA: Study of 132 cases of heterochromic cyclitis of Fuchs, *Arq Bras Oftalmol* 51:160-162, 1988.

92. Smith RE, O'Connor R: Cataract extraction in Fuchs syndrome, *Arch Ophthalmol* 91:39-41, 1974.

93. Stave J, Schulze F, Rothe M: Examinations of the endothelium in patients with uveitis, *Folia Ophthalmol* 10:167-169, 1985.

94. Stefani FH: Befunde bei Fuchsscher Heterochromie-Zyklitis, *Ber Dtsch Ophthalmol Ges* 78:57-63, 1981.

95. Strieff EB: Sur l'hèrèditè de l'hètèrochromie, *Arch Klaus-Stiflung Vererb-Forsch* 22:256-260, 1947.

96. Tabbut BR, Tessler HH, Williams D: Fuchs heterochromic iridocyclitis in blacks, *Arch Ophthalmol* 106:1688-1690, 1988.

97. Turut P, Carballet L: Intraocular lens in Fuchs syndrome, *J Fr Ophtalmol* 11:651-656, 1988.

98. Vadot E: La cyclitè de Fuchs: aspects ètiologiques et cliniques, *Bull Soc Ophthalmol Fr* 90:861-864, 1990.

99. Van der Gaag R, Broersma L, Rothova A et al.: Immunity to a corneal antigen in Fuchs heterochromic cyclitis patients, *Invest Ophthalmol Vis Sci* 30:443-448, 1989.

100. Verma LV, Arora R: Clinico-pathologic correlates in Fuchs heterochromic iridocyclitis—an iris angiographic study, *Indian J Ophthalmol* 38:159-161, 1990.

101. Wacker WB, Donoso LA, Kalsow CM et al.: Experimental allergic uveitis: isolation, characterization and localisation of a soluble uveitopathogenic antigen from bovine retina, *J Immunol* 119:1949-1958, 1977.

102. Ward DM, Hart CT: Complicated cataract extraction in Fuchs heterochromic uveitis, *Br J Ophthalmol* 51:530-538, 1967.

103. Weill G: Uber heterophthalmus, *Z Augenheilkd* 11:165-176, 1904.

104. Weiner A, BenEzra D: Clinical patterns and associated conditions in chronic uveitis, *Am J Ophthalmol* 112:151-158, 1991.

105. Wobmann P: Fuchs heterochromic cyclitis: electron microscopic study of nine iris biopsies, *Albrecht von Graefes Arch Ophthalmol* 199:167-178, 1976.

106. Zygulska-Machowa H, Starzycka M, Przepiorkowski R: Cataract extraction in cases of Fuchs heterochromia, *Klin Oczna* 44:375-380, 1974.

42 Lens-Associated Uveitis

SCOTT W. COUSINS, ELLEN KRAUS-MACKIW

Lens-associated uveitis (LAU) represents a group of disorders with varied clinical features, pathogenic mechanisms, and histologic appearances. The cardinal feature common to all forms of LAU is a mixture of acute and chronic inflammation directed against released or residual lens protein within the anterior chamber (AC) or vitreous, usually in a setting of a traumatized, operated, or congenitally abnormal eye. Although LAU can be suspected on clinical grounds, its confirmation remains a pathologic diagnosis. Classically, the pathologic criterion for LAU is zonal inflammation centered around the lens, characterized by an inner zone of neutrophils invading the lens substance, a secondary zone of granulomatous inflammation surrounding the capsule injury site, and an outer zone with nongranulomatous inflammation and fibrotic granulation response. Many cases of LAU, however, vary significantly from the classic description. Experimental evidence indicates that antilens autoimmunity is one potential mechanism for triggering and sustaining inflammation, although other mechanisms no doubt contribute in some cases.

Surprisingly, many aspects of LAU (including not only its pathogenesis but also its classification and name) remain highly controversial in spite of nearly a century of interest in the disorder. Is LAU more than one entity? If so, how should these different entities be designated? Are all cases of LAU caused by autoimmunity, or are multiple pathogenic mechanisms involved with similar presentation? Are atypical cases of LAU fundamentally different from the classic phacoanaphylactic endophthalmitis? Is hypopyon uveitis that is associated with retained nucleus in the vitreous after cataract surgery an immunologic disease? Can ocular infection trigger inflammation directed at the lens?

The literature describing lens inflammation uses colorful but often contradictory and confusing terminology that represents historic carryovers from days past. In this chapter the term *phacoanaphylactic endophthalmitis* (PE) will designate the specific pathologic entity described by Verhoeff and Lemoine.[130] Although the term "phacoanaphylaxis" is a misnomer, the name has become entrenched in the literature and refers to a distinct "histopathologic" entity. Nevertheless, even though PE represents the classic manifestation of LAU, some of the variant forms of LAU probably share the same pathogenesis (see the following). Therefore, this chapter will support the concept that LAU is a "syndrome" rather than a discrete entity of uniform and unique clinical, histologic, and pathophysiologic features. The terms "phacogenic," "phacotoxic," "phacoallergic," or "phacoantigenic" will be avoided in this text, because they are vague; they imply a specific pathogenic mechanism; or they have been used differently by various authors in the past. In fact, the term "lens-*associated* uveitis" will be used rather than "lens-*induced* uveitis" to avoid the presumption that the lens is always the "inducer" of LAU.

The confusing nature of the terminology is reflected in the inconsistency of most classification schemes. The clinical appearance is rarely diagnostic, because few clinical signs readily differentiate the classic form of LAU from its variants. Schemes based on the presumed pathophysiology (for example, toxicity versus immunity) are not useful, because the pathogenic mechanism remains unknown in the vast majority of cases. Perhaps classification systems based on histologic criteria are the most useful, because at least reproducible criteria can be applied to the diagnosis and inferences made pertaining to the mechanism. Even pathology-based schemes are problematic, because the variability of the pathology might represent a spectrum of changes. Additionally, an absolute correlation between the histologic pattern and a specific pathogenic mechanism has not been established. Finally, in the modern era, with the availability of vitrectomy and improved surgical techniques, specimens for the pathologic diagnosis of LAU are rarely obtained, except in the most devastating cases.

For the purposes of this chapter, six categories will be distinguished:[95] (1) classic lens-associated endophthalmitis (phacoanaphylactic endophthalmitis); (2) variants of lens-associated inflammation (including granulomatous lens-induced uveitis or GLU); (3) infection-related lens-associated inflammation; (4) nonspecific infiltration and macrophage reactions toward lens material; (5) phacolytic responses; and (6) fibrosis and residual nonspecific changes. This classification scheme is not dependent on pathogenic mechanisms, but merely on histologic features. In this way, a consistent classification can be applied to both human and experimental studies. Thus the term "lens-associated uveitis" will be applied to three categories: classic phacoanaphylactic endophthalmitis, variants of lens-associated inflammation (including GLU), and infection-related lens-associated inflammation (categories 1, 2, and 3). Nonspecific infiltration and macrophage reactions (category 4) and phacolytic responses (category 5) probably represent disorders that are quite different from LAU, but they will be included for completeness. Finally, fibrosis and residual nonspecific changes (category 6) may represent the end stage for these other forms of LAU, but they can also occur in the absence of preexisting inflammation.

HISTORICAL BACKGROUND

Cataract Surgery and Lens Inflammation

The notion that the lens can act as a source of inflammation is as old as cataract surgery itself. A cataract is an age-related clouding of the natural, crystalline lens of the eye.[19] The crystalline lens (hereafter simply called the "lens") is a unique structure. It is an optically clear tissue that is required to supply controlled variations in optical power to the eye. Suspended by zonules from the ciliary body of the eye, the lens consists of a capsule (actually a secreted basement membrane) lined anteriorly by cuboidal epithelium. During development (and continuing throughout life), the epithelia elongate, migrate posteriorly, and ultimately fill their cytoplasm with specialized structural proteins called crystallins. A key feature of crystallins is their chemical inertness. This property prevents covalent interactions, thereby allowing the fibers to retain flexibility and optical clarity.[44] The central collection of fibers forms a dense core called the nucleus; the zone of fibers surrounding the nucleus is called the cortex. During aging, a number of biologic modifications to the crystallins occur, including denaturization, nonenzymatic glycosylation, oxidation of amino acids, and other covalent reactions that result in darkening and opacification of the lens (that is, a cataract).[103] Visually, catastrophic cataracts are among the most important causes of blindness worldwide, and they probably have been so among the elderly for millennia. The only treatment for cataracts is surgery.

Historically, the practice of couching (the intentional surgical dislocation of the lens into the vitreous cavity) was used by ancient Hindus and Romans for treatment of cataracts. The practice was immortalized in lithographs depicting itinerant "couchers" travelling among medieval villages offering their services for a fee.[23] Although dramatic successes were promised (and possibly realized immediately after surgery), failure was often the long-term outcome, apparently attributable to postoperative inflammation. One observer estimated that over 30% of eyes might have been lost as a result of the procedure.[147] Although in some eyes the postoperative inflammation was probably caused by infectious endophthalmitis or trauma, the idea that the contents of the injured lens might be "toxic" to the eye was considered.

The potential toxic nature of the lens figured into the controversy during emergence of the extracapsular cataract surgical technique that was popularized by Daviel[17] in 1753. This technique involved removal of the nucleus via an incision in the cornea and anterior capsule of the lens, although the lens cortex and posterior capsule remained in the eye. Postoperative inflammation was also commonly observed following this procedure, and various authors during the early 1800s argued over the relative merits of couching versus extraction.[42]

A competing surgical technique, known as intracapsular extraction, was introduced during the late 1700s by Sharp and associates.[23] During this procedure, the entire lens was removed with the capsule intact. By the early 1900s, this technique had been perfected to the point at which reasonable success rates for visual rehabilitation were achieved. Accordingly, because the entire lens was removed at the time of surgery, LAU became a rare entity that was associated only with ocular trauma and complicated surgery. The superiority of this surgical approach was verified by the longevity of its use. Only since the 1980s has the intracapsular technique been replaced by two new variants of Daviel's original extracapsular procedure.

Recognition of Lens-Associated Uveitis

The transition into the modern era of the understanding of LAU can probably be traced to two publications that appeared near the turn of the century. In 1899 Schirmer[116] was the first investigator to propose that lens inflammation was a consequence of toxicity. It was a monograph by Straub[124] (published posthumously in 1919), however, that provided the first comprehensive clinical and pathologic evidence that lens proteins could be "toxic"; that is, lens proteins could directly trigger inflammation via an unknown mechanism. This book was highly influential in stimulating support for the "toxicity" theory of pathogenesis for LAU.[148]

The early twentieth century was an exciting period for immunology, and new ideas were being confirmed regularly. The realization that the immune system could go awry and result in autoimmune attack against "self" had been postulated by Ehrlich and Morgenroth.[25] Clinical examples were sought, and the eye was one of the first organs to confirm the principle. Indeed, involvement of the second eye in sympathetic ophthalmia was one of the first recognized autoimmune diseases. The lens became another ocular example of autoimmunity.[122] Experiments by Uhlenhuth[129] in 1903 indicated that lens antigens could initiate an immune response. Clinical support was offered by Verhoeff and Lemoine,[130] who published a manuscript in 1922 suggesting that LAU might have an immunologic basis. These authors described (and named) the classic syndrome of phacoanaphylactic endophthalmitis in patients who had suffered traumatic injury to the lens of the eye, and the histopathologic features described in this publication are still accurate today. In addition, this publication described clinical manifestations, immunologic studies, and confirmatory animal experiments. Additional clinical evidence for the autoimmune nature of this form of LAU was provided by case reports that recognized a high association between LAU and the spontaneous development of sympathetic ophthalmia.[11,24] Finally, a series of animal studies performed in the 1970s confirmed that autoimmunity to the lens could reproduce PE experimentally (see the following).

Relationship to Modern Cataract Surgery

In the 1970s plastic intraocular lens implants were introduced to correct the visual deficit caused by surgical removal of the crystalline lens.[103] This advancement in technology compelled ophthalmic surgeons to seek another surgical technique for cataract extraction in which the lens capsule might be retained by the eye. For this reason, the extracapsular procedure was reintroduced. In the modern version of the standard extracapsular procedure, a limbal incision is used to remove the nucleus; but the cortical remnants are removed by a variety of aspiration devices, leaving the residual lens capsule intact to serve as a support for the plastic intraocular lens implant (used to replace the optical power of the surgically removed natural lens).[103] Yet another technique for cataract extraction was introduced by Kelman[51,52] in the 1960s, although it did not gain popularity until the 1980s. Termed phacoemulsification, this procedure involves the in situ emulsification of the nucleus by ultrasonic vibrations using a specialized instrument, followed by aspiration of the nuclear and cortical remnants as in standard extracapsular techniques. Both techniques allow the intraocular retention of small residual amounts of lens cortex and significant numbers of lens epithelial cells.[52,101] In fact, these epithelia continue to proliferate in the eye postoperatively where they probably synthesize crystallins and represent a cause of postoperative opacification (or "fibrosis") of the posterior capsule.[4,140]

Interestingly (and thankfully), the vast majority of patients who undergo modern cataract surgery fail to develop clinically significant LAU. Yet a small subset of patients ultimately develop a chronic granulomatous inflammatory process directed against the residual lens material that exhibits elements of PE. Other patients develop inflammation secondary to complicated surgery because modern surgery carries with it the risk of complications that include incomplete removal of the nucleus.[34] The associated inflammation is usually sight-threatening and requires a second operation to remove the stimulating nidus. Because over 1.3 million cataract operations are performed each year in the United States alone[103] (and probably an equal number are performed worldwide), a small fraction of surgically related cases can therefore affect a large number of people. Although an epidemic of LAU never materialized, the issues pertaining to a role for lens proteins as a nidus for inflammation have nonetheless become relevant once more.

Reemergence of Variant Forms of LAU

A review of the literature for clinical cases of inflammation related to lens surgery or injury during the 1980s leads to an interesting observation. Although classic PE might not be common, other less typical forms of LAU have not been infrequently encountered in clinical practice. Several new syndromes with features resembling PE have been identified. Of special interest is the syndrome of *Propionibacterium acnes* endophthalmitis, in which the anaerobic bacterium replicates in a sequestered pocket formed by the residual leaflets of the lens capsule.[5,83,84,111] Another syndrome has been reported after nuclear fragments are lost in the vitreous cavity during complicated cataract surgery.[47] In these eyes, a severe inflammatory reaction occurs, mimicking infectious endophthalmitis; but the vitreous is sterile and the inflammation resolves after removal of the fragments. Even though it is unlikely that either of these two syndromes are mediated by autoimmunity to the lens, the importance of the many variants of LAU has not been appreciated. Indeed, close scrutiny of the published cases, even some that appeared in Verhoeff's original series, reveals that not all of the cases meet the classic criteria for PE. Variants of LAU, even infection-related cases, might be more frequent than currently suspected.[85] The possibility that immunity contributes to the inflammation in many of these cases should at least be reconsidered.

PATHOGENESIS

Immunology of the Lens

Major misconceptions about the immunology of the lens continue to appear in textbooks and other references.[28,32,54] Perhaps the most notorious misunderstanding is the belief that lens proteins are sequestered from the immune system, and in this regard, they are treated differently by the immune system than are self proteins. In fact the opposite is true.

Firstly, most lens proteins are not sequestered. Secondly, active immunity to most lens protein is present, but this immunity produces tolerance and noninflammatory immunity.

Upon immunization with any antigen (foreign or self), one of three outcomes is possible: (1) nonresponsiveness (failure of the immune system to recognize and respond); (2) immune responsiveness that triggers inflammation; or, (3) immune responsiveness that is tolerizing and noninflammatory (indicating the distinction between inflammatory and noninflammatory immunity). Historically, the first possibility was assumed to explain the lack of inflammation upon exposure to autoantigens, including after lens injury or extracapsular surgery. In addition, lens antigens were presumed to enjoy an added layer of protection, because they were (supposedly) sequestered from the immune system. A great number of experimental data support the existence of active tolerance to autoantigens, however. This chapter will reinterpret the literature to demonstrate that this possibility is also most consistent with both clinical and experimental observations that relate to the lens and the immune response of the eye.

Lens Antigens Are Not Sequestered. The classic explanation for LAU that follows capsule injury was attributed to "sequestering" of lens protein by the intact lens capsule that forms early during embryogenesis of the lens.[28,32,54,65,117] Injury to the capsule was hypothesized to result in release of lens that, according to this theory, then acted as a "neoantigen," provoking a de novo primary immune response. Intuitively, this theory fails to make sense, and modern clinical experience and experimental data indicate it is indeed incorrect. The sequestered antigen theory leads to four testable predictions that have been evaluated experimentally: (1) lens crystallins must be organ-restricted to the lens; (2) basement membranes (that is, lens capsule) must be impermeable to lens crystallins; (3) the immune system of normal individuals with intact lens should not have encountered lens antigens; and (4) LAU should occur after any injury to the lens capsule because of the induction of antilens immunity. Experimental results have proven that all four predictions are incorrect.

Recent studies investigating the molecular biology of the lens have demonstrated that the synthesis of lens proteins is not organ-restricted. The major proteins of the lens, the crystallins, have been carefully characterized at the molecular level, and at least three classes of crystallins (alpha, beta, and gamma) have been recognized in humans.[44,106] Crystallins are actually complex molecules assembled from smaller subunits. For example, the alpha crystallins are composed of polymers of two subunits—A and B—each encoded by a separate gene.[44] The concept that lens protein is organ-specific is partially supported by molecular studies examining alpha-A crystallin promoter, which have revealed that this gene is active in the lens but not in other ocular or nonocular tissues.[106] Alpha-B crystallin gene, however, is expressed in many different tissues (including heart and skeletal muscle), indicating that alpha-B proteins (and therefore antigens) are not lens-restricted.[44]

Even if the synthesis of lens proteins was restricted to the lens, the lens capsule would not be an absolute barrier to leakage from the lens. Basement membranes can be relatively permeable to some water-soluble proteins, and therefore, the capsule itself is not an absolute sequestering barrier. Indeed, crystallins can be identified in the aqueous humor of many normal individuals.[16,112] In addition, lens proteins actually reside within the lens fibers that also possess a plasma membrane. This barrier might be more impenetrable than the capsule, but swelling of the fibers with increased permeability characterizes many different pathophysiologic insults to the lens that might produce leakage of lens protein.[16]

Antigenically, lens proteins are neither organ-restricted nor species-restricted. Alpha crystallin appears to be the most antigenic of the lens proteins, and it is believed to be the principal autoantigen (although the actual antigenic determinants for B cell or T cell responses have not been mapped as have other ocular autoantigens such as S antigen).[73] Additionally, the antigenicity of other lens proteins, including those in the capsule or new antigens formed by denatured crystallins, has not been well-characterized. Nonetheless, antisera raised against lens proteins cross-reacts with the retina, the iris, and various nonocular tissues.[60] Studies using immunostaining with anticrystallin antibodies have detected the presence of alpha crystallin antigens (against both A and B subunits) in many organs.[44] Thus lens antigens are present within ocular and nonocular tissues, disproving the concept of organ-specificity.

Studies analyzing the molecular evolution of the crystallins also indicate that lens proteins are not unique to the lens.[146] Some crystallins are probably inactive enzymes, retained from the phylogenetic past, but they have been subverted from a functional purpose in lower organisms to a structural purpose in humans.[145] For example, one of the alpha crystallin subunits resembles a small heat shock protein.[46,55] Some lens proteins therefore share a high degree of molecular homology (and hence antigenicity) with other nonlens proteins. A high degree of molecular homology exists among lens crystallins of different species, indicating regions of probable antigenic identity. Nevertheless, most lens proteins can be demonstrated to be immunogenic in other species.[146] It is therefore important to recognize that xenogeneic (derived from a foreign species) lens, when used as an antigen to immunize the host, contains both foreign and self antigenic determinants.

Based on the previous discussion, it is clear that lens antigens have ample opportunity to gain access to the immune system. Over the past 20 years, a large body of work has definitively demonstrated that the immune system has indeed recognized and responded to lens antigens in normals. Antilens antibodies can be demonstrated in many normal individuals if sensitive assays are used.* Antibodies to lens proteins have been identified in the serum of 50% of normal subjects, and in higher frequency in the serum and aqueous humor of cataract or diabetic patients prior to surgery. In addition, titers of antibodies to lens proteins often increase after extracapsular cataract surgery without appreciable increase in inflammation.[144] Thus the immune system has already recognized and processed lens antigens prior to any injury or surgery to the lens; and in fact, antilens immunity is a normal response in the general population.[7] Conversely, antilens immune-triggered inflammation is not normal. The maintenance of this subtle but physiologically crucial distinction is the direct consequence of active intervention by the immune system, an immune function called tolerance (see the following).

Finally, the prediction that LAU should routinely occur after capsule injury is readily dispelled. Injection of a large dose of protein antigen, such as albumin, into the vitreous produces a pattern of severe immune-mediated uveitis 7 days later. Thus according to the sequestered antigen theory, injury to the lens capsule should be an analogous situation. When the lens capsule is injured, large amounts of lens proteins are released that should serve as putative neoantigens. Experiments performed in rats, mice, rabbits, and even humans (extracapsular surgery), however, demonstrate that spontaneous inflammation after lens capsule injury is rare.[93] Even the intravitreal injection of lens protein after prior immunization usually produces minimal inflammation.[9,38,88]

Mechanisms of Immunologic Tolerance Relevant to the Lens. A central theme in immunology is the ability of the immune response to differentiate between self and foreign. The paradox was eloquently recognized by Erlich who coined the term ''horror autotoxicus'' to incorporate the idea that a sophisticated mechanism must exist to prevent the immune system from attacking normal tissues.[25,122] Subsequently, Billingham, Brent and Medawar enunciated the formal concept of self tolerance.[122] This chapter proposes that *tolerance* to the lens is the *sum total* of the mechanisms by which the immune system differentiates self from foreign to prevent *inflammation-triggering* immune responses against self antigens. Tolerance is especially relevant to understanding the immunology of the lens, because cataract surgery (or any type of lens injury) and the ensuing release of lens protein intuitively suggests an event that should initiate such an autoimmune attack. Yet the relative rarity of true autoimmune uveitis directed against the lens indicates the power of the protective tolerance to self.

Recent advances in immunology have clarified various mechanisms of immunologic tolerance that prevent widespread autoimmune inflammation. Although a detailed de-

scription of these mechanisms is beyond the scope of this chapter, a brief overview of three classic mechanisms (clonal deletion, anergy, and suppression) is directly relevant to understanding the immunology of the lens. The reader is referred to other recent reviews of tolerance for more specific details.* In addition, new immunologic insights into immunoregulation have clarified yet another proposed mechanism for tolerance (noninflammatory immunity) that will be discussed in some detail. It is noteworthy that these mechanisms of immunologic tolerance can operate independently and simultaneously.

Classic Mechanisms for Tolerance.

Clonal Deletion. Clonal deletion results from the ability of the thymus to destroy autoreactive T cells during T cell maturation,[132] and represents a mechanism for immunologic unresponsiveness that provides a ''hole'' in the repertoire of potential antigens (presumably self) against which the immune response can recognize. In principle, clonal deletion has been demonstrated to occur in mice using several different experimental approaches.[49,100] Intriguingly, alpha crystallin protein has been detected within the thymus, suggesting the possibility of crystallin-specific deletion of T cells.[50] The mechanism has not yet been demonstrated, however, to operate for relevant autoantigens, including lens proteins. Although clonal deletion would predict the absence of lens-responsive T cells during LAU, lens-responsive T cells can indeed be demonstrated under certain experimental conditions, indicating that clonal deletion, if present, is incomplete. Thus the precise role of clonal deletion in immunologic tolerance to the lens remains uncertain.

Anergy. Anergy, clonal inactivation, and other terms have been used to describe the situation in which antigen-specific T cells or B cells are rendered incapable of mounting a normal inflammation-triggering response to that antigen.[1,100] For example, when B cells of mice are exposed to antigen early in the developmental process, they are rendered unresponsive to the antigen after maturation.[1] Similarly, several different mechanisms that ''tolerize'' T cells have been demonstrated.[100,118] When T cells are presented antigen by nonprofessional antigen-presenting cells such as endothelium or Mueller cells, they are inactivated from further differentiation into inflammatory effector cells.[92,118] Although these T cells survive, they are incapable of initiating inflammatory immune responses. Anergy therefore provides another mechanism for immunologic unresponsiveness.

Suppression. Suppression, the third classic mechanism for tolerance, postulates that a population of downregulatory T cells exists to balance the population of helper and inflammation-enhancing T cells.[1] These downregulatory T cells modulate and diminish the level of activation by the effector or helper T cell. Whereas clonal deletion or anergy proposes immunologic unresponsiveness, suppression indicates an

---

*References 9, 40, 53, 63, 87, 105, 113, 114, 126, 144.

*References 86, 89, 99, 100, 131, 135.

active (but tolerizing) immune response to the antigen in question. The best-characterized mechanism is through the release of immunosuppressive cytokines,[12] but many other mechanisms have also been supported by experimental data.[1] The physiologic importance and mechanism(s) by which suppression is induced and regulated have been challenged, however.[120] Nonetheless, suppression is clearly an important regulatory mechanism for the immune system in general,[6] and for ocular immune responses in particular.[98,125] Although suppression has not been evaluated in terms of the lens, it is likely to exist.

Noninflammatory Immunity. How can immunity to an autoantigen exist in most individuals in the absence of inflammation? Evidence exists for many organ systems that autoimmunity (the presence of specific antibody or autoantigen-specific T cells) is common in normal individuals, yet autoimmune inflammation rarely develops.[14,32] An explanation for this apparent paradox is that the immune system has already recognized and responded to the autoantigen, but that the type of immune response that occurs does so in the absence of inflammation.[14,32] In fact, the relevant target organ might even be protected from future immune-mediated inflammation. A concept called *noninflammatory immunity* (as compared to *inflammatory immunity*) can therefore be invoked to explain this form of tolerance. Four experimental observations that support this concept follow.

Potential Role of Antibody Isotype. The concept of clonal inactivation of B cells would predict that autoantibodies should not be demonstrable in normals; yet, anti-self antibodies to many major autoantigens can be demonstrated in sera of normal individuals.[14] Why don't these autoantibodies cause inflammation? It has been known for many years that the specific inflammatory effects of antibody responses can be correlated with the isotype (or class) of antibody. The major inflammation-inducing mechanism of antibody is caused by complement activation, which in turn is a function of the isotype of the antibody molecule itself. Two antibodies with identical capacity to bind to an antigen will therefore have different inflammatory outcomes dependent upon their isotype.[31] For example, human IgM and IgG3 are good complement activators, but IgG4 is not. Similarly, mouse IgG2 is a good complement activator, but IgG1 and IgG3 are not (although they are efficient at agglutinization). Preferential activation of B cells that produce complement-fixing antibodies will result in inflammation-inducing immunity, because complement activation will be initiated after immune complex formation. Conversely, preferential activation of noncomplement-fixing antibodies will result in high antibody titers, but not in severe inflammation. Immune complexes will opsonize or agglutinate the antigen, but complement will not be activated. Therefore, the key to B cell effector function is determined by the regulation of the class switch from an IgM-synthesizing B cell to one produc-

ing an antibody of the other isotypes. This switch is controlled by different T cell-derived cytokines (see Snapper[123] for a review). By inference, the regulation of this form of B cell tolerance is passive and under the control of T helper signals.

T Cell Cross-Regulation. Recent advances in understanding T cell helper responses suggest how more subtle forms of regulation of T cell activation can lead to tolerance via noninflammatory immunity.[12] Mosmann and associates[91] have demonstrated that upon activation, T cells differentiate from a universal precursor subset, T helper 0 (Th0), into one of two functional subsets, T helper 1 (Th1) or T helper 2 (Th2)—a distinction valid for both mice and humans. Th1 cells secrete one specific panel of lymphokines (IL-2, TNF-β, IL-12, and IFN-γ), whereas Th2 cells secrete a different panel of lymphokines (IL-4, IL-5, and IL-10). Of importance, Th1 cytokines contribute significantly to inflammation, either (1) by mediating delayed hypersensitivity (DH), (2) by activating macrophages, or (3) by inducing B cells to switch into complement-fixing, IgG2-producing B cells (as occurs in the mouse). Conversely, Th2 cytokines are much less inflammatory, inducing B cells to produce IgE, IgA, and other noncomplement-fixing isotypes. In general, Th2 cytokines do not mediate DH or classic macrophage activation. Finally, Th2-derived cytokines suppress the activation of Th1, and conversely, Th1-derived cytokines suppress the activation of Th2. Although this subdivision is without doubt overly simplistic, it does provide a conceptual framework for an immunologic mechanism whereby immunity might be predominated selectively by noninflammatory effectors (Th2-mediated) versus inflammatory effectors (Th1-mediated). In some respects, suppression can be considered a sophisticated variation of this effect. For example, CD8 suppressor T cells secrete yet another pattern of cytokines (especially TGF-β), resulting in the cross-regulation of both T helper cells and B cells by suppressor T cell-derived cytokines.

In Vivo Examples. Experimentally, a phenomenon known as "split tolerance" or "immune deviation" can be demonstrated. Under various conditions, upregulation of a specific immunologic effector mechanism (antibody responses) can occur in the absence of elicitation of other effector mechanisms (T cell-mediated DH). By way of example, intravenous immunization with a soluble, nonaggregated protein antigen often produces increased antibody titers, but prevents the elicitation of cell-mediated DH (so-called intravenous immune deviation).[134] In fact, suppressor T cells are often induced during immune deviation that function to downregulate T cell-mediated immunity, but not necessarily downregulate all B cells. Thus "low-zone tolerance" (defined as the inability to elicit T cell-mediated immune-triggered inflammation after intravenous administration of low doses of antigen) can be explained in part by such a phenomenon.

Oral tolerance is another form of acquired tolerance that is related to the concept of noninflammatory immunity.[1] Upon feeding animals a variety of autoantigens (including retinal S antigen), a tolerizing immune response is initiated that probably depends on the induction of suppressor T cells in the spleen and demonstrates other components of "noninflammatory" immunity. If such an animal is subsequently immunized with the same autoantigen via a cutaneous immunization, autoimmune disease fails to develop in the relevant target organ.

Immune Privilege of the Eye. Investigations in several laboratories have developed the general hypothesis that the AC of the normal eye is an immunologically-privileged site on the basis of enhanced survivability of incompatible tissue grafts implanted within the AC. This immune privilege imparts onto the eye a powerful defensive mechanism that protects the delicate visual structures from autoimmune inflammation. In contrast, eyes experiencing uveitis (immunogenic inflammation) must have lost this protective mechanism, thereby becoming susceptible to immunologic attack. The physiologic mechanism of immune privilege is described in detail elsewhere (Chapters 3 and 7), but immunosuppressive cytokines produced by normal tissues within the anterior segment, such as transforming growth factor-β and neuropeptides, are crucial regulators.[15]

Phenomenologically, immune privilege can be demonstrated to operate on both the afferent (or immunization) and efferent (or elicitation) limbs of the ocular immune response. Intuitively, immunization (such as with lens protein or other autoantigens) via the AC should result in the same pattern of systemic immunity as immunization by any other route. Experimentally, however, this is not the case. Immunization via an AC injection results in an altered form of systemic immunity to that antigen as compared to the immune response following conventional cutaneous immunization. This immune response is noninflammatory, characterized by a selective deficiency of antigen-specific DH and a selectively diminished production of the IgG2 isotype (the complement-fixing isotype in the mouse). The other antibody isotypes and cytotoxic T cell precursors are the same as after conventional immunization.[136-139] The hallmark of this unique immune response (called *anterior chamber associated immune deviation* or ACAID) is the production of effector suppressor T cells that downregulate DH responses to the immunizing antigen at all body sites.[125] This pattern of immunity would result in noninflammatory immunity to the antigen. ACAID has not been evaluated with respect to lens antigens, but it can influence the immune response to other ocular autoantigens. Rats immunized via the AC with the retinal autoantigen S-antigen develop ACAID, as do mice immunized with the autoantigen interphotoreceptor retinol binding protein.[41,90] Both rats and mice with ACAID are protected from experimental autoimmune uveitis in the contralateral eye after subsequent conventional immunization. Thus ACAID may be yet another physiologic mechanism for regulating tolerance to the lens.

Summary of Mechanisms for Tolerance. Tolerance is the result of one or both of two immunologic outcomes after exposure to autoantigen (Table 42-1). In some cases, the immune system is *nonresponsive* (fails to recognize or respond to antigen), usually the result of clonal deletion and/or inactivation. In other cases, however, the immune system does recognize self antigens, but the resultant immune response is *noninflammatory*. Noninflammatory effectors are those capable of producing some (protective) immune functions in the absence of significant inflammation. These include noncomplement-fixing, agglutinizing antibodies; suppressor T cells; cytotoxic T cells; and perhaps, Th2 subset of helper cells. Conversely, a third immunologic outcome upon exposure to antigen, *inflammatory immunity,* leads to the production of immunologic effectors that induce and amplify inflammation, specifically complement-fixing antibodies and Th1 subset of DH T cells. The predominance of nonresponsiveness or noninflammatory immune response results in maintenance of tolerance to autoantigens. Conversion of nonresponsiveness or noninflammatory immunity to inflammatory immunity results in loss of tolerance.

The controlling factors that determine this regulation are complex, and they are related to the nature of the antigen, the site of immunization, the type of antigen-presenting cell, and the immunologic microenvironment in which induction or elicitation occurs. Phenomenologically, certain routes of

TABLE 42-1 POTENTIAL CONSEQUENCES OF IMMUNOLOGIC EXPOSURE TO LENS ANTIGENS

Tolerance		Inflammation
Nonresponsiveness	Noninflammatory Immunity	Inflammatory Immunity
Clonal deletion of lens-reactive T cells	Lens-specific suppressor T cells	Complement-fixing antibodies
Clonal inactivation of lens-reactive B cells or T cells	Agglutinizing, but noncomplement-fixing antibodies	Delayed hypersensitivity T cells with high inflammatory potential
	Helper T cells with low inflammatory potential	

immunization favor the production of inflammatory (versus noninflammatory) immunity. Conventional immunizations (intradermal or cutaneous) with adjuvant usually produce inflammatory effectors. Intravenous, oral, AC, or even cutaneous immunizations without adjuvant often result in tolerance with noninflammatory immunity. Physiologically, regulation of T cell subset activation and cytokine production is probably the crucial determinant. The particular type of antigen-presenting cell and the microenvironment at the site where antigen presentation occurs appear to be important determinants. Similar mechanisms probably determine the noninflammatory autoimmune response to the lens in normal individuals when compared with the inflammatory immune response of those individuals who suffer with some forms of LAU.

Conclusions, Speculations, and Evidence Supporting Immunologic Tolerance to the Lens. In actuality, immunologic tolerance to the lens has not been directly evaluated, but it can be inferred to exist from the experimental literature. Because the regulation of tolerance to the lens is likely to be highly complex, the following discussion is speculative. Nevertheless, it is consistent with current concepts of both systemic immunoregulation and ocular immunology. Thus the following speculations on tolerance to lens antigens probably explain the development of mild phacolytic responses or nonspecific inflammation rather than LAU after most lens injuries (Fig. 42-1).

B cell tolerance to the lens is probably indirect, controlled at the level of the helper T cell. Thus functional lens-specific B cells certainly exist, because serum antibody can be identified in normal individuals, and antibody titers can be stimulated in all animals by most routes of immunization.[62,64,65,87] The capacity of antilens B cells to become activated, mature, and differentiate is regulated by T helper cells, however. If these helper cells are absent as a result of clonal deletion, anergy, and/or suppression, the B cell will remain inactive unless the requirement for help is circumvented by a nonspecific B cell-stimulating signal. The isotype of antibody produced by the mature B cell will be similarly regulated. It is important to recognize, however, that an increase in the titer of antilens antibody after immunization does not necessarily indicate loss of tolerance and the induction of inflammatory immunity. Few, if any, studies have carefully evaluated antibody effector activities and the isotypes in normal individuals after various manipulations. As long as the antibody titers are predominated by noncomplement-fixing isotypes, tolerance can be maintained.

Marak[66,71] has suggested that profound T cell tolerance exists to native lens, both at the level of T cell help and T cell effectors. The nature of the T cell tolerance (cross-regulation, clonal deletion, anergy, and/or suppression) is unknown. Clonal deletion or anergy cannot be complete, however, because helper T cell responses can be demonstrated under certain experimental conditions.[33,37] The large increase in antibody titer that develops after immunization with homologous lens is unlikely to represent a nonspecific polyclonal response (see the following). In those individuals with antilens antibodies, noninflammatory immunity might exist, mediated by helper T lymphocytes for B cells (perhaps Th2 subset), but not effector T cells (Th1 subset). Thus experiments designed to identify Th1-type antigen-specific T cell responses in (immunized) normal individuals without LAU would be predicted to fail. This prediction is consistent with the inability to detect proliferating T cells within lymph nodes of animals immunized to homologous lens protein.

Interestingly, immunization with xenogeneic lens activates both effector T cells and proliferating T cells in the lymph nodes.[33,37] The ability of these activated T cells to respond to antigenic determinants on self lens, or merely to antigenic differences expressed by the foreign lens protein, has not yet been thoroughly investigated. It is therefore possible that immunization to xenogeneic lens activates Th1-type of T helper/effector cells that respond only to antigenic determinants contained in the foreign lens antigen; however, these activated T cells would provide helper signals to amplify and differentiate "self" lens-responsive B cells into complement-fixing antibody producers in the lymph node. Yet these xenogeneic-responsive T cells would not contribute effector T cell activity to inflammation within the eye, because they would not be able to respond to self lens antigens (see the following controversies section).

The preceding scenario is highly speculative. The crucial element of tolerance to the lens predicted by this hypothesis would lie at the regulation of helper T cells (Fig. 42-1), however. Antilens T cells are probably present and activated in normal individuals, but these T cells would belong to a subset of "noninflammatory" helper cells. For instance, preferential activation of Th2 cells in normal individuals would allow an increase in antilens antibody titer, but these antibodies would be noninflammatory. Suppressor T cells would contribute similarly. This pattern of T cell activation is not inconsistent with immune deviation, perhaps induced by low doses of circulating lens antigen, or by the specific effects of anterior chamber immunization from the natural leakage of lens crystallins.

On the other hand, loss of tolerance would be manifested by the inappropriate coactivation of the Th1 cell subset, in which B cells would be directed to mature into plasma cells capable of synthesizing complement-fixing antibodies (Fig. 42-2). Adjuvants are good activators of Th1-type T cells, but relevant in vivo stimuli for Th1 cells are still being sought. The additional protective role of ocular immune privilege might be to provide an alternative mechanism for tolerance. An ACAID-like pattern of immune responses would therefore reinforce noninflammatory immunity. If Th1 cells, or even B cells, were to become activated and recruited to the normal eye, the intrinsic immunosuppressive microenvironment of the normal AC would also downregulate DH or

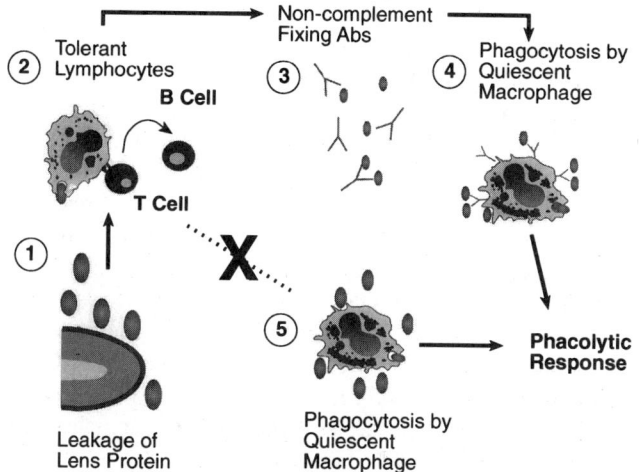

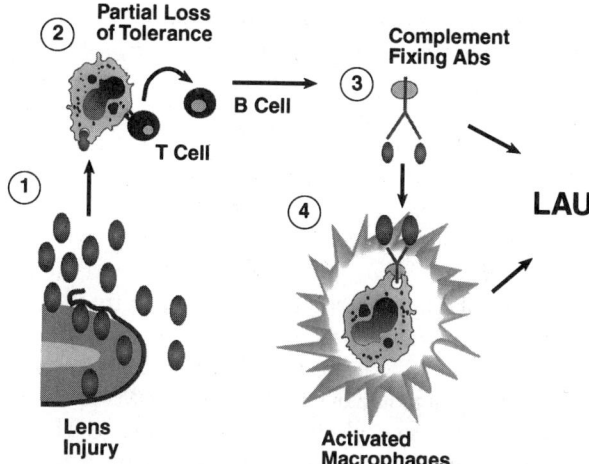

Fig. 42-1. Schematic representation of hypothetic immunologic events that produce a mild nonspecific or phacolytic response in most normal eyes with lens injury. Upon leakage of lens protein from an intact capsule or an eye with mild trauma, **(1)**, tolerant T cells (caused by anergy, suppression, cross-regulation, or immune privilege) are presented with lens antigen **(2)**. The tolerant T cells either remain unresponsive or provide "noninflammatory" helper cytokines to lens-specific B cells that result in the production of noncomplement fixing, lens-reactive antibodies **(3)**. In the absence of complement activation, "quiescent" phagocytosis of lens protein by ocular macrophages is enabled by these immune complexes **(4)**, without significant inflammation, thereby resulting in a phacolytic pattern. Also, because tolerant T cells do not produce macrophage-activating factors or delayed hypersensitivity **(5)**, other alternative pathways for macrophage activation and inflammation are also absent.

Fig. 42-2. Schematic representation of hypothetic immunologic events that might result in autoimmune LAU. Upon release of lens proteins after injury **(1)**, an undefined event (perhaps severe trauma or genetic predisposition) leads to partial loss of T cell tolerance to lens antigens **(2)**, resulting in "inflammation-enhancing" T helper signals that cause B cells to produce lens-reactive complement-fixing antibodies **(3)**. Inflammatory products of complement activation directly initiate the pattern of LAU **(3)**. Alternatively, complement and phagocytosis of complement-coated, lens/anti-lens immune complexes can activate ocular macrophages **(4)**, that, in turn, contribute to the pattern of LAU. Additionally, macrophage-activating factors released from activated inflammatory T cells might also participate.

macrophage responses locally, thereby diminishing local inflammation in the eye. Perhaps studies using transgenic mice, genetically modified to express membrane-bound or soluble foreign antigens within the lens, will better characterize the mechanisms of lens tolerance.[58a,149a]

Evidence that Inflammatory Autoimmunity to the Lens Causes LAU

Clinical Evidence for Autoimmunity in LAU. Clinical evidence for the role of complement-fixing antibodies causing human LAU, especially PE, has not been reported. Although serum titers of antibodies to lens proteins have been demonstrated in some patients with LAU,[144] they also occur in sera of patients without LAU. As discussed previously, qualitative differences in the functional capacity of antibodies might be one focus of future studies. Some studies have examined skin testing as an indicator of cell-mediated immunity to lens. Verhoeff and Lemoine[130] reported 12 patients who had positive skin tests. Unfortunately, this study failed to differentiate between cell-mediated DH or antibody-mediated Arthus reaction as the cause for a positive skin response. Furthermore, this study did not use control tests, nor did it differentiate between xenogeneic or homolo-

gous lenses in the challenge reagents. Similar limitations are found in other skin test studies.[9] Several investigators, however, have reported positive lymphocyte proliferation tests of peripheral blood cells in cases of LAU.[9] Nevertheless, preliminary reports from Opremcak[102] indicate that many patients with chronic uveitis (not LAU) also have lens-responsive T cells in the blood, suggesting that lens-specific T cells might become activated in nonspecific uveitis. Thus no solid evidence supports or refutes a role for autoantibodies, DH, or cell-mediated immunity to the lens in human LAU.

The best evidence supporting the premise that LAU is an autoimmune disorder is found in case reports of bilaterality. Over the years, at least 38 cases of bilateral PE have been described in the literature (reviewed in Woods[149]). Very few of these case reports actually document the classic pathology of PE in the sympathizing eye, relying instead on clinical findings. Furthermore, many of the bilateral cases either revealed pathologic signs of sympathetic ophthalmia in the exciting eye, or they were not described in sufficient detail to ensure a diagnosis of PE. Because diagnosis of LAU is on the basis of histologic findings, it cannot be concluded with certainty that all bilateral cases represent LAU and not sympathetic ophthalmia. Moreover, bilateral PE is rare, occurring in only one out of 144 cases examined in a recent series.[127]

Experimental Models for Autoimmune LAU. *Experimental Lens-Induced Granulomatous Endophthalmitis.* Experimental lens-induced granulomatous endophthalmitis (ELGE), the best-characterized animal model for autoimmune LAU, has been developed in Lewis, Wistar, or Sprague Dawley rats that have been immunized against whole xenogeneic or homologous lens proteins.[66,67,71-77,79] After three to six repeated immunizations, the lens is surgically injured. Uveitis ultimately develops over the next three to ten days, exhibiting a spectrum of severity. Thirty to eighty percent of rats immunized to *homologous* lens (lens from the same species, in this case rat) develop severe disease associated with a granulomatous infiltrate and histology similar to classic phacoanaphylactic endophthalmitis.[74] The remainder of animals, however, develop a pattern of atypical inflammation, characterized by a neutrophilic and monocytic infiltrate without giant cells. Rats receiving lens injury without immunization develop a pattern of nonspecific macrophage infiltration.

In contrast, immunization with *xenogeneic* lens (lens from a foreign species) increases the frequency of the PE-like pattern.[77] Under some conditions, rats hyperimmunized similarly develop a severe panuveitis associated with retinitis, vasculitis, and choroiditis in addition to lenticular inflammation.[72] A strain-dependence is observed, with a range in susceptibility and variation in histologic findings. For example, Brown Norway rats do not develop the characteristic PE-like pattern; these rats instead develop a necrotizing vasculitis of the retina and uvea without the prominent neutrophilic reaction.[76]

The immunopathogenesis of the autoimmune response in experimental LAU has been partially characterized. ELGE can be transferred with hyperimmune antisera.[71] The role of lymph node cells in transferring uveitis has not been fully examined using modern methodology, but preliminary results indicate that direct transfer of lymphocytes fails to induce LAU.[67] Cutaneous DH reactions, however, can be demonstrated after immunization with xenogeneic lens, but not after homologous lens.[96] In addition, T helper cell responses for B cell activation appear to be required. Presumably, B cell activation and antibody production to lens proteins can occur when helper T cell tolerance is abolished by the immunization protocol. Bypassing the requirement for antigen-specific T helper signals with polyclonal B cell activation, such as bacterial lipopolysaccharide[75] or allogeneic lymphocytes,[78] also allows induction of uveitis.

The pathophysiology of the ocular inflammation has been thoroughly evaluated (Fig. 42-2). Studies by Marak and associates[69,71] have indicated that complement-fixing antibodies specific for lens protein are sufficient to cause a PE-like pattern,[69,71] and the prevention of complement activation diminishes the inflammatory infiltration.[68] Presumably, generation of complement-dependent inflammatory mediators, such as the anaphylatoxin C5a, by complement-activating

immune complexes within the lens substance explains the neutrophil infiltration into the lens. Diffusion of these mediators into the AC probably results in a chemotactic gradient, yielding a zonal pattern. In some eyes with a severe panuveitis pattern, widespread complement activation is proposed to occur within the uveal tract itself. Activated macrophages must also contribute, because epithelioid and giant cells (subsets of activated, differentiated macrophages) are classic features. The mechanism for giant cell formation has not been totally resolved. Phagocytosis of immune complexes coated with complement can contribute to macrophage activation, and it might induce giant cell formation in some models for nonocular inflammation.[115] IL-4, a Th2-derived cytokine, is also a giant cell-inducing factor in vitro.[94] Although granulomatous inflammation is believed to be dependent on a Th1 T cell, DH-related mechanism in other experimental animals models,[2,8,121] granuloma formation in ELGE might be mediated by immune complexes, complement activation, and Th2 T cells. Injury to retina or other tissues is probably exacerbated by toxic oxygen radicals, because antioxidant enzymes or free-radical scavengers appear to diminish the severity of the disease.[70,107,108]

Another model for autoimmune LAU that is similar to ELGE has been developed in the rat. Termed experimental ophthalmia (EO), this disease is produced in CAP rats immunized to homogenates of guinea pig eyes, which is followed by lens capsule injury.[57] Approximately 30% of rats develop histopathologic changes consistent with PE, and these changes are associated with neovascularization and other abnormalities of the anterior segment prior to the onset of LAU. In contrast, Lewis rats fail to develop characteristic histologic changes. Of interest, 5% of CAP rats develop PE-like changes after lens injury, but in the absence of presensitization. This model for LAU therefore suggests that certain rat strains such as CAP, that are especially sensitive to the reparative response after nonspecific ocular inflammation, might be predisposed to the characteristic changes of LAU.

Other Models Based on Autoimmunity. Several mouse models for autoimmune LAU have also been developed. Immunization of BALB/c mice with *xenogeneic* lens results in severe granulomatous inflammation resembling PE in 30% of animals following lens capsule injury.[79] Another model for LAU has been attempted following immunization with homologous or autologous lens.[36,37] This approach, however, was less successful in producing the characteristic pattern of inflammation. Following injury to one lens of a BALB/c mouse, the fellow lens was injured 3 weeks later. Histologic evaluation of the fellow eye performed 1 week after injury revealed that 60% of eyes developed nonspecific infiltration, but approximately 40% of eyes developed a mild variant of LAU. The exciting eyes developed minimal nonspecific infiltration. Antibodies to lens proteins were formed in all mice, but serum titers were not related to onset or severity of disease; T cell proliferative responses were minimal. It is unknown whether this mild variation of LAU represents a different pathophysiologic process distinct from ELGE, or whether it is merely a less severe form of the classic autoimmune disease.

Several investigators have attempted to elicit autoimmune LAU in rabbits, but this species fails to develop the distinctive features of LAU.[9,38,88] Although immunization with homologous or xenogeneic lens results in high titers of antibodies to lens proteins, lens injury is defined by an atypical histologic pattern characteristic of nonspecific infiltration. In comparison, guinea pigs that have been immunized to xenogeneic lens develop LAU.[79]

Controversies with the Autoimmune Hypothesis. *How Is Tolerance to the Lens Lost? What Is the Role of Ocular Trauma?* The mechanism whereby tolerance is lost in LAU is uncertain. In experimental animal models, immunization with xenogeneic lens apparently activates helper T cells, but the analogous event in humans remains unclear (as it is in other human autoimmune disorders). Genetic susceptibility has been suggested by some animal studies, but it has not been rigorously examined.

Perhaps the traumatic insult itself contributes to the pathogenesis. LAU rarely occurs in normal eyes in humans.[127] In contrast to all other models for autoimmune disease, experimental LAU does not develop spontaneously after immunization, but must be initiated by injury to the lens capsule. In humans, however, other cofactors are required, including the near universal presence of an abnormal eye caused by surgery, trauma, or developmental anomalies. In the setting of these abnormalities, immune privilege of the eye might be neutralized or abrogated. Although speculative, Lewis rats, which is one of the most susceptible strains for ELGE, appear to have a defect in immune privilege; injury to one eye produces an acute bilateral infiltration with inflammatory cells.[27] CAP rats also appear to develop LAU in association with anterior segment neovascularization,[56] a phenomenon that has been associated with loss of immune privilege of the eye.

Several authors have noted a relationship between trauma, sympathetic ophthalmia, and LAU.[11,24,61] Sympathetic ophthalmia is probably a T cell-mediated disease (see Chapter 57 by Chan and Roberge). Because PE is postulated to be an autoantibody mediated disease, co-occurrence of the two disorders would not be predicted, even though the predisposing risk factors and setting (trauma and surgery) are similar. In cases in which the primary diagnosis was sympathetic ophthalmia, approximately 25% to 46% of eyes also revealed PE or variants of LAU.[11,24,61] Conversely, if the primary diagnosis was PE, only a few eyes exhibited sympathetic ophthalmia.[127] Thus the development of PE does not necessarily predispose to sympathetic ophthalmia; however, the occurrence of sympathetic ophthalmia might predispose to PE. It is possible that lens injury occurring in a setting of cell-mediated immunity directed against retinal or uveal antigens might result in LAU by a different pathogenesis from that of isolated, classic LAU. Perhaps LAU in sympathetic ophthalmia occurs via a bystander mechanism in which inflammation directed against retinal/uveal antigens indirectly and nonspecifically involves the lens (see the following).

Are T Cells Involved in Disease Pathogenesis? Several observations have suggested a more complicated relationship between autoimmunity and lens inflammation than indicated by the classic autoantibody hypothesis. First, serum antibody titers do not correlate with disease onset or severity in experimental animals, with the exception of rats. Mice, guinea pigs, and rabbits fail to develop classic granulomatous disease after homologous lens immunization in spite of high titers of antibody. Marak[66] argues, however, that intraocular antibody formation may be important in this model and that serum titers do not reflect local ocular conditions. In addition, the effector function of antibodies that is produced in these animal models has not been well characterized. It is possible that titers of complement-fixing antibodies would correlate better.

A second line of reasoning implicates the role of T cells in LAU. Manipulations that enhance the severity of LAU are often associated with the enhancement of T cell dependent responses. Interestingly, immunization with xenogeneic lens protein prior to lens injury is required to induce LAU in most species, especially mice and guinea pigs. A similar dependence on immunization with xenogeneic autoantigen has been observed for experimental autoimmune uveitis and experimental allergic encephalomyelitis, two authentic T cell dependent models. In these models, immunization with foreign autoantigen has been noted to abrogate tolerance and induce immunoreactivity (both humoral and cellular) against the self autoantigen. Similarly, immunization with xenogeneic lens activates antilens T lymphocyte proliferative responses and positive cutaneous DH reactions to lens proteins.

Similarities between experimental LAU and experimental autoimmune thyroiditis (EAT) suggest that the same inflammatory mechanisms may be shared by these two autoimmune diseases. Advances in our understanding of the pathogenesis of EAT now indicate that T cells are crucial for disease induction in most experimental systems, especially in the mouse.[109,133,135] Thyroglobulin and lens crystallins are both large, relatively tissue-specific proteins formed by polymerization of smaller polypeptide chains. Both proteins, however, can be detected in low levels in the blood. The systemic autoimmune response to thyroglobulin is very similar to the systemic response to lens crystallin. Evidence suggests that both T cells and antibody effectors contribute to pathogenesis of the severest form of inflammation.[133] If the analogy between EAT and LAU is correct, then a role for T cell responses (in the form of T cell help, T cell regulation, and even effector T cells) would be predicted.

Evidence that Infection or Immunity to Infection Causes LAU

Clinical Evidence that Infection Contributes to Some Cases of LAU. Certain clinical observations suggest that intraocular infection might contribute to LAU in humans. Many of the original cases presented at the turn of the century occurred in the presence of prominent purulent infection. Infection was, therefore, one of the proposed causes of this disorder, and it was postulated by Verhoeff and associates that infection (either ''latent'' or active) at the time of surgery or trauma could initiate PE.[23,149] In a recent review, at least 5% of cases of PE were associated with obvious bacterial infection.[127] A number of cases of suspected LAU over the past 10 years have been found to be associated with a concomitant infection of the AC and residual lens material (after cataract surgery) with the anaerobic organism *Propionibacterium acnes*.[5,83,84,111] This bacterium, presumably introduced at the time of surgery, replicates very slowly within the eye and fails to produce a significant purulent infection. Thus the presence of infection is clinically undetectable. Some clinical event, however, such as additional surgery (YAG laser) or other unknown trigger, results in inflammation apparently related to enhanced replication or release of the bacterium.[5] Granulomatous inflammation ultimately develops in response to the bacterium that spreads to involve the residual lens.

Two popular concepts regarding the pathogenesis of this syndrome pertain to the physiologic side effects of the ocular infection. Some investigators favor the notion that this disease represents an infectious endophthalmitis and that the living organism initiates an acute inflammatory reaction as in other forms of endophthalmitis.[30,111,143] Many aspects of *P. acnes* infection, however, suggest a unique pathophysiology. In many eyes infected with *P. acnes,* the bacterium replicates without inciting inflammation. Conversely, in eyes with the full syndrome, the inflammation seems to persist long after the eye has been sterilized, suggesting an immunologic or inflammatory contribution by even dead organisms.

Other investigators have postulated that *P. acnes* infection acts as an adjuvant that results in the abrogation of immunologic tolerance to the lens and the emergence of antilens autoimmunity.[82] In fact, *P. acnes* can substitute for *Mycobacteria* sp. in Freund adjuvant during the immunization of rats to xenogeneic lens.[119] The lack of contralateral involvement in *P. acnes* syndrome, however, fails to support the hypothesis that autoimmunity to the lens is an important pathogenic mechanism.[150]

A third explanation is offered by animal experiments described in the next section, in which a T cell-mediated immune response to the infective organism indirectly involves the residual lens in a granulomatous reaction. A recent observation that most patients with ocular *P. acnes* infection share homology in the antigen-binding site of the class II,

HLA DR molecule might support the idea of an immunogenic pathogenesis.[18] Nevertheless, a clear explanation for the pattern of inflammation in the *P. acnes* syndrome is presently unavailable.

Animal Models Based on Infective Mechanisms. Several investigators have attempted to reproduce LAU using animal models based on intraocular infection. Neubauer and associates[97] have demonstrated in rabbits that AC injections of live *Staphylococcus aureus* coupled with simultaneous lens injury produced a histologic pattern similar to that observed in PE.[3,96] Although these investigators found that the live organisms were cleared from the eyes by day 10 postinoculation, they were unable to distinguish between the effects of bacterial infection and the effects of immunity to the bacterial antigens. The possibility was raised that coexisting infection and lens injury can produce the distinctive pattern of LAU in the absence of an obvious purulent infection, but these studies could not determine if an immune response in the absence of infection can produce characteristic LAU.

Other investigators have postulated that immunity to bacterial antigens can indirectly result in the pattern of LAU in the setting of lens capsule injury (Fig. 42-3). Lyda and Lippincott[64] immunized rabbits to extracts of *S. aureus,* followed several weeks later by intraocular injection with antigen at the time of lens injury. The histology that developed, however, was more consistent with nonspecific infiltration

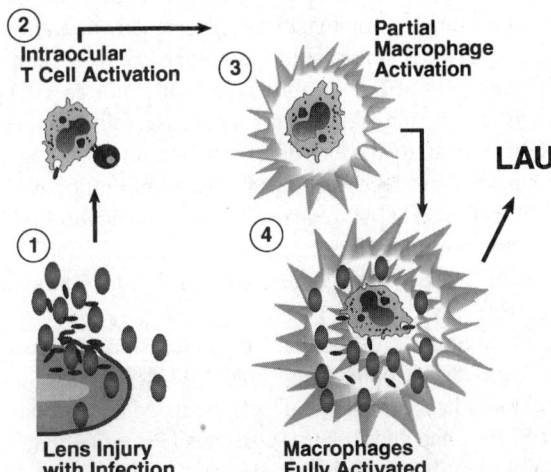

Fig. 42-3. Schematic representation of hypothetic immunologic events that might result in infection-related LAU. Upon release of lens protein in the presence of bacterial infection or residual bacterial antigens (1), bacteria-specific T cells recognize and respond to the bacterial antigens (2), producing a typical T cell-mediated immune response to the bacteria. Macrophage-activating factors (cytokines such as interferon-gamma) lead to the partial activation of intraocular macrophages (3). Bacterial toxins and cell wall products (4), however, provide additional macrophage activational signals. Phagocytosis of lens proteins by fully activated macrophages leads to LAU. Note that though antibacteria antibodies might contribute, immunity to the lens is not involved in this schema.

than LAU. Unfortunately, this study was flawed by the route of immunization (intravenous) that might have resulted in T cell tolerance to the challenge antigen. Ishimoto and associates[48] were able to produce LAU as a consequence to immunogenic inflammation directed against a third-party antigen. These investigators observed that in guinea pigs previously sensitized to porcine albumin, intravitreal injections of porcine albumin at the time of lens injury produced a histologic pattern resembling PE, including giant cell formation. Thus intravitreal inflammation to a third-party antigen resulted in a pattern of LAU.

A murine model for LAU supports the concept of indirect involvement of the lens during immune-mediated inflammation directed against bacterial antigens.[59] In mice immunized to *Mycobacterium tuberculosis,* intraocular (intralenticular) injection of high doses of antigen simultaneously with lens capsule injury produces LAU in 80% of eyes, and 20% of eyes develop a PE-like pattern. The proposed pathogenetic mechanism invokes a role for effector T cells directed against the bacterial antigen, resulting in the release of T cell-derived cytokines that activate macrophages within the eye.[142] These activated macrophages, upon interaction with residual bacterial antigen and/or toxins in the lens substance, mediate the infiltration of the lens with neutrophils via the release of neutrophil chemotactic mediators such as IL-8.

A number of studies have attempted to determine if the adjuvant properties of bacterial antigens or extracts in the setting of lens injury might induce autoimmunity to the lens. Intravenous administration of various bacterial extracts or adjuvants were reported to have no significant effect upon the ocular pathology.[9] Intraocular injection of these at the time of lens injury generally enhanced the inflammation, but in all cases the pattern resembled nonspecific infiltration and not LAU. Thus the ability of bacterial toxins to act as an intraocular adjuvant and stimulate antilens autoimmunity has not been confirmed.

Evidence that Toxicity to Lens Protein Causes LAU

Until the 1920s, toxicity was accepted as the foremost mechanism for LAU, and some advocates (especially Woods[149]) defended the existence of the toxic pathogenesis until the 1960s. It is often misconstrued that proponents of this mechanism believed that all lens proteins were themselves toxic. To the contrary, the advocates of this theory knew from clinical experience that lens proteins were usually nontoxic, but believed that they could become toxic under certain conditions. The transformation was not clearly articulated, but two factors (degradation byproducts and absorption of toxic substances from the blood) probably were considered.

Current investigators tend to dismiss the toxic mechanism, but perhaps it should be reconsidered from a perspec-

tive of modern revisionism (Fig. 42-4). Toxicity can be redefined in modern terms as the capacity to directly trigger inflammation in the absence of preexisting immunity or trauma. In light of this definition, lens protein might contribute to "toxic inflammation" by several mechanisms. First, Rosenbaum[110] has demonstrated that lens proteins, or their apparent degradation products, can be chemotactic for monocytes. Thus lens byproducts can attract inflammatory cells into the eye. Second, it is now accepted that extracellular matrix and other gels are sequestering reservoirs for cells, cytokines, growth factors, and other biologic response modifiers. Perhaps the retained lens proteins "adsorb" cytokines in a similar manner. Indeed, lens contains fibronectin and laminin—powerful matrix components for cell attachment.[104] Furthermore, lens can store iron, an important cofactor for production of many mediators by inflammatory cells.[81] Third, bacterial toxins might contribute to LAU in another way, because systemic exposure to bacterial LPS has been reported to enhance or induce LAU in rabbits or rats.[27] Importantly, lipopolysaccharide produces transient localized inflammation in the eye (see Chapter 5 by Cousins and Rouse). Perhaps LPS-related LAU is another example of bystander involvement. Lens injury in an eye with preexisting inflammation caused by bacterial toxins, antiretinal autoimmunity, immunity to bacterial antigens, or even severe posttraumatic inflammation, might result in a pattern of LAU.

How nonspecific inflammation would induce the specific pattern of LAU is unknown. In a quiet eye with a normal immunosuppressive microenvironment, resident ocular

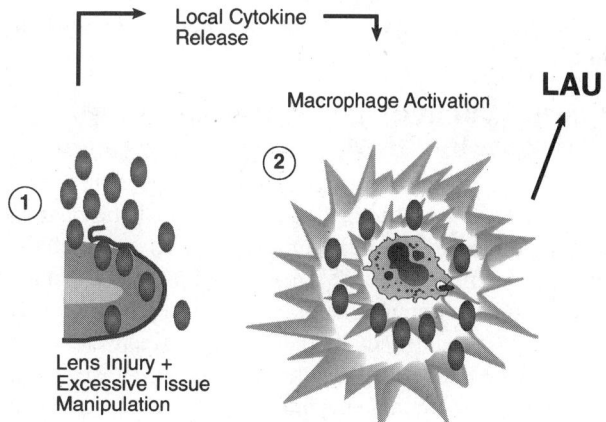

Fig. 42-4. Schematic representation of hypothetic inflammatory events that might result in toxin-related LAU. Upon the release of lens protein in the setting of excessive tissue manipulation **(1)** (such as after trauma or complicated surgery), persistent local production of inflammatory cytokines (interleukin-1) by injured ocular tissue and loss of immune privilege results in inappropriate ocular macrophage activation **(2).** Chemotactic activity of lens proteins, cell adhesion molecules within lens capsule, and adsorption of cytokines by the lens itself might enhance and direct inflammation to the lens.

macrophages (which richly invest the iris and ciliary body) are significantly inhibited by TGF-β and other immunosuppressive factors in the eye from becoming activated. Thus phagocytosis of lens proteins by these inhibited macrophages would simply produce clearance of excessive lens protein without significant inflammation. Even the formation of immune complexes between noncomplement-fixing antibody and lens antigens would only serve to enhance phagocytosis of lens protein by inactive macrophages. This sequence of events would result in a phacolytic response or nonspecific infiltration.

It is possible that following various insults (including accidental trauma or complicated surgery), nonspecific inflammation alters the immunologic microenvironment of the eye in such a way that macrophages are partially activated (see Chapter 5 by Cousins and Rouse). Proinflammatory cytokines (such as IL-1 or IL-6) or bacterial toxins (such as LPS or others) that are released in such a microenvironment are well known macrophage-activating stimuli. Furthermore, noncomplement-fixing antibodies directed against the lens might contribute to the pathogenesis of LAU. In a "hot" eye that possesses a proinflammatory microenvironment, partially activated macrophages might become fully activated into inflammatory effector cells upon recognition of noncomplement-activating immune complexes. Phagocytosis of immune complexes by activated macrophages might also produce additional activation in the absence of complement. The subsequent release of IL-8 or other chemokine mediators would recruit neutrophils into the lens, thereby producing LAU. Although this scenario is speculative, it could explain the pathogenesis of some cases of LAU in the absence of infection or loss of immunologic tolerance to the lens.

Conclusions and Speculations about the Pathogenesis of LAU

Is LAU caused by one or multiple pathogenic mechanisms? From the preceding discussion, it should be clear that no single mechanism satisfactorily explains every clinical case or experimental model of LAU. Importantly, both infective and autoimmune animal models can produce a spectrum of histologic findings that range between classic PE and variant LAU. Also, histopathology is not always an ideal indicator of immunopathogenesis, because identical histologic manifestations do not always follow from identical immunogenic stimuli among different species. Cousins and Kraus-Mackiw[14a] therefore believe that LAU represents a pathologic syndrome in which various triggering mechanisms, including autoimmunity, infection, and perhaps toxic mechanisms, could contribute.

How can the inflammatory response to dislocated lens fragments after cataract surgery be explained? Because the most severe cases of LAU observed in modern practice occur in this setting, it is important to understand whether the inflammation generated against retained lens fragments in the vitreous is autoimmune, infective, or toxic. Each explanation would have different implications for treatment of the inflamed eye, as well as for recommendations about surgery on the fellow eye. It is unclear whether the autoimmune or infective models apply to this disorder.

Could some of the classic cases of PE represent occult infection? It is not likely that active purulent infection is present in most cases of PE. Subclinical infection with organisms like *P. acnes*, however, would be difficult to identify retrospectively in pathologic specimens. Molecular studies using polymerase chain reaction for detection of DNA of various microorganisms in fixed tissue specimens could be used to examine this issue retrospectively.

Does a common final denominator link the pathophysiology of these different pathogenic mechanisms? In many ways, all three of the pathogenic mechanisms share significant similarities. The major differences are actually linked to the specific triggering mechanism initiating the inflammation. The possibility that the activated macrophage is the central regulatory effector cell is attractive, because a key role for its participation could be envisioned in autoimmune, infective, or even toxic scenarios.

CLINICAL FEATURES

LAU is a relatively rare disorder, although its variants are being seen more commonly as a result of the changing nature of cataract surgery. Accordingly, the peak age of onset ranges between 50 and 70 years of age (the age of patients usually undergoing surgery).[127] LAU can occur at any age, however, in the appropriate setting.[141] In general, the diagnosis of LAU is often missed clinically,[21] being suspected in less than 5% of the cases in a recent review.[127] Nevertheless, because the confirmation of LAU is a pathologic diagnosis, a definitive series outlining the clinical features and natural history of the entire spectrum of LAU is lacking.

LAU characteristically presents in one of three settings. The most serious cases present as a panuveitis or endophthalmitis, associated with a history of recent surgery or injury.[43,47] A history of retained lens fragments lost in the vitreous may be obtained from the operating surgeon, but this occurrence is sometimes unrecognized. In spontaneous cases, preexisting developmental abnormalities of the eye might be present, such as microphthalmia or persistence and hyperplasia primary vitreous (PHPV).[127] Eyes with severe LAU are usually painful, hyperemic, and possess poor vision. Clinically, hypopyon uveitis can be present, and the posterior segment is often not visible (Fig. 42-5). Onset can occasionally occur months after surgery, and the association between the lens and inflammation may be forgotten. Nevertheless, the clinical findings cannot be differentiated reliably from infective endophthalmitis. These eyes rapidly deteriorate without treatment.

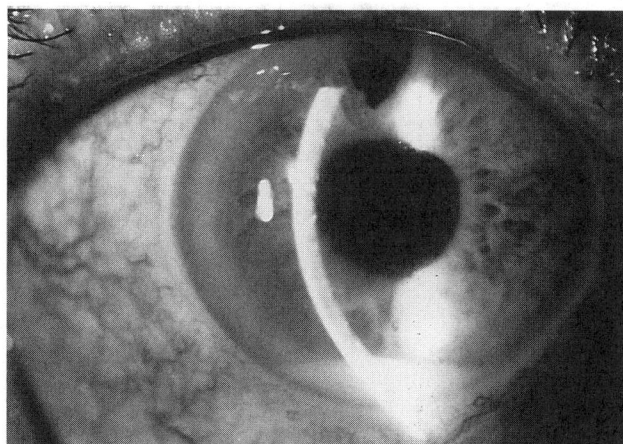

Fig. 42-5. Hypopyon uveitis in a patient with severe LAU, several months following dislocation of the nucleus into the vitreous during cataract surgery.

A second typical presentation is the setting of smoldering anterior segment inflammation, usually following cataract surgery.[66,127] Although clinical signs of granulomatous inflammation often include synechiae, keratic precipitates, aqueous cell, and flare, these signs are not diagnostic (Fig. 42-6). The inflammation can be partially diminished with topical corticosteroids, but it will persist until the residual lens is resorbed. A reparative response, ranging from iris neovascularization to cyclitic membrane formation, can ultimately develop if definitive treatment is not instituted. Differential between LAU and other forms of anterior uveitis (perhaps exacerbated by the surgery) can be difficult in this setting.

In addition, a chronic indolent infection associated with *P. acnes, S. epidermidis,* various fungi, or other low-virulence organisms can provoke inflammation against residual lens material and may be confused with LAU.[30] The appearance of a white plaque on the posterior capsule is typical for these cases, especially during *P. acnes* infection.[83,84,111,151] Inflammation caused by the intraocular lens (IOL) itself should also be differentiated from LAU. The uveitis-glaucoma-hyphema (UGH) syndrome appears to represent postoperative inflammation related to chafing or trauma to the iris caused by the lens.[58] Although UGH syndrome was more common when rigid anterior chamber lenses were used during the early 1980s, this syndrome has also been reported with posterior chamber lenses.[22] Toxicity caused by contaminants on the lens surface have become rare. Nevertheless, many eyes with IOL's can develop histologic evidence of low-grade foreign body reactions.[13]

A third presentation is similar, but it occurs bilaterally and often follows surgery or injury in the fellow eye after prior surgery in the first eye. The smoldering inflammation that results can therefore resemble sympathetic ophthalmia.

LAU, however, is also associated with sequential bilaterally, the second eye becoming inflamed long after the first. Conversely, bilateral simultaneous inflammation is common in sympathetic ophthalmia.[66,149]

LABORATORY INVESTIGATIONS

Diagnostic Approaches

Because LAU is a pathologic diagnosis, a secure diagnosis cannot be made on clinical grounds. In the cases of LAU presenting as endophthalmitis, ultrasound can occasionally be useful in detecting the presence of residual lens in the vitreous cavity.[43] Although analysis of vitreous aspirates can sometimes suggest the diagnosis,[39,80] cytopathologic evaluation is rarely definitive. Additionally, the cytologic differentiation between LAU and infective endophthalmitis can be very difficult. Bacterial cultures of aspirates, however, can help to rule out an infectious cause. In the most severe cases, the patient should be evaluated and treated for suspected infection.[30,47] In less severe cases, in which retained lens fragments are thought to be the cause, vitrectomy with bacterial cultures can be performed. In some cases, intraoperative antibiotics can be withheld until after vitrectomy, while the patient is closely observed for improvement—pending negative culture results.

In the cases in which the eye has smoldering inflammation (especially in the fellow eye), an ultrasound of the posterior segment can occasionally confirm the diagnosis of sympathetic ophthalmia through findings of choroidal thickening and serous retinal detachment. Aspiration of aqueous fluid or vitreous for cytopathology might be helpful in bilateral cases (especially in the fellow eye) because the predominance of neutrophils would suggest LAU, whereas the predominance of lymphocytes would suggest sympathetic ophthalmia.

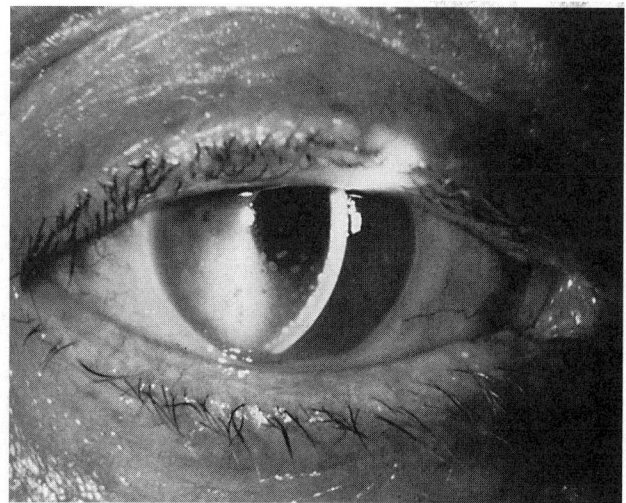

Fig. 42-6. Granulomatous uveitis in a patient with chronic LAU.

PATHOLOGY

Although the histopathology of classic PE has been firmly established, the pathology of the variants of LAU has not been as clearly defined in the literature. Only blind eyes generally become available for pathologic examination. A selection bias is therefore evident, as these cases often represent severe or end stage manifestations, and examples of early stage or mild-to-moderate disease are not readily available. Many eyes that would have become available for pathologic study in the past now undergo operation by vitrectomy, further obscuring the natural evolution of the disease. Finally, the ability to locate and analyze cases histopathologically in a retrospective fashion is dependent upon the cataloging system used to retrieve the specimen. If an atypical case were not cataloged as LAU, it might not be identified for the purposes of analysis. A clinical series is therefore unavailable to elucidate the frequency and pattern of the entire spectrum of PE and the LAU variants. For the purposes of this chapter, a classification scheme modified from that of Muller-Hermelink and Daus[95] will be used.

Classic Phacoanaphylactic Endophthalmitis. The classic histologic features of PE were defined by Straub[124] in 1919 and by Verhoeff and Lemoine[130] in 1922. JA deVeer[20] further refined the criteria in 1953 to include five zones of inflammation or fibrosis. A recent series of 144 cases by Thatch, Marak, McLean, and Green[127] has provided an excellent modern clinicohistopathologic characterization of PE. The pathologic criteria for classic PE includes inflammation centered around the lens that is characterized by three distinct zones: an inner zone of neutrophils invading the lens substance; a secondary zone of monocytes, macrophages, epithelioid cells, and/or giant cells surrounding the capsule injury site; and an outer zone of fibrotic reparative or granulation tissue infiltrated with nongranulomatous inflammation and plasma cells (Fig. 42-7). A nongranuloma-tous infiltrate within the iris and ciliary body varies from minimal to severe, but it is never granulomatous. Vitreous infiltration is often present if lens material is admixed with vitreous. Fifty percent of the eyes demonstrate retinal inflammation (especially perivasculitis), and eighty percent of the eyes also demonstrate mild choroidal involvement with focal nongranulomatous infiltration. Sequelae of chronic inflammation are common and include retinal detachment, iris neovascularization, optic atrophy, and phthisis. In the series by Thatch, only one case was bilateral.

Variants of LAU. Many cases of LAU, including some classified as PE in various series, fail to fit the classic criteria described previously, but nevertheless demonstrate acute inflammation centered around the lens.[66] In the past, some of these cases were designated "phacotoxic uveitis."[149] In an attempt to avoid controversy that often diverts attention from more important considerations, these nonclassic cases will be designated as "variant forms of LAU" in this chapter. Thus histologic variants of LAU can incorporate a variety of cases that demonstrate inflammation centered around lens injury, but that might not be considered classic PE by strict application of histologic criteria. It is important to recognize, however, that these variants still belong to the spectrum of LAU, and many of them might actually have the same pathogenesis as PE.

Usually, variant cases demonstrate significant neutrophil invasion of the lens and nongranulomatous inflammation in the ciliary body, but they lack one or more of the other classic features of PE (Fig. 42-8). Hence, in variant cases, the prominent granulomatous component, the definite zonal character,[66] or the fibrotic reparative response may not be present. Alternatively, some variant cases lack the intense neutrophil component. For example, Muller-Hermelink[95] has described a pathologic variant of LAU, termed granulomatous lens-induced uveitis (GLU), in which the histologic pattern is predominated by the granulomatous response

Fig. 42-7. Zonal pattern of inflammation in an eye with phacoanaphylactic endophthalmitis.

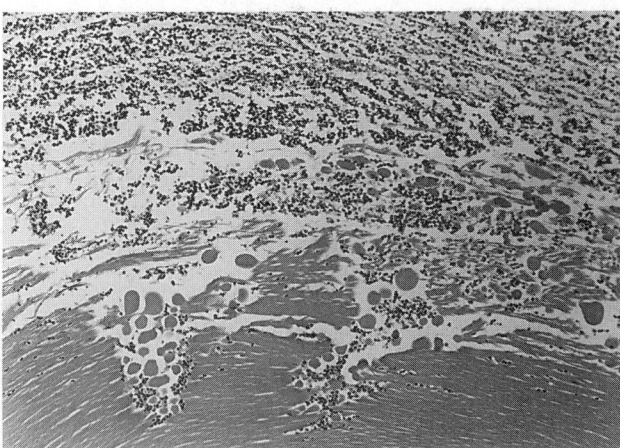

Fig. 42-8. Variant form of LAU demonstrating marked neutrophil infiltration into the nucleus in the absence of granulomatous inflammation.

around the lens, within the anterior uvea, and even within the choroid. Conspicuous is the absence of a neutrophilic invasion of the lens substance.

One additional variant of LAU includes the cases of acute inflammation following dislocated lens fragments after cataract surgery.[47] Very little has been published concerning the pathology of these eyes. A review of five cases of retained or removed nuclear fragments evaluated in the pathology laboratory at Bascom Palmer Eye Institute revealed surprisingly mild neutrophil and macrophage infiltration within the fragments (Fig. 42-9), in spite of the fact that all eyes demonstrated moderately severe inflammation clinically.

Infection-Related Lens-Associated Inflammation. Some cases that include either classic PE or its variants demonstrate the presence of obvious infective organisms. In Thatch's series,[127] 5% of cases revealed obvious signs of infection. The inflammation may be centered around the infective agent within the retained lens. Alternatively, the residual antigenic material may not be visible upon histopathologic analysis if the pathogen is dead. Marak,[66] however, has indicated that none of the published cases of *P. Acnes* syndrome, or those that he has examined personally, demonstrate the typical pathologic features of PE.[66]

Nonspecific Infiltration and Macrophage Reactions. Mild infiltration centered around the lens is observed in some specimens, but the histologic pattern is predominated by macrophage invasion and mild nongranulomatous inflammation in the "absence" of prominent neutrophil infiltration or significant uveal inflammation.[95] An occasional giant cell may be present, but extensive granulomatous changes are absent. Nonspecific reactions occur in nearly all eyes with lens injury, including those that have been subjected to routine cataract surgery.

Phacolytic Response. This pattern represents a variant of nonspecific infiltration described by Flocks[29] in 1955 in which glaucoma occurs in the setting of a hypermature cataract that leaks lens protein through an "intact" capsule. Lens-engorged macrophages are present in the AC, and glaucoma develops as a consequence of these cells blocking the trabecular meshwork outflow channels (Fig. 42-10). Other signs of LAU are conspicuously absent. Sometimes, lens-engorged macrophages can infiltrate the lens after capsular injury in the absence of LAU.[130,149]

Fibrosis and Residual Nonspecific Changes. In some eyes, the histologic pattern is dominated by the reparative response in the absence of prominent, active inflammation.[95] This pattern is a separate entity, even though it may be the end stage for "burnt-out" cases of LAU. The fibrotic response can range from localized proliferation of lens epithelium to cyclitic membrane formation. The reparative response often appears to be an attempt to seal off the rent in the capsule.

THERAPY

It has been known for nearly 150 years that inflammation persists as long as the residual lens persists.[35] In 1919, Straub reported several cases that improved upon surgical removal of the residual lens fragments, thereby suggesting the therapeutic role for the surgical removal of the residual lens.[148,149] Because LAU is now encountered in various clinical settings, management can be considered as follows.

Management of Presumed LAU

Medical management of presumed LAU with topical, periocular, or systemic corticosteroids should only be used as a temporizing therapy prior to definitive surgery.[66] Because the inflammation may only partially respond, surgical removal of the residual lens is the definitive procedure. If the posterior capsule is intact, aspiration of the residual cortex can be achieved via a limbal incision using a manual aspiration canula or similar device. For complete removal of lens

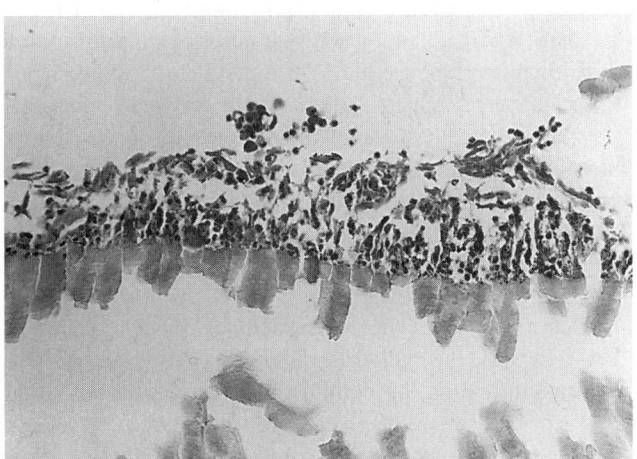

Fig. 42-9. Neutrophil and macrophage infiltration into lens fragment that had been dislocated into the vitreous.

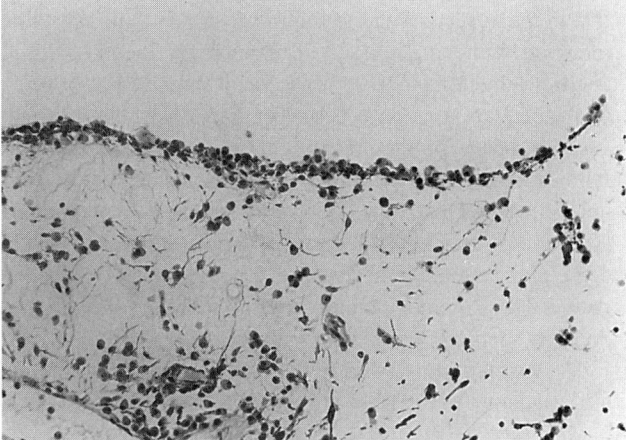

Fig. 42-10. Macrophages lining the anterior iris in an eye with a phacolytic response to lens protein.

remnants and capsule, however, a standard three-port pars plana vitrectomy (PPV) is often an excellent procedure.[47] Infective causes should always be considered in the treatment plan, and severe cases that resemble acute postoperative infective endophthalmitis should be evaluated and treated as any other form of postoperative endophthalmitis.

Prevention of LAU by Management of Retained Lens Fragments

Nucleus fragments and cortex lost in the vitreous cavity at cataract surgery are probably the most common settings for LAU in current practice. The prevention of LAU by surgical and/or medical management of residual lens is therefore often indicated. Various authorities disagree as to the best management of chips or pieces of lens in the vitreous, and no definitive management scheme has been proven superior. Some surgeons advocate surgical removal of any retained lens, and contraindicate an IOL.* Others advocate a conservative approach based on close clinical observation of the patient and treatment with topical corticosteroids.[66]

At the Bascom Palmer Eye Institute (BPEI), some retinal surgeons advocate a tailored approach that is based on presentation.[10,34,45,122a] Small chips or pieces of lens (representing less than 25% of the nucleus) usually can be observed and treated medically. A thorough anterior vitrectomy should be performed at the time of cataract surgery, with certainty that vitreous is not incarcerated in the wound or adherent to the IOL. Good cortical cleanup should be performed, but removal of every bit of cortex is not necessary. Topical corticosteroids and cyclo-oxygenase inhibitors should be employed postoperatively, and cystoid macular edema (CME) is a common complication. Delayed-onset LAU is possible up to many months later, so close monitoring of the patient is necessary. If elevated intraocular pressure, aqueous cell infiltrate, or CME persists, consideration of PPV should be undertaken to remove the retained-lens fragments.

At times, a large piece of lens (> 25% of the nucleus) is lost in the vitreous, but the fragments are soft enough to be removed with vitrectomy instrumentation. In this setting, anterior vitrectomy and cortex cleanup should be performed by the cataract surgeon as described previously. The cataract surgeon, however, should avoid excessive surgical manipulation and try to leave as much residual capsule as is reasonable. Placement of a posterior chamber IOL in the sulcus (with suture fixation if necessary) can be attempted, but in some cases, an anterior chamber IOL is a reasonable alternative. The patient should be referred to a vitreoretinal surgeon as soon as possible for removal of retained lens and PPV. A watertight wound free of vitreous and clear cornea are requisites for PPV. Techniques for removing retained lens fragments have been well-described in the literature.[10,26,45] IOL placement can be safely performed at the time of PPV, if not done at the time of cataract extraction.

In rare cases, a large fragment of retained lens is present (> 25% of the nucleus), but the fragment is "rock hard." Anterior vitrectomy plus cortex cleanup should be performed at the time of cataract surgery, but no IOL should be placed. The "rock hard" lens fragment probably will require removal via the limbus after a complete posterior vitrectomy. Any existing IOL would therefore need to be explanted prior to the vitrectomy, increasing the difficulty of the surgery.

Lens disruption associated with penetrating trauma is relatively frequent, occurring in 43% of eyes observed at BPEI with open globes caused by laceration with sharp objects.[128] These eyes have a worse outcome than those eyes without lens disruption, especially those demonstrating an increased risk for endophthalmitis. Because differentiation between infection versus sterile lens-associated inflammation is extremely difficult in these seriously injured eyes, some surgeons perform vitrectomy/lensectomy at the time of initial wound repair in cases in which corneoscleral laceration is associated with lens injury.

Management of Suspected *P. Acnes* or Other Indolent Infections

An algorithm for the treatment of this disorder has been advocated by some surgeons.[143,151] In mild cases, topical and intraocular antibiotics alone cure some eyes, but the infection can recur. For smoldering cases with predominantly anterior segment inflammation, pars plana vitrectomy for the removal of posterior capsule, any residual lens remnants, and the nidus of bacteria are usually effective. A limbal approach, however, can also be used, especially if an IOL exchange is planned. Removal of the capsule with its bacterial colonization is the only definitive way to prevent recurrence.[143] Bacterial cultures should be sent to the clinical laboratory with a specific request for anaerobes. The IOL can be secured with a fixation suture if necessary. Postoperative inflammation is controlled with topical corticosteroids, although some cases demonstrate severe persistent inflammation even after sterilization of the eye. Severe cases that resemble postoperative infective endophthalmitis should be evaluated and treated as any other form of postoperative endophthalmitis.[30,143]

PROGNOSIS

Determination of the prognosis is extremely difficult in LAU. Because the diagnosis of definite LAU requires histologic confirmation, by definition, the prognosis for visual recovery and saving the eye is probably extremely poor in the classic, well-documented cases. In addition, most series include cases from the pre-1970s, prior to the advent of sophisticated microsurgical techniques for repairing traumatic

---

*T.H. Neuhann, personal communication.

or surgical wounds. In modern practice, however, it is highly likely that milder, presumed (but unverified) cases respond relatively well to modern surgical therapy, and in general, the prognosis for saving the eye is excellent if timely surgical intervention is performed.

The visual prognosis probably remains guarded in eyes with established LAU, but good vision can be recovered in some cases if severe LAU is prevented by timely intervention. In a review (between 1990 and 1992) of 59 patients at BPEI who were undergoing surgical management for dislocated lens fragments after cataract surgery, 70% of eyes recovered at least 20/40 vision.* Of eyes with sterile hypopyon uveitis associated with retained lens fragments after cataract surgery, however, only two of four eyes achieved visual acuity better than 20/40—although inflammation subsided in all eyes after vitrectomy.[47] Retinal detachment is a frequent complication, and other problems including corneal edema, cystoid macular edema, and glaucoma can persist even after surgical therapy and cessation of acute inflammation. In cases of chronic LAU associated with trauma, long-term visual prognosis can be quite poor.

REFERENCES

1. Abbas AK, Lichtman AH, Pober JS: *Molecular and cellular immunology,* Philadelphia, 1991, WB Saunders.
2. Adams DO: The granulomatous response, *Am J Pathol* 84:164-191, 1976.
3. Adams H, Daus W, Neubauer G: Phacogenic reactions in animal experiments. In First International Symposium on Uveitis, Hanasarri, Espoo, Finland, 1984, Excerpta Medica.
4. Apple DJ, Solomon DD, Tetz MR: Posterior capsule opacification, *Surv Ophthalmol* 37:73-116, 1992.
5. Apple DJ, Tetz MR, Legler UFC: Localized endophthalmitis. In Bialasiewicz AA, editor: *Fortschr ophthalmology* 378, 1991.
6. Arnon R, Teitelbaum D: On the existence of suppressor cells, *Int Arch Allergy Immunol* 100:2-7, 1993.
7. Aronson S: Annual review: The uvea, *Arch Ophthalmol,* 79:495, 1968.
8. Asano M, Nakane A, Minagawa T: Endogenous gamma interferon is essential in granuloma formation induced by glycolipid-containing mycolic acid in mice, *Infect Immun* 61:2872-2878, 1993.
9. Bloch-Michel E: Autoimmunity to the lens. In Campinchi R, Faure JP, Haut J, editors: *Uveitis: immunologic and allergic phenomena,* Springfield, 1973, Charles C. Thomas.
10. Blodi BA, Flynn HW Jr, Blodi CF et al.: Retained lens nuclei after cataract surgery, *Ophthalmology* 99:41-44, 1992.
11. Blodi FC: Sympathetic uveitis as an allergic phenomenon: with a study of its association with phacoanaphylactic uveitis and a report on the pathologic findings in sympathizing eyes, *Trans Am Acad Ophthalmol Otolaryngol* 63:642-649, 1959.
12. Bloom BR, Salgame P, Diamond B: Revisiting and revising suppressor T cells, *Immunol Today* 13:131-136, 1992.
13. Champion R, McDonnell PJ, Green WR: Intraocular lenses: histopathologic characteristics of a large series of autopsy eyes, *Surv Ophthalmol* 30:1-32, 1985.
14. Cohen IR, Young DB: Autoimmunity, microbial immunity and the immunologic homunculus, *Immunol Today* 12:105-110, 1991.
14a. Cousins SW, Kraus-Mackiw E: Unpublished data.
15. Cousins SW, Streilein JW: Immune privilege and its regulation by immunosuppressive growth factors in aqueous humor. In Usui M, Ohno S, Aoki K, editors: *Ocular immunology today,* 81-84, Amsterdam, 1990, Excerpta Medica.
16. D'Ermo F, Secchi AG, Segato T et al.: Immunopathology of the lens. II. 86Rb efflux and protein leakage from normal lenses exposed to antilens and antiuveoretina antibodies, *Ophthalmologica* 176:230-237, 1978.
17. Daviel J, editor: *Sur une nouvelle method de guerir la cataracte par l'extraction du crystalin,* Paris, 1753, Academe Royale.
18. Davis JL, Winward KR, Lonardo EC et al.: Association of *P. acnes* endophthalmitis with HLA type, *Invest Ophthalmol Vis Sci* 33(suppl):1421, 1992.
19. Davson H: *Physiology of the eye,* New York, 1990, Pergamon Press.
20. deVeer JA: Bilateral endophthalmitis phacoanaphylactica, *Arch Ophthalmol* 49:607-632, 1953.
21. Domarus von D, Hinzpeter EN, Naumann GOH: Klinik der "Endophthalmitis phacoanaphylactica," *Klin Mbl Augenheilk* 166:637-644, 1975.
22. Doren GS, Stern GA, Driebe WT: Indications for and results of intraocular lens explanation, *J Cataract Refract Surg* 18:79-85, 1992.
23. Duke-Elder WS: *Diseases of the lens and vitreous: glaucoma and hypotony,* St Louis, 1969, Mosby.
24. Easom HA, Zimmerman LE: Sympathetic ophthalmia and bilateral phacoanaphylaxis, *Arch Ophthalmol* 72:9-16, 1964.
25. Ehrlich P, Morgenroth J: Uber Hamolysine. III. Mitteilung, *Berlin Klinische Wschr,* 37:453-458, 1900.
26. Fastenberg DM, Schwartz PL, Shakin JL, Gloub BM: Management of dislocated nuclear fragments after phacoemulsification, *Am J Ophthalmol* 112:535-562, 1991.
27. Ferrick MR, Thurau SR, Oppenheim MH et al.: Ocular inflammation stimulated by intravitreal interleukin-8 and interleukin-1, *Invest Ophthalmol Vis Sci* 32:1534-1539, 1991.
28. Fiedlander MH: *Allergy and immunology of the eye,* Cambridge, 1986, Harper & Row.
29. Flocks M, Littwin CS, Zimmerman LE: Phacolytic glaucoma: a clinicopathologic study of 138 cases of glaucoma associated with hypermature cataract, *Arch Ophthalmol* 54:541-547, 1955.
30. Fox GM, Joondeph BC, Flynn HW et al.: Delayed onset pseudophakic endophthalmitis, *Am J Ophthalmol* 111:163-171, 1991.
31. Frank MM, Fries LF: Complement. In Paul WE, editor: *Fundamental immunology,* 679-702, New York, 1989, Raven Press.
32. Gammon G, Sercarz E: Does the presence of self-reactive T cells indicate the breakdown of tolerance? *Clin Immunol Immunopath* 56:287-297, 1990.
33. Gery I, Nussenblatt R, BenEzra D: Dissociation between humoral and cellular immune responses to lens antigens, *Invest Ophthalmol Vis Sci* 20:32, 1981.
34. Gilliland GD, Hutton WL, Fuller DG: Retained intravitreal lens fragments after cataract surgery, *Ophthalmology* 99:1263-1269, 1992.
35. Girin L: *De l'inflammation de l'oeil qui suit l'operation de la cataract par abaissement,* Paris, 1836, La Faculté de Médecine.
36. Goldschmidt L, Goldbaum M, Walker SM, Weigle WO: The immune response to homologous lens crystallin. I. Antibody production after lens injury, *J Immunol* 129:1652-1657, 1982.
37. Goldschmidt L, Goldbaum M, Walker SM, Weigle WO: The immune response to homologous lens crystallin. II. A model of ocular inflammation involving eye injuries at separate times, *J Immunol* 129:1658-1662, 1982.
38. Goodner EK: Lens-induced uveitis in rabbits. In Maumenee AE, Silverstein AM, editors: *Immunopathology of uveitis,* 233-242, Baltimore, 1964, Williams & Wilkins.
39. Green WR: Diagnostic cytopathology of ocular fluid specimens, *Ophthalmology* 91:726-749, 1984.
40. Hackett E, Thompson A: Anti-lens antibody in human sera, *Lancet* 663, 1964.
41. Hara Y, Caspi RR, Wiggert B et al.: Suppression of experimental autoimmune uveitis in mice by induction of ACAID with interreceptor retinol binding protein, *J Immunol* 148:1685-1692, 1992.
42. Hirschberg J: *The renaissance of ophthalmology in the eighteenth century (part one),* 143-222, Bonn, 1984, Wayenborgh.

*H. Flynn, personal communication.

43. Hodes BL, Stern G: Echographic diagnosis of phacoanaphylactic endophthalmitis, *Ophthalmic Surg* 7:60-65, 1976.
44. Horwitz J: The function of alpha-crystallin, *Invest Ophthalmol Vis Sci* 34:10-22, 1993.
45. Hutton WL, Snyder WB, Vaiser A: Management of surgically dislocated intravitreal lens fragments by pars plana vitrectomy, *Trans Am Acad Ophthalmol Otolaryngol* 85:176-181, 1978.
46. Ingolia TD, Craig EA: Four small Drosophila heat shock proteins are related to each other and to mammalian alpha-crystallin, *Proc Natl Acad Sci* 79:2360-2364, 1982.
47. Irvine WD, Flynn HW, Murray TG, Rubsamen PE: Retained lens fragments after phacoemulsification manifesting as marked intraocular inflammation with hypopyon, *Am J Ophthalmol* 114:610-614, 1992.
48. Ishimoto SI, Sanui H, Ishibashi T, Inomata H: Experimental lens-induced granulomatous endophthalmitis in guinea pigs. In Usui M, Ohno S, Aoki K, editors: *Ocular immunology today,* 167-170, Amsterdam, 1990, Excerpta Medica.
49. Kappler JW, Roehm N, Marrack P: T cell tolerance by clonal elimination in the thymus, *Cell* 49:273-280, 1987.
50. Kato K, Shinohara H, Kurobe N et al.: Immunoreactive αA-crystallin in rat nonlenticular tissues detected with a sensitive immunoassay, *Biochem Biophys Acta* 1080:173-180, 1991.
51. Kelman CD: Phacoemulsification and aspiration: a new technique of cataract removal: a preliminary report, *Am J Ophthalmol* 64:23-25, 1967.
52. Kelman CD: History of phacoemulsification. In Phacoemulsification and Aspiration of Cataracts. (Emory JM, Little JH, eds.) C.V. Mosby, St. Louis, 1979.
53. Khalil MK, Lorenzetti DW: Lens-induced inflammations, *Can J Ophthalmol* 21:96, 1986.
54. Klein J: *Immunology,* Boston, 1990, Blackwell Scientific.
55. Klemenz R, Frohli E, Steiger RH et al.: αB-crystallin is a small heat shock protein, *Proc Natl Acad Sci* 88:3652-3656, 1991.
56. Kraus-Mackiw E: Immunophthalmalogische Untersuchungen mit Hetero- und Auto-Antiseren. Ein kritischer Beitrag zur Autoimmunpathogenese von Augenerkrankungen. In Bargmann W, Doerr W, editors: *Normale und pathologische Anatomie,* Stuttgart, 1972, Thieme.
57. Kraus-Mackiw E, Buttner K, Muller-Ruchholtz W: Lens-induced uveitis: further immunologic studies in an experimental model, *Graefes Arch Klin Exp Ophthalmol* 202:297-303, 1977.
58. Kraus-Mackiw E, Coles RS: Exogenous uveitis: sympathetic ophthalmia and toxic lens syndrome. In Kraus-Mackiw E, O'Connor GR, editors: *Uveitis: pathophysiology and therapy,* Stuggart, 1986, Goerg Thieme Verlag.
58a. Lai JC, Wawrousek EF, Lee RS, Chan C-C, Whitcup SM and Gery I. Analysis of peripheral tolerance to autologous antigens expressed in an immunologically privileged site. In: Nussenblatt RB, Whitcup SM, Caspi RR, Gery I, editors. Adv Ocular Immunol., Amsterdam, 1994, Elsevier.
59. Lane C, Streilein JWS, Cousins SW: Lens-induced uveitis associated with intraocular delayed hypersensitivity to bacterial antigens, *Invest Ophthalmol Vis Sci* 32:936, 1991.
60. Little J: 1963.
61. Lubin JR, Alber DM, MW: Sixty-five years of sympathetic ophthalmia: a clinicopathologic review of 105 cases (1913-1978), *Ophthalmology* 87:109-121, 1980.
62. Luntz MH: Experimental endophthalmitis phacoanaphylactica, *Exp Eye Res* 3:166-168, 1964.
63. Luntz MH: Anti-uveal and anti-lens antibodies and their significance, *Exp Eye Res* 7:561-569, 1968.
64. Lyda W, Lippincott SW: Lens-induced endophthalmitis, *Am J Ophthalmol* 40:120, 1955.
65. Manski W, Wirostko E, Halbert SP, Hofeldt AJ: Autoimmune phenomena in the eye. In Mieschner PA, Müller Eberhard HJ, editors: *Immunopathology,* 877, San Francisco, 1976, Grune & Strattner.
66. Marak GE: Phacoanaphylactic endophthalmitis, *Surv Ophthalmol* 36:325-339, 1992.
67. Marak GE, Font RA, Alepa P: T-cell function in lens-induced endophthalmitis. In *XXIII Concilium Ophthalmologicum Acta,* 1978, Kyoto.
68. Marak GE, Font RL, Alepa FP, Ward PA: Effects of C3 inactivator factor on the development of experimental lens-induced granulomatous endophthalmitis, *Ophthalmol Res* 9:416-420, 1979.
69. Marak GE, Font RL, Ward PA: Fluorescent antibody studies in experimental lens-induced granulomatous endophthalmitis, *Ophthalmol Res* 9:317-320, 1977.
70. Marak GE, Rao NA, Scott JM et al.: Antioxidant modulation of phacoanaphylactic endophthalmitis, *Ophthalmol Res* 17:297-301, 1985.
71. Marak GE, Font RL, Alepa FP: Experimental lens-induced granulomatous endophthalmitis: passive transfer with serum, *Ophthalmic Res* 8:117-122, 1976.
72. Marak GE, Font RL, Alepa FP: Arthus-type panophthalmitis in rats sensitized to heterologous lens protein, *Opthalmic Res* 9:162-170, 1977.
73. Marak GE, Font RL, Alepa FP: Immunopathogenicity of lens crystallins in the production of experimental lens-induced granulomatous endophthalmitis, *Ophthalmic Res* 10:30-36, 1978.
74. Marak GE, Font RL, Czawlytko LN, Alepa FP: Experimental lens-induced granulomatous endophthalmitis: preliminary histopathologic observations, *Exp Eye Res* 19:311-316, 1974.
75. Marak GE, Font RL, Rao NA: Abrogation of tolerance to lens protein. I. Effects of lipopolysaccharide, *Ophthalmol Res* 11:192, 1979.
76. Marak GE, Font RL, Rao NA: Strain differences in autoimmunity to lens protein, *Ophthalmol Res* 13:320-329, 1981.
77. Marak GE, Font RL, Weigle WO: Pathogenesis of lens-induced endophthalmitis. In Silverstein AM, O'Connor GR, editors: *Immunology and immunopathology of the eye,* New York, 135, 1979 Masson.
78. Marak GE, Lim LY, Rao NA: Abrogation of tolerance to lens protein: II. Allogeneic effect, *Ophthalmic Res* 14:176-181, 1982.
79. Marak GE, Rao NA, Antonakou G, Sliwinski A: Experimental lens-induced granulomatous endophthalmitis in common laboratory animals, *Ophthalmol Res* 14:292-297, 1982.
80. McDonnell PJ, Green WR, Champion R: Pathologic changes in pseudophakia, *Semin Ophthalmol* 1:80-103, 1986.
81. McGahan MC: Does the lens serve as a 'sink' for iron during ocular inflammation? *Exp Eye Res* 54:525-530, 1992.
82. Meisler DM, Mandelbaum S: Propionibacterium associated endophthalmitis after extracapsular cataract extraction: a review of reported cases, *Ophthalmology* 98:56-61, 1989.
83. Meisler DM, Palestine AG, Vastine DW, Demartini DR: Chronic propionibacterium endophthalmitis after extracapsular cataract extraction and intraocular lens implantation, *Am J Ophthalmol* 102:733-739, 1986.
84. Meisler DM, Zakov ZN, Bruner WE et al.: Endophthalmitis associated with sequestered intraocular propionibacterium acnes, *Am J Ophthalmol* 10:428, 1987.
85. Menikoff JA, Speaker MG, Marmor M, Raskin EM: A case-control study of risk factors for postoperative endophthalmitis, *Ophthalmol* 98:1761-1768, 1991.
86. Miller JFA, Morahan G: Peripheral T cell tolerance, *Ann Rev Immun* 10:51-70, 1992.
87. Misra RN, Rahi AHS, Morgan G: Immunopathology of the lens. II. Humoral and cellular immune responses to homologous lens antigens and their roles in ocular inflammation, *Br J Ophthalmol* 61:285, 1977.
88. Misra RN, Rahi AHS, Morgan G: Immunopathology of the lens. III. Humoral and cellular immune responses to autologous lens antigens and their roles in ocular inflammation, *Br J Ophthalmol* 61:371-379, 1977.
89. Mitchison NA: Specialization, tolerance, memory, competition, latency and strife among T cells, *Ann Rev Immun* 10:1-12, 1992.
90. Mizuno K, Clark AF, Streilein JW: Anterior chamber associated immune deviation induced by soluble antigens, *Invest Ophthalmol Vis Sci* 30:1112-1119, 1989.
91. Mosmann T, Coffman RC: TH1 and TH2 cells: different patterns of lymphockine secretion lead to different functional properties, *Ann Rev Immun* 7:145-173, 1989.
92. Mueller DL, Jenkins MK, Schwartz RH: Clonal expansion vs functional clonal inactivation, *Ann Rev Immun* 7:445-479, 1989.
93. Muller H: Phacolytic glaucoma and phacogenic ophthalmia (lens-induced uveitis), *Trans Ophthalmol Soc UK* 83:689-704, 1963.
94. Muller KM, Jaunin F, Masouye I et al.: Th2 cells mediate IL-4 dependent local tissue inflammation, *J Immunol* 150:5576-5584, 1993.

95. Muller-Hermelink HK, Daus W: Recent topics in the pathology of uveitis. In Kraus-Mackiw E, O'Connor GR, editors: *Uveitis: pathophysiology and therapy,* 155-203, Stuttgart, 1986, Thieme.

96. Muller-Hermelink HK, Kruas-Mackiw E, Daus W, Adams H: Lens as inducer and target in uveitis: comparison of different types of naturally occurring and experimentally induced phacogenic reactions. In Kraus-Mackiw E, O'Connor GR, editors: *Uveitis: pathophysiology and therapy,* 155, Stuttgart, 1986, Thieme.

97. Neubauer G, Kraus-Mackiw E: Inflammation after intraocular surgery and IOL implant in inbred rats. In Usui M, Ohno S, Aoki K, editors: *Ocular immunology today,* Amsterdam, 1990, Excerpta Medica.

98. Niederkorn JY: Immune privilege and immune regulation of the eye, *Adv Immunol* 48:191, 1990.

99. Nossal GJV: Immunologic tolerance. In Paul WE, editor: *Fundamental immunology,* 571-586, New York, 1989, Raven Press.

100. Nossal GJV: Immunologic tolerance: collaboration between antigen and lymphokines, *Science* 245:147-153, 1989.

101. Ohrloff C, Dardenne MU, Konen C, Sherif A: Erfahrungen mit den ersten 1400 Hinterkammerlinsenimplantationen nach Phako-emulsifikation, *Klin Mbl Augenheilk* 181:253-256, 1982.

102. Opremcak ME, Scales DK: Enumeration of autoreactive, cytokine secreting T cells by LDA in patients with uveitis, *Invest Ophthalmol Vis Sci* 33(suppl):931, 1992.

103. Panel CMG: *Management of functional impairment due to cataracts in adults,* Rockville, 1993, U.S. Department of Health and Human.

104. Parmigiani CM, McAvoy JW: The roles of laminin and fibronectin in the development of the lens capsule, *Curr Eye Res* 10:501-511, 1991.

105. Patel M, Shine B, Muuray PI: Antilens antibodies in cataract and inflammatory eye disease: an evaluation of a new technique, *Int Ophthalmol* 14:97-100, 1990.

106. Pitatigorsky J: Gene expression and genetic engineering in the lens, *Invest Ophthalmol Vis Sci* 28:9, 1987.

107. Rao NA: Role of oxygen free radicals in retinal damage associated with experimental uveitis, *Trans Am Ophthalmol Soc* 89:797-850, 1990.

108. Rao NA, Calandra AJ, Sevanian A et al.: Modulation of lens-induced uveitis by superoxide dismutase, *Ophthal Res* 18:41-46, 1986.

109. Rose NR: Pathogenic mechanisms in autoimmune diseases, *Clin Immunol Immunopath* 53:S7-S16, 1989.

110. Rosenbaum JT, Samples JR, Seymour B et al.: Chemotactic activity of lens proteins and the pathogenesis of phacolytic glaucoma, *Arch Ophthalmol* 105:1582, 1987.

111. Roussel TJ, Culbertson WW, Jaffe NS: Chronic postoperative endophthalmitis associated with propionibacterium acnes, *Arch Ophthalmol* 104:1199, 1987.

112. Sandberg HO: The alpha crystallin content of aqueous humor in cortical, nuclear and complicated cataracts, *Exp Eye Res* 22:75-84, 1976.

113. Sandberg HO, Closs O: The humoral response to alpha, beta and gamma crystallins of the human lens, *Scand J Ophthalmol* 10:549-554, 1979.

114. Sandberg HO, Closs O: The immune response to lens antigens. In Silverstein AM, O'Conner GR, editors: *Immunology and immunopathology of the eye,* 151-154, 1979, Mason Press. New York

115. Scherzer H, Ward PA: Lung injury produced by immune complexes of varying composition, *J Immunol* 121:947-952, 1978.

116. Schirmer O: Ueber eine benigne postoperative Cyklitis auf infectioser Basis. In Straub M, editor: *Acta IX. Congres International d'ophthalmologie d'Utrecht, du 14-18 Aout, 1899,* Amsterdam, 1900, Bergmann van Rossen.

117. Schlaegel TF, Coles RS: Uveitis and miscellaneous general diseases. In Duane TD, editor: *Clinical ophthalmology,* Philadelphia, 1983, Harper & Row.

118. Schwartz RH: Acquisition of immunologic self-tolerance, *Cell* 57:1073-1081, 1989.

119. Semel J, Bowe B, Guo A et al.: Propionibacterium acnes-enhanced lens-induced granulomatous uveitis in the rat, *Invest Ophthalmol Vis Sci* 33:1766-1770, 1992.

120. Sercarz E, Oki A, Gammon G: Central versus peripheral tolerance: clonal inactivation versus suppressor T cells, the second half of the "Thirty Years War," *Immunology* 2:9-14, 1989.

121. Sheffield EA: The granulomatous inflammatory response, *J Pathol* 160:1-2, 1990.

122. Silverstein AM: The history of immunology. In Paul WE, editor: *Fundamental immunology,* New York, 1989, Raven Press.

122a. Smiddy WE, Flynn HW Jr: Management of retained lens nuclear fragments and dislocated posterior chamber intraocular lenses after cataract surgery, *Semin Ophthalmol* 8:96-103, 1993.

123. Snapper CM, Mond JJ: Towards a comprehensive view of immunoglobulin class switching, *Immunol Today* 14:15-17, 1993.

124. Straub M: *Over Ontsteikingen van het Oog veroorzaakt door oplossing van lens massa in de Oog Lymphe,* Amsterdam, 1919, DeBussy.

125. Streilein JW: Immune regulation and the eye: a dangerous compromise, *FASEB* 1:199, 1987.

126. Sunakawa M, Yoshida H, Arai I, Okinami S: Anti-lens crystallin antibodies in human sera. II. Uveitis, *Acta Soc Ophthalmol Jpn* 91:699, 1987.

127. Thatch AB, Marak GEJ, McLean IW, Green WR: Phacoanaphylactic endophthalmitis: a clinicopathologic review, *Int Ophthalmol* 15:271-279, 1991.

128. Thompson WS, Rubsamen PE, Schiffman J, Cousins SW: Risk factors for the development of endophthalmitis following penetrating ocular trauma, *Invest Ophthalmol Vis Sci* 34:1113, 1993.

129. Uhlenhuth P: Zur Lehre von der Unterscheidung verschiedener Eiweißarten mit Hilfe spezifischer Sera. In Festschrift zum 60., Jena, 1903, Fischer.

130. Verhoeff FH, Lemoine AN: Endophthalmitis phacoanaphylactica, *Am J Ophthalmol* 5:737-745, 1922.

131. von Boehmer H, Kisielow P: How the immune system learns about self, *Sci Am* 74-81, 1991.

132. von Boehmer H, Teh HS, Kisielow P: The thymus selects the useful, neglects the useless and destroys the harmful, *Immunol Today* 10:57-61, 1989.

133. Weetman AP, McGregor AM: Autoimmune thyroid disease: developments in our understanding, *Endocr Rev* 5:309-355, 1984.

134. Weigle WO: Immunological unresponsiveness, *Adv Immunol* 16:61-122, 1973.

135. Weigle WO: Analysis of autoimmunity through experimental models of thyroiditis and allergic encephalomyelitis, *Adv Immunol* 30:159-273, 1980.

136. Wilbanks GA, Mammolenti MM, Streilein JW: Studies on the induction of Anterior Chamber Associated Immune Deviation (ACAID). II. Eye-derived cells participate in generating blood-borne signals that induce ACAID, *J Immunol* 146:3018, 1991.

137. Wilbanks GA, Mammolenti MM, Streilein JW: Studies on the induction of Anterior Chamber Associated Immune Deviation. III. Induction of anterior chamber associated immune deviation depends upon intraocular transforming growth factor-B, *Eur J Immunol* 22:165, 1992.

138. Wilbanks GA, Streilein JW: Characterization of humoral immune responses following anterior chamber and intravenous administration of soluble antigen: B-cell secretion of complement-fixing antibody is selectively and actively suppressed. In Usui M, Ohno S, Aoki K, editors: *Ocular immunology today,* Amsterdam, 1990, Excerpta Medica.

139. Wilbanks GA, Streilein JW: Distinctive humoral responses following anterior chamber and intravenous administration of soluble antigen. Evidence for active suppression of IgG_{2a}-secreting B cells, *Immunology* 71:566, 1990.

140. Wilhelmus K, Emery J: Posterior capsule opacification following phacoemulsification, *Ophthalmic Surg* 11:264-267, 1980.

141. Wilson-Holt N, Hing S, Taylor DSJ: Bilateral blinding uveitis in a child after secondary intraocular lens implantation for unilateral cataract, *J Pediatr Ophthalmol Strabismus* 28:116-118, 1991.

142. Winton A, Eshbaugh C, Roth E, Cousins SW: Intraocular macrophage activation and lens-associated uveitis, 34(suppl):1482, 1993.

143. Winward KE, Pflugfelder SC, Flynn HW et al.: Postoperative propionibacterium endophthalmitis. Treatment strategies and long-term results, *Ophthalmology* 100:447-451, 1993.

144. Wirostko E, Spalter HF: Lens-induced uveitis, *Arch Ophthalmol* 78:1, 1967.

145. Wistow GJ, Piatigorsky J: Recruitment of enzymes as lens structural proteins, *Science* 236:1554-1556, 1987.

146. Wistow GJ, Piatigorsky J: Lens crystallins: the evolution and expression of proteins for a highly specialized tissue, *Ann Rev Biochem* 57:479-504, 1987.
147. Wood CA: *The American encyclopedia and dictionary of ophthalmology,* Chicago, 1913, Cleveland Press.
148. Woods AC: An adventure in ophthalmic literature: Manuel Straub and the tradition of toxicity in lens protein, *Am J Ophthalmol* 48:463-472, 1959.
149. Woods AC: Lens-induced uveitis. In *Endogenous inflammations of the uveal tract,* 211-236, Baltimore, 1961, Williams & Wilkins.

149a. Woodward JG, Martin WD, Stevens JL, Egan RL: Immunological recognition of transgene encoded MHC class I alloantigen in the lens. In Nussenblatt RB, Whitcup SM, Caspi RR, Gery I, editors: *Adv Ocular Immunol,* Amsterdam, 1994, Elsevier.
150. Yang CM, Cousins SW: Fate of the fellow eye in *Probionibacterium acnes* infection, *Am J Ophthalmol* 68:99-100, 1992.
151. Zambrano W, Flynn HW, Pflugfelder SC et al.: Management options for *Propionibacterium acnes* endophthalmitis, *Opthalmology* 96:1100-1105, 1989.

43 Posner-Schlossman Syndrome

CARL B. CAMRAS, DAVID M. CHACKO, ABRAHAM SCHLOSSMAN, ADOLPH POSNER

The syndrome of recurrent glaucomatocyclitic crises, or the Posner-Schlossman syndrome, is a rare and poorly understood clinical entity that typically occurs in young to middle-aged adults. The symptoms include a history of intermittent episodes of mild ocular discomfort and slightly blurred vision in one eye. Patients with Posner-Schlossman syndrome have very high intraocular pressure (IOP), with open angles and minimal evidence of anterior segment inflammation. The level of IOP, typically at 40 to 60 mm Hg, is out of proportion to the minimal symptomatology and inflammatory findings. These patients respond well to medical therapy with ocular hypotensive agents and topical corticosteroids. They have an excellent long-term prognosis, with very few developing evidence of permanent functional visual loss.

HISTORICAL BACKGROUND

In 1929 Terrien and Veil[59] described seven patients with uveitis and glaucoma. Several of these patients had persistent inflammation, rather than acute recurrent attacks, and two were found to have syphilis. Of these seven cases, three or four had a clinical picture resembling glaucomatocyclitic crises. Only one of these four patients was followed long enough to verify that recurrent attacks occurred.

In 1935 Kraupa[30] described four patients with a distinct clinical entity characterized by recurrent episodes of uniocular inflammation and glaucoma. All four patients had iris heterochromia. Kraupa felt that the underlying pathogenesis was related to the sympathetic nervous system. He labeled this syndrome "glaucoma allergicum," without precisely describing the patients' allergies.

In 1944 Kronfeld[31] reported a group of "cases of acute elevation of IOP occurring simultaneously with mild recurrent cyclitis." He felt that these patients represented a "clinical entity," but gave no detailed description of this syndrome.

In 1948 Posner and Schlossman[43] provided a precise, detailed description of the clinical entity that has come to bear their name. A series of nine patients had the clinical features that they described (see box). Although three of their original nine patients exhibited iris heterochromia,[43] they did not observe heterochromia in any of their patients subsequently diagnosed with glaucomatocyclitic crises;[45] therefore, despite their original description, they decided that heterochromia was not characteristic of this syndrome.[45]

EPIDEMIOLOGY

Glaucomatocyclitic crises tend to occur in young adults, usually in the age range of 20 to 50 years, and rarely occur in patients older than 60 years. There is no apparent racial or ethnic predilection. Although only five of the nine patients originally described by Posner and Schlossman[43] were men, all subsequent series of substantial size have demonstrated a preponderance of men as follows (number of men per total number of patients): nine of 11,[19] six of seven,[18] nine of 11,[27] 10 of 11,[36] 17 of 17,[5] and 19 of 32.[28] The incidence or prevalence of Posner-Schlossman syndrome in the general population or as a subset of patients in a uveitis or glaucoma practice is unknown. Nevertheless, it is a rare disease that is seldom diagnosed in the practicing lifetime of a general ophthalmologist.

Although Posner's and Schlossman's original description[43] and follow-up report[45] emphasized that the disease was unilateral, with each recurrent attack in the same eye of an individual patient, several subsequent series have reported bilateral involvement in some patients.* In a series of 11 patients described by Higgitt,[19] one patient exhibited attacks in both eyes, but never simultaneously. Brooks and associates[5] found that seven of 17 patients had both eyes affected, with attacks often occurring simultaneously, but asymmetrically. These patients with bilateral involvement tended to have more severe disease, with each attack lasting longer and occurring more frequently, over a greater number

---

*References 5, 11, 19, 28, 32, 37, 40, 42, 47.

of years. Of 32 patients described by Knox,[28] six exhibited bilateral involvement. Two of these six occasionally experienced simultaneous attacks in both eyes.

CLINICAL FEATURES

Patients with glaucomatocyclitic crises typically have symptoms of mild ocular discomfort. The few, mild symptoms are surprising in view of the extreme elevation of IOP. Some patients are totally asymptomatic. In view of the minimal symptomatology, it seems possible that undiagnosed attacks may occasionally occur in some patients. Photophobia rarely occurs. Because corneal edema may be induced by the very high IOPs, some patients report mildly blurred vision and colored halos around lights. Although symptomatology is usually strikingly slight or absent, a few case reports describe more severe symptoms, including a single patient who experienced severe ocular pain,[33] and another who had projectile vomiting.[46]

In Posner's and Schlossman's[43] original series of nine patients, three had a pupil that was slightly dilated and sluggishly reactive to light in the affected eye. Rarely, the anisocoria persisted between the attacks.

Despite the high IOP, the conjunctiva usually is not injected and does not exhibit ciliary flush. Occasionally, very mild injection occurs. In contrast, several case reports describe severe conjunctival hyperemia.[1,24,26,37,63]

The acute, abrupt rise in IOP to the levels characteristic of glaucomatocyclitic crises will occasionally result in mild microcystic edema of the cornea. Keratic precipitates may precede, occur simultaneously with, or follow the onset of the IOP rise by a few days. The keratic precipitates are small, discrete, well defined, flat, round, and without pigmentation.[43] They vary in number from 0 to 25 and usually appear in the lower one third of the cornea. They may disappear and then reappear at some later time during the attack.

Brooks and associates[5] found no change in the endothelial cell counts in patients with the Posner-Schlossman syndrome. On the other hand, Setala and Vannas[52] found a reduced central endothelial cell count in 16 of 16 patients having several attacks, two of three patients with two attacks, and none of four patients with a single attack. During attacks, no more than trace aqueous flare and rare anterior chamber cells are present.

Although heterochromia was present in several of the patients described by Kraupa[30] and in three of the original nine patients described by Posner and Schlossman,[43] it has not been a feature of most cases reported subsequently. Several other authors, however, also reported heterochromia.* Sugar[58] found heterochromia in 5 of 11 patients in his series, and in 16 of 119 from the literature at that time. Hollwich[21] found that 30% to 40% of the patients in his series had obvious heterochromia. Sokolic[55] felt that the heterochromia was a developmental defect, as he found it at the time of a patient's first attack. On the other hand, Sugar[58] felt that the heterochromia was acquired as a result of recurrent attacks leading to iris stromal atrophy, with the presence and degree of heterochromia related to the degree and total duration of the cyclitic episodes. Adamantiadis[2] described a case in which heterochromia occurred only after 8 years of observation.

In a study evaluating iridial vasculature by fluorescein angiography,[49] focal, segmental iridial ischemia was noted during attacks of glaucomatocyclitic crises. Immediately following the attacks, congestion was noted with profuse leakage of vessels around the pupillary border. This leakage often occurred during a period of extreme ocular hypotony following the IOP elevation. During the intervals between attacks, a rich vascular pattern was observed with tortuous vascular tufts. Some eyes showed iris stromal and sphincter

---

*References 2, 10, 16, 21, 50, 51, 55, 58, 63.

atrophy between attacks, which were considered secondary to the marked IOP elevation.[49] Another study using iris fluorescein angiography demonstrated hypoperfusion with attenuated vessels.[5]

The rise in IOP may precede, occur simultaneously with, or follow the mild iridocyclitis by a few days. The IOP is often in the 40- to 60-mm Hg range during the attacks, but has been reported as high as 90 mm Hg.[44,45] The level of IOP does not appear to be related to the degree of inflammation. Acute attacks with very high IOP are often followed by a period of relative hypotony.

Most studies describe normal open angles during the attacks and during the intervals between attacks. Occasionally, a few tiny precipitates are noted in the angle. Others describe an anomalous angle believed by some to be related to the pathogenesis of the disease (see Pathogenesis section).

Despite the recurrent iridocyclitis, neither posterior synechiae nor peripheral anterior synechiae form in patients with recurrent glaucomatocyclitic crises, as originally noted by Posner and Schlossman.[43] Nevertheless, although distinctly uncharacteristic of the syndrome, posterior synechiae have been described in two patients.[26,33] In view of this unusual finding in these two patients, the validity of the diagnosis of the Posner-Schlossman syndrome comes into question, especially since these patients also had severe pain and intense conjunctival congestion (additional features that are rarely found in this syndrome).

Attacks of glaucomatocyclitic crises usually last 1 to 3 weeks, regardless of treatment. The length varies from as short as a few hours to as long as 1 month. The attacks rarely last longer than 2 weeks. Obvious precipitating events are not apparent in most patients. Of the seven patients followed by Hart and Weatherill,[18] however, one had recurrent attacks apparently associated with the onset of menstruation, and one had attacks that appeared to be seasonal.

Most reports describe completely normal eyes during the intervals between attacks. During these periods, provocative tests for glaucoma are usually negative, and symptoms and signs of iridocyclitis or glaucoma are absent.[43] Higgitt,[19] however, reported that in seven of 11 patients, IOP in the affected eye was consistently lower (by a few mm Hg) than in the contralateral eye during the interval between attacks. On the other hand, Kass, Becker, and Kolker[27] found that the IOP was above 21 mm Hg between attacks in 8 of 11 of their patients (see Pathogenesis section).

Most studies report that the contralateral, unaffected eyes of patients with Posner-Schlossman syndrome are totally normal. In contrast, Kass and associates[27] found increased IOP in the contralateral eye in nine of 11 patients.

COMPLICATIONS

Despite the extreme elevation of IOP during the attacks of glaucomatocyclitic crises, optic disc cupping and visual field loss rarely occur. Nevertheless, two of the nine patients

originally described by Posner and Schlossman[43] demonstrated permanent visual field loss. Some patients had transient enlargement of their blind spot during the episodes of extremely elevated IOP. Mattsson[37] reported a patient who developed optic disc atrophy. Iwata, Takahashi, and Kojima[25] also reported a patient who developed disc pallor, moderate glaucomatous excavation, and pronounced concentric constriction of the visual field. In a series of eleven patients reported by Kass and associates,[27] four developed asymmetric enlargement of their cup and five showed glaucomatous visual field loss in the affected eye. Hung and Chang[23] reported three patients with glaucomatocyclitic crises who developed optic disc cupping and visual field loss. In seventeen patients followed by Brooks and associates,[5] two developed visual field loss.

PATHOGENESIS

Although many studies allude to possible causes of Posner-Schlossman syndrome (see box), very little information exists that elucidates its pathogenesis or defines its pathologic features.

Aqueous Humor Dynamics

Several studies evaluated aqueous humor dynamics in patients with the Posner-Schlossman syndrome. All studies reported a reduction of outflow facility during attacks of glaucomatocyclitic crises.* In studies discussing the rate of aqueous humor formation, most described values in the low-to-normal range,[15,18,35] although two studies suggested an increase.[57,58] The rate of aqueous humor formation was not directly measured in any of these studies. Instead, it was indirectly calculated by the Goldmann equation, using the values for IOP and outflow facility and assuming that episcleral venous pressure was normal. At the time of these indirect calculations, factors such as uveoscleral outflow were not considered. Possible errors in concluding that hypersecretion exists have been previously discussed.[18] Considering all available information, it is unlikely that aqueous formation increases.

During the interval between attacks, most studies find outflow facility to be normal, or at times increased, compared with that in the contralateral unaffected eye.[15,19,35,57] On the other hand, Kass and associates[27] found reduced outflow facility in both affected and contralateral unaffected eyes in six of 11 patients.

Developmental Angle Anomaly

Several reports[18,40,54-56] describe angle anomalies in patients with the Posner-Schlossman syndrome and postulate that the syndrome represents a variant of developmental

---

*References 11, 15, 18, 19, 27, 35, 57, 58, 61.

POSSIBLE CAUSAL FACTORS IN THE PATHOGENESIS OF GLAUCOMATOCYCLITIC CRISES

Abnormalities in aqueous humor dynamics
Developmental angle anomaly
Sympathetic nervous system defect
Allergy
Gastrointestinal disturbances and emotional distress
Primary vascular abnormality
Immunogenetic disorder
Inflammation
Virus
Prostaglandins
Variant of primary open-angle glaucoma

---

glaucoma. Features on gonioscopy include the following: a thickened, anteriorly-displaced Schwalbe line, an abnormally wide trabecular meshwork, an irregular or anterior insertion of the iris, an indistinguishable scleral spur, absence of a normal angle recess, transparent fibers or cellophane tissue bridging the angle, many fine iris processes adhering to the trabecular meshwork, and fine irregular vessels in the angle.[18,40,55] The appearance of the angle was no different during the attacks of glaucomatocyclitic crises as compared to the intervals between attacks. Iris anomalies thought consistent with a developmental defect include heterochromia[55] or segmental hypoplasia of the iris stroma associated with microaneurysm.[56]

Hart and Weatherill[18] described angle anomalies mentioned previously in seven of seven patients with the Posner-Schlossman syndrome. They felt that the reduced outflow facility noted during attacks was explained by the angle anomalies,[18] but no explanation was offered to account for the normal outflow facility between attacks, despite the anomalous angles. The angle anomaly was usually felt to be more pronounced in the affected eye of patients with glaucomatocyclitic crises.[18] On histopathologic evaluation of a trabeculectomy specimen obtained from an eye with glaucomatocyclitic crises, a homogeneous, osminophilic membranous structure was observed on the surface of the trabecular meshwork.[34]

In the series of seven patients described by Hart and Weatherill,[18] two were brothers who had a family history of glaucoma. This family provided evidence for a recessive inheritance, similar to other types of developmental glaucoma. On the other hand, Levatin[32] described a patient with the Posner-Schlossman syndrome whose identical twin did not exhibit the syndrome.

The theory of a developmental glaucoma with an associated angle anomaly does not account for the episodic nature of the acute attacks of glaucomatocyclitic crises characteristic of this syndrome, or for the unilaterality of the attacks in patients with bilateral angle anomalies.

Sympathetic Nervous System

Involvement of the sympathetic nervous system in patients with the Posner-Schlossman syndrome with some type of autonomic imbalance has been suggested on the basis of the iris heterochromia that is occasionally present.[10,21,30,43] Posner and Schlossman[43] initially hypothesized that the syndrome resulted from a "central disturbance in the hypothalamus, superimposed on a labile peripheral autonomic nervous system," involving the sympathetic center in the diencephalon. With the exception of the iris heterochromia noted in a minority of patients, little evidence supports a causal role for the sympathetic nervous system.

Allergic Factors

Several studies suggest that an allergic factor is involved in the pathogenesis of the glaucomatocyclitic crises.[10,12,28-30,60] Kraupa[30] labeled the four patients in his series with the term "glaucoma allergicum," even though he did not precisely describe his patients' allergies. In a series of eight patients reported by Theodore,[60] two had hay fever and one had repeated episodes of vasomotor rhinitis, which often preceded the attacks of glaucomatocyclitic crises. A single patient described by Kornzweig[29] underwent a complete workup by an allergist, who suggested that the syndrome may represent "angioneurotic edema" of the eye. The patient received injections for ragweed and grasses, with an apparent reduction in the severity and frequency of attacks.

All 13 patients reported by Demailly, Zaegel, Blamoutier, and Abadie[12] had an atopic history. Immunity tests demonstrated positive responses to pneumallergens and to *Streptococcus hemolyticus*. Specific desensitization in early cases led to a reduced frequency and eventual resolution of recurrent attacks.[12]

Thirteen of 20 patients (65%) with the Posner-Schlossman syndrome reported by Knox[28] had a history of "major" allergies including hay fever, asthma, and eczema. Likewise, the International Uveitis Study Group found 55% of 90 patients with nonspecific uveitis had allergic symptoms.[28] Because allergic symptoms are very common and nonspecific, the ability to elicit an allergic history in a patient depends on the effort expended. Proper control groups are required before concluding that allergies occur at a greater frequency in patients with recurrent glaucomatocyclitic crises.

Gastrointestinal Disturbances and Emotional Distress

Several reports described an association of glaucomatocyclitic crises with gastrointestinal disturbances and emotional distress.[28,30,53] Kraupa[30] described his patients as "neurasthenic, angiopathic, and heavy cigarette smokers." One of his four patients had "spastichen darmsturungen," or a spastic intestinal disturbance. Simpson[53] described a single patient with "nervous tension" as a causal factor.

Knox[28] felt that his patients were intense and hyperactive, with attacks occurring during physical, emotional, and intellectual stress. Two of his 32 patients were emphatic that emotional distress was temporally associated with their recurrent attacks of glaucomatocyclitic crises. Eleven of his 32 patients had proven peptic ulcer disease, and another seven were suspects for this disease. Overall, 68% of the men and 38% of the women in his series had peptic ulcer disease, compared with a normal incidence of 10% to 20% and 5% in men and women, respectively.[28] In addition to the high incidence of peptic ulcer disease, 11 of his 32 patients had gastrointestinal disorders other than peptic ulcer disease.[28]

Primary Vascular Abnormality

A few studies suggest that the Posner-Schlossman syndrome may be caused by a primary vascular abnormality.[30,40,49] Iris fluorescein angiography demonstrated hypoperfusion with attenuated vessels.[5] Raitta and Vannas[49] felt that acute attacks of glaucomatocyclitic crises were due to abnormal reactivity of the autonomically-innervated vessels in the ciliary body. Initial ischemia of the ciliary vessels was followed by dilation and leakage. The extreme ocular hypotony that occasionally followed the hypertensive attacks was thought to be due to the collapse of ciliary secretion.[49] These vascular-induced episodes were similar to migraines. Naveh-Floman and associates[40] reported a single patient with an apparent retinal periphlebitis.

Immunogenetics

Using a standard microlymphocytotoxicity technique, Hirose, Ohno, and Matsuda[20] found HLA-Bw54 to be positive in 41% (9 out of 22) of Japanese patients with the Posner-Schlossman syndrome, but in only 8% of 195 unrelated, healthy controls. This finding suggests an immunogenetic factor that is closely associated with the major histocompatibility complex. Without providing direct evidence, Dernouchamps[13] also suggested that glaucomatocyclitic crises may represent the clinical expression of an immunologic reaction of the anaphylactoid type, in connection with a viral infection in genetically predisposed patients.

Inflammation

Although inflammatory signs are disproportionately minimal compared with the severe IOP elevation during attacks of glaucomatocyclitic crises, inflammation remains an important clinical feature of this syndrome. It is conceivable that the inflammation is extremely localized to the trabecular meshwork in glaucomatocyclitic crises. Therefore minimal inflammation spills over as a cellular response in the anterior chamber or causes a breakdown of the blood-aqueous barrier. This localized inflammatory reaction in the trabecular meshwork, or trabeculitis, may acutely and severely reduce outflow facility to cause high spikes in IOP. This hypothesis is difficult to prove, but seems logical. In a tissue specimen obtained from a patient with glaucomatocyclitic crises undergoing trabeculectomy, Harstad and Ringvold[17] found numerous mononuclear cells in the trabecular interspaces and a lack of vacuoles in the endothelium of the Schlemm canal.

Virus

Bloch-Michel, Dussaix, Cerqueti, and Patarin[4] found cytomegalovirus antibodies in the aqueous humor of seven of 11 patients with the Posner-Schlossman syndrome, but in only three of 379 control eyes with other uveitides. Dernouchamps[13] agreed with a possible viral cause, without providing direct evidence.

Prostaglandins

Masuda, Izawa, and Mishima[36] found significantly elevated prostaglandin (PG) E levels in the aqueous humor of seven patients during attacks of glaucomatocyclitic crises, compared with levels found in five patients (with normal IOPs) undergoing cataract extraction. Although the authors described a "probable" direct correlation between the IOP levels and the PGE levels, the actual results[36] do not appear to support such a correlation. Two of the seven patients also had aqueous humor samples assessed for PG levels during intervals between attacks, at which time lower values were found.

Eight patients were treated with indomethacin, an inhibitor of PG synthesis, administered orally during the attacks of glaucomatocyclitic crises for an average of 12 days.[36] Three of these patients were thought to exhibit a faster reduction of IOP than after previous episodes treated with acetazolamide, epinephrine, and/or topical dexamethasone. The patients were not randomized or masked, however, and historic controls were used for comparison. In three patients, subconjunctival injection of polyphloretin phosphate, a presumed PG inhibitor, resulted in a reduction of IOP in a few hours, but no controls were used.

Nagataki and Mishima[38] found that the transfer coefficient of fluorescein into the anterior chamber by flow or by diffusion was increased in the affected eye as compared to the contralateral control eye of patients during glaucomatocyclitic crises, or as compared to the same eye during remission. This effect is somewhat comparable to the effect of high doses of PGE administered to rabbit eyes, leading to an increase in blood-aqueous barrier permeability, ultrafiltration, and IOP.[41,64]

Several inconsistencies exist in the hypothesis proposing a causal relationship between PGs and glaucomatocyclitic crises. Although high doses of PGs cause an initial elevation of IOP in rabbits for a few hours,[8] most PGs result in a pronounced reduction—rather than elevation—of IOP in humans.[7,9] Only two PG types have been demonstrated to raise IOP in humans, but the rise is sustained for no longer than a few hours with either type.[14,39] During glaucomatocyclitic crises the IOP is elevated because of a marked reduction of outflow facility (see previous section on Aqueous

Humor Dynamics).* Thus far all PGs studied appear to increase uveoscleral outflow, and some occasionally increase outflow facility.[7,61] None have been shown to reduce outflow facility.

These observations make a causal relationship between glaucomatocyclitic crises and PGs most unlikely. Although elevated PG levels are associated with attacks of glaucomatocyclitic crises, they are not likely to contribute to the rise in IOP. On the contrary, PGs may be locally produced by ocular tissues to help counteract the rise in IOP that occurs during the attacks. Moreover, PGs probably mediate the ocular hypotony that often accompanies chronic uveitis.[8]

Variant of Primary Open-Angle Glaucoma

Several studies report a relationship between glaucomatocyclitic crises and primary open-angle glaucoma (POAG).† Posner and Schlossman[43] noted that two of their nine patients with glaucomatocyclitic crises had a positive family history for POAG. Hart and Weatherill[18] reported two brothers with glaucomatocyclitic crises, who had a positive family history for POAG. Sokolic[54] reported a patient with unilateral recurrent glaucomatocyclitic crises with POAG in the opposite eye. Varma, Katz, and Spaeth[62] reported a patient that seemed to have coexisting glaucomatocyclitic crises and POAG. In the 10 patients with glaucomatocyclitic crises studied by Raitta and Vannas,[49] one had concomitant POAG and two additional patients were suspects for POAG.

In fifteen patients with the Posner-Schlossman syndrome reported by Raitta and Klemetti,[48] a topical corticosteroid provocative test was positive in four (27%) affected eyes. When combined with water provocative testing, 33% of affected eyes and 47% of contralateral eyes showed a positive response to at least one of the two provocative tests.

Kass and associates[27] found that four of five patients with unilateral glaucomatocyclitic crises were high responders to topical corticosteroids in their contralateral eyes. Furthermore, the contralateral eye had abnormally low outflow facility values in six of their 11 patients. Outflow facility was low in all affected eyes tested during glaucomatocyclitic crises, and remained below normal in six of the 11 affected eyes tested during the interval between crises. Three of these 11 patients reported a positive family history for POAG in close relatives. Five of the 11 had glaucomatous visual field loss in the contralateral eye. Four of the seven patients tested with a glucose tolerance test were classified as having diabetes mellitus.[27]

Overall, a relationship between the Posner-Schlossman syndrome and POAG is suggested by the following: increased IOP, reduced outflow facility, and enlarged cup:disc ratio. Other evidence for such a relationship includes visual field loss in affected eyes (during intervals between attacks) and in contralateral eyes, positive corticosteroid and water-drinking provocative tests in affected and contralateral eyes, positive family history of POAG, and relatively high incidence of diabetes mellitus.

DIFFERENTIAL DIAGNOSIS

Common clinical entities in the differential diagnosis of recurrent glaucomatocyclitic crises are indicated in Table 43-1.

As with the Posner-Schlossman syndrome, patients with acute primary angle-closure glaucoma have acute elevations of IOP at very high levels in one eye. The corneas may be edematous, albeit more frequently with acute angle-closure glaucoma; and the pupils are often larger in the affected eye, with either clinical entity. Symptomatology, however, is often much more severe with acute angle-closure glaucoma; with patients complaining of severe pain, headaches, and photophobia. The conjunctiva is usually severely injected in angle-closure glaucoma. The diagnosis is established by gonioscopy, which shows a closed angle in the affected eye and a narrow angle in the contralateral eye of patients with acute primary angle-closure glaucoma. The angles are open in glaucomatocyclitic crises. Acute angle-closure glaucoma, but not glaucomatocyclitic crises, responds well to laser iridectomy.

Similarities between Fuchs uveitis syndrome and glaucomatocyclitic crises include minimal or absent symptomatology in the presence of very low-grade inflammation and iris heterochromia (more common with Fuchs uveitis syndrome). Fuchs uveitis syndrome produces chronic, low-grade inflammatory findings, whereas glaucomatocyclitic crises occur episodically. The IOP is much higher during attacks of glaucomatocyclitic crises than with Fuchs uveitis syndrome. Cataracts commonly occur with Fuchs uveitis syndrome. Rouher[50] described a patient with recurrent glaucomatocyclitic crises that seemed to transform into a case of Fuchs uveitis syndrome. Likewise, Sugar[58] reported three cases of glaucomatocyclitic crises that seemed to become cases of Fuchs uveitis syndrome. He concluded that "clinical separation of glaucomatocyclitic crises, heterochromic cyclitis [Fuchs uveitis syndrome], and mild uveitis glaucoma is difficult."

Patients with a nonspecific iridocyclitis usually have more symptomatology and inflammatory signs than those with glaucomatocyclitic crises. With a nonspecific iridocyclitis, IOP is not as elevated and may in fact be normal or reduced. The pupil may be smaller, rather than larger, in the affected eye. Posterior synechiae and peripheral anterior synechiae may develop. Differential features may be blurred, however, occasionally making the distinction between these entities very difficult.[50,58]

Similar to patients with glaucomatocyclitic crises or

---

*References 11, 15, 18, 19, 27, 35, 57, 58.
†References 18, 27, 43, 48, 49, 54, 62.

TABLE 43-1 CLASSICAL CLINICAL FEATURES OF GLAUCOMATOCYCLITIC CRISIS AND OF OTHER CLINICAL ENTITIES IN ITS DIFFERENTIAL DIAGNOSIS

	Glaucomatocyclitic Crisis	Acute Angle-Closure Glaucoma	Fuchs Uveitis Syndrome	Nonspecific Iridocyclitis	Neovascular Glaucoma
Unilateral	+	+	−	±	+
Episodic	+	±	−	+	−
Pain	±	+++	−	++	+++
Photophobia	±	+++	−	++	+++
Halos	±	+++	−	−	+
Reduced visual acuity	±	++	±	++	+++
Pupil size	↑	↑	−	↓	−
Ciliary flush	±	+++	−	+++	+++
Corneal edema	±	+++	−	−	+++
Keratic precipitates	±	−	+	+++	−
Flare	±	±	+	+++	+++
Cells	±	−	+	+++	±
Heterochromia	±	−	+	−	−
Iris nodules	−	−	−	±	−
Rubeosis	−	−	±	±	+++
Posterior synechiae	−	−	−	±	−
Intraocular pressure	↑↑↑	↑↑↑	↑	↑-↓	↑↑↑
Narrow angles	−	+	−	−	−
Peripheral anterior synechiae	−	±	−	±	+
Cataract	−	−	+	±	−
Retinal pathology	−	−	±	±	+
Pathologic signs between attacks	−	±	+	+	+
Visual field loss	−	±	+	±	++
Optic disc cupping	−	±	+	±	++
Benefit of iridectomy	−	+	−	±	−
Benefit of chronic medical therapy	−	±	±	+	+
Benefit of filtering surgery	−	−	±	±	+

Key: − Absent or No Change or No   ± Present or Absent   + Present or Mild or Yes   ++ Moderate   +++ Severe
↓ Decrease   ↑ Mild Increase   ↑↑ Moderate Increase   ↑↑↑ Severe Increase

acute angle-closure glaucoma, patients with neovascular glaucoma often have extremely elevated IOPs in one eye. Unlike patients with glaucomatocyclitic crises, those with neovascular glaucoma usually have severe pain, photophobia, blurred vision, and conjunctival injection. Also, the iris of patients with neovascular glaucoma shows rubeosis, and the angle has neovascularization—occasionally with severe peripheral anterior synechiae, which are not features of Posner-Schlossman syndrome. The patient with neovascular glaucoma usually has retinal pathology, including proliferative diabetic retinopathy or a central retinal vein occlusion.

THERAPY

In view of this definitive evidence that optic disc cupping and/or visual field loss occur in some patients, treatment for the elevated IOP during attacks of glaucomatocyclitic crises is advisable, especially as it cannot be predicted a priori which patients will develop neuronal loss. In general, treatment is not required between attacks of glaucomatocyclitic crises, when aqueous humor dynamic measurements usually return to normal.

Ocular Hypotensive Agents

As with any glaucoma associated with uveitis, treatment primarily involves topically-applied medications, including beta-adrenergic blockers as a first-line agent, apraclonidine, epinephrine or dipivefrin, and possibly low concentrations of pilocarpine.

Apraclonidine has recently been shown especially effective in acutely reducing IOP in patients with glaucomatocyclitic crises.[22] When measured four hours after application, apraclonidine 1% was found to reduce IOP by 50% in 13 patients with glaucomatocyclitic crises, compared to 25% in 13 patients with primary open-angle glaucoma. Although epinephrine was commonly used before the advent of beta-blockers, its additivity with beta-blocker therapy is not expected to be substantial. Nevertheless, either epinephrine or dipivefrin may be tried, especially if beta-blockers are contraindicated for systemic, medical reasons. Although miotic agents, such as pilocarpine, are usually contraindicated in uveitic glaucomas, lower concentrations of 0.25% to 2% may be helpful, especially since inflammatory signs are minimal during glaucomatocyclitic crises.[44,60] Pilocarpine-induced posterior synechiae are not likely to occur, as sometimes happens with other uveitic glaucomas.

If needed for further IOP control, orally-administered carbonic anhydrase inhibitors are usually well tolerated and effective for the self-limited attacks of glaucomatocyclitic crises. Although these agents are not well tolerated by many patients with primary open-angle glaucoma who require treatment for many years, oral carbonic anhydrase inhibitor therapy for several days or weeks during glaucomatocyclitic crises is usually accepted. In the rare circumstance that topical ocular hypotensive medications and carbonic anhydrase inhibitors are not sufficient, oral hyperosmotic agents, such as glycerol or isosorbide, may be considered on a short-term basis.

Surgical Management

Medical treatment for elevated IOP is preferable and usually effective in Posner-Schlossman syndrome. Argon laser trabeculoplasty or filtering surgery is usually not recommended or necessary. It is not logical to perform a procedure to maintain a prolonged reduction of IOP for a disease that produces only intermittent IOP elevations. Under the rare circumstances in which a more prolonged reduction of IOP is required, however, argon laser trabeculoplasty may be considered, despite its known reduced efficacy in other types of uveitic glaucomas. Laser iridectomy has no role in glaucomatocyclitic crises, since the angles are open and pupillary block does not occur.

Despite the rare need for filtering surgery in patients with Posner-Schlossman syndrome, several studies describe cases with mixed results.* Whereas most series of patients with the Posner-Schlossman syndrome do not include any patients who have undergone glaucoma surgery, filtering procedures were performed in two of four patients reported by Kraupa,[30] one of 11 by Sugar,[58] three of five by Hung and Chang,[23] and eight of 32 by Knox.[28] Some of these authors described consistent IOP control[23,50,58,62] after filtering procedures, despite recurrent attacks of cyclitis; whereas others reported no effect on the subsequent course of the disease, including the IOP spikes.[3,30,32] Lowe[33] described a patient who was free of recurrent attacks of glaucomatocyclitic crises following filtering surgery, until failure of the filter occurred 10 years later.

Antiinflammatory Agents

Whereas most types of anterior uveitis require antiinflammatory treatment to prevent posterior synechiae, pe-

---

*References 3, 17, 23, 28, 30, 32, 33, 50, 58, 62.

ripheral anterior synechiae, inflammatory membranes, and cataracts, these sequelae are not usually associated with the Posner-Schlossman syndrome. As a result, antiinflammatory treatment is justified only on the basis of its potential to shorten the ocular hypertensive episodes. Although no controlled studies have been performed to verify the benefit of topical corticosteroids in the Posner-Schlossman syndrome, most authors feel that they are useful.[3,21,45,60] In view of the possible role of prostaglandins in this syndrome (see Pathogenesis section), some ophthalmologists have advocated the use of cyclo-oxygenase inhibitors, which block prostaglandin synthesis. The cyclo-oxygenase inhibitors available for topical application in the United States include flurbiprofen, suprofen, ketorolac, and diclofenac. Unlike topical corticosteroids, these agents seem to have less potential for raising IOP and producing cataracts. Nevertheless, as previously discussed, the role for prostaglandins and these nonsteroidal antiinflammatory drugs is controversial in the Posner-Schlossman syndrome. Furthermore, the use of these agents to prevent recurrent attacks has not been verified.

Cycloplegic agents are used in uveitis therapy to relieve ciliary spasm and help prevent posterior synechiae. Because ciliary spasm and posterior synechiae usually do not occur in Posner-Schlossman syndrome, cycloplegic agents are not required, nor are they especially useful.[3,21,44]

PROGNOSIS

The attacks of glaucomatocyclitic crises recur at varying frequencies, but usually recur at intervals of every few months to every 1 to 2 years. The range of intervals between attacks is a couple of months to 5 years. Some patients experience a single episode without recurrences. Repeated attacks occur for 15 to 25 years in many patients, with the frequency of attacks decreasing with increasing age. Because attacks rarely occur in the elderly, it is assumed that the recurrent attacks eventually stop in most patients before causing permanent visual loss.

REFERENCES

1. Abboud IA: Glaucomato-cyclitic crises: Posner Schlossman syndrome, *Ophthalmol Soc Egypt* 47:151-153, 1954.
2. Adamantiadis B: Sur un cas type de syndrome de Posner et Schlossman (crises glaucomatocyclitiques), *Arch Ophthalmol* 17:573-574, 1957.
3. Billet E: Syndrome of glaucomato-cyclitic crises, *Am J Ophthalmol* 35:214-216, 1952.
4. Bloch-Michel E, Dussaix E, Cerqueti P, Patarin D: Possible role of cytomegalovirus in the etiology of the Posner-Schlossman syndrome, *Int Ophthalmol* 11:95-96, 1987.
5. Brooks AM et al.: Cyclitic glaucoma, *Aust N Z J Ophthalmol* 17:157-164, 1989.
6. Burton EW: Glaucomatocyclitis crises, *South Med J* 50:257-258, 1957.
7. Camras CB: Mechanism of the prostaglandin-induced reduction of intraocular pressure in humans. In Samuelsson B, Paoletti R, Ramwell PW, editors: *Advances in prostaglandin, thromboxane, and leukotriene research, vol 23*, 519-525, New York, 1995, Raven Press.
8. Camras CB, Bito LZ, Eakins KE: Reduction of intraocular pressure by prostaglandins applied topically to the eyes of conscious rabbits, *Invest Ophthalmol Vis Sci* 16:1125-1134, 1977.

9. Camras CB, Podos SM: Reduction of intraocular pressure by exogenous and endogenous prostaglandins in monkeys and humans. In Drance S, Van Buskirk EM, Neufeld A, editors: *Pharmacology of the glaucomas,* 175-183, Baltimore, 1992, Williams and Wilkins.

10. Curschmann V: Etiological and therapeutic observations in glaucomatocyclitic crises, *Klin Monatsbl Augenheilkd* 136:678-680, 1960.

11. Delmarcelle MY: Un glaucome secondaire souvent meconnu: le syndrome de Posner-Schlossman, *Bull Soc Belge Ophtalmol* 114:566-574, 1957.

12. Demailly P, Zaegel R, Blamoutier J, Abadie P: Syndrome de Posner Schlossman et allergie, *J Fr Ophtalmol* 8:773-777, 1985.

13. Dernouchamps JP: The Posner-Schlossman syndrome, *Bull Soc Belge Ophtalmol* 230:13-17, 1989.

14. Flach JG, Eliason JA: Topical prostaglandin E$_2$ effects on normal human intraocular pressure, *J Ocular Pharm* 4:13-18, 1988.

15. Grant WM: Clinical measurements of aqueous outflow, *Arch Ophthalmol* 46:113-131, 1951.

16. Harris JL: Glaucomato-cyclic crises: report of two cases, *J Med Soc N J* 50:453-455, 1953.

17. Harstad HK, Ringvold A: Glaucomatocyclitic crises (Posner-Schlossman syndrome), *Acta Ophthalmol* 64:146-151, 1986.

18. Hart CT, Weatherill JR: Gonioscopy and tonography in glaucomatocyclitic crises, *Br J Ophthalmol* 52:682-687, 1968.

19. Higgitt AC: Secondary glaucoma, *Trans Ophthalmol Soc UK* 76:73-82, 1956.

20. Hirose S, Ohno S, Matsuda H: HLA-Bw54 and glaucomatocyclitic crisis, *Arch Ophthalmol* 103:1837-1839, 1985.

21. Hollwich F: Zur klinik und therapie des Posner-Schloβman syndroms, *Klin Monatsbl Augenheilkd* 172:736-744, 1978.

22. Hong C, Song KY: Effect of apraclonidine hydrochloride on the attack of Posner-Schlossman syndrome, *Korean J Ophthalmol* 7:28-33, 1993.

23. Hung PT, Chang JM: Treatment of glaucomatocyclitic crises, *Am J Ophthalmol* 77:169-172, 1974.

24. Israel EB: The syndrome of glaucomato-cyclitic crises, *S Afr Med J* 26:809-810, 1952.

25. Iwata K, Takahashi K, Kojima M: Prognosis of the Posner-Schlossman's syndrome, *Acta Soc Ophthalmol Jpn* 74:110-112, 1970.

26. Jain NS: Glaucomatocyclitic crisis (Posner-Schlossman syndrome), *J All-India Ophthalmol Soc* 1:119-121, 1954.

27. Kass MA, Becker B, Kolker AE: Glaucomatocyclitic crisis and primary open-angle glaucoma, *Am J Ophthalmol* 75:668-673, 1973.

28. Knox DL: Glaucomatocyclitic crises and systemic disease: peptic ulcer, other gastrointestinal disorders, allergy and stress, *Trans Am Ophthalmol Soc* 86:473-495, 1988.

29. Kornzweig AL: Glaucomatous cyclic crises, *Am J Ophthalmol* 36:123-124, 1953.

30. Kraupa E: Die drucksteigerung bei akuter angioneurose des ciliarkörpers (''glaucoma allergicum'') in ihren beziehungen zum zyklitischen und heterochromieglaukom, *Arch Augenheilkd* 109:416-433, 1935.

31. Kronfeld PC: Gonioscopic correlates of responsiveness to miotics, *Arch Ophthalmol* 32:447-455, 1944.

32. Levatin P: Glaucomatocyclitic crises occurring in both eyes, *Am J Ophthalmol* 41:1056-1059, 1956.

33. Lowe RF: Glaucomato-cyclitic crises, *Trans Ophthalmol Soc Aust* 13:168-171, 1954.

34. Maezawa N, Maezawa Y, Kohda N, Tsukahara S: Glaucomatocyclitic crises, *Folia Ophthalmol Jpn* 28:1130-1135, 1977.

35. Mansheim BJ: Aqueous outflow measurements by continuous tonometry in some unusual forms of glaucoma, *Arch Ophthalmol* 50:580-587, 1953.

36. Masuda K, Izawa Y, Mishima S: Prostaglandins and glaucomatocyclitic crisis, *Jpn J Ophthalmol* 19:368-375, 1975.

37. Mattsson R: Ueber glaukomatozyklitische krisen, *Acta Ophthalmol* 32:523-533, 1954.

38. Nagataki S, Mishima S: Aqueous humor dynamics in glaucomatocyclitic crisis, *Invest Ophthalmol* 15:365-370, 1976.

39. Nakajima M, Goh Y, Azuma I, Hayaishi O: Effects of prostaglandin D$_2$ and its analogue, BW245C, on intraocular pressure in humans, *Graefes Arch Clin Exp Ophthalmol* 229:411-413, 1991.

40. Naveh-Floman N et al.: Protein glaucoma as a possible mechanism in a case of glaucomatocyclitic crisis and periphlebitis, *Metab Pediatr Syst Ophthalmol* 7:85-88, 1983.

41. Neufeld AH, Sears ML: Prostaglandin and eye, *Prostaglandins* 4:157-175, 1973.

42. Posner A: Present status of the syndrome of glaucomatocyclitic crises, *EENT Monthly* 37:402-403, 1958.

43. Posner A, Schlossman A: Syndrome of unilateral recurrent attacks of glaucoma with cyclitic symptoms, *Arch Ophthalmol* 39:517-535, 1948.

44. Posner A, Schlossman A: Treatment of glaucoma associated with iridocyclitis, *JAMA* 139:82-86, 1949.

45. Posner A, Schlossman A: Further observations on the syndrome of glaucomatocyclitic crises, *Trans Am Acad Ophthalmol Otolaryngal* 57:531-536, 1953.

46. Pratt-Johnson JA: The phenomenon of glaucomatocyclitic crises, *S A Tydskrif Geneeskunde* 23:595-597, 1956.

47. Pur S: Syndrom glaukomatocyklitickych krisi (Kraupa-Posner-Schlossman), *Czechoslov Ophthalmol* 9:534, 1953.

48. Raitta C, Klemetti A: Steroidbelastung bei Posner-Schlossmanschem syndrom, *Graefes Arch Clin Exp Ophthalmol* 174:66-71, 1967.

49. Raitta C, Vannas A: Glaucomatocyclitic crisis, *Arch Ophthalmol* 95:608-612, 1977.

50. Rouher F: Syndrome de Posner-Schlossman, *Bull Soc Ophtalmol Fr* 55:534-540, 1955.

51. Rouher F, Cantat: L'hypertension oculaire paroxystique benigne (syndrome de Posner et Schlossman), *Arch Ophthalmol* 16:798-810, 1956.

52. Setala K, Vannas A: Endothelial cells in the glaucomato-cylitic crisis, *Adv Ophthalmol* 36:218-224, 1978.

53. Simpson DG: Glaucomatocyclitic crises, *Am J Ophthalmol* 50:163-165, 1960.

54. Sokolic P: Observation of glaucomatocyclitic crisis associated with developmental glaucoma: contribution to the etiology, *Acta Ophthalmol* 44:607-612, 1966.

55. Sokolic P: Another case with recurrent glaucomatocyclitic crisis and anomalies in chamber angle, observed during and between hypertensive episodes contribution to etiology, *Acta Ophthalmol* 47:1129-1134, 1969.

56. Sokolic P: Developmental factor in the etiopathogenesis of glaucomatocyclitic crisis, *Ophthalmologica* 161:446-450, 1970.

57. Spivey BE, Armaly MF: Tonographic findings in glaucomatocyclitic crises, *Am J Ophthalmol* 55:47-51, 1963.

58. Sugar HS: Heterochromia iridis, with special consideration of its relation to cyclitic disease, *Am J Ophthalmol* 60:1-18, 1965.

59. Terrien F, Veil P: De certains glaucomes soi-disant primaties, *Bull Soc Ophtalmol Fr* 42:349-368, 1929.

60. Theodore FH: Observations on glaucomatocyclitic crises; Posner-Schlossman syndrome, *Br J Ophthalmol* 36:207-210, 1952.

61. Toris CB, Camras CB, Yablonski ME: Effects of PhXA41, a new prostaglandin F$_{2\alpha}$ analog, on aqueous humor dynamics in human eyes, *Ophthalmology* 100:1297-1304, 1993.

62. Varma R, Katz LJ, Spaeth GL: Surgical treatment of acute glaucomatocyclitic crisis in a patient with primary open-angle glaucoma, *Am J Ophthalmol* 105:99-100, 1988.

63. Vouters J: Une forme d'uvéite hypertensive mal connue: la cyclite hypertensive à repetition. Relation de quatre cas, *Bull Soc Ophtalmol Fr* 695-702, 1951.

64. Whitelocke RAF, Eakins KE: Vascular changes in the anterior uvea of the rabbit produced by prostaglandins, *Arch Ophthalmol* 89:495-499, 1973.

44 Retinal Vasculitis

ELIZABETH M. GRAHAM, MILES R. STANFORD, SCOTT M. WHITCUP

Inflammatory involvement of the retinal vessels occurs in many cases of intermediate uveitis, posterior uveitis, and panuveitis. Whereas vasculitis elsewhere in the body is generally confirmed and classified based on histopathologic findings, the ophthalmologist's diagnosis of retinal vasculitis must rely on biomicroscopic examination, which can be complemented by fluorescein angiography. Retinal vasculitis can be defined as vascular leakage and staining of vessel walls seen on fluorescein angiography[37] in association with intraocular inflammation.

This inflammation, when severe, can lead to occlusion of the vessel lumen and retinal ischemia. Any of the retinal vessels can be involved, including arterioles, venules, and capillaries. Many of the retinal vasculitides are associated with underlying systemic diseases that may be life-threatening if unrecognized and untreated.[74] In addition, sight-threatening complications of retinal vasculitis include macular edema, retinal ischemia, and new vessel formation.[37a,72,73]

The exact cause of retinal vasculitis is not well defined. The term *retinal vasculitis* suggests that disease is due to a type III hypersensitivity reaction with deposition of immune complexes in the vessel wall. The presence of circulating immune complexes alone does not prove a causal role for immune complexes in the pathogenesis of the vasculitis, however. In addition, many cases of presumed retinal vasculitis are more accurately termed *perivasculitis,* with inflammation surrounding vessels but not actually involving the vessel wall.

A variety of noninflammatory diseases can cause retinal vascular abnormalities;[70a] they include diabetes mellitus, atherosclerosis, and congenital disorders such as Coats disease. Vascular involvement with these disorders may lead to sclerosis of vessels (or other clinically apparent vascular anomalies), hemorrhage, and ischemia. Systemic vasculitides that have associated retinal vascular lesions, but not necessarily intraocular inflammation, include Wegener granulomatosis, polyarteritis nodosa, polymyositis, and dermatomyositis. Other diseases in which noninflammatory

retinal vasculopathy occurs are Buerger disease, Sjögren syndrome, Takayasu disease, and Cogan syndrome. In some cases eyes become inflamed secondarily if vasculopathy is sufficiently severe to cause ischemia or tissue necrosis; intraocular inflammation is not a primary feature of these conditions, however. Nevertheless, these vasculopathies are sometimes inappropriately referred to as "retinal vasculitis," leading to confusion in the literature.

This chapter deals only with those disorders fulfilling the diagnostic criteria for retinal vasculitis described previously. Disorders that cause retinal vasculitis are listed in Table 44-1. They are divided into conditions associated with systemic disease, conditions caused by infectious agents, and diseases limited to the eye. Sarcoidosis, multiple sclerosis, and Behçet disease are three of the systemic diseases most commonly associated with retinal vasculitis. Frequently, ocular disease can be the first sign of these systemic diseases, and the ophthalmologist should be diligent in establishing the diagnosis so these potentially life-threatening diseases can be expediently treated. Similarly, it is important to recognize an infectious cause for retinal vasculitis. First, subsequent treatment with corticosteroids alone may cause exacerbation of infectious diseases, and in cases like tuberculosis could lead to significant morbidity. Second, appropriate antimicrobial therapy is often curative, and the sooner that therapy is started, the less chance there is of permanent retinal damage. In many cases, retinal vasculitis remains an isolated finding of unknown cause. Much of the material in this chapter deals with such cases of idiopathic retinal vasculitis.

EPIDEMIOLOGY

The basic epidemiologic features (e.g., age, sex, race) of isolated, idiopathic retinal vasculitis remain poorly understood, probably because of the lack of any formal definition of this disease in past studies. Indeed there are both fluorescein angiographic[52,69] and electrophysiologic[12] overlaps between this disease and pars planitis syndrome.

TABLE 44-1 DISORDERS ASSOCIATED WITH RETINAL VASCULITIS

Systemic Diseases	Infectious Diseases	Primary Ocular Diseases
Behçet disease	Syphilis	Birdshot retinochoroidopathy
Wegener granulomatosis	Lyme borreliosis	Pars planitis syndrome
Systemic lupus erythematosus	Toxoplasmosis	Eales disease
Polyarteritis nodosa	Toxocariasis	Retinal arteritis and macroaneurysms
Polymyositis	Coccidioidomycosis	Fuchs uveitis syndrome
Dermatomyositis	Tuberculosis	Malignancy
Whipple disease	Cytomegalovirus retinitis	Ocular ischemia
Crohn disease	Herpes simplex virus retinitis	Multifocal choroiditis and panuveitis
Sarcoidosis	Varicella-zoster virus retinitis	syndrome
Multiple sclerosis	Zoster ophthalmicus	Frosted branch angiitis
Postvaccination syndrome	Candidiasis	
Buerger disease	Brucellosis	
Takayasu disease	Leptospirosis	
Cogan syndrome	Rickettsial infection	
Sjögren syndrome	Amebiasis	
Allergic granulomatosis	Mononucleosis	
	Epstein-Barr virus infection	

Idiopathic retinal vasculitis usually occurs in young people, with an equal male/female ratio, and causes significant visual morbidity in this age group. In 75% of cases it presents before 40 years of age and usually disappears by the age of 50.

Figures pertaining to the incidence and prevalence of disease must be interpreted against the background that this disorder is a rare disease, that mild cases may be missed, and that the figures produced from tertiary referral centers will certainly not reflect the frequency of disease seen in the general population. In a prospective epidemiologic study in the Savoy region of France, the prevalence of uveitis as a whole was 38/100,000 and the incidence 17/100,000 per year.[84] Closer examination of these figures shows that only 13% of the described cases could possibly refer to retinal vasculitis using the International Uveitis Study Group classification,[7] and it is likely that the true prevalence in this region was 4/100,000 and the incidence 2/100,000 per year. Similar figures may be derived from other centers,* most recently from Rotterdam, a tertiary referral center in which only 4% of uveitis cases were ascribed to retinal vasculitis.[4]

In a series of 150 patients with retinal vasculitis seen over 10 years at St. Thomas' Hospital in London, UK, the disease was confined to the eye in 67 patients (40%).[37a] In this group 27 patients were male and 40 were female, and 72% of them were between 15 and 40 years of age. In general these findings are in agreement with the results from other referral centers with a predominantly Caucasian population, but differ markedly from the incidence of disease seen in Brazil

or Japan,[56] where underlying environmental and/or genetic factors are relevant. The incidence and prevalence of different types of retinal vasculitis (see next section) have also not been properly documented, although a study from Essen showed that Eales disease was more common and more often bilateral in men.[78]

CLINICAL FEATURES

Patients with retinal vasculitis often complain of blurred or decreased vision. A study of 150 patients with vasculitis showed two thirds to have corrected visual acuities of 6/18 or better on presentation, and 20% had an acuity worse than 6/18 in both eyes.[37a] Retinal ischemia may lead to scotoma formation, and associated vitritis often causes floaters. Some patients report distortion of color vision, difficulty with reading or metamorphopsia if the macula is involved. Many cases of retinal vasculitis are associated with a scleritis, and these patients may complain of pain and redness. Symptoms or signs relating to systemic disease (e.g., orogenital ulceration, arthritis, skin rashes, signs of recent sexually transmitted disease, thrombosis, chest and neurologic symptoms) should be sought from patients routinely. Occasionally, patients with retinal vasculitis, especially with mild peripheral involvement only, may have no ocular symptoms at all. This situation is quite characteristic for the vascular involvement associated with multiple sclerosis.

Signs in the anterior segment are of little overall diagnostic value. Cellular infiltration of the vitreous humor may be very severe, but usually there is sufficient clarity to make out retinal details. Vitreous snowballs are often present inferiorly, and the majority of patients have detachment of the posterior vitreous face.

*References 15, 41, 55, 57, 67, 86.

Vascular sheathing is a characteristic ophthalmoscopic feature of retinal vasculitis. "Skip areas" are common, and vessels in the periphery are frequently involved. Many cases of retinal vasculitis are associated with a prominent vitritis, optic disc edema, optic disc pallor, or cystoid macular edema. Although these signs can be observed ophthalmoscopically, fluorescein angiography is useful in evaluating these patients. Staining of the vessel wall occurs along inflamed retinal vessels. In addition, the degree of retinal ischemia and presence of cystoid macular edema can also be evaluated on the angiogram. If retinal vasculitis results in vascular occlusion, then retinal hemorrhage, cotton-wool spots, or white areas of retinal swelling caused by ischemia can be seen. Neovascularization may result from chronic retinal ischemia. Central retinal artery and vein occlusions as well as microaneurysms are rare complications. These signs of severe disease are more likely to occur with the retinal vasculitis associated with systemic disorders, such as Behçet disease, than with idiopathic retinal vasculitis.

A review of the retinal signs in 67 patients with idiopathic retinal vasculitis showed that the most common retinal sign in this group was peripheral vascular sheathing (64%) followed by macular edema (60%). One third of patients had an associated anterior uveitis, but this feature was usually asymptomatic. One third of patients had associated retinal pigment epithelial disease or choroiditis (Fig. 44-1). Retinal neovascularization (16%) (Fig. 44-2), periphlebitis (15%), and retinal vein occlusions (10%) were rarer. Retinal infiltrates were not seen in any patients in this study, making that sign a valuable diagnostic marker to differentiate patients with idiopathic retinal vasculitis from those with Behçet disease.[37a] Fluorescein angiography revealed capillary leakage in 80% of patients and capillary closure in the remainder. Optic disc or peripheral neovascularization occurs in a mi-

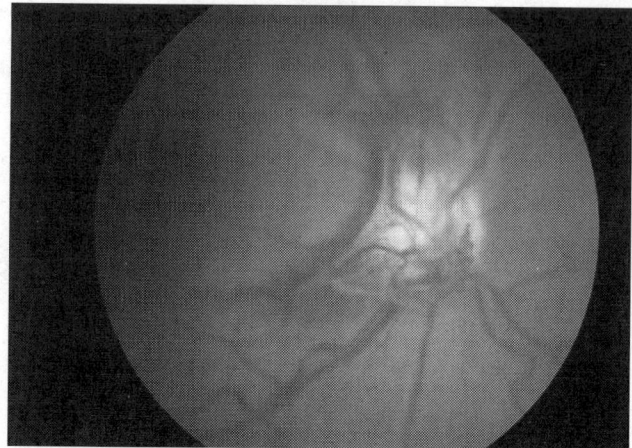

Fig. 44-2 Photograph of the optic disc of a 30-year-old woman with optic disc neovascularization secondary to nonischaemic retinal vasculitis. Despite the presence of fibrovascular elements, active neovascularization resolved with medical control of her inflammation.

nority of patients, but often neovascularization is not associated with significant capillary closure.

Three main clinical categories of idiopathic retinal vasculitis can be identified: a nonocclusive "leaky" or edematous type, an occlusive ischemic type, and retinal vasculitis associated with choroiditis.

Nonocclusive Edematous Retinal Vasculitis

Most patients fall into this category. Their disease is characterized by leakage from retinal veins and capillaries on fluorescein angiography, and the main cause of vision loss is from cystoid macular edema (Fig. 44-3). The response to treatment is generally good in the early stage of

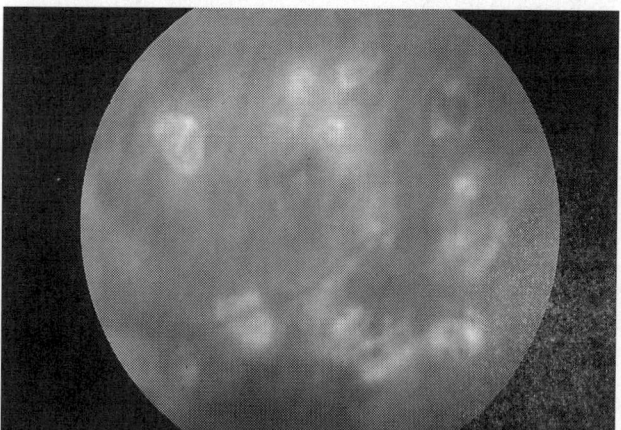

Fig. 44-1 A 35-year-old African male with poor vision had a mild panuveitis and fundus examination showing multiple areas of pigment epithelial atrophy suggestive of retinal vasculitis with choroiditis. Investigations for sarcoidosis, tuberculosis, and toxoplasmosis were not helpful.

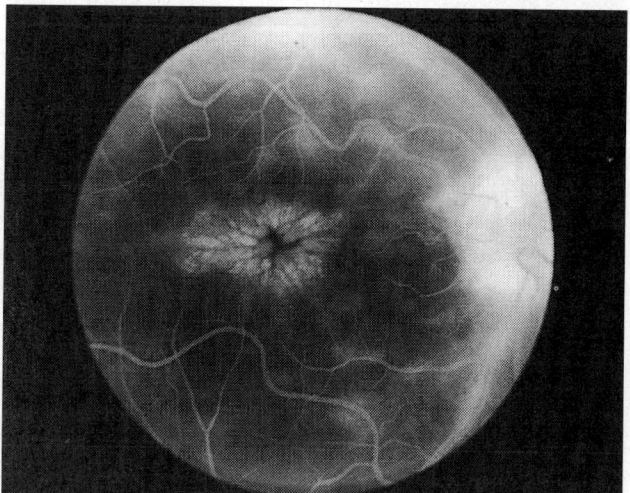

Fig. 44-3 A 34-year-old woman complained of central vision loss in both eyes. A fluorescein angiogram (late phase) shows classical cystoid macular edema.

disease, but vision loss may arise from persistent macular problems.

Occlusive Ischemic Retinal Vasculitis

In 20% of patients disease is dominated by the appearance of peripheral retinal hemorrhages and capillary nonperfusion on fluorescein angiography (Fig. 44-4 and 44-5), with only mild cellular infiltration of the vitreous humor. The main clinical features in these patients are neovascularization, intraretinal hemorrhages, obliterated vessels, and peripheral vascular sheathing.[78]

A subgroup of these patients were described as multifocal hemorrhagic retinal vasculitis; the patients developed a pattern of disease very similar to that seen in Behçet disease, with a comparable visual prognosis, although no patient ever developed systemic features.[8] Patients with Eales disease also fall into this category; this term is not favored by many investigators, however, since most patients with idiopathic occlusive disease have not suffered with constipation or epistaxis, which were included in Eales' original description of the disease.[27d] Vision loss may arise from macular edema, which is sometimes complicated by macular ischemia with a poor visual prognosis.

Retinal Vasculitis with Choroiditis

The syndrome of multifocal choroiditis and panuveitis was described as a separate clinical entity in 1984,[23] although it had been recognized for many years before. The

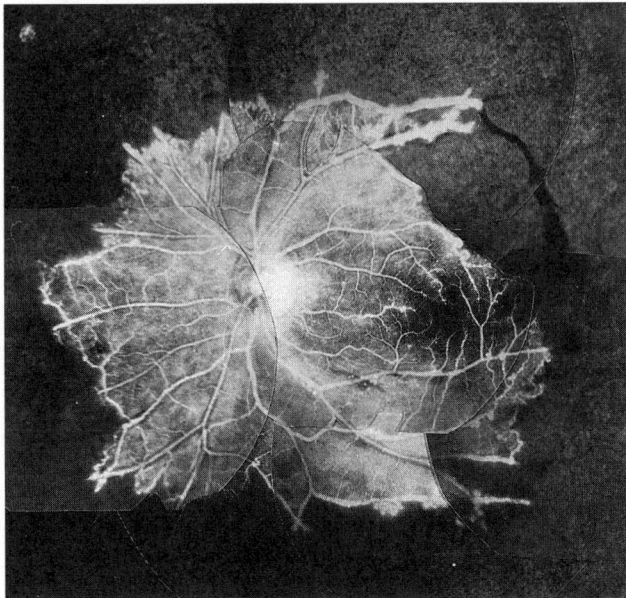

Fig. 44-4 A 30-year-old Mauritian man with blurred vision was found to have early rubeosis. A composite fluorescein angiogram (venous phase) shows the dramatic large vessel and capillary closure, venous beading and leakage, and optic disc neovascularization. His Mantoux reaction was positive, and he was treated with antituberculosis chemotherapy.

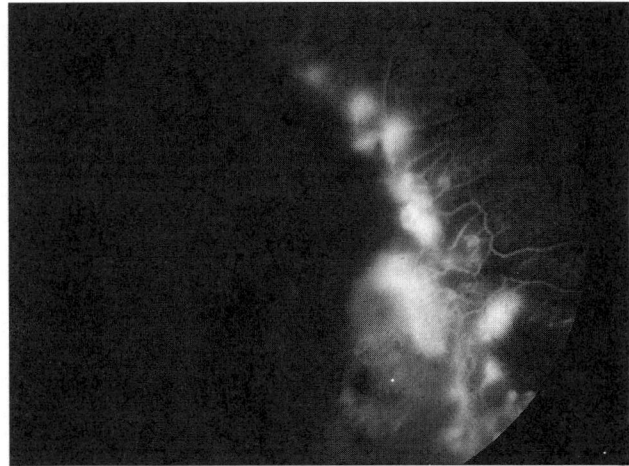

Fig. 44-5 Fluorescein angiogram of the peripheral retina of a 40-year-old lady with a panuveitis and a vitreous hemorrhage. Neovascularization has developed at the border of nonischemic and ischemic retina.

differential diagnosis of this disorder includes the white dot syndromes (Chapters 46, 47, 48). The main causes of diagnostic confusion are presumed ocular histoplasmosis syndrome (POHS) (Chapter 90), in which intraocular inflammation is unusual, and birdshot retinochoroidopathy (Chapter 47), in which the lesions are more superficial and the visual prognosis is poor with a relentless downhill course. The main differential diagnosis, however, is subclinical sarcoidosis, since many patients show a mild-to-moderate elevation of serum angiotensin converting enzyme with a negative Mantoux reaction.[71]

PATHOLOGY

The main problem associated with studying the pathogenesis of retinal vasculitis is the lack of suitable pathologic material, particularly from eyes with early disease. The few cases of active, retinal vasculitis studied at autopsy by histopathology or immunopathology have revealed T-lymphocytes in blood vessel walls, some of which were positive for the interleukin-2 (IL-2) receptor activation marker.[52a,77a,77b] Generally the histopathologic findings are nonspecific. The degree of pathologic damage to intraocular structures is proportional to the severity and duration of disease, but is not as severe as that seen in suppurative disease. Infiltrating inflammatory cells in and surrounding the retinal vessel walls are mainly T-lymphocytes; B-lymphocytes, cells, plasma cells, monocytes, and epithelioid or giant cells are rare.

The ocular media may contain a fibrinous exudate with lymphocytes and macrophages. Focal aggregates of monocytes on the corneal endothelium (keratic precipitates) as well as both anterior and posterior synechiae may be present. The choroid may have diffuse or focal aggregates of lymphocytes or may be normal. The retinal veins characteristically show perivascular lymphocytic cuffing, but retinal infiltration and actual retinal necrosis are rare. After active disease has resolved, focal areas of retinal pigment epithelial atrophy and gliosis may be apparent.

COMPLICATIONS

Neovascularization is an unusual but well recognized complication of retinal vasculitis[37] that affects about 10% of patients, their eyes usually showing a moderate vitritis and posterior vitreous detachment. Vitreous hemorrhage absorbs quickly, usually without the propensity for traction retinal detachment seen in other ischemic retinopathies such as diabetic retinopathy. Fluorescein angiography commonly reveals diffuse microvascular leakage rather than capillary closure (Fig. 44-6).

The new vessels probably arise in response to the inflammatory process, and most of the vessels will regress with adequate control of the inflammation. Treatment should aim to suppress the inflammation, with laser photocoagulation reserved for patients with recurrent vitreous hemorrhages, despite full immunosuppression or significant capillary closure of more than one quadrant on fluorescein angiography. Inflammation must be maximally suppressed prior to laser photocoagulation whenever possible, since preliminary evidence shows it may induce cystoid macular edema.[37]

Macular ischemia, defined as closure of perifoveal capillaries and identified by an enlarged and/or irregular foveal avascular zone on fluorescein angiography (Fig. 44-7), occasionally occurs in patients with retinal vasculitis.[6]

This inflammatory disease may be active or quiescent, and, on close inspection, the ischemic macula may be identified in the capillary phase of the angiogram, even in the presence of cystoid macular edema. A specific search for this complication at 1 month is advisable if the ocular media

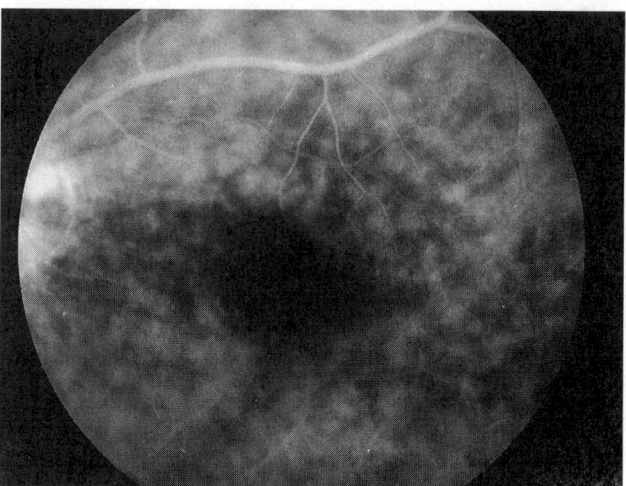

Fig. 44-7   A 26-year-old man who experienced vision loss caused by cystoid macula edema. The vision did not improve despite high doses of systemic corticosteroids. The fluorescein angiogram shows macular ischemia with an enlarged foveal avascular zone, perifoveal capillary dilatation, and loss of the perifoveal ring nasally.

has cleared in response to immunosuppression but the vision is still poor, since an angiogram at this time may give much better definition of the capillary phase than one before treatment is begun.

Retinal detachment is a relatively uncommon complication of retinal vasculitis, but when it does occur in an eye with active inflammation, proliferative vitreoretinopathy may develop very rapidly. Patients with this complication should therefore be treated with systemic corticosteroids in the perioperative period during retinal detachment repair.[11]

PATHOGENESIS

The cause of idiopathic retinal vasculitis is presumedly related to a disorder of autoimmunity, possibly triggered by an unknown infectious agent in which T-lymphocytes play a predominant role.[35] Several lines of evidence support a role for T-lymphocytes. They include the response of the disease to specific immunosuppression; study of occasional pathologic material; and the study of well-characterized animal models in which disease may be adoptively transferred. It has been difficult to demonstrate consistently the presence of T-lymphocyte abnormalities in peripheral blood, however, unless extraocular disease is also present.[31] Retinal biopsy is not yet practical in an eye with potential vision, and no methods of localized blood sampling (for instance, cannulation of the vortex veins) have yet been devised, so the main hypotheses about disease pathogenesis come from the study of animal models.[30,35]

The exact contribution of humoral, immune complex, or cellular immunity to the initiation, perpetuation, relapse, or burnout of disease are unknown. The reasons underlying

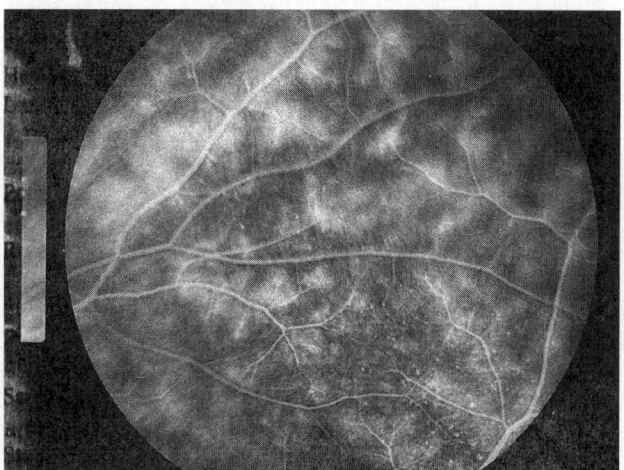

Fig. 44-6   A young man complained of floaters caused by vitreous humor cells. Fluorescein angiography in the midvenous phase of the retinal periphery shows diffuse microvascular leakage characteristic of nonocclusive retinal vasculitis.

different patterns of disease and responses to therapy remain obscure. Patients with secondary vascular occlusion, for example, do not improve with systemic immunosuppression. This lack of improvement may reflect the fact that microvascular damage is not primarily caused by lymphocytic infiltration, but rather to thrombosis associated with procoagulant changes in the vascular endothelium.

Cell Adhesion Molecules

Vasculitis is characterized histologically by the presence of infiltrating inflammatory cells at the site of vascular damage. Over the last decade investigators have come to understand the mechanisms governing the interaction between leukocytes and the vascular endothelium. Cell adhesion molecules are surface proteins important for cell migration and adhesion. There are three major families of cell adhesion molecules: selectins, integrins, and the immunoglobulin supergene family.[78a]

Expression of members of the selectin family is important for the initial adhesion and rolling of leukocytes along the vascular endothelium at sites of inflammation. Expression of P-selectin (CD62) is rapidly upregulated by inflammatory mediators such as histamine, and mediates the initial binding and rolling of leukocytes along the inflamed vascular endothelium.[34b] Similarly, E-selectin (CD62E) is not normally expressed on the vascular endothelium, but is upregulated in the presence of cytokines including IL-1, interferon-gamma, and tumor necrosis factor (TNF)-alpha.[52c,67a] E-selectin binds to CD15, a carbohydrate moiety on leukocytes, and also fosters the rolling of inflammatory cells along vascular endothelium.[49c,67a] Studies have also demonstrated expression of E-selectin on the vascular endothelium of the ciliary body in Lewis rats within 12 hours after endotoxin injection, before the binding of neutrophils to inflamed ocular tissues.[87a]

Transmigration of leukocytes across the inflamed vascular endothelium is mediated by members of the integrin and immunoglobulin supergene families. Vascular cell adhesion molecule-1 (VCAM-1, CD106) is a member of the immunoglobulin supergene family that binds to the integrin called very late antigen-4 (VLA-4, CD49d) on leukocytes.[34a,69a] Likewise, the immunoglobulin supergene family member intercellular adhesion molecule-1 (ICAM-1, CD54) binds to the integrins lymphocyte function molecule-1 (LFA-1, CD11a/CD18) and Mac-1 (CD11b/CD18).[27a,49a] The expression of ICAM-1 and VCAM-1 on endothelium is upregulated by cytokines including IL-1, TNF-alpha, and interferon-gamma.[27b,78a] The increased expression of these cell adhesion molecules is critical to the development of vasculitis.

In vitro studies have demonstrated that ICAM-1 is expressed on the retinal pigment epithelium at low levels constitutively, but is only expressed on retinal vascular endothelial cells after induction with interferon-gamma.[52a] In vivo studies showed that ICAM-1 is expressed on the vascular endothelium of the retina in animal eyes with experimental autoimmune uveitis (EAU) (Fig. 44-8).[87c] ICAM-1 expression was strongest in those eyes with the most severe vasculitis, and inflammatory cell infiltration into the retina was limited to areas where ICAM-1 was expressed. ICAM-1 expression preceded the migration of inflammatory cells into the eye, and monoclonal antibodies against either ICAM-1 or its counter-receptor LFA-1, inhibited the development of retinal vasculitis and uveitis in mice.

Studies have also shown that ICAM-1 is expressed on the vascular endothelium in human eyes with uveitis.[87b] ICAM-1 is expressed on the retinal and choroidal vascular endothelium in areas of active inflammation and vasculitis, suggesting that cytokine-mediated upregulation of cell adhesion molecule expression may be a critical event in the pathogen-

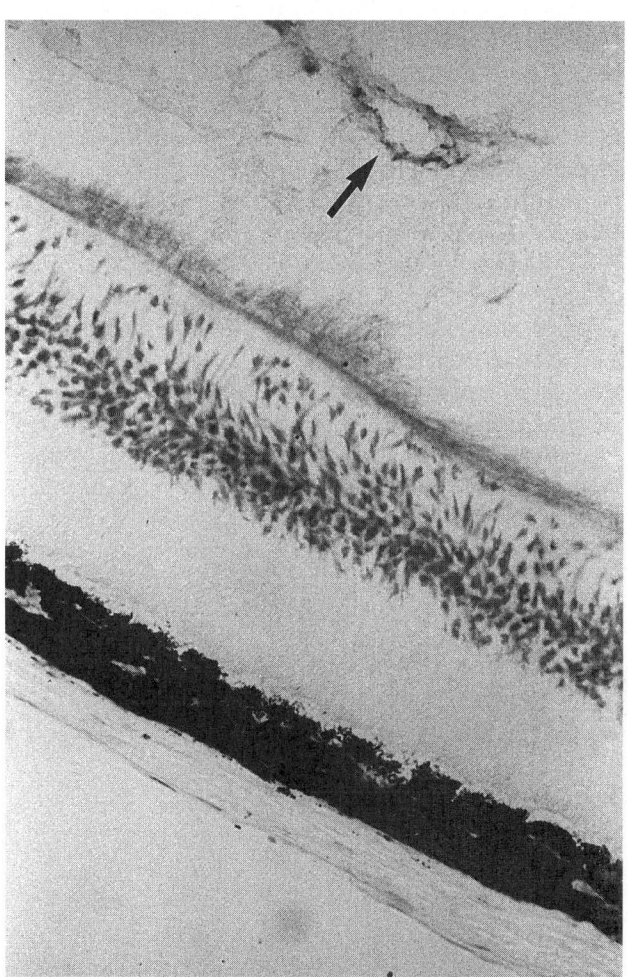

Fig. 44-8 Immunohistochemical staining of the retina from a mouse with experimental autoimmune uveoretinitis shows strong expression of ICAM-1 on the vascular endothelium (arrow) 7 days after immunization with interphotoreceptor retinoid-binding protein (IRBP). ICAM-1 expression preceded the infiltration of inflammatory cells into the retina. (Original magnification × 400.)

esis of retinal vasculitis. In fact, treatment with immunosuppressive agents including corticosteroids, cyclosporine, and tacrolimus (FK506) has been shown to inhibit the expression of cell adhesion molecules in the eye,[49b,52b] and may be an important therapeutic action for these drugs.

Antibody-Mediated Mechanisms

Humoral reactivity against retinal components can be detected in the serum of patients with retinal vasculitis either by indirect immunofluorescence, or by specific reactivity with purified retinal proteins shown to be uveitogenic in experimental models.* The main criticisms of these studies has been the inability to discriminate between patients and controls without eye disease,[33] the failure of antibody levels to correlate with the clinical course of disease, and the failure to transfer disease experimentally by passive immunization.

Immunofluorescence studies do not show any distinctive pattern of staining in various forms of retinal vasculitis, and Western blotting of patients' sera against extracts of human retina do not reveal any diagnostic patterns of reactivity with retinal proteins.[22] Furthermore, raised antibody levels have been found in both infectious retinal diseases (toxoplasmosis,[38] onchocerciasis[13]) and after panretinal photocoagulation, indicating these levels are probably the result of retinal damage rather than of primary pathogenic significance.[39] Nevertheless, patients with retinal vasculitis may be differentiated from healthy controls by the affinity of their antiretinal antibody. Antibody affinity against retinal S-antigen, as measured by sodium thiocyanate dissociation on standard ELISA plates, was significantly lower in patients than in healthy controls who expressed antibody. The authors postulated that this finding might represent a failure of immunoregulation leading to retinal disease.[48] In animal studies it has been found that complement depletion may modify S-antigen-induced disease,[53a] and there is some evidence that antibody affinity is lower in animals genetically susceptible to EAU compared to those that are resistant.[49]

Immune Complex Mechanisms

The role of immune complexes in retinal tissue damage is still controversial. Pathologic specimens taken from eyes of patients with retinal vasculitis do not consistently show evidence of immune complex deposition (fibrinoid necrosis, complement fixation) in vessel walls or in Bruch membrane. Raised titres of circulating immune complexes in both peripheral blood and aqueous humor have been demonstrated,[14] but their presence may represent a response to injury rather than be a cause of it; such immune complexes may be formed as a protective response.[26,27,47,80] In both point prevalence and longitudinal studies it has been shown that patients with severe disease had high titres of antiretinal antibody in the absence of circulating immune complexes, whereas those with mild disease showed a reversal of this pattern;[26,27,47,80] similar findings were noted during disease relapse.[80] These findings may be explained by the hypothesis that the complexes are composed of idiotypic-antiidiotypic antibody, and serve to mop up pathogenic antibody and thus protect the retina.[26]

Cell-Mediated Mechanisms

T-lymphocytes play a central role in the pathogenesis of retinal vasculitis. In experimental models disease may be adoptively transferred by retinal antigen-specific T-lymphocytes and, in both animals and man, the histopathologic picture and response to specific immunosuppression strongly implicates the operation of cellular mechanisms.* As with humoral immunity, however, the exact mechanisms involved are still unknown, and the relative roles of the various cytokines produced by these cells require further evaluation.[19,85] Lymphocyte reactivity to retinal antigens, or the production of macrophage inhibitory factor in response to these antigens, has been shown in patients with retinal vasculitis and healthy controls.[18,22] Similar findings, however, have also been shown in patients with retinal detachments,[10] retinitis pigmentosa,[42] and ocular toxoplasmosis,[63] indicating that, in part, this reactivity is an epiphenomenon to retinal damage.

The results of current studies to identify markers of recent lymphocyte activation (soluble IL-2 receptors, T-lymphocytes bearing IL-2 receptors, HLA-DR or CD45Ro[31]) in peripheral blood, in an attempt to identify patients in remission, require further evaluation. Similarly, although the markers of endothelial cell activation and damage (von Willebrand factor, ICAM-1,[3] ELAM-1, and anti-endothelial cell antibodies[28a]) in isolated idiopathic retinal vasculitis are abnormal, longitudinal studies have not yet been completed to assess the significance of these findings.

HLA Associations

A major role for T-lymphocyte-mediated autoimmune processes can be postulated when there are significant HLA associations for a disease. One of the most striking is the association between HLA A29 and birdshot choroidopathy, although this association has only been reported in European and North American populations.[51,61,68] Significant, but less marked, associations have also been reported with Behçet disease (HLA-B51), multiple sclerosis (HLA-B7;DR2) and sarcoidosis (HLA-B8), although there are major variations in different racial groups.

Although the cause of pars planitis syndrome remains unknown, findings suggest that the disease is immune-

---

*References 22, 26, 30, 33, 38, 47, 80.

*References 18, 22, 32, 35, 43, 60, 61.

TABLE 44-2 RELATIVE FREQUENCIES OF HLA HAPLOTYPES FOUND IN RETINAL VASCULITIS*

Disease Type	Number	HLA	% Patients	% Controls	P Value (Chi-Square)
All	73	B44	38	23	0.002
Occlusive, ischemic	22	C5	45	19	0.005
		B44	55	23	0.0009
		A2,B44,C5	41	19	0.027
Nonocclusive, edematous	36	A29	17	7	0.04
With choroiditis	15	B7	45	27	0.025

*Adapted from Edelsten C, Stanford MR, Graham EM, Welgh K: HLA Class I associations of idiopathic retinal vasculitis, *Br J Ophthalmol* 1995 (in press).

mediated. Multiple sclerosis is associated with uveitis, and the most common ocular findings are intermediate uveitis with periphlebitis. Recently Malinowski and associates[53] found an association between HLA-B8, -B51, -DR2, and multiple sclerosis in patients with intermediate uveitis. HLA-B8 was present in 15 (37.5%) of 40 patients versus 85 (19.7%) of 431 controls (relative risk = 2.16; $P = 0.49$). HLA-DR2 was present in 27 patients (67.5%) versus 121 (28.0%) controls (relative risk = 5.32; $P < .0001$).

Few studies exist that have examined the associations of idiopathic retinal vasculitis. No class I associations were found in a group of 52 consecutive patients presenting with intermediate uveitis and retinal vasculitis in Austria,[2] and a weak association was found with the class II haplotype DR2/DQw1 in 43 Caucasian patients presenting with the same diagnosis in Miami, Florida, USA.[17]

A recent review of class I specificities in 75 patients with retinal vasculitis attending the Medical Eye Unit, St. Thomas' Hospital, London, UK, showed a significant increase in HLA-B44 compared to local controls (Table 44-2).[28a] When these patients were analyzed in terms of the pattern of posterior segment involvement, the association was found, particularly in patients with ischemic disease rather than in those with diffuse leakage or choroiditis. Furthermore, there was also an unexpected increase in HLA-A29 in those patients with nonischemic disease, some of whom might go on to develop birdshot retino-choroidopathy.[77]

DIFFERENTIAL DIAGNOSIS

The main differential diagnosis of idiopathic retinal vasculitis includes conditions that also give rise to retinal vasculitis, but which have not declared themselves systemically. Systemic disease may be missed, because lesions in other organ systems are in clinically silent areas (for instance, enhancing lesions seen in the central nervous system on magnetic resonance imaging in patients with early demyelination), or the systemic involvement of a disease has evaded identification as can occur with sarcoidosis or tuberculosis. Conditions that may present with retinal vasculitis are listed in Table 44-1.

Systemic Diseases

In the majority of cases, systemic disease may be excluded on symptomatic grounds, but certain ophthalmologic signs are useful. The presence of either retinal infiltrates or branch retinal vein occlusions with a marked vitritis distinguishes patients with Behçet disease from all other groups.[37a] Periphlebitis in the presence of choroidal or retinal pigment epithelial disease points strongly toward sarcoidosis. Although sarcoidosis is not categorized as a systemic vasculitis, it is probably the most common systemic disease associated with ocular inflammation and retinal vasculitis. Behçet disease may involve systemic vasculitis and have frequent and often devastating ocular involvement. In a review of 49 patients with Behçet disease who were evaluated at the National Eye Institute, 28 of 98 eyes with retinal vascular involvement had vision of 20/400 or worse.[58a]

Retinal vasculitis may occur in patients with multiple sclerosis. Multiple sclerosis was first associated with inflammatory eye disease in the early 1900s, and Breger and Leopold found uveitis in 14 of 52 patients with multiple sclerosis.[9b] The most common ocular findings in patients with multiple sclerosis include intermediate uveitis and periphlebitis, and the uveitis may precede or follow the development of multiple sclerosis.

Inflammatory bowel disease can involve the eyes in a number of ways; intermediate uveitis, retinitis, scleritis, and keratitis have all been described. Duker and associates[25a] reported a patient with Crohn disease who had a severe bilateral obliterative retinal arteritis and phlebitis that appeared to respond to treatment with corticosteroids and cyclophosphamide. Another bowel disease associated with retinal vasculitis is Whipple disease. Patients with this disorder have malabsorption with diarrhea, and PAS-positive material, probably bacterial, can be identified on biopsy of the intestine or vitreous humor. Fluorescein angiography shows diffuse vasculitis with hemorrhages, exudates, retinal capillary occlusion, and choroidal folds.[3b]

Noninflammatory Retinal Vasculopathies

As stated earlier, a group of noninflammatory retinal vasculopathies are often confused with the retinal vasculitis. It is appropriate to consider them in the differential diagnosis of idiopathic retinal vasculitis, however, since certain signs overlap. The lack of obvious intraocular cellular reactions is an important differentiating feature, however.

Wegener Granulomatosis. Wegener granulomatosis is a systemic vasculitis characterized by a necrotizing granulomatous vasculitis of the upper and lower respiratory tracts, a focal necrotizing glomerulonephritis, and systemic small vessel vasculitis involving a number of organ systems. Ocular involvement, including uveitis, scleritis, and retinal vasculopathy, occurs in about 16% of patients.[11a,29b] The antineutrophil cytoplasmic antibody (ANCA) test is useful in diagnosing and following the clinical course of patients with Wegener granulomatosis.[14a,57b] Young[89] described 98 patients tested for the presence of ANCA by an indirect immunofluorescence method and found a positive ANCA in patients with chronic uveitis of various causes. A cytoplasmic pattern of staining (cANCA) is more specific for Wegener granulomatosis than a peripheral pattern (pANCA). Soukasian and associates[77a] reported that ANCA tests, positive in seven patients with scleritis caused by Wegener granulomatosis, were negative in 54 patients with other ocular inflammatory diseases, suggesting the test is both sensitive and specific. High specificity of the cANCA for Wegener granulomatosis in patients with ocular inflammatory disease has been reported by other investigators as well.[57a]

Polyarteritis Nodosa. Polyarteritis nodosa is classified as a necrotizing vasculitis involving medium-size muscular arteries and smaller arterioles. Polyarteritis nodosa may involve the eye in up to 20% of patients,[81a] and patients can present with bilateral iritis, vitritis, and retinal vasculitis involving both the arterioles and venules.[1,56a]

Similar to Wegener granulomatosis, polyarteritis nodosa is a potentially fatal disease, but therapy (including corticosteroids and cyclophosphamide) can substantially improve the prognosis.[1,29a] Cogan syndrome, which consists of a nonsyphilitic interstitial keratitis and hearing loss, is associated with retinal vasculitis and may be a variant of polyarteritis nodosa.

Systemic Lupus Erythematosis. Systemic lupus erythematosis (SLE) is a systemic collagen vascular disease diagnosed by both clinical and laboratory criteria. The eye can be involved in patients with SLE, and the retinal vasculature is frequently affected. Severe retinal vasoocclusive disease has been described and may be associated with central nervous system involvement.[44b] In most cases, the retinal vascular disease of SLE is not associated with an inflammatory cell infiltrate.[36a] Less frequently, a retinal vasculitis with perivascular inflammatory sheathing will be seen.[9a,21,84a]

Relapsing Polychondritis. Relapsing polychondritis is a systemic inflammatory disease that causes inflammatory destruction of the cartilage of the nose and ear lobes. Involvement of the trachea with respiratory compromise can be fatal. In a review of 112 patients, Isaak[44a] noted ocular disease in 21 patients at the time of diagnosis. Although scleritis and episcleritis were the most common findings, retinal vasculitis occurred in 9% of patients.

Infectious Diseases

As in the case with systemic disease causing retinal vasculitis, it is important to diagnose promptly and accurately infectious causes of retinal vasculitis so that appropriate therapy can be initiated (Table 44-1).

Although tuberculosis was considered one of the most common causes of both uveitis and retinal vasculitis in the early part of this century, toxoplasmosis is probably the most common infectious cause of retinal vascular disease today. In cases of ocular toxoplasmosis, retinal vasculitis occurs in association with discrete foci of retinochorioiditis at the site of infection. Patients with florid retinal vasculitis and peripheral capillary closure, particularly those from the Indian subcontinent of other endemic areas, should always be suspected of harboring tuberculosis.[70] Rarely, analysis of intraocular fluids may provide evidence of unsuspected infection such as toxoplasmosis.[4] Syphilis and herpetic viral infections of the retina (herpes simplex virus, varicella-zoster virus, and cytomegalovirus infections) are also frequent causes of retinal vasculitis.

Primary Ocular Diseases

A number of diseases limited to the eye are associated with retinal vasculitis. Intermediate uveitis of the pars planitis syndrome subtype occurs without associated systemic disease. Frequently, pars planitis syndrome occurs with a prominent vasculitis requiring therapy. Birdshot choroidopathy is characterized not only by circular, white-yellow, deep choroidal lesions, but also with narrowing of the retinal vessels with occasional retinal vasculitis.

Eales Disease

Henry Eales[27c,27d] described five young men with recurring vitreous and retinal hemorrhages associated with constipation and epistaxis. Although in India many patients with Eales disease were reported to have reactive skin tests to PPD,[3a] patients in the United States are less likely to have this history and do not respond to antituberculosis therapy. Therefore, to many investigators, the disease represents an idiopathic form of retinal vasculitis in younger patients that often occurs without systemic associations, and the term *Eales disease* is not used.

LABORATORY INVESTIGATIONS

The most important investigation in any patient who presents with apparently isolated retinal vasculitis is a full general medical history and examination. The principles of investigation of patients with retinal vasculitis are to identify any underlying systemic disease, to elicit the extent and severity of disease, and to ensure no other medical problems exist that might interfere with immunosuppressive therapy.

The weight and blood pressure of the patient is routinely

recorded. Depending on history, review of systems, and physical findings, appropriate tests may include a full blood count, erythrocyte sedimentation rate, blood sugar, blood urea nitrogen, electrolytes, liver function tests, and serum angiotensin converting enzyme level, as well as syphilis serology. A chest x-ray may reveal bilateral hilar adenopathy consistent with sarcoidosis or may show changes compatible with tuberculosis. If the patient is to be started on cyclosporine, a creatinine clearance is obtained. Routine skin tests are not necessary, although a Mantoux test (starting at 1 : 10,000 then 1 : 1,000) may be very useful in differentiating sarcoidosis from tuberculosis, particularly in patients with ischemic or choroidal forms of disease. Coagulation studies (fibrinogen, prothrombin time, thrombin time, activated partial thromboplastin time, and protein S, protein C, and antithrombin three levels) are performed in patients with ischemic retinal vasculitis.

Serologic investigations for Epstein-Barr virus,[82] *Brucella* sp.,[87] and *Borrelia* sp. infections[9] are not routinely performed. Although a chest x-ray is appropriate, other imaging studies are only performed if clinically indicated. The role of HLA typing has yet to be critically evaluated, but it appears that (1) HLA B-7 may be predictive of demyelinating disease, particularly in female patients,[29] and (2) the presence of HLA A-29 should raise the possibility of birdshot chorioretinopathy in patients in whom the typical features of depigmented lesions and electroretinogram (ERG) changes have not yet developed.[77]

Good quality stereoscopic fluorescein angiograms are essential in the evaluation and management of retinal vasculitis,[52] but technically high-quality angiograms are often hard to obtain. The pupil may be small, with posterior synechiae making pupil dilatation difficult; the vitreous humor may be opaque with inflammatory cells and debris; and peripheral views under these conditions may be impossible. The main purpose of fluorescein angiography is to ascertain the state of the macula. A cystoid appearance must be interpreted with care, as it may be compatible with a good visual acuity.[62] When the capillary phase of the angiogram is not initially visualized, and when the patient's vision does not improve as expected on immunosuppressive therapy, the angiogram should be repeated to look for underlying macular ischemia.[6] Characteristic features of retinal vasculitis seen on fluorescein angiography include optic disc leakage, diffuse or focal microvascular leakage or staining, peripheral capillary closure, and new vessel formation.

Little work has been carried out on the electrophysiology of human eyes with retinal vasculitis. Measurement of the electrooculogram (EOG) and ERG is particularly useful in monitoring progression of disease when retinal pigment epithelial pathology is present.[44] Findings in most human studies have shown subnormal ERG responses proportional to the degree of retinal damage.[12,34,50] One study looked at both EOG and ERG in patients with retinal vasculitis at different stages of disease. Those patients with early disease (vitreous

humor cells only) showed enhanced EOG with little change in the ERG; both parameters were similarly depressed in patients with more destructive disease.[44] There was no change in the b wave:a wave ratio, indicating that most of the changes were occurring at the level of the outer blood retinal barrier; similar findings have been seen in multifocal choroiditis and panuveitis syndrome.[23]

Experimental studies have consistently shown that the ERG has three phases in relation to the development of EAU;[50,79] there is an initial supernormal phase prior to disease onset, which has been linked to circulating antiretinal antibodies,[81] followed by a subnormal phase during active inflammation, with some recovery when disease settled. Again, these studies reported no change in the b wave:a wave ratio, indicating primary photoreceptor pathology.

THERAPY

Over the last century many different treatment regimens have been tried in patients with idiopathic retinal vasculitis. These treatments have ranged from protein shock therapy (intravenous injection of milk products or diphtheria antitoxin), deliberate infection with malaria, surgical removal of supposed infective foci (dental clearance or appendectomy), to the encouragement of antibodies to enter the eye by repeated paracentesis or by direct inoculation with blood.[16,25] The introduction of corticosteroid therapy in the 1950s was a major step forward in the management of this condition. These and newer immunosuppressive agents have become the mainstay of treatment,[40] although no appropriate randomized double-blind, placebo-controlled studies have ever been reported.

Not all patients require treatment. In many cases ocular inflammation is relatively mild, visual function is good, and patients may simply be observed, treated with topical agents to prevent anterior segment complications, or maintained with intermittent injections of periocular corticosteroids.[46] It is important to remember that, once started, systemic treatment may be required for several years, so the potential toxicity of the agents used becomes increasingly significant. Fortunately, idiopathic retinal vasculitis tends to burn out in middle age, so the principles of management involve suppressing intraocular inflammation with a minimum of side effects, while retaining good vision until resolution.

Medical Treatment

Many investigators reserve systemic treatment for patients with a vision of 6/12 or worse, when visual changes can be attributed to inflammation or macular edema. Most episodes of vision loss with relapse of disease can be managed using systemic corticosteroids alone; patients are started on prednisolone (80 mg/day or 1-2 mg/kg in children) for 4 days, 60 mg for 4 days, and then 40 mg/day for 1 month with the dose adjusted thereafter according to the clinical and angiographic signs of inflammation. One of the most common reasons for therapeutic failure is undertreatment. Patients may not show improvement with this regimen until the third or fourth week, which emphasizes the importance of continuing with a high dose of corticosteroids for a long time. A recent study of this regimen, which followed 23 patients with retinal vasculitis for a year, showed that resolution could be achieved in 80% of the subjects without recourse to other immunosuppressive agents; in fact half of the patients were off treatment within 12 months.[43a] Minor side effects occurred in 50% of the patients, but only two required further medical intervention.

Pulsed methylprednisolone (1 g alternate days for 3 pulses) may be used in very severe cases, although there is no evidence that this treatment is more effective than an equivalent dose of oral corticosteroids. Azathioprine is a useful additional drug since it allows both a reduction in corticosteroid dosage and reduces the frequency of relapse. This drug is usually well tolerated, but patients on azathioprine should have their white cell count monitored every 6 weeks, since pancytopenia caused by a genetically determined enzyme deficiency may develop.[1a]

The value of cyclosporine in the management of idiopathic retinal vasculitis has not been fully established.[20,59,64] Cyclosporine may be used as an antiinflammatory drug or a corticosteroid-sparing agent in patients who require more than 40 mg prednisolone daily to achieve remission. It is not known, however, whether it is better than azathioprine in this respect. Initial trials using 10 mg/kg caused considerable side effects, particularly renal damage, with severe rebound disease when the dose was tapered.[40,59] Trials using low-dose cyclosporine (5 mg/kg) are currently being evaluated;[83] the drug is effective, but on its own is no better than an equivalent dose of systemic corticosteroids. Only a few patients appear to benefit from being transferred to cyclosporine if appropriate doses of corticosteroids have failed.[64] In cases in which all of these therapeutic maneuvers have failed, plasma exchange has proved successful,[88] and early results with low-dose methotrexate appear promising;[75] further clinical trials are necessary.

Laser Treatment

Laser photocoagulation is rarely required in patients with retinal vasculitis. The main indication, as mentioned previously, is in the management of persistent neovascularization resulting in recurrent vitreous hemorrhage or in rubeotic glaucoma. It is worth repeating that before photocoagulation the eye must be made as quiet as possible by medical means to avoid inducing cystoid macula edema.[37]

Surgical Treatment

Surgical treatment is reserved for the complications of retinal vasculitis that do not respond to medical therapy. In practically all cases it is advisable to reduce the amount of intraocular inflammation as much as possible in the perioperative period.[58] Raised intraocular pressure[65] unresponsive to medical agents may require drainage surgery. Unfortu-nately, in the presence of peripheral anterior synechiae or rubeosis, tube drainage may be needed. The results of trabeculectomy in this situation (particularly in aphakic eyes) are often poor, with filter failure within months; the addition of 5-fluorouracil may be necessary, and preliminary results have been encouraging.[45,66]

Removal of the vitreous humor has been advocated to reduce intraocular inflammation, to enhance the penetration of corticosteroids, and to improve macular edema unresponsive to corticosteroids.[24] The benefits of vitrectomy for reduction of intraocular inflammation on a sustained basis have not been verified. Indications for vitrectomy also include persistent dense vitreous humor inflammation, vitreous hemorrhage, traction retinal detachment, and epiretinal membrane formation.[54,58]

PROGNOSIS

The natural history of the condition has been poorly documented, particularly since it responds well to systemic immunosuppression. Patients seem to fall into two groups: those that do well, retaining a vision of 6/12 or better, and those that do poorly, despite adequate and intensive immunosuppression. The ability to distinguish between these two groups has been the goal of investigators for many years. In terms of visual prognosis, severity of disease seems to be more important than duration of disease.[76] In one study the visual outcome in 26 patients with retinal vasculitis was followed for a mean of 2 years; half the patients had a visual acuity of 6/18 or better at the end of the study. This outcome, however, was unrelated to relapse rate or changes in immunologic markers (circulating immune complexes or antiretinal antibodies).[80]

SUMMARY

Improvements in the understanding and management of retinal vasculitis must arise from increased knowledge of the underlying immunopathology of the condition. Improvements can be envisaged in three main areas: etiology, diagnosis, and treatment.

Easy access to tissue samples from the eye should revolutionize the understanding of retinal vasculitis with improved techniques of chorioretinal biopsy, immunocytology, and molecular microbiology. Immunogenetic studies may elucidate what factors govern disease pattern, relapse, and visual prognosis. Rheologic studies must be developed to distinguish nonocclusive from ischemic retinal vasculitis.

Further improvements in the diagnosis of systemic disorders will probably show that many of the idiopathic cases are *formes frustes* of generalized diseases (such as sarcoidosis). The ability to image the eye, in particular the choroidal circulation, may throw light on the early stages of disease with implications for management.

The treatment of retinal vasculitis will come to rely on more specific pharmacologic and immunologic intervention than is presently available. Modification of the immune response either systemically (anti-CD4 antibody, cytokine infusions, or idiotypic manipulation) or at the local level (anti-ICAM antibody) theoretically should be much more successful than the treatments currently used. The results of active immunization programs in animal models, including the dosed administration of oral antigens to induce immunologic tolerance, have shown some success in both ameliorating and preventing disease and hold much hope for the future treatment of human idiopathic retinal vasculitis.

REFERENCES

1. Akova A et al.: Ocular presentations of polyarteritis nodosa, *Ophthalmology* 100:1775-1781, 1993.
1a. Anstey A et al.: Pancytopenia related to azathioprine—an enzyme deficiency caused by a common genetic polymorphism: a review, *J R Soc Med* 85:752-755, 1992.
2. Arocker-Mettinger E et al.: Intermediate uveitis: do HLA antigens play a role? *Dev Ophthalmol* 23:15-19, 1992.
3. Arocker-Mettinger E et al.: Circulating ICAM-1 levels in serum of uveitis patients, *Curr Eye Res* 11(suppl):161-166, 1992.
3a. Ashton N: Pathogenesis and aetiology of Eales's disease. In Pandit YK, editor: 19th International Congress of Ophthalmology, Bombay, 1962, The Time of India Press.
3b. Avila MP, Jalkh AE et al.: Manifestations of Whipple's disease in the posterior segment of the eye, *Arch Ophthalmol* 102:384-390, 1984.
4. Baarsma GS: The epidemiology and genetics of endogenous uveitis: a review, *Curr Eye Res Suppl* 11:1-9, 1992.
5. Baarsma GS et al.: Analysis of local antibody production in the vitreous humour of patients with severe uveitis, *Am J Ophthalmol* 112:147-150, 1991.
6. Bentley CR et al.: Macular ischaemia in posterior uveitis, *Eye* 7:411-414, 1993.
7. Bloch-Michel E, Nussenblatt RB: International Uveitis Study Group recommendations for the evaluation of intraocular inflammatory disease, *Am J Ophthalmol* 103:234-235, 1987.
8. Blumenkranz MS et al.: Acute multifocal haemorrhagic retinal vasculitis, *Ophthalmology* 95:1663-1672, 1988.
9. Bodine SR et al.: Multifocal choroiditis with evidence lyme disease, *Ann Ophthalmol* 24:169-173, 1992.
9a. Böke W, Bäumer A: Klinische und histopathologische Augenbefunde beim akuten Lupus Erythematodes disseminatus, *Klin Monatsbl Augenheilkd* 146:175-187, 1965.
9b. Breger BC, Leopold IH: The incidence of uveitis in multiple sclerosis, *Am J Ophthalmol* 62:540-545, 1966.
10. Brinkman CJ, Roekhuyse RM: Cell-mediated immunity after retinal detachment as determined by lymphocyte stimulation, *Am J Ophthalmol* 86:260-265, 1978.
11. Brockhurst RJ, Schepens CL: Uveitis 4. Peripheral uveitis: the complication of retinal detachment, *Arch Ophthalmol* 80:747-753, 1986.
11a. Bullen CL et al.: Ocular complication's of Wegener's granulomatosis, *Ophthalmology* 90:279-290, 1983.
12. Cantrill HL et al.: Electrophysiologic changes in chronic pars planitis, *Am J Ophthalmol* 91:305-312, 1981.
13. Chan CC et al.: Immunopathology of ocular onchocerciasis. 2. Antiretinal autoantibodies in serum and ocular fluids, *Ophthalmology* 94:439-443, 1987.
14. Char DH et al.: Immune complexes in uveitis, *Am J Ophthalmol* 87:678-681, 1979.
14a. Cohen Tervaert JW et al.: Association between active Wegener's granulomatosis and anticytoplasmic antibodies: *Arch Int Med* 149:2461-2465, 1989.
15. Darrell RW, Wagener HP, Kurland LT: Epidemiology of uveitis, *Arch Ophthalmol* 68:502-515, 1962.
16. Davis AE: Uveitis, *JAMA* 73:1331-1335, 1919.
17. Davis JL, Mittal KK, Nussenblatt RB: HLA in intermediate uveitis, *Dev Ophthalmol* 23:35-38, 1992.
18. de Smet MD et al.: Cellular immune responses of patients with uveitis to retinal antigens and their fragments, *Am J Ophthalmol* 110:135-142, 1990.
19. de Vos AK, Hoekzema R, Kijlstra A: Cytokines and uveitis: a review, *Curr Eye Res* 11:581-597, 1992.
20. de Vries J et al.: Cyclosporin in the treatment of severe chronic idiopathic uveitis, *Br J Ophthalmol* 74:344-349, 1990.
21. Diddie KR, Ernest JT, Aronson AJ: Chorioretinopathy in a case of systemic lupus erythematosus. *Trans Am Ophthalmol Soc* 75:122-131, 1975.
22. Doekes G et al.: Humoral and cellular immune responsiveness to human S-antigen in uveitis, *Curr Eye Res* 6:909-919, 1987.
23. Dreyer RF, Gass DM: Multifocal choroiditis and panuveitis, *Arch Ophthalmol* 102:1776-1784, 1984.
24. Dugel PU et al.: Pars plana vitrectomy for inflammation-related cystoid macular edema unresponsive to corticosteroids, *Ophthalmology* 99:1535-1541, 1992.
25. Duke-Elder S, editor: *System of ophthalmology,* vol IX, London, 1966, Henry Kempton.
25a. Duker JS, Brown GC, Brooks L: Retinal vasculitis in Crohn's Disease, *Amer J Ophthalmol* 103:664-668, 1987.
26. Dumonde DC et al.: Anti-retinal autoimmunity and circulating immune complex in patients with retinal vasculitis, *Lancet* 2:787-792, 1982.
27. Dumonde DC et al.: Autoimmune mechanisms in inflammatory eye disease, *Trans Ophthalmol Soc UK* 104:232-238, 1985.
27a. Dustin ML, Springer TA: Lymphocyte function-associated antigen-1 (LFA-1) interaction with intercellular adhesion molecule-1 (ICAM-1) is one of at least three mechanisms for lymphocyte adhesion to cultured endothelial cells, *J Cell Biol* 107:321-331, 1988.
27b. Dustin ML et al.: Induction by LI 1 and interferon-γ: tissue distribution, biochemistry, and function of a natural adherence molecule (ICAM-1), *J Immunol* 137:245-254, 1986.
27c. Eales H: Cases of retinal hemorrhage associated with epistaxis and constipation; *Birmingham Med Rev* 9:262-273, 1880.
27d. Eales H: Primary retinal haemorrhage in young men, *Ophthal Rev* 1:41, 1882.
28. Edelsten C, Stanford MR, Graham EM, Welgh K: HLA Class I associations of idiopathic retinal vasculitis, *Br J Ophthalmol* 1995 (in press).
28a. Edelsten C et al.: Antiendothelial cell antibodies in retinal vasculitis, *Curr Eye Res* 11:203-208, 1992.
29. Edelsten C et al.: Prevalence of HLA B7 in MS patients with symptomatic uveitis, *Lancet* 339:942, 1992.
29a. Fauci AS, Doppman JL, Wolff SM: Cyclophosphamide-induced remissions in advanced polyarteritis nodosa, *Am J Med* 64:890-894, 1978.
29b. Fauci AS, Haynes BF, Katz P et al.: Wegener's granulomatosis: prospective clinical and therapeutic experience with 85 patients for 21 years, *Ann Intern Med* 98:76-85, 1983.
30. Faure JP: Autoimmunity and the retina, *Curr Top Eye Res* 2:215-302, 1980.
31. Feron EJ, Calder VL, Lightman SL: Distribution of IL-2R and CD45Ro expression on D4+ and CD8+ T-lymphocytes in the peripheral blood of patients with posterior uveitis, *Curr Eye Res* 11(suppl):167-172, 1992.
32. Forrester JV: Uveitis: pathogenesis, *Lancet* 338:1498-1501, 1991.
33. Forrester JV, Stott DI, Hercu KM: Naturally occurring antibodies to bovine and human retinal S-antigen: a comparison between uveitis patients and healthy controls, *Br J Ophthalmol* 73:155-159, 1989.
34. Francois J: L'electroretinographie dans les uveitis, *Ophthalmologica* 125:137-143, 1953.
34a. Freedman AS et al.: Adhesion of human B cells to germinal centers in vitro involves VLA-4 and IN CAM-110, *Science* 249:1030-1033, 1990.
34b. Geng JC et al.: Rapid neutrophil adhesion to activated endothelium mediated by GMP-140, *Nature* 343:757-760, 1990.
35. Gery I, Mochizuki M, Nussenblatt RB: Retinal specific antigens and immunopathogenic processes they provoke. In Osborne N, Chader J, editors: *Progress in retinal research,* Oxford, 1986, Pergamon Press.
36. Graham E, Spalton DJ, Sanders MD: Immunological investigations in retinal vasculitis, *Trans Ophthalmol Soc UK* 101:12-16, 1980.
36a. Graham EM et al.: Cerebral and retinal vascular changes in systemic lupus erythematosis, *Ophthalmology* 92:444-448, 1985.
37. Graham EM et al.: Neovascularization associated with posterior uveitis, *Br J Ophthalmol* 71:826-833, 1987.
37a. Graham EM et al.: A point prevalence study of 150 patients with idiopathic retinal vasculitis. 1. Diagnostic value of ophthalmological features, *Br J Ophthalmol* 73:714-721, 1989.

38. Gregerson DS, Abrahams IW, Thirkill CE: Serum antibody levels of uveitis patients to bovine retinal antigens, *Invest Ophthalmol Vis Sci* 21:669-680, 1981.

39. Gregerson DS, Abrahams WI, Pucklin JE: Serum antibody responses to bovine retinal S-antigen and rod outer segments in proliferative diabetic retinopathy before and after argon laser photocoagulation, *Ophthalmology* 89:767-771, 1982.

40. Hemady R, Tauber J, Foster CS: Immunosuppressive drugs in immune and inflammatory ocular disease, *Surv Ophthalmol* 35:369-385, 1991.

41. Henderly DE et al.: Changing patterns of uveitis, *Am J Ophthalmol* 103:131-136, 1987.

42. Hendricks RL, Rishman GA: Lymphocyte subpopulations and S-antigen reactivity in retinitis pigmentosa, *Arch Ophthalmol* 103:61-65, 1985.

43. Hirose S et al.: Lymphocyte responses to retinal-specific antigens in uveitis patients and healthy subjects, *Curr Eye Res* 7:393-402, 1988.

43a. Howe L, Stanford MR, Edelsten C, Graham EM: The efficacy of systemic corticosteroids in sight threatening retinal vasculitis, *Eye* 8:443-447, 1994.

44. Ikeda H et al.: Electroretinography and electro-oculography to localize abnormalities in early-stage inflammatory eye disease, *Doc Ophthalmol* 73:387-394, 1990.

44a. Isaak BI, Liesegang TJ, Michet CJ: Ocular and systemic findings in relapsing polychondritis, *Ophthalmology* 93:681-689, 1986.

44b. Jabs DA, Fine SL, Hochberg MC et al.: Severe retinal vaso-occlusive disease in systemic lupus erythematosis, *Arch Ophthalmol* 104:558-563, 1986.

45. Jampel HD, Jabs DA, Quigley HA: Trabeculectomy with 5-fluorouracil for adult inflammatory glaucoma, *Am J Ophthalmol* 9:168-173, 1990.

46. Jennings T et al.: Posterior sub-Tenons injections of corticosteroids in uveitis patients with cystoid macular oedema, *Jpn J Ophthalmol* 32:385-391, 1988.

47. Kasp E et al.: A point prevalence study of 150 patients with idiopathic retinal vasculitis. 2. Clinical relevance of antiretinal autoimmunity and circulating immune complexes, *Br J Ophthalmol* 73:722-730, 1989.

48. Kasp E et al.: Antibody affinity to retinal S-antigen in patients with retinal vasculitis, *Am J Ophthalmol* 113:697-701, 1992.

49. Kasp E et al.: Circulating immune complexes may play a regulatory and pathogenic role in experimental autoimmune uveoretinitis, *Clin Exp Immunol* 88:307-312, 1992.

49a. Kishimoto TK et al.: The leukocyte integrins, *Adv Immunol* 46:149-182, 1989.

49b. Lai J et al.: Treatment with corticosteroids and cyclosporine A inhibits the expression of cell adhesion molecules in experimental autoimmune uveitis (EAU), *Invest Ophthalmol Vis Sci* 34(suppl):1206, 1993.

49c. Lawrence MB, Springer TA: Leukocytes roll on a selectin at physiological flow rates: distinction from and prerequisite for adhesion through integrins, *Cell* 65:859-873, 1991.

50. Lawwill T, Wacker W, Macdonald R: The role of electroretinography in evaluating posterior uveitis, *Am J Ophthalmol* 74:1086-1093, 1972.

51. LeHoang P et al.: HLA-A29.2 subtype associated with birdshot retinochoroidopathy, *Am J Ophthalmol* 113:33-35, 1992.

52. Listhaus AD, Freeman RW: Fluorescein angiography in patients with posterior uveitis, *Int Ophthalmol Clin* 30:297-308, 1990.

52a. Liversidge J, Sewell HF, Forrester JV: Interactions between lymphocytes and cells of the blood-retina barrier: mechanisms of T lymphocyte adhesion to human retinal capillary endothelial cells and retinal pigment epithelial cells in vitro, *Immunology* 71:390-396, 1990.

52b. Liversidge JA, Thomson AW, Forrester JV: FK 506 modulates accessory cell adhesion molecule expression and inhibits CD4 lymphocyte adhesion to retinal pigment epithelial cells in vitro: implications for therapy of uveoretinitis, *Transplant Proc* 23:3339-3342, 1991.

52c. Luscinskas FW et al.: Cytokine-activated human endothelial cell monolayers support enhanced neutrophil transmigration via a mechanism involving both endothelial-leukocyte adhesion molecule-1 and intercellular adhesion molecule-1, *J Immunol* 146:1617-1625, 1991.

53. Malinowski SM et al.: The association of HLA-B8, B-51, DR2, and multiple sclerosis in pars planitis, *Ophthalmology* 100:1199-1205, 1993.

53a. Marak G: Effects of complement depletion on experimental uveitis, *Ophthalmic Res* 11:97-107, 1979.

54. Mieler WF et al.: Vitrectomy in the management of peripheral uveitis, *Ophthalmology* 95:859-864, 1988.

55. Miettinen R: Incidence of uveitis in Northern Finland, *Acta Ophthalmol* 55:252-260, 1977.

56. Mishima S et al.: Behçet's disease in Japan: ophthalmological aspects, *Trans Am Ophthalmol Soc* 76:225-229, 1979.

56a. Morgan CM, Foster CS, Gragoudas ES: Retinal vasculitis in polyarteritis nodosa, *Retina* 6:205-209, 1986.

57. Mortensen K, Sjolie AK, Goldschmidt E: Uveitis: eine epidemiologische untersuchung, *Ber Dtsch Ophthalmol Ges* 78:97-100, 1981.

57a. Nolle B, Coners H, Guncker G: ANCA in ocular inflammatory disorders, *Adv Exp Med Biol* 336:305-307, 1993.

57b. Nolle B, Specks U, Ludemann J et al.: Anticytoplasmic autoantibodies: their immunodiagnostic value in Wegener's granulomatosis, 111:28-40, 1989.

58. Nolthenuis PA, Deutman AF: Surgical treatment of the complications of chronic uveitis, *Ophthalmologica* 186:11-16, 1983.

58a. Nussenblatt RB, Palestine AG: Uveitis in fundamentals and clinical practice, Chicago, 1989, Yearbook Medical Publishers, 216.

59. Nussenblatt RB, Palestine AG, Chan CC: Cyclosporin A therapy in the treatment of intraocular inflammatory disease resistant to systemic corticosteroids and cytotoxic agents, *Am J Ophthalmol* 96:275-282, 1983.

60. Nussenblatt RB et al.: Cellular immune responsiveness of uveitis patients to retinal S-antigen, *Am J Ophthalmol* 89:173-179, 1980.

61. Nussenblatt RB et al.: Birdshot retinochoroidopathy associated with HLA-A29 antigen and immune responsiveness to retinal s-antigen, *Am J Ophthalmol* 94:147-158, 1982.

62. Nussenblatt RB et al.: Macular thickening and visual acuity: measurement in patients with cystoid macular edema, *Ophthalmology* 94:1134-1139, 1987.

63. Nussenblatt RB et al.: Lymphocyte proliferative responses of patients with ocular toxoplasmosis to parasite and retinal antigen, *Am J Ophthalmol* 107:632-641, 1989.

64. Nussenblatt RB et al.: Randomized, double-masked study of cyclosporine compared to prednisolone in the treatment of endogenous uveitis, *Am J Ophthalmol* 112:138-146, 1991.

65. Panek WC et al.: Glaucoma in patients with uveitis, *Br J Ophthalmol* 74:223-227, 1990.

66. Patitsas CJ et al.: Glaucoma filtering surgery with postoperative 5-fluorouracil in patients with inflammatory disease, *Ophthalmology* 99:594-599, 1992.

67. Perkins ES, Folk J: Uveitis in London and Iowa, *Ophthalmologica* 189:36-40, 1984.

67a. Picker LJ et al.: ELAM-1 is an adhesion molecule for skin homing T-cells, *Nature* 349:796-799, 1991.

68. Priem HA et al.: HLA typing in birdshot chorioretinopathy, *Am J Ophthalmol* 105:182-185, 1988.

69. Pruett RC, Brockhurst RJ, Letts NF: Fluorescein angiography of peripheral uveitis, *Am J Ophthalmol* 77:448-453, 1974.

69a. Rice GE, Munro JM, Bevilaqua MP: Inducible cell adhesion molecule 110 (IN CAM-110) is an endothelial receptor for lymphocytes, *J Exp Med* 171:1369-1374, 1990.

70. Rosen PH, Spalton DJ, Graham EM: Intraocular tuberculosis, *Eye* 4:486-492, 1990.

70a. Rosenbaum JT, Robertson JE Jr, Satzke RC: Retinal vasculitis-a primer, *West J Med* 154:182-185, 1991.

71. Rothova A et al.: Risk factors for ocular sarcoidosis, *Doc Ophthalmol* 72:287-296, 1989.

72. Sanders MD: Retinal vasculitis: a review, *J R Soc Med* 72:908-915, 1979.

73. Sanders MD: Retinal arteritis, retinal vasculitis and autoimmune retinal vasculitis, *Eye* 1:441-465, 1987.

74. Sanders MD, Graham EM: Retinal vasculitis, *Postgrad Med J* 64:488-496, 1988.

75. Shah SS et al.: Low dose methotrexate therapy for ocular inflammatory disease, *Ophthalmology* 99:1419-1423, 1992.

76. Smith RE, Godfrey WA, Kimura SS: Chronic cyclitis. 1. Course and visual prognosis, *Trans Am Acad Ophthalmol Otolaryngol* 77:760-767, 1973.

77. Soubrane G, Bokobza R, Coscas G: Late developing lesions in birdshot retinochoroidopathy, *Am J Ophthalmol* 109:204-210, 1990.

77a. Soukasian SH et al.: Diagnostic value of antineutrophil cytoplasmic antibodies in scleritis associated with Wegener's granulomatosis, *Ophthalmology* 99:125-132, 1992.

77b. Spencer WH: *Ophthalmic pathology,* ed 3, 1985, WB Saunders.

78. Spitznas M, Meyer-Schwiekerath, Stephan B: The clinical picture of Eales' disease, *Graefes Arch Clin Exp Ophthalmol* 194:73-85, 1975.

78a. Springer TA: Adhesion receptors of the immune system, *Nature* 346:425-434, 1990.

79. Stanford MR, Robbins J: Experimental posterior uveitis. 2. Electroretinographic studies, *Br J Ophthalmol* 72:88-96, 1988.

80. Stanford MR et al.: A longitudinal study of clinical and immunological findings in 52 patients with relapsing retinal vasculitis, *Br J Ophthalmol* 72:442-447, 1988.

81. Stanford MR et al.: Passive administration of antibody against retinal S-antigen induces electroretinographic supernormality, *Invest Ophthalmol Vis Sci* 33:30-35, 1992.

81a. Stillerman ML: Ocular manifestations of duffuse collagen disease, *Arch Ophthalmol* 45:239-250, 1951.

82. Tiedeman JS: Epstein-Barr antibodies in multifocal choroiditis and panuveitis, *Am J Ophthalmol* 103:659-663, 1987.

83. Towler H et al.: Low dose cyclosporin A therapy in chronic posterior uveitis, *Eye* 3:282-287, 1989.

84. Vadot E: Epidemiology of intermediate uveitis: a prospective study in Savoy. In Boke W, Manthey K, Nussenblatt R, editors: *Intermediate uveitis,* Basel, 1990, Karger.

84a. Vine AK, Barr CC: Proliferative lupus retinopathy, *Arch Ophthalmol* 102:852-854, 1984.

85. Wakefield D, Lloyd A: The role of cytokines in the pathogenesis of inflammatory eye disease, *Cytokine* 4:1-5, 1992.

86. Wakefield D et al.: Uveitis: aetiology and disease associations in an Australian population, *Aust N Z J Ophthalmol* 14:181-187, 1986.

87. Walker J, Sharma OP, Rao NA: Brucellosis and uveitis, *Am J Ophthalmol* 114:374-375, 1992.

87a. Whitcup SM et al.: Endothelial leukocyte adhesion molecule-1 in endotoxin-induced uveitis, *Invest Ophthalmol Vis Sci* 33:2626-2630, 1992.

87b. Whitcup SM et al.: Expression of cell adhesion molecules in posterior uveitis, *Arch Ophthalmol* 110:662-666, 1992.

87c. Whitcup SM et al.: Monoclonal antibodies against ICAM-1 (CD-54) and LFA-1 (CD11a/CD18) inhibit experimental autoimmune uveitis, *Clin Immunol Immunopathol* 67:143-150, 1993.

88. Wizemann AJ, Wizemann V: Therapeutic effects of short-term plasma exchange in endogenous uveitis, *Am J Ophthalmol* 97:565-572, 1984.

89. Young DW: The antineutrophil antibody in uveitis. *Br J Ophthalmol* 75:208-211, 1991.

45 Cystoid Macular Edema

HOWARD TESSLER, SHERIDAN LAM

Cystoid macular edema (CME) is a common cause of decreased vision in various inflammatory or noninflammatory ocular disorders. The inflammatory disorders include chronic iridocyclitis, intermediate uveitis (which consists of chronic cyclitis, pars planitis, and idiopathic age-related vitreitis), retinochoroiditis, and retinal vasculitis. Cystoid macular edema following intraocular surgery (cataract extraction and vitrectomy) is also believed to have an inflammatory component. Noninflammatory disorders include diabetic retinopathy, central retinal vein occlusion, branch retinal vein occlusion, retinitis pigmentosa, radiation retinopathy, hypotony, and dominantly inherited CME. This chapter will concentrate on CME secondary to intraocular inflammation and occurring after cataract extraction.

EPIDEMIOLOGY

Cystoid macular edema in uveitis is usually the sequela of long-standing intraocular inflammation. It is rarely seen in acute uveitides, such as acute iritis and iridocyclitis, in which the intraocular inflammation lasts from 2 to 6 weeks.

The incidence of CME associated with various uveitides is not well documented. The occurrence of CME is between 28% and 52% in pars planitis.[14,15,42] In Behçet disease with ocular involvement, the occurrence of CME is 24%[2]; and in intermediate uveitis, the incidence of CME is 30%.[1]

In aphakic or pseudophakic eyes, visually significant CME with reduced acuity occurs 6 weeks to 6 months after surgery and commonly lasts 3 to 6 months. Although CME can take place after uncomplicated cataract extraction, it happens more often and is more persistent in complicated cases (those with vitreous loss and vitreous wound incarceration).

The occurrence rate of CME in patients who have undergone cataract extraction varies, depending on the method of cataract extraction, the type of intraocular implant, and the procedure used to detect CME. Not all cases of CME lead to decreased vision, and CME is more commonly seen on the fluorescein angiograms than with ophthalmoscopy. Clini-

cally significant CME after cataract extraction is considered to be CME with decreased vision to 20/40 or worse.

Angiographic evidence of CME after cataract extraction can be present in more than 50% of patients in the immediate postoperative period, whereas CME with reduced visual acuity exists in up to 8% of victims after cataract extraction.[46] Only 1% to 3% of patients develop persistent CME with reduced vision.[30] The incidence of CME with decreased visual acuity after intracapsular cataract extraction (ICCE) alone is 2%,[47] but for ICCE with an iris-support intraocular lens (IOL), the incidence of CME with decreased visual acuity is between 6.7% and 23%.[6,26,44,45,47] Following ICCE with an anterior chamber IOL, the occurrence of CME with decreased visual acuity is 5% to 13%,[12,32] and the incidence of CME with decreased vision is between 1.2% and 2.3% for extracapsular cataract extraction (ECCE) with a posterior chamber IOL.[6,44,45,47] The occurrence of angiographic evidence of CME after phacoemulsification has been reported to be similar to that after ECCE.[3]

PATHOGENESIS

The exact pathogenesis of CME remains uncertain. Chronic intraocular inflammation leads (it is generally believed) to the disruption of the blood-retinal barrier located at the endothelium of the retinal vessels. It is hypothesized that the anterior segment inflammation releases inflammatory mediators that reach the posterior pole and induce CME. An intact posterior capsule can act as a barrier to these mediators and can explain the lower incidence of CME after ECCE as compared with ICCE. Between 3 and 6 months after ECCE with IOL's, the incidence of angiographic CME was 21.5% in eyes that had primary capsulotomy as compared with 5.6% in eyes in which the capsule remained intact.[24]

Free radicals, prostaglandins, and other inflammatory mediators (serotonin, bradykinin, histamine, substance P, and leukotrienes) may also be important factors in the development of CME.[31,52] Use of nonsteroidal antiinflammatory eyedrops preoperatively and postoperatively prevents CME after cataract extraction,[18,20,23,31] and this indirectly supports the theory that prostaglandins are important mediators. The prostaglandins are believed to come from iris because of chronic irritation by vitreous or the IOL.[31] An intact lens capsule can theoretically prevent vitreous from touching the iris, thus explaining the lower incidence of CME associated with ECCE. The level of prostaglandins is elevated after ICCE and ECCE, and the topical indomethacin lowers the aqueous level of prostaglandins.[31]

Vitreous Traction

Vitreous traction at the macula has been proposed as a mechanism of CME.[38,39] Vitreous fibers connecting to the Müller cells in the macular area have been documented histologically[39] and may be an important finding if Müller cell decompensation is an early finding in CME. Theoretically, Müller cells act as a metabolic pump to dehydrate the macula, and their decompensation can lead to macular swelling. In a national, prospective, randomized study, Fung[9] reported that only 4% of eyes with aphakic CME showed vitreous traction on the macula.

Loss of vitreous or vitreous wound incarceration could lead to traction on the macula and contribute to the development of CME. Loss of vitreous during cataract extraction increases the incidence of CME with decreased vision.[17] Hirokawa and associates[16] showed that uveitic eyes with complete vitreous detachment tend to have fewer macular changes and better visual acuities than those eyes without complete vitreous detachment. This observation seems to imply that vitreous traction on the macula may also be detrimental to the macular function in eyes with uveitis.

Uveitis

Perivascular sheathing by inflammatory cells of the retinal vessel are present in certain uveitides (Behçet disease) and may contribute to the disruption of retinal vascular endothelium. Retinal phlebitis has also been documented in Irvine-Gass syndrome.[28] In Vogt-Koyanagi-Harada disease and sympathetic ophthalmia, however, choroidal inflammation may lead to macular edema resulting from disruption of the blood-retinal barrier located at the level of the retinal pigment epithelium.

Phototoxicity

Light toxicity from the operating microscope may also contribute to the development of CME. Removal of the cataract exposes the macula to the ultraviolet light that was filtered previously by the cataract.[19] Ultraviolet light can generate free radicals that can then lead to production of prostaglandins.[19] Breakdown of the blood-retinal barrier at the level of the retinal pigment epithelium has been reported in retinal photic injury.[49] Ultraviolet-filtering intraocular lenses may be beneficial in preventing CME, and after ECCE, angiographic evidence of CME is present in 9.5% of eyes receiving ultraviolet-filtering IOL's as compared with 18.8% of eyes receiving nonfiltering IOL's.[25]

PATHOLOGY

The cystoid spaces observed clinically in CME are located in the outer plexiform layer and may extend into the inner nuclear layer.[13,21] The cystoid spaces may coalesce to form large macular cysts; full-thickness and lamellar macular holes may also develop.[13] There may be concomitant hypertrophy and hyperplasia of the retinal pigment epithelium.[13] Retinal glial cells may also migrate to the inner surface of the retina.[13]

Swelling and degeneration of the Müller cells is present in early CME, indicating that dysfunction of Müller cell may lead to accumulation of extracellular fluid in the retina.[48] It has been contended that the cystoid spaces seen in CME actually represent swelling and degeneration of Müllers cells,[8,54] which are glial cells that transport fluid between the vitreous and the subretinal space.[48] The accumulation of extracellular fluid probably represents chronic changes resulting from prolonged intracellular swelling and cell death.[54] Other concomitant histopathologic findings with CME include severe damage to the microvasculature and swelling of the glial cells of the lamina choroidalis of the optic nerve with compression of the axons.[54]

CLINICAL FEATURES

The main complaint of patients with CME is decreased or blurred vision. Often they state that certain letters are clearer than others and that they have to scan a line to read it. Edema spreading apart the cone photoreceptors may cause micropsia. In eyes with uveitis, there may be accompanying signs of intraocular inflammation, such as keratic precipitates, cells and flare in the anterior chamber, and vitreous cells. In some cases, fundus lesions and vasculitis may also be present, such as in birdshot retinochoroidopathy and Behçet disease. In eyes with CME after cataract extraction, a mild anterior chamber reaction usually exists.

Classic CME involves the presence of small intraretinal cysts around the fovea, arranged in a petaloid pattern that is often incomplete (Fig. 45-1). A halo of retinal edema with increased retinal thickness may surround the cysts. In mild cases, intraretinal cysts may not be visible clinically and only blunting of the foveal reflex is present. Moreover, if there is significant cataract or opacification of the vitreous, visualization of the macula may be compromised.

The macula is best examined stereoscopically with a Hruby lens, a contact lens, or a 78- or 90-diopter lens. Direct ophthalmoscopy is also a useful way to examine the macula; however, it does not give a stereoscopic view of the macula, and the examiner cannot judge the retinal thickness.

It is important to note that in patients with uveitis, media haze (vitreal cells and cataracts) may not be responsible for

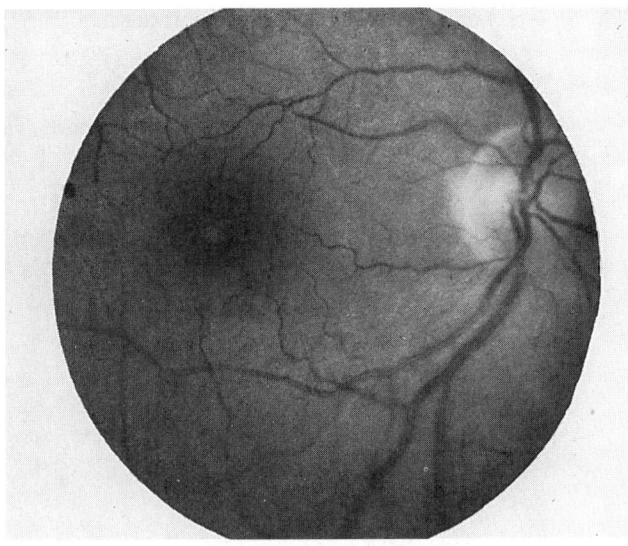

A

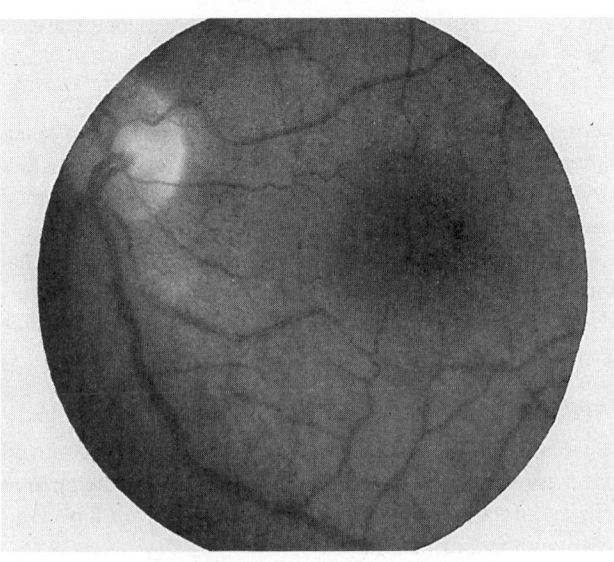

B

Fig. 45-1. Bilateral cystoid macular edema in a patient with chronic iridocyclitis associated with sarcoidosis. Mild vitreous haze is also present in both eyes.

much diminution of vision, and CME should be suspected as the major problem.

Clinical Course

Cystoid macular edema is usually the result of chronic intraocular inflammation. The severity of CME may wax and wane with the severity of the intraocular inflammation. Once the CME has caused permanent structural damage, however, the fluctuation in vision will lessen. On occasion, the amount of CME does not correlate with the visual acuity.

The onset of CME after cataract extraction is usually within the first 6 months after surgery. In most cases of CME after cataract extraction, the visual loss is transient, and the

macular edema resolves spontaneously. The incidence of CME is lower after ECCE than after ICCE.[17] According to Stark and associates,[46] transient CME associated with decreased visual acuity is noted in 10% of ICCE cases with IOL's and 2% of ECCE cases with IOL's, whereas persistent CME with decreased visual acuity occurs in 1% of ICCE cases with IOL's and 0.3% of ECCE cases with IOL's.

DIFFERENTIAL DIAGNOSIS

Entities that mimic CME include X-linked retinoschisis, nicotinic maculopathy, and Goldmann-Favre syndrome. In these disorders, cysts are seen in the macular area; however, they do not stain on fluorescein angiogram.[11] In cases of long-standing inactive CME, the macular cysts may not stain after the blood-retinal barrier has been reestablished.

LABORATORY INVESTIGATIONS

On a fluorescein angiogram, CME can be demonstrated by accumulation of fluorescein in the macular cysts (Fig. 45-2). Leakage from the perifoveal capillaries can also be present. Staining of the optic disc and leakage from the capillaries of the optic disc may also take place.[38]

Fluorescein angiography is more sensitive in detecting CME than is ophthalmoscopic examination, and CME is more frequently seen with fluorescein angiogram than with clinical ophthalmoscopy. The amount of leakage on fluorescein angiogram frequently correlates poorly with visual acuity, however.[35] In some cases, CME can be demonstrated only on fluorescein angiogram and is not suspected clinically.

CME detectable with fluorescein angiogram can be present in the early postoperative period in more than 50% of the patients who underwent cataract extraction with or without implants.[46] An incidence is noted of 24% of angiographic evidence of CME after ECCE with primary capsulotomy and 16% of angiographic evidence of CME after ECCE without capsulotomy 6 weeks after surgery. Six months after surgery, angiographic evidence of CME persists, present in 4% in both groups, and there was no statistical difference between the two groups.[51]

In a study, 20% of patients with intermediate uveitis had edema of the macula, the optic disc, or both that was undetected by ophthalmoscopy.[37]

By using stereoscopic fluorescein angiogram to estimate retinal thickness, retinal thickness correlated better with visual acuity than the amount of fluorescein leakage.[35] Direct retinal thickness measurement may potentially be the most sensitive method of detecting early macular edema; however, the current method can be limited by opacification of the ocular media (cataracts and vitreous debris) that may hinder the visibility of the macula.[55]

Vitreous fluorophotometry measures the permeability of the blood-retinal barrier and can also locate the area of blood-retinal barrier breakdown.[5] In pars planitis, greater

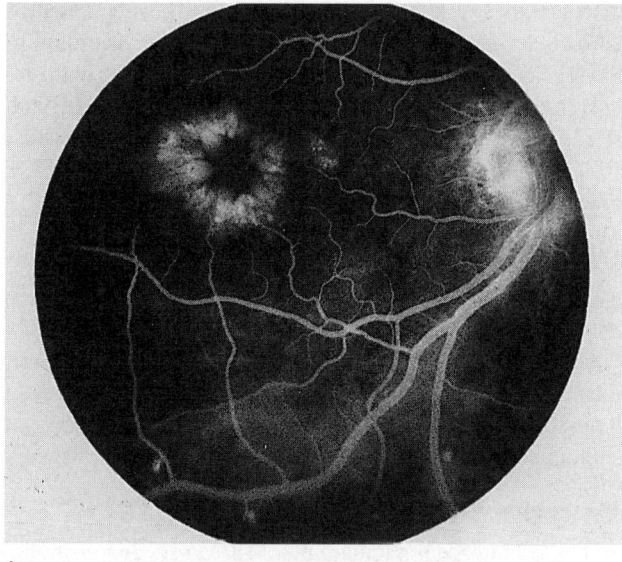

A

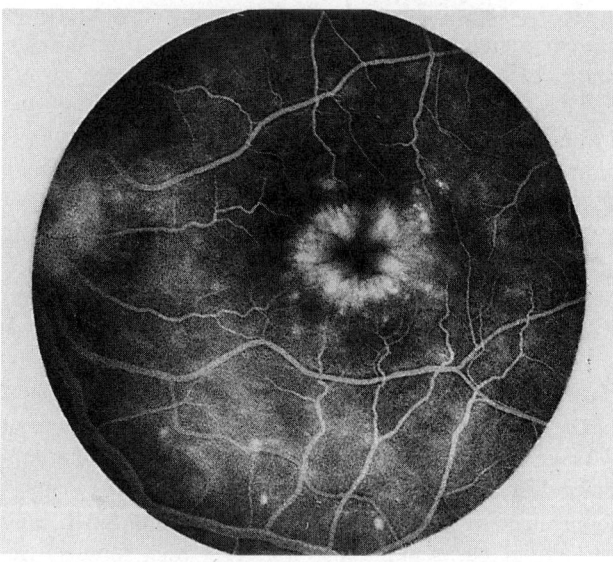

B

Fig. 45-2. Fluorescein angiogram showing staining of the retinal cysts surrounding the fovea. The optic discs also appear hyperfluorescent.

leakage takes place in the midperipheral and equatorial regions.[5] In aphakic eyes with vitreous loss, leakage from the anterior chamber through the ruptured anterior hyaloid face is present, whereas in aphakic eyes with intact vitreous, the leakage is concentrated on the posterior pole.[5]

THERAPY

In CME in which there is significant loss of vision, therapy should be instituted (Figs. 45-3 and 45-4). In pars planitis, patients with visual acuity worse than 20/40 should be treated.[36,43] As for determining the visual acuity at which cataract surgery should be performed, however, the need for

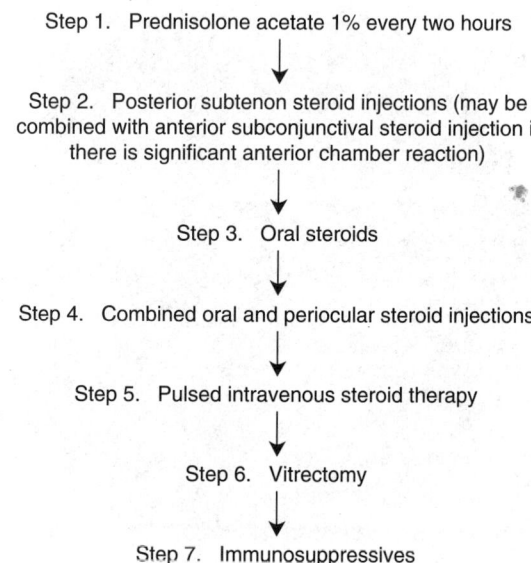

Step 1. Prednisolone acetate 1% every two hours

Step 2. Posterior subtenon steroid injections (may be combined with anterior subconjunctival steroid injection if there is significant anterior chamber reaction)

Step 3. Oral steroids

Step 4. Combined oral and periocular steroid injections

Step 5. Pulsed intravenous steroid therapy

Step 6. Vitrectomy

Step 7. Immunosuppressives

Fig. 45-3. Flow chart in the treatment of uveitic CME. (This serves as a guide to therapy but is not an absolute routine, and each patient must be treated individually).

therapy in CME should be assessed individually; in some patients, a visual acuity less than 20/20 may be unsatisfactory. Patients with visually demanding occupations may even require a visual acuity of 20/15.

Manifest refraction may change frequently in patients with CME, because hyperopia and a small amount of astigmatism may develop with macular swelling. Meticulous refraction should be performed in patients with CME.

Medical Therapy

Because CME is a self-varying phenomenon, randomized and masked studies are needed to determine the therapeutic efficacy of various medications. Many studies are flawed by small numbers of patients.

Nonsteroidal Antiinflammatory Drugs. Studies on topical nonsteroidal antiinflammatory eyedrops (indomethacin and

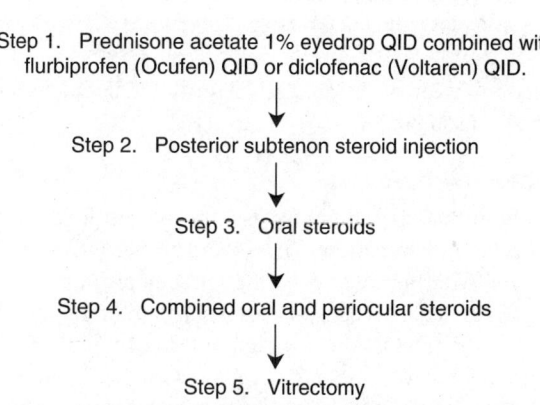

Step 1. Prednisone acetate 1% eyedrop QID combined with flurbiprofen (Ocufen) QID or diclofenac (Voltaren) QID.

Step 2. Posterior subtenon steroid injection

Step 3. Oral steroids

Step 4. Combined oral and periocular steroids

Step 5. Vitrectomy

Fig. 45-4. Flow chart in the treatment of aphakic/pseudophakic CME. (This serves as a guide to therapy but is not an absolute routine, and each patient must be treated individually).

fenoprofen) have shown that they help prevent angiographic findings of CME but do not necessarily improve the long-term visual outcome.[18] Topical antiprostaglandins (flurbiprofen [Ocufen] and diclofenac [Voltaren]) are effective in treating CME in aphakic patients.[26a] A prescription usually consists of topical flurbiprofen 0.03% or diclofenac 0.1% four times a day for 2 to 3 weeks; if the condition responds, the regimen is continued for another 12 weeks. Topical antiprostaglandins are not useful in treating uveitic CME.[26a]

Systemic use of nonsteroidal antiinflammatory drugs has not been proved effective in preventing or treating CME after cataract extraction. Yannuzzi and associates[53] demonstrated the ineffectiveness of oral indomethacin in treating CME after cataract extraction that had lasted for 4 months or more. Sholiton and associates[41] did not find preoperative and postoperative use of oral indomethacin to be beneficial in CME after cataract extraction. Aspirin was pronounced ineffectual as prophylaxis against CME after cataract extraction by Shammas and Milkie.[40] Nevertheless, there are anectodal reports of patients with aphakic CME whose vision improved after the use of oral fenoprofen (Nalfon), indomethacin, or both.

Corticosteroids. Topical corticosteroids can reduce the inflammation in the anterior segment of the eye and may be helpful in treating (1) postcataract CME with significant anterior chamber reaction and (2) CME caused by chronic iritis or iridocyclitis. On occasion, CME secondary to intermediate uveitis may also respond to topical corticosteroids. Prednisolone acetate 1% four times a day for 2 to 3 weeks should be long enough for the clinician to evaluate the efficacy of this regimen and to check for steroid-induced elevation of intraocular pressure. If the condition responds, the regimen is continued and then slowly tapered. If elevated intraocular pressure develops, topical beta-blockers are frequently prescribed. Often the intraocular pressure increases as the visual acuity improves. Elevated intraocular pressure may indicate better function of the ciliary body, and it has been hypothesized that elevated intraocular pressure drives fluid out of the macula.[29] In some patients, topical prednisolone acetate may have to be discontinued and fluorometholone (which causes less elevation of intraocular pressure) used instead.

Periocular corticosteroids are the choice of treatment in cases of CME in which topical corticosteroids are ineffective. One ml (40 mg) of triamcinolone diacetate (Aristocort) is injected using the technique described by Nozik.[33] A 25-gauge needle, 5/8-inch in length, is inserted below Tenon capsule at the superotemporal conjunctival fornix with the bevel kept up for direct visualization. Longer 25-gauge needles should not be used because they are too flexible and too long. After the needle is inserted, the bevel is turned down by rotating the needle and the syringe 180 degrees, so that the medication can be injected toward the globe. The needle is then slowly advanced posteriorly toward the macula with

a side-to-side sweeping or wiping motion to prevent perforation of the globe. Attention is directed toward the movement of the globe. If the globe moves as much as the side-to-side motion of the needle, indicating that the needle tip is engaging the sclera, the needle is withdrawn slightly and redirected. After the entire length of the needle is inserted, the medication is slowly injected. If properly administered, no periocular steroid should be visible. Injections can be given every 3 weeks, and periocular corticosteroids are deemed ineffective if there is no response after 3 consecutive injections.[26a] If a longer-acting steroid is needed, 1 ml of triamcinolone acetonide (Kenalog, 40 mg/ml) is given; or if stronger corticosteroids are desired, 1 ml of methylprednisolone acetate (Depo-Medrol, 80 mg/ml) can be given. Ocular complications associated with periocular corticosteroids include elevation of intraocular pressure and cataract formation.

Oral prednisone is usually prescribed in patients whose condition is unresponsive to periocular corticosteroids or who cannot receive periocular corticosteroids. The average adult dosage is 80 mg of prednisone once a day for 1 to 2 weeks, then rapid tapering of the dosage to every other day. Some patients may need about 10 to 20 mg of prednisone every other day for several years to keep CME stable. In patients receiving long-term corticosteroids (for more than 1 year), administration of calcium supplements and vitamin D should be considered to prevent osteoporosis and vertebral collapse.

In children, the dosage should be adjusted for body weight. Young children should not, however, be given oral corticosteroids for more than 6 months because of the possibility of growth retardation associated with long-term steroid use. After 6 months of oral steroid treatment, periocular injection of corticosteroids is given to the patient under general anesthesia.

In certain cases unresponsive to oral corticosteroids alone, a combination of oral steroid and posterior sub-Tenon injection of corticosteroids (below Tenon capsule and against sclera and toward the macula) is given for additive effects. Also, periodic sub-Tenon injections (every 4 to 12 weeks) of corticosteroids allow reduction in the dosage of the oral corticosteroids.

Pulse intravenous corticosteroids may be tried with patients for whom periocular and oral corticosteroids are ineffective.[50] A dosage of 1 g of methylprednisolone is given initially on an outpatient basis 4 times a week for the first week, tapered to 500 mg of methylprednisolone weekly for 3 weeks, 250 mg weekly for 2 weeks, and then to a maintenance dosage of 125 mg weekly.[50] Occasionally, intravenous steroid treatment can improve visual acuity when oral or periocular corticosteroids do not.

Diuretics. Acetazolamide is effective in treating uveitic CME.[4] A double-masked study was recently completed on acetazolamide in the treatment of uveitic CME, in which acetazolamide was shown to be more effective than placebo.[7] It seems that acetazolamide is more effectual in mild to moderate CME and in younger patients.[7] The patient should initially be treated with 500 mg once a day for about 2 to 3 weeks; if there is clinical response, the treatment is continued and then tapered. In some cases, the CME can be controlled with as low a dosage as 125 mg once every other day. Methazolamide (Neptazane) can also be used with an initial dosage of 25 to 50 mg twice a day and then tapered to 25 mg once every other day. Patients' conditions can be maintained with acetazolamide or methazolamide for a long period.

Because of the rare complication of aplastic anemia secondary to acetazolamide,[56] a complete blood cell count is recommended for all patients about 6 weeks after therapy begins.

Immunosuppressives. In severe uveitides (such as Behçet disease, sympathetic ophthalmia, or pars planitis with severe CME) unresponsive to conventional treatment, immunosuppressives (cyclosporine, azathioprine, cyclophosphamide, chlorambucil, and methotrexate) may be needed to reduce intraocular inflammation and CME.[1,34] Immunosuppressive medications can induce serious side effects, and the risks associated with their use must be carefully explained to the patient. For ophthalmologists who are not familiar with their use, consultation with a hematology/oncology specialist is recommended.

Hyperbaric Oxygen. Hyperbaric oxygen can improve vision in about half of the patients with uveitic CME,[22] although changes have not been documented with fluorescein angiography or fluorophotometry. Improvement in vision has also been reported in aphakic patients with long-standing CME after treatment with hyperbaric oxygen. It is believed that hyperbaric oxygen increases the delivery of oxygen to the macula, thus improving macular function, although the macula may remain edematous. Hyperbaric oxygen treatment is time consuming, however, requiring 2 hours a day for 3 to 4 weeks; and the improvement in vision may be transient, with vision returning to the pretreatment level in about 2 to 4 weeks. Hyperbaric oxygen is not a practical therapeutic modality in the treatment of uveitic CME.[26a]

Surgical Therapy

Laser Photocoagulation. Grid laser photocoagulation has no role in the treatment of uveitic, pseudophakic, or aphakic patients with CME, except in cases in which there is concomitant diabetic macular edema. In these combined cases, it may be difficult to determine whether the CME is secondary to uveitis or to diabetic retinopathy. The presence of multiple microaneurysms supports the hypothesis that the diabetic component could be important. Pharmacologic treatment of any uveitic CME is usually tried before attempting laser therapy.[26a]

Vitrectomy. Vitrectomy may be beneficial in some cases of CME.[27] Vitrectomy may lessen or stabilize the amount of CME in patients with uveitis whose condition is unresponsive to any other treatment, especially in chronic iridocyclitis, pars planitis, and vitritis. The exact role remains to be determined, however. Vitrectomy may be indicated in cases in which the patients are unresponsive to medical treatments.[26] Vitrectomy may be a safer approach than immunosuppressive therapy when corticosteroids fail. Clinical judgment in each individual patient should be the guide, however; and there is no absolute treatment routine.

The goal of vitrectomy in the treatment of aphakic patients with CME is to remove all vitreous from the anterior segment, to restore the normal anatomy of the pupil and iris, and to remove the vitreous strands incarcerated in the wound.[9] A pars plana approach may be more efficacious because it can remove vitreous behind the iris that cannot be removed via a limbal approach. The surgery should be done early, before there is permanent alteration of the macula. Alternatively, the vitreous strands to the wound can be severed with neodymium:YAG laser. Vitreous strands frequently are resistant to complete severance with the neodymium:YAG laser, but improvement has been seen with partial neodymium:YAG vitreolysis.[26]

Fung[10] recommended that vitrectomy be performed for CME in aphakic patients if the vision is stable for 2 to 3 months and the visual acuity has been 20/80 or worse for 2 years or less.

It is uncertain how vitrectomy improves CME. It has been hypothesized that vitrectomy relieves macular traction or removes antigenic factors from the vitreous. Patients with uveitis who have total vitreous detachment are more responsive to anti-CME therapy than are patients with partial vitreous detachment.[16] Vitrectomy may induce a complete vitreous detachment and thus make the macula more responsive to medical treatment.

Removal of Intraocular Implant. A poorly positioned IOL that incarcerates the iris or touches the ciliary body may lead to chronic intraocular inflammation and CME. A malpositioned IOL should be removed or replaced if medical management is ineffective.

PROGNOSIS

Most cases of CME after cataract extraction are transient, whereas uveitic CME tends to be more persistent and may vary with the severity of intraocular inflammation. With proper and prompt treatment and careful follow-up, many uveitic patients with CME will regain or retain good visual acuity.

REFERENCES

1. Arocker-Mettinger E, Grabner G: Intermediate uveitis: clinical findings and treatment, *Klin Monatsbl Augenheilkd* 194:249-251, 1989.
2. Atmaca LS: Fundus changes associated with Behçet's disease, *Graefes Arch Clin Exp Ophthalmol* 227:340-344, 1989.
3. Colin J, Bonnet P: Comparison of phacoemulsification and manual extracapsular extraction of the lens, *Ophtalmologie* 3:233-234, 1989.

4. Cox SN, Hay E, Bird AC: Treatment of chronic macular edema with acetazolamide, *Arch Ophthalmol* 106:1190-1195, 1988.
5. Cunha-Vaz JG, Travassos A: Breakdown of the blood-retinal barriers and cystoid macular edema, *Surv Ophthalmol* 28(suppl):485-492, 1984.
6. Fagadau WR, Maumenee AE, Stark WJ Jr, Datiles M: Posterior chamber intraocular lenses at the Wilmer Institute: a comparative analysis of complications and visual results, *Br J Ophthalmol* 68:13-18, 1984.
7. Farber MD, Tessler HH, Jennings TJ et al.: Acetazolamide reduction of macular edema in uveitis patients: a prospective crossover study, *Ophthalmology* 99(suppl):96, 1992 (abstract).
8. Fine BS, Brucker AJ: Macular edema and cystoid macular edema, *Am J Ophthalmol* 92:466-481, 1981.
9. Fung WE: The national, prospective, randomized vitrectomy study for chronic aphakic cystoid macular edema: progress report and comparison between the control and nonrandomized groups, *Surv Ophthalmol* 28(suppl):569-575, 1984.
10. Fung WE, Vitrectomy—ACME Study Group: Vitrectomy for chronic aphakic cystoid macular edema: results of a national, collaborative, prospective, randomized investigation, *Ophthalmology* 92:1102-1111, 1985.
11. Gass JDM: *Stereoscopic Atlas of macular diseases: diagnosis and treatment,* ed 3, St Louis, 1987, Mosby.
12. Girard LJ, Madero R, Monasterio R: Complications of the Simcoe flexible loop phacoprosthesis in the anterior chamber, *Ophthalmic Surg* 14:332-335, 1983.
13. Green WR: Retina. In Spencer WH, editor: *Ophthalmic pathology: an atlas and textbook,* ed 3, vol 2, 589-1291, Philadelphia, 1985, WB Saunders.
14. Henderly DE, Genstler AJ, Rao NA, Smith RE: Pars planitis, *Trans Ophthalmol Soc UK* 105:227-232, 1986.
15. Henderly DE, Haymond RS, Rao NA, Smith RE: The significance of the pars plana exudate in pars planitis, *Am J Ophthalmol* 103:669-671, 1987.
16. Hirokawa H, Takahashi M, Trempe CL: Vitreous changes in peripheral uveitis, *Arch Ophthalmol* 103:1704-1707, 1985.
17. Jaffe NS, Clayman HM, Jaffe MS: Cystoid macular edema after intracapsular and extracapsular cataract extraction with and without an intraocular lens, *Ophthalmology* 89:25-29, 1982.
18. Jampol LM: Pharmacologic therapy of aphakic cystoid macular edema: a review, *Ophthalmology* 89:891-897, 1982.
19. Jampol LM: Aphakic cystoid macular edema: a hypothesis, *Arch Ophthalmol* 103:1134-1135, 1985.
20. Jampol LM: Pharmacologic therapy of aphakic and pseudophakic cystoid macular edema: 1985 update, *Ophthalmology* 92:807-810, 1985.
21. Jampol LM: Macular edema. In Ryan SJ, editor: *Retina,* vol 2, 81-88, St Louis, 1989, Mosby.
22. Jennings T, Tessler H, Zanetti C: *Hyperbaric oxygen therapy and ophthalmology.* In Belfort R, Petrili AMN, Nussenblatt R, editors: World Uveitis Symposium, Sao Paulo, Brazil, 1989, ROCA.
23. Kraff MC, Sanders DR, Jampol LM et al.: Prophylaxis of pseudophakic cystoid macular edema with topical indomethacin, *Ophthalmology* 89:885-890, 1982.
24. Kraff MC, Sanders DR, Jampol LM, Lieberman HL: Effect of primary capsulotomy with extracapsular surgery on the incidence of pseudophakic cystoid macular edema, *Am J Ophthalmol* 98:166-170, 1984.
25. Kraff MC, Sanders DR, Jampol LM, Lieberman HL: Effect of an ultraviolet-filtering intraocular lens on cystoid macular edema, *Ophthalmology* 92:366-369, 1985.
26. Krause U: Eight years experience with the Worst Medallion two loop lens, *Acta Ophthalmol* 61:655-661, 1983.
26a. Lam S, Tessler H: Unpublished data.
27. Limon SY, Bloch-Michel E, Furia M: 100 vitrectomies in uveitis. In Saari KM, editor: *Uveitis Update,* Proceedings of the First International Symposium on Uveitis, Espoo, Finland, 1984, Amsterdam, Excerpta Medica.
28. Martin NF, Green WR, Martin LW: Retinal phlebitis in the Irvine-Gass syndrome, *Am J Ophthalmol* 83:377-386, 1977.
29. McEntyre JM: A successful treatment for aphakic cystoid macular edema, *Ann Ophthalmol* 10:1219-1224, 1978.
30. Milch FA, Yannuzzi LA: Medical and surgical treatment of aphakic cystoid macular edema, *Int Ophthalmol Clin* 27:205-217, 1987.
31. Miyake K: Indomethacin in the treatment of postoperative cystoid macular edema, *Surv Ophthalmol* 28(suppl):554-568, 1984.
32. Moses L: Complications of rigid anterior chamber implants, *Ophthalmology* 91:819-825, 1984.
33. Nozik RA: Periocular injection of steroids, *Trans Am Acad Ophthalmol Otolaryngol* 76:695-705, 1972.
34. Nussenblatt RB: Macular alterations secondary to intraocular inflammatory disease, *Ophthalmology* 93:984-988, 1986.
35. Nussenblatt RB, Kaufman SC, Palestine AG et al.: Macular thickening and visual acuity: measurement in patients with cystoid macular edema, *Ophthalmology* 94:1134-1139, 1987.
36. Nussenblatt RB, Palestine AG: *Uveitis: fundamentals and clinical practice,* 185-197, Chicago, 1989, Mosby.
37. Schenck F, Böke W: Angiographic findings in intermediate uveitis, *Klin Monatsbl Augenheilkd* 193:261-265, 1988.
38. Schepens CL, Avila MP, Jalkh AE, Trempe CL: Role of the vitreous in cystoid macular edema, *Surv Ophthalmol* 28(suppl):499-504, 1984.
39. Sebag J, Balazs EA: Pathogenesis of cystoid macular edema: an anatomic consideration of vitreoretinal adhesions, *Surv Ophthalmol* 28(suppl):493-498, 1984.
40. Shammas HJF, Milkie CF: Does aspirin prevent postoperative cystoid macular edema? *J Am Intraocul Implant Soc* 5:337, 1979.
41. Sholiton DB, Reinhart WJ, Frank KE: Indomethacin as a means of preventing cystoid macular edema following intracapsular cataract extraction, *J Am Intraocul Implant Soc* 5:137-140, 1979.
42. Smith RE, Godfrey WA, Kimura SJ: Chronic cyclitis. I. Course and visual prognosis, *Trans Am Acad Ophthalmol Otolaryngol* 77:760-768, 1973.
43. Smith RE, Nozik RA: *Uveitis: a clinical approach to diagnosis and management,* ed 2, 166-170, Baltimore, 1989, Williams & Wilkins.
44. Stark WJ, Maumenee AE, Dangel ME et al.: Intraocular lenses: experience at the Wilmer Institute, *Ophthalmology* 89:104-108, 1982.
45. Stark WJ, Maumenee AE, Fagadau WR et al.: Intraocular lenses: experience at the Wilmer Institute, *Aust J Ophthalmol* 11:95-102, 1983.
46. Stark WJ Jr, Maumenee AE, Fagadau W et al.: Cystoid macular edema in pseudophakia, *Surv Ophthalmol* 28(suppl):442-451, 1984.
47. Taylor DM, Sachs SW, Stern AL: Aphakic cystoid macular edema: longterm clinical observations, *Surv Ophthalmol* 28(suppl):437-441, 1984.
48. Tso MOM: Cystoid macular edema. In Tso MOM, editor: *Retinal diseases: biomedical foundations and clinical management,* 215-241, Philadelphia, 1988, JB Lippincott.
49. Tso MOM, Woodford BJ: Effect of photic injury on the retinal tissues, *Ophthalmology* 90:952-963, 1983.
50. Wakefield D, McCluskey P, Penny R: Intravenous pulse methylprednisolone therapy in severe inflammatory eye disease, *Arch Ophthalmol* 104:847-851, 1986.
51. Wright PL, Wilkinson CP, Balyeat HD et al.: Angiographic cystoid macular edema after posterior chamber lens implantation, *Arch Ophthalmol* 106:740-744, 1988.
52. Yannuzzi LA: A perspective on the treatment of aphakic cystoid macular edema, *Surv Ophthalmol* 28(suppl):540-553, 1984.
53. Yannuzzi LA, Klein RM, Wallyn RH et al.: Ineffectiveness of indomethacin in the treatment of chronic cystoid macular edema, *Am J Ophthalmol* 84:517-519, 1977.
54. Yanoff M, Fine BS, Brucker AJ, Eagle RC Jr: Pathology of human cystoid macular edema, *Surv Ophthalmol* 28(suppl):505-511, 1984.
55. Zeimer RC, Shahidi M, Mori MT, Benhamou E: In vivo evaluation of a noninvasive method to measure the retinal thickness in primates, *Arch Ophthalmol* 107:1006-1009, 1989.
56. Zimran A, Beutler E: Can the risk of acetazolamide-induced aplastic anemia be decreased by periodic monitoring of blood cell counts? *Am J Ophthalmol* 104:654-658, 1987.

46 White Dot Syndromes

HILEL LEWIS, LEE M. JAMPOL

Many infectious and noninfectious inflammatory diseases of the eye are characterized by the presence of white lesions in the choroid, the retinal pigment epithelium, and/or the sensory retina. These diseases are commonly grouped under the umbrella term *white dot syndromes,* which helps to generate appropriate differential diagnoses in the evaluation of patients with fundus lesions. White dot syndrome itself is therefore, not a specific diagnosis.

A list of these diseases is presented in Table 46-1. It is important to differentiate between them accurately because their treatments and prognoses vary. To reach the correct diagnosis, the ophthalmologist has to consider the age of the patient at the onset of the disease, the gender of the patient, the symptoms, the distribution and shape of the white lesions, the associated ocular findings, any associated systemic disease, the fluorescein angiographic features, the laboratory findings, and the clinical course of the disease (see Table 46-2 on page 563).

ACUTE MACULAR NEURORETINOPATHY

Acute macular neuroretinopathy is a very rare disease, first described by Bos and Deutman[2] in 1975. It is seen in young adults, mostly women. It may be unilateral or bilateral. The patients complain of decreased vision and paracentral scotomata. Examination reveals an absence of anterior chamber or vitreous cellular reaction. Multiple dark red or brown lesions are seen in the parafoveal area[1] (Fig. 46-1). These lesions may be circular or wedge-shaped. They appear to be present at the level of the deep retina or pigment epithelium, although there is some controversy about the exact level of involvement. The fluorescein angiographic picture, however, is usually normal, or there may be slight hypofluorescence in the areas of involvement. The electroretinogram is normal. Following the disease onset, the patients have symptomatic scotomata for periods of weeks or months followed by a gradual improvement in the visual acuity and the scotoma size and density. The ophthalmoscopically visible lesions disappear as symptomatic improvement occurs.

One patient had multiple recurrences affecting both eyes.* Although the lesions in this condition are not white, it is grouped with the white dot syndromes because its discrete spots share other characteristics and possibly pathogenesis with other diseases in this group.

The cause of acute macular neuroretinopathy remains uncertain. It has been associated in some patients with the administration of sympathomimetic medications. The similarity of the lesions to the depression sign seen with inner retinal infarction is striking.[8,23] With the resolution of acute inner retinal ischemia, a concavity or depression in the retina develops that mimics the lesions of acute macular neuroretinopathy. In contrast, though, during the acute phase of inner retina ischaemia, cotton wool spots are usually observed. Recently it has been suggested by investigators at the Mayo Clinic that the lesions represent occlusive disease of the deep layer of retinal capillaries.† This hypothesis remains unsubstantiated.

A very interesting association of this condition with multiple evanescent white dot syndrome (MEWDS) (see the following) has been noted. Gass and Hamed[16] described two patients who demonstrated both diseases at different times in their clinical courses. Although both diseases are seen primarily in young females, the absence of intraocular inflammation with acute macular neuroretinopathy and the very marked difference in the clinical appearances makes a causal association difficult to see. An additional patient with MEWDS and reddish lesions in the macula that resembled acute macular retinopathy has been observed, but the macular lesions were asymptomatic.‡

ACUTE POSTERIOR MULTIFOCAL PLACOID PIGMENT EPITHELIOPATHY

Acute posterior multifocal placoid pigment epitheliopathy (APMPPE) was first described by Gass[14] in 1968.

---

*Unpublished data.

†H. Buettner, MD and D. Robertson, MD, unpublished data.

‡Unpublished data.

TABLE 46-1   WHITE DOT SYNDROMES

Listed below are infectious and inflammatory diseases that may produce white lesions of the choroid, retinal pigment epithelium, and/or sensory retina, and are commonly included in the differential diagnosis of white dot syndromes. Highlighted disorders are discussed in this chapter. Major discussions of other entities are found in the indicated chapters.

1. **Acute macular neuroretinopathy**
2. **Acute posterior multifocal placoid pigment epitheliopathy**
3. **Acute retinal pigment epitheliitis**
4. AIDS-related retinal microvasculopathy (cotton-wool spots) (Ch. 22)
5. **Bacterial chorioretinitis**
6. Behçet disease (Ch. 54)
7. Birdshot retinochoroidopathy (Ch. 47)
8. Cytomegalovirus retinitis (Ch. 81)
9. Diffuse unilateral subacute neuroretinitis (Ch. 88)
10. Fungal chorioretinitis (Chs. 90, 91, 103)
11. Herpes simplex virus retinitis (Ch. 83)
12. **Multifocal choroiditis and panuveitis**
13. **Multiple evanescent white dot syndrome**
14. Presumed ocular histoplasmosis syndrome (Ch. 90)
15. **Punctate inner choroidopathy**
16. Sarcoidosis (Ch. 59)
17. Serpiginous choroiditis (Ch. 48)
18. **Subacute sclerosing panencephalitis**
19. Sympathetic ophthalmia (Ch. 57)
20. Syphilis (Ch. 104)
21. Toxocariasis (Ch. 86)
22. Toxoplasmosis (Ch. 85)
23. Tuberculosis (Ch. 101)
24. **Unilateral acute idiopathic maculopathy**
25. Varicella-zoster virus retinitis (Ch. 82)
26. Vogt-Koyanagi-Harada syndrome (Ch. 58)

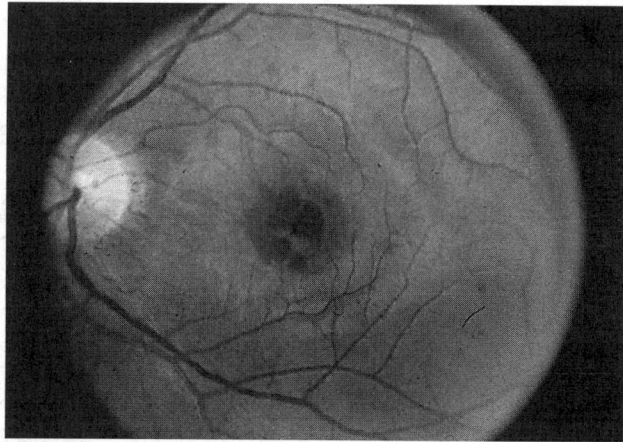

Fig. 46-1.   Acute macular neuroretinopathy. (Figure also in color insert.)

initial hypofluorescence and then late staining. This hypofluorescence has been attributed to either hypoperfusion of the underlying choriocapillaris or swelling and opacification of the overlying retinal pigment epithelium with blockage of choroidal fluorescence. Controversy regarding this distinction continues. Indocyanine green angiography also demonstrates hypofluorescence of the lesions.[7]

The patients may show scleritis, iritis, and vitritis. Optic disc edema and retinal vascular sheathing may also be seen.

The patients rarely show signs of systemic vasculitis. They may develop meningeal symptoms, elevated protein levels, and cells in the cerebrospinal fluid. Rarely central nervous system involvement has produced death. Patients may also show evidence of vasculitis elsewhere, including abnormal urinary sediment from renal involvement.

In general, the electroretinogram and electrooculogram are normal. A rapid resolution of the placoid lesions is seen with a decreasing thickness of the lesions and the development of irregular pigmentation at the level of the retinal pigment epithelium. The amount of pigmentary and choroidal atrophy is considerably less than with the similar-appearing lesions of serpiginous choroiditis. Even when the fovea is involved, central visual acuity usually recovers—although recovery may take months. Rarely does choroidal neovascularization develop. In some cases, the central vision does not recover. In patients who have unilateral involvement, recurrences, or permanent severe loss of vision, the differential diagnosis of serpiginous choroiditis should be carefully considered.

The cause of APMPPE remains uncertain. A viral cause has been suggested, but not confirmed. It has been suggested that the disease represents a systemic vasculitis with the choroidal findings corresponding to choroidal vascular occlusion. This hypothesis remains unsubstantiated. Besides the rare patient with central nervous system or renal vasculitis, the patients are otherwise healthy. Although some clini-

The disease is seen in young patients and is often preceded by a flulike illness. It is equally common in males and females, and both eyes are usually affected. The clinical course is usually monophasic; rarely have recurrences been reported. Patients with APMPPE have multiple, cream-colored, placoid lesions that appear to be at the level of the outer retina and pigment epithelium (Fig. 46-2, A,B). These lesions are often geographic and are scattered throughout the posterior pole. The fovea may or may not be involved. The patients complain of central vision loss and scotomata. Fluorescein angiography has a characteristic appearance with

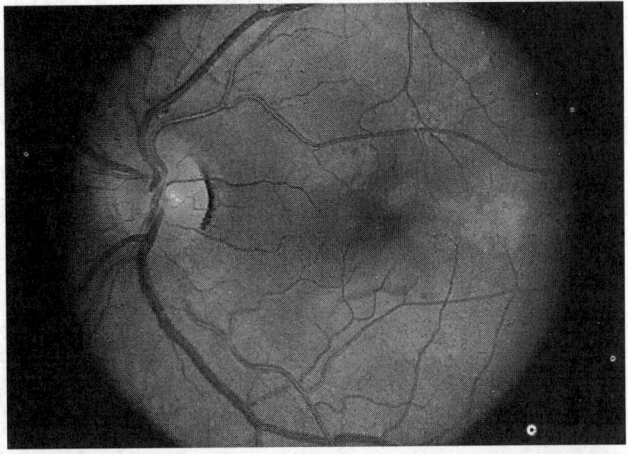

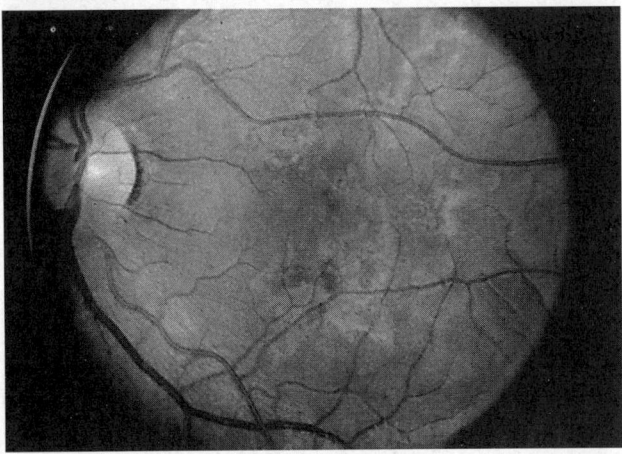

Fig. 46-2. A, APMPPE: Acute grey geographic lesions. **B,** APMPPE: Several weeks later, lesions have pigmented. (Figure also in color insert.)

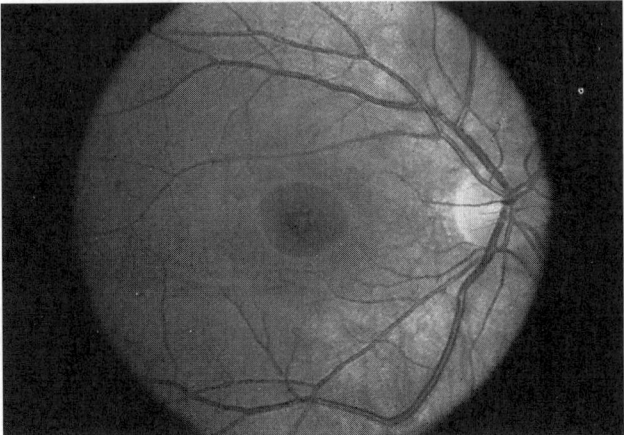

Fig. 46-3. Possible case of acute retinal pigment epitheliitis. Small yellow lesions are seen in the fovea. (Figure also in color insert.)

lesion and a surrounding halo of hyperfluorescence. The electroretinogram and visual evoked response were normal. The electrooculogram was subnormal. The lesions were noted to evolve over a several-month period, with a return of central visual acuity and a less-prominent clinical appearance.

The exact nature of this entity remains undetermined. It may be that some of these patients are showing macular changes similar to those seen with MEWDS or multifocal choroiditis and panuveitis syndrome. Further clinical investigations should establish whether acute retinal pigment epitheliitis is a separate and specific disorder.

BACTERIAL CHORIORETINITIS

Bacterial chorioretinitis can occur in immunocompetent and immunosuppressed patients and should be considered in patients with AIDS who have posterior segment lesions unresponsive to treatment for suspected viral, fungal, or protozoan infections.[1,5,19,20,22]

Host factors in patients with metastatic bacterial chorioretinitis include intravenous drug use, diabetes mellitus, recent surgery or trauma, cardiac abnormality, malignancy, and corticosteroid treatment.[4]

Infections of the retina and/or choroid with mycobacteria and *Treponema pallidum* are described in Chapters 101 and 104 respectively.

Bacterial organisms can infect primarily the retina, primarily the choroid, or both. In most cases, the patients have endogenous ocular involvement. The high rate of blood flow in the choriocapillaries probably explains why endogenous blood-bone infections commonly localize to the choroid and posterior retina.[10]

Bacterial infections can appear as an inflammatory choroidal mass with or without overlying subretinal fluid and intraretinal hemorrhage (Fig. 46-4), or as a slowly progressive retinitis with multifocal white-yellow retinal lesions associated with lipid, hemorrhage (which can have a white

cians treat patients with systemic corticosteroids, there is no evidence that this treatment affects the short-term or long-term outcome. In most cases the visual outcome is good without therapy.

ACUTE RETINAL PIGMENT EPITHELIITIS

Acute retinal pigment epitheliitis is a rare macular disease first described in 1972.[26] Whether it represents a truly unique disease entity remains uncertain. Krill[26] described the disorder in young adults who developed acute vision loss varying from minimal to the level of 20/100. Both unilateral and bilateral cases were seen. Patients had normal eye examinations except for small discrete clusters of two to four small, brown or grayish spots seen in the involved macula (Fig. 46-3). The spots were often surrounded by a small, yellow or white halo. Fluorescein angiography in the acute stage showed hypofluorescence of the central part of the

TABLE 46-2 DIFFERENTIATING FEATURES OF WHITE DOT SYNDROMES

Disease	Age	Gender Predominance	Unilateral or Bilateral	Vitreous Humor Cells	ERG	Retinal Findings	Level of Retinal Involvement	Treatment	Outcome	Recurrences or Exacerbations
Acute macular neuroretinopathy	Young adults	Female	U or B	No	Normal	Red or brown wedge-shaped or circular lesions in macula	Controversial	None	Partial or complete recovery	Very rare
APMPPE	Young adults	None	Usually B	Yes	Usually normal	Multiple, cream colored placoid lesions	Outer retina, RPE	Corticosteroids (?)	Recovery	Rare
Acute retinal pigment epitheliitis	Young adults	Too few cases	U or B	No	Normal	Small discrete clusters of spots in macula	RPE (?)	None	Recovery	No
Multifocal choroiditis and panuveitis syndrome	Young adults	Female	U or B	Often	Normal or decreased	Multiple foci of choroiditis, posterior or peripheral	RPE, choroid	Corticosteroids	Lesions heal; CNV may develop	Yes
MEWDS	Young adults	Female	U, occasionally B	Yes	Decreased acutely with recovery	Multiple white dots, granular macula	Outer retina, RPE	None	Recovery; CNV may rarely develop	Occasional
Unilateral Acute Idiopathic Maculopathy (UAIM)	Young adults	None	U	Sometimes	Unknown	Macular neurosensory detachment with RPE thickening and intraretinal hemorrhage	RPE	None	Recovery; CNV may develop	No
Birdshot retinochoroidopathy	Middle-aged adults	None	Usually B	Yes	Often decreased	Deep indistinct scattered lesions, cream-colored; CME	Choroid, outer retina, RPE	Corticosteroids; cyclosporine	Chronic course	Yes
Serpiginous choroiditis	Usually middle-aged adults	None	Usually B	Yes	Normal unless advanced disease	Geographic areas of choroiditis; peripapillary or macular	Choroid, outer retina, RPE	Corticosteroids; immunosuppression	Healing of acute lesion; CNV may develop	Yes
DUSN	Children, young adults	None	U	Yes	Decreased with retinal damage	Optic disc swelling, evanescent crops of grey-white lesions. End stage: optic atrophy, pseudo-retinitis pigmentosa	Outer retina	Laser; antihelminthic drugs	Chronic course	No (indolent course)

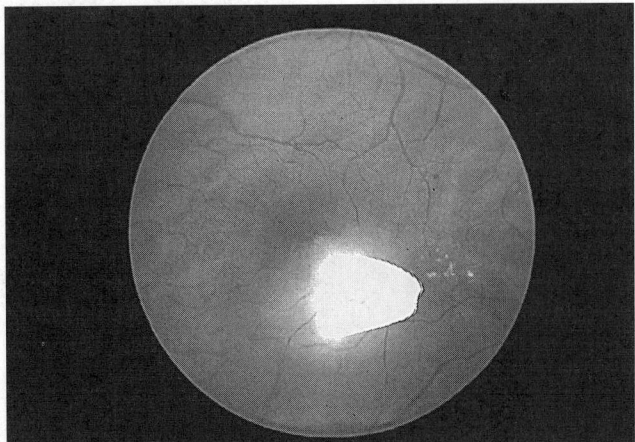

Fig. 46-4. Metastatic choroidal abscess secondary to staphylococcus aureus.

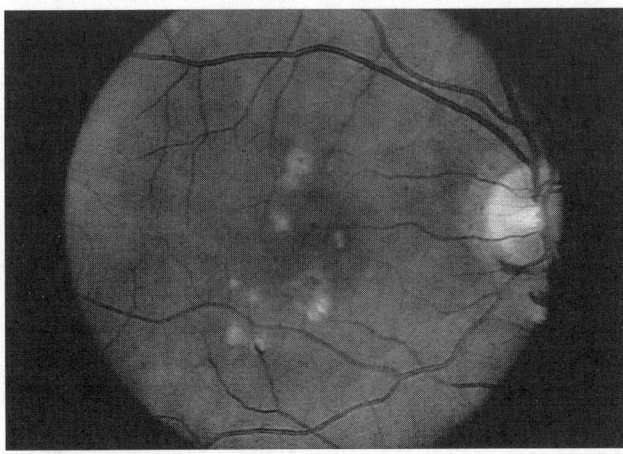

Fig. 46-5. Multifocal choroiditis and panuveitis syndrome. Lesions are clustered in the macula.

center), subsensory fluid, and/or vitreous humor cells.* Most cases of metastatic septic bacterial chorioretinitis progress to endopthalmitis (see Chapter 92) as a result of a delay in treatment and the virulence of the organism.[4,17] Thus early, accurate diagnosis and prompt treatment are important. Coll and Lewis[4] reported a case of an intravenous heroin user who developed a choroidal abscess in the macula after *Staphylococcus aureus* endocarditis. This patient also developed a subfoveal choroidal neovascular membrane at the site of active bacterial choroidal infection. Systemic antibiotic therapy successfully eradicated the choroidal infection, prevented progression to endophthalmitis, and improved visual acuity.

If the diagnosis of bacterial chorioretinitis is not made clinically and the patient does not respond to treatment, retinal or choroidal biopsy will frequently demonstrate the organisms in stain and culture.

Treatment with antibiotics should be directed at the specific causative organism based on the result of systemic and/or ocular cultures and sensitivities.[4,17] If the patient develops endophthalmitis, prompt vitrectomy with intravitreous injection of antibiotics is mandatory.

Uncommon causes of bacterial chorioretinitis include *Borrelia burgdorfi* (multifocal, monocular chorioretinitis), *Nocardia* sp. (associated with lung and liver involvement), and *Salmonella typhi* (bilateral chorioretinitis with monocular stellate maculopathy).[13,28,30]

MULTIFOCAL CHOROIDITIS AND PANUVEITIS SYNDROME

In recent years, many publications have described a group of young patients who demonstrate multifocal choroiditis of unknown cause.[9,29] These patients have intraocular inflammation, usually with vitreous cellular reaction.

Retinal vascular sheathing may be seen, but, the predominant findings in these patients are multiple foci of choroiditis scattered in the posterior, midperipheral, or peripheral retina (Fig. 46-5). Subretinal fibrosis is often seen (Fig. 46-6) and may be severe.[29] Some of the patients have lesions that resemble those seen with the presumed ocular histoplasmosis syndrome (POHS), but patients with POHS do not have vitreous humor cells, whereas many of these patients with multifocal choroiditis and panuveitis syndrome do. Studies by Spaide and associates[33] have shown that patients with multifocal choroiditis and panuveitis syndrome do not have a predominance of HLA-DR2, as seen with POHS. The lesions of multifocal choroiditis and panuveitis syndrome may be totally "inactive" or may show a variable amount of fluorescein dye staining and leakage. Cystoid macular edema or neurosensory retinal elevation may be present. The lesions may involve the fovea and the parafoveal area or may be restricted to the peripheral retina. The variable clinical appearance suggests several causes. Recently optic nerve

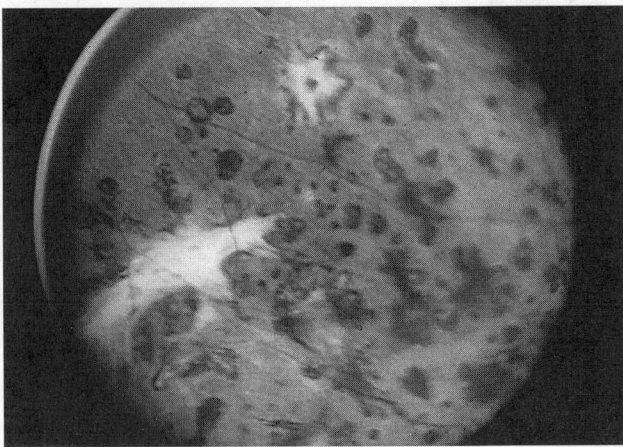

Fig. 46-6. Multifocal choroiditis and panuveitis syndrome. Peripheral lesions with subretinal fibrosis.

*References 4, 13, 17, 28, 30, 32.

changes[8,25] in patients with multifocal choroiditis and pan-uveitis syndrome have been emphasized. The patients may have optic disc edema, enlarged blind spots, temporal photopsias, and temporal visual field loss. Peripapillary scarring may develop. The similarity of some symptoms to those in patients with MEWDS is noteworthy. The patients may have recurrent episodes of blind spot enlargement with photopsias but without disc edema. Choroidal neovascularization is a common late complication of multifocal choroiditis and panuveitis syndrome. Indocyanine green angiography can distinguish patients with multifocal choroiditis and panuveitis syndrome from patients with POHS. The latter disease shows predominantly hyperfluorescent lesions, whereas the lesions of multifocal choroiditis and panuveitis syndrome are hypofluorescent on indocyanine green angiography.*

Another entity that may represent part of the spectrum of multifocal choroiditis and panuveitis syndrome is punctate inner choroidopathy (PIC).[37] This disease is seen in myopic women who have blurred vision and either unilateral or bilateral paracentral scotomata. Small, yellow-white macular lesions are seen at the level of the choroid and retinal pigment epithelium. During the acute phase of the disease, overlying serous elevation of the retina with fluorescein dye leakage may be seen. Choroidal neovascularization is common. At present, many clinicians believe that punctate inner choroidopathy and multifocal choroiditis and panuveitis syndrome are the same entity. As originally described, punctate inner choroidopathy has less vitreous humor cellular involvement, and the lesions are restricted to the posterior pole, particularly the macular area. These patients may simply represent a subset of patients with multifocal choroiditis and panuveitis syndrome.

Patients with multifocal choroiditis and panuveitis syndrome may have vision loss from active choroiditis or from choroidal neovascularization. The best treatment of the choroidal neovascular membranes remains uncertain. Laser photocoagulation may be effective, but spontaneous resolution of the active neovascularization may occur. The exact role of antiinflammatory therapies, such as periocular or systemic corticosteroids, in treating the choroiditis and choroidal neovascularization remains undetermined. When patients demonstrate active choroiditis (and perhaps choroidal neovascularization) near the fovea, systemic or periocular corticosteroids may be helpful in protecting central vision.

The cause of the multifocal choroiditis and panuveitis syndrome is uncertain. The intriguing similarity to POHS remains. The changes may also resemble the multifocal choroiditis seen with sarcoidosis or other granulomatous diseases such as Vogt-Koyanagi-Harada syndrome, sympathetic ophthalmia, or tuberculosis. Linear circumferential areas of scarring in the periphery, sometimes called Schlae-

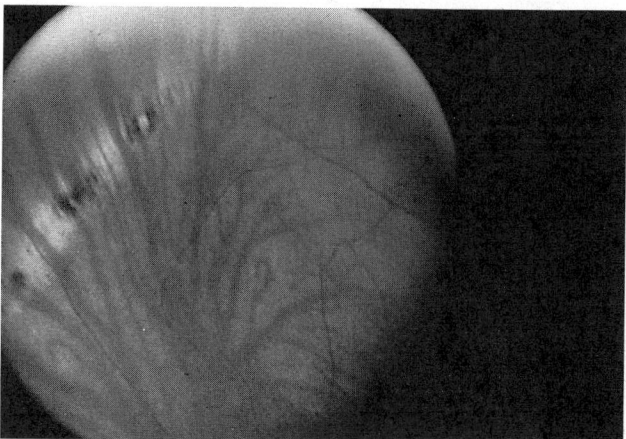

Fig. 46-7. Multifocal choroiditis and panuveitis syndrome. Linear peripheral scar.

gel lines, are seen with both POHS and multifocal choroiditis and panuveitis syndrome (Fig. 46-7). The exact mechanisms whereby choroiditis can produce these linear lesions remain uncertain.

Tiedemann,[35] based on serologic testing, suggested that multifocal choroiditis can be a manifestation of Epstein-Barr virus infection in the retina and choroid. Spaide and associates[34] could not corroborate these findings. At present, the role of Epstein-Barr virus remains uncertain.

Gass[16] has recently suggested that the entities of MEWDS, multifocal choroiditis and panuveitis syndrome, and acute idiopathic blind spot enlargement syndrome may be the same disease. Acute idiopathic blind spot enlargement has been described in young females, with enlargement of the blind spot but without associated retinal, choroidal, or optic disc findings.[11] Several investigators suggested that these patients might have MEWDS with resolution or absence of the white dots and a protracted course of blind spot enlargement with photopsias. It is now clear that at least some cases of acute idiopathic blind spot enlargement syndrome do have MEWDS. The similar temporal scotomata and photopsias with multifocal choroiditis and panuveitis syndrome suggests that this disorder is also a cause of acute idiopathic blind spot enlargement syndrome.

Some patients with multifocal choroiditis and panuveitis syndrome may show areas of whitening of the outer retina in association with activity. These white spots are transitory and Callanan and Gass[3] believe they are similar to those seen with MEWDS. In contrast, experience with other patients has shown that these white spots are often larger, less uniform, less discrete, and different in appearance from the white spots of MEWDS.* The classic granular macular changes of MEWDS have not been documented with multifocal choroiditis and panuveitis syndrome. Callanan and

---

*J. Slakter and L. Yannuzzi, unpublished data.

*Lee M Jampol, MD, unpublished data.

Gass[3] also noted some chorioretinal scars with MEWDS that they believe show overlap between these two entities.

In addition to the previous entities, Gass[15] has also described acute zonal occult outer retinopathy (AZOOR). Patients are young healthy individuals who develop unilateral or bilateral, large areas of dysfunction of the outer retina with photopsias, initially associated with a normal-appearing retina. Presumably the photoreceptors are dysfunctional, which causes visual field loss. Electroretinopathy in the involved eyes is often abnormal. Many of the patients show recurrences and progression. There may be severe peripheral visual field and central visual loss. Eventually the areas of retina involved may show thinning and pigmentary changes at the level of the retinal pigment epithelium with bone spiculelike pigment extending into the retina. Gass[15] believes that AZOOR is also part of a spectrum of diseases that includes the clinical appearances of MEWDS, acute idiopathic blind spot enlargement, multifocal choroiditis and panuveitis syndrome, and acute macular neuroretinopathy. To date, this hypothesis has not been verified.

MULTIPLE EVANESCENT WHITE DOT SYNDROME

Multiple evanescent white dot syndrome (MEWDS), first described in 1984, is an acute, multifocal retinopathy that involves primarily the retinal pigment epithelium and the outer retina.[24] The disease may lead to unilateral or, rarely, bilateral vision loss in young patients. The vast majority of patients are females. Affected individuals may notice the onset of vision loss, temporal or paracentral scotomata, or photopsias—often in the temporal visual field. The characteristic appearance in the fundus includes multiple, small (100 to 200 micron) white dots that appear to be at the level of the outer retina and retinal pigment epithelium (Fig. 46-8). These dots usually appear in the perimacular area and become less prominent outside of the vascular arcades. In

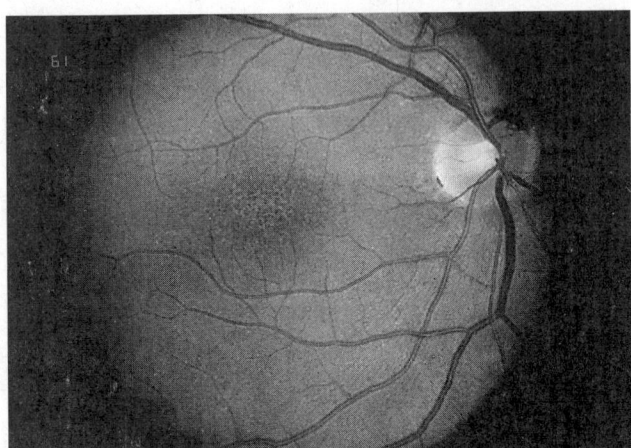

Fig. 46-9. MEWDS: Granular macula is apparent. (Figure also in color insert.)

severe cases, the white spots become almost confluent. The lesions in these patients may be up to 500 microns or more in size. A common, but not invariable, finding is granularity of the macula characterized by multiple, small yellow, orange or white granules in the fovea (Fig. 46-9). The foveal reflex is distorted or absent. Patients may show intraocular inflammation with vitreous humor cells. Additional findings may include retinal vascular sheathing (especially involving venules), optic disc edema, and opacification of local areas of the nerve fiber layer. An afferent pupillary defect and substantial temporal visual field loss may be present. Fluorescein angiography shows focal areas of punctate hyperfluorescence that correspond to the white dots (Fig. 46-10). Indocyanine green angiography shows hypofluroescence of the lesions, with more and larger lesions than observed clinically.[21] The lesions on indocyanine green angiography often cluster around the optic nerve. With fluorescein dye, but not with indocyanine green, staining and leakage from the optic disc may be observed (Fig. 46-10). Fluorescein leakage from deep retinal capillaries and the retinal pigment epithelium is also observed. In the acute phase, the electroretinogram and the early receptor potential are usually diminished and then show recovery.

MEWDS is usually monophasic, unilateral, and self-limited. Rare patients may show simultaneous or sequential bilateral involvement. A few patients may show a chronic form of the disease with multiple exacerbations affecting both eyes.[36] Despite the chronic course, these patients have a good visual outcome. The remarkable feature of MEWDS is the dramatic resolution of visual symptoms. Over a period of several weeks to months, central visual acuity recovers either to normal or close to normal. The enlargement of the blind spot often improves, although there may be some residual enlargement. Photopsias improve, although again, persistence of the photopsias for prolonged periods is occasionally seen. With resolution of the process, some patients may show mild pigmentary changes in the macula and elsewhere at the level of the retinal pigment epithelium. Choroi-

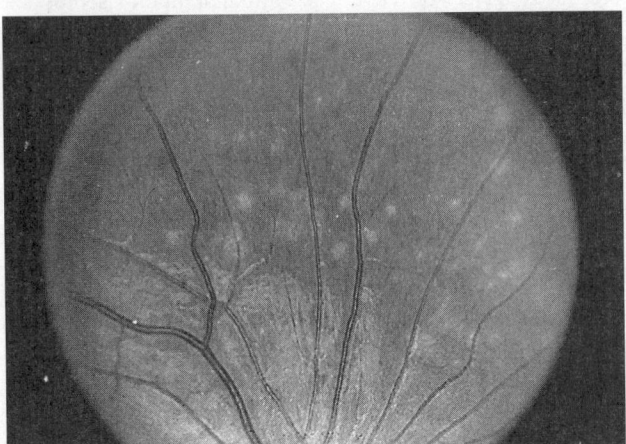

Fig. 46-8. MEWDS: Multiple white dots are seen in the midperiphery. (Figure also in color insert.)

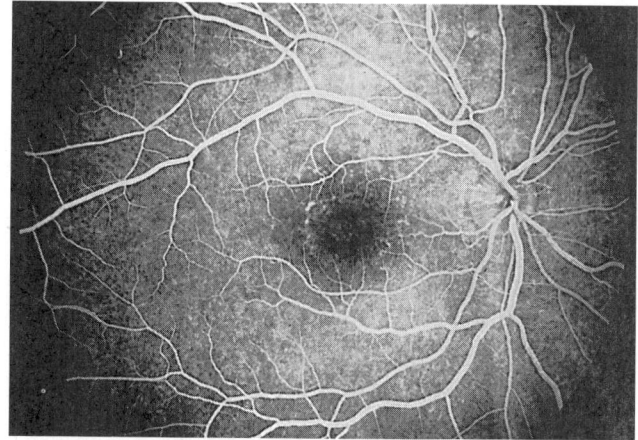

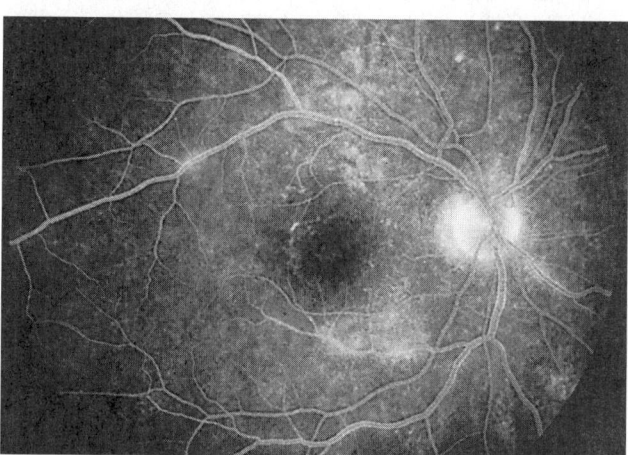

Fig. 46-10. **A,** MEWDS: Early stage angiogram. Punctate hyperfluorescent spots are seen in the macula and elsewhere. **B,** Late phase shows staining of the disk, retinal veins and focal areas away from the fovea.

dal neovascularization in the macula may develop as a late complication of MEWDS.[38]

The cause of MEWDS is unknown. The possible association of this condition with acute macular neuroretinopathy and multifocal choroiditis and panuveitis syndrome has been described previously. No effective therapy for MEWDS has been described, but the natural course has an excellent outcome in most cases.

SUBACUTE SCLEROSING PANENCEPHALITIS

Subacute sclerosing panencephalitis (SSPE) is a rare, progressive, and usually fatal neurodegenerative disease of childhood that is believed to be caused by a persistent measles virus infection. As a result of a nationwide immunization program against measles in the United States, the incidence of SSPE has decreased considerably, coexistent with the decline in natural measles infection. Nevertheless, the disease still represents a great international problem.

Ocular changes, frequently a macular chorioretinopathy, occur in up to 50% of patients with SSPE.[18] The typical lesion of SSPE chorioretinitis consists of superficial retinal hemorrhages in the macula region associated with edema and retinal folds.[6,27,31,40] Other changes in the fundus include macular pigmentary changes, papilledema, and optic atrophy.[31] In most patients the visual symptoms and ocular changes occur at the same time as other neurologic signs.[40] It is believed that the retinal lesions are caused by actual viral invasion.[27] Measles antigen has been found in the infected retinal cells by immunofluorescence.[12] Treatment of SSPE has been disappointing.

UNILATERAL ACUTE IDIOPATHIC MACULOPATHY

Unilateral acute idiopathic maculopathy (UAIM) is a recently described disorder seen in young patients.[39] The patients experience unilateral, marked loss of central vision. They demonstrate neurosensory detachment of the macular

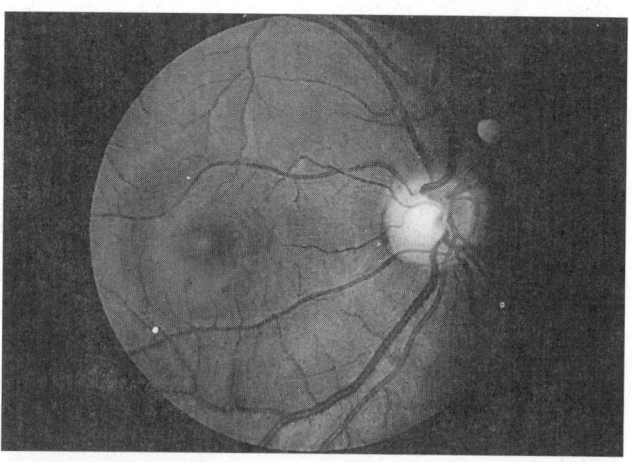

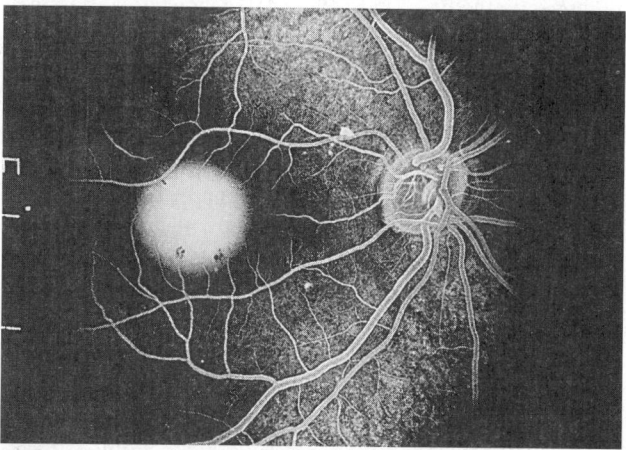

Fig. 46-11. A patient with UAIM. **A,** Acute elevation of the fovea with intraretinal hemorrhage. **B,** Angiogram shows intense leakage.

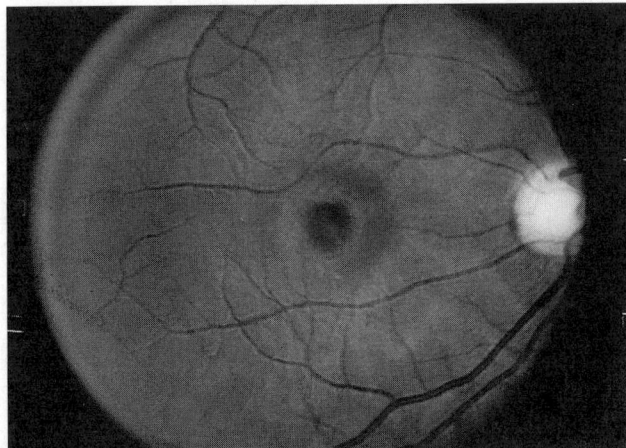

A

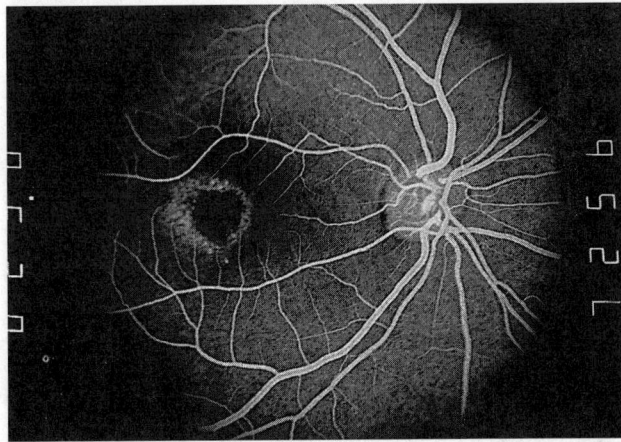

B

Fig. 46-12. The same patient with UAIM illustrated in Fig. 46-11, taken several weeks later. **A,** Bull's eye lesion. **B,** All fluorescein leakage is gone.

area with thickening at the level of the underlying retinal pigment epithelium (Fig. 46-11, *A*). Punctate intraretinal hemorrhages are often seen, which suggests choroidal neovascularization, but neovascularization is not identified. Vitreous humor inflammation is sometimes present. Fluorescein angiography is remarkable for very intense hyperfluorescence corresponding to the area of retinal neurosensory detachment (Fig. 46-11, *B*). The patients show a rapid evolution (several weeks) of the lesion, with a disappearance of the neurosensory elevation and the development of a bull's-eye pattern of pigmentation (Fig. 46-12). The visual outcome is usually excellent. The late development of choroidal neovascularization has been seen. To date, 10 cases of this syndrome have been reported.[39]

The cause of unilateral acute idiopathic maculopathy is uncertain. Some of the patients have had a flulike illness. Bilateral involvement or recurrences have not been seen. If choroidal neovascularization develops, the visual outcome is much worse.

REFERENCES

1. Ai E, Wong KL: Ophthalmic manifestations of AIDS, *Ophthalmol Clin N Am* 1:53, 1988.
2. Bos PJM, Deutman AF: Acute macular neuroretinopathy, *Am J Ophthalmol* 80:573-584, 1975.
3. Callanan D, Gass JDM: Multifocal choroiditis and choroidal neovascularization associated with the multiple evanescent white dot syndrome and acute idiopathic blind spot enlargement syndrome, *Ophthalmology* 99:1678-1685, 1992.
4. Coll GE, Lewis H: Metastatic choroidal abscess and choroidal neovascular membrane associated with staphylococcus aureus endocarditis in a heroin user, *Retina* 14:256-259, 1994.
5. Davis JL et al.: Endogenous bacterial retinitis in AIDS, *Am J Ophthalmol* 107:613, 1989.
6. DeLaey JJ et al.: Subacute sclerosing panencephalitis: fundus changes and histopathology correlations, *Doc Ophthalmol* 56:11-21, 1983.
7. Dhaliwal RS et al.: Acute posterior multifocal placoid pigment epitheliopathy: an indocyanine green angiographic study, *Retina* 13:317-325, 1993.
8. Dodwell DG et al.: Optic nerve involvement associated with the multiple evanescent white dot syndrome, *Ophthalmology* 97:862-868, 1990.
9. Dreyer RF, Gass JDM: Multifocal choroiditis and panuveitis: a syndrome that mimics ocular histoplasmosis, *Arch Ophthalmol* 102:1776-1784, 1984.
10. Eagle RC: Mechanisms of maculopathy, *Ophthalmology* 91:613-625, 1984.
11. Fletcher WA et al.: Acute idiopathic blind spot enlargement: a big blind spot syndrome without optic disc edema, *Arch Ophthalmol* 106:44-49, 1988.
12. Font RL, Jenis EH, Ruck KD: Measles maculopathy associated with subacute sclerosing panencephalitis, *Arch Pathol* 96:168-174, 1973.
13. Fusco R, Magli A, Gvacci P: Stellate maculopathy due to salmonella thyphi, *Ophthalmologica* 192:154-158, 1986.
14. Gass JDM: Acute posterior multifocal placoid pigment epitheliopathy, *Arch Ophthalmol* 80:177-185, 1968.
15. Gass JDM: Acute zonal occult outer retinopathy, *J Clin Neuroophthalmol* 13:79-97, 1993.
16. Gass JDM, Hamed LM: Acute macular neuroretinopathy and multiple evaenescent white dot syndrome occurring in the same patients, *Arch Ophthalmol* 107:189-193, 1989.
17. Greenwald MJ, Wohl LG, Sell CH: Metastatic endophthalmitis: a contemporary reappraisal, *Surv Ophthalmol* 32:81-101, 1986.
18. Hiatt RL et al.: Ophthalmologic manifestations of subacute sclerosing panencephalitis (Dawson's encephalitis), *Trans Am Acad Ophthalmol Otolaryngol* 75:344-350, 1971.
19. Holland GN: AIDS: retinal and choroidal infections. In Lewis H, Ryan SJ, editors: *Medical and surgical retina: advances, controversies and management,* 415-433, St Louis, 1994, Mosby.
20. Holland GN et al.: Acquired immune deficiency syndrome: ocular manifestations, *Ophthalmology* 90:859-873, 1983.
21. Ie D et al.: Indocyanine green angiography in multiple evanescent white-dot syndrome, *Am J Ophthalmol* 117:7-12, 1994.
22. Jabs DA, Green WR, Fox R: Ocular manifestations of acquired immune deficiency syndrome, *Ophthalmology* 96:1092-1099, 1989.
23. Jampol LM: Arteriolar occlusive disease of the macula, *Ophthalmology* 90:534-539, 1983.
24. Jampol LM et al.: Multiple evanescent white dot syndrome, *Arch Ophthalmol* 102:671-674, 1984.
25. Khorram KD, Jampol LM, Rosenberg MA: Blind spot enlargement as a manifestation of multifocal choroiditis, *Arch Ophthalmol* 108:1403-1407, 1991.
26. Krill AE, Deutman AF: Acute retinal pigment epitheliitis, *Am J Ophthalmol* 74:193-205, 1972.
27. Nelson DA et al.: Retinal lesions in subacute sclerosing panencephalitis, *Arch Ophthalmol* 84:613-621, 1970.
28. Niutta A, Barcaroli I, Palombi E: Monolateral chorioretinitis with multiple foci in one case of lyme disease, *Am J Ophthalmol* 25:257-261, 1993.
29. Palestine AG et al.: Progressive subretinal fibrosis and uveitis, *Br J Ophthalmol* 68:667-673, 1984.
30. Price NC, Frith PA, Awdry PN: Intraocular nocardiosis: a further case and review, *Int Ophthalmol* 13:177-180, 1989.

31. Robb RM, Watters GV: Ophthalmic manifestations of subacute sclerosing panencephalitis, *Arch Ophthalmol* 83:426-435, 1970.
32. Savir H: Septic retinitis, *Can J Ophthalmol* 22:171-172, 1987.
33. Spaide RF et al.: Lack of the HLA-DR2 specificity in multifocal choroiditis and panuveitis, *Br J Ophthalmol* 74:536, 1990.
34. Spaide RF et al.: Epstein-Barr virus antibodies in multifocal choroiditis and panuveitis, *Am J Ophthalmol* 112:410-413, 1991.
35. Tiedemann JS: Epstein-Barr viral antibodies in multifocal choroiditis and panuveitis, *Am J Ophthalmol* 103:659-663, 1987.
36. Tsai L et al.: Chronic recurrent multiple evanescent white dot syndrome, *Retina* (in press).
37. Watzke RC et al.: Punctate inner choroidopathy, *Am J Ophthalmol* 98:572-584, 1984.
38. Wyhinny GJ et al.: Subretinal neovascularization following multiple evanescent white-dot syndrome, *Arch Ophthalmol* 108:1384-1385, 1990.
39. Yannuzzi LA et al.: Unilateral acute idiopathic maculopathy, *Arch Ophthalmol* 109:1411-1416, 1991.
40. Zagami AS, Lethlean AK: Chorioretinitis as a possible very early manifestation of subacute sclerosing panencephalitis, *Aust NZ J Med* 21:350-352, 1994.

47 Birdshot Retinochoroidopathy

PHUC LEHOANG, STEPHEN J. RYAN

Birdshot retinochoroidopathy is a chronic intraocular inflammatory disease affecting mainly the posterior segment of the eye. It is distinct from other forms of posterior uveitis because of a very characteristic clinical presentation and a strong association with HLA-A29.2 antigen. The cause of birdshot retinochoroidopathy is unknown, but autoimmune mechanisms are presumed to play a role in its pathogenesis.

HISTORICAL BACKGROUND

The earliest report of this disease was probably by Franceschetti and Babel[18] in 1949, who named it *chorioretinopathie en taches de bougies,* as pointed out by Priem and Oosterhuis.[42] It has been called by a variety of names since it became accepted as a distinct entity in the early 1980s. The term *vitiliginous chorioretinitis* was chosen by Gass[20] because of the depigmented nature of the fundus lesions, which were reminiscent of vitiligo, and the association in some patients of a cutaneous vitiligo.[20] Other descriptive terms have included *salmon patch choroidopathy,* used by Aaberg,[1] and *chorioretinopathie en grains de riz,* used by Amalric and Cuq.[3] *Birdshot retinochoroidopathy* however, is the most commonly used term to describe this uveitic entity. This name was chosen by Ryan and Maumenee[44] because the fundus develops ''multiple, small white spots that frequently have the pattern seen with birdshot in the scatter from a shotgun.''

EPIDEMIOLOGY

Birdshot retinochoroidopathy is a rare disease. In the United States only seven cases of birdshot retinochoroidopathy were identified among a population of 600 patients in one specialized uveitis clinic.[22] In Europe 102 cases of birdshot retinochoroidopathy were collected from 14 eye clinics between 1980 and 1986.[42]

Birdshot retinochoroidopathy is found more frequently in Caucasians of Northern European extraction than in other ethnic or racial groups.[20,27,42,44] Unlike other uveitic entities that typically occur in younger patients, birdshot retinocho-roidopathy occurs during the third to the sixth decades with an average age of 50 years and a range of 35 to 70 years.[20,27,42,44] The reason for its occurrence during middle age is unclear. Patients who have birdshot retinochoroidopathy are otherwise healthy individuals. Women represent approximately 70% of the reported patients in the literature,[20,44] but this gender predilection for development of the disease is not observed in all studies.[8,11,31,32]

RISK FACTORS

The association between birdshot retinochoroidopathy and HLA-A29 antigen is the strongest known disease association with an HLA-A locus. About 80% to 98% of the patients with birdshot retinochoroidopathy are HLA-A29 positive compared to 7% of controls, and the presence of HLA-A29 antigen increases the risk of developing the disease approximately 50- to 224-fold.[4,5,32,35,41] The serologically defined HLA-A29 specificity can be split using immunoelectrofocusing into two subtypes: A29.1 and A29.2. In normal populations, the distribution of HLA-A29 subtypes varies with different ethnic groups. In the Caucasian population, among those who are HLA-A29-positive, the HLA-A29.2 subtype is found in approximately 80% to 90% of healthy individuals.[11,52] Birdshot retinochoroidopathy susceptibility appears to be exclusively linked to the HLA-A29.2 molecule.[32]

The exact mechanism by which the presence of HLA-A29.2 confers susceptibility to birdshot retinochoroidopathy remains unknown. HLA-A29.2 may alter antigen presentation or share common epitopes with an unidentified responsible agent. In Europe birdshot retinochoroidopathy seems to be located preferentially in some areas of Belgium, France, the Netherlands, and Switzerland, suggesting a possible infectious origin. An intercurrent infection might facilitate the presentation of self-peptides to T-lymphocytes by the HLA-A29 molecule. Although birdshot retinochoroidopathy was reported possibly to occur in HLA-A29-positive monozygotic twins,[17] no strong familial association can be observed; it is clearly not a heriditary disease with a recognizable mode of inheritance. No differences in the apparent electrophoretic migration and in the sequences of the HLA-A29.2 molecules from patients with birdshot retinochoroidopathy and healthy subjects have been observed.

HLA-A29.1 subtype is mainly found in populations from Southeast Asia where birdshot retinochoroidopathy has never been reported. Only one patient with birdshot retinochoroidopathy was stated to be HLA-A29.1 positive, but the corresponding cDNA sequencing could not be performed.[11]

Comparison of the HLA-A29.1 and HLA-A29.2 sequences shows a single difference in the extracellular domains between the two subtypes. The mutation exhibited by HLA-A29.1 is unique to that molecule, suggesting that the ancestral type is HLA-A29.2. Whereas the HLA-A29.2 molecule confers susceptibility to development of birdshot retinochoroidopathy, the more recently mutated HLA-A29.1 molecule appears to confer resistance to birdshot retinochoroidopathy. The unique amino acid sequence of HLA-A29.1 may influence the binding of CD8 or another accessory molecule and thus interfere with T-lymphocyte activation.[49]

CLINICAL FEATURES

Patients generally complain of floaters with variable degrees of decreased vision. Photophobia, difficulty with color distinction, and some evidence of night blindness are frequently reported. Visual complaints are often out of proportion to measured central visual acuity, indicating diffuse dysfunction of the retina.

In the original description by Ryan and Maumenee[44] diagnostic criteria included (1) a quiet nonpainful eye, (2) minimal anterior segment inflammation, (3) vitritis without snowballs or snowbanks, which differentiated birdshot retinochoroidopathy from pars planitis syndrome, (4) retinal vascular leakage leading to cystoid macular edema, often associated with optic disc edema, and (5) distinctive, discrete, cream-colored or depigmented spots scattered throughout the postequatorial fundus.

There may be a mild anterior chamber cellular reaction, but clinical examination shows few other signs of anterior segment inflammation. Irido-capsular synechiae are never observed. Patients do not complain of pain in the majority of cases, and the anterior segment is clear of any inflammation. The disease is usually bilateral and is characterized by the appearance of disseminated cream-colored spots throughout the postequatorial fundus at the level of the retinal pigment epithelium or choroid (Fig. 47-1). The spots are often more easily seen in the inferior nasal area of the fundus. They can have a variable distribution pattern in the posterior pole and the midperiphery. Lesions may be either diffuse or asymmetric with a concentration of spots, particularly inferiorly. Also, there may be either macular sparing or a macular predominance of lesions.[19] Some of the peripheral lesions are

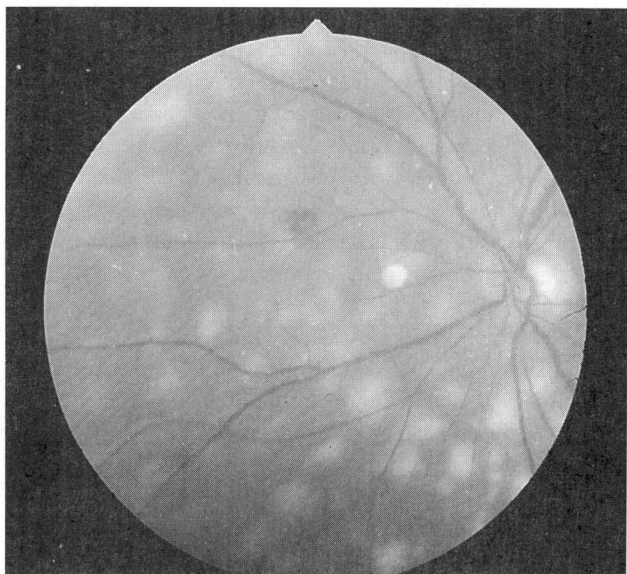

Fig. 47-1. Scattered cream-colored spots located predominantly in the nasal area of the fundus. A retinal hemorrhage can be seen. (Figure also in color insert.)

elongated and are distributed along the large choroidal vessels.[19,38,42] They may appear to radiate from the optic disc.[44] The lesions are usually oval with no reactive hyperpigmentation. They measure a quarter or three fourths of the optic disc diameter in size. Occasionally these lesions become confluent.[43]

A few eyes can show a peculiar evolution with the appearance of hypopigmented spots several years after the onset of intraocular inflammation consisting of papillitis, vitritis, and retinal vasculitis.[42,46] In long-standing inflammation of the retinal vessels and uvea, the HLA-A29 antigen must be assessed, because the development of cream-colored lesions of birdshot retinochoroidopathy can be delayed, and consequently the patients may be misdiagnosed as idiopathic retinal vasculitis.[46]

A vitreous humor cellular reaction is present in all patients, but its severity may vary between patients and from one examination to another; cellular infiltrates of the vitreous humor are usually diffuse or more marked in the posterior portion. They are often more numerous and severe during the early stages of the disease,[43] sometimes associated with vitreous strands. The cells may collect on the posterior vitreous face to form vitreous precipitates.[20]

Other clinical features may include narrowing of the retinal arterioles, vascular tortuosity,[43,44] retinal and preretinal neovascularization,[6,42] perivascular hemorrhages in the nerve fiber layer,[43] and epiretinal membranes that can threaten the macula.[42] Vasculitis involving the retinal venules can result in subtle sheathing that appears gray in contrast to the thick yellowish cuffing in other types of retinal vasculitis (sarcoidosis, for example). Retinal vasculitis and diffuse inflammation of the posterior segment can cause macular edema, either focally or diffusely, often leading to cystoid macular edema. Papillitis with optic disc swelling can be progressively replaced by optic atrophy. In many patients fundus spots are adjacent to the optic disc, giving a petaloid appearance.[42] Acute anterior ischemic optic neuropathy was reported in one patient with birdshot retinochoroidopathy.[9]

In rare cases patients can be left with peripheral chorioretinal scarring after many years of disease.

Natural History

Birdshot retinochoroidopathy is a slowly progressive disease. It is characterized by a chronic course of exacerbations and remissions with a progressive decrease of vision. Vision loss is related to cystoid macular edema or to an optic atrophy related to nerve fiber layer damage.[43] Although two thirds of the reported patients maintained a visual acuity better than 20/40 without treatment during the course of the disease in one study,[42] other experience shows a higher frequency of severely impaired vision (45% of patients having visual acuity less than 20/40) with an inexorable decline of vision during the natural course of the disease without adequate treatment (P. LeHoang, MD, unpublished data). Active birdshot retinochoroidopathy leads to severe visual impairment within the first few years of follow-up, if no treatment is administered.

In 20% of cases a self-limited form of birdshot retinochoroidopathy can be observed in which patients maintain 20/20 vision, with spontaneous regression of the intraocular inflammation and persistence of rather atrophic disseminated spots throughout the fundus.

After 7 to 10 years, while the disease process is becoming inactive, the fundus lesions may become partially pigmented* centrally, rather than at their periphery. At the advanced stages of the disease, optic atrophy and diffuse depigmentation of the fundus are often observed.

PATHOLOGY

An enucleated, phthisical eye from a patient with birdshot retinochoroidopathy in the other eye has been examined histopathologically.[35] It showed a moderate focal infiltration of lymphocytes and plasma cells of the iris and ciliary body. There was diffuse granulomatous inflammation in the outer retinal layers with giant cells, epithelioid cells, and plasma cells. The choroid was less inflamed, with a moderate number of epithelioid and giant cells.[35]

COMPLICATIONS

Chronic cystoid macular edema is the most common complication of the disease, occurring in 62.6% of cases.[42] It threatens central vision and indicates a need for therapy. If started early, before cystoid macular degeneration has developed, the treatment can reduce retinal edema and restore good central vision.

Epiretinal membranes and cellophane maculopathy are frequent complications, occurring in nearly 10% of cases.[42] Interestingly, the macular pucker can enlarge and progress as a cicatricial phenomenon while the intraocular inflammation (vitritis and retinal vasculopathy) resolves on treatment.[31]

Subretinal neovascular membranes occurred infrequently during the course of birdshot retinochoroidopathy (approximately 6% of cases) in the series reported by Priem and Oosterhuis.[42] In some patients there is a relationship between a fundus lesion and the development of subretinal new vessels arising from an atrophic retinochoroidal scar. Subretinal neovascular membranes can develop adjacent to fundus lesions from 6 months to 5 years after the onset of the disease.[8] Subretinal neovascular membranes can also involve the juxtapapillary area or threaten central vision in the juxtafoveal region. Fluorescein and indocyanine green (ICG) angiographies are essential to identify neovascular membranes and to guide the laser photocoagulation that can prevent the loss of central vision.[8,42,47]

Peripheral retinal and optic disc neovascularization occur in 7% of cases and can occur in the absence of retinal capillary nonperfusion.[42] Peripheral preretinal neovascularization can be induced by a local inflammation in the retinal vascular bed without evidence of retinal capillary closure. This form of neovascularization can lead to vitreous hemorrhage.

Optic atrophy represents a severe sequela of long-standing inflammation but can also occasionally be related to an acute anterior ischemic optic neuropathy.[9]

Patients with birdshot retinochoroidopathy have a high incidence of cardiovascular disease (systemic hypertension, coronary artery disease, strokes, retinal vein occlusion) and of open angle glaucoma.[42]

PATHOGENESIS

The cause of birdshot retinochoroidopathy is unknown. Birdshot retinochoroidopathy is probably an acquired inflammatory disease that shares some clinical aspects and possibly some pathogenic mechanisms with Vogt-Koyanagi-Harada disease and sympathetic ophthalmia. In predisposed HLA-A29-positive individuals, retinal autoimmunity seems to play a role in the pathogenesis of the disease, particularly in the perpetuation of intraocular inflammation. The histopathologic study of an eye from a patient with birdshot retinochoroidopathy revealed a granulomatous inflammation in and under the retina.[35] The patient also had a positive proliferative response of peripheral blood lymphocytes to retinal S antigen in vitro.

The retina can be destroyed progressively by the inflammation, leaving areas of residual retina with foci of granulomatous cells. The adjacent choroid is diffusely infiltrated with lymphocytes, in which there are foci of granulomatous

---

*Howard Tessler, MD and J. Donald M. Gass, MD personnal communications, also see reference 29.

inflammation. A granulomatous inflammation may also be observed in the vitreous humor, with large macrophage and multinucleated giant cells.[14]

These general pathologic features are similar to those observed in S-antigen-induced experimental autoimmune uveoretinitis (EAU) in monkeys with granulomatous inflammation in the retina around and under retinal veins and in the underlying choroid.[16,34] The same genetic predisposition, histopathologic findings, and evidence of sensitization against retinal antigens are also found in the animal model of EAU.[15] The numerous similarities between birdshot retinochoroidopathy and EAU may indicate that retinal autoimmunity represents a possible pathogenic mechanism for development of the disease.

The trigger and the precise pathogenic role of retinal autoimmunity are unknown. Retinal autoimmunity may simply represent an epiphenomenon that develops after retinal damage caused by an unrelated insult; alternatively, it is possible that although autoimmunity does not initiate ocular inflammation, it may perpetuate and maintain the inflammatory state and produce further damage to ocular tissues. The study of the anchoring characteristics of the endogen peptides present within the HLA-A29 molecule pouch may help to find analogous peptides of various origins (viral, bacterial, or other unknown antigens) capable of inducing an autoimmune reaction in the altered self or receptor theory. Interesting preliminary results on the serology of various infectious agents, including *Borrelia burgdorferi* in patients carrying the HLA-A29 antigen, warrant further studies in that direction.[28,48] It is interesting to note that in a population of patients with vitiligo, 39% had discrete areas of depigmentation of the retinal pigment epithelium and choroid and 4.8% to 8% had uveitis.[2] Conversely, 5.4% of 129 patients with uveitis of unknown origin also had cutaneous depigmentation, poliosis, or early grey hair. These observations suggest that Vogt-Koyanagi-Harada syndrome, sympathetic ophthalmia, birdshot retinochoroidopathy, and the other diseases included in this spectrum may be more related than previously thought.

Because the pineal gland and the retina have a common embryologic origin, they share common antigens[26] and can both be involved in the autoimmune inflammatory reactions induced in experimental models by immunization with retinal extracts or purified proteins such as retinal S-antigen, rhodopsin, or interphotoreceptor retinoid binding protein (IRBP). The pineal inflammatory syndrome observed in experimental autoimmune uveoretinitis can also be suspected in chronic posterior uveitis in humans. Alterations of the pineal function and circadian rhythms may result in depression and disruption of the sleep-wake cycle. The pineal gland is responsible for melatonin secretion that controls the dermal pigmentation and might play a role in the development of the vitiliginous birdshot retinochoroidopathy lesions—as suggested by Opremcak.[39] Nighttime peak levels of plasma melatonin are significantly decreased by

about 45% in patients with chronic posterior uveitis, particularly in patients suffering from birdshot retinochoroidopathy. This observation may indicate that a systemic immune inflammatory reaction also involves the pineal gland in patients with birdshot retinochoroidopathy, considering that the main source of plasma melatonin is pineal synthesis of the hormone.[50] In addition, the measurement of elevated levels of soluble IL-2 receptor in the serum of patients with active birdshot retinochoroidopathy compared to serum from normal controls suggests a possible systemic component to this disease.*

DIFFERENTIAL DIAGNOSIS

Birdshot retinochoroidopathy shares some features with a variety of disorders including pars planitis syndrome, various other white dot syndromes, sarcoidosis, and infectious and noninfectious uveitis.

The pars planitis syndrome variant of intermediate uveitis tends to occur in a younger age group and presents with bilateral vitritis, predominantly in the anterior vitreous humor, without cream-colored spots at fundus examination. Patients with pars planitis syndrome have changes in the vitreous base, peripheral retina, and pars plana that give the appearance of "snowballs and snowbanks."

Multiple evanescent white dot syndrome (MEWDS) is seen in younger patients (average age of onset 28 years) and is characterized by acute vision loss in association with white dots at the retinal pigment epithelial level. This syndrome is usually unilateral. Vitreous humor inflammation is minimal, and in most cases a spontaneous improvement occurs within 6 weeks. Patients suffering from multifocal choroiditis and panuveitis syndrome also tend to be younger than birdshot retinochoroidopathy patients. They have unilateral disease, greater degrees of inflammation, and are less likely to have night blindness or electroretinographic abnormalities. The lesions tend to become hyperpigmented, and they are smaller and better defined than those seen with birdshot retinochoroidopathy.

Patients with sarcoidosis can develop choroidal granulomata presenting as white or yellowish lesions that can be confused with the fundus lesions of birdshot retinochoroidopathy, particularly when other signs of granulomatous uveitis (mutton fat keratitic precipitates and iris nodules in the anterior segment, or "candle wax drippings" and thick sheathing of the retinal vessels in the posterior segment) are missing, as is often the case when sarcoidosis patients have deep foci of choroidal involvement. In the literature some patients described as having birdshot retinochoroidopathy in fact showed systemic signs of sarcoidosis.[42,53] Sarcoidosis must therefore be ruled out before a diagnosis of birdshot retinochoroidopathy is made.[7]

Other diseases that might be confused with birdshot ret-

---

*F. G. Roberge MD, personnal communication.

inochoroidopathy include tuberculosis, syphilis, histoplasmosis, choroidal pneumocystosis, intraocular lymphoma, sympathetic ophthalmia, Vogt-Koyanagi-Harada syndrome, and acute posterior multifocal placoid pigment epitheliopathy (APMPPE).

LABORATORY INVESTIGATIONS

The diagnosis of birdshot retinochoroidopathy is based on clinical findings. HLA typing can support the diagnosis because HLA-A29 antigen is present in 80% to 90% of cases.[4,5,32,35,42] HLA-A29 subtyping does not contribute further to the diagnosis.[32] As in other chronic posterior uveitides, positive humoral and cellular immune reactions to retinal S antigen and IRPB have been reported,[13,25] but these findings are nonspecific. An appropriate workup to rule out other disorders in the differential diagnosis can include serum angiotensin converting enzyme, lysozyme, and gallium scan for sarcoidosis, and FTA-Abs testing for syphilis.

For intraocular lymphoma, a systemic workup consisting of hematology testing, magnetic resonance imaging (MRI), lumbar puncture, and computed tomography should be performed. Diagnostic vitrectomy may be the crucial means of making that diagnosis. Invasive retinochoroidal biopsy is rarely needed and should be proposed only when there is a strong suspicion of intraocular lymphoma and when other disorders have been ruled out.

Fluorescein Angiography

Most of the cream-colored lesions remain silent during the whole course of a fluorescein angiogram. Thus in the majority of cases the spots are more visible by indirect ophthalmoscopy than by fluorescein angiography.[43] Nevertheless, careful study of the fluorescein angiogram may reveal early hypofluorescence and late hyperfluorescence of some of the active fundus lesions.[20,43,44] The presence of lesions of different ages in the same fundus can explain the angiographic heterogeneity of the spots. Moreover, the early hypofluorescent area and the late hyperfluorescent area are not exactly superimposable, either to each other or to the visible spots on the red-free photographs, suggesting a complex nature of a single lesion. The early hypofluorescent surface, when present, can be smaller than the surface of the corresponding visible spot. In some of the early hypofluorescent lesions, large choroidal vessels are visible; this hypofluorescence in the early phase is not caused by a yellow filtering effect but seems to be related to the nonperfusion of the choriocapillaris associated with an atrophic or depigmented retinal pigment epithelium.

Depending on the stage of the disease, two categories of fundus lesions can be roughly distinguished on the fluorescein angiogram. First, the fresh lesions appear as cream-colored spots on the colored and red-free photographs (Fig. 47-1). Many of these cream-colored spots can remain silent during all the phases of the angiogram showing neither early

hypofluorescence nor late-phase hyperfluorescence; they correspond to either "very early" lesions or to deeper lesions that do not yet affect the choriocapillaris and the retinal pigment epithelium. On the other hand, the early phase of the angiogram can reveal a small area of hypofluorescence within the surface of some cream-colored spots; this early hypofluorescence can correspond to some degree of alteration of the retinal pigment epithelium associated with a nonperfusion of the choriocapillaris. Slight diffuse hyperfluorescence may be present in the late phase. Second, the advanced lesions appear as well-delineated, whitish, atrophic spots on the red-free photograph; the whole surface of the lesion becomes hypofluorescent in the early phase of the angiogram, with visibility of large choroidal vessels through an atrophic or depigmented retinal pigment epithelium and a nonperfused choriocapillaris. In the late phase they appear diffusely hyperfluorescent, sometimes with a lighter peripheral halo. These advanced lesions are often adjacent to the optic disc, giving the appearance of petals or of "Mickey Mouse" ears.

Hyperfluorescence of the optic disc is a common finding. Variable degrees of macular edema can precede cystoid changes. Diffuse retinal vascular leakage and diffuse hyperfluorescence of the fundus, particularly along the major retinal vessels, may be easily noted at the late phase of the angiogram (Fig. 47-2).

Indocyanine Green Angiography

Indocyanine green angiography shows a vasotropic orientation of choroidal hypofluorescent lesions, as originally reported by Yannuzzi and Slakter.[45] Their location also corresponds to the cream-colored lesions and they are generally greater in number than the spots seen on the color and red-free fundus photographs (Fig. 47-3,A and Fig. 47-3,B). Thus ICG angiography can reveal unsuspected lesions that may represent an early stage of the cream-colored fundus lesions. ICG angiography gives a better estimate of the severity of the choriocapillary and choroidal involvement and of the actual number of spots during the course of the disease. The surface area of the ICG angiogram dark lesions is equal to or larger than the surface of the fundus lesions visible on red-free photographs. These dark spots identified on ICG angiography are most often located between large choroidal vessels; they also appear to follow the main choroidal vascular pathways and may represent an equivalent of some type of granulomatous choroidal vasculitis. This pattern is similar to the one seen in Vogt-Koyanagi-Harada syndrome. The explanation of the dark appearance of the lesions is not clear. It may be related to many factors including (1) the presence of nonvascularized granulomatous infiltrates located in the outer choroid or between large choroidal vessels, (2) the possible hypoperfusion of the choriocapillaris and of the choroidal vessels, and (3) the abnormal visibility (in some cases) of the sclera through atrophic lesions (Fig. 47-4).

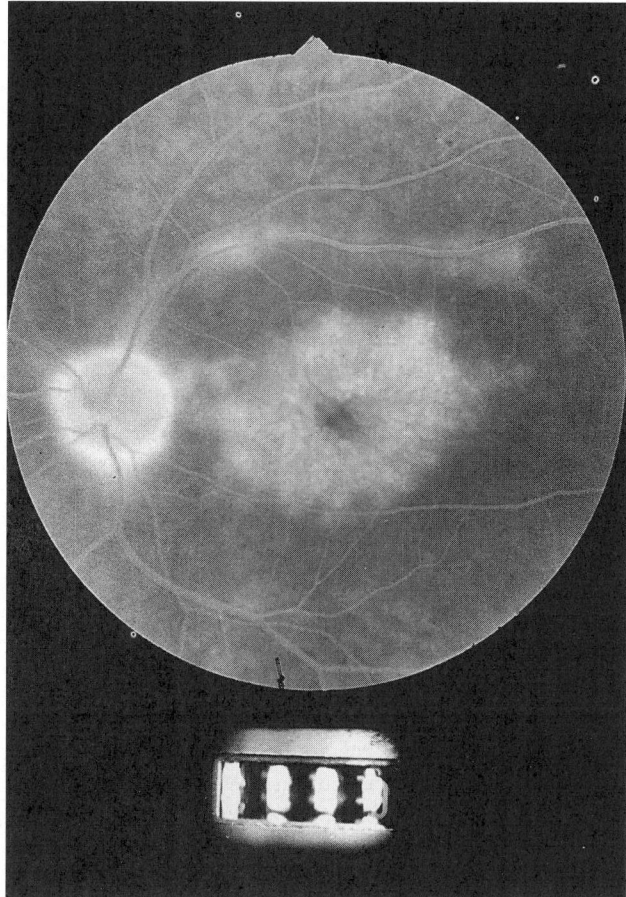

Fig. 47-2. Fluorescein angiogram (late phase) showing vascular leakage and cystoid macular edema.

Electrophysiology

Alterations of the electroretinogram[23,27,40] in patients with birdshot retinochoroidopathy suggest an impairment of the inner neural layer rather than involvement of the photoreceptor-retinal pigment epithelium-choroid complex; they can give evidence for the severity of the disease. The "a" wave of the electroretinogram is well preserved, in contrast to a reduced amplitude and an increased latency time of the "b" wave. The oscillatory potentials may be the only abnormal findings.

Abnormalities on the electrooculogram have been observed with a subnormal ratio of slow oscillations (L/D ratio) in 71% of the cases. There is no correlation between the abnormality of slower oscillations and choroidal disease, as measured by the number of fundus spots, but there is a strong correlation with retinal vasculopathy.[42] Conversely, the fast oscillation ratio (D/L ratio) is normal in the majority of cases.

Increased latency or abnormal amplitudes of the pattern-evoked potentials are frequently observed; the flash visual-evoked cortical potential amplitudes and wave forms are

within normal limits. The dark adaptation threshold is elevated in 70% of cases.[42]

Laser Flare Photometry

Whereas a profound breakdown of the blood-retinal barrier can be observed on fluorescein angiography, there is little impairment of the blood-aqueous barrier as measured by laser flare photometry. Patients with birdshot retinochoroidopathy have been found to have mean ($\pm$ standard error) values of 5.7 $\pm$ 1.1 photons/ms, compared to 4.7 $\pm$ 0.16 photons/ms for controls.[21] More recent studies have found slightly different results (13.0 $\pm$ 5.7 photons/ms for patients with birdshot retinochoroidopathy, 4.0 $\pm$ 0.8 photons/ms

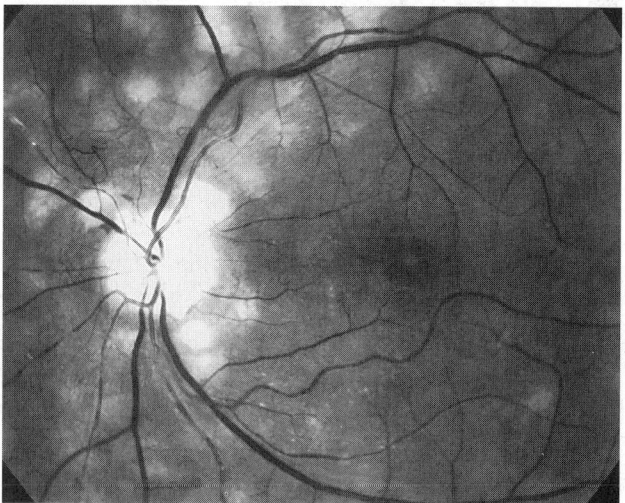

A

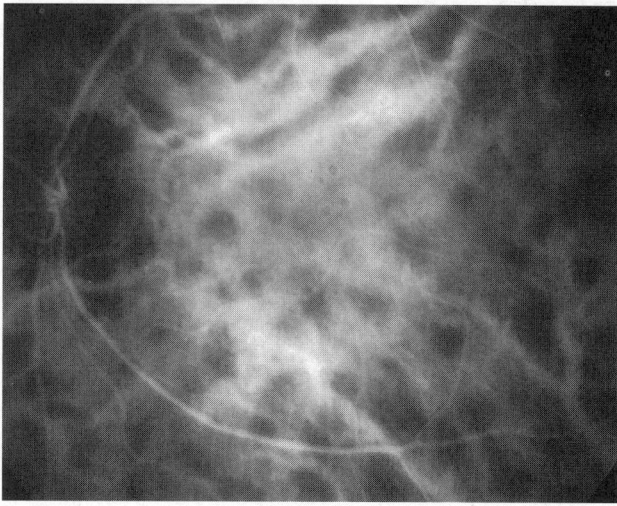

B

Fig. 47-3. **A,** Red-free fundus photograph showing only few choroidal lesions. **B,** Indocyanine green (ICG) angiogram revealing numerous dark spots that were absent on red-free photograph. (Courtesy of Dr. G. Quentel.)

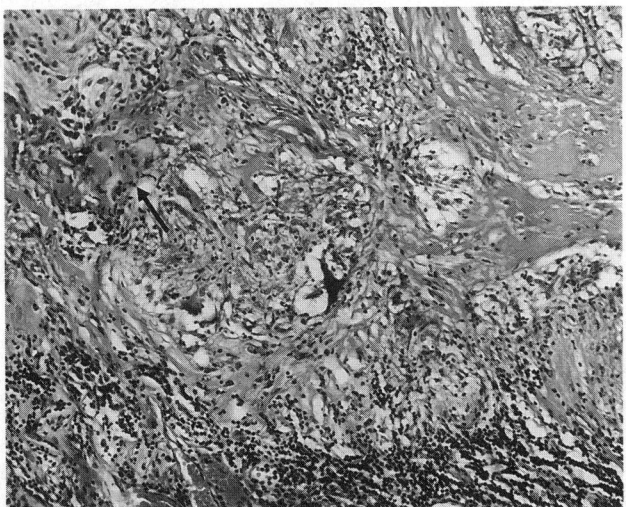

Fig. 47-4. Focus of granulomatous cells (arrow) in area of residual retina. Diffuse infiltration of lymphocytes in the adjacent choroid in which there are foci of granulomatous inflammation. (Hematoxylin and eosin, ×140)

for controls), but confirm the minimal disruption of the blood-aqueous barrier.* These findings are reflected in the minimal amount of flare seen by slit lamp biomicroscopic examination.

Other Tests

Central or paracentral scotomata, depression or constriction of the visual field, or enlarged blind spot may be noted.[19,20] Color vision abnormalities consist of acquired dyschromatopsia of the blue-yellow type. Some patients have both blue-yellow and red-green defects.[42]

THERAPY

Because the number of patients with birdshot retinochoroidopathy is small, and because intraocular inflammation can sometimes resolve spontaneously, there have been no randomized trials of therapy and therefore no specific therapeutic regimen has emerged as the best method for treating patients with birdshot retinochoroidopathy.

Corticosteroids

Periocular and systemic corticosteroids have not shown consistent efficacy.† High dosages of prednisone (1 mg/kg/day) can initially cause improvement in vision, but patients can become rapidly dependent on dosages of prednisone above 20 to 30 mg/day, which cannot be tolerated as a prolonged treatment. Although fewer than 15% of patients achieve a good clinical response and can be maintained on

*P. LeHoang, MD, unpublished data.
†References 19, 20, 27, 35, 42, 44.

moderate to low dosages of prednisone, an initial trial on prednisone is indicated.[39]

Immunosuppression

Various cytotoxic agents (azathioprine, cyclophosphamide, chlorambucil) have been used without proven efficacy. Cyclosporine is a fungal metabolite that inhibits helper T-lymphocyte function by preventing the production of interleukin-2. Cyclosporine can control experimental EAU induced by immunization with retinal autoantigens.[33,37] Because T-lymphocyte-mediated retinal autoimmunity is thought to play an important role in the pathogenesis of both EAU[10] and birdshot retinochoroidopathy and because the efficacy of corticosteroids is inconsistent in this disease, the use of cyclosporine in the treatment of birdshot retinochoroidopathy was justified and appears to be effective.[31,36,51] As a result of cyclosporine-induced nephrotoxicity at higher dosage (10 mg/kg/day), low-dosage cyclosporine (5 mg/kg/day) has been used in the management of the disease, either alone or combined with low-dosage corticosteroids (oral prednisone, less than 20 mg/day).[31,51] Although it is better tolerated, the use of low-dosage cyclosporine alone or in combination with low-dosage prednisone does not prevent the occurrence of systemic hypertension in 81% of patients with birdshot retinochoroidopathy who have healthy native kidneys.[12] One study showed that vision preservation is possible with very low initial dosages of cyclosporine (2.5 mg/kg/day) alone or in combination with azathioprine (1.5 to 2 mg/kg/day) as another corticosteroid-sparing agent. This favorable visual outcome could be obtained without any demonstrable cyclosporine-associated nephrotoxicity nor secondary side effects; furthermore, improvement or stabilization of visual acuity occurred in 20 of 24 eyes (83.3%) in patients receiving cyclosporine therapy alone or in combination with azathioprine, whereas six of 11 eyes (54%) in patients receiving only periocular corticosteroids had a significant decrease in visual acuity.[51]

Other Therapies

Nonsteroidal antiinflammatory agents and radiation therapy have been used[24,35,44] but have not proved effective and are not recommended.

An experimental approach to treatment has been to manipulate the idiotypic network through repeated infusions of high doses of normal polyspecific immunoglobulins; such therapy has been successfully used in a number of organ-specific and systemic autoimmune conditions for which there is evidence of a primary pathogenic role of autoantibodies or of autoaggressive T-lymphocytes. Preliminary results for birdshot retinochoroidopathy have been encouraging (P. LeHoang, unpublished data).

Laser photocoagulation may be necessary in cases where subretinal neovascularization threatens central vision.

PROGNOSIS

The clinical course of birdshot retinochoroidopathy is marked by sequences of exacerbations and remissions. The prognosis is variable; without treatment, the vision usually worsens progressively and the disease process remains active for 2 to 5 years or longer.[19] Useful central vision in at least one eye is often retained.[20] Few untreated patients maintain good visual acuity.

PREVENTION

There is no way to prevent development of birdshot retinochoroidopathy; prevention efforts are aimed at avoiding permanent, vision-threatening complications of the disease. All the patients with birdshot retinochoroidopathy who complain only of floaters should have repeated ophthalmologic examinations and fluorescein angiograms even if their central vision remains good. The detection of increasing intraocular inflammation, macular edema, or gradual decrease of vision warrants the initiation of therapy to prevent vision loss.

REFERENCES

1. Aaberg TM: *Diffuse inflammatory salmon patch choroidopathy syndrome.* Paper presented at the International Fluorescein Macula Symposium, Carmel, CA, 1979.
2. Albert DM, Nordlund JJ, Lerner AB: Ocular abnormalities occurring with vitiligo, *Ophthalmology* 86:1145-1158, 1979.
3. Amalric P, Cuq G: Une forme très particulière de choriorétinopathie en grains de riz, *Bull Soc Ophtalmol Fr* 81:131-134, 1981.
4. Baarsma GS, Kijlstra A, Oosterhuis JA et al.: Association of birdshot retinochoroidopathy and HLA-A29 antigen, *Doc Ophthalmol* 61:267-269, 1986.
5. Baarsma GS, Priem HA, Kijlstra A: Association of birdshot retinochoroidopathy and HLA-A29 antigen, *Curr Eye Res* 9:63-68, 1990.
6. Barondes MJ, Fastenberg DM, Schwartz PL et al.: Peripheral retinal neovascularization in birdshot retinochoroidopathy, *Ann Ophthalmol* 21:306-308, 1989.
7. Brinkman CJ, Rothova A: Fundus pathology in neurosarcoidosis, *Int Ophthalmol* 17:23-26, 1993.
8. Brucker AJ, Deglin EA, Bene C et al.: Subretinal choroidal neovascularization in birdshot retinochoroidopathy, *Am J Ophthalmol* 99:40-44, 1985.
9. Caballero-Presencia A, Diaz-Guia E, Lopez-Lopez JM: Acute anterior ischemic optic neuropathy in birdshot retinochoroidopathy, *Ophthalmologica* 196:87-91, 1988.
10. Caspi RR, Roberge FG, McAllister CG et al.: T cell lines mediating experimental autoimmune uveoretinitis (EAU) in the rat, *J Immunol* 136:928-933, 1986.
11. de Waal LP, Lardy NM, van der Horst AR et al.: HLA-A29 subtypes and birdshot chorioretinopathy, *Immunogenetics* 35:51-53, 1992.
12. Deray G, Benhmida M, LeHoang P et al.: Renal function and blood pressure in patients receiving long-term, low-dose cyclosporine therapy for idiopathic autoimmune uveitis, *Ann Intern Med* 117:578-583, 1992.
13. de-Smet MD, Yamamoto JH, Mochizuki M et al.: Cellular immune responses of patients with uveitis to retinal antigens and their fragments, *Am J Ophthalmol* 110:135-142, 1990.
14. Engel HM, Green WR, Michels RG et al.: Diagnostic vitrectomy, *Retina* 1:121-149, 1981.
15. Faure JP: Autoimmunity and the retina, *Curr Top Eye Res* 2:215-302, 1980.
16. Faure JP, LeHoang P, Takano S et al.: Uvéo-rétinite expérimentale induite par l'antigène S rétinien chez lz singe, *J Fr Ophtalmol* 4:465-472, 1981.
17. Fich M, Rosenberg T: Birdshot retinochoroidopathy in monozygotic twins, *Acta Ophthalmol* 70:693-697, 1992.
18. Franceschetti A, Babel J: La chorio-rétinite en "tâches de bougie", manifestation de la maladie de Besnier-Boeck, *Ophthalmologica* 118:701-710, 1949.
19. Fuerst DJ, Tessler HH, Fishman GA et al.: Birdshot retinochoroidopathy, *Arch Ophthalmol* 102:214-219, 1984.
20. Gass JD: Vitiliginous chorioretinitis, *Arch Ophthalmol* 99:1778-1787, 1981.
21. Guex-Crosier Y, Pittet N, Herbort CP: Evaluation of laser flare-cell photometry in the appraisal and management of intraocular inflammation in uveitis, *Ophthalmology* 101:728-735, 1994.
22. Henderly DE, Genstler AJ, Smith RE et al.: Changing patterns of uveitis, *Am J Ophthalmol* 103:131-136, 1987.
23. Hirose T, Katsumi O, Pruett RC et al.: Retinal function in birdshot retinochoroidopathy, *Acta Ophthalmol* 69:327-337, 1991.
24. Hofmann HM, Feicht B: Birdshot chorioretinopathy: systemic therapy with corticosteroids and nonsteroidal anti-inflammatory drugs, *Klin Monatsbl Augenheilkd* 197:159-161, 1990.
25. Jobin D, Thillaye B, de-Kozak Y et al.: Severe retinochoroidopathy: variations of humoral and cellular immunity to S-antigen in a longitudinal study, *Curr Eye Res* 9:91-96, 1990.
26. Kalsow CM, Wacker WB: Pineal reactivity of anti-retina sera, *Invest Ophthalmol Vis Sci* 16:181-184, 1977.
27. Kaplan HJ, Aaberg TM: Birdshot retinochoroidopathy, *Am J Ophthalmol* 90:773-782, 1980.
28. Kuhne F, Morlat P, Riss I et al.: Is A29, B12 vasculitis caused by the Q fever agent? (Coxiella burnetii), *J Fr Ophtalmol* 15:315-321, 1992.
29. Lam S, Tessler HH: Birdshot retinochoroidopathy (vitiliginous chorioretinitis). In Nozik RA, Michelson JB, editors: *Uveitis,* 81-84, Philadelphia, 1993, WB Saunders.
30. LeHoang P, Donnefort N, Foucault C et al.: Association between HLA-A29 antigen and birdshot retinochoroidopathy. In Blodi F, Brancato R, Cristini G et al., editors: *Acta XXV Concilium Ophthalmologicum,* 45-46, Amsterdam, 1987, Kugler & Ghedini.
31. LeHoang P, Girard B, Deray G et al.: Cyclosporine in the treatment of birdshot retinochoroidopathy, *Transplant Proc* 20(3 suppl 4):128-130, 1988.
32. LeHoang P, Ozdemir N, Benhamou A et al.: HLA-A29.2 subtype associated with birdshot retinochoroidopathy, *Am J Ophthalmol* 113:33-35, 1992.
33. Nordmann JP, De-Kozak Y, LeHoang P et al.: Cyclosporine therapy of guinea-pig autoimmune uveoretinitis induced with autologous retina, *J Ocul Pharmacol* 2:325-333, 1986.
34. Nussenblatt RB, Kuwabara T, deMonasterio F et al.: S-antigen uveitis in primates: a new model for human disease, *Arch Ophthalmol* 99:1090-1092, 1981.
35. Nussenblatt RB, Mittal KK, Ryan S et al.: Birdshot retinochoroidopathy associated with HLA-A29 antigen and immune responsiveness to retinal S-antigen, *Am J Ophthalmol* 94:147-158, 1982.
36. Nussenblatt RB, Palestine AG, Chan CC: Cyclosporine A: therapy in the treatment of intraocular inflammatory disease resistant to systemic corticosteroids and cytotoxic agents, *Am J Ophthalmol* 96:275-282, 1983.
37. Nussenblatt RB, Rodrigues MM, Wacker WB et al.: Cyclosporin A: inhibition of experimental autoimmune uveitis in lewis rats, *J Clin Invest* 67:1228-1231, 1981.
38. Oosterhuis JA, Baarsma GS, Polak BC: Birdshot chorioretinopathy—vitiliginous chorioretinitis, *Int Ophthalmol* 5:137-144, 1982.
39. Opremcak EM: Birdshot retinochoroiditis. In Albert DM, Jakobiec FA, editors: *Principles and practice of ophthalmology,* 475-480, Philadelphia, 1994, WB Saunders.
40. Priem HA, De-Rouck A, De-Laey JJ et al.: Electrophysiologic studies in birdshot chorioretinopathy, *Am J Ophthalmol* 106:430-436, 1988.

41. Priem HA, Kijlstra A, Noens L et al.: HLA typing in birdshot chorioretinopathy, *Am J Ophthalmol* 105:182-185, 1988.
42. Priem HA, Oosterhuis JA: Birdshot chorioretinopathy: clinical characteristics and evolution, *Br J Ophthalmol* 72:646-659, 1988.
43. Ryan SJ: Birdshot retinochoroidopathy. In Ryan SJ, editor: *Retina,* vol 2, *Medical retina,* 671-677, St Louis, 1989, CV Mosby.
44. Ryan SJ, Maumenee AE: Birdshot retinochoroidopathy, *Am J Ophthalmol* 89:31-45, 1980.
45. Slakter JS: Indocyanine green videoangiography in inflammatory diseases. In Yannuzzi L, Flower R, Slakter J, editors: *Indocyanine green videoangiography* St Louis, CV Mosby (in press).
46. Soubrane G, Bokobza R, Coscas G: Late developing lesions in birdshot retinochoroidopathy, *Am J Ophthalmol* 109:204-210, 1990.
47. Soubrane G, Coscas G, Binaghi M et al.: Birdshot retinochoroidopathy and subretinal new vessels, *Br J Ophthalmol* 67:461-467, 1983.
48. Suttorp-Schulten MS, Luyendijk L, van-Dam AP et al.: Birdshot chorioretinopathy and Lyme borreliosis, *Am J Ophthalmol* 115:149-153, 1993.
49. Tabary T, Prochnicka-Chalufour A, Cornillet P et al.: HLA-A29 subtypes and "birdshot" choroido-retinopathy susceptibility: a possible "resistance motif" in the HLA-A29.1 molecule, *C R Acad Sci III* 313:599-605, 1991.
50. Touitou Y, LeHoang P, Claustrat B et al.: Decreased nocturnal plasma melatonin peak in patients with a functional alteration of the retina in relation with uveitis, *Neurosci Lett* 70:170-174, 1986.
51. Vitale AT, Rodriguez A, Foster CS: Low-dose cyclosporine therapy in the treatment of birdshot retinochoroidopathy, *Ophthalmology* 101:822-831, 1994.
52. Yang SY: Population analysis of class I HLA antigens by one-dimensional isoelectric focusing gel electrophoresis: workshop summary report. In Dupont B, editor: *Immunobiology of HLA,* 309-331, New York, 1989, Springer-Verlag.
53. Yoshioka T, Yoshioka H, Tanaka F: Birdshot retinochoroidopathy as a new ocular sign of the sarcoidosis, *Nippon Ganka Gakkai Zasshi* 87:283-288, 1983.

48 Serpiginous Choroiditis

PHILIP L. HOOPER, ANTONIO G. SECCHI, HENRY J. KAPLAN

Serpiginous choroiditis is a rare disease that results in a progressive loss of the retinal pigment epithelium and choriocapillaris. The disease has been known for over 60 years and has been referred to by several names including geographic helicoid peripapillary choroidopathy and geographic choroidopathy.[15a] Its course is variable between individuals, and there may be months or years of inactivity between episodes of disease. As a result, little is known about its cause or pathogenesis, and assessment of therapeutic regimens is difficult.

EPIDEMIOLOGY

Serpiginous choroiditis usually occurs as a bilateral disorder in the fourth to sixth decades of life, although lesions may develop at an earlier age.[3,36] The disorder is most prevalent in Caucasians, and in some series a male preponderance has been observed.[36] Familial clusters have not been described.[15] Aside from a single report of serpiginous choroiditis developing in association with extra pyramidal dystonia, no association with systemic disease has been noted.[11,30]

CLINICAL FEATURES

Patients typically have a unilateral decrease in central vision, metamorphopsia, or scotoma.[3,11,16,33,36] On examination, the anterior segment of the involved eye usually appears quiet, although patients who have an associated nongranulomatous uveitis have been described.[12,23] Fine pigmented cells within the vitreous humor have been seen in up to 50% of eyes in some series.[3,11] The fundus lesions themselves range in size from one to several disc diameters and have a variable distribution. Lesions classically develop first in a peripapillary location and spread centrifugally.[3,12,33] New lesions may develop in the macula in the absence of peripapillary scars, and isolated peripheral lesions have been described.[13,15,22] There is usually evidence of inactive disease in the asymptomatic eye.[3,11,16,33,36] Most patients, however, will eventually develop active disease in this eye as

well. Disease progression is markedly asymmetric (Fig. 48-1, *A*, *B*).

The lesions themselves develop deep to the retina and appear gray-white to yellow with irregular, ill-defined edges. The overlying retina usually appears edematous.[3,12] An associated serous neurosensory retinal detachment may occur.[3,33] Multiple areas of activity may be seen, most frequently at the distal edges of inactive scars. Over a 2- to 3-month period, the edema resolves and atrophy of the retinal pigment epithelium and choriocapillaris is observed.[3,36] In time, coarse irregular clumps of retinal pigment epithelial hyperpigmentation develop within the lesions, and the large choroidal vessels become increasingly prominent. Lesions at varying stages of evolution are usually seen within the same eye. Months or years may elapse between episodes of active disease (Fig. 48-2, *A*, *B*).[3,11,17,33,36]

As the disease progresses, a multitongued area of chorioretinal atrophy is produced that may extend into the far retinal periphery. Skip areas of normal retina completely surrounded by disease may be seen. These areas often are spared as the disease progresses peripherally, but they can become involved by recurrent disease.[33] Subretinal fibrosis may develop within the atrophic scars.[3,33] This process occurred in one half of the eyes in one series.[3]

The lesions are associated with a variable disturbance in the visual field. Acute lesions usually produce absolute scotomata, although minimal field change has been reported.[36] As the lesions become atrophic, relative scotomata (often with sloping margins) are frequently observed. Central vision is unaffected unless foveal involvement is present, in which case it will be markedly decreased, frequently to finger counting.[3,12,17,36] Recovery of vision following foveal involvement by an active lesion is variable, with a few patients demonstrating complete recovery and others showing partial improvement of one or two lines of acuity.[16,17,36] Visual recovery may be delayed by 1 year or more and does not appear to correlate with the degree of initial vision loss nor with the appearance of the lesion. A

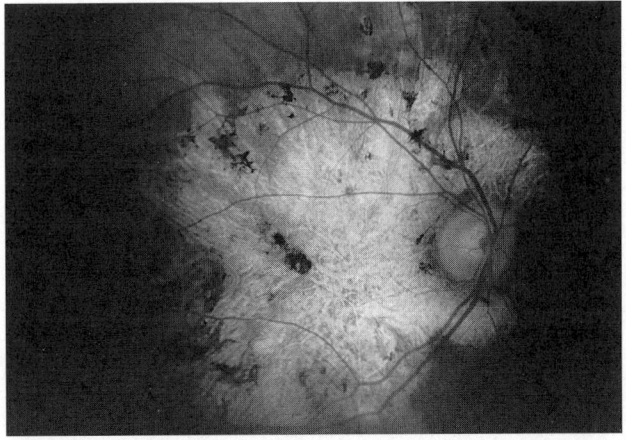
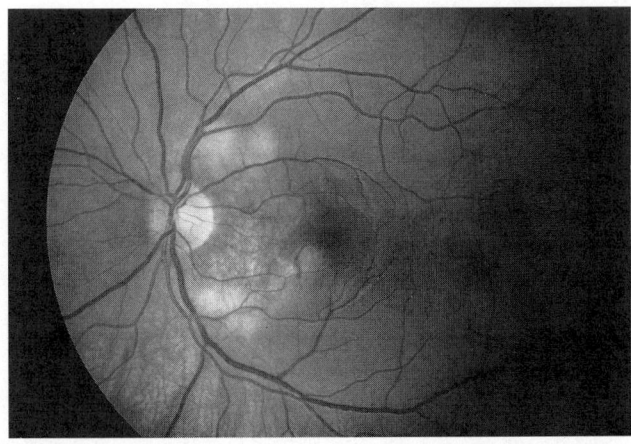

A   B

Fig. 48-1. **A,** Marked asymmetry is seen between the two eyes of a patient with serpiginous choroiditis. **B,** Disease activity is shown by the indistinct border of the lesion in the left eye at its superior and inferior poles.

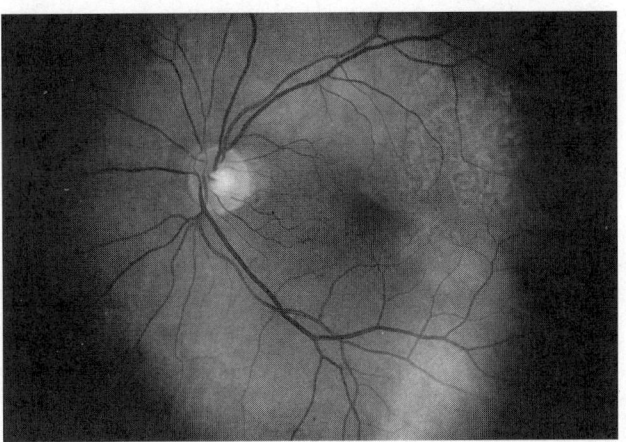
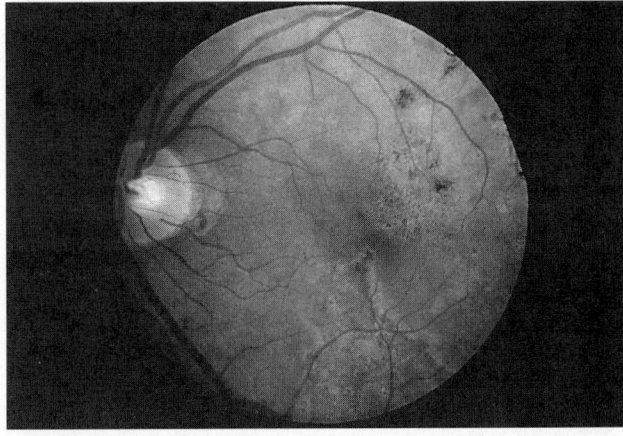

A   B

Fig. 48-2. **A,** An active lesion of serpiginous choroiditis is seen immediately inferior to a mature quiescent scar. **B,** One year later the previously active area has become quiescent and a new lesion has developed in the inferior macula.

majority of eyes retain poor vision following foveal disease, however.[3,16,17,33,36]

PATHOLOGY

Few eyes with serpiginous choroiditis and no eyes in the acute phase of the disorder have been studied histopathologically. In eyes that have been examined, a diffuse and focal accumulation of lymphocytes in the choroid has been seen.[11,38] This accumulation was greatest at the margins of the atrophic scars. Within the scars themselves, the retinal pigment epithelium and the photoreceptor layers were lost with focal defects of the underlying Bruch membrane occurring at various sites within the lesions. Fibroglial scar tissue was seen on the inner surface of Bruch membrane in one eye and in another, similar tissue was observed migrating through breaks in Bruch membrane into the choroid.

COMPLICATIONS

Subretinal neovascularization has been described in 13% to 20% of eyes with serpiginous choroiditis in long-term studies.[2,11,13,15,18] This neovascularization usually develops at the border of an old scar and, if subfoveal, may result in permanent loss of vision. The clinical appearance of a subretinal neovascular membrane can appear quite similar to that of the acute lesion of serpiginous choroiditis, but associated subretinal hemorrhage or exudate is more likely to be seen with a neovascular membrane. Fluorescein angiography allows subretinal neovascular membranes to be differentiated from active disease in most patients.[2,15,18] Rarely, neovascular membranes may develop adjacent to active serpiginous choroiditis, and in one reported case the neovascularization resolved as the acute lesion became atrophic.[18]

Retinal vasculitis and inflammation of the optic disc during active serpiginous choroiditis have been described infrequently.[3,16,36,37] There are also case reports depicting patients who developed retinal pigment epithelial detachments, branch retinal vein or artery occlusions, and neovascularization of the optic disc in association with active serpiginous choroiditis.[2,9,23,37]

PATHOGENESIS

The recurrent, episodic nature of the disease activity in serpiginous choroiditis, the presence of vitreous and anterior segment inflammation at times of disease activity, and the histologic finding of diffuse lymphocytic infiltration of the choroid are all suggestive of an inflammatory basis for the disorder and its manifestations. This supposition is also supported by a study that demonstrated an increased prevalence of HLA-B7 specificity in patients with serpiginous choroiditis, when compared to a control population.* No consistent association with prior exposure to viral or bacterial pathogens has been identified serologically, and there has been no clear demonstration of an association with antecedent illnesses or chemical exposures.[7,12] As additional pathologic material becomes available for study and more sophisticated techniques are employed in diagnostic studies, our understanding of the pathogenesis of serpiginous choroiditis may improve.

DIFFERENTIAL DIAGNOSIS

The clinical diagnosis of serpiginous choroiditis is relatively straightforward when a patient of the appropriate age has acute disease in one eye in conjunction with a characteristic bilateral distribution of inactive scars. When the disease develops in the absence of previous lesions, diagnosis is more difficult.

A number of infectious, inflammatory, and hereditary disorders may produce a clinical picture that is similar to serpiginous choroiditis (Table 48-1). The disease most likely to be confused with an acute presentation of serpiginous choroiditis is acute posterior multifocal placoid pigment epitheliopathy (APMPPE), because the acute lesions of APMPPE involve the retinal pigment epithelium and choriocapillaris and have similar coloration.[4,31] Multiple clinical differences between the two diseases exist, however. Bilateral simultaneous onset of disease is usual with APMPPE and its lesions are round, more widely distributed, and do not tend to coalesce as with serpiginous choroiditis. The lesions of APMPPE regress in unison over a period of 1 to 2 weeks, leaving scars that are more highly pigmented and less atrophic than those of serpiginous choroiditis. Although occasional recurrences of APMPPE have been described, multiple recurrences developing over a span of years have not been seen.[21]

Outer retinal toxoplasmosis may also mimic serpiginous choroiditis. Lesions in this disorder do not coalesce and are virtually always unilateral. Vitreous inflammation usually develops and the overlying retina eventually becomes involved.[5,10] Multifocal choroiditis and panuveitis syndrome are less likely to be confused with serpiginous choroiditis. The multifocal choroidal lesions are smaller and more widely distributed. Significant vitreous inflammation is seen in over 90% of the patients. The peak incidence of this disorder occurs at a younger age and patients are most often female.[6,24,27]

In older patients, metastatic tumors and non-Hodgkin lymphoma may mimic the appearance of the acute unilateral lesion of serpiginous choroiditis. Stepwise progression with severe loss of the retinal pigment epithelium and choriocapillaris is unusual in these disorders, however. Various hereditary retinal and choroidal dystrophies may produce a fundus appearance that is similar to the chronic lesions of serpiginous choroiditis; however, these disorders are most often bilaterally symmetrical and do not progress in a stepwise fashion.

LABORATORY INVESTIGATIONS

The fluorescein angiographic appearance of serpiginous choroiditis is distinctive.* Acute lesions block fluorescence early and show progressive late staining. As the lesions resolve, the blockage lessens. Atrophic lesions demonstrate early hypofluorescence, secondary to a loss of the choriocapillaris, and progressive hyperfluorescence develops from staining at the borders of the lesions. Diffuse late staining is eventually seen. In eyes with early disease activity, the two patterns may be superimposed, producing Bernard sign (which is a focal clouding of the hyperfluorescent border of the lesion). This subtle sign may be the first objective indication of disease reactivation. Late staining of the retinal vasculature may occur, particularly in the presence of active disease (Fig. 48-3, A, B).[16]

Electrophysiologic testing is frequently normal in serpiginous choroiditis. Abnormalities may be present in patients with extensive disease and correlate with the degree of retinal damage.[3,12,16] This pattern differs from that seen in the hereditary dystrophies, where electrophysiologic abnormalities are frequently found and the degree of dysfunction is often greater than expected from the clinical appearance.

Visual field testing in serpiginous choroiditis often demonstrates relative scotomata that correlate with the visible lesions.[3,36] For this reason, regular use of the Amsler grid may be helpful to follow the central progression of disease. Nevertheless, patients have been found to have progression of macular disease without developing an altered Amsler field. Fundus photographs may be used to document subclinical progression of disease.

---

*References 3, 7, 11, 16, 23, 36, 38.

*References 3, 11, 12, 13, 16, 22, 33, 36.

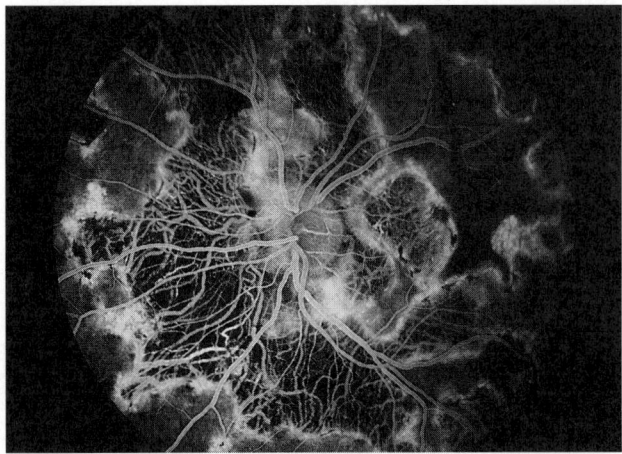

A

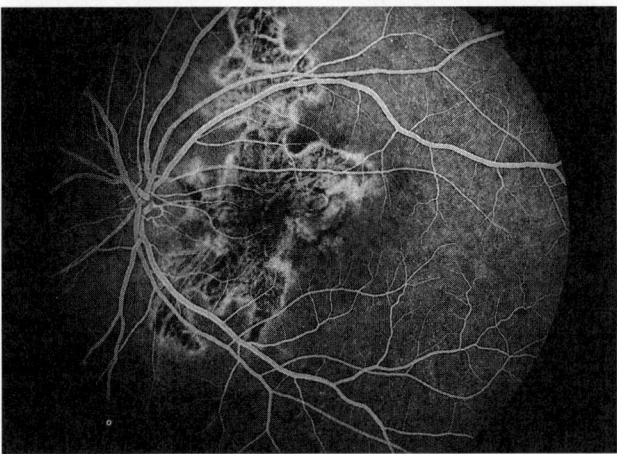

B

Fig. 48-3. **A,** The angiographic appearance of a mature inactive lesion of serpiginous choroiditis is shown. Note the prominence of the large choroidal vessels within the center of the lesion. A ring of late onset hyperfluorescence demarcates the lesion border. **B,** The uniform hyperfluorescence on the border of this lesion of serpiginous choroiditis is interrupted at its temporal margin just above the fovea. This change may be a subtle indicator of early reactivation.

THERAPY

Active Disease

At the present time, there is no consensus regarding the efficacy of therapeutic intervention in serpiginous choroiditis. Inflammatory components of the disorder, such as vitritis and anterior segment inflammation, appear to respond well to treatment with topical, periocular, or systemic corticosteroid.[11,16,23,29] The reported results of oral or periocular corticosteroid treatment of acute choroidal lesions have been conflicting, with some authors reporting a beneficial effect and others unable to demonstrate a response.* Because most

---

*References 3, 12, 13, 14, 16, 17, 29, 33, 36.

of the choroidal lesions that respond to corticosteroid treatment became inactive over the same 1- to 2-month period as did untreated lesions in other studies, the effect of corticosteroid treatment remains unclear. There is some evidence that active lesions in the subgroup of patients who have observable inflammation in the anterior chamber or vitreous humor may respond better to corticosteroid treatment, with some eyes showing resolution of inflammatory activity within 10 days of initiating therapy.[29] This conclusion is also controversial.

Treatment with cyclosporine also has produced mixed results. Both disease progression and continued disease activity have been reported following cyclosporine treatment.[19,28,29,34] One group has reported favorable results following the treatment of patients with cyclosporine, with both disease regression and visual improvement being observed.[34] In this study, 8 patients were followed for 33 to 73 months. Patients received cyclosporine for periods ranging from 6 to 21 months, in doses ranging from 4 to 7 mg/kg/day. Patients entered within the last 2 years received no more than 5 mg/kg/day and remained on the drug for less than 1 year. A response to treatment was generally seen within 1 month of initiation. Eighty percent of the patients maintained vision equal to or better than baseline, while twenty percent of patients lost vision. This result compares favorably with the average rate of vision loss of 36% reported in the literature for patients treated with corticosteroids alone or in combination with immunosuppressive agents.

Experience with the use of antimetabolites alone in the treatment of serpiginous choroiditis is limited, with no reports of an apparent benefit.[1,26] These drugs have been successfully used in combination with cyclosporine and prednisone in transplantation to reduce the incidence of side effects while maintaining adequate immunosuppression.[8,20,25,35] Synergism of effect between these drugs has also been demonstrated in animal models of transplantation.[32] Azathioprine (2 mg/kg/day), cyclosporine (5 mg/kg/day), and prednisone (1 mg/kg/day) were used to treat five eyes with active serpiginous choroiditis. All five eyes demonstrated a resolution of activity within 2 weeks of beginning therapy. Vision remained stable in three eyes and improved in two, as edema and subretinal fluid resolved. A recurrence developed in one eye following discontinuation of therapy and in another, when the drugs were rapidly weaned. All recurrences responded promptly to reinstitution of therapy and remained inactive over 18 months of follow-up. Two of the five eyes had received unsuccessful treatment with corticosteroids alone prior to beginning combination therapy.[14]

Clear confirmation of a definitive treatment effect in serpiginous choroiditis will require long-term prospective study of a comparatively large group of patients, because of the disorder's variable and idiosyncratic course. In the interim, it would seem reasonable to reserve the use of treatment for eyes with active lesions in close proximity to the

TABLE 48-1 DISORDERS THAT PRODUCE A CLINICAL PICTURE SIMILAR TO SERPIGINOUS CHOROIDITIS

	Serpiginous Choroiditis	APMPPE	Multifocal Choroiditis and Panuveitis Syndrome	Outer Retinal Toxoplasmosis
Average Age of Onset	30-50	20-30	20-40 (variable)	7-50 (variable)
Gender	male = female	male = female	female (80%)	male = female
Laterality	usually bilateral (asymmetric)	usually bilateral (symmetric)	usually bilateral (asymmetric)	unilateral
Lesion Characteristics	grey-white irregular edge, often peripapillary, active and inactive lesions coexist	grey-white, round, one disc diameter or larger, multiple, coalescence unusual	grey-yellow, small round, often greater in periphery, variable pigmentation of old lesions	multifocal, small grey-white, often in posterior pole
Angiographic Characteristics	acute: block early, hyperfluoresce late; chronic: hypofluoresce early, late edge staining	hypofluorescent early, late hyperfluorescence	acute: block early, stain late, chronic: window defect	acute: may hyperfluoresce or block, chronic: variable
Associated Inflammation	fine cells in vitreous humor (50%), papillitis, retinal vasculitis described occasionally	usually quiet, low-grade iritis and vitritis occasionally seen; rarely, papillitis, retinal vasculitis	mild iritis (60%), vitritis (90%), macular edema may occur	mild iritis common, vitritis mild or absent initially, vasculitis common, may occur remote from lesion
Complications	SRNVM in 13-20%; pigment epithelial detachment, vein and artery occlusions described	SRNVM very rare, neurosensory retinal detachment unusual	SRNVM in over 50%, subretinal fibrosis may occur, peripapillary atrophy occasionally seen	SRNVM may occur, involvement of overlying retina common, macular edema may develop
Clinical Course	multiple recurrences variably spaced over many years, visual prognosis variable	recurrences uncommon, visual prognosis good but permanent loss may be seen after foveal involvement	new lesions common over time, may coalesce, vision loss common, particularly if SRNVM present	new lesions may develop with time, often in proximity to old lesions; vision loss variable
Treatment	controversial—some may respond to corticosteroids, some to cyclosporine or therapy with azathioprine, cyclosporine, and prednisone	none demonstrated to be effective	corticosteroids decrease inflammation, effect on long-term prognosis unclear	lesions respond to anti-*T. gondii* therapy, response often slow

SRNVM = subretinal neovascular membrane.

fovea or optic nerve. An initial period of intensive oral and periocular corticosteroid treatment should be tried in unilateral disease demonstrating vitreous humor cells and/or anterior chamber inflammation. In patients who have only one eye with good vision or who have bilateral sight-threatening lesions, careful consideration of prolonged therapy with triple-agent immunosuppression should be given.

Treatment of Associated Subretinal Neovascular Membranes

Although reports of spontaneous involution of subretinal neovascular membranes associated with serpiginous choroiditis exist, in most instances these membranes will grow slowly or resolve with subretinal scar formation.[2,11,15,18] No convincing response of the neovascularization to antiinflammatory treatment has been reported, but laser treatment was effective in some studies in ablating the neovascular membranes when it was applied in the manner used for the treatment of neovascular membranes from other causes.[15] For this reason, consideration should be given to laser treatment of all macular subretinal neovascular membranes that are not subfoveal. Because of the difficulties encountered in distinguishing neovascularization clinically from acute disease recurrence, all lesions that are sight-threatening should be investigated angiographically. Lesions not studied angiographically should be monitored closely for changes suggestive of the presence of a neovascular membrane, such as the development of subretinal blood or exudate.

PROGNOSIS

Despite many years of experience with serpiginous choroiditis, it remains an enigma in many respects. Because the course of disease is highly variable, even between eyes of the same individual, the ultimate severity of vision loss is difficult to predict. On the basis of data from multiple published reports, between 12% and 38% of eyes will have central vision reduced to less than 20/200 over time—in many cases to the level of counting fingers. Conversely, fewer than 5% of patients will have vision reduced to less than 20/200 in both eyes.* Although medical therapy for the active phase of disease remains a subject of controversy, evidence increasingly suggests that many patients will respond to treatment. Also, early detection and treatment of associated neovascular membranes can be effective in preserving central vision. For these reasons, long-term, careful follow-up of patients with serpiginous choroiditis is necessary. Patients should be encouraged to monitor their central vision for the development of scotomata or metamorphopsia and to report such changes immediately.

REFERENCES

1. Andrasch RH, Pirofsky B, Burns RP: Immunosuppressive therapy for severe chronic uveitis, *Arch Ophthalmol* 96:247-251, 1978.
2. Blumenkranz MS, Gass JDM, Clarkson JG: Atypical serpiginous choroiditis, *Arch Ophthalmol* 100:1773-1775, 1982.
3. Chisholm IH, Gass JDM, Hutton WL: The late stage of serpiginous (geographic) choroiditis, *Am J Ophthalmol* 82:343-451, 1982.
4. Deutman AF, Lion F: Choroicapillaris nonperfusion in acute multifocal placoid pigment epitheliopathy, *Am J Ophthalmol* 84:652-657, 1977.
5. Doft BH, Gass JD: Outer retinal layer toxoplasmosis, *Graefes Arch Clin Exp Ophthalmol* 224:78-82, 1986.
6. Dreyer RF, Gass JDM: Multifocal choroiditis and panuveitis: a syndrome that mimics ocular histoplasmosis, *Arch Ophthalmol* 102:1776-1784, 1984.
7. Erkkila H, Laatikainen L, Jokinen E: Immunological studies on serpiginous choroiditis, *Graefes Arch Clin Exp Ophthalmol* 219:131-134, 1982.
8. First MR et al.: The use of low doses of cyclosporin, azathioprine, and prednisone in renal transplantation, *Transplant Proc* 18(suppl 1):132-135, 1986.
9. Friberg TR: Serpiginous choroiditis with branch vein occlusion and bilateral periphlebitis, *Arch Ophthalmol* 106:585-587, 1988.
10. Friedman CT, Knox DL: Variations in recurrent active toxoplasmic retinochoroiditis, *Arch Ophthalmol* 81:481-493, 1969.
11. Gass JDM: *Stereoscopic atlas of macular diseases: diagnosis and treatment,* ed 3, vol 1, 136-144, St Louis, 1987, Mosby.
12. Hamilton AM, Bird AC: Geographical choroidopathy, *Br J Ophthalmol* 58:784-797, 1974.
13. Hardy RA, Schatz H: Macular geographic helicoid choroidopathy, *Arch Ophthalmol* 105:1237-1242, 1987.

14. Hooper PL, Kaplan HJ: Triple agent immunosuppression in serpiginous choroiditis, *Ophthalmol* 98:944-952, 1991.
15. Jampol LM et al.: Subretinal neovascularization with geographic (serpiginous) choroiditis, *Am J Ophthalmol* 88:663-689, 1979.
15a. Junius P: Seltene augenspeilgelbilder zum klinischen phanomen der retinitis exsuditiva coats und der retinochoroiditis "parapapillaris," *Arch Augenheilkunde* 106:475-478, 1932.
16. Laatikainen L, Erkkila H: Serpiginous choroiditis, *Br J Ophthalmol* 58:777-783, 1974.
17. Laatikainen L, Erkkila H: A follow-up study on serpiginous choroiditis, *Acta Ophthalmol* 59:707-718, 1981.
18. Laatikainen L, Erkkila H: Subretinal and disc neovascularization in serpiginous choroiditis, *Br J Ophthalmol* 66:326-331, 1982.
19. Laatikainen L, Tarkkanen A: Failure of cyclosporine A in serpiginous choroiditis, *J Ocular Ther Surg* 3:280-283, 1984.
20. Lorber MI et al.: Cyclosporine toxicity: the effect of combined therapy using cyclosporin, azathioprine, and prednisone, *Am J Kidney Dis* 9:476-484, 1987.
21. Lyness AL, Bird AC: Recurrences of acute posterior placoid pigment epitheliopathy, *Am J Ophthalmol* 98:263-267, 1984.
22. Mansour AM et al.: Macular serpiginous choroiditis, *Retina* 8:125-131, 1988.
23. Masi RJ, O'Connor GR, Kimura SJ: Anterior uveitis in geographic or serpiginous choroiditis, *Am J Ophthalmol* 86:228-232, 1978.
24. Morgan CM, Schatz H: Recurrent multifocal choroiditis, *Ophthalmology* 93:1138-1147, 1986.
25. Mourad G et al.: Triple drug immunosuppression (cyclosporin, azathioprine and low-dose prednisolone): a safe and effective regimen in first-cadaver kidney transplantation, *Transplant Proc* 19:3672-3673, 1987.
26. Newell FW, Krill AE, Thomson A: The treatment of uveitis with six-mercaptopurine, *Am J Ophthalmol* 61:1250-1255, 1966.
27. Nozik RA, Dorsch W: A new chorioretinopathy associated with anterior uveitis, *Am J Ophthalmol* 76:758-762, 1973.
28. Nussenblatt RB, Palestine AG, Chan CC: Cyclosporine A therapy in the treatment of intraocular inflammatory disease resistant to systemic corticosteroids and cytotoxic agents, *Am J Ophthalmol* 96:275-282, 1983.
29. Nussenblatt RB, Palestine AG: *Uveitis: fundamentals and clinical practice,* 309-314, Chicago, 1989, Mosby.
30. Richardson RR, Cooper IS, Smith JL: Serpiginous choroiditis and unilateral extrapyramidal dystonia, *Ann Ophthalmol* 13:15, 1981.
31. Ryan SJ, Maumenee AE: Acute posterior multifocal placoid pigment epitheliopathy, *Am J Ophthalmol* 74:1066-1074, 1972.
32. Schareck WD et al.: Reduction of nephrotoxicity and improvement of immunosuppression by combination of cyclosporin A and azathioprine, *Transplant Proc* 19:1937-1939, 1987.
33. Schatz H, Maumenee AE, Patz A: Geographic helicoid peripapillary choroidopathy: clinical presentation and fluorescein angiographic findings, *Trans Am Acad Ophthalmol Otolaryngol* 78:747-760, 1974.
34. Secchi AG, Tognon MS, Moro F: Cyclosporin A in the treatment of serpiginous choroiditis. In Belfort R Jr, Petrelli AM, Nussenblatt RB, editors: *World uveitis symposium: proceedings of the first world uveitis symposium,* Sao Paulo, 1989, Livraria Roca.
35. Squifflet JP, Sutherland DER, Rynasiewicz JJ: Combined immunosuppressive therapy with cyclosporin A and azathioprine, *Transplantation* 34:315-318, 1982.
36. Weiss H et al.: The clinical course of serpiginous choroidopathy, *Am J Ophthalmol* 87:133-142, 1979.
37. Wojno T, Meredith TA: Unusual findings in serpiginous choroiditis, *Am J Ophthalmol* 94:650-655, 1982.
38. Wu JS et al.: Clinicopathologic findings in a patient with serpiginous choroiditis and treated choroidal neovascularization, *Retina* 9:292-301, 1989.

*References 3, 12, 13, 17, 33, 36.

49 Cancer-Associated Retinopathy

JOSEPH F. RIZZO III, NICHOLAS J. VOLPE

The devastation wrought by cancer is usually the result of local invasion, metastases, or the consequences of asthenia. Peculiar instances of organ failure also can develop as a remote effect of cancer in which the affected organ remains free of invasion by either the primary tumor or metastases. Dysfunction of any organ system, particularly the nervous system (see box), can either herald or occur together with a neoplasm (''para'' neoplasia). Aside from scientific curiosity, early recognition of this class of disease is important so that appropriate therapy can be instituted. Paraneoplastic syndromes present diagnostic challenges and provide insight into the behavior of malignancies and their effects on the host immune system.

HISTORICAL BACKGROUND

Visual loss associated with malignancy usually results from metastases to the brain, meninges, optic nerve, choroid, retina, or orbit. Sawyer, Selhorst, Zimmermann, and Hoyt[115] were the first to recognize the unusual characteristics of a retinopathy occurring as a remote effect of cancer. It is instructive to reflect on the sequence of events that led to the recognition of the syndrome of paraneoplastic retinopathy.

ANATOMY OF A DISCOVERY

A Conversation with Ralph Sawyer, MD

''. . . A 65 year old white woman complained of hoarseness and bilateral episodic dimming of vision. Bilateral dimness of vision would occur suddenly. It seemed like 'the lights were turned down low.' . . . She complained of 'seeing only parts of things,' she missed some of the numbers on a clock or portions of a picture. Several weeks later she began experiencing bizarre images in her visual field like 'floating spaghetti or tissue paper.' Initial general physical exam was normal except for partial paralysis of the vocal cord and ocular examination revealed 20/25 acuity, mild dyschromatopsia and bilateral arcuate scotomas with normal appearing discs and scattered retinal drusen. Within two months vision was hand motions and oat cell

carcinoma of the lung was discovered. Ocular examination now demonstrated narrowed retinal arterioles, peripheral retinal pigmentary flecks and a yellowish pale disc. Electroretinogram was almost flat with a scotopic response that was 10% of normal and no photopic response. No improvement occurred with a ten day course of 100-mg prednisone.

The patient died one year later and her son, who was grateful for the medical attention shown to his mother, called the ophthalmology resident to inquire whether a post mortem examination was desired in view of the intense interest and dilemma surrounding her process. Necropsy revealed only minimal pathology to explain this visual perplexity. Extensive histological study of the entire visual pathway from globe to visual cortex was otherwise normal.

Drs. Sawyer and Selhorst surmised that this process was similar to the distant effects of cancer that caused peripheral neuropathy or cerebellar degeneration. 'Our patient seemed like a one-of-a-kind, with a devastating process and no identifiable cause. We continued to ask, share the case and probe the literature for any similar signs or symptoms that might suggest a clue to act upon.' Her case was presented to numerous consultants and at various conferences looking for clues to a missed diagnosis or a colleague with a similar patient. Was the rapidly progressive visual loss secondary to drug effect, toxic neuropathy, a cancer producing chemical process, or an auto-immune process? The search continued.

Dr. Selhorst was then taking a neuro-ophthalmology fellowship with Dr. William Hoyt. During daily discussions this unusual case was presented to Dr. Hoyt who recalled a similar case. Hoyt had previously reported a patient with a diagnosis of carcinomatous optic neuropathy and bizarre symptoms that were remarkably similar to those of the woman who had just died. The pathology from this other case was sent to Dr. Zimmerman at the Armed Forces Institute of Pathology who reported identical retinal findings to those described above.

The third case was jointly suspected by Drs. Sawyer and Zimmerman while attending a local conference given by a visiting professor from Scotland who discussed choroidal vasculopathies. He shared an unusual case for which he had

585

PARANEOPLASTIC SYNDROMES

Brain, brainstem
    brainstem encephalomyelitis
    subacute cerebellar degeneration
    opsoclonus/myoclonus
    limbic encephalitis
Spinal cord
    necrotizing myelopathy
    subacute motor/sensory neuronopathy
Peripheral nerve
    sensorimotor peripheral neuropathy
    mononeuritis multiplex
    autonomic neuropathy
    myeloma peripheral neuropathy
Neuromuscular junction
    myasthenia gravis
    Lambert-Eaton myasthenic syndrome
Muscle
    dermatomyositis
Eye
    photoreceptor degeneration
    optic neuritis
    uveal melanocytic proliferation

no clear answer. Dr. Zimmermann acknowledged his familiarity with this presentation and he reviewed this patient's retinal pathology which mimicked those of the two prior patients.

We had something new indeed. Visual loss in three patients with symptoms before the diagnosis of cancer and identical retinal pathology of photoreceptor degeneration and pigmentary migration without the presence of cancer cells. A distant effect of cancer was suggested, the pathogenesis unclear.''

Paraneoplastic retinopathy (PR) or cancer-associated retinopathy (CAR) refers to a syndrome characterized by acute or subacute deterioration of vision resulting from a nonmetastatic, remote effect of a systemic malignancy. The syndrome was first recognized by Sawyer and associates[115] in 1976 and has been reported in 45 cases (Table 49-1) as of 1994.* Seven of these cases were reported in abstract form at the 1993 meeting of the American Academy of Ophthalmology,[53,71] and ten were reported in tabular form.[123] The prevalence of cancer associated retinopathy is unknown, but the syndrome is now well recognized and is seen periodically by neuro-ophthalmologists and ophthalmologists who study retinal degenerations.

---

*References 2, 3, 7, 12, 19, 21, 25, 28, 45, 51-53, 55, 63, 69, 71, 73, 75, 76, 88, 91, 98, 101, 102, 110, 111, 122, 123, 124, 130, 131.

EPIDEMIOLOGY

Nervous system dysfunction and visual loss usually result from metastatic disease, but the incidence of paraneoplastic disease has been estimated to be as high as 10% to 15% with certain types of tumors.[99,118] The incidence of paraneoplastic syndromes is highest among patients with small cell tumors of the lung and ovary, with about 50% of paraneoplastic nervous system dysfunction occurring in patients with primary tumors in the lung. Carcinomas of breast, stomach, uterus, kidney, cervix, larynx, and Hodgkin disease and cancers of neural crest origin have also been associated with paraneoplastic disease of the nervous system.[132,133] Cerebrospinal fluid analysis shows no malignant cells, although mild pleocytosis and mild elevation of protein are frequently observed. Histopathologically, the affected part of the neuraxis has perivascular cuffing with lymphocytes and plasma cells, neuronal loss, and microglial proliferation. There is ample evidence that these syndromes do not result from the toxic effects of tumor therapy.

Most paraneoplastic neurologic syndromes are manifested by encephalomyelitis either in the cerebrum, cerebellum, brainstem, or spinal cord. Patients may have features of disease in more than one location. Paraneoplastic cerebellar cortical degeneration (PCD) produces limb and truncal ataxia, dysarthria, and nystagmus.[16] This clinical picture is often so characteristic that the clinician suspects a paraneoplastic cause. Until 1982, Henson and Urich[59] were able to identify only 50 pathologically proved cases. Despite this, these authors noted that 50% of the middle-aged patients that have subacute cerebellar degeneration will have cancer.[59] PCD subdivides into several disorders that can be distinguished clinically and immunologically. Patients fall into both neuronal antibody seropositive and neuronal antibody seronegative subgroups.[54] Syndromes differ based on the most commonly associated primary malignancy and autoantibody identified. For instance, breast and gynecologic malignancies are associated with anti-Yo antibodies[54,103] (see the following), and PCD associated with a more widespread encephalomyelitis and small cell carcinoma of the lung is linked with anti-Hu antibodies.[5,31] PCD with Hodgkin disease is not associated with either anti-Yo or anti-Hu.[56] Pathologic findings include loss of Purkinje cells from the cerebellar cortex and, occasionally, perivascular lymphocytic infiltration in the cerebellar white matter and brainstem. Often the primary malignancy can be identified early enough (especially with anti-Yo[103]) so that the patient can be cured of the malignancy, but the neurologic deficits persist.

Another more widely known cerebellar syndrome of opsoclonus and myoclonus occurs in about 7% of children with neuroblastoma.[17] Patients with opsoclonus develop large amplitude saccades (without intersaccadic intervals) in all directions, often associated with excessive blinking. The

TABLE 49-1 SUMMARY OF THE CLINICAL, ELECTROPHYSIOLOGIC, AND LABORATORY FINDINGS OF REPORTED CASES OF PARANEOPLASTIC RETINOPATHY

Author	Age Sex	Tissue Diagnosis	Retinal Immunohistochemistry	Western Blot	Pathology	ERG
Sawyer	62F	Oat cell	—	—	PR degeneration	Flat/reduced
	65F	Oat cell	—	—	PR degeneration	—
	76F	Small cell, lung	—	—	PR degeneration	—
Kornguth[a,b,c]	72M	Oat cell	Large ganglion cell staining	20/65		Flat/reduced
	68M	Oat cell, lung	Nonspecific nuclear staining	—	—	—
Keltner[d]	61F	Small cell ca, cervix	Diffuse staining	23	PR degeneration	Flat
Buchanan	66M	Oat cell	—	—	PR degeneration	Flat ERG, reduced VEP
Klingele	43F	Adeno ca, breast				Flat ERG
Grunwald[b,e,f]	72M	Oat cell	Inner retinal staining	145/205[g]	Ganglion cell loss	Abnormal VEP
Thirkill	71M	Nonsmall cell, lung	—	23	—	Flat ERG
	64M	Oat cell lung		23/48	—	Flat ERG
van der Pol	37M	Oat cell lung	—	—	—	Flat ERG
Vargas Nunez	68F	Oat cell lung	—	—	—	Flat ERG
Berson	69M	Melanoma				Selective loss of ERG b wave
Crofts	64F	Endometrial ca		50		Flat ERG
Thirkill	60W	Oat cell lung	Diffuse staining of nuclei in all layers	23		Reduced[h]
Jacobson	67M	Oat cell lung		23/48		Almost flat ERG
	71M	Oat cell lung		23		Flat ERG
Rizzo	67M	Oat cell lung	Selective staining of outer retina	none		Predominant rod dysfunction
	59M	Oat cell lung	Selective staining of outer retina	48	Patchy PR loss, sparring of cones	Flat ERG
Rush	50M	Melanoma		no 23[j]		Extinguished rod response
Cogan	72W	Uterine carcinoma			Photoreceptor loss, especially cones in macula and elsewhere	Suppression of cone response on ERG
Hammerstein[k]	6M	Embryonal rhabdo				
Campo	72W	Endometrial small cell			PR degeneration	Suppression of cone response
Matsui	67W	Unknown				Nonrecordable
	68M	Prostate bladder larynx				Marked reduction of both a and b wave
Alexander	58M	Melanoma				Selective loss of ERG b wave
Adamus	64W	Oat cell lung		23 kD, 65kD and others	PR degeneration, inflammatory cells	No response

Continued

TABLE 49-1 SUMMARY OF THE CLINICAL, ELECTROPHYSIOLOGIC, AND LABORATORY FINDINGS OF REPORTED CASES OF PARANEOPLASTIC RETINOPATHY cont'd

Author	Age Sex	Tissue Diagnosis	Retinal Immunohistochemistry	Western Blot	Pathology	ERG
Pepkowitz[l]	55W	Breast		Antirhodopsin		Normal
Oohira	62M	Lung, adeno ca				Barely detectable
Ohnishi	50M	Small cell lung	Ganglion cell layer staining	24, 48	PR degeneration	—
Gehrs	69M	Squamous cell lung				No rod and gross atten. of cone
Andreasson	48M	Melanoma				Normal cone, absent rod
Milam	36M	Melanoma	Bipolar cell staining			Decreased rod normal cone
Guy[l]	5 pts	Lung, breast, bladder, prostate		46, all patients		Markedly reduced
Kim[l]	2 pts	Melanoma				Selective loss of ERG b wave
Thirkill	10 pts	Small cell ca lung		All 23 kD		All reduced or nonreactive

PR—photoreceptor, ERG—electroretinogram, VEP—visual evoked potential

References 2, 3, 7, 12, 19, 21, 25, 28, 45, 51, 52, 53, 55, 63, 69, 71, 73, 75, 76, 88, 91, 98, 101, 102, 110, 111, 115, 122, 123, 124, 130, 131.

[a]also described as case 1 in Grunwald (1985) and case 1 in Kornguth (1986)
[b]western blot data found in Kornguth 1986
[c]retinal immunochemistry provided in Grunwald 1985
[d]also described as case 1 in Thirkill, 1987
[e]case 1 also described as case 1 in Kornguth, 1982
[f]case 2 also described as case 4 in Thirkill, 1987 and as case 2 in Kornguth, 1986 and the autopsy findings are described in the case report section of Grunwald, 1987.
[g]western blot data on same patient also reported in Thirkill, 1987 (case 4) and in the latter report 23 kD binding was observed instead of 145/205 kD binding.
[h]reported later in (143)
[j]other antibodies to human optic nerve and retina identified
[k]maybe different disease, given reported presence of RPE changes, vitreous opacities and optic atrophy
[l]to date only reported in abstract form

condition results from loss of the Purkinje cells and, to a lesser extent, the granular cells and dentate nuclei. Opsoclonus has also been seen in association with breast, uterine, and lung carcinoma. Paraneoplastic myoclonic encephalopathy is frequently observed in previously healthy children without known malignancy and is characterized by ataxia, polymyoclonus, and opsoclonus.

Paraneoplastic myelopathy is a rare syndrome that begins with the rapid onset of pain and paresthesias in the lower limbs, with progression to paraparesis and urinary sphincter dysfunction. The cervical spinal cord often becomes involved. Pathologically, there is necrosis of all tracts within the spinal cord.

Various motor and sensory syndromes have been ascribed to paraneoplasia that affects the central and/or peripheral nervous systems. Subacute sensory neuronopathy is

a purely sensory syndrome (seen in patients with lung cancer) that results from inflammation of the dorsal root ganglia. Pathologically, there is inflammatory infiltrate and loss of neurons in the dorsal root ganglia, and degeneration of posterior nerve roots, sensory nerves, and posterior columns of the spinal cord. An antibody directed against the sensory neurons in the dorsal root ganglia has been identified.[46] The antibody, which is species-specific but reacts with other CNS neurons, is found only in patients with lung cancer and cross-reacts with identical antigens found in the primary tumor.[46]

Peripheral sensorimotor polyneuropathy occurs in 5% of patients with lung cancer and is thus probably the most common neurologic paraneoplastic syndrome.[133] Nerve conduction studies of asymptomatic patients with a variety of cancers have found abnormalities in 35% to 50% of patients.[133] A striking association between solitary plasmacytoma and this type of peripheral neuropathy is characterized by weakness, numbness, paresthesia, and pain.[67,68,108] Reflexes are diminished or absent and there is often distal muscle atrophy. Nerve biopsy reveals segmental demyelination and axonal degeneration. Occasionally, a lymphocytic infiltration is noted.[26] An immune mechanism has been postulated for the paraneoplastic sensorimotor neuropathy because patients contract a syndrome that may appear identical to idiopathic inflammatory polyneuropathy (Guillain-Barré syndrome), although the latter is believed to be primarily cell-mediated. Antibody (IgM) and complement deposition on peripheral nerve myelin have been demonstrated,[33,65] but it is unclear whether this is the cause of nerve damage or the reaction to nerve injury.

Of final consideration is the neuromuscular junction. The Lambert-Eaton Myasthenic Syndrome (LEMS) is an autoimmune paraneoplastic syndrome that usually occurs with oat cell carcinoma of the lung[80] but has also been found with other malignancies and rarely occurs in isolation. The syndrome is characterized by weakness and fatigability of the proximal muscles (particularly the pelvic girdle), and occasionally, paresthesias and autonomic dysfunction may be present. Unlike myasthenia gravis, involvement of the extraocular muscles is uncommon and usually mild. Nerve conduction studies reveal subnormal release of acetylcholine from motor nerve terminals, which correlates with the known loss of membrane particles in the presynaptic nerve terminals. Several patients with LEMS and PCD have been identified.[24] Some of these patients were found to have antibodies to voltage-gated calcium channels.[24] LEMS has been passively transferred to mice with immunoglobulins from affected patients.[80] It has also been shown that when these antibodies are injected into mice, they can deplete calcium channels[42] and block bovine voltage-dependent calcium channels.[72] Treatment with immunosuppressives is occasionally effective. Myasthenia gravis is an autoimmune disease that may have a paraneoplastic association with malignant thymoma.

Finally, muscles can be affected by paraneoplastic processes, either as a primary myopathy or as a polymyositis with dermatomyositis. The pathogenesis is believed to be inflammatory, and the condition may respond to immunosuppressive therapy.

PATHOGENESIS

Paraneoplastic Neurologic Disease

The central nervous system paraneoplastic syndromes were the first to be recognized. Compromised immunologic status and opportunistic infection with a virus[58] were postulated to be the pathogenic sequence of events, and on two occasions virus-like particles were found on electron microscopy in patients with paraneoplastic myelitis.[97] Alternative explanations of pathogenesis focused on the known examples of tumors that could produce biologically active substances, such as ACTH, in patients who develop Cushing syndrome. Especially notable is the disproportionate number of paraneoplastic neurologic syndromes found in patients with oat (small) cell carcinoma of the lung. These tumors are believed to arise in Kulchitsky cells of the tracheal bronchial mucosa that possess neuroendocrine properties linking them to the nervous system.[57] These tumors are unique in their ability to synthesize small biologically active peptides,[48] however, it is still not known why these tumors cause paraneoplastic nervous system disease.

Most of the CNS paraneoplastic syndromes are associated with elevated protein and immunoglobulins in the CSF.[16,121] Protein elevation is mild and generally does not reach the high levels seen in the Guillain-Barré syndrome. Jaeckle,[64] Trotter,[129] and Greenlee[49,50] demonstrated complement-fixing, IgG antibodies to Purkinje cells in the serum and CSF of patients with ovarian, breast, and lung primaries and cerebellar degeneration. The immunohistochemical pattern of staining in these cases suggested that the Purkinje cell antigen was located in the rough endoplasmic reticulum.

Antineuronal antibodies (directed against Purkinje cell antigens) are found in most patients with paraneoplastic cerebellar disease, however, their role in disease pathogenesis remains unclear.[6,29] There seems to be a more inexorable and steady progression of these diseases in patients who are identified as antibody positive. The condition was therefore postulated to result from a cross-reactivity between an antigenic stimulus in the tumor and the Purkinje cell antigen. The antigens have molecular weights of 62 to 64 (anti-Yo)[54,103] and 34 to 38 (anti-Hu)[5,31] kilodaltons. The antibodies have been found in patients with several different primary tumors, as well as in patients who have carcinoma and are neurologically normal.[6,14,18] These antibodies have been identified in the brains of affected patients by immunohistochemistry[30]; and the antigens recognized by these antibodies have been cloned, but their role in disease pathogenesis remains uncertain.[35,37,113,114] In addition, antineuronal antibodies have been detected in the serum of patients with carcinoma,[135] and lymphocytes have been found to be sensitized to myelin basic protein.[39] Despite the presence of presumed autoantibodies, there have been no successful attempts to reproduce this syndrome in animals. The various syndromes may have very different mechanisms of disease (as in one patient with both LEMS and PCD in whom only the LEMS responded to plasmapheresis and treatment of the primary malignancy).[13] In some of the syndromes, such as opsoclonus/myoclonus, antibodies are less commonly identified.[20] Most autopsy studies fail to demonstrate inflammation around degenerated Purkinje cells.

Paraneoplastic Photoreceptor Degeneration

Sawyer and associates[115] recognized that the syndrome observed in the original three patients (see previous section) did not correlate with any known hereditary, toxic, or pigmentary retinopathy. Histopathologic evaluation of their first patient showed degeneration of the rods, cones, and the outer nuclear layer. They concluded that a hormonelike substance was capable of causing damage to photoreceptors and may have been produced by the small cell lung carcinomas. Toxins or hormonelike products were believed to be responsible for the visual loss in the setting of cancer.[19] Other cases of meningeal carcinomatous and visual loss have had seemingly little optic nerve involvement, and these authors have postulated a toxic effect or impairment of axonal flow as a cause of visual loss.*

Autoantibodies

Paraneoplastic retinopathy is now believed to result, at least in part, from an antibody-mediated loss of photoreceptors. Several steps are required for an autoimmune paraneoplastic process to cause disease. First, antibody production must occur. Generally, the antibody is believed to form as part of the autoimmune reaction to tumor antigens. These antigens may show cross-reactivity with retinal antigens because of shared epitopes (antigenic mimicry), or the tumor may produce the retinal antigen itself. Tumor necrosis can expose antigens to immunologic surveillance and result in antibody production, or an antigen or homologue in photoreceptors (or other tissues) can be exposed to the immune systems because of the altered immune status caused by the tumor. It is also possible that some undefined, presumably tumor-related, antigenic stimulus mobilizes the more soluble interleukins or cytokines (produced in peripheral lymphoid tissue) that subsequently enter the central nervous system and cause release and exposure to immune surveillance of retinal antigens.[127] Components of the activated immune response must then be able to cross the blood-retinal barrier, presumably altered by focal or general cellular inflammation, and react with a photoreceptor antigen. Still another possibility is that the antibodies are synthesized in the central nervous system. Based on simultaneous measurement of antibody levels in CSF and serum in patients with paraneoplastic neurologic disease, Furneaux and associates[43] have shown that antibodies are produced in the CNS. Finally, the tissue-bound antibody-antigen complex must result in cell death or apoptosis. The antibody-antigen complex itself may be sufficient to poison the cell's energy system, or these immune complexes may bind complement and activate the complement cascade. A summary follows of the direct and indirect evidence to support this theoretical mechanism of disease.

*References 9, 27, 40, 66, 85, 100.

In 1982 Kornguth and associates[76] reported antiretinal ganglion cell antibodies in the serum of a patient with blindness and oat cell carcinoma. Later these authors showed antigens of similar molecular weight in both the retina and the small cell lung tumor that reacted with the abnormal serum antibody.[51,76] One antigen had the same molecular weight as neurofilament triplet protein and the other was a 20- to 24-kD protein. The apparent inconsistency of an abnormal electroretinogram (a test that does not measure activity of retinal ganglion cells) being caused by an antiganglion cell antibody was not explained. Nonetheless, further support for the role of antiganglion cell antibodies came from Grunwald and associates,[52] who reported histopathologic findings in one of the original oat cell carcinoma patients of Kornguth.[76] The patient had undergone retinal detachment surgery and developed decreased acuity, visual field loss, and subsequent optic atrophy. Fluorescent antibodies directed against human immunoglobulins demonstrated specific staining of large cells in the ganglion cell and inner nuclear layers of the patient's retina. Histopathologic evaluation showed diffuse loss of ganglion cells and preservation of photoreceptors. This is in contrast to the original description by Sawyer,[115] in which the inner retinal layers had been preserved. Recently another case with immunofluorescence demonstrating staining of the ganglion cell layer was reported.[98] Interestingly, although this patient did not have an ERG and there was some reduction in the number of ganglion cells found on histopathology, the primary histopathologic finding was photoreceptor loss.

In 1983 Keltner and associates[69] demonstrated antiretinal antibodies in a patient with cervical carcinoma. Unlike the previously described antiganglion cell antibodies, these antibodies reacted with photoreceptors from normal human retina. Based on this finding, Keltner and associates[69] were the first to propose an autoimmune pathogenesis. In 1987 Thirkill, Roth, and Keltner[124] performed ELISA and Western blot testing in four patients with cancer-associated retinopathy and found a serum antibody that bound a 23-kD retinal antigen, which they termed the cancer-associated retinopathy (CAR) antigen. In 1989 Thirkill and associates[122] reported another case with an extinguished ERG,[125] no autopsy findings, and antibodies that stained all three retinal nuclear layers, nuclei of the retinal pigment epithelium, and choroidal blood vessels. This lack of specificity differed significantly from results of autopsied cases that have shown selective loss photoreceptor outer segments.[69,110,115]

Excluding the cases described previously with histopathologic evidence of retinal ganglion cell or optic nerve disease, the majority of cases have been associated with photoreceptor dysfunction. This is supported both by an abnormal ERG and immunohistochemical studies that have shown binding of serum antibodies to outer retinal layers. The mechanisms that give rise to these antibodies and result in photoreceptor death are not clear, however. The antibodies could be an epiphenomenon that occurs in response to retinal damage initiated by some other mechanism. For instance, Thirkill[126] has recently demonstrated antiretinal antibodies in patients with retinitis pigmentosa.

The presence of abnormal antiretinal antibodies in patients with PR is inarguable. These antibodies may develop as a result of the primary malignancy and affect the retina by means of molecular mimicry. In this scenario, antibodies may be generated against a tumor antigen that is coincidentally similar to retinal antigens. Alternatively, the immune system may become "turned on" by the tumor with a resultant nonspecific production of antibodies, some of which may cross-react with retinal antigens. Adamus and associates[2] found antibodies to retinal photoreceptors, optic nerve, small cell lung tumors, and normal lung tissue in their patient with paraneoplastic retinopathy. Finally, it is also possible that the tumor cells themselves contain a retinal antigen (recoverin, see the following) that becomes exposed to immune surveillance.[2]

One study[122] showed, by Western blot analysis, a cross-reactivity between antibodies from a patient with PR and a small cell carcinoma of the lung antigen of molecular weight 65 kD. Adamus and associates,[2] however, were unable to demonstrate such a cross-reactivity between recoverin and a lung cancer antigen, although serum antibodies cross-reacted with the 65-kD antigen. Thirkill and associates[128] demonstrated that ascites-propagated, small cell carcinoma of the lung cells in rats will express a cancer-associated gene that encodes for a protein that is antigenically similar to the 23-kD retinal CAR antigen. This supports the hypothesis that the carcinoma-retina immunologic cross-reaction is responsible for the induction of the antibody response. It is unclear as to whether the tumor produces recoverin itself or an antigenically similar protein that incites the immunologic reaction.

How the antibodies reach the photoreceptors and cause cellular dysfunction is unsolved. The blood-retinal barrier would normally prevent serum antibodies from reaching photoreceptors. The presence of immunoglobulins in the CSF of patients with paraneoplastic neurologic syndromes, however, indicates that the blood-brain barrier is compromised in some instances. Cancer-associated retinopathy may be associated with uveitis,* which increases blood vessel permeability, and it is therefore possible that antibodies gain access to the photoreceptors via abnormally permeable vasculature. Several authors have shown that antibodies can cross the CNS blood barrier[82,119] and that anti-S antigen antibodies can cross the blood retinal barrier in rats and acutely alter the ERG without evidence of inflammation.[119]

These findings provide theoretic explanations for two of the three criteria that must be satisfied to establish the au-toimmune nature of paraneoplastic retinopathy. The final criterion regards the mechanism by which the antiphotoreceptor antibody causes cell death. Immunologic attack and destruction usually involve the participation of inflammatory cells, whether they are called into action by the humoral or cell-mediated components of the immune system. Inflammatory cells, although not a prominent feature, have been identified in some of the autopsied cases (see the following).* Adamus and associates[2] identified inflammatory cells from the subretinal space to the nerve fiber layer, whereas Rizzo and Gittinger[110] found very little inflammation.

Retinal Antigens

Recoverin. If patients with PR are presumed to have antibody-mediated disease, then the involved antigen must play an important role in the biochemical function of the retina. Several authors have defined retinal antigens against which serum antibodies from PR patients have reacted. Although it was originally thought to be visinin,[106] the 23-kD antigen is now thought to be recoverin.[107] Polans and associates[107] found that antibodies in patients with paraneoplastic retinopathy reacted with recoverin, a calcium channel photoreceptor protein (in the calmodulin family). In addition, serum antibodies from CAR patients have been used to isolate the gene encoding the CAR antigen from a cDNA library of human retina, and the resultant nucleotide sequence was shown to be 90% homologous to the published sequence of bovine recoverin.[127] Recoverin is the CAR antigen in most patients.

Antibodies to the CAR antigen have been found in most patients with paraneoplastic retinopathy, especially in those with small cell carcinoma of the lung.[34,106,107,123] Antibodies produced to the CAR antigen (recoverin) are not found in patients with other retinopathies.[123] A recent study has shown that the major binding site of antibody to recoverin is a unique sequence that suggests a high degree of immunospecificity.[2] Although recoverin was initially thought to only be in rod outer segments,[34,79,106] it has been shown that recoverin, or a nearly identical protein, is also present in mammalian cones,[107] retina from multiple species,[120] optic nerve,[122] pineal body,[34] a subpopulation of cone bipolar cells,[91] and the chick optic tectum.[81] This suggests that recoverin may play a broader role beyond the visual transduction system in photoreceptors.

Initially, recoverin was considered to be important in the regulation of the biochemical recovery of photoreceptors after exposure to light.[34,127] Recoverin was thought to function in the activation and regulation of guanylate cyclase, which regulates the level of cyclic guanylate monophosphate (cGMP) in photoreceptor outer segments[34,79]—

---

possibly through calcium binding.[41] Increasing cGMP opens calcium channels that participate in the phototransduction process initiated by a conformation change in rhodopsin.[34,38,74] Very recent data suggests, however, that recoverin may have no role in photoreceptor function.[47,61] Immunologic inactivation of recoverin in some way results in photoreceptor dysfunction, cytolysis, and death (see the following).

Another theory for the mechanism of CAR-induced cell damage is based on a single mutational event in primary tumor cells.[89] Recoverin maps to mouse chromosome 11, which is syntenic with human chromosome 17. This mouse gene is positioned very near to a well-known tumor-suppresser gene, Trp 53.[10] Depending on how close the two genes are positioned, a single mutational event—either a translocation or deletion in the primary tissue cells (lung, ovary, and so on), could affect recoverin production and the tumor-suppressor gene. This could inactivate the tumor-suppressor gene and allow for growth of abnormal tumor cells. At the same time, the mutation could join the recoverin gene to the coding sequence of another transcriptionally active gene, thereby causing abnormal production of recoverin outside of the immunologically isolated retina and brain. This ectopic protein could incite the development of an antibody that would cross-react with the retina. This theory offers another plausible explanation (in addition to the theory of antigenic similarity of tumor cells and recoverin) for how antiretinal antibodies could develop without some other toxin or destructive force releasing the retinal antigens outside of the eye.

In summary, the CAR antigen seems to be recoverin. The classic immune-mediated form of destruction that includes lymphocytic cellular infiltration is not observed in most cases but may play some role in cell destruction.[2] Alternatively, antibody binding to recoverin may be sufficient to cause photoreceptor death, but by some still unknown mechanism. Although not specifically put forth to explain PR, a recent hypothesis suggested by Fain and Lisman[36] suggests a final common pathway for photoreceptor death in many different conditions. In this "equivalent light hypothesis," a "disease" of the photoreceptor excites photoreceptors (photopsias in PR), simulating a continuous light stimulus (a well-known cause of photoreceptor damage). This may cause photoreceptor death by interfering with the normal circadian processes in the photoreceptors, which include protein synthesis and disc shedding.

Other Antigens. Not all patients with paraneoplastic retinopathy have antibodies against the 23-kD retinal antigen and others have additional antibodies.[2,53,110,111] Patients reported by Crofts and associates,[28] Jacobson,[63] Rush,[111] Rizzo,[110] Adamus,[2] Thirkill,[123] Guy,[53] and Ohnishi[98] were studied immunologically (Table 49-1). Crofts' patient had antibodies to a 50-kD antigen found in human retina and optic nerve. Jacobson reported one patient with antibodies to

48-kD and 23-kD retinal antigens and a second patient with just the latter antibody. One patient reported by Rizzo had an antibody only to a 48-kD antigen, and initial testing showed no antibody to the 23-kD protein.[110] Repeat assays with more sensitive Western blot analyses (using the product of a gene that encodes for the CAR antigen) showed "significant, although low," CAR antibody levels.[125]

Rush's patient with primary malignant melanoma had antiretinal and antioptic nerve antibodies that were not specific for the 23-kD CAR antigen.[111] The patients with paraneoplastic retinopathy associated with cutaneous melanoma probably represent a distinct subset and have been further subcharacterized as melanoma-associated retinopathy (MAR).[3,12,71,92,111] The condition is frequently nonprogressive and ERG findings (Table 49-1, description follows) are different than in other PR patients. Immunofluorescence studies demonstrated staining of bipolar cells (not photoreceptors) by sera and IgG fractions from patients with MAR. The involved retinal antigen and syndrome of PR in melanoma patients appear to be distinct.[71,92]

Recently Guy and associates[1,53] reported five patients with primary tumors in the lung, breast, bladder, or prostate —none of which had antibodies to the 23-kD antigen. All patients had antibodies to a 46-kD protein that Guy and associates identified as enolase, which subsequently was found in photoreceptor outer segments. Another patient with invasive ductal breast carcinoma had vision loss with a normal ERG. Serum antibodies were identified to a protein that migrated electrophoretically as rhodopsin.[102] Given the diversity and specificity of the immune system, it is likely that several different antigens can elicit an immune response capable of causing retinal damage. For instance, in addition to several possible photoreceptor antigens, there are well-documented cases in which paraneoplastic visual loss occurred as a result of ganglion cell loss[27,52] and "optic neuritis."[14,105] These facts support the notion that visual loss may result from immune attack directed against more than one retinal or optic nerve antigen.

The absence of an antibody to the 23-kD CAR antigen in some patients may also be analogous to myasthenia gravis, an autoimmune disease mediated by antibodies against acetylcholine receptors.[84] Antibodies are not detectable in all patients with myasthenia gravis, and there is no correlation between the severity of disease and presence of antibody.[117] Cases of seronegative paraneoplastic cerebellar degeneration have been described as well.[6,54] This inconsistency may result from an insufficiently sensitive assay for the offending antibody. It is also possible that the antibody is bound to receptors and therefore not detectable in the serum. Recent advances in the sensitivity of the diagnostic tests for the CAR antigen will undoubtedly reduce the number of false negative results. As valuable as these tests are, the diagnosis of paraneoplastic retinopathy should still be based on clinical criteria.

CLINICAL FEATURES

Patients with paraneoplastic retinopathy often display symptoms before recognition of the malignancy. The symptoms are fairly uniform, quite typical, and include vision loss, night blindness, and reduced ERG.[23,123] The primary visual complaint is usually decreased vision or a halo of missing peripheral vision. Positive visual phenomena (like sparkles or ''dancing lights'') are often observed. Some patients will report difficulty with night vision,[25,63] glare, or sensitivity to light (day blindness or hemeralopia).[45,63] These symptomatic differences may correlate with the degree to which the rods versus cones are affected.

Ocular symptoms may vary between the eyes. Acuity at presentation can range from 20/20 to hand motions. Progression typically occurs rapidly, with patients losing significant vision within days or weeks. Abnormal color vision and prolonged photostress recovery time (time for visual recovery following exposure to bright light) also occur. An afferent pupil defect may be present in cases with asymmetric ocular involvement. The visual fields (Fig. 49-1) initially show midperipheral scotomas or paracentral defects that eventually connect to form a classic ring scotoma. The arcuate defects do not typically respect the horizontal meridian because they result from damage to the outer retina near the vascular arcades. This outer retina does not have an anatomic demarcation along the horizontal meridian like the nerve fiber layer.

Ocular examination may show a mild vitreitis,[28,63,98] and although the retina may appear normal, there is usually a mild-to-moderate attenuation of retinal vessels (Fig. 49-2).* Peripheral retinal pigmentation,[115] mild optic disc pallor,[63,115,117,124] and a ''beaten metal''[69] or granular[25] appearance of the retina have also been described. Fluorescein angiography does not contribute to the diagnosis of this condition but may help to document the gross status of the blood-ocular barrier and identify periphlebitis.[98,101] One patient had progressive diminution of peripheral blood flow and slowed perfusion.[101]

The diagnosis of paraneoplastic retinopathy is usually missed at initial presentation. Important clues include symptoms of positive visual phenomena (flashing lights, sense of movement, and so on) and a ring scotoma or midperipheral defects on visual field testing.[63,110] The condition should be suspected in older patients who have positive visual phenomena and ring scotomata on Goldmann visual field testing, and in whom there is a paucity of findings compared to the symptoms and level of disability. An electroretinogram will reveal evidence of retinal dysfunction (see the following). The diagnosis of paraneoplastic retinopathy can be made with confidence if an abnormal ERG is found in a patient who experienced relatively precipitous visual loss

*References 19, 25, 55, 63, 73, 76, 88, 111, 124.

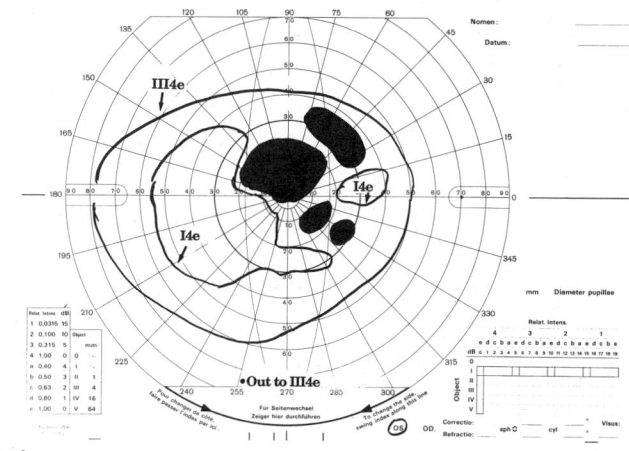

Left

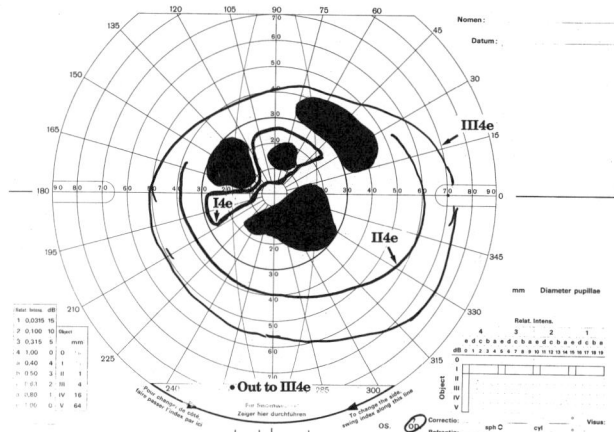

Right

Fig. 49-1. Goldmann visual field test results in a patient with paraneoplastic retinopathy. Left (left eye) and right (right eye) revealing midperipheral scotomas and constriction of the peripheral isopters. (Rizzo JF III, Gittinger J Jr: Selective immunohistochemical staining in the paraneoplastic retinopathy syndrome, *Ophthalmology* 99:8, 1992.)

(most abnormal ERG's are found in patients with chronic retinal degenerations like retinitis pigmentosa). At this point the medical history should be reviewed and questions should be asked in an attempt to identify an underlying malignancy. A chest x-ray should be obtained. Approximately one half of the cases of paraneoplastic retinopathy will occur prior to the discovery of the malignancy.[23,69,115,124] To date, paraneoplastic retinopathy has not been reported to occur in conjunction with other neurologic disease. One patient with undifferentiated carcinoma, posterior uveitis, and paraneoplastic encephalomyelitis was found to have serum antibodies reacting with retina and brain.[8] This patient's clinical course was not that of paraneoplastic retinopathy, and histopathologic evaluation of the eyes was not performed.

As with other paraneoplastic syndromes, small cell carcinoma of the lung is the most common primary tumor in patients with paraneoplastic retinopathy and is found in

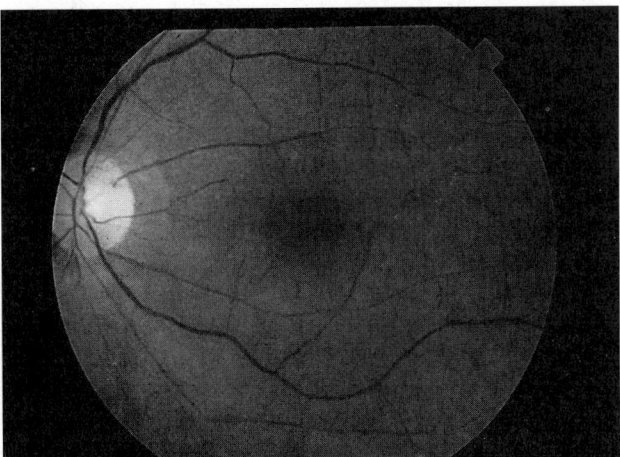

Fig. 49-2. Fundus photograph of the left eye of a patient with paraneoplastic retinopathy. Note the vessel attenuation, especially inferotemporally.

roughly two thirds of these patients (Table 49-1). Other primary tumors associated with paraneoplastic retinopathy include melanoma,[7,12,71,111] uterine carcinoma,[21,25,28] rhabdomyosarcoma,[55] breast carcinoma,[73] cervical carcinoma,[69] and unknown primary tumor.[88] One case had three primary tumors (prostate, bladder, larynx).[88] Interestingly, despite the fact that they are among the most common malignancies, gastrointestinal carcinomas have never been reported to cause paraneoplastic retinopathy.

LABORATORY INVESTIGATIONS

The electroretinogram (ERG) is a measure of the electrical activity of the retina that is elicited by stimulation with light. The wave form has two components: an a wave that reflects activity of the photoreceptors and a b wave that is believed to reflect activity of Müller cells as neural impulses move through the retina. The ERG largely measures the function of the rods when it is gauged in the dark-adapted state (scotopic ERG). Cone function can be isolated by stimulation with a 30-Hz flickering light.

The ERG can produce variable findings in paraneoplastic retinopathy. In cases with light-induced glare, photosensitivity, decreased acuity, and dyschromatopsia (all of which suggest dysfunction of cones), an abnormal cone ERG is found. In patients with nyctalopia and peripheral or ring scotomas (which suggest rod dysfunction), an abnormal scotopic ERG is found. In the majority of cases (Table 49-1), the amplitude of both the a and b wave of the ERG are very attenuated or nonrecordable. An abnormal electrooculogram also has been reported.[69,76,88,130]

Progressive visual loss has been correlated with progressive reduction of ERG amplitudes.[69] A more selective ERG pattern, typical of congenital stationery night blindness (absence of b wave under dark-adapted conditions and normal-cone ERG amplitudes), has been described in patients with cutaneous melanoma.[3,7,12,71,111] One patient tested with pro-

longed flashes showed a loss of the cone ERG "on" response with relative preservation of the cone "off" response.[3] This suggests that the visual impairment in this setting does not result from a defect in photoreceptor outer segment function but from a defect in signal transmission from the photoreceptor to the second order neuron (bipolar cell).

DIFFERENTIAL DIAGNOSIS

Conditions that appear clinically similar but are not associated with systemic malignancy, conditions secondary to a direct effect of spread of the tumor, and toxic effects of chemotherapy must be excluded before a diagnosis of paraneoplastic retinopathy is made. In the setting of a normal-appearing fundus, acute and subacute visual losses in adults usually result from retrobulbar optic neuropathy (provided that functional visual loss is excluded). Attenuation of retinal vessels may be a clue to the diagnosis of paraneoplastic retinopathy, but this is often a subtle finding. Decreased acuity, dyschromatopsia, relative afferent pupil defect, and visual field defects are commonly seen with both retinopathies and neuropathies, but positive visual phenomena more commonly occur with retinal disease. The visual field defects observed in retinopathy and optic neuropathy also overlap; however, patients with paraneoplastic retinopathy typically have midperipheral defects that cross the vertical meridian.

Compressive lesions of the anterior visual pathway or inflammatory optic neuritis must be considered in instances of subacute visual loss. Optic neuritis is a common initial diagnosis in patients ultimately shown to have paraneoplastic retinopathy.[88,110] In addition, nearly all of the reported cases undergo neuroimaging of the anterior visual pathway to rule out a compressive lesion prior to diagnosis. Historical information usually uncovers less common causes of subacute visual loss such as toxic, hereditary, and nutritional optic neuropathy. Although ischemic optic neuropathy may be progressive, it is almost always associated with a swollen optic nerve. Further, simultaneous involvement of both eyes would be unusual for ischemic optic neuropathy, except in the setting of giant cell arteritis. Symptoms of inflammatory optic neuritis (secondary to demyelination, lupus or sarcoid) can include subacute bilateral visual loss and normal-appearing fundus. Ultimately, the ERG will distinguish paraneoplastic retinopathy from optic neuropathy.

The relatively fast tempo of visual loss distinguishes paraneoplastic retinopathy from other more common retinal degenerations like retinitis pigmentosa. Visual loss from hereditary retinal degeneration occurs over many years, whereas with paraneoplastic retinopathy it occurs over weeks to months. Otherwise, the two conditions are very similar, because both result from photoreceptor dysfunction. Although most cases of retinitis pigmentosa have abnormal fundi, some victims do not have pigmentary deposition.

There are other mechanisms by which subacute visual

loss may occur in the setting of cancer. Metastatic disease may occur as carcinomatous meningitis and cause an optic neuropathy. Cuffing or infiltration of the optic nerve by neoplastic cells (carcinomatous meningitis) can cause an optic neuropathy, which usually occurs with an edematous optic disc. Metastases can invade the optic nerve proper, the orbit, or orbital bones, which can cause a compressive optic neuropathy. In these conditions the neuroimaging and/or spinal fluid analysis will be abnormal.

Visual loss may occur as a consequence of the toxic effects of chemotherapy.[95] BCNU has been associated with acute optic neuropathy[90,104] and vincristine with photoreceptor dysfunction[109] and optic atrophy.[116] Cis-platinum is believed to cause optic neuropathy, maculopathy, and pigmentary retinopathy.[78,93] Radiation therapy around the eye, optic nerves, or chiasm may cause retinopathy or optic neuropathy months to years after treatment.

Two other paraneoplastic syndromes are noteworthy. Paraneoplastic optic neuropathy (PON) has been described in patients with small cell carcinoma of the lung,* Hodgkin disease,[62] and lymphoma.[77] Patients can have unilateral visual loss (bilateral cases have been depicted) and a swollen optic nerve. Based on histopathologic demonstration of perivascular lymphocytic infiltration, gliosis, and demyelination of the optic nerves,[14,105] the condition is thought to be inflammatory and might be more accurately termed paraneoplastic optic neuritis. Abnormal serum antibodies against cytoplasm of the central neurons and glia of the central nervous system were found in one patient.[86]

Diffuse uveal melanocytic proliferation is another paraneoplastic syndrome that causes painless, subacute loss of vision that typically occurs prior to diagnosis of the primary tumor.† Carcinoma of the reproductive tract in women and cancers of the retroperitoneal area and the lungs in men are the most common primary tumors associated with this syndrome. Examination is notable for bilateral proliferation of subretinal pigment (that appears similar to choroidal nevi) and yellow-orange lesions at the level of the retinal pigment epithelium, which may be associated with serous detachments of the retina. Fluorescein angiography in the early phase shows a striking pattern of hyperfluorescence, which corresponds to the abnormalities observed at the level of the retinal pigment epithelium. Frequently, uveitis and rapid progression of cataract occur. Pathologic studies have shown proliferation of nonmalignant cells, and metastases have never been reported.[15,44,83]

The pathogenesis of the uveal melanocytic syndrome is unknown, but one possibility is melanocytic proliferation in response to a common oncogenic stimulus or as a response to some hormonal factor secreted by the visceral malignancy. Another possibility is that these patients have congenital hypopigmented choroidal nevi that undergo transformation under the influence of some tumor-secreted factor.[112] The causes of the uveitis, rapidly progressive cataract, and RPE lesions are unknown. Serous retinal detachments of this type may be responsive to systemic corticosteroids or radiation. Treatment of the primary tumor may not alter the course of the progressive visual loss.

PATHOLOGY

Most standard laboratory investigations (blood chemistries and serum immunoglobulins) have no role in the diagnosis of paraneoplastic retinopathy. Identification of serum antiretinal antibodies has recently become an important diagnostic aid, however. Thirkill and associates[124] reported four patients whose sera were studied by ELISA and Western blot analysis. Serum immunoglobulins bound a 23-kD retinal antigen, which they called the cancer-associated retinopathy antigen. Antibodies against CAR antigen were found only in cancer patients who experienced visual loss and not in normal control patients or cancer patients who did not have visual loss.[124] Another report from the University of California at Davis group demonstrated antibodies to the CAR antigen, optic nerve antigens, and small cell carcinoma antigens.[122] As summarized previously, most patients have antibodies to the 23-kD antigen, and others have antiretinal antigens. Immunologic studies to date do not prove that paraneoplastic retinopathy results from damage caused by antibodies against a single specific retinal antigen. The possibility that more than one antigen may be associated with PR is analogous to cases of paraneoplastic cerebellar degenerations in which multiple distinct antibodies have been demonstrated.[5,31,54,103]

A total of 11 patients with paraneoplastic retinopathy had undergone post-mortem examinations of the eyes.* In all but one of these cases,[52] findings were very similar to those found in the original description of the condition by Sawyer and associates.[115] As might be expected (based on the clinical finding of decreased ERG amplitude), loss of photoreceptor inner and outer segments was present in each case. The degree of macular involvement has been variable,[21,25] and generally there has been more rod than cone involvement.[19,110] Disintegration of the outer nuclear layer and variable presence of inflammatory infiltrate are other notable features. Several patients have had lymphocytic infiltration,[2,19,52,69,115] but only one case had more than scattered foci of lymphocytes.[2] Retinal vasculature was normal, except in one case with phlebitis.[98] Barring one patient,[52] all cases have had relative sparing of the inner nuclear layer. In areas of photoreceptor loss, scattered melanophages and disruption of the retinal pigment epithelium have been observed.[19,21,98,115] Buchanan[19] found normal-appearing RPE with light microscopy, but on ultrastructural analysis with electron microscopy premelanosomes, melanolysosomes

*References 14, 32, 86, 94, 105, 134.
†References 11, 15, 44, 83, 87, 96, 112, 146.

*References 2, 19, 21, 25, 52, 69, 98, 110, 115.

and giant melanolysosomes were identified, suggesting abnormal melanin synthesis and resorption.

Immunohistochemistry has also helped to characterize the nature of the serum antiretinal antibodies. Keltner and associates[69] demonstrated "diffuse hyperfluorescence more intense in the outer retinal layers" when their patient's serum was incubated with normal human retina. Selective immunohistochemical staining confined to the outer retina has also been demonstrated.[110] This latter staining pattern respects the anatomic boundary between the outer plexiform and the inner nuclear layers, and within the outer retina (the rods stained more diffusely than cones).[110] A similar immunohistochemical staining pattern occurs with antibodies directed against recoverin. Correlation between this immunohistochemical staining and pathology, both of which are confined to the outer retina, supports the concept that these antibodies have a role in the pathogenesis of the disease. Other immunohistochemical studies have shown staining of the ganglion cell layer,[76,98] supporting a role for other antibodies. One of these patients,[76] however, had an abnormal ERG (which is inconsistent with ganglion cell dysfunction), dysfunction and the second patient showed predominant loss of photoreceptors on histopathology.[98]

THERAPY

In general, patients with paraneoplastic retinopathy progress to severe visual loss over a period of several months. Because of the presumed autoimmune mechanism, the mode of therapy most frequently recommended has been systemic immunosuppression to reduce the level of antiretinal antibody. Treatment of the primary malignancy, together with radiation or chemotherapy, may be associated with stabilization of the retinopathy[76,130]—an effect that could result from a decreased antigenic load or destruction of circulating lymphocytes. Therapy directed against the primary tumor without immunosuppression is ineffective in stabilizing vision.

The mainstay of therapy is with systemic corticosteroids.[70] Alternative drugs for immunosuppression have not been systematically applied or reported on. Improvement of acuity and visual fields in paraneoplastic retinopathy patients has been reported with the use of corticosteroids.[63,70,73,98,101] In one case, visual acuity decreased each time the corticosteroids were tapered and improved when they were reinstated.[69] Other patients have failed to improve with corticosteroids.[28,115] Antineoplastic therapy with immunosuppressive drugs and plasma exchange has been shown to reverse other paraneoplastic neurologic deficits and probably does not adversely affect the treatment of the primary tumor.[4,22,54,60] To date, these types of therapy have not been systematically applied to the treatment of paraneoplastic retinopathy. Plasmapheresis was tried unsuccessfully in one case.[122] It was successful in another, although this patient had antirhodopsin antibodies and the authors postu-

lated that plasmapheresis was more likely to work in a situation in which antibody was directed against a replenishable pigment.[102]

Recently, Keltner and associates[70] reported a case in which the titer of serum antibodies to retinal antigens correlated with increasing immunologic response and preceded subsequent visual deterioration. They found that antiretinal antibody titers could be reduced to normal levels with prednisone therapy. In addition, they were able to maintain useful vision in one eye for a year after diagnosis. Patients should be followed closely with serial acuities, visual fields, ERG's, and antiretinal antibody titers. Exacerbations of visual loss should be treated with prednisone or intravenous pulse corticosteroids. Rising antiretinal antibody titers could be a precursor of visual loss, but this has not been conclusively demonstrated in a series of patients. Recently a laboratory test that measures antiretinal antibodies has become commercially available.*

PROGNOSIS

The clinical course of paraneoplastic retinopathy is variable, but frequently there is progression to profound bilateral loss of vision within weeks to months. Visual acuities range from 20/25 to no light perception.[69,110] Central (Snellen) acuity may be lost early or late. Many patients die before they become totally blind. Visual field loss is progressive and often results in a ring scotoma. Retinal arterioles become progressively attenuated, and ERG responses progressively decline. Central acuity can be maintained or improved in some patients with systemic corticosteroids. The serum level of serum antiretinal antibodies may correlate with success of treatment and severity of disease (see Therapy section). Treatment of the primary malignancy does not seem to alter the course of visual loss, although one patient improved slightly in this setting.[101]

REFERENCES

1. Adamus G, Aptsiauri N, Guy J et al.: Anti-enolase antibodies in cancer associated retinopathy, *Invest Ophthalmol Vis Sci* 34:1485, 1993.
2. Adamus G, Guy J, Schmied J et al.: Role of Anti-Recoverin autoantibodies in cancer-associated retinopathy, *Invest Ophthalmol Vis Sci* 34:2626-2633, 1993.
3. Alexander KR, Fishman GA, Peachey NS et al.: "On" response defect in paraneoplastic night blindness with cutaneous malignant melanoma, *Invest Ophthalmol Vis Sci* 33:477, 1992.
4. Anderson NE: Anti-neuronal autoantibodies and neurological paraneoplastic syndromes, *Aust NZ J Med* 19:379, 1989.
5. Anderson NE, Rosenblum MK, Graus F et al.: Autoantibodies in paraneoplastic syndromes associated with small-cell lung cancer, *Neurology* 38:1391, 1988.
6. Anderson NE, Rosenblum MK, Posner JB: Paraneoplastic cerebellar degeneration: clinical-immunological correlations, *Ann Neurol* 24:559, 1988.

---

*Genica Pharmaceuticals, Worcester, Mass.

7. Andreasson S, Ponjavic V, Ehinger B: Full-field electroretinogram in a patient with cutaneous melanoma-associated retinopathy, *Acta Ophthalmol* 71:487-490, 1993.

8. Antoine JC et al.: Posterior uveitis, paraneoplastic encephalomyelitis and auto-antibodies reacting with developmental protein of brain and retina, *J Neurol Sci* 117:215-223, 1993.

9. Appen RE, DeVenecia G, Sellikan J et al.: Meningeal carcinomatosis with blindness, *Am J Ophthalmol* 86:661-665, 1978.

10. Ashworth A et al.: Chromosomal localization of zinc finger protein genes in man and mouse, *Genomics* 4:323-327, 1989.

11. Barr CC, Zimmerman LE, Curtin VT, Font RL: Bilateral diffuse uveal tumors associated with systemic malignant neoplasms: a recently recognized syndrome, *Arch Ophthalmol* 100:249, 1982.

12. Berson EL, Lessell S: Paraneoplastic night blindness with malignant melanoma, *Am J Ophthalmol* 106:307, 1988.

13. Blumenfeld AM et al.: Coexistence of Lambert-Eaton myasthenic syndrome and subacute cerebellar degeneration: differential effects of treatment, *Neurology* 41:1682-1685, 1991.

14. Boghen D, Sebag M, Michaud J: Paraneoplastic optic neuritis and encephalomyelitis: report of a case, *Arch Neurol* 45:353, 1988.

15. Borruat FX, Othenin-Girard P, Uffer S et al.: Natural history of diffuse uveal melanocytic proliferation, *Ophthalmology* 99:1698, 1992.

16. Brain L, Wilkinson M: Subacute cerebellar degeneration associated with neoplasms, *Brain* 88:465-478, 1965.

17. Brain WR, Norris FH, editors: *The remote effects of cancer on the nervous system,* New York, 1965, Grune & Stratton.

18. Brashear HR et al.: Anticerebellar antibodies in neurologically normal patients with ovarian neoplasms, *Neurology* 39:1605-1609, 1989.

19. Buchanan TAS, Gardiner TA, Archer DB: An ultrastructural study of retinal photoreceptor degeneration associated with bronchial carcinoma, *Am J Ophthalmol* 97:277, 1984.

20. Budde-Stefan C et al.: An antineuronal antibody in paraneoplastic opsoclonus, *Ann Neurol* 23:528-531, 1988.

21. Campo E, Brunier MN, Merino MJ: Small cell carcinoma of the endometrium with associated ocular paraneoplastic syndrome, *Cancer* 69:2283, 1992.

22. Chalk CH, Murray NM, Newsom-Davis J et al.: Response of the Lambert-Eaton myasthenic syndrome to treatment of associated small-cell lung carcinoma, *Neurology* 40:1152, 1990.

23. Chung SM, Selhorst JB: Cancer-associated retinopathy, *Ophthalmol Clin N Am* 5:3, 1992.

24. Clouston PD et al.: Paraneoplastic cerebellar degeneration. III. Cerebellar degeneration, cancer and the Lambert-Eaton myasthenic syndrome, *Neurology* 42:1944-1950, 1992.

25. Cogan DG, Kuwabara T, Currie J, Kattah J: Paraneoplastische retinopathie unter dem klinischen bild einer zapfendystrophie mit achromatopsie, *Klin Monatsbl Augenheilkd* 197:156, 1990.

26. Croft PB, Urich H, Wilkinson M: Peripheral neuropathy of the sensoriomotor type associated with malignant disease, *Brain* 90:31-66, 1967.

27. Croft PB, Wikinson M: Carcinomatous neuromyopathy: its incidence in patients with carcinoma of the lung and carcinoma of the breast, *Lancet* 1:184-188, 1963.

28. Crofts JW, Bachynski BN, Odel JG: Visual paraneoplastic syndrome associated with undifferentiated endometrial carcinoma, *Can J Ophthalmol* 23:128, 1988.

29. Cunningham J et al.: Partial characterization of the purkinje cell antigens in paraneoplastic cerebellar degeneration, *Neurology* 36:1163-1168, 1986.

30. Dalamu J et al.: Detection of the anti-Hu antibody in specific regions of the nervous system and tumor from patients with paraneoplastic encephalomyelitis/sensory neuronopathy, *Neurology* 41:1757-1764, 1991.

31. Dalamu J et al.: Anti-Hu associated paraneoplastic encephalomyelitis/sensory neuronopathy: a clinical study of 71 patients, *Medicine* 71:59-72, 1992.

32. Davies PDB: Carcinomatous neuropathy with papilloedema, *Proc Roy Soc Med* 54:236, 1961.

33. DeVisser BW, Feltkamp-Vroom TM, Feltkamp CA: Sural nerve immune deposits in polyneuropathy as a remote effect of malignancy, *Ann Neurol* 14:261-266.

34. Dizhoor AM, Ray S, Kumar S et al.: Recoverin: a calcium sensitive activator of retinal rod guanylate cyclase, *Science* 251:915, 1991.

35. Dropcho EJ et al.: Cloning of a brain protein identified by autoantibodies from a patient with paraneoplastic cerebellar degeneration, *Proc Natl Acad Sci USA* 84:4552-4556, 1987.

36. Fain GL, Lisman JE: Photoreceptor degeneration in vitamin A deprivation and retinitis pigmentosa: the equivalent light hypothesis, *Exp Eye Res* 57:335-340, 1993.

37. Fathallah-Shaykh H et al.: Cloning of a leucine-zipper protein recognized by the sera of patients with antibody associated paraneoplastic cerebellar degeneration, *Proc Natl Acad Sci USA* 88:3451-3454, 1991.

38. Fesenko EE, Kolesnikov SS, Lyubarsky AL: Induction by cyclic GMP of cationic conductance in plasma membrane of rod retinal outer segment, *Nature* 313:310-312, 1985.

39. Field EJ, Caspary EA: Lymphocyte sensitization: an in vitro test for cancer? *Lancet* ii:1337-1341, 1970.

40. Fischer-Williams M, Bosanquet F, Daniel PM: Carcinomatosis of the meninges: a report of three cases, *Brain* 78:42-58, 1955.

41. Flaherty KM, Zozulya S, Stryer L: Three-dimensional structure of recoverin, a calcium sensor in vision, *Cell* 75:709-716, 1993.

42. Fukunaga H, Engel AG, Lang B et al.: Passive transfer of Lambert-Eaton myasthenic syndrome with IgG from man to mouse depletes the presynaptic membrane active zones, *Proc Natl Acad Sci* 80:7636, 1983.

43. Furneaux HF, Reich L, Posner JB: Autoantibody synthesis in the central nervous system of patients with paraneoplastic syndromes, *Neurology* 40:1085, 1990.

44. Gass JDM, Gieser RG, Wilkinson CP et al.: Bilateral diffuse uveal melanocytic proliferation in patients with occult carcinoma, *Arch Ophthalmol* 108:527, 1990.

45. Gehrs K, Tiedeman J: Hemeralopia in an older adult, *Surv Ophthalmol* 37:185-189, 1992.

46. Graus F, Elkon KB, Cordon-Cardo C: Sensory neuropathy and small cell lung cancer. Antineuronal antibody that also reacts with the tumor, *Am J Med* 80:45-52, 1986.

47. Gray-Keller MP et al.: The effect of recoverin-like calcium binding proteins on the photoresponse of retinal rods, *Neuron* 10:523-531, 1993.

48. Greco FA, Hainsworth J, Sismani A et al.: Hormone production and paraneoplastic syndromes. In *Small cell lung cancer,* 177-224, 1981, Greco and Stratton.

49. Greenlee JE, Brashear HR: Antibodies to cerebellar Purkinje cells in patients with paraneoplastic cerebellar degeneration and ovarian cancer, *Ann Neurol* 14:609-613, 1983.

50. Greenlee JE, Lipton HL: Anticerebellar antibodies in serum and cerebrospinal fluid of a patient with oat cell carcinoma of the lung and paraneoplastic cerebellar degeneration, *Ann Neurol* 19:82, 1986.

51. Grunwald GB, Klein R, Simmonds MA, Kornguth SE: Autoimmune basis for visual paraneoplastic syndrome in patients with small-cell lung carcinoma, *Lancet* 1:658, 1985.

52. Grunwald GB, Kornguth SE, Towfighi J et al.: Autoimmune basis for visual paraneoplastic syndrome in patients with small cell lung carcinoma: retinal immune deposits and ablation of retinal ganglion cells, *Cancer* 60:780, 1987.

53. Guy JR, Adamus G, Aptsiauri N et al.: Cancer associated retinopathy: a new antibody, *Suppl Ophthalmol* 100:116, 1993.

54. Hammack JE, Kimmel DW, O'Neill BP, Lennon VA: Paraneoplastic cerebellar degeneration: a clinical comparison of patients with and without Purkinje cell cytoplasmic antibodies, *Mayo Clin Proc* 65:1423, 1990.

55. Hammack J et al.: Paraneoplastic cerebellar degeneration. II. Clinical and immunologic findings in 21 patients with Hodgkin's disease, *Neurology* 42:1938-1943, 1992.

56. Hammerstein W, Jurgens H, Gobel U: Retinadegeneration und embryonales rhabdomyosarkom des thorax, *Fortschr Ophthalmol* 88:463, 1991.

57. Haveman K, Luster W, Gropp C et al.: Peptide hormone production associated with small cell lung cancer. In Seeber S, editor: *Recent advances in cancer research: small cell lung cancer,* 65-76, Berlin, 1985, Springer-Verlag.

58. Henson RA, Russell DS, Wilkinson M: Carcinomatous neuropathy and myopathy: a clinical and pathological study, *Brain* 77:82-121, 1954.
59. Henson RA, Urich H: *Cancer and the nervous system,* Oxford, 1982, Blackwell Scientific.
60. Hetzel DJ, Stanhope CR, O'Neill BP, Lennon VA: Gynecologic cancer in patients with subacute cerebellar degeneration predicted by anti-Purkinje cell antibodies and limited in metastatic volume, *Mayo Clin Proc* 65:1558, 1990.
61. Hurley JB et al.: Recoverin's role: conclusion withdrawn, *Science* 260:740, 1993.
62. Hutchinson EC et al.: Neurological complications of the reticuloses, *Brain* 81:75-92, 1958.
63. Jacobson DM, Thirkill CE, Tipping SJ: A clinical triad to diagnose paraneoplastic retinopathy, *Ann Neurol* 28:162, 1990.
64. Jaeckle KA, Graus F, Houghton A: Autoimmune response of patients with paraneoplastic cerebellar degeneration to a Purkinje cell cytoplasmic protein antigen, *Ann Neurol* 18:592-600, 1985.
65. Julien J, Vital C, Vallat JM et al.: Polyneuropathy in Waldenstrom's macroglobulinemia—Deposition of M component on myelin sheaths, *Arch Neurol* 35:423-425, 1978.
66. Katz JL, Valsamis MP, Jampel RS: Ocular signs in diffuse carcinomatous meningitis, *Am J Ophthalmol* 22:681-690.
67. Kelly JJ, Kyle RA, Miles JM et al.: The spectrum of peripheral neuropathy in myeloma, *Neurology* 31:24-31, 1981.
68. Kelly JJ, Kyle RA, Miles JM et al.: Osteosclerosis myeloma and peripheral neuropathy, *Neurology* 33:202-210, 1983.
69. Keltner JL, Roth AM, Chang RS: Photoreceptor degeneration: possible autoimmune disorder, *Arch Ophthalmol* 101:564, 1983.
70. Keltner JL, Thirkill CE, Tyler NK, Roth AM: Management and monitoring of cancer-associated retinopathy, *Arch Ophthalmol* 110:48, 1992.
71. Kim RY, Retas s, Arden G et al.: Melanoma associated retinopathy, *Ophthalmology* 100(suppl):141, 1993.
72. Kim YI, Neher E: IgG from patients with Lambert-Eaton syndrome blocks voltage-dependent calcium channels, *Science* 239:405, 1988.
73. Klingele TG, Burde RM, Rappazzo JA et al.: Paraneoplastic retinopathy, *J Clin Neuro Ophthalmol* 4:239, 1984.
74. Koch KW, Stryer L: Highly cooperative feedback control of retinal rod guanylate cyclase by calcium ions, *Nature* 334:64-66, 1988.
75. Kornguth SE, Kalinke T, Grunwald GB et al.: Antineurofilament antibodies in the sera of patients with small cell carcinoma of the lung and with visual paraneoplastic syndrome, *Cancer Res* 46:2588, 1986.
76. Kornguth SE, Klein R, Appen R, Choate J: Occurrence of antiretinal ganglion cell antibodies in patients with small cell carcinoma of the lung, *Cancer* 50:1289, 1982.
77. Krauss AM, O'Rourke J: Lymphomatous optic neuropathy, *Arch Ophthalmol* 70:173-175, 1963.
78. Kupersmith MJ et al.: Maculopathy caused by intraarterially administered cisplatin and intravenously administered carmustine, *Am J Ophthalmol* 113:435-438, 1992.
79. Lambrecht HG, Koch CW: A 26 kD calcium binding protein from bovinerod outer segments as modulator of photoreceptor guanylate cyclase, *EMBO J* 10:793-798, 1991.
80. Lang B, Newsom-Davis J, Wray D: Autoimmune aetiology for myasthenic (Eaton-Lambert) syndrome, *Lancet* ii:224-226, 1981.
81. Lenz SE, Henschel Y, Zopf D et al.: VILIP, a cognate protein of the retinal calcium binding proteins visinin and recoverin is expressed in the developing chicken brain, *Mol Brain Res* 15:133-140, 1992.
82. Levine B, Hardwick JM, Trapp BD et al.: Antibody-mediated clearance of alphavirus infection from neurons, *Science* 254:856-860, 1991.
83. Leys AM, Dierick HG, Sciot RM: Early lesions of bilateral diffuse melanocytic proliferation, *Arch Ophthalmol* 109:1590, 1991.
84. Lindstrom J, Shelton D, Fujii Y: Myasthenia gravis, *Adv Immunol* 42:233, 1988.
85. Little J, Dale AJ, Okazaki H: Meningeal carcinomatosis: clinical manifestations, *Arch Neurol* 30:138-143, 1974.
86. Malik S, Furlan AJ, Sweeney PJ et al.: Optic neuropathy: a rare paraneoplastic syndrome, *J Clin Neuro Ophthalmol* 12:137, 1992.

87. Margo CE, Pavan PR, Gendelman D, Gragoudas E: Bilateral melanocytic uveal tumors associated with systemic nonocular malignancy: malignant melanomas or benign paraneoplastic syndrome, *Retina* 7:137, 1987.
88. Matsui Y, Mehta MC, Katsumi O et al.: Electrophysiological findings in paraneoplastic retinopathy, *Graefes Arch Clin Exp Ophthalmol* 230:324, 1992.
89. McGinnis JF, Lerious V, Pazik J, Elliott RW: Chromosomal assignment of the recoverin gene and cancer-associated retinopathy, *Mamm Genome* 4:43-45, 1993.
90. McLennan R, Taylor HR: Optic neuroretinitis in association with BCNU and procarbazine therapy, *Med Pediatr Oncol* 4:43-48, 1978.
91. Milam AH, Dacey DM, Dizhoor DM: Recoverin immunoreactivity in mammalian cone bipolar cells, *Vis Neurosci* 10:1-2, 1992.
92. Milam AH, Saari JC, Jacobson SG et al.: Autoantibodies against retinal bipolar cells in cutaneous melanoma-associated retinopathy, *Invest Ophthalmol Vis Sci* 34:91-100, 1993.
93. Miller DF et al.: Ocular and orbital toxicity following intracarotid injection of BCNU (carmustine) and cis platinium for malignant gliomas, *Ophthalmology* 92:402-406, 1985.
94. Miller NR: Paraneoplastic syndromes. In Walsh, Hoyt, editors: *Clinical neuroophthalmology,* vol 3, ed 4, 1735-1739, Baltimore, 1988, Williams and Wilkins.
95. Miller NR: Retrobulbar toxic and deficiency optic neuropathies. In Walsh, Hoyt, editors: *Clinical neuroophthalmology,* vol 1, ed 4, 289-308, Baltimore, 1988, Williams and Wilkins.
96. Mullaney J, Mooney D, O'Connor M, McDonald GSA: Bilateral ovarian carcinoma with bilateral uveal melanoma, *Br J Ophthalmol* 68:261, 1984.
97. Norris FH Jr, McMenemey WH, Barnard RO: Unusual particles in a case of carcinomatous neuronal disease, *Acta Neuropathol* 14:350-353, 1970.
98. Ohnishi Y, Ohara S, Sakamoto T et al.: Cancer-associated retinopathy with retinal phlebitis, *Br J Ophthalmol* 77:795-798, 1993.
99. Ojeda VJ: The classification of spinal chord disorders in patients with cancer, *Pathology* 5:122-124, 1973.
100. Olson M, Chernik N, Posner J: Infiltration of the leptomeninges by systemic cancer, *Arch Neurol* 30:122-137, 1974.
101. Oohira A, Tamaki Y, Nagahara K: A case of paraneoplastic retinopathy, *Jpn J Ophthalmol* 37:28-31, 1993.
102. Pepkowitz S, Reader A, Jacobs A et al.: Paraneoplastic retinopathy: resolution with plasmapheresis, *Transfusion* 33(suppl):71s, 1993.
103. Peterson K et al.: Paraneoplastic cerebellar degeneration. I. A clinical analysis of 55 anti-Yo antibody positive patients, *Neurology* 42:1931-1937, 1992.
104. Pickrell L, Purvin V: Ischemic optic neuropathy secondary to intracarotid infusion of BCNU, *J Clin Neuro Ophthalmol* 7:87, 1987.
105. Pillay N, Gilbert JJ, Ebers GC, Brown JD: Internuclear ophthalmoplegia and "optic neuritis": paraneoplastic effects of bronchial carcinoma, *Neurology* 34:788, 1984.
106. Polans AS, Buczylko J, Crabb J, Palczewski K: A photoreceptor calcium binding protein is recognized by autoantibodies obtained from patients with cancer-associated retinopathy, *J Cell Biol* 112:981, 1991.
107. Polans AS, Burton MD, Haley TL et al.: Recoverin, but not visinin, is an autoantigen in the human retina identified with a cancer-associated retinopathy, *Invest Ophthalmol Vis Sci* 34:81, 1993.
108. Read D, Warlow C: Peripheral neuropathy and solitary plasmacytoma, *J Neurol Neurosurg Psychiatry* 41:177-184, 1978.
109. Ripps H et al.: Functional abnormalities in vincristine induced night blindness, *Invest Ophthalmol Vis Sci* 25:787, 1984.
110. Rizzo JF III, Gittinger JW: Selective immunohistochemical staining in the paraneoplastic retinopathy syndrome, *Ophthalmology* 99:1286, 1992.
111. Rush JA: Paraneoplastic retinopathy in malignant melanoma, *Am J Ophthalmol* 115:390, 1993.
112. Ryll DL, Campbell RJ, Robertson DM, Brubaker SJ: Pseudometastatic lesions of the choroid, *Ophthalmology* 87:1181, 1980.
113. Sakai K et al.: Isolation of a complementary DNA clone encoding an autoantigen recognized by an anti-neuronal cell antibody from a patient with paraneoplastic cerebellar degeneration, *Ann Neurol* 28:692-698, 1990.

114. Sakai K et al.: Analysis of auto antibody binding to 52-kd paraneo-plastic cerebellar degeneration-associated antigen expressed in recombinant proteins, *Ann Neurol* 33:373-380, 1993.

115. Sawyer RA, Selhorst JB, Zimmerman LE, Hoyt WF: Blindness caused by photoreceptor degeneration as a remote effect of cancer, *Am J Ophthalmol* 81:606, 1976.

116. Shurin SB, Rekate HL, Annable W: Vincristine optic atrophy, *Pediatrics* 70:288-291, 1982.

117. Soliven BC, Lange DJ, Penn AS et al.: Seronegative myasthenia gravis, *Neurology* 38:514.

118. Spence AM, Sumi SM, Ruff R: Paraneoplastic syndromes that involve the nervous system, *Curr Probl Cancer* 8:4-43, 1983.

119. Stanford MR, Robbins J, Kasp E, Dumonde DC: Passive administration of antibody against retinal s-antigen induces electroretinographic supernormality, *Invest Ophthalmol Vis Sci* 33:30, 1992.

120. Stepanik PL, Lerious V, McGinnis JF: Developmental appearance, species and tissue specificity of mouse 23-k-Da, a retinal calcium-binding protein (recoverin), *Exp Eye Res* 57:189-197, 1993.

121. Steven MM, Mackay JR, Carnegie PR et al.: Cerebellar cortical degeneration with ovarian carcinoma, *Postgrad Med J* 58:47-51, 1982.

122. Thirkill CE, Fitzgerald P, Sergott RC et al.: Cancer-associated retinopathy (CAR syndrome) with antibodies reacting with retinal, optic-nerve, and cancer cells, *N Engl J Med* 321:1589-1594, 1989.

123. Thirkill CE, Keltner JL, Tyler NK et al.: Antibody reactions with retina and cancer-associated antigens in 10 patients with cancer associated retinopathy, *Arch Ophthalmol* 111:931-937, 1993.

124. Thirkill CE, Roth AM, Keltner JL: Cancer-associated retinopathy, *Arch Ophthalmol* 105:372-375, 1987.

125. Thirkill CE, Roth AM, Keltner JL: Paraneoplastic retinopathy syndrome, *Ophthalmology* 100:147, 1993.

126. Thirkill CE, Roth AM, Takemoto DJ et al.: Antibody indications of secondary and superimposed retinal hypersensitivity in retinitis pigmentosa, *Am J Ophthalmol* 112:132-137, 1991.

127. Thirkill CE, Tait RC, Tyler NK et al.: The cancer-associated retinopathy antigen is a recoverin-like protein, *Invest Ophthalmol Vis Sci* 33:2768-2772, 1992.

128. Thirkill CE, Tait RC, Tyler NK et al.: Intraperitoneal cultivation of small-cell carcinoma induces expression of the retinal cancer-associated retinopathy antigen, *Arch Ophthalmol* 111:974-978, 1993.

129. Trotter JL, Hendin BA, Osterland CK: Cerebellar degeneration with Hodgkin's disease: An immunological study, *Arch Neurol* 33:660-661, 1976.

130. van der Pol BAE, Planten JTh: A non-metastatic remote effect of lung carcinoma, *Doc Ophthalmol* 67:89-94, 1987.

131. Vargas Nunez JA, Bonilla Velasco F, Cases Fernandez-Tejerina J, Vaquero Ruano M: Degeneracion retiniana paraneoplasica, *Med Clin* 88:431, 1987.

132. Walsh JC: Neuropathy associated with lymphoma, *J Neurol Neurosurg Psych* 34:42-50, 1971.

133. Walton JN, Tomlinson BE, Pearce GW: Subacute "poliomyelitis" and Hodgkin's disease, *J Neurol Sci* 6:435-445, 1968.

134. Waterston JA, Gilligan BS: Paraneoplastic optic neuritis and external ophthalmoplegia, *Aust NZ J Med* 16:703-704, 1986.

135. Wilkinson P, Zeromski J: Immunofluorescent detection of antibodies against neurons in sensory carcinomatous neuropathy, *Brain* 88:529-538, 1965.

50 Neuroretinitis

NANCY WILLIAMS, NEIL R. MILLER

HISTORICAL BACKGROUND

In 1916 Theodore Leber[23] described a condition characterized by acute unilateral visual loss that was associated with an exudative maculopathy consisting of hard exudate arranged in a star figure around the fovea. Leber believed that this state was a primary retinal process and called it a "stellate maculopathy." The condition subsequently became known as Leber stellate maculopathy until 1977, when Gass[17] reported that victims showed swelling of the optic disc before and often concurrent with the appearance of the star figure. The optic disc swelling then resolved, leaving the maculopathy as the primary or sole ophthalmoscopic abnormality. Gass performed fluorescein angiography in several of the afflicted patients and showed that there was no leakage from retinal vessels surrounding the macula. He thus concluded that the condition was not a primary maculopathy, but rather a form of optic neuritis. Because this form of optic neuritis affected both the optic nerve and the retina, he called it *neuroretinitis*.

Gass emphasized that the condition occurred commonly in children and young adults—up to 50% of whom had an antecedent viral illness (usually affecting the respiratory tract) a few weeks before the onset of visual symptoms. It has subsequently become clear that some cases of neuroretinitis are associated with particular infectious diseases, whereas others occur as apparently isolated phenomena.[11,25] In the latter setting, the condition has been called *Leber idiopathic stellate neuroretinitis.*[7,11,22,31]

EPIDEMIOLOGY

Neuroretinitis affects persons of all ages, although it occurs most often in the third and fourth decades of life. There is no sex predilection, and both the right and left eyes are equally involved.

CLINICAL FEATURES

The condition usually is painless, but some patients complain of an aching sensation behind the affected eye or eyes, and the discomfort occasionally may worsen with eye movements. Afflicted patients complain of visual blurring that progresses as the maculopathy evolves. Visual acuity at the time of initial examination may range from 20/20 to light perception. A patient has never been observed who lost all perception of light during the course of this condition. Color vision is variably affected, and the degree of color deficit is usually significantly worse than the degree of visual loss would suggest.

The most common field defect is a cecocentral scotoma, but central scotomas, arcuate defects, and even altitudinal defects may be present, and the peripheral field may be nonspecifically constricted. A relative afferent pupillary defect occurs in most patients, unless the condition is bilateral, in which case even patients with clinically asymmetric visual loss may have no evidence of a relative afferent pupillary defect.

The degree of disc swelling ranges from mild to severe, depending in part on the point in time that the patient is first examined (Fig. 50-1). In severe cases, splinter hemorrhages may occur. Segmental disc swelling has been reported, but is uncommon. A macular star figure composed of lipid (hard exudates) may not be present when the patient is examined soon after visual symptoms begin, but it becomes apparent within days to weeks and tends to become more prominent even as the optic disc swelling is resolving (Figs. 50-2, 50-3).[11,17,25,30] Small, discrete chorioretinal lesions have been described in idiopathic cases in both the symptomatic and asymptomatic eyes.[7,11,25,38] Posterior inflammatory signs consisting of vitreous cells and venous sheathing, as well as occasional anterior chamber cell and flare also have been described in patients with neuroretinitis.[11,25]

Fluorescein angiography in patients with acute neuroretinitis demonstrates diffuse disc swelling and leakage of dye from vessels on the surface of the discs (Fig. 50-4).[17] The retinal vessels may show slight staining in the peripapillary region; however, the macular vasculature is entirely normal. Chorioretinal lesions, when present, show late hyperfluorescence and exhibit progressive scarring on follow-up examinations.[11,25]

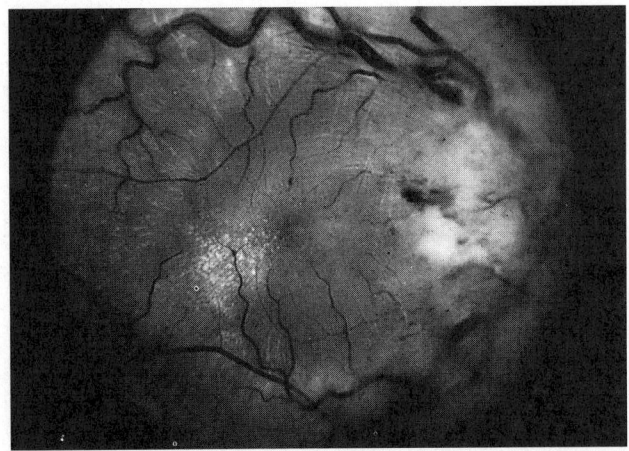
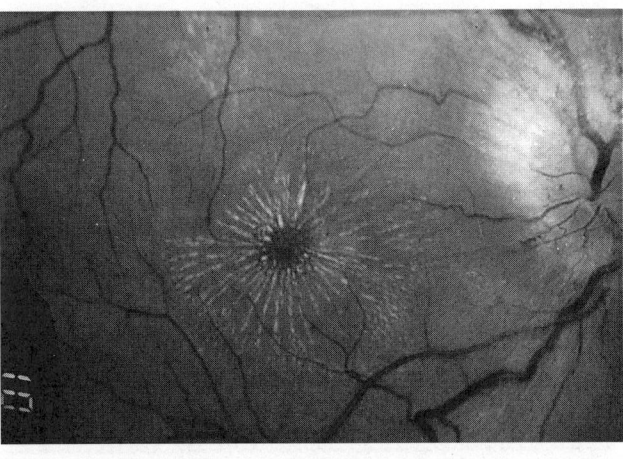

A   B

Fig. 50-1.   Variable severity of optic disc swelling in acute neuroretinitis. **A,** the patient has severe optic disc swelling associated with a macular star figure, hemorrhages, exudates, and moderate edema of the retina in the posterior pole. **B,** in this patient with neuroretinitis, there is only mild swelling of the optic disc, primarily superiorly, despite the presence of star figure surrounding the macula.

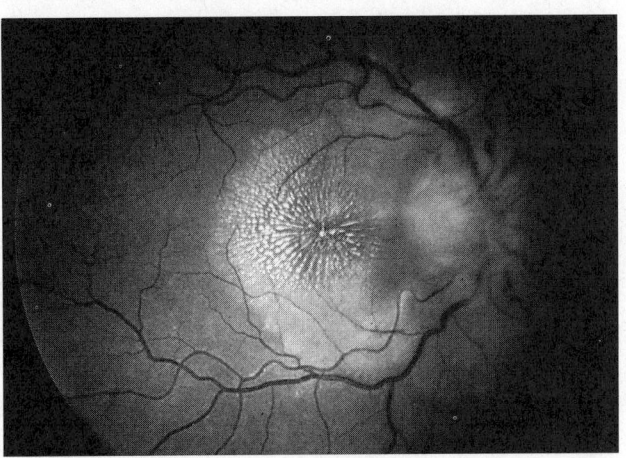
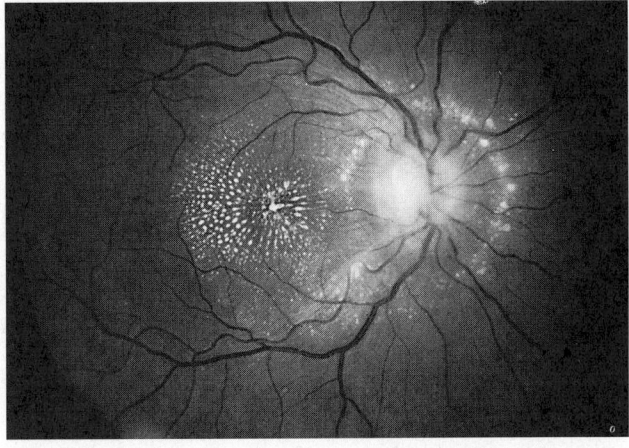

A   B

Fig. 50-2.   Increase of macular exudate despite resolution of optic disc swelling in neuroretinitis. **A,** in acute phase of disorder, the right optic disc is severely swollen, and there is edema in the papillomacular bundle. A macular star figure surrounds the fovea. **B,** 5 weeks later, the optic disc swelling and macular edema have improved, but the star figure is more prominent, and there is now lipid surrounding the optic disc as well.

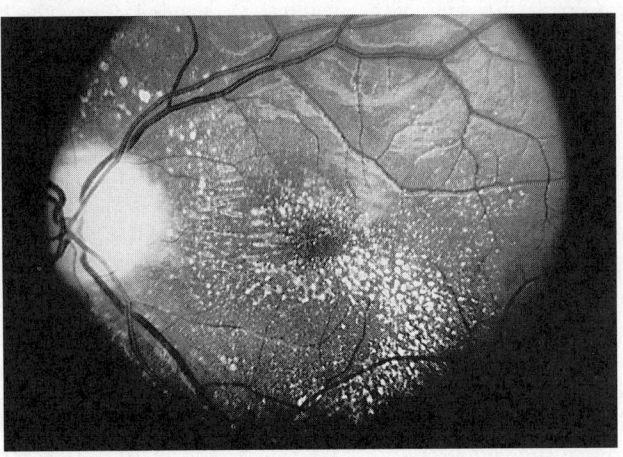

Fig. 50-3.   Extensive macular and posterior pole lipid after an episode of neuroretinitis. Note that the optic disc swelling has subsided, and the optic disc is pale.

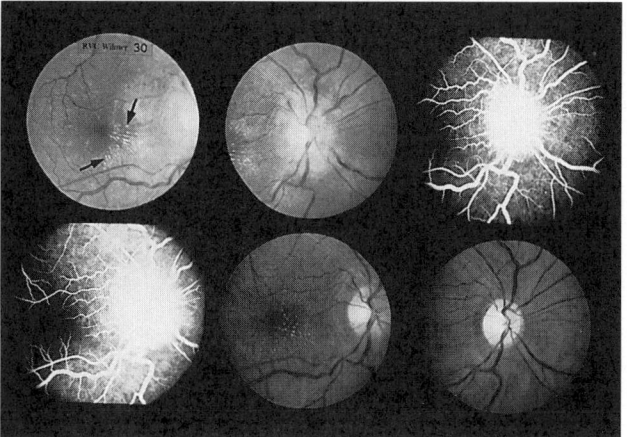

Fig. 50-4. Evolution of neuroretinitis including results of fluorescein angiography. *Top left and top center,* right optic disc is swollen and there is a beginning star figure in the right macula *(arrows). Top right,* fluorescein angiogram, early arteriovenous phase, shows diffuse leakage from the right optic disc. *Bottom left,* late arteriovenous phase shows both leakage and staining of the right optic disc. *Bottom center and bottom right,* 6 weeks later, the right optic disc is no longer swollen, although there is still hard exudate in the macula. (From NR Miller, SL Fine: The ocular fundus in neuro-ophthalmologic diagnosis, St Louis, 1977, Mosby.)

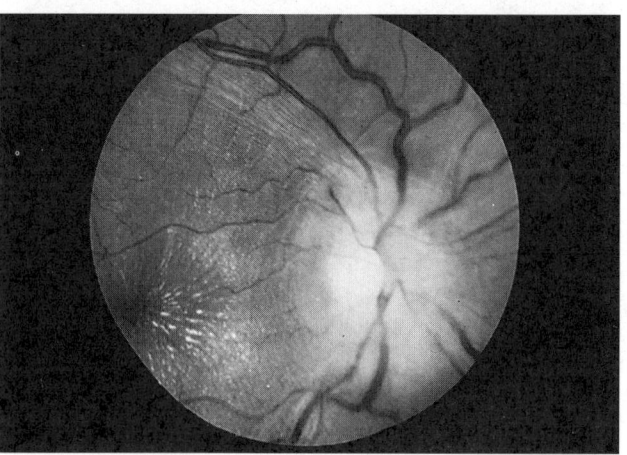

A

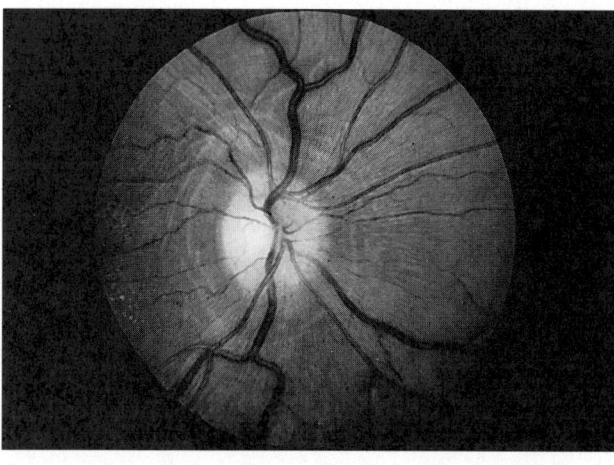

B

Fig. 50-5. Resolution of optic disc swelling in neuroretinitis. **A,** in the acute phase, there is diffuse swelling of the right optic disc. **B,** 6 weeks later, the swelling has largely resolved. Note Paton lines surrounding the disc and persistence of macular star figure.

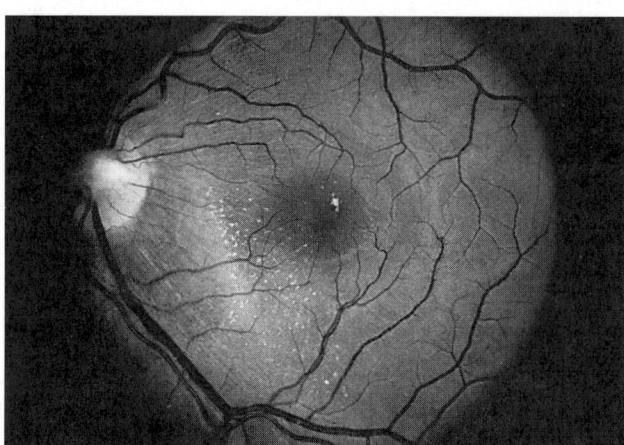

Fig. 50-6. Persistent macular lipid 6 months after an attack of neuroretinitis in the left eye. Note normal appearance of left optic disc.

Resolution

Neuroretinitis is a self-limited disorder. With time (usually over 6 to 8 weeks), the optic disc swelling resolves, and the appearance of the disc becomes normal—or nearly so (Fig. 50-5).[11,17,25,30] The macular exudate progresses over about 7 to 10 days. It then remains stable for several weeks before gradual resolution occurs (Figs. 50-3, 50-4, 50-6). Resolution may take 6 to 12 months, but the lipid eventually disappears. Most patients ultimately recover good visual acuity, although some complain of persistent metamorphopsia or nonspecific blurred vision from mild disruption of the macular architecture, despite disappearance of the macular exudate. Ophthalmoscopy and fluorescein angiography usually reveal defects in the retinal pigment epithelium of the macula in such cases (Fig. 50-7). Patients rarely develop moderate to severe visual loss, and one patient had bilateral loss of vision down to 20/400 OU. Such patients invariably have evidence of optic atrophy (Figs. 50-8, 50-9).

Recurrence

Most patients who develop neuroretinitis do not experience a subsequent attack in the same eye, and only a small percentage of patients who have experienced an attack in one eye subsequently develop a similar attack in the opposite eye. Nevertheless, several patients have been examined who had recurrent episodes of neuroretinitis in one or both eyes (Fig. 50-10). Such patients almost always suffer significant visual loss associated with optic atrophy and permanent macular pigmentary disturbances.

DIFFERENTIAL DIAGNOSIS

Neuroretinitis is thought to be an infectious or immune-mediated process that may be precipitated by a number of different agents. Numerous authors[11,17,19,25] have empha-

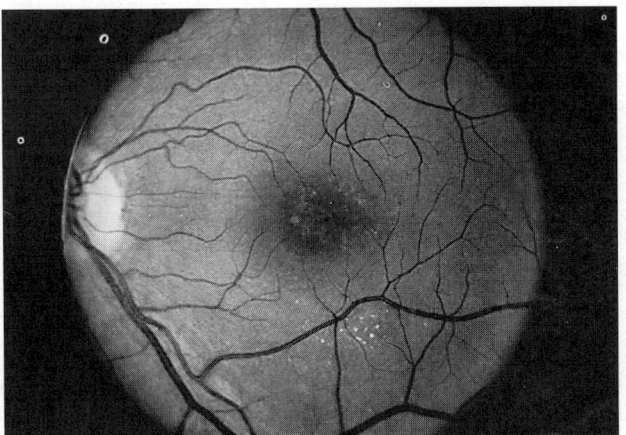

Fig. 50-7. Macular pigmentary disturbance after episode of neuroretinitis in the left eye. The optic disc swelling has resolved, and most of the macular star has resolved with only a small amount of exudate remaining inferior to the macula; however, the patient complains of persistent visual distortion in the left eye. Note macular pigmentary changes responsible for visual distortion.

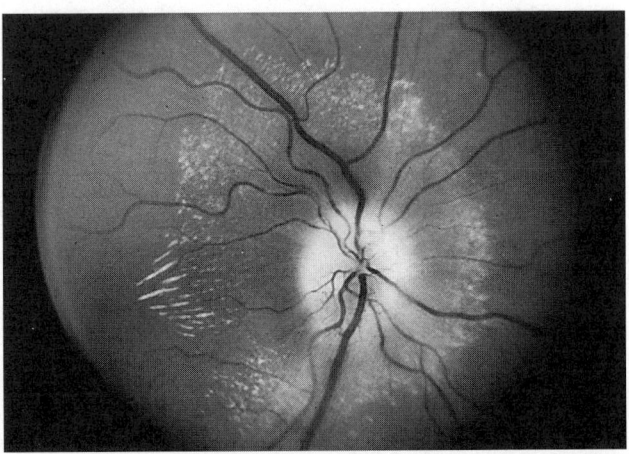

Fig. 50-8. Optic atrophy after a severe attack of neuroretinitis. **A,** in the acute phase of the illness, the right optic disc is swollen and is surrounded by edematous retina. There is a mild star figure nasal to the macula. Visual acuity is 20/400 in this eye; there is diminished color vision, a cecocentral scotoma, and a relative afferent pupillary defect. **B,** 2 months later, visual acuity remains 20/400. The optic disc swelling has completely resolved, leaving severe optic atrophy with focal narrowing of retinal arteries. Note persistent remnants of macular star figure.

sized the common occurrence of an antecedent viral syndrome in patients with neuroretinitis, suggesting a possible viral cause for up to 50% of cases. Viruses, however, are rarely cultured from the cerebrospinal fluid of such patients, and serologic evidence of a concomitant viral infection is usually lacking.[11,17,25,29] One case of neuroretinitis associated with herpes simplex encephalitis has been reported,[21] as has a case of bilateral neuroretinitis associated with serologic evidence of hepatitis B virus infection.[12] Foster and associates[16] described a case of neuroretinitis that occurred in association with mumps in a young man. In addition, Margolis and associates[27] reported the occurrence of an "arcuate neuroretinitis" associated with optic disc swelling in a

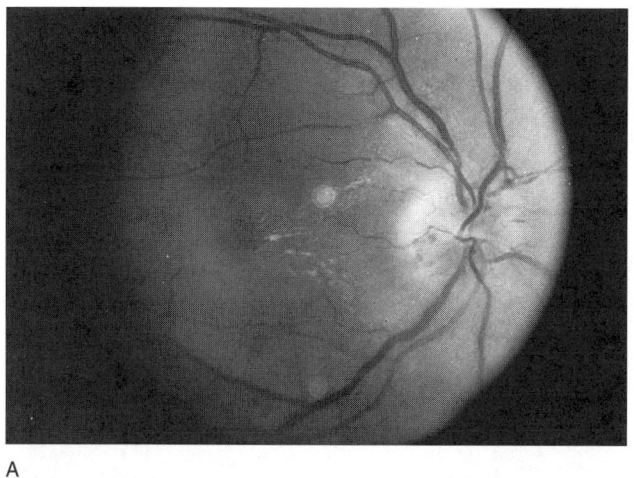

A

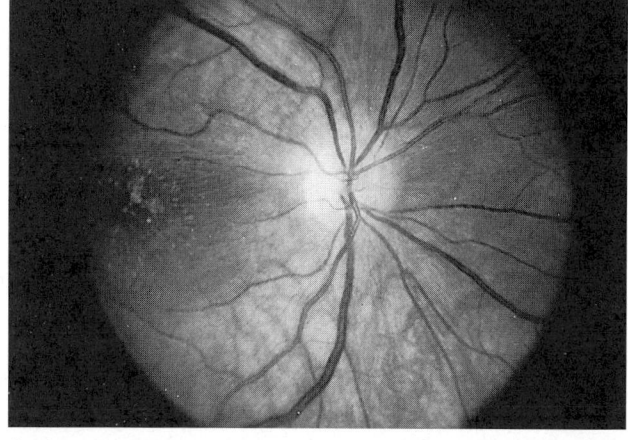

A

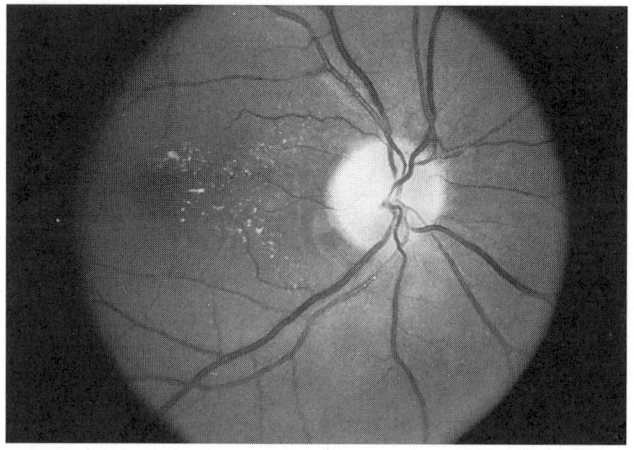

B

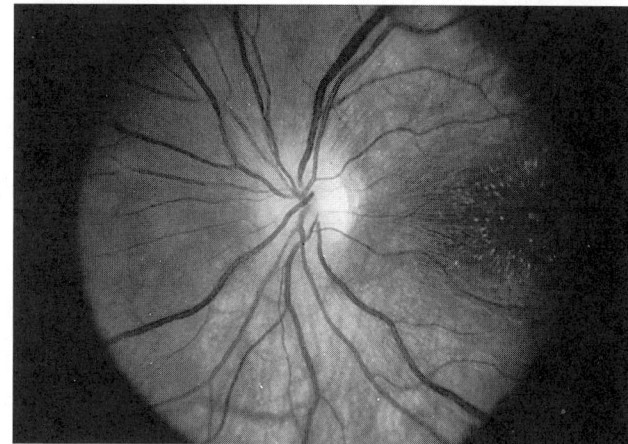

B

Fig. 50-9. Optic atrophy after neuroretinitis. **A,** 1 week after the onset of visual symptoms in the right eye, the optic disc is mildly swollen, and there is a mild hemistar figure in the right macula. **B,** 6 months later, visual acuity has improved several lines but is still reduced. The right optic disc is diffusely pale, and there is persistent lipid in the macula.

Fig. 50-10. Bilateral, simultaneous, recurrent neuroretinitis. Both optic discs are mildly swollen and pale. Both maculas show star figures. The patient's visual acuity was 20/200 OU. **A,** right fundus; **B,** left fundus.

patient with the acute retinal necrosis (ARN) syndrome, a condition thought to be caused by one or more of the herpesviruses.

Neuroretinitis may occur in patients with evidence of infectious disease caused by organisms other than viruses. Gass[17] described neuroretinitis associated with cat scratch disease (CSD), a systemic infection of presumed proteobacterial origin, in 1977. Since then, numerous similar cases of neuroretinitis have been described in patients with clinical manifestations consistent with CSD,[5,11,38] some of whom have had positive cat scratch antigen skin tests.[2,9]

Perhaps the most common conditions that seem to cause neuroretinitis are the spirochetoses. Neuroretinitis frequently occurs in patients with secondary and tertiary (late) syphilis. It may develop in patients with secondary syphilis as part of the syndrome of syphilitic meningitis.[1] In such cases, it is usually bilateral and associated with evidence of

meningeal irritation and multiple cranial neuropathies. It may also occur as an isolated phenomenon in patients with secondary syphilis, in which case it is often associated with uveitis and may be either unilateral or bilateral.* Graveson[18] described a 37-year-old man with a previous history of a transient oculomotor nerve paresis at age 21, who subsequently developed acute visual loss in the right eye that never improved. He then lost his sense of smell, developed bilateral facial weakness, and began to experience left-sided facial spasms. Three weeks before admission, he abruptly lost vision in the left eye. On examination, the patient had bilateral anosmia, bilateral facial paresis, and left hemifacial spasm. Visual acuity was hand motions in the right eye and 20/600 in the left eye. The right optic disc was "dead white." The left optic disc showed "enormous swelling" with peripapillary hemorrhages and exudates, and there was

*References 1, 13, 15, 20, 28, 32, 37.

extension of edema into the posterior pole associated with a macular star figure of hard exudate. The patient subsequently developed a patch of choroiditis adjacent to the left optic disc. Serologic tests for syphilis were positive, and the patient was treated with procaine penicillin daily for 3 weeks. Over the next 5 months, the vision in the left eye gradually improved to 20/40, the optic disc swelling resolved, and the hemorrhages and exudates disappeared. Neuroretinitis occasionally occurs in patients with late syphilis, usually in victims with meningovascular neurosyphilis.[1] The condition is indistinguishable from that which affects patients with secondary syphilis.

Lyme disease is another spirochetosis that is associated with neuroretinitis. Almost all cases occur in patients with stage II Lyme disease.[3,24,35,36] Like the neuroretinitis that occurs in syphilis, the neuroretinitis of Lyme disease may be unilateral or bilateral—but when bilateral, it is usually simultaneous and symmetric. Also, like the neuroretinitis of syphilis, the neuroretinitis that occurs in Lyme disease may recover spontaneously, but it also resolves rapidly once the patient is treated with appropriate antibiotics.[1]

Leptospira were identified in the cerebrospinal fluid in one of three patients with neuroretinitis who all had unilateral visual loss and bilateral small, deep, intraretinal lesions consistent with septic retinitis.[11] The patient in whom the leptospira were detected had no evidence of leptospirosis. No infectious agent was identified in blood or CSF in the remaining two patients.

Patients with toxoplasmosis, toxocariasis, and histoplasmosis may develop an acute anterior optic neuritis that, in rare cases, may be associated with a macular star figure.[4,6,10,14,26] Whether or not such conditions are truly examples of neuroretinitis is unclear. Any presumed or known inflammatory or infectious optic neuropathy that is characterized by optic disc swelling and the eventual development of a macular star figure should be defined as neuroretinitis.[39] Thus these cases fit that description. On the other hand, there are noninfectious or noninflammatory conditions that should not be called neuroretinitis, even though they are characterized by optic disc swelling that may occasionally be associated with the development of a macular star figure. These mimicking conditions include papilledema, anterior ischemic optic neuropathy, infiltration of the optic disc by tumor (Fig. 50-11), and peripapillary subretinal angioma.[11,25,31] Systemic hypertension may cause both optic disc swelling and a macular star figure, but fluorescein angiography in such cases shows leakage from macular vessels. A similar phenomenon may occur in diffuse unilateral subacute neuroretinitis (DUSN), thought to be caused by one or more types of helminths.

One condition that is **not** associated with neuroretinitis is multiple sclerosis. A valid assumption is that because neuroretinitis is a form of optic neuritis, the likelihood of developing multiple sclerosis after an attack of neuroretinitis is as high as it seems to be after an attack of straightforward optic

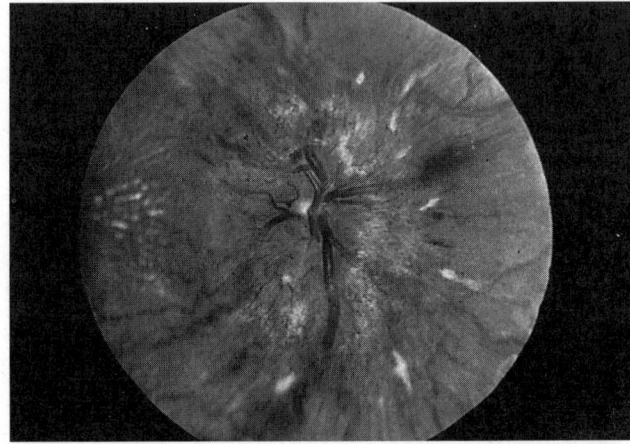

A

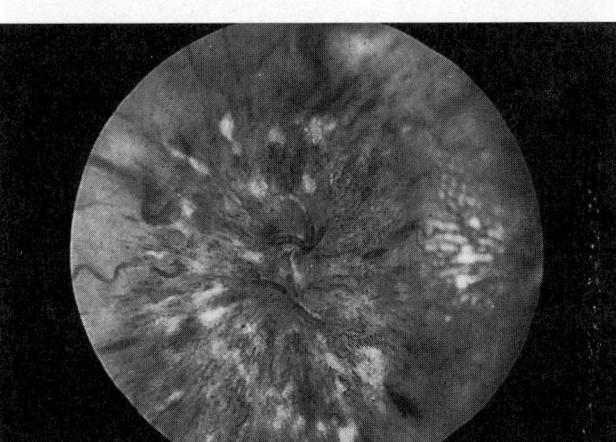

B

Fig. 50-11. Bilateral, severe papilledema associated with lipid star figures in the macula. This patient had symptoms of increased intracranial pressure, and an evaluation revealed pseudotumor cerebri. The papilledema (and the exudate) resolved once intracranial pressure was normalized. **A,** right fundus; **B,** left fundus.

neuritis. In fact, although the rate of development of multiple sclerosis after an attack of anterior or retrobulbar optic neuritis is about 70% over 15 years,[34] there is no increased tendency for patients who experience an attack of neuroretinitis to develop multiple sclerosis.[33] The rate of development of multiple sclerosis in such patients is the same as that in the normal population, about 6 to 80 per 100,000. Thus the designation of an attack of acute optic neuropathy as an episode of neuroretinitis rather than anterior optic neuritis substantially alters the systemic prognosis in the patient being evaluated.

LABORATORY INVESTIGATIONS

Investigation into the cause of neuroretinitis should have a systematic approach. A careful history is crucial and should include questioning regarding sexually transmitted diseases, skin rashes, and viral exanthema. Complete physical and ocular examinations are also essential, and a neurologic examination may be required.

Patients with secondary or tertiary syphilis, for example, usually provide a history of previous sexual contact; and they may have had a chancre in the past. They may also complain of arthralgias and myalgias, and some have symptoms of meningitis or encephalopathy. Many of these patients have been treated for syphilis or some other sexually transmitted disease in the past.

Patients with stage 2 Lyme disease usually live or work in an endemic area and may even give a history of a tick bite within the last 6 months. They often have cutaneous, cardiac, or neurologic manifestations in addition to visual complaints. The most common cutaneous manifestation is a solitary red or violaceous abnormality that ranges in size from a small nodule to a plaque that is several centimeters in diameter. The lesion is called a "lymphocytoma" or "lymphadenosis benigna cutis." It may appear at the site of the tick bite or remote from it. Typical remote sites are the ear lobe in children and the nipple in adults. Cardiac manifestations occur in about 5% to 8% of patients with stage 2 Lyme disease. The most common abnormality is fluctuating atrioventricular block that may progress to asystole. Other cardiac disorders that may occur in patients with stage 2 Lyme disease include myocarditis, cardiomyopathy, and pericarditis. Such patients may complain of chest pain, difficulty breathing, or episodic fainting spells. Neurologic manifestations occur in 10% to 15% of cases of stage 2 Lyme disease and include meningitis, myelitis, encephalitis, cranial neuropathies, meningoradiculitis, and peripheral neuropathies. Patients with these disturbances may have a variety of complaints. More than one of these disturbances may develop in a single patient who is often said to have neuroborreliosis. Some patients with neuroretinitis caused by Lyme disease have other ocular disturbances including unilateral or bilateral granulomatous iridocyclitis, choroiditis, pars planitis, vitritis, and panophthalmitis. Intraocular vascular disturbances, such as retinal perivasculitis, branch retinal artery occlusion, recurrent vitreous hemorrhage, sheathing of retinal vessels, and intraretinal hemorrhages are also common in such patients. Fluorescein angiography may reveal areas of nonperfusion in one or both eyes in these patients.

Patients with cat scratch fever usually have a history of contact with a cat. They complain of malaise, fever, muscle aches, and headache. Examination typically reveals local lymphadenopathy. Rarely, patients may also have symptoms of arthritis, hepatitis, meningitis, or encephalitis.

If there is no history suggesting an underlying inflammatory or infectious disease, and the patient has no clinical evidence of such a process; it probably is inappropriate to perform any serologic testing, analysis of cerebrospinal fluid, neuroimaging, or other evaluation. On the other hand, specific patients may require lumbar puncture, magnetic resonance imaging, or computed tomographic scanning, and serologic tests for syphilis, Lyme disease, toxoplasmosis,

histoplasmosis, or toxocariasis; whereas others should undergo serologic and/or skin testing for cat scratch disease. The use of molecular biologic techniques to identify viral nucleic acids in various body tissues and fluids may eventually result in identification of specific viruses that cause the condition in otherwise normal persons or in persons who have recently suffered what seems to be a viral illness. At this time, however, a recommendation cannot be made to use such techniques on a regular basis, because they are both time consuming and expensive. Patients in whom neuroretinitis is accompanied by diffuse retinal or choroidal lesions suggesting septic retinitis or choroiditis may require a complete evaluation for systemic infection, including blood cultures and cardiac echography.[38]

THERAPY

Treatment of neuroretinitis depends on whether or not there is an underlying infectious or inflammatory condition that requires therapy. Cat scratch disease is thought to be caused by a pleomorphic gram-negative bacillus, and patients with CSD are usually treated with antibiotics such as trimethoprim-sulfamethoxazole, ciprofloxacin, rifampin, doxycycline, or tetracycline. Such treatment is almost always associated with improvement of the associated neuroretinitis, although whether or not the neuroretinitis would resolve spontaneously without treatment is unknown.[5,38] Patients with neuroretinitis who have secondary or late syphilis should be treated with intravenous penicillin as recommended by the Centers for Disease Control,[8] and patients with neuroretinitis that occurs in the setting of Lyme disease should also be treated with appropriate antibiotics such as ceftriaxone, amoxacillin, or tetracycline.[24] Patients in whom neuroretinitis is found to be associated with evidence of toxoplasmosis, toxocariasis, or histoplasmosis should likewise undergo treatment specific for their underlying systemic disease.

Patients with presumed viral or idiopathic neuroretinitis may or may not require treatment. Some authors have advocated the use of systemic corticosteroids or adrenocorticotrophic hormone (ACTH) to treat isolated neuroretinitis, but there is no definite evidence that such treatment alters either the speed of recovery of the condition or the ultimate outcome. Interestingly, Weiss and Beck[38] reported a case of idiopathic neuroretinitis that did not respond to treatment with oral prednisone but improved rapidly and dramatically when intravenous corticosteroids were given.

PROGNOSIS

As noted previously, the ultimate prognosis for most cases of Leber's idiopathic neuroretinitis is excellent. The majority of patients achieve good visual recovery, although there is a subgroup of sufferers who develop optic atrophy and poor vision. These patients typically have very poor visual acuity from the beginning of the process, significant visual field loss at presentation, and a marked, relative, afferent, pupillary defect if the condition is unilateral or asymmetric.[25] Nevertheless, even patients with profound loss of visual function may recover normal or near normal vision over time.

REFERENCES

1. Arruga J, Valentines J, Mauri F et al.: Neuroretinitis in acquired syphilis, *Ophthalmology* 92:262-270, 1985.
2. Bar S, Segal M, Shapira R, Savir H: Neuroretinitis associated with cat scratch disease, *Am J Ophthalmol* 110:703-705, 1990.
3. Bialiasiewicz AA, Huk W, Druschky KF, Naumann GOH: Borrelia burgdorferi-Infektion mit beidseitiger Neuritis nervic optici und intrazerebralen Demyelinisierungsherden, *Klin Monatsbl Augenheilkd* 195:91-94, 1989.
4. Bird AC, Smith JL, Curtin VT: Neomatode optic neuritis, *Am J Ophthalmol* 69:72-77, 1984.
5. Brazis PW, Stokes HR, Ervin FR: Optic neuritis in cat scratch disease, *J Clin Neuroophthalmol* 6:172-174, 1986.
6. Brown GC, Tasman WS: Retinal arterial obstruction in association with presumed toxocara canis neuroretinitis, *Ann Ophthalmol* 13:1385-1387, 1981.
7. Carroll DM, Franklin RM: Leber's idiopathic stellate retinopathy, *Am J Ophthalmol* 93:96-101, 1982.
8. Centers for Disease Control: 1989 Sexually transmitted diseases treatment guidelines, *MMWR* 38(suppl 8):9, 1989.
9. Chrousos GA, Drack AV, Young M et al.: Neuroretinitis in cat scratch disease, *J Clin Neuroophthalmol* 10:92-94, 1990.
10. Cox TA, Haskins GE, Gangitano JL et al.: Bilateral toxocara optic neuropathy, *J Clin Neuroophthalmol* 3:267-274, 1983.
11. Dreyer RF, Hopen G, Gass DM, Smith JL: Leber's idiopathic stellate neuroretinitis, *Arch Ophthalmol* 102:1140-1145, 1984.
12. Farthing CF, Howard RS, Thin RN: Papillitis and hepatitis B, *BMJ* 292:1712, 1986.
13. Fewell AG: Unilateral neuroretinitis of syphilitic origin with a striate figure in the macula, *Arch Ophthalmol* 8:615, 1932.
14. Folk JC, Lobes LA: Presumed toxoplasmic papillitis, *Ophthalmology* 91:64-67, 1984.
15. Folk JC, Weingeist TA, Corbett JJ et al.: Syphilitic neuroretinitis, *Am J Ophthalmol* 95:480-496, 1983.
16. Foster RE, Lowder CY, Meisler DM et al.: Mumps neuroretinitis in an adolescent, *Am J Ophthalmol* 110:91-93, 1990.
17. Gass JDM: Diseases of the optic nerve that may simulate macular disease, *Trans Am Acad Ophthalmol Otolaryngol* 83:766-769, 1977.
18. Graveson GS: Syphilitic optic neuritis, *J Neurol Neurosurg Psychiatr* 13:216-224, 1950.
19. Guillaume J-B, Risse JF, Rovira JC: Neurorétinite aigue: discussion nosologique à propos d'un cas chez un adulte jeune, *Bull Soc Ophthalmol Fr* 91:39-42, 1991.
20. Halperin LS: Neuroretinitis due to seronegative syphilis associated with human immunodeficiency virus, *J Clin Neuroophthalmol* 12:171-172, 1992.
21. Johnson BL, Wisetzley HM: Neuroretinitis associated with herpes simplex encephalitis in an adult, *Am J Ophthalmol* 83:481-489, 1977.
22. King MN, Cartwright MJ, Carney MD: Leber's idiopathic neuroretinitis, *Arch Ophthalmol* 23:58-60, 1991.
23. Leber T: Pseudonephritic retinal disease, stellate retinitis; the angiopathic retinal affections after severe skull injury. In Graefe-Saemisch Handb Ges Augenheilkd 7:1319, 1916.
24. Lesser RL, Kornmehl EW, Pachner AR et al.: Neuro-ophthalmologic manifestations of Lyme disease, *Ophthalmology* 97:699-706, 1990.
25. Maitland CG, Miller NR: Neuroretinitis, *Arch Ophthalmol* 102:1146-1150, 1984.
26. Manschot WA, Daamen CBF: Connatal ocular toxoplasmosis, *Arch Ophthalmol* 74:48, 1965.
27. Margolis T, Irvine AR, Hoyt WF, Hyman R: Acute retinal necrosis syndrome presenting with papillitis and acute neuroretinitis, *Ophthalmology* 95:937-940, 1988.
28. McLeish WM, Pulido JS, Holland S et al.: The ocular manifestations of syphilis in the human immunodeficiency virus type 1—infected host, *Ophthalmology* 97:196-203, 1990.
29. Miller NR: *Walsh and Hoyt's clinical neuro-ophthalmology,* ed 4, 234-235, vol 1, Baltimore, 1982, Williams and Wilkins.
30. Miller NR, Fine SL: The ocular fundus in neuro-ophthalmologic diagnosis, St Louis, 1977, Mosby.
31. Neetens A, Smets RM: Leber's neurogenic stellate maculopathy, *Neuro-ophthalmology* 6:315-328, 1987.
32. Ninomiya H, Hamada T, Akiya S, Kazama H: Three cases of acute syphilitic neuroretinitis, *Folia Ophthalmol Jpn* 41:2088-2094, 1990.
33. Parmley VC, Schiffman JS, Maitland CG et al.: Does neuroretinitis rule out multiple sclerosis? *Arch Neurol* 44:1045-1048, 1987.
34. Rizzo JF, Lessell S: Risk of developing multiple sclerosis after uncomplicated optic neuritis: a long-term prospective study, *Neurology* 38:185-190, 1988.
35. Schönherr U, Lang GE, Meythaler FH: Bilaterale Lebersche Neuroretinitis stellata bei Borrelia burgdorferi-Serokonversion, *Klin Monatsbl Augenheilkd* 198:44-47, 1991.
36. Schönherr U, Wilk CM, Lang GE, Naumann GOH: Intraocular manifestations of Lyme borreliosis. Presented at the Fourth International Conference on Borreliosis, Stockholm, Sweden, June 18-21, 1990.
37. Veldman E, Bos PJM: Neuroretinitis in secondary syphilis, *Doc Ophthalmol* 64:23-29, 1986.
38. Weiss AH, Beck RW: Neuroretinitis in childhood, *J Pediatr Ophthalmol* 26:198-203, 1989.
39. Williams N, Miller, N: Unpublished data.

51 Orbital Inflammatory Disease

LYNN K. GORDON, ROBERT A. GOLDBERG, HOWARD R. KRAUSS

Many authors have attempted to characterize the orbital inflammatory syndromes according to various parameters. One classification by Rootman and Nugent[98] differentiated these lesions on the basis of orbital location. They reviewed the histories of 484 patients with orbital disease who were seen at the University of British Columbia Orbital Clinic over a 6-year period. Of these, only 23 patients had orbital inflammatory disease, excluding Graves related orbitopathy. These patients were then classified on the basis of location within the orbit including anterior, diffuse, posterior, lacrimal, and myositic.[72,98] A different classification was proposed by Kennerdell and Dresner.[60] They divided these patients into acute and chronic forms, and then further classified them according to predominant tissue involvement including myositis, dacryoadenitis, periscleritis, and perineuritis. Other classifications have been made on the basis of histopathology including lymphocytic, granulomatous, or sclerosing.[37,81] There is value to all of these systems and a combined approach is used in this text.

HISTORICAL BACKGROUND

Orbital pseudotumor is a term first used by Birch-Hirschfeld in the early 1900s to describe nonneoplastic causes of orbital lesions that simulated tumors. Since that time there have been great advances in laboratory diagnosis and radiologic imaging techniques that permit specific diagnoses in cases of orbital "pseudotumor." A better term is *orbital inflammatory disease*. This encompasses idiopathic orbital inflammation, orbital inflammation associated with systemic disease, the spectrum of lymphoid-related inflammatory orbital disease, and infectious causes of orbital inflammation. These disease syndromes, with the exception of infectious orbital cellulitis and Graves related orbitopathy, are the subject of this chapter.

CLINICAL APPROACH

Orbital inflammatory disease occurs in every age group, in men and women, and in every race. Bilateral involvement

is seen but may indicate a young age-of-onset or an underlying systemic illness.[120] The differential diagnosis of idiopathic orbital inflammatory disease includes Graves disease, orbital cellulitis, fungal infections, lymphoma or leukemia, vasculitides, periorbital sinus disease, primary tumors, metastatic tumors, ruptured dermoid cysts, retained foreign body, eosinophilic granuloma, and sarcoidosis.* Intraocular melanomas have been shown to occasionally present with orbital inflammation.[99]

In any patient with an acute orbital inflammatory process, orbital cellulitis must be considered, and aggressive therapy for possible infection may be instituted while proceeding with a complete diagnostic evaluation. Acute idiopathic orbital inflammation is characterized by the sudden onset of pain, periorbital swelling, erythema, proptosis, possible limitation in ocular movement, and chemosis. Intraocular changes may accompany the orbital signs. These include uveitis, papillitis, and exudative retinal detachment. In posterior acute inflammatory processes optic nerve dysfunction may be an early finding. Patients with the chronic form of nonspecific orbital inflammation often have severe visual loss and ophthalmoplegia. Chronic periorbital edema may be the predominant sign in chronic lesions.[69] Recurrence of disease may occur over a time period of many years.[15]

The evaluation of patients with orbital inflammatory disease includes a careful history and physical examination, laboratory evaluation, and diagnostic imaging. Prompt and appropriate therapy is then chosen in response to these examinations. The history should include antecedent trauma, a history of possible sinus disease, known systemic illnesses, constitutional symptoms, and known malignancy. The details of the chief complaint must be elucidated including rapidity of onset, duration, bilateral or unilateral symptoms, presence of diplopia, and possible alteration in visual func-

---

*References 14, 15, 27, 37, 48, 57, 60, 69, 72, 79, 96, 98, 99, 119, 121, 123, 128, 129, 130.

tion. The physical examination is a thorough ocular and orbital evaluation. Blood work might include a complete blood count, erythrocyte sedimentation rate, angiotensin-converting enzyme, serum lysozyme, rheumatoid factor, antinuclear antibody screen, antineutrophil cytoplasmic antibodies (ANCA), serum protein electrophoresis, and serum cryoglobulin.[48,55,60,82] Evaluation of the cerebrospinal fluid may be required.

Diagnostic imaging is a critical portion of the evaluation and is invaluble in the differential diagnosis.* Ultrasonography typically identifies inflammatory changes that produce low internal reflectivity and poorly delineated margins. Sub-Tenon fluid may be identified in patients with anterior orbital inflammations. The tendinous insertions of the extraocular muscles are often involved in myositic inflammatory disease in contrast to the more posterior myositic involvement in Graves-related orbitopathy. Computed tomography or magnetic resonance imaging are helpful in the evaluation of orbital inflammations.[36,112] These tests can fully image the involvement of adjacent sinuses, can demonstrate bony changes, and can identify which orbital structure (or structures) are predominantly involved. Bony erosion and or sinus involvement is not a typical sign of idiopathic inflammation but may indicate bacterial or fungal cellulitis, vasculitis, an infected mucocele, malignancy, or a ruptured dermoid cyst.[132] One interesting case of orbital inflammation had a soft-tissue density in the sphenoid sinus without other sinus-related complaints.[81] This patient had an aspergilloma of the sphenoid sinus and required surgical removal of this abnormal material with complete resolution of the orbital disease. Neuroradiologic imaging is also critical in evaluating the extent of posterior or apical orbital inflammatory changes. Frohman and associates[36] described three patients who had diffuse, posterior orbital inflammation with intracranial extension and associated bony changes.

THERAPEUTIC APPROACH

The acute orbital inflammations are generally exquisitely sensitive to oral corticosteroids, often given in a dosage of 1 mg per kg of oral prednisone per day as a starting dose. Some patients are steroid intolerant, are refractory to corticosteroids, become steroid dependent, or have frequent or severe recurrent disease. These patients usually need a different treatment modality. Radiotherapy in low doses has been used to successfully treat some patients with orbital inflammatory disease of several histologic types.[61,66,104] Low-dose radiotherapy is well tolerated and usually does not produce ocular complications. There are occasional patients with orbital inflammatory disease who are refractory to both corticosteroids and radiation therapy. These patients may be treated with pulsed-chemotherapy consisting of cyclophosphamide or chlorambucil with prednisone.[91] Low-dose methotrexate has also been used.[105] This type of combination pharmacologic therapy has produced encouraging results with low morbidity in refractory patients.[35]

LYMPHOID LESIONS

Clinical Features

Accurate diagnosis of predominantly lymphoid lesions in association with orbital inflammatory disease is critical.[52,53] Specifically, neoplastic lesions must be differentiated from nonneoplastic lesions for the patient to receive the appropriate systemic evaluation and therapeutic intervention. Three categories of lymphoid lesions have been identified in association with an orbital inflammatory appearance. The first is reactive lymphoid hyperplasia, which occurs in both a diffuse and a follicular pattern. These lesions show mature lymphocytes, increased vascularity, and (possibly) germinal center formation. Second, there are lesions with atypical lymphocytic infiltration. Patients with this diagnosis have a higher frequency of subsequent malignancy than the patients with reactive hyperplasia. Third, there are lymphocytic lymphomas that initially present in association with an inflammatory appearance. These demonstrate a monomorphic collection of cells and are not the topic for this discussion.

These lesions can occur anywhere in the orbit but are particularly prevalent in the lacrimal gland and orbital fat. A number of cases have also been described with primary involvement of the extraocular muscles.[49] Rarely, lymphoid disease may be associated with systemic illness, for example myasthenia gravis.[119]

The evaluation usually includes a systemic lymphoma evaluation with the coordinated efforts of the oncologist. Ultrasonography characteristically shows a low reflective lesion with indistinct margins that often molds to the globe and associated structures. Neuroimaging also confirms the location of the orbital pathology.

The histopathology of these lesions may present challenges to the accurate pathologic diagnosis. Often these lesions need to be evaluated with immunologic techniques to check for clonality and expression of particular cell markers on T cells and kappa and lambda light chain markers on B cells.[54,119] Fine needle aspiration cytology is often quite accurate in making the appropriate diagnosis, but a larger sample of abnormal tissue, obtained either with multiple fine needle passes or with incisional biopsy, may be required for complete immunologic analysis.[7] Whereas monoclonal lesions are malignant, genetic analysis suggests the presence of malignant transformation-producing small clones of monoclonal B cells within some lesions that are grossly polyclonal on immunocytologic study.[53a]

Sixty patients with orbital lymphoid abnormalities were

---

*References 20, 40, 77, 85, 89, 112, 114, 136.

reviewed by Knowles and Jacobiec.[65] They found that 15% were benign, 29% had an atypical lymphoid hyperplasia, and the majority had a form of lymphoma. The large number of patients in this series with lymphoma may represent a particular tertiary care-referral pattern. Thirty-seven patients with lymphoid orbital disease were reviewed by Barthold II and associates.[10] Almost 80% of these patients had benign disease at the time of presentation. There has been a concern regarding the possible progression of benign lymphoid lesions to frank lymphoma. Evidence in the literature suggests that this transition occurs in a small percentage of patients.

Therapy

Treatment of the benign form of lymphoid-related orbital inflammatory disease consists of a trial of oral corticosteroids with supplemental radiotherapy.[5,8,10,117] Lower doses of radiotherapy are required to achieve a complete therapeutic response in benign lesions. Malignant lymphomas require more aggressive therapy. The dose of radiotherapy is quite important because of the potential for complications such as dry eyes, cataract, retinal vascular lesions, and optic neuropathy.

SCLEROSING ORBITAL INFLAMMATION

Clinical Features

Idiopathic sclerosing orbital inflammation (orbital cementum) is a distinct diagnosis that often results in significant and permanent alterations in visual function and ocular motility. As such, it is critical to make a timely and accurate diagnosis for the initiation of early aggressive treatment.*

The largest series of patients with this disorder was recently reported.[99] The authors found that 16 patients had idiopathic sclerosing orbital inflammation over the period of 1979 to 1991, and that these patients represented 7.8% of the total number of patients with orbital inflammatory disease. In addition, they reviewed the data from 19 other cases reported in the literature. The typical presentation of a patient with this form of orbital inflammation includes a chronic, insidious, and progressive course of pain, exophthalmos, variable inflammation, restriction of extraocular movements, and visual loss (Fig. 51-1). Bilateral disease was present in 12.5% of patients. The age-of-onset ranged from 12 to 72 years and there was no sexual predilection. They found that most disease began either in the lacrimal region or in the apical region of the orbit, with relative sparring of the inferior and medial compartments. One case of sclerosing orbital inflammation of the lacrimal gland also involved ectopic lacrimal gland tissue of the orbit.[71] In late stages of the

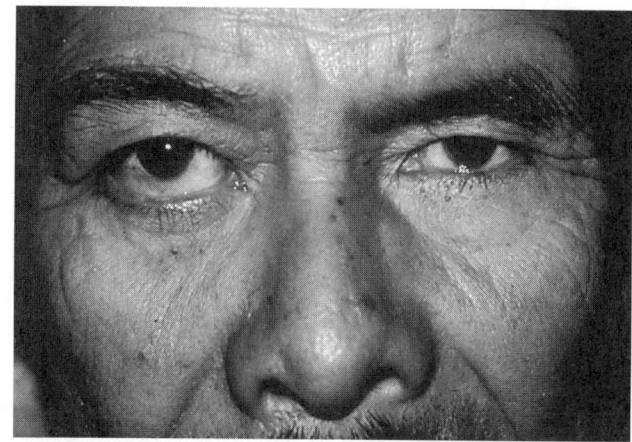

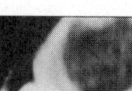

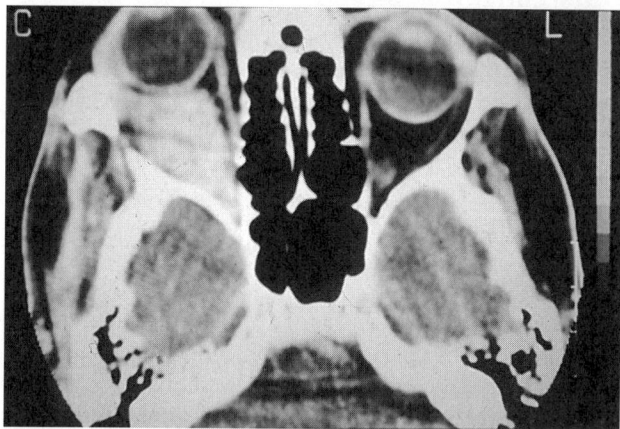

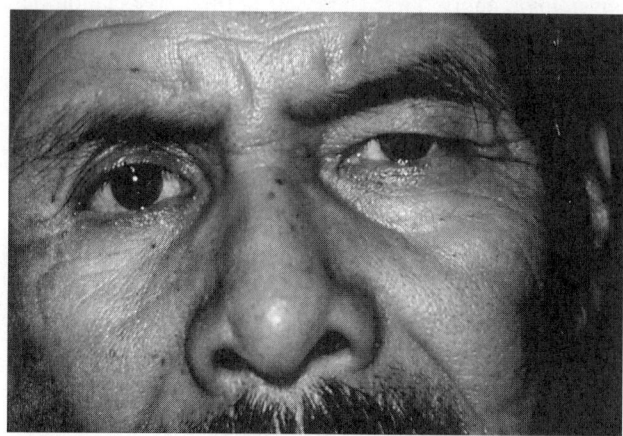

Fig. 51-1. **A,** Idiopathic sclerosing orbital inflammation presenting as a slowly growing, mildly painful orbital mass in an otherwise healthy 55-year-old man. **B,** Computed tomography (CT) demonstrates a localized "moulding" mass in the inferolateral orbit. **C,** The mass decreased in size and stabilized following surgical debulking, steroid therapy, and radiotherapy 2500 cGy.

---

*References 1, 24, 73, 95, 97, 103, 125, 127, 133.

disease there can be extensions into other vital tissues, and there may even be extension of disease along the tissue planes into the intracranial space. Bony involvement is rare and is more typically found in ruptured dermoids, Wegener granulomatosis reactive giant-cell lesion, or mucormycosis.[89]

Neuroradiologic imaging is often helpful in evaluation of sclerosing orbital inflammation. Computed tomography (CT) demonstrates a homogeneously enhancing mass with irregular borders and involvement of multiple orbital tissues. When located in the orbital apex there have been neuroradiologic misdiagnoses of meningiomas.[1] MRI imaging also shows the irregular nature of this disease and often has an intermediate signal intensity on T1 weighted images.

Differential Diagnosis

The differential diagnosis of sclerosing orbital inflammation is large and includes Wegener granulomatosis, tuberculosis, neoplasms, lymphoma, and Graves related orbital disease. Orbital biopsy is needed to establish the correct diagnosis. Histologic evaluation of sclerosing inflammatory lesions reveals significant fibrosis with an associated paucicellular, lymphoplasmacytic infiltrate.[73]

Pathogenesis

In early papers authors suggested that sclerosing orbital inflammation was not a distinct clinical entity but rather a common end-stage pattern after a chronic lymphocytic inflammatory process.[6,13,37,47] Several features of this disease, however, are more compatible with it as a unique pathophysiologic entity. First, there has been an association between orbital inflammatory disease of the sclerosing variant and systemic sclerosing diseases. A particularly interesting family was described in 1966[24] in which two family members were affected with a variety of illnesses including retroperitoneal fibrosis, mediastinal fibrosis, sclerosing cholangitis, Riedel's thyroiditis, and orbital inflammatory disease. The association between orbital inflammation and retroperitoneal fibrosis has subsequently been confirmed in other patients.[67,95,103] Second, the histopathology of sclerosing orbital pseudotumor closely resembles retroperitoneal fibrosis.[73] Immunohistochemistry was used to evaluate specimens from sclerosing orbital inflammation and retroperitoneal fibrosis patients. The cellular pattern seen in these specimens consisted variably of plasma cells, T-lymphocytes, B-lymphocytes, histiocytes, and HLA-DR positive cells. A similar cellular pattern has been seen in specimens from patients with retroperitoneal fibrosis. The plasma cells showed positivity for IgG, IgM, and IgA with equal amounts of both kappa and lambda light chain. This observation invokes the possibility of an immune-mediated inflammatory process, however; the driving antigenic stimulus and precise pathophysiology are obscure. An immunohistologic study of orbital pseudotumor revealed eosinophil infiltration in asso-

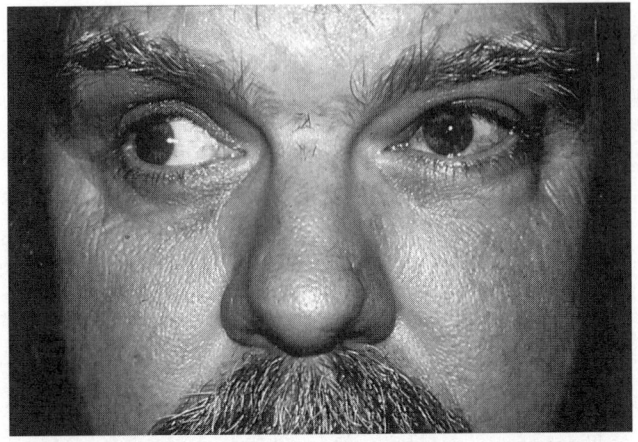

A

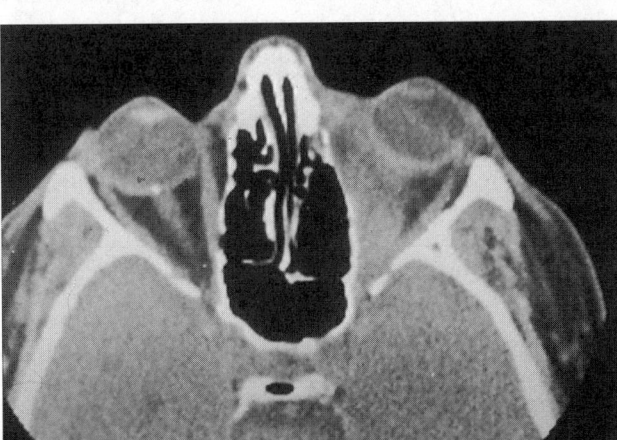

B

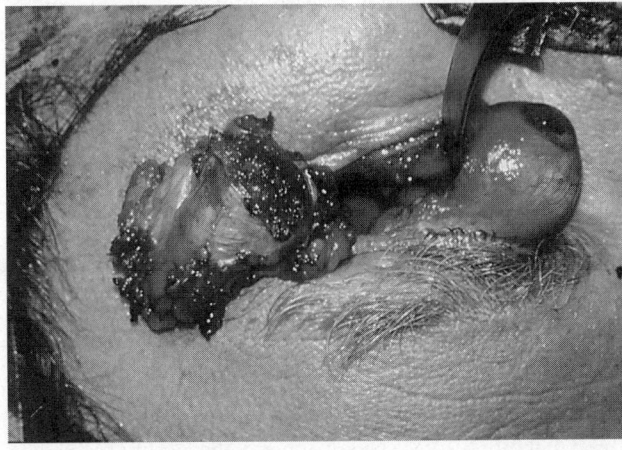

C

Fig. 51-2. **A,** Idiopathic sclerosing orbital inflammation presenting as a relentlessly progressing orbital apical mass. **B,** CT demonstrates an infiltrative lesion of the medial orbit and apex. **C,** Despite high-dose steroid therapy, radiotherapy, and cytotoxic drug therapy, the tumor continued to grow, resulting in intractable pain and orbital apical dysfunction with loss of vision. Globe-sparing exenteration was required for pain control and to prevent spread into the cavernous sinus.

ciation with neutrophils and plasma cells as well as evidence of eosinophil degranulation (cytotoxic extracellular eosinophil granule major basic protein in inflamed areas with degrees of fibrosis).[81] Eosinophil infiltration may be a selective response to local chenio-tactic stimuli and that the toxic effect of eosinophil degranulation is associated with subsequent fibrosis.

Therapy

Treatment of sclerosing orbital inflammation is difficult because of the poor response to traditional therapy (Fig. 51-2). Surgical excision of the lesion is appropriate if the lesion is well demarcated, but most sclerosing orbititis involves a diffuse, poorly delineated process. Steroid therapy yields a significant, stable response in less than 30% of patients.* Of the patients that failed steroid therapy, 50% responded to orbital irradiation in the series described by Rootman.[97] Five additional patients have been described who have received radiotherapy for this process, with significant response in two and a partial response in two others. Aggressive treatment of sclerosing orbital inflammation has been suggested using other immunosuppressives such as azathioprine or cyclophosphamide. The underlying rationale was that these agents are successful in the treatment of retroperitoneal fibrosis and should be equally effective in the orbital form of the disease. They have only been occasionally successful, however, in the few patients described in the ophthalmologic literature. Approximately 20% of patients lost visual functioning to the level of legal blindness. Early, aggressive treatment may provide a better visual and functional outcome.

ORBITAL MYOSITIS

Clinical Features

Idiopathic orbital myositis is a common presentation of orbital inflammatory disease. The characteristic symptom of these patients is an acute or, less commonly, a subacute or chronic inflammation primarily affecting the extraocular muscles.† There is usually pain on extraocular movement with diplopia and limitation of ocular excursions in the direction of the affected muscle or muscles (Fig. 51-3). There may be proptosis, chemosis, lid edema, and ptosis. Unilateral or bilateral involvement is observed.

Differential Diagnosis

The diagnosis is based on clinical examination, ultrasonography, neuroradiologic imaging, and a dramatic therapeutic response to oral corticosteroids. Biopsy is usually un-

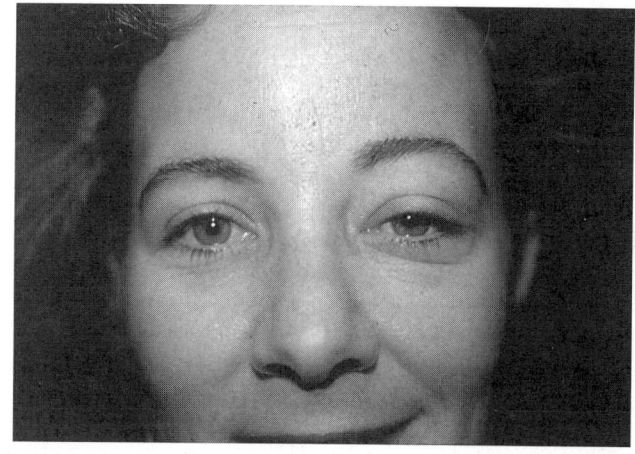
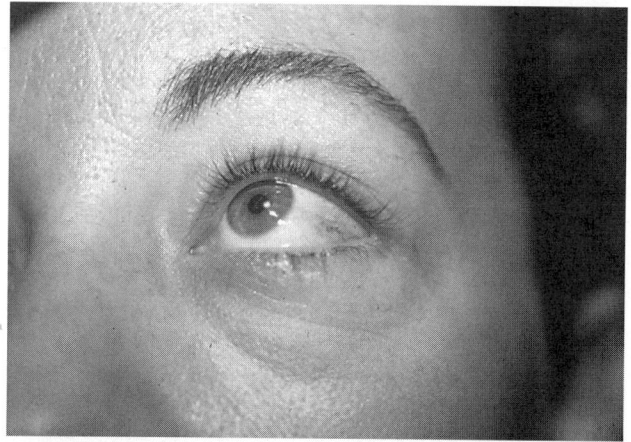
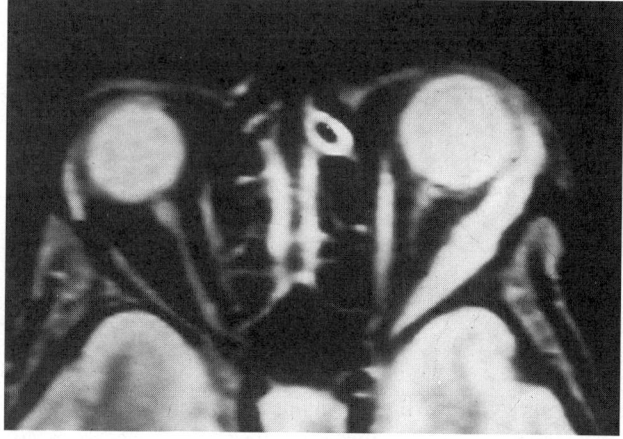

Fig. 51-3. A, Left lateral rectus myositis presenting with proptosis, lid edema and erythema, and decreased ductions. **B,** Ocular examination shows localized inflammatory changes in association with the insertion of the tendon. **C,** CT demonstrates involvement of the entire lateral rectus muscle with involvement of the tendon.

*References 1, 22, 36, 37, 42, 58, 59, 80, 104, 124.
†References 18, 70, 96, 101, 106, 109.

necessary in orbital myositis. The differential diagnosis includes Graves-related orbital disease, arteriovenous fistula, Tolosa-Hunt syndrome, orbital metastasis, trichinosis, Whipple disease, myositis associated with HIV or herpes zoster virus infections, and giant cell polymyositis.[32,54,86,122] One interesting patient with underlying chronic progressive external ophthalmoplegia developed orbital myositis involving the levator palpebrae, which caused proptosis, lid swelling, and elevation of the eyelid.[128] Laboratory evaluation should be considered and might include complete blood count with differential, erythrocyte sedimentation rate, immunologic tests for *Trichinella,* thyroid function tests, serum muscle enzymes, serum complement, cryoglobulins, antinuclear antibodies, and rheumatoid factor.

Ultrasonography is a useful tool in the evaluation of muscular involvement in orbital inflammatory diseases. A-scan imaging allows the measurement of the thickness of the extraocular muscle and the identification of the characteristics of internal reflectivity. B-scan imaging allows the topographic assessment of the extraocular muscle and its insertion into the globe. Comparison of the two orbits using B-scan technology allows for the analysis of relative size discrepancies of the extraocular muscles and insertions. It also is helpful in identifying enlargements of the superior ophthalmic vein. In orbital myositis there is enlargement of the involved muscle with a low internal reflectivity and involvement of the tendinous insertion. There may be associated chorioretinal thickening and edema of the orbital tissue. Ultrasonography is also helpful in differentiating orbital myositis from Graves-associated orbitopathy in which the muscles usually show no involvement of the tendinous insertion and a normal internal reflectivity.

On computed tomographic imaging of these cases the involved muscle or muscles show a diffuse enlargement with irregular margins and involvement of the tendinous insertion. These features help to distinguish this process from Graves-related orbital disease because the enlargement of muscle in Graves disease is usually fusiform with relative sparing of the tendinous insertion. Magnetic resonance imaging may be more sensitive than CT when evaluating patients with orbital myositis involving the oblique muscles.

Pathogenesis

Histology shows both lymphocytic and polycellular infiltrations in orbital myositis. The cause of this disease is not known, but there are many immunologic clues suggestive of an autoimmune-triggered disease. In several series of patients orbital myositis followed upper respiratory infections and was postulated to be immune-mediated.[74,75,93] In at least one patient there was marked elevation of IgG, IgM, and immune complexes by cryoprecipitation.[70] The majority of patients with idiopathic orbital myositis do not undergo extensive immunologic testing prior to initiation of therapy, and it is possible that increased testing may yield other clues about the pathogenesis of this fascinating disease.

Therapy

Initial treatment of orbital myositis consists of high-dose corticosteroids, which usually produce a dramatic improvement in both signs and symptoms, with complete recovery. There are special cases, however, which either do not adequately respond to steroid treatment or relapse.[70] In refractory cases, low-dose radiotherapy with protection of the globe has been successful. Other pharmacologic agents, such as cyclosporin[101] and low-dose methotrexate,[105] have also been reported effective in patients refractory to corticosteroids. In patients who do not follow the usual clinical course or therapeutic response, orbital biopsy should be considered.

TROCHLEITIS

Clinical Features

A subgroup of patients with inflammations involving ocular muscles have isolated trochleitis with associated superior oblique myositis.[118,134] This group of patients generally complain of a generalized aching sensation of the orbit with accompanying headache and occasional stabbing pains. In less than 50% of patients the pain is aggravated by eye movement. Diplopia is an uncommon complaint. On examination these patients may have localized injection in the region of the superior oblique insertion. Typically there is exquisite tenderness on orbital palpation in the region of the trochlea. Systemic association is occasionally seen with rheumatoid arthritis.

Ultrasonography may show thickening of the superior oblique tendon and a low internal acoustic reflectivity.[118] There is sometimes asymmetric enhancement in the region of the trochlea on computed tomography. Laboratory evaluation is usually unrevealing but may show an elevated rheumatoid factor.

Pathology

Histology was obtained on two patients with a diagnosis of trochleitis and anophthalmia secondary to distant (greater than 7 years) enucleation. These biopsies demonstrated perivascular and muscular infiltration of lymphocytes, thus suggestive of an inflammatory process.

Therapy

Trochleitis is extremely responsive to systemic or locally injected corticosteroids. It is often self-limited within several months of onset if untreated; and despite differing treatment regimens, it may recur. There is no long-term morbidity associated with this process.

DACRYOADENITIS

Clinical Features

Orbital inflammatory disease involving the lacrimal gland (Fig. 51-4) characteristically presents with the sudden onset of pain, tenderness, and injection and edema of the lateral upper eyelid with associated S-shaped ptosis.[29,30,60,98] This process accounted for approximately 25% of the patients with orbital inflammatory disease in the experience at the Vancouver General Hospital. These patients usually have a downward displacement of the globe and may have normal or mildly affected ocular motility. An associated optic neuropathy is rare in these patients. Generally there is no sign of systemic illness such as fever or lymphocytosis. Rarely, there may be bilateral involvement. A subgroup of patients with inflammatory disease centered in the region of the lacrimal gland experience a chronic course with scant inflammation.

Differential Diagnosis

The differential diagnosis includes infections, specific inflammatory syndromes, and either primary or metastatic neoplasia. Infections involving the lacrimal gland may include viruses such as mumps, mononucleosis, and herpes zoster and, less commonly, bacteria. These illnesses are usually associated with fever, leukocytosis, and may have associated purulence. Ruptured dermoid cysts may present with localized inflammation in the region of the lacrimal gland. These cysts have a characteristic appearance on fine needle aspiration cytology. Sarcoid may present with localized enlargement of the lacrimal gland but is usually not associated with a significant inflammatory component. Sjögren disease may also present with a localized lacrimal gland inflammation or mass. Tumors may grow in the region of the lacrimal gland and may be associated with severe pain, particularly in cases of adenoid cystic carcinomas.

Laboratory evaluation should include a complete blood count. Ultrasonography is extremely helpful in the evaluation of the lacrimal gland. In inflammatory lesions, ultrasonography will demonstrate a mass in the region of the lacrimal fossa with reduced internal reflectivity. Computed tomography usually shows enlargement of the lacrimal gland without associated bony changes. The gland usually enhances with contrast and there is often edema that involves Tenon space. Bony erosion or changes may indicate a neoplastic process.

Biopsy of the lacrimal gland using either fine needle aspiration or open techniques may be critical in defining the diagnosis and should definitely be considered in patients with atypical presentations, recurrent disease, or poor response to initial therapy. Incisional biopsy should be avoided in cases of suspected pleomorphic adenoma (benign mixed tumor) or primary malignancy of the lacrimal gland.

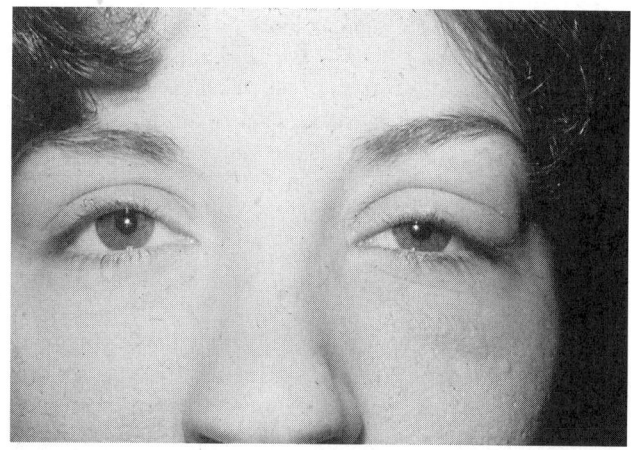

A

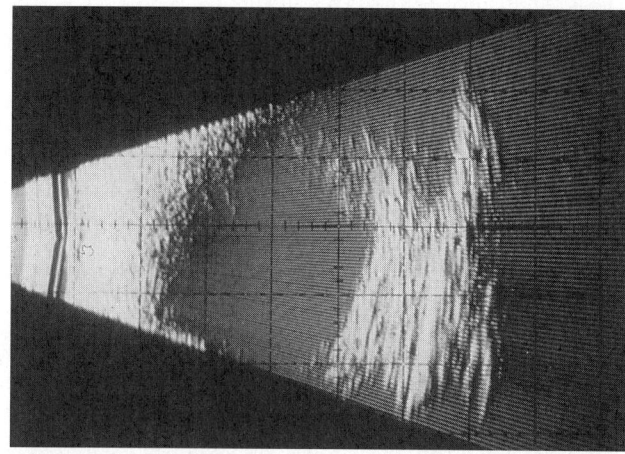

B

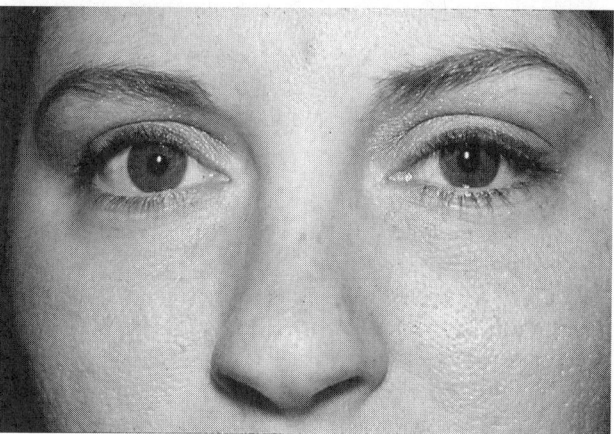

C

Fig. 51-4. **A,** Dacryoadenitis presenting with left upper lid edema and erythema in association with the typical S-shaped ptosis associated with lacrimal gland enlargement. **B,** B-mode ultrasonography demonstrating the enlarged lacrimal gland with a low internal reflectivity. **C,** Clinical photograph demonstrates the complete response to oral steroid therapy.

The acute nonspecific inflammatory process shows a polymorphous cellular infiltrate with edema and vascular dilatation. In addition, destruction of the glandular tissues is seen in cases of chronic or subacute inflammatory disease. Patterns of inflammation consisting of primarily sclerosing changes have also been seen and were discussed under a separate heading. Primary lymphocytic inflammatory disease is also considered in a separate category.

Dacryoadenitis has also been observed in association with systemic diseases. Bilateral acute inflammation of the lacrimal glands has been described in a patient with a concurrent exacerbation of Crohn disease.[30] Crohn disease is probably an immune-mediated disease, and it is possible there is an antigen that is cross-reactive in ocular and gastrointestinal tissues and is a critical factor in the propogation of the inflammatory process. HIV infection has also been associated with acute lacrimal gland inflammatory changes in at least one patient.[12] In this case a 22-year-old woman had typical acute orbital inflammatory disease with radiographic evidence of an enhancing lesion in the lacrimal fossa and involvement of the soft tissue and sclera. The initial response to systemic corticosteroids was dramatic, but within several months she developed active systemic HIV disease.

Therapy

Treatment of orbital inflammatory disease of the lacrimal gland consists of oral corticosteroids in a moderate dosage. Orbital inflammatory disease is generally extremely sensitive to systemic corticosteroids, and complete resolution is seen within 1 to 4 months. Inflammation may recur but should alert the clinician to consider other underlying diagnoses.

SCLERITIS

Clinical Features

A variant of nonspecific orbital inflammatory disease involves the sclera and has been called periscleritis.[60] This disease probably represents a continuum from posterior scleritis to periscleritis to orbital inflammatory disease.[20,78] The typical presentation involves severe pain with variable complaints of alteration in visual acuity. Associated findings may include periorbital edema, conjunctival inflammation, and uveitis (Fig. 51-5). Choroiditis, retinal edema, and retinal striae may also be seen in these patients. The disease is usually unilateral; however, bilateral cases have been reported, and recurrences are possible.

Differential Diagnosis

The differential diagnosis includes episcleritis, systemic vasculitis, infection, and herpes zoster. Careful physical and laboratory examination will help to identify the diagno-

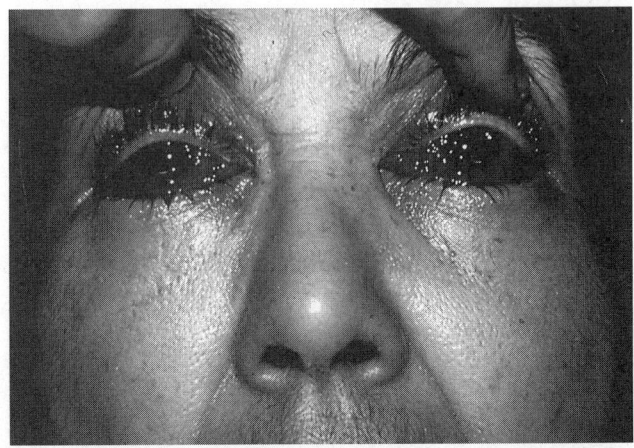

A

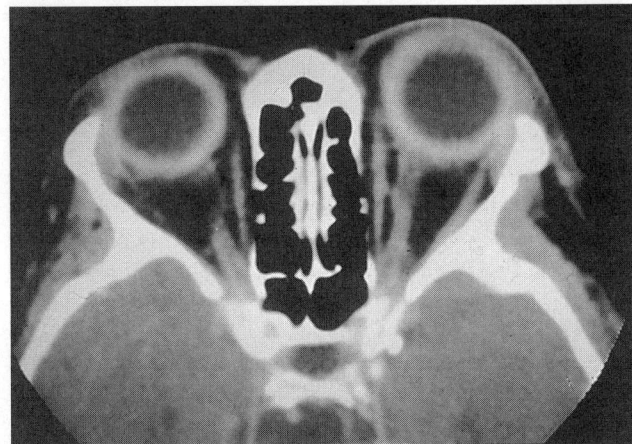

B

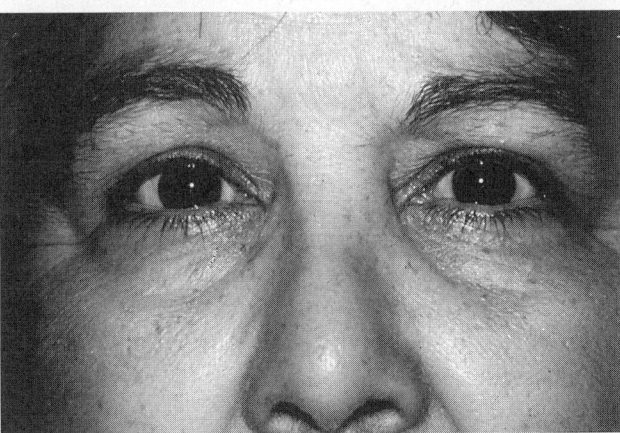

C

Fig. 51-5. **A,** Idiopathic scleritis presenting as a rapidly developing bilateral orbital cellulitis in a 68-year-old woman. The patient had pain, decreased ocular ductions, and choroidal folds. **B,** Axial CT scan demonstrating diffusely thickened and enhancing sclera bilaterally. **C,** The patient responded well to IV and then oral prednisone. Systemic workup was negative.

sis. Ultrasonography is often quite useful in these patients and shows thickening of the posterior sclera and edema or fluid in Tenon space. This is one of the most sensitive techniques for establishing the diagnosis. Neuroradiologic imaging using either computed tomography or magnetic resonance imaging also demonstrates scleral changes and may show a more diffuse orbital inflammatory process.[20]

Therapy

Therapy consists of a trial of nonsteroidal antiinflammatories or high-dose steroids, with prompt response in most patients. Spontaneous improvement may also be seen.

PERINEURITIS

An unusual variant of orbital inflammatory disease has been recognized as a predominantly perineural location of inflammation.[60] This process typically simulates optic neuritis with orbital pain that is exacerbated by ocular movement, decreased visual acuity, and optic disc edema. It is distinct from optic neuritis in that exophthalmos and pain on ocular displacement are usually present (Fig. 51-6). Computed tomography demonstrates a ragged inflammatory process located adjacent to the optic nerve. Systemic associations have not been identified. Oral corticosteroids usually produce dramatic resolution of the signs and symptoms; however, there may be recurrent disease.

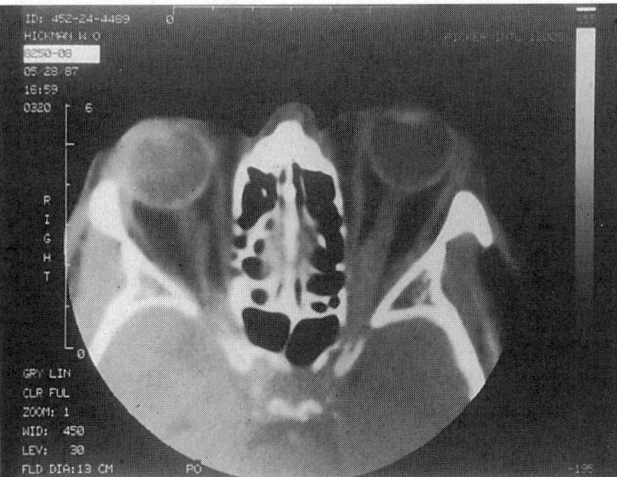

Fig. 51-6. Clinical presentation of this elderly patient with perineuritis consisted of pain, proptosis, reduced visual function, and enhancement of pain on ocular movement. CT demonstrates the diffuse thickening of the orbital portion of the left optic nerve. CT-guided fine needle aspiration biopsy confirmed the inflammatory nature of this lesion and the patient responded to steroid therapy.

GRANULOMATOUS INFLAMMATORY ORBITAL DISEASE

Granulomatous inflammatory orbital diseases represent a heterogeneous group of diseases sharing a common histopathologic finding of epithelioid cellular infiltration.[89,102] These diseases range from foreign body reactions, to endogenous inflammatory disease such as sarcoid or Wegener granulomatosis, to reactions to infections such as tuberculosis or cysticercosis.

Among 1900 patients with orbital lesions evaluated in Vancouver, 2.2% had granulomatous disease.[102] Thirty-seven percent of patients with granulomatous orbital disease experienced a subacute, tender inflammatory process. The diagnoses of these patients include ruptured dermoid cyst, Wegener granulomatosis, sarcoidosis, foreign body granuloma, zygomycosis, cysticercosis, and necrobiotic granuloma.

Ruptured dermoid cysts can present as a chronic, painless mass or as an acute inflammatory process with multiple recurrences or fistula formation. Some patients will give a history of antecedent trauma. Neuroradiologic imaging is helpful because fat may be pathognomonic for dermoid lesions.[85,89] Additional features include orbital expansion, usually in the lacrimal fossa, and evidence of a bony defect. These lesions are amenable to surgical excision with a good prognosis.

TOLOSA-HUNT SYNDROME

Clinical Features

The Tolosa-Hunt syndrome is a variant of granulomatous inflammatory disease that may occur in the cavernous sinus, superior orbital fissure, and/or orbital apex.[40,50,64,113,136] It is characterized by a painful ophthalmoplegia that lasts for days to weeks, with occasional spontaneous remissions, periodic recurrences, and an exquisite response to systemic corticosteroids. On examination proptosis and occlusion of the superior ophthalmic vein may be seen in addition to the classic findings of ophthalmoplegia and hypoesthesia.

Differential Diagnosis

The differential diagnosis includes sarcoid, infections such as syphilis or tuberculosis, lymphoma, meningioma, or other neoplasia. Several cases of meningioma mimicking Tolosa-Hunt have been described.[135] One patient complained of a 6-month history of pain, blurred vision, and episodic diplopia. Computed tomography showed enlargement of the optic nerve and ultimately revealed an abnormal tissue density in the orbital apex. Pain was promptly relieved with intravenous corticosteroids, however, the pain was steroid-dependent and eventually was not controllable. Biopsy at that time demonstrated a meningioma. This case indicates the importance of histologic diagnosis in cases that do not behave in a classic pattern.

Neuroradiologic imaging using computed tomography may show an enlarged cavernous sinus or abnormal soft-tissue densities in the orbital apex. Alternatively, CT may be within normal limits. MRI imaging is more sensitive in examining the region of the cavernous sinus. Abnormal signals may be seen on intermediate and T1 images. Lesions of Tolosa-Hunt often are isointense with muscle on short TR/TE images and isointense with fat on long TR/TE images.

Pathology

Histologic evaluation of lesions of Tolosa-Hunt classically showed a granulomatous periarteritis or a proliferation of fibroblasts, lymphocytes, and plasma cells within the vascular adventitia. Nonspecific inflammation is also observed in these patients.

Therapy

Treatment is systemic corticosteroids with prompt response to therapy.

SARCOIDOSIS

Clinical Features

Sarcoidosis is a multisystem granulomatous disease that produces subcutaneous nodules, erythema nodosum, polyarthritis, hilar adenopathy, pulmonary fibrosis, hepatosplenomegaly, and ocular disease. It may affect any age group (including children) but is more common in the second and third decades. It has a strong predilection for blacks and is more common in women than in men. Ocular involvement includes uveitis, chorioretinitis, conjunctival nodules, lacrimal gland enlargement, optic neuropathy, and (rarely) lesions in the deep orbit.*

Orbital involvement may occasionally be the presenting symptom of sarcoid (Fig. 51-7). One patient had bilateral lid and orbital masses diffusely involving the rectus muscle, with inflammatory periocular changes on computed tomography, and thickening of the optic nerve sheath.[51] On systemic evaluation, bilateral hilar lymphadenopathy, a positive gallium scan, erythema nodosum, and cutaneous anergy were found consistent with the diagnosis. In a study of 15 patients with biopsy-confirmed orbital or lacrimal gland involvement by sarcoid, the orbital disease preceded systemic identification in 11 patients, thus confirming the importance of a thorough systemic evaluation in patients with suspected sarcoidosis.[23]

*References 11, 23, 51, 62, 88, 96.

Differential Diagnosis

Laboratory findings in sarcoidosis include an increased serum calcium in 10%, increased serum lysozyme (which is nonspecific), and increased angiotensin-converting enzyme (ACE). The ACE level is thought to reflect the activity of T-lymphocytes, and decreasing levels are used as a marker for therapeutic response to treatment. Immunologically there is deficient delayed hypersensitivity causing cutaneous anergy. On systemic evaluation the gallium scan shows increased uptake in granulomata and may even identify involved lacrimal glands. The combination of an elevated ACE and abnormal gallium scan is usually diagnostic for sarcoid.

Pathology

Histologically there is a granulomatous inflammation with dense accumulations of epithelioid cells sparsely surrounded by lymphocytes. There is no caseation and little

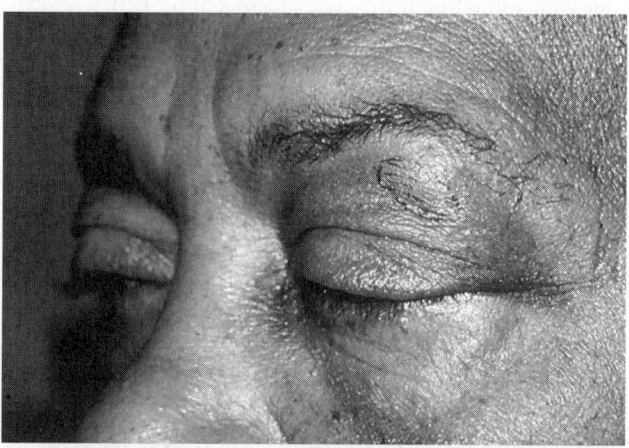

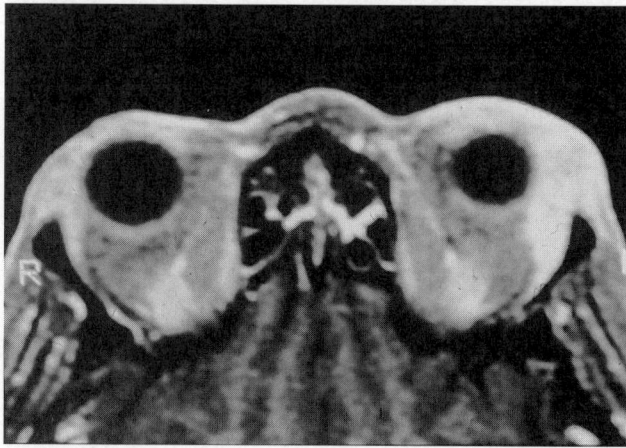

Fig. 51-7. A, Sarcoidosis with lacrimal gland involvement (firm nodular enlarged lacrimal gland outlined with skin marker). B, Axial MRI demonstrating homogeneous-enhancing enlargement of the lacrimal gland.

fibrosis. Giant cells are present and are of the foreign body or Langhan variety. Inclusions may be present. The histopathology is nondiagnostic, and the differential includes sarcoid, bacterial infection (tuberculosis or leprosy), fungal infection, or draining lymph nodes.

Therapy

Therapy usually consists of systemic corticosteroids with prompt resolution of signs and symptoms.

WEGENER GRANULOMATOSIS

Clinical Features

Wegener granulomatosis is a multisystem disease that frequently has ophthalmologic manifestations.* Two forms of the disease exist; the first is a classic form, which is rapidly fatal if untreated; the second is a limited form, with a mortality of 20% over 5 years. Ophthalmic involvement is common, occurring in up to 80% of cases, and may occur in either the classic or limited form (Fig. 51-8). Thus it is critical for the ophthalmologist to recognize the ocular and orbital manifestations of this serious, but potentially treatable, disease.

Orbital involvement is only slightly less common than ocular involvement and includes orbital inflammatory disease and nasolacrimal obstruction.† A chronic form of ophthalmic disease has been described and usually causes sclerouveitis and marginal keratitis preceding the orbital involvement.[25] The largest series of patients with orbital involvement from Wegener granulomatosis was from the Mayo Clinic.[17] In this series, the histories of 140 patients with Wegener granulomatosis were reviewed for ophthalmic involvement. Forty patients had ophthalmologic disease, and of these, 45% had orbital involvement, 25% had nasolacrimal involvement, and 20% had dysfunction of the optic nerve. Bilateral orbital involvement was seen in only two patients.

Patients with orbital inflammatory disease associated with Wegener granulomatosis usually have pain, proptosis, restriction of extraocular movements, and eyelid edema. The optic nerve may be affected either by mechanical forces causing a compressive optic neuropathy or by vasculitic causes of localized ischemia. In patients with nasolacrimal obstruction, epiphora may be the prominent complaint. Surgical management of nasolacrimal duct obstruction may be successful in a quiescent phase of the disease.[43]

Laboratory Investigations

Laboratory evaluations may be helpful in diagnosis of this systemic illness. Nonspecific indicators such as an elevated erythrocyte sedimentation rate and an elevated serum IgE may be observed in this group of patients. A more specific indicator for a group of autoimmune diseases has been the presence of antineutrophil cytoplasmic antibodies (ANCA). ANCA has been associated with Wegener granulomatosis, ulcerative colitis, sclerosing cholangitis, and autoimmune hepatitis. In Wegener granulomatosis ANCA are positive in 96% of patients with generalized disease and in 67% of patients with limited disease.[83] Two patterns of staining, one that targets the cytoplasm or c-ANCA and one that targets the nucleus and perinuclear region or p-ANCA, have been observed. Nolle and associates[83] have reported a high specificity for c-ANCA in patients with ocular inflammation secondary to Wegener. The presence of ANCA has been shown to be helpful in the diagnosis of patients with Wegener granulomatosis-associated ophthalmologic disease.[107,110]

Pathology

The diagnosis of Wegener granulomatosis is best supported by histopathologic criteria in association with the

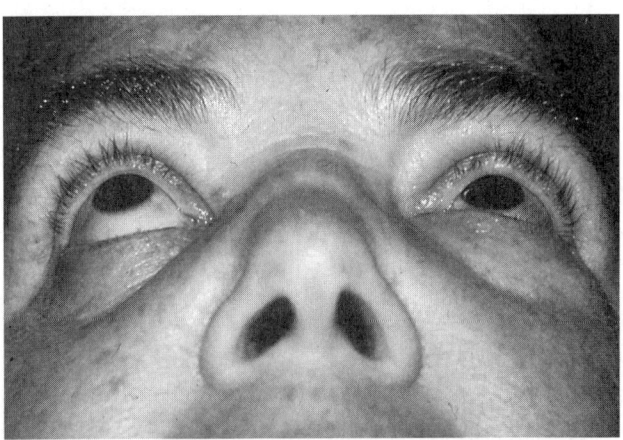

A

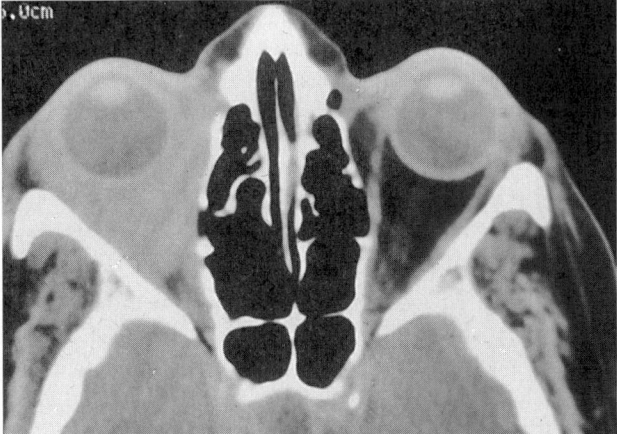

B

Fig. 51-8. A, Wegener granulomatosis: proptosis, "frozen orbit," and nasal deformity. **B,** Axial CT scan demonstrating diffuse infiltration of the entire orbit.

---

*References 3, 17, 26, 44, 68, 112, 126.
†References 17, 25, 44, 108, 110, 111.

clinical course.[56,116] Classically, these patients demonstrate a granulomatous inflammation within an arteriole wall or perivascular area that is a necrotizing, granulomatous inflammation. In a review of the pathologic data from 13 patients at the Mayo Clinic with orbital involvement from Wegener granulomatosis, however, these classic changes were observed in only 7 specimens.[56] Vasculitis in association with other findings was seen in four specimens. Perivascular infiltrates and chronic inflammatory cells were seen as the only orbital pathologic alteration in three specimens. In addition, intact eosinophils and neutrophils with significant extracellular eosinophil major basic protein and neutrophil elastase were observed in orbital tissues. These have been postulated to cause local cytotoxic effects. The disease is thought to be autoimmune-mediated but the exact antigenic stimulus is not understood.

Therapy

The prompt recognition and treatment of the disease is critical to reduce morbidity and mortality. Treatment consists of cytotoxics such as cyclophosphamide and chlorambucil.[84] There may be a role for systemic corticosteroids in some patients as a combined therapy, and high-dose intravenous corticosteroids have been used in patients with acute exacerbations of orbital disease.[4,100]

SYSTEMIC LUPUS ERYTHEMATOSUS

Systemic lupus erythematosus is associated with ocular involvement in 3% to 30% of patients. Orbital involvement is a rare but important complication of the disease.* These patients are often taking oral prednisone or other immunosuppressive or antiinflammatory medications. Thus the differential diagnosis of an acute orbital inflammation must include infectious disease of traditional and opportunistic origins, neoplastic disease, and lupus-related orbital inflammatory disease. It is critical to make the correct diagnosis to properly treat the patient. In these cases blood work, cultures, and biopsy may be indicated early in the course of the disease. In patients with lupus-related orbital inflammation, intravenous steroid treatments are usually required for adequate therapy.

ORBITAL VASCULITIS

Clinical Features

Orbital vasculitis may present as an acute or chronic inflammatory orbital disease.[38,46,52] This is a disease that can occur at any age and may have a relapsing, remitting course with a delay between onset of disease and accurate diagnosis. It may be independent from systemic vasculitides or may be the first manifestation of a systemic illness.

The onset often involves multiple orbital structures such as extraocular muscle involvement with associated soft tissue lesions and optic neuropathy. The disease may become bilateral in up to 20% of patients as reported in the literature.[38,45,46] Lesions are identified on neuroradiologic imaging as soft tissue masses.

Differential Diagnosis

Diagnosis is by biopsy and proper pathologic evaluation. Many cases in the literature were initially misdiagnosed as nonspecific pseudotumor or sclerosing pseudotumor. The primary vasculitic process is defined as an angiocentric and angiodestructive process.[52] Histologically, intramural or transmural polymorphonuclear leukocytes can be identified in the vasculature with associated perivascular eosinophils.

Therapy

Orbital vasculitis is rare and the therapeutic control of the disease is controversial. Corticosteroids may help alleviate pain and acute swelling but may be ineffective for long-term control. Low-dose radiation therapy may be successful in control of this process.[63] Alternatively, cyclophosphamide has been used successfully in some patients whose disease was refractory to other modalities.[38] Early diagnosis and aggressive therapeutics may produce more favorable outcomes.

SINUS DISEASE

Idiopathic orbital inflammation may occasionally be associated with simultaneous inflammation of the sinuses.* The typical signs and symptoms include pain, proptosis, and periorbital swelling. In addition, many of these patients have a history of acute or chronic nasal discharge, congestion of the nose and nasophanynx, or a clinical diagnosis of a sinus infection. There is usually indication of sinus involvement with sinus series radiographs, computed tomography, magnetic resonance imaging, or ultrasonography. In some cases these findings may be coincidental. There are several examples from the literature, however, that clearly indicate a single, combined sinus and orbital inflammatory process.

The orbit and paranasal sinuses are in close proximity, and an incomplete bony barrier is often along the medial orbital wall. There may be congenital absences of part of the medial wall; there are numerous perforations by vasculature in the medial wall; and the ophthalmic venous vasculature is valveless, allowing for extensive communication. In many cases orbital cellulitis and orbital abscesses are a result of extension of infection from contiguous sinuses into the orbit. Additionally, some tumors that originate in the sinuses subsequently involve the orbit by producing bony erosion into it. The primary differential in the diagnosis of sinus and

---

*References 2, 9, 16, 19, 28, 33, 39, 41, 132.

*References 21, 31, 34, 87, 92, 94, 124.

orbital inflammatory disease is either infection or neoplasia. It has been suggested that patients with questionable diagnoses of inflammatory disease receive an initial course of antibiotics prior to steroid therapy.[21]

One interesting case documents the initial presentation of a patient with infectious orbital cellulitis and subperiosteal abscess, who developed an aggressive inflammatory reaction that caused proptosis, loss of vision, and optic atrophy.[94] The proptosis was steroid-sensitive; however, the resolution of proptosis was also dependent on the continued use of corticosteroids. Biopsy of the ethmoid and maxillary sinuses and from the orbit demonstrated a dense collagenous tissue with scant chronic inflammatory cells without granuloma or significant perivascular inflammation.

Other cases from the literature document a combined orbital and sinus inflammatory process without antecedent infection.[31,92] In some of these patients the initial radiographic or ultrasonographic evaluation suggested bony erosion of the orbital floor or medial orbital wall. Biopsies were performed to evaluate for a neoplasia.[31] Histology showed inflammation without evidence of neoplasia. These patients typically respond to oral corticosteroids.

PEDIATRIC ORBITAL INFLAMMATION

Clinical Features

Orbital inflammatory diseases are also seen in the pediatric age group. Although this constellation of diseases is similar to that found in the adult population, there are enough distinctions to make it worthwhile to separately consider the pediatric group.[42,75,76,90] The usual presentation is one of the acute or subacute onset of pain, proptosis, and soft tissue involvement with accompanying ocular signs of chemosis and injection (Fig. 51-9). Orbital inflammatory disease is often associated with an antecedent trauma; however, this is a common association in many childhood illnesses and may

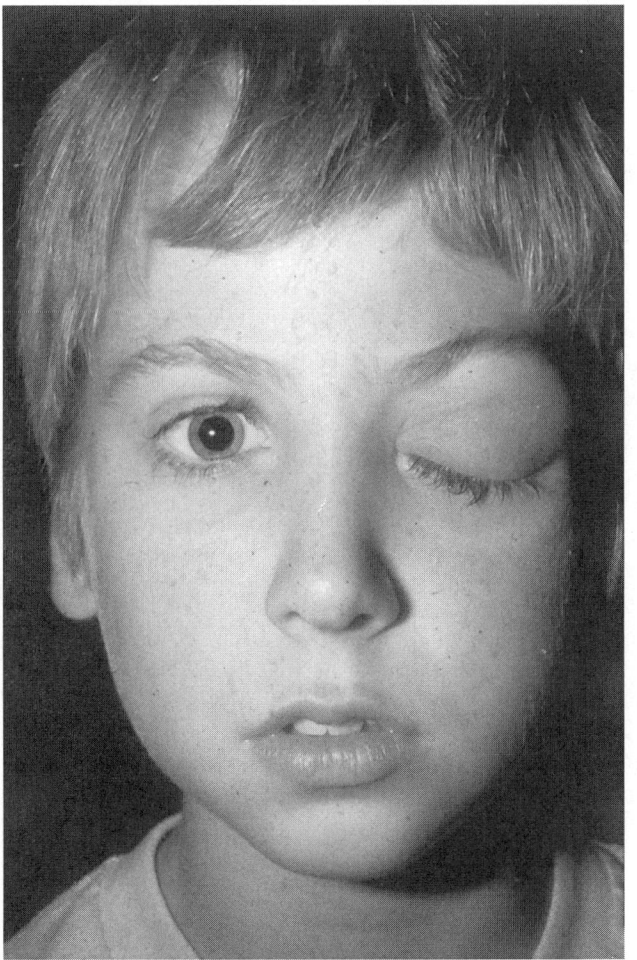

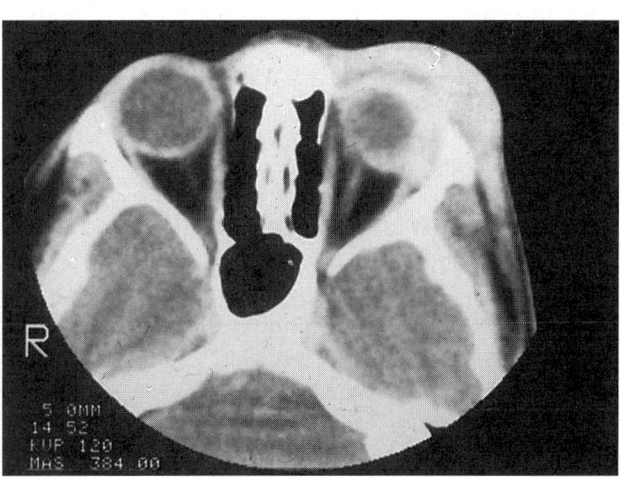

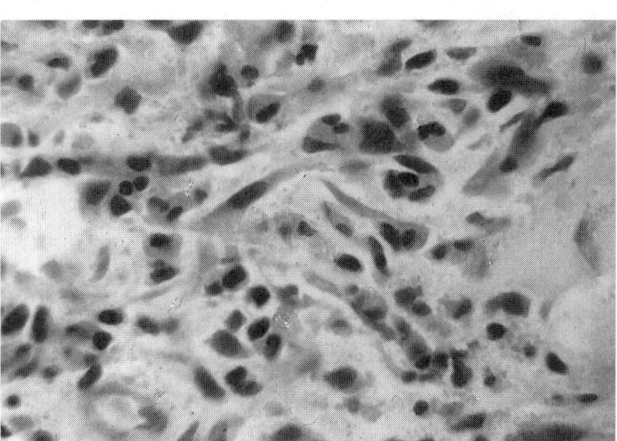

Fig. 51-9. **A,** Juvenile patient with a severely inflamed and edematous upper eyelid. **B,** CT demonstrates diffuse soft tissue swelling with localized enlargement of the lacrimal gland. **C,** Histopathology shows a chronic inflammatory mass with prominent eosinophils.

not be causally related. It may be bilateral in almost half of the patients and, unlike the adult population, there may be an accompanying uveitis.[42]

Several categories of patients were described by Mattow and Jakobiec[75] in 1978 after the review of 29 cases of pediatric orbital inflammatory disease. First, there was a group of children with one episode of a unilateral inflammatory disease. These patients often had residual motility disturbances or proptosis. A second group had multiple unilateral episodes and, although some had residual proptosis, they tended to recover full motility. A third group had multiple bilateral episodes. These patients had associated intraocular inflammation, and a significant number developed visual loss. A small group of patients had a form of Tolosa-Hunt.

Differential Diagnosis

The differential diagnosis includes infection, thyroid-related orbitopathy, Wegener granulomatosis, lymphoma, neoplasia, sarcoidosis, and histiocytosis. The infections can include fungal etiologies such as aspergillosis.[130] It is therefore critical that prompt clinical evaluation, laboratory analysis, and neuroradiologic imaging be performed to obtain an accurate diagnosis and allow for the timely initiation of appropriate therapy. Timely therapy is likely to reduce the long-term morbidity of this disease.

Laboratory Investigations

In the pediatric group of patients with idiopathic orbital inflammations, several important observations were made.[75,76] First, almost one third of the patients had an elevated level of eosinophils. The majority of patients had an elevated erythrocyte sedimentation rate ranging from 20 to 116. Several patients had hypercomplementemia, positive ANA, or elevated α-2-globulin, β-globulin, or γ-globulin. The significance of these findings is not yet understood. Spinal fluid analysis revealed a mild lymphocytic pleocytosis in two out of six patients that were tested. Thus a complete blood count with absolute eosinophil counts must be performed in all pediatric patients, and other blood or spinal fluid analysis needs to be considered.

Ultrasonography is often helpful in the demonstration of sub-Tenon fluid, evaluation of the characteristics of involved muscles, and observation of changes in the optic nerve outline. Neuroradiologic imaging is particularly useful in identifying the involved structures.

Therapy

Inflammatory orbital disease in children is generally quite sensitive to oral steroid therapy. A definitive clinical response within 48 hours of the initiation of treatment usually allows for confidence in the clinical diagnosis. If the disease or response to treatment is atypical, however, then biopsy is necessary. Histopathology of the acute disease shows lymphocytic, eosinophilic, and plasmacytic infiltra-

tion with pericapillary and perivenular collections of inflammatory cells and sparse fibroblastic proliferation. In late biopsies there are prominent changes in the connective tissue with increased collagen deposition.

HISTIOCYTOSIS X

Histiocytosis X may initially have signs and symptoms suggestive of orbital inflammatory disease.[115,129] Three forms of the disease are recognized, but they may represent the disease spectrum instead of distinct clinical entities. These forms are eosinophilic granuloma, Hand-Schüller-Christian disease, and Letterer-Siwe disease; the latter being the most aggressive, with soft tissue and visceral involvement. This disease usually occurs in childhood. Two patients were identified at the Mayo Clinic with presentations of a subacute orbital inflammatory disease; both had a 2-month history of swelling and tenderness of the superotemporal orbit with or without associated erythema. In both patients computed tomography revealed a lytic bone lesion, and definitive diagnosis was made on orbital biopsy. Prompt diagnosis and radiation therapy to the lesions resulted in resolution of the disease without recurrence.

REFERENCES

1. Abromovitz JN, Kasdon DL, Sutula F et al.: Sclerosing orbital pseudotumor, *Neurosurgery* 12:463-467, 1983.
2. Aiello JS: Ocular findings in lupus erythematosus, *Am J Ophthalmol* 35:837-843, 1952.
3. Allen JC, France TD: Pseudotumor as the presenting sign of Wegener's granulomatosis in a child, *J Pediatr Ophthalmol* 14:158-159, 1977.
4. Alloway JA, Cupps TR: High dose methylprednisolone for retroorbital Wegener's granulomatosis, *J Rheumatol* 20:752-754, 1993.
5. Ampil FL, Bahrassa FS: Primary orbital lymphomapseudotumor (pseudolymphoma): case reports and review of radiotherapy literature, *J Surg Oncol* 30:91-95.
6. Arnott EJ, Greaves DD: Orbital involvement in Reidel's thyroiditis, *Br J Ophthalmol* 49:1-5, 1965.
7. Arora R, Rewari R, Betharia SM: Fine needle aspiration cytology of orbital and adnexal masses, *Acta Cytol* 36:483-491, 1992.
8. Austin-Seymour MM, Donaldson SS, Egbert PR et al.: Radiotherapy of lymphoid diseases of the orbit, *Int J Radiat Oncol Biol Phys* 11:371-379, 1985.
9. Bankhurst AD, Carlow TJ, Reidy RW: Exophthalmos in systemic lupus erythematosus, *Ann Ophthalmol* 16:669-671, 1984.
10. Barthold HJ II, Harvey A, Markoe AM et al.: Treatment of orbital pseudotumors and lymphoma, *Am J Clin Oncol* 9:527-532, 1986.
11. Barzel US, Kolbert GS, Edberg SC et al.: Ocular sarcoidosis and Graves ophthalmopathy, *Ann Ophthalmol* 18:186-187, 1986.
12. Benson WH, Linberg JV, Weinstein GW: Orbital pseudotumor in a patient with AIDS, *Am J Ophthalmol* 105:697-698, 1988.
13. Blodi FC, Gass JDM: Inflammatory pseudotumor of the orbit, *Trans Am Acad Ophthalmol Otolaryngol* 71:303-323, 1967.
14. Blodi FC, Gass JDM: Inflammatory pseudotumor of the orbit, *Br J Ophthalmol* 52:79-93, 1968.
15. Braig RF, Romanchuk KG: Recurrence of orbital pseudotumor after 10 years, *Can J Ophthalmol* 23:187-189, 1988.
16. Brenner EH, Shock JP: Proptosis secondary to systemic lupus erythematosus, *Arch Ophthalmol* 91:81-82, 1974.
17. Bullen CL, Liesegang TJ, McDonald TJ, DeRemee RA: Ocular complications of Wegeners granulomatosis, *Ophthalmology* 90:279-290, 1983.
18. Bullen CL, Younge BR: Chronic orbital myositis, *Arch Ophthalmol* 100:1749-1751, 1982.

19. Burkhalter E: Unique presentation of systemic lupus erythematosus, *Arthritis Rheum* 16:428, 1973.

20. Chaques VJ, Lam S, Tessler HH, Mafee MF: Computed tomography and magnetic resonance imaging in the diagnosis of posterior scleritis, *Ann Ophthalmol* 25:89-94, 1993.

21. Chawla HS, Goodwin JA, Ticho BH, Feist RM: Orbital and sinus inflammation with secondary optic neuropathy, *Ann Ophthalmol* 23:231-233, 1991.

22. Colley T: A case of inflammatory pseudo-tumor of the orbit, *Br J Ophthalmol* 19:93-95, 1935.

23. Collison JM, Miller NR, Green WR: Involvement of orbital tissues by sarcoid, *Am J Ophthalmol* 102:302-307, 1986.

24. Comings DE, Skubi KB, Van Eyes J, Motulsky AG: Familial multifocal fibrosclerosis, *Ann Intern Med* 66:884-887, 1967.

25. Coppeto JR, Yamase H, Monteiro MLR: Chronic ophthalmic Wegener's granulomatosis, *J Clin Neuroophthalmol* 5:17-25, 1985.

26. Coutu RE, Klein M, Lessell S et al.: Limited form of Wegener's granulomatosis: eye involvement as a major sign, *JAMA* 233:868-871, 1975.

27. Curtin HD: Pseudotumor, *Radiol Clin North Am* 25:583-599, 1987.

28. Dubois EL, Tuffanelli DL: Clinical manifestations of systemic lupus erythematosus: computor analysis of 520 cases, *JAMA* 190:104-111, 1964.

29. Dunnington JH, Berke RN: Exophthalmos due to chronic orbital myositis, *Arch Ophthalmol* 30:446-465, 1943.

30. Dutt S, Cartwright MJ, Nelson C: Acute dacryoadenitis and Crohn's disease: findings and management, *Ophthalmic Plast Reconstr Surg* 4:295-299, 1992.

31. Eshagian J, Anderson RL: Sinus involvement in inflammatory orbital pseudotumor, *Arch Ophthalmol* 99:627-630, 1982.

32. Fabricus EM, Hoegl I, Pfaefel W: Ocular myositis as first presenting symptom of HIV-1 infection and its response to high-dose cortisone treatment, *Br J Ophthalmol* 75:696-697, 1991.

33. Feinfield RE, Hesse RJ, Rosenberg SA: Orbital inflammatory disease associated with systemic lupus erythematosus, *South Med J* 84:98-99, 1991.

34. Fortson JK, Shapshay SM, Weiter JJ et al.: Otolaryngologic manifestations of orbital pseudotumors, *Otolaryngol Head Neck Surg* 88:342-348, 1980.

35. Foster CS: Immunosuppressive therapy for external ocular inflammatory disease, *Ophthalmology* 87:140-150, 1980.

36. Frohman LP, Kupersmith MJ, Lang J et al.: Intracranial extension and bone destruction in orbital pseudotumor, *Arch Ophthalmol* 104:380-384, 1986.

37. Fujii H, Fujisada H, Kondo T et al.: Orbital pseudotumor: histopathological classification and treatment, *Ophthalmologica* 190:230-242, 1985.

38. Garrity JA, Kennerdell JS, Johnson BJ, Ellis LD: Cyclophosphamide in the treatment of orbital vasculitis, *Am J Ophthalmol* 102:97-103, 1986.

39. Gold DH, Morris DA, Henkind P: Ocular findings in systemic lupus erythematosus, *Br J Ophthalmol* 56:800-804, 1972.

40. Goto Y, Hosokawa S, Goto I et al.: Abnormality in the cavernous sinus in three patients with Tolusa-Hunt syndrome: MRI and CT findings, *J Neurol Neurosurg Psych* 53:231-234, 1990.

41. Grimson BS, Simmons KB: Orbital inflammation, myositis, and systemic lupus erythematosis, *Arch Ophthalmol* 101:736-738, 1983.

42. Grossniklaus HE, Lass JH, Abramowsky CR, Levine MR: Childhood orbital pseudotumor, *Ann Ophthalmol* 17:372-377, 1985.

43. Hardwig PW, Bartley GB, Garrity JA: Surgical management of nasolacrimal duct obstruction in patients with Wegener's granulomatosis, *Ophthalmology* 99:133-139, 1992.

44. Haynes BF, Fishman ML, Fauci AS, Wolff SM: The ocular manifestations of Wegener's granulomatosis. Fifteen years experience and review of the literature, *Am J Med* 63:131-141, 1977.

45. Heersink B, Rodrigues MR, Flanagan J: Inflammatory pseudotumor of the orbit, *Ann Ophthalmol* 9:17, 1977.

46. Henderson JW: *Orbital tumors,* ed 2, New York, 1980, Thieme-Stratton.

47. Henderson JW, Farrow GM: Inflammatory pseudotumor and orbital sarcoid. In *Orbital tumors,* 555-588, Philadelphia, 1973, WB Saunders.

48. Hopfner J, Ganser G, Schmidt H, Clemons S: Unilateral pseudotumor of the orbit—an autoimmune disease? *Monats Kinderheilkunde* 134:43-45, 1986.

49. Hornblass A, Jakobiec FA, Reifler DM, Mines J: Orbital lymphoid tumors located predominantly within extraocular muscles, *Ophthalmology* 94:688-697, 1987.

50. Hunt WE, Meagher JN, LeFever HE, Zeman W: Painful ophthalmoplegia: its relation to indolent inflammation of the cavernous sinus, *Neurol* 11:56-62, 1961.

51. Imes RK, Reifschneider JS, O'Connor LE: Systemic sarcoidosis presenting initially with bilateral orbital and upper lid masses, *Ann Ophthalmol* 20:466-467, 1988.

52. Jakobiec FA, Jones IS: Orbital inflammations. In Duane TD, Jaeger FA, editors: *Clinical ophthalmology,* 1-16, 26-35, Philadelphia, 1985, Harper and Row.

53. Jakobiec FA, Lefkowich J, Knowles DM: B- and T-lymphocytes in ocular disease, *Ophthalmology* 91:635-654, 1984.

53a. Jakobiec FA, Neri A, Knowles DM II: Genotypic monoclonlity in immunophenotypically polyclonal orbital lymphoid tumors. A model of tumor progression in the lymphoid system, *Ophthalmology* 94:980-994, 1987.

54. Jampol LM, West C, Goldberg MF: Therapy of scleritis with cytotoxic agents, *Am J Ophthalmology* 86:266-271, 1978.

55. Kalina PH, Garrity JA, Herman DC et al.: Role of testing for anticytoplasmic autoantibodies in the differential diagnosis of scleritis and orbital pseudotumor, *Mayo Clin Proc* 65:1110-1117, 1990.

56. Kalina PH, Lie JT, Campbell RJ, Garrity JA: Diagnostic value and limitations of orbital biopsy in Wegener's granulomatosis, *Ophthalmology* 99:120-124, 1992.

57. Kattah JC, Zimmerman LE, Kolsky MP et al.: Bilateral orbital involvement in fatal giant cell polymyositis, *Ophthalmology* 97:520-525, 1990.

58. Kaye AH, Hahn JF, Craciun A et al.: Intracranial extension of inflammatory pseudotumor of the orbit: case report, *J Neurosurg* 60:625-629, 1984.

59. Kennerdell JS: The management of sclerosing nonspecific orbital inflammation, *Ophthalmic Surg* 22:512-518, 1991.

60. Kennerdell JS, Dresner SC: The nonspecific orbital inflammatory syndromes, *Surv Ophthalmol* 29:93-103, 1984.

61. Kennerdell JS, Johnson BL, Deutsch M: Radiation treatment of orbital lymphoid hyperplasia, *Ophthalmology* 86:942-947, 1979.

62. Khan JA, Hoover DL, Giangiacomo J, Singsen BH: Orbital and childhood sarcoidosis, *J Pediatr Ophthalmol Strabismus* 23:190-194, 1986.

63. Kin RY, Roth RE: Radiotherapy of orbital pseudotumor, *Radiology* 127:507-509, 1978.

64. Kline LB: The Tolusa-Hunt syndrome, *Surv Ophthalmol* 27:79-95, 1982.

65. Knowles DM, Jakobiec FA: Orbital lymphoid neoplasms: a clinicopathologic study of 60 patients, *Cancer* 46:576-589, 1980.

66. Lanciano R, Fowble B, Sergott RC et al.: The results of radiotherapy for orbital pseudotumor, *Int J Radiat Oncol Biol Phys* 18:407-411, 1990.

67. Levine MR, Kaye L, Mair S, Bates J: Multifocal fibrosclerosis: report of a case of bilateral idiopathic sclerosing pseudotumor and retroperitoneal fibrosis, *Arch Ophthalmol* 111:841-843, 1993.

68. Levitt RA, Fauci AS, Bloch DA et al.: The American College of Rheumotology 1990 criteria for the classification of Wegener's granulomatosis, *Arthritis Rheum* 33:1101-1107, 1990.

69. Li JT, Garrity JA, Kephart GM, Gleich GJ: Refractory periorbital edema in a 29 year old man, *Ann Allergy* 69:101-105, 1992.

70. Ludwig I, Tomsak RL: Acute recurrent orbital myositis, *J Clin Neuroophthalmol* 3:41-47, 1983.

71. Margo CE, Naugle TC Jr, Karcioglu ZA: Ectopic lacrimal gland tissue of the orbit and sclerosing dacryoadenitis, *Ophthalmol Surg* 16:178-181, 1985.

72. Mauriello JA, Flanagan JC: Management of orbital inflammatory disease, *Protocol Surv Ophthalmol* 29:104-116, 1984.

73. McCarthy JM, White VA, Harris G et al.: Idiopathic sclerosing inflammation of the orbit: immunohistologic analysis and comparison with retroperitoneal fibrosis, *Mod Pathol* 6:581-587, 1993.

74. Mejlszenkier JD, Safran AP, Healy JJ: Myositis of influenza, *Arch Neurol* 29:441-443, 1973.

75. Mottow LS, Jakobiec FA: Idiopathic inflammatory pseudotumor in childhood: clinical characteristics, *Arch Ophthalmol* 96:1410-1417, 1978.

76. Mottow-Lippa L, Jakobiec FA, Smith M: Idiopathic inflammatory orbital pseudotumor in childhood, *Ophthalmology* 88:565-574, 1981.

77. Munk P, Downey D, Nicolle D et al.: The role of color flow doppler ultrasonography in the investigation of disease in the eye and orbit, *Can J Ophthalmol* 28:171-176, 1993.

78. Munk P, Nicolle D, Downer D et al.: Posterior scleritis: ultrasound and clinical findings, *Can J Ophthalmol* 28:177-180, 1993.

79. Nielsen EW, Weisman RA, Savino PJ, Schatz NJ: Aspergillosis of the sphenoid sinus presenting as orbital pseudotumor, *Otolaryngol Head Neck Surg* 91:699-703, 1983.

80. Noble SC, Chandler WF, Lloyd RV: Intracranial extension of orbital pseudotumor: a case report, *Neurosurgery* 18:798-801, 1986.

81. Noguchi H, Kephart GM, Campbell RJ et al.: Tissue eosinophilia and eosinophil degranulation in orbital pseudotumor, *Ophthalmology* 98:928-932, 1991.

82. Nolle B, Coners H, Duncker G: ANCA in ocular inflammatory disorders, *Adv Exp Med Biol* 336:305-307, 1993.

83. Nolle B, Specks U, Ludemann J et al.: Anticytoplasmic autoantibodies: their immunodiagnostic value in Wegener's granulomatosis, *Ann Intern Med* 111:28-40, 1989.

84. Novack SN, Pearson CM: Cyclophosphamide therapy in Wegener's granulomatosis, *New Eng J Med* 284:938-942, 1971.

85. Nugent RA, Lapointe JS, Rootman J et al.: Orbital dermoids: features on CT, *Radiology* 165:475-478, 1987.

86. Orssaud C, Poisson M, Gardeur D: Orbital myositis, recurrence of Whipple's disease, *J Fr Ophthalmol* 15:205-208, 1992.

87. Osguthorpe JD, Hochman M: Inflammatory sinus disease affecting the orbit, *Otolaryngol Clin North Am* 26:657-671, 1993.

88. Osguthorpe JD, Weisman RA, Tapert MJ: Management of lacrimal fossa masses, *Arch Otolaryngol Head Neck Surg* 112:164-167, 1986.

89. O'Sullivan RM, Nugent RA, Satorre J, Rootman J: Granulomatous orbital lesions: computed tomographic features, *Can Assoc Radiol J* 43:349-358, 1992.

90. Parelhoff ES, Chavis RM, Friendly DS: Wegener's granulomatosis presenting as orbital pseudotumor in children, *J Pediatr Ophthalmol Strabismus* 22:100-104, 1985.

91. Paris GL, Waltuch GF, Egbert PR: Treatment of refractory orbital pseudotumors with pulsed chemotherapy, *Ophthal Plast Reconstr Surg* 6:96-101, 1990.

92. Pillai P, Saini JS: Bilateral sino-orbital pseudotumor, *Can J Ophthalmol* 23:177-180, 1988.

93. Purcell JJ, Taulbee WA: Orbital myositis after upper respiratory tract infection, *Arch Ophthalmol* 99:437, 1981.

94. Reidy JJ, Giltner J, Apple DJ, Anderson RL: Paranasal sinusitis, orbital abscess, and inflammatory tumors of the orbit, *Ophthalmol Surg* 18:263-366, 1987.

95. Richards AB, Skalka HW, Roberts FJ, Flint A: Pseudotumor of the orbit and retroperitoneal fibrosis, *Arch Ophthalmol* 98:1617-1620, 1980.

96. Rootman J: *Diseases of the orbit,* Philadelphia, 1988, JB Lippincott.

97. Rootman J, McCarthy M, White V et al.: Idiopathic sclerosing inflammation of the orbit, *Ophthalmology* 101:570-584, 1994.

98. Rootman J, Nugent R: The classification and management of acute orbital pseudotumors, *Ophthalmology* 89:1040-1048, 1982.

99. Rose GE, Hoh HB, Harrad RA, Hungerford JL: Intraocular malignant melanomas presenting with orbital inflammation, *Eye* 7:539-541, 1993.

100. Rothwell RS, Percy JS: Adjunctive corticosteroids to treat Wegener's granulomatosis of the eye, *J Rheumatol* 6:721, 1979.

101. Sanchez-Roman J, Varela-Aguilar JM, Bravo-Ferrer J et al.: Idiopathic orbital myositis: treatment with cyclosporin, *Ann Rheum Dis* 52:84-85, 1993.

102. Satorre J, Antle CM, O'Sullivan R et al.: Orbital lesions with granulomatous inflammation, *Can J Ophthalmol* 26:174-195, 1991.

103. Schonder AA, Clift RC, Brophy JW, Dane LW: Bilateral recurrent orbital inflammation associated with retroperitoneal fibrosclerosis, *Br J Ophthalmol* 69:783-787, 1984.

104. Sergott RC, Glaser JS, Charyulu K: Radiotherapy for idiopathic inflammatory pseudotumor: indications and results, *Arch Ophthalmol* 99:853-856, 1981.

105. Shah SS, Lowder CY, Schmitt MA et al.: Low-dose methotrexate therapy for ocular inflammatory disease, *Ophthalmology* 99(9):1419-1423, 1992.

106. Slavin ML, Glaser JS: Idiopathic orbital myositis, *Arch Ophthalmol* 100:1261-1265, 1982.

107. Soukiasian SH, Foster CS, Niles JL, Raizman MB: Diagnostic value of antineutrophil cytoplasmic antibodies in scleritis associated with Wegener's granulomatosis, *Ophthalmology* 99:125-132, 1992.

108. Spalton DJ, Graham EM, Page NGR, Sanders MD: Ocular changes in limited forms of Wegener's granulomatosis, *Br J Ophthalmol* 65:553-563, 1981.

109. Spoor TC, Hartel WC: Orbital myositis, *J Clin Neuroophthalmol* 3:67-74, 1983.

110. Stavrou P, Deutsch J, Rene C et al.: Ocular manifestations of classical and limited Wegener's granulomatosis, *Q J Med* 86:719-725, 1993.

111. Straatsman BR: Ocular manifestations of Wegener's granulomatosis, *Am J Ophthalmol* 44:789-799, 1957.

112. Sullivan JA, Haras SE: Characterization of orbital lesions by surface coil MR imaging, *Radiographics* 7:9-28, 1987.

113. Tolusa EJ: Periarteritic lesions of the carotid siphon with clinical features of carotid intraclinoid aneurysms, *J Neurol Neurosurg Psychiatry* 17:300-302, 1954.

114. Trikel SL, Hilal SK: Submillimeter resolution CT scanning of orbital diseases, *Ophthalmology* 87:412-417, 1980.

115. Trocme SD, Baker RH, Bartley GB et al.: Extracellular deposition of eosinophil major basic protein in orbital Histiocytosis X, *Ophthalmology* 98:353-356, 1991.

116. Trocme SD, Bartley GB, Campbell RJ et al.: Eosinophil and neutrophil degranulation in ophthalmic lesions of Wegener's granulomatosis, *Arch Ophthalmol* 109:1585-1589, 1991.

117. Turner RR, Egbert P, Warnke RA: Lymphocytic infiltration if the conjunctiva and orbit: immunohistochemical staining of 16 cases, *Am J Clin Pathol* 81:447-452, 1984.

118. Tychsen L, Tse DT, Ossoinig K, Anderson RL: Trochleitis with superior oblique myositis, *Ophthalmology* 91:1075-1079, 1984.

119. Van de Mosselaer G, Van Deuren H, Dewolf-Peters C, Missotten L: Pseudotumor orbitae and myasthenia gravis, *Arch Ophthalmol* 98:1621-1622, 1980.

120. Verma N, Singh J: Bilateral idiopathic inflammatory pseudotumor of the orbits, *Ann Ophthalmol* 16:1076-1080, 1984.

121. Vestal KP, Bauer TW, Berlin AJ: Nodular fasciitis presenting as an eyelid mass, *Ophthal Plast Reconstr Surg* 6:130-132, 1990.

122. Volpe NJ, Shore JW: Orbital myositis associated with herpes zoster, *Arch Ophthalmol* 109:471-472, 1991.

123. Weinstein JM, Koch K, Lane S: Orbital pseudotumor in Crohn's colitis, *Ann Ophthalmol* 16:275-278, 1984.

124. Weisberger EC, Zauel DW, Gilmor RL, Yune H: Otolaryngologists' role in diagnosis and treatment of orbital pseudotumor, *Otolaryngol Head Neck Surg* 93:536-549, 1985.

125. Weissler MC, Miller E, Fortune MA: Sclerosing orbital pseudotumor: a unique clinicopathologic entity, *Ann Otol Rhinol Laryngol* 98:496-501, 1989.

126. Weiter J, Farkas TG: Pseudotumor of the orbit as a presenting sign in Wegener's granulomatosis, *Surv Ophthalmol* 17:106-119, 1972.

127. Wenger J, Gingrinch GW, Mendeloff J: Sclerosing cholangitis: a manifestation of systemic disease, *Arch Intern Med* 116:509-514, 1965.

128. Wesley RE, Cheij G, Bond JB, Davis WG: Orbital pseudotumor of the levator muscle, *Ophthalmic Plast Reconstr Surg* 2:139-142, 1986.

129. Wesley RE, Cooper J, Litchford DW: Orbital inflammatory pseudotumor associated with multifocal systemic neoplastic incompetence, *Ann Ophthalmol* 20:150-152, 1988.

130. Whitehurst FO, Liston TE: Orbital aspergillosis: report of a case in a child, *J Ped Ophthalmol Strabismus* 18:50-54, 1981.

131. Whyte IF, Young JDH, Guthrie W, Kemp EG: Orbital inflammatory disease and bone destruction, *Eye* 6:662-666, 1992.
132. Wildinson LS, Panush RS: Exophthalmos associated with systemic lupus erythematosus, *Arthritis Rheum* 18:188-189, 1975.
133. Woolner LB, McConahey WM, Beahrs OH: Invasive fibrosis thyroiditis (Reidel's struma), *J Clin Endocrinol Metab* 17:201-220, 1957.
134. Wright KW, Silverstein D, Marrone AC, Smith RE: Acquired inflammatory superior oblique tendon sheath syndrome; a clinicopathologic study, *Arch Ophthalmol* 100:1752-1754, 1982.
135. Wroe SJ, Thompson AJ, McDonald WI: Painful intraorbital meningiomas, *J Neurol Neurosurg Psychiatry* 54:1009-1010, 1991.
136. Yousen DM, Atlas SW, Grossman RC et al.: MR imaging of Tolusa-Hunt syndrome, *Am J Radiol* 154:167-170, 1990.

52 Dysthyroid Orbitopathy

JOHN S. KENNERDELL, EDWARD BARON, ANNA TYUTYUNIKOV,
JACK R. WALL, CHRISTINE GENOVESE

Graves ophthalmopathy is the most frequent orbital disorder, heading the list of differential diagnoses of both uni- and bilateral exophthalmos in the adult population.[48]

HISTORICAL BACKGROUND

In the Anglo-Saxon literature this disease is named after Robert Graves,[32] but in the German-speaking countries it is referred to by the name of Carl von Basedow.[94] It was Caleb Parry, however, who was the first (in 1786) to focus attention on the association of goiter and exophthalmos.[12]

Major research activities over the past 3 decades have focused on the thyroid component and have advanced knowledge in the pathogenesis of Graves disease, Hashimoto thyroiditis, and other thyroid dysfunctions. Graves disease comprises hyperthyroidism, diffuse goiter, and ophthalmopathy. Other characteristic features, such as dermopathy (pretibial myxedema) and acropachy, add to the spectrum of the clinical manifestations of the disease but occur much less frequently. Until recently, investigations of the eye manifestations of Graves disease have been rather sporadic, and there was little communication and collaboration between the major subspecialists involved, namely the endocrinologist and the ophthalmologist.

Remarkably, there is no general agreement as to what the disease should be called. Numerous labels, including Graves ophthalmopathy, Graves eye disease, endocrine ophthalmopathy, thyroid eye disease, dysthyroid eye disease, exophthalmic goiter, and immune thyroid-associated ophthalmopathy, exophthalmos, have been advocated. This chapter uses dysthyroid orbitopathy to describe this disease.

PATHOGENESIS

Thyroid-associated ophthalmopathy has become the major research focus of an increasing number of clinicians and scientists worldwide, and the idea that a multidisciplinary and coordinated approach to all facets of the disease is needed is gradually gaining ground. Substantial progress has been achieved in recent years, but many old but pertinent questions remain. What is the cause of Graves ophthalmopathy? How and why is this disorder related to the thyroid gland and autoimmune disease? To what extent and by what methods should patients be investigated and assessed? What is the treatment of choice for the various manifestations of the disease, especially severe progressive ophthalmopathy and vision-threatening optic neuropathy? There is growing evidence that thyroid-associated ophthalmopathy is an autoimmune disease in which the target appears to be the extraocular muscle cells and/or the orbital fibroblasts.

Evidence for Extraocular Muscle Damage in Thyroid-Associated Ophthalmopathy. Although earlier electron microscopy studies of a few cases of thyroid-associated ophthalmopathy failed to reveal extraocular muscle damage,[11,43] preliminary studies of eye muscle from patients with thyroid-associated ophthalmopathy[108] have shown clear evidence of muscle fiber damage. The main abnormalities include dissolution of the Z-bands, abnormalities of the mitochondria, enlargement and displacement of the nuclei, and lipid vacuoles. These changes range from mild damage to massive necrosis and destruction with collagen replacement (Fig. 52-1). There is some evidence that extraocular muscle fibers may differ from other skeletal muscle in respect to their myosin isotypes and enzyme profiles.[61,62] Studies correlating electron microscopic parameters of extraocular muscle cell damage with in vitro expression of extraocular muscle autoantigens suggest that these muscles are more susceptible.

Extraocular Muscle Autoantigens. Several extraocular muscle-reactive autoantibodies are detectable in the serum of patients with thyroid-associated ophthalmopathy. A variety of antibody assays are used, including enzyme-linked immunosorbent assay (ELISA),[4,47,69] immunofluorescence,[67] protein A binding,[21] and SDS polyacrylamide gel electrophoresis (SDS-PAGE) with Western blotting.[1,80] Little is known, however, about the molecular structure, subcellular distribution, tissue specificity, or function of the target autoantigens.

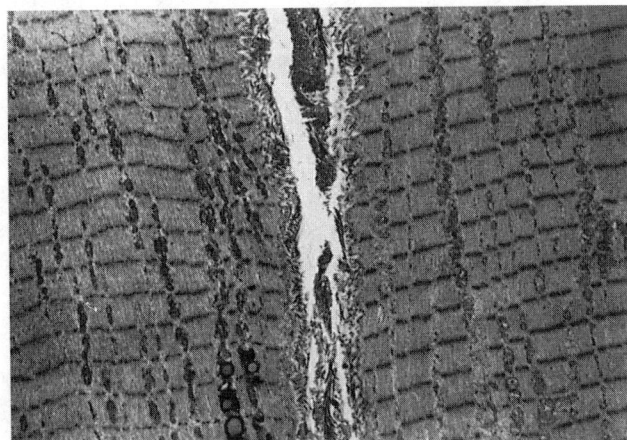

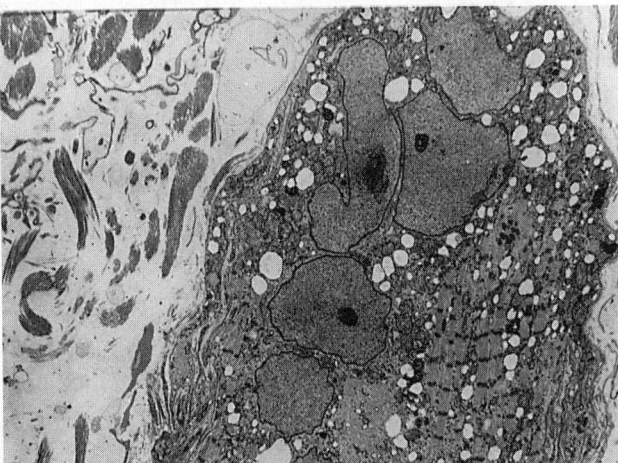

Fig. 52-1. Electron micrographs of extraocular muscle from: **A,** a normal individual showing two muscle fibers separated by a small amount of interstitial connective tissue with clear preservation of Z-band striation; **B,** a patient with thyroid-associated ophthalmopathy showing a fiber with partially preserved Z-band striation on one edge, numerous abnormal nuclei with prominent nucleoli, and complete loss of the normal striation in the middle.

The best candidate antigens for the early inflammatory reaction in patients with thyroid autoimmunity appear to be proteins of 64 kDa expressed in the membrane fraction of human extraocular muscle and thyroid cells. Two such 64-kDa antigens have been partially characterized, namely a membrane protein identified in immunoblotting and a recombinant protein, called $_1$D, recently cloned from a thyroid cDNA expression library. A 64-kDa antigen identified in Western blotting by reactivity with autoantibodies in the serum of patients with thyroid-associated ophthalmopathy has been extensively studied.[70,80,81] Antibodies reactive with this protein are early and reliable markers for the development of ophthalmopathy in patients with Graves hyperthyroidism.[70]

Immunoprecipitation of a 64-kDa antigen in cultured eye muscle and thyroid cells by antibodies in the serum from patients with thyroid-associated ophthalmopathy has been achieved.[106] On the other hand, this was not the case for human skeletal muscle cells in which a different antigen, of 66 kDa, was precipitated by antibodies in the serum of patients with thyroid autoimmunity, with or without ophthalmopathy, as well as normal subjects[107] (Fig. 52-2). Supportive findings were reported recently,[40] in which the use of SDS-PAGE of rat extraocular muscle membranes showed that although only thyroid-associated ophthalmopathy sera reacted with a 64-kDa protein in extraocular muscle membranes, sera from patients with thyroid-associated ophthalmopathy and from normal subjects reacted nonspecifically with a 66-kDa protein in both extraocular muscle and skeletal muscle membranes. These workers measured antibody reactivity as an index calculated by comparing the density of the 64-kDa band with that at 66 kDa, showing much higher indices in patients with thyroid-associated ophthalmopathy compared to control subjects.[40]

A prospective study of patients with Graves hyperthyroidism without apparent eye disease showed that antibody reactivity to a 64-kDa protein in human and pig eye muscle membranes predicted the development of eye disease in all patients who developed clinically overt ophthalmopathy.[17] Orbital CT scan of these patients—and the others who did not have evident eye disease—carried out at the end of the 24- to 36-month observation period demonstrated increased eye muscle swelling.* The high prevalence of antibodies to a recombinant 64-kDa eye muscle antigen in patients with Graves hyperthyroidism (see the following) further suggests that antibodies reactive with 64-kDa antigens may be early markers of ophthalmopathy in patients with thyroid autoimmunity. This theory is reminiscent of the natural history of islet cell antibodies in Type I diabetes mellitus.[5]

A second 64-kDa antigen has been cloned from a thyroid cDNA expression library by screening a pool of Hashimoto thyroiditis patients' sera.[18,20] The initial clone, D$_1$, encoded a 98 amino acid fragment of a full-length 562 amino acid protein, called $_1$D, corresponding to a molecular weight of 63 to 64 kDa. D$_1$-affinity purified autoantibodies reacted with a 64-kDa eye muscle membrane protein in SDS-PAGE[18] (Fig. 52-3).

Reactivity to the full-length molecule D$_1$, expressed in transfected Chinese hamster ovary cells, is much more closely associated with the ophthalmopathy. This reactivity is detected in approximately 50% of patients with active ophthalmopathy and in 73% of those with Graves hyperthyroidism without evident eye disease, but in only 20% of patients with Hashimoto thyroiditis without ophthalmopathy and in 17% of controls.†

*Wall and Salvi, unpublished observations.
†Bernard and associates, submitted.

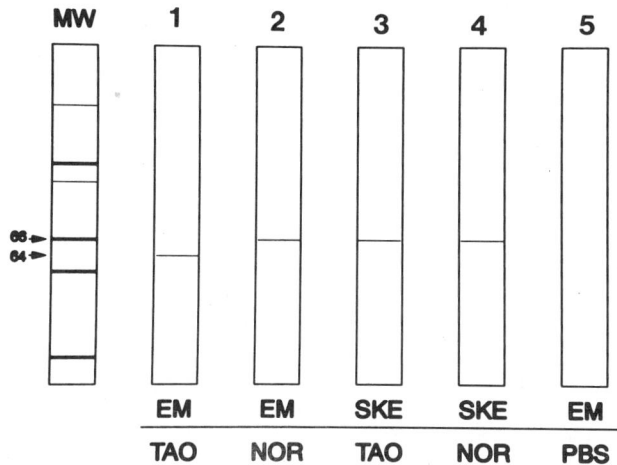

Fig. 52-2. Immunoprecipitation of antigens of 64 and 66 kDa from human eye muscle (EM) and skeletal muscle (SKE) by sera from patients with thyroid-associated ophthalmopathy (TAO) and normals (NOR). Whereas the TAO patient serum precipitates a 64-kDa protein from EM *(lane 1)*, that from a normal subject does not *(lane 2)*. On the other hand, both sera precipitate a 66-kDa protein from SKE *(lanes 3 and 4 respectively)*. MW = molecular weight standards. PBS = phosphate buffered saline *(lane 5)*.

The development of ophthalmopathy in patients with thyroid autoimmunity is best explained by B and T lymphocyte immunoreactivity against a 64-kDa extraocular muscle and thyroid-shared membrane autoantigen[97] — although extensive study is necessary to confirm this. Whereas such cross-reactive antibodies are expected to be cytotoxic to both human extraocular muscle and thyroid cells,[37,38,40,100] there is no close relationship between antibodies that are cytotoxic to the two targets in antibody-dependent, cell-mediated cytotoxicity (ADCC) and reactivity to either a 64-kDa protein in immunoblotting[106] or to $_1$D. By using Chinese hamster ovary cells expressing $_1$D on their surface as targets in ADCC, serum cytotoxic activity can be compared with reactivity against a 64-kDa antigen in ELISA and Western blotting.

Extraocular Muscle-Specific Autoantigens. Extraocular muscle-specific autoantigens (those not expressed in other skeletal muscle) are expected to exist, but it has been difficult to demonstrate such antigens with certainty. Extraocular muscles express an autoantigen of 25 kDa[96]; all other antigens, including those of 55, 70, and 95 kDa, are expressed by other skeletal muscles. Autoantibodies have also been found that react with another, lower molecular-weight (~ 35 kDa) antigen and are associated with late stage, progressive ophthalmopathy in patients with autoimmune thyroid disease.[82] Thus there is good evidence for humoral immunity against extraocular muscle and orbital connective tissue antigens in thyroid-associated ophthalmopathy.

Few studies of T cell reactivity to orbital antigens have been undertaken. Lymphokines produced by T cells sensitized to specific antigens in crude orbital extracts and mem-

brane fractions were measured by their effects on mononuclear cell proliferation, migration, and adherence. Macrophage inhibitory factor (MIF) is produced in response to crude human retrobulbar tissue antigens, as well as thyroid antigens, in patients with thyroid-associated ophthalmopathy.[32] MIF is present in all patients with thyroid-associated ophthalmopathy and in one third of patients with Graves disease without ophthalmopathy.[72] Studies using the lymphocyte transformation test and the leukocyte adherence test have yielded equivocal results, however.[95]

Material from retrobulbar tissues obtained from patients with thyroid-associated ophthalmopathy shows that the majority of infiltrating mononuclear cells are T cells.[101] The leukocyte procoagulant activity (LPCA) assay has been used to measure cellular immunity in autoimmune disease. The LPCA assay is based on the cellular collaboration between lymphocytes and monocytes, with the elaboration of a procoagulant factor by the latter cells. When cultured in the presence of appropriate antigen, CD4 lymphocytes produce a lymphokine that interacts with monocytes to elaborate LPCA (thought to be thromboplastin). In these studies, the test was found to be more sensitive and specific than other tests of cell-mediated immunity.

An LPCA assay was used to test for cellular immunity against extraocular muscle, orbital connective tissue membrane, and soluble fractions in patients with thyroid-associated ophthalmopathy and with autoimmune thyroid disorders without evident eye disease. These studies confirmed earlier findings using lymphocyte transformation, leukocyte

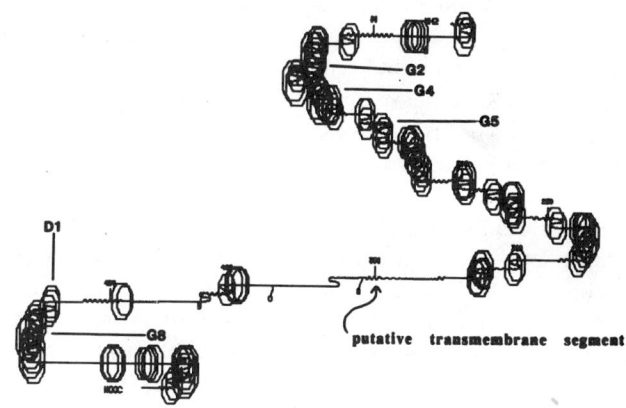

Fig. 52-3. Proposed model and predicted antigenicity profile for D_1, a 64-kDa eye muscle and thyroid protein cloned from a thyroid cDNA expression library. The molecule comprises a long extracellular and short intracellular segment with a short transmembrane domain. Identified antibody reactive epitopes are indicated; G_2, G_4, G_5, and G_8 were derived from a sublibrary of random 100 to 200 bp fragments of D_1 by screening with TAO sera. D_1 is the portion of the molecule originally isolated from the thyroid cDNA library and used to obtain the full length molecule. Potential antigenicity is represented by the open circles.

0 = antigen index $\geq$ 1.2.

adherence inhibition, and the MIF assay. The lack of significant immunoreactivity to OCT fractions in patients with thyroid-associated ophthalmopathy supports the theory that the extraocular muscle is the more important target in this disorder. Significant LPCA induced by thyroid membrane is consistent with similar degrees of thyroid autoimmunity in Graves disease and in Hashimoto thyroiditis. The finding of significant LPCA in response to extraocular muscle membrane in patients with Graves hyperthyroidism without evident ophthalmopathy is further reinforcement for the theory that perhaps all patients with Graves hyperthyroidism have an associated ophthalmopathy. Although, because of the lack of a precise clinical test for ophthalmopathy, it is difficult to prove this contention. Because the mean LPCA levels for groups of patients with and without evident ophthalmopathy were similar, this apparent discrepancy could be explained if (1) ophthalmopathy occurs in the great majority of patients with Graves hyperthyroidism, and (2) cell-mediated immunity is an early event in the course of the eye disease, as has been shown for antibodies to the 64-kDa extraocular muscle antigen.

Whereas antibodies against eye muscle and OCT antigens may be important as markers for the orbital autoimmune process, most workers believe that T cell responses to candidate antigens represent the primary immune abnormality in autoimmune disorders.[97] The failure to demonstrate an association between T cell reactivity to extraocular muscle membranes and antibodies to a 64-kDa eye muscle membrane antigen suggests that B and T cell reactivities may be directed against different target antigens. This finding would be consistent with the immunologic abnormalities identified in other organ-specific autoimmune disorders. The possibility that ophthalmopathy and autoimmune thyroid disorders are associated because of immunoreactivity against shared antigens has been extensively studied in antibody testing and absorption.[97] There is a significant positive correlation between LPCA induction by both pig and human extraocular muscle membrane and that to thyroid membrane. Although this does not prove that T cell reactivity was against a common antigen, the findings support such a hypothesis. A role of cellular immunoreactivity against shared thyroid and extraocular muscle antigens in the association of autoimmune thyroid disorders and ophthalmopathy can be further studied with the availability of recombinant extraocular muscle proteins.

Hypothesis. The relationship of thyroid eye disease and autoimmunity remains open. Current understanding postulates that mild extraocular muscle inflammation occurs in an unknown, but probably large, proportion of patients with Graves hyperthyroidism and in a small proportion of those with Hashimoto thyroiditis. This orbitopathy is associated with autoantibodies and sensitized T cells reactive with extraocular muscle membrane antigens of 64 kDa. Later, immunoreactivity against extraocular muscle-specific proteins of 25 to 35 kDa, perhaps shed as a result of the extraocular

muscle damage, induces progressive disease in approximately 25% of patients with Graves hyperthyroidism and in 2% of those with Hashimoto thyroiditis. Identifying patients at risk for progressive ophthalmopathy could be possible by carrying out immunoblotting with extraocular muscle membranes in patients with Graves hyperthyroidism at the onset of their illness.

CLINICAL FEATURES

The evaluation of a patient with orbitopathy must first establish the exact diagnosis of thyroid-associated ophthalmopathy by ruling out such masqueraders as nonspecific orbital inflammation, neoplasms, orbital cellulitis, carotid-cavernous fistula, and axial myopia. The ophthalmologist plays a key role in staging the disease and determining the effect of orbitopathy on ocular structures, so as to advise when medical management and surgical intervention are indicated.

Classification

In 1969 Werner, as chairman of a special committee of the American Thyroid Association, introduced the NOSPECS classification to describe and grade the eye changes of a patient with Graves ophthalmopathy.[103] NOSPECS is an acronym, in which NO (classes: 0 and 1) refers to 'noninfiltrative' ophthalmopathy, and SPECS (classes: 2-6) represents the major classes of symptoms (infiltrative ophthalmopathy). Although by no means ideal, this scheme with its modifications[93,104] has been generally adopted and can be used to assess severity, to evaluate the natural history of the disease, and to judge its response to treatment.[45]

An alternative classification is based on identifying four classes of disease activity (Table 52-1). This four-point classification is useful in characterizing patients with regard to clinical characterization and treatment. Additionally, the active stage of dysthyroid orbitopathy may be subcategorized into mild, moderate, and severe disease.[92]

External Examination

The clinical evaluation of staging of patients begins with the external examination. The congestive signs of dysthyroid orbitopathy are of special importance. Eyelid and conjunctival edema and chemosis vary from very mild to severe with extensive swelling of both upper and lower lids as well as secondary prolapse of orbital fat if swelling is prolonged and severe (Fig. 52-4). It has been postulated that increased orbital compliance caused by inflammation, edema, extraocular muscle enlargement, or crowding of the fibrous septa may lead to venous obstruction, which in turn may cause the lid and conjunctival edema often associated with dysthyroid orbitopathy.[22]

Associated with retraction of the upper eyelids is eyelid lag on downgaze, both of which are characteristics of dysthyroid orbitopathy. Proposed mechanisms for this have included increased sympathetic tone of Müller muscle, fibrotic

TABLE 52-1 GROUPING OF PATIENTS WITH THYROID-ASSOCIATED OPHTHALMOPATHY

Group	Description
1. Stable	No change in signs and symptoms for at least 6 months.
2. Acute active	Actively worsening disease characterized by increasing proptosis, worsening restrictive myopathy and/or visual impairment. Signs of conjunctival chemosis and eyelid edema.
3. Chronic	Signs and symptoms similar to, but generally milder than, those of the active group. Signs and symptoms progressing more slowly than those of group 2 (i.e., change not clearly noted within 1 month but apparent over a period of 1 year).
Recurrent	Increasing signs and symptoms as described above noted after a period of apparent inactivity.
4. Myopathy	Rapid onset and spontaneous stabilization. Primary sign: abnormal positioning of eyeball with severe motility restriction. No evidence of congestive signs or optic neuropathy.

changes within the levator muscle itself, as well as changes in the levator aponeurosis and superior rectus complex secondary to inflammation. When occurring as an early sign of dysthyroid orbitopathy, which is often the case, it must be distinguished from other causes of lid retraction such as aberrant regeneration of the third nerve, midbrain disease, lid retraction associated with contralateral ptosis (caused by Hering law), and lid retraction from the use of sympathomimetic and chronic steroid therapy.[29]

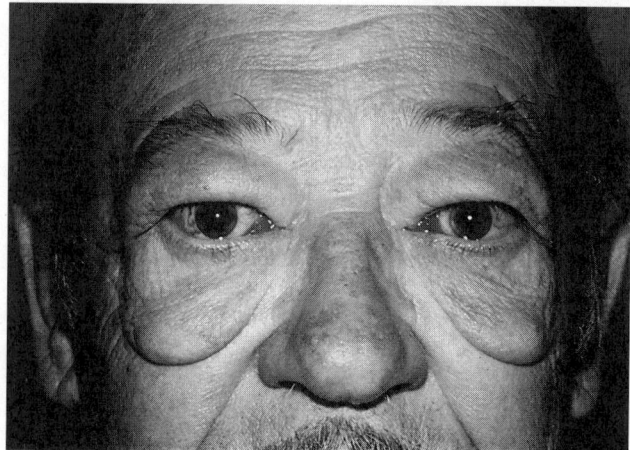

Fig. 52-4. 61-year-old man demonstrates the acute congestive phase of thyroid-associated ophthalmopathy with severe swelling of lids and fat prolapse.

Measurement of Exophthalmos

Proptosis, when it occurs, may be unilateral or bilateral in thyroid-associated ophthalmopathy. It is caused by increased orbital volume as a result of enlargement of the extraocular muscles and increased compliance of the orbital fat. A difference of 2 mm or greater between the two eyes is usually considered an abnormal asymmetry. A reading of greater than 21 mm on exophthalmometry may also represent proptosis, although this is variable between gender and race. The mean normal protrusion of globes is 15.4 mm in white females, 16.5 mm in white men, 17.8 mm in black females, and 18.4 mm in black males.[68] The upper limit of normal among black males was 25 mm.[68]

Proptosis is assessed using Hertel exophthalmometry and by viewing the cornea from above the brow or below looking upwards, allowing a comparative view of the degree of proptosis as well as observation of the temporal fossa to check for bossing (Figs. 52-5, *A*, 52-5, *B*). Digital ballotment assessing resistance to retropulsion is performed to rule out an orbital mass. Palpation of the periorbital tissue can rule out periorbital diseases such as metastatic orbital disease. Auscultation is performed to identify a bruit that might suggest a carotid-cavernous sinus fistula.

Extraocular Muscles

Patients with dysthyroid orbitopathy and extraocular muscle involvement often have diplopia and motility disturbance. This may be demonstrated on ultrasound, computerized tomography, or magnetic resonance imaging. Typically, the belly of the extraocular muscle is enlarged, but the tendon is spared. (In myositis, the tendon is usually involved.) The pattern of extraocular muscle involvement in order of frequency is inferior rectus, medial rectus, superior rectus, and, rarely, lateral rectus.[79] The most typical pattern is upgaze restriction (Fig. 52-6). A few patients may have superior rectus involvement, including bilateral superior rectus involvement, associated with predominant downgaze restriction (Fig. 52-7). It is unknown why some muscles are involved more than others, and why the oblique muscles are apparently never clinically involved.

The single most common ocular motility abnormality encountered is a unilateral elevator palsy or hypodeviation that increases in upgaze, causing vertical diplopia. This is a result of fibrotic shortening of the inferior rectus muscle causing restricted elevation. Such upgaze palsy must be clinically distinguished from other inflammations affecting the inferior rectus, namely myositis, restriction caused by blowout fracture, partial third nerve palsy with superior rectus involvement, myasthenia gravis, and Brown superior oblique tendon syndrome, as well as brainstem lesions. Additionally, when medial rectus fibrosis occurs, a six-nerve palsy may be mimicked.[29]

In evaluating vertical and horizontal deviations, quantitative measurements must be made with simultaneous prism cover testing and by measurement of ductions from the pri-

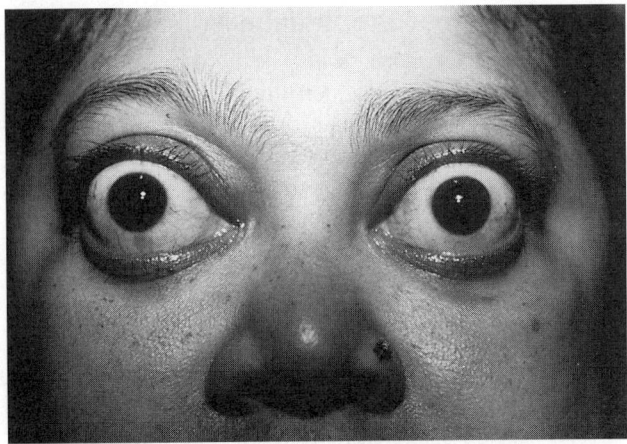

A

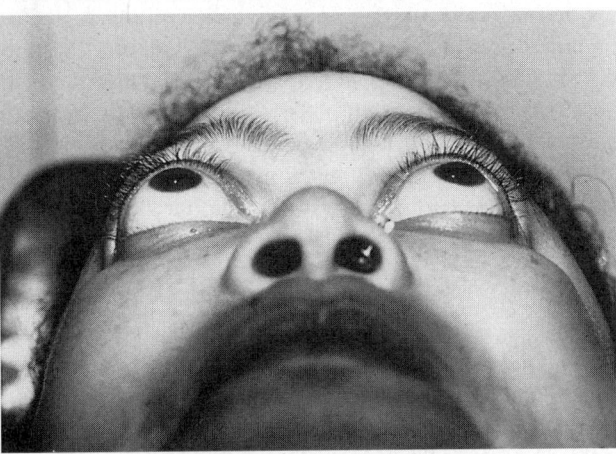

B

Fig. 52-5. A, Proptosis and lid retraction of both upper and lower lids. (Hertel exophthalmometry: right eye, 28 mm; left eye, 27 mm.) **B,** Proptosis viewed from below, with patient looking up.

mary position to compare excursions between each eye. Quantitation of ocular misalignment and degree of restriction are important baseline data to determine whether the disease is worsening and to evaluate response to treatment such as orbital decompression (which may initially worsen such misalignment). Such restrictive myopathy may be caused by fibrosis or entrapment and can be confirmed by forced duction testing (which will distinguish restrictive from paretic abnormality of the muscle).

There are rare cases of end-stage myopathy, with paretic rather than restrictive function, that will have a negative forced duction test and abnormal electromyography.[36]

Cornea

The slit-lamp examination provides an opportunity to observe whether corneal exposure is causing superficial punctate keratopathy from eyelid retraction, lid lag, or proptosis. Corneal exposure can rapidly lead to abrasion and ulcer-

ation. Corneal damage is a significant cause of visual impairment in this condition.

Intraocular Pressure

The inelasticity and fibrosis of the inferior rectus muscle are believed to produce pressure against the globe itself in elevation. It was shown that patients with Graves disease and significant proptosis had a mean intraocular pressure rise on upgaze of 9 mm Hg compared to 5 mm in those without exophthalmos.[25] Controls, on the other hand, showed an average of < 1 mm Hg rise of pressure on upgaze. Therefore those patients with orbitopathy and vertical deviation who have developed a chin-up position as compensation will often show false intraocular pressure elevations that can lead to a misdiagnosis of primary glaucoma.

Prolonged rises in intraocular pressure caused by orbitopathy can potentially cause glaucomatous cupping of the nerve as well. A diagnostic dilemma is to distinguish glaucomatous optic nerve damage from true optic neuropathy related to dysthyroid orbitopathy. If the extraocular muscles are enlarged but associated with only minimal proptosis, orbital decompression may relieve the pressure exerted by the extraocular muscles on the globe and have a positive effect lowering the intraocular pressure.[49] Similarly, a decrease in the congestive phase of the orbitopathy can also result in the lowering of intraocular pressure. Despite appropriate therapy for dysthyroid orbitopathy, some patients will have prolonged elevation of intraocular pressure and require antiglaucoma therapy.

Optic Nerve

It is reported that 3% to 8.6% of patients with dysthyroid orbitopathy can develop optic neuropathy. In the evaluation of such patients, visual acuity testing should be performed along with color plate testing and color comparison, as well

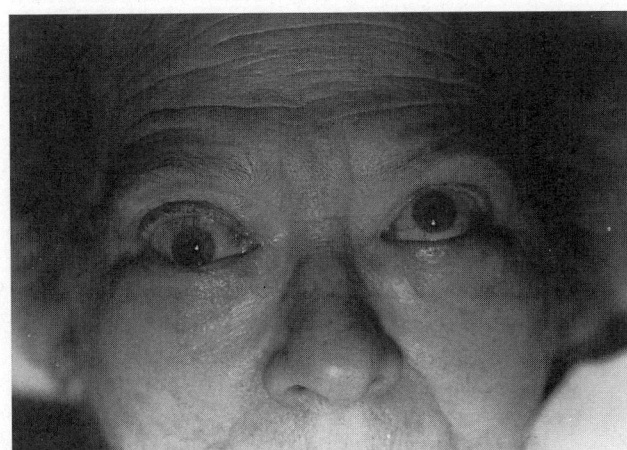

Fig. 52-6. 53-year-old woman with thyroid-associated ophthalmopathy and inferior rectus muscle restriction as demonstrated by the absence of elevation of the right globe in up-gaze.

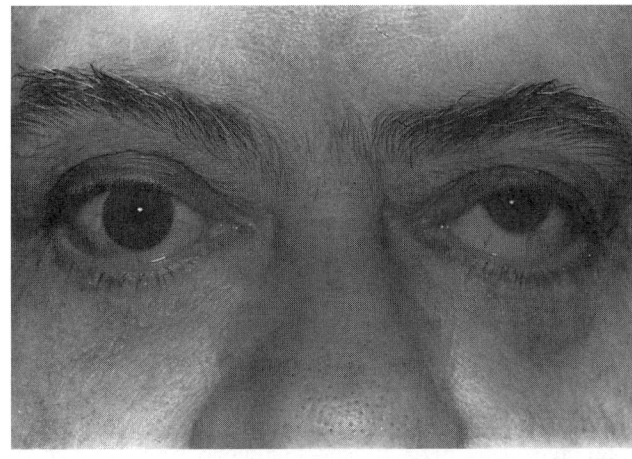

A

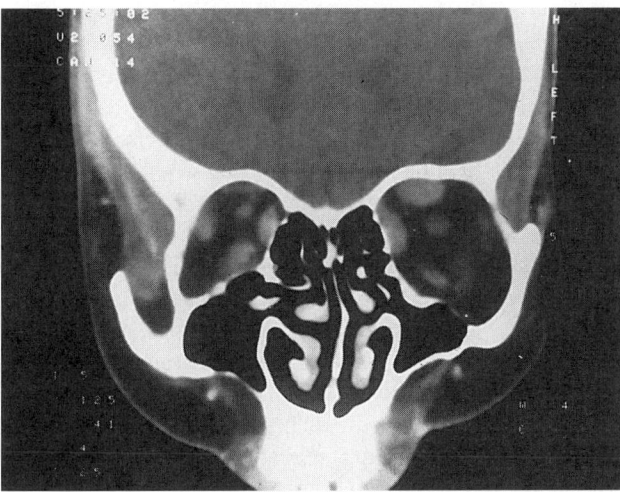

B

Fig. 52-7. **A,** 65-year-old woman with thyroid-associated oph- thalmopathy and left superior rectus muscle involvement. **B,** Corresponding coronal CT scan.

as assessment of pupillary responses, visual field testing, and ophthalmoscopy to evaluate optic nerve function. In pa- tients who perform poorly with subjective testing, visual- evoked potentials can be checked.[79] Optic neuropathy is most often caused by compression of the optic nerve (near the annulus of Zinn at the orbital apex) by enlarged extraoc- ular muscles.

Support for a compressive mechanism in Graves disease is confirmed by CT studies of the extraocular muscles at the orbital apex.[23,53,91] Extraocular muscle volume studies have demonstrated a quantitative increase in the extraocular mus- cle volume within those orbits of patients suffering from dysthyroid optic neuropathy.[23] The muscular index can be expressed as a percentage of orbital width—horizontally and vertically.[7] These studies suggest impingement of the optic nerve near the orbital apex.

Not all optic nerve dysfunction in dysthyroid orbitopathy has been attributed to a compressive cause. Progressive vi- sual field loss has occurred without enlargement of the ex- traocular muscles in dysthyroid orbitopathy (in which ante- rior to posterior stretching of the optic nerve was the only proposed mechanism for peripheral field constriction).[3] An- other case has been reported with an enlarged optic nerve sheath in the absence of extraocular muscle involve- ment (suggested to be an optic neuritislike association caused by an inflammatory infiltrate related to dysthyroid orbitopathy).[7] It is not clear whether this represented coin- cident, unrelated optic neuritis in a patient with dysthy- roid orbitopathy, or inflammatory perineuritis symboliz- ing a distinct entity related to autoimmune dysthyroid disease.

The natural history of optic neuropathy is one of a slow insidious visual loss preceded by congestive symptoms such as lid fullness, conjunctival injection, diplopia, and a rela- tively mild degree of proptosis. Visual field defects most commonly show central scotomas, although paracentral scotomas and inferior nerve fiber bundle defects associated with increased blindspot or generalized constriction have been reported. The optic nerve may appear to be normal, pale, or swollen at any stage of optic neuropathy. Usually optic neuropathy is bilateral, but occasionally it may be uni- lateral. A relative lack of proptosis, associated with sym- metric motility restriction, is a hallmark of the subgroup of patients that develop optic neuropathy. It is assumed that these patients have not compensated for their increased or- bital compliance and volume by developing proptosis. Overall, optic neuropathy occurs slightly more often in fe- males than in males, compared to thyroid disease, in which there is a heavy female predominance. Some authors have noted a greater prevalence of diabetes in patients with optic neuropathy and a more severe loss of vision.[14,35,74,79,89]

LABORATORY INVESTIGATIONS

Clinical diagnosis is easy in patients with bilateral ex- ophthalmos, lid retraction, and myopathy who have a history of hyper- or hypothyroidism. In euthyroid individuals with unilateral proptosis, however, the differentiation from other orbital disorders (tumors, orbital myositis) can still be trou- blesome. Diagnostic methods such as ultrasonography, computed tomography (CT), and magnetic resonance imag- ing (MRI) are helpful.

Ultrasonography

Orbital ultrasonography has proved very useful in the diagnosis of Graves ophthalmopathy. In A-scan ultrasonog- raphy, a beam of sound waves is directed perpendicularly to the extraocular muscle of interest within the orbit. The sound waves reflected from the muscle denote the cross-sectional diameter of the muscle.[85]

B-scan ultrasonography can produce a two-dimensional

image of the extraocular muscle. The qualitative increase in diameter of the extraocular muscle is easily seen by the experienced ultrasonographer[75]; however, quantitation and differentiation are more difficult than with the A-scan technique.

The advantages of ultrasound for diagnosis and management of Graves ophthalmopathy are (1) an absence of radiation, (2) the availability of equipment within the ophthalmologist's office, (3) the relatively low cost of initial and follow-up examinations, (4) quantitative capability, and (5) "tissue diagnosis." On the other hand, ultrasound may miss enlargement of the muscles at the orbital apex. Also, a considerable degree of expertise is required to use and interpret the test.

Radiographic Imaging

The greatest radiologic advance in orbital imaging is computed tomographic scanning. Late model CT scanners can generate serial two-dimensional images with high resolution and minimal volume averaging. The extraocular muscles, optic nerve, lacrimal gland, and bony orbit are easily differentiated from adjacent orbital fat in both axial and coronal sections.

Features of Graves ophthalmopathy can be readily distinguished by CT scan.[91] Enlargement of the extraocular muscles is the characteristic finding. As with ultrasound, the near normal size and configuration of the tendinous muscle insertions are helpful in the differential diagnosis. Computed tomography has the advantage of giving superb anatomic detail, including the orbital apex. Unfortunately, the test is relatively expensive and the patient is exposed to ionizing radiation (although the amount is well below that known to cause cataracts).

The newest radiologic technique applicable to the orbit is magnetic resonance imaging. Unlike CT scanning, MRI does not require ionizing radiation. Images are produced by electronically monitoring the behavior of the hydrogen nucleus under influence of high magnetic and radio frequency fields. The major benefit of MRI is improved differentiation of adjacent tissues. As previously described, however, the orbital fat serves to clearly separate other soft tissue and bony structures on CT scan. Patients sensitive to confined spaces and noise may be unable to complete this test.

THERAPY

Local measures can provide considerable relief from mild symptoms in many cases. Ocular discomfort (described as "grittiness" by the vast majority of patients) is probably secondary to corneal exposure with resulting tear film abnormalities and corneal surface damage.[28] Corneal exposure responds to both artificial tear (1% methylcellulose or equivalent) and to other maneuvers designed to protect the cornea. These measures include (1) using darkened glasses with side shields—which also reduce epiphora (the use of protective eye patches by day is rarely necessary), (2) applying ocular ointment, and (3) taping of lids at night. Diplopia, usually a consequence of impaired compliance of swollen or fibrosed extraocular muscles, can be managed in mild cases by use of corrective prisms, which may require frequent revision during the course of active disease to optimize binocular vision. Unfortunately, prismatic correction is not tolerated by most of the patients.

Corticosteroids

Medical management is usually considered the first modality of treatment for the acute, congestive phase of dysthyroid orbitopathy. Steroids in modest doses (equivalent to oral prednisone 20 to 30 mg per day) may be considered for recent onset of soft tissue signs, with slow tapering. In the case of acute, severe congestion with rapid proptosis, periorbital edema, ophthalmoplegia, or compressive optic neuropathy, high corticosteroid doses (equivalent to oral prednisone 80 to 120 mg per day) for 1 to 2 weeks with slow tapering thereafter has been the mainstay of medical therapy in the literature.[15,76,79,89] Many patients respond with a reduction in periorbital edema, chemosis, and hyperemia. In those with compressive optic neuropathy, permanent improvement is noted in about 33% of eyes. Most patients with optic neuropathy improve with oral corticosteroids, but approximately 20% relapse.[76] In severe cases, higher doses of intravenous corticosteroids (1 gm/day methylprednisolone for 3 days) have been advocated by some authors.[34] In these patients, remission can be maintained with 80 to 120 mg of oral prednisone, tapering by 10 mg/week combined with supervoltage orbital external beam radiation.

Corticosteroid therapy, despite its efficiency in the acute congestive phase of the disease in most of the patients, has numerous shortcomings. These include a high prevalence of recurrent disease in treated eyes, even with slow tapering and numerous side effects (such as myopathy and psychosis). Steroid therapy has a minimal influence on lid retraction and on chronic disease of longer than one year's duration. This finding is best explained by the fact that corticosteroids effect early mononuclear cell infiltration but not chronic fibrotic changes.[13] Corticosteroids are most efficient in acute congestive orbitopathy, when dose reduction is performed slowly over 2 to 3 months. For those failing corticosteroid therapy, either because of lack of outcome, a rebound result after taper down, or severe side effects, radiation therapy in association with a maintenance dosage of corticosteroids is an excellent choice of therapy.[51a]

Radiotherapy

Radiation therapy has received more popularity in the last decade as an effective means of controlling the acute inflammatory response in dysthyroid ophthalmopathy. Super-

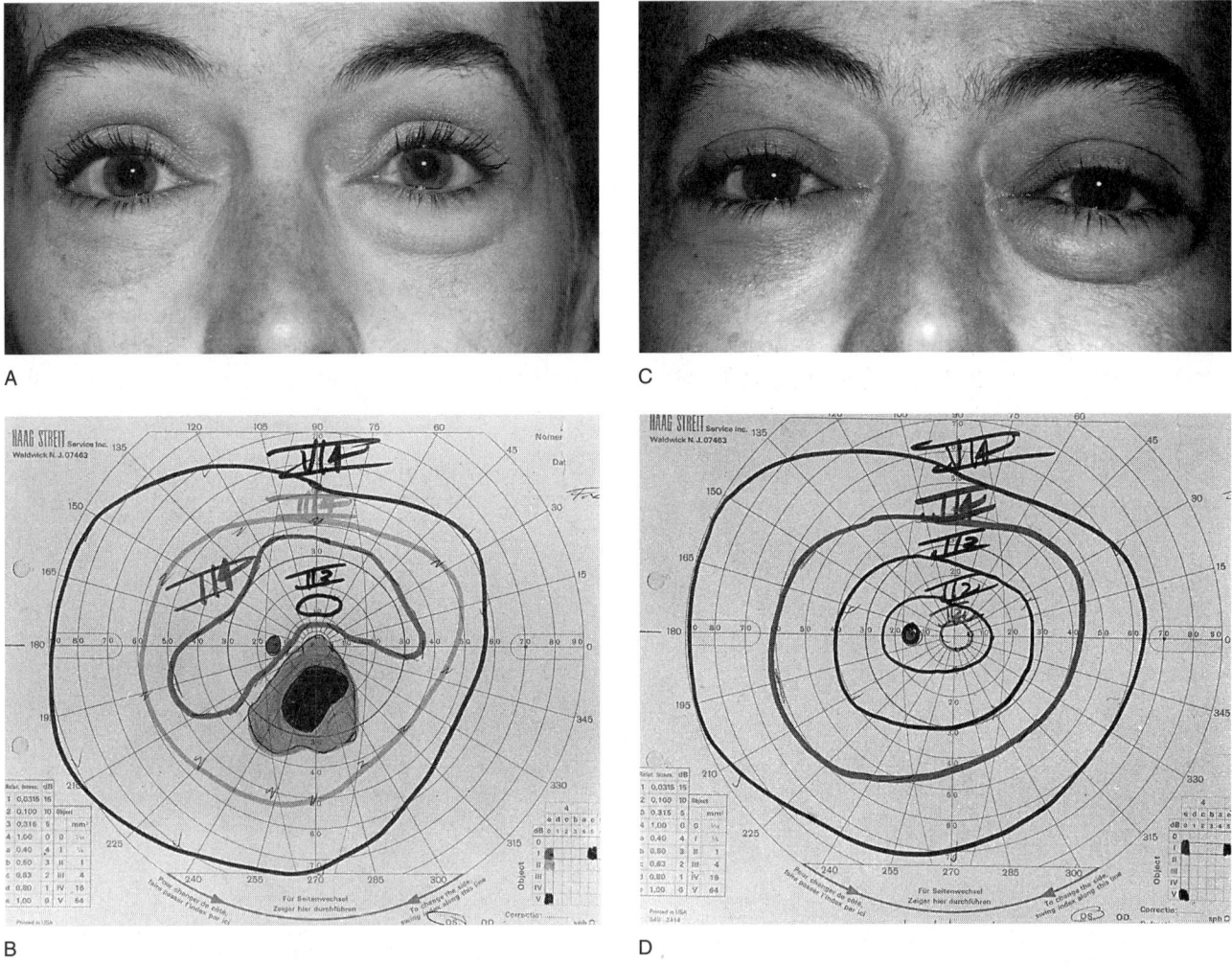

Fig. 52-8. 42-year-old woman with acute congestive phase of thyroid eye disease **A,** and visual field loss **B**. Same patient after radiation therapy with resolution of acute symptoms **C,** and resolved optic neuropathy demonstrated by visual field improvement **D**.

voltage irradiation therapy of 2000 rads (1000 rads from each lateral port) in 200 rad doses over 10 days and delivered in a columnated beam, has been shown to be most effective in this regimen.[51a] Patients with acute inflammation respond best. Improvement in soft tissue signs is usually seen within 1 month after treatment, but there may be an initial period of up to 2 weeks after treatment during which the inflammatory response worsens. This can be minimized by maintaining patients on an appropriate dose of corticosteroids. Response rates of 70% or better are reported in most large series with few side effects, although radiation retinopathy and optic neuropathy have been reported.

Side effects are much less prevalent than with corticosteroids. In most published series, radiation therapy has little effect on proptosis, ophthalmoplegia, and chronic disease.[8,10,17] Reduction of soft tissue inflammation is measured by 1- to 3-mm reduction in proptosis, although radiation may have little effect on myopathy.[10] Fig. 52-8, *A* shows a photograph of a patient suffering from the acute congestive phase of orbitopathy, who developed psychosis and improved little when treated with corticosteroids. Her postradiation treatment response showed disappearance of all congestive signs (Fig. 52-8, *B*). Her visual fields improved dramatically, indicating that there is a subgroup of patients with optic neuropathy who respond to radiation therapy. Such treatment is considered in selected subgroups of patients before surgery.

Immunosuppressive Agents

Cyclosporine, an agent that reversibly inhibits immunocompetent lymphocytes, has been used as an alternative to prednisone. Initially, beneficial effects on Graves ophthalmopathy were described,[102,105] but soon additional case reports indicated that cyclosporine was not effective[9] or even

caused deterioration of eye disease.[42] Long-term maintenance therapy with cyclosporine, continued after high-dose
corticosteroids, is considered to be beneficial by some authors.[46]

A number of cytotoxic drugs, including methotrexate,
azathioprine, and cyclophosphamide have been tried. Their
effect on Graves ophthalmopathy is doubtful, and their side
effects are often very serious.[6]

The rationale for plasma exchange therapy in Graves eye
disease is based on the assumption that circulating antibodies play a role in the pathogenesis of the disease. Incidental
beneficial effects have been reported,[30,83] but rebound phenomena after discontinuation underline the need of subse-

quent immunosuppressive drug therapy. Fatal complications
have been described.[86]

Surgical Management

Although medical therapy has a role in the treatment of
dysthyroid optic neuropathy, failure of corticosteroids and/
or irradiation to halt the progression of visual field loss or
acute visual loss with signs of optic nerve dysfunction during the course of treatment are indications for immediate
orbital decompression. The majority of such patients will
have demonstrable orbital apical crowding seen on CT scan.
Because both corticosteroids and irradiation have been
shown to have a limited effect on the underlying myopathy,
surgical decompression of the orbital apex can be the defini-

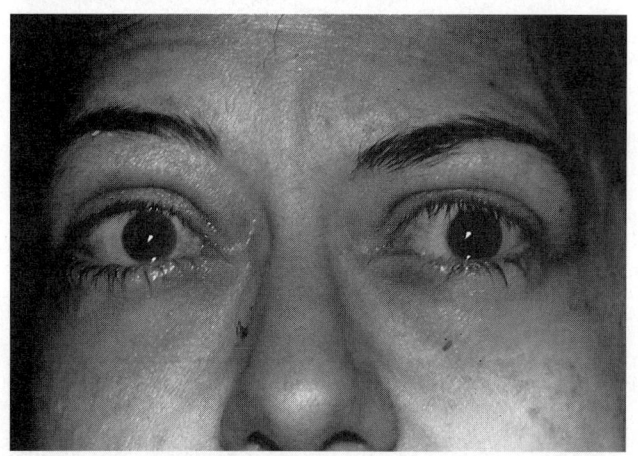

A

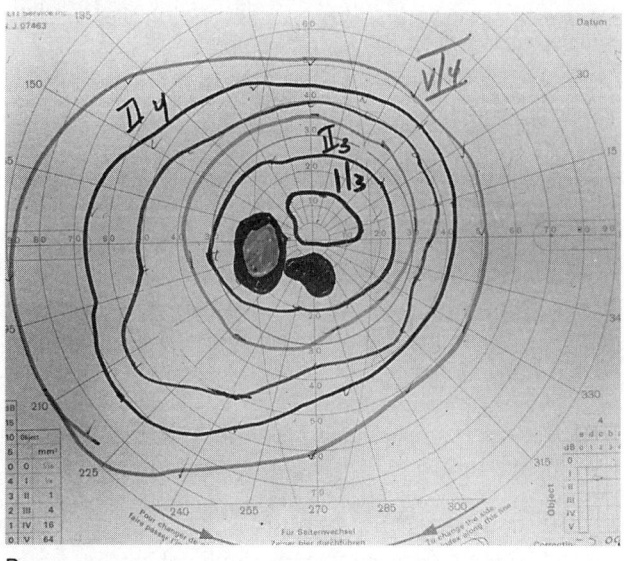

B

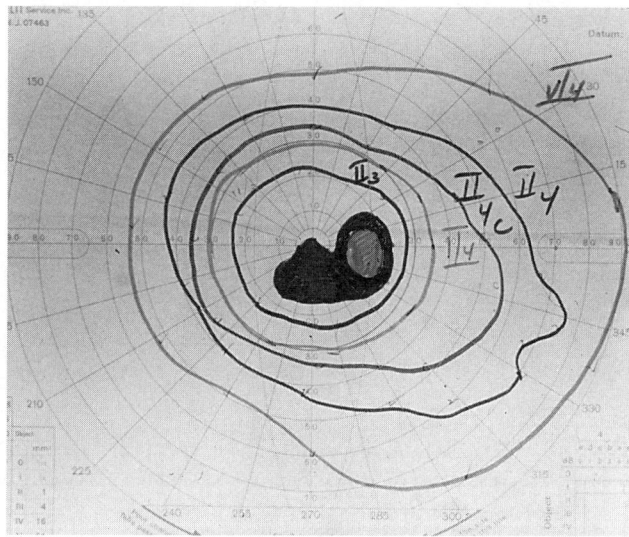

C

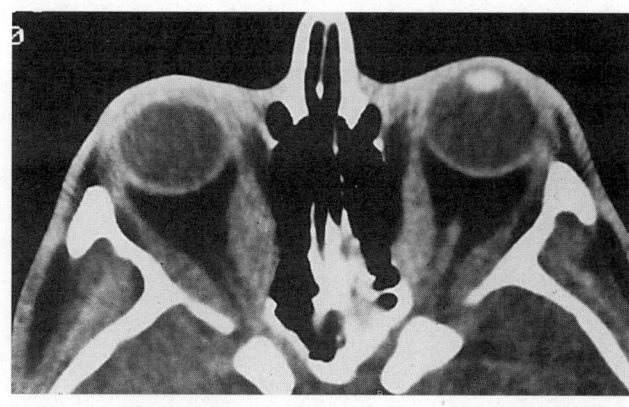

D

Fig. 52-9. **A,** 48-year-old patient with compressive optic neuropathy who did not respond to a course of corticosteroids. Note the lack of
exophthalmos. Visual fields show bilaterally enlarged blindspots with cecocentral scotoma of right eye **B,** and paracentral scotoma of left
eye, **C.** Axial **D,** CT scans confirm crowding at the orbital apex with enlargement of extraocular muscles.

tive solution for this mechanical problem once other therapy has failed (Fig. 52-9, *A-D*).

Orbital Decompression. Orbital decompression has primarily been used as a treatment for thyroid-associated ophthalmopathy when corticosteroids and radiation fail to decompress the orbital contents. Though the natural course of the disease may be self-limited, it may run a more malignant protracted course—leaving patients with optic neuropathy, lid retraction, exophthalmos, and extraocular muscle restriction. The primary indication for orbital decompression has traditionally been compressive optic neuropathy, unresponsive to medical management. In addition, corneal decompensation secondary to exposure from severe proptosis, cosmetic deformity, and restrictive myopathy with diplopia may also be indications for surgical decompression—as surgical techniques have improved. Among ophthalmic plastic surgeons, 61% of orbital decompressions were performed for mild to severe exophthalmos to correct corneal exposure and/or cosmetic disfigurement, 33% were performed for mild proptosis, and 39% were performed for the more traditional indication of optic neuropathy.[64]

Numerous attempts have been made to expand the confinement of the bony orbit and to allow tissues to expand outward. In the early part of the twentieth century Kronlein[55]

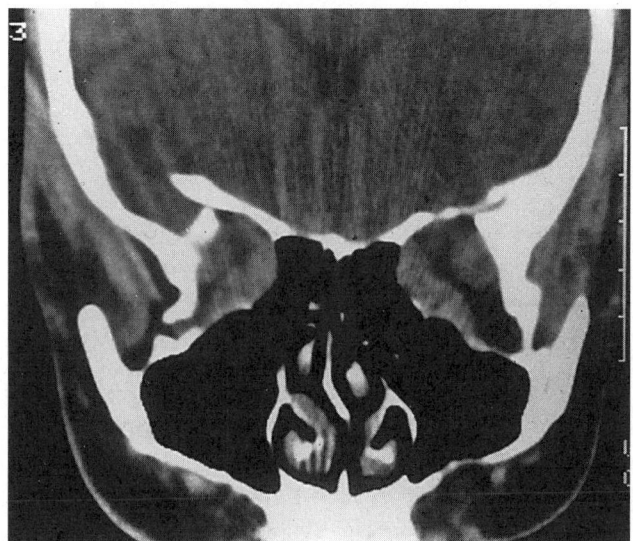

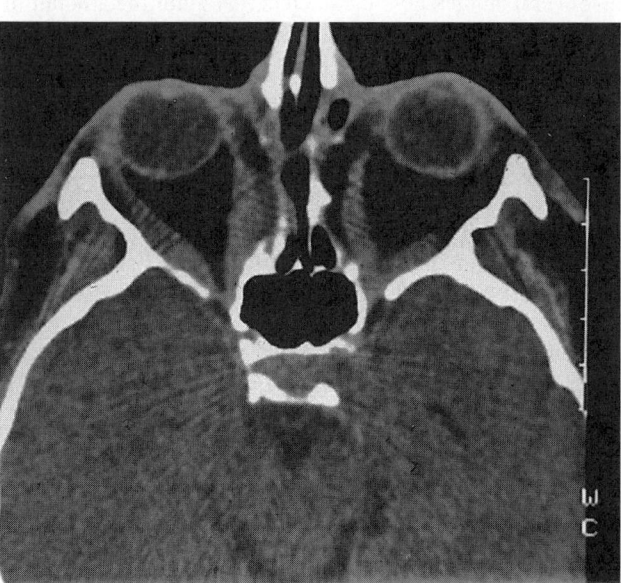

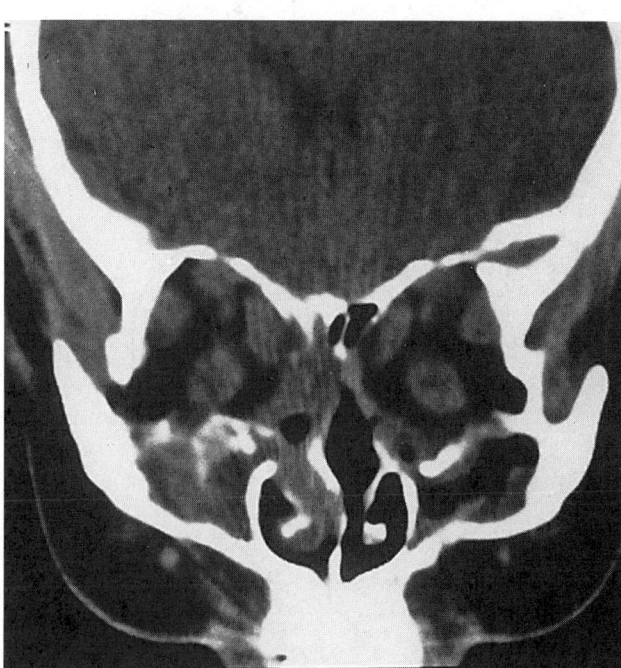

Fig. 52-9, cont'd.   Coronal **E,** CT scans confirm crowding at the orbital apex with enlargement of extraocular muscles. Postoperational axial **F,** and coronal **G,** CT scans demonstrate decompression into sinuses at the orbital apex. Approach was via bilateral medial Lynch incision with medial wall and inferior medial floor removal.

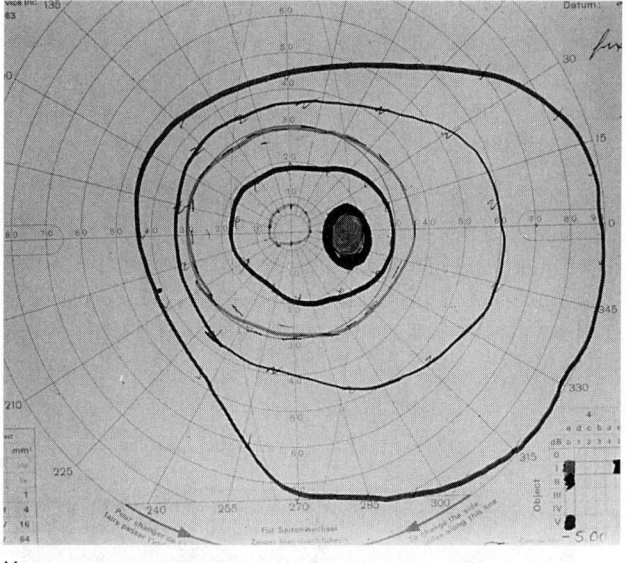

H

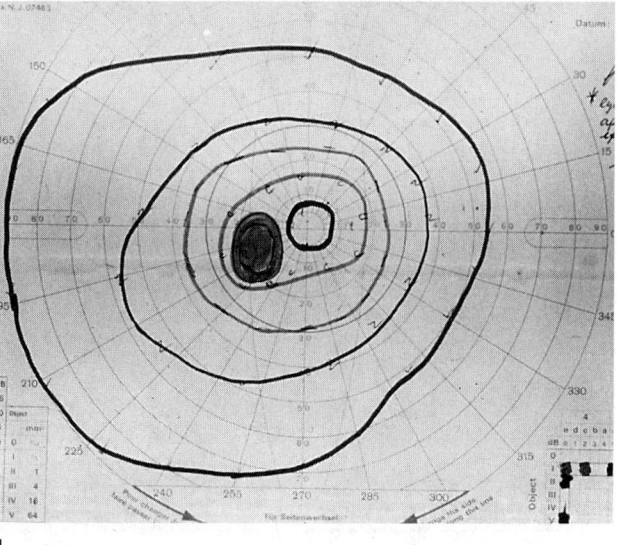

I

Fig. 52-9, cont'd.   Postoperational visual fields of right **H,** and left **I,** eyes show marked improvement.

and Dollinger[16] advocated lateral orbitotomy, offering the temporal fossa as a space for expansion of orbital volume. The major limitation with this approach is that the temporalis muscle rests within the temporal tossa and limits volume expansion. Naffziger[73] described a neurosurgical approach in 1930, whereby the orbital roof was removed from the border of the frontal sinus back to the optic foramen. A high morbidity with meningitis and pulsating exophthalmos were the natural consequences of this approach to decompression. The degree of decompression was limited by the fact that the space between the frontal lobe and the orbital contents left minimal room for volume expansion. This was also true for the lateral decompression.

The currently preferred concept of decompression with

orbital volume expansion into the aerated sinuses was pioneered by Hirsch and Sewall,[41,82] whereby Hirsch advocated decompression of the orbital floor through the maxillary-sinus, and Sewall through the medial wall via the ethmoid sinus. These procedures tended to offer more open volume for the expansion of the orbital contents. In 1957 Walsh and Ogura[99] reported successful results with transantral decompression, through a Caldwell-Luc approach that removed the inferior and medial orbital walls, allowing decompression into the maxillary and ethmoid sinuses. Several cases in their series involved successful decompression in the setting of dysthyroid optic neuropathy—where other procedures had failed.

Anterior approaches to orbital decompression have been advocated by ophthalmic surgeons. These include variations of transconjunctival approaches to the orbit for floor and medial wall decompression,[63,64,65,71] subciliary incisions with and without extension laterally,[58,90] and skin incisions at the orbital rim to reach the medial wall and orbital floor.[2,59] Combined translid and transantral methods have been proposed in a team approach.[56,87]

Goal-oriented orbital decompression allows flexibility of approach.[45,52] In patients with compressive optic neuropathy, decompression near the orbital apex is best qualified to deal with the pathophysiologic changes in the crowded orbital apex. This not only includes posterior orbital floor removal, but also medial wall decompression carried far posteriorly to allow the frequently enlarged medial rectus muscle to fall into the ethmoid sinus. If disfiguring or symptomatic proptosis are the pressing issues in a given case, then multiple wall decompressions (2, 3, or 4) must be planned to allow enough volume expansion with prolapse of orbital contents to reduce the degree of proptosis.

Several studies give parameters that tailor the amount of wall removal with needed volume expansion and reduction of proptosis. Stabile and Trokel[88] systematically studied the absolute volumes expected from decompression of each wall using dried skulls and dental moldings. They found that floor removal medial to the infraorbital groove added 7 cc of volume to the orbit, but removal of the medial wall alone added less volume. Removal of both of those walls added a combined 13 to 14 cc volume expansion. Of significance was the observation that lateral floor removal provided only 1 cc and the lateral wall only 2 cc of additional volume. Similarly, McCord and associates[66] studied orbital pressure and volume relationships using saline-filled balloons in the anterior and posterior orbit. He found orbital apical pressures reduced by 52% with antral-ethmoidal decompression, 60% with three-wall decompression when the lateral wall was added, and 80% with four-wall decompression.[50] In another cadaver study,[52] removal of the orbital floor reduced proptosis the most—an average of 3.7 mm, followed by the roof—averaging 2.7 mm, lateral wall—2.0 mm, and the medial wall—1.7 mm.

Medial wall and medial floor decompression are most commonly required. A Lynch incision is made medially with periosteal elevation along the medial wall for medial wall and floor decompression. A transconjunctival approach via lateral canthotomy and inferior fornix incision with detachment of refractors is used to further expose the orbital floor for decompression when necessary. The transconjunctival incision can also be extended medially to remove the inferior part of the medial wall. For more severe exophthalmos, a lateral orbitotomy is added with removal of the lateral wall and sphenoid. A portion of the lateral roof can be removed in a 4-wall decompression.[50] Endoscopic transnasal decompression is employed for optic neuropathy caused by prominent medial rectus involvement.[51] Complications following decompression include the degenerating of motility dysfunction, hypoglobus, and deteriorated lid malposition.

Corrective Surgery. After the need for decompression is addressed, motility dysfunction and lid malposition are assessed. For restrictive myopathy, extraocular muscle recessions with an adjustable suture technique can attain ocular alignment.[26] Botulinum toxin treatment for thyroid-associated ophthalmopathy patients with myopathy is not indicated. Criteria for surgery include diplopia in the primary position and a constant angle of deviation for at least 6 months. Success after surgery is defined as single vision in primary and reading positions. Long-term satisfactory results of extraocular muscle surgery in patients with stable dysthyroid orbitopathy can be achieved in almost 90% of the cases, although sometimes repeated surgery is required. Eyelid malposition should be corrected after orbital decompression and strabismus surgery, if those operations are necessary. Stabilization of the disease process is essential before eyelid correction is attempted, and a period of at least 6 months should be documented before trying a surgical correction.

Müller muscle excision,[98] levator stripping,[78] levator marginal myotomy,[32] levator recession,[31] and spacers[24] have all been described to adequately deal with upper lid retraction. Müller muscle excision with a graduated levator myotomy is preferred for greater than 2 mm of lid retraction. Lower lid retraction is dealt with by the placement of spacers between the lower lid retractors and the tarsal plate. Banked sclera,[19] ear cartilage,[77] hard palate mucosal grafts,[54] and free tarsal conjunctival grafts[27] are other alternatives. A lateral tarsorrhaphy can also be used to protect the exposed cornea.

REFERENCES

1. Ahmann A et al.: Antibodies to porcine eye muscle in patients with Graves ophthalmopathy: identification of serum immunoglobulins directed against unique determinants by immunoblotting and enzyme-linked immunosorbent assay, *J Clin Endocrinol Metab* 64:454-460, 1987.
2. Anderson RL, Linberg JV: Transorbital approach to decompression in Graves' disease, *Arch Ophthalmol* 99:120-124,1981.
3. Anderson RL et al.: Dysthyroid optic neuropathy without extraocular muscle involvement, *Ophthalmic Surg* 20:568-574, 1989.
4. Atkinson S, Holcombe M, Kendall-Taylor P: Ophthalmopathic immunoglobulin in patients with Graves' ophthalmopathy, *Lancet* ii:374-376, 1984.
5. Baekkeskov S et al.: Antibodies to a 64,000 Mr human islet cell antigen precede the clinical onset of insulin dependent diabetes, *J Clin Invest* 79:926-934, 1987.
6. Bahn RS, Gorman CA: Choice of therapy and criteria for assessing treatment outcome in thyroid-associated ophthalmopathy, *Endocrinol Metab Clin North Am* 16:391-407, 1986.
7. Barrett L et al.: Optic nerve dysfunction in thyroid eye disease, *CT Radiology* 167:503-507, 1988.
8. Bartalena L et al.: Orbital cobalt irradiation combined with systemic corticosteroids for Graves' ophthalmopathy: comparison with systemic cortiscosteroids alone, *J Clin Endocrinol Metab* 56:1139-1144, 1983.
9. Brabant G et al.: Cyclosporin in infiltrative eye disease, *Lancet* 1:515-516, 1984.
10. Brennan MW, Leone CR, Janaki L: Radiation therapy for Graves' disease, *Am J Ophthalmol* 96:195-199, 1983.
11. Campbell RJ: Pathology of Graves' ophthalmopathy, Eye Orbit Thyroid Dis 25-31, 1984.
12. Char DH: Introduction. In Gardner J, Vayghn V, Powell L, editors: *Thyroid eye disease*, 1-4, Baltimore, 1985, Williams & Wilkins.
13. Char DH: *Thyroid eye disease*, Baltimore, 1985, Williams and Wilkins.
14. Day RM, Carroll FD: Optic nerve involvement associated with thyroid dysfunction, *Arch Ophthalmol* 67:289-297, 1962.
15. Day RM, Carroll FD: Corticosteroids in the treatment of optic nerve involvement associated with thyroid dysfunction, *Trans Am Ophthalmol Soc* 65:41-51, 1967.
16. Dollinger J: Dracken thlastund der Augenhohle durch Eatfernung der qusseren orbital wand bet hoch gradigem exophthalmus (Morbus Basedowin) und Konsekutiver Hornhauter Krankung, *Dtsch Med Wochenschr* 37:1888-1890, 1911.
17. Doneldson SS et al.: Supervoltage orbital radiotherapy for Graves' ophthalmopathy, *J Clin Endocrinol Metab* 37:276-285, 1973.
18. Dong Q, Ludgate M, Vassart G: Cloning and sequencing of a novel 64 kDa autoantigen recognized by patients with autoimmune thyroid disease, *J Clin Endocrinol Metab* 72:1375-1381, 1991.
19. Dryden RM, Soll DB: The use of scleral transplantation in cicatricial entropion and eyelid retraction, *Trans Am Head Ophthalmol Otolarying* 83:669-678, 1977.
20. Elisei R, Dong Q, Ludgate M: Cloning and sequencing of candidate eye muscle antigens in Graves' ophthalmopathy. In Gordon A, Gross, Hennemann G, editors: *Progress in thyroid research*, Proceedings of the 10th International Thyroid Congress, The Hague, 1991.
21. Faryna M, Nauman T, Gordon A: Measurement of autoantibodies against human eye muscle membranes in Graves' ophthalmopathy, *Br Med J* 290:191-192, 1985.
22. Feldon SE, Weiner JM: Clinical significance of extraocular muscle volumes in Graves ophthalmopathy: a quantitative computed tomography study, *Arch Ophthalmol* 100:1266-1269, 1982.
23. Feldon SE et al.: Quantitative computed tomography of Graves' ophthalmopathy, extraocular muscle, and orbital fat in development of optic neuropathy, *Arch Ophthalmol* 103:213-215, 1985.
24. Flanagan JC: Eye bank sclera in oculoplastic surgery, *Ophthalmic Surg* 5:45-53, 1974.
25. Gamblin GT et al.: Prevalence of increased intraocular pressure in Graves' disease. Evidence of frequent subclinical ophthalmopathy, *New Eng J Med* 308:420-424, 1983.
26. Gardner TA, Kennerdell JS: Treatment of dysthyroid myopathy with adjustable suture recession, *Ophthalmic Surg* 21:519-521, 1990.
27. Gardner TA, Kennerdell JS, Buerger GF: Treatment of dysthyroid lower lid retraction with autogenous tarsus transplants, *Ophthalmic Plast Reconstr Surg* 8:26-31, 1992.
28. Gilbard JP, Farris RL: Ocular surface drying and tearfilm osmolarity in thyroid eye disease, *Acta Ophthalmol* 61:108-116, 1983.
29. Glaser JS: *Neuroophthalmology*, ed 2, 398-402, Philadelphia, 1990, JB Lippincott.

30. Glinoer D et al.: Beneficial effects of intensive plasma exchange followed by immunosuppressive therapy in severe Graves ophthalmopathy, *Metab Pediatr Syst Ophthalmol* 11:133-140, 1988.

31. Goldstein J: Recession of the levator muscle for lagophthalmos in exophthalmic goiter, *Arch Ophthalmol* 11:389-393, 1934.

32. Graves RJ: Newly observed affection of the thyroid gland in females, *London Med Surg J* 7:516-520, 1835.

33. Grove AS: Upper eyelid retraction and Graves' disease, *Ophthalmology* 88:499, 1981.

34. Guy JR et al.: Methylprednisolone pulse therapy in severe dysthyroid optic neuropathy, *Ophthalmology* 96:1046-1053, 1987.

35. Hedges TR Jr, Scherer HG: Visual field defects in exophthalmos with thyroid disease, *Arch Ophthalmol* 54:885-892, 1955.

36. Hermann JS: Paretic thyroid myopathy, *Ophthalmology* 89:473-478, 1982.

37. Hiromatsu Y et al.: Antibody-dependent cell-mediated cytotoxicity against human eye muscle cells and orbital fibroblasts in Graves' ophthalmopathy—roles of class II MHC antigen expression and γ-interferon action on effector and target cells, *Clin Exp Immunol* 70:597-603, 1987.

38. Hiromatsu Y et al.: A thyroid cytotoxic antibody that cross-reacts with an eye muscle cell surface antigen may be the cause of thyroid-associated ophthalmopathy, *J Clin Endocrinol Metab* 67:565-570, 1988.

39. Hiromatsu Y et al.: Significance of cytotoxic eye muscle antibodies in patients with thyroid-associated ophthalmopathy, *Autoimmunity* 5:205-213, 1990.

40. Hiromatsu Y et al.: Significance of anti-eye muscle antibody in patients with thyroid-associated ophthalmopathy by quantitative Western blot, *Autoimmunity* 14:1-8, 1993.

41. Hirsch O: Surgical decompression of malignant exophthalmos, *Arch Otolaryngol* 51:325-334, 1950.

42. Howlett TA et al.: Deterioration of severe Graves' ophthalmopathy. In Schindler R, editor: *Cyclosporine in autoimmune disease,* 229-234, Berlin, 1985, Springer-Verlag.

43. Hufnagel TJ et al.: Immunohistochemical and ultrastructural studies on the exenterated orbital tissues of a patient with Graves' disease, *Ophthalmology* 91:1411-1419, 1984.

44. Hurwitz JJ, Birt D: An individualized approach to orbital decompression in Graves' orbitopathy, *Arch Ophthalmol* 103:660-665, 1985.

45. Jacobson DH, Gorman CA: Endocrine ophthalmopathy: current ideas concerning etiology, pathogenesis and treatment, *Endocr Rev* 5:200-220, 1984.

46. Kahaly G et al.: Ciclosporin and prednisone vs. prednisone in treatment of Graves' ophthalmopathy: a controlled, randomized and prospective study, *Eur J Clin Invest* 16:415-422, 1986.

47. Kapusta M et al.: Eye muscle membrane reactive antibodies are not detected in the serum or immunoglobulin fraction of patients with thyroid-associated ophthalmopathy using an ELISA and crude membranes, *Autoimmunity* 7:33-40, 1990.

48. Katowitz JA et al.: Classification and management of orbital disorders. In ed *Orbit, Eyelids and Lacrimal System,* 76, San Francisco, 1988, The American Academy of Ophthalmology.

49. Kazim M, Kennerdell JS: Elevated intraocular pressure in dysthyroid orbitopathy, *Orbit* 10:211-215, 1991.

50. Kennedy DW et al.: An orbital decompression for severe dysthyroid exophthalmos, *Ophthalmology* 89:467-472, 1982.

51. Kennedy DW et al.: Endoscopic transnasal orbital decompression, *Arch Otolaryngol Head Neck Surg* 116:275-282, 1990.

51a. Kennerdell JS, Baron EM, Tyutyunikov A, Wall JR, Genovese C: Unpublished data.

52. Kennerdell JS, Maroon JB, Buerger GF: Comprehensive surgical management of proptosis in dysthyroid orbitopathy, *Orbit* 6:153-179, 1989.

53. Kennerdell JS, Rosenbaum AE, El-Hoshy MH: A typical optic nerve compression of dysthyroid optic neuropathy on computed tomography, *Arch Ophthalmol* 99:807-809, 1981.

54. Kersten RC et al.: Management of lower lid retraction with hard-palate mucosa grafting, *Ophthalmology* 108:1339-1343, 1990.

55. Kronlein R: Zur Pathologic und operativen Behandlung der Dermoidcysten der Orbita, *Beitr Kein Chir* 4:149-163, 1888.

56. Kulwin DR, Cotton RT, Kersten RC: Combined approach to orbital decompression, *Otolaryngol Clin North Am* 23:381-390, 1990.

57. Leone CR: The management of ophthalmic Graves' disease, *Ophthalmology* 770-779, 1984.

58. Leone CR, Bajandas FJ: Interior orbital decompression for thyroid ophthalmology, *Arch Ophthalmol* 98:890-892, 1980.

59. Linberg JV, Anderson RL: Transorbital decompression indications and results, *Arch Ophthalmol* 99:113-114, 1981.

60. Mahieu P, Winand R: Demonstration of delayed hypersensitivity to retrobulbar and thyroid tissues in human exophthalmos, *J Clin Endocrinol Metab* 34:1090-1092, 1972.

61. Martinez AJ, Hay S, McNeer KW: Extraocular muscles, light microscopy and ultrastructural features, *Acta Neuropathol* 34:237-253, 1976.

62. Martinez AJ et al.: Extraocular muscles: morphogenetic study in humans: light microscopy and ultrastructural features, *Acta Neuropathol* 38:87-93, 1977.

63. McCord CD: Orbital decompression for Graves' disease, *Ophthalmology* 88:533-541, 1981.

64. McCord CD: Current trends in orbital decompression, *Ophthalmology* 92:21-33, 1885.

65. McCord CD, Moses JL: Exposure of the inferior orbit with fornix incision and lateral canthotomy, *Ophthalmic Surg* 10:53-63, 1979.

66. McCord CD, Putnam JR, Ugland DN: Pressure-volume orbital measurement comparing decompression approaches, *Ophthalmic Plast Reconstr Surg* 1:55-63, 1985.

67. Mengistu M et al.: Clinical significance of a new autoantibody against a human eye muscle soluble antigen detected by immunofluorescence, *Clin Exp Immunol* 65:19-27, 1986.

68. Migliori ME, Gladstone GF: Determination of the normal range of exophthalmometric values for black and white adults, *Am J Ophthalmol* 398:438, 1984.

69. Miller A et al.: Evaluation of an enzyme-linked immunosorbent assay for the measurement of autoantibodies against eye muscle membrane antigens in Graves ophthalmopathy, *Acta Endocrinol* 113:514-522, 1986.

70. Miller A et al.: Significance of antibodies reactive with a 64 kDa eye muscle membrane antigen in patients with thyroid autoimmunity, *Thyroid* 2:197-202, 1992.

71. Moses JL, McCord CD: Orbital decompression, *Am Surg* 45:608-611, 1979.

72. Munro RE et al.: Cell-mediated immunity in exophthalmos of Graves' disease as demonstrated by the migration inhibition factor (MIF) test, *J Clin Endocrinol Metab* 37:286-292, 1973.

73. Naffziger HC: Progressive exophthalmos following thyroidectomy: its pathology and treatment, *Ann Surg* 94:582-586, 1931.

74. Neigel J et al.: Dysthyroid optic neuropathy—the crowded orbital apex syndrome, *Ophthalmology* 95:1515-1521, 1988.

75. Ossoinig KC: Ultrasonic diagnosis of Graves ophthalmopathy. In Gorman CA, Waller RR, Dyer JA, editors: *The eye and orbit in thyroid disease,* 185-211, New York, 1984, Raven Press.

76. Panzo GJ, Tomsak RL: A retrospective review of 26 cases of dysthyroid optic neuropathy, *Am J Ophthalmol* 96:190-194, 1983.

77. Putterman AM: Surgical treatment of dysthyroid eyelid retraction and orbital fat hernia, *Otolaryngol Clin North Am* 13:39-51, 1980.

78. Putterman AM, Urist M: Surgical treatment of upper eyelid retraction, *Arch Ophthalmol* 87:401-405, 1972.

79. Rootman J: *Diseases of the orbit,* 241-280, Philadelphia, 1988, JB Lippincott.

80. Salvi M, Miller A, Wall JR: Human orbital tissue and thyroid membranes express a 64 kDa protein which is recognized by autoantibodies in serum of patients with thyroid-associated ophthalmopathy, *FEBS Lett* 232:135-139, 1988.

81. Salvi M et al.: Prevalence of antibodies reactive with a 64 kDa eye muscle membrane antigen in thyroid-associated ophthalmopathy, *Thyroid* 1:207-213, 1991.

82. Sato M et al.: Antibodies reactive with eye muscle and thyroid antigens in early and late thyroid-associated ophthalmopathy, Proc Intl Symposium on Hashimoto's Thyroiditis, Fukuoka, December 2-5, 1992.

83. Schrooyen M, Winand R, Glinoer D: Plasma exchange therapy for severe Graves' ophthalmopathy, *Orbit* 5:105-110, 1986.

84. Sewall EC: Operative control of progressive exophthalmos, *Arch Otolaryngol* 24:621-624, 1936.

85. Shammas HJF, Minckler DS, Ogden C: Ultrasound in early thyroid orbitopathy, *Arch Ophthalmol* 98:277-279, 1980.

86. Shumak KH, Rock GA: Therapeutic plasma exchange, *New Eng J Med* 310:762-771, 1984.

87. Small RG, Meiring LN: A combined orbital and antral approach to surgical decompression of the orbit, *Ophthalmology* 88:542-547, 1981.

88. Stabile JR, Trokel SM: Increase in orbital volume obtained by decompression in dried skulls, *Am J Ophthalmol* 95:329-331, 1983.

89. Trobe J, Glaser JS, Laflamme P: Dysthyroid optic neuropathy, *Arch Ophthalmol* 96:1199-1209, 1978.

90. Trokel SL, Cooper WC: Orbital decompression: effect on motility and globe position, *Ophthalmology* 86:2064-2070, 1979.

91. Trokel SL, Jacobiec FA: Correlation of CT scanning and pathologic features of ophthalmic Graves' disease, *Ophthalmology* 88:553-564, 1981.

92. Tyutyunikov A et al.: Re-examination of peripheral blood T cell subsets in dysthyroid orbitopathy, *Invest Ophthalmol Vis Sci* 33:2299-2303, 1992.

93. van Dijk HJL: Orbital Graves' disease: a modification of the ''NO SPECS'' - classification, *Ophthalmology* 88:479-484, 1981.

94. von Basedow CA: Exophthalmos durch Hypertrophie des Cellgewebes in der Agenhohle, *Wochenschr Ges Meilk* 6:197-120, 1840.

95. Wall JR, Trewin A, Joyner DM: Peripheral blood lymphocyte transformation in response to human thyroid fractions in patients with Graves hyperthyroidism and ophthalmopathy, *Acta Endocrinol* 93:419-423, 1980.

96. Wall JR et al.: Antibody cross-reactivity may explain the association of ophthalmopathy and thyroid autoimmunity, *Clin Res* 38:(abstract), 1990.

97. Wall JR et al.: Thyroid-associated ophthalmopathy—a model for the association of organ-specific autoimmune disorders, *Immunol Today* 12:150-153, 1991.

98. Waller RR: Eyelid malpositions in Graves' ophthalmopathy, *Trans Am Ophthalmol Soc* 80:855-930, 1982.

99. Walsh TE, Ogura JH: Transantral orbital decompression of malignant exophthalmos, *Laryngoscope* 67:544-568, 1957.

100. Wang PW et al.: Immunologically mediated cytotoxicity against human eye muscle cells in Graves' ophthalmopathy, *J Clin Endocrinol Metab* 63:316-320, 1986.

101. Weetman AP: Thyroid-associated ophthalmopathy, *Autoimmunity* 12:215-222, 1992.

102. Weetman AP et al.: Cyclosporine improves Graves' ophthalmopathy, *Lancet* 2:486-489, 1983.

103. Werner SC: Classification of the eye changes of Graves' disease, *Am J Ophathalmol* 68:646-649, 1969.

104. Werner SC: Modification of the classification of the eye changes of Graves' disease, *Am J Ophthalmol* 83:725-727, 1977.

105. Witte A et al.: Treatment of Graves' ophthalmopathy with cyclosporin A, *Klin Wochenschr* 63:1000-1004, 1985.

106. Zhang ZG et al.: Studies of cytotoxic antibodies against eye muscle antigens in patients with thyroid associated ophthalmopathy. Proc Intl Symposium on Graves' ophthalmopathy, Helsinki, May 1989. *Acta Endocrinologica* 21(2):23-30, 1989.

107. Zhang ZG et al.: Restricted tissue reactivity of autoantibodies to a 64 kDa eye muscle membrane antigen in thyroid-associated ophthalmopathy, *Clin Immunol Immunopathol* 62:183-189, 1992.

108. Zhang ZG et al.: Molecular characterization of 64 kDa eye muscle membrane autoantigens and significance of the corresponding autoantibodies, Proceedings of the 66th Meeting of the American Thyroid Association, Rochester, Minn, September 1992, *Thyroid* 2 (suppl 1) (abstract).

53 Scleritis and Episcleritis

PETER J. McCLUSKEY, DENIS WAKEFIELD

Scleritis is a chronic, painful, destructive, potentially blinding, inflammatory process involving the sclera. It is commonly associated with systemic disease and requires systemic therapy to control the inflammation. Scleritis may be the presentation of a potentially life-threatening systemic disease.

Episcleritis (which involves the episclera) is acute in nature and mild in severity. It is not a threat to vision, is infrequently linked with systemic disease, and usually responds to topical therapy.

The differentiation of scleritis from episcleritis is essential to allow correct management decisions. Whereas severe necrotizing scleritis presents a highly characteristic clinical picture, milder forms of scleritis may be difficult to distinguish from episcleritis unless careful attention is paid to the history and clinical signs.

HISTORICAL BACKGROUND

Scleritis has been recognized since the time of Galen. It was first described as a distinct clinical entity by William Read in the early eighteenth century and was initially considered a manifestation of rheumatic disease.[48] By the nineteenth century, advances in pathology and microbiology allowed the classification of rheumatic diseases into gout, rheumatoid arthritis, tuberculous arthritis, and syphilis. Scleritis was linked with each of these diseases.

Scleritis is now recognized as a distinct inflammatory disease that may occur in isolation or in association with a variety of immune and rheumatic diseases. Scleral inflammation may also result from microbial infection of the sclera or from infiltration by neoplasms.

The careful observations and clinical research of Watson have added to the knowledge of the pathology, clinical features, and treatment of scleral inflammation. His numerous publications on scleral disease form the basis of many of the current concepts of scleritis. In recent years the techniques of immunopathology have added significantly to the understanding of scleral inflammation, but the precise cause and pathogenesis remain obscure in many patients.

ANATOMY

The sclera is a highly organized, opaque tissue composed of precisely arranged, interlacing collagen fibrils. Collagen comprises approximately 80% of the sclera by weight and is arranged in bundles that vary in diameter from 30 to 300 microns. The collagen bundles are often quite convoluted within the sclera.[48] The collagen of the sclera is predominantly type I, and there are small amounts of type II and type III collagen. Collagen bundles may contain mixtures of different collagen types or a single collagen type. The collagen is strengthened by the addition of elastin fibers. A proteoglycan matrix completes the microstructure of the sclera.[11,15]

The unique arrangement of collagen and elastin in the sclera produces maximal rigidity and stability, providing a stable environment for vision during ocular rotations and fluctuations of intraocular pressure.[48] The collagen fibers are densest and the sclera is thickest posteriorly. The sclera thins toward the equator and is thinnest posterior to the insertions of the extraocular muscles. It increases significantly in thickness at the muscle insertions and in the limbal area.

The sclera is richly innervated by branches from the short and long ciliary nerves. Anteriorly, the branches of the long ciliary nerves form a dense network supplying the perilimbal sclera, ciliary body, and cornea. The posterior sclera is supplied by branches from the short posterior ciliary nerves.

The blood supply of the anterior segment of the eye (including the sclera) is derived from the long posterior ciliary arteries and the anterior ciliary arteries that accompany the rectus muscles. These arteries run forward from the muscle insertions within Tenon capsule, giving off branches within the episclera. These branches give rise to three vascular arcades that lie in the episclera and conjunctiva, forming a richly anastomotic network of vessels to supply the conjunctiva, cornea, iris, and ciliary body.[29,45] The sclera itself is poorly vascularized. Sandwiched between the highly vascular episclera and choroid, its metabolic requirements are met by diffusion.

The most superficial vascular layer of the anterior segment is the conjunctival plexus, a dense network of fine vessels in the substantia propria of the conjunctiva that is easily moved over the underlying structures during examination of the globe. This superficial layer of vessels dilates readily and can obscure the deeper tissues. The vessels can be blanched with the topical application of dilute solutions of phenylephrine or adrenaline. The superficial episcleral plexus is a radially oriented layer of larger vessels that are readily visible when dilated. There is a dense anastomosis of these vessels at the limbus that, together with vessels from the other vascular layers, forms the anterior episcleral arterial circle whose branches supply the episclera, anterior conjunctiva, limbus, and iris. The third and deepest layer, the episcleral plexus, is an interlacing network of blood vessels adherent to the superficial sclera.

The blood vessels of the episclera and conjunctiva are visible on slit-lamp examination and can be imaged accurately with videoangiography and high-speed, external, anterior segment, fluorescein angiography. The vascular plexuses of the anterior segment are most clearly defined in the arterial circulation. The venous pattern is far more variable but tends to parallel the arterial circulation. Correctly identifying the relationship between the various vascular networks and the underlying sclera is crucial to the correct differentiation of episcleral from scleral inflammation.

The posterior sclera is supplied by a fine plexus of vessels derived from the short posterior ciliary arteries. These have a variable anastomosis with the blood vessels that supply the anterior segment of the sclera.

Classification of Scleral and Episcleral Inflammations

The morphologic classification of scleral inflammation developed by Watson[47] is the most widely used system for assessing the site and severity of scleral inflammation. This classification divides episcleritis into simple and nodular varieties, and scleritis into anterior and posterior types. Anterior scleritis is further subdivided into diffuse, nodular, necrotizing with inflammation, and necrotizing without inflammation (Table 53-1). Diffuse anterior scleritis is the mildest form, and necrotizing scleritis is the most severe form. The cornea is frequently involved in scleral inflammation, and some authors include various types of sclerokeratitis within the spectrum of scleral disease.[27]

Watson's classification has stood the test of time, and he has shown that the majority of patients do not change from one type of scleritis to another during the course of their disease.[39] The crucial issue with the use of this classification is to interpret the patient's clinical signs correctly and thus classify the disease accurately at the initial assessment. It is then possible to formulate a rational management plan.

TABLE 53-1   CLASSIFICATION OF SCLERAL INFLAMMATION

Episcleritis	Scleritis
Simple	**Anterior**
	Diffuse
	Nodular
Nodular	Necrotizing
	-with inflammation
	-without inflammation
	(scleromalacia perforans)
	Posterior

EPISCLERITIS

The term episcleritis refers to inflammation of the episclera, the loose, highly vascular, connective tissue that lies deep to Tenon capsule and superficial to the sclera. Episcleritis is abrupt in onset, acute in its course, and recurrent in nature. It may be localized or diffuse in extent and is classified as simple or nodular in type.

Epidemiology

Episcleritis occurs in all parts of the world. There is no known racial predilection and no known genetic association. This inflammation is seen more often in spring and autumn.

Episcleritis is a common disease affecting all age groups that most frequently occurs in young and middle-aged adults.[45] It is more prevalent in females.

Natural History

Episcleritis is usually mild, transient, and recurrent. Patients with mild disease often do not seek nor need medical intervention, as the episcleritis subsides rapidly without treatment. Episcleritis severe enough to require treatment responds to topical antiinflammatory therapy. Most attacks of simple episcleritis resolve within 2 to 21 days with or without treatment. Many patients have numerous, frequent recurrences. Patients who have prolonged attacks of episcleritis are more resistant to treatment, and an associated disease is more likely to be present.[48]

Nodular episcleritis tends to be the most severe and persistent clinical form of the disease. It may take several weeks to resolve and usually requires topical and systemic treatment. It has a marked tendency to recur.

Pathogenesis

Episcleritis may be produced by a variety of immune and nonimmune mechanisms. Immune mechanisms may involve acute hypersensitivity responses (type I hypersensitivity), presumably caused by Ig E-mediated degranulation of tissue mast cells. Immune complex-mediated reactions (type III hypersensitivity) may occur in vasculitic diseases involving the episclera. Delayed-type hypersensitivity reactions (type IV) are characteristic of granulomatous diseases such as sarcoidosis, tuberculosis, and syphilis.

Episcleritis is usually idiopathic in nature but may be associated with a range of systemic diseases. Diffuse episcleritis may occasionally occur as a result of allergic, infectious, and drug-induced diseases. It is also seen in association with seronegative arthropathies (such as Reiter syndrome and enteropathic arthritis) and vasculitic diseases (such as erythema multiforme and erythema nodosum). Histologically, diffuse episcleritis is an example of acute inflammation with widespread vasodilatation, oedema, and a diffuse lymphocytic infiltrate.[50] Healing occurs without significant scarring.

Nodular episcleritis is most frequently idiopathic but may be associated with granulomatous conditions, connective tissue diseases, and vasculitis. Histologically, episcleral nodules are composed of a chronic inflammatory cell infiltrate with mononuclear cells and giant cells.[50] Granulomata may have a central area of necrosis surrounded by a zone of epithelioid cells, giant cells, lymphocytes, and plasma cells. This chronic inflammatory response may be associated with syphilis, tuberculosis, gout, foreign-body reactions, and vasculitic syndromes such as polyarteritis nodosa and giant-cell arteritis.

Clinical Features

Episcleritis takes the form of an acute inflammatory response and its onset is typically abrupt. It is frequently bilateral. Patients complain of redness and irritation of the affected eye and note burning, hot, irritating ocular discomfort; and watering (rather than the severe pain of scleritis). Pain is uncommon but when present is always localized to the eye. In patients with chronic or nodular episcleritis, pain can be significant enough to be the presenting complaint.

Vasodilatation of the superficial episcleral vessels and edema of the episclera are the cardinal signs of episcleral inflammation. The degree of injection can range from a mild pink discoloration to intense redness. On careful examination there is no deep bluish discoloration as is observed in scleritis; however, an examination in natural daylight may be necessary to appreciate this distinction. The area of episcleritis may be diffuse and involve the entire globe, or it may be localized and sectorial in extent. Episcleral edema and thickening are usually readily identifiable as superficial to the sclera proper, and any nodules or localized areas of swelling can be moved over the sclera.

The location of the tissue edema and maximal vessel injection are the keys to the diagnosis of episcleritis. The sclera is not involved, and there is no displacement of the deep episcleral vascular plexus. Blanching the conjunctival vascular plexus with the topical application of 10% phenylephrine allows the underlying vessels to be seen more easily.

The use of red-free light and diffuse slit-lamp illumination is very helpful for studying the relationship of the vascular layers.

The globe is not tender to palpation in patients with episcleritis. Vision is not affected. Keratitis, uveitis, and other intraocular inflammation is usually absent. Intraocular pressure is normal. External eye examination is otherwise normal except for signs of allergic disease that may be seen in patients with episcleritis.

Laboratory Investigations

Investigations are not usually necessary in patients with episcleritis, as the majority of patients have idiopathic disease on clinical assessment. The crucial investigations are to take a full medical history, to examine the eye carefully, and to undertake a review of systems to ascertain clues that may point to the need for further selective investigation. It is inappropriate and unrewarding to order a large battery of tests in patients with episcleritis. Selective investigations (Table 53-2) are performed to rule out specific disease entities in patients with an atypical clinical course, symptoms suggestive of an associated systemic disease, or severe nonresponsive recurrent episcleritis.

Therapy

Episcleritis is a benign, episodic, self-limiting process causing irritating symptoms to the patient rather than destructive changes to the globe. It responds rapidly to local antiinflammatory therapy in the vast majority of patients who require treatment. Patients not responding to topical treatment will usually respond to oral, nonsteroidal, antiin-

TABLE 53-2 LABORATORY INVESTIGATIONS FOR ASSESSING PATIENTS WITH EPISCLERITIS OR SCLERITIS

Tests	Episcleritis	Scleritis
Blood & serologic tests	Antinuclear antibody MHA-TP Uric acid	Antinuclear antibody (ANA) Antineutrophil cytoplasmic antibody (ANCA) Angiotensin-converting enzyme Calcium Complete blood count Erythrocyte sedimentation rate MHA-TP Rheumatoid factor Uric acid
Skin tests	Allergy tests	Tuberculin skin test
Radiologic tests		Chest x-ray Sacroiliac joint x-rays

flammatory drugs (NSAID) such as naproxen, indometha-cin, and flurbiprofen (Fig. 53-1).

Episcleritis may be so mild and evanescent that no treat-ment is necessary. A short, intensive course of topical corti-costeroids is sufficient therapy for most patients with either simple or nodular episcleritis. A small number of patients, particularly those with nodular episcleritis, require an oral NSAID to control the inflammation. Persistent or frequently recurrent episcleritis can often be controlled by the pro-longed use of oral NSAID. Failure to respond to this regimen of treatment should lead to questioning of the diagnosis of episcleritis and to consideration of the possi-bility that the patient may have an associated systemic dis-ease, scleritis rather than episcleritis, or a masquerade syn-drome.

Surgery has no place in the management of episcleritis except in the rare circumstance of diagnostic uncertainty or when a masquerade syndrome is suspected. An episcleral biopsy may then be indicated. Patients with episcleritis do not require any special perioperative treatment when under-going ocular surgery.

Complications

Peripheral corneal stromal opacities occur in up to 10% of patients with episcleritis. These changes are small, local-ized, nonprogressive, and do not affect vision. Patients may also develop transient low-grade anterior uveitis with severe attacks.[48]

Watson has observed mild, superficial, scleral thinning and pigmentary changes in the pars plana in a small number of patients after many years of recurrent nodular episcleritis, but these have not been progressive and have not affected vision.[48]

EPISCLERITIS: THERAPEUTIC APPROACH

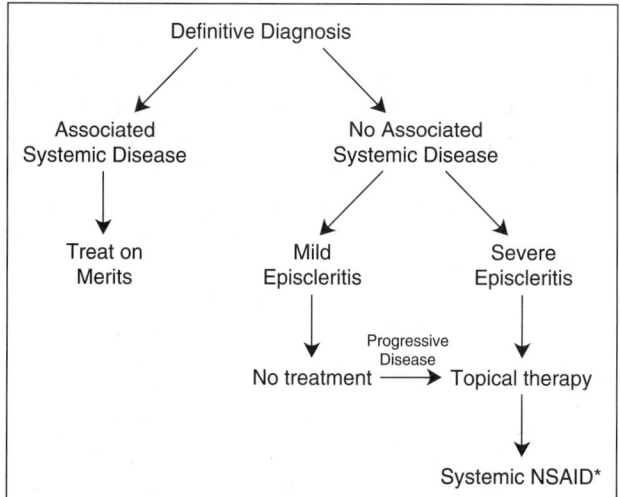

*NSAID = Nonsteroidal antiinflammatory drug

Fig. 53-1.   Therapeutic approach to episcleritis.

Prognosis

Episcleritis does not produce significant ocular compli-cations and does not impair vision. Episcleritis is typically idiopathic and usually responds rapidly to topical therapy. Although some patients have recurrent episodes (particu-larly those with gout), the disease gradually becomes quies-cent after a period of years.

SCLERITIS

Scleritis is a severe, chronic, destructive inflammation of the sclera and is symptomatic, except for scleromalacia per-forans, which is an uncommon but asymptomatic form of severe scleritis.

Scleritis is classified clinically into anterior and posterior types, with anterior scleritis further subclassified into dif-fuse, nodular, necrotizing with inflammation, and necrotiz-ing without inflammation (scleromalacia perforans).[45]

Differential Diagnosis

Whereas scleritis may have signs and symptoms sugges-tive of a neoplastic lesion, the opposite situation in which a malignancy appears as an inflammatory scleritis has been rarely reported. Eyes with malignant melanoma have an in-flammatory syndrome in 5% of cases, which is episcleritis in nearly two thirds of the patients.[9] Choroidal melanoma has also rarely presented as posterior scleritis.[5,51] In these pa-tients, the diagnosis of choroidal melanoma was mistakenly excluded by the initial, and sometimes prolonged, response to systemic corticosteroids.

Invasive squamous cell carcinoma of the limbus may also rarely masquerade as necrotizing scleritis.[22,23,38] One case that presented as necrotizing anterior scleritis associated with a scleral perforation was correctly diagnosed by histo-logic examination of specimens taken at the time of scleral patch grafting.

It is difficult to give precise guidelines that will alert the clinician to the possibility of a masquerade syndrome in pa-tients with scleritis. Clearly, all tissue removed at the time of surgery should be examined pathologically. Consideration of a diagnosis of a neoplasm should be given in patients who have an atypical clinical course or who do not respond to seemingly adequate antiinflammatory therapy. When the diagnosis is not certain initially, the patient must be followed closely and reevaluated regularly. A biopsy may be appro-priate.

Infective scleritis caused by bacteria, fungi, or viruses is the other form of scleral inflammation that may masquerade as inflammatory scleritis.[1,20,31,34]

Epidemiology

Scleritis occurs in all age groups and is most common in the fourth to sixth decades. The age range of patients is from 12 to 77 years with a mean age of onset of about 48 years.[2] Scleritis is rare in children. There is a variable female preponderance of patients with scleritis and the female-to-male ratio is about 1.5 to 1. No known geographic or racial predisposition toward scleritis exists, nor is there a recognized association of any HLA phenotype with scleritis.

Scleritis usually involves the anterior sclera (85% to 90%) but may also involve the posterior sclera, either in isolation or as spread from the anterior sclera.[45] Posterior scleritis is a frequently underdiagnosed complaint because of its diverse clinical manifestations. Its true incidence is undoubtedly higher than in most reported series.[45] Up to 50% of patients with scleritis develop bilateral disease, with about 50% of these patients having a simultaneous onset and the remaining 50%, a delay in disease onset. Bilateral involvement occurs nearly twice as frequently in patients with systemic disease when compared to patients with idiopathic disease.[2,39,45]

Risk Factors

Scleritis is commonly associated with systemic disease, with approximately 50% of scleritis patients having an identifiable underlying or associated systemic disease, of which rheumatoid arthritis is the most common.[45] Systemic vasculitic syndromes such as Wegener granulomatosis and polyarteritis nodosa; granulomatous diseases such as sarcoidosis; and infective diseases including syphilis, tuberculosis, and ophthalmic zoster are frequent associations. Ocular surgery and bacterial, protozoal, or fungal infections may also result in scleritis.[1,20,31,32,34] Table 53-3 details the recognized systemic disease associations of scleritis.

Inflammation of the sclera may be confined either to the anterior segment or the posterior segment, or it may involve both. The area of scleral inflammation is usually thickened and clearly demarcated from the adjacent normal tissue; although in necrotizing scleritis and scleromalacia perforans, the sclera can be extremely thin or perforated.

In anterior scleritis, the cornea may be involved with central or peripheral opacification and thinning. A descemetocele may form as a result of severe keratitis. Uveitis is uncommon unless scleral inflammation extends to the ciliary body. Staphylomas may occur as a result of elevated intraocular pressure. The inflammatory response may be confined to the sclera and episclera or may extend to involve the entire eye wall from episclera to retina. This is particularly prominent in posterior scleritis, in which there is inflammation of adjacent intraocular structures including the choroid, retina, and optic nerve. This spread of inflammation may result in significant choroiditis, retinal detachment, retinal vasculitis, and optic disc swelling.

Pathology

Information on the histopathology of scleritis has been limited in the past, as it was derived largely from surgical specimens obtained either at the time of surgery for perforations of the globe or from enucleation of blind eyes.[10,16,50,53]

TABLE 53-3 SCLERITIS: ASSOCIATED DISEASES

1. Rheumatic diseases	Gout
	Juvenile chronic arthritis
	Reiter syndrome
	Rheumatoid arthritis
	Seronegative polyarthritis
2. Connective-tissue diseases	IgA nephropathy
	Polymyositis
	Relapsing polychondritis
	Systemic lupus erythematosus
3. Systemic vasculitides	Behçet syndrome
	Giant-cell arteritis
	Polyarteritis nodosa
	Takayasu disease
	Wegener granulomatosis
4. Granulomatous diseases	Lyme disease
	Sarcoidosis
	Syphilis
	Tuberculosis
5. Cutaneous diseases	Varicella-zoster
	Porphyria
	Pyoderma gangrenosum
	Rosacea
6. Enteropathies	Crohn disease
	Ulcerative colitis

Until recently, episcleral and scleral biopsies were considered extremely hazardous because of the risks of subsequent scleral perforation, and they were rarely performed. Only lately have investigators begun to perform deep episcleral biopsies in patients with active scleritis and only recently have the techniques of modern immunohistochemistry been applied to the study of scleritis specimens.[7,33a] These strategies have resulted in valuable insights into the pathologic features of this enigmatic disease.

Histologically, the changes of anterior and posterior scleritis are identical, and early histologic studies emphasized several important features now recognized to be common to chronic inflammatory and immune diseases.[10,48,53] These include a proliferative inflammatory cell infiltrate composed principally of lymphocytes, plasma cells, macrophages, and occasionally, granulomata. Associated with this cellular response, fibrinoid necrosis and fibrin deposition are usually evident.

Episcleral biopsies have revealed a variety of vascular anomalies characteristic of chronic inflammatory disease processes. The most important of these processes is vasculitis, which is believed to be the basic pathologic lesion in most types of scleritis.[7,33] Fibrinoid necrosis and neutrophil leucocyte invasion of the vessel wall are detected in 75% of the scleral and 50% of the conjunctival biopsies from patients with severe scleritis.[7] Immunofluorescent studies demonstrate the presence of immunoglobulin and/or complement in most of these scleral and conjunctival tissues. Circulating immune complexes are often found in patients with scleral vasculitis. CD4 lymphocytes and some B cells and macrophages are present in inflamed sclera. These findings parallel the immunopathologic changes in the joints of patients with rheumatoid arthritis.

Pathogenesis

There is evidence that scleritis is primarily an immune-mediated vasculitis. Clinical studies showing that scleritis responds to cyclosporine is indirect evidence that immune mechanisms are important in the causation and perpetuation of this disease. Anterior-segment fluorescein angiography of scleritis lesions reveals a widespread disturbance of the microcirculation involving the capillaries and venules, with characteristic patterns of capillary closure and shunt vessel formation as the earliest signs of the disease. Such changes are present angiographically in areas that later develop clinical scleritis.[29,44] Other studies have documented a spectrum of systemic immunologic abnormalities including elevated levels of circulating immune complexes and elevated autoantibody titres in patients with scleritis.[7,44] A specific immune response may be directed toward scleral antigens in patients with scleritis.[52]

Thus, recent evidence strongly indicates that necrotizing scleritis is the result of an immune complex-mediated vasculitis leading to fibrinoid necrosis of the vessel wall, thrombotic occlusion of vessels, and the generation of a chronic inflammatory response in the sclera. Scleritis is a granulomatous inflammation adjacent to or involving the scleral and episcleral blood vessels and is a cell-mediated response to local antigens or immune complex deposition (Fig. 53-2). The antigens responsible for such immune complex formation are unknown.

Considerable knowledge has been gained into the pathogenesis of scleritis as a result of studies in connective-tissue and autoimmune diseases such as rheumatoid arthritis and vasculidites such as Wegener granulomatosis. The immunopathogenesis of these pathologic processes give insight into the mechanisms likely to be involved in the production of scleral inflammation.

Rheumatoid Arthritis. Rheumatoid arthritis is a common systemic inflammatory disease in which the basic pathologic process is produced by immune complex-mediated inflammation. The local formation of immune complexes or the deposition of immune complexes in a variety of tissues leads to activation of the complement pathway and the subsequent generation of an inflammatory response. The tissue damage generated as a result of this inflammation is caused by a combination of cellular and biochemical mediators. The pathogenesis of rheumatoid lesions involves complex interactions between acute and chronic inflammatory cells as well as a variety of other mediators including prostaglandins, complement, coagulation pathways, metalloproteinases, cytokines, and tissue enzymes (Fig. 53-3).

Histopathologic examination of the synovial membrane

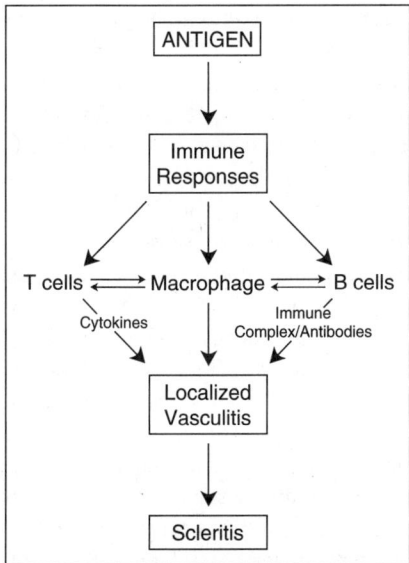

Fig. 53-2. Pathogenesis of scleritis.

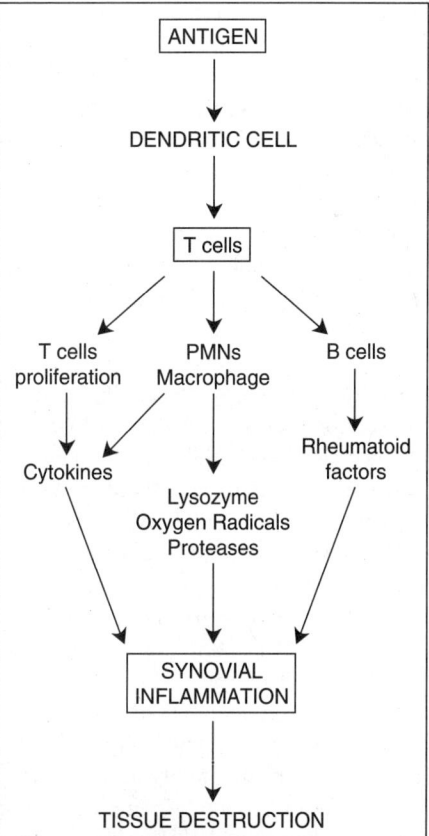

Fig. 53-3. Pathogenesis of rheumatoid arthritis.

in rheumatoid arthritis shows microvascular endothelial cell injury. Small blood vessels are obliterated by inflammatory cells and thrombus; synovial lining cells are observed to be proliferating; and there is evidence of polymorphonuclear leucocyte infiltration. Later, an invasive and proliferative synovitis develops with pannus formation, prominent villi, hyperplasia, and hypertrophy of synovial lining cells. A dense subsynovial cellular infiltrate consists predominantly of CD4 lymphocytes and plasma cells. Immunoglobulins and IgG rheumatoid factor, produced locally by plasma cells, may polymerize or interact with antigenic components of the joint tissue or other inflammatory blood products, resulting in local immune complex formation with subsequent complement activation and augmentation of the inflammatory response.

Leukotrienes, vasoactive amines, oxygen radicals, and platelet-activating factor contribute to the synovitis. Cytokines (including IL-2, IL-6, GM-CSF, TNF, IL-1, PDGF, ILGF, and TGF) stimulate T and B cell proliferation and differentiation and activate neutrophils and monocytes.[41] These cytokines are probably responsible for the activation of proteinases, collagenases, sulphatases, elastases, and other enzymes that are released into the joint cavity and contribute to the destruction of the cartilage and supporting joint structures.

Extracellular matrix degradation is a hallmark of chronic rheumatoid arthritis and is responsible for the characteristic destruction of the cartilage, ligaments, and bone observed in patients with rheumatoid arthritis.[6] This process is mediated by a family of enzymes known as metalloproteinases that includes collagenases, gelatinases, and stromelysin.[6] Metalloproteinases are proenzymes that are activated after proteolytic cleavage by enzymes (such as trypsin, plasmin, and tryptase) and contain an activated zinc cation. The matrix proteins digested by members of the metalloproteinase family are variable; collagenases degrade only triple helix type 1, 2, 3, 7, and 10 collagen, whereas gelatinase is able to degrade native collagen. Stromelysin has broader specificity and is also able to cleave activated collagenase. The activity of these metalloproteinases is balanced by a system of inhibitors known as tissue inhibitors of metalloproteinases (TIMP). Two members of this family of inhibitors have been identified to date (TIMP1 and TIMP2). These proteins are able to bind to the activated enzymes and block their proteolytic activity. Immunohistochemical studies of rheumatoid arthritis synovial tissue demonstrated abundant stromelysin, collagenase, and TIMP1 within the synovium.

The histologic appearance of the sclera would indicate that there is a chronic granulomatous cellular infiltrate similar to that observed in rheumatoid arthritis, and that cytokine-mediated mechanisms involving macrophages and fibroblasts play an important role in the pathogenesis of scleritis. Scleritis is most likely an immune complex-mediated vasculitis.

Wegener Granulomatosis. Wegener granulomatosis is a clinicopathologic syndrome of unknown cause characterized by a granulomatous vasculitis involving the upper and lower respiratory tracts and by glomerulonephritis. Virtually any organ system can be affected. Eye disease has been reported in up to 58% of patients with Wegener granulomatosis, and it is the presenting manifestation in approximately 16% of patients.[4,15] Although scleritis is the most common type of ocular involvement, a variety of ocular manifestations have been described including conjunctivitis, keratitis, episcleritis, scleritis, uveitis, retinal vasculitis, optic neuropathy, and orbital infiltration.

Recognition of the presence of antineutrophil cytoplasmic antibodies (ANCA) in the sera of patients with Wegener granulomatous has helped to establish the diagnosis in patients with atypical presentations. Antineutrophil cytoplasmic autoantibodies are a useful diagnostic serologic marker for a variety of vasculitic syndromes including Wegener granulomatosis, polyarteritis nodosa (especially microscopic polyarthritis nodosa), Churg-Strauss syndrome, and pulmonary renal syndrome with alveolar capillaritis.[18] Cytoplasmic ANCA is associated with Wegener granulomatosis, and perinuclear ANCA staining is linked with polyarteritis nodosa. Idiopathic scleritis has also been reported to be associated with the presence of ANCA antibodies.[37]

The histopathologic features of ANCA-associated diseases are characterized by focal distribution, infiltration by granulocytes during the acute phase, necrosis, and the absence of immunohistologic evidence of immune complex deposition or direct antibody binding to tissue.[18] Some ANCA-associated vasculidities have additional features such as granulomatous inflammation in Wegener granulomatosis and tissue eosinophilia in Churg-Strauss syndrome.

As well as being a useful serologic marker for certain forms of vasculitis, ANCA may be directly involved in the immunopathogenesis of vasculitis.[18] ANCA activate neutrophils, resulting in dose-dependent degranulation and the release of reactive oxygen metabolites. It has recently been shown that ANCA-activated, cytokine-primed neutrophils can kill endothelial cells in vitro. It has been hypothesized that ANCA is a necessary, but not sufficient, pathogenic factor for ANCA-associated diseases. For circulating ANCA to activate neutrophils and monocytes, a synergistic primary event must occur, such as the release of leucocyte-stimulating products from microorganisms or the release of leucocyte-stimulating cytokines (Fig. 53-4). Thus a preceding infection may give the initial stimulus to prime neutrophils and other inflammatory cells to respond to ANCA-producing vascular inflammation and damage. Although the role of ANCA in the pathogenesis of scleral lesions is yet to be examined, these antibodies may be partly responsible for the vascular damage associated with scleral inflammation.

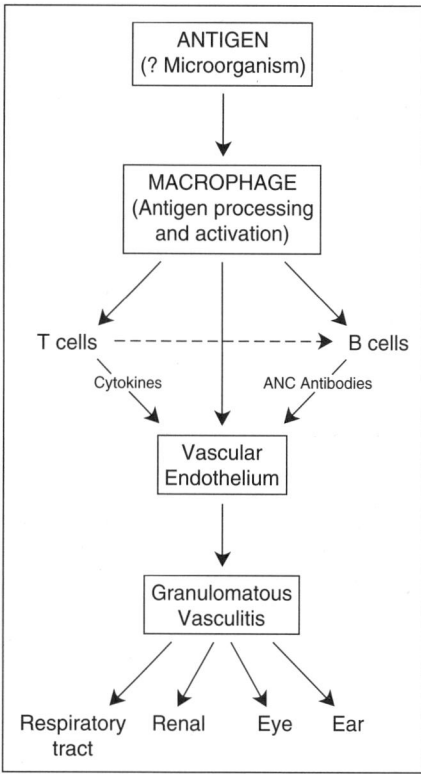

Fig. 53-4. Pathogenesis of Wegener granulomatosis.

Clinical Features

Scleritis is a painful disease. Other symptoms are watering, and redness, but the severe and constant pain that worsens in the early morning is the typical presentation of the illness. There is also a largely asymptomatic form of scleritis, scleromalacia perforans, that is pain-free and occurs in patients with advanced rheumatoid arthritis.

The presentation of scleritis differs from episcleritis. Patients with scleral disease, such as those with rheumatoid arthritis, may already be on systemic corticosteroids or other immunosuppressive drugs that can mask the pain and tenderness so typical of active scleritis. Intensive topical corticosteroid therapy may also ameliorate some of the signs and symptoms of mild scleritis. The ophthalmologist must therefore actively exclude scleritis by careful examination of the patient rather than inferring that inflammation without severe pain represents episcleritis.

The hallmark of scleritis is pain; its severity, characteristic boring nature, facial radiation, and nocturnal worsening have been recognized since the earliest descriptions of the disease.[48] The pain of scleritis presents a characteristic pattern involving the eye and spreading to the periorbital region. The pain typically radiates to involve the brow, forehead, temple, ear, and jaw. The pain is dull, aching, and boring in nature; is severe enough to limit activity and to prevent sleep; and characteristically increases in severity at night, typically awakening the patient from sleep in the early

hours of the morning. In patients with necrotizing disease the pain may be so excruciating that it is totally disabling. The severity of the pain in patients with scleritis may appear quite disproportionate to the clinical signs, and patients with severe scleritis have undergone extensive neurologic evaluation for pain prior to the diagnosis of scleritis.

Patients may also note other symptoms including ocular redness, photophobia, lacrimation, and epiphora. Corneal or posterior segment involvement may result in a change in vision. The signs present in individual patients depend on the location and severity of the scleritis and the presence or absence of complications. The essential sign of scleritis is scleral edema, usually accompanied by intense injection and tenderness of the globe. Maximal dilatation of the deep episcleral vascular plexus and the presence of underlying scleral edema allow the diagnosis of scleritis to be made. Severity is graded by the presence of nodules or signs of scleral necrosis.

Careful examination of the blood vessels of the ocular surface and anterior segment are key for optimal diagnosis. As all patients with scleral inflammation have an overlying episcleritis, the presence or absence of scleral edema is the key sign enabling the differentiation of scleritis from episcleritis. Therefore attention must be paid to the location of the deep episcleral vascular plexus in relation to the location of the underlying sclera and the superficial episcleral plexus. In episcleritis, there is no scleral edema, and there is separation of the superficial and deep episcleral plexuses. In scleritis, there is intense dilatation of the deep episcleral vascular plexus and outward displacement of these vessels by scleral edema. It is essential to carefully examine the involved areas for capillary closure—the earliest sign of necrotizing scleritis.[44] Red-free light and diffuse slit-lamp illumination are helpful for studying the vascular layers of the episclera in detail. It may be necessary to blanch the vascular plexuses of the conjunctiva and Tenon capsule with topical phenylephrine or adrenaline to appreciate these signs in some patients.

Tenderness of the globe to palpation is a valuable sign of scleral inflammation, and areas of involvement by anterior scleritis are exquisitely tender. Scleral tenderness can be graded and is a most useful sign for the assessment of scleritis severity and its response to treatment.[26]

A grading system for the assessment of scleritis severity is useful in the management of patients with scleritis (Table 53-4).[26] Clinical parameters include degree of scleral tenderness, area of involvement by scleritis, presence of scleral nodules or necrosis, presence of corneal infiltrates, degree of anterior and posterior uveitis, and presence of retinal detachment. A severity score is calculated at the initial clinical assessment and at subsequent reexaminations to provide evidence of the course and response of the scleritis to treatment over time.

Diffuse Anterior Scleritis. Diffuse anterior scleritis is the most common and least severe form of scleritis and accounts

TABLE 53-4 DIAGNOSTIC CRITERIA AND MAJOR CLINICAL FEATURES OF SYSTEMIC DISEASES ASSOCIATED WITH SCLERITIS

Syndrome	Diagnostic Criteria and Major Features	
Rheumatoid arthritis	1. Morning stiffness > 1 hr 2. Arthritis > 3 joints 3. Arthritis of hand joints 4. Symmetric polyarthritis	5. Rheumatoid nodules 6. Serum rheumatoid factor 7. Radiographic changes—erosions, decalcification (>4 criteria necessary for diagnosis)
Wegener granulomatosis	1. Nasal or oral inflammation 2. Abnormal chest radiograph 3. Abnormal urinary sediment	4. Granulomatous vascular inflammation on biopsy
Polyarteritis nodosa	1. Weight loss > 4 kg 2. Livedo reticularis 3. Testicular pain or tenderness 4. Myalgias, weakness, or leg tenderness 5. Mononeuropathy or polyneuropathy 6. Diastolic BP > 90 mm Hg	7. Elevated BUN or creatinine 8. Hepatitis B virus antigen 9. Arteriographic abnormalities 10. Biopsy of small- or medium-sized artery containing PMN's
Relapsing polychondritis	1. Tender auricular and nasal cartilage 2. Tracheal and laryngeal pain and collapse 3. Polyarthritis 4. Fever	5. Raised ESR 6. Systemic vasculitis 7. Serous otitis media 8. Valvular heart disease
Churg-Strauss syndrome	1. Asthma 2. Eosinophilia 3. History of allergy 4. Mononeuropathy or polyneuropathy	5. Pulmonary infiltrates: migratory or transient 6. Paranasal sinus abnormalities 7. Extravascular eosinophils on biopsy
Henoch-Schönlein purpura	1. Palpable purpura on extensor surfaces 2. Age < 20 years at disease onset	3. Bowel angina 4. Vessel wall granulocytes on biopsy
Reiter syndrome	1. Arthritis—asymmetric, sacroiliitis, enthesitis 2. Urethritis	3. Conjunctivitis, iritis 4. Keratoderma blenorrhagica, circinate balanitis
Giant-cell arteritis	1. Age at disease onset > 50 years 2. Headache 3. Temporal artery tender or decreased pulse	4. Elevated erythrocyte sedimentation rate 5. Abnormal artery biopsy-vasculitis, giant cells
Systemic lupus erythematosus	1. Malar rash 2. Discoid rash 3. Photosensitivity 4. Oral or nasapharyngeal ulcers 5. Arthritis—nonerosive 6. Pleurisy, pericarditis, serositis 7. Proteinuria/casts	8. Seizures/psychosis 9. Hemolytic anemia, leukopenia, thrombocytopenia 10. ANA, DNA, Sm antibodies, LE cells, false positive syphilis serology (>4 criteria necessary for diagnosis)
Behcet syndrome	1. Oral ulcers—recurrent 2. Genital ulcers 3. Cutaneous vasculitis	4. Arthritis 5. Uveitis 6. Meningoencephalitis
Takayasu arteritis	1. Age at disease onset < 40 years 2. Claudication of extremities 3. Decreased brachial pulses 4. BP difference > 10 mm Hg between arms	5. Bruit over subclavian arteries or aorta 6. Arteriogram abnormalities—narrowing or occlusion

for 25% to 50% of patients.[2] Diffuse anterior scleritis occurs at a younger age than other forms of scleritis and is equally prevalent in females and males. This disease usually involves relatively large areas of the sclera, but uncommonly small localized areas may be affected. Widespread, severe, diffuse anterior scleritis has been referred to as brawny scleritis when there is intense overlying injection, redness, and chemosis.

Patients with diffuse anterior scleritis have dilated superficial and deep episcleral vascular plexuses with some distortion of the normal vascular pattern caused by the formation of large vascular channels in areas affected by scleritis.

There is edema of the sclera and overlying episcleral tissue with outward displacement of the blood vessels. There is no evidence of vascular closure clinically or angiographically (Fig. 53-5).

Resolution of diffuse anterior scleritis results in subtle but permanent changes to the sclera. Although there is no loss of scleral collagen, it is rearranged to increase scleral translucency, producing a slight, bluish discoloration. There is also a permanent alteration of the vasculature in the affected area of the sclera that causes vascular beading or focal, aneurysmal dilatations.

Only a small number of patients with diffuse anterior scleritis progress to more aggressive forms of scleritis. This tends to occur in the 25% of patients who develop multiple attacks.[39] From this group, one half progress to nodular or necrotizing scleritis. Conversely, of patients with recurrent nodular or necrotizing scleritis, less than 5% change the pattern of their disease to diffuse scleritis.

Nodular Anterior Scleritis. Nodular scleritis is the second most common form of anterior scleritis and accounts for 20% to 40% of patients.[2] Nodular anterior scleritis is 50% more prevalent in women than in men. Multiple attacks of scleritis are most frequent in patients with this type of scleritis and occur in approximately 50% of patients. Nodular anterior scleritis is characterized by the presence of single or multiple, localized elevations of the sclera that may coalesce in some patients. Nodules are typically found posterior to the limbus and are localized, nonmobile areas of firm, tender scleral edema associated with intense dilatation of the deep

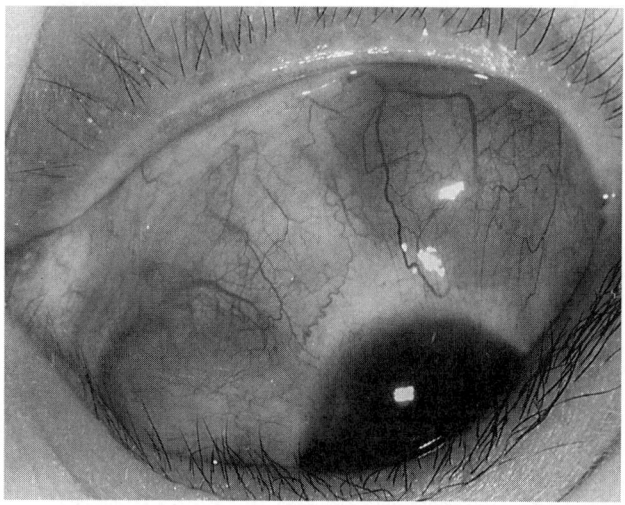

Fig. 53-6. Nodular scleritis in a patient with relapsing polychondritis.

episcleral vessels (Fig. 53-6). There is overlying episcleral edema. Extensive areas of nodular scleritis may elevate the intraocular pressure until the scleritis is controlled.

With treatment, the pain and scleral tenderness resolve rapidly; however, the nodules may persist for months. Nodular scleritis usually does not result in a loss of scleral thickness, but there is often a bluish-grey discoloration of the previously affected sclera as a result of rearrangement of scleral collagen and altered opacification.

Of patients with multiple attacks of nodular scleritis, approximately 20% progress to necrotizing disease.[39]

Necrotizing Anterior Scleritis. Necrotizing scleritis is the least common, but most severe, form of scleritis and represents up to 25% of cases.[2] It occurs more frequently in women, has an older mean age of onset (average of 66 years), and is more frequently associated with systemic disease than diffuse or nodular scleritis. Bilateral disease develops in up to 25% of patients. Approximately 25% of patients develop multiple attacks, but less than 15% of these patients change to less aggressive forms of scleritis.[39]

Necrotizing anterior scleritis occurs in two distinct clinical forms: necrotizing anterior scleritis with inflammation and necrotizing anterior scleritis without inflammation.

With Inflammation. Necrotizing anterior scleritis with inflammation produces the classical clinical features of severe scleritis. The patient has severe ocular and periocular pain that steadily worsens over days or weeks to excruciating levels if appropriate treatment is not started. The pain worsens in the early morning and has a dull, boring quality.

On examination, there is scleral edema and intense vasodilation of the deep episcleral plexus and superficial vessels; however, the areas of scleritis are less injected centrally and careful slit-lamp examination will detect that these less in-

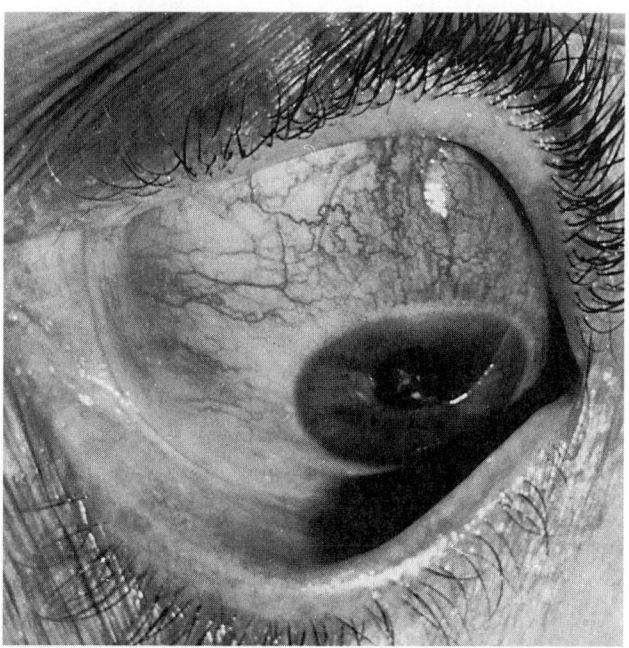

Fig. 53-5. Vascular dilatation of the episcleral plexus during diffuse anterior scleritis.

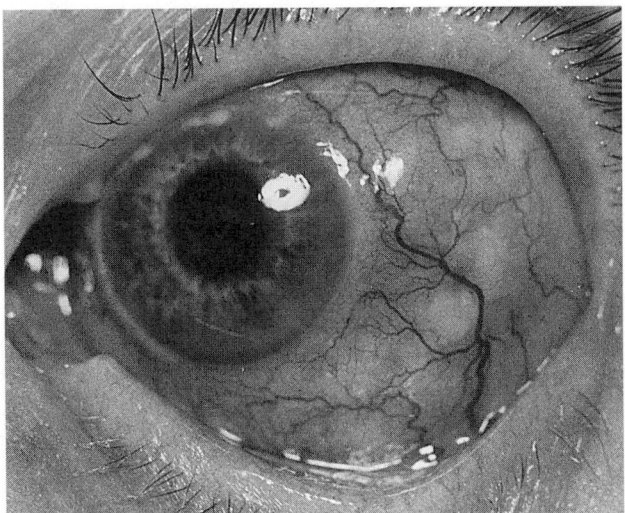

Fig. 53-7.   Early capillary closure during necrotizing scleritis.

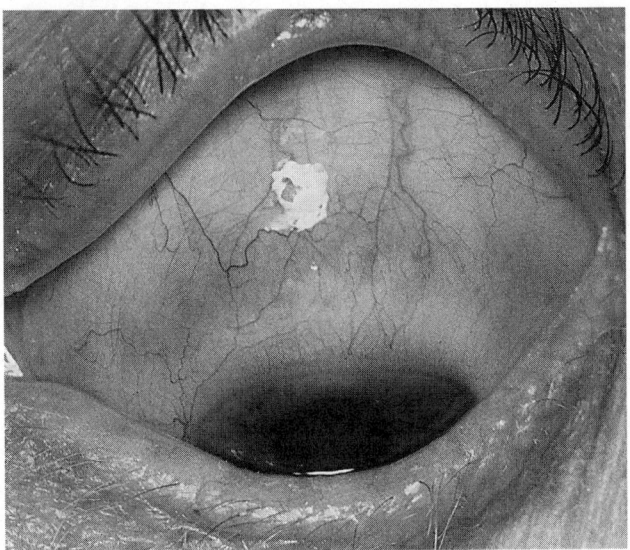

Fig. 53-9.   Residual scleral and vascular changes following resolution of necrotizing scleritis.

jected areas are foci of capillary closure in the episcleral vasculature (Fig. 53-7). In early necrotizing disease these areas may be so subtle that they are only discernible with the use of fluorescein angiography.[28,44,45] In advanced disease there is clinically obvious blood vessel closure associated with (1) thinning and color change of the sclera, (2) parchment-white, avascular areas of necrotic sclera, and (3) blue, thinned areas of sclera where the underlying choroid is easily visible (Fig. 53-8).

The affected eye is exquisitely tender, and there is often reflex withdrawal of the patient's head from attempted palpation of the globe. Without treatment, the edges of the scleritis lesions enlarge and will progress to eventually encircle the globe.

Scleral thinning is an inevitable result of scleral necrosis unless the earliest signs of necrotizing scleritis are recog-

nized and adequate treatment is given (Fig. 53-9). The severity of the loss of sclera varies from localized thinning to massive infarction and loss of scleral tissue. If there is profound elevation of the intraocular pressure, staphylomas may form in areas of thinned sclera (Fig. 53-10). Spontaneous perforation of the globe is rare—even in patients with widespread necrotizing scleritis—although these eyes are quite susceptible to traumatic rupture.

Patients with necrotizing scleritis may develop corneal ulceration and inflammation. Necrotizing scleritis involving the cornea has a very high association with systemic vascu-

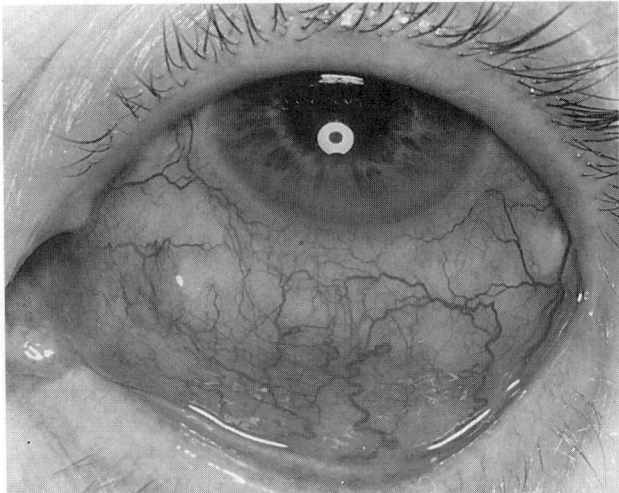

Fig. 53-8.   Necrotizing scleritis in a patient with rheumatoid arthritis.

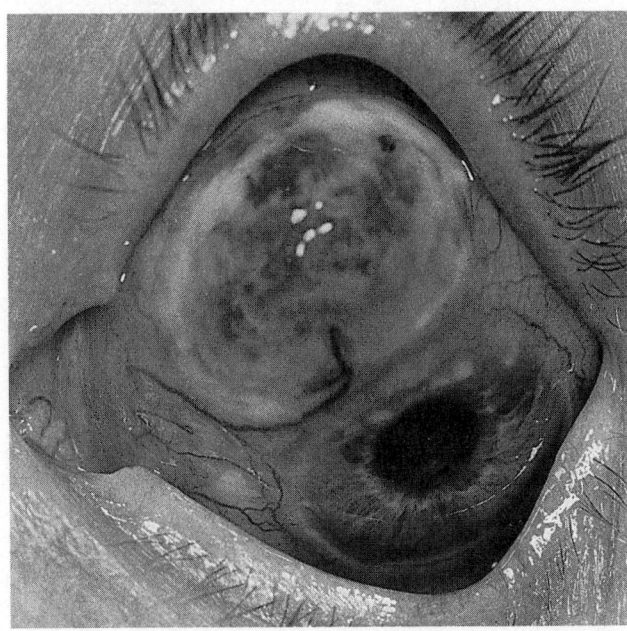

Fig. 53-10.   Scleral staphyloma from severe necrotizing scleritis.

litic syndromes, especially Wegener granulomatosis. Even in the absence of other evidence of systemic vasculitis, this type of scleritis is often considered to be a localized form of Wegener granulomatosis and is managed in a similar way.[4,15]

Without Inflammation. Necrotizing anterior scleritis without inflammation is a rare form of severe scleritis that is commonly bilateral, usually occurs in females, and is observed almost exclusively in patients with rheumatoid arthritis.[45,48] It is widely known by the term scleromalacia perforans, although this label is often used inappropriately to describe any type of scleritis in a patient with rheumatoid arthritis.

Scleromalacia perforans is characterized by its almost complete lack of symptoms. Patients remain totally asymptomatic and have the lesions brought to their attention at the time of an eye examination. Patients may notice either a change in color of the sclera or reduced vision from induced astigmatism.

Slit-lamp examination reveals thinning and atrophy of the episclera and loss of the normal episcleral vasculature. The anterior sclera develops localized areas of yellow-white, infarcted tissue. These lesions are not associated with vascular dilatation, tenderness, or other signs of inflammation. Slowly, over many months, these areas of sclera become demarcated from the surrounding tissue and are reabsorbed, leaving exposed choroid in contact with conjunctiva. Corneal astigmatism may result in reduced vision. Spontaneous perforation is rare, although areas affected by scleromalacia perforans are susceptible to trauma. Staphylomas do not form unless the intraocular pressure is elevated.

Surgically Induced. Surgically induced necrotizing scleritis is a rare type of anterior scleritis that occurs following ocular surgery and is more frequent after multiple surgical procedures.[12,21,32,33a] Like other forms of necrotizing scleritis, it is more common in females and has a high association with underlying systemic disease. It usually begins within 6 months of surgery but has occurred in adult life, decades after childhood strabismus surgery. Although it is usually necrotizing in type, surgically induced scleritis may present initially as a milder form of scleritis and then progress to necrotizing disease. The pathogenesis of this form of scleritis is unknown. Surgically induced necrotizing scleritis is treated like other forms of necrotizing scleritis, except that in patients who have undergone retinal detachment surgery, the buckle material must be removed to gain control of the inflammation.[32]

Posterior Scleritis. Posterior scleritis is inflammation involving the sclera posterior to the ora serrata, occurring in isolation or in association with anterior scleritis. Posterior scleritis has protean clinical manifestations and a variable and changeable clinical course that may lead to diagnostic difficulty.

Posterior scleritis is often misdiagnosed and its occurrence is higher than the proportion listed in published series might suggest. In a 1976 report, posterior scleritis accounted for only 2% of scleritis patients; however, by 1990, 12% of patients at the same hospital had a diagnosis of posterior scleritis. This increase probably reflected raised clinical awareness of the disease and more accurate diagnosis from the use of ultrasonography.[40,48] Pathologic studies, in which up to 62% of enucleated eyes had histologic evidence of posterior scleritis, suggest that posterior scleritis is more prevalent than its clinical recognition.[10]

Posterior scleritis may be unilateral, but up to 33% of patients develop bilateral disease.[2] It affects females more often than males, although annular choroidal detachments may be more prevalent in males. Posterior scleritis occurs in all age groups but is most common in the fourth to sixth decades and has a mean age of onset of approximately 50 years. The symptoms of posterior scleritis are variable and usually consist of a combination of ocular pain, reduced vision, and ocular redness. Diplopia and pain on eye movement are also frequent.

Pain is the predominant symptom of posterior scleritis and is severe and similar in its characteristics to that of anterior scleritis. Vision may be normal, but more typically, is reduced from posterior pole changes. Redness of the globe may be mild and unnoticed by the patient, but a large number of patients have anterior scleral involvement. Redness and injection of the anterior segment reflect the spread of inflammation to the anterior sclera, but these symptoms may be sufficiently subtle to be missed on cursory examination. It is important, therefore, to look critically at the episcleral vessels near the extraocular muscle insertions for evidence of dilatation and to carefully inspect the fornices for areas of episcleral injection suggesting anterior extension of scleritis.

The signs of posterior scleritis reflect the range of possible clinical presentations and are highly variable in type and severity.[17] The common signs of posterior scleritis are the consequence of posterior scleral inflammation on the choroid and retina, and include exudative retinal detachment (which is either localized to the posterior pole or peripheral retina, or generalized, involving most of the retina), annular choroidal detachment, optic disc edema, retinal folds, choroidal folds, a subretinal mass lesion, maculopathy, uveitis, retinal vasculitis, and elevated intraocular pressure. Exudative retinal detachment is the most common presentation (40%), followed by retinal and/or choroidal folds (32%), annular choroidal detachment (16%), and a circumscribed mass lesion (12%).[2] Table 53-5 details the differential diagnosis of the common ocular manifestations of posterior scleritis. Uveitis occurs frequently but is of variable severity in patients with posterior scleritis. Intraocular pressure may become elevated by a number of mechanisms and is raised most often by ciliochoroidal effusion with an annular cho-

TABLE 53-5 POSTERIOR SCLERITIS: DIFFERENTIAL DIAGNOSIS

Presenting Feature of Posterior Scleritis	Causes Other than Posterior Scleritis
1. Exudative detachment	Sympathetic ophthalmia
	Neoplasm
	Central serous retinopathy
	Punctate inner choroidopathy
	Rhegmatogenous retinal detachment
	Vogt-Koyanagi-Harada disease
2. Retinal folds	Orbital mass lesion
	Papilledema
	Hypotony
	Graves disease
	Subretinal neovascular membrane
	Scleral buckle
3. Annular choroidal detachment	Uveal effusion syndrome
	Rhegmatogenous retinal detachment
	Intraocular surgery
	Ring melanoma
4. Fundus mass	Melanoma
	Metastatic carcinoma
	Choroidal hemangioma
	Lymphoma
	Orbital mass

roidal detachment that rotates the ciliary body and iris forward to produce angle closure.

Other less common signs of posterior scleritis represent the spread of inflammation from the posterior sclera and Tenon capsule into the adjacent orbital tissue.[2,17] When this occurs, the clinical features can mimic those of idiopathic inflammatory orbital pseudotumour and may include proptosis, severe pain, pain on eye movement, limitation of eye movement, ptosis, and chemosis. In the past, labels such as sclerotenonitis and acute periscleritis have been applied to combinations of these signs and the intraocular signs of posterior scleritis, depending on the dominant clinical features.[2,17] There is clearly clinical overlap between posterior scleritis and idiopathic inflammatory orbital pseudotumor, and the clinical picture depends on the dominant clinical signs. There are sufficient clinical and pathologic similarities that, in the absence of an orbital mass lesion, posterior scleritis, acute periscleritis, sclerotenonitis, and idiopathic inflammatory orbital pseudotumor should be considered a spectrum of the same disease process.

Laboratory Investigations

The initial step in the management of patients with scleritis is to make the correct diagnosis. This is based on a careful history, detailed examination, and appropriate investigations. The aims of investigation in the patient with scleritis are to evaluate the severity and extent of the scleritis and to exclude the presence of an associated systemic disease or infiltrative process (Table 53-4). Approximately 50% of patients with scleritis have an associated systemic disease, and it is well recognized that scleritis may be the presentation of a potentially fatal illness.[25,45] The clinician must therefore carefully exclude associated disease by clinical assessment and appropriate selective further investigation. A complete medical history, comprehensive ocular examination, and a careful review of systems—particularly directed toward symptoms of clinical entities associated with scleritis—are the essential first steps in the investigation and management of the patient with scleritis.

Anterior scleritis is usually clinically apparent and can be diagnosed and classified on the basis of its clinical features. External fluorescein angiography is potentially very useful in the assessment of the severity of scleritis. It is, however, a demanding technique requiring considerable expertise to obtain good quality, high-speed images of the episcleral vasculature.[28] In selected patients there is no doubt that external angiography can identify subtle signs of necrotizing scleritis that would be missed on clinical examination.

Posterior scleritis has variable clinical manifestations that may overlap with other clinical entities. Ultrasonography can confirm the scleral thickening that is the hallmark of the disease.[25,39,44] Computerized tomography and magnetic resonance imaging may be needed to exclude orbital lesions, and scleral biopsy may be used to exclude the presence of an infiltrative disease.

Investigations are selected on the results of the clinical assessment to rule out specific disease entities.[25] Although it is clearly essential not to miss treatable infective causes of scleritis, such as syphilis and Lyme disease, there is no place for ordering an undirected large battery of tests in all patients with scleritis. Investigations useful in patients with symptoms suggestive of an associated systemic disease are detailed in Table 53-2. Investigation of patients with scleritis often involves consultation with other specialities and may require biopsy of other organs such as kidney, nasal or pharyngeal mucosa, or skin to obtain a diagnosis (Table 53-5).

Therapy

Medical Management. The treatment of scleritis always requires systemic therapy with either nonsteroidal antiinflammatory agents, corticosteroids, or other immunosuppressive drugs. This treatment must be individualized according to the severity of the patient's disease, response to treatment, side effects, and the presence of associated disease. The medical therapy of a patient with scleritis can be conveniently divided into four phases: remission induction, consolidation, maintenance, and treatment withdrawal (Table 53-6). It is important to have clearly defined therapeutic objectives before starting a patient on systemic immunosuppressive therapy: preservation of vision, relief of

TABLE 53-6 SCLERITIS: APPROACH TO THERAPY

Stages in Treatment	NSAID*	Corticosteroids	Cytotoxic Drugs**
1. Remission induction	First-line treatment for mild disease (scleritis score < 11)	High-dose oral prednisolone or I.V. methylprednisolone for severe disease (scleritis score > 11) Consider risks of adverse effects	Severe disease not controlled by corticosteroids alone Consider risks of adverse effects
2. Consolidation	Continue NSAID for mild disease	Slowly decrease dosage to maintenance level (< 15 mg/day)	Continue or add second-line immunosuppressive agent early in course of disease
3. Withdrawal	Scleritis in remission for 6 weeks, stop NSAID and observe	Decrease dosage over 4–8 week period after scleritis in remission for 3 months	Withdrawal after decreasing corticosteroids to maintenance dosage and scleritis in remission for 6–12 weeks
4. Relapse	Restart NSAID at original dosage Consider use of corticosteroid	Restart oral or I.V. steroids and/or add second-line immunosuppressive drug	Reintroduce at remission/induction dosage with corticosteroids

* NSAID: Nonsteroidal antiinflammatory drug
** Cyclophosphamide, Cyclosporine, Azathioprine, Methotrexate, Chlorambucil

symptoms, prevention of scleritis complications, and prevention of treatment complications.

Careful pretreatment evaluation and rational planning of immunosuppression will avoid many of the pitfalls encountered in the use of cytotoxic and other immunosuppressive drugs. Three issues are important in the pretreatment phase of the management of the patient with scleritis. These are the exclusion of latent or active infection and evaluation of infection risk, careful evaluation for the presence of coexisting local and systemic disease, and consideration of the potential for drug side effects and interactions. About 50% of patients with scleritis have an associated systemic disease

that should be treated on its merits, as the treatment of this disease may well provide adequate therapy for the associated scleritis. Table 53-7 outlines a recommended pretreatment evaluation for patients with scleritis prior to the use of systemic therapy. Table 53-8 lists the principal agents used in the medical management of scleritis.

Necrotizing scleritis must be identified as early in its course as possible so that intensive therapy can be instituted, because these patients are at high risk of a poor outcome if not treated aggressively.[44,45] Immunosuppressive drugs in patients with necrotizing scleritis improve the ocular outcome and decrease the mortality from associated systemic

TABLE 53-7 PRETREATMENT ASSESSMENT AND PREVENTION OF SIDE EFFECTS IN SCLERITIS PATIENTS

Drug	Pretreatment Assessment	Prevention of Side Effects
Nonsteroidal antiinflammatory agents	Urinalysis, urea, creatinine, history of allergy, bleeding disorder, peptic ulceration, asthma	Medication to be taken on full stomach
Corticosteroids	Glucose, U/E/Cr, BSL Calcium, uric acid, lipids, chest x-ray, Mantoux test, blood pressure History or family history of osteoporosis, especially postmenopausal women Psychologic assessment	Restrict caloric intake Exercise, sunlight, high-calcium diet Estrogen replacement Avoidance of infections, no live vaccines Treat raised blood pressure and BSL Psychologic support
Cytotoxics	Blood count, platelets, ESR, urinalysis, U/E/creatinine, liver function tests, chest x-ray, Mantoux test FSH/LH levels Sperm count Exclude evidence of malignant or premalignant disease, cervical smear, EPG/IEPG	Adequate fluid intake and diuresis Mesna with alkylating agents Hormone replacement therapy Sperm bank storage 6 monthly check for evidence of malignancy Avoid infections, no live vaccines

TABLE 53-8   DRUGS COMMONLY USED IN TREATING SCLERITIS

Drug	Mechanisms	Major Adverse Effects	Monitoring
Cyclooxygenase inhibitors	Inhibit prostaglandin production, leukotriene synthesis and superoxide generation Decrease lysosomal enzyme and release WBC adhesion and lymphocyte function decreases	Peptic ulceration, fluid retention, renal failure, papillary necrosis, interstitial nephritis, hepatitis	Clinical assessment, urinalysis Serum creatinine—3 monthly
Corticosteroids	Increase lipocortin levels, inhibition of phospholipase A Reduced cytokine production Inhibit Fc receptor expression Suppress lymphocyte function Redistribute circulating leukocytes	Weight gain, bruising, fluid retention, hypertension, diabetes, osteoporosis, acne Muscle weakness, growth retardation (children), infections Psychologic disturbances	Blood glucose, urinalysis—monthly Blood pressure monitoring—monthly Bone density Psychologic assessment
Cyclophosphamide	Crosslinks DNA leading to cell death Decreases circulating T and B cells	Cystitis, neoplasms, infections, infertility, alopecia, pneumonitis	Blood count and urinalysis monthly after initial weekly tests
Azathioprine	Interferes with DNA synthesis Inhibits lymphocyte proliferation	Nausea, oncogenicity, cytopenias, hepatitis	Blood count 1-2 weekly initially, then 1-3 monthly Liver function tests 1-3 monthly
Cyclosporine	Blocks synthesis/release of IL-2 Potentiate corticosteroids effects	Renal impairment, hypertension, tremor, hirsutism, gingivitis	Blood count, serum creatinine, blood pressure weekly, then 2-4 weekly on maintenance dose
Methotrexate	Decreases thymiolate synthetase activity and subsequent DNA synthesis Diminishes PMN chemotaxis	Hepatic fibrosis, nausea, cytopenias, pneumonitis	Blood count and liver function tests second weekly, then 1-3 monthly
Chlorambucil	Similar to cyclophosphamide	Leukemia, infections, cytopenias, infertility, alopecia	Blood count monthly initially, then 3 monthly

disease.[8] A treatment protocol can be planned that uses a scleritis scoring system to determine severity.[26] Mild cases of idiopathic scleritis usually respond to treatment with nonsteroidal antiinflammatory agents or systemic corticosteroids alone. Patients with severe disease usually require therapy with multiple immunosuppressive agents to control the inflammatory response (Fig. 53-9). A response of scleritis to therapy is evidenced initially by resolution of pain, which can be rapid and quite dramatic. Scleral tenderness and injection are the next to resolve, whereas scleral nodules, uveitis, and raised intraocular pressure respond over a slower time course of weeks to even months.

Cyclooxygenase Inhibitors. Nonsteroidal antiinflammatory drugs are useful for the management of mild forms of nonnecrotizing scleritis such as low-grade diffuse or nodular disease.[25] Such patients are given a two-week course of an oral, nonsteroidal, antiinflammatory drug such as naproxen, indomethacin, or flurbiprofen. Unfortunately, cyclooxygenase inhibitors can have serious side effects in patients with rheumatic disease.[3] If there is no response, systemic corticosteroids are added.[30] Orbital-floor corticosteroids may also

be useful in selected patients to minimize the need for systemic corticosteroids; however, their effect is short-lived.[14]

Corticosteroids. High-dose systemic corticosteroids are the most useful and effective form of therapy in patients with scleritis and are the preferred initial treatment for severe scleritis.[25,45] Corticosteroids may be given orally on a daily or alternate-day basis, or as intermittent intravenous or oral pulse doses. Corticosteroid therapy is often associated with side effects that limit their ability to induce a remission in patients with severe scleritis. Side effects are most frequently seen in patients treated with daily oral corticosteroids. High-dose, intermittent intravenous methylprednisolone is safe and effective in inducing remission in patients with scleritis.[24,29,43] Pulse methylprednisolone therapy has advantages similar to those of alternate-day oral corticosteroids in reducing the side effects of corticosteroids (Table 53-9).

Side effects associated with corticosteroid therapy are numerous, and several are potentially life-threatening. Corticosteroid complications are dependent on the dosage, frequency, route of administration, and duration of therapy. In

TABLE 53-9 CORTICOSTEROID ADMINISTRATION: ADVANTAGES AND DISADVANTAGES

	Daily Oral	Alternate-Day Oral	Intravenous
Advantages	Early remission Ease of administration	Maintenance therapy Few side effects Less HPA suppression Less growth retardation Less infections	Rapid remission induction Relatively few side effects Control of steroid dosage No problems with compliance Less infections Less HPA suppression
Disadvantages	Side effects common Growth retardation Compliance difficult to monitor Increased infections	Loss of disease control Relapse on "off day"	IV injection Vascular access Acute side effects Arrhythmias Hypotension Relapse between injections

general, short-term therapy with low-dose corticosteroids is well tolerated with few adverse effects; whereas high-dose corticosteroid administration (such as oral prednisone greater than 1 mg/kg/day), frequent oral corticosteroid administration using multiple doses per day, or high-dose intravenous steroid (such as methylprednisolone greater than 250 mgm/day) are often complicated by side effects. Some of these adverse effects (such as weight gain, fluid retention, cushingoid habitus, and myopathy) are predictable, as they are the direct result of the physiologic effects of corticosteroids. Others, such as aseptic necrosis of the femur, psychosis, and reactivation of latent infection, are less common or idiosyncratic in nature and are much less predictable. Patients at increased risk of developing corticosteroid side effects are the elderly, patients with diabetes, patients who are hypoalbuminaemic (from the nephrotic syndrome or liver disease), patients with a history of psychologic illness, and pregnant women.

Corticosteroid side effects, particularly osteoporosis, weight gain, diabetes, and hypertension, can be reduced by regular exercise, adequate sunshine, calcium supplements, appropriate diet, and weight control. Blood pressure monitoring, control of diabetes, and plasma lipid control are also important.

Immunosuppressive Agents. Patients whose scleritis is not controlled with high-dose oral corticosteroids or intravenous pulse therapy require additional immunosuppressive therapy (Fig. 53-10). It is important to realize that immunosuppression itself can produce complications, and these forms of therapy should be managed by physicians experienced in the use of such drugs. Hematologic, biochemical, and liver function assessments are mandatory. The decision to use potentially hazardous drugs should only be made after careful consultation and consideration (Fig. 53-11). In particular, the risk of permanent visual loss must be balanced against the risks of immunosuppressive therapy in each patient (Table 53-10).

A number of cytotoxic drugs are effective in treating oc-

TABLE 53-10 COMPARISON OF RELATIVE FREQUENCY OF SIDE EFFECTS OF IMMUNOSUPPRESSIVE DRUGS IN THE TREATMENT OF SCLERITIS

Side Effects	Cyclophosphamide	Azathioprine	Cyclosporine	Methotrexate
Gastrointestinal intolerance	+	++	+	+
Hair loss	++	−	−	+
Hirsutism	−	−	++	−
Cystitis	++	−	−	−
Hepatic damage	−	+	+	++
Lung damage	+	−	−	++
Renal damage	−	−	+	−
Gonadal damage	++	−	+	+
Bone marrow depression	++	+	−	+
Oncogenesis	++	+	++	++
Teratogenicity	++	−	+	+

SCLERITIS: THERAPEUTIC APPROACH

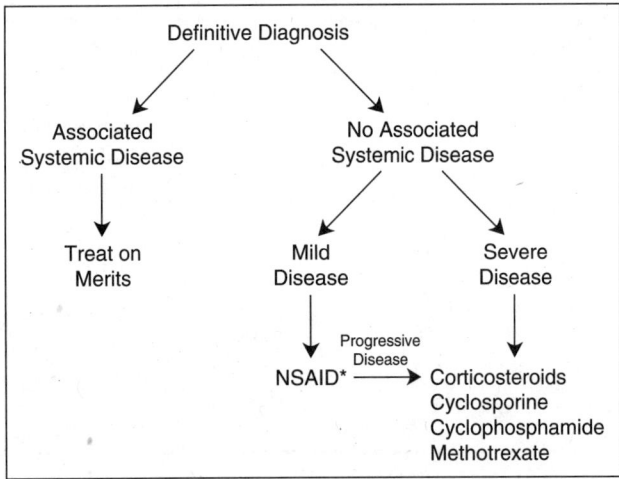

*NSAID = Nonsteroidal antiinflammatory drug

Fig. 53-11. Therapeutic approach to scleritis.

ular inflammatory disease, including azathioprine, cyclophosphamide, chlorambucil, methotrexate, and cyclosporine.[25] Complications of these drugs include bone marrow suppression, oncogenesis, gonad failure, vital organ damage, and infection. Azathioprine is useful as an adjunct to corticosteroids in the treatment of scleritis and allows the use of low-dose corticosteroids while still maintaining disease remission. Although azathioprine is usually well tolerated and has relatively fewer side effects than other immunosuppressive agents, it is less effective than cyclophosphamide and cyclosporine in the control of severe scleritis.

Cyclophosphamide is one of the more effective drugs for the treatment of systemic vasculitic syndromes and for severe scleritis.[8,25,29] Cyclophosphamide may be used as a single daily oral dosage (1 to 3 mg/kg/day) or as intermittent, intravenous pulse therapy. Oral cyclophosphamide should be administered as a single morning dose, and the patient should be encouraged to drink at least 3 liters of fluid per day to ensure adequate urine output and to minimize the risk of hemorrhagic cystitis. Cyclophosphamide may be used as a steroid-sparing agent or as additional immunosuppressive therapy to aid disease control. The long-term complications of cyclophosphamide, particularly infertility and oncogenesis (which are of great concern in young patients), can be minimized to a certain extent by limiting the duration of therapy to 6 to 12 months (which tends to be the duration of therapy required in patients with scleritis).

Cyclosporine has been used in the treatment of scleritis.[13,42] These patients had severe disease that failed to improve with other immunosuppressive drugs or developed unacceptable side effects. Cyclosporine was effective in controlling the inflammatory response in severe scleritis, although its use was associated with significant side effects.

Attempts to withdraw cyclosporine often resulted in disease relapse in patients who had previously responded to this form of therapy. Cyclosporine has been beneficial in young patients with scleritis that could not be controlled by corticosteroids alone.

Other cytotoxic drugs such as chlorambucil and methotrexate may be useful in the management of patients with severe scleritis. Experience with these drugs is limited, but they may be beneficial in selected patients.[36]

Follow-up. The decision to cease treatment is often difficult and should not be made in haste. Scleritis should be quiescent for a minimum of 6 to 12 weeks, and there should be no evidence of associated systemic disease activity. Immunosuppressive drugs, including corticosteroids, should be withdrawn slowly over a 6- to 12-week period, and the patient should be carefully assessed for evidence of disease relapse. The patient should be given a detailed outline of the proposed sliding scale to be used during the withdrawal of immunosuppressive therapy and should be instructed to report any evidence of disease recurrence. If disease relapse occurs, the dosage of corticosteroids should be doubled and the dose of additional immunosuppressive agents returned to maintenance levels until disease control is regained. It is essential to carefully consider the potential risks of continuing immunosuppressive therapy against the potential for saving useful vision.

Stopping corticosteroid therapy may rarely produce signs and symptoms related to drug withdrawal, with the most important being the steroid withdrawal syndrome and adrenal gland failure. An Addisonian crisis is an acute life-threatening medical emergency and is treated by the use of intravenous corticosteroids, cardiovascular support, and other resuscitative measures. The steroid withdrawal syndrome is characterized by severe polyarthralgia and polymyalgia, which can be confused with a systemic rheumatic syndrome, autoimmune disease, or sarcoidosis. Recognition of the benign self-limiting nature of steroid withdrawal will prevent unnecessary investigations or reinstitution of therapy. It is usually not seen in patients treated with alternate-day steroid therapy.

Surgical Management. Surgical intervention is rarely required in patients with scleritis, as the management is primarily medical in nature. Surgical procedures may be necessary for diagnosis, to repair scleral and corneal defects, to repair globe perforations, or to treat complications of scleritis. Surgery in patients with scleritis should not be performed until appropriate medical therapy has been commenced, otherwise the surgery will be complicated by the effects of unchecked inflammation on the eye. In patients with large scleral defects or perforations and severe necrotizing scleritis this often necessitates the use of pulsed intravenous corticosteroids and cyclophosphamide.[29,33b,44]

Diagnostic surgery is usually an episcleral biopsy to exclude a neoplastic process masquerading as an inflammatory scleritis. Episcleral biopsy should not be approached lightly, as interference to the episclera and its vasculature can accelerate significantly the intensity of scleritis.[48]

Intensive immunosuppressive therapy for severe scleritis has improved the outlook for such patients and decreased the frequency of massive scleral necrosis and globe perforation. There are, however, patients who have large areas of scleral or corneal stromal loss who require tectonic grafting to prevent perforation until immunosuppressive therapy becomes effective (which may take from 4 to 8 weeks). Such patients require surgical reconstruction using fresh or preserved donor sclera or lamellar cornea. In brief, the necrotic host tissue should be excised and a bed prepared into which the donor sclera or cornea can be sutured. Scleral perforations are managed by vitrectomy to excise prolapsed vitreous, and the host bed is then treated with cryotherapy or diathermy.[4b] The scleral or corneal graft can then be sutured into place. Corneal perforations should be treated with lamellar grafting where appropriate. It is essential that patients with severe, active scleritis who require surgery be treated with aggressive antiinflammatory therapy, otherwise the graft will be destroyed by uncontrolled inflammation.[33b]

Surgical intervention may become necessary for patients with scleritis to deal effectively with complications such as cataract and glaucoma. This surgery should only be undertaken once the scleritis is controlled medically, and patients should be covered perioperatively with corticosteroids to minimize the risk of a relapse precipitated by the surgical procedure.

Complications

Scleritis is a severe, destructive inflammatory disease that often spreads to adjacent intraocular structures (Table 53-11). Corneal complications are the most frequent, and posterior-segment complications the most serious. Complications may occur at any time during the course of scleritis and depend on the type and location of scleral inflammation. Visual loss occurs in approximately 10% of patients with anterior diffuse scleritis, 25% of those with nodular scleritis, and 75% to 85% of individuals with necrotizing scleritis or posterior scleritis.[39]

Corneal Changes. The type and severity of corneal involvement tend to parallel the severity of the scleritis. Stromal keratitis occurs in approximately one third of patients with scleritis.[45] Different clinical types of scleritis are associated with a number of different corneal lesions. Corneal changes occur in approximately 50% of patients with nodular scleritis, 40% of patients with necrotizing scleritis, 20% of patients with diffuse scleritis, and 5% of patients with posterior scleritis.[39] Nodular scleritis tends to be associated with localized corneal changes adjacent to areas of scleral inflammation in contrast to the more diffuse corneal infiltrates seen with other types of scleritis.

A classification is based on the morphology of the corneal lesions and the severity of the scleritis[48]:

1. Diffuse scleritis:
   Stromal keratitis
   Sclerosing keratitis
   Peripheral corneal guttering
2. Nodular scleritis:
   Localized stromal keratitis
   Localized sclerosing keratitis
3. Necrotizing scleritis:
   Sclerosing keratitis
   Peripheral corneal guttering
   Keratolysis

Stromal keratitis is typically acute in onset, may be localized or diffuse in extent, and usually begins near the limbus as areas of infiltration and edema that form focal corneal stromal opacities. The opacities may remain multiple and discrete or coalesce to result in large areas of diffuse corneal opacification. Corneal vascularization accompanies the opacities. The inflammation of severe stromal keratitis may be sufficient to produce stromal loss (keratolysis). There may be corneal ulceration, and there is usually an associated anterior uveitis. Stromal keratitis occurs with severe scleritis and is seen most commonly in necrotizing scleritis. Its presence therefore signals the need for intensive antiinflammatory therapy. If treated early, the opacification will usually resolve without loss of corneal substance, although corneal scarring frequently follows resolution of stromal keratitis.

Keratolysis is a rare but devastating form of acute stromal keratitis that occurs in severe necrotizing scleritis and results in massive corneal stromal lysis and descemetocele formation. Perforation of the globe may occur and result in loss of

TABLE 53-11   COMPLICATIONS OF SCLERITIS

1. Cornea	Stromal keratitis
	Sclerosing keratitis
	Keratolysis
	Peripheral corneal melting
	Perforation
2. Sclera	Scleral thinning
	Scleral necrosis
	Staphyloma
	Perforation
3. Uvea	Uveitis (anterior or posterior)
	Choroidal granuloma
4. Ciliary Body	Glaucoma
5. Lens	Cataract
6. Retina	Exudative detachment
	Macula edema
	Vasculitis
7. Optic Nerve	Disc edema
	Optic atrophy

the eye. This type of corneal disease, like other destructive corneal lesions with scleritis, signifies the presence of a systemic vasculitis and requires intensive immunosuppressive therapy, as well as tectonic grafting, to control the inflammatory process.

Sclerosing keratitis is the most prevalent corneal infiltration associated with scleritis and may be localized or diffuse. It consists of a full-thickness coarsening and edema of the corneal stroma with the formation of multiple small discrete white opacities in the stroma that are crystalline and similar to cotton candy in appearance. Corneal vascularization occurs in the involved cornea. With treatment the keratitis stops progressing, and the edema resolves, but the stromal opacification is permanent.

Peripheral corneal melting can occur in association with scleritis. In patients with scleritis, it is most common in necrotizing disease in which up to 40% of patients develop a degree of peripheral corneal melting.[39] It begins adjacent to the limbus as a localized area of grey opacified edematous cornea that thins, resulting in a peripheral area of stromal loss with well-demarcated edges. The thinned areas become vascularized. The degree of stromal loss is variable. The lesions extend circumferentially rather than centrally and may involve 360° of the cornea. Mild forms of this limbal guttering without severe accompanying scleritis resemble the isolated peripheral corneal thinning seen in patients with rheumatoid arthritis and run a similar course. Severe forms of corneal melting associated with florid scleritis may closely resemble Mooren ulcer and have a similar progressive clinical course requiring aggressive treatment.[46]

Uveitis. Uveitis occurs in up to 50% of patients with scleritis.[49] Anterior uveitis may occur in any type of anterior scleritis. Posterior uveitis is rare in patients with isolated anterior scleritis, and its presence usually signifies posterior segment involvement.[45] Vitreous inflammation is very typical in posterior scleritis and often accompanies elevated intraocular pressure. In general, although the uveitis accompanying scleritis is not severe, its chronicity may allow the development of complications such as synechiae, raised intraocular pressure, and cataract—unless it is recognized and treated appropriately.

Glaucoma. The incidence of glaucoma complicating scleritis has fallen dramatically with better understanding of scleritis and the advent of effective treatment for scleritis. In 1965 45% of eyes with scleritis had secondary glaucoma, whereas by 1991, only 9% of patients developed glaucoma.[35,39]

Glaucoma is most prevalent in posterior and nodular scleritis and occurs the least in diffuse scleritis. Approximately 20% of patients with nodular scleritis and 15% of patients with posterior scleritis develop raised intraocular pressure. Glaucoma in patients with scleritis can be classified in the following manner:

1. Open angle:
   Blockage by debris
   Trabecular inflammation
   Raised episcleral venous pressure
   Primary open-angle glaucoma
   Steroid-induced glaucoma
2. Closed angle:
   Ciliary body rotation
   Pupil block from posterior synechiae
   Angle closure from peripheral anterior synechiae

In patients with anterior scleritis, involvement of the perilimbal sclera may result in trabecular inflammation and/or elevated episcleral venous pressure. This will result in raised intraocular pressure that can be quite refractory to medical therapy until the scleritis is controlled.[45]

Uveitis may lead to trabecular obstruction from inflammatory debris, but more frequently the development of synechiae leads to closure of the angle either directly from peripheral anterior synechiae or from iris bombé as a result of pupil block caused by posterior synechiae.

Posterior scleritis resulting in annular choroidal detachment may produce a ciliochoroidal effusion that rotates the ciliary body and iris forward to produce angle closure and elevated intraocular pressure.[2,10]

Both primary open-angle glaucoma and steroid-induced glaucoma are common entities. There are patients who develop scleritis who (1) have primary glaucoma, (2) are susceptible to the effects of corticosteroids on intraocular pressure, or (3) have both problems.

Clearly there is the potential for multiple mechanisms to be operational in a disease such as scleritis, with the net result being a moderate to severe elevation of the intraocular pressure. It is essential to monitor the intraocular pressure regularly in patients with scleritis and to pay careful attention to the gonioscopic findings in patients with elevated intraocular pressures. In general, the management of the intraocular pressure should treat the underlying scleritis and any associated uveitis. Medical therapy using topical beta-blockers and an oral carbonic anhydrase inhibitor may not be effective until the scleritis is controlled. It is unusual for patients to require surgery for pressure control, but filtration surgery can be safely performed once the scleritis is controlled.

Cataract. Cataract is a complication related to the severity of the scleritis and occurs frequently only in necrotizing scleritis, where its incidence is 20%.[39] Its incidence is less than 5% in other types of scleritis. Visually significant lens opacities may develop in patients with necrotizing scleritis, as a result of corticosteroid therapy, or because of accelerated progression of preexisting lens opacities.

When necessary, cataract surgery is safe, provided the

scleritis is in remission. The patient is covered perioperatively with systemic corticosteroids and is warned that cataract surgery may precipitate a relapse of the scleritis. A corneal wound for cataract surgery is safe and effective.

Scleral Thinning. Loss of scleral collagen is a common result of severe scleritis and occurs typically in patients with necrotizing scleritis. Patients with diffuse anterior scleritis have mild disease and rarely develop substantial loss of sclera, although about 12% may develop mild scleral thinning as distinct from the increased scleral transparency that is common. In nodular scleritis, up to 50% of patients have evidence of scleral thinning.[45] Scleral necrosis leads to loss of scleral substance even with early effective treatment; therefore, all patients with necrotizing scleritis will have some degree of scleral thinning.

Scleral thinning results in a bluish discoloration to the affected sclera caused by increased visibility of the underlying choroid and decreased thickness of the sclera in involved areas. Scleral thinning may result in clinically significant astigmatism.

Posterior Segment Complications. Most of the posterior-segment manifestations of scleritis discussed in the section on posterior scleritis could be equally considered as complications, as they represent the effects of scleral inflammation on ocular structures adjacent to the sclera. With appropriate treatment they resolve without sequelae, except for exudative retinal detachment. Exudative retinal detachments that involve the macula result in permanent visual loss despite resolution of the detachment and are responsible for the high rate of visual loss in patients with posterior scleritis. Peripheral detachments result in the formation of small punctate areas of retinal pigment epithelial cell clumping and hyperplasia that lead to tide marks and scattered focal areas of pigmentation in areas of previous detachment.[48]

Prognosis

Scleritis is a highly destructive inflammatory process commonly associated with systemic disease. The prognosis depends on the severity of the scleritis and the prognosis of any associated disease. Some of the systemic diseases that produce scleritis can be fatal. Treatment with aggressive immunosuppression in patients with rheumatoid arthritis who develop necrotizing scleritis improves the ocular outcome and reduces the mortality rate from associated systemic vasculitis.[8]

Scleritis may cause profound morbidity from pain, and the inflammation is sufficient to frequently produce visual loss from complications. Untreated, necrotizing scleritis (the most aggressive form of scleritis) tends to be relentlessly progressive until the sclera is largely destroyed. Nodular and diffuse scleritis are more benign forms and will eventually resolve but will leave areas of altered sclera or scleral thinning without effective treatment. Posterior scleritis often

produces exudative retinal detachments that lead to severe visual loss if unrecognized. Necrotizing scleritis may result in loss of the affected eye. Correct diagnosis and management will avoid the hazards of immunosuppression, will prevent visual loss in the majority of eyes, and will identify associated systemic disease.

REFERENCES

1. Altman AJ, Cohen EJ, Berger ST, Mondino BJ: Scleritis and *Streptococcus pneumoniae, Cornea* 10:341-345, 1991.
2. Benson WE: Posterior scleritis, *Surv Ophthalmol* 32:297, 1988.
3. Brooks PM: Clinical management of rheumatoid arthritis, *Lancet* 341:286, 1993.
4. Charles SJ, Meyer PA, Watson PG: Diagnosis and management of systemic Wegener's granulomatosis presenting with anterior ocular inflammatory disease, *Br J Ophthalmol* 75:201-207, 1991.
5. Finger PT et al.: Posterior scleritis as an intraocular tumour, *Br J Ophthalmol* 74:121, 1990.
6. Firestein GS: Mechanisms of tissue destruction and cellular activation in rheumatoid arthritis, *Curr Opin Rheumatol* 4:348, 1992.
7. Fong LP et al.: Immunopathology of scleritis, *Ophthalmology* 98:472, 1991.
8. Foster CS, Forstot SL, Wilson LA: Mortality rate in rheumatoid arthritis patients developing necrotizing scleritis or peripheral ulcerative keratitis: effects of systemic immunosuppression, *Ophthalmology* 91:1253, 1984.
9. Fraser DJ Jr, Font RL: Ocular inflammation and haemorrhage as initial manifestations of uveal malignant melanoma: incidence and prognosis, *Arch Ophthalmol* 97:1482, 1979.
10. Fraunfelder F, Watson PG: Evaluation of eyes enucleated for scleritis, *Br J Ophthalmol* 60:227, 1976.
11. Freeman IL: The eye. In Weiss JB, Jaycon MI: *Collagen in health and disease,* London, 1982, Churchill Livingstone.
12. Glasser DB, Bellor J: Necrotizing scleritis of scleral flaps after transscleral suture fixation of an intraocular lens, *Am J Ophthalmol* 113:529-532, 1992.
13. Hakin KN, Ham J, Lightman SL: Use of cyclosporin in the management of steroid dependent non-necrotizing scleritis, *Br J Ophthalmol* 75:340, 1991.
14. Hakin KN, Ham J, Lightman SL: Use of orbital floor steroids in the management of patients with uniocular non-necrotizing scleritis, *Br J Ophthalmol* 75:337, 1991.
15. Hakin KN, Watson PG: Systemic associations of scleritis, *Int Ophthalmol Clin* 31:111, 1991.
16. Hogan MJ, Zimmerman LE: *Ophthalmic pathology,* New York, 1964, WB Saunders.
17. Jakobiec FA, Jones IS: Orbital inflammations. In Duane TD: *Clinical ophthalmology,* vol 2, Hagerstown MD, 1984, Harper and Row.
18. Jennette JC, Falk RJ: Disease associations and pathogenic role of anti neutrophil cytoplasmic autoantibodies in vasculitis, *Curr Opin Rheumatol* 4:9, 1992.
19. Karma A et al.: Phenotypes of conjunctival inflammatory cells in sarcoidosis, *Br J Ophthalmol* 76:101, 1992.
20. Kattan HM, Pflugfelder SC: *Nocardia* scleritis, *Am J Ophthalmol* 110:446, 1990.
21. Kaufman LM et al.: Necrotizing scleritis following strabismus surgery for thyroid ophthalmopathy, *J Pediatr Ophthalmol Strabismus* 26:236, 1989.
22. Kim RY et al.: Necrotizing scleritis secondary to conjunctival squamous cell carcinoma in acquired immunodeficiency syndrome, *Am J Ophthalmol* 109:231, 1990.
23. Lindenmuth KA et al.: Invasive squamous cell carcinoma of the conjunctiva presenting as necrotizing scleritis with scleral perforation and uveal prolapse, *Surv Ophthalmol* 33:50, 1988.
24. McCluskey PJ, Wakefield D: Intravenous pulse methylprednisolone in scleritis, *Arch Ophthalmol* 105:793, 1987.

25. McCluskey P, Wakefield D: Current concepts in the management of scleritis, *Aust NZ J Ophthalmol* 16:169, 1988.

26. McCluskey P, Wakefield D: Prediction of response to treatment in patients with scleritis using a standardized scoring system, *Aust NZ J Ophthalmol* 19:211, 1991.

27. McCluskey PJ, Wakefield D, Penny R: Scleritis and the spectrum of external inflammatory eye disease, *Aust NZ J Ophthalmol* 13:159, 1985.

28. Meyer PAR: Patterns of blood flow in episcleral vessels studied by low dose fluorescein videoangiography, *Eye* 2:533, 1988.

29. Meyer PAR et al.: Pulsed immunosuppressive therapy in the treatment of immunologically induced corneal and scleral disease, *Eye* 1:487, 1987.

30. Mondino BJ, Phinney RB: Treatment of scleritis with combined oral prednisone and indomethacin therapy, *Am J Ophthalmol* 106:473, 1988.

31. Nanda M, Pflugfelder SC, Holland S: Mycobacterium tuberculosis scleritis, *Am J Ophthalmol* 108:736, 1989.

32. O'Donoghue E et al.: Surgically induced necrotizing sclerokeratitis (SINS)-precipitating factors and response to treatment, *Br J Ophthalmol* 76:17, 1992.

33. Rao NA, Marak GE, Hidayat AA: Necrotizing scleritis: a clinicopathological study of 41 cases, *Ophthalmology* 92:1542, 1985.

33a. Sainz de la Maza M, Foster CS: Necrotizing scleritis after ocular surgery. A clinicopathologic study, *Ophthalmology* 98:1720, 1991.

33b. Sainz de la Maza M, Tauber J, Foster CS: Scleral grafting for necrotizing scleritis, *Ophthalmology* 96:306, 1989.

34. Schuman JS et al.: Toxoplasmic scleritis, *Ophthalmology* 95:1399, 1988.

35. Sevel D: Rheumatoid nodule of the sclera, *Trans Ophthalmol Soc UK* 85:357, 1965.

36. Shah SS et al.: Low dose methotrexate therapy for ocular inflammatory disease, *Ophthalmology* 99:1419, 1992.

37. Soukiasian SH et al.: Diagnostic value of anti-neutrophil cytoplasmic antibodies in scleritis associated with Wegener's granulomatosis, *Ophthalmology* 99:125, 1992.

38. Stokes JJ: Intraocular extension of epibulbar squamous cell carcinoma of the limbus, *Trans Am Acad Ophthalmol Otolaryngol* 59:143, 1955.

39. Tuft SJ, Watson PG: Progression of scleral disease, *Ophthalmology* 98:467, 1991.

40. Wakefield D, Hawkins N: Sarcoidosis: current concepts of pathogenesis, *Saudi Med J* 73:92, 1992.

41. Wakefield D, Lloyd A: The role of cytokines in the pathogenesis of inflammatory eye disease, *Cytokine* 4:1, 1992.

42. Wakefield D, McCluskey PJ: Cyclosporin therapy for severe scleritis, *Br J Ophthalmol* 73:743, 1989.

43. Wakefield D, McCluskey PJ, Penny R: Intravenous pulse methylprednisolone therapy in severe inflammatory eye disease, *Arch Ophthalmol* 104:847, 1986.

44. Watson PG: The nature and treatment of scleral inflammation (Doyne memorial lecture), *Trans Ophthalmol Soc UK* 99:257, 1982.

45. Watson PG: Diseases of the sclera and episclera. In Duane TD: *Clinical ophthalmology,* vol 4, Hagerstown, Md, 1984, Harper and Row.

46. Watson PG: Vascular changes in peripheral corneal destructive disease, *Eye* 4:65, 1990.

47. Watson PG, Hayreh SS: Scleritis and episcleritis, *Br J Ophthalmol* 60:163, 1976.

48. Watson PG, Hazleman BL: *The sclera and systemic disorders,* London, 1976, WB Saunders.

49. Wilhelmus KR, Watson PG, Vasavada AR: Uveitis associated with scleritis, *Trans Ophthalmol Soc UK* 101:351, 1981.

50. Yanoff M, Fine B: *Ocular pathology: a text and atlas,* Hagerstown, Md, 1975, Harper and Row.

51. Yap E-Y, Robertson DM, Buettner H: Scleritis as an initial manifestation of choroidal malignant melanoma, *Ophthalmology* 99:1693, 1992.

52. York LJ, McCluskey PJ, Wakefield D: Scleral autoantibodies in external eye disease, *Proc Aust Soc Exp Pathol* 17:17, 1985.

53. Young RD, Watson PG: Microscopical studies of necrotizing scleritis. I. Cellular aspects, *Br J Ophthalmol* 68:770, 1984.

54 Behçet Disease

MANABU MOCHIZUKI, LEVENT AKDUMAN, ROBERT B. NUSSENBLATT

HISTORICAL BACKGROUND

Behçet disease bears the name of Hulusi Behçet, a Turkish dermatologist. Although this disease was probably known to the ancients (Hippocrates described a disease quite similar to the one we now call Behçet disease) Behçet's 1937 report[5] of this entity engendered enormous interest in the disorder. Adamantiades also described a group of such patients in 1931,[1] as did Shigeta from Japan in 1924.[81]

EPIDEMIOLOGY

The disease, though found worldwide, has a distinctly high incidence among certain groups of people. It is seen relatively often in Asians, North Africans, and Europeans living between latitudes 30° and 45° N. Behçet disease is the leading cause of endogenous uveitis and one of the major causes of acquired blindness in Japan and Turkey. The prevalence rate has been reported as 80 to 300 per 100,000 in Turkey and 7 to 8.5 per 100,000 in Japan.[51,84,93,97] It is also a very common entity in countries around the Mediterranean basin and in areas extending through the Middle East into Iran. There is no evidence that the disease is either increasing or decreasing in frequency. It has been suggested that Behçet disease, or at least an immunogenetic predisposition to it, was distributed throughout the ancient world by merchants who plied the old silk trading routes.

Many reports have suggested that the disease is more prevalent in males. More recent evidence, however, suggests a more even distribution of the disease between the sexes. Although the discrepancies in reported male to female ratios might reflect a change in the nature of the disease, it is more likely that in previous years, women in many countries were embarrassed to see a physician with complaints related to the cluster of signs and symptoms that make up Behçet disease. Male patients, as well as young individuals 15 to 25 years of age, experience a more protracted and severe form of the disease.[95]

The disease has an interesting distribution even within countries where it is prevalent. The disorder occurs more frequently in patients living in the northern parts of Japan than in those from the southern areas. Because there is no known HLA or other genetic difference between Japanese living in the north and south, this finding suggests that an exogenous agent may play a role in the induction of the disease. Of interest as well is a report from Hawaii[31] that could not document a case of Behçet disease in the Nisei population; this observation also supports the concept that an exogenous factor found in parts of Japan may play a part in the development of the disease. Although several familial cases[15,90] and a pair of monozygotic brothers[27] concordant for the syndrome have been reported, no consistent inheritance pattern has been noted.[52,86]

CLINICAL FEATURES

Behçet disease is a multisystem inflammatory illness characterized by intraocular inflammation, oral and mucosal ulcerations, skin lesions, and a variety of other disorders involving multiple organ systems in the body. It may involve the joints, the intestine, the epididymis, the vascular system, and the central nervous system. Behçet disease is characterized by recurrent episodes of inflammation involving one or more organ systems. The onset of these episodes is generally sudden. Inflammation then subsides over a period of several weeks. These clinical features constitute criteria on which a diagnosis of Behçet disease is based.

The Behçet Disease Research Committee, organized by the Ministry of Health and Welfare of Japan in 1972, proposed a Guide for the Diagnosis of Behçet Disease,[83] which has been used throughout the world. The International Study Group for Behçet Disease proposed another set of diagnostic criteria in 1990.[36] Although there are basic similarities between these criteria, the Behçet Disease Research Committee places more importance on ocular findings, whereas the International Study Group for Behçet Disease gives more emphasis to the presence of oral aphthous ulcers in confirming a diagnosis. The Behçet Disease Research Committee classifies symptoms of Behçet disease into major and minor diagnostic criteria. Behçet disease itself is divided into complete and incomplete types. A brief summary of the most recent version of the committee's diagnostic criteria, presented in 1987,[53] appears in Table 54-1. The committee also identified several special clinical types of Behçet disease: intestinal Behçet disease, vasculo-Behçet disease, and neuro-Behçet disease, based on the most prominent manifestations of the disease.

The diagnostic criteria proposed by the International Study Group for Behçet Disease[34] are listed in Table 54-2. By these criteria, oral aphthous ulcers must be present for a diagnosis of Behçet disease.

Lesions involving the joints, the intestine, the epididymis, the vascular system and the central nervous system are called the "minor criteria" with respect to their importance in making a diagnosis of Behçet disease, but some of the minor criteria can be markedly troublesome—or even life-threatening—for patients. The most severe of these disorders are joint, vascular, and central nervous system lesions.

Ocular Disease

The ocular manifestations of Behçet disease have serious implications for patients. In a recent, large epidemiologic survey of patients with Behçet disease carried out in Japan, ocular involvement was seen in 69.1% of 3316 patients; iridocyclitis was present in 59.7% of patients; and uveoretinitis was present in 54.0%.[59] Visual prognosis, particularly for patients having inflammation of the posterior segment, is poor. An analysis of long-term visual acuity outcomes disclosed that a good visual acuity (> 20/40) was retained for almost 10 years in all the eyes that had anterior

TABLE 54-1 DIAGNOSTIC CRITERIA FOR BEHÇET DISEASE PROPOSED BY THE BEHÇET DISEASE RESEARCH COMMITTEE OF JAPAN

CRITERIA

Major

1. Recurrent oral aphthous ulcers
2. Skin lesions:
   Erythema nodosumlike lesions
   Acneiform lesions
   Folliculitis
   Thrombophlebitis
   Cutaneous hypersensitivity
3. Genital ulcers
4. Ocular disease:
   Iridocyclitis typically with hypopyon
   Chorioretinitis

Minor

1. Arthritis
2. Epididymitis
3. Intestinal symptoms attributed to multiple ulcers in the ileocecal region
4. Vascular symptoms:
   Obliterative thrombophlebitis
   Arterial occlusion
   Aneurysm
5. Neurologic symptoms attributed to nervous system lesions

DIAGNOSIS

Complete Type

1. The presence of all four major criteria either simultaneously or at different times during the course of the disease

Incomplete Type

1. The presence of three major criteria or two major criteria plus two minor criteria, either simultaneously or at different times during the clinical course
2. Ocular disease criteria plus another major criterion or ocular disease criterion plus two minor criteria, either simultaneously or at different times during the clinical course

From Mizushima Y, Inaba G, Mimura Y et al.: *Guide for the diagnosis of Behçet disease, report of Behçet disease research committee,* Japan, 1987, Ministry of Health and Welfare.

TABLE 54-2 DIAGNOSTIC CRITERIA FOR BEHÇET DISEASE PROPOSED BY THE INTERNATIONAL STUDY GROUP FOR BEHÇET DISEASE

Recurrent oral ulceration:	Minor aphthous ulcers, major aphthous ulcers, or herpetiform lesions observed by physician or patient that have recurred at least 3 times in one 12-month period

Plus two of the following:

1. Recurrent genital ulceration:	Aphthous ulceration or scarring, observed by physician or patient
2. Eye lesions:	Anterior uveitis, posterior uveitis, or cells in vitreous humor on slit lamp examination; or retinal vasculitis observed by ophthalmologist
3. Skin lesions:	Erythema nodosum observed by physician or patient, pseudofolliculitis, or papulopustular lesions; or acneiform nodules observed by physician in postadolescent patients not on corticosteroid treatment
4. Positive pathergy test:	Read by a physician at 24-48 hours

From International Study Group for Behçet Disease: Criteria for diagnosis of Behçet disease, *Lancet* 335:1078-1080, 1990.

uveitis alone, whereas only one quarter of the eyes with posterior involvement retained good visual acuity 5 years after the onset of uveitis.[51]

Although the disease can affect the anterior and posterior portions of the eye separately, the majority of patients have panuveitis or posterior uveitis; only a small portion (~10%) of patients have only anterior uveitis. Ocular disease usually develops 2 to 3 years after the initial lesions of Behçet disease, which in most patients are oral aphthous ulcerations. Ocular disease is the initial manifestation of Behçet disease in about 20% of cases,[33] however. The disease is almost always bilateral; only rarely does uveitis develop in a single eye. A long-term study in Japan found that 93.6% of patients have bilateral disease, but in some cases, the interval between involvement of the two eyes was more than 5 years.[33]

Anterior Uveitis. Behçet disease is characterized by explosive attacks of intraocular inflammation. These episodes resolve spontaneously over several weeks with or without treatment. Patients can have many recurrent episodes of uveitis, which result in irreversible damage to intraocular tissues. Anterior uveitis is characterized by gross hypopyon formation in about one third of cases[51] (Fig. 54-1). The hypopyon is composed primarily of neutrophils.[82] In eyes with severe iridocyclitis in which no hypopyon is seen by direct examination with the slit lamp biomicroscope, a small layering of leukocytes can be observed in the angle by gonioscopy (''angle hypopyon''). The iridocyclitis is nongranulomatous in nature, and cells move freely in the currents of the aqueous humor. A characteristic feature of the hypopyon of Behçet disease is that it shifts with gravity as the patient changes head positions. The hypopyon resolves spontaneously after several days, without sequelae. Posterior synechiae, iris atrophy, and peripheral anterior synechiae may develop during the course of repeated ocular inflammatory attacks. Peripheral anterior synechiae or iris bombé from

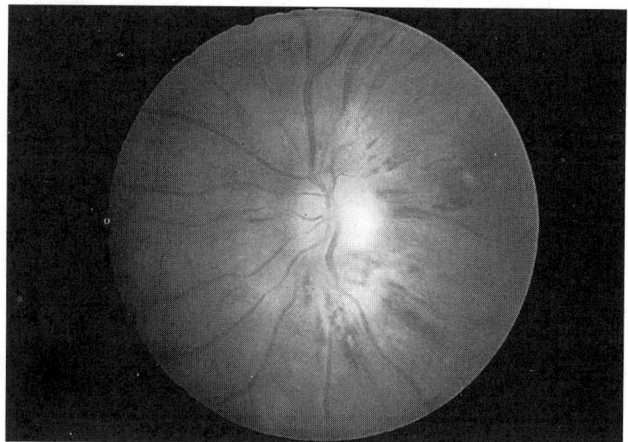

Fig. 54-2. Papillitis in a patient with Behçet disease. (From Washington University, St. Louis.)

pupillary seclusion may cause secondary glaucoma. An isolated vitreous inflammatory reaction is not characteristic of Behçet disease.

Retinal Disease. Retinal disease is the most serious complication of Behçet disease. Recurrent retinal vascular occlusive episodes can ultimately lead to irreversible alterations in the sensory retina with severe visual impairment. Funduscopic examination reveals venous engorgement, retinal hemorrhages, yellow-white exudates, retinal infiltrates, intense retinal edema, and hyperemia and edema of the optic disc. Retinal infiltrates have been reported as pathognomonic findings.[25] Optic disc edema may be secondary to inflammation or increased intracranial pressure that develops subsequent to cerebral vein thrombosis and can be the initial manifestation.[16,38,75] Papillitis may be observed (Fig. 54-2). There is an accompanying vitreous inflammatory response. Retinal vasculitis is very intractable to treatment and rarely disappears completely (Fig. 54-3). Patients with chronic posterior uveitis and retinal vasculitis may have anterior uveitis attacks with variable frequency; often the periods of remission in their anterior uveitis are longer in the late stages of the disease, possibly because of intense medications directed to the posterior disease.

In the very late stages the fulminant picture of active retinal disease, with intraretinal edema, hemorrhage, infiltrates, and venous engorgement, is replaced with an atrophic retina and optic disc, sheathed arteries and veins, and a variable degree of chorioretinal scars and retinal pigment epithelial alterations with trace to mild vitreous inflammation (Fig. 54-4). The incidence of anterior uveitis attacks is also greatly reduced in this very late stage even without treatment, as observed in some patients unable to use medications. Retinal neovascularization, secondary to either retinal vein occlusions, inflammation, or both, results in retinal or vitreous hemorrhage and is occasionally observed. Neovascular glaucoma occurs in as many as 6% of patients and

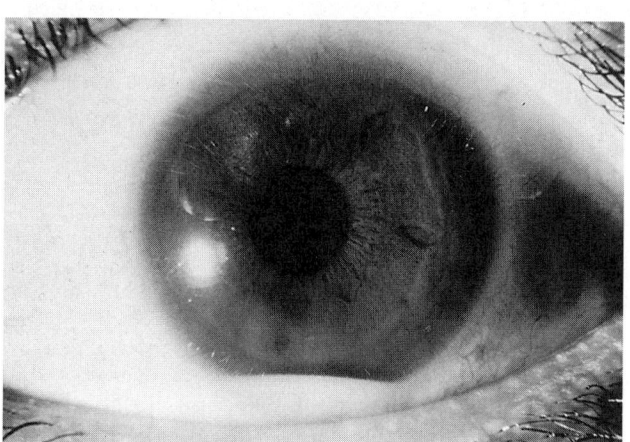

Fig. 54-1. Hypopyon in a patient with Behçet disease. (From Kurume University, Kurume, Japan.)

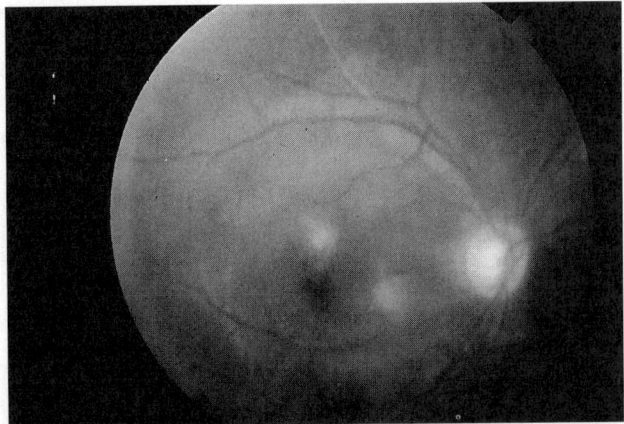

A

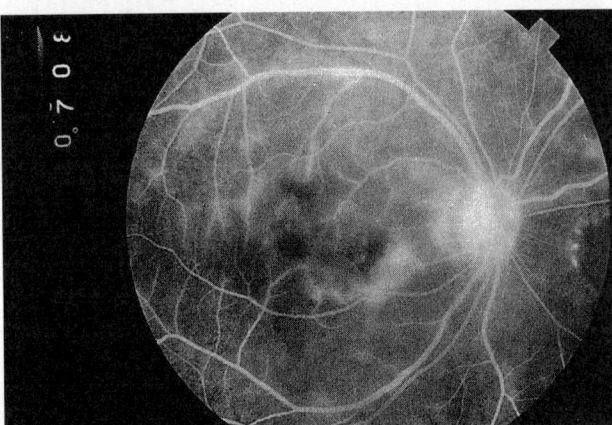

B

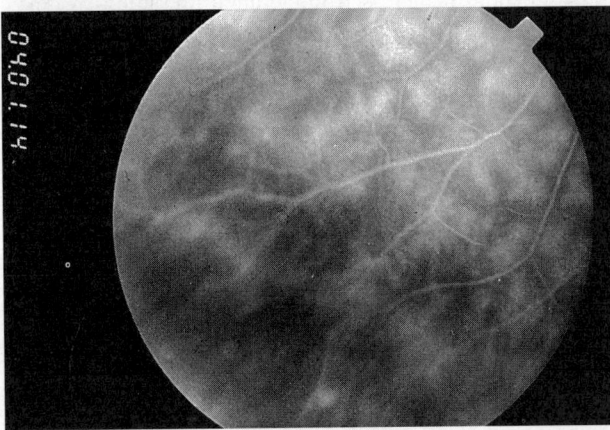

C

Fig. 54-3.   A. The fundus after an acute episode of chorioretinitis with white exudates in a patient with Behçet disease. **B.** The fluorescein angiogram of the same fundus showing retinal vasculitis. **C.** The fluorescein angiogram in another patient with Behçet disease demonstrating marked leakage from the retinal vessels, particularly from the capillaries. (From Kurume University, Kurume, Japan)

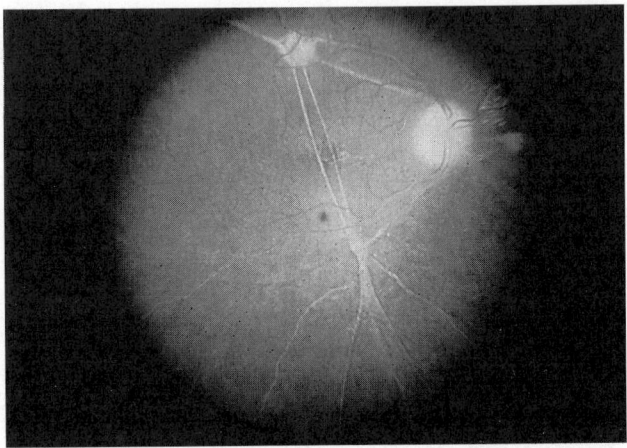

Fig. 54-4.   Retinal vasculitis in a late stage of Behçet disease revealing vascular obliteration, sheathing, and retinal and optic nerve atrophy. (From Gazi University, Ankara, Turkey.)

often results in phthisis bulbi. Central retinal artery and/or vein occlusions can, on rare occasions, result in no light perception vision (Fig. 54-5).

Fluorescein angiography demonstrates marked dilatation and occlusion of the retinal capillaries. Diffuse dye leakage from the capillaries, from larger engorged vessels, and from the optic disc also occurs. Persistent, diffuse leakage of dye is seen even with resolution of inflammatory episodes. Macular ischemia, which may be responsible for poor vision, can be revealed by fluorescein angiography[7] (Fig. 54-6). Fluorescein angiography may also detect cystoid macular edema secondary to inflammation. Evidence of choroidal or retinal pigment epithelial involvement (Fig. 54-7) is rarely seen in this disorder.

Retinal atrophy with or without optic atrophy is the end result of repeated episodes of posterior segment inflamma-

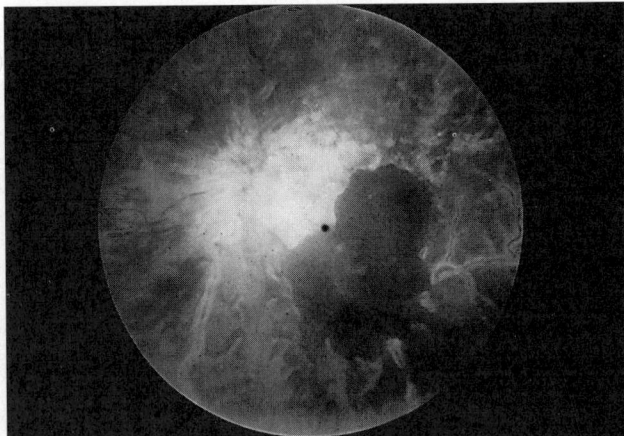

Fig. 54-5.   A 30-year-old Turkish male patient with combined central retinal artery and vein occlusion as a rare manifestation of Behçet disease. The patient progressed rapidly to no light perception vision. (From Gazi University, Ankara, Turkey.)

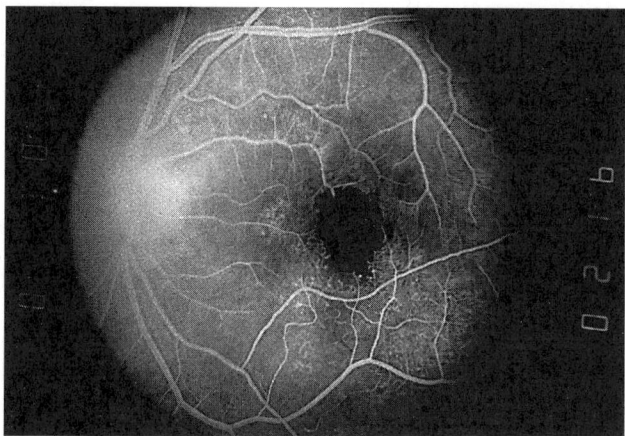

Fig. 54-6. Capillary dropout with irregularly enlarged foveal avascular zone demonstrating macular ischemia in fluorescein angiography of a patient with Behçet disease. (From Washington University, St. Louis.)

tion. If extensive areas of the retina are involved or retinal vein occlusions are complicated, retinal neovascularization with or without rubeosis iridis can occur, leading to severe and repeated vitreous hemorrhages, subsequent vitreous humor contraction, retinal detachment, and phthisis bulbi.

Nonocular Disease

Skin and Mucous Membrane Findings. The most common nonocular manifestations of Behçet disease are recurrent oral aphthous ulcers. According to a 1991 nationwide survey of Behçet disease in Japan, 3239 of 3316 patients with the disease (97.7%) had recurrent aphthous ulcers.[59] The oral aphthous ulcers can be found not only on the gums, but also on the lips, posterior pharynx, uvula, hard palate, and tongue (Fig. 54-8). The ulcers are painful, round or oval, and usually small and sharply defined. They ordi-

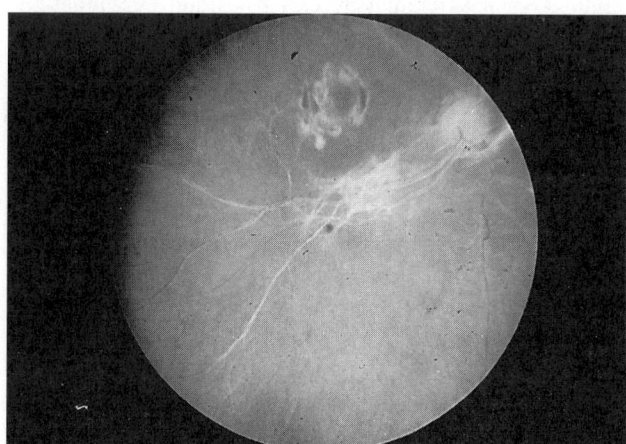

Fig. 54-7. Sheathed vessels and macular chorioretinal scar in late stage of Behçet disease. (From Gazi University, Ankara, Turkey.)

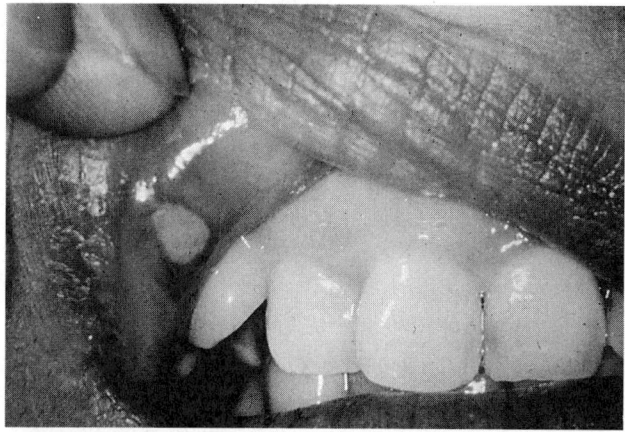

A

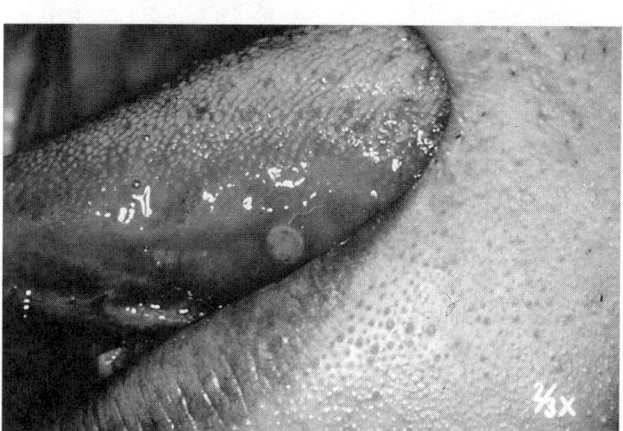

B

Fig. 54-8. A, B, Oral aphthous lesions in a patient with Behçet disease. (From Kurume University, Kurume, Japan)

narily heal in 7 to 10 days. Scarring occurs only with particularly large ulcers.

A variety of skin lesions can occur in patients with Behçet disease. Erythema nodosumlike lesions are noted frequently on the anterior surface of the legs, but they can also be seen on various body surfaces including the face, neck, and buttocks. The lesions are slightly raised, tender red nodules. They involute after several weeks without ulceration (Fig. 54-9). Acneiform lesions or folliculitis are common on the backs and faces of the patients. Because corticosteroid therapy can induce similar skin lesions, acneiform lesions in patients receiving corticosteroids have no diagnostic meaning. Thrombophlebitis is less common than the former two skin lesions. It usually occurs in the extremities and can be migratory. It can also develop after an injection or following venipuncture for blood sampling (Fig. 54-10). The reported proportions of patients having erythema nodosumlike lesions, acneiform lesions, and thrombophlebitis are 70.7%, 57.7%, and 15.8% of 3316 patients, respectively.[18]

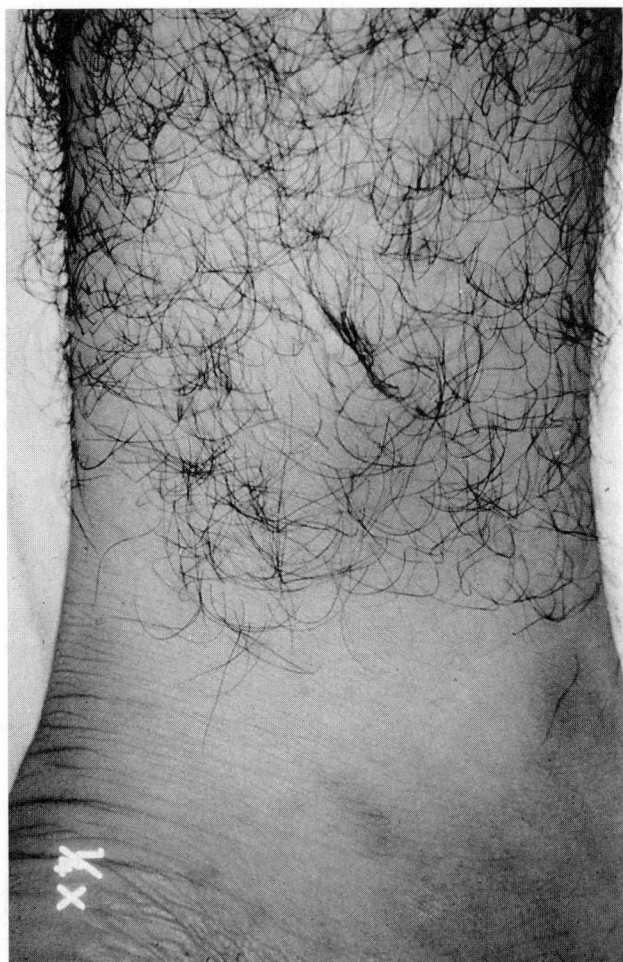

Fig. 54-9. Erythema nodosum-like skin lesion in a patient with Behçet disease. (From Kurume University, Kurume, Japan)

"Cutaneous hypersensitivity" is a characteristic feature of Behçet disease. A clinical manifestation of cutaneous hypersensitivity in male patients is hyperreaction of the skin after shaving. Cutaneous hypersensitivity can be tested with the "prick" test, in which a pustule forms after scratching the skin with a needle. In 1972 this phenomenon of pathergy occurred in 70% of the patients in Japan,[47] whereas a 1991 study found it to be much less common, with only 23.8% of patients having a positive test.[59] On the other hand, another recent study from Turkey reported a positive pathergy test in 78.9% of patients with—and 56.6% of patients without— vascular system disease, indicating a significant association of positive pathergy tests with vascular involvement.[44] A reduced prevalence of positive pathergy tests following surgical cleaning of the skin implicates factors other than disruption of the structural integrity of dermis and epidermis in this phenomenon.[20] The test is believed to be commonly positive among patients from the Mediterranean basin but is uncommonly positive among patients in the United States.[62]

Genital ulcers in male patients may appear on the scrotum and penis and are therefore easily identified. In female patients, lesions can develop on the vulva or the vaginal mucosae. The genital ulcers can be deep and can leave scars. An examination of the genital region can therefore be useful in a suspected Behçet disease patient, because signs of old disease may be present.

Arthritis. At least half of Behçet disease patients are affected by a nonmigratory and nondestructive arthritis. The nationwide survey conducted in Japan revealed that 1730 of 3316 patients (52.2%) had arthritis.[59] The most commonly affected joint was the knee. Arthritis usually reflects the level of systemic disease activity and is occasionally linked to ocular lesions.

Vascular Disease. Vessels of all sizes can be affected in Behçet disease. Those patients who develop vasoocclusive inflammatory changes in large vessels, with aneurysm or thrombus formation, are considered to have the "vasculo-Behçet," "angio-Behçet," or "cardio-Behçet" disease variant. Each of these variants has a poor prognosis, because infarction or rupture of an aneurysm can be life-threatening. In these patients, both the arterial and venous systems can be involved, although the latter is more frequently affected. The prevalence of the angio-Behçet disease variant in a large series of Behçet disease patients was 259 of 3316 patients (7.8%) in Japan[59]; this prevalence has been constant for the last 20 years. Other studies have reported vascular system involvement in up to 27.7% of patients.[44]

Central Nervous System Disease. Involvement of the central nervous system is seen in 8% to 10% of Japanese patients with Behçet disease, with a predominance of male patients.[35] It is noteworthy that Inaba[34] reported the majority of his patients with central nervous system involvement (90.4%) did not have ocular disease. In 68 autopsy cases studied by Inaba, multiple lesions in the central nervous system were found, particularly in the thalamus, basal ganglia, and the brainstem. In addition to a variety of neurologic findings such as cranial nerve palsies and pyramidal and

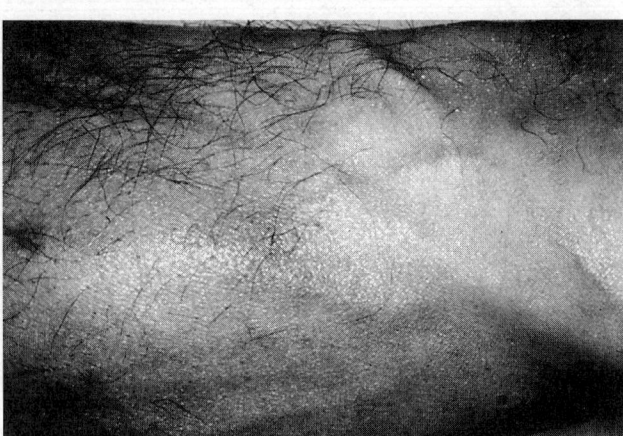

Fig. 54-10. Thrombophlebitis seen at the lower extremity in a patient with Behçet disease. (From Kurume University, Kurume, Japan)

extrapyramidal signs, psychiatric disorders may appear. Behçet disease has also been implicated as a cause of vertigo and hearing loss; these changes are believed to have a vasculitic cause.[9]

Examination of the cerebrospinal fluid during the acute stage of neuro-Behçet disease discloses a pleocytosis with neutrophils as the predominant cellular component.

PATHOLOGY

Few eyes with active disease have been examined histologically. The anterior segment may initially show the presence of a large number of neutrophils, consistent with the increased chemotactic activity of neutrophils reported in Behçet disease.[51] In other specimens taken from the anterior chamber, T-lymphocytes have been found.[10a] The underlying lesion in the eye was postulated by Winter and Yukins[92] to be an obliterative vasculitis. Most specimens show a perivasculitis with fibrinoid necrosis rather than a true vasculitis. Nevertheless, vasculitis is a key feature of the disease.[68] Arterial and venous lymphocytic and plasma cell infiltrates, disrupted elastic lamina, aneurysms, thromboses, and vasculitis (which is of recent onset, necrotic, or fibrotic) have also been described.[17,68,78,84] In one report by Mullaney and Collum[58] mural IgA, IgG, and C3 deposits were found in the veins of the episclera and choroid of an eye, but not in the retina.

PATHOGENESIS

Immunogenetics

The fact that certain racial groups appear to be at increased risk for Behçet disease suggests a genetic predisposition to the disease. Indeed, HLA-B5 has been found in a significantly higher proportion of patients suffering with Behçet disease than in the general population. The antisera denoting HLA-B5 has since been found to cross-react with at least two different antigens that were similar in structure: HLA-B51 and HLA-B52. Subsequent testing has identified that HLA-B51 is the antigen associated with this disorder. In one study from Japan, 58% of patients with the complete Behçet disease were HLA-B51-positive in contrast to 12% of Japanese controls, resulting in a calculated relative risk of 9.4 for this marker.[72] Godeau and associates[23] also identified an association between HLA-B5 and Behçet disease in patients of Mediterranean origin. Others have corroborated a similar association in patients from the Mediterranean basin and found HLA-B5 to be more frequently positive only in severely affected individuals, indicating that HLA-B5 is associated with a poor visual prognosis.[18,74,97] In contrast, studies performed in North America with patients from other ethnic groups have not found such an association. One of the studies, by Ohno and associates,[70] included six Caucasian patients who had "atypical" disease. Another, by O'Duffy and associates,[69] did not identify this association in 26 patients.

The reason for the association between HLA-B51 and Behçet disease is not known. Because HLA antigens are encoded by the same genomic region that controls the immune response, it is possible that the HLA specificity is a marker for an altered immune response in these patients. Another hypothesis suggests that HLA antigens may function as targets themselves, either for exogenous agents or for endogenous autoimmune reactions. It is interesting to reflect on the aforementioned report[31] that no Hawaiian residents of Japanese ancestry were found to have Behçet disease, despite the fact that they would presumably have the same genetic backgrounds as individuals in Japan, and therefore would theoretically also be at higher risk than other Hawaiians for development of this disease. The absence of disease suggests that in addition to a specific HLA-associated genetic predisposition, an exogenous stimulus is needed for development of the disease.

By polymerase chain reaction-restriction fragment link polymorphism (PCR-RFLP) genotyping, no significant difference was seen in any class II alleles between patients with Behçet disease and controls.[52] In an analysis of the tumor necrosis factor-ß (TNF-ß) gene, the frequency of the NcoI 5.5 kb homozygote was decreased in patients with the disease, however.[52]

Humoral Immunity

Initial concepts of immune alterations in patients with Behçet disease concerned immune complexes. Circulating immune complexes have been associated with uveitis[10] and found in ocular specimens.[14] The finding of circulating immune complexes in patients with Behçet disease supports such an association for its ocular complications.[45] An eye examined by Mullaney and Collum[58] was found to have deposition of IgA, IgG, and C3 in the walls of some episcleral and choroidal vessels, but not in the retina. Neutrophils have been found in the aqueous of patients and an increase in chemotactic activity has also been reported.[85] There is little other evidence to support a type III hypersensitivity reaction in the eye, however. Furthermore, Kasp and associates[39] have evaluated the question of immune complexes in the context of retinal vasculitis.[39] They have reported that patients with immune complexes have a better visual prognosis than individuals without circulating immune complexes. Kasp and associates have theorized that immune complexes may have a protective value, as opposed to a destructive role, because they help to eliminate potentially harmful initiators of the immune reaction.

Circulating antibodies found in patients with Behçet disease have been used in an attempt to define the disease itself. Klok and associates[43] used an indirect immunofluorescence assay with the external surface of the guinea pig lip as a substrate and sera from patients with different types of uveitis, and found that patients with Behçet disease had antibodies to this substrate more often than patients of the same ethnic origin with other forms of uveitis (70% versus 19%, p < 0.05). Of interest was the fact that they found no antibodies directed against the iris, the cornea, or the retina, but did find antibodies against the episclera. This finding was reminiscent of those reported by Mullaney and Collum.[58] Michaelson and associates,[50] using the same test, found that each of the eight American patients tested had antibodies that cross-reacted to guinea pig lip, but that only 10 of 16 Turkish patients with Behçet disease had such antibodies.

The existence of both IgM and IgG type antiendothelial cell antibodies in sera of patients with Behçet disease and active thrombophlebitis or retinal vasculitis has been shown.[4] Antiendothelial cell antibodies may also be detected in patients with various rheumatologic and vasculitic diseases such as systemic lupus erythematosus and rheumatoid arthritis; however, whether their presence reflects the cause or the result of the disease is unknown.

Cellular Immunity

More recent evaluations have suggested that various arms of the immune response are altered in Behçet disease. Of particular interest are alterations of T-lymphocyte circuitry. Sakane and associates[79] reported a defect in the T-lymphocyte-mediated suppressor system and alterations in the CD4-CD8 ratio of circulating cells of patients with Behçet disease, which can be explained by an increase in the CD8 fraction of T-lymphocytes.[42,89]

Other observations also support the concept of altered T-lymphocyte function. Ohno and associates[71] noted high amounts of interferon-gamma in the sera of patients with Behçet disease during their periods of disease quiescence. T-lymphocytes were found in the hypopyon,[62] and large numbers of cells were found infiltrating the mouth ulcers of this disorder.[77] In another study of the oral lesions in patients with Behçet disease, Fortune and associates[19] looked at the number of IgA-bound T-lymphocyte and the expression of gamma delta T-lymphocyte receptors. There was a very sharp upregulation of gamma-delta T-lymphocyte receptors in the CD8+ subset of cells. Also a significant increase of cytophilic IgA1 was found in T-lymphocytes.

Immunomodulation

Others have investigated the underlying mechanisms that lead to the state of immune activity. Delilbasi and associates[13] evaluated selenium levels, which can have an effect on the development and expression of humoral and cell-mediated responses. Mean selenium levels were significantly lower in patients with Behçet disease when compared to controls. This decrease in circulating selenium levels led the authors to suggest that selenium deficiency may lead to a defect in the humoral immune response, since their patients with Behçet disease also demonstrated a decrease in circulating IgM and IgG levels.

It has been suggested that infectious agents such as some strains of streptococci, viruses, chlamydia, or *Candida* species trigger the immune system and activate the disease.[29,54,60,84] Most of those studies are circumstantial, at best.

The pathergy phenomenon has been studied with respect to disease pathogenesis. Wechsler and associates[91] injected sterile water intradermally and used immunofluorescence techniques to demonstrate the deposition of complement and/or IgM. They found that 60% of patients with Behçet disease have positive staining, as opposed to 14% of controls. Gihar and associates[22] performed further tests evaluating skin hyperreactivity. They did not find a deposition of immunoglobulin, nor of complement, 4 hours after an injection of histamine or saline into the skin of patients with Behçet disease that they evaluated. Nevertheless, 10 of 11 patients tested had positive staining after 24 hours, but only two had evidence of vasculitis. They concluded that any cutaneous response, though nonspecific, may be a good way to evaluate for pathergy, but little or no evidence exists to support the notion that pathergy is immune-complex driven.

Recent work has centered around the presence of adhesion molecules in the eye of patients with Behçet disease. These molecules are expressed during an inflammatory event and may act as a "beacon" for inflammatory cells that invade the tissue. ICAM-1 was expressed in dramatic fashion in the retina of the one eye studied.*

DIFFERENTIAL DIAGNOSIS

In patients with incomplete forms of Behçet disease and mild or atypical presentations, it is important to consider other forms of uveitis in the differential diagnosis, since other diseases may have ocular findings similar to those in Behçet disease. The anterior uveitis related to HLA-B27 can be a severe, recurrent iridocyclitis with hypopyon. In contrast to Behçet disease, however, the uveitis is usually unilateral and the hypopyon may be less mobile, presumably because it is associated with increased fibrinous reaction. Sarcoidosis may have posterior pole lesions similar to those in Behçet disease, but sarcoidosis is generally indolent in contrast to the explosive nature of uveitis with Behçet disease. Furthermore, although vasculitis can occur with sarcoidosis, it is usually not occlusive in nature and often involves the veins in a segmentary manner. Behçet disease involves both arteries and veins (the latter being more intense) in a diffuse manner.[80] Retinal infiltrates seen in the retinitis of Behçet disease—in its most severe form—can be remarkably similar to a viral retinitis (such as the acute retinal necrosis syndrome), except they do not progress to coalescence.

LABORATORY INVESTIGATIONS

There are no laboratory findings specific for Behçet disease; therefore careful assessment of a patient's clinical findings and history are critical for diagnosis. There are some laboratory tests that are useful adjuncts in the evaluation of patients with Behçet disease, however.

Patients may have high erythrocyte sedimentation rates,

---

*Unpublished data.

high C-reactive protein levels, or increased numbers of peripheral leukocytes during the active stage of disease. Without such changes during episodes of acute inflammation, the diagnosis of Behçet disease should be questioned. The presence of autoantibodies or extremely high values of immunoglobulin are not compatible with a diagnosis of Behçet disease; instead they suggest collagen vascular diseases.

As discussed previously, HLA-B51 antigen is strongly associated with the disease. HLA typing may help to support a clinical diagnosis, although it alone is not diagnostic of Behçet disease.

The pathergy test can be useful in patient evaluations. In fact, a positive pathergy test is one of the diagnostic criteria suggested by the International Study Group for Behçet Disease, although the Behçet Disease Research Committee of Japan considers it only one of the tests that may be supportive of the diagnosis. The test is discussed in the Clinical Features section.

Imaging studies using computed tomographic scanning or magnetic resonance imaging are useful for identifying central nervous system lesions.

THERAPY

Behçet disease is characterized by abnormal functioning of leukocytes, particularly in the acute phase of the disease; there is an increase in the number of peripheral leukocytes, high chemotactic activity of peripheral leukocytes, and migration of cells to the eyes. Based on these findings, Matsumura and Mizushima[49] first used colchicine to inhibit such migration and found an associated decrease in the number of inflammatory attacks. Its use by most practitioners is intended to prevent recurrences of inflammation, not to treat the active lesions of inflammation. Hijikata and Masuda[30] found that patients treated with colchicine had better long-term visual prognoses than those receiving systemic corticosteroids.[30] The optimum dosage of colchicine is 0.5 to 1.0 mg/day. Colchicine therapy has been used as the treatment of choice by some investigators in Japan, but the efficacy of colchicine for treatment of Behçet disease seems to vary among races. A masked, randomized study in Turkey, in which patients received either colchicine or a placebo, demonstrated no differences between groups.[2]

Immunosuppressive Drug Therapy

Various immunosuppressive agents have been used. Among them, azathioprine, chlorambucil, and cyclophosphamide had favorable therapeutic effects. In a double-blind study from Turkey, azathioprine was not effective in restoring compromised vision, but was superior to the placebo in maintaining visual acuity in those with established disease or in retarding the emergence of new eye disease.[94] Azathioprine has been found effective in oral and genital ulcers and in arthritis.[94] Cyclophosphamide has been used widely in Japan with considerable efficacy in preventing ocular attacks and maintaining good visual acuity for long periods.[30]

Because of cyclophosphamide's profound effect on bone marrow, some investigators have suggested other agents of the same family. Godfrey and associates[24] reported the effectiveness of chlorambucil in the treatment of many noninfectious ocular disorders, including Behçet disease. The rationale behind its use was that it was slower acting than cyclophosphamide and could be administered more safely on an outpatient basis. The drug usually is reasonably well tolerated. Ultimately, its side effects, including bone marrow suppression, are the same as with cyclophosphamide. Pivetti-Pezzi and associates[76] reported that early intervention with chlorambucil produced a better outcome than corticosteroid therapy. A high-dose, short-term chlorambucil regimen for Behçet disease has also produced a favorable outcome.[88] In contrast, Tabbara[87] reported that the long-term results with chlorambucil were not particularly encouraging, with 75% of eyes having a visual acuity of 20/200 or less when this agent was used as the sole therapy. The fact that the agent is slow to act on the immune system would seem to be a disadvantage, since a rapid therapeutic response is usually desirable when treating patients with Behçet disease. Because of their cytotoxicity, these drugs may affect reproductive organs, resulting in azoospermia in males and amenorrhea in females.

Cyclosporine. The need to develop safer and more effective therapies for this condition is evident to all clinicians who treat the disease. Experimental autoimmune uveoretinitis (EAU) is an animal model of human intraocular inflammatory disease that has permitted an in-depth study of the mechanisms that may underlie many forms of endogenous uveitis[61] and that has shown the potential benefit of cyclosporine for control of severe intraocular inflammation. In the EAU model immune complexes do not appear to play an important role; a growing body of evidence suggests the same is true for Behçet disease. The model (which is induced by injecting uveitogenic antigen mixed with adjuvant at a site remote from the globe) has some features in common with the ocular manifestations of Behçet disease, although they may not share a common pathogenesis. An intense vitreous inflammation ensues with retinal and subretinal infiltrates as well as retinal hemorrhage. The fluorescein angiogram of subhuman primates with EAU demonstrates a profound retinal vasculitis.

The model demonstrates the important role of T-lymphocytes in disease pathogenesis, supporting a therapeutic role for cyclosporine, a medication with an effect on T-lymphocytes. Cyclosporine's effect appears to be on cells that have the binding molecule cyclophilin. The agent appears to prevent the activation of T-lymphocytes by interfering with early activation signals. The drug is not cytotoxic and therefore presumably cannot induce clonal deletion of autoaggressive cells. Because cyclosporine was efficient in preventing the expression of EAU,[67] it was used soon thereafter in the treatment of ocular diseases of noninfectious origin.[64,66]

In one early study, cyclosporine was used successfully in the treatment of 10 patients with the ocular manifestations of Behçet disease.[65] The explosive recurrent ocular attacks, which are characteristic of the disorder, were either abolished or were dramatically decreased in number. There was also amelioration of the other manifestations of the disease, such as mouth ulcers. It is also interesting to note that the level of circulating immune complexes did not dramatically change in these patients when cyclosporine was administered, despite improvement of clinical symptoms. Subsequent to these initial findings, several randomized studies were performed[48,73] in which cyclosporine was found more effective for prevention of ocular recurrences than colchicine or cyclophosphamide.

The initial starting dosage in most of the previously mentioned studies was 10 mg/kg/day. Because of the risk of inducing renal toxicity with this dosage, it has been recommended that the starting dose be reduced to 5 mg/kg/day.[6] At the lower dose of cyclosporine, few complications have been noted (aside from a decreased, but ever-present possibility of renal toxicity and hypertension); no increased numbers of opportunistic infections or tumors have been noted in these patients. Development of disease resembling neuro-Behçet disease has been noted in some Japanese patients taking cyclosporine long-term, but this occurrence has not been noted in the patients treated at the National Eye Institute.* In Israel cyclosporine was exceptionally efficient in treating the neurologic manifestations of the disease.†

Cyclosporine therapy is generally limited to bilateral sight-threatening cases of Behçet disease. Serum creatinine, and if possible creatinine clearance, must be followed closely. The goal of any therapy for this disease is to prevent the recurring explosive episodes of ocular inflammatory disease. Cyclosporine therapy is usually not well suited to patients with long-standing renal disease or uncontrolled hypertension because these disorders will limit the possibility of long-term treatment. Patients will need to be treated for a long period of time (years) since cyclosporine does not appear to induce immunologic tolerance, and a very slow taper of the medication must be initiated. A ''rebound'' phenomenon has been seen with cyclosporine therapy, as with corticosteroids, in which disease recurs as therapy is withdrawn.

Tacrolimus. Tacrolimus (FK506) is a newly developed immunosuppressive drug isolated from fermentation broth of *Streptomyces tsukubaensis*. Its immunologic activity is very similar to that of cyclosporine; it selectively suppresses CD4+ T-lymphocytes. A series of studies using tacrolimus for treatment of EAU in rats[40,41,55] and monkeys[21] demonstrated that tacrolimus (1) prevents the development of EAU

at doses 10 to 30 times lower than cyclosporine when it is given from the day of immunization with retinal uveitogenic antigen; (2) reduces the intensity of EAU when it is given only after the animals develop EAU, indicating a therapeutic effect of the drug; and (3) inhibits the induction of EAU in primates. Recently a multicenter clinical open-labelled trial of tacrolimus for refractory uveitis was performed by the Japanese FK506 Study Group on Refractory Uveitis.[56,57] Fifty-three patients with refractory uveitis, including 41 with Behçet disease, were treated with tacrolimus (0.05 to 0.2 mg/kg/day). These patients were previously treated with either systemic corticosteroid, colchicine, cyclophosphamide, or cyclosporine. The therapy was converted to tacrolimus because of therapeutic failures or adverse side effects with the previous medications. Tacrolimus was felt to have very favorable effects in 75% of the cases. The adverse effects of the drug observed in the study were renal impairment, neurologic symptoms, gastrointestinal symptoms, and hyperglycemia. It has been suggested that neurological side effects are related to increased permeability of the blood-brain barrier caused by tacrolimus, which then results in increased cerebrospinal fluid levels of drug.[32] The rate of these adverse effects was dependent on the dosage and blood trough level of the agent. According to the study, the optimum dosage of tacrolimus for uveitis is between 0.10 and 0.15 mg/kg/day. Much longer observation, as well as evaluation of tacrolimus by a masked randomized study, will be needed to confirm whether the drug is truly beneficial.

Corticosteroids

Corticosteroids can be used concurrently with other immunosuppressive drugs. The addition of corticosteroid to a therapeutic regimen for treatment of the ocular manifestations of Behçet disease is not well accepted in Japan. Nevertheless, this medication is used in the United States in combination with other modalities and is felt to have a positive effect on the course of disease by many investigators.

Both prednisone and cytotoxic agents, particularly cyclophosphamide, have been used in a pulse mode to treat Behçet disease. The concept behind this approach is to treat the patient with an exceedingly high dose of medication, followed by a relatively long therapy-free period (assuming that the aggressive therapy renders the disease quiescent until the next pulsing). More experience has been accrued with pulse corticosteroid therapy than with pulse cytotoxic therapy. Although therapeutic protocols may vary, the basic approach calls for a bolus of corticosteroid, frequently 1 g of prednisone given intravenously over a period of 1 hour and repeated 3 days in a row. Usually the pulses are repeated every month or as needed. This approach has been quite effective in rapidly reversing ocular inflammatory crises in some diseases, but has not been especially effective in treating the recurring episodes of Behçet disease at the Na-

---

*Unpublished data.

†David BenEzra, M.D., personal communication.

tional Eye Institute.* A more recent approach has been to use pulse cyclophosphamide, usually a dose of 750 mg/m^2 intravenously, followed by a repeat therapy about 1 month later. Although more beneficial than bolus corticosteroids,[28] this approach has not proved to be especially effective, with ocular attacks breaking through before the next therapeutic intervention.

Plasmapheresis

The concept that circulating molecules, such as antibodies or immune complexes, can produce disease helped to develop methods to remove these offending materials from the blood. Plasmapheresis is such a technique, in which the noncellular component of the blood is cleansed of some molecules. This approach to therapy has been used in certain systemic autoimmune conditions with variable results. The shifts of fluids and electrolytes that potentially occur in this procedure are associated with risks to the patient. Plasmapheresis is usually coupled with concomitant immunosuppressive therapy. Bonnet and associates[8] attempted plasma exchange therapy accompanied with acyclovir in seven Behçet disease patients, with discouraging results.

Management of Ocular Complications

An important aspect of therapy for patients with Behçet disease is treatment of its ophthalmic complications such as cystoid macular edema, glaucoma, neovascularization, vitreous hemorrhage, and cataract. Uveitic cystoid macular edema resolves following sub-Tenon injection of corticosteroids in approximately 50% of the cases.[96] Management of pseudophakic cystoid macular edema associated with Behçet disease, on the other hand, is more difficult. The presence of neovascular glaucoma is a most ominous sign, often leading to the loss of the eye. Aggressive evaluation of the retina for the presence of capillary dropout is important.

Patients with severe, recurrent disease of the retina risk developing large areas of capillary dropout with hypoperfusion and secondary neovascularizations of the optic disc, retina, or iris. Secondary neovascularization may also result from retinal vein occlusions. Intense antiinflammatory treatment may result in regression of neovascularization, via the possible mechanism of decreased angiogenic factors from the inflammatory cells or better retinal perfusion following the suppression of vasculitis.[3] Cases refractory to antiinflammatory treatment have been successfully treated with panretinal or sectorial retinal laser treatment.[26] Laser treatment in a uveitic eye may also precipitate or aggravate macular edema.[3] Concern has been expressed that laser photocoagulation will release antigens from the retina, thus permitting systemic sensitization. This concern may be justified since recurrences of disease temporally related to such

*Unpublished data.

therapy have been seen. Patients are therefore followed carefully for any signs of a recurrence of their disease and are treated vigorously if such signs are noted.

As with other forms of uveitis, preoperative control of inflammation in patients with Behçet disease is critical before cataract extraction. Topical, periocular, and oral corticosteroids are used for this purpose. Principles of cataract surgery for patients with uveitis, including the decision whether or not to implant an intraocular lens, have been reviewed elsewhere.[11] An in-depth evaluation of visual potential is particularly important in patients with Behçet disease, since they may have multiple reasons for their decrease in vision. Fluorescein angiography and an electroretinogram may be indicated, but it should be pointed out that the eyes with dense cataracts may have markedly abnormal electroretinograms despite potentially good central vision. The postoperative period is very critical. Patients with Behçet disease need to be followed closely for any signs of active inflammatory disease, because aggressively treating the activity can frequently end the episode at that point.

Although not commonly employed in clinical practice for Behçet disease, flash electroretinography and pattern visually evoked potentials have been suggested as ways to (1) monitor posterior segment changes, (2) indicate visual prognoses, and (3) establish the efficacy of therapy.[12,46]

Vitreous hemorrhage is a common complication of the severe retinal disease observed in patients with Behçet disease. Blood may clear with observation alone, but in some cases, repeated vitreous hemorrhages necessitate a vitrectomy. The patient should be prepared for surgery with antiinflammatory medications. Ideally, the patient's inflammatory disease should be in a quiescent state, as before cataract surgery. If bleeding has been a major problem, endolaser can be considered at the time of vitrectomy. Visual outcome following vitrectomy may be disappointing because of existing macular damage.[37]

Patients who have had multiple attacks of vasoocclusive retinitis develop remarkably thin areas in the retina. Retinal detachments are therefore common in the later stages of the disease. Phthisis bulbi with or without iris neovascularization usually follows retinal detachment. It is not yet known whether cryoablation or laser ablation of the retina enhances or decreases the chance that these patients will develop recurrent ocular inflammatory attacks.

REFERENCES

1. Adamantiadis B: Sur un cas d'iritis à hypopyon récidevante, *Ann Ocul* 168:271-274, 1931.
2. Aktulga E, Altac M, Muftuoglu A et al.: A double blind study of colchicine in Behçet disease, *Haematologica* 65:399-402, 1980.
3. Atmaca L: Experience with photocoagulation in Behçet disease, *Ophthalmic Surg* 21:571-576, 1990.
4. Aydintug AO, Tokgoz G, D'Cruz DP et al.: Antibodies to endothelial cells in patients with Behçet disease, *Clin Immunol Immunopathol* 67:157-162, 1993.

5. Behçet H: Uber die rezideivierende, aphthose, durch ein Virus verur-. sachte Geschwure am Mund, am Auge und an den Genitalen, *Dermatol Wochenschr* 46:414-419, 1937.
6. BenEzra D, Nussenblatt RB, Timonen P: *Optimal use of sandimmun in endogenous uveitis,* Berlin Heidelberg, 1988, Springer-Verlag.
7. Bentley CR, Stanford MR, Shilling JS et al.: Macular ischemia in posterior uveitis, *Eye* 7:411-414, 1993.
8. Bonnet M, Ouzan D, Trepo C: Plasma exchange and acyclovir in Behçet disease, *J Fr Ophtalmol* 9:15-22, 1986.
9. Brama I, Fainaru M: Inner ear involvement in Behçet disease, *Arch Otolaryngol* 106:215-217, 1980.
10. Char DH, Stein P, Masi R et al.: Immune complexes in uveitis, *Am J Ophthalmol* 87:678-681, 1979.
10a. Charteris DG, Barton K, McCartney ACE, Lightman SL: CD4+ lymphocyte involvement in ocular Behçet's disease, *Autoimmunity* 12:201-206, 1992.
11. Chung YM, Yeh TS: Intraocular lens implantation following extracapsular cataract extraction in uveitis, *Ophthalmic Surg* 21:272-276, 1990.
12. Cruz RD, Adachi-Usami E, Kakisu Y: Flash electroretinograms and pattern visually evoked cortical potentials in Behçet disease, *Jpn J Ophthalmol* 34:142-148, 1990.
13. Delilbasi E, Turan B, Yucel E et al.: Selenium and Behçet disease, *Biol Trace Elem Res* 28:21-25, 1991.
14. Dernouchamps JP, Vaerman JP, Michels J et al.: Immune complexes in the aqueous humor and serum, *Am J Ophthalmol* 84:24-31, 1977.
15. Dundar SV, Gencalp U, Simsek H: Familial cases of Behçet disease, *Br J Dermatol* 113:319-321, 1985.
16. El-Ramahi KM, Al-Kawi MZ: Papilledema in Behçet disease: value of MRI in diagnosis of dural sinus thrombosis, *J Neurol Neurosurg Psychiatry* 54:826-829, 1991.
17. Enoch BA, Castillo-Olivares JK, Khoo TCL et al.: Major vascular complications in Behçet syndrome, *J Postgrad Med* 44:453-459, 1968.
18. Ersoy F, Berkel A, Firat T et al.: HLA antigens associated with Behçet disease. In Dausset J, Svejgaard A, editors: *HLA and disease,* 100, Paris, 1976, PUB.
19. Fortune F, Walker J, Lehner T: The expression of gamma delta T cell receptor and the prevalence of primed, activated and IgA-bound T cells in Behçet syndrome, *Clin Exp Immunol* 82:326-332, 1990.
20. Fresco I, Yazici H, Bayramicli M et al.: Effect of surgical cleaning of skin on the pathergy phenomenon in Behçet syndrome, *Ann Rheum Dis* 52:619-620, 1993.
21. Fujino Y, Chan CC, de Smet MD et al.: FK506 treatment of experimental auroimmune uveoretinitis in primates, *Transplant Proc* 23:3335-3338, 1991.
22. Gihar A, Winterstein G, Turani H et al.: Skin hyperreactivity response (pathergy) in Behçet disease, *J Am Acad Dermatol* 21:547-552, 1989.
23. Godeau P, Torre D, Campanchi R et al.: HLA-B5 and Behçet disease. In Dausset J, Svejgaard A, editors: *HLA and disease,* 101, Paris, 1976.
24. Godfrey WA, Epstein WV, O'Connor GR et al.: The use of chlorambucil in intractable idiopathic uveitis, *Am J Ophthalmol* 78:415-428, 1974.
25. Graham EM, Stanford MR, Sanders MD et al.: A point prevalence study of 150 patients with idiopathic retinal vasculitis. I. Diagnostic value of ophthalmological features, *Br J Ophthalmol* 73:714-721, 1989.
26. Graham EM, Stanford MR, Shilling JS et al.: Neovascularisation associated with posterior uveitis, *Br J Ophthalmol* 71:826-833, 1987.
27. Hamuryudan V, Yurdakul S, Ozbakir F et al.: Monozygotic twins concordant for Behçet syndrome, *Arthritis Rheum* 34:1071-1072, 1991.
28. Hamza M, Meddeb S, Mili I et al.: Les bolus de cyclophosphamide et de methylprednisolone dans l'uveite de la maladie de Behçet: resultats preliminaires comportant l'utilisation de nouveaux criteres d'evalation, *Ann Med Interne (Paris)* 143:438-441, 1992.
29. Hayasaka S, Noda S, Setogawa T: Increased D-arabinitol/creatinine ratio in sera of patients with Behçet disease during an active phase, *Br J Ophthalmol* 77:39-40, 1993.
30. Hijikata K, Masuda K: Visual prognosis in Behçet disease: effects of cyclophosphamide and colchicine, *Jpn J Ophthalmol* 16:284-329, 1978.
31. Hirohata T, Kuratsume M, Nomura A: Prevalence of Behçet syndrome in Hawaii, *Hawaii Med J* 34:244-246, 1975.
32. Igarashi T, Ishigatsubo Y, Ohno S et al.: Central nervous system toxicity related to FK506 in patients with Behçet disease, *Ann Rheum Dis* 53:350-351, 1994.
33. Imai Y: Studies on prognosis and symptoms of Behçet disease in longterm observation, *Jpn J Clin Ophthalmol* 25:661-694, 1971.
34. Inaba G: Clinical features of neuro-Behçet syndrome. In Lehner T, Barnes CC, editors: *Recent advances in Behçet disease,* London, 1986, Royal Society of Medical Services.
35. Inaba G: Behçet disease. In McKendall RR, editor: *Handbook of clinical neurology,* vol 6, *Viral disease,* 593-610, Amsterdam, 1989, Elsevier.
36. International Study Group for Behçet Disease: Criteria for diagnosis of Behçet disease, *Lancet* 335:1078-1080, 1990.
37. James CR, Jacobs PM, Leaver PK et al.: Closed microsurgery for sequelae of neovascularisation from veno-occlusive retinopathies, *Eye* 1:106-114, 1987.
38. Kalbian VV, Challis MT: Behçet disease: report of twelve cases with three manifesting as papilledema, *Am J Med* 49:823-829, 1970.
39. Kasp E, Graham EM, Stanford MR et al.: Retinal autoimmunity and circulating immune complexes in ocular Behçet disease. In Lehner T, Barnes CG, editors: *Recent advances in Behçet disease,* 67-72, London, 1986, Royal Society of Medicine Services.
40. Kawashima H, Fujino Y, Mochizuki M: A new immunosuppressive agent, FK506, on experimental autoimmune uveitis in rats, *Invest Ophthalmol Vis Sci* 29:1265-1271, 1988.
41. Kawashima H, Mochizuki M: Effects of a new immunosuppressive agent, FK506, on the efferent limb of the immune responses, *Exp Eye Res* 51:565-572, 1990.
42. Kikkawa T, Shirotsuki H: Imbalance in T lymphocyte subsets in panuveitis type of Behçet disease, *J Eye* 1:1007-1010, 1984.
43. Klok AM, de Vries J, Rothova A et al.: Antibodies against ocular and oral antigens in Behçet disease associated with uveitis, *Curr Eye Res* 8:957-962, 1989.
44. Koc Y, Gullu I, Akpek G et al.: Vascular involvement in Behçet disease, *J Rheumatol* 19:402-410, 1992.
45. Levinsky RJ, Lehner T: Circulating soluble immune complexes in recurrent oral ulceration and Behçet syndrome, *Clin Exp Immunol* 32:193-198, 1978.
46. Martenet AC, Niemeyer G: Interet de l'electroretinographie dans les uveites, *Ophtalmologie* 4:69-72, 1990.
47. Masuda K, Inaba G, Mizushima H et al.: A nation-wide survey of Behçet disease in Japan, *Jpn J Ophthalmol* 19:276-285, 1975.
48. Masuda K, Nakajima A: A double masked study of ciclosporin treatment in Behçet disease. In Schindler R, editor: *Ciclosporin in autoimmune diseases,* 162-164, Berlin, 1985, Springer-Verlag.
49. Matsumura N, Mizushima Y: Leukocyte movement and colchicine treatment in Behçet disease, *Lancet* ii:813, 1975.
50. Michaelson JB, Chisari FV, Kansu T: Antibodies to oral mucosa in patients with ocular Behçet disease, *Ophthalmology* 92:1277-1281, 1985.
51. Mishima S, Masuda K, Izawa Y et al.: Behçet disease in Japan: ophthalmologic aspects, *Trans Am Ophthalmol Soc* 77:225-279, 1979.
52. Mizuki N, Ohno S, Tanaka H et al.: Association of HLA B-51 and lack of association of class II alleles with Behçet disease, *Tissue Antigens* 40:22-30, 1992.
53. Mizushima Y, Inaba G, Mimura Y et al.: *Guide for the diagnosis of Behçet disease,* Report of Behçet Disease Research Committee, 8-17, Japan, 1987, Ministry of Health and Welfare.
54. Mizushima Y, Matsuda T, Hoshi K et al.: Induction of Behçet disease symptoms after dental treatment and streptococcal antigen skin test, *J Rheumatol* 15:1029-1030, 1988.
55. Mochizuki M, Kawashima H: Effects of FK506, 15-deoxyspergulin, and cyclosporine on experimental autoimmune uveoretinitis in the rat, *Autoimmunity* 8:37-41, 1990.
56. Mochizuki M, Masuda K, Sakane T et al.: A multicenter trial of FK506 in refractory uveitis, including Behçet disease, *Transplant Proc* 23:3343-3346, 1991.
57. Mochizuki M, Masuda K, Sakane T et al.: A clinical trial of FK506 in refractory uveitis, *Am J Ophthalmol* 115:763-769, 1993.
58. Mullaney J, Collum LM: Ocular vasculitis in Behçet disease: a pathologic and immunohistochemical study, *Int Ophthalmol* 7:183-191, 1985.

59. Nakae K, Masaki F, Hashimoto T et al.: A nation-wide epidemiological survey on Behçet disease, report 2: association of HLA-B51 with clinic-epidemiological features, *Report of Behçet Disease Research Committee,* Japan, 1992, Ministry of Health and Welfare, pp. 70-82 .

60. Namba K, Ueno T, Okita M: Behçet disease and streptococcal infection, *Jpn J Ophthalmol* 30:385-401, 1986.

61. Nussenblatt RB: Experimental autoimmune uveitis: mechanisms of disease and clinical therapeutic indications (Proctor Lecture), *Invest Ophthalmol Vis Sci* 32:3131-3141, 1991.

62. Nussenblatt RB, Palestine AG: Behçet disease and other retinal vasculitis. In Nussenblatt RB, Palestine AG, editors: *Uveitis: fundamentals and clinical practice,* 212-247, Chicago, 1989, Mosby.

63. Reference deleted in proof.

64. Nussenblatt RB, Palestine AG, Chan CC: Cyclosporine therapy in the treatment of intra-ocular disease resistant to systemic corticosteroids or cytotoxic agents, *Am J Ophthalmol* 96:275-282, 1983.

65. Nussenblatt RB, Palestine AG, Chan CC et al.: Effectiveness of cyclosporine therapy for Behçet disease, *Arthritis Rheum* 28:671-679, 1985.

66. Nussenblatt RB, Palestine AG, Rook AH et al.: Cyclosporine therapy for intra-ocular inflammatory disease, *Lancet* ii:235-238, 1983.

67. Nussenblatt RB, Rodrigues MM, Wacker WB et al.: Cyclosporine A: inhibition of experimental autoimmune uveitis in Lewis rats, *J Clin Invest* 67:1228-1231, 1981.

68. O'Duffy JD: Vasculitis in Behçet disease, *Rheum Dis Clin North Am* 16:423-431, 1990.

69. O'Duffy, Taswell HF, Elveback LR: HL-A antigens in Behçet disease, *J Rheumatol* 3:1-3, 1976.

70. Ohno S, Char DH, Kimura SJ et al.: Studies on HLA antigens in American patients with Behçet disease, *Jpn J Ophthalmol* 22:58-61, 1978.

71. Ohno S, Kato F, Matsuda H et al.: Studies on spontaneous production of gamma-interferon in Behçet disease, *Ophthalmologica* 185:187-192, 1982.

72. Ohno S, Matsuda H: Studies of HLA antigens in Behçet disease in Japan. In Lehner T, Barnes CGT, editors: *Recent advances in Behçet disease,* 11-16, London, 1986, Royal Society of Medicine Services.

73. Ozyazgan Y, Yurdakul S, Yazici H et al.: Low dose cyclosporine A versus pulsed cyclophosphomide in Behçet syndrome: a single masked trial, *Br J Ophthalmol* 76:241-243, 1992.

74. Palimeris G, Papakonstantinoy P, Mantas M: The Adamantiades-Behçet syndrome in Greece. In Saari KM, editor: *Uveitis update,* 321, Amsterdam, 1984, Excerpta Medica.

75. Pamir MN, Kansu T, Erbengi A et al.: Papilledema in Behçet syndrome, *Arch Neurol* 38:643-645, 1981.

76. Pivetti-Pezzi P, Gasparri V, De Liso P et al.: Prognosis in Behçet disease, *Ann Ophthalmol* 17:20-25, 1985.

77. Poulter LW, Lehner T, Duke O: Immunohistological investigation of recurrent oral ulcers and Behçet disease. In Lehner T, Barnes CG, editors: *Recent advances in Behçet disease,* London, 1986, Royal Society of Medicine Services.

78. Raz I, Okon E, Chajek-Shaul T: Pulmonary manifestations in Behçet syndrome, *Chest* 95:585-589, 1989.

79. Sakane T, Kotani H, Takada S et al.: Functional aberration of T cell subsets in patients with Behçet disease, *Arthritis Rheum* 25:1343-1351, 1982.

80. Sanders MD: Duke Elder lecture: retinal arteritis, retinal vasculitis and autoimmune retinal vasculitis, *Eye* 1:441-465, 1987.

81. Shigeta T: Recurrent iritis with hypopyon and its pathologic findings, *Acta Soc Ophthalmol Jpn* 28:516-521, 1924.

82. Shimada K, Yaoita H, Shikano S: Chemotactic activity in the aqueous humor in patients with Behçet disease, *Jpn J Ophthalmol* 16:84-92, 1972.

83. Shimizu T: Behçet disease, *Jpn J Ophthalmol* 18:291-294, 1974.

84. Shimizu T, Ehrlich GE, Inaba G et al.: Behçet disease (Behçet syndrome), *Semin Arthritis Rheum* 8:223-260, 1979.

85. Sobel JD, Haim S, Obedeanu N et al.: Polymorphonuclear leucocyte function in Behçet disease, *J Clin Pathol* 30:250-253, 1977.

86. Stewart B: Genetic analysis of families of patients with Behçet syndrome: data incompatible with autosomal recessive inheritance, *Ann Rheum Dis* 45:265-268, 1986.

87. Tabbara KF: Chlorambucil in Behçet disease: a reappraisal, *Ophthalmology* 90:906-908, 1983.

88. Tessler HH, Jennings T: High-dose short-term chlorambucil for intractable sympathetic ophthalmia and Behçet disease, *Br J Ophthalmol* 74:353-357, 1990.

89. Valesini G, Pivetti-Pezzi P, Manstrandrea F et al.: Evaluation of T cell subsets in Behçet syndrome using anti-T cell monoclonal antibodies, *Clin Exp Immunol* 60:55-60, 1985.

90. Villanueva JL, Gonzalez-Dominguez J, Gonzale-Fernandez R and associates: HLA antigen familial study in complete Behçet syndrome affecting three sisters, *Ann Rheum Dis* 52:155-157, 1993.

91. Wechsler J, Wechsler B, Herreman G et al.: *An immunofluorescent study of intradermal distilled water injection by studying 48 patients—value for diagnosis.* Presented at the International Academy of Pathology, Paris, 1980.

92. Winter FC, Yukins RE: The ocular pathology of Behçet disease, *Am J Ophthalmol* 62:257-262, 1966.

93. Yazici H: Behçet syndrome. In Klippel JH, Dieppe PA, editors: *Rheumatology,* 6.20.1-6.20.6, London, 1994, Mosby.

94. Yazici H, Pazarli H, Barnes CG et al.: A controlled trial of azothioprine in Behçet syndrome, *New Eng J Med* 322:281-285, 1990.

95. Yazici H, Tuzun Y, Pazarli H et al.: Influence of age of onset and patient's sex on the prevalence and severity of Behçet syndrome, *Ann Rheum Dis* 43:783-789, 1984.

96. Yoshikawa K, Ichiishi A, Kotake S et al.: Posterior sub-Tenon's space injections of repository corticosteroids in uveitis patients with cystoid macular edema, *Nippon Ganka Gakkai Zasshi* 97:1070-1074, 1993.

97. Yurdakul S, Gunaydin I, Tuzun Y et al.: The prevalence of Behçet syndrome in a rural area in Northern Turkey, *J Rheumatol* 15:820-822, 1988.

55 Intermediate Uveitis

JANET L. DAVIS, ETIENNE BLOCH-MICHEL

Intermediate uveitis is one of four major categories of uveitis in the classification scheme proposed by the International Uveitis Study Group.[15] This classification scheme subdivides intraocular inflammatory disease into anterior, intermediate, posterior, and panuveitis, based on the principal anatomic site of inflammation. Intentionally imprecise, *intermediate uveitis* encompasses a large number of former terms such as hyalitis, posterior cyclitis, basal retinouveitis, senile vitritis, and pars planitis. It refers to inflammation in the region of the posterior ciliary body, anterior retina and choroid, and vitreous. It is unknown how many separate disease entities are included in the category of intermediate uveitis. The distinctive triad of vitritis, peripheral retinal vasculitis, and pars plana exudation (commonly known as pars planitis) may be a specific subtype of intermediate uveitis or may simply be a more intense manifestation of nonspecific inflammation in those regions of the eye. Most authors of clinical and pathologic descriptions cited in this chapter refer to *pars planitis* or other historic terms because *intermediate uveitis* has only recently come into use. Intermediate uveitis is the preferred term for disorders characterized predominantly by vitreous humor inflammation accompanied by minimal or no anterior or chorioretinal inflammatory signs. This preference holds true regardless of whether the inflammatory disorders are idiopathic or associated with systemic disease (such as sarcoidosis and multiple sclerosis).*

HISTORICAL BACKGROUND

Detailed knowledge of intermediate uveitis was not possible until the binocular indirect ophthalmoscope revealed the distinctive inflammatory signs in the region of the ora serrata.[120] *Peripheral uveitis* was the first name applied,[22,120] but it was later criticized because uveal tissue does not have a "periphery" that corresponds to the pars plana.[11] *Posterior cyclitis* or *chronic cyclitis*[67,132] were other early names. *Pars planitis* was introduced by Welch[146] in 1960. This term was adopted both by other authors[27,38,87] and by practicing ophthalmologists—despite objections that the term was grammatically incorrect and inaccurate (as the pars plana was not uniformly involved).[11] Other authors have used *vitritis*[19] or *hyalitis*[51] to refer to what is probably the same disease.

Bec and associates[11] attempted to formalize the nomenclature by dividing the periphery into three anatomic zones. Only those inflammations centered over the region of the vitreous base were called "l'uvéo-rétinite basale" (basal uveoretinitis); other peripheral inflammations were classified as either anterior or posterior uveitis (depending on their relation to the vitreous base). The idea is similar to the recommendations of the International Uveitis Study Group,[15] but it is uncertain whether a disease exists that is confined entirely to this narrow region. A general term such as intermediate uveitis appears to be all that is warranted by current knowledge.

---

*Use of the terms *intermediate uveitis* and *pars planitis* remains confusing. There is general agreement among uveitis specialists that all cases formerly designated pars planitis can be classified as intermediate uveitis, as defined by the International Uveitis Study Group in their classification scheme. That designation does not imply a single disease entity or known cause. There is less agreement whether patients with a specific group of signs, including vitreous inflammatory reaction, peripheral retinal vasculitis, inferior vitreous inflammatory condensates ("snowballs"), and pars plana exudations ("snowbanks"), have a distinctive and specific subtype of intermediate uveitis called *pars planitis, pars planitis syndrome,* or *intermediate uveitis, pars planitis subtype.* The International Uveitis Study Group has recommended the term *intermediate uveitis* be used for all forms of intermediate uveitis, and the term *pars planitis* be dropped altogether. Nevertheless, some investigators prefer to retain a subgroup designation for such patients to facilitate research and teaching, and because of its possible implications for therapy and prognosis. The terms *pars planitis* (or its variants) and *intermediate uveitis* are not interchangeable, however. In cases in which intermediate uveitis is associated with a systemic disease, such as sarcoidosis, it is inappropriate to refer to findings as *pars planitis syndrome,* which (if it is used at all) should be reserved for idiopathic disease.

Pars planitis has persisted as the most recognized and accepted of the various terms, particularly in the American literature, despite its unproven implication concerning the principal site of inflammation.[11] The term's popularity may pertain to its descriptive power.[146] Inflammatory exudates over the inferior pars plana region, associated with retinal periphlebitis and cystoid macular edema, form one of the classic images of ophthalmology. At present the term designates a subgroup of intermediate uveitis with definite peripheral inflammatory exudation. This subgroup may or may not turn out to be a distinct entity.

EPIDEMIOLOGY

A 2-year survey to determine the incidence of uveitis was conducted from 1982 to 1984 among 16 ophthalmologists in Savoy, France. There were 215 cases of uveitis, of which 19 were intermediate uveitis, in the population of 323,675 during those 2 years. The prevalence of intermediate uveitis was estimated to be 5.9 per 100,000 population or roughly 1 in 15,000. A total of 127 new cases of uveitis were diagnosed; 9 were intermediate uveitis. The annual incidence of new cases of intermediate uveitis was therefore only 1.4 per 100,000, with a confidence interval of 0.64 to 2.64.[139] There are no comparative figures in other population groups; however, the yearly incidence of all types of uveitis in Savoy is in close agreement with that reported in other epidemiologic studies, suggesting that the incidence of intermediate uveitis should be similar in other regions.

Most tabulations of the frequency of intermediate uveitis are expressed relative to the total number of uveitis patients seen in a particular practice (or group of practices), rather than in relation to the general population. Older studies use terminology such as chronic cyclitis or peripheral uveitis and may therefore not be strictly comparable to newer ones. Nevertheless, the frequency of intermediate uveitis is similar among different uveitis clinics. In the United States an early survey recorded 250 of 3085 uveitis patients (8%) as having chronic cyclitis.[132] A later series from the same western region noted that 92 of 600 patients had intermediate uveitis (15.4%).[63] In France Martenet[88] had 75 chronic cyclitis cases among 615 total uveitis cases (12%) from 1968 to 1972; from 1986 to 1987 there were 89 intermediate uveitis cases out of 492 cases (18%).[89] The proportion of intermediate uveitis cases may have increased with time because of referral or diagnostic trends. When only more recent studies are compared, the prevalence of intermediate uveitis appears remarkably constant among different countries. In Korea 107 of 683 uveitis patients (15.7%) were diagnosed as having intermediate uveitis from 1978 to 1987.[28] Weiner and BenEzra[145] reported a 15.3% prevalence in Israel (61 of 400 uveitis clinic patients). Table 55-1 summarizes the percentages of intermediate uveitis cases reported in various surveys.

Most of the larger published series report an average patient age of 23 to 28 years.[27,64,133] It is not always made clear

whether these figures refer to the age of onset (or diagnosis) or simply to the prevalent age of the patients in the series. A review of the reported age distribution reveals that the majority of patients are less than 40 years of age.* The recent broadening of the definition of intermediate uveitis to include cases without characteristic pars plana exudation may increase the proportion of older people with this diagnosis and raise the average age.[89] Senile vitritis, as described by Gass,[54] would currently be classified as an intermediate uveitis.

Despite the perception that intermediate uveitis is primarily a young person's disease, its prevalence in pediatric uveitis surveys is similar to that recorded among all age groups. Thus in the Korean study cited previously, 14.8% of 81 uveitis patients under the age of 20 had intermediate uveitis compared to 15.7% of all uveitis patients.[28] Bloch-Michel and associates[13,98] reported 28% prevalence among adult uveitis patients and 15% among children up to 16 years of age. Table 55-2 summarizes the cases of intermediate uveitis reported in pediatric series. Intermediate uveitis is an important, but not major, cause of childhood uveitis.

Most studies report a slight male preponderance. The average calculated from several different European and American studies is 54% male and 46% female.† Chung's Korean study[28] is atypical in reporting 83% male intermediate uveitis patients compared to 66% males in the general uveitis clinic population.

Several families have been described in which multiple members are affected with pars planitis.‡ No definite inheritance pattern exists; identical twins, siblings, and a parent and child of both sexes have been affected. Simultaneous onset in two siblings of different ages suggests that an environmental factor may play a role.[29]

Typing for DR locus histocompatibility leukocyte antigens in two separate families revealed all four affected members to be HLA-DR2 positive.[42,147] There were no shared A and B locus antigens between these four cases and the other cases in which HLA typing has been reported.[8,29,40]

Two studies of HLA antigens in intermediate uveitis patients show conflicting results. In one study 52 consecutive patients with intermediate uveitis underwent HLA typing by standard microcytotoxicity assay; increases in A31, B5, B17, C7, B22, and DR1 were found but were not considered statistically significant.[7] In another study 43 Caucasians with intermediate uveitis of the pars planitis subtype were typed in another laboratory.[31] HLA-DR2 and DQ1 were felt to be significantly increased in patients with intermediate uveitis, but the increase was modest, as the two antigens were present in only about 50% of patients. Other investiga-

*References 4, 11, 27, 79, 84, 88, 123, 133, 146.
†References 7, 10, 11, 22, 27, 55, 84, 120, 123, 133.
‡References 8, 29, 40, 42, 56, 67, 79, 147, 150.

TABLE 55-1 INTERMEDIATE UVEITIS AS A PERCENTAGE OF UVEITIS CASES

Study	Country	Intermediate Uveitis Cases (%)	Total Uveitis Cases
Smith 1973[132]	United States	250 (8%)	3085
Martenet 1968-1972[88]	France	75 (12%)	615
Bec 1977[11]	France	19 (12.8%)	149
Abrahams 1986[3]	China	16 (22%)	72
Martenet 1986-1987[89]	France	89 (18%)	492
Chung 1978-1987[28]	Korea	107 (15.7%)	683
Henderly 1987[63]	United States	92 (15.4%)	600
Weiner 1991[145]	Israel	61 (15.3%)	400

TABLE 55-2 INTERMEDIATE UVEITIS AS A PERCENTAGE OF UVEITIS CASES IN CHILDREN

Study	Age	Intermediate Uveitis Cases (%)	Total Pediatric Uveitis Cases
Hogan 1965[67]	Up to 21 years	16% (estimate)	243
Witmer 1966[150]	Not stated	32 (38%)	84
Niessen 1981[98]	Up to 16 years	15 (14.4%)	104
Chung 1989[28]	Up to 20 years	12 (14.7%)	81
Althaus 1992[4]	Up to 14 years	25%	258

tors have confirmed a statistically significant increase in HLA-DR2 among patients with pars planitis compared to race-matched controls.[86] HLA-DR2 was present in 27 of 40 patients (67.5%); HLA-B8 and B51 were also increased. If there are HLA associations with intermediate uveitis, it is possible that they are present only for certain subtypes; resolution of this issue will require further study.

CLINICAL FEATURES

Most patients with symptomatic intermediate uveitis complain of blurred vision. Another typical symptom is floaters, although they are less commonly reported.[28] The onset is typically insidious and only vague responses can be made to questions regarding the duration of symptoms.[11,13,89] The exception is the occasional patient who seems to present at the time of posterior vitreous humor detachment and, occasionally, the onset is marked by typical anterior segment inflammatory signs of pain, redness, and sensitivity to light.[130] Children may be more prone to develop anterior segment inflammation including posterior synechiae,[22,146] band keratopathy,[22,55,133] and a peculiar, linear, white deposit along the inferior corneal endothelium.[78,136] Despite these inflammatory signs, the amount of anterior segment inflammatory cell is usually minimal after onset, particularly in adults.[11,67,146]

Vitreous humor inflammation is the most consistent sign of intermediate uveitis. The vitreous humor cellular reaction has the appearance of "dust" at the slit lamp biomicroscope.[67] Retraction of the vitreous architecture with strand-

ing and other alterations (such as posterior vitreous humor detachment) are commonly noted.[11,65] Vitreous humor bands were noted in 3 of 28 eyes in one series and may extend to the optic disc.[11] Examination of the posterior vitreous humor is necessary to evaluate fully the degree of vitritis, as it is usually more prominent posteriorly.[89] Characteristic mobile, round, white, focal vitreous humor opacities, dubbed "oeufs de formi" (ants' eggs) in French,[87] can be seen in the peripheral vitreous humor in approximately one third of patients.[11,67] Brockhurst[22] interpreted these focal opacities as the equivalent of the pars plana exudate in the vitreous cavity, although this interpretation has been proved incorrect histologically, as they are clusters of cells rather than collections of protein.[59] In English the colloquial name for the opacities is nevertheless "snowballs" by analogy to the pars plana "snowbank."

Presence of the characteristic peripheral retina and pars plana exudate facilitates diagnosis (Fig. 55-1). In children exuberant exudates, which extend onto the back of the crystalline lens, can be easily seen by looking into the pupil as the patient looks down through an indirect ophthalmoscope without a hand lens.[105] Scleral depression aids detection of the pars plana exudate. Estimates of the number of eyes with peripheral exudation ranges from 100%[11] to about 50%, depending in part on the definition of a "case."[67,123] A series of patients with intermediate uveitis defined according to current terminology has not appeared and might show a lower rate, as older patients may not form exudates.[27]

Bec[11] described the pars plana exudate as a white, well-

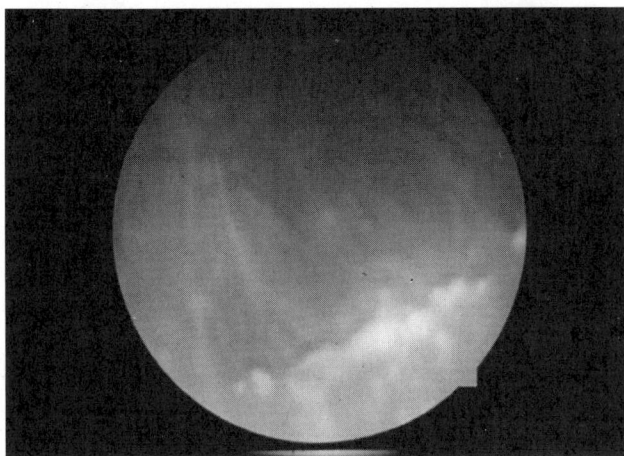

Fig. 55-1. Peripheral exudates in intermediate uveitis. The inflammatory deposits are preretinal, peripheral, typically inferior, and sometimes abundant, as shown here. This appearance is characteristic of active inflammatory exudation as opposed to the linear, smooth appearance of collagenous ''snowbanks.'' From the Laboratory of Immunology, National Eye Institute, National Institutes of Health. (Figure also in color insert.)

The significance of the pars plana exudate is unclear. Henderly and associates[64] compared eyes with exudates to fellow eyes without exudates in 61 patients with intermediate uveitis. There was no statistical difference in the severity of the vitritis, the visual acuity, or the degree of vascular leakage in eyes with or without exudates, but there was a clinical impression (as has been asserted by others) that eyes with exudates were more severely involved.[131] Okinami and associates[111] reported in 1991 that 17 of 17 eyes with small snowbanks demonstrated visual acuity greater than or equal to 20/25, compared to only 7 of 11 eyes with large snowbanks.

Cuffing of retinal vessels with inflammatory cells is a common feature, and there is occasionally obliterative vasculitis.[13] These changes are most common in the terminal branches of retinal veins adjacent to the peripheral exudate[22] but may extend posteriorly.[13] Arterioles are rarely involved.[22] Clinically detectable vascular involvement occurs in 10% to 32% of eyes.[11,114,123] Veins were abnormally dilated or tortuous in 30 of 34 eyes,[114] and dilated venules were noted in early series of ''chronic cyclitis.''[67] Examination with red-free filters[114] or fluorescein angiography[5,114,119,123] may show more extensive vascular anomalies.

Cases may be unilateral, bilateral, or asymmetric. Of Schepens' early cases,[120] 70% were bilateral at presentation, but 25% of these cases had only minimal involvement of the second eye. Other estimates of bilaterality range from about 70%[139] to about 90% in both adults[22,133] and children.[67] The experience of Chung[28] is atypical in that intermediate uveitis was unilateral in 101 of 107 cases (94.4%). Despite the contention of Hogan[67] that unilateral cases remain unilateral, subsequent involvement of fellow eyes may occur in about 10% of patients.[64,133]

delimited, condensation in the vitreous, located at the ora serrata with extension onto pars plana or onto the peripheral retina. It usually involves the inferior peripheral retina, but it may also be superior or divided into multiple foci. Fingerlike extensions into vitreous humor may occur. Thin vitreous humor condensations, oriented circumferentially and overlying the peripheral retina, are sometimes seen instead of the thick, yellow-white exudates. Chronicity seems to produce gliosis and collagen deposition similar to that seen in preretinal membranes.[59,77]

TABLE 55-3 AVERAGE DURATION OF INTERMEDIATE UVEITIS AMONG PATIENTS ATTENDING THE CENTRE HOSPITALIER DE BICÉTRE, PARIS, COMPARED TO PATIENTS WITH OTHER TYPES OF UVEITIS

Type of Uveitis	Number of Patients	Average Follow-up in Years	Number Resolved (%)
Anterior uveitis			
1972-1979	18	8	11 (61%)
1981-1987	20	4.8	6 (30%)
Intermediate uveitis			
1972-1979	**21**	**8**	**9 (42.8%)**
1981-1987	**20**	**3**	**0 (0%)**
Posterior uveitis			
1972-1979	21	9	19 (76%)
1981-1987	20	4.3	15 (75%)
Panuveitis			
1972-1979	16	7.8	7 (43.7%)
1981-1987	18	5	3 (16.6%)

Course of Disease

Most series describe a chronic course that may have periodic exacerbations and remissions.[67] Smith[132] found that 16 of 173 eyes (10%) improved over time, 98 of 173 eyes (59%) had a prolonged (but relatively stable) course without exacerbations, and 51 of 173 eyes (31%) had one or more periods of exacerbation. Exacerbations were more common in patients with severe disease.[132] As a result, the number of patients with severe disease changed little with length of follow-up.[132] Durations of active disease up to 15 to 20 years are not uncommon.[84,132] Compared to other types of uveitis, the duration of intermediate uveitis is among the longest (Table 55-3).

Brockhurst[22] noted a benign course in 28% of his series; some patients cleared the peripheral exudates within a few months, but 48% had a chronic, smoldering course and were considered at risk for secondary complications.[22] Only 6 patients, all 15 years of age or younger, were felt to have a malignant course with the formation of massive peripheral exudates.[22] In another series a grading scheme based on the degree of inflammation categorized 33 of 173 eyes (19%) as mild inflammation, 73 of 173 (42%) as moderate inflammation, and 67 of 173 (39%) as severe inflammation.[132]

PATHOLOGY

Pathologic studies have been hampered by the advanced stages of disease in most specimens. Nevertheless, some useful observations have been made. Both chronic low-grade inflammation in the ciliary body and perivascular infiltration of retinal vessels were reported in an eye enucleated for retinal detachment 10 years after onset of intermediate uveitis.[79] The posterior choroid contained only mild diffuse lymphocytic infiltration. An eye enucleated for glaucoma showed a few chronic inflammatory foci in the ciliary body and lymphocytic infiltration of retinal veins with arteriolar sparing.[77] A thick connective tissue mass with nonfenestrated blood vessels was present; on the vitreous humor side, the mass contained probable fibrous astrocytes. No significant choroidal inflammation was noted.

Green and associates[59] described seven eyes from six patients; five eyes were enucleated for uveitic complications, and two were obtained at autopsy from a patient with disease for 4 years and 20/60 visual acuity. The autopsy eyes showed minimal uveal inflammation and inflammatory cells in the walls of retinal vessels and the vitreous cavity. Fibrous organization at the vitreous base and retinal inflammation, including phlebitis, periphlebitis, and edema of the optic nerve and macula, were the main features noted in the enucleated eyes.

Three years after the onset of uveitis, inflammatory cell infiltration of the ciliary body was also noted in an eye enucleated for rubeosis and vitreous hemorrhage.[147] Contrary to the prior reports of minimal uveal inflammation, Wetzig and associates[147] noted mild-to-moderate lymphocytic infiltration in the pars plana and a scattered lymphocytic infiltrate in the peripheral choroid. Focal lymphocytic infiltration of the peripheral choroid was also noted in an evisceration specimen from an eye with traction retinal detachment.[154] Perivascular lymphocytic infiltration in the detached retina was noted. Furthermore, venules with isolated enlarged endothelial cells were found in the pars plana region. This specialized modification, known as a high endothelial venule, is thought to play a role in lymphocyte trafficking. It was therefore hypothesized that the pars plana venules might be active in recruitment of cells into the pars plana inflammatory reaction.

The characteristic yellow-white pars plana exudate has been identified as organized collagen, fibroblasts, fibrous astrocytes, nonpigmented ciliary epithelium, with scattered plasma cells, macrophages, and lymphocytes.[154] Immunohistochemical staining has further identified Type IV collagen and laminin as the major glycoproteins in the exudate.[147] These glycoproteins are products of glial cells, not fibroblasts. Additionally, in one case the pars plana exudate was shown to stain heavily for glial fibrillary acid protein and for Müller cells, suggesting that the glial cells of the retina are major contributors to its formation.[147]

There is no general agreement as to the meaning of these observations. Retinal perivasculitis is a prominent finding in all eyes. The degree of uveal inflammation is more variable and has been absent in some cases. An inflammatory reaction primarily centered in the peripheral retinal and pars plana blood vessels is one possible explanation. Recruitment of inflammatory cells into the vitreous cavity and a reactive gliosis by the peripheral retina would explain most of the other pathologic features. In cases in which reactive gliosis does not develop, the characteristic pars plana exudate would be absent.

COMPLICATIONS

Cataract formation is common among patients with intermediate uveitis, but it is unclear whether cataract is the result of treatment with corticosteroids or of the inflammation itself. Estimates of the percentage of eyes affected with cataract range from 13% to 61% of eyes[11,67,85,133] and from 15% to 54% of patients.[22,79,85,120] One series recorded cataracts in 11 of 60 pediatric patients (18%).[54] Most cataracts are posterior subcapsular[55,67,120,133] or posterior cortical.[22,120,133] In Smith's series[133] of complications of chronic cyclitis, only half of the cataracts became visually significant. Cataracts were twice as common in the group with severe inflammation.[133] In a small group of eight patients with intermediate uveitis undergoing cataract surgery, the cataracts were posterior subcapsular with additional nuclear sclerosis, which may have made them more visually significant.[93]

Glaucoma

Increased intraocular pressure occurs in patients with intermediate uveitis, but its frequency is low. Brockhurst[22] noted open-angle glaucoma in 8 of 100, angle-closure glaucoma in 2 of 100, and "secondary" glaucoma in 6 of 100 patients. Smith[57,133] found glaucoma in 15 of 182 eyes; in 11 of these eyes the increased pressure was felt to be due to corticosteroid use.

Macular Edema

Macular and optic disc edema occur in all but about 12% of eyes with intermediate uveitis.[146] The edema appears to be caused by small vessel leakage similar to the large vessel leakage noted angiographically.[53] Although blood vessel leakage is most likely secondary to the inflammatory process, a predilection for leakage where vitreous humor attachments are strongest has been noted.[124]

Macular changes increase with severity and duration of disease.[133] The prevalence of macular edema in various studies is high. An update of Hogan's original series[79] recorded 62 of 136 patients to have macular edema when first examined. Of the 62 cases, 26 were of the cystoid type; all of these patients had had active disease for several years.[79] Other series have recorded ophthalmoscopically visible macular edema or degenerative changes secondary to edema in about 20% to 50% of eyes.[11,22,85,114,133] Optic disc edema is recorded less often and is less likely to be visually significant.[11,67,79] When fluorescein angiography is performed, more eyes are found to have posterior edema.[114,119]

Neovascularization and Vitreous Hemorrhage

Clinically important neovascularization of the posterior segment probably occurs in no more than about 5% to 15% of patients with intermediate uveitis.[32,85] A few small series have been published. Felder and Brockhurst[47] described 15 patients with pars planitis; 11 with neovascularization of the peripheral exudate, 3 with neovascularization of the optic disc, and 1 with neovascularization of the retina elsewhere. This distribution is assumed to be typical of the sites usually affected.

In a series limited to neovascularization of the optic disc, 1 eye each in 9 of 163 patients with pars planitis was affected (5.5%).[72] Each case was associated with an exacerbation. Two patients also had neovascularization of the iris and two had peripheral retinal neovascularization.[72] Capillary nonperfusion nasal to the optic disc was noted in one case. It was the opinion of the authors that more nonperfusion would have been detected had peripheral angiograms routinely been obtained. Slezak[128] also ascribed neovascularization to ischemia of the peripheral retina, and Schepens[120] felt that the end result of the vascular inflammation was vascular obliteration. A report of four cases of neovascularization of the optic disc without evidence of retinal ischemia suggests that neovascularization may also arise from angiogenic stimuli liberated by the inflammatory process itself.[126] The good response to antiinflammatory treatment alone[72] would also seem to suggest the importance of inflammatory stimuli to neovascularization.

A single case of peripapillary choroidal neovasculariza-

tion has been described in intermediate uveitis.[6] Chronic optic disc edema was proposed as a mechanism by which a break in the Bruch membrane and subsequent neovascularization could occur.[6]

Vitreous hemorrhage probably occurs in less than 5% of cases; it was noted in 6 of 182 eyes in the series of Smith[133] (3.3%) and in 3 of 100 in the series of Brockhurst[22] (3%). Hemorrhage is strongly associated with neovascularization. About two thirds of patients with neovascularization in two small series had vitreous hemorrhage at some point.[47,72] Martenet[89] also attributed some vitreous hemorrhages to traction by the pars plana membranes on normal retinal vessels.

Retinal Detachment

Referral patterns and interpretation of the peripheral retinal findings vary among different authors, leading to wildly different estimates of the frequency of retinal detachment as a complication. In the original descriptions of Schepens,[120] subclinical detachments were found in 34 of 47 cases (72%), although retinal breaks were found in only about half the cases. Schepens[120] was so enthused by this discovery he hypothesized that the majority of aphakic detachments probably were caused by old uveitis. Other early series with high estimates of the frequency of retinal detachment may have been influenced by the retinal surgical orientation of the authors. For example, Brockhurst[21] reported 13 retinal detachments in 31 patients with "benign" pars planitis (of which 4 were not treated), 21 detachments in 49 patients with mild uveitis (of which 9 spontaneously reattached), and 9 retinal detachments in 15 patients with severe neovascular exudation. Other series have been more moderate in their estimates of the rate of detachment, which is ordinarily cited in the range of 5% to 17% of patients.[10,11,85,114,133]

Peripheral exudates in intermediate uveitis may induce retinal elevation without retinal breaks or rhegmatogenous retinal detachment. Subretinal exudation may occur on an ischemic or inflammatory basis and is not accompanied by choroidal leaks, swelling, or detachment, as is usual for inflammatory exudative detachments.[22] In two series retinoschisis was described in less than 5% of patients.[20,133] Retinal folds and distortion of retinal vessels caused by vitreous humor traction bands have also been described.[133] If retinal breaks are not seen, caution should be used in interpreting peripheral retinal elevations as rhegmatogenous detachments in need of surgical repair.

In addition to severity of inflammation,[21] risk factors for rhegmatogenous retinal detachment may include performance of cryotherapy at the time of pars plana vitrectomy,[151] neovascularization of the peripheral exudate,[72] and cryotherapy or vitrectomy alone.[10]

Other Retinochoroid Changes

Peripheral retinal degeneration can result from the inflammation of intermediate uveitis. Pigmentary changes have ordinarily been confined to the areas of peripheral exudation. Schepens[120] ascribed the peripheral chorioretinal atrophy to resolution of the exudate with irregularity of pigmentation and pigmentary hyperplasia.[120] Bec[11] described chorioretinal scarring as being "hidden" under the exudate in 21 of 28 eyes. In 1 series of 51 patients, 6 patients with retinitis pigmentosa (4 with family histories) were included as cases of intermediate uveitis.[27] The principal features of these cases were vitreous humor cellular reaction and cystoid macular edema; one illustrated case had peripheral exudates.[27]

Although it is unlikely that cases of retinitis pigmentosa will be mistaken for intermediate uveitis, cases with prominent retinal pigmentary changes have been reported, some of which have been associated with changes in the electroretinogram (ERG).[24] The occurrence of excessive pigmentary change seems low; Smith[133] reported pigmentary changes similar to retinitis pigmentosa in only 2 of 182 eyes. Despite the inclusion of 24 patients with chorioretinal lesions posterior to the equator in Brockhurst's series[22] of 100, most experts would consider postequatorial fundus lesions exclusionary for the diagnosis of intermediate uveitis.[38]

PATHOGENESIS

Except for the few cases of systemic disease with inflammation confined to the intermediate anatomic zone, the causes of intermediate uveitis are unknown. No microbiologic associations have been consistently found. Anatomic, pathologic, and immunologic studies have been undertaken in an effort to understand its pathogenesis.

The predisposition for involvement of the pars plana region prompted anatomic studies. Gärtner[51,52] used electron microscopy to examine eyes enucleated with other diseases such as tumors. Damaged cells with liberated cell organelles, cell remnants, and basement membrane deposits were found in the pars plana region, particularly at younger ages. Gärtner proposed that the cell breakdown products in the vitreous base region (possibly from the embryonic vitreous humor) might be antigenic, or that basement membrane fragments might act as a trap for circulating antigen-antibody complexes, which would then stimulate inflammation.

Gross, light microscopic description of the peripheral retinal region supported Bec's theories[11] of pathogenesis and his uveitis classification scheme (vide supra). He noted progressive thinning of the retina and choroid from the posterior pole to the ora serrata, with the choriocapillaris as such ending at the ora serrata. The retinal vascular arcades terminated 1 mm posterior to the ora serrata, which suggested a relative ischemia contributing to chronic inflammation. Like Gärtner, Bec found the vitreous base rich in cellular elements and debris that might act as antigenic stimuli.

Lütjen-Drecoll[83] has described other anatomic features that might promote inflammation. Like Bec, she emphasized the relative ischemia of the region. Venous capillaries of posterior pars plana are perfused with partially deoxygenated blood from the ciliary muscles; arterial capillaries are found only in the transition zone of the ora serrata. A candidate antigen for autoimmune attack was suggested by the demonstration of production of hyaluronic acid in the posterior pars plana. The specialized pars plana pigment epithelium also was found to contain enzymes capable of active fluid transport. Metabolic perturbation by inflammation might therefore result in peripheral serous retinal detachments, as seen in some cases of intermediate uveitis.

Anatomic studies show the pars plana to be a region of relatively low oxygen tension, with specialized molecules and functions that might make it prone to nonspecific inflammation or to specific immunologic attack.

Determination of the type of cells infiltrating the vitreous humor cavity is an obvious first step in the immunologic characterization of intermediate uveitis. In histologic studies focal vitreous humor opacities were noted to contain degenerating and intact macrophages consistent with epithelioid granulomata.[59] Lymphocytes, plasma cells, histiocytes, and giant cells were noted in other vitreous humor specimens.[45,59]

More precise characterization of the vitreous humor inflammatory cells based on their immunologic function has produced contradictory results. Kaplan and associates[74] found primarily B-lymphocytes in 10 uveitis patients, including 2 patients with pars planitis. The B-lymphocytes were detected by adherence to beads coated with antiheavy chain antibody. The same group later corroborated the finding that B-lymphocytes were the predominant vitreous humor cell type by fluorescence-activated cell sorting in 24 uveitis patients.[75] Only the aqueous humor of one patient with pars planitis was studied with this technique, however.[75]

In contrast, fluorescent-labeled monoclonal antibodies against cell-surface molecules identified T-lymphocytes as the predominant vitreous humor cell in 15 eyes of 13 patients with intermediate uveitis.[101] T-lymphocytes accounted for 11% to 95% of all vitreous humor cells, with median counts of 52% to 57%, depending on the exact antibody used. T-helper or T-inducer cells made up 5% to 73% of the total (median 36%). Macrophages were the second most common cell type (median 27%). B-lymphocytes were scarce (median 2%). Lymphocytes with cell-surface HLA-DR, a marker considered a sign of immunologic activation, were present in a range of 8% to 65%, with a median of 30%. Three vitreous humor biopsy specimens from intermediate uveitis patients were studied with similar techniques and showed comparable results.[33] Of vitreous humor cells, 50% to 95% were T-lymphocytes; 35% to 90% were T-helper or T-inducer subclass; and 5% to 50% were T-suppressor or T-cytotoxic cells. Low levels of B-lymphocytes and macrophages were present. In two of the three cases, the cells were HLA-DR positive. The finding of T-helper lymphocytes in the vitreous humor is consistent with data from other uveitis patients.[33] It is also consistent with the mild infiltrate of

T-helper lymphocytes (Leu 4 positive) found in a case of intermediate uveitis in which the posterior segment was examined with immunohistochemical techniques.[147]

Abnormalities in the immune system have been difficult to demonstrate. Yokoyama and associates[153] noted mild elevations of serum IgD in nine patients. Antiganglioside antibody was found in four. Levels of inflammatory molecules such as α-2 microglobulin, β-2 microglobulin, and complement components were normal. Absolute numbers of T- and B-lymphocytes in the peripheral blood were also normal. An increased ratio of T-helper to T-suppressor lymphocytes was found in six other patients with the pars planitis subtype, however.[110]

Retinal autoantibodies have been found in Behçet disease, Vogt-Koyanagi-Harada syndrome, sympathetic ophthalmia,[25] retinal vasculitis,[43] and in normal controls.[102] The sera of 58 patients with intermediate uveitis, 256 normal controls, and 685 patients with autoimmune diseases without eye involvement were studied with an indirect immunofluorescence assay to detect reactivity against frozen human retinal sections.[100] Staining patterns specific for the photoreceptor layer were found with the same low frequency in all three groups. Antibodies against Müller cells were present in 10% of intermediate uveitis patients versus 2.3% of healthy controls and 7.4% of other autoimmune controls. Using a slightly different assay with an avidin-biotin-peroxidase reaction to detect serum immunoglobulin bound to frozen human retinal sections, staining of the inner retina was detected in the sera of 8 of 12 intermediate uveitis patients; staining of retinal vessel walls was present in 5 of the 12.[30] The importance of humoral antiretinal antibodies in the pathogenesis of intermediate uveitis is unclear and may simply reflect a response to tissue damage from other causes.

Evidence of immunologic defense against retinal S-antigen has been sought because of this photoreceptor protein's uveitogenic potential in animal models.[141] The same percentage of anterior and intermediate uveitis patients, posterior uveitis patients, and normal controls had anti-S-antigen antibodies in one study.[39] Lymphocyte proliferation indicative of cellular immunity against retinal S-antigen and interphotoreceptor retinol-binding protein was demonstrated in one fourth to one third of patients with intermediate uveitis in each of three separate studies.[35,39,110] More posterior and panuveitis patients than intermediate uveitis patients were responders to S-antigen. If cell-mediated immune responses against known uveitogenic retinal photoreceptor proteins exist, they seem to occur in a minority of patients with intermediate uveitis.

Some experimental models of uveitis have been proposed that might have relevance for intermediate uveitis. Primate models of experimental autoimmune uveitis resemble intermediate uveitis in having retinal vascular leakage, but the retinal and choroidal infiltrates are atypical.[66] Aggregates of cells were produced in the anterior vitreous humor by multiple injections of hyaluronic acid into the vitreous cavity of owl monkeys.[69] The deposits were more numerous inferiorly, mimicking the typical appearance of pars planitis. Injections of endotoxin, although inflammatory, did not produce a similar picture. A model of intravitreous injections of crystalline egg albumin in rabbits produced infiltration of iris, choroid, and blood vessels, but not the characteristic peripheral vitreous humor infiltrates.[156]

The proliferation of Müller (retinal glial) cells in vitro in the presence of soluble products from activated lymphocytes and macrophages[115] suggests that Müller cells, present in the pars plana exudate,[147] may be stimulated in vivo by inflammatory cells.[82] It is unknown why this proliferation of Müller cells should be relatively specific for intermediate uveitis and for the pars plana region.

Anatomic studies cited previously show that the peripheral retina and pars plana region has a distinctive blood supply that may render it prone to ischemia and nonspecific inflammation.[83] Retinal vascular inflammatory changes are a consistent feature of pathologic studies of intermediate uveitis.[59,77,79,147,154] There is evidence that the retinal vessels may be modified in active disease to foster lymphocytic infiltration.[154] These factors suggest that intermediate "uveitis" may be a disease of the retinal vasculature. The contribution of T-lymphocytes to disease pathogenesis, as in other types of uveitis, seems clear, however. Glial proliferation by Müller cells may be the distinctive clinical feature by which the disease is recognized.

There is no good evidence linking idiopathic intermediate uveitis to any of the known uveitogenic proteins, to infection, or to systemic immunologic disturbances. Antigens specific to the vitreoretinal interface, the peripheral retina, or the retinal vasculature, however, have not been tested for possible involvement in intermediate uveitis; and specific, immunologically-mediated "autoimmune" attack against an ocular antigen cannot be excluded. If such an antigen exists, the vitreoretinal interface or the peripheral retina and pars plana are its likely sites of localization. An immune-mediated attack against hyaluronic acid, a principal vitreous humor protein, could be implicated, although the experimental work in models of intermediate uveitis is quite preliminary.

DIFFERENTIAL DIAGNOSIS

Consideration of infectious causes is an important part of the evaluation of intermediate uveitis, as specific treatment and cure may be achieved. Intermediate uveitis may occur with spirochetal infections caused by *Treponema pallidum*[135] or *Borrelia burgdorferi*.[17] Perivasculitis may occur with toxoplasmic retinochoroiditis[144] or tuberculosis.[80] Fairly typical intermediate uveitis, which responds to corticosteroids, has also been reported with human immunodeficiency virus (HIV) infection.[90] Another retrovirus, human T-lymphotrophic virus-I (HTLV-1), has been associated with an intermediate uveitis in Japan, where the virus is endemic.[95] Severe vitritis may also be seen in endogenous fungal and bacterial endophthalmitis; sudden onset and a compatible history are helpful in making a correct diagnosis.[91]

Whereas toxoplasmosis and tuberculosis can produce distinctive ocular manifestations that facilitate diagnosis, and syphilis is easily excluded by laboratory tests, the diagnosis of borrelial infection may be difficult unless other signs and symptoms of Lyme disease, such as cranial nerve palsy, chronic meningitis, migratory arthralgias, or erythematous skin rash, are present.[129] Breeveld[17] reported a woman diagnosed with the classic features of pars plana exudation and cystoid macular edema, with an immunofluorescent antibody titer of 1:320 against *B. burgdorferi,* who responded promptly to antibiotic therapy despite failure of corticosteroids and cryotherapy to control her disease during a 10-year course. Vitreous humor "clouding" in a patient with typical systemic signs of Lyme disease also responded to antibiotic therapy after an initial exacerbation on treatment.[81]

Lyme disease may present with intermediate uveitis.[60] In a small series of six patients with positive Lyme disease serology and ocular complaints, five had vitritis and iridocyclitis.[149] One case had typical peripheral exudates and two others had preretinal cellular aggregates overlying the vitreous base inferiorly. These cases were different from the typical pars planitis subtype of intermediate uveitis in having a vigorous anterior segment inflammatory response; for example, three of the five had posterior synechiae. All five patients responded to antibiotic therapy, although two later relapsed.

Peripheral granulomata from *Toxocara canis* infection might be mistaken for a unilateral case of the pars planitis subtype of intermediate uveitis, as the granuloma may simulate a peripheral exudate and vitreous humor bands to the optic disc can occur in both diseases.[125] The age of presentation of this form overlaps with that of pars planitis.[143] In very young children the alternate diagnoses of retinoblastoma and Coats disease also may need to be considered.[125,143]

Multiple Sclerosis

Patients with multiple sclerosis may develop ocular disease resembling other forms of intermediate uveitis. Retinal vascular sheathing, dubbed periphlebitis retinae, has been reported to occur in 5% to more than 20% of multiple sclerosis patients.[18,46,58,155] Vitreous humor cells may be present as well, fulfilling the criteria for an intermediate uveitis. Macular edema is uncommon.[9] Breger[18] prospectively studied 52 patients with the diagnosis of multiple sclerosis for evidence of peripheral uveitis. Nine of the fifty-two had bilateral uveitis, and five had unilateral inflammation for an incidence of 27%. Breger suggested an autoimmune disorder directed against an unknown antigen common to both eye and myelin nerve sheath.[18] Conversely, Chester[27] noted a 17% incidence of multiple sclerosis in his series of 51 pars planitis patients. Although a shared HLA-DR2 phenotype has been proposed as the common feature in both pars planitis and multiple sclerosis, in one study[86] only three of five intermediate uveitis patients who later developed multiple sclerosis were HLA-DR2 positive.[86]

Engell[46] attempted to confirm an association between intermediate uveitis and multiple sclerosis by correlating vascular sheathing with stages of activity of multiple sclerosis. Of 303 patients, 27 (9%) had sheathing of the retinal veins. All but 1 of these 27 patients had active disease, and the rate of involvement was 21% in patients who became wheelchair-bound within 5 years versus 7.3% of patients with a benign course. Moreover, periphlebitis was found in 43% of patients who were having rapid progression or an attack.

Graham and associates[58] confirmed the association between periphlebitis and progressive multiple sclerosis in 50 multiple sclerosis patients who had no prior ocular illness other than optic neuritis. Three of the fifty patients had venous sheathing, and four had focal venous cuffing. The rate of involvement was 31.3% in patients with progressive disease but only 11.6% in patients with remitting multiple sclerosis. Better vision in eyes with periphlebitis was ascribed to a negative correlation between prior optic neuritis and retinal vascular changes. The authors hypothesized that with optic atrophy there was less retinal vascularity or less neural tissue to serve as a target for immunologic attack.

Multiple sclerosis does not have to be active for intermediate uveitis to be present. Intermediate uveitis may precede multiple sclerosis by more than 7 years.[86,155] A case report of a woman with severe intermediate uveitis and myelin basic protein in the cerebrospinal fluid suggests that a subset of intermediate uveitis patients may be at risk for the subsequent development of multiple sclerosis.[99] During long-term follow-up, 8 of 54 patients (14.8%) with intermediate uveitis in 1 series developed multiple sclerosis, and an additional 4 patients developed optic neuritis.[85]

Sarcoidosis

Some patients with sarcoidosis (probably a small number) meet the diagnostic criteria for intermediate uveitis. In a series of 183 patients with known sarcoidosis referred for ophthalmologic examination, 47 (26%) had ocular involvement.[71] Eleven of the forty-seven had intraocular inflammation consistent with intermediate uveitis. One had exudative retinal detachment and periphlebitis; six of the remaining ten had vitritis, and seven had periphlebitis. Sarcoidosis was ultimately diagnosed in about 2% to 10% of patients with intermediate uveitis in various series.[27,88,155]

Periodic examination for sarcoidosis may be warranted because uveitis may precede the other systemic manifestations by years.[118,155] Unlike pars planitis, sarcoid uveitis is slightly more common in females than males, with an older average age of presentation.[118] Anterior uveitis is more common than posterior uveitis, and anterior segment signs are usually more pronounced in patients with sarcoidosis and intermediate uveitis than in patients with idiopathic pars planitis.[70,118] In the series of Jabs[71] only one patient had vitritis and periphlebitis without anterior segment inflammatory signs.

Lymphoma

Vitritis without fundus lesions, which can mimic intermediate uveitis, has been reported with intraocular lymphoma.[26,92,116,127,148] Because intraocular lymphoma can occur at any age,[34] consideration of this diagnosis should not be limited to the elderly. Poor response to corticosteroids, lack of vitreous destruction by the cellular infiltrate, and lack of macular edema may be helpful diagnostic features.

Other Uveitis Syndrome

Rarely, other forms of uveitis may be mistaken for intermediate uveitis.[91] Fuchs uveitis syndrome can produce a unilateral, chronic, low-grade anterior segment inflammation with spillover of cells into the vitreous cavity. A chronic, bilateral, low-grade iridocyclitis might have the same appearance. The vitreous humor cells are ordinarily confined to the anterior vitreous humor in these cases. Mild Vogt-Koyanagi-Harada syndrome, a form of panuveitis, might also simulate intermediate uveitis alone if the choroidal involvement was not detected. Vitritis with arteriolar vasculitis overlaps with Behçet disease and other retinal vasculitides. Prominent vascular occlusive disease may suggest Eales disease. Arteritic or nonarteritic ocular ischemia may show a "hot" anterior segment with excessive flare and high-or-low intraocular pressure, that may have microangiopathic or neovascular complications in addition to vitritis. Perfusion defects in both the choroidal and retinal circulations suggest this diagnosis.

LABORATORY INVESTIGATIONS

There is no confirmatory test for diagnosis of the pars planitis subtype of intermediate uveitis; the diagnosis is based on clinical findings. Laboratory investigations and ancillary ocular testing are used to exclude other more specific diagnoses and to define the extent of ocular involvement. Table 55-4 lists the principal diagnoses, which may present as intermediate uveitis, and summarizes the clinical and laboratory studies that may be helpful.

The initial battery of examinations is based on the likely differential diagnosis. In adults it may include an RPR and FTA-ABS, Lyme disease antibody titers, complete blood count, erythrocyte sedimentation rate, and chest X-ray. A tuberculin skin test and antinuclear antibodies have very low predictive value given the current low prevalence of tuberculosis and systemic lupus erythematosus as causes of uveitis.[117] Fluorescein angiography is useful to check for unsuspected pigment epithelial or choroidal disease, subclinical

macular edema, and retinal vascular staining or capillary nonperfusion.

Anterior segment inflammation that seems equal to or out of proportion to the vitreous reaction may suggest sarcoidosis or a chronic iridocyclitis. Testing (other than a chest X-ray) may not be warranted if there are no systemic symptoms, even if a diagnosis of sarcoidosis is suspected; however, some centers perform a full battery of tests for sarcoidosis.[155] Periodic reevaluation with a chest X-ray is appropriate, and more thorough evaluation of patients with ocular features suggestive of sarcoidosis who may require systemic immunosuppression is also desirable. A confirmed diagnosis of sarcoidosis requires a biopsy that shows noncaseating granulomata in lung or extrapulmonary granulomata and chest X-ray abnormalities.[155] Retinal vascular inflammation that involves the arteries[89] or is associated with capillary nonperfusion warrants testing for collagen vascular disease and other causes of retinal vasculitis such as Behçet disease (Table 55-4).

If toxocariasis is considered in cases of unilateral inflammation, serologic studies are of limited value because 20% to 30% of young children have evidence of prior infection.[44] A negative serum titer does not exclude this diagnosis, as only the intraocular fluid may contain detectable antibody.[12]

Fluorescein angiography is useful diagnostically because of the high rate of vascular abnormalities in intermediate uveitis. Pruett[114] noted patchy staining of major veins in 34 of 34 eyes. Segmental hyperfluorescence of retinal veins was also noted by Bec.[11] Other studies have shown leakage of retinal blood veins or venules on angiography in greater than 40% to 50% of eyes.[119,123] Diffuse retinal edema was seen in 4 of 68 eyes in 1 series.[123]

Arellanes and associates[5] recently cataloged the findings present on fluorescein angiography in 52 eyes of 26 patients from 4 to 29 years of age. All had focal vitreous humor opacities or a peripheral exudate. Only 2 eyes were normal angiographically; 28 eyes showed capillary hyperfluorescence, 25 eyes optic disc hyperfluorescence, and 17 eyes staining of the vessel walls.[5] Eleven eyes exhibited a "fern" pattern of radial hyperfluorescence in the small vessels surrounding the optic disc.[5] Subretinal leaks or abnormal choroidal fluorescence are not described in intermediate uveitis and should call the diagnosis into question. Extensive capillary nonperfusion or large vessel occlusions posterior to the equator are also atypical for intermediate uveitis.

Echographic studies showing a solid, highly reflective peripheral mass with a vitreous humor band and a retinal fold (or traction detachment) between the mass and the optic nerve are useful in confirming the diagnosis of toxocariasis.[143] Echography can also demonstrate ciliochoroidal detachments and scleral and choroidal thickening indicative of various posterior uveitides. It is not routinely needed in the evaluation of intermediate uveitis.

Fluorophotometry can detect abnormal leakage at an ear-

TABLE 55-4 PRINCIPAL DIFFERENTIAL DIAGNOSES FOR INTERMEDIATE UVEITIS

Disorder	Distinguishing Features	Diagnostic Tests
Infections		
Syphilis	Marked anterior inflammation, may have posterior polar choroidal and RPE infiltrates	RPR, FTA-ABS
Lyme disease	Systemic and CNS signs, anterior inflammation, response to antibiotics	Lyme antibody titer, confirmatory physical findings
Toxocariasis	Unilateral, vitreous humor bands, retinal folds or detachments	Serology, echography, antibody titer
Endogenous endophthalmitis	Acute and subacute onset, intense inflammation, focal retinochoroidal lesions, compatible history	Vitreous or aqueous humor culture, cultures of other body sites
Systemic and CNS Diseases		
Multiple sclerosis	Neurologic findings, optic neuritis	Brain imaging studies, cerebrospinal fluid studies
Sarcoidosis	Anterior segment inflammation, choroidal granulomata, "candlewax" periphlebitis	Chest X-ray, tissue biopsy, gallium scan, pulmonary function tests, angiotensin-converting enzyme
Lymphoma	Vitreous cell without destruction of vitreous architecture or macular edema	Vitreous humor cytology and immunophenotyping, brain imaging studies
Other Ocular Diseases		
Fuchs uveitis syndrome	Unilateral, chronic, low-grade, anterior location of vitreous humor cell, frequent cataract and glaucoma, white fibrillary and round keratic precipitates	Clinical diagnosis
Chronic iridocyclitis of unknown cause	Anterior location of vitreous humor cell, exacerbations with prominent anterior segment inflammatory signs	Clinical diagnosis
Vogt-Koyanagi-Harada syndrome	Choroidal infiltrates, posterior exudative detachments, prominent anterior segment inflammatory signs, acute onset	Fluorescein angiography, ethnic and genetic associations
Retinal vasculitis (Behçet disease, Eales disease, collagen-vascular disease)	Usually with arterial involvement causing retinal whitening, systemic features of Behçet disease	Fluorescein angiography, ANA, other specific autoantibodies, complement studies, sedimentation rate, chest X-ray, urinanalysis, renal and liver function studies, HLA-B51$_{PPD}$, cardiolipin antibodies, tissue biopsy
Ocular ischemia	Anterior segment inflammatory signs especially flare, hypotony or glaucoma, microangiopathy, neovascularization	Ophthalmodynamometry, fluorescein angiography, noninvasive ocular blood flow studies, sedimentation rate

lier stage of disease than fluorescein angiography.[84] Although it is not used clinically on a routine basis, this sensitive technique can deduce the principal breakdown site of the blood-retinal barrier in intermediate uveitis. Schlaegel[121] reported that the greatest leakage was into the anterior and inferior vitreous humor. Mahlberg[84] later studied 23 eyes in 12 patients with pars planitis. All eyes leaked abnormal amounts of fluorescein into the vitreous humor. No pattern of excessive inferior leakage was observed. In addition, the leakage at 15 minutes was greater in the posterior vitreous than the anterior vitreous in 18 of 23 eyes. Inferior-anterior leakage was more pronounced in those eyes that had the greatest posterior leakage overall. These results have been interpreted as a generalized permeability disturbance with somewhat greater leakage in the equatorial and midperipheral regions.[84] Peaks of fluorescein leakage in the posterior vitreous and anterior chamber in early disease (Fig. 55-2), with a more uniform, diffuse leak in later disease (Fig. 55-3), were demonstrated by Bloch-Michel.[13] The diffuse type of leak diminished in chronic cases but did not completely resolve with recovery (Fig. 55-4), suggesting a secondary scarring change of the blood-ocular barriers with chronicity.[14,61]

The importance of retinovascular leakage to the pathophysiology of intermediate uveitis is underscored by a good correlation between the amount of cystoid macular edema and the fluorophotometric values.[84] Vitreous humor haze,

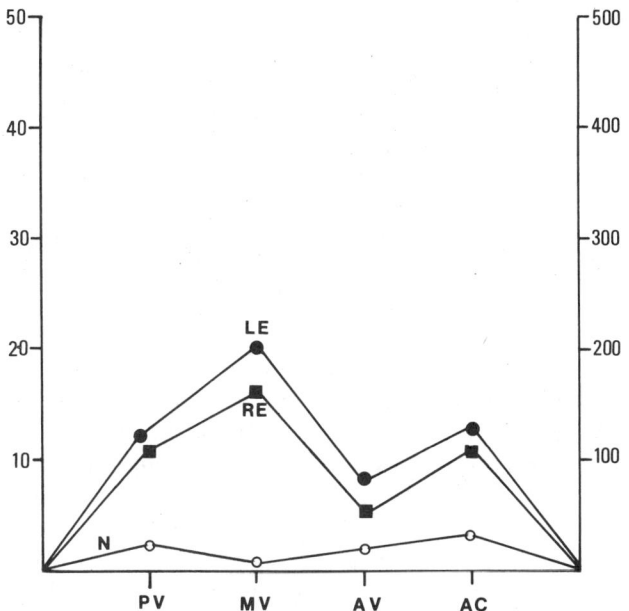

Fig. 55-2. Fluorometric curve in intermediate uveitis of recent onset. The scale for the posterior segment is on the left Y axis, 0 to 50 ng/ml. The scale for the anterior segment is on the right Y axis, 0 to 500 ng/ml. Notice the biphasic curve. PV = posterior vitreous. MV = mid-vitreous. AV = anterior vitreous. AC = anterior chamber. N = normal curve. RE = right eye. LE = left eye.

size of the pars plana exudate, and visual acuity also correlated well with the degree of fluorescein leakage.[84] The fluorophotometric findings have also been used to support the opinion that the preferential inferior localization of the pars plana exudate is due to a gravitational effect.[84]

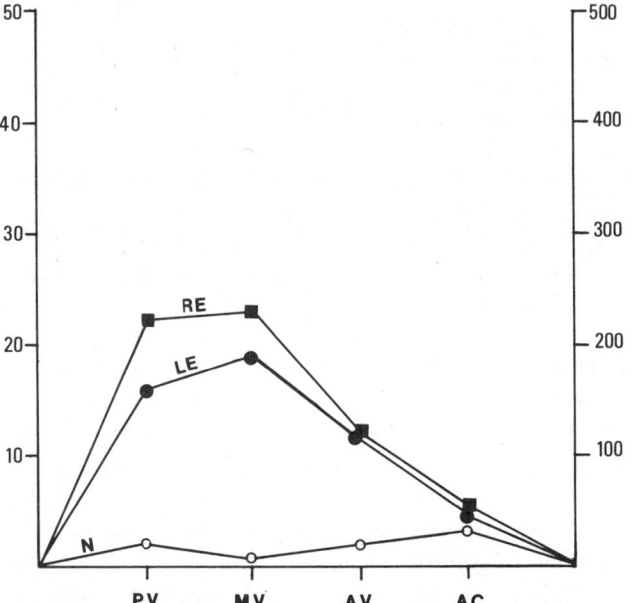

Fig. 55-3. Fluorometric curve in intermediate uveitis of moderate duration. The curve has lost its biphasic nature and has become a "dome." Scale markings and abbreviations as in Fig. 55-2.

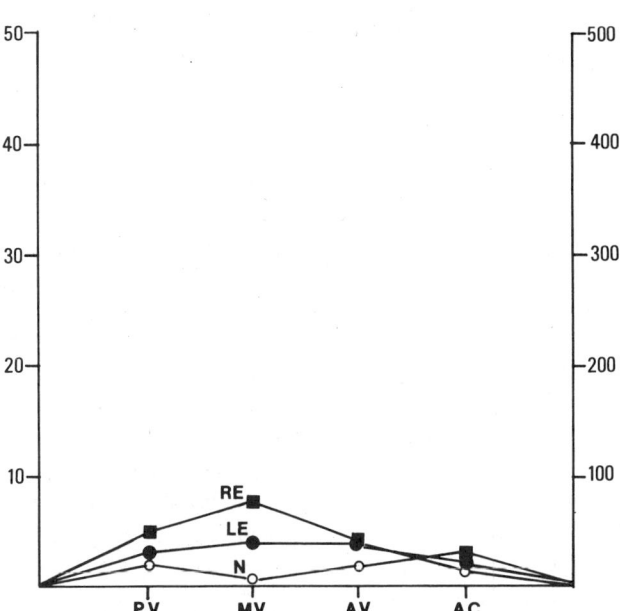

Fig. 55-4. Fluorometric curve in chronic intermediate uveitis. The domed curve has flattened into a "plateau." Low levels of blood-ocular barrier breakdown persist even with clinical recovery. Scale markings and abbreviations as in Fig. 55-2.

Electrophysiologic studies may detect widespread dysfunction of the retina in some patients with intermediate uveitis. Thirteen patients with typical pars plana exudates and duration of disease over 2 years were studied by Cantrill and associates.[24] Most of the changes were fairly mild: 11 of 13 had abnormal b-wave implicit times on the ERG, and there was reduction or absence of scotopic b-wave oscillations in 12 of 13 patients; however, reduced b-wave amplitudes were present in 3 patients with complaints of night blindness who had retinal pigmentary changes. Similarly, nonrecordable (or nearly nonrecordable) amplitudes occurred in two patients with (1) pigmentation in a pattern consistent with burned-out uveitis, and (2) disease durations of 7 and 15 years, respectively.[137] Cone and rod a and b waves were equally impaired. In this series oscillatory potentials were reduced in 10 of the 14 eyes with a recordable ERG.

In mild disease b-wave amplitude has been reported to be increased.[24,112] The supernormal ERG seen in some patients may indicate active retinal inflammation.[137] Alternatively, supernormal ERG may occur in patients receiving oral corticosteroids.[157]

Cytologic or immunohistochemical examination of the infiltrating vitreous humor cells can establish the diagnosis of intraocular lymphoma.[92,113] The efficiency is limited by cell number, cell viability, and the experience of the laboratory handling the specimen. Flow cytometry has been used in a small number of cases.[148] Vitreous humor cultures are a reliable means of confirming bacterial or fungal intraocular infection as a cause for vitritis.[48] Even "negative" biopsies can have diagnostic value if the immunohistochemical staining of the cells confirms an inflammatory infiltrate with T-helper lymphocyte predominance (as is usual in uveitis).[33]

THERAPY

If a specific cause (such as syphilis or Lyme disease) can be identified in cases of intermediate uveitis, then treatment is directed against these disorders. The following discussion deals with the nonspecific antiinflammatory therapy of idiopathic intermediate uveitis.

Schlaegel[122] recommended treating patients with pars planitis only to "prevent or handle important complications," not to get rid of all the vitreous humor cell or snowbank. Although others have articulated more aggressive approaches in which absolute clarity of the media is the goal, particularly before intraocular surgery,[49] most would limit therapy to severe vision loss (defined as vision less than or equal to 20/40) caused by macular edema or vitreous opacity. Some clinicians treat symptomatic patients with visible macular cysts at any level of visual acuity. Topical corticosteroids are reserved for clinically important anterior segment inflammation,[55] as they do little to decrease posterior segment inflammation in phakic eyes and may enhance the rate of cataract formation. Systemically administered immunosuppressive agents, including corticosteroids, are generally reserved for bilateral, severe disease.[105,107]

Periocular Corticosteroid Injections

The use of periocular corticosteroid injections was reported early for this disorder.[67,150] Although Chester[27] stated that corticosteroid therapy was not effective for reducing macular edema, others have emphasized the need to continue treatment for a series of up to eight injections before abandoning it as not efficacious.[55,76] Schlaegel[122] noted that most patients took up to 2.5 months to improve with treatment. A more recent series showed improvement of at least 2 Snellen lines in 12 of 18 patients, at a median of 3 weeks after injection, although vision subsequently declined in 4.[62]

Godfrey and associates[57] studied the effects of treatment on cystoid macular edema in 100 patients with adequate treatment histories and follow-up. Visual results were analyzed after 1 or 2 months of treatment. Seven of 74 eyes received only topical corticosteroids, 22 eyes oral corticosteroids, and 38 eyes periocular corticosteroid injections. Seven eyes were untreated. Untreated eyes or eyes receiving only topical corticosteroids did not improve visually, whereas 41% of the orally treated eyes and 71% of the periocularly treated eyes did improve. Angiographic improvement in cystoid macular edema has also been noted after treatment with corticosteroids.[114]

Periocular corticosteroid injection schedules of roughly every 3 to 5 weeks have been recommended,[57,62,79,150] although it is now common for injections to be spaced at 2- to 3-week intervals during initial treatment. Either the depot,

long-acting form of methylprednisolone (40 mg) or depot triamcinolone acetonide (20 to 40 mg) is typically used. Injection given superotemporally in the sub-Tenon capsule space as far posteriorly and close to the globe as possible results in a deposit of drug closer to the macula, which is possibly more effective than injections in the inferotemporal quadrant or in the retrobulbar space.[50] Side-to-side movement of the needle tip during penetration reduces the risk of globe entry.[50] Posterior injection may also reduce the risk of intraocular pressure rise.

Some toxicity to the orbital tissues probably occurs from the repeated injection of long-acting preparations.[107] Histologic examination shows crystalline inclusions in fibroblasts and macrophages with degeneration of collagen.[103] With repeated injections, orbital scarring and enophthalmos have been noted.[106] Other complications of periocular corticosteroid injection include allergic reactions with breakdown of the conjunctiva,[56] intraocular pressure increase,[62] and cataract.[57] Intraocular pressure rises may be severe enough to require filtration surgery.[62] In children the risks of general anesthesia must also be considered, although with proper coaching and good topical conjunctival anesthesia, even very young children can be injected without being put to sleep.

Oral Corticosteroid Therapy

Oral corticosteroids are probably the safest of the systemic immunosuppressive drugs and are generally the next step for severe, bilateral disease when a series of periocular corticosteroid injections has failed.[76] Initial dosages of 1 to 1.5 mg per kg daily followed by dosage reductions every 3 to 4 weeks allow many patients to stabilize at a daily dosage in the 15 to 20 mg range, which can be maintained for months with minimal side effects. Wakefield and associates[142] reported a regimen of high-dose, intermittent ("pulse") intravenous corticosteroids, which is purported to have fewer side effects than chronic oral corticosteroid administration. One patient with pars planitis was included among the 17 patients with inflammatory disease treated in this fashion. None experienced the serious potential complications of seizures, death, or anaphylaxis. Corticosteroids are also useful in the treatment of neovascularization in intermediate uveitis.[47,72]

Immunosuppressive Drugs

In a series of 52 patients treated with cyclosporine, all 11 intermediate uveitis patients achieved therapeutic success.[109] Reduction in vitreous humor haze was noted after 3 months.[108] Visual acuity also improved in the majority of eyes treated with low-dose cyclosporine and prednisone in a series of 13 patients, including 4 with intermediate uveitis.[138] Because of elevations in serum creatinine with a starting dosage of 10 mg per kg per day, a regimen of cyclosporine 5 mg per kg per day, with 0.2 to 0.4 mg per kg per day prednisone has been recommended.[108] Increases in dosage are possible after 4 to 6 weeks if no clinical response is seen.[108] For children requiring chronic immunosuppression, cyclosporine may be a better choice than prednisone because of the possible growth retardation with prednisone.[41] Side effects of hypertension, hirsutism, hypomagnesemia, taste disturbance, rashes, paresthesias, and gingivitis are common.[138]

A series of 16 patients with "peripheral uveitis" had good responses to 2- to 3-month courses of cyclophosphamide, although follow-up was short.[23] Ten patients with intermediate uveitis were included among 20 patients treated with azathioprine—a less toxic alternative to 6-mercaptopurine.[96,97] Use of azathioprine allowed reduction of the corticosteroid dosage and resulted in visual improvement in 10 of 15 eyes with macular involvement.[96] In 4 of 10 patients the pars plana exudation decreased as well. Methotrexate has also been reported in the treatment of intermediate uveitis.[152]

Cyclophosphamide is ordinarily started at about 2 mg per kg daily by mouth and is titrated to a white blood cell count of 3000 to 5000. Concomitant use of corticosteroids can increase the tolerance of high dosages of cyclophosphamide. Azathioprine is usually started at 1 to 2.5 mg per kg daily and may also be combined with corticosteroids. Both agents are best administered by physicians familiar with their actions, side effects, and the realization that they are not labeled for the treatment of uveitis. Use in children for uveitis should be avoided whenever possible.[104] Risks include infertility, teratogenicity, and secondary malignancies as well as the expected bone marrow toxicity. With the exception of methotrexate and azathioprine, other cytotoxic agents are probably not indicated for the treatment of uveitis because of greater risks and less familiarity.[134]

Diflunisal (500 mg twice daily) has been used (1) as an adjunct in the control of intraocular inflammation following cataract extraction in intermediate uveitis and (2) as a second-line agent if periocular corticosteroids are ineffective.[76]

Surgical Management

Cryotherapy and vitrectomy have been employed to treat patients with intermediate uveitis.[73] In 1973 Aaberg[1] reported decreased inflammation in 23 eyes of 14 patients with intermediate uveitis who were treated with cryotherapy. Eight eyes appeared to go into complete remission and required no further corticosteroid therapy. Nine patients with bilaterally progressive disease showed decreased inflammation in treated eyes, but untreated fellow eyes deteriorated. With longer follow-up of an average 52 months and with an additional 14 patients, the initial 92% success rate after a single treatment fell to 42%.[2] All but two of the patients who required retreatment achieved control without corticosteroid use. Initial patient selection was based more on inflammatory signs, including the presence of neovascularization, than on visual acuity, which was often good before treatment.

Other series have reported successful results with cryotherapy. Devenyi and associates[36] treated 27 eyes of 18 patients, all of which had neovascularization and were resistant to corticosteroid treatment. With a median follow-up of 4.5 years, 23 of 27 eyes required only 1 treatment before regression of neovascularization was achieved. Of 27 eyes, 21 eyes had no active anterior chamber or vitreous reaction following treatment, and 18 eyes had improvement in visual acuity. Similarly, the series of Okinami[111] had a 61% regression rate after a single session of cryotherapy. Verma and associates[140] randomly chose patients to continue corticosteroid therapy or to receive cryotherapy. Patients were not limited to those with neovascularization of the vitreous base. Four of eight eyes had improved vision after cryotherapy compared to only one eye after corticosteroids. A principal advantage of cryotherapy may be that it places patients in long-term remission following a single treatment (Fig. 55-5).

Cryotherapy appeared safe in these series. Three of twenty-seven eyes in which vision became worse after cryotherapy had epiretinal membrane, cataract and macular edema, or traction retinal detachment with subsequent atrophia bulbi.[36] Tractional retinal detachment was also mentioned in 1 of 28 eyes in another series.[111] Five of seven rhegmatogenous retinal detachments in a series of 55 intermediate uveitis patients followed vitrectomy with cryotherapy for neovascularization of the vitreous base, and one followed cryotherapy alone.[151] These rates of retinal detachment are not higher than that reported for intermediate uveitis patients as a group.[10,11,114,133]

The mechanism of cryotherapy remains unclear. Chester,[27] who also felt that corticosteroids were not useful, stated that cryotherapy was not effective because deposits were gravitational. Verma[140] hypothesized that cryotherapy worked by ablating ischemic tissue. Destruction of high endothelial venules in the peripheral uvea and retina would result in less lymphocyte traffic into the eye and decreased inflammation.[154]

Although vitrectomy is usually performed for complications of intermediate uveitis (such as vitreous humor or lenticular opacity, tractional retinal detachment, vitreous hemorrhage, or epiretinal membrane),[94] the procedure itself has also been advocated as potentially having an antiinflammatory effect in patients who have failed to respond to periocular corticosteroids or cryotherapy. Vitrectomy is believed by some to be "more benign" than systemic immunosuppression.[73] Even when performed for complications, visual results have been good following vitrectomy. In one series 6 of 12 eyes attained 20/40 or better, with the remainder 20/100 or better.[94] Eyes with no active neovascularization or with treated, inactive neovascularization of the vitreous base appeared to have a better visual prognosis.[94] No severe increase in inflammation was noted after surgery in this series. In another series of 11 eyes, 10 had improved vision following surgery, although visual improvement was slight in

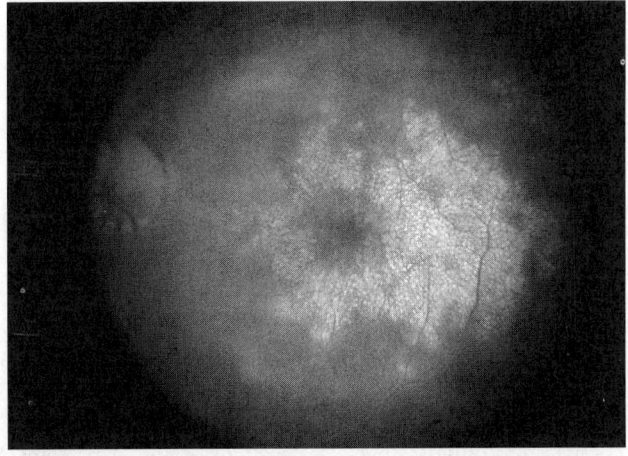

A

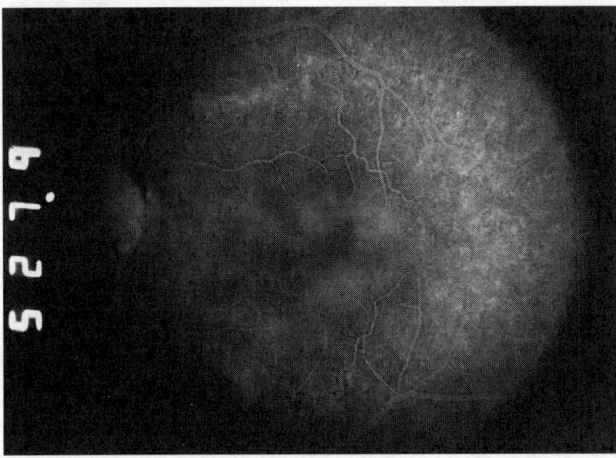

B

Fig. 55-5. **A,** Late fluorescein angiographic appearance in a patient with intermediate uveitis prior to treatment of peripheral exudative detachments with cryoretinopexy. A Lyme disease antibody test was positive. Multiple treatment courses with antibiotics and periocular corticosteroids and pars plana vitrectomy and lensectomy had been undertaken without sustained visual improvement. Vision was 20/200. The right macula had a similar appearance with 20/80 visual acuity. **B,** Late fluorescein angiographic appearance 9 months after cryotherapy. There is minimal residual edema. Vision is 20/60. The right eye was treated with cryotherapy and improved to 20/25. Visual improvement was sustained in both eyes on follow-up of 2 years without further treatment.

some cases because of macular edema.[16] Vitrectomy was felt to be of no benefit in ameliorating the activity of the uveitis or the macular edema.

Four intermediate uveitis patients were included in Diamond and Kaplan's report[37] of pars plana lensectomy and vitrectomy for uveitic cataracts. Three achieved vision of 20/40 or better. Successful extracapsular cataract extraction with intraocular lens implantation has also been described in intermediate uveitis patients with controlled inflammation.[49]

If vitreous humor inflammation is present, uveitis patients undergoing cataract surgery may benefit from vitrectomy as well.[68] In a series of 15 eyes of 8 patients with pars planitis (which received intraocular lens implants after extracapsular cataract extraction), 5 eyes required multiple laser or surgical discissions of posterior membranes and two eyes required explantation of the intraocular lens.[93] Nevertheless, 60% of eyes achieved vision of 20/40 or better, a rate similar to the 13 of 20 eyes that achieved this level of vision after cataract extraction with no intraocular lens.[133] Fifteen of seventeen eyes (88%), in which all active inflammation was suppressed prior to surgery, were 20/40 or better following cataract extraction; most eyes received intraocular lens implantation and some had pars plana vitrectomies performed, which may have improved visual results.[76]

PROGNOSIS

The current clinical treatment practice of ameliorating secondary complications rather than attempting to eradicate all inflammatory signs is supported by the strong relationship between ocular complications and visual prognosis. The most important factor for visual prognosis is macular status, which may account for three fourths of the cases in which vision was less than 20/40.[133] Vitreous opacification contributes to vision loss early in the course of disease; later, cataract becomes an important factor.[132] All complications are more common in severe disease.[79] Although only 6% of eyes with mild disease have vision less than or equal to 20/200, this level of vision is seen in 18% with severe disease.[132]

The chronicity of the disease may adversely affect outcome. A decreasing percentage of eyes have good vision as duration of disease increases.[79,133] Nevertheless, half to three fourths of eyes have vision of at least 20/40 with long-term follow-up.[64,85,88,123,132] Completion of the posterior vitreous detachment may be associated with less macular edema and better vision.[65]

It is unclear whether aggressive treatment of inflammation in the earliest stages would shorten the disease course and result in excellent visual outcomes for more patients. Changes in the ERG in some patients[24] suggest that insidious damage to the retina may occur as the result of long-standing retinovascular or vitreous humor inflammation. It is also possible that allowing the inflammation to persist in the early stages of disease may impair the "immune privilege" of the eye and permit unchecked leukocyte trafficking. Some eyes that improve after onset will be free of disease in a relatively short period of time,[132] possibly because the protective ocular barriers are restored.[61] Although cures of immunologically-mediated disorders are not generally expected with the current methods of management, treatment before ocular complications arise might allow ocular healing before secondary chronic inflammation is established. More aggressive and earlier treatment of this disorder, which has a relatively good visual prognosis, should be subjected to clinical trials before widespread use.

REFERENCES

1. Aaberg TM, Cesarz TJ, Flickinger RR: Treatment of peripheral uveoretinitis by cryotherapy, *Am J Ophthalmol* 75:685-688, 1973.
2. Aaberg TM, Cesarz TJ, Flickinger RRJ: Treatment of pars planitis. I. Cryotherapy, *Surv Ophthalmol* 22:120-130, 1977.
3. Abrahams IW, Jiang Y: Ophthalmology in China, *Arch Ophthalmol* 104:444-446, 1986.
4. Althaus C, Sundmacher R: Intermediate uveitis: epidemiology, age and sex distribution, *Dev Ophthalmol* 23:9-14, 1992.
5. Arellanes L, García LM, Morales V and associates: Report of characteristic angiographic findings in a series of pars planitis patients, *Invest Ophthalmol Vis Sci* 33:743, 1992.
6. Arkfeld DF, Brockhurst RJ: Peripapillary subretinal neovascularization in peripheral uveitis, *Retina* 5:157-160, 1985.
7. Arocker-Mettinger E, Georgiew L, Grabner G, Mayr WR: Intermediate uveitis: do HLA antigens play a role? *Dev Ophthalmol* 23:15-19, 1992.
8. Augsberger JJ, Annesley WH, Sergott RC et al.: Familial pars planitis, *Ann Ophthalmol* 13:553-557, 1981.
9. Bamford CR, Ganley JP, Sibley WA, Laguna JF: Uveitis, perivenous sheathing and multiple sclerosis, *Neurology* 28:119-124, 1978.
10. Bazard MC, Bouvier P, Berrod JP, Raspiller A: Les pars planites: problèmes thérapeutiques, *Bull Soc Ophtalmol Fr* 92:453-456, 1992.
11. Bec P, Arne JL, Philippot V et al.: L'uvéo-rétinite basale et les autres inflammations de la périphérie rétinienne, *Arch Ophthalmol* (Paris) 37:169-196, 1977.
12. Biglan AW, Glickman LT, Lobes LAJ: Serum and vitreous *Toxocara* antibody in nematode endophthalmitis, *Am J Ophthalmol* 88:898-901, 1979.
13. Bloch-Michel E: Uvéite intermédiaire. In Faure JP, editor: *L'immunologie de l'Oeil,* 342-347, Paris, 1988, Masson.
14. Bloch-Michel E: Introduction a la table ronde sur l'uvéite intermediare, *Bull Soc Belge Ophtalmol* 230:49-51, 1989.
15. Bloch-Michel E, Nussenblatt RB: International uveitis study group recommendations for the evaluation of intraocular inflammatory disease, *Am J Ophthalmol* 103:234-235, 1987.
16. Bovey EH, Gonvers M, Herbort CP: Vitrectomie par la pars plana au cours des uveites, *Klin Monatsbl Augenheilkd* 200:464-467, 1992.
17. Breeveld J, Rothova A, Kuiper H: Intermediate uveitis and Lyme borreliosis, *Br J Ophthalmol* 76:181-182, 1992.
18. Breger BC, Leopold IH: The incidence of uveitis in multiple sclerosis, *Am J Ophthalmol* 62:540-545, 1966.
19. Brinton GS, Osher RH, Gass JDM: Idiopathic vitritis, *Retina* 3:95-98, 1983.
20. Brockhurst RJ: Retinoschisis: complication of peripheral uveitis, *Arch Ophthalmol* 100:750-754, 1981.
21. Brockhurst RJ, Schepens CL, Okamura ID: Uveitis. II. Peripheral uveitis: clinical description, complications and differential diagnosis, *Am J Ophthalmol* 49:1257-1266, 1960.
22. Brockhurst RJ, Schepens CL: Uveitis. IV. Peripheral uveitis: the complication of retinal detachment, *Arch Ophthalmol* 80:747-753, 1968.
23. Buckley CE, Gills JP: Cyclophosphamide therapy of peripheral uveitis, *Arch Intern Med* 124:29-35, 1969.
24. Cantrill HL, Ramsay RC, Knobloch WH, Purple RL: Electrophysiologic changes in chronic pars planitis, *Am J Ophthalmol* 91:505-512, 1981.
25. Chan CC, Palestine AG, Nussenblatt RB et al.: Anti-retinal auto-antibodies in Vogt-Koyanagi-Harada syndrome, Behçet's disease, and sympathetic ophthalmia, *Ophthalmology* 92:1025-1028, 1985.
26. Char DH, Ljung BM, Miller T, Phillips T: Primary intraocular lymphoma (ocular reticulum cell sarcoma) diagnosis and management, *Ophthalmology* 95:625-630, 1988.
27. Chester GH, Blach RK, Cleary PE: Inflammation in the region of the vitreous base. Pars planitis, *Trans Ophthalmol Soc UK* 96:151-157, 1976.
28. Chung H, Choi DG: Clinical analysis of uveitis, *Korean J Ophthalmol* 3:33-37, 1989.
29. Culbertson WW, Giles CL, West C, Stafford T: Familial pars planitis, *Retina* 3:179-181, 1983.
30. Davis JL, Chan CC, Nussenblatt RB: Immunology of intermediate uveitis, *Dev Ophthalmol* 23:71-85, 1992.
31. Davis JL, Mittal KK, Nussenblatt RB: HLA in intermediate uveitis, *Dev Ophthalmol* 23:35-37, 1992.
32. Davis JL, Palestine AG, Nussenblatt RB: Neovascularization in uveitis, *Ophthalmology* 95:171, 1988.
33. Davis JL, Solomon D, Nussenblatt RB et al.: Immunocytochemical staining of vitreous cells: indications, techniques, and results, *Ophthalmology* 99:250-256, 1992.
34. deSmet MD, Nussenblatt RB, Davis JL, Palestine AG: Large cell lymphoma masquerading as a viral retinitis, *Int Ophthalmol* 14:413-417, 1990.
35. deSmet MD, Yamamoto JH, Mochizuki M et al.: Cellular immune responses of patients with uveitis to retinal antigens and their fragments, *Am J Ophthalmol* 110:135-142, 1990.
36. Devenyi RG, Mieler WF, Lambrou FH et al.: Cryopexy of the vitreous base in the management of peripheral uveitis, *Am J Ophthalmol* 106:135-138, 1988.
37. Diamond JG, Kaplan HJ: Lensectomy and vitrectomy for complicated cataract secondary to uveitis, *Arch Ophthalmol* 96:1798-1804, 1978.
38. Dinning WJ: Intermediate uveitis: history, terminology, definition pars planitis: systemic disease associations, *Dev Ophthalmol* 23:3-8, 1992.
39. Doekes G, vanderGaag R, Rothova A et al.: Humoral and cellular immune responsiveness to human S-antigen in uveitis, *Curr Eye Res* 6:909-919, 1987.
40. Doft BH: Pars planitis in identical twins, *Retina* 3:32-33, 1983.
41. *Drug information for the health care professional,* The United States Pharmacopeia Convention, Rockville, MD, 1992.
42. Duinkerke-Eerola KU, Pinckers A, Cruysberg JRM: Pars planitis in father and son, *Ophthalmic Pediatr Genet* 11:305-308, 1990.
43. Dumonde DC, Kasp-Grochowska E, Graham E et al.: Anti-retinal autoimmunity and circulating immune complexes in patients with retinal vasculitis, *Lancet* ii:787-792, 1982.
44. Ellis GS, Pakalnis VA, Worley G et al.: *Toxocara canis* infestation: clinical and epidemiological associations with seropositivity in kindergarten children, *Ophthalmology* 93:1032-1037, 1986.
45. Engel HM, Green WR, Michels RG et al.: Diagnostic vitrectomy, *Retina* 1:121-149, 1981.
46. Engell T: Neurological disease activity in multiple sclerosis patients with periphlebitis retinae, *Acta Neurol Scand* 73:168-172, 1986.
47. Felder KS, Brockhurst RJ: Neovascular fundus abnormalities in peripheral uveitis, *Arch Ophthalmol* 100:750-754, 1982.
48. Forster RK, Abbott RL, Gelender H: Management of infectious endophthalmitis, *Ophthalmology* 87:313-319, 1980.
49. Foster CS, Fong LP, Singh G: Cataract surgery and intraocular lens implantation in patients with uveitis, *Ophthalmology* 96:281-287, 1989.
50. Freeman WR, Green RL, Smith RE: Echographic localization of corticosteroids after periocular injection, *Am J Ophthalmol* 103:281-288, 1987.
51. Gärtner J: The fine structure of vitreous base of the human eye and pathogenesis of pars planitis, *Am J Ophthalmol* 71:1317-1327, 1971.
52. Gärtner J: The vitreous base of the human eye and ''pars planitis'', *Mod Probl Ophthalmol* 10:250-255, 1972.
53. Gass JDM: Fluorescein angiography in endogenous intraocular inflammation. In Aronson SB, Gamble CN, Goodner EK, O'Connor GR, editors: *Clinical methods in uveitis,* St Louis, 1968, Mosby.
54. Gass JDM: *Stereoscopic atlas of macular disease: diagnosis and treatment,* St Louis, 1987, Mosby.
55. Giles CL: Pediatric intermediate uveitis, *J Pediatr Ophthalmol Strabismus* 26:136-139, 1989.
56. Giles CL, Tanton JH: Peripheral uveitis in three children of one family, *J Pediatr Ophthalmol Strabismus* 17:297-299, 1980.
57. Godfrey WA, Smith RE, Kimura SJ: Chronic cyclitis: corticosteroid therapy, *Trans Am Ophthalmol Soc* 74:178-188, 1976.

58. Graham EM, Francis DA, Sanders MD, Rudge P: Ocular inflammatory changes in established multiple sclerosis, *J Neurol Neurosurg Psychiatry* 52:1360-1363, 1989.

59. Green WR, Kincaid MC, Michels RG et al.: Pars planitis, *Trans Ophthalmol Soc UK* 101:361-367, 1981.

60. Guex-Crosier Y, Herbort CP: Maladie de Lyme en Suisse: atteintes oculaires, *Klin Monatsbl Augenheilkd* 200:545-546, 1992.

61. Hamel C, Bloch-Michel E, Offret M and associates: Fluorométrie et uvéite, *Ophthalmologie* 2:249-252, 1988.

62. Helm CJ, Holland GN: The effects of posterioir sub-Tenon injection of triamcinolone acetonide in patients with intermediate uveitis, *Am J Ophthalmol* 120:55-64, 1995.

63. Henderly DE, Genstler AJ, Smith RE, Rao NA: Changing patterns of uveitis, *Am J Ophthalmol* 103:131-136, 1987.

64. Henderly DE, Haymond RS, Rao NA, Smith RE: The significance of the pars plana exudate in pars planitis, *Am J Ophthalmol* 103:669-671, 1987.

65. Hikichi T, Trempe CL: Role of the vitreous in the prognosis of peripheral uveitis, *Am J Ophthalmol* 116:401-405, 1993.

66. Hirose S, Kuwabara T, Nussenblatt RB et al.: Uveitis induced in primates by interphotoreceptor retinoid-binding protein, *Arch Ophthalmol* 104:1698-1702, 1986.

67. Hogan MJ, Kimura SJ, O'Connor GR: Peripheral retinitis and chronic cyclitis in children, *Trans Ophthalmol Soc UK* 85:39-51, 1965.

68. Hooper PL, Rao NA, Smith RE: Cataract extraction in uveitis patients, *Surv Ophthalmol* 35:120-144, 1990.

69. Hultsch E: Peripheral uveitis in the owl monkey: experimental model, *Mod Probl Ophthalmol* 18:247-251, 1977.

70. Jabs DA, Green WR, Fox R et al.: Ocular manifestations of acquired immune deficiency syndrome, *Ophthalmology* 96:1092-1099, 1989.

71. Jabs DA, Johns CJ: Ocular involvement in chronic sarcoidosis, *Am J Ophthalmol* 102:297-301, 1986.

72. Kalina PH, Pach JM, Buettner H, Robertson DM: Neovascularization of the disc in pars planitis, *Retina* 10:269-273, 1990.

73. Kaplan HJ: Intermediate uveitis (pars planitis, chronic cyclitis)—A four step approach to treatment. In Saari KM, editor: *Uveitis update,* 169-172, Amsterdam, 1984, Excerpta Medica.

74. Kaplan HJ, Aaberg TM, Keller RH: Recurrent clinical uveitis: cell surface markers on vitreous lymphocytes, *Arch Ophthalmol* 100:585-587, 1982.

75. Kaplan HJ, Waldrep JC, Nicholson JKA, Gordon D: Immunologic analysis of intraocular mononuclear cell infiltrates in uveitis, *Arch Ophthalmol* 102:572-575, 1984.

76. Kaufman AH, Foster CS: Cataract extraction in patients with pars planitis, *Ophthalmology* 100:1210-1217, 1993.

77. Kenyon KR, Pederson JE, Green WR, Maumenee AE: Fibroglial proliferation in pars planitis, *Trans Ophthalmol Soc UK* 95:391-397, 1975.

78. Khodadoust AA, Attarzadeh A: Presumed autoimmune corneal endotheliopathy, *Am J Ophthalmol* 93:718-722, 1982.

79. Kimura SJ, Hogan MJ: Chronic cyclitis, *Trans Am Ophthalmol Soc* 61:397-413, 1963.

80. Knox DL: Syphilis and tuberculosis. In Ryan SJ, editor: *Retina,* 647-654, St Louis, 1989, Mosby.

81. Kuiper H, Koelman JHTM, Jager MJ: Vitreous clouding associated with Lyme borreliosis, *Am J Ophthalmol* 108:453-454, 1989.

82. Lightman S, Chan CC: Immune mechanisms in choroido-retinal inflammation in man, *Eye* 4:345-353, 1990.

83. Lütjen-Drecoll E: Morphology of the pars plana region, *Dev Ophthalmol* 23:50-59, 1992.

84. Mahlberg PA, Cunha-Vaz JG, Tessler HH: Vitreous fluorophotometry in pars planitis, *Am J Ophthalmol* 95:189-196, 1983.

85. Malinowski SM, Pulido JS, Folk JC: Long-term visual outcome and complications associated with pars planitis, *Ophthalmology* 100:818-824, 1993.

86. Malinowski SM, Pulido JS, Goeken NE et al.: The association of HLA-B8, B-51, DR2, and multiple sclerosis in pars planitis, *Ophthalmology* 100:1199-1205, 1993.

87. Martenet AC: A propos d'un terme nouveau dans le cadre uvéites: La "pars planitis", *Ophthalmologica* 147:282-290, 1964.

88. Martenet AC: Les cyclites chroniques, *Arch Ophtalmol* (Paris) 33:533-540, 1973.

89. Martenet AC: Uvéites intermédiares, *Bull Soc Belge Ophtalmol* 230:33-39, 1989.

90. Martenet AC: Unusual ocular lesions in AIDS, *Int Ophthalmol* 14:359-363, 1990.

91. Martenet AC: Diseases masquerading intermediate uveitis, *Dev Ophthalmol* 23:38-40, 1992.

92. Michels RG, Knox DL, Erozan YS, Green WR: Intraocular reticulum cell sarcoma. Diagnosis by pars plana vitrectomy, *Arch Ophthalmol* 93:1331-1335, 1975.

93. Michelson JB, Friedlaender MH, Nozik RA: Lens implant surgery in pars planitis, *Ophthalmology* 97:1023-1026, 1990.

94. Mieler WF, Will BR, Lewis H, Aaberg TM: Vitrectomy in the management of peripheral uveitis, *Ophthalmology* 95:859-864, 1988.

95. Mochizuki M, Watanabe T, Yamaguchi K et al.: Uveitis associated with human T-cell lymphotropic virus type I, *Am J Ophthalmol* 114:123-129, 1992.

96. Newell FW, Krill AE: Treatment of uveitis with azathioprine (Imuran), *Trans Ophthalmol Soc UK* 87:499-511, 1967.

97. Newell FW, Krill AE, Thomson A: The treatment of uveitis with six-mercaptopurine, *Am J Ophthalmol* 61:1250-1255, 1966.

98. Niessen F, Campinchi R, Bloch-Michel E: Etiology of endogenous uveitis in childhood, *Ber Dtsch Ophthalmol Ges* 78:209-213, 1981.

99. Nissenblatt MJ, Masciulli L, Yarian DL, Duvoisin R: Pars planitis—a demyelinating disease? *Arch Ophthalmol* 99:697, 1981.

100. Nölle B: Antiretinal autoantibodies in intermediate uveitis, *Dev Ophthalmol* 23:94-98, 1992.

101. Nölle B, Eckardt C: Cellular phenotype of vitreous cells in intermediate uveitis, *Dev Ophthalmol* 23:145-149, 1992.

102. Nölle B, Müller-Ruchholtz W: Fluorescent serology of the retina: patterns of retinal layer reactivity. In Secchi AG, Fregona IA, editors: *Modern trends in immunology and immunology of the eye,* 441-451, Milano, 1989, Masson.

103. Noye JF, George JL, Aymard B et al.: Evaluation des effets histopathologiques secondaires aux injections sous- conjonctivales de corticoïdes en formes immédiates et retard, *J Fr Ophtalmol* 12:587-594, 1989.

104. Nussenblatt RB, Palestine AG: *Uveitis, fundamentals and clinical practice,* Chicago, 1989, 104, Mosby.

105. Nussenblautt RB, Palestine AG: *Uveitis, fundamentals and clinical practice,* 188, Chicago, 1989, Mosby.

106. Nussenblautt RB, Palestine AG: *Uveitis, fundamentals and clinical practice,* 114, Chicago, 1989, Mosby.

107. Nussenblautt RB, Palestine AG: *Uveitis, fundamentals and clinical practice,* 106, 114, Chicago, 1989, Mosby.

108. Nussenblatt RB, Palestine AG: *Ciclosporin (Sandimmun®) therapy: experience in the treatment of pars planitis and present therapeutic guidelines,* Basel, 1992, Karger.

109. Nussenblatt RB, Palestine AG, Chan CC: Cyclosporine therapy for uveitis: long-term followup, *J Ocul Pharmacol* 1:369-382, 1985.

110. Nussenblatt RB, Salinas-Carmona M, Leake W, Scher I: T lymphocyte subsets in uveitis, *Am J Ophthalmol* 95:614-621, 1983.

111. Okinami S, Sunakawa M, Arai I et al.: Treatment of pars planitis with cryotherapy, *Ophthalmologica* 202:180-186, 1991.

112. Ortega C, Jimenez JM, Arellanes L, Angel E: Electrophysiologic changes in chronic pars planitis, *Invest Ophthalmol Vis Sci* 33:743, 1992.

113. Parver LM, Font RL: Malignant lymphoma of the retina and brain: initial diagnosis by cytologic examination of vitreous aspirate, *Arch Ophthalmol* 97:1505-1507, 1979.

114. Pruett RC, Brockhurst RJ, Letts NF: Fluorescein angiography of peripheral uveitis, *Am J Ophthalmol* 77:448-453, 1974.

115. Roberge F, Caspi R, Chan C et al.: Long term culture of Müller cells from adult rats in the presence of activated lymphocyte/monocyte products, *Curr Eye Res* 4:975-982, 1985.

116. Rockwood EJ, Zakov ZN, Bay JW: Combined malignant lymphoma of the eye and CNS (reticulum-cell sarcoma), *J Neurosurg* 61:369-374, 1984.

117. Rosenbaum JT, Wernick R: The utility of routine screening of patients with uveitis for systemic lupus erythematosus or tuberculosis: a Bayesian analysis, *Arch Ophthalmol* 108:1291-1293, 1990.

118. Rothova A, Alberts C, Glasius E et al.: Risk factors for ocular sarcoidosis, *Doc Ophthalmol* 72:287-296, 1989.

119. Schenck F, Böke W: Fluoreszenzangiographische Befunde bei intermediärer Uveitis, *Klin Monatsbl Augenheilkd* 193:261-265, 1988.

120. Schepens CL: L'inflammation de la région de l'"ora serrata" et ses séquelles, *Bull Soc Ophthalmol Fr* 73:113-124, 1950.

121. Schlaegel TF: *Ocular toxoplasmosis and pars planitis,* 263-360, New York, 1978, Grune and Stratton.

122. Schlaegel TF, Weber JC: Treatment of pars planitis. II. Corticosteroids, *Surv Ophthalmol* 22:120-130, 1977.

123. Schmidt F: Fluorescein angiography in intermediate uveitis, *Dev Ophthalmol* 23:139-144, 1992.

124. Schubert HD: Cystoid macular edema: the apparent role of mechanical factors, *Prog Clin Biol Res* 312:277-291, 1989.

125. Shields JA: Ocular toxocariasis: a review, *Surv Ophthalmol* 28:361-381, 1984.

126. Shorb SR, Irvine AR, Kimura SJ, Morris BW: Optic disc neovascularization associated with chronic uveitis, *Am J Ophthalmol* 82:175-178, 1976.

127. Siegel MJ, Dalton J, Friedman AH et al.: Ten-year experience with primary ocular 'reticulum cell sarcoma' (large cell non-Hodgkin's lymphoma), *Br J Ophthalmol* 73:342-346, 1989.

128. Slezak H, Kenyeres P: Vasoproliferative intermediäre Uveitis, *Klin Monatsbl Augenheilkd* 179:231-233, 1981.

129. Smith JL: Neuro-ocular Lyme borreliosis, *Neurol Clin* 9:35-53, 1991.

130. Smith RE: *Intermediate uveitis: pars planitis.* Proceedings of the World Uveitis Symposium, 251-257, Guarujá, Sao Paulo, 1989, Roca.

131. Smith RE: Intermediate uveitis: what is the significance of the pars plana exudate in 'pars planitis'?: a summary, *Dev Ophthalmol* 23:48-49, 1992.

132. Smith RE, Godfrey WA, Kimura SJ: Chronic cyclitis. I. Course and visual prognosis, *Trans Am Acad Ophthalmol Otolaryngol* 77:760-768, 1973.

133. Smith RE, Godfrey WA, Kimura SJ: Complications of chronic cyclitis, *Am J Ophthalmol* 82:277-282, 1976.

134. Tabbara K: Chlorambucil in Behçet's disease: a reappraisal, *Ophthalmology* 90:906-908, 1983.

135. Tamesis RR, Foster CS: Ocular syphilis, *Ophthalmology* 97:1281-1287, 1990.

136. Tessler HH: Pars planitis and autoimmune endotheliopathy, *Am J Ophthalmol* 103:599, 1987 (letter).

137. Tetsuka S, Katsumi O, Mehta MC et al.: Electrophysiological findings in peripheral uveitis, *Ophthalmologica* 203:89-98, 1991.

138. Towler HMA, Whiting PH, Forrester JV: Combination low dose cyclosporin A and steroid therapy in chronic intraocular inflammation, *Eye* 4:514-520, 1990.

139. Vadot E: Epidemiology of intermediate uveitis: a prospective study in Savoy, *Dev Ophthalmol* 23:33-34, 1992.

140. Verma L, Kumar A, Garg S et al.: Cryopexy in pars planitis, *Can J Ophthalmol* 26:313-315, 1991.

141. Wacker WB, Donoso LA, Kalsow CM et al.: Experimental allergic uveitis: isolation, characterization, and localization of a soluble uveitopathogenic antigen from bovine retina, *J Immunology* 119:1949-1958, 1977.

142. Wakefield D, McCluskey P, Penny R: Intravenous pulse methylprednisolone therapy in severe inflammatory eye disease, *Arch Ophthalmol* 104:847-851, 1986.

143. Wan WL, Cano MR, Pince KJ, Green RL: Echographic characteristics of ocular toxocariasis, *Ophthalmology* 98:28-32, 1991.

144. Webb RM, Tabbara KF, O'Connor GR: Retinal vasculitis in ocular toxoplasmosis in nonhuman primates, *Retina* 4:182-188, 1984.

145. Weiner A, BenEzra D: Clinical patterns and associated conditions in chronic uveitis, *Am J Ophthalmol* 112:151-159, 1991.

146. Welch RB, Maumenee AE, Wahlen HR: Peripheral posterior segment inflammation, vitreous opacities and edema of the posterior pole: pars planitis, *Arch Ophthalmol* 64:540-549, 1960.

147. Wetzig RP, Chan CC, Nussenblatt RB et al.: Clinical and immunopathological studies of pars planitis in a family, *Br J Ophthalmol* 72:5-10, 1988.

148. Wilson DJ, Braziel R, Rosenbaum JT: Intraocular lymphoma. Immunopathologic analysis of vitreous biopsy specimens, *Arch Ophthalmol* 110:1455-1458, 1992.

149. Winward KE, Hamed LM, Glaser JS: The spectrum of optic nerve disease in human immunodeficiency virus infection, *Am J Ophthalmol* 107:373-380, 1989.

150. Witmer VR, Körner G: Uveitis im Kindesalter, *Ophthalmologica* 152:277-282, 1966.

151. Wolf MD, Mieler WF: Retinal detachment after cryotherapy for peripheral uveitis, *Ophthalmology* 99:100, 1992.

152. Wong VG: Imunosuppressive therapy of ocular inflammatory diseases, *Arch Ophthalmol* 81:628-637, 1969.

153. Yokoyama MM, Matsui Y, Yamashiroya HM et al.: Humoral and cellular immunity studies in patients with Vogt-Koyanagi-Harada syndrome and pars planitis, *Invest Ophthalmol Vis Sci* 20:364-370, 1981.

154. Yoser SL, Forster DJ, Rao NA: Pathology of intermediate uveitis, *Dev Ophthalmol* 23:60-70, 1992.

155. Zierhut M, Foster CS: Multiple sclerosis, sarcoidosis and other diseases in patients with pars planitis, *Dev Ophthalmol* 23:41-47, 1992.

156. Zimmerman LE, Silverstein AM: Experimental ocular hypersensitivity: histopathologic changes observed in rabbits receiving a single injection of antigen into the vitreous, *Am J Ophthalmol* 48:447-465, 1959.

157. Zimmerman MD, Dawson WW, Fitzgerald CR: Part I: electroretinographic changes in normal eyes during administration of prednisone, *Ann Ophthalmol* 5:757-765, 1973.

56 Multiple Sclerosis

ROBERT C. SERGOTT, ROY W. BECK, ROBERT P. LISAK,
ANTHONY C. ARNOLD

Multiple sclerosis (MS) is a confounding disease in terms of its pathogenesis and clinical course. Debates about the cause of MS have invoked viral hypotheses, genetic theories, and cell-mediated, antibody-induced, and cytokine-amplified immune reactions. Most investigations postulate a role for an aberrant immunologic response, but the etiology of MS has so far eluded the unravelling of its origins.

EPIDEMIOLOGY

Multiple sclerosis is most common among white people living in the Northern United States, Canada, Europe, and southern Australia[165]; however, some geographic and genetic populations, such as the Bantu, Inuit, Hungarian Gypsy, and Mongolian ethnic groups, rarely develop optic neuritis and MS.

World War II provided two unplanned epidemiologic studies about MS. The United States Congress legislated that MS was a "service-connected" illness when the symptoms of demyelination developed during World War II or up to 7 years after discharge. Because of this legislation, the 16.5 million Americans serving in World War II and the 5 million involved in the Korean conflict were followed meticulously in terms of the development of central nervous system (CNS) disease. Kurtzke, Beebe, and Norman[168] identified 5305 "service-connected" MS cases that were compared to the military control group in terms of age, dates of military service, and survival.[166,168] This analysis showed that military personnel from states at or above the 37° of latitude had a higher incidence of MS compared to soldiers from states below 37° latitude. A gradient of high prevalence (30 cases per 100,000) at more northern latitudes to lower prevalence (20 per 100,000) at more southern latitudes was found for individuals living within a specific area until age 15. But if a person moved before age 15, he assumed the risk of the new location.[65,169]

The unlikely geographic location of the Faeroe Islands, a small land cluster off the coast of Iceland, provided the set-ting for the second unplanned MS epidemiologic experiment of World War II. This small chain of islands between Iceland and Norway was of strategic importance for North Atlantic shipping; and on April 13, 1940, 4 days after Denmark fell to the German blitzkrieg, the British occupied the Faeroes. Prior to 1939, inhabitants of the Faeroes were said to have no MS. Between 1943 and 1960, however, 24 inhabitants of the Faeroes developed MS. This outbreak of MS fulfilled the requirements of a "point source" epidemic traceable to an event before 1943. The British occupation was the only unusual event that could be identified, and it was concluded that the troops in someway "brought" MS to the Faeroes where it affected a genetically susceptible Scandinavian ethnic group. Kurtzke and Hyllested[170,171] have extended their initial observations in the Faeroes and believe the data are consistent with MS being an infectious transmissible disease.[170,171] Lending some additional support to the infectious disease theory is the fact that only one case of MS has been documented in the Faeroes since 1960. Kurtzke and associates[165-171] believe that a virus is the likely infectious agent. It is possible, however, that an infectious agent such as a parasite or bacterium is localized at another anatomic site, and the CNS demyelination represents a secondary immunologic attack.

Epidemiologic data have also implicated a genetic influence for developing MS. Despite the latitude of 43° and 42° north, Sapparo, Japan, has a MS prevalence rate of 2 per 100,000 compared to Boston, Massachusetts with a rate of 44 per 100,000. Therefore, the Oriental genotype was thought to have limited the MS prevalence, despite the similar latitude as the northeastern United States.

Two racially and genetically well-differentiated subpopulations were studied in Hungary. The native white Hungarian population demonstrated a 37 per 100,000 MS prevalence, the rate expected at that latitude. In comparison, only two cases of MS have been identified in the Gypsy population that migrated to Hungary from Northern India.[236]

CLINICAL FEATURES

Multiple Sclerosis

A detailed description of the signs and symptoms of MS along with the clinical course is outside the scope of this chapter.[211] A few general statements may prove useful for consideration of different proposed treatments. The clinical manifestations are related to involvement of CNS myelin, which is found predominantly in white matter. The symptoms and signs are also the result of loss of normal function of myelin, either from actual demyelination or effects of cytokines or other factors (such as antibodies) on myelin and axonal function at the nodes of Ranvier. Negative symptoms such as weakness, ataxia, loss of normal perception of sensation, diplopia, and increased tone (spasticity) secondary to loss of normal inhibitory influences from higher centers result from conduction block, slow conduction, and temporal dispersion (lack of synchronous conduction by adjacent nerve fibers). Positive symptoms such as paresthesias, dysesthesias, and paroxysmal attacks result from impulse reflection, stimulation of adjacent fibers (cross talk), ectopic impulse generation, and increased mechanosensitivity.[362]

As noted from the earliest pathologic reports and confirmed by modern magnetic resonance imaging (MRI) studies, there are many more lesions than clinical attacks, symptoms, and signs.[240] Although there are clearly prognostic factors, there is no single (or even multivariant) analysis that predicts the clinical course in individual patients, especially over the relatively short periods of time involved in well-controlled (and even most poorly controlled) clinical trials.[211,365] The relatively benign course in thc long term for many patients as well as in the short run for a large percentage of patients makes toxic and life-threatening therapies inappropriate. Such treatment should certainly be limited to a small population of patients and to agents shown to be effective in prospective, randomized, placebo-controlled trials.

Optic Neuritis

Because of its frequency, its possible poor visual outcome, and its role as a harbinger to widespread MS, optic neuritis is the most important demyelinating syndrome for ophthalmologists. Neuropathologic specimens fail to show any difference between the histopathology of optic neuritis compared to demyelination in the brain and spinal cord.

The diagnosis of optic neuritis rests on clinical grounds.[243] Thus an understanding of the expected clinical profile is imperative. Patients developing isolated (or MS-related) optic neuritis are usually between the ages of 15 and 45 years. Females are affected more commonly than males by a ratio of about 3 : 1. In children developing optic neuritis, the pathogenesis is often related to a viral syndrome rather than a primary demyelinating disease. Although optic neuritis can occur in adults older than 45 years, it is sufficiently uncommon that unless a patient has previously been diagnosed as having multiple sclerosis, other causes of optic neuropathy must be investigated and ruled out before a diagnosis of demyelinative optic neuritis is considered.

The tempo of visual loss and recovery is a key feature of the disorder. Typically, visual loss is sudden and may progress for several days. Progression for a longer period of time is possible but should make the clinician suspicious of an alternative cause. Pain is present to some degree in more than 90% of patients. It may precede or occur concurrently with visual loss, usually is exacerbated by eye movement, and generally lasts no more than a few days. In most cases the visual loss is monocular but in a small percentage of cases both eyes will be simultaneously affected.

Examination of the patient with acute optic neuritis will demonstrate evidence of optic nerve dysfunction. Visual acuity is reduced in most cases but varies from a mild reduction to severe loss (no light perception is possible). Color vision and contrast sensitivity are impaired in almost all cases, often out of proportion to acuity. Even when visual acuity is 20/20 or better, these measures are abnormal in more than 90% of cases.[232]

Almost any type of visual field defect is possible with optic neuritis.[156] In most cases there is at least some degree of central field loss commensurate with the decrease in visual acuity; however, the classically described field change of a central scotoma with an intact peripheral field is present in only a minority of patients.[156,232] Field defects (including altitudinal type defects) occur in a nerve fiber bundle distribution with sufficient frequency to limit the value of the field loss pattern in differentiating between optic neuritis and anterior ischemic optic neuropathy. Even unilateral hemianopic defects can occur in optic neuritis without evidence of apparent chiasmal involvement.[156]

A relative afferent pupillary defect will be detectable in almost all unilateral cases. If such a defect is not present, a preexisting optic neuropathy in the fellow eye should be suspected.

The optic disc may appear normal (retrobulbar neuritis) or swollen (papillitis) in the acute phase (Table 56-1). Clinical features are similar in both forms, including the expected course and the response to corticosteroid treatmcnt.[21,232]

Retinal Vasculitis and Retinitis

Retinal venous "sheathing," originally described by Rucker[280] in 1944, encompasses both active periphlebitis and chronic venous sclerosis.[13] It has been reported in 10% to 36% of MS cases studied clinically.[19,84,340] The periphlebitic lesion appears as a focal whitish or yellowish opacity with feathered margins, obscuring or surrounding a length of vein wall, often located equatorially in the retina (Fig. 56-1). There may be associated constriction and dilation of the veins, with occasional retinal hemorrhage. In up to 35% of acute cases, the lesion may focally extend into the overlying

TABLE 56-1 CHARACTERISTICS OF PATIENTS WITH ACUTE OPTIC NEURITIS (Experience of the Optic Neuritis Treatment Trial)

Characteristic	
Female gender	77%
Age (mean ± SD)	31.8 ± 6.7
Ocular pain	92%
Worsened by eye movement	87%
Visual acuity	
20/40 or better	35%
20/50‑20/190	29%
20/200 or worse	36%
Optic disc swollen	35%
Patterns of visual field loss	
Diffuse	48%
Central/centrocecal	8%
Altitudinal/arcuate	18%
Hemianopic	4%
Other	22%
Fellow eye abnormalities	
Visual acuity	14%
Contrast sensitivity	16%
Color vision	22%
Visual field	48%
MRI of brain abnormal	49%

vitreous; these lesions have been termed ''Rucker bodies.''[281] Focal whitish lesions of the retina, isolated from periphlebitic lesions and consistent with inflammation, have also been described. The chronic form of sheathing appears typically as dense, white linear stripes following the course of a longer portion of vein; in some cases, thickening or obscuring the vessel wall (Fig. 56-2). Most authorities feel

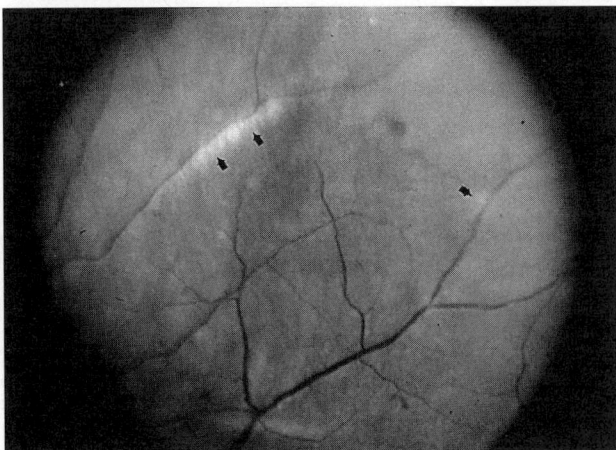

Fig. 56-1. Fundus photograph, active periphlebitis, showing focal regions *(arrows)* of fluffy perivenous infiltrate. (Photo courtesy of Dr. Ronald Klein.)

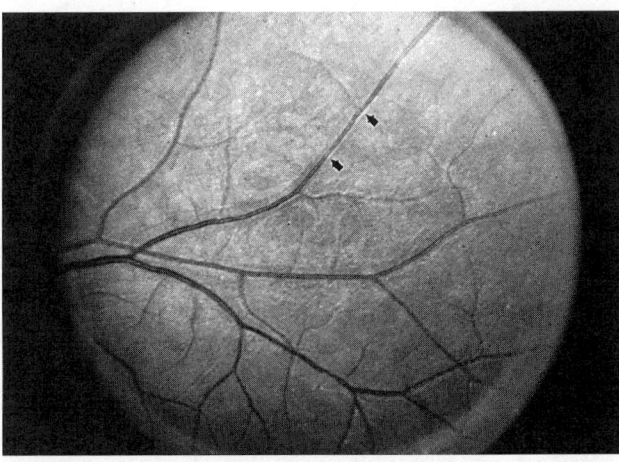

Fig. 56-2. Fundus photograph, with chronic venous sclerosis, showing linear white opacity *(arrows)* along vein wall. Focal narrowing and irregularity of vein caliber is seen. (Photo courtesy of Dr. Brian Younger.)

that venous sclerosis is the result of persistent inflammation. Retinal arteriolar involvement has not been consistently documented clinically; visible sheathing has not been reported, although one case of arteriolar occlusion, located in a region of concurrent venous involvement, has been described.[244]

Periphlebitis in MS is not clearly associated with optic neuritis, systemic exacerbations, or severity of disease. It typically is mild, transient, and not secondary to active uveitis. It differs from that seen with pars planitis and Eales disease in that it may be more posteriorly located and is only rarely associated with macular edema[19] or severe retinal vascular occlusive disease, with neovascularization and its sequelae.[359] It does not assume the ''candlewax drippings'' appearance observed in sarcoidosis. When seen in conjunction with isolated optic neuritis, it does appear to predict a significantly higher rate of development of MS. In one series, periphlebitis was seen in 28% of 50 cases of isolated optic neuritis; of them, 57% had developed other clinical evidence of MS by the mean follow-up of 3.5 years, compared to 16% of subjects without sheathing.[181]

Fluorescein angiography of active periphlebitis demonstrates delayed filling, persistence of dye, staining, and leakage from affected vessels; all indicating both flow impedance and breakdown of the blood-retinal barrier (BBB).[377] Some vessels show staining or leakage in regions without visible periphlebitis. Venous sclerosis may show either late staining or normal appearance on angiography. Immunopathologic studies similarly have revealed abnormal vascular permeability, both in areas of visible infiltrates and those that appear clinically normal.[13] The fluorescein and immunopathologic data suggest that vein wall abnormalities are more widespread than detectable clinically. Although it is suspected, there is not clear documentation of the evolution of periphlebitis to sclerosis.

Histopathologic studies have confirmed that the sheathing in MS represents periphlebitis in the active phase[13] and venous sclerosis in the chronic phase.[314] The periphlebitis consists of a lymphoplasmacytic infiltrate within and surrounding vein walls (Fig. 56-3), occasionally showing granulomatous characteristics. Venous sclerosis is characterized by hyalinization of the vein wall with material consistent with laminated collagen; cellular infiltrate is minimal. The appearance of both lesions corresponds to that seen in CNS perivenular lesions in MS.[4] In the most comprehensive study of the active lesions,[13] seven eyes with active periphlebitis were studied in detail. Five had no evidence of associated uveitis, and two of three cases with meningeal evaluation showed no visible cellular reaction there, indicating that the retinal lesions were not a secondary phenomenon to other inflammation. Sections through retinal lesions consistent with the isolated white inflammatory foci seen clinically revealed similar chronic infiltrates in the inner retina and overlying vitreous in three cases (Fig. 56-4), one of which showed granulomatous features. One case of periarteriolar inflammation was documented. The presence of perivenous and retinal inflammation in tissue without myelin has prompted investigation as to the inciting antigenic stimulus, particularly as it may relate to the pathogenesis of MS.[201] Immunocytologic studies performed on retinal tissue from autopsy cases of MS have shown no herpes simplex, varicella-zoster, or cytomegalovirus antigens. Immunoperoxidase studies did, however, show cross-reactivity between myelin-associated glycoprotein and Müller cells. Additionally, tissue-bound IgG, IgA, and IgM were demonstrated on retinal ganglion cells of patients with MS, although not directly correlated with detectable periphlebitis or retinitis. The studies suggest that a retinal target tissue other than myelin, but with cross-reactive properties, may be involved in the immune response in MS.

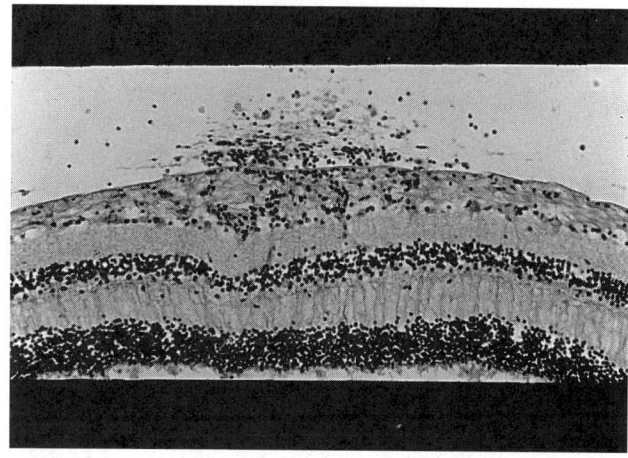

Fig. 56-4.   Photomicrograph of retina in case of retinitis, showing similar infiltrate involving the inner retina and overlying vitreous (Hematoxylin-eosin ×250). (Photo courtesy of Dr. Robert Foos.)

Uveitis

Uveitis is more common in patients with MS than in the general population, but the incidence varies widely (2.4% to 27%) between reports, attributable to varying patient populations, examination techniques, and criteria for diagnosis.[19,41,119,248] Peripheral uveitis is most commonly described, ranging from mild vitreous cellular reaction to overt pars planitis; in most cases, the inflammatory process is mild, without associated macular edema or peripheral retinal neovascularization, and does not require therapy. The relation of uveitis activity to the course of MS exacerbations is unclear; although many authors noted intraocular inflammation most frequently associated with active CNS disease[83,119]; others have not seen a consistent correlation.[10,19] The HLA-DR2 antigen, strongly associated with MS, is associated with pars planitis as well.[204]

Although anterior chamber reaction is commonly (40% to 67%) seen with peripheral uveitis in MS,[16,41,248] it rarely has been noted without posterior involvement. In two recent reports, however, anterior granulomatous uveitis has been documented as the prominent inflammatory finding,[182] in some cases preceding general neurologic involvement or diagnosis of MS.

Eye Movement Abnormalities

Internuclear ophthalmoplegia (INO) is the most common eye movement abnormality and the most common cause of diplopia in MS, occurring in 53% of cases in one report.[285] The syndrome, which results from involvement of the medial longitudinal fasciculus (MLF) in the demyelinative process, classically includes impaired adduction of the eye ipsilateral to the MLF lesion, with dissociated nystagmus of the contralateral eye ("abduction nystagmus"). The adduction deficit may be manifest as a limitation of range, but in less severe cases may show only slowing of adducting saccades, with full ocular versions. Nystagmus in the abducting eye is

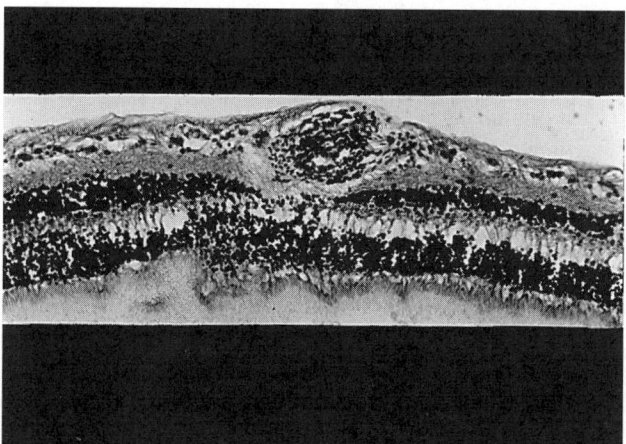

Fig. 56-3.   Photomicrograph of retina in case of active periphlebitis, with lymphoplasmacytic infiltration of vein wall (Hematoxylin-eosin ×250). (Photo courtesy of Dr. Robert Foos.)

a horizontal, jerk form, with fast phase laterally, and may be associated with a milder gaze-evoked nystagmus of the weakened adducting eye. Overshooting of abducting saccades (dysmetria) may be seen on eye movement recordings.[18] Quantitative eye movement analysis has documented frequencies of occurrence for the four characteristic abnormalities: (1) slowed adducting saccades in 100%, (2) limited adducting range in 58%, (3) dissociated nystagmus in 91%, and (4) dysmetria in 82%.[61] Subtle abnormalities of saccadic velocity might not be detected by simple clinical tests of ocular versions; evaluation of voluntary saccades, optokinetic nystagmus, or quantitative saccadic velocity measurements may be required to demonstrate the lag of ipsilateral adducting saccades behind corresponding contralateral abducting movements. In some cases, medial rectus function may be spared in convergence; it has been suggested that this finding localizes the lesion more caudally in the MLF and may aid in the distinction of INO from partial oculomotor palsy. Although most cases of bilateral INO are related to MS,[57] demyelination is a common cause of unilateral involvement as well (38% of the series of Crane and associates; 1983); conversely, ischemia, usually reported as the most common cause of unilateral INO, produces bilateral involvement in a significant percentage of cases.

Additional eye movement abnormalities, such as skew deviation and upgaze maintenance weakness with gaze-evoked nystagmus, may be the result solely of MLF lesions and do not necessarily imply a multifocal neurologic process; similarly, associated abducens or conjugate gaze paresis may be the result of a single lesion and does not confirm multiple foci of involvement. Other lesions of the brainstem and cerebellar oculomotor pathways, however, are commonly seen in MS and may produce a variety of nonspecific eye movement abnormalities. Nystagmus has been reported in up to 67% of patients with MS, and may be gaze-evoked jerk nystagmus, pendular, or torsional. Saccadic abnormalities, fixation instability, and impaired pursuit and visuo-vestibular interactions all may relate to lesions in the cerebellum or brainstem. Although MS is a relatively uncommon cause of cranial nerve palsies, the frequency of this cause increases in younger patients. Abducens involvement is most common, followed in frequency by oculomotor palsy; trochlear lesions are rare.[151,286]

PATHOLOGY

The hallmark neuropathologic lesion of MS is demyelination of central nervous system axons.[53,54] Myelin sheaths in the CNS exhibit bilamellar glycolysed membranes concentrically surrounding axon cylinders. The myelin sheath is elaborated and maintained by the oligodendrocyte, a specific glial cell within the CNS, as an extension and modification of its plasma membrane. Numerous cytoplasmic "arms" extend from the oligodendrocyte cell body, encircle the axon with a tongue of cytoplasm termed the "internal meraxon," and envelope the axons with myelin. Compared to the peripheral nervous system (PNS), where myelin-producing Schwann cells subserve an individual internode of a single axon, oligodendrocytes connect with numerous axons, some of which are frequently a considerable distance away from the oligodendrocyte cell body. The segment of myelin along an axon produced by a single oligodendrocyte is termed the "internode." At the termination of the internode, a specialized histologic region of astrocyte foot plates attach to the axon leading to an unmyelinated segment called the node of Ranvier.

MS is considered a "primary" demyelinating disease. The classification primary means that the myelin is damaged and destroyed without disruption of the axon. In "secondary" demyelinating disease, the axon is the initial site of injury and the myelin is disrupted as a consequence of the axonal pathology. In primary demyelinating diseases, axonal loss may occur, but generally axons are spared in the typical MS lesion or "plaque."

Within the brain, plaques are found preferentially in the periventricular regions adjacent to the lateral and fourth ventricles in over 90% of MS cases.[202] In the brain, spinal cord, and optic nerve, plaques often encircle a small vein (venule), a relationship that extends along the longitudinal course of venules as shown by serial histopathologic sections.[88,89]

Although the hallmark lesion in MS is one of demyelination, secondary axonal loss is seen, especially in long-standing lesions. The MS plaque contains demyelinated axons, with varying degrees of axonal loss.[251,252] Although the gliosis has been attributed to actual astrocyte proliferation, there is no evidence that astrocytes proliferate; however, they enlarge and become very prominent, and the amount of glial fibrillary acidic protein (GFAP) increases. Oligodendrocytes are reduced in number in many of the plaques.[251,261] In other areas, especially at the periphery of lesions, there seems to be an increase in the number of oligodendrocytes.[253,261] It is not clear if this increase represents proliferation of remaining mature oligodendrocytes or proliferation of oligodendrocyte precursors.[254,258,261] There is still controversy as to whether the initial lesion is an attack on myelin[258] or the oligodendrocyte.[274]

The other important feature of the MS lesion is the presence of inflammatory cells, with mononuclear cells, lymphocytes, and monocyte/macrophages making up the vast majority.[251] The inflammatory cells are prominently located in a perivascular pattern, although studies using monoclonal antibodies demonstrate lymphocytes in the parenchyma at the leading edge of the areas of demyelination and some cells in areas of myelin that show no evidence of demyelination.[34,118,345] Macrophages are found in lesions and can be shown to be ingesting myelin.[251] It is not known if the macrophages are (1) simply ingesting myelin damaged by a nonimmunopathologic process or a macrophage-independent immunopathologic process, or (2) actively involved in the immunologic process demonstrated in certain antibody-mediated or cell-mediated immune mechanisms. The presence of "coated pits" may indicate that some of the macrophage activity relates to direct involvement of these cells in an antibody-triggered reaction.[252] It is possible, even probable, the macrophages present in the lesions are participating in several immune and nonspecific phagocytic reactions. In addition to macrophage involvement in the pathologic process, it is also likely that microglia, which probably originate from narrow cells during development, are also participants in the development of the MS lesion. These cells have many similarities to other cells of the monocyte/macrophage lineage (see the following).

Because isolated optic neuritis and MS have identical light and electron microscopic features, it has been postulated that optic neuritis is a limited form of MS.[167] This relationship is supported by the observation that 13% to 85% of patients with an episode of isolated optic neuritis eventually develop MS. The relationship between optic neuritis and MS can be approached electrophysiologically, as more than 50% of MS patients will have delayed visually evoked responses.[299] Neuroradiologic observations further support the interrelationship of MS and optic neuritis, with 58% of patients with isolated optic neuritis demonstrating abnormal magnetic resonance imaging.[137,143]

For years it was widely held that although remyelination occurs in the peripheral nervous system, it does not occur within the CNS. This theory was frequently ascribed to differences in the capacity to remyelinate of the Schwann cell in the PNS when compared to the oligodendrocyte in the CNS. Although the PNS remyelination might not be totally normal, it was sufficient to allow for recovery from disorders of the PNS, such as Guillain-Barré syndrome, as long as there was not too much secondary axonal degeneration. The lack of CNS remyelination was held to explain residual deficits in MS, even when there was not extensive secondary axonal degeneration. It is now clear that some attempts at remyelination do occur in the CNS in MS, although they are incomplete.[252,258,261] Most of this remyelination is oligodendrocyte-produced myelin, although Schwann cells also contribute to this remyelination at entry and exit zones in the spinal cord and elsewhere.[251,252] As it now seems certain that oligodendrocytes can remyelinate to some extent, the question is why they do not do so to a clinically useful degree. One difference could still be that the Schwann cell, which is a simpler cell responsible for the myelination of one internode of one axon in the PNS, is more capable of remyelination. A second factor is that in MS, the most common demyelinating disease of the CNS, the oligodendrocyte and its myelin are under repeated or constant immunologic assault. In Guillain-Barré syndrome the subsidence of a single immunopathologic event leaves the remaining Schwann cells

and Schwann cell precursors able to remyelinate. In chronic inflammatory demyelinating neuropathy (CIDP), constant immunomodulatory therapy is necessary in two thirds to three quarters of patients to prevent further demyelination as well as further axonal damage. In MS there is no effective immunomodulatory therapy to prevent recurrent or chronic damage to CNS myelin. Whether the gliosis resulting from astrocytic hypertrophy inhibits remyelination attempts in MS is controversial. Interestingly, a component of CNS myelin is able to inhibit neurite outgrowth,[298] but Schwann cells allow for neurite outgrowth.

It is also not known what occurs at the tissue level to cause an exacerbation. In the era before MRI and evoked responses, it was assumed that an exacerbation was due to a new lesion when the exacerbation was manifested by a new symptom or sign. Worsening or a relapse with reappearance of old signs was thought an extension of an old lesion. It is now clear that some exacerbations representative of clinically new areas of disease can be related to lesions already present on MRI scan or evoked potentials. Some of the symptoms may be from inflammatory mediators and edema, especially early in an exacerbation before extensive demyelination (with or without axonal damage) can occur. Recovery from exacerbations is also not well understood. It seems unlikely that rapid remyelination, which is so often incomplete, can explain the frequently rapid recovery seen in some exacerbations. Inhibitory cytokines may block the effect of the more proinflammatory cytokines (see Cytokines and Mononuclear Cell Subsets), and repair of the blood brain barrier (BBB), which unfortunately is not permanent, may also lead to symptomatic improvement, as toxic and demyelinating factors no longer have free access to the CNS parenchyma. The symptomatology of exacerbations could partly represent (1) edema related to new or increased inflammation or (2) pathophysiologic effects of antibodies to myelin/oligodendrocytes or of cytokines that do not cause demyelination but cause pathophysiologic changes (especially in an already partly demyelinated area of CNS). A combination of these may cause deterioration in CNS function.

Many investigators have attempted to distinguish between "early" and "late" histopathologic lesions in the hope of deciphering the initial pathophysiologic insult in MS. The differentiation between "early" and "late" depends totally on retrospective clinical and pathologic correlation, a difficult (if not impossible) task, as an acute MS lesion is rarely complicated by sudden death. Patients with acute MS who progress to early death (Marburg and other variants) are sometimes used as a model of the acute lesion of classical relapsing-remitting MS, but this reasoning may not be totally appropriate. In addition, a lesion arbitrarily termed "early" may not necessarily be "early" in relationship to the initiation of myelin damage.

PATHOGENESIS

Epidemiologic data have provided the strongest current evidence that an infectious agent is involved in the pathogenesis of MS. A virus has been thought the likely pathogen, and several studies have reported slightly elevated antibody titers to measles virus in the serum and CSF of patients with MS.[94,115] Elevated serum and CSF titers to other viruses such as mumps, herpes simplex, and rubella have been reported in MS patients.[221,223] But the significance of these elevated titers is uncertain, as an individual patient may have increased antibody titers to more than one virus reflecting polyclonal B-cell activation.

Viruses and Multiple Sclerosis

The hypothesis that MS has an infectious cause is not new. Bacteria, including spirochetes, and viruses have been considered. Reports of (1) elevated antibody titers in serum and CSF to particular viruses; (2) abnormally low in vitro cell-mediated immune responses to different candidate viruses; (3) cytopathic effect in CNS cultures incubated with MS tissue extracts, (4) passive transfer to experimental animals, (5) viral-like particle inclusions seen with immunohistochemistry or electron microscopy, and (6) presence of viral genomic material employing modern molecular biologic techniques abound in the literature.[35,64,147] Invariably these reports cannot be confirmed by different laboratories or are found not to be specific for MS. Viral studies are often done with tissue obtained at autopsy as many as 20 to 40 years after onset of the disease. In addition, if epidemiologic data claiming exposure to the triggering environmental factor occurs even earlier (prior to or during the second decade of life) are correct, it may not be surprising that viruses cannot be isolated at autopsy.

Several animal models of MS following viral infections after a latent period are mediated by an immunologic reaction either to the virus or to a CNS antigen in which viruses either are undetectable or are present in very low titer during the immune/demyelinating reaction.[64] It is possible that a viral infection could infect cells within the CNS and form a neoantigen. A viral infection could also have some of its DNA incorporated into the CNS cell genome, resulting in the expression of the viral protein or other antigen by the CNS cell, making the CNS cell a target for an immunologic reaction.

Another mechanism would be an immune reaction against a viral antigen that shares sequences with oligodendrocyte/myelin. Antibodies or cell-mediated immunity would then develop against the cross-reactive epitope. This phenomenon is called molecular mimicry.[97,139,193,239] Several sequences of viruses have strong homology with nervous system components.[97,98] It is also possible that a viral infection could serve as adjuvant or otherwise activate lymphocytes that enter the CNS and by chance happen to include cells that express a myelin antigen. Those cells could then

remain to trigger an immunopathologic reaction in the CNS. Certainly acute disseminated encephalomyelitis (ADEM) can result from viral infections or immunizations, even with killed viruses, in which there is no evidence for even a transient CNS infection.[59,148,188]

It is of some interest that transgenic mice made to carry the appropriate T cell receptor gene and HLA develop spontaneous experimental allergic encephalomyelitis (EAE) if they are kept in an open colony, but not if they are kept in a germ-free environment with little or no exposure to infectious agents that could serve as pathogens or activators of the immune system.[109] These observations are certainly compatible with an infection triggering an acute monophasic inflammatory/demyelinating disorder such as acute disseminated encephalomyelitis, the first attack of MS, and/or an exacerbation of MS. There seems to be a statistically significant association between a recent viral illness and exacerbations of MS,[237,317,319] in contradistinction to physical trauma in which such associations have not been demonstrated.[318,324]

A transient infection of the nervous system could release a nervous system (NS) antigen and stimulate a reaction directed at the nervous system (NS)[135,193] even if the virus is no longer present in the NS or present in extremely low copy. It is clear that the late demyelinating phase of infection of certain strains of mice with certain strains of Thieler virus, which in the acute phase causes a polioencephalomyelitis, is immunologically mediated.[64] It has also been shown that lymphocytes obtained from the CNS of rats with a coronovirus have myelin basic protein reactive cells that can in turn passively transfer EAE to naive animals in the absence of transferring the triggering viral infection.[361] It is also possible there is a persistent infection of the CNS with an unidentified virus, perhaps in an incomplete form, that serves as a stimulus for the immune system, which in an attempt to destroy or otherwise control the virus, also injures the host cell (such as an oligodendrocyte) with its myelin.[370]

Attempts to identify a specific virus in the CNS of patients with MS using molecular biologic techniques have failed to define a causative agent.[35,147] Although there is a possibility that a direct infection of the CNS with a virus (including a retrovirus) is directly responsible for MS, the initial serologic and molecular biologic studies[110,161,226,263] as well as other studies have not confirmed HTLV-1 as an etiologic agent.[197,249,267] Retroviruses, however, are attractive candidate viruses,[56] as several of them can cause neurologic disease with involvement of white matter/myelin, including HTLV-1,[102,164,235,275] and HIV in humans.[250] There is no question that there are naturally occurring chronic inflammatory/demyelinating diseases of animals and humans strongly associated with a viral cause, including ''tropical spastic paraparesis'' caused HTLV-1 and some CNS manifestations of HIV infection. There is evidence in these two disorders that some of the pathology is not the result of direct viral-induced oligodendrocyte damage, but rather is the result of cytokine or other immune mediator-induced damage. Cytokines are able to directly affect glial cells of the CNS and PNS, including TNF-α, which can cause in vitro demyelination.[305] These cytokines are found in MS lesions and certainly support a major role for cell-mediated immunity in the pathogenesis of MS.[258] The question is whether the stimulus for the immune reaction is directly or indirectly caused by a virus or whether it is triggered to an autoantigen independent of any viral infections, systemic or localized to the CNS.

Humoral Immunity

Much of the early work on the immunopathogenesis of MS centered on the humoral portion of the immune system, that is, antibodies to myelin and/or oligodendrocytes. The evidence for involvement of an antibody-mediated autoimmune reaction as the primary pathogenic mechanism is indirect and includes (1) evidence of increased intra-CNS synthesis of immunoglobulins,[343] (2) relative restriction of the immunoglobulin repertoire within the CSF and the CNS lesions (oligoclonal bands),[343] (3) demonstration of antibodies to myelin, oligodendrocytes, and components of myelin and other central nervous system components in the serum and CSF of patients with MS,[1,185,196] (4) serum or immunoglobulins (from animals sensitized with whole CNS or unfractionated myelin who develop EAE, an inflammatory/demyelinating disease of the CNS) that bind to myelin and oligodendrocytes, and induce complement-mediated demyelination and oligodendrocyte toxicity,[36,37,300,301] (5) serum and CSF from patients with MS that also have the capacity to induce demyelination of organotypic CNS cultures,[37,300] and (6) evidence for activation of the complement system in the CSF of patients with MS.[295]

Because of the possibility that MS is either caused by an antibody-mediated reaction, or more likely, that an antibody-mediated reaction may serve to cause or enhance demyelination initiated by a cell-mediated reaction, it is useful to consider experimental antibody-induced demyelination. Local injection of antibodies to galactocerebroside (GalC), a major CNS and PNS glycolipid, into optic nerves results in ultrastructural evidence of demyelination.[63,308,309] Using the same technique, demyelination has been induced by the immunoglobulin-containing fraction of serum from patients with MS and optic neuritis, although a lesser effect is occasionally seen after injection of serum from controls.[309] The ultrastructural pattern of myelin injury induced by anti-GalC appears to primarily affect oligodendrocytes rather than directly affecting myelin. Such an oligodendrocytopathy might be expected to adversely affect the most distal part of a myelin-forming cell, which is at the node of Ranvier. Such early changes could lead to alterations in the electrophysiologic properties and ion channels in the bared axon in this region and to loss of normal saltatory conduction as well as

conduction block, a hallmark of demyelination.[362] In contrast, antibodies to myelin-associated glycoprotein (MAG) result in several different changes including (1) vesiculation, (2) widening of the myelin lamellae (a finding in the peripheral nerves of patients with anti-MAG-associated demyelinating neuropathy,[174] and (3) monocyte and neutrophil attacks on both damaged and normal-appearing myelin compatible with an antibody-dependent cell-mediated (ADCC) immunopathologic reaction. Because of technical differences in tissue handling it is difficult to directly compare these patterns with those seen in autopsy- or even biopsy-obtained areas of demyelination acquired from patients with MS.

These humoral immune reactions are probably not the initiating immune reaction and are either epiphenomenon or secondary reactions that amplify the primary, cell-mediated reaction. The increase in the intra-CNS synthesis of immunoglobulin (Ig) likely represents chronic inflammation and is also seen in infections of the CNS such as syphilis, cryptococcus, subacute sclerosing panencephalitis (SSPE), HTLV-1, HIV, and Lyme disease. In most of these disorders, and others, much of the immunoglobulin can be specifically absorbed by the infectious agent, suggesting the vast majority of the IG, including that in the predominate oligoclonal bands, is antibody to the inciting agent.[185,247,357] Oligoclonal bands can be demonstrated in the CSF of animals with EAE induced by purified antigen myelin basic protein (MBP), which is a T cell-mediated disease.[279] The specificity of the vast majority of the immunoglobulin in the CSF and extracts from the plaques in MS patients is unknown.[185] It may be that a relatively restricted population of B cells penetrate the blood brain barrier, as T cells, at least when activated, cross the blood brain barrier more readily than B cells. If inflammation persists, the restricted population of B cells can be stimulated by cytokines (secreted by T cells, macrophages, and perhaps glial cells such as microglia and astrocytes) that stimulate this relatively limited repertoire of B cells to make immunoglobulin in a restricted pattern. The other possible explanations for the persistence of the restricted pattern are (1) there is specific antigenic drive stimulated by either an infectious agent (discussed previously) or by an autoantigen, (2) some component of the CNS itself acts as a B cell mitogen and/or maturation factor, or (3) the oligoclonal bands represent an antiidiotypic response to other immunoglobulins or to specific T cell populations. Although all of these explanations are plausible, there is no proof for any of them.

Although there are a myriad of papers demonstrating antibodies to myelin, oligodendrocytes, and myelin components [including known experimental autoantigens such as myelin basic protein (MBP), proteolipid protein (PLP), and galactocerebroside (GalC)], there are at least an equal number that either fail to demonstrate higher antibody titers than normals or (more often) do not demonstrate specificity of the reaction or significant differences in titers when compared to neurologic disease controls.[30,185,193,196] Although the serum or serum Ig of animals with EAE (induced with whole CNS or unfractionated myelin) induces demyelination, and oligodendrocyte toxicity in vitro is not capable of passively transferring disease when given systemically, in experimental autoimmune myasthenia gravis, serum immunoglobulins passively transfer disease.[344] Moreover, animals in which EAE was induced by sensitization with the purified antigen MBP develop EAE, and their serum has neither the capacity to cause in vivo or in vitro demyelination or oligodendrocyte toxicity.[300,301] Admittedly there are some reports of toxicity induced by passive transfer of serum Ig from whole CNS-sensitized EAE animals when the blood brain barrier was bypassed by intraventricular injections.[140] Demyelination by injection of serum into tadpole eye[336] or into guinea pig optic nerve[308] has not been unequivocally demonstrated to be caused by antimyelin antibodies or even by IgG or IgM fractions from serum or CSF.

In vitro demyelination can be induced by serum from normal subjects and individuals with neurologic diseases other than MS. It now seems that much, if not all, of the in vitro demyelinating effect in human serum and CSF results at least in part from nonspecific antibody-independent activation of the complement system through alternate pathways[322] or via classical pathways (even in the absence of antimyelin antibodies.[358] It has also been demonstrated that the complement pathway may be somehow involved in antigen-specific T cell-mediated cytotoxicity, perhaps contributing to chemotaxis. Therefore some of the activation of the complement system reported in the CSF of patients with MS may represent such cell-mediated cytotoxicity.

Recently, experimental evidence for an enhancing role for antibodies directed at components of myelin and oligodendrocytes[173,176,183,297,375] raised the possibility that antibodies to myelin, even if not the initiating event in the development of MS or in individual relapses, may be important in the evolution of the fully developed demyelinating lesion. Animals developing a single episode of EAE after active sensitization with antigen in complete adjuvant (''acute EAE'') have lesions of the CNS marked by inflammation and edema, but in general these animals have little (e.g. rat) or sometimes no (e.g. guinea pig) demyelination. Similar pathology can be induced by passive transfer of activated lymphocytes or antigen-specific [myelin basic protein (MBP) or proteolipid protein (PLP)] cell lines or clones to histocompatible naive animals. Serum immunoglobulins from animals sensitized with myelin oligodendrocyte protein (MOG) or GalC with high titer of antibodies to these antigens are incapable of transfer of either inflammation or demyelination to naive recipients. Combining the inflammatory cell-mediated reaction with passive transfer of antiserum results, however, in a lesion that is both inflammatory and demyelinative. This fact suggests that lesions in the CNS of patients with MS, and perhaps in the nerves of pa-

tients with Guillain-Barré syndrome and CIDP as well, are the result of more than one type of immunopathologic reaction and perhaps directed at more than one myelin/glial cell antigen. The change in the BBB caused by the inflammatory cells via systemically and locally produced cytokines is probably the initial event in an exacerbation (as demonstrated by enhanced CT and MRI scans) that then leads to humoral factors, such as antibodies, and complement access to the tissue (see Cell-Mediated Immunity). These humoral factors, as well as some of the factors released by the inflammatory cells themselves, likely cause demyelination and damage to oligodendrocytes.

There has been recent interest in the possible role of antibodies to one or more myelin components in enhancing CNS remyelination.[259,273] It is not clear how these antibodies work, and there is said to be some enhancement of remyelination with normal (non-CNS) directed Ig.

Cellular Immunity

The current pathogenic view of MS is that it is a cell-mediated disease of myelin or at least the initiation of the immune process is cell-mediated. There is some evidence from animal models [such as experimental (allergic) autoimmune encephalomyelitis (EAE)] and from patient studies that humoral mechanisms may be involved in enhancing lesions that commence as a result of a cell-mediated reaction. Much of the emphasis on cell-mediated immunity, the role of cytokines, cell-mediated and cytokine-induced changes in blood brain barrier via adhesion molecule induction at the endothelial cell level, the imbalance between subsets of T-helper cells and T-cytotoxic/suppressor cells, the important role of macrophages as both antigen-presenting cells (APCs) and effector cells, and the possible enhancing role of humoral factors is based on the extensive work on experimental models such as EAE and the similarities between animal models and immunopathologic findings in MS lesions.

Experimental Autoimmune Encephalomyelitis. EAE can be induced in many species of animals by sensitization of animals with whole CNS or CNS myelin. Disease induction is made more efficient by the use of adjuvants.[206,207] For many years only myelin basic protein (MBP), a major CNS myelin protein, was the only well-established component of myelin that could be shown to consistently induce EAE. Extensive studies in different species and different inbred strains of guinea pigs, mice, and rats have demonstrated that particular peptide sequences of MBP served as encephalitogenic epitopes for different species and even for different inbred strains within a species.[206,207] With continued duration of disease, however, more parts of the antigen become antigenic and even encephalitogenic or ''epitope spreading.''[63,178,179,217] Exploration of the different genes controlling these responses may be of importance in understanding susceptibility to MS, which also seems to be multigenetic.[78] In addition to EAE induction by active sensitization, induction of EAE can be accomplished by passive transfer of mononuclear cells, activated mononuclear cells, CD4+ MBP-specific T cell lines, or MBP-specific clones to naive inbred recipients.[200,206,207]

The control of susceptibility for the development of EAE is highly dependent on both the major histocompatibility complex (MHC) as well as specific T cell receptor (TCR) families.[206,207,341] The specific inducing peptide epitope (encephalitogenic epitope), the specific MHC molecule, and the specific TCR are called the trimolecular complex. Interfering with one or more components of the trimolecular complex provides the most specific inhibition of the development of EAE. Blocking the trimolecular complex is the theoretic underpining for some of the current strategies for treatment of MS (see the following).

More recently, other myelin components have been identified that are capable of induction of pathologic or clinical EAE. These include proteolipid protein (PLP),[348,351] myelin associated glycoprotein (MOG),[176,297] and most recently, S-100 protein,[160] which is not a constituent of myelin. In the instance of PLP, epitopes that are T cell reactive have been identified,[242] and passive transfer of disease has been clearly demonstrated. Similar studies are underway for myelin oligodendrocyte-associated protein (MOG).[7] Rabbits repeatedly sensitized with a major myelin glycolipid, galactocerebroside (GalC), develop high titers of anti-GalC antibodies. A third to one half of the animals develop PNS demyelination and weakness.[289] The demyelination, which is relatively acellular, does not affect the CNS. As previously noted, however, the antibodies can induce demyelination in vivo when injected directly into either the sciatic[288] or optic[309] nerves. In addition, such antibodies can cause in vitro demyelination of both PNS[291] and CNS[290] organotypic cultures and lytic reactions to Schwann cells[12] and oligodendrocytes.[125] In the absence of complement, anti-GalC can also dramatically alter the phenotype of oligodendrocytes in culture.[28] Antibodies to the carbohydrate determinant on MAG have been reported to cause in vivo demyelination after intraneural injection (as noted earlier), but to date, active sensitization of animals has not been reported to cause either an antibody or mediated disease in these animals.

Acute EAE is an excellent model for an acute monophasic inflammatory/demyelinating disease of humans seen after systemic viral infections and immunizations (such as postrabies vaccination) called acute disseminated encephalomyelitis (ADEM).[59,148,188] The two major criticisms of acute EAE as a model for MS were (1) relatively limited demyelination, and (2) acute EAE is a monophasic disease, and MS is a relapsing remitting and/or progressive disease. In some species, such as mice and nonhuman primates, however, significant demyelination is seen with active or passive transfer induction of EAE.[200] Of even more importance as a model of MS, chronic/relapsing EAE with demyelination can be induced with active sensitization in cer-

tain strains of guinea pigs[260,333,369] and with both active and passive induction of EAE in mice.[200]

Blood Brain Barrier (BBB) and Adhesion Molecules. It is now clear that local alterations in the BBB comprise a pivotal event in the development of EAE lesions and in the evolution of new lesions and reactivation of already existent lesions in MS. It is also clear that the cells of the microvessels of the CNS, especially the vascular endothelial cells and the pericytes and/or microglia, are actively involved in changes in the barrier.* Changes in the astrocytes adjacent to the vessels, which also contribute to the integrity of the BBB, may also be important. B cells do not normally enter the CNS through an intact BBB with any particular efficiency, nor do nonactivated T cells. Activated T cells do cross the vessels into the CNS but do not remain there unless they encounter a cognate antigen.[123] The presence of adhesion molecules on the T cells as part of activation is very important for the entry of the T cells into the CNS.[20] If T cells do enter the CNS, they can proliferate and secrete various lymphokines that can further break down the BBB and attract other T cells, lymphocytes, and macrophages. These can then form the characteristic inflammatory lesions of EAE. The cells that specifically recognize the sensitizing CNS antigen do not themselves constitute a large percentage of mononuclear cells in the lesion[59] and do not migrate out of the perivascular cuff,[62] at least in EAE. Whether both of these observations pertain to MS is not known, as the antigen of MS is unknown. Serial MRI studies of patients with MS has also confirmed the fact that MS is a chronic continuous disease with evidence of changes in the BBB, changes in the size of lesions, and the accumulation of new lesions occurring even during periods of apparent clinical quiescence.[240]

In EAE the CNS vascular endothelial cells become activated in parallel with or even slightly before inflammatory cells accumulate in the perivascular region.[50,67] All three types of adhesion molecules are induced generally with the sequence of the selectins, integrins, and members of the immunoglobulin superfamily such as ICAM-1. MHC molecules, which would allow vascular cells to present antigen, are upregulated later than the adhesion molecules. Pericytes and microglia also are induced to bear these molecules and may actually be the antigen-presenting cells within the CNS in vivo as opposed to the astrocytes, which likewise can be induced to upregulate these molecules and present antigen in vitro. The various cytokines secreted by activated inflammatory cells, microglia, and astrocytes in the lesion can further contribute to the changes in the BBB. It is not known how the initial activation of cells occurs or whether systemic activation or activation by inflammatory cells in the CNS or CNS vessels leads to the initial endothelial cell activation

---

*References 50, 67, 70, 121, 346, 360.

and breach in the BBB. Treatment of animals with antibodies to various adhesion molecules inhibits the development of EAE.[11,52,376] Such inhibition could occur during either the affector or effector stage of the autoimmune reaction. Administration of antiinflammatory cytokines or the production of such cytokines in the animal can inhibit the disease process.

As noted studies in MS patients likewise suggest, changes in the BBB are important in MS. The strongest evidence involves serial MRI studies in patients, including those with administration of gadolinium, which crosses open or incompetent BBB. Immunohistologic studies of MS lesions as well as cultures of intact microvessels from MS brains demonstrate the presence of activation of endothelial cells that have upregulated adhesion and MHC molecules. In addition, there are some reports that the serum and (especially) the CSF of patients with active MS show increased levels of adhesion molecules, as well as of activating proinflammatory cytokines and products associated with mononuclear cell activation.[69,117,270,312,350]

Cytokines and Mononuclear Cell Subsets. The presence of a mononuclear cell infiltrate in the CNS of patients with MS has long been recognized as a hallmark of the pathology of MS. The advent of specific phenotypic markers (generally monoclonal antibodies to different subsets of T cells, B cells, and monocyte/macrophages) has lead characterization of the cell types involved in the lesion and their putative roles. There has not always been agreement between these studies as to the predominant T cell subclass in MS lesions. Increased CD4+ and/or CD8+ have both been reported in the perivascular cuff and in the parenchyma (including at the leading edge of plaques).[34,118,345] Some of the problems in interpreting these studies and explaining the differences lie in accurately staging individual lesions and even parts of the same plaque in a chronic and/or relapsing disorder.[381] In both EAE and MS there is indication that many of these cells are activated as judged by the presence of cytokines, receptors for cytokines, and evidence of increased message for cytokines within the cells and lesions as well as evidence in most studies of activation in the CSF and CSF cells.* In addition, several cytokines have been shown to interact with glial cells, including oligodendrocytes, astrocytes, and microglia.† Moreover, it has also been demonstrated that the glial cells can produce various cytokines as well as other inflammatory mediators.‡ As in the instance of induction of MHC antigens on glial cells, there may be differences between in vitro and in vivo studies. In addition to evidence of increased levels of cytokines within the CNS, there is clear-cut evidence that peripheral blood mononuclear cells are activated and secreting increased levels of cytokines in patients with MS, especially during periods of clinical disease activity.*

In EAE the makeup of lesions varies with time, CD4+ cells predominating early after disease onset and C8+ cells later.[58] This pattern has been interpreted as a CD8 T cell-mediated suppressor shutting down a CD4+-initiated response. It is of some importance, therefore, that inhibition of EAE can be mediated by Th2 CD4+ T cells, likely as a result of secretion of the "antiinflammatory" cytokines IL-4, IL-10, and (especially) TGF-β.† TGF-β likely inhibits production and some of the biologic activities of the proinflammatory cytokines at the level of inflammatory cells and the blood brain barrier.[17] It is also of note that CD8+ cells in animals with EAE do not seem to inhibit CD4+ proliferative responses in vitro to the antigen-inducing MBP.[86] Although CD8- mice have a decreased mortality but an increased relapse rate of EAE,[159] and antibodies to CD8 modify EAE,[141] it is not known what turns off EAE and what reactivates relapsing EAE. There is evidence of cytokine and adhesion molecule activation in recurrent disease.[50,51,67] In addition to suppressive effects of certain cytokines, there is also evidence of lymphocyte death in these lesions, including evidence of apoptosis.[327] The regulatory control of EAE and relapsing EAE is therefore complex, and the control mechanisms in MS are at least as complicated and multifactorial.

Although originally thought of as exclusively products of immune system cells, it has become clear that cytokines are synthesized and secreted by many cell types and are important in communication between cells generally acting at a local level (autocrine or paracrine). However, certain cytokines, such as interleukin-1 (IL-1) and tumor necrosis factor-α (TNF-α), released during systemic infections and inflammatory reactions can affect sleep and appetite as well as the neuroendocrine system either by directly crossing into the CNS at regions where the BBB does not exist and/or by indirectly stimulating other cells to secrete these cytokines within the CNS.[66] It is also clear that when given in pharmacologic doses, cytokines can act systemically on inflammatory/immune cells as well as on other cell types. Even if cytokines cannot cross an intact BBB, they can cause CNS or PNS side effects by activating a large number of inflammatory cells, vascular endothelial cells, or other BBB-related cells, which in turn may secrete cytokines into the nervous system. The cytokines could effect neuronal and glial cell functions. Administration of interferon-γ (IFN-γ) to patients with MS was associated with an increase in exacerbations (relapses).[238] Animals manipulated to have the appropriate TCR α and β families to recognize an encephalito-

---

*References 92, 100, 120, 127, 128, 198, 199, 258, 303.
†References 29, 90, 186, 190, 210, 272, 305.
‡References 72, 91, 112, 132, 177, 180, 186.

*References 25, 68, 198, 199, 284, 304, 305.
†References 142, 153, 157, 255, 256, 257, 332, 354.

genic MBP epitope can develop EAE without exogenous sensitization with MBP. This occurs more frequently in animals not housed in a germ-free environment, suggesting that systemic infections leading to activation of inflammatory cells can alter the CNS vascular endothelial cells and the BBB, and lead to a CNS-specific autoimmune disorder.[108] Several studies have demonstrated that viral infections in MS patients are associated with an increase in relapses. Cytokines are important in the afferent phase of immunologic reactions by activating, recruiting, and otherwise enhancing the cellular reaction. They are involved in the efferent phase as well by mediating trafficking to the CNS as well as altering the BBB. Inhibition of certain "proinflammatory" cytokines inhibits the development of EAE,[282,306] although the timing of the administration of the antibodies may be critical to the observed effect. Furthermore, cytokines and chemokines recruit nonspecific cells to the lesion and may also cause neurologic symptoms (see the following). If antibodies to constituents of myelin are also involved in the pathogenesis of EAE and MS, then cytokines that enhance B cell proliferation, maturation, and Ig secretion would also be important in development of disease.

Administration of IFN-α, IFN-β, and IL-2 as therapeutic agents in immune diseases and in patients with neoplastic disorders results in neurologic side effects.[310] These side effects can occur without apparent crossing of the BBB and can affect patients with and without CNS disease. The ability of different cytokines to produce neurologic symptoms (including somnolence) also raises the possibility that local production of cytokines, such as IL-1 and TNF-α, could be responsible for some of the fatigue seen in MS patients, especially fatigue associated with exacerbations. In addition, certain cytokines can cause electrophysiologic abnormalities that precede histologic evidence of demyelination, inflammation, or toxic effects on glial or neuronal cells.[44] Thus it is possible that some of the symptoms during exacerbations are related to neurophysiologic and other effects of cytokines rather than new or increased demyelination. Animals with EAE, particularly guinea pigs and rats, can become severely ill and die despite having little or no demyelination. Edema and toxic effects of locally released cytokines could mediate and be responsible for the neurologic symptoms in these animals. The release of nitric oxide (NO) and free oxygen radicals and the activations of proteases by macrophages, microglia, and macroglia are also likely to be important in generation of the inflammatory and demyelinating lesions as well as symptoms of inflammation and demyelination.[144,209]

Much has been made of an apparent division of cytokines into proinflammatory and antiinflammatory cytokines as well as the differences in the types of T cells and macrophages that secrete them. CD4+ T cells have been recently viewed as either Th1, which secrete cytokines that enhance delayed hypersensitivity cell-mediated reactions such as IL-2, TNF-α, and IFN-γ, or Th2, which secrete "antiinflam-

matory" cytokines such as IL-4, IL-5, IL-10, and transforming growth factor-β (TGF-β).[219,335] Although this scheme has some validity and advantages, there are clearly problems with such a simplistic view in EAE and (especially) in MS. Although a cytokine such as IL-4 may tend to inhibit cell-mediated reactions, it may potentiate B cell reactions. IL-6 shares many actions with IL-1, a proinflammatory monocyte product, and is secreted by both monocytes and Th2 cells. Monocytes secrete both antiinflammatory cytokines, such as IFN-α and IFN-β, but also proinflammatory cytokines, such as IL-1. Different prostaglandins have various effects in the immune reactions. In addition, cytokines that may enhance immune reactions and help mediate demyelination can cause myelin-forming cells to proliferate. This reaction could likewise either inhibit or help recovery, depending on when in the recovery process the secretion of a particular cytokine occurs. Even TGF-β, which seems to be basically downregulatory, can stimulate proliferation of certain glial cells.[79,192,262,268,316]

CD8+ cells are present in MS lesions and some researchers have speculated that these cells are the more important in the evolution of MS lesions, or at least at certain phases of the disease.[118] The presence of MHC class I in MS lesions would allow for CD8+-mediated antigen-specific T cell reactions. Lymphotoxin or perforin is secreted by these cells that mediate cytotoxic reactions including those directed against myelin and myelin-forming cells. CD4+ cells are also capable of causing cytotoxic reactions, which likely include roles for monocyte/macrophages.

T Cell Receptor. The T cell receptor is a glycoprotein heterodimer with both peptide chains members of the immunoglobulin superfamily. They are in either an α/β—or γ/δ—configuration. As members of the immunoglobulin superfamily, the chains have common (C), variable (V), as well as joining (J) regions. The specificity of recognition and interaction with a specific epitope resides in the V, J, and diversity (D) regions. These proteins are formed as a result of alternate gene rearrangements, allowing for a relatively modest number of genes to provide antigenic recognition for an almost infinite number of epitopes. The interaction of the TCR with a specific epitope occurs in the context of epitope presentation by MHC molecules and with the modulation of T cell activation, which is partly caused by accessory molecules both on the T cell and the antigen-presenting cell. It is also possible to nonspecifically activate T cells that are non-TCR dependent. Differences in the V region in the TCR peptides allow the classification groups of β—or α—proteins into various "families." The α/β—TCR are found on mature T cells, whereas the γ/δ—configuration is generally associated with immature (CD4− CD8−) T cells. It is of some interest that such cells are found in the muscle of some patients with polymyositis[129] and in some MS lesions.[303,307] Such cells can be toxic for human glial cells in culture.[95] Attempts to demonstrate restriction in the use of different γ—or δ—families in MS patients, similar to the following described studies with α—and β—, have failed to reveal a consistent pattern.[133,371] γ/δ—TCR T cells have been reported to be colocalized with heat shock proteins (HSP), which in turn have been demonstrated in both astrocytes and oligodendrocytes in MS lesions.[303,371] The age of a multiple sclerosis lesion may be important in the proportion of γδ-bearing cells.[315] Heat shock proteins are an interesting family of proteins that are extremely well conserved evolutionary that can be upregulated in cells undergoing stress. Their complete function is not fully understood, but some HSP may protect cells by acting as chaperones for other proteins within the threatened cell.[101] They have also been shown to cross-react with microbial antigens and, more recently, with some constituents of myelin.[33] Moreover, CSF lymphocytes from patients with MS seem to react to some heat shock proteins in vitro.[32]

Much of the interest in TCR in MS patients relates to the very interesting finding that both Lewis rats and certain strains of mice use the Vβ8 family exclusively in mounting the response to encephalitogenic epitopes of MBP, although different sequences of MBP are encephalitogenic in the two species.[2,45,122,353] Because there was no agreement on the predominance of a specific MBP epitope for bulk lymphocyte cultures, T cell lines, or clones from patients compared with controls,[185,353] it was hoped that a predominate Vβ or Vα— family could be identified for MBP-responsive clones from blood, CSF, brain, or at least an increased frequency of activated T cells bearing a particular TCR Vβ or Vα family. This approach was potentially important because it was possible (1) to inhibit the development of EAE by vaccinating with altered encephalitogenic T cell clones[27,130] or administering antibodies to the appropriate Vβ family[378] or (2) to induce antibodies to a peptide from the variable portion of that family by sensitizing the animal itself.[356] This raised the possibility, currently being tested, that patients could be immunized to such a peptide, specifically inhibiting only that V family and leading to inhibition of disease with virtually no risk of broad-based immunosuppression.

At first, two groups reported that T cells bearing one or two TCR families were present in increased frequency, either activated in the blood or from within the nervous system.[114,162,373] It soon became clear different groups were identifying different predominate families and others could not identify a predominate family from blood, CSF, or CNS, even in the same individual patient.[26,103,150,205-207] This might represent a response to different epitopes of the same myelin antigen or even to different antigens in different patients. The lack of excessive useage of a particular TCR family could also represent involvement of a wider range of epitopes with longer duration of disease or even with influx of additional lymphocytes in a single lesion as it evolved.[334] This phenomenon is referred to as epitope or determinant spreading.[179]

More recently, one group has reported an increase in a particular segment of a particular sequence from TCR, obtained from the brains of MS patients from two different geographic areas, California and Australia. Thus this particular hypervariable region (CDR3) might be the important epitope-recognizing region independent of which individual TCR families are represented or which epitope of which antigen was the important inducer of disease.[227,229] Independent verification of this finding with a larger number of normal and disease controls, including inflammatory CNS disease controls, is needed to judge if this will be a helpful clue as to the cause and treatment of MS.[353,372]

Immunogenetics

It has been known for some time that there is a genetic component involved in susceptibility to developing MS. There is an increased incidence of MS in some families, and the presence of MS in a first-degree relative increases the risk of developing MS by 10- to 25-fold.[78] There is concordance of MS in identical twins of up to 30%,[77,78] and if one accepts abnormalities on MRI scan or the presence of oligoclonal bands in the clinically nonaffected twin as evidence of subclinical disease, perhaps 50 or more percent of such twins are concordant.[77,225,374] The concordance of MS in dizygotic twins is essentially the same as in nontwin siblings.[77,78] Even the geographic distribution of the prevalence of MS may in part be related to genetics, and the different prevalence rates in different ethnic and racial groups clearly suggest a strong genetic influence on disease susceptibility and resistance.

It became clear that the development of immunologic reactions to different antigens was under genetic control, with the MHC class I and class II antigens playing major roles along with other genes that control nonantigen-specific reactions, including complement components. This led to the study of the frequency of MHC class I and II alleles in patients with putative, immunopathologically mediated, and autoimmune diseases.

The other related impetus for frequency studies of MHC alleles in MS patients was the demonstration that susceptibility to MS in developing EAE, the model for MS, was different in various inbred strains of guinea pigs, rats, and mice. In rats and mice this susceptibility seems to map to different MHC antigens. With the use of backcrossed mice as well as congenic and recombinant animals, however, it became clear that susceptibility to the development of EAE was not entirely controlled by the MHC.[330,341] In addition, it was possible to overcome resistance to development of EAE by manipulating suppressor cell circuits[14,216] and sensitizing schedules.[313] Thus EAE susceptibility is polygenetic.

In MS there seemed to be an increase in certain MHC class I (HLA-A and HLA-B) antigens defined serologically, and class II (HLA-D) antigens defined by mixed lymphocyte reactions. In Caucasian populations, especially Scandinavian and other Nordic populations, HLA-A3, HLA-B7, and HLA-D2 seemed to be overrepresented, although a large number of normal individuals in those populations had an increased frequency of the same alleles.[60] With a better definition of MHC molecules using molecular biologic techniques, more specific haplotypes, such as DR15, DQ6, Dw2 in Caucasians, have been identified in these same populations.[124,339] There still is no single haplotype, however, that is specific for MS. Moreover, there seem to be different associations in different ethnic and racial groups,[228,341] and it has been suggested that there is a genetic influence on clinical course as well. In addition, as monozygotic twins are genetically identical, including MHC antigens, the MHC cannot be the only determinant for development of MS, even in individual population studies. Although group data shows increased susceptibility to MS of individuals with certain MHC molecules, studies do not demonstrate absolute tracking with these particular alleles in individual families. It is of some interest then that the TCR usage, a product of somatic cell gene rearrangements, need not be identical in identical twins. It has been recently suggested that there is a general skewing of TCR usage for the immune response to several antigens in the affected member of noncondordant monozygotic twinships.[352] The consensus view of MS is that it is polygenetic, and that although MHC is probably the most important of these factors, it is not the only genetic factor; environmental factors are also likely to be important.

The Antigens of MS. Because CNS myelin bears the brunt of the pathologic changes in MS, much of the effort to identify a target antigen for an autoimmune reactions has been centered on myelin/oligodendrocyte constituents.[185,196,265] Several CNS molecules have been demonstrated to cause inflammatory and/or demyelinating disorders (resembling MS) in experimental animals. There are also many constituents of myelin to which one can raise antibodies and/or induce cell-mediated T cell (CD4 or CD8) immunity that are not accompanied by any evident clinical or pathologic disease. Although these myelin constituents are somewhat unlikely candidates as the target antigens in MS, they cannot be absolutely dismissed, as it is possible they are pathogenic in man but not in experimental animals. Conversely, a demonstration of pathogenesis is still needed, as is an identification of the disorders. As an example, there is no proof that antibodies to galactocerebroside are associated with any immunologic disorders of the CNS or PNS in humans,[276] although animals can be immunized to develop a demyelinating neuropathy by sensitization with GalC, and when antibodies to GalC gain access to the CNS and PNS they can mediate demyelination. Moreover, the anti-GalC antibodies can mediate demyelination in vitro as well as induce cytotoxic and other changes in glial cells.

There have been innumerable studies attempting to demonstrate that one particular antigen is the target antigen for patients with MS and that one particular immunopathologic

reaction to that antigen explains the pathogenesis of MS. Many of these studies have focused on antibody-mediated reactions; however, other studies using different techniques have attempted to identify a specific antigen for a T cell-mediated autoimmune reaction.* This has not been possible, perhaps because this is not the case. The data with animal studies suggests that there may be different antigens capable of inducing similar, if not identical, clinical-pathologic pictures. Based on animal studies it is also likely that more than one immunopathologic process is involved in the full evolution of the disease. In addition, based on animal models of MS as well as other experimental autoimmune diseases, different epitopes of the same antigen may be important in disease induction in different patients.

An additional problem in unequivocally demonstrating that a particular antigen or peptide sequence of an autoantigen is causative for a T cell-mediated disease is that it is well established that normal individuals have circulating T cells that react specifically with such antigens and peptides.[48,245] Therefore patients may differ from controls not in the absolute sense but rather in the frequency of such autoreactive cells, the compartmentalization of these cells, the state of activation, and/or the cytokine profile of the reactive cells.†

If MS is due to a virus, a viral antigen incorporated into the host cell or as a part of an ongoing infection might also serve as the target of an immune reaction in which the cell is damaged, because it now bears a foreign or modified neoantigen or because it is an innocent bystander in the reaction mounted by the host organism as part of homeostatic defense.

Passive Transfer of MS. The first obstacle in proving that MS is caused by a cell-mediated reaction is the difficulty in passively transferring disease in vitro or even testing for a cytotoxic effect on oligodendrocytes in vitro. This is partly because foreign cells are rejected by the host experimental animals, and inhibition of this rejection involves the use of agents that inhibit the very cells involved in the development of an immune reaction. The second problem is that CD4+ cells react to antigen in the context of the appropriate MHC class II antigen, and CD8+ cells—in the context of MHC class II antigens, although there are cytotoxic cell-mediated reactions that can occur outside the restrictions of the MHC. In the case of antibody-mediated reactions, this restriction does not exist and accelerated immune clearance of foreign immunoglobulins such as IgG can be inhibited by immunosuppressive agents as mononuclear cells are not required to mediate certain type II immunopathologic reactions. The passive transfers of myasthenia gravis[344] and Lambert-Eaton myasthenic syndrome[99] to mice are examples of this passive transfer, and in vitro effects of myasthenic[189] and LEMS

---

*References 145, 185, 196, 242, 265, 328, 342, 379.
†References 6, 55, 194, 230, 231, 328, 380.

patients'[85] serum can be demonstrated using muscle or nervous system origin cells without the concern for MHC restriction. The BBB (or blood nerve barrier in the case of PNS demyelinating diseases) can be circumvented with direct injections into the brain or nerves of the experimental animals. In the instance of MS, MHC matched oligodendrocytes would be necessary for in vitro antigen-specific reactions or cells would have to be passively transferred to an MHC matched human recipient, a clearly unethical experiment. Killing of human oligodendrocytes in a nonantigen restricted fashion can be accomplished in vitro.[95] In addition, there is a problem of access to tissue caused by the BBB.

In an attempt to demonstrate that cells from patients with MS can passively transfer an inflammatory demyelinating disorder to animals, investigators have turned to the use of severe combined immunodeficient (SCID) mice. These animals have a severe defect in both T cell- and antibody-mediated immunity and do not reject foreign cells with any efficiency. Myasthenia gravis has been transferred to such animals by intraperitoneal inoculation of B cells.[208] The donor cells of such animals do not circulate in the normal way, but as the myasthenic deficit is mediated by antibodies to acetylcholine receptor, antibodies secreted by the human plasma cells in the peritoneum of the SCID mouse enter the circulation and come into contact with the neuromuscular junction of the host animal. Intracisternal inoculation of CSF mononuclear cells obtained from patients with active disease, but from controls or patients with MS in "remission," have been reported by one group to induce an inflammatory demyelinating disease (accompanied by astrocytic hypertrophy) in mice. In addition, these mice develop neurologic signs.[287] It has been argued that this experiment may not represent passive transfer of a cell-mediated immunopathologic reaction, but rather an enzoosis.[184] Other groups have been unable to confirm the passive transfer of any disease.[116,149,175]

Abnormalities in Immunoregulation

If MS is an immunopathologically mediated disease, especially a true autoimmune disease directed against myelin, it is likely abnormalities in regulatory mechanisms allow the emergence and persistence of the immune reaction.[185] Many studies (qualitative and quantitative) employing various in vitro techniques have shown the blood cells of MS patients do not have normal suppressor activity, especially during periods of exacerbation or progression.* The exact relationships between these abnormalities and in vivo effects, if any, are not clear. There have been therapeutic strategies designed to correct the imbalances of help and suppression, including treatment of patients with antibodies to helper T cells. It is also possible that one of the effects of IFN-β and

IFN-α in MS is to help reestablish balance between help and suppression.

DIFFERENTIAL DIAGNOSIS

There are a number of possible causes for optic neuritis, but in most cases the diagnosis connotes demyelination of the optic nerve, regardless of whether multiple sclerosis has been diagnosed. In a small percentage of cases, primary demyelination is not the cause, and another cause such as syphilis, sarcoidosis, a viral or postviral syndrome, systemic lupus erythematosus, or another autoimmune disease is identified.

Optic neuritis can occur in systemic lupus erythematosus (SLE), polyarteritis nodosa, and other vasculitides. Involvement of the optic nerve occurs in about 1% of patients with SLE.[135a] Rarely is the optic neuropathy the presenting sign of the disease. The term *autoimmune optic neuritis* has been suggested for cases of optic neuritis in which there is (1) serologic evidence of vasculitis, such as a positive antinuclear antibody (ANA), but no signs of systemic involvement other than the optic neuropathy, and (2) progressive visual loss, which tends to be steroid responsive and often steroid dependent (flares when steroids are tapered).[75,163a] Megadose intravenous steroids have been recommended as treatment. The existence of autoimmune optic neuritis as an entity distinct from either SLE or multiple sclerosis has not been proved. Some patients with multiple sclerosis manifest positive ANAs. As noted earlier, in the Optic Neuritis Treatment Trial (ONTT), patients with positive ANAs received randomized treatment allocations, and to date there is no evidence that the corticosteroid-treated patients fared better than the placebo-treated patients.

Parainfectious optic neuritis typically follows the onset of a viral infection by 1 to 3 weeks.[86a,163,302] It has been associated with rubeola, rubella, mumps, varicella-zoster virus, infectious mononucleosis, enterovirus, other viruses, and as a postvaccination phenomenon. The optic neuritis occurs on an immunologic basis, producing demyelination of the optic nerve. An immune-mediated meningoencephalitis is frequently associated and may be asymptomatic.

Parainfectious optic neuritis is more common in children than in adults. The optic neuritis may be unilateral but often is bilateral. The optic discs may appear normal or swollen. Retinal involvement is common when the disc is swollen (called neuroretinitis). Initially it may be in the form of diffuse edema involving the macula. Within days, hard exudates form in the macula, frequently in a star-shaped pattern. Deep whitish lesions occasionally are noted scattered throughout the retina at the level of the retinal pigment epithelium. Recognizing either type of retinal involvement is important because it virtually rules out multiple sclerosis as the cause.[71,203]

It is not unusual for the optic neuritis to be associated with meningeal inflammation as well as inflammation and

---

*References 8, 9, 15, 107, 155, 218, 264, 266.

perhaps demyelination in the brain [part of the acute disseminated encephalomyelitis, (ADEM)]. Thus changes in the brain or MRI may be seen, and cerebrospinal fluid (CSF) pleocytosis is possible. Visual recovery following parainfectious optic neuritis is usually excellent without any treatment. Whether or not corticosteroids hasten recovery is unknown, but this treatment is reasonable to consider, particularly in cases in which visual loss is bilateral and severe.

As discussed previously, the diagnosis of optic neuritis and other ocular findings in MS are based on clinical grounds. If the patient's clinical course is typical for optic neuritis and there is no historical or examination evidence of a systemic disease other than multiple sclerosis, serologic studies, such as an antinuclear antibody determination (ANA) and rapid plasma reagin (RPR) test, chest x-ray, computed tomography (CT), magnetic resonance imaging (MRI), lumbar puncture, and evoked potentials, generally are of limited utility and not necessary for diagnosis.[232] A work-up might further define a diagnosis of multiple sclerosis; however, at the present time this will not alter patient management. If the course becomes atypical—visual loss progresses for more than 10 days, pain persists or other symptoms develop—then an ancillary work-up should be undertaken in an attempt to make a more definitive diagnosis.

LABORATORY INVESTIGATIONS

Serologic Studies

Serologic studies such as an ANA and FTA were not shown to be of value in the ONTT.[232] Of the 457 patients entered into the ONTT, 16.3% had a positive ANA (3.4% with a titer $\geq 1:320$), but after the first year of follow-up only 1 patient had developed clinical signs of connective tissue disease. Response to corticosteroid treatment was not affected by ANA status. The FTA-ABS test was positive in six patients, but in all of them either a repeat test or a rapid plasma reagin test was negative, and none of these patients were diagnosed as having syphilis.

With an atypical course such as progressive visual loss, frequent recurrent attacks, or apparent steroid responsiveness, an autoimmune basis for the optic neuritis should be considered and appropriate serologic studies obtained.
Radiographic Studies. A chest x-ray could be considered to evaluate for sarcoidosis. In the ONTT, the chest x-ray was not suggestive of sarcoidosis in any patients.[232]

Lesions of the type seen in multiple sclerosis are frequently identified on brain MRIs in patients with isolated optic neuritis (i.e. monosymptomatic patients meaning no clinical historic or examination evidence of MS). In the ONTT, 27% of the 277 patients with isolated optic neuritis had an abnormal brain MRI (two or more lesions).[23] Other studies have reported the prevalence of abnormal brain MRIs in isolated optic neuritis to be 48 to 70%.[94a,138,143,213,234] Two or more lesions on brain MRIs of patients with isolated optic neuritis were reported by Miller and associates[214] (1988) in 64% of 53 patients under 50 years old scanned 1 to 40 weeks after onset; by Frederiksen and associates[49a] (1989) in 62% of 50 patients aged 12 to 53 years scanned after 3 to 49 days; and by Jacobs and associates (1991) in 40% of 48 patients aged 12 to 61 years scanned after 3 weeks to 7 years.

MRIs of the optic nerve can identify an area of inflammation[113,213] but this is only confirmatory of the clinical diagnosis and is not necessary in most cases.

Cerebrospinal Fluid Examination

Cerebrospinal fluid abnormalities of the type seen in multiple sclerosis are also seen with isolated optic neuritis, although with lower prevalence. Cerebrospinal fluid pleocytosis (> 5 cells/mm³) has been reported to occur in 32% to 60%,[220,293,294] elevated total protein concentration in 24% to 29%,[220,293] elevated relative immunoglobulin G concentration in 16% to 36%,[220,293] and oligoclonal banding in 24% to 46%.[220,293,294,331]

Visually Evoked Potentials

Visually evoked potential testing (VEP) can be used to assess optic nerve conduction. It is abnormal in virtually all cases of acute optic neuritis and remains abnormal in most cases even after vision has been recovered.[52a] This test is not of value in diagnosing optic neuritis, as it merely confirms the examination evidence for optic nerve dysfunction. Whether it is of any value to perform VEP on the fellow eye in unilateral cases to attempt to identify a conduction delay is not known. Visual function deficits in the fellow eye in apparent unilateral optic neuritis are common[23]; however, whether the presence of these deficits or of a delayed VEP is predictive of the development of MS is unknown.

THERAPY

Multiple Sclerosis

At this time there are four general approaches to the management of patients with MS. The first relates to the general care and preventive medicine for these individuals. Because there is little effect on longevity and many patients will have only mild-to-moderate disability, patients should be encouraged to maintain their general health, including the usual attention to blood pressure, cholesterol levels, mammography, Pap smears, avoiding smoking, and so on.

The second approach asserts that symptomatic therapy (therapy aimed at improvement of neurologic dysfunction) is very important in patients with MS.[311,326,327] Treatment of spasticity, when necessary, with physical therapy and pharmacologic agents such as baclofen or diazepam, management of neurogenic bladder and bowel, treatment of pain, occupational therapy, speech and swallowing therapy, energy conservation and treatment of fatigue, therapy for sexual dysfunction, and so on are often highly effective and can lead to major improvements in the patient's life and ability to perform activities of daily living. As some individuals with MS show extraordinary sensitivity to even modest elevations of body temperature or increases in environmental temperatures, aggressive therapy of febrile illness, with emphasis on antipyretic therapies and hydration, is often an important part of symptomatic management.

The third component of MS management is related to the disease process itself, the treatment of patients in exacerbation. At the current time the preponderance of evidence suggests that treatment of exacerbations with short-term large doses of corticosteroids, generally administered as intravenous methylprednisilone[74,215] and often followed by a tapering dose of oral corticosteroids, leads to a more rapid recovery than nontreatment of such exacerbations and is also quicker in comparison to more traditional oral doses of corticosteroids or ACTH. The mechanisms responsible for such improvement are likely multiple, but normalization of the changes in the BBB, as demonstrated on double-dose CT[347] scans and (more recently) on gadolinium-enhanced MRI, seems to be among the most important.

Corticosteroids. The capacity of corticosteroids to help repair alterations in the BBB is not limited to inflammatory/demyelinating diseases and likely involves actions at several points. Among these are direct inhibition of the effects of proinflammatory cytokines at the BBB, suppression of the synthesis and secretion of proinflammatory cytokines, alteration of lymphocyte compartmentalization with induction of margination, and so on. In addition, the broad-based antiinflammatory effects of corticosteroids on other functions of T cells, monocytes, and (eventually) B cells may also play a role in the therapeutic effects of the use of these drugs in exacerbations of MS.

As there is no evidence that treatment of exacerbations of established MS results in less long-term disability, it is not necessary or even advisable to treat every exacerbation. Corticosteroids are associated with innumerable side effects, even when given short term, and MS is a chronic disease with exacerbations that are not life-threatening. Because it is possible that secondary progression does not differ in the basic mechanism of relapsing-remitting disease, periods of rapid progression are often treated with short-term corticosteroids as well, although there are no studies to support this practice.

The last general area of management that is also directed at the disease itself attempts to alter the "natural history" of MS.[187,366] Until recently there was no therapy shown in a rigorous, double blind, prospective, randomized placebo-controlled trial to alter the natural course of the disease, even over the relatively brief period of a clinical trial. Although there have been studies purporting beneficial effects of different immunosuppressive agents: (1) the effects were often modest*; (2) the toxicities were unacceptable[283]; (3) the studies were small[323]; (4) the patient populations were "mixed"[367]; (5) the outcome measures were not always "ideal"[323]; (6) there were no true placebo controls[119,131,152]; or the results have not been confirmed in placebo-controlled trials.[41a,80,82,320] It must be realized that it is extraordinarily difficult to design and carry out a randomized blinded controlled study of therapy in multiple sclerosis. There are many problems including how to determine a successful outcome in different studies.[81,224,367]

It has recently been suggested that treatment of acute optic neuritis with very high doses of corticosteroids in high risk patients (those with a large number of lesions by MRI scan) may delay the clinical progression to MS.[232] This theory needs to be confirmed in a larger study in which this outcome measure is planned before the study[321] and extended to examine other isolated syndromes that may be the first attack of MS (such as myelitis and brainstem syndromes like internuclear ophthalmoplegia). If this theory is confirmed, it should also be determined if intermittent immunomodulating therapy in such patients would be even more effective (delay of clinical MS or new MRI lesions) than treatment of only the first acute attack. Although it is difficult to think of a specific mechanism by which short-term therapy could have such a prolonged effect, perhaps delaying epitope determinant spread, or effects on the vascular endothelium could be invoked.[349]

Immunosuppression and Immunomodulation. The basic premise for recent clinical trials in MS is that MS is an immunopathologically mediated autoimmune disease to one (or more) specific antigens of myelin/oligodendrocytes. In addition, it is assumed, with some supporting evidence, that there are similarities in the disease mechanisms in MS and different stages of EAE. Even if the antigen is a viral-induced neoantigen or a viral antigen incorporated into a cell without casing direct cytotoxicity, this would be a reasonable starting point. If MS is actually caused by an active, albeit slow, infectious process, then the appropriate strategy should be directed toward eradicating or slowing the viral infection and altering the destructive immune process it elicits, without allowing a wider dissemination of the occult infection.

Immunologic therapy in MS can be thought of as interfering with the afferent and/or efferent portions of the immunopathologic reaction.[187] It can also be thought of as being completely nonspecific, relatively specific, or specific; that is, directed at the response to the specific antigen.[366] The afferent portion of the response is the interaction between antigen-specific cells and antigen-presenting cells leading to an increased number and frequency of activated

---

*References 42, 82, 106, 219a, 320, 325.

antigen-specific T cells and, in some immunologic reactions, B cells. The further increase in cell numbers, the trafficking of these cells to the CNS, the crossing of the BBB, the secreting of cytokines and chemokines and attracting and expanding other cells to the immune reaction, the demyelination and/or toxic reactions against glial cells, the binding of antibodies to target antigens, and so on are all components of the efferent phase.

Two other stages can also be added, (1) the systemic and local inhibition, however temporary in multiple sclerosis, of this immunopathologic reaction and (2) attempts to induce remyelination or to enhance the electrophysiologic properties of the demyelinated CNS axons. It should also be remembered that some agents will have an effect in more than one stage of the immunologic response and that certain targets of immunomodulatory therapies (such as subsets of T cells, B cells, and monocytes as well as cytokines) can be involved in more than one stage of the immune response. Moreover, some cytokines may be deleterious and pathogenic at one phase of an immunopathologic reaction but could be important in recovery or remyelination at later stages. Thus although administration of IL-1 receptor antagonist (IL-1Ra) could inhibit the proinflammatory effects of IL-1, it might also inhibit the effect of IL-1 on glial cell proliferation and the stimulatory effect of IL-1 on glial cell secretion of nerve growth factor.[191] Indeed it has been shown that inhibition of IL-1 by IL-1Ra inhibits recovery of the PNS from traumatic injuries in experimental animals[112] and that it also markedly inhibits proliferation of Schwann cells induced by a mixture of cytokines.[188]

Broad-based therapies include corticosteroids and some of the cytotoxic/cytostatic immunosuppressive immunomodulatory agents such as cyclophosphamide, azathioprine, and methotrexate, although these agents do differ somewhat in their spectrum of immunosuppressive and antiinflammatory effects as well as their mechanisms of action. Cyclosporine would be considered more specific than these other agents, because it primarily affects the secretion and response to IL-2; however, as IL-2 can hardly be considered exclusively involved in immunopathologic reactions, this is not specific, or even truly selective, immunotherapy. Plasma exchange, not useful in MS, is broad-based passive inhibition of humoral immune responses and is not selective, because it normally removes all immunoglobulins (not just autoantibodies) as well as other circulating factors.

Blocking the secretion or the effects of proinflammatory cytokines would be relatively selective but not truly selective or specific, because it would block the effects of such cytokines in normal protective immunologic reactions. One strategy is to only inhibit cells that are immunologically activated and have upregulation of high avidity receptors for different cytokines such as IL-2R. Linking IL-2 to a toxin would then only damage cells with upregulated high avidity receptors for IL-2.[278] These would include those cells ac-

tively involved in the immunopathologic reaction, especially as IL-2 is such a key cytokine for T and B cell reactions. It would, however, also damage any cells with upregulated IL-2 receptors involved in "normal" immune reactions. Photopheresis is another technique designed to preferentially affect activated T cells and has recently been tested in MS.[277]

Therapy designed to interfere with the efferent phase, the putative immunopathologic reaction in MS, offers multiple points for modulation. Inhibition of pathologic T cells with monoclonal antibodies such as anti-CD3 or anti-CD4 would inhibit (or potentially destroy) these cells so as to reduce their number and their ability to circulate and/or to secrete cytokines that upregulate adhesion molecules.[126] This would inhibit the changes in the BBB that allow activated cells to leave the circulation and enter the perivascular space, where they can attract additional cells and form the classic perivascular and parenchymal lesions. This is more selective than pan immunosuppressive agents but would potentially make the patient at least partially immunodeficient. Another strategy would be to inhibit the cytokines that upregulate the changes in the vasculature or to administer antibodies to one or more of the adhesion molecules. This would only affect ongoing immune reactions that require upregulation of these molecules. If adhesion molecules specific for or active in the CNS or CNS vessels could be detected, then one would have a relatively specific, albeit not antigen-specific, reaction. So-called antiinflammatory cytokines would have the same potential, and it has been suggested that some of the activity of the IFN-α[73] and IFN-β—[134,136,241] in MS may relate to the capacity to inhibit the secretion of or the activities of IFN-γ.[73,222,246] Other "antiinflammatory" cytokines such as IL-4, IL-10, IL-13, and TGF-β might also have this effect. Indeed, there is currently consideration of a treatment study with TGF-β. It has also been suggested that TGF-β may be important in oral tolerization[158,296] in the inhibition of EAE by CD4 Th2 cells by countering the effects of IFN-γ and TNF-α. Downregulation of cytokines would also interfere with evolution of the lesion in the perivascular space and parenchyma. Since the final step in the evolution of the lesion is demyelination, inhibition of toxic cytokines, proteases, or enzymes that also enhance nitric oxide (NO) formation might inhibit the lesion and help lessen the disease.

If antibodies are involved in the demyelination, then inhibiting antibody formation with immunosuppressive agents, inhibiting T cell B cell interactions, inhibiting B cells, or inhibiting complement cascade would all have the potential to inhibit disease. Of course one would wish to inhibit only those B cells making the specific autoantibody and would have to inhibit the reaction in the CNS. At this time, the antigen is not known. Even when a specific antigen is known, such as antiacetylcholine receptor in myasthenia gravis, there still is no specific immunotherapy.

Virtually all of the previously discussed therapeutic approaches, modulating the afferent or efferent phase, are either broad-based or only relatively selective. Highly specific therapy would be aimed at interfering with the specific reactions to the autoantigen or, even more specifically, the critical epitope of the autoantigen. There are three components of the trimolecular complex, the MHC molecule, the antigen (epitope peptide), and the TCR. There are also other adhesion/accessory molecules that enhance interactions between the components of the trimolecular complex. Inhibition of the accessory molecules, some of which are involved in BBB, also inhibits the immune reactions, which, as noted, are not specific for a particular antigenic specificity as these molecules are accessories for many immune reactions.

Monoclonal Antibodies. Antibodies to the MHC molecule will block those immune reactions controlled by the particular MHC molecule. Antibodies to the specific MHC inhibit EAE.[330] The second way to inhibit the trimolecular complex is to inhibit the specific TCR $V\beta$ or $V\alpha$ family or the specific TCR (the variable, diversity or joining regions) that recognizes the pathogenic peptide. In EAE this inhibition has been accomplished by either administering antibodies to the TCR[378] or immunizing animals to their own TCR, using peptide sequences for the specific TCR.[356] In humans the use of any experimentally produced monoclonal antibodies is limited by the immune response to the foreign mouse protein. This response can be overcome by creating human-mouse hybrid antibodies in which the specific antibody-binding portion of the molecule is from the mouse and the rest of the Ig molecule is of human origin, reducing the chances of rejection (enhanced clearance and/or inactivation).[269,368] There is currently an ongoing trial of immunization of patients of synthetic peptides identical to the MBP-epitope-reacting predominate TCR V sequence to see if patients will make antibodies to the peptide and the TCR as well as to see if there is any effect on the clinical course. Although some patients seem to make antibodies to some of the peptides, there is a problem in inducing antibodies to the peptides in other patients, which is not surprising as it is harder to induce antibodies to self-antigens than to allogenic, heterologous, or xenogenic antigens.[40] In addition, the patients in this study are not in a randomized controlled prospective blinded trial, and there will be no way to assess clinical efficacy. There are other serious limitations of this strategy. It has now become clear that there is not predominate useage of one or two TCR $V\beta$ or $V\alpha$ for particular MBP epitopes in patients with MS. Indeed, individual patients may use several TCR $V\beta$ and $V\alpha$ in responding to the same epitopes. There is the problem of determinant or epitope spreading which would mean additional TCR useage in patients with disease duration. Thus peptides would have to be customized for individual patient immunizations and those might have to be changed with time. Moreover, it is not clear that MBP is the inducing autoantigen in any patients with MS. Even choosing the TCR on the basis of analysis of the in vivo activated T cells from blood or CSF may not work.

Antigenic Tolerance. The final strategy is to specifically administer the specific antigen in protocol that would desensitize or block, rather than enhance, reactivity to the protein (such as a nondisease-inducing peptide complexed to the MHC molecule[292]) or to administer a peptide that simulates the antigen and takes its place in the complex without activating the immune response to the antigen. There are problems with this strategy as well, which are related to not knowing the antigen of MS, with the further possibility that there may be different epitopes and antigens of importance in different patients with MS. Injection of MBP has been used with no clinical success.[49,104] Administration of oral MBP or myelin inhibits EAE and chronic relapsing EAE, but once again the antigen of MS is not known. It has been argued that using whole myelin obviates the need for specific identification of the MS antigen and that the inhibitory effect is at least partially mediated by suppressor cells secreting TGF-β.[158,212,296] The one published report of oral tolerization in MS with oral myelin really had very little (if any) hint of clinical efficacy and in a rather selected subpopulation of patients (DR2-negative men with relapsing-remitting disease).[364]

Copolymer. Copolymer-1, a synthetic polymer of L-alanine, L-glutamic acid, L-lysine, and L-tyrosine, synthesized to simulate MBP, was shown to inhibit both acute EAE and chronic EAE.[154,195,338] The basis of this inhibition is controversial, with suggestions that there is cross-reactivity with MBP at the level of both cell-mediated and humoral immunity.[337,363] It has also been reported by the same group that copolymer-1 induces suppressor cells[5,172] and specifically replaces MBP in the trimolecular complex.[337] Animals with copolymer-1 modified EAE, however, mount a normal in vitro response to MBP,[195] and copolymer-1 seems to be able to compete with antigens other than MBP for binding in the trimolecular complex.[96,255,257] In humans there is little proof of cross-reactivity to MBP,[46,47] and it is possible that the inhibitory effect relates to interference with less specific efferent phases of the immune response in EAE and presumably in MS.[43,195] It is also possible that interference with the trimolecular complex could be the result of a superantigen-like effect of copolymer-1. Copolymer-1 was reported to reduce the frequency of relapses in patients with mild-to-moderately disabling MS[38] but had little effect in progressive MS.[39] More recently it has been reported in a larger study that copolymer-1 reduces relapses and may have a salutary effect on accumulated neurologic disability as measured by the expanded disability scale (EDSS).[146]

Therefore at the current time and with the current imperfect understanding of the immunology of MS relatively specific therapy, perhaps a safe technique to inhibit adhesion molecules or inhibit activated Th1 helper T cells is the most likely approach to lead to a more striking improvement in the course of patients with MS. The more specific therapy may be premature. Eventually the use of more than one agent, with different actions, may emerge as treatment for MS.

Agents to Improve Neuronal Function. A final area of potential therapeutic benefit is the attempt to improve conduction in demyelinated fibers. This approach employs agents that affect ion channels and currently centers around the use of 4-aminopyridine or 3,4-diaminopyradine that inhibits slow K+ channels.[31,329] Remyelination, as noted, is not effective in the CNS. Antibodies to one or more components of myelin have been reported to enhance remyelination in models of MS.[259,273] CNS myelin, but not PNS myelin, has also been reported to inhibit neurite outgrowth as well.[298] Normal Ig has also been reported to have some effect, but not as much as the immune Ig. This report has lead to the suggestion that intravenous immunoglobulin be tried as a potential treatment of stable MS,[224,355] although others have suggested the use of IV Ig on the basis of immunomodulation.[3]

Optic Neuritis

Corticosteroids. The efficacy of corticosteroids as treatment for optic neuritis was investigated in a multicenter clinical trial.[21] To be eligible for the study a patient had to be between the ages of 18 and 46 years, have a history and examination consistent with acute unilateral optic neuritis with visual symptoms lasting 8 days or less, and have no evidence of a systemic disease other than multiple sclerosis that could cause optic neuritis. Patients with a past history of optic neuritis in the currently affected eye or a past history of corticosteroid treatment of multiple sclerosis or optic neuritis in the fellow eye were excluded.

Two treatment regimens were evaluated in comparison with oral placebo: (1) intravenous methylprednisolone 250 mg every 6 hours for 3 days followed by oral prednisone 1 mg/kg/day for 11 days, and (2) oral prednisone 1 mg/kg/day for 14 days. Both regimens were followed by a short taper.

The study found that vision recovered faster, but at 6 months was only slightly better, in the intravenous group compared to the placebo group. The benefit of the intravenous regimen after 6 months was most apparent in patients whose baseline visual acuity was 20/200 or worse. Even in this subgroup, however, the benefit at 6 months was slight and was principally seen in a higher percentage of patients in the intravenous group recovering to better than 20/20 than in the placebo group. With starting vision of 20/200 or worse, 91% of the patients in the placebo group recovered to 20/40 or better compared to 85% in the intravenous group.

For the regimen of oral prednisone alone, no benefit was found either in the rate of recovery of the 6-month outcome. In addition, patients in this group had a higher rate of new attacks of optic neuritis in both the affected and fellow eyes than patients in the placebo group.

From the results of the ONTT, it is apparent that there is no role for oral prednisone in standard doses in the treatment of acute demyelinative optic neuritis. The higher-dose intravenous regimen should be considered particularly when visual loss is severe. The clinician must remember, however, that the main benefit is in the rate of recovery and that the benefit after 6 months is slight. No treatment at all also is a viable therapeutic option.

Other Treatments. No other treatments for optic neuritis have been systematically studied. Numerous treatment modalities have been evaluated for multiple sclerosis, such as imuran, cytoxan, and plasma exchange.[105] Most of the studies have evaluated patients with chronic progressive MS and are not directly applicable to the treatment of optic neuritis. No studies on any treatments have demonstrated clear-cut benefits in altering the course of MS.[105] Ongoing trials are investigating interferon and copolymer.

PROGNOSIS

Visual Outcome

Regardless of the degree of impairment of vision, visual function in most cases of optic neuritis begins improving one to several weeks after the onset (without any treatment). Based on the ONTT results from placebo-treated patients, about 95% of patients will have visual acuity of better than 20/50, and 60%—acuity better than 20/20 after 6 months.[21] Even when the presenting visual acuity is 20/200 or worse, 90% still recover to better than 20/50 and 33% to better than 20/20.[21] Despite good recovery of acuity, however, there may still be significant optic nerve damage. Residual deficits in color vision, contrast sensitivity, light brightness sense, stereopsis, and other measures are frequent.[21,87] On examination, a relative afferent pupillary defect is detectable in most cases, and the optic disc usually has evidence of pallor.[87]

The relationship between optic neuritis and MS has been further emphasized by the results of the Optic Neuritis Treatment Trial (ONTT).[233] The ONTT has now reported that high-dose intravenous methylprednisolone (250 mg IV Q6H) followed by a short course of oral corticosteroids reduced the risk for the development of MS during a 2-year follow-up period.[21] Abnormal MRI scans were a strong indicator for developing MS, and corticosteroid treatment had the most benefit for patients with abnormal MRI scans.[24] Therefore, although corticosteroid therapy may not change the ultimate visual outcome of optic neuritis,[22] its use may be helpful in delaying or perhaps even reducing the risk of repeat episodes of widespread demyelination. This possibility and the effects of treatment of other "first attack" syndromes require evaluation.

Development of Multiple Sclerosis

Optic neuritis occurs in about 50% of patients with multiple sclerosis, and it is the presenting sign in about 20%. The course of optic neuritis tends to be the same, whether or not MS is present.

There is no evidence to suggest that the pathogenesis of isolated optic neuritis is different than that of MS. In fact a strong case can be made that optic neuritis is a "forme fruste'' of multiple sclerosis based on similarities in demographic characteristics such as age and gender distributions, geographic differences in incidence rates, histocompatibility antigen associations, family history, as well as CSF and MRI findings.[76] Both optic neuritis and multiple sclerosis are more common in northern latitudes, in females, and in young adults. Ebers and associates[76] described 10 patients with isolated optic neuritis who had a family member with MS, which also suggests an etiologic association between the two.

Previous studies have reported the risk of developing multiple sclerosis after optic neuritis to be as low as 13% and as high as 88%.[167] In the most statistically sound study, Rizzo and Lessell[271] reported that 58% of patients with optic neuritis developed MS during an average follow-up of 14.9 years. Life table analysis indicated that at 15 years follow-up, 74% of women and 34% of men would be expected to develop MS. The average time to the development of MS was 7.8 years. The risk for MS was greater, the earlier the age of onset of the optic neuritis. This study, surprisingly, did not find that recurrent attacks of optic neuritis increased the risk. Although most other studies have shown a similar risk for younger ages, not all have demonstrated such a difference in the risk of developing MS between men and women nor the lack of risk with recurrent attacks.[93,294] The presence of HLA haplotype DR2 has also been identified as a risk factor.[220]

Whether the identification of lesions in the brain consistent with demyelination is predictive of which patients with isolated optic neuritis will develop clinical MS is not certain. Miller and associates[214] followed 53 patients with isolated optic neuritis, 34 of whom had an initial MRI that was abnormal and 19 a scan that was normal. Of the 34 with an abnormal MRI, 12 developed clinical MS in a mean follow-up of 12.3 months (range 6 to 23 months), and 7 others without new symptoms developed new lesions on MRI. Of the 19 patients with an initial normal scan, none developed clinical MS in 12.1 months of follow-up (range 5 to 30 months), and 3 without new symptoms developed new lesions on MRI. Frederiksen and associates[94a] reported that 7 of 31 patients with isolated optic neuritis with initially abnormal MRIs developed clinical MS with median follow-up of all months (range 1 to 20 months) compared to none of 19 patients with an initial normal scan. Contrary to these two reports, Jacobs and associates[137] reported that MRI changes in patients with isolated optic neuritis were not a good predictor of the development of MS. With mean follow-up of 4 years (range 2 months to 15.5 years), clinical MS developed in 6 of 23 patients with an initial abnormal MRI and 3 of 25 with normal MRI. All of these studies lacked sufficiently long follow-up to fully assess the predictive value of MRI for the development of MS in patients with isolated optic neuritis. Miller and associates[213] and Frederiksen and associates[94a] data provide compelling evidence that MRI may be predictive of the early development of MS. Jacobs and associates' study,[138] despite a number of design problems, raises questions about the long-term predictive value.

Patients with isolated optic neuritis and abnormal CSF are more likely to develop definite multiple sclerosis; however, patients with normal CSF are still at risk. Sandberg-Wolheim and associates[294] reported that of 31 patients with isolated optic neuritis who had normal CSF, only 7 were diagnosed with MS during median follow-up of 12.9 years, compared to 26 of 55 patients with abnormal CSF who developed MS. Stendahl-Brodin and Link[331] reported that after 6 years of follow-up, 9 of 11 patients with isolated optic neuritis and oligoclonal bands present in the CSF developed MS, compared to 1 of 19 with normal CSF who developed MS. Nikoskelainen and associates[220] reported that 6 of 8 patients with isolated optic neuritis and oligoclonal bands developed MS after 7 to 10 years, compared to 9 of 19 with no oligoclonal bands.

REFERENCES

1. Abramsky O, Lisak RP, Silberberg DH, Pleasure DE: Antioligodendroglia antibodies in patients with multiple sclerosis, *N Engl J Med* 297:850-853, 1977.
2. Acha-Orbea H, Mitchell DJ, Timmermann L et al.: Limited heterogeneity of T-cell receptors from lymphocytes mediating autoimmune encephalomyelitis allows specific immune interventions, *Cell* 54:263-273, 1988.
3. Achiron A, Gilad R, Margalit R et al.: Intravenous gammaglobulin treatment in multiple sclerosis and experimental autoimmune encephalomyelitis: delineation of useage and mode of action, *J Neurol Neurosurg Psychiatry* 57(suppl):57-61, 1994.
4. Adams CWM, Poston RN, Buk SJ et al.: Inflammatory vasculitis in multiple sclerosis, *J Neurol Sci* 69:269-283, 1985.
5. Aharoni R, Teitelbaum D, Arnon R: T suppressor hybridomas and interleukin-2-dependent lines induced by copolymer 1 or spinal cord homogenate down-regulate experimental allergic encephalomyelitis, *Eur J Immunol* 23:17-25, 1993.
6. Allegretta M, Nicklas J, Sriram S, Albertini R: T cell responsive to myelin basic protein in patients with multiple sclerosis, *Science* 247:718-721, 1990.
7. Amor S, Groome N, Linington C et al.: Identification of epitopes of myelin oligodendrocyte protein for the induction of experimental allergic encephalomyelitis in SJL and Biozzi AB/H mice, *J Immunol* 153:4349-4356, 1994.
8. Antel JP, Arnason BGW, Medof ME: Suppressor cell function in multiple sclerosis-correlation with clinical disease activity, *Ann Neurol* 5:338-342, 1979.
9. Antel JP, Oger Jackevicius S, Kuo HH et al.: Modulation of T lymphocyte differentiation antigens: potential relevance for multiple sclerosis, *Proc Natl Acad Sci USA* 79:3330-3334, 1982.
10. Archambeau PL, Hollenhorst RW, Rucker CW: Posterior uveitis as a manifestation of multiple sclerosis, *Mayo Clin Proc* 40:544-551, 1965.
11. Archelos JJ, Jung S, Mauarer M et al.: Inhibition of experimental autoimmune encephalomyelitis by an antibody to the intercellular adhesion molecule ICAM-1, *Ann Neurol* 34:145-154, 1993.
12. Armati-Gulson PJ, Lisak RP, Kuchmy D, Pollard J: 51Cr release cytotoxicity radioimmunoassay to rat Schwann cells in vitro, *Neurosci Lett* 35:321-326, 1983.
13. Arnold AC, Pepose JS, Hepler RS, Foos RY: Retinal periphlebitis and retinitis in multiple sclerosis: pathologic characteristics, *Ophthalmology* 91:255-262, 1984.
14. Arnon R: Experimental allergic encephalomyelitis: susceptibility and suppression, *Immunol Rev* 55:5-30, 1981.

15. Bach MA, Phan-Dinh F, Tournier E et al.: Deficit of suppressor T cells in active multiple sclerosis, *Lancet* 2:1221-1224, 1980.

16. Bachman DM, Rosenthal AR, Beckingsale AB: Granulomatous uveitis in neurological disease, *Br J Ophthalmol* 69:192-196, 1985.

17. Balabanov R, Dore-Duffy P: Recovery in acute EAE in rats is associated with endothelial unresponsiveness, *J Neuroimmunol* 54:151, 1994.

18. Baloh RW, Yee RD, Honrubia V: Internuclear ophthalmoplegia. I. Saccades and dissociated nystagmus, *Arch Neurol* 35:484-489, 1978.

19. Bamford CR, Ganley JP, Sibley WA, Laguna JF: Uveitis, perivenous sheathing and multiple sclerosis, *Neurology* 28:119-124, 1978.

20. Barron J, Madri J, Ruddle N et al.: Surface expression of $\alpha4$—integrin by CD4 T cells is required for their entry into the brain, *J Exp Med* 177:57-68, 1993.

21. Beck RW, Cleary PA, Anderson MA et al.: A randomized controlled trial of corticosteroids in the treatment of acute optic neuritis, *N Engl J Med* 326:581-588, 1992.

22. Beck RW, Cleary PA, Trobe JD et al.: The effect of corticosteroids for acute optic neuritis in the subsequent development of multiple sclerosis, *N Engl J Med* 329:1764-1769, 1993.

23. Beck RW, Kupersmith MJ, Cleary PA et al.: Fellow eye abnormalities in acute unilateral optic neuritis: experience of the Optic Neuritis Treatment Trial (submitted for publication).

24. Beck RW, Murtagh FR, Arrington J et al.: Optic Neuritis Study Group. Brain MRI in Acute Optic Neuritis: experience of the Optic Neuritis Study Group (submitted for publication).

25. Beck J, Rondot P, Catinot L et al.: Increased production of interferon gamma and tumor necrosis factor precedes clinical manifestation in multiple sclerosis: do cytokines trigger off exacerbations? *Acta Neurol Scand* 78:318-323, 1988.

26. Ben Nun A, Liblau RS, Cohen L et al.: Restricted T-cell receptor V beta gene useage by myelin basic protein-specific T-cell clones in multiple sclerosis: predominant genes vary in individuals, *Proc Natl Acad Sci USA* 88:2466-2470, 1991.

27. Ben Nun A, Wekerle H, Cohen I: Vaccination against autoimmune encephalomyelitis with T-lymphocyte line cells reactive against myelin basic protein, *Nature* 292:60-61, 1981.

28. Benjamins JA, Dyer CA: Glycolipids and transmembrane signaling in oligodendroglia, *Ann NY Acad Sci* 605:90-100, 1990.

29. Benveniste EN, Merrill JE: Stimulation of oligodendroglial proliferation and maturation by interleukin-2, *Nature* 321:610-613, 1986.

30. Bernard CCA, Kerlero de Rosbo N: Multiple sclerosis: an autoimmune disease of multifactorial etiology, *Curr Opin Immunol* 4:760-765, 1992.

31. Bever CT: The current status of studies of aminopyridines in patients with multiple sclerosis, *Ann Neurol* 36(suppl):S118-S121, 1994.

32. Birnbaum G, Kotilinek L, Albrecht L: Spinal fluid lymphocytes from a subgroup of multiple sclerosis patients respond to mycobacterial antigens, *Ann Neurol* 34:18-24, 1993.

33. Birnbaum G, Kotilnek L, Schlievert P, Clark HB: Immunologic cross-reactivity between a mycobacterial heat shock protein and the myelin protein $2'3'$ cyclic nucleotide $3'$ phosphodiesterase, *Neurology* 44(suppl 2):A146, 1994.

34. Booss J, Esiri M, Tourtellotte WW, Mason DY: Immunohistological analysis of T lymphocyte subsets in the central nervous system in chronic progressive multiple sclerosis, *J Neurol Sci* 62:219-232, 1993.

35. Booss J, Kim JH: Evidence for a viral etiology of multiple sclerosis. In Cook SD, editor: *Handbook of multiple sclerosis,* 41-62, New York, 1990, Marcel Dekker.

36. Bornstein MB, Appel SH: The application of tissue culture to the study of experimental ''allergic'' encephalomyelitis. I. Patterns of demyelination, *J Neuropathol Exp Neurol* 20:141-157, 1961.

37. Bornstein MB, Appel SH: Tissue culture studies of demyelination, *Ann NY Acad Sci* 122:280-286, 1965.

38. Bornstein MB, Miller A, Slagle S et al.: A pilot trial of Cop 1 in exacerbating-remitting multiple sclerosis, *N Engl J Med* 317:408-414, 1987.

39. Bornstein MB, Miller A, Slagel S et al.: A placebo-controlled, double-blind, randomized, two-center, pilot trial of Cop 1 in progressive multiple sclerosis, *Neurology* 41:533-539, 1991.

40. Bourdette DN, Whitham RH, Chou YK et al.: Successful immunization of multiple sclerosis patients with synthetic TCR Vβ—peptides, *J Neuroimmunol* 54:154, 1994.

41. Breger BC, Leopold IH: The incidence of uveitis in multiple sclerosis, *Am J Ophthalmol* 62:540-545, 1966.

42. British and Dutch Multiple Sclerosis Trial Group: Double masked trial of azathioprine in multiple sclerosis, *Lancet* 2:179-183, 1988.

43. Brosnan CF, Litwak M, Neighbour PA et al.: Immunogenic potentials of copolymer I in normal human lymphocytes, *Neurology* 35:1754-1759, 1985.

44. Brosnan CF, Litwak MS Schroeder CE et al.: Preliminary studies of cytokine-induced functional effects on the visual pathways in the rabbit, *J Neuroimmunol* 25:227-239, 1989.

45. Burns FR, Li X, Shen N et al.: Both rat and mouse T cell receptors specific for the encephalitogenic determinant of myelin basic protein use similar Vα—and Vβ—cahin genes even though the major histocompatibility complex and encephalitogenic determinant being recognized are different, *J Exp Med* 169:27-39, 1988.

46. Burns J, Krasner J, Guerro F: Human cellular immune response to copolymer 1 and myelin basic protein, *Neurology* 36:92-94, 1986.

47. Burns J, Littlefield K: Failure of copolymer 1 to inhibit the human T-cell response to myelin basic protein, *Neurology* 41:1317-1319, 1991.

48. Burns JB, Rosenzweig A, Zweiman B, Lisak RP: Isolation of myelin basic protein reactive T-cell lines from normal human blood, *Cell Immunol* 81:435-440, 1983.

49. Campbell B, Vogel PJ, Fisher E, Lorenz R: Myelin basic protein administration in multiple sclerosis, *Arch Neurol* 29:10-15, 1973.

49a. The Canadian Cooperative Multiple Sclerosis Study Group: The Canadian cooperative trial of cyclophosphamide and plasma exchange in progressive multiple sclerosis, *Lancet* 2:441-446, 1991.

50. Cannella B, Cross AH, Raine CS: Upregulation and coexpression of adhesion molecules correlate with relapsing autoimmune demyelination in the central nervous system, *J Exp Med* 172:1521-1524, 1990.

51. Cannella B, Cross AH, Raine CS: Adhesion molecules in the central nervous system: upregulation correlates with inflammatory cell influx during relapsing experimental autoimmune encephalomyelitis, *Lab Invest* 65:23-31, 1991.

52. Cannella B, Cross AH, Raine C: Anti-adhesion molecule therapy in experimental autoimmune encephalomyelitis, *J Neuroimmunol* 46:43-55, 1993.

52a. Celesia GG, Kaufman DI, Brigel M et al.: Optic neuritis: a prospective study, *Neurology* 40:919-923, 1990.

53. Charcot JM: Histologic de la sclerose en plaques, *Gazette des Hopitaux Civils et Militaries* (Paris) 41:554-556, 1868.

54. Charcot JM: Lectures on the diseases of the nervous system (English translation by G. Sigerson), First series, 157, London, 1877, New Sydenham Society.

55. Chou Y, Bourdette D, Offner H et al.: Frequency of T cells specific for myelin basic protein and myelin proteolipid protein in blood and cerebrospinal fluid in multiple sclerosis, *J Neuroimmunol* 38:105-114, 1992.

56. Christensen T, Moller-Larsen A, Haar S: A retroviral implication in multiple sclerosis, *Trends Microbiol* 2:332-336, 1994.

57. Cogan DG: Internuclear ophthalmoplegia, typical and atypical, *Arch Ophthalmol* 84:583-589, 1970.

58. Cohen JA, Essayan DM, Zweiman B, Lisak RP: Frequency analysis of antigen-reactive lymphocytes in the lesions of animals with experimental allergic encephalomyelitis, *Cell Immunol* 108:203-213, 1987.

59. Cohen JA, Lisak RP: Acute disseminated encephalomyelitis. In Aarli JA, Behan WMH, Behan PO, editors: *Clinical neuroimmunology,* 192-203, Oxford, 1987, Blackwell Scientific Publications.

60. Compston DAS: Genetic factors in the aetiology of multiple sclerosis. In McDonald WI, Silberberg DH, editors: *Multiple sclerosis,* 56-73, London, 1986, Butterworths.

61. Crane TB, Yee RD, Baloh RW, Hepler RS: Analysis of characteristic eye movement abnormalities in internuclear ophthalmoplegia, *Arch Ophthalmol* 101:206-210, 1983.

62. Cross AH, Cannella B, Ptosnan CF, Raine CS: Homing to central nervous system vasculature by antigen-specific lymphocytes. I. Localization of 14C-labelled cells during acute, chronic, and relapsing experimental autoimmune encephalomyelitis, *Lab Invest* 2:162-170, 1990.

63. Cross A, Tuohy VK, Raine CS: Development of reactivity to new myelin antigens during chronic relapsing autoimmune demyelination, *Cell Immunol* 146:261-269, 1993.

64. DalCanto MC: Experimental models of viral-induced demyelination. In Cook SD, editor: *Handbook of multiple sclerosis,* 63-100, New York, 1990, Marcel Dekker.

65. Dean G, Kurtzke JF: On the risk of multiple sclerosis according to age at immigration to South America, *BMJ* 3:725-729, 1971.

66. Dinarello CA, Wolff SM: The role of inter leukin-1 in disease, *N Engl J Med* 328:106-113, 1993.

67. Dopp JM, Breneman SM, Olschowka JA: Expression of ICAM-1, VCAM-1, L-selectin, and leukosialin in the mouse central nervous system during the induction and remission stages of experimental allergic encephalomyelitis, *J Neuroimmunol* 54:129-144, 1994.

68. Dore-Duffy P, Donaldson JO, Koft T et al.: Prostaglandin release in multiple sclerosis: correlation with disease activity, *Neurology* 36:1587-1590, 1986.

69. Dore-Duffy P, Newman W, Balabanov R et al.: Evaluation of circulating soluble adhesion proteins in CSF and serum of patients with multiple sclerosis: correlation with clinical activity, *Ann Neurol* 37:55-62, 1995.

70. Dore-Duffy P, Washington R, Dragovic L: Expression of endothelial cell activation in microvessels from patients with multiple sclerosis, *Adv Exp Med Biol* 331:243-248, 1993.

71. Dreyer RF, Hopen G, Gass DM, Smith JL: Leber's idiopathic stellate neuroretinitis, *Arch Ophthalmol* 102:1140-1145, 1984.

72. DuBois JH, Bolton C, Cuzner ML: The production of prostaglandin and the regulation in neonatal primary mixed glial cell cultures, *J Neuroimmunol* 11:277-285, 1986.

73. Durelli L, Bongioanni MR, Cavallo R el al.: Chronic systemic high-dose recombinant α-2a reduces exacerbation rate, MRI signs of disease activity, and γ interferon production in relapsing-remitting multiple sclerosis, *Neurology* 44:406-413, 1994.

74. Durelli L, Cocito D, Riccio A et al.: High-dose intravenous methylprednisolone in the treatment of multiple sclerosis: clinical-immunologic correlations, *Neurology* 36:238-243, 1986.

75. Dutton JJ, Burde RM, Klingele TG: Autoimmune retrobulbar optic neuritis, *Am J Ophthalmol* 94:11-17, 1982.

76. Ebers GC: Optic neuritis and multiple sclerosis, *Arch Neurol* 42:702-704, 1985.

77. Ebers GC, Bulman DE, Sadovnick AD et al.: A population-based twin study in multiple sclerosis, *N Engl J Med* 315:1638-1642, 1986.

78. Ebers GC, Sadovnick AD: The role of genetic factors in multiple sclerosis susceptibility, *J Neuroimmunol* 54:1-18, 1994.

79. Eccleston PA, Jessen KR, Mirsky R: Transforming growth factor-β— and α- interferon have dual effects of growth of peripheral glia, *J Neurosci* 13:49-60, 1989.

80. Ellison GW: Steroids and immunosuppressive drugs. In Cook SD, editor: *Handbook of multiple sclerosis,* 371-402, New York, 1990, Marcel Dekker.

81. Ellison GW, Myers LW, Leake BD et al.: Design strategies in multiple sclerosis clinical trials, *Ann Neurol* 36(suppl):S108-S113, 1994.

82. Ellison GW, Myers LW, Mickey MR et al.: Clinical experience with azathioprine: The pros, *Neurology* 38(suppl 2):20-23, 1988.

83. Engell T: Neurological disease activity in multiple sclerosis patients with periphlebitis retinae, *Acta Neurol Scand* 73:168-172, 1986.

84. Engell T, Andersen PK: The frequency of periphlebitis retinae in multiple sclerosis, *Acta Neurol Scand* 65:601-608, 1982.

85. Erlington G, Newsom-Davis J: Clinical presentation and current immunology of the Lambert-Eaton myasthenic syndrome. In Lisak RP, editor: *Handbook of myasthenia gravis and myasthenic syndromes,* 81-102, New York, 1994, Marcel Dekker.

86. Essayan DC, Cohen JA, Zweiman B, Lisak RP: Effects of OX8+ lymphocytes on in vitro lymphocyte reactivity during experimental allergic encephalomyelitis, *J Neuroimmunol* 16:53, 1987.

86a. Farris BK, Pickard DJ: Bilateral postinfectious optic, *Ophthalmology* 97:339-345, 1990.

87. Fleishman JA, Beck RW, Linares OA, Klein JW: Deficits in visual function after resolution of optic neuritis, *Ophthalmology* 94:1029-1035, 1987.

88. Fog T: The topography of plaques in multiple sclerosis, *Acta Neurol Scand* 41(suppl 15):1-162, 1965.

89. Fog T: Vessel plaque relations and cerebrospinal fluid and brain tissue changes in multiple sclerosis, *Acta Neurol Scand* 40(suppl 100):9-15, 1964.

90. Fontana A, Fierz W, Wekerle H: Astrocytes present myelin basic protein to encephalitogenic T-cell lines, *Nature* 307:276, 1984.

91. Fontana A, Kristensen F, Dubs R et al.: Production of prostaglandin E and interleukin-1 like factors by cultured astrocytes and C-6 glioma cells, *J Immunol* 129:2413-2419, 1982.

92. Franciotta DM, Grimaldi LME, Martino GV et al.: Tumor necrosis factor in serum and cerebrospinal fluid of patients with multiple sclerosis, *Ann Neurol* 26:787-789, 1989.

93. Francis DA, Compston DA, Batchelor JR et al.: A reassessment of the risk of multiple sclerosis developing in patients with optic neuritis after extended follow up, *J Neurol Neurosurg Psychiatry* 50:758-765, 1987.

94. Fraser KB: Multiple sclerosis. A virus disease? *BMJ* 33:34-39, 1977.

94a. Frederiksen JL, Larsson HBW, Henriksen O, Olesen R: Magnetic resonance imaging of the brain in patients with acute monosymptomatic optic neuritis, *Acta Neurol Scand* 80:512-517, 1989.

95. Freedman M, Ruijs T, Selin L, Antel J: Peripheral blood γδ—T cells lyse fresh human brain-derived oligodendrocytes, *Ann Neurol* 30:794-800, 1991.

96. Fridkis-Hareli M, Teitelbaum D, Gurevitch E et al.: Direct binding of myelin basic protein and synthetic copolymer 1 to class II major histocompatibility complex molecules on living antigen presenting cells—specificity and promiscuity, *Proc Natl Acad Sci USA* 91:4872-4876, 1994.

97. Fujinami RS, Oldstone MBA: Amino acid homology between the encephalitogenic site of myelin basic protein and virus: a mechanism for autoimmunity, *Science* 230:1043-1045, 1985.

98. Fujinami RS, Oldstone MBA, Wroblewska Z et al.: Molecular mimicry in virus infection: crossreaction of measles virus phosphoprotein or of herpes simplex virus protein with human intermediates filaments, *Proc Natl Acad Sci USA* 80:2346-2350, 1983.

99. Fukunaga H, Engel AG, Lang B et al.: Passive transfer of Lambert-Eaton myasthenic syndrome with IgG from man to mouse depletes the presynaptic active zones, *Proc Natl Acad Sci USA* 80:7636-7640, 1983.

100. Gallo P, Piccinno MG, Krzalic L, Tavolato B: Tumor necrosis factor alpha (TNFα) in the cerebrospinal fluid from patients with multiple sclerosis, AIDS dementia complex, and brain tumors, *J Neuroimmunol* 23:41-44, 1989.

101. Georgopoulos C, McFarland HF: Heat shock proteins in multiple sclerosis and other autoimmune diseases, *Immunol Today* 14:373-375, 1993.

102. Gessain A, Barin F, Vernant JC et al.: Antibodies to HTLV-1 in patients with tropical spastic paraparesis, *Lancet* II:407-409, 1985.

103. Giegerich G, Pette M, Meinl E et al.: Diversity of T cell receptor α—and β—chain genes expressed by human T cells specific for similar myelin basic protein peptide/major histocompatibility complexes, *Eur J Immunol* 22:753-758, 1992.

104. Gonsette RE, Delmotte P, Demonty L: Failure of basic protein therapy for multiple sclerosis, *J Neurol* 216:27-31, 1977.

105. Goodin DS: The use of immunosuppressive agents in the treatment of multiple sclerosis: a critical review, *Neurology* 41:980-1005, 1991.

106. Goodkin DE, Rudick RA, Medendrop SV et al.: Low-dose (7.5mg) oral methotrexate reduces the rate of progression in chronic progressive multiple sclerosis, *Ann Neurol* 37:30-40, 1995.

107. Goust J-M, Hogan EL, Arnaud P: Abnormal regulation of IgG production in multiple sclerosis, *Neurology* 32:228-234, 1982.

108. Goverman J, Woods A, Larson L et al.: Transgeneic mice that express a myelin basic protein-specific T cell receptor develop spontaneous autoimmunity, *Cell* 72:551-560, 1993.

109. Graham EM, Francis DA, Sanders MD, Rudge P: Ocular inflammatory changes in established multiple sclerosis, *J Neurol Neurosurg Psychiatry* 52:1360-1363, 1989.

110. Greenberg SJ, Ehrlich GD, Abbott MA et al.: Detection of sequences homologous to human retroviral DNA in multiple sclerosis by gene amplification, *Proc Natl Acad Sci USA* 86:2878-2882, 1989.

111. Guenard V, Dinarello CA, Weston PJ, Aebischer P: Peripheral nerve regeneration is impeded by interleukin-1 receptor antagonist released from a polymeric guidance channel, *J Neurosci Res* 29:396-400, 1991.

112. Guilian D, Lachman LB: Interleukin-1 stimulation of astroglial proliferation after brain injury, *Science* 228:497-499, 1985.

113. Guy J, Mancuso A, Quisling RG et al.: Gadolinium-DPTA-enhanced magnetic resonance imaging in optic neuropathies, *Ophthalmology* 97:592-600, 1990.

114. Hafler DA, Duby AD, Lee SJ et al.: Oligoclonal T lymphocytes in the cerebrospinal fluid of patients with multiple sclerosis *J Exp Med* 167:1313-1322, 1988; (published erratum in *J Exp Med* 168:459, 1989).

115. Haire M: Significance of virus antibodies in multiple sclerosis, *Br Med Bull* 33:40-44, 1977.

116. Hao Q, Saida T, Nishimura M et al.: Failure to transfer multiple sclerosis into severe combined immunodeficiency mice by mononuclear cells from CSF of patients, *Neurology* 44:163-165, 1994.

117. Hartung H-P, Michels M, Reiners K et al.: Soluble ICAm-1 serum levels in multiple sclerosis and viral encephalitis, *Neurology* 43:2331-2335, 1993.

118. Hauser SL, Bhan AK, Giles F et al.: Immunocytochemical analysis of the cellular infiltrates in multiple sclerosis lesions, *Ann Neurol* 19:578-587, 1986.

119. Hauser SL, Dawson DM, Lehrich JR et al.: Intensive immunosuppression in progressive multiple sclerosis: a randomized, three-armed study of high-dose intravenous cyclophosphamide, plasma exchange and ACTH, *N Engl J Med* 308:173-180, 1983.

120. Hauser SL, Doolittle TH, Lincoln R et al.: Cytokine accumulations in CSF of multiple sclerosis patients: frequent detection of interleukin 1 and tumor necrosis factor but not interleukin 6, *Neurology* 40:1735-1739, 1990.

121. Hayashi T, Morimoto C, Burks JS et al.: Dual-label immunohistochemistry of the active multiple sclerosis lesion: major histocompatibility complex and activation antigens, *Ann Neurol* 24:523-531, 1988.

122. Heber-Katz E, Acha-Oreba H: The V-region disease hypothesis: evidence from auto-immune encephalomyelitis, *Immunol Today* 10:164-169, 1989.

123. Hickey WF: Migration of hematogenous cells through the blood-brain barrier and the initiation of CNS inflammation, *Brain Pathol* 1:97-105, 1991.

124. Hillert J, Olerup O: Multiple sclerosis is associated with genes within or close to the HLA-DR-DQ subregion on a normal DR15,DQ6, Dw2 haplotype, *Neurology* 43:163-168, 1993.

125. Hirayama M, Silberberg DH, Lisak RP, Pleasure DE: Long-term culture of oligodendrocytes isolated from rat corpus callosum by Percoll density gradient, *J Neuropathol Exp Neurol* 42:16-28, 1983.

126. Hodgkinson SJ, Steinman L: Monoclonal antibodies for treatment of multiple sclerosis. In Cook SD, editor: *Handbook of multiple sclerosis,* 481-492, New York, 1990, Marcel Dekker.

127. Hofman FM, Hinton DR, Johnson K, Merrill JE: Tumor necrosis factor identified in multiple sclerosis brain, *J Exp Med* 170:607-612, 1989.

128. Hofman FM, von Hanwehr RI, Dinarello CA et al.: Immunoregulatory molecules and IL-2 receptors identified in multiple sclerosis brain, *J Immunol* 136:3239-3245, 1986.

129. Hohlfeld R, Engel AG, Li K, Harper MC: Polymyositis mediated by T lymphocytes that express the γ/δ receptor, *N Engl J Med* 324:877, 1991.

130. Holoshitz J, Frenkel A, Ben Nun A, Cohen IR: Autoimmune encephalomyelitis (EAE) mediated or prevented by T lymphocyte lines directed against diverse antigenic determinants of myelin basic protein: vaccination is determinant specific, *J Immunol* 131:2810-2813, 1983.

131. Hommes OR, Lamers KJ, Reekers P: Effect of intensive immunosuppression on the course of chronic progressive multiple sclerosis, *J Neurol* 123:1616-1618, 1980.

132. Hulkower K, Brosnan CF, Aquino DA et al.: Expression of CSF-1, c-Fms, and MCP-1 in the central nervous system with experimental allergic encephalomyelitis, *J Immunol* 150:2525-2533, 1993.

133. Hvas J, Oksenberg JR, Fernando R et al.: Gamma delta T cell receptor repertoire in brain lesions of patients with multiple sclerosis, *J Neuroimmunol* 46:225-234, 1993.

134. The IFNB Multiple Sclerosis Study Group: Interferon β-1b is effective in relapsing-remitting multiple sclerosis. I. Clinical results of a multicenter, randomized, double-blind, placebo controlled trial, *Neurology* 43:655-661, 1993.

135. Isaacson P: Myxoviruses and autoimmunity, *Prog Allergy* 10:256, 1967.

135a. Jabs DA, Miller NR, Newman SA et al.: Optic neuropathy in systemic lupus erythematosus, *Arch Ophthalmol* 104:564-568, 1986.

136. Jacobs L, Cookfair D, Rudick R et al.: Results of a phase III trail of IM recombinant beta interferon as treatment for MS, *J Neuroimmunol* 54:170, 1994.

137. Jacobs L, Kinkel PR, Kinkel WR: Silent brain lesions in patients with isolated idiopathic optic neuritis: a clinical and nuclear magnetic resonance imaging study, *Arch Neurol* 43:452-455, 1986.

138. Jacobs L, Manschauer FE, Kaba SE: Clinical and magnetic resonance imaging in optic neuritis, *Neurology* 41:15-19, 1991.

139. Jahnke U, Fischer EH, Alvord EC: Sequence homology between viral proteins and proteins related to encephalomyelitis and neuritis, *Science* 229:282-284, 1985.

140. Jankovic BD, Draskaci M, Janjic M: Passive transfer of ''allergic'' encephalomyelitis with antibrain serum injected into the lateral ventricle of the brain, *Nature* 207:428, 1965.

141. Jiang H, Zhang SI, Pernis B: Role of CD8+ T cells in murine experimental allergic encephalomyelitis, *Science* 256:1213-1215, 1992.

142. Johns L, Flanders K, Ranges G, Sriram S: Successful treatment of experimental allergic encephalomyelitis with transforming growth factor -β1, *Immunol* 147:1792-1796, 1991.

143. Johns K, Lavin P, Elliot JH, Partain CL: Magnetic resonance imaging of the brain in isolated optic neuritis, *Arch Ophthalmol* 104:1486-1488, 1986.

144. Johnson AW, Land JM, Thompson EJ et al.: Evidence for increased nitric oxide production in multiple sclerosis, *J Neurol Neurosurg Psychiatry* 58:107, 1995.

145. Johnson D, Hafler DA, Fallis RJ et al.: Cell-mediated immunity to myelin-associated glycoprotein, proteolipid protein and myelin basic protein, *J Neuroimmunol* 13:99-108, 1986.

146. Johnson KP, Brooks BR, Cohen J et al.: Copolymer 1 (Cop 1) positively influences the relapse rate and progression of disability in relapsing-remitting multiple sclerosis: clinical results of a multi-center, placebo-controlled, double-blind trial, *Neurology* (in press).

147. Johnson RT: The virology of demyelinating diseases, *Ann Neurol* 36(suppl):S54-S60, 1994.

148. Johnson RT, Griffin DE: Post-infectious encephalomyelitis. In Kennedy PGE, Johnson RT, editors: *Infections of the nervous system,* 209-226, London, 1987, Butterworths.

149. Jones RE, Chou Y, Young A et al.: T cells with encephalitogenic potential from multiple sclerosis patients and Lewis rats do not induce disease in SCID mice following intracisternal injection, *Neurology* 44(suppl 2):A301-A302, 1994.

150. Joshi N, Usuku K, Hauser SL: The T-cell response to myelin basic protein in familial multiple sclerosis: diversity of fine specificity, restricting elements, and T-cell receptor useage, *Ann Neurol* 34:385-393, 1993.

151. Kahana E, Liebowitz U, Alter M: Brainstem and cranial nerve involvement in multiple sclerosis, *Acta Neurol Scand* 49:269-279, 1973.

152. Kappos L, Patzold U, Dommasch D et al.: Cyclosporine versus azathioprine in the long-term treatment of multiple sclerosis: results of the German multicenter study, *Ann Neurol* 23:56-63, 1988.

153. Karpus W, Gould K, Swanborg R: Suppressor cells of autoimmune encephalomyelitis respond to T cell receptor-associated determinants on effector cells by interleukin-4 secretion, *Eur J Immunol* 22:1757-1763, 1993.

154. Keith AB, Arnon R, Teitelbaum D et al.: The effect of Cop-1, a synthetic polypeptide, on chronic relapsing experimental allergic encephalomyelitis in guinea pigs, *J Neurol Sci* 42:267-274, 1979.

155. Kelley RE, Ellison GW, Myers LW et al.: Abnormal regulation of in vitro IgG production in multiple sclerosis, *Ann Neurol* 9:267-272, 1981.

156. Keltner JL, Johnson CA, Spurr JO, Beck RW: Optic Neuritis Study Group: baseline visual field profile of optic neuritis. The experience of the Optic Neuritis Treatment Trial (submitted for publication).

157. Kennedy M, Torrance D, Picha K, Mohler K: Analysis of cytokine mRNA expression in the central nervous system of mice with experimental autoimmune encephalomyelitis reveals that IL-10 mRNA correlates with recovery, J Immunol 2496-2515, 1992.

158. Khoury SJ, Hancock WW, Weiner HL: Oral tolerance to myelin basic protein and natural recovery from experimental autoimmune encephalomyelitis is associated with downregulation of inflammatory cytokines and differential upregulation of transforming growth factor β, —interleukin 4, and prostaglandin E expression in the brain, J Exp Med 176:1355-1364, 1992.

159. Koh D-R, Fung-Leung W-P, Ho A et al.: Less mortality but more relapses in experimental allergic encephalomyelitis in CD8—mice, Science 256:1210-1213, 1992.

160. Kojima K, Linington C, Lassmann H, Wekerle H: Induction of experimental allergic encephalomyelitis (EAE) by S100β—: an autoantigen expressed in both the CNS and thymus, J Neuroimmunol 54:176, 1994.

161. Koprowski H, DeFreitas EC, Harper ME et al.: Multiple sclerosis and human T-cell lymphotropic viruses, Nature 318:154-160, 1985.

162. Kotzin B, Karuturi S, Chou YK et al.: Preferential T-cell receptor β-chain variable gene use in myelin basic protein-reactive T-cell clones from patients with multiple sclerosis, Proc Natl Acad Sci USA 88:9161-9165, 1991.

163. Kriss A, Francis DA, Cuendet F et al.: Recovery after optic neuritis in childhood, J Neurol Neurosurg Psychiat 51:1253-1258, 1988.

163a. Kupersmith MJ, Burde RM, Warren FA et al.: Autoimmune optic neuropathy: evaluation and treatment, J Neurol Neurosurg Psychiatry 51:1381-1386, 1988.

164. Kuroda Y, Matsui M, Kikuchi M et al.: In situ demonstration of the HTLV-1 genome in the spinal cord of a patient with HTLV-1-associated myelopathy, Neurology 44:2295-2299, 1994.

165. Kurtzke JF: Further consideration on the geographic distribution of multiple sclerosis, Acta Neurol Scand 43:283-297, 1967.

166. Kurtzke JF: Data registries on selected segments of the population. In Schoenberg BS, editor: Veterans in neurologic epidemiology, principles and clinical applications, 55-67, New York, 1978, Raven Press.

167. Kurtzke JF: Optic neuritis or multiple sclerosis, Arch Neurol 42:704-710, 1985.

168. Kurtzke JF, Beebe GW, Norman JE: Epidemiology of multiple sclerosis in US veterans: 1. Race, sex, and geographic distribution, Neurology 29:1228-1235, 1979.

169. Kurtzke JF, Dean G, Botha DRJ: A method of estimating the age at immigration of white immigrants to South Africa with an example of its importance, S Afr Med J 44:663-669, 1970.

170. Kurtzke JF, Hyllested K: Multiple sclerosis in the Faeroe Islands. I. Clinical and epidemiologic features, Ann Neurol 5:6-21, 1979.

171. Kurtzke JF, Hyllested K: Multiple sclerosis in the Faeroe Islands. II. Clinical update, transmission, and the nature of MS, Neurology 36:307-328, 1986.

172. Lando Z, Teitelbaum D, Arnon R: Effect of cyclophosphamide on suppressor cell activity in mice unresponsive to EAE, J Immunol 123:2156-2160, 1979.

173. Lassman H, Linington C: The role of antibodies against myelin surface antigens in demyelination in chronic EAE. In Crescenzi GS, editor: A multidisciplinary approach to myelin diseases, 219-225, New York, 1987, Plenum.

174. Latov N: Neuropathic syndromes associated with monoclonal gammopathies. In Waksman BH, editor: Immunologic mechanisms in neurologic and psychiatric disease, vol 68, 221-232, New York, 1990, Association for Research in Nervous and Mental Disease, Raven Press.

175. Lavi E, Burns JB, Rostami A: Transfer of multiple sclerosis (MS) peripheral blood lymphocytes (PBL) into severe combined immunodeficiency (SCID) mice, Neurology 44(suppl 2):A302, 1994.

176. LeBar R, Lubetski C, Vincent C et al.: The M2 autoantigen of central nervous system myelin, a glycoprotein present in oligodendrocyte membrane, Clin Exp Immunol 66:423-443, 1986.

177. Lee SC, Liu W, Roth P et al.: Macrophage colony stimulating factor (CSF-1) in human fetal astrocytes and microglia: differential regulation by cytokines and LPS, and modulationclass II MHC on microglia, J Immunol 150:594-604, 1992.

178. Lehmann PV, Forsthuber T, Miller A, Sercaz EE: Spreading of T-cell autoimmunity to cryptic determinants of an autoantigen, Nature 358:155-157, 1992.

179. Lehmann PV, Sercarz EE, Forsthuber R et al.: Determinant spreading and the dynamics of the autoimmune T-cell repertoire, Immunol Today 14:203-208, 1993.

180. Lieberman AP, Pitha PM, Shin H, Shin ML: Production of tumor necrosis factor and other cytokines by astrocytes stimulated with lipopolysaccharide or a neurotropic virus, Proc Natl Acad Sci USA 86:6348-6352, 1989.

181. Lightman S, McDonald WI, Bird AC et al.: Retinal venous sheathing in optic neuritis: its significance for the pathogenesis of multiple sclerosis, Brain 110:405-414, 1987.

182. Lim JI, Tessler HH, Goodwin JA: Anterior granulomatous uveitis in patients with multiple sclerosis, Ophthalmology 98:142-145, 1991.

183. Linington C, Lassmann H: Antibody responses in chronic relapsing experimental allergic encephalomyelitis: correlation of serum demyelinating activity with antibody titre to the myelin/oligodendrocyte glycoprotein (MOG), J Neuroimmunol 17:61-69, 1987.

184. Lipton HL: Transfer of multiple sclerosis into severe combined immunodeficiency mice, Ann Neurol 34:115, 1993.

185. Lisak RP: Immunological abnormalities. In McDonald IA, Silberberg DH, editors: Multiple sclerosis, 74-98, London, 1986, Butterworths.

186. Lisak RP: Glial cells and products of activated inflammatory cells: implications of pathogenesis and treatment of multiple sclerosis. In Cassullo CL, Caputo D, Ghezzi A, Zaffaroni M, editors: Virology and immunology in multiple sclerosis: rationale for therapy, 13-20, Heidelberg, 1988a, Springer-Verlag.

187. Lisak RP: Overview of the rationale for immunomodulating therapies in multiple sclerosis (MS), Neurology 38(suppl2):5-8, 1988b.

188. Lisak RP: Immune-mediated parainfectious encephalomyelitis. In McKendell RR, Stroop WG, editors: Handbook of neurovirology, 173-186, New York, 1994, Marcel Dekker.

189. Lisak RP, Barchi RL: Myasthenia gravis, 128-131; 134-137, Philadelphia, 1982, WB Saunders.

190. Lisak RP, Bealmear B: Antibodies to interleukin-1 inhibit cytokine induced proliferation of neonatal rat Schwann cells in vitro, J Neuroimmunol 31:123-132, 1991.

191. Lisak RP, Bealmear B, Ragheb S: Antibodies to interleukin-1α,—but not interleukin-1β,—is a co-mitogen for neonatal rat Schwann cells in vitro and acts via interleukin-1 receptors, J Neuroimmunol 55:171-178, 1994.

192. Lisak RP, Bealmear B: Transforming growth factor-β—(TGF-β) is co-mitogenic for Schwann cells (SC) with interleukin-1—(IL-1α), Neurology (in press).

193. Lisak RP, Heinze RG, Falk GA, Kies MW: Search for antiencephalitogenic antibodiesin human demyelinating diseases, Neurology 18(part 2):122-128, 1968.

194. Lisak RP, Zweiman B: In vitro cell mediated immunity of cerebrospinal fluid lymphocytes to myelin basic protein in primary demyelinating diseases, N Engl J Med 297:850-853, 1977.

195. Lisak RP, Zweiman B, Blanchard N, Rorke LB: Effect of treatment with copolymer 1 (Cop1) on the in vivo and in vitro manifestations of experimental allergic encephalomyelitis (EAE), J Neurol Sci 62:281-293, 1983.

196. Lisak RP, Zweiman B, Burns JB et al.: Immune response to myelin antigens in multiple sclerosis, Ann NY Acad Sci 436:221-230, 1984.

197. Lisby G: Search for an HTLV-1-like retrovirus in patients with MS by enzymatic DNA amplification, Acta Neurol Scand 88:385-387, 1993.

198. Lu C-Z, Fredrickson S, Xiao B-G, Link H: Interleukin-2 secreting cells in multiple sclerosis and controls, J Neurol Sci 120:99-106, 1993.

199. Lu C-Z, Jensen MA, Arnason BGW: Interferon γ—and interleukin-4-secreting cells in multiple sclerosis, J Neuroimmunol 46:123-128, 1993.

200. Lublin F: Relapsing experimental allergic encephalomyelitis—an autoimmune model of multiple sclerosis, Springer Semin Immunopathol 8:197-208, 1985.

201. Lucarelli MJ, Pepose JS, Arnold AC, Foos RY: Immunopathologic features of retinal lesions in multiple sclerosis, *Ophthalmology* 98:1652-1656, 1991.

202. Lumsden CE: The pathology of multiple sclerosis. In Virken PV, Bruyn GW, editors: *Clinical neurology,* vol 9, 217-309, Amsterdam, North Holland, 1970.

203. Maitland CG, Miller NR: Neuroretinitis, *Arch Ophthalmol* 102:1146-1150, 1984.

204. Malinkowski SM, Pulido JS, Goeken NE et al.: The association of HLA-BB, B51, DR2, and multiple sclerosis, *Ophthalmology* 100:1199-1205, 1993.

205. Martin R, Howell MD, Jaraquemada D et al.: A myelin basic protein peptide is recognized by cytotoxic T cells in the context of four HLA-DR types associated with multiple sclerosis, *J Exp Med* 173:19-24, 1991.

206. Martin R, McFarland HF, McFarlin DE: Immunological aspects of demyelinating diseases, *Annu Rev Immunol* 10:153-187, 1992a.

207. Martin R, Utz U, Coligan JE et al.: Diversity in fine specificity and T cell receptor useage of the human CD4+ cytotoxic T cell response specific for the immunodominant myelin basic protein peptide 87-106, *J Immunol* 148:1359-1366, 1992b.

208. Martino G, DuPont BL, Wollmann RL et al.: The human-severe combined immunodeficiency myasthenia mouse model: a new approach for the study of myasthenia gravis, *Ann Neurol* 34:48-56, 1993.

209. Merrill JE, Ignarro IJ, Sherman MP et al.: Migroglial cell cytotoxicity of oligodendrocytes is mediated through nitric oxide, *J Immunol* 151:2132-2141, 1993.

210. Merrill JE, Kutsunai S, Mohlstrom C et al.: Proliferation of astroglia and oligodendroglia in response to human T-cell derived factors, *Science* 224:1428, 1984.

211. Miller AE: Clinical features. In Cook SD, editor: *Handbook of multiple sclerosis,* 169-186, New York, 1990, Marcel Dekker.

212. Miller A, Al-Sabbagh A, Santos LMB et al.: Epitopes of myelin basic protein that trigger TGF-β—release after oral tolerization are distinct from encephalomyelitis epitopes and mediate epitope-driven bystander suppression, *J Immunol* 151:7307-7315, 1993.

213. Miller DH, Newton MR, van der Poel JC et al.: Magnetic resonance imaging of the optic nerve inoptic neuritis, *Neurology* 38:175-179, 1988.

214. Miller DH, Ormerod IEC, McDonald WI et al.: The early risk of multiple sclerosis after optic neuritis, *J Neurol Neurosurg Psychiatry* 51:1569-1571, 1988.

215. Milligan NM, Newcomb R, Compston DAS: A double blind controlled trial of high dose methylprednisolone in patients with multiple sclerosis. 1. Clinical effects, *J Neurol Neurosurg Psychiatry* 50:511-516, 1987.

216. Montgomery IN, Rauch HC: Experimental allergic encephalomyelitis in mice: adoptive transfer of disease is modulated by the presence of natural suppressor cells, *Neurochem Res* 9:1399-1406, 1984.

217. Mor F, Cohen I: Shifts in the epitopes of myelin basic protein recognized by Lewis rat T cells before, during and after the induction of experimental autoimmune encephalomyelitis, *J Clin Invest* 92:2199-2206, 1993.

218. Morimoto C, Hafler DA, Weiner HL: Selective loss of suppressor inducer T cell subset in progressive multiple sclerosis, *N Engl J Med* 316:67-72, 1988.

219. Mossman T, Moore K: The role of IL-10 in cross regulation of Th1 and Th2 responses, *Immunol Today* 12:A49-A53, 1991.

219a. The Multiple Sclerosis Study Group: Efficacy and toxicity of cyclosporine in chronic progressive multiple sclerosis: a randomized, double-blind, placebo-controlled clinical trial, *Ann Neurol* 27:591-605, 1990.

220. Nikoskelainen E, Frey H, Salmi A: Prognosis of optic neuritis with special reference to cerebrospinal fluid immunoglobulins and measles virus antibodies, *Ann Neurol* 9:545-550, 1981.

221. Nordal HJ, Vnadvick B, Norrby E: Multiple sclerosis: local synthesis of electrophoretically restricted measles, rubella, mumps, and herpes simplex virus antibodies in the central nervous system, *Scand J Immunol* 7:473-479, 1978.

222. Norhona A, Toscas A, Jensen MA: Interferon β—decreases T cell activation and interferon γ—production in multiple sclerosis, *J Neuroimmunol* 46:145-154, 1993.

223. Norrby E, Link H, Olsson JE: Measles virus antibodies in multiple sclerosis, comparison of antibody titers in cerebrospinal fluid and serum, *Arch Neurol* 30:285-292, 1974.

224. Noseworthy JH, O'Brien PC, van Engelen BGM: Intravenous immunoglobulin therapy in multiple sclerosis: progress from remyelination in the Thieler's virus model to a randomized, double-blind, placebo-controlled trial, *J Neurol Neurosurg Psychiatry* 57(suppl):11-14, 1994.

225. Nuwer MR, Visscher BR, Packwood JW, Namerow NS: Evoked potential testing in relatives of multiple sclerosis patients, *Neurology* 18:30-34, 1985.

226. Ohta M, Ohta K, Mori F et al.: Sera from patients with multiple sclerosis react with human T cell lymphotropic virus-1 GAG proteins but not ENV proteins: western blotting analysis, *J Immunol* 137:3440-3443, 1986.

227. Oksenberg JR, Panzara MA, Begovitch AB et al.: T-cell receptor V beta-D beta-J beta gene rearrangements with specificity for a myelin basic protein peptide in brain lesions of multiple sclerosis, *Nature* 362:68-70, 1993a.

228. Oksenberg JR, Panzara MA, Steinman L: Multiple sclerosis: from immunogenetics to immunotherapy, *J Neurol Sci* 115(suppl 1):S29-S37, 1993b.

229. Oksenberg JR, Stuart S, Begovich AB et al.: Limited heterogeneity of rearranged T-cell receptor V alpha transcripts in brains of multiple sclerosis patients, *Nature* 345:344-346, 1990 (published erratum *Nature* 353:94, 1991).

230. Olsson T, Sun J, Hillaert J et al.: Increased numbers of T cells recognizing multiple myelin basic protein epitopes in multiple sclerosis, *Eur J Immunol* 22:1083-1087, 1992.

231. Olsson T, Wang WZ, Zhi WW et al.: Autoreactive T lymphocytes in multiple sclerosis determined by antigen induced secretion of interferon-gamma, *J Clin Invest* 86:981-985, 1990.

232. Optic Neuritis Study Group: The clinical profile of optic neuritis: experience of the Optic Neuritis Study Group, *Arch Ophthalmol* 109:1673-1678, 1991.

233. Optic Neuritis Study Group: The effect of corticosteroids for acute optic neuritis on the subsequent development of multiple sclerosis, *N Engl J Med* 329:1764-1769, 1993.

234. Ormerod IEC, McDonald WI, du Boulay GH et al.: Disseminated lesions at presentation in patients with optic neuritis, *J Neurol Neurosurg Psychiatry* 49:124-127, 1986.

235. Osame M, Matsumoto M, Usuku K et al.: Chronic progressive myelopathy associated with elevated antibodies to human T-lymphotropic virus type and adult T-cell leukemia like cells, *Ann Neurol* 21:117-122, 1987.

236. Palffy G: MS in Hungary including the gypsy population. In Kuroiwa Y, Kurland LT, editors: *Multiple sclerosis east and west,* 149-157, Karger, Basel.

237. Panitch H: Influence of infection on exacerbations of multiple sclerosis, *Ann Neurol* 36(suppl):S25-S28, 1994.

238. Panitch HS, Hirsch RL, Schindler J, Johnson KP: Exacerbations of multiple sclerosis in patients treated with gamma interferon, *Lancet* I:893-895; Panel discussion, 1984, *Ann NY Acad Sci* 436:291-293, 1987.

239. Panitch HS, Swoveland P, Johnson KP: Antibodies to measles virus react with myelin basic protein, *Neurology* 29:548-549, 1979.

240. Paty DW: Neuroimaging in multiple sclerosis. In Cook SD, editor: *Handbook of multiple sclerosis,* 291-316, New York, 1990, Marcel Dekker.

241. Paty DW, Li DK, UBC MS/MRI Study Group, and the IFNB Multiple Sclerosis Study Group: Interferon beta-1b is effective in relapsing-remitting multiple sclerosis. II. MRI analysis results of a multicentre, randomized, double, placebo-controlled trial, *Neurology* 43:662-667, 1993.

242. Pelfrey CM, Trotter JL, Tranquill LR, McFarland HF: Identification of a second T cell epitope of human proteolipid protein (residues 89-106) recognized by proliferative and cytolytic CD4+ T cells from multiple sclerosis patients, *J Neuroimmunol* 53:153-161.

243. Perkin GD, Rose FC: *Optic neuritis and its differential diagnosis,* Oxford, 1979, Oxford University Press.

244. Perry HD, Mallen FJ, Wright GD Jr, Maris PJG: Retinal arteriolar occlusion in multiple sclerosis, *Ann Ophthalmol* 18:168-170, 1986.

245. Pette M, Fujita K, Kitze B et al.: Myelin basic protein specific T lymphocyte lines from MS patients and healthy individuals, *Neurology* 40:1770-1776, 1990.

246. Porrini AM, Reder AT: IFN-γ—, IFN-β, and PGE₁ affect monokine secretion: relevance to monocyte activation in multiple sclerosis, *Cell Immunol* 157:428-438, 1994.

247. Porter KG, Sinnamon DG, Gilles RR: Cryptococcus neoformans-specific oligoclonal bands in cerebrospinal fluid in cryptococcal meningitis, *Lancet* 1:1262, 1977.

248. Porter R: Uveitis in association with multiple sclerosis, *Br J Ophthalmol* 56:478-481, 1972.

249. Prayoonwiwat MD, Pease LR, Rodriguez M: Human T-cell lymphotropic virus type I sequences detected by nested polymerase chain reactions are not associated with multiple sclerosis, *Mayo Clin Proc* 66:665-680, 1991.

250. Price RW, Brew BJ, Rosenbaum M: The AIDS dementia complex and HIV-1 brain infection: a pathogenetic model of virus-immune interaction. In Waksman BH, editor: *Immunologic mechanisms in neurologic and psychiatric disease,* vol 68, 269-290, New York, 1990, Association for Research in Nervous and Mental Disease, Raven Press.

251. Prineas JW: The neuropathology of multiple sclerosis. In Vinken PJ, Bruyn GW, Klawans, Koetsier JC, editors: *Demyelinating diseases: handbook of clinical neurology,* vol 47, *rev ser 3,* 213-258, Amsterdam, 1985, Elsevier.

252. Prineas JW: The pathology of multiple sclerosis. In Cook SD, editor: *Handbook of multiple sclerosis,* New York, 1990, Marcel Dekker.

253. Prineas JW, Barnard RO, Kwon EE et al.: Multiple sclerosis: remyelination of nascent lesions, *Ann Neurol* 33:137-151, 1993.

254. Prineas JW, Kwon EE, Goldenberg PZ et al.: Multiple sclerosis: oligodendrocytes proliferation and differentiation in fresh lesions, *Lab Invest* 61:489-503, 1989.

255. Racke MK, Cannella B, Albert P et al.: Evidence of endogenous regulatory function of transforming growth factor β1 in experimental allergic encephalomyelitis, *Int Immunol* 4:615-620, 1992a.

256. Racke MK, Dhib-Jalbut S, Cannella B et al.: Prevention and treatment of chronic relapsing experimental allergic encephalomyelitis by transforming growth factor β1, *J Immunol* 146:3012-3017, 1991.

257. Racke MK, Martin R, McFarland H, Fritz RB: Copolymer-1-induced inhibition of antigen-specific T-cell activation: interference with antigen presentation, *J Neuroimmunol* 37:75-84, 1992b.

258. Raine CS: Multiple sclerosis: immune system expression in the central nervous system, *J Neuropathol Exp Neurol* 53:328-337, 1994.

259. Raine CS, Hintzen R, Traugott U, Moore GR: Oligodendrocyte proliferation and enhanced CNS remyelination after therapeutic manipulation of chronic relapsing EAE, *Ann NY Acad Sci* 540:712-714, 1988.

260. Raine CS, Stone SH: Animal model for multiple sclerosis—chronic experimental allergic encephalomyelitis in inbred guinea pigs, *NY State J Med* 77:1693-1696, 1977.

261. Raine CS, Wu E: Multiple sclerosis: remyelination in acute lesions, *J Neuropathol Exp Neurol* 52:199-205, 1993.

262. Ransohoff R, Hamilton T, Tani M et al.: Astrocyte expression of mRNA encoding cytokines IP-10 and JE/MCP-1 in experimental autoimmune encephalomyelitis, *FASEB J* 7:592-602, 1993.

263. Reddy EP, Sandberg-Wollheim M, Mettus RV et al.: Amplification and molecular cloning of HTLV-1 sequences from DNA of multiple sclerosis patients, *Science* 243:529-533, 1989.

264. Reder AT, Antel JP, Oger J et al.: Low T8 antigen density on lymphocytes in active multiple sclerosis, *Ann Neurol* 16:242-249, 1984.

265. Reder AT, Arnason BGW: Immunology of multiple sclerosis. In Vinken PJ, Bruyn GW, Klawans HL, Koestsier JC, editors: *Handbook of clinical neurology,* vol 47, rev series 3, *Demyelinating diseases,* 337-396, Amsterdam, 1985, Elsevier.

266. Reinherz EL, Weiner SL, Hauser SL et al.: Loss of suppressor T cells in active multiple sclerosis: analysis with monoclonal antibodies, *N Engl J Med* 303:125-129, 1980.

267. Rice GPA: Virus-induced demyelination in man: models for multiple sclerosis, *Curr Opin Neurol* 5:188-194, 1992.

268. Ridley AJ, Davis JB, Stroobant P, Land H: Transforming growth factors β1—and β2—are mitogens for Schwann cells, *J Cell Biol* 109:3419-3424, 1989.

269. Riechmann L, Clark M, Waldmann H, Winter G: Reshaping human antibodies for therapy, *Nature* 332:323-327, 1988.

270. Rieckmann P, Martin S, Weichselbraun I et al.: Serial analysis of circulating adhesion molecules and TNF receptor in serum from patients with multiple sclerosis: cICAM-1 is an indicator for relapse, *Neurology* 44:2367-2372, 1994.

271. Rizzo JF, Lessell S: Risk of developing multiple sclerosis after uncomplicated optic neuritis: a long term prospective study, *Neurology* 38:185-190, 1988.

272. Robbins DS, Shirazi Y, Drysdale BE et al.: Production of cytotoxic factor for oligodendrocytes by stimulated astrocytes, *J Immunol* 139:2593-2597, 1987.

273. Rodriguez M, Lennon VA: Immunoglobulins promote remyelination in the central nervous system, *Ann Neurol* 27:12-17, 1990.

274. Rodriguez M, Scheithauer BW, Forbes T, Kelley PJ: Oligodendrocyte injury is an early event in lesions of multiple sclerosis, *Mayo Clin Proc* 68:627-636, 1993.

275. Rogers-Johnson PEB, Ono SG, Asher DM, Gibbs CJ Jr: Tropical spastic paraparesis and HTLV-1 myelopathy: clinical features and pathogenesis. In Waksman BH, editor: *Immunologic mechanisms in neurologic and psychiatric disease,* vol 68, 117-130, New York, 1990, Association for Research in Nervous and Mental Disease, Raven Press.

276. Rostami AM, Burns JB, Eccelston PA et al.: Search for antibodies to galactocerebroside in the sera and cerebrospinal fluid in human demyelinating disorders, *Ann Neurol* 22:381-383, 1987.

277. Rostami AM, Galetta S, Farber RE et al.: A double-blind clinical trial of extracorporeal photopheresis in chronic progressive multiple sclerosis, *Neurology* 40(suppl 1):393-394, 1990.

278. Rostami AM, Hilliarrd BA, Ventura ES, Phillips SM: Suppression of experimental autoimmune encephalomyelitis (EAE) by diphtheria-IL-2 fusion toxin, *Neurology* 44(suppl 2):A326-A327, 1994.

279. Rostami AM, Lisak RP, Blanchard N et al.: Oligoclonal IgG in the cerebrospinal fluid of animals with acute experimental allergic encephalomyelitis, *J Neurol Sci* 53:433-441, 1982.

280. Rucker CW: Sheathing of the retinal veins in multiple sclerosis, *Proc Staff Mg Mayo Clin* 19:176-178, 1944.

281. Rucker CW: Sheathing of the retinal veins in multiple sclerosis: review of pertinent literature, *Mayo Clin Proc* 47:335-340, 1972.

282. Ruddle NH, Beyman CM, McGrath Grunett ML et al.: An antibody to lymphotoxin and tumor necrosis factor prevents transfer of experimental allergic encephalomyelitis, *J Exp Med* 172:1193-1200, 1990.

283. Rudge P, Koetsier JC, Mertin J et al.: Randomized double blind controlled trial of cyclosporin in multiple sclerosis, *J Neurol Neurosurg Psychiatry* 52:559-565, 1989.

284. Rudick RA, Ransohoff RM: Cytokine secretion by multiple sclerosis monocytes: relationship to disease activity, *Arch Neurol* 49:265-270, 1992.

285. Ruelen JPH; Sanders EACM, Hogenhuis LAH: Eye movement disorders in multiple sclerosis and optic neuritis, *Brain* 106:121-140, 1983.

286. Rush JA, Younge BR: Paralysis of cranial nerves III, IV, and VI: cause and prognosis in 1000 cases, *Arch Ophthalmol* 99:76-79, 1981.

287. Saeki Y, Mima R, Sakoda S et al.: Transfer of multiple sclerosis into severe combined immunodeficiency mice by mononuclear cells from cerebrospinal fluid of the patients, *Proc Natl Acad Sci USA* 89:6157-6161, 1992.

288. Saida K, Saida T, Brown MJ, Silberberg DH: In vivo demyelination by intraneural injection of antigalactocerebroside serum: a morphologic study, *Am J Pathol* 95:99-116, 1979.

289. Saida T, Saida K, Dorfman SH et al.: Experimental allergic neuritis induced by sensitization with galactocerebroside, *Science* 204:1103-1106, 1979a.

290. Saida T, Saida K, Silberberg DH: Demyelination produced by experimental allergic neuritis serum and antigalactocerebroside antiserum in CNS cultures: an ultrastructural study, *Acta Neuropathol* 48:19-25, 1979b.

291. Saida T, Silberberg DH, Fry JM, Manning MC: Demyelinating antigalactocerebroside antibodies in EAN and EAE, *J Neuropath Exp Neurol* 36:627, 1977.

292. Sakai K, Mitchell DJ, Hodgkinson SJ et al.: Prevention of experimental encephalomyelitis with peptides blocking T cell-MHC interaction, *Proc Natl Acad Sci USA,* 1992.

293. Sandberg M, Bynke H: Cerebrospinal fluid in 25 cases of optic neuritis, *Acta Neurol Scand* 49:443-452, 1973.

294. Sandberg-Wolheim M, Bynke H, Cronzvist S et al.: A long-term prospective study of optic neuritis: evaluation of risk factors, *Ann Neurol* 27:386-393, 1990.

295. Sanders ME, Koski CL, Robbins D et al.: Terminal complement pathway activation in cerebrospinal fluid in Guillain-Barre Syndrome and multiple sclerosis, *J Immunol* 136:4456-4459, 1986.

296. Santos LMB, Al-Sabbagh A, Londono A, Weiner HL: Oral tolerance to myelin basic protein induces regulatory TGF-β—secreting cells in Peyer's patches of SJL mice, *Cell Immunol* 157:439-447, 1994.

297. Schluesener HJ, Sobel RA, Linington C, Weiner HL: A monoclonal antibody against a myelin oligodendrocyte glycoprotein induces relapses and demyelination in central nervous system autoimmune disease, *J Immunol* 139:4016-4021, 1987.

298. Schwab ME, Kapfhammer JP, Bandtolow CE: Inhibitors of neurite growth, *Annu Rev Neurosci* 16:565-595, 1993.

299. Sedwick EM: Pathophysiology and evoked responses in multiple sclerosis. In Hallpike JF, Adams CWM, Tourtellotte WW, editors: *Multiple sclerosis,* 177-201, Baltimore, 1983, Williams and Wilkins.

300. Seil FJ: Tissue culture studies of demyelinating disease: a critical review, *Ann Neurol* 2:345-355, 1977.

301. Seil FJ, Falk GA, Kies MW, Alvord EC Jr: The in vitro demyelinating activity of sera from guinea pigs sensitized with whole CNS and with purified encephalitogen, *Exp Neurol* 22:545-555, 1968.

302. Selbst RG, Selhorst JB, Harbison JW, Myer EC: Parainfectious optic neuritis: report and review following varicella, *Arch Neurol* 40:347-350, 1983.

303. Selmaj K, Brosnan CF, Raine CS: Co-localization of lymphocytes bearing $\gamma\delta$—T-cell receptor and heat shock protein hsp65$^+$ oligodendrocytes in multiple sclerosis, *Proc Natl Acad Sci USA* 88:6452-6456, 1991a.

304. Selmaj K, Nowak Z, Tchorzewski H: Interleukin 1 and interleukin 2 production by peripheral blood mononuclear cells in multiple sclerosis patients, *J Neurol Sci* 85:67-76, 1988.

305. Selmaj K, Raine CS: TNF mediates myelin and oligodendrocyte damage in vitro, *Ann Neurol* 23:339-346, 1988.

306. Selmaj K, Raine CS: Anti-tumor necrosis factor therapy abrogates autoimmune demyelination, *Ann Neurol* 30:694-700, 1991.

307. Selmaj K, Raine CS, Cannella B, Brosnan CF: Identification of lymphocytotoxin and tumor necrosis factor in multiple sclerosis, *J Clin Invest* 87:949-954, 1991b.

308. Sergott RC, Brown MJ, Lisak RP, Silberberg DH: Optic nerve demyelination induced by human serum: patients with multiple sclerosis or optic neuritis and normal subjects, *Neurology* 35:1438-1442, 1985.

309. Sergott RC, Brown MJ, Silberberg DH, Lisak RP: Anti-galactocerebroside serum demyelinates optic nerve in vivo, *J Neurol Sci* 64:297-303, 1984.

310. Shah A, Lisak RP: Neurologic complications of immunomodulating therapies. In Vinken PJ, Bruyn GW, Klawans HL, editors: *Handbook of clinical neurology: intoxications of the nervous system,* Amsterdam, Elsevier, (in press).

311. Shapiro RT: Symptom management in multiple sclerosis, *Ann Neurol* 36:S12-129, 1994.

312. Sharief MK, Noori MA, Ciardi M et al.: Increased levels of circulating ICAM-1 in serum and cerebrospinal fluid of patients with active multiple sclerosis: correlation with TNF-α—and blood brain barrier damage, *J Neuroimmunol* 43:15-22, 1993.

313. Shaw MK, Kim C, Ho K-L et al.: A combination of adoptive transfer and antigenic challenge induces consistent murine experimental autoimmune encephalomyelitis in C57BL/6 mice and other reputed resistant strains, *J Neuroimmunol* 39:139-150, 1992.

314. Shaw PJ, Smith NM, Ince PG, Bates D: Chronic periphlebitis retinae in multiple sclerosis: a histopathological study, *J Neurol Sci* 77:147-152, 1987.

315. Shimonnkevitz R, Colburn C, Burnham JA et al.: Clonal expansions of activated gamma/delta T cells in recent-onset multiple sclerosis, *Proc Natl Acad Sci USA* 90:923-927, 1993.

316. Shubert D: Synergistic interactions between transforming growth factor beta and fibroblast growth factor regulate Schwann cell mitosis, *J Neurobiol* 23:143-148, 1992.

317. Sibley WA, Bamford CR, Clark K: Clinical viral infections and multiple sclerosis, *Lancet* 1:1313-1315, 1985.

318. Sibley WA, Bramford CR, Clark K et al.: A prospective study of physical trauma and multiple sclerosis, *J Neurol Neurosurg Psychiatry* 54:584-589, 1991.

319. Sibley WA, Foley JM: Infection and immunization in multiple sclerosis, *Ann NY Acad Sci* 122:457-468, 1965.

320. Silberberg DH: Azathioprine in multiple sclerosis: the cons, *Neurology* 38(suppl 2):24-27, 1988.

321. Silberberg DH: Corticosteroids and optic neuritis, *N Engl J Med* 326:1810-1810, 1993.

322. Silberberg DH, Manning MC, Schreiber AD: Tissue culture demyelination by normal human serum, *Ann Neurol* 15:575-580, 1984.

323. Sipe JC, Romine JS, Koziol JA et al.: Cladribine in treatment of chronic progressive multiple sclerosis, *Lancet* 334:9-13, 1994.

324. Siva A, Radhakrishnan K, Kurland LT et al.: Trauma and multiple sclerosis: a population-based cohort study from Olmsted County, Minnesota, *Neurology* 43:1878-1882, 1993.

325. Smith CR, Aisen ML, Scheinberg LC: Symptomatic management of multiple sclerosis. In McDonald WI, Silberberg DH, editors: *Multiple sclerosis,* 166-183, London, 1986, Butterworths.

326. Smith CR, Scheinberg LC: Symptomatic treatment and rehabilitation in multiple sclerosis. In Cook SD, editor: *Handbook of multiple sclerosis,* 327-330, New York, 1990, Marcel Dekker.

327. Smith T, Schmeid M, Lassman H, Cuzner ML: The HPA-axis and T-cell apoptosis during EAE, *J Neuroimmunol* 54:198, 1994.

328. Soderstrom M, Link H, Sun J-B et al.: T cells recognizing multiple peptides of myelin basic protein are found in blood and enriched in the cerebrospinal fluid in optic neuritis and multiple sclerosis, *Scand J Immunol* 37:355-268, 1993.

329. Stefoski D, Davis FA, Faut M, Schauf CL: 4-aminopyridine in patients with multiple sclerosis, *Ann Neurol* 21:71-81, 1987.

330. Steinman L: Multiple sclerosis and its animal models: the role of the major histocompatibility complex and the T cell receptor repertoire, *Springer Semin Immunopathol* 14:79-93, 1992.

331. Stendahl-Brodin L, Link H: Optic neuritis: oligoclonal bands increase the risk of multiple sclerosis, *Acta Neurol Scand* 67:301-304, 1983.

332. Stevens DB, Gould KE, Swanborg RH: Transforming growth factor-$\beta1$ inhibits tumor necrosis factor-α/lymphotoxin production and adoptive transfer of disease by effector cells of autoimmune encephalomyelitis, *J Neuroimmunol* 51:77-83, 1994.

333. Stone SH, Lerner EM II: Chronic disseminated allergic encephalomyelitis in guinea pigs, *Ann NY Acad Sci* 122:227-238, 1965.

334. Sun D, Le J, Malotkey M, Coleclough C: Major role of antigen-presenting cells in the response of rat encephalitogenic T cells to myelin basic proteins, *J Immunol* 151:111-118, 1993.

335. Swain SL, Bradley LM, Croft M et al.: Helper T-cell subsets: phenotype, function and the role of lymphokines in regulating their development, *Immunol Rev* 123:115-144, 1991.

336. Tabira T, Webster H deF, wary SH: Multiple sclerosis cerebrospinal fluid produces myelin lesions in tadpole optic nerves, *N Engl J Med* 295:644-649, 1976.

337. Teitelbaum D, Aharoni R, Sela M, Arnon R: Cross-reactions and specificities of monoclonal antibodies against myelin basic protein and against the synthetic copolymer 1, *Proc Natl Acad Sci USA* 88:9528-9532, 1991.

338. Teitelbaum D, Meshorer A, Hirshfeld T et al.: Suppression of experimental allergic encephalomyelitis by a synthetic polypeptide, *Eur J Immunol* 1:242-248, 1971.

339. Tienari P, Wilkstrom J, Koskimies S et al.: Reappraisal of HLA in multiple sclerosis: close linkage in multiplex families, *Eur J Hum Genet* 1:257-268, 1993.

340. Tola MR, Granieri E, Casetta I et al.: Retinal periphlebitis in multiple sclerosis: a marker of disease activity? *Eur Neurol* 33:93-96, 1993.

341. Tournier-Lasserve E, Bach J-F: The immunogenetics of myasthenia gravis, multiple sclerosis and their animal models, *J Neuroimmunol* 47:103-114, 1993.

342. Tournier-Lasserve E, Hashim GA, Bach MA: Human T cell response to myelin basic protein in multiple sclerosis patients and healthy subjects, *J Neurosci Res* 19:149-156, 1988.

343. Tourtellotte WW: The cerebrospinal fluid in multiple sclerosis. In Vinken PJ, Bruyn GW, Klawans HL, Koestier JC, editors: *Handbook of clinical neurology: demyelinating diseases,* vol 47, rev ser 3, 79-130, Amsterdam, 1985, Elsevier.

344. Toyka KV, Drachman DB, Pestronk A, Kao I: Myasthenia gravis: passive transfer from man to mouse, *Science* 190:397-399, 1975.

345. Traugott U, Reinherz EL, Raine CS: Multiple sclerosis: distribution of T cell subsets within active chronic lesions, *Science* 219:308-310, 1983.

346. Traugott V, Scheinberg LC, Raine CS: On the presence of Ia-positive endothelial cells and astrocytes in multiple sclerosis lesions and its relevance to antigen presentation, *J Neuroimmunol* 8:1-14, 1985.

347. Troiano R, Hafstein M, Ruderman M et al.: Effect of high-dose intravenous steroid administration on contrast enhancing computed tomographic scan lesion in multiple sclerosis, *Ann Neurol* 15:257-263, 1984.

348. Trotter JL, Clark HB, Collins KG et al.: Myelin proteolipid protein induces demyelinating disease in mice, *J Neurol Sci* 79:173-178, 1987.

349. Tselis AC, Lisak RP: Acute disseminated encephalomyelitis and isolated CNS demyelinative syndromes 1993-1994, *Curr Opin Neurol* (in press).

350. Tsukuda N, Miyagi K, Matsuda M, Yanagisawa N: Increased levels of intercellular adhesion molecule-1 in multiple sclerosis and human T-lymphotrophic virus type 1-associated myelopathy, *Ann Neurol* 33:646-649, 1993.

351. Tuohy VK, Sobel RA, Lees MB: Myelin proteolipid protein-induced experimental allergic encephalomyelitis: variations of disease expression in different strains of mice, *J Immunol* 140:1868-1873, 1988.

352. Utz U, Biddison WE, McFarland HF et al.: Skewed T-cell repertoire in genetically identical twins correlates with multiple sclerosis, *Nature* 364:243-247, 1993.

353. Utz U, McFarland HF: The role of T cells in multiple sclerosis: implications for therapies targeting the T cell receptor, *J Neuropathol Exp Neurol* 53:351-358, 1994.

354. van den Veen R, Stohlman S: Encephalitogenic Th1 cells are inhibited by Th2 cells with related peptide specificity: relative roles of interleukin (IL)-4 and IL-10, *J Neuroimmunol* 48:213-220.

355. van Engelen BGM, Hommes OR, Pinckers A et al.: Improved vision after intravenous immunoglobulin in stable demyelinating optic neuritis, *Ann Neurol* 32:835-836, 1992.

356. Vandenbark AA, Hashim G, Offner H: Immunization with a synthetic T-cell receptor V-region peptide protects against experimental autoimmune encephalomyelitis, *Nature* 341:541-544, 1989.

357. Vandvick G, Norrby E, Nordal JH, Degre M: Oligoclonal measles virus-specific IgG antibodies isolated from cerebrospinal fluids, brain extracts, and sera from patients with subacute sclerosing panencephalitis and multiple sclerosis, *Scand J Immunol* 5:979-992, 1976.

358. Vanguri P, Koski CL, Silverman B, Shin ML: Complement activation by isolated myelin: activation of the classical pathway in the absence of myelin-specific antibody, *Proc Natl Acad Sci USA* 79:3290-3291, 1982.

359. Vine AK: Severe periphlebitis, peripheral retinal ischemia, and preretinal neovascularization in patients with multiple sclerosis, *Am J Ophthalmol* 113:28-32, 1992.

360. Washington R, Burton J, Todd RF et al.: Expression of immunologically relevant endothelial cell activation antigens on isolated central nervous system microvessels from patients with multiple sclerosis, *Ann Neurol* 35:89-97, 1994.

361. Watanabe R, Wege H, ter Meulen V: Adaptive transfer of EAE-like lesions from rats with corona virus induced demyelinating encephalomyelitis, *Nature* 305:150-153, 1983.

362. Waxman SG: Structure and function of the myelinated fiber. In Vinken PJ, Bruyn GW, Klawans HL, Koestier JC, editors: *Handbook of clinical neurology: demyelinating diseases,* vol 47, rev ser 3, 1-28, Amsterdam, 1985, Elsevier.

363. Webb C, Teitelbaum D, Arnon R, Sela M: In vivo and in vitro immunological cross-reactions between basic encephalitogen and synthetic basic polypeptides capable of suppressing experimental allergic encephalomyelitis, *Eur J Immunol* 3:279-286, 1973.

364. Weiner HL, Macklin GA, Matsui M et al.: Double-blind pilot trial of oral tolerization with myelin antigens in multiple sclerosis, *Science* 259:1321-1324, 1993.

365. Weinshenker BG: Natural history of multiple sclerosis, *Ann Neurol* 36(suppl):S6-S11, 1994.

366. Whitaker JN: Rationale for immunotherapy in multiple sclerosis, *Ann Neurol* 36(suppl):S103-S107, 1994.

367. Whitaker JN, Mitchell GW, Cutter GR: Clinical outcomes and documentation of partial beneficial effects of immunotherapy for multiple sclerosis, *Ann Neurol* 37:5-6, 1995.

368. Winter G, Milstein C: Man made antibodies, *Nature* 349:293-299, 1991.

369. Wisniewski HM: Immunopathology of demyelination, *Br Med Bull* 33:54-59, 1977.

370. Wisniewski HM, Keith AB: Chronic relapsing experimental allergic encephalomyelitis—an experimental model of multiple sclerosis, *Ann Neurol* 1:144-147, 1977.

371. Wucherpfennig KW, Newcombe J, Li H et al.: Gamma delta T cell receptor repertoire in acute multiple sclerosis lesions, *Proc Natl Acad Sci USA* 89:4588-4592, 1992a.

372. Wucherpfennig KW, Newcomb J, Li H et al.: T cell receptor $V\alpha$-$v\beta$—repertoire and cytokine gene expression in active multiple sclerosis, *J Exp Med* 175:993-1002, 1992b.

373. Wucherpfennig KW, Ota K, Endo N et al.: Shared human T cell receptor $V\beta$ usage to immunodominant regions of myelin basic protein, *Science* 248:1016-1019, 1990.

374. Xian-hao X, McFarlin DE: Oligoclonal bands in CSF: twins with MS, *Neurology* 34:769-774, 1984.

375. Yamada M, Zurbriggen A, Fujinami RS: Monoclonal antibody to Theiler's murine encephalomyelitis virus defines a determinant on myelin and oligodendrocytes and augments demyelination in experimental allergic encephalomyelitis, *J Exp Med* 171:1893-1907, 1990.

376. Yednock TA, Cannon C, Fritz LC et al.: Prevention of experimental autoimmune encephalomyelitis by antibodies to $\alpha4\beta$ integrin, *Nature* 356:63-66, 1990.

377. Younge BR: Fluorescein angiography and retinal venous sheathing in multiple sclerosis, *Can J Ophthalmol* 11:31-36, 1976.

378. Zaller DM, Osman G, Kanagawa O, Hood L: Prevention and treatment of murine experimental allergic encephalomyelitis with T cell receptor $V\beta$-specific antibodies, *J Exp Med* 171:1943-1955, 1990.

379. Zhang Y, Burger T, Saruhan G et al.: The T-lymphocyte response against myelin-associated glycoprotein and myelin basic protein in patients with multiple sclerosis, *Neurology* 43:403-407, 1993.

380. Zhang J, Markovic-Plese S, Lacet B et al.: Increased frequency of interleukin 2-responsive T cells specific for myelin basic protein and proteolipid protein in peripheral blood and cerebrospinal fluid of patients with multiple sclerosis, *J Exp Med* 179:973-984, 1994.

381. Zweiman B, Lisak RP: Lymphocyte phenotypes in the MS lesion: what do they mean? *Ann Neurol* 19:588-589, 1986.

57 Sympathetic Ophthalmia

CHI-CHAO CHAN, FRANÇOIS G. ROBERGE

Sympathetic ophthalmia is a bilateral granulomatous panuveitis that follows a penetrating injury (produced by either accidental trauma or surgery) involving the uvea of one eye. The traumatized eye is called the exciting or sympathogenic eye, and the fellow eye is qualified as sympathizing.

HISTORICAL BACKGROUND

The concept that injury to one eye can lead to disease in the other eye can be traced back to the teachings of Hippocrates.[1] The first written reference to sympathetic ophthalmia (according to Woods,[137] and Duke-Elder and Perkins[42]) was the note from Agathias in the anthology compiled from Constantius Cephalis in 1000 AD stating that "The right eye when diseased often gives its suffering to the left." In the first German textbook of ophthalmology (*Augendienst,* published in 1583), Bartisch said that after injury to one eye, "the other good eye is besides also in great danger."[123] During the eighteenth and early nineteenth centuries, Duddell (in 1729), Le Dran (in 1737), Wardrop (in 1818), and Demours (in 1818) also recognized and reported this disease.[1,42]

The first full clinical description of sympathetic ophthalmia, however, should be credited to William Mackenzie,[83] who also gave the entity its current name in 1840. Mackenzie presented six illustrative cases. In all of them one eye had a penetrating and lacerating wound. Within 3 weeks to 1 year, the fellow eye also developed photopsia, iritis, amaurosis, and atrophy. Mackenzie observed that no treatment was effective and that the vision was lost to recurrent attacks.

Schirman's critical survey and experiments in 1892 and 1905 provided complementary information about sympathetic ophthalmia.[1,42] The classic histopathologic description by Ernest Fuchs[50] in 1905 established sympathetic ophthalmia as a separate disease-entity, distinct from any other ocular disorder. In the 35 cases studied by Fuchs, a nodular or diffuse nonnecrotizing infiltration of the entire uveal tract, particularly in the choroid, was observed. It was composed of round cells with a preponderance of epithelioid cells and some giant cells among lymphocytes. A cellular infiltrate was also frequently present around the retinal vessels.

EPIDEMIOLOGY

The prevalence of sympathetic ophthalmia is difficult to assess because of the relative rarity of the disease. On average, the older literature reported a prevalence of about 2% following a penetrating ocular wound.[42] Accidental perforation of an eye was the leading cause. Before Fuchs' histopathologic characterization of the disease, bilateral ocular inflammation was often considered to be sympathetic ophthalmia. *History of the American Civil War (1861-1865)* relates that as many as 16.14% of all ocular injuries led to presumed sympathetic ophthalmia. In contrast, only a few cases were reported during World War I (1914-1918) and World War II (1939-1945). None were reported in the Korean War (1950-1953), the Vietnam War (1966-1975), or the Middle East War (1967).* In surveys unrelated to warfare, Von Holland[131] found sympathetic ophthalmia in 0.7% of 838 cases of unspecified ocular trauma, and Allen[3] reported a rate of 0.3% among 348 cases of ocular perforating injuries. In Canada the incidence of sympathetic ophthalmia following intraocular penetrating trauma was 0.19% from 1960 to 1970.[79] In Germany sympathetic ophthalmia developed in 0.1% of 3,323 cases of traumatic eye perforation and in 0.015% of 21,638 cases of intraocular surgery.[72]

A surgical wound is the second most important cause of sympathetic ophthalmia. In the United States a combined histopathologic series from the Armed Forces Institute of Pathology (AFIP) and the Wilmer Institute identified that 43% out of a total of 257 cases of sympathetic ophthalmia occurred following a surgical penetrating wound.[134] Allen[3] observed one case (0.015%) of sympathetic ophthalmia in a survey of 6613 cases of ocular surgery (5325 cataract ex-

---

*References 1, 3, 54, 60, 61, 129.

tractions and 1288 glaucoma operations). Gass[51] reported that sympathetic ophthalmia occurred in 2 of every 1000 accidentally traumatized globes examined at 26 eye pathology laboratories from 1975 to 1980. In 99 histopathologic cases of sympathetic ophthalmia, Lubin and associates[81] found that traumatic perforating wounds accounted for 53.5% of sympathetic ophthalmia and operative wounds accounted for 40.4%. Of the 40 postsurgical cases of sympathetic ophthalmia, 28 followed cataract extraction; 7 followed iridencleisis; 4 followed iridectomy; and one followed a trephine glaucoma procedure. In the series from Shanghai by Kuo and associates,[74] only 10% of 50 cases of sympathetic ophthalmia occurred after ocular surgery; the rest were caused by accidental trauma or infectious perforation. With the development of vitreoretinal surgical procedures for the management of ocular trauma, the occurrence of sympathetic ophthalmia seems to have slightly increased. In 1978 Smith and associates[118] reported sympathetic ophthalmia as an extremely rare complication of vitrectomy. Since then, more isolated cases of sympathetic ophthalmia following multiple intraocular surgeries, including pars plana vitrectomy, have been described.* Gass,[51] in a collected series of 14,915 vitrectomies, reported an incidence of sympathetic ophthalmia of 0.01% after vitrectomy alone, but found a rate of 0.06% when the vitrectomy was associated with other penetrating wounds. Other intraocular procedures that induce sympathetic ophthalmia include iridectomy,[16,35,81] iridencleisis,[81,134] paracentesis,[134] trabeculectomy,[81,116] evisceration,[55] cyclocryotherapy,[15,44,58,110] cyclodialysis,[42,134] retinal detachment repair,[64,77,84,100,133] keratectomy,[42,81,134] laser photocoagulation,[24,76] laser cyclotherapy,[8] and local irradiation.[49,89]

In uveitis clinics the disease is encountered more often. At the Illinois Eye and Ear Infirmary, Jennings and Tessler[66] diagnosed sympathetic ophthalmia in 1.4% (20 cases) of the total number of referred uveitis patients seen over an 11-year period. At the National Eye Institute (NEI) 32 cases of sympathetic ophthalmia (1.4%) were seen from 1982 to 1992 out of a total 2287 referred uveitic patients.[25a] Twenty-three cases occurred following accidental ocular injury, and nine developed after multiple intraocular surgeries.

Males have a higher prevalence of sympathetic ophthalmia than females, but this observation is probably related to a higher injury rate in males.[42,52,54,81] For postsurgical cases, the rates are equal.[52] Among the 32 cases examined at the NEI, 16 were male and 16 were female.

The disease is considered age independent, although it appears to occur more often in children because of their higher accident rate, and in the elderly because of surgery.[1,42,134] In the NEI series of 32 cases, 6 patients were under 20 years of age, 11 were over 56, and 15 were between 20 and 55 years of age.

---

*References 1, 32, 51, 54, 78, 122, 125.

No significant predilection with regard to race or endemic area has been observed.[1,52] It is interesting to note, however, that sympathetic ophthalmia was not seen in the Southwest Pacific after untreated perforating injuries with uveal prolapse.[42] If this geographic variation is real, it may be related to the genetic makeup of the population.[86] In this regard an association between the HLA type and sympathetic ophthalmia has been recognized in the United Kingdom,[31] in the United States,[34,108] and in Japan.[95]

Many authors have reported a remarkable decrease in the incidence of sympathetic ophthalmia during this century.[98,112] This decline began after Fuchs[50] defined the disease histopathologically and provided a better objective basis for its diagnosis.[86] In addition, there was a tenfold decrease in sympathetic ophthalmia incidence in the last three decades, probably because of better medications (such as corticosteroids and antibiotics) and improved management techniques.[79,99,138]

CLINICAL FEATURES

The interval between ocular injury and the onset of sympathetic ophthalmia is important. It can be as short as 5 days,[81,127] or as long as 66 years.[90,140] The earliest case recorded with adequate clinical and histopathologic data had an interval of 10.5 days.[121] For the long intervals, it is difficult to exclude a fortuitous ocular inflammation or the possibility of another unnoticed injury. In general 65% of sympathetic ophthalmia cases occur from 2 weeks to 2 months after ocular injury; 70% occur before 3 months; and 90% occur within 1 year.[42,52,81]

The onset of sympathetic ophthalmia is usually insidious and the presenting symptoms are slight pain, photophobia, and a decrease of vision in both the sympathizing and the exciting eye. The exciting eye is usually chronically inflamed, painful, and often phthisical.[90,140] The disease course is prolonged and marked by repeated exacerbations of inflammation.[137]

Sympathetic ophthalmia is a bilateral panuveitis. The severity of the inflammation usually ranges from a moderate to a marked level, but may be mild. Except for stigmata of the previous trauma in the exciting eye, the clinical presentation is similar in both eyes.[42,86] A forewarner is the persistence of a sustained inflammatory reaction in the eye, despite the progressive recovery from the damage related to the wound. Early in the presentation of sympathetic ophthalmia there is a cyclitis with ciliary injection and pain, accompanied by blurred vision in the sympathizing eye. In the absence of therapy, the disease usually progresses into granulomatous panuveitis characterized by mutton-fat keratic precipitates on the corneal endothelium, ciliary injection, aqueous cells and flare, a thickened iris, posterior synechiae, vitreous cells and haze, choroidal infiltration and thickening, retinal vascular sheathing, and papilledema.[42,52,66,85,86] The typical diagnostic feature of sympathetic ophthalmia is the presence of Dalén-Fuchs nodules—small yellowish-white infiltrates,

60 to 700 μm in size—at the level of the retinal pigment epithelium. These nodules are most commonly located in the midperiphery of the fundus and best observed by indirect ophthalmoscopic examination.[42,86] Among the 32 cases seen at the NEI, Dalén-Fuchs nodules were present in 15 and papilledema in 3 (Fig. 57-1).

Cataract, rubeosis iridis, secondary glaucoma, pupillary membrane formation, macular edema, and exudative retinal detachment can complicate the disease process.[18,38,71,85] Chorioretinal scarring may eventually form and the eyes may become phthisical. Isolated cases of sympathetic ophthalmia with subretinal choroidal neovascularization have been reported.[17,27]

Sometimes patients with sympathetic ophthalmia have only a mild and transient nongranulomatous inflammation.[41,71,81,86,101] This atypical clinical presentation may be caused by early enucleation of the exciting eye or ongoing immunosuppressive therapy.[24,80,86,101]

Uncommon extraocular manifestations of sympathetic ophthalmia include vitiligo, poliosis, alopecia, dysacusia, and meningeal irritation.[42,52,102] An increased number of cells (mostly lymphocytes) can be observed in the cerebrospinal fluid.

The evolution of sympathetic ophthalmia is variable; but without adequate treatment, the disease usually runs an unrelenting course marked with frequent episodes of exacerbation.[24,38,42,66,85] Blindness often ensues. There may be recurrent bouts of painful inflammation—even in the blind eye—that may necessitate removal of the eye. Occasionally a rapid recovery has been observed.[27,42,69]

Fluorescein angiography typically shows multiple areas of leakage at the level of the retinal pigment epithelium and the choroid.[52,69,86,120] If there is a serous retinal detachment, pooling of dye in the late stage will be observed.[19,78,86,117,120] Areas of early hypofluorescence followed by increased fluorescence late in the venous phase of the angiogram indicate either the obliteration of the choriocapillaris or the presence of Dalén-Fuchs nodules and choroidal granulomata.[4,78,117] Among cases at the NEI, the angiogram was characterized by persistent irregular choroidal filling, patchy choroidal staining, and leakage from the optic nerve in the absence of involvement of the retinal vasculature.

PATHOLOGY

Apart from the changes related to the wound, the histopathology of the inflammation in the exciting eye is similar to that of the sympathizing eye.[42,43,50,52,54] The main feature is diffuse nonnecrotizing granulomatous inflammation in the uvea. This inflammation is characterized by a massive lymphocytic infiltrate with superimposed nests of macrophages, epithelioid cells, and giant cells. Phagocytosis of pigment granules by the epithelioid cells and giant cells is a unique finding and correlates with both the magnitude of the inflammation and the visual outcome in the sympathizing eye.[33,48,81,88,134] The uveal tract, especially the posterior choroid, is markedly thickened (Fig. 57-2). In the iris the infil-

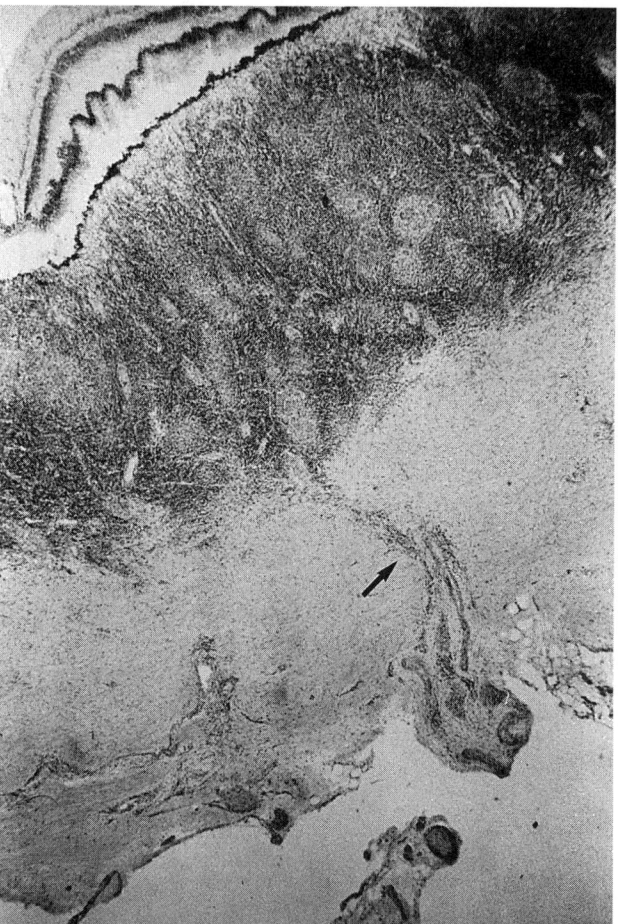

Fig. 57-2. Photomicrograph of the posterior pole of an exciting eye with marked granulomatous inflammation in the thickened choroid and the scleral emissaries *(arrow)* (hematoxylin and eosin, × 60).

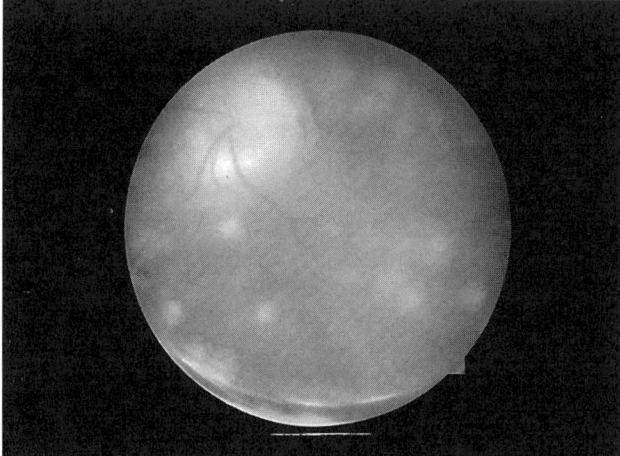

Fig. 57-1. Fundus photograph of a sympathizing eye with vitreous haze, disc swelling, and multiple subretinal yellowish infiltrates. (Figure also in color insert.)

tration usually begins in the posterior stroma. Infiltrate containing chronic or granulomatous inflammation around scleral emissaries, particularly along the vortex veins, is common in the sympathizing eye.[42,50,130] Eosinophils and plasma cells may be present in the infiltrates and may be associated with the severity of inflammation.[33,43,88,130] In the choroid of black patients Marak,[86] but not Lubin and associates,[81] observed a large number of eosinophils.

Other classic histopathologic features of sympathetic ophthalmia include the relative lack of retinal involvement, sparing of the choriocapillaris, and the formation of Dalén-Fuchs nodules.[43,50] Dalén-Fuchs nodules occur mostly in the midperiphery and consist mainly of epithelioid cells located between the Bruch membrane and the retinal pigment epithelium (Figs. 57-3 and 57-4). These hemispheric nodules are a characteristic feature of sympathetic ophthalmia, but they are not pathognomonic. Fuchs observed the presence of these nodules in approximately 25% of eyes with sympa-

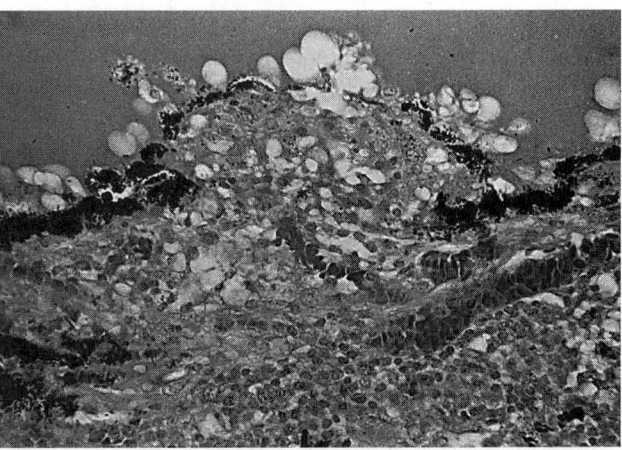

Fig. 57-4. Photomicrograph of a Dalén-Fuchs nodule composed of epithelioid cells, lymphocytes, and RPE cells. The choroid is filled with lymphocytes (hematoxylin and eosin; × 400).

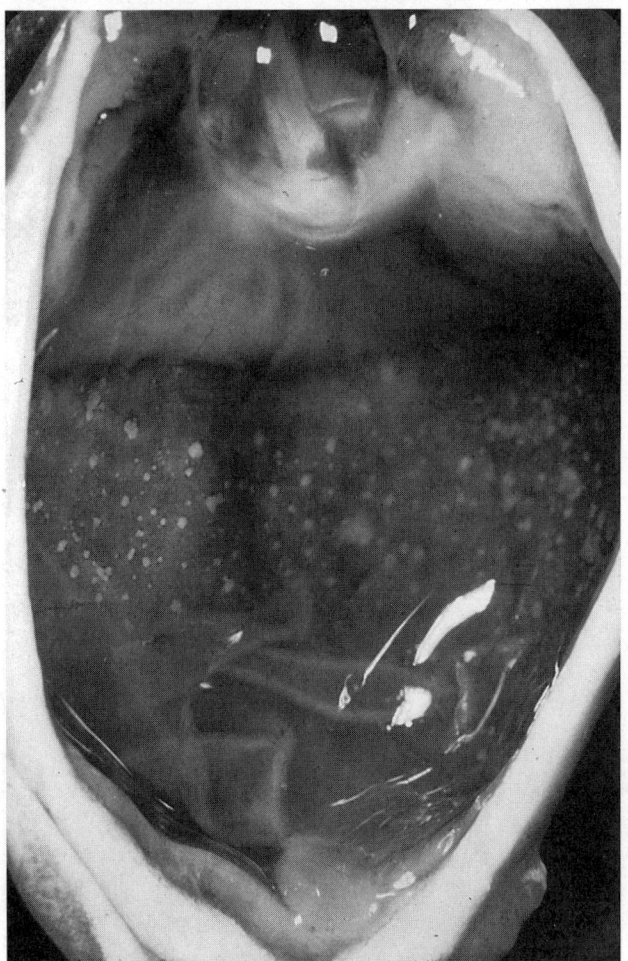

Fig. 57-3. Macroscopic photograph showing numerous subretinal discrete yellowish lesions at the RPE level in an eye that had a penetrating injury through the anterior segment and prolapse of the vitreous.

thetic ophthalmia.[50] Lubin and associates[81] reported more than 1 nodule in 33 of 93 cases (35.5%). Reynard and associates[107] examined 50 eyes with sympathetic ophthalmia and identified Dalén-Fuchs nodules in 18.[107] Kuo and associates[74] reported the presence of Dalén-Fuchs nodules in each of 50 severe cases of sympathetic ophthalmia in China. Fuchs[50] and Friedenwald[48] considered these nodules to be derived from a transformed retinal pigment epithelium. This notion was further supported by the electron microscopic studies of Ishikawa and Ikui,[63] and by the studies of Font and associates.[47] Immunohistochemical and ultrastructural analyses, however, revealed Dalén-Fuchs nodules to be composed of a mixture of primarily histiocytes-macrophages, some retinal pigment epithelial cells, and a few T lymphocytes.[21,22,24,65]

Cases with a classic history of sympathetic ophthalmia, but atypical histopathologic features, have been reported in the literature.* These features include focal nongranulomatous (instead of diffuse granulomatous) inflammation of the uvea, involvement of the retina and choriocapillaris, and optic atrophy. Focal nongranulomatous inflammation was recognized as early as Fuchs' original article. Friedenwald[48] prepared serial sections of flat preparations of the choroid and found small foci of epithelioid cells in cases in which granulomatous inflammation was not identified by conventional histologic sections. Various degrees of retinal involvement, including retinal perivasculitis, retinitis, detachment, and gliosis, have been documented in the literature: in 30% of cases by Winter,[134] in 42.2% by Lubin and associates,[81] and in 55% by Croxatto and associates.[33] The choriocapillaris was focally obliterated in 40% of 100 eyes with a clinical diagnosis of sympathetic ophthalmia, and chorio-

---

*References 24, 33, 74, 81, 86, 102.

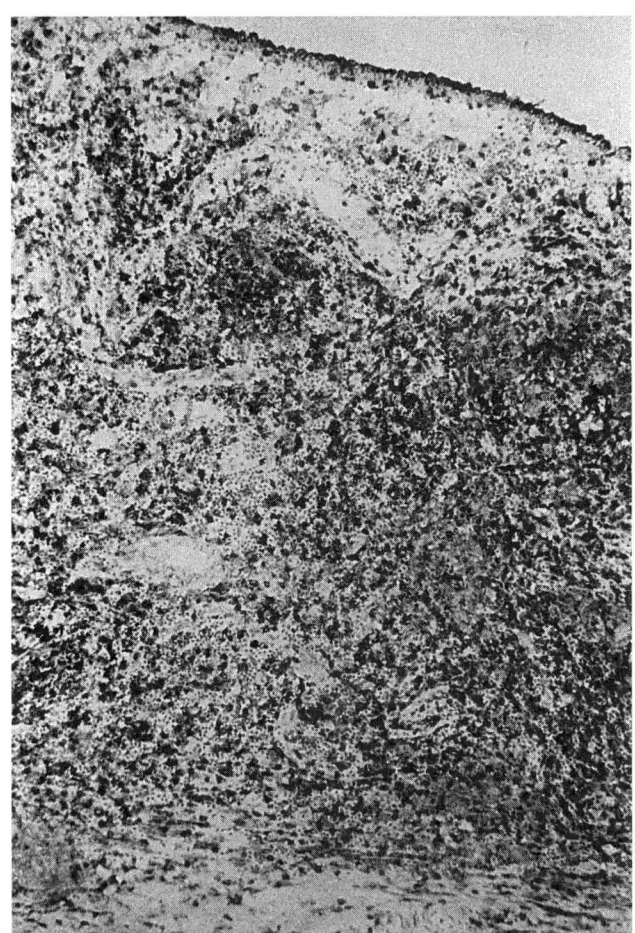

Fig. 57-5. Photomicrograph of the choroid infiltrated with numerous T lymphocytes in an exciting eye (avidin-biotin peroxidase complex, anti-CD3 monoclonal antibody, ×60).

retinal scarring was found in 7% of these cases.[33] There may also be involvement of the optic nerve and meninges. Optic nerve inflammation and atrophy were observed in 25% to 66% of the eyes.[33,74,81] These so-called atypical features in the choriocapillaris, retina, and optic nerve seem to be associated with the most severe inflammation and advanced stage of the disease.

Immunohistopathologic studies of sympathetic ophthalmia demonstrate that choroidal infiltrates are composed predominantly of T lymphocytes (CD3+) in both classic and atypical cases (Fig. 57-5).* With the exception of one case,[91] a predominance of T helper-inducer lymphocytes (CD4+) has been seen in the early stages of the disease, compared with a relatively larger number of T suppressor-cytotoxic cells (CD8+) in the later stages. Less than 5% to 15% of the choroidal infiltrate is composed of B lymphocytes. Shah and associates[115] reported a higher percentage of B lymphocyte

*References 22, 24, 65, 67, 91, 104.

infiltration in 4 out of 29 eyes with sympathetic ophthalmia obtained from the Armed Forces Institute of Pathology (AFIP). These authors interpreted the prevalence of B lymphocytes in these four cases as representing the end stage of the disease process, or reflecting the association of a secondary pathologic process.[115] Even though a large accumulation of T lymphocytes is observed in the eyes with sympathetic ophthalmia, an increase of T lymphocytes in the peripheral blood of these patients has not been documented, with the exception of one case reported by Kaplan and associates.[67] Bone marrow-derived macrophages and histiocytes (CD68+, CD11c/18+) are the main cellular components of the granuloma (Fig. 57-6). Expressions of adhesion molecules and major histocompatibility class II molecules are observed on the ocular resident cells of the eyes with active sympathetic ophthalmia.[24,75] The immunopathologic findings of sympathetic ophthalmia indicate that T lymphocyte-mediated delayed hypersensitivity

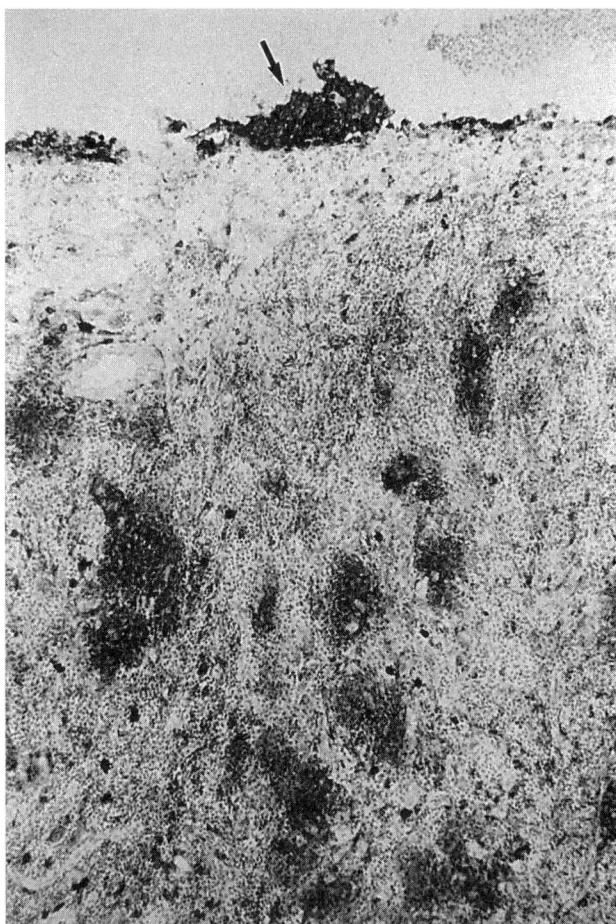

Fig. 57-6. Photomicrograph of the choroid interspersed with nests of mostly bone marrow-derived histiocytes (CD68+). A Dalén-Fuchs nodule *(arrow)* is also composed mainly of CD68+ cells (avidin-biotin peroxidase complex, anti-CD68 monoclonal antibody, ×60).

plays an important role in the pathogenesis of this disease.[20,65]

PATHOGENESIS

The definite cause of sympathetic ophthalmia is still unknown. The possibility of an infectious origin has been raised but has not been proved. Schreck,[113] in Germany, reported the presence of *Mycoplasma* organisms in three human eyes with sympathetic ophthalmia, two of which were sympathizing nontraumatized eyes. Schreck claimed he could induce bilateral uveitis in laboratory animals by injecting culture of these organisms in one eye. There was no independent confirmation of these observations. The presence of *Mycoplasma* organisms was not reported in other electron microscopy studies of sympathetic ophthalmia. Claims of viral infection have not been substantiated.[105] Since its formulation at the beginning of this century,[45] the autoimmune hypothesis has, on the other hand, received increasing support from clinical observations and from experimental studies. The current dominant view is that the penetrating trauma to one eye creates the necessary conditions for an immune reaction to be generated against uveal self-antigen.

There are numerous reports of cellular immune reactivity of peripheral blood lymphocytes from sympathetic ophthalmia patients to various uveoretinal extracts.[70,87,101,136] Circulating antiretinal antibodies were also detected in patients' serum.[25] In some patients, the association of peripheral signs (such as vitiligo, poliosis, and dysacusia) suggests a more generalized sensitization against melanin pigment-containing tissues.

In animals the original experiments of Collins[28,29] showed that an ocular inflammation resembling sympathetic ophthalmia could be produced by sensitization of guinea pigs with whole uvea homogenate in adjuvant. The concept of self-ocular tissue sensitization was further developed by Aronson and associates[5,6] using crude uveal extract. The nature of the antigen contained in these preparations has been the subject of intensive study. Three immunogenic proteins from the retina have been identified: S-antigen, interphotoreceptor retinoid binding protein (IRBP), and rhodopsin.[14,36,111,132] It was felt for a time that contamination of uveal preparations with these antigens probably explained earlier reports of uveal tissue sensitization. Indeed, IRBP was found to produce a disease that shared histopathologic similarities with sympathetic ophthalmia in monkeys.[59] Broekhuyse,[12,13] however, recently described a partially purified uveal melanin preparation that produces an inflammation limited to the uvea in immunized animals.[12,13] Chan and associates[23] also reported that spontaneous recurrence occurred in this experimental model. Such a role for a uveal antigen is more consistent with clinical data because sympathetic ophthalmia usually follows uveal tissue trauma, often without any retinal involvement.

The manner in which the immune system would be sensitized to intraocular antigens following trauma has been studied by Rao and associates[103] and by Roberge and associates.[109] These investigators were unable to induce a contralateral uveitis by injecting the retinal S-antigen mixed with adjuvant into one eye; injections under the conjunctiva were, on the other hand, very effective. They concluded that the introduction in the eye (at the time of trauma) of a contaminant playing the role of adjuvant would be insufficient to produce sympathetic ophthalmia, probably because of the absence of lymphatic drainage of the interior of the eye. The most probable scenario for sympathetic ophthalmia induction appears to be that the extrusion of intraocular tissue allows for sensitization to liberated antigens via the lymph nodes draining the conjunctiva. In addition, bacterial contamination of the wound could play the role of adjuvant to reinforce sensitization. In this paradigm some points remain to be explained: the rare occurrence of sympathetic ophthalmia despite the presence of extruded intraocular tissue in many cases of trauma; the rarity of sympathetic ophthalmia in patients with filtering surgery in which uveal tissue is exposed to conjunctival lymphatics; and the occasional long delay between trauma and disease onset.

In response to the frequency question, there appears to be a genetic predisposition to the disease. HLA-A11, HLA-B40, HLA-DR4/DRw53, and HLA-DR4/DQw3 haplotypes are all associated with sympathetic ophthalmia.[7,31,34,95,108]

The low incidence of sympathetic ophthalmia after filtering procedures would be better explained by the known inhibitory property of aqueous humor on the function of immune cells.[9] This property was recently ascribed to the presence of transforming growth factor beta.[30,53] The suppressive property of aqueous humor was shown by BenEzra and Sachs[9] to be abolished when it was collected from inflamed eyes. This reversal of inhibition could explain the increased incidence of sympathetic ophthalmia in delayed repair of ocular wounds and after repeated ocular surgery. This mechanism is also possibly involved in the recently described triggering of sympathetic ophthalmia by Nd:YAG cyclotherapy in eyes that had previously undergone surgical procedures.[8,15,44,76] The sometimes long delay between trauma and the beginning of sympathetic ophthalmia is harder to understand. Presumably, a break might occur in the central suppressive mechanism that the immune system established at the time of the insult to control the initial response against self-antigens. A reduced suppressive function is one of the contributing factors in many autoimmune disorders.

DIFFERENTIAL DIAGNOSIS

The clinical diagnosis of sympathetic ophthalmia depends essentially on the history of ocular injury by trauma or surgery, and on bilateral granulomatous uveitis. The pathologic diagnosis depends mainly on the predominant T lymphocytic infiltration in the uvea, the early phagocytosis of pigment granules, and the presence of Dalén-Fuchs nodules. Sympathetic ophthalmia may, however, need to be differentiated from some bilateral noninfectious uveitides, such as Vogt-Koyanagi-Harada (VKH) syndrome, phacoanaphylactic endophthalmitis, and ocular sarcoidosis.

The similarities between sympathetic ophthalmia and VKH syndrome have been well described both clinically and histopathologically.[46,102] The ocular manifestations and fluorescein angiography of sympathetic ophthalmia and VKH syndrome can be difficult to differentiate.[20,42,86] The clinical signs of vitiligo, alopecia, dysacousia, and central nervous system disturbances are more characteristic of VKH syndrome. A history of trauma is more indicative of sympathetic ophthalmia. The complications of both sympathetic ophthalmia and VKH syndrome are also similar and include cataract, secondary glaucoma, optic neuritis, retinal detachment, and chorioretinal scarring. Makley and Azar[85] reported that 4 out of 17 patients with sympathetic ophthalmia developed choroidal scarring; in contrast, chorioretinal scarring is seen in most cases of VKH syndrome.[96] Histopathologic comparison of these two entities also shows similarities characterized by granulomatous and nongranulomatous inflammation of the uveal tract and the formation of Dalén-Fuchs nodules.[46,97,102,139] Unlike sympathetic ophthalmia, VKH syndrome is frequently accompanied by the obliteration of the choriocapillaris, focal active chorioretinitis, chorioretinal scarring, migration of pigment granules into the retina, and marked retinal pigment epithelial disturbance. On histology, a very close contact between infiltrating lymphocytes and necrotizing melanocytes is more characteristic of VKH syndrome than of sympathetic ophthalmia.[62,124] Among the infiltrating cells, B lymphocytes and plasma cells are relatively more prominent in VKH syndrome.[20,97] It should be taken into consideration, however, that most of the eyes with VKH syndrome that were studied histopathologically were in the late stage of the disease, and were from patients who had received long-term treatment, particularly with corticosteroids. In contrast, eyes with sympathetic ophthalmia were often studied at an earlier stage, after only a short course of treatment. A similar genetic background between patients with sympathetic ophthalmia and VKH syndrome has been reported among Japanese and American patients.[34,95] The frequency of HLA-DR4 and HLA-DRw53 was high in patients with VKH syndrome in Japan and the United States as well as in Japanese patients with sympathetic ophthalmia, whereas the occurrence of HLA-DR4 and HLA-DQw3 was significantly elevated in American patients with sympathetic ophthalmia. The similarities between sympathetic ophthalmia and VKH syndrome suggest that their antigens may be closely related and may involve a similar immune mechanism.[20,86]

Phacoanaphylactic endophthalmitis was associated with sympathetic ophthalmia in 14% to 46% of the cases.[10,33,81]

The coexistence of these two conditions in the sympathizing eyes has been emphasized in the literature.[2,37,43,56] A marked decline in this association has occurred in the last three decades because of the improved management of traumatized eyes in which the lenticular material is usually removed at the time of repair.[86,135] Indeed, in the series studied by Lubin and associates[81] only 1 of 31 cases of phacoanaphylactic endophthalmitis occurred with sympathetic ophthalmia after 1949. Croxatto and associates[33] reported an association rate of 22% before 1950, but only a rate of 7% after 1950.[81] Only 1 patient had phacoanaphylactic endophthalmitis among the 32 cases of sympathetic ophthalmia seen at the NEI. A zonal granulomatous inflammation surrounding the ruptured lens is characteristic of phacoanaphylactic endophthalmitis. Polymorphonuclear neutrophils and cellular debris gather at the margin of the disrupted lens. A zone of granulomatous infiltration, composed mainly of macrophages, epithelioid cells, and giant cells, surrounds the neutrophils. The outermost inflammatory cell layer is lymphoplasmacytic. The iris and ciliary body are inflamed, but unlike the findings in sympathetic ophthalmia, the choroid is usually not involved.

Ocular sarcoidosis may resemble sympathetic ophthalmia by clinical and histopathologic features.[92,93] Both diseases are characterized by a granulomatous panuveitis with mutton-fat keratic precipitates, iridocyclitis, retinal perivenous sheathing, and Dalén-Fuchs nodules. On the other hand, intense vitritis with "snowball" opacities; extensive retinal involvement including macular edema, periphlebitis, and subretinal neovascularization; and frequent optic disc changes are more commonly seen in ocular sarcoidosis.[94,119] Involvement of the lungs, skin, and joints is seen in sarcoidosis. An immunopathologic study showed that the granulomata in sympathetic ophthalmia and sarcoidosis are mainly composed of bone marrow-derived monocytes.[21] In ocular sarcoidosis the T helper-inducer (CD4+) lymphocyte is more often found in an activated stage, and the various cellular subsets are characteristically compartmentalized.[26] In the 32 cases of sympathetic ophthalmia at the NEI, two had originally been diagnosed as having ocular sarcoidosis and one was considered to have VKH syndrome.

THERAPY

Enucleation of Exciting Eye

The classic and only known prevention for sympathetic ophthalmia is enucleation of the traumatized eye before the sympathizing eye develops the disease. As a principle, because sympathetic ophthalmia is an extremely rare disease (with a prevalence of 0.1% to 0.2% following penetrating ocular trauma) and because of the actual surgical success in the repair of wounds, every attempt should be made to save the injured eye. Brackup and associates[11] reviewed 50 ruptured eyes collected from 1975 to 1987. The eyes had not been removed within 2 weeks of injury and the visual acuity was less than hand motion. Seventeen of the fifty eyes were later removed due either to pain (9 eyes) or because of phthisis or as prophylaxis against sympathetic ophthalmia (8 eyes). The other 33 eyes, which were not removed, remained comfortable over a follow-up period of at least 1 year (12 to 61 months). Sympathetic ophthalmia did not occur in any of these 50 patients. This suggests that even the most severely traumatized eyes will not require removal. On the other hand, when the traumatic eye becomes blind and painful, the rapid and cost-effective rehabilitation afforded by enucleation may be considered to avoid the delayed onset of sympathetic ophthalmia.[39]

There has been some controversy regarding the indication for enucleating the exciting eye once sympathetic ophthalmia has developed.[86,134] Lubin and associates,[82] in their statistical analysis of 55 patients without medical treatment, came to the conclusion that enucleation within 2 weeks after the onset of symptoms might improve the visual prognosis (p value of 0.007). In the 50 Chinese cases studied by Kuo and associates,[74] there was a significant decrease in the recurrence rate in the group enucleated early, but there was no improvement in the final visual acuity. In a retrospective, clinicopathologic study of 30 cases by Reynard and associates,[106] early enucleation of the exciting eye was associated with a visual acuity better than 20/50 and with fewer and milder relapses (p ≤ 0.008). Even when corticosteroid-treated patients were excluded, the association of early enucleation with a benign clinical course remained significant (p ≤ 0.018). These observations demonstrated that early enucleation of the exciting eye had an important impact on the outcome of sympathetic ophthalmia, yet the authors still emphasized that an eye with potential useful vision should not be enucleated in a patient with sympathetic ophthalmia.[82,106] In addition, sympathetic ophthalmia in the sympathizing eye has been documented even after enucleation of the exciting eye.[40,68] One of 18 patients with sympathetic ophthalmia at Moorfields Eye Hospital was enucleated before the onset of disease, and in a recent AFIP study two of the 29 cases of sympathetic ophthalmia occurred after enucleation of the traumatized eye.[57,115]

Immunosuppressive Agents

Corticosteroids. Antiinflammatory therapy has had a great influence in both the visual outcome and the recurrence of sympathetic ophthalmia.* Systemic and topical corticosteroids are the most commonly used agents. High-dose corticosteroid therapy should be given at the onset of the disease and maintained until the inflammation is under control. A starting dose of at least 1.0 to 1.5 mg/kg/day of oral prednisone is suggested.[93] The dose should be gradually tapered down as the inflammation subsides, usually within 3 months. Topical corticosteroids and cycloplegic agents are

*References 42, 57, 73, 74, 81, 85, 86, 106.

used in conjunction with the systemic therapy. Published long-term results of corticosteroid therapy for sympathetic ophthalmia from several groups show that a visual acuity of 20/60 or better can be preserved in a majority of patients.[57,81,85,106] Nevertheless, an awareness must be maintained of the side effects of corticosteroids. Along with secondary glaucoma and cataract formation, complications of corticosteroids include deterioration of diabetic control, vascular hypertension, myopathy, bone resorption, and peptic ulceration. It is also important to note that patients on low doses of systemic corticosteroids are not necessarily protected from developing sympathetic ophthalmia. Several instances of sympathetic ophthalmia appearing despite prophylactic corticosteroid therapy after ocular trauma have been reported.[42,68]

Cyclosporine. Based on the critical role of activated T lymphocytes in sympathetic ophthalmia,[22,65,67,91,104] cyclosporine, a potent inhibitor of T lymphocyte function, is used as a second-line medication in the treatment of this disease. Cyclosporine use is recommended after corticosteroids and before cytotoxic agents.[93] Renal function should be closely monitored because of the high degree of nephrotoxicity of cyclosporine. In a study conducted in Aberdeen,[128] 13 patients with chronic uveitis, which had not been controlled with oral prednisone alone, were treated with oral cyclosporine (mean 4.1 mg/kg/day) combined, when required, with oral prednisone (15 mg/day or less). The mean duration of treatment was 26 months (range 8 to 44) over a mean follow-up of 29 months (range 8 to 49). The average serum creatinine level had increased significantly by 26% after 6 months and by 32% after 1 year, but remained stable during the subsequent 18 months. On cessation of cyclosporine, the serum creatinine returned to the upper limit of normal. An appropriate combination dosage is cyclosporine 3 to 5 mg/kg/day with prednisone 15 to 20 mg/day. Thirty-two patients with sympathetic ophthalmia were followed for treatment at the NEI from 1982 to 1992. Of these patients, seven required combined treatment with corticosteroids and cyclosporine to control their disease.[25a]

Immunosuppressive Drugs. Other immunosuppressive agents, such as chlorambucil, cyclophosphamide, or azathioprine, may be used in cases with failure of, or intolerable side effects of, the noncytotoxic immunosuppressants.[52,57,93,114] When cytotoxic drugs are used, it is advisable to enlist the assistance of an internist, because these agents have serious complications such as bone marrow toxicity, neoplasms, and sterility. Tessler and Jennings[126] reported the short-term treatment of five patients with chlorambucil. Three of the patients had a final visual acuity of 20/25 or better; the other two patients both had 20/200 visual acuity.[126] Azathioprine, at a dose of 50 mg three times a day, has also been used in combination with low-dose corticosteroids.[57] Only one patient required corticosteroid and cyclophosphamide in the NEI series. The combination of short-term cytotoxic agents with low-dose corticosteroids may allow control of the intraocular inflammation with concomitant reduction in the side effects.

Surgical treatment of ocular complications of sympathetic ophthalmia, such as cataract and glaucoma, should be done under the cover of short-term systemic corticosteroids or immunosuppressants.

PROGNOSIS

Sympathetic ophthalmia remains a very serious disease that can result in a poor visual outcome. The relapsing nature of sympathetic ophthalmia commands a careful, long-term follow-up, even in those patients who have been free of ocular inflammation for several years.[42,86] Spontaneous improvement has rarely been observed.[69]

The use of systemic corticosteroids and immunosuppressants has improved the prognosis of sympathetic ophthalmia, and good visual acuity in the sympathizing eye can now be expected. In 65% of 17 cases of sympathetic ophthalmia treated with corticosteroids, Makley and Azar[85] reported that visual acuity of 20/60 or better was retained with follow-up for as long as 23 years. In a recent series a visual acuity between 20/20 to 20/60 was achieved in 14 of 18 patients treated with prednisolone, cyclosporine, and azathioprine—alone or in combination.[57] Complications such as cataract, macular edema, and secondary glaucoma are the major causes for the visual deficit. Today, with prompt diagnosis and early and sufficient treatment, the prognosis of sympathetic ophthalmia is greatly improved. Tomorrow, with advances in the understanding of its pathogenesis, it is hoped that sympathetic ophthalmia will be completely preventable.

REFERENCES

 1. Albert DM, Diaz-Rohena R: A historical review of sympathetic ophthalmia and its epidemiology, *Surv Ophthalmol* 34:1-14, 1989.
 2. Allen JC: Sympathetic uveitis and phacoanaphylaxis, *Am J Ophthalmol* 63:280-283, 1967.
 3. Allen JC, Ho JK: Sympathetic ophthalmia: a disappearing disease, *JAMA* 209:1090, 1969.
 4. Allinson RW, Le TD, Kramer TR et al.: Fluorescein angiographic appearance of Dalen-Fuchs nodules in sympathetic ophthalmia, *Ann Ophthalmol* 25:152-156, 1993.
 5. Aronson SB, Hogan MJ, Zweigart P: Homoimmune uveitis in the guinea pig. I. General concepts of auto- and homoimmunity, methods, and manifestations, *Arch Ophthalmol* 69:105-109, 1963.
 6. Aronson SB, Hogan MJ, Zweigart P: Homoimmune uveitis in the guinea pig. III. Histopathologic manifestations of the disease, *Arch Ophthalmol* 69:208-219, 1963.
 7. Azen SP, Marak Jr GE, Minckler DS et al.: Histocompatibility antigens in sympathetic ophthalmia, *Am J Ophthalmol* 98:117-119, 1984.
 8. Bechrakis NE, Müller-Stolzenburg NW, Helbig H et al.: Sympathetic ophthalmia following laser cyclocoagulation, *Arch Ophthalmol* 112:80-84, 1994.
 9. BenEzra D, Sachs U: Growth factors in aqueous humor of normal and inflamed eyes of rabbits, *Invest Ophthalmol* 13:868-870, 1974.
10. Blodi FC: Sympathetic ophthalmia as an allergic phenomenon: with a study of its association with phacoanaphylactic uveitis and a report on the pathological findings in sympathizing eyes, *Trans Am Acad Ophthalmol Otolaryngol* 63:642-649, 1959.
11. Brackup AB, Carter KD, Nerad JA et al.: Long-term follow-up of severely injured eyes following globe rupture, *Ophthal Plast Reconstr Surg* 7:194-197, 1991.
12. Broekhuyse RM, Kuhlmann ED, Winkens HJ et al.: Experimental autoimmune anterior uveitis (EAAU), a new form of experimental uveitis. I. Induction by a detergent-insoluble, intrinsic protein fraction of the retinal pigment epithelium, *Exp Eye Res* 52:465-474, 1991.
13. Broekhuyse RM, Kuhlmann ED, Winkens HJ: Experimental autoimmune anterior uveitis (EAAU). II. Dose-dependent induction and adoptive transfer using a melanin-bound antigen of the retinal pigment epithelium, *Exp Eye Res* 55:401-411, 1992.
14. Broekhuyse RM, Winkens HJ, Kuhlmann ED: Induction of experimental autoimmune uveoretinitis and pinealitis by IRBP. Comparison to uveoretinitis induced by S-antigen and opsin, *Curr Eye Res* 5:231-240, 1986.
15. Brown SVL, Higginbotham E, Tessler H: Sympathetic ophthalmia following Nd:YAG cyclotherapy, *Ophthalmic Surg* 21:736-737, 1990.
16. Burns DMJ, Ainley RH: Sympathetic ophthalmia after glaucoma surgery, *Trans Ophthalmol Soc UK* 86:757-761, 1966.
17. Carney MD, Tessler HH, Peyman GA et al.: Sympathetic ophthalmia and subretinal neovascularization, *Ann Ophthalmol* 22:184-186, 1990.
18. Castier P, Six A, Ernould F: Ophtalmie sympathique. Evolution à long terme, *Bull Soc Ophtalmol Fr* 88:1503-1504, 1988.
19. Castier P, Six A, Prin L: Ophtalmie sympathique à forme postérieure, *Bull Soc Ophtalmol Fr* 85:47-51, 1985.
20. Chan C-C: Relationship between sympathetic ophthalmia, phacoanaphylaxic endophthalmitis, and Vogt-Koyanagi-Harada disease, *Ophthalmology* 95:619-624, 1988.
21. Chan C-C, BenEzra D, Hsu S-M et al.: Granulomas in sympathetic ophthalmia and sarcoidosis: immunohistochemical study, *Arch Ophthalmol* 103:198-202, 1985.
22. Chan C-C, BenEzra D, Rodrigues MM et al.: Immunohistochemistry and electron microscopy of choroidal infiltrates and Dalén-Fuchs nodules in sympathetic ophthalmia, *Ophthalmology* 92:580-590, 1985.
23. Chan C-C, Hikita N, Dastgheib K et al.: Experimental melanin-protein induced uveitis in the Lewis rat: immunopathological process, *Ophthalmology* 101:1275-1280, 1994.
24. Chan C-C, Nussenblatt RB, Fujikawa LS et al.: Sympathetic ophthalmia: immunopathological findings, *Ophthalmology* 93:690-695, 1986.
25. Chan C-C, Palestine AG, Nussenblatt RB et al.: Anti-retinal autoantibodies in Vogt-Koyanagi-Harada syndrome, Behçet's disease, and sympathetic ophthalmia, *Ophthalmology* 92:1025-1028, 1985.
25a. Chan C-C, Roberge FG, Whiteup SM et al.: Thirty-two cases of sympathetic ophthalmia: a retrospective study at the National Eye Institute, USA, from 1982-1992, *Arch Ophthalmol*, 1995 (in press).
26. Chan C-C, Wetzig RP, Palestine AG et al.: Immunohistopathology of ocular sarcoidosis. Report of a case and discussion of immunopathogenesis, *Arch Ophthalmol* 105:1398-1402, 1987.
27. Chew EY, Crawford J: Sympathetic ophthalmia and choroidal neovascularization, *Arch Ophthalmol* 106:1507-1508, 1988.
28. Collins RC: Experimental studies on sympathetic ophthalmia, *Am J Ophthalmol* 32:1687-1699, 1949.
29. Collins RC: Further experimental studies on sympathetic ophthalmia, *Am J Ophthalmol* 36:150-161, 1953.
30. Cousins SW, McCabe MM, Danielpour D et al.: Identification of transforming growth factor-β as an immunosuppressive factor in aqueous humor, *Invest Ophthalmol Vis Sci* 32:2201-2211, 1991.
31. Crews SJ, MacKintosh P, Barry DR et al.: HLA antigen and certain types of uveitis, *Trans Ophthalmol Soc UK* 99:156-159, 1979.
32. Croxatto JO, Galentine P, Cupples HP et al.: Sympathetic ophthalmia after pars plana vitrectomy-lensectomy for endogenous bacterial endophthalmitis, *Am J Ophthalmol* 91:342-346, 1981.
33. Croxatto JO, Rao NA, McLean IW et al.: Atypical histopathologic features in sympathetic ophthalmia. A study of a hundred cases, *Int Ophthalmol* 4:129-135, 1981.
34. Davis JL, Mittal KK, Freidlin V et al.: HLA association and ancestry in Vogt-Koyanagi-Harada disease and sympathetic ophthalmia, *Ophthalmology* 97:1137-1142, 1990.
35. Daxecker F, Kieselbach G: Sympathische ophthalmie nach eingriffen wegen eines hämorrhagischen glaukoms, *Klin Monatsbl Augenheilkd* 188:601-603, 1986.

36. de Kozak Y, Sakai J, Thillaye B et al.: S-antigen-induced experimental autoimmune uveoretinitis in rats, *Curr Eye Res* 1:327-337, 1981.

37. deVeer JA: Bilateral endophthalmitis phacoanaphylactica: pathologic study of the lesion in the eye first involved and, in one instance, the secondarily implicated, or "sympathizing," eye, *Arch Ophthalmol* 49:607-632, 1953.

38. DeVoe AG: A ten-year follow-up on a case of sympathetic ophthalmia., *Trans Am Ophthalmol Soc* 68:105-112, 1970.

39. Drew RC: Delayed onset of sympathetic ophthalmia, *Ophthalmic Surg* 25:62-63, 1994.

40. Dreyer WB Jr, Zegarra H, Zakov ZN et al.: Sympathetic ophthalmia, *Am J Ophthalmol* 92:816-823, 1981.

41. Dubois C, Kantelip P, Bacin F: L'ophtalmie sympathique: Données clinique actuelles à propos de 3 cas, *Bull Soc Ophtalmol Fr* 88:725-730, 1988.

42. Duke-Elder S, Perkins ES: Sympathetic ophthalmitis. In Duke-Elder S, editor: *Diseases of the uveal tract*, 558-593, St Louis, 1966, Mosby.

43. Easom HA, Zimmerman LE: Sympathetic ophthalmia and bilateral phacoanaphylaxis, *Arch Ophthalmol* 72:9-15, 1964.

44. Edward DP, Brown SVL, Higginbotham E et al.: Sympathetic ophthalmia following neodymium: YAG cyclotherapy, *Ophthalmic Surg* 20:544-546, 1989.

45. Elschnig A: Studien zur sympathischen Ophthalmie. I. Wirkung von antigen vom augeninnern aus, *Arch Ophthalmol* 75:459-473, 1910.

46. Fine BS, Gilligan JH: The Vogt-Koyanagi-Harada syndrome, a variant of sympathetic ophthalmia: report of two cases, *Am J Ophthalmol* 43:433-440, 1957.

47. Font RL, Fine BS, Messmer E et al.: Light and electron microscopic study of Dalén-Fuchs nodules in sympathetic ophthalmia, *Ophthalmology* 90:66-75, 1983.

48. Friedenwald JS: Notes on the allergy theory of sympathetic ophthalmia, *Am J Ophthalmol* 17:1008-1018, 1934.

49. Fries PD, Char DH, Crawford JB et al.: Sympathetic ophthalmia complicating helium ion irradiation of a choroidal melanoma, *Arch Ophthalmol* 105:1561-1564, 1987.

50. Fuchs E: Über sympathisierende Entzündung zuerst Bemerkungeen über seröse traumatische Iritis, *Albrecht von Graefes Arch Ophthalmol* 61:365-456, 1905.

51. Gass JD: Sympathetic ophthalmia following vitrectomy, *Am J Ophthalmol* 93:552-558, 1982.

52. Goto H, Rao NA: Sympathetic ophthalmia and Vogt-Koyanagi-Harada syndrome, *Int Ophthalmol Clin* 30:280-285, 1990.

53. Granstein RD, Staszewski R, Knisely TL et al.: Aqueous humor contains transforming growth factor-β and a small (<3500 Daltons) inhibitor of thymocyte proliferation, *J Immunol* 144:3021-3027, 1990.

54. Green WR: The uveal tract. In Spencer W, editor: Ophthalmic pathology, 1913-1956, Philadelphia, 1986, WB Saunders.

55. Green WR, Maumenee AE, Sanders TE et al.: Sympathetic ophthalmia following evisceration, *Trans Am Acad Ophthalmol Otolaryngol* 76:625-644, 1972.

56. Haik GM, Waugh RL Jr, Lyda W: Sympathetic ophthalmia: similarity to bilateral endophthalmitis phacoanaphylactica; new therapeutic methods, *Arch Ophthalmol* 47:437-453, 1952.

57. Hakin KN, Pearson RV, Lightman SL: Sympathetic ophthalmia: visual results with modern immunosuppressive therapy, *Eye* 6:453-455, 1992.

58. Harrison TJ: Sympathetic ophthalmia after cyclocryotherapy of neovascular glaucoma without ocular penetration, *Ophthalmic Surg* 24:44-46, 1993.

59. Hirose S, Kuwabara T, Nussenblatt RB et al.: Uveitis induced in primates by interphotoreceptor retinoid-binding protein, *Arch Ophthalmol* 104:1698-1702, 1986.

60. Hoefle FB: Initial treatment of eye injuries, *Arch Ophthalmol* 79:33-35, 1968.

61. Hull FE: Management of eye casualties in the far east command during the Korean Conflict, *Trans Am Acad Ophthalmol Otolaryngol* 55:885-891, 1951.

62. Inomata H: Necrotic changes of choroidal melanocytes in sympathetic ophthalmia, *Arch Ophthalmol* 106:239-242, 1988.

63. Ishikawa T, Ikui H: The fine structure of the Dalén-Fuchs nodule in sympathetic ophthalmia, *Jpn J Ophthalmol* 16(4):34-45, 1972.

64. Jain IS, Gangwar DN, Kaul RL et al.: Sympathetic ophthalmitis simulating Vogt-Koyanagi-Harada disease after retinal detachment surgery, *Ann Ophthalmol* 11:1121-1123, 1979.

65. Jakobiec FA, Marboe CC, Knowles II D et al.: Human sympathetic ophthalmia: an analysis of the inflammatory infiltrate by hybridoma-monoclonal antibodies, immunochemistry, and correlative electron microscopy, *Ophthalmology* 90:76-95, 1983.

66. Jennings T, Tessler HH: Twenty cases of sympathetic ophthalmia, *Br J Ophthalmol* 73:140-145, 1989.

67. Kaplan HJ, Waldrep JC, Chan WC et al.: Human sympathetic ophthalmia: immunologic analysis of the vitreous and uvea, *Arch Ophthalmol* 104:240-244, 1986.

68. Kay ML, Yanoff M, Katowitz JA: Development of sympathetic uveitis in spite of corticosteroid therapy, *Am J Ophthalmol* 78:90-94, 1974.

69. Kayazama F: A case of sympathetic uveitis, *Ann Ophthalmol* 12:1106-1108, 1980.

70. Kincses E, Török M: Study on cellular immune response after complicated cataract operations and in sympathetic ophthalmia, *Albrecht von Greafes Arch Klin Exp Ophthalmol* 204:149-152, 1977.

71. Kinyoun JL, Bensinger RE, Chuang EL: Thirty-year history of sympathetic ophthalmia, *Ophthalmology* 90:59-65, 1983.

72. Kraus-Mackiw E, Müller-Ruchholtz W: Sympathetic eye diseases: diagnosis and therapy, *Klin Monatsbl Augenheilkd* 176:131-139, 1980.

73. Kraus-Mackiw E: Prevention of sympathetic ophthalmia: state of the art 1989, *Int Ophthalmol* 14:391-394, 1990.

74. Kuo PK, Lubin JR, Ni C et al.: Sympathetic ophthalmia: a comparison of the histopathological features from a Chinese and American series, *Int Ophthalmol Clin* 22(3):125-139, 1982.

75. Kuppner MC, Liversidge J, McKillop-Smith S et al.: Adhesion molecule expression in acute and fibrotic sympathetic ophthalmia, *Curr Eye Res* 12:923-934, 1993.

76. Lam S, Tessler HH, Lam BL et al.: High incidence of sympathetic ophthalmia after contact and noncontact neodymium: YAG cyclotherapy, *Ophthalmol* 99:1818-1822, 1992.

77. Laroche L, Pavlakis C, Saraux H et al.: Ocular findings following intravitreal silicone injection, *Arch Ophthalmol* 101:1422-1425, 1983.

78. Lewis ML, Gass DM, Spencer WH: Sympathetic uveitis after trauma and vitrectomy, *Arch Ophthalmol* 96:263-267, 1978.

79. Liddy BSTL, Stuart J: Sympathetic ophthalmia in Canada, *Can J Ophthalmol* 7:157-159, 1972.

80. Lubin JR, Albert DM: Sympathetic ophthalmia: ample room for controversy, *Surv Ophthalmol* 24:137-140, 1979.

81. Lubin JR, Albert DM, Weinstein M: Sixty-five years of sympathetic ophthalmia: a clinicopathologic review of cases (1913-1978), *Ophthalmology* 87:109-121, 1980.

82. Lubin JR, Albert DM, Weinstein M: Letters to the editor, *Ophthalmology* 89:1291-1292, 1982.

83. Mackenzie W: A practical treatise on the diseases of the eye, 523-534, London, 1840, Longman Group.

84. Maisel JM, Vorwerk PA: Sympathetic uveitis after giant tear repair, *Retina* 9:122-125, 1989.

85. Makley Jr TA, Azar A: Sympathetic ophthalmia, *Arch Ophthalmol* 96:257-262, 1978.

86. Marak GE Jr: Recent advances in sympathetic ophthalmia, *Surv Ophthalmol* 24:141-156, 1979.

87. Marak GE Jr, Font RL, Johnson MC et al.: Lymphocyte-stimulating activity of ocular tissues in sympathetic ophthalmia, *Invest Ophthalmol* 10:770-774, 1971.

88. Marak GE Jr, Font RL, Zimmerman LE: Histologic variations related to race in sympathetic ophthalmia, *Am J Ophthalmol* 78:935-938, 1974.

89. Margo CE, Pautler SE: Granulomatous uveitis after treatment of a choroidal melanoma with proton-beam irradiation, *Retina* 10:140-143, 1990.

90. McClellan KA, Billson FA, Marijan F: Delayed onset sympathetic ophthalmia, *Med J Aust* 147:451-454, 1987.

91. Müller-Hermelink HK, Kraus-Mackiw E, Daus W: Early stage of human sympathetic ophthalmia: histologic and immunopathologic findings, *Arch Ophthalmol* 102:1353-1357, 1984.
92. Nussenblatt RB, Palestine AG: Sarcoidosis. In Nussenblatt RB, Palestine AG, editors: *Uveitis. Fundamentals and clinical practice,* Chicago, 1989, Year Book Medical.
93. Nussenblatt RB, Palestine AG: Sympathetic ophthalmia. In Nussenblatt RB, Palestine AG, editors: *Uveitis. Fundamentals and clinical practice,* Chicago, 1989, Mosby.
94. Obenauf CD, Shaw HE, Sydnor CF et al.: Sarcoidosis and its ophthalmic manifestations, *Am J Ophthalmol* 86:648-655, 1978.
95. Ohno S: *Immunogenetic studies on ocular diseases.* In Blodi F, editor: The XXVth International Congress of Ophthalmology, Rome, 1986, Kugler and Ghedini.
96. Ohno S, Char DH, Kimura SJ et al.: Vogt-Koyanagi-Harada syndrome, *Am J Ophthalmol* 83:735-740, 1977.
97. Perry HD, Font RL: Clinical and histopathologic observations in severe Vogt-Koyanagi-Harada syndrome, *Am J Ophthalmol* 83:242-254, 1977.
98. Pietruschka G, Schill J: Zur gegenwärtigen klinischen Bedeutung und Häufigkeit der sympathischen ophthalmie, *Klin Monatsbl Augenheilkd* 162:451-456, 1973.
99. Punnonen E: Pathological findings in eyes enucleated because of perforating injury, *Acta Ophthalmol* 68:265-269, 1990.
100. Pusin SM, Green WR, Tasman W et al.: Simultaneous bacterial endophthalmitis and sympathetic uveitis after retinal detachment surgery, *Am J Ophthalmol* 81:57-61, 1976.
101. Rahi A, Morgan G, Levy I et al.: Immunological investigations in post-traumatic granulomatous and non-granulomatous uveitis, *Br J Ophthalmol* 62:722-728, 1978.
102. Rao NA, Marak GE: Sympathetic ophthalmia simulating Vogt-Koyanagi-Harada's disease: a clinico-pathologic study of four cases, *Jpn J Ophthalmol* 27:506-511, 1983.
103. Rao NA, Robin J, Hartmann D et al.: The role of penetrating wound in the development of sympathetic ophthalmia, *Arch Ophthalmol* 101:102-104, 1983.
104. Rao NA, Xu S, Font RL: Sympathetic ophthalmia: an immunohistochemical study of epithelioid and giant cells, *Ophthalmology* 92:1660-1662, 1985.
105. Redslob E: Considérations anciennes et nouvelles sur la pathologie et la pathogénie de l'ophtalmie sympathique, *Ophthalmologica* 118:483-495, 1949.
106. Reynard M, Riffenburgh RS, Maes EF: Effect of corticosteroid treatment and enucleation on the visual prognosis of sympathetic ophthalmia, *Am J Ophthalmol* 96:290-294, 1983.
107. Reynard M, Riffenburgh RS, Minckler DS: Morphological variation of Dalén-Fuchs nodules in sympathetic ophthalmia, *Br J Ophthalmol* 69:197-201, 1985.
108. Reynard M, Shulman IA, Azen SP et al.: Histocompatibility antigens in sympathetic ophthalmia, *Am J Ophthalmol* 95:216-221, 1983.
109. Roberge FG, de Kozak Y, Utsumi T et al.: Immune response to intraocular injection of retinal S-antigen in adjuvant, *Graefes Arch Clin Exp Ophthalmol* 227:67-71, 1989.
110. Sabates R: Choroiditis compatible with the histopathologic diagnosis of sympathetic ophthalmia following cyclocryotherapy of neovascular glaucoma, *Ophthalmic Surg* 19:176-182, 1988.
111. Schalken JJ, Winkens HJ, Van Vugt AHM et al.: Rhodopsin-induced experimental autoimmune uveoretinitis in monkeys, *Br J Ophthalmol* 73:168-172, 1989.
112. Schmidt U, Murken J, Klauss V: Change in the course of blindness in childhood, *Klin Monatsbl Augenheilkd* 193:457-464, 1988.
113. Schreck E: Further investigations for the demonstration of a specific microorganism in sympathetic ophthalmia, *Albrecht von Graefes Arch Klin Exp Ophthalmol* 193:229-243, 1975.
114. Schwartzenberg T, Cahnita M: Ophtalmie sympathique associée à une invasion épithéliale kystique de la chambre antérieure. Considérations sur un cas clinique, *J Fr Ophtalmol* 5:831-837, 1982.
115. Shah DN, Piacentini MA, Burnier Jr MN et al.: Inflammatory cellular kinetics in sympathetic ophthalmia: a study of traumatized (exciting) eyes, *Ocul Immunol Inflamm* 1:255-262, 1993.
116. Shammas HF, Zubyk NA, Stanfield TF: Sympathetic uveitis following glaucoma surgery, *Arch Ophthalmol* 95:638-641, 1977.
117. Sharp D, Bell RA, Patterson E et al.: Sympathetic ophthalmia. Histopathologic and fluorescein angiographic correlation, *Arch Ophthalmol* 102:232-235, 1984.
118. Smith RS, Webb R, van Heuven WAJ: Sympathetic ophthalmia as a complication of pars plana vitrectomy, *Perspect Ophthalmol* 2:117-120, 1978.
119. Spalton DJ, Sanders MD: Fundus changes in histologically confirmed sarcoidosis, *Br J Ophthalmol* 65:348-358, 1981.
120. Spitznas M: Fluoreszenzangiographie der sympathischen ophthalmie, *Klin Monatsbl Augenheilkd* 169:195-200, 1976.
121. Stafford WR: Sympathetic ophthalmia, *Arch Ophthalmol* 74:521-524, 1965.
122. Stern WH: Complications of vitrectomy, *Int Ophthalmol Clin* 32:205-212, 1992.
123. Straub W: The first German textbook of ophthalmology "Augendienst" by G. Bartisch, 1583, *Doc Ophthalmol* 68:105-114, 1988.
124. Sugiura S: Vogt-Koyanagi-Harada disease, *Jpn J Ophthalmol* 22:9-35, 1978.
125. Tamai M, Obara J, Mizuno K et al.: Sympathetic ophthalmia induced by vitrectomy not by trauma, *Jpn J Ophthalmol* 28:75-79, 1984.
126. Tessler HH, Jennings T: High-dose short-term chlorambucil for intractable sympathetic ophthalmia and Behçet's disease, *Br J Ophthalmol* 74:353-357, 1990.
127. Thies O: Gedanken über den Ausbruch der sympathetischen ophthalmie, *Klin Monatsbl Augenheilkd* 112:185-187, 1947.
128. Towler HMA, Whiting PH, Forrester JV: Combination low-dose cyclosporin A and steroid therapy in chronic intraocular inflammation, *Eye* 4:514-520, 1990.
129. Treister G: Ocular casualties in the six-day war, *Am J Ophthalmol* 68:669-675, 1969.
130. Trowbridge DH Jr: Sympathetic ophthalmia: a study of some clinical and pathological factors in thirty-two cases, *Am J Ophthalmol* 20:135-148, 1937.
131. Von Holland G: Über indikation und zeitpunkt der entfernung eines verletzten auges, *Klin Monatsbl Augenheilkd* 145:732-740, 1964.
132. Wacker WB, Donoso LA, Kalsow CM et al.: Experimental allergic uveitis: isolation, characterization and localization of a soluble uveitopathogenic antigen from bovine retina, *J Immunol* 119:1949-1958, 1977.
133. Wang WJ: Clinical and histopathological report of sympathetic ophthalmia after retinal detachment surgery, *Br J Ophthalmol* 67:150-152, 1983.
134. Winter FC: Sympathetic uveitis: a clinical and pathologic study of the visual field, *Am J Ophthalmol* 39:340-347, 1955.
135. Wohl LG, Lucier AC, Kline OR et al.: Pseudophakic phacoanaphylactic endophthalmitis, *Ophthalmol Surg* 17:234-237, 1986.
136. Wong VG, Anderson R, O'Brien PJ: Sympathetic ophthalmia and lymphocyte transformation, *Am J Ophthalmol* 72:960-966, 1971.
137. Woods AC: Sympathetic ophthalmia, *Am J Ophthalmol* 19:9-15, 1936.
138. Wykes WN: A 10-year survey of penetrating eye injuries in Gwent, 1976-85, *Br J Ophthalmol* 72:607-611, 1988.
139. Yuge T: The relation between Vogt-Koyanagi syndrome and sympathetic ophthalmia: report of a case of Vogt-Koyanagi syndrome, *Am J Ophthalmol* 43:735-744, 1957.
140. Zaharia MA, Lamarche J, Laurin M: Sympathetic uveitis 66 years after injury, *Can J Ophthalmol* 19:240-243, 1984.

58 Vogt-Koyanagi-Harada Syndrome

NARSING A. RAO, HAJIME INOMATA, RAMANA S. MOORTHY

Vogt-Koyanagi-Harada (VKH) syndrome is characterized by a severe bilateral panuveitis, signs of meningeal irritation, and integumentary changes. Hallmarks of the uveitis are bilateral serous retinal detachments. Other ocular manifestations include iridocyclitis, diffuse choroidal thickening, and hyperemia of the optic disc.[6] The meningeal or neurologic manifestations usually occur in the initial stage of the disorder and consist of headache, meningismus, and, occasionally, focal neurologic signs. There may be auditory disturbances, including tinnitus, hearing loss, and vertigo.[32] Integumentary signs include patchy alopecia; poliosis of lashes, eyebrows, and scalp hair; and patchy vitiligo (see box).

Typical cases of VKH syndrome show all of these ocular and extraocular manifestations; however, such cases are relatively rare. Most patients have severe bilateral uveitis associated with exudative retinal detachment and signs of meningismus. As a result of wide variation in clinical presentation, the American Uveitis Society adopted the following criteria for the diagnosis of VKH syndrome in 1978:[101] (1) the patient should have no history of ocular trauma or surgery, and (2) at least three of the following four signs should be present: (a) bilateral chronic iridocyclitis, (b) posterior uveitis, including exudative retinal detachment, *retinal pigment epithelial changes that can be considered* a forme-fruste of exudative retinal detachment, disc hyperemia or edema, or "sunset-glow" fundus, (c) neurologic signs of tinnitus, neck stiffness, cranial nerve or central nervous system problems, or cerebrospinal fluid pleocytosis, and (d) cutaneous findings of alopecia, poliosis, or vitiligo. These guidelines serve as a cornerstone in the diagnosis and subsequent management of VKH syndrome (see box).

The course of the syndrome follows four stages. Initially there is a prodromal stage that mimics a viral illness and is associated with fever, nausea, and neurologic signs and symptoms. It is followed in 3 to 5 days by an active uveitic phase, which may last for several weeks. The convalescent or chronic phase is manifested by gradual depigmentation of the integumentary system and uvea.[32] This phase may last for several months to years, depending on the timing and course of therapeutic intervention. If the convalescent phase is interrupted by recurrent uveitis, the disease is considered in a recurrent phase.

HISTORICAL BACKGROUND

Poliosis in association with uveitis was initially reported in 1873 by Schenkl.[19] In 1892 Hutchinson[38] first described the rudiments of VKH syndrome in a patient with "blanched eyelashes" and bilateral uveitis. Vogt[110] confirmed Hutchinson's observations in 1906 by reporting a similar case. In 1926 a Japanese army surgeon, Einosuke Harada,[33] described a primarily posterior uveitis associated with exudative retinal detachments and accompanied by cerebrospinal fluid pleocytosis. Koyanagi,[58] in 1929, described six patients with bilateral chronic exudative iridocyclitis associated with patchy depigmentation of the skin (vitiligo), patchy loss of hair (alopecia), and whitening of hair, especially of the eye lashes (poliosis). These patients also had deafness and tinnitus. These neurologic, integumentary, and ocular manifestations were termed "uveitis with alopecia, vitiligo, poliosis, and dysacousia."[19]

Babel,[3] in 1932, and later Bruno and McPherson,[11] in 1949, unified the disorders described by Vogt, Koyanagi, and Harada. They suggested that these seemingly disparate entities were a continuum of the same disease process. Since then, this uveomeningoencephalitic syndrome has been known as Vogt-Koyanagi-Harada syndrome.

EPIDEMIOLOGY

VKH syndrome occurs mainly in Asians, Hispanics, Native Americans, and Asian Indians. It is distinctly uncommon in whites.[103] The incidence of VKH syndrome is variable worldwide. Uveitis clinics in Japan report that VKH syndrome accounts for 6.8% to 9.2% of all uveitis referrals,[67,97] whereas in the United States VKH syndrome accounts for only 1% to 4% of all uveitis clinic referrals.[81,101] Ohno and associates[81] reported the following about patients

734

TYPICAL CLINICAL MANIFESTATIONS OF VOGT-KOYANAGI-HARADA SYNDROME

1. Bilateral panuveitis
2. Central nervous system manifestations
   a. Meningismus
   b. Headache
   c. CSF pleocytosis
3. Auditory manifestations
   a. Hearing loss
   b. Tinnitus
4. Cutaneous manifestations
   a. Vitiligo
   b. Alopecia
   c. Poliosis

---

in northern California with VKH syndrome: 41% were Asian, 29% were white, 16% were Hispanic, and 14% were black. In contradistinction, Hispanics accounted for 75% of cases in a report from southern California.[6] In this study whites accounted for 10% of cases, Asians 10%, and blacks 4%.[6] Nussenblatt[75] noted that 50% of VKH syndrome patients at the National Eye Institute considered themselves Caucasian, 35% black, and 13% Hispanic. A majority of these patients, however, reported at least remote Native American ancestry.

Women seem to be affected more often than men. Studies reveal that 60% to 69% of those affected are females.[6,81] Most patients are in their second to fifth decades of life at the onset of the illness,[6] although a few cases in young children have been reported. Forster, Green, and Rao[22] described a case of VKH syndrome in a 7-year-old boy, who was the youngest patient reported to date. Similarly, Weber and Kazdan[113] reported two children with VKH syndrome: a 9-year-old Asian Indian boy with neurologic symptoms and exudative retinal detachments and a 12-year-old black girl with chronic diffuse uveitis. Thus VKH syndrome appears

---

CLINICAL COURSE OF VOGT-KOYANAGI-HARADA SYNDROME

1. Prodromal stage: symptoms of headache, nausea, vertigo, fever, meningismus, orbital pain
2. Uveitic stage: blurred vision, serous retinal detachments, iridocyclitis
3. Chronic stage:
   a. Sunset-glow fundus (choroidal depigmentation)
   b. Retinal pigmentary disturbances
   c. Dalen-Fuchs nodules
   d. Sugiura sign (perilimbal vitiligo)
   e. Integumental changes (poliosis, vitiligo)
4. Recurrent stage: usually anterior uveitis only

---

to more commonly affect pigmented races, women, and individuals in the second to fifth decades of life.

CLINICAL FEATURES

VKH syndrome can be categorized clinically into the prodromal, uveitic, chronic, and recurrent phases[103] (see box).

Prodromal Stage

The prodromal stage consists of headache, nausea, vertigo, fever, meningismus, and orbital pain, all of which are present for only a few days.[32] Photophobia and tearing may follow within 1 to 2 days of the prodrome.[103] More specific neurologic signs (such as cranial nerve palsies and optic neuritis) may occur, but these manifestations are rare. In addition to the neurologic signs and symptoms, the cerebrospinal fluid may reveal pleocytosis.

Uveitic Stage

The uveitic stage quickly follows the prodromal stage and is accompanied by acute blurring of vision in both eyes in 70% of patients.[103] About 30% of patients experience a delay of 1 to 3 days before involvement of the second eye, and in a few cases this interval may be up to 10 days.[118] Despite this delay in symptomatology, careful examination reveals bilateral posterior uveitis, the first signs of which include a fullness to the choroid, hyperemia and edema of the optic disc, and circumscribed retinal edema.[32] The choroidal inflammation eventually becomes multifocal and is

---

IMMUNOSUPPRESSIVE/CYTOTOXIC AGENTS USED IN THE MANAGEMENT OF VOGT-KOYANAGI-HARADA SYNDROME

1. Corticosteroids
   a. 100 to 200 mg of prednisone
   b. Pulse therapy up to 1 gm
   c. Topical medications
2. Cytotoxic agents
   a. Cyclophosphamide
      1. 1 to 2 mg/kg/day
   b. Chlorambucil
      1. 0.1 mg/kg/day
      2. Dose adjust every 3 weeks to maximum of 18 mg/day.
   c. Azathioprine
      1. 1 to 2.5 mg/kg/day
3. Immunosuppressives
   a. Cyclosporine
      1. Dose 5 mg/kg/day
      2. Maintain trough 0.1 to 0.4 mcg/ml
   b. Tacrolimus (FK506)
      1. Dose 0.1 to 0.15 mg/kg/day
      2. Maintain trough < 20 ng/ml

associated with alterations of the overlying retinal pigment epithelium, best seen on fluorescein angiography. The retinal pigment epithelial barrier to the subretinal space breaks down, resulting in multiple areas of subretinal fluid accumulation and, ultimately, serous retinal detachments occur (Fig. 58-1). These features form the characteristic picture of the Harada form of VKH syndrome.

Inflammation eventually involves the anterior segment, with the development of anterior chamber flare and cell. Occasionally, mutton-fat keratic precipitates and nodules on the iris surface and pupillary margin may be seen. These findings led many early observers to believe that VKH syndrome was primarily a granulomatous uveitis. The anterior chamber may initially be shallow as a result of edema and inflammatory cell infiltration of the ciliary body, which leads to forward displacement of the lens-iris diaphragm.[107] Intraocular pressure is often elevated in these cases. Indeed, acute angle closure glaucoma has been reported as an initial sign of VKH syndrome.[98]

Chronic Stage

The chronic or convalescent phase follows after several weeks of the inflammatory, uveitic phase and is characterized by depigmentation of the integument and choroid. Perilimbal vitiligo, also known as Sugiura sign, is the earliest depigmentation and is often seen within 1 month of the onset of the uveitis, particularly in Japanese patients.[27,103] Depigmentation of the choroid occurs 2 to 3 months after the uveitic phase, and the fundus exhibits an orange-red color that simulates the appearance of sunset. This characteristic appearance is known as "sunset-glow" fundus (Fig. 58-2). At this stage of the disease, indirect ophthalmoscopy may reveal a pale disc with a bright orange-red choroid. This appearance is more common in Asian patients than in Cauca-

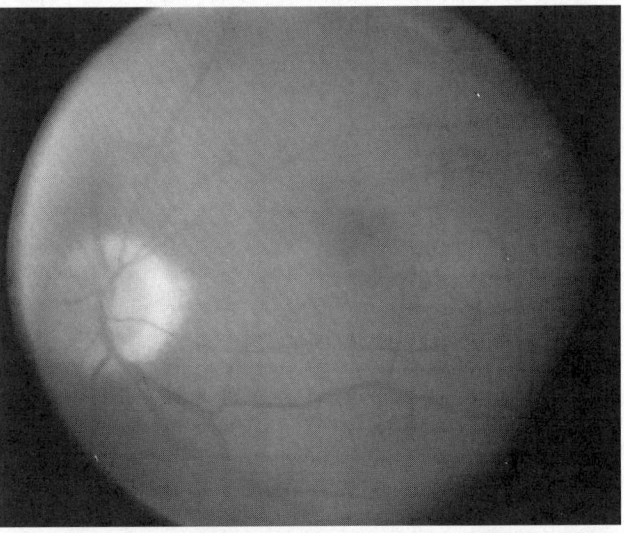

Fig. 58-2. "Sunset-glow" fundus appearance in the convalescent phase of VKH syndrome. (Figure also in color insert.)

sians.[32] As with Asian patients, Hispanics tend to show a sunset-glow fundus, but the latter exhibit foci of hyperpigmentation, which reflect alterations in retinal pigment epithelium.[52] Multiple small, yellow, well-circumscribed Dalen-Fuchs nodules appear in the midperiphery of the fundus (Fig. 58-3), and retinal pigment epithelial migration occurs (Fig. 58-4). The posterior uveitis reaches a smoldering stage as more melanocytes disappear from the choroid. The convalescent phase may last from 3 months to many years.[89]

Recurrent Stage

The recurrent phase is characterized by panuveitis, typically with exacerbations of acute anterior uveitis that are

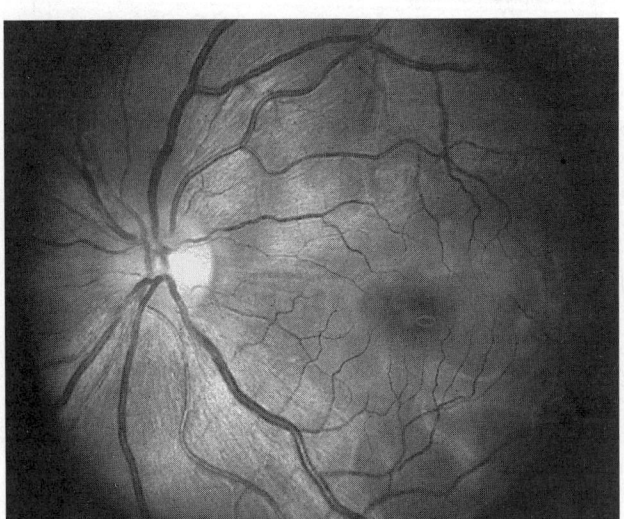

Fig. 58-1. Multiple serous retinal detachments during the acute phase of VKH syndrome.

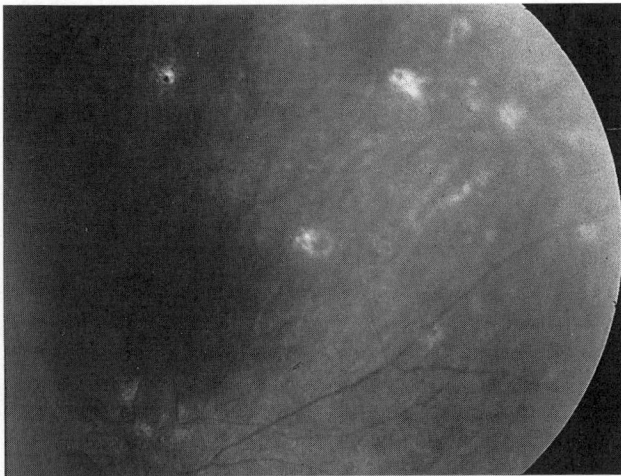

Fig. 58-3. RPE alterations from resolved Dalen-Fuchs nodules in the midperiphery of the fundus in the convalescent phase of VKH syndrome.

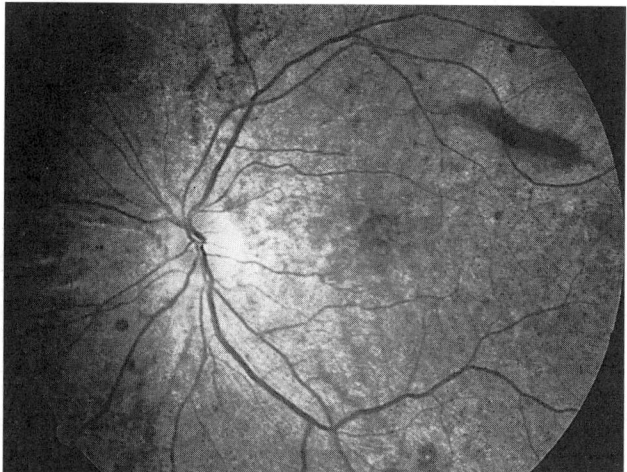

Fig. 58-4. RPE migration and clumping in the convalescent phase of VKH syndrome.

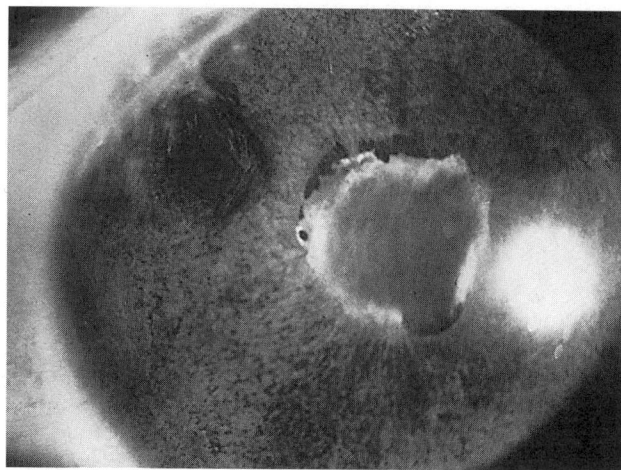

Fig. 58-6. Focal areas of atrophy of the iris stroma. There is also extensive posterior synechiae formation at the pupillary margin.

often unresponsive to treatment with systemically administered corticosteroids. Recurrent posterior uveitis is distinctly uncommon during this phase. Another characteristic finding in the chronic recurrent phase is iris nodules; these are round, whitish, well-circumscribed, fluffy nodules on a background of atrophic iris stroma (Fig. 58-5). Focal atrophy of the iris with loss of pigment may occur (Fig. 58-6), and pigment pearls may be found in the angle on gonioscopy (Fig. 58-7). Complications of chronic inflammation may also be seen during this phase, the most visually debilitating of which are choroidal neovascular membranes.[89] These neovascular membranes can be macular, juxtapapillary, or peripapillary. They appear as whitish, raised lesions and can be associated with hemorrhage (Fig. 58-8). Posterior subcapsular cataracts, inflammatory glaucoma associated with either angle closure or an open angle, and posterior synechiae may also be seen. These complications will be discussed in detail in a later subsection of this chapter. Other

pathologic changes of the fundus can include arteriovenous anastomoses and linear streak lesions of the fundus that simulate presumed ocular histoplasmosis syndrome.[16,63]

Extraocular Manifestations

Extraocular signs involving the integumentary system and central nervous system are seen at various stages of the disease. Sensitivity of the hair and skin to touch occurs early in the prodromal phase.[103] Poliosis, involving the eyebrows, eyelashes, and scalp hair (Fig. 58-9), and vitiligo occur during the convalescent stage and correspond closely with fundus depigmentation. The vitiligo often has a symmetric

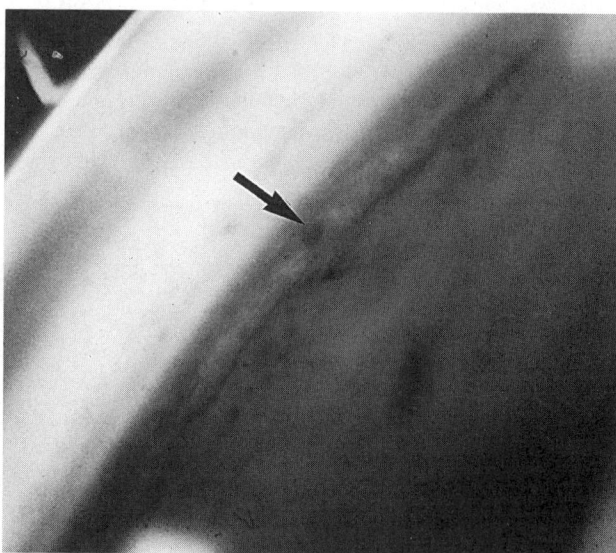

Fig. 58-7. A goniophotograph of the chamber angle of a patient with VKH syndrome in the late convalescent stage. Note pigment "pearl" or "bead" in the angle *(arrow)*. Ciliary body band appears to be less pigmented because of the disappearance of uveal melanocytes.

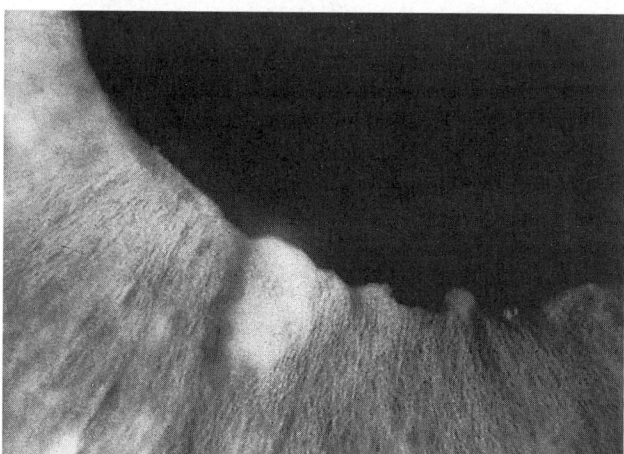

Fig. 58-5. Iris nodules and stromal atrophy in the convalescent phase of VKH syndrome.

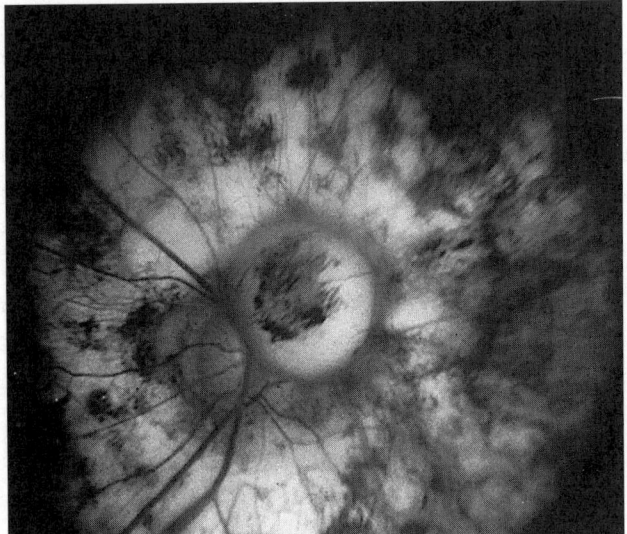

Fig. 58-8.   Peripapillary choroidal neovascular membrane in the recurrent phase of VKH syndrome.

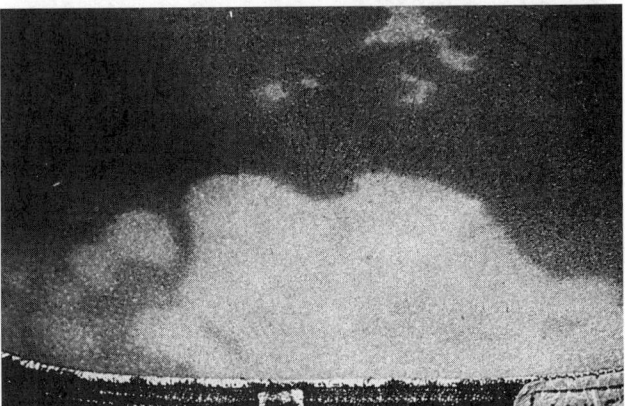

Fig. 58-10.   Sacral vitiligo in the convalescent phase of VKH syndrome.

Inner ear problems are seen in up to 75% of patients[68,88]; dysacusis and vertigo are common.[76] The patterns of hearing loss are similar in both ears (typical cochlear hearing loss of up to 30 dB occurs, mainly in the high-frequency range), although all frequencies may be affected in early stages of the disease.[37] The inner ear dysfunction improves within 2 to 3 months.[103] Vestibular dysfunction is uncommon in VKH syndrome.[32]

Beniz and associates[6] reported several atypical features of VKH syndrome among patients from southern California, of whom 75% were Hispanic, 10% white, 10% Asian, and 4% black. In this population meningismus occurred in 66% of the patients, but tinnitus and dysacusis occurred in 17% and 13% of patients, respectively. Dermatologic changes were also rare. Vitiligo occurred in 10%, alopecia in 13%, and poliosis in 6% of the patients (Table 58-1). Despite fewer extraocular manifestations, the ocular disease in these patients had a typical course, and complications were similar to those reported in Asian patients.

distribution over the head, eyelids, and trunk, and especially over the sacrum[103] (Figs. 58-9 and 58-10). Depending on race, 10% to 63% of patients with VKH syndrome will develop vitiligo.[6,88] Hispanics tend to have a low incidence of these skin and hair changes,[6] but they still display the typical ocular and neurologic manifestations.

Neurologic signs are most common in patients with VKH syndrome during the prodromal stage. Meningeal signs include neck stiffness, headache, and mild confusion. More than 80% of patients develop cerebrospinal fluid lymphocytic pleocytosis,[81,103] which may persist for as long as 8 weeks. Marked meningoencephalitic impairment has been reported with VKH syndrome.[108] Focal neurologic signs such as cranial neuropathies, hemiparesis, aphasia, transverse myelitis, and ciliary ganglionitis have been described,[60] but these signs and symptoms respond well to systemic corticosteroid therapy.

TABLE 58-1   VARIATIONS IN CLINICAL FINDINGS BETWEEN HISPANIC AND ASIAN PATIENTS WITH VKH SYNDROME

	Beniz and associates		Sugiura
	Hispanic (n = 36)	Non-Hispanic (n = 12)	Japanese (%)
Meningism	25(69%)	7(58%)	97
Dysacusis	4(11%)	2(17%)	80
Tinnitus	5(14%)	3(25%)	NA*
Vitiligo	3(8%)	2(17%)	25
Alopecia	6(17%)	0(0%)	60
Poliosis	2(6%)	1(8%)	60

Adapted from Beniz J and associates: Variations in clinical features of the Vogt-Koyanagi-Harada syndrome, *Retina* 11:275-280, 1991, and Sugiura S: Vogt-Koyanagi-Harada disease, *Jpn J Ophthalmol* 22:9-35, 1978.
*NA = Not available.

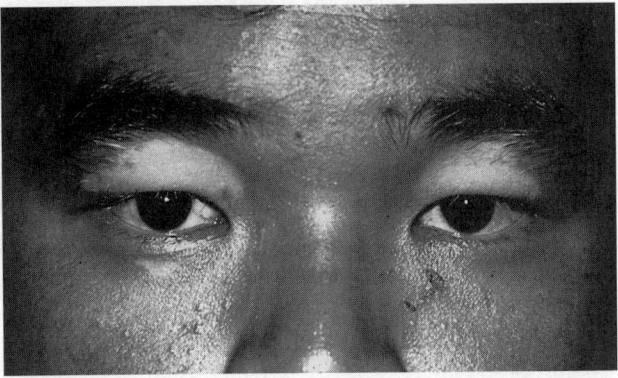

Fig. 58-9.   Poliosis and vitiligo in the convalescent phase of VKH syndrome.

PATHOLOGY

There have been only a few published reports describing the histopathologic findings of VKH syndrome. These reports emphasize the presence of a granulomatous panuveitis. In 1952 Ikui and associates[40] described two VKH syndrome patients with uveal inflammation (similar to sympathetic ophthalmia) consisting of a diffuse, nonnecrotizing granulomatous process that spared the choriocapillaris. Boniuk,[9] in 1971, described a 49-year-old black patient (diagnosed with chronic VKH syndrome) who had a choroid with a diffuse lymphocytic infiltration that spared the choriocapillaris; this infiltrate involved the iris, ciliary body, and scleral emissary canals. The largest series of eyes with chronic VKH syn-

drome was reported by Perry and Font.[85] In that study five of the nine eyes had nongranulomatous infiltration, primarily plasma cells, in the uvea. The other four eyes demonstrated diffuse granulomatous inflammation of the uvea consisting of epithelioid cells, lymphocytes, a few plasma cells, and multinucleated giant cells (Fig. 58-11). Many of the epithelioid cells and giant cells contained melanin pigment. There was a relative sparing of the choriocapillaris from inflammation.[85] In another report Dalen-Fuchs nodules consisting of macrophages, epithelioid cells, lymphocytes, and altered retinal pigment epithelium (Fig. 58-12) were noted in the chronic stage.[61] In the chronic stage the melanocytes tend to disappear from the choroid (Fig. 58-13). In long-standing cases, inflammation may extend into the choriocapillaris and retina, resulting in chorioretinal adhesions.[86,102] Interestingly, a clinicopathologic correlation of Sugiura sign by Friedman and Deutsch-Sokol[27] revealed absence of pigment in the basal epithelial layer at the limbus. Similarly, biopsy of the vitiliginous skin shows loss of melanocytes along the basal epithelium and focal lymphocytic infiltration in the superficial layers. Among the complications of VKH syndrome, Inomata and associates[42] reported evidence of multifocal choroidal neovascularization in eyes with long-standing VKH syndrome (Figs. 58-14 and 58-15), and suggested that chronic inflammation in the choroid may cause breaks in Bruch membrane, leading to choroidal angiogenesis.

COMPLICATIONS

Long-term complications of VKH syndrome include cataract, secondary glaucoma, subretinal neovascular membranes, optic atrophy, and chronic pigmentary changes in the fundus. The first three sequelae are the most important and require surgery or other methods of intervention. Optic atrophy develops during the chronic phase of the disease, particularly following the resolution of optic disc edema. Pigmentary changes of the fundus, which occur during the convalescent phase of VKH syndrome, have been discussed; these are usually not associated with significant loss of vision.

Cataract

Posterior subcapsular cataracts develop because of long-standing inflammation and corticosteroid therapy. Cataracts have been reported to occur in approximately 10% to 35% of patients with VKH syndrome.[6,68,81,89,103] Surgery for cataracts in patients with VKH syndrome has not been well studied, but there is general agreement that the uveitis should be inactive prior to surgery, and that extracapsular cataract extraction can be successfully performed in such patients. The perioperative management of inflammation in uveitis patients undergoing cataract extraction and surgical techniques appropriate for such cases has been reviewed elsewhere.[24,25,36]

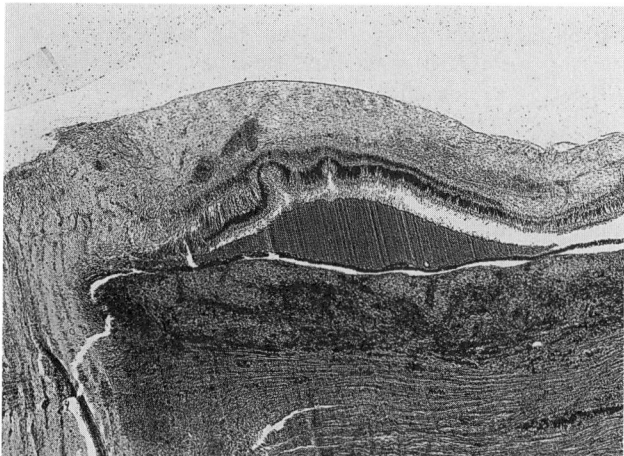

Fig. 58-11. Light micrograph of an eye with VKH syndrome in the early active phase. The choroid is markedly thickened with granulomatous inflammation. The neurosensory retina is detached, and the subretinal space contains exudate. (Hematoxylin and eosin; ×50)

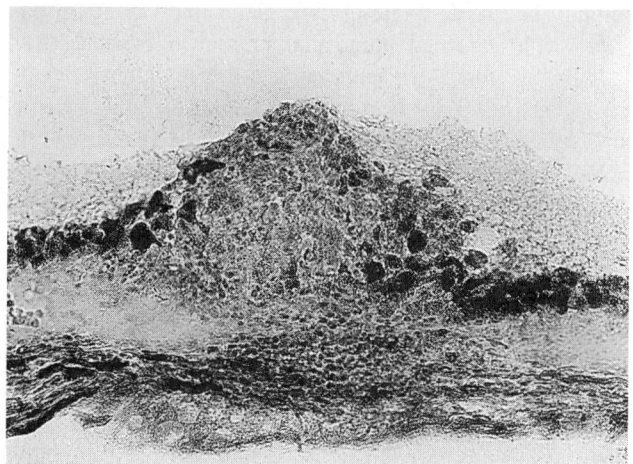

Fig. 58-12. Light micrograph of Dalen-Fuchs nodule in an eye with VKH syndrome in the early active phase. There is degeneration and reactive proliferation of the RPE cells. (Hematoxylin and eosin; ×300)

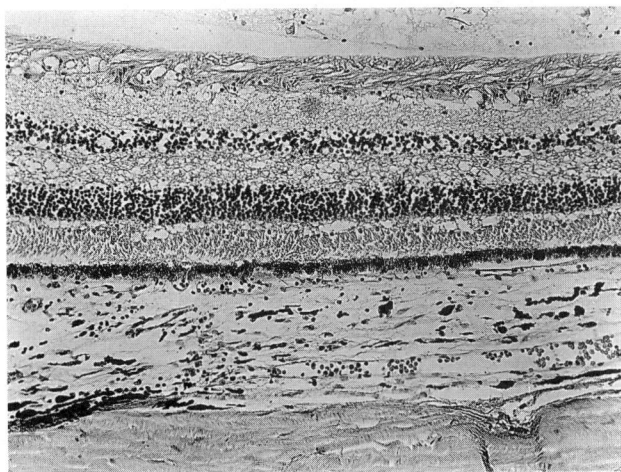

Fig. 58-13. Light micrograph of an eye that clinically showed "sunset-glow" fundus. Note disappearance of melanocytes in the choroid. A few inflammatory cells, mostly lymphocytes, have infiltrated the choroid. The inflammation is nongranulomatous. (Hematoxylin and eosin; ×210)

Glaucoma

Intraocular pressure elevation in patients with uveitis can occur from inflammation of the trabecular meshwork, inflammatory cells blocking the trabecular meshwork, peripheral anterior synechiae, and pupillary block with angle closure. Acute angle closure is a sign of VKH syndrome.[98] Shirato and associates[98] described two patients with shallow anterior chambers, elevated intraocular pressures, myopic refractive error shifts, and intraocular inflammation. Both of these patients had resolution of the angle closure following treatment with systemic corticosteroids. It has been postu-

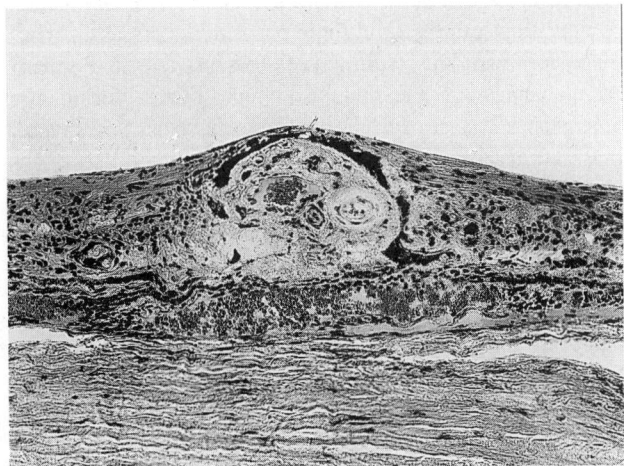

Fig. 58-14. Light micrograph of an eye with long-standing VKH syndrome. There is choroidal neovascularization forming a large fibrovascular nodule beneath the RPE. The fibrovascular nodule protrudes toward the neural retina, causing pronounced atrophy of the overlying tissue. (Hematoxylin and eosin; ×180) (From Inomata H and associates: *Jpn J Ophthalmol* 27:9-26, 1983.)

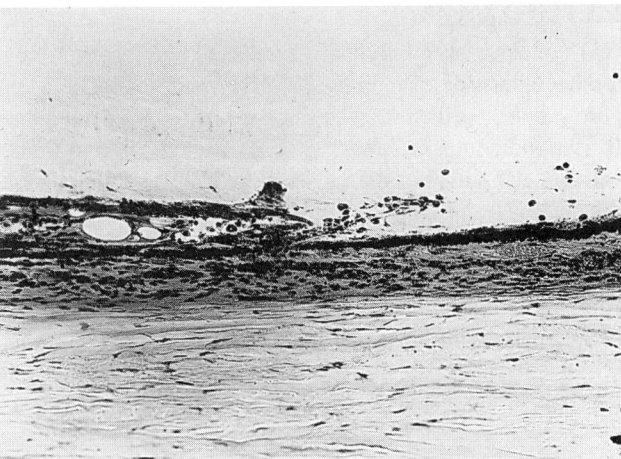

Fig. 58-15. Light micrograph of the ora serrata seen in a long-standing case of VKH syndrome. Note choroidal neovascularization at the ora serrata. (Hematoxylin and eosin; ×200)

lated that acute edema of the ciliary body results in forward transposition of the lens-iris diaphragm, which produces angle closure.[98] This mechanism is different from the progressive development of peripheral anterior synechiae with chronic angle closure, a more common cause of glaucoma in patients with VKH syndrome. Glaucoma secondary to angle closure from peripheral anterior synechiae or from posterior synechiae with iris bombe has been reported in 6% to 29% of patients with VKH syndrome.[6,68]

In a retrospective study of patients with VKH syndrome, 23 (55%) of 42 patients had elevated intraocular pressure during the course of their disease,[23] although 7 of these patients had only transient pressure elevations. The remainder required medical or surgical intervention. Nine patients had open anterior chamber angles on gonioscopy, and seven had pupillary block with secondary angle closure; four patients initially had acute angle closure glaucoma. Of the 16 patients with sustained intraocular pressure elevations, five (31%) were controlled with medical therapy alone, including the use of topical beta blockers, dipivifrin, and carbonic anhydrase inhibitors. Pilocarpine was not used because of its potential for causing an exacerbation of intraocular inflammation. After a mean follow-up period of 40 months, 11 (69%) of the 16 patients required one or more surgical procedures. Laser peripheral iridectomy was performed in nine eyes of five patients. Three of these eyes required repeat laser iridotomies after only two weeks, and another three eyes required trabeculectomy or an implanted filtering valve (Molteno implant) after a mean period of eleven months. Primary surgical iridectomy was performed on four eyes of three patients; in three of the eyes the iridectomy remained open after nine and a half months. Trabeculectomy was performed on six patients (10 eyes): three had a functioning filter bleb at 24 months, but in seven eyes this procedure failed. Repeat surgery usually consisted of placing a Molteno implant or performing a trabeculectomy with adjunctive use of 5-fluorouracil (5FU). Of these two procedures, only the Molteno implant provided adequate control of intraocular pressure in 100% of eyes after 18 months of follow-up. Thus surgical iridectomy for pupillary block was more successful than laser iridotomy. Molteno implant and trabeculectomy with the use of 5FU were more successful than standard trabeculectomy when filtering surgery was required.[23] The use of 5FU in inflammatory glaucoma has been associated with a greater than 80% success rate in some studies.[49] Weinreb[114] noted also that when 5FU was used, lower dosages of corticosteroids were required for control of inflammation, suggesting that 5FU had an antiinflammatory effect. This benefit , however, has not been confirmed for the management of uveitis in general or VKH syndrome specifically.

Choroidal Neovascularization

Another major cause of visual loss with VKH syndrome is choroidal neovascularization. Rubsamen and Gass[89] described this complication, which occurred in 9% of their patients, as an important predictor of final visual acuity in patients with VKH syndrome. In 1977 Carlson and Kerman[14] reported hemorrhagic macular detachment with VKH syndrome. Ober and associates[79] documented four cases of choroidal neovascular membranes (CNVM), one of which had bilateral peripapillary CNVM. Another patient had disciform macular lesions with fluorescein angiographic findings compatible with CNVM. The peripapillary nets can appear white and fluffy, and retinochoroidal anastomoses are often associated with these nets.[79] None of the patients reported by Ober and associates[79] could be treated with laser photocoagulation. Inomata and associates[42] concluded that the peripapillary and macular areas were the most common sites of CNVM because inflammatory foci appeared to concentrate in these areas, as noted on fluorescein angiography. Based on histopathologic evidence, Inomata and associates[42] suggested that CNVM may develop from inflammatory damage to Bruch membrane and the choriocapillaris, which leads to choroidal and outer retinal ischemia; the ischemia may then act as a stimulus for proliferation of endothelium of the choriocapillaris.

The use of scanning laser ophthalmoscopy may facilitate the treatment of CNVM.[93] Anecdotally, an 18-year-old patient with chronic VKH syndrome had a temporal peripapillary CNVM in her left eye that bled into the maculopapillary bundle, causing visual acuity to drop from 20/20 to 20/70.* Using the scanning laser ophthalmoscope, indocyanin green (ICG) angiography delineated the CNVM, and semiconductor diode laser photocoagulation of the net was performed. The subretinal hemorrhage resolved within 2 weeks and her

---

*Narsing A Rao, MD, unpublished case report.

vision improved to 20/30. ICG angiography revealed no peripapillary hyperfluorescence. Four weeks after the first photocoagulation session, however, she again experienced a decrease in visual acuity to 20/60. Repeat ICG angiography demonstrated a recurrence of the peripapillary CNVM, and diode laser photocoagulation of the net was repeated. The patient's condition has since remained stable. Her vision at the 2-month follow-up was 20/50, and there was no evidence of recurrent CNVM. This case illustrates the utility of ICG angiography and photocoagulation in the treatment of CNVMs. Despite their rarity, choroidal neovascular membranes are an important cause of late visual loss in patients with VKH syndrome.

PATHOGENESIS

Although more than 100 years have passed since the first description of VKH syndrome, its cause still remains unclear. Because VKH syndrome has symptoms with diverse clinical manifestations, it is logical to assume that a unifying mechanism accounts for the ocular, central nervous system, dematologic, and auditory signs and symptoms. Histopathologic studies have revealed inflammation and loss of melanocytes in the uveal tract and skin, and similar changes could be present in the meninges of the central nervous system and in the inner ear, at the site of melanin-containing cells. The mechanism for such selective damage of melanocytes and distribution of inflammation is believed to be related to either an infectious or an autoimmune process. The latter process could be initiated by an infectious agent in a genetically susceptible individual.

It was initially proposed in two studies that viral infections played a role in the pathogenesis of VKH syndrome.[19,71] Neither of these studies provided convincing evidence of a viral causation, however. Recent molecular studies using polymerase chain reaction (PCR) have shown the presence of the Epstein-Barr virus genome in the cerebrospinal fluid of VKH patients.[109] Additional studies are required, however, to confirm this observation and to evaluate the specificity and significance of detecting viral genome by the PCR method, when limited numbers of nucleotides are used as primers for the amplification process.

Autoimmunity

At present, the ocular inflammatory aspect of VKH syndrome is believed to reflect a hypersensitivity or autoimmunity, in particular cellular immunity, against melanocytes.[74,91,103,105,117] Using electron microscopic studies, Matsuda and Sugiura[65] demonstrated close contact between lymphocytes and melanocytes and showed an absence of intercellular spaces and basement membranes of the uveal melanocytes at the site of contact. The "trigger" that initiates this autoimmune process is still unknown, however.[65] The continuing search for an autoimmune pathogenesis led to the isolation of antiretinal antibodies directed against photoreceptor outer segments and Muller cells in sera of patients with VKH syndrome.[15] This antibody response could, however, be a nonspecific epiphenomenon secondary to the damage of retinal tissue in these patients. Studies of in vitro lymphocyte proliferation in the presence of retinal antigens have yielded contradictory results. Lymphocytes from some patients in the chronic stage of VKH syndrome showed no response, whereas those from other patients at the acute stage and without treatment exhibited a positive response to retinal S antigen and/or interphotoreceptor retinoid binding protein.[18,73]

Immunohistochemical studies have recently shed new light on the autoimmune pathogenesis of VKH syndrome. Okubo and associates[83] reported that the percentages of OKT3, OKT4, and OKT11 lymphocytes in the peripheral blood of patients with VKH syndrome were significantly lower than in normal subjects. More importantly, the percentage of OKIa1+ cells, which are activated T lymphocytes, was greater than in normal subjects. Furthermore, OKIa1+ cells were found in even greater numbers during episodes of active uveitis, indicating a possible autoimmune pathogenesis to the disease. The cytotoxic activity of peripheral blood lymphocytes on various antigens has also been studied. Norose and associates[74] documented that peripheral blood lymphocytes and cerebrospinal fluid lymphocytes of patients with VKH syndrome have a cytotoxic effect on the B36 melanoma cell line. McClellan and associates[66] identified antibodies to melanoma cells in a cytotoxic assay of one patient with VKH syndrome; in another patient they found IL-2-dependent T lymphocytes with specificity for normal melanocytes and for melanoma cells in cytotoxic and proliferation assays.[66] These findings lend credence to the belief that autoimmunity to melanocytes is responsible for the inflammation seen in the skin, uvea, and meninges of patients with VKH syndrome.

Immunohistochemical studies on eyes of patients with active VKH syndrome revealed (1) an increased ratio of T-helper to T-suppressor cells, (2) the presence of activated T-lymphocytes expressing CD25 (an antigen to the IL-2 receptor and a marker of early T lymphocyte activation), and (3) CD26 (an antigenic marker of late T lymphocyte activation) on their surfaces.[91] Sakamoto, Murata, and Inomata[91] also found that class II major histocompatibility complex (MHC) antigens were expressed on choroidal melanocytes and on the endothelium of the choriocapillaris. These authors suggested that T lymphocyte-mediated, delayed-type hypersensitivity against choroidal melanocytes that aberrantly express class II MHC antigens is responsible for the autoimmune inflammatory process in the VKH syndrome. In the convalescent phase of VKH syndrome, Inomata and Sakamoto[43] found immunohistopathologic evidence of ongoing active inflammation, with a CD4 to CD8 T-lymphocyte ratio of 2 to 3, lymphocytic infiltration consisting primarily of T-lymphocytes, and disappearance of

choroidal melanocytes. Their findings suggest that melanocytes may indeed be the target cells of the immune system in VKH syndrome patients, and that inflammation is active even in what appears to be the convalescent phase of the illness. Thus even at the target tissue level, evidence exists for the role of autoimmunity in the pathogenesis of VKH syndrome. Choroidal melanocytes are the target of the inflammatory cascade, and a cell-mediated immune response sustains and amplifies the inflammatory cascade that results ultimately in tissue destruction.

Genetics

The role of genetics in patients with VKH syndrome was studied extensively in Japan. Among Japanese, HLA-DR4 and HLA-Dw53 have a strong association with the disease. Chinese also have this same HLA association, with a relative risk of 16.0 for HLA-DR4 (or a 16-times-greater likelihood of expressing HLA-DR4 than the population at large), and 34.2 for HLA-DRw53.[119] These HLA associations were also found in American patients with VKH syndrome and sympathetic ophthalmia.[17] In comparing racially matched controls without disease, the strongest HLA association was found with HLA-DQw3, which is in positive linkage equilibrium with DR4.[17] Also, an association has been found between VKH syndrome and HLA-DR1 and HLA-DR4 specificities.[114a] These two HLA specificities have been shown by PCR analysis to share a critical sequence in the DR-β 1 genome, which defines gene variants of the DR4 molecule.[74a]

Recently Martinez and associates[64] detected the HLA-DRw52 haplotype in seven patients of Cherokee Indian ancestry who had VKH syndrome. Five of these patients were homozygous for this allele, suggesting that a class II HLA antigen may predispose to the development of VKH syndrome in some patients. The role of genetics in the pathogenesis of VKH syndrome is strengthened by reports of familial cases of this disease. Itho, Kurimoto, and Kouno[45] reported VKH syndrome in monozygotic twins with HLA-A2, A26, B51, B7, Cw7, DR1, and DR4.

Animal Models

Several disorders in other species have features resembling VKH syndrome. A mutant, delayed amelanotic strain of domestic chickens exists that develops cutaneous and plumage depigmentation after birth. They develop diffuse choroiditis and a loss of choroidal melanocytes that is histopathologically similar to that of VKH syndrome.[100] Uveodermatologic syndrome in dogs is similar to VKH syndrome; it is characterized by uveitis, poliosis, and vitiligo.[2] Kern and associates[54] reported the histopathologic findings in six dogs with uveitis, vitiligo, and poliosis. They found diffuse infiltration of the uvea with plasma cells, histiocytes, and small lymphocytes; in addition, many of the animals had retinal detachments, as well as infiltration of lymphocytes, plasma cells, and macrophages in the vitreous and anterior chamber. Lindley and associates[59] described an Akita dog with a similar syndrome. On histologic examination, they found the iris, ciliary body, and choroid to be thickened by macrophages, plasma cells, lymphocytes, and a few polymorphonuclear leukocytes. The inflammatory cells seemed to surround and sequester the remaining uveal melanocytes, and the inflammation extended to the optic chiasm. No Dalen-Fuchs nodules were found, in contrast to the study of dogs by Asakura and associates.[2] These similar uveitic syndromes in other species point to autoimmune destruction of melanocytes as the cause of VKH syndrome. Both the dogs and the chickens exhibited cutaneous findings comparable to those seen in humans.

DIFFERENTIAL DIAGNOSIS

The differential diagnosis of VKH syndrome includes other causes of posterior uveitis and panuveitis, particularly sympathetic ophthalmia, large-cell lymphoma, ocular Lyme borreliosis, and sarcoidosis. Sympathetic ophthalmia should be considered in the differential diagnosis, although it does not occur without a history of previous penetrating trauma to the eye or surgery. The chronic stages of sympathetic ophthalmia have clinical and pathologic features similar to those of VKH syndrome, although granulomatous inflammation in the anterior segment is more common with sympathetic ophthalmia than with VKH syndrome. Optic disc edema and hyperemia, choroidal thickening, Dalen-Fuchs nodules, and serous retinal detachments can be seen in either condition. Extraocular manifestations, such as dysacusis, vitiligo, poliosis, and alopecia can occur in sympathetic ophthalmia but are rare.[86]

Intraocular large-cell lymphoma has presenting symptoms of chronic uveitis associated with neurologic signs and symptoms. Fundus examination typically reveals multifocal raised, lobulated, yellowish, subretinal and subretinal pigment epithelial (RPE) lesions involving the posterior pole. Satellite lesions may also be present,[57] some of which may simulate resolved Dalen-Fuchs nodules. The choroid is usually thickened and may be associated with a retinal detachment.[57] Fluorescein angiography shows blockage of choroidal fluorescence with late staining at the site of infiltrative lesions.[57] VKH syndrome, however, has symptoms of punctate hyperfluorescent dots that more intensely stain the surrounding subretinal fluid. Unlike patients with VKH syndrome, who are usually between 20 and 50 years of age, patients with large-cell lymphoma tend to be over 60 years of age (although patients in their forties have been reported).[57] Because central nervous system involvement is present in over 50% of the patients with large-cell lymphoma, this entity must be carefully excluded in older patients who have uveitis and central nervous system symptoms.[4] Neurologic studies, including lumbar puncture and magnetic resonance imaging, are helpful in arriving at the

diagnosis, and large-cell lymphoma can usually be confirmed by vitreous or chorioretinal biopsy.[57]

Ocular Lyme borreliosis was characterized by Winward and associates[115] as a bilateral granulomatous iridocyclitis and vitritis. In some cases it may resemble pars planitis syndrome, although it more typically shows granulomatous keratic precipitates and posterior synechiae. Occasionally, Lyme disease can have presenting symptoms of severe bilateral panuveitis associated with exudative retinal detachment. Recently Isogai and associates[44] found elevated antibody titers to *Borrelia burgdorferi* in patients with VKH syndrome, Behçet syndrome, sarcoidosis, and HLA-B27-associated anterior uveitis, suggesting that some cross-reactivity exists between anti-*B. burgdorferi* antibodies and those produced in patients with various uveitis syndromes. Indeed, the 60-KD common antigen (heat shock protein) that is expressed by *B. burgdorferi* has been shown to be involved in the pathogenesis of autoimmune arthritis.[95] Despite these immunologic similarities, Lyme disease may have focal neurologic signs, such as cranial nerve palsies and optic neuritis,[115] that are unusual with VKH syndrome (nonlocalizing neurologic signs and symptoms are the norm). Unlike ocular Lyme borreliosis, in which corticosteroids are of questionable value,[115] VKH syndrome responds well to systemic corticosteroid therapy. Ocular Lyme borreliosis does, however, respond to systemic antibiotics.[115]

Sarcoidosis must also be considered in the differential diagnosis of VKH syndrome. Sixty percent of patients with ocular sarcoidosis have chronic granulomatous uveitis.[47] Isolated anterior uveitis is more common in sarcoidosis. Posterior uveitis is much less common, occurring in 6% to 33% of patients,[47] and serous retinal detachment is unusual in sarcoidosis. Additionally, retinal vasculitis with venous sheathing and "candlewax drippings," the classic findings in patients with sarcoidosis, is not seen in VKH syndrome. Dalen-Fuchs nodules, which are seen in VKH syndrome, can also occur in ocular sarcoidosis but tend to be larger.[12] Large sarcoid granulomata of the choroid are also present,[12] which are not seen in VKH syndrome. Sarcoid meningoencephalitis occurs in 5% of patients. Neurologic signs tend to be localizing and include cranial nerve palsies, peripheral neuropathies, and aseptic meningitis.[99] Computerized tomography, magnetic resonance imaging, and lumbar puncture can be helpful in the diagnosis of sarcoid meningoencephalitis.[99] Serologic markers include angiotensin-converting enzyme and lysozyme. Biopsy of suspected granulomata of conjunctiva, skin, lacrimal gland, or lymph nodes and pulmonary evaluation may be helpful in the patient with suspected sarcoidosis.

Acute posterior multifocal placoid pigment epitheliopathy (APMPPE) can also be confused with VKH syndrome.[30] APMPPE patients develop sudden loss of central vision following a viral prodrome. Multiple, white-yellow, flat-to-placoid lesions are present at the level of the RPE.

There is minimal-to-no vitreous inflammation. Both eyes eventually became involved, but spontaneous and rapid resolution of the lesions with return of vision is the norm, despite the prominent RPE alterations. On fluorescein angiography, the lesions show early blocking of background choroidal fluorescence, followed by late staining of the lesions. Subretinal fluid or punctate hyperfluorescent dots seen in VKH syndrome, are not present in APMPPE. Kayazawa and Takahashi[53] emphasized the similarity of APMPPE to VKH syndrome by describing two patients who had similar presentations. One, however, had clinical and angiographic signs of APMPPE, whereas the other manifested typical fluorescein angiographic signs of VKH syndrome. The prodromal symptoms can mimic VKH syndrome, but the absence of anterior segment inflammation and the absence of cells in the vitreous in APMPPE are very helpful in establishing the diagnosis. Rarely, there may be a few cells in the vitreous of patients with APMPPE.

The retinal lesions of multiple evanescent white dot syndrome (MEWDS) may initially mimic VKH syndrome. This disorder is usually unilateral, affects young women, and is characterized by a sudden drop in vision to about the 20/200 level, often with an afferent pupillary defect.[50] The disease is self-limiting, unlike VKH syndrome, and visual acuity returns to the 20/20 to 20/40 range within a few weeks.[50] The anterior chamber reaction seen in VKH syndrome is absent in MEWDS. Vitreous cells may be present in MEWDS, but choroidal thickening and fullness are absent. Fluorescein angiographic findings include multiple ''wreathlike'' areas of hyperfluorescence around the periphery of each of the white dots, which fill in centrally in the late phases of the angiogram; staining of the disc; and, occasionally, perivascular sheathing. Recurrences are uncommon.[50]

Bilateral diffuse melanocytic hyperplasia is a rare but clearly defined entity that affects primarily middle-aged white females. Patients experience rapid loss of vision, aqueous cell and flare, and cataract formation. Other symptoms include multiple pigmented and nonpigmented placoid iridic and choroidal nodules and serous retinal detachments. This form of melanocytic hyperplasia is seen only in patients with metastatic malignant neoplasms, especially carcinoma of the bowel, squamous cell carcinoma of the lung, pancreatic adenocarcinoma, and ovarian carcinoma.[5] Histopathologically, the melanocytic hyperplasia results in the uvea being thickened by aggregates of melanocytes, with features of a nevus; in some cases the choroid exhibits epithelioid melanoma cells. There is often scleral extension of this tumor, but despite this finding, these tumors do not metastasize.[5] The similarity of these findings to those of VKH syndrome makes it worth considering bilateral diffuse melanocytic hyperplasia in the differential diagnosis of VKH syndrome. In patients with bilateral diffuse melanocytic hyperplasia, ultrasonography of the globe shows diffusely thickened choroid, measuring 1 to 2 mm. The fluorescein angiographic qualities have not been well characterized but may include mottled choroidal fluorescence.[87] The occurrence of bilateral diffuse melanocytic hyperplasia in older patients and its association with systemic malignancy, however, differentiate it clinically from VKH syndrome.

Choroidopathy associated with systemic lupus erythematosus presents with multiple serous RPE and retinal detachments,[46] but they are rare manifestations of that disease. Patients with severe vascular and renal complications of systemic lupus erythematosus, especially those with hypertension, can experience visual loss. The anterior segment is usually quiet, but the fundus examination reveals multiple serous RPE and retinal detachments (Fig. 58-16). Fluorescein angiography discloses multiple areas of dye leakage at the level of the RPE; the dye accumulates in the subretinal or sub-RPE space. Ultrasonography demonstrates the serous retinal detachments; the choroid, however, is not thickened, which distinguishes lupus choroidopathy from VKH syndrome. The findings in systemic lupus erythematosus are thought to be caused by immune complex-mediated choroidal vasculitis, secondary RPE damage, and subsequent subretinal fluid leakage. With treatment of the systemic vasculitis, the serous retinal and RPE detachments resolve.[46] Despite fluorescein angiographic similarities to VKH syndrome, the clinical history of systemic lupus erythematosus and the ultrasonographic evidence of a lack of choroidal thickening are helpful in excluding this entity from the differential diagnosis.

Uveal effusion syndrome can mimic VKH syndrome both angiographically and clinically. On fluorescein angiography, numerous fluorescent blotches in the subretinal space during the serous detachment phase and subsequent pigment migration resulting in mottled fluorescence during the convalescent phase of the uveal effusion syndrome may appear similar to VKH syndrome. The onset of serous retinal detachments in uveal effusion syndrome, however, is subacute and chronically progressive.[52,94] In addition, there is minimal intraocular inflammation. The disease involves both

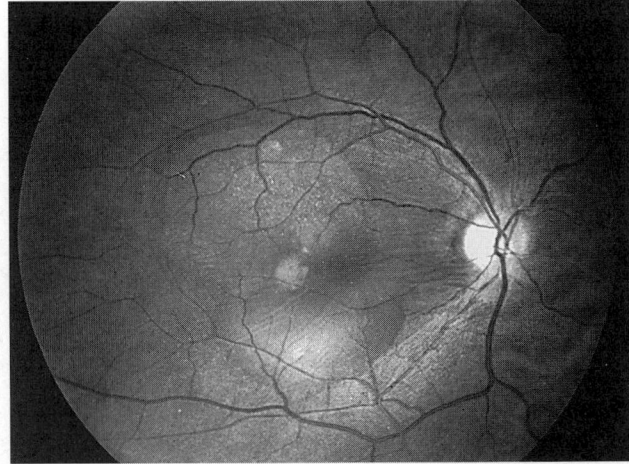

Fig. 58-16. Lupus choroidopathy with serous detachment of the macula mimicking VKH syndrome.

eyes, although not simultaneously. Spontaneous reattachment of the serous retinal detachments occurs in 1 to 2 years.[52] Thus the progressive clinical course and lack of intraocular inflammation in uveal effusion syndrome help to differentiate it from VKH syndrome.

Posterior scleritis must also be included in the differential diagnosis of VKH syndrome. It usually affects women and is often bilateral. There is a strong association with systemic rheumatologic disorders, especially in patients who have bilateral involvement. Patients with posterior scleritis may experience ocular pain, photophobia, and loss of vision. Cells are often seen in the vitreous. Fundus signs include a circumscribed fundus mass, choroidal folds, retinal striae, disc edema, annular choroidal detachment, exudative macular detachment, cystoid macular edema, and localized peripheral retinal detachment.[7] Ultrasound examination of the globe reveals flattening of the posterior aspect of the globe, thickening of the posterior coats of the eye, retrobulbar edema, and high internal reflectivity of the thickened sclera.[7,13] In VKH syndrome the sclera is often secondarily thickened by contiguous inflammation. Similarly, in posterior scleritis the choroid may be thickened by adjacent scleral inflammation. The choroidal thickening in posterior scleritis can be either diffuse or localized, however, and it is highly reflective on ultrasonography, unlike VKH syndrome.[8] Fluorescein angiographic findings may, in some instances, be similar to those of sympathetic ophthalmia, with the initial appearance of mottled choroidal fluorescence followed by multiple hyperfluorescent pinpoint dots in the early phases. The middle and late phases of the angiogram show the spread of fluorescence from these dots to the subretinal fluid.[7] Ultrasonography, however, can easily differentiate posterior scleritis from sympathetic ophthalmia and VKH syndrome.

In addition to the disorders noted previously, numerous systemic conditions can cause serous retinal detachments that mimic the Harada form of VKH syndrome. These include toxemia of pregnancy and renal disease associated with anasarca.[31,84] The history and clinical examination easily differentiate these disorders from VKH syndrome.

Despite a wide array of disorders that may, on cursory examination, appear similar, VKH syndrome is a distinct clinical entity with some unique features. Careful review of the patient's medical history and physical findings (as well as pertinent laboratory, angiographic, and ultrasound evaluations) should clearly confirm or exclude other conditions, thereby strongly supporting the clinical diagnosis of VKH syndrome.

LABORATORY INVESTIGATIONS

In the majority of cases the diagnosis of VKH syndrome is based on clinical findings, although fluorescein angiography and lumbar puncture with examination of the cerebrospinal fluid can provide additional data to support the diagnosis. Other laboratory investigations are useful as adjuncts

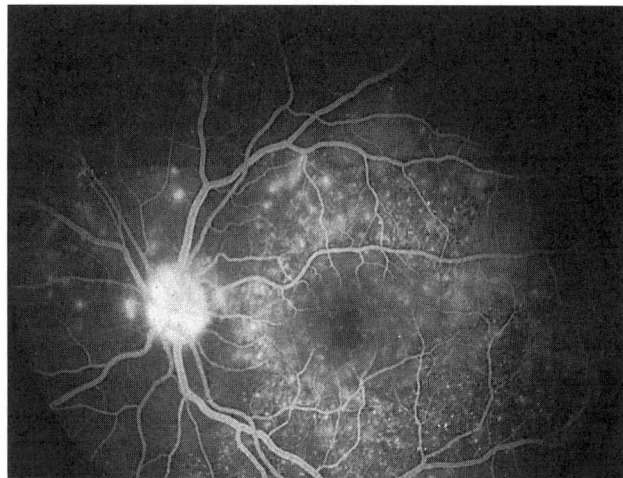

Fig. 58-17. Mid-arteriovenous phase of a fluorescein angiogram showing disc staining and multiple hyperfluorescent dots (at the level of the RPE) that progressively stain fluid in the subretinal space.

to aid in the diagnosis of VKH syndrome; they include echography of the globe, electrooculography, electroretinography, and magnetic resonance imaging.

Fluorescein Angiography

Fluorescein angiography in the acute phase of VKH syndrome characteristically has the appearance of numerous punctate hyperfluorescent dots at the level of the RPE; these foci of hyperfluorescence overlie areas of choroiditis. These dots gradually enlarge and, ultimately, staining of the surrounding subretinal and sub-RPE fluid is seen (Figs. 58-17 and 58-18). The dye travels from the choriocapillaris,

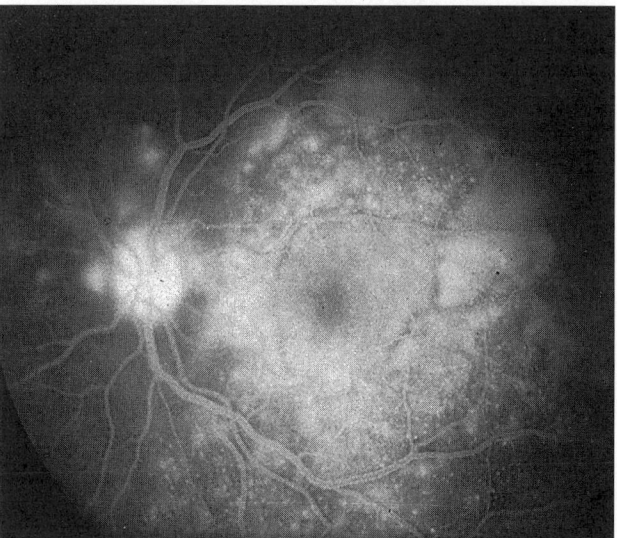

Fig. 58-18. Late arteriovenous phase fluorescein angiogram showing increased fluorescence of the dots and staining of subretinal fluid.

through Bruch membrane and the altered RPE, and enters the subretinal space, where it delineates the multiple exudative retinal detachments (Fig. 58-19). Another characteristic finding on fluorescein angiography of VKH syndrome patients in the uveitis phase is radial, alternating dark and light bands of choroidal fluorescence, created by folding of the swollen choroid.

In a recent review of the fluorescein angiograms of 43 patients with VKH syndrome, several characteristic features were reported by Brinkley, Dugel, and Rao.[10] Patients were classified by the phases of their disease: acute, recovery, chronic, and relapse. The acute and recovery phases in that report corresponded to the uveitic phase described previously; the chronic and relapse phases corresponded to the convalescent and recurrent phases, respectively. Pooling of dye under the sensory retina or focal leaks at the level of the retinal pigment epithelium were seen on the angiograms of all patients in the acute phase, and it was suggested that, together, these signs may be diagnostic.[10] These signs did not occur in the late stages. Nearly 70% of patients had leakage of dye in the area of the optic disc during the acute phase of the disease.[10] Greater than normal permeability of optic disc capillaries resulted in optic disc staining.[97] Punctate hyperfluorescent spots that did not leak were found in 9% to 17% of the patients, depending on the phase of the disease. They were more common in the acute phase of uveitis, but had no funduscopic correlate.[10]

One report suggested that there is no retinal vascular extravasation or sheathing in the acute phase of the VKH syndrome.[32] Nevertheless, periphlebitis in the posterior pole was documented by Okamura,[82] and peripapillary venous sheathing was seen angiographically in 35% of the VKH syndrome patients in the series reported by Snyder and Tessler.[101] More recently, Brinkley and associates[10] reported

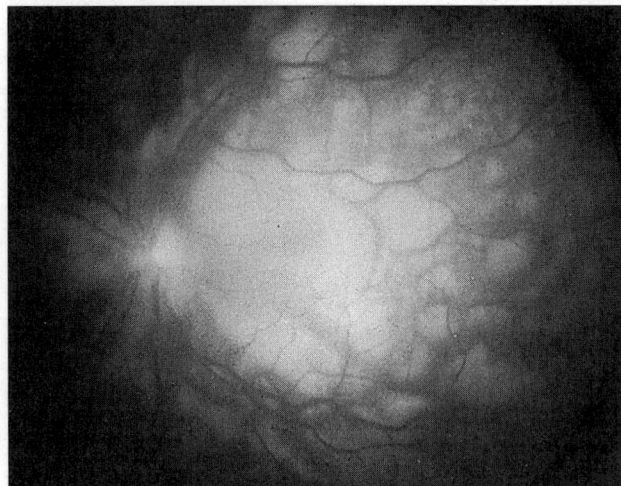

Fig. 58-19. Late phases of fluorescein angiogram showing multiple serous retinal detachments with pooling of dye in the subretinal space.

that, among 43 patients with VKH syndrome, only 2 (5%) had evidence of retinal vascular leakage attributable to the uveitis. It thus appears that retinal vascular sheathing and extravasation do occur, albeit rarely, in VKH syndrome.

After treatment with corticosteroids, inflammation subsides, abnormal leakage of dye at the level of RPE ceases, exudative retinal detachments resolve, and vision improves. These occurrences are the hallmarks of the recovery phase, although other features of this phase include optic disc staining, seen in 29% of patients, and punctate hyperfluorescent dots that represent leaks in 14% of the patients.[10] RPE alterations, consisting of window defects and mottled background fluorescence, are less common than in the chronic phase of the illness.[10]

In chronic VKH syndrome, diffuse pigment "migration" occurs at the level of the RPE. The fluorescein angiogram takes on a "moth-eaten" appearance,[52] and multiple, hyperfluorescent RPE window defects are seen, without progressive staining. Brinkley and associates[10] reported that fluorescein angiographic signs of RPE atrophy are universal in the chronic phase but are rare in the acute phase. These signs include window defects, RPE "mottling" from peripheral yellow-white spots, and alternating hyperfluorescence and hypofluorescence reflecting the "salt-and-pepper" fundus appearance caused by diffuse RPE alterations.

The relapse or recurrent phase consists of recurrence of intraocular inflammation and reduction in visual acuity. Intraocular inflammation is usually of the anterior uveitis type, and fluorescein angiographic changes are thus the same as in the chronic phase. Brinkley and associates[10] reported that one of the two patients in their series who was in the recurrent phase also had optic disc staining.

Complications of chronic VKH syndrome visible on fluorescein angiography include subretinal neovascularization and retinochoroidal and arteriovenous anastamoses, which represent collateral vessels overlying areas of damaged RPE cells.[63] Neovascularization of the disc has been reported also.[52,106] Inflammation may play a role in the pathogenesis of optic disc neovascularization, because it is also seen in sarcoidosis, toxoplasmosis, birdshot retinochoroidopathy, and other uveitic entities.[106] Focal areas of nonperfusion of the choriocapillaris, blockage of choroidal fluorescence by whitish placoid lesions at the level of the RPE, linear pigment accumulations, and choroidal neovascular membranes have also been documented by Brinkley and associates.[10]

History and clinical examination are the most important tools for the diagnosis of VKH syndrome, but if the diagnosis remains in doubt, the fluorescein angiogram is sufficiently characteristic to differentiate VKH syndrome from other disorders. In the acute phase, pooling of dye in the subretinal space, focal leaks at the level of the RPE, and leakage from the disc are the most common signs. In the chronic and recovery phases, window defects and alternating areas of hyperfluorescence and hypofluorescence caused by alterations in RPE are the most common findings.[10]

Cerebrospinal Fluid

Lumbar puncture is a useful diagnostic test in atypical VKH syndrome, but it is rarely required in a typical case, particularly when angiography reveals characteristic changes. In a study by Ohno and associates[81] more than 80% of VKH syndrome patients who underwent lumbar puncture had cerebrospinal fluid pleocytosis; all but one of these patients had signs of meningeal irritation. The pleocytosis associated with VKH syndrome consists mostly of lymphocytes[103] possessing cytotoxic activity against the B36 melanoma cell line.[74] Cerebrospinal fluid pleocytosis is transient, occurring in 89% of patients within 1 week after the onset of symptoms and in 97% of patients within 3 weeks.[103] It resolves in 8 weeks, despite recurrences of intraocular inflammation.[76] In more recent studies, however, lumbar puncture has not been used routinely to establish the diagnosis of VKH syndrome, since noninvasive testing with ultrasonography and fluorescein angiography is usually sufficient to confirm a diagnosis of VKH syndrome.[26]

Ultrasonography

Ultrasonography can also be helpful in diagnosis, especially in cases where inadequate pupillary dilation caused by posterior synechiae or dense vitritis obscures the view of the fundus. It is also helpful in cases with an atypical presentation, such as an absence of extraocular manifestations.[6] Forster and associates[21] described in detail the echographic manifestations of VKH syndrome. They include (1) diffuse, low-to-medium reflective thickening of the posterior choroid, (2) serous detachments of the retina found in the posterior pole or located inferiorly, (3) some vitreous opacities with no posterior vitreous detachment, and (4) posterior thickening of the sclera or episclera (Fig. 58-20).[21] Ultrasonography can also monitor the ophthalmic therapy response in patients who have media opacities and atypical features.

The ultrasonographic features of VKH syndrome, although distinct, must be differentiated from other disorders. For example, posterior scleritis has presenting symptoms of optic disc edema, vitreous cells, and serous retinal detachments[7]; echography shows flattening of the posterior aspect of the globe, thickening of the posterior sclera and episclera, and retrobulbar edema.[13] In contradistinction, eyes with VKH syndrome show diffuse scleral thickening with low-to-medium reflective choroidal thickening, unlike the high reflective choroidal thickening seen in posterior scleritis.[8] The symptoms of benign reactive lymphoid hyperplasia of the uvea include diffuse lymphocytic infiltration of the iris, the choroid, and the ciliary body. As in VKH syndrome, anterior uveitis, serous retinal detachments, and RPE changes can also be seen in this disorder.[90] Approximately 90% of patients with benign reactive lymphoid hyperplasia,

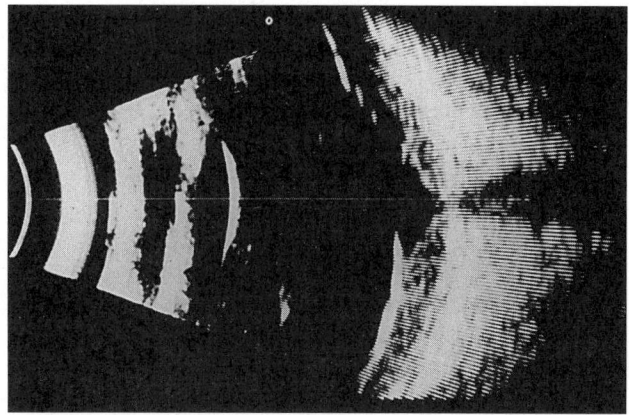

Fig. 58-20. B-mode ultrasonogram of a patient with VKH syndrome showing diffuse low reflective choroidal thickening and serous retinal detachment. (Courtesy Ronald L. Green, MD, Los Angeles CA)

however, have unilateral involvement,[21] and the inflammation may extend to retrobulbar structures.[48] Echography shows low reflective choroidal thickening with sonolucent retrobulbar extension in most cases.[48] Diffuse malignant melanoma of the choroid is rare but usually presents with low reflective thickening of the choroid on echography, similar to that of VKH syndrome.[21] Again, however, unlike VKH syndrome, most cases are unilateral.[21] Choroidal involvement occurs in 85% of eyes with leukemia or lymphoma infiltration.[1] Abramson and associates[1] reported that even subtle, 1- to 2-mm choroidal thickening can be seen with echography of eyes with intraocular lymphoma or leukemia. Kincaid and associates[55,56] highlighted the difficulty in differentiating neoplastic infiltration from VKH syndrome, however. They presented a patient with bilateral serous retinal detachments, changes in mental status, and fluorescein angiographic findings consistent with VKH syndrome. This patient subsequently died of leukemia and was found at autopsy to have choroidal leukemic infiltrates. Thus leukemic infiltrates may closely resemble the choroidal thickening of VKH syndrome on echography. Intraocular large-cell lymphoma is often characterized by irregular medium-to-high reflective choroidal thickening, but the lesions appear more like metastatic tumors to the choroid than VKH syndrome.[21] Sympathetic ophthalmia may result in ultrasonographic features that are virtually identical to those of VKH syndrome, but this disorder is seen only in patients with a history of penetrating eye injury or surgery.[21] Chronic long-standing uveitis is associated with high reflective choroidal thickening, unlike VKH syndrome. Despite rare instances of diagnostic confusion, all of these disorders can usually be differentiated by appropriate history and laboratory evaluations.

Other granulomatous disorders of the choroid, such as tuberculosis and sarcoidosis, tend to cause more nodular choroidal thickening, unlike the diffuse thickening of VKH syndrome. Hence the echographic features of VKH syndrome are unique, especially when applied in context with the history and other physical findings. Echography is therefore an invaluable adjunct for the diagnosis and management of patients with VKH syndrome.

Electroencephalography

Electroencephalographic abnormalities have been recognized in approximately 66% of patients with VKH syndrome.[41] The most common changes include a slowing of the dominant rhythm or a mixing in of theta activity with the background activity. The theta activity may be diffuse or localized, and may occur sporadically or in bursts. These findings are temporally variable.[104]

Magnetic Resonance Imaging

Magnetic resonance imaging has been utilized recently to differentiate choroiditis in VKH syndrome from scleritis.[51] Special surface coils are used to superbly reproduce ophthalmic anatomic detail. Ikeda and Tsukagoshi[39] recently documented multifocal lesions of the brain parenchyma on T1-weighted magnetic resonance images in VKH syndrome.[39] The clinical significance of these lesions remains unclear.

Electrophysiology

Electrooculograms (EOGs) can be useful in diagnosing and monitoring the progression of Harada disease (posterior segment component of VKH syndrome).[72] The electroretinogram (ERG) a-waves and b-waves may be mildly depressed initially and may remain depressed for long periods; the light peak of the EOG may be simultaneously depressed in the initial prodromal and uveitic phases of the disease. Eventually the EOG light peak and ERG amplitudes return toward normal in the chronic phases of the disease.[72] The hyperosmolarity response of the ocular standing potential remains normal during the active inflammatory phase of VKH syndrome; however, in the chronic phase of VKH syndrome a decrease in sensitivity to osmotic stress occurs in the RPE when depigmentation begins.[62] Unfortunately, this change cannot be evaluated by standard electrooculographic techniques. Thus electrooculography and electroretinography demonstrate only nonspecific changes in VKH syndrome. Although these electrophysiologic tests may be helpful in monitoring the disease course in patients with cloudy media, ultrasonography may be more useful by following choroidal inflammation in these situations.

Blood Tests

There are no specific serologic investigations that help to establish the diagnosis of VKH syndrome. Antiganglioside antibodies have been detected in 12 (71%) of 17 patients tested in one study.[80] Antiphotoreceptor outer segment and anti-Müller cell antibodies have also been found in sera of patients with VKH syndrome,[15] and serum IgD has been reported to be elevated. Although some of these tests are promising, they have neither the sensitivity nor the specificity to be clinically practical. Among Asian patients, HLA-DR4 and HLA-Dw53 are associated with a high relative risk,[119] but these HLA specificities are not diagnostic of the syndrome. Ohno[80] also reported increased gamma interferon levels in patients with VKH syndrome.

THERAPY

The principle of treatment for VKH syndrome is to suppress the acute intraocular inflammation with early and aggressive use of systemic corticosteroids, followed by slow tapering over 3 to 6 months, depending on the clinical response. Such early treatment may shorten the duration of the disease, may prevent progression into the chronic stage, and may reduce the incidence of extraocular manifestations.[32] If there is disease exacerbation because the corticosteroids are tapered too rapidly, recurrences may become increasingly corticosteroid-resistant and respond only to cytotoxic/immunosuppressive agents.

The associated anterior uveitis should be treated additionally with topical corticosteroid, with dosage based on the intensity of the inflammation. Use of a cycloplegic/mydriatic agent is recommended to reduce ciliary spasm and to prevent formation of posterior synechiae.

Corticosteroids

Systemic corticosteroids are the mainstay of therapy for the VKH syndrome, although there is a report of good visual outcome without the use of corticosteroids.[116] Nevertheless, systemic administration of corticosteroids can significantly alter the course and prognosis of VKH syndrome when used properly. Rubsamen and Gass,[89] in their recent series of 26 patients with VKH syndrome, treated all of the patients with systemic corticosteroids at an average initial dosage of 80 to 100 mg per day. Approximately 66% (17) of their patients had visual acuity of 20/30 or better at the latest examination.[89] Similarly, in a series of 48 patients seen at the Doheny Eye Institute, Los Angeles, California, USA, 60% had vision of 20/40 or better after initial treatment with high dosages of corticosteroids.[6] Early aggressive use of oral corticosteroids followed by slow tapering of the drugs may reduce the incidence of chronic inflammation in these patients.[32]

Slow tapering of corticosteroids over a 3-month period is recommended, as Rubsamen and Gass[89] found that recurrences occurred in 43% and 52% of patients in the first 3 and 6 months of the disease, respectively; these recurrences were usually associated with too rapid tapering of the corticosteroids.[89] Fujioka and associates[29] noted the average duration of the uveitis to be 3 to 8 months in patients treated within 2 weeks of onset of the disease, but if therapy were delayed, corticosteroids were required for up to 45 months. Hayasaka and associates[34] found that patients required less than 100 mg of prednisone daily for adequate suppression of the inflammation in the Harada form of VKH syndrome, but those patients with severe anterior uveitis in association with exudative retinal detachments (the Vogt-Koyanagi form of disease) were more resistant to treatment, requiring 200 mg or more of intravenous prednisone therapy daily.[81] Based on their own classification, Ohno and associates[81] treated patients with high-dose corticosteroids and reported that 83% of patients with type 3 disease (ocular involvement with skin, hair, or ear changes) had vision of 20/50 or better, compared with 42% of type 2 patients (ocular disease with at least one skin manifestation), and 50% of type 1 patients (ocular signs and symptoms without ear or skin changes). Sasamoto and associates[92] reported 47 new patients treated with pulse doses of corticosteroids (up to 1 gm intravenously of methylprednisolone daily for 3 days followed by a slow oral taper), high-dose corticosteroid therapy (200 mg of methylprednisolone intravenously for 3 days followed by slow oral taper), or no corticosteroid therapy. Both the pulse and the high-dose corticosteroid therapy groups showed improvement in both anterior chamber inflammation and visual acuity.

Among Hispanics, recurrences of inflammation tend to be of the anterior uveitis type and are usually resistant to topical and systemic corticosteroid therapy.[6] In these instances oral cytotoxic agents, such as cyclophosphamide, or azathioprine, or potent immunosuppressive agent, cyclosporine, may be useful as described in the next section.

Immunosuppressive Therapy

Cytotoxic/immunosuppressive agents may be used when corticosteroids alone cannot control intraocular inflammation or when a patient cannot tolerate the side effects of corticosteroids (see box). Cyclophosphamide, chlorambucil, and azathioprine have all been used to treat VKH syndrome and sympathetic ophthalmia.[35] Cyclophosphamide, a potent alkylating agent, may be given intravenously or orally at dosages of 1 to 2 mg/kg/day. Its major side effects include alopecia, anemia, and sterile hemorrhagic cystitis. Chlorambucil, the slowest-acting nitrogen mustard, may be started orally at 0.1 mg/kg/day, with the dosage adjusted upward every 3 weeks to a maximum of 18 mg/day. Irreversible azoospermia and myelosuppression complicate its use. Both cyclophosphamide and chlorambucil can cause secondary systemic malignancies. Azathioprine, an inhibitor of purine synthesis, may be used in orally administered divided dosages totaling 1 to 2.5 mg/kg/day. Unfortunately, myelosuppression and leukopenia may appear rapidly with the use of this agent; other side effects include gastrointestinal distress, alopecia, stomatitis, and secondary infections.[35] All of these medications have toxic side effects that can cause a significant morbidity and, in rare cases, death. In place of these cytotoxic agents, cyclosporine may be used; it is a cytostatic agent with relatively less systemic toxicity, particularly on the bone marrow.

Cyclosporine is generally preferred when corticosteroid-resistant therapy is required for inflammation or when the patient has intolerable or life-threatening side effects from long-term corticosteroid use. As discussed earlier, the T-helper and cytotoxic lymphocyte-mediated damage to the choroid is probably the immunopathologic basis of this disease, so it is appropriate to consider suppression of cell-mediated immune events by using cyclosporine in the treatment of VKH syndrome. In 1988 Wakatsuki and associates[111] successfully treated a case of VKH syndrome resistant to corticosteroid therapy alone by using cyclosporine and corticosteroids. Rubsamen and Gass[89] treated 2 of 26 patients who had VKH syndrome with oral cyclosporine. Each of these patients had inflammation that was refractory to corticosteroid therapy, and each had a final visual acuity of 20/50 or better. In a study performed by Wakefield and associates[112] in Australia, three cases of VKH syndrome that were refractory to corticosteroid therapy were treated with initial pulse dosages of cyclosporine at 10 mg/kg/day; the dosage was reduced to 3 to 5 mg/kg/day when the inflammation subsided. Two of the three patients had a partial response, with improvement in visual acuity; the other patient had no improvement in inflammation, and the disease followed a smoldering course. Nussenblatt and associates[77] used cyclosporine to treat 16 patients who had bilateral, noninfectious posterior uveitis and had not responded to corticosteroid and cytotoxic immunosuppressive therapy, or who had intolerable side effects to the corticosteroids. Although only one of the patients had VKH syndrome, this study gives some insight into its mechanism of action for inflammation of the choroid. Each of these patients initially received 10 mg/kg/day of cyclosporine. After a follow-up period ranging from 2 to 18 months, 15 of the 16 patients had a reduction in inflammation and an improvement in vision. The most common side effect to the cyclosporine was nephrotoxicity with increased serum creatinine levels and decreased creatinine clearance, which occurred in five (30%) of the patients. Renal function improved with a reduction in cyclosporine dosage. Reversible hepatotoxicity with mildly elevated serum glutamic oxaloacetic transaminase and glutamic pyruvate transaminase levels was also reported.[77] In an earlier report[78] eight of these patients had OKT4 and OKT8 counts performed on peripheral blood. In all of these cases the OKT4 cells eventually decreased with therapy, and thus the OKT4/OKT8 ratio also decreased. Cyclosporine did not seem to influence natural killer cell activity.

It is now recommended that cyclosporine dosages be no higher than 5 mg/kg/day.[20] Furthermore, increases in serum creatinine of greater than 30% above the patient's baseline value must be avoided to prevent irreversible, focal proximal tubular and glomerular changes.[20] Serum trough levels measured by radioimmunoassay should lie between 0.1 and 0.4 mg/μl.[35] In addition to dose-dependent nephrotoxicity and hepatotoxicity, cyclosporine can cause neurologic symptoms such as tremors and myopathy, integumentary changes such as hirsutism, and systemic hypertension.[20]

Tacrolimus (also known as FK506), a new cellular immunosuppressant isolated from the broth of *Streptomyces tsukubaensis,* has been found effective in the treatment of both transplant rejection and experimental autoimmune uveitis. Like cyclosporine, tacrolimus operates as a prodrug that binds endogenous intracellular receptors, the immunophilins, and the target protein complexes—protein phosphatase and calcineurin.[96] Tacrolimus has been used in the treatment of S antigen-induced uveitis in primates,[28] and was found to prevent the development of uveitis even 3 weeks after immunization with S antigen, when immunopathogenic mechanisms of uveitis had developed fully. In addition, inflammation in primates was inhibited at dosages of less than 0.125 mg/kg/day,[28] and was shown to be even more potent than cyclosporine because it suppressed experimental autoimmune uveitis in rats at much lower dosages.[69] An initial multicenter clinical trial of tacrolimus has yielded promising results.[70] Twenty-nine patients were enrolled in the study: 25 had Behçet syndrome, 3 had idiopathic retinal vasculitis, and 1 had VKH syndrome. Patients were treated with a twice-daily regimen of 0.05, 0.1, or 0.2 mg/kg/day for 12 weeks. Nine patients received the 0.05 mg/kg/day dose; thirteen received 0.1 mg/kg/day; and seven received 0.2 mg/kg/day. Intraocular inflammation improved clinically in 62% of the patients overall, and vision remained stable or improved in over 80%. An initial dosage of 0.05 mg/kg/day of tacrolimus reduced inflammation in 22% of the cases; 0.1 mg/kg/day reduced inflammation in 50% of the cases; and 0.2 mg/kg/day reduced inflammation in all cases receiving this dosage, but was associated with nephrotoxicity. Renal impairment was seen in 30% of the patients, most of whom were receiving 0.2 mg/kg/day of tacrolimus. In nearly half of the cases of nephrotoxicity, the increase in serum creatinine was dose-dependent and reversible. Other side effects included tremor in 10% of the patients, nausea in 6%, hyperglycemia in 3%, and chest discomfort in 3%. Nearly 70% of the patients receiving tacrolimus had no side effects. Overall, in 62% of the patients (18) uveitis activity improved with tacrolimus therapy. In the remaining 38% of patients (19) uveitis activity remained unchanged.[70] Currently a daily dosage of 0.1 to 0.15 mg/kg is considered appropriate for treatment of intraocular inflammation. Trough levels of the drug in whole blood should be less than 20 ng/ml.[70] Further clinical studies are needed to determine the role of tacrolimus in the treatment of uveitis.

PROGNOSIS

The use of systemic corticosteroids has improved the visual prognosis of VKH syndrome, which was originally de-

TABLE 58-2 VISUAL OUTCOME IN VKH SYNDROME AFTER CORTICOSTEROID TREATMENT

Visual Acuity	Initial Number of Eyes (n = 95 eyes)	Final Number of Eyes (n = 95 eyes)
20/20 to 20/40	16(17%)	57(59%)
20/50 to 20/100	18(19%)	27(28%)
20/200 or less	49(51%)	8(8%)
Not Available	12(13%)	4(4%)

From Beniz J and associates: Variations in clinical features of the Vogt-Koyanagi-Harada syndrome, *Retina* 11:275-280, 1991.

scribed as a disorder with a guarded visual prognosis.[85] Beginning in 1978, reports from Japan indicated the impact of corticosteroid therapy on the disease outcome. Sugiura[103] reported that among his patients, 70% had vision of 20/50 or better and only 20% had vision of 20/200 or less. Snyder and Tessler[101] recounted that 80% of their patients had 20/70 or better vision in at least one eye after follow-up of 2 to 5 years, and Minnakawa and associates[68] reported vision of 20/40 or better in 158 (85%) of their 186 cases. Beniz and associates[6] stated that in their series of 48 patients, 20 (41%) had visual acuity of 20/200 or less; however, 28 (59%) had 20/40 or better vision after treatment with systemic corticosteroids (Table 58-2).[1] Nevertheless, 21 (44%) of the patients had at least one recurrence of inflammation, and five required cytotoxic/immunosuppressive agents. Rubsamen and Gass[89] recently showed that 66% of patients had visual acuity of 20/30 or better after treatment with corticosteroids and/or immunosuppressives; only 7% had severe visual loss to a level of 20/400 or less.

In most cases the intraocular inflammation of VKH syndrome diminishes markedly in 1 month and invariably improves in 6 months, when treated with corticosteroids. In the cases reported by Rubsamen and Gass,[89] corticosteroid therapy was continued for an average of 6 months, with some patients being treated for up to 48 months. They reported three factors that are predictive of poor visual prognosis: older age of the patient at the onset of inflammation, chronic ocular inflammation requiring long-term treatment with corticosteroids, and subretinal neovascular membranes. They emphasized the importance of early and prolonged high-dose systemic corticosteroid therapy in preventing poor visual outcome.[89]

SUMMARY

In conclusion, the VKH syndrome is a bilateral, diffuse granulomatous uveitis associated with poliosis, vitiligo, alopecia, and auditory and other central nervous system signs. These manifestations are variable and race-dependent. This inflammatory syndrome is probably the result of autoimmune mechanisms influenced by genetic factors, and it appears to be directed against melanocytes. Histopathologically, typical cases show nonnecrotizing diffuse granulomatous panuveitis with sparing of the choriocapillaris and formation of Dalen-Fuchs nodules virtually identical to the findings of sympathetic ophthalmia. The only distinguishing feature appears to be the absence of penetrating injury in VKH syndrome. Fluorescein angiography, lumbar puncture, and echography are useful adjuncts in its diagnosis and management. The syndrome is treated with high-dose systemic corticosteroids or, when necessary, with cyclosporine or other immunosuppressive cytotoxic agents. The prognosis of patients with VKH syndrome is fair, with nearly 60% of patients retaining vision of 20/50 or better.

The complications of VKH syndrome that lead to visual loss include cataracts, in about 25% of patients; glaucoma, in about 33% of patients; and choroidal neovascular membranes, in less than 10% of patients. The latter are important causes of late visual loss. These complications usually require medical and/or surgical intervention, including photocoagulation. It appears the initial treatment with high-dose corticosteroids followed by prolonged therapy with maintenance doses of this antiinflammatory agent may minimize these complications and improve visual prognosis.

REFERENCES

1. Abramson DH, Jereb B, Wollner N et al.: Leukemic ophthalmopathy detected by ultrasound, *J Pediatr Ophthalmol Strabismus* 20:92-97, 1983.
2. Asakura S, Takashi T, Onishi T: Vogt-Koyanagi-Harada syndrome (uveitis diffusa acuta) in the dog, *Jpn J Vet Med* 673:445-455, 1977.
3. Babel J: Syndrome de Vogt-Koyanagi (Uveite bilaterale, poliosis, alopecie, vitiligo et dysacousie), *Schweiz Med Wochenschr Nr* 44:1136-1140, 1932.
4. Barr CC, Green WR, Payne JW et al.: Intraocular reticulum-cell sarcoma: clinico-pathologic study of four cases and review of the literature, *Surv Ophthalmol* 19:224-239, 1975.
5. Barr CC, Zimmerman LE, Curtin VT, Font RL: Bilateral diffuse melanocytic uveal tumors associated with systemic malignant neoplasms: a recently recognized syndrome, *Arch Ophthalmol* 100:249-255, 1982.
6. Beniz J, Forster DJ, Lean JS et al.: Variations in clinical features of the Vogt-Koyanagi-Harada syndrome, *Retina* 11:275-280, 1991.
7. Benson WE: Posterior scleritis, *Surv Ophthalmol* 32:297-316, 1988.
8. Benson WE, Shields JA, Tasman W, Crandall AS: Posterior scleritis: a cause of diagnostic confusion, *Arch Ophthalmol* 97:1482-1486, 1979.
9. Boniuk M: *Skin lesions in Vogt Koyanagi Harada syndrome.* Case presented at the joint meeting of the Verhoeff Society and European Ophthalmic Pathology Society, London, April 25-28, 1971.
10. Brinkley JR, Dugel PU, Rao NA: *Fluorescein angiographic findings in the Vogt-Koyanagi-Harada syndrome.* Annual meeting American Academy of Ophthalmology, Dallas, 1992.
11. Bruno MG, McPherson Jr SD: Harada's disease, *Am J Ophthalmol* 32:513-522, 1949.
12. Campo RV, Aaberg TM: Choroidal granuloma in sarcoidosis, *Am J Ophthalmol* 97:419-427, 1984.
13. Cappaert WE, Purnell EW, Frank KE: Use of B-sector scan ultrasound in the diagnosis of benign choroidal folds, *Am J Ophthalmol* 84:375-379, 1977.
14. Carlson MR, Kerman BM: Hemorrhagic macular detachment in the Vogt-Koyanagi-Harada syndrome, *Am J Ophthalmol* 84:632-635, 1977.
15. Chan CC, Palestine AG, Nussenblatt RB et al.: Anti-retinal auto-antibodies in Vogt-Koyanagi-Harada syndrome, Behçet's disease, and sympathetic ophthalmia, *Ophthalmology* 92:1025-1028, 1985.
16. Chung YM, Yeh TS: Linear streak lesions of the fundus equator associated with Vogt-Koyanagi-Harada syndrome, *Am J Ophthalmol* 109:745-746, 1990.
17. Davis JL, Mittal KK, Freidlin V et al.: HLA associations and ancestry in Vogt-Koyanagi-Harada disease and sympathetic ophthalmia, *Ophthalmology* 97:1137-1142, 1990.
18. DeSmet MD, Yamamoto JH, Mochizuki M et al.: Cellular immune responses of patients with uveitis to retinal antigens and their fragments, *Am J Ophthalmol* 110:135-142, 1990.
19. Duke-Elder S, Perkins ES: *System of ophthalmology,* vol X, *Diseases of the uveal tract,* 373-375, London, 1966, Henry Kimpton Pub.
20. Feutren G, Mihatsch MJ: For the int. kidney biopsy registry of cyclosporine in autoimmune diseases: risk factors for cyclosporine-induced nephropathy in patients with autoimmune diseases, *N Engl J Med* 326:1654-1660, 1992.
21. Forster DJ, Cano MR, Green RL, Rao NA: Echographic features of the Vogt-Koyanagi-Harada syndrome, *Arch Ophthalmol* 108:1421-1426, 1990.
22. Forster DJ, Green RL, Rao NA: Unilateral manifestation of the Vogt-Koyanagi-Harada syndrome in a 7-year-old child, *Am J Ophthalmol* 111(3):380-382, 1991.
23. Forster DJ, Rao NA, Hill RA et al.: Incidence and management of glaucoma in Vogt-Koyanagi-Harada syndrome, *Ophthalmology* 100:613-618, 1993.
24. Foster CS, Fong LP, Singh G: Cataract surgery and intraocular lens implantation in patients with uveitis, *Ophthalmology* 96:281-288, 1989.
25. Foster RE, Lowder CY, Meisler DM, Zakov ZN: Extracapsular cataract extraction and posterior chamber intraocular lens implantation in uveitis patients, *Ophthalmology* 99:1234-1241, 1992.
26. Franklin RM: Systemic disease-related and noninfectious uveitis, *Curr Opin Ophthalmol* 3:512-518, 1992.
27. Friedman AH, Deutsch-Sokol H: Sugiura's sign: perilimbal vitiligo in the Vogt-Koyanagi-Harada syndrome, *Ophthalmology* 88:1159-1165, 1981.
28. Fujino Y, Mochizuki M, Chan CC et al.: FK506 treatment of S antigen induced uveitis in primates, *Curr Eye Res* 10(7):679-690, 1991.
29. Fujioka T, Fukuda M, Okinami S: A statistic study of Vogt-Koyanagi-Harada syndrome, *Acta Soc Ophthalmol Jpn* 84:1979-1982, 1980.
30. Gass JDM: Acute posterior multifocal placoid pigment epitheliopathy, *Arch Ophthalmol* 80:177-185, 1968.
31. Gitter KA et al.: Toxemia of pregnancy: an angiographic interpretation of fundus changes, *Arch Ophthalmol* 80:449-454, 1968.
32. Goto H, Rao NA: Sympathetic ophthalmia and Vogt-Koyanagi-Harada syndrome, *Int Ophthalmol Clin* 30(4):274-285, 1990.
33. Harada Y: Beitrag zur klinischen kenntnis von nichteitriger Choroiditis (Choroiditis diffusa acta), *Acta Soc Ophthalmol Jpn* 30:356-378, 1926.
34. Hayasaka S, Okabe H, Takahashi J: Systemic corticosteroid treatment in Vogt-Koyanagi-Harada disease, *Graefes Arch Clin Exp Ophthalmol* 218:913, 1982.
35. Hemady R, Tauber J, Foster CS: Immunosuppressive drugs in immune and inflammatory ocular disease, *Surv Ophthalmol* 35:369-385, 1991.
36. Hooper PL, Rao NA, Smith RE: Cataract extraction in uveitis patients, *Surv Ophthalmol* 35:120-144, 1990.
37. Hoshi H, Tamada Y, Murata Y et al.: Changes in audiogram in the course of Harada's disease, *Jpn J Clin Ophthalmol* 31:23-30, 1977.
38. Hutchinson J: A case of blanched eyelashes, *Arch Surg* 4:357, 1892.
39. Ikeda M, Tsukagoshi H: Vogt-Koyanagi-Harada disease presenting meningoencephalitis: report of a case with magnetic resonance imaging, *Eur Neurol* 32:835, 1992.
40. Ikui H, Hiroshi M, Furuyoshi Y: Histologic investigation of idiopathic uveitis (Vogt-Koyanagi-Harada syndrome): report of two cases, *Acta Soc Ophthalmol Jpn* 56:1089-1096, 1952.
41. Inomata H, Kato M: Vogt-Koyanagi-Harada disease: viral disease. In McKendall RR, editor: *Handbook of clinical neurology,* 1989, Elsevier Scientific Publishers B.V., pp. 611-626.

42. Inomata H, Minei M, Taniguchi Y, Nishimura F: Choroidal neovascularization in long-standing case of Vogt-Koyanagi-Harada disease, *Jpn J Ophthalmol* 27:9-26, 1983.

43. Inomata H, Sakamoto T: Immunohistochemical studies of Vogt-Koyanagi-Harada disease with sunset sky fundus, *Curr Eye Res* 9(suppl):35-40, 1990.

44. Isogai E, Isogai H, Kotake S et al.: Detection of antibodies against Borrelia Burgdorferi in patients with uveitis, *Am J Ophthalmol* 112:23-30, 1991.

45. Itho S, Kurimoto S, Kouno T: Vogt-Koyanagi-Harada disease in monozygotic twins, *Int Ophthalmol* 16:49-54, 1992.

46. Jabs DA, Hanneken AM, Schachat AP, Fine SL: Choroidopathy in systemic lupus erythematosus, *Arch Ophthalmol* 106:230-234, 1988.

47. Jabs DA, Johns CJ: Ocular involvement in chronic sarcoidosis, *Am J Ophthalmol* 102:297-301, 1986.

48. Jakobiec FA, Sacks E, Kronish JW et al.: M: Multifocal static creamy choroidal infiltrates: an early sign of lymphoid neoplasia, *Ophthalmology* 94:397-406, 1987.

49. Jampel HD, Jabs DA, Quigley HA: Trabeculectomy with 5-fluorouracil for adult inflammatory glaucoma, *Am J Ophthalmol* 109:168-173, 1990.

50. Jampol LM, Sieving PA, Pugh D et al.: Multiple evanescent white dot syndrome. I. Clinical findings, *Arch Ophthalmol* 102:671-674, 1984.

51. Johnston CA, Teitelbaum CS: Magnetic resonance imaging in Vogt-Koyanagi-Harada syndrome, *Arch Ophthalmol* 108:783-784, 1990.

52. Kanter PJ, Goldberg MF: Bilateral uveitis with exudative retinal detachment: angiographic appearance, *Arch Ophthalmol* 91:13-19, 1974.

53. Kayazawa F, Takahashi H: Acute posterior multifocal placoid pigment epitheliopathy and Harada's disease, *Ann Ophthalmol* 15:58-62, 1983.

54. Kern TJ, Walton DK, Riis RC et al.: Uveitis associated with poliosis and vitiligo in six dogs, *JAMA* 187(4):408-414, 1985.

55. Kincaid MC, Green WR: Ocular and orbital involvement in leukemias, *Surv Ophthalmol* 27:211-232, 1983.

56. Kincaid MC, Green WR, Kelley JS: Acute ocular leukemia, *Am J Ophthalmol* 87:698-702, 1979.

57. Kirmani MH, Thomas EL, Rao NA, Laborde RP: Intraocular reticulum cell sarcoma: diagnosis by choroidal biopsy, *Br J Ophthalmol* 71:748-752, 1987.

58. Koyanagi Y: Dysakusis, Alopecia und Poliosis bei schwerer Uveitis nicht traumatischen Ursprungs, *Klin Monatsbl Augenheilkd* 82:194-211, 1929.

59. Lindley DM, Boosinger TR, Cox NR: Ocular histopathology of Vogt-Koyanagi-Harada-like syndrome in an akita Dog, *Vet Pathol* 27:294-296, 1990.

60. Lubin JR, Loewenstein JI, Frederick AR Jr: Vogt Koyanagi Harada syndrome with focal neurologic signs, *Am J Ophthalmol* 91:332-341, 1981.

61. Lubin JR, Ni C, Albert DM: A clinicopathological study of the Vogt Koyanagi Harada syndrome, *Int Ophthalmol Clin* 22(3):141-156, 1982.

62. Madachi-Yamamoto S, Kawasaki K, Yonemura D: Retinal pigment epithelium disorder in Vogt-Koyanagi-Harada disease revealed by hyperosmolarity response of ocular standing potential, *Jpn J Ophthalmol* 28:362-369, 1984.

63. Manger CC III, Ober RR: Retinal arteriovenous anastomoses in the Vogt-Koyanagi-Harada syndrome, *Am J Ophthalmol* 89:186-191, 1980.

64. Martinez JA, Lopez PF, Sternberg Jr P et al.: Vogt-Koyanagi-Harada syndrome in patients with Cherokee Indian ancestry, *Am J Ophthalmol* 114:615-620, 1992.

65. Matsuda H, Sugiura S: Ultrastructural changes in the melanocyte in Vogt-Koyanagi-Harada syndrome and sympathetic ophthalmia, *Jpn J Ophthalmol* 15:69-80, 1971.

66. McClellan KA, MacDonald M, Hersey P, Billson FA: Vogt-Koyanagi-Harada syndrome — isolation of cloned T cells with specificity for melanocytes and melanoma cells, *Aust N Z J Ophthalmol* 17:347-352, 1989.

67. Mimura Y: Vogt-Koyonagi-Harada disease. In Uyama M, editor: *Ganka Mook,* vol 12, 116-144, Tokyo, 1980, Kanehara.

68. Minnakawa R, Ohno S, Hirose S et al.: Clinical manifestations of Vogt Koyanagi Harada disease, *Jpn J Clin Ophthalmol* 39:1249-1253, 1985.

69. Mochizuki M, Kawashima H: Effects of FK506, 15deoxy spergualin, and Cyclosporine on experimental autoimmune uveoretinitis in the rat, *Autoimmunity* 8(1):37-41, 1990.

70. Mochizuki M, Masuda K, Sakane T et al.: A multicenter clinical open trial of FK506 in refractory uveitis, including Behçet's disease: Japanese FK506 study group on refractory uveitis, *Transplant Proc* 23(6):3343-3346, 1991.

71. Morris WR, Schlaegel Jr TF: Viruslike inclusion bodies in subretinal fluid in uveo-encephalitis, *Am J Ophthalmol* 58:940-944, 1969.

72. Nagaya T: Use of the electrooculogram for diagnosing and following the development of Harada's disease, *Am J Ophthalmol* 74:99-109, 1972.

73. Naidu YM, Pararajasegaram G, Sun Y et al.: Predominant expression of T-cell antigen receptor (TCR) V Alpha 10 in Vogt-Koyanagi-Harada (VKH) syndrome, *Invest Ophthalmol Vis Sci* 32:934, 1991.

74. Norose K, Yano A, Aosai F, Segawa K: Immunologic analysis of cerebrospinal fluid lymphocytes in Vogt-Koyanagi-Harada disease, *Invest Ophthalmol Vis Sci* 31:1210-1216, 1990.

74a. Numaga J, Matsuki K, Tokunaga K et al.: Analysis of human leukocyte antigen HLA-DR-beta amino acid sequence in Vogt-Koyanagi-Harada syndrome, *Invest Ophthalmol Vis Sci* 32:1958-61, 1991.

75. Nussenblatt RB: Clinical studies of Vogt-Koyanagi-Harada's disease at the National Eye Institute, *Jpn J Ophthalmol* 32:330-333, 1988.

76. Nussenblatt RB, Palestine AG: Vogt-Koyanagi-Harada syndrome (uveomeningitic syndrome). In Ryan SJ, editor: *Retina,* vol 2, 723-728, St Louis, 1984, Mosby.

77. Nussenblatt RB, Palestine AG, Chan CC: Cyclosporin A therapy in the treatment of intraocular inflammatory disease resistant to systemic corticosteroids and cytotoxic agents, *Am J Ophthalmol* 96:275-282, 1983.

78. Nussenblatt RB, Palestine AG et al.: Treatment of intraocular inflammatory disease with cyclosporin A, *Lancet* 2:235-238, 1983.

79. Ober RR, Smith RE, Ryan SJ: Subretinal neovascularization in the Vogt-Koyanagi-Harada syndrome, *Int Ophthalmol* 6:225-234, 1983.

80. Ohno S: Vogt-Koyanagi-Harada disease. In Saari KM, editor: *Uveitis update,* 735-740, Proceedings of the first international symposium on uveitis held in Hanasaari, Amsterdam, 1984, Excerpa Medica.

81. Ohno S, Char DH, Kimura SJ, O'Connor GR: Vogt-Koyanagi-Harada syndrome, *Am J Ophthalmol* 83:735-740, 1977.

82. Okamura S: Harada's disease, *Acta Soc Ophthalmol Jpn* 42:196, 1938.

83. Okubo K, Kurimoto S, Okubo K et al.: Surface markers of peripheral blood lymphocytes in Vogt-Koyanagi-Harada disease, *J Clin Lab Immunol* 17:49-52, 1985.

84. Paris GL, Macoul KL: Reversible chronic retinal detachments in chronic renal disease, *Am J Ophthalmol* 67:249-251, 1969.

85. Perry HD, Font RL: Clinical and histopathologic observations in severe Vogt-Koyanagi-Harada syndrome, *Am J Ophthalmol* 83:242-254, 1977.

86. Rao NA, Marak GE: Sympathetic ophthalmia simulating Vogt Koyanagi Harada's disease: a clinico-pathologic study of four cases, *Jpn J Ophthalmol* 27:506-511, 1983.

87. Rohrbach JM, Roggendorf W, Thanos S et al.: Simultaneous bilateral diffuse melanocytic uveal hyperplasia, *Am J Ophthalmol* 110:49-56, 1990.

88. Rosen E: Uveitis, with poliosis, vitiligo, alopecia and dysacusia (Vogt-Koyanagi syndrome), *Arch Ophthalmol* 33:281-292, 1945.

89. Rubsamen PE, Gass JDM: Vogt-Koyanagi-Harada syndrome: clinical course, therapy, and longterm visual outcome, *Arch Ophthalmol* 109:682-687, 1991.

90. Ryan SJ, Zimmerman LE, King FM: Reactive lymphoid hyperplasia: an unusual form of intraocular pseudotumor, *Trans Am Acad Ophthalmol Otolaryngol* 76:652-671, 1972.

91. Sakamoto T, Murata T, Inomata H: Class II major histocompatibility complex on melanocytes of Vogt-Koyanagi-Harada disease, *Arch Ophthalmol* 109:1270-1274, 1991.

92. Sasamoto Y, Ohno S, Matsuda H: Studies on corticosteroid therapy in Vogt-Koyanagi-Harada disease, *Ophthalmologica* 201:162-167, 1990.

93. Scheider A, Kaboth A, Neuhauser L: Detection of subretinal neovascular membranes with indocyanine green and an infrared scanning laser ophthalmoscope, *Am J Ophthalmol* 113:45-51, 1992.

94. Schepens CL, Brockhurst RJ: Uveal effusion. I. Clinical picture, *Arch Ophthalmol* 70:189-201, 1963.

95. Schoenfeld Y, Isenberg DA: Mycobacteria and autoimmunity, *Immunologic Today* 9:178-182, 1988.

96. Schreiber SL, Crabtree GR: The mechanism of action of cyclosporin A and FK506, *Immunol Today* 13:136-142, 1992.

97. Shimizu K: Harada's, Behcet's, Vogt-Koyanagi syndromes—are they clinical entities? *Trans Am Acad Ophthalmol Otolaryngol* 77:OP281-OP290, 1973.

98. Shirato S, Hayashi K, Masuda K: Acute angle closure glaucoma as an initial sign of Harada's disease—report of two cases, *Jpn J Ophthalmol* 24:260-266, 1980.

99. Siltzbach LE, James DG et al.: Course and prognosis of sarcoidosis around the world, *Am J Med* 57:847-852, 1974.

100. Smyth JR Jr, Boissy RE, Fite KV et al.: Retinal dystrophy associated with a postnatal amelanosis in the chicken, *Invest Ophthalmol Vis Sci* 20:799-803, 1981.

101. Snyder DA, Tessler HA: Vogt-Koyanagi-Harada syndrome, *Am J Ophthalmol* 90:69-75, 1980.

102. Spencer WH: *Ophthalmic pathology: an atlas and textbook,* vol 3, 1956-1966, Philadelphia, 1985, WB Saunders.

103. Sugiura S: Vogt-Koyanagi-Harada disease, *Jpn J Ophthalmol* 22:9-35, 1978.

104. Suzuki T, Tanaka N: EEG of the Patients with uveomeningoencephalitic (Vogt-Koyanagi-Harada) syndrome, *Clin Psychiatry* 19:1173-1179, 1977.

105. Tagawa Y: Lymphocyte-mediated cytotoxicity against melanocyte antigens in Vogt-Koyanagi-Harada disease, *Jpn J Ophthalmol* 22:36-41, 1978.

106. To KW, Nadel AJ, Brockhurst RJ: Optic disc neovascularization in association with Vogt-Koyanagi-Harada syndrome, *Arch Ophthalmol* 108:918-919, 1990.

107. Tomimori S, Uyama M: Shallow anterior chamber and transient myopia as initial signs of Harada's disease, *Jpn J Clin Ophthalmol* 31:1271-1273, 1977.

108. Trebini F, Appiotti A, Bacci R et al.: Vogt-Koyanagi-Harada syndrome: clinical and instrumental contribution, *Ital J Neurol Sci* 12(5):479-484, 1991.

109. Usui M, Usui N, Goto H et al.: Detection of Epstein Barr virus DNA by polymerase chain reaction in cerebrospinal fluid from patients with Vogt-Koyanagi-Harada disease, *Invest Ophthalmol Vis Sci* 32:807, 1991.

110. Vogt A: Frühzeitiges Ergrauen der Zilien und Bemerkungen über den sogenannten plötzlichen Eintritt dieser Veränderung, *Klin Monatsbl Augenheilkd* 4:228-242, 1906.

111. Wakatsuki Y, Kogure M, Takahashi Y, Oguro Y: Combination therapy with cyclosporin A and steroid in severe case of Vogt-Koyanagi-Harada's disease, *Jpn J Ophthalmol* 32:358-360, 1988.

112. Wakefield D, McCluskey P, Reece G: Cyclosporin therapy in Vogt Koyanagi Harada disease, *Aust N Z J Ophthalmol* 18:137-142, 1990.

113. Weber SW, Kazdan JJ: The Vogt-Koyanagi-Harada syndrome in children, *J Pediatr Ophthalmol* 14:96-99, 1977.

114. Weinreb RN: Adjusting the dose of 5-fluorouracil after filtration surgery to minimize side effects, *Ophthalmology* 94:564-570, 1987.

114a. Weisz JM, Holland GN, Roer LN et al.: An association between Vogt-Koyanagi-Harada syndrome and HLA-DR1 and DR4 in Hispanic patients living in Southern California, *Opthalmology* (in press).

115. Winward KE, Smith JL, Culbertson WW, Paris-Hamelin A: Ocular Lyme Borreliosis, *Am J Ophthalmol* 108:651-657, 1989.

116. Yamamoto T, Sasaki T, Saito H et al.: Visual prognosis in Harada's disease: a reevaluation of massive systemic corticosteroid therapy, *Jpn J Clin Ophthalmol* 40:461-464, 1986.

117. Yokoyama MM, Matsui Y, Yamashiroya HM et al.: Humoral and cellular immunity studies in patients with Vogt-Koyanagi-Harada syndrome and pars planitis, *Invest Ophthalmol Vis Sci* 20:364-370, 1981.

118. Yoshioka H: Early fundus changes in Harada's syndrome, *Jpn J Clin Ophthalmol* 21:135-141, 1967.

119. Zhao M, Jiang Y, Abrahams IW: Association of HLA antigens with Vogt-Koyanagi-Harada syndrome in a Han Chinese population, *Arch Ophthalmol* 109:368-370, 1991.

59 Sarcoidosis

ROBERT HAIMOVICI, C. STEPHEN FOSTER

Sarcoidosis is a chronic granulomatous inflammation that can affect nearly every organ system, but particularly the lungs, thoracic lymph nodes, skin, and eyes.[84a] The lack of an identifiable causal agent triggering sarcoidosis has hindered the ability to define the disease. It is still characterized in terms of its multisystem involvement, its clinical and radiographic appearance, and the presence of epithelioid-cell noncaseating granulomata on tissue biopsy.[94,96,174] Many patients with sarcoidosis develop symptomatic eye disease. In some patients ocular findings are the sole initial manifestation of the disease.[53,84] Regrettably, permanent vision loss as a result of ocular inflammation associated with sarcoidosis is much more common than is generally appreciated. An understanding of the systemic manifestations of sarcoidosis can help the ophthalmologist uncover clues that can lead to early diagnosis and to the initiation of proper treatment.[84a]

HISTORICAL BACKGROUND

In the late 1860s Jonathan Hutchinson, an English physician and ophthalmologist, and Carl William Boeck, a Norwegian dermatologist, independently described cutaneous lesions that possibly represented chronic cutaneous sarcoidosis.[131,175] In 1889 Bresnier described the raised violaceous lesions of the nose, ear lobe, and fingers as "lupus pernio," which 3 years later were demonstrated histopathologically to consist of epithelioid and giant cells.[95] Caesar Boeck (the nephew of Carl William) studied the clinical and histopathologic features of the disorder and introduced the term "sarkoid" to depict the sarcoma-like histologic appearance of the skin lesions.

The multisystem nature of the disorder was recognized by Schaumann in 1914 and Kuznitski and Bittorf in 1915.[48,175] Heerfordt, a Danish ophthalmologist, described the clinical association of uveitis and enlargement of the parotid glands accompanied by cranial nerve palsies, especially of the seventh cranial nerve. Schumacher in 1909 and Bering in 1910 depicted iritis in association with cutaneous lesions.[175]

EPIDEMIOLOGY

Sarcoidosis affects individuals of both sexes and of a wide variety of ages, races, and geographic locations. Epidemiologic data suggest considerable inconsistency in the prevalence of the disease among ethnic and racial groups. These data are imprecise, however, because of the variability in suveillance and diagnostic criteria from country to country.[16,82,180] In the United States most patients are between 20 and 40 years of age at the time of diagnosis, although children and the elderly may also be affected. Blacks outnumber whites by approximately 15 to 1. The age-adjusted annual incidence in blacks is 82 per 100,000. In U.S. whites, the prevalence is 8 per 100,000. Puerto Rican and Mexican Americans are more commonly affected than U.S. whites.

Outside the United States, the incidence is reported to peak bimodally from age 20 to 30 and age 50 to 60. In Europe most affected patients are white. The reported prevalence throughout the world varies markedly. The disease is rare in Spain (0.04 per 100,000) and Japan (0.2 per 100,000) and is much more common in the United Kingdom (20 per 100,000) and Sweden (64 per 100,000). Women outnumber men 2:1 in some studies, whereas the sex distribution is equal in others.[82,174,180] Little reliable information is available on mortality from sarcoidosis. The sarcoidosis-related mortality rate in a clinic population has been estimated to be between 0.5% and 5%.[16]

Cases of familial sarcoidosis and sarcoidosis in both monozygotic and dizygotic twins are well recognized and suggest genetic influences. Familial sarcoidosis occurs more frequently in monozygotic than in dizygotic twins, females, and maternal offspring. The disease has also been recorded in husband-wife pairs and in unrelated individuals living in close proximity. These later findings are probably best explained by an environmental factor. There is no consistent association with any HLA phenotype, although it has been suggested that HLA-B8 may be associated with early resolution of sarcoidosis.[16,182] HLA-B8 occurs frequently in patients with erythema nodosum,[16,70] and HLA-B27 phenotype occurs in Swedish patients with advanced sarcoidosis. Sarcoidosis has rarely been reported in HIV-infected patients.[4,127]

Epidemiologic studies have attempted to link sarcoidosis to various infectious, environmental, occupational, allergic, or dietary factors—some of which cause chronic granulomatous disease and may be difficult to distinguish clinically from sarcoidosis. No association has been conclusively proved.[16,82] The association, if any, between sarcoidosis and malignancy remains unclear.[18,191,202] There is new evidence, however, to suggest that sarcoidosis may be associated with *Mycobacterium tuberculosis*. Mycobacterial DNA was detected by the polymerase chain reaction technique in 10 of 20 patients with radiographic evidence consistent with sarcoidosis, negative cultures, and biopsy-proven noncaseating granulomata.[169] Mycobacterial rRNA hybridization detected from the spleens of 5 sarcoidosis patients using liquid phase DNA/RNA hybridization (with a DNA probe specific for the rRNA of *Mycobacterium tuberculosis*) was 4.8 times greater than that detected from the spleens of controls.[142]

Ocular Disease

There is a high rate of ocular involvement in patients with sarcoidosis. Depending on the demographic and diagnostic criteria, 25% to 75% of patients with known sarcoidosis have ocular involvement on examination.[157,180] Despite the presence of objective physical findings, many of these patients are visually asymptomatic. Among patients with ocular manifestations of sarcoidosis, most will have systemic evidence of the disease, although many will be asymptomatic except for the eyes. Sarcoidosis is diagnosed in a relatively small proportion of patients with uveitis. Retrospective studies indicate that 3.9% to 5.5% of patients with uveitis later develop biopsy-proven sarcoidosis (Table 59-1). In a large recent prospective study of patients with uveitis, 59 of 865 (or 7%) were found to have sarcoidosis proved by biopsy.[165] Of these patients, 15 (25%) were known to have sarcoidosis prior to the onset of uveitis. In the other 44 (75%), the diagnosis was established after the onset of the uveitis.[165] Black patients are more likely to have ocular manifestations of sarcoidosis than are white patients.[96,157]

CLINICAL FEATURES

The initial presentation of sarcoidosis may vary dramatically. The clinical course may be acute, subacute, or chronic and may affect virtually any single organ or combination of organs (Table 59-2). About 15% to 40% of patients with sarcoidosis initially have respiratory symptoms. A large proportion (12% to 35%) are asymptomatic at the time of diagnosis. Some patients (15% to 40%) have generalized complaints such as fever, malaise, or weight loss. A small proportion (5% to 10%) have other specific extrathoracic symptoms. Making a correct diagnosis of sarcoidosis when the disease affects uncommon sites or unusual combinations of organs continues to challenge clinicians.

Acute (or "subacute") disease develops over a few weeks and is associated with constitutional symptoms in 25% to 50% of patients. Lofgren syndrome and Heerfordt-Waldenstrom syndrome are two classic acute presentations of sarcoidosis. Lofgren syndrome consists of the acute onset of fever, erythema nodosum, bilateral hilar adenopathy, and (often) arthralgias. Heerfordt-Waldenstrom syndrome (uveoparotid fever) is the combination of fever, parotid enlargement, and uveitis. Seventh cranial nerve palsy with other neurologic involvement may be present. Acute symptoms may resolve with minimal residual damage or in some cases may progress to chronic sarcoidosis. In one large series,

TABLE 59-2 ORGAN INVOLVEMENT IN PATIENTS WITH SARCOIDOSIS

Organ	Involvement
Lungs	90%-94%
Lymph nodes	28%-73%
Skin	18%-32%
Eyes	21%-22%
Liver	21%
Spleen	10%-18%
Bones	14%
Salivary glands	6%
Heart	5%
Nervous system	5%
Joints	6%
Endocrine system	5%
Kidney	4.3%
Lacrimal gland	3%
Tonsil	2.4%
Breast	1%
Gastrointestinal tract	0.7%
Uterus	0.7%

Adapted from Maycock RL, Bertand P, Morrison CE et al.: Manifestations of sarcoidosis, *Am J Med* 35:67-89, 1963 and Siltzbach LE, James DG, Neville E et al.: Course and prognosis of sarcoidosis around the world, *Am J Med* 57:847-852, 1974.

TABLE 59-1 PATIENTS WITH UVEITIS: PROPORTION OF CASES ATTRIBUTED TO SARCOIDOSIS

Investigators	Number of Patients	Percentage Developing Uveitis
Karma et al[105]	7,970	5%
Perkins[158]	1,890	4%–5%
Henderly[76]	600	3.9%
Rosenbaum[162]	236	5.5%
Rothova[165]	865	7%

uveitis and parotid enlargement were both present in only 6 of 185 (3%) patients with ocular sarcoidosis.[39]

In 40% to 70% of patients, sarcoidosis develops insidiously over a period of months. These patients usually have respiratory complaints without constitutional symptoms. Patients with chronic sarcoidosis may develop permanent parenchymal destruction and protracted extrathoracic complications.

Nonocular Disease

Thorax. Thoracic manifestations of sarcoidosis are the hallmarks of the disease, and staging is based on radiologic assessment of both parenchymal and lymphatic involvement.[94,96,174,175] Bilateral hilar adenopathy (stage 1) is the most common presenting form of pulmonary sarcoidosis (Fig. 59-1). Hilar adenopathy, particularly in association with erythema nodosum, may be an acute and self-limited form of the disease.[175] Patients may also have pulmonary parenchymal involvement in association with hilar adenopathy (stage 2) or without hilar adenopathy (stage 3) (Fig. 59-2). Pulmonary fibrosis with bullae formation and bronchiectasis (stage 4) represents the end stage of the disorder and may lead to cor pulmonale (Fig. 59-3).

About 90% of patients will have symptoms of respiratory involvement in the course of their disease, although up to 20% will be asymptomatic at the time of diagnosis. About 33% to 50% of patients that have respiratory symptoms will develop permanent pulmonary abnormalities. These abnormalities include dyspnea (especially on exertion), dry cough, and chest pain. Dyspnea is usually caused by parenchymal disease, but sometimes results from granulomatous obstruction of upper airways. On physical examination, dry rales are occasionally heard in acute and subacute cases. Wheezing is less common. Hemoptysis may occur if there is hemorrhage from mycetoma in cavitary lesions. Productive cough and pleural effusions are rare. Pneumothorax may occasionally develop in patients with advanced fibrotic disease. The diagnosis and treatment of pulmonary sarcoidosis is discussed later in this chapter.

Skin. Erythema nodosum is the most common skin manifestation of sarcoidosis. These red, tender nodules appear on the anterior surface of both legs and occasionally on the buttocks and arms. Biopsy of these nodules reveals a septal panniculitis. The onset is usually sudden, and it is often accompanied by constitutional symptoms such as polyarthralgias, acute uveitis, and hilar adenopathy. The lesions are self-limited and do not usually recur. Erythema nodosum is not specific for sarcoidosis and can also be seen in infections, drug reactions, and other inflammatory disorders such as tuberculosis, inflammatory bowel disease, and lymphoma. Cutaneous granulomata may be maculopapular, raised, or nodular and are seen on the face, buttocks, and extremities (Fig. 59-4). Transient maculopapular or vesicular eruptions may coincide with acute uveal or parotid in-

volvement and usually resolve spontaneously. They are most common in black patients.[175]

Subcutaneous skin nodules are easily biopsied but are detectable only by palpation. They are present in about 5% of patients and are associated with acute forms of the dis-

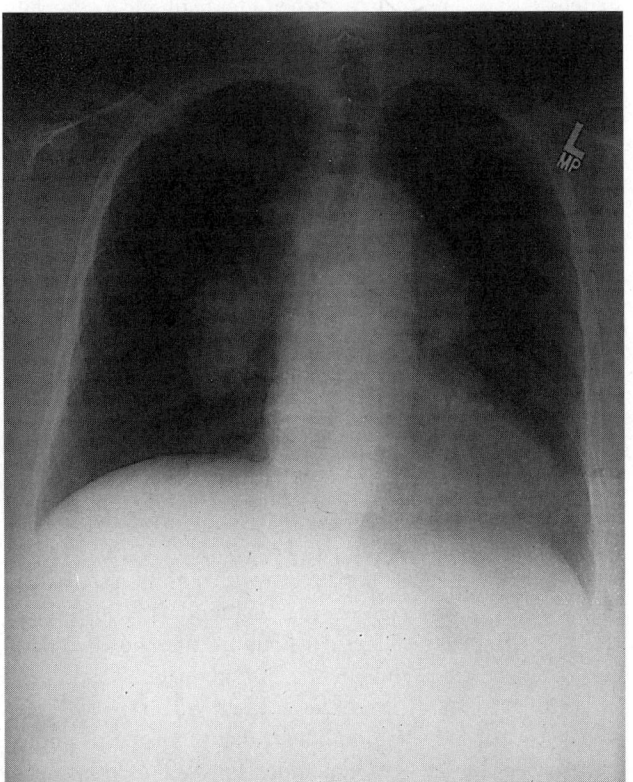

A

B

Fig. 59-1.   Chest x-ray **A,** and CT scan **B,** showing bilateral hilar, paratrachial and subcarinal lymphadenopathy in a patient with sarcoidosis. (Courtesy of Jo-Anne Shepard MD)

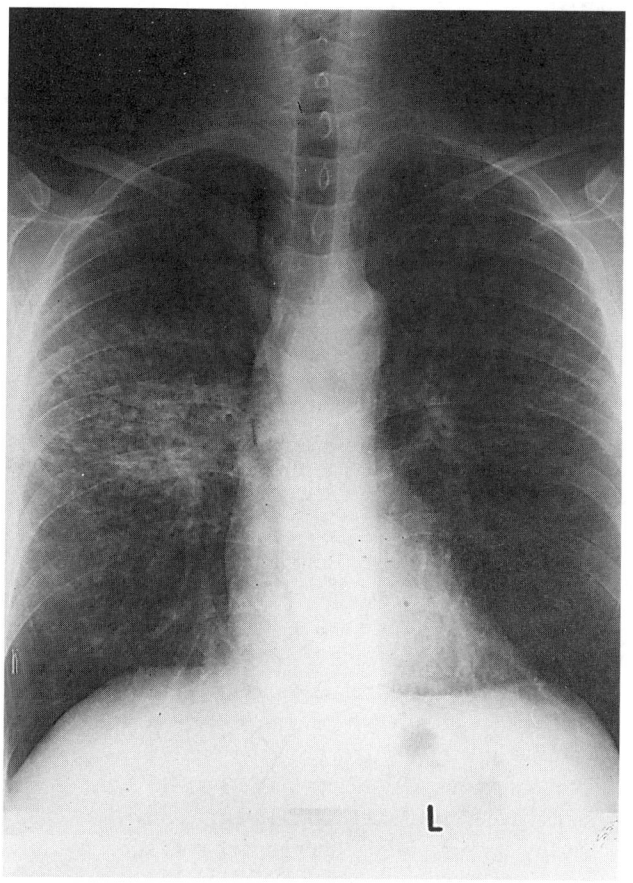

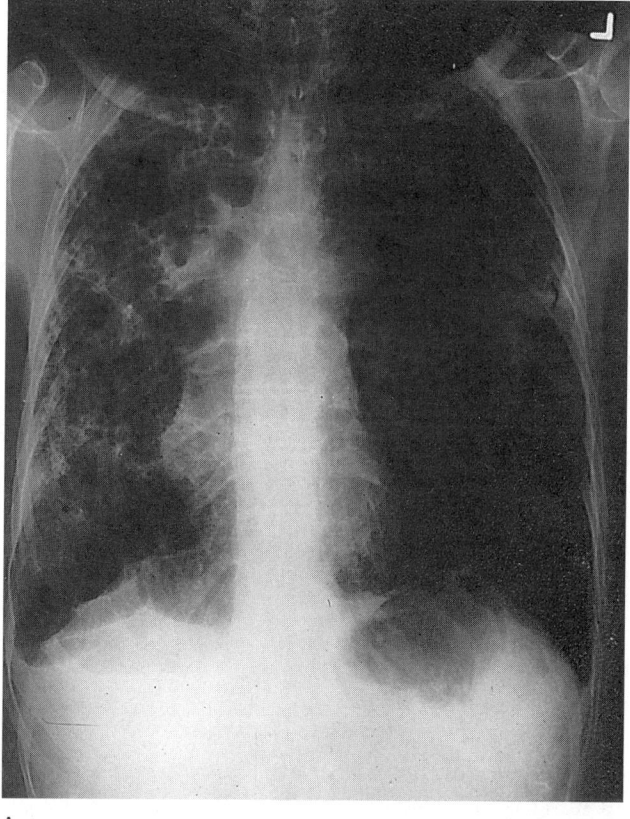

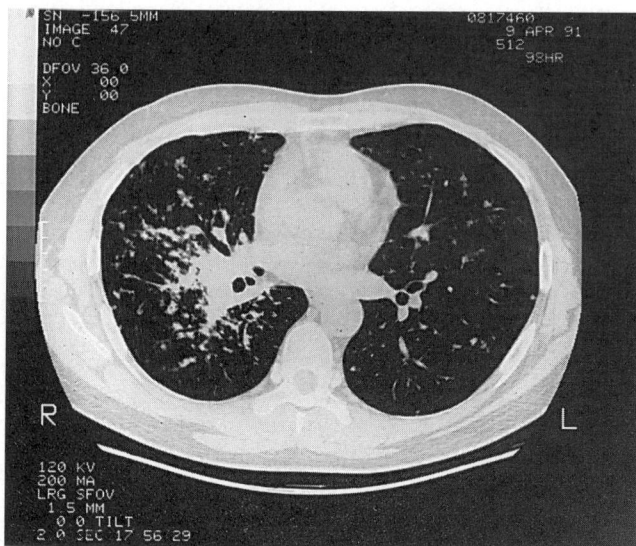

Fig. 59-2. Chest x-ray **A,** and CT scan **B,** showing bilateral retic-ular-nodular interstitial opacities in a patient with sarcoidosis. (Courtesy of Dr. Jo-Anne Shepard MD)

Fig. 59-3. Chest x-ray **A,** and CT scan **B,** showing end stage fibrosis, cystic changes, and volume loss in the upper lobes in a patient with sarcoidosis. (Courtesy of Jo-Anne Shepard MD)

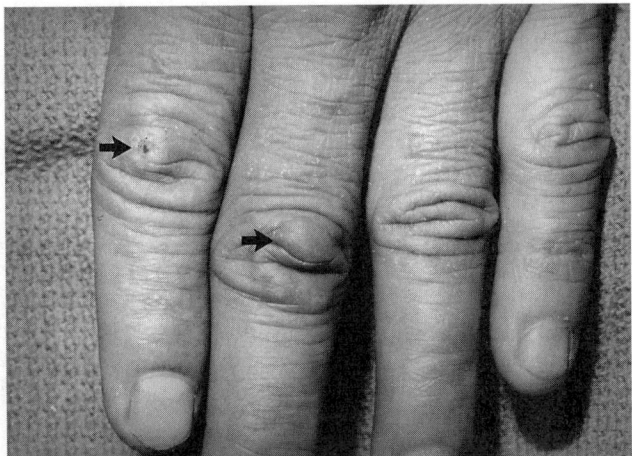

Fig. 59-4.   Subcutaneous nodules in a patient with sarcoidosis.

ease.[99] Cutaneous scars can suddenly become activated with granulomata coincident with disease elsewhere in the body. Lupus pernio (''purple lupus'') represents a classic cutaneous granulomatous manifestation specific for sarcoidosis. These chronic, indurated, blue-purple, shiny lesions occur on the nose, eyelids, cheeks, lips, ears, fingers, and knees. Resolved granulomatous skin lesions may produce hypopigmented macules, but with the exception of lupus pernio, scarring is uncommon.[205] Perforating sarcoid skin lesions are occasionally seen and may be confused with generalized perforating granuloma annulare.[172]

Lymph Nodes. Peripheral lymphadenopathy is usually bilateral and occurs in 75% of patients. Involved lymph nodes are usually firm, painless, and mobile. Cervical, axillary, epitrochlear, and inguinal lymphadenopathy occur in decreasing frequency. Gallium scanning allows detection of enlarged mesenteric and retroperitoneal lymph nodes not detectable clinically. Biopsy of palpable lymph nodes usually reveals granulomata. Massive peripheral lymphadenopathy may be disfiguring but rarely causes functional deficits.

Nervous System.* About 5% of patients with sarcoidosis develop neurologic manifestations.[65] At the onset of neurosarcoidosis, about 60% of patients have pulmonary involvement.[139] Cranial neuropathies develop in almost three quarters of patients with neurologic disease and may affect any of the cranial nerves. Many of these patients have multiple, bilateral, or recurrent cranial neuropathies. The facial nerve is the most commonly affected. The optic nerve is discussed under Ocular Disease. The third, fourth, or sixth cranial nerves may also be involved.[33,167] A sixth cranial nerve palsy may be associated with raised intracranial pressure or aseptic meningitis, or (rarely) it may be the sole manifestation of sarcoidosis.[170] Dyphagia and dysphonia are seen with involvement of the ninth and tenth cranial nerves.

---

*References 15, 32, 33, 41, 65, 74, 132, 159, 189.

Hearing loss may be caused by reversible neuropathy or a permanent vasculitic insult to the neuroepithelium.

Aseptic meningitis may be chronic and insidious. Isolated meningeal infiltration may masquerade as a meningioma. Intracranial hypertension, hydrocephalus, and hypothalamic dysfunction may occur.[28,73,139] Intracranial and intraspinal granulomata may produce space-occupying lesions with focal neurologic deficits.[27] Seizures and neuropsychiatric and personality disturbances may occur in as many as 20% of patients with neurosarcoidosis.[27,139] Peripheral mononeuropathies or polyneuropathies and, rarely, a Guillain-Barre type of polyradiculitis may occur. Neurosarcoidosis has a significant morbidity and mortality and should be promptly treated with systemic corticosteroids. Neurologic deterioration in corticosteroid-dependent patients with neurosarcoidosis should alert the clinician to the possibility of secondary infections.[159]

Musculoskeletal System. Bone involvement is seen in 5% of patients, almost always in conjunction with chronic sarcoidosis. It is rarely observed in the absence of skin or pulmonary involvement. Bone lesions are cystic and usually occur in the hands and feet. Osseous lesions in patients with sarcoidosis are usually lytic and involve the peripheral skeleton. Osteosclerosis, a less common presentation, is most often found in the axial skeleton.[71] Between 15% and 40% of patients have involvement of bone marrow; this involvement is usually asymptomatic, although it can occasionally cause hematologic abnormalities.[50,94,96,175] Bone density, as measured by vertebral cancellous mineral content, is normal in early untreated sarcoidosis but declines in many long-standing cases.[144] Osteoporosis is also potentiated by glucocorticoid therapy. These factors may lead to an increased risk of fractures in elderly sarcoidosis patients with or without corticosteroid therapy.

Although intramuscular granulomata are seen in most patients with sarcoidosis, they are usually asymptomatic. A painless, slowly progressive myopathy leading to weakness and wasting is the most common symptomatic form of muscular involvement. These patients have elevated muscle enzymes and an abnormal electromyogram. An acute painful myopathy or tender muscle nodules are less common.

Connective Tissues. Acute arthritis in sarcoidosis is usually symmetric and may involve the ankles, knees, elbows, wrists, and hands. It may be associated with fever, hilar lymphadenopathy, uveitis, and erythema nodosum. Joint symptoms remit, either spontaneously or with therapy. In chronic sarcoidosis synovial thickening, granulomata, and cystic changes may be demonstrated histologically.[51,94,96,175] Degenerative articular and subchondral bone changes may occur. Arthritis also develops in most children with sarcoidosis who are under the age of five years.[83,163]

Both sarcoidosis patients and those with autoimmune diseases may have keratoconjunctivitis sicca, weight loss, fever, lymphadenopathy, pulmonary complaints, and skin lesions.[50] Both groups may have elevated rheumatoid factor and antinuclear antibodies. Biopsy for pathologic confirmation may be required to distinguish them. New, unexplained symptoms in patients with sarcoidosis warrant careful investigation as sarcoidosis and other autoimmune disorders may occasionally coexist.[50]

Heart.[51,94,96,175] Cor pulmonale is a common finding in patients with severe pulmonary disease (including those with sarcoidosis) and is not caused by direct sarcoid infiltration. Clinically evident cardiac dysfunction caused by direct cardiac involvement is seen in 5% of patients with sarcoidosis. Serious conduction abnormalities include ventricular tachycardia, bundle branch and complete heart block, and sudden death. Other abnormalities include a myocardopathy, papillary muscle dysfunction, pericarditis, and pericardial effusion that can lead to congestive heart failure. The diagnosis is particularly difficult as a result of the frequent lack of involvement elsewhere in the body. Thallium perfusion scanning and endometrial biopsy may be useful in confirming the diagnosis. Patients with sarcoid myocarditis should be treated with systemic corticosteroids.

Kidneys. Renal insufficiency may develop secondary to granulomatous nephritis, hypercalcemia, or (more rarely) from renal glomerulonephritis or arteritis.[137] Hypercalcemia and hypercalcinuria are probably caused by elevated levels of 1,25-dihydroxy vitamin D and increased intestinal calcium reabsorption, which if left untreated, may result in nephrocalcinosis and nephrolithiasis.[94] Administration of systemic corticosteroids may lead to normalization of serum calcium and creatinine levels—at least early in the disease process.

Gastrointestinal System. Gastrointestinal sarcoidosis is uncommon but may display oral, esophageal, or gastric symptoms and may simulate peptic ulcer disease.[57,155] Small bowel sarcoidosis rarely simulates Crohn disease and is characterized by folate deficiency anemia.[129] Crohn disease and Whipple disease may be confused with sarcoidosis, but patients usually have a normal chest x-ray, angiotensin converting enzyme, and Kveim-Siltzbach reaction.[175] Sclerosing peritonitis with exudative ascites has also been described.[153] The liver is palpably enlarged in 20% of sarcoidosis patients, and hepatic granulomata are present in 60% to 90% of these patients. Although elevations of the alkaline phosphatase and bilirubin are common, patients are usually asymptomatic. The prevalence of splenomegaly is about 10% to 15%, with massive enlargement seen in only 3%.[53] When splenic biopsy is performed, granulomata are present in a majority of patients. Massive splenomegaly may be associated with pancytopenia, and although it is treated with corticosteroids, a splenectomy may be required.

Endocrine and Reproductive Systems. Endocrine abnormalities in patients with sarcoidosis may be caused by glandular infiltration. Involvement of the pituitary and hypothalamus may lead to diabetes insipidus, polydipsia, polyphagia, impotence, decreased libido, or amenorrhea.[28] Involvement of the pancreas, thyroid, and adrenals less commonly leads to hypofunction.[73] Isolated sarcoid infiltration of the male and female reproductive organs[147,168] is uncommon but may masquerade as a primary malignancy.[48a] Treatment with corticosteroids is indicated to preserve gonadal function. Nodular sarcoidosis of the breasts is rare, and carcinoma must be excluded by biopsy.[58] Infertility is rare, and pregnancy is usually not affected.

Head and Neck. Sarcoidosis of the upper respiratory tract affects 2% to 6% of patients.[26] Symptoms of nasal mucosal involvement include epistaxis, congestion, or discharge.[26] Dyspnea, stridor, or hoarseness may indicate upper airway or laryngeal involvement. Isolated sarcoidosis of the cervical nodes in association with hypercalcemia may simulate parathyroid adenoma by clinical, sonographic, and scintillographic criteria.[150] Parotid enlargement is usually bilateral and painless, and is seen in about 6% to 10% of patients.[174] Patients with salivary gland involvement may develop xerostomia. Asymptomatic parotid enlargement may be demonstrated by gallium-67 scanning in up to 75% of patients.

Sarcoidosis in Childhood. Sarcoidosis occurs less often in children than in adults.[79,199] There appear to be 2 distinct subsets of childhood sarcoidosis, one in patients 5 years of age or younger and another in older children (8 to 15 years of age).[81] Sarcoidosis in children younger than 5 years of age is characterized by eye, skin, and joint disease. It has also (less frequently) been characterized by lung involvement (33%) and has been designated childhood sarcoid arthritis (see the following). Sarcoidosis in older children resembles adult sarcoidosis but shows an increased incidence of lymphadenopathy, hepatomegaly, and splenomegaly.[81] Unlike adults, hilar and parenchymal disease (stage 2) is the most common presenting chest x-ray finding in pediatric sarcoidosis. Pediatric sarcoidosis is often self-limited, with resolution of active disease over 2 to 3 years. Chest x-ray abnormalities resolve in about 70% of patients. With long-term (> 20 year) follow-up, a minority will develop moderate-to-severe loss of lung function.[133] Overall, the prognosis for childhood sarcoidosis is better than for the adult disease.[6]

Ocular Disease

The ophthalmologist may be asked to evaluate patients with known or suspected sarcoidosis, or they may make the initial diagnosis based on the ocular findings. The ocular abnormalities reported in large retrospective series vary according to the demographic and diagnostic criteria employed. In general, uveitis (either anterior or posterior) and glaucoma are the most common vision-threatening manifestations of sarcoidosis. Conjunctival granulomata may be helpful diagnostically but do not contribute to the ocular morbidity associated with the disease. Lacrimal involvement is common and may lead to tear deficiency. Optic nerve involvement is relatively uncommon but may lead to substantial vision loss. Comprehensive reviews of ocular involvement in sarcoidosis are summarized in Table 59-3.

TABLE 59-3 PREVALENCE OF OCULAR FINDINGS IN PATIENTS WITH SARCOIDOSIS*

Investigator	Crick et al[39] N = 115	James et al[93] N = 542	Obenauf et al[157] N = 202	Jabs & Johns[88] N = 47	Karma et al[102] N = 79	Rothova et al[164] N = 50	Angi et al[6] N = 308	Quigley et al[160] N = 260
Uveitis								
Anterior	14%	66%	53%	70%	22%	28%	5%	21%
Anterior or posterior	66%	80%		74%	28%	58%		26%
Posterior	3%	14%	25%	28%	10%	30%		2%
Panuveitis	23%						0.3%	5%
Anterior segment								
Conjunctival involvement	31%	25%	7%	17%	47%	46%	17%	
Glaucoma	3%			23%	14%	12%		
Cataract		7%	8%	17%	14%	12%		
Posterior segment								
Chorioretinitis			11%	4%	6%		14%	
Periphlebitis or vasculitis	0%		10%	17%				5%
Retinal neovascularization			2%			4%		
Lacrimal system								
Keratoconjunctivitis sicca	42%	5%		11%	38%		18%	7%
Lacrimal disease				28%	51%	38%		32%
Lacrimal enlargement			16%	17%	8%			
Optic nerve disease		2%	7%	2%			0.3%	0.7%

Adapted from Hunter DG, Foster CS: Ocular manifestations of sarcoidosis. In Jakobiec F, Albert DM, editors: *Principles and Practice of Ophthalmology*, Philadelphia, 1994, WB Saunders.
* Space left blank if data not included or insufficient for calculation.

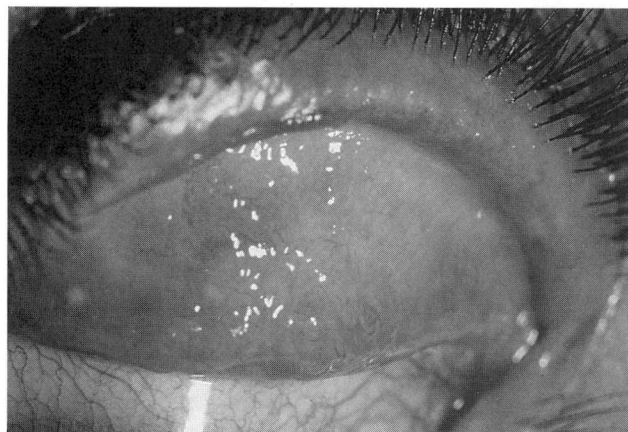

Fig. 59-5. Conjunctival nodules in a patient with sarcoidosis. (Figure also in color insert.)

Anterior Segment

Conjunctiva. Conjunctival nodules may occur and usually involve the fornix or palpebral conjunctiva (Fig. 59-5). Patients may be asymptomatic or complain of foreign body sensation. Biopsy of conjunctival nodules often reveals noncaseating granulomata, although granulomata may also be seen histologically in clinically unaffected areas. Cicatrizing conjunctivitis and symblepharon formation are rare and may partially respond to subconjunctival corticosteroids.[52,60] Keratoconjunctivitis sicca may result from granulomatous infiltration of the major and minor lacrimal glands.[88,103,164] Inferior corneal thickening is said to be the most common corneal finding in patients with sarcoidosis.[135] Scleritis is a rare manifestation of sarcoidosis.[93,203]

Uvea. Patients with acute anterior uveitis usually complain of blurred vision, pain, photophobia, or red eyes. On examination, there are conjunctival or perilimbal injection, pigmented ("granulomatous") keratic precipitates (Fig. 59-6), and aqueous cells and proteinaceous flare in the anterior chamber. There may be nodules on the iris surface, either at the pupillary margin (Koeppe nodules) or the iris surface

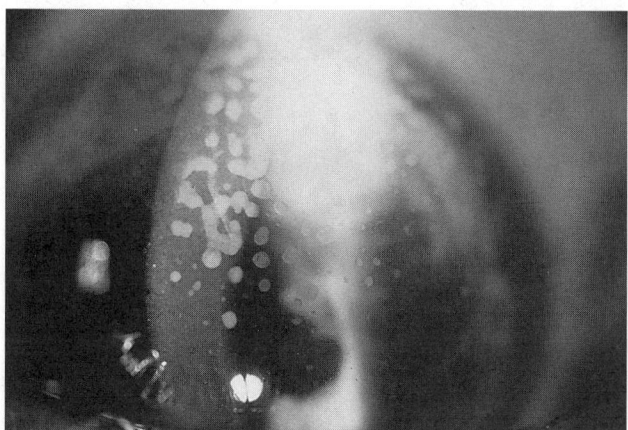

Fig. 59-6. Keratic precipitates in a patient with sarcoidosis-associated iridocyclitis.

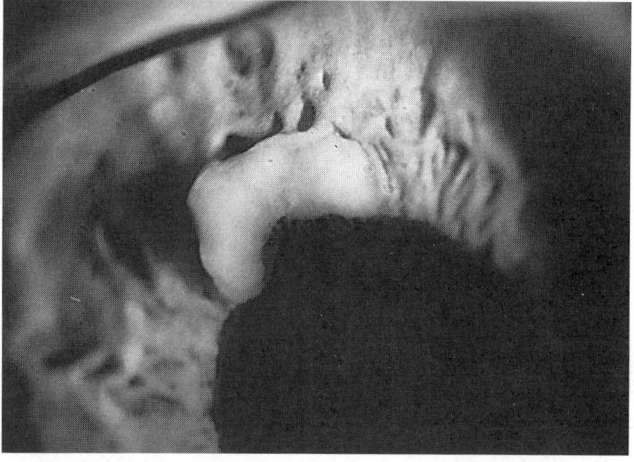

A

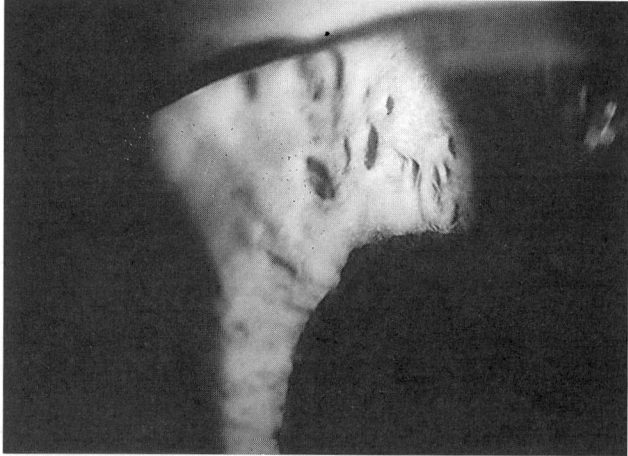

B

Fig. 59-7. Koeppe nodules in the eye of a patient with sarcoidosis seen before **A,** and after **B,** topical corticosteroid therapy.

(Busacca nodules) (Fig. 59-7). Posterior synechiae may also form (Fig. 59-8). Massive iris granulomata may lead to anterior synechiae and sector cataracts. One such lesion responded to subconjunctival corticosteroids.[130] Acute anterior uveitis may be associated with systemic features, such as erythema nodosum or bilateral hilar adenopathy, and may be self-limited.[88,91]

Chronic anterior uveitis is usually insidious in onset. Patients may have anterior synechiae, posterior synechiae (Fig. 59-8), or cataract in addition to keratic precipitates and aqueous cell and flare. Chronic anterior uveitis may be more common than acute uveitis in patients with sarcoidosis.[93,103,157] Some investigators claim that patients with uveitis and histologically confirmed sarcoidosis are most likely to have panuveitis.[45,76,185] Patients with panuveitis typically have posteror synechiae, retinal vasculitis, and macular edema.[45] Both acute and chronic anterior uveitis are treated with topical corticosteroids and cycloplegic agents. The frequency of corticosteroid therapy is determined by the sever-

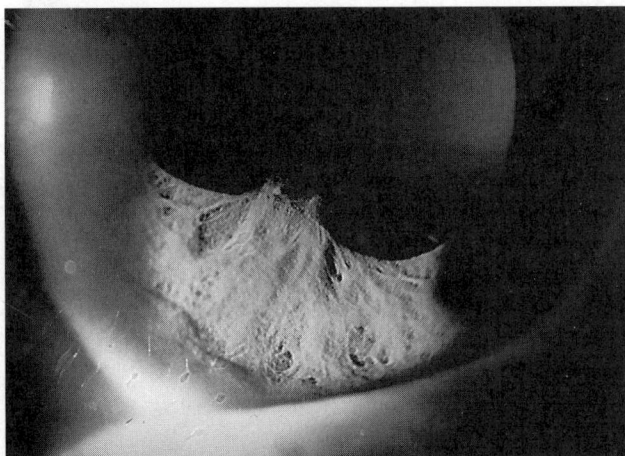

Fig. 59-8. Posterior synechiae in a patient with resolved sarcoid iridocyclitis.

ity of inflammation. Systemic corticosteroids may be required in particularly severe cases. Treatment is continued until the anterior chamber reaction has resolved, and therapy is then tapered. Recurrent bouts of inflammation are common.

Vitreous Humor. Cellular infiltration of the vitreous is a major manifestation of posterior segment involvement in sarcoidosis. These cells may be evenly dispersed within the vitreous gel or may aggregate into clumps ("snowballs") in the inferior vitreous. When these clumps occur in chains ("string of pearls"), they may cast a shadow on the retina.[118] Vitreous snowballs are characteristic, but not diagnostic, of sarcoidosis and may occur in a variety of other uveitic syndromes. Vitritis in patients with sarcoidosis may occur with or without focal pars plana, retinal, or choroidal lesions. Vitreous biopsy is not routinely performed but may reveal activated T-lymphocyte subsets suggestive of sarcoidosis. Low-grade vitritis, which is not visually symptomatic or associated with either cystoid macular edema or optic disc edema, may not require therapy but must be observed closely. Vitreous hemorrhage may occur from optic disc or retinal neovascularization. In these patients, panretinal photocoagulation and/or vitrectomy may be necessary.

Pars Plana. Anterior vitreous cells and pars plana exudation in patients with sarcoidosis may cause a clinical picture indistinguishable from idiopathic pars planitis syndrome.[66,220] Clinical signs of sarcoidosis may be seen at presentation or may be delayed by several years.[220] The indications for periocular or systemic corticosteroid treatment include elevated intraocular pressure, visually significant vitreous opacities, and cystoid macular or optic disc edema.

Posterior Segment. Posterior segment involvement in sarcoidosis occurs in 14% to 43% of patients and may be the only ocular manifestation of the disease.[36,119,157,185] Involvement of the fundus in sarcoidosis is thought to be associated with an increased risk of central nervous system involvement,[64,119,161,185] although this view has been disputed.[173]

Retina and Retinal Pigment Epithelium. Periphlebitis is the most common posterior pole fundus lesion seen in patients with sarcoidosis.[63,185] Rarely, periarteritis is observed. Acute periphlebitis may be accompanied by retinal hemorrhage and edema. Retinal pigment epithelial atrophy may later develop beneath these periphlebitic lesions.[185] Systemic corticosteroids may lead to substantial resolution of the periphlebitis, but some residual vascular sheathing may remain. Dilation and tortuosity of the retinal veins or frank retinal venous obstruction may occur,[58,112,173] and sometimes resolve, after corticosteroid treatment. Some uncommon but well recognized manifestations of sarcoidosis are the yellow perivenous exudates ("taches de bougie" or "candle wax drippings") usually associated with periphlebitis. They represent perivascular granulomatous tissue with associated exudation.[59,119] Intravitreous, preretinal, and intraretinal granulomata may also occur.[59] Subretinal pigment epithelial granulomata may clinically resemble Dalen-Fuchs nodules seen in sympathetic ophthalmia. Fluorescein angiography in patients with sarcoidosis may reveal retinal vascular staining[3,36,161] or more nonspecific diffuse staining with macular edema consistent with breakdown of the blood-ocular barrier. Retinal neovascularization may occur, usually with evidence of capillary dropout on fluorescein angiography.[47,185,188] Panretinal photocoagulation usually leads to regression of neovascularization.

Choroid. Solitary choroidal granulomata often have an overlying sensory retinal detachment and may exist without signs of anterior segment or vitreous inflammation[24,134,200] (Fig. 59-9). These lesions may simulate metastatic choroidal carcinoma and usually disappear or decrease in size after corticosteroid therapy.[24,134] Nevertheless, solid choroidal lesions in patients with known systemic sarcoidosis cannot be assumed to represent granulomata, as metastatic carcinoma has also been reported in this situation.[43a]

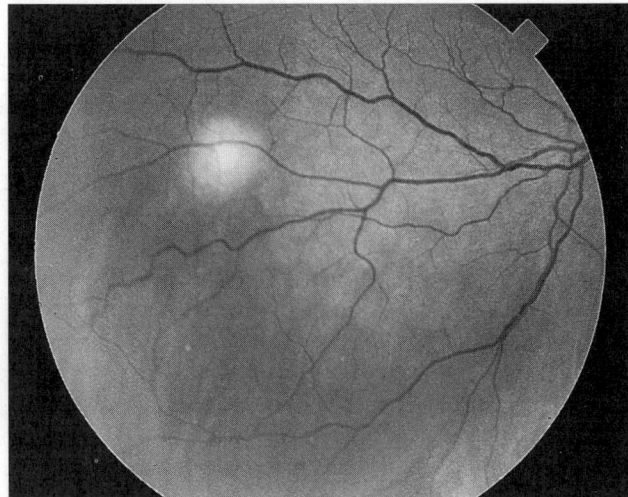

Fig. 59-9. Solitary choroidal granuloma in a patient with sarcoidosis.

central nervous system lesions. They may resolve spontaneously but should be treated with corticosteroids if vision is affected.[9] Optic atrophy is an unusual presenting sign but a common sequela of optic nerve involvement in patients with sarcoidosis.[205] Neovascularization of the optic disc may occur even without manifest capillary nonperfusion but must be differentiated from optociliary shunts, which have also been described.[132] Optic disc neovascularization may respond to corticosteroids or require panretinal photocoagulation.[46]

Orbit. The lacrimal gland is the orbital tissue most commonly involved in patients with sarcoidosis (Fig. 59-10).[157] Asymptomatic involvement can be demonstrated by gallium scanning, which indicates lacrimal gland involvement in 60% to 87% of patients with sarcoidosis.[39,88,103,212] Palpable bilateral enlargement is usually painless but may cause diminished basal and/or reflex tearing.

Involvement of other orbital structures by sarcoidosis is uncommon (Fig. 59-11).[89,138,157] An orbital inflammatory syndrome with variable features including proptosis, eyelid swelling, pain, decreased vision, and (occasionally) diplopia or ptosis has been described (Fig. 59-12).[111] Almost all patients with biopsy-proven orbital sarcoidosis have evidence of systemic sarcoidosis.[38] The orbital connective tissues may also become involved by contiguous spread from adjacent sinuses.[20] Direct involvement of the extraocular muscles and Tenon capsule may be characterized by focal subconjunctival thickening and erythema.[187] Orbital sarcoidosis lesions usually regress after treatment with corticosteroids, although spontaneous regression may occur.[111] Eyelid lesions include nodular elevations, papular eruptions, and (less commonly) lupus pernio. When these lesions are disfiguring, they may

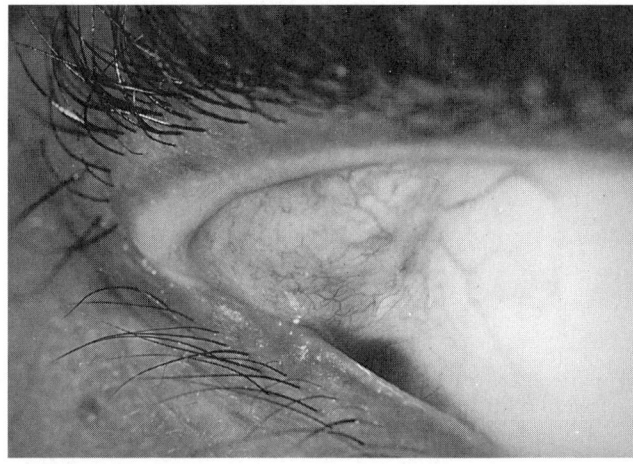

A

B

Fig. 59-10. **A,** Enlarged lacrimal gland in patient with sarcoidosis. **B,** Axial CT scan with soft tissue windows illustrating bilateral symmetric enlargement of both palpebral and orbital lobes of the lacrimal gland from another patient with sarcoidosis. (Courtesy of Jurij Bilyk MD and Peter A. D. Rubin MD)

Multiple flat depigmented choroidal lesions may simulate birdshot retinochoroidopathy,[19,115,185] acute multifocal placoid pigmentary retinopathy,[44] or multifocal choroiditis.[79] Peripapillary choroidal neovascularization has also been recorded.[64,161]

Optic Nerve. After the facial nerve, the optic nerve is the next most frequently involved cranial nerve in patients with sarcoidosis.[108] Optic nerve involvement may take many forms.[9] Optic disc edema may occur as a sole finding or may be associated with active posterior uveitis.[56,185] Optic disc swelling has also been associated with increased intracranial pressure or a granulomatous infiltration of the optic nerve or central nervous system.[216] Optic disc granulomata are a striking finding, and although uncommon, are characteristic of the disorder. These lesions are usually solitary and are sometimes associated with other posterior pole findings or

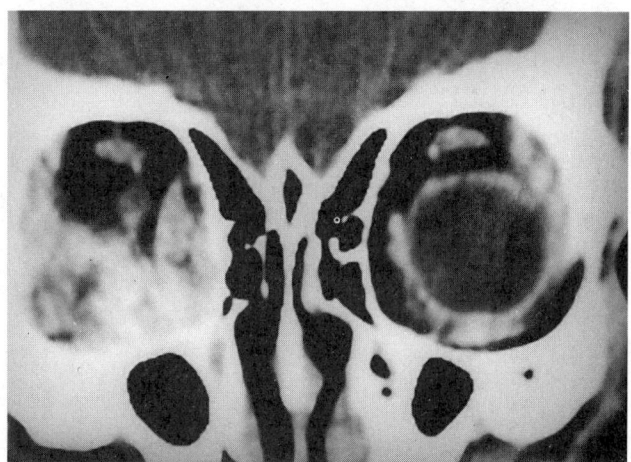

Fig. 59-11. Coronal CT scan of the orbit with soft tissue windows from a 16-year-old black male patient with bilateral hilar lymphadenopathy, elevated ACE, and diffuse, poorly circumscribed, opacification of the inferior orbit with involvement of the inferior and lateral rectus muscles presumed secondary to sarcoidosis. (Courtesy of John W. Shore MD)

TABLE 59-4 COMPARISON OF CLINICAL FEATURES IN PATIENTS WITH CHILDHOOD SARCOID ARTHRITIS AND JUVENILE RHEUMATOID ARTHRITIS

	Childhood Sarcoid Arthritis	Juvenile Rheumatoid Arthritis
Presence of uveitis	Majority (80%-90%)	Minority (10%-20%)
Location	Anterior (80%-90%)	Anterior (almost 100%)
Arthritis onset	Polyarticular	Pauciarticular
Rash	Usually present (77%)	Uncommon (1-6%)
Erythema nodosum	18%	Rare
Elevation of ANA	Uncommon	Usually elevated
Elevation of ACE	40%	Rare
Noncaseating granulomata	All	Rare

Adapted from Khan JA, Hoover DL, Giangiacomo J et al.: Orbital and childhood sarcoidosis, *J Ped Ophthalmol Strab* 23:190-194, 1983 and Hoover DL, Khan JA, Giangiacomo J: Pediatric ocular sarcoidosis, *Surv Ophthalmol* 30:215-228, 1986.

be treated with systemic or intralesional corticosteroids or antimalarials.[12,22,85] Sarcoidosis involving the lacrimal sac is rare. Obstruction of the nasolacrimal duct or lacrimal sac involvement[72] with noncaseating granulomata may lead to acute or chronic dacryocystitis,[37,72] which can recur after initially responding to antibiotics. The correct diagnosis is usually made at the time of dacryocystorhinostomy.[37,72,151]

Ocular Sarcoidosis in Children. Childhood sarcoid arthritis (CSA)—consisting of a granulomatous anterior uveitis, a characteristic polyarticular arthritis, and a rash—is usually seen in children aged 5 years or less.[163] Anterior uveitis occurs in 77% to 95% of cases, and posterior uveitis occurs in about 14%. The arthritis involves primarily the knees and wrists and consists of nontender effusions and synovial thickening. Erythema nodosum is frequently seen in CSA. Biopsy of the rash may be nonspecific or may show noncaseating granulomata. It may be misdiagnosed as juvenile rheumatoid arthritis (JRA), as both disorders share a high prevalence of arthritis and anterior uveitis (Table 59-4).[111,171] In JRA the arthritis is usually pauciarticular and a rash is relatively uncommon. In CSA the arthritis is predominantly polyarticular and a rash is present in about 75% of those afflicted.[111] Other differentiating features include a positive antinuclear antibody (ANA), which is present in

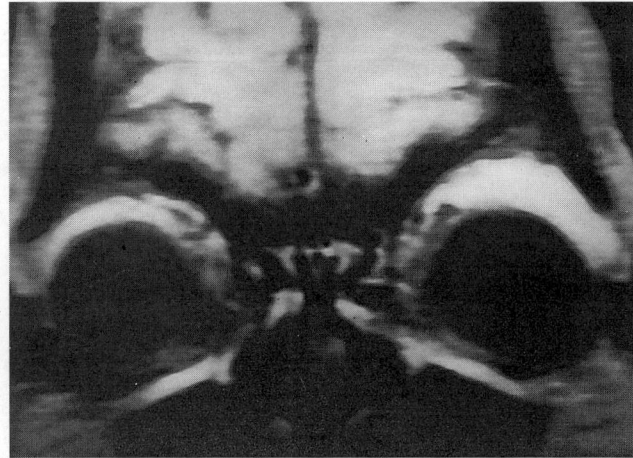

A   B

Fig. 59-12. **A,** Ptosis secondary to infiltration of the preaponeurotic fat pad caused by sarcoidosis. **B,** T1-weighted coronal magnetic resonance image with gadolinium shows enhancement in the area of the preaponeurotic fat pad. (Courtesy of Francis C. Sutula MD)

most patients with JRA but in very few with CSA. The angiotensin converting enzyme (ACE) is elevated in up to 40% of patients with CSA and rarely with JRA. The pattern of ocular involvement of older children with sarcoidosis is similar to that of adults.[62,80,106] Sequelae of chronic anterior uveitis in children include band keratopathy, anterior and posterior synechiae, cataract, glaucoma, and phthisis bulbi. Children with sarcoidosis may be visually asymptomatic, despite severe ocular disease, and require frequent ophthalmic examinations.

PATHOLOGY

The initial lesion of pulmonary sarcoidosis is an interstitial pneumonitis composed of lymphocytes, monocytes, and macrophages. The epithelioid granuloma, which develops following—or in conjunction with—the initial pneumonitis, is nevertheless considered the characteristic lesion of sarcoidosis.[84a,89,96,197,215] The granuloma is a cluster of closely packed epithelioid histiocytes, macrophages, and multinucleated giant cells[31] intermingled with—and surrounded by—a thin rim of lymphocytes, monocytes, and fibroblasts.[143] Epithelioid histiocytes are derived from monocytes that originate in the bone marrow. They contain abundant eosinophilic cytoplasm and vesicular nuclei. In mature granulomata, epithelioid cells may fuse, leading to the formation of (Langhans) giant cells. These cells have an eosinophilic granular cytoplasm surrounded by a ring of nuclei. The giant cells are active secretory cells that contain a syncytium of dense lysozyme granules.

Three types of inclusion bodies have been observed within the sarcoid granuloma.[23,84a,113] Schaumann (lamellated, conchoidal) bodies are calcium- and phosphorus-containing intracellular structures with concentrically arranged lamellae of basophilic mineral deposits.[113] Crystalline inclusions are birefringent, irregularly shaped, calcium carbonate crystals. Asteroid bodies are star-shaped structures predominantly composed of vimentin intermediate filaments and, to a lesser extent, microtubules.[23] They are found exclusively in multinucleated giant cells and possibly represent local aggregation of preexisting cytoskeletal components.[23] These inclusions are not diagnostic of sarcoidosis and may be seen in granulomata in other conditions.

T-helper cells and macrophage-derived cells are distributed in the center of the granuloma, whereas T-suppressor cells are more prevalent in the periphery.[175] Activated lymphocytes surround granulomata and are most numerous with newly formed granulomata. In the initial phases, the lymphocytes are primarily T-helper cells, although B-lymphocytes are also present. With maturation of the granuloma, the lymphocyte population diminishes and consists primarily of T-suppressor cells. Fibroblasts are seen at the periphery of these mature granulomata. Sarcoid granulomata are usually nonnecrotizing, but small areas of fibrinoid necrosis may develop. No histopathologic feature of a sarcoid granuloma allows it to be distinguished from granulomata of other causes. Stains and cultures for acid-fast bacilli and fungi should always be performed, and a search for foreign bodies helps to exclude other diseases. Granulomata may resolve without fibrotic changes or may undergo an obliterative fibrosis. Fibrotic granulomata in the lung are associated with interstitial fibrosis and may be seen in chronic sarcoidosis.[51,96] Vasculitis is seen in 42% to 67% of lung biopsies in patients with sarcoidosis, although it is rarely a prominent feature clinically.[199]

Ocular Disease

Noncaseating granulomata of the iris, ciliary body, retina, choroid, sclera, optic nerve, and extraocular muscles have all been demonstrated histopathologically.[38a,59,109] Vaso-occlusive disease with peripheral retinal neovascularization[6a] and choroidal neovascularization[55a] have also been recognized.

COMPLICATIONS

Chronic posterior uveitis and its sequelae are a major cause of ocular morbidity associated with sarcoidosis. Untreated or inadequately treated posterior uveitis may lead to macular and optic disc edema with subsequent atrophy.[185] Treatment with periorbital or systemic corticosteroids is generally required. Large areas of capillary nonperfusion may develop in eyes with chronic uveitis leading to optic nerve and retinal neovascularization, which sometimes result in vitreous hemorrhage and subsequent vision loss.[46,173,188] These new vessels may regress with corticosteroid therapy or may require photocoagulation.[112] Chronic uveitis with cataract and vitreous opacification may require pars plana lensectomy and vitrectomy. Other vision-threatening sequelae of chronic intraocular inflammation include band keratopathy and secondary angle closure glaucoma, which may eventually lead to phthisis bulbi.[135,157]

Glaucoma

Glaucoma is a major cause of permanent vision loss in patients with sarcoid uveitis.[88,157] A secondary open angle glaucoma may occur in acute or chronic sarcoid cyclitis or iridocyclitis.[21] Postulated mechanisms include increased aqueous production, decreased aqueous outflow, or trabecular meshwork dysfunction. In chronic iridocyclitis, secondary angle closure may result from peripheral anterior synechiae formation or from iris bombé (caused by posterior synechiae).

Uveitic glaucoma is initially treated with corticosteroids or other agents required to control active inflammation. Initial medical therapy of uveitic glaucoma includes topical beta-blockers and epinephrine. Miotics are relatively contraindicated. Laser trabeculoplasty and conventional filtering surgery are not generally effective. Uveitic glaucoma has been treated successfully in some patients with trabeculodialysis—a modified goniotomy procedure.[78,100,214] One such histologic specimen revealed a non-healed incision between the anterior chamber and the canal of Schlemm.[78] Filtering surgery with antimetabolites, cyclo-destructive procedures, or seton valve surgery may be required in some instances. Insidious and chronic elevation of intraocular pressure may lead to the formation of a perilimbal anterior staphyloma.[218]

PATHOGENESIS*

The harvesting and isolation of inflammatory cells using the technique of bronchoalveolar lavage (BAL) has changed the understanding of the immunologic cascade responsible for the formation of the sarcoid granuloma.[95] Rather than being a disease characterized by depressed immunity, sarcoidosis shows heightened cellular and humoral immunity that is at least partially limited to the sites of inflammation.[83]

The first step in this process in the lung is the development of inflammatory alveolitis. The (unknown) inciting agent of sarcoidosis induces alveolar macrophages to secrete interleukin-1 (IL-1), resulting in an increase in the accumulation and proliferation of T-helper cells (CD4+).[96,143] These T-helper cells release mediators, such as interleukin-2 (IL-2), leading to further clonal proliferation of T-lymphocytes and gamma interferon, which may activate alveolar macrophages. Chemotaxis and migration inhibition factors released by T-helper cells also lead to increased numbers of mature and immature newly formed macrophages that demonstrate increased expression of HLA-DR (class II) antigens. Interleukin-1, fibronectin, and other growth factors are secreted by macrophages and stimulate fibroblast activity. Gamma interferon also increases HLA-DR (class II) glycoprotein expression on resident ocular tissue cells that do not ordinarily express these molecules, resulting in amplification of the inflammatory response. Antibodies to various infectious agents may be produced and are thought to result from nonspecific polyclonal stimulation of B-lymphocytes by T-helper cells (CD4+) at the site of inflammation.

Immunohistopathologic study of an eye with active ocular sarcoidosis has demonstrated the presence of activated T-lymphocytes, macrophages, epithelioid cells, and lymphokine production.[30] Increased CD4/CD8 ratios have been reported in the aqueous humor and conjunctiva of patients with active sarcoid uveitis as well as in conjunctival sarcoid follicles.[6]

DIFFERENTIAL DIAGNOSIS

The differential diagnosis of pulmonary sarcoidosis in listed in the first box. The ocular differential diagnosis depends on the site of primary involvement in the eye. The differential diagnosis of anterior uveitis, posterior uveitis, or panuveitis associated with sarcoidosis is listed in the second box.

---

*References 5, 83, 91, 123, 143, 197, 211.

DIFFERENTIAL DIAGNOSIS OF PULMONARY SARCOIDOSIS
HYPERSENSITIVITY PNEUMONITIS
Diffuse idiopathic pulmonary fibrosis
Pneumoconiosis
Berylliosis
Asbestosis
Silicosis
INFECTIOUS PNEUMONIA
Tuberculosis
Histoplasmosis
Coccidioidomycosis
Cryptococcosis
Brucellosis
Pneumocystosis
DRUG REACTIONS[177]
Autoimmune disease[50]
Rheumatoid arthritis
Scleroderma
Systemic lupus erythematosis
Ankylosing spondylitis
LYMPHOMA AND LEUKEMIA

Modified from Sharma OP: Sarcoidosis, *Dis Mon* 36:469-535, 1990.

LABORATORY INVESTIGATIONS

The definitive diagnosis of sarcoidosis requires both a consistent clinical or radiologic appearance and histologic confirmation of noncaseating granulomata in association with negative bacterial and fungal studies in the biopsy specimen. Other tests, which are discussed in the following section, may support a clinical suspicion or may be useful in following the disease course.

Radiologic Studies

About 90% of patients with sarcoidosis have an abnormal chest x-ray at some time in the course of their disease.* Characteristic chest x-ray abnormalities are almost always bilateral and symmetric. In stage 0, the chest x-ray is normal, but there is evidence of extrathoracic disease. In stage I, the most common presenting form, there is bilateral bronchopulmonary, tracheobronchial, or paratracheal lymphadenopathy, which is characteristic (although not diagnostic) of sarcoidosis (Fig. 59-1). Unilateral anterior or posterior mediastinal lymphadenopathy is rare in patients with sarcoidosis and should suggest other diagnoses. Stage II is hilar lymphadenopathy with parenchymal infiltration, and stage III is pulmonary infiltration without hilar lymphadenopathy (Fig. 59-2). Parenchymal abnormalities may assume a re-

---

*References 51, 67, 94, 96, 175.

<table>
<tr><td colspan="1">DIFFERENTIAL DIAGNOSIS OF VARIOUS UVEITIC SYNDROMES ASSOCIATED WITH SARCOIDOSIS</td></tr>
</table>

ANTERIOR UVEITIS
Idiopathic iridocyclitis
HLA-B27-associated iridocyclitis
Juvenile rheumatoid arthritis
Fuchs uveitis syndrome
Herpes simplex virus-associated iridocyclitis
Herpes zoster virus-associated iridocyclitis
Ankylosing spondylitis
Intraocular lens-associated uveitis
Reiter syndrome
Syphilitic iridocyclitis
Tuberculous iridocyclitis
Inflammatory bowel disease
Glaucomatocyclitic crisis

POSTERIOR UVEITIS
Idiopathic
Toxoplasmosis
Toxocariasis
Histoplasmosis
Tuberculosis
Syphilis
Cytomegalovirus retinitis
HIV-associated disease
HTLV-1 associated disease
Birdshot retinochoroiditis
Serpiginous choroidopathy
Lupus retinitis
Acute retinal necrosis syndrome
Lymphoma/leukemia
Ocular candidiasis
Whipple disease

PANUVEITIS
Idiopathic
Vogt-Koyanagi-Harada syndrome
Behçet disease
Phacogenic
Sympathic ophthalmia
Brucellosis

Modified from Henderly DE, Genstler AJ, Smith RE and associates: Changing patterns of uveitis, *Am J Ophthalmol* 103:131-136,1987.

ticulonodular, alveolar, or nodular pattern. Parenchymal infiltrates that precede hilar lymphadenopathy or paratracheal lymphadenopathy in the absence of hilar lymphadenopathy also are less consistent with sarcoidosis. Stage IV represents end stage, irreversible pulmonary fibrosis (Fig. 59-3).

In East India, patients with sarcoidosis are more likely to demonstrate fibrotic changes on chest x-rays, possibly reflecting a longer time interval prior to diagnosis.[69a] Abnor-mal chest x-rays may normalize after treatment, particularly in children.[133]

Lytic bone lesions in patients with sarcoidosis may be demonstrated radiographically. Because bone involvement is primarily seen with chronic sarcoidosis, skeletal x-rays are not usually required to make the diagnosis.

Computed tomography (CT) scanning is useful in assessing the extent of mediastinal and hilar involvement. Magnetic resonance imaging (MRI) may also further delineate pulmonary lesions and may be particularly useful in detecting neurosarcoidosis lesions.[68,110] Gadolinium injection demonstrates lesions not visible on conventional T1 and T2 weighted spin-echo sequences.[49,221] Gadolinium-enhanced fat suppression MRI has documented isolated sarcoid lesions in the optic nerve without chiasmal involvement.[49]

Nonspecific Tests

Gallium Scan. After intravenous injection, gallium-67 citrate localizes to areas of active inflammation as well as to the liver, spleen, and bone. In sarcoidosis, gallium scanning may be more sensitive than chest x-ray in detecting pulmonary involvement.[149] It is not specific for sarcoidosis, however, because pulmonary uptake is increased in lymphoma, carcinoma, tuberculosis, silicosis, and most other conditions confused with sarcoidosis. Some features of the gallium scan may improve its specificity. In a recent study bilateral hilar uptake was very common (47%) in sarcoidosis but was not seen in lymphoma; whereas peripheral lymph node uptake was observed in only 5% of patients with sarcoidosis but was noted in 57% of patients with lymphoma.[2]

Gallium scanning can also be used to identify increased metabolic activity in lacrimal and parotid glands. Lacrimal gland uptake is increased in 60% to 87% of sarcoidosis patients and may be present even in the absence of other manifestations.[104,212] The distinctive appearance of lacrimal, parotid, and submandibular gland gallium uptake is known as the "Panda sign".[193] Disorders causing lacrimal gland inflammation such as Sjogren syndrome, orbital pseudotumor, and collagen vascular disease may also show increased lacrimal-gland uptake.

It has been suggested by some researchers that the results of gallium scanning correlate with disease activity, although this view is disputed.[96,98] Uptake of gallium is suppressed by corticosteroids. Gallium scintilography should not be performed in nursing mothers because gallium is excreted in human breast milk.[166] Gallium scanning has a role in the evaluation of patients with normal or equivocal chest x-rays and suspicious clinical findings. It can also be used to assess disease activity, choose a biopsy site, or follow a therapeutic response.[124] The diagnostic specificity of a positive gallium scan for the diagnosis of sarcoidosis is increased from 38% to 83% to close to 99% when combined with an elevated serum ACE level.[156,192] The combination of these two tests is a valuable part of the diagnostic evaluation of sarcoidosis.

Gallium Scan in Ocular Disease. Gallium uptake in the lacrimal and parotid glands is markedly increased in patients with newly diagnosed active sarcoidosis as compared with patients with chronic sarcoidosis and with controls.[104] Despite increased uptake, most of these patients are visually asymptomatic. The gallium scan showed increased lacrimal uptake in 19 of 24 patients with ocular sarcoidosis and in 7 of 18 with ocular disease but without sarcoidosis.[212] Provided other causes of increased gallium uptake are excluded, in patients with eye disease consistent with sarcoidosis and other equivocal findings, gallium scanning may identify lacrimal gland or subclinical pulmonary involvement or suggest a definitive candidate biopsy site.[208]

Angiotensin Converting Enzyme. ACE is a peptidyldipeptide hydrolase that cleaves the terminal dipeptide histidine-leucine from the C-terminus of angiotensin I, converting it to the vasopressor octapeptide angiotensin II. ACE is present in the luminal surface of vascular endothelial cells and in cells from the monocyte-macrophage system.[11] ACE levels vary according to age and sex and also depend on the method of determination.[11] In normal subjects serum ACE level is elevated in childhood but then remains relatively constant throughout life.[84a] In disease states elevation of ACE reflects the total body mass of ACE-producing granulomata.

In 1975 Lieberman[120] reported that serum ACE was elevated in sarcoidosis patients. The serum ACE was subsequently found to be elevated in 41% to 80% of patients with active sarcoidosis[121] and in a smaller percentage of patients with chronic, quiescent, or extrapulmonary disease. The serum ACE may be elevated in a variety of other diseases, some of which share clinical features with sarcoidosis (Table 59-5).

Corticosteroid treatment depresses ACE activity, and falsely low values are caused by ACE inhibitors.[122,190] Decreased ACE levels may be seen in patients with endothelial abnormalities (such as deep vein thrombosis) and after chemotherapy or radiation treatments.[11] The serum ACE may be normal in patients with acute sarcoidosis and erythema nodosum.[35] For these reasons, a normal serum ACE may not rule out sarcoidosis. ACE levels are more variable in children and are not as helpful in cases of possible childhood sarcoidosis.[81,190]

The specificity of the serum ACE is about 90% with a positive predictive value of 84% to 90%.[35,190] Although not 100% specific for sarcoidosis, the serum ACE is a valuable test when interpreted in the appropriate clinical context. There is controversy regarding the ability to follow disease activity with ACE levels.[96,190] Nevertheless, many investigators feel that serum ACE levels roughly correlate with disease activity. The combination of serum ACE and gallium scanning in a patient with suspected sarcoidosis can increase diagnostic specificity of both tests.[93,156]

ACE in Ocular Disease.[98,211] The differential diagnosis of elevated serum ACE levels in patients with uveitis is largely limited to sarcoidosis, leprosy, histoplasmosis, and

TABLE 59-5 ELEVATION OF SERUM ACE* IN CONDITIONS OTHER THAN SARCOIDOSIS

	Percentage of Patients with Elevated ACE Levels
Infectious	
Miliary tuberculosis	89%
Active tuberculosis	4%-7%
Treated tuberculosis	10%
Mycobacterium leprae infection	18%
Atypical mycobacterial infection	13%
Coccidioidomycosis	6%
Pneumocystis carinii pneumonia[181]	†
Occupational	
Asbestosis	19%
Berylliosis	12%
Silicosis	45%
Coal mining[198]	†
Inflammatory	
Allergic alveolitis	4%
Pulmonary fibrosis	5%
Primary biliary cirrhosis	20%
Neoplastic	
Hodgkin disease	6%
Lung carcinoma	1%-3.6%
Metabolic	
Gaucher disease	80%
Hyperthyroidism	62%
Diabetes mellitus	18%
Cirrhosis	11%-28%
Familial[77]	†

Modified from Studdy PR, Bird R: Serum angiotensin converting enzyme in sarcoidosis—its value in present clinical practice, *Ann Clin Biochem* 26:13-18, 1989, and Lieberman J: Elevation of serum angiotensin-converting-enzyme (ACE) level in sarcoidosis, *Am J Med* 59:365-372, 1975.
* ACE = angiotensin converting enzyme
† Association has been reported.

tuberculosis (Table 59-5).[7] Mean serum ACE levels are higher in a group of patients with granulomatous uveitis and systemic sarcoidosis than without systemic disease.[209] The ACE activity in the aqueous humor of patients with granulomatous uveitis and probable sarcoidosis may be significantly elevated.[210] Measuring the aqueous ACE may be beneficial in patients with granulomatous uveitis, equivocal laboratory and radiographic analyses, and normal serum ACE. For patients with uveitis and serum ACE levels above 50 units/liter, the sensitivity for detecting ocular sarcoidosis was 84%, specificity was 85%, and predictive value was 47%.[7] Tear ACE levels may also be elevated in patients with granulomatous uveitis and sarcoidosis.[178] Cerebrospinal fluid ACE is frequently elevated in patients with neurosarcoidosis.[32]

Lysozyme. Lysozyme is a low-molecular-weight enzyme produced by epithelioid and histiocytic cells, and levels are elevated in patients with sarcoidosis.[156] Serum lysozyme usually parallels ACE activity, but it is less specific than ACE. Serum lysozyme activity is also suppressed by corticosteroids. Unlike ACE, lysozyme levels are not elevated in children.

Lysozyme in Ocular Disease. Serum lysozyme levels may be elevated in patients with active sarcoidosis and uveitis.[206] This finding is not specific for sarcoidosis, as patients with acute or chronic idiopathic iritis may have serum lysozyme levels higher than patients with inactive or treated sarcoidosis.[206] In one study patients with uveitis had lysozyme levels above 8 mg/l that were 60% sensitive and 76% specific for sarcoidosis. The predictive value of the serum lysozyme test was only 12%.[7] The usefulness of this test would be increased if it were carried out only on patients with a high clinical suspicion of sarcoidosis. The combination of elevated serum lysozyme and ACE may carry a higher predictive value in diagnosing sarcoidosis than an elevated lysozyme alone.

Aqueous lysozyme levels are elevated in experimental uveitis in rabbits despite normal serum levels.[195] Tear lysozyme may be elevated in patients with sarcoidosis and keratoconjunctivitis sicca.[43]

Other Serum Markers. A variety of other biochemical markers of sarcoid activity such as beta-2-microglobulin, thermolysin-like serum metalloendopeptidase, transcobalamin, serum immunoglobulin, and urinary neopterin have been studied but do not appear to have any advantages over ACE assays.[114,117] Hyperglobulinemia and circulating immune complexes are produced in about 50% of patients with acute sarcoidosis.[175] Soluble mediators of inflammation (such as interleukin-2 receptors) in serum and other tissues are presently under investigation as indices of disease activity.

Elevation of the erythrocyte sedimentation rate (ESR), eosinophilia, and leukopenia are common, but not in a pattern or frequency to be diagnostic. Anemia is relatively uncommon.[175] Hypercalcemia is found in 9% to 24% of patients with sarcoidosis.[136] Hypercalcemia tends to be episodic in patients with acute sarcoidosis and persistent in patients with chronic sarcoidosis. Hypercalcemia is probably the result of increased production of 1,25-dihydroxy vitamin D by macrophages within granulomata, which increases intestinal calcium absorption.[1b] Hypercalciuria occurs in 15% to 60% of patients, and if severe, may lead to nephrolithiasis and nephrocalcinosis. Hypercalcemia may be treated with corticosteroids or chloroquine.[1a,175] Oral ketoconazole was successfully used to treat hypercalcemia in a patient who refused a second course of corticosteroids.[13]

HLA Typing. HLA-B8 has been associated with acute arthritis,[92] anterior uveitis, erythema nodosum,[70] and spontaneous remission of the disease.[182] HLA-B13 is associated with chronic sarcoidosis,[17] and lack of HLA-BW15 is associated with increased risk of disease.[1c] HLA-B8 and DR3 have been connected with neurosarcoidosis.[139] No HLA association was reported in black patients with ocular sarcoidosis from North Carolina.[141] HLA testing is not currently performed in the management of sarcoidosis patients.

Skin Tests

Cutaneous anergy to such antigens as *Candida* sp., mumps, and *Trichophyton* sp. is present in approximately 50% of patients with sarcoidosis but is not diagnostic of the disorder. Tuberculin skin tests should be performed and are usually negative.[136] Although a patient with sarcoidosis has impaired cutaneous delayed type hypersensitivity reaction, this patient does not have altered susceptibility to infection.

The Kveim-Siltzbach Reaction. In 1935 Williams and Nickerson discovered that intradermal injection of a sarcoid tissue suspension into the skin of sarcoidosis patients resulted in the development of red papules. Kveim demonstrated that these papules contained sarcoid granulomata.[51,67,94,96,175] In the Kveim-Siltzbach reaction (as it is now termed), a sterile particulate suspension of spleen from a sarcoidosis patient (K-S antigen) is injected intracutaneously into a patient with suspected sarcoidosis. In patients with a positive test, a nodule forms 2 to 6 weeks after injection. The skin lesion is biopsied and in a positive test, T-helper lymphocytes, monocytes, macrophages, and noncaseating epithelioid granulomata are seen. The mechanism of the Kveim-Siltzbach reaction is unknown, but chemical fractionation of the active agent may diminish granulocyte-generating activity.[128] The Kveim test is positive in about 80% of patients with clinically obvious sarcoidosis, and false positive Kveim tests are seen in 0.7% to 2% of healthy controls.[51,67,146] The incidence of a positive Kveim test declines to between 25% and 50% in patients with extrathoracic sarcoidosis and a normal chest x-ray. A positive Kveim test has been reported in a patient with AIDS and in another with asymptomatic HIV infection.[4] Drawbacks of this test include unavailability of the antigen, lack of standardization, delay in the time to diagnosis, and the inability to administer corticosteroids in the interim. In the United States the Kveim test is almost never performed. Recently a skin test prepared from autologous bronchoalveolar lavage cells was positive for granulomata in 41% of patients with a positive Kveim test.

Pulmonary Function Tests*

Spirometry and carbon monoxide diffusion capacity may be normal in the face of radiographic findings or abnormal even before abnormalities are apparent on chest x-ray. Early abnormalities seen in sarcoidosis patients are decreased lung volumes and diffusing capacity,[176] but later, patients may

---

*References 51, 67, 94, 96, 175.

develop restrictive changes. Occasionally, patients may have findings consistent with airway obstruction or bronchial hyperreactivity. Pulmonary function tests are useful for characterizing the extent of pulmonary involvement before, during, and after therapy.

Bronchoalveolar Lavage

In bronchoalveolar lavage (BAL), normal saline is instilled into a distal airway via a fiberoptic bronchoscope and is then recovered by suction. Normal bronchoalveolar lavage fluid contains 90% alveolar macrophages and 10% lymphocytes, with less than 1% neutrophils. Sarcoidosis patients have a relative lymphocytosis of the bronchoalveolar lavage fluid with an increased number of activated T-helper cells.[40] A high lymphocyte count is not specific for sarcoidosis and can also be seen in patients with lymphoma, tuberculosis, hypersensitivity pneumonitis, metastatic lung disease, and other conditions. An increase in bronchoalveolar lavage CD4/CD8 ratio may be more useful than T-lymphocyte count alone in predicting the subsequent clinical course.[67] The roles of non-T-lymphocyte and noncellular elements of the BAL fluid are under intensive investigation.[114] Although it is performed in a large number of centers, the role of bronchoalveolar lavage in routine clinical practice is not yet established. It has been suggested that the results of BAL fluid analysis are useful in monitoring disease activity and progression, and response to treatment.[51]

Tissue Diagnosis

The definitive diagnosis of sarcoidosis requires histologic confirmation of noncaseating granulomata in the absence of other causes of granulomatous inflammation. In general, suspicious cutaneous sites, enlarged peripheral lymph nodes, or other accessible clinically involved sites such as the conjunctiva, lacrimal glands, or salivary glands should be biopsied.[152,207,211] Otherwise, transbronchial biopsy or mediastinoscopy is usually performed. The positive yield of transbronchial biopsy is about 90% in patients with radiologic evidence of parenchymal disease and 50% to 60% in those without x-ray findings.[51] Step sectioning of transbronchial biopsies increases the diagnostic yield.[194] Although thoracotomy and open-lung biopsy give the highest yields of sarcoid granulomata, they are rarely necessary.

Ocular Tissue Diagnosis of Sarcoidosis. Patients with suspected sarcoidosis are often referred to the ophthalmologist for assessment of ocular findings and assistance in confirming the diagnosis. Among ocular tissues affected by this disorder, the conjunctiva and lacrimal gland are the most accessible and most likely to be affected.[211] Biopsy of these tissues can sometimes obviate the need for other more invasive procedures.

Conjunctival Biopsy. Conjunctival biopsy is an easily performed diagnostic test that may be helpful in the diagnosis of sarcoidosis.[140] In patients with biopsy-proven sarcoid-

osis elsewhere, the positive yield of conjunctival biopsies varies from 20% to 71%.[39,101,111,154,184] Technical factors such as the number of biopsies, serial sectioning, and length of tissue submitted may affect the yield substantially. Eyes with conjunctival follicles or other ocular abnormalities are most likely to have a positive biopsy. There is little reason to perform a conjunctival biopsy in patients with biopsy-proven sarcoidosis elsewhere. There is controversy about the efficacy of random biopsies of clinically uninvolved conjunctiva in confirming the diagnosis in patients with presumptive clinical sarcoidosis. The incidence of a positive random conjunctival biopsy in these patients ranges from only about 10% to about 31%, depending on the study.[39,101,184] The relatively low yield of this procedure must be weighed against the possibility of obviating a more invasive clinical procedure.[101]

An increased ratio of T-helper to T-suppressor cells, macrophages, and HLA-DR positivity was seen by immunohistopathologic study of conjunctival biopsies from sarcoidosis patients. The number of immunocompetent cells in the conjunctiva declines in chronic disease.[105]

Lacrimal Gland Biopsy. Biopsy of the lacrimal gland is a relatively simple outpatient procedure that can confirm a tissue diagnosis of sarcoidosis. It may be performed using either a transconjunctival or eyelid-crease approach. Transconjunctival biopsy of the palpebral lobe has the potential for injuring the lacrimal gland ductules, thus leading to a dry eye syndrome. This is a particular concern in patients with sarcoidosis who have an increased incidence of keratoconjunctivitis sicca. Modification of the transconjunctival technique to minimize the risk of dry eye has been described.[211] Lacrimal biopsy through a lid-crease incision provides superior hemostasis and may allow for a larger specimen. Patients with clinically enlarged lacrimal glands or increased uptake on gallium scan are candidates for this procedure.

Chorioretinal Biopsy. This diagnostic modality has a potential role in the characterization of choroidal and chorioretinal inflammations that eludes diagnosis by other less invasive means.[134a]

THERAPY

In sarcoidosis the decision to treat must be an individualized one that depends on the potential for life-threatening or permanent structural damage to the involved organ and on patient symptoms.[8]

Corticosteroids

Sarcoidosis is very responsive to administration of systemic corticosteroids, which is the primary therapy in sarcoidosis, when treatment is indicated.[149] Asymptomatic patients with isolated hilar lymphadenopathy (stage 1) and normal pulmonary function tests do not generally require treatment, but must be followed serially. Patients with stage 2 to 4 disease and symptomatic or progressive pulmonary disease (or other organ-threatening disease) receive moderate- (½ mg/kg) to high-dosage (1 mg/kg) oral prednisone, which is continued until a clinical response is observed (usually by 2 to 4 weeks). After a period of months, the dosage is slowly tapered over many weeks to months until the lowest maintenance dosage that controls the disease is attained. Reactivation is common and usually requires increasing the dosage. Therapy may be required for years. Lack of improvement after 6 weeks suggests the possibility of pulmonary fibrosis, and therapy should be discontinued. Inhaled corticosteroids are generally not effective but may cause symptomatic improvement in pulmonary disease.

The most common indication for corticosteroid therapy of eye disease is for the treatment of uveitis. Patients with mild anterior uveitis are treated with topical corticosteroids and cycloplegics, but may require periorbital or systemic corticosteroids if the uveitis is not responsive. Intermediate and posterior uveitis, which is unilateral or asymmetric, may be initially treated with periocular corticosteroid preparations, but systemic corticosteroids are usually required if there is bilateral or sight-threatening disease. Systemic chemotherapy may occasionally be required in patients with severe complications of corticosteroid therapy.[55,75]

Cytotoxic and Chemotherapeutic Agents[75]

Chronic corticosteroid treatment may produce disabling side effects that require tapering or discontinuation of the drugs. In such situations and when corticosteroids are ineffective, the addition of other immunosuppressive drugs may be necessary.[148] The use of immunosuppressive agents in patients with sarcoidosis is generally based on uncontrolled studies. With all such agents the white cell, granulocyte, and platelet count must be monitored closely and kept within appropriate parameters.

Patients with acute exudative sarcoid skin lesions not responsive to corticosteroids have been treated successfully with oxyphenylbutazone or thymopoietin pentapeptide (TP5).[90,196] Chronic fibrotic sarcoidosis not responsive to corticosteroids is usually treated with courses of chloroquine or hydroxychloroquine.[97,145] Therapy with either agent requires regular ophthalmologic consultation to minimize the risk of retinal toxicity.[219] Methotrexate has been used successfully to treat skin lesions refractory to chloroquine and/or corticosteroids.[116,205a] Oral methotrexate for refractory pulmonary sarcoidosis allows reduction of corticosteroid dose and is correlated with improved pulmonary function tests.[125,126,201] Methotrexate has also been used with some success in patients with refractory neurosarcoidosis.[183]

Chlorambucil has also been used with variable success to treat patients unresponsive to—or intolerant of—systemic corticosteroids.[87,107] Prolonged therapy in reduced dosage is required to prevent relapse.[87] Both chlorambucil and azathioprine have been used to treat patients with severe neurosarcoidosis unresponsive to corticosteroids and radiotherapy.[61]

Corticosteroid-resistant or corticosteroid-intolerant, sight-threatening ocular sarcoidosis has been treated successfully with azathioprine.*

Cyclosporine is useful in some patients with either refractory pulmonary sarcoidosis,[217] neurosarcoidosis,[14,41] or sight-threatening ocular disease, who have failed other immunosuppressive therapy.[204] Nephrotoxicity is the most serious adverse effect of systemic cyclosporine use and is more frequent at higher dosages (10 mg/kg/day). Lower-dosage (2 to 5 mg/kg/day) therapy may limit this toxicity. Three patients with sarcoidosis of the anterior visual pathways were successfully treated with low-dosage cyclosporine.[14] Corticosteroid-resistant or corticosteroid-intolerant sight-threatening ocular sarcoidosis has been treated successfully with low-dosage (2 to 5 mg/kg/day) cyclosporine.†

Radiation

Central nervous system sarcoidosis, which is unresponsive to high-dosage corticosteroid therapy, may respond to irradiation. A wide variety of dosages (1000 to 4500 rads) have been used.[10,61,69] Patients with parenchymal, meningeal, and optic nerve involvement have all been treated with at least temporary success.

PROGNOSIS

Most patients with sarcoidosis in a given population are asymptomatic. Of symptomatic patients with known sarcoidosis, two thirds will improve substantially or be cured within 2 to 3 years. In those in whom the disease persists, disease activity may continue for long periods of time. A minority of patients in this subgroup eventually develop fatal complications such as generalized pulmonary insufficiency, cor pulmonale, renal failure, cardiac arrest (from myocardial involvement), or massive hemoptysis caused by bronchiectasis or aspergilloma. The prognosis is influenced by the extent of pulmonary involvement at the time of diagnosis and the extent of extrapulmonary involvement. Patients with hilar adenopathy alone (stage 1), have the best prognosis, and those with evidence of pulmonary fibrosis (stage 3) have the worst. Patients with hilar adenopathy and parenchymal involvement have an intermediate prognosis but may respond to corticosteroids. The prognosis is worse in blacks who may have an increased prevalence of chronic persistent disease.

The clinical course of ocular sarcoidosis is variable, and the prognosis depends in part on the ocular structures involved. In general, patients with chronic uveitis who remain untreated or inadequately treated are at risk for developing synechiae, cataracts, and optic disc or macular edema.

*Unpublished data.
†Unpublished data.

Sarcoidosis is an idiopathic multisystem disorder that has ophthalmic manifestations in about one third to one half of patients. Patients frequently develop acute or subacute anterior uveitis, posterior uveitis, or panuveitis, which is often associated with vasculitis. Other manifestations are conjunctival and iris nodules, vitreous snowballs, and retinal, choroidal, and optic nerve granulomata. The systemic manifestations of sarcoidosis often provide the ophthalmologist with a clue to the presence of the disease. Typical symptoms include fever, malaise, weakness, weight loss, dry cough, chest pain, or dyspnea. In patients in whom the diagnosis is suspected, physical examination should include auscultation of the lungs, examination of the skin, and a search for peripheral lymphadenopathy. Initial laboratory investigation should include a chest x-ray and a serum ACE determination. Skin tests for anergy should be performed. A gallium scan of the head and chest may be helpful. Biopsy of suspicious and clinically accessible lesions should be performed. Serum lysozyme and immunoelectrophoresis, serum and urine calcium levels, and liver function tests are adjunctive tests that are not performed routinely.

Although the definitive diagnosis of sarcoidosis requires histologic confirmation, patients with characteristic findings on chest x-ray, elevated ACE levels or abnormal gallium scan findings and mild disease who do not require corticosteroids, are sometimes followed without biopsy. If the eye or any other organ system is threatened, or if systemic corticosteroid therapy is to be instituted, tissue diagnosis should be obtained. Conjunctival, minor salivary gland, or lacrimal gland biopsies are sometimes useful. If diagnostic confirmation remains elusive, bronchoscopy with transbronchial biopsy should be performed. Corticosteroids remain the mainstay of therapy, but in patients with intolerable side effects or in those in whom corticosteroids are ineffective, other immunosuppressive agents may be required.

REFERENCES

1a. Adams J, Diz MM, Sharma OP: Effective reduction in the serum 1,25-dihydroxy-vitamin D and calcium concentration in sarcoidosis associated hypercalcemia with short course chloroquine therapy, *Ann Intern Med* 111:437-438, 1989.

1b. Adams JS, Sharma OP, Gacad MA, Singer FR: Metabolism of 25-hydroxyvitamin D3 by cultured pulmonary alveolar macrophages in sarcoidosis, *J Clin Invest* 72:1856-1860, 1983.

1c. Al-Arif L, Goldstein RA, Affronti LF et al.: *HLA antigens in sarcoidosis in North American black population.* In Williams W, Davis B, editors: Proceedings of the 8th International Conference on Sarcoidosis and other Granulomatous Diseases, 206-211, Cardiff, 1980, Alpha Omega.

2. Albertine KH, Park CH, Patrick H: Whole body gallium 67 scans: role in diagnosis of sarcoidosis, *Am Rev Respir Dis* 144:1182-1186, 1991.

3. Algvere P: Fluorescein studies of retinal vasculitis, *Acta Ophthalmol* 48:1129-1139, 1970.

4. Amin DM, Sperber K, Brown LK et al.: Positive Kveim test in patients with coexisting sarcoidosis and human immunodeficency virus infection, *Chest* 101:1454-1456, 1992.

5. Angi MR, Forattini F, Chilosi M et al.: Immunopathology of sarcoidosis, *Int Ophthalmol* 14:1-11, 1990.

6. Angi MR, Forattini F, Cipriani A et al.: Ophthalmic changes in sarcoidosis: a prospective study of 308 patients. In Grassi C, Rizzato G, Pozzi E, editors: *Sarcoidosis and other granulomatous disorders,* Proceedings of the XI World Congress, 493-497, Amsterdam, 1988, Experta Medica.

6a. Asdourian GK, Goldberg MF, Busse BJ: Peripheral retinal neovascularization in sarcoidosis, *Arch Ophthalmol* 93:787-791, 1975.

7. Baarsma GS, La Hey E, Glasius E et al.: The predictive value of serum angiotensin converting enzyme and lysozyme levels in the diagnosis of ocular sarcoidosis, *Am J Ophthalmol* 104:211-217, 1987.

8. Bascom R, Johns CJ: The natural history and management of sarcoidosis, *Adv Intern Med* 31:213-241, 1986.

9. Beardsley TL, Brown SWL, Snydnor CF et al.: Eleven cases of sarcoidosis of the optic nerve, *Am J Ophthalmol* 97:62-77, 1984.

10. Bejar JM, Kerby GR, Ziegler DK et al.: Treatment of central nervous system sarcoidosis with radiotherapy, *Ann Neurol* 18:258, 1985.

11. Beneteau-Burnat B, Baudin B: Angiotensin converting enzyme: clinical applications and laboratory investigations on serum and other biological fluids, *Crit Rev Clin Lab Sci* 28:337-356, 1991.

12. Bersani TA, Nichols CW: Intralesional triamcinolone for cutaneous palpebral sarcoidosis, *Am J Ophthalmol* 99:561-562, 1985.

13. Bia MJ, Insogna K: Treatment of sarcoidosis-associated hypercalcemia with ketoconazole, *Am J Kidney Dis* 18:702-705, 1991.

13a. Bielory L, Frohman LP: Low-dose cyclosporine therapy of granulomatous optic neuropathy and orbitopathy, *Ophthalmology* 98:1732-1736, 1991.

14. Bielory L, Holland C, Gascon P et al.: Uveitis, cutaneous and neurosarcoid: treatment with low-dose cyclosporine A, *Trans Proc* 20(suppl 4):144-148, 1988.

15. Boruch SJ, Nguyen BV, Ladoulis CT et al.: Cerebrospinal fluid immunoglobulin abnormalities in neurosarcoidosis, *Arch Neurol* 46:270-273, 1989.

16. Bresnitz EA, Strom BL: Epidemiology of sarcoidosis, *Epidemiol Rev* 5:124-156, 1983.

17. Brewerton DA, Cockburn C, James DCO et al.: HLA antigens in sarcoidosis, *Clin Exp Immunol* 27:227-229, 1977.

18. Brincker H: Coexistence of sarcoidosis and myeloproliferative disease: a case of sarcoidosis preceding polycythemia vera with a literature review, *J Int Med* 225:355-357, 1989.

19. Brod RD: Presumed sarcoid choroidopathy mimicking birdshot retinochoroidopathy, *Am J Ophthalmol* 109:357, 1990.

20. Bronson L, Fisher T: Sarcoidosis of the paranasal sinuses with orbital extension, *Arch Ophthalmol* 94:243, 1976.

21. Brooks AMV, Gillies WE: Fluorescein angiography of the iris and specular microscopy of the corneal endothelium in some cases of glaucoma secondary to chronic cyclitis, *Ophthalmology* 95:1624-1630, 1988.

22. Brownstein S, Liszauer AD, Carey WD, Nicolle DA: Sarcoidosis of the eyelid skin, *Can J Ophthalmol* 25:256-259, 1990.

23. Cain H, Kraus B: Immunofluorescence microscopic demonstration of vimentin filaments in asteroid bodies of sarcoidosis, *Virchows Archiv B Cell Pathol* 42:213-226, 1983.

24. Campo RV, Aaberg TM: Choroidal granuloma in sarcoidosis, *Am J Ophthalmol* 97:419-427, 1984.

25. Reference deleted in proofs.

26. Case records of the Massachusetts General Hospital: Case 2-1990, *N Engl J Med* 322:116-123, 1990.

27. Case records of the Massachusetts General Hospital: Case 6-1990, *N Engl J Med* 322:388-397, 1990.

28. Case records of the Massachusetts General Hospital: Case 10-1991, *N Engl J Med* 324:677-687, 1991.

29. Reference deleted in proofs.

30. Chan CC, Wetzig RP, Palestine AG et al.: Immunohistopathology of ocular sarcoidosis, *Arch Ophthalmol* 105:1398-1402, 1987.

31. Chan Chi-Chao, BenEzra D, Hsu Su-Ming et al.: Granulomas in sympathetic ophthalmia and sarcoidosis, *Arch Ophthalmol* 103:198-202, 1985.

32. Chan Seem CP, Norfok G, Spokes EG: CSF angiotensin-converting enzyme in neurosarcoidosis, *Lancet* 1:456-457, 1985.

33. Chapelon C, Ziza JM, Piette JC et al.: Neurosarcoidosis: signs, course and treatment in 35 confirmed cases, *Medicine* (Baltimore) 69:261-276, 1990.

34. Chen RC, McLeod JG: Neurological complications of sarcoidosis, *Clin Exp Neurol* 26:99, 1989.

35. Chretien J: Assessment of sarcoid activity: state of the art. In Grassi C, Rizzato G, Pozzi E, editors: *Sarcoidosis and other granulomatous disorders,* Proceedings of the XI World Congress, 525-540, Amsterdam, 1988, Excerpta Medica.

36. Chumbley LC, Kearns TP: Retinopathy of sarcoidosis, *Am J Ophthalmol* 73:123-131, 1972.

37. Coleman SL, Brull S, Green WR: Sarcoid of the lacrimal sac and surrounding area, *Arch Ophthalmol* 88:645-646, 1970.

38. Collison JMT, Miller NR, Green WR: Involvement of orbital tissues by sarcoid, *Am J Ophthalmol* 102:302-307, 1986.

38a. Cornblath WT, Elner V, Rolfe M: Extraocular muscle involvement in sarcoidosis, *Ophthalmology,* 100:501-505, 1993.

39. Crick RP, Hoyle C, Smellie H: The eyes in sarcoidosis, *Br J Ophthalmol* 45:461-481, 1961.

40. Crystal RG, Roberts WC, Hunninghake GW et al.: Pulmonary sarcoidosis: a disease characteristic and perpetuated by activated lung T-lymphocytes, *Ann Intern Med* 94:73-94, 1981.

41. Cunnah D, Chew S, Wass J: Cyclosporine for central nervous system sarcoidosis, *Am J Med* 85:580-581, 1988.

42. Dacso CC, Bortz DL: Significance of the Argyll Robertson pupil in clinical medicine, *Am J Med* 86:199-202, 1989.

43. deLuise VP, Tabbara KF: Quantitation of tear lysozyme levels in dry eye disorders, *Arch Ophthalmol* 101:634-635, 1983.

43a. De-Potter P, Shields JA, Shields CL et al.: Unusual MRI findings in metastatic carcinoma to the choroid and optic nerve: a case report, *Int Ophthalmol* 16:39-44, 1992.

44. Dick DJ, Newman PK, Richardson J et al.: Acute posterior multifocal placoid pigment epitheliopathy and sarcoidosis, *Br J Ophthalmol* 72:74-77, 1988.

45. Dinning WJ: Sarcoidosis—a serious enigma, *Int Ophthalmol* 14:389-390, 1990.

46. Doxanas MT, Kelley JS, Prout TE: Sarcoidosis with neovascularization of the optic nerve head, *Am J Ophthalmol* 90:347-351, 1980.

47. Duker JS, Brown GC, McNamara JA: Proliferative sarcoid retinopathy, *Ophthalmology* 95:1680-1686, 1988.

48. Elias JA, Daniele RP: Systemic sarcoidosis. In Baum GL, Wolinsky E, editors: *Textbook of pulmonary diseases,* ed 4, 663-688, Boston, 1989, Little Brown.

48a. Emberton M, Ellis BW, Duchesne GM: Seminoma or sarcoid? *Clin Oncol* 4:56-57, 1992.

49. Engelken JD, Yuh WT, Carter KD, Nerad JA: Optic nerve sarcoidosis: MR findings, *Am J Neuroradiol* 13:228-230, 1992.

50. Enzenauer RJ, West SG: Sarcoidosis in autoimmune disease, *Semin Arthritis Rheum* 22:1-17, 1992.

51. Fanburg BL: *Sarcoidosis and other granulomatous diseases of the lung,* ed 1, New York, 1983, Marcel Dekker.

52. Flach A: Symblepharon formation in sarcoidosis, *Am J Ophthalmol* 85:210-214, 1978.

53. Fordice J, Katras T, Jackson RE et al.: Massive splenomegaly in sarcoidosis, *South Med J* 85:775-778, 1992.

54. Foster CS: Ocular manifestations of sarcoidosis preceding systemic manifestations. In Grassi C, Rizzato G, Pozzi E, editors: *Sarcoidosis and other granulomatous disorders,* Proceedings of the XI World Congress, 177-181, Amsterdam, 1988, Excerpta Medica.

55. Foster CS, Regan CDJ: Retinal vascular diseases: management, *Int Ophthalmol Clin* 26:55-71, 1986.

55a. Frank KW, Weis H: Unusual clinical and histopathologic findings in ocular sarcoidosis, *Br J Ophthalmol* 77:8-16, 1983.

56. Galetta S, Schatz NJ, Glaser JS: Acute sarcoid optic neuropathy with spontaneous recovery, *J Clin Neuroophthalmol* 9:27-32, 1989.

57. Gallagher P, Harris M, Turhbull FW et al.: Gastric sarcoidosis, *J R Soc Med* 77:837-839, 1984.

58. Ganster TS, Wheeler JE: Mammary sarcoidosis: two cases and literature review, *Arch Pathol Lab Med* 108:673-675, 1984.

59. Gass JDM, Olson CL: Sarcoidosis with optic nerve and retinal involvement, *Arch Ophthalmol* 94:945-950, 1976.

60. Geggel HS, Mensher JH: Cicatricial conjunctivitis in sarcoidosis: recognition and treatment, *Ann Ophthalmol* 21:92-94, 1989.

61. Gelwan MJ, Kellen RI, Burde RM et al.: Sarcoidosis of the anterior visual pathway: successes and failures, *J Neurol Neurosurg Psychiatry* 51:1473-1480, 1988.

62. Giles CL, Handleman J: Panuveitis—presenting symptom of systemic sarcoidosis in a child, *J Pediatr Ophthalmol* 13:189-191, 1976.

63. Gould H, Kaufman HE: Sarcoid of the fundus, *Arch Ophthalmol* 65:161-164, 1961.

64. Gragoudas ES, Regan CDJ: Peripapillary subretinal neovascularization in presumed sarcoidosis, *Arch Ophthalmol* 99:1194-1197, 1981.

65. Graham E, James DG: Neurosarcoidosis, *Sarcoidosis* 5:125-131, 1988.

66. Graham EM, Edelsten C: Intermediate uveitis and sarcoidosis, *Dev Ophthalmol* 23:106-110, 1992.

67. Grassi C, Rizzato G, Pozzi E, editors: *Sarcoidosis and other granulomatous disorders,* Proceedings of the XI World Congress, Amsterdam, 1988, Excerpta Medica.

68. Greco A, Steiner R: Magnetic resonance imaging in neurosarcoidosis, *Magn Reson Imaging* 5:15-21, 1987.

69. Grizzanti JN, Knapp AB, Schecter AJ et al.: Treatment of sarcoid meningitis with radiotherapy, *Am J Med* 73:605-608, 1982.

69a. Gupta SK, Gupta S: Sarcoidosis in India: a review of 125 biopsy-proven cases from eastern India, *Sarcoidosis* 7:43-49, 1990.

70. Guyatt GH, Bensen WG, Stolman LP et al.: HLA-B8 and erythema nodosum, *Can Med Assoc J* 127:1005-1006, 1982.

71. Hall FM, Shmerling RH, Aronson M, Faix JD: Case report 705: osteosclerotic sarcoidosis, *Skeletal Radiol* 21:182-185, 1992.

72. Harris GJ, Williams GA, Clarke GP: Sarcoidosis of the lacrimal sac, *Arch Ophthalmol* 99:1198-1201, 1981.

73. Hayashi H, Yamada K, Kuroki T et al.: Lymphocytic hypophysitis and pulmonary sarcoidosis: report of a case, *Am J Clin Pathol* 95:506-511, 1991.

74. Heck AW, Phillips LH: Sarcoidosis and the nervous system, *Neurol Clin* 7:641-654, 1989.

75. Hemady R, Tauber J, Foster CS: Immunosuppressive drugs in immune and inflammatory ocular disease, *Surv Ophthalmol* 35:369-389, 1991.

76. Henderly DE, Genstler AJ, Smith RE et al.: Changing patterns of uveitis, *Am J Ophthalmol* 103:131-136, 1987.

77. Henze T, Bardosi A, Reichmann HR: Familial myopathy with elevated serum angiotensin-converting enzyme, creatine kinase and lactate dehydrogenase isoenzyme 5, *J Neurol* 238:265-270, 1991.

78. Herschler J, Davis EB: Modifed goniotomy for inflammatory glaucoma: histologic evidence for the mechanism of pressure reduction, *Arch Ophthalmol* 98:684-687, 1980.

79. Hershey JM, Pulido JS, Massicotte SJ et al.: Noncaseating conjunctival granulomas in patients with multifocal choroiditis and panuveitis, *Invest Ophthalmol Vis Sci* 32(suppl):681, 1991.

80. Hetherington S: Sarcoidosis in young children, *Am J Dis Child* 136:13-15, 1982.

81. Hoover DL, Khan JA, Giangiacomo J: Pediatric ocular sarcoidosis, *Surv Ophthalmol* 30:215-228, 1986.

82. Hosoda Y: Epidemiology of sarcoidosis: state of the art. In Grassi C, Rizzato G, Pozzi E, editors: *Sarcoidosis and other granulomatous disorders,* Proceedings of the XI World Congress, 279-290, Amsterdam, 1988, Excerpta Medica.

83. Hunninghake GW, Crystal RG: Pulmonary sarcoidosis—a disorder mediated by excess helper T-lymphocyte activity at sites of disease activity, *New Engl J Med* 305:429-434, 1981.

84. Hunter DG, Foster CS: Isolated ocular sarcoidosis: late development of systemic manifestations in uveitis patients, *Invest Ophthalmol Vis Sci* 32(suppl):681, 1991.

84a. Hunter DG, Foster CS: Ocular manifestations of sarcoidosis. In Jakobiec F, Albert DM, editors: *Principles and practice of ophthalmology,* Philadelphia, 1994, WB Saunders.

85. Imes RK, Reifschneider JS, O'Connor LE: Systemic sarcoidosis presenting initially with bilateral orbital and upper lid masses, *Ann Ophthalmol* 20:466-469, 1988.

86. Israel HL, Albertine KH, Park CH, Patrick H: Whole body gallium scans: role in diagnosis of sarcoidosis, *Am Rev Resp Dis* 144:1182-1186, 1991.

87. Israel HL, McComb BL: Chlorambucil treatment of sarcoidosis, *Sarcoidosis* 8:35-41, 1991.

88. Jabs DA, Johns CJ: Ocular involvement in chronic sarcoidosis, *Am J Ophthalmol* 102:297-301, 1986.

89. Jakobiec F, Jones I: Orbital inflammations. In Jakobiec F, Jones I, editors: *Diseases of the orbit,* Hagerstown, 1979, Harper & Row.

90. Reference deleted in proofs

91. James DG, Graham E, Hamblin A: Immunology of multisystem ocular disease, *Surv Ophthalmol* 30:155-167, 1985.

92. James DG, Neville E: Pathology of sarcoidosis, *Pathobiol Annu* 7:31-36, 1977.

93. James DG, Neville E, Langley DA: Ocular sarcoidosis, *Trans Ophthalmol Soc UK* 96:133-139,1976.

94. James DG, Williams WJ, editors: *Sarcoidosis and other granulomatous disorders,* ed 1, Philadelphia, 1985, WB Saunders.

95. Johns CJ: Sarcoidosis. In Fishman AP, editor: *Pulmonary diseases and disorders,* vol 1, 619-644, New York, 1992, McGraw Hill.

96. Johns CJ, Scott PP, Schonfeld SA: Sarcoidosis, *Ann Rev Med* 40:353-371, 1989.

97. Jones E, Callen JP: Hydroxychloroquine is effective therapy for control of cutaneous sarcoidal granulomas, *J Am Acad Dermatol* 23:487-489, 1990.

98. Jordan DR, Anderson RL, Nerad JA et al.: The diagnosis of sarcoidosis, *Can J Ophthalmol* 23:203-207, 1988.

99. Kalb RE, Epstein W, Grossman ME: Sarcoidosis with subcutaneous nodules, *Am J Med* 85:731-736, 1988.

100. Kanski JJ, McAllister JA: Trabeculodialysis for inflammatory glaucoma in children and young adults, *Ophthalmology* 92:927-930, 1985.

101. Karcioglu ZA, Brear R: Conjunctival biopsy in sarcoidosis, *Am J Ophthalmol* 99:68-73, 1985.

102. Karma A: Ophthalmic changes in sarcoidosis, *Acta Ophthalmol* 141(suppl):1-94, 1979.

103. Karma A, Huhti E, Poukkula A: Course and outcome of ocular sarcoidosis, *Am J Ophthalmol* 106:467-472, 1988.

104. Karma A, Poukkula AA, Ruokonen AO: Assessment of activity of ocular sarcoidosis by gallium scanning, *Br J Ophthalmol* 71:361-367, 1987.

105. Karma A, Taskinen E, Kainulainen H, Partanen M: Phenotypes of conjunctival inflammatory cells in sarcoidosis, *Br J Ophthalmol* 76:101-106, 1992.

106. Kataria S, Trevathan GE, Holland JE et al.: Ocular presentation of sarcoidosis in children, *Clin Pediatr* 22:793-797, 1983.

107. Kataria YP: Chlorambucil in sarcoidosis, *Chest* 78:36-43, 1980.

108. Katz B: Disc edema, transient obscurations of vision, and a temporal fossa mass, *Surv Ophthalmol* 36:133-139, 1991.

109. Kelley JS, Green WR: Sarcoidosis involving the optic nerve head, *Arch Ophthalmol* 89:486-488, 1973.

110. Ketonen L, Oksanen V, Kuuliala I: Preliminary experience of magnetic resonance imaging in neurosarcoidosis, *Neuroradiology* 29:127-129, 1987.

111. Khan JA, Hoover DL, Giangiacomo J et al.: Orbital and childhood sarcoidosis, *J Pediatr Ophthalmol Strabismus* 23:190-194, 1983.

112. Kimmel AS, McCarthy MJ, Blodi CF: Branch retinal vein occlusion in sarcoidosis, *Am J Ophthalmol* 107:561-562, 1989.

113. Kirkpatrick CJ, Curry A, Bisset DL: Light- and electron-microscopic studies on multinucleated giant cells in sarcoid granuloma: new aspects of asteroid and Schaumann bodies, *Ultrastruct Pathol* 12:581-597, 1988.

114. Klech H: Clinical risk assessment in sarcoidosis. In Grassi C, Rizzato E, Pozzi E, editors: *Sarcoidosis and other granulomatous disorders,* Amsterdam, 1988, Excerpta Medica.

115. Kuboshiro T, Yoshioka H: Birdshot retinochoroidopathy—a possible relationship to ocular sarcoidosis, *Kurume Med J* 35:193, 1988.

116. Lacher MJ: Spontaneous remission of response to methotrexate in sarcoidosis, *Ann Int Med* 63:1247-1248, 1968.

117. Lacronique J, Auzeby A, Valeyre D et al.: Urinary neopterin in pulmonary sarcoidosis—relationship to clinical and biologic assessment of the disease, *Am Rev Respir Dis* 139:1474-1478, 1989.

118. Landers PH: Vitreous lesions observed in Boeck's sarcoid, *Tr Am Ophthalmol Soc* 32:1740-1741, 1949.

119. Letocha CE, Shields JA, Goldberg RE: Retinal changes in sarcoidosis, *Can J Ophthalmol* 10:184-192, 1975.

120. Lieberman J: Elevation of serum angiotensin-converting-enzyme (ACE) level in sarcoidosis, *Am J Med* 59:365-72, 1975.

121. Lieberman J: Enzymes in sarcoidosis: angiotensin-converting-enzyme (ACE), *Clin Lab Med* 9:745-755, 1989.

122. Lieberman J, Sastre A: An angiotensin-converting enzyme (ACE) inhibitor in human serum: increased sensitivity of the serum ACE assay for detecting sarcoidosis, *Chest* 90:869-875, 1986.

123. Lightman S, Chan CC: Immune mechanisms in choroido-retinal inflammation in man, *Eye* 4:345-353, 1990.

124. Line BR, Hunninghake GW, Keogh BA et al.: Gallium-67 scanning as an indicator of the activity of sarcoidosis. In Fanburg BL, editor: *Sarcoidosis and other granulomatous diseases of the lung,* 287-322, New York, 1983, Marcel Dekker.

125. Lower EE, Baughman RP: The use of low dose methotrexate in refractory sarcoidosis, *Am J Med Sci* 299:153-157, 1990.

126. Lower EE, Baughman RP, Winget D: The long term use of methotrexate in patients with chronic symptomatic sarcoidosis, *Sarcoidosis* 9(suppl 1):465-466, 1992.

127. Lowery WS, Whitlock WL, Dietrich RA et al.: Sarcoidosis complicated by HIV infection: three case reports and a review of the literature, *Am Rev Respir Dis* 142:887-889, 1990.

128. Lyons DJ, Donald S, Mitchell DN, Asherson GL: Chemical inactivation of the Kveim reagent, *Respiration* 59:22-26, 1992.

129. MacRury SM, McQuaker G, Morton R, Hume R: Sarcoidosis: association with small bowel disease and folate deficiency, *J Clin Pathol* 45:823-825, 1992.

130. Mader TH, Chismire KJ, Cornell FM: The treatment of an enlarged sarcoid iris nodule with injectable corticosteroids, *Am J Ophthalmol* 106:365-366, 1988.

131. Mandel W, Thomas JH, Carmen CT et al.: *Bibliography on sarcoidosis* 1878-1963, Public Health Service Publication No. 1213, Washington, D.C., 1964.

132. Mansour AM: Sarcoid optic disc edema and optociliary shunts, *J Clin Neuroophthalmology* 6:47-52, 1986.

133. Marcille R, McCarthy M, Barton JW et al.: Long-term outcome of pediatric sarcoidosis with emphasis on pulmonary status, *Chest* 102(5):1444-1449, 1992.

134. Marcus DF, Bovino JA, Burton TC: Sarcoid granuloma of the choroid, *Ophthalmology* 89:1326-1330, 1982.

134a. Martin DF, Chan C-C, deSmet MD et al.: The role of chorioretinal biopsy in the management of posterior uveitis, *Ophthalmology* 10:705-714, 1993.

135. Mayers M: Ocular sarcoidosis, *Int Ophthalmol Clin* 30:257-263, 1990.

136. Mayock RL, Bertand P, Morrison CE et al.: Manifestations of sarcoidosis, *Am J Med* 35:67-89, 1963.

137. McCurley T, Salter J, Glick A: Renal insufficiency in sarcoidosis: a clinical and pathologic study, *Arch Pathol Lab Med* 114:488-492, 1990.

138. Melmon K, Goldberg J: Sarcoidosis with bilateral exophthalmos as the presenting symptom, *Am J Med* 33:158-160, 1962.

139. Mende D, Suchenwirth RM: Neurosarcoidosis: comparative analysis of the clinical profile based on 537 cases from the world literature up to 1963 and from 1976-1988, *Fortschr Neurol Psychiatr* 58:7-18, 1990.

140. Merritt JC, Lipper SL, Peiffer RL et al.: Conjunctival biopsy in sarcoidosis, *J Nat Med Assoc* 72:347-349, 1980.

141. Merritt JC, Whitsett CF, Daffin L, Mower P: HLA-A, -B, and DR antigenic factors in ocular sarcoidosis, *Am J Ophthalmol* 96:296-397, 1983.

142. Mitchell IC, Turk JL, Mitchell DN: Detection of mycobacterial rRNA in sarcoidosis with liquid-phase hybridization, *Lancet* 339:1015-1017, 1992.

143. Mondlin RL, Hofman FM, Sharma OP et al.: Demonstration *in situ* of subsets of T-lymphocytes in sarcoidosis, *Am J Dermatopathol* 6:423-427, 1984.

144. Montemurro L, Fraioli P, Rizzato G: Bone loss in untreated long-standing sarcoidosis, *Sarcoidosis* 8:29-34, 1991.

145. Morse SI, Cohn ZA, Hirsch JG et al.: The treatment of sarcoidosis with chloroquine, *Am J Med* 30:779-784, 1961.

146. Munro CS, Mitchell DN: The Kveim response: still useful, still a puzzle, *Thorax* 42:321-331, 1987.

147. Murphy O, Hogan J, Bredin CP: Endometrial and pulmonary sarcoidosis, *Ir J Med Sci* 161:14-15, 1992.

148. Muthiah MM, Macfarlane JT: Current concepts in the management of sarcoidosis, *Drugs* 40:231-237, 1990.

149. Myslivecek M, Husak V, Koek V et al.: Absolute quantitation of gallium-67 citrate accumulation in the lungs and its importance for the evaluation of disease activity in pulmonary sarcoidosis, *Eur J Nucl Med* 19:1016-1022, 1992.

150. Nabriski D, Bendahan J, Shapiro MS et al.: Sarcoidosis masquerading as a parathyroid adenoma, *Head Neck* 14:384-386, 1992.

151. Neault R, Riley FC: Report of a case of dacryocystitis secondary to Boeck's sarcoid, *Am J Ophthalmol* 70:1011-1013, 1970.

152. Nessan VJ, Jacoway JR: Biopsy of minor salivary glands in the diagnosis of sarcoidosis, *N Engl J Med* 301:922-924, 1979.

153. Ngo Y, Messing B, Marteau P et al.: Peritoneal sarcoidosis. An unrecognized cause of sclerosing peritonitis, *Dig Dis Sci* 37:1776-1780, 1992.

154. Nichols CW, Eagle RC Jr, Yanoff M, Menocal NG: Conjunctival biopsy as an aid in the evaluation of the patient with suspected sarcoidosis, *Ophthalmology* 87:287-291, 1980.

155. Nidiry JJ, Mines S, Hackney R, Nabhani H: Sarcoidosis: a unique presentation of dysphagia, myopathy, and photophobia, *Am J Gastroenterol* 86:1679-1682, 1991.

156. Nosal A, Schleissner L, Mishkin F et al.: Angiotensin converting enzyme and gallium scan in noninvasive evaluation of sarcoidosis, *Ann Int Med* 90:328-331, 1979.

157. Obenauf CD, Shaw HE, Sydnor CF, Klintworth GK: Sarcoidosis and its ophthalmic manifestations, *Am J Ophthalmol* 86:648-655, 1978.

158. Perkins ES, Folk J: Uveitis in London and Iowa, *Ophthalmologica* 189:36-40, 1984.

159. Poropatich R, Phillips YY: Listerial brain abscess in long-standing sarcoidosis, *South Med J* 85:554-556, 1992.

160. Quigley C, Blake MA, Ward K et al.: Eye disease in 260 consecutive patients attending an Irish sarcoidosis clinic, *Sarcoidosis* 1(suppl):363-364, 1992.

161. Regan CDJ, Foster CS: Retinal vascular diseases: clinical presentation and diagnosis, *Int Ophthalmol Clin* 26:25-53, 1986.

162. Rosenbaum JT: Uveitis—an internist's view, *Arch Intern Med* 149:1173-1176, 1989.

163. Rosenberg AM, Yee EH, MacKenzie JW: Arthritis in childhood sarcoidosis, *J Rheumatol* 10:987-990, 1983.

164. Rothova A, Alberts C, Glasius E et al.: Risk factors for ocular sarcoidosis, *Doc Ophthalmol* 72:287-296, 1989.

165. Rothova A, Buitenhuis HJ, Meenken C et al.: Uveitis and systemic disease, *Br J Ophthalmol* 76:137-141, 1992.

166. Rubow S, Klopper J, Scholtz P: Excretion of gallium 67 in human breast milk and its inadvertent ingestion by a 9-month-old child, *Eur J Nucl Med* 18:829-833, 1991.

167. Rush JA, Younge BR: Paralysis cranial nerves III, IV, and VI, *Arch Ophthalmol* 99:76-79, 1981.

168. Ryan DM, Lesser BA, Crumley LA et al.: Epididymal sarcoidosis, *J Urol* 149:134-136, 1993.

169. Saboor SA, Johnson N McI, McFadden J: Detection of mycobacterial DNA in sarcoidosis and tuberculosis with polymerase chain reaction, *Lancet* 339:1012-1015, 1992.

170. Sachs R, Kashii S, Burde RM: Sixth nerve palsy as the initial manifestation of sarcoidosis, *Am J Ophthalmol* 110:438-440, 1990.

171. Sahn EE, Hampton MT, Garen PD et al.: Preschool sarcoidosis masquerading as juvenile rheumatoid arthritis: two case reports and a review of the literature, *Pediatr Dermatol* 7:208-213, 1990.

172. Samlaska CP, Sandberg GD, Maggio KL, Sakas EL: Generalized perforating granuloma annulare, *J Am Acad Dermatol* 27:319-322, 1992.

173. Sanders MD, Shilling JS: Retinal, choroidal, and optic disc involvement in sarcoidosis, *Trans Ophthal Soc UK* 96:140-144, 1976.

174. Sharma OP, editor: *Sarcoidosis: clinical management,* London, 1984, Butterworths & Co.

175. Sharma OP: Sarcoidosis, *Dis Mon* 36:469-535, 1990.

176. Sharma OP, Colp C, Williams MH Jr: Pulmonary function studies in patients with bilateral sarcoidosis of hilar lymph nodes, *Arch Intern Med* 117:436-439, 1966.

176a. Sharma OP: Sarcoidosis of the skin. In Fitzpatrick TB, Eisen AZ, Wolff K et al., editors: *Dermatology in general medicine,* New York, 1993, McGraw-Hill.

177. Sharma OP, Kalkat G: Drug induced clinical syndromes mimicking sarcoidosis, *Sarcoidosis* 8:3-5, 1991.

178. Sharma OP, Vita JB: Determination of angiotensin-converting enzyme activity in tears: a noninvasive test for evaluation of ocular sarcoidosis, *Arch Ophthalmol* 101:559-561, 1983.

179. Siltzbach LE, Greenberg GM: Childhood sarcoidosis—a study of 18 patients, *N Engl J Med* 279:1239-1245, 1968.

180. Siltzbach LE, James DG, Neville E et al.: Course and prognosis of sarcoidosis around the world, *Am J Med* 57:847-852, 1974.

181. Singer F, Talavera W, Zumoff B: Elevated levels of angiotensin-converting enzyme in *pneumocystis carinii* pneumonia, *Chest* 95:803-806, 1989.

182. Smith MJ, Turton CW, Mitchell DN et al.: Association of HLA-B8 with spontaneous resolution in sarcoidosis, *Thorax* 36:296-298, 1981.

183. Soriano FG, Caramelli P, Nitrini R et al.: Neurosarcoidosis: therapeutic success with methotrexate, *Postgrad Med J* 66:142-143, 1990.

184. Spaide RF, Ward DL: Conjunctival biopsy in the diagnosis of sarcoidosis, *Br J Ophthalmol* 74:469-471, 1990.

185. Spalton DJ, Sanders MD: Fundus changes in histologically confirmed sarcoidosis, *Br J Ophthalmol* 65:348-358, 1981.

186. Spiteri MA, Newman SP, Clarke SW et al.: Inhaled corticosteroids can modulate the immunopathogenesis of pulmonary sarcoidosis, *Eur Respir J* 2:218-224, 1989.

187. Stannard K, Spalton DJ: Sarcoidosis with infiltration of the external ocular muscles, *Br J Ophthalmol* 69:562-566, 1985.

188. Steahly LP: Sarcoidosis and peripheral neovascularization, *Ann Ophthalmol* 20:426-427, 1988.

189. Stern BJ, Krumholz A, Johns C et al.: Sarcoidosis and its neurological manifestations, *Arch Neurol* 42:909-917, 1985.

190. Studdy PR, Bird R: Serum angiotensin converting enzyme in sarcoidosis—its value in present clinical practice, *Ann Clin Biochem* 26:13-18, 1989.

191. Suen JS, Forse MS, Hyland RH et al.: The malignancy-sarcoidosis syndrome, *Chest* 8:1300-1302, 1990.

192. Sulavick B, Weed D, Spencer R et al.: A combinatorial analysis of ^{67}Ga scanning of the head and thorax in the diagnosis of sarcoidosis —The *Panda* sign. In Grassi C, Rizzato G, Pozzi E, editors: *Sarcoidosis and other granulomatous disorders,* Proceedings of the XI World Congress, 517-518, Amsterdam, 1988, Excerpta Medica.

193. Sulavik SB, Spencer RP, Weed DA et al.: Recognition of distinctive patterns of gallium-67 distribution in sarcoidosis, *J Nucl Med* 31:1909-1914, 1990.

194. Takayama K, Nagata N, Miyagawa Y et al.: The usefulness of step sectioning of transbronchial lung biopsy specimen in diagnosing sarcoidosis, *Chest* 102:1441-1443, 1992.

195. Tessler HH, Weinberg RS: Aqueous and serum lysozyme values in experimental uveitis in rabbits, *Invest Ophthalmol* 14:953-956, 1975.

196. Thivolet J, Faure M, Nicolas JF et al.: Therapeutic use of TPS (thymopoietin 3236) in sarcoidosis of the skin, *Clin Immunol Immunopathol* 26:350, 1983.

197. Thomas PD, Hunninghake GW: Current concepts of the pathogenesis of sarcoidosis, *Am Rev Respir Dis* 135:747-760, 1987.

198. Thompson AB, Cale WF, Lapp NL: Serum angiotensin-converting enzyme is elevated in association with underground coal mining, *Chest* 100:1042-1045, 1991.

199. Thrasher DR, Briggs DD: Pulmonary sarcoidosis, *Clin Chest Med* 3:537-563, 1982.

200. Tingey DP, Gonder JR: Ocular sarcoidosis presenting as a solitary choroidal mass, *Can J Ophthalmol* 27:25-29, 1992.

201. Toews GB, Lynch III JP: Methotrexate in sarcoidosis, *Am J Med Sci* 300:33-36, 1990.

202. Toner GC, Bosl GJ: Sarcoidosis, "Sarcoid-like lymphadenopathy," and testicular germ cell tumors, *Am J Med* 89:651-656, 1990.

203. Tuft SJ, Watson PG: Progression of scleral disease, *Ophthalmology* 98:467-471, 1991.
204. Wakefield D, McCluskey P: Cyclosporine: a therapy in inflammatory eye disease, *J Ocular Pharmacol* 7:221-226, 1991.
205. Wall M: Optic atrophy, *Surv Ophthalmol* 36:51-58, 1991.
205a. Webster GF, Razsi LK, Sanchez M, Shupack JL: Weekly low-dose methotrexate therapy for cutaneous sarcoidosis, *J Am Acad Dermatol* 24:451-454, 1991.
206. Weinberg RS, Tessler HH: Serum lysozyme in sarcoid uveitis, *Am J Ophthalmol* 82:105-108, 1976.
207. Weinreb RN: Diagnosing sarcoidosis by transconjunctival biopsy of the lacrimal gland, *Am J Ophthalmol* 97:573-576, 1984.
208. Weinreb RN, Barth R, Kimura SJ: Limited gallium scans and angiotensin converting enzyme in granulomatous uveitis, *Ophthalmology* 87:202-209, 1980.
209. Weinreb RN, Kimura SJ: Uveitis associated with sarcoidosis and angiotensin converting enzyme, *Am J Ophthalmol* 89:180-185, 1980.
210. Weinreb RN, Sandman R, Ryder MI et al.: Angiotensin-converting enzyme activity in human aqueous humor, *Arch Ophthalmol* 103:34-36, 1985.
211. Weinreb RN, Tessler H: Laboratory diagnosis of ophthalmic sarcoidosis, *Surv Ophthalmol* 28:653-664, 1984.
212. Weinreb RN, Yavitz EQ, O'Connor GR, Barth RA: Lacrimal gland uptake of gallium citrate Ga 67, *Am J Ophthalmol* 92:16-20, 1981.
213. Reference deleted in proofs.
214. Williams RD, Hoskins HD, Shaffer RN: Outcome of trabeculodialysis for inflammatory glaucoma: a review of 25 cases, *Invest Ophthalmol Vis Sci* 32(suppl):742, 1991.
215. Williams WJ, Erasmus DA, Valerie James EM et al.: The fine structure of sarcoid and tuberculous granulomas, *Postgrad Med J* 46:496-500, 1970.
216. Yohai RA, Bullock JD, Margolis JH: Unilateral optic disc edema and a contralateral temporal fossa mass, *Am J Ophthalmol* 115:261-262, 1993.
217. York EL, Kovithavongs T, Man SF et al.: Cyclosporine and chronic sarcoidosis, *Chest* 98:1026-1029, 1990.
218. Zeitar JH, Bhavsar A, McDermott ML et al.: Ocular sarcoidosis manifesting as an anterior staphyloma, *Am J Ophthalmol* 112:345-347, 1991.
219. Zic JA, Horowitz DH, Arzubiaga C, King LE Jr: Treatment of cutaneous sarcoidosis with chloroquine. Review of the literature, *Arch Dermatol* 127:1034-1040, 1991.
220. Zierhut M, Foster CS: Multiple sclerosis, sarcoidosis and other diseases in patients with pars planitis, *Dev Ophthalmol* 23:41-47, 1992.
221. Zouaoui A, Maillard JC, Dormont D et al.: MRI in neurosarcoidosis, *J Neuroradiol* 19:271-284, 1992.

SECTION

V

INFECTIOUS OCULAR DISEASES

---

60 Preseptal Cellulitis

PAUL R. BADENOCH, DOUGLAS J. COSTER

Preseptal (periorbital) cellulitis refers to infection of the eyelids and to the soft tissue of the periocular region anterior to the orbital septum. Preseptal infection is more common than postseptal (orbital) cellulitis.[17,29,49,60,66] These conditions often progressed to blindness or the death of patients prior to the antibiotic era. Preseptal cellulitis is still a medical emergency in children and must be treated immediately in patients of all ages. The frequency of subdural abscesses, brain abscesses, or meningitis as complications of preseptal cellulitis is approximately 3%, similar to that of orbital cellulitis.[33] To minimize the risk of central nervous system involvement or visual loss, the clinician must have (1) an understanding of the pathogenesis of preseptal cellulitis and (2) the ability to recognize the clinical features, to initiate diagnostic investigations, and to deliver appropriate antimicrobial and surgical therapy.

ANATOMY

The orbital septum (palpebral fascia) is a continuation of the periosteum. It emerges from a thickening, the arcus marginale, near the orbital rim. The superior orbital septum attaches to the levator aponeurosis either above (in Occidentals) or below (in Orientals) the superior tarsal border.[16] The inferior orbital septum connects with the lower border of the inferior tarsal plate.[33]

Rather than a dense, impenetrable structure, the septum should be thought of as a thin anterior seal to the orbital cavity. This flexible membrane participates in all movements of the eyelids. The septum consists of two layers of fibers running in arcades and crossing each other at right angles. It is pierced by a number of structures: the lacrimal vessels and nerves, the supraorbital and supratrochlear vessels and nerves, the infratrochlear nerve, the anastomosis between the angular and ophthalmic veins, and the palpebral arteries juxtaposed to the medial palpebral ligament.[37] Despite this apparent fragility, the septum impedes the spread of infection posteriorly. In the absence of treatment, the likelihood and celerity of orbital invasion through the sep-

tum depends on the virulence of the organism. The structures involved in preseptal cellulitis include the tarsi, the pretarsal space, the preseptal space, and the preseptal muscles and fat.

EPIDEMIOLOGY AND RISK FACTORS

Preseptal cellulitis typically is characterized by a unilateral infection in children and young adults. A summary of common predisposing events and the microbial agents found is given in Table 60-1. In a retrospective study the principal risk factors were found to be trauma, skin infection, and age less than 6 years.[32]

Organisms gain access to preseptal tissue by several pathways. The route of infection influences the clinical signs, the range of organisms responsible, the methods of investigation, and the treatment.

Trauma

Organisms can be inoculated directly by trauma. This can occur from lacerations, insect bites, and puncture wounds with or without deposition of a foreign body. Infection has followed surgical procedures such as septorhinoplasty.[47] The flora of the wound depends on the mode of infliction, the environment, and the degree of contamination of adjacent areas of skin. Traumatic injuries are often complicated by indigenous, facultatively anaerobic bacteria such as *Staphylococcus aureus* and Lancefield group A streptococci *(Streptococcus pyogenes)*. In cases involving the latter, an acute subcutaneous cellulitis known as erysipelas may result. Clostridia are prominent among the obligate anaerobes associated with traumatic wounds, leading to gas gangrene or tetanus under certain conditions. These organisms and *Bacillus cereus* should be considered if the wound has been contaminated with soil. Other anaerobic bacteria such as *Bacteroides* and *Peptostreptococcus* may contaminate animal bites. Infection with anaerobes is suggested by a foul-smelling discharge, necrosis, gas, or severe toxemia.

TABLE 60-1 PREDISPOSING CONDITIONS AND ORGANISMS ASSOCIATED WITH PRESEPTAL CELLULITIS

Predisposing Event	Principal Responsible Organisms	Usual Age Group
Trauma	*Staphylococcus aureus*	Any
	Streptococcus pyogenes	
Erysipelas	*Streptococcus pyogenes*	Infants, the elderly
Ruptured dacryocele	*Staphylococcus aureus*	Neonates
	Streptococcus pyogenes	
Impetigo	*Staphylococcus aureus*	Children
	Streptococcus pyogenes	
Herpetic diseases	Herpes simplex virus type 1	Adults, children
	Herpes simplex virus type 2	Neonates
	Varicella-zoster virus	Elderly
Upper respiratory tract infection/otitis media	*Haemophilus influenzae* type b	Children
	Streptococcus pneumoniae	

Preseptal cellulitis can occur after blunt trauma without an apparent entry wound. Subsequent inflammation and bruising may contribute to the breakdown of preseptal integrity and allow access of sinusal organisms.

Contiguous Infection

Preseptal cellulitis may result from the spread of infection from skin or adjacent tissue such as an inflamed eyelid margin or lacrimal gland. For example, the rupture of a dacryocele can lead to preseptal cellulitis in neonates.[45] In this age group, *S. aureus, S. pyogenes,* and other organisms found on the skin are responsible for most preseptal infections. The distribution and appearance of any skin lesions suggest the cause of the preseptal inflammation. Three major diseases are commonly involved: impetigo, herpes simplex virus, and varicella-zoster virus.[33]

Impetigo is a dermatitis caused by *S. aureus* or *S. pyogenes.* Often complicating other skin conditions such as eczema, it is most commonly found in children less than 6 years of age who are subjected to poor hygiene.

Herpes simplex virus type 1 may induce preseptal cellulitis either as a consequence of primary infection or as a recurrence in adults or children. Herpes simplex virus type 2 is sometimes transmitted to the eyelids of neonates from an infected birth canal.

The reactivation of latent varicella-zoster virus may occur in adults (commonly of middle-age) or children, thus giving rise to shingles. Vesicular eruption in the periocular region is known as herpes zoster ophthalmicus. This is accompanied by severe preseptal inflammation and edema. Secondary bacterial infection is unusual but may occur in immunocompromised patients.

Sinusitis and Otitis Media

Preseptal cellulitis can occur without prior trauma or skin disease. Bacteria are believed to migrate to preseptal tissue

from the paranasal sinuses or the middle ear via veins and lymphatics.[28,30] The condition resulting from such endogenous spread of organisms has been termed "nonsuppurative" preseptal cellulitis.[33] The mean age of patients who have this condition is 30 months. It is most often associated with upper respiratory tract infection during cold weather,[60] but in many children the site of primary infection is not identified. Most cases are caused by *Haemophilus influenzae* type b (Hib); *Streptococcus pneumoniae* is also commonly found.[28] Other streptococci, *Neisseria meningitidis* group B[18] or *S. aureus* are less frequently implicated. A mixed infection may occur.

Preseptal cellulitis and other infections caused by Hib are most frequently seen in male infants 4 to 12 months of age from poor families.[15,49,65,67] This is consistent with the finding that serum of children aged 3 months to 3 years lacked bactericidal activity against the type b strain.[20] Type-specific antibody is important in resistance to Hib, and the type b capsule is antiphagocytic.[1] Presumably, the antibody detected in neonates has been maternally transferred. Its appearance in later childhood is less well understood, occurring in the apparent absence of exposure to Hib. It has been proposed that antibody develops from the interaction with cross-reacting antigens present in food or commensal bacteria, for example, *Escherichia coli.*[57]

Nonsuppurative preseptal cellulitis in adults is extremely rare. Presumably, the pathogenesis is the same as in children. *S. pneumoniae, S. pyogenes,* and *S. aureus* are the principal organisms found. *H. influenzae* preseptal cellulitis has not been reported in adults. Noninfectious causes such as allergic blepharodermatitis, dacryoadenitis, and dacryocystitis should be considered in the differential diagnosis.

PATHOGENESIS

Four bacterial species, *S. aureus, H. influenzae, S. pneumoniae,* and *S. pyogenes,* are responsible for more than 95%

of the cases of preseptal cellulitis.[28] This reflects their common colonization of the skin or upper respiratory tract. The adherence to human tissue, release of toxic substances, and strategies for avoiding the host response of these organisms are subject to continuing investigation. Many possible mechanisms may play a role in the pathogenesis of preseptal cellulitis.

Staphylococcus aureus

Several cell wall components of S. aureus have been implicated in virulence. One, peptidoglycan, elicits the production of endogenous pyrogen from human monocytes, induces a local Swartzmann reaction, and activates complement.[35] Another, protein A, binds the F_c terminal of human IgG, rendering such antibodies ineffective as opsonins.[19] In addition, most clinical isolates of S. aureus are encapsulated. The capsule is a secreted polysaccharide that covers the cell wall and renders the organism less susceptible to recognition and attack by the host immune system. Certain S. aureus capsular serotypes correlate with virulence.[38] S. aureus also has a fibronectin receptor on its cell surface.[34] The fibronectins are a class of matrix glycoproteins that (1) promote cell adhesion to fibrous collagens and other connective-tissue components and (2) protect against attachment by many bacteria. For example, the high incidence of respiratory infection caused by Pseudomonas aeruginosa in cystic fibrosis patients correlates with a high level of protease in their sputum, leading to degradation of fibronectin on the epithelial cells lining the respiratory tract with subsequent attachment of bacteria.[69] S. aureus circumvents this defense by adhering directly to fibronectin, which facilitates tissue invasion.

S. aureus produces a number of enzymes and toxins, some clearly implicated in pathogenesis and others in which the association remains theoretical. The production of catalase correlates with pathogenicity by counteracting hydrogen peroxide-mediated killing by polymorphonuclear leukocytes.[42] The production of another enzyme, coagulase, is a marker of virulence in staphylococci. This causes a layer of fibrin to be deposited around the bacteria, perhaps restricting access of phagocytes or concealing the organisms from the immune system. In addition, S. aureus secretes hyaluronidase and a lipase that are believed to be factors in dissemination of the organism.[59,61] S. aureus also expresses five cytolytic toxins: α, β, δ, γ, and leukocidin.[46] α-Toxin permeabilizes a wide variety of cell membranes by inducing pores of uniform size.[43] β-Toxin has an associated sphingomyelinase activity.[11] This is potentially harmful to lipids of the plasma membrane and disruptive to the transduction of intracellular signals.[3] δ-Toxin has unusual hydrophobicity properties and disrupts biologic membranes with a detergent-like action. γ-Toxin and leukocidin are structurally related;[13] the former lyses erythrocytes from many species including humans, whereas the latter kills human phago-

cytes.[14] Another toxin that may play a role in the pathology of preseptal cellulitis is exfoliatin, the causal agent of staphylococcal scalded skin syndrome.[41] This condition is seen most commonly in neonates and is caused by the toxin-mediated splitting of epidermal cell junctions.

Haemophilus influenzae

The composition of the capsule is the major determinant of virulence for H. influenzae.[70] Of the six antigenically distinct capsular types,[52] type b is present on more than 95% of strains isolated from invasive infections including meningitis and preseptal cellulitis.

The adherence of Hib to human mucosa is believed to be pili-mediated.[51] A Hib outer membrane protein contributing to transepithelial invasion has recently been described.[9] As with other gram-negative bacteria, the release of lipopolysaccharides (endotoxins) from the cell wall of Hib induces a number of complex and interrelated biologic effects. Endotoxin activates the complement, coagulation, and fibrinolytic pathways. Endotoxin also triggers enzymatic reactions leading to the release of bradykinins and other vasoactive peptides that cause hypotension.

Streptococcus pneumoniae

Capsular polysaccharide is also an important determinant of virulence in S. pneumoniae. Encapsulated bacteria, particularly serotypes 1, 2, 3, 4, 7, 8, 12, and 14, are virulent in humans, whereas bacteria without polysaccharides ("rough" strains) are not. As well as having antiphagocytic properties, capsular polysaccharides may consume antibodies when released from the cell.[44]

The adherence of S. pneumoniae is mediated by amino sugars, and pneumococcal neuraminidase activity correlates with virulence.[63] The mechanism may involve the exposure of receptor sites on both the bacterial and host surfaces.[40] An important toxin of this organism is pneumolysin. It is dermotoxic and haemolytic in experimental animals and has been demonstrated to play a role in the pathogenesis of pneumococcal keratitis.[31]

Streptococcus pyogenes

S. pyogenes has a formidable array of tissue-damaging enzymes and toxins of which only a small number are well characterized. Its capsule contains hyaluronic acid apparently identical to that found in human connective tissue. This is nonantigenic and hinders recognition of the bacterium by the host.

M protein is the major virulence antigen of S. pyogenes. It assembles into coiled fibrils protruding from the cell surface and mediates resistance to phagocytosis by binding mammalian proteins such as fibrinogen and complement factor H. This prevents effective opsonization by the alternative complement pathway.[54] Adherence of S. pyogenes is mediated by lipoteichoic acids on fimbriae.[6] Distinct IgA and

IgG F_c-binding proteins are recognized.[7] The organism produces at least three pyrogenic exotoxins (scarlet fever toxins) that seem to exert their effect, in part, by polyclonal activation of T-lymphocytes[8] and modulation of inflammatory mediator release from neutrophils.[25] *S. pyogenes* also produces two haemolysins: streptolysins O and S. These are toxic to erythrocytes, granulocytes, and a variety of tissue culture cells. A number of other extracellular products may be important in tissue digestion and bacterial dissemination including proteinases, amylases, esterases, hyaluronidase, and streptokinase. The last of these promotes the dissolution of blood clots by activation of plasminogen.

CLINICAL FEATURES

The patient with preseptal cellulitis usually has an acute onset of unilateral pain, is febrile, and has periocular swelling and erythema. An eyelid abscess may be present. Orbital involvement is usually excluded by the absence of proptosis and normal motility, but radiographic studies are often performed.

In preseptal cellulitis following trauma, the clinical signs are most pronounced when the injury has occurred along the superior orbital rim (Fig. 60-1). The upper eyelid becomes edematous, and the swelling may extend to the eyebrow and forehead. Subcutaneous edema and hematoma predispose to abscess formation. The skin becomes taut and inflamed. It is often impossible to open the eyelids in severe cases. Pus may drain spontaneously from the wound. The lower eyelid of the infected eye or the periocular tissue of the other eye may also become swollen as the result of lymphoedema. In general, the patient is mildly feverish and has leukocytosis. If not involved in the injury, the globe will remain normal. Vision, pupillary reaction, motility, corneal sensation, and ophthalmoscopy are unaffected.[58] Orbital pain should not be present, whether the eye is in motion or at rest.

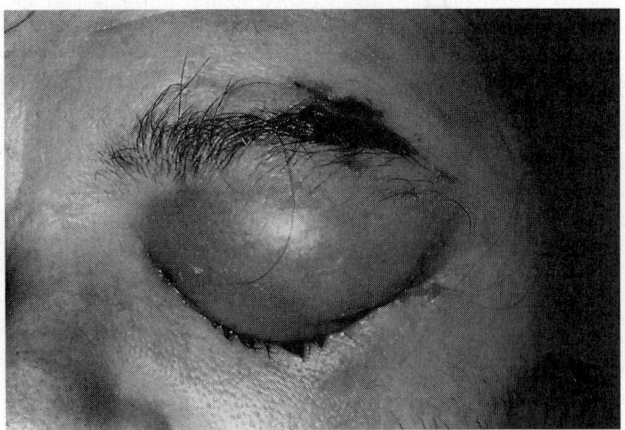

Fig. 60-1. Preseptal cellulitis in a 42-year-old man following a wound above the eyebrow. *S. aureus* and *S. pyogenes* were cultured from periorbital pus.

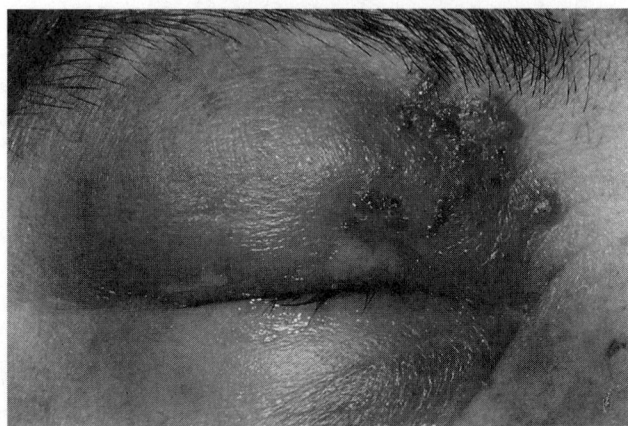

Fig. 60-2. Preseptal cellulitis in a 53-year-old woman as a complication of herpes simplex type 1 blepharoconjunctivitis. Both pustular and crusted vesicles are present. (Figure also in color insert.)

Preseptal cellulitis caused by impetigo is characterized by marked erythema of the eyelids, edema of the preseptal spaces, and vesicular rupture whereby a serous, purulent material is released. This dries to a thick, yellow crust. Regional lymphadenopathy is common. Fever and leukocytosis are usually mild. No clinical features distinguish staphylococcal and streptococcal infections in these cases.

In herpes simplex blepharodermatitis, preseptal cellulitis may develop during primary or recurrent disease. Eyelid vesicles progress to pustular and crusted stages (Fig. 60-2). In herpes zoster ophthalmicus, preseptal inflammation and edema can be severe (Fig. 60-3). Periorbital vesicles, usually confined to the upper eyelid and the medial and lateral canthal areas, are recognizable by the accompanying clinical findings.

Erysipelas is most common in very young children and in the elderly. Antecedent streptococcal respiratory tract infection occurs in about 30% of patients, but bacteria may no longer be recoverable by the time the skin lesion has devel-

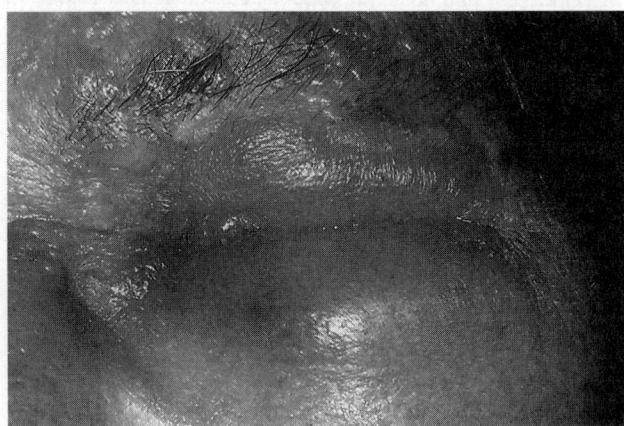

Fig. 60-3. Herpes zoster ophthalmicus in a 63-year-old man.

oped. The lesion begins as an elevated plaque that enlarges to sharply demarcated erythema with edema of the eyelids and associated pain and tenderness.[33] Vesicle formation is uncommon. There may be no demonstrable entry site. Orbital tissue often becomes involved; and the patient may show chemosis, mild proptosis, and limitation of motion. Presumably, these effects are caused by diffusion of toxins and an associated accumulation of pus rather than postseptal spread of streptococci. A temperature of up to 40° C (104° F), leukocytosis, chills, and malaise are common. Usually, a diagnosis can be made by recognizing typical skin lesions and finding preseptal cellulitis with orbital congestion.

Nonsuppurative preseptal cellulitis is characterized by tender, red-violet periorbital swelling and concurrent bacteremia.[2,10,48] Because of Hib, the disease is typically preceded by a mild upper respiratory tract infection. This progresses to unilateral hyperemia, chemosis, and eyelid edema with continuing fever and leukocytosis. A sharply demarcated,

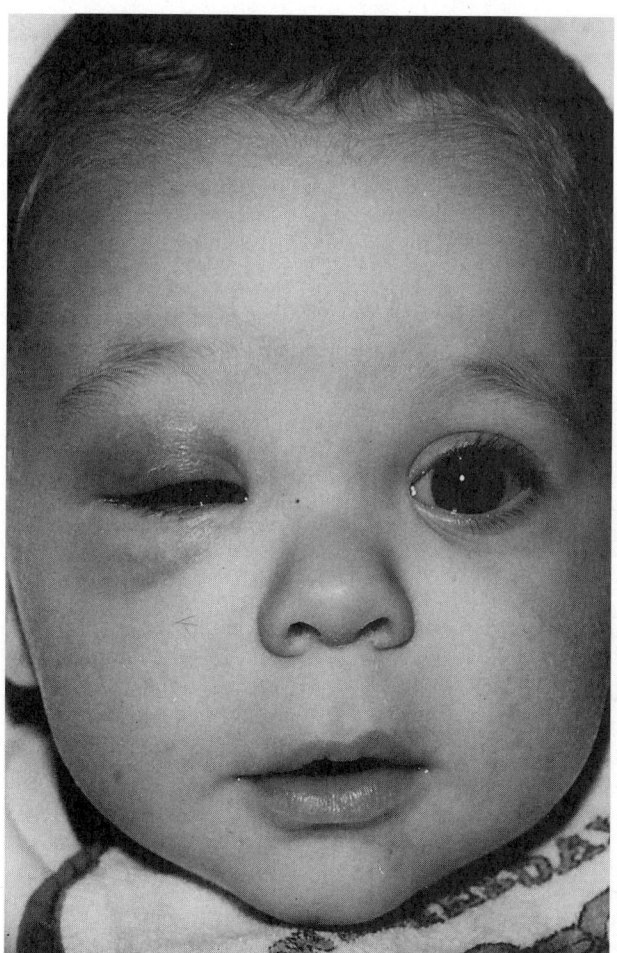

Fig. 60-4. Nonsuppurative preseptal cellulitis in a 7-month-old infant. *H. influenzae* type b was isolated from blood cultures. (Courtesy of Dr. Timothy Blackmore).

dark purple discoloration of the lids is characteristic (Fig. 60-4). The vision remains normal, and there is no orbital congestion. This entity should be distinguished from preseptal cellulitis secondary to severe bacterial or chlamydial conjunctivitis or adenoviral pharyngoconjunctival fever.[26] It is advisable to admit children under 5 years of age to the hospital, as a number of them will progress to meningitis[56] and other complications (such as subperiosteal abscess, which requires ethmoidectomy). Preseptal cellulitis with negative blood cultures is usually secondary to upper respiratory tract infection, whereas positive blood cultures are normally found in preseptal cellulitis secondary to sinusitis.

DIFFERENTIAL DIAGNOSIS

A number of conditions may be mistaken for preseptal cellulitis. These include eyelid lymphoma, dacryocystitis with secondary inflammation of the lids, angioneurotic edema, swelling secondary to bone marrow transplantation, allergy to atropine, contact allergies to topical medication, and acute myeloblastic leukemia.[24,27]

LABORATORY INVESTIGATIONS

In general, computerized tomography (CT) should be performed (1) in cases of posttraumatic preseptal cellulitis in which the septum has likely been penetrated, (2) in erysipelas, (3) as an aid to localize a foreign body, and (4) in patients with preseptal cellulitis in whom the globe cannot be examined. CT will also yield information on the extent of any sinus involvement. It is recommended that both axial and coronal views be obtained using thin (2.5 mm) cuts.[68] Orbital ultrasound and magnetic resonance imaging may then be considered, if additional information is required.

As in other ocular infections, the isolation of the causative organism and the determination of antibiotic susceptibility are important in the management of patients with preseptal cellulitis. Indeed, as the disease is periorbital and systemic treatment is advocated, the standard methods for antimicrobial susceptibility testing[4,55] are arguably more relevant to an agent's clinical effectiveness in this situation than for an anterior segment infection requiring topical treatment or an intraocular infection in general. If possible, specimens should be collected prior to commencement of antimicrobial therapy. Although the infectious agent can usually be isolated from periorbital pus, sampling from this region is contraindicated in some situations, and the organism may prove elusive. In the absence of pus, aspirates from periorbital soft tissue are of little value.

As drainage is part of the management of posttraumatic preseptal cellulitis, the exudate should be collected for microbiologic examination. Pus, collected with a sterile needle and syringe, is sent to the laboratory without delay. Routinely, a Gram stain is prepared and samples are assayed using agars and broths incubated both aerobically and anaerobically. For the cultivation of aerobes, a liquid medium (such as brain-heart infusion broth supplemented with nicotinamide adenine dinucleotide, hemin, and vitamin K[50]) and a chocolate agar plate are recommended. These media are suitable for the culture of the more fastidious bacteria and are incubated in 5% CO_2/air at 35° C. For the cultivation of anaerobes, cooked meat medium[50] and a blood agar plate are incubated at 35° C in an anaerobic chamber. After 48 hours, whether turbid or not, the broths should be subcultured onto agar.

For erysipelas or nonsuppurative preseptal cellulitis, needle aspiration of pus should be avoided because of the possibility of spreading the infection. Blood cultures may be useful in these cases to confirm the suspected clinical diagnoses of S. pyogenes and Hib respectively. The rate of a positive blood culture (which is more likely in young children) during preseptal cellulitis varies from 11% to 53%.[5,22] Serologic evidence of recent streptococcal infection by antideoxyribonuclease B assay or other methods may be helpful in erysipelas.[39] Latex particle agglutination for Hib capsular polysaccharide is a useful serologic assay.[64] For impetigo, material may be collected from the surface of denuded skin with a moist swab or, preferably, vesicle fluid may be collected with a dry swab. Blood and chocolate agar are inoculated, and a Gram stain is prepared. For confirmation of herpes simplex virus or varicella-zoster infection, the base of a new vesicle may be scraped for viral culture or a rapid detection assay.

THERAPY

For preseptal cellulitis following trauma, the important steps in treatment are skin incision, drainage, and systemic antibiotics based on the Gram stain and culture. The patient will probably require hospitalization. Tetanus prophylaxis should be considered, depending on the patient's immunization history. The skin incision may be performed in the clinic, although general anaesthesia is usually necessary with children. Local infiltrative anaesthesia should not be used. The skin is swabbed with a povidone-iodine preparation. The site of incision should be along the lateral third of the superior orbital rim.[33]

The choice of antibiotic depends on the initial suspicion of a particular organism, any subsequent isolation and susceptibility tests, and the clinical course. Antibiotics are usually given for 7 to 10 days or until the suppuration has waned. Oral administration may be substituted for intravenous treatment after 2 to 3 days if the patient is improving. An adult can be given outpatient treatment with oral antibiotics but must be considered as having a low threshold for hospital admission. Recommended agents are given in Table 60-2.

An appropriate antibiotic for severe preseptal cellulitis caused by S. aureus is intravenous flucloxacillin. If the patient is allergic to penicillin, intravenous cephalothin may be substituted. If there is a history of severe penicillin hypersensitivity, intravenous vancomycin by slow (2-hour) infusion should be used. In less severe cases of S. aureus preseptal cellulitis, oral flucloxacillin or cephalexin may be given. For severe preseptal cellulitis caused by S. pyogenes, intravenous benzylpenicillin is the treatment of choice. In less severe cases, intramuscular procaine penicillin or oral phenoxymethylpenicillin can be used. Erysipelas may require several weeks to resolve. In penicillin-sensitive patients, cephalothin or vancomycin may be administered as for S. aureus. If obligate anaerobic bacteria are isolated or suspected, intravenous benzylpenicillin, chloramphenicol, or cefuroxime is recommended. Any patient who does not improve after 2 to 3 days of supposedly appropriate antibiotics should have the drainage and exploration of the area repeated. A hot compress helps to localize the inflammation. A CT scan is advisable to examine for sinusitis, progression of inflammation to the orbit, or noninfectious causes of preseptal cellulitis such as retinoblastoma, rhabdomyosarcoma, and inflammatory pseudotumor. If sinusitis is present, nasal decongestants and vasoconstrictors help the drainage of paranasal sinuses.

For impetigo, the lesions should be washed two or three times a day with soap and water and treated with a topical antibiotic ointment such as bacitracin 0.5% or ciprofloxacin 0.3%. An antiseptic agent such as chlorhexidine or povidone-iodine may be preferred. In severe cases requiring a systemic antimicrobial agent, a 10-day course of oral flucloxacillin or erythromycin is suitable.

The skin lesions of herpes simplex preseptal infection can be treated with 3% vidarabine or 5% acyclovir ointment. The skin lesions of varicella-zoster ophthalmicus may be benefited by a moisturizing cream or ointment. In immunocompetent patients, a 10-day course of oral acyclovir is useful if started within 3 days of the onset of skin lesions. Immunodeficient patients may require hospitalization and intravenous acyclovir by slow (1-hour) infusion.

Because of the risk of meningitis, young children with nonsuppurative preseptal cellulitis should be hospitalized. The selection of an initial antibiotic is based on the likelihood that the causative organism is Hib. Suggested agents are a third-generation cephalosporin, for example, cefotaxime or ceftriaxone. The total duration of treatment should be 7 to 10 days. These agents cross the blood-brain barrier effectively. Another option is chloramphenicol.[21] An assay of serum chloramphenicol concentration should be considered in high-dosage treatment regimens to avoid dose-related toxicity. These regimens will also cover other organisms implicated in nonsuppurative preseptal infection: S. pneumoniae, S. aureus, and S. pyogenes. If pneumococci are identified, amoxicillin is preferred. Mild pneumococcal infection in older children can be treated with oral cotrimoxazole or a cephalosporin.

TABLE 60-2 DOSAGES OF ANTIMICROBIAL AGENTS USED IN THE SYSTEMIC TREATMENT OF PRESEPTAL CELLULITIS

Antimicrobial Agent	Route of Administration	Dosage		
		Neonates	Children	Adults
Acyclovir	Oral	—	—	0.2-0.8 g, 4-hourly while awake
	I.V.*	—	—	5-10 mg/kg, 8-hourly
Amoxicillin	I.V.	Not recommended	25-50 mg/kg/day, 6-hourly	—
Benzylpenicillin	I.V.	$50\text{-}150 \times 10^3$ U/kg/day, 8 to 12-hourly	$100\text{-}250 \times 10^3$ U/kg/day, 2 to 12-hourly	$1.2\text{-}2.4 \times 10^6$ U/day, 2 to 12-hourly
Cefotaxime	I.V.	25-50 mg/kg, 12-hourly	50-180 mg/kg/day, 4 to 6-hourly	—
Ceftriaxone	I.V.	50 mg/kg/day	50-100 mg/kg/day, 12-hourly	—
Cefuroxime	I.V.	—	50-240 mg/kg/day, 6 to 8-hourly	0.75-1.5 g, 8-hourly
Cephalexin	Oral	—	6.25-25 mg/kg, 6-hourly	0.25-1 g, 6-hourly
Cephalothin	I.V.	40 mg/kg/day, 8 to 12-hourly	75-160 mg/kg/day, 4 to 6-hourly	0.5-2 g, 4 to 6-hourly
Chloramphenicol	I.V.	25 mg/kg/day	12.5-25 mg/kg, 6-hourly	12.5-25 mg/kg, 6-hourly
Cotrimoxazole	Oral, I.V.	—	4-5 mg/kg, 6 to 12-hourly	—
Erythromycin	Oral	—	7.5-12.5 mg/kg, 6-hourly	250-500 mg, 6-hourly
Flucloxacillin	Oral	Not recommended	12.5-25 mg/kg, 6-hourly	0.5-1 g, 6-hourly
	I.V.	Not recommended	75-160 mg/kg/day, 4 to 6-hourly	0.5-2 g, 4 to 6-hourly
Phenoxymethyl-penicillin	Oral	—	6.25-12.5 mg/kg, 6-hourly	250-500 mg, 6-hourly
Procaine penicilin G	I.M.†	—	25×10^3 U/kg, 12 to 24-hourly	$0.3\text{-}4.8 \times 10^6$ U/day
Vancomycin	I.V.	15 mg/kg, 12-hourly	10 mg/kg, 6-hourly	15 mg/kg, 12-hourly

* I.V., intravenous
† I.M., intramuscular
Based on the tables of Norris S, Nightingale CH, Mandell GL: Tables of antimicrobial agent pharmacology. In Mandell GL, Douglas Jr RG, Bennett JE, editors: *Principles and practice of infectious diseases,* ed 3, New York, 1990, Churchill Livingstone.

PREVENTION

As preseptal cellulitis has a number of causes and its occurrence is often related to economic status, it is not a problem that will disappear in the near future. The continued development of bacterial vaccines and their effective delivery to children will impact on the incidence of preseptal infection, however. A new vaccine for Hib has recently become available, vaccines for *S. pneumoniae* are being improved, and the search for a group A streptococcal vaccine is continuing.

The Hib vaccine consists of capsular polyribophosphate conjugated with diphtheria toxoid. This is recommended for children at 18 months of age.[12]

The currently used multivalent pneumococcal vaccine consisting of capsular polysaccharides of 23 serotypes is not particularly effective in young children, with the exception of certain high-risk populations.[53] A strategy of broadening the serotypic base of the vaccine and combining the immunogens with a carrier protein (as for the Hib vaccine) to improve responses in children, is promising but not yet vindicated.[23]

The continuing problem of rheumatic fever is spurring research toward a group A streptococcal vaccine. Two major problems must be overcome, however, to achieve the goal of developing an M protein-based vaccine, known to be the major protective antigen.[36] These are (1) the serologic diversity of the protein and (2) its ability to elicit antibodies that are cross-reactive with host tissue and are believed to induce poststreptococcal autoimmune diseases.[62]

Vaccines are expected to decrease the incidence of invasive bacterial infections such as preseptal cellulitis in children. It will be interesting to see what effect the new vaccines have on the incidence of ocular infections such as conjunctivitis and keratitis. Neonates and infants too young to be vaccinated should also benefit from a decreased pool of pathogenic bacteria in older children.

REFERENCES

1. Alexander HE, Heidelberger M, Leidy G: The protective or curative element in type b *H. influenzae* rabbit serum, *Yale J Biol Med* 16:425-434, 1944.
2. Baker RC, Bausher JC: Meningitis complicating acute bacteremic facial cellulitis, *Pediatr Infect Dis J* 5:421-423, 1986.
3. Ballou LR: Sphingolipids and cell function, *Immunol Today* 13:339-341, 1992.
4. Barry AL, Thornsberry C: Susceptibility tests: diffusion test procedures. In Balows A et al., editors: *Manual of clinical microbiology,* ed 5, Washington DC, 1991, American Society for Microbiology.
5. Barson WJ et al.: Cefuroxime therapy for bacteremic soft-tissue infections in children, *Am J Dis Child* 139:1141-1144, 1985.
6. Beachey EH, Ofek I: Epithelial cell binding of group A streptococci by lipoteichoic acid on fimbriae denuded of M protein, *J Exp Med* 143:759-771, 1976.
7. Bessen D, Fischetti V: Nucleotide sequences of two adjacent M or M-like protein genes of group A streptococci: different RNA transcript levels and identification of a unique immunoglobulin A-binding protein, *Infect Immun* 60:124-135, 1992.
8. Braun MA et al.: Stimulation of human T cells by streptococcal "superantigen" erythrogenic toxins (scarlet fever toxins), *J Immunol* 150:2457-2466, 1993.
9. Chanyangam M et al.: Contribution of a 28-kilodalton membrane protein to the virulence of *Haemophilus influenzae, Infect Immun* 59:600-608, 1991.
10. Chartrand SA, Harrison CJ: Buccal cellulitis reevaluated, *Am J Dis Child* 140:891-893, 1986.
11. Coleman DC et al.: Cloning and expression in *Escherichia coli* and *Staphylococcus aureus* of the beta-lysin determinant from *Staphylococcus aureus:* evidence that bacteriophage conversion of beta-lysin activity is caused by insertional inactivation of the beta-lysin determinant, *Microb Pathog* 1:549-564, 1986.
12. Committee on Infectious Diseases: *Haemophilus influenzae* type b conjugate vaccine, *Pediatrics* 81:908-911, 1988.
13. Cooney J et al.: The gamma-hemolysin locus of *Staphylococcus aureus* comprises three linked genes, two of which are identical to the genes for the F and S components of leukocidin, *Infect Immun* 61:768-771, 1993.
14. Cribier B et al.: *Staphylococcus aureus* leukocidin: a new virulence factor in cutaneous infections: an epidemiological and experimental study, *Dermatology* 185:175-180, 1992.
15. Dajani AS, Asmar BI, Thirmoorthi MC: Systemic *Haemophilus influenzae* disease: an overview, *J Pediatr* 94:355-364, 1979.
16. Doxanas MT, Anderson RL: Oriental eyelids: an anatomic study, *Arch Ophthalmol* 102:1232-1235, 1984.
17. Eustis HS et al.: Staging of orbital cellulitis in children: computerized tomography characteristics and treatment guidelines, *J Pediatr Ophthalmol Strabismus* 23:246-251, 1986.
18. Ferson MJ, Shi E: Periorbital cellulitis with meningococcal bacteremia, *Pediatr Infect Dis J* 7:600-601, 1988.
19. Forsgren A, Sjöquist J: "Protein A" from *S. aureus.* I. Pseudo-immune reaction with human γ-globulin, *J Immunol* 97:822-827, 1966.
20. Fothergill LD, Wright J: Influenzal meningitis: the relationship of age incidence to the bactericidal power of blood against causal organism, *J Immunol* 24:273-284, 1933.
21. Gans LA, Shackelford PG: Ocular infections. In Feigin RD, Cherry JD, editors: *Textbook of pediatric infectious diseases,* ed 2, Philadelphia, 1987, WB Saunders.
22. Gellady AM, Shulman ST, Ayoub EM: Periorbital and orbital cellulitis in children, *Pediatrics* 61:272-277, 1978.
23. Giebink GS et al.: Pneumococcal capsular polysaccharide-meningococcal outer membrane protein complex conjugate vaccine: immunogenicity and efficacy in experimental pneumococcal otitis media, *J Infect Dis* 167:347-355, 1993.
24. Grossniklaus HE, Wojno TH: Leukemic infiltrate appearing as periorbital cellulitis, *Arch Ophthalmol* 108:484, 1990.
25. Hensler T et al.: *Staphylococcus aureus* toxic shock syndrome toxin 1 and *Streptococcus pyogenes* erythrogenic toxin A modulate inflammatory mediator release from human neutrophils, *Infect Immun* 61:1055-1061, 1993.
26. Herman J, Katzuni E: Periorbital cellulitis complicating adenovirus infection, *Am J Dis Child* 140:745, 1986 (letter).
27. Hirst LW: Ocular and periocular infections. In *Sights and sounds in ophthalmology,* vol 6, A slide-tape presentation of the Wilmer Institute, St Louis, 1985, Mosby.
28. Israele V, Nelson JD: Periorbital and orbital cellulitis, *Pediatr Infect Dis J* 6:404-410, 1987.
29. Jackson K, Baker SR: Clinical implications of orbital cellulitis, *Laryngoscope* 96:568-574, 1986.
30. Jackson K, Baker SR: Periorbital cellulitis, *Head Neck Surg* 9:227-234, 1987.
31. Johnson MK et al.: Confirmation of the role of pneumolysin in ocular infections with *Streptococcus pneumoniae, Curr Eye Res* 11:1221-1225, 1992.
32. Jones DB, Steinkuller PG: Strategies for the initial management of acute preseptal and orbital cellulitis, *Trans Am Ophthalmol Soc* 86:94-108, 1988.
33. Jones DB, Steinkuller PG: Microbial preseptal and orbital cellulitis. In Tasman W, Jaeger EA, editors: *Duane's clinical ophthalmology,* Philadelphia, 1992, JB Lippincott.
34. Kanzaki H, Arata J: Role of fibronectin in the adherence of *Staphylococcus aureus* to dermal tissues, *J Dermatol Sci* 4:87-94, 1992.
35. Kaplan MH, Tenenbaum MJ: *Staphylococcus aureus:* cellular biology and clinical application, *Am J Med* 72:248-258, 1982.
36. Kehoe MA: Group A streptococcal antigens and vaccine potential, *Vaccine* 9:797-806, 1991.
37. Last RJ: *Eugene Wolff's anatomy of the eye and orbit,* ed 6, London, 1968, HK Lewis and Co.
38. Lee JC et al.: Virulence studies, in mice, of transposon-induced mutants of *Staphylococcus aureus* differing in capsule size, *J Infect Dis* 156:741-750, 1987.
39. Leppard BJ et al.: The value of bacteriology and serology in the diagnosis of cellulitis and erysipelas, *Br J Dermatol* 112:559-567, 1985.
40. Linder TE, Lim DJ, DeMaria TF: Changes in the structure of the cell surface carbohydrates of the chinchilla tubotympanum following *Streptococcus pneumoniae*-induced otitis media, *Microb Pathog* 13:293-303, 1992.
41. Lyell A: The staphylococcal scalded skin syndrome in historical perspective: emergence of dermopathic strains of *Staphylococcus aureus* and discovery of the epidermolytic toxin, *J Am Acad Dermatol* 9:285-294, 1983.
42. Mandell GL: Catalase, superoxide dismutase, and virulence of *Staphylococcus aureus:* in vitro and in vivo studies with emphasis on staphylococcal-leukocyte interaction, *J Clin Invest* 55:561-566, 1975.
43. Menestrina G et al.: Structural features of the pore formed by *Staphylococcus aureus* alpha-toxin inferred from chemical modification and primary structure analysis, *FEMS Microbiol Immunol* 5:19-28, 1992.
44. Mims CA: *The pathogenesis of infectious disease,* ed 3, London, 1987, Academic Press.
45. Molarte AB, Isenberg SJ: Periorbital cellulitis in infancy, *J Pediatr Ophthalmol Strab* 26:232-234, 1989.
46. Möllby R: Isolation and properties of membrane damaging toxins. In Easmon CSF, Adlam C, editors: *Staphylococci and staphylococcal infections,* vol 2, London, 1983, Academic Press.
47. Moscona R, Ullmann Y, Peled I: Necrotizing periorbital cellulitis following septorhinoplasty, *Aesthetic Plast Surg* 15:187-190, 1991.
48. Nelson JD, Ginsburg CM: An hypothesis on the pathogenesis of *Haemophilus influenzae* buccal cellulitis, *J Pediatr* 88:709-710, 1976.

49. Noel LP, Clarke WN, Peacocke TA: Periorbital and orbital cellulitis in childhood, *Can J Ophthalmol* 16:178-180, 1981.
50. *The Oxoid manual,* ed 6, Basingstoke, England, 1990, Unipath.
51. Pichichero ME: Adherence of *Haemophilus influenzae* to human buccal and pharyngeal epithelial cells: relationship to piliation, *J Med Microbiol* 18:107-116, 1984.
52. Pittman M: Variation and type specificity in the bacterial species *Haemophilus influenzae, J Exp Med* 53:471-492, 1931.
53. Riley ID et al.: Pneumococcal vaccine prevents death from acute lower-respiratory-tract infections in Papua New Guinean children, *Lancet* 2:877-881, 1986.
54. Robinson JH, Kehoe MA: Group A streptococcal M proteins: virulence factors and protective antigens, *Immunol Today* 13:362-367, 1992.
55. Sahm DF, Washington JA II: Antibacterial susceptibility tests: dilution methods. In Balows A et al., editors: *Manual of clinical microbiology,* ed 5, Washington DC, 1991, American Society for Microbiology.
56. Sankrithi UM, LiPuma JJ: Clinically inapparent meningitis complicating periorbital cellulitis, *Pediatr Emerg Care* 7:28-29, 1991.
57. Schneerson R, Robbins JB: Induction of serum *Haemophilus influenzae* type b capsular antibodies in adult volunteers fed cross-reacting *Escherichia coli* 075.K.100.H5, *New Eng J Med* 292:1093-1096, 1975.
58. Sinnott JT, Rodnite JA, Ruland RT: Is this orbital or periorbital cellulitis, *Postgrad Med* 85:267-269, 1989.
59. Smeltzer MS, Hart ME, Iandolo JJ: Quantitative spectrophotometric assay for staphylococcal lipase, *Appl Environ Microbiol* 58:2815-2819, 1992.
60. Spires JR, Smith RJ: Bacterial infections of the orbital and periorbital soft-tissues in children, *Laryngoscope* 96:763-767, 1986.
61. Steiner B, Cruce D: A zymographic assay for detection of hyaluronidase activity on polyacrylamide gels and its application to enzymatic activity found in bacteria, *Anal Biochem* 200:405-410, 1992.
62. Stollerman GH: Rheumatogenic streptococci and autoimmunity, *Clin Immunol Immunopathol* 61:131-142, 1991.
63. Vishniakova LA, Reztsova IuV: The virulence of *Streptococcus pneumoniae* strains-the causative agents of pneumococcal infection at different sites, *Zh Mikrobiol Epidemiol Immunobiol* 9:26-29, 1992.
64. Ward JI et al.: Rapid diagnosis of *Haemophilus influenzae* type b infections by latex particle agglutination and counterimmunoelectrophoresis, *J Pediatr* 93:37-42, 1978.
65. Watters EC et al.: Acute orbital cellulitis, *Arch Ophthalmol* 94:785-788, 1976.
66. Weiss A et al.: Bacterial orbital and periorbital cellulitis in childhood, *Ophthalmology* 90:195-203, 1983.
67. Weizman Z, Mussaffi H: Ethmoiditis-associated periorbital cellulitis, *Int J Pediatr Otorhinolaryngol* 11:147-151, 1986.
68. Westfall CT, Shore JW, Sullivan Baker A: Orbital infections. In Gorbach SL, Bartlett JG, Blacklow NR, editors: *Infectious diseases,* Philadelphia, 1992, WB Saunders.
69. Woods DE et al.: Role of salivary protease activity in adherence of gram-negative bacilli to mammalian buccal epithelial cells *in vivo, J Clin Invest* 68:1435-1440, 1981.
70. Zwahlen A et al.: The molecular basis of pathogenicity in *Haemophilus influenzae:* comparative virulence of genetically-related capsular transformants and correlation with changes at the capsulation locus cap, *Microb Pathog* 7:225-235, 1989.

61 Staphylococcal Blepharitis

DAVID V. SEAL, LINDA A. FICKER, PETER WRIGHT

Staphylococcal blepharitis is a common disease affecting the anterior eyelid margin. Predisposing factors are incompletely understood but involve chronic bacterial colonization and immunologic susceptibility.

HISTORICAL BACKGROUND

Staphylococcal blepharitis has a long history, summarized in a review of blepharitis in 1929.[3]

Besides staphylococcal infection, alternative causes have included allergy, seborrhea, vitamin deficiency, and endocrine disorders. In an effort to establish the clinical features and cause of blepharitis, during the 1940s Thygeson studied a large cohort of otherwise healthy young soldiers.[37,38] This research resulted in the classification of blepharitis into three major clinical groups: staphylococcal, seborrheic, and diplobacillary. Thygeson found that, of consecutive cases of blepharitis, there were ulcerative and nonulcerative forms corresponding to staphylococcal and seborrheic types (Table 61-1), with many patients exhibiting mixed staphylococcal and seborrheic features. There was a strong association between microbial colonization and clinical features: coagulase-positive staphylococci with ulcerative disease, *Pityrosporum ovale* with nonulcerative disease, and both organisms with the "mixed picture." Staphylococcal blepharitis was different from meibomian gland dysfunction.

Thygeson defined staphylococcal blepharitis as chronic inflammation of the lids with colonization by large numbers of *Staphylococcus aureus* and *Staphylococcus albus*. The presence of both gram-positive cocci and polymorphonuclear leukocytes in lid margin smears was a reliable indicator of the disease. Although normal lid margins were colonized by pathogenic staphylococci in up to 10% of cases, only a few colonies grew on culture plates; and confluent growth on agar was typical of patients with blepharitis. Thygeson stressed the importance of biomicroscopic examination of the eyelids in cases of chronic conjunctivitis.

The association between clinical disease and colonization by large numbers of *S. aureus* resulted in the introduction of antibiotic therapy for this disorder. In an uncontrolled clinical study, treatment with a topical steroid-antibiotic preparation was usually effective, but long-standing disease was less responsive.[40] The observation that early disease was more easily treated was not readily explained, but immunologic studies were later to reveal the importance of exposure to staphylococcal antigens, as may occur during lid colonization. Steroid was included to suppress the frequently associated keratitis, including superficial punctate keratopathy and marginal infiltrates. The infiltrates were sterile and presumed to be an immunologic response to the presence of staphylococci.

Experimental Studies

The concept of staphylococcal blepharitis was supported by immunologic studies that linked lid and corneal inflammation to the presence of *S. aureus*. Cell-mediated immunity as the mechanism for hypersensitivity to *S. aureus* provided an immunologic explanation for the ocular surface manifestations of staphylococcal blepharitis.[15,29] Exposure to relatively small numbers of bacteria in the rabbit was demonstrated to have the potential for generating an amplified inflammatory response.

The observation that some patients with staphylococcal blepharitis developed phlyctenular keratoconjunctivitis further implicated the immune system in this disease.[28,39] These individuals gave a strong positive skin reaction to staphylococcal toxoid, but were tuberculin-negative and seemed to improve by desensitization using the toxoid. Corneal infiltration could be elicited by the intracorneal injection of staphylococcal cell-wall antigen in rabbits that were immunized subcutaneously with *S. aureus*,[14] although this was not a true model of disease.

Mondino[23,25] was the first to create experimental models of marginal keratitis and ulcerative staphylococcal blepharitis by exploiting cell-mediated immunity. Marginal infiltrates and ulcerative blepharitis occurred, providing there had been immunization followed by topical exposure to via-

TABLE 61-1 THYGESON'S CLASSIFICATION OF STAPHYLOCOCCAL AND SEBORRHEIC BLEPHARITIS

Characteristic	Staphylococcal	Seborrheic
Presence of seborrhea	Occasional	Always
Associated dermatoses	Rosacea, impetigo	Seborrheic dermatitis of brows and external ear
Site	Unilateral or bilateral	Bilateral
Ulceration of lid margin	Frequent	Absent
Stye	Frequent	Rare
Associated conjunctivitis	Frequent	Minimal or absent
Associated keratitis	Punctate epithelial erosions Marginal infiltrates and ulcers common	Absent
Scales and crusting	Hard, tenacious	Greasy
	Removed with difficulty	Easily removed
Microbiology of lid margin	*Staphylococcus aureus*	*Pityrosporum ovale*

ble *S. aureus*. This finding supported the importance of *S. aureus* in the pathogenesis of blepharitis and its sequelae. It was also consistent with the recurrent nature of the clinical disease and the observation that *S. aureus* are intermittent colonizers of the lid margin.

Classification Schemes

The classification of blepharitis has been revised with the introduction of new investigative methods. McCulley[20] classified patients with chronic blepharitis into six subgroups that included Thygeson's staphylococcal, seborrheic, and mixed staphylococcal/seborrheic groups. In addition, he further identified three subgroups of meibomian dysfunction: seborrheic with meibomian seborrhea, seborrhea with meibomitis, and meibomitis alone. These latter groups were characterized by excessive meibomian secretion and inflamed meibomian orifices that were plugged in some cases. Patients with staphylococcal blepharitis were more frequently colonized by *S. aureus* than both normals and patients with meibomian gland dysfunction. The original observations made by Thygeson were essentially unchanged as *S. aureus* colonization was dissociated from meibomian disease.

Whether different forms of blepharitis are distinct entities or represent a continuum is controversial. The in vitro lipolytic activity of some staphylococci includes the ability to hydrolyse cholesteryl oleate and behenyl oleate.[8,9] Thus alterations of meibomian secretion by staphylococci can mimic some of the features of meibomian gland dysfunction. The associated tear-film instability could explain the symptoms of burning and dryness typical of patients with staphylococcal blepharitis.

Staphylococcal blepharitis is now considered a subgroup of the blepharitides associated with cell-mediated immunity.

Although coagulase-negative staphylococcal strains have the potential to alter the tear film and to generate symptoms related to meibomian gland dysfunction, this is a distinct entity that should not be confused with staphylococcal blepharitis.

EPIDEMIOLOGY

S. aureus colonizes the nares, axillary and perineal skin, and the gastrointestinal tract. This colonization is transient so that, at any one time, approximately one third of the normal population will be colonized at one of these sites, thereby providing sources for recolonization of other sites. The skin, lids, and nares are permanently colonized with *S. aureus* in 70% of atopic patients.

In the normal population, staphylococci on the lid margin do not usually result in disease, and their presence remains subclinical. For the individual with enhanced cell-mediated immunity to the organism there is a greater likelihood of local inflammation. Although cross-infection with *S. aureus* is not recognized in patients with blepharitis, repeated infection by *S. aureus* may be acquired either from the patient's own flora or from other colonized individuals.

Coagulase-negative staphylococci constitute part of the resident bacterial flora of the skin, including that of the eyelid margin. The pathogenic role of these staphylococci is therefore difficult to assess. Resistant strains occur with selective pressure by intensive use of antibiotics. A consequence of permanent colonization is that eradication with antibiotics usually fails. Resistant strains also occur in patients on long-term antibiotic treatment for blepharitis.

Risk Factors

S. aureus colonization of the lid margin has been quantified for normal volunteers using soluble alginate swabs.[4] *S.*

TABLE 61-2 MICROBIOLOGY OF STAPHYLOCOCCI AND MICROCOCCI

	Staphylococci						Micrococci	
	I	II	III	IV	V	VI	1–4	5–8
Growth on 7.5 percent salt	+	+	+	+	+	+	+	+
Anaerobic growth	+ +	+ +	+ +	+ +	+ +	+ +	+/−	+/−
Coagulase/Staphaurex	+	−	−	−	−	−	−	−
Novobiocin	S	S	S	S	S	S	R	S
Voges-Prausker (tube test)	+	+	−	+	+	+	+	−
Phosphatase (plate)	+	+	+	−	−	−	−	(V)
Mannitol (plate)	+	−	(+)*	−	−	+	(V)	(V)
Lactose (tube)	.	.	.	−	+	(V)†	.	.
Maltose (tube)	.	.	.	.	.	(V)	.	.

	VI (1)	VI (2)	VI (3)
Lactose	+	−	−
Maltose	+	+	−

* (+) = occasionally positive.
† (V) = variable.

aureus counts greater than 15 colony-forming units/ml swab eluate are considered greater than normal. The expected number of coagulase-negative staphylococci colonizing the normal lid margin has also been assessed in normal volunteers using soluble alginate swabs.[4] These staphylococci were isolated from 88% of lid margins in numbers up to 100 colony-forming units/ml swab eluate. Values greater than 1000 colony-forming units/ml swab eluate are considered greater than normal for coagulase-negative staphylococci.

In acute lid folliculitis, *S. aureus* are isolated in numbers between 45 and 400 colony-forming units/ml swab eluate, indicating active infection.[10] Semiquantitative lid "scrub" cultures yield a "heavy" growth of *S. aureus* on standard solid agar. In chronic blepharitis, *S. aureus* is not necessarily isolated from the lid margin in numbers greater than normal. Such observations need to be considered in relation to the patient's disease, in particular the presence of marginal keratitis and whether topical antibiotic therapy is being used.

Bacterial isolates are often identified biochemically using a simplified version (Table 61-2) of the Baird-Parker scheme[5,33] devised for ocular staphylococci. An alternative biochemical identification system, adopted by manufacturers of kit tests, is based on the Kloos and Schleifer scheme[17] but does not differentiate staphylococci from micrococci. Isolates have not been successfully correlated with pathogenicity for ocular infection using the Kloos scheme.

Using a "lid scrub method" and the modified Baird-Parker identification scheme, the normal distribution of coagulase-negative staphylococcal strains was found to be 74% type II/III, 14% type IV/V, and 5% type VI.[31] This was repeated with the "soluble swab method" in different volunteers, with results of 74% II/III, 11% IV/V, and 3% VI for staphylococci and 9% for micrococci.[4] For chronic blepha-ritis of mixed cause, coagulase-negative staphylococci were isolated from 63% of the patients using the soluble swab method, and there was a type distribution of 70% II/III, 17% IV/V, and 4% VI among staphylococci and 6% micrococci.[33] This distribution suggests that there are no particular biotypes of coagulase-negative staphylococci associated with chronic blepharitis.

Other studies comparing the lid flora of normal controls with patients suffering from chronic blepharitis of mixed cause show that coagulase-negative staphylococci are isolated from 90% of normal lids and from 95% of lids of blepharitic patients classified clinically as staphylococcal, seborrheic, or meibomian dysfunction.[7,13] The proportions of various colony types do not differ between the patients and normals, but higher counts of coagulase-negative staphylococci and *Propionibacterium acnes* are sometimes found on the lids of patients with blepharitis of mixed cause than on controls.[13]

PATHOGENESIS

Staphylococcal Toxins

Toxin production by *S. aureus* has been investigated as a possible cause of blepharitis.[2,32,42] Alpha-lysin, the most lethal staphylococcal toxin, is produced by all isolates of *S. aureus,* including those colonizing the lids of normal, atopic, and blepharitic patients. It is not produced by coagulase-negative staphylococci. Isolates vary in the quantity of alpha-lysin they produce in the laboratory. Alpha-lysin has membrane-damaging activity and is a potent inducer of acute inflammation, resulting in tissue necrosis and smooth muscle paralysis (including capillary vessel walls).[11] It is lethal when injected intravenously into laboratory animals.[6]

It appears unlikely that production of alpha-lysin by *S. aureus* is the principal cause of blepharitis.

Other *S. aureus* toxins include beta- and delta-lysins, which are much less cytotoxic. Different isolates of *S. aureus* produce various combinations of toxins. A recent study showed 12% of isolates from blepharitic lids produced alpha-lysin alone, 41% alpha- and beta-lysins, and 47% alpha-, beta- and delta-lysins.[32] This compares with 10% of isolates from normals producing delta-lysin. The increased likelihood of delta-lysin production with bacterial keratitis and in sepsis is interesting, but its precise role in suppuration is not clear.[1]

Lipase is produced by *S. aureus,* cultured from the lids of normal volunteers and of patients with chronic blepharitis of mixed cause.[8] All isolates hydrolyze triolein, behenyl, and cholesteryl oleate, and there is no difference between isolates from normals and those with blepharitis.

Toxins of *S. epidermidis* have also been incriminated in blepharitis.[42] Dermonecrosis toxin, different from *S. aureus* alpha-lysin, is detected in isolates from blepharitis patients—but not from controls. Another toxin has also been described.[32] A role for hemolytic toxin production or lipase production[8] by *S. epidermidis* has not been identified as a cause of blepharitis.

Staphylococcal Cell-Wall Antigenicity

Isolates of *S. aureus* vary in the production of cell-wall protein A.[27] This protein has a molecular weight of 42,000 daltons and is composed of an alpha-helix (31%), a beta structure (16%), and a random coil (53%). Although protein A is of pathogenic significance and binds nonspecifically to antibody at the F_c site, it may not always play a role in disease.[41] Approximately 10% of *S. aureus* isolates from blepharitic lids lack protein A, and coagulase-negative staphylococci and micrococci have never been found to produce cell-wall protein A.

S. aureus and coagulase-negative staphylococci have a cell-wall structure that includes repeating peptidoglycan units together with teichoic acid.[27] For *S. aureus,* this teichoic acid contains ribitol, and that of coagulase-negative staphylococci contains glycerol. Micrococci contain two teichoic acids and a mixture of both sugars.

Cellular and Humoral Immunity

Cell-mediated immunity to *S. aureus* was first demonstrated in 1929 by dermal immunization of rabbits.[29] After repeated challenge, the inflammatory effect of a large subcutaneous inoculum of *S. aureus* was considerably reduced, but inocula diluted 100-fold and 1000-fold gave rise to inflammatory skin lesions where no such effect had occurred prior to challenge.

This mechanism of delayed hypersensitivity to *S. aureus* was further shown by passive transfer. Homogenized spleen cells transferred staphylococcal cell-mediated immunity to normal rabbits with negative skin tests.[15] Furthermore, rabbits with cell-mediated immunity to *S. aureus* have an increased susceptibility to, and mortality from, intravenous challenge.[15]

Dermal immunization to *S. aureus* is ineffective in establishing cell-mediated immunity within the anterior chamber of the eye. Although more severe infections are elicited by inoculating *S. aureus* into the knee joints of sensitized animals than in controls without cell-mediated immunity, no such differences were found by anterior-chamber challenge.[16] By contrast, corneal infiltrates are elicited in immunized rabbits by injection of staphylococcal cell-wall antigen into the corneal stroma.[14]

Phlyctenules and corneal infiltrates can be produced in rabbits previously immunized with either whole cells of *S. aureus* or with cell-wall ribitol teichoic acid.[24,25] Topical application of viable *S. aureus* six times daily for five weeks resulted in corneal vascularization and elevated nodular infiltrates, often separated from the limbus by a clear zone. By modifying the interval between immunization and challenge, acute ulcerative blepharitis could be produced in the same model.[23] Rabbits developed crusting around the lashes with lash loss and chronic corneal infiltrates, but retained normal meibomian glands.

Similar experiments with coagulase-negative staphylococci resulted in cell-mediated immunity being gained in the rabbit, but acute ulcerative blepharitis could not be produced.[21] This finding suggests that *S. aureus* protein A may be the antigenic determinant for the cell-mediated immune response causing acute disease.

Studies of animal models have shown that the clinical features of *S. aureus* blepharitis and associated corneal disease do not occur in the absence of cell-mediated immunity. When this immunity is induced by *S. aureus* in the rabbit, humoral immunity is manifested by the production of IgG antibodies to cell-wall ribitol teichoic acid.[22] Such IgG antibody diffuses from serum into the cornea at a low titer and with an even lower titer in tears.

After subconjunctival immunization of the rabbit with *S. aureus* cell walls, or topical conjunctival immunization with viable *S. aureus* cells, IgG titers to ribitol teichoic acid in corneas are higher than both tears and serum, suggesting local production of antibody.[22] IgA titers to ribitol teichoic acid are found in tears, but not in serum, and only occasionally in the cornea. The role of humoral immunity alone is not known, as passive transfer experiments in rabbits have not been performed in the absence of a cell-mediated immune response.

The response to intradermal inoculation of killed *S. aureus* cells[10] and protein A has also been studied. Normal subjects give no significant induration response to either *S. aureus* or coagulase-negative staphylococci.

Folliculitis occurs more commonly among patients with cell-mediated immunity, and grittiness and morning stickiness are more frequent among patients without cell-mediated immunity. Marginal keratitis occurs equally among patients with and without enhanced systemic cell-mediated immunity, but those with an enhanced response require more steroid therapy. There is no difference in isolation rates of *S. aureus* for patients with and without enhancement, consistent with transient colonization.

Antibodies to *S. aureus* and coagulase-negative staphylococci teichoic acids are found in normals and in patients with chronic blepharitis. They can be found in tears in 20% of normals and patients. No difference exists between those with and without enhanced cell-mediated immunity to *S. aureus.*

Patients with chronic blepharitis have an incidence of atopy similar to the normal population (28%). Atopy has not been correlated with cell-mediated immunity to *S. aureus* in chronic blepharitis. Differences have not been found between atopes with and without keratoconjunctivitis with respect to their serum IgG and IgE antibodies to *S. aureus* ribitol teichoic acid.[41]

Host Susceptibility

S. aureus is a pyogenic organism that has an antigenic cell wall. The relative importance of toxin production and immunoreactivity depends on individual host susceptibility. Children with malfunctioning neutrophils, such as the "lazy leukocyte" syndrome or congenital neutropenia, are more prone to recurrent acute pyogenic episodes, including blepharitis. Deficiencies in production of complement factors, opsonic antibody (including IgG subclass 2), or gamma globulins can also lead to acute pyogenic infection that can be managed by monthly injections of normal human immunoglobulin. These diseases can be expected to result in an increased concentration of *S. aureus* cell-wall antigens in the macrophage system, which may in turn lead to enhancement of cell-mediated immunity.[34]

Some patients have enhanced cell-mediated immunity to *S. aureus.*[26] There are two populations with marginal keratitis—those with an enhanced systemic reaction to *S. aureus* and those without—each representing a different expression of immunity. These patients are particularly susceptible to *S. aureus* antigens that trigger a cell-mediated response resulting in marginal keratitis or ulcerative blepharitis. Host susceptibility to coagulase-negative staphylococci is not thought to be involved.

Total IgA production by the lacrimal gland has not been shown to differ between normals and those with chronic blepharitis.[31] The presence of chronic conjunctival inflammation allows serum IgG to leak into the tears. The role of these humoral antibodies in the production and maintenance of blepharitis and marginal keratitis is not known, but they are not neutralizing antibodies and do not prevent colonization of the lid margin by *S. aureus.* Opsonic antibodies will,

however, specifically enhance phagocytosis of acute infection by binding to the cell wall (F_{ab} antibody site) with the F_c site binding to polymorphonuclear cells.

CLINICAL FEATURES

Thygeson's original descriptions[37,38] of staphylococcal blepharitis remain applicable. Symptoms include soreness, watering, photophobia, and blurred vision. Acute infective episodes cause purulent discharge with ulcerative blepharitis. Recent-onset cases may be unilateral, but chronic staphylococcal blepharitis is typically bilateral.

Pustular folliculitis (Fig. 61-1) is characteristic of staphylococcal blepharitis and tends to localize to a portion of the lid, causing ulceration with adherent fibrinous scales. If abscess formation involves a sebaceous gland, it can cause an external hordeolum. Chronic inflammation accounts for the eventual lash loss and entropion with trichiasis that occurs in some cases.

Corneal signs include punctate epithelial keratitis with staining of the inferior cornea. Marginal infiltrates are usually unilateral (Fig. 61-2) and culture-negative, and they may be recurrent, leading to marginal thinning (Fig. 61-3). Phlyctenular keratitis (Fig. 61-4) is more commonly bilateral. In children the central cornea can be affected, with potentially serious consequences for visual prognosis.

Dermatologic disease, often with colonization by *S. aureus,* is frequent and includes rosacea (Fig. 61-5), acne vulgaris, and infectious eczematoid dermatitis. The posterior lid margin is infrequently involved in the absence of hordeola and chalazia.

A scoring system has been devised to permit comparisons between examiners (Table 61-3). The following signs can be quantified as to severity: lash collarettes, folliculitis, lash misdirection, lash loss, telangiectasis, lid margin thickening, entropion, corneal epitheliopathy, marginal keratitis, corneal vascularization, and phlyctenule formation.

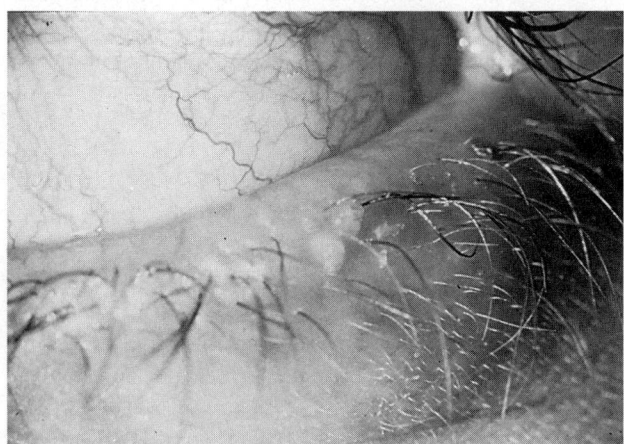

Fig. 61-1. Pustular folliculitis.

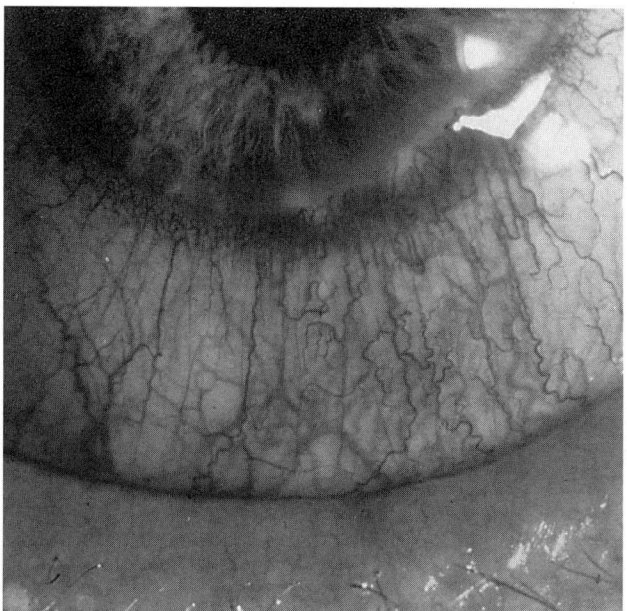

Fig. 61-2. Marginal corneal infiltrates.

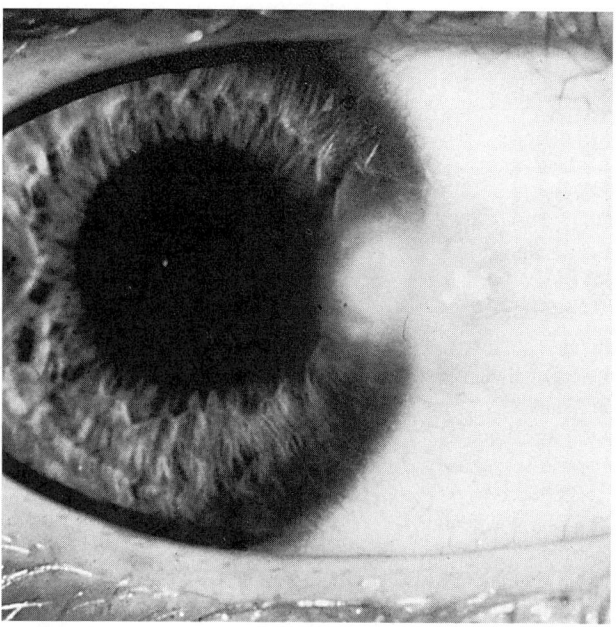

Fig. 61-4. Phlyctenular keratitis.

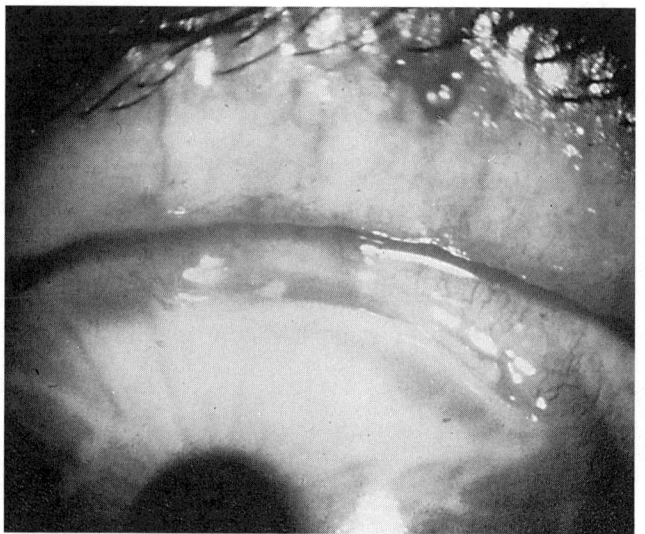

Fig. 61-3. Marginal corneal thinning following recurrent marginal keratitis.

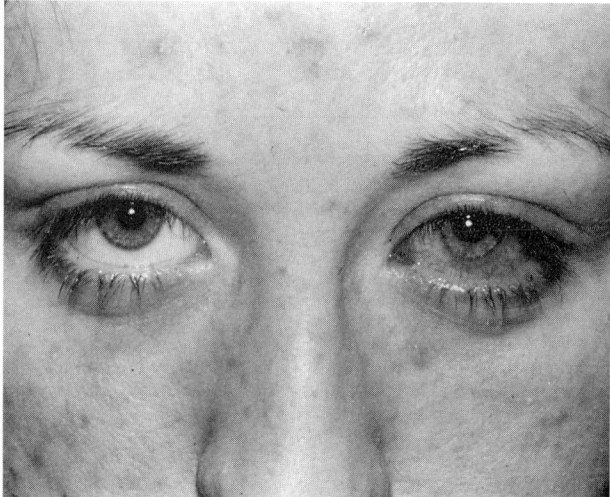

Fig. 61-5. Staphylococcal blepharitis complicated by marginal keratitis and associated with rosacea.

TABLE 61-3   SCORING SYSTEM FOR BLEPHARITIS

	Right Eye				Left Eye			
Symptoms								
Redness	0	1	2	3	0	1	2	3
Watery	0	1	2	3	0	1	2	3
Blurred vision	0	1	2	3	0	1	2	3
Photophobia	0	1	2	3	0	1	2	.3
Sore	0	1	2	3	0	1	2	3
AM stickiness	0	1	2	3	0	1	2	3
Signs								
Lash collarettes	0	1	2	3	0	1	2	3
Folliculitis	0	1	2	3	0	1	2	3
Lash misdirection	0	1	2	3	0	1	2	3
Lash loss	0	1	2	3	0	1	2	3
Telangiectasis	0	1	2	3	0	1	2	3
Marginal thickening	0	1	2	3	0	1	2	3
Entropion	0	1	2	3	0	1	2	3
Corneal epitheliopathy	0	1	2	3	0	1	2	3
Marginal keratitis	0	1	2	3	0	1	2	3
Marginal vascularization	0	1	2	3	0	1	2	3
Phlyctenule	0	1	2	3	0	1	2	3

Treatment

Lid scrubs with _____

Topical antibiotic _____

Topical steroid _____

Topical tear supplement _____

Systemic antibiotic _____

Systemic steroid _____

DIFFERENTIAL DIAGNOSIS

A cause other than staphylococcal blepharitis should be borne in mind when dealing with asymmetric or unilateral inflammatory lesions of the lids. Inflammatory signs may be caused by tumors such as sebaceous carcinoma and squamous cell carcinoma. Biopsy should be considered in chronic, atypical, or unresponsive lid disease.

Blepharitis may be associated with microbial colonization by other organisms including *Malassezia furfur* (associated with seborrhoeic skin disease), *Demodex* sp., and gram-negative bacteria.

Meibomian gland dysfunction and the dry eye are major causes of ocular discomfort. Clinical examination is generally effective in establishing the cause of symptoms. A diagnostic algorithm can assist with the clinical diagnosis of recalcitrant blepharitis and serves to distinguish ''staphylococcal'' from other causes of blepharitis.

LABORATORY INVESTIGATIONS

Lid hygiene and antibiotics may be advised for uncomplicated blepharitis in the absence of investigations. Unresponsive disease may benefit from special studies. As fur-

ther understanding of the cause of staphylococcal blepharitis emerges, the status of patients with respect to cell-mediated immunity may become important in establishing host susceptibility and in guiding therapy.

Culture

Qualitative culture is used to demonstrate the presence of a pathogenic organism and is best achieved by the lid scrub technique. Swabs are dipped into tryptic digest broth and rubbed along the lid margin. They can be sent to the laboratory in bacterial transport media, where they are cultured for 18 hours on 4% horse blood agar at 37° C in 4% CO_2, as some strains of *S. aureus* are capnophilic. Colonies are identified by standard laboratory techniques.

The soluble swab method demonstrates the presence of *S. aureus* quantitatively.[4] A calcium alginate swab, which dissolves in saline on shaking, is rubbed once along the everted lid margin. The swab is placed in 3 mls Ringer saline and transported directly to the laboratory or held at + 4° C. At the laboratory it is shaken for 2 minutes and 0.5 mls of the swab eluate is spread onto 4% horse blood agar. Plates are incubated for 18 hours at 37° C in 4% CO_2. Bacteria are identified by standard methods. The bacterial count from the lid is expressed in colony-forming units per ml swab eluate.

Methods of examining isolates of *S. aureus* for cell-wall protein A have been described elsewhere,[41] as have methods for hemolytic toxin production by *S. aureus* and coagulase-negative staphylococci.[32] Biotyping isolates of coagulase-negative staphylococci can be useful for comparing strains among different groups of patients. Antibiotic sensitivity tests are performed by standard disc-diffusion methods. Phage-typing of staphylococcal isolates is available in reference laboratories but is only useful for epidemiologic purposes.

Immunologic Studies

Patients can be tested for cell-mediated immunity to *S. aureus* and coagulase-negative staphylococci antigens by intradermal injection of 0.1 ml preparations[10] containing 5×10^8 staphylococcal cells per ml. It is necessary to prepare or purchase heat-killed cultures of *S. aureus* and coagulase-negative staphylococci and preserve them with 0.5% phenol. Intradermal injections are given on the internal surface of the forearm at 2 cm intervals, starting 2 cm below the cubital fossa. Reactions are read at 15 minutes for the type I wheal and flare response (Fig. 61-6) and at 48 hours for the type IV cell-mediated immune response (Fig. 61-7) of induration. A flare sometimes occurs at 48 hours but is considered negative unless induration is present.

Patients can be tested for cell-mediated immunity to staphylococcal protein A with a 0.05 ml intradermal injection containing 50 nanograms per ml (total dose of 2.5 nanograms). This should be freshly prepared and diluted in sterile saline. If this solution has been preserved with thio-

Fig. 61-6. Type I wheal and flare response to intradermal injection of protein A.

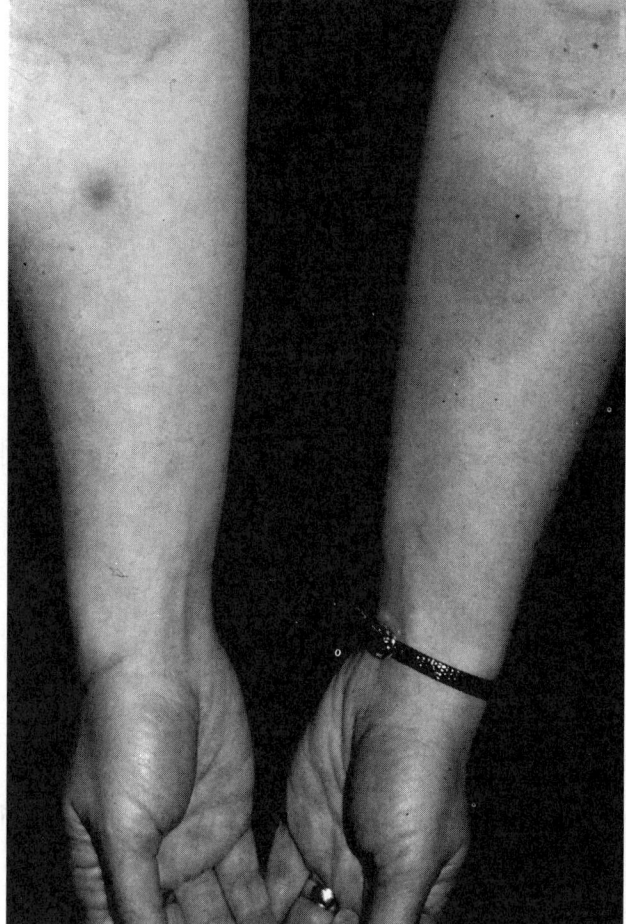

Fig. 61-7. Type IV induration response to intradermal injection of protein A (left arm) and killed *S. aureus* (right arm).

mersal, an additional control injection is required with the preserved saline. These injections should be given in the other forearm if *S. aureus* and coagulase-negative staphylococcal cells are to be injected. Because a large induration reaction (up to 10 cm) can occur with protein A, this antigen is best placed in the left arm if the patient is right-handed, or vice versa. A wheal and flare reaction always occurs at 15 minutes, the result of histamine release caused by protein A cross-binding F_c receptors of IgE on mast cells.

An enzyme immunoassay for detecting antibodies to teichoic acid of *S. aureus* and coagulase negative staphylococci has been studied.[10] Teichoic acid antigen has to be produced in the laboratory, as it is not available commercially. Assay of antibody titers to these teichoic acids has not been found of value diagnostically in blepharitis.

Tests of cell-mediated immunity can be relevant for some patients with recurrent marginal corneal ulceration. If such patients exhibit an enhanced reaction, they are likely to require local steroid treatment. Desensitization of this type of cellular immune reaction may prove useful in the future.

Investigation of Differential Diagnoses

The marginally dry eye can produce symptoms similar to chronic blepharitis—from which it must be differentiated. Lacrimal function is assessed crudely by observation of the tear margin meniscus, the tear film, or by the Schirmer test (filter paper strip). If there is no wetting after 2 minutes, the strip is moved to another site to eliminate false-positive results.[18] Five minutes should be allowed before measuring tear flow along the strip. The wetting of the strip is influenced by the temperature and humidity of the test environment and decreases with age. Lacrimal gland function is also assessed by assaying tear lysozyme[18,35] or lactoferrin[31] concentration and by measuring tear osmolarity, by freezing point depression.[19]

Meibomian gland dysfunction is diagnosed by clinical examination. The lower lid meibomian glands can be assessed by infrared transillumination.[19] The lid is folded over a fiberoptic light probe and photographed using high-speed, black-and-white infrared film. The expected total number of glands in the normal lid is 20. The photographs can be analyzed for the following features: loss of glands, duct dilatation, translucent cysts, and obscuration by chalazia. This technique, however, requires specialized equipment, and practical alternatives provide functional information about meibomian secretions and their effects on the tear film.

THERAPY

Lid Hygiene

Daily lid margin scrubs with sodium bicarbonate have a weak antibacterial effect, augmenting the influence of antimicrobials. Soaps containing antiseptics (hexachlorophene, chlorhexidine) and pads with mild detergents are alternatives.

If there is associated tear-film instability or deficiency, artificial tears or topical lubricants are indicated. Punctal

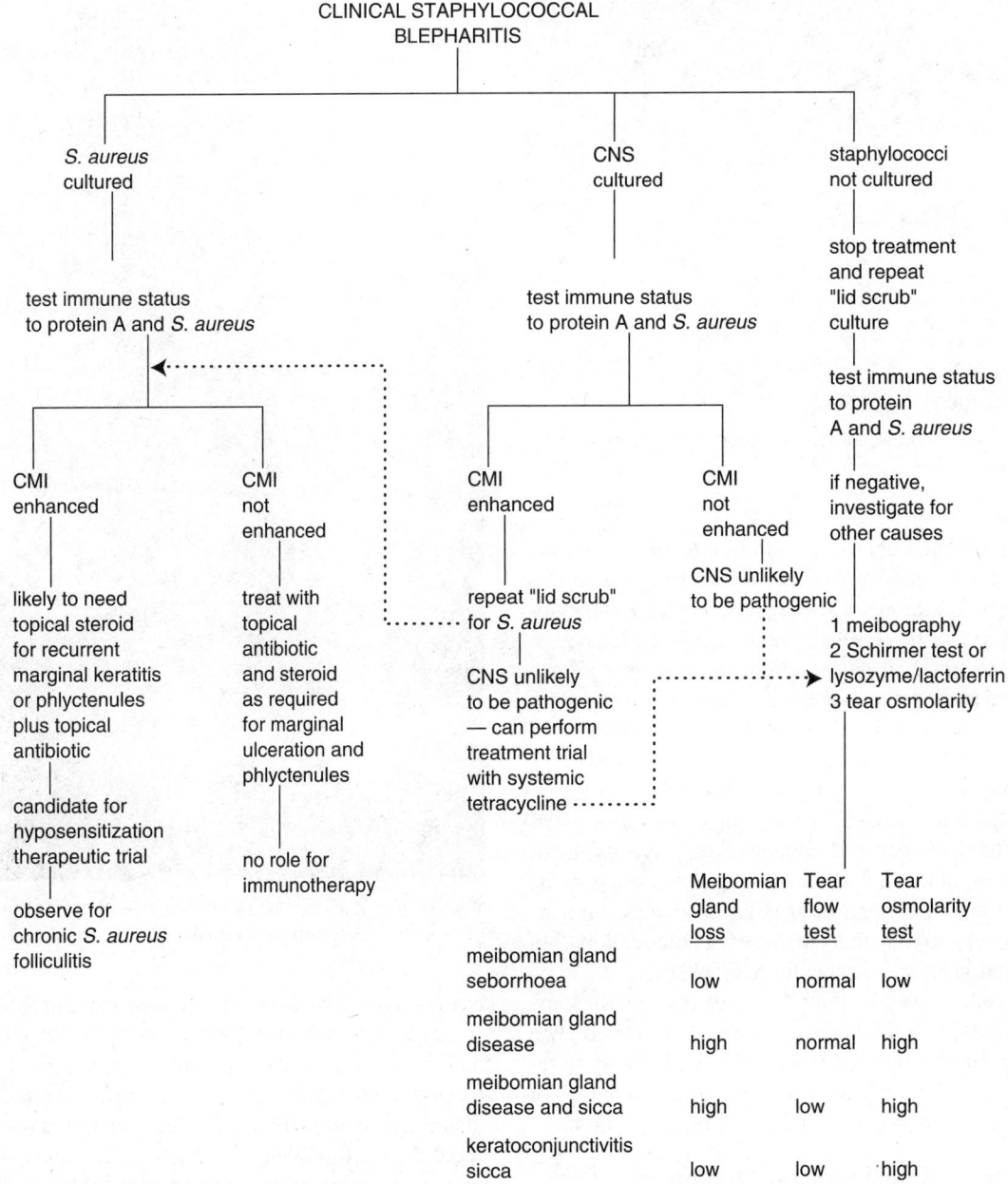

CLINICAL STAPHYLOCOCCAL
BLEPHARITIS

S. aureus cultured | CNS cultured | staphylococci not cultured

test immune status to protein A and *S. aureus*

stop treatment and repeat "lid scrub" culture

test immune status to protein A and *S. aureus*

if negative, investigate for other causes

CMI enhanced | CMI not enhanced

likely to need topical steroid for recurrent marginal keratitis or phlyctenules plus topical antibiotic

candidate for hyposensitization therapeutic trial

observe for chronic *S. aureus* folliculitis

treat with topical antibiotic and steroid as required for marginal ulceration and phlyctenules

no role for immunotherapy

CMI enhanced | CMI not enhanced

repeat "lid scrub" for *S. aureus*

CNS unlikely to be pathogenic — can perform treatment trial with systemic tetracycline

CNS unlikely to be pathogenic

1 meibography
2 Schirmer test or lysozyme/lactoferrin
3 tear osmolarity

	Meibomian gland loss	Tear flow test	Tear osmolarity test
meibomian gland seborrhoea	low	normal	low
meibomian gland disease	high	normal	high
meibomian gland disease and sicca	high	low	high
keratoconjunctivitis sicca	low	low	high

Fig. 61-8. Therapeutic decision-making in the management of chronic blepharitis.

occlusion may be required to supplement tear replacement. Trichiasis may be a problem (resulting from aberrant lashes or entropion) and is managed by lash removal, follicle destruction (by electrolysis or modified cryotherapy), or surgical lid eversion.

Topical Therapy

Antibacterial Agents. Acute folliculitis caused by *S. aureus* responds readily to topical antibiotics. Effective ointments include bacitracin, erythromycin, chloramphenicol, chlortetracycline, gentamicin, neomycin, dibromopropamidine, and fucidin. Effective drops include 0.5% chloramphenicol,

0.3% gentamicin, 0.5% neomycin, 0.1% propamidine isethionate, and 0.3% ciprofloxacin. Contact dermatitis may, however, be a problem with some of these agents.

Chronic folliculitis or chronic blepharitis (with the occasional isolation of *S. aureus*) is more difficult to treat. Long-term use of topical antibiotics is not recommended. Intermittent use may be indicated if there is associated recurrent marginal ulceration or phlyctenulosis. Such treatment achieves suppression of *S. aureus,* the antigenic stimulus, on the lid margin. Antistaphylococcal antibiotic ointments and gels are preferred to drops, as there is a longer contact time between the lid-margin bacteria and the antibiotic. Rotation of different antibiotics helps to prevent the emergence of resistant staphylococci. Topical fusidic acid (fucidin) is effective for relieving symptoms of blepharitis in patients with concomitant rosacea.[36]

Corticosteroids. The role of topical corticosteroids in blepharitis should be limited to specific complications such as marginal keratitis (Fig. 61-8). The dosage of steroid may initially be high (dexamethasone 0.1%) to suppress inflammation and cytokine release. A concurrent antibiotic reduces bacterial cell-wall antigen and thereby contributes to the control of inflammation. After initial control, the dosage of steroid is tapered. There may be a continued need for topical steroid for some months, especially in children, to prevent recurrent episodes of marginal keratitis. Nonsteroidal antiinflammatory drugs may be effective, but clinical experience is limited.

Systemic Therapy

Long-term systemic antibiotics to eradicate *S. aureus* from the lid margin are not usually effective. Systemic therapy does play a role in acute folliculitis, and oral flucloxacillin or trimethoprim (for penicillin-allergy) can augment topical antistaphylococcal drugs.

The role of systemic tetracycline is controversial. Oral tetracycline has antiinflammatory activity for rosacea,[12,36] a condition associated with *S. aureus* blepharitis and *S. aureus*[12,36] lid colonization. Because bacterial lipases can convert meibomian lipids into toxic fatty acids, the effect of systemic tetracycline on lipase production by staphylococci has been investigated.[9] Tetracycline causes a significant decrease in the production of lipase by sensitive and resistant stains of coagulase-negative staphylococci at concentrations that do not inhibit bacterial growth. A subinhibitory effect does not occur with *S. aureus,* however, for which inhibition of lipase production only occurs with inhibition of growth.

REFERENCES

1. Adlam C, Ward PD, Turner WH: Effect of immunisation with highly purified Panton-Valentine leucocidin and delta-toxin on staphylococcal mastitis in rabbits, *J Comp Pathol* 90:265-274, 1980.
1a. Adlam C, Ward PD, Turner WH: Effect of immunisation with highly purified Panton-Valentine leucocidin and delta-toxin on staphylococcal mastitis in rabbits, *J Comp Pathol* 86:581-593, 1980.
2. Allen JH: Staphylococcic conjunctivitis: experimental reproduction with staphylococcus toxin, *Am J Ophthalmol* 20:1025-1031, 1937.
3. Aubaret E: Etiologie et traitement des blépharities, *Bull Mem Soc Fr Ophtalmol* 42:1-23, 1929.
4. Badiani D, Bron A, Elkington A et al.: Use of a novel transport method for the normal flora of the external eye, *Microb Ecol Health Dis* 1:57-59, 1988.
5. Baird-Parker AC: A classification of micrococci and staphylococci based on physiological and biochemical tests, *J Gen Microbiol* 30:409-427, 1963.
6. Burnet FM: The exotoxins of *Staphylococcus aureus, J Pathol* xxxii:717-734, 1929.
7. Dougherty JM, McCulley JP: Comparative bacteriology of chronic blepharitis, *Br J Ophthalmol* 68:524-528, 1984.
8. Dougherty JM, McCulley JP: Bacterial lipases and chronic blepharitis, *Invest Ophthalmol Vis Sci* 27:486-491, 1986.
9. Dougherty JM, McCulley JP, Silvany RE, Meyer DR: The role of tetracycline in chronic blepharitis, *Invest Ophthalmol Vis Sci* 32:2970-2975, 1991.
10. Ficker L, Ramakrishnan M, Seal D, Wright P: Role of cell-mediated immunity to staphylococci in blepharitis, *Am J Ophthalmol* 111:473-479, 1991.
11. Freer J, Arbuthnott JP: Toxins of *Staphylococcus aureus, Pharmacol Ther* 19:55-106, 1983.
12. Freinkel RK, Strauss JS, Yip SY, Pochi PE: Effect of tetracycline on the composition of sebum in acne vulgaris, *N Engl J Med* 273:850-854, 1965.
13. Groden LR, Murphy B, Rodnite J, Genvert GS: Lid flora in blepharitis, *Cornea* 10:50-53, 1991.
14. Hogan MJ, Diaz-Bonnet V, Okumoto M, Kimura SJ: Experimental staphylococcic keratitis, *Invest Ophthalmol Vis Sci* 1:267-272, 1962.
15. Johanovsky J: Role of hypersensitivity in experimental staphylococcal infection, *Nature* 182:1454, 1958.
16. Johnson JE, Cluff LE, Goshi K: Studies on the pathogenesis of staphylococcal infection, *J Exp Med* 113:235-247, 1960.
17. Kloos WE, Schleifer KH: Simplified scheme for routine identification of human staphylococcus species, *J Clin Microbiol* 1:82-88, 1975.
18. Mackie IA, Seal DV: The questionably dry eye, *Br J Ophthalmol* 65:2-9, 1981.
19. Mathers WD, Shields WJ, Suchelev MS et al.: Meibomian gland dysfunction in chronic blepharitis, *Cornea* 10:277-285, 1991.
20. McCulley JP, Dougherty JM, Deneau DG: Classification of chronic blepharitis, *Ophthalmology* 89:1173-1180, 1982.
21. Mondino BJ, Adamu S: Ocular immune response to *S. epidermidis.* In Cavanagh III Dwight H, editor: *The cornea: transactions of the World Congress on the cornea,* 431-433, New York, 1988, Raven Press.
22. Mondino BJ, Brawman-Mintzev O, Adamu S: Corneal antibody levels to ribitol teichoic acid in rabbits immunised with staphylococcal antigens using various routes, *Invest Ophthalmol Vis Sci* 28:1553-1558, 1987.
23. Mondino BJ, Caster AI, Dethlefs B: A rabbit model of staphylococcal blepharitis, *Arch Ophthalmol* 105:409-412, 1987.
24. Mondino BJ, Dethlefs B: Occurrence of phlyctenules after immunisation with ribitol teichoic acid of *S. aureus, Arch Ophthalmol* 102:461-463, 1984.
25. Mondino BJ, Kowalski R, Ratajczak HV et al.: Rabbit model of phlyctenulosis and catarrhal infiltrates, *Arch Ophthalmol* 99:891-895, 1981.
26. Mudd S, Taubler JH, Baker AG: Delayed-type hypersensitivity to *S. aureus* in human subjects, *J Reticuloendothel Soc* 8:493-499, 1970.
27. Oeding P: Taxonomy and identification. In Easmon CSF, Adlam C, editors: *Staphylococci and staphylococcal infections,* vol 1, 1-31, London, 1983, Academic Press.
28. Ostler BH: Corneal perforation in non-tuberculous (staphylococcal) phlyctenular keratoconjunctivitis, *Am J Ophthalmol* 79:446-448, 1975.
29. Panton PN, Valentine FCO: Staphylococcal infection and reinfection, *Br J Exp Pathol* 10:257-262, 1929.
30. Parfentjev IA, Clapp FL, Waldschmidt A: Staphylococcal toxoid prepared by peptic digestion, *J Immunol* 40:189-199, 1941.
31. Seal DV: *Pathophysiology of bacterial infection in the external eye,* MD thesis, University of London, 1984.
32. Seal DV, Ficker L, Ramakrishnan M, Wright P: Role of staphylococcal toxin production in blepharitis, *Ophthalmology* 97:1684-1688, 1990.
33. Seal DV, Ficker L, Wright P: Role of coagulase-negative staphylococci in chronic blepharitis, *Microb Ecol Health Dis* 5:69-75, 1992.
34. Seal DV, Lightman S: Immunodeficiency, immunity and staphylococcal infection, *Lancet* ii:1522, 1991.
35. Seal DV, Mackie IA, Coakes RL, Farooqi B: Quantitative tear lysozyme assay: a new technique for transporting specimens, *Br J Ophthalmol* 64:700-704, 1980.
36. Seal DV, Wright P, Ficker L et al.: Placebo-controlled trial of fusidic acid gel and oxytetracycline for recurrent blepharitis and rosacea. *Br J Ophthalmol,* 79:42-45, 1995.
37. Thygeson P: The etiology and treatment of blepharitis: a study in military personnel, *Mil Surg* 98:191-203, 1946.

38. Thygeson P: Marginal corneal infiltrates and ulcers, *Trans Am Acad Ophthalmol Otolaryngol* 51:198-209, 1946.
39. Thygeson P: Observations on non-tuberculous kerato-conjunctivitis, *Trans Am Acad Ophthalmol Otolaryngol* 58:128-133, 1954.
40. Thygeson P: Complications of staphylococcic blepharitis, *Am J Ophthalmol* 68:446-449, 1969.
41. Tuft SJ, Ramakrishnan M, Seal DV et al.: Role of *S. aureus* in chronic allergic conjunctivitis, *Ophthalmology* 99:180-184, 1992.
42. Valenton MJ, Okumoto M: Toxin-producing strains of *S. epidermidis:* isolates from patients with staphylococcic blepharo-conjunctivitis, *Arch Ophthalmol* 89:186-189, 1973.

62 Bacterial Conjunctivitis

DAVID G. HWANG

Bacterial conjunctivitis is characterized by an overgrowth of bacteria on the conjunctival surface that leads to acute or chronic mucosal inflammation. Although most cases of bacterial conjunctivitis are benign and self-limited, it is essential for the clinician to recognize the types of conjunctivitis that can lead to serious ocular morbidity or even death, if not properly treated.

HISTORICAL BACKGROUND

Acute conjunctivitis was recognized by the ancients, and accurate descriptions of this illness have been found among the earliest medical writings extant. An Egyptian papyrus of 1550 BC gave accurate descriptions of the cardinal signs of conjunctivitis (redness, secretion, and edema) and provided topical remedies for various forms of conjunctivitis.[61] The pre-Alexandrian Greek physicians of the Hippocratic school (fourth century BC) described several forms of conjunctivitis including *taraxis,* or mild mucopurulent conjunctivitis; *psorophthalmia,* or ulcerative blepharoconjunctivitis; *sycosis* and *tylosis,* two forms of trachoma; and epidemic conjunctivitis.[61] Descriptions of conjunctivitis are also found in ancient Indian and Chinese manuscripts. The Sui-Tang Dynasty compendium *General Treatise on the Causes and Symptoms of Diseases* (610 AD) detailed the presenting symptoms and presumed pathogenesis of a variety of ocular disorders, including purulent conjunctivitis.[19]

The contagious nature of conjunctivitis was formally suggested by the German medical professor Quelmalz (1696-1758), who postulated that neonatal conjunctivitis was caused by contact with purulent gonorrheal vaginal secretions from the mother.[62] Bacteria were not recognized as a cause of conjunctivitis until the discovery in 1879 by Neisser of diplococci in the secretions of ophthalmia neonatorum.[25] The causative agent of "Egyptian ophthalmia," *Haemophilus aegyptius,* was seen on smears by Koch in 1883 and isolated in culture by Weeks in 1886.[35]

Over the centuries, a variety of remedies have been recommended for the treatment of acute conjunctivitis. Ancient Indian, Aramaic, and Roman medical texts recognized the value of topical treatment of acute conjunctivitis and recommended the compounding of poultices and collyria (powders dissolved in water before ocular instillation). Some of these formulations included substances with known therapeutic activity such as milk (which contains the antibacterial substance lactoferrin) and bacteriostatic metals (such as zinc and copper).[49] An assortment of collyria discovered in an 1854 excavation of a Roman tomb included some labeled *collyrium penicillum,* an ocular compound made from a soft fungus (possibly bread mold). Despite the apparent validity of some of these remedies, superstitious and unscientific approaches to the treatment of conjunctivitis often prevailed.[49] The encyclopedic medical text *Corpus Hippocraticum* (circa 300 BC) recommended the sufferer ingest a diet of bread and water and lie in a darkened room with the eyes open to avoid prolonged exposure to noxious "hot tears."[79]

This emphasis on a systemic rather than topical approach to the treatment of acute conjunctivitis persisted in medieval and Renaissance medicine. A rational approach to the treatment of bacterial conjunctivitis would have to await the development of the germ theory of disease by Pasteur and Koch in the latter half of the nineteenth century. Credé's 1881 introduction of silver nitrate drops for the prophylaxis of ophthalmia neonatorum[24] heralded the modern conception of topical antimicrobial therapy that reached its contemporary fruition with the introduction of antibiotics some 60 years later.

EPIDEMIOLOGY

Incidence

Although bacterial conjunctivitis is acknowledged to be an extremely common disorder, the precise incidence in the general population is not known. The incidence is higher among children and young adults than among older individuals.[96] Among neonates the overall incidence of culture-proven conjunctivitis caused by bacteria of all types was reported to be 4.6% in the United Kingdom,[106] where Credé prophylaxis is not routinely practiced, compared to 0.6% in the United States,[2] where neonatal antimicrobial prophylaxis is mandatory. Among male military recruits, a weekly case incidence of nonepidemic conjunctivitis was found to be 0.01%, of which 25% were culture-positive for bacteria.[59] A seasonal variation in attack rates of acute conjunctivitis has been observed, with an incidence peaking in the late summer to fall among neonates in Atlanta, Georgia,[2] and a peak in the spring and autumn among children and adults in northern Egypt.[96] The relative incidence of viral and bacterial conjunctivitis also shows a seasonal variation, with bacterial causes predominating in the winter and spring and viral causes predominating in the summer.[36]

Transmission

The predominant mode of transmission in bacterial conjunctivitis is hand-to-eye contact. In certain settings, however, other routes of transmission may occur (see box). Contiguous spread may occur from the nasopharynx, as in the case of *Haemophilus influenzae* or *Staphylococcus aureus*. Other sources of contiguous spread include the lids; the cornea, as can occasionally occur in cases of bacterial keratitis leading to secondary conjunctival infection; or the nasolacrimal system, as can occur in dacryostenosis or dacryocystitis. In rare instances transmission from the oral cavity has been implicated.[138] An uncommon mode of endogenous transmission is hematogenous spread. Blood-borne spread

---

MODES OF TRANSMISSION OF BACTERIAL CONJUNCTIVITIS

ENDOGENOUS
Contiguous
　Lids
　Cornea
　Nasolacrimal drainage system
Hematogenous
Hand-to-eye
　Oculogenital
　Cross-inoculation from opposite eye
Factitious
EXOGENOUS
Hand-to-eye
Oculogenital
　Sexual intercourse
　Vaginal delivery
Fomites
　Eye drops
　Contact lenses
　Microscopes
　Eye makeup
Insect-borne
Nosocomial

---

can occur in immunocompromised hosts or in immunocompetent persons with certain types of infections, such as meningococcemia.[3] Oculogenital routes of transmission may occur from sexual intercourse, vaginal delivery, or self-inoculation from contact with genital secretions. Deliberate self-inoculation of contaminated oral or fecal material may occur as part of an ocular Munchausen syndrome and can manifest as a chronic or recurrent mixed bacterial conjunctivitis. Contaminated eye drops, contact lenses, microscopes,[30,103] eye makeup,[117] or other fomites have been implicated in some cases of bacterial conjunctivitis. Insect vectors are an important cause of transmission of bacterial and chlamydial conjunctival pathogens in arid regions of the developing world. Insect-borne transmission has also been reported in certain less-developed regions of industrialized countries.[143] Nosocomial outbreaks of bacterial conjunctivitis have been reported in nurseries,[58] inpatient wards,[75] intensive care units,[60] and long-term care facilities.[10] Iatrogenic transmission can also occur in the outpatient setting (usually through contact of the examiner's hand and the patient's eye), but also through the use of contaminated drops, tonometer tips, contact lenses, or ophthalmic instruments.

Sporadic versus Epidemic Cases

Most cases of bacterial conjunctivitis are sporadic. Epidemic spread occurs most commonly in settings in which susceptible individuals are congregated in close quarters, such as day-care centers,[133] boarding schools,[117] military camps,[2,129] or college dormitories. Another factor predisposing to epidemic spread is an increased susceptibility to bacterial ocular infection in the population at risk. Examples include hospitalized immunocompromised patients who are at risk for nosocomial conjunctivitis,[60] and patients with epidemic viral conjunctivitis who are predisposed to bacterial superinfection.[97]

Risk Factors

Variations in the age and immune status of the bacterial conjunctivitis patient affect the relative frequency of most commonly cultured pathogens. Children under the age of 5 years with bacterial conjunctivitis have a much higher incidence of *Haemophilus influenzae* than older children and adults.[14,15,102,139] Among all age groups, infants under the age of 1 year have the highest frequency of enterococcal and coliform bacterial conjunctivitis.[118] Alcoholics and immunocompromised adults have an increased susceptibility to bacterial conjunctivitis, especially that caused by *Moraxella*[4] spp. or gram-negative bacteria.

PATHOGENESIS

Normal conjunctival health is maintained when host defense mechanisms sustain a conjunctival surface that is either sterile or colonized with low numbers of bacteria. Bacterial conjunctivitis results when resident or deposited bacteria on the conjunctival surface are able to (1) overcome host mucosal defenses, (2) penetrate the epithelial layer, (3) multiply in large numbers, and (4) evoke a conjunctival inflammatory response characterized by signs of epithelial toxicity and necrosis, vascular hyperemia, and exudative discharge. Key factors in the pathogenesis of bacterial conjunctivitis are invasion of bacteria beyond the epithelial barrier and pathogen evasion of host defenses. The balance between host defense mechanisms and bacterial virulence factors governs whether conjunctival health or disease prevails.

Host Defenses

Normal host systemic immunity is an important defense against bacterial invasion and proliferation. Compromise of systemic immunity may result in a predilection to bacterial conjunctivitis. Hypogammaglobulinemia has been associated with an increased incidence of infections caused by *Haemophilus influenzae.*[55] Combined deficiency of humoral and cell-mediated immunity, such as can occur in bone marrow transplant recipients, also predisposes to bacterial conjunctival infections.

In addition to systemic humoral and cellular immunity, local defenses play a major role in guarding against the development of bacterial conjunctivitis. The eyelids serve as a barrier to the entry of microorganisms, and the tear film and blink reflex provide a protective flushing of the ocular surfaces. The intact epithelium provides an important mechanical barrier to the entry of bacteria. Experimental studies have shown that direct inoculation of large numbers of bacteria onto the intact conjunctival surface of rabbits often fails to produce conjunctivitis.[5] However, if the conjunctiva is incised prior to inoculation of *S. aureus* onto the conjunctival surface, experimental bacterial conjunctivitis readily develops.[5]

The mucus component in tears may interfere with bacterial attachment to the epithelium. The tears also contain a number of secreted factors with antibacterial properties, including lysozyme, lactoferrin, beta-lysin, secretory IgA, other immunoglobulins, and complement. Lysozyme comprises 20% to 40% of the proteins found in human tears and exerts its antibacterial action by enzymatic degradation of the mucopeptides of bacterial cell walls, particularly those of gram-positive bacteria.[119] Lactoferrin, first isolated from milk, is an iron-binding protein that disrupts bacterial growth by complexing free iron ions requisite for bacterial metabolism.[12] The low-molecular-weight protein beta-lysin disrupts bacterial cytoplasmic membranes and may work in concert with lysozyme, which acts on cell walls.[38,44] Secretory IgA is the major immunoglobulin found in tear fluid.[88] It is a noncomplement-fixing immunoglobulin product that is elaborated on the surface of all mucosal tissue, including the conjunctiva. Secretory IgA is formed from a complex of conjunctival epithelial cell-derived secretory peptide and immunoglobulin A produced by plasma cells in the substantia propria.[137] Secretory IgA blocks the adherence of bacteria to conjunctival epithelial cells[144] and may interfere with bacterial growth.[8] Other immunoglobulins, particularly IgG,[88] and complement components[146] are present in the tears and may play important roles in mucosal immunity via antibody-dependent cytoxicity and complement activation cascades.

Cellular mucosal immunity also plays an important part in the defense against bacterial pathogens. In addition to providing a physical barrier to bacterial entry, the epithelium can phagocytize and destroy bacterial pathogens. For example, guinea pig conjunctival epithelial cells phagocytize *Listeria monocytogenes* within 30 minutes after inoculation onto the conjunctival surface.[149] After endocytosis the bacteria enter phagosomes, whereupon they are inactivated and digested by various enzymes, including peroxidase[69] and acid phosphatase.[80] *Salmonella typhimurium* takes advantage of this cellular uptake mechanism as a means to penetrate intact conjunctival cells. Although the majority of organisms are destroyed within phagosomes, a sufficient number can survive to produce experimental *S. typhimurium* keratoconjunctivitis in a guinea pig model.[81] Bacteria that invade beyond the epithelial layer into the substantia propria are met by macrophages and Langerhans cells that specialize in phagocytosis, antigen processing, and antigen presentation to T cells. The substantia propria underlying the epithelium is also rich in other types of inflammatory cells, including lymphocytes that participate in cell-mediated immunity and plasma cells that produce antibodies.[1]

Disruption of the epithelial barrier and impairment of nonspecific or specific local defenses may lead to an increased risk of developing bacterial conjunctivitis. The protective function of the lids and tears may be compromised by chronic entropion, lagophthalmos, or keratoconjunctivitis sicca. Loss of epithelial integrity may occur with antecedent viral conjunctivitis, chlamydial conjunctivitis, chemical burns, or Stevens-Johnson syndrome. Local immunosuppression from topical corticosteroid use can predispose to the development of bacterial, fungal, and viral infections of the conjunctiva and cornea.[32]

A summary of epidemiologic and host-specific risk factors for the development of bacterial conjunctivitis in different age groups is listed in the box.

Normal Bacterial Flora

A heterogeneous population of microbial flora may be found on the conjunctival surface of approximately two thirds of normal individuals (see box).[91,92,105,121,147] In children (age > 1 year) and adults the most common bacteria isolated are *Staphylococcus epidermidis, Corynebacterium* spp., and *Propionibacterium acnes.* Neonates have a different composition of ocular flora, varying according to the route of birth delivery. In vaginally delivered newborns,

```
┌─────────────────────────────────────────────┐
│   IMPORTANT RISK FACTORS FOR THE              │
│   DEVELOPMENT OF BACTERIAL                    │
│   CONJUNCTIVITIS (BY AGE)                     │
├─────────────────────────────────────────────┤
```

INFANTS (AGE < 1 YEAR)
Vaginal delivery in mother with colonized or infected birth canal
Concomitant bacterial otitis media or pharyngitis
Chronic nasopharyngeal bacterial carriage
Nasolacrimal duct obstruction
Sporadic or epidemic person-to-person contact
Superinfection following viral or chlamydial conjunctivitis

CHILDREN
Sporadic or epidemic person-to-person contact
Concomitant bacterial otitis media, sinusitis, or pharyngitis
Chronic nasopharyngeal bacterial carriage
Superinfection following viral conjunctivitis
Spread via fomites (for example, eye makeup)
Oculogenital spread

ADULTS
Sporadic or epidemic person-to-person contact
Concomitant blepharitis
Superinfection following viral or chlamydial conjunctivitis
Oculogenital spread
Concomitant sinusitis or pharyngitis
Chronic nasopharyngeal bacterial carriage
Tear deficiency
Lid malposition
Use of contaminated eye drops or contact lenses
Local or systemic immunosuppression
Immunodeficiency
Nosocomial spread

80% of conjunctival cultures are positive, predominantly composed of facultatively and obligately anaerobic bacterial species characteristic of the vaginal tract (*Lactobacillus* spp. and *Bifidobacterium* spp.).[67,68] Among neonates delivered by cesarean section, the incidence of positive conjunctival cultures is only 20%, and the principal isolates are those found on the skin, including *S. epidermidis, P. acnes,* and *Corynebacterium* spp.[68]

Although the role of the normal microbial flora in host defenses has not been clearly established, the colonization of the conjunctival surface by these organisms may prevent attachment or overgrowth of more pathogenic bacteria inoculated onto the conjunctiva. In addition to competing with pathogenic bacteria for available space and nutrients on the conjunctival surface, the normal microbial flora of the conjunctiva may produce natural antibiotic-like products that inhibit the growth of foreign bacteria.[64]

Bacterial Virulence Factors

Inoculum size and bacterial virulence factors presumably play important roles in the establishment of bacterial infection of the conjunctiva. From the few available animal models of bacterial conjunctivitis, it appears that even virulent bacteria require relatively large inocula to establish infection. Studies of other mucosal infections indicate that bacteria with a lower predilection for attachment and invasion require a larger inoculum to establish infection than species or strains that possess these virulence factors.

Bacterial virulence factors may potentiate the establishment of infection at any number of stages including attachment, adhesion, invasion, multiplication, toxin production, protease release, and evasion of host defenses. Pili, glycocalyx, and adhesins are a few of the bacterial factors that mediate attachment and adhesion to cells, thereby promoting infection.[140] With most bacterial species, invasion requires disruption of the epithelial layer. Certain bacterial species, however, including *Listeria monocytogenes*,[146] *Salmonella typhimurium*,[80] *Corynebacterium diphtheriae*,[66] *Haemophilus* spp.,[34] and *Neisseria* spp.,[66] are able to directly invade intact epithelia. Release of exotoxins may play an important role in modulating the severity of tissue damage, particularly in membranous conjunctivitis caused by *Streptococcus pyogenes* and *Corynebacterium diphtheriae*. Bacterial proteases may mediate tissue spreading, as in the case of *Pseudo-*

```
┌─────────────────────────────────────────────┐
│   NORMAL BACTERIAL FLORA OF THE               │
│   CONJUNCTIVA IN ADULTS AND                   │
│   CHILDREN (AGE > 1 YEAR)[91,92,105,121,147]  │
├─────────────────────────────────────────────┤
```

STERILE (9%-47%)
POSITIVE CONJUNCTIVAL CULTURES (53%-91%)
Present in over 25% of cultures
  Staphylococcus epidermidis
  Corynebacterium spp.
Present in 5%-25% of cultures
  Propionibacterium acnes
  Staphylococcus aureus
Present in 1%-5% of cultures
  Branhamella catarrhalis
  Haemophilus influenzae
  Proteus spp.
  Streptococcus pneumoniae
  Viridans streptococci
Present in < 1% of cultures
  Moraxella spp.
  Klebsiella pneumoniae
  Serratia marcescens
  Bacillus subtilis
  Micrococcus spp.
  Peptococcus spp.

monas elastase, or inactivate host immune factors, such as the IgA protease produced by certain strains of *Neisseria* spp. and *Haemophilus* spp.[34] Other pathogenic factors include the ability to evade immune defenses, an example of which is the polysaccharide encapsulation of certain bacteria (e.g., *Streptococcus pneumoniae*), which interferes with phagocytosis by host immune cells.

BACTERIAL ETIOLOGY

Many pathogenic bacteria can cause conjunctivitis, and the list of reported causal agents is long and continues to expand (see box).[14,118] In temperate latitudes bacterial conjunctivitis in nonimmunocompromised adults is most frequently caused by *Streptococcus pneumoniae, Staphylococcus aureus, Staphylococcus epidermidis,* and viridans streptococci.[15,118] In tropical climates *Haemophilus influenzae* biogroup aegyptius (formerly known as *Haemophilus aegyptius* or Koch-Weeks bacillus) predominates as a cause of bacterial conjunctivitis.[96]

Staphylococcus epidermidis is the most frequent isolate from cases of bacterial conjunctivitis, but its pathogenic significance is unclear because it can be recovered at a similar rate from normals.[105] If the criterion of moderate to heavy

growth is used to define clinically significant *S. epidermidis* recovery,[124] *S. epidermidis* is reported to cause only 2% of cases of bacterial conjunctivitis.[36] *Corynebacterium* spp. and *Propionibacterium* spp. (often grouped together under the term "diphtheroids" based on their similar morphologic appearance on smears) are also isolated with moderate frequency, but are generally considered nonpathogenic resident flora.[15] In epidemic conjunctivitis, *Haemophilus influenzae* biogroup aegyptius, *Staphylococcus aureus,* and *Moraxella* spp. are frequently implicated. Less common, but clinically important aerobic bacterial pathogens in adults include *Neisseria gonorrhoeae, Neisseria meningitidis, Haemophilus influenzae, Branhamella catarrhalis, Corynebacterium diphtheriae, Listeria monocytogenes, Escherichia coli, Proteus* spp., *Klebsiella* spp., *Serratia marcescens,* and *Pseudomonas aeruginosa.*[15,125]

Anaerobic bacteria are uncommon as sole causal agents but can be isolated in conjunction with aerobic species in 35% to 65% of cases of bacterial conjunctivitis.[14,15,105] *Propionibacterium acnes* and *Peptococcus* spp. are among the anaerobic isolates most frequently found,[15] but their significance is unclear because they are recovered at a comparable frequency from normal conjunctivae.[105] A significantly increased rate of recovery of *Peptostreptococcus* spp. from eyes with acute conjunctivitis as compared to normal eyes (29% versus 6%, respectively[105]) suggests a potential pathogenic role for these anaerobes, however.

CLINICAL FEATURES

Sufferers of bacterial conjunctivitis typically complain of redness, tearing, and discharge. Irritation and foreign body sensation are also frequent symptoms. Pain is a distinctly uncommon finding in conjunctivitis, and its presence suggests an alternative or concurrent diagnosis of episcleritis, scleritis, keratitis, or uveitis. Mild photophobia is not uncommon and may suggest a modest degree of associated keratitis. Vision is generally normal or minimally affected.

Although the clinical presentation of bacterial conjunctivitis may vary according to chronicity, severity, and age of the patient, certain clinicopathologic hallmarks remain constant. These include conjunctival hyperemia, chemosis, and exudation.

Hyperemia results from inflammatory engorgement of the vasculature of the palpebral and bulbar conjunctiva. The conjunctival vessels are dilated and tortuous, and the conjunctiva assumes a characteristic reddened appearance. In bacterial conjunctivitis this inflammatory vascular dilatation is limited to the conjunctiva, sparing the deeper episcleral and scleral layers. On the bulbar conjunctiva the conjunctival vasculature arborizes in a radial, branching pattern and can be readily mobilized with a swab brushed gently against the anesthetized conjunctival surface. In contrast, the deeper episcleral and scleral vascular beds assume a plexiform or

---

COMMON ISOLATES IN BACTERIAL CONJUNCTIVITIS IN ADULTS AND CHILDREN (AGE > 1 YEAR)[15,118]

FREQUENT ISOLATES (>5% OF CASES)
  Usually considered nonpathogenic
    Staphylococcus epidermidis
    Corynebacterium spp.
    Propionibacterium acnes
    Peptococcus spp.
  Usually of pathogenic significance
    Staphylococcus aureus
    Streptococcus pneumoniae
    Viridans streptococci
    Peptostreptococcus spp.
    Haemophilus influenzae
    Haemophilus influenzae biogroup aegyptius *(Haemophilus aegyptius)*
LESS-FREQUENT ISOLATES (<5% OF CASES)
    Bacteroides spp.
    Branhamella catarrhalis
    Escherichia coli
    Klebsiella spp.
    Moraxella spp.
    Neisseria gonorrhoeae
    Neisseria meningitidis
    Peptostreptococcus
    Proteus spp.
    Pseudomonas spp.
    Streptococcus pyogenes

netlike configuration and cannot easily be mobilized with a swab or microsponge. Topical vasoconstrictors are sometimes helpful in differentiating bulbar conjunctival vascular engorgement from episcleral or scleral vascular dilatation. In response to an alpha-adrenergic agonist such as phenylephrine, the conjunctival vasculature will blanch more rapidly and to a greater degree than vessels in the episclera or sclera.

In addition to causing vascular engorgement, the autacoids, cytokines, and other mediators released during the inflammatory cascade also produce increased vascular permeability. The resultant chemosis, or conjunctival edema, is manifest clinically as conjunctival thickening and translucent waxiness of the conjunctiva that tends to obscure vascular detail. If severe, chemosis may result in grossly swollen lids and secondary ptosis.

The exudate of bacterial conjunctivitis is a composite of inflammatory cells (mostly polymorphonuclear leukocytes),[130] epithelial cell remnants, bacteria, protein, fibrin, mucus, and serous fluid. Depending on the relative proportions of these components, the exudate may appear purulent, mucoid, or serous, although a mucopurulent consistency is most common. Despite the fact that bacteria are generally confined to exudative debris and necrotic superficial epithelium, in severe cases of conjunctivitis, bacteria may be found invading the substantia propria.[31]

In addition to these cardinal manifestations, associated findings may be present. Persistent dilatation of palpebral conjunctival vessels frequently manifests in the formation of fine (~ 0.1 mm) bumps on the mucosal surface (papillae), each of which has at its center a dilated terminal conjunctival vessel seen in end-on fashion. Each papilla is the result of focal perivascular transudation of proteinaceous fluid and infiltration of inflammatory cells arising from the core conjunctival vessel. The boundaries of the papillae are formed by the fine fibrous septations of the connective tissue bridging the tarsus and the conjunctival epithelium.[123] Subconjunctival hemorrhages may develop as the result of breakage of dilated conjunctival vessels.

There may be an associated lid infection or inflammation (blepharoconjunctivitis) or keratitis (keratoconjunctivitis). The keratitis is usually manifest as a punctate epithelial keratopathy, presumably resulting from a toxic response to the admixture of bacterial exoproducts, proteases, and inflammatory mediators present in the conjunctival exudate.

An uncommon finding that often indicates severe disease is the presence of a pseudomembrane or membrane. Pseudomembranes are formed from an exuberant exudate of fibrin and inflammatory cells that coalesces and adheres in sheetlike fashion to the conjunctival surface. Membranes, a hallmark of severe conjunctivitis associated with coagulative necrosis of the superficial conjunctival layers, represent avascular plaques of fibrinous inflammatory exudate enmeshed with sheets of sloughened epithelial cells. Pseudo-

membranes usually detach from the conjunctival surface in a well-defined plane without significant bleeding, whereas the removal of membranes is usually difficult and accompanied by bleeding from the subepithelial conjunctival vasculature. Although mild subepithelial scarring may occur with pseudomembranous conjunctivitis, more marked degrees of subepithelial scarring and late symblepharon formation are seen primarily in association with membranous conjunctivitis.

Acute Mucopurulent Conjunctivitis

The most common form of bacterial conjunctivitis is the acute mucopurulent form (Fig. 62-1). Among adults, acute mucopurulent conjunctivitis is usually caused by *Staphylococcus aureus, Streptococcus pneumoniae,* or viridans group streptococci.[36] Two to three days after inoculation, patients develop the acute onset of conjunctival hyperemia and mucopurulent conjunctival discharge. If the fellow eye is initially unaffected, it often becomes involved from cross-inoculation within 2 to 3 days. Symptoms of foreign body sensation, irritation, tearing, and eyelid stickiness are frequent. Vision is usually unaffected. In addition to conjunctival hyperemia and a mild-to-moderate conjunctival discharge, there may be associated findings of subconjunctival hemorrhages, tarsal papillary reaction, conjunctival chemosis with secondary lid swelling, mechanical ptosis, and mild punctate epithelial keratopathy. Preauricular adenopathy is uncommon. These cases are usually self-limited, showing spontaneous resolution within 10 to 12 days (in most cases) if left untreated.

In children, nontypable *Haemophilus influenzae, Staphylococcus aureus,* and *Streptococcus pneumoniae* are the most frequent isolates.[14,47] The subgroup of children under the age of 5 has a particularly high incidence of *Haemophilus influenzae* conjunctivitis.[139] These children may be susceptible to recurrent episodes of acute conjunctivitis,[133] sometimes in association with concurrent *Haemophilus* spp.

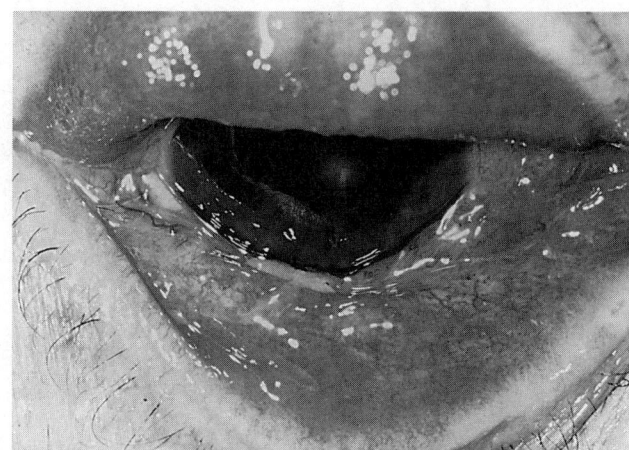

Fig. 62-1. Acute mucopurulent conjunctivitis caused by *Proteus.* (Courtesy of John P. Whitcher, MD.)

...)

otitis media (conjunctivitis-otitis syndrome).[7] *Haemophilus influenzae* conjunctivitis is generally similar to acute mucopurulent conjunctivitis caused by other organisms, but may be differentiated by its longer duration (10 to 15 days) and the characteristic findings in some cases of petechial conjunctival hemorrhages and perilimbal corneal infiltrates. *Haemophilus* spp. conjunctivitis in children is usually associated with nontypable, unencapsulated *H. influenzae*.[111] Children with conjunctivitis caused by encapsulated *Haemophilus influenzae* (particularly *H. influenzae* group b) may be at risk for periocular or disseminated infection including sinusitis, periorbital cellulitis, sepsis, and meningitis.[86] Although nontypable *Haemophilus* spp. are generally not associated with severe disseminated infections, a specific, virulent clone of *Haemophilus influenzae* biogroup aegyptius has been identified as the causative agent in outbreaks of conjunctivitis followed by fulminant purpuric sepsis in Brazilian children (Brazilian purpuric fever).[57,127] Because topical therapy in these cases does not prevent subsequent disseminated *Haemophilus* spp. sepsis, it is probable that the conjunctivitis is simply an index of underlying carriage of the organism in the nasopharynx, which is the likely source of bacteremic spread.[9]

There are a number of entities that can produce acute conjunctivitis, the most important of which are viruses (including adenovirus, enterovirus, Coxsackie virus, and herpes simplex virus). Clinical differentiation between bacterial and viral conjunctivitis is often difficult. Features that are sometimes helpful in differentiating bacterial from viral conjunctivitis include the presence or absence of systemic symptoms, the character of the discharge, the type of conjunctival reaction, the involvement of the cornea, and the presence or absence of preauricular adenopathy (Table 62-1.) Nevertheless, because of considerable clinical overlap between bacterial and viral conjunctivitis, the predictive value of any single clinical symptom or sign for differentiating between bacterial and viral causes is low.[36]

Hyperpurulent Conjunctivitis

Hyperpurulent conjunctivitis (sometimes termed acute purulent conjunctivitis) is used to describe acute conjunctivitis associated with a profuse, purulent discharge, often with severe chemosis of the lids (Fig. 62-2). Although initial symptoms are similar to those seen in acute mucopurulent conjunctivitis, they crescendo rapidly in severity within a few days of onset. The conjunctiva is chemotic and densely hyperemic, and the lids frequently become tensely swollen. Thick, purulent exudate is present in large amounts in the cul-de-sac and overlying the ocular surface, reaccumulating rapidly after irrigation. Preauricular adenopathy is often present. Prolonged contact of the corneal surface with a copious exudate containing microorganisms and proteases can lead to the formation of peripheral corneal infiltrates. In untreated cases, this can rapidly progress to a ring infiltrate,

TABLE 62-1 DIFFERENTIATING CHARACTERISTICS OF BACTERIAL VERSUS VIRAL ETIOLOGIES OF ACUTE MUCOPURULENT CONJUNCTIVITIS

	Bacterial Conjunctivitis	Viral Conjunctivitis
Foreign body sensation	Less common	Common
Systemic symptoms	Usually none	May have symptoms of respiratory or systemic viral illness
Character of discharge	Usually mucopurulent, but may be watery	Usually watery, but may be mucopurulent
Conjunctival reaction	Papillary or mixed papillary/follicular	Follicular or mixed papillary/follicular
Superficial Corneal infiltrates	Uncommon	Common in adenoviral keratoconjunctivitis
Preauricular adenopathy	Infrequent	Common but not universally present

abscess formation, and corneal perforation. Other, less common sequelae include dacryadenitis, lid abscesses, and bacteremic dissemination. Prompt diagnosis and therapy are necessary to minimize the incidence of these potentially severe complications.

Neisseria gonorrhoeae is the major causative agent of hyperpurulent conjunctivitis.[135] Symptoms of cervicitis or urethritis and a history of exposure to sexually transmitted disease can be elicited in some cases. The diagnosis can usually be easily made on conjunctival scrapings that show

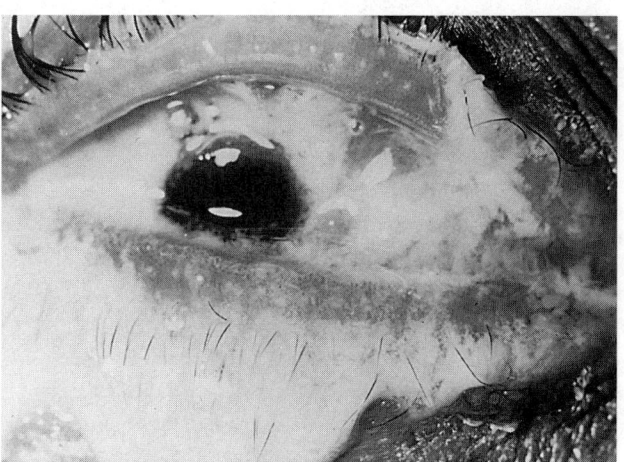

Fig. 62-2. Severe hyperpurulent conjunctivitis caused by *Neisseria gonorrhoeae*.

gram-negative diplococci within both epithelial cells and polymorphonuclear leukocytes (Fig. 62-3). *Neisseria meningitidis* is a less-frequent cause of hyperpurulent conjunctivitis but can also lead to disseminated bacteremia, meningitis, and sepsis.[3,101,129] Rarely, hyperpurulent conjunctivitis can result from species of bacteria that are usually responsible for milder forms of acute conjunctivitis, such as staphylococci and streptococci.

Membranous and Pseudomembranous Conjunctivitis

Membranous conjunctivitis is a severe form of conjunctivitis characterized by necrosis and sloughing of the conjunctival epithelium, producing a membrane of cellular debris and fibrin that is firmly adherent to the underlying substantia propria. *Corynebacterium diphtheriae* is classically associated with membranous conjunctivitis. However, in countries where passive diphtheria immunization is widely practiced, *Streptococcus pyogenes* is a more frequent cause of membranous conjunctivitis. The diffusible extracellular proteases and toxins produced by *C. diphtheriae* and *S. pyogenes* can cause widespread necrosis of the epithelial layers of the ocular surface, leading to subsequent development of conjunctival membranes. The infection begins with several days of severe conjunctival inflammation and marked chemosis, progressing to formation of plaquelike, avascular, yellow-gray membranes on the palpebral conjunctival surface (Fig. 62-4).[39] With *S. pyogenes,* membranes may form on both the palpebral and bulbar conjunctival surfaces. Corneal involvement may occur with both *C. diphtheriae* and *S. pyogenes* membranous conjunctivitis, sometimes in the form of corneal infiltrates[22] but more commonly manifest as epithelial sloughing. In the recovery stages of membranous conjunctivitis, subepithelial fibrosis,

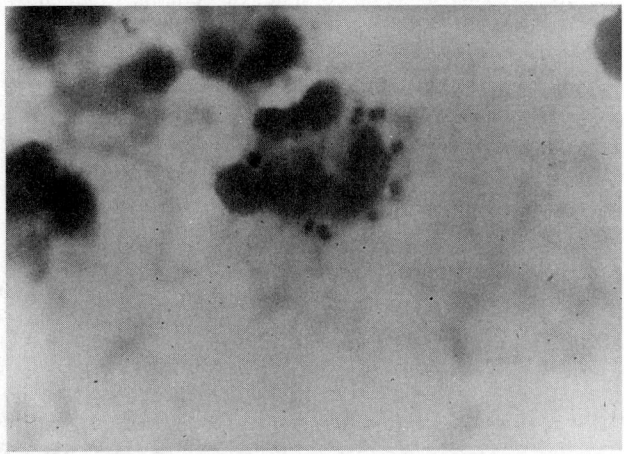

Fig. 62-3. Conjunctival smear from a case of hyperpurulent conjunctivitis, showing the characteristic gram-negative diplococci of *N. gonorrhoeae* within polymorphonuclear leukocytes.

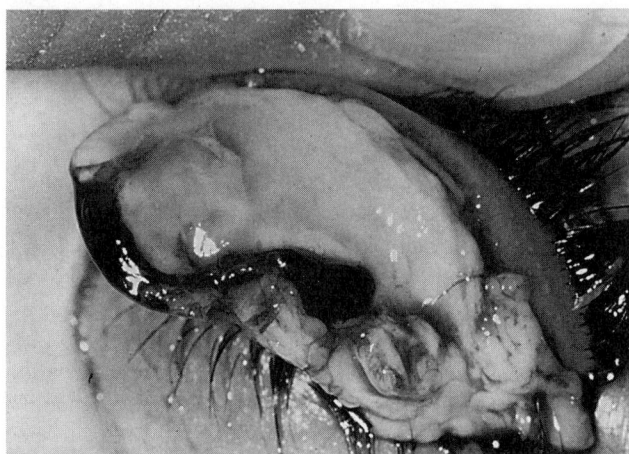

Fig. 62-4. Membranous conjunctivitis caused by *Corynebacterium diphtheriae.* (Courtesy of John P. Whitcher, MD.)

corneal scarring, symblepharon formation, tear deficiency, and trichiasis may be found.

Systemic involvement is a frequent accompaniment of membranous conjunctivitis. In the case of *C. diphtheriae,* diphtheritic membranes may be found concomitantly in the oral cavity or nasopharynx. Systemic diffusion of diphtheria toxin in untreated cases can result in fatal involvement of the myocardium and peripheral nerves. Patients with *S. pyogenes* membranous conjunctivitis may be febrile and toxic, and they may be susceptible to complications of bacteremic dissemination.

Pseudomembranous bacterial conjunctivitis is produced by infectious and inflammatory processes similar to those causing membranous conjunctivitis, but less severe in intensity and without epithelial and subepithelial necrosis. Pseudomembranous bacterial conjunctivitis may be produced by any severe form of acute conjunctivitis, but it is most commonly associated with *Streptococcus pyogenes* and *Neisseria gonorrhoeae.* Other causes include *Corynebacterium diphtheriae, Haemophilus influenzae* biogroup aegyptius, *Neisseria meningitidis, Branhamella catarrhalis, Streptococcus pneumoniae,* and *Staphylococcus aureus.*

The differential diagnosis of membranous and pseudomembranous bacterial conjunctivitis includes neonatal chlamydial conjunctivitis,[115] adenoviral conjunctivitis (for example, epidemic keratoconjunctivitis), herpes simplex conjunctivitis, *Candida* conjunctivitis, ligneous conjunctivitis, Stevens-Johnson syndrome, and chemical burns.

Neonatal Conjunctivitis

Neonatal conjunctivitis (or ophthalmia neonatorum) is the most common infectious disease of the first 6 weeks of life.[18] This condition affects 1.6% to 19% of newborns in industrialized countries[2,26,106] and up to 24% of neonates in developing countries.[40] Bacterial causes account for approximately half of the cases of neonatal conjunctivitis.[109]

In industrialized countries the most common causes of neonatal bacterial conjunctivitis are *Staphylococcus* spp., viridans streptococci, *Haemophilus influenzae*, *Haemophilus parainfluenzae*, *Streptococcus pneumoniae*, *Branhamella catarrhalis*, enterococci, *Escherichia coli*, and *Klebsiella pneumoniae*.[18,71,109] These bacterial species generally cause a mild, acute mucopurulent conjunctivitis beginning 3 to 5 days after birth. Serious complications are few, except in the case of nosocomial infections caused by *Pseudomonas aeruginosa*, which can lead to sepsis and death.[16] Although a century ago gonococcal conjunctivitis was the leading cause of ophthalmia neonatorum and childhood blindness, it now accounts for less than 3% of the cases of neonatal conjunctivitis in Europe[27,106] and the United States.[71,109] Despite the decline in gonococcal neonatal conjunctivitis in industrialized countries to the current level of 0.01% to 0.04% of live births,[42,71] *Neisseria gonorrhoeae* neonatal conjunctivitis remains a significant and pressing health problem in many developing nations. In Kenya 12% of the cases of neonatal conjunctivitis were reported to be caused by *N. gonorrhoeae*,[77] and half of the gonococcal isolates were penicillinase-producing strains.[41]

Gonococcal ophthalmia neonatorum appears 2 to 4 days after birth as an acute mucopurulent or hyperpurulent conjunctivitis (Fig. 62-5). Hyperemia, chemosis, and lid swelling are prominent. Corneal involvement may begin as a diffuse punctate keratopathy progressing to peripheral corneal infiltration and ulceration, intrastromal abscess formation, and perforation. Prompt recognition and combined local and

CAUSES OF NEONATAL CONJUNCTIVITIS

CHEMICAL
Silver nitrate
Erythromycin
CHLAMYDIAL
Chlamydia trachomatis
BACTERIAL
Staphylococcus aureus
Staphylococcus epidermidis
Viridans group streptococci
Streptococcus pneumoniae
Group D streptococci
Haemophilus influenzae
Haemophilus parainfluenzae
Haemophilus haemolyticus
Neisseria gonorrhoeae
Neisseria meningitidis
Branhamella catarrhalis
Escherichia coli
Klebsiella pneumoniae
VIRAL
Herpes simplex virus
NOSOCOMIAL
Staphylococcus aureus
Pseudomonas aeruginosa
IRRITATIVE
Birth trauma
OTHER
Mycoplasma hominis (?)
Ureaplasma urealyticum (?)

References 2, 16, 27, 42, 51, 58, 71, 72, 74, 86, 94, 106, 107, 109, 115, 116.

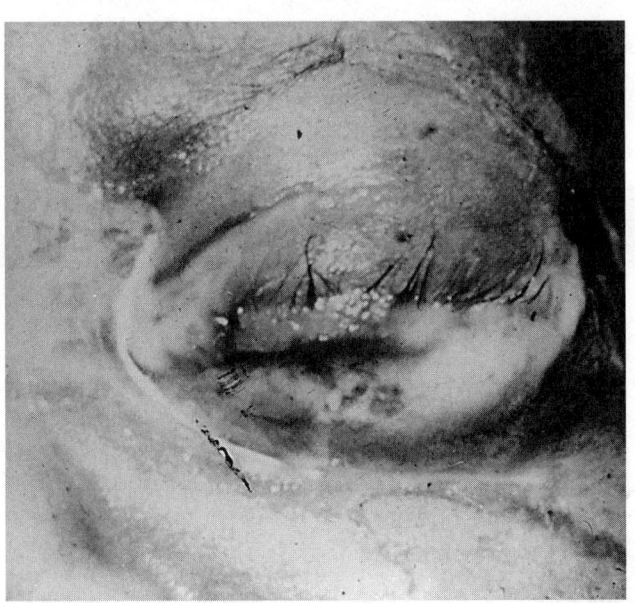

Fig. 62-5. Gonococcal neonatal conjunctivitis.

systemic therapy are essential for preventing blinding complications of this disease.

There are a number of other causes of neonatal conjunctivitis (see box),* the most common of which are chemical conjunctivitis and chlamydial conjunctivitis. A transient chemical conjunctivitis lasting 24 to 48 hours is seen in up to 90% of infants receiving Credé prophylaxis with silver nitrate,[51] and a persistent chemical conjunctivitis is seen in 5% to 7%.[2,71] The incidence of chlamydial neonatal conjunctivitis varies depending on the demographic and socioeconomic characteristics of the population at risk. In a Baltimore inner-city hospital, 46% of the cases of neonatal conjunctivitis were positive for *Chlamydia trachomatis*.[108] In contrast, 6% of cultures performed in Northern Norway for

*References 2, 16, 27, 42, 51, 58, 71, 72, 74, 86, 94, 106, 107, 109, 115, 116.

neonatal conjunctivitis showed *Chlamydia* spp.[27] In developing nations where gonococcal conjunctivitis is prevalent, there is a high rate of concomitant *N. gonorrhoeae* and *C. trachomatis* infection.[77]

Chronic Mucopurulent Conjunctivitis

Chronic mucopurulent conjunctivitis is the term used to designate cases of conjunctivitis with active signs of hyperemia and discharge of greater than 4 weeks in duration. Symptoms include chronic mucoid discharge, sticky lids upon awakening, hyperemic conjunctivae, reddened lid margins, and irritation. The condition is usually bilateral. In contrast to most cases of acute conjunctivitis, the discharge in chronic cases is generally reduced in quantity and more mucoid than purulent. There is frequently an associated chronic blepharitis, manifest as hyperemic and slightly thickened lid margins with pouting meibomian gland orifices. Preauricular adenopathy is generally absent.

The organisms most frequently responsible for chronic mucopurulent conjunctivitis are *Staphylococcus aureus* and *Moraxella lacunata*. Chronic conjunctivitis caused by *S. aureus* is often accompanied by blepharitis and punctate epithelial keratopathy (Fig. 62-6). In some instances, noninfectious marginal infiltrates or phlyctenules can be seen. *Moraxella* spp. (often *lacunata*) can produce an acute mucopurulent conjunctivitis,[136] a chronic follicular conjunctivitis[76] (often epidemic),[110,117] or a chronic blepharoconjunctivitis affecting the medial and lateral canthi *(angular blepharoconjunctivitis)*.[93] In the latter instance there is a low-grade chronic mucoid discharge with maceration and madarosis of the lid margins at the canthal regions (Fig. 62-7). Some cases of angular blepharoconjunctivitis may show a mixed infection with both *Moraxella* spp. and *Staphylococcus aureus*.[131] Other bacterial causes of chronic mucopurulent conjunctivitis include *Streptococcus* spp.,

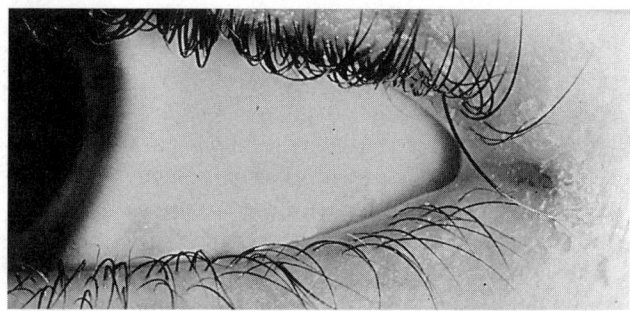

Fig. 62-7.   Angular blepharoconjunctivitis caused by *Moraxella.*

Haemophilus spp., *Proteus* spp., and other organisms that more frequently cause acute mucopurulent conjunctivitis.

DIFFERENTIAL DIAGNOSIS

A number of entities should be considered in the differential diagnosis of the patient with suspected chronic mucopurulent bacterial conjunctivitis. Parinaud oculoglandular conjunctivitis is a regional manifestation of cat-scratch disease characterized by unilateral chronic granulomatous conjunctivitis and visible, chronic ipsilateral preauricular and/or submandibular adenopathy.[128] The regional adenopathy and conjunctival granulomata (Fig. 62-8) of this entity distinguish it from mucopurulent bacterial conjunctivitis. Children and young adults with a history of exposure to cats are usually affected. Although a number of pathogens can cause Parinaud oculoglandular syndrome, the causative agents appear to be *Bartonella henselae* in the majority of cases[29a] and possibly *Afipia felis* in a minority of instances.[11,101] These bacilli are fastidious, pleiomorphic gram-negative rods that can be isolated in tissue culture[141] but grow poorly on artificial media. Biopsy of the conjunctival granulomata or the involved lymph nodes may show the characteristic slender bacilli on Warthin-Starry silver stain.[6] Symptomatic

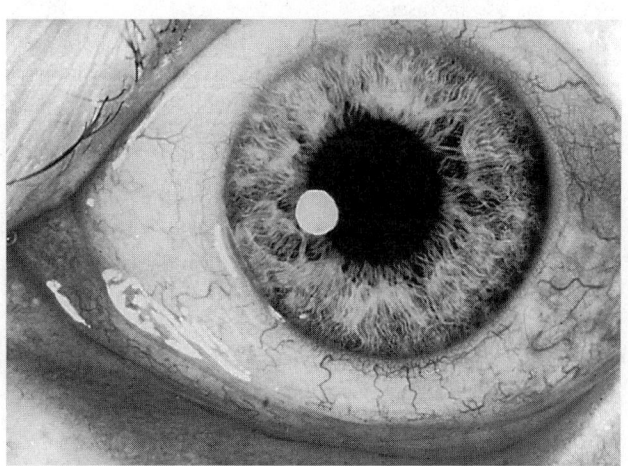

Fig. 62-6.   Chronic blepharoconjunctivitis caused by *Staphylococcus aureus.*

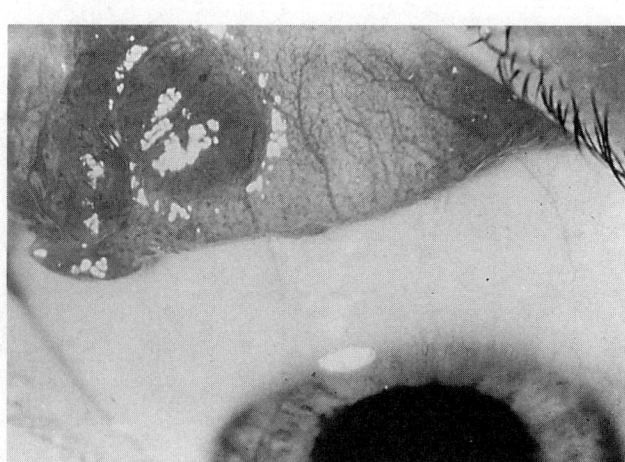

Fig. 62-8.   Upper tarsal conjunctival granulomata in a patient with Parinaud oculoglandular conjunctivitis.

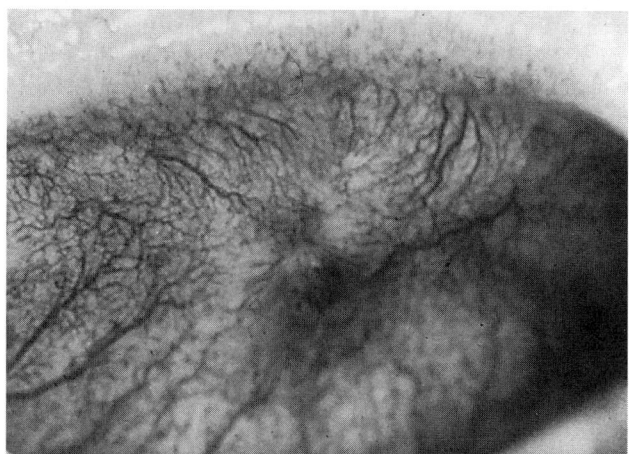

Fig. 62-9. Meibomian gland carcinoma masquerading as a chronic blepharoconjunctivitis.

cases can be treated systemically with fluoroquinolones, rifampin, or trimethoprim/sulfamethoxazole.[87]

Sebaceous gland carcinoma and other malignancies of the lid and conjunctiva should always be excluded as potential causes of chronic blepharoconjunctivitis or conjunctivitis (Fig. 62-9). A lid biopsy should be performed to rule out the possibility of malignancy in any case of chronic unexplained conjunctivitis not responding to therapy.

Nonbacterial infectious causes of chronic conjunctivitis include adult chlamydial conjunctivitis, molluscum contagiosum-associated conjunctivitis, and some cases of prolonged viral conjunctivitis. Other common noninfectious causes of subacute conjunctivitis include hayfever conjunctivitis, vernal keratoconjunctivitis, atopic keratoconjunctivitis, giant papillary conjunctivitis, floppy lid syndrome, mucus fishing syndrome,[90] toxic conjunctivitis, keratoconjunctivitis sicca, exposure keratoconjunctivitis, graft-vs.-host disease, and bullous oculocutaneous disorders. Although these entities can usually be differentiated from chronic mucopurulent bacterial conjunctivitis on the basis of history and physical findings, bacterial cultures may be of value in doubtful cases.

LABORATORY INVESTIGATIONS

Microbiologic studies have a limited role in the management of routine cases of suspected bacterial conjunctivitis.[84] In uncomplicated acute mucopurulent conjunctivitis, conjunctival smears often yield false positive readings and very frequently yield false negatives when compared to results of conjunctival cultures.[48,84] Microbial identification and antibiotic susceptibility testing, which may take 48 to 72 hours to obtain, may be of limited value in a disease in which 85% to 95% of the cases respond to empiric broad-spectrum therapy within 5 days.[48,85,132] Although antibiotics have no beneficial effect in the remaining 50% to 60% of cases that rep-

resent viral conjunctivitis,[36] the risk/benefit ratio for empiric therapy remains favorable because of the extremely low incidence of serious side effects from commonly used topical antimicrobials.

Although of limited benefit for most routine cases of acute conjunctivitis, bacteriologic studies are mandated in certain clinical settings (see box). Smears and cultures should be performed in all cases of neonatal conjunctivitis, hyperpurulent conjunctivitis, membranous conjunctivitis, pseudomembranous conjunctivitis, nosocomial conjunctivitis, or conjunctivitis in an immunocompromised host. Because these patients are at high risk for developing serious ocular and systemic complications, establishment of a microbiologic diagnosis (when possible) can aid in timely selection and refinement of an appropriate antibiotic regimen. Additional indications for microbiologic studies may include chronic mucopurulent conjunctivitis, recurrent or relapsing acute mucopurulent conjunctivitis, or acute muco-

---

INDICATIONS FOR MICROBIOLOGIC STUDIES IN SUSPECTED BACTERIAL CONJUNCTIVITIS

ACUTE MUCOPURULENT CONJUNCTIVITIS IN CHILDREN AND ADULTS
Systemic immunocompromise
  Debilitating illness
  Children < 1 year of age
  Inherited or acquired immunodeficiency
  Immunosuppression
Local immunocompromise
  Recent ocular surgery
  Presence of a filtering bleb or seton valve
  Topical corticosteroid use
  Chronic antibiotic use
  Contact lens or prosthesis wear
  Corneal or conjunctival surface disease
Transmission in special clinical settings
  Nosocomial transmission
  Household contact with individuals with known carriage or infection with *Neisseria meningitidis* or *Haemophilus influenzae* type b
  Sexual contact with individuals with known or suspected *Neisseria gonorrhoeae* infection
  Children in high-risk regions during epidemics of Brazilian purpuric fever
Relapsing or recurring acute mucopurulent conjunctivitis
Acute mucopurulent conjunctivitis that fails to improve after 7 to 10 days of empiric treatment
HYPERPURULENT CONJUNCTIVITIS
MEMBRANOUS CONJUNCTIVITIS
PSEUDOMEMBRANOUS CONJUNCTIVITIS
NEONATAL CONJUNCTIVITIS
CHRONIC MUCOPURULENT CONJUNCTIVITIS

purulent conjunctivitis showing no signs of resolution after 7 to 10 days of empiric therapy.

Specimen Collection

Because even partial antibiotic treatment can markedly reduce the yield of subsequent cultures, if bacteriologic studies are indicated, they should be performed prior to initiating topical or systemic antibiotics. If antibiotic therapy has already been initiated, antibiotics should be discontinued for a minimum of 36 hours before cultures are performed. If only a limited quantity of material is available for sampling, priority should be given to securing material for cultures before performing smears.

Conjunctival cultures should be performed by vigorously swabbing the unanesthetized conjunctiva with a sterile calcium alginate or dacron swab slightly moistened with either liquid broth or nonbacteriostatic saline. Calcium alginate or dacron swabs are preferred over cotton swabs, which contain fatty acids that may inhibit bacterial growth.[112] To maximize recovery, cultures should be inoculated directly into final culture media rather than into transport media.

At a minimum, both blood agar and chocolate agar plates should be inoculated. Blood agar, an excellent general-purpose medium for supporting the growth of bacteria at 37°C (and many fungi at 25°C), has the advantage of facilitating rapid identification of various groups of streptococci on the basis of their differing hemolytic properties. Chocolate agar contains supplemental factors that aid in the growth of Neisseria spp., Haemophilus spp., and Moraxella spp. If transport to the microbiology laboratory is delayed for any length of time, the inoculated plates should be held in a 37°C incubator. Chocolate agar plates additionally require placement in a CO_2-enriched atmosphere, like that of a candle jar. In special instances other media can be inoculated, such as mannitol salt agar (for rapid identification of Staphylococcus spp.), Thayer-Martin medium (for Neisseria spp.), cyclo-heximide-free Sabouraud agar at 25°C (for fungi), thioglycolate broth (for anaerobic bacteria), or brain-heart infusion broth (for fastidious bacteria). If viral or chlamydial cultures are to be taken, separate calcium alginate or dacron swabs should be employed for brushing the conjunctival surface and inoculating the appropriate media.

Depending on the clinical presentation, additional cultures of sites other than the conjunctiva may be indicated. Cultures should be taken from the lid margins in cases of blepharoconjunctivitis. If meibomitis is present, meibum should be gently expressed from the meibomian orifices and cultured. The same media plate may be used for cultures of both the conjunctiva and lids if conjunctival swabs are streaked in the pattern of rows of C's and lid swabs streaked with rows of L's. (The additional prefix of R or L can be used to designate right or left, respectively.) In cases of hyperpurulent conjunctivitis, cervical or urethral cultures for both Neisseria gonorrhoeae and Chlamydia trachomatis should

be performed. Similarly, cervical cultures of the mother should be performed in cases of neonatal conjunctivitis with culture-proven recovery of gonococci or chlamydia. Nasopharyngeal cultures of the patient and contacts should be considered in cases of conjunctivitis caused by Neisseria meningitidis, Haemophilus influenzae type b, or nosocomially transmitted Staphylococcus aureus. In cases of recurrent conjunctivitis a latent infectious focus (for example, chronic dacryocystitis) should be sought and cultured if present. If contact lenses, ocular prostheses, topical medications, or eye makeup have been in use at the onset of conjunctivitis, appropriate cultures of these materials should also be performed.

If smear examination is indicated, conjunctival scrapings should be performed after cultures have been taken. A flame-sterilized platinum spatula (Kimura or Lindner) is used to gently, but firmly, stroke the topically anesthetized palpebral conjunctival surface. Excessive trauma to the congested and friable tissues should be avoided, because any bleeding that may be induced can interfere with subsequent smear interpretation. A sufficient amount of material should be thinly spread onto three clean glass slides.

Slides should immediately be fixed in methanol (or heat-fixed, if methanol is not available), then air-dried. Two slides should be retained for examination by the microbiology laboratory (one slide for Gram stain and the other for Giemsa stain or special studies such as immunofluorescent labeling). The third slide can be Gram-stained and examined in the office.

The slide should initially be scanned at 100× to 400×, then examined at 1000× under oil-immersion for detailed study of the morphology of any identified intracellular or extracellular bacteria. The number of epithelial cells present on the smear will give an indication of the adequacy of the scraping. Cytologic examination of the epithelial and inflammatory cells can be helpful in characterizing the nature and degree of the conjunctival inflammatory response.[130] For example, a smear predominated by polymorphonuclear leukocytes is consistent with acute mucopurulent bacterial conjunctivitis and correlates with a high probability of bacterial recovery by culture.[134]

Interpretation of Smears

The reliability and diagnostic utility of a smear examination depends on the adequacy of sampling, quantity and uniformity of organisms recovered, quality of fixation and staining, thoroughness of inspection, and diagnostic experience of the examiner. Deficiencies in one or more of these areas may yield incomplete or inaccurate information. Several studies have shown that false positive readings and false negative readings in particular are common.[48,84] Conversely, false positive readings may occur in culture-negative cases.[84]

The interpretation of a smear is generally more reliable when numerous organisms of a single morphology can be identified in the presence of a background of numerous epithelial cells and inflammatory cells. In this regard smears of pneumococcal and gonococcal conjunctivitis are often diagnostic because of the appearance of morphologically uniform microorganisms (gram-positive lancet-shaped diplococci and gram-negative diplococci, respectively) that are frequently found in abundant numbers both intracellularly and extracellularly. More frequently, the smear may show moderate to numerous inflammatory cells, but bacteria are absent, scanty, or heterogeneous in morphology or staining characteristics. Smears with these features are likely to be unreliable and should be interpreted with great caution, preferably with the assistance of an experienced microbiologist. Thus unless a smear is unequivocally positive, it should not be relied on for guiding therapy.

Interpretation of Culture Results

Although the evaluation of culture results is generally straightforward, interpretive difficulties can arise for a number of reasons. A negative culture may indicate a viral or other nonbacterial cause, but also may represent a false negative result. False negatives can result from prior antibiotic treatment, inadequate sampling or inoculation technique, delayed specimen transport, use of inappropriate media, or laboratory errors in specimen processing. On the other hand, a positive culture result may also require caution in interpretation.[84,125] A bacterial isolate recovered on culture may be a contaminant or represent part of the normal resident flora. To differentiate colonization from pathogenic overgrowth, cultures of Staphylococcus epidermidis, Corynebacterium spp., and Propionibacterium spp. are generally considered nondiagnostic, unless the initial sample contains a moderate-to-heavy initial inoculum of bacteria.[82,114] A qualitative estimate of inoculum size can be acquired by examining the density of colonies obtained on a streaked media plate. A semiquantitative determination of inoculum size can be performed by dilutional plating of a known volume of sample,[17,52] but this method is laborious and therefore is generally reserved for research studies.

An additional interpretive issue arises in relation to the analysis of antibiotic susceptibility testing. Kirby-Bauer disk diffusion tests and other methods of antibiotic susceptibility testing define susceptibility breakpoints on the basis of tissue or body fluid antibiotic levels typically achieved after systemic antibiotic administration. Because topical administration can produce antibiotic tissue levels greatly in excess of those achievable from systemic routes,[89] an organism that is resistant to a particular antibiotic based on conventionally defined criteria may in fact be highly susceptible when the same antimicrobial is given topically. In circumstances in which resistance can be overcome by increasing the antibiotic concentration several-fold (as is often the case with aminoglycoside-resistant Pseudomonas aeruginosa),[104] topical antibiotic therapy may be successful. With high-level

antibiotic resistance (for example, chromosomal or plasmid-mediated expression of beta-lactamase), however, increases in antibiotic concentration are likely to have little appreciable effect. Establishment of more precise guidelines for defining susceptibility breakpoints relevant to ophthalmic infections are clearly needed, but will not be possible until systematic studies of the ocular pharmacokinetics and pharmacodynamics of topically administered antimicrobials are undertaken.

THERAPY

There are two types of approaches to the treatment of ocular infections: specific therapy and empiric therapy. Serious ophthalmic infections such as bacterial keratitis, endophthalmitis, or complicated cases of bacterial conjunctivitis mandate specific therapy, usually divided into two stages. The first step entails culture of relevant sites and the initiation of an empiric regimen of bactericidal antimicrobials designed to provide coverage for a broad range of potential pathogens. In designing empiric antimicrobial therapy, priority is given to covering the most likely pathogens as well as the less likely (but highly virulent) organisms. In the second stage the regimen is then modified according to culture and sensitivity results to provide therapy that is narrower in spectrum but of equal or greater efficacy.

In routine, uncomplicated cases of bacterial conjunctivitis appearing within 7 days of onset, an empiric approach to therapy is usually justified on several grounds. Approximately half of the cases of acute mucopurulent conjunctivitis are bacterial in cause,[36] and 85% to 95% will respond to an empiric 7- to 10-day course of any number of nonfortified bacteriostatic or bactericidal antimicrobials.[48,82,85,131] Antibiotic treatment shortens the duration of symptoms[48] and may reduce the potential for communicable spread to the opposite eye or other persons. Treatment is generally performed with broad-spectrum antimicrobials that are established, inexpensive, and well-tolerated to avoid problems relating to antibiotic overusage, cost containment, and safety. In the remaining 5% to 15% of bacterial conjunctivitis cases that do not respond to empiric therapy and in cases of viral conjunctivitis, the consequence of treatment failure is negligible because the disease usually resolves spontaneously and without sequelae within 10 days of onset. By empirically treating routine cases of acute mucopurulent conjunctivitis and reserving cultures for the small fraction of atypical, complicated, or unresponsive cases, uncomplicated acute conjunctivitis in adults and children can be managed in a cost-effective manner.

Certain cases may require no treatment whatsoever. In a nonimmunocompromised patient with resolving acute mucopurulent conjunctivitis of 7 or more days' duration, treatment would be marginally beneficial and is therefore best withheld. Cases of acute nonmucopurulent conjunctivitis with classic hallmarks of viral conjunctivitis and no signs of

TABLE 62-2   SELECTED COMMERCIALLY AVAILABLE ANTIBACTERIALS FOR FIRST-LINE THERAPY OF UNCOMPLICATED BACTERIAL CONJUNCTIVITIS

Generic Name	Concentration	Formulation	Common Trade Name(s)* (Manufacturer)	Comment
Bacitracin +Polymyxin B	500 U/g 10,000 U/ml	Ointment	Polysporin (Burroughs Wellcome)	Not available in solution form
Chloramphenicol	0.5% 1.0%	Solution Ointment	Chloromycetin (Parke-Davis) Chloroptic (Allergan) Ophthochlor† (Parke-Davis)	Rare occurrence of aplastic anemia
Neomycin +Polymyxin B +Bacitracin	1.75 mg/g 10,000 U/g 400 U/g	Ointment	Neosporin (Burroughs Wellcome)	Neomycin sensitivity not infrequent
Neomycin +Polymyxin B +Gramicidin	3.5 mg/ml 10,000 U/ml 0.025 mg/ml	Solution	Neosporin (Burroughs Wellcome)	Neomycin sensitivity not infrequent
Polymyxin B +Trimethoprim	10,000 U/ml 0.1%	Solution	Polytrim (Allergan)	Higher in cost than generically available alternatives
Sulfacetamide	10%, 15%, 30% 10%	Solution Ointment	Bleph-10 (Allergan) Sodium Sulamyd (Schering)	Rare occurrence of Stevens-Johnson syndrome in setting of prior systemic sulfa exposure

* Name applies to both solution and ointment formulations, unless otherwise specified.
† Preservative-free; solution formulation only.

bacterial conjunctivitis are also likely not to benefit from antibiotic therapy.

There is no single antibiotic regimen that is best for all cases of bacterial conjunctivitis. Antibiotic selection and dosing should be based on a number of factors: the nature and severity of the infection, antibiotic susceptibility patterns of the most likely causative organisms, host immune status, patient compliance, antimicrobial activity spectrum, adverse effect profile, cost, and antibiotic resistance considerations. A number of nonfortified bacteriostatic or bacteri-

cidal antimicrobials (discussed in the next section) are equally effective for uncomplicated bacterial conjunctivitis (Table 62-2). Agents that are generally inappropriate for empiric or primary therapy of routine bacterial conjunctivitis include the aminoglycosides and the fluoroquinolones (Table 62-3). Although aminoglycosides such as gentamicin and tobramycin provide excellent coverage against *Staphylococcus aureus* and gram-negative bacilli,[33] their activity against *Streptococcus* spp. is variable.[142] Another disadvantage of aminoglycosides is the corneal and conjunctival epi-

TABLE 62-3   SELECTED COMMERCIALLY AVAILABLE ANTIBACTERIALS FOR SECOND-LINE THERAPY OF BACTERIAL CONJUNCTIVITIS*

Generic Name	Concentration	Formulation	Common Trade Name† (Manufacturer)	Comment
Bacitracin	500 U/g	Ointment	Bacitracin (Bausch & Lomb)	Not active against gram-negative bacilli Not available in solution form
Ciprofloxacin	0.3%	Solution	Ciloxan (Alcon)	Overuse may promote resistance, esp. among staphylococci
Gentamicin	0.3% 0.3%	Solution Ointment	Garamycin (Schering) Genoptic (Allergan)	Can cause toxic keratoconjunctivitis Variable activity against streptococci
Norfloxacin	0.3%	Solution	Chibroxin (Merck)	Overuse may promote resistance Less effective than ciprofloxacin against *Pseudomonas*
Ofloxacin	0.3%	Solution	Ocuflox (Allergan)	Overuse may promote resistance
Tobramycin	0.3% 0.3%	Solution Ointment	Tobrex (Alcon)	Same as for gentamicin

* Reserved for cases in which a first-line agent (such as those in Table 62-2) cannot be used because of documented or suspected drug resistance or because of drug hypersensitivity
† Name applies to both solution and ointment formulations, unless otherwise specified.

thelial toxicity that can accompany their use. Fluoroquinolones, such as ciprofloxacin, have an excellent safety profile and a broad spectrum of activity, particularly against staphylococci and *Pseudomonas aeruginosa*.[63] Their activity against streptococci is generally only fair to moderate.[63] Fluoroquinolones should be reserved for empiric therapy of serious infections like bacterial keratitis[83] or for second-line therapy in cases of documented resistance to first-line agents. Indiscriminate use of fluoroquinolones for less severe infections such as blepharitis or conjunctivitis should be strongly discouraged so that the usefulness of these agents can be prolonged. Resistance to topical ciprofloxacin has already been reported, less than 3 years after its introduction in the United States.[122] Preliminary evidence suggests that the incidence of ciprofloxacin resistance among ocular isolates increased in the first 2 years after the introduction of ciprofloxacin.[95] It remains to be seen whether this possible trend of increasing resistance among ocular isolates will continue in a fashion similar to that observed after the introduction of systemic fluoroquindones.[28]

The problems of antibiotic overusage and antibiotic resistance are urgent issues with profound implications for the future of antimicrobial therapy. In the current era of antibiotic usage, the dissemination of antibiotic resistance occurs rapidly because of heavy antibiotic selection pressure. This fact has been exemplified in recent decades by the rapid rise in prevalence of methicillin-resistant *Staphylococcus aureus*, penicillinase-producing *Neisseria gonorrhoeae*, penicillin-resistant *Streptococcus pneumoniae*, and multidrug resistant *Pseudomonas aeruginosa*.[98] Although the traditional solution to the problem of drug resistance has been the synthesis of new antimicrobials, the rate of introduction of new classes of antimicrobials has been slowing in recent years.[120] Unless measures are taken to control the usage of newly developed antimicrobials, the rapid evolutionary pace of new bacterial resistance mechanisms may soon outstrip the chemist's ability to synthesize new antimicrobials. A concern for the future is the possible scenario of a "post-antimicrobial era" in which the majority of antimicrobials will have been rendered ineffective because of widespread multidrug resistance.[23]

Selection of Topical Antibiotics for Uncomplicated Bacterial Conjunctivitis

Routine cases of acute bacterial conjunctivitis respond equally well to a 7- to 10-day course of any of a number of broad-spectrum antibiotics including chloramphenicol, sulfacetamide, neomycin-polymyxin B, and trimethoprim-polymyxin B[46,85] (see Table 62-2).

Chloramphenicol, though highly effective for most cases of bacterial conjunctivitis,[13,46] is currently not in wide use. This low usage is mainly the result of concerns over the rare incidence of idiosyncratic aplastic anemia following topical chloramphenicol use,[43] although the strength of this association is unclear.

Sulfacetamide is inexpensive and effective in shortening the duration of symptoms in acute mucopurulent conjunctivitis caused by the most commonly encountered pathogens.[85] Adverse effects to sulfacetamide occur uncommonly. Although Stevens-Johnson syndrome (erythema multiforme major) has been frequently associated with systemic sulfonamide use, there are only three case reports of its occurrence following topical sulfonamide administration.[45,50,113] In all three cases there had been previous exposure to systemic sulfa drugs, suggesting a possible role for presensitization in the pathogenesis of these Stevens-Johnson reactions.[126] Although there is no evidence that the risk of Stevens-Johnson syndrome is higher with the use of topical sulfonamides than with other topical antimicrobials, it is reasonable to consider alternative antimicrobials if there has been a prior history of systemic sulfonamide use.

Other agents to consider include neomycin-polymyxin B-gramicidin, an inexpensive, well-established antibiotic combination that is effective in the majority of cases of bacterial conjunctivitis.[70] Its only significant drawback is a not infrequent (~ 10%) incidence of neomycin allergy, typically manifest as a periocular contact dermatitis.[145]

Trimethoprim-polymyxin B is a combination antimicrobial with an activity profile similar to that of neomycin-polymyxin B-gramicidin,[99] but without the potential for neomycin exposure. It can also be safely used in patients with sulfa allergies, because trimethoprim is structurally distinct from the sulfonamide drugs.[46] Trimethoprim-polymyxin B has the drawback of costing considerably more than neomycin-polymyxin B-gramicidin, sulfacetamide, or chloramphenicol.

Selection of Topical Antibiotics for Complicated Bacterial Conjunctivitis

If a case of suspected bacterial conjunctivitis fails to respond to initial therapy with one of the above-described broad-spectrum antimicrobials, a number of potential causes should be considered before making a potentially unwarranted change in the antibiotic regimen. A common reason for an apparent non-response to treatment is that the conjunctivitis is not bacterial in etiology. In this circumstance, discontinuation of antibiotic therapy and observation is the appropriate course. Other potential factors include patient noncompliance, inadequate dosing or duration of therapy, secondary conjunctivitis due to drug toxicity, or antimicrobial resistance. Culture and susceptibility testing may be helpful in differentiating among these varying causes.

If a change in antibiotic therapy is indicated, an attempt should first be made to select another first-line, broad-spectrum antimicrobial or antimicrobial combination such as those listed in Table 62-2. If an appropriate alternative in this category is not available, other antibiotics may be considered. These second-line antimicrobials (see Table 62-3), which include the aminoglycosides, fluoroquinolones, and bacitracin, are best reserved for circumstances in which drug hypersensitivity, drug toxicity, or antimicrobial resistance limits the use of any of the recommended first-line agents. These antimicrobials are generally not advised for empiric therapy of uncomplicated bacterial conjunctivitis because of one or more potential disadvantages, including increased cost (fluoroquinolones), important gaps in antimicrobial spectrum (bacitracin, fluoroquinolones, and aminoglycosides), higher toxicity (aminoglycosides), or promotion of antimicrobial resistance (fluoroquinolones and possibly aminoglycosides).

Indications for Systemic Antibiotic Treatment of Bacterial Conjunctivitis

Although topical routes of antibiotic delivery are preferred for most cases of bacterial conjunctivitis, systemic treatment may be necessary in selected instances. These include *Neisseria gonorrhoeae* conjunctivitis, *Neisseria meningitidis* conjunctivitis, conjunctivitis-otitis syndrome caused by *Haemophilus influenzae,* conjunctivitis resulting from the Brazilian purpuric fever variant of *Haemophilus influenzae* biogroup aegyptius, membranous or pseudomembranous conjunctivitis caused by *Corynebacterium diphtheriae* or *Streptococcus pyogenes,* and *Pseudomonas* conjunctivitis in immunocompromised patients.

Gonococcal conjunctivitis in neonates, children, and adults is currently treated with parenteral administration of ceftriaxone,[53,78] a long-acting third-generation cephalosporin with excellent activity against penicillinase-producing *N. gonorrhoeae.* Because of the high frequency of concomitant chlamydial infection,[73] empiric treatment with an oral tetracycline (or erythromycin in children or pregnant women) should be simultaneously administered. Patients with gonococcal conjunctivitis should be admitted to a hospital for close observation and frequent lavage of purulent material from the ocular surface to guard against secondary keratitis and corneal perforation. Although adjunctive therapy with topical bacitracin or penicillin G is often prescribed, it is generally not necessary because parenteral antibiotic therapy is sufficient to eradicate all viable organisms. Adjunctive systemic treatment is similarly indicated in all cases of primary *Neisseria meningitidis* conjunctivitis to reduce the risk of systemic dissemination.[29,100] At present penicillin G remains the drug of choice for *N. meningitidis.*

Systemic therapy for *Haemophilus influenzae* is indicated in conjunctivitis-otitis syndrome[56] and the Brazilian purpuric fever variant of *Haemophilus influenzae* biogroup aegyptius.[127] At present the majority of strains of *Haemophilus influenzae* are responsive to treatment with either amoxicillin or trimethoprim-sulfamethoxazole. If microbial resistance to these agents is documented on susceptibility testing or widely prevalent in a particular community, therapy with a second-generation cephalosporin (cefuroxime axetil or cefaclor) or third-generation cephalosporin (cefixime) should

be considered. Adjunctive therapy with rifampin can be helpful in eradicating nasopharyngeal carriage in refractory cases.[65]

Systemic penicillin G should be administered in membranous conjunctivitis caused by either *Streptococcus pyogenes* or *Corynebacterium diphtheriae.* If diphtheritic conjunctivitis is suspected, diphtheria antitoxin should immediately be administered systemically.

A final indication for systemic treatment is gram-negative bacillary conjunctivitis (particularly *Pseudomonas aeruginosa*) in premature infants or severely immunocompromised patients. Because of the potential risk of fatal bacteremic dissemination in these patients, adjunctive therapy with an appropriately chosen antimicrobial agent should be considered.

Because antibiotic treatment recommendations are in a state of constant evolution, current guidelines should be consulted before prescribing treatment for these frequently serious conditions.

PREVENTION

Efforts to prevent bacterial conjunctivitis have primarily focused on the prophylaxis of gonococcal neonatal conjunctivitis, which was once among the most common causes of childhood blindness.[37] Topically applied silver nitrate solution, erythromycin ointment, or tetracycline ointment is each highly effective in reducing the incidence of bacterial conjunctivitis (including gonococcal conjunctivitis), but none of them can prevent chlamydial conjunctivitis.[54,148] The declining incidence of gonococcal conjunctivitis in many parts of Europe has led to a discontinuation of Credé prophylaxis in these regions.[106] Nevertheless, because gonococcal conjunctivitis remains a problem in certain population subgroups of the United States and in many developing nations, prophylaxis remains essential in most parts of the world.[20]

Simple hygienic measures such as handwashing and avoidance of hand-to-eye contact are the most effective means of preventing person-to-person transmission of acute bacterial conjunctivitis in adults and children. During outbreaks of bacterial conjunctivitis occurring in specific groups, it may be possible to identify and eliminate a specific source of transmission (microscope oculars in a manufacturing facility[30] or eye makeup in a boarding school[117]).

REFERENCES

1. Allansmith MR, Kajiyama G, Abelson MB et al.: Plasma cell content of main and accessory lacrimal glands and conjunctiva, *Am J Ophthalmol* 82:819, 1976.
2. Armstrong JH, Zacarias F, Rein MF: Ophthalmia neonatorum: a chart review, *Pediatrics* 57:884, 1976.
3. Barquet N et al.: Primary meningococcal conjunctivitis: report of 21 patients and review, *Rev Infect Dis* 12:838, 1990.
4. Baum J, Fedukowicz HB, Jorda A: A survey of *Moraxella* corneal ulcers in a derelict population, *Am J Ophthalmol* 90:476, 1980.
5. Behrens-Baumann W, Begall T: Reproduzierbares Modell einer bakteriellen Konjunktivitis, *Ophthalmologica* 206:69, 1993.

6. Birkness KA, George VG, White EH et al.: Intracellular growth of *Afipia felis*, a putative etiologic agent of cat scratch disease, *Infect Immun* 60:2281, 1992.

7. Bodor FF, Marchant CD, Shurin PA et al.: Bacterial etiology of conjunctivitis-otitis syndrome, *Pediatrics* 76:26, 1985.

8. Brandtzaeg P, Fjellanger I, Gjeruldseu ST: Adsorption of immunoglobulin A onto oral bacteria *in vivo*, *J Bacteriol* 96:242, 1968.

9. Brazilian Purpuric Fever Study Group: *Haemophilus aegyptius* bacteremia in Brazilian purpuric fever, *Lancet* 2:761, 1987.

10. Brennen C, Muder RR: Conjunctivitis associated with methicillin-resistant *Staphylococcus aureus* in a long-term-care facility, *Am J Med* 88:14, 1990.

11. Brenner DJ, Hollis DG, Moss CW et al.: Proposal of *Afipia* gen. nov., with *Afipia felis* sp. nov. (formerly the cat scratch disease bacillus), *Afipia clevelandensis* sp. nov. (formerly the Cleveland Clinic Foundation strain), *Afipia broomeae* sp. nov., and three unnamed genospecies, *J Clin Microbiol* 29:2450, 1991.

12. Broekhuyse RM: Tear lactoferrin: a bacteriostatic and complexing protein, *Invest Ophthalmol Vis Sci* 13:550, 1974.

13. Bron AJ, Leber G, Rizk SN et al.: Ofloxacin compared with chloramphenicol in the management of external ocular infection, *Br J Ophthalmol* 75:675, 1991.

14. Brook I: Anaerobic and aerobic bacterial flora of acute conjunctivitis in children, *Arch Ophthalmol* 98:833, 1980.

15. Brook I, Pettit TH, Martin WJ, Finegold SM: Anaerobic and aerobic bacteriology of acute conjunctivitis, *Ann Ophthalmol* 11:389, 1979.

16. Burns RP, Rhodes DH: *Pseudomonas* eye infection as a cause of death in premature infants, *Arch Ophthalmol* 65:517, 1961.

17. Cagle GD, Abshire RL: Quantitative ocular bacteriology: a method for the enumeration and identification of bacteria from the skin-lash margin and conjunctiva, *Invest Ophthalmol Vis Sci* 20:751, 1981.

18. Centers for Disease Control: A technique for rapid epidemiologic assessment, *MMWR* 31:61, 1982.

19. Chan E: The general development of Chinese ophthalmology from its beginnings to the 18th century, *Doc Ophthalmol* 68:177, 1988.

20. Chandler JW: Controversies in ocular prophylaxis of newborns, *Arch Ophthalmol* 107:814, 1989.

21. Chusid MJ, Davis SD: Pathogenesis of corneal and conjunctival infections. In Tabbara KF, Hyndiuk RA, editors: *Infections of the eye*, ed 2, Boston, 1986, Little, Brown.

22. Coachman EH: Bilateral circumlimbal ulcers from malignant diphtheria, *Am J Ophthalmol* 34:1176, 1951.

23. Cohen ML: Epidemiology of drug resistance: implications for a post-antimicrobial era, *Science* 257:1050, 1992.

24. Credé CSF: Die Verhutung der Augenentzundung der Neugeborenen, *Arch Gynäkol* 18:367, 1881.

25. Credé CSF: The prophylactic treatment of ophthalmia neonatorum. In Lebensohn JE, editor: *An anthology of ophthalmic classics*, Baltimore, 1969, Williams and Wilkins.

26. Dannevig L, Straume B, Melby K: Ophthalmia neonatorum in Northern Norway. I: Epidemiology and risk factors, *Acta Ophthalmol* 70:14, 1992.

27. Dannevig L, Straume B, Melby K: Ophthalmia neonatorum in Northern Norway. II: Microbiology with emphasis on *Chlamydia trachomatis*, *Acta Ophthalmol* 70:19, 1992.

28. Daum TE, Schaberg DR, Terpenning MS et al.: Increasing resistance of *Staphylococcus aureus* to ciprofloxacin, *Antimicrob Agents Chemother* 34:1862, 1990.

29. Dillman CE: Meningococcemia following meningococcal conjunctivitis, *South Med J* 60:456, 1967.

29a. Dolan MJ, Wong MT, Regnery RL et al.: Syndrome of *Rochalimaea henselae* adenitis suggesting cat-scratch disease, *Ann Intern Med* 118:331, 1993.

30. Doyle L, Gallagher K, Heath BS, Patterson WB: An outbreak of infectious conjunctivitis spread by microscopes, *J Occup Med* 31:758, 1989.

31. Duke-Elder S: Diseases of the outer eye. In Duke-Elder S, editor: *System of ophthalmology*, vol 8, St Louis, 1965, Mosby.

32. Easty DL: Infection in the compromised eye, *Trans Ophthalmol Soc UK* 105:61, 1986.

33. Edson RS, Terrell CL: The aminoglycosides, *Mayo Clin Proc* 66:1158, 1991.

34. Farley MM, Whitney AM, Spellman P et al.: Analysis of the attachment and invasion of human epithelial cells by *Haemophilus influenzae* biogroup aegyptius, *J Infect Dis Suppl* 165:S111, 1992.

35. Feldman M: The Koch-Weeks bacillus and John Weeks, M.D., *Arch Ophthalmol* 70:430, 1963.

36. Fitch CP, Rapoza PA, Owens S et al.: Epidemiology and diagnosis of acute conjunctivitis at an inner-city hospital, *Ophthalmology* 96:1215, 1989.

37. Flach AJ: Ophthalmia neonatorum. In Tabbara KF, Hyndiuk RA, editors: *Infections of the eye*, ed 2, Boston, 1986, Little, Brown.

38. Ford LC, DeLange RJ, Petty RW: Identification of a nonlysozymal bactericidal factor (beta lysin) in human tears and aqueous humor, *Am J Ophthalmol* 81:30, 1976.

39. François J: Catarrhal diphtheritic conjunctivitis, *Br J Ophthalmol* 19:1, 1935.

40. Fransen L, Klauss V: Neonatal ophthalmia in the developing world, *Int Ophthalmol* 11:189, 1988.

41. Fransen L, Nsanze H, Klauss V et al.: Ophthalmia neonatorum in Nairobi, Kenya: the roles of *Neisseria gonorrhoeae* and *Chlamydia trachomatis*, *J Infect Dis* 153:862, 1986.

42. Fransen L, Van den Berghe P, Mertens A et al.: Incidence and bacterial aetiology of neonatal conjunctivitis, *Eur J Pediatr* 146:152, 1987.

43. Fraunfelder FT, Bagby GC, Kelly DJ: Fatal aplastic anemia following topical administration of ophthalmic chloramphenicol, *Am J Ophthalmol* 93:356-360, 1982.

44. Friedland BR, Anderson DR, Forster RK: Non-lysozyme antibacterial factor in human tears, *Am J Ophthalmol* 74:52, 1972.

45. Genvert GI, Cohen EJ, Donnenfeld ED, Blecher MH: Erythema multiforme after use of topical sulfacetamide, *Am J Ophthalmol* 99:465, 1985.

46. Gibson JR: Trimethoprim-polymyxin B ophthalmic solution in the treatment of presumptive bacterial conjunctivitis—a multicentre trial of its efficacy versus neomycin-polymyxin B-gramicidin and chloramphenicol ophthalmic solutions, *J Antimicrob Chemother* 11:217, 1983.

47. Gigliotti F, Williams WT, Hayden FG et al.: Etiology of acute conjunctivitis in children, *J Pediatr* 98:531, 1981.

48. Gigliotti F, Hendley JO, Morgan J et al.: Efficacy of topical antibiotic therapy in acute conjunctivitis in children, *J Pediatr* 104:623, 1984.

49. Gorin G: *History of ophthalmology*, Wilmington, Del, 1982, Publish or Perish.

50. Gottschalk HR, Stone OJ: Stevens-Johnson syndrome from ophthalmic sulfonamide, *Arch Dermatol* 112:513, 1976.

51. Grosskreutz C, Smith LBH: Neonatal conjunctivitis, *Int Ophthalmol Clin* 32:71-79, 1992.

52. Hadley WR, Aronson SB, Goodner EK: Quantitative conjunctival bacteriology, *Arch Ophthalmol* 90:386, 1973.

53. Haimovici R, Roussel TJ: Treatment of gonococcal conjunctivitis with single-dose intramuscular ceftriaxone, *Am J Ophthalmol* 107:511, 1989.

54. Hammerschlag MR et al.: Efficacy of neonatal ocular prophylaxis for the prevention of chlamydial and gonococcal conjunctivitis, *N Engl J Med* 318:653, 1988.

55. Hansel TT et al.: Infective conjunctivitis and corneal scarring in three brothers with sex linked hypogammaglobulinaemia (Bruton's disease), *Br J Ophthalmol* 74:118, 1990.

56. Harrison CJ, Hedrick JA, Block SL, Gilchrist MJ: Relation of the outcome of conjunctivitis and the conjunctivitis-otitis syndrome to identifiable risk factors and oral antimicrobial therapy, *Pediatr Infect Dis J* 6:536, 1987.

57. Harrison LH, daSilva GA, Vranjac A, Broome CV: Brazilian purpuric fever: an epidemiologic and clinical summary, *Pediatr Infect Dis J* 8:239, 1989.

58. Hedberg K, Ristinen TL, Soler JT et al.: Outbreak of erythromycin-resistant staphylococcal conjunctivitis in a newborn nursery, *Pediatr Infect Dis J* 9:268, 1990.

59. Heggie AD: Incidence and etiology of conjunctivitis in navy recruits, *Mil Med* 155:1, 1990.

60. Hilton E, Adams AA, Vliss A et al.: Nosocomial bacterial eye infections in intensive-care units, *Lancet* 1:1318, 1983.

61. Hirschberg J: *The history of ophthalmology*, vol 1, *The history of ophthalmology in antiquity*, Bonn, 1982, JP Wayenborgh (Translated by FC Blodi).

62. Hirschberg J: *The history of ophthalmology,* vol 4, *The renaissance of ophthalmology in the eighteenth century,* part 2, Bonn, 1984, JP Wayenborgh (Translated by FC Blodi.)

63. Hooper DC, Wolfson JS: Fluoroquinolone antimicrobial agents, *N Engl J Med* 324:384, 1991.

64. Hsu C, Wiseman GM: Antibacterial substances from staphylococci, *Can J Microbiol* 13:947, 1967.

65. Hwang DG: Systemic therapy for relapsing *Haemophilus influenzae* conjunctivitis, *Am J Ophthalmol* 115:814, 1993.

66. Hyndiuk RA, Skorich DN, Burd EM: Bacterial keratitis. In Tabbara KF, Hyndiuk RA, editors: *Infections of the eye,* 305, ed 2, Boston, 1986, Little, Brown.

67. Isenberg SJ et al.: Bacterial flora of the conjunctiva at birth, *J Pediatr Ophthalmol Strabismus* 23:284, 1986.

68. Isenberg SJ et al.: Source of the conjunctival bacterial flora at birth and implications for ophthalmia neonatorum prophylaxis, *Am J Ophthalmol* 106:458, 1988.

69. Iwata T: Cytochemical studies on endogenous peroxidase in conjunctival and corneal epithelial cells, *Invest Ophthalmol Vis Sci* 15:235, 1976.

70. Jarudi N, Golden B, Joyme J et al.: Comparison of antibiotic therapy in presumptive bacterial conjunctivitis, *Am J Ophthalmol* 79:790, 1975.

71. Jarvis VN, Levine R, Asbell PA: Ophthalmia neonatorum: study of a decade of experience at the Mount Sinai Hospital, *Br J Ophthalmol* 71:295, 1987.

72. Jones DM, Tobin B: Neonatal eye infections due to *Mycoplasma hominis,* *BMJ* 3:467, 1968.

73. Judson FN: The importance of coexisting syphilitic, chlamydial, mycoplasmal, and trichomonal infections in the treatment of gonorrhea, *Sex Transm Dis* 6(suppl):112, 1979.

74. Kenny JF: Meningococcal conjunctivitis in neonates, *Clin Pediatr* 26:473, 1987.

75. King S et al.: Nosocomial *Pseudomonas aeruginosa* conjunctivitis in a pediatric hospital, Infect Control Hosp Epidemiol 9:77, 1988.

76. Kowalski RP, Harwick MD: Incidence of *Moraxella* conjunctival infection, *Am J Ophthalmol* 101:437, 1986.

77. Laga M et al.: Epidemiology of ophthalmia neonatorum in Kenya, *Lancet* 2:1145, 1986.

78. Laga M et al.: Single dose therapy of gonococcal ophthalmia neonatorum with ceftriaxone, *N Engl J Med* 315:1382-1385, 1986.

79. Lascaratos J, Marketos S: Ophthalmological lore in the *Corpus Hippocraticum,* *Doc Ophthalmol* 68:35, 1988.

80. Latkovic S: Cytochemical localisation of acid phosphatase in the phagocytic conjunctival epithelium of the guinea pig, *Histochemistry* 8:395, 1985.

81. Latkovic S, Wrigstad A: Early morphological changes of intracellular bacteria in *Salmonella typhimurium* infection of the guinea pig conjunctival epithelium, *Acta Ophthalmol* 67:69, 1989.

82. Leibowitz HM: Antibacterial effectiveness of ciprofloxacin 0.3% ophthalmic solution in the treatment of bacterial conjunctivitis, *Am J Ophthalmol* 112(suppl):S29, 1991.

83. Leibowitz HM: Clinical evaluation of ciprofloxacin 0.3% ophthalmic solution for treatment of bacterial keratitis, *Am J Ophthalmol* 112(suppl):S34, 1991.

84. Leibowitz HM et al.: Human conjunctivitis. I. Diagnostic evaluation, *Arch Ophthalmol* 94:1747, 1976.

85. Lohr J et al.: Comparison of three topical antimicrobials for acute bacterial conjunctivitis, *Pediatr Infect Dis J* 7:626, 1988.

86. Londer L, Nelson DL: Orbital cellulitis due to *Haemophilus influenzae,* *Arch Ophthalmol* 91:89, 1974.

87. Margileth AM: Antibiotic therapy for cat-scratch disease: clinical study of therapeutic outcome in 268 patients and a review of the literature, *Pediatr Infect Dis J* 11:474, 1992.

88. McClellan BH et al.: Immunoglobulins in tears, *Am J Ophthalmol* 76:89, 1973.

89. McCloskey RV: Topical antimicrobial agents and antibiotics for the eye, *Med Clin North Am* 72:717, 1988.

90. McCulley JP, Moore MB, Matoba AY: Mucus fishing syndrome, *Ophthalmology* 92:1262, 1985.

91. McGill J et al.: Pathophysiology of bacterial infection in the external eye, *Trans Ophthalmol Soc UK* 102:7, 1982.

92. McNatt J et al.: Anaerobic flora of the normal human conjunctival sac, *Arch Ophthalmol* 96:1448, 1978.

93. Mitsui Y, Hinokuma S, Tanaka C: Etiology of angular conjunctivitis, *Am J Ophthalmol* 34:1579, 1951.

94. Mølgaard I-L, Nielsen PB, Kaern J: A study of the incidence of neonatal conjunctivitis and of its bacterial causes including *Chlamydia trachomatis,* *Acta Ophthalmol* 62:461, 1984.

95. Nakamura T, Trousdale MD, Hwang DG: Ciprofloxacin resistance among ocular staphylococcal and streptococcal isolates: potential role of newer generation fluoroquinolones, *Invest Ophthalmol Vis Sci* 34(4):847, 1993.

96. Nakhla LS, Al-Hussaini MK, Shokeir AAW: Acute bacterial conjunctivitis in Assiout, upper Egypt, *Br J Ophthalmol* 43:540, 1970.

97. Ndinya-Achola JO, Nsanzumuhire H, Mnjalla ND: Role of bacterial superinfection during an outbreak of acute haemorrhagic conjunctivitis, *East Afr Med J* 61:184, 1984.

98. Neu HC: The crisis in antibiotic resistance, *Science* 257:1064, 1992.

99. Nozik RA et al.: Trimethoprim-polymyxin B ophthalmic solution in treatment of surface ocular bacterial infections, *Ann Ophthalmol* 17:746, 1985.

100. Nushbaum E, Jeyaranjan T, Feldman F: Primary meningococcal conjunctivitis followed by meningitis, *J Pediatr* 92:784, 1978.

101. Odegaard A: Primary meningococcal conjunctivitis followed by meningitis and septicaemia, *NIPH Ann* 6:55, 1983.

102. Olafsen LD, Storvøld G, Melby K: A microbiological study of conjunctivitis with emphasis on *Chlamydia trachomatis,* in Northern Norway, *Acta Ophthalmol* 64:463, 1986.

103. Olcerst RB: Microscopes and ocular infections, *Am Ind Hyg Assoc J* 48:425, 1987.

104. Ormerod LD et al.: Gentamicin-resistant pseudomonal infection: rationale for a redefinition of ophthalmic antimicrobial sensitivities, *Cornea* 8:195, 1989.

105. Perkins RE et al.: Bacteriology of normal and infected conjunctiva, *J Clin Microbiol* 1:147, 1975.

106. Pierce JM, Ward ME, Seal DV: Ophthalmia neonatorum in the 1980s: incidence, aetiology and treatment, *Br J Ophthalmol* 66:728, 1982.

107. Prentice MJ, Hutchinson GR, Taylor-Robinson D: A microbiological study of neonatal conjunctivae and conjunctivitis, *Br J Ophthalmol* 61:601, 1977.

108. Rapoza PA et al.: Assessment of neonatal conjunctivitis with a direct immunofluorescent monoclonal antibody stain for *Chlamydia,* *JAMA* 255:3369, 1986.

109. Rapoza PA et al.: Epidemiology of neonatal conjunctivitis, *Ophthalmology* 93:456, 1986.

110. Ringvold A, Vik E, Bevanger LS: *Moraxella lacunata* isolated from epidemic conjunctivitis among teen-aged females, *Acta Ophthalmol* 63:427, 1985.

111. Roberts MC et al.: Characterisation of *Haemophilus* spp. isolated from infant conjunctivitis, *J Med Microbiol* 21:219, 1986.

112. Rubbo SD, Benjamin M: Some observations on the survival of pathogenic bacteria on cotton wool swabs, *BMJ* 1:983, 1951.

113. Rubin R: Ophthalmic sulfonamide-induced Stevens-Johnson syndrome, *Arch Dermatol* 113:235, 1977.

114. Rubinfeld RS et al.: Diphtheroids as ocular pathogens, *Am J Ophthalmol* 108:251, 1989.

115. Sandström I: Etiology and diagnosis of neonatal conjunctivitis, *Acta Pediatr Scand* 76:221, 1987.

116. Sandström KI et al.: Microbial causes of neonatal conjunctivitis, *J Pediatr* 105:706, 1984.

117. Schwartz B et al.: Investigation of an outbreak of *Moraxella* conjunctivitis at a Navajo boarding school, *Am J Ophthalmol* 107:341, 1989.

118. Seal DV, Barrett SP, McGill JI: Aetiology and treatment of acute bacterial infection of the external eye, *Br J Ophthalmol* 66:357, 1982.

119. Selinger DS, Selinger RC, Reed WP: Resistance to infection of the external eye: the role of tears, *Surv Ophthalmol* 24:33, 1979.

120. Shlaes DM: Editorial. Vancomycin-resistant bacteria, *Infect Control Hosp Epidemiol* 13:193, 1992.

121. Singer TR, Isenberg SJ, Apt L: Conjunctival anaerobic and aerobic bacterial flora in paediatric versus adult subjects, *Br J Ophthalmol* 72:448, 1988.
122. Snyder ME, Katz HR: Ciprofloxacin-resistant bacterial keratitis, *Am J Ophthalmol* 114:336, 1992.
123. Spencer WH, Zimmerman LE: Conjunctiva. In Spencer WH, editor: *Ophthalmic pathology: an atlas and textbook,* 109-228, vol 1, ed 3, Philadelphia, 1985, WB Saunders.
124. Stenson S: Acute conjunctivitis, *Arch Ophthalmol* 101:667, 1983 (letter to the editor).
125. Stenson S, Newman R, Fedukowicz H: Laboratory studies in acute conjunctivitis, *Arch Ophthalmol* 100:1275, 1982.
126. Stern GA, Killingsworth DW: Complications of topical antimicrobial agents, *Int Ophthalmol Clin* 29:137, 1989.
127. Swaminathan B et al.: Microbiology of Brazilian Purpuric fever and diagnostic tests, *J Clin Microbiol* 27:605, 1989.
128. Tabbara KF: Parinaud's oculoglandular conjunctivitis. In Tabbara KF, Hyndiuk RA, editors: *Infections of the eye,* 469-475, ed 2, Boston, 1986, Little, Brown.
129. Theodore FH, Kost PF: Meningococcic conjunctivitis, *Arch Ophthalmol* 31:245, 1944.
130. Thygeson P: The cytology of conjunctival exudates, *Am J Ophthalmol* 29:1499, 1946.
131. Thygeson P, Kimura S: Chronic conjunctivitis, *Trans Am Acad Ophthalmol Otolaryngol* 67:494, 1963.
132. The Trimethoprim-Polymyxin B Sulphate Ophthalmic Ointment Study Group: Trimethoprim-polymyxin B sulphate ophthalmic ointment versus chloramphenicol ophthalmic ointment in the treatment of bacterial conjunctivitis—a review of four clinical studies, *J Antimicrob Chemother* 23:261, 1989.
133. Trottier S, Stenberg K, von Rosen IA et al.: *Haemophilus influenzae* causing conjunctivitis in day-care children, *Pediatr Infect Dis J* 10:578, 1991.
134. Ugomori S, Hayasaka S, Setogawa T: Polymorphonuclear leukocytes and bacterial growth of the normal and mildly inflamed conjunctiva, *Ophthalmic Res* 23:40, 1991.
135. Ullman S, Roussel TJ, Culbertson WW et al.: *Neisseria gonorrhoeae* keratoconjunctivitis, *Ophthalmology* 94:525, 1987.
136. van Bijsterveld OP: Acute conjunctivitis and *Moraxella, Am J Ophthalmol* 63:1702, 1967.
137. van Haeringen NJ: Clinical biochemistry of tears, *Surv Ophthalmol* 26:84, 1981.
138. van Winkelhoff AJ et al.: Chronic conjunctivitis caused by oral anaerobes and effectively treated with systemic metronidazole plus amoxicillin, *J Clin Microbiol* 29:723, 1991.
139. Vichyanond P, Brown Q, Jackson D: Acute bacterial conjunctivitis: bacteriology and clinical implications, *Clin Pediatr* 25:506, 1986.
140. Watt PJ: Pathogenic mechanisms of organisms virulent to the eye, *Trans Ophthalmol Soc UK* 105:26, 1986.
141. Wear DJ et al.: Cat-scratch disease in the conjunctiva of patients with Parinaud's oculoglandular syndrome, *Ophthalmology* 92:1282, 1985.
142. Weidemann B, Atkinson BA: Susceptibility to antibiotics: species incidence and trends. In Lorian V, editor: *Antibiotics in laboratory medicine,* 962-1062, ed 3, Baltimore, 1991, Williams and Wilkins.
143. Weinstein P: The Australian bushfly (*Musca vetustissima* Walker) as a vector of *Neisseria gonorrhoeae* conjunctivitis, *Med J Aust* 155:717, 1991.
144. Williams RC, Gibbons RJ: Inhibition of bacterial adherence by secretory immunoglobulin A: a mechanism of antigen disposal, *Science* 177:697, 1972.
145. Wilson FM: Adverse external ocular effects of topical ophthalmic medications, *Surv Ophthalmol* 24:57-88, 1979.
146. Yamamoto GK, Allansmith MR: Complement in tears from normal humans, *Am J Ophthalmol* 88:758, 1979.
147. Yamazaki T: Bacterial examination of conjunctival-sac by thioglycolate medium and human-blood agar, *Acta Soc Ophthalmol Jpn* 62:1291, 1958.
148. Zanoni D, Isenberg SJ, Apt L: A comparison of silver nitrate with erythromycin for prophylaxis against ophthalmia neonatorum, *Clin Pediatr* 31:295, 1992.
149. Zimianski MC, Dawson CR, Togni B: Epithelial cell phagocytosis of *Listeria monocytogenes* in the conjunctiva, *Invest Ophthalmol Vis Sci* 13:623, 1974.

63 Chlamydial Keratoconjunctivitis

CHANDLER R. DAWSON, JULIUS SCHACHTER, RICHARD S. STEPHENS

Human chlamydial infections include a wide spectrum of diseases. Blinding trachoma is still highly endemic in some developing countries, where it affects approximately 500 to 600 million people and has caused blindness in at least 6 million. Sexually transmitted chlamydial infections are common in the urban populations of industrialized and developing countries and are a frequent cause of neonatal conjunctivitis and pneumonia. *Chlamydia pneumoniae* which often results in lower respiratory tract infections, was initially isolated from the eyes of children in developing countries.

The major syndromes associated with *Chlamydia trachomatis* eye infections occur in two distinct epidemiologic patterns. One pattern is classic blinding endemic trachoma of developing countries, which is spread "eye-to-eye" and is usually associated with infections by serotypes A, B, Ba, or C.

The second major pattern of eye infection (also known as inclusion conjunctivitis or paratrachoma) is caused by sexually transmitted *C. trachomatis* serovars D through K, which produce an eye disease resembling the early inflammatory phases of endemic trachoma but (usually) without the severe conjunctival scarring. These sexually transmitted strains also infect the eyes of newborns and cause neonatal ophthalmia, pneumonia, and gastrointestinal infection. Although these sporadic chlamydial infections of the eye rarely cause permanent visual loss, the involvement of other sites produces other diseases in adults and neonates.

Other uncommon chlamydial eye diseases are caused by lymphogranuloma venereum (LGV) agent, *C. pneumoniae,* and *C. psittaci.* The *C. trachomatis* serovars of LGV (L1, L2, and L3) are more invasive than the A through K serovars. LGV serovars rarely infect the eye but are a cause of Parinaud oculoglandular syndrome with conjunctivitis and massive preauricular and cervical lymphadenopathy. *C. pneumoniae* causes lower respiratory infections in young adults. Although it was initially isolated from the eyes of children with trachoma, laboratory infections have resulted

in a follicular conjunctivitis. Avian strains of *C. psittaci* can also infect the human eye to produce follicular conjunctivitis.

HISTORICAL BACKGROUND

Trachoma

Trachoma has been described since antiquity. Chinese texts from the twenty-seventh century BC described treatments for trichiasis. Between 1900 BC and 1200 BC, eight medical papyri in Egypt, including the Ebers papyrus (1500 BC), identified eye diseases such as granulations, trichiasis, and entropion—all signs of trachoma. Eye cosmetics from ancient Egyptian tombs included galena (lead sulfide), hematite (ferric oxide), and copper sulfate. All remain in use in current Egyptian ethnomedical practice to treat eye infections.

The Hippocratic corpus (430 BC to 330 BC) described trachoma as a conjunctivitis with the appearance of a fig; indeed, the cut surface of a black fig with white seeds in a deep red pulp resembles trachomatous follicles with severe papillary infiltration. The Hippocratic texts prescribed cutting the veins of the temple and rubbing the conjunctiva of the everted upper lid with Milesian wool on a wood spindle, treatments still used in Egyptian villages today.

The Sicilian physician Pedonius Discorides, first used the term "trachoma" (Greek for "rough swelling") in 60 AD. Heliodorus of Alexandria (circa 100 AD) wrote a book on trachoma and recommended scraping the lid to remove ingrowing cilia. Galen (circa 130-200 AD), Aëtius of Amida (502-575), and Paula of Agina (circa 650) described the progressive stages of the disease from granular conjunctivitis to scarring and trichiasis. In Egypt the Unani medical system, based on Galen and other Greek medical texts, was ascendant from the ninth to thirteenth centuries AD. Treatments for trachoma included scraping the inside of the upper tarsus with the bone of a cuttlefish or squid and rubbing on powdered hematite.

European invasions of the Eastern Mediterranean during the Crusades of the twelfth and thirteenth centuries AD led to the spread of eye infections among European invaders and pilgrims. (After his return from the Holy Land, St. Francis of Assisi developed an ocular disease that scarred his upper lid and led to marked loss of vision by his death 8 years later.) The British and French invasions of Egypt (1798 to 1799) led to disastrous epidemics in the armies and to the wide dissemination of trachoma in Western Europe. Both the French and British armies suffered from the disease; Vetch described how 636 of 700 men in a single battalion developed "Egyptian ophthalmia," with 50 blinded in both eyes and 40 in 1 eye. With the return of the armies to Europe and disruptions of the Napoleonic wars, the disease spread in Europe and persisted in some parts well into the twentieth century (western Ireland and Bosnia-Herzogovina).

During his visit to Egypt in 1883, Koch studied smears from cases of purulent conjunctivitis and described both the slender rod of the Koch-Weeks bacillus *(Haemophilus aegyptius)* and a gonococcus-like bacteria now known to be a unique species, *Neisseria kochii.* In 1907 Halberstaedter and von Prowazek[28,29] identified the causative agent of trachoma by inoculating scrapings from a trachoma patient onto the conjunctiva of an orangutan and finding granular, cytoplasmic inclusions in conjunctival epithelial cells. Similar inclusions were soon identified in conjunctival cells of newborns with nongonococcal neonatal conjunctivitis[35,41] and nongonococcal urethritis.[36] These trachoma inclusions were identified as the causative agent of trachoma despite a later claim for a bacterial cause, *Bacterium granulosis.*[48] Thygeson[68,69] confirmed the causative role of chlamydial elementary bodies by inoculating human volunteers and nonhuman primates with bacteria-free filtrates to produce the typical eye disease and new inclusions in conjunctival epithelial cells.

In 1957 T'ang and associates[62] in Beijing first isolated the agent of trachoma in the yolk sac of embryonated eggs. This isolation of *C. trachomatis* was soon repeated in other countries, and isolation of *C. trachomatis* in cell culture is now a standard diagnostic procedure.

The modern era of chemotherapy began with the use of oral sulfonamides in 1938 in American Indians. Oral sulfa drugs were widely used for individual and "blanket" treatment of whole villages and individual families. The high rate of untoward reactions to sulfonamides motivated a change to topical tetracycline or erythromycin ointment (daily or intermittently) for trachoma.[52] Oral tetracyclines or doxycycline has been used to treat children over the age of 7 years and adults, except for nursing mothers.

Chlamydial Keratoconjunctivitis

In nineteenth century Europe a mild type of "trachoma" that occurred in epidemics among the clients of swimming pools[53] was described as "endemische Bad Konjunktivitis."[20] The chlamydial agent was first reported from an af-

flicted adult in 1913. It was later proved that infection of the eye occurred through genital discharges coming in contact with the eye.

In parallel, a form of ophthalmia neonatorum without apparent bacterial infection[34] was recognized and labeled "conjonctivite amicrobienne" by Morax.[41] By 1909 the typical cytoplasmic inclusion was found in conjunctival scrapings from newborns,[35,55] from the genital tract of their mothers, and from the urethras of their fathers.[23,37] Material from infants with inclusion conjunctivitis inoculated into primates produced follicular conjunctivitis[23] identical to that obtained with material from adults with follicular conjunctivitis.[32] Thus the etiology and epidemiology of the disease were established soon after the disease in infants was clinically defined.

Much of the research on extraocular infection was done by ophthalmologists who reported the apparently self-limited nature of the genital infection. There were occasional infections of gynecologists from patients' genital material, and eye-to-eye transmission by tonometry in a glaucoma clinic.[67]

Isolation of the chlamydial agent led to the observations in England that some genitally transmitted chlamydial infections met the criteria for the diagnosis of trachoma; namely, presence of lymphoid follicles on the upper tarsal plate, pannus formation, and presence of an agent causing trachoma inclusion conjunctivitis (TRIC) in conjunctival scrapings.[33] These observations caused a revival of Lindner's term "paratrachoma" for any sexually transmitted chlamydial infection of the eye or genital tract.

During the 1960s and 1970s the rapid evolution of methods of serotyping chlamydial isolates led to the observation that isolates from patients with trachoma in endemic trachoma areas were largely limited to serotypes A, B, Ba, and C, whereas isolates from the genital tract were, for the most part, serotypes D through K with a few types of B and Ba strains. Primate inoculations were first performed with material from human cases,[66] and later with isolated chlamydial strains. These experiments showed that the genital chlamydial strains appeared to be more pathogenic for the eyes of monkeys and other subhuman primates than did classic trachoma strains.[19,26] In the 1980s repeated inoculation of primates (rhesus monkeys) with serotypes B or E serovars produced a follicular, then cicatricial, conjunctivitis but no corneal lesions or corneal vascularization.[63]

EPIDEMIOLOGY

Trachoma has a worldwide distribution, and blinding trachoma is still a major public health problem in parts of Africa, Southwest Asia (the Middle East), Southeast Asia, and in limited areas of Latin America, Australasia, and the Pacific Islands. Nonblinding trachoma is present in a much larger region of these same areas that includes most of the drier subtropical and tropical countries. Trachoma was once prevalent and severe in many countries of Europe, North America, and northern Asia, but it regressed and disappeared with rising living standards that accompanied industrialization and economic development.

Under the prevailing living conditions in developed countries and in many urban communities of developing countries, trachoma is rarely transmitted and, if acquired, it is mild. In persons with healed trachoma, however, there may be recurrences of active disease, (1) following treatment with topical corticosteroids, (2) with recurrent atopic conjunctivitis, and (3) in old age. This recurrent adult disease usually does not present a significant public health risk.

In endemic communities most children are infected by the age of 1 or 2 years (infectious trachoma is most prevalent in 2- to 5-year-olds), then the prevalence of active disease declines steadily, although some adults continue to have signs of active disease. Because children constitute such a large proportion of the population in developing countries with endemic trachoma, those with active disease are the chief reservoir of trachomatous infection in the community. Blinding lesions (trichiasis/entropion and corneal scarring) are the outcome of earlier severe or moderate intensity inflammatory disease. These blinding sequelae are generally observed in adults but may occur in childhood as the result of very severe inflammatory disease.

Adult inclusion conjunctivitis is relatively uncommon and occurs in about 1 in 300 cases of genital chlamydial infection in the United Kingdom.[70] Eye infection occurs by the transfer of infectious genital discharges during oral-genital sexual activities or by the fingers. Most patients who have the acquired chlamydial infection of the eye are between the ages of 15 and 30. Sexually transmitted chlamydia were once thought to be the common cause of swimming pool conjunctivitis. There has also been some family spread of disease from infected newborns. Gynecologists have rarely acquired chlamydial eye infection by accidental ocular inoculation with genital material while performing surgery.

RISK FACTORS

Trachoma is associated with poverty. Economic development appears to eliminate or reduce the severity of the disease. Transmission of the disease is by direct or indirect contact with infected material (hands, clothing, towels) and by flies.[8] Among the environmental features of greatest importance are the presence of young children in the household, crowding, and the unavailability of safe water and household latrines.[13,76] The behavioral risk factors associated with the severity of trachoma are primarily the lack of face washing of young children and the lack of latrines in households.

In many endemic areas the open disposal of human and animal wastes contributes to an increase in the fly population. The flies that cluster on children's eyes to feed on

ocular discharges transfer these discharges to the eyes of other children in the same family within 15 to 30 minutes. Children with endemic trachoma also harbor *C. trachomatis* in the upper respiratory and gastrointestinal tracts. Thus transmission may also occur by aerosol droplet spread and fecal contamination of fomites, as well as by flies.

CLINICAL FEATURES

Trachoma

In communities with endemic trachoma the disease often has inapparent or gradual onset. Initially, trachoma is a conjunctivitis characterized by the formation of lymphoid follicles in the subconjunctival tissue and inflammatory infiltration (papillary hypertrophy) of the conjunctiva (Fig. 63-1). In children under 2 years of age the papillary reaction with inflammatory thickening of the conjunctiva may be the predominant sign, and follicles may not be a prominent sign. The disease involves the entire conjunctiva, but its effects are most noticeable on the upper tarsus, which has been selected as a convenient area of examination to represent the degree of trachomatous inflammation and scarring.

Trachoma is a chronic disease, and as the disease progresses it causes scarring of the conjunctiva (Fig. 63-2)—with fine linear and small stellate scars in milder cases, or broad confluent or synechial scars in severe cases.[65] This scarring causes distortion of the lids, particularly of the upper tarsus, to produce trichiasis and entropion (Fig. 63-3). The disease also can destroy the goblet cells and injure the lacrimal glands and tear ducts. Thus constant corneal abrasion by the inturned eyelashes and deficient tear secretion can lead to corneal ulceration followed by opacification and visual loss. The deep trachomatous scarring in the upper tarsus and fornix may also produce defects in lid closure,

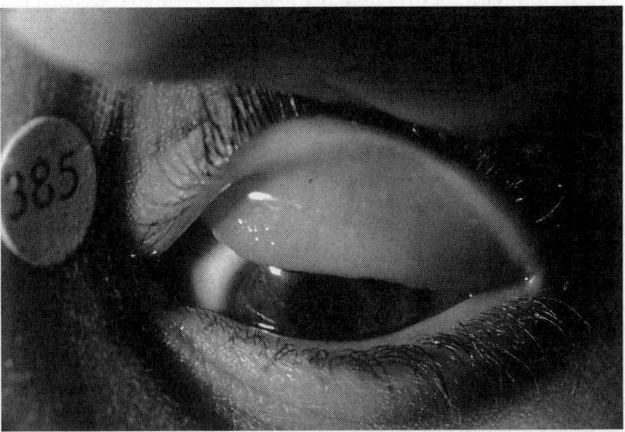

Fig. 63-1. Active infectious trachoma. The presence of lymphoid follicles (white spots) and papillary infiltration on the upper tarsal conjunctiva indicates active, presumably infectious, trachoma in this Tunisian child. The numbered label was used to identify the child in a therapy trial.

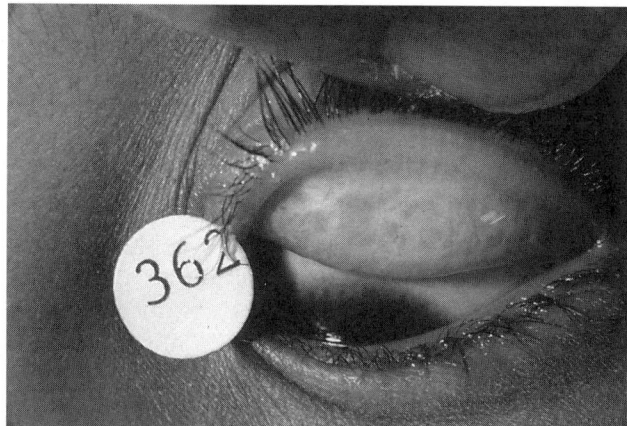

Fig. 63-2. Trachoma scarring and Herbert pits. The presence of diffuse scarring in the absence of active inflammation indicates a case of healed trachoma. The presence of Herbert pits, seen here as notches or punched out lesions in the conjunctival limbus, is a specific sign of trachoma.

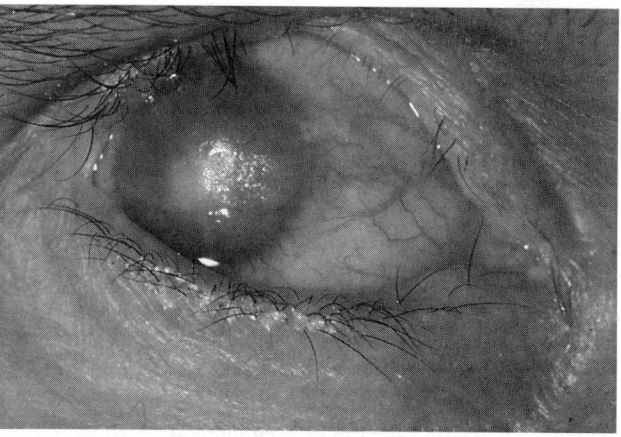

Fig. 63-4. Corneal scarring, trichiasis, and exposure in trachoma. Distortion of the lids has produced trichiasis and corneal exposure leading to corneal opacity in this 48-year-old Tunisian woman.

which predispose to traumatic and infectious damage to the cornea (Fig. 63-4).

During its inflammatory infectious phases, trachoma produces lesions of the cornea ranging from epithelial keratitis (usually in the upper portions of the cornea), to anterior stromal infiltrates and superficial neovascularization (vascular pannus). A unique characteristic of trachoma is the formation of lymphoid follicles in the limbal conjunctiva, which on resolution leave characteristic depressions at the limbus called Herbert peripheral pits. Vascular pannus is usually twice as extensive at the upper limbus as it is at the inferior limbus.

The degree of conjunctival scarring is directly proportional to the intensity and duration of inflammation.[18] Very

severe scarring occurs in children as young as 4 or 5 years of age. Inturned eyelids are uncommon at this age, however, and tend to occur in late adolescence and early adult life, long after the active inflammatory disease subsided. This late onset of inturned lids is due to gradual contraction of the scars, particularly deeper scars close to the lid margin.

Because trachoma is so widespread, standardized descriptions have been developed for public health control programs. The clinical descriptions now in use include two related systems recommended by the World Health Organization and the older MacCallan classification. For the clinical evaluation of trachoma, disease of the upper tarsal conjunctiva is used as a convenient index of the disease process. These conjunctival signs include lymphoid follicles, diffuse inflammation and papillary hypertrophy, inturned lashes, and corneal opacity.

In the 1936 MacCallan classification, trachoma cases are classified in "stages" by the findings in the conjunctiva alone (Table 63-1). This classification describes the evolution of the disease but does not have prognostic value. The

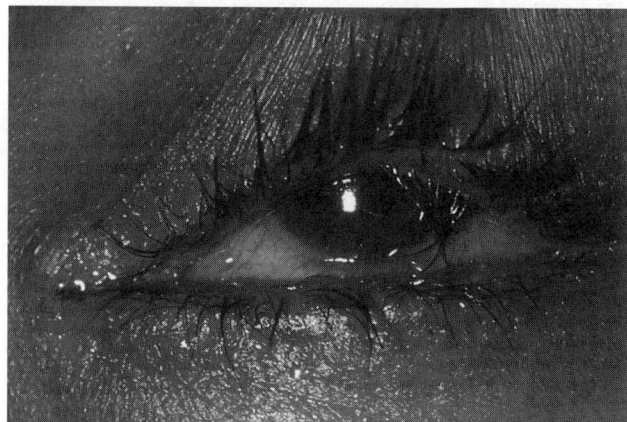

Fig. 63-3. Trachomatous trichiasis. Conjunctival scarring acquired in childhood causes gradual contraction of the lid margins, producing trichiasis and entropion as in this 32-year-old Tunisian woman.

TABLE 63-1 MacCALLAN CLASSIFICATION OF TRACHOMA

Stage I:	Small follicles on the upper tarsal conjunctiva
Stage II:	Characteristic conjunctival scarring but no signs described in the following:
Stage IIA:	Large ("mature") follicles in the tarsal conjunctiva
Stage IIB:	Diffuse infiltration and papillary hypertrophy obscuring the follicles
Stage III:	The signs of Stages I and II with conjunctival scarring
Stage IV:	Noninfectious disease, although changes in scars may occur

MacCallan classification does not describe the inflammatory intensity or severity, nor does it identify cases with visually disabling lesions.

A simplified description system was introduced in 1987 by WHO for use by primary health-care workers (Table 63-2). This simplified system was developed for use by non-specialized health workers in developing countries, using a handlight and loupe for examination. A specific series of interventions is linked to the clinical findings.

A more comprehensive WHO descriptive system empha-sized the grading of the intensity of inflammatory disease on the basis of tarsal follicles (F) and diffuse inflammation and papillary hypertrophy (P) (Table 63-3). This system also graded the relative degree of conjunctival scarring (C), an important indicator of blinding complications, and distin-guished the degree of corneal scarring and lid deformity. This more detailed description has been useful for field studies.[77]

To identify the presence or absence of trachoma in a community, individual cases must have at least two of the following signs: (1) follicles in the upper tarsal conjunctiva, (2) limbal follicles or their sequelae, Herbert pits, (3) typical conjunctival scarring, and (4) vascular pannus marked at the superior limbus. To these criteria, another criterion for tra-choma should be added: (5) the presence of a positive test for C. trachomatis infection in a substantial proportion (20% to 50% depending on the severity of the disease) of active cases.

A community with blinding trachoma can be recognized by the presence of persons with severe visual loss caused by corneal opacity and a substantial prevalence of potentially disabling trachomatous lesions, particularly trichiasis/entro-pion. These irreversible changes appear as the long-term outcome of prolonged or recurrent inflammatory disease of moderate or severe intensity. Communities with nonblinding trachoma may have a low incidence of potentially blinding

TABLE 63-2 SIMPLIFIED DESCRIPTION OF TRACHOMA FOR PRIMARY EYE CARE

Trachoma follicles (TF):	Five or more lymphoid follicles on the central area of the upper tarsal conjunctiva
Trachomatous inflammation (TI):	Diffuse inflammation of the tarsal conjunctiva, which obscures 50% or more of the normal deep tarsal vessels
Trachomatous scarring (TS):	Any characteristic scarring of the conjunctiva
Trichiasis or entropion (TT):	Deviated lashes touching the eyeball
Corneal opacity (CO):	Any opacity or scarring of the cornea

TABLE 63-3 CLINICAL SCORING OF INFLAMMATORY SIGNS FOR EPIDEMIOLOGIC AND THERAPEUTIC STUDIES OF TRACHOMA

The intensity of trachoma correlates well with the presence of the chlamydial agent and is a good prognostic sign. Intensity can be determined by the examiner at the time of clinical examination or by data analysis from the follicle and papillae scores.

The scores for upper tarsal follicles (F) are:
F0 No follicles
F1 Follicles present, but no more than 5 in the central tarsus
F2 5 or more follicles on the central tarsal conjunctiva
F3 10 or more follicles on the central tarsus

The scores for upper tarsal papillary hypertrophy and diffuse in-filtration (P) are:
P0 Absent: normal appearance
P1 Minimal: vessels on the tarsus not obscured
P2 Moderate: normal vessels appear hazy
P3 Pronounced: conjunctiva thickened, normal vessels on the tarsus are hidden over more than half of the surface

Intensity	Key Sign	Follicles	Papillae
Severe	P3	F3 (or F2 or F1)*	P3
Moderate	F3	F3	P2
Mild	F2	F2	P0, P1 or P2
Trivial (insignificant or absent)	F2 or F1	F0 or F1	P0, P1 or P2

From WHO "Guide to Trachoma Control"
* The follicles may be obscured by severe papillary hypertrophy and dif-fuse infiltration.

lesions, but not a substantial prevalence of trachomatous visual loss.

In communities with blinding trachoma, chlamydial in-fection is always present, but other ocular microbial patho-gens appear to contribute significantly to the intensity of trachoma and to the lesions that impair vision.

Adult Chlamydial Keratoconjunctivitis

In adults "paratrachoma" presents as a follicular con-junctivitis of acute onset (Fig. 63-5) with a preauricular node on the side of the involved eye.[70,72] Unlike acute adenovirus follicular conjunctivitis, chlamydial conjunctivitis may per-sist for many months if untreated. There is a scanty muco-purulent discharge. Corneal involvement includes epithelial keratitis, marginal and central infiltrates,[15] and subepithelial opacities like those of adenoviral keratoconjunctivitis.[56] Conjunctival scarring has been reported in chronic cases, and there may be corneal vascularization (micropannus) in others. In naturally occurring and experimentally induced disease, anterior uveitis is an uncommon complication, whereas otitis media is a regular feature.

The subconjunctival lymphoid follicles are most promi-nent in the lower conjunctiva but may be present in the upper

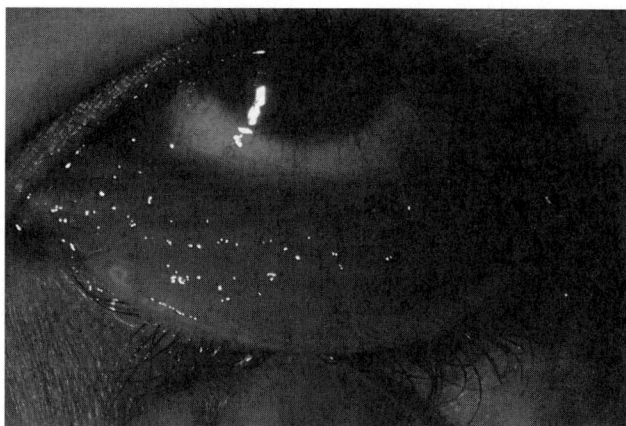

Fig. 63-5. Adult inclusion conjunctivitis. This 26-year-old woman has had follicular conjunctivitis for 4 weeks. The follicles are most prominent in the lower fornix.

tarsus. Tarsal follicles, infiltration with corneal vascularization, and the rare occurrence of conjunctival scarring have led to a confusion in the clinical diagnosis. As a result of this confusion some acute cases have been classified as "acute trachoma", although the infections were clearly with sexually transmitted C. trachomatis.

In adult inclusion conjunctivitis there is evolution of the clinical appearance of the disease during the course of the infection, which may last from 3 to 12 months if untreated. During the first 2 weeks hyperemia, infiltration, and discharge of the conjunctiva dominate the clinical picture. After 2 weeks the conjunctival lymphoid follicles and superficial keratitis become more prominent features. In cases that have persisted for several months the follicles may be less prominent. Corneal vascularization, keratitis, and conjunctival scarring may occur.

Neonatal Chlamydial Conjunctivitis

This disease usually appears 5 to 19 days after birth, but earlier infection can result if the placental membranes have ruptured before delivery.

The diagnosis of chlamydial neonatal ophthalmia is relatively easy (even with Giemsa-stained conjunctival smears), because there are large numbers of inclusions. C. trachomatis neonatal conjunctivitis is also common in some developing countries. As in all cases of neonatal ophthalmia, gonococcal infection must be excluded by the use of appropriate cultures and smears.

Neonatal inclusion conjunctivitis is characterized by a swelling of the lids, hyperemia and infiltration of the conjunctiva, and a purulent discharge. Keratitis has been reported in some cases, and newborns who are treated late (or not at all) develop conjunctival scarring and superficial corneal vascularization. Respiratory tract involvement occurs in 35% to 50% of infected infants, so systemic antibiotic treatment is necessary.

Untreated cases of neonatal inclusion blennorrhea will run a course of 3 to 12 months. The eye disease clears slowly with ocular antibiotic treatment alone but responds promptly to oral erythromycin (40 mg per kg body weight per day in 4 divided doses) for 2 weeks, which is indicated to treat extraocular infection and prevent pneumonia. Ocular antibiotic treatment alone is not sufficient to cure the conjunctival disease. Parents should also be treated with systemic tetracyclines or erythromycin for their genital tract infection.

Ocular Lymphogranuloma Venereum

Eye infection with the LGV serovars (L1, L2, and L3) of C. trachomatis can present as Parinaud oculoglandular conjunctivitis (conjunctival inflammation associated with massive preauricular, submandibular, and cervical lymphadenopathy). The LGV biovars appear to be less common causes of genital tract infection than the other C. trachomatis serotypes. LGV infection of the rectum and lower bowel may be relatively common in male homosexuals,[52] but manifest eye involvement is very rare.

Ocular Infection with *Chlamydia psittaci* and *Chlamydia pneumoniae*

Conjunctivitis has been reported in association with infection by the agent of feline pneumonitis and by an avian C. psittaci strain. Feline pneumonitis is a chlamydial infection of cats that causes conjunctivitis and pneumonia in kittens.

Guinea pig inclusion conjunctivitis (GPIC) is a C. psittaci strain that is a naturally occurring disease of guinea pig herds. This disease has been studied extensively as a model of human trachoma. The agent infects the mucosal epithelium of the conjunctiva, genital tract, and rectum. Experimental infection of the eye produces a severe conjunctivitis that resolves in 3 to 4 weeks and leaves the animal relatively resistant to reinfection.

Human cases have presented as a follicular conjunctivitis with a subacute onset and minimal mucopurulent discharge. One case persisted for 3 months without treatment, the other for 4 weeks. There was a small, slightly tender, preauricular node on the side of the involved eye. In addition to lymphoid follicles on the palpebral conjunctival, they were also present on the bulbar conjunctiva. There was no pannus in either case, but there was diffuse epithelial keratitis. Prolonged and intense antimicrobial treatment with tetracycline led to resolution of the disease.

In one well-documented case of laboratory infection with an avian strain of C. psittaci, a unilateral subacute conjunctivitis developed with a minimal amount of mucopurulent discharge and a small preauricular node. There was no corneal vascularization, but there was a diffuse superficial keratitis with subepithelial infiltrates. The infection responded slowly to treatment with oral tetracycline for 6 weeks. The C. psittaci strain was isolated from the eye before treatment and after 2 weeks of oral tetracycline.

A single laboratory eye infection has been reported with *C. pneumoniae* (I0L 207), a strain similar to the first isolate of this species. A papillary and follicular conjunctivitis occurred without keratitis, but with a mild rhinitis. The disease resolved on treatment with systemic doxycycline and topical chlortetracycline. *C. pneumoniae* appears to be a common cause of respiratory disease in adults and children, but naturally occurring eye infection has not been demonstrated since the original isolations in Taiwan and Iran. In guinea pigs, *C. pneumoniae* produces a papillary conjunctivitis and does not appear to infect epithelial cells; however, the organism can be re-isolated from the conjunctiva.

PATHOLOGY

The host response of the human conjunctiva infected with *C. trachomatis* is characterized both clinically and histologically by the presence of lymphoid follicles with germinal centers. In the early stages of trachoma the epithelial and subepithelial tissues are infiltrated with lymphocytes and polymorphonuclear leukocytes. Where the conjunctiva is bound down over the tarsal plate, it is thrown up in villous processes to form papillae with a central vascular tuft and folds of epithelium between the elevations.

Early in the disease, collections of lymphocytes are seen in the submucosa either just beneath the epithelium or deeper within the connective tissue. These early follicles do not have germinal centers and appear to consist mostly of small lymphocytes. As the disease progresses, the collections of lymphocytes develop a structure like that of lymphoid follicles, with an outside layer of small, dense lymphocytes and an inner center of lighter-staining cells with more cytoplasm—the germinal center. Unlike central lymph nodes, the germinal center is displaced toward the surface. The lymphocytes of the subepithelial follicles appear to be infiltrating the conjunctival epithelium, which is flattened and loosened over the follicle itself, allowing ready access of foreign material into the follicle. This structure may be analogous to Peyer patches in the intestinal tract. Lymphoid follicles in the conjunctiva can also occur deeper in the connective tissue and are not necessarily adjacent to the conjunctival epithelium.

In more advanced stages of trachoma the follicle itself or the germinal center of the follicle becomes necrotic and connective tissue forms around the follicles, producing scarring. The formation of Herbert pits by follicles at the corneal-scleral junction is evidence that the follicle (during its formation in this confined space) can erode the connective tissue without causing any overt ulceration or connective tissue reaction with scarring.

Macrophages are frequently found in the epithelium and in the follicles themselves. Plasma cells appear to be distributed throughout the conjunctiva. Between the follicles there is marked lymphocytic infiltration. In addition, the capillaries appear to be dilated, and the whole conjunctival layer can be considerably thickened by the cellular infiltration with the formation of papillary villae or fronds. As scarring takes place, the islands of epithelium between the elevated papillae may become trapped and form epithelial-lined cysts, which are identified clinically as "post-trachomatous degeneration". Progressive scarring produces entropion and trichiasis.[1]

PATHOGENESIS

Chlamydiae are eubacteria but do not have any identified close relatives. Chlamydiae have been placed in their own order, Chlamydiales, with one genus, *Chlamydia,* and several species (*C. trachomatis, C. psittaci,* and *C. pneumoniae*).[47] In nature and in the laboratory, chlamydiae can only grow within eukaryotic host cells. Thus chlamydial survival is strictly dependent on attachment to host cell surfaces, invasion of the target cell, and survival and growth inside the mammalian cell.[46] Although chlamydia can be grown in the laboratory using a wide range of mammalian cell lines, the human portal of entry for *C. trachomatis* is the columnar epithelial cell at mucosal surfaces. Once inside the host cell, chlamydiae grow within a host membrane vacuole-like structure called an "inclusion" and acquire nutrients and energy compounds from their eukaryotic host. How chlamydiae compete with their host cells and acquire essential metabolites is unknown. It appears that chlamydiae are unable to produce net energy and require host-derived ATP.[30] Thus chlamydiae have been aptly called "energy parasites."[45]

The biosynthetic capabilities of chlamydiae are not well defined; however, chlamydiae have one of the smallest bacterial chromosomes with approximately one-fourth the protein-coding capacity of their free-living counterparts (such as *Escherichia coli*).[57] Although it is evident that chlamydiae derive many of their nutrients and precursors for macromolecular synthesis of nucleic acids, polysaccharides, lipids, and proteins from their eukaryotic host cells, chlamydiae are nevertheless independently capable of synthesis of these complex macromolecules.[30]

There are two primary biochemical differences used to differentiate between *C. trachomatis* and *C. psittaci* isolates. One is that all *C. trachomatis* (and, with a few exceptions, none of the *C. psittaci*) synthesize folic acid and are thus sensitive to sulfonamides. The other is that *C. trachomatis* strains produce large quantities of glycogen released from the chlamydial cell into the intracellular inclusion. This glycogen can be readily detected in infected tissue culture cells by staining with iodine and thus has also served to detect inclusions of *C. trachomatis* for diagnostic purposes. The morphology of *C. trachomatis* and *C. psittaci* inclusions are quite distinct and have served as additional criteria for species differentiation. *C. trachomatis* inclusions are round or oval and sufficiently rigid to displace and deform the nucleus to the cell periphery, whereas *C. psittaci* inclusions are pleomorphic and tend to follow the cellular and nuclear contour.

Developmental Cycle

One of the unique biologic properties of *Chlamydia* is its developmental cycle. Chlamydiae have two basic developmental and morphologic forms that differ structurally and metabolically. The elementary body (EB) is the extracellular and infectious developmental form. The EB is metabolically inactive and its outer membrane is highly resistant to osmotic and sonic stress. The three major proteins that make up the outer membrane are cysteine-rich and highly disulfide cross-linked.[49] Two of these proteins are only present in the EB developmental form; the other, the major outer membrane protein (MOMP), is the dominant surface exposed protein and is present during all stages of development. Another prominent morphologic feature of the EB is that the chromosome is highly compacted and appears very dense[39] by electron microscopy. The chromosome compaction is mediated by DNA-binding proteins that are only present in the EB developmental stage, and it is thought that the highly condensed DNA represents an efficient mechanism for preventing metabolic activity in the extracellular EB.[74]

The other developmental stage is called the reticulate body (RB) or initial body in the older literature. This stage is the vegetative form of the organism that is metabolically active and divides by binary fission. The RB does not have the electron dense chromosome structure and is three to four times larger in diameter than the EB (300 nm versus 1000 nm). The RB also differs from the EB by sensitivity of the RB to sonic or detergent lysis. This difference is related to the presence of the two cysteine-rich proteins in the outer membrane of EBs that are not present in RBs. The outer membrane of the EB is highly disulfide cross-linked and dependent on these EB-specific cysteine-rich proteins and MOMP, which is also relatively cysteine-rich. The consequence of this disulfide cross-linked outer membrane organization is an environmentally resistant extracellular form of the organism. EBs can readily be solubilized by the use of chemical reducing reagents, however.

The microbiology of persistent chlamydial infections is not understood. Clinical persistence could represent a low-grade infection from which isolation of infectious EB is unlikely, or it could represent a defined developmental pathway without production of infectious progeny. In vitro observations have shown that RB to EB transitions are inhibited by a variety of factors such as deprivation of essential amino acids (cysteine) or by the presence of penicillin and penicillin-related antibiotics.[46] Following addition of the essential amino acid or removal of the antibiotic, RBs can then complete the developmental cycle and produce infectious EBs.[30] Interferon-gamma, often elicited during chlamydial infection, has also been shown to reversibly inhibit chlamydial development, presumably by limiting tryptophan.[9] The consequence of these findings is there appear to be several mechanisms for promoting persistent infection in vivo.

Immunogenicity

Human strains of *C. trachomatis* have been classified into over 18 serovariants (serovars) and 2 biovariants (biovars): (1) trachoma biovar (serovars A-K and type-variants) and (2) lymphogranuloma vereneum (LGV) biovar (serovars L1-L3). The trachoma biovar strains cause ocular infections, inclusion conjunctivitis, and trachoma, as well as genital tract infections. Serovars A, B, Ba, and C are typically associated with trachoma, whereas all the serovars have been found in the genital tract (although generally with preponderance of serovars D and E). Virulence differences have yet to be identified that could account for this distribution of serovars. The LGV biovar strains cause much more invasive infection than the trachoma biovar strains. The LGV biovar strains also show considerable differences in tissue culture that appear related to their virulence properties—hence the biovar distinction. Even between the biovariants, however, the molecular basis of virulence differences is unknown.

All chlamydiae share a common lipopolysaccharide (LPS), which is similar in structure but less complex than LPS from gram-negative bacteria.[49] Significantly, the chlamydial LPS is antigenically distinct from most other bacteria and represents an important target for culture-independent diagnostic assays. Another essential antigenic component is the surface-exposed MOMP.[10] The MOMP is antigenically complex and displays both serovar-specific antigens and antigens shared by *C. trachomatis* strains that cause human infection.[59] The latter antigen is also used for culture-independent detection of *C. trachomatis*. Consequently, diagnostic assays that detect LPS will identify all chlamydial species, whereas, assays that detect MOMP will not identify *C. psittaci* or *C. pneumoniae*. Unlike the LPS antigens, the MOMP antigens are thought to be targets of host immunity. This theory has been supported by an association of immune protection with serovar specificity and by in vitro neutralization of infectivity using anti-MOMP monoclonal antibodies.[81]

Cellular Adherence and Invasion

Humans are the only known reservoir for *C. trachomatis*. A newly defined chlamydial species, *C. pneumoniae*, is considered a natural pathogen of humans and a common cause of acute respiratory infections.[24] These strains were originally isolated from ocular sites in trachoma patients[22,25]; thus ocular infection may also represent an important site for *C. pneumoniae*.

As chlamydia must attach to and enter eukaryotic cells to propagate, understanding the molecular basis of host cell attachment and entry will provide important insights into the microbiology of these unique organisms to serve as a basis to develop new intervention strategies. Until recently, little was known about the chlamydial molecules that bind host cells and those that promote entry into host cells. It has recently been proposed that chlamydial EBs display heparan sulfatelike adhesion molecules on their surfaces that mediate attachment of EBs to host cells.[80] Because eukaryotic cells bind and endocytose heparan sulfate, it is likely that binding of the chlamydial adhesion is sufficient to mediate uptake into host cells. Such a novel mechanism of attachment and means of cellular invasion offers several potential benefits. Synthesis by *C. trachomatis* of a unique sulfated glycosaminoglycan should provide a new diagnostic marker and, depending on its quantity and longevity, could offer more sensitive assays than currently available. Synthesis of sulfated polysaccharides is extremely rare among bacteria, thus providing the opportunity to develop chlamydia-specific antimicrobial agents. As the chlamydial adhesion is the primary functional molecule for host-cell interactions, it represents an important target for immune-mediated intervention by vaccination.

Host Immune Responses

Disease caused by chlamydial infections is the result of the host inflammatory responses to the presence of the organism.[12] The host immune response to reinfection is the most important component to the production of the severe inflammatory responses leading to conjunctival scarring.[27] Thus persistent infection or frequent re-infection causes chronic mucosal inflammation. The subsequent scarring leads to corneal blindness and, in women, infertility. Although immune-mediated pathogenesis is the mechanism for chlamydial disease,[31] there is little understanding of the chlamydial components or the immune mechanisms involved.

Two lines of evidence implicate the chlamydial groEL analog, called heat shock protein hsp60, as at least one mediator of pathogenesis. In an ocular guinea pig model, Triton X-100 detergent extracts of a *C. psittaci* strain that contain this protein elicit conjunctival inflammatory responses.[42,43] Using *C. psittaci* hsp60 cloned and expressed in *E. coli*, it was demonstrated that this material could also elicit ocular inflammatory responses; however, eliciting this response required Triton X-100, which itself is quite toxic. A second line of evidence is that strong serologic responses to *C. trachomatis* hsp60 are detected in patients with severe pathology, such as ectopic pregnancy caused by *C. trachomatis*.[11,73] In contrast, in the face of strong serologic responses to other chlamydial proteins, no serologic response to hsp60 is observed from most *C. trachomatis*-infected patients without severe pathology. As heat shock proteins are antigenically highly conserved between bacteria and humans, eliciting immune responses to this bacterial protein in human hosts might facilitate pathologic processes that endure even following resolution of infection.

An alternative cause of inflammation is direct attachment of organisms to immune cells thereby eliciting immune mediators. Chlamydiae attach to T cells, macrophages, and B cells and elicit cellular responses that generate a variety of cytokines, some of which are mediators of inflammation.[21] This mitogenic activity associated with intact organisms could provide the stimulus for the acute inflammation observed following infection and set the stage for later immune dysregulation by uncontrolled elaboration of immune regulating cytokines.

LABORATORY INVESTIGATIONS

Cytologic examination of conjunctival swabbings or scrapings can reveal a typical inflammatory reaction of lymphocytes, macrophages, plasma cells, and immature mononuclear cells.[78,79] Giemsa staining can sometimes reveal intracytoplasmic inclusions within conjunctival epithelial cells (Fig. 63-6). Inclusions are not commonly seen in chronic trachoma[2] or adult chlamydial conjunctivitis but are often present in specimens from neonatal chlamydial conjunctivitis. Extracellular elementary bodies can be identified with immunofluorescent methods.[5,40,54] Other antigen-detection techniques include enzyme immunoassays.[6] Nucleic acid probes, along with amplification by the polymerase chain reaction, are under development for clinical use.[61]

Definitive diagnosis is made by isolating *C. trachomatis* in a cell-culture system.[16] Conjunctival scrapings or swabs are usually inoculated into a transport medium, and then sent to the laboratory. Nasal and urethral swabs are not usually obtained.[44] It is difficult to isolate chalmydiae in the late, chronic stages of trachoma.[64]

Serologic tests are not useful in diagnosing chlamydial keratoconjunctivitis, as many individuals have preexisting circulating antibodies. Antibodies in tears may correlate with disease severity.

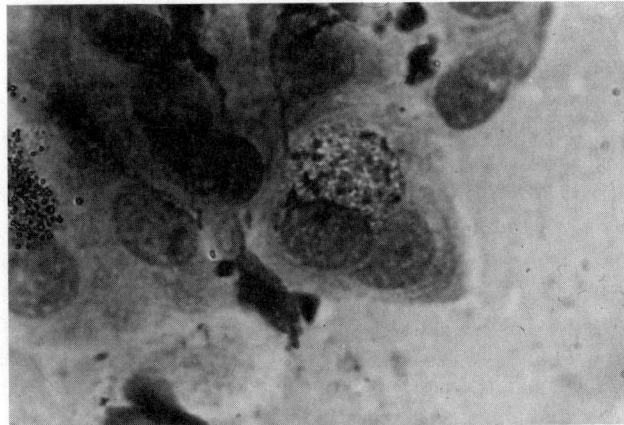

Fig. 63-6. Chlamydial inclusion in a conjunctival epithelial cell. The chlamydial agent is seen here as a micro colony of discrete particles in the cytoplasm of this conjunctival epithelial cell (Giemsa, × 500).

THERAPY

Trachoma

In trachoma-endemic regions, treatment is based on public health efforts to prevent blindness. Programs to control trachoma include both chemotherapy and surgical intervention of lid deformities.

In communities with severe blinding endemic trachoma, the objectives of chemotherapy are (1) reduction in the intensity of trachoma, and thence of the risk of blindness in the individual, and (2) reduction in transmission of infection from one individual to another.

Sulfonamides, tetracyclines, erythromycin, other macrolides and azalides, and rifampin are effective in treating active trachoma. Topical tetracyclines (eye ointments or suspensions) are still recommended for large-scale treatment of trachoma. When patients can be screened and those with severe or moderate intensity disease identified, systemic antibiotics may be appropriate, and are potentially much more effective than topical application.

Current trachoma control programs are based on the mass application of locally applied antibiotics. In theory, initial intensive large-scale chemotherapy is intended to reduce the ocular reservoir of chlamydia in the population and should be followed by intermittent, family-based topical treatment to control further eye-to-eye transmission. This strategy has not been effective in endemic areas, except when accompanied by economic development.[75]

Systemic antibiotic treatment is more effective than topical treatment in children with severe-intensity infectious trachoma and should eliminate the extraocular reservoirs of *C. trachomatis*. At present, WHO recommends systemic antibiotics for individuals with severe- and moderate-intensity trachoma. This "selective" therapy involves screening of the affected population for disease and assumes monitoring of treated children for side effects.

Oral doxycycline given once daily to 6- to 8-year-olds by the intermittent schedule significantly reduced trachoma intensity. In theory, oral erythromycin in four divided doses can be used to treat younger children. Oral sulfonamides were once used, but they had an unacceptably high rate of untoward reactions, some of them very serious. A study with the new long-acting azalide, azithromycin, has shown that a single dose is as effective for active trachoma as 30 doses of topical tetracycline.[3] This erythromycin-like drug could well be the drug of choice for childhood trachoma. Azithromycin is advantageous in that it can be administered to children as young as 4 months of age.

The surgical correction of trichiasis and/or entropion (lid deformities) has an immediate impact on preventing blindness. These simple procedures can be carried out in affected communities by mobile teams. When ophthalmologists are not available, general physicians or auxiliary personnel can be trained to do these lid operations.[7] In general, lid rotation procedures have been most successful.[14,50,51]

Keratopathy has a poor outcome in patients with trachoma. The reduced flow of aqueous tears, loss of mucus from goblet cell destruction, and poor mechanical surfacing by distorted lids all contribute to corneal opacification.

Adult Chlamydial Keratoconjunctivitis

The adult disease usually responds promptly to 3 weeks of treatment with full doses of systemic tetracyclines or erythromycin.[60,71] Sexual consorts should be treated at the same time. Topical application of tetracycline or erythromycin is marginally effective when given alone,[17] and does not improve outcome when systemic antibiotics are given.

The sexually transmitted *Chlamydia trachomatis* serovars are a major cause of genital tract disease such as nongonococcal urethritis in both men and women, as well as endometritis and salpingitis in women (which may be followed by fallopian tube scarring and infertility). Women can also develop perihepatitis by an ascending infection into the peritoneum (Fitz-Hugh–Curtis syndrome). Prompt systemic antibiotic treatment of patients with chlamydial eye infections and their sexual consorts is indicated.

PREVENTION

Trachoma control is based on the mass treatment of all affected individuals within a community. Improved living conditions provide the most effective prevention. Reducing the transmission of genital infection, such as by barrier contraception, can minimize the occurrence of adult and neonatal chlamydial keratoconjunctivitis.

Experimental vaccines can induce a short-lived immune response. Unfortunately, humoral immunity is not protective[4] and can cause more severe disease. Understanding how the host responds to chlamydial infection will offer future opportunities for prevention.[58]

REFERENCES

1. al Rajhi AA, Hidayat A, Nasr A, al-Faran M: The histopathology and the mechanism of entropion in patients with trachoma, *Br J Ophthalmol* 100:1293-1296, 1993.
2. Babalola OE, Bage SD: The persistence of chlamydial inclusions in clinically quiescent trachoma, *West Afr J Med* 11:55-61, 1992.
3. Bailey RL, Arullendran P, Whittle HC, Mabey DC: Randomized controlled trial of single-dose azithromycin in treatment of trachoma, *Lancet* 342:453-456, 1993.
4. Bailey RL, Kajbaf M, Whittle HC et al.: The influence of local antichlamydial antibody on the acquisition and persistence of human ocular chlamydial infection: IgG antibodies are not protective, *Epidemiol Infect* 111:315-324, 1993.
5. Bialasiewicz AA, Jahn GJ: Evaluation of diagnostic tools for adult chlamydial keratoconjunctivitis, *Ophthalmology* 94:532-537, 1987.
6. Bobo L, Munoz B, Viscidi R et al.: Diagnosis of *Chlamydia trachomatis* eye infection in Tanzania by polymerase chain reaction/enzyme immunoassay, *Lancet* 338:847-850, 1991.
7. Bog H, Yorston D, Foster A: Results of community-based eyelid surgery for trichiasis due to trachoma, *Br J Ophthalmol* 77:81-83, 1993.
8. Brechner RJ, West S, Lynch M: Trachoma and flies: individual *vs* environmental risk factors, *Arch Ophthalmol* 110:687-689, 1992.

9. Byrne GI, Lehmann LK, Altera KP: Induction of tryptophan catabolism is the mechanism for gamma interferon-mediated inhibitions of intracellular *Chlamydiae psittaci* replication in T24 cell, *Infect Immun* 53:347, 1986.

10. Caldwell HD, Kromhout J, Schachter J: Purification and partial characterization of the major outer membrane protein of *Chlamydia trachomatis, Infect Immun* 31:1161, 1981.

11. Cerrone M, Ma J, Stephens RS: Cloning, sequencing, and immunological specificity of the *Chlamydia trachomatis* groEL homolog, *Infect Immun* 59:79-90, 1990.

12. Courtright P, Lewallen S, Howe R: Cell-mediated immunity in trachomatous scarring: evidence from a leprosy population, *Ophthalmology* 100:94-104, 1993.

13. Courtright P, Sheppard J, Lane S et al.: Latrine ownership as a protective factor in inflammatory trachoma in Egypt, *Br J Ophthalmol* 75:322-325, 1991.

14. Cruz AA, Moribe I, Sakuma JT, Neto JM: Surgical correction of trachoma-related upper eyelid cicatricial entropion utilizing the Barbera-Carre technique, *Ophthal Plast Reconstr Surg* 7:269-272, 1991.

15. Darougar S, Viswalingam ND: Marginal corneal abscess associated with adult chlamydial ophthalmia, *Br J Ophthalmol* 72:774-777, 1988.

16. Darougar S, Forsey T, Jones BR et al.: Isolation of *Chlamydia trachomatis* from eye secretion (tears), *Br J Ophthalmol* 63:256-258, 1979.

17. Darougar S, Viswalingam N, El-Sheikh H et al.: A double-blind comparison of topical therapy of chlamydial ocular infection (TRIC infection) with rifampicin or chlortetracycline, *Br J Ophthalmol* 65:549-552, 1981.

18. Dawson CR, Juster R, Marx R et al.: Limbal disease in trachoma and other ocular chlamydial infections: risk factors for corneal vascularization, *Eye* 3:204-209, 1989.

19. Dawson CR, Mordhorst C, Thygeson P: Infection of rhesus and cynomolgus monkeys with egg-grown viruses of trachoma and inclusion conjunctivitis, *Ann NY Acad Sci* 98:167-176, 1962.

20. Fehr T: Endemische Bad Konjunktivitis, *Berl Klin Wochenschr* 37:10-11, 1900.

21. Fitzpatrick DR, Wie J, Webb D et al.: Preferential binding of *Chlamydia trachomatis* to subsets of human lymphocytes and induction of interleukin-6 and interferon-γ, *Immunol Cell Biol* 69:337-348, 1991.

22. Forsey T, Darougar S, Treharne JD: Prevalence in humans of antibodies to chlamydia IOL207, an atypical strain of chlamydia, *J Infect* 12:145, 1986.

23. Fritsch H, Hofstätter K, Lindner K: Experimentelle Studien zur Trachomfrage, *Graefes Arch Ophthalmol* 76:547-558, 1910.

24. Grayston JT, Kuo CC, Campbell LA, Wang SP: *Chlamydia pneumoniae* sp. nov. for *Chlamydia* sp. strain TWAR, *Int J Syst Bacteriol* 39:88-90, 1990.

25. Grayston JT, Kuo CC, Wang SP, Altman J: A new *Chlamydia psittaci* strain, TWAR, isolated in acute respiratory tract infections, *New Eng J Med* 315:161, 1986.

26. Grayston JT, Wang S-P: New knowledge of chlamydiae and the diseases they cause, *J Infect Dis* 132:87-105, 1975.

27. Grayston JT, Wang SP, Yeh LJ, Kuo CC: Importance of reinfection in the pathogenesis of trachoma, *Rev Infect Dis* 7:717-725, 1985.

28. Halberstaedter L, von Prowazek S: Über Zelleinschlüsse parasitärer Natur beim Trachom, *Arb Gesundheitsa* 26:44-47, 1907.

29. Halberstaedter L, von Prowazek S: Zur Ätiologie des Trachoms, *Dtsch Med Wochenshr* 33:1285-1287, 1909.

30. Hatch TP: Metabolism of chlamydia. In Barron AL, editor: *Microbiology of chlamydia,* 97, Boca Raton, Fla., 1988, CRC Press.

31. Holland MJ, Bailey RL, Hayes LJ et al.: Conjunctival scarring in trachoma is associated with depressed cell-mediated immune responses to chlamydial antigens, *J Infect Dis* 168:1528-1531, 1993.

32. Huntmüller and Padderstein: Befunde bei Schwimmbadkonjunktivitis, *Dtsch Med Wochenschr* 39:63-66, 1913.

33. Jones BR: Ocular syndromes of TRIC virus infection and their possible genital significance, *Br J Vener Dis* 40:3-18, 1964.

34. Kroner T: Zur Ätiologie der Ophthalmoblennorrhoea neonatorum, *Zentralbl Gynaekol* 8:643-645, 1884.

35. Linder K: Uebertragungsversuche von gonokokkenfreien Blennorrhoea neonatorum auf Affen, *Wien Klin Wochenschr* 22:1555, 1909.

36. Linder K: Zur Ätiologie der gonokokkenfreien Urethritis, *Wien Klin Wochenschr* 23:283-284, 1910.

37. Linder K: Gonoblennorrhöe, Einschlussblennorhoe, und Trachoma, *Graefes Arch Ophthalmol* 78:380, 1911.

38. Mark DB, McCulley JB: Reiter's keratitis, *Arch Ophthalmol* 100:781-784, 1982.

39. Matsumoto A: Structural characteristics of chlamydial bodies. In Barron AL, editor: *Microbiology of chlamydia,* 39, Boca Raton, Fla., 1988, CRC Press.

40. Milano F, Gorini G, Olliatro P et al.: Evaluation of diagnostic procedures in chlamydial eye infection, *Ophthalmologica* 203:114-117, 1991.

41. Morax V: Sur l'étiologie des ophtalmies du nouveau-né et la déclaration obligatoire, *Ann Ocul* 129:346-363, 1895.

42. Morrison RP, Belland RJ, Lyng K, Caldwell HD: Chlamydial disease pathogenesis: the 57-kD chlamydial hypersensitivity antigen is a stress response protein, *J Exp Med* 170:1271-1283, 1989.

43. Morrison RP, Lyng K, Caldwell HD: Chlamydial disease pathogenesis: ocular hypersensitivity elicited by a genus-specific 57k-D protein, *J Exp Med* 169:663-675, 1989.

44. Morton CE, Mallinson H, Clearkin LG et al.: Per-nasal swabbing as an aid to the diagnosis of chlamydial and adenovirus conjunctivitis, *Eye* 4:510-513, 1990.

45. Moulder JW: *The biochemistry of intracellular parasitism,* Chicago, 1962, The University of Chicago Press.

46. Moulder JW: Intracellular parasitism: life in an extreme environment, *J Infect Dis* 130:300-306, 1974.

47. Moulder JW: Order *Chlamydiales* and family *Chlamydiaceae.* In Kreig NR, editor: *Bergey's manual of systematic bacteriology,* vol 1, 729, Baltimore, 1984, Williams and Wilkins.

48. Noguchi H: The etiology of trachoma, *J Exp Med* 48:1-53, 1928.

49. Newhall WJ: Macromolecular and antigenic composition of chlamydiae. In Barron AL, editor: *Microbiology of chlamydia,* Boca Raton, Fla., 1988, CRC Press.

50. Reacher MH, Huber MJ, Canagaratnam R, Alghassany A: A trial of surgery for trichiasis of the upper lid from trachoma, *Br J Ophthalmol* 74:109-113, 1990.

51. Reacher MH, Munoz B, Alghassany A et al.: A controlled trial of surgery for trachomatous trichiasis of the upper lid, *Arch Ophthalmol* 110:667-674, 1992.

52. Reinhards J, Weber A, Maxwell-Lyons F: Collective antibiotic treatment of trachoma, *Bull WHO* 21:665-702, 1959.

53. Schultz P: Eine hiesige Badeanstalt, der Infektionsort verschiedener Trachomerkrankungen, *Berl Klin Wochenschr* 36:865-866, 1899.

54. Sheppard JD, Kowalski RP, Meyer MP et al.: Immunodiagnosis of adult chlamydial conjunctivitis, *Ophthalmology* 95:434-442, 1988.

55. Stargardt K: Über Epithelzellveränderungen beim Trachom und andern Konjunctivalerkrankugen, *Graefes Arch Ophthalmol* 69:525-542, 1909.

56. Stenson S: Adult inclusion conjunctivitis: clinical characteristics and corneal changes, *Arch Ophthalmol* 99:605-608, 1981.

57. Stephens RS: Chlamydial genetics. In Barron AL, editor: *Microbiology of chlamydia,* 111, Boca Raton, Fla., 1988, CRC Press.

58. Stephens RS: Challenge of *Chlamydia* research, *Infect Agents Dis* 1:279, 1993.

59. Stephens RS, Wagar EA, Schoolnik G: High resolution mapping of serovar-specific and common antigenic determinants of the major outer membrane protein for *Chlamydia trachomatis, J Exp Med* 167:817-831, 1988.

60. Sternberg K, Mardh PA: Treatment of concomitant eye and genital chlamydial infection with erythromycin and roxithromycin, *Acta Ophthalmol* 71:332-335, 1993.

61. Talley AR, Garcia-Ferrer F, Laycock KA et al.: The use of polymerase chain reaction for the detection of chlamydial keratoconjunctivitis, *Am J Ophthalmol* 114:685-692, 1992.

62. T'ang F-F, Chang H-L, Huang Y-T, Wang K-C: Trachoma virus in chick embryo, *Natl Med J China* 43:81-86, 1957.

63. Taylor HR, Prendergast RA, Dawson CR et al.: An animal model for cicatrizing trachoma, *Invest Ophthalmol Vis Sci* 21:422-433, 1981.

64. Taylor HR, Siler JA, Mkocha HA et al.: Longitudinal study of the microbiology of endemic trachoma, *J Clin Microbiol* 29:1593-1595, 1991.

65. Taylor HR, Siler JA, Mkocha HA et al.: The natural history of endemic trachoma: a longitudinal study, *Am J Trop Med Hyg* 46:552-559, 1992.

66. Thygeson P, Crocker T: Observations on experimental trachoma and inclusion conjunctivitis, *Am J Ophthalmol* 42:76-83, 1956.

67. Thygeson P, Mengert WF: The virus of inclusion conjunctivitis: further observations, *Arch Ophthalmol* 15:377-410, 1936.

68. Thygeson P, Proctor FI: Etiological significance of the elementary body in trachoma, *Am J Ophthalmol* 18:811-813, 1935.

69. Thygeson P, Richards P: Nature of the filterable agent of trachoma, *Arch Ophthalmol* 20:569-584, 1938.

70. Tullo AB, Richmond SJ, Easty DL: The presentation and incidence of paratrachoma in adults, *J Hyg* 87:63-69, 1981.

71. Viswalingam ND, Darougar S, Yearsley P: Oral doxycycline in the treatment of adult chlamydial ophthalmia, *Br J Ophthalmol* 70:301-304, 1986.

72. Viswalingam ND, Wishart MS, Woodland RM: Adult chlamydial ophthalmia (paratrachoma), *Br Med Bull* 39:123-127, 1983.

73. Wagar EA, Schachter J, Baviol P, Stephens RS: Differential human serological response to two 60,000 m.w. *Chlamydia trachomatis* antigens, *J Infect Dis* 162:922-927, 1990.

74. Wagar EA, Stephens RS: Developmental-specific DNA-binding proteins of *Chlamydia, Infect Immun* 56:1678-1684, 1988.

75. West S, Munoz B, Bobo L et al.: Nonocular *Chlamydia* infection and risk of ocular reinfection after mass treatment in a trachoma hyperendemic area, *Invest Ophthalmol Vis Sci* 34:3194-3198, 1993.

76. West SK, Congdon N, Katala S, Mele L: Facial cleanliness and risk of trachoma in families, *Arch Ophthalmol* 109:855-857, 1991.

77. West SK, Taylor HR: Reliability of photographs for grading trachoma in field studies, *Br J Ophthalmol* 74:12-13, 1990.

78. Wilhelmus KR, Robinson NM, Tredici LL, Jones DB: Conjunctival cytology of adult chlamydial conjunctivitis, *Arch Ophthalmol* 104:691-693, 1986.

79. Yoneda C, Dawson CR, Daghfous T et al.: Cytology as a guide to the presence of chlamydial inclusions in Giemsa-stained conjunctival smears in severe endemic trachoma, *Br J Ophthalmol* 59:116-124, 1975.

80. Zhang JP, Stephens RS: Mechanism of attachment of *Chlamydia trachomatis* to eukaryotic host cells, *Cell* 69:861-869, 1992.

81. Zhang YX, Stewart SJ, Caldwell HD: Protective monoclonal antibodies to *Chlamydia trachomatis* serovar- and serogroup-specific major outer membrane protein determinants, *Infect Immun* 57:636-638, 1989.

64 Neonatal Conjunctivitis

MARGARET R. HAMMERSCHLAG, PETER A. RAPOZA

Neonatal conjunctivitis is conjunctival inflammation with discharge occurring within the first 24 days of life.[90] It is the most common ocular disorder of the postnatal period. Causative organisms vary in relative importance over time and by geographic location.

Ophthalmia neonatorum is an ocular emergency. Treatment must be directed at a specific cause. Optimal management requires knowledge of the responsible agents and the availability of diagnostic assays.

HISTORICAL BACKGROUND

At the beginning of the twentieth century there was no screening of expectant mothers for sexually transmitted diseases, no instillation of prophylactic eyedrops, and no antibiotic treatment for ocular infections. In this period neonatal conjunctivitis meant, for all practical purposes, gonococcal conjunctivitis. Prevalence studies in the early twentieth century indicated that 20% to 79% of children residing in European institutions for the blind had lost their vision as a result of infection by *Neisseria gonorrhoeae*.[15]

Credé's introduction of the practice of instillation of topical silver nitrate solution onto the ocular surface at birth reduced the incidence of gonococcal ophthalmia neonatorum from 10% to 0.3%.[67] The most visually threatening cause of neonatal infection came under control with silver nitrate prophylaxis.

Soon afterward, the importance of another form of ophthalmia neonatorum termed *inclusion blennorrhea* was noted. The relationship between maternal urethral infection and conjunctivitis of the newborn associated with inclusion bodies within epithelial cells was established.[39] Subsequently, in the 1950s *Chlamydia trachomatis* was isolated from an infant with inclusion blennorrhea.[33] Chlamydial infection remains the most common cause of infectious neonatal conjunctivitis in developed countries.

Numerous other bacteria were reported to be associated with neonatal conjunctivitis, but they were not usually associated with serious sequelae.[3,52,53] Viral causes of neonatal conjunctivitis are uncommonly detected. Herpes simplex virus is a potentially devastating cause of ophthalmia neonatorum and can result in morbidity and mortality.[47]

EPIDEMIOLOGY

Infectious conjunctivitis occurs in up to 12% of neonates in developed countries and 23% of neonates in developing nations.[34,53] The introduction of neonatal ocular prophylaxis and the routine screening and treatment of pregnant women for gonorrhea has altered the epidemiology of neonatal conjunctivitis, especially in the United States and other industrialized countries.

The relative importance of the various causes of conjunctivitis of the newborn has varied over time. Within the same decade, estimates of the prevalence of neonatal conjunctivitis have been reported to range between 1.6% to 23%.[3,34,41,53] Much of the disparity is attributable to differences between countries and (sometimes) between regions and cities. The incidence of gonococcal conjunctivitis varies from 0.04 per 1000 live births in Belgium to 40 per 1000 live births in Kenya.[17] For chlamydial conjunctivitis the incidence varies from 5 to 60 per 1000 live births in the United States to 80 per 1000 live births in Kenya.[17]

These international differences mirror the generally increased prevalence of sexually transmitted diseases among the poor. For example, the disadvantaged have a 26% prevalence of chlamydial genital infections,[56] and in an American inner-city population, neonatal chlamydial conjunctivitis is statistically associated with lower socioeconomic status.[60]

PATHOGENESIS

Microbiology

Chlamydia trachomatis. *Chlamydia trachomatis* is the most commonly identified infectious cause of ophthalmia neonatorum. It has been isolated from 10% to over 55% of neo-

TABLE 64-1 PREVALENCE OF *C. TRACHOMATIS* AND *N. GONORRHOEAE* AMONG INFANTS WITH NEONATAL CONJUNCTIVITIS

Author, Country, Year	Percentage with	
	C. trachomatis	*N. gonorrhoeae*
Rowe and associates, USA, 1979	32	0
Sandström and associates, USA, 1984	14	0
Hammerschlag and associates, USA, 1985	44	0
Rapoza and associates, USA, 1986	46	0
Barry and associates, UK, 1986	42	1
Fransen and associates, Kenya, 1986	17	46
Laga and associates, Kenya, 1986	34	15
Sandström and associates, Sweden, 1987	12	0
Fransen and associates, Belgium, 1987	10	0
Mabey and associates, The Gambia, 1987	36	27
Winceslaus and associates, UK, 1987	55	9
Isenberg and associates, Kenya, 1995	8	1

nates with conjunctivitis.* *C. trachomatis* is an obligate intracellular parasite with a complex life cycle involving infectious (elementary bodies) and replicative forms (reticulate bodies). Chlamydial infections are the most prevalent sexually transmitted diseases in the United States.[7,21]

Neisseria gonorrhoeae. Numerous bacterial species have been implicated as causes of ophthalmia neonatorum. It is difficult to ascertain the importance of particular species, as many of these bacteria have been isolated from the eyes of infants with conjunctivitis and from controls in equal frequency.

Neisseria gonorrhoeae is the most important bacterial cause of neonatal conjunctivitis, if not by frequency, then by the organism's potential to damage the eye. *N. gonorrhoeae* accounts for less than 1% of cases of ophthalmia neonatorum in the United States and many European countries.[19,59,68,69,79] In contrast, 12% of the newborns with conjunctivitis in Gambia and 15% in Kenya have *N. gonorrhoeae* isolated from their conjunctivae.[34,41]

A major problem has been the spread of resistance to penicillin and tetracycline by gonococci. The first isolates of plasmid-mediated, penicillinase-producing *N. gonorrhoeae* (PPNG) occurred in the Far East. Studies from Singapore demonstrated a steady rise in cases of gonorrhea in adults caused by PPNG from 0.1% in 1976 to 30% in 1980.[83] This rise was paralleled by an increase in the number of cases of neonatal conjunctivitis caused by PPNG from 0% in 1976 to 35% in 1980. In Kenya 52% of gonococcal isolates were found to be PPNG.[34] By 1989 the incidence of PPNG among adults with gonorrhea in Brooklyn, New York, exceeded 24%, and the incidence of infections caused by PPNG in children, including ophthalmia neonatorum, was 26.5%[63] (Table 64-1).

Other Bacteria. Other bacterial organisms implicated as causes of ophthalmia neonatorum include those commonly responsible for bacterial conjunctivitis in older children: *Streptococcus pneumoniae* and *Haemophilus influenzae.* The latter was once designated *H. aegypticus* but is now recognized to be nontypable *H. influenzae.* Several recent studies of neonatal conjunctivitis (Table 64-2) found the prevalence of *S. pneumoniae* to extend to 11% and the prevalence of *H. influenzae* to range up to 22%.* These organisms are isolated from 1% of infants without conjunctivitis. These data confirm that *S. pneumoniae* and *H. influenzae* are pathogens, but they account for a small number of the total cases of neonatal conjunctivitis.

Viridans streptococci, including *Streptococcus viridans*, *Streptococcus mitis*, *Streptococcus sanguis*, and other species, are sometimes associated with neonatal conjunctivitis. They have been isolated in up to 54% of infants examined. *S. viridans* is often present in association with other organisms and can be isolated from the eyes of up to 5% of infants without conjunctivitis. Its exact role in conjunctivitis of the newborn remains to be determined.

Various gram-negative enteric rods such as *Enterobacter* species, *Eschericia coli*, *Klebsiella* species, *Proteus* species, and (rarely) *Pseudomonas* species are infrequently associated with neonatal conjunctivitis. *Pseudomonas* conjunctivitis may progress to corneal ulceration with perforation.

The role of *Staphylococcus aureus* in neonatal conjunctivitis is controversial. Although the organism has been isolated from the conjunctiva of 8% to 46% of infants with conjunctivitis, it has also been isolated from the conjunctiva of 3% to 10% of age-matched controls without conjunctivitis (Table 64-3). The presence of *S. aureus* on an eye with

---

*References 4, 18, 19, 24, 26, 27, 34, 41, 59, 65, 68, 69, 71, 89.

*References 19, 34, 53, 55, 59, 68, 69, 71.

TABLE 64-2 BACTERIAL CAUSES OF NEONATAL CONJUNCTIVITIS

Author, Country, Year	S. pneumoniae	H. influenzae	S. viridans	E. coli
Prentice and associates, UK, 1977	1%	0	16%	5%
Rowe and associates, USA, 1979	7%	5%	NS*	NS
Pierce and associates, UK, 1982	0	5%	17%	2%
Sandström and associates, USA, 1982	11%	17%	NS	NS
Laga and associates, Kenya, 1986	11%	13%	2%	2%
Rapoza and associates, USA, 1986	11%	22%	54%	2%
Fransen and associates, Belgium, 1987	NS	NS	14%	0
Sandström, Sweden, 1987	6%	3%	9%	1%

* NS: Not stated.

conjunctivitis may be secondary to the wetter environment of the infected eye rather than a direct cause of the infection. It is frequently isolated in conjuction with other pathogens, especially *C. trachomatis.*

Other bacteria that are infrequent causes of neonatal conjunctivitis are *Moraxella catarrhalis* and various *Neisseria* species, including *N. cinerea* and *N. meningitidis.* These organisms are gram-negative diplococci and can be confused with *N. gonorrhoeae* if appropriate culture methods are not used. Anaerobic bacteria have only occasionally been isolated in cases of neonatal conjunctivitis, and their significance is uncertain.[59] *Mycoplasma* species have not been demonstrated to be associated with neonatal conjunctivitis.

The cause of the conjunctivitis cannot be determined in a sizable proportion of the infants, ranging from 27% to 60%. This may be due in part to differences in culture techniques and populations.

Viruses. Viruses are uncommon causes of neonatal conjunctivitis, although few studies have obtained viral cultures.

Herpes simplex virus infection is acquired during delivery, and the conjunctiva may be the portal of entry for disseminated infection. Conjunctivitis as the only manifestation of neonatal herpes is rare. Less than 1% of infants with neonatal herpes simplex infection have conjunctivitis alone.[46] Of the studies summarized in Table 64-2, only two obtained viral cultures. Herpes simplex virus was isolated from the eye of 1 of 61 infants with conjunctivitis.[71]

TABLE 64-3 ROLE OF *S. AUREUS* IN NEONATAL CONJUNCTIVITIS

Author, Country, Year	% Infants with S. aureus	
	Cases	Controls
Prentice and associates, UK, 1977	8%	3%
Pierce and associates, UK, 1982	10%	5%
Sandström and associates, USA, 1984	17%	2%
Sandström, Sweden, 1987	46%	8%
Fransen and associates, Belgium, 1987	19%	10%

Coxsackievirus A9 was isolated from 1 of 100 neonates, with the positive culture occurring in a patient with concurrent chlamydial conjunctivitis.[59]

Toxicology

Chemical conjunctivitis occurs most commonly following the instillation of prophylactic drops or ointments. Silver nitrate inactivates gonococci by agglutination but can injure epithelial cells. Up to 90% of neonates receiving silver nitrate 1% solution develop conjunctivitis.[49] High concentrations can cause corneal opacification and narrowing or occlusion of the lacrimal puncta. Conjunctivitis is uncommon when erythromycin, tetracycline, or povidone iodine are employed.

Transmission

The primary means of inoculation of the newborn's conjunctiva is via vertical transmission from mother to child during vaginal delivery. This is particularly the case for the sexually transmitted pathogens *N. gonorrhoeae, C. trachomatis,* and herpes simplex virus. Of infants born to mothers with culture-proven gonococcal cervicitis at the time of delivery, gonococcal cultures were positive from the conjunctiva of 42% and from the oropharynx of 7% of the newborns.[34] The disease can also occur in infants born by cesarean section in which rupture of membranes has occurred.[13,84]

The risk to an infant born to a mother with active cervical chlamydial infection ranges from 20% to 50%.[2,21] In infants born to mothers with culture-documented chlamydial infection, conjunctival cultures were positive in 31% and oropharyngeal cultures positive in 2% of the infants.[34] Chlamydial pneumonitis, another manifestation of neonatal chlamydial infection, may develop in 8% to 20% of newborns whose mothers have chlamydial infection.[9,22,75] Ascending infection has been documented in a mother with chlamydial cervicitis despite cesarian section.[29] This usually occurs with premature rupture of membranes, but there are rare reports of chlamydial infection developing with intact membranes at the time of delivery. Chlamydial neonatal conjunctivitis must be considered, regardless of the means of delivery.

The infant can be exposed to herpes simplex virus during passage through the birth canal. The skin, eyes, mouth, and respiratory tract are the usual portals of entry for this virus that may cause localized or disseminated disease.[47] The risk of acquiring a neonatal herpes infection in the presence of active maternal genital herpes is estimated to be up to 40%.[48]

There are no convincing data supporting horizontal transmission of sexually transmitted pathogens from the mother or other family members after delivery, although the newborn's eyes could conceivably be inoculated by hands or fomites carrying genital secretions. Other bacterial species causing neonatal conjunctivitis, such as *Staphylococcus* spp., *Haemophilus* spp., *Pseudomonas* spp., and gram-negative enterics, are nosocomial agents associated with the newborn nursery.

Host Susceptibility

Conjunctivitis occurs when an organism is able to overcome the defenses of the ocular surface, a process dependent on both the status of the host defenses and the virulence of the organism.

The eye has a wide variety of defense mechanisms against the acquisition of infection via an external route.[43] Eyelid closure normally serves to spread ocular lubricants and to protect the ocular surface from abrasion. Delivery through the uterus can lessen this protection and expose the surface of the eye to inoculation by flora of the mother's vagina.

In the neonate specific immunity has not developed and plays little part in combating the primary acquired infection. The intact conjunctival epithelium is the principal barrier to penetration of infectious organisms. The normal flora of the conjunctiva can inhibit colonization in the postnatal period but probably does not paly a role in infections acquired at (or soon after) birth.

Microbial Virulence Factors

Organisms have a variety of virulence factors that contribute to their ability to colonize and infect the ocular surface of the newborn. *N. gonorrhoeae* possess pili that may be responsible for the adherence of gonococci to epithelial and cell surfaces.[86] Pili may also be an important virulence factor for gram-negative bacilli.[50]

Gram-positive bacteria produce toxins and enzymes that aid the establishment of infection by direct effects on the host tissue. *S. aureus*, for example, produces hemolysins, coagulase, leukocidin, hyaluronidase, staphylokinase, epidermolytic toxins, pyogenic toxin, and enterotoxins.[32]

Chlamydia are prokaryotes and obligate intracellular parasites. They have a unique reproductive cycle initiated by internalization by cells, possibly in a receptor-determined fashion.[45] Within host cells, chlamydial phagosomes are protected against fusion with lysosomes by an undetermined mechanism.[91] Elementary bodies differentiate into reticulate bodies that divide by binary fission within the phagosome, producing the characteristic intracytoplasmic inclusion. The reticulate bodies condense into elementary bodies by 48 hours after infection. Mature elementary bodies are released by autolysis of endosomes and host cytoplasmic membranes or exocytosis without causing death to the host cell.[85]

CLINICAL FEATURES

All infants developing conjunctivitis during the neonatal period should undergo a prompt, systematic, and comprehensive evaluation including histories of the infant and mother, ocular and general examination of the infant, and preparation of appropriate laboratory studies.[57,90] In selected cases evaluation of the mother may be required, particularly a pelvic examination to monitor for sexually transmitted diseases.[8]

Presentation

Although it is rarely possible to establish the cause of a particular case of neonatal conjunctivitis through history alone, the collection of appropriate information may lead the clinician toward increasing or decreasing the index of suspicion for certain organisms. In addition to the usual demographic information gathered, the clinician should inquire into the duration of ocular and (possibly) systemic signs, the type of ocular prophylaxis administered, and prior therapy for the conjunctivitis. The mother should be questioned regarding the extent of prenatal care, prior or current sexually transmitted diseases, and treatments. The clinician should be aware of any ongoing infections within the newborn nursery or carried by caretakers.

Chlamydial Conjunctivitis. The incubation period of chlamydial conjunctivitis is usually 4 to 14 days, with clinical signs of conjunctivitis appearing about 1 week after birth.[18,34,60,69] Conjunctivitis is often present for several days prior to the infant's evaluation by a health professional.

Gonococcal Conjunctivitis. Gonococcal neonatal conjunctivitis has typically been described as a "hyperacute" conjunctivitis. The incubation period is usually 1 to 7 days.[34,40] Up to 9% of cases occur after 14 days of age, especially if a topical antibiotic has been used.[18] Inadequate prenatal care and a history of drug abuse are risk factors associated with gonococcal neonatal conjunctivitis.[21]

Bacterial Conjunctivitis. Infants with nongonococcal bacterial neonatal conjunctivitis tend to exhibit signs of infection later than those with either chlamydial or gonococcal disease. On average, signs of conjunctivitis are noted by parents when the infants in this group reach 2 weeks of age.[60]

Herpes Simplex Virus Keratoconjunctivitis. A high degree of suspicion should be maintained for herpes simplex infections of the newborn in mothers with a history of genital herpes infections. The absence of visible active genital lesions does not preclude the possibility of viral transmission to the newborn, as asymptomatic shedding of herpes simplex virus (HSV) can occur in 4% to 14% of women tested.[1,62] A history of prior herpes infection or suspicious genital lesions in a mother or skin or ocular lesions in the newborn mandate assessment for a viral cause of conjunctivitis.

Toxic Conjunctivitis. Chemical conjunctivitis typically develops within hours of birth and follows the instillation of antimicrobial agents used at delivery. Although a transient conjunctivitis usually accompanies the use of silver nitrate, it is uncommonly observed following the application of erythromycin or tetracycline.[49]

Physical Examination

Physical examination may aid in establishing a causal diagnosis in neonatal conjunctivitis, but few findings are pathognomonic (Fig. 64-1). The severity of the conjunctivitis cannot be relied on to indicate a causative agent, as a wide range of severity of presentation exists for bacterial, chlamydial, and viral infections. Coinfection sometimes occurs and may require more than one treatment regimen for adequate therapy.[64]

Chlamydial Conjunctivitis. The presentation of chlamydial neonatal conjunctivitis ranges from mild hyperemia with scant mucoid discharge to severe hyperemia, copious purulent discharge, chemosis, and pseudomembrane formation. Bilateral infections are present in two thirds of cases.[60] Asymptomatic eye infection with *C. trachomatis* has been reported in several European and African studies. In one study from Kenya, many of these ocular infections were detected when the infants were more than 2 months of age.[36] This finding is in variance with the experience in the United States, where asymptomatic ocular chlamydial infection has been uncommon.[21,25] A follicular reaction is not seen, because infants less than 3 months of age do not have the

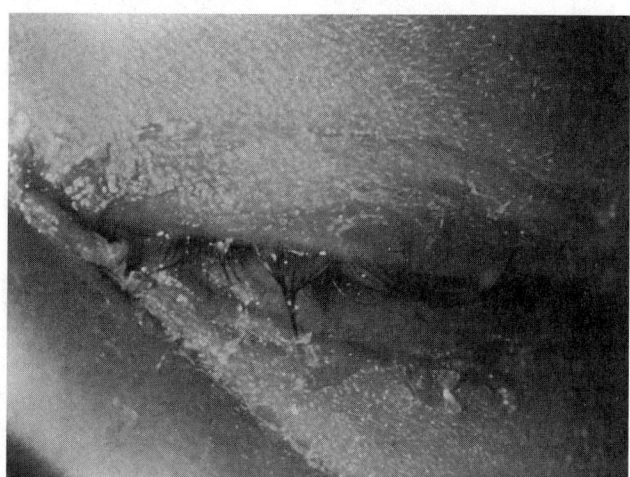

Fig. 64-1. Chlamydial neonatal conjunctivitis.

requisite lymphoid tissue present in the conjunctiva. The conjunctiva may be very friable, resulting in a bloody discharge, and may bleed when stroked with a swab. Eyelid erythema and edema are frequently present. Although uncommon, chlamydial neonatal conjunctivitis has been noted to induce long-term sequelae of corneal neovascularization and scarring.[16,44]

Gonococcal Conjunctivitis. The signs of gonococcal conjunctivitis are typically more severe than nongonococcal bacterial infections, but they may be minimal in selected cases.[34,54] The infection is usually bilateral.[90] Eyelid edema, erythema, conjunctival injection, and chemosis may be pronounced. Corneal involvement has been noted in up to 16% of cases of gonococcal neonatal conjunctivitis.[18] The corneal epithelium may be disrupted, allowing for the development of stromal edema possibly followed by ulceration. If the cornea perforates, the anterior chamber may be shallowed and the pupil displaced, as iris plugs the perforation site. Endophthalmitis and phthisis can rapidly ensue. Septicemia with arthritis and meningitis are potential systemic complications.

Other Bacterial Conjunctivitis. Nongonococcal bacterial conjunctivitis usually does not produce systemic manifestations, with the exception of meningococci, some gram-negative bacilli, and most importantly *Pseudomonas* spp. and *Haemophilus* spp. The degree of clinical signs varies, but it is usually less than that seen with *N. gonorrhoeae* and not substantially different from *C. trachomatis*.[34] A purulent discharge is variably present.

Herpes Simplex Virus Keratoconjunctivitis. Conjunctivitis caused by herpes simplex virus begins with the onset of conjunctival injection and chemosis, which may be accompanied by an outbreak of cutaneous vesicles on the eyelids or elsewhere. Corneal findings include dendritic and geographic epithelial keratitis, stromal keratitis, and eventually corneal neovascularization and opacification. Uveitis, cataract, vitreitis, retinitis, retinal detachment, and optic neuritis are found in a minority of cases.

Toxic Conjunctivitis. Except for mild edema, eyelid findings are uncommon in chemical conjunctivitis. Conjunctival injection is minimal to moderate, and the discharge is typically watery and not purulent. The conjunctivitis reduces rapidly without treatment to resolution within 1 to 2 days.

LABORATORY INVESTIGATIONS

Laboratory testing is needed to identify a specific agent as the cause of a case of neonatal conjunctivitis. Conjunctival cytology can enable preliminary management. Definitive diagnosis and modification of the treatment plan is based on the results of cultures and other assays for specific organisms.

Conjunctival Cytology

Application of a topical anesthetic is generally used for obtaining conjunctival scrapings or swabbings for smears

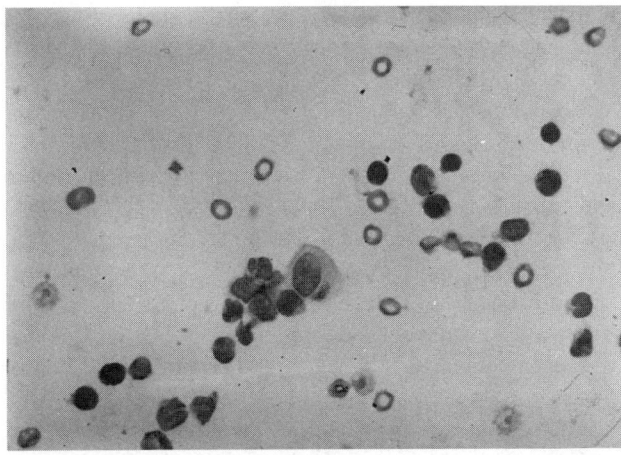

A

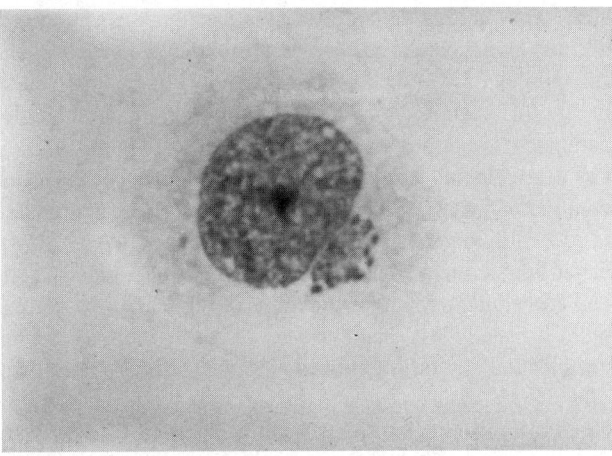

B

Fig. 64-2. **A,** Giemsa-stained conjunctival smear demonstrating a mixed inflammatory cell infiltrate in a patient with chlamydial neonatal conjunctivitis. Numerous epithelial cells, neutrophils, and lymphocytes are present. **B,** Giemsa-stained conjunctival smear showing a typical basophilic intracytoplasmic inclusion in chlamydial neonatal conjunctivitis.

and rapid diagnostic tests. Although the morphology of stained cells is best when a metal spatula is used, an adequate smear can be prepared with a swab.[58] Obtaining the specimen may produce bleeding, and parents should be forewarned that this will not damage their child's eyes. Smears should be prepared for Giemsa, Gram, and (in selected cases) Papanicolaou staining.

Giemsa Stain. Examination of a Giemsa-stained conjunctival smear allows an assessment of the types of inflammatory cells present (Fig. 64-2, *A*). General patterns exist but are not diagnostic in most cases[57,88] (Table 64-4). A pathognomonic finding is the presence of characteristic basophilic intracytoplasmic Halberstaedter-von Prowazek inclusions[20] (Fig. 64-2, *B*). The correlation of cytology and chlamydial culture in chlamydial conjunctivitis ranges from 39% to more than 90%.[59,69,74] Success of the method is highly dependent on the

TABLE 64-4 PRELIMINARY CAUSAL DIAGNOSIS BASED ON CYTOLOGIC CHARACTERISTICS OF GIEMSA-STAINED CONJUNCTIVAL SMEARS

Cause	Cytologic Characteristics
Bacterial	Neutrophils, bacteria
Chemical	Neutrophils, occasional lymphocytes
Chlamydial	Neutrophils, lymphocytes, plasma cells, Leber cells, basophilic intracytoplasmic inclusions
Viral	Lymphocytes, plasma cells, multinucleated giant cells, occasional eosinophilic intranuclear inclusions

manner in which the scraping is obtained and the experience of the microscopist in evaluating the specimen. In many settings Giemsa staining can be performed at the time of presentation, so the results may provide the examiner with valuable information upon which to initiate therapy.

Gram Stain. The Gram stain is widely available as a standard laboratory test for detection of bacterial organisms in the initial evaluation of infection. It can provide important information to the examiner at the patient's initial examination, so that appropriate treatment is started promptly. The presence of gram-negative diplococci in a conjunctival smear, particularly if the bacteria are within polymorphonuclear leukocytes, guides initiation of systemic antibiotics (Fig. 64-3). The Gram stain may be positive in up to 100% of the cases of gonococcal conjunctivitis, so its inclusion in the laboratory evaluation of neonatal conjunctivitis is important.[18,89] Proper staining technique and the availability of a well-trained microscopist are pivotal to the success of the test.

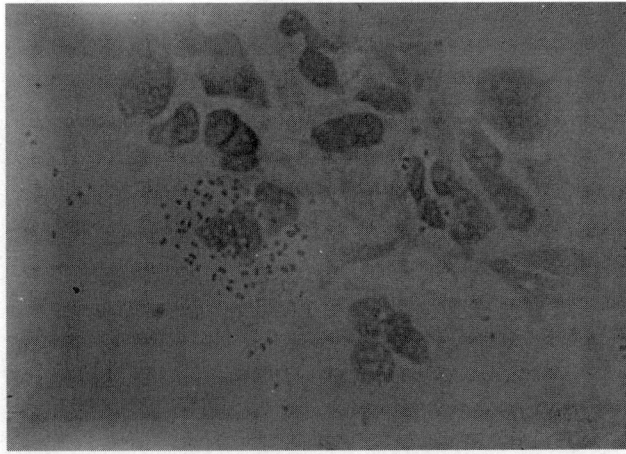

Fig. 64-3. Gram-stained conjunctival smear depicting multiple gram-negative diplococci within a neutrophil. *Neisseria gonorrhoeae* was isolated. (Reprinted with permission from Rapoza PA, Chandler JW: *Focal points: clinical modules for ophthalmologists* 6(1), San Francisco, 1988, American Academy of Ophthalmology.)

Papanicolaou Stain. Preparation of a conjunctival smear or a sample of fluid from a vesicle may demonstrate the presence of multinucleated giant cells and/or intranuclear inclusions of herpes simplex virus. The smear is usually processed by a central laboratory, so it is not as useful as the Giemsa or Gram stain in guiding initial therapy.

Rapid Diagnostic Tests

Several types of nonculture tests are available for rapid detection of chlamydial antigens or nucleic acid. These tests were primarily developed and evaluated for use in diagnosing chlamydial genital infections in adults. Few have been tested or have regulatory approval for the diagnosis of chlamydial conjunctivitis in infants. The types of tests that are available include direct fluorescent antibody tests (Syva MicroTrak, Kallestad Pathfinder, and others); enzyme immunoassays (EIA) (Chlamydiazyme, Abbott, Kallestad, Ortho, Syva MicroTrak EIA, and others); rapid macro EIAs (Kodak SureCell); and nucleic acid probes (GenProbe PACE II). A DNA amplification test using the polymerase chain reaction (Amplicor, Roche Molecular Diagnostics) is approved for chlamydial genital infections.

The conjunctiva is an ideal site for the use of these antigen tests because it is relatively free of other bacteria that can interfere and the number of organisms is high. The performance with conjunctival specimens has been superior to every other anatomic site, including the endocervix and urethra in adults and the nasopharynx in infants. These tests may give positive results based on the presence of nonviable organisms. Caution must be used to correlate their results with the clinical examination and/or the review of a Giemsa-stained conjunctival smear to test for the presence of an ongoing inflammatory response, if the tests are performed during or following antibiotic therapy.

Direct Fluorescent Antibody. Direct fluorescent antibody (DFA) testing identifies *C. trachomatis* elementary bodies morphologically in a specimen smear. The most extensively evaluated tests in infants have been Syva MicroTrak and Kallestad Pathfinder. Both tests have received FDA approval for detection of chlamydia in neonatal conjunctivitis. Both assays use a species-specific monoclonal antibody directed against the major outer membrane protein (MOMP) of *C. trachomatis*. Specimens are obtained by vigorously rubbing the papebral conjunctiva of the involved eye. It is useful to use one swab to remove surface mucus and debris prior to specimen collection with a second swab, as the appropriate specimen contains a large number of epithelial cells infected by chlamydia. Slides are air-dried, then fixed with methanol or acetone supplied with the kit. Antibody is applied to the specimen, then rinsed. The slides are read under oil immersion by fluorescence microscopy.[80] An adequate specimen should contain numerous epithelial cells in the field. The elementary bodies should be disc-shaped, bright, apple-green fluorescing particles with smooth edges (Fig. 64-4). To be considered positive, there should be at least 5 to 10 elementary bodies in the smear as well as intact epithelial cells. Whole inclusions are seen occasionally in conjunctival specimens.

Several studies comparing the DFA to culture for the diagnosis of neonatal chlamydial conjunctivitis have found sensitivities of 81% to 100%[59,65,79] (Table 64-5). A DFA takes only 15 to 20 minutes to perform, is widely available to practitioners who may not have access to chlamydial culture facilities, and provides a means to assess the quality of a specimen. The test requires a fluorescence microscope and a trained technologist to properly read the smears. Interpretation of smears can be subjective, which is a drawback to the test. Although the DFA is a rapid diagnostic test, the facilities for processing and reading the smear are seldom available in the practitioner's office or emergency room, so results may not be available for 1 day or longer.

Enzyme Immunoassay. Enzyme immunoassays detect chlamydial antigen by color change, either in solution or solid phase. These tests use polyclonal or genus-specific monoclonal antibodies, are not species specific, and can detect *C. pneumoniae*. Tests can take from 3 to 5 hours to run. Specimens are usually processed at central laboratories, so results may not be available for 1 or more days. Processing of enzyme immunoassays is semiautomated, allowing for testing of large numbers of specimens without technician fatigue or subjectivity that may accompany techniques using microscopy. Disadvantages include difficulties in assessing the adequacy of the specimen and in determining if the positive result is caused by the presence of cross-reacting bacteria. The performance of standard enzyme immunoassays (Abbott Chlamydiazyme and Kallestad Pathfinder) for the diagnosis of chlamydial ophthalmia neonatorum has been

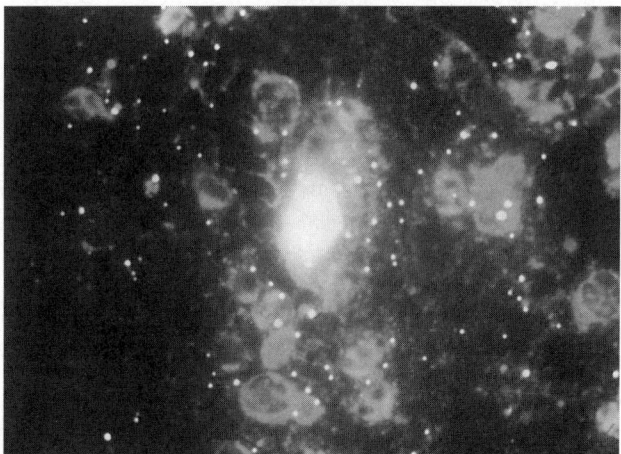

Fig. 64-4. Conjunctival smear stained with monoclonal antibody to *Chlamydia trachomatis*. Elementary bodies are evident as small, round, apple-green fluorescing particles.

TABLE 64-5 PERFORMANCE OF ANTIGEN DETECTION TESTS COMPARED TO CULTURE FOR THE DIAGNOSIS OF NEONATAL CHLAMYDIAL CONJUNCTIVITIS

Author, City, Year	Test (Brand)	No. Infants	% with Chlamydial Infection	% Sensitivity	% Specificity
Hammerschlag and associates, Brooklyn, 1985	EIA* (Chlamydiazyme)	90	44	93	98
Rapoza and associates, Baltimore, 1986	DFA† (MicroTrak)	100	43	100	94
Roblin and associates, Brooklyn, 1990	DFA (MicroTrak)	56	32	88	95
Stenberg and associates, Uppsala, 1990	EIA (Chlamydiazyme)	117	47	88	99
	DFA (Chlamyset)	107	43	81	98
	(MicroTrak)	118	47	87	97
Hammerschlag and associates, Brooklyn, 1990	EIA (Chlamydiazyme) (Pathfinder)	97	30	97	100
				97	99
Hammerschlag and associates, Brooklyn, 1991	EIA (SureCell)	75	40	97	93
Dumornay and associates Brooklyn, 1992	CIA‡ (MagicLite)	71	31	84	100

* EIA = Enzyme immunoassay
† DFA = Direct fluorescent antibody
‡ CIA = Chemiluminometric immunoasay

compared to culture, and sensitivities range from 88% to 93%[24,26,79] (Table 64-5).

The only macro enzyme immunoassay approved for the diagnosis of chlamydial conjunctivitis in infants is SureCell (Kodak). This test is self-contained with positive and negative controls. It requires no special equipment and the endpoints can be easily read with the naked eye. The test takes approximately 10 minutes to perform and is, perhaps, the first chlamydial antigen detection test that can be performed in a physician's office. The performance of SureCell has been similar to standard EIAs with a sensitivity of 97% and specificity of 93%[27] (Table 64-5).

Another recently introduced assay is the chemiluminometric immunoassay (MagicLite, Ciba-Corning). Instead of a color change, which is read in a spectrophotometer, this test uses a chemiluminescent reaction, which is read in a luminometer. In the only study of the use of this immunoassay for the diagnosis of chlamydial conjunctivitis, the sensitivity was 83% and specificity was 100%[14] (Table 64-5).

Nucleic Acid Probes. Nucleic acid probes take advantage of nucleic acid hybridization technology in diagnosing the presence of organisms within a specimen. Preliminary work has revealed an RNA probe useful in detecting chlamydia in a monkey model of trachoma, but it has not been tested in chlamydial neonatal conjunctivitis.[31]

The only clinically available DNA probe (Pace II, Gen-Probe) is FDA approved for use in cervical specimens only. A DNA probe has been successfully used to diagnose trachoma with sensitivity of 87% and specificity of 97%.[12]

Culture

Solid and Liquid Media. Recommended culture media include reduced blood agar, a medium suitable to support growth of *H. influenzae* and *N. gonorrhoeae* (such as chocolate agar or Thayer-Martin media), and cooked meat or thioglycolate broth. Prewetting the swab and avoiding topical anesthetic may increase the yield of the test.

Tissue-Culture Media. Culture still remains the "gold standard" for the diagnosis of chlamydial infections.[72] Because the organism is an obligate intracellular parasite, isolation is done in tissue culture. Specimens should be collected with wire shafted dacron-tipped swabs vigorously rubbed along the palpebral conjunctiva and then placed into appropriate transport media.[82] If not processed immediately, specimens for culture may be refrigerated for up to 48 hours or frozen at −70°C for longer periods. Cell lines used include McCoy and HeLa 229. The tissue-culture monolayers need to be pretreated with cycloheximide, and the inoculum must be centrifuged onto the cells to enhance absorption and infection.

After 48 to 72 hours of incubation, the cultures are fixed and stained, preferably with a fluorescein-conjugated monoclonal antibody, and examined microscopically for the presence of the characteristic intracellular inclusions.[9] The Centers for Disease Control and Prevention strongly recommends that culture confirmation be performed with visual identification of chlamydial inclusions.

The culture test has the important advantage of being the sole assay to detect the presence of viable chlamydial organisms in the conjunctiva. Disadvantages include the lack of availability in many settings, the requirement for meticulous specimen handling (including dependence on a ''cold chain'' in settings where immediate inoculation of tissue culture is not present), and the delay inherent in obtaining a test result. Culture may, on occasion, fail to be positive in some cases of chlamydial conjunctivitis in neonates and adults.[59,61]

In cases where a viral cause is suspected, the palpebral conjunctiva should be swabbed and the specimen placed in viral transport media for subsequent inoculation into appropriate cell lines. Cutaneous or mucosal vesicles may also be sampled.

THERAPY

Initial treatment is based on a systematic approach to history, clinical examination, and interpretation of Gram- and Giemsa-stained conjunctival smears. Therapy is altered based on the results of rapid diagnostic studies and/or the isolation of specific organisms.

Chlamydial Conjunctivitis. Topical sulfonamides were formerly the recommended treatment for neonatal chlamydial conjunctivitis, but several studies have conclusively demonstrated that topical therapy, including sulfacetamide, erythromycin, tetracycline, and chloramphenicol, is often inadequate.[23,30,51,53] More than 50% of infants with chlamydial conjunctivitis will also be infected at other sites including the nasopharynx, vagina, or rectum. Systemic therapy is indicated.

The only antibiotics that have been investigated so far are erythromycin estolate and erythromycin ethylsuccinate suspensions. Studies have demonstrated that a 10- to 14-day course of either preparation of erythromycin administered 2 or 4 times a day will eliminate both conjunctival and nasopharyngeal infection in approximately 80% of infants.[23,30,51] A Swedish study demonstrated a 100% cure rate following a twice daily dosing schedule.[70] The CDC recommends a 14-day course of erythromycin at a dosage of 50 mg/kg/day orally, 4 times a day.[7] There are no data to support the use of topical therapy in addition to the oral therapy. The efficacy of this dosing regimen was evaluated in an inner-city American population, and a 19% treatment failure rate was found.[59]

Patients not responding to the first course of erythromycin should be administered a second course at the same dosage. Treatment failure may be the result of poor compliance with antibiotic administration, insufficient absorption of the drug, reinfection, or resistance of the organism to the antibiotic. If failure again occurs, a treatment of trimethoprim-sulfamethoxazole pediatric suspension 0.5 mL/kg/day in 2 doses a day for 2 weeks should be considered. The patient should be examined following the conclusion of treatment.

Several new macrolide and azalide antibiotics have been introduced. Azithromycin has been approved for use in chlamydial infections of adults in the United States. Others, including roxithromycin, are available in Europe and Japan. These drugs have superior tissue penetration and improved pharmacokinetic profiles and patient tolerance as compared to erythromycin, and they are more active against *C. trachomatis* in vitro.[77,87] Roxithromycin can be administered twice a day, but requires a 10-day course of therapy. Azithromycin has a 30-hour halflife in serum and greater than a 5-day halflife in tissue, which allows for once-a-day dosing and a shorter course of therapy. Azithromycin as a single 1-gram oral dose has been shown effective for the treatment of genital chlamydial infection in adolescents and adults.[28,42] These drugs may prove very effective for the treatment of neonatal chlamydial conjunctivitis, offering improved efficacy with a shorter course of treatment. Only roxithromycin has been studied so far and appears to be equivalent to erythromycin for the treatment of neonatal chlamydial conjunctivitis.[78]

Gonococcal Conjunctivitis. As a result of the significant increase in the prevalence of infections caused by PPNG in the United States, the Centers for Disease Control and Prevention recommends the use of a penicillinase-resistant antibiotic in any area that is hyperendemic for PPNG. A hyperendemic area is defined as a >3% prevalence of gonococcal infections caused by PPNG over a 3-month period.

Ceftriaxone is the first-line drug recommended for treatment of gonococcal conjunctivitis at a dosage of 50 mg/kg/day (IV or IM, once a day for 7 days) or as a single dose of up to 125 mg.[7,35] Cefotaxime is an alternative drug, at a single dose of 100 mg/kg.[38] The World Health Organization (WHO) recommends 100 mg cefotaxime or kanamycin, 25 mg/kg as a single IM dose.[37,38] Additional topical antibiotic therapy is not needed when ceftriaxone or cefotaxime is used, but the infant's eyes should be irrigated with saline hourly until the discharge is eliminated. Careful followup of patients with gonococcal neonatal conjunctivitis is necessary because of the high degree of morbidity associated with the infection. Infants born to mothers with active gonorrhea should receive treatment regardless of whether conjunctivitis is present.[7,90]

Nongonococcal Bacterial Conjunctivitis. The data available on treatment of neonates with conjunctivitis caused by other bacterial organisms are limited. Considering the wide range of potential organisms, it is difficult to recommend one antibiotic over another. Once gonococcal and chlamydial infection have been ruled out, gram-positive cocci can be treated with erythromycin ointment, and gram-negative bacilli can be treated with gentamicin or tobramycin ointment applied every 4 hours for 1 week.[57] This therapy is usually sufficient for these generally self-limited, nondisseminated infections. Oral erythromycin has been advocated as treatment for nongonococcal bacterial neonatal conjunctivitis, but this therapy has not been widely accepted.[70] Conjunctivitis caused by *Haemophilus* spp., *Neisseria* spp., or *Pseu-*

domonas spp. should be treated with appropriate topical and systemic antibiotics because of the risk of disseminated disease. A followup examination should be performed at the conclusion of the treatment regiment.

Viral Conjunctivitis and Toxic Conjunctivitis. The only viral cause of ophthalmia neonatorum requiring specific treatment is herpes simplex virus. Trifluridine 1% solution should be instilled every two hours up to nine times per day. In addition, most pediatricians use intravenous acyclovir 10 mg/kg or 500 mg/M² IV every 8 hours for 10 days.[57]

No treatment is necessary for toxic conjunctivitis because of the self-limited nature of chemical conjunctivitis.

PREVENTION

Antimicrobial Prophylaxis

Ocular prophylaxis for gonococcal ophthalmia neonatorum is required by law or by health department regulations in most of the United States. The use of silver nitrate drops is specified by approximately half of the states. The CDC recommends the use of ointments containing either tetracycline or erythromycin or 1% silver nitrate drops for neonatal ocular prophylaxis.[7] Bacitracin ointment is not recommended. All three endorsed preparations have demonstrated efficacy for the prevention of gonococcal ophthalmia in high-risk populations.[25,36,66] Tetracycline and erythromycin ophthalmic ointments also appear to be effective in the prevention of gonococcal ophthalmia caused by PPNG and tetracycline-resistant *Neisseria gonorrhoeae* (TRNG), probably because of the high concentration of antibiotic in the ointments.[36] The prophylactic preparation should be instilled into the eyes of the neonate within 1 hour of birth to ensure efficacy.[90] To minimize cross-contamination, single-use tubes or ampules are preferable and are available for erythromycin and silver nitrate.

Prevention of chlamydial infections of the newborn requires the combined approach of maternal screening with contact tracing and provision of effective systemic antibiotic treatment.[73] Neonatal ocular prophylaxis with either erythromycin or tetracycline does not appear to be effective for the prevention of chlamydial conjunctivitis.[5,21] Neonatal ocular prophylaxis should therefore be directed primarily toward preventing gonococcal conjunctivitis, which poses the greatest risk of eye injury to the newborn.

Povidone-iodine is effective in vitro against *N. gonorrhoeae, C. trachomatis,* and herpes simplex virus.[6] Povidone-iodine is inexpensive and is generally widely available in both developed and developing countries.[31a]

Maternal Screening and Contact Tracing

The use of neonatal ocular prophylaxis for the prevention of gonococcal conjunctivitis is not a universal practice. Several western countries, including Great Britain and Denmark, do not mandate neonatal ocular prophylaxis. They depend instead on universal prenatal care and intensive contact tracing to control maternal and neonatal gonococcal infections. The highest risk of gonococcal ophthalmia occurs in infants born to mothers who have not received any prenatal care.[25] There is an association of gonococcal neonatal conjunctivitis with maternal substance abuse, specifically the use of "crack" cocaine. Although prenatal screening and treatment of maternal gonorrhea have a major effect on the prevention of neonatal gonococcal ophthalmia, neonatal ocular prophylaxis remains warranted in many populations because of the inadequate level of prenatal care.

All pregnant women should be cultured for gonorrhea at the first prenatal-care visit. For women at high risk of sexually transmitted diseases, a second culture should be obtained late in the third trimester. The CDC recommendation for treatment of uncomplicated gonorrhea in pregnant women is ceftriaxone, 250 mg IM once plus erythromycin base 500 mg orally 4 times a day for 7 days for possible coexisting chlamydial infection.[7] Cefixime, a new expanded-spectrum cephalosporin antibiotic, is also effective as a single oral dose but has not as yet been approved for use during pregnancy. Pregnant women with gonorrhea who are allergic to beta-lactam antibiotics can be treated with spectinomycin 2 g IM once, followed by erythromycin at the previous dosing schedule.

Contact tracing should be initiated for all consorts. The diagnosis of chlamydial conjunctivitis in an infant implies infection in the mother and father or mother's sexual partner. Treatment should be offered presumptively, even if both partners are asymptomatic. Many genital chlamydial infections in men and women are asymptomatic. Given the apparent ineffectiveness of ocular prophylaxis with silver nitrate or antibiotics in the prevention of neonatal chlamydial conjunctivitis, the most effective means of control for chlamydial disease may be screening and treatment of pregnant women.[25]

Screening for *C. trachomatis* is more feasible since the introduction of nonculture methods. Unfortunately, the treatment of maternal chlamydial infection is more complicated than that for gonorrhea for the following reasons: (1) the need for multiple doses and (2) only erythromycin is FDA-approved for use in pregnancy.

Treatment with oral erythromycin has resulted in 75% to 92% cure rates for pregnant women.[10,11,76] The CDC currently recommends four different erythromycin regimens: (1) erythromycin base, 500 mg orally 4 times a day for 7 days; or, if not tolerated, (2) 250 mg 4 times a day for 14 days; or (3) erythromycin ethylsuccinate 800 mg orally 4 times a day for 7 days; or, if not tolerated, (4) 400 mg orally 4 times a day for 14 days.[7] Tolerance and compliance are problematic with these dosing schedules, which require frequent daily administration over a long period of time.

Other antibiotics are being evaluated as alternative therapies. Results of one study suggest that amoxicillin, 500 mg orally 3 times a day for 7 days, was as effective and better tolerated than erythromycin.[11] The available published studies demonstrate efficacy ranging from 75% to over 90% in eliminating *C. trachomatis* from the genital tract. Even if the mother of an infant with conjunctivitis claims she was treated for chlamydia infection during pregnancy, the diagnosis should not be excluded by history alone, as reinfection or inadequate treatment may have occurred. As for gonorrhea, consorts of the mother should be referred for evaluation and treatment of presumed genital tract infection.

REFERENCES

1. Adam E et al.: Persistence of virus shedding in aymptomatic women after recovery from herpes genitalis, *Obstet Gynecol* 54:171-173, 1979.
2. Alexander ER, Harrison HR: Role of *Chlamydia trachomatis* in perinatal infection, *Rev Infect Dis* 5:713-719, 1983.
3. Armstrong JH, Zacarias F, Rein MF: Ophthalmia neonatorum: a chart review, *Pediatrics* 57:884-892, 1976.
4. Barry WC et al.: *Chlamydia trachomatis* as a cause of neonatal conjunctivitis, *Arch Dis Child* 61:797-799, 1986.
5. Bell TA et al.: Comparison of ophthalmic silver nitrate solution and erythromycin ointment for prevention of natally acquired *Chlamydia trachomatis*, *Sex Transm Dis* 14:195-200, 1987.
6. Benevento WJ: The sensitivity of Neisseria *gonorrhoeae, Chlamydia trachomatis,* and herpes simplex virus type II to disinfection with povidone-iodine, *Am J Ophthalmol* 109:329-333, 1990.
7. Centers for Disease Control and Prevention: 1993 sexually transmitted diseases treatment guidelines, *MMWR* 42:1-102, 1993.
8. Chandler JW, Rapoza PA: Ophthalmia neonatorum, *Int Ophthalmol Clin* 30:36-38, 1990.
9. Chandler JW et al.: Ophthalmia neonatorum associated with maternal chlamydial infections, *Trans Am Acad Ophthalmol Otolaryngol* 83:302-308, 1977.
10. Cohen I et al.: Improved pregnancy outcome following successful treatment of chlamydial infection, *JAMA* 263:3160-3163, 1990.
11. Crombleholme WR et al.: Amoxicillin therapy for *Chlamydia trachomatis* in pregnancy, *Obstet Gynecol* 75:752-756, 1990.
12. Dean D et al.: Use of a *Chlamydia trachomatis* DNA probe for detection of ocular chlamydiae, *J Clin Microbiol* 27:1062-1067, 1989.
13. Diener B: Cesarean section complicated by gonococcal ophthalmia neonatorum, *J Fam Pract* 13:739-744, 1981.
14. Dumornay W et al.: Comparison of a chemiluminometric immunoassay with culture for the diagnosis of chlamydial infections in infants, *J Clin Microbiol* 30:1867-1869, 1992.
15. Forbes GB, Forbes GM: Silver nitrate and the eye of the newborn: Credé's contribution to preventative medicine, *Am J Dis Child* 121:1-3, 1971.
16. Forster RK, Dawson CR, Schachter J: Late follow-up of patients with neonatal inclusion conjunctivitis, *Am J Ophthalmol* 69:467-472, 1970.
17. Fransen L, Volker K: Neonatal ophthalmia in the developing world, *Int Ophthalmol* 11:189-196, 1988.
18. Fransen L et al.: Ophthalmia neonatorum in Nairobi, Kenya: the roles of Neisseria *gonorrhoeae* and *Chlamydia trachomatis, J Infect Dis* 153:862-869, 1986.
19. Fransen L et al.: Incidence and bacterial aetiology of neonatal conjunctivitis, *Eur J Pediatr* 146:152-155, 1987.
20. Halberstaedter L, von Prowazek S: Über chlamydozoenbefunde bei: blenorrhoea neonatorum non gonorrhoica, *Berl Klin Wochenschr* 41:1839-1840, 1909.
21. Hammerschlag MR: Chlamydial infections, *J Pediatr* 114:727-734, 1989.
22. Hammerschlag MR et al.: Prospective study of maternal and infantile infection with *Chlamydia trachomatis, Pediatrics* 64:142-148, 1979.
23. Hammerschlag MR et al.: Longitudinal studies of chlamydial infections in the first year of life, *Pediatr Infect Dis* 1:395-401, 1982.
24. Hammerschlag MR et al.: Enzyme immunoassay for the diagnosis of neonatal chlamydial conjunctivitis, *J Pediatr* 107:741-743, 1985.
25. Hammerschlag MR et al.: Efficacy of neonatal ocular prophylaxis for the prevention of chlamydial and gonococcal coniunctivitis, *New Eng J Med* 320:769-772, 1989b.
26. Hammerschlag MR et al.: Comparison of two enzyme immunoassays to culture for the diagnosis of chlamydial conjunctivitis and respiratory infections in infants, *J Clin Microbiol* 28:1725-1727, 1990.
27. Hammerschlag MR et al.: Office diagnosis of neonatal chlamydial infection, *Pediatr Infect Dis J* 10:540-541, 1991.
28. Hammerschlag MR et al.: Chlamydia trachomatis in children, *Pediatr Ann* 23:349-353, 1994.
29. Harrison HR, Alexander ER: *Chlamydia trachomatis* infections in infants and children. In Holmes KK, March PA, Sparling PF, Wiesner PJ, editors: *Sexually transmitted diseases,* New York, 1990, McGraw-Hill Information Services.
30. Heggie AD et al.: Topical sulfacetamide vs oral erythromycin for neonatal chlamydial conjunctivitis, *Am J Dis Child* 139:564-566, 1985.
31. Hudson et al.: A molecular hybridization study of ocular chlamydial infection in cynomolgus monkeys, *Abstract Program,* Annual Spring Meeting, April-May, 1990, Association for Research in Vision and Ophthalmology.
31a. Isenberg SJ, Apt L, Wood M: A controlled trial of povidone-iodine as prophylaxis against opthalmia neonatorum, *N Engl J Med* 332:562-566, 1995.
32. Johnson MK: Toxins and enzymes in ocular disease caused by gram-positive bacteria. In Duane TD, Jaeger EA, editors: *Biomedical foundations of ophthalmology,* Philadelphia, 1991, JB Lippincott.
33. Jones BR, Collier LH, Smith CH: Isolation of virus from inclusion blenorrhoea, *Lancet* i:902-905, 1959.
34. Laga M et al.: Epidemiology of ophthalmia neonatorum in Kenya, *Lancet* ii:1145-1149, 1986.
35. Laga M et al.: Single-dose therapy of gonococcal ophthalmia neonatorum with ceftriaxone, *New Eng J Med* 315:1382-1385, 1986.
36. Laga M et al.: Prophylaxis of gonococcal and chlamydial ophthalmia neonatorum, *New Eng J Med* 318:653-657, 1988.
37. Latif A et al.: Management of gonococcal ophthalmia neonatorum with single-dose kanamycin and ocular irrigation with saline, *Sex Transm Dis* 15:108-109, 1988.
38. Lepage P, Kestelyn P, Bogearts J: Treatment of gonococcal conjunctivitis with a single intramuscular injection of cefotaxime, *J Antimicrob Chemother* 26(suppl A):23-27, 1990.
39. Lindner K: Gonoblennorrhoe, einschlussblenorrhoe und trachom, *Albrecht von Grafes Arch Klin Exp Ophthalmol* 78:345-380, 1911.
40. Lossick JGL: Prevention and management of neonatal gonorrhea, *Sex Transm Dis* 6:192, 1979.
41. Mabey D et al.: Chlamydial and gonococcal ophthalmia neonatorum in The Gambia, *Ann Trop Paediatr* 7:177-180, 1987.
42. Martin DM et al.: A controlled trial of a single dose of azithromycin for the treatment of chlamydial urethritis and cervicitis, *New Eng J Med* 327:921-925, 1992.
43. Mondino BJ: Host defense against bacterial and fungal disease. In Duane TD, Jaeger EA, editors: *Biomedical foundations of ophthalmology,* Philadelphia, 1991, JB Lippincott.
44. Mordhorst CH, Dawson C: Sequelae of neonatal inclusion conjunctivitis and associated disease in parents, *Am J Ophthalmol* 71:861-867, 1971.
45. Moulder JW: Intracellular parasitism: life in an extreme environment, *J Infect Dis* 130:300-306, 1974.
46. Nahmias AJ, Alford CA, Korones GR: Infection of the newborn with *Herpesvirus hominis, Adv Pediatr* 17:185, 1970.
47. Nahmias AJ, Josey WE, Naib ZML: Neonatal herpes simplex infections, *JAMA* 199:164-168, 1967.
48. Nahmias AJ et al.: Perinatal risk associated with maternal herpes simplex virus infection, *Am J Obstet Gynecol* 110:825-837, 1971.
49. Nishida H, Risenberg HM: Silver nitrate ophthalmic solution and chemical conjunctivitis, *Pediatrics* 56:368-373, 1975.
50. Otto TCG: Ecology, physiology, and genetics of fimbriae and pili, *Ann Rev Microbiol* 29:79, 1975.
51. Patamasucon P et al.: Oral v topical erythromycin therapies for chlamydial conjunctivitis, *Am J Dis Child* 136:817-821, 1982.

52. Persson K et al.: Neonatal chlamydial eye infection: an epidemiological and clinical study, *Br J Ophthalmol* 67:700-704, 1983.
53. Pierce JM, Ward ME, Seal DVL: Ophthalmia neonatorum in the 1980s: incidence, aetiology and treatment, *Br J Ophthalmol* 66:728-731, 1982.
54. Podgore JK, Holmes KK: Ocular gonococcal infection with minimal or no inflammatory response, *JAMA* 246:242-243, 1981.
55. Prentice MJ, Hutchinson GR, Taylor-Robinson D: A microbiological study of neonatal conjunctiva and conjunctivitis, *Br J Ophthalmol* 61:601-607, 1977.
56. Quinn TC et al.: The prevalence and detection of *Chlamydia trachomatis* in an inner city population: a comparison of diagnostic methods, *J Infect Dis* 152:419-423, 1985.
57. Rapoza PA, Chandler JW: Neonatal conjunctivitis: diagnosis and treatment. In *Focal points 1988: clinical modules for ophthalmologists*, vol VI, module 1, San Francisco, 1988, American Academy of Ophthalmology.
58. Rapoza PA, Johnson S, Taylor HR: Platinum spatula vs dacron swab in the preparation of conjunctival smears, *Am J Ophthalmol* 102:400-401, 1986.
59. Rapoza PA et al.: Assessment of neonatal conjunctivitis with a direct immunofluorescent monoclonal antibody stain for *Chlamydia, JAMA* 255:3369-3373, 1986.
60. Rapoza PA et al.: Epidemiology of neonatal conjunctivitis, *Ophthalmology* 93:456-461, 1986.
61. Rapoza PA et al.: A systematic approach to the diagnosis and treatment of chronic conjunctivitis, *Am J Ophthalmol* 109:138-142, 1990.
62. Rattray MC et al.: Recurrent genital herpes among women: symptomatic v asymptomatic viral shedding, *Br J Vener Dis* 54:262-265, 1978.
63. Rawstron SA et al.: Ceftriaxone treatment of penicillinase-producing Neisseria *gonorrhoeae* infections in children, *Pediatr Infect Dis J* 8:445-448, 1989.
64. Rees E et al.: Neonatal conjunctivitis caused by Neisseria *gonorrhoeae* and *Chlamydia trachomatis, Br J Vener Dis* 53:173-179, 1977.
65. Roblin PM et al.: Comparison of two rapid microscopic methods to culture for the detection of *Chlamydia trachomatis* in ocular and nasopharyngeal specimens from infants, *J Clin Microbiol* 27:968-970, 1989.
66. Rothenberg R: Ophthalmia neonatorum due to Neisseria *gonorrhoeae*: prevention and treatment, *Sex Transm Dis* 6:S-187-191, 1979.
67. Rothenberg R: Ophthalmia neonatorum in the 1980s: incidence, aetiology and treatment, *Br J Ophthalmol* 66:728-731, 1982.
68. Rowe DS et al.: Purulent ocular discharge in neonates: significance of *Chlamydia trachomatis, Pediatrics* 63:628-632, 1979.
69. Sandström I: Etiology and diagnosis of neonatal conjunctivitis, *Acta Paediatr Scand* 76:221-227, 1987a.
70. Sandström I: Treatment of neonatal conjunctivitis, *Arch Ophthalmol* 105:925-928, 1987b.
71. Sandström I et al.: Microbial causes of neonatal conjunctivitis, *J Pediatr* 105:706-709, 1984.
72. Schachter J: Overview of human diseases. In Barron AL, editor: *Microbiology of Chlamydia,* Boca Raton, 1988, CRC Press.
73. Schachter J: Why we need a program for the control of *Chlamydia trachomatis, New Eng J Med* 320:802-803, 1989.
74. Schachter J et al.: Evaluation of laboratory methods for detecting acute TRIC agent infection, *Am J Ophthalmol* 70:375-380, 1970.
75. Schachter J et al.: Prospective study of chlamydial infections in neonates, *Lancet* ii:377-379, 1979.
76. Schachter J et al.: Experience with the use of erythromycin for chlamydial infections in pregnancy, *New Eng J Med* 314:276-279, 1986.
77. Segreti J et al.: In vitro activity of A-5628 (TE-031) and four other antimicrobial agents against *Chlamydia trachomatis, Antimicrob Agents Chemother* 31:100-101, 1987.
78. Stenberg K, Mardh P-A: Treatment of chlamydial conjunctivitis in newborns and adults with erythromycin and roxythromycin, *J Antimicrob Chemother* 28:301-307, 1991.
79. Stenberg K et al.: Culture, ELISA and immunofluorescence tests for the diagnosis of conjunctivitis caused by *Chlamydia trachomatis* in neonates and adults, *APIMS* 98:514-520, 1990.
80. Tam MR et al.: Culture-independent diagnosis of *Chlamydia trachomatis* using monoclonal antibodies, *New Eng J Med* 310:1146-1150, 1984.
81. Taylor HR, Agarwala N, Johnson SL: Detection of experimental *Chlamydia trachomatis* eye infection in conjunctival smears and in tissue culture by use of a fluorescein-conjugated monoclonal antibody, *J Clin Microbiol* 27:968-970, 1984.
82. Taylor HR et al.: The diagnosis and treatment of chlamydial conjunctivitis, *Int Ophthalmol* 12:95-99, 1988.
83. Thirumoorthy T, Rajan VS, Goh CL: Penicillinase-producing *Neisseria gonorrhoeae* ophthalmia neonatorum in Singapore, *Br J Vener Dis* 58:308-310, 1982.
84. Thompson TR, Swanson RE, Wiesner PF: Gonococcal ophthalmia neonatorum: relationship of time of infection to relevant control measures, *JAMA* 228:186-188, 1974.
85. Todd WJ, Caldwell HD: The interaction of *Chlamydia trachomatis* with host cells: ultrastructural studies of the mechanism of release of a biovar II strain from HeLa 229 cells, *J Infect Dis* 151:1037-1044, 1985.
86. Ward ME, Watt PJ: Adherence of Neisseria gonorrhoea to urethral mucosal cells: an electron microscopic study, *J Infect Dis* 126:601, 1972.
87. Welsh LE, Gaydos CA, Quinn TC: In vitro evaluation of azithromycin, erythromycin and tetracycline against *Chlamydia trachomatis* and *Chlamydia pneumoniae, Antimicrob Agents Chemother* 36:291-294, 1992.
88. Wilhemus KR, Robinson NM, Tredici LL: Conjunctival cytology of adult chlamydial conjunctivitis, *Arch Ophthalmol* 104:691-693, 1986.
89. Winceslaus J et al.: Diagnosis of ophthalmia neonatorum, *Br Med J* 295:1377-1379, 1987.
90. World Health Organization: *Conjunctivitis of the newborn: prevention and treatment at the primary health care level,* Geneva, 1986, WHO.
91. Zeichner SL: Isolation and characterization of macrophage phagosomes containing infectious and heat-inactivated *Chlamydia psittaci:* two phagosomes with different intracellular behaviors, *Infect Immun* 40:956-966, 1983.

65 Lice Infestation of the Eyelids

ISAAC ASHKENAZI

Phthiriasis palpebrarum is an odd and uncommon dermato-ophthalmologic condition encountered in children and young adults. Eyelash infestation is caused by the crab louse *Phthirus pubis* and its ova.

EPIDEMIOLOGY

The incidence of pubic louse infestation is as high as approximately 5 per 1000 army recruits[8] and 10 per 1000 individuals attending a sexually transmitted disease clinic.[11] Sexual activity with multiple partners[11] and low socioeconomic status[9] are principal risk factors, and the incidence increases slightly during warmer months.[8] The proportion of individuals with pubic infestation who develop eyelash involvement is not known with certainty, but it appears low. Eyelash infestation alone may also occur.

CLINICAL FEATURES

Clinical characteristics of phthiriasis palpebrarum include itching and irritation of the eyelid margins. These features of blepharoconjunctivitis are not invariable, for lice are initially found on noninflamed palpebral margins during early infection. Frequent scratching and rubbing lead to inflammation, which may be intense and persistent.

The crab louse has three sets of legs attached to the anterior part of the abdomen (Fig. 65-1). The middle and hind sets are wider, with a stout claw and an opposing tibial thumb on each leg. Four sets of small conical feet are present on the posterior part of the abdomen. Two segmented antennae protrude from the lateral aspect of the cylindrical head. Deeply pigmented digestive material can be seen dispersed throughout the broad oval abdomen, extending to the posterior aspect of the louse.

The adult louse grips the roots of the lashes or brows with its claws (Fig. 65-2). Nits and empty nit shells, adherent to the base of the cilia, may be deposited in great numbers (Fig. 65-3). Adult lice may be transparent and difficult to see, but the telltale nits on the lashes are readily visible.

PATHOGENESIS

Pediculosis and phthiriasis occur in humans from close physical contact and inadequate sanitary conditions. *Phthirus pubis* is typically found in the hair of pubic and inguinal regions, whereas *Pediculus capitis* occurs in scalp hair and *Pediculus corporis* clings to body hair and the seams of clothing. Despite the remoteness of the eyelashes, the pubic louse is the most common cause of eyelash "pediculosis." The head louse, frequently seen in children, is usually restricted to the scalp, and involvement of the eyelids is extremely rare.[14]

The pubic louse dies quickly when separated from its host, its transmission from person to person usually being by sexual contact. The pubic area is the most frequently affected. An infected person may transfer the organism from one hairy area to another, resulting in infestation of axillary hair, beard, eyebrows, and eyelashes. Phthiriasis palpebrarum can occur in infants who are usually infested by direct passage of the lice from the axillary or chest hair of the parents, nurse, or attendant.[16]

DIFFERENTIAL DIAGNOSIS

Pediculus corporis and *Pediculus capitis* can be easily distinguished from *Phthirus pubis* by their larger size (2 to 4 mm), their flattened, elongated, triple-segmented, fused thoraces, and their long slender legs. In contrast, *Phthirus pubis* is usually 2 mm or less, has a broad oval abdomen, and possesses stout legs resembling a crab's claws. Crab lice are better suited for grasping the shafts of hairs and remaining more localized.[7]

THERAPY

The effective management of phthiriasis palpebrarum requires thorough investigation and treatment of contacts. Treatment consists of delousing the patient, other family members, clothing, and bedding. Reinfestation can be prevented by sterilizing clothing, linen, brushes, and combs at a temperature of 50°C for 30 minutes. Contaminated cosmet-

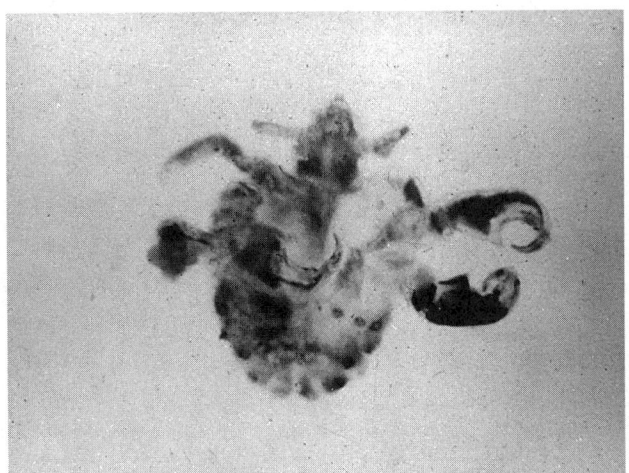

Fig. 65-1. Adult crab louse removed from lower eyelid. (Unstained, ×72.)

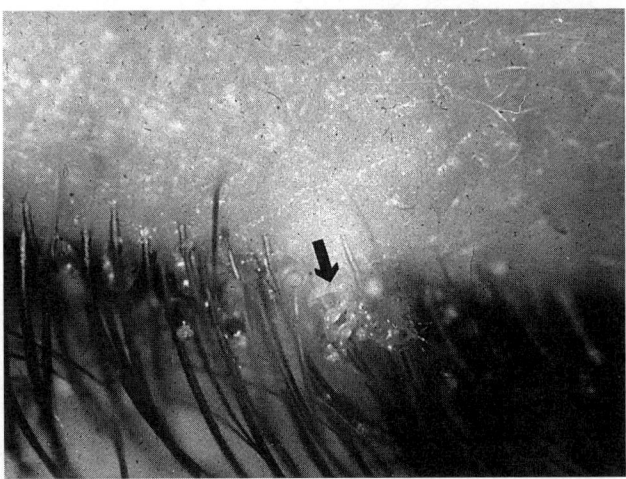

Fig. 65-3. Numerous *Phthirus pubis* eggs (nits) adherent to eyelashes of the upper eyelid and a transparent pubic louse *(arrow)* attached to the lashes.

ics should be destroyed. The epidemic spread of *Phthirus pubis* can be prevented by proper hygiene.

The most popular ocular treatment is the removal of the parasites with forceps.[14,16] "The infant's head is held as firmly as possible with the help of assistants. In spite of batting eyelids, screams, and tears, the struggle will be a brief one and end to everybody's satisfaction."[16] In cooperative patients it is possible to remove the adult parasites with forceps at the slit-lamp biomicroscope. This procedure is not without discomfort for both the doctor and patient, however, and the use of anesthesia or sedation may be necessary.[10]

A single application of gamma benzene hexachloride with careful nit removal is usually adequate to eradicate the lice. Disadvantages include the high potential for ocular irritation and epithelial toxicity.[5,15] In view of reports of possible toxicity to the central nervous system, this agent should

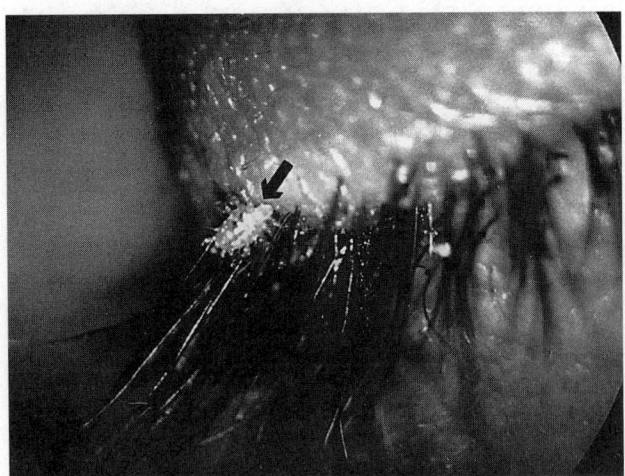

Fig. 65-2. Phthiriasis palpebrarum. One adult crab louse *(arrow),* with its stout claws gripping onto the roots of two eyelashes.

be used with caution in infants, children, and pregnant women.

Good results may be obtained by anticholinesterase agents, when applied in standard concentrations used in the treatment of glaucoma.[6] The additional unwanted ocular symptoms of physostigmine may be prohibitive, and it does not affect the nits themselves. Anticholinesterase insecticides may be useful. Malathion 1% aqueous shampoo can be applied to the eyelashes, then rinsed off after a few minutes to eradicate lice infestation.[18]

Cryotherapy has been used in the management of phthiriasis palpebrarum.[3] It is advantageous in that it provides a fast cure and alleviates the need for repeated visits to the doctor. This treatment may be very uncomfortable and potentially dangerous for the young uncooperative patient, and it is not generally accepted as a primary mode of treatment.

Argon laser phototherapy has the advantage of being a quick and effective method of treatment that can be performed in one sitting.[4] Its disadvantages include occasional, but tolerable, stinging and slicing of eyelash stems carrying the nits. Cut eyelashes regain their normal length within a few days. This method cannot be used to treat young children because of poor patient cooperation.

Yellow mercuric oxide ointment is an effective, safe, and "patient-friendly" form of treatment. A regimen of 1% yellow oxide of mercury ointment 4 times daily is used for 14 days.[2] Complete resolution of signs and symptoms rapidly occurs. Known side effects of 1% yellow oxide of mercury ointment include irritation to the eyelid, conjunctiva, and cornea, and possible lens discoloration.[1] The patient may complain of photophobia, blurred visual sensation, mucous discharge, itching, burning, tearing, or gritty feeling. These side effects are uncommon,[12] and this agent is a cheap, simple, safe, and effective form of treatment for phthiriasis palpebrarum, especially for children. Petrolatum is not specifically pediculocidal but has also been used to smother lice on the eyelashes.

PROGNOSIS

Topical treatment to the eyelids and lashes is curative, and no permanent lid margin changes occur. Antiparasitic therapy for concurrent pubic louse infestation should be provided.[17] Screening for other sexually transmitted diseases is indicated.[13]

REFERENCES

1. Abramomicz I: Deposition of mercury in the eye, *Br J Ophthalmol* 30:696-697, 1946.
2. Ashkenazi I, Desatnik HR, Abraham FA: Yellow mercuric oxide: a treatment of choice for phthiriasis palpebrarum, *Br J Ophthalmol* 75:356-358, 1991.
3. Awan KJ: Cryotherapy in phthiriasis palpebrarum, *Am J Ophthalmol* 83:906-907, 1977.
4. Awan KJ: Argon laser phototherapy of phthiriasis palpebrarum, *Ophthalmic Surg* 17:813-814, 1986.
5. Ben-Ezra D, Paez JH, Almeida C et al.: Keratoconjunctivitis following pediculocides, *Harefuah* 104:96-98, 1983.
6. Cogan DG, Grant WM: Treatment of pediculosis ciliaris with anticholinesterase agents, *Arch Ophthalmol* 41:627-628, 1949.
7. Couch JM, Green WR, Hirst LW, de la Cruz SC: Diagnosing and treating *Phthirus pubis* palpebrarum, *Surv Ophthalmol* 26:219-225, 1982.
8. Gillis D, Slepon R, Karsenty E, Green M: Seasonality and long-term trends of pediculosis capitis and pubis in a young adult population, *Arch Dermatol* 126:638-641, 1990.
9. Gillis D, Slepon R, Karsenty E, Green MS: Sociodemographic factors associated with pediculosis capitis and pubis among young adults in the Israel Defense Forces, *Public Health Rev* 18:345-350, 1991.
10. Goldman L: *Phthirus pubis* infestation of the scalp and cilia in young children, *Arch Dermatol* 57:274-276, 1954.
11. Hart G: Factors associated with pediculosis pubis and scabies, *Genitourin Med* 68:294-295, 1992.
12. Kastl PR, Zulfigar A, Mather F: Placebo-controlled double-blind evaluation of the efficacy and safety of yellow mercuric oxide in suppression of eyelid infections, *Ann Ophthalmol* 19:376-379, 1987.
13. Opaneye AA, Jayaweera DT, Walzman M, Wade AA: Pediculosis pubis: a surrogate marker for sexually transmitted diseases, *J R Soc Health* 113:6-7, 1993.
14. Perlman HH, Fraga S, Medina M: Phthiriasis palpebrarum, *J Pediatr* 49:88-90, 1956.
15. Reinecke RD, Kinder RSL: Corneal toxicity of the pediculocide A-200 pyrinate, *Arch Ophthalmol* 68:36-38, 1962.
16. Ronchese F: Treatment of pediculosis ciliarum in an infant, *New Eng J Med* 249:897-898, 1953.
17. Rufli T: Domestic ectoparasitoses: a review, *Schweiz Med Wochenschr* 123:1268-1273, 1993.
18. Rundle PA, Hughes DS: *Phthirus pubis* infestation of the eyelids, *Br J Ophthalmol* 77:815-816, 1993.

66 Molluscum Contagiosum, Orf, and Vaccinia

JAY S. PEPOSE, JOSEPH J. ESPOSITO

Of the nine poxviruses that cause disease in humans,[100] four are associated with ocular or eyelid infections: variola virus, vaccinia virus, orf virus, and molluscum contagiosum virus, the latter being the most common poxvirus to cause ocular infection (Table 66-1). Variola virus was the cause of smallpox, previously a disease of epidemic proportions with major ocular sequelae including ulcerative keratitis, and (rarely) blindness. Ocular sequelae afflicted as many as 1% of survivors, generally malnourished individuals of underdeveloped countries.[29] Smallpox was eradicated from the world by 1977 after widespread vaccination and epidemiologic intervention. Excellent reviews are available[29,82,100] on this now extinct disease entity. Several reviews of poxvirus features are also available,[28,72] and methods of clinical laboratory diagnosis for various human poxvirus infections have been summarized.[27] This chapter focuses on molluscum contagiosum, orf, and vaccinia virus infections of the eye.

VIROLOGY

Poxviruses are large, morphologically complex virions that contain a virtually complete transcription system in the particle. This system includes a DNA-dependent RNA polymerase for production of primary transcripts, a transcript poly-A polymerase, a capping enzyme, and methylating enzymes for converting transcripts into messenger RNAs (mRNAs). Virions contain a covalently closed, linear, double-stranded genome DNA molecule ranging in size from 130 to 300 kilobase pairs. Members of different genera have different guanosine and cytosine content, ranging from approximately 25% to 65%. All members share a similar DNA molecule architecture. Generally, the DNA contains hairpinlike ends adjacent to one or more arrays of variable-size clusters of tandem repeat elements; transcripts of unresolved function arise from the hairpin-end sequences. The hairpin-ends and the tandem repeat clusters compose an inverted terminal repeat region (ITR) that may also contain DNA coding for proteins, thereby enabling certain genes to be diploid. The ITRs flank the central coding region of DNA,

which contains about 200 closely spaced open reading frames, each preceded by a transcriptional promoter element.

Poxviruses grow in the cell cytoplasm with virtually no nuclear involvement. The poxvirus life cycle can be summarized as follows. Virions attach to the cell membrane and become uncoated in a two-stage process upon entering the cytoplasm. Poxvirus infection rapidly shuts down virtually all host cell protein synthesis. During penetration of the cell membrane and entry into the cytoplasm, transcription occurs in the virus core. Discrete cytoplasmic inclusions termed *virus factories* or basophilic (B type) inclusions begin to develop early in infection. Functional, capped, and polyadenylated mRNAs are made and translated on cell ribosomes during a temporally regulated system of gene expression that proceeds through distinctive early, intermediate, and late stages. Translation of the mRNAs results in the production of approximately 200 proteins including (1) enzymes such as viral DNA polymerase for DNA replication, (2) proteins for virion structure, and (3) proteins that define host-range and mediate virus survival against particular host defense mechanisms.

During virus particle assembly, a core membrane and virion outer membrane enclose the genome, which is contained in a nucleosome. Most of the infectious particles remain cell-associated and are released upon cell lysis; however, a small proportion, ranging to about 10% (depending on host cell type and virus strain), is released by exocytosis through the Golgi apparatus. Such particles, termed *extracellular enveloped virions* (EEVs), obtain an antigenically distinctive envelope containing a variety of viral glycoproteins.

Growth of the virus in tissue culture produces a characteristic cell-rounding cytopathic effect.[28] Vertebrate poxviruses in vivo induce hyperplastic responses in the skin, and it is reasonable to assume that this effect results from activity of viral isologs of growth factors. For example, vaccinia virus and various other poxvirus-infected cells produce an isolog of epidermal and transforming growth factors. Orf virus contains a gene that encodes an isolog of vascular en-

TABLE 66-1 MEMBERS OF THE POXVIRIDAE FAMILY ASSOCIATED WITH OCULAR DISEASES

Genus	Type Species	Disease	Host Range
Orthopoxvirus	Vaccinia	Smallpox vaccination complications	Broad experimental host range; no natural reservoir except buffalopox subspecies
	Variola	Smallpox (eradicated)	Human beings
Parapoxvirus	Orf	Contagious pustular dermatitis	Humans and certain ungulates (sheep, goats, musk oxen, deer)
Molluscipoxvirus	Molluscum contagiosum	Molluscum contagiosum	Human beings

dothelial growth factor,[63] and variola and vaccinia virus DNAs have vestiges of this gene.[67]

MOLLUSCUM CONTAGIOSUM

Historical Background

In 1817 Thomas Bateman[4] described the clinical aspects of molluscum contagiosum disease and used the word *molluscum* to signify a pedunculated lesion and *contagiosum* to stress its transmissibility, which he postulated was caused by "milky fluid" expressed from the lesion. In 1841 William Henderson[43] and Robert Patterson[80] independently described hyaline-like eosinophilic intracellular inclusions within the milky exudate, and these inclusions became known as "molluscum bodies" or Henderson-Patterson bodies (Fig. 66-1). Patterson believed that the milky substance with globular bodies was a parasitic infection that caused what was referred to as the "entirely British disease" of molluscum contagiosum. In 1907 Lipschütz[62] described spherical elementary bodies (Lipschütz granules) within the Henderson-Patterson bodies, which are now known to be poxvirus particles; they are large enough to be just visible with a light microscope. In 1905 Juliusberg and later Wile and Kingery[110] established the viral causation of molluscum contagiosum by transmitting the disease with a filtrate of lesion material,[21] although other attempts at such transmission were unsuccessful.[33] In the 1930s the coincidence of cellular inclusion bodies and virus particle "elementary bodies" in molluscum contagiosum, vaccinia, and fowlpox infections was recognized by Goodpasture,[36] who concluded that the three diseases were caused by members of the same virus family.

Epidemiology

In children, molluscum contagiosum infection is spread by direct contact with lesions or through contact with fomites or contaminated water, as in public baths and swimming pools.[6] Lesions develop predominantly on the face, extremities, and trunk. A linear pattern of lesions is common in young patients, indicating that autoinoculation occurs by scratching. In adults, the disease appears to be increasing in frequency, with peak occurrence in patients 20 to 29 years of

age.[27] The disease generally is spread sexually, and therefore lesions in adults are most commonly located in the lower abdomen, pubis, genitalia, and inner thigh. Infection sometimes involves the eye or adnexa, however, because of autoinoculation by digitogenital contact transmission. There also have been reports of nonsexual transmission of molluscum contagiosum in teenagers and adults including wrestlers,[66] cross-country runners,[70] and patients of a surgeon who had a hand lesion.[79] The incubation period

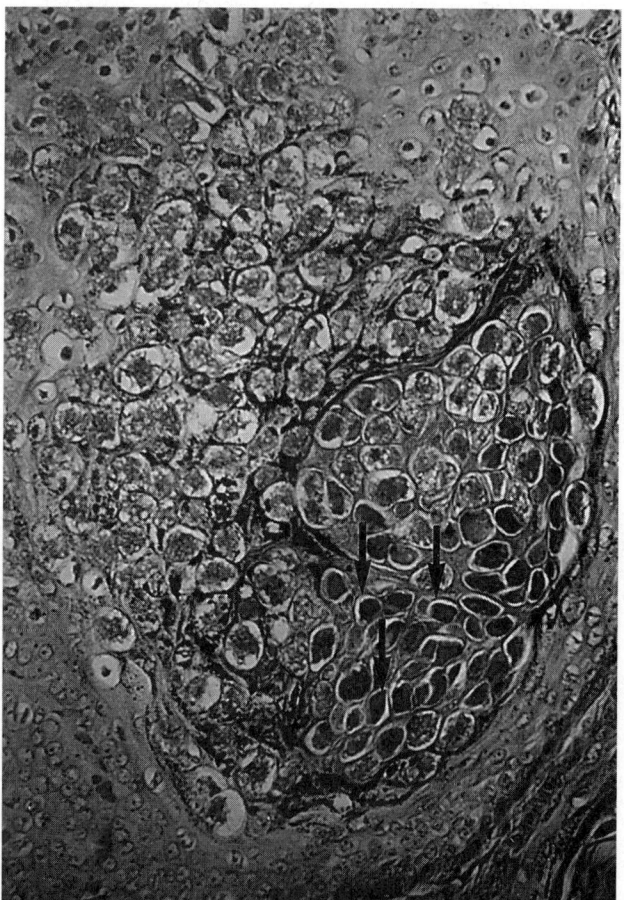

Fig. 66-1. Histologic section of a molluscum contagiosum lesion with numerous hyaline-like intracellular inclusions *(arrows)* known as molluscum bodies. (Hematoxylin and eosin, × 250.)

of molluscum contagiosum ranges from 1 week to 2 to 3 months.

Molluscum contagiosum lesions may be more common and more severe in immunocompromised patients, including those with acquired immunodeficiency syndrome (AIDS) and AIDS-related complex (ARC). The presentation of multiple, disseminated lesions has led to the diagnosis of human immunodeficiency virus (HIV) infection in selected cases (Fig. 66-2).[65] Different studies have reported a prevalence of molluscum contagiosum ranging from 9.4% to 18% in patients with AIDS or ARC, compared with 1% in a matched HIV-seronegative group.[19,20,35,68]

Clinical Features

Molluscum contagiosum (Fig. 66-3) presents as round, pearly white or flesh-colored lesions that are smooth and centrally umbilicated papules on an erythematous base. Lesions contain a central viscous core of virus-infected cells. Generally, more than one lesion is present and ocular involvement is unilateral or (less commonly) bilateral. Skin lesions in immunocompetent patients are generally 2 mm to 4 mm in diameter; however, reports have described unusually large molluscum contagiosum lesions on the eyelids of some infected persons.[25,88,104] Lesions are more likely to be larger in immunocompromised patients. The lesions are generally painless, inconspicuous, not inflamed, and sometimes obfuscated by cilia. Baterial superinfection of lesions is common. Rare primary conjunctival or caruncular[16,105] lesions may exist that appear as pinkish or yellow nodules with a central umbilication; they are usually not associated with follicular conjunctivitis. Such lesions often can be excised with no adverse sequelae.[15] Follicular conjunctivitis and an erosive superficial keratitis appear to be toxic reactions to molluscum contagiosum involving the eyelid margins. Focal eczema may also appear on the eyelid, and each of the aforementioned manifestations can produce photophobia, foreign body sensation, epiphora, and/or burning.

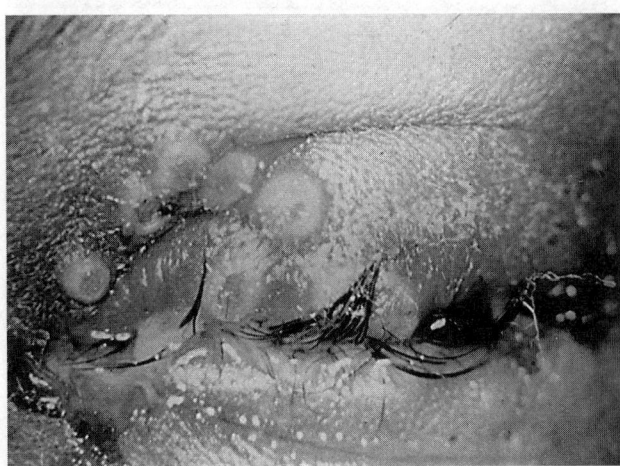

Fig. 66-2. Multiple molluscum contagiosum lesions involving the upper eyelid in an AIDS patient.

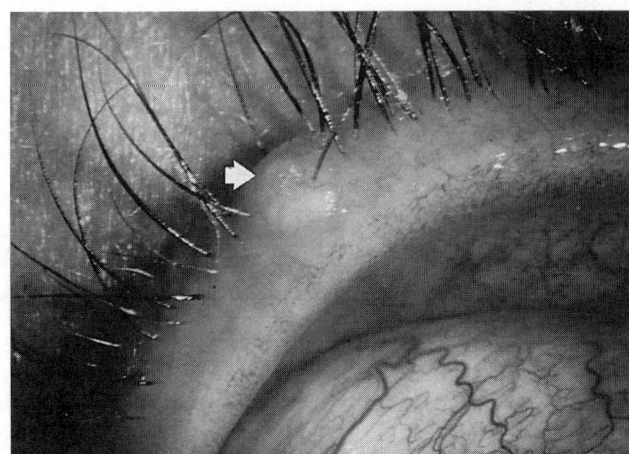

Fig. 66-3. Molluscum contagiosum lesion (nodule) appears as a round, centrally umbilicated papule on an erythematous base. The lesion contains a central viscous infiltrate material *(arrow)* comprised of virus-infected cells.

Periocular skin infection can also result in secondary chronic follicular conjunctivitis, superficial keratitis, or punctal occlusion. Corneal involvement can range from a fine-grouped epithelial keratitis with superior superficial pannus formation (mimicking trachoma), to pseudodendrites with intraepithelial and subepithelial infiltrates, to keratinization and/or ulceration.

Pathogenesis

Virologic Aspects. Molluscum contagiosum virus (MCV) appears to be strictly a human poxvirus. MCV produces benign lesions of the skin, ocular surface, and adnexa that are characterized by epithelial hypertrophy and hyperplasia. There is no experimental animal model for the disease, and the virus has not yet been grown in tissue culture (although infected cell cultures sometimes show cytopathic or cytotoxic effects,[20] and the production of interferon and abortive infection have been described).[69]

Ultrastructural studies have demonstrated a brick-shaped virus particle, $300 \times 220 \times 100$ nm in size, containing a biconcave core enclosed by a core membrane, around which is an outer membrane (Fig. 66-4). The MCV genome DNA contains about 178 kilobase pairs, including ITRs.[18] Molecular studies of MCV isolates have shown three primary DNA restriction map types, which have been classified as MCV-I, MCV-II, and MCV-III; a candidate MCV-IV DNA type has been described in Japan.[106] Within the DNA genome groups, there may be additional variants based on minor differences in DNA restriction cleavage patterns.[93] No correlations exist between the restriction map type and the anatomic location of lesions, the age or gender of the patient, the distribution of lesions, the clinical features, or the strains more likely to afflict HIV-infected individuals. In a small number of HIV-infected and non-HIV-infected molluscum contagiosum patients, coinfection of a single lesion

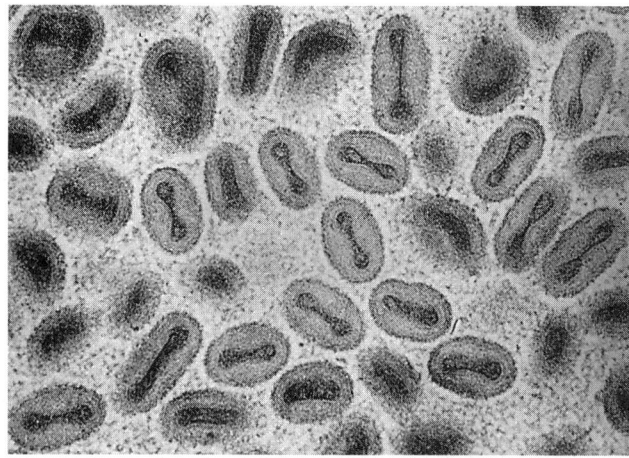

Fig. 66-4. Brick-shaped poxvirus with biconcave and outer membrane core apparent. (Uranyl acetate and lead citrate stain, ×86,000.)

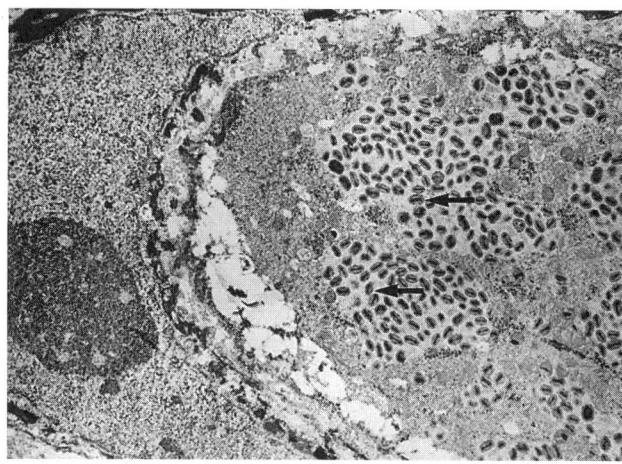

Fig. 66-5. Numerous dark-stained molluscum contagiosum virus particles *(arrows)* restricted to the cytoplasm of the cell. (Uranyl acetate and lead citrate stain, ×33,000.)

with multiple types of MCV has been documented,[102] suggesting generation of DNA polymorphisms during infection. There seems to be a large variation in the geographic distribution of different MCV DNA types.[94,102,106]

Replication of MCV appears to be limited to epidermal layers. Focal areas of hyperplastic epidermis surround cyst-like lobules filled with degenerating molluscum bodies and keratinized debris. Mitotic figures are localized to basal keratinocytes. In the spindle layer, cells show vacuolization in the cytoplasm and eosinophilic molluscum bodies, the latter displacing the cell nuclei to the periphery. As cells progress into the granular layer, the molluscum bodies become more homogeneous with further degeneration of the surrounding cellular components. The molluscum bodies are then desquamated into the cystic lobules. Virus cores can be seen by electron microscopy in all layers of epidermis. The second stage of uncoating and release of virus DNA into the cytoplasm does not occur until cells progress upward into the spindle and granular cell layers. Replication of virus DNA and establishment of electron-dense virus factories in the cytoplasm of these cells (Fig. 66-5) lead to development of the molluscum bodies with numerous maturing virions in these layers.[89]

As mentioned previously, recent studies of poxvirus-encoded cellular growth factor cognates have revealed a vaccinia virus 19 kilodalton polypeptide isologous to epidermal growth factor and alpha-transforming growth factor. On the basis of DNA sequencing, MCV also appears to encode a protein related to the conserved domain of epidermal growth factor (EGF).[86] Epidermal growth factor receptor has been demonstrated in basal keratinocytes of molluscum lesions[75,81]; however, there are conflicting reports about the presence of EGF and transferrin growth factor receptors on virus-inclusion-bearing cells within the lesions.[107]

Immunologic Aspects. Molluscum contagiosum lesions are often atypically large, severe, multiple, and persistent in im-

munocompromised individuals such as the following: HIV-infected patients; patients with selective IgM deficiency, thymoma, acute lymphocytic or myelogenous leukemia, non-Hodgkin lymphoma, sarcoidosis, systemic lupus erythematosus, mycosis fungoides, atopy, or congenital immunodeficiency syndromes; patients who have had splenectomy; and patients receiving chemotherapy and/or corticosteroids.[41,44,61,91] The incidence and severity of infection in immunocompromised individuals likely relates to poorly understood roles of humoral and cellular immune responses in controlling and preventing the spread of lesions. Interestingly, adults with HIV infection often develop molluscum contagiosum lesions in a distribution similar to that seen in infected children, such as on the face, neck, scalp, upper trunk, and legs.

Individual lesions in HIV-infected patients range from 1 cm to 2 cm in diameter, appearing as nodules. Patients with AIDS sometimes have hundreds of molluscum contagiosum lesions,[90] and it has been reported that an inverse relationship exists between the CD4+ T-lymphocyte cell count and the number of lesions.[95] It seems reasonable to assume that a decrease in cutaneous Langerhans cells and T-helper lymphocytes may affect the outcome of the disease in patients with AIDS, because Langerhans cells are bone marrow-derived, HLA-DR-positive dendritic cells capable of antigen presentation to T-lymphocytes. A study of molluscum contagiosum in five apparently healthy persons showed an absence of Langerhans cells within molluscum contagiosum lesions, with a normal or increased number in the perilesional skin.[7] Studies of 10 immunocompetent children showed no T-lymphocytes, beta-2-macroglobulin, or Langerhans cells associated with molluscum contagiosum lesions, however.[84]

Spontaneous regression of individual molluscum contagiosum lesions apparently can occur with or without a surrounding inflammatory infiltrate. Molluscum contagiosum dermatitis, a localized eczematous reaction that is sometimes observed around molluscum contagiosum lesions in seemingly immunocompetent persons,[42,54] has not been reported in patients with AIDS. Spontaneous regression of lesions in these and other immunocompromised patients generally does not occur. If present, inflammation surrounding molluscum contagiosum lesions is generally composed of neutrophils, lymphocytes, and macrophages; sometimes, atypical lymphoblasts are seen adjacent to molluscum bodies and zones of epithelial hyperplasia or erosion. Cell necrosis is often seen in the peripheral epithelium. Regression of the lesions (with or without inflammation) is associated with proliferation of endothelial cells and fibroblasts in the adventitial dermis and with a new steady state between epidermal hyperplasia and cell loss.[84] Clinically, inflammatory dermatitis is commonly seen with disruption of these lesions[42,54]; however, it is unclear whether the infiltrate is the primary effector or a secondary response in the regression of molluscum contagiosum. Low levels of antibodies to MCV have been noted in patients, regardless of disease duration, suggesting that a poor humoral immune response occurs during infection. Virus-specific antibodies have been reported as undetectable in up to 30% of infected patients,[98] however.

Differential Diagnosis

The differential diagnosis of molluscum contagiosum includes infection by varicella zoster virus, herpes simplex virus, or papilloma virus, keratoacanthoma, infected follicular keratosis, epithelioma, pyoderma, syringoma, basal cell carcinoma, and cutaneous cryptococcosis. Giant molluscum contagiosum lesions must be differentiated from epidermal inclusion cysts, chalazia, and furuncles.

Laboratory Investigations

Biopsy specimens of molluscum contagiosum lesions show eosinophilic hyaline cytoplasmic inclusions (molluscum bodies) eccentrically displacing the nuclei. Thinly spread smears of expressed material from the core of the lesion show numerous infected, inclusion-bearing cells after staining with Papanicolaou, Wright, Giemsa, or Gram stains. A squash preparation stained with a supravital dye enables visualization of the molluscum contagiosum virions, which are in the range of 0.3 μm and just visible by light microscopy.[97] MCV infection can also be demonstrated by immunocytochemical methods[81] and in situ or dot-blot hybridization.[45,101]

Therapy

Several therapies for molluscum contagiosum lesions have been reported including incision and/or curettage,[34] surgical excision, cryotherapy alone or with curettage, electrodessication, and caustic chemical applications, such as 0.9% cantharidin.[38] Not all of these treatments may be suitable for eyelid or periorbital MCV infections. For example, cryotherapy may lead to madarosis or depigmentation of dark skin, and caustic chemicals applied to the eyelids may cause corneal scarring and scarring of the eyelid. The goal of incision and curettage is removal of the fibrous capsule containing the central core of malpighian cells, which is the site of virus replication. This treatment often does not result in scar formation. In the immunocompetent individual lesions may eventually regress spontaneously, but new lesions may crop up, with an average overall duration of approximately 2 years if left untreated.[40,87] Bacterial superinfection could require local or systemic antibiotic therapy. Lesions in patients with AIDS can become confluent and involve an entire eyelid border; such lesions are often recalcitrant to many forms of therapy, including excision.[90]

HUMAN ORF

Historical Background

Although the parapoxviruses that cause milker's nodule (pseudocowpox, paravaccinia) and bovine pustular stomatitis can infect humans as occupational diseases, they are less common than infections with the parapoxvirus orf virus. Orf is a word derived from the ancient Anglo-Saxon name for cattle. The disease orf (contagious pustular dermatitis, ecthyma contagiosum, contagious ecthyma, scabby mouth) is an endemic poxvirus disease of sheep and goats. It can be transmitted to humans by direct contact with infected animals.[8,14,64] The vesiculopapular eruption of orf was first reported in sheep by Steeb[58] in 1787, and in goats in 1879 by the Norwegian veterinarian Hansen.[39] In 1923 the cause of orf was proved to be a filterable agent,[2] which was later immunologically distinguished from vaccinia and variola viruses.[10] The first defined human orf infection was reported in the United States in 1934; the disease was reproduced in sheep by inoculation of material from the human lesion.[77]

Epidemiology

The vesiculopapular eruption in its natural hosts, lambs and young goats, primarily affects the limbs, gums, lips, nose, and groin. Humans can contract orf by direct contact either with an infected animal or with contaminated objects. The average incubation time for orf infection is 3 to 6 days. Orf virus is relatively resistant to heat and drying, a feature that may account for its rather prolonged existence in the environment. Human-to-human transmission of orf virus is poor and therefore is not well documented. Most cases involve veterinarians, sheep ranchers, farmers, and occasionally laboratory workers.[71] Immunity is partial in humans and animals, and reinfection can occur.[5,8]

Clinical Features

Orf virus produces 1-cm to 3-cm epidermal skin lesions that go through well-defined stages. Before regression and clearing, lesions progress from the maculopapular stage, to the bullseyelike stage (red center, white ring, red halo), to a stage of vascularized ulcerated nodular lesions with central umbilication, to a crusted eschar with regenerating epidermis. Some lesions advance to a discrete papillomatous stage. Eruptions usually involve the hand, one or more digits, or the forearm; and infections of the face and (rarely) the eye have been reported. Regional lymphadenopathy is common, but most patients do not develop fever or constitutional symptoms.

Ocular Findings. Ocular involvement generally appears to be quite rare in orf infections; however, involvement of the eye in conjunction with skin lesions may occur, often with preauricular and/or submandibular lymphadenopathy. Canthal lesions that may become ulcerated and nodular with crusting have been reported.[31] Swelling with follicular and papillary conjunctivitis may be present. Conjunctival vesicles and papulovesicles have been described.[111] A case of blindness, caused by bacterial superinfection of an orf lesion, has been reported.[92]

Laboratory Investigations

The diagnosis of orf infection is primarily a clinical one, based on the characteristic lesion, the marked lymphadenopathy, and the history of contact with an infected animal. The skin lesion can be differentiated clinically from cutaneous anthrax, keratoacanthoma, pyogenic granuloma, and from large lesions of molluscum contagiosum. The diagnosis can be confirmed by electron microscopic examination of scrapings of lesions, by biopsy, by complement-fixation serology,[109] or by virus isolation in tissue culture followed by more-specific identification tests such as DNA assay or immunofluorescence assays with orf virus antiserum.[10] By electron microscopy, the virus can be observed in various stages in the epithelial cell cytoplasm, with the mature, 325 nm × 135 nm, cylindrical, ovoid-shaped particles containing electron dense centers. Biopsies show intracytoplasmic eosinophilic inclusions in vacuolated epidermal cells; infiltrates of histiocytes, macrophages, lymphocytes, and plasma cells may also develop.

In addition to transmission by inoculation of nonimmune sheep or goats, there have been inconsistent reports of experimental transmission of some strains of orf virus to rabbits, guinea pigs, and embryonated chicken eggs.[74] Orf virus has been propagated in primary human amniotic cells[85]; however, selected laboratory strains and clinical samples are usually isolated and cultured in primary cells derived from sheep, goats, or oxen.[83] Primary embryonic ovine kidney cell cultures are often used. Once isolated, the virus generally will pass into human embryonic fibroblasts (HELF cells), monkey kidney cell lines (LLC-MK2 cells), and certain other cell lines.[30]

OCULAR VACCINIA

Historical Background

In 1798 Edward Jenner[49] proved by immunization and challenge of a young boy that the folk practice of inoculation with cowpox material[49] provided resistance to challenge with the orthopoxvirus variola virus—the cause of smallpox. This method of disease prevention supplanted a practice known as *variolation*, which involved either the inoculation of smallpox vesicle fluid (or scab material) into the skin or the nasal insufflation of dried smallpox scab material. The disease induced by variolation was relatively mild (with a 1% to 2% fatality rate) compared with naturally acquired smallpox infection (which had a fatality rate as high as 40% in some outbreaks). Jenner's method, which he termed *cowpoxing,* rapidly gained widespread favor among physicians. (Given the terminology used in his writings, Jenner is thought to have used authentic cowpox virus.) By the mid-1950s smallpox was eradicated from most industrialized countries by using a liquid vaccine containing vaccinia virus. The origin of vaccinia virus and the history of the transition from the use of authentic cowpox virus to the use of vaccinia virus in vaccine manufacture is unclear. Cowpox and vaccinia are orthopoxviruses that cross-react serologically, but have rather different biologic properties and DNA restriction endonuclease maps.[26]

The concept of eradication of smallpox was first proposed by the Soviet Union and adopted by the World Health Organization (WHO) in the mid-1950s; however, it was not until 1967 that sufficient funding and administrative details enabled the establishment of a WHO Smallpox Eradication Unit that began an intensified program of smallpox eradication. By using a disease control strategy based on active surveillance and containment and by vaccinating all who entered or left an outbreak area (creating a "zone sanitaire" around outbreaks), the WHO was able to achieve global eradication of smallpox by the late 1970s. The last known natural case occurred in a nomadic cook in Somalia in October 1977, although in 1978 a laboratory-associated fatal infection occurred in a scientific photographer in Birmingham University, England, with subsequent transmission to her mother. In 1979 the world was certified "free of smallpox" by a global commission established by the World Health Organization,[112] and in May 1980 eradication worldwide was officially acknowledged by the World Health Assembly.

Epidemiology

During the era of routine smallpox vaccination, ocular vaccinia sometimes occurred by transmission from the vaccination lesion of another individual or by autoinoculation from the vaccinee's own lesion. Spread of virus to the eye was mainly by digital contact after rubbing the vaccination site. The incidence of ocular vaccinia was approximately one per 40,000 primary vaccinations[56]; it was far more common in primary vaccinees than revaccinees.[108] Nonocular complications of vaccination included progressive vaccinia, usually occurring in patients with depressed cellular immunity; eczema vaccinatum, usually occurring in eczematous children by vaccination or contact with vaccinees; and postvaccinal encephalitis, which was fatal in as many as 30% of cases.

Immunization with vaccinia is still practiced in special circumstances. The Advisory Committee on Immunization Practices (ACIP) of the United States recommends that only laboratory and health-care workers at high risk of contracting human orthopoxviruses (vaccinia, cowpox, buffalopox, monkeypox, recombinant vaccinia viruses) be vaccinated (within 10 years of potential exposure). Vaccinia infection should therefore be considered in the differential diagnosis of infectious keratouveitis, conjunctivitis, and eyelid lesions in selected cases. Considering the potential for serious complications of vaccinia infection, routine vaccination of civilians and military personnel is highly limited and no longer recommended by the WHO. Smallpox vaccination is not licensed for the treatment of other diseases, such as herpesvirus infections, and it is contraindicated in immunocompromised individuals.

Vaccinia virus is an orthopoxvirus containing a ca. 190 kilobase pair DNA genome with covalently closed ends and tandem repeats within large ITRs that contain coding and noncoding sequences.[3,72] It is a laboratory and vaccine virus that has no known natural reservoir; however, buffalopox virus is now recognized, after DNA analysis, as a subspecies of vaccinia virus.[28,29] Buffalopox virus infections of dairy cattle and milking water buffalo are often transmitted to humans either by direct contact or by drinking virus-infected milk. Infections commonly occur in the springtime after calving, mainly in India. Outbreaks have also been reported in Egypt, Afganistan, Pakistan, and Indonesia.[28,29] The epidemiology, clinical picture, and natural history of human buffalopox virus infection is largely unstudied; however, it seems reasonable to assume that the virus is a residue from the mass smallpox vaccination era and that the disease in humans is similar to vaccinia infection. Similarly, cowpox virus is endemic in Europe; it is transmitted mainly to cattle, and on occasion to humans. A reservoir cycle for transmission has been implicated that involves rodents and cats that prey on rodents. Human cowpox virus infection is similar to vaccinia infection, although it may sometimes produce a comparatively more severe lesion.

Clinical Features

Clinical manifestations of ocular vaccinia (as well as buffalopox and cowpox infections) vary depending on the specific immune status of the host. In previously vaccinated individuals, accidental vaccinia inoculation into the eye following contact with a recent vaccinee often resulted in mucopurulent blepharoconjunctivitis.[96] Severe ocular manifestations could occur upon primary vaccination or accidental primary inoculation. Vaccinia infection of the eyelid, conjunctiva, or ocular surface leads to formation of vesicles, and then white pustules that umbilicate and indurate. Single or multiple lesions produce eyelid swelling and periorbital erythema with signs resembling orbital cellulitis. Tender preauricular and/or submandibular lymphadenopathy is common.[24,108] The eyelid or conjunctival lesions go through a transformation similar to the successful vaccine "take" on the skin following primary vaccination. Ocular infection can lead to eyelid scarring, madarosis, and symblepharon formation. In the majority of cases ocular vaccinia is confined to the eyelid and conjunctiva. Corneal involvement following autoinoculation is uncommon, with approximately 1.2 cases per million primary vaccinations.[57] Other studies report postvaccinal keratitis in 6% to 37% of vaccinia cases with ocular involvement; keratitis appears more often in primary vaccinees than revaccinees.[57,96,108]

Corneal manifestations of ocular vaccinia range from mild superficial punctate keratitis, to interstitial or stromal keratitis, to disciform endotheliitis with keratic precipitates, to necrosis with perforation in those patients without preexisting immunity. Epithelial lesions stain with rose bengal early in the course of infection. Multiple, fine, focal, epithelial lesions may later coalesce to form a geographic pattern mimicking herpes simplex virus keratitis. Stromal involvement, which initially appears as scattered subepithelial opacities similar to those seen in epidemic keratoconjunctivitis, occurs along with corneal ring formation, ulceration, and/or stromal necrosis. Long-term sequelae are more common in cases with corneal manifestation (18%) than in ocular vaccinia without keratitis (2%).[108]

Pathogenesis

Virus entry into cells results in the uncoating of virions with accompanying activity of a virion RNA polymerase and other enzymes that lead to production of mRNAs. After expression of an early class of genes, virus DNA replication signals a shift to expression of intermediate and late classes of genes.[72,73] Virus assembly and maturation begins at select, granular, electron-dense regions of the cell cytoplasm. The virus acquires one or more lipoprotein membranes upon maturation into intracellular nonenveloped virions (INVs) or EEVs, both of which are infectious.[17,72] Vaccinia virus infection in tissue culture produces profound cytopathic effects with changes in cell membrane permeability and virtually complete shut off of host protein, DNA, and RNA synthesis to enable cellular machinery to produce viral particles.

Infected cells secrete a vaccinia growth factor (VGF) that is synthesized early in infection.[9,11,12,13,99] This glycosylated protein can bind to EGF-receptor, stimulating EGF-receptor autophosphorylation and an anchorage-independent cell growth.[103] It is known that expression of VGF coincides with cell proliferation in experimental systems; thus VGF may be largely responsible for the hyperplastic response seen during vaccinia infection of the skin or eyelid.

Studies, mainly with vaccinia virus, have indicated that poxviruses have evolved several mechanisms to impede the host inflammatory and immune response. For example, vaccinia virus infection of cell culture has been shown resistant to the action of interferon.[78] In addition, a 35-kilodalton major secreted protein of vaccinia virus-infected cells binds to derivatives of the fourth component of complement. The virus may thereby evade the consequences of complement activation by the protein-inhibition of the classic complement cascade.[55] Vaccinia virus has also been shown to encode an inhibitor of the lipoxygenase pathway, which produces chemotactic signals for the inflammatory response. An abundant, secretory glycoprotein has been described that may function in the infected host as a soluble interleukin-1 receptor[1]; it has been suggested that this secretion can block interleukin-1β, a proinflammatory cytokine produced in response to infection and tissue injury. Diminishing the inflammatory response reduces the host's acute phase response to infection, thus enhancing virus proliferation.

Differential Diagnosis

The differential diagnosis of vaccinia lesions of the eyelid or ocular adnexae includes molluscum contagiosum, keratoacanthoma, papilloma, staphylococcal eyelid infection, and infection with herpes simplex or varicella-zoster viruses. Postvaccinal keratitis or keratouveitis (Fig. 66-6) must be differentiated from herpes simplex virus or varicella-zoster keratitis, epidemic keratoconjunctivitis, and Acanthamoebic keratitis. The history of recent vaccination or exposure to a recent vaccinee is very useful supporting information.

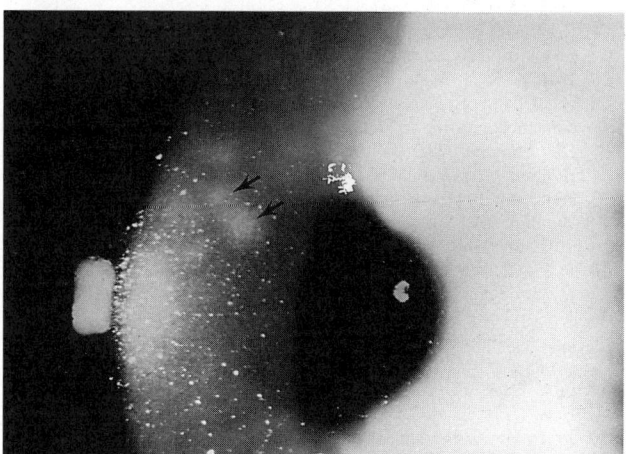

Fig. 66-6. Vaccinia virus keratouveitis from accidental autoinoculation. Grouped subepithelial and anterior stromal opacities are apparent *(arrows)*.

Laboratory Investigations

Histopathologic smears of the mucopurulent discharge observed in ocular vaccinia show numerous polymorphonuclear cells. Eosinophilic cytoplasmic inclusion bodies known as Guarneri bodies are often observed histologically in the scrapings of vaccinia lesions. The virus can be propagated in a wide variety of tissue cultures, including HeLa cells, primary or continuous rabbit or monkey kidney cells, MRC-5 human embryonic lung fibroblasts, and human embryonic kidney cells.[24] Vaccinia virus also grows on the chorioallantoic membrane (CAM) of 12-day-old fertile chicken eggs and in mouse brain,[100] although the latter is not recommended because of potential contamination with ectromelia mousepox virus, an orthopoxvirus.

By electron microscopy of thin sections of infected cells, the virus has a characteristic brick-shaped morphology, measuring 300×200 nm; particles are usually restricted to the cell cytoplasm. The identification of vaccinia virus isolates can be confirmed by restriction endonuclease analysis of infected cell DNA extracts.[26,27]

Therapy

Because ocular vaccinia virus infections are generally self-limited, treatment should be directed toward shortening the course and limiting the severity of disease. Corneal involvement may render a less favorable prognosis, necessitating more aggressive therapy. Treatments that have been used for ocular vaccinia include intramuscular injections of vaccinia immune globulin[23,32] (available through the Centers for Disease Control and Prevention), vidarabine,[46] idoxuridine,[32,48,53,60] cytosine arabinoside,[37] topical monkey or human leukocyte interferon,[51,76] or trifluridine.[47] Acyclovir has not been shown effective against vaccinia by in vitro antiviral screening.[22]

Whereas there are several reports suggesting successful treatment of vaccinia infection of the eyelids, conjunctiva, and cornea by topical and/or intramuscular injections of vaccinia immune globulin, intramuscular treatment has been shown in one study to increase corneal scarring in active experimental vaccinia keratitis.[32] Intramuscular human vaccinia immune globulin may therefore be contraindicated for patients if signs of keratitis have developed. Experimental studies in rabbits have shown that topical trifluridine is more effective than idoxuridine for reducing virus shedding and the clinical severity of postvaccinal keratitis.[47] Following initiation of topical antiviral therapy and the resolution of epithelial disease, judicious use of a tapering course of topical corticosteroids might be useful (1) for the treatment of disciform disease[50] or (2) if anterior chamber inflammation or stromal inflammation is severe. Corticosteroid treatment should be administered while maintaining topical antiviral coverage and mydriatic treatment. In cases with ulcerative keratitis, topical antibiotic therapy to prevent bacterial superinfection may be indicated. For end stage disease with a visually disabling scar or leukoma, lamellar or penetrating keratoplasty has a generally favorable prognosis, assuming that corneal neovascularization is not prominent.

REFERENCES

1. Alcami A, Smith GL: A soluble receptor for interleukin-1β encoded by vaccinia virus: a novel mechanism of virus modulation of the host response to infection, *Cell* 71:153-167, 1992.
2. Aynaud M: La stomatite pustuleuse contagieuse des ovins (Chancre du mouton), *Ann Inst Pasteur* 37:498, 1923.
3. Baroudy BM, Venkatesan S, Moss B: Incompletely base-paired flip-flop terminal loops link the two DNA strands of the vaccinia virus genome into one uninterrupted polynucleotide chain, *Cell* 28:315-324, 1982.
4. Bateman T: *Delineation of cutaneous diseases,* London, 1817, Paternoster-Row.
5. Beck CC, Taylor WB: Orf: It's awful, *Vet Med/Small Anim Clin* 69:1413, 1974.
6. Becker TM, Blount JH, Douglas J, Judson FN: Trends in molluscum contagiosum in the United States, 1966-1983, *Sex Trans Dis* 13:88-92, 1986.
7. Bhawan J, Dayal Y, Bhan AK: Langerhans cells in molluscum contagiosum, verruca vulgaris, plantar wart, and condyloma acuminatum, *J Am Acad Dermatol* 15:645-649, 1986.
8. Blakemore F, Abdussalam M, Goldsmith WN: A case of orf (contagious pustular dermatitis): identification of the virus, *Br J Dermatol Syphilis* 60:404, 1948.
9. Blomquist MC, Hunt LT, Barker WC: Vaccinia virus 19-kilodalton protein: relationship to several mammalian proteins including two growth factors, *Proc Natl Acad Sci USA* 81:7363-7367, 1984.
10. Broughton IB, Hardy WT: Contagious ecthyma (sore mouth) of sheep and goats, *J Am Vet Med Assoc* 85:150, 1934.
11. Brown JP, Twardzik DR, Marquardt H, Todaro GJ: Vaccinia virus encodes a polypeptide homologous to epidermal growth factor and transforming growth factor, *Nature* 313:491-492, 1985.
12. Buller RM, Chakrabarti S, Cooper JA et al.: Deletion of the vaccinia virus growth factor gene reduces virus virulence, *J Virol* 62:866-874, 1988.
13. Buller RM, Chakrabarti S, Moss B, Frederickson T: Cell proliferative response to vaccinia virus vs mediated by VGF, *Virology* 164:182-192, 1988.
14. Carne HR et al.: Infection of man by the virus of contagious pustular dermatitis of sheep, *Aust J Sci* 9:73, 1946.
15. Charles WC, Friedberg DN: Epibulbar molluscum contagiosum in acquired immune deficiency syndrome: case report and review of the literature, *Ophthalmology* 99:1123-1126, 1992.
16. Cotton DWK, Cooper C, Barrett DF, Leppard BJ: Severe atypical molluscum contagiosum infection in an immunocompromised host, *Br J Dermatol* 116:871-876, 1987.
17. Dales S, Pogo BGT: Biology of poxviruses. In Kingsbury DW, zur Hausen H, editors: *Virology monographs,* vol 18, New York, 1981, Springer-Verlag.
18. Darai G et al.: Analysis of the genome of molluscum contagiosum virus by restriction endonuclease analysis and molecular cloning, *J Med Virol* 18:29-37, 1986.
19. Delescluse J, Goens J: Multiple mollusca contagiosa revealing HTLV-III infection, *Dermatologica* 172:283-285, 1986.
20. Dennis J, Oshiro LS, Bunter JW: Molluscum contagiosum, another sexually transmitted disease: its impact on the clinical virology laboratory, *J Infect Dis* 151:376, 1985.
21. Douglas JM: Molluscum contagiosum. In Holmes KK, Märdh P, Sparling PF et al., editors: *Sexually transmitted diseases,* ed 2, New York, 1990, McGraw Hill.
22. Elion GB, Rideout JL, de Miranda P et al.: Biological activities of some purine arabinosides, *Ann NY Acad Sci* 255:468-480, 1975.
23. Ellis PP, Winograd LA: Ocular vaccinia: a specific treatment, *Arch Ophthalmol* 68:600-609, 1962.
24. Ellis PP, Winograd LA: Current concepts of ocular vaccinia, *Trans Proc Coast Otoophthalmol Soc* 44:141-148, 1963.
25. Emaugler RB, Henkind P: Molluscum contagiosum of the eyelids: an interesting case, *J Pediatr Ophthalmol Strabismus* 5:201-203, 1968.
26. Esposito JJ, Knight JC: Orthopoxvirus DNA: a comparison of restriction profiles and maps, *Virology* 143:23-51, 1985.
27. Esposito JJ, Massung RF: Poxviruses infecting humans. In Murray PR, Tenover F et al., editors: *Manual of clinical microbiology,* ed 6, Washington, DC, 1994, American Society for Microbiology (in press).
28. Fenner F: Poxviruses. In Fields BN, Knipe DM et al., editors: *Virology,* ed 2, 2113-2133, New York, 1990, Raven Press.
29. Fenner F, Henderson DA, Arita I et al.: *Smallpox and its eradication,* Geneva, 1988, World Health Organization.
30. Fenner F, Nakano JH: Poxviridae: the poxviruses. In Lennette EH, Halonen P, Murphy FA, editors: *The laboratory diagnosis of infectious diseases: principles and practice,* vol II. *Viral, rickettsial and chlamydial diseases,* 177-210, New York, 1988, Springer-Verlag.
31. Freeman G, Bron AJ, Juel-Jensen B: Ocular infection with orf virus, *Am J Ophthalmol* 97:601, 1984.
32. Fulginiti VA, Winograd LA, Jackson M, Ellis P: Therapy of experimental vaccinial keratitis. Effect of iodoxuridine and VIG, *Arch Ophthalmol* 74:539-544, 1965.
33. Goldfschmidt H, Kligman AM: Experimental inoculation of human with ectodermotropic viruses, *J Invest Dermatol* 31:175, 1958.
34. Gonnering RS, Kronish JW: Treatment of periorbital molluscum contagiosum by incision and curettage, *Ophthalmic Surg* 19:325-327, 1988.
35. Goodman DS, Teplitz ED, Wishner A et al.: Prevalence of cutaneous disease in patients with acquired immunodeficiency syndrome (AIDS) or AIDS related complex, *J Am Acad Dermatol* 17:210-220, 1989.
36. Goodpasture EW: Borreliotoses: fowlpox, molluscum contagiosum and variola-vaccinia, *Science* 77:119-123, 1933.
37. Gordon DM, Advocate S: Vaccinial blepharokeratitis, treated with cytosine arabinoside, *Am J Ophthalmol* 59:480, 1965.
38. Groden LR, Arentsen JJ: Molluscum contagiosum. In Fraunfelder FT, Roy FH, Meyer SM, editors: *Current ocular therapy,* ed 3, 87-88, Philadelphia, 1990, WB Saunders.
39. Hansen G: Om en egen sygdom (Kopper?) hos Geden: Norge, *Tidsskrift for Veterinairer* 9:298, 1879.
40. Hawley TG: The natural history of molluscum contagiosum in Fijiian children, *J Hyg (Camb)* 68:631-637, 1970.
41. Hellier FF: Profuse Mollusca contagiosa of the face induced by corticosteroids, *Br J Dermatol* 85:398, 1971.
42. Henas M, Freeman RG: Inflammatory molluscum contagiosum, *Arch Dermatol* 90:479-482, 1964.
43. Henderson W: Notice of the molluscum contagiosum, *Edinb Med Surg J* 56:213-218, 1841.
44. Hughes WT, Parham DM: Molluscum contagiosum in children with cancer or acquired immunodeficiency syndrome, *Pediatr Infect Dis J* 10:152-156, 1991.
45. Hurst JW, Forghani B, Chan CS et al.: Direct detection of molluscum contagiosum virus in clinical specimens by dot blot hybridization, *J Clin Microbiol* 29:1959-1962, 1991.
46. Hyndiuk RA, Okumoto M, Damiano R et al.: Treatment of vaccinial keratitis with vidarabine, *Arch Ophthalmol* 94:1363-1364, 1976.
47. Hyndiuk RA, Seideman S, Leibsohn JM: Treatment of vaccinial keratitis with trifluorothymidine, *Arch Ophthalmol* 94:1785, 1976.
48. Jack MK, Sorenson RW: Vaccinial keratitis treated with IDU, *Arch Ophthalmol* 69:730, 1963.
49. Jenner E: An inquiry into the causes and effects of the variolae vaccinae, a disease discovered in some of the western counties of England, particularly Gloucestershine, and known by the name of cowpox, *Classics of Medicine and Surgery* Dover, Dover Publications, New York, 1759 (1798 reprinted in CNB Comac).
50. Jones BR, Al-Hussaini MK: Therapeutic considerations in ocular vaccinia, *Trans Ophthalmol Soc UK* 83:613-631, 1964.
51. Jones BR, Galbraith JEK, Al-Hussaini MK: Vaccinial keratitis treated with interferon, *Lancet* 1:875, 1962.

52. Julianelle LA, James WM: Molluscum contagiosum of the eye, its clinical course and transmissibility and the cultivability of the virus, *Am J Ophthalmol* 26:565-570, 1943.
53. Kaufman HE, Nesburn AB, Maloney ED: Cure of vaccinia infection by 5-iodo-2 deoxyuridine, *Virology* 18:567-578, 1962.
54. Kipping HF: Molluscum dermatitis, *Arch Dermatol* 103:106-108, 1971.
55. Kotwal GJ, Isaacs SN, McKenzie R et al.: Inhibition of the complement cascade by the major secretory protein of vaccinia virus, *Science* 250:827-830, 1990.
56. Lane JM, Ruben FL, Neff JM, Millar JD: Complications of smallpox vaccination, 1968: national survey in the United States, *N Engl J Med* 281:1201-1208, 1969.
57. Reference deleted in proofs.
58. Leavell VW, McNamara MJ, Muelling R et al.: Orf. Report of 19 human cases with clinical and pathological observations, *JAMA* 204:109, 1968.
59. Lee OS Jr: Keratitis with molluscum contagiosum, *Arch Ophthalmol* 31:64-67, 1944.
60. Lepu G, Parducci F: Iodo-deoxyuridine in experimental vaccinia keratitis, *Ann Ophthalmol Otolaryngol* 88:44307, 1962.
61. Linberg JV, Blaylock WK: Giant molluscum contagiosum following splenectomy, *Arch Ophthalmol* 108:1076, 1990.
62. Lipschütz B: *Wien Klin Wehnschr* 20:253, 1907.
63. Little DJ, Fraser KM, Fleming SB et al.: Homologues of vascular endothelial growth factor are encoded by the poxvirus, orf virus, *J Virol* 68:84-92, 1994.
64. Lloyd GM, McDonald A, Glover RE: Human infection with the virus of contagious pustular dermatitis, *Lancet* 1:720, 1951.
65. Lombardo PC: Molluscum contagiosum and the acquired immune deficiency syndrome, *Arch Dermatol* 121:834-835, 1985.
66. Low RC: Molluscum contagiosum, *Edinb Med J* 53:657-661, 1944.
67. Massung RF, Esposito JJ et al.: Potential virulence determinants in terminal regions of variola smallpox virus genome, *Nature* 366:748-751, 1993.
68. Matis WL, Triana A, Shapiro R et al.: Dermatologic findings associated with human immunodeficiency virus infection, *J Am Acad Dermatol* 17:746-751, 1987.
69. McFadden G et al.: Biogenesis of pox-viruses: transitory expression of molluscum contagiosum early functions, *Virology* 4:297-303, 1979.
70. Mobacken H, Nordin P: Molluscum contagiosum among cross-country runners, *J Am Acad Dermatol* 17:519-520, 1987.
71. Moore RM Jr: Human orf in the United States, 1972, *J Infect Dis* 127:731, 1973.
72. Moss B: Poxviridae and their replication. In Fields BN, Knipe DM, editors: *Virology,* ed 2, 2079-2111, New York, 1990, Raven Press.
73. Moss B, Salzman NP: Sequential protein synthesis following vaccinia virus infection, *J Virol* 2:1016-1027, 1968.
74. Nagington J, Whistle CH: Human orf isolation of the virus by tissue culture, *BMJ* 2:1324, 1961.
75. Nanney LB, Ellis DL, Levine J, King LE: Epidermal growth factor receptors in idiopathic and virally induced skin diseases, *Am J Pathol* 140:915-925, 1992.
76. Neuman-Haeflin D, Sundmacher R, Sauter B: Effect of human leukocyte interferon cultures and monkey corneas, *Infect Immun* 12:148-155, 1975.
77. Newson IE, Cross F: Sore mouth transmissible to man, *J Am Vet Med Assoc* 84:799, 1934.
78. Paez E, Esteban M: Resistance of vaccinia virus to interferon is related to an interference phenomenon between the virus and the interferon system, *Virology* 134:12-28, 1984.
79. Paton EP: Seven cases in which operation wounds were infected with molluscum contagiosum, *Westminister Hosp Report* 16:11-15, 1909.
80. Patterson R: Causes and observations on the molluscum contagiosum of Bateman with an account of the minute structure of the tumours, *Edinb Med Surg J* 56:279-288, 1841.
81. Penney NS, Matsuo S, Mogollon R: The identification of molluscum infection by immunohistochemical means, *J Cutan Pathol* 13:97-101, 1986.
82. Pettit TH: The poxviruses: vaccinia and variola, *Int Ophthalmol Clin* 15:203-210, 1975.
83. PHLS Communicable Disease Surveillance Centre and Communicable Diseases (Scotland) Unit: Orf paravaccinia infectious, British Isles, 1975-81. Epidemiological report, *Br Med J* 284:1958, 1982.
84. Pierard-Franchimont C, Legrain A, Pierard GE: Growth and regression of molluscum contagiosum, *J Am Acad Dermatol* 9:669-672, 1983.
85. Plowright W: Studies with a strain of contagious pustular dermatitis virus in tissue culture, *Arch Ges Virusforsch* 9:214, 1959.
86. Porter CD, Archard LC: Characterization and physical mapping of molluscum contagiosum virus DNA and location of a sequence capable of encoding a conserved domain of epidermal growth factor, *J Gen Virol* 68:673-682, 1987.
87. Postlethwaite R et al.: Features of molluscum contagiosum in the north-east of Scotland and in Fijiian village settlements, *J Hyg (Lond)* 65:281-289, 1967.
88. Rao VA, Baskaran RK, Krishnam MM: Unusual cases of molluscum contagiosum of eye, *Indian J Ophthalmol* 33:263-265, 1985.
89. Reed RJ, Parkinson RP: The histogenesis of molluscum contagiosum, *Am J Surg Pathol* 1:161-169, 1977.
90. Robinson MR, Udell IJ, Garber PF et al.: Molluscum contagiosum of the eyelids in patients with acquired immune deficiency syndrome, *Ophthalmology* 99:1745-1747, 1992.
91. Rosenberg EW, Yusk JW: Molluscum contagiosum: eruption following treatment with prednisone and methotrexate, *Arch Dermatol* 101:439-441, 1970.
92. Royer J, Joubert L, Prave M: Grave ocular damage in man due to ovine contagious pustular dermatitis. Bull Soc Sci Vét Med Comp Lyon 72:93, 1970.
93. Scholz J, Rösen-Wolff A, Burgert J et al.: Molecular epidemiology of molluscum contagiosum, *J Infect Dis* 158:898-900, 1988.
94. Scholz J, Rösen-Wolff A, Bugert J et al.: Epidemiology of molluscum contagiosum using genetic analysis of the viral DNA, *J Med Virol* 27:87-90, 1989.
95. Schwartz JJ, Myskowski PL: Molluscum contagiosum in patients with human immunodeficiency virus infection. A review of twenty-seven patients, *J Am Acad Dermatol* 27:583-588, 1992.
96. Sedan J, Ourgaud AG, Guillot P: Les accidents oculaires dòrigine vaccinale observés daub le département de bouches-du-rhone au cours de lèpidemie variolique de l'hiver 1952, *Ann Oculist* 186:34-61, 1953.
97. Shelley WB, Burmeister V: Office diagnosis of molluscum contagiosum by light microscopic demonstration of virions, *Cutis* 36:465-466, 1985.
98. Shirodaria PV, Matthews RS: Observation on the antibody responses in molluscum contagiosum, *Br J Dermatol* 96:29-34, 1977.
99. Stroobant P, Rice AP, Gullick WJ et al.: Purification and characterization of vaccinia virus growth factor, *Cell* 42:383-393, 1985.
100. Sugar A, Meyer RF: Smallpox and vaccinia. In Darrell RW, editor: *Viral diseases of the eye,* 121-127, Philadelphia, 1985, Lea and Febiger.
101. Thompson CH, Biggs IM, de Zwart-Steffe RT: Detection of molluscum contagiosum virus DNA by in situ hybridization, *Pathology* 22:181-186, 1990.
102. Thompson CH, Zwart-Steffe RT, Biggs IM: Molecular epidemiology of Australian isolates of molluscum contagiosum, *J Med Virol* 32:1-9, 1990.
103. Twardzik DR, Brown JP, Ranchalis JE et al.: Vaccinia virus-infected cells release a novel polypeptide functionally related to transforming and epidermal growth factors, *Proc Natl Acad Sci USA* 82:5300-5304, 1985.
104. Van der Meer Maastricht BCJ, Gomperts CE: Molluscum contagiosum giganteum, *Am J Ophthalmol* 33:965-967, 1950.
105. Vannas S, Lapinleimu K: Molluscum contagiosum in the skin, caruncle and conjunctiva: detection of a cytopathic agent in tissue culture, *Acta Ophthalmol* 45:314-321, 1967.
106. Vemura T: Molecular epidemiologic study of molluscum contagiosum, *Jpn J Dermatol* 101:689-695, 1991.

107. Viac J, Chardonnet Y: Immunocompetent cells and epithelial cell modifications in molluscum contagiosum, *J Cutan Pathol* 17:202-205, 1990.
108. Waddington E, Bray PT, Evans AD: Cutaneous complications of mass vaccination against smallpox in South Wales, 1962, *St John Hosp Derm Soc* 50:22-42, 1964.
109. Wheeler CE, Potter M, Cawley EP: Experimental ecthyma contagiosum (orf), *J Invest Dermatol* 26:275, 1956.
110. Wile VJ, Kingery LB: Etiology of molluscum contagiosum, *J Cutan Dis* 37:431-435, 1919.
111. Wilkinson JD: Orf: a family with unusual complications, *J Dermatol* 97:447, 1977.
112. World Health Organization: The global eradication of smallpox. *Final report of the global commission for the certification of smallpox eradication* (History of international public health, No 4), Geneva, 1980, World Health Organization.

67 Human Papillomavirus Diseases

JAN M. McDONNELL, JONATHAN H. LASS

Human papillomavirus (HPV) is a relative newcomer to textbooks of ocular disease, and the understanding of its epidemiology as an ocular infection, symptomatic or otherwise, is rudimentary. The virus deserves attention at this time for three very important reasons. First, a small number of reports from a variety of investigators indicate this virus finds the ocular surface a hospitable site for growth.* There is also a high prevalence of HPV type 6/11 in conjunctival papillomas† as well as a high incidence of HPV type 16 and 18 infection in conjunctival dysplasia and carcinoma.[82,84] One group identified HPV type 16 DNA in over 85% of 60 conjunctival epithelial neoplasias using the polymerase chain reaction (PCR) (see Laboratory Investigations and Pathology sections).[80,82] In two smaller series others have confirmed the finding.[69,102] HPV DNA was found in each of a group of three lacrimal sac papillomas and three lacrimal sac carcinomas.[74] Thus both adnexal and ocular surface neoplasms have developed with associated HPV DNA. Second, HPV-associated lesions, predominantly mucosal warts, in nonocular sites are considered by the National Institutes of Health and the Centers for Disease Control and Prevention to be an epidemic worldwide.[94] And third, aside from the direct morbidity of genital warts and of their treatment, rapidly mounting epidemiologic and molecular evidence point to HPV as a major factor in the development of carcinomas of the anogenital tract and, to a lesser extent, other mucosal carcinomas.[136] Certain HPV types are strongly associated with dysplasias and carcinomas of the anogenital region. Over 90% of invasive carcinomas of the uterine cervix, penis, and anus can be shown to contain HPV DNA, usually of type 16 or 18.[136] HPV-related cervical carcinoma is the second leading cause of cancer deaths among the women of the world. It is imperative that the relationship between virus

and tumor in the development of adnexal and ocular surface neoplasms be clarified.

VIROLOGY

Human papillomavirus is a member of the Papovavirus family. The first HPV to be identified and to have its DNA cloned was HPV 6.[79] Papillomaviruses are icosahedral, and their genetic material consists of a circular, supercoiled double-stranded DNA molecule approximately 8 kilobases long. The genome is organized into open reading frames (ORFs) that are all found on the same strand of DNA. The other strand is presumed to be noncoding. These ORFs are divided into early (E) and late (L) regions, with E designation assigned to sequences that encode proteins associated with viral replication and transformation functions, and L assigned to two large ORFs (L1 and L2) that encode structural proteins. There is extensive conservation of genomic organization and sequence among the different HPV types.

HPV exists in over 60 known types. Although these may differ from one another by relatively few nucleotides, it is clear that different types have vastly different potentials as infectious agents for a particular epithelium, and as factors in the development of invasive carcinoma. Table 67-1 illustrates the preferred epithelial target and resulting lesions for some of the more common HPV types. Of note, HPV 6 and 11 prefer mucous membranes, including the conjunctiva, and most HPV 6- or 11-associated lesions are papillomata or condylomata. HPV 16 and 18, although also preferring to grow in mucous membranes, are seldom found in benign lesions, but are the types most often present in dysplasias or carcinomas. These four types, 6, 11, 16 and 18, are the only HPV types so far identified in lesions of the conjunctiva. Because of these type-specific behaviors in the face of a basic genetic similarity of HPV types, explanations of HPV-related neoplasia must explain not only the steps between infection and the development of lesions, but also the differences in lesions according to HPV type.

---

*References 68, 69, 74, 80, 81, 82, 85, 92, 96, 102.
†References 68, 80, 81, 85, 92, 102.

TABLE 67-1 HPV TYPE AND TYPICAL ASSOCIATED LESIONS

HPV Type	Lesion
1	Cutaneous wart
6, 11	Respiratory papilloma
	Anogenital condyloma (condyloma accuminata)
	Conjunctival papilloma
16, 18	Squamous dysplasia and carcinoma of anogenital area, upper respiratory tract, conjunctiva; other mucosal dysplasias
18	Adenocarcinoma, uterine cervix
31, 33, 35, and others	Cervical carcinoma (minus common HPV types)

EPIDEMIOLOGY

There is no published study that outlines the prevalence of ocular surface HPV in a cross section of the population. Studies from other sites are more abundant, however. In the last 2 decades HPV has assumed major importance as a cause of anogenital tumors in both men and women. If the prevalence of HPV infection is measured only by the incidence of HPV-related lesions, there are now over 14 million infected patients in the United States alone, and new infections (that is, new patients with anogenital condylomata or dysplasia) are appearing at a rate of 1 million per year.[94]

The number of patients with HPV-related lesions at any given time is probably a gross underestimate of the actual prevalence of HPV infection, however. Molecular studies and routine cytopathologic screening have identified patients who have HPV infection without overt lesions. The rate of HPV positivity varies with the demographics of the study group and the body site evaluated.

Genital and Oral HPV

The best-studied body site is the female genital tract. In a study of adolescents (defined by the authors as women aged 14 to 23) going to a private suburban adolescent health clinic, Fisher, Rosenfeld, and Burk[34] found that 34 of 106 (32%) had cervical swabs that contained HPV DNA. A full 21% had DNA from HPV types most commonly associated with cervical carcinoma, HPV 16, 18, or 31. HPV DNA was present in the cervices of 34% of a group of women in the Bronx with no gross culposcopic abnormalities.[5] In a study of 505 women in Norway applying for a first trimester abortion, 31 (6.1%) had HPV DNA in cervical swabs.[27] Among women aged 65 or older, HPV DNA was found in 3.5% of a group of 232 patients, and the crude odds ratio for cervical neoplasia among HPV DNA-positive patients was 18.3 (adjusted odds 12.2).[76]

Men have also been studied and found to carry HPV

DNA. HPV 16 DNA was found in the semen of 85% of a series of men with genital warts, but also in 33% of men attending the same infertility clinic who had no history or clinical manifestations of genital lesions.[43] Among 105 heterosexual men (without clinical anogenital warts) who attended a genitourinary medical clinic, 28 (27%) had cytologic evidence of HPV infection, and 21 (20%) had HPV DNA by hybridization studies of exfoliated cells, yielding a total of 42 (40%) patients with occult HPV infection identified with either technique.[75] Samples of anal mucosa from a cohort of homosexual men had a positivity rate of up to 53% for HPV 16 or 18 DNA in one study,[16] and the prevalence was as high as 65% in another.[70] The presence of HIV infection is associated with an increased prevalence of HPV and dysplasia on anal smears in men,[62] who have much more rapid progression to anal carcinoma than HIV-negative, HPV-positive patients.[98] HIV infection is also associated with an increase in cervical HPV infection and carcinoma among women.[65]

Swabs from the oral mucosa of asymptomatic subjects have also yielded HPV DNA. Forty-three percent of 62 patients studied by Jalal and associates[52] had HPV 16 DNA present in buccal mucosa, epithelium of the dorsal tongue and hard palate.

Sexual partners of patients with genital HPV infection have a greater likelihood than a comparable population of sexually active adults of becoming infected,[6] further confirming that HPV is a sexually transmitted infection. But it may also be possible for patients with anogenital infection to have HPV DNA in other mucosal sites, including the oral cavity[56,99] and concomitant nasal papillomas.[37] Genital tract papillomavirus may also spread to neonates passing through an infected birth canal[116]; polymerase chain reaction studies identified HPV DNA in swabs of maternal cervical smears and neonatal buccal mucosal smears, and infection persisted in the children for at least 6 weeks.[36] The conjunctiva was not studied in these patients.

Conjunctival HPV

HPV DNA has been identified in the majority of conjunctival papillomata[84] and in up to 85% of conjunctival dysplasias and carcinomas,[82,84] described in greater detail in the next section. But conjunctival papillomata, dysplasia, and carcinoma are uncommon lesions, and HPV is a common infection in extraocular sites. Is HPV common as an asymptomatic ocular infection?

Not surprisingly, HPV DNA can be identified in asymptomatic conjunctivae.[80,82,83] There are no epidemiologic studies of HPV and the ocular surface, but there is evidence to suggest that people without ocular lesions may harbor the infection. In the first report linking HPV DNA with conjunctival carcinoma, a patient with unilateral corneal neoplasia had HPV DNA in swabs from both conjunctivae.[80] In a later report 5 of 6 (83.3%) patients with unilateral conjunctival or corneal neoplasia, some of whom were studied up to 8 years after the original excision, had demonstrable HPV DNA in bilateral ocular swabs, and the same HPV type was present in both swabs and tissue samples from the 5 patients from whom both types of specimen were available for study.[82] In another study a group of 17 women with biopsy-proven HPV-associated cervical dysplasias were evaluated following eradication of their cervical lesions. During the same clinic visit, cervical and bilateral ocular surface swabs were obtained and examined for the presence of HPV DNA. The overall recovery rate of conjunctival HPV 16 or 18 DNA in these patients was 76.5%,[83] and none of the patients had ocular surface lesions by slit lamp examination.

In a study of patients at a public, urban, general ophthalmology clinic, 60% had HPV 16 DNA present in conjunctival swabs from one or both eyes, and 24% harbored HPV 18 DNA. These patients ranged in age from 3 to 87 years, and 53% were females.* But the prevalence of HPV infection in a cross section of the population has not been described. Should the study ever be done, longitudinal data will need to be added to prevalence data before the significance of the findings can be determined, as the clinical significance of a single positive test for HPV DNA is unknown.

What happens when other mucosal surfaces become infected with HPV? Once acquired, the infection may not be curable in some patients; although lesions may be eradicated, in many patients lesions will recur because of persistent viral infection.[32] Two reported patients suggest that a similarly variable clinical course may occur with conjunctival HPV infection. One patient with conjunctival dysplasia remained tumor-free, but positive for HPV type 16 DNA 8 years after excision of her lesion. Another patient with HPV DNA-positive carcinoma in situ of the conjunctiva remained DNA positive at 12 months and developed recurrence at 15 months.[82]

As the number of people with ocular HPV infection is unknown, knowledge of the epidemiology of ocular HPV must be acquired in another way. How often do patients have lesions that are probably ocular manifestations of HPV? There are two types of lesions that are HPV-associated: benign, that is, noninvasive epithelial proliferations included in the generic ophthalmologic term "papilloma"; and a spectrum of lesions in which the capacity to invade is potential or realized, the dysplasias and carcinomas. The counterparts to these lesions in the anogenital tract are condyloma and dysplasia/carcinoma. (A discussion of the proposed mechanisms by which HPV causes epithelial proliferation follows in the section entitled Pathogenesis.) The type of lesion varies with the HPV type, described in Laboratory Investigations and Pathology.

---

*Sun YY, Carpenter JD, McDonnell J, *Prevalence of Human Papillomavirus DNA in Asymptomatic Patients.*

Conjunctival Papilloma. Conjunctival papillomata are relatively rare, benign stratified squamous epithelial tumors. Ash[2] found 13 papillomata among 174 epibulbar lesions (7%) in persons under the age of 20 years. Papillomata accounted for 12% (126 of 1016) of all epibulbar lesions he reported from the collection at the Armed Forces Institute of Pathology. A similar percentage of papillomata, 8%, was found in another series of 298 histopathologic specimens of epibulbar tumors in children.[95] At the Mayo Clinic only 27 papillomata were excised over a 64-year period.[118] From a histopathologic collection of 2455 conjunctival lesions removed from patients over the age of 15 years, Grosniklaus, Green, Luckenbach, and Chan[44] found 93 (4%) papillomata. They also noted that papillomata was the fourth most common acquired epithelial lesion in their patient group, accounting for 15% of 641 epithelial lesions. The average age of patients with papillomata in their series was 40 years.

Many authors have separated papillomata into three categories: infectious, limbal, and inverted.[118] The classifications are based on clinical features such as appearance, location, age of onset, tendency to recur, and histopathology. Although these designations are still used clinically, evidence from HPV studies (which were not a part of the classic papers on papillomata) suggests that all of the lesions are, in fact, "infectious," whether they occur in a child or adult, at the limbus or elsewhere.

In the classic reports papillomata categorized as infectious occur in children and young adults. They are usually pedunculated and may occur on the bulbar or palpebral conjunctivae, the semilunar fold, the caruncle, or even at the limbus. They are fleshy lesions, often with a prominent vascularity (Figs. 67-1 to 67-3). Recurrence may be associated with extensive spread of the tumor (Fig. 67-4). Rarely, infectious papillomata extend into the nasolacrimal duct,[87] de-

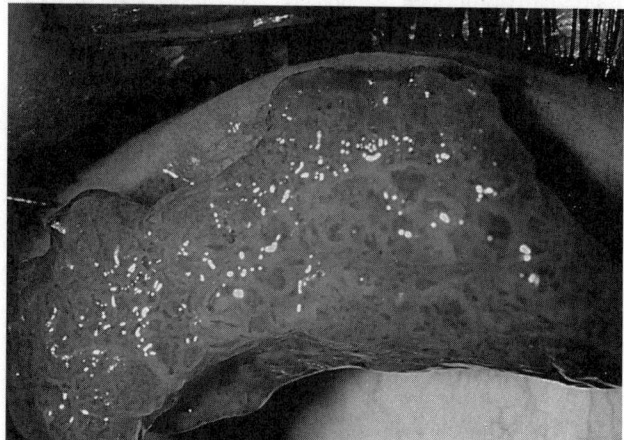

Fig. 67-1.   Tarsal conjunctival papilloma in a 28-year-old woman. The lesion is raised and nonkeratinized, with the subepithelial vascular network readily apparent. The fleshy appearance is typical of papillomata.

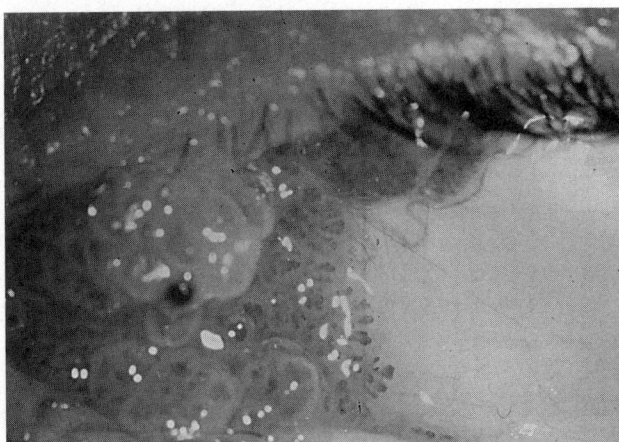

Fig. 67-2. Recurrent, extensive papilloma involving left caruncle, medial bulbar conjunctiva, and medial, upper and lower tarsal conjunctivae in a 31-year-old man. The arborizing vessels at the ledge of the lesion are prominent.

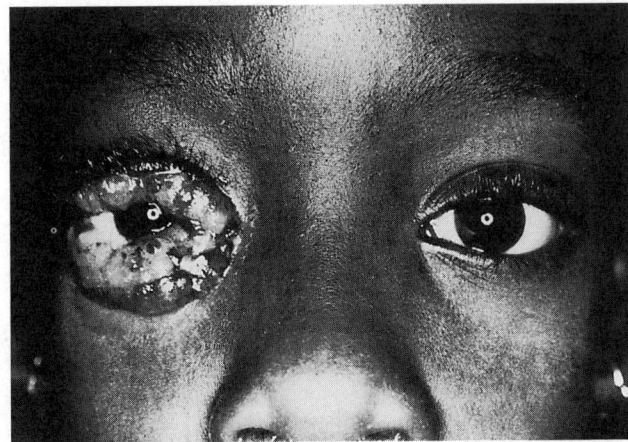

Fig. 67-4. One of multiple, progressive recurrences for this 9-year-old girl, with extensive involvement of upper and lower, tarsal and bulbar conjunctivae. This lesion was positive for HPV 6/11 DNA by in situ hybridization.

velop in the canaliculus,[127] or originate in the lacrimal sac.[74] The recurrence rate, in various series, hovers around 40%.[2,44,46,95,118]

Lesions categorized as limbal papillomata include all those papillomata located at the limbus that have a sessile configuration and occur in adults. They also have a recurrence rate of around 40%.[118] They were, until recently, thought to be entirely due to sun exposure because of their tendency to occur in older adults and their typical location within the interpalpebral zone.

The final category of papilloma, the inverted papilloma, is the least common form on the bulbar or tarsal conjunctiva.[121] Inverted papillomata, that grow by invagination into the underlying stroma, are the most common form of papilloma to occur in the lacrimal sac, however.[109]

This chapter will attempt to prove that nearly all conjunctival papillomata, dysplasias, and carcinomas are associated with human papillomavirus infection. It may be time

to remove the qualifier ''infectious'' to describe one of the clinical varieties of papilloma, as it is not only redundant, but implies that the other two varieties are noninfectious.

Conjunctival Neoplasia. Dysplasia and carcinoma of the conjunctiva comprise a spectrum of neoplastic proliferations of the squamous mucosal cells of any of the conjunctival surfaces. They often arise at the limbus and are classically described as occurring in the interpalpebral zone.* The pathogenesis of conjunctival dysplasia and carcinoma has not been determined, but these lesions are referred to in the literature as conditions of older, predominantly Caucasian, men.[15,31,129] The lesions were thought by some researchers to be a consequence of sun exposure,[31,103] perhaps in some cases through transformation of a benign squamous proliferation or papilloma.[128] The only case-control study in the literature discounted the role of sun exposure and identified cigarette smoking as the only factor that increased the risk of conjunctival dysplasia in the population studied.[93]

The incidence of ocular surface neoplasia has not been established. According to the LAC/USC Cancer Surveillance Program (the cancer registry covering Los Angeles County), the sex-specific average annual age-adjusted incidence rates of squamous cell carcinoma of the conjunctiva in Los Angeles County between 1980 and 1989 were 0.18 per 100,000 in men and 0.05 per 100,000 in women. In a study that simply counted the number of histopathologic diagnoses of conjunctival dysplasia and carcinoma in all 10 hospital pathology labs in Brisbane, Australia over a 10-year period, Lee and Hirst[72] reported incidence of 1.9 per 100,000 per year averaged over 10 years, and a male-to-female ratio of 2.3 to 1. Their study is the only systematic approach in the literature to the epidemiology of the conjunctival neoplasia,

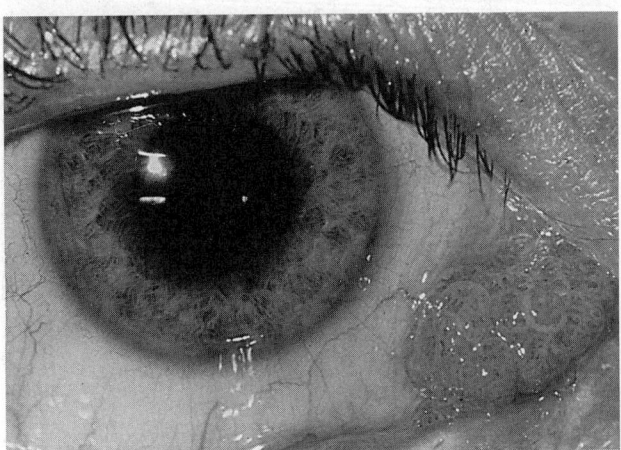

Fig. 67-3. Papilloma of the caruncle in a 10-year-old boy.

---

*References 15, 31, 51, 81, 93, 103, 129.

and it does not address the role of HPV. The authors do point out, however, that the incidence of conjunctival neoplasia is not on the rise, in contrast with cutaneous melanoma. Their data, like those of Napora, Cohen, Genvert and associates,[93] suggest a cause other than sun exposure for these lesions.

The recurrence rate has been reported to vary from 33% to 40%,[15,103,129] and recurrence may be associated with more severe disease, although in general the growth of these lesions is slow.[103]

RISK FACTORS

Although ultraviolet light exposure has long been considered the cause of conjunctival neoplasia, a single case-control study of patients with and without conjunctival dysplasia or carcinoma found no increased risk in those who worked out-of-doors.[93] These researchers did not determine the HPV status of the patients, nor did Lee and Hirst,[72] who reported the incidence of ocular surface neoplasia over a 10-year period in Brisbane, Australia. They found no increase in incidence over the study period, unlike the dramatic increases in cutaneous melanoma attributed to UV light in recent years. The only risk factor documented in these (albeit scant) studies was cigarette smoking; smokers had an increased risk of conjunctival dysplasia by a factor of 2.[93]

Cigarette smoking is also a risk factor for HPV-related cervical carcinoma.[5] Other risk factors have been proposed, including reduced plasma levels of ascorbic acid and beta-carotene.[5] Reduced red blood cell folate levels were found in patients with cervical dysplasia, and it was postulated that these levels could be attributed to cigarette smoking, which might alter the local immune system and permit HPV-related neoplasia to develop.[13] Focal breakdown of the immune system was postulated as a cofactor for HPV infection by another group, who found viral DNA in 90% of tumor samples of cervical dysplasia, but also in 46% of secondary biopsies from grossly normal areas from the same patients.[104] Global immune deficiency, such as found in HIV infection and AIDS, is associated with an increase in HPV infection and HPV-related lesions.[54,61,122]

CLINICAL FEATURES

Papillomas

Conjunctival papilloma is a soft, usually pedunculated, grayish-red elevation with an irregular surface that may or may not be keratinized. There is often a prominent vascular pattern. Papillomata may occur unilaterally or bilaterally, and may be multifocal within the same eye. They may be in the palpebral area (Fig. 67-1), fornix (Fig. 67-2), semilunar fold, caruncle (Fig. 67-3), or limbus. Involvement may be extensive (Fig. 67-4). A sessile papilloma that occurs at the limbus in an older adult may be indistinguishable from a limbal dysplasia (Fig. 67-5). The inverted papilloma, al-

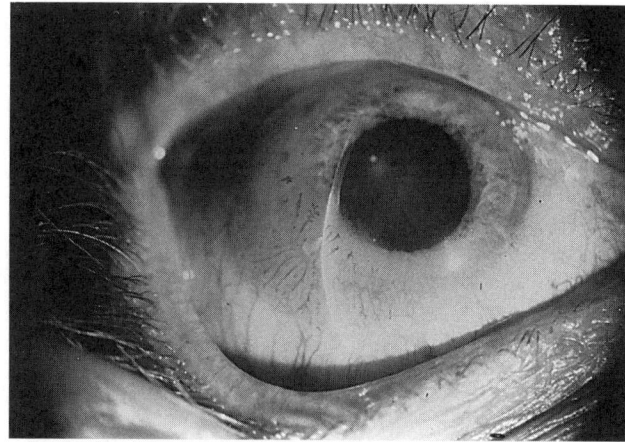

Fig. 67-5. This raised limbal lesion in a 56-year-old man is non-keratinized and has the prominent vascular pattern seen with papillomata. Vessels can be seen extending out onto the cornea. The lesion, a moderate dysplasia by light microscopy, was HPV 16 DNA-positive by polymerase chain reaction (PCR), and has since recurred.

though rare in the conjunctiva, is the most common configuration found in the lacrimal sac. It typically invaginates into the underlying stroma rather than growing in an exophytic pattern.[109]

Dysplasia and Carcinoma

Dysplasia and carcinoma of the conjunctiva exist as a spectrum of abnormal proliferations of the corneal or conjunctival squamous mucosa.* Over the years these lesions have been called, among other names, intraepithelial epithelioma,[85] Bowens disease,[40] and, in an attempt to simplify the matter, precancerous epithelioma of the limbus.[40] The clinical appearances of lesions along the spectrum are so similar that clinical appearance alone is insufficient to determine the severity of a given lesion. These lesions can be pedunculated, but are much more likely to be sessile thickenings of the conjunctival or corneal epithelium.[124] They may be white or yellow with keratinization, or have a gelatinous fleshy-gray appearance. Most dysplasias and carcinomas are vascular and contain multiple tiny vessels in addition to an associated increase in vessels adjacent to the lesions. Although usually solitary, dysplasia or carcinoma may be multiple and can be located anywhere on the bulbar or tarsal conjunctiva. In lesions of the bulbar conjunctiva, there may be underlying degeneration of the connective tissue suggestive of pterygium or pingueculum. Figs. 67-5, 67-6, and 67-7 illustrate the clinical appearance of two dysplasias and carcinomas, each of which has been shown to contain HPV DNA.

As can be seen from Figs. 67-5 through 67-7, and has long been noted in the literature, the majority of lesions

---

*References 15, 31, 51, 81, 85, 93, 103, 129.

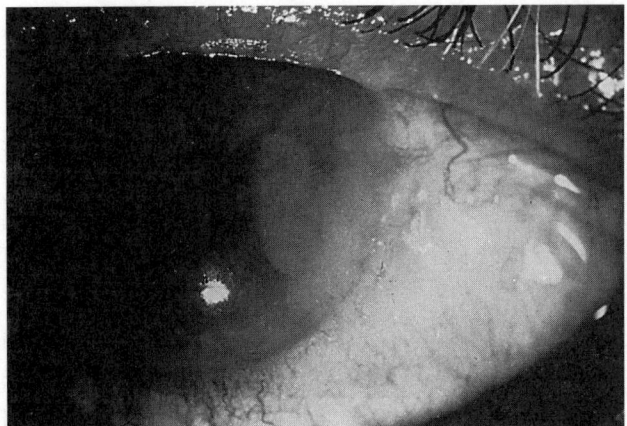

Fig. 67-6. A severe dysplasia-carcinoma in situ from the limbal region of a 42-year-old woman. Although the lesion has not recurred, conjunctival swabs remain positive for HPV 16 DNA by PCR 8 years after the original excision.[82]

involve the corneoscleral limbus, the junction between corneal and conjunctival epithelium.[103,124] As authors have pointed out the histopathologic similarities between conjunctival, corneal, and uterine cervical dysplasia,[103,124] so have they pointed out that uterine cervical dysplasias most often occur at a transition zone, the uterine cervical squamo-columnar junction. Earlier papers postulated that it was the juxtaposition of two different epithelial types that explained the propensity for lesions to develop in these regions, one stating that " . . . a transition zone in epithelial cell type confers an instability that is conducive to dysplasia,"[103] but later it was proposed that the limbus and cervical transition zone are both sites of high mitotic activity relative to neighboring sites in the same epithelium, and this higher mitotic rate puts these regions at increased risk.[124] For the cervix, the higher mitotic rate is due in part to squamous metaplasia of more delicate columnar epithelium in response to physical

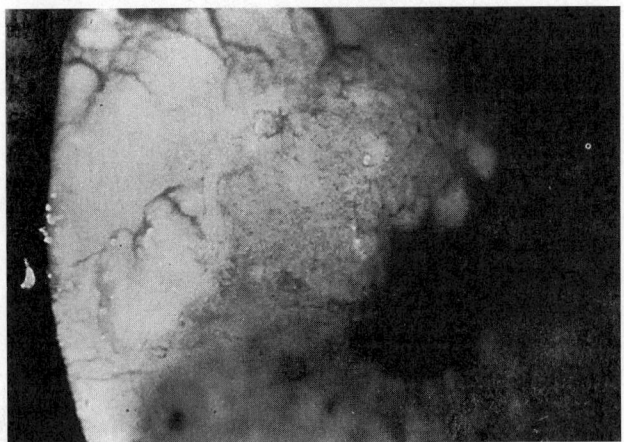

Fig. 67-7. Rose bengal staining of a severe dysplasia in an 86-year-old man. The tumor was positive for HPV 16 DNA by PCR.

trauma and other factors; for the cornea and conjunctiva, there is evidence that the limbus serves at the main source of stem cells that may differentiate and migrate centripetally to the basal epithelium, where they remain mitotically active.[114] It seems clear that HPV must also be factored into the equation for both sites.

PATHOLOGY

It was the histopathologic appearance of conjunctival papilloma, dysplasia, and carcinoma—more than any other feature—that first led to the suspicion that they were HPV-associated lesions. They are virtually indistinguishable from epithelial lesions of the uterine cervix, with papillomata from both exhibiting acanthosis of benign, well-organized epithelium, thrown into folds and fronds supported by fibrovascular pegs (Fig. 67-8). Dysplasias and carcinomas of the cervix and the ocular surface have, in addition, varying degrees of loss of organization of the epithelial layers, mitotic figures above the basal layer of the epithelium, variability in size, shape, and staining characteristics of the cells, and occasional large, bizarre mononuclear cells or multinucleated cells. One of the first histopathologic features to be associated with HPV infection was *koilocytosis,* a term used to describe epithelial cells with a hyperchromatic, shrunken nucleus and cytoplasmic clearing.[64]

Koilocytosis has been identified in the majority of conjunctival lesions by authors seeking to demonstrate an HPV association,[68,80,81,92,102] but perhaps even more suggestive, a biopsy with features strongly resembling koilocytosis was published as part of a series on corneal neoplasia by authors who did not associate the lesions they described with HPV[124] (Fig. 67-9). Although those lesions were not studied for the presence of HPV, koilocytosis is often found in both benign

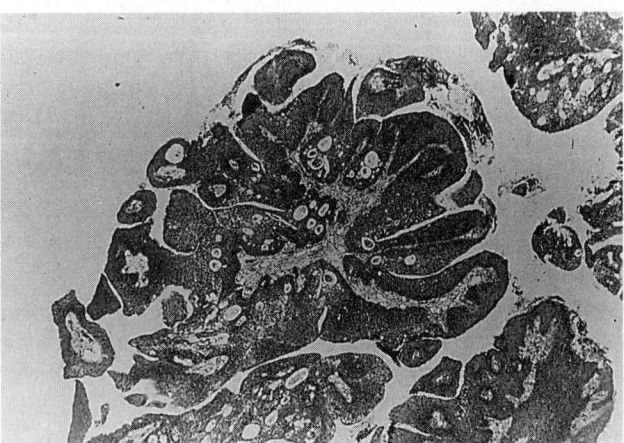

Fig. 67-8. A typical conjunctival papilloma is pedunculated, with a prominent underlying vascular network. Within papillomata, there can be preservation of some goblet cells, and mucous secretion sometimes results in the formation of cysts within the papilloma. (Hematoxylin and eosin, ×20.)

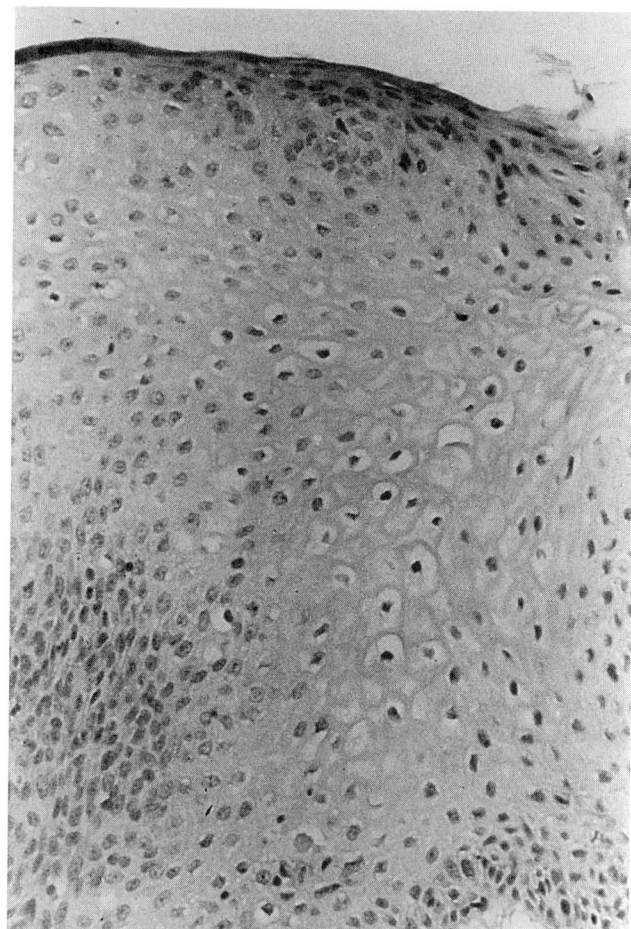

Fig. 67-9. Koilocytosis in a conjunctival papilloma, positive for HPV 6/11 DNA by in situ hybridization. Infected cells can be identified by their shrunken or pyknotic nuclei and the surrounding cytoplasmic vacuoles. Adjacent, nonkoilocytotic cells may also be infected; koilocytosis is strongly suggestive of HPV infection but is not a sine qua non (H and E × 200).

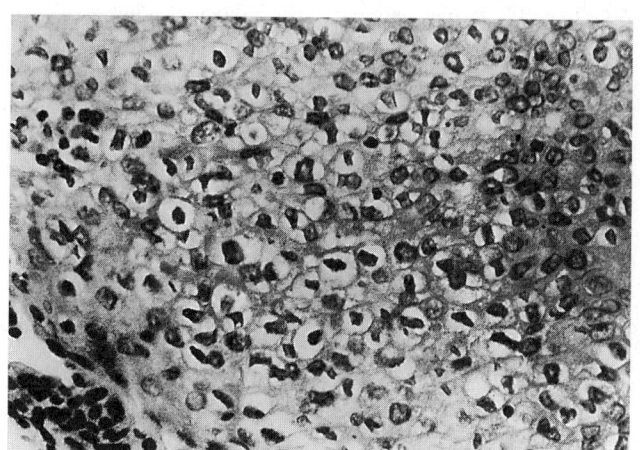

Fig. 67-10. Koilocytosis in a conjunctival dysplasia, positive for HPV 16 DNA by PCR (H and E × 200).

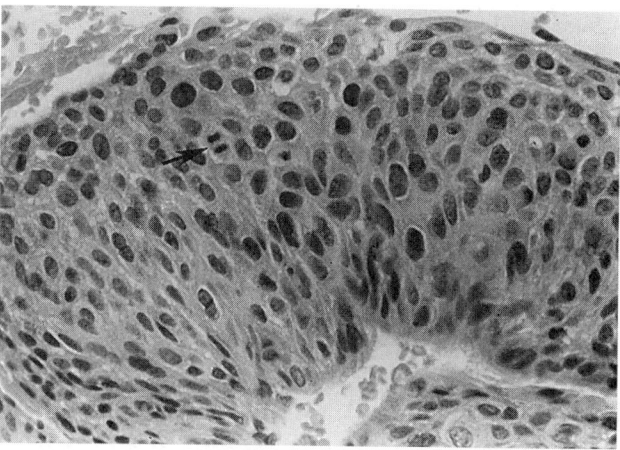

Fig. 67-11. Severe dysplasia-carcinoma in situ of the conjunctiva. There is squamous metaplasia and complete loss of maturation of the epithelium. Mitotic figures are present *(arrow)* (Hematoxylin and eosin, × 400).

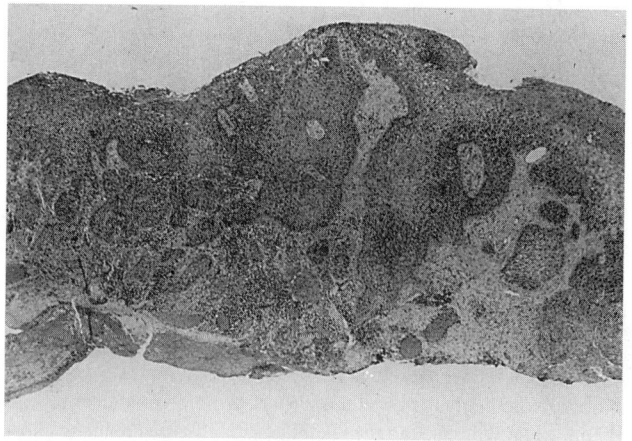

A

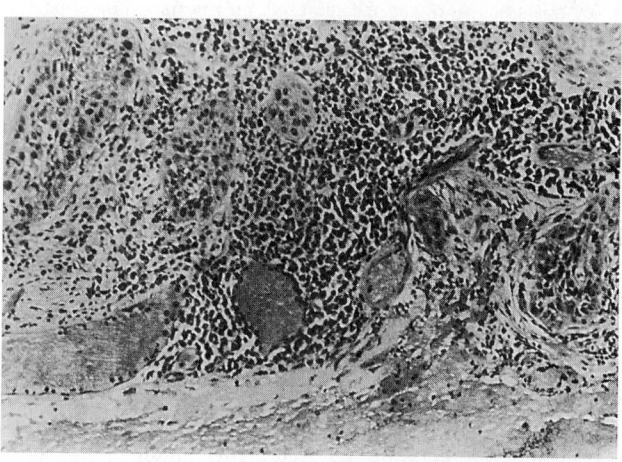

B

Fig. 67-12. Invasive squamous carcinoma of the conjunctiva, positive for HPV 16 DNA by PCR. Islands of carcinoma cells infiltrate the substantia propria (H and E × 100, × 400).

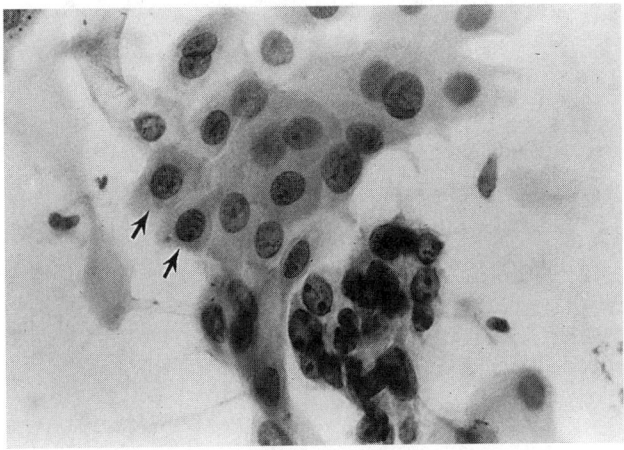

A

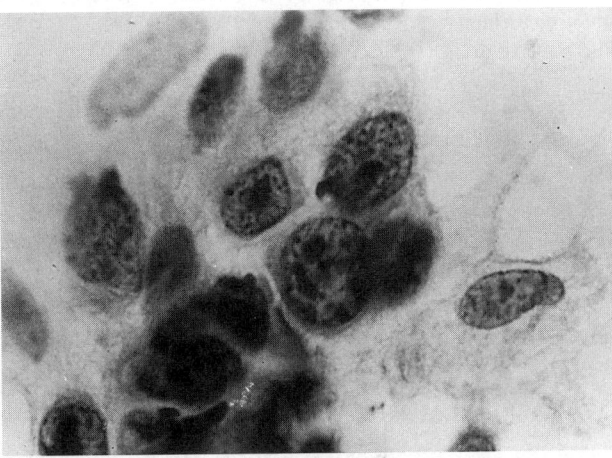

B

Fig. 67-13. Cytopathologic smear of conjunctival dysplasia. Normal conjunctival epithelium has a low ratio of nuclear size to cytoplasmic volume, and the nuclei are small with a delicate chromatin pattern *(small arrows)*. Dysplastic cells have a high nucleus-to-cytoplasmic ratio, and the enlarged, pleomorphic nuclei have a coarse chromatin pattern. If effective nonsurgical treatments are developed, diagnosis based on cytopathology may become routine for the conjunctiva as it is for the uterine cervix (Papanicolaou ×400, ×1000).

and dysplastic lesions that are, with molecular methods, shown to be HPV-positive (Fig. 67-10).

Conjunctival dysplasia is graded in a system identical to that of the cervix, with designations of mild, moderate, and severe carcinoma in situ. Some authors have even used the same acronym, CIN, for conjunctival (cervical) intraepithelial neoplasia[103]. The grading system is based on the combination of the level within the epithelial thickness of disorganized maturation, and the maximum height within the epithelium at which mitotic figures are identified. Mild dysplasia has mitotic figures present above the basal layer but confined to the lower ⅓ of the epithelial thickness, and shows maturation (that is, flattening out of more superficial

cells) of the upper ⅔ of the epithelium. Moderate dysplasia has mitotic figures up as high as ⅔ of the epithelial thickness, and shows less maturation. Severe dysplasia is interchangeable with carcinoma in site. At this grade, mitotic figures are present full-thickness within the epithelium, and there is no maturation of the superficial cells. Lesions at any grade may have multinucleated cells or large, bizarre nuclei, and mitotic figures may appear to have extra chromosomes. Finding a multipolar mitotic figure, even in a lesion that otherwise appears to be low-grade, is an ominous discovery and usually earns a diagnosis of carcinoma in situ (Fig. 67-11). Microinvasion, with cells adherent to the epithelium but penetrating the basement membrane, may be found, as may frankly invasive squamous carcinoma (Fig. 67-12). Although these lesions are usually removed as excisional biopsies because of the possibility they are dysplastic (see Therapy section), cytopathologic studies of scrapings are also diagnostic (Fig. 67-13).

PATHOGENESIS

One way by which HPV is known to influence proliferation of the host cell is through insertion of the HPV genome into the host cell DNA. It is extremely unusual for HPV types usually associated with benign lesions to insert into the host genome at all, and this difference was among the first to be found between dysplasia-associated or "high-risk" types and papilloma or condyloma-associated "low-risk" HPV types. In less severe dysplasias, as it does in benign lesions, HPV DNA exists exclusively as an extrachromosomal fragment. In more severe dysplasias, HPV integrates into the genome, as it does in carcinomas.[29,30] In all cell lines studied so far, that insertion has been clonal, indicating that HPV DNA insertion occurred very early in the development of the malignant proliferation.[29,123] Initial studies proposed that the inserted HPV DNA "relates the papillomavirus in a formal sense to a tumor promoter,"[30] and in some cervical carcinoma cell lines HPV was found inserted close to known oncogenes.[29] It has become clear, however, that it is not simply the phenomenon of insertion of the HPV DNA into the host genome, nor is it the site of insertion within the host genome that provides the molecular trigger for promoting tumor development. Rather, it is the insertion into the host of a particular type of HPV DNA that itself contains a disrupted HPV genome.[136] Disruption of a regulatory portion of the HPV genome, the E2 gene, or open reading frame is present in all tumors studied so far that have HPV DNA integration.

HPV E2 is an important controller of HPV proliferation. E2 disruption allows for overproduction of the E6 and E7 ORFs. The E6 and E7 gene products of high-risk HPV types, unlike those of low-risk HPV types, are capable of inducing malignant growth in vitro[136] (see the following section). So the high-risk and low-risk capacities of different viral types appear to hinge at least in part on the ability of the DNA to integrate: high-risk types integrate into the host and low-risk types do not. Integration allows for E2 disruption, and resulting E6 and E7 protein overproduction. A second factor in the ability of each particular HPV type's oncogenic potential lies in the type-determined abilities of E6 and E7 proteins to disrupt normal controls of cell proliferation.

One mechanism by which E6 and E7 disrupt normal cell growth is through interaction with important cellular regulatory proteins or tumor suppressors. The retinoblastoma gene product, Rb, was the first to be identified among a growing number of human regulatory proteins known as tumor suppressor genes or, formerly, antioncogenes.[125] The list now includes the neurofibromatosis tumor suppressor gene (NF-1), the deleted-in-colon-carcinoma gene (DCC), the Wilms tumor gene (WT), and p53.[49,73,125] Each of these genes encodes for a protein that is vital for normal cell proliferation. For most of these important genes, individuals are homozygous for the wild-type gene, even though heterozygotes are capable of producing enough of the protein for normal function with their one wild-type gene. Homozygosity of mutant genes appears to be incompatible with life. Each of these conditions may be familial, that is, inherited in Mendelian autosomal dominant fashion, and result in somatic and germline cells that are heterozygous for the tumor suppressor gene. In patients who are heterozygous as a germline condition, that is, every cell in their body contains only one wild-type copy of the tumor suppressor gene, there is great likelihood that, through the normal minor inaccuracies of DNA replication, the one wild-type copy may become lost or undergo mutation. Without a functional copy of this protein, individual cells will develop malignant clones and progress to clinically detectable malignancy. In the case of the Rb protein, retinoblastoma and osteosarcoma will ensue with loss of both functioning Rb genes. With loss of both NF-1 genes, neurogenic sarcoma results. Loss of the WT gene is associated with the development of Wilms tumor, a primitive tumor of renal origin. Only in cells that have lost the one functioning copy of that gene—through mitotic recombination, chromosomal nondysfunction, point mutation, or some other mechanism—does a tumor develop. It is this loss of heterozygosity (LOH) that provides the molecular trigger for oncogenesis.[29] In wild-type homozygous patients, it is the same molecular event—lack of a functioning tumor suppressor protein—that leads to the development of, for example, retinoblastoma. But these patients must inactivate both wild-type genes in a single somatic cell, and that event is statistically much less likely. Patients who must take two "hits" in the same somatic cell are also much less liable to have multiple or bilateral tumors, unlike patients with, for example, heritable retinoblastoma. The classic 1972 paper by Knudson,[63] when read assuming each hit is loss of a functioning tumor suppressor gene, is an elegant explanation of this molecular genetic phenomenon.

The most frequently mutated gene in human cancer appears to be the p53 gene.[49,73,125] It has been mutated in carci-

nomas of the bladder, breast, lung, liver, and colon, hematopoietic tumors, brain tumors, and rhabdomyosarcoma.[125] An important role is played by p53 in the repression of DNA transcription and regulation of the cell cycle.[71] Many people are heterozygous for p53, possessing both a wild-type and a mutant gene. When there is loss of the gene encoding for wild-type p53, or loss of heterozygosity, only the gene for the mutant protein remains, and the control exercised on cellular proliferation by wild-type p53 is lost.[49,86]

Mutation or loss of heterozygosity is one way to eliminate a functioning p53 protein from a cell. But it is not the only way employed in nature or in the lab. The p53 genes may remain normal and produce normal protein, but a foreign protein may interfere with p53 protein function by forming a complex. Some proteins with which wild-type p53 has been demonstrated to interact include those of transforming viruses such as the large T antigen of simian virus 40 (SV40), and adenovirus E1B. In some instances the complex leads to rapid destruction of wild-type p53 protein.[38,50,111,113,126]

Human papillomavirus appears to intervene in the ability of wild-type p53 to control cellular growth. The E6 protein of HPV 16 and HPV 18 forms complexes with wild-type p53 protein and targets it for early degradation.[38,50,111,113,126] Expression of HPV 16 E6 gene appears to interfere with p53-mediated cellular response to DNA damage.[57] In contrast, the E6 protein of low-risk HPV types, such as 6 and 11, does not appear to bind to p53, providing a possible explanation for the different oncogenic risk potential of the HPV 16 versus the HPV 6 and HPV 11 types.[38]

High-risk HPV E7 product may also contribute to the development of neoplasia, through inactivation of the retinoblastoma gene product, pRB. HPV 16 E7 binding to pRB prevents pRB from binding cellular proteins and inhibits its growth-suppressing activity. E7 binding to pRB also prevents pRB-DNA binding.[120] E7 proteins of oncogenic HPV 16 bind to pRB more strongly than do E7 proteins of nononcogenic HPV 6, suggesting another molecular difference that might explain the variance in behavior of the lesions.[48,111] E7 from HPV 18, another of the major oncogenic HPV types, also has a high affinity for binding pRB.[112]

In carcinomas most commonly associated with HPV, such as those of the anus and of the uterine cervix, both p53 degradation and p53 mutation appear to be important, albeit in different tumors. HPV-positive carcinomas of the anus[25] and uterine cervix[26,111,132] retain wild-type p53, whereas HPV-negative carcinomas of those same sites exhibit loss of wild-type p53 function.[24,25,26,111,132] But the relationship between HPV and p53 is slightly more complicated than initial studies disclosed. In a group of HPV-positive anogenital cancers initially possessing wild-type p53 genes, metastases developed. Point mutations were found in the metastases, which suggested that p53 mutation is associated with a greater likelihood of developing metastases,[23] whether or not the original carcinoma contained HPV DNA.

Over time, it appears that HPV infection may clear, persist, or progress. The risk of progression to cervical intraepithelial neoplasia (CIN) or carcinoma in women with HPV-positive smears but normal cytology at initial exam has been estimated by one study as 0.082% (annual frequency), with a lifetime risk of 3.7% (G28). Simple presence of HPV infection does not, then, automatically progress to any lesion, much less dysplasia and carcinoma. Molecular studies suggest that another step in the process involves actual expression of HPV genes, especially E6 and E7, and interaction with host proteins. Mutation of host tumor suppressor genes also occurs in some patients, with associated tumor development or progression.

Where is the immune system while all of this is going on? Using enzyme-linked immunosorbent assay (ELISA) or Western blot, it can be shown that patients with condyloma acuminatum, laryngeal papillomata, and cervical carcinoma develop serum antibodies to various HPV proteins that do not appear in the sera of controls (which have included people with HPV negative cervical carcinoma).* The antibodies to some proteins are type-specific, but there is cross-reaction among minor capsid proteins. Antibody status does not appear to correlate with severity. Although antibodies may help identify HPV type, DNA analysis appears to be a more accurate method of identification (see the following section). Because lesions may occur and recur—even metastasize—with serum antibodies present, the current understanding of the relationship between HPV and the humoral immune system does not permit speculation on the development of vaccine.

Are there immune system interactions occurring at the epithelium that offer insights into the pathogenesis of HPV-related neoplasia? Uterine cervical HPV infection is associated with a significant decrease in the number of intraepithelial Langerhans cells, the main antigen-processing cells of squamous epithelia.[89] With examination of sheets of epithelium from HPV-positive cervical lesions, HPV-negative lesions, and epithelium from culposcopically normal regions from the same patients, Morelli and associates[89] found that Langerhans cells were decreased in all tissues with lesions, whether or not the lesions were HPV-positive with their methods (they postulated that most of the HPV-negative cases were false negatives). Higher-grade lesions had more residual cells than lower-grade lesions, but all had fewer cells than normal. The role of Langerhans cells in HPV infection and neoplasia is yet to be elucidated.

LABORATORY INVESTIGATIONS

Initial laboratory studies of HPV in the uterine cervix and other extraocular sites (such as the respiratory tract) relied on histopathology or cytopathology. In the early 1980s the focus turned to immunohistochemical studies, and the finding of papillomavirus-specific capsid antigens further strengthened the association between HPV and these epithelial lesions.[10,21,66,90,131] At nearly the same time, however, DNA-based technology rapidly took over on the research front, and the earliest papers demonstrating an association between HPV and conjunctival papillomata used both immunohistochemistry and DNA-based techniques, including Southern blot analysis and in situ hybridization.[68,85,92,102,136] Although immunohistochemistry suggested that conjunctival dysplasias and carcinomas were also HPV-related, initial in situ hybridization was negative.[84] With the advent of the polymerase chain reaction, a highly sensitive DNA amplification technique, HPV DNA could be identified in small ocular samples,[69,74,80,82,96] and the association between HPV and conjunctival dysplasia and carcinoma was further strengthened.

Although immunohistochemical studies demonstrate that a papillomavirus is present, important information is added with DNA studies—HPV type. Among the over 62 known HPV types, most differ from one another in relatively small ways in DNA sequences. Specific HPV types are associated with very different lesions. HPV types 6 and 11 are predominantly associated with papillomata of the respiratory tract and conjunctival, anogenital condylomata, and benign HPV-related epithelial lesions of other mucosal surfaces. HPV types 16, 18, 31, 33, and 35, in order of diminishing frequency, are most commonly found in dysplasias, carcinomas in situ, and invasive carcinomas of these same sites.[135] There are now commercially-available DNA-based techniques that permit identification of HPV type from fresh, frozen, or formalin-fixed, paraffin-embedded tissues or swabs of cervical samples (for example, Virapap,* in addition to the PCR-based DNA studies that dominate the ophthalmology HPV literature. Although PCR is most reliable when done by an experienced laboratory because of the danger of contamination, information about HPV type could, in theory, be ascertained for every lesion suspected of being HPV-related.

Is there any point to establishing that a specific patient's conjunctival or corneal lesion is HPV-associated, or to doing HPV typing? The most persuasive argument for doing HPV typing is that it may help in understanding the epidemiology of ocular HPV infection. For individual patients the value of any HPV information is less clear. The presence or absence of HPV in ocular lesions does not, at this point, help predict whether or not the lesion will recur. When and if more patients are studied, and long-term follow-up studies that include HPV information are performed, HPV-associated lesions may be found to have a different course from those that are HPV-negative. But in the absence of data, there seems to

---

*References 7, 8, 19, 41, 53, 55, 77, 91, 133.

*Life Technology Industries, Gaithersberg, Maryland.

be no reason to note whether or not a given patient's lesion is HPV-associated.

If a more specific approach is taken and HPV type is noted, will that information be of value in predicting outcome? Again, probably not for individual patients. Although the small number of conjunctival lesions reported to date appear to conform exactly to the high-risk and low-risk designations correlating HPV type and severity of lesions, there are enough exceptions reported in the cervix that HPV type alone should not be used to predict outcome. There are HPV 11 positive invasive carcinomas and HPV 16 positive papillomata. Lesions must be treated according to their grade, rather than according to the presence or type of HPV. This conclusion has been reached for treating cervical lesions,[135] and, it seems logical to extend it to the conjunctiva and cornea.

THERAPY

The treatment of choice for conjunctival papillomas and dysplasia/carcinoma has always been surgical, with various suggested treatments to "sterilize" the base of the lesions such as cryotherapy, cautery, diathermy, irradiation, and keratolytics.* Surgery remains the treatment of choice, although up to 40% of HPV-related ocular lesions recur.[103]

There are reports of other modalities to treat ocular disease, such as carbon dioxide laser.[9,110] As might be predicted from their relative frequency, anogenital lesions have been much more extensively studied, and a variety of other therapies have been tried, with about the same rate of success as surgery. Carbon dioxide laser has been used to treat cervical HPV,[107,108] but the same group whose initial report identified a marked improvement in treatment with laser over "routine" surgery, could find no difference between the two therapies in a later report. In addition, intact, therefore potentially infectious, HPV DNA has been recovered from the laser vapor following treatment of skin warts.[39] As HPV can infect the respiratory tract and other mucous membranes of any person in the operating room, caution in the use of CO_2 laser to treat HPV-related lesions was suggested.

Topical Antimetabolites

5-FU is an antimetabolite known to inhibit fibroblast proliferation, and it has been used to increase the success of filtering surgery in the treatment of glaucoma.[3] Topical 5-FU has been used as an adjunct to CO_2 laser ablation in the treatment of HPV-associated lesions of the uterine cervix and vagina. Weekly applications for 8 weeks in a group of 20 patients resulted in normal vaginal biopsies in 88% (15 of 17) and normal cervical biopsies in 59% (10 of 17), with treatment failures confined to the patients with HPVs of a high-risk type.[11] A 5% solution of 5-FU applied to intact corneal epithelium of rabbits delayed epithelial healing,[1] suggesting that HPV-related conjunctival lesions might also

respond to 5-FU. Studies of 5-FU and fellow antimetabolite mitomycin C have concentrated on avoiding ocular epithelial injury, which with mitomycin C can be quite severe.[1] These compounds might be considered in investigations of the treatment for conjunctival dysplasia and papilloma (to follow surgery), but studies addressing the issue have not been done.

Another topical treatment that has been tried in ocular disease is dinitrochlorobenzene (DNCB).[12,33,101] The few case reports have not been followed by larger studies, so the status of DNCB as a treatment is unclear.

Interferon

The endogenous eukaryotic reactive-protective proteins and interferons have been studied in a number of ways as possible anti-HPV treatment. Systemic injections with human leukocyte-derived interferon-alpha were initially thought to control the growth of HPV-associated laryngeal papillomas,[45] but in all studies, lesions recurred rapidly after cessation of interferon injections.[22,115] Interferon injections were accompanied in some patients by side effects such as fever, chills, myalgias, and rare neurotoxicity.[22] Psychiatric complications were also noted in patients treated with alpha-interferon for chronic viral hepatitis; it is of note that the hepatitis patients were treated with recombinant alpha-interferon, which had been expected to cut down on some of the side effects that occurred with the use of alpha-interferon extracted from human leukocytes.[106] A long-term study that evaluated patients over a 2-year period concluded that systemic interferon was "neither curative nor of substantial value as an adjunctive agent in the long-term management of recurrent respiratory papillomatosis."[47]

Interferon was also evaluated in the treatment of anogenital HPV-related lesions. In the hands of some investigators, systemic interferon appeared to diminish the recurrence rate when administered following debulking surgery.[105] In a randomized, double-blind placebo-controlled trial of patients with cervical lesions caused by a variety of HPV types, however, systemic injections with interferon-alpha (recombinant) did not show a significant therapeutic effect when compared with placebo.[134]

Some investigators tried other routes of interferon administration. Intralesional injections of recombinant interferon alfa-2b, thought to have potentially broader antiviral activity with fewer side effects, continued to result in side effects in the majority (20 of 24, 83%) of women who received them in lesions of cervical intraepithelial neoplasia. The response rate offered no advantages over the standard treatments of surgery/cryosurgery/lasersurgery.[119] Topical administration of beta-interferon in the form of a cream was reported to lead to regression in nearly 80% of patients whose culposcopic abnormalities were treated, and who were followed for up to 24 months. This study was neither blinded nor placebo-controlled, however, so the value of the information is uncertain.[20]

---

*References 15, 31, 35, 46, 51, 103, 124, 129.

There is a single report of the use of alpha-interferon in the treatment of ocular lesions. Five patients with multiple, recurrent conjunctival papillomas were identified, and HPV 11 DNA was found in tissues from three of the patients. All 5 were treated with surgical excision followed by daily injections of purified human leukocyte interferon-alpha for 1 month, then 2 to 3 injections weekly for 6 months. Treatment was then tapered or discontinued, and the patients were followed for from 1 to 4 years. Two of the five had no further recurrences, and the remainder had recurrences, one of which occurred during therapy. The other two recurrences developed after interferon treatment was stopped. All patients experienced some side effects, though none were so debilitating that treatment had to be stopped. The authors concluded that ''A regimen of interferon therapy appears to be tumor suppressive, but not curative.'' They nonetheless suggested randomized, controlled clinical trials, which, because of the rarity of papillomas, are yet to be carried out by any group.[67] There is a single additional case report of interferon use in a 4-year-old girl.[18]

The only FDA-approved treatment with interferon for HPV disease is the use of intralesional interferon-alpha for anogenital condyloma. In addition, interferons of all types are extremely expensive. The available information suggests that the enthusiasm for interferons as a treatment for ocular HPV-related disease should, at present, be tepid.

Retinoids

Are there other possible treatment modalities for HPV that can be suggested by basic studies of viral growth or proliferation? Retinoic acid is one. Retinoic acid (vitamin A) is a regulator of epithelial cell differentiation, and it has been shown to inhibit the growth of HPV 18-positive immortalized cervical carcinoma cells, HeLa cells.[4] Retinoic acid-receptors may be negative regulators for the expression of HPV 18 E6 and E7 genes, mentioned previously as key elements in the development of malignancy.[4] HPV 16-infected human keratinocytes (squamous epithelial cells) are also inhibited in their production of E6 and E7 when treated with retinoic acid, and HPV-infected cells are more sensitive to the effects on growth of retinoic acid than are noninfected cells.[59]

Retinoic acid ointment has been tested in the treatment of dry eye, for which it was ultimately found no more effective than placebo.[42] It was nontoxic in the concentrations used in the study ranging from 0.01% to 0.1% up to 4 times daily. Topical application of retinoic acid to ocular HPV-related lesions might be a fruitful area of investigation.

Steroids

Another avenue for HPV treatment may also show promise. Following up on studies suggesting that HPV infections could be influenced by sex steroid hormones, Monsonego and associates[88] studied anogenital HPV-related lesions and found that cervical dysplasias and carcinomas positive for HPV 16 and 18 DNA contained high levels of progesterone receptors. HPV 16-positive cervical carcinoma cells also have glucocorticoid receptors, and glucocorticoid administration (as dexamethasone) leads to enhanced transcription rates of E6 and E7 in some HPV-positive cervical carcinoma cell lines.[28] The drug RU-486 is an antiprogesterone and an antiglucocorticoid. In an experimental system in which HPV 16-transforming genes were used to transform primary baby rat kidney cells, RU-486 led to severe growth inhibition and cell death when administered to cells initially transformed in the absence of RU-486.[100] In other experiments studying HPV-positive cervical carcinoma cell lines, RU-486 interfered with cellular response to progesterone and glucocorticoids.[17] Unfortunately, the noncervical, HPV-positive lesions studied by one group of investigators did not contain progesterone receptors,[88] making the relevance of this work to the eye unclear.

PREVENTION

Are people with known HPV-related disease of the anogenital or respiratory tracts at risk of developing ocular infection and ocular lesions? Are people with ocular disease capable of passing their infections on to others as ocular or nonocular infections? Will the current epidemic of anogenital HPV infection be followed by an epidemic of ocular HPV-related lesions? This has been the case with other sexually transmitted organisms that are capable of involving the eye. Historically, the rates of adult inclusion conjunctivitis, and syphilitic ocular disease were directly related to prior increases in the incidence of venereal infections with chlamydia[78] and syphilis,[117] respectively. Autoinoculation by genito-ocular or genito-digital-ocular routes is an important mechanism by which herpes simplex, another epidemic sexually transmitted disease,[117] reaches the eye.[97] There are groups one would expect to be most vulnerable to HPV-related lesions, such as people with HIV infection and AIDS, and there are a few case reports of conjunctival dysplasia and carcinoma in HIV-positive or AIDS patients.[58,60,130] But in spite of the large number of AIDS patients with cervical or anal dysplasias and carcinomas, widespread ocular HPV-related lesions have not occurred.

This discussion has come full circle. To recap: first, HPV is an epidemic, and it plays an important, direct role in the development of some mucosal carcinomas. Second, HPV can grow in the eye. Yet most ophthalmologists have never seen ocular manifestations of HPV and even fewer have considered the possibility that they might represent viral lesions.[119] Given the difficulty in treating HPV in other, less-delicate body sites, it is hoped that HPV-related ocular lesions will remain unusual.

REFERENCES

1. Ando H, Ido T, Kaway Y et al.: Inhibition of corneal epithelial wound healing: a comparative study of mitomycin C and 5-fluorouracil, *Ophthalmology* 99:1809-1814, 1992.

2. Ash JE: Epibulbar tumors, *Am J Ophthalmol* 33:1203-1219, 1950.

3. Avinoam O, Ticho U: A randomized study of trabeculectomy and subconjunctival administration of fluorouracil in primary glaucomas, *Arch Ophthalmol* 110:1072-1075, 1992.

4. Bartsch D, Boye B, Baust C et al.: Retinoic acid-mediated repression of human papillomavirus 18 transcription and different ligand regulation of the retinoic acid receptor beta gene in non-tumorigenic and tumorigenic HeLa hybrid cells, *EMBO J* 11:2283-2291, 1992.

5. Basu J, Palan PR, Vermund SH et al.: Plasma ascorbic acid and beta-carotene levels in women evaluated for HPV infection, smoking, and cervix dysplasia, *Cancer Detect Prev* 15:165-170, 1991.

6. Bergman A, Nalick R: Prevalence of human papillomavirus infection in men: comparison of the partners of infected and uninfected women, *J Reproduct Med* 37:710-712, 1992.

7. Bonnez W, DaRin C, Rose RC et al.: Evolution of the antibody response to human papillomavirus type 11 (HPV-11) in patients with condyloma acuminatum according to treatment response, *J Med Virol* 39:340-344, 1993.

8. Bonnez W, Kashima HK, Leventhal B et al.: Antibody response to human papillomavirus (HPV) type 11 in children with juvenile-onset recurrent respiratory papillomatosis (RRP), *Virology* 188:384-387, 1992.

9. Bosniak SL, Novick NL, Sachs ME: Treatment of recurrent squamous papillomata of the conjunctiva by carbon dioxide laser vaporization, *Ophthalmology* 93:1078-1082, 1986.

10. Braun L, Kashima H, Eggleston J et al.: Demonstration of papillomavirus antigen in paraffin sections of laryngeal papillomas, *Laryngoscope* 92:640-643, 1982.

11. Brodman M, Dottine P, Frieddman Jr F et al.: Human papillomavirus-associated lesions of the vagina and cervix, *J Reprod Med* 37:453-456, 1992.

12. Burns RP, Wankum G, Giangiacoma J, Anderson PC: Dinitrochlorobenzene and debulking therapy of conjunctival papilloma, *J Pediatr Ophthalmol Strabismus* 20:221-226, 1983.

13. Butterworth CE, Hatch KD, Macaluso M et al.: Folate deficiency and cervical dysplasia, *JAMA* 276:528-533, 1992.

14. Cameron JA, Hidayat AH: Squamous cell carcinoma of the cornea, *Am J Ophthalmol* 111:571-574, 1991.

15. Carroll JM, Kuwabara T: A classification of limbal epitheliomata, *Arch Ophthalmol* 73:545-551, 1965.

16. Caussy D, Goedert JJ, Palefsky J: Interaction of human immunodeficiency and papillomaviruses: association with anal epithelial abnormality in homosexual men, *Int J Cancer* 214-219, 1990.

17. Chan W-K, Klock G, Bernaard H-U: Progesterone and glucocorticoid response elements occur in the long control regions of several human papillomaviruses involved in anogenital neoplasia, *J Virol* 63:3261-3269, 1989.

18. Chiemchaisri Y, Wasi C, Tuchinda C et al.: The regression of recurrent conjunctival papillomas by lymphoblastoid interferon treatment, *J Med Assoc Thai* 73:406-413, 1990.

19. Chrestensen ND, Kreider JW, Shah KV, Rando RF: Detection of human serum antibodies that neutralize infectious human papillomavirus type 11 virions, *J Gen Virol* 73:1261-1267, 1992.

20. Cinel A, Wittenberg L, Minucce D: Beta-interferon topical treatment in low and high risk cervical lesions, *Clin Exp Obstet Gynecol* 18:911-917, 1991.

21. Costa J, Howley PM, Bowling MC et al.: Presence of human papilloma viral antigens in juvenile multiple laryngeal papilloma, *Am J Clin Pathol* 75:194-197, 1981.

22. Crockett DM, McCabe BF, Lusk RP, Mixon JH: Side effects and toxicity of interferon in the treatment of recurrent respiratory papillomatosis, *Ann Otol Rhinol Laryngol* 96:601-607, 1987.

23. Crook T, Vousden KH: Properties of p53 mutations detected in primary and secondary cervical cancers suggest mechanisms of metastasis and involvement of environmental carcinogens, *EMBO J* 11:3935-3940, 1992.

24. Crook T, Wrede D, Tidy JA et al.: Clonal p53 mutation in primary cervical cancer: association with human-papillomavirus-negative tumours, *Lancet* 339:1070-1073, 1992.

25. Crook T, Wrede D, Tidy J et al.: Status of c-myc, p53 and retinoblastoma genes in human papillomavirus positive and negative squamous cell carcinomas of the anus, *Oncogene* 6:1251-1257, 1991.

26. Crook T, Wrede D, Vousden KH: p53 point mutation in HPV negative human cervical carcinoma cell lines, *Oncogene* 6:873-875, 1991.

27. Csango PA, Skuland J, Nilsen A et al.: Papillomavirus infection amount abortion applicants and patients at a sexually transmitted disease clinic, *Sex Transm Dis* 19:149-153, 1992.

28. Doeberitz MVK, Bauknecht T, Bartsch D, zur Hausen H: Influence of chromosomal integration on glucocorticoid-regulated transcription of growth-stimulating papillomavirus genes E6 and E7 in cervical carcinoma cells, *Proc Natl Acad Sci USA* 88:1411-1415, 1991.

29. Durst M, Croce CM, Gissmann L et al.: Papillomavirus sequences integrate near cellular oncogenes in some cervical carcinomas, *Proc Natl Acad Sci USA* 84:1070-1074, 1987.

30. Durst M, Kleinheinz A, Hotz M, Gissmann L: The physical state of human papillomavirus type 16 DNA in benign and malignant genital tumours, *J Gen Virol* 66:1515-1522, 1985.

31. Erie JC, Campbell RJ, Liesegang TJ: Conjunctival and corneal intraepithelial and invasive neoplasia, *Ophthalmology* 93:176-183, 1986.

32. Ferenczy A, Mitao M, Nagai N et al.: Latent papillomavirus and recurring genital warts, *N Engl J Med* 313:784-788, 1985.

33. Ferry AP, Meltzer MA, Taub RN: Immunotherapy with dinitrochlorobenzene for recurrent squamous cell tumor of conjunctiva, *Trans Am Ophthalmol Soc* 74:154-171, 1976.

34. Fisher M, Rosenfeld WD, Burk RD: Cervicovaginal human papillomavirus infection in suburban adolescents and young adults, *J Pediatr* 119:821-825, 1991.

35. Fraunfelder FT, Wingfield D: Management of intraepithelial conjunctival tumors and squamous cell carcinomas, *Am J Ophthalmol* 95:359-363, 1983.

36. Fredericks BD, Balkin A, Daniel HW et al.: Transmission of human papillomaviruses from mother to child, *Aust NZ J Obstet Gynaecol* 33:30-32, 1993.

37. Fu Y-S, Hoover L, Franklin M et al.: Human papillomavirus identified by nucleic acid hybridization in concomitant nasal and genital papillomas, *Laryngoscope* 102:1014-1019, 1992.

38. Gage JR, Meyers C, Wettstein FO: The E7 proteins of the nononcogenic human papillomavirus type 6b (HPV-6b) and of the oncogenic HPV-16 differ in retinoblastoma protein binding and other properties, *J Virol* 64:723-730, 1990.

39. Garden JM, O'Banion MK, Shelnitz LS et al.: Papillomavirus in the vapor of carbon dioxide laser-treated verrucae, *JAMA* 259:1199-1202, 1988.

40. Reference deleted in proofs.

41. Ghosh AK, Smith NK, Stacey SN et al.: Serological response to HPV 16 in cervical dysplasia and neoplasia: correlation of antibodies to E6 with cervical cancer, *Int J Cancer* 53:591-596, 1993.

42. Gilbard JP, Huang AJW, Belldegrun R et al.: Open-label crossover study of vitamin A ointment (all-trans retinoic acid) as a treatment for keratoconjunctivitis sicca, *Ophthalmology* 96:244-246, 1989.

43. Green J, Monteiro E, Bolton VN et al.: Detection of human papillomavirus DNA by PCR in semen from patients with and without penile warts, *Genitourin Med* 67:207-210, 1991.

44. Grosniklaus HE, Green WR, Luckenbach M, Chan CC: Conjunctival lesions in adults, *Cornea* 6:78-116, 1987.

45. Haglund S, Lundquist P-G, Cantell K, Strander H: Interferon therapy in juvenile laryngeal papillomatosis, *Arch Otolaryngol* 107:327-332, 1981.

46. Harkey ME, Metz HS: Cryotherapy of conjunctival papillomata, *Am J Ophthalmol* 66:872-874, 1968.

47. Healy BG, Gelber RD, Trowbridge AL et al.: Treatment of recurrent respiratory papillomatosis with human leukocyte interferon, results of a multicenter randomized clinical trial, *New Eng J Med* 391:401-407, 1988.

48. Hech DV, Yee CL, Howley PM, Munger K: Efficiency of binding the retinoblastoma protein correlates with the transforming capacity of the E7 oncoproteins of the human papillomaviruses, *Proc Natl Acad Sci USA* 89:4442-4446, 1992.

49. Hollstein M, Sidransky D, Vogenstein B, Harris CC: p53 mutations in human cancers, *Science* 253:49-53, 1991.
50. Hubbert NL, Sedman SA, Schiller JT: Human papillomavirus type 16 E6 increases the degradation rate of p53 in human keratinocytes, *J Virol* 66:6237-6241, 1992.
51. Irvine AR Jr: Dyskeratotic epibulbar tumors, *Trans Am Ophthalmol Soc* 61:243-273, 1963.
52. Jalal H, Sanders CA, Prime SS et al.: Detection of human papilloma virus type 16 DNA in oral squames from normal young adults, *J Oral Pathol Med* 21:465-470, 1992.
53. Jochmus I, Bouwes-Bavinck JN, Gissman L: Detection of antibodies to the E4 or E7 proteins of human papillomaviruses (HPV) in human sera by western blot analysis: type-specific reaction of ando-HPV-16 antibodies, *Mol Cell Probes* 6:319-325, 1992.
54. Johnson JC, Burnett AF, Willet GD et al.: High frequency of latent and clinical human papillomavirus cervical infections in immunocompromised human immunodeficiency virus-infected women, *Obstet Gynecol* 79:321-327, 1992.
55. Kanda T, Onda T, Zanma S et al.: Independent association of antibodies against human papillomavirus type 16 E1/E4 and E7 proteins with cervical cancer, *Virology* 190:724-732, 1992.
56. Kellokoski J, Syrjaenen S, Yliskoski M, Syrjaenen K: Dot blot hybridization in detection of human papillomavirus (HPV) infections in the oral cavity of women with genital HPV infections, *Oral Microbiol Immunol* 7:19-23, 1992.
57. Kessis TD, Slebos RJ, Nelson WB et al.: *Proc Natl Acad Sci USA* 90:3988-3992, 1993.
58. Kesthlyn P, Stevens A-M, Ndayambaje A et al.: HPV and conjunctival malignancies, *Lancet* 336:51-52, 1990.
59. Khan MA, Jenkins GR, Tollesion WH et al.: Retinoic acid inhibition of human papillomavirus type 16-mediated transformation of human keratinocytes, *Cancer Res* 53:905-909, 1993.
60. Kim RY, Selff SR, Howos HL, O'Donnell JJ: Necrotizing scleritis secondary to conjunctival squamous cell carcinoma in acquired immunodeficiency syndrome, *Am J Ophthalmol* 109:231-233, 1990.
61. Kivaty N, Rompalo A, Bowden R et al.: Anal human papillomavirus infection among human immunodeficiency virus-seropositive and -seronegative men, *J Infect Dis* 162:358-361, 1990.
62. Kiviat NB, Critchlow CW, Holmes KK et al.: Association of anal dysplasia and human papillomavirus with immunosuppression and HIV infection among homosexual men, *AIDS* 7:43-49, 1993.
63. Knudson A Jr: Genetics of tumors of the head and neck, *Arch Otolaryngeal Head Neck Surg* 119:735-737, 1993.
64. Koss LG, Durfee GR: Unusual patterns of squamous epithelium of the uterine cervix and pathologic study of kiolocytotic atypia, *Ann NY Acad Sci* 63:1245-1261, 1956.
65. Laga M, Icenogle JP, Marsella R et al.: Genital papillomavirus infection and cervical dysplasia—opportunistic complications of HIV infection, *Int J Cancer* 50:4a5a-8, 1992.
66. Lancaster W, Jenson AB: Evidence for papillomavirus genus-specific antigen and DNA in laryngeal papillomas, *Intervirology* 15:204-212, 1981.
67. Lass JH, Foster CS, Grove AS et al.: Interferon-alpha therapy of recurrent conjunctival papillomas, *Am J Ophthalmol* 103:294-301, 1987.
68. Lass JH, Grove AS, Papale JJ et al.: Detection of human papillomavirus DNA sequences in conjunctival papilloma, *Am J Ophthalmol* 96:670-674, 1983.
69. Lauer SA, Malter JS, Meier JR: Human papillomavirus type 18 in conjunctival intraepithelial neoplasia, *Am J Ophthalmol* 110:23-27, 1990.
70. Law CL, Qassim M, Thompson CH et al.: Factors associated with clinical and sub-clinical anal human papillomavirus infection in homosexual men, *Genitourin Med* 67:92-98, 1991.
71. Lechner MS, Mack DH, Finicle AB et al.: Human papillomavirus E6 proteins bind p53 in vivo and abrogate p53-mediated repression of transcription, *EMBO J* 11:3045-3052, 1992.
72. Lee GA, Hirst LW: Incidence of ocular surface epithelial dysplasia in metropolitan Brisbane: a 10-year study, *Arch Ophthalmol* 110:525-527, 1992.
73. Levine AJ, Momand J, Finlay CA: The p53 tumour suppressor gene, *Nature* 351:453-456, 1991.
74. Madreperla SA, Green WR, Daniel R, Shah KV: Human papillomavirus in primary epithelial tumors of the lacrimal sac, *Ophthalmology* 100:569-573, 1993.
75. Mandal D, Haye KR, Ray TK et al.: Prevalence of occult human papillomavirus infection, determined by cytology and DNA hybridization, in heterosexual men attending a genitourinary medicine clinic, *Int J STD AIDS* 2:351-355, 1991.
76. Mandelblatt J, Richart R, Thomas L et al.: Is human papillomavirus associated with cervical neoplasia in the elderly? *Gynecol Oncol* 46:6-12, 1992.
77. Mandelson MT, Jenison SA, Sherman KJ et al.: The association of human papillomavirus antibodies with cervical cancer risk, *Cancer Epidemiol Biomarkers Prev* 1:281-286, 1992.
78. Mannis MJ: Chlamydial disease. In *The cornea*, Kaufman HE, Barron BA, McDonald MB, Waltman SR, editors: 201-216, New York, 1988, Churchill Livingston.
79. Matlashewski G: The cell biology of human papillomavirus transformed cells, *Anticancer Res* 1447-1556, 1989.
80. McDonnell JM, Mayr AJ, Martin WJ: DNA of human papillomavirus type 16 in dysplastic and malignant lesions of the conjunctiva and cornea, *N Engl J Med* 320:1442-1446, 1989.
81. McDonnell JM, McDonnell PJ, Mounts P et al.: Demonstration of papillomavirus capsid antigen in human conjunctival neoplasia, *Arch Ophthalmol* 104:1801-1805, 1986.
82. McDonnell JM, McDonnell PJ, Sun YY: Human papillomavirus DNA in tissues and ocular surface swabs of patients with conjunctival epithelial neoplasia, *Invest Ophthalmol Vis Sci* 33:184-189, 1992.
83. McDonnell JM, Wagner D, Ng ST et al.: Human papillomavirus type 16 DNA in ocular and cervical swabs of women with genital tract condylomata, *Am J Ophthalmol* 112:61-66, 1991.
84. McDonnell PJ, McDonnell JM, Kessis T et al.: Detection of human papillomavirus type 6/11 DNA in conjunctival papillomas by in situ hybridization with radioactive probes, *Hum Pathol* 18:1115-1119, 1987.
85. McGavic JS: Intraepithelial epithelioma of the corneal and conjunctival (Bowen's disease), *Am J Ophthalmol* 25:167-176, 1942.
86. Meltzer SJ, Yin J, Huang Y et al.: Reduction to homozygosity involving p53 in esophageal cancers demonstrated by the polymerase chain reaction, *Proc Nat Acad Sci USA* 88:4976-4980, 1991.
87. Migliori ME, Putterman AM: Recurrent conjunctival papilloma causing nasolacrimal duct obstruction, *Am J Ophthalmol* 110:17-22, 1990.
88. Monsonego J, Magdelenat H, Catalan F et al.: Estrogena and progesterone receptors in cervical human papillomavirus related lesions, *Int J Cancer* 48:533-539, 1991.
89. Morelli AE, Sananes C, Di Paola G et al.: Relationship between types of human papillomavirus and Langerhans' cells in cervical condyloma and intraepithelial neoplasia, *Am J Clin Pathol* 99:200-206, 1993.
90. Mounts P, Shah KV, Kashima H: Viral etiology of juvenile and adult onset squamous papilloma of the larynx, *Proc Natl Acad Sci USA* 79:5425-5429, 1982.
91. Mueller M, Viscidi RP, Sun Y et al.: Antibodies to HPV-16 E6 and E7 proteins as markers for HPV-16 associated invasive cervical cancer, *Virology* 187:508-514, 1992.
92. Naghashfar Z, McDonnell PJ, McDonnell JM et al.: Genital tract papillomavirus type 6 in recurrent conjunctival papilloma, *Arch Ophthalmology* 104:1814-1815, 1986.
93. Napora C, Cohen EJ, Genvert GI et al.: Factors associated with conjunctival entraepithelial neoplasia: a case control study, *Ophthalmic Surg* 21:27-30, 1990.
94. National Institute of Allergy and Infectious Disease: *Fact sheet on sexually transmitted disease,* 1989.
95. Nicholson DH, Green WR: Tumors of the eye, lids, and orbit in children. In Nelson LB, Calhoun JH, Harley RH, editors: *Pediatric ophthalmology,* ed 3, 923-1067, Philadelphia, 1991, WB Saunders.
96. Odrich MG, Jakobiec FA, Lancaster WD et al.: A spectrum of bilateral squamous conjunctival tumors associated with human papillomavirus type 16, *Ophthalmology* 98:628-635, 1991.
97. Oh J: Ocular infections of herpes simplex virus type 2 in adults. In Darrell RW, editor: *Viral diseases of the eye,* 59-62, Philadelphia, 1985, Lea and Febiger.

98. Palefsky JM, Holly EA, Gonzales J et al.: Natural history of analy cytologic abnormalities and papillomavirus infection among homosexual men with group IV HIV disease, *J AIDS* 5:1258-1265, 1992.

99. Panici PB, Scambia G, Perrone L et al.: Oral condyloma lesions in patients with extensive genital human papillomavirus infection, *Am J Obstet Gynecol* 167:451-458, 1992.

100. Pater MM, Pater A: RU486 inhibits glucocorticoid hormone-dependent oncogenesis by human papillomavirus type 16 DNA, *Virology* 183:799-802, 1992.

101. Petrelli R, Cotlier E, Robins S, Stoessel K: Dinitrochlorobenzene immunotherapy of recurrent squamous papilloma of the conjunctival, *Ophthalmology* 88:1221-1225, 1981.

102. Pfister H, Fuchs PG, Volcker HE: Human papillomavirus DNA in conjunctival papilloma, *Graefes Arch Clin Exp Ophthalmol* 223:164-167, 1985.

103. Pizzarello LD, Jakobiec FA: Bowen's disease of the conjunctiva: a misnomer. In Jakobiec FA, editor: *Ocular and adnexal tumors,* 553-671, Birmingham, 1978, Aesculapius Publishing.

104. Reid R, Greenberg M, Jenson AB et al.: Sexually transmitted papillomaviral infections. I. The anatomic distribution and pathologic grade of neoplastic lesions associated with different viral types, *Am J Obstet Gynecol* 156:212-222, 1987.

105. Reid R, Greenberg MD, Pizzuti DJ et al.: Superficial laser vulvectomy. V: surgical debulking is enhanced by adjuvant systemic interferon, *Am J Obstet Gynecol* 166:815-820, 1992.

106. Renault PF, Hoofnagle JH, Park Y et al.: Psychiatric complications of long-term interferon alpha therapy, *Arch Intern Med* 147:1577-1580, 1987.

107. Ruge S, Felding C, Skouby SO et al.: CO_2-laser vaporization of human papillomavirus (HPV)-induced abnormal cervical smears: a simple and effective solution to a recurrent clinical problem, *Clin Exp Obstet Gynecol* 18:99-101, 1991.

108. Ruge S, Felding C, Skouby SO et al.: CO_2 laser vaporization in the treatment of cervical human papillomavirus infection in women with abnormal Papanicolaou smears, *Gynecol Obstet Invest* 33:172-176, 1992.

109. Ryan SJ, Font RL: Primary epithelial neoplasms of the lacrimal sac, *Am J Ophthalmol* 76:73-88, 1973.

110. Schachat A, Illiff WJ, Kashima HK: Carbon dioxide laser therapy of recurrent squamous papilloma of the conjunctiva, *Ophthalmic Surg* 13:916-918, 1982.

111. Scheffner M, Muenger K, Byren JC, Howley PM: The state of the p53 and retinoblastoma genes in human cervical carcinoma cell lies, *Proc Natl Acad Sci USA* 88:5523-5527, 1991.

112. Scheffner M, Muenger K, Huibregtse JM, Howley PM: Targeted degradation of the retinoblastoma protein by human papillomavirus E6-E7 fusion proteins, *EMBO J* 11:2425-2431, 1992.

113. Scheffner M, Werness BA, Huibregtse JM et al.: The E6 oncoprotein encoded by human papillomavirus types 16 and 18 promotes the degradation of p53, *Cell* 63:1129-1136, 1990.

114. Scherner A, Galvin S, Sun TT: Differentiation-related expression of a major 64K corneal keratin in vivo and in culture suggests limbal location of corneal epithelial stem cells, *J Cell Biol* 103:49-63, 1986.

115. Schouten TJ, Weimar W, Bos JH et al.: Treatment of juvenile laryngeal papillomatosis with two types of interferon, *Laryngoscope* 92:686-688, 1982.

116. Smith EM, Johnson SR, Cripe TP et al.: Perinatal vertical transmission of human papillomavirus and subsequent development of respiratory tract papillomatosis, *Ann Otol Rhinol Laryngol* 100:479-483, 1991.

117. Smith RE, Nozik RA: Syphilis, tuberculosis and miscellaneous infections. In Smith RE, Nozik RA, editors: *Uveitits: a clinical approach to diagnosis and management,* 213-221, Baltimore, 1989, Williams and Wilkins.

118. Spencer WH, Zimmerman LE: Conjunctiva. In Spencer WH, editor: *Ophthalmic pathology,* ed 3, 109-228, Philadelphia, 1985, WB Saunders.

119. Stellato G: Intralesional recombinant alpha 2B interferon in the treatment of human papillomavirus-associated cervical intraepithelial neoplasia, *Sex Transm Dis* 19:124-126, 1992.

120. Stirdivant SM, Huber HE, Patrick DR et al.: Human papillomavirus type 16 E7 protein inhibits DNA binding by the retinoblastoma gene product, *Mol Cell Biol* 12:1905-1914, 1992.

121. Streeten BW, Carrillo R, Jamison R et al.: Inverted papilloma of the conjunctiva, *Am J Ophthalmol* 88:1062-1066, 1979.

122. Vermund SH, Kelley KF, Klein RS et al.: High risk of human papillomavirus infection and cervical squamous intraepithelial lesions among women with symptomatic human immunodeficiency virus infection, *Am J Obstet Gynecol* 165:382-400, 1991.

123. Wagatsuma M, Hashimoto K, Matsukura T: Analysis of integrated human papillomavirus type 16 DNA in cervical cancers: amplification of viral sequences together with cellular flanking sequences, *J Virol* 64:813-821, 1990.

124. Waring GO, Roth AM, Elkins MB: Clinical and pathologic description of 17 cases of corneal intraepithelial neoplasia, *Am J Ophthalmol* 97:547-559, 1984.

125. Weinberg RA: Tumor suppressor genes, *Science* 254:1138-1146, 1991.

126. Werness BA, Levine AJ, Howley PM: Association of human papillomavirus types 16 and 18 E6 proteins with p53, *Science* 248:76-79, 1990.

126a. Weskamp C: Bowen's disease of the cornea, *Arch Ophthalmol* 31:310-315, 1944.

127. Williams R, Ilsar M, Welham RAN: Lacrimal canalicular papillomatosis, *Br J Ophthalmol* 69:464-467, 1985.

128. Wilson II FM, Ostler HB: Conjunctival papillomas in siblings, *Am J Ophthalmol* 77:103-107, 1974.

129. Winter FC, Kleh TR: Precancerous epithelioma of the limbus, *Arch Ophthalmol* 64:208-215, 1960.

130. Winward KE, Curtin VT: Conjunctival squamous cell carcinoma in a patient with human immunodeficiency virus infection, *Am J Ophthalmol* 107:554-555, 1989.

131. Woodruff JD, Braun L, Cavalieri R et al.: Immunologic identification of papillomavirus antigen in condyloma tissues from the female genital tract, *Obstet Gynecol* 56:727-732, 1980.

132. Wrede D, Tidy JA, Crook T et al.: Expression of RB and p53 proteins in HPV-positive and HPV-negative cervical carcinoma cell lines, *Mol Carcinog* 4:171-175, 1991.

133. Yaegashi N, Jenson SA, Batra M, Galloway DA: Human antibodies recognize multiple distinct type-specific and cross-reactive regions of the minor capsid proteins of human papillomavirus types 6 and 11, *J Virol* 66:2008-2019, 1992.

134. Yliskoski M, Syrjaenen K, Syrjaenen S et al.: Systemic alpha-interferon (Wellferon) treatment of genital human papillomavirus (HPV) type 6, 11, 16, and 18 infections: double-blind, placebo-controlled trial, *Gynecol Oncol* 43:55-60, 1991.

135. Young LS, Tierney RJ, Ellis JR et al.: PCR for the detection of genital human papillomavirus infection: a mixed blessing, *Ann Med* 24:215-219, 1992.

136. Zur Hausen H: Viruses in human cancers, *Science* 254:1167-1173, 1991.

68 Newcastle Disease

T. RODMAN WOOD

Newcastle disease virus, an important cause of morbidity and mortality among poultry throughout the world, causes a brief infection of the external eye in humans, presenting as an acute follicular conjunctivitis. The disease is occupationally related and occurs predominantly in poultry workers, veterinarians, and laboratory workers.

HISTORICAL BACKGROUND

Newcastle disease in chickens first appeared in England, Java, and Korea in 1926, and the first description was given in the Dutch East Indies by Kraneveld.[10] The viral cause of the disease was proved by Doyle[4] during an outbreak at Newcastle-upon-Tyne, England, in 1927. That city's name was given to the illness by Doyle to avoid confusion with other fowl diseases.

Newcastle disease spread to many countries of the world. In 1944 it was reported on both coasts of the United States.[1] By 1948 Newcastle disease was established in poultry flocks throughout the United States.

The first human infection was reported by Burnet[2] in 1943 and resulted from a laboratory accident in which the virus was splashed into an eye. The first human cases in the United States were reported in 1948.[6,8] The pertinent ophthalmologic literature was reviewed by Duke-Elder[5] in 1965.

EPIDEMIOLOGY

Strains of Newcastle disease virus vary widely in virulence and in the severity of disease they cause. Lentogenic pathotypes are mildly pathogenic, mesogenic pathotypes are moderately pathogenic, and velogenic pathotypes are markedly pathogenic. The milder lentogenic and mesogenic strains are endemic in the United States and are controlled by frequent vaccination of chicken and turkey flocks. The velogenic pathotype, particularly in its viscerotropic form, is the most serious disease of poultry throughout the world. Infected birds shed large amounts of virus from the respiratory and digestive tracts. The disease is transmitted by direct contact, the fecal-oral route, aerosols produced by coughing, and contaminated watering equipment. The virus may be spread to other flocks by contaminated equipment and personnel such as vaccination teams.[1]

Newcastle disease is considered exotic to the United States and is usually introduced by caged birds or fighting cocks, often illegally imported. Traffic in pet birds has been implicated in several outbreaks in the United States including the 1971 to 1973 epizootic.

Human infections frequently occur in clusters paralleling avian epizootics. Human conjunctival infection may be acquired from infected birds or flocks by aerosols or dust of respiratory or fecal origin, by the hand-to-eye route, or from live vaccine sprays. Conjunctivitis in humans has been reported in poultry farmers,[14] vaccination teams, veterinarians,[9,14] feed salesmen,[9] poultry processors,[6,12] kitchen personnel,[9] and laboratory workers.[1,11,14] Infection occurs by inoculation onto the ocular surface, where the disease remains localized. A transient viremia occurs in most cases,[9] producing mild systemic signs but no extraocular sequelae. Human-to-human spread is rare, but cases occurring in family members of patients suggest that it can occur.[12,14] No case of human infection has been caused by consumption of poultry products.[1]

PATHOGENESIS

Virology

Newcastle disease is caused by a member of the virus family Paramyxoviridae, which consists of three genera. The genus *Paramyxovirus* includes nine serotypes of avian viruses, of which Newcastle disease virus is the prototype, as well as mumps virus and the human parainfluenza viruses. Related genera are *Morbillivirus,* which includes the agent of measles, and *Pneumovirus* which contains the respiratory syncytial virus.

Paramyxoviruses are pleomorphic when viewed by negative-contrast electron microscopy. They range from 100 to 500 nm in diameter and are round, with a loose lipoprotein envelope enclosing a helical nucleocapsid that has "herringbone" morphology. The genome is a single molecule of single-strand RNA with a molecular weight of 5 × 10⁶ daltons. The virion is susceptible to heat, desiccation, and freezing—thawing. Specimens for culture must be kept at 4°C and transported to the laboratory promptly.[13]

The ability of Newcastle disease virus to agglutinate red blood cells is due to the HN surface protein, which forms projections on the surface of the virus particles as seen by electron microscopy. The inhibition of this reaction by antisera is a valuable tool in the diagnosis of Newcastle disease; a rising convalescent titer is diagnostic. An enzyme-linked immunosorbent assay (ELISA) technique is superior to the hemagglutination inhibition test for demonstrating antibodies to the virus.[3]

The virus multiplies readily in a variety of avian and nonavian species; the chicken is the most frequently used laboratory animal. Although the virus will grow in a wide range of cell-culture systems, embryonated hen's eggs are the preferred medium for virus isolation and culture because of their availability and the high titers that can be obtained.[1]

Avian Newcastle Disease

Newcastle disease occurs in all poultry-producing countries of the world and is endemic in Asia, Africa, and Central and South America. Most bird species are susceptible. Morbidity and mortality vary among species and by viral pathotype. Chickens are the most susceptible species, with morbidity and mortality rates of up to 100% in epizootics. Turkeys and waterfowl have a milder form of the disease. Psittacine and passerine birds may be inapparent carriers and shedders of the virus.

The pet bird trade has contributed to the spread of Newcastle disease worldwide. Three worldwide panzootics have occurred during this century. The first started in Southeast Asia in 1926 and took 30 years to spread to the rest of the world. The second panzootic started in the Middle East in the late 1960s and had spread to most countries by 1973. The virus that caused this panzootic was associated with caged psittacine birds. The third panzootic arose in the Middle East in the late 1970s and by 1981 reached Europe, where it affected mainly pigeons and doves. In 1971 to 1973 an extensive outbreak occurred in chickens and pet birds in California, Florida, and Puerto Rico; the outbreak was controlled by destroying 12,000,000 birds. As a result of these epizootics, most countries have instituted vaccination and quarantine programs to limit the importation and spread of Newcastle disease.[1]

The clinical signs of avian Newcastle disease are variable, depending on the species, age, vaccination status, and virulence of the infecting strain. The incubation period in chickens is usually 2 to 6 days. Susceptible young chickens infected with a viscerotropic, velogenic strain may die suddenly with few signs or symptoms. Commonly there is a period of listlessness with diarrhea, fever, and loss of appetite. Egg laying is severely curtailed. Chickens may have edema of the neck and periorbital area, exudate from the mouth and nares, and neurologic symptoms such as (1) torticollis with unusual positions of the head ("star-gazer" posture) and (2) paralysis.

Pathologically there is focal hemorrhage and ulceration throughout the intestinal mucosa, especially in lymphoid foci. The trachea and air sacs are inflamed.

Laboratory confirmation is imperative at the start of an outbreak. Material from cloacal or tracheal swabs is inoculated into the allantoic sacs of 8- to 11-day-old embryonated hens' eggs. Virus is found in the amniotic and allantoic fluids of killed embryos and will agglutinate avian erythrocytes, a reaction that is titrable with Newcastle disease antisera. Isolates can be inoculated into susceptible chickens. Infected chickens die within 10 days.

Vaccines, both live and inactivated, do not prevent infection but may reduce severity. They are less effective against the viscerotropic, velogenic form of Newcastle disease than against milder strains. Present policy for control and eradication of Newcastle disease requires immediate depopulation of infected flocks. Treatment is of no value and is precluded by the policy of quick eradication of flocks.

Since 1973 all poultry and birds imported into the United States from countries endemic for Newcastle disease are required to be held in quarantine for 30 days until determined to be free of poultry pathogens. Imported eggs for hatching must be hatched and brooded for 30 days in quarantine.

CLINICAL FEATURES

The most important diagnostic feature of Newcastle conjunctivitis is the history of occupational exposure to the agent. During an epidemic, the clinical diagnosis is usually readily apparent.

After a brief incubation period of 18 to 48 hours, an acute follicular conjunctivitis appears, usually unilateral. A palpable, tender preauricular lymph node is a constant finding and subsides within a week. The conjunctiva shows papillary and follicular hypertrophy with edema and congestion that is most marked in the lower fornix (Fig. 68-1). Secretion is scanty and nonpurulent. Chemosis and subconjunctival hemorrhage have been reported. A transient, mild keratitis is common, consisting of fine punctate epithelial keratitis that resolves in 3 or 4 days. Superficial infiltrates may occur,[9] and residual subepithelial opacities have been seen.[6]

Systemic signs are mild. Fever, headache, and malaise occur at the onset and disappear within a day or two. Cervical adenopathy can occur. The conjunctiva returns to normal within 7 to 10 days.

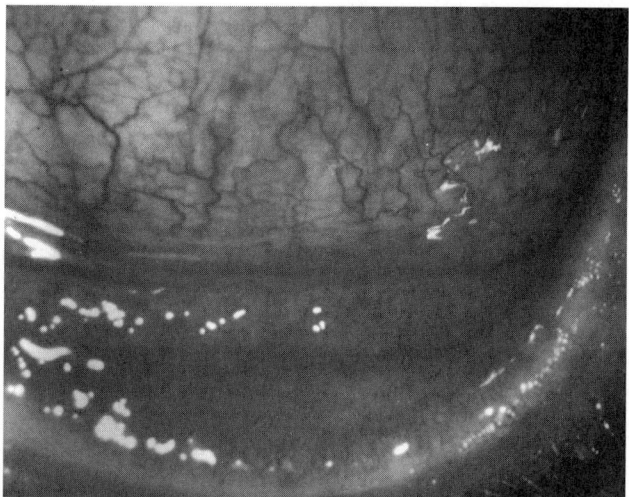

Fig. 68-1. Newcastle conjunctivitis in a veterinarian. Lower fornix shows edema, congestions, and follicular hypertrophy.

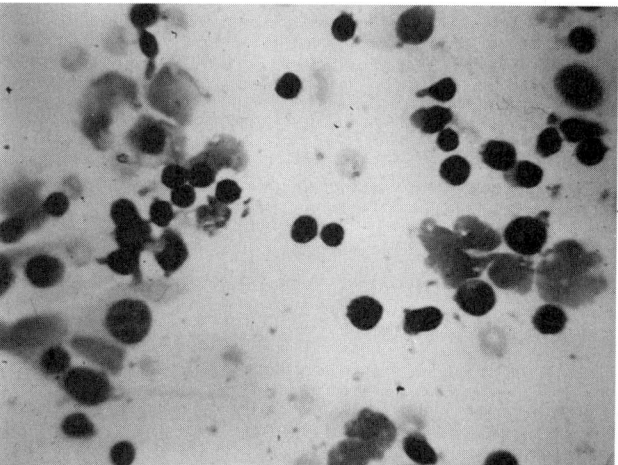

Fig. 68-2. Newcastle conjunctivitis. Conjunctival scraping stained with Giemsa stain. Inflammatory cells are almost entirely lymphocytes. (Original magnification ×1000.)

DIFFERENTIAL DIAGNOSIS

The differential diagnosis of Newcastle conjunctivitis includes other causes of acute follicular conjunctivitis. Adenoviral conjunctivitis with pharyngoconjunctival fever may be differentiated by the pharyngitis, but the onset and brief course may be otherwise quite similar. Adenoviral keratoconjunctivitis is usually more severe than Newcastle conjunctivitis with pseudomembrane formation and a longer course, with characteristic subepithelial infiltrates appearing at the end of the second week.

Adult chlamydial conjunctivitis usually presents with more follicles, coarser punctate epithelial keratitis, and a prolonged course that may become chronic. Inclusion conjunctivitis and Newcastle disease may be easily separated by the cytology of Giemsa-stained conjunctival smears: inclusion conjunctivitis has a characteristic cytologic finding of polymorphonuclear leukocytes, plasma cells, Leber cells, and epithelial inclusions, whereas Newcastle disease shows a lymphocytic exudate.

Newcastle conjunctivitis can be differentiated from acute bacterial conjunctivitis by the absence of purulence and by the systemic signs, conjunctival follicles, and preauricular adenopathy, which are not a feature of bacterial infection. Conjunctival scrapings show masses of polymorphonuclear leukocytes in bacterial cases.

LABORATORY INVESTIGATIONS

Human infection with Newcastle disease virus can be diagnosed by an increase in neutralizing or hemagglutination-inhibition antibodies or preferably by the ELISA technique. The virus can be cultured from conjunctival swabs or washings; the preferred medium is embryonated hens' eggs. Specimens for culture must be kept at 4°C in ice packs and transported to the laboratory promptly. If transport time will be prolonged, specimens should be frozen.

Conjunctival smears stained with Wright or Giemsa stain show a typical viral type of cytologic finding with an inflammatory cell component consisting almost entirely of lymphocytes (Fig. 68-2). Keeney and Hunter[9] described basophilic cytoplasmic inclusions in conjunctival epithelial cells stained with Giemsa stain but were unable to demonstrate them in scrapings from experimentally infected rabbits. Other investigators have not duplicated this observation.

THERAPY

No specific treatment is available. Since human infection with Newcastle disease virus is restricted to the external eye and is brief and nondisabling, treatment is usually unnecessary. Decongestant drops may provide some symptomatic relief.[12]

PROGNOSIS

Newcastle disease conjunctivitis usually heals in 7 days without sequelae. Subepithelial opacities disappear within 18 months and leave no trace.[6]

PREVENTION

Preventive measures for human infection include universal precautions. Protective eyewear should be worn when working with the virus in the laboratory, when administering live vaccine, and when coming in contact with infected birds.

REFERENCES

1. Alexander DJ: Newcastle disease. In Calnek BW and associates, editors: *Diseases of poultry,* ed 9, 496-519, Ames, Iowa, 1991, Iowa State University Press.
2. Burnet FM: Human infection with the virus of Newcastle disease of fowls, *Med J Aust* 2:313-314, 1943.
3. Charan S, Rai A, Mahajan VM: Comparison of enzyme-linked immunosorbent assay and hemagglutination inhibition test for the detection of Newcastle disease virus antibodies in human sera, *J Clin Pathol* 34:90-92, 1981.

4. Doyle TM: A hitherto unrecorded disease of fowls due to a filter-passing virus, *J Comp Pathol Ther* 40:144-169, 1927.

5. Duke-Elder S: *System of ophthalmology,* vol 8, *Diseases of the outer eye,* Part 1, 369-372, St Louis, 1965, Mosby.

6. Freymann MW, Bang FB: Human conjunctivitis due to Newcastle virus, *Bull Johns Hopkins Hosp* 84:409-413, 1949.

7. Hales RH, Ostler HB: Newcastle disease conjunctivitis with subepithelial infiltrates, *Br J Ophthalmol* 57:694-697, 1973.

8. Ingalls WI, Mahoney A: Isolation of Newcastle virus from humans, *Am J Public Health* 39:73740, 1949.

9. Keeney AH, Hunter MC: Human infection with the Newcastle virus of fowls, *Arch Ophthalmol* 44:573-580, 1950.

10. Kraneveld FC: Over een in Ned-Indie heerochende ziekte onder het pluimyes, *Ned Indisch Blad Diergeneesk* 38:448-450, 1926.

11. Mustaffa-Babjee A, Ibrahim AL, Khim TS: A case of human infection with Newcastle disease virus, *Asian J Trop Med Public Health* 7(4):622-624, 1976.

12. Trott DG, Pilsworth M: Outbreaks of conjunctivitis due to Newcastle disease among workers in chicken broiler factories, *BMJ* 5477:1514-1517, 1965.

13. White DO, Fenner F: *Medical virology,* ed 3, Orlando, Florida, 1986, Academic Press, Inc.

14. Wood TR, Story RF: Unpublished observations, 1971.

69 Adenovirus Keratoconjunctivitis

Y. JEROLD GORDON, KOKI AOKI, PAUL R. KINCHINGTON

Adenoviral ocular infections occur worldwide in community- and office-based epidemics. Although usually self-limited, these eye infections may be associated with significant patient morbidity and major socioeconomic consequences caused by absenteeism from work and school. Adenovirus keratoconjunctivitis is the most common viral infection of the ocular surface in many parts of the world.[6,19,30,89]

HISTORICAL BACKGROUND

In 1889 an epidemic of ocular infection spread throughout Austria, and the doctors of the day reported their findings. Adler described a "subepithelial keratitis," Fuchs observed a "superficial punctate keratitis," and Van Ruess commented on a "macular keratitis."[77] These reports provide the earliest descriptions of epidemic keratoconjunctivitis (EKC) in Western literature. Over the next fifty years reports from the United Kingdom, India, Japan, Palestine, and the United States[30] confirmed two important characteristic features of EKC: worldwide distribution and community-based epidemics.

In the late 1930s epidemics of EKC passed by maritime travel from the Far East to Hawaii, where 10,000 cases were documented in naval shipyards, and then to the shipyards of the West Coast of the United States, where cases were so numerous that the disease was called "shipyard eye". During the 1940s it was named "epidemic keratoconjunctivitis,"[53] and outbreaks were most commonly reported from industries associated with the war effort such as shipbuilding, automotive manufacture, construction, and boiler making.[26]

A single case of "superficial punctate keratitis" was reported in the United States in 1909.[118] The first epidemic associated with a medical facility involved 16 cases and was reported by Hobson[52] in 1936 at the Veterans Administration Hospital in San Fernando, Calif. The characteristic association between EKC epidemics and medical facilities (eye clinics, eye hospitals, and ophthalmologists' offices)

has continued despite considerable efforts to eliminate medical facilities as sites of transmission. EKC epidemics also generally occur at schools, camps, and military bases.

The most common adenovirus serotypes that cause EKC, in order of frequency, are adenovirus types 8, 19, 37, and 5. AD8 was first recovered from a sailor in 1955, AD19 was isolated from a Saudi Arabian child in 1959, AD37 was cultured from a Dutch patient in 1976,[30] and AD5 was isolated in tissue culture from the adenoids of a 4-year-old girl in 1953.[94]

EPIDEMIOLOGY

The epidemiology of adenoviral ocular infections is well characterized. The human ocular serotypes are host- and organ-specific with no known animal reservoirs. Patients of all ages are at risk, but most cases occur in those between 20 and 40 with no differentiation by sex, race, or socioeconomic or nutritional status. In temperate climates seasonal variation has been reported with peaks in midwinter associated with acute respiratory diseases and in midsummer associated with swimming pool use. All epidemics of ocular infection may be classified as either community-based or medical facility-based with some overlap.[82,117]

The principal mode of transmission of ocular disease is direct contact with virus in ocular secretions or on shared fomites (towels, linens, soap, eyeglasses). Crowding of infected patients and susceptibles enhances transmission. Other conditions contributing to spread in ophthalmologists' offices and other health-care facilities include infectious adenovirus on the fingers of patients[7] and health professionals, contaminated instruments, and infected eye drops. Ocular disease transmission also is facilitated by microtrauma following ocular manipulation. The acquisition of infection from desiccated adenovirus on shared surfaces in the waiting room also may be an important risk factor in iatrogenic spread.[36,78]

Other reservoirs of adenovirus infection that could be

sources of community outbreaks of eye disease include asymptomatic ocular shedding,[82] concurrent gastrointestinal infections,[61] or possibly even genital tract infections.[47,95,106] Rare cases of viral persistence associated with chronic papillary conjunctivitis also have been described.[16,20,87,112]

The incubation period before the onset of clinical symptoms is 4 to 10 days (mean = 7 days) for most ocular adenoviral serotypes. The usual course of ocular replication on the eye is less than 14 days but may extend to 21 days depending on serotype, isolate virulence, inoculation dose, and host immune status.[21,92]

Molecular Epidemiology

Advances in molecular virology and diagnostic immunology have been important in defining the relatively new field of molecular epidemiology. Molecular epidemiology identifies the particular isolate involved in office-based and community epidemics and traces the evolution and spread of new variants and serotypes around the world.

Adenoviruses are serologically typed into 47 serotypes determined by specific antigens on the virus particle. The penton fibers, protein spikes that project outward from 12 vertices (Fig. 69-1), carry these serotype-specific antigenic determinants, and type-specific monoclonal antibodies have been important in typing and identifying isolates in clinical settings and in epidemiologic tracing studies.

Another important tool in epidemiologic tracing studies is restriction enzyme analysis, which is based on the variations within the DNA genome of the various serotypes. Restriction enzyme analysis distinguishes among serotypes, an important feature because only about 10% to 15% of the DNA is highly conserved in all serotypes, although up to 80% may be shared among the members of a group.

In restriction enzyme analysis, adenovirus DNA, which is easily obtained from tissue culture, is digested with one or more restriction enzymes that digest the DNA at specific sequences. Changes within the DNA of different serotypes occasionally result in the loss (or gain) of a restriction enzyme site, causing the generation of different size DNA fragments. These fragments are resolved by agarose gel electrophoresis, and the DNA fragments are visualized by ethidium bromide staining or Southern blotting and hybridization (Fig. 69-2). The characteristic pattern of bands on the gel (DNA fingerprint) facilitates tracing of a particular virus, because loss or gain of restriction sites is usually genetically stable. Therefore variations from the prototype serotype could indicate the evolution of sequential variants and new genome types. Over 200 principal genome types have been identified for the 47 known serotypes, and many minor variations probably arise in the human population.

The techniques just discussed have been used extensively for epidemiologic tracing of adenoviruses as agents of conjunctivitis. The paragraphs that follow summarize some of the information gained from studies about the serotypes.

Adenovirus Type 3. Originally recovered from 80 patients in 1955,[11] adenovirus type 3 is frequently isolated from patients with acute respiratory illness and conjunctivitis. Its distribution appears to be worldwide based on reports from the United States, England, Japan, and Australia. In some cases little variation among AD3 isolates was observed, but in others several genome type of variants were found in epidemiologically related outbreaks. Yearly alternation between two or three different genome types has been described, suggesting a cyclic effect of subgenome type survival. Furthermore, variations that localize to specific regions may occur more frequently.[41,59,83]

Adenovirus Type 4. Adenovirus type 4, originally isolated from military recruits in the United States, was quickly rec-

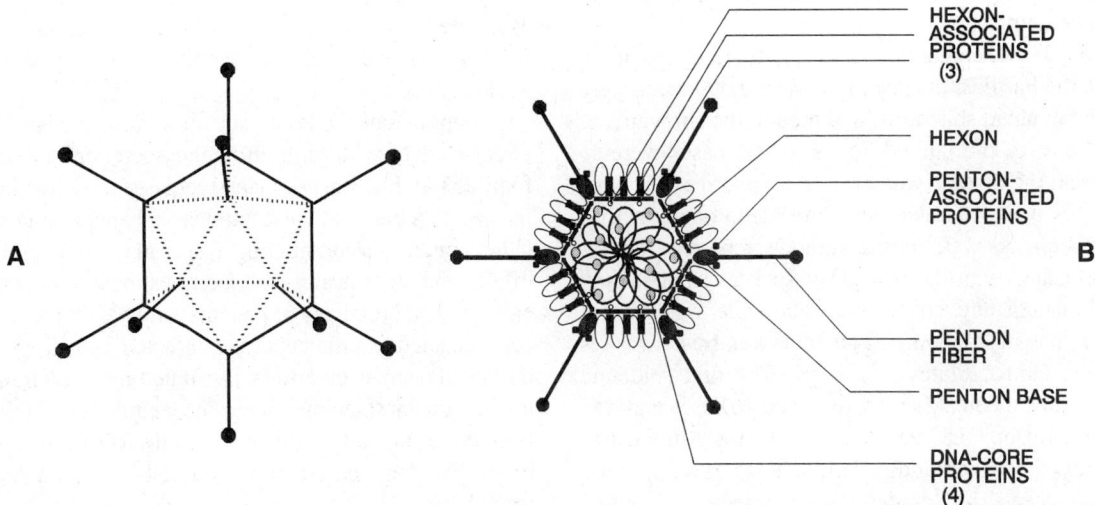

Fig. 69-1. **A,** Representative adenovirus particle with 20 identical faces comprising the nonenveloped icosahedral shell. **B,** The principal components of an adenovirus particle: hexons, pentons, and the penton fibers (or spikes).

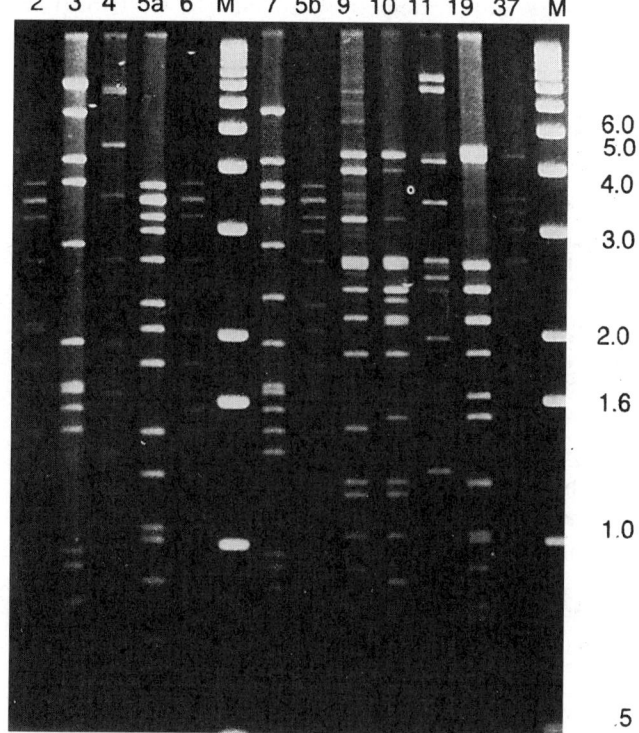

2 3 4 5a 6 M 7 5b 9 10 11 19 37 M

6.0
5.0
4.0
3.0

2.0

1.6

1.0

.5

Fig. 69-2.   Restriction enzyme analysis of adenovirus serotypes. Patterns of DNA fragments following digestion of serotypes DNAs with PstI, separation by gel electrophoresis, and staining with ethidium bromide. Horizontal numbers designate adenoviral serotypes. Vertical numbers represent known reference size markers (M).

ognized as an agent that also caused pharyngeal conjunctival fever (PCF) in children. PCF is characterized in the pediatric age group by an acute onset of conjunctivitis in association with fever and sore throat.[33] In 1979 a variant identified as AD4A was isolated, and current strains similar or identical to this variant now account for many conjunctivitis cases seen worldwide.[34]

Adenovirus Type 7. Adenovirus type 7, originally isolated from the pharynx in 1955, has been associated with PCF epidemics and mild conjunctival infections, although it is considerably rarer than other types.[3] It is closely related to AD3. Adenovirus type 11, originally isolated from a stool and urine specimen,[65] is one of the most common causes of acute hemorrhagic conjunctivitis (AHC) in East Asian countries. For example up to 45% of AHC in Taiwan is caused by type 11.[51]

Adenovirus Type 8. Adenovirus type 8, the serotype originally associated with shipyard eye, appears to be the most common worldwide cause of EKC.* It was clearly the main cause of EKC in the United States until 1973, when AD19A became more prevalent. Recently, however, AD8 has again

emerged as the serotype most commonly reported as causing epidemics around the world.[56,73,77]

Based on data from serotyping and restriction enzyme analysis, it appears that AD8 originated in Asia. Asia appears to serve as the major reservoir for the continuing evolution of new variants of AD8.[98] There are nine known genomic variants of AD8.[73] Epidemiologically, EKC caused by AD8 and other serotypes passes through the susceptible homogeneous Asian population in "epidemic waves".[63] In contrast, AD8 continues to circulate in the large diverse population of the United States with little genetic variation from the prototypic type 8 strain.[63] The reasons for these epidemiologic differences are not known. In western countries AD8 is often associated with transmission at medical facilities, most notably the ophthalmologist's office.[117]

Adenovirus Type 19. Adenovirus type 19 (AD19), first isolated in 1955 and identified in 1959, was the main cause of EKC (35% of total cases encountered) in the United States from 1973 to 1976 and later spread in epidemics to become the major cause of EKC in Canada and Eastern Europe. A new variant, 19A, was identified by differential agglutination of dog red cells, and this variant is still frequently isolated.[64] Many cases of EKC attributed to type 19, however, were later shown to be caused by type 37, a main serotype in the late 1970s.[64]

Adenovirus Type 37. Adenovirus type 37, recognized only relatively recently, was reported as the major cause of EKC in the United States from 1977 to 1983.[64] A study by Aoki and associates[6] proved AD37 a major cause of EKC in Japan. EKC caused by AD37 is clinically indistinguishable from AD8 and AD19, and together they account for the majority of cases of EKC in the United States. It has been proposed that these three viruses should be subgrouped in a separate pathogenic grouping.[58]

Serotype Variations

Epidemiologic and molecular studies of clinical adenoviral isolates suggest that specific adenovirus groups continually change and evolve. DNA restriction enzyme profiles vary most for subgroup D, which includes serotypes that are major causes of EKC. Virus genome types and serotypes associated with EKC also change over time, with a predominant serotype becoming superseded by a second serotype or variant. For example, before 1973 AD8 was the major cause of EKC, but later was superseded by AD19 and AD37. AD8 again appears to be the main cause of EKC.[56,73,77] This variation is due to sequence changes generated by a low-fidelity polymerase in the copying of critical genes or through recombination with other serotypes to give partial in vivo-generated recombinants. Evidence implicates both mechanisms.[2,81,119] A number of adenoviruses that have been isolated may be intermediates of two adenovirus serotypes. For example, some isolates associated with EKC in the United States have a neutralizing epitope characteristic of

---

*References 40, 56, 60, 73, 77, 117.

type 9 but have hemagglutination properties of type 15.[2] Similarly, recent adenovirus isolates in Japan have a serum neutralization serotype of 22 but have hemagglutination properties of type 10, 19, or 37.[81] The existence of these intermediate phenotypes led to the belief that recombination was the chief mechanism of variation, but in only a few cases has restriction enzyme analysis (REA) supported recombination as a mechanism. Few intermediate viruses possess fragments diagnostic of two serotypes.[119] This finding implies that recombination may not be as important as previously assumed. It appears more probable that continual changes occur within the genome of adenoviruses, but the viruses are maintained within the population at a clinically asymptomatic level. Occasionally a change in the genotype enhances its pathogenicity and a clinical epidemic ensues.

PATHOGENESIS

Microbial Mechanisms

Adenoviruses were named after their discovery as infectious agents that could be consistently isolated from tissue culture cells derived from the adenoids or tonsils.[94] This virus group includes many viruses isolated not only from humans but also from many other animals; it includes viruses from simian, bovine, equine, porcine, ovine, canine and opossum species and also many avian species. Adenoviruses are highly species-specific, and animal adenoviruses do not cause human disease or act as reservoirs for human adenoviruses.

As a group the adenoviruses possess a unique structure containing a large DNA genome. They have a complex genetic organization of gene expression with a unique set of viral-specified enzymes and functions that facilitate proliferation and spread. Compared to the mammalian cell, however, adenoviruses are relatively simple in their molecular organization and therefore have been very important biologic models for studying events that occur in the normal cell. Many principles underlying basic concepts of molecular and cellular biology have been derived from studies on the adenoviruses, including the following: the mechanisms of RNA processing, particularly its splicing and polyadenylation, the basis for DNA replication and its control; the complex interplay of conditions that result in the control of gene expression; and the principal mechanisms and proteins involved in the action through which a DNA gene is transcribed into mRNA. Many of the techniques used in investigative molecular biology were developed to characterize the adenoviruses.

To understand the molecular basis for pathogenesis, it is important to understand some of the salient features of this virus group. It is beyond the scope of this chapter, however, to review the molecular biology of this virus extensively. The reader is referred to a more comprehensive source,[54] if desired.

Structure and Principles of Adenovirus Classification. Adenoviruses are differentiated from other viruses mainly by the classic characteristic shape of the virus particle. Figure 69-1 shows the structure of a typical adenovirus. The particle is a nonenveloped icosahedral shell with 20 identical faces and an overall hexagonal shape. Figure 69-1, *A,* depicts a virus particle as seen by looking directly at one face. Each particle is composed of 240 units called hexons, which form the faces and edges of the particle, and 12 units called pentons, at the vertices. From the twelve pentons, fibers or spikes project outward from the particle. Within the outer shell is a protein core containing the viral genome and core proteins. As a nonenveloped virus, adenovirus lacks a lipid membrane common to herpesviruses and HIV, and this fact may partly explain its resistance to most disinfecting agents and its ability to withstand desiccation.

The hexons, pentons, and penton fibers (Fig. 69-1, *B*) are the principal components of the virus that initially interact with a susceptible cell. The capsid proteins are also those which principally interact with the immune system. The hexon protein possesses a common group antigen that cross-reacts with all human adenoviruses. This antigen reflects a highly conserved and evolutionary constrained part of the protein. The hexon protein is also the preponderant target antigen for complement fixation tests and many immunofluorescent assays used in the diagnosis and typing of adenoviruses. In contrast, proteins that form the penton fiber, the principal means by which a virus attaches to the host cell, are highly variable and possess unique antigens representing the 47 serotypes as defined by neutralization.

Within the icosahedral shell is the adenovirus genome, a 36,000 bp linear double-stranded DNA molecule sufficient to encode a large number of viral-specific proteins. Its composition can vary (48% to 61% G + C content), indicating the underlying variation among serotypes. An unusual feature of the adenovirus genome is the presence of a protein covalently attached to the ends of the DNA genome, which plays important roles in the replication and stability of the genome. The complete DNA sequence for two serotypes (AD2 and AD5) has been derived,[17] and partial DNA sequences for several other serotypes (3, 4, 7, 12, 40 and 41) are known, providing a basis for comparisons of the virus genes.

Classification of the 47 adenovirus serotypes that infect humans is based on a combination of several biologic, immunologic, and pathogenic properties (Table 69-1). Historically, groupings based on hemagglutination of erythrocytes of different animals were used. Groupings based on other criteria (G + C content, antigenic cross-reactivity, and oncogenicity in rodents) have generally been consistent with the original groupings, and six groups, A through F, are defined for human adenoviruses.

One of the most important differentiating features in classification is the ability of a human adenovirus to cause

TABLE 69-1 CLASSIFICATION SCHEMES FOR 47 HUMAN ADENOVIRUS SEROTYPES

S	Serotypes	Tumors in Animals	Cellular Transformation	Hemagglutination Group*
A	12, 18, 31	High	+	IV
B	3, 7, 11, 14, 16, 21, 34, 35	Moderate	+	I
C	1, 2, 5, 6	Low or none	+	III
D	8, 9, 10, 13, 15, 17, 19, 20, 22-30, 32, 33, 36-39, 42-47	Low or none	+	II
E	4	Low or none	+	III
F	40, 41	NK	NK	III

Modified from Horwitz MS: In Fields and associates, editors: *Virology,* ed 2, New York, 1990, Raven Press.
* = Hemagglutination; I = complete agglutination of monkey erythrocytes; II = complete agglutination of rat erythrocytes; III = partial agglutination of rat erythrocytes; IV = little or no agglutination.
NK = not known.

tumors in animals. Despite the benign nature of adenoviruses in humans, members of the adenovirus group A are highly tumorigenic in certain rodents, such as newborn hamsters. Subgroup B viruses are somewhat less tumorigenic, with long periods occurring between infection and tumor appearance. Members of subgroups C and D rarely cause tumors. Some serotypes, most notably AD12, are also documented as fully transforming retinal cells and of causing retinoblastoma-like disease after intraocular injection.[4,75] It is important to emphasize, however, that no human malignancy has been proved to be associated with a human adenovirus.

The Adenovirus Infectious Cycle. An adenovirus-infected cell is a prolific replication machine. For example, for the Group C adenoviruses, each infected cell may produce as many as 10,000 virions in a single cycle of 30 to 36 hours.[43] The consequences of such proliferation include death at the cellular level and/or an induced inflammatory and immune response at the tissue level that accounts for observable clinical disease.

Upon entry of the virus into the cell, a complex process occurs in which the virus takes over the cellular machinery. First, normal cellular operations are shut down, partly by the action of one of the incoming adenovirus structural proteins that form the penton base. This protein alone causes rapid onset of cytopathic (cell-killing) effects, resulting in rounding up of cells in tissue culture.[110] In fact adenovirus penton base protein has been found in the blood of patients with adenovirus-induced pneumonia and may well be defined as a viral toxin.[69] Furthermore, a second protein from the E1a region of the adenoviral genome is responsible for programmed cell death.[88]

Adenoviruses code for many proteins necessary for the efficient production of more virus. Not all of the adenovirus proteins are made at once, however, but rather particular proteins are made at particular stages of the infectious cycle. This phenomenon is known as a transcriptional cascade.

First a limited set of genes is made into proteins; these genes in turn switch on additional genes so that they are made into proteins. Transcriptional cascades are common to most complex viruses (for example, herpesviruses). Generally control of the time at which a particular protein is made is mediated at the transcriptional, or RNA synthesis level. Analysis of the transcription from these genes has shown that each gene can be defined as belonging to a particular transcriptional class, referred to as early, delayed early, and late, depending on the requirements for transcription.

The adenovirus genes transcribed first into RNA, the early genes, are made immediately upon infection, relying almost exclusively on cellular transcriptional machinery for their synthesis. The DNA regions controlling their transcription are very similar to those controlling the expression of cellular genes and thus are appropriate models for the study of gene function of a normal human cell.

The main region of the adenovirus genome (expressed immediately on infection) is referred to as Ela and is found at the extreme left-hand end of the genome. The E1a region serves as a template for multiple RNA species that encode two different proteins that are expressed throughout the adenovirus life cycle and are in part responsible for normal cell shutdown. Furthermore, the products of the E1a region (in addition to the products of the adjacent region referred to as E1b) are the principal means by which adenoviruses transform cells and cause tumors. The E1a proteins interact with an important cellular growth control factor known as the retinoblastoma gene product or RB.[27] Similarly, E1b proteins interact with a gene product known as p53. Both RB and p53 are cellular factors known as tumor suppressor genes, which normally regulate and control the division of a cell. When they interact with the E1a proteins in rodents, however, the outcome is a loss of this control, resulting in abnormal cell division.[114]

The next adenovirus genes expressed, the delayed early genes, come from five regions of the genome referred to as

E1b, E2a and E2b, E3, and E4. These gene products further adapt the infected cell to the replication of adenovirus and replicate the adenoviral genome (encoded proteins include viral DNA polymerase and DNA-binding protein). Viral-encoded DNA polymerase represents a prime target for the development of antivirals directed against the adenoviruses. S-HPMPC, which has shown promise in in vitro[8,39] and in vivo animal studies,[38] appears to inhibit this polymerase. The E3 region encodes several proteins that modulate the immune status of the cell.[124] One of these proteins stimulates the response of cells to epidermal growth factors, making the cell more efficient for virus growth.

The final class of adenovirus genes, the late genes, encodes mostly those proteins involved in the assembly and structure of the virion particle. They are made in a unique mechanism of expression. In the late phase a single promoter makes a single RNA, which is then differentially spliced and rearranged to give 16 to 18 different RNAs that encode the structural proteins. It was the study of these genes and the mechanism by which the RNAs were processed that clarified the mechanism of RNA splicing and processing, now known to occur in virtually all human genes.[14]

Immune Avoidance and Viral Persistence. An important pathogenic feature of many adenovirus serotypes is their ability to persist in a host and avoid destruction by an active immune system. They persist in asymptomatic individuals by replicating chronically at low levels in various host tissues (adenoids, tonsils).[94] It has been suggested that adenoviruses, like herpesviruses, enter a latent state in which adenovirus DNA maintains itself in particular tissues including B cells and the adenoids.[29,80]

Adenoviruses have developed evasive molecular mechanisms by which an infected cell is overlooked by the hosts' immune surveillance.[76,124] The E3 region of the genome encodes several proteins with activities that promote survival despite an active immune system. The first mechanism involves the normal ability of an infected cell to signal the presence of a foreign antigen to the immune system. To appreciate this phenomenon, it is important to understand the mechanisms underlying the normal cellular immune response.[103]

In a normal host, antigens can be divided into two groups: intracellular antigens and extracellular antigens. Although the groups are not mutually exclusive, each evokes a specific cellular immune response. Antigens made within a cell, such as a viral protein, induce a response known as a class I response. The "foreign" viral proteins within the cell are processed by it into short peptides through mechanisms as yet unclear. Some of these peptides become associated with a group of host proteins known as type I Major Histocompatibility antigens (MHC-I), which migrate to the cell surface and present antigens to T cells.

MHC-I–presented antigens are recognized by T cells bearing the marker antigen CD8; these cells elicit a cyto-

toxic immune response. MHC-I antigens are made by most, but not all, nucleated cells. In contrast, soluble extracellular antigens generally elicit a type II response, which is more restricted to macrophages and lymphocytes. Extracellular antigens are first internalized and then, as with the class I response, antigens are processed into short peptides and presented in association with host proteins. The latter, however, are type II MHC molecules, which present the antigen to lymphocytes bearing the CD4 marker antigen. The major function of such lymphocytes is not cytotoxic (like the CD8 cells) but as helper cells that aid in inducing the humoral and complement components of the immune response.

Adenoviruses have evolved a mechanism to suppress the MHC type I immune response. In an adenovirus-infected cell, a viral-specific protein encoded by the E3 region is able to prevent type I MHC presentation by interfering with the proper processing and glycosylation of the MHC-I antigen proteins. The MHC-I antigen is trapped within the cell and little reaches the cell surface, and the consequence is that foreign antigens are not presented or recognized.

The second mechanism of immune evasion is via the action of the E1a proteins of some serotypes, which act to suppress the transcription of the cellular genes-encoding components of the MHC-I complex. A third mechanism is the function of another protein from the E3 region, which acts to prevent lysis of cells by the potent lymphokine tumor necrosis factor.[35]

Host Immunologic Defenses and Immunogenic Disease

The immune system plays a dichotomous role in the pathogenesis and control of ocular adenoviral infections. As in most viral infections, the immune system provides the host with a complex defense to limit replicating virus by direct neutralization with circulating antibodies and the cell-mediated lysis of virus-infected cells.[122]

Usually ocular and systemic adenoviral infections are readily controlled by the immune system of an immuno-competent host. Severe immunosuppression, however, as seen in patients following organ transplantation, cancer chemotherapy, and in acquired immunodeficiency syndrome (AIDS), may result in a fatal generalized infection in 10% of cases. In these immunosuppressed populations, various serotypes of adenovirus have been recovered from the central nervous system (CNS), and the respiratory, urinary, and gastrointestinal systems.[48,51]

Although the beneficial effects of the host immune system in the control of ocular adenoviral infections are generally recognized, the negative pathogenic effects and the role of "immunogenic disease" in prolonging patient morbidity through the formation of subepithelial infiltrates deserve special attention. The clinical significance of corneal subepithelial infiltrates and the dilemma of their management are described in detail in a later section, Clinical Presentation. Figure 69-3 presents a model of their pathogenesis that relates possible roles for the host immune system, viral factors, and the corneal target tissue.

To understand the negative effects of immunogenic disease in EKC, one can consider the importance of corneal transparency as an essential requirement for good vision. Following external infection the host inflammatory and immune responses normally are beneficial in clearing pathogens from most tissues or organs. These host defenses become particularly destructive, however, when the transmission of light through the cornea is altered by scarring or surface irregularity. Similar mechanisms underlie immunogenic diseases of the cornea caused by herpes simplex, herpes zoster, Epstein-Barr virus, *Acanthamoeba* species, and *Borrelia burgdorferi* (Lyme disease).

Jones[62] first proposed that subepithelial infiltrates (Fig. 69-4) represent a delayed immune response to viral antigen that was "blotted" by the cornea during acute infection. The model of pathogenesis of subepithelial infiltrates (Fig. 69-3), based on this hypothesis, helps explain the following: (1) observed differences in the severity of ocular disease among patients, (2) the unpredictable clinical response in a patient to treatment with topical corticosteroids, and (3) the potential benefits of antiviral therapy to reduce an immunogenic disease (that is, subepithelial infiltrates).

The severity of clinical disease varies according to differences in viral genetics that defines the virulence of the infecting serotype and of that specific isolate. Viral genetics determines the replicative capacity (that is, efficiency of replication) of the virus, which in turn determines the total epithelial antigen load that is deposited at the level of the Bowman membrane. Topical corticosteroids administered during acute infection may enhance the total antigen load through mechanisms of local immunosuppression and thereby promote adenoviral replication.

Significant host factors that define the immune response and the efficiency of viral clearance have been discussed

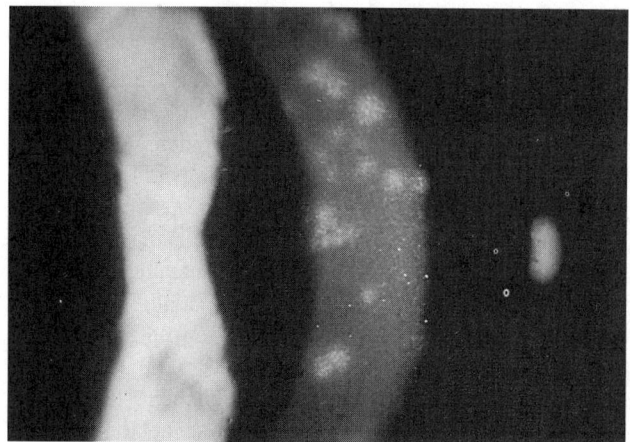

Fig. 69-4. Corneal subepithelial infiltrates: multiple small greyish-white opacities of presumed immune origin distributed over the entire cornea.

briefly. The extent of immune induction of subepithelial infiltrates varies according to the total corneal antigenic load and the immunogenicity of the viral antigen(s), which is serotype- and isolate-dependent, with a possible role for cell adhesion molecules. Adhesion molecules encompass a group of cellular glycoproteins that regulate lymphocyte binding to cells and extracellular matrix, facilitate bidirectional transmission of information across the cell membrane,[24] and thereby promote immune responses including site-specific targeting of cells for destruction by activated leukocytes.[28]

Aggressive initial treatment with topical corticosteroids always inhibits the immune effector response and prevents the formation of subepithelial infiltrates, but the response to corticosteroid withdrawal varies clinically. Subepithelial infiltrates always appear (or reappear) if sufficient viral antigen was deposited and remains trapped within the cornea. Therefore the dilemma facing the ophthalmologist when deciding to treat with topical corticosteroids is that the factors that determine clinical outcome (total antigen load, immunogenicity, infecting serotype, and isolate virulence) cannot be known, and the decision always remains a guess.

The model in Fig. 69-3 predicts that early treatment of EKC with an effective antiviral will reduce the total antigen load and thereby reduce or prevent the formation of clinically significant subepithelial infiltrates. Progress in developing an effective antiviral is summarized under a later section, Future Directions.

Adenoviral Serotypes and Clinical Syndromes

Of the 47 human adenoviral serotypes, about one half have been demonstrated to cause human disease spontaneously.[12,25,54] These pathogenic serotypes have shown a definite tendency to infect mucosal cells lining the ocular sur-

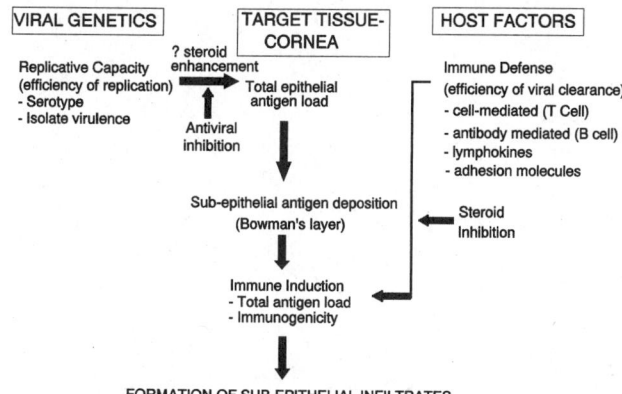

Fig. 69-3. Theoretical model of pathogenesis of corneal subepithelial infiltrates.

face and the respiratory, gastrointestinal, and genitourinary tracts (Table 69-2).

Ocular adenoviral infections manifest themselves in three common presentations: follicular conjunctivitis (FC), pharyngeal conjunctival fever (PCF), and epidemic keratoconjunctivitis (EKC).[112] Mild, nonspecific follicular conjunctivitis is the most common presentation of ocular adenoviral infection. FC can be caused by any of the ocular serotypes, but AD1, 2, 4, 5, and 6 are the most frequent agents. Children are affected more commonly than adults, and ocular infection is often associated with an acute respiratory infection. The disease is characterized by its mild, self-limited nature and absence of any corneal involvement. There is no specific therapy and there are no ocular sequelae following acute infection.

Pharyngeal conjunctival fever was first described by Beale[10] in 1906. It is most commonly caused by adenovirus types 3 and 7, but types 4, 1, 14, and others also have been reported.[91] The epidemiology of PCF includes both sporadic cases and clustered epidemics associated with schools in the winter and camps in the summer. Inadequately chlorinated swimming pools and contaminated small lakes have resulted in transmission of the virus to produce outbreaks of "swimming pool conjunctivitis."[100]

Clinically, PCF is characterized by an abrupt onset of systemic illness consisting of high fever, pharyngitis, and bilateral follicular conjunctivitis. As with follicular conjunctivitis, children are more commonly affected than adults. In young children PCF may be associated with more severe signs (high fever, general malaise, nausea, vomiting, and diarrhea), but the disease usually runs its course over 10 to 14 days and resolves without complications.

In PCF, ocular involvement usually is restricted to an acute bilateral follicular conjunctivitis with small petechial hemorrhages occurring on the bulbar conjunctiva. During the acute disease keratitis is usually mild, and the delayed appearance of corneal subepithelial infiltrates is much less common than in epidemic keratoconjunctivitis (EKC). EKC, the most prevalent form of adenoviral ocular infection, is discussed in a later section, Clinical Presentation.

In addition to ocular infections, various adenoviral serotypes commonly infect the mucosal cells lining the respiratory tract to produce both upper and lower respiratory illnesses, including coinfection in pertussis syndrome in

TABLE 69-2 ADENOVIRUS INFECTIONS AND SEROTYPES INVOLVED

Syndrome	Signs and Symptoms	Serotypes Involved	
		Frequently	Infrequently
Upper respiratory illness	Coryza, pharyngitis, fever, tonsillitis, diarrhea	1-3, 5, 7	4, 6, 11, 18, 21, 29, 31
Lower respiratory illness	Bronchitis, pneumonia, fever, coryza, cough	3, 4, 7, 21	1, 2, 5, 35
Pertussis syndrome	Paroxysmal cough, vomiting, fever, upper respiratory illness	5	1-3
Acute respiratory disease	Tracheobronchitis, fever, myalgia, coryza, pneumonia	4, 7	3, 14, 21, 35
Acute follicular conjunctivitis	Lid edema, follicles, petechial hemorrhage, preauricular nodes, URI	1-11, 19	14-17, 20, 22, 26
Pharyngoconjunctival fever	Pharyngitis, conjunctivitis, fever, coryza, headache, diarrhea, rash, nodes	3, 4, 7	1, 11, 14, 16, 19, 37
Epidemic keratoconjunctivitis	Keratitis, headache, preauricular nodes, coryza, pharyngitis, diarrhea	8, 19, 37	3, 4, 7, 10, 11, 21
Acute hemorrhagic conjunctivitis	Chemosis, follicles, subconjunctival hemorrhage, preauricular nodes, fever	11	2-8, 14, 15, 19, 37
Cystitis	Cystitis (usually hemorrhagic), fever, pharyngitis	11	7, 21, 34, 35
Immunocompromised host disease	Diarrhea, rash, upper respiratory illness, pneumonia, hepatitis, cystitis, otitis media	11, 34, 35	1, 2, 5, 7, 21, 29, 31, 37-39
Gastroenteritis (infant)	Diarrhea, fever, nausea, vomiting, mild upper respiratory illness	31, 40, 41	1, 2, 12-17, 21, 25, 26, 29
Central nervous system disease	Meningitis, encephalitis, Reye syndrome	7	3, 32
Venereal disease	Ulcerative genital lesions, urethritis, cervicitis	2, 19, 37	1, 5, 7, 11, 18, 31

Modified from Hierholzer JC: In Balows A, editor: *Manual of clinical microbiology,* Washington, DC, 1991, American Society for Microbiology.

children and acute respiratory disease in military recruits (Table 69-2). As noted previously the capacity of different adenoviral serotypes to establish latent and chronic infections in the respiratory tract and adjacent lymphoid tissue (tonsils and adenoids) is well known.[29,80,94] Persistent shedding of adenovirus in asymptomatic individuals has been demonstrated by serial positive cultures of respiratory secretions and stool specimens.[29,31,91]

Adenoviruses play an important role in respiratory infections in children. Approximately 10% of all children under the age of 5 are seropositive, and types 1, 2, 3, 5, and 6 are thought to be endemic. The most common clinical presentation in both children and adults is as an exudative pharyngitis mimicking streptococcal tonsillitis with fever, chills, and cervical lymphadenopathy. Milder cases may present with common cold symptoms and signs of afebrile rhinitis, mild pharyngitis, and myalgias. These acute presentations usually run their clinical course over 1 to 2 weeks and resolve without complications.

More significantly, adenovirus types 1, 2, 3, 5, 6, and 7 have been implicated in mild cases of acute laryngotracheitis (croup), childhood bronchiolitis (5% of cases), and childhood pneumonias (10% of cases). Adult pneumonia in immunocompetent adults has also been reported for types 3 and 7. Most cases of lower respiratory infections resolve without serious complications, but chronic bronchiectasis (AD7) and even death has been reported in vulnerable patient populations (malnourished young children and immunosuppressed patients).[91] A recent study in children[79] demonstrated an association between *Bordetella pertussis* (the agent that causes whooping cough) and acute adenoviral infection (AD5, 1, 2, and 3), suggesting concurrent infection following reactivation of adenovirus from latently infected tonsils or adenoids.

Acute respiratory disease has been a significant cause of morbidity among military recruits in training camps,[74] especially during the winter. Types 4 and 7 produce an influenza-like syndrome of pharyngitis, lymphadenitis, tracheobronchitis, fever, myalgias, and diarrhea, requiring hospitalization in up to 20% of cases. Additional risk factors include crowding and fatigue. To combat this threat to military preparedness, the U.S. and Canadian military have introduced a specific oral, live virus vaccine that is thought to be effective in reducing the incidence of this disease.[102]

The role of adenoviruses as causal agents of gastrointestinal diseases has recently been clarified. Previously the demonstration of chronic shedding of different adenoviral serotypes in both symptomatic and asymptomatic individuals confused the issue, but it now appears that two fastidious serotypes, AD40 and AD41, are the causal agents of diarrhea in 5% to 12% of pediatric cases,[22,120] and these cases are often accompanied by a concurrent respiratory illness. Adenoviral gastroenteritis occurs both as community-based epidemics and in hospital environments (nosocomial spread). The association between adenoviruses and intussusception, mesenteric adenitis, appendicitis, and celiac disease has been reported, but proof of a causative role awaits confirmation.[54,91]

Adenoviral infections of the genitourinary tract are less common but have been documented. Acute hemorrhagic cystitis was first reported in Japan to be a self-limited infection of the bladder (5 days) associated with gross hematuria and dysuria but without renal involvement.[13] Causative serotypes include AD11 and AD21. Ocular adenoviral serotypes associated with sexually transmitted diseases (genital lesions, urethritis, cervicitis) include AD2, 19, and 37. Central nervous system infections by adenoviruses are rare, but meningoencephalitis (AD7) and Reye syndrome (AD3) have been reported.[48,97]

As previously discussed, severely immunocompromised patients are at greater risk for serious complications of adenoviral infections. The current view of disease pathogenesis in these vulnerable patients is that immunosuppression promotes reactivation and replication of latent and persistent adenoviruses (AD11, AD34, AD35) in a manner similar to latent herpesviruses (cytomegalovirus, herpes zoster, and herpes simplex). The serotypes isolated from AIDS patients include five newly described viruses (AD42 to AD47) of subgroup D, and they are of particular scientific interest in the study of the formation of new adenoviral serotypes.[51]

CLINICAL FEATURES

The symptoms and signs of acute epidemic keratoconjunctivitis result from the replication of virus in the conjunctiva and corneal epithelial cells and the induced host inflammatory and immune responses. EKC usually is a bilateral disease characterized by rapid onset of symptoms in the first eye with subsequent development of similar but milder symptoms in the fellow eye within 2 to 7 days. The principal symptoms associated with adenoviral ocular infection include significant tearing, redness, foreign body sensation, photophobia, lid swelling, and visual disturbances.[21,30,70] Replication of the virus in the palpebral and bulbar conjunctiva is always associated with follicular hypertrophy, edema, and hyperemia, and small petechial hemorrhages are common. Upon inspection, lid edema with narrowing of the palpebral fissure is also often present (Fig. 69-5). The tarsal conjunctiva usually manifests both a follicular and papillary inflammatory response to replicating virus (Fig. 69-6).

The occurrence of associated preauricular and submandibular lymphadenopathy is variable (15% to 94%). Severe cases of adenoviral infection may present with chemosis, iritis, inflammatory pseudomembranes (Fig. 69-7), and early symblepharon formation. Rarely, EKC may be associated with subconjunctival hemorrhage,[6,49] disciform keratitis,[15] increased intraocular pressure,[46] and Stevens-Johnson syndrome.[66]

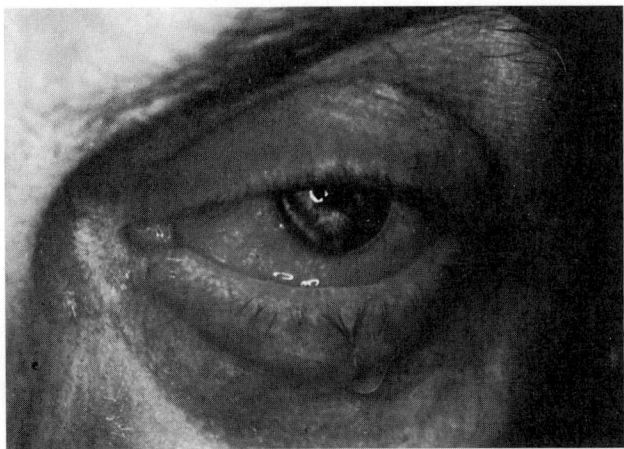

Fig. 69-5. Acute adenoviral infection with lid edema, narrowed palpebral fissure, bulbar conjunctival swelling and lacrimation.

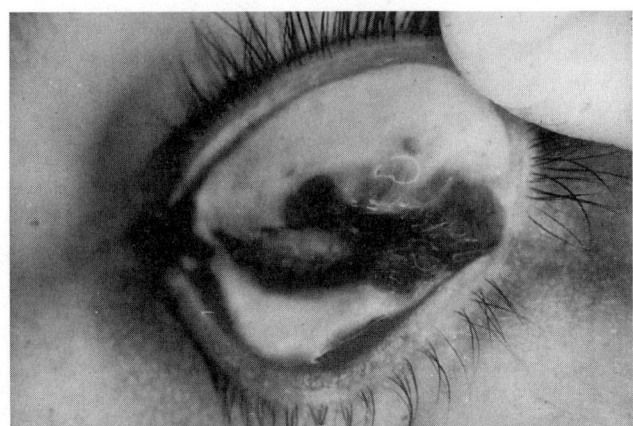

Fig. 69-7. Severe adenoviral infection with inflammatory pseudomembranes on the upper and lower tarsal conjunctivae.

The natural history of adenoviral infection in the first eye is approximately 14 days, with the delayed course in the second eye often extending the total duration to 18 to 21 days. Adenenovirus type 8 can be recovered from the ocular surface for up to 2 weeks in most cases,[68,121] and decline in titers during the second week usually is associated with resolution of inflammation of the conjunctiva and ocular adnexae.

The corneal response to adenovirus replicating in the surface epithelium follows a well-documented clinical pattern of characteristic sequential changes[21,70] (Fig. 69-8). Three or four days after the onset of clinical symptoms caused by follicular conjunctivitis, viral replication produces a very fine, diffuse punctate keratitis on the corneal surface. This keratitis may be associated with a foreign body sensation or may be entirely asymptomatic. At about 1 week, the diffuse pinpoint spots begin to coalesce to form multiple focal areas of raised irregular epithelium that stain with fluorescein.

These focal lesions are usually symptomatic (irritation, tearing, photophobia) and persist through the second week. Between the second and third week host inflammatory and immune cells invade the cornea beneath the focal epithelial lesions to form characteristic subepithelial infiltrates (Fig. 69-4). The subepithelial infiltrates are thought to be induced by viral antigen that has filtered down from the overlying epithelium and is fixed at the level of the Bowman membrane.[62] A hypothetical model of the essential factors required for the formation of subepithelial infiltrates (Fig. 69-3) was discussed in a previous section, Pathogenesis.

On slit-lamp examination, these subepithelial infiltrates appear as 30 to 50 greyish-white dots (1 to 2 mm in diameter) that are distributed superficially over the entire cornea (Fig. 69-4). Affected patients may experience reduction in several lines of vision if the visual axis is involved. Furthermore, direct sunlight may produce disabling photophobia, and glare from oncoming headlights may make night driving

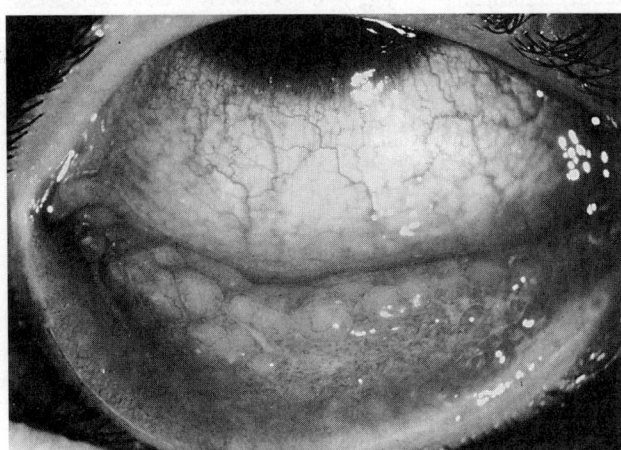

Fig. 69-6. Acute follicular conjunctivitis common to all adenoviral ocular infections. Note large follicules in the inferior fornix and conjunctival hyperemia.

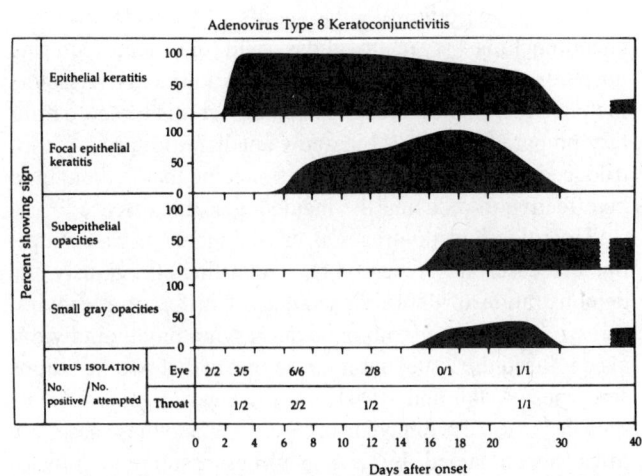

Fig. 69-8. Natural history of epidemic keratoconjunctivitis (EKC) caused by adenovirus type 8. (Published with permission from Dawson CA et al.: *Am J Ophthalmol* 69:473–480, 1970.)

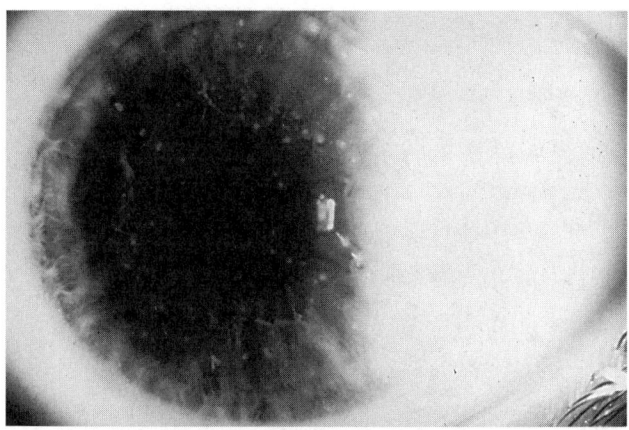

Fig. 69-9. Thygeson superficial punctate keratitis with multiple, greyish-white opacities in central cornea. Note absence of inflammation of bulbar conjunctiva.

hazardous. The natural history of these presumed immune-mediated subepithelial infiltrates is gradual resolution over weeks to months, but the literature documents persistence up to 16 years in rare cases.[70]

Clinically the appearance of longstanding subepithelial infiltrates caused by EKC may be confused with Thygeson superficial punctate keratitis (Thygeson SPK)[101] because they both appear as small, superficial greyish-white corneal dots in the absence of conjunctival inflammation (Fig. 69-9). The cause of Thygeson SPK is unknown.[84] Generally these two entities can usually be distinguished by history, clinical course, and slit lamp examination. Thygeson SPK differs from EKC in that there is no antecedent episode of acute follicular conjunctivitis. Instead there is an insidious onset of foreign body sensation, photophobia, tearing, and minimal visual disturbances in the absence of significant conjunctivitis. The clinical course of Thygeson SPK usually includes numerous episodes of remission and exacerbation over 2 to 4 years. Whereas EKC, without topical steroid therapy, is almost always characterized by gradual fading and resolution of infiltrates over months. The corneal opacities of Thygeson SPK are always central and restricted to the epithelium. The lesions frequently are raised and look like bread crumbs or snowflakes; they often stain centrally with fluorescein. In contrast the infiltrates of EKC may be either central or diffusely spread over the entire corneal surface, are usually subepithelial, and do not stain with fluorescein late in the course of the disease. Infiltrates of both diseases are exquisitely sensitive to low dose topical corticosteroids, and EKC, when treated, may have the same clinical course as Thygeson SPK of remissions and exacerbations following unsuccessful attempts at corticosteroid withdrawal.

DIFFERENTIAL DIAGNOSIS

The differential diagnosis of acute adenoviral infection includes other infectious diseases associated with follicular conjunctivitis and keratitis, such as the following: herpes simplex virus keratitis, herpes zoster ophthalmicus, and chlamydial conjunctivitis. Less common causes include epidemic hemorrhagic conjunctivitis caused by picornaviruses (EV70 and Coxsackie A24), Newcastle disease, *Moraxella* conjunctivitis, influenza type A infection, molluscum contagiosum, cat-scratch fever and other causes of Parinaud syndrome, and medicamentosum. Appropriate history, clinical examination, diagnostic testing, and clinical course allow the clinician to distinguish these diseases from EKC in the majority of cases.

LABORATORY INVESTIGATIONS

The clinical diagnosis of acute adenoviral infection usually is not difficult, especially if there is a history of recent exposure at work, school, or eye clinic, along with clinical findings of follicular conjunctivitis, regional lymphadenopathy, and corneal infiltrates. In cases with atypical presentations, the diagnostic laboratory may prove useful in identifying adenovirus as the causal agent.

Viral Culture

Historically, growth in cell culture has provided the definitive diagnosis. The patient's inferior fornix is swabbed with a sterile cotton-tipped applicator that is placed in a tube of Chlamydial Transport Media* and stored in the refrigerator (4°C). All swabs are inoculated within 18 hours onto monolayers of A-549 cells and MRC-5 cells, and the cells are examined daily for viral cytopathic effect (CPE). CPE is characterized by the rounding up and sloughing of infected cells, producing a focal break in the cell monolayer called a plaque. No inclusions are seen in living cells. CPE may be seen as early as 1 day following inoculation and is usually present within 7 days (95% of cases) if the infected eye was swabbed within 1 week of the onset of clinical symptoms. Swabs taken after 7 days from the onset of symptoms may be positive for up to 4 weeks.

Rapid Diagnostic Tests

Although a positive adenoviral culture is definitive when confirmed by EIA testing, it is of no use to the clinician in making the correct diagnosis at the time of the initial examination. Therefore there is a need for an accurate, rapid diagnostic test for office use. Adenoclone† is an enzyme immune assay (EIA) test that detects adenoviral antigen from direct conjunctival swabs.[68,121] It is simple to perform, rapid (1 hour), requires no expensive equipment, and is suitable for office use (Fig. 69-10). Compared to the standard of a positive cell culture, Adenoclone demonstrated a sensitivity of 81% and a specificity of 100% when samples were collected within 1 week of the onset of clinical symptoms. Swabs taken after 1 week were negative.[68]

*Bartels Immunodiagnostic Supplies, Bellevue, Wash.
†Cambridge BioScience, Cambridge, Mass.

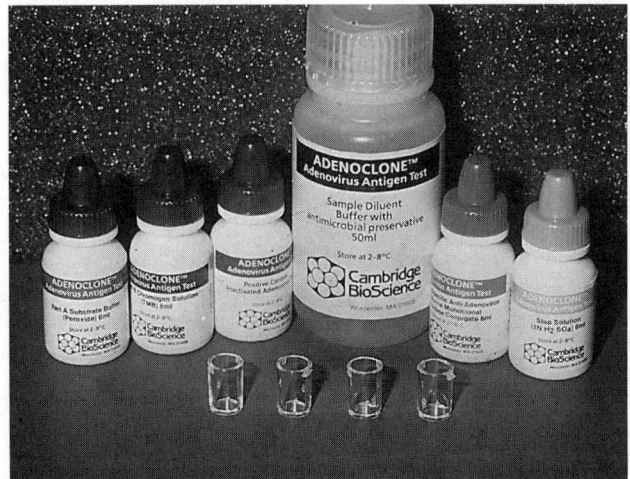

Fig. 69-10. Adenoclone Assay (Cambridge BioScience, Cambridge, Mass). Enzyme immune assay (EIA) useful for rapid detection of adenoviral hexon antigen from direct conjunctival swabs.

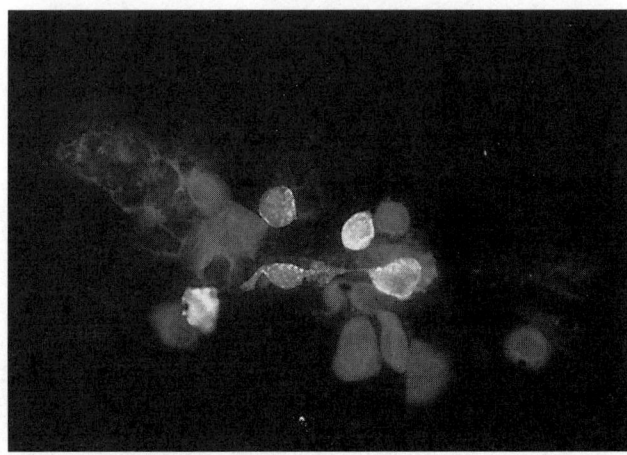

Fig. 69-12. Direct fluorescent antibody assay for detection of adenoviral antigen in infected conjunctival cells. Note that the bright fluorescence denotes antigen-positive cells.

Future diagnostic tests will be based on the detection of organism-specific nucleic acid sequences, which will be amplified millions of times until they are detectable by specific probes. The polymerase chain reaction (PCR), a prototype of this test, has already been successfully applied to the diagnosis of adenovirus[5,108] (Fig. 69-11). PCR is experimental and expensive, however, and requires skilled personnel and expensive equipment. It is limited to central diagnostic laboratories and takes longer than Adenoclone (1 to 2 days compared to 1 hour), but may be considerably more sensitive.

In the past both direct[45,109,113] and indirect fluorescent antibody tests[96,115] have generally proved to be accurate, reliable methods of detecting adenoviral antigen both experimentally and in clinical diagnostic laboratories (Fig. 69-12). While the methods are reasonably rapid, sensitive and specific, they require an expensive fluorescent microscope and skilled personnel to perform the tests and interpret the re-

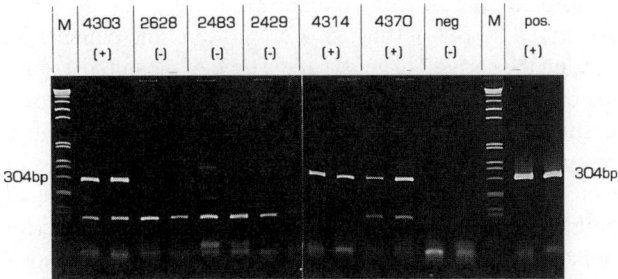

Fig. 69-11. Diagnosis of adenovirus from clinical ocular swabs based on polymerase chain reaction (PCR). DNA was extracted from clinical samples, amplified, and probed with common hexon-based probe. Positive results are demonstrated by 304 base-pair band on agarose gels. Top row represents clinical samples, positive and negative controls, and reference size markers (M). Second row indicates positive or negative culture for adenovirus.

sults. Fluorescent antibody tests are also difficult for a central laboratory to automate and generally are not suited to a busy office practice.

Other diagnostic tests for adenovirus based on cytology,[67] electron microscopy,[111] and in situ hybridization[55] proved to be unreliable and/or impractical in a clinical setting. Complement fixation and other serologic tests have proved useful in the study of the epidemiology of adenoviral infections but have little direct clinical application.[32]

PATHOLOGY

Because adenoviral ocular infections are generally non-blinding and self-limiting, pathologic specimens are rarely obtained. Specimens have been examined from two patients, however, who underwent lamellar graft surgery because of persistent visual loss following documented adenoviral ocular infections two years previously. Lymphocytes, histiocytes, and fibroblasts were found in the deep layers of the epithelium and in the anterior corneal stroma associated with breaks in the Bowman membrane. Normal collagen layers were disrupted in the anterior stroma. Adenovirus was not demonstrated by culture, electron microscopy, or indirect immunofluorescence.[72,107] The pathologic findings generally support the theory that subepithelial infiltrates represent a host immune and inflammatory response to viral antigen that is deposited at the level of the Bowman membrane during acute infection.[62] Studies in New Zealand rabbits infected with a clinical isolate of human adenovirus type 5 demonstrated subepithelial infiltrates with similar pathologic findings.[37]

In contrast to the paucity of pathologic specimens, cytologic documentation of acute adenoviral infection is well documented. A conjunctival smear taken from an acutely infected patient usually shows a marked lymphocytic inflammatory response with degenerated epithelial cells and some polymorphonuclear leukocytes.[112] If inflammatory psuedomembranes are present clinically, numerous polymorphonuclear leucocytes may be found. Within lymphocytic nuclei two characteristic alterations have been described: intranuclear inclusions and a ground-glass nuclear appearance.[67] The presence of giant cells on smear may be useful in establishing the cause of an unknown ocular infection. Although giant cells are commonly seen following infection by the herpes viruses, they are rarely seen in adenoviral infections.

THERAPY

Previous attempts to treat adenoviral ocular infections with topical antiherpetic antivirals (idoxuridine,[23] adenine arabinoside,[86] trifluridine[116]) proved unsuccessful. Some clinical studies with interferon were promising,[57,99] but critical analysis of other studies[1,90,123] failed to demonstrate convincing efficacy. Because no specific antiviral treatment is presently available, the principles of therapy of adenoviral ocular infection remain as follows: (1) symptomatic treatment of the affected individual and (2) prevention of spread to others by isolation of the affected individual from susceptibles at work, school, and within the family.

During the first 2 weeks, treatment of the acutely infected patient includes cold compresses for comfort, dark glasses for photophobia, mild vasoconstrictors, and reassurance. There is no indication for treatment with potent topical antibiotics such as the aminoglycosides or fluoroquinolones, because secondary bacterial infection is very rare. Furthermore, these antibiotics are expensive and potentially toxic to the inflamed eye, and indiscriminate usage will select for resistant bacteria in the community. In rare cases of virulent infection with disabling vision loss, pseudomembrane formation, iridocyclitis, and corneal edema, a combined antibiotic–low-dose corticosteroid combination and cycloplegic may be used and tapered over the first 7 days.

Antiinflammatory Agents

The role of topical corticosteroid therapy following the appearance of subepithelial infiltrates at 10 to 14 days remains controversial. The empirical clinical experience suggests that treatment with topical corticosteroids may spare some patients with subepithelial infiltrates considerable morbidity (visual loss, discomfort, photophobia, and glare), and tapering them off corticosteroids over several weeks can be accomplished without consequences. On the other hand, the clinical experience also clearly demonstrates that many other patients cannot be tapered off corticosteroids without the return of disabling symptoms. This undesirable situation of "steroid addiction" can prolong a normally self-limiting disease for months or even years[71] and expose the patient to the risks of glaucoma, cataracts, and other microbial superinfections.

As previously discussed, the dilemma faced by the treating ophthalmologist is that, at the time of decision, the doctor does not know which clinical course the patient will follow. The pathogenic factors (Fig. 69-3) that determine the clinical outcome (total antigen load, immunogenicity, infecting serotype and isolate virulence) cannot be known. Therefore initiating treatment with topical corticosteroids at 10 to 14 days, when subepithelial infiltrates first appear, generally is to be discouraged. Instead continuing supportive therapy (reassurance, sunglasses, artificial tears, vasoconstrictors) is recommended because the natural history of subepithelial infiltrates is gradual resolution over time. Topical nonsteroidal antiinflammatory drugs (NSAIDs)—for example, diclofenac (Voltaren) and ketorolac (Acular)—may prove useful and should also be considered.

Significant patient morbidity (visual loss, inability to drive safely, loss of time from work) may persuade the doctor to treat subepithelial infiltrates with topical corticosteroids. In this case a fully informed consent of the risks and benefits should be obtained from the patient and documented in the record.

Surgery

Prolonged and significant visual loss because of permanent scarring in the visual axis from subepithelial infiltrates is a very rare outcome of adenoviral ocular infection. In the past, surgical procedures including superficial keratectomy and lamellar keratoplasty have been performed.[72,107] In the future, excimer laser may prove useful in the treatment of these rare cases.

Prevention of Spread

In addition to treatment of the affected individual, therapy includes the prevention of spread to others by isolation of the affected individual from susceptibles at work and school and within the family. Because ocular shedding of infectious adenovirus continues for up to 2 weeks from the onset of symptoms in the second eye, infected individuals should be excused from work or school for that period. The secondary attack rates in institutions and households range from 5 to 32%[30] and may be dependent on serotype and isolate virulence. Because the virus is spread by direct contact, the ophthalmologist should instruct the patient that transmission within the family can be minimized by careful adherence to the following guidelines of personal hygiene. The family should not share eyeglasses, sunglasses, towels, washcloths, linens, or bars of soap.[30,85] Sexual intimacy should be avoided, and infected family members should avoid direct physical contact with other family members during the period of communicability.

Infected individuals should wash their hands frequently to avoid spreading the virus to common surfaces; a recent study demonstrated that infectious adenovirus could be cultured from the hands of 46% of patients during the period of active ocular infection.[7] Contact lens wearers should use heat sterilization whenever possible, because a contaminated lens case was the apparent source of repeated episodes of adenovirus keratoconjunctivitis in a wearer of soft contact lenses.[9]

PROGNOSIS

Most cases of acute ocular adenovirus infection resolve without significant sequelae within 2 to 3 weeks. Most cases with symptomatic delayed-onset subepithelial corneal infiltrates also resolve within weeks or months in the absence of topical corticosteroid therapy. Even those eyes in which subepithelial infiltrates persist for years rarely experience prolonged photophobia and visual loss.

The problems encountered in certain patients following the initial successful treatment of subepithelial infiltrates with topical corticosteroids have already been discussed. The inability to taper patients off corticosteroids without the immediate return of subepithelial infiltrates and associated disabling symptoms (visual loss, glare, and photophobia) may prolong patient morbidity for months to years. Furthermore the enhanced corticosteroid-related risks of glaucoma and cataracts create a frustrating dilemma for both patient and doctor. After several failed attempts to wean the patient from topical corticosteroids, it is sometimes necessary just to stop the corticosteroid treatment abruptly ("cold turkey"), and to reassure the patient over the next several months as the infiltrates and their associated symptoms undergo natural resolution. Alternatively the use of topical NSAIDs such as diclofenac (Voltaren) or ketorolac (Acular) may help wean a patient from chronic corticosteroid therapy.

Most episodes of ocular adenoviral infection resolve without problems, but occasionally, virulent isolates and serotypes (AD5, AD8, AD19)[25] may cause permanent conjunctival scarring, symblephara, blepharoptosis,[18] and vision loss.[72,107] Furthermore, months after documented adenoviral infection, chronic recurrent papillary conjunctivitis with keratitis has been reported with recovery on rare occasions by culture of AD2, AD3, AD4, AD5, and AD19.[112]

PREVENTION

Preventive measures to reduce the spread of ocular adenoviral infection within households have already been discussed in the section on therapy. Prevention of community epidemics is based on the general principle of isolating infected individuals from susceptibles. Because the general population of the United States and Europe has a relatively low level of natural immunity (<10% for AD8 based on serology),[44,50] the availability of unprotected individuals within the community remains high. Therefore, as previously recommended, infected individuals should be sent home and thus removed from the workplace, school, and camp during the period of communicability (2 weeks after the onset of clinical symptoms in the second eye).

In the military, epidemics of ocular and respiratory adenoviral infections have had a major negative impact on military preparedness. A recent epidemic of EKC at Clark Air Base affected 18% of military personnel, persisted for 6 months, and resulted in the loss of 9038 workdays.[85] Live virus vaccines have been developed against AD4 and AD7 and their efficacy has been demonstrated against ARD,[93,102] but unfortunately these serotypes are not the most common serotypes that cause ocular infection (that is, AD8, AD19). Even so, interest in the use of adenovirus vaccines has recently been stimulated by proposals to use the current vaccine as a delivery vector for other vaccines.[42] Vaccines for rabies, hepatitis, cytomegalovirus, herpesvirus and several other important viral diseases are currently undergoing testing in the laboratory and in clinical trials.

Prevention guidelines to reduce the spread of ocular adenoviral infections at health care facilities is of special interest to the ophthalmologist. Over the past 50 years the role of the ophthalmologist as vector and his or her office as transmission site has been well documented.[30,117] These epidemics occur because infected patients are brought into contact with susceptible patients and office personnel, and viral spread occurs through direct contact of shared surfaces.

Recent laboratory experiments suggest another possible reason why office-based transmission continues despite all educational efforts to eliminate it. It now appears that some of the more common ocular serotypes (AD8, AD19, AD5) are much hardier than previously suspected. Under experimental conditions desiccated virus could be recovered from nonporous surfaces in infectious doses for up to 4 to 5 weeks.[36,78] The possibility that transmission occurs in the waiting room via AD-infected tear secretions deposited on shared surfaces (door handles, chairs, magazines, public telephones, common bathrooms) deserves further consideration.

The general principles involved in preventing office-based epidemics include (1) triage to separate infected individuals from susceptibles and (2) specific preventive measures to eliminate viral spread by direct contact on shared surfaces. Practical measures include the prompt identification by knowledgeable staff of "red-eyed" patients and separating them quickly from other patients in the waiting area. These patients should be taken directly to a dedicated "red-eye" examining room. These measures diminish direct spread of virus in the waiting area by reducing deposits of infected secretions, eliminating crowding, and reducing exposure time between infected and susceptibles. Initiating and following these measures diligently, however, require considerable organization and commitment by the average office practice.

In the examining area, spread by direct contact is eliminated by careful handwashing by all health personnel who come in contact with the patient, sterilization of all instruments that touch the eye (tonometers, contact lenses for laser and gonioscopy, scleral depressors, etc.), and the use of unit dose solutions of topical anesthetics, mydriatics, and sterile fluorescein strips. All bathroom areas serving both patients and staff should have hot-air dryers and soap dispensers to avoid spread by common cloth dryers and bars of soap. Strict adherence to all of these preventive measures is effective in preventing office-based epidemics.[30,117] Occasional lapses in following all of these guidelines in a busy office practice may contribute to the continuing problem of office-based epidemics, however.

Terminating established epidemics within an office practice can be difficult. In addition to strict adherence to the above guidelines, infected personnel should be removed from the office, all elective procedures should be postponed, and consultation with appropriate infectious disease specialists and epidemiologists should be obtained. Despite adherence to all of these rigorous measures, an epidemic of AD8 involving 110 patients at the Illinois Eye and Ear Infirmary required more than 4 months to eradicate completely.[117]

FUTURE DIRECTIONS

There is no clinically effective antiviral that inhibits the many serotypes of adenovirus that replicate on the ocular surface and produce clinical disease. The development of such a drug is highly desirable to reduce patient morbidity and to reduce absenteeism in the workplace, the classroom, and the military. An antiviral that inhibits viral replication would shorten the duration of ocular viral shedding and reduce the total antigen load in the cornea. Not only would the duration of acute disease be reduced, but the number and severity of subepithelial infiltrates would also be diminished, thereby shortening the course of the disease. The reduced duration of viral shedding would also reduce the number and duration of community and office-based epidemics because the time for transmission to susceptibles would be shortened. Furthermore, antiviral prophylaxis to the fellow eye and to family members at risk would also reduce the epidemic spread of virus within the family and community.

In vitro cell culture studies have demonstrated a number of promising compounds that inhibit some or all of the ocular serotypes known to produce human ocular disease. The most effective compounds to date include the nucleoside analogs: HPMPC, HPMPA, 2'-nor-cGMP and ganciclovir.[8,39] Reliable models of adenoviral replication have been developed in the New Zealand (NZ) rabbit[37] and cotton rat.[104,105] Because these animal models of ocular adenoviral replication mimic human infection, their availability will accelerate the testing of promising antiviral compounds. One ocular model is based on the ocular inoculation of NZ rabbits with a clinical isolate, AD5 McEwen, that subsequently replicates in 100% of eyes, reaches peak titers of 10^4 pfu/ml by day 4, and clears completely by day 14.[37] In this NZ rabbit model, topical 0.2% HPMPC was effective in reducing viral titers and duration of viral shedding in both treatment and pretreatment studies.[38] Further studies with HPMPC and other promising compounds (for example, ganciclovir in the cotton rat[104]) will probably soon lead to the development of an effective antiviral for the treatment of adenoviral ocular infections.

Clinical testing and further development of topical non-steroidal antiinflammatory drugs to treat established subepithelial infiltrates also may prove useful. Direct inhibition of the inflammatory and/or immune response by topical medications that act against mononuclear cells (for example, FK 506) or decrease adhesion molecule expression may be productive avenues of future research.

Another area of research that is likely to affect office-based and community epidemics is the development of rapid, accurate diagnostic kits for detecting adenovirus in the office. Rapid, accurate diagnosis in atypical clinical cases would enable the ophthalmologist to advise the patient appropriately, to limit the spread within families and to remove the patient from school or the workplace to reduce community epidemics. Furthermore, rapid diagnosis would enable the doctor to clean the red-eye room, sterilize his instruments, wash his hands, and further protect himself and office personnel from an office-based epidemic. In the future when effective antivirals are available, rapid diagnosis will allow for the immediate initiation of therapy and prophylaxis of individuals at risk.

REFERENCES

1. Adams CP et al.: Interferon treatment of adenoviral conjunctivitis, *Am J Ophthalmol* 98:429-432, 1984.
2. Adrian T, Bastian B, Wagner V: Restriction site mapping adenovirus type 9 and 15 and genomic types of intermediate A15/H19, *Intervirol* 30:169-176, 1989.
3. Adrian T, Becker M, Hierholzer JC et al.: Molecular epidemiology and restriction site mapping of adenovirus type 7 genome types, *Arch Virol* 106:73-84, 1989.
4. Albert DM et al.: In vitro neoplastic transformation of uveal and retinal tissue by oncogenic DNA viruses, *Int Ophthalmol Clin* 7:357-375, 1968.
5. Allard A et al.: Polymerase chain reaction for detection of adenoviruses in stool samples, *J Clin Microbiol* 28:2659, 1990.
6. Aoki K et al.: Viral conjunctivitis with special reference to adenovirus type 37 and enterovirus 70 infection, *Jpn J Ophthalmol* 30:158-164, 1986.
7. Azar M et al.: The recovery of adenovirus from the hands of EKC patients, *Invest Ophthalmol Vis Sci* 34(suppl):1003, 1993.
8. Baba M et al.: Selective inhibitory effect of (S)-9-(3-Hydroxy-2-Phosphonylmethoxypropyl) Adenine and 2'-nor-cyclic GMP on adenovirus replication in vitro, *Antimicrob Agents Chemother* 31:337-339, 1987.
9. Balyeat HD, Bowman J, Rowsey JJ: Adenoviral keratoconjunctivitis associated with chemical disinfection of a flexible lens, *Contact Intraocular Len Med J* 4:68-69, 1978.
10. Beale R: Sur une forme particuliere de conjunctivite aigue avec follicules, *Ann Oculist* 87:1, 1907.
11. Bell JA, Rowe WP, Engler JI et al.: Pharyngo-conjunctival fever: epidemiological studies of a recently recognized disease entity, *JAMA* 175:1083-1092, 1955.
12. Bell SD et al.: Adenovirus isolated from Saudi Arabia—six new serotypes, *Am J Trop Med Hyg* 9:523-526, 1960.

13. Belshe RB, Mufson MA: Identification of immunofluorescence of adenoviral antigen in exfoliated bladder epithelial cells from patient with acute hemorrhagic cystitis, *Proc Soc Exp Biol Med* 146:754-758, 1974.

14. Berget SM, Moore C, Sharpe PA: Spliced segments at the 5′ terminus of adenovirus type 2 late mRNA, *Proc Soc Natl Acad Sci USA* 74:3171-3175, 1977.

15. Bietti GB, Bruna F: Epidemic keratoconjunctivitis in Italy, some contributions to its clinical aspects, epidemiology and etiology, *Am J Ophthalmol* 43:50-57, 1957.

16. Boniuk M et al.: Chronic adenovirus type 2 keratitis in man, *New Eng J Med* 273:924-925, 1965.

17. Chroboczek J, Bieber F, Jackrot B: The sequence of the genome of adenovirus type 5 and its comparison with the genome of AD type 2, *Virol* 186:280-285, 1992.

18. Corin S, Harvey J: Epidemic keratoconjunctivitis associated with blepharoptosis, *Am J Ophthalmol* 106:360-361, 1968.

19. Culliver AB: Clinical and epidemiological features of adenovirus keratoconjunctivitis, *Trans Ophthalmol Soc UK* 100:263-267, 1980.

20. Darougar S et al.: Epidemic keratoconjunctivitis and chronic conjunctivitis in London due to adenovirus type 19, *Br J Ophthalmol* 61:76-85, 1977.

21. Dawson CR et al.: Adenovirus type 8 kerato-conjunctivitis in the United States, *Am J Ophthalmol* 69:473-480, 1970.

22. deJong JC, Wigand R, Kidd AH et al.: Candidate adenoviruses 40 and 41: fastidious adenoviruses from human infant stool, *J Med Virol* 11:215-231, 1983.

23. Dudgeon J et al.: Treatment of adenovirus infection of the eye with 5-iodo-2′-deoxyuridine, *Br J Ophthalmol* 53:530-533, 1969.

24. Dustin ML, Springer TA: Role of lymphocyte adhesion receptors in transient interactions and cell locomotion, *Ann Rev Immunol* 9:27-66, 1991.

25. Editorial: Adenovirus keratoconjunctivitis, *Br J Ophthalmol* 61:73-75, 1977.

26. Editorial: Epidemic keratoconjunctivitis, *JAMA* 156:1503, 1954.

27. Egan D, Bayley ST, Branton PE: Binding of the Rb1 protein to E1A products is required for adenovirus transformation, *Oncogene* 4:383-388, 1989.

28. Elner VM et al.: Intercellular adhesion molecule-1 (ICAM-1) and HLA-DR antigens in herpetic keratitis, *Ophthalmology* 99:1400-1407, 1992.

29. Evans AS: Latent adenovirus infections of the human respiratory tract, *Am J Hyg* 67:256-266, 1958.

30. Ford E, Nelson KE, Warren D: Epidemiology of epidemic keratoconjunctivitis, *Epidemiol Rev* 9:244-261, 1987.

31. Fox JP, Brand CD, Wasserman FE et al.: The Virus Watch Program: a continuing surveillance of viral infections in metropolitan New York families. VI. Observation of adenovirus infections, *Am J Epidemiol* 89:25-50, 1969.

32. Gibson JA et al.: Comparative sensitivity of a cultural test and the complement fixation test in the diagnosis of adenovirus ocular infection, *Br J Ophthalmol* 63:617-620, 1979.

33. Gitliotti F et al.: Etiology of acute conjunctivitis in children, *J Pediatr* 98:531-536, 1981.

34. Gomes SA, Gabbay YB, Nascimento JP et al.: Genome analysis of adenovirus 4a, a causative agent of pharyngoconjunctival fever and respiratory diseases, *J Med Virol* 26:453-459, 1988.

35. Gooding LR, Elmore LW, Tollefson AE et al.: A 14.700 Mw protein from the E3 region of adenovirus inhibits cytolysis by tumor necrosis factor, *Cell* 53:341-346, 1991.

36. Gordon R et al.: Prolonged recovery of desiccated adenovirus 5, 8, and 19 in vitro may partially explain clinical epidemics, *Ophthalmology* 99(suppl):83, 1992.

37. Gordon YJ et al.: An ocular model of adenovirus type 5 infection in the NZ rabbit, *Invest Ophthalmol Vis Sci* 33:574-580, 1992.

38. Gordon YJ et al.: Pre-treatment with topical 0.1% S-HPMPC inhibits adenovirus type 5 replication in the NZ rabbit ocular model, *Cornea* 11:529-533, 1992.

39. Gordon YJ et al.: Inhibitory effect of (S)-HPMPC, (S)-HPMPA and 2′-nor cyclic GMP on clinical ocular adenoviral isolates is serotype-dependent in vitro, *Antiviral Res* 16:11-16, 1991.

40. Gordon YJ et al.: Replication of ocular isolates of human adenovirus is serotype-dependent in rabbit corneal organ culture, *Curr Eye Res* 10:267-271, 1991.

41. Guo D, Shibita R, Sinagawa M et al.: Genomic comparison of adenovirus type 3 isolates from patients with acute conjunctivitis in Japan, Australia and the Phillipines, *Microbiol Immunol* 32:833-842, 1988.

42. Graham FL, Prevec L: Adenovirus based expression vectors and recombinant vaccines, *Biotechniques* 20:363-390, 1992.

43. Greene M, Daesch GE: Biochemical studies on adenovirus multiplication I Kinetics of nucleic acid and protein synthesis in suspension cultures, *Virol* 13:169-176, 1961.

44. Guyer B et al.: Epidemic keratoconjunctivitis a community outbreak of mixed adenovirus type 8 and type 19 infection, *J Infect Dis* 132:142-150, 1975.

45. Hallsworth, McDonald PJ: Rapid diagnosis of viral infections with fluorescent antisera, *Pathology* 17:629-632, 1985.

46. Hara J et al.: Adenovirus type 10 keratoconjunctivitis with increased intraocular pressure, *Am J Ophthalmol* 90:481-484, 1980.

47. Harnett GB, Newnham WA: Isolation of adenovirus type 19 from the male and female genital tracts, *Br J Vener Dis* 57:55-57, 1981.

48. Hierholzer JC: Adenoviruses. In Balows A, editor: *Manual of clinical microbiology,* Washington, D.C., 1991, American Society for Microbiology.

49. Hierholzer JC, Hatch MH: Acute hemmorhagic conjunctivitis. In Darrell RW, editor: *Viral diseases of the eye,* 165-196, Philadelphia, 1985, Lea & Feiberger.

50. Hierholzer JC, Sprague JB: Five-year analysis of adenovirus 8 antibody levels in an industrial community following an outbreak of keratoconjunctivitis, *Am J Epidemiol* 110:132-140, 1979.

51. Hierholzer JC et al.: Adenovirus from patients with AIDS: a plethora of serotypes and a description of five new serotypes of subgenus D (types 43-47), *J Infect Dis* 158:804-813, 1988.

52. Hobson LC: Acute epidemic superficial punctate keratitis, *Am J Ophthalmol* 21:1153-1155, 1938.

53. Hogan MJ, Crawford JW: Epidemic keratoconjunctivitis (superficial punctate keratitis, keratitis subepithelialis, keratitis maculosa, keratitis nummularis), *Am J Ophthalmol* 25:1059-1078, 1942.

54. Horwitz MS: Adenoviruses. In Fields BN, Knipe DM et al., editors: *Virology,* 1723-1740, New York, 1990, Raven.

55. Huang G, Deibel R: Nucleic acid hybridization for detection of cell culture-amplified adenovirus, *J Clin Microbiol* 26:2652-2656, 1988.

56. Insler MS, Kern MD: Keratoconjunctivitis due to adenovirus type 8, *South Med J* 82:159-160, 1989.

57. Isacsohn M et al.: Human fibroblast interferon in treatment of viral diseases of the skin and mucous membranes, *Isr J Med Sci* 19:959-962, 1983.

58. Ishii K, Nakazono N, Fujinaga K et al.: Comparative studies on the aetiology and epidemiology of viral conjunctivitis in three countries of East Asia and Japan, Taiwan and South Korea, *Int J Epidemiol* 16:98-103, 1987.

59. Itakura S, Aoki K, Sawada H et al.: Analysis with restriction endonucleases recognizing 4 and 5 base pair sequences of human adeonivirus type 3 isolated from ocular diseases in Sapporo, Japan, *J Clin Microbiol* 28:2365-2369, 1990.

60. Jawatz E, Kimura SJ, Hanna L et al.: Studies on the etiology of epidemic keratoconjunctivitis, *Am J Ophthalmol* 40:200-211, 1955.

61. Jones BR: Adenovirus infections of the eye in London, *Trans Ophthalmol Soc UK* 88:621-640, 1962.

62. Jones BR: The clinical features of viral keratitis and a concept of their pathogenesis, *Proc Roy Soc Med* 51:13-20, 1958.

63. Kemp MC, Hierholzer JC: Three adenovirus type 8 genome types defined by restriction enzymes: prototype stability in geographically separated populations, *J Clin Microbiol* 23:469-474, 1986.

64. Kemp MC, Hierholzer JC, Cabradilla CP et al.: The changing etiology of epidemic keratoconjunctivitis; antigenic and restriction enzyme analysis of adenovirus types 19 and 37 isolated over a 10 year period, *J Infect Dis* 148:24-33, 1983.

65. Kibrick S, Melengez L, Enders JF: Clinical association of enterovirus with particular reference to agents exhibiting properties of the ECHO group, *Am NY Acad Sci* 67:311, 1957.

66. Kiernan JP: Stevens-Johnson syndrome associated with adenovirus keratoconjunctivitis, *Am J Ophthalmol* 92:543-5455, 1981.

67. Kobayashi TK et al.: Cytological evaluation of adenoviral follicular conjunctivitis by cytobrush, *Ophthalmologica* 202:156-160, 1991.

68. Kowalski RP, Gordon YJ: Comparison of direct rapid tests for the detection of adenovirus antigen in routine conjunctival specimens, *Ophthalmology* 96:1106-1109, 1989.

69. Ladisch S, Lovejoy FH, Hierholzer JC et al.: Extrapulmonary manifestations of the adenovirus type 7 pneumonia simulating Reyes syndrome and the possible role of adenovirus toxin, *J Pediatr* 95:348-355, 1979.

70. Laibson PR: Ocular adenoviral infections, *Int Ophthalmol Clin* 24:49-64, 1984.

71. Laibson PR et al.: Corneal infiltrates and epidemic keratoconjunctivitis: response to double blind corticosteroid therapy, *Arch Ophthalmol* 84:36-40, 1987.

72. Lund O, Stefani FD: Corneal histology after epidemic keratoconjunctivitis, *Arch Ophthalmol* 96:2085-2088, 1978.

73. McMinn PC et al.: A community outbreak of epidemic keratoconjunctivitis in central Australia due to adenovirus type 8, *J Infect Dis* 164:1113-1117, 1991.

74. Mogabgab WJ: Mycoplasma pneumonia and adenovirus respiratory disease in military and university personnel, 1959-1966, *Am Rev Respir Dis* 97:345-358, 1968.

75. Mukai N et al.: A DNA virus-induced model of retinoblastoma, *Int Ophthalmol Clin* 20:2233-245, 1980.

76. Mullbacher A: Virus escape from immune recognition; multiple strategies of adenoviruses, *Immunol Cell Biol* 70:59-63, 1992.

77. Murrah WF: Epidemic keratoconjunctivitis, *Am Ophthalmol* 20:36-38, 1988.

78. Nauheim RC et al.: Prolonged recovery of desiccated adenovirus type 19 from various surfaces, *Ophthalmology* 97:1450-1453, 1990.

79. Nelson KE et al.: The role of adenoviruses in the pertussis syndrome, *J Pediatr* 86:335-341, 1975.

80. Neummann R, Genersch E, Eggers HJ: Detection of adenovirus nucleic acid sequences in human tonsils in the absence of infectious virus, *Virus Res* 7:93-97, 1987.

81. Noda M et al.: Intermediate human adenoviruses type 22/H10, 19, 37 as a new etiological agent of conjunctivitis, *J Clin Microbiol* 29:1286-1289, 1991.

82. O'Day DM, Guyer B: Clinical and laboratory evaluation of epidemic keratoconjunctivitis due to adenovirus types 8 and 19, *Am J Ophthalmol* 81:207-215, 1976.

83. O'Donnell B, Bell E, Payne SP et al.: Genomic analysis of species 3 adenoviruses isolated during the summer outbreaks of conjunctivitis and pharyngo-conjunctival fever in the Glasgow and London areas in 1981, *J Med Virol* 18:213-227, 1986.

84. Ostler HB: Suspected infectious etiology. In Thoft RA, Smolin G, editors: *The cornea,* ed 2, 299-302, Boston, 1994, Little, Brown.

85. Paparello SF et al.: Epidemic keratoconjunctivitis at a U.S. military base: Republic of the Phillipines, *Mil Med* 156:256-259, 1991.

86. Pavan-Langston D, Dohlman CH: A double-blind clinical study of adenine arabinoside therapy of viral conjunctivitis, *Am J Ophthalmol* 74:81-88, 1972.

87. Pettit TH, Holland GN: Chronic keratoconjunctivitis associated with ocular adenovirus infection, *Am J Ophthalmol* 88:748-751, 1979.

88. Rao L, Debbas M, Sabbatini P et al.: The adenovirus E1A protein induces apoptosis, which is inhibited by the E1B 19Kda and Bcl-2 proteins, *Proc Soc Natl Acad Sci USA* 89:7742-7746, 1992.

89. Rapoza PR et al.: Epidemiology and diagnosis of acute conjunctivitis at an inner-city hospital, *Ophthalmology* 96:1215-1220, 1989.

90. Reilly S et al.: Adenovirus type 8 keratoconjunctivitis–an outbreak and its treatment with topical human fibroblast interferon, *J Hyg* 96:557-575, 1984.

91. Rivadeneira ED, Henshaw NG: Adenoviruses and adeno-associated viruses. In Joklik WK, Willet HP, Amos DB, Wilfert CM, editors: *Zinsser microbiology,* ed 20, 968-974, Norwalk, 1992, Appleton & Lange.

92. Roba L et al.: How long are patients with epidemic keratoconjunctivitis infectious?, *Invest Ophthalmol Vis Sci* 34(suppl):848, 1993.

93. Rose HM et al.: Adenoviral infection in military recruits: emergence of type 7 and 21 infections in recruits immunized with type 4 oral vaccine, *Arch Environ Health* 21:356-361, 1970.

94. Rowe WP, Huebner RJ, Gilmore LK et al.: Isolation of a cytopathogenic agent from human adenoids undergoing spontaneous degeneration in tissue culture, *Proc Soc Exp Biol Med* 84:570, 1953.

95. Schaap GJ et al.: A new intermediate adenovirus causing conjunctivitis, *Arch Ophthalmol* 97:2336-2338, 1979.

96. Schwartz HS et al.: Immunofluorescent detection of adenovirus antigen in epidemic keratoconjunctivitis, *Invest Ophthalmol Vis Sci* 15:199-207, 1976.

97. Simila S et al.: Encephalomeningitis in children associated with an adenovirus type 7 epidemic, *Acta Pediatr Scand* 59:310-316, 1970.

98. Sprague JB, Hierholzer JC, Gurrier RW II et al.: Epidemic keratoconjunctivitis; a severe industrial outbreak due to adenovirus type 8, *New Eng J Med* 289:1341-1345, 1973.

99. Sundmacher R et al.: The value of exogenous interferon in adenovirus keratoconjunctivitis, *Graefes Arch Clin Exp Ophthalmol* 218:139-140, 1982.

100. Tanaka C: Epidemic keratoconjunctivitis in Japan and the Orient, *Am J Ophthalmol* 43:46-49, 1957.

101. Thygeson P: Further observations on superficial punctate keratitis, *Arch Ophthalmol* 66:158-162, 1961.

102. Top FH: Control of adenovirus acute respiratory disease in US Army trainees, *Yale J Biol Med* 48:185-195, 1975.

103. Townsend A, Bodmer H: Antigen recognition by class I restricted T lymphocytes, *Ann Rev Immunol* 7:601-624, 1989.

104. Trousdale MD, Goldschmidt PL, Nobrega R: Activity of ganciclovir against human adenovirus type-5 infection in cell culture and cotton rat eyes, *Invest Ophthalmol Vis Sci* 34(suppl):848, 1993.

105. Tsai JC et al.: An experimental animal model of adenovirus-induced ocular disease, the cotton rat, *Invest Ophthalmol Vis Sci* 110:1167-1170, 1992.

106. Tullo AB: Shipyard eye, *Br Med J* 283:1056-1057, 1981 (letter).

107. Tullo AB, Higgins PG: An outbreak of adenovirus keratoconjunctivitis in Bristol, *Br J Ophthalmol* 63:621, 1979.

108. Turse SE et al.: Development of P.C.R. for the detection of adenovirus in clinical ocular samples, *Invest Ophthalmol Vis Sci* 34(suppl):1349, 1993.

109. Uchida Y, Inoue S: Fluorescent antibody studies of epidemic keratoconjunctivitis, *Jpn J Ophthalmol* 11:17-22, 1967.

110. Valentine RC, Pereira HG: Antigens and structure of the adenoviruses, *J Mol Biol* 13:13-20, 1965.

111. Van Rij G et al.: Immune electron microscopy and cultural test in the diagnosis of adenovirus ocular infection, *Br J Ophthalmol* 66:317-319, 1982.

112. Vastine DW: Adenoviruses and miscellaneous viral infections. In Thoft RA, Smolin G, editors, *The cornea,* ed 2, 267, Boston, 1988, Little, Brown.

113. Vastine DW et al.: Cytologic diagnosis of adenoviral epidemic keratoconjunctivitis by direct immunofluorescence, *Invest Ophthalmol Vis Sci* 16:195-200, 1977.

114. Wagner S, Green MR: A transcriptional tryst, *Nature* 352:189, 1991.

115. Walpita P, Darougar S: Double-label immunofluorescence method for simultaneous detection of adenovirus and herpes simplex virus from the eye, *J Clin Microbiol* 27:1623-1625, 1989.

116. Ward JB, Siojo LG, Waller SG: A prospective masked clinical trial of trifluridine, dexamethasone, and artificial tears in the treatment of epidemic keratoconjunctivitis, *Cornea* 12:216-221, 1993.

117. Warren D et al.: A large outbreak of epidemic keratoconjunctivitis: problems in controlling nosocomial spread, *J Infect Dis* 160:938-943, 1989.

118. Wiener M: Keratitis punctata superficialis, with the report of a case, *Arch Ophthalmol* 38:120-124, 1909.

119. Wigand R, Brian T: Intermediate adenovirus strains of subgroup D occur in extensive variety, *Med Microbiol Immunol* 178:45-57, 1989.

120. Wigand R et al.: Isolation and identification of enteric adenoviruses, *J Med Virol* 11:233-240, 1983.

121. Wiley L et al.: Rapid diagnostic test for ocular adenovirus, *Ophthalmology* 95:431-433, 1988.

122. Wilfert CM, Joklik WK: Pathogenesis of viral infection. In Joklik WK, Willet HP, Amos DB, Wilfert CM, editors: *Zinsser microbiology,* ed 20, 935, Norwalk, 1992, Appleton & Lange.

123. Wilhelmus KR et al.: Topical human fibroblast interferon for acute adenoviral conjunctivitis, *Graefes Arch Clin Exp Ophthalmol* 225:461-464, 1987.

124. Wold WSM, Gooding LR: The region E3 of adenovirus; a cassette of genes involved in host immunosurveillance and virus cell interactions, *Virol* 184:1-8, 1991.

70 Enterovirus Keratoconjunctivitis

ROBERT H. ROSA JR., EDUARDO C. ALFONSO

Ocular enterovirus infection is classically associated with acute hemorrhagic conjunctivitis (AHC), which is most often caused by enterovirus 70 and coxsackievirus A24. AHC is characterized by the acute onset of periorbital pain and/or foreign body sensation, subconjunctival hemorrhages, diffuse fine superficial punctate erosions, lid edema, and profuse watery discharge. Rapid resolution of symptoms typically occurs within 3 to 5 days without significant ocular sequelae. The short incubation period, rapid time course, and absence of subepithelial infiltrates are distinctly different from the typical presentation of patients with epidemic keratoconjunctivitis (EKC) caused by adenovirus.

EPIDEMIOLOGY

Acute hemorrhagic conjunctivitis, also known as Apollo 11 disease, epidemic hemorrhagic conjunctivitis, Singapore epidemic conjunctivitis, Joy Bangla disease, and picornavirus epidemic conjunctivitis, was first recognized in Accra, Ghana on the western coast of Central Africa in June 1969.[18,19,83,86,114] AHC was subsequently reported between 1969 and 1971 in other mainly coastal African countries including Nigeria, Morocco, Algeria, Sierra Leone, Senegal, and Tunisia.[10,43,80] In Asia a very similar epidemic was seen in Java, Djakarta, and Bali in Indonesia in 1970.[75]

Enterovirus Conjunctivitis

Enterovirus 70 was identified as the causative agent of AHC.[44,73] Large epidemics of AHC were reported during 1971 in Japan, Singapore, Malaysia, Korea, Thailand, Vietnam, Cambodia, Laos, Hong Kong, Taiwan, the Philippines, Burma, India, and Pakistan.[17,40,65,86] Small outbreaks of EV70 AHC were observed in London, Moscow, France, and Yugoslavia in the early 1970s.[35,64,66] Serologic surveys indicate that EV70 was not prevalent before this pandemic and that antibodies in the populations involved appeared after the outbreak of AHC.[42,47,50,72]

After an apparent absence of several years, AHC reappeared and spread widely in Africa and Asia. Until 1981 virtually no EV70 infection had been found in the Americas.[29] Between July and September of 1980, an epidemic of AHC occurred in several refugee camps and transit centers in Southeast Asia. Following the creation of a conjunctivitis-free transit center and the institution of preembarkation screening procedures, relatively few cases were imported, and only one possible secondary case was reported.[11] In 1981 AHC spread extensively in the Caribbean and Central and South America including Panama, Colombia, Guyana, Surinam, Honduras, Puerto Rico, Belize, and Trinidad.[8,13,90,108] In August and September 1981 the first outbreaks of EV70 AHC occurred concurrently in Key West and Miami, Florida.[12,28] In Key West 989 cases of AHC were identified.[68] In Miami the outbreak involved 800 documented cases and more than 2500 suspected cases.[84,98] Since 1981 several small outbreaks of EV70 AHC have been reported in the United States, in North Carolina, Minnesota, California, and New York.[12,54,110] The enterovirus 70 isolates from widely separated regions during the same pandemic period (1980 to 1981) were closely related by ribonuclease T1 oligonucleotide fingerprinting.[39]

Coxsackievirus Conjunctivitis

In 1970, soon after the first reports of AHC, a large epidemic of acute conjunctivitis occurred in Singapore in which the causal agent identified was a variant of coxsackievirus A24.[65,74,112] The distinction between coxsackievirus A24 (CA24) and EV70 as separate enteroviruses causing identical clinical presentations was made by serologic characterization and nucleotide sequence homology.[47,79,117] Other coxsackievirus A24 outbreaks have been reported subsequently in Hong Kong in 1971 and 1975, and in Singapore in 1975 and 1985.[17,25,116] Neighboring Taiwan first reported the virus in October, 1985, and Japan suffered an outbreak during 1985 and 1986.[6,21] In 1986 CA24 was isolated for the first time in the Western hemisphere. Large outbreaks of coxsackievirus infection were reported in Trinidad, Jamaica, St. Croix, and Puerto Rico.[14,15] Three outbreaks of CA24

AHC occurred during 1987 and 1988 in the Yucatan Peninsula, Delicias, and Tampico, Mexico.[16]

Mixed Viral Conjunctivitis

Adenovirus (AV) type 11 is said to produce an illness clinically indistinguishable from AHC caused by EV70 or CA24.[7] Mixed epidemics caused by EV70 and AV11 have occurred in Taiwan and Singapore.[103,113] EV70 and CA24 have occurred together in mixed epidemics in Hong Kong and Singapore.[31,74]

Manifestations other than Conjunctivitis

Although ocular enteroviral infection is classically associated with AHC, other manifestations of ocular enteroviral infection appear to be extant. Culture-positive enterovirus cases seen at the Bascom Palmer Eye Institute between January 1986 and December 1992 were reviewed to determine the clinical diagnoses that prompted viral culture. In 18 cases with the typical enterovirus cytopathic effect, the following clinical findings were observed: AHC, nonhemorrhagic conjunctivitis, herpetiform dermatoblepharoconjunctivitis, and dendritic epithelial keratitis. Enterovirus was also cultured from the vitreous in one patient with suspected endophthalmitis with immunosuppression secondary to mycosis fungoides and systemic corticosteroid therapy. Of thirteen patients whose isolates were typed by indirect immunofluorescence, an enterovirus 70/71 blend was positive in two cases of nonhemorrhagic conjunctivitis, both of which were negative for EV70. Echovirus was found in six cases, five with conjunctivitis and one with dermatoblepharoconjunctivitis. Coxsackievirus A24 was isolated from one patient with nonhemorrhagic conjunctivitis (in whom echovirus was also isolated) and from a case of AHC with stromal keratitis in an AIDS patient.

Other investigators have documented infections with some coxsackieviruses and echoviruses that have been accompanied by conjunctivitis. In Sweden in 1973,[2] during an epidemic of meningoencephalitis caused by echovirus type 7 and coxsackievirus type B5, numerous cases of conjunctivitis were observed. In Finland in 1975 echovirus type 7 was isolated from the conjunctiva during an epidemic of meningoencephalitis caused by the same virus.[92] In the former Soviet Union Malanova and associates[67] observed an epidemic outbreak of conjunctivitis caused by coxsackievirus B1. Lemp and associates[63] described a case of chronic cyclical cystic conjunctivitis thought to be caused by coxsackievirus B2. Several authors from the former Soviet Union believe that echovirus 11 is responsible for outbreaks of anterior uveitis in newborns and infants.*

---

*References 36, 52, 53, 62, 97, 104.

PATHOGENESIS

The family of Picornaviridae consists of ribonucleic acid-containing (RNA) viruses and includes the genera of *Enterovirus, Rhinovirus, Aphthovirus,* and *Cardiovirus.* The genus *Enterovirus* spp. consists of polioviruses, echoviruses, enteroviruses of humans, coxsackievirus groups A and B, and enteroviruses of species other than humans. Enterovirus virions are made up of single-stranded RNA and four structural proteins. The epitopes responsible for inducing neutralizing antibodies to the various serotypes are located on the structural proteins. Even within a single recognized serotype (EV70), antigenic differences may occur between different isolates.[70]

Enterovirus 70 was first classified as the causal agent of acute hemorrhagic conjunctivitis in 1973, and cross-neutralization tests showed that the viruses isolated during the 1971 epidemics in Japan, Singapore, and Morocco were distinct from all other known human enterovirus immunotypes.[73] Further studies have characterized the viral isolates into three antigenic subgroups: prototype J670/71-like, intermediate G-10/72-like, and prime variant G2/74-like. Antigenic drift may have occurred by immunologic pressure during the process of transmission from eye to eye of the host.[23,38] EV70 isolates obtained in Asia and the Americas during the 1980 to 1981 epidemics of AHC were found to be very closely related by RNase T1 oligonucleotide fingerprinting.[35] An evolutionary study of EV70 in which a phylogenetic tree was constructed indicates that all isolates were derived from a common ancestor that probably emerged in 1967 ± 15 months.[77] EV70 may actually represent a zoonotic picornavirus that has extended its host range to encompass humans.[91] This hypothesis is supported by seroepidemiologic studies in West Africa that have demonstrated the existence of a virus-neutralizing substance against EV70 in cattle, swine, and sheep.[51] EV70 neutralizing IgM and IgG in animal sera was also found in Japan.[47,93]

A variant of coxsackievirus A24 is the causal agent of an AHC syndrome clinically indistinguishable from EV70 AHC.[74] The complete nucleotide sequence of the EH 24/70 strain of CA24 was determined and indicates that the overall structure and organization of the RNA genome is typical for an enterovirus; however, it is distinguished serologically and genetically from EV70.[79,102] An evolutionary study employing a phylogenetic tree for the CA24 variant indicated that the common ancestral virus appeared in July 1968 ± 25 months.[76] Another study in which a phylogenetic tree was constructed suggests that CA24 evolved from a common ancestor that appeared in November 1963 ± 21 months—7 years before the first isolation of CA24 in Singapore—and that recent epidemic isolates diverged from each other after 1981.[34]

The transmission of enteroviral infection is typically by the fecal-oral route.[70] In contrast to other enteroviruses,

EV70 is spread by fomites and direct inoculation of the conjunctiva from contaminated fingers.[42,94] The conjunctiva is believed to be the primary replication site of both EV70 and CA24. EV70 has been found almost exclusively in conjunctival and throat specimens, but a few fecal isolations have been reported.[70] The incubation period is short, ranging from 12 to 48 hours, and averaging 24 hours. The virus replicates preferentially at 33°C to 35°C, perhaps an adaptation to conjunctival rather than gastrointestinal temperatures.[94,100] Experiments have shown that ultrahigh levels of relative humidity can prolong EV70 survival even at higher air temperatures, apparently because of the lack of drying of the virus inoculum. The presence of moisture in porous fomites (towels) may enhance virus transmission by the inanimate object. Higher levels of skin moisture resulting from increased perspiration under hot, humid conditions may prolong EV70 survival on the hands.[94] The results of these laboratory investigations are very consistent with, and even predictive of, the epidemiologic characteristics of AHC. For example, the incidence of AHC is highest in overcrowded familial settings, among schoolchildren, and in warm, humid tropical environments.*

An epidemic may be triggered when the "herd immunity" of the population falls below a critical level.[26] The number of "susceptible" individuals increases between epidemics. An example of the preceding is the recurrence of multiple epidemics of both EV70 and CA24 in Singapore. During such an epidemic, what host factors are involved in combating enteroviral infections? Virus-specific, early appearing neutralizing activity (ENA) and interferon (IFN) have been detected in tears collected from patients during AHC epidemics.[59] ENA to EV70 was detected by Langford and associates[59] in 6 of 11 patients 1 to 6 hours before the onset of AHC. Sixty-eight percent of patients seen on the first day of symptoms had tears containing ENA to EV70. Fibroblast IFN was also detected in 30% of tear samples collected from patients on the day of onset of EV70 AHC. Langford and associates[57] also found high concentrations of specific anti-CA24 neutralizing activity (NA) in tears collected very early in the infectious process. This finding suggests that biologically, NA may be a factor in the short duration of the disease, the localization of viral damage to the superficial epithelial cells of the conjunctivae and cornea, the recovery without sequelae, the ability to isolate virus for only a short period of time after the onset of illness, the variability in serum antibody responses, and the recurrent epidemics. Langford and associates[58] also detected human fibroblast interferon in the tears of patients very early after the onset of CA24 AHC. This finding suggests that the early signs and symptoms in ocular enteroviral infections are primarily caused by virus implantation and replication in conjunctival and corneal epithelial cells rather than an immunopathologic process as might be triggered by human immune interferon. Virus-specific serum antibody production is not detectable until 7 to 10 days after the onset of AHC, and these levels are inconsistent with some patients who remain seronegative and others who have only a minimal antibody response.[47,107]

Rarely, neurologic complications including an acute lumbar radiculomyelopathy or polio-like syndrome and cranial nerve involvement have been observed during epidemics of EV70 AHC.[20,33,105,107] Motor paralysis resembling poliomyelitis is the most striking feature, and in some patients there is residual paralysis and muscle atrophy. The neurologic manifestations will be characterized in a later section on clinical findings. The neurovirulence of EV70 was demonstrated in cynomolgus monkeys by Kono and associates[45] upon inoculation of the spinal cord and thalamus simultaneously with virus-containing African green monkey kidney-cell cultures. The virus could not be recultured from the central nervous system (CNS) after inoculation. Subsequent studies to date have failed to isolate virus from the CNS or cerebrospinal fluid.[37,48,106] Neutralizing antibodies to EV70, however, have been found in a significant portion of the patients with neurologic complications.[20,44,48,106,107] To date, no neurologic complications have been reported with CA24 AHC.

CLINICAL FEATURES

Ocular Manifestations

The first description of the clinical manifestations of AHC was reported in 1970 by Chatterjee, Quarcoopome, and Apenteng.[18,19] The patients typically complained of severe ocular pain, marked swelling of the lids, tearing, and discharge. Subsequent studies added the following common symptoms: redness, irritation, foreign body sensation, photophobia, itching, burning, and blurry or decreased vision.* Much less common complaints included general malaise, headache, rhinorrhea, cough, general body pains, fever, and sore throat[8,57,68,83] (Table 70-1). Two studies reported upper eyelid pain and frontal headaches that were aggravated or worsened by bending over.[8,98] Onset of the symptoms is usually unilateral with rapid involvement of the second eye —most often within 12 to 24 hours. Resolution of symptoms typically occurs within 3 to 5 days after onset.[98,109] Gangwar and associates[24] compared the clinical picture of sporadic cases of AHC to epidemic cases and found that in sporadic cases redness and watering were the commonest symptoms, whereas itching and irritation were the commonest presenting symptoms in epidemic cases.

---

*References 27, 29, 32, 42, 81, 84, 95.

*References 5, 9, 71, 81, 96, 112.

TABLE 70-1 SYMPTOMS OF AHC AND FREQUENCY OF OCCURRENCE (IN ORDER OF DECREASING FREQUENCY)

Symptom	Average Frequency and Range (%)*
Redness	97 (92-100)
Foreign body sensation	95 (91-100)
Discharge	91 (77-97)
Lacrimation/tearing	88 (70-97)
Bilateral involvement	81 (58-98)
Pain	79 (72-85)
Itching (late)	75 (73-77)
Swelling	62 (33-80)
Photophobia	44 (7-88)
Burning	43 (15-82)
Rhinorrhea†	30 (13-46)
Itching (early)	19 (17-20)
URI or systemic symptoms‡	16
Sore throat‡	16
Headache	15 (1-23)
Cough‡	3
Fever	3 (0-6)
Body aches/pain‡	3

*The frequency of distribution of each symptom was determined by averaging the percentage of patients reported from various series in the literature.[8,9,24,68,81,96,98,109]
†Reported in only two studies.[68,81]
‡Each reported in only one study.[68,81,96,109]

The most characteristic clinical feature of AHC is the appearance of subconjunctival hemorrhages associated with conjunctival injection.[19] These hemorrhages vary from minute pinpoint petechiae to large blotches of frank hemorrhages almost invariably involving the superior temporal bulbar conjunctiva[19,96,109,112] (Figs. 70-1 and 70-2). The inferior bulbar conjunctiva and palpebral conjunctiva are more variably affected. These hemorrhages begin to resolve at

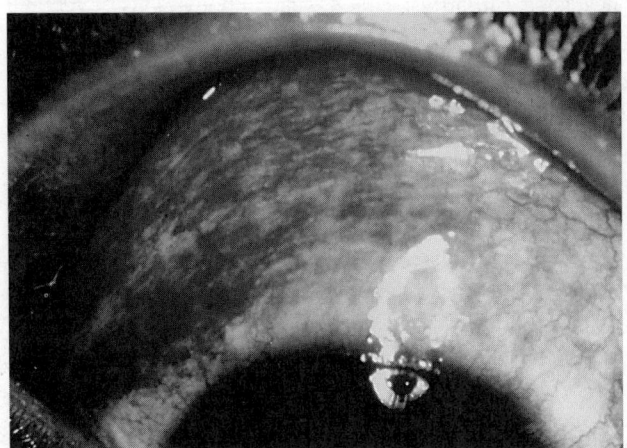

Fig. 70-1. Petechial conjunctival hemorrhages.

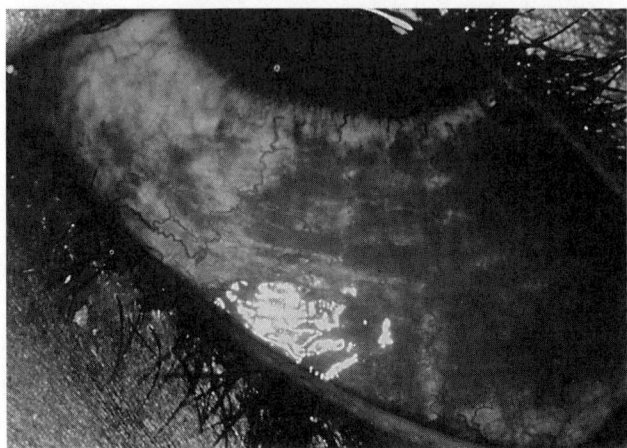

Fig. 70-2. Large patch of frank conjunctival hemorrhage.

approximately day 4 to 5 after onset of the disease, with nearly complete resolution within 7 to 10 days.[19] Conjunctival congestion with follicular hypertrophy involving mostly the lower fornix and chemosis can be quite marked. Mixed papillary and follicular reactions have been reported as common[9,98] (Fig. 70-3).

Chatterjee and associates[19] initially felt that corneal involvement was not characteristic of *epidemic hemorrhagic conjunctivitis*. Quarcoopome,[87] however, subsequently reported fine punctate epithelial and subepithelial erosions and corneal infiltrates involving predominantly the lower half of the cornea in patients with AHC. He found that these lesions cleared completely in the majority of patients in 7 to 14 days without residual corneal opacities. Numerous clinical studies have since documented a rather high incidence of diffuse fine superficial punctate erosions in patients with AHC.* The subepithelial infiltrates characteristic of epidemic keratoconjunctivitis (EKC) are generally not seen in AHC. Some reports have documented only minimal to no corneal epithelial involvement.[96,98,101]

Eyelid edema with a variable degree of puffiness is often seen in patients with AHC. Only rarely is the lid edema severe enough to shut the eye(s).[71] Periorbital ecchymoses are occasionally observed in the acute phase of infection.[8]

At the initial examination the majority of patients with AHC have a profuse, watery discharge. A mucoid to mucopurulent discharge may also be seen in the later stages of the disease.[9,98,112] A pseudomembrane-like appearance was reported in one series.[8]

In the initial description of the clinical findings in AHC, Chatterjee and associates[19] reported a significant percentage (64%) of patients with enlarged preauricular lymph nodes. In other earlier studies, regional lymphadenopathy was not observed.[83,86] Numerous studies have since documented the

*References 5, 8, 75, 81, 109, 112.

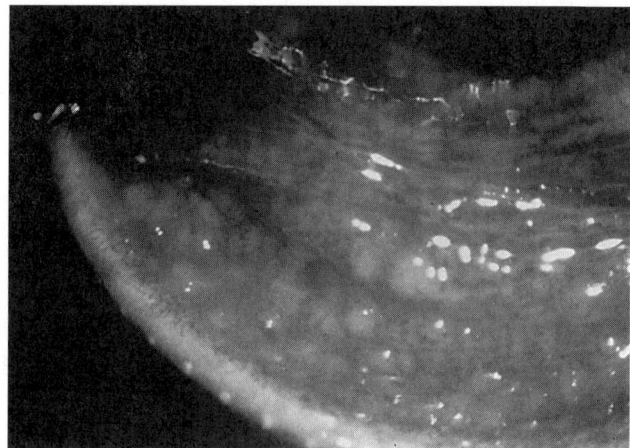

Fig. 70-3. Follicular conjunctival reaction.

prevalence of preauricular lymphadenopathy in patients with AHC.* In 15% to 38% of the patients with AHC the preauricular lymph nodes may actually be quite tender[8,96,112] (Table 70-2).

The clinical syndrome of acute hemorrhagic conjunctivitis that is caused by a variant of coxsackievirus A24 is indistinguishable from AHC caused by enterovirus 70. Some studies indicate that the course of conjunctivitis with CA24 is milder, with less bilaterality than EV70.[6,116] A higher incidence of upper respiratory tract symptoms including nasal discharge, fever, cough, and sore throat, as well as headaches, is reported among patients with CA24 AHC.[6,95,116] Yin-Murphy and associates[116] reported herpeslike vesicles in the conjunctiva and skin of the eyelids in a patient with CA24 AHC.

Neurologic Manifestations

In addition to the potential for bacterial suprainfection, perhaps a more grave difficulty that has been reported is the rare neurologic complication of EV70 AHC occurring in 1 in 10,000 to 20,000 patients. This rare complication has not been reported with CA24 AHC. In 1973 Wadia and associates[105] reported 19 patients who developed an acute neurologic syndrome after having had, or been exposed to, AHC. Males appear to be affected more often than females.† A latent period between the onset of AHC and the onset of neurologic symptoms varies between 5 days and 8 weeks, the majority of patients having neurologic symptoms between 1 to 5 weeks. Wadia and associates[107] saw four patients with neurologic disease and high antibody titers to EV70, who had an exposure to AHC but no personal history of conjunctivitis. Patients may complain of prodromal symptoms such as fever, malaise, myalgias, limb or nerve

root pains, headache, dizziness, and sometimes vomiting before the onset of the neurologic deficit. Intramuscular drug administration and undue physical exertion during the prodromal phase of the illness should be avoided because they seemed to precipitate muscular paralysis in seven patients reported by Phuapradit and associates.[85] Three main forms of neurologic disease have been described: spinal, cranial nerve, and combined.[106,107] The spinal form usually begins with a backache and severe muscular or root pains lasting up to 3 weeks. Most patients then develop an acute, often asymmetric, proximal, areflexic, flaccid paralysis of the lower limbs usually within 4 days of the onset of pains. The iliopsoas, adductor longus, and quadriceps are most often involved, followed by the lower paraspinal and abdominal muscles.[3,106,107] The limb involvement is often asymmetric, with the upper limbs affected less often. Muscle wasting follows the paralytic phase, with the degree of atrophy dependent on the severity and duration of paralysis. The pattern of distribution of flaccid paralysis, the early development of muscle wasting, and the absence of sensory loss during the paralytic stage indicate that the principal lesion is in the anterior horn cells of the spinal cord. This paints a clinical picture that is very similar to poliomyelitis, however, adults rather than children are predominately affected.[33]

The interval between the peak neurologic deficit and the onset of recovery varies from less than a week to 10 weeks, with the majority of patients starting to recover within 3 weeks.[20] As time passes, wasting becomes more prominent,

TABLE 70-2 SIGNS OF AHC AND FREQUENCY OF OCCURRENCE (IN ORDER OF DECREASING FREQUENCY)

Sign	Average Frequency and Range (%)*
Conjunctival injection	99 (95-100)
Follicular reaction	81 (60-100)
Subconjunctival hemorrhage	77 (46-100)
Serous (watery) discharge	76 (45-97)
Superficial punctate staining/erosions	72 (40-100)
Lid edema	57 (4-87)
Papillary reaction	54†
Watery and mucopurulent discharge	51‡
Preauricular lymphadenopathy	49 (7-98)
Chemosis	48 (16-100)
Mucopurulent discharge	23 (13-33)
Pseudomembranes	20‡

*The frequency of distribution of each sign was determined by averaging the percentage of patients reported from various series in the literature.[5,8,9,19,24,68,81,96,98,101,109,112]

†Frequency reported in only one study, however three other studies described the occurrence of a papillary and/or mixed papillary-follicular reaction.[9,69,98,109]

‡Each reported in only one study.[8,9]

---
*References 9, 75, 81, 98, 101, 109.

†References 20, 33, 37, 48, 105, 106, 107.

and functional recovery is based on the severity of paralysis. Chopra and associates[20] followed 38 patients for 3 to 15 months and found complete functional recovery in 3 patients, good functional recovery in 18 patients, a severely handicapped condition in 15 patients, and no recovery in 2 patients.

Unilateral cranial motor nerve palsies are also seen, with the facial nerve the most commonly affected.[33,81,98,107] Trigeminal nerve involvement with masseter weakness, as well as rare cases of abducens and bulbar palsies have been reported.[20,37,106] Numerous reports of palato-pharyngeal weakness or palsy (vagus nerve) have been described.[20,33,96] A combination of spinal and cranial nerve involvement usually indicates a more serious outcome, whereas the prognosis for complete recovery with lone cranial nerve involvement is good.

DIFFERENTIAL DIAGNOSIS

The differential diagnosis of an acute conjunctivitis with subconjunctival hemorrhage includes trauma, toxic or chemical conjunctivitis, allergic conjunctivitis, bacterial conjunctivitis *(Chlamydia trachomatis, Neisseria gonorrhoeae, Hemophilus influenzae, Streptococcus pneumoniae),* and viral conjunctivitis (adenoviruses types 3, 7, 8, 11, 19, herpes simplex, and enteroviruses).[4,89,110] Epidemic keratoconjunctivitis and pharyngoconjunctival fever are adenoviral conjunctivitides with fairly characteristic clinical findings that usually can be differentiated quite easily from the findings in AHC. A purulent discharge would suggest a bacterial cause and further laboratory investigation (cultures) would be warranted. Alfonso and associates[1] reported ten patients with gonococcal conjunctivitis during an epidemic of AHC. These patients applied urine to their eyes as a folk remedy for the symptoms of AHC. Other reports of self-treatment with folk remedies such as human breast milk, an extract of tree bark, and other tribal medicines have been published.[35,81]

LABORATORY INVESTIGATIONS

Viral Culture

Enterovirus 70 has been isolated mainly from conjunctival swabs and scrapings, much less commonly from throat swabs or feces, and never from the cerebrospinal fluid (CSF). In a number of studies during various epidemics of EV70, the yield of viral cultures has been rather small, especially in more recent years. The short incubation period, rapidity of the disease process, and changes in the characteristics of the virus may all contribute to the relatively low isolation rate of EV70.

To isolate enterovirus, specimens must be obtained very early in the course of AHC (within 1 to 2 days after the onset of symptoms). Primary cell cultures of human origin (HEK, HEL, WF), established continuous cell lines of human origin (HeLa, HeLa-53, HEp-2, KB, RD, WI-38), primary cell cultures of simian origin (MK), and organ cultures (human embryonic ciliated respiratory epithelium, conjunctiva, small intestine) have all been employed in the isolation of EV70 and CA24.[30,78] Nakazono and Kondo[78] recommend primary cell cultures such as HEK, HEL, or MK cells and continuous cell lines such as HeLa, HEp-2, or human diploid cells for the isolation of EV70 and CA24. Yin-Murphy[115] feels that the HeLa cell line is most suitable for CA24 virus isolation.

Suckling mice are the isolation system of choice for the coxsackievirus A group; however, tissue cell cultures (HeLa) are more sensitive for the isolation of CA24. Stanton and associates[100] reported EV70 isolates that replicated in mouse L cells. Ramia and Arif[88] showed that the diploid cell lines MRC-5 and HSF were quite sensitive for the isolation of EV70. Langford and Stanton[56] showed that EV70 isolates grow readily in monkey, rabbit, and mouse conjunctival and corneal (C/C) cells, whereas CA24 isolates replicate in monkey C/C cells only. The same group[60] later reported an animal model of conjunctivitis in rabbits that was caused by EV70. Bilateral infections, subconjunctival hemorrhage, corneal lesions, and CNS disease were not observed in the rabbits, however.

Interestingly, during an epidemic of CA24 AHC in Singapore, Yin-Murphy and associates[116] reported five poliovirus isolates, three of which were isolated in conjunction with CA24. Apparently two virus strains from the 1971 and 1975 AHC epidemics in Calcutta and one isolate from the 1984 epidemic in Malaysia were identified as polioviruses. Yin-Murphy and associates[116] proposed that rare cases of polio-like paralysis following AHC may be caused by concurrent infections with a poliovirus and an EV70 or CA24 virus.

Serology

Serologic diagnosis by a virus neutralization test or hemagglutination-inhibition test is the only practical and available means of confirmation for cases with neurologic complications, as well as patients with AHC and negative viral cultures.[3,49] A titer equal to or above 1:16 is of diagnostic value, but it only indicates that the patient has had EV70 infection in the past.[33,46] A fourfold or greater rise in antibody titers between paired acute and convalescent sera can be regarded as confirmative evidence of the observed AHC or paralytic symptoms.[48,106,107] Kono and associates[46] found that the results of neutralization tests against three types of poliovirus clearly showed that poliovirus had nothing to do with the neurologic/paralytic disease that was seen in Bombay as a complication of AHC.

Rapid Diagnostic Testing

Andersson and associates[3] reported the use of monoclonal antibodies in the detection of EV70 by employing virus neutralization, indirect immunofluorescence, and enzyme-linked immunosorbent assay (ELISA). By choosing the appropriate monoclonal antibody or mixture of monoclonal antibodies with the aforementioned techniques, isolates of EV70 can be typed. Pal, Szucs, and Melnick[82] described a method of rapid diagnosis of AHC caused by EV70 by indirect immunofluorescence. In developing countries lacking virus isolation facilities, this technique is a promising method for use with direct smear preparations. Virus-specific, early appearing neutralizing activity to EV70 detected in tears may be useful diagnostically in identifying the etiologic agent of AHC.[59] Wulff and associates[111] developed an EV70 IgM ELISA based on the capture antibody technique and the use of monoclonal antibodies to EV70 to diagnose outbreaks in a simple, rapid manner with relatively high specificity and sensitivity. The capture antibody technique eliminates the need to separate IgM from IgG, minimizes false-positive results caused by rheumatoid factor, and requires only very small volumes of serum.

Cerebrospinal Fluid Analysis and Electrophysiology

Laboratory investigations in patients with neurologic complications following AHC have included CSF analysis, serology, electromyography, and nerve conduction studies. CSF protein is variably elevated with a nonspecific, lymphocytic pleocytosis of 10 to 200 cells/cubic mm.[20,37,85,106,107] Viral cultures of the CSF have not isolated EV70 to date. Significant antibody titers against EV70 have been demonstrated in the serum, and perhaps more relevantly, in the CSF.[106,107] Wadia and associates[107] reported 36 of 38 CSF specimens from patients with spinal (or a combination of spinal and cranial) motor paralysis associated with AHC that had neutralizing antibody titers ranging from 1:2 to 1:256. In the same study no neutralizing antibody was detected in CSF specimens from patients with AHC alone or from noninfected controls. The preceding findings suggest that intrathecal synthesis of antibody occurred in response to direct invasion of the central nervous system by EV70.

The electrophysiologic observations included prolonged terminal latencies, normal-to-mild slowdown of motor conduction velocities, reduction in the amplitude of motor action potentials associated with normal sensory conduction, and the electromyographic finding of active denervation and fallout of motor units with ongoing reinnervation in some patients. These findings suggest a proximal lesion at the anterior horn cells or motor roots.[20,37,106]

Ancillary Tests

Chopra and associates[20] did HLA studies to determine whether or not genetic factors might play a role in host susceptibility to EV70. They found a significantly decreased HLA B15 in patients with AHC, irrespective of neurologic complications, which suggests a protective role of HLA B15 against AHC. A very significant decrease of HLA A2 was seen among AHC cases without neurologic complications.

Even though HLA A2 appeared to protect against AHC, the HLA A2-positive patients who developed AHC appeared to develop the neurologic complications with increased frequency. This study indicates that perhaps HLA-linked genetic factors contribute to host resistance against EV70 infections.

THERAPY

In the early epidemics of AHC, numerous modalities of treatment were employed including normal saline eyewashes, moist hot compresses, antibiotics (topical and/or oral), and analgesics.[18,85,86] Erythromycin and tetracycline were the most commonly used oral antibiotics, and sulfacetamide and chloramphenicol were the most common topical antibiotics. Saxena, Bhatia, and Chaturvedi[96] first reported the use of tetrahydrozoline hydrochloride (Visine) and phenylephrine hydrochloride for symptomatic relief during an epidemic of AHC. Bacterial suprainfection, if encountered, must be addressed and treated appropriately with antibiotic therapy.

Symptomatic Control

Upon the introduction of AHC into the United States, Sklar and associates[98] in Miami, Florida obtained data on various treatment methods for 100 consecutive patients who were examined within 24 hours of the onset of symptoms. The patients were divided into 5 groups with 20 patients in each group. Group 1 only applied cold compresses four times each day. The other four groups were treated with artificial tears (Group 2), Vasocon A—a decongestant (Group 3), prednisolone acetate 1% (Group 4), or a combination of decongestant and prednisolone acetate 1% (Group 5). All topical medications were applied four times daily to both eyes. The time course of AHC infection was not significantly altered by any of the topical therapeutic regimens. Regardless of the treatment modality, most patients were totally asymptomatic within 4 to 5 days. Treatment with simple cold compresses appears to afford adequate temporary relief in a very short-lived viral infection. Stanton and associates[100] found that isolates of EV70 and CA24 replicate well between 33°C and 37°C, and that above 37°C there is a rapid decline of viral replication. Their results suggest that the application of hot packs, rather than cold packs, to the eye may help control the infection more effectively.

Infection Control

Another very important means of interrupting viral spread during an epidemic is to decrease exposure to the virus by hygienic precautions and by excluding children or employees from school and the workplace. Patients should be instructed to avoid touching their eyes, to wash their hands frequently, and to use separate towels and utensils in the home. These precautions are especially important in crowded familial settings. Health-care workers seeing patients with AHC during an epidemic must prevent cross-infection by washing their hands rigorously before examining each patient, using gloves, and sterilizing instruments.[22] Another possible approach is to establish a separate clinic in which patients with AHC or "conjunctivitis suspects" are directed and seen.[98] Several groups recommended that patients with AHC stay home for 7 days after the onset of symptoms.[68,84] The number of reported cases in various communities steadily declined after the exclusion of symptomatic children from school for a period of 7 days.

Neurologic Management

Although AHC itself is a benign eye disease, the rare paralytic neurologic complications that may occur in some adult patients can be quite seriously incapacitating. No specific therapy is available to prevent the progression of motor weakness once it appears. Corticosteroids can produce dramatic relief of the root pains and sensory phenomena but do not apparently affect the muscular weakness.[33,85,105] Physiotherapy should be started as soon as the root pains subside and the progression of motor paralysis stops. Crutches and orthopedic braces can facilitate ambulation in patients with severe paralysis involving the lower limbs.

Antiviral Agents

Experimental treatment modalities against EV70 and CA24 have been investigated, including reports in the literature of recombinant and natural interferon-α and interferon-β and arildone. Stansfield and associates[99] used a randomized, double-blind study method to investigate the effect of human leukocyte interferon (HLI) in the treatment and prophylaxis of AHC. The clinical course of AHC in their patients was not different in the HLI and saline placebo-treated groups. A significant effect was observed on intrahousehold spread of infection to unaffected nonparticipant household members; however, this may actually have been caused by the hygienic practices provided to the families involved in the study. Langford and associates[61] found that natural and recombinant IFN-α and IFN-β were generally equally effective in inhibiting CA24 infection.[61] The antiviral activity of IFN against AHC in vivo may actually vary with the size of the inoculum of CA24, the type of IFN, and the time of infection with respect to the start of IFN treatment. Langford and associates[55] also investigated the use of arildone, which is a broad-spectrum antiviral agent that can selectively inhibit the replication of picornaviruses.[41] The mechanism of action involves inhibition of the uncoating process. Arildone can inhibit AHC virus spread in cell cultures, without affecting macromolecular synthesis or cellular transport systems. The combined inhibitory effect of arildone and IFN against AHC viruses was found to be additive rather than synergistic.[55]

PROGNOSIS

Acute hemorrhagic conjunctivitis caused by enterovirus 70 and coxsackievirus A24 is generally a rather benign eye disease of short duration and without significant ocular sequelae. Rarely, neurologic complications may be seen with EV70, ranging in severity from an acute cranial nerve palsy that resolves spontaneously to a polio-like syndrome that can cause a severe handicap. It is impossible to predict which patients will develop the neurologic complications associated with EV70 AHC. To date, a polio-like syndrome following AHC has not been reported in the Americas. The best means to prevent such a complication is to limit the spread of the virus during an epidemic by educating the public in hygienic measures and by excluding symptomatic children and adults from school and the workplace. The development of a vaccine has been recommended, especially following the numerous reports of "radiculomyelitis" from India; however, no vaccine is available presently.

REFERENCES

1. Alfonso E et al.: Neisseria gonorrhoeae conjunctivitis—an outbreak during an epidemic of acute hemorrhagic conjunctivitis, *JAMA* 250:794, 1983.
2. Anderson SO, Bjorksten B, Burman LA: A comparative study of meningoencephalitis epidemics caused by echovirus type 7 and Coxsackievirus type B5, *Scand J Infect Dis* 7:233, 1975.
3. Andersson LJ et al.: Detection of enterovirus 70 with monoclonal antibodies, *J Clin Microbiol* 20:405, 1984.
4. Aoki K et al.: Viral conjunctivitis with special reference to adenovirus type 37 and enterovirus 70 infection, *Jpn J Ophthalmol* 30:158, 1986.
5. Aoki K et al.: An epidemic of acute hemorrhagic conjunctivitis in the city of Sao Paulo, *Jpn J Ophthalmol* 31:532, 1987.
6. Aoki K et al.: An outbreak of acute hemorrhagic conjunctivitis due to Coxsackie virus type A24 variant in Japan, *Jpn J Ophthalmol* 32:1, 1988.
7. Arnow PM et al.: Acute hemorrhagic conjunctivitis—a mixed virus outbreak among Vietnamese refugees on Guam, *Am J Epidemiol* 105:68, 1977.
8. Asbell PA et al.: Acute hemorrhagic conjunctivitis in Central America—first enterovirus epidemic in the Western Hemisphere, *Ann Ophthalmol* 17:205, 1985.
9. Babalola OE et al.: An outbreak of acute haemorrhagic conjunctivitis in Kaduna, Nigeria, *Br J Ophthalmol* 74:89, 1990.
10. Bagar B, Cummings ES, Mayerova A: Epidemic of acute hemorrhagic conjunctivitis in Freetown, Sierra Leone, in 1970, *J Hyg Epidemiol Microbiol Immunol* 23:135, 1979.
11. Bernard KW et al.: Acute hemorrhagic conjunctivitis in Southeast Asian refugees arriving in the United States—isolation of enterovirus 70, *Am J Trop Med Hyg* 31:541, 1982.
12. Centers for Disease Control: Acute hemorrhagic conjunctivitis—Florida, North Carolina, *MMWR* 30:501, 1981.
13. Centers for Disease Control: Acute hemorrhagic conjunctivitis—Latin America, *MMWR* 30:450, 1981.
14. Centers for Disease Control: Acute hemorrhagic conjunctivitis caused by Coxsackie virus A24—Caribbean, *MMWR* 36:245, 1987.
15. Centers for Disease Control: Acute hemorrhagic conjunctivitis caused by Coxsackie A24 variant—Puerto Rico, *MMWR* 37:123, 1988.
16. Centers for Disease Control: Acute hemorrhagic conjunctivitis—Mexico, *MMWR* 38:327, 1989.
17. Chang WK et al.: Acute hemorrhagic conjunctivitis in Hong Kong 1971-1975, *Southeast Asian J Trop Med Public Health* 8:1, 1977.

18. Chatterjee S, Quarcoopome CO, Apenteng A: An epidemic of acute conjunctivitis in Ghana, *Ghana Med J* 9:9, 1970.

19. Chatterjee S, Quarcoopome CO, Apenteng A: Unusual type of epidemic conjunctivitis in Ghana, *Br J Ophthalmol* 54:628, 1970.

20. Chopra JS et al.: Neurological complications of acute haemorrhagic conjunctivitis, *J Neurol Sci* 73:177, 1986.

21. Chou M, Malison MD: Outbreak of acute hemorrhagic conjunctivitis due to Coxsackie A24 variant—Taiwan, *Am J Epidemiol* 127:795, 1988.

22. Dawson CR, Whitcher JP, Schmidt NJ: Acute hemorrhagic conjunctivitis, *JAMA* 230:727, 1974.

23. Esposito JJ et al.: Characterization of four virus isolates obtained during acute haemorrhagic conjunctivitis outbreaks, *Microbios* 11:215, 1974.

24. Gangwar DN et al.: Enterovirus 70 acute hemorrhagic conjunctivitis —sporadic cases, *Jpn J Ophthalmol* 28:183, 1984.

25. Goh KT, Doraisingham S: An epidemiological study of five families in the 1975 conjunctivitis epidemic, *Singapore Med J* 17:225, 1976.

26. Goh KT et al.: Acute haemorrhagic conjunctivitis—seroepidemiology of Coxsackievirus A24 variant and enterovirus 70 in Singapore, *J Med Virol* 31:245, 1990.

27. Grist NR, Bell EJ, Assaad F: Enteroviruses in human disease, *Prog Med Virol* 24:114, 1978.

28. Hatch MH, Malison MD, Palmer EL: Isolation of enterovirus 70 from patients with acute hemorrhagic conjunctivitis in Key West, Florida, *N Engl J Med* 305:1648, 1981.

29. Hierholzer JC, Hilliard KA, Esposito JJ: Serosurvey for "acute hemorrhagic conjunctivitis" virus (enterovirus 70) antibodies in the Southeastern United States—with review of the literature and some epidemiologic implications, *Am J Epidemiol* 102:533, 1975.

30. Higgins PG, Scott RJD: The isolation of enterovirus from cases of acute conjunctivitis, *J Clin Pathol* 26:706, 1973.

31. Higgins PG et al.: A comparative study of viruses associated with acute hemorrhagic conjunctivitis, *J Clin Path* 27:292, 1974.

32. Hossain MM et al.: Outbreak of enterovirus 70 conjunctivitis in Bangladesh—1981, *Trans R Soc Trop Med Hyg* 77:217, 1983.

33. Hung TP: A polio-like syndrome in adults following acute hemorrhagic conjunctivitis, *Int J Neurol* 15:266, 1981.

34. Ishiko H et al.: Phylogenetic analysis of a Coxsackievirus A24 variant —the most recent worldwide pandemic was caused by progenies of a virus prevalent around 1981, *Virology* 187:748, 1992.

35. Jones BR: Epidemic haemorrhagic conjunctivitis in London 1971—a conjunctival picornavirus infection, *Trans Ophthalmol Soc UK* 92:625, 1972.

36. Katargina LA, Koroleva GL, Khvatova AV: Role of enterovirus infection in the etiology of uveitis in children, *Vestn Oftalmol* 107:40, 1991.

37. Katiyar BC et al.: Adult polio-like syndrome following Enterovirus 70 conjunctivitis—natural history of the disease, *Acta Neurol Scand* 67:263, 1983.

38. Kawamoto H: Antigenic analysis of acute hemorrhagic conjunctivitis viruses (enterovirus type 70), *Microbiol Immunol* 23:859, 1979.

39. Kew OM et al.: Oligonucleotide fingerprint analysis of enterovirus 70 isolates from the 1980 to 1981 pandemic of acute hemorrhagic conjunctivitis—evidence for a close genetic relationship among Asian and American strains, *Infect Immun* 41:631, 1983.

40. Kim JH et al.: Epidemic hemorrhagic conjunctivitis in Korea, *J Korean Ophthalmol Soc* 13:17, 1972.

41. Kim KS, Sapienza VJ, Carp RI: Antiviral activity of arildone on deoxyribonucleic acid and ribonucleic acid viruses, *Antimicrob Agents Chemother* 18:276, 1980.

42. Kono R: On the causative agent of acute haemorrhagic conjunctivitis and its epidemiology, *Acta Soc Ophthalmol Jpn* 78:333, 1974.

43. Kono R: Apollo 11 disease or acute hemorrhagic conjunctivitis—a pandemic of a new enterovirus infection of the eyes, *Am J Epidemiol* 101:383, 1975.

44. Kono R et al.: Pandemic of new type of conjunctivitis, *Lancet* 2:1191, 1972.

45. Kono R et al.: Neurovirulence of acute haemorrhagic conjunctivitis virus in monkeys, *Lancet* 1:61, 1973.

46. Kono R et al.: Neurologic complications associated with acute hemorrhagic conjunctivitis virus infection and its serologic confirmation, *J Infect Dis* 129:590, 1974.

47. Kono R et al.: Serologic characterization and sero-epidemiologic studies on acute hemorrhagic conjunctivitis (AHC) virus, *Am J Epidemiol* 101:444, 1975.

48. Kono R et al.: Virological and serological studies of neurological complications of acute hemorrhagic conjunctivitis in Thailand, *J Infect Dis* 135:706, 1977.

49. Kono R et al.: Hemagglutination and hemagglutination inhibition tests with enterovirus type 70, *J Clin Microbiol* 7:595, 1978.

50. Kono R et al.: Seroepidemiologic studies of acute hemorrhagic conjunctivitis virus (enterovirus type 70) in West Africa. II. Studies with human sera collected in West African countries other than Ghana, *Am J Epidemiol* 114:274, 1981.

51. Kono R et al.: Seroepidemiologic studies of acute hemorrhagic conjunctivitis virus (enterovirus type 70) in West Africa. III. Studies with animal sera from Ghana and Senegal, *Am J Epidemiol* 114:362, 1981.

52. Koroleva GA, Lashkevich VA, Savinov AP: Lesions of the vascular tract of the eye (uveitis) caused by enteroviruses in man and monkeys, *Vaprosy Virusol* 29:447, 1984.

53. Koroleva GA et al.: Echo-11 virus—the pathogen of the third outbreak of uveitis in children in Kransnoyarsk, 1986, *Vaprosy Virusol* 34:55, 1989.

54. Kuritsky JN et al.: An outbreak of acute hemorrhagic conjunctivitis in central Minnesota, *Am J Ophthalmol* 96:449, 1983.

55. Langford MP, Carr DJJ, Yin-Murphy M: Activity of arildone with or without interferon against acute hemorrhagic conjunctivitis viruses in cell culture, *Antimicrob Agents Chemother* 28:578, 1985.

56. Langford MP, Stanton GJ: Replication of acute hemorrhagic conjunctivitis viruses in conjunctival-corneal cell cultures of mice, rabbits, and monkeys, *Invest Ophthalmol Vis Sci* 19:1477, 1980.

57. Langford MP et al.: Early-appearing antiviral activity in human tears during a case of picornavirus epidemic conjunctivitis, *J Infect Dis* 139:653, 1979.

58. Langford MP et al.: Human fibroblast interferon in tears of patients with picornavirus epidemic conjunctivitis, *Infect Immun* 29:995, 1980.

59. Langford MP et al.: Virus-specific, early appearing neutralizing activity and interferon in tears of patients with acute hemorrhagic conjunctivitis, *Curr Eye Res* 4:233, 1985.

60. Langford MP et al.: Conjunctivitis in rabbits caused by enterovirus type 70 (EV70), *Invest Ophthalmol Vis Sci* 27:915, 1986.

61. Langford MP et al.: Inhibition of epidemic isolates of Coxsackievirus type A24 by recombinant and natural interferon alpha and interferon beta, *Intervirology* 29:320, 1988.

62. Lashkevich VA et al.: Outbreak of enteroviral uveitis in children in Omsk in 1987-88, *Vaprosy Virusol* 35:33, 1990.

63. Lemp MA, Chambers RW, Tio F: Chronic cyclic conjunctivitis associated with enterovirus infection, *Ann Ophthalmol* 4:381, 1972.

64. Likar M, Talanyi-Pfeifer L, Marin J: An outbreak of acute hemorrhagic conjunctivitis in Yugoslavia in 1973, *Pathol Microbiol* 42:29, 1975.

65. Lim KH, Yin-Murphy M: An epidemic of conjunctivitis in Singapore in 1970, *Singapore Med J* 12:247, 1971.

66. Maitchuk YF et al.: An outbreak of a new type of epidemic conjunctivitis, *Vestn Oftalmol* 1:66, 1973.

67. Malanova NL et al.: An epidemic outbreak of conjunctivitis induced by Coxsackie B1 enterovirus, *Vestn Oftalmol* 101:31, 1985.

68. Malison MD et al.: Acute hemorrhagic conjunctivitis, Key West, Florida, *Am J Epidemiol* 120:717, 1984.

69. McMoli TE et al.: Epidemic acute haemorrhagic conjunctivitis in Lagos, Nigeria, *Br J Ophthalmol* 68:401, 1984.

70. Melnick JL: Enteroviruses: Polioviruses, Coxsackieviruses, Echoviruses, and newer enteroviruses. In Fields BN et al., editors: *Virology*, New York, 1990, Raven-Press.

71. Metselaar D, Awan AM, Ensering HL: Acute haemorrhagic conjunctivitis and enterovirus 70 in Kenya, *Trop Geogr Med* 28:131, 1976.

72. Minami K et al.: Seroepidemiologic studies of acute hemorrhagic conjunctivitis virus (enterovirus type 70) in West Africa. I. Studies with human sera from Ghana collected eight years after the first outbreak, *Am J Epidemiol* 114:267, 1981.

73. Mirkovic RR et al.: Enterovirus type 70—the etiologic agent of pandemic acute haemorrhagic conjunctivitis, *Bull World Health Organ* 49:341, 1973.

74. Mirkovic RR et al.: Enterovirus etiology of the 1970 Singapore epidemic of acute conjunctivitis, *Intervirology* 4:119, 1974.

75. Mitsui Y et al.: Haemorrhagic conjunctivitis—a new type of epidemic viral keratoconjunctivitis, *Jpn J Ophthalmol* 16:33, 1972.

76. Miyamura K et al.: Evolution of enterovirus 70 in nature—all isolates were recently derived from a common ancestor, *Arch Virol* 89:1, 1986.

77. Miyamura K et al.: Evolutionary study on the Coxsackievirus A24 variant causing acute hemorrhagic conjunctivitis by oligonucleotide mapping analysis of RNA genome, *Arch Virol* 114:37, 1990.

78. Nakazono N, Kondo K: Virus isolation of enterovirus 70. In Uchida E et al., editors: *Acute hemorrhagic conjunctivitis,* Tokyo, 1989, University of Tokyo Press.

79. Natori K et al.: Genetic relationship between two enteroviruses causing the acute hemorrhagic conjunctivitis syndrome, *Intervirology* 22:97, 1984.

80. Nejmi S et al.: Isolation of virus responsible for an outbreak of acute haemorrhagic conjunctivitis in Morocco, *J Hyg* 72:181, 1974.

81. Onorato IM et al.: Acute hemorrhagic conjunctivitis caused by enterovirus type 70—an epidemic in American Samoa, *Am J Trop Med Hyg* 34:984, 1985.

82. Pal SR, Szucs G, Melnick JL: Rapid immunofluorescence diagnosis of acute hemorrhagic conjunctivitis caused by enterovirus 70, *Intervirology* 20:19, 1983.

83. Parrott WF: An epidemic called Apollo—an outbreak of conjunctivitis in Nigeria, *Practitioner* 206:253, 1971.

84. Patriarca PA et al.: Acute hemorrhagic conjunctivitis—Investigation of a large-scale community outbreak in Dade County, Florida, *JAMA* 249:1283, 1983.

85. Phuapradit P et al.: Radiculomyelitis complicating acute haemorrhagic conjunctivitis, *J Neurol Sci* 27:117, 1976.

86. Pramanik DD: Joy Bangla, an epidemic of conjunctivitis in India, *Practitioner* 206:805, 1971.

87. Quarcoopome CO: Epidemic haemorrhagic conjunctivitis in Ghana, *Br J Ophthalmol* 57:692, 1973.

88. Ramia S, Arif M: Isolation of enterovirus 70 (EV70) from patients with acute haemorrhagic conjunctivitis in two areas of Saudi Arabia, *Trans R Soc Trop Med Hyg* 84:139, 1990.

89. Reed K: Epidemic viral keratoconjunctivitis diagnosis and management, *J Am Optom Assoc* 54:141, 1983.

90. Reeves WC et al.: Acute hemorrhagic conjunctivitis epidemic in Colon, Republic of Panama, *Am J Epidemiol* 123:325, 1986.

91. Ryan MD et al.: The complete nucleotide sequence of enterovirus type 70—relationships with other members of the Picornaviridae, *J Gen Virol* 71:2291, 1990.

92. Sandelin K, Tuomioja M, Erkkila H: Echovirus type 7 isolated from conjunctival scrapings, *Scand J Infect Dis* 9:71, 1977.

93. Sasagawa A, Miyamura K, Kono R: Enterovirus type 70 neutralizing IgM in animal antisera, *Jpn J Med Sci Biol* 35:63, 1982.

94. Sattar SA et al.: Spread of acute hemorrhagic conjunctivitis due to enterovirus 70—effect of air, temperature, and relative humidity on virus survival on fomites, *J Med Virol* 25:289, 1988.

95. Sawyer LA et al.: An epidemic of acute hemorrhagic conjunctivitis in American Samoa caused by Coxsackievirus A24 variant, *Am J Epidemiol* 130:1187, 1989.

96. Saxena RC, Bhatia M, Chaturvedi UC: Recent epidemic conjunctivitis in Lucknow—a clinical study, *Orient Arch Ophthalmol* 10:253, 1972.

97. Shatilova RI et al.: Enteroviral uveitis in children—results of five-year observations, *Oftalmol Zhurnal* 2:79, 1986.

98. Sklar VEF et al.: Clinical findings and results of treatment in an outbreak of acute hemorrhagic conjunctivitis in Southern Florida, *Am J Ophthalmol* 95:45, 1983.

99. Stansfield SK et al.: Human leukocyte interferon in the treatment and prophylaxis of acute hemorrhagic conjunctivitis, *J Infect Dis* 149:822, 1984.

100. Stanton GJ, Langford MP, Baron S: Effect of interferon, elevated temperature, and cell type on replication of acute hemorrhagic conjunctivitis viruses, *Infect Immun* 18:370, 1977.

101. Sugiura S et al.: Outbreak of acute haemorrhagic conjunctivitis (AHC) in Hokkaido, *Acta Soc Ophthalmol Jpn* 76:424, 1972.

102. Supanaranond K, Takeda N, Yamazaki S: The complete nucleotide sequence of a variant of Coxsackievirus A24—an agent causing acute hemorrhagic conjunctivitis, *Virus Genes* 6:149, 1992.

103. Tai FH et al.: A new form of acute conjunctivitis epidemic in Taiwan. A simultaneous outbreak of adenovirus type 11 and "acute hemorrhagic conjunctivitis" virus infections, *Chin J Microbiol* 7:79, 1974.

104. Umanskaya SV et al.: Echo-11 virus-induced enteroviral uveitis, *Vestn Oftalmol* 107:65, 1991.

105. Wadia NH, Irani PF, Katrak SM: Lumbosacral radiculomyelitis associated with pandemic acute haemorrhagic conjunctivitis, *Lancet* 1:350, 1973.

106. Wadia NH et al.: A study of the neurological disorder associated with acute haemorrhagic conjunctivitis due to enterovirus 70, *J Neurol Neurosurg Psych* 46:599, 1983.

107. Wadia NH et al.: Polio-like motor paralysis associated with acute haemorrhagic conjunctivitis in an outbreak in 1981 in Bombay, India—clinical and serologic studies, *J Infect Dis* 147:660, 1983.

108. Waterman SH et al.: Acute hemorrhagic conjunctivitis in Puerto Rico, 1981-1982, *Am J Epidemiol* 120:395, 1984.

109. Whitcher JP et al.: Acute hemorrhagic conjunctivitis in Tunisia, *Arch Ophthalmol* 94:51, 1976.

110. Wright PW, Strauss GH, Langford MP: Acute hemorrhagic conjunctivitis, *Am Fam Phys* 45:173, 1992.

111. Wulff H et al.: Diagnosis of enterovirus 70 infection by demonstration of IgM antibodies, *J Med Virol* 21:321, 1987.

112. Yang YF et al.: Epidemic hemorrhagic keratoconjunctivitis, *Am J Ophthalmol* 80:192, 1975.

113. Yin-Murphy M, Kim KH, Chua PH: Adenovirus type 11 epidemic conjunctivitis in Singapore, *Southeast Asian J Trop Med Public Health* 5:333, 1974.

114. Yin-Murphy M: An epidemic of picornavirus conjunctivitis in Singapore, *Southeast Asian J Trop Med Public Health* 3:303, 1972.

115. Yin-Murphy M: Diagnosis of Coxsackievirus A24 variant. In Uchida, E et al., editors: *Acute hemorrhagic conjunctivitis,* Tokyo, 1989, University of Tokyo Press.

116. Yin-Murphy M et al.: A recent epidemic of Coxsackie virus type A24 acute hemorrhagic conjunctivitis in Singapore, *Br J Ophthalmol* 70:869, 1986.

117. Yin-Murphy M: Viruses of acute haemorrhagic conjunctivitis, *Lancet* 1:545, 1973.

71 Herpes Simplex Virus Diseases: Anterior Segment of the Eye

JAY S. PEPOSE, DAVID A. LEIB, P. MICHAEL STUART, DAVID L. EASTY

Herpes simplex virus eye disease is the most common infectious cause of corneal blindness in industrialized nations and the most common cause of unilateral infectious corneal blindness in the world. Epidemiologic studies estimate that there are approximately 400,000 cases of ocular herpes simplex in the United States.[155]

HISTORICAL BACKGROUND

The word *herpes* has its derivation in a Greek verb meaning "to creep or crawl" and has been used in medicine for at least 25 centuries to describe spreading cutaneous lesions. The earliest descriptions of herpetic disease date back to antiquity and can be found in the writings of Hippocrates.[316]

Cold sores were described by the Roman physician Herodotus in 100 AD,[316] and aphthous ulcers in children were discussed by Celsus in 1516 and by Cooke in 1676.[295] Pringe[235] in 1890 differentiated herpes catarrhalis (herpes simplex) into two types—herpes facialis and herpes genitalis. In 1830 MacKenzie described a disease termed "erysipelatous ophthalmia" that meets the description of herpetic vesicular blepharitis with conjunctivitis.

MacKenzie was one of the first to distinguish herpetic corneal disease. In his text *A Practical Treatise on Diseases of the Eye,* clinical features consistent with herpes simplex keratitis are described under the heading "Catarrhorheumatic Ophthalmia." Horner described herpes corneae febrilis in 1871, and the term *dendritic keratitis* was coined by Grut in 1885. Disciform keratitis as a manifestation of vaccinia was described by Ernest Fuchs in 1901 and was later applied to other viral infections of the cornea including herpes simplex. Rabbit corneal inoculations from material taken from clinical herpes keratitis lesions were performed by Grüter beginning in 1912. These experiments were confirmed by Kraupa and extended to include scarification from genital lesion inoculum by Löwenstein in 1919, definitively establishing the infectious nature of herpes simplex virus (HSV). Doerr and Vöchting first recognized the central nervous system involvement that frequently followed experimental corneal inoculation with the virus.

The development of the electron microscope and appreciation that nucleic acid represented the genetic material in the 1940s and the availability of tissue culture and viral propagation techniques in the 1950s set the stage for more sophisticated characterization of herpes simplex virus. The first plaque assay for HSV was described in 1957.[117] The ultrastructural components of the virion consisting of an envelope, central core, and icosahedral capsid were established by Wildy and associates[318] in 1960, and Russell[254] gave unequivocal proof that the HSV genome is comprised of DNA in 1962. That same year Kaufman[122] reported that idoxuridine, the first topical antiviral, was active against herpes simplex keratitis in rabbits and humans. It was later shown by Kaufman and Heidelberger[124] that trifluridine was more active than idoxuridine in treating herpes keratitis when used in equal concentration. Nahmias and Dowdle,[193] in 1968, demonstrated well-defined antigenic and biologic differences between herpes simplex virus type 1 and type 2. The complete DNA nucleotide sequence of the 17-syn⁺ strain of herpes simplex virus type 1 was determined by McGeoch and associates.[170,171,172,229]

The astute observations of numerous scientists and clinicians helped formulate the concept of latent herpes simplex infection. The viral genome persists in an apparently inactive state in the nervous system of the host for prolonged periods of time, later to be reactivated by a provocative stimulus. Goodpasture[85] suggested in 1929 that HSV was in some way persistently associated with trigeminal ganglia. In 1905 Cushing[49] noted that patients with trigeminal neuralgia treated by sectioning a branch of the trigeminal nerve developed herpetic lesions along the innervated dermatome. Andrews and Carmichael[3] demonstrated in 1930 that patients can reactivate latent HSV despite the presence of neutralizing antibodies. Landmark studies in the early 1970s by Baringer[6] and by Stevens and Cook[42] demonstrated that the sites of HSV latency include the trigeminal, sacral, and vagal ganglia; and that following acute infection the virus is transported from the periphery to the neuronal soma of the sensory nerve via retrograde axoplasmic flow. There the virus

905

establishes latent infection, in which no viral structural proteins or components are synthesized and only selected latency-associated transcripts are transcribed.[47,53,106,245]

EPIDEMIOLOGY

Herpes simplex type 1 can be transmitted to a susceptible individual following close contact with the secretions, skin, or mucous membranes of a person shedding virus at a peripheral site. Infection occurs via the mucosal surfaces or through small cracks in the skin of the susceptible person. The levels of HSV seropositivity greatly exceed the low incidence of clinically apparent infection, indicating that in the vast majority of instances primary herpetic infection occurs subclinically.

Although numerous animal models of herpetic disease have been created, humans are the only natural reservoir of HSV. Laboratory studies in animals have shown that primary herpetic infection of the area innervated by the second or third division of the trigeminal ganglia can lead to replication within the ganglia and establishment of HSV latency in other divisions of the trigeminal ganglia itself.[298] Thus primary infection of a child when kissed on the cheek by a relative with a cold sore could lead to the establishment of viral latency in the ophthalmic as well as the maxillary division of the child's trigeminal ganglia. This could theoretically result in recurrent herpes keratitis later in life, without the eye having been the site of primary infection.

Primary Infection and Latency

Studies using restriction endonuclease fingerprinting of HSV have shown that individuals can be infected with different strains of the same type of HSV at various sites, although the rate of exogenous reinfection in immunocompetent individuals appears to be extremely low.[20] In general, primary infection and establishment of latency in the trigeminal ganglia with a particular strain of herpes simplex results in immunity from exogenous reinfection; and serial recurrences of herpes keratitis show the same viral restriction endonuclease profile.[4] There is, however, a report of herpes simplex type 1 and type 2 simultaneously isolated from the cornea of an AIDS patient with keratitis.[251]

Ocular herpes simplex virus type 2 infection is thought to spread predominantly via oculogenital or digito-oculogenital routes, although hematogenous dissemination has been proposed in selected cases. Nonimmunocompromised patients who are first infected with herpes simplex type 2 are relatively immune to subsequent infection with herpes simplex virus type 1. Patients colonized with herpes simplex virus type 1 in the trigeminal ganglia are only partially immune and may remain susceptible to genital infection and subsequent latency in the sacral ganglia with herpes simplex type 2. Similarly, in experimental animals vaccination with subunit vaccines (containing the herpes simplex type 2 glycoprotein D and adjuvants) partially protects against the establishment of trigeminal latency with herpes simplex type 1 following ocular challenge; it also reduces both primary and recurrent ocular disease.[129]

In the United States antibodies against HSV type 1 are generally detected in about 50% of high-status and 80% of low-status socioeconomic persons by the age of 30.[194] Seroconversion generally occurs earlier in less-developed countries.

Ocular Herpes

One fifth of patients with ocular herpes develop some form of stromal disease.[25,154] The odds of developing stromal disease are three times greater following recurrent herpetic keratitis than following the first clinical episode. Of patients with stromal disease, between 44% and 90% contract disciform keratitis (frequently within a month following resolution of the original ulcer), and the remainder contract stromal opacities, particularly patients treated originally with topical corticosteroids. Ocular herpes simplex results in frequent office visits and time lost from work. In one study there were, on average, four visits to the ophthalmologist for the primary ocular episode and six for each recurrent attack. The average length of active disease for the first attack was 18 days and for recurrent episodes, 28 days.[321] Permanent structural damage from ocular herpes is the cause of approximately 3% of the 43,000 penetrating keratoplasties performed annually in the United States.[16,161,188]

A study[154,155] in a predominantly Caucasian middle-class population in the northern United States revealed 8.4 new cases of ocular herpes per 100,000 person years. The incidence of all episodes of ocular herpes was 20.7 per 100,000 person years. The overall prevalence of ocular herpes in this community was 149 cases per 100,000 people, similar to the estimate of ocular herpes in Tunisia, a developing nation.[322] If the results of this sampling of this stable community in the northern United States were extrapolated to the general U.S. population, 20,000 new cases of ocular herpes could be projected each year, 84,000 episodes per year and 400,000 affected individuals in the United States. In this community, the ratio of the annual incidence of ocular herpes simplex as compared to zoster ophthalmicus was 0.7:1. Nonophthalmic zoster occurred with 14.9 times the incidence of ocular herpes, and genital herpes had 15.2 times the incidence. The mean age for the initial episode of ocular herpes was 37 years, with a trend toward an older mean age over the 33-year study period. This trend could possibly imply later primary infection in this particular population.

The visual prognosis for ocular herpes is good in the modern era of antivirals and corticosteroids. Approximately 90% to 94% of individuals maintain 20/40 vision or better, and about 3% develop vision of 20/100 or worse. In some,[321] but not all studies,[154] patients with geographic ulcers with concomitant steroid use or keratouveitis were more likely to lose vision.

Herpes Simplex Virus Type 2

Most cases of herpes simplex virus type 2 (HSV-2) are sexually acquired. Antibodies to HSV-2 are therefore not generally detected in sera until puberty, with prevalence rates correlating with history of sexual activity. Seroprevalence to HSV-2 is somewhat higher in women than men and ranges between 20% to 40% of Caucasians and 30% to 60% of non-Caucasians in the general U.S. population.[194] Approximately 80% of genital infections are due to HSV type 2 and 20% from HSV type 1. Genitoocular spread of infection with HSV-2 in adults has been reported[209] and may be severe (Fig. 71-1), but the majority of ocular infection in adults is due to HSV type 1. HSV-1 appears to reactivate less frequently than HSV-2, whether the site of latency is the trigeminal or sacral ganglia.

Maternal genital herpes simplex infection with HSV type 2 and (less frequently) type 1 can be transmitted to the neonate, with the estimated frequency in the United States of approximately 1 in 7500 live births or about 700 cases per year. From the mid-1960s until the onset of the AIDS epidemic, genital herpes simplex infection was the sexually transmitted disease with the fastest documented growth.[25] There has been a concomitant increase in the incidence of neonatal HSV infection. These babies may show signs of herpetic chorioretinitis and/or keratoconjunctivitis, among other findings discussed in detail in later sections. In utero transmission of infection can occur via transplacental or ascending infection, with the frequency of occurrence estimated at 1 in 100,000 deliveries.[286] Long-term follow-up of patients with a history of anterior segment involvement alone showed that all had resulting vision of 20/40 or better. Obviously, those cases with chorioretinitis, encephalitis, or optic atrophy (more common with HSV type 2 than type 1) had a far worse visual prognosis.[62a]

As opposed to transplacental infection, neonates are more frequently infected intrapartum via contact of the fetus with maternal genital secretions, although the mothers often show no symptoms or signs of HSV infection at delivery. The risk of transmitting HSV to the fetus appears to depend on a number of factors,[314] including the following: (1) whether the genital infection is recurrent or primary (the latter associated with higher viral excretion), and (2) the level of maternal antibody against HSV at the time of delivery (which can help protect the infant by transplacental transfer, and which may be low if primary infection occurred late in gestation). The risk is also increased if there is prolonged rupture of membranes and use of fetal scalp monitors.[221] The increasing frequency of neonates with HSV type 1 infection (in disproportion to the prevalence of HSV-1 genital infection), suggests that postnatal transmission of HSV-1 to the neonate has also become significant.[5]

RISK FACTORS

Many factors have been associated with herpes simplex reactivation including stress, ultraviolet radiation, menses, surgery, and trauma. The likelihood of recurrence increases with the number of episodes of recurrence. With further recurrences there is a trend toward a shorter interval between recurrences. In Liesegang's study there was a 10% risk of recurrence of some form of ocular herpes 1 year after the initial episode; this recurrence risk rose to 23% at 2 years, and 50% at 10 years. Other studies have found recurrence rates closer to 25% within the first 1 to 2 years.[8,203,320] For patients with primary disease the likelihood of recurrence doubled if the primary episode had corneal involvement as opposed to isolated lid and conjunctival involvement alone. In 28% of cases the patient could identify a triggering stimulus associated with the recurrence.

Up to 12% of patients have bilateral ocular or periocular HSV, either at the same time or consecutively. Atopy was a significant risk factor for developing bilateral disease and has been reported in 25% to 40% of bilateral cases. Other risk factors for bilateral disease include antecedent systemic illnesses such as malaria, pulmonary tuberculosis, lumbar zoster, and gastric carcinoma.[320] Depressed cellular immune function caused by cytotoxic agents for malignancy, organ transplantation, malnutrition, burns, atopy, and inherited cellular immune defects makes these individuals more likely to contract bilateral and/or more severe recurrent disease.[224] Measles infection has been associated with severe unilateral and bilateral ulcerative herpes keratitis,[74,301] noted particularly in malnourished children in Africa who may also have vitamin A deficiency. Although it is unclear whether the constellation of immune defects seen in AIDS patients is associated with a higher incidence of HSV keratitis, once reactivation has occurred, the course of HSV keratitis is generally prolonged and recurrences are frequent (Fig. 71-2).[267]

There are some conflicting data in various epidemiologic studies regarding the influence of sex, season, and age on ocular herpes. In the studies of Liesegang[154,155] and Shuster

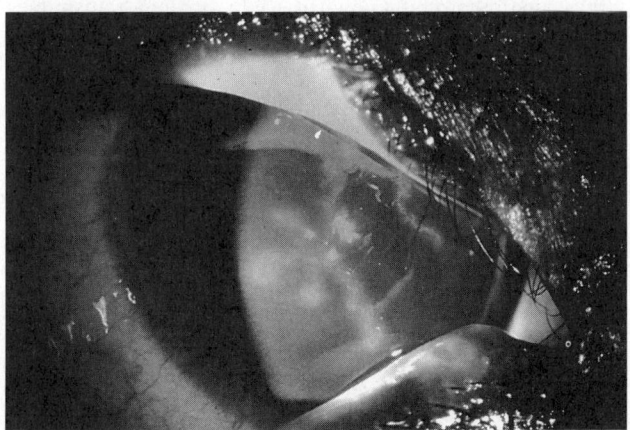

Fig. 71-1. Dendritic epithelial keratitis caused by HSV-2 with marked subepithelial infiltration. (Figure also in color insert.)

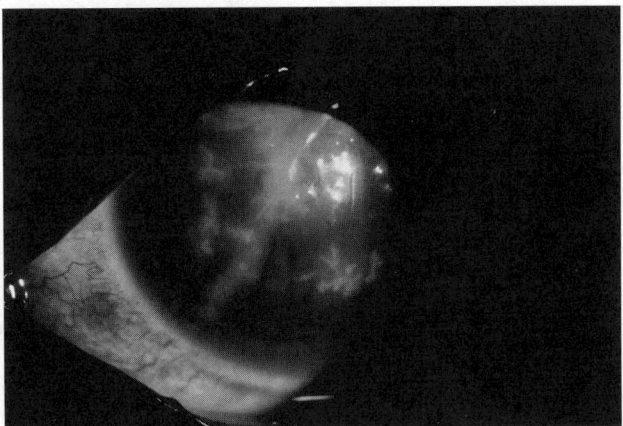

Fig. 71-2. An extensive herpes simplex dendrite extending to the limbus and several adjacent dendrites are seen in a patient with AIDS.

and associates,[268] age-adjusted rates of herpes keratitis by sex were comparable, and there were no seasonal trends noted, nor an influence of previous therapy on recurrence. Studies by Wilhelmus and associates,[321] Bell and associates,[8] and Norn[203,204] showed a higher ratio of male to female patients, particularly those over the age of 40. In the study by Bell and associates, there were more herpetic recurrences (although not primary disease) in the fall and winter, raising the possibility that unrelated viral upper respiratory tract infections could play a role in triggering herpetic reactivation.

PATHOGENESIS

Viral Life Cycle

Observations from animal models and studies of HSV-1 infections in humans have led to the classical theory of the pathogenesis of alphaherpesviruses,[278,317] which include herpes simplex types 1 and 2, and varicella-zoster virus, among others. According to this theory there are four stages that characterize an HSV infection (Fig. 71-3). *Entry* into the host occurs at the time of a primary infection, and HSV replicates at peripheral sites such as the eyes, skin, or mucosae. *Spread* to the axonal terminae of sensory neurons is followed by retrograde intraaxonal transport to neuronal cell bodies in sensory and autonomic ganglia (trigeminal and ciliary), where further viral replication may occur. *Establishment of latency* then occurs, at which time lytic gene expression is repressed. At this stage no infectious virus can be detected, but the viral genome persists in the neuron in a transcriptionally active state. *Reactivation* occurs when certain poorly defined stimuli such as stress, menstruation, or sunlight cause the controls responsible for maintaining latency to break down. This breakdown leads to the production of infectious virus in the ganglion, followed by anterograde transport to the periphery which, following further

replication, may be manifested by lesions at or near the site of primary infection. The molecular mechanisms involved in the repression of lytic gene expression during the establishment and maintenance of latency, and the derepression of lytic gene expression that occurs during reactivation, are not understood.

Herpes Simplex Virus Structure

Membership into the Herpesviridae is based solely on the architecture of the virus[318] (Fig. 71-4). The electron-dense viral core contains a double-stranded linear DNA, surrounded by an icosahedral capsid of approximately 100 nanometers diameter made up of 162 capsomers. Surrounding the capsid, and located between the envelope and the capsid, is an amorphous, asymmetric-appearing structure called the tegument that contains a number of virion structural and regulatory proteins, including the virion host shut-off protein and the alpha-transinducing factor. The outermost component of the virion is a lipid envelope derived from altered cellular membranes, which contains spikes of viral glycoproteins on its surface. The herpes simplex type 1 and 2 genomes are comprised of approximately 152 kilobase pairs, with a high guanine-cytosine base composition of 67% to 69%. The genome consists of two covalently linked components designated as L (long) and S (short). Each component is made up of unique sequences bracketed by inverted repeats.[247]

Lytic Gene Expression

Viral gene expression is tightly regulated during the viral life cycle. According to the manner in which they are expressed, viral genes can be divided into three temporal classes: immediate-early, early, and late.[104] Broadly speaking, the immediate-early class consists of regulatory genes, the early class of genes encode viral DNA replication functions, and the products of late genes are the structural proteins of the virus. Soon after infection of a cell, the cascade of viral gene expression is initiated, and it is enhanced by a viral structural protein known as VP16, or alpha-transinducing factor (alpha-TIF), that is brought into the nucleus with the viral genome.[24,223] VP16 transactivates immediate-early genes as part of a complex with the cellular transcription factor Oct-1 and other proteins.[277] Immediate-early gene products then activate early gene expression with resultant initiation of HSV DNA replication.

The DNA replication mechanism is not completely understood, but it is likely to involve a rolling circle type of mechanism with a replicative intermediate consisting of a linear head-to-tail concatemer of the viral genome.[280] Viral DNA replication is mediated by a large number of virally-encoded proteins. A subset of these proteins is essential for viral DNA replication (viral DNA polymerase, origin-binding protein, helicase-primase complex), whereas others (thymidine kinase, ribonucleotide reductase) are involved in

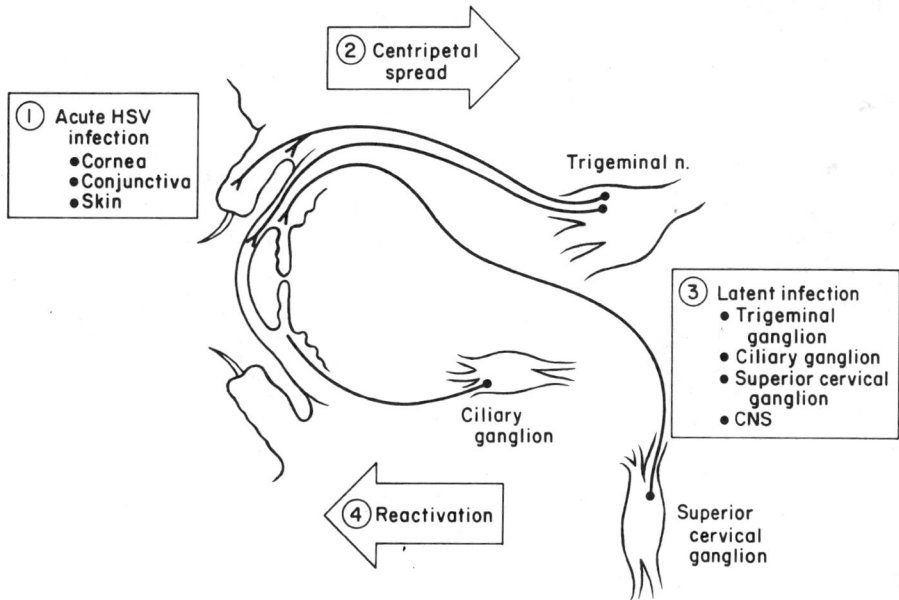

Fig. 71-3.   Acute infection of the ocular surface leads to centripetal axonal spread to sensory and autonomic ganglia, where latency is established. Various factors may later stimulate viral reactivation.

DNA metabolism and are required only in nondividing cells.[248] Following DNA synthesis, late genes are expressed that lead to the assembly of capsids in the nucleus. A series of cleavage and packaging events occur that require a specific viral DNA signal known as the "a" sequence, and the capsid is filled with a unit length of linear DNA.[306,307] The viral capsid then acquires its envelope as it buds through the nuclear membrane. Finally, the entire lytic pathway culminates with lysis of the host cell and release of newly synthesized and assembled virus particles.

Viral Gene Expression

HSV has a broad host range and can lytically infect a wide variety of cell types. The peripheral nervous system (PNS) neuron, however, is unique in that it can support ei-

HERPES SIMPLEX VIRUS

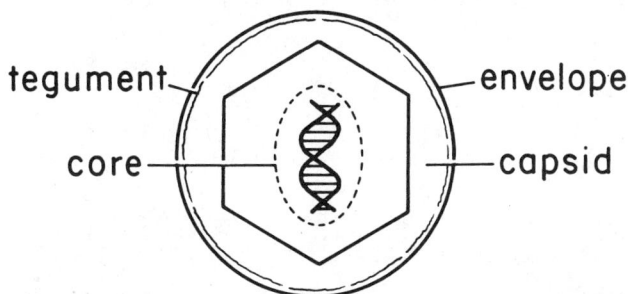

Fig. 71-4.   The herpes simplex virion contains double-stranded linear DNA, surrounded by an icosahedral capsid, amorphous tegument, and lipid envelope.

ther a lytic (Figs. 71-5 and 71-6) or a latent mode (Figs. 71-5 and 71-7) of HSV gene expression, and it is the only cell type that has been unequivocally shown to support latency.[212] Although the lytic pathway has been extensively studied and characterized in cultured nonneuronal cells, it is not known whether this conventional cascade of gene expression occurs in neurons.[134,135]

To date, two nonmutually exclusive hypotheses have been proposed to explain the downregulation of viral gene expression during the establishment of latency in neurons. The first of these hypotheses has focused on cellular factors and proposes that there are specific transcription factors in neurons (Oct-2), which can bind and downregulate HSV immediate-early genes and other octamer-containing promoters.[130,156] The primary evidence for this idea comes from a series of experiments in which co-transfection of an Oct-2 expression plasmid led to a dose-dependent decrease in VP16 activation of immediate-early gene promoter CAT activity in neuronal cells. Furthermore, specific binding of Oct-2 to immediate-early promoters was demonstrated. These findings are consistent with the observations that, at least in vitro, nerve growth factor (NGF) is essential for the establishment and maintenance of latency and that expression of Oct-2 mRNA is strongly induced by NGF.[315,324] A variation on this hypothesis is that it is the lack of a stimulatory factor in neurons (Oct-1), rather than the presence of an inhibitor (Oct-2), which leads to the observed reduced level of viral gene expression.[105]

The second hypothesis focuses on viral factors and proposes that viral DNA replication represents a "decision point" at which the virus becomes committed to either latent

LYTIC [INFECTION] LATENT

NEURONS AND NONNEURONS   **NEURONS ONLY**

[Entry of virus into nucleus]

① Transactivation by VP16 etc.   ⑦

[Immediate-early gene expression]   [Reduced immediate-early gene expression]

②Transactivation   ⑧

[Early gene expression]   ⑥   [Shutoff of lytic genes]

③DNA synthesis   ⑨

[Late gene expression]

[LATENCY:
• Viral DNA persistence
• LATs expression
• No virus production
• Cell survival]

④ Assembly

[Virus release]   ⑩

⑤

[Cell death]   Reactivation

Fig. 71-5. Early in neuronal infection is a "decision point" at which the virus becomes committed to either latent or lytic infection.[212]

or lytic infection (Fig. 71-5). This idea originates from trigeminal ganglia examination using in situ hybridization during acute infection with wild-type virus in the presence of DNA-replication inhibitors or with viruses mutated in thymidine kinase.[134,135] In both cases, prevention of early gene expression (DNA replication) led to a profound decrease in immediate-early gene expression.

Given that immediate-early gene expression occurs before early gene expression in tissue culture, these results are surprising; two basic models have been proposed. First, the temporal regulation of gene expression in neurons may not be recapitulated in tissue culture. Second, DNA replication is required for optimal immediate-early and early viral gene

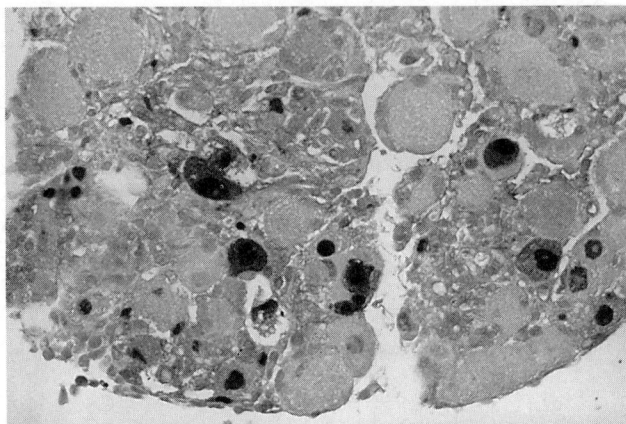

Fig. 71-6. Shortly following acute infection of the ocular surface, lytic viral infection of selected neurons in the trigeminal ganglia occurs. The darkly stained neurons in this immunoperoxidase-processed section are expressing the herpes simplex infected cell protein (ICP) 4.

expression in neurons. If the second model is correct, it is possible that DNA replication leads to the limiting titration of cellular inhibitor factors away from parental DNA molecules, leading to enhanced gene expression. Alternatively, expression of early genes may lead to expression of stimulatory late genes (VP16), which can in turn feed back and stimulate immediate-early expression.

Latency-Associated Gene Expression

During lytic infection, nearly all viral genes are expressed. In contrast, during latency in neurons, viral gene expression is almost completely repressed. During latency, however, the viral genome remains in a transcriptionally active state. Transcription occurs from one region of the viral genome and results in a family of RNA molecules known as latency-associated transcripts (LATs).[279] It has not

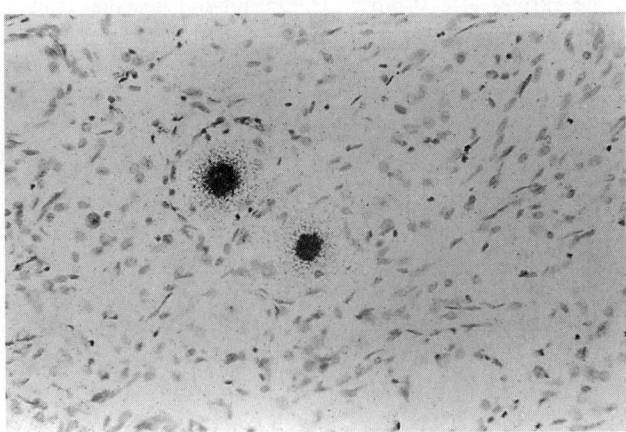

Fig. 71-7. During the period of neuronal latency, selected viral gene expression occurs. Silver grains are localized over selected neuronal nuclei in the trigeminal ganglia following in situ hybridization for latency-associated transcripts.

been demonstrated in vivo that the LATs encode a protein, and their function is not understood.[80] The LATs are abundant, largely poly (A)⁻ transcripts and have been observed in the neuronal nuclei of latently infected sensory ganglia both in man and experimental animals.[47,279] It has been shown that the LATs' promoter is responsive to cAMP and other second messengers, is neuron-specific, and contains a conventional TATA box.[152,237,330] The precise nature of the promoter, however, is yet to be determined. Latency-related RNA transcription has been reported in bovine herpesvirus type 1 latency in a rabbit model,[244] pseudorabies virus latency in swine,[246] and varicella-zoster virus latency in man,[48] implying a possible common pattern of viral gene expression in latency of neurotropic herpesviruses.

Four LATs have now been demonstrated for HSV-1,[308,330] although the precise function of any of these transcripts is unclear. Examination of the sequences specifying the HSV-1 LATs reveals the presence of at least two potential open reading frames (ORFs). One group has demonstrated a latency-associated antigen derived from the LATs in latently infected neuronal cell cultures, although the significance of this finding remains to be determined.[56] Deletion mutant analyses have shown unequivocally that the LATs of HSV-1 are not essential for the establishment or reactivation of viral latency.[150,276] The reactivation phenotypes of such HSV mutants, however, have varied widely, depending on the nature of the mutation, virus strain, and animal model.[15,55] Most studies have indicated that the LATs are important either for efficient establishment of latency or for reactivation from the latent state.[99,256,297] Consistent with this idea, a recent study has shown that the LATs may play a role in the efficient egress of virus from infected cells, especially in older monolayers.[14] In contrast, other studies have indicated that the LATs play no role in reactivation, at least from explant cultures.[13,101,110] Overall, the function of the LATs remains obscure, in spite of much work by many laboratories.

Cellular and Viral Gene Expression

No unifying hypothesis has been proposed for the variety of stimuli known to induce reactivation in humans and animal models. However, a number of reactivation stimuli, including UV irradiation, iontophoresis of epinephrine, and trauma, are likely to raise cAMP levels in neurons either directly or indirectly through prostaglandin release.[98,100,146,263] This is consistent with the observation that cAMP analogs can significantly accelerate reactivation, and prostaglandin synthesis inhibitors such as indomethacin can inhibit reactivation from explanted latently infected ganglia.[52,138,152] In addition, as mentioned previously, deprivation of NGF from latently infected neurons induces reactivation,[318] although the effect of NGF on intracellular cAMP levels is controversial.

Many viral mutants have now been tested for their ability

to establish and reactivate from latency. It has been shown that viral replication is not necessary for the establishment of latency, as judged by the presence of viral DNA within sensory neurons (demonstrated using DNA PCR technology).[120] Many of these viruses fail to reactivate simply by virtue of their inability to replicate efficiently in neuronal cells. Exceptions to this rule are mutants in infected cell protein (ICP) 0 and the LATs, in which specific roles in reactivation (as distinct from replication) have been shown.[23,30,55,151,276] The LATs of HSV-1 are derived from the DNA strand opposite that which encodes the mRNA specifying ICP0, which is an immediate-early regulatory protein. Although dispensable for growth in cell culture,[255,281] ICP0 is a potent transactivator of all three classes of viral genes[65,81,210,211] and is essential for efficient reactivation of virus from latency. This finding supported the idea that the LATs may act by antisense repression of ICP0 during the establishment and maintenance of latency, consistent with the idea that ICP0 may act as an "initiator protein" during reactivation.[279] Observations, however, that LATs mutants often reactivate less efficiently than wild-type means that antisense repression of ICP0[150,276] must be an oversimplistic view of LATs function.

Attempts to unify observations of cAMP-induction of reactivation with the role of ICP0 and the LATs in reactivation have yielded interesting results. Both genes are responsive to cAMP in transient transfection assays and bind CREB, a cAMP-responsive transcription factor.[152,311] The cAMP-responsiveness of the LATs has been addressed in vivo, and it has been shown that acceleration of reactivation by cAMP is independent of the LATs. The possibility of ICP0 being responsive to cAMP in reactivation has not been directly addressed, although it has been shown that a neuroblastoma-neuron fusion cell line is more permissive for infection in the presence of cAMP.

These findings suggest important roles by both viral and cellular factors in the reactivation of latency. The elucidation of such factors will lead to a better understanding of the latency process and ultimately to the development of novel therapeutic agents, which may prevent reactivation of HSV.

PATHOGENESIS OF HSV KERATITIS

Immune Response to Viral Infection

The immune response plays a central role in the pathogenesis of HSV keratitis, however, the specific mechanisms remain a complicated and controversial subject.[295,316] Although it is clear the genetics of the infecting virus can, to some degree, determine the pattern of infection, it is equally clear the genetics of the host, through its ability to actively resist infection, also impacts HSV-induced disease. The immune system has a number of effects on the clinical course of herpetic infections of the eye. Viral-induced immune responses directed against this pathogen clearly restrict the spread of HSV and, to some extent, probably facilitate the establishment of latency. The immune state may also play a role in allowing activation of latent virus, and it certainly influences the extent of the active recurrent infection.

There are three general types of herpes simplex virus corneal disease. The first involves lytic viral infection of the epithelium, which tends to be self-limiting and typically effects no permanent damage to the cornea (Fig. 71-8). Dendritic lesions form when localized productive viral infection of corneal epithelial cells results in cell lysis, with release and spread of virus to adjacent cells. These microloci coalesce, first forming dendrites which, if untreated, can combine to produce a map-shaped, "geographic" ulcer.

The second results in disciform endotheliitis with accompanying stromal edema. Several theories have been proposed to explain this phenomenon. Sundmacher and associates[289] have cultured infectious HSV from the aqueous humor of several patients with disciform disease. They have postulated (although they have not demonstrated directly) that viral infection of the corneal endothelium results in endothelial cell lysis caused by the viral infection alone or in combination with immune mechanisms. Resultant endothelial dysfunction or abnormalities lead to stromal edema (Fig. 71-9).[191,304] An alternative, and not mutually exclusive, theory is that stromal edema seen in disciform keratitis may reflect a delayed type of hypersensitivity reaction to herpes antigens within the stroma or endothelium. This theory is also consistent with the rapid response observed clinically to topical corticosteroids in patients with HSV disciform keratitis. Animal studies show that animals presensitized to HSV produce disciform disease following intrastromal injection of antigen.[290] In addition, the disease could be ameliorated in rabbits by depletion of polymorphonuclear cells.[182]

The third disease pattern is HSV stromal keratitis, a form of stromal opacification produced by immunologically mediated mechanisms.[51,179,182] Recurrent episodes of viral pro-

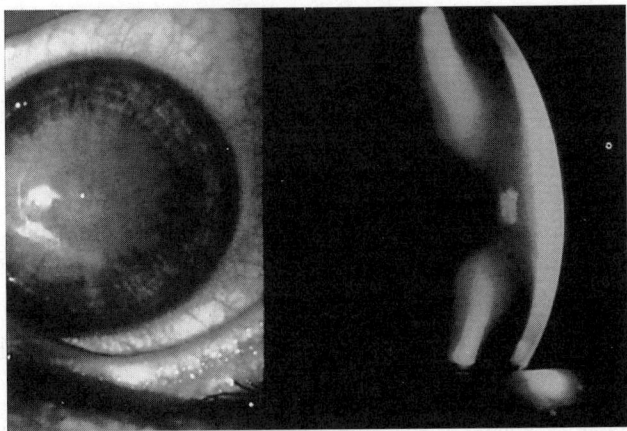

Fig. 71-9.   Disciform herpes simplex keratitis presents with central inflammation edema seen with diffuse illumination on the left and in optical section on the right. (Figure also in color insert.)

duction lead to stromal inflammation and progressive corneal scarring with possible loss of vision. Pannus formation, fragmentation of Bowman membrane, scarring, and stroma necrosis are common. Retrocorneal membranes, duplications of Descemet membrane, and a granulomatous reaction around Descemet membrane (Fig. 71-10) or in the stroma have been described. Detection of viral profiles and antigens in keratoplasty buttons have been variable[103,148,225] and probably reflect the different stages of the disease at the time of keratoplasty, as well as the use of corticosteroids and antivirals. There appears to be a wide spectrum of clinical disease produced by different isolates of HSV. In comparing clinical isolates of HSV from patients with dendritic keratitis to those with stromal keratitis, the latter strains released larger amounts of soluble glycoprotein D into the media when the viruses were propagated in vitro.[269] The authors postulated that a similar release of viral antigens into the stroma could occur in clinical disease. Others have claimed increased levels of glycoprotein C, rather than D, released into the culture fluid of cells infected with strains causing stromal (as compared to epithelial) disease.[299] Glycoprotein C is the immunodominant antigen for HSV-specific memory cytotoxic cells, whereas envelope glycoprotein D elicits neutralizing antibody binding and high levels of lymphocyte proliferation in vitro. Immunogenetic background of the host, as well as the viral strain, may also produce a broad spectrum of disease.

Herpes simplex virus may produce an iritis that may accompany the keratitis, or more rarely, occur independently. The iritis is frequently granulomatous in nature, and there may be keratic precipitates scattered on the corneal endothelium. Lytic infection of the iris may result in tissue destruction and transillumination defects, and the anterior chamber inflammation and/or trabeculitis may produce elevated intraocular pressure.[68] Herpesvirus particles have been demonstrated in the posterior synechiae from the iridectomy

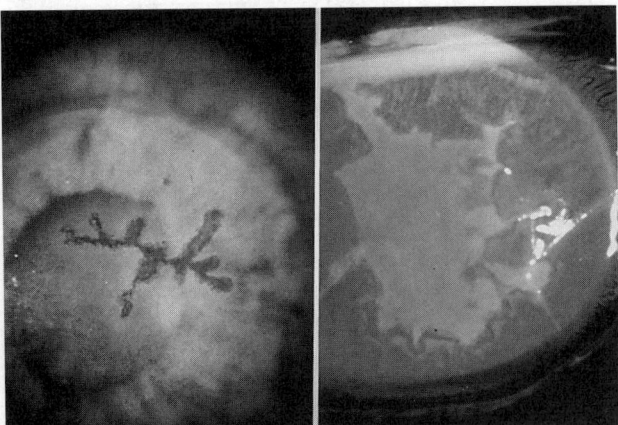

Fig. 71-8.   A herpes simplex dendrite stained with rose bengal is seen on the left, and a geographic herpes ulcer stained with fluorescein is shown on the right. (Figure also in color insert.)

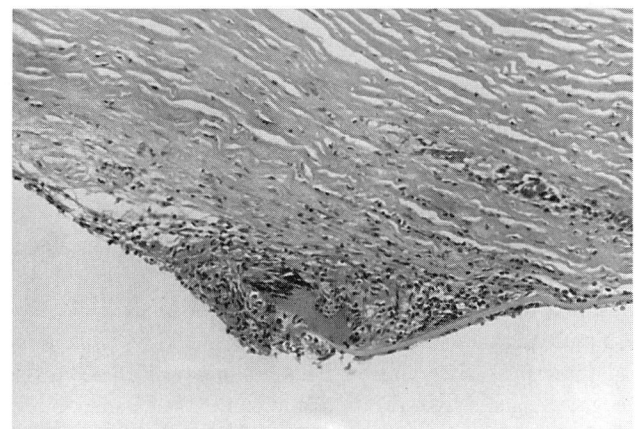

Fig. 71-10. A granulomatous reaction made up of lymphocytes, macrophages, histiocytes, plasma cells, and giant cells is seen adjacent to Descemet membrane in the posterior cornea of a patient transplanted for herpes simplex keratitis.

specimen of a patient treated for painful secondary glaucoma.[323]

Experimental studies by Oh[207] showed that infectious HSV could be isolated from rabbit eyes with primary herpetic uveitis during the acute stages of disease, but virus could not be isolated in secondary uveitis. This observation was thought to be due to high levels of neutralizing intraocular antibody that persisted long after recovery from the primary infection. There has been some disparity in the abilities of various investigators to isolate infectious herpes simplex virus from aqueous taps from patients with uveitis,[131,289] which may reflect differences in the relative concentrations of antibody to virus, different viral titers, or antibody neutralization effects. Further studies by Oh[208] demonstrated that primary uveitis requires infectious virus for its production, whereas either live or inactivated virus is sufficient to produce secondary disease. It was concluded that primary herpetic uveitis is mediated initially by infection of uveal tissue by live virus and later by various immune-mediated mechanisms. It is possible that the adherence of keratic precipitates on the corneal endothelium relates to the upregulation of adhesion molecules on these cells by inflammatory cytokines, as seen in several studies.[63,84]

Immunopathology

The cellular infiltrate of the stromal inflammatory response is composed of polymorphonuclear cells, macrophages, lymphocytes, and plasma cells.[51,94,179,182,225] Studies designed to quantitate these cells have demonstrated that the majority are macrophages or express T cell determinants, with the macrophages typically outnumbering those cells expressing T cell markers (Fig. 71-11). Analysis of cells expressing T cell markers (Leu-1) indicates that those expressing CD4 (Leu-3a +), which phenotypically represent helper-inducer cells, are the most numerous; followed by

CD8 (Leu-2a +) expressing cells, which phenotypically represent primarily cytotoxic T cells; and then a minor component that expresses natural killer cell markers.[225,327,328] Several reports have indicated that cells isolated from patients with HSV keratitis are capable of both HSV-specific cytotoxic activity[92,258,296,328] (mediated by T lymphocytes) and HSV-nonspecific cytotoxic activity (mediated by natural killer cells).[92]

Early in the inflammatory response there is induction of intercellular adhesion molecule-1 (ICAM-1) expression on basal epithelium, stromal keratocytes, and corneal endothelial cells.[63,84] This cell-surface molecule is involved in facilitating leukocyte-endothelial adhesion and regulates extravascular trafficking of immunocompetent cells.[158,270] Following ICAM-1 expression, major histocompatibility (MHC) HLA-DR antigens are detected within the epithelium, anterior stroma, and endothelium of the cornea[1,63,84,168]; and they are found on cells that morphologically appear to be epithelial cells, keratocytes, and endothelial cells.[291] HLA-DR antigens are required for proper antigen presentation to T lymphocytes, which is a necessary step in the activation of these T lymphocytes.[262] The mechanism for increased expression of these cell-surface molecules appears to be due to the release of cell-free factors termed cytokines, which are known to regulate the activity and function of immunocompetent cells.[61]

Studies have demonstrated that corneal ICAM-1 expression is rapidly upregulated by tumor necrosis factor-alpha (TNF-α), interleukin-1 beta (IL-1-β), and interferon-gamma (IFN-γ).[112,220] HLA-DR could only be induced on these cells by IFN-γ,[60,73] however. Once activated, these T-lymphocytes release more cytokines, further inducing ICAM-1 and HLA-DR expression on corneal cells,[329] which only serves to further increase the intensity of the inflammatory response. One study that attempted to determine whether the level of MHC class II expression in the cornea correlated

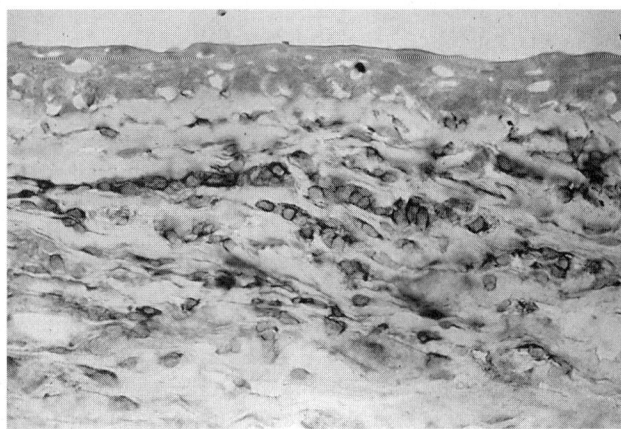

Fig. 71-11. Many of the mononuclear cells infiltrating a herpetic cornea stain with immunocytologic techniques for the CD4 T-helper cell-surface marker.

with the severity of disease reported that the frequency and density of HLA-DR expression, particularly in the corneal stroma, was more pronounced in those cases with severe corneal disease.[291]

The mechanism that is responsible for the immunopathology seen in human herpes simplex keratitis is unknown, although both delayed type of hypersensitivity (DTH) and cytotoxic T lymphocyte (CTL) responses may be involved differentially in response to various strains of HSV. Typically, DTH responses are mediated by T cells that express the CD4+ phenotype, whereas CTL activity is most often mediated by T cells that express the CD8+ phenotype.[217] It is, however, interesting to note that nonocular infections of HSV-1 generate CTLs, some of which express CD4 and some that express CD8 cell-surface markers.[296] In fact, some studies have indicated that the primary T cell involved in lysis of HSV-1 infected targets is a MHC class II restricted T cell that is CD4+, CD8-.[258]

Studies designed to directly measure the production of cytokines have found that HSV-1 can weakly induce peripheral blood lymphocytes to produce the proinflammatory cytokines IL-1 beta, TNF-α, and IL-6.[86] In addition, Oakes and associates[205] have reported that HSV-1 induces IL-8 when corneal keratocytes, but not corneal epithelial cells, are infected with HSV-1. IL-8 is particularly interesting in that it is known to be an important proinflammatory cytokine that acts as a potent chemoattractant for neutrophils and lymphocytes.[7] In addition to acting as a chemoattractant, IL-8 also activates neutrophils, which could play a role in the damage associated with this disease.

There is a whole body of research describing the inhibitory activity that HSV has on immunocompetent cell activation and function. Infection of monocytes with HSV leads to a significant reduction in the ability of these cells to present antigen to T cells.[89] Natural killer cell and cytotoxic cell lytic function are inhibited when exposed to fibroblasts or epithelial cells infected with HSV.[41,234]

Persistence of HSV Nucleic Acid in Corneal Tissues

Several laboratories have demonstrated persistent HSV DNA in humans and animals during quiescent stromal keratitis,[127,148,249] however; LATs transcription (or lytic transcription) has not been demonstrated.[148] Thus persistent HSV DNA in corneal tissue differs from neuronal latency in that it does not appear to be transcriptionally active for LATs (at the limits of detection of in situ hybridization). Easty and associates[62] isolated HSV by organ cultures from 10 of 34 corneal buttons from chronic HSV stromal keratitis that had been previously treated with corticosteroids. Similarly, HSV has been recovered from a limited number of explanted rabbit and mouse corneal tissues 6 to 8 weeks following corneal inoculation. In summary, the understanding of HSV persistence in corneal tissue is limited, but it is unlikely that LATs

are made in abundance in human cornea after resolution of acute infection. This theory is also consistent with the finding that the LATs promoter appears to be neuron specific.[330]

One explanation of the data, suggested by Hill and Blyth, is that infectious particles are periodically produced in the trigeminal ganglia and transported to the cornea via retrograde axoplasmic flow. Following transport, if virus resides in the cornea in a nonreplicating form but does not establish latency, then no viral transcripts will be expressed or detected. Following explantation, however, corneal cells may be more permissive for viral infection and allow replication of these passenger viruses. This action would resolve the negative in situ hybridization studies for viral transcripts[148] with the recovery of virus in corneal explant cultures.[62,127] Recent studies suggest that a similar situation could exist in selected eye bank corneas maintained at 34°C in organ culture, in which HSV infection of selected donor corneas appeared to be the cause of endothelial loss and possible graft failure.[29] Whether similar replication of HSV could occur in explanted corneal tissue following short- or intermediate-term storage at 4°C deserves further study.

Animal Models of HSV-1 Keratitis

Much of the early literature on experimental herpes keratitis employed rabbits. The rabbit model is particularly useful for studying the basic histopathology of primary and recurrent disease, testing the effects of various drug treatments on the course of disease, and studies of disciform endotheliitis and both induced and spontaneous viral reactivation. It has proved, however, more difficult to study immunopathologic aspects of herpetic eye disease in outbred rabbits. Consequently, a number of investigators have turned to murine models, which, because of the existence of genetically defined strains and the ready availability of immunologic reagents, provide an excellent model system to determine the role that immune responses play in the development of HSV-mediated tissue damage. Another consideration is the possibility that the immune cells mediating disease in mice and in rabbits may not be the same. In the rabbit, the disease typically resembles the necrotizing form of human herpetic keratitis.[59] The dominant cells found in these lesions are polymorphonuclear neutrophils (PMNs).[182] In fact, if animals are depleted of PMNs or the complement system is inhibited, the disease is markedly suppressed.[182] This observation suggests that stromal disease may, in part, be the result of immune complex-driven immunopathology.[252] Because of the lack of immunologic reagents specific for the rabbit, it is difficult to resolve the exact mechanisms responsible for herpetic keratitis in these animals.

Mice have proved a useful model for herpetic keratitis because of their defined genetics and immune system and because researchers are able to study both primary and recurrent disease following induced reactivation. As is the case for many diseases, certain mouse strains are more susceptible for developing herpetic keratitis (BALB/c, A/J, NIH), whereas other strains tend to resist the development of disease (C57BL/6, C3H).[283] To date, the vast majority of reports examining herpetic keratitis in mice have focused on the events following primary HSV infection. The cellular infiltrate observed in primary HSV keratitis consists primarily of lymphocytes and mononuclear cells when certain strains of virus are employed, whereas infection with other strains of HSV leads to a cellular infiltrate that is primarily PMNs.[94,214] One potential problem with extrapolating data from primary HSV infection in mice is that the diffuse, often exuberant blepharokeratoconjunctivitis may not mimic many of the clinical signs characteristic of human herpetic primary or recurrent keratitis, such as focal opacification, neovascularization, and endotheliitis.[240] Recently, however, investigators have developed[264,266] and characterized[147,185] a murine model for recurrent herpes keratitis using NIH strains of mice. The features of herpetic keratitis manifested in these animals more closely resemble the clinical signs and immunopathology seen in human disease and thus should prove an informative model for future studies.[147,185,264,266]

As is the case in human disease, the exact mechanism for primary herpetic keratitis (primary HSK) in animal models has not been conclusively determined. It is believed, however, that the disease is predominantly the result of the interaction of virus and host immune cells and components and not the result of direct viral cytolysis of corneal cells.[94] Evidence supporting the role that immunologic responses play in herpetic keratitis includes the fact that neither SCID or nude mice develop the disease following corneal infection with the virus.[17,160,177,178,253] These mouse strains are immunodeficient because of mutations that either (1) do not allow for the expression of antigen-specific receptors—leading to a lack of functional T and B lymphocytes (severe combined immunodeficiency or SCID mice)[160]—or (2) lack a thymus (nude mice), which is necessary for the proper maturation and development of T cells, and thus do not possess functional T cells.[325] When these immunodeficient mice are reconstituted by adoptive transfer of spleen cells (from mice exposed to HSV) and then infected intraocularly with HSV, they develop signs characteristic of primary HSK.[177,253] These studies clearly demonstrate the requirement of immunocompetent cells for the development of HSV-induced corneal keratitis.

These findings were further extended by Russell and associates,[253] who deleted T cells from the HSV immune spleen cells prior to adoptive transfer into nude mice. Their results indicated that only one mouse in seven developed primary HSK, whereas all seven mice that received unfractionated immune spleen cells developed disease. As a result of these and other studies, most investigators agree that primary HSK is T cell-mediated disease. Ksander and Hendricks[137] went on to show that when cell-mediated immunity

was inhibited by HSV-1 injection into the anterior chamber of the eye, both anti-HSV-1 cell-mediated immune responses, as well as primary HSK, were inhibited. There is some dispute, however, as to which subset of T cell, CD4[+] or CD8[+], is the primary mediator of disease process. It is generally held, though there are many exceptions, that CD8[+] cells are the primary mediators of cytotoxic T lymphocyte (CTL) activity; and that CD4[+] cells, by the release of various cytokines, mediate delayed type of hypersensitivity (DTH) responses.[217]

The concept that CD4[+] cells are the primary mediators of primary herpetic keratitis has been put forward by many investigators. The studies that have supported this belief have used an adoptive transfer model in which nude[17,178,253] or SCID mice[177] are reconstituted with either CD4[+] or CD8[+] T cells prior to infection with HSV-1. These studies demonstrated that only those mice reconstituted with CD4[+] T cells developed primary HSK. Likewise, when normal mice were depleted of CD4[+]-bearing T cells and then challenged with HSV-1 (RE strain), HSK immunopathology was either markedly reduced or eliminated. Conversely, when these mice were treated with anti-CD8 antibody, HSK was more severe and the incidence of encephalomyelitis increased. It was concluded from these experiments that CD4[+] cells are responsible for HSK, and CD8[+] cells appear to play a protective role against viral infections.[58,199,200] When corneal sections were immunochemically stained for T cell markers or mononuclear cells removed from the cornea were subjected to microfluorimetric analysis, only CD4[+] cells could be detected.[58] Further evidence supporting the role that CD4[+] cells play in primary HSK comes from a study by Opremcak and associates.[214] This study demonstrated that the ratio of CD4[+] to CD8[+] T cells found in the cornea of HSK-susceptible mouse strain, C.AL-20, following HSV-1 infection was 7 : 1, whereas the ratio for the resistant C.B-17 mouse strain was 1 : 8 in the cornea. Furthermore, when the draining lymph nodes were analyzed, both CD8[+] and CD4[+] T cells were found to have anti-HSV-1 cytolytic activity, with the CD4[+] component making up approximately 30% of the anti-HSV-1 cytotoxic T cell response.[58,201] These results were confirmed by Niemialtowski and Rouse,[132] who demonstrated that only CD4[+] cells could be isolated from the eyes of mice with primary HSK, whereas the draining lymph node had both CD4[+] and CD8[+] anti-HSV CTLs. Additionally, they showed that the anti-HSV CTL-precursor in the eye was 20 or less, suggesting that CTL activity probably is not the principal mechanism for this disease.[132]

The evidence supporting a dominant role for CD8[+] CTLs comes from work by Hendricks and associates.[90,93] Their studies took advantage of the fact that injection of certain mutant gC virus into the anterior chamber leads only to impaired CTL responses (and not DTH responses). This observation has not been duplicated by other investigators and is contrary to what is typically seen for anterior chamber injection of antigen, namely that antigen-specific DTH (and not CTL) responses are impaired.[108,118,282] Hendricks and associates[94] have modified and extended these findings to demonstrate that the subpopulation of T lymphocytes that mediates stromal inflammation is dependent on the strain of HSV-1 used. They show that infections with the RE strain of HSV-1 require the presence of $CD4^+$ T cells, whereas those that employ the KOS strain of HSV-1 require the presence of $CD8^+$ T cells in the injected mice.

B lymphocytes, which are not a prominent feature of the mononuclear cell infiltrate, are also not considered a major factor in the development of this disease. It has been reported, however, that genes linked to the Igh-1 locus on chromosome 12 play an important role in determining which strains of mice are resistant and which strains are susceptible to the development of primary HSK.[77] In addition, it is well documented that passive treatment of mice with high-titered anti-HSV monoclonal antibody directed against the various glycoproteins of herpes simplex type 1 virus prevent the development of primary HSK in mice.[144,180,238,265] It also appears that the ability of these monoclonal antibody preparations to protect mice against the development of primary HSK does not require the presence of $CD4^+$, $CD8^+$, or asialo $GM1^+$ cells.[275] The mechanism for protection against primary HSK by monoclonal antibody treatment has not been conclusively determined, though it is thought to involve both viral neutralization and antibody-dependent cellular cytotoxicity (ADCC).[109] In contrast to the results reported for HSV-1-induced primary HSK, when mice are treated with monoclonal antibodies against HSV type 2 glycoproteins, there is no reduction of HSV type 2-induced primary HSK.[241] The reason for this differential effect of monoclonal antibody treatment is unknown, but it has been speculated to be due to differences in either (1) the levels of cytokine production following infection with these two types of herpes viruses or (2) the levels of glycoprotein found on infected cells.[241]

The role that monocytes, and in particular Langerhans cells (LC), play in this disease also appears to be very important (Fig. 71-12). LC are the only corneal cells that constitutively express MHC class II antigens and are normally not found in the central corneal region.[90,153,185] When the cornea is subjected to a variety of insults, however, LC migrate from the peripheral cornea and contiguous conjunctiva to the central regions of the cornea, and various corneal epithelial and stromal cells are induced to express MHC class II antigens.[90,153,185] Activation of $CD4^+$ T cells requires the antigen-presenting function of Langerhans cells and other MHC class II^+ cells, which typically include macrophages and B cells (though corneal epithelial cells are also capable of antigen presentation to T cells).[66,302] When migration of LC to the central cornea precedes HSV-1 infection, it has been shown that DTH responses to HSV-1 are enhanced and the severity of corneal inflammation is increased.[176] These studies suggest that when DTH appears to mediate primary HSK, LC probably play a major role. This theory was tested by Hendricks and associates,[91] who showed that when mice were irradiated with ultraviolet-B (UV-B) light, prior to infection with HSV-1, there was no migration of LC to the central cornea following HSV-1 infection. They went on to show that if the RE strain of HSV-1 was used, exposure to UV-B, the mice displayed significantly reduced incidence and severity of corneal stromal disease. If the KOS strain was used, however, there was no change in corneal stromal disease. These studies demonstrate that when pathology is associated with $CD4^+$-me-

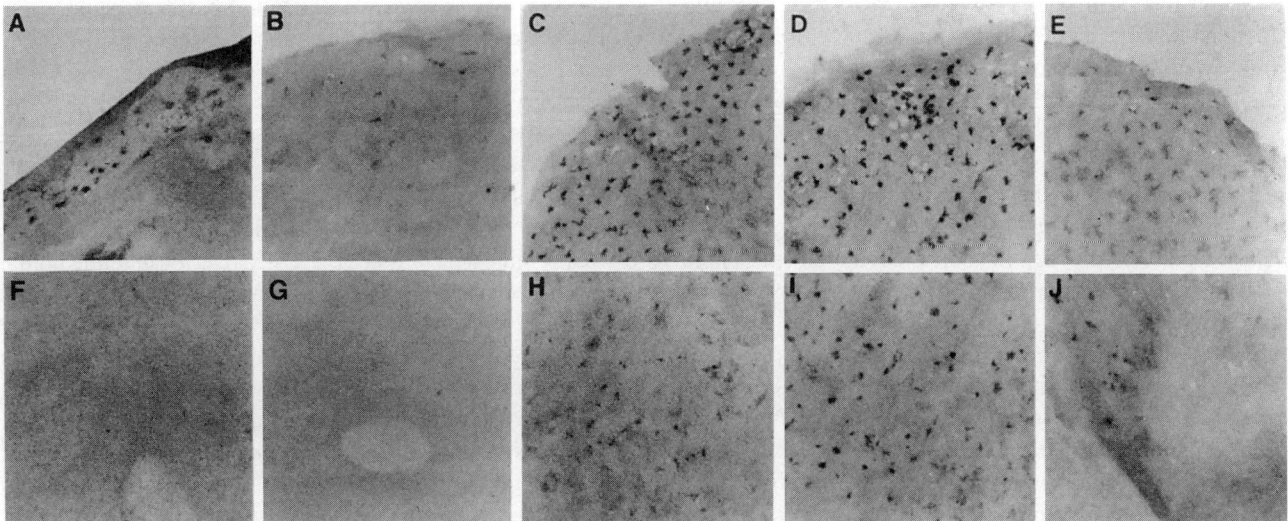

Fig. 71-12. Dendritic-appearing Langerhans cells, normally restricted to the corneal limbus (left), may migrate toward the central and paracentral cornea following primary or recurrent herpes simplex keratitis (right). The darkly stained Langerhans cells are readily discerned in these corneal and conjunctival epithelial sheets.

diated antiviral DTH reactions (RE strain), the presence of LC in the central cornea is critical to disease. Conversely, when pathology is associated with CD8[+] T cells (KOS strain), the presence of LC in the central cornea is not required for primary HSK disease. Jager and associates[111] used a different strategy to monitor the importance of Langerhans cells in the central cornea. They found that if they elicited Langerhans cell migration to the central cornea prior to HSV-1 infection, the disease was much more severe, indicating that these cells are very important to disease development. Furthermore, LC migration to central cornea has also been shown to correlate with the degree of persistent stromal opacification seen in a murine model of recurrent HSK.[128,185] This migration is also the observation in human corneas during primary and recurrent HSK.[83]

Cytokines

The role that cytokine production plays in primary herpetic keratitis has been addressed using a variety of techniques. Several investigators have demonstrated that particular cytokines are associated with protection of mice from primary HSV-1-induced corneal keratitis. Two studies have reported that corneal infection with particular strains of HSV-1 rarely, if ever, results in corneal keratitis. When the mechanism for the inability of these HSV-1 strains to induce primary HSK was examined, it was discovered to be particularly sensitive to the presence of IFN-α or IFN-β.[145,284] When mice were treated with anti-IFN-α or anti-IFN-β monoclonal antibody prior to infection with these viruses, they developed moderate-to-severe stromal keratitis.[284] A separate study by Hendricks and associates[97] demonstrated that mice injected with UV-treated HSV-1 prior to corneal infection with HSV-1 did not develop primary HSK. Hendricks and associates[97] determined that serum levels of IFN-α were elevated and that anti-IFN-α or anti-IFN-β reversed the protective effects of preinjection with UV-treated HSV-1. They also demonstrated that treatment of mice with recombinant IFN-α, prior to corneal infection with the KOS strain of HSV-1, did not lead to corneal stromal keratitis disease.[253] These data indicate that, at least for the particular strains of HSV-1 tested, IFN-α prevents the development of primary HSV-1-induced corneal keratitis.

Studies have also been performed to evaluate the cytokine profile of ocular cells removed following infection with HSV-1. It is generally held that there are two types of T helper cells. These cells are differentiated on the basis of the types of cytokines they produce. Those that produce IFN-γ, IL-2, and TNF-α or TNF-β are considered Th1 cells and mediate responses such as DTH, whereas those T cells that produce IL-4, IL-6, and IL-10 are designated Th2 cells and favor certain antibody responses.[190] Niemialtowski and Rouse[202] discovered that the predominant cytokines produced were IFN-γ, IL-2, and TNF-α or TNF-β. At the same time they were unable to detect the production of IL-4 or

IL-10, suggesting that the major CD4[+] cell in the eye is of the Th1 type. Similar conclusions were derived when Hendricks and associates[95] treated mice with antibodies directed against IFN-γ, IL-2, and IL-4. Their results indicated that mice, which were treated with anti-IFN-γ and anti-IL-2 antibodies, which would block a Th1-mediated response, did not develop primary HSK disease. However, those mice that were treated with anti-IL-4 antibodies, which will inhibit Th2-mediated responses, demonstrated a normal disease course.

In contrast to these reports, when Staats and Lausch[274] attempted to directly detect cytokines in eyes following HSV-1 infection, they were only able to detect increased levels for IL-1-α and IL-6. Levels for both of these cytokines were either reduced or undetectable when mice were given an anti-HSV antibody that blocks disease. Interestingly, although the levels of IL-10 increased dramatically following viral infection, anti-HSV antibody treatment did not significantly alter IL-10 levels. However, administration of exogenous IL-10, a pleomorphic cytokine, ameliorated the onset of herpes simplex stromal disease.[300] In addition, these workers were unable to detect IFN-γ, IL-4, or GM-CSF; and levels of TNF-α were unchanged over naive control mice. Recently published data from Jayaraman and associates[113] have further complicated the issue of what cytokines, and therefore what T cells, are involved in primary HSK. Jayaraman and associates have developed a long-term glycoprotein D-specific CD4[+] T cell line, which responds to an amino terminal peptide of gD in the context of I-E[d]. The dominant cytokine produced by these cells is IL-4, indicating that this cell line belongs to the Th2 subtype of T cells.[190] When these cells were adoptively transferred into HSK-susceptible mice (BALB/c), the onset of disease was shortened and the severity increased. Furthermore, when adoptively transferred into normally resistant mice (C.B-17), they developed a transient stromal keratitis following infection with HSV-1.[274] It should be kept in mind, however, that these results are best considered indirect evidence implicating the possible role of Th2 cells in primary HSK. The fact that they can, by in vitro culturing, develop a Th2 T cell line capable of enhancing the disease-producing potential of HSV-1, does not mean that this is necessarily the primary mechanism whereby HSV-1 infection leads to the development of HSK disease.

Various types of therapeutic modalities have been employed to reduce clinical symptoms in both human herpetic stromal keratitis and in animal models of primary HSV keratitis. Therapies targeting the virus alone have not proved consistently effective in treatment of HSV-1 corneal stromal disease,[239] though there are studies in which the use of antivirals, such as trifluridine, reduces the severity of the HSV-1-induced stromal keratitis.[18] Limitations to the use of antiherpetic drugs alone may reflect the immunopathologic nature of the disease, which is initiated by T cell responses to

HSV-1 antigens in the cornea* is not a target of antiviral agents. To better control stromal disease, steroidal antiinflammatory compounds have been tested for their ability to modulate disease. These studies have not proved consistently beneficial to treated patients. In many cases, topical treatment with corticosteroids reduces the inflammation and scarring that cause vision impairment, but in other patients the result of such treatment is an exacerbation of herpetic corneal keratitis.[294] These results may be due, not only to the fact that antiviral responses are inhibited, but also to the observation that corticosteroids enhance HSV-1 replication.[309] More recently, Hendricks and associates[96] tested the efficacy of the nonsteroidal antiinflammatory drug, flurbiprofen on their murine model of primary HSV corneal keratitis. They compared this drug (flurbiprofen) to the corticosteroid, dexamethasone. The effects of dexamethasone in these mice were very similar to those observed in human studies with this drug; namely, some mice displayed a significant reduction in severity of disease, whereas most had a significant exacerbation of corneal stromal opacity. In contrast, flurbiprofen, although it did not consistently lead to significant reduction of the intensity of corneal stromal opacity, also did not exacerbate the disease in any of the treated animals. Another drug that has been tested in this model is cylosporine. The antiinflammatory effects of this drug are well documented, and therefore it is a logical candidate for the treatment of this disease. Because cylosporine has such a strong immunosuppressive effect, however, there are concerns that, as with corticosteroids, treatment with this drug might only exacerbate the viral component of the disease, leading to an uncontrolled viral infection. When Naito and associates[196] tested the efficacy of this drug, along with the antiherpetic drug ganciclovir, in a rabbit model of herpetic stromal keratitis, they observed that treatment with cyclosporine alone was not particularly effective in treating the disease. When ganciclovir and cyclosporine were used together, however, there was significant lessening of the corneal stromal keratitis.

CLINICAL FEATURES

Neonatal Infection

Neonates acquiring herpes simplex in utero or from maternal infection can manifest conjunctivitis (Fig. 71-13), keratitis (Fig. 71-14), microphthalmia, cataract, iridocyclitis, iris atrophy, posterior synechiae, optic neuritis, retinitis, chorioretinitis with subsequent scarring, or encephalitis leading to cortical blindness.[192] Whereas 80% of neonatal herpes is caused by HSV type 2, both HSV types 1 and 2 have been associated with neonatal ocular infection. Neonatal infection can either (1) remain localized to the skin, eye,

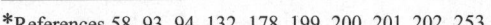

*References 58, 93, 94, 132, 178, 199, 200, 201, 202, 253.

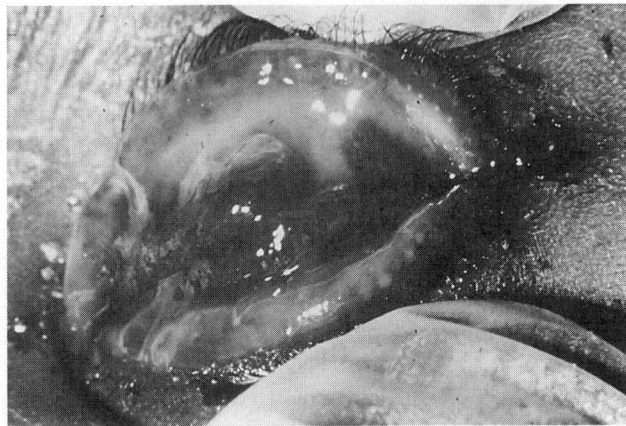

Fig. 71-13. Neonatal herpes simplex pseudomembranous conjunctivitis of everted upper and lower lids presenting with an exudative mucoid discharge, hyperemia, and diffuse injection.

or mouth, (2) infect the central nervous system with or without skin, eye, or mouth involvement, or (3) disseminate to multiple viscera and organs, of which the eye may be one. These differences may relate to a number of factors, including the timing and route of infection (in utero versus intrapartum), the site of inoculation, the degree of passive and endogenous immunity, and the hematogenous dissemination of virus to multiple organs via mononuclear cells. The reported incidence of keratitis (which may appear as microdendrites, dendrites, or punctate keratitis) among newborns with HSV infection is 6% to 7%. Most of these patients with pathology limited to the anterior segment generally retain good vision, perhaps in part because neonates are naturally immunocompromised, limiting the immunopathologic destruction of the cornea sometimes seen in stromal keratitis. Much of the corneal opacity in these newborns, in fact, appears to be reversible edema. Herpes simplex can also infect other anterior segment tissues and has been isolated from the lens of an infected infant who developed cataracts several months after the acute infection.[28] The more common late

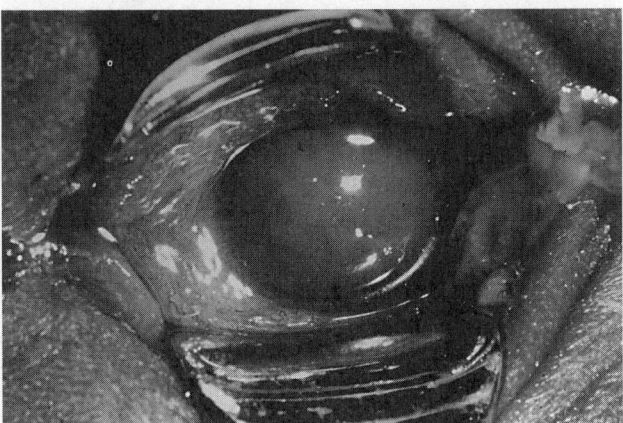

Fig. 71-14. Neonatal herpes simplex stromal keratitis.

ophthalmologic sequelae following neonatal herpes simplex infection include oculomotility disorders (44%), chorioretinal scars (28%), optic atrophy (22%), and cortical blindness (which harbors a worse visual prognosis and occurs more frequently in neonates with central nervous system involvement from HSV type 2).

Primary Ocular Infection

Primary HSV infection beyond the neonatal period is more commonly subclinical, and in some cases may be detected only by seroconversion. It is relatively common in children from ages 1 to 5, after maternal antibody protection has waned. Most commonly, subclinical, primary HSV may manifest as a gingivostomatitis, pharyngitis, rhinitis, or tonsillitis, which may be accompanied by fever, chills, and myalgias.[215] Regional lymphadenopathy is common, and a vesicular eruption may involve the skin of the lid and periorbital region (Fig. 71-15).

Vesicular skin lesions generally clear within 7 to 10 days and do not result in permanent scarring. A follicular or pseudomembranous conjunctivitis may be present alone or accompanied by an ulcerative keratitis, which may be punctate, dendritic, or geographic in appearance. The border cells of the corneal ulcers often stain with rose bengal, and the central ulcer base stains with fluorescein.

Individuals with or without a history of ocular herpes have been found periodically to have herpes simplex virus or nucleic acid in the tear film,[123,126] reflecting asymptomatic viral shedding. Secretory IgA, IgA, and IgG directed against herpes simplex in the tears of infected individuals have been found in significantly higher concentrations than in accompanying saliva or sera, consistent with local antibody production in the lacrimal and accessary lacrimal glands.[45,79,169,222] Antibodies to herpes simplex, as well as to other viruses, have also been detected in the tears of individuals with no history of ocular herpetic disease.

The initial clinical episode of ocular herpes involves the superficial cornea (63%) ten times more frequently than the deep cornea (6%), and accompanying iridocyclitis is also less common. Subepithelial footprints of the overlying lesion may be seen and probably represent an inflammatory response to HSV antigens that have permeated the stroma. A disciform endotheliitis may produce stromal edema and Descemet folds, along with focal keratic precipitates. Herpes labialis may occur before, after, or during (Fig. 71-16) the initial ocular infection.

Recurrent Disease

Recurrent herpes keratitis has been reported in response to a wide variety of nonspecific stress stimuli including trauma, fever, menses, and ultraviolet B light exposure. Viral recurrence has been documented following a wide range of ocular surgery including cataract, keratoplasty, radial keratotomy, and excimer laser procedures.[228] Recur-

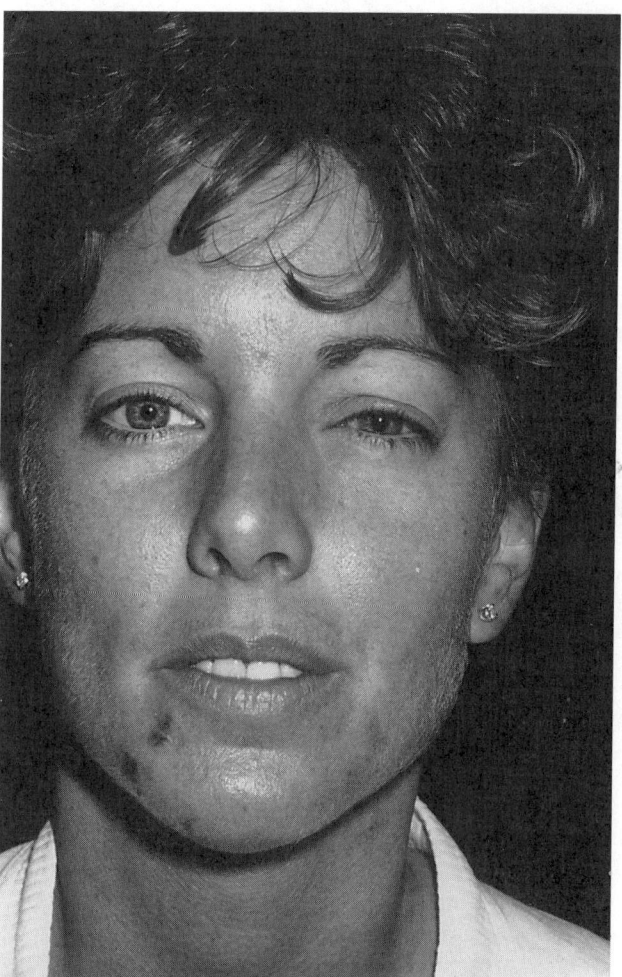

Fig. 71-16. A patient with herpes simplex shown in the distribution of the third division of the trigeminal nerve on the right, along with a dendritic herpes simplex keratitis on the left.

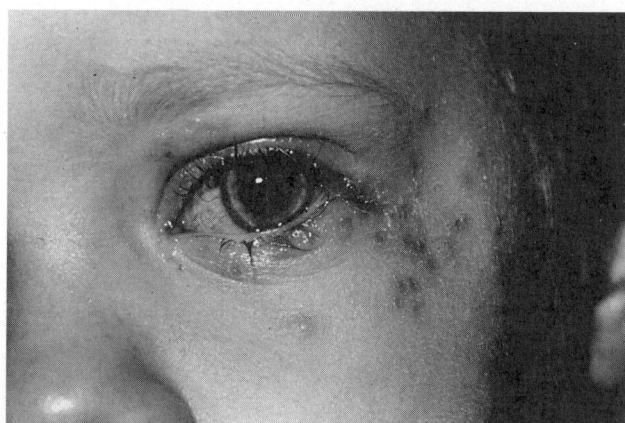

Fig. 71-15. Primary herpes simplex in a child is characterized by a vesicular periocular eruption, which may be accompanied by preauricular lymphadenopathy.

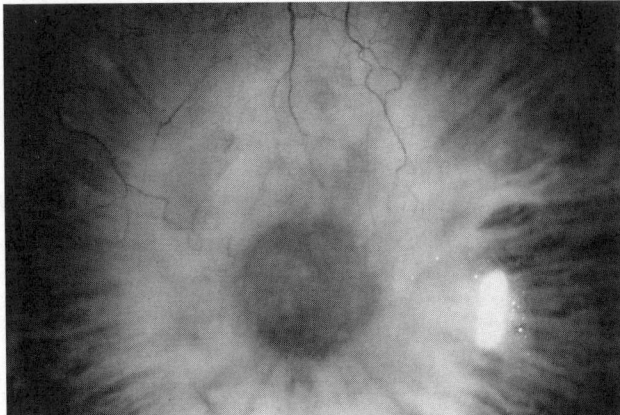

Fig. 71-17. Corneal neovascularization and opacification has resulted from herpes simplex keratitis.

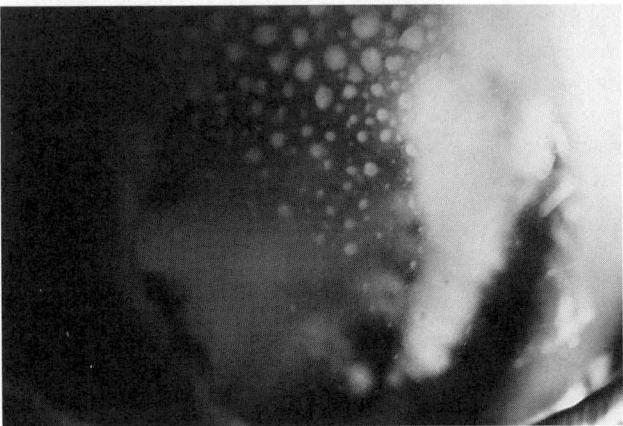

Fig. 71-19. Granulomatous-appearing herpes simplex iridocyclitis is seen in a patient with recurrent herpes simplex eye disease. Posterior synechiae are present.

rences are more common in patients with a history of herpetic corneal ulcers. Multiple recurrences can lead to a hypoesthetic cornea caused by herpetic damage to corneal sensory nerves. In recurrent disease the lids and conjunctiva are less commonly involved than in primary disease, in which there is more superficial corneal and (considerably more) corneal stromal involvement. Stromal disease may present as disciform (disk-shaped) inflammatory edema, comprised of localized keratic precipitates on the endothelium, underlying a zone of stromal edema and striae. Stromal (interstitial) keratitis, in contrast, presents as stromal opacification as a result of cellular immune infiltrates. A subset of patients with stromal keratitis may demonstrate frank stromal necrosis or permanent scarring, which is more common following recurrent HSV. Herpetic stromal keratitis may produce neovascularization (Fig. 71-17), secondary lipid deposition, stromal edema, as well as stromal melting with descemetocele production and corneal perforation (Fig. 71-18). Granulomatous iridocyclitis (Fig. 71-19) and trabec-

ulitis may lead to the formation of posterior synechiae and increased intraocular pressure, requiring therapy. Productive iris infection with HSV may leave patchy iris transillumination defects (Fig. 71-20), and spontaneous hyphemas may occur. Wessley immune rings (Fig. 71-21) may form as a result of immune complex deposition, cytotoxic antibodies, complement activation, and antibody dependent cellular cytotoxicity.[181,183]

A number of cases of linear endotheliitis have been associated with herpes simplex virus.[213,243,285] This disorder presents clinically as a line of keratic precipitates on the corneal endothelium that progresses centrally and is accompanied by peripheral, stromal, and epithelial edema. Cases may be bilateral or unilateral, and some have followed cataract surgery. A small subset of patients with this disease entity had accompanying dendritis or evidence of herpes antibodies in aqueous. All of these patients had unilateral findings and several had antecedent cataract surgery, suggesting reactivating HSV in some cases. Successful treat-

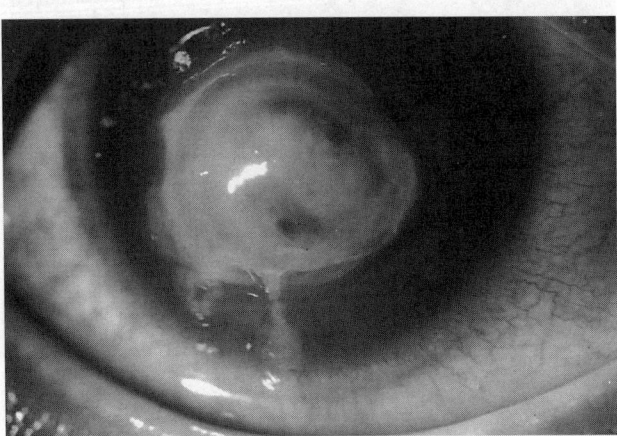

Fig. 71-18. Necrotizing stromal keratitis producing a descemetocele with impending corneal perforation in a young patient with recurrent herpes simplex.

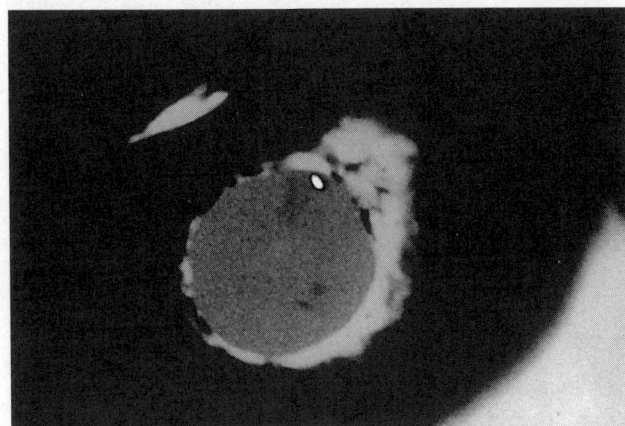

Fig. 71-20. Patchy iris transillumination defects, especially at papillary border, can be seen in this patient with a history of herpetic keratouveitis.

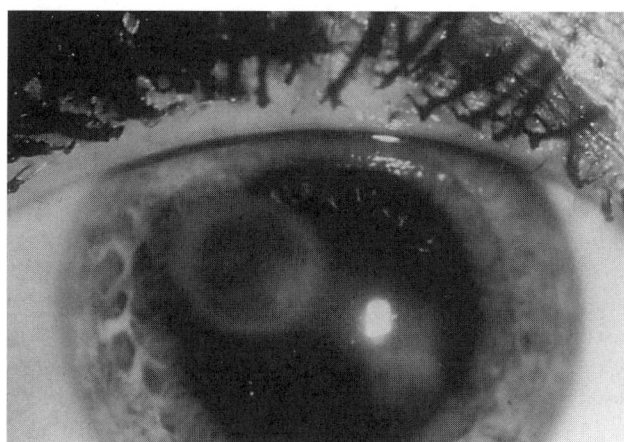

Fig. 71-21. Partial or complete Wessley immune rings may form as a result of immune complex deposition.

ment of patients with linear endotheliitis required topical antivirals and topical corticosteroids, sometimes accompanied by oral acyclovir. Those patients treated with corticosteroids alone had a poor outcome and often were left with residual corneal edema.

Metaherpetic Disease

Not to be confused with active herpetic disease—epithelial erosions, defects, or granularity may be seen in the healing phases of dendritic or geographic disease. These manifestations of nonactive or metaherpetic disease may result from the presence of a damaged basement membrane and stroma, a neurotrophic component, as well as prolonged use of toxic antiviral medications. The lesions may appear as nonhealing, gray-bordered epithelial defects with characteristic rolled-up edges (Fig. 71-22). A generalized lackluster appearance of the corneal epithelium may be the effect of neurotrophic damage.

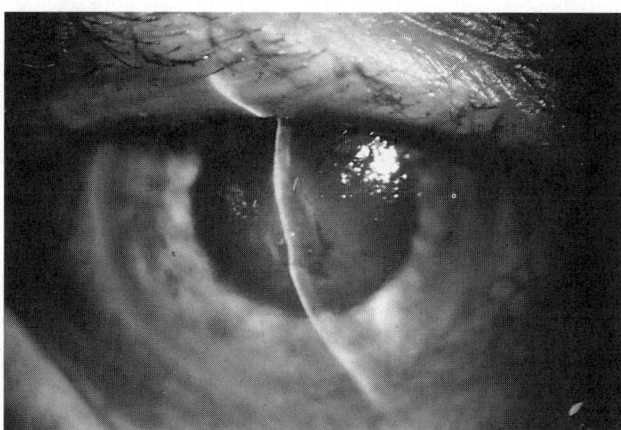

Fig. 71-22. An indolent (metaherpetic) corneal ulcer with characteristic rolled edges and gray borders. (Figure also in color insert.)

Herpes Simplex Retinitis

Herpes simplex may be a cause of viral retinitis and/or encephalitis in both immunologically competent and incompetent adults[226,227] (see Chapter 83). The full-thickness necrotizing retinitis presents as diffuse retinal opacification and edema, with perivascular inflammation. In AIDS patients, selected rampant cases of cytomegalovirus retinopathy and encephalitis have been documented to be co-infected with HSV[163] and/or HIV-1. There are also a few isolated reports of the acute retinal necrosis syndrome linked to HSV types 1 and 2.[163,230]

DIFFERENTIAL DIAGNOSIS

Neonatal herpes simplex keratoconjunctivitis must be differentiated from other forms of microbial keratoconjunctivitis in the newborn, including bacterial and chlamydial keratoconjunctivitis. Leukoma, in this setting, includes the differential diagnosis of dermoid, Peters anomaly, congenital hereditary endothelial dystrophy, sclerocornea, and tears in Descemet membrane secondary to forceps injury. Primary or recurrent herpetic epithelial lesions should be discerned from abrasions, as well as acanthamoeba, zoster, bacterial, or fungal keratitis. Stromal herpetic inflammation and opacification can mimic that seen in connective tissue disorders or Cogan syndrome, as well as stromal or disciform keratitis resulting from mumps, varicella zoster, vaccinia, Epstein-Barr virus, syphilis, or acanthamoeba, and fungal or bacterial infection. It may be difficult to differentiate graft rejection from recurrent herpes in patients after penetrating keratoplasty. Dendrites or persistent epithelial defects in corneal allografts, even defects not clinically suggestive of herpes simplex keratitis, have proved HSV culture positive in some cases.[9,162] Granulomatous keratic precipitates on the corneal endothelium crossing the graft-host interface may also be a sign of recurrent herpes simplex, whereas the precipitates in graft rejection may be more localized to within the corneal button itself.

LABORATORY INVESTIGATIONS

Viral Blepharitis, Conjunctivitis, and Epithelial Keratitis

Scrapings of corneal or conjunctival epithelial lesions can be stained with Giemsa or Papanicolaou stain to look for multinuclear giant cells and eosinophilic intranuclear inclusions. Conjunctival impression smears generally show an even distribution of polymorphonuclear cells and monocytes.[50]

Viral isolation in tissue culture can be accomplished on a wide range of primary or diploid cells and cell lines, including Vero cells, MRC-5 cells, rabbit skin and kidney cells, and human embryonic lung and kidney and foreskin cells. Depending on the viral inoculum, typical cytopathic effects comprised of rounded-up, refractile cells and plaques can be discerned in 24 to 48 hours. HSV type 1 versus type 2 can be differentiated by using monoclonal antibodies or restriction endonuclease analysis. The use of topical rose bengal prior to obtaining viral cultures should be avoided, if possible, to maximize the sensitivity of viral isolation. Rose bengal has antiviral activity against extracellular HSV via photoinactivation, and this antiviral effect is further exacerbated by intense light exposure. In comparative animal studies, the percentage of HSV-culture-positive eyes was significantly reduced by the application of rose bengal to the ocular surface prior to culture.[19]

In partially treated or atypical cases of ocular herpes, rapid diagnosis can be facilitated by use of the Herpchek ELISA test (Dupont) that does not depend on recovery of infectious virus, but rather viral antigens. Field testing with ocular specimens shows this assay to have comparable sensitivity and specificity as tissue culture isolation.[141] Direct immunofluorescence for HSV antigen is a very rapid test, with considerably lower sensitivity than tissue culture or ELISA.[149] The polymerase chain reaction represents a sensitive research laboratory tool, that with standardization and conversion to a colorimetric ELISA readout, could prove useful for diagnosing ocular HSV from corneal swabs[136] or tear film.[326]

Stromal Keratitis and Uveitis

The diagnosis of herpes simplex stromal keratitis is predominantly a clinical one. In atypical cases, other forms of stromal keratitis should be ruled out by appropriate laboratory testing, such as the use of the MHA-TP testing for syphilis. Cases that are recalcitrant to therapy may require corneal biopsy for investigating an alternate diagnosis, with tissue sent for viral isolation, immunocytochemical staining for herpes simplex antigens, as well as culture for isolation of other pathogens (if appropriate), such as acanthamoeba.

Corneal epithelium and stromal tissue have been shown to harbor herpes simplex DNA by polymerase chain reaction in the absence of active viral infection, thus limiting its diagnostic significance. The demonstration of active herpes simplex RNA transcripts by RT-PCR would be of more potential diagnostic value. Although of epidemiologic interest, serologic testing for herpes simplex antibodies is rarely clinically useful in daily patient management. As much of the adult population is seropositive, a positive test is not necessarily diagnostic of herpetic keratitis. Different serologic assays for HSV antibodies have different levels of sensitivity. In addition, there is a time period required for seroconversion following primary infection. Although it is possible to have past or current ocular herpes in the presence of negative HSV serology, this uncommon finding should motivate a search for other potential etiologic diagnoses.

THERAPY

Antiviral Agents

Idoxuridine. The first antiviral used for the clinical treatment of herpes simplex keratitis was idoxuridine (IDU). This thymidine analogue was synthesized by Prusoff[236] in 1959. It is incorporated into the viral DNA and inhibits thymidine monophosphate kinase as well as viral-encoded thymidine kinase and DNA polymerase.[54] Kaufman,[122] in 1962, showed that experimental and clinical herpes simplex keratitis responded to topical idoxuridine therapy. This was confirmed in some,* but not all,[22,114,157] subsequent placebo-controlled trials. It is often difficult to compare clinical trials of antivirals in humans with efficacy evaluations in laboratory models of herpes keratitis, unless such models are already immune at the time of corneal inoculation. This difficulty occurs because the immune response itself is a potent viral inhibitor and disguises the true efficacy of topical antiviral therapy.[164] Idoxuridine is available as a 0.1% drop.

Vidarabine. This purine nucleoside acts by incorporation into viral DNA and inhibition of viral DNA polymerase. It is available as a 5% ophthalmic ointment, as well as in a preparation for intravenous use. Vidarabine ointment has been investigated in a number of trials comparing it with IDU, with which it has a comparable effect.[139,173,219] Similar comparisons have been made with trifluorothymidine.[43,173,218]

Trifluridine. The low solubility of IDU and adenine arabinoside prevented good penetration into the stroma, a limiting factor in their effectiveness. Trifluorothymidine is 10 times more soluble in water that IDU and does not produce toxic effects to such a high degree when used topically for long periods. Comparative trials have generally not demonstrated a superior effect of 1% trifluorothymidine drops over other antivirals such as IDU[218,310] or adenine arabinoside.[218,310] Corneal epithelial dysplasia has been reported after prolonged use.[167]

Acyclovir. Acycloguanosine (acyclovir, Zovirax) is the generic term for 9-(2-hydroxyethoxymethyl)guanine. Acyclovir acts through inhibition of the herpes virus-encoded DNA polymerase. To become active, acyclovir is first phosphorylated selectively by viral thymidine kinase. Cellular enzymes then convert the monophosphate form to the active triphosphate. Acyclovir triphosphate acts as a guanosine analogue and is a potent inhibitor of herpes simplex virus DNA polymerase.[57] In addition, acyclovir triphosphate lacks a 3'-hydroxyl group and therefore causes chain termination of the growing viral DNA strand.[313] Acyclovir is available as a 3% ophthalmic ointment (for investigational use in the United States), for oral administration as 200 mg and 500 mg capsules, and as a 200 mg/5 ml suspension, in addition to a powder to be used for intravenous infusions.

A major advantage of this drug is its ability to penetrate the corneal epithelial barrier and reach the stroma and anterior chamber in therapeutic amounts. Antiviral activity was first described by Schaeffer and associates.[257] Plaque inhibition assays showed that acyclovir is more active than IDU, trifluorothymidine, vidarabine, and phosphonoacetic acid.[37] Clinical studies in man soon confirmed in vitro find-

---

*References 88, 116, 122, 125, 140, 216.

ings,[38,115,174] and it was shown that toxicity was low in comparison to the first generation of antivirals. Introduction of the drug as a therapeutic agent in patients with systemic herpes simplex infection in a dosage of 5 mg per kg every 8 hours demonstrated minimal toxicity with good efficacy.[233] A number of investigators have reported (in uncontrolled studies) a therapeutic effect of systemic acyclovir with topical corticosteroid in treatment of stromal keratouveitis.[36,259]

Other Antivirals. The discovery of acyclovir led to other compounds such as 9-(1,3-dihydroxy-2-propoxymethyl) guanine (ganciclovir, DHPG), which is a potent inhibitor of viruses of the herpes family. Like acyclovir, topical ganciclovir penetrates the stromal and anterior chambers.[260] Studies have shown that ganciclovir is effective in laboratory models of herpes simplex keratitis.[196] In a viscotear suspension, it is effective in human herpes simplex keratitis[102] and has the singular advantage that it is not used in ointment form.

Whereas most nucleoside analogues with antiherpes activity (acyclovir, ganciclovir) are selectively phosphorylated by the virus-encoded thymidine kinase (TK), acyclic nucleotide phosphonate analogues that are phosphorylated by cellular enzymes have been recently designed and shown to have antiherpes activity. HPMPC (Cidofovir) is a compound in this group with in vitro activity against TK^+ and TK^- strains of herpes simplex virus (HSV), human cytomegalovirus (HCMV), adenovirus, and varicella zoster virus. HPMPC eyedrops were efficacious in the treatment of experimental herpes simplex keratitis in rabbits and may be a candidate drug for future clinical studies.[166]

Antiviral Resistance. To date there have been a limited number of reports of clinical and in vitro acyclovir resistance in herpetic eye disease.[27,175,187,271] Most, but not all, resistant isolates have been from patients with deficiencies in cell-mediated immunity.[133,269] Some strains have proved resistant in vitro and in vivo to multiple antiviral agents.[69,187] Several reports have shown a benefit to topical interferon-α and/or interferon-γ in combination with antivirals for resistant mucocutaneous[11] or corneal herpes simplex infection.[288,292]

Resistance to acyclovir may develop in several ways. Mutations in the viral thymidine kinase gene can result in abolished activity, decreased enzyme activity, or lowered affinity for its natural substates or acyclovir. The thymidine kinase gene mutations are the most common acyclovir-resistant herpes simplex virus isolates, and the majority of these should be responsive to drugs that are not dependent on thymidine kinase for activation, such as idoxuridine, trifluridine, vidarabine, and foscarnet. Alternatively, mutations in the viral DNA polymerase may alter its function so that it is less inhibited by acyclovir triphosphate.[32] Although rare, herpes simplex virus strains harboring viral DNA polymerase mutations have been known to complement sensitive viruses to allow acyclovir resistance, and acyclovir-sensitive viruses may complement drug-resistant strains for pathogenicity.

Although widely popularized, the concept of slowly tapering corticosteroids while concurrently tapering topical antivirals for stromal or disciform herpes keratitis may allow long periods of subtherapeutic antiviral levels, which could theoretically select for antiviral resistant strains of herpes simplex in the event of a recurrence.

Antiviral Toxicity. Most of the existing antivirals work on the basis of selective phosphorylation by the viral (as opposed to cellular) thymidine kinase or higher affinity of antiviral metabolites for the HSV DNA polymerase than cellular DNA polymerase. This selectivity, however, is not absolute, and antiviral drug toxicity may result. Toxicity is more common after prolonged antiviral use, and with the exception of corneal epitheliopathy, is a rare problem after short-term use, as in treatment of recurrent ulcerative disease. Toxic effects include follicular conjunctivitis, bulbar conjunctival chemosis and hyperemia, punctal stenosis, superficial punctate keratitis, chronic epithelial keratopathy, reduced tear secretion, and keratinization of tarsal plates.[67] Patients have also shown hypersensitivity reactions to thimerosal, which is the preservative used in trifluridine drops. Toxic reactions appear to be quite low with topical acyclovir ointment.[87]

Systemic acyclovir may be associated with renal insufficiency, gastrointestinal distress, and headache. Less-common side effects include encephalopathy, nausea and vomiting, urticaria, and phlebitis. Acyclovir has been assigned an FDA pregnancy category C status, indicating that safety in human pregnancies has not been determined. Comparison of the acyclovir in Pregnancy Registry with birth defects surveillance data of the Centers for Disease Control and Prevention indicated no increase in the risk of birth defects among infants born to women exposed to acyclovir during pregnancy.[26]

Medical Management

The different clinical manifestations of herpes simplex eye disease dictate different medical and surgical therapies. The underlying principle of treatment is to inhibit viral replication and, at the same time, reduce the inflammatory reaction that can lead to irreversible structural damage to the corneal parenchyma.

Herpes Simplex Blepharitis. Herpes simplex blepharitis generally resolves without scarring. Prophylactic treatment of the eye with a topical antiviral seems prudent in this setting to prevent the corneal epithelium from becoming infected.

Herpes Simplex Conjunctivitis. Primary or recurrent herpes simplex infection may produce a follicular conjunctivitis, with or without involvement of the cornea or deeper structures. Occasionally, dendritic or geographic ulcers can be seen on the conjunctivae. Topical antiviral drops or ointment should be used until the lesions resolve.

Epithelial Herpes Simplex Keratitis. Epithelial herpetic ulcers without stromal involvement should be treated with debridement along with topical antiviral therapy using initially acyclovir ointment or trifluridine drops.[303] A cycloplegic should be considered if there is iritis. Oral acyclovir provides therapeutic levels of drug in the tear film and is an effective treatment for epithelial herpes simplex keratitis.[10,40,75,184,261]

Cautery and Debridement. Before the appearance of antivirals, dendritic ulcers were treated by cautery using carbolic acid, ether, or iodine. Although this resulted in resolution of the ulceration, it was associated with stromal scarring,[44] damaged basement membranes, and recurrent erosions. Cryotherapy, like cautery techniques, carries risks of severe stromal reactions. It lacks precision and appears to have a lasting influence on the stroma and endothelium.[2]

Epithelial keratitis can be managed with gentle debridement along with the use of topical antivirals. Minimal-wiping debridement can be accomplished using a sterile cotton-tipped applicator to gently remove the loose epithelium, or by application of a sterilized cellulose acetate filter strip to the epithelial lesion, in a manner similar to impression cytology. Removal of loosely adherent, damaged, and infected epithelial cells via debridement reduces the inoculum of the virus, as well as viral antigens that can consequently be absorbed into the stroma, eliciting a cell-mediated immune response. This treatment is reasonably successful as inferred from clinical trials in which debridement has been compared with idoxuridine.[159,310,312]

Photodynamic Inactivation. Herpes simplex virus particles are rendered noninfective by a number of heterotricyclic dyes when exposed to visible light.[242] The technique, known as photodynamic inactivation, is a process of photo-autooxidation. The first step is the binding of a photoactive dye to specific sites on viral DNA, probably guanine in the case of herpes simplex virus. Proflavine dye has been investigated in human disease, but its use is complicated by severe corneal epitheliopathy, and occasionally, iritis.[206]

Trophic Keratopathy. Ocular herpes simplex may damage the corneal nerves, basement membrane, and anterior stroma, leading to noninfectious, metaherpetic disease. This damage may consist of corneal thinning or recurrent erosions caused by difficulties in reforming the epithelial anchoring complex. This condition should be treated with copious lubrication with nonpreserved artificial tears and ointment, soft bandage contact lenses of high water content, conjunctival flap, or tarsorrhaphy. It should be noted that recurrent herpes simplex can occur in a conjunctival flap.[250]

In the event of progressive corneal thinning or melting, a cyanoacrylate tissue adhesive can be applied, followed by a bandage lens. This procedure may allow lamellar or penetrating keratoplasty to be delayed and performed on a more elective basis. In this clinical setting, however, the diagnosis of metaherpetic disease must be correct, as active epithelial keratitis would benefit from antiviral application.

HSV Endotheliitis, Iridocyclitis, and Trabeculitis. As mentioned previously, patients with linear HSV endotheliitis, iridocyclitis, and/or trabeculitis may respond to treatment with a topical trifluridine or acyclovir ointment and topical corticosteroid, with or without oral acyclovir. Severe iridocyclitis may be the principal manifestation of herpetic eye disease, sometimes appearing with stromal keratitis or with no active corneal inflammation. Cycloplegia should be provided by use of homatropine and elevated intraocular pressure treated medically. The Herpetic Eye Disease Study (which has enrolled patients with herpetic iridocyclitis) is comparing oral acyclovir and placebo to test the null hypothesis that oral acyclovir (at 400 mg 5 times daily) does not increase the time to treatment failure during a 16-week trial interval. This dose of acyclovir was based on a study that showed adequate antiviral levels in serum and aqueous.[107]

Disciform Keratitis. Disciform keratitis should be treated with a topical antiviral agent and the minimal dose of topical corticosteroid required to reduce the edema and inflammation. The steroid should then be gradually tapered. Reduction from 1% prednisolone acetate to ⅛% prednisolone acetate to 0.1% fluoromethalone may be required, increasing the frequency of drops when going to the less-potent steroid. Rebound disciform keratitis requires going back to the more potent steroid, with initiation of a slower taper. Prospective, randomized studies by Collum and associates[39] demonstrated that topical antiviral acyclovir alone, without concomitant corticosteroids, was not an effective treatment of disciform endotheliitis. Another study[35] suggested that topical trifluorothymidine or acyclovir with topical corticosteroids was superior to topical vidarabine in combination with corticosteroids for treatment of disciform disease.

The National Eye Institute recently sponsored a prospective, randomized, multicentered trial regarding the treatment of herpes simplex stromal keratitis patients who had not received any corticosteroids for at least 10 days and did not have epithelial disease. The trial showed that topical trifluorothymidine and a tapering dosage of corticosteroids was significantly better than trifluorothymidine and placebo in reducing progression or persistence of stromal inflammation and in shortening the duration of stromal keratitis.[319] Another arm of this trial demonstrated that oral acyclovir did not show a significant beneficial effect in the treatment of HSV stromal keratitis in patients receiving topical corticosteroids and trifluridine with regard to time to treatment failure, proportion of patients who failed treatment or whose keratitis resolved, time to resolution, or 6-month best-corrected visual acuity. Whether patients with necrotizing herpetic keratitis would benefit from oral acyclovir will require further study.

Herpes Simplex Retinitis. Herpes simplex retinitis, with or without encephalitis, is treated with intravenous acyclovir until there is no progression of lesions, followed by oral acyclovir at 500 mg 5 times daily, with doses adjusted for renal failure.

Studies suggest that 3-year graft survival is in the range of 75% in eyes without an early HSV recurrence, and drops to 53% in eyes with an early recurrence.[231] Further risks to graft survival include preoperative cataract, glaucoma, and anterior vitrectomy[64]; regrafts appear to have a worse prognosis than first corneal allografts.[70]

Surgical Management of Herpes Simplex Keratitis

In the past, many cases of corneal scarring or opacification were treated with lamellar keratoplasty. This was due, in part, to the poor prognosis for penetrating keratoplasty in treating herpes simplex prior to the availability of antivirals. There appears to be an improved prognosis in recent years for penetrating keratoplasties for HSV keratitis, perhaps relating to the use of prophylactic antivirals and topical corticosteroids during rejection episodes. Studies concur that penetrating keratoplasty in acutely inflamed eyes with active herpes and neovascularization has a poor prognosis.[76,232] In 1980 a study at Moorfields Eye Hospital reported a 79% graft failure rate after rejection episodes in eyes grafted for herpes keratitis. There was a 32% recurrence rate within 4 months of a graft rejection treated with topical corticosteroids and no antiviral cover.[31] In addition, early recurrence of herpes keratitis was associated with a significant decrease in long-term graft survival, perhaps because of endothelial damage.[31,33]

Studies* suggest that the recurrence rate of herpes keratitis in corneal allografts for herpes ranges from 6% to 18% at 2 to 3 years, with or without routine prophylactic topical antiviral therapy. Overall, long-term graft survival in herpes may be currently greater than 70%, in part, because of the detection of early rejection signs and the appreciation that rejection episodes require antiviral treatment along with intense corticosteroids. These changes increased the success rate in grafting inflamed eyes to one comparable for uninflamed eyes. Early recurrence tends to localize to the graft-host interface epithelium, consistent with the pattern of graft re-innervation. It may be difficult to differentiate allograft rejection from recurrent herpes simplex, as both may be interrelated and associated with anterior chamber inflammation. In vitro studies have shown that interferon-γ produced by lymphocytes responding to HSV can induce Class II major histocompatability antigens in the cornea, a finding common to corneal allograft rejection and herpes keratitis.[329]

PREVENTION

Prophylaxis

The use of oral acyclovir prophylactically in patients with a history of frequent recurrences of herpes simplex keratitis or postoperative occurrences following penetrating kerato-

---

*References 31, 33, 71, 72, 76, 143, 232.

plasty for herpes may have promise, but will require prospective, multicentered trials for proof of efficacy. Chronic oral acyclovir use at a dosage of 400 mg twice daily has been shown effective in reducing recurrences of genital and labial herpes in immunocompetent and immunocompromised patients.[119,273] Blatt and associates[12] showed that prophylactic acyclovir could limit herpes simplex reactivation following ultraviolet B exposure in a murine model.

Beyer and associates[10] demonstrated the efficacy of oral acyclovir in reducing viral shedding and recurrent epithelial and stromal herpes keratitis after penetrating keratoplasty in latently infected rabbits treated with topical and subconjunctival corticosteroids. An unmasked, retrospective study suggested a significant decrease in recurrent rate and graft failure in patients with a history of recurrent herpes simplex keratitis given oral acyclovir, trifluridine, idoxuridine, or vidarabine. This decrease was associated with a decline in allograft rejection episodes and clinical herpetic recurrences.[184] The potential benefit of chronic topical antiviral prophylaxis must be weighed against side effects such as epithelial toxicity and delayed wound healing.[142]

Vaccination

Attempts have been made to generate antigen-specific protective immune responses that do not lead to stromal keratitis in experimental models. The most commonly used techniques involved the vaccination of animals with live or attenuated virus.[21] Although some success has been seen in animal models using UV-inactivated virus[97,293] or purified glycoprotein D,[78] there are currently no FDA licensed herpes simplex vaccines. Clinical trials are underway, however, for treatment of genital herpes testing several different adjuvant-associated vaccines containing glycoprotein D2 alone or in combination with glycoprotein B2.[34] Recently replication-defective mutants of HSV-1 have been used for immunization in murine models of primary HSK. Results from these studies have indicated that such immunization leads to protection of the animal from acute and latent infection of the nervous system and inhibits the development of primary HSK.[189] Recombinant baculoviruses expressing HSV glycoproteins gB, gC, gD, gE, and gI resulted in production of higher neutralizing antibody titers to HSV-1 and protection against intraperitoneal and ocular lethal challenges with HSV-1.[82] Periocular vaccination of latently infected rabbits with recombinant HSV-2 glycoproteins D and B plus adjuvant significantly reduced spontaneous ocular viral shedding, supporting the concept that vaccination may have potential in a therapeutic as well as prophylactic mode.[198] Immunotherapy of acute and recurrent vaginal herpes simplex virus type 2 infection was recently accomplished in a guinea pig model with an adjuvant-free form of recombinant glycoprotein D-interleukin 2 fusion protein.[197] This immunotherapeutic agent has not yet been tested in a comparable ocular model of acute and recurrent HSV. Interestingly, it has also been reported that Fischer rats receiving topical application of soluble glycoprotein D (2 hours prior to infection with HSV-1) displayed reduced incidence (44% versus 100%) of ocular infection leading to the death of the animal.[165] In addition, for those rats that survived the infection, only 3 of 14 displayed any corneal opacity, and those that did, demonstrated only mild corneal opacity. The authors demonstrated that the protective effect of glycoprotein D was not mediated by inducing the production of IFN-α. They also proposed that soluble glycoprotein acted primarily by inhibiting entry of HSV-1 into corneal cells by blocking potential viral receptors on the surface of these cells.[165] Other routes of vaccine delivery, such as via intranasal and intragastric administration, have been studied in experimental systems to see if they can better produce local mucosal immunity. Whether any of these vaccine strategies can prevent infection and the establishment of latency, in distinction to disease amelioration, remains to be determined.

Disinfection

Although there are no reports documenting direct transmission of herpes simplex keratitis from patient to patient via the practice of ophthalmology, recovery of infectious herpesvirus from the tears of asymptomatic patients as well as the viability of herpes simplex on applanation tonometer tips raises this possibility. Ophthalmologists should practice handwashing before and after examination of every patient. In addition, applanation tonometers should be wiped with a 70% isopropyl alcohol swab to inactivate this enveloped virus.[305] At least 1 minute should be allowed for the tip to air dry, lest the alcohol lead to corneal opacification.[272]

REFERENCES

1. Abu El-Asrar AM et al.: Expression of MHC class II antigens and immunoglobulin M by the corneal epithelial cells in herpetic keratitis, *Int Ophthalmol* 14:233-239, 1990.
2. Amolis SP, Maier G: Cryosurgery and immunotherapy in herpes keratitis, *Br J Ophthalmol* 57:809-814, 1973.
3. Andrews CH, Carmichael EA: A note on the presence of antibodies to herpesvirus in post-encephalitic and other human sera, *Lancet* 1:857, 1930.
4. Asbell P, Centifano-Fitzgerald Y, Chandler J et al.: Analysis of viral DNA in isolettes from patients with recurrent herpetic keratitis, *Invest Ophthalmol Vis Sci* 25:951, 1984.
5. Baldwin S, Whitley RJ: Intrauterine HSV infection, *J Teratology* 39:1-10, 1988.
6. Baringer JR: The biology of herpes simplex virus infections in humans, *Surv Ophthalmol* 21(2):171, 1976.
7. Barker JNWN et al.: Modulation of keratinocyte-derived interleukin-8 which is chemotactic for neutrophils and T lymphocytes, *Am J Pathol* 139:869-876, 1991.
8. Bell DM et al.: Herpes simplex keratitis: epidemiologic aspects, *Ann Ophthalmol* 14:421, 1982.
9. Berger CF et al.: Herpes simplex virus and persistent epithelial defects after penetrating keratoplasty, *Am J Ophthalmol* 109:95-96, 1990.
10. Beyer CF, Arens MQ, Hill GA et al.: Oral acyclovir reduces the incidence of recurrent herpes simplex keratitis in rabbits after penetrating keratoplasty, *Arch Ophthalmol* 107:1250-1255, 1989.
11. Birch CJ, Tyssen DP, Tachedjian G et al.: Clinical effects and in vitro studies of trifluorothymidine combined with interferon-alpha for treatment of drug-resistant and drug-sensitive herpes virus infections, *J Infect Dis* 166:108-112, 1992.

12. Blatt AN, Laycock KA, Brady RH et al.: Prophylactic acyclovir effectively reduces herpes simplex virus type 1 reactivation after exposure of latently infected mice to ultraviolet B, *Invest Ophthalmol Vis Sci* 34:3459-3651, 1993.
13. Block TM et al.: A herpes simplex type 1 latency-associated transcript mutant reactivates with normal kinetics from latent infection, *J Virol* 64:4317-4326, 1990.
14. Block TM et al.: An HSV LAT null mutant reactivates slowly from latent infection and makes small plaques on CV-1 monolayers, *Virology* 192:618-630, 1993.
15. Bloom DC et al.: Molecular analysis of herpes simplex virus type 1 during epinephrine-induced reactivation of latently infected rabbits in vivo, *J Virol* 68:1283-1292, 1994.
16. Brady SE et al.: Clinical indications for and procedures associated with penetrating keratoplasty, 1983-1988, *Am J Ophthalmol* 108:118-122, 1989.
17. Brandt CR: Susceptibility of $+/+$, $+/v$, and v/v BALB/c mice to ocular herpes simplex virus infection, *Ophthalmic Res* 24:332-337, 1992.
18. Brandt CR, Coakley LM, Grau DR: A murine model of herpes simplex virus-induced ocular disease for antiviral drug testing, *J Virol Methods* 36:209-222, 1992.
19. Brooks SE, Kaza V, Nakamura T, Trousdale MD: Photo inactivation of herpes simplex virus by rose bengal and fluorescein. In vitro and in vivo studies, *Cornea* 13:43-50, 1994.
20. Buchman TG et al.: Demonstration of exogenous reinfection with herpes simplex virus type-2 by restriction endonuclease fingerprinting of viral DNA, *J Infect Dis* 140:295, 1979.
21. Burke RL: Contemporary approaches to vaccination against herpes simplex virus, *Curr Top Microbiol Immunol* 179:137-174, 1992.
22. Burns RP: A double-blind study of IDU in human herpes simplex keratitis, *Arch Ophthalmol* 70:318-324, 1963.
23. Cai W et al.: The herpes simplex virus type regulatory protein ICP0 enhances viral replication during acute infection and reactivation from latency, *J Virol* 67:7510-7512, 1993.
24. Campbell MEM, Palfreyman JW, Preston CM: Identification of herpes simplex virus DNA sequences which encode a trans-acting polypeptide responsible for stimulation of immediate-early transcription, *J Mol Biol* 180:1-19, 1984.
25. Centers for Disease Control: Genital herpes infection—United States, 1966-1984, *MMWR* 35:402-404, 1986.
26. Centers for Disease Control: Pregnancy outcome following systemic prenatal acyclovir exposure—June 1, 1984-June 30, 1993, *MMWR* 42:390-393, 1993.
27. Charles SJ, Gray JJ: Ocular herpes simplex virus infection: reduced sensitivity to acyclovir in primary disease, *Br J Ophthalmol* 74:286-288, 1990.
28. Cibis A, Burde R: Herpes simplex virus induced congenital cataracts, *Arch Ophthalmol* 85:220-223, 1971.
29. Cleator GM, Klapper PE, Dennett C et al.: Corneal donor infection by herpes simplex virus: herpes simplex virus DNA in donor corneas, *Cornea* 13:294-304, 1994.
30. Clements GB, Stow ND: A herpes simplex virus type 1 mutant containing a deletion within immediate early gene 1 is latency-competent in mice, *J Gen Virol* 70:2501-2506, 1989.
31. Cobo LM, Coster DJ, Rice NSC, Jones BR: Prognosis and management of corneal transplantation for herpetic keratitis, *Arch Ophthalmol* 98:1755-1759, 1980.
32. Coen DM, Schaffer PA: Two distinct loci confer resistance to acycloguanosine in herpes simplex type 1, *Proc Natl Acad Sci* 77:2265-2269, 1980.
33. Cohen EJ, Laibson PR, Arentsen JJ: Corneal transplantation for herpes simplex keratitis, *Am J Ophthalmol* 95:645-650, 1983.
34. Cohen J: Vaccines get a new twist, *Science* 264:503-505, 1994.
35. Colin J, Mazet D, Chastel C: Treatment of herpetic keratouveitis: comparative of vidarabine, trifluorothymidine and acyclovir in combination with corticoids. In Maudgal PC, Missotten L, editors: *Herpetic eye diseases,* 227-232, Dordrecht, 1985, Junk.
36. Colin J, Malet F, Chestel C et al.: Acyclovir in herpetic anterior uveitis, *Ann Ophthalmol* 23:28-30, 1991.
37. Collins P, Bauer DJ: The activity in vitro against herpes of 9-(2-hydroxyethoxymethyl)guanine (acycloguanosine), a new antiviral agent, *J Antimicrob Chemother* 5:431-436, 1970.

38. Collum LMT, Benedict-Smith A, Hillary IB: Acyclovir in dendritic corneal ulceration. In Roper P Trevor, editor: *The corneal health and disease*, RSM International Congress Series No 40, London, 1980, RSM/Academic Press.

39. Collum LMT, Logan P, Ravenscroft T: Acyclovir (Zovirax) in herpetic disciform keratitis, *Br J Ophthalmol* 67:115-118, 1983.

40. Collum LMT, McGettrick P, Akhau J et al.: Oral acyclovir (Zovirax) in herpes simplex dendritic corneal ulceration, *Br J Ophthalmol* 70:435-438, 1986.

41. Confer DL et al.: Herpes simplex virus-infected cells disarm killer lymphocytes, *Proc Natl Acad Sci USA* 87:3609, 1990.

42. Cook ML, Stevens JG: Pathogenesis of herpetic neuritis and gangliomites in mice: evidence of intra-axonal transport of infection, *Infect Immun* 7:272-288, 1973.

43. Coster DJ, McKinnon JR, McGill JI et al.: Clinical evaluation of adenine arabinoside and tribluorothyumidine in the treatment of corneal ulcers caused by herpes simplex virus, *J Infect Dis* 133(suppl A):173-177, 1976.

44. Coster DL, Jones BR, Falcon MC: Role of debridement in the treatment of herpetic keratitis, *Trans Ophthalmol Soc UK* 97:314-317, 1977.

45. Coyle P, Sibony P, Sibony P: Viral antibodies in normal tears, *Invest Ophthalmol Vis Sci* 29:1552-1558, 1988.

46. Reference deleted in proofs.

47. Croen KD et al.: Latent herpes simplex virus in human trigeminal ganglia: detection of an immediate-early gene "anti-sense" transcript by in situ hybridization, *New Engl J Med* 317:1427-1432, 1987.

48. Croen KD et al.: Patterns of gene expression and sites of latency are different for varicella-zoster and herpes simplex viruses, *Proc Natl Acad Sci USA* 85:9773-9777, 1988.

49. Cushing H: Surgical aspects of major neuralgia of trigeminal nerve: report of 20 cases of operation upon the Gasserian ganglion with anatomic and physiologic notes on the consequence of its removal, *JAMA* 44:1002, 1905.

50. Darougar S et al.: Acute follicular conjunctivitis and keratoconjunctivitis due to herpes simplex virus in London, *Br J Ophthalmol* 62:843-847, 1978.

51. Dawson CR, Togni B: Herpes simplex eye infections: clinical manifestations, pathogenesis and management, *Surv Ophthalmol* 21:121-135, 1976.

52. de la Maza MS, Wells PA, Foster CS: Cyclic nucleotide modulation of herpes simplex virus latency and reactivation, *Invest Ophthalmol Vis Sci* 30:2154-2159, 1989.

53. Deatly AM et al.: RNA from an immediate-early region of the type 1 herpes simplex virus genome is present in the trigeminal ganglia of latently infected mice, *Proc Natl Acad Sci USA* 84:3204-3208, 1987.

54. Delamore IW, Prusoff WH: Effect of 5-iodo-2'-deoxyuridine on the biosynthesis of phosphorylated derivates of thymidine, *Biochem Pharmacol* 11:101-112, 1962.

55. Devi-Rao GB, Bloom DC, Stevens JG, Wagner EK: Herpes simplex virus type 1 DNA replication and gene expression during explant-induced reactivation of latently infected murine sensory ganglia, *J Virol* 68:1271-1282, 1994.

56. Doerig C, Pizer LI, Wilcox CL: An antigen encoded by the latency-associated transcript in neuronal cell cultures latently infected with herpes simplex virus type 1, *J Virol* 65:2724-2727, 1991.

57. Dorsky DI, Crumpacker CS: Drugs five years later: acyclovir, *Ann Intern Med* 107:859-874, 1987.

58. Doymaz MZ, Rouse BT: Herpetic stromal keratitis: an immunopathologic disease mediated by CD4$^+$ T lymphocytes, *Invest Ophthalmol Vis Sci* 33:2165-2173, 1992.

59. Doymaz MZ, Rouse BT: Immunopathology of herpes simplex virus infections, *Curr Top Microbiol and Immunol* 179:121-136, 1992.

60. Dreizen NG, Whitsett CF, Stulting RD: Modulation of HLA antigen expression on corneal epithelial and stromal cells, *Invest Ophthalmol Vis Sci* 29:933-939, 1989.

61. Durum SK, Oppenheim JJ: Macrophage-derived mediators: interleukin-1 tumor necrosis factor, interleukin-6, interferon, and related cytokines. In Paul WE, editor: *Fundamental immunology*, ed 2, 639-661, New York, 1989, Raven Press.

62. Easty DL et al.: Herpes simplex virus isolation in chronic stromal keratitis, human and laboratory studies, *Curr Eye Res* 6:69-74, 1987.

62a. el Azazi M et al.: Late ophthalmologic manifestations of neonatal herpes simplex virus infection, *Am J Ophthalmol* 109:1-7, 1990.

63. Elner VM et al.: Intercellular adhesion molecule-1 (ICAM-1) and HLA-DR antigens in herpes keratitis, *Ophthalmology* 99:1400-1407, 1992.

64. Epstein RJ, Seedor JA, Dreisen NG et al.: Penetrating keratoplasty for herpes simplex keratitis and keratoconus: allograft rejection and survival, *Ophthalmology* 94:935-942.

65. Everett RD: Transactivation of transcription by herpes virus product: requirement for two HSV-1 immediate-early polypeptides for maximum activity, *EMBO J* 3:3135-3141, 1984.

66. Fahy GT, Hooper DC, Easty DL: Antigen presentation of herpes simplex virus by corneal epithlium—an in vitro and in vivo study, *Br J Ophthalmol* 77:440-444, 1993.

67. Falcon MG, Jones BR, Willams HP et al.: Adverse reactions in the eye from topical therapy with idoxuridine, adenine arabinoside and trifluorothymidine. In Sundmacher R, editor: *Herpetic eye diseases*, 263, Munich, JF Bergmann Verlag, 1981.

68. Falcon MG, Williams HP: Herpetic simplex kerato-uveitis and glaucoma, *Trans Ophthalmol Soc UK* 98:101-104, 1978.

69. Fardeau C, Langlois M, Nugier F et al.: Cross-resistances to antiviral drugs of IUDR-resistant HSV 1 in rabbits and in vitro, *Cornea* 12:19-24, 1993.

70. Ficker LA, Kirkness CM, Rice NSC, Steel ADMcG: Long term prognosis for corneal grafting in herpes simplex keratitis, *Eye* 2:400-408, 1988.

71. Ficker LA, Kirkness CM, Rice NSC, Steele AD: The changing management and improved prognosis for corneal grafting in herpes simplex keratitis, *Ophthalmology* 96:1587-1596, 1989.

72. Fine M, Cignetti FE: Penetrating keratoplasty in herpes simplex keratitis recurrence in grafts, *Arch Ophthalmol* 95:613-616, 1977.

73. Foets BJJ, van den Oord JJ, Billau A et al.: Heterogeneous induction of major histocompatibility complex class II antigens on corneal endothelium by interferon gamma, *Invest Ophthalmol Vis Sci* 32:341-345, 1991.

74. Foster A, Sommer A: Corneal ulceration, measles, and childhood blindness in Tanzania, *Br J Ophthalmol* 71:331-343, 1987.

75. Foster CS, Barney NP: Systemic acyclovir and penetrating keratoplasty for herpes simplex keratitis, *Doc Ophthalmol* 80:363-369, 1992.

76. Foster CS, Duncan J: Penetrating keratoplasty for herpes simplex keratitis, *Am J Ophthalmol* 92:336-343, 1981.

77. Foster CS et al.: Genetic studies on murine susceptibility to herpes simplex keratitis, *Clin Immunol Immunopathol* 40:313-325, 1986.

78. Foster CS et al.: Immunomodulation of experimental herpes simplex keratitis. II. Glycoprotein D protection, *Curr Eye Res* 7:1051-1061, 1988.

79. Fox PD, Khaw PT, McBride BW et al.: Tear and serum antibody levels in ocular herpetic infection: diagnostic precision of secretary IgA, *Br J Ophthalmol* 70:584-589, 1986.

80. Fraser NW, Block TM, Spivack JG: The latency associated transcripts of herpes simplex virus: RNA in search of function, *Virology* 191:1-8, 1992.

81. Gelman IH, Silverstein S: Identification of immediate-early genes from herpes simplex virus that transactivate the viral thymidine kinase gene, *Proc Natl Acad Sci USA* 82:5265-5269, 1985.

82. Ghiasi H et al.: Expression of seven herpes simplex virus type 1 glycoproteins (gB, gC, gD, gE, gG, gH, and gI): comparative protection against lethal challenge in mice, *J Virol* 68:2118-2126, 1994.

83. Gillette TE, Chandler JW, Greiner JV: Langerhans cells of the ocular surface, *Ophthalmology* 89:700-711, 1982.

84. Goldberg MF, Feguson TA, Pepose JS: Detection of cellular adhesion molecules in inflamed human corneas, *Ophthalmology* 101:161-168, 1994.

85. Goodpasture EW: Herpetic infections with special reference to involvement of the nervous system, *Medicine* 8:223, 1929.

86. Gosselin J et al.: Modulatory effects of Epstein-Barr, herpes simplex, and human herpes-6 viral infections and co-infections on cytokine synthesis: a comparative study, *J Immunol* 149:181-187, 1992.

87. Grant DM: Acyclovir (Zovirax) ophthalmic ointment: a review of clinical tolerance, *Curr Eye Res* 6:231-235, 1987.

88. Hart DRL et al.: Treatment of human herpes simplex keratitis with idoxuridine, *Arch Ophthalmol* 73:623-634, 1965.

89. Hayward AR, Read GS, Cosyns M: Herpes simplex virus interferes with monocyte accessory cell function, *J Immunol* 150:190-196, 1993.

90. Hendricks RL, Epstein RJ, Tumpey T: The effect of cellular immune tolerance to HSV-1 antigens on the immunopathology of HSV-1 keratitis, *Invest Ophthalmol Vis Sci* 30:105-115, 1989.

91. Hendricks RL, Janowicz M, Tumpey TM: Critical role of corneal Langerhans cells in the CD4- but not CD8-mediated immunopathology in herpes simplex virus-1 infected mouse corneas, *J Immunol* 148:2522-2529, 1992.

92. Hendricks RL, Sugar J: Lysis of herpes simplex virus (HSV) infected targets. IV. HSV-induced change in the effector population, *Invest Ophthalmol Vis Sci* 26:208-213, 1985.

93. Hendricks RL, Tao MSP, Glorioso JC: Alterations in the antigenic structure of two major HSV-1 glycoproteins, gC and gB, influence immune regulation and susceptibility to murine herpes keratitis, *J Immunol* 142:263-269, 1989.

94. Hendricks RL, Tumpey T: Contribution of virus and immune factors to herpes simplex virus type 1 induced corneal pathology, *Invest Ophthalmol Vis Sci* 31:1929-1939, 1990.

95. Hendricks RL, Tumpey TM, Finnegan A: IFN-gamma and IL-2 are protective in the skin but pathologic in the corneas of HSV-1-infected mice, *J Immunol* 149:3023-3028, 1992.

96. Hendricks RL et al.: The effect of flurbiprofen on herpes simplex virus type 1 stromal keratitis in mice, *Invest Ophthalmol Vis Sci* 31:1503-1511, 1990.

97. Hendricks RL et al.: Endogenously produced IFN alpha protects mice from herpes simplex virus type 1 corneal disease, *J Gen Virol* 72:1601-1610, 1991.

98. Hill JH, Rayfield MA, Haruta Y: Strain specificity of spontaneous and adrenergically induced HSV-1 ocular reactivation in latently infected rabbits, *Curr Eye Res* 6:91-97, 1987.

99. Hill JM et al.: Herpes simplex virus latent phase transcription facilitates in vivo reactivation, *Virology* 174:117-125, 1990.

100. Hill TJ, Blyth WA, Harbour DA: Trauma to the skin causes recurrence of herpes simplex in the mouse, *J Gen Virol* 39:21-28, 1978.

101. Ho DY, Mocarski ES: Herpes simplex virus latent RNA (LAT) is not required for latent infection in the mouse, *Proc Natl Acad Sci USA* 86:7596-7600, 1989.

102. Hoh HB, Goldschmidt P, Easty DL: Comparative efficacy of ganciclovir and acyclovir ointment in the treatment of herpes simplex dendritic keratitis, *Curr Eye Res* 101:68-72, 1992.

103. Holbach LM et al.: HSV antigens and HSV DNA in avasular and vascularized lesions of human herpes simplex keratitis, *Curr Eye Res* 10(suppl):63-68, 1991.

104. Honess RW, Roizman B: Regulation of herpesvirus macromolecular synthesis. I. Cascade regulation of the synthesis of three groups of viral proteins, *J Virol* 14:8-19, 1974.

105. Howard MK et al.: Transactivation by the herpes simplex virus virion protein Vmw65 and viral permissivity in a neuronal cell line with reduced levels of the cellular transcription factor Oct-1, *Exp Cell Res* 207:194-196, 1993.

106. Hung SO, Patterson A, Clark DI, Rees PJ: Oral acyclovir in the management of herpetic corneal ulceration, *Br J Ophthalmol* 68:398-400, 1984.

107. Hung SO, Patterson A, Rees PJ: Pharmakokinetics of oral acyclovir (Zovirax) in the eye, *Br J Ophthalmol* 68:192-195, 1984.

108. Igietseme JV et al.: Protection of mice from herpes simplex virus-induced retinitis by in vitro activated immune cells, *J Virol* 63:4808-4813, 1989.

109. Inoue Y et al.: Protective effects of anti-glycoprotein D monoclonal antibodies in murine herpetic keratitis, *Curr Eye Res* 11:53-60, 1991.

110. Izumi KM et al.: Molecular and biologic characterization of a type 1 herpes simplex virus (HSV-1) specifically deleted for expression of the latency-associated transcript (LAT), *Microb Pathog* 7:121-134, 1989.

111. Jager MJ et al.: Presence of Langerhans in the central cornea linked to the development of ocular herpes in mice, *Exp Eye Res* 54:835-841, 1992.

112. Jayaraman S, Martin CA, Dorf ME: Enhancement of in vivo cell-mediated immune responses by three distinct cytokines, *J Immunol* 144:942-951, 1990.

113. Jayaraman S et al.: Exacerbation of murine herpes simplex virus-mediated stromal keratitis by Th2 type T cells, *J Immunol* 151:5777-5789, 1993.

114. Jepson CN: Treatment of herpes simplex of the cornea with IDU, *Am J Ophthalmol* 57:213-217, 1964.

115. Jones BR, Coster DJ, Fison PN et al.: Efficacy of acycloguanosine (Wellcome 248u) against herpes simplex corneal ulcers, *Lancet* 1:243-244, 1979.

116. Juel-Jensen BE, MacCallum FO: Treatment of herpes simplex lesion of the face with idoxuridine: results of a double-blind controlled trial, *Br Med J* 2:987-988, 1964.

117. Kaplan AS: A study of the herpes simplex-rabbit kidney cell system by the plaque technique, *Virology* 4:435, 1957.

118. Kaplan HJ, Streilein JW: Immune response to immunization via the anterior chamber of the eye. I. F1 lymphocyte induce immune deviation, *J Immunol* 118:809-814, 1977.

119. Kaplowitz LG, Baker D, Gelb L: Prolonged continuous acyclovir treatment of normal adults with frequently recurring genital herpes simplex virus infection, *JAMA* 265:747-753, 1991.

120. Katz JP, Bodin ET, Coen DM: Quantitative polymerase chain reaction analysis of herpes simplex virus DNA in ganglia of mice infected with replication incompetent mutants, *J Virol* 64:4288-4295, 1990.

121. Reference deleted in proofs.

122. Kaufman HE: Clinical cure of herpes simplex keratitis by 5-iodo-2'-deoxyuridine, *Proc Soc Exp Biol* (NY) 109:251-252, 1962.

123. Kaufman HE, Brown DC, Ellison EM: Recurrent herpes in the rabbit and man, *Science* 156:1628-1629, 1967.

124. Kaufman HE, Heidelberger C: Therapeutic antiviral action of 5-trifluoromethyl-2'deoxyuridine in herpes simplex keratitis, *Science* 145:585, 1964.

125. Kaufman HE, Nesburn AB, Maloney ED: IDU therapy of herpes simplex, *Arch Ophthalmol* 67:583-591, 1962.

126. Kaye S, Madan N, Dowd T et al.: Ocular herpes virus shedding, *Br J Ophthalmol* 74:114-119, 1990.

127. Kaye SB et al.: Evidence for herpes simplex viral latency in the human cornea, *Br J Ophthalmol* 75:195-200, 1991.

128. Keadle TL et al.: Clinical features and immunologic mechanisms of recurrent versus primary herpes simplex keratitis in inbred mice, *Invest Ophthalmol Vis Sci* 34(suppl):901, 1993.

129. Keadle T et al.: Efficacy of two HSV-2 glycoprotein D vaccines against acute and recurrent ocular herpes simplex virus type 1 infection in mice, *Invest Ophthalmol Vis Sci* 35(suppl):1333, 1994.

130. Kemp LM, Dent CL, Latchman DS: Octamer Motif mediates transcriptional repression of HSV immediate-early genes and octamer-containing cellular promoters in neuronal cells, *Neuron* 2:215-222, 1990.

131. Kimura SJ: Herpes simplex uveitis: a clinical and experimental study, *Trans Am Ophthalmol Soc* 60:440-470, 1962.

132. Kolaitis G, Doymaz M, Rouse BT: Demonstration of MHC class II-restricted cytotoxic T lymphocytes in mice against herpes simplex virus, *Immunology* 71:101-106, 1990.

133. Kost RG, Hill EL, Tigges M, Straus SE: Recurrent acyclovir-resistant genital herpes in an immunocompetent patient, *New Engl J Med* 329:1777-1782, 1993.

134. Kosz-Vnenchak M, Coen DM, Knipe DM: Restricted expression of herpes simplex virus lytic genes during the establishment of latent infection by thymidine kinase-negative mutant viruses, *J Virol* 64:5396-5402, 1990.

135. Kosz-Vnenchak M, Jacobson J, Coen DM, Knipe DM: Evidence for a novel regulatory pathway for herpes simplex virus gene expression in trigeminal ganglion neurons, *J Virol* 67:5383-5393, 1993.

136. Kowalski RP et al.: A comparison of enzyme immunoassay and polymerase chain reaction with the clinical examination for diagnosing ocular herpetic disease, *Ophthalmology* 100:530-533, 1993.

137. Ksander BR, Hendricks RL: Cell-mediated immune tolerance to HSV-1 antigens associated with reduced susceptibility to HSV-1 corneal lesions, *Invest Ophthalmol Vis Sci* 28:1986-1993.

138. Kurane I, Tsuchiya Y, Sekizawa T, Kumagai K: Inhibition by indomethicin of in vitro reactivation of latent herpes simplex virus type 1 in murine trigeminal ganglia, *J Gen Virol* 65:1665-1674, 1984.

139. Laibson PR, Kratchmer JH: Controlled comparison of adenine arabinoside and iodoxyuridine therapy of human superficial dendritic keratitis. In Pavan-Langston D, Buchanan RA, Alford GA, editors: *Adenine arabinoside: an antiviral agent,* 323, New York, 1976, Raven Press.

140. Laibson PR, Leopold IH: An evaluation of double-blind IDU therapy in 100 cases of herpetic keratitis, *Trans Am Acad Ophthalmol Otolaryngol* 68:22-34, 1965.

141. Langston DP, Dunkel EC: A rapid clinical diagnostic test for herpes simplex infectious keratitis, *Am J Ophthalmol* 107:675-677, 1989.

142. Langston RHS, Pavan-Langston D, Dohlman CH: Antiviral medication and corneal wound healing, *Arch Ophthalmol* 92:509-513, 1974.

143. Langston RHS, Pavan-Langston D, Dohlman CH: Penetrating keratoplasty for herpetic keratitis: prognostic and therapeutic determinants, *Trans Am Acad Ophthalmol Otolaryngol* 79:577-583, 1975.

144. Lausch RN et al.: Quantitation of purified monoclonal antibody needed to prevent HSV-1 induced stromal keratitis in mice, *Curr Eye Res* 8:499-506, 1989.

145. Lausch RN et al.: Evidence endogenous interferon production contributed to the lack of ocular virulence of an HSV intertypic recombinant, *Curr Eye Res* 10:39-45, 1991.

146. Laycock KA, Lee SF, Brady RH, Pepose JS: Characterization of a murine model of recurrent herpetic keratitis induced by ultraviolet B radiation, *Invest Ophthalmol Vis Sci* 32:2741-2746, 1991.

147. Laycock KA et al.: Characterization of a murine model of recurrent herpes simplex viral keratitis induced by ultraviolet-B radiation, *Invest Ophthalmol Vis Sci* 32:2741-2746, 1991.

148. Laycock KA et al.: Herpes simplex virus type 1 transcription is not detectable in quiescent human stromal keratitis by in situ hybridization, *Invest Ophthalmol Vis Sci* 34:285-292, 1993.

149. Lee SF et al.: Comparative laboratory diagnosis of experimental herpes simplex keratitis, *Am J Ophthalmol* 109:8-12, 1990.

150. Leib DA et al.: A deletion mutant of the latency-associated transcript of herpes simplex virus type 1 reactivates from the latent state with reduced frequency, *J Virol* 63:2893-2900, 1989.

151. Leib DA et al.: Immediate-early regulatory gene mutants define different stages in the establishment and reactivation of herpes simplex virus latency, *J Virol* 63:759-768, 1989.

152. Leib DA et al.: The promoter of the latency-associated transcripts of herpes simplex virus type 1 contains a functional cAMP-response element: role of the latency-associated transcripts and cAMP in reactivation of latency, *Proc Natl Acad Sci USA* 88:48-52, 1991.

153. Lewkowicz-Moss SJ et al.: Quantitative studies on Langerhans cells in mouse corneal epithelium following infection with herpes simplex virus, *Exp Eye Res* 45:127-140, 1987.

154. Liesegang TJ: Epidemiology of ocular herpes simplex: natural history in Rochester Minn 1950 through 1982, *Arch Ophthalmol* 107:1160-1165, 1989.

155. Liesegang TJ et al.: Epidemiology of ocular herpes simplex. Incidence in Rochester Minn 1950 through 1982, *Arch Ophthalmol* 107:1155-1159, 1987.

156. Lillycrop KA et al.: The octamer-binding protein Oct-2 represses HSV immediate-early genes in cell lines derived from latently infectable sensory neurons, *Neuron* 3:381-390, 1991.

157. Luntz MH, MacCallum FO: Treatment of herpes simplex keratitis with 5-iodo-2'deoxyuridine, *Br J Ophthalmol* 47:449-456, 1963.

158. Luscinskas FW et al.: Cytokine-activated human endothelial monolayers support enhanced neutrophil transmigration via a mechanism involving both endothelial-leukocyte adhesion molecule-1 and intercellular adhesion molecule-1, *J Immunol* 146:1617-1625, 1991.

159. Mackenzie AD: A comparison of IDU solution, IDU ointment, and carbolisation in the treatment of dendritic corneal ulcer, *BJO* 48:274-276, 1964.

160. Malynn BA et al.: The scid defect affects the final step of the immunoglobulin VDJ recombinase mechanism, *Cell* 54:453-460, 1988.

161. Mamalis N et al.: Changing trends in the indications for penetrating keratoplasty, *Arch Ophthalmol* 110:1409-1411, 1992.

162. Mannis MJ et al.: Herpes simplex dendritic keratitis after keratoplasty, *Am J Ophthalmol* 111:480-484, 1991.

163. Margolis T et al.: Acute retinal necrosis presenting with papillitis and acute neuroretinitis, *Ophthalmology* 95:937-940, 1988.

164. Markham RHC, Carter C, Scobie MA et al.: Double-blind clinical trial of adenine arabinoside and idoxuridine in herpetic corneal ulcers, *Trans Ophthalmol Soc UK* 333-340, 1977.

165. Martin LB, Montgomery PC, Holland TC: Soluble glycoprotein D blocks herpes simplex virus type 1 infection of rat eyes, *J Virol* 66:5183-5189, 1992.

166. Maudgal PC, De Clercq E: (S)-1-(3-Hydroxy-2-phosphonyl-methoxypropyl) cytosine in the therapy of thymidine kinase-positive and -deficient herpes simplex experimental keratitis, *Invest Ophthalmol Vis Sci* 32:1816-1820, 1991.

167. Maudgal PC, Van Damme B, Missotten L: Corneal epithelial dysplasia after trifluridine use, *Graefes Arch Clin Exp Ophthalmol* 22:6-12, 1983.

168. McBride BW, McGill JI, Smith JL: MHC class 1 and class II antigen expression in normal human corneas and in corneas from cases of herpetic keratitis, *Immunology* 65:583-587.

169. McBride BW, Ward KA: Herpes simplex-specific IgG subclass response in herpetic keratitis, *J Med Virol* 21:179-185, 1987.

170. McGeoch DJ, Dalrymple MA, Davison AJ et al.: The complete DNA sequence of the long unique region in the genome of herpes simplex virus type 1, *J Gen Virol* 69:1531-1574, 1988.

171. McGeoch DJ, Dolan A, Donald S, Brauer DHK: Complete DNA sequence of the short repeat region in the genome of the herpes simplex type 1, *Nucleic Acids Res* 14:1727-1745, 1986.

172. McGeoch DJ, Dolan A, Donald S, Rixon FJ: Sequence determination and genetic content of the short unique region of the genome of herpes simplex virus type 1, *J Mol Biol* 181:1-13, 1985.

173. McGill JI, Holt Wilson AD, McKinnon JR et al.: Some aspects of the clinical use of trifluorothymidine in the treatment of herpetic ulceration of the cornea, *Trans Ophthalmol UK* 94:342-352, 1974.

174. McGill JI, Tormey P: The clinical use of acyclovir in the treatment of herpes simplex corneal ulceration. In Sundmacher R, editor: *Herpetic eye disease* Munich, 1981, JF Bergmann Verlag.

175. McLeish W, Pflugfelder SC, Rabinowitz S et al.: Interferon treatment of herpetic keratitis in a patient with acquired immunodeficiency syndrome, *Am J Ophthalmol* 109:93-94, 1990.

176. McLeish W et al.: Immunobiology of Langerhans cells on the ocular surface. II. Role of central cornea Langerhans cells in stromal keratitis following experimental HSV-1 infection in mice, *Reg Immunol* 2:236, 1989.

177. Mercadal CM et al.: Herpetic stromal keratitis in the reconstituted scid mouse model, *J Virol* 67:3404-3408, 1993.

178. Metcalf JF, Hamilton DS, Reichert RW: Herpetic keratitis in athymic (nude) mice, *Infect Immunol* 26:1164-1171, 1979.

179. Metcalf JF, Kaufman HE: Herpetic stromal keratitis—evidence for cell-mediated immunopathogenesis, *Am J Ophthalmol* 82:827-834, 1976.

180. Metcalf JF et al.: Passive immunization with monoclonal antibodies against herpes simplex virus glycoproteins protects mice against herpetic ocular disease, *Curr Eye Res* 6:173-177, 1987.

181. Meyers RL, Chitjian PA: Immunology of herpes virus infection: immunity to herpes simplex virus in eye infections, *Surv Ophthalmol* 21:194-203, 1976.

182. Meyers-Elliott RH, Chitjian PA: Immunopathogenesis of corneal inflammation in herpes simplex virus stromal keratitis: role of the polymorphonuclear leukocyte, *Invest Ophthalmol Vis Sci* 20:784-798, 1981.

183. Meyers-Elliott RH et al.: Viral antigens in the immune ring of herpes simplex stromal keratitis, *Arch Ophthalmol* 98:897-904, 1980.

184. Meyes AL, Sugar A, Musch DC, Barnes RD: Antiviral therapy after penetrating keratoplasty for herpes simplex keratitis, *Arch Ophthalmol* 112:601-607, 1994.

185. Miller JK et al.: Corneal Langerhans cell dynamics after herpes simplex virus reactivation, *Invest Ophthalmol Vis Sci* 34:2282-2290, 1993.

186. Reference deleted in proofs.

187. Minkovitz JB, Pepose JS: Interferon alpha-2a treatment of herpes simplex keratitis resistant to multiple antiviral medications in an immunosuppressed patient, *Cornea* 14:326-30, 1995.

188. Mohamadi P et al.: Changing indications for penetrating keratoplasty, *Arch Ophthalmol* 107:550-552, 1989.

189. Morrison LA, Knipe DM: Immunization with replication-defective mutants of herpes simplex virus type 1: sites of immune intervention in pathogenesis of challenge virus infection, *J Virol* 68:689-696, 1994.

190. Mosmann TR et al.: Two types of murine helper T cell clones. I. Definition according to profiles of lymphokine activities and secreted proteins, *J Immunol* 136:2348-2357, 1986.

191. Nagy RM et al.: Scanning electron microscope study of herpes simple virus experimental disciform keratitis, *Br J Ophthalmol* 62:838-842, 1978.

192. Nahmias AJ et al.: Eye infections with herpes simplex viruses in neonates, *Surv Ophthalmol* 21:100-105, 1976.

193. Nahmias AJ, Dowdle WR: Antigenic and biologic difference in herpesvirus hominis, *Prog Med Virol* 10:110, 1968.

194. Nahmias AJ et al.: Sero-epidemiological and sociological patterns of herpes simplex virus infection in the world, *Scand J Infect Dis* (suppl)69:19-36, 1990.

195. Reference deleted in proofs.

196. Naito T et al.: Effects of 9-(1,3-dihydroxy-2-propoyxymethyl) guanine (DHPG) eye drops and cyclosporine eye drops in the treatment of herpetic stromal keratitis in rabbits, *Curr Eye Res* 10(suppl):201-203.

197. Nakao M et al.: Immunotherapy of acute and recurrent herpes simplex virus type 2 infection with an adjuvant-free form of recombinant glycoprotein D-interleukin-2 fusion protein, *J Infect Dis* 169:787-791, 1994.

198. Nesburn AB, Burke RL, Ghiasi H et al.: Vaccine therapy for ocular herpes simplex virus (HSV) infection periocular vaccination reduces spontaneous ocular HSV type 1 shedding in latently infected rabbits, *J Virol* 68:5084-5092, 1994.

199. Newell CK, Senele D, Rouse BT: Effect of CD4+ and CD8+ T-lymphocyte depletion on the induction and expression of herpes simplex stromal keratitis, *Reg Immunol* 2:366, 1989.

200. Newell CK et al.: Herpes simplex virus-induced stromal keratitis: role of T-lymphocyte subsets in immunopathology, *J Virol* 63:769-775, 1989.

201. Niemialtowski MG, Rouse BT: Phenotype and functional studies on ocular T cells during herpetic infections of the eye, *J Immunol* 148:1864-1870, 1992.

202. Niemialtowski MG, Rouse BT: Predominance of Th1 cells in ocular tissues during herpetic stromal keratitis, *J Immunol* 149:3035-3039, 1992.

203. Norn MS: Dendritic (herpetic) keratitis. I. Incidence, seasonal variation, recurrent rate, visual impairment, therapy, *Acta Ophthalmol* 48:91-107, 1970.

204. Norn MS: Dendritic (herpetic) keratitis. II. Follow-up examination of corneal opacity, *Acta Ophthalmol* 48:214, 1970.

205. Oakes JE et al.: Induction of interleukin-8 gene expression is associated with herpes simplex virus infection of human corneal keratocytes but not human corneal epithelial cells, *J Virol* 67:4777-4784, 1993.

206. O'Day DM, Jones BR, Poirier R et al.: Proflavine photodynamic viral inactivation in herpes simplex keratitis, *AJO* 79:941-948, 1975.

207. Oh JO: Primary and secondary herpes simplex uveitis in rabbits, *Surv Ophthalmol* 21:178-184, 1976.

208. Oh JO: The role of immunity in the pathogenesis of herpes simplex uveitis. In Silverstein AM, O'Connor R, editors: *International Symposium on Immunology and Immunopathology of the Eye*, New York, 1979, Masson.

209. Oh JO et al.: Oculogenital transmission of type 2 herpes simplex virus in adults, *Surv Ophthalmol* 21:106-109, 1976.

210. O'Hare P, Hayward GS: Evidence for direct role for both 175K and 110K immediate-early proteins of herpes simplex virus in the transactivation of delayed-early promoters, *J Virol* 53:751-760, 1985.

211. O'Hare P, Hayward GS: Three trans-acting regulatory proteins of herpes simplex virus modulate immediate-early gene expression in a pathway involving positive and negative feedback regulation, *J Virol* 56:723-733, 1985.

212. Olivo PD, Leib DA: Gene delivery neurons: Is herpes simplex virus the right tool for the job? *Bio Essays* 15:547-554, 1993.

213. Olsen TW et al.: Linear endotheliitis, *Am J Ophthalmol* 117:468-474, 1994.

214. Opremcak EM et al.: Histology immunohistology of Igh-1 restricted herpes simplex keratitis in BALB/c congenic mice, *Invest Ophthalmol Vis Sci* 31:305-312, 1990.

215. Osler HB: Herpes simplex: the primary infection, *Surv Ophthalmol* 21:91-99, 1976.

216. Patterson A et al.: Controlled studies of IDU in the treatment of herpetic keratitis, *Trans Ophthalmol Soc UK* 83:583-591, 1963.

217. Paul WE: The immune system: an introduction. In Paul WE, editor: *Fundamental immunology*, 1-10, New York, 1993, Raven Press.

218. Pavan-Langston D: Trifluorothymidine and idoxuridine therapy of ocular herpes, *AJO* 84:818-825, 1977.

219. Pavan-Langston D, Dohlman CH: A double blind clinical study of adenine arabinoside therapy of viral keratoconjunctivitis, *AJO* 74:81-88, 1972.

220. Pavilack MA et al.: Differential expression of human corneal and perilimbal ICAM-1 by inflammatory cytokines, *Invest Ophthalmol Vis Sci* 33:564-573, 1992.

221. Pawey LS, Chien LT: Neonatal herpes simplex virus infection introduced by fetal monitor scalp electrode, *Pediatrics* 65:1150, 1980.

222. Pederson B, Moller Andersen S, Klauber A et al.: Secretary IgA specific for herpes simplex virus in lacrimal fluid from patients with herpes keratitis—a possible diagnostic parameter, *Br J Ophthalmol* 66:648-653, 1982.

223. Pellett PE, McKnight JLC, Jenkins FJ, Roizman B: Nucleotide sequence and predicted amino acid sequence of a protein encoded in a small herpes simplex virus DNA fragment capable of trans-inducing a genes, *Proc Natl Acad Sci USA* 82:5870-5874, 1985.

224. Pepose JS: External ocular herpesvirus infections in immunodeficiency, *Curr Eye Res* 10:87, 1991.

225. Pepose JS: Herpes simplex keratitis: role of viral infection versus immune response, *Surv Ophthalmol* 35:345-352, 1991.

226. Pepose JS et al.: Immunocytologic localization of herpes simplex type 1 viral antigens in herpetic retinitis and encephalitis in an adult, *Ophthalmology* 92:160-166, 1985.

227. Pepose JS et al.: Concurrent herpes simplex and cytomegalovirus retinitis and encephalitis in the acquired immune deficiency syndrome, *Ophthalmology* 91:1669-1677, 1989.

228. Pepose et al.: Reactivation of latent herpes simplex virus by excimer laser photokeratectomy, *Am J Ophthalmol* 114:45-50, 1992.

229. Perry LJ, McGeoch DJ: The DNA sequences of the long repeat region and adjourning parts of the long unique region in the genome of herpes simplex virus type 1, *J Gen Virol* 69:28-31, 1988.

230. Peyman G et al.: Vitrectomy and intravitreal antiviral drug therapy in acute retinal necrosis syndrome. Report of two cases, *Arch Ophthalmol* 102:1618-1621, 1984.

231. Pfister RR, Richards JSF, Dohlman CH: Recurrence of herpetic keratitis in corneal grafts, *Am J Ophthalmol* 73:192-196, 1972.

232. Polack FM, Kaufman HE: Penetrating keratoplasty in herpetic keratitis, *Am J Ophthalmol* 73:908-913, 1972.

233. Porter SM, Patterson A, Kho P: A comparison of local and systemic acyclovir in the management of herpetic disciform keratitis, *Br J Ophthalmol* 74:283-285, 1990.

234. Posavad CM, Newton JJ, Rosenthal KL: Inhibition of human CTL-mediated lysis by fibroblasts infected with herpes simplex virus, *J Immunol* 151:4865-4873, 1993.

235. Pringe JJ: Herpes. In Fowler JK, editor: *A dictionary of practical medicine*, 344, London, 1890, J and A Churchill.

236. Prusoff WH: Synthesis and biologic activities of isododeoxyuridine, an analogue of thymidine, *Biochem Biophys Acta* 32:295-302, 1959.

237. Rader KA et al.: In vivo characterization of site-directed mutants in the promoter of the latency-associated transcripts, *J Gen Virol* 74:1859-1869, 1993.

238. Raizman MB, Foster CS: Passive transfer of anti-HSV-1 1 gG protects against stromal keratitis in mice, *Curr Eye Res* 7:823-829, 1988.

239. Rheines ED, Gross PA: Antiviral agents, *Med Clin North Am* 72:691, 1988.

240. Rinne JR, Abghari SZ, Stulting RD: The severity of herpes simplex virus keratitis in mice does not reflect the severity of disease in humans, *Invest Ophthalmol Vis Sci* 33:268-272, 1992.

241. Ritchie MH, Oakes JE, Lausch RN: Passive transfer of anti-herpes simplex virus type 2 monoclonal and polyclonal antibodies protect against herpes simplex virus type 1-induced but not herpes simplex type 2-induced stromal keratitis, *Invest Ophthalmol Vis Sci* 34:2460-2468, 1993.

242. Roat MI, Romanowski E, Araullo-Cruz T, Gordon YJ: The antiviral effects of rose bengal and fluorescein, *Arch Ophthalmol* 105:1415-1417, 1987.

243. Robin JB, Steigner JB, Kaufman HE: Progressive herpetic corneal endotheliitis, *Am J Ophthalmol* 100:336, 1985.

244. Rock DL, Beam SL, Mayfield JE: Mapping bovine herpesvirus type 1 latency-related RNA in trigeminal ganglia of latently infected rabbits, *J Virol* 61:3827-3831, 1987.

245. Rock DL et al.: Detection of latency-related viral RNAs in trigeminal ganglia of rabbits latently infected with herpes simplex virus type 1, *J Virol* 61:3820-3826, 1987.

246. Rock DL et al.: Transcription from the pseudorabies virus genome during latent infection, *Arch Virol* 98:99-106, 1988.

247. Roizman B: The structure and isomerization of herpes simplex virus genomes, *Cell* 16:481-494, 1979.

248. Roizman B, Sears AE: Herpes simplex viruses and their replication. In Fields BN, Knipe DM and associates, editors: *Virology,* ed 2, vol 2, 1875-1941, New York, 1990, Raven Press.

249. Rong BL et al.: Detection of herpes virus thymidine kinase and latency-associated transcript gene sequences in human herpetic cornea by polymerase chain reaction amplification, *Invest Ophthalmol Vis Sci* 32:1808-1815, 1991.

250. Rosefeld SI, Alfonso EC, Gollamudi S: Recurrent herpes simplex infection in a conjunctival flap, *Am J Ophthalmol* 116:242-243, 1993.

251. Rosenwasser GOD, Greene WH: Simultaneous herpes simplex type 1 and 2 keratitis in acquired immunodeficiency syndrome, *Am J Ophthalmol* 113:102-103, 1992.

252. Rouse BT: Immunopathology of herpes virus infections. In Roizman B, Lopez C, editors: *Herpes-viruses,* vol 4, New York, 1985, Plenum.

253. Russell RG et al.: Role of T-lymphocytes in the pathogenesis of herpetic stromal keratitis, *Invest Ophthalmol Vis Sci* 25:938-944, 1984.

254. Russell WC: Herpesvirus nucleic acid, *Virology* 16:355, 1962.

255. Sacks WR, Schaffer PA: Deletion mutants in the gene encoding the herpes simplex virus type 1 immediate-early protein ICP0 exhibit impaired growth in cell culture, *J Virol* 61:829-839, 1987.

256. Sawtell NM, Thompson RL: Herpes simplex virus type 1 latency-associated transcription unit promotes anatomic site-dependent establishment and reactivation from latency, *J Virol* 66:2157-2169, 1992.

257. Schaeffer HJ, Beauchamp L, De Miranda P et al.: 9-(2-hydroxyethoxymethyl)guanine activity against viruses of the herpes group, *Nature* 272:583, 1978.

258. Schmid DS: The human MHC-restricted cellular response to herpes simplex virus type 1 is mediated by CD4$^+$, CD8$^-$ T cells restricted to the DR region of the MHC complex, *J Immunol* 140:3610-3616, 1988.

259. Schulman J, Peyman GA, Horton MB et al.: Intraocular penetration of new antiviral agent, hydroxyacyclovir (BW-B759U), *Jpn J Ophthalmol* 30:116-124, 1986.

260. Schulman J et al.: Intraocular penetration of a new antiviral agent, hydroxyacyclovir (BW-B759U), *Jpn J Ophthalmol* 30:116-124, 1986.

261. Schwab IR: Oral acyclovir in the management of herpes simplex ocular infection, *Ophthalmology* 95:423-430, 1988.

262. Schwartz RH: T-lymphocyte recognition of antigen in association with gene products of the major histocompatibility complex, *Ann Rev Immunol* 3:237-261, 1985.

263. Shimeld C, Hill TJ, Blyth WA, Easty DL: Reactivation of latent infection and induction of recurrent herpetic eye disease in mice, *J Gen Virol* 71:397-404, 1990.

264. Shimeld C et al.: An improved model of recurrent herpetic eye disease in mice, *Curr Eye Res* 8:1193-1205, 1989.

265. Shimeld C et al.: Passive immunization protects the mouse eye from damage after herpes simplex virus infection by limiting spread of virus in the nervous system, *J Gen Virol* 71:681-687, 1990.

266. Shimeld C et al.: Reactivation of latent infection and induction of recurrent herpetic eye disease in mice, *J Gen Virol* 71:397-404, 1990.

267. Shuler JD et al.: External ocular disease and anterior segment disorders associated with AIDS, *Int Ophthalmol Clin* 29:98-104, 1989.

268. Shuster JJ et al.: Statistical analysis of the rate of recurrence of herpes virus ocular epithelial disease, *Am J Ophthalmol* 91:328-331, 1981.

269. Smeraglias R et al.: The role of herpes simplex virus secreted glycoproteins in herpetic keratitis, *Exp Eye Res* 35:443-459, 1982.

270. Smith CW et al.: Cooperative interactions of LFA-1 and Mac-1 with intercellular adhesion molecule-1 in facilitating adherence and transendothelial migration of human neutrophils in vitro, *J Clin Invest* 83:2008-2017, 1989.

271. Sonkin PL, Baratz KH, Frothingham R, Cobo LM: Acyclovir-resistant herpes simplex virus keratouveitis after penetrating keratoplasty, *Ophthalmology* 99:1805-1808, 1992.

272. Soukiasian SH, Asdourian GK, Weiss JS, Kachakosian HA: A complication from alcohol-swabbed tonometer tips, *Am J Ophthalmol* 105:424-425, 1988.

273. Spruance SL, Stewart JC, Rowe NH et al.: Treatment of recurrent herpes simplex labialis with oral acyclovir, *J Infect Dis* 161:185-189, 1990.

274. Staats HF, Lausch RN: Cytokine expression in vivo during murine herpetic stromal keratitis, *J Immunol* 151:277-283, 1993.

275. Staats HF, Oakes JE, Lausch RN: Anti-glycoprotein D monoclonal antibody protects against herpes simplex type-1-induce diseases in mice functionally depleted of selected T-cell subsets or asialo GM1+ cells, *J Virol* 65:6008-6014, 1991.

276. Steiner I et al.: Herpes simplex virus type 1 latency-associated transcripts are evidently not essential for latent infection, *EMBO J* 8:505-511, 1989.

277. Stern S, Tanaka M, Herr W: The Oct-1 homeodomain directs formation of a multiprotein-DNA complex with the HSV transactivator VP16, *Nature* 341:624-630, 1989.

278. Stevens JG: Latent herpes simplex and the nervous system, *Curr Top Immunol* 70:31, 1975.

279. Stevens JG et al.: RNA complementary to a herpesvirus alpha-gene mRNA is prominent in latently infected neurons, *Science* 235:1056-1059, 1987.

280. Stow ND: Localization of an origin of DNA replication within the TRs/IRs repeated region of the herpes simplex virus type 1 genome, *EMBO J* 1:863-867, 1982.

281. Stow ND, Stow EC: Isolation and characterization of a herpes simplex type 1 mutant containing a deletion within the gene encoding the immediate-early polypeptide Vmw 110, *J Gen Virol* 67:2571-2585, 1986.

282. Streilein JW: Immune regulation and the eye: a dangerous compromise, *FASEB J* 1:199-208, 1987.

283. Stulting RD, Kindle JC, Nahmias AJ: Patterns of herpes simplex keratitis in inbred mice, *Invest Ophthalmol Vis Sci* 26:1360-1367, 1985.

284. Su Y-H, Oakes JE, Lausch RN: Ocular avirulence of a herpes simplex virus type 1 strain is associated with heightened sensitivity of alpha/beta interferon, *J Virol* 64:2187-2192.

285. Sugar A, Smith T: Presumed autoimmune corneal endotheliopathy, *Am J Ophthalmol* 94:689, 1982.

286. Sullivan-Bolyai J et al.: Neonatal herpes simplex virus infection in King County, Washington: increasing incidence and epidemiological correlates, *J Am Med Assoc* 250:3059, 1983.

287. Reference deleted in proofs.

288. Sundmacher R, Mattes A, Neumann-Haefelir D et al.: The potency of interferon-alpha 2 and interferon-gamma in a combination therapy of dendritic keratitis. A controlled clinical study, *Curr Eye Res* 6:273-276, 1987.

289. Sundmacher R, Neumann-Haefelin D: Herpes simplex virus—positive and negative keratouveitis. In Silverstein AM, O'Connor R, editors: *Immunology and immunopathology of the eye,* 225-229, New York, 1979, Masson.

290. Swyers JS et al.: Corneal hypersensitivity to herpes simplex, *Br J Ophthalmol* 51:843-846, 1967.

291. Tang S, Scheiffarth OF, Stefani FH: Clinical and immunohistochemical correlation of herpetic keratitis with the expression of HLA-DR antigen, *Graefes Arch Clin Exp Ophthalmol* 231:162-165, 1993.

292. Taylor JL, Punda-Polic V, O'Brien WJ: Combined anti-herpes virus activity of nucleoside analogs and interferon, *Curr Eye Res* 10(suppl):205-210, 1991.

293. Thompson P et al.: Immunomodulation of experimental herpes simplex keratitis. I. UV-HSV protection, *Curr Eye Res* 7:1043-1049, 1988.

294. Thygeson P: The unfavorable role of corticosteroids in herpetic keratitis. In Boruchoff SA, Hutchinson BR, Lessel S, editors: *Controversy in ophthalmology,* 450-469, Philadelphia, 1970, Saunders.

295. Thygeson P: Historical observations on herpetic keratitis, *Surv Ophthalmol* 21:82-90, 1976.

296. Topey DJ, Lindsey MD, Rinaldo CR: HLA restricted lysis of herpes simplex virus infected monocytes and macrophages mediated by CD4+ and CD8+ T lymphocytes, *J Immunol* 142:1325-1332, 1989.

297. Trousdale MD et al.: In vivo and in vitro reactivation impairment of a herpes simplex virus type 1 latency-associated transcript variant in a rabbit eye model, *J Virol* 65:6989-6993, 1991.

298. Tullo AB, Shimeld C, Blyth WH et al.: Latent infection following ocular herpes simplex in non-immune and immune mice, *J Gen Virol* 63:95-101, 1982.

299. Tullo AB et al.: Analysis of glycoproteins expressed by isolates of herpes simplex virus causing different forms of keratitis in man, *Curr Eye Res* 6:33-38, 1987.

300. Tumpey TM et al.: Interleukin-10 treatment can suppress stromal keratitis induced by herpes simplex virus type 1, *J Immunol* 153:2258-2265, 1994.

301. Ukety TO, Maertens K: Ocular ulcerative herpes following measles in Kinshasa, Zaire, *Curr Eye Res* 10:131, 1991.

302. Unanue ER: Macrophages, antigen-presenting cells, and the phenomena of antigen handling and presentation. In Paul WE, editor: *Fundamental immunology,* 111-144, New York, 1993, Raven Press.

303. Van Bijsterveld OP, Post HJ: Trifluorothymidine and adenine arabinoside in the treatment of dendritic keratitis. In Sundmacher R, editor: *Herpetic eye diseases,* Nunich, 1980, JF Bergmann Verlag.

304. Vannas A et al.: Corneal endothelium in herpetic keratouveitis, *Arch Ophthalmol* 101:913-915, 1983.

305. Ventura LM, Dix RD: Viability of herpes simplex virus type 1 on the applanation tonometer, *Am J Ophthalmol* 103:48-52, 1987.

306. Vlazny DA, Frenkel N: Replication of herpes simplex virus DNA: location of replication recognition signals within defective virus genomes, *Proc Natl Acad Sci USA* 78:742-746, 1981.

307. Vlazny DA, Kwong A, Frenkel N: Site specific cleavage packaging of herpes simplex virus DNA and the selective maturation of nucleocapsids containing full length viral DNA, *Proc Natl Acad Sci USA* 79:1423-1427, 1982.

308. Wechsler SL et al.: Fine mapping of the latency-related gene of herpes simplex virus type 1:alternative splicing produces distinct latency-related RNAs containing open reading frames, *J Virol* 62:4051-4058, 1988.

309. Weinstein BL et al.: Characterization of a glucocorticoid receptor and the direct effect of dexamethasone on herpes simplex virus infection of rabbit corneal cells in culture, *Invest Ophthalmol Vis Sci* 28:651, 1982.

310. Wellings C, Awdry PN, Bors FH et al.: Clinical evaluation of trifluorothyumidine in the treatment of herpes simplex corneal ulcers, *Am J Ophthalmol* 73:932-942, 1972.

311. Wheatley SC, Dent CL, Wood JN, Latchman DS: Elevation of cyclic AMP levels in cell lines derived from latently infectable sensory neurons increases their permissivity for herpes virus infection by activating the viral immediate-early 1 gene promoter, *Mol Brain Res* 12:149-154, 1992.

312. Whitcher JP, Dawson CR, Hoshiwara I et al.: Herpes simplex keratitis in a developing country, *Arch Ophthalmol* 94:587-592, 1976.

313. Whitley RJ, Gnann JW: Acyclovir: a decade later, *New Engl J Med* 327:782-789, 1992.

314. Whitley RJ et al.: Changing presentation of neonatal herpes simplex virus infection, *J Infect Dis* 158:109, 1988.

315. Wilcox CL, Johnson EM: Nerve growth factor deprivation results in the reactivation of latent herpes simplex virus in vitro, *J Virol* 61:2311-2315, 1987.

316. Wildy P: Herpes history and classification. In Kaplan AS, editor: *The herpes viruses,* 1-25, New York, 1973, Academic.

317. Wildy P, Field HJ, Nash AA: Classical herpes latency revisited. In Mahy BWJ, Minson AC, Darby GK, editors: *Virus persistence,* Cambridge UK, 1982, Cambridge University Press.

318. Wildy P et al.: The morphology of herpes virus, *Virology* 12:204, 1960.

319. Wilhelmus KR, Gee L, Lauck WW et al.: Herpetic eye disease study (HEDS): a controlled trial of topical corticosteroids for herpes simplex stromal keratitis, *Ophthalmology* 101:1883-1896, 1994.

320. Wilhelmus KR et al.: Bilateral herpetic keratitis, *Br J Ophthalmol* 65:385-387, 1981.

321. Wilhelmus KR et al.: Prognostic indicators of herpetic keratitis: analysis of a five-year observation period after corneal ulceration, *Arch Ophthalmol* 99:1578-1582, 1981.

322. Witcher JP et al.: Herpes simplex keratitis in a developing country, *Arch Ophthalmol* 94:587-592, 1976.

323. Witmer R, Iwamato T: Electron microscopic observations of herpes-like particles in the iris, *Arch Ophthalmol* 79:331-337, 1968.

324. Wood JN et al.: Regulation of expression of the neuronal POU protein Oct-2 by nerve growth factor, *J Biol Chem* 267:17787-17791, 1992.

325. Wortis HH: Immunological responses of ''nude'' mice, *Clin Exp Immunol* 8:305, 1971.

326. Yamomoto S et al.: Detection of herpes simplex viral DNA in human tear film by polymerase chain reaction, *Am J Ophthalmol* 100:530-533, 1993.

327. Youinou P, Colin J, Ferec C: Monoclonal antibody analysis of blood and cornea T lymphocyte subpopulations in herpes simplex keratitis, *Graefes Arch Clin Exp Ophthalmol* 224:131-133, 1985.

328. Youinou P, Colin J, Mottier D: Immunological analysis of the cornea in herpetic stromal keratitis, *J Clin Lab Immunol* 17:105-106, 1985.

329. Young E, Pepose JS: Class II induction of human corneal fibroblasts by cell-free supernatants from HSV stimulated lymphocytes, *Curr Eye Res* 6:141-144, 1987.

330. Zwaagstra JC et al.: Activity of herpes simplex virus type 1 latency-associated transcript (LAT) promoter in neuron-derived cells: evidence for neuron specificity and for a large LAT transcript, *J Virol* 64:5019-5028, 1990.

72 Varicella-Zoster Virus Diseases: Anterior Segment of the Eye

DEBORAH PAVAN-LANGSTON, EDMUND DUNKEL

The varicella-zoster virus (VZV) is the etiologic agent of the most common of childhood primary infectious diseases, chickenpox. In its recurrent form it may cause a far more devastating disease, herpes zoster (shingles or zona), as it reactivates from the latent state established during the primary illness. Because of the fastidious nature of the VZV agent, it has been a far more difficult organism to investigate, and animal models have been less than satisfactory.

VIROLOGY AND MOLECULAR BIOLOGY

VZV is a member of the herpesvirus family, which also includes herpes simplex virus (HSV) type 1, HSV type 2, Epstein-Barr virus (EBV), cytomegalovirus (CMV), B cell lymphotropic virus (herpes virus 6), and herpes virus 7. Of all of these, VZV is the most closely related to the HSV viruses and is thought to have descended from a common ancestral virus strain.[28,95] VZV and the HSVs are subclassified as alpha herpesviruses, a group characterized by rapid growth and spread, destruction of infected cells, a variety of susceptible hosts, and the ability to establish latent infection primarily in ganglionic tissue (neurotropism). These characteristics are comparable with the beta herpesviruses (such as CMV and lymphotropic virus), that are slow to grow and spread, and become latent within lymphoreticular and secretory gland cells. Gamma viruses such as EBV also remain latent within the lymphoreticular system but have a host range restricted to humans.

Morphologically, all viruses are infectious agents that are both acellular and incapable of sustaining "life" outside of living host cells. VZV is 150 to 200 nm in diameter with double-stranded DNA (MW 83 to 86 × 10^6 daltons)[28] (Fig. 72-1). This DNA protein center is protected by a protein capsid made of repeated polypeptide chains and is symmetric in the shape of an icosahedron with 20 equilateral triangular faces. Outside the capsid is an amorphous protein tegument that is key to shutting down host cell protein production and inducing active viral transcription in the nucleus. Surrounding the tegument is the lipid bilayer envelope derived from the nuclear membrane of the host cell. It is modified by the addition of VZV-encoded glycoprotein peptomers that project from the outer surface. The specific antigenicity of the virus is conferred by the protein capsid, and the glycoprotein peptomers and host antibodies are formed against these antigens.

The entire VZV genome has been sequenced and found to vary in size from 124,000 to 126,000 base pairs (bp), which code for about 68 genes and 80 proteins.[29,133] These genes and proteins are organized into two primary fragments, a unique long region (U_L, about 105,000 bp) and a unique short region (U_s, about 5200 bp) (Fig. 72-2). On either side of each region are inverted repeat elements of shorter bps. During replication, two isomeric forms of VZV DNA are produced as the U_s and its repeats invert. This isomerization results in about half of the new organisms having the U_s oriented in a direction opposite that of the other new VZVs produced. In addition, there is evidence that about 5% of the new viruses have the U_L inverted as well.[133] Each VZV replicative cycle, then, produces four DNA isomers, two major and two minor.

Analysis of HSV and VZV DNA sequencing and identification of open reading frames, coding proteins, and numerous transcriptional regulatory sequences have revealed a sufficiently close relationship between these viruses. Therefore assumptions can be made about many VZV gene functions based on information derived from the better-characterized HSV gene function.[29,115] Determination of gene function and localization of protein and other coding sites may be critical to developing target sites for future antiviral drugs. The locations of the genetic coding sites for the major glycoprotein families (that are key to immune recognition and potential vaccine production) have been most extensively studied. Glycoproteins confer antigenicity through their incorporation into the viral external membrane, and they are the primary contact points between virus and cell as infection is initiated.[28] Similarly, the genomes for the origin of replication have been mapped in both HSV and VZV as

933

Glycoprotein spikes —

Tegument

Envelope

Core protein

Nucleocapsid

Viral DNA —

Fig. 72-1. Diagram of varicella-zoster virus. This agent is morphologically indistinguishable from herpes simplex virus. Viral DNA is wrapped around a protein core that lies within an icosahedal protein capsid. Together these form the nucleocapsid. The tegument, an amorphous protein structure, lies between the outer phospholipoprotein membrane and the nucleocapsid.

homologous sequences, with HSV having two such sequences and VZV just one. The VZV origin of replication gene site is about 60 kilobases downstream from gene 29. In situ hybridization and polymerase chain reaction (PCR) using cloned fragments of both VZV genome sites serve as useful molecular biologic tools for detecting the presence of latent VZV DNA. The detection of both genetic sites within the same human ganglia indicates that more than one region of the viral genome is retained in the latent state.[26,103]

Because of the fastidious nature of the organism and its strong cell association, it has not yet been possible to determine the exact order of appearance of VZV proteins as they are transcribed from the genetic coding sites during replication. Comparison with HSV replication gives some indication, however. HSV-1 DNA replication appears to require involvement of seven genes, each of which has a homologue in the VZV genome. VZV has analogues to four of the five immediate early genes expressed at the initiation of HSV replication, thus suggesting, but not proving, that VZV may have an HSV-like cascade of events programmed by immediate early genes, early genes, and late genes.[28]

Animal Models of Disease

Because of the fastidious nature of VZV, the development of animal models of disease has been slow and usually unsatisfactory. Intranasal inoculation of adapted VZV in weanling guinea pigs produces nasal viral replication, seroconversion to VZV, generalized viremia, and animal-to-animal viral transmission—but no discernible clinical disease.[129] The delta herpesvirus is immunologically related to VZV and may be used to create (and is recovered from) an exanthematous disease in nonhuman primates.[145] Viremia may be demonstrated prior to the onset of exanthem, but persistence and reactivation of the viral infection has not been demonstrated. There are numerous other reports in the literature on partial success in creating animal models of VZV infection.[56,61,111,128,130]

In ocular studies VZV inoculation of the corneal stroma produced seroconversion (but no ocular disease) in one

study, and no ocular disease (but VZV genome in the trigeminal ganglia by PCR) in another.[56,111] In a newly developed model of ocular VZV infection in guinea pigs and rabbits, a high titer (10^{4-5} PFU Oka and MSD strains respectively) was used for both superficial and deep stromal

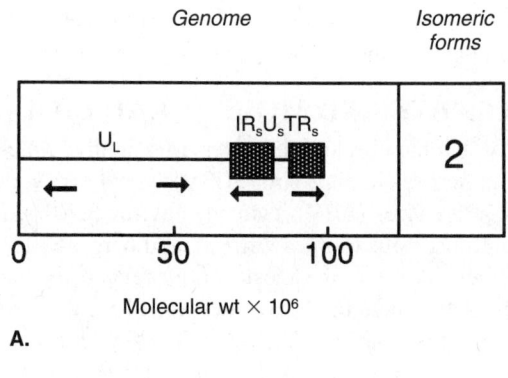

A.

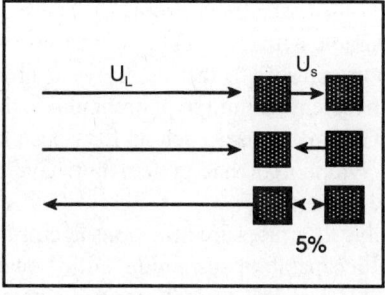

B.

Fig. 72-2. **A,** Schematic diagram of the varicella-zoster genome showing the unique long and short regions (U_L, U_s) flanked by series of bases that form the terminal or internal repeat zones. Heavy arrows indicate areas of the genome most actively transcribed during latent infection. **B,** The major and minor isomeric forms result from inversion of the U_s and U_L. The U_L inverts only about 5% of the time. The two major isomers are produced by inversion of U_s in either direction. Adapted from Liesegang, T.[95]

injection of the corneas under the operating microscope.[43,140] In the more superficial injections multiple dendritiform epithelial lesions develop from day 3 to day 7 postinoculation (PI) and stromal edema and haze progress from day 3 to day 12 PI before all disease spontaneously regresses. In the animals receiving deep corneal injections, stromal edema, haze, and severe iritis predominate, with little to no epithelial disease. About 20% of animals also develop a typical viral interstitial pneumonitis. Viral recovery is unreliable, using external swabbing techniques with only about 10% of cultures from guinea pig epithelial lesions yielding virus. In situ hybridization with a radiolabeled DNA probe in the rabbit model has, however, revealed VZV DNA not only in the vast majority of corneas but in the corresponding and contralateral trigeminal ganglia as well. This finding has been confirmed by PCR detection of DNA fragment, gene 29. Replication of VZV in the cornea has also been demonstrated by finding VZV RNA using PCR techniques. Detection of VZV RNA in the ganglia is equivocal and still under study. Nonetheless, the rabbit model has already proved useful in evaluating systemic antiviral therapy of VZV infection of the eye.[43]

Humoral Immune Response to VZV Infection

In 1965 Hope-Simpson[67] first hypothesized that continued immunity to VZV is the result of intermittent reemergence of the latent original chickenpox strain and/or subsequent contact with another exogenous VZV strain. Either strain induces a brief, usually subclinical, infection that augments the VZV-immune status of the host. Subsequent studies have supported this hypothesis and have identified various antibodies as markers for times and types of infection. In an early study, increases in VZV IgA, IgG, and IgM were detectable within 5 days of onset of varicella rash, but only IgG persisted longer than a few weeks to months.[12] Subsequent household exposure to zoster or varicella resulted in no clinical disease or change in IgG levels, but IgA titers increased 2 to 4 times within 2 to 4 weeks before returning gradually to baseline. This fluctuation in IgA titers indicated a subclinical reinfection.

The VZV genome codes for more than 30 structural and nonstructural proteins including 16 known immunogenic components.[163] Weigle and Grose[190] have studied the temporal pattern of the antibody response to molecularly defined VZV proteins during primary varicella infection, quiescence, subclinical reinfection, and overt zoster. In chickenpox the first antibodies produced were against the virion envelope structural glycoproteins, gp66, gp118, gp98, and gp62, and the nucleocapsid protein, p155. One to two months later antibodies to a wider variety of viral glycosylated and nonglycosylated proteins appeared. As most of these antibodies became undetectable by 3 to 4 months after infection, their presence indicated recent VZV infection. Antibodies to the immunodominant gp66, gp118, and p155,

however, were still present for years after infection, constituted excellent markers for previous VZV infection, and remained unchanged during quiescence. During subclinical reinfection after exogenous exposure to VZV, there was an overall rise in glycoprotein antibody level, with the greatest rise in gp98 and gp62, and their subsequent decrease over the following 2 years. This subclinical response was more restricted and of lesser magnitude than that noted after endogenous reactivation of zoster.

In contrast to all the preceding immune patterns, zoster was characterized by the presence of antibodies against virtually all VZV glycoproteins within a week, if not at onset. In addition to this quantitative and temporal difference, another striking difference between chickenpox and zoster was the rapid appearance of antibody to p32 in the latter, but not in the former. The p32 humoral response abates over the ensuing weeks to months, but its presence in a patient's serum indicates recent zoster.

Immunocompromised children (cancer) with varicella developed antibodies to gp66 and gp118 similar to healthy children but had less antibodies to gp98 and gp62 than did normals. In hypogammaglobulinemia, despite disseminated disease, there is very little detectable VZV antibody by 3 weeks after onset.

VARICELLA

Epidemiology

Varicella (chickenpox) and herpes zoster (shingles, zona) are two distinct clinical diseases caused by the same organism, the varicella-zoster virus (VZV).[191,192] With a peak incidence in the spring, an estimated 2,800,000 cases of varicella occur annually in the United States alone, with approximately 90% of the population having seroconverted by age 60 years.[50,171] The major complications, pneumonia and encephalitis, account for 100 to 200 deaths per year and occur primarily in normal or immunosuppressed adults, immunosuppressed children, and the fetuses of nonimmune women.[2,45,147,148,171]

Varicella represents primary infection with the VZV and, unlike primary HSV, is a disseminated disease. Spread is by direct skin contact with a chicken pock or zoster lesion or by inhaling infectious respiratory secretions from a patient with varicella.[94,134] The period of contagion extends from 2 days before the appearance of the rash until all sores have crusted over. The virus replicates locally and then spreads by viremia and the lymphatics to be taken up by the reticuloendothelial system. Here multiple replicative cycles occur during the incubation period, which may be as long as 17 days before the second viremia occurs. The widespread skin and mucous membrane lesions of chickenpox are a result of this secondary viremia. The virus then spreads from the peripheral lesions centripetally via the contiguous nerves (and rarely, hematogenously) to the dorsal root (sensory) ganglia of the corresponding dermatomes. Here it enters the latent state in nearly 100% of those patients primarily infected with VZV.*

Clinical Features

Ocular manifestations of varicella may be either those of congenital varicella syndrome or of disseminated varicella most commonly seen in young children.†

Congenital varicella syndrome is fortunately quite rare and results from maternal varicella infection during pregnancy, most frequently during the first or second trimester.[86] Systemic findings may include hemiparesis, bulbar palsies, dermatomal distribution of cicatricial skin lesions, delayed development, and learning disorders. Ocular abnormalities include chorioretinitis, optic nerve atrophy or hypoplasia, congenital cataract, and Horner syndrome. There is no definitive therapy for congenital varicella syndrome. As 5% to 16% of women of child-bearing age are susceptible to VZV, until a varicella vaccine is in wider use, these infections will continue to occur during pregnancy, albeit rarely, and cause the unfortunate congenital malformations that appear to be largely the result of VZV's high affinity for the nervous system.[49,86]

Classical varicella is characterized by fever, malaise, and an infectious mucocutaneous exanthem. This maculopapulovesicular rash appears in successive crops such that lesions in various stages are present simultaneously. All lesions ultimately crust over and few leave scars after healing.[50] The rash may involve the lid margins and, more rarely, vesicular lesions may appear on the conjunctiva. These are most often unilateral, small phlyctenular-like lesions that erupt most at the corneal limbus.[84,194] It is unclear whether these are caused by a live virus, an immune phlyctenule-like reaction, or both. These lesions usually resolve without sequelae. Rarely, they become pustular, punched out, dark red painful ulcers with swollen margins and secondary intraocular inflammation.

Varicella keratitis may present as an infectious superficial punctate keratitis or as branching dendritiform lesions.[132,179] Varicella dendrites may be distinguished from those of herpes simplex virus in that the former are fine, linear lesions that lack the classic swollen endings (terminal bulbs) of HSV dendrites and appear to be heaped up on intact underlying epithelium.[84,135,141] Gentle debridement of these varicella lesions will commonly leave no underlying ulcer, whereas removal of HSV dendrites will leave a full thickness epithelial defect. There is local anesthesia in the area of the varicella dendrite.

Weeks to months after primary infectious varicella, a patient may develop infectious varicella dendritic keratitis that may run a course of successive crops of dendrites similar to the successive crops of lesions seen during the acute mucocutaneous disease.[30] In the same time frame, an immune disciform keratitis similar to that seen in HSV disease may develop independent of, or in conjunction with, varicella dendritic keratitis.[30,193] This disciform reaction is usually mild and responsive to topical corticosteroids. Rarely, however, it may cause a severe fibrotic scar before resolving over a several-month period.

Fortunately, other manifestations of ocular varicella are less frequently seen including lid necrosis, interstitial keratitis with neovascularization, neurotrophic ulceration with corneal melting, iritis (occasionally fibrinous), extraocular muscle palsies, internal ophthalmoplegia, cataract, chorioretinitis, and optic neuritis.*

Therapy of Ocular Varicella

The FDA has recently approved oral acyclovir, 800 mg qid for 5 days, as routine treatment of chickenpox in children 2 years or older. No data are yet available as to whether this will prevent or curb ocular disease, but common sense would dictate that less virus means less disease. There are also no data available concerning the effect of acyclovir on ocular disease (once it has developed), but anything greater than a mild and transient lesion might most prudently be treated with the systemic drug.

As a result of this data void, definitive therapy of varicella lid lesions, conjunctival phlyctenules, or epithelial keratitis is not conclusively established, but the current recommendation is vidarabine ointment 5 times daily for 10 to 14 days or until any external ocular lesion has resolved. In Deborah Pavan-Langston's personal experience treating primary or recurrent varicella dendritic ulcers, vidarabine appeared to be more effective than trifluridine in resolving the lesions, but it is also likely that the lesions resolved independent of any treatment.[30] Steroids should not be used during the primary infectious disease, as this may only serve to worsen the viral process. The disciform keratitis or iritis is commonly managed with mild topical steroid, 1/8% prednisolone, once to four times daily with tapering over a several-week to 2- to 3-month period. In general, the disciform disease of varicella does not have as great a preponderance for recurrence in comparison to HSV.

Prevention

Gershon and associates[51] have reported the use of live, attenuated varicella (Oka strain) vaccine in 307 children with leukemia in remission and in 86 healthy adults. The vaccine was effectively immunogenic and well tolerated. In the children 89% developed protective levels of VZV antibodies after the first vaccination, and 95% developed them

---

*References 19, 50, 84, 140, 171, 194.
†References 19, 38, 50, 84, 148, 171, 191, 192, 194.

*References 30, 38, 82, 84, 132, 152, 169, 174, 178, 193.

after the second injection (given 3 months after the first) including 17 who did not seroconvert after the first dose. VZV cell-mediated immunity (CMI) developed in 93% of vaccinees after a single injection. Adverse side effects included a transient maculopapular or vesiculopapular rash in 6% of those not on chemotherapy and in 42% of those in whom chemotherapy had been suspended for 2 weeks. Vaccine virus was recovered from the rash. There were also occasional transient fever, local reaction, and respiratory symptoms. There was no increased relapse in leukemia caused by the interruption of chemotherapy compared to nonvaccinated leukemic children.

Eight percent (23) of the children developed varicella between 6 weeks and 3 years after vaccination. Serum antibodies and CMI were variably present in all children, and the severity of disease was significantly less than that noted in unvaccinated leukemic children who developed varicella. Nonvaccine virus was isolated from five patients. One patient developed self-limited zoster at the vaccination site 21 months after injection; vaccine virus was cultured from the lesions.

VZV antibodies gradually waned over the ensuing 3 years. At 1 year 75% were seropositive, at 2 years 71% were seropositive, and after 3 years only 66% had detectable antibodies. Similarly, CMI decreased over this same period. These figures suggested that booster doses of vaccine might be advisable, particularly in immunocompromised or other high-risk individuals (nonimmune adults).

In the 86 vaccinated healthy adults, 58% seroconverted and 83% were CMI positive with 1 dose; 92% seroconverted with 2 doses. Adverse side effects were almost nonexistent (1 mild rash, 1 mild local reaction). No VZV was isolated from any adult subject. Antibodies waned to a lesser degree than in children, with 88% of healthy adults remaining seropositive after 4 years. Although the majority of the adults were exposed to VZV, only 6 cases of mild varicella occurred between 4 and 72 months after vaccination. Nonvaccine VZV was isolated from two cases.

Subsequent studies using restriction endonuclease analysis in vaccinated immunocompromised and healthy patients have revealed that rashes occurring during the first 6 weeks after injection are always caused by the vaccine virus, and that true breakthrough wild-type (nonvaccine) infections may occur.[48] Five cases of zoster were noted in vaccinated leukemic children in remission; vaccine virus was isolated from one and wild-type virus from another. Previous infection with one strain of VZV did not prevent establishment of latency with a different strain of VZV. Two different strains could be latent simultaneously, with either capable of reactivating later as herpes zoster. Nonetheless, existing studies on VZV vaccination indicate that this approach confers protection from severe varicella in high-risk populations and that booster doses should be given every 2 to 4 years to maintain immunity.

HERPES ZOSTER OPHTHALMICUS

Whereas primary VZV is a disseminated disease (varicella), recurrent disease caused by reactivation of latent ganglionic virus is largely a focal infection of one or more dermatomes. Although the thoracic and lumbar dermatomes are the most frequently affected clinically, the trigeminal ganglia are involved in about 15% of cases, reflecting the frequent infection with latent virus (87%) as determined by PCR.[103] Ophthalmic zoster is potentially the most devastating form of recurrent VZV disease.*

Epidemiology

Herpes zoster is a disease international in scope and without seasonal variation. The annual incidence in the American and British populations falls within a range of 2% to 4%.[67,149,177,191,192] Hope-Simpson's British study[67] revealed that the annual attack rate increases between 0 and 19 years of age, stabilizes at $\frac{3}{1000}$ between ages 20 and 49, and then rises steadily to $\frac{10}{81000}$ by the eighth decade of life. Based on the U.S. Bureau of Census 1984 figures, this translates to 312,800 new cases per year of zoster of any dermatome in the 20- to 49-year age group and 306,800 cases in the 50- to 89-year-old group.[177] This increased incidence in the older age groups agrees with a Mayo Clinic population-based finding of 1.3 cases/1000 person years. Ragozzino and associates[149] estimated 300,000 new zoster cases annually in the United States.

The incidence of trigeminal zoster varies considerably with different studies. Two Mayo Clinic studies reported incidences of trigeminal nerve zoster (herpes zoster ophthalmicus, HZO) of 9.3% and 16%, both of which are at the low end of the 8% to 56% range in other studies.[32,67,75] In an 86-case study of HZO from 1975 to 1980, Womack and Liesegang[195] noted a predominance in female patients and in the left eye, and a peak incidence in the seventh and eighth decades of life. Other series show a male predominance or equal distribution between the sexes and a peak incidence in the fourth or fifth decade through the seventh decade of life.[14,34,36,78,161] In the Mayo Clinic series of 64 patients with acute HZO, 72% had ocular involvement, a figure significantly higher than the 50% usually noted in the literature.[149]

Pathogenesis

Latency and Reactivating Factors. During the primary disease, varicella, the virus migrates centripetally from the skin lesions and gains access to the sensory ganglia where, like HSV, it enters a latent state. A disturbance of the host-parasite relationship is capable of reactivating the latent VZV DNA to the infectious state years to decades after the original infection. Unlike HSV, VZV cannot be isolated by co-cultivation of the ganglia unless active zoster infection

---

*References 84, 91, 92, 93, 103, 136, 140.

has been recent.[53-55,149,181] Molecular biologic techniques used in the aforementioned studies included DNA dot-blot and in situ nucleic acid hybridization, however, and demonstrated the VZV genome in acutely infected and in "normal" ganglia. Using the polymerase chain reaction, Mahalingham and associates[103] showed that the viral gene for origin of replication is present in 87% of trigeminal and 53% of thoracic ganglia of seropositive cadavers, a finding that reflects the relative severity of dermatomal involvement during varicella.

The site of latency within the ganglion appears to differ in HSV and VZV. Some reports suggest that the neuronal cells may harbor both, but the most definitive work (in situ hybridization studies) has shown HSV only in the neuronal cells, and RNA in situ hybridization studies have localized latent VZV only within the satellite cells that lie adjacent to and support the neuronal cells.[26,55,71] Between 0.01% and 0.15% of nonneural cells exhibited VZV transcripts. Conversely, during reactivation of VZV, both the satellite and neuronal cells (0.6%) expressed VZV RNA for several regions of the genome.[26] This ability of VZV to reactivate in satellite cells, spread to both other satellites, and infect neuronal cells may account for the more widespread and destructive ganglionitis seen with VZV compared to HSV. This widespread ganglionitis may, in turn, account for the greater pain and more severe and widespread dermatomal involvement seen with zoster.

VZV reactivates as zoster in one out of five people during the course of a lifetime.[171] Studies done during the pre-AIDS era reveal that within that group there is a 20% chance of a second recurrence of this disease.[134] When the acute, often necrotic ganglionitis develops upon reactivation of latent virus, the newly manufactured viruses travel centrifugally back down the axones to cause an infectious, inflammatory vesicular dermatitis in the affected dermatome. Viral particles have been detected by electron microscopy in neurones following VZV infection, and biopsy of an involved dermatome on the first day of eruption has shown loss of nerve fiber staining. Both of these findings suggest that nerve involvement precedes that of the skin.[7,41,60,126]

The disease is rare in children, with 7% of HZO occurring in childhood.[153] Varicella infection of the mother during gestation probably results in neuronal latency in the fetus.[11] Infantile or childhood zoster appears to be the reactivation of that latent VZV. The disease tends to be short-lived, not as painful as in adults, and leaves little-to-no dermal scarring. Short of overt immunosuppression, the precipitating factors in children have not been well defined.

Advancing age and other factors contributing to a depressed immune response greatly enhance the risk of developing zoster in the adult population.[123] Immunologic studies imply that reactivation of the VZV genome may be a frequent and dynamic process, with overt disease held in check by the host cell-mediated immune defense system.[94] A breakdown of this system ultimately allows productive viral replication in the ganglion, resulting in a destructive ganglionitis and spread of infectious virus down the axones to the affected dermatome(s). There is now a worldwide increasing incidence of this disease caused by the growing numbers of immunosuppressed patients infected with the AIDS who are iatrogenically immunosuppressed because of organ transplantation, neoplasia, or blood dyscrasia.[36] Scheie noted that among hospitalized patients, zoster occurred in 0.2% of those without malignant disease and in 0.85% of those with malignancy.[159] Scheie's figures do not take into account, however, the many thousands of patients with zoster who are not hospitalized and who do not have malignant disease. The alleged relationship with occult malignancy has never been adequately demonstrated, although there is an increased incidence in those patients with overt malignant disease such as leukemia or lymphoma. This finding is discussed further in the next section. Other factors related to the development of zoster in patients are emotional or physical trauma, debilitating systemic disease of any type (tuberculosis, malaria, syphilis), chemotherapy, surgery, and trauma to the involved ganglion.*

Neuronal Relationships. The trigeminal dermatomes are the most commonly affected by clinically manifest VZV.[67,103] The ophthalmic division of this nerve is involved about 20 times more often than is the second or third division and, within that division, the frontal nerve is the most commonly involved. Via its supraorbital and supratrochlear branches, the frontal nerve innervates the upper lid, forehead, and some superior conjunctiva. The nasociliary branch is the primary sensory nerve to the eyeball; it supplies the lacrimal sac, conjunctiva, skin of both lids, and the root of the nose via the infratrochlear nerve. The nasal branches of this nerve, however, along with the sympathetic branches from the ciliary ganglion, innervate the sclera, cornea, iris, ciliary body, and choroid via the long and short ciliary nerves (as well as the diagnostically useful side of the tip of the nose). Involvement of the tip of the nose is called Hutchinson sign, a sign taken to indicate that the eye may be seriously involved by VZV because of the involvement of the nasal branch of the nasociliary nerve.[77] Clinically, however, it is highly variable in its reliability.

These direct neural connections allow VZV access to the many external and internal ocular structures. Additional damage is caused by direct viral spread through the orbital tissues to other cranial and autonomic nerves, and to the central nervous system nuclei of ocular and orbital nerves. So many routes of travel lend themselves to a wide variety and severity of VZV-induced disease. Table 72-1 gives a more complete listing of the complications of HZO, but in brief the most common include cicatricial lid retraction or

---

*References 36, 63, 75, 84, 140, 191, 192, 194.

TABLE 72-1   INCIDENCE OF COMPLICATIONS IN HERPES ZOSTER OPHTHALMICUS*

Complication	Percent
1. Lids	13
2. Canalicular occlusion	2
3. Cornea	22
4. Sclera	4
5. Iridocyclitis	57
6. Glaucoma (Secondary)	12
7. Cataract	8
8. Neuro-ophthalmic	7
9. Postherpetic neuralgia	17

*Based on a total of 86 HZO patients.
Adapted from Womack L, Liesegang T: Complications of herpes zoster opthalmicus, *Arch Ophthalmol* 101:42, 1983.

loss, paralytic ptosis, conjunctivitis, scleritis, episcleritis, keratitis (infectious or immune), iridocyclitis, Argyll Robertson pupil, glaucoma, retinitis, choroiditis, optic neuritis, optic atrophy, retrobulbar neuritis, exophthalmos, and extraocular muscle palsies.[37,84,136,159,196]

Pathology

Viral proliferation causes inflammatory and hemorrhagic destruction of the sensory ganglion and perineural tissues. VZV particles have been demonstrated in acute disease in central nervous system (CNS) tissues, the trigeminal ganglion, its nerve axons, and in the arterial walls of ocular and CNS tissues by electron microscopy and immunofluorescence.[41,101] The associated cellular infiltrate is primarily monocytic, and eosinophilic intranuclear inclusions may be seen in satellite and neuronal cells during the acute infectious process.[7,52,60,63] The affected peripheral nerves ultimately undergo demyelinization and cellular infiltration, which resolves to leave scarring and fibrosis.[197] In addition to traveling along the trigeminal sensory nerves, the VZV may also travel via the affected sensory nerve roots to the brainstem or spinal cord to cause necrosis in the corresponding sensory nuclei.[96,154]

Hedges and Albert's study[63] on the histopathology of acute (2 weeks post onset) and subacute (6 weeks post onset) HZO revealed, in the acute cases, mild episcleral round cell inflammation, normal corneal stroma with pigment-laden macrophages in the endothelium, nongranulomatous lymphocytes and plasma cell infiltration of the iris and ciliary body with extension into the choroid, macrophage, and other inflammatory cell infiltration of the trabecular meshwork.[63] Many of these acute changes appeared to be reversible. In the subacute specimens, the cornea and sclera were still minimally involved, but from the iridocyclitic structures and back, inflammation was nongranulomatous, granulomatous (epithelioid and giant cells), or mixed. The process was

more destructive and involved many types of tissues in disease processes such as retinitis, choroiditis, and hemorrhagic vasculitis. The trigeminal ganglia were diffusely and intensely infiltrated by lymphocytes and plasma cells; occasional giant cells were seen.

These changes were also noted in chronic cases (>2 years post onset), but anterior segment disease included granulomatous and nongranulomatous infiltrates, scleral thinning, corneal perforation, neovascularization, retrocorneal membrane, and synechial angle closure. Additionally, the central retinal vessels, optic nerve, posterior ciliary arteries and nerves, and meninges could be involved in a severe granulomatous or lymphocytic-plasma cell inflammation with some vessels being occluded. A granulomatous intracranial arteritis was also noted and has been reported by others.[33,96,154] Such findings indicate that the damage wrought by zoster is caused both by chronic inflammation and vasculitic ischemia in response to direct viral invasion of a multitude of tissues.

Disciform keratitis similar to that seen in HSV appears to work by a mechanism of delayed hypersensitivity as manifested by the chronic lymphocytic infiltrate.[92,116] Other studies by Greene and Zimmerman,[57] and Naumann, Gass, and Font's study[131] on chronic HZO have described a keratitis characterized by giant cell reaction to Descemet membrane.[57,131] Additionally, these studies reported a lymphocytic-plasma cell infiltration of the posterior ciliary nerves and vessels that appears to be unique to zoster ophthalmicus. There was also chronic inflammation and vasculitis of the iris and ciliary body with patchy necrosis of the iris and pars plicata, perivascular cuffing by chronic inflammatory cells in the retina, and granulomatous choroiditis with one case involving a giant cell granulomatous arteritis. It has also been suggested that the extraocular muscle palsies, orbital myositis, and orbital edema seen in HZO may be the result of perineuritis and perivasculitis associated with the generalized orbit inflammation[91,94,131] (Fig. 72-3).

Clinical Features

There appear to be two mechanisms by which ocular zoster infections may occur: (1) reactivation of latent virus in the trigeminal sensory ganglion or, (2) reintroduction of exogenous virus through direct or indirect contact with either a chickenpox or zoster patient. The former mechanism is, by far, the most common of the two possibilities. The incubation for endogenous zoster is not known, but in those patients exposed to chickenpox, incubation varied from a few days to 2 weeks.[175] Analysis of viral DNA recovered from clinical isolates of varicella patients with subsequent zoster reveals a slight variation in the mobility of some DNA fragments, indicating some genome instability compared to outbreaks of varicella in which all patients in a given cohort exhibit stability of the genome.[170]

The illness may begin with headache, fever, malaise, and

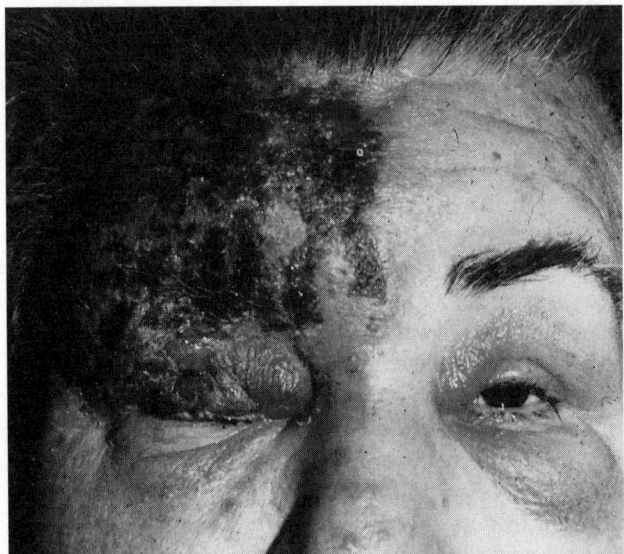

Fig. 72-3. Acute herpes zoster ophthalmicus in its hemorrhagic phase in immunocompetent patient. Transient extraocular muscle palsy and iritis developed within 2 weeks of onset but no recurrence occurred during 3 years of follow-up and remarkably little scarring remained over the dermatome.

chills, preceded or followed by neuralgic dermatomal pain in the distribution of the first division of the trigeminal nerve. This neuralgia may be lancinating, itching, tingling, burning, or deep boring, as well as either intermittent or continuous. If the virus spreads centrally along the posterior nerve roots to the meninges, central nervous system, or spinal cord; the severe headache, nuchal rigidity, focal weakness, hemiplegia, or cognitive disturbance of a leptomeningitis, cerebral necrotizing angiitis, or segmental myelitis may ensue. Spinal fluid pleocytosis is noted in these cases.[65,101] Because there is no respiratory infection and skin involvement is localized, patients with zoster are not as contagious as those with varicella.

Dermatitis and Lid Damage. Rarely, the dermatitis may never materialize (zoster sine herpete), but typical neuralgia and ocular disease may develop.[90,179] More commonly, however, within 2 to 3 days hot, flushed hyperesthesia develops along with edema of the dermatomes, which then erupts into multiple crops of clear, grouped vesicles from which virus may be cultured for approximately 3 to 5 days (and even longer in immunocompromised patients). The vesicles become turbid and hemorrhagic by about day 4 and crust over by day 10. Unlike herpes simplex, zoster involves the subdermal tissues forming deep eschars that frequently leave behind permanent pitted scars over the involved dermatome. The acute inflammatory period lasts 8 to 14 days, with the lesion groups considered infectious until they have scabbed over. A tender focal lymphadenopathy is often present during the early phases of the disease. The deep skin ulceration may take many weeks to heal and result either in

little scarring or the equivalent of third-degree burns with significant loss and scarring of tissues.[37,84,136]

Pigmentation or hyperemia may be present in the early phase of dermal scarring; the derma later becomes more pale and white or silvery in advanced cases. These scarred areas are anesthetic to pinprick, although paradoxically the area is often hyperesthetic. This increased sensitivity to tactile stimulus often causes the patient difficulty in contact with clothing or care of the skin or hair.

Permanent lid damage secondary to the dematitis is all too common. There may be major cicatricial lid retraction, entropion, ectropion, or trichiasis. The vasculitic ischemia may cause partial lid sloughing and permanent lash loss. Epicanthal scarring and paralytic ptosis are also common.

Conjunctivitis, Episcleritis, and Scleritis. Conjunctival inflammation is extremely common and characterized by watery hyperemia, occasionally with clear vesicles, petechial hemorrhages, follicular hypertrophy with or without regional adenopathy, and (rarely) severe necrotizing membranous inflammation. The episcleritis is often sectoral and may be flat or nodular. Similarly, the scleritis tends to be focal and may involve several areas, particularly in the perilimbal region, either as a flat or nodular process [Fig. 72-4A]. The episcleritis or scleritis may occur during the acute disease or several months after the cutaneous eruption has cleared. As the scleritis resolves, scleral thinning is frequently noted. About 1% of patients may develop a striking complication of HZO characterized by 360° of perilimbal vasculitis that results in anterior segment ischemic necrosis. This apparent immune reaction may occur months after the initial acute disease. The episcleritis, scleritis, and vasculitis all appear to be variably responsive to topical or, if necessary, systemic corticosteroids. The nodular scleritis may also respond dramatically to long-term therapy with nonsteroidal antiinflammatory agents such as ibuprofen, 300 mg po tid.*

Keratitis. Keratitis develops in nearly two thirds of HZO patients.[72,92] This fact is very often associated with marked corneal hypesthesia caused either by significant corneal damage or, more commonly, the widespread necrotic ganglionitis associated with this illness. The keratitis may precede or follow the neuralgia or skin lesions by several days and may assume a variety of forms, infectious and immune, as noted in Table 72-2. The infectious forms of epithelial keratitis may present as a fine or course punctate epithelial keratitis with or without stromal edema and give the cornea a ground glass appearance. There may be group vesicle formation, dendritiform in pattern, that appears to be layered superficially on the corneal surface but may be easily mistaken for HSV keratitis.[46] These lesions may be differentiated from HSV dendrites in that VZV dendrites lack the rounded terminal bulbs at the end of the branches and when

---

*References 21, 25, 92, 106, 141, 144, 159.

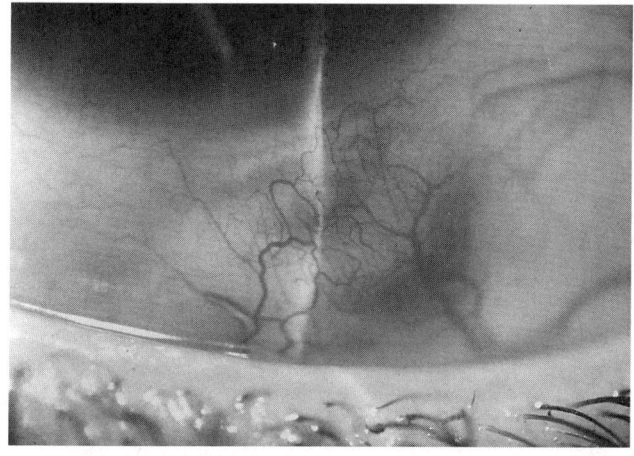

A

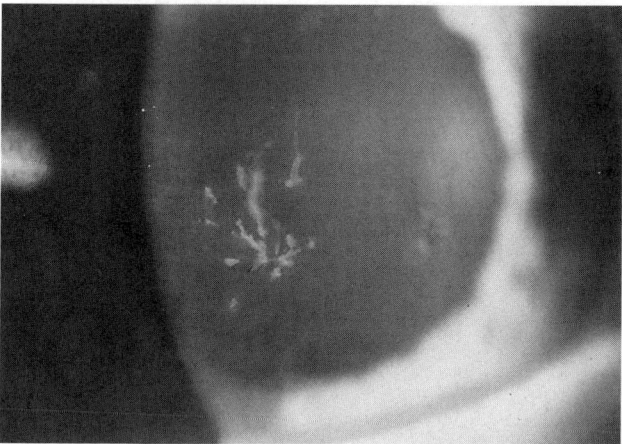

B

Fig. 72-4. A, Nodular scleritis in 16-year-old herpes zoster ophthalmicus patient. Lesion persisted despite topical corticosteroids but was responsive to ibuprofen and resolved with slight scleral thinning after several months. **B,** Acute herpes zoster dendritic keratitis showing thready superficial lesion lacking terminal bulbs, which distinguishes it from herpes simplex dendritic ulcers. (Figure also in color insert.)

wiped from the corneal epithelium tend to leave behind a layer of intact epithelium rather than the full thickness ulcers noted with HSV [Fig. 72-4B].

Pavan-Langston and McCulley[141] have isolated VZV from these dendritic lesions and Uchida, Kaneko, and Hayashi[178] have demonstrated VZV by immunofluorescence. The former investigators described the lesions as medusa-like in pattern, grey and linear with tapering ends, and appearing to be "painted on" the surface of the cornea. These zoster dendrites cleared rapidly on either idoxuridine (IDU) or steroid therapy alone, leaving no or mild anterior stromal nebulae, suggesting that they would have cleared with no therapy whatsoever. Piebenga and Laibson[144] described similar lesions in HZO patients, noting the superficial

plaquelike formations without terminal bulbs that stained poorly with fluorescein. Similarly, Liesegang[92] has reported "pseudodendrites" in HZO patients, noting lesions similar to those described previously that appeared 2 to 15 days after the onset of acute illness. The location of the lesions was usually peripheral, with only moderate staining with rose bengal or fluorescein. They were also broader and more plaquelike than HSV dendrites without central ulceration and were frequently stellate. Liesegang was also able to culture VZV from four of nine cases. Multinucleated giant cells and intranuclear inclusions were noted on cytologic study of corneal scrapings from these lesions. Topical antiviral agents were not used and corticosteroids were ineffective. The lesions, as in all other reports, were self-limited and cleared within a few days. Mild anterior stromal infiltrates remained in 52% of patients.

Delayed pseudodendrites or "delayed corneal mucous plaques" as described by Liesegang,[92,93] and Marsh and Cooper[107] appear in about 13% of patients, usually 8 to 12 weeks after the acute event. Foreign body sensation is common and the lesions are elevated coarse grey-white swollen epithelial cells piled in plaques or dendritiform shape on the surface of the cornea. Delayed pseudodendrites are both migratory and transitory, often associated with a neurotrophic keratitis (75%) or previous corneal inflammation (100%). The tear film is unstable. Viral cultures are negative and cytologic study shows ballooning degeneration of the epithelial cells, with occasional giant cells. The plaques do not respond to most therapy (steroid, soft contact lens, acetylcysteine, or lubrication; antivirals equivocal), but they are self-limited as in the case of the early pseudodendrites.

Anterior stromal infiltrates, single or multiple, are the next most common corneal findings and usually appear between the second and third weeks after onset of acute dis-

TABLE 72-2   FORMS AND INCIDENCE OF ZOSTER KERATITIS*

Clinical Presentation	Percent
1. Pseudodendrites	51
2. Punctate epithelial keratitis	51
3. Anterior stromal infiltrates	41
4. Keratouveitis-endotheliitis	34
5. Neurotrophic keratitis	25
6. Delayed mucous plaques	13
7. Exposure keratitis	11
8. Disciform keratitis	10
9. Serpiginous ulceration	7
10. Sclerokeratitis	1
11. Delayed limbal vasculitis	<1

*61 of 94 patients (65%) had corneal involvement.
Adapted from Liesegang T: Corneal complications from herpes zoster opthalmicus, *Ophthalmol* 92:316, 1985.

ease.[72,92] These infiltrates are almost invariably associated with a preceding infectious epithelial keratitis and probably represent an immune response to soluble viral antigen diffusing into the anterior stroma. Keratouveitis is seen in about one third of patients and may have its onset immediately (with acute disease) or several weeks later. There is frequently an endotheliitis with focal or diffuse keratic precipitates, folds in Descemet membrane, and diffuse or focal stromal edema. The endotheliitis may result in significant loss of endothelial cells, with permanent corneal decompensation.[112,151] Intraocular pressure is elevated in one third of these patients presumably because of an associated trabeculitis with inflammatory cells clogging the meshwork. A severe vasculitis with hypopyon or hyphema and pars plicata ischemia may develop, leading to anterior segment ischemia.[25,92] Viral particles at the endothelial level have been identified by immunofluorescent staining in at least one case of permanent corneal edema following HZO.[112] A necrotic interstitial keratitis or Wessley ring consisting of antigen-antibody complement-mediated reaction with polymorphonuclear neutrophil leukocytes (PMN) infiltration may be seen. This keratitis resolves to leave white patches of lipid deposition and fibrovascular scarring, often with deep neovascularization [Fig. 72-5A].

Disciform immune keratitis resembles focal endotheliitis and corneal edema but lacks the keratic precipitates. It may occur at any time after the acute event, most commonly after 3 or 4 months. There may be full thickness stromal edema and associated necrotic interstitial keratitis, Wessley rings, or vasculitis. PMNs, lymphocytes, and macrophages infiltrate these corneas, indicating a delayed hypersensitivity cell-mediated response to residual viral antigen and to antigenic alteration of host cell membranes in the cornea. This immune reaction is responsive to corticosteroids, but drug tapering is frequently slow, with many patients requiring minimal daily doses to prevent rebound immune disease. An associated interstitial keratitis increases the incidence of deep neovascularization with lipid deposition and fibrovascular scarring.[57,63,131]

Peripheral ulcerative keratitis (PUK) is commonly associated with collagen vascular disease. Liesegang,[92] however, has reported PUK in 7% of his HZO patients. The peripheral cornea may develop an acute stromal edema (with an overlying crescent-shaped ulcer with smooth edges and a grey-white base) within the first 5 months of the acute disease. The cornea is almost invariably markedly hypesthetic, and there may be a mild-to-marked uveitis. Three quarters of these ulcers are thin and vascularized and one quarter perforate if untreated. A delayed Arthus reaction similar to that of limbal vasculitis or to a cell-mediated immune disease of the limbal vessels is the proposed mechanism of disease[74,124] [Fig. 72-5B]. Fortunately, PUK is responsive to topical steroid therapy, but some ulcers may require tissue adhesive and a therapeutic soft lens to enhance healing.

Neurotrophic keratopathy is seen in nearly 50% of pa-

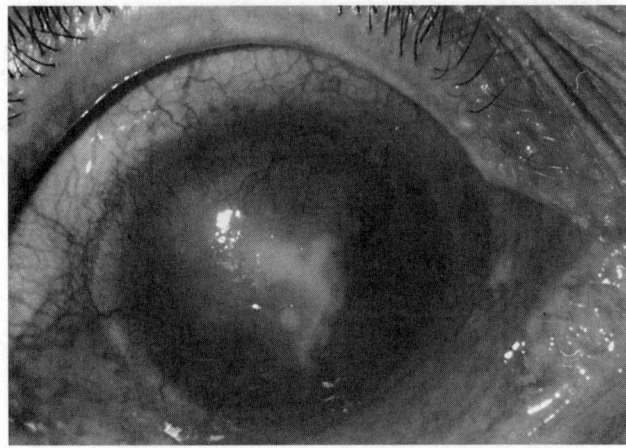

A

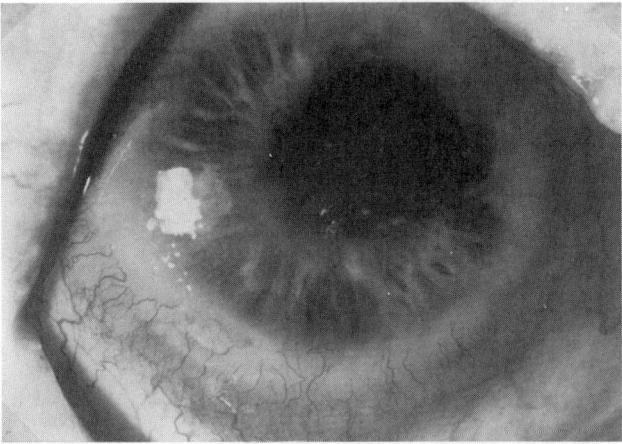

B

Fig. 72-5. **A,** Chronic herpes zoster ophthalmicus necrotic white interstitial keratitis with dense neovascular pannus invading 360 degrees. Pannus covered cornea by 9 months and became quiescent. **B,** Inferior zoster immune limbal vasculitis associated with healing peripheral ulcerative keratitis. Keratic precipitates are present centrally and iris sphincter atrophy distorts pupil. (Figure also in color insert.)

tients, the result of corneal anesthesia secondary to the destructive VZV ganglionitis.[72,92,195] Corneal anesthesia may be evident at the onset of HZO or develop over the next 2 to 3 weeks. Fortunately, 60% of those patients with anesthesia will recover protective sensitivity within 2 to 3 months. About 10% to 25% of all HZO patients will, however, develop clinical signs of neurotrophic keratitis caused by permanent corneal anesthesia.[20,92] Initial clinical findings include a hazy or irregular corneal surface with a coarse punctate epithelial keratitis, which evolves into a grey diffuse epithelial haze or edema with fine intraepithelial vesicles. The condition is further aggravated as the tear film is highly unstable, and blink frequency is reduced in these anesthetic eyes.

If the condition progresses, oval epithelial defects frequently develop in the palpebral fissure area or lower cornea with subsequent melting and corneal thinning (Fig. 72-6).

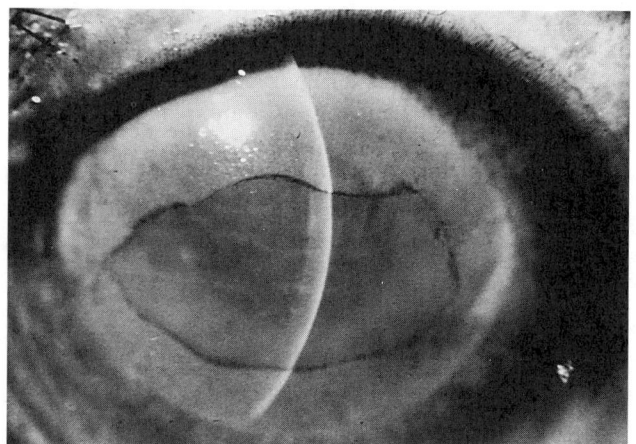

Fig. 72-6. Large zoster indolent trophic ulcer in totally anesthetic cornea. No thinning occurred and ulcer healed slowly under a therapeutic soft contact lens over an 8-month period. Lateral tarsorrhaphy was performed shortly after ulcer appeared.

This complication of neurotrophic keratitis is frequently seen in patients who had previous keratouveitis (80%). In Liesegang's study[92] there was an accompanying exposure pattern in 40% of patients so affected.

Neuroparalytic ulcerations of the type seen after trigeminal nerve ablation may develop slowly, without any spontaneous cicatrization. In the absence of this fibrous scarring, corneal thinning and perforation may ensue. Alternatively, a neovascular pannus, which heals but also severely scars the cornea, may grow in and prevent perforation. Factors enhancing the chance of ulceration in the anesthetic cornea include lid structural abnormalities with exposure or trichiasis, meibomian gland destruction with tear dysfunction, decreased blink frequency, abnormal epithelial cell turnover in denervated eyes, reduced cell wetability, and probably reduced availability of neurotransmitter substances necessary for epithelial healing.*

Therapy of the anesthetic eye with unhealthy epithelium includes an early lateral tarsorrhaphy and copious lubrication with artificial tears and ointments. High water content soft therapeutic contact lenses should be used only if the epithelium has actually ulcerated. Application of these lenses to an unhealthy (but intact) epithelium may induce, rather than prevent, the development of an epithelial defect. Vascularization occurring under the soft contact lens (SCL) should probably be allowed to progress, as it may slow corneal melting and aid in healing the defect. Topical corticosteroids are probably ill-advised, as they inhibit collagen synthesis and the growth of healing neovascular pannus. A melting corneal ulcer may require application of Nexacryl† tissue adhesive under a therapeutic lens [Fig. 72-7A and B].

---

*References 18, 91, 92, 102, 106, 186.
†Tri-Point Medical L.P., Raleigh, North Carolina, under FDA-Investigational New Drug study.

Over several weeks to months the stroma and epithelium should heal in underneath the tissue adhesive and dislodge it spontaneously, leaving behind a scarred but intact cornea.

Exposure keratitis is often a complicating factor in patients with neurotrophic keratitis and may develop anywhere from the period of the acute illness to several months later. Cicatricial retraction of the upper lid makes blinking ineffective and complete lid closure impossible. If there is also a poor Bell reflex, there will be constant corneal exposure, especially in sleep. The lower lid may be similarly involved. Additional keratopathy-aggravating changes in either or both lids, as noted previously, include thickening, irregular

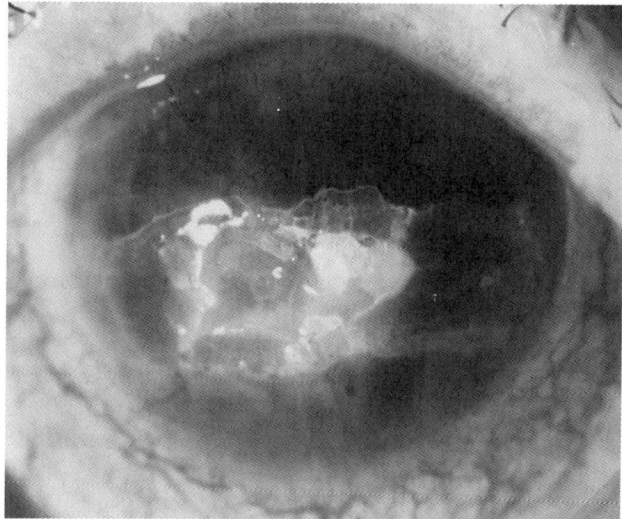

A

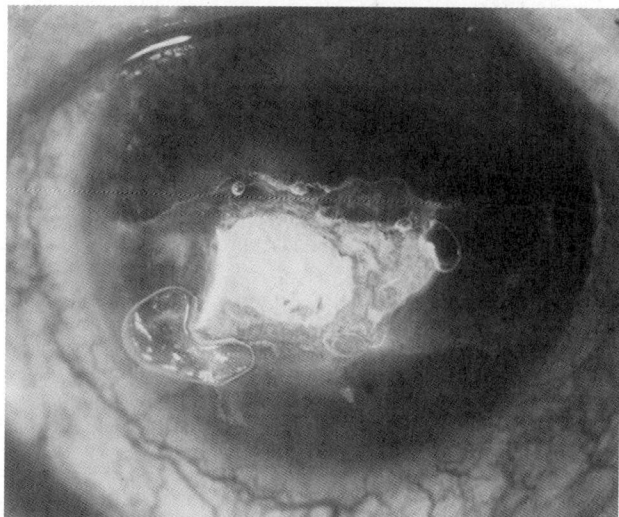

B

Fig. 72-7. **A,** Deep stromal focal thinning in band keratopathy of chronic herpes zoster neurotrophic keratopathy. **B,** Ulcer bed has been debrided and filled with sterile tissue adhesive. Cornea healed over 6 months and adhesive dislodged spontaneously under the therapeutic soft contact lens.

margins, meibomian gland dysfunction, trichiasis, punctal occlusion, ectropion, or entropion.

The application of warm wet compresses and an antibiotic ointment to the ulcerated skin may help reduce local cellulitis and secondary infection, with consequent decreased scarring of the periocular skin and lids. In severe cases cicatricial retraction of the lids may require full thickness skin grafts or tarsorrhaphy for the protection of the ocular structures.[102,186]

Iridocyclitis. According to Womack and Liesgang's studies[195] uveitis was seen in 43% of their patients, a figure that generally agrees with other HZO reports.[20] Other characteristic findings were vascular dilatation, posterior synechiae, striate keratopathy, pigment iris atrophy, sectoral pigment iris atrophy, and sphincter damage.[20,106,110,195] Fluorescein angiography revealed occlusion of iris vessels, presumably by vasculitis, at the sites of atrophy. This occlusion differs from the iris atrophy seen with HSV, which causes sharply defined borders and scalloped margins with the iris arterioles patent in the involved areas. Sectoral iris atrophy occurs in 17% to 25% of HZO patients.* Involvement may occur early or many months or years after the onset of acute disease and independent of corneal activity. The pathogenesis appears to be immune reaction in response to direct invasion of the uveal tract by infectious VZV. Late-onset uveitis may be a response to the antigenic residua of this invasion.

The iridocyclitis may be characterized clinically simply by photophobia in a white and quiet eye with just a few cells and flare in the anterior chamber. More severe acute disease will involve ciliary flush, miosis, deep ocular pain, visual decrease, keratic precipitates, iris edema and hyperemia, and anterior and posterior synechiae secondary to a fibrinous exudate.

Zoster iritis differs from HSV iritis in that the former is chiefly a plasma cell-lymphocyte vasculitis, whereas the latter is primarily a diffuse lymphocytic infiltrate of iris stroma. The iris focal or sector atrophy seen in HZO is the result of the localized ischemic necrosis resembling that resulting from excessive diathermy and muscle detachment in retinal surgery.

Hyphema, hypopyon, glaucoma, and ultimate phthisis bulbi may all result from this severe zoster iridovasculitis.[63,95,131,195]

As with HZO immune keratitis, this uveal inflammatory reaction is responsive to topical and, if needed, systemic steroid therapy. The usual gradual tapering regimen must be used once disease is under control to avoid rebound intraocular reaction. It is not unusual for a patient to require indefinite treatment with ⅛% prednisolone daily, or even every 2 to 3 days, to prevent recurrent disease.

Glaucoma. Intraocular pressure may be markedly elevated in 10% to 43% of patients.[20,91,92] Peripheral endotheliitis with an associated trabeculitis, isolated trabeculitis with no corneal involvement, or secondary to cicatricial closure of

---

*References 20, 91, 110, 135, 136, 195.

the angle are all mechanisms of HZO glaucoma. Necrosis of the pars plicata of the ciliary body with subsequent decreased aqueous production may occasionally result in a marked decrease in intraocular pressure. This decrease may be more than counterbalanced by impairment of outflow facility caused by clogging of the trabecular meshwork with inflammatory cellular debris. Depending on the balance between decreased aqueous production and decreased outflow, the intraocular pressure(IOP) may be low, normal, or elevated.[91,131,195]

Miotics should not be used in HZO glaucoma of an inflammatory nature. They may be useful, however, in an uninflamed secondary angle closure. Beta blockers, epinephrine or its prodrug, iopidine, and/or carbonic anhydrase inhibitors may all be used effectively to treat both the acute and chronic aspects of both inflammatory and synechial closure glaucoma.

Cranial Nerve Palsies. Partial or even complete paralysis of the extraocular muscles (EOM) is uncommon and generally appears within the first week of the dermatitis. Involvement of the third, fourth, or sixth nerves has been reported by Hunt[69] in 14% of 158 patients studied. The pupil may or may not have been spared in third nerve paresis. Marsh, Dudley, and Kelly[109] have noted an even higher incidence of 33% in a prospective study of 77 HZO patients. There was an increased incidence of paresis in the elderly and in patients with more severe disease, especially those with iritis and iris atrophy, but not in those with lid and corneal involvement alone. Although EOM paresis is thought to result primarily from the spread of virus through the orbit to involve the cranial nerves III, IV, and/or VI, this latter study noted that 12% of patients had contralateral muscle palsies and 6% had bilateral palsies. This finding suggests a CNS disturbance caused by retrograde migration of the VZV. Total ophthalmoplegia associated with proptosis or even complete facial paralysis may occur in a few patients, and isolated fourth or sixth nerve palsies are less frequent than involvement of the third nerve. All palsies may occur together in varying degrees of severity.[16,84,125,139,183] Fortunately, EOM palsies are self-limited. Even complete ophthalmoplegia will resolve within a year to 18 months.[84,109,198]

Posterior Segment. Involvement of the posterior segment by VZV is detailed in Chapter 82. Clinical manifestations include optic neuritis, central retinal vein occlusion, central retinal artery occlusion, necrotizing retinitis, delayed thrombophlebitis, optic neuropathy, and localized arteritis with or without exudates and acute retinal necrosis (ARN).[27]

Neuralgia. Pain experienced by patients during the early phases of HZO is attributed to acute swelling and lymphocytic infiltration of the trigeminal nerve as well as the pain of inflammatory reaction in and around the eye itself.[59] Patients in pain often display sympathetic hyperactivity such as tachypnea, tachycardia, diaphoresis, mydriasis, and an effect characterized by anxiety.

DeMoragas and Kierland,[32] in a 1957 study of 916 zoster

patients seen from the years 1935 through 1949, reported a 12.5% incidence of acute neuralgia in patients under 20 years of age, approximately 40% in those 30 to 50 years of age, and only 20% in those in the sixth and seventh decades. In contrast, within this same population the incidence of chronic postherpetic neuralgic pain lasting more than 1 year fell to less than 4% in the youngest age group and to about 10% in those patients in the middle group, but rose to nearly 50% in those patients in the 60- to 80-year age group. Similarly, Womack and Liesegang[195] noted postherpetic neuralgia persisting in 17% of their patients, with the most severe cases involving those patients in the sixth through eighth decades of life. Four of their patients had been treated with prednisone in the course of disease. Ragozzino and associates[149] reported a lower incidence of 9.3%, which was also in the older patient population.

Long-term, postherpetic neuralgia (PHN), which manifests different clinical findings, has been defined variably as pain after the crusting has ceased, pain persisting longer than 1 month, or pain after the skin has healed.[14,37,159] Perhaps the most encompassing definition of PHN is "that which lasts longer than six months or that which persists for more than a month beyond the usual healing of an inciting lesion."[188,189] This chronic pain is associated with quiescent behavior, which is often overlooked by the treating physician. Such behavior includes sleep disturbance, lassitude, anorexia, weight loss, constipation, and (in place of anxiety) depression. Watson's report[189] of 100 patients with HZO indicated that approximately 10% will have severe pain for 1 month, 5% will have severe pain for 3 months, and 2% to 3% will be in severe pain for more than 1 year after the acute episode. It has been noted that PHN is most common in the elderly, the immunocompromised, and those with more severe pain or rash at the time of onset of the illness.[59] The pathophysiology of postherpetic neuralgia is not clearly defined. Fibrosis occurs in the peripheral nerve and, in advanced cases, does not appear to be inflammatory. There is also fibrosis in the dorsal root ganglion. The structure of the dorsal horn of the spinal cord is disordered without atrophy. There is also an increase in the small nerve fibers and a reduction in large fibers that may allow increased transmission through the unopposed smaller nerve fibers.[146,188] It is known that the small fibers are excitory, transmit pain, and contain substance P, a tachykinin amenable to therapy as noted in the next section. Postherpetic neuralgia, then, appears to be the result of disordered fiber input into a diseased dorsal root ganglion and dorsal horn rather than an inflammatory fibrotic scarring disease of the peripheral nerve axons.[5,146,188,196,197]

HZO in AIDS and Other Immunocompromised Patients

VZV infections have long been a major complication of immunocompromised patients.[66,143] Although recurrent clinically apparent cases of varicella are rare, reinfection in immunocompromised patients may occur subclinically or overtly after exposure to exogenous VZV.[76,190] The effect of increasing age on decreasing CMI and humoral response has already been noted, although the latter is of considerably less importance in preventing or minimizing the ravages of zoster.[15,149] Although the occurrence of zoster is not a predictor of increased risk of subsequent malignancy, preexistent cancer does increase the risk of subsequent zoster. In patients with solid tumors the incidence is 1% to 3%, in those with non-Hodgkin lymphoma 7% to 9%, and in Hodgkin disease 13% to 15%, of which up to 30% will disseminate.[66] Depending on the severity of impairment of CMI, cutaneous dissemination will occur in 6% to 26% of patients within 4 to 11 days after localized zoster appears, and half of these will have ocular, visceral, or neurologic involvement. Such dissemination is unaffected by administration of high doses of either normal serum globulin or zoster immune globulin.[167] Local factors such as tumor site and irradiation also predispose to occurrence of zoster at the affected region.[4]

Children who contract chickenpox and undergo a primary immune response prior to developing leukemia appear to have immunologic protection against subsequent zoster, as opposed to children who contract varicella after developing leukemia. It is notable, however, that VZV seropositive children with leukemia are 30 times more likely to develop zoster than are healthy children.[58] Chemotherapy in childhood cancer patients also presents significant added risk. Of 77 such patients off all therapy for at least 3 months, none died or developed visceral involvement after contracting varicella. Of 60 such patients still on therapy, 32% had visceral involvement and 7% died.[44]

In bone marrow and organ transplant patients lymphocyte transformation to VZV antigen is depressed for up to 100 days after surgery, whereas HSV response is maximally depressed immediately after the procedure. This depression of CMI matches the temporal recurrence of activity for each virus, that is, zoster may be delayed and occur later than disease caused by HSV.[122,155]

The increasing incidence of HZO in apparently healthy young patients has heralded the advent of the AIDS epidemic. This pandemic retroviral disease that cripples the cell-mediated immune response has resulted in physicians seeing increasing numbers of herpes zoster patients in the younger age groups than ever previously reported. In 1984 Cole and associates[24] reported four cases of zoster ophthalmicus in four males with AIDS ranging in age from 26 to 41. One of these patients required treatment with systemic antiviral therapy (IV vidarabine), all received topical corticosteroids for ocular immune reactions, and one received systemic prednisone therapy; yet all recovered without immediate adverse consequences of the HZO. In 1988 Seiff and associates[161] reported HZO in two AIDS patients, 24 and 49 years of age, both successfully treated with IV acyclovir. As the reactivation of VZV in immunocompetent individuals under the age of 50 is uncommon, the presence of zoster in patients under age 50 must alert the physician to the possible coexistence of HIV infection.

A report by Freidmann-Kein and associates[47] noted that 8% of AIDS patients with Kaposi sarcoma had a past history of herpes zoster, an incidence seven times that of age-matched controls (ages 24 to 52). In a prospective study by Sandor and associates[155] on herpes zoster patients under the age of 45, 75% had AIDS risk factors, altered T cell subsets, and polyclonal increases in serum gamma globulin; and all tested positive for HIV antibody. They concluded that for any patient in a high-risk group [homosexual, intravenous drug abuser, Haitian with hemophilia A or having received other blood products, (and in this day and age, anyone with a history of sexual exposure to persons in these categories)], acyclovir therapy should not be delayed in the face of VZV infection and IV therapy, 30 mg/kg for 7 days, should be initiated immediately. In other studies in young adults, there was a 23% incidence of AIDS within 2 years of zoster and 46% within 4 years.[120]

Zoster ophthalmicus, as most forms of zoster disease, is normally considered an illness with little tendency for rapid or frequent recurrence. In the face of AIDS, however, recurrence may be more frequent than previously seen. Litoff and Catalano[97] reported treating a 40-year-old HIV-positive woman with zoster ophthalmicus with a 10-day course of IV acyclovir (10 mg/kg q8h). There was complete resolution of disease, but 3 weeks later the patient re-presented with recurrence of her dendritic lesions ou and another vesicular eruption in the trigeminal dermatome. Additionally, she had a marked zoster vasculitis and retinitis. She underwent a repeat 10-day course of IV acyclovir and a 5-day course of IV methylprednisolone sodium succinate (250 mg/q6h). The ocular lesions gradually resolved, although visual acuity remained poor in the eye with severe retinitis. She was discharged on maintenance therapy with oral acyclovir, 800 mg 5 times daily and topical cycloplegics and fluorometholone. She remained asymptomatic in the 6 weeks of follow-up.

Another report exemplifies the chances of misdiagnosis because of the potential for atypical presentation. The majority of HZO cases in HIV patients are characterized by severe and enduring cutaneous lesions, epithelial and stromal keratitis, and anterior uveitis.[24] Engstom and Holland[40] have reported a patient with active perianal herpes simplex lesions, who developed vesicles on the left brow, side of the nose, and upper lip, as well as left dendriform keratitis with only mild stromal haze. HSV keratitis was diagnosed. In the face of 6 weeks of intensive topical trifluridine and oral acyclovir, the skin sores healed, but the corneal epithelial lesions progressed, became geographic, and sensation was lost. VZV, not HSV, was cultured from the cornea. Healing was achieved within 5 days with topical acyclovir ointment alone.

Kestelyn and associates[80] have also reported the greater difficulties encountered in HIV-positive HZO patients. Of 19 HIV-HZO patients (the mean age was 28 years) 80% were otherwise totally healthy, 89% developed punctate keratitis and anterior stromal infiltrates, 53% had iritis, and 42% contracted PHN. It was noted that the presence of peripheral retinal perivasculitis and sheathing greatly raised the index of suspicion for coexisting HIV infection in HZO patients. In general, this category of patients with combined infection requires prolonged therapy for chronic morbidity of disease.[160]

Although prolonged therapy is often a necessity, it also increases the chance of resistant virus emerging. Jacobson and associates[73] have reported 4 patients with HIV treated for 1 to 5 months with oral acyclovir dosages of 400 to 4000 mg/day for suppression of chronic HSV or VZV disease. All four patients developed persistent disseminated zoster lesions from VZV, which is highly resistant to acyclovir but, fortunately, sensitive to vidarabine and foscarnet. To decrease such emergence of acyclovir-resistant strains, it was recommended that persistent or disseminated zoster be treated aggressively with a minimum course of 7 to 10 days of high-dose oral or IV acyclovir. This treatment could possibly continue a few days after the healing of lesions, but avoiding long-term oral suppressive therapy should be avoided.

Laboratory Investigations

The diagnosis of herpes zoster is almost always based on clinical findings alone. There are, however, occasions when objective laboratory data are essential to making the diagnosis and for differentiating this disease from those that mimic it. Such illnesses include zosteriform HSV, hypersensitivity reactions, vesicular enteroviral infections, and contact dermatitis. The many laboratory tests available are very nicely discussed by Liesegang,[94] Solomon,[165] and Koneman, Allen, and Dowell[83] and will be more briefly summarized here.

The five general categories of laboratory tests for VZV are viral isolation, morphologic and immunomorphologic tests, cellular immunity assessment, and serologic tests.

Viral isolation remains the most definitive diagnostic test, but it lacks the sensitivity of the viral antigen detection tests. Virus is present in highest titers in the clear vesicle stage. Fluid should be aspirated and scrapings taken to obtain cells from the base of two or three lesions (VZV is strongly cell-associated). The scrapings and fluid are inoculated immediately into human, primate, or guinea pig monolayer tissue cultures, as VZV will not long survive at room temperature. Focal and linear cytopathic effects (CPE) develop slowly over a 3- to 5-day period in about 40% to 50% of such cultures taken. Even if no CPE appears, antigen detection tests discussed in the following section may be used to confirm diagnosis.

Of the morphologic tests, the most simple is the Tzanck

technique. This involves smearing the scraping (not just fluid) taken from the base of a recent vesicle on a slide and staining it with Giemsa, Wright hematoxylin-eosin, Papanicolaou, methylene blue, or Paragon multiple stain. A positive light microscopic exam will reveal multinucleated giant cells, a mononuclear cellular reaction, eosinophilic intranuclear inclusion bodies, and margination of nuclear chromatin. This technique is positive in about 70% of vesicles and 55% of pustules, and is almost always negative in crusts.[83,165] Another drawback seen with this technique, with similar tests on skin biopsies, or with electron microscopic exam of tissue specimens is that the tests can only confirm the presence of HSV or VZV, but they cannot distinguish between these two morphologically identical viruses.

Immunofluorescent and immunoenzyme stains (immunoperoxidase, enzyme-linked immunosorbent assays [ELISA]) for viral antigen are more sensitive than viral isolation because the antigens are present later in the disease when virus is no longer in the lesions. The availability of monoclonal antibodies derived from cloned hybridoma cell lines now provides a reliable, stable source of diagnostic antibody capable of detecting very small fragments of antigen. The wide variety of immunologic tests now available in sophisticated state, private, and major medical center laboratories are listed in the box.

Cell-mediated immunity to VZV is far more critical than humoral response, both clinically and diagnostically. Immunosuppressed patients tend to develop clinical zoster of a severity commensurate with their diminished CMI.[66,134] Evaluation of peripheral lymphocyte VZV antigen-stimulated proliferative response and evaluation of the host response to the VZV antigen skin test are both useful in distinguishing between immune and immunoincompetent patients.[3,173] The lymphocyte test is reliable but requires a sophisticated laboratory. The skin test is easy but its significance is not well established.[142,172]

The significance of the humoral response in reactivated VZV is also not fully understood. Unless there is marked immunosuppression, patients previously infected with varicella will have an anamnestic humoral and CMI when reexposed to VZV or endogenous virus reactivates.[3,173] Normally about 90% of the adult population have detectable titers of VZV antibodies, but only about 5% have titers of 1:640 or higher in the absence of disease. Failure to detect high VZV antibody titers a week or two after onset of VZV-like disease suggests that it is not caused by this virus, whereas high titers suggest that VZV is the causative agent. Although IgM indicates a recent infection, not all patients will demonstrate more than a mild rise in titer, whether stimulated by exogenous exposure to new virus or endogenous reactivation of latent VZV. High IgG titers, then, may be a more reliable indicator of the cause of illness than the presence or absence of IgM.[159]

DIAGNOSTIC TESTS FOR VARICELLA-ZOSTER VIRUS

Vesicular Scrapings
1. Viral isolation on tissue culture
2. Morphology: Tzanck staining techniques, for example, Giemsa, Wright, Papanicolaou, light and electron microscopy
3. Immunologic tests: direct immunofluorescence or immunoperoxidase stains, radioimmunoassay, ELISA (enzyme-linked immunosorbent assay), agar gel immunodiffusion, immunoelectrophoresis
4. Molecular biology of VZV DNA: in situ hybridization, polymerase chain reaction

Cell-mediated Immunity
1. VZV antigen skin test
2. VZV lymphocyte proliferation

Serology
1. Neutralizing or complement fixing antibody titers
2. ELISA
3. Radioimmunoassay
4. Membrane antigen immunofluorescence
5. Immune adherence hemagglutination

Therapy of Ophthalmic Zoster

Antiviral Agents. Despite in vitro susceptibility HZO is clinically unresponsive to the commercially available topical antiviral medications idoxuridine, vidarabine, and trifluridine. McGill and associates[117-119] have reported several studies indicating that topical 5% acyclovir ointment five times daily was highly effective in resolving HZO epithelial keratitis and in preventing recurrent disease, in comparison to control patients receiving topical corticosteroids.[159] Additionally, acyclovir alone was more effective than combined topical acyclovir and steroid. There was no significant difference, however, in resolution of stromal keratitis, iritis, scleritis, or secondary glaucoma among any treatment groups (acyclovir alone or acyclovir-steroid combination).

Conversely, Marsh and associates noted a more rapid trend toward resolution of inflammation in zoster patients treated with topical acyclovir-steroid combination compared to the progressive ocular disease noted in patients receiving acyclovir alone.[106] They concluded that topical corticosteroids were of use in management of the inflammatory aspects of HZO, and that there were no clear benefits from use of topical acyclovir alone. Perhaps more pertinent is the use of systemic antivirals in therapy of VZV infections. Such agents include IV vidarabine, interferon, and acyclovir.[171]

Acyclovir. Systemic acyclovir is significantly better than IV vidarabine in treatment of zoster infections of immunocompromised patients.[6,164] A guanosine analogue, acyclovir is activated via phosphorylation by viral-specific thymidine kinase.[137,138] It works by selective inhibition of viral DNA polymerase and by DNA chain termination. Whereas IV acyclovir may cause renal toxicity by crystallizing within the collecting tubules, the elevated creatinine levels noted in one quarter of the acyclovir patients may, in fact, have been caused by concomitant cyclosporine therapy. Lethargy, nervousness, tremor, and disorientation were occasionally reported, especially in patients with renal compromise.[62,176] In general, however, acyclovir toxicity was minimal, with frequent reversible hematologic changes, but not enough to necessitate a change in therapy.

Oral acyclovir is one therapeutic mainstay of zoster (see Addendum for famciclovir). Absorption from the GI tract is only 10% to 20% and is occasionally erratic. The drug is well tolerated, however, and only rarely produces nausea or diarrhea at high doses.[62] Plasma levels after oral dosing range from means of 4.0 to 5.75 um/l to 8.74 um/l with the ID_{50} for zoster reaching a high of 6.4 um/l for some strains, although the majority of strains are well within the therapeutic range.[31,68] Tear and aqueous levels 4 hours after a 400-mg oral dose are in excess of the minimal inhibitory concentration of VZV (mean = 3.28 μm, range = 0.96 to 8.8 μm).

The occurrence of distressing gastrointestinal upset, particularly diarrhea, with the use of oral acyclovir may indicate a lactose intolerance. This intolerance is found in North American adults; approximately 75% of native Americans and blacks, 51% of hispanics, and 21% of whites.[185] Oral acyclovir tablets contain lactose and intolerance to this is caused by a lack of the intestinal enzyme lactase. Manka[105] has reported reversal of acyclovir intolerance by administration of oral lactase in the form of one Lactaid™ caplet five times daily po.

Masked control studies by Cobo and associates[22,23] in a clinical trial of 55 immunocompetent patients with acute HZO revealed that acyclovir therapy (600 mg po 5 times daily for 10 days) was significantly better than placebo. Although benefit was not confined to the early treatment group, the patients responding most dramatically were those whose treatment began within 72 hours of the onset of disease. There was complete cessation of acute pain, a prompt resolution of skin rash, more rapid healing, reduced duration of viral shedding, reduced duration of new lesion formation, and a marked reduction in the incidence of episcleritis, keratitis, and iritis. Systemic and local toxicity were insignificant. Long-term follow-up on this patient cohort indicated no beneficial effect, however, on postherpetic neuralgia at these dosage levels. Forty-one percent of drug-treated patients had persistent pain. This latter finding differed from the controlled study of Harding,[59] who noted a statistically significant reduction in incidence and severity of PHN to 13% in the acyclovir group over 2 to 6 months of follow-up. Dosage was higher at 800 mg and had been given 5 times daily for 10 days during the acute disease, compared to that used in the Cobo and associates study.[23,35]

Herbort and associates[64] prospectively treated 48 HZO patients with 800 mg acyclovir po 5 id for 7 days, specifically excluding anyone who had had steroid therapy within a week of disease onset, and compared their results retrospectively with a cohort of nonacyclovir-treated HZO patients. They noted comparable acute ocular involvement (67% versus 59%, respectively) but a significantly lower incidence of longer term (> 2 months) complications, primarily keratitis and uveitis, in the acyclovir group (4%) as opposed to the untreated group (21%). No acyclovir patient required steroid therapy. Herbort and associates pointed out that acyclovir therapy heralded the end of the steroid era in management of HZO. PHN was not addressed.

In a double-blind placebo controlled study, Hoang-Xuan and associates[66a] combined oral acyclovir, 800 mg 5 times daily for 7 or 14 days, with topical 3% acyclovir ointment, 5 times daily for 7 days, in 86 immunocompetent patients with herpes zoster.[62] They confirmed the preceding clinical findings and noted late ocular inflammatory complications such as keratitis or iritis reduced to 29% in acyclovir-treated patients compared to 50% in the placebo group. They also noted a reduced prevalence of localized zoster-associated neurologic symptoms such as paresthesia, dysesthesia, or hyperesthesia, as well as long-term postherpetic neuralgia (0% severe, 13% mild neuralgia for 2 years).[62] It was difficult to compare this research to other studies on the incidence of PHN in untreated patients, as the incidence range was 10% to 52%, but severity of pain was not reported.[20,146] Current evidence suggests, however, that high-dose oral acyclovir (800 mg 5 times a day for 7 to 10 days) may truly lower the incidence of debilitating PHN.

Famciclovir. Recently, an important new antiviral drug was FDA approved for therapy of varicella-zoster: famciclovir.[154a] This orally administered drug is the diacetyl ester of 6-deoxy-penciclovir, similar in structure to acyclovir.[35a] In vitro it is effective against HSV-1, HSV-2, VZV, and Epstein-Barr virus. The activity against VZV equals that of acyclovir with a mean EC_{50} in tissue culture of 3 to 4 μg/ml.[185a]

Famciclovir is highly absorbed from the gastrointestinal tract (77%) and rapidly hydrolyzed to penciclovir. The intracellular duration of active penciclovir is 9 times that of acyclovir (10 to 20 hours for HSV-infected cells and 9 hours for VZV-infected cells).[177a] It is a nonobligate chain terminator and inhibits DNA polymerase-mediated viral DNA elongation. For two reasons—(1) penciclovir is preferentially phosphorylated in herpesvirus-infected cells (far in excess of acyclovir) but minimally phosphorylated in uninfected cells, and (2) the low activity of penciclovir triphosphate (PCV-TP) against cellular DNA polymerases—this agent has little-to-no toxicity in cell culture and in clinical studies.[10a,148a,185a]

Famciclovir is FDA approved for therapy of acute infectious varicella-zoster at dosages of 500 mg/day for 7 days.

In clinical studies famciclovir (500 or 750 mg PO TID) was compared to placebo in treating 323 immunocompetent zoster patients.[177a] Both dosage groups had similar results, indicating famciclovir (1) accelerates cutaneous healing, (2) lowers the time to vesicle loss from 6 to 5 days, and (3) decreases the time to full crusting from 7 to 6 days. Of note was the significant effect on reduction of postherpetic neuralgia. The median time to resolution of the neuralgia was 55 and 62 days in the famciclovir groups compared to 128 days in the placebo group. These data on PHN are more favorable than those seen in acyclovir-treated patients.

Other clinical trials comparing famciclovir in masked doses of 250 mg, 500 mg, or 750 mg PO TID against acyclovir (800 mg PO 5 times a day) were done in 544 immunocompetent zoster patients.[52a] There was no difference among any famciclovir doses nor between the two drugs in rate of cutaneous healing, resolution of acute pain, or safety and tolerance. Postherpetic neuralgia data in this study are not reported.

BV Ara-U. Bromovinyl arabinosyl uracil (BV Ara-U) is an experimental drug with marked in vitro efficacy against HSV-1 and VZV, but particularly VZV.[99,100] It is currently under clinical evaluation in Japan, Europe, and the United States for management of zoster in normal and immunocompromised patients. BV Ara-U's advantages over acyclovir include a higher therapeutic efficacy and longer duration of action allowing once daily dosing.

Corticosteroids. The successful treatment of zoster dendritic keratitis with topical corticosteroids by Pavan-Langston and McCulley[141] and Piebenga and Laibson[144] would suggest that, unlike HSV disease, their use for immune zoster keratouveitis will not aggravate the presence of an infectious epithelial keratitis. Forrest and Kaufman[46] have, however, reported four cases in which zoster ophthalmicus was confused with herpes simplex keratitis and subsequent steroid therapy exacerbated the disease. If the diagnosis of HZO is secure, then antivirals topically appear to be optional. If a doubt exists, however, it is probably more prudent to include full topical antiviral therapy along with topical corticosteroids to ensure coverage of possible HSV.

In therapy of immune keratitis Berghaust and Westby[9] reported 45 cases of HZO treated with topical corticosteroids and antibiotics. There was a marked reduction in corneal infiltrates and anterior uveitis in the steroid-treated group in comparison to 25 untreated controls. No adverse side effects were noted. Liesegang[92] has also reported rapid response to topical corticosteroids of HZO anterior segment inflammatory disease: disciform keratitis, keratouveitis/endotheliitis, sclerokeratitis, and serpiginous ulcerations. Delayed corneal mucous plaques (late pseudodendrites) did not respond to any therapy, steroid or antiviral, but self-resolved.

The personal experience of Deborah Pavan-Langston is similar to the preceding. Topical steroid therapy at whatever dosage is required to bring the inflammatory process under control is initiated, usually at levels of dexamethasone 0.1% qid for more severe disease and prednisolone 0.12% tid-qid for milder disease. This treatment is slowly tapered over a period of several weeks to a month, extending taper time the lower the dosage becomes and not decreasing by more than 50% at any given time. Appropriate antibiotic coverage should be used, but topical antivirals may only cause toxicity and have no effect on the zoster inflammatory process. There are a few patients who will require low-dose corticosteroids indefinitely (for example, prednisolone 0.12% qd or qod), or immune-inflammatory rebound will occur.

Systemic corticosteroids are more controversial in the therapy of VZV. In general, the literature pertinent to the use of corticosteroids systemically in zoster disease is favorable. Scheie[159] has reported treating 93 HZO patients, 6 of whom were immunosuppressed, with topical corticosteroids and intravenous adreno-corticotrophic hormone or systemic corticosteroids. Compared to untreated patients corticosteroids were more effective in the rapid control of pain and in reducing the incidence and severity of keratitis, uveitis, and secondary glaucoma. No patient disseminated infection, but recurrent steroid-sensitive keratitis developed in four patients and postherpetic neuralgia developed in 18% of patients. Carter and Royd noted similar efficacy using systemic prednisone in HZO to reduce edema and scarring, but they also did not succeed in reducing the incidence of postherpetic neuralgia.

Elliott[39] used high doses of systemic prednisone in zoster in an open study of efficacy on acute and long-term disease. Sixteen patients (3 HZO, 2 geniculate, and 11 thoracic) received 60 mg prednisone po qd for 10 days immediately after the onset of rash. In comparison to 10 untreated control zoster patients, the pain was significantly reduced from a mean of 3½ weeks to 3½ days. There were no cases of postherpetic neuralgia in the treated group as opposed to two cases in the controls (too small for statistical analysis), and there was no dissemination of disease. Elliott further noted that use of low doses of corticosteroids was of no value, and the earlier treatment was begun the better, preferably within 2 weeks of onset of disease.

The major study in favor of systemic corticosteroids for the prevention of postherpetic neuralgia was a masked controlled evaluation published by Keczkes and Basheer.[79] Therapy was begun immediately after onset of rash. Forty immunocompetent zoster patients were treated with 40 mg prednisone po daily, tapered over a 4-week period. Control patients received carbamazepine in a similar regimen. Sixty-five percent of the control group developed postherpetic neuralgia lasting up to 2 years, whereas only 15% of the prednisone-treated group developed neuralgia, which lasted only up to 6 months. There was no dissemination of disease.

An equally convincing study by Esmann and associates[42] contradicted these findings. These investigators reported that high-dose oral prednisolone, even in combination with oral acyclovir, did not prevent postherpetic neuralgia. Seventy-eight patients (60 years or older) with acute VZV infections of less than 4 days duration were treated prospectively in a double-masked study. Patients received either 225 mg prednisolone or calcium lactate over a 10-day period plus acyclovir, 300 mg po 5 times daily for 7 days. Twelve of these patients had HZO. Although the acute pain was relieved in the steroid group during the first 3 days of treatment, the long-term results were not significantly different between treatment groups. Approximately 23% of both placebo and steroid-acyclovir-treated patients had persistent neuralgia at 6 months time. Of the 78 patients entering the study, 29% of the HZO patients, but only 22% of the nonocular patients, still suffered pain. Pain did not develop in several patients until 1 to 2 weeks after entry into the study; there was no difference between treatment groups in this respect.

Those who cite the increased chance of systemic dissemination of VZV are also aligned against the proponents of systemic corticosteroids. Merselis, Kaye, and Hook[121] reported disseminated zoster with the use of systemic corticosteroids. A closer look at the figures, however, reveals that 11 of these patients were immunocompromised (leukemia, lymphoma). Of six patients with no underlying illness, only two had actually received any systemic steroid. The six basically healthy patients all underwent an illness similar to chickenpox and recovered without sequelae.

Nonetheless, times have changed with the advent of the AIDS epidemic and the fact that zoster ophthalmicus may be an early presenting sign in this immunosuppressive disease. In the absence of a clear-cut benefit from the use of systemic corticosteroids and the availability of a safe and effective antiviral acyclovir, which appears to accomplish the same end, the use of corticosteroids systemically has become less necessary and more controversial. The now added risk of potentiating VZV infectious disease in an unrecognized AIDS patient mandates an ever-increasing need to evaluate patient immunocompetence, avoid the use of corticosteroids in those patients manifesting immunodeficiency of whatever cause, infectious or iatrogenic, and carefully weigh the risk-benefit ratio before starting steroid therapy—even in immunocompetent zoster patients.[24,155,156] At this time the place of systemic corticosteroids in zoster would be in the therapy of the inflammatory vasculitic complications such as severe scleritis, keratitis, uveitis, and orbital apex syndrome. Systemic acyclovir should be given concomitantly to control the infectious component of the disease.

Cimetidine (Tagamet™). Cimetidine, the histamine-2 blocker, is marketed commercially for therapy of gastrointestinal ulcers. Two uncontrolled studies have reported relief of discomfort, edema, and erythema of acute HZO. Presumably the mechanism of action is caused by the histamine blockade of receptors in the skin.

In two open studies cimetadine (300 to 400 mg po qid for 7 days starting within 72 hours of onset of acute disease) resulted in rapid relief of pain, itching, and erythema, and in the resolution of vesicles. The drug appeared effective in both immunocompromised and immunocompetent patients. A third controlled study, however, noted no significant effect of the drug on these parameters, although dosage was somewhat lower and follow-up of patients less complete.[89,113,182] Further controlled studies are needed to ascertain the exact role, if any, of cimetidine in therapy of zoster disease. As with systemic corticosteroids, the availability of acyclovir makes the benefits of cimetidine dubious at best.

Capsaicin (Zostrix-HP™). Capsaicin is a vanillyl alkaloid extracted from red peppers and related plants.[1,10,13] This substance relieves both acute and chronic pain by depleting substance P from the small sensory peripheral and central neurones and preventing its reaccumulation at these sites. Substance P is a tachykinin peptide, which is an important neurotransmitter in transmission of peripheral pain impulses. In vitro, it opens channels allowing sodium and calcium ions into the sensory dorsal root ganglia cells, causing sustained depolarization as long as it is present. Its depletion from the C fibers does not interfere with the sensations of pressure, touch, or vibration. Watson[189] has reported an open label capsaicin study on 31 men and women with a median age of 71 years and median duration of severe postherpetic neuralgia of 2 years. Four-times daily application of 0.025% capsaicin cream (Zostrix-HP) for 4 weeks resulted in a positive response rate in 76% of patients. One third of these patients reported an excellent-to-good response, and an additional 16% reported feeling 50% to 60% better but still having some pain.

Bernstein's review[10] of a multicenter, double-blind clinical trial with a higher concentration of drug noted that 77% of 16 elderly patients with 6 months or longer postherpetic neuralgia reported pain relief by 6 weeks under treatment with 0.075% capsaicin.[166] This was in comparison to relief noted in only 31% of 16 patients treated with vehicle alone. Burning, stinging, or erythema occurred in 30% of capsaicin-treated patients but only in 12% of the vehicle control group.

In Deborah Pavan-Langston's own experience with this drug in 28 patients with chronic zoster neuralgia, pain was markedly diminished in 75% of patients with qid use. More remarkably, four patients were able to maintain suppression of pain (on a prn basis using the ointment tid for about 1 week), as the neuralgia began to return several weeks after discontinuing the mediation.[10b]

Based on experience with capsaicin cream the following guidelines have evolved:

1. 0.075% cream must be applied three to four times daily on a continuous basis for several weeks. Maintenance may be just a few doses weekly.

2. Pain relief will be noted between 2 and 6 weeks after initiation of treatment.

3. In patients less than 55 years of age with pain of less than 3 months duration, treatment may be stopped after 3 to 5 months of pain relief.

4. In patients greater than 70 years of age with chronic pain of more than 6 months duration treatment may need to be continued for several years at doses considerably less frequent than those required initially.

5. Recurrence of pain after discontinuation of capsaicin is responsive to resumption of capsaicin treatment.

Antidepressants in Postherpetic Neuralgia. Psychotrophic medication has become an integral part of the multimodal treatment of chronic neuralgia of any cause.* In a placebo controlled study Watson, Evans, and Reed[188] reported the significant clinical value of the tricyclic antidepressant (TCA), amitriptyline hydrochloride (HCL) (25 to 150 mg po qd), in elderly patients suffering long-term postherpetic neuralgia.† The drug response rate was 60%, with the most severe pain becoming mild but not entirely relieved. In two thirds of the patients pain was reduced from severe to mild within 3 weeks, yet serum amitriptyline levels were well below those associated with antidepressant activity. A therapeutic window for the analgesic dosage of the TCAs exists, however, as increased dosage produces increased pain in some patients. Kvinesdal and associates[85] have reported similar successful clinical responses using imipramine IICL, 100 mg po daily, in nondepressed patients with severe diabetic neuropathy of greater than 2 years duration. Analgesia was achieved at levels half of that required for antidepressant effect and occurred within 2 weeks of initiating treatment. There are also reports that the combination of either doxepin or amitriptyline with a low-dose narcotic analgesic reduced pain intensity more than either an antidepressant or a narcotic drug alone in patients suffering chronic neuralgic pain.[88,181]

The exact mechanism of action of the TCAs is not well established, but those proposed include (1) alteration of transport or activity of substances involved in inflammation at the tissue level, for example, serotonin; (2) inhibition of prostaglandin synthetase, an enzyme crucial to inflammation; and (3) modification of blood protein binding capacity, a property shared with conventional antiinflammatory drugs.[114,157,185]

The several TCAs in use for control of pain include amitriptyline, desipramine, doxepin, imipramine, and nortriptyline. Because there is little data suggesting notable differences among these drugs for treatment of pain, selection of one or more of these drugs may depend on the side effects. The tertiary amines, amitriptyline, imipramine, and doxepin have more anticholinergic, cardiac, and CNS effects than the demethylated secondary amines, nortriptyline and desipramine. Therefore in the more vegetative patient desipramine may be the least sedating, whereas an agitated patient may benefit more from amitriptyline or doxepin. Nortriptyline is the drug of choice in patients with bradycardia or heart block.[157] Common dosage administration is amitriptyline, doxepin, or desipramine, 25 to 50 mg po qhs with increasing increments every 3 to 4 days to a stable dosage of 75 to 100 mg daily. The drugs are usually given at bedtime to take advantage of the sedating effect.

Neuroleptic agents are also useful as alternative therapy. These include the combination of such drugs as perphenazine, a tranquilizer, and amitriptyline (Triavil 2-10 or Estrafon 2-10 tablets), 3 to 4 times daily for those chronic pain patients with a mixture of anxiety and agitation with symptoms of depression. This combination therapy is particularly effective in patients under the age of 60. Irreversible tardive dyskinesia (involuntary movements of the face or extremities) and other extrapyramidal reactions such as motor restlessness, oculogyrocrisis, or opisthotonos may occasionally occur in older patients.[70,127,157] Medication should be stopped immediately upon the appearance of any suggestion of these symptoms. Despite the preceding side effects, the use of antidepressants or antidepressant-antianxiety combination medications have proved highly effective in situations in which other medical management or even neurosurgical therapy has failed.

The all-too-common severe lancinating pain of zoster is often controlled by the anticonvulsant carbamazepine (Tegretol), 100 mg po qd increased by 200 mg weekly to qid or lower if therapeutic effect is achieved.[81] Other anticonvulsants such as phenytoin and valproic acid may also be of use. Patients suffering both PHN and lancinating pain appear to respond to combined TCA and anticonvulsant therapy.[146]

Surgical Procedures. There are numerous surgical procedures for the various complications of HZO: lateral tarsorrhaphy for neurotrophic keratitis, stellate ganglion block for acute severe uncontrolled pain, cryotherapy or hyfrecation for trichiasis, entropion or ectropion repair, dacryocystorhinostomy with placement of a Jones tube for canaliculus obstruction, conjunctival transplant, conjunctival flap or tissue adhesive for corneal melting, and penetrating keratoplasty.[136,195]

The most common surgical procedure performed for HZO is lateral tarsorrhaphy for exposure or neurotrophic keratopathy of the anesthetic cornea. If lid structures are basically intact, but closure is incomplete because of scarring, a 3- to 4-mm lateral tarsorrhaphy coupled with lubricating artificial tears will frequently suffice to protect the anterior segment.[8,84,98,108,136] In the event lid tissue has been

---

*References 84, 94, 114, 136, 157, 187-189.

†References 84, 94, 114, 135, 157.

lost, plastic reconstruction involving the swinging of flaps may be required. This procedure is often difficult, as the remaining tissues are often friable and hold tissues poorly.

Lateral tarsorrhaphy should also be performed in the anesthetic eye, which may not be exposed, but which, because of a state of poor innervation, manifests grey unhealthy epithelium with impending breakdown. The physician should probably not use a therapeutic soft contact lens in these eyes, as the lens itself may induce a surface breakdown in an eye that may have remained intact if tarsorrhaphy alone with artificial tear lubricants and ointments had been used. About 3% of chronic HZO keratitis patients will develop ulceration, however.[106] If an epithelial defect does develop, a therapeutic SCL such as a plano Permalens or Sauflon lens with artificial tear lubrication and antibiotic cover is indicated to aid in healing.

In the event of an epithelial break and corneal thinning, sealing the defect with sterile tissue adhesive* will frequently suffice to allow healing, ultimate dislodging of the adhesive, and, in all likelihood, significant scarring but an intact globe.[87] A multicenter study on such use of tissue adhesive is currently under review by the FDA. Alternatives in this situation include the pulling down of a conjunctival flap or conjunctival transplantation.[98]

Penetrating keratoplasty (PK) has a limited role in HZO. As the majority of these eyes are anesthetic, the cornea will heal poorly and transplanted eyes are prone to melting, superinfection, and wound dehiscence.[104] A scarred cornea that has retained a reasonable amount of sensation may be considered a candidate for such a surgical procedure in an effort to restore vision. If this is done, however, a lateral tarsorrhaphy should be placed at the same time to protect the new graft. In a study by Reed, Joyner, and Knauer[150] 12 HZO patients, 5 with neurotrophic ulcers, underwent PK. Ten patients had lateral tarsorrhaphies placed, which were beneficial in preventing postoperative breakdown of the corneal epithelium. At 3 years average follow-up 83% of the grafts were clear, and 75% had vision of 20/80 or better.

Marsh and Cooper[108] have reviewed the outcome of several surgical procedures in HZO patients. With the exception of more prolonged inflammation in the postoperative period, recovery and outcome were similar to those of non-HZO patients. Forty patients underwent lateral tarsorrhaphy for neurotrophic ulceration, corneal anesthesia, exposure keratitis, and chronic edema. Although reoperation was necessary in 33% of patients because of failure of the tarsorrhaphy, the remaining patients began to recover within 2 weeks of surgery, demonstrating good epithelial healing. Of the nine patients undergoing penetrating keratoplasty for disciform

scarring, seven had successful outcomes. Only one of these patients had significant corneal anesthesia, however. Anesthesia bodes poorly for a successful outcome of keratoplasty in HZO patients.

Stellate ganglion block may be useful in acute severe pain uncontrolled by medical management. A 10-ml mixture of plain 1% xylocaine and 0.5% bupivicaine is injected at the C5-C6 vertebrae level with the head extended. An anesthesiologist or neurosurgeon experienced in such techniques should perform the procedure.

Summary of Therapeutic Approaches. Management of the acute and chronic disease resulting from reactivated VZV may be briefly summarized as follows:

A. Acute HZO

1. All patients, regardless of the severity of their disease, should have the following: acyclovir (Zovirax), 200 mg 4 tablets po 5 times daily for 7 to 10 days or famciclovir (Famvir) 500 mg po TID for 7 days, preferably (but not necessarily) starting within 72 hours of the onset of acute disease in immunocompetent patients. In immunocompromised patients intravenous acyclovir, 10 mg/kg q8h for 7 days in adults and 500 mg/m^1 q8h for children under 12 years of age (FDA approved dosages) should be used. Immunocompromised patients should have continued treatment with 1 to 3 weeks of oral acyclovir at full dosage after completion of the IV course of therapy.

2. For dermatitis—warm wet compresses should be applied, possibly followed by Betadine gel (not near eyes) to keep involved skin clean and minimize scarring.

3. For punctate or dendritic keratitis, the treatment should consist of gentle debridement with sterile applicator tip or no debridement and topical antibiotic ointment tid. Antivirals are optional (efficacy has not been proved).

4. Moderate-to-severe corneal disciform disease with intact epithelium or iritis should be treated with topical corticosteroids (⅛% prednisolone bid to qid up to 0.1% dexamethasone) in the same frequency as warranted by disease.

5. Antiviral ointments or drops are the best option if diagnosis is not secure as HZO versus HSV disease.

6. Topical antibiotics bid should be administered in the presence of epithelial defects.

7. Cycloplegics should be dispensed as needed for iritis (homatropine, atropine).

8. Nonnarcotic or narcotic analgesics are advised for acute neuralgia on days 1 through 7-10.

---

*Nexacryl, Tri-Point Medical L.P., Raleigh, North Carolina.

9. If there is no resolution of pain or increasing uncontrolled neuralgia, ocular inflammatory disease, or orbital apex syndrome, the institution of a systemic steroid program for the immunocompetent patient should be considered. The dosage is prednisone 20 mg po tid for 7 days, 15 mg bid for 7 days, then 15 mg po qd for 7 days. Cycloplegics and topical corticosteroids should be continued as needed, and the patient monitored for disseminated infection by an internist or dermatologist. The patient should be preevaluated for immunosuppression before systemic corticosteroids are initiated. Systemic corticosteroids are not FDA approved for this condition.

10. Artificial tears and ointment are appropriate for unstable tear film or exposure to keratitis.

11. Optional cimetidine, 300 mg po qid for 10 days, should preferably be started within 72 hours of the onset of disease; it is not FDA approved for zoster infections, however.

12. Stellate ganglion block is the treatment for uncontrolled acute pain.

B. Long-term or chronic problems

1. Lateral tarsorrhaphy is advised for exposure or anesthetic corneas.

2. Therapeutic SCL with or without tissue adhesive (FDA-IND), conjunctival flap, or transplant (as described) are treatments for exposure or corneal thinning.

3. For chronic postherpetic neuralgia, the advised treatment is tricyclic antidepressants (amitriptyline, desipramine, doxepin, imipramine, nortriptyline) alone or in combination with perphenazine as described in text tid to qid.

4. Capsaicin (Zostrix-HP) cream applied 3 to 6 times daily to skin should provide relief for postherpetic neuralgia. Treatment should continue for several months to several years per text description.

5. For lancinating pain carbamazepine or perphenazine-amitriptyline combination should be considered as noted in text.

6. Sympathetic blockade or invasive pain management techniques should be used if all preceding treatments fail to control incapacitating chronic pain, for example, trigeminal ganglion ablation.

Prognosis

The key to prognosis in herpes zoster ophthalmicus appears to be directly related to the immunologic competence of the patient, in particular, the competence of cell-mediated immunity. Latent virus remains clinically in check as long as CMI is fully functional. As host factors such as increasing age or HIV infection interfere with this function the virus reactivates and causes an infectious-inflammatory disease that is more devastating as CMI is more depressed. Although there are no studies yet available on the effect of immune-stimulating agents in controlling or preventing HZO, an excellent antiviral agent is available in oral and intravenous acyclovir with other agents not far behind. The long-term prognosis depends on the extent of damage done to ganglion and end organ during the acute disease. Damage control in these areas will prevent much of the chronic morbidity that all too frequently characterizes varicella-zoster infection of the eye and periocular structures.

REFERENCES

1. Abramowicz M, editor: Capsaicin—a topical analgesic, *The Med Lett on Drugs Therapeu* 34.873:62, 1992.
2. Centers for Disease Control: Annual Summary: Reported morbidity and mortality in the United States, *MMWR*, 1981.
3. Arvin AM, Koropchak CM, Wittek AE: Immunologic evidence of reinfection with varicella-zoster virus, *J Infect Dis* 148:200-205, 1983.
4. Arvin AM et al.: Cellular and humoral immunity in the pathogenesis of recurrent herpes viral infections in patients with lymphoma, *J Clin Invest* 65:869-878, 1980.
5. Asbury AK, Fields HL: Pain due to peripheral nerve damage: an hypothesis, *Neurology* 34:1587-1590, 1984.
6. Balfour H Jr et al.: Acyclovir halts progression of herpes zoster in immunocompromised patients, *New Eng J Med* 308:1448, 1983.
7. Bastian F et al.: Herpes virus varicella isolated from human dorsal root ganglia, *Arch Pathol* 97:331, 1973.
8. Baum J: Advantages of partial patching or tarsorrhaphy over complete eyelid closure, *Am J Ophthalmol* 103:339, 1987.
9. Bergaust B, Westby R: Zoster ophthalmicus: local treatment with cortisone, *Acta Ophthalmol* 45:787, 1967.
10. Bernstein JE et al.: Treatment of chronic postherpetic neuralgia with topical capsaicin: a preliminary report, *J Am Acad Dermatol* 17:93-96, 1987.
10a. Boyd M, Safrin S, Kern E: Penciclovir: a review of spectrum of activity, selectivity, and cross-resistance pattern, *Antiviral Chem Chemother* 4(suppl 1):25-36, 1993.
10b. Brody J, Pavan-Langston D: Decreasing dose regimen for capsaicin in postherpetic neuralgia, *Ophthalmology* 99:126(suppl), 1994.
11. Brunell PA, Kotchmar GS Jr: Zoster in infancy: failure to maintain virus latency following intrauterine infection, *J Pediatr* 98:71-73, 1981.
12. Brunell PA et al.: Varicella-zoster immunoglobulins during varicella, latency, and zoster, *J Infect Dis* 132.1:49-54, 1975.
13. Bucci Jr FA, Gabriels CF, Krohel GB: Successful treatment of postherpetic neuralgia with capsaicin, *Am J Ophthalmol* 106:758-759, 1988 (letter).
14. Burgoon Jr C, Burgoon J, Baldridge G: The natural history of herpes zoster, *JAMA* 164:265, 1957.
15. Burke B et al.: Immune responses to varicella-zoster in the aged, *Arch Intern Med* 142:291-293, 1982.
16. Carmody RF: Herpes zoster ophthalmicus complicated by ophthalmoplegia and exophthalmos, *Arch Ophthalmol* 18:707-711, 1937.
17. Carter A, Royds J: Systemic steroids in herpes zoster, *Br Med J* 2:746, 1957.
18. Cavanagh C, Colley A, Pihlaja D: Persistent corneal epithelial defects, *Int Ophthal Clin* 19:197, 1979.
19. Cherry J: Chickenpox transmission, *JAMA* 250:2060, 1983.
20. Cobo LM, Foulks GN, Liesegang T: Observations on the natural history of herpes zoster ophthalmicus, *Curr Eye Res* 6:195-199, 1987.

21. Cobo L et al.: Prognosis and management of corneal transplantation for herpetic keratitis, *Arch Ophthalmol* 98:1755, 1980.

22. Cobo L et al.: Oral acyclovir in the therapy of acute herpes zoster ophthalmicus: an interim report, *Ophthalmology* 92:1574, 1985.

23. Cobo L et al.: Oral acyclovir in the treatment of acute herpes zoster ophthalmicus, *Ophthalmology* 93:763, 1986.

24. Cole E et al.: Herpes zoster ophthalmicus and acquired immune deficiency syndrome, *Arch Ophthalmol* 102:1027, 1984.

25. Crock G: Clinical syndromes of anterior segment ischaemia, *Trans Ophthalmol Soc UK* 87:513, 1967.

26. Croen K et al.: Patterns of gene expression and sites of latency in human ganglia are different for varicella-zoster and herpes simplex viruses, *Proc Natl Acad Science USA* 85:9773-9777, 1988.

27. Culbertson WW et al.: Varicella-zoster virus as a cause of the acute retinal necrosis syndrome, *Ophthalmology* 93:559-569, 1986.

28. Davison A: Varicella-zoster virus: the fourteenth Fleming lecture, *J Gen Virol* 72:475-486, 1991.

29. Davison A, Scott J: The complete DNA sequences of varicella-zoster virus, *J Gen Virol* 67:1759-1816, 1986.

30. deFreitas D, Sato E, Pavan-Langston D: Delayed onset varicella keratitis, *Cornea* 11:471-474, 1992.

31. deMiranda P, Blum MR: Pharmacokinetics of acyclovir after intravenous and oral administration, *J Antimicrob Chemother* 12(suppl B):29-37, 1983.

32. deMoragas J, Kierland R: The outcome of patients with herpes zoster, *Arch Dermatol* 75:193, 1957.

33. Doyle PW, Gibson G, Dohlman CH: Herpes zoster ophthalmicus with contralateral hemiplegia: identification of cause, *Ann Neurol* 14:84-85, 1983.

34. Duke-Elder S: *System of ophthalmology*, 342, 808, St Louis, 1963, Mosby.

35. Dunkel E et al.: Rapid detection of herpes simplex virus antigen in human ocular infections, *Curr Eye Res* 7:661, 1988.

35a. Earnshaw D, Bacon T, Darlison S et al.: Mode of antiviral action of penciclovir in MRC-5 cells infected with herpes simplex virus type 1 (HSV-1), HSV-2, and varicella-zoster virus, *Antimicrob Agents Chemother* 36:2747-2757, 1992.

36. Edgerton A: Herpes zoster ophthalmicus: report of cases and review of literature, *Arch Ophthalmol* 34:40-62, 1945.

37. Edgerton A: Herpes zoster ophthalmicus: report of cases and review of literature, *Arch Ophthalmol* 34:114-153, 1945.

38. Edwards T: Ophthalmic complications of varicella, *J Pediatr Ophthalmol* 2:37, 1965.

39. Elliott R: Treatment of herpes zoster with high doses of prednisone, *Lancet* 2:610, 1964.

40. Engstrom RE, Holland GN: Chronic herpes zoster virus keratitis associated with the acquired immunodeficiency syndrome, *Am J Ophthalmol* 105:556-559, 1988.

41. Esiri M, Tomlinson A: Herpes zoster: demonstration of virus in trigeminal nerve and ganglion by immunofluorescence and electron microscopy, *J Neurol Sci* 15:35-38, 1972.

42. Esmann V et al.: Prednisolone does not prevent post-herpetic neuralgia, *Lancet* 2:126, 1987.

43. Fedukowicz HB: *External infections of the eye: bacterial, viral and mycotic*, ed 2, 191, New York, 1978, Appleton-Century-Crofts.

44. Feldman S, Hughes WT, Daniel B: Varicella in children with cancer: seventy-seven cases, *Pediatrics* 56.3:388-396, 1975.

45. Fleisher G et al.: Life threatening complications of varicella, *Am J Dis Child* 135:896, 1981.

46. Forrest W, Kaufman H: Zosteriform herpes simplex, *Am J Ophthalmol* 81:86, 1976.

47. Freidmann-Kein A et al.: Herpes zoster: a possible clinical sign for development of acquired immune deficiency syndrome in high risk individuals, *J Am Acad Dermatol* 14:1023-1028, 1986.

48. Gelb LD et al.: Molecular epidemiology of live, attenuated varicella virus vaccine in children with leukemia and in normal adults, *J Infect Dis* 155.4:633-640, 1987.

49. Gershon A: Varicella in mother and infant. In Krugman S, Gershon A, editors: *Infections of the fetus and the newborn infant*, 79, New York, 1975, Alan R. Liss.

50. Gershon A, Steinberg S: Antibody responses to varicella-zoster virus and the role of antibody in host defense, *Am J Med Sci* 282:12-17, 1981.

51. Gershon A, Steinberg S, Gelb L: Live attenuated varicella vaccine use in immunocompromised children and adults, *Pediatrics* 78(suppl):757-762, 1986.

52. Ghatak NR, Zimmerman HM: Spinal ganglion in herpes zoster, *Arch Pathol* 95:411-415, 1973.

52a. Gheeraert P, The Famciclovir Herpes Zoster Clinical Study Group: Efficacy and safety of famciclovir in the treatment of uncomplicated herpes zoster. *Program and abstracts, 32nd ICAAC, Washington DC, American Society for Microbiology* Abstract 1108, 1992.

53. Gilden D et al.: Varicella-zoster virus DNA in human sensory ganglia, *Nature* 306:478-480, 1983.

54. Gilden D et al.: *Detection of varicella-zoster virus nucleic acids in human thoracic ganglia and leukocytes*, 206, Ann Arbor, 1985.

55. Gilden DH et al.: Detection of varicella-zoster virus nucleic acid in neurons of normal human thoracic ganglia, *Ann Neurol* 22:377-380, 1987.

56. Grant S, Edmond S, Syme J: A prospective study of cytomegalovirus infection in pregnancy. I. Laboratory evidence of congenital infection following maternal primary and reactivated infection, *J Infec* 3:24, 1981.

57. Green W, Zimmerman L: Granulomatous reaction of Descemet's membrane, *Am J Ophthalmol* 64:555, 1967.

58. Grose C, Giller RH: Varicella-zoster virus infection and immunization in the healthy and the immunocompromised host, *Crit Rev Oncol Hematol* 8:27-64, 1988.

59. Harding SP, Lipton JR, Wells JCD: Natural history of herpes zoster ophthalmicus: predictors of postherpetic neuralgia and ocular involvement, *Br J Ophthalmol* 71:353-358, 1987.

60. Hassegawa T: Further electron microscopic observations on herpes zoster virus, *Arch Dermatol* 103:45, 1970.

61. Hayward A et al.: Major histocompatibility complex restriction of T-cell responses to varicella-zoster virus of guinea pigs, *J Virol* 65:1491-1495, 1991.

62. Hazeltine W: Silent HIV infections, *New Eng J Med* 320:1487, 1989.

63. Hedges T III, Albert D: The progression of the ocular abnormalities of herpes zoster: histopathologic observations of nine cases, *Ophthalmology* 89:169-177, 1982.

64. Herbort CP et al.: High-dose oral acyclovir in acute herpes zoster ophthalmicus: the end of the corticosteroid era, *Curr Eye Res* 10(suppl):171-175, 1991.

65. Hilt DC et al.: Herpes zoster ophthalmicus and delayed contralateral hemiparesis caused by cerebral angiitis: diagnosis and management approaches, *Ann Neurol* 14:543-553, 1983.

66. Hirsch M: Herpes group in the immunocompromised host. In Rubin R, Young L, editors: *Clinical approach to infection in the compromised host*, 347-365, New York, 1988, Plenum Publishers.

66a. Hoang-Xuan T, Buchi E, Herbert C et al.: Oral acyclovir for herpes-zoster ophthalmicus, *Ophthalmology* 99:1062-1071, 1992.

67. Hope-Simpson R: The nature of herpes zoster: a long term study and a new hypothesis, *Proc Soc Exp Biol Med* 58:9, 1965.

68. Hung SO, Patterson A, Rees PJ: Pharmacokinetics of oral acyclovir (Zovirax) in the eye, *Br J Ophthalmol* 68:192-195, 1984.

69. Hunt JR: The paralytic complications of herpes zoster of the cephalic extremity, *JAMA* 53:1456-1457, 1909.

70. Hurtig H: Fluphenazine and post-herpetic neuralgia, *JAMA* 263:2750, 1990.

71. Hyman R, Ecker J, Tenser R: Varicella-zoster virus RNA in human trigeminal ganglia, *Lancet* 2:814-816, 1983.

72. Hyndiuk R, Glasser D: Herpes simplex keratitis. In Tabbara KF, Hyndiuk RA, editors: *Infections of the eye*, ed 1, 343, Boston, 1986, Little, Brown.

73. Jacobson MA et al.: Acyclovir-resistant varicells zoster virus infection after chronic oral acyclovir therapy in patients with the acquired immunodeficiency syndrome (AIDS), *Ann Intern Med* 112:187-191, 1990.

74. Jones D: Herpes zoster ophthalmicus. In Golden B, editor: *Ocular inflammatory disease*, 198, IL, 1974, Charles C. Thomas.

75. Juel-Jensen B, MacCallum F: *Herpes simplex, varicella and zoster: clinical manifestations and treatment,* Philadelphia, 1972, JB Lippincott.

76. Junker K et al.: Reinfection with varicella-zoster virus in immunocompromised patients, *Curr Probl Dermatol* 18:152-157, 1989.

77. Kanski JJ: *Clinical ophthalmology,* ed 2, 101-105, London, 1989, Butterworth-Heinemann.

78. Kass E, Aycock R, Finland M: Clinical evaluation of aureomycin and chloramphenicol in herpes zoster, *New Eng J Med* 246:167, 1952.

79. Keczkes K, Basheer A: Do corticosteroids prevent post-herpetic neuralgia?, *Br J Dermatol* 101:551, 1980.

80. Kestelyn P et al.: Severe herpes zoster ophthalmicus in young African adults: a marker for HTLV-III seropositivity, *Br J Ophthalmol* 71:806-809, 1987.

81. Killian JM, Fromm GH: Carbamazepine in the treatment of neuralgia: use and side effects, *Arch Neurol* 19:129-136, 1968.

82. Knoll L, Watson A: Internal ophthalmoplegia following chickenpox, *Can J Ophthalmol* 11:267, 1976.

83. Koneman EW, Allen SD, Dowell VR Jr: *Color atlas and textbook of diagnostic microbiology,* 691-764, Philadelphia, 1988, JB Lippincott.

84. Kowalski R, Gordon YJ: Evaluation of immunologic tests for the detection of ocular herpes simplex virus, *Ophthalmology* 96:1583, 1989.

85. Kvinesdal B et al.: Imipramine treatment of painful diabetic neuropathy, *JAMA* 251:1727, 1984.

86. Lambert S et al.: Ocular manifestations of the congenital varicella syndrome, *Arch Ophthalmol* 107:52, 1989.

87. Lee S et al.: Comparative laboratory diagnosis of experimental herpes simplex keratitis, *Am J Ophthalmol* 109:8, 1990.

88. Levin J et al.: Desipramine enhances opiate postoperative analgesia, *Pain* 27:45, 1986.

89. Levy D, Banerjee A, Glenny H: Cimetidine in the treatment of herpes zoster, *J R Coll Physicians Lond* 19:96, 1985.

90. Lewis G: Zoster sine herpete, *Br Med J* 2:418, 1958.

91. Liesegang T: Varicella-zoster virus: systemic and ocular features, *J Am Acad Dermatol* 11:165, 1984.

92. Liesegang T: Corneal complications from Herpes zoster ophthalmicus, *Ophthalmology* 92:316, 1985.

93. Liesegang T: Herpes zoster ophthalmicus, *Int Ophthalmol Clin* 25(1):77-96, 1985.

94. Liesegang T: Diagnosis and therapy of herpes zoster ophthalmicus, *Ophthalmology* 98:1216-1229, 1991.

95. Liesegang T: The biology and molecular aspects of herpes simplex and varicella zoster virus infections, *Ophthalmology* 99:781-799, 1992.

96. Linnemann Jr C: Pathogenesis of varicella-zoster angiitis in the CNS, *Arch Neurol* 37:239, 1980.

97. Litoff D, Catalano R: Herpes zoster optic neuritis in human immunodeficiency virus infection, *Arch Ophthalmol* 108:782, 1990.

98. Lugo M, Arentsen J: Treatment of neurotrophic ulcers with conjunctival flaps, *Am J Ophthalmol* 103:711, 1987.

99. Machida H: Comparison of susceptibilities of varicella-zoster virus and herpes simplex virus to nucleoside analogs, *Antimicrob Agents Chemother* 29:524-526, 1986.

100. Machida H, Sakata S: In vitro and in vivo antiviral activity of 1-B-D-darabinofuranosyl-E-(2-bromovinyl) uracil (BV-ara U) and related compounds, *Antiviral Res* 4:135-141, 1984.

101. MacKenzie RA, Forbes GS, Karnes WE: Angiographic findings in herpes zoster arteritis, *Ann Neurol* 10:458-461, 1981.

102. Mackie I: Role of the corneal nerves in destructive disease of the cornea, *Trans Ophthalmol Soc UK* 98:343, 1978.

103. Mahalingam R et al.: Latent varicella-zoster viral DNA in human trigeminal and thoracic ganglia, *New Eng J Med* 323:627-631, 1990.

104. Makensen G, Sundmacher R, Witschel D: Late wound complications after circular keratotomy for zoster keratitis, *Cornea* 3:95, 1984.

105. Manka R: Exogenous lactase in the treatment of oral acyclovir intolerance, *Am J Ophthalmol* 108:733, 1989.

106. Marsh RJ: Ophthalmic herpes zoster, *Br J Hosp Med* 15:609-618, 1976.

107. Marsh RJ, Cooper M: Ophthalmic zoster: mucous plaque keratitis, *Br J Ophthalmol* 71:725-728, 1987.

108. Marsh RJ, Cooper M: Ocular surgery in ophthalmic zoster, *Eye* 3:313-317, 1989.

109. Marsh RJ, Dudley B, Kelly V: External ocular motor palsies in ophthalmic zoster: a review, *Br J Ophthalmol* 61:677-682, 1977.

110. Marsh RJ, Easty D, Jones B: Iritis and iris atrophy in herpes zoster ophthalmicus, *Am J Ophthalmol* 78:255, 1974.

111. Matsunaga Y, Yamanishi K, Takahashi M: Experimental infection and immune response of guinea pigs with varicella-zoster virus, *Infect Immun* 27:407-412, 1982.

112. Maudgal P et al.: Varicella-zoster virus in the human corneal endothelium: a case report, *Bull Soc Belge Ophtalmol* 190:71, 1980.

113. Mavligit G, Talpaz M: Cimetidine for herpes zoster, *New Eng J Med* 310:318, 1984.

114. Max MB et al.: Amitriptyline, but not lorazepam, relieves postherpetic neuralgia, *Neurology* 38:1427-1432, 1988.

115. McGeoch D et al.: The complete DNA sequence of the long unique region in the genome of herpes simplex virus type 1, *J Gen Virol* 69:1531-1574, 1988.

116. McGill, J: The enigma of herpes stromal disease, *Br J Ophthalmol* 71:118-125, 1987.

117. McGill J, Chapman C: Comparison of topical acyclovir with steroids in the treatment of herpes zoster keratouveitis, *Br J Ophthalmol* 67:746, 1983.

118. McGill J et al.: Intravenous acyclovir in acute herpes zoster infection, *J Infect* 6:157, 1983.

119. McGill J et al.: Review of acyclovir treatment of ocular herpes zoster and skin infections, *J Antimicrob Chemother* 12(suppl B):45, 1983.

120. Melbye M et al.: Risk of AIDS after herpes zoster, *Lancet* i:728-730, 1987.

121. Merselis J, Kaye D, Hook E: Disseminated herpes zoster, *Arch Intern Med* 113:679, 1961.

122. Meyers JG, Flournoy N, Thomas ED: Cell-mediated immunity to varicella-zoster virus after allogeneic marrow transplantation, *J Infect Dis* 141:479-487, 1980.

123. Miller A: Selective decline in cellular immune response to varicella-zoster in the elderly, *Neurology* 30:582, 1980.

124. Mondino B, Brown S, Mondzelewski J: Peripheral corneal ulcers with herpes zoster ophthalmicus, *Am J Ophthalmol* 86:611, 1978.

125. Montgomery DW: Zoster ophthalmicus with paresis of the facialis, *Times* 14:189, 1904.

126. Muller S, Winklemann R: Cutaneous nerve changes in zoster, *J Invest Dermatol* 52:71, 1969.

127. Murphy T: Post-herpetic neuralgia, *JAMA* 262:3478, 1989.

128. Myers MG, Connelly BL, Stanberry LR: Varicella in hairless guinea pigs, *J Infect Dis* 163:746-751, 1991.

129. Myers MG, Duer HL, Hausler CK: Experimental infection of guinea pigs with varicella-zoster virus, *J Infect Dis* 142:414-420, 1980.

130. Myers MG, Stanberry LR: Drug testing for activity against varicella-zoster virus in hairless guinea pigs, *Antiviral Res* 15:341-344, 1991.

131. Naumann G, Gass J, Font R: Histopathology of herpes zoster ophthalmicus, *Am J Ophthalmol* 65:533, 1968.

132. Nesburn A et al.: Varicella dendritic keratitis, *Invest Ophthalmol* 13:764, 1974.

133. Ostrove J: Molecular biology of varicella-zoster virus, *Adv Virus Res* 38:45-98, 1990.

134. Oxman MN: Varicella and herpes zoster. In Fitzpatrick TB et al., editors: *Dermatology in general medicine: textbook and atlas,* ed 2, New York, 1979, McGraw-Hill.

135. Pavan-Langston D: Varicella-zoster ophthalmicus, *Int Ophthalmol Clin* 15(4):171-185, 1975.

136. Pavan-Langston D: Herpes zoster ophthalmicus: medical and surgical management. In Spaeth G, Katz L, editors: *Current therapy in ophthalmic surgery,* 99, Philadelphia, 1989, BC Decker.

137. Pavan-Langston D: Viral keratitis and conjunctivitis. Clinical disease. Herpetic infections. In Smolin G, Thoft R, editors: *The cornea,* ed 3, 240, Boston, 1994, Little, Brown.

138. Pavan-Langston D, Dunkel E: Principles of antiviral chemotherapy. In Duane T, editor: *Biomedical foundations of ophthalmology,* vol 2, chapter 100; 1-17, Philadelphia, 1986, Harper and Row.

139. Pavan-Langston D, Dunkel E: Herpes zoster ophthalmicus, *Compr Ther* 3-9, 1988.

140. Pavan-Langston D, Dunkel E: Ocular varicella-zoster virus infection in the guinea pig, *Arch Ophthamol* 107:1068-1072, 1989.

141. Pavan-Langston D, McCulley J: Herpes zoster dendritic keratitis, *Arch Ophthalmol* 89:25, 1973.

142. Pepose JS: Skin test with varicella-zoster virus antigen for ophthalmic herpes zoster, *Am J Ophthalmol* 98:825-826, 1984.

143. Pepose JS: External ocular herpesvirus infections in immunodeficiency, *Curr Eye Res* 10(suppl):87-95, 1991.

144. Piebenga L, Laibson P: Dendritic lesions in herpes zoster ophthalmicus, *Arch Ophthalmol* 90:268, 1973.

145. Plotkin J, Reynaud A, Okumoto M: Cytologic study of herpetic keratitis, *Arch Ophthalmol* 85:597, 1971.

146. Portenoy RK, Duma C, Foley KM: Acute herpetic and postherpetic neuralgia: clinical review and current management, *Ann Neurol* 20:651-664, 1986.

147. Preblud S: Age specific risks of varicella complication, *Pediatrics* 68:14, 1981.

148. Preblud S, D'Angelo I: Chickenpox in the United States, 1972-1977, *J Infect Dis* 140:257, 1979.

148a. Pue M, Benet L: Pharmacokinetics of famciclovir in man, *Antiviral Chem Chemother* 4(suppl 1):47-55, 1993.

149. Ragozzino M et al.: Population based study of herpes zoster and its sequellae, *Medicine* 61:310, 1982.

150. Reed J, Joyner S, Knauer W III: Penetrating keratoplasty for herpes zoster keratopathy, *Am J Ophthalmol* 107:257, 1989.

151. Reijo A, Antti V, Jukka M: Endothelial cell loss in herpes zoster keratouveitis, *Br J Ophthalmol* 67:751, 1983.

152. Robb R: Cataracts acquired following varicella infection, *Arch Ophthalmol* 87:352, 1972.

153. Rogers RS, Tindall JP: Geriatric herpes zoster, *J Am Geriatr Soc* 19:495, 1971.

154. Rosenblum W, Hadfield M: Granulomatous angiitis of the nervous system in cases of herpes zoster and lymphosarcoma, *Neurology* 22:348, 1972.

154a. Saltzman R, Jurewicz R, Boon R: Safety of famciclovir in patients with herpes zoster and genital herpes. *Antimicrob Agents Chemother* 38:2454-2457, 1994.

155. Sandor E et al.: Herpes zoster ophthalmicus in patients at risk for the acquired immune deficiency syndrome (AIDS), *Am J Ophthalmol* 101:153, 1986.

156. Sandor E et al.: Herpes zoster ophthalmicus in young patients and its correlation with HTLV-III sensitivity, *ARVO* (abstracts) 28:46, 1987.

157. Satterthwaite J, Tollison C, Kriegel M: Use of tricyclic antidepressants for the treatment of intractable pain, *Comp Ther* 16(4):10, 1990.

158. Sauer GC: Herpes zoster, *Arch Dermatol* 71:488-491, 1955.

159. Scheie H: Herpes zoster ophthalmicus, *Trans Ophthalmol Soc UK* 90:899, 1970.

160. Schulman JS et al.: Acquired immunodeficiency syndrome (AIDS), *Surv Ophthalmol* 31:384-410, 1987.

161. Scott T: Epidemiology of herpetic infections, *Am J Ophthalmol* 43:134, 1957.

162. Seiff S et al.: Use of intravenous acyclovir for treatment of herpes zoster ophthalmicus in patients at risk for AIDS, *Ann Ophthalmol* 20:480, 1988.

163. Shemer Y, Leventon-Kriss S, Sarov I: Isolation and polypeptide characterization of varicella-zoster virus, *Virology* 106:133-140, 1980.

164. Shepp D, Dandliker P, Meyers J: Treatment of varicella-zoster infection in severely immunocompromised patients, *New Eng J Med* 314:208, 1986.

165. Solomon AR: New diagnostic tests for herpes simplex and varicella zoster infections, *J Am Acad Dermatol* 18:218-221, 1988.

166. Stagno S, Whitley R: Herpes virus infections of pregnancy. Part I, Cytomegalovirus and Epstein-Barr virus infections, *New Eng J Med* 313:1270, 1985.

167. Stagno S, Whitley R: Herpes virus infections of pregnancy. Part II, Herpes simplex virus and varicella zoster virus infections, *New Eng J Med* 313:1327, 1985.

168. Stevens D, Merigan TC: Zoster immune globulin prophylaxis of disseminated zoster in compromised hosts, *Arch Intern Med* 140:52-54, 1980.

169. Strachman J: Uveitis associated with chickenpox, *J Pediatr* 46:327, 1955.

170. Straus S et al.: Endonuclease analysis of viral DNA from varicella and subsequent zoster infection in the same patient, *New Eng J Med* 311:1362-1364, 1984.

171. Straus S et al.: NIH conference varicella-zoster virus infections: biology, natural history, treatment, and prevention, *Ann Intern Med* 108:221-237, 1988.

172. Tanaka Y et al.: Reply to 826-7. Pepose JS: Skin test with varicella-zoster virus antigen for ophthalmic herpes zoster, *Am J Ophthalmol* 98:825-826, 1984.

173. Tanaka Y et al.: Skin test with varicella-zoster virus antigen for ophthalmic herpes zoster, *Am J Ophthalmol* 98:7-10, 1984.

174. Taylor D, Ffytche T: Optic disc pigmentation associated with a field defect following chickenpox, *J Pediatr Ophthalmol* 13:80, 1976.

175. Thomas M, Robertson W: Dermal transmission of a virus as a cause of shingles, *Lancet* 2:1349, 1968.

176. Tilson HH: Monitoring the safety of antivirals: the example of the acyclovir experience, *Am J Med* 85(suppl 2A):116-122, 1988.

176a. Tyring S, Nahlik J, Cunningham A et al.: Efficacy and safety of famciclovir in the treatment of patients with herpes zoster. *Program and abstracts, 33rd ICAAC, Washington DC, American Society for Microbiology,* Abstract 1540, 1993.

177. U.S. Department of Commerce, Bureau of Census: United States population, *Federal Census Bureau Publication,* 1984.

178. Uchida Y, Kaneko M, Hayashi K: Varicella dendritic keratitis, *Am J Ophthalmol* 89:259, 1980.

179. Uchida Y, Kaneko M, Onishi Y: Ophthalmic herpes zoster without eruption. In Henkind P, editor: *Acta: XXIV International Congress of Ophthalmol,* 876, Philadelphia, 1983, Lippincott.

180. Urban B et al.: Longer term use of narcotic/antidepressant medication in the management of phantom limb pain, *Pain* 24:191, 1986.

181. Vafai A et al.: Expression of varicella-zoster virus and herpes simplex virus in normal human trigeminal ganglia, *Proc Natl Acad Sci USA* 85:2362-2366, 1988.

182. van der Spuy S, Levy D, Levin W: Cimetidine in the treatment of herpesvirus infections, *S Afr Med J* 58:112, 1980.

183. Vargha P: Facial paralysis as rare complication, *Orvosi Gyak* 15:196, 1938.

184. Vastine V: Adenoviruses and miscellaneous viral infections. In Smolin G, Thoft R, editors: *The cornea,* ed 2, 266, Boston, 1987, Little, Brown.

184a. Vere Hodge R, Cheng Y-C: The mode of action of penciclovir, *Antiviral Agents Chemother* 4(suppl 1):13-24, 1993.

185. Walsh TD: Antidepressants in chronic pain, *Clin Neuropharmacol* 6:271-295, 1983.

186. Waring G, Ekins M: Corneal perforation in herpes zoster ophthalmicus caused by eyelid scarring with exposure keratitis. In Sundmacher R, editor: *Herpetic eye disease,* 469, Munich, 1981, JF Bergman.

187. Watson C, Evans R, Reed K: Amitriptyline vs placebo in postherpetic neuralgia, *Neurology* 32:671, 1982.

188. Watson PN, Evans RJ: Postherpetic neuralgia: a review, *Arch Neurol* 43:836-840, 1986.

189. Watson P et al.: Therapeutic advances in the management of postherpetic neuralgia, *Geriatr Med Today* 70:20, 1988.

190. Weigle KA, Grose C: Molecular dissection of the humoral immune response to individual varicella-zoster viral proteins during chickenpox, quiescence, reinfection, and reactivation, *J Infect Dis* 149:741-749, 1984.

191. Weller T: Varicella and herpes zoster: changing concepts of the natural history, control, and importance of a not so benign virus. Part I, *New Eng J Med* 309:1362-1368, 1983.

192. Weller T: Varicella and herpes zoster: changing concepts of the natural history, control, and importance of a not so benign virus. Part II, *New Eng J Med* 309:1434-1440, 1983.

193. Wilhelmus K, Hamill M, Jones D: Varicella disciform stromal keratitis, *Am J Ophthalmol* 111:575-580, 1991.
194. Wilson II F: Varicella and herpes zoster ophthalmicus. In Tabbara K, Hyndiuk R, editors: *Ocular infections,* 369, Boston, 1986, Little, Brown.
195. Womack L, Liesegang T: Complications of herpes zoster ophthalmicus, *Arch Ophthalmol* 101:42, 1983.

196. Zacks SI, Langfitt HM: Spinal ganglion in herpes zoster, *Arch Pathol* 95:411-415, 1973.
197. Zacks SI, Langfitt TW, Elliott FA: Herpetic neuritis: a light and electron microscopic study, *Neurology* 14:744-750, 1964.
198. Zentmayer W: A case of herpes zoster ophthalmicus complicated by oculomotor palsy, *Am J Med* 4:1007-1008, 1902.

73 Epstein-Barr Virus Diseases

ALICE Y. MATOBA

HISTORICAL BACKGROUND

In 1962 Burkitt[17] suggested that a lymphoma prevalent in East African children might be caused by a virus. In 1964 Epstein and Barr[33] and Pulvertaft[120] established continuous lymphoblastoid cell lines from explants of Burkitt lymphoma. Ultrastructural studies of these cell lines revealed viral profiles with characteristics consistent with a member of the herpesvirus family. Epstein-Barr virus (EBV) was thereby first discovered in 1964 in cultured lymphoblasts from a patient with Burkitt lymphoma.[32]

In 1968 its association with infectious mononucleosis was reported,[56,104] and in 1973 its etiologic role was established.[58] The EBV is the most common causative agent of infectious mononucleosis. EBV has been seroepidemiologically associated with nasopharyngeal carcinoma[100]; and EBV DNA, viral transcripts, and selected viral proteins have been found in these carcinomas.[155] In patients with acquired or congenital forms of immunodeficiency, EBV has been linked to a variety of lymphoproliferative syndromes including lymphoma. In AIDS patients EBV-associated lesions include diffuse polyclonal lymphomas, lymphocytic intestinal pneumonitis, and hairy oral leukoplakia of the tongue.[51] Finally, cumulative seroepidemiologic, in situ hybridization, antigen staining, and polymerase chain reaction studies have linked EBV infection with the pathogenesis of some cells of aqueous tear deficiency and Sjögren syndrome (see Chapter 23).

EPIDEMIOLOGY

Geographic and socioeconomic class-related variations exist in the incidence of EBV seropositivity, although the mechanisms by which these factors influence transmission remain unclear. The virus is transmitted to all individuals in all climates throughout the world and appears endemic even among isolated tribes in New Guinea and the Amazon River basin.

Acquisition of the virus occurs at a younger age in persons of lower socioeconomic class, with 50% to 85% of children acquiring antibodies by age 4. In some populations, particularly in tropical regions, infants appear to become infected soon after the disappearance of transplacentally-acquired antibodies. For those not infected in infancy or early childhood, susceptibility to EBV infection may decline or change, corresponding to the increasing age of the host. This change in communicability may reflect variations in exposure to the virus, differences in inherent host susceptibility, or geographic variables such as climate and temperature.[37,57,103]

The occurrence of seropositivity to EBV varied from 26% to 87% among different groups of New England college students studied between 1958 and 1963; the infection rate as measured by seroconversion was 11.1% per year in the susceptible groups.[103]

In a more recent study of sera from 2000 pregnant women in 1980 to 1981, only 0.6% of women attending an obstetrical clinic were seronegative, whereas 2.9% of women attending a private practice were seronegative.[42] The overall incidence of seropositivity in this population was surprisingly high (98.7%). A 1988 study of 40 normal individuals detected EBV-specific antibodies in 65% of tear and 87.5% of serum samples.[23]

PATHOGENESIS

EBV is transmitted principally via saliva, although transmission can also follow blood transfusion.[49] Continual low-level replication of virus is likely in the oropharynx. Over 85% of acute infectious mononucleosis patients demonstrate continuous or intermittent oropharyngeal excretion of EBV for many months.[88] Immunosuppressed patients, such as allograft or chemotherapy recipients, also have a high rate of oropharyngeal secretion of EBV.[18] It is unknown whether EBV can be transmitted by all patients who excrete virus. Recently EBV was isolated from the uterine cervix[135] and vulvovaginal ulcers in young adult females,[119] and detected in urethral discharges of men attending a clinic for sexually transmitted diseases.[70] These observations raise the possibil-

958

ity of venereal transmission of EBV, although no epidemiologic studies support this contention.

Acute Infection

The major established routes of EBV transmission are exposure to saliva and blood transfusion.[60] EBV usually initiates human infection in the oropharyngeal epithelium. EBV exhibits narrow tropism, and oropharyngeal epithelium, which is permissive for virus replication, probably provides the source of virus for B cell infection in which latent infection is established.[136,144] However, EBV replication has recently been demonstrated in cervical epithelium,[138] and viral genome has been identified in a variety of T cell proliferations including T cell lymphoma,[72] thymic carcinoma,[77] as well as benign polyclonal and monoclonal T cell proliferations.[68,169] Detection of EBV DNA in corneal epithelium[24] and lacrimal gland ductal epithelium[113] suggests that infection of ocular and adnexal epithelium may play a role in the pathogenesis of diseases such as keratitis and tear deficiency. Recently EBV tissue tropism was found to be altered by interaction with the human immune system.[139] When bound to polymeric IgA, EBV entered epithelial cells through secretory component-mediated IgA transport, but it could no longer infect B lymphocytes. These findings suggest one mechanism by which EBV could pass from trafficking B lymphocytes to mucosal epithelium, providing (1) a route by which epithelium other than nasopharyngeal cells, such as ocular or adnexal epithelium, could become infected, and (2) a mechanism by which epithelial infection could "reactivate."

EBV attachment to B lymphocytes is mediated by CR2 (now renamed CD21), an integral B cell membrane glycoprotein of approximately 145 kDa,[21] which is also the receptor for the C3d component of human complement.[39] The protein in the virion envelope that attaches to CR2 is the EBV glycoprotein gp 350/220,[148] which is a product of the BLLF 1 gene.[11] Human B lymphocytes express the C3d receptor prominently,[50] and affinity of gp 350/220 for CR2 in solution is high, exceeding the affinity of C3d for the same protein.[67,93] Recently molecules that share epitopes with the B cell CR2 have been demonstrated on oropharyngeal, nasopharyngeal, and cervical epithelial cells,[147,170,171] as well as peripheral T cells[41] and human follicular dendritic cells.[124] In addition, investigators have shown immunoreactivity with anti-CD21 antibodies in human lacrimal gland ductal epithelia, suprabasal conjunctival and corneal epithelia,[75,76] retinal pigment epithelia, and portions of the ciliary body.[158]

Entry of EBV into B cells occurs either by direct fusion with cell membranes or endocytosis, with direct fusion occurring primarily in lymphoblastoid lines and endocytosis in infection of normal B cells.[67,102,164] Internalization is triggered by the binding of gp 350/220 to CR2. Fusion of the endosome is partially mediated by another membrane glycoprotein, gp 85.[89] The mechanisms of EBV entry and fusion in epithelial cells are poorly understood. Entry of EBV into epithelial cells may occur by direct fusion at the cell surface.[90]

Following penetration of the B lymphocyte, the EBV capsid dissolves, the genome is transported to the cell nucleus, and the DNA circularizes into episomes physically distinct from cellular chromatin.[50] Circularization of the EBV genome is required for establishment of latency and/or transformation of B cell growth to perpetual proliferation.[144]

Latency and Reactivation

Latent infection in in vitro-maintained B cells is characterized by expression of at least 11 viral proteins.[127,130] The six nuclear proteins expressed are numbered EBNA (Epstein-Barr nuclear antigen) 1, 2, 3A, 3B, 3C, and 4, although the nomenclature varies.[127]

EBNA 1 is the most well characterized of the latent infection proteins. It is required to maintain the viral genome in a circular form and may function to initiate DNA replication at *ori* P, the episomal origin of replication.[127,130] EBNA 2 is essential for immortalization of B cells by EBV.[116,119]

EBNA 2 activates a variety of cellular genes including CD23, a B cell activation marker and proposed B cell growth factor; c-fgr, a tyrosine kinase proto-oncogene; and CD21, the EBV receptor.[119]

The functions of EBNA 3A, 3B, and 4 are not well understood. EBV membrane proteins expressed during latency include LMP-1 (latency membrane protein), an integral membrane protein believed to play a role in B cell immortalization,[130] as well as TP 1 (terminal protein, also called LPM 2A), and TP 2 (also called LMP 2B), whose functions are not well understood.[127]

Two other proteins identified in latency are two small polymerase transcripts (EBERs) that localize to the nucleus and associate with the autoantigen La.[130] The function of EBERs in EBV biology is unknown; however, extensively homologous adenovirus VAI RNAs promote efficient protein synthesis.[127,130]

Recently evaluation of viral mRNA sequences in purified uncultured peripheral blood lymphocytes revealed consistent TP 1 gene expression, but no evidence of EBNA or LMP gene expression.[122] The polymerase chain reaction primers used for this study were developed on the basis of structures known from cultured B cells, so that the viral gene expression in uncultured B cells was studied only in terms of the latent states observed in classical tumors and in vitro immortalized cells. Despite this limitation, the consistent expression of TP 1 suggests that the TP gene may have an important role in the latency of EBV, and the lack of EBNA gene expression suggests one mechanism by which latently infected B cells may escape immune surveillance by antigen-specific cytotoxic T cells.

The activation to replication of latent EBV genome is

believed to be mediated by the EBV ZEBRA (Z EB replication activator) gene (BZLF1), which is located within the *Bam* HI Z fragment.[87] Neither BZLF1 mRNA nor the ZEBRA protein is detected in cells that are latently infected.[150] When cells are stimulated by an inducing agent such as butyrate or a phorbol ester, however, both the BZLF1 mRNAs and ZEBRA protein appear.[87] The ZEBRA protein turns on the expression of other EBV genes that encode proteins involved in viral replication. It is not yet clear whether ZEBRA expression is obligatory for entry into the replication pathway or whether other mechanisms for initiation of replication exist. It is believed that (1) additional transcriptional transactivators are needed for activation of the full replication cycle, and (2) the permissivity factors are closely related to cell differentiation, as epithelial cells are much more permissive of replication than lymphocytes.[87]

Humoral and Cellular Immunity

The EBV-infected host mounts both humoral and cellular immune responses. The relative importance of humoral (as opposed to cellular) immunity is still not clearly defined. Following initial infection, which usually occurs in the nasopharyngeal epithelium, viral replication occurs in the nasopharynx, and latent infection of B-lymphocytes develops. Antibody responses are initially directed against antigens associated with the replication cycle, such as viral capsid antigen (VCA) and early antigen (EA). During the convalescent phase antibodies to EBNA and membrane proteins develop. Antibodies directed against glycoproteins of the membrane antigens are virus-neutralizing, and they are believed to be clinically significant in limiting dissemination of virus.[29,50] Antibodies to this group of viral antigens may also mediate antibody-dependent cellular cytotoxicity (ADCC).[111]

Cell-mediated immune responses in primary EBV infection are composed largely of CD8 positive T cells.[30] The early proliferative T cell response appears to be a polyclonal T cell activation,[50] with participation of natural killer cells that mediate relatively nonspecific lysis of EBV-infected cells.[82] Within weeks, development of cytotoxic as well as suppressor T lymphocyte responses directed against virus-infected B cells occurs.[153,161] Following clinical recovery, EBV-specific memory T cells are believed to control the level of EBV-positive B lymphocytes.[97,125] These CTLs are predominantly CD8, MHC class I restricted,[125] although CD4, class II restricted CTLs have been also described.[91] Many of the EBNAs are effective targets for specific CTL lysis.[97,98] In view of recent evidence that many noncultured latently infected B-lymphocytes may not express EBNAs,[122] however, it seems likely that other sites of EBV-specific CTL epitopes exist and may be more clinically significant.

It is evident that EBV is a ubiquitous virus that can survive long-term in human hosts and has the capability of producing wide-ranging disease, despite narrow tissue tropism. Recent studies have shed further light on mechanisms by which EBV may enhance its survival, despite vigorous immune capabilities of the host. Human IL-10, cytokine synthesis inhibiting factor (CSIF), with many immunosuppressive properties including inhibition of IFN 2 by Th1 subset of CD4 T-lymphocytes[40] and T cell activation by monocytes,[142] has been noted to exhibit marked homology to an open reading frame in the EBV genome, BCRF1.[92] BCRF 1 exhibits CSIF activity.[65] The BCRF 1 gene is transcribed during the late phase of the EBV replicative cycle[66] and theoretically may promote infection by inhibition of T lymphocytes. An ancestor of BCRF1 may have been a captured, processed host IL-10 gene,[92] which was retained to enable the virus to employ cytokine mimicry as a survival strategy.

Another example of viral adaptation is the recent finding that peptide residues 416 to 424 of the EBV nucleus antigen-4, which is recognized by (HLA)-A11-restricted CTLs, carry a mutation that abrogates CTL recognition and binding in strains isolated from New Guinea, where A11 positivity is prevalent.[27] In EBV strains from Caucasian and central African populations in which A11 is relatively rare, the epitope is conserved. Thus there is evidence for evolutionary influence by pressure from MHC-restricted CTL responses.

CLINICAL FEATURES

Ocular diseases attributed to EBV infection involve all segments of the eye. Prior to the availability of EBV-specific serologic tests, the association of EBV with ocular disease was documented with hemagglutination tests and the presence of clinical signs compatible with infectious mononucleosis. Infectious agents other than EBV, including cytomegalovirus, adenovirus, *Toxoplasma gondii,* and human herpesvirus 6,[1,59] can produce infectious mononucleosis syndrome, however. Differential absorption, which renders the hemagglutination tests more specific, was not always performed. Therefore early reports of EBV-associated eye disease must be reviewed critically.

Anterior segment diseases reported prior to the availability of virus-specific tests include conjunctivitis,* episcleritis,[71,78] dacryoadenitis,[71] dacryocystitis,[8] keratitis, and iritis.[110,149] Conjunctivitis was frequently noted; however, the possible heterogeneous nature of the patients is suggested by the variability of the clinical descriptions, which ranged from dry, granular[46,54,149] to follicular[71,163] in appearance, with a reported incidence of 5%[163] to 38%.[7]

Neurologic complications documented only by clinical signs and/or hemagglutination tests were reported in 1% to 23%[14,73] of patients with infectious mononucleosis, with approximately 45% having ocular manifestations.[14] Major findings include disturbance of ocular motility,[25,52,101] papilledema or optic neuritis,[15,43,116,149] impaired accommoda-

---

*References 7, 14, 71, 78, 149, 163.

tion,[151] and a peripheral facial nerve palsy.[14] Retinitis described as edema of the macula[73] or retinitis with hemorrhages and perivasculitis[71] has also been reported.

Conjunctiva and Lacrimal System

EBV-associated external ocular diseases documented by EBV-specific serologic tests include acute dacryocystitis,[143] Parinaud oculoglandular syndrome,[86] conjunctival mass, and Sjögren syndrome.[47,115,165] Steele and Meyer[143] described an 8-year-old boy who developed bilateral lacrimal sac distention in conjunction with acute infectious mononucleosis. The conjunctival injection preceded the onset of systemic signs by 2 weeks. Steele and Mayer speculated that the Epstein-Barr virus may have invaded the nasal lacrimal duct or junctional nasal epithelium with resultant nasolacrimal duct obstruction and secondary bacterial infection. Culture of the right lacrimal sac discharge grew coagulase-negative *Staphylococcus* spp. The patient improved with antibiotic therapy.

In 1981 Meisler and associates[86] reported that an 11-year-old boy developed infectious mononucleosis concomitantly with (1) oculoglandular syndrome with marked preauricular and cervical lymphadenopathy, (2) conjunctivitis, and (3) a firm, nontender mass of the right superior tarsal conjunctiva. Biopsy of the conjunctival mass revealed "fibrous tissue heavily infiltrated with mature and immature lymphoid cells in a perivascular distribution," with large multinucleated cells. The conjunctivitis and lymphadenopathy resolved with resolution of the systemic disease.

Gardner and associates[46] described a 38-year-old man who developed primary EBV infection documented by (1) a positive IgM titer to VCA and (2) a negative titer to Epstein-Barr nuclear antigen. Eleven days after system signs and symptoms developed, a painless, 1×2-cm salmon-colored mass appeared on the supranasal bulbar conjunctiva of the left eye. No keratitis, diffuse conjunctivitis, or iritis was present. Pathologic evaluation revealed an extensive cellular infiltrate consisting primarily of mature lymphocytes and plasma cells. Immunocytologic analysis of the biopsy specimen disclosed the presence of Epstein-Barr latent membrane protein and nuclear protein 2, associated with a small percentage of the lymphocytes. Control specimens failed to stain with either antiserum. The conjunctival mass and cervical lymphadenopathy resolved over the following 3 weeks with only supportive therapy.

Sjögren syndrome has been rarely reported following infectious mononucleosis.[48,105,115,165] Whittingham and associates[165] described an 18-year-old woman who had contracted Sjögren syndrome (confirmed by labial salivary gland biopsy), along with Raynaud phenomenon and immune-mediated thrombocytopenic purpura, 4 years following a protracted course of clinical infectious mononucleosis (IM). Specific cytotoxic T lymphocyte responses to Epstein-Barr virus-infected cells were defective. In 1987

Pflugfelder and associates[115] described two patients with biopsy-confirmed Sjögren syndrome, whose symptoms developed within 1 to 2 months following the onset of infectious mononucleosis. One patient had serologic evidence of a recent primary EBV infection, and the second patient had EBV titers consistent with a viral carrier state. A potential role of Epstein-Barr virus in the pathogenesis of Sjögren syndrome is discussed in detail in Chapter 23.

Cornea and Sclera

Epstein-Barr virus has been implicated as a cause of several forms of corneal disease. A patient with multifocal epithelial dendritic keratitis in association with infectious mononucleosis was described by Wilhelmus.[166] Epstein-Barr virus was cultured from conjunctival and tear samples. The corneal lesions healed within 2 days with topical acyclovir therapy. In 1990 Pflugfelder and associates[114] reported that a 66-year-old woman contracted bilateral multifocal dendritic keratitis 4 days after undergoing a chemical facial peel. An impression cytology specimen of the corneal epithelium exhibited strong staining by an immunoperoxidase technique with a monoclonal antibody to Epstein-Barr virus early antigen. EBV DNA was also detected by polymerase chain reaction. Pflugfelder and associates suggested that the phorbol esters contained in the chemical peel may have induced Epstein-Barr virus replication in latently infected cells. The dendrites resolved in 4 weeks with topical trifluridine therapy, although it is uncertain if this agent has any clinical antiviral activity against EBV. EBV DNA has also been demonstrated by polymerase chain reaction in a number of intraocular tissues including iris, ciliary body, retina, retinal pigment epithelium, and choroid; although it is not possible to discern the specific cellular source of EBV in these locations.[159]

Corneal stromal disease associated with EBV infection involves all layers.[83,84,117,154] Subepithelial infiltrates resembling lesions associated with adenoviral keratoconjunctivitis have been described in two patients.[83] In one patient the infiltrates occurred at the time of acute primary infection with EBV, whereas the second patient had a 23-month history of recurrent subepithelial infiltration in both eyes. Serologic tests indicated acute or previous EBV infection and negative antibody titers for adenovirus.

Multifocal nonsuppurative stromal keratitis has been described by several authors.[84,117] Pinnolis and associates[117] described discrete, translucent, gray-white, coin-shaped lesions involving 360 degrees of the peripheral cornea, at all levels of depth. The patient was a 16-year-old boy with severe infectious mononucleosis treated with oral prednisone. The lesions were noted 2 weeks following discontinuation of the prednisone.

Matoba and associates[84] reported three patients with discrete, sharply demarcated, multifocal, pleomorphic or ring-shaped, granular anterior stromal opacities with clear intervening stroma as well as one patient with multifocal midstromal nondiscrete infiltrates[84] (Fig. 73-1). The association with EBV infection was based on (1) positive serologic tests for Epstein-Barr virus-specific antigens and (2) negative titers for antibodies against other potential causes of multifocal stromal keratitis, including adenovirus and herpes simplex virus.

Peripheral infiltrative keratitis has been recounted by several authors[84,98,108,150,166] (Fig. 73-2). The infiltrates are associated with stromal vascularization and may involve the deep stroma or full-thickness cornea in a confluent fashion. In one patient nodular scleritis was noted 6 weeks following discontinuation of topical corticosteroids to which the keratitis was responsive.[84] Associated clinical and laboratory profiles varied from symptomatic primary EBV infection or chronic severe Epstein-Barr virus disease to asymptomatic with serologic evidence of past infection.

A 71-year-old woman had bilateral necrotizing scleritis with peripheral corneal ulcers. Serology revealed elevated levels of anti-VCA and anti-early antigen. Immunofluorescence testing of conjunctival squamous epithelium showed staining for VCA.[45]

Recently elevated titers of IgG antibodies to EBV capsid antigen were noted in patients with iridocorneal endothelial syndrome.[154] The serologic profiles suggest that patients with iridocorneal endothelial syndrome have a cellular immune abnormality sufficient to permit reactivation of latent EBV infection. The significance of this finding to the pathogenesis of iridocorneal endothelial syndrome is not clear.

Posterior Segment

Posterior segment diseases reported in patients with acute EBV infection include retinitis,[74,123] uveitis,[74,123,134,167] and choroiditis.[167] Raymond and associates[123] described a patient who had EBV-associated infectious mononucleosis with

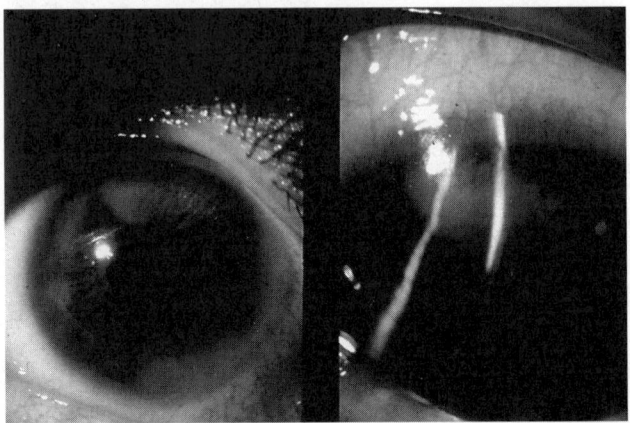

Fig 73-2. Peripheral infiltrative keratitis in a patient with serologic evidence of recent infection with Epstein-Barr virus and absent antibodies against herpes simplex virus and *Treponema pallidum*.

"punctate outer retinitis" characterized by gray-white deep retinal lesions (measuring 50 to 75 μm in diameter). Vitritis was also noted. Kelly and associates[74] depicted a 17-year-old male patient with retinitis of the posterior pole, with retinal hemorrhages, vascular sheathing, and vitritis. Optic disc edema was also noted. Primary EBV infections were well documented serologically; however, antibody to toxoplasma was also detected. The patients improved following antitoxoplasma therapy. It is not clear whether the retinitis was caused directly by EBV or by reactivation of infection with *Toxoplasma gondii*. Usui and associates[157] postulated that EBV plays a role in the pathogenesis of Vogt-Koyanagi-Harada (VKH) syndrome, following amplification of EBV genomic sequences in 75% of cerebrospinal fluid of VKH patients, but not in controls with other disorders.[157]

X-linked lymphoproliferative disease is an inherited disorder rendering affected males susceptible to fatal infectious mononucleosis, aplastic anemia, malignant lymphoma, and hypogammaglobulinemia after EBV infection. Retinal necrosis was seen in a fatal case of X-linked lymphoproliferative disease, but it is unknown whether the retinal necrosis was due to active EBV infection or to a host inflammatory response.[53]

Uveitis

Uveitis ranging from an anterior uveitis (responsive to topical steroid therapy) to a severe panuveitis with vitritis and macular edema (responsive only to topical and systemic steroids and acyclovir with pars plana vitrectomy) has been noted in three patients with well-documented atypical EBV infections.[167] The infections were characterized by persistent severe systemic manifestations and high antibody titers to EBV-specific antigens. Another three cases of EBV-associated uveitis were characterized by a common flulike prodrome, bilateral involvement, severe acute anterior uveitis

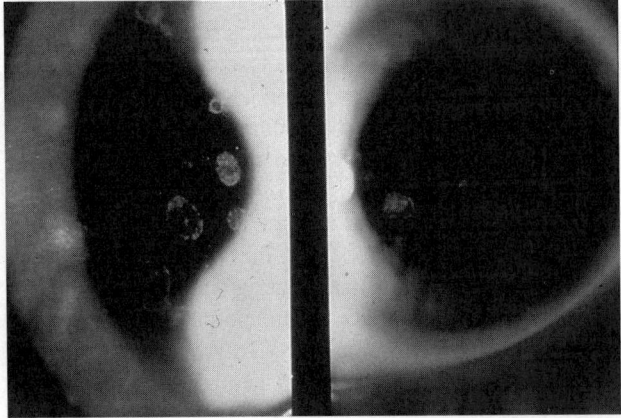

Fig 73-1. Anterior and midstromal, granular, sharply demarcated, pauciinflammatory lesions in a patient with serologic evidence of EBV infection and absent antibodies against herpes simplex virus, adenovirus, and *Treponema pallidum*.

with fibrinous exudate, granulomatous anterior uveitis in the chronic stage, disc hyperemia edema, and a sunset glow fundus.[156]

In 1987 Tiedeman[152] reported positive antibody titers to viral capsid antigen IgM (or early antigen) in 10 patients with multifocal choroiditis, whereas all 8 control patients had nondetectable antibody levels. He suggested that multifocal choroiditis might be associated with an active or a persistent state of EBV infection with incomplete immunologic resolution of the infection. Details of the evaluation of the study group to rule out other potential causes of choroiditis were not provided, however. Subsequently Spaide and associates[141] found that neither their group of 11 patients with multifocal choroiditis nor the control group had increased antiviral capsid antigen IgM titers. No difference could be detected in the serologic profiles between the two groups. Spaide and associates concluded that their study did not support the hypothesis that patients with multifocal choroiditis and panuveitis have serologic evidence of atypically active Epstein-Barr virus infection.

Central Nervous System

Approximately 5% of patients with infectious mononucleosis develop neurologic complications.[134] Neuro-ophthalmologic manifestations of EBV infection documented by EBV-specific serologic tests include optic nerve edema in association with retinitis or uveitis,[167] abducens nerve palsy,[146] ophthalmoplegia as a manifestation of Fisher syndrome,[69,140] opsoclonus,[28] and optic neuritis.[121,145]

Isolated abducens nerve delay palsy has been reported in children aged 3½ to 5 years, in association with primary Epstein-Barr viral infection.[146] Spontaneous recovery was noted in one case, but persistent esotropia requiring surgical correction was also documented.

Fisher syndrome, characterized by acute ophthalmoplegia, ataxia, and areflexia, is believed related to Guillain-Barré syndrome or acute idiopathic polyradiculopathy. The course of development of the ophthalmoplegia was rapid in all cases, but the time of onset varied from immediately following a flulike illness[140] to a 2-month delay.[69] Most patients recovered fully following systemic corticosteroid therapy. In one patient persistent deficiency of smooth pursuit was documented.[69] Opsoclonus was noted in a 71-year-old woman with acute onset of vertigo, tremulousness, unsteadiness, and oscillopsia.[28] Antibody titers to EBV viral capsid antigen and early antigen were elevated in both the serum and cerebral spinal fluid. The authors believed that the patient had acute central nervous system infection with EBV. The patient had a complete recovery over several weeks without any treatment.

Retrobulbar pain and blurred vision developed in a 13-year-old boy 2 weeks following the onset of an influenzalike illness.[121] Chiasmal neuritis was diagnosed based on characteristic visual field defects and the absence of other lesions on a CT scan of the head and orbits. Serum antibody levels were compatible with primary EBV infection; however, cerebrospinal fluid antibodies were nondetectable. Following institution of systemic corticosteroid therapy the visual field defects resolved, but persistently reduced contrast sensitivity was noted in one eye. Optic neruritis was reported in an 8-year-old boy with encephalitis. Titers of antibodies for Epstein-Barr viral capsid antigen and nuclear antigen were diagnostic of recent primary infection. The patient recovered fully following systemic dexamethasone therapy.[145]

Systemic Disease

The clinical features of systemic primary Epstein-Barr virus infection include the classic triad of fever, sore throat, and lymphadenopathy with frequent enlargement of the spleen and liver. Prodromal symptoms include chills, sweats, anorexia, malaise, headache, arthralgia, and myalgia.[13]

VIROLOGY

Epstein-Barr virus is a member of the genus *Lymphocryptovirus*, which belongs to the subfamily Gammaherpesvirinae.[75] EBV has a protein core encased in DNA, a nucleocapsid with 162 capsomeres, a protein tegument surrounding the nucleocapsid, and an outer envelope with external glycoprotein spikes.

The EBV genome is a linear, double-stranded, 172-kilobase-pair DNA. The EBV genome was the first herpesvirus whose genome was completely cloned and sequenced.[9] Comparison of the EBV genome to other herpesvirus genes reveals regions with distant homology at the DNA or protein level.[9,22,26] Major replication-cycle EBV genes are located in relatively conserved domains. Antigenic cross-reactivity between EBV and other human herpesviruses is rare, however.[75]

Two EBV types have been identified, EBV-1 and EBV-2 (or EBV-A, EBV-B), based primarily on differences in the latent infection genes.[6,162] The two types of EBV encode antigenically distinct Epstein-Barr nuclear antigens called EBNAs 2, 3, and 4;[129,133] the B type of strains show a reduced efficiency of transformation of B lymphocytes.[126]

Traditionally, it was believed that the geographic distribution of the two types of EBV was quite different, with EBV-2 primarily segregated to equatorial Africa and Papua, New Guinea; and EBV-1 predominantly in the United States and Europe.[173] A recent study of subjects in Memphis, Tennessee, however, identified EBV-2 in 41% of 157 healthy adults, with 9% carrying both types of EBV.[137] Therefore there is evidence for worldwide distribution of both EBV-1 and EBV-2.

LABORATORY INVESTIGATIONS

The laboratory diagnosis of primary Epstein-Barr viral infection is made on the basis of compatible hematologic findings and appropriate serology. In approximately 70% of cases a relative and absolute lymphocytosis occurs, peaking during the second or third week of illness. Atypical lymphocytes account for about 30% of the differential.[13,85] Other laboratory abnormalities include mild granulocytopenia, elevation of liver transaminases, and mild elevation of bilirubin.[13]

Traditionally, serologic diagnosis of Epstein-Barr viral infection has depended on the detection of heterophile antibodies, which are predominantly IgM antibodies that act with antigens on horse and sheep red blood cells. These antibodies are present in 80% to 90% of patients with acute infectious mononucleosis,[37] peaking between the second and third week of illness and detectable for up to 1 year.[59] The monospot is a rapid slide agglutination test that uses stabilized horse red blood cells as the agglutinating antigen. This test is highly specific for EBV infection, with a low frequency of false positive results (< 3%)[10,59]; however, the antibody remains undetectable in 10% to 20% of individuals with acute infection.[36] Recently a commercially available rapid immunochromatographic test has also been shown to accurately detect infectious mononucleosis-associated heterophile antibodies (sensitivity 91%, specifically 100%).[38] EBV-specific antiviral antibody tests are useful for diagnosis of (1) patients with suspected EBV infection with negative heterophile antibody tests, (2) patients suspected of past EBV infection, and (3) subjects with an atypical immunologic response to EBV.

The most clinically useful EBV-specific serologic tests are measurements of antibody levels against viral capsid antigen, Epstein-Barr nuclear antigen, and early antigen. Patients with acute infectious mononucleosis usually have elevated IgM and IgG antibodies against VCA.[59] The IgM component becomes nondetectable 4 to 8 weeks after the onset of symptoms, but the IgG component persists for life.[61] EBV EAs are detectable 2 to 4 weeks after the onset of symptoms of acute IM.[1] Two of the EA antigens are differentiated based on their distribution within the host cell: early antigen-diffuse (EA-D) and early antigen-restricted (EA-R).[13] In most cases antibodies to EAs become nondetectable within 2 to 6 months. Persistence of both EA-R and EA-D antibodies has been described in patients with atypical or severe infections[64]; however, asymptomatic subjects also have persistence of elevated antibodies to EA.[63] Anti-EBNA antibodies are absent until several weeks or months after the onset of clinical disease, but remain detectable for life.[59,61] The presence of elevated VCA IgM or IgG antibodies in association with rising (fourfold increase) EBNA antibodies is diagnostic of recent EBV infection.[59,61] Elevated VCA IgM antibodies with nondetectable EBNA antibodies are also consistent with acute EBV infection. Long-term persistence of antibodies against EA in conjunction with clinical features consistent with persistent active infection may suggest an atypical course with inadequate or inappropriate immune responses of the host.

THERAPY

Epstein-Barr virus can cause productive infection in epithelial cells and a mainly latent, persistent infection in lymphoid cells. Inhibitors of viral replication include nucleoside analogs such as acyclovir [9-(2-hydroxyethoxy-methyl)-guanine],[128] bromovinyldeoxyuridine,[79] and 9-[(1,3-dihydroxy-2-propoxy) methyl] guanine (ganciclovir).[19] Acyclovir, a synthetic acyclic nucleoside compound, has potent inhibitory activity against herpes simplex virus (types 1 and 2) and less activity against other herpesviruses (including varicella-zoster virus, cytomegalovirus, and Epstein-Barr virus).[128] Bromovinyldeoxyuridine is a stronger inhibitor of EBV replication in vitro, however, it is more toxic than acyclovir.[79] Ganciclovir has substantial bone marrow toxicity at potentially effective doses.[19] Zidovudine (AZT), a potent inhibitor of human immunodeficiency virus and other retroviruses, also has significant activity against Epstein-Barr virus.[44] In combination with either IFN-α or IFN-γ, zidovudine can inhibit transformation of human umbilical cord lymphocytes by Epstein-Barr virus.[80] Recently 28-mer phosphorothioate oligodeoxynucleotides (S-oligos) were reported to have a potent inhibitory effect on EBV replication in cell culture.[168] They may constitute a new class of drug with potential efficacy against replicating EBV. None of these drugs have been demonstrated to affect EBV genome in the latent state, however.[20,132]

Acyclovir has been used most extensively to treat patients with EBV infection. Both intravenous and oral administration can achieve significant serum and tissue levels.[106] Ocular penetration of acyclovir following local administration has been studied in rabbits. Subconjunctival injection of 25 mg acyclovir led to aqueous levels that can inhibit DNA replication in vitro,[131] but topical application of 3% acyclovir ointment led to low aqueous concentrations.[118] Ocular formulations of acyclovir are not commercially available in the United States.

Management of Acute Infection

Infectious mononucleosis is usually a self-limited illness requiring little more than bed rest during the acute phase. Supportive measures such as saline gargles and oral nonsteroidal antiinflammatory drugs may be useful.[8] Four double-masked controlled clinical studies[3,5,107] demonstrated no significant effect of systemic acyclovir on clinical symptoms. Both intravenous acyclovir (10 mg/kg 3 times a day) and oral acyclovir (800 mg 5 times per day for 7 days) produced inhibition of oropharyngeal EBV replication, but viral shedding resumed after cessation of therapy.[3,5,107] Systemic corticosteroid therapy reduces both fever and pharyngitis in young adults with infectious mononucleosis.[12,16] Steroid therapy, however, is not recommended in the routine management of patients with IM. In patients with fulminant disease, combined therapy with intravenous acyclovir (10 mg/kg thrice daily) and prednisolone (0.7 mg/kg tapered for 10 days) may reduce the duration of fever and oropharyngeal symptoms.[4] Currently the effects of combined therapy with systemic acyclovir, corticosteroids, and interferon-α are being studied.[2]

Management of Ocular Disease

Guidelines for the therapy of EBV-associated ocular disease are not well established because of the small number of reported cases. The patient with lacrimal duct obstruction and secondary bacterial infection responded well to antibiotic therapy directed against the bacterial infectious component of the disease.[143] Tarsal and bulbar conjunctival lesions have resolved following excisional biopsy[86] or spontaneously.[46]

Long-term follow-up of patients with Sjögren syndrome following infectious mononucleosis has not been described. Because there is evidence of more extensive infection of lacrimal gland ductal epithelium in patients with Sjögren syndrome compared to patients with no symptoms of tear deficiency,[112] systemic therapy with acyclovir and possibly corticosteroids may theoretically be of benefit, however, there are no clinical data to support this possibility.

Epithelial keratitis, which is presumably caused by replicative infection of the epithelium, is self-limited in the course of infectious mononucleosis,[166] but it may have a prolonged course if inciting factors (such as exposure to phorbol esters) are involved.[114] Oral acyclovir (800 mg 5 times daily) is appropriate therapy, although there are no reports of proven efficacy or benefit. Stromal inflammatory disease attributed to EBV infection responds to topical corticosteroid therapy. Prednisolone acetate or prednisolone phosphate 1% (1 drop 4 times daily or every 2 hours) is recommended. Concurrent antiviral therapy is not necessary if other potential etiologic agents (such as herpes simplex) have been excluded. Other systemic infections (such as lues) should be considered and excluded in the deep stromal infiltrative form of the keratitis.

Posterior segment diseases (such as panuveitis, choroiditis, and papillitis) in patients with persistently symptomatic EBV infection have been reported to improve with acyclovir and corticosteroid therapy administered systemically and topically.[167] Neither therapy appeared to induce long-term remission reliably, however. In patients with retinitis, infection with *Toxoplasma gondii* should be excluded.

Neuro-ophthalmologic complications associated with EBV infection are usually self-limited and/or responsive to systemic corticosteroid therapy.[69,121,145] Neurologic disease should be managed in cooperation with a neurologist.

PREVENTION

Epstein-Barr virus is a ubiquitous virus that infects more than 95% of the human population worldwide; therefore, avoidance of exposure is not feasible. The severity of disease associated with EBV depends on the status of the host. Infection at an early age most frequently leads to seroconversion without symptoms, and infection at adolescence or in adulthood leads to infectious mononucleosis syndrome in approximately 50% of cases.[94] The vast majority of patients recover clinically, although the infection persists for life. In patients with immune deficiency, however, EBV-associated lymphomas occur with a high incidence. Organ transplant recipients, patients with acquired immunodeficiency syndrome, and patients with Duncan syndrome (an X-linked disorder characterized by defective cellular immune responses) are particularly vulnerable.[55,99] Endemic Burkitt lymphoma, the commonest childhood tumor in Africa, and undifferentiated nasopharyngeal carcinoma, the commonest tumor of men in Southern China,[109] have both been linked to EBV infection.[81,172,174] Recent studies also suggest that Hodgkin lymphoma may be connected with EBV infection.[62] The association of EBV with lymphoid and epithelial cell malignancies has provided an impetus to develop a vaccine.

Antibodies directed against viral cell-surface membrane antigen complex are virus-neutralizing in vitro.[29] The membrane antigen complex consists of three envelope glycoproteins: gp 350, gp 220, and gp 85.[105] Gp 350 and gp 220 are encoded by the same open reading frame.[11] Gp 350 is the virus ligand that binds to its host cell receptor.[148]

In the cottontop tamarin model of EBV-induced B cell tumors, gp 350 is an effective vaccine.[34] The efficacy, however, is dependent on the degree and mode of purification.[35,91] Recombinant-derived gp 350 vaccine is protective in the marmoset EBV-induced infectious mononucleosis model.[31] Although subunit vaccines do not generate as broad-ranging an immune response as attenuated, live, recombinant virus vaccines, they have the advantages of (1) no risk of serious infection in immune-compromised individuals, (2) absence of potential virus reverters, and (3) lack of potentially oncogenic EBV DNA.[95,96] The gp 350 subunit EBV vaccine is considered a promising candidate for use in human trials.[95,96]

REFERENCES

1. Akashi K, Eizuru Y, Sumiyoshi Y et al.: Brief report: severe infectious mononucleosis-like syndrome and primary human herpesvirus 6 infection in an adult, *N Engl J Med* 329:168-171, 1993.
2. Andersson JP: Clinical aspects of Epstein-Barr virus infection, *Scand J Infect Dis Suppl* 78:94-104, 1991.
3. Andersson J, Britton S, Ernberg I et al.: Effect of acyclovir on infectious mononucleosis: a double-blind, placebo-controlled study, *J Infect Dis* 153:283-290, 1986.
4. Andersson J, Ernberg I: Management in Epstein-Barr virus infections, *Am J Med* 88(suppl 2A):108-115, 1988.
5. Andersson J, Sköldberg B, Henle W et al.: Acyclovir treatment in infectious mononucleosis: a clinical and virological study, *Infection* 15(suppl 1):14-21, 1987.
6. Arrand JR, Young LS, Tugwood JD: Two families of sequences in the small RNA-encoding region of Epstein-Barr virus (EBV) types A and B, *J Virol* 63:983-986, 1989.
7. Ash HH, Arbogast JL: Infectious mononucleosis, *J Indiana Med Assoc* 35:562-564, 1942.
8. Atkinson PL, Ansons AM, Patterson A: Infectious mononucleosis presenting as bilateral acute dacryocystitis, *Br J Ophthalmol* 74:750, 1990.

9. Baer R, Bankier AT, Biggin MD et al.: DNA sequence and expression of the B95-8 Epstein-Barr virus genome, *Nature* 310:207-211, 1984.

10. Basson V, Sharp AA: Monospot: a differential slide test for infectious mononucleosis, *J Clin Pathol* 22:324-325, 1969.

11. Beisel B, Tanner JT, Matsuto T et al.: Two major outer envelope glycoproteins of Epstein-Barr virus are encoded by the same gene, *J Virol* 54:665-674, 1985.

12. Bender CE: The value of corticosteroids in the treatment of infectious mononucleosis, *JAMA* 199:529-531, 1967.

13. Benson CA, Kessler HA: Update: Epstein-Barr virus-related disease, *Compr Ther* 14(3):58-64, 1988.

14. Bernstein TC, Wolfe HG: Involvement of the nervous system in infectious mononucleosis, *Ann Int Med* 33:1120-1138, 1950.

15. Blaustein A, Caccavo A: Infectious mononucleosis complicated by bilateral papilloretinal edema, *Arch Ophthalmol* 43:853-856, 1950.

16. Bolden KJ: Corticosteroids in the treatment of infectious mononucleosis, *J R Coll Gen Pract* 22:87-95, 1972.

17. Burkitt D: Determining the climatic limitations of a children's cancer common in Africa, *Br Med J* 2:1019-1023, 1962.

18. Chang RS, Lewis JP, Abildgaard CF: Prevalence of oropharyngeal excretes of leukocyte-transforming agents among a human population, *New Eng J Med* 289:1325-1329, 1973.

19. Cheng YC, Huang ES, Lin J-C et al.: Unique spectrum of activity of 9-[(1,3-dihydroxy-2-propoxy) methyl]-guanine against herpes-viruses in vitro and its mode of action against herpes simplex type 1, *Proc Natl Acad Sci USA* 80:2767-2770, 1983.

20. Colby BM, Shaw JE, Elion GB et al.: Effect of acyclovir [9-(2-hydroxyethoxy methyl) guanine] on Epstein-Barr virus DNA replication, *J Virol* 34:560-568, 1980.

21. Cooper NR, Moore MD, Nemerow NR: Immunobiology of CR2, the B lymphocyte receptor for Epstein-Barr virus and the C3d complement fragment, *Ann Rev Immunol* 6:85-113, 1988.

22. Cossta RH, Draper KG, Kelly TJ, Wagner EK: An unusual HSV-1 transcript with sequence homology to EBV DNA, *J Virol* 54:317-328, 1985.

23. Coyle PK, Sibony PA: Viral antibodies in normal tears, *Invest Ophthalmol Vis Sci* 29:1552-1558, 1988.

24. Crouse CA, Pflugfelder SC, Pereira I et al.: Detection of herpes viral genomes in normal and diseased corneal epithelium, *Curr Eye Res* 9:569-581, 1990.

25. Davie JC, Ceballos R, Little SC: Infectious mononucleosis with fatal neuronitis, *Arch Neurol* 9:265-272, 1963.

26. Davison AJ, Taylor P: Genetic relations between varicella-zoster virus and Epstein-Barr virus, *J Gen Virol* 68:1067-1079, 1987.

27. de Campos-Lima P-O, Gavioli R, Zhang Q-J et al.: HLA-A11 epitope loss isolates of Epstein-Barr virus from a highly A11+ population, *Science* 260:98-100, 1993.

28. Delreux V, Kevers L, Callewaert A, Sindic C: Opsoclonus secondary to an Epstein-Barr virus infection, *Arch Neurol* 46:480-481, 1989.

29. de Schryver A, Klein G, Hewetson J et al.: Comparison of EBV neutralization tests based on abortive infection or transformation of lymphoid cells and their relation to membrane reactive antibodies (anti-MA), *Int J Cancer* 13:353-362, 1974.

30. de Waele M, Thielemans C, Van Camp BKG: Characterization of immunoregulatory T cells in EBV-induced infectious mononucleosis by monoclonal antibodies, *New Eng J Med* 304:460-462, 1981.

31. Emini EA, Schleit WA, Siberklang M et al.: Vero cell-expressed Epstein-Barr virus (EBV) gp 350/220 protects marmosets from EBV challenge, *J Med Virol* 27:120-123, 1989.

32. Epstein MA, Achong BG, Barr YM: Virus particles in cultured lymphoblasts from Burkitt's lymphoma, *Lancet* i:702-703, 1964.

33. Epstein MA, Barr YM: Cultivation in vitro of human lymphoblasts from Burkitt's malignant lymphoma, *Lancet* 1:252-253, 1964.

34. Epstein MA, Morgan AJ, Finerty S et al.: Protection of cotton top tamarins against Epstein-Barr virus-induced malignant lymphoma by a prototype subunit vaccine, *Nature* 318:287-289, 1985.

35. Epstein MA, Randle BJ, Finerty S, Kirkwood JK: Not all potently neutralizing, vaccine-induced antibodies to Epstein-Barr virus ensure protection of susceptible experimental animals, *Clin Exp Immunol* 63:485-490, 1986.

36. Erlich KS: Laboratory diagnosis of herpesvirus infections, *Clin Lab Med* 7:759-776, 1987.

37. Evans AS, Niederman JC, Cenabre LC et al.: A prospective evaluation of heterophile and Epstein-Barr virus specific IgM antibody tests in clinical and subclinical infectious mononucleosis. Specificity and sensitivity of the tests and persistence of antibody, *J Infect Dis* 132:546-554, 1975.

38. Farhat SE, Finn S, Chua R et al.: Rapid detection of infectious mononucleosis-associated heterophile antibodies by a novel immunochromato-graphic assay and a latex agglutination test, *J Clin Microbiol* 31:1597-1600, 1993.

39. Fingeroth JD, Weiss JJ, Tedder TF et al.: Epstein-Barr virus receptor of human B lymphocytes is the C3d receptor CR2, *Proc Natl Acad Sci USA* 81:4510-4514, 1984.

40. Fiorentino DF, Zlotnik A, Vieria P et al.: IL-10 acts on the antigen-presenting cell to inhibit cytokine production by th1 cells, *J Immunol* 146:3444-3451, 1991.

41. Fischer E, Delibrias C, Kazatchkine MD: Expression of CR2 (the C3 dg/EBV receptor CD21) on normal human peripheral blood T lymphocytes, *J Immunol* 146:865-869, 1991.

42. Fleisher GR, Bolognese R: Seroepidemiology of Epstein-Barr virus in pregnant women, *J Infect Dis* 145:537-541, 1982.

43. Frey T: Optic neuritis in children. Infectious mononucleosis as an etiology, *Doc Ophthalmol* 34:183-188, 1973.

44. Furman PA, Barry DW: Spectrum of activity antiviral activity and mechanism of action of zidovudine, *Am J Med* 85(suppl 2A):176-181, 1988.

45. Furukawa H, Hamada T, Nagaya K et al.: A case of necrotizing scleritis associated with Epstein-Barr virus infection, *J Jpn Ophthalmol Soc* 97:1337-1342, 1993.

46. Gardner BP, Margolis TP, Mondino BJ: Conjunctival lymphocytic nodule associated with the Epstein-Barr virus, *Am J Ophthalmol* 112:567-571, 1991.

47. Reference deleted in proofs.

48. Gaston JSH, Rowe M, Bacon P: Sjögren's syndrome after infection by Epstein-Barr virus, *J Rheumatol* 17:558-561, 1990.

49. Gerber P, Walsh JN, Rosenblun EN, Purcell PH: Association of EB-virus infection with the post perfusion syndrome, *Lancet* 1:593-596, 1969.

50. Giller RH, Grose C: Epstein-Barr virus: the hematologic and oncologic consequences of virus-host interaction, *Crit Rev Oncol Hematol* 9:149-195, 1989.

51. Greensparre JS, Greeneparr D, Lennette ET et al.: Replication of Epstein-Barr virus within the lesions of oral "hairy" leukophakia, an AIDS-associated lesion, *New Eng J Med* 313:1564-1571, 1985.

52. Grose C, Henle W, Henle G, Feorino PM: Primary Epstein-Barr virus infections in acute neurologic diseases, *N Engl J Med* 292:392-395, 1975.

53. Grossnilaus HE, Aaberg TM, Purmell EW et al.: Retinal necrosis in x-linked kynphoproliferative disease, *Ophthalmology* 101:705-709, 1994.

54. Guthrie CC, Pessel JF: An epidemic of "grandular fever" in a preparatory school for boys, *Am J Dis Child* 29:492-496, 1925.

55. Hanto DW, Frizzera G, Gajl-Peczalska KJ et al.: Epstein-Barr virus-induced B-cell lymphoma after renal transplantation: acyclovir therapy and transition from polyclonal to monoclonal B0-cell proliferation, *New Eng J Med* 306:913-918, 1982.

56. Henle G, Henle W, Diehl V: Relation of Burkitt's tumor-associated Herpestype virus to infectious mononucleosis, *Proc Natl Acad Sci USA* 59:94-101, 1968.

57. Henle W, Henle G: Observations on childhood infections with the Epstein Barr virus, *J Infect Dis* 121:303-310, 1970.

58. Henle W, Henle G: Epstein-Barr virus and infectious mononucleosis, *N Engl J Med* 288:263-264, 1973.

59. Henle W, Henle G: Serodiagnosis of infectious mononucleosis, *Resident Staff Physician* 27:37-43, 1981.

60. Henle W, Henle G, Harrison FS et al.: Antibody responses to the Epstein-Barr virus and cytomegaloviruses after open-heart and other surgery, *New Eng J Med* 282:1068-1074, 1968.

61. Henle W, Henle GE, Horwitz CA: Epstein-Barr virus specific diagnostic tests in infectious mononucleosis, *Hum Pathol* 5:551-565, 1974.

62. Herbst H, Niedobitek G, Kneba M et al.: High incidence of Epstein-Barr virus genomes in Hodgkin's disease, *Am J Pathol* 137:13-18, 1990.

63. Horwitz CA, Henle W, Henle G et al.: Long-term serological follow-up of patients for Epstein-Barr virus after recovery, from infectious mononucleosis, *J Infect Dis* 151:1150-1153, 1985.

64. Horwitz CA, Henle W, Henle G, Schmitz H: Clinical evaluation of patients with infectious mononucleosis and component of the Epstein-Barr virus-induced early antigen complex, *Am J Med* 58:330-338, 1975.

65. Hsu DH, de Waal Malefyt R, Fiorentino DF et al.: Expression of IL-10 activity by Epstein-Barr virus protein BCRF1, *Science* 250:830-832, 1990.

66. Hudson GS, Bankier AT, Satchwell SC, Barrell BG: The short unique region of the B95-8 Epstein-Barr virus genome, *Virology* 147:81-98, 1985.

67. Hutt-Fletcher L: Epstein-Barr virus tissue tropism: a major determinant of immunopathogenesis, *Springer Semin Immunopathol* 13:117-131, 1991.

68. Ishihara S, Tawa A, Yamura-Yagi M et al.: Clonal T-cell lymphoproliferation containing Epstein-Barr (EB) virus in a patient with chronic active EB virus infection, *Jpn J Cancer Res* 80:99-103, 1989.

69. Ishikawa H, Wakakura M, Ishikawa S: Enhanced ptosis in Fisher's syndrome after Epstein-Barr virus infection, *J Clin Neuroophthalmol* 10(3):197-200, 1990.

70. Israele V, Shirley P, Sixbey JW: Excretion of the Epstein-Barr virus from the genital tract of men, *J Infect Dis* 163:1341-1343, 1991.

71. Jones BR, Howie JB, Wilson RP: Ocular aspects of an epidemic of infectious mononucleosis, *Pro Univ Otago Med Sch* 30:1-4, 1952.

72. Jones JF, Shurim S, Abramowsky C et al.: T-cell lymphomas containing Epstein-Barr virus DNA in patients with chronic Epstein-Barr virus infections, *New Eng J Med* 318:733-741, 1988.

73. Karpe G, Wising P: Retinal changes with acute reduction of vision as initial symptoms of infectious mononucleosis, *Acta Ophthalmol* 26:19-24, 1948.

74. Kelly SP, Rosenthal AR, Nicholson KG, Woodward CG: Retinochoroiditis in acute Epstein-Barr virus infection, *Br J Ophthalmol* 73:1002-1003, 1989.

75. Kieff E, Liebowitz D: Epstein-Barr virus and its replication. In Fields BN, Knipe DM, editors: *Virology,* 1889-1920, New York, 1990, Raven Press.

76. Leine J, Pflugfelder SC, Yen M et al.: Detection of the complement (CD21)/EBV receptor in human lacrimal gland and ocular surface epithelia, *Reg Immunol* 3:164-170, 1990.

77. Leyvraz S, Henle W, Chahinian AP et al.: Association of Epstein-Barr virus with thymic carcinoma, *N Engl J Med* 312:1296-1299, 1985.

78. Librach IM: Ocular symptoms in glandular fever, *Br J Ophthalmol* 40:619-621, 1956.

79. Lin JC, Machida H: Comparison of two bromovinyl nucleoside analogs, 1-beta-D-arabino-furanosyl-E-5-(2-bromovinyl) uracil and E-5 (2-bromovinyl)-2'-deoxyuridine, *Antimicrob Agents Chemother* 32:1068-1072, 1988.

80. Lin J-C, Zhang Z-Xi, Chou T-C et al.: Synergistic inhibition of Epstein-Barr virus: transformation of B lymphocytes by α- and γ-interferon and by 3'-azido-3'-deoxy-thymidine, *J Infect Dis* 159:248-254, 1989.

81. Magrath I: The pathogenesis of Burkitt's lymphoma, *Adv Cancer Res* 55:133-270, 1990.

82. Masucci MG, Bejarano MT, Masucci G, Klein E: Large granular lymphocytes inhibit the in vitro growth of autologous Epstein-Barr virus infected B cells, *Cell Immunol* 76:311-321, 1983.

83. Matoba AY, Jones DB: Corneal subepithelial infiltrates associated with systemic Epstein-Barr viral infection, *Ophthalmology* 94:1669-1671, 1987.

84. Matoba AY, Wilhelmus KR, Jones DB: Epstein-Barr viral stromal keratitis, *Ophthalmology* 93:746-751, 1986.

85. Mauer AM: Mononucleosis and lymphocytosis. In Stein JH, editor: *Internal medicine,* 1086-1090, Boston, 1987, Little, Brown.

86. Meisler DM, Bosworth DE, Krachmer JH: Ocular infectious mononucleosis manifested as Parinaud's oculoglandular syndrome, *Am J Ophthalmology* 92:722-726, 1981.

87. Miller G: The switch between latency and replication of Epstein-Barr virus, *J Infect Dis* 161:833-844, 1990.

88. Miller G, Niederman JC, Andrews LL: Prolonged oropharyngeal excretion of EB virus following infectious mononucleosis, *New Eng J Med* 288:229-232, 1973.

89. Miller N, Hutt-Fletcher LM: A monoclonal antibody to glycoprotein gp inhibits fusion but not attachment of Epstein-Barr virus, *J Virol* 62:2366-2372, 1988.

90. Miller N, Hutt-Fletcher LM: Epstein-Barr virus enters B cells and epithelial cells by different routes, *J Virol* 66:3409-3414, 1992.

91. Misko IS, Pope JH, Hutter R et al.: HLA-DR-antigen-associated restriction of EBV-specific-T-cell colonies, *Int J Cancer* 33:239-243, 1984.

92. Moore KW, Rousset F, Banchereau J: Evolving principles in immunopathology: interleukin 10 and its relationship to Epstein-Barr virus protein BCRF1, *Springer Semin Immunopathol* 13:157-166, 1991.

93. Moore MD, DiScipio RG, Cooper NR, Nemerow GR: Hydrodynamic, electron microscopic and ligand-binding analysis of the Epstein-Barr virus/ C3 dg receptor (CR2), *J Biol Chem* 34:20576-20582, 1989.

94. Morgan AJ: Control of viral disease: the development of Epstein-Barr virus vaccines, *Springer Semin Immunopathol* 13:249-262, 1991.

95. Morgan AJ: Epstein-Barr virus vaccines, *Vaccine* 10:563-571, 1992.

96. Morgan AJ, Allison AC, Finerty S et al.: Validation of a first-generation Epstein-Barr virus vaccine preparation suitable for human use, *J Med Virol* 29:74-78, 1989.

97. Moss DJ, Misko IS, Sculley TB et al.: Immune regulation of Epstein-Barr virus (EBV): EBV nuclear antigen as a target for EBV-specific T cell lysis, *Springer Semin Immunopathol* 13:147-156, 1991.

98. Moss DJ, Rickinson AB, Pope JH: Long-term T-cell mediated immunity to Epstein-Barr virus in man. I. Complete regression of virus-induced transformation in cultures of sero-positive donor leukocytes, *Int J Cancer* 22:662-668, 1978.

99. Nalesnik MA: Lymphoproliferative disease in organ transplant recipients, *Springer Seminars in Immunopathol* 13:199-216, 1991.

100. Neel HB, Person GR, Weiland LH and associates: Application of Epstein-Barr virus serology to the diagnosis and staging of North America patients with nasopharyngeal carcinoma, *Otolaryngol Head Neck Surg* 91:255-262, 1983.

101. Nelhaus G: Isolated oculomotor nerve palsy in infectious mononucleosis, *Neurology* 16:221-224, 1966.

102. Nemerow GR, Cooper Nr. Early events in the infection of human B lymphocytes by Epstein-Barr virus: the internalization process, *Virology* 132:186-198, 1984.

103. Niederman JC, Evans AS, Subrahmanyan MS, McCollum RW: Prevalence, incidence and persistence of EB virus antibody in young adults, *New Eng J Med* 282:361-365, 1970.

104. Niederman JC, McCollum RW, Henle G and associates: Infectious mononucleosis: clinical manifestations in relation to EB virus antibodies, *JAMA* 203:205-209, 1968.

105. North JR, Morgan AJ, Epstein MA: Observation on the EBV envelope and virus-determined membrane antigen (MA) polypeptides, *Int J Cancer* 26:231-240, 1980.

106. O'Brien JJ, Campoli-Richards DM: Acyclovir: an updated review of its antiviral activity, pharmacokinetic properties and therapeutic efficacy, *Drugs* 37:233-309, 1989.

107. Pagano JS, Sixbey JW, Lin J-C: Acyclovir and Epstein-Barr virus infection, *J Infect Dis* 153:283-290, 1986.

108. Palay DA, Litoff D, Krachmer JH: Stromal keratitis associated with Epstein-Barr virus infection in a young child, *Arch Ophthalmol* 111:1323-1324, 1993.

109. Parkin DM, Stjemsward J, Muir CS: Estimates for the worldwide frequency of twelve major cancers, *Bull WHO* 62:163-182, 1984.

110. Payrau P, Höel J: Mononucleose infectieuse et keratitis, *Bull Soc Ophtalmol Fr* 5-6:381-384, 1958.

111. Pearson GR: In vitro and in vivo investigations on antibody-dependent cellular cytotoxicity, *Curr Top Microbiol Immunol* 80:65-96, 1978.

112. Pflugfelder SC, Crouse CA, Atherton SS: Ophthalmic manifestations of Epstein-Barr virus infection, *Int Ophthalmol Vis Sci* 33:95-101, 1993.

113. Pflugfelder SC, Crouse CA, Pereira I, Atherton SS: Amplification of Epstein-Barr virus genomic sequences in blood cells, lacrimal glands, and tears from primary Sjögren's syndrome patients, *Ophthalmology* 97:976-984, 1990.

114. Pflugfelder SC, Huang A, Crouse C: Epstein-Barr virus keratitis after a chemical facial peel, *Am J Ophthalmology* 110:571-573, 1990.

115. Plugfelder SC, Roussel TJ, Culbertson WW: Primary Sjögren's syndrome after infectious monoclueosis, *JAMA* 257:1049-1050, 1987 (letter).

116. Piel JJ, Thelander HE, Shaw EB: Infectious mononucleosis of the central nervous system with bilateral papilledema, *J Pediatr* 37:661-665, 1950.

117. Pinnolis M, McCulley JP: Nummular keratitis associated with infectious mononucleosis, *Am J Ophthalmol* 89:791-794, 1980.

118. Poirier RH, Kingham JD, de Miranda P et al.: Intraocular antiviral penetration, *Arch Ophthalmol* 100:1694-1967, 1982.

119. Portnoy J, Ahronheim GA, Ghibu F et al.: Recovery of Epstein-Barr virus from genital ulcers, *New Eng J Med* 311:966-968, 1984.

120. Pulvertaft RJV: Cytology of Burkitt's tumor (African lymphoma), *Lancet* 1:238-240, 1964.

121. Purvin V, Herr GJ, DeMyer W: Chiasmal neuritis as a complication of Epstein-Barr virus infection, *Arch Neurol* 45:458-460, 1988.

122. Qu L, Rowe DT: Epstein-Barr virus latent gene expression in uncultured peripheral blood lymphocytes, *J Virol* 66:3715-3724, 1992.

123. Raymond LA, Wilson CA, Linnemann CC et al.: Punctate outer retinitis in acute Epstein-Barr virus infection, *Am J Ophthalmol* 104:424-426, 1987.

124. Reynes M, Albert JP, Cohen JHM et al.: Human follicular dendritic cells express CR 1, CR 2, CR 3 complement receptor antigens, *J Immunol* 135:2687-2694, 1985.

125. Rickinson AB, Moss DJ, Wallace LE et al.: Long term cell-mediated immunity to Epstein-Barr virus, *Cancer Res* 41:4216-4221, 1981.

126. Rickinson AB, Young LS, Rowe M: Influence of the Epstein-Barr virus nuclear antigen. EBNA 2 on the growth phenotype of virus-transformed B cells, *J Virol* 61:1310-1317, 1987.

127. Rogers RP, Strominger JL, Speck SH: Epstein-Barr virus in B lymphocytes: viral gene expression and function in latency, *Adv Cancer Res* 58:1-26, 1992.

128. Rosenberry KR, Bryan CK, Soln CA: Acyclovir: evaluation of a new antiviral agent, *Clin Pharm* 1:399-406, 1982.

129. Rowe M, Young LS, Cadwallader K et al.: Distinction between Epstein-Barr virus type A (EBNA 2A) and type B (EBNA 2B) isolates extend to the EBNA 3 family of nuclear proteins, *J Virol* 63:1031-1039, 1989.

130. Sample C, Kieff E: Molecular basis for Epstein-Barr virus induced pathogenesis and disease, *Springer Semin Immunopathol* 13:133-146, 1991.

131. Schulman J, Peyman GA, Fiscella R et al.: Intraocular acyclovir levels after subconjunctival and topical administration, *Br J Ophthalmol* 70:138-140, 1986.

132. Schuster V, Kreth HW: Epstein-Barr virus infection and associated diseases in children. II. Diagnostic and therapeutic strategies, *Eur J Pediatr* 151:794-798, 1992.

133. Sculley TB, Apolloni A, Moss DJ et al.: Expression of Epstein-Barr nuclear antigens 3, 4, and 6 are altered in cell lines containing B type virus, *Virology* 171:401-408, 1989.

134. Silverstein A, Steinberg G, Nathanson M: Nervous system involvement in infectious mononucleosis, *Arch Neurol* 26:352-358, 1972.

135. Sixbey JW, Lemon SM, Pagano JS: A second site for Epstein-Barr virus shedding: the uterine cervix, *Lancet* 2:1122-1124, 1986.

136. Sixbey JW, Nedrud JG, Raab-Traub N et al.: Epstein-Barr virus replication in oropharyngeal epithelial cells, *N Engl J Med* 310:1225-1230, 1984.

137. Sixbey JW, Shirley P, Chesney PJ et al.: Detection of a second widespread strain of Epstein-Barr virus, *Lancet II:* 761-765, 1989.

138. Sixbey JW, Vesterinen EH, Nedrud JG et al.: Replication of Epstein-Barr virus in human epithelial cells infected in vitro, *Nature* 306:480-483, 1983.

139. Sixbey JW, Yao Q-Y: Immunoglobulin A-induced shift of Epstein-Barr virus tissue tropism, *Science* 255:1578-1580, 1992.

140. Slavick HE, Shapiro RA: Fisher's syndrome associated with Epstein-Barr virus, *Arch Neurol* 38:134-135, 1981.

141. Spaide RF, Sugin S, Yannuzzi LA, deRosa JT: Epstein-Barr virus antibodies in multifocal choroiditis and panuveitis, *Am J Ophthalmol* 112:410-413, 1991.

142. Spits H, de Waal Malefyt R: Functional characterization of human IL-10, *Int Arch Allergy Immunol* 99:8-15, 1992.

143. Steele RJ, Meyer DR: Nasolacrimal duct obstruction and acute dacryocystitis associated with infectious mononucleosis (Epstein-Barr virus), *Am J Ophthalmol* 115:265-266, 1993.

144. Stevens JG: Human herpesviruses: a consideration of the latent state, *Microbiol Rev* 53:318-332, 1989.

145. Straussberg R, Amir J, Cohen HA et al.: Epstein-Barr virus infection associated with encephalitis and optic neuritis, *J Pediatr Ophthalmol Strabismus* 30:262-263, 1993.

146. Straussberg R, Cohen AH, Amir J, Varsano I: Benign abducens palsy associated with EBV infection, *J Pediatr Ophthalmol Strabismus* 30:60, 1993.

147. Talacko AA, Teo CG, Griffin BE, Johnson NW: Epstein-Barr virus receptors but not viral DNA are present in normal and malignant oral epithelium, *J Oral Pathol Med* 20:20-25, 1991.

148. Tanner J, Weis J, Fearon D et al.: Epstein-Barr virus gp 350/220 mediates absorption, capping and endocytosis, *Cell* 50:202-213, 1987.

149. Tanner OR: Ocular manifestations of infectious mononucleosis, *Arch Ophthalmol* 51:229-241, 1952.

150. Taylor N, Countryman J, Rooney C et al.: Expression of the BZLF1 latency-disrupting gene differs in standard and defective Epstein-Barr viruses, *J Virol* 63:1721-1728, 1989.

151. Thal LS, Phillip SR, Stark L: Paralysis of accommodation in infectious mononucleosis, *Am J Optom Physiol Optics* 54:19-26, 1977.

152. Tiedeman JS: Epstein-Barr viral antibodies in multifocal choroiditis and panuveitis, *Am J Ophthalmol* 103:659-663, 1987.

153. Tosato GI, Magrath I, Koski I et al.: Activation of suppressor T cells during Epstein-Barr virus induced infectious mononucleosis, *New Eng J Med* 301:1133-1137, 1979.

154. Tsai CS, Ritch R, Strauss SE et al.: Antibodies to Epstein-Barr virus in iridocorneal endothelial syndrome, *Arch Ophthalmol* 108:1572-1576, 1990.

155. Tugwood JD, Lau WH, Sai-kio SY: Epstein-Barr virus-specific transformation in normal and malignant nasopharyngeal biopsies and in lymphocytes from healthy donor and infectious mononucleosis patients, *J Gen Virol* 68:1081-1091, 1987.

156. Usui M, Sakai J: Three cases of Epstein-Barr virus-associated uveitis, *Int Ophthalmol* 4:371-376, 1990.

157. Usui M, Usui N, Goto H et al.: Detection of Epstein-Barr virus DNA by polymerase chain reaction in cerebral spinal fluid from patients with Vogt-Koyanagi-Harada disease, *Invest Ophthalmol Vis Sci* 32:807, 1991.

158. Usui N, Sakai J, Usui M et al.: Expression of the Epstein-Barr virus receptors in normal human intraocular tissue, *J Eye* (Atarashii Granka) 10(3):435-440, 1993.

159. Usui N, Sakai J, Usui M et al.: Detection of herpesvirus DNA in intraocular tissues, *J Jpn Ophthalmol Soc* 98(5):443-448, 1994.

160. Van der Horst C, Joncas J, Ahronheim G et al.: Lack of effect of peroral acyclovir for the treatment of acute infectious mononucleosis, *J Infect Dis* 164:788-792, 1991.

161. Wallace LE, Rickinson AB, Rowe M, Epstein MA: Epstein-Barr virus specific cytotoxic T cell clones are restricted through a single HLA antigen, *Nature* 297:413-415, 1982.

162. Wang F, Petti L, Braun D et al.: A bicistronic Epstein-Barr virus mRNA encodes two nuclear proteins in latently infected, growth transformed lymphocytes, *J Virol* 61:945-954, 1987.

163. Weschler HF, Rosenblum AH, Sills AT: Infectious mononucleosis: report of an epidemic in an army post, part II, *Ann Int Med* 25:236-260, 1946.

164. White J, Kielian K, Helenius A: Membrane fusion proteins of enveloped animal viruses, *Q Rev Biophys* 16:151-195, 1983.

165. Whittingham S, McNeilage J, Mackay IR: Primary Sjögren's syndrome following infectious mononucleosis, *Ann Int Med* 102:490-493, 1985.

166. Wilhelmus KR: Ocular involvement in infectious mononucleosis, *Am J Ophthalmol* 91:117-118, 1981.

167. Wong KW, D'Amico DJ, Hedges III TR et al.: Ocular involvement associated with chronic Epstein-Barr virus infection, *Br J Ophthalmol* 73:1002-1003, 1989.

168. Yao G-Q, Grill S, Egan W, Cheng Y-C: Potent inhibition of Epstein-Barr virus replication by phosphorothioate oligodeoxynucleotides with sequence specification, *Antimicrob Agents Chemother* 37:1420-1425, 1993.

169. Yoneda N, Tatsumi E, Kawanishi M et al.: Detection of Epstein-Barr virus genome in benign polyclonal proliferative T cells of a young male patient, *Blood* 76:172-177, 1990.
170. Young LS, Clark D, Sixbey JW, Rickinson AB: Epstein-Barr virus receptors on human pharyngeal epithelial, *Lancet* I:240-242, 1986.
171. Young LS, Dawson CW, Rickinson AB: Epstein-Barr virus/complement receptor and epithelial cells, *Lancet* II:448-450, 1989.

172. Zeng Y: Seroepidemiological studies on nasopharyngeal carcinoma in China, *Adv Cancer Res* 44:121-138, 1985.
173. Zimber U, Aldinger HK, Lenoir GM et al.: Geographic prevalence of two Epstein-Barr virus types, *Virology* 154:56-66, 1986.
174. zur Hausen H, Schulte-Holthausen H, Klein G et al.: EBV-virus DNA in biopsies of Burkitt tumors and anaplastic carcinomas of the nasopharynx, *Nature* 228:1956-1958, 1970.

74 Bacterial Keratitis

KIRK R. WILHELMUS

Corneal infection is a leading cause of visual loss. Multiple microorganisms, varying by geography and risk factors, can produce microbial keratitis. Bacterial keratitis is the most common cause of suppurative corneal ulceration.

Local and systemic factors that predispose to corneal infection involve a breakdown of defense mechanisms. Once bacteria enter the cornea, microbial virulence factors direct the pathogenic potential of individual species. The subsequent interplay between bacterial proliferation and tissue inflammation leads to the clinical picture of bacterial keratitis. Understanding how bacteria invade the cornea and how the host responds provides the basis for appropriate diagnosis and management.

HISTORICAL BACKGROUND

The diagnosis of bacterial infection of the cornea, as distinguished from other ocular inflammatory disorders, has been possible only within the past 100 years. Microbial keratitis, however, has undoubtedly occurred throughout history and can be inferred by reexamining past texts from a more recent perspective.[175]

The Ancient World

The Ebers Papyrus, written in Egypt in approximately 1550 B.C., mentions eye pain and opacification for which an ointment, containing antimony sulfide imported from the Arabian Peninsula and thickened with honey, was used. Sanskrit manuscripts originating in India around 500 B.C. differentiate superficial, peripheral corneal ulcers that were potentially curable from central, deep, and extensive ulcerations or perforations that were not.

The Hippocratic books of approximately 400 B.C. cautioned that treatment was not generally effective for purulent eye conditions, especially those that progressed to perforation and iris prolapse. These sources mentioned hypopyon as a sign of advanced disease and noted that the severity of corneal inflammation correlated with the extent of subsequent scarring, graded according to density as fog, nebula,

macula, and leukoma. Except for warm compresses and drinking wine, Hippocrates offered little in the way of therapy for ocular inflammation, although the ancient Greeks did have topical copper-containing compounds. Surgical puncturing of the eye was mentioned as a treatment option to evacuate anterior-chamber pus, but visual loss generally followed.

Celsus (25 B.C.-58 A.D.), Galen (129-199 A.D.), and many subsequent authors restated the Hippocratic findings that appear to pertain to corneal infection. Galen advised zinc oxide, antimony compounds, copper derivatives, and astringents derived from plant extracts (e.g., myrrh, frankincense, and saffron). Arabic texts recommended that medications for topical ophthalmic use be diluted with egg white, sap, or human milk and suggested pain relief with belladonna or mandrake extracts. Patients were warned not to cry out, sneeze, or vomit lest perforation occur.

The Middle Ages

Few improvements in the management of microbial keratitis were made over the next several centuries, although various remedies were apparently tried. One of the first published ophthalmic texts, written by a 12th century oculist, warned "against nostrums that only aggravate the sufferings of the patient, in consequence of which the eyes are bleached so that they never return to their normal condition. In many instances the ocular humors are destroyed by severe pain, the result of improper applications, the contents of the eyes run out between the eyelids, and this misfortune is followed by total loss of sight."[149]

Bloodletting by peripheral venesection and the application of leeches was frequently used, sometimes to the point of patient unconsciousness. Reaching a peak in the early 19th century, bleeding for corneal ulceration sometimes included conjunctival scarification. The practice was based on the belief that blood "is the fuel by which the fire is kept up"[3] but abated during the mid1800s when better observers noted no benefit from this practice. Laxatives, emetics, diuretics, and a strict diet were often recommended. Poultices were made from warm water, bread and milk, egg yolks, egg whites, the pulp of roasted apples, tobacco infusion, poppy tea, camomile tea, or rose water. Their frequent application was advised as a soothing and antiphlogistic emollient. In retrospect, egg white contains lysozyme and milk has lactoferrin, substances that might have had a beneficial antibacterial effect; but ingredients such as pigeon's dung were probably injurious. Some thought the whole idea of herbal compresses was absurd, being "at a loss to conceive how persons who know so much of this part of medicine, should persist in such ridiculous trifling." [242]

Various topical agents were tried (Table 74-1), administered with an eyecup or other device. Spicy infusions and wine were used to dissolve certain ingredients. Lotions and ointments were thickened with various substances ranging from butter and sugar to the fat of vipers and baked millipedes. Irrigation of the eye was done with an animal's bladder or undine. Continuous immersion of the eye in an antiseptic solution was achieved by molding clay around the eye.

The term *ophthalmia* was originally used by Hippocrates principally to denote conjunctivitis but came to be applied to various ocular inflammatory disorders, including bacterial keratitis. Acute "hot" ophthalmia was distinguished from "cold" ophthalmia by its symptoms and signs of pain, light sensitivity, tearing, discharge, and hyperemia. Ophthalmitis sclerotica designated eyeball inflammation that sometimes led to corneal ulceration and hypopyon, but differentiating infectious from noninfectious disorders in retrospect is problematic. Before the discovery of microorganisms, ophthalmias were attributed to various physical stimulants and viewed as varying in severity but not necessarily cause.

Trauma was particularly likely to lead to corneal inflammation that could rapidly spread from the injured site to involve the entire eye. Stromal destruction usually proceeded rapidly but seemed to slow as the Descemet membrane was exposed. Subsequent perforation with leakage of aqueous humor and iris prolapse was not uncommon. The resemblance of the dark, exposed iris to a housefly's head produced the short-lived term *myocephalon*. Because of the common occurrence of various ophthalmias, specialized textbooks detailing these entities were compiled during the late 18th century. [307,457]

The Age of Experimentation

The first clear description of keratitis was by Wardrop in the early 19th century. Rather than grouping ocular inflammatory disorders under the nonspecific term "ophthalmia," Wardrop used a topographic description based upon the involved tissue. He clearly summarized the typical symptoms of suppurative keratitis: "Inflammation of the cornea is . . . accompanied by more or less general fever, pain in the eye extending to the head, intolerance of light, increased

TABLE 74-1 TREATMENT OPTIONS FOR BACTERIAL KERATITIS BEFORE THE ANTIBIOTIC ERA

Topical Agents	Surgical Techniques
Antiseptics and astringents	Cauterization and debridement
Boric acid	Caustics (absolute alcohol, bile,
Camphor	carbolic acid, hydrogen
Cupric sulfate	peroxide, iodine tincture,
Cupric tartrate	lactic acid, silver nitrate,
Formol	trichloroacetic acid, zinc
Hydrogen peroxide	sulfate)
Iodine compounds	Cryotherapy
Lead acetate	Curettage
Mercuric cyanide	Thermal cautery (diathermy,
Mercuric chloride	direct heat, electrocautery,
Mercuric muriate	proximal heat, steam, hot air)
Silver nitrate	Conjunctival surgery
Zinc carbonate	Conjunctival flap
Zinc chloride	Conjunctival transplant
Zinc oxide	Peritomy
Zinc sulfate	Tarsorrhaphy
Extracts	Corneal surgery
Lysozyme	Corneal incision
Optochin	Lamellar keratectomy
Pyocyanin	Paracentesis
Resorcin	Trephination
Trypsin	Irradiation
Subconjunctival injection	Beta-irradiation
Oxygen	Phototherapy
Saline	Radiotherapy
Mercuric chloride	Ultrasound
Sublimate	Ultraviolet light
Miscellaneous agents	Fever therapy
Antipneumococcal serum	Pyrogen injection (blood,
Antidiphtheritic serum	endotoxin, milk, typhoid
Blood and plasma	vaccine)
Carotene	Passive heating or steam bath
Cod-liver oil	Turpentine seton
Coffee	Miscellaneous
Hypertonic glucose	Blockage of ciliary or stellate
Honey	ganglion
Insulin	Bloodletting: leeches, wet-
Placental extract	cupping
Quinine	

secretion of tears, and impaired vision. . . . It most frequently arises from wounds and other external causes. . . . During the progress of the violent inflammation, purulent matter is formed between the lamellae of the cornea, which by ulceration either discharges itself internally into the anterior chamber or externally, leaving an ulcer of the cornea." [456]

This mistaken belief that hypopyon was due to a posterior rupture of a corneal abscess persisted into the early 20th century and probably contributed to the idea for therapeutic corneal surgical incisions.[217] Further impetus for surgery arose from the observation that "if the anterior chamber be opened simply by the ulcerative process, the efforts of nature may succeed in repairing the injury."[374] The technique of paracentesis had changed little since the time of Hippocrates. Based on recommendations of Paré, a medieval ophthalmic text advised the surgeon to retract the lids with one hand and "with the other hand with the pointe of a launcet hee shall finally and cunningly picke the hornie membrane untill hee come to the slimie matter."[155] Surgical recommendations varied from draining the hypopyon or aqueous humor via the uninvolved limbal cornea to directly incising the ulcer bed. A small wound was usually advised "or the crystalline lens, on the sudden discharge of the matter and aqueous humor, may likewise protrude and be discharged."[361] Additional techniques aimed to reduce iris adhesions at the incision site.

Keratocentesis was believed to stimulate healing, to prevent a large spontaneous perforation, and to alleviate the pain from secondary glaucoma. Even so, various opinions were aired regarding whether paracentesis helped or worsened keratitis. For example, Scarpa, writing during the same era as Wardrop, correctly deduced that a hypopyon was an exudate of the uveal tract rather than internal rupture of a corneal abscess and felt that paracentesis was ill-advised because it "frequently gives rise to evils of greater magnitude than the hypopyon itself."[375]

Despite paracentesis, debridement, cauterization,[353a] and other medical and surgical modalities (Table 74-1), severe corneal infection frequently progressed. Many developed increased intraocular pressure. Occasional patients healed with an adherent leukoma and corneal staphyloma, but many ended in perforation and phthisis bulbi. Sympathetic ophthalmia of the other eye was a rare but feared event.

Scientific developments of the late 19th century led to improved understanding of the nature of bacterial keratitis. The microscopic appearance of microbial keratitis was first described in 1875, and Uhthoff and Axenfeld[438] subsequently detailed the histopathologic features. Clinicopathologic investigations also clarified the nature of the hypopyon. The finding of pigment granules within leukocytes from the hypopyon correctly identified its iris origin as opposed to intracameral rupture of a corneal abscess.[244]

Clinical descriptions gradually became more detailed. Gonorrheal eye disease with corneal involvement is one of the first causes of bacterial keratitis that was clearly delineated. Various terms came into use such as *hypopyon keratitis,*[358] *torpid corneal infiltrate, serpiginous* or *creeping corneal ulcer,*[367] *suppurative keratitis,*[452] and *septic ulcer.* Texts tried to distinguish between corneal ulcers and corneal abscesses,[138] but the emphasis gradually changed from clinical classifications to the infecting agents.

The Antibiotic Era

The development of microbiology during the late 19th and early 20th centuries led to our current understanding of bacterial keratitis. Gradle,[148] a German-American ophthalmologist, wrote the first work in English on the new germ theory. Pneumococci, first identified in a human keratitis case in 1893[140] and later confirmed by Axenfeld,[438] were found to account for most cases of human bacterial keratitis at the turn of the century. *Pseudomonas,*[373] *Moraxella,*[41,333] and multiple other microorganisms[17,264] were soon identified as specific causes of bacterial keratitis in humans and animals. As a result, by 1910 Gram staining and cultures of corneal scrapings were recommended to establish a bacteriologic diagnosis.[265]

Medical management remained problematic. Ophthalmic practitioners relied on medications used during the Middle Ages. Silver preparations had been mentioned in Arabic and medieval European texts; and silver nitrate, introduced into ophthalmic practice in the early 19th century, became a standard treatment. Chemical cauterization with a silver nitrate stick or solution came into use. Other forms of chemical debridement and disinfection were later tried, such as holding a swab soaked in an antiseptic solution onto the cornea. Unfortunately, antiseptic agents such as iodine-based preparations are not very effective in curing bacterial keratitis.

With few choices of topical antimicrobial agents, subconjunctival injection of antiseptic substances was tried with some success. One practitioner, however, noted that some patients were "so frightened by the swelling that I did not venture to continue it, and I am afraid that many patients will revolt against the injection."[49] Better agents were needed that could be safely applied to the eye.

Following Fleming's legendary discovery of penicillin in 1928, its preliminary use was evaluated during 1930 in patients with eye infections in Sheffield, England.[453] Subsequent clinical studies of penicillin at Oxford included a patient with a corneal ulcer.[1] Other agents were soon to be applied to corneal infections. The clinical efficacy of sulfonamides was shown during the mid1930s, and Dubos first published on gramicidin in 1939. By innovative approaches using soil and marine microorganisms, Waksman discovered streptomycin and neomycin and coined the term *antibiotic.* Experimental and clinical demonstrations of newly developed drugs, such as polymyxins for pseudomonal keratitis,[468] led to the concept of selecting antibiotics for bacterial keratitis based on spectrum of activity.

Before the antibiotic era visual loss was common. For example, before 1930 in an English industrial city, posttraumatic keratitis resulted in enucleation or visual loss worse than 20/200 in more than half of affected patients. In comparison, soon after the introduction of sulfacetamide in this community, the incidence of significant visual loss was reduced to less than 10%.[384] The development of chemotherapeutic drugs with specific antimicrobial properties revolutionized the management of bacterial keratitis.

As new antibacterial agents were developed, topical administration was tried not only with eyedrops and ointments, but with innovative drug-delivery techniques such as dry powders, iontophoresis, and soaked cotton or other material. With increasing choices of drugs and vehicles, ophthalmologists learned to determine treatment by deducing the bacterial cause based on the typical morphology and clinical course of various types of bacterial keratitis.[110,123] Empiric recommendations for antimicrobial therapy included ophthalmic products fortified to a higher concentration and topical antibiotic solutions formulated from systemic preparations.[200] The expansion of hospital microbiology laboratories allowed a standardized, procedural approach for laboratory diagnosis.[199]

Current knowledge regarding the pathogenesis and management of bacterial keratitis is based on collective clinical experiences and studies of experimental animal models.[23] During the 20th century terminology evolved from *central corneal ulcer*[427] to the more descriptive *microbial keratitis*.[203] The emphasis is shifting to an approach based on understanding the molecular biology of bacterial keratitis and the effects of treatment on outcome. Areas of ongoing concern are the increasing resistance of bacterial corneal isolates and the emergence of previously unrecognized species as corneal pathogens.

EPIDEMIOLOGY

Incidence

The incidence of bacterial keratitis is not accurately known. In a single northern U.S. county, the incidence of ulcerative keratitis increased from approximately 2 per 100,000 in the 1950s and 1960s to 11 per 100,000 in the 1980s.[120] Contact lens wear was the most important reason accounting for this increase. In the late 1980s an estimated 10 to 30 individuals per 100,000 contact lens wearers developed ulcerative keratitis annually in the U.S.[266,341] Extrapolations of these figures to the U.S. population suggest that about 25,000 Americans currently get bacterial keratitis each year, with current estimated costs of approximately $20 million annually in medical expenditures for diagnosis and treatment. Similar estimates for Great Britain show approximately 1500 annual cases of microbial keratitis from all causes.[94]

Epidemiologic information is more limited for developing countries. Using an incidence rate of 2 per 100,000 population, an estimated 100,000 people worldwide develop bacterial keratitis annually. Continued changes in the patterns of risk factors and causal microorganisms will influence these extrapolations.

Except for certain entities such as neonatal keratoconjunctivitis, gonococcal infection, meningococcal disease, diphtheria, and nosocomial infections, bacterial keratitis is not a reportable infectious disease in the U.S. or other countries. Some professional organizations (e.g., the Contact Lens Association of Ophthalmologists and the Eye Bank Association of America) collect information on cases associated with specific risk factors. More data are needed to learn the relative importance of bacterial keratitis as a cause of human disability.

Blindness Statistics

The impact of bacterial keratitis on corneal blindness is substantial. Recent survey data show that bacterial keratitis is a leading cause of corneal blindness in developing nations.[71,125] Usually occurring because of trauma,[442] corneal infection may also be the most important reason for visual loss after trachoma and xerophthalmia. Despite medical therapy, permanent corneal opacification frequently results. Globally several hundred thousand people have a vision-limiting corneal opacity because of bacterial keratitis.

Destructive corneal infection occasionally requires surgery. U.S. eyebanking statistics identify microbial keratitis as a reason for keratoplasty in approximately 1% of all corneal transplants. When compared to the annual incidence of bacterial keratitis, approximately 0.5% to 1% of U.S. cases of corneal infection become surgical candidates.

RISK FACTORS

The corneal surface is awash with multiple microorganisms of the normal flora. Understanding how the cornea is protected helps in ascertaining how certain factors put it at risk for infection.

Normal Corneal Defense Mechanisms

The eyelids and eyelashes provide a first level of defense against exogenous microbes. The rinsing action of the tear film and the protective effects of its constituents provide additional safeguards.[399] Basal tear production is 1 to 2 μL/minute, but with an irritative stimulus the total tear volume is replaced every 15 seconds.

Among more than 60 proteins identified in the tear film, several have antibacterial effects[387] (see Chapter 13). Lysozyme influences the bacterial population of the ocular surface by cleaving the $\beta(1,4)$-linkages of the cell-wall peptidoglycan of susceptible bacteria[471] and by promoting microbial aggregation.[290] Tear lactoferrin and ceruloplasmin bind metallic ions necessary for microbial growth. Lactoferrin also has a direct bactericidal effect, can interact with specific antibodies, and may affect the superoxide-producing system of the tear-film's mucin component. Immunoglobulins, including secretory IgA directed against components of the conjunctival flora,[135] and complement components are normally present in the tear film.

The normal conjunctival flora is modulated not only by tear-film components but also by microbial metabolic products such as the bacteriocins, a group of high-molecular-weight proteins that affect the growth of pneumococci and gram-negative bacilli.[263] The conjunctival flora includes both planktonic bacteria suspended in the tears and sessile bacteria attached to the ocular surface (see Chapter 14). The tear film and other limiting factors regulate this conjunctival ecosystem, suppressing microbial activity to a relatively low population density. Furthermore corneal epithelial cells are capable of phagocytosis and intercellular transport of ingested particles, potentially providing a way to eradicate adherent microbes.

Impaired Corneal Defense Mechanisms

Aging contributes to alterations of eyelid skin flora. Streptococci and enteric gram-negative rods become relatively more common on the senescent cutaneous surface, partially because of reduced sweat and sebum that normally inhibit bacterial growth. Chronic colonization or infection of the eyelid margin or lacrimal outflow system can, in turn, predispose to bacterial keratitis when minor trauma occurs. Lacking protective blinking reflexes or an adequate Bell phenomenon, debilitated older individuals and unconscious patients are at particular risk for bacterial keratitis.

Prolonged epiphora can lead to reduced concentrations of certain tear-film antibacterial substances.[195] More commonly a dry eye predisposes to secondary infection.[252] Reduced lacrimal gland function from rheumatologic disorders, HIV infection, and conjunctival scarring leads to reduced antimicrobial protection.[385] Loss of the mucin[404] or oily[297] layers of the tear film from congenital or acquired disorders can also result in bacterial keratitis.

The presence of a suitable substrate that allows bacterial adhesion permits formation of a biofilm, a slimy layer composed of an organic polymer matrix produced by embedded bacteria.[69] Natural biofilms form on mucous membranes such as the conjunctiva by the normal microbiota. Biofilm on contact lenses can protect adherent bacteria from antibacterial substances[287] and provides a nidus for infection. The use of topical medications that alter the normal flora also predisposes to corneal infection, particularly when combined with corneal disease or trauma.

Ocular surface diseases such as cicatricial pemphigoid, Stevens-Johnson syndrome, atopic keratoconjunctivitis, radiation and chemical injuries, and vitamin A deficiency alter the normal tear film and can cause intrinsic corneal changes. Disruption of the normal epithelial glycocalyx leads to a breakdown of surface integrity that permits bacterial adherence.[229] Trauma and surgery can directly bypass the protective epithelial barrier and inoculate microorganisms into the corneal stroma. When the normal corneal surface is breached, the typically avascular stroma provides a substrate for microbial proliferation, although the Descemet membrane seems to be an effective barrier to intraocular extension of bacterial keratitis. The defense mechanisms of the healthy cornea minimize the occurrence of microbial invasion, but bacterial keratitis is one of the most important causes of corneal ulceration.[300]

Specific Risk Factors

An anterior route of microbial access accounts for practically all cases of suppurative bacterial keratitis. Any impairment in the integrity of the tear film and corneal epithelium can provide a portal of entry for microorganisms. Rarely do bacteria invade the cornea by other routes, although isolated cases have occurred by way of the limbal blood vessels during sepsis, from contiguous spread of infectious scleritis, and through the corneal endothelium during intraocular infection.

Trauma, ocular surface disorders, corneal surgery, and other local and systemic changes bypass the natural resistance of the cornea to infection (Table 74-2).[233] These risk factors vary by locale.* Predisposing causes are similar for children,[78,91,319] with trauma and systemic illness being common.

Trauma. Trauma is one of the most common predisposing factors to bacterial keratitis. Posttraumatic infection occurred in 6% of occupational anterior-segment eye injuries in one series[365] and in 5% of rural corneal abrasions in another,[444] but the incidence of bacterial keratitis following corneal trauma is not known.

Trauma predisposes to corneal infection by various means: corneal surface injuries that permit invasion of the normal flora, foreign-body injuries that inoculate exogenous microorganisms into the cornea, and nonmechanical injuries that compromise the structure or function of the cornea. The clinical presentation is often determined by the nature of the injury, ranging from minute particles that superficially abrade the corneal epithelium to perforating corneal lacerations.

Epithelial Trauma. Epithelial injuries expose the corneal stroma to the normal microflora of the ocular surface. A corneal abrasion may occur by means of numerous objects in daily use in domestic life and industrial surroundings. Following abrasive trauma, epithelial regeneration is generally rapid, but secondary infection can occur.[18] Posttraumatic recurrent erosions and persistent, nonhealing epithelial defects are predisposed to secondary infection by prolonging the duration of exposure to the conjunctival flora. Microorganisms in the tear film, particularly if chronic blepharitis or lacrimal infection is present, provide a readily available inoculum source.

---

*References 63, 88, 93, 154, 189, 257, 286, 313, 318, 442, 483.

TABLE 74-2 PREDISPOSING FACTORS FOR BACTERIAL KERATITIS

Risk Factors	Relative Frequency*	
	Developed Countries	Developing Countries
A. Trauma	20%	50-70%
1. Abrasion		
2. Foreign body		
3. Toxic agents		
B. Contact lens wear	25-50%	0-5%
C. Preexisting ocular surface disease	25-50%	20-30%
1. Eyelid and tear-film dysfunction		
a. Dry eye syndrome		
b. Eyelid malposition and eyelash problems		
c. Exposure		
2. Corneal epithelial disorders		
a. Corneal edema		
b. Corneal erosions		
c. Persistent epithelial defect		
D. Corneal surgery	5-10%	<1%
1. Penetrating or lamellar keratoplasty		
2. Keratorefractive procedures		
3. Limbal wounds		
4. Corneal sutures		
E. Associated conditions	0-5%	5-10%
1. Local infection		
2. Systemic conditions		

* Frequency estimates pertain to adult patients and are based on multiple sources including literature reports from North America, Europe, and Australia for developed countries and from selected areas of Asia and Africa for the developing world. In children of both developed and developing nations, trauma is the major risk factor for bacterial keratitis, followed by preexisting corneal disease and associated conditions such as malnutrition.

Microbes may also be introduced by the injuring agent or by contaminated objects or solutions if the eye is rubbed or irrigated. Infection can follow a superficial corneal scratch by a fingernail or animal claw. Contact with animals provides a source for uncommon microbes.[5,177,330] Accidents with dental instruments can inoculate the oral flora into the cornea,[188] and superficial corneal injury with a mascara brush can lead to secondary infection, particularly with *Pseudomonas aeruginosa*.[487] Preservatives in ocular cosmetics may be inadequate to prevent microbial contamination;[486] for example, 5% of shared sample products in U.S. retail stores are contaminated.

When proprietary eyedrops came into widespread commercial use during the 1940s, many cases of bacterial, especially pseudomonal, keratitis occurred from contaminated ophthalmic solutions, such as fluorescein eyedrops.[449] Guidelines for preparing topical solutions under sterile conditions[425] were subsequently adopted, and preservatives are routinely added to multiuse ophthalmic solutions and suspensions. Even so, in-use contamination of topical medications and the eyedropper bottle can still occur and lead to corneal infection.[380,423]

Stromal Trauma and Foreign Bodies. A corneal laceration can inoculate microorganisms into the stroma. Nonperforating wounds may develop superficial or deep bacterial keratitis by organisms of the tear film or on the foreign body.

Corneal injury can occur from a wide variety of metallic, vegetative, and other foreign bodies. Because certain microorganisms such as *Pseudomonas* sp. survive longer in aqueous environments, a working rule-of-thumb is that wet injuries tend to produce gram-negative bacterial infections whereas dry accidents are likely to yield gram-positive bacterial infections.

Corneal foreign bodies may be complicated by infection from three potential sources:

1. The foreign body. A foreign body can carry microorganisms on its surface or in its substance. Approximately 15% of removed corneal foreign bodies carry bacterial contaminants.[103] The premise that solid foreign bodies, particularly metallic particles that generate heat when traveling at high speed, are less likely to be contaminated than porous materials has not been proved. Metal is as likely to be contaminated as other materials. Chips of stone and pieces of vegetable or other organic matter are frequently contaminated. Bacterial keratitis following corneal trauma is typically more likely in an agricultural[443] or mining setting than in an industrial factory. Foreign-body injuries tend to involve the lower, usually inferonasal, cornea and are more likely to injure the nonamblyopic eye. Bacterial keratitis usually begins around the foreign body; multiple fine foreign bodies may rarely develop one or more foci of infection. Some foreign bodies elicit irritative and inflammatory reactions that can mimic bacterial keratitis. For example, copper can cause focal necrosis, and vegetable matter frequently induces acute sterile inflammation followed by a granulomatous reaction.

2. Contaminated solutions or instruments. Eye rubbing can enlarge an epithelial defect and inoculate microorganisms from a dirty handkerchief or other fomites. Solutions, including tap water, that are used to irrigate the ocular surface may also harbor potential pathogens. Trauma associated with contaminated water or other solutions can lead to bacterial keratitis. Keratitis caused by *Bacillus thuringiensis* has developed after this biologic insecticide was accidentally splashed in the eye.[369] Tearing is only partially protective in rinsing con-

taminants from the ocular surface, especially for organisms that produce IgA proteases. Contaminated instruments used to extract a foreign body may convert a simple injury to a severe infectious complication.

3. Conjunctival flora. The conjunctival surface and preocular tear film harbor multiple bacteria. A foreign body may carry these microorganisms into the corneal stroma.

Perforating injuries can lead to combined corneal and intraocular infection. Peripheral corneal infiltration, sometimes called a ring abscess, is a sterile corneal reaction frequently associated with severe intraocular infection caused by *Bacillus cereus* or gram-negative bacteria.

Nonmechanical Trauma. Trauma from chemicals (especially alkalis), radiation, and other nonmechanical events can lead to acute and chronic ocular surface changes. Some corneal injuries, such as thermal burns, infrequently lead to secondary infection unless there is concomitant eyelid injury with exposure, whereas other causes of keratopathy appear more likely to do so. The chronic abuse of any topical agent, such as an anesthetic,[357] that disrupts the corneal surface places it at risk for microbial adherence and invasion. Smoking crack cocaine has been identified as a risk factor for corneal infection, probably by disruption of corneal epithelium through cellular and neuronal toxicity.[366,453a]

Contact Lens Wear. Contact lenses were identified as a risk factor for bacterial keratitis in the 1960s. The subsequent association with soft contact lens wear, first recognized in the 1970s, gained in importance with their widespread use. On the average individuals have a 1.5% chance of developing infectious keratitis during a lifetime of contact lens use. In countries such as the United States and Great Britain where contact lenses account for a substantial market share of optical corrective devices, contact lens use is the most common cause of bacterial keratitis.

During the early years of contact lens production, a few were found to be contaminated by *Pseudomonas* sp. or fungi when received from the distributor. Better industrial standards and improved manufacturing and packaging now ensure sterile lenses in unopened containers. Subsequent contamination during improper lens handling commonly takes place, however. Bacteria can adhere to a contact lens regardless of composition, hydration, or surface ionic charge.[241] Worn lenses with surface deposits or irregularities are susceptible to bacterial adhesion.[58,59] Multiple microorganisms can contaminate contact lenses and cause corneal infection (see Chapter 16), but *Pseudomonas* sp. is the organism most commonly isolated from bacterial keratitis associated with contact lens wear (Fig. 74-1).[105,232,379]

Incidence. All types of refractive, cosmetic, and therapeutic contact lenses, including hard, gas-permeable, and soft lenses, have been implicated in microbial keratitis.[473] A

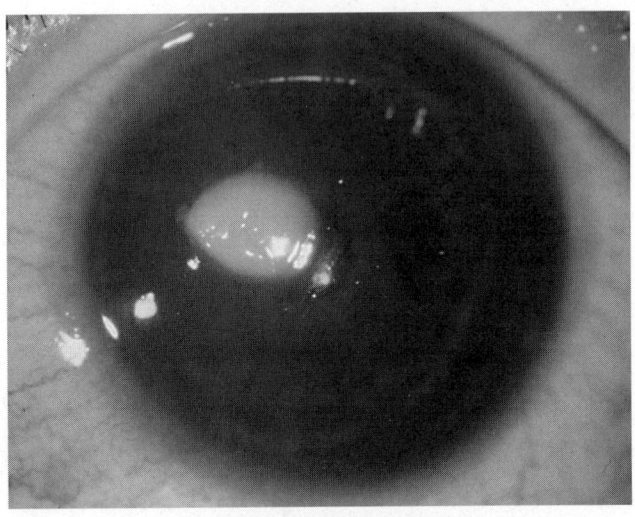

A

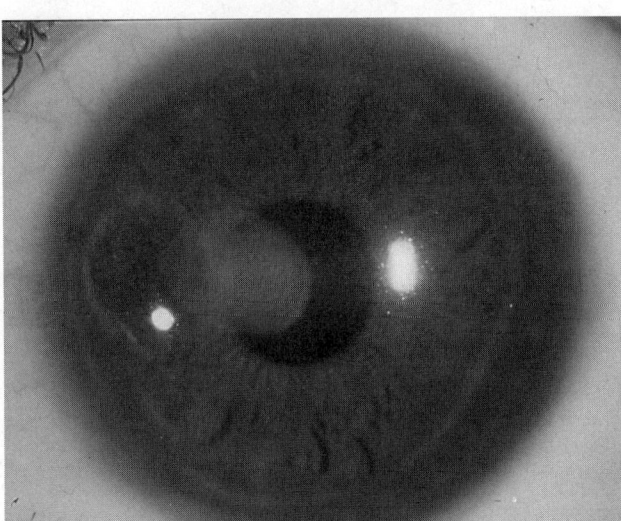

B

Fig. 74-1. Bacterial keratitis. **A,** *Pseudomonas aeruginosa* keratitis associated with extended-wear soft contact lens. **B,** Residual corneal opacity after three weeks of topical ceftazidime therapy.

national survey in the United States during the 1960s found an incidence of ulcerative keratitis in 0.03% of contact lens wearers.[108] A subsequent survey in England during the 1970s suggested that the risk had increased to approximately 0.9% as a result of the incremental use of soft contact lenses.[362] In the 1980s, U.S. data showed incidence rates of about 0.05% for soft daily-wear lens wearers and 0.2% for soft extended-wear lens users.[266] An incidence study conducted during 1987 in New England[341] provides current estimates of the annual incidence of ulcerative keratitis in U.S. contact lens wearers: 0.02% for hard (PMMA) lenses, 0.04% for rigid gas-permeable lenses, 0.04% for daily-wear soft lenses, and 0.2% for extended-wear soft lenses.

Bacterial keratitis also occurs with disposable soft contact lenses.[83,196,340] Extended wear of disposable lenses is about 10 times more likely to result in ulcerative keratitis than conventional soft contact lenses.[52,282] Whether lens fit, hygiene, or other factors account for the apparent increased risk associated with disposable soft contact lenses remains to be determined.

Three patient groups that carry an increased risk of contact lens-related bacterial keratitis are aphakes, patients with a corneal transplant, and patients wearing a bandage lens because of chronic keratopathy. The rate of ulcerative keratitis is proportionally greater in aphakic compared to cosmetic contact lens wearers.[144] Case series reporting one or more culture-proved cases of bacterial keratitis showed an incidence of approximately 1% to 5% among aphakic extended-wear soft contact lens wearers,[475] and current incidence estimates suggest that 0.5% of all aphakic contact lens wearers develop ulcerative keratitis.[144]

Contact lenses increase occasions for bacterial keratitis in patients who have corneal edema or who have undergone corneal transplantation. A compilation of case series evaluating extended-wear contact lens use following penetrating keratoplasty implies that the incidence of microbial keratitis is increased in these patients to approximately 2%.[475]

Preexisting keratopathy with therapeutic contact lens wear predisposes to infection by less common microorganisms.[218] Bacterial keratitis has been reported to occur in 1% to 5% of therapeutic soft contact lens wearers.[475]

Contamination of Contact Lenses. The risk of bacterial keratitis during contact lens wear is related to the multiple ways that contact lenses may become contaminated and can affect the cornea. Case-control studies[96,377] show that overnight lens use is a principal risk factor of soft contact lens-related keratitis. Continuous lens wear increases the chance of corneal infection by approximately tenfold, and the risk of infection rises incrementally with each additional consecutive night of lens wear.

Many patients who develop contact lens–associated bacterial keratitis fail to follow recommended lens care practices,[46] and the same organism is often found conjointly from corneal scrapings and the contact lens case. Recent lens manipulation, particularly if there is a break in lens care technique with reinsertion of a contaminated lens, is a common occurrence that precipitates an infectious complication.[284] In other cases an environmental source rather than contaminated lens care materials appears more likely.[93] Although hospital workers do not necessarily have an altered conjunctival flora,[67] contact lens–wearing health-care workers can develop infection caused by resistant bacteria.[47] Contact lens wear may or may not affect the normal conjunctival flora,[119] although some lens disinfection systems may have an effect on the microbial population.[128]

Organisms causing contact lens–related bacterial keratitis may originate from the ocular surface or from contaminated paraphernalia. Smoking is an important risk factor in contact lens–associated ulcerative keratitis,[377] perhaps because tobacco smoke selectively inhibits gram-positive cocci more than gram-negative rods, thereby altering the conjunctival flora. *Pseudomonas aeruginosa* and other microorganisms have been recovered from tap and bottled water formerly used to prepare contact lens saline solutions, and microbes can survive in the moist chamber of a contact lens case. Isolating the same bacterial species from a contact lens case as the organism that is identified from corneal material does not necessarily prove a cause-and-effect association but does raise suspicion about the route of infection.

The polysaccharide slime layer that coats encapsulated bacteria facilitates hydrophobic colonization of the contact lens surface. A biofilm provides a protective environment that enables bacteria to persist even in the presence of antibacterial agents. Irregularities of the lens surface along with deposition of protein and mucin further enhance bacterial adherence.[409,415] Extended-wear contact lenses facilitate infection by their accumulated coatings and adherent bacteria, by the prolonged entrapment of debris under the lens,[15] and by enhancing bacterial adherence to corneal epithelial cells.[129]

Corneal Effects of Contact Lens Wear. An altered corneal surface can multiply the relative risk of bacterial keratitis associated with contact lens wear. A seasonal variation in the incidence of contact lens–associated bacterial keratitis might be due to summertime activities such as swimming[345] that affects the superficial cornea. More important is the intrinsic health of the ocular surface. A dry-eye syndrome, corneal anesthesia, and thimerosal epitheliopathy are some examples of conditions that increase the cornea's susceptibility to infection during contact lens wear.

Contact lens wear can also adversely affect the healthy cornea. Accidental epithelial abrasion may occur during lens insertion or removal. Epithelial thinning, epithelial microcysts, decreased epithelial mitosis and exfoliation, enhanced anaerobic metabolism, and endothelial cell changes are among the morphologic and physiologic changes induced by contact lenses. Other metabolic effects are induced by tear-film stagnation or hypotonicity and the use of topical solutions containing a preservative or other surface-acting agent. Furthermore an improperly fitted lens exacerbates these changes. A tight-lens syndrome can be precipitated by lens dehydration, limited oxygen permeability of the contact lens polymer, and repeated overnight hypoxic stress. Epithelial hypoxia and transient endothelial dysfunction result in acute epithelial edema that provides opportunities for bacterial adherence and invasion.

Ocular Surface Disorders. *Eyelid and Tear-Film Dysfunction.* Dry eyes caused by Sjögren syndrome or conjunctival scarring disorders (including Stevens-Johnson syndrome, pemphigoid, radiation, and trachoma) are predisposed to secondary infection.[315] Because the conjunctival flora of the dry eye is not substantially different from normal,[386] any increased susceptibility is probably due to the likelihood of epithelial defects. Bacterial keratitis can, therefore, complicate graft-versus-host disease after bone-marrow transplantation. Patients with vitamin A deficiency are especially at risk because epithelial keratinization caused by xerophthalmia[104] encourages bacterial adherence that can precipitate keratomalacia and bacterial keratitis.[446]

Eyelid malposition from ectropion or seventh cranial nerve palsy can lead to corneal exposure with focal desiccation. Lagophthalmos may also occur from a variety of orbital disorders. Prolonged proptosis can result in exposure keratopathy and secondary infection. Eyelash abnormalities such as trichiasis, distichiasis, and broken eyelashes[311] can predispose to epithelial surface defects that can become secondarily infected. Bacterial keratitis related to entropion is a major pathway to corneal blindness in trachoma.[73] Chronic bacterial colonization of the eyelid margins during blepharitis and other disorders may also affect corneal health.

Corneal Epithelial Disorders. Punctate epithelial erosions, microcystic epithelial edema, and persistent epithelial defects may predispose to bacterial keratitis. One example of preexisting corneal disease that can be complicated by secondary bacterial infection is herpes simplex virus keratitis,[45,305,469] including dendritic and geographic epithelial keratitis, disciform stromal keratitis, and neurotrophic keratopathy.[460] Besides the disruption of the corneal epithelium that occurs during herpetic keratitis, antiviral agents such as idoxuridine can lead to cytotoxic effects that contribute to the occurrence of bacterial keratitis.[109,490] Furthermore topical corticosteroid use for herpetic eye disease might directly modify microbial replication, alter host resistance to opportunistic infections,[428] and delay recognition of secondary infection by reducing the symptoms and signs of corneal inflammation. Patients with devitalized corneal tissue and corneal hypesthesia from prior herpes simplex virus or varicella-zoster virus[262] eye disease may be particularly susceptible to secondary infection.

Bacterial keratitis, most commonly due to staphylococci or streptococci, can complicate a corneal epithelial erosion associated with corneal epithelial basement membrane dystrophy,[260a] climatic droplet keratopathy,[107] lattice dystrophy, vernal or atopic keratoconjunctivitis,[220] and blepharokeratoconjunctivitis. Bacterial keratitis has been recognized in association with corneal edema from a variety of causes such as Fuchs dystrophy, aphakic and pseudophakic corneal edema, and permanent endothelial dysfunction associated with chronic glaucoma.[474] Any persistent, nonhealing epithelial defect is vulnerable to bacterial infection.

Corneal Surgery. *Corneal Transplantation.* Bacterial keratitis in a corneal transplant can occur in the early postoperative period, which has been linked with contamination of the donor cornea, but is more likely during subsequent follow-up and rehabilitation (Fig. 74-2). Retrospective series

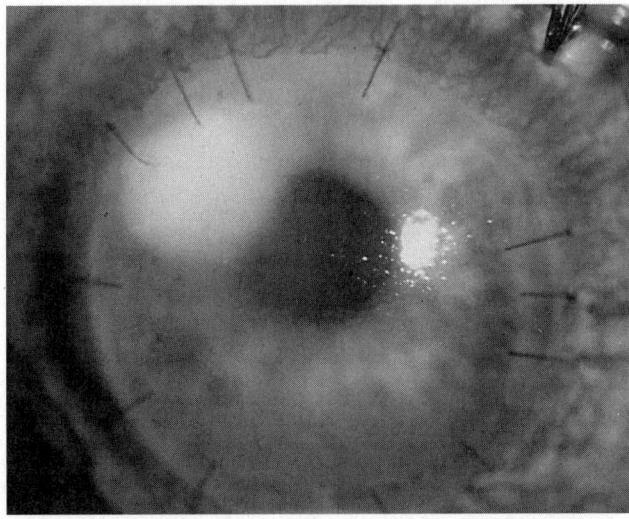

Fig. 74-2. *Streptococcus pneumoniae* keratitis occurring in a corneal transplant.

evaluating the occurrence of bacterial keratitis following corneal transplantation show an incidence of approximately 2% to 5%.[65,216,359,435] The use of extended-wear soft contact lenses has been the single most common predisposing factor.[368,398] Other risk factors for infection of a corneal graft are concurrent dry-eye syndrome, chronic epithelial defects, the frequent application of topical corticosteroids and other agents, and suture-related problems.* Loose, broken, and exposed sutures can harbor microorganisms and permit an entry site for microbes; suture removal can drag surface microorganisms into the corneal stroma. Inflammation beginning in the peripheral corneal graft tends to progress into the graft-host junction or along a lamellar wound interface.

Keratorefractive Surgery. Bacterial keratitis has been reported after radial and transverse keratotomy[279,347,477] and is estimated to occur in approximately 0.01% to 0.05% of refractive keratotomy procedures.[89,272,275] Corneal infection may begin shortly after surgery or occur several years postoperatively.[272,393] Early-onset keratitis typically begins in a keratotomy incision, sometimes deep in the cornea. Intraoperative factors, including nonsterile surgical instruments, have been implicated in some cases. Delayed-onset keratitis has occurred from six months to five years after radial keratotomy. Infection in these late cases usually begins superficially in a keratotomy scar, predominately in the lower cornea; approximately half are associated with contact lens wear. Epithelial ridges, tear-film irregularities, wound gape, recurrent erosions, and corneal hypesthesia presumably increase the susceptibility of these corneas to infection. *S. aureus* is most common, but many bacterial species have been found. Bacterial keratitis has rarely occurred after other types of keratorefractive procedures, including postkerato-

---

*References 6, 26, 112, 130, 158, 243.

plasty relaxing incisions, epikeratoplasty,[146] hydrogel lamellar implantation, and excimer laser photorefractive keratectomy.[368a]

Other Procedures. Limbal incisions, such as cataract and keratocentesis wounds, can become infected and subsequently involve the peripheral cornea.[69a] Medical-grade tissue adhesive has a partial antibacterial effect,[118] but infection has followed the application of glue used to treat corneal perforation.[66,464]

Spread from Adjacent Structures. Most forms of bacterial keratitis begin with a corneal epithelial defect initiated by trauma or a preexisting ocular disorder. Selected microorganisms, such as *Neisseria gonorrhoeae, N. meningitidis, Corynebacterium diphtheriae, Listeria monocytogenes, Shigella sonnei,* and *Haemophilus influenzae,* are said to be able to penetrate intact corneal epithelium during acute conjunctivitis. Severe blepharitis can also predispose to corneal infection by providing a large potential inoculum and opportunities for corneal epithelial disruption. Dacryocystitis can be complicated by bacterial, usually pneumococcal, keratitis following minor corneal trauma.

Bacterial keratitis may be a component of bacterial scleritis and is often referred to as sclerokeratitis. The spread of infection may be from the limbus into the adjacent cornea and sclera, from the cornea into the sclera, or from the anterior sclera into the peripheral cornea.

Bacterial keratitis may coexist with bacterial endophthalmitis, but both are usually due to simultaneous seeding of the cornea and intraocular structures by trauma or surgery. Occasionally progressive corneal infection with perforation can lead to endophthalmitis; the converse, intraocular infection causing corneal infection, seldom happens. A suppurative hypopyon can sometimes permeate into the cornea, but bacteria causing endophthalmitis do not spread across an intact endothelial surface. Some forms of endophthalmitis may result in a sterile ring infiltrate of the peripheral cornea from exudation of the limbal blood vessels.

Hematogenous Spread. Dissemination of spirochetes or mycobacteria may result in stromal keratitis or scleritis, but endogenous suppurative keratitis from blood-borne bacteria is essentially unheard-of. Premature infants are susceptible to corneal involvement during pseudomonal sepsis. Colonization of the ocular surface by *P. aeruginosa* in the nursery rather than hematogenous spread to the cornea, however, is probably the usual route.

Bacteria causing systemic infection do not typically involve the cornea but can transiently pass through the ocular blood vessels or tissues. Because microorganisms may be present on or in the clinically normal cornea or sclera during sepsis, eyebanks screen potential donors to minimize transmitting an infection to recipients.

Systemic Conditions. Patients with chronic alcoholism,[317] dementia, parkinsonism, and other debilitating or aging changes[314] may have altered host defenses such as reduced blinking, decreased tear flow, lowered tear lysozyme, cor-

neal hypesthesia, chronic blepharitis, and eyelid malposition with exposure (Fig. 74-3). Experimental studies suggest that parental alcohol consumption increases a newborn's susceptibility to bacterial keratitis.[38] For elderly adults poor personal hygiene and other social factors, the nursing home or hospital environment, and a reluctance or delay in seeking medical aid are possible predisposing factors to bacterial keratitis. These conditions also probably play a role in the spectrum of bacteria responsible for keratitis in the elderly: coagulase-negative staphylococci, *Moraxella* spp., and enteric gram-negative bacilli.

Whether immunity plays a clinically important role in bacterial keratitis has not been determined. Systemic immunosuppression and neutropenia may determine severity if not susceptibility.[166] Patients with the acquired immunodeficiency syndrome or other immunocompromised state who develop bacterial keratitis sometimes have a fulminant or more prolonged course.[11,170,301,429] Malnutrition and vitamin deficiency, particularly xerophthalmia and scurvy, can also impair host defenses to posttraumatic infection.[389,446] Systemic endocrinologic conditions such as diabetes mellitus might affect epithelial healing, which could possibly lead to corneal infection.

Serious illness and hospitalization can predispose to corneal infection in children[9,78,91] and adults. Nosocomial corneal infections have occurred in stuporous patients and burn victims[342] as a result of lagophthalmos and corneal exposure, especially in the setting of a tracheostomy or respiratory infection. Inadvertent contamination of the eyes can occur by the catheter used for tracheal suctioning.[173] Impairment of the normal corneal reflex during general anesthesia and coma[187] are additional risk factors in hospitalized patients.

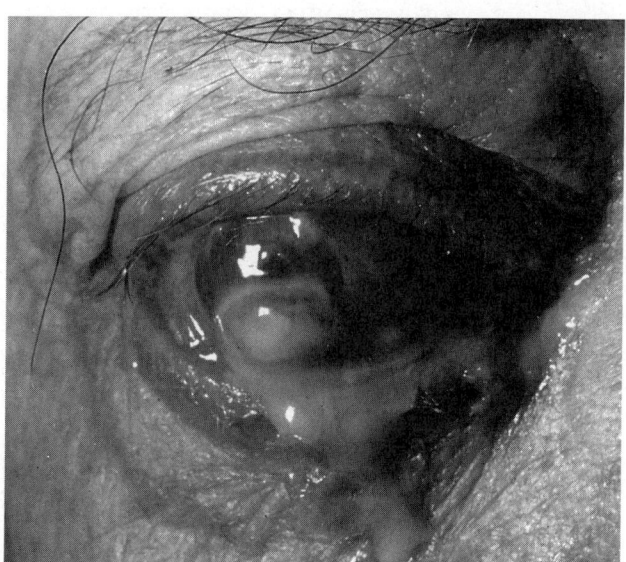

Fig. 74-3. Suppurative microbial keratitis caused by chronic exposure in cachectic septuagenarian.

CLINICAL FEATURES

The evaluation of a patient with suppurative or ulcerative keratitis should include a careful history and anterior-segment examination to evaluate possible predisposing factors. The acute symptoms of pain, photophobia, lacrimation, blepharospasm, and blurred vision are typical of bacterial keratitis but nonspecific. Disorders other than bacterial keratitis are frequently encountered as causes of corneal ulceration.[300]

During the initial clinical examination pertinent ocular abnormalities must be accurately identified and recorded. A detailed drawing should be made of the corneal changes, especially the size and shape of the epithelial defect and the area, depth, and density of the stromal infiltrate. Both frontal and slit sections are sketched with descriptive labeling. Different colors,[458] shadings,[400] or lines[231] help to illustrate how different corneal layers are involved (Table 74-3). Accurate measurements are simplified with a slit-beam ruler (Fig. 74-4)[61] or eyepiece reticule. Besides the pen or pencil drawing, photographic documentation is useful for subsequent comparisons. Examination techniques such as confocal microscopy may provide additional information.[70] Ultrasonography can help if intraocular abnormalities are suspected and when corneal opacification prevents direct visualization of the posterior segment.

Using qualitative and quantitative measures, the overall severity should be judged. A grading scheme[160,204] should consider the location, extent, and depth of stromal suppuration and ulceration; the pace of progression; the perceived risk of perforation or scleral involvement; and the amount of intraocular inflammation. This global clinical evaluation

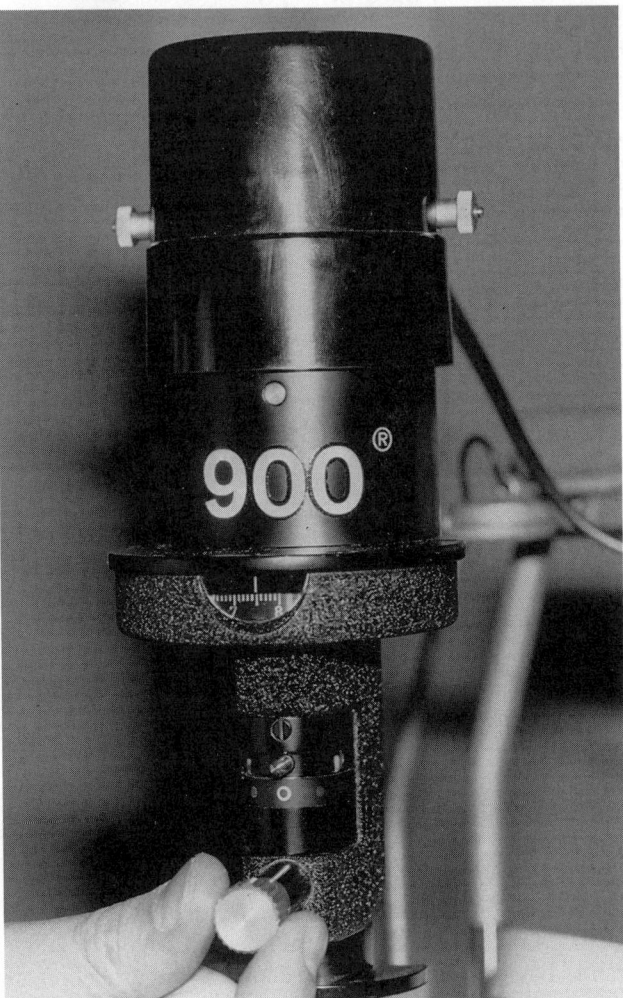

Fig. 74-4. Slit-beam ruler for corneal measurement. Eyepiece reticules are also available that are either calibrated to standard ruler at a given magnification or used on a single biomicroscope for repetitive measurements.

helps decide the need for treatment beyond intensive topical antibacterial therapy.

Suppurative Keratitis

The presenting clinical features of bacterial keratitis are determined by the interaction of the responsible microorganisms and the host's inflammatory response. The signs of bacterial keratitis are also modulated by any predisposing factors that might be present; the duration of infection; the cornea's structural status; and the prior use of antibacterial, antiinflammatory, and other medications. The combination of these multiple determinants leads to a spectrum of symptoms and signs.

Nonspecific signs include limbal and conjunctival hyperemia, sometimes with marked episcleral injection and papillary conjunctivitis. Eyelid edema sometimes appears more marked because of secondary ptosis. The conjunctival dis-

TABLE 74-3 GUIDELINES FOR DRAWING FRONTAL AND SLIT DIAGRAMS OF MICROBIAL KERATITIS

Characteristic	Black and White	Color
Edge of epithelial defect	Line	Black
Epithelial edema	Stipple or small circles	Blue
Stromal infiltrate	Crosshatched grid or shade	Orange
Stromal edema	Diagonals	Blue
Striae	Wavy lines	Blue
Stromal vessels	Branching lines	Red
Superficial	Slender lines	
Deep	Thicker lines	
Ghost	Dashed lines	
Hypopyon and keratitic precipitates	Solid or asterisks	Orange
Hyphema	Solid	Red
Pigment and iris	Solid	Brown
Lens	Solid	Green

charge varies according to bacterial virulence and tends to stick to the ulcerated area.

The hallmark of early, untreated microbial keratitis is focal stromal suppuration. Slit-lamp biomicroscopy typically reveals a dense yellow-white or grey-white stromal infiltrate with an overlying epithelial defect and an adherent mucopurulent exudate. Infants typically exhibit less corneal inflammation than others.[53] Multiple infiltrates are sometimes seen in association with contact lens wear, several corneal foreign bodies, or polymicrobial infection. Stromal ulceration and liquefactive necrosis can occur during progression of more severe disease. Diffuse cellular infiltration in the adjacent stroma occurs by the active migration of inflammatory cells between lamellae that blur the margins of the focal infiltrate. Stromal edema and striae usually surround this area because of localized endothelial dysfunction as manifested by endothelial pseudoguttata. A crescentic or ring-shaped infiltrate may suggest an immunogenic reaction to gram-negative organisms such as *P. aeruginosa.* Infiltration around peripheral corneal nerves, called radial keratoneuritis, has infrequently been identified in gram-negative bacterial keratitis.[124,418] Various microorganisms produce a wide range of clinical changes. Bacterial keratitis should be suspected in a patient with focal suppurative and ulcerative keratitis.

Intraocular inflammation may vary from mild aqueous cells and flare to marked hypopyon formation and accumulation of an inflammatory plaque on the posterior corneal surface underlying the area of bacterial keratitis. This anterior chamber reaction often correlates with the intensity of iris vascular congestion. The hypopyon is typically more voluminous centrally than at its edges. Accumulated inflammatory cells can sometimes affect the endothelial cells locally, resulting in mild edema or permitting ingress of inflammatory cells into the posterior cornea. The range of pupillary reactivity is diminished, and iris synechiae may occur. Secondary glaucoma may ensue by several different mechanisms, including inflammatory blockage of the anterior-chamber angle, formation of peripheral anterior synechiae and iridocorneal adhesions, and pupillary block. Apart from anterior vitreous cells, changes do not usually occur in the posterior segment, although mild retinal perivasculitis and optic disc edema are rarely noted.

The causative microorganisms cannot be decided by the clinical examination alone. Some bacteria can cause distinctive, although not pathognomonic, corneal changes, however (Fig. 74-5).

Distinctive Features of Specific Bacteria

Staphylococcus aureus. Staphylococcal keratitis often presents as a well-defined, white-gray or creamy stromal infiltrate. Patients with a persistent epithelial defect, especially those on prolonged corticosteroids, sometimes develop staphylococcal infection beginning as multifocal, su-

perficial stromal opacities consisting largely of bacteria with few inflammatory cells. The infected area is surrounded by mild stromal edema and superficial stromal cells. Gradual progression typically occurs by circumferential enlargement and extension into the deeper stromal layers. Some cases go on to rapid suppuration and form a dense stromal abscess whereas others take a more indolent course. Intraocular inflammation is usually slight but can occasionally be out of proportion to the amount of corneal involvement.

Streptococcus pneumoniae. Pneumococcal keratitis typically begins with a focal suppurative stromal infiltrate that has a tendency for superficial spread, forming a serpiginous leading edge. Irregular enlargement makes the progressive changes look as if there is an advancing margin that burrows under an overhanging edge with epithelium heaping up on the other side of the ulcer. This apparent directional or creeping pattern is short-lived. Enlarging necrosis can involve a large area of the cornea and progress to thinning or perforation. Cellular infiltration into the deeper stroma with localized edema can lead to stretching of the Descemet membrane with radiating folds. An inflammatory plaque or clot is typically present on the underlying posterior corneal surface, sometimes visible as a ringlike pattern on the endothelium. Uncontrolled iritis causes anterior and posterior synechiae. Beta-hemolytic streptococci and other species may present with a similarly severe appearance, whereas viridans streptococci usually cause a more localized ulceration.

Pseudomonas aeruginosa. *Pseudomonas aeruginosa* is a common organism associated with bacterial keratitis, especially in more tropical climates, in contact lens wearers, and in debilitated or hospitalized patients. *P. aeruginosa,* like most other microorganisms, typically requires a preexisting corneal surface injury for corneal invasion, although the neonatal cornea seems to be especially susceptible to penetration.[167] *P. aeruginosa* has few nutritional requirements and can adapt to various ecologic conditions such as nonpreserved ophthalmic solutions and the hospital environment. Pseudomonal and other gram-negative bacterial corneal infections typically present as a rapidly evolving, suppurative stromal infiltrate with a marked mucopurulent exudate. Pseudomonal strains produce a pigment that fluoresces under ultraviolet light but not with the cobalt-blue filter of the slit-lamp biomicroscope. Yellowish coagulative necrosis surrounded by inflammatory epithelial edema is distinctive. Circumferential enlargement, progressive suppuration, and stromal ulceration can lead to substantial stromal loss. A ring infiltrate may appear in the surrounding, paracentral cornea. A hypopyon or dense inflammatory coagulum is usually present. Stromal destruction with descemetocele formation or perforation is not uncommon. Extension into the adjacent sclera has occurred. *Serratia* spp. and various enteric bacilli, such as *Enterobacter* spp.[153] and *Klebsiella* spp.,[194] frequently show similar characteristics of progressive suppurative keratitis.

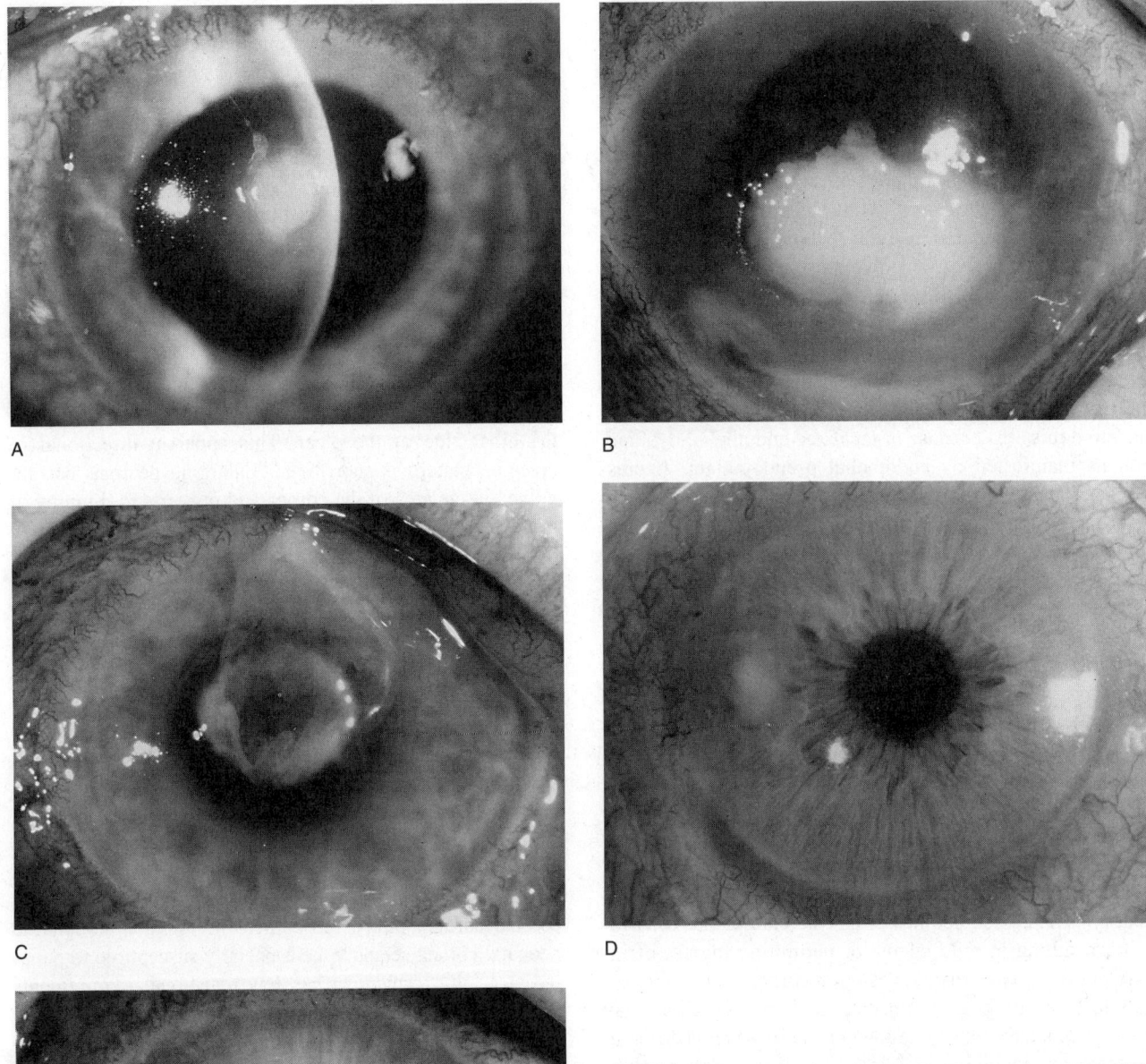

Fig. 74-5. Differential clinical features of common causes of bacterial keratitis. **A,** *Staphylococcus aureus* keratitis showing round, creamy-white infiltrate and mild iritis. **B,** *Streptococcus pneumoniae* keratitis presenting as large suppurative infiltrate with serpiginous border advancing centrally. **C,** *Pseudomonas aeruginosa* keratitis presenting as focal necrotic infiltrate with surrounding ring-shaped inflammation and mucopurulent discharge adherent to epithelial ulceration. **D,** *Moraxella lacunata* keratitis presenting as round indolent infiltrate with minimal iritis. **E,** *Propionibacterium acnes* keratitis with granular, slowly evolving infiltrate that extends into deeper stroma. (Figures **A, B** also in color insert.)

Neisseria gonorrhoeae. Gonococcal conjunctivitis occurs in neonates and in sexually active adults. Initial signs are marked conjunctival hyperemia and chemosis, copious purulent discharge, preauricular lymphadenitis, and, less commonly, dacryoadenitis. The conjunctival exudate can cause punctate epithelial erosions and intracellular edema that give the corneal surface a dull appearance. Keratitis may occur early in the disease but becomes more likely with prolonged, untreated conjunctivitis. Transient subepithelial infiltrates, usually appearing peripherally with or without epithelial ulceration, are probably due to a marginal hypersensitivity reaction.[440] An epithelial defect with stromal infiltration and thinning suggests corneal infection.[383,454] Rapid stromal necrosis can lead to a large perforation with endophthalmitis. *N. meningitidis*[22] and *Acinetobacter calcoaceticus* (formerly *A. anitratus, Mima polymorpha,* and *Herellea vaginicola*)* resemble gonococci on smear and can cause acute keratoconjunctivitis, including corneal necrosis and perforation.

Moraxella species. *Moraxella* sp. keratitis generally begins with a superficial focal infiltrate that may have irregular margins but can lead to deep stromal involvement.[274] Some cases progress slowly with round indolent ulceration[80] and a peripheral clear cornea, whereas other cases show dense focal suppuration that can perforate.[408] Iritis is usually mild, and any hypopyon is small. Species with low pathogenicity, such as *M.* (formerly *Branhamella*) *catarrhalis,*[168,267,478] are occasional opportunistic pathogens of an immunologically compromised or structurally altered cornea. A related organism, *Kingella kingae,* has caused childhood infection.[293]

Clostridium species. Clostridial keratitis can present with a frothy, bullous keratitis caused by accumulation of subepithelial or intrastromal air produced by these gas-producing microorganisms.[271,412]

Bacillus species. Bacillus keratitis can begin with multifocal epithelial opacities that lead to a focal stromal infiltrate. Failure of contact lens disinfection to kill spores can predispose to infection by these organisms,[111,448] and trauma has been implicated in other cases.[420]

Corynebacterium diphtheriae. Patients with nasopharyngeal or cutaneous diphtheria can develop a membranous or pseudomembranous conjunctivitis with preauricular lymphadenopathy. Corneal involvement begins with a diffuse epithelial haze that rapidly progresses to stromal dissolution with necrosis and suppuration.[68] Other *Corynebacterium* spp.,[169,363] including *C.* (formerly *Bacterionema*) *matruchotii,*[480] cause less virulent disease similar to other causes of bacterial keratitis. *Listeria monocytogenes* can be confused with diphtheroids on smear and cause necrotizing keratitis[182,183,493] and colonize a persistent epithelial defect.[114]

Haemophilus influenzae. *H. influenzae,* including a biotype formerly called *H. aegyptius,* is an occasional cause of conjunctivitis that can be complicated by corneal infection. These gram-negative coccobacilli have also caused bacterial keratitis during therapeutic contact lens wear, dry-eye syndromes, corneal transplantation, and chronic corneal disorders.

Azotobacter species. *Azotobacter* spp. are aerobic bacteria found in soil and water. These pleomorphic, gram-negative rods are uncommon causes of human disease but can cause suppurative keratitis.[258] Other unusual soil and water contaminants, such as *Aeromonas hydrophila*[63a,122] and *Comamonas acidovorans*[418] are known causes of corneal disease. Many of these organisms do not produce unique or distinctive clinical changes and resemble other causes of bacterial keratitis.

Anaerobes. Nonsporeforming anaerobic bacteria such as *Peptococcus* spp.,[332] *Peptostreptococcus* spp.,[117,208] and *Propionibacterium acnes*[208,332,492] may cause a focal, stromal infiltrate that may be indistinguishable from other causes of bacterial keratitis or that may be more indolent, sometimes with healing of the overlying epithelium. *P. acnes* releases a polysaccharide that is a chemoattractant for neutrophils, and the organism can survive intracellularly. Underlying corneal disease, prior corneal trauma or surgery, contact lens wear, and chronic topical corticosteroid use are the most common predisposing factors. Trauma can inoculate organisms into the deeper cornea where an anaerobic bacterial abscess can form.[414] Some facultative anaerobes such as *Capnocytophaga* spp.,* *Stenotrophomonas* (formerly *Xanthomonas*) *maltophilia,* and *Eikenella corrodens*[215,228] are opportunists that can cause a chronic, smoldering, deep keratitis or perforation that may be difficult to cure medically. When anaerobes are a component of polybacterial infection, the clinical appearance may present as a typical suppurative keratitis or as lobulated or multifocal infiltrates.

Indolent or chronic keratitis is an unusual but possible presentation of bacterial corneal infection (Fig. 74-6). Organisms of low virulence can replicate within the posterior cornea and cause mild inflammation.[260] For example, *Capnocytophaga* spp.[106] and *S. maltophilia* can produce deep stromal infection that persists for weeks or months.

Antecedent corneal disease, prior corneal transplantation, and topical corticosteroid use enhance the opportunity for infection by opportunistic microorganisms and can alter the typical clinical signs. Persistent ulceration and other forms of chronic keratopathy may make the diagnosis of bacterial keratitis difficult.[461] Inadequate antibacterial therapy can also mask the typical features of bacterial keratitis. Enlarging stromal infiltration or ulceration and nonspecific inflammation in the aqueous humor may be the first signs of secondary infection in eyes with preexisting corneal disease.

---

*References 156, 171, 283, 343, 455, 491.

*References 116, 130a, 221, 316, 325, 360.

Infectious Crystalline Keratopathy

With a suppressed or impaired inflammatory response, bacteria can proliferate between stromal lamellae to form focal accumulations of bacterial colonies with minimal inflammation under an intact epithelium. Bacterial growth between stromal lamellae produces the characteristic arborescent opacities of infectious crystalline keratopathy.[350,351] The borders of these opacities resemble needles or fern-like networks (Fig. 74-7).

Viridans streptococci (*S. mitis, S. salivarius,* and *S. sanguis*) account for most cases of pauciinflammatory keratitis. *S. pneumoniae, Gemella morbillorum, Enterococcus* spp., *S. epidermidis, Haemophilus aphrophilus, Peptostreptococcus* spp., *Acinetobacter calcoaceticus, Pseudomonas aeruginosa, Propionibacterium acnes,* diphtheroids, and other microorganisms have also caused intrastromal crystalline changes. Less common causes include *Mycobacterium chelonae, Mycobacterium fortuitum, Candida albicans, Candida tropicalis,* and *Alternaria* spp.

The use of topical corticosteroid therapy in many cases of intrastromal crystalline infection accounts for the initial lack of corneal suppuration, because abrupt discontinuation of corticosteroids can provoke stromal inflammation. Reduced inflammation during bacterial keratitis can also be partially due to engulfment of bacteria within a fibrin meshwork or inside keratocytes.[288] Some bacteria can produce capsular exopolysaccharide and other material that allow proliferation without the usual host inflammatory response.[278a,320] Anatomic factors may also play a role, because many cases have occurred within a corneal graft, by the graft-host junction, or along suture tracks. Incisional keratotomy,[224] epikeratophakia, chemical burns, corneal edema, contact lens wear, topical anesthetic abuse,[225] and 5-fluorouracil use[329] have been also implicated. Intrastromal bacterial growth has

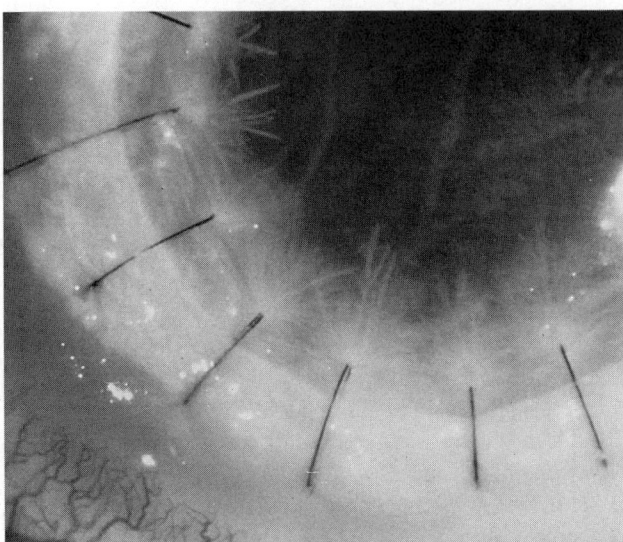

Fig. 74-7. Infectious crystalline keratopathy caused by streptococci presenting as arborescent opacities around multiple sutures following penetrating keratoplasty.

occurred in the setting of herpes simplex virus keratitis, varicella-zoster virus keratitis, and acanthamoebic keratitis. The diagnosis of infectious crystalline keratopathy can be delayed because the usual signs of inflammation are absent.

Exercise caution in interpreting clinical features without laboratory confirmation of a specific microbe. Many microorganisms causing bacterial keratitis produce nondistinctive changes, and clinical features can be unreliable in establishing a specific cause. Because the diagnosis of bacterial keratitis cannot be made with certainty based on the clinical features alone, laboratory evaluation is necessary to distinguish bacterial keratitis from other causes of focal corneal inflammation.

COMPLICATIONS

Most of the complications of bacterial keratitis are structural alterations of the cornea. Other sight-threatening problems include secondary glaucoma and cataract.[259] These consequences are largely caused by the host's inflammatory response, but the influence of bacterial toxins and treatment toxicity, including corticosteroid effects, may also be important.

Persistent Epithelial Defect

Corneal epithelial toxicity from various topical antimicrobial agents is related to their concentration and frequency of use[484] and possibly to any included preservatives. In experimental animals topical aminoglycoside antibiotics can slow epithelial wound healing when administered in frequent, fortified dosages.[334,414] Toxic conjunctival ulceration and necrosis, usually of the lower bulbar conjunctiva, can occur with the use of topical and fortified aminoglycosides

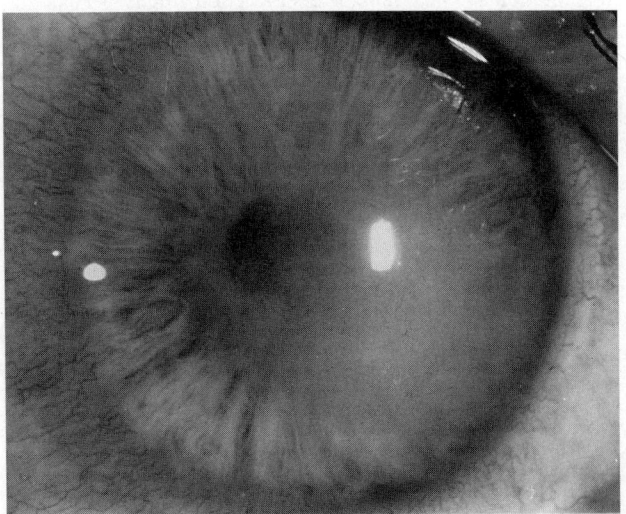

Fig. 74-6. Chronic posttraumatic inflammation caused by *Staphylococcus haemolyticus* mimicking noninfectious keratitis.

within 1 week.[102] Corneal ulceration with stromal keratitis mimicking bacterial infection has occurred as a result of corneal toxicity from prolonged use of topical antibiotics. Some antimicrobial agents, such as ciprofloxacin, can precipitate or crystallize within an epithelial defect. Because all topical antimicrobial agents are potentially toxic and can retard corneal wound healing, therapy should be reduced after the first definite signs of clinical improvement.

Corneal Thinning and Perforation

Structural alterations of the cornea can occur as a result of bacterial keratitis. A persistent epithelial defect predisposes to stromal collagen loss.[40] Progressive inflammation could be due to necrotizing enzymes and other exotoxins, continued microbial replication because of suboptimal antimicrobial therapy, or other disease entities. Rescrapings may be indicated for continued corneal inflammation with ongoing tissue destruction.

The appearance of radiating striae from a point of stromal thinning suggests tension of Descemet membrane as a sign of impending perforation.[147] With severe corneal thinning or descemetocele formation, a protective eye shield is useful to prevent inadvertent ocular trauma and corneal rupture. Likewise, if a subconjunctival injection is given in the presence of a descemetocele, eyelid akinesia can prevent extreme eyelid squeezing that could dangerously raise the intraocular pressure and lead to dehiscence.

Bacterial keratitis with corneal perforation can progress to endophthalmitis and result in expulsive hemorrhage.[276] Blindness and enucleation may be the final outcome. Definitive surgical and medical management is needed to save these eyes.

PATHOGENESIS

Multiple microorganisms are capable of causing bacterial keratitis (Table 74-4). Streptococci, particularly *S. pneumoniae,* are a predominant cause of bacterial keratitis in many developing nations* and were formerly the most common cause of bacterial keratitis in industrialized countries.[450] With changing risk factors[324] most series from Europe and North America now identify *Staphylococcus* species or *P. aeruginosa* in at least 50% of infected patients.[13] Regional variations reflect diverse patient populations, climatic conditions, and risk factors (Table 74-5).[141a,470]

The smallest inoculum that produces infection in the human cornea is not known. A single viable organism can theoretically initiate corneal infection. Only one clone predominates in most human infections. Quantitative experiments show that only about 50 *P. aeruginosa* or 100 *S. aureus* are needed to initiate corneal infection.[235,236] Animal models of bacterial keratitis are produced by topical appli-

cation of bacteria after scratching or abrading the epithelium,[190] by intrastromal inoculation, and by placement of a contaminated suture or contact lens to the cornea. These studies have led to current understanding of the mechanisms of corneal inflammation during bacterial keratitis (Fig. 74-8).

Bacterial Adherence

Bacterial keratitis results when microbial virulence factors overcome host defense mechanisms. The successful corneal pathogen attaches to the corneal surface and avoids the clearance mechanisms of the tear film. Some bacteria secrete IgA proteases that cleave the proline-rich hinge region of IgA, thereby allowing microbial colonization and attachment. Within approximately 15 to 30 minutes after injury, viable bacteria adhere to the damaged edge of basal corneal epithelial cells (Fig. 74-9),[346,413,422] occasionally to older cells near a traumatized area, and to the basement membrane or the bare stroma near the wound edge.[406] Some bacteria adhere predominantly to areas without microvilli or microplicae,[402] and the glycocalyx of injured epithelium is particularly susceptible to attachment by microorganisms. In the neonate, bacteria can adhere without prior trauma by preferentially attaching to superficial epithelial cells.[167] The molecular changes of the corneal surface or extracellular matrix that predispose to bacterial infection in the wounded or immature cornea remain to be elucidated.

Microbial attachment is initiated by the interaction of bacterial adhesins with glycoprotein receptors of the ocular surface.[42,328,349,396] Different bacterial genera, species, and

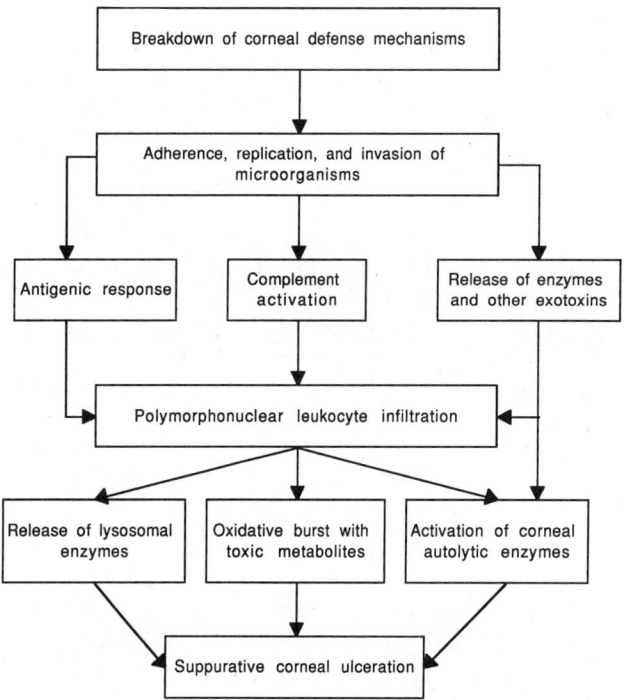

Fig. 74-8. Pathogenetic mechanisms of bacterial keratitis.

---

*References 7, 63, 211, 269, 442, 482, 483.

TABLE 74-4 REPORTED CAUSES OF BACTERIAL KERATITIS

Taxonomic Group	Family	Genus and Species
Aerobic or facultatively anaerobic gram-positive cocci	Micrococcaceae	*Micrococcus kristinae*
		Micrococcus luteus
		Micrococcus roseus
		Micrococcus sedentarius
		Micrococcus varians
	Micrococcaceae	*Stomatococcus mucilaginosus*
	Micrococcaceae	*Planococcus citreus*
		Planococcus halophilus
	Micrococcaceae	*Staphylococcus aureus*
		Staphylococcus capitis
		Staphylococcus ohnii
		Staphylococcus epidermidis
		Staphylococcus haemolyticus
		Staphylococcus hominis
		Staphylococcus hyicus
		Staphylococcus lentus
		Staphylococcus simulans
		Staphylococcus warneri
		Staphylococcus xylosus
	Nonspecified	*Streptococcus acidominimus*
		Streptococcus agalactiae
		Streptococcus pneumoniae
		Streptococcus pyogenes
		Streptococcus anginosus ⎫
		Streptococcus mitis ⎪
		Streptococcus mutans ⎬ "viridans"
		Streptococcus salivarius ⎪
		Streptococcus sanguis ⎭
		Enterococcus durans
		Enterococcus faecalis
		Enterococcus faecium
		Pedicoccus damnosus
		Pedicoccus parvulus
		Aerococcus viridans
Anaerobic gram-positive cocci	Nonspecified	*Gemella morbillorum*
	Nonspecified	*Peptococcus niger*
	Nonspecified	*Peptostreptococcus anaerobius*
		Peptostreptococcus asaccharolyticus
		Peptostreptococcus magnus
		Peptostreptococcus prevotii
	Nonspecified	*Coprococcus eutactus*
Aerobic or facultatively anaerobic gram-positive rods	Nonspecified	*Listeria monocytogenes*
	Nonspecified	*Erysipelothrix rhusiopathiae*
	Nonspecified	*Kurthia zopfii*
	Nonspecified	*Corynebacterium diphtheriae*
		Corynebacterium jeikeium
		Corynebacterium matruchotii
		Corynebacterium minutissimum
		Corynebacterium mycetoides
		Corynebacterium pseudodiphtheriticum
		Corynebacterium striatum
		Corynebacterium xerosis
		Arcanobacterium haemolyticum
	Nonspecified	*Propionibacterium acnes*
		Propionibacterium avidum
		Propionibacterium granulosum

TABLE 74-4   REPORTED CAUSES OF BACTERIAL KERATITIS   cont'd

Taxonomic Group	Family	Genus and Species
	Nonspecified	*Eubacterium lentum*
	Nonspecified	*Bifidobacterium dentium*
Aerobic or spore-forming facultatively anaerobic gram-positive rods	Nonspecified	*Bacillus brevis*
		Bacillus cereus
		Bacillus circulans
		Bacillus coagulans
		Bacillus laterosporus
		Bacillus licheniformis
		Bacillus megaterium
		Bacillus polymyxa
		Bacillus pumilus
		Bacillus sphaericus
		Bacillus subtilis
		Bacillus thuringiensis
Anaerobic spore-forming gram-positive rods	Nonspecified	*Clostridium perfringens*
		Clostridium septicum
		Clostridium sputigena
		Clostridium tetani
Aerobic gram-negative rods and cocci	Pseudomonadaceae	*Pseudomonas acidovorans*
		Pseudomonas aeruginosa
		Pseudomonas alcaligenes
		Pseudomonas diminuta
		Pseudomonas fluorescens
		Pseudomonas mallei
		Pseudomonas mendocina
		Pseudomonas paucimobilis
		Pseudomonas pickettii
		Pseudomonas pseudoalcaligenes
		Pseudomonas putida
		Pseudomonas stutzeri
		Pseudomonas vesicularis
	Pseudomonadaceae	*Burkholderia cepacia*
	Pseudomonadaceae	*Stenotrophomonas maltophilia*
	Pseudomonadaceae	*Comamonas acidovorans*
	Pseudomonadaceae	*Flavimonas oryzihabitans*
	Pseudomonadaceae	*Chryseomonas luteola*
	Azotobacteraceae	*Azomonas agilis*
	Azotobacteraceae	*Azotobacter beijerinkii*
		Azotobacter chroococcum
		Azotobacter paspali
		Azotobacter vinelandii
	Methylococcaceae	*Methylobacterium extorquens*
		Methylobacterium mesophilicum
	Neisseriaceae	*Neisseria cinerea*
		Neisseria flavescens
		Neisseria gonorrhoeae
		Neisseria lactamica
		Neisseria meningitidis
		Neisseria mucosa
		Neisseria sicca
		Neisseria subflava
	Neisseriaceae	*Moraxella atlantae*
		Moraxella catarrhalis
		Moraxella lacunata
		Moraxella nonliquefaciens
		Moraxella osloensis

Continued

TABLE 74-4 REPORTED CAUSES OF BACTERIAL KERATITIS cont'd

Taxonomic Group	Family	Genus and Species
	Neisseriaceae	*Acinetobacter baumannii*
		Acinetobacter calcoaceticus
		Acinetobacter johnsonii
		Acinetobacter junii
	Neisseriaceae	*Kingella denitrificans*
		Kingella kingae
	Nonspecified	*Flavobacterium breve*
		Flavobacterium indologenes
		Flavobacterium meningosepticum
		Flavobacterium multivorum
		Flavobacterium odoratum
		Flavobacterium spiritovorum
	Nonspecified	*Alcaligenes denitrificans*
		Alcaligenes faecalis
		Alcaligenes odorans
		Alcaligenes xylosoxidans
	Nonspecified	*Paracoccus denitrificans*
Facultatively anaerobic gram-negative rods	Enterobacteriaceae	*Escherichia coli*
		Escherichia hermanii
	Enterobacteriaceae	*Shigella flexneri*
		Shigella sonnei
	Enterobacteriaceae	*Citrobacter amalonaticus*
		Citrobacter diversus
		Citrobacter freundii
	Enterobacteriaceae	*Klebsiella oxytoca*
		Klebsiella ozaenae
		Klebsiella pneumoniae
	Enterobacteriaceae	*Enterobacter aerogenes*
		Enterobacter agglomerans
		Enterobacter amnigenus
		Enterobacter cloacae
		Enterobacter gergoviae
		Enterobacter sakazakii
	Enterobacteriaceae	*Serratia liquefaciens*
		Serratia marcescens
		Serratia plymuthica
		Serratia rubidaea
	Enterobacteriaceae	*Edwardsiella tarda*
	Enterobacteriaceae	*Proteus mirabilis*
		Proteus vulgaris
	Enterobacteriaceae	*Providencia rettgeri*
		Providencia stuartii
	Enterobacteriaceae	*Morganella morganii*
	Enterobacteriaceae	*Tatumella ptyseos*
	Enterobacteriaceae	*Yersinia enterocolitica*
		Yersinia ruckeri
	Vibrionaceae	*Aeromonas hydrophila*
		Aeromonas salmonicida
		Aeromonas sobria
	Vibrionaceae	*Shewanella putrefaciens*
	Pasteurellaceae	*Pasteurella multocida*
	Pasteurellaceae	*Haemophilus aphrophilus*
		Haemophilus haemolyticus
		Haemophilus influenzae
		Haemophilus parahaemolyticus
		Haemophilus parainfluenzae
		Haemophilus paraphrophilus

TABLE 74-4 REPORTED CAUSES OF BACTERIAL KERATITIS cont'd

Taxonomic Group	Family	Genus and Species
	Cytophagaceae	*Capnocytophaga canimorsus*
		Capnocytophaga ochracea
		Capnocytophaga sputigena
	Nonspecified	*Eikenella corrodens*
Anaerobic gram-negative rods	Bacteroidaceae	*Bacteroides fragilis*
		Bacteroides melaninogenicus
	Bacteroidaceae	*Fusobacterium nucleatum*
Anaerobic gram-negative cocci	Veillonellaceae	*Veillonella parvula*

Compiled from literature reports and ocular microbiology laboratory sources. Other causes of bacterial keratitis include the nontuberculous mycobacteria and the actinomycetes (Chapters 75 and 76).

TABLE 74-5 PREDOMINANT MICROORGANISMS CAUSING BACTERIAL KERATITIS

	Relative Frequency		
	Developed Countries		
Bacteria	Adults	Children	Developing Countries
Staphylococcus species	30-50%	25%	15-25%
Streptococcus species	15%	40%	30-50%
Pseudomonas species	15-30%	20%	10-20%
Enteric gram-negative rods	10%	5-10%	5%
Corynebacterium species	5%	5%	10%
Moraxella and related species	5%	5%	5%

Compiled from multiple sources.

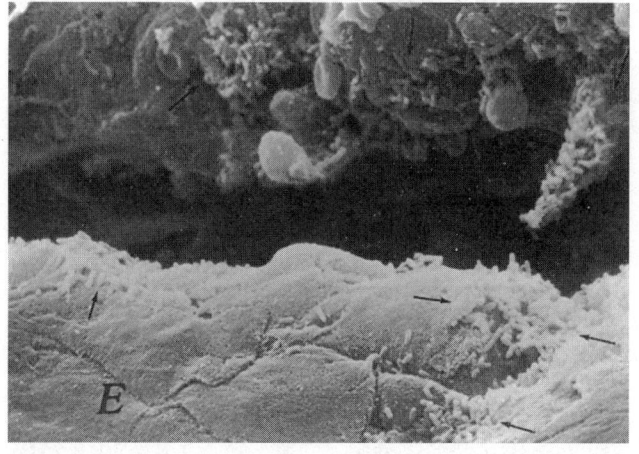

Fig. 74-9. Electron micrograph showing bacteria adherent to damaged edge (*arrows*) of corneal epithelium rather than to intact surface (*E*). (Reprinted with permission from Stern GA, Weitzenkorn D, Valenti J: Adherence of *Pseudomonas aeruginosa* to the mouse cornea: epithelial *v* stromal adherence. *Arch Ophthalmol* 100:1956-1958, 1982.)

strains have various mechanisms for adherence[164,197] and disparate binding affinities for corneal epithelial cells.[327] Many bacterial surface proteins serve as adhesins and mediate colonization to components of the cornea's extracellular matrix, such as fibronectin, fibrinogen, collagen, laminin, and elastin. Bacterial binding proteins are present within the outer membrane of many bacteria and on the fimbriae (pili) of gram-negative rods (see Chapter 15).

Adherence Mediated by Nonpilar Adhesins. Cell-surface integrins such as fibronectin act as receptors for lipoteichoic acid of *S. aureus*. Hydrophobic interactions might also be important during adherence.[230] The ability of certain bacteria to adhere to an epithelial defect may account for the frequent occurrence of *S. aureus, S. pneumoniae,* and *P. aeruginosa* infection.[348] Biofilm production enhances bacterial aggregation, protects adherent microorganisms, and helps growth during these early stages of infection.[190]

Adherence Mediated by Pili. *P. aeruginosa* can bind to epithelium by pili via the carboxy-terminal region of the pilin subunit. Glycoproteins, including galactose- and mannose-containing glycoconjugates,[165,364] and other substances[459] have been identified as molecular receptors for *P. aeruginosa. Moraxella* sp., another common cause of bacterial keratitis, formerly associated with poor hygiene and malnutrition[33] and more recently with various causes of corneal epithelial changes,[80,274] attaches to a damaged corneal surface with pili. Pili also facilitate adherence of *Neisseria* sp.

Entry into surface epithelial cells is partially mediated by the production of a bacterial cell-surface protein called invasin that binds to epithelial cell-surface proteins known as integrins. This tight interaction triggers phagocytosis of the bacterium by the epithelial cell through stimulation of cytoskeletal processes normally involved in cell motility. Other mechanisms involved in epithelial cell penetration involve the release of a protease. *N. gonorrhoeae,*[431] *N. meningitidis,*[22] *Corynebacterium diphtheriae, Haemophilus influenzae, Shigella* spp.,[432] and *Listeria monocytogenes* could penetrate the intact corneal epithelial surface by these types of mechanisms.

Bacterial Invasion

As fusion begins between the bacterial and epithelial cell membranes, shallow pit-like depressions appear in the corneal epithelial cell. As more bacteria are engulfed with progressive intracellular invasion, granular elevations of the corneal epithelium may be the presenting sign of early bacterial keratitis.[356] Bacteria multiply by binary fission and gradually migrate across the epithelial barrier into the anterior stroma. Some bacteria invade intercellularly by separating apical tight junctions, and others proliferate on the bare stromal surface of a corneal wound. Some bacterial strains are cytotoxic whereas others can persist within epithelial cells. The effect on bacterial growth of a reduction in anti-

bacterial proteins associated with increased tearing is difficult to determine.[237a] The attachment and invasion processes will become better characterized as the bacterial binding epitopes and the corneal surface receptors are better identified.

Colonization on the corneal surface sometimes precedes stromal invasion. The colony-like proliferation of bacteria within a macroulcerative epithelial defect has been called an "agar-plate phenomenon" (Fig. 74-10). These microsatellites can evolve to a variant of infectious crystalline keratopathy. Without antibiotics or other modulating factors, bacteria invade, survive, and replicate in the corneal stroma.

The bacterial capsule and other surface components are important in corneal invasion. For example, some bacteria avoid activation of the alternate complement pathway because of their capsular polysaccharide. It is the subcapsular cell-wall constituents, namely lipopolysaccharide, however, that are the major determinants of corneal inflammation. Experimental intrastromal inoculation of endotoxin shows a dose- and time-dependent inflammatory response.[434]

Keratocytes are capable of phagocytosis,[238] but the exposed, avascular corneal stroma has little protection. Microorganisms insinuate between the anterior stromal lamellae and produce extracellular enzymes that destroy corneal ground substance and collagen fibrils. Invasion begins within one hour after exogenous contamination of a corneal wound[190] and within several hours after the application of a heavily contaminated contact lens.[240] The largest relative increase in the bacterial population occurs within the first one to two days of stromal infection.[235]

Soon after inoculation bacteria infiltrate under the surrounding epithelium and into the deeper stroma around

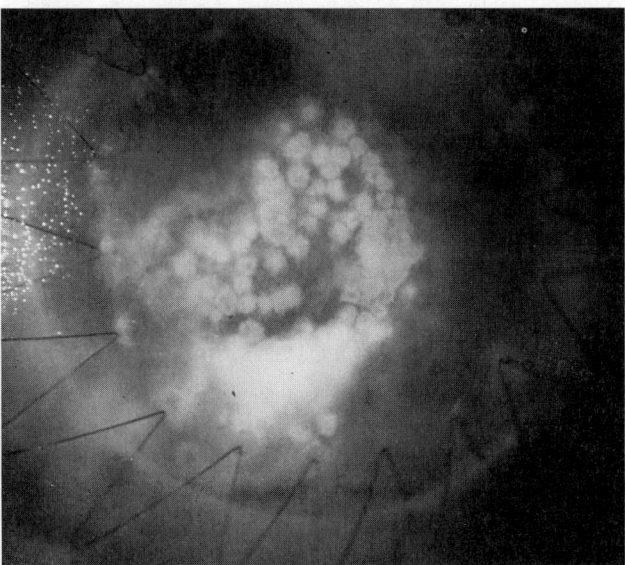

Fig. 74-10. *Staphylococcus aureus* keratitis occurring in corneal transplant as superficial, multifocal, pauciinflammatory infiltrates.

the initial site of infection. Whereas no single strain of a bacterial species accounts for most infections, a single clone probably predominates in a given patient.[52a] Special stains can reveal microorganisms throughout the area of focal inflammation, but viable bacteria tend to be more likely found at the peripheral margins of the infiltrate or deep within a central ulcer crater. Rods align parallel to the long axis of collagen fibrils. Unchecked invasion and multiplication of bacteria in the corneal stroma result in progressive enlargement or extension of infectious foci into the surrounding cornea (Fig. 74-11).

Host Response

Corneal inflammation results from various soluble mediators and inflammatory cells. Some of these components are

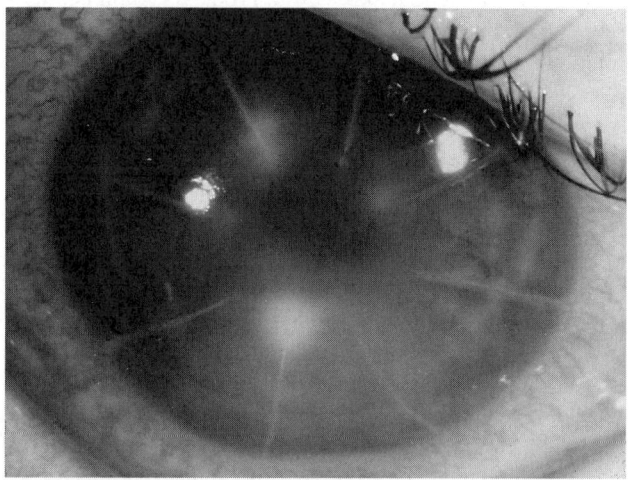

A

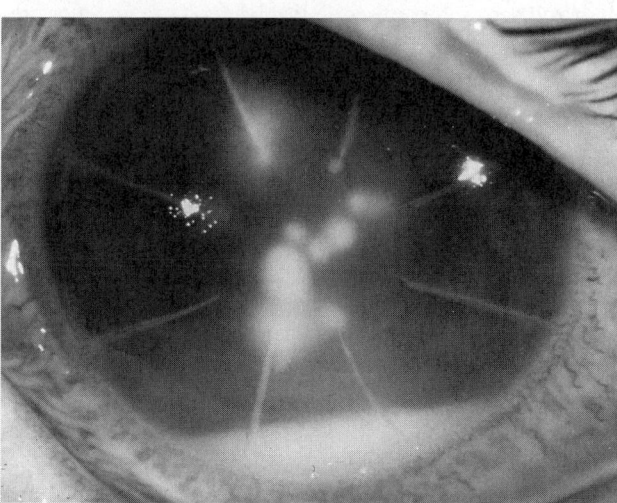

B

Fig. 74-11. Worsening of pneumococcal keratitis. **A,** Suppurative infiltrates deep within radial keratotomy incisions. **B,** Two days later, infiltrates have enlarged, and "satellite lesions" have appeared in deep stroma.

endogenously present in the normal cornea, others are locally produced, and the remainder are brought to the cornea by the vascular and lymphatic systems. Soluble mediators of inflammation include the kinin-forming system, the clotting and fibrinolytic systems, immunoglobulins, complement components, vasoactive amines, eicosanoids, neuropeptides, and cytokines (see Chapter 17). The relative importance of these substances remains to be clarified.

The complement cascade can be triggered to kill bacteria by three different molecules: C3 that binds directly to exposed bacterial proteins, mannose-binding protein (secreted by the liver in response to interleukin-6 released by stimulated macrophages) that binds to the bacterial capsule, and antibodies that bind to bacterial antigens and activate C1q. The role of the complement system in bacterial keratitis remains uncertain,[451] but complement-dependent chemotaxins[296] can initiate focal inflammation.

The production of polypeptide cytokines such as tumor necrosis factor and interleukin-1[390] results in the adherence and transendothelial passage of neutrophils in limbal blood vessels. This process is mediated by cell adhesion molecules. These glycoproteins include integrins and selectins on vascular endothelial cells and on leukocytes and members of the immunoglobulin superfamily such as intercellular adhesion molecules. During bacterial keratitis, intercellular adhesion molecule-1 (ICAM-1, a ligand for a β2 integrin on leukocytes) is expressed on limbal vascular endothelial cells and is focally increased on corneal cells.[339] Selectin, a lectin-like surface glycoprotein, mediates adhesion between neutrophils and cytokine-stimulated sialomucin receptors on vascular endothelium. A complex but coordinated sequence of events leads to neutrophil diapedesis (Fig. 74-12).

Vascular dilatation of the conjunctival and limbal blood vessels is associated with increased permeability, leading to an inflammatory exudate in the tear film and peripheral cornea. Neutrophils adhere to the capillary vascular endothelium of many vessels of the anterior segment and interpose between these endothelial cells. Polymorphonuclear leukocytes can enter the injured cornea anteriorly through an epithelial defect, but most migrate from the limbus.[74] Factors that delay the initial inflammatory response, such as contact lens wear and aging, can facilitate bacterial growth.

Recruitment of acute inflammatory cells occurs within a few hours after bacterial inoculation, particularly in the corneal quadrant closest to the infected area. For superficial infections, neutrophils insinuate between the anterior stromal lamellae. This influx of neutrophils is chemotactically directed toward the area of microbial proliferation by bacterial proteins. One of these chemotactic factors has been identified as a protein ending in the tripeptide formylmethionyl-leucyl-phenylalanine. As neutrophils accumulate at the infected site, host substances such as leukotrienes and complement components are presumably released that attract additional leukocytes. Macrophages subsequently

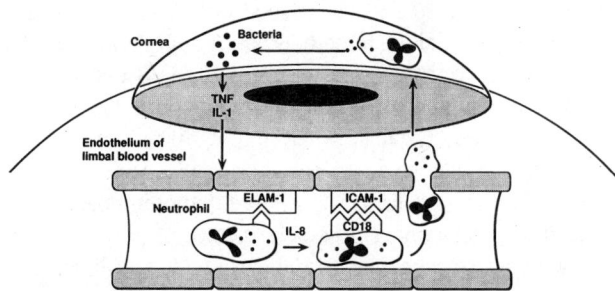

Fig. 74-12. Schematic model of neutrophil recruitment into corneal stroma during bacterial keratitis. Replicating bacteria induce production of chemoattractants and cytokines such as interleukin-1 (IL-1) and tumor necrosis factor (TNF) by corneal epithelial and stromal cells. These polypeptides result in expression of selectin molecules, such as endothelial leukocyte-adhesion molecule-1 (ELAM-1), on vascular endothelium that bind to specific carbohydrate component of neutrophil surface glycoproteins. Soon thereafter cytokines increase expression of integrins (CD18) on neutrophils and intercellular adhesion molecule-1 (ICAM-1) on endothelial cells. Following adherence, neutrophils migrate between endothelial cells into peripheral cornea. Cytokines and other stimuli result in degranulation and release of toxic oxygen metabolites and vasoactive lipid autacoids, such as leukotrienes and prostaglandins. Expression of ELAM-1 on corneal endothelial cells may account for appearance of inflammatory plaque on posterior cornea.

begin to migrate to the cornea toward the area of bacterial proliferation, ingesting invading microorganisms and degenerating neutrophils.[185]

The overlying epithelium becomes edematous and necrotic then sloughs. Iris vascular dilatation with increased vascular permeability and exudation of proteins and inflammatory cells into the anterior chamber occurs, leading to an inflammatory plaque on the endothelial surface under the infected zone and to a hypopyon.

Progression: Bacterial Factors

Many manifestations of bacterial keratitis involve microbial constituents and products. Different bacteria have different pathogenic effects.[2,212] Proliferating microorganisms liberate a variety of extracellular toxins capable of corneal destruction.[201,205,459] Bacterial exoenzymes such as elastase and alkaline protease degrade proteoglycans such as lumican and decorin, types III and IV collagens, and gelatins (denatured collagen). Despite the presence of protease inhibitors in tears[494] and the cornea, these and other bacterial cell components are important factors in the pathogenesis of bacterial keratitis.

The effect of bacterial enzymes is magnified by their various actions. By activating the kallikrein-kinin cascade that enhances vascular permeability,[281] proteases released from bacteria such as *P. aeruginosa* and *Serratia marcescens* can produce as much corneal damage as live organisms.

Other bacteria that produce extracellular proteases include *S. aureus, S. pyogenes, Bacillus* spp., *Bacteroides* spp., and *Neisseria* spp. Hyaluronidase released by several microorganisms can directly digest the mucopolysaccharide ground substance of the corneal stroma. Both nuclear and plasmid-encoded cytolysins include several substances, especially phospholipases, that destroy cellular membranes and produce corneal destruction. Some extracellular compounds, such as exotoxin A produced by *P. aeruginosa,* are directly cytotoxic to corneal cells.[162]

Unlike exotoxins, which are generally proteins, endotoxins are lipopolysaccharides of the outer bacterial cell membrane. Released upon bacterial death, bacterial lipopolysaccharide complexes with lipopolysaccharide-binding protein and binds to either soluble or membrane-bound CD14 receptors on macrophages. This results in a transmembrane signal for stimulated leukocytes to produce certain peptides (e.g., tumor necrosis factor, interleukin-1, interleukin-6, and interleukin-8), lipids (e.g., prostaglandin E_2, thromboxane A_2, leucotriene B_4, and platelet-activating factor), and oxides (including O_2-, H_2O_2, and NO). While these substances facilitate bacterial killing, they also contribute to corneal destruction. Platelet-activating factor, for example, activates the expression of certain metalloproteinases that may promote corneal ulceration.

Endotoxin, liberated after the death of gram-negative bacteria, can activate the alternate complement pathway and is believed to be involved in the appearance of the ring infiltrate induced by *P. aeruginosa, E. coli,* and other gram-negative bacteria.[295,298] Complement components that mediate leucocyte chemotaxis initiate this annular accumulation of neutrophils. Complement can also induce the release of lysosomal enzymes that exacerbate the inflammatory response.

Virulence factors of individual bacteria of known or presumed importance for corneal infection are summarized as follows:

Staphylococci. *Staphylococcus aureus* produces coagulase and lysozyme, but staphylococcal species that lack these traits are also occasional pathogens. Most *S. aureus* strains contain protein A, a cell-wall component lacking in other staphylococcal species. Protein A appears to protect the bacterium from phagocytosis by binding immunoglobulin but is not a major virulence factor for bacterial keratitis. Other virulence factors produced by *S. aureus,* and also some strains of *S. epidermidis* and other species, include lipoteichoic acid, the capsule, and extracellular enzymes such as hyaluronidase, lipase, staphylokinase, and DNAse. Staphylococcal alpha-toxin and, to a lesser extent, beta-hemolysin are involved in stimulating necrosis and inflammation during bacterial keratitis. Staphylococcal strains that produce exoenzymes generally cause more severe corneal inflammation.[270]

Streptococci. Pneumococci can proliferate in the presence of neutrophils as peptidoglycan and M protein inhibit opsonization, impair complement activation, and reduce leukocyte migration. This action by M protein is further enhanced by the fibrinogen degradation products produced in infected tissue from the activation of plasminogen by streptokinase. During established infection, pneumolysin, a cytolytic protein that can activate complement, attracts polymorphonuclear leukocytes.[198] Bacterial collagenase, hyaluronidase, streptodornase, and streptokinase exacerbate stromal suppurative necrosis and help bacteria to invade.

Gram-Negative Rods. *Pseudomonas* spp. and other gram-negative rods contain endotoxin, a cell-wall lipopolysaccharide that can activate the kinin, fibrinolytic, and complement systems that enhance corneal inflammation.[337] The lipid component, called lipid A, is embedded in the outer membrane and is responsible for many of the biologic effects of endotoxin. Its rigid structure makes the membrane less permeable and partially accounts for the difficulty of gram-negative bacteria to absorb and retain crystal violet in the Gram stain. This substance results in the poor penetration and ineffectiveness of many antibiotics against these organisms. Attached to lipid A is a polysaccharide that protrudes externally. The outermost string of sugars varies between bacterial species and produces antigenic specificity. Lipopolysaccharide aids in attachment of gram-negative bacteria to the cornea through hydrophobic effects and is involved in intraepithelial entry. These and other substances of the bacterial cell surface, such as ferripyochelin,[403] are involved in virulence.

Pseudomonas sp. produces extracellular metalloenzymes such as elastase, alkaline protease,[184] and other proteinases that digest corneal glycosaminoglycans.[233] Bacterial metalloproteinases can degrade immunoglobulins and cytokines, inhibit neutrophils and lymphocytes, and aid bacterial invasion through the corneal basement membrane and stroma. These proteases are the major initiators of corneal destruction during pseudomonal[95,489] and serratial[209,261] keratitis and can activate corneal metalloproteases through limited proteolysis.

Other exoenzymes include lipolytic hemolysins, predominantly phospholipases, that degrade cellular membranes. Exotoxin A is a nonenzymatic polypeptide that inhibits protein biosynthesis through inactivation of elongation factor 2 by adenosine diphosphate ribosylation. Whereas other bacterial proteases are more important in producing keratitis, exotoxin A can affect corneal cells,[162,191] damage the stromal proteoglycan ground substance, and produce a cataract, without stimulating rapid neutrophil infiltration.[161]

Progression: Host Factors

Progressive corneal ulceration occurs by enzymes liberated from bacteria, from corneal epithelial and stromal cells, and from inflammatory cells.[201,219] Exoenzymes released from proliferating bacteria are responsible for the initial pathogenic events of bacterial keratitis, but sequential tissue destruction is largely due to the release of lysosomal contents from stimulated leukocytes.[417] In *P. aeruginosa* keratitis, pseudomonal elastase is involved in the early stages of invasion and inflammation; but while it initially inactivates leukocytic enzymes, progressive suppurative ulceration is due to ongoing recruitment of neutrophils.

Corneal Enzymes. Activation of corneal proenzymes can exacerbate corneal damage during bacterial keratitis. Corneal cells can produce matrix metalloproteinases (MMPs, matrixins), including an interstitial collagenase (MMP1), a stromelysin (MMP3), a gelatinase (MMP2), and a serine proteinase (MMP9). Some of these enzymes are produced constitutively while others require induction. Cleaving a cysteine-containing propeptide from the NH_2-terminal end yields the active enzyme with a zinc-binding catalytic domain. Enzyme production is genetically regulated, and these corneal proteases are controlled by endogenous protein inhibitors, the tissue inhibitor of metalloproteinases (TIMP) family. The cornea also produces serine proteinase inhibitors, α_1-proteinase inhibitor, plasminogen activator inhibitors 1 and 2, and α_2-macroglobulin that may help protect the cornea from proteolytic degradation by bacterial enzymes. Corneal production of acid proteases (e.g., cathepsins B and D), plasminogen activator, urokinase, and calpain may also play roles in bacterial keratitis.

Bacterial exoenzymes, such as pseudomonal elastase and pneumococcal pneumolysin, stimulate the production and activation of endogenous corneal metalloproteases.[280,437] Collagenase is activated about 3 days after inoculation. Collagenases cleave collagen molecules and disrupt their helical structure, allowing other proteases to disrupt the glycoprotein stromal matrix. Collagen degradation products are chemotactic for polymorphonuclear leukocytes.

Leukocytic Enzymes. Bacterial eradication by polymorphonuclear leukocytes involves phagocytosis and lysosomal degranulation. Within the phagolysosome, digestive enzymes and an acidic pH kill bacteria. Phagocytosis and intracellular degranulation by polymorphonuclear leukocytes also involve oxidative attack with the production of toxic oxygen metabolites. Triggering of the phagocyte's respiratory burst by bacterial engulfment, as well as by an endogenous corneal protein stimulant,[335] results in the biosynthesis of superoxide anions and other oxidizing agents such as hydrogen peroxide and taurine chloramine.

Phagocytic secretion and lysis result in extracellular lysosomal enzymes, such as proteoglycanase, elastase, collagenases, cathepsins, and myeloperoxidase. These enzymes and the oxygen-derived free radicals cause stromal destruction by breaking collagen strands, digesting glycosaminoglycans, and disrupting keratocytes.[10] Nitric oxide also mediates vasodilatation and can function as a neurotransmitter. These and other substances released from activated neutrophils are responsible for stromal necrosis and corneal edema[75] during bacterial keratitis.

Immune Mediators. The importance of humoral and cellular immunity during bacterial keratitis has not been determined. Immune recognition seems to play a role in effective phagocytosis by polymorphonuclear leukocytes.[436] Antibodies might speed resolution during reinfection but are probably not important in bacterial clearance during the initial infection.[344] Langerhans cells are found in the corneal epithelium,[338] but the functional importance of these antigen-presenting cells during bacterial keratitis is unclear.

Bacterial endotoxin and exotoxins can stimulate macrophages to release several biologically active substances including interleukin-1, interleukin-6, and cachectin, cytokines that act synergistically to elicit inflammatory reactions. Selected cytokines, certain eicosanoids, and other molecular mediators are involved in ulceration and angiogenesis during bacterial keratitis. CD8 + T cells are possibly involved in the successful resolution of bacterial keratitis.

Tissue Damage

Extensive inflammatory necrosis leads to a necrotic and disorganized stroma. If superficial, stromal ulceration appears; if deep, an abscess forms. Corneal inflammation may remain localized, expand into the surrounding cornea, extend in a crescentic distribution from a peripheral focus, or advance into the deeper stroma. With progression, liquefactive stromal necrolysis occurs. Extension into the adjacent sclera is unusual unless there has been prior trauma or surgery.

As inflammatory cells spread diffusely throughout the corneal stroma, macrophages begin to encircle the area. The pattern of inflammatory spread depends upon microbial virulence and proliferation, the inflammatory response, the anatomy of the host cornea, and the efficacy of antimicrobial therapy. Clinical variations are due to differences in one or more of these factors. For example, phagocytic function impaired by aging[163,178] or disease can result in reduced stromal inflammation.

Gradually a distinct line of demarcation encircles the zone of ulceration or abscess. With increasing edema the Descemet membrane may stretch into undulating folds. As the cornea weakens from progressive stromal ulceration, the Descemet membrane may then bulge forward. With persistent thinning and stretching, a descemetocele is liable to perforate from accidental trauma. Extensive tissue loss may lead to corneal perforation with iris prolapse that may either seal the wound and prevent intraocular progression or provide a portal of entry for intraocular invasion leading to bacterial endophthalmitis.

Neovascularization. Limbal vascular dilatation is common. Persistent inflammation may produce corneal neovascularization.[254] Peripheral corneal neovascularization may appear within one to two weeks. Capillary budding is first noted as tufts in the palisades of Vogt near the infectious focus. These vascular sprouts gradually lengthen, invading the subepithe-lial cornea and sometimes the mid or deeper corneal stroma. Neovascularization can advance to, and even beyond, the infected site.

Intraocular Inflammation. The sterile anterior-chamber inflammatory reaction consists predominantly of polymorphonuclear leukocytes. Nonspecific phagocytosis of iris pigment granules occurs. Sometimes macrophages and giant cells are present. Since the iris blood vessels are usually dilated, erythrocytes may be admixed in the hypopyon, but a visible hyphema rarely appears unless iris neovascularization is present from prior disease. Fibrinous strands tend to form between apposed tissues, leading to peripheral iris adhesions and posterior synechiae. Leukocytes accumulate in a gravity-dependent hypopyon in the lower angle and are sometimes enmeshed in a fibrinous coagulum on the iris and in the pupil. Severe anterior-chamber inflammation can lead to secondary ocular hypertension.

Recovery

After the initial proliferation of bacteria, the number of organisms soon plateaus at several million.[447] Polymorphonuclear leukocytes play a major role in limiting bacterial multiplication. Granulocyte phagocytosis can be mediated by bacterial surface lectins recognized by specific sugar subunits of surface glycoproteins on leukocytes. This process of lectinophagocytosis acts in reverse when lectins on macrophages interact with bacterial carbohydrates.

Bacteria are eliminated by both pharmacologic and inflammatory mechanisms. Within one week of effective topical bactericidal therapy, all viable bacteria are usually killed. Undigested bacteria can sometimes survive within degranulated neutrophils or in sequestered, necrotic stroma. The optimal duration of antibacterial therapy has not been determined.

With control of bacterial proliferation, healing and reparative processes begin as the acute inflammatory reaction subsides. The overlying epithelium gradually regenerates, and epithelial cells fill stromal depressions. Langerhans cells appear in the central cornea during epithelial healing.[139] Complete reepithelialization can be followed by partial regression of corneal neovascularization. A damaged Bowman layer is replaced by a fibrovascular pannus, and necrotic tissue sloughs. Local fibroblastic transformation lays down fibrous tissue in the affected stroma, occasionally causing an elevated outgrowth.

Fibrogenesis in response to corneal inflammation is mediated by cytokines such as transforming growth factor β (TGF-β). Tissue injury upregulates the TGF-β-1 gene of corneal epithelial cells to synthesize precursors that are proteolytically cleaved and then activated. TGF-β-1 acts on keratocytes to induce the deposition of extracellular matrix through increased protein synthesis and inhibition of stromal collagenase synthesis.

The opaque scar is composed predominantly of disorga-

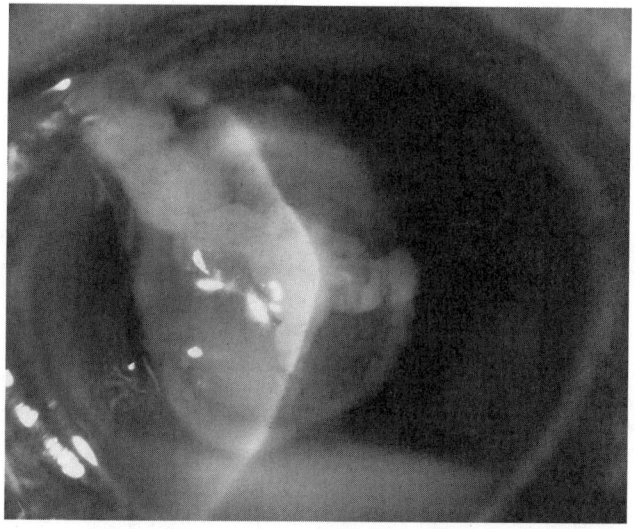

A

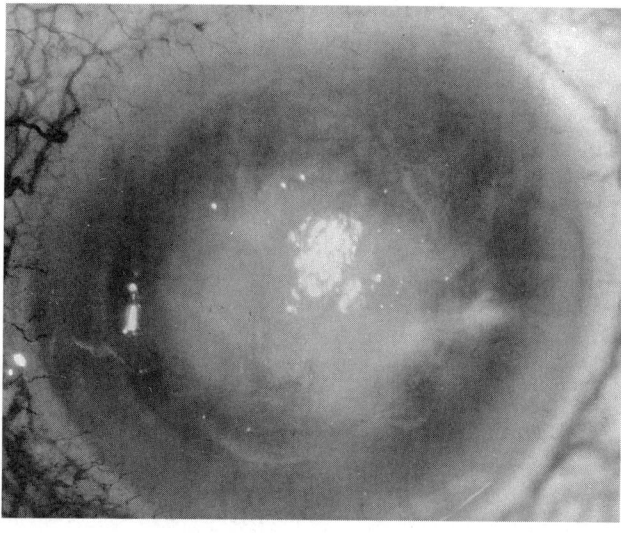

B

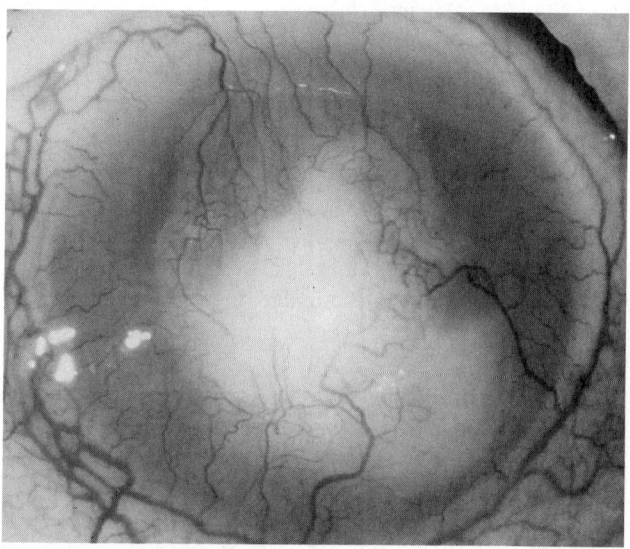

C

Fig. 74-13. Resolution of *Pseudomonas aeruginosa* keratitis. **A,** Bacterial keratitis occurred in patient with end-stage neovascular glaucoma. **B,** Residual corneal scarring followed one month of topical antibacterial therapy. **C,** Three years later vascularized corneal opacification has resulted. (Figure **A** also in color insert.)

nized collagen fibrils that can gradually remodel over the subsequent months (Fig. 74-13). The density of scar tissue can fade with time, especially in younger patients. Older individuals seem more likely to have a denser corneal scar (perhaps because during early infection they have enhanced bacterial growth and delayed neutrophil influx as a result of impaired upregulation of leukocyte adhesion molecules[178a]). A corneal staphyloma may follow a descemetocele, particularly if the intraocular pressure increased because of inflammatory blockage of the anterior-chamber angle. An adherent leukoma is evidence that corneal perforation occurred.

DIFFERENTIAL DIAGNOSIS

A suppurative stromal infiltrate raises the suspicion of bacterial keratitis, but the differentiation of microbial from nonmicrobial keratitis may be difficult. Certain clinical fea-

tures (Table 74-6) aid in distinguishing a microbial process from a sterile inflammatory reaction.[407]

Sterile corneal infiltrates occurring during contact lens wear[27,407] are commonly associated with poor contact lens hygiene and lens case contamination.[205] Gram-negative bacterial contamination of a soft contact lens can initiate a sterile, endotoxin-induced keratitis.[35] Punctate infiltrates are also associated with staphylococcal blepharitis and acute bacterial conjunctivitis[85] and typically appear as transient marginal subepithelial infiltrates. Similar antigenic reactions can follow foreign-body injuries.

Ocular surface disorders such as toxic keratopathy associated with chemical injury or overuse of topical drugs can cause epithelial ulceration and stromal keratitis. Dry-eye syndromes can also be associated with macroulcerative epithelial defects and a sterile inflammatory reaction. White

TABLE 74-6   CLINICAL COMPARISONS BETWEEN BACTERIAL KERATITIS
AND NONINFECTIOUS KERATITIS

Feature	Bacterial Keratitis	Noninfectious Keratitis
Onset	Usually acute	Subacute or acute
Predisposing factors	Various, including trauma, contact lens wear, and prior ocular surface disease	Various, including corneal foreign-body soft contact wear, blepharoconjunctivitis, herpetic eye disease, topical medications, etc.
Symptoms	Increasing pain and light sensitivity	Variable; usually initial mild discomfort or foreign-body sensation
Eyelids	Lid edema	Pseudoptosis
Conjunctiva	Marked hyperemia with episcleral injection and mucopurulent discharge	Mild hyperemia with mucoid discharge
Corneal epithelium	Usually ulcerated	Usually intact with punctate erosions
Corneal stroma	White-yellow suppurative infiltrate with blurred margins and surrounding inflammatory cells and edema	White-gray superficial infiltrate
Corneal endothelium	Pseudoguttata with occasional inflammatory plaque or ring under stromal infiltrate	Minimal changes
Anterior chamber	Variable; hypopyon common	Mild flare and cells, hypopyon uncommon

deposits in the anterior stroma of a corneal transplant can mimic some features of bacterial keratitis.[463]

Multiple other causes of acute and chronic corneal diseases may present with a persistent epithelial defect and stromal inflammation. Many of these causes of focal infiltration and necrosis, such as necrotizing stromal keratitis due to herpes simplex or varicella-zoster viruses, may resemble bacterial infection. Because various corneal stimuli can lead to hypopyon formation, the anterior-chamber inflammatory reaction is not a reliable sign in detecting the presence or absence of infection.

Intrastromal crystalline deposits occurring from several degenerative and traumatic conditions can resemble in-

fectious crystalline keratopathy. After penetrating keratoplasty, crystalline-like changes can follow stromal allograft rejection, presumably because of immune-complex deposition. Calcific degeneration can also take on a branching, needlelike appearance. Granular or crystalline foreign bodies may be mistaken as corneal infection if there is associated ulceration.[251]

Clinical indicators that help to distinguish bacterial keratitis from an underlying disease process are the following: an abrupt change in symptoms, the onset of a purulent discharge, an increase in the signs of corneal inflammation, the rapid enlargement of a suppurative infiltrate, and progressive stromal ulceration (Fig. 74-14). Daily observation may

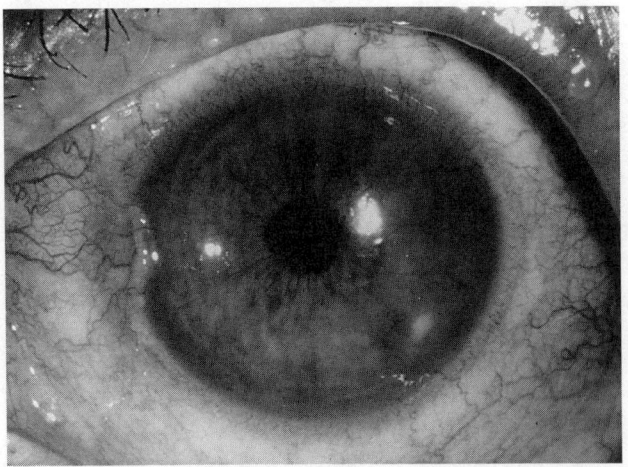
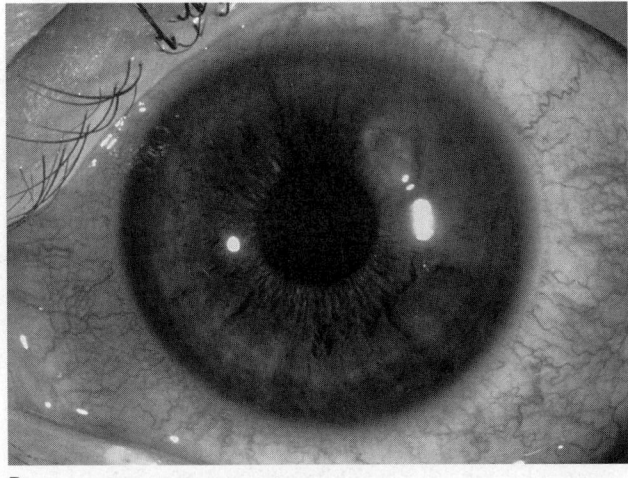

A   B

Fig. 74-14.   Comparison of noninfected and infected corneal infiltrates associated with soft contact lens wear. **A,** Sterile, nonnecrotic, nonulcerated, peripheral corneal infiltrate. **B,** Focal, suppurative ulceration with surrounding edema caused by *Pseudomonas aeruginosa.*

be an option in nonsevere cases because without treatment the natural courses of infected and sterile infiltrates differ. When two suspicions become one, then is the time to act.

LABORATORY INVESTIGATIONS

The diagnosis of bacterial keratitis cannot be established with certainty by the clinical features alone. Because distinguishing infectious from noninfectious causes of corneal inflammation can be difficult, diagnosis is based not only on clinical appearance but on definitive laboratory methods. Microbiologic evaluation can also guide appropriate therapy.

Specimen collection should try to get material directly from the infected site for smears and for inoculation to a transport system or, preferably, directly to culture media. Laboratory methods should isolate all potentially responsible microorganisms, including aerobic, facultatively anaerobic, and anaerobic bacteria, and fungi. A similar, thorough plan for specimen collection and inoculation should be applied to all cases of suspected microbial keratitis.[481a] Necessary materials and media (see box) are assembled and organized.[159] Additional selective media may be chosen to encourage the isolation of microorganisms that are less frequently encountered such as atypical mycobacteria and amoebae.

MATERIALS FOR LABORATORY INVESTIGATIONS OF SUSPECTED BACTERIAL KERATITIS

Items for Specimen Collection
Proparacaine hydrochloride 0.5%
Metallic spatula
Sterile calcium alginate swabs
Coplin jar with 95% methanol
Alcohol lamp with lighter
Glass slides with slide holders
Wax pencil or labels
Trypticase soy broth

Routine Media
Blood agar plate
Chocolate agar plate
Thioglycollate broth tube
Sabouraud dextrose agar plate with antibiotic (e.g., gentamicin 50 µg/ml)

Special Media
Brain-heart infusion broth with antibiotic (e.g., gentamicin 50 µg/ml)
Brucella blood agar plate
Thayer-Martin agar plate or slant
Löwenstein-Jensen agar slant
Middlebrook-Cohn agar slant
Nonnutrient agar plate with bacterial (e.g., *E. coli*) overlay
Tissue culture medium

Specimens should be collected directly from the infected corneal tissue. The value of material obtained from the eyelid margins and conjunctiva has not been clearly determined. If available, cultures can be taken from the traumatizing agent such as a foreign body, the contact lens, or an eyedropper bottle. Specimen containers must be properly labeled with the patient's name, collection date, and source. Information about the working diagnosis and recent medications should be provided. The type and duration of topical antibiotics can aid subsequent interpretation because prior antibacterial therapy can impair recovery.[181] Universal precautions should be followed in all phases of collection and transportation of infectious material, and all specimens must be treated as potentially hazardous.

Specimen Collection

Eyelid Margins and Conjunctiva. Swabbings may be done to evaluate the ocular flora of the eyelid margins, conjunctiva, and tear film.[121] Polyester and rayon swabs are adequate, but calcium alginate applicators are preferred because of their solubility in liquid media. Cotton-tipped swabs are acceptable but may contain fatty acids that inhibit bacterial growth. Unfortunately conjunctival and eyelid flora do not usually establish which bacteria are infecting the cornea.

Cornea. Before corneal scrapings or biopsy are started adequate anesthesia is usually administered. Ideally a sterile, unopened or unit-dose, nonpreserved topical anesthetic is used. Proparacaine hydrochloride 0.5% has less antibacterial properties than other commonly available topical anesthetic agents.[19] Sedation (e.g., oral chloral hydrate 50 to 100 mg/kg) is useful for children, particularly those younger than 5 years of age,[91] and mentally impaired adults.

An assistant or speculum can help hold the eyelids widely apart to reduce inadvertent contamination by the lid margins or eyelashes. Because the mucopurulent discharge may not contain viable bacteria, adherent exudate is removed before obtaining corneal scrapings.

Corneal Scrapings. A heat-sterilized Kimura spatula, bent needle,[397] rounded surgical knife, or similar instrument is used to perform corneal scrapings using slit-lamp biomicroscopic visualization (Fig. 74-15). Alternate collection methods include corneal swabbing,[36] rubbing with a cellulose sponge, and impression with sterile filter paper. These techniques can collect more bacteria than scraping. The metal spatula is heated to a bright orange with an alcohol lamp flame and allowed to cool. An assistant can speed the procedure by having several spatulas ready for use each time the cornea is scraped. A disposable cautery[312] that self-sterilizes between scrapings would be useful as a collection instrument if a proper tip were fashioned.

The ulcerated or infiltrated area is scraped by firmly but gently stroking and restroking without touching the eyelashes or eyelid margins. Both the central and peripheral margins of the infiltrated area are sampled to obtain material

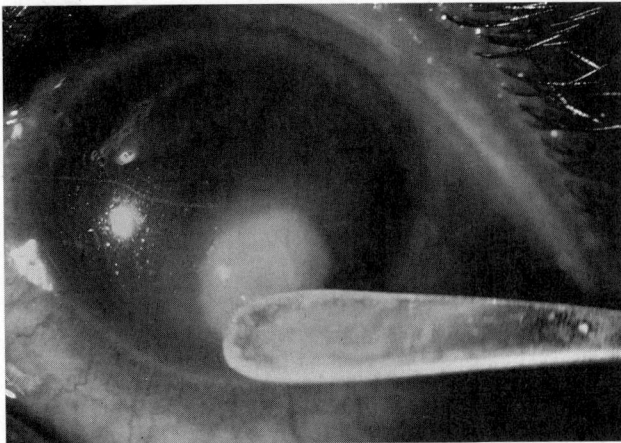

Fig. 74-15. Technique of corneal scrapings using metallic spatula to sample suppurative infiltrate directly.

for smears and for inoculation onto various media (Fig. 74-16). Viable organisms may be present throughout the inflamed area or localized to one zone such as the advancing margin or deep in the ulcer crater. For infections confined to the deep cornea, a vertical or oblique incision can permit sampling with a needle or minispatula.

After each set of scrapings, material is smeared onto a clean glass slide or is inoculated to a culture medium. Smears are prepared from all representative areas of suppuration, and multiple samples are obtained for each culture medium. Rescrapings are done after reflaming and cooling the spatula in order to obtain additional material from multiple areas of corneal suppuration. If material is limited, high priority should be given to inoculating the blood agar and chocolate agar plates and to preparing one or two smears. A purposeful order of specimen collection (Table 74-7) requires about 20 separate sets of corneal scrapings. Inoculation directly to growth media is preferred, but a reduced transport medium at room temperature can be used if delivered to the microbiology laboratory within a half hour.

Corneal Biopsy. Besides corneal scrapings, surgery can procure adequate material for laboratory evaluation.[304] Cor-

TABLE 74-7 SUGGESTED SEQUENCE OF CORNEAL SCRAPINGS FOR MICROBIAL KERATITIS

Step	Media and Smears	No. of Separate Sets of Scrapings*
1	Blood agar	1-4
2	Smear: acridine orange or Gram	1
3	Chocolate agar	1-4
4	Smear: acridine orange or Gram	1
5	Sabouraud agar	1
6	Thioglycollate broth	1
7	Smear: Giemsa or calcofluor white	1
8	Brain-heart infusion broth	1
9	Anaerobic agar	1-4
10	Smear: reserve (acid-fast, methenamine-silver, etc.)	1
11	Optional media (Löwenstein-Jensen agar, nonnutrient agar, etc.)	1-4
12	Optional tests (*Limulus* lysate assay, immunoassays, etc.)	1-4

* Each solid medium is inoculated with up to 4 rows of C-streaks; each row is obtained from a single set of corneal scrapings. If insufficient material exists, then a single row is inoculated and the next sequential medium or smear is prepared. The entire sequence is repeated until all inoculations are completed or no more material is available.

neal biopsy is performed with a disposable skin punch or small (i.e., 2-mm to 4-mm diameter) corneal trephine.[136] After marking and incising the superficial cornea the incision is deepened with a surgical blade to approximately 0.2 mm. Lamellar dissection is performed with a sharp, spatula-like knife or microsurgical scissors. The biopsy is then carefully excised, avoiding tissue crushing with a fine-toothed forceps. The intact specimen is placed in a sterile Petri dish where sectioning can be done to provide tissue for histopathologic and microbiologic processing.[245]

A freehand lamellar dissection with a diamond blade[467] or superficial keratectomy can excise a single specimen or small fragments that can be placed onto culture media. A method for obtaining material from the deeper stroma is to pass a 6-0 silk suture through the involved area, then cut it into separate sections for inoculation onto appropriate culture media. A corneal button obtained by lamellar or penetrating keratoplasty is bisected for microbiologic and pathologic evaluations.

Corneal tissue is transported to the microbiology laboratory in a sterile liquid medium such as trypticase soy broth. Tissue grinding or chemical digestion permits smears and inoculation of multiple media. Additional corneal scrapings can be obtained from the base of a partial-thickness corneal biopsy.

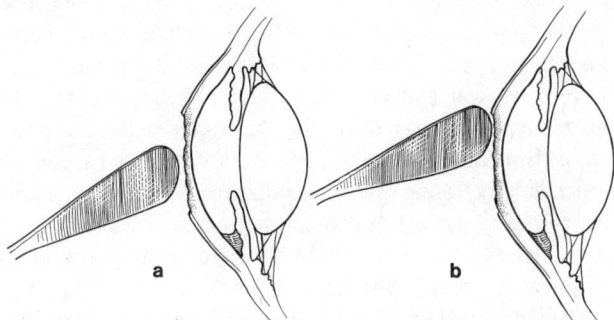

Fig. 74-16. To maximize microbial isolation multiple areas are scraped, including central infiltrate (**A**) and its borders (**B**).

Intraocular Sampling. Rarely is it necessary to obtain a specimen from an approach through the anterior chamber. One possible reason might be a case of perforating corneal trauma in which there is a deep focus of corneal suppuration. Opening a corneal wound is usually safer than obtaining a retrocorneal specimen, however. Aspiration of aqueous humor or of a hypopyon is not indicated, because this inflammatory reaction is usually sterile. One exception is the patient with bacterial keratitis who has progressed to endophthalmitis; sampling of intraocular fluids is considered if the responsible microorganism is not known.

Serum and Tears. Serum[237] and tear[135,388] total immunoglobulin levels remain unchanged during bacterial keratitis. Specific antibody responses are detectable during the first few weeks after experimental bacterial keratitis,[37] and the amount of tear IgA increases during corneal infection. Although serologic assays to detect antibodies to several bacterial antigens are available,[344] tests for specific antibodies in serum or tear fluid are not used clinically for evaluating bacterial keratitis.

Other Material. Nonocular specimens incriminated in causing corneal infection may be submitted for laboratory evaluation. Foreign bodies, sutures, and similar material are either divided and distributed to individual media or cultured by sweeping the object across agar plates. Material is collected from contact lens cases, eyedropper bottles, and other containers by swabbing the internal surfaces or caps with a premoistened swab. Because residual preservatives or disinfectants can inhibit growth of contaminating bacteria, the specimen can be either diluted in a broth medium or processed with an antimicrobial removal device before inoculation. Multiple media should be inoculated because of possible high microbial density and the likelihood of multiple species. Solutions are handled in a similar manner;

TABLE 74-8 STAINING METHODS FOR SMEARS OF CORNEAL SCRAPINGS OBTAINED FROM BACTERIAL KERATITIS

Staining	Accuracy*	Technique
Acridine orange	70%	1. Apply acidic (pH 3.5) acridine orange for 2 minutes. 2. Rinse with tap water and dry. 3. Examine by fluorescent microscopy.
Gram	60-70%	1. Apply crystal violet for 1 minute, then rinse with tap water. 2. Apply Gram iodine for 1 minute, then rinse with tap water. 3. Decolorize with a few drops of ethanol-acetone or 95% ethanol-acetone or 95% ethanol until no further violet stain eludes from smear, then rinse with tap water. 4. Apply safranin (or basic fuchsin) for 1 minute, then rinse with tap water. 5. Examine by light microscopy.
Giemsa	ND	1. Prepare fresh Giemsa stain by mixing 47 ml distilled water, 2 ml buffer (pH 6.5), and 1 ml Giemsa stain. 2. Immerse slide into staining jar for 45-60 minutes. 3. Rinse in 95% ethanol. 4. Examine by light microscopy.
Fluorescein-conjugated lectins	ND	1. Prepare buffered dilution at 0.02 mg/ml by mixing 495 ml hydroxymethyl-aminomethane and 5 ml of 2 mg/ml lectin solution. 2. Flood slide with buffer albumin diluent for 5 minutes. 3. Rinse with TRIS buffer. 4. Flood slide with fluoresceinated lectin solution for 20 minutes in dark. 5. Rinse with TRIS buffer and apply coverslip. 6. Examine by fluorescent microscopy.
Fluorescein-conjugated antibodies	ND	1. Use slide fixed in cold acetone. 2. Apply either fluoresceinated antibody (for direct test) or unlabeled antibody (for indirect test). 3. Incubate slide at 35-37°C for 30 minutes. 4. Rinse with distilled water and air dry. 5. For direct test examine with fluorescent microscopy. For indirect test apply fluorescein-labeled antibody, incubate 30 minutes at 35-37°C, rinse, air dry, and examine by a fluorescent microscopy.

* The ability to identify gram-positive bacteria accurately is generally greater than that for gram-negative species. Correct identification of polymicrobial keratitis is less accurate than with single-organism infections. Accuracy is reduced by prior antibacterial therapy. ND, not determined.

large volumes can be concentrated by filtration or centrifugation.

Stains

Multiple smears should be obtained by directly transferring corneal specimens onto clean glass slides. The inoculation site is identified with an etched mark on the glass or with a wax pencil. Accurate interpretation of stained smears is fostered by rigorous attention to specimen collection and preparation. Unclean instruments that contain carbon particles, talcum powder, or salt crystals can lead to staining artifacts. Corneal scrapings should be smeared in a thin film to distribute microorganisms evenly rather than clustering them at a single location. If the smear is too thick, precipitated or crystallized stain can accumulate that can resemble bizarre bacterial shapes or mask recognition of microorganisms. Excessive smearing, on the other hand, can fragment inflammatory cells and lead to extracellular granules and pyknotic nuclei that can be confused with bacteria. Prior antibiotic use, inadequate sampling, poor fixation, improper staining, and incomplete smear examination impair reliability of laboratory results.

After brief air drying the slide is flooded or immersed in 95% methanol or another cytologic fixative for approximately 5 minutes. For fluorescent antibody staining, smears should be fixed in methanol or cold acetone. Heat fixation can alter staining characteristics and cytomorphology. Because unstained bacteria cannot be easily seen with conventional light microscopy, staining is used to increase the optical contrast.

Different staining techniques are useful in interpreting smears of corneal material (Table 74-8). Acridine orange is a suitable initial screening stain to detect the presence of most microorganisms. Gram staining is routinely done on a parallel smear or directly onto the acridine orange-stained smear. Giemsa staining can help in bacterial recognition but is generally reserved to identify fungi and to distinguish cytologic details. When fungal or amoebic keratitis is suspected, calcofluor white, methenamine silver, and trichrome stains may be helpful. Acid-fast stains are used to screen for mycobacterial infections. Immunofluorescent stains are currently under development for many causes of microbial keratitis.

Interpretation of the stained smear begins with recognizing the nature of the inflammatory reaction. The presence of many polymorphonuclear leukocytes suggests infection. Clumps of neutrophils and degenerating epithelial cells can give a clue where to search for microorganisms on the smear. An occasional epithelial cell can sometimes be found with many adherent bacteria. A few randomly scattered organisms originating from the normal tear-film microflora may be seen. The presence of multiple similar bacteria with acute inflammatory cells suggests the responsible microorganism (Fig. 74-17). In streptococcal infections there are typically many proliferating microorganisms. For most other causes of bacterial keratitis fewer numbers are usually present, making bacteria difficult to locate and to identify.

Acridine Orange. Acridine orange is a diphenylmethane derivative initially used as a dye in the textile industry. After the invention of the fluorescent microscope this fluorochrome was introduced into cytopathology. Optical activity is apparently due to intercalation of acridine orange into double-stranded nucleic acids to form a green-fluorescing complex. At neutral pH, viable cell nuclei fluoresce green

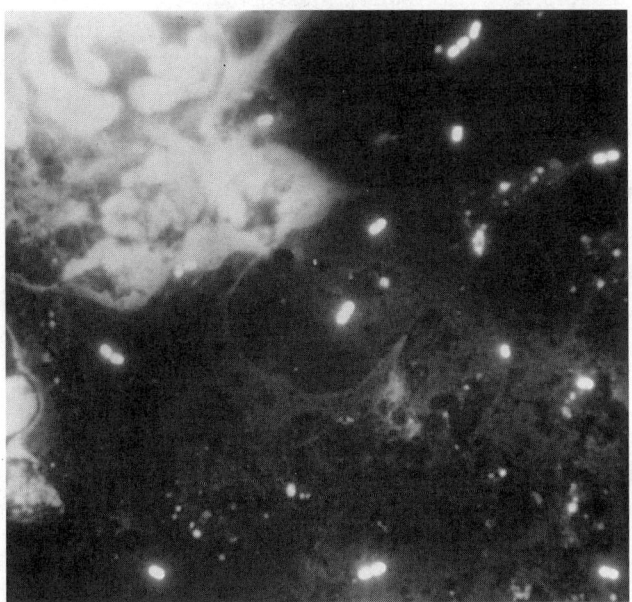

A

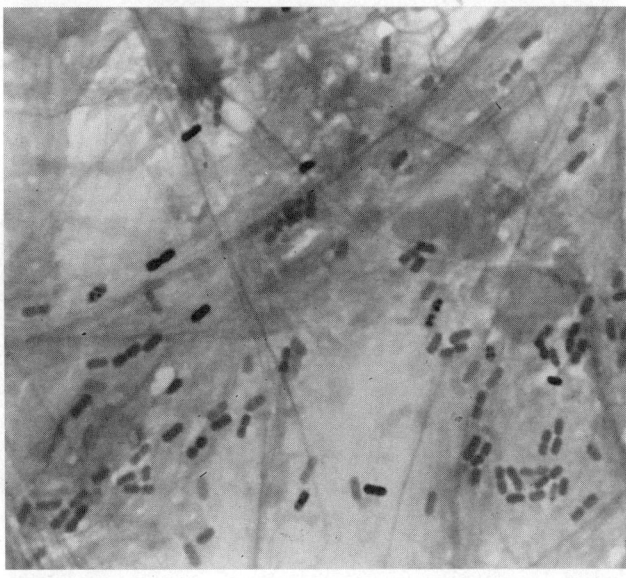

B

Fig. 74-17.   Smears of corneal scrapings from *Moraxella* keratitis. **A,** Acridine orange stain highlights yellow-orange bacteria against dark background. **B,** Gram stain shows gram-negative diplobacilli with inflammatory cells and necrotic debris.

whereas dead cells stain red-orange. With an acidic buffer, acridine orange results in orange fluorescence of bacteria and green-yellow fluorescence of human cells and background material (Fig. 74-18).

Acidic acridine orange is more sensitive than the Gram stain in detecting low amounts of bacteria on corneal scrapings.[152,433] Most viable bacteria typically stain orange (although atypical mycobacteria stain a pale yellow-orange), and dying or dead bacteria stain light yellow-green. Possible staining artifacts include faint yellow-orange granules from disintegrating leukocytes. Because staining intensity fades with time, smears should be examined soon after initial staining, preferably with a small diaphragm opening of the fluorescent microscope. Chemofluorescent dyes such as acridine orange enhance microbial identification by staining bacteria more brightly than the darker background. Bacterial morphology can be determined, but acridine orange does not help in classification as much as the Gram stain. Acridine orange-stained smears can be Gram-stained without an intervening decolorization step to detect the Gram reaction of bacteria.

Gram Stain. Originally described by Gram in Denmark during 1884 for distinguishing bacteria in histologic sections, the Gram stain is a standard technique in ocular bacteriology.[479] Dyes commonly used in the Gram stain include aromatic derivatives of coal tar with color-producing chromophoric groups and other side-chain radicals called auxochromes. Many changes have been proposed to simplify the use of the Gram stain, and modifications such as the Brown-Hopps stain are applicable to histopathologic sections.

The Gram stain produces distinctive color changes and allows morphologic classification by light microscopy. The chemical composition and structural organization of the viable bacterial cell wall is the basis why gram-positive bacteria stain violet and gram-negative appear pink-red. Gram-positive bacteria are usually more numerous and easier to detect than gram-negative bacteria. Lysis of the cell wall results in a loss of the "positive" Gram stain characteristic. Microorganisms that show both color characteristics are sometimes termed gram-variable.

Giemsa Stain. The detection of slender gram-negative bacteria is sometimes difficult because of their similar coloration with background material. The Giemsa stain may be useful to enhance microscopic detail. Although Giemsa staining colors all material blue, microscopic details can be enhanced and bacteria easier to see. For example, Giemsa staining provides better morphologic details of bacteria such as *Haemophilus* spp. and *Azotobacter* spp. than does the Gram stain. The Giemsa stain takes longer to do than acridine orange and Gram stains and, in the evaluation of microbial keratitis, is generally reserved as an ancillary stain especially when fungal keratitis is suspected. Other methylene blue-based stains, such as the Wright and Wayson stains, can also be used.

Other Microbial Detection Methods. Antigen-detection tests are routinely done on specimens from bacterial meningitis but are not commonly used for bacterial keratitis. The clinical utility of these tests in diagnostic ocular microbiology remains to be determined. Because these assays detect antigen and do not necessarily require viable bacteria, test results may remain positive for several days during initial therapy. Rather than supplanting staining and culture, they will probably be most useful as supplements to standard procedures. For specimens that are to be stored for future evaluation, refrigeration at $\leq 4°C$ is recommended to reduce breakdown of bacterial polysaccharide antigens.

Limulus Amoebocyte Lysate Assay. As a result of research in marine biology circulating blood elements, called

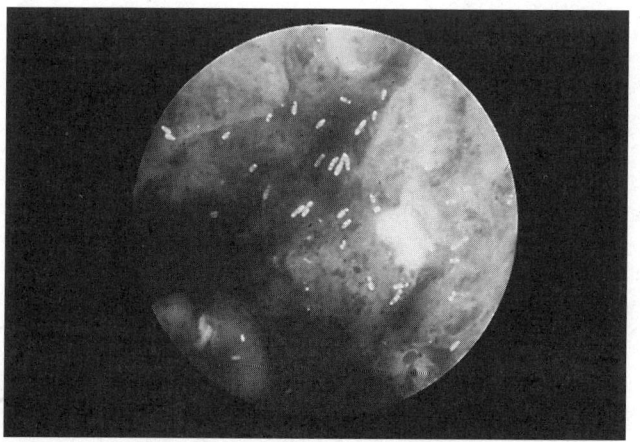
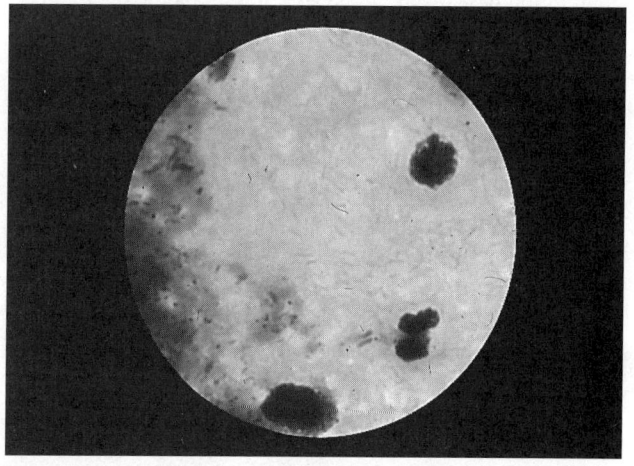

A   B

Fig. 74-18. Smears of corneal scrapings from *P. aeruginosa* keratitis. **A,** Acridine orange stain with fluorescent microscopy reveals yellow-orange bacilli against dark green background. **B,** Gram stain with light microscopy shows slender gram-negative rods that can be difficult to discern against pink background.

amoebocytes, of the horseshoe crab *Limulus polyphemus* were found to coagulate when exposed to gram-negative bacteria. Standardized lysates of *Limulus* amoebocytes are now available with sensitivity expressed as endotoxin units. The reaction takes place when bacterial endotoxin activates a proclotting enzyme to produce a turbid gel or, with a chromogenic substrate, a yellow solution. For use in bacterial keratitis, corneal scrapings are directly inoculated into pyrogen-free water; an aliquot is added to the test reagents to detect clot formation, turbidity, or a color reaction. The test is reported to have an overall accuracy of approximately 90% for gram-negative bacterial keratitis[4] but is limited to gram-negative bacteria, does not differentiate among these organisms, and is not necessarily more accurate than Gram staining.

Quellung Procedure. Rarely used, the quellung capsular reaction procedure can confirm the presence of certain bacteria such as *S. pneumoniae* and *H. influenzae* type b. Antisera specific for individual capsular polysaccharides are mixed with the specimen along with methylene blue. The formation of an antigen-antibody complex changes the refractive index of the capsule, making it look clear and swollen by direct microscopy.

Fluoresceinated Lectins. Lectins are glycoproteins that bind to individual polysaccharides, including microbial cell-wall carbohydrates. Fluorescein-conjugated lectins enable visualization by fluorescent microscopy of various microorganisms, especially fungi and parasites.[353] Examples of lectins capable of binding to several species of aerobic and anaerobic bacteria include wheat-germ agglutinin that binds to polymers of N-acetylglucosamine and concanavalin A that binds to alpha-D-mannose and alpha-D-glucose. Limitations exist because the sugar composition of bacterial cell walls varies with growth phase and environmental factors.

Fluoresceinated Antibodies. Direct and indirect fluorescent antibody tests are applicable to the diagnosis of bacterial keratitis.[273] For fluorescent antibody staining, the smear should be fixed in 100% cold acetone. The antibody test reagent is applied to the smear and incubated for approximately 30 minutes. For the indirect test the fluorescein-labeled antibody is subsequently added and allowed to incubate. The smear is then examined by fluorescent microscopy to detect apple-green microbial staining. Depending on the specificity of the antibody, either whole cells or cell sections will fluoresce.

Counterimmunoelectrophoresis. In this assay an electric current is applied to immunodiffusion agar to speed diffusion of the test specimen and specific antibodies toward each other. Immunoprecipitation confirms the presence of individual bacteria. This cumbersome procedure has been replaced by faster and easier immunoassays.

Immunoassays. Various immunologic antigen-detection methods are becoming available, including agglutination assays and enzyme immunoassays.[401] Preliminary experience suggests that these rapid diagnostic tests are useful for identifying specific causes of bacterial keratitis. By detecting species-specific antigens these assays are promising, but limited experience and expense restrict routine clinical use at this time.

Manufacturers' directions are followed for commercially available coagglutination and latex agglutination kits. Coagglutination reagents are composed of *S. aureus* coated with specific immunoglobulin. This IgG molecule adheres to staphylococcal protein A, leaving its immunoreactive end free to bind specific antigen. A positive reaction results in visible agglutination of staphylococci. Latex agglutination utilizes polystyrene beads with adsorbed IgG. Commercial assays based on these methods are available for common causes of bacterial meningitis, including *H. influenzae* type b, *S. pneumoniae,* group B streptococci, and *N. meningitidis.*

Enzyme immunoassays use immobilized specific antibody that binds bacterial antigen, followed by an enzyme-labeled antibody that binds to the bound antigen. Addition of the enzyme's substrate yields a colored product, showing the presence of a specific bacterial antigen in the specimen. Commercial enzyme immunoassay kits are currently under development for a variety of common microorganisms.

Nucleic Acid Probes. DNA and RNA hybridization reactions are becoming available as potential diagnostic tests for certain microbes of ophthalmic importance. The application of these developments in molecular biology to bacterial keratitis is underway. Amplification by the polymerase chain reaction (PCR) might be useful for detecting microbial DNA in culture-negative corneal specimens. By detecting specific nucleic acid sequences, these assays can identify specific microorganisms and can potentially reveal the presence of genes encoding antimicrobial resistance.

Enzyme Detection. Bacteria and leukocytes release several enzymes during keratitis. Fibronectin, plasmin, and other proteins involved in inflammation are detectable in tear fluid during bacterial keratitis.[21,424,495] Finding one or more of these or other substances suggests acute infection or inflammation.[308,354]

Cultures

Corneal scrapings should ideally be inoculated directly onto culture media. Whereas waiting for refrigerated media to warm to room temperature (which can take nearly 1 hour) is not needed for recovering common corneal bacteria; all media should be sufficiently fresh and not allowed to dry out. Agar plates and broth tubes (Table 74-9) recommended for routine use in isolating most bacteria and fungi known to cause corneal infections include the following:

1. blood agar plate
2. chocolate agar plate
3. thioglycollate broth tube
4. anaerobic agar plate
5. Sabouraud agar plate
6. brain-heart infusion broth.

TABLE 74-9 CULTURE MEDIA FOR INOCULATION OF CORNEAL SCRAPINGS FROM BACTERIAL KERATITIS

Medium (Alternatives)	Constituents	Bacterial Isolation
Blood agar plate	Heart infusion agar (infusion from beef heart, peptic digest of animal tissue, agar, sodium chloride, water) Horse, sheep, or rabbit blood (5%)	Aerobes and facultative anaerobes (exceptions: *Haemophilus* sp., *Neisseria gonorrhoeae*, *Bordetella pertussis*, *Calymmatobacterium granulomatis*, *Francisella tularensis*, *Mycobacteria* spp., and *Legionella* spp.)
Chocolate agar plate (modified Thayer-Martin agar, Transgrow agar, Martin-Lewis agar)	Heart infusion agar (or similar) Heated blood (5-10%)	Aerobes and facultative anaerobes (including *Haemophilus* spp. and *Neisseria* spp.)
Thioglycolate broth tube (thiol broth, chopped meat-glucose broth)	Pancreatic digest of milk casein Papain digest of soybean Glucose Sodium chloride Sodium thioglycolate Water Supplements (hemin, polysorbate, vitamin K)	Aerobes, facultative anaerobes, and aerotolerant anaerobes
Brucella agar plate (Anaerobic blood agar, Schaedler agar)	Pancreatic digest of milk casein Peptic digest of animal tissue Yeast extract Sodium chloride Glucose Sodium bisulfite Agar Water Supplements (hemin, vitamin K)	Anaerobes
Trypticase soy broth tube (brain-heart infusion broth without antibiotic, minimal essential medium)	Pancreatic digest of milk casein Papain digest of soybean Sodium chloride Potassium phosphate Glucose Water Supplements (polysorbate, fetal calf serum)	Most bacteria

Solid media are directly inoculated by making a single row of inoculation marks with each collected scraping. Small C-streak marks are made by lightly sweeping both sides of the spatula on the surface of the agar plate without gouging (Fig. 74-19). Each row of inoculation marks is from one set of scrapings; 3 to 4 rows of C-streaks are applied to each plate. The thioglycollate broth tube is inoculated by grasping the shaft of a sterile calcium alginate swab near its end, transferring the specimen from the spatula onto the moistened swab tip, inserting the swab into the bottom of the culture tube (taking care not to accidentally contaminate the shaft of the swab during inoculation), and breaking and discarding the swab's proximal end. Thioglycollate tubes are not shaken; otherwise the aerobic-to-anaerobic gradient would be disturbed. After inoculation the cap is flamed and replaced. Other liquid media such as brain-heart infusion broth are directly inoculated, then gently agitated.

Media plates are transported to the laboratory in their prepared Petri dishes with the surface facing down to prevent condensation within the plate from dripping onto the medium. Broth tubes are maintained in an upright position during transportation.

Additional media are selected if more fastidious microorganisms are suspected. Nontuberculous mycobacteria can be isolated on a Löwenstein-Jensen, Middlebrook-Cohn, or Pctragnani agar slant. A nonnutrient agar plate with a live or killed bacterial overlay can support the growth of *Acanthamoeba* species. Minimal essential medium or other tissue-culture substrates without antibiotics might prove helpful to isolate unusual organisms with anomalous growth requirements. The laboratory should be familiar with the need to

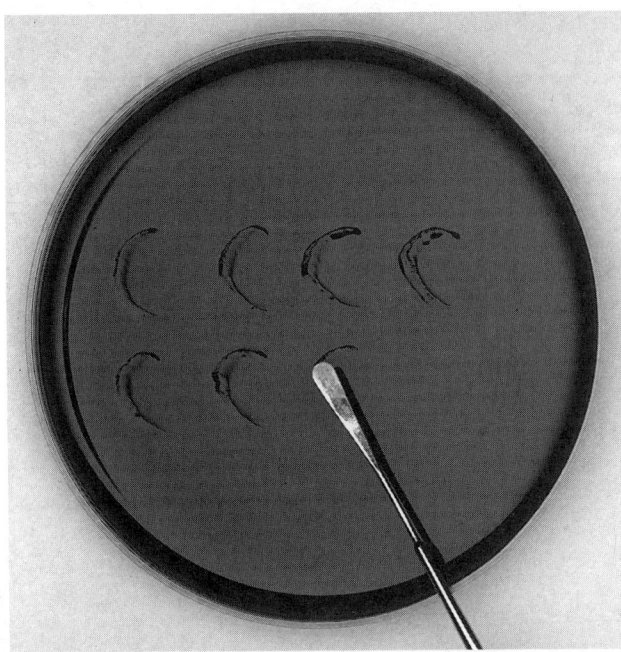

Fig. 74-19. Corneal specimen is directly inoculated onto solid agar plate by making multiple C-streaks.

identify all isolates and must not ignore the growth of a few colonies or misclassify them as possible contaminants.

Media. *Trypticase Soy Broth.* A tube containing soybean casein digest broth or a similar liquid medium is useful for moistening swabs used to collect ocular surface specimens. Corneal scrapings are transferred to a saturated calcium alginate swab for optimal inoculation of thioglycollate broth.

Blood Agar Plate. This nonselective medium is used for the primary isolation of most aerobic microorganisms including bacteria, fungi, and amoebae, although some microorganisms such as *Haemophilus* spp. and *Neisseria* spp. will not grow well without additional supplementation. Blood agar can be prepared using red blood cells from several animals such as sheep, rabbits, and horses. Horse blood agar is preferred by some microbiologists because it contains adequate nutrient supplements for fastidious organisms like *Haemophilus* spp. and because hemolysis is easily detectable. Enteric gram-negative rods grow well on certain selective media, such as a MacConkey agar plate or an eosin-methylene blue agar plate, but these are not usually used for primary isolation from the eye. After inoculation the blood agar plate is incubated at 35°C to 37°C, usually in a candle jar that provides a partial CO_2 environment. An additional blood agar plate can be incubated anaerobically for isolation of most anaerobic organisms.

Chocolate Agar Plate. Containing hemolyzed sheep erythrocytes, this medium supports growth of most aerobic bacteria including *Haemophilus, Neisseria,* and *Moraxella* species. The inoculated chocolate agar plate is incubated at 35°C to 37°C under 5% to 10% CO_2. Similar media, such as

Thayer-Martin medium, contain vancomycin, colistin, and nystatin to favor growth of *Neisseria* spp. from a contaminated specimen. The use of a candle jar or a plastic bag with a CO_2 generator aids recovery of both aerobic and facultatively anaerobic microorganisms and reduces evaporation.

Thioglycollate Broth. Thioglycollate and thiol broths are similar media that provide an adequate growth environment for aerobic and microaerophilic bacteria, but these media are not optimal for the isolation of strict anaerobic bacteria. Thioglycollate is a sulfur-containing, oxygen-reducing agent that permits isolation of aerotolerant and facultatively anaerobic bacteria. Supplements can be added to thicken the medium, to improve the recovery of certain microorganisms, and to inactivate residual antibiotics present in the clinical specimen. Instead of thioglycollate or thiol tubes, some laboratories provide fresh chopped-meat broth, brain-heart infusion broth without antibiotic supplementation, or a similar enrichment broth for anaerobic incubation. The inoculated broth tube should be transported in an upright position and incubated at 35°C to 37°C.

Brucella Blood Agar or Schaedler Agar Plates. These prereduced, anaerobically sterilized media contain sheep blood, hemin, vitamin K, reducing agents, and other compounds that aid in the isolation of anaerobic bacteria. Growth on solid rather than liquid media can be easier to interpret, because contamination can be monitored, overgrowth of competing organisms is restricted, and growth can be quantified. Although these enriched media will allow growth of aerobic bacteria when incubated in an aerobic environment, they are designed to enhance recovery of anaerobic bacteria in an anaerobic chamber, jar, or bag system. Brewer anaerobic agar and other prereduced solid and liquid media are also available for anaerobic cultures.

Sabouraud Agar Plate. This acidic, nutritionally deficient medium favors fungal growth. An antibiotic, usually gentamicin or chloramphenicol, is added to reduce bacterial contamination. Cycloheximide-supplemented Sabouraud plates are available in many microbiology laboratories to prevent growth of saprophytic fungi, but because these fungi can cause corneal disease cycloheximide should be excluded from plates used in ocular microbiology. The plate is incubated in a room-temperature incubator at 25°C and, as growth may take weeks, should be partially sealed to reduce evaporation.

Brain-Heart Infusion (BHI) Broth. BHI broth is composed of calf brain and beef heart extracts with neopeptone and other supplements that favor fungal growth. Gentamicin 50 μg/ml is generally added to inhibit bacterial replication. This liquid medium is incubated in a rotary shaker at room temperature.

Antimicrobial Removal Device. For patients using an antibacterial medication before specimen collection, an antimicrobial removal device might be helpful to improve the chances for microbial recovery. This patented mixture contains sodium polyanethol sulfonate and two resins that bind many antimicrobial agents such as beta-lactams, aminoglycosides, and imidazoles. The commercial suspension can be put into smaller test tubes that are more appropriate for corneal scrapings. Corneal scrapings are directly introduced into the liquid, and aliquots are reinoculated onto appropriate laboratory media. Trypticase soy broth or thioglycollate broth can be added to the residual resinous material for incubation.

Tissue-Culture Medium. While most bacteria known to cause microbial keratitis can be isolated on routine culture media, extremely fastidious microorganisms might require special supplements. Modified essential medium contains 10% fetal calf serum with buffer, amino acids, and vitamins. Without antibiotics this medium can support bacterial growth. After inoculation this medium is incubated under 5% to 10% CO_2 at 35°C to 37°C.

Minimal Nutrient Agar. While amoebae can be isolated on blood agar plates and other media, concomitant bacterial growth can mask their presence. Bacterial growth is inhibited on minimal nutrient agar. The presence of amoebic trophozoites are detected by trails on the agar surface, although leukocytes and other tissue cells can mimic this appearance. The surface of this agar can be preinoculated with an overlay of live or dead microorganisms such as *Escherichia coli, Enterobacter cloacae, Burkholderia cepacia,* or *Stenotrophomonas maltophilia* to enhance recovery of *Acanthamoeba* species. Live microorganisms can enhance amoebic excystation and shorten their recovery period, but subsequent reisolation of the amoebae in pure culture is difficult because of bacterial proliferation. The use of a dead bacterial overlay is more common. Ideally duplicate plates should be inoculated for incubation at both 30°C and 35°C to 37°C.

Other Media. Other special media are rarely used. One exception might be infectious crystalline keratopathy in which nutritionally deficient streptococci have been incriminated. A hypertonic medium or media supplemented with pyridoxal hydrochloride or L-cysteine might be useful. The lysis-centrifugation method might be considered for cases in which an unusual microorganism has eluded detection.

Bacterial Identification Methods. All routine bacteriologic media are observed daily for at least one week. Within 12 to 24 hours early growth on solid media plates can be detected with a dissecting microscope as small colonies on the C-streak marks. Valid growth appears as colonies on the scratched C-streaks; other colonies usually represent plate contaminants (Fig. 74-20). The number of identical colonies is counted, and the colony morphology is described. A representative sample from a selected colony is transferred to differential media. Liquid media tubes are observed daily for turbidity, and aliquots can be plated onto nutrient and differential media for isolation and identification. Anaerobes may take one week or longer to grow, typically beginning as a globular haze around the swab deep in the thioglycollate broth tube or as small colonies on the anaerobic plate.

The number of colonies on solid media is counted, and representative samples of colonies of different morphology are selected for Gram staining and biochemical testing. Normal flora from the tear film can sometimes grow on the culture media. Laboratory criteria (Table 74-10) that help to substantiate an isolated microorganism as the specific cause of bacterial keratitis include (a) growth in at least two media or (b) growth in only one medium of bacteria present on the initial smear of corneal scrapings. At least 10 colonies should be present on several C-streaks of a solid medium plate to prove a definitive cause. Lack of growth may mean a nonmicrobial cause but can be due to prior antibiotic treatment or inadequate sampling techniques. Fastidious microorganisms or corneal scrapings obtained from patients with a small amount of material may also result in lesser amounts of growth. Semiquantitative growth interpretation has not yet been correlated with smear microscopy or with clinical severity or outcome.

Species identification is based on Gram staining characteristics, colony morphology, biochemical reactivity, and analysis of cellular constituents by standard laboratory methods. Methods that are available for epidemiologic in-

TABLE 74-10 SEMIQUANTITATIVE INTERPRETATION OF SMEARS AND MEDIA RESULTS*

Test	Indeterminate	Definite
Smear	< 10 organisms per slide	≥ 1 organism per high-power field
Media†	< 10 colonies on only one solid medium or Growth in liquid medium only	Growth on at least 2 solid media or Growth on both solid and liquid media or Growth on at least one medium of organism identified on smear

* Interpretation not valid for patients with recent antimicrobial therapy, for cases of incomplete specimen collection, or for fastidious microorganisms.
† Growth on each solid medium is recorded as the number of colonies or is semiquantified according to the following scale: 1+(< 50 colonies), 2+(coalescent colonies), and 3+(mass growth).

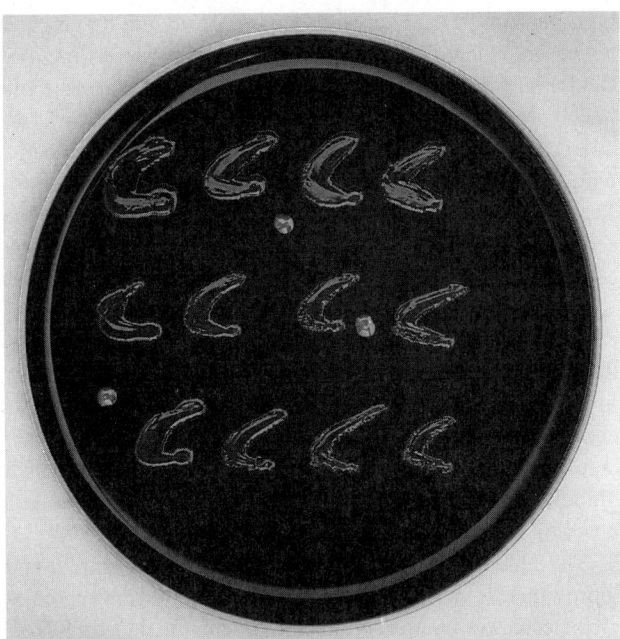

Fig. 74-20. Bacterial growth *(P. aeruginosa)* on inoculation marks indicates responsible microorganisms. Colonies *(S. aureus)* on other areas of the agar surface are presumed contaminants.

vestigation of several bacteria of ophthalmic importance include serologic phenotyping, antibiotic-resistance profile comparison, plasmid-profile analysis, and genomic fingerprinting (including restriction-endonuclease analysis, electrophoretic typing, Southern hybridization, and PCR amplification with DNA sequencing).

Even if bacterial growth is identified, all media should continue to be examined for at least one week. Larger corneal infiltrates are more likely to be culture-positive. Approximately 8% to 15% of cases of bacterial keratitis are polymicrobial.[154,206] Mixed infections are frequently caused by two or more gram-positive cocci, a combination of aerobic gram-positive cocci and gram-negative rods, fungi with gram-positive bacteria, or *Acanthamoeba* spp. with streptococci.

Antibacterial Susceptibility Testing. Rapid identification of the presence of antibiotic-inhibiting enzymes, such as beta-lactamase, can be detected by macroscopic methods. Commercial methods for detecting beta-lactamase production are based on either an acidometric or chromogenic assay in which a positive reaction entails a color change. Beta-lactamase testing is most useful for gram-positive cocci and *Neisseria* spp. A similar assay for the detection of chloramphenicol acetyltransferase is also available. Other rapid diagnostic tests for detecting bacterial enzymes (or their genes) that inactivate several antibacterial agents are under development. DNA probes will potentially be able to detect bacterial gene sequences coding for antimicrobial resistance.

Antibacterial susceptibility testing for both minimal inhibitory (bacteristatic) concentrations (MIC) and minimal lethal (bactericidal) concentrations (MLC) can be performed for most bacterial isolates. The MIC is measured by disc-diffusion and serial-dilution methods. Commercially prepared batteries of common antibacterial agents are available to test gram-positive bacteria and gram-negative bacilli. Because chemically related compounds have similar activity, a class representative is chosen. For example, cephalothin and cefazolin are essentially interchangeable for susceptibility purposes, and oxacillin substitutes for methicillin. Several different representatives are selected for other drug clusters, such as the third-generation cephalosporins, that differ in their spectra of activity. The most correlative results are obtained when the clinically used drug is tested, but laboratories are economically limited in their flexibility to provide custom-designed susceptibility test panels.

Although pharmacokinetic data are available for many antibacterial agents, direct correlations between achievable corneal levels and in vitro sensitivity values are not available for most ophthalmic antibacterial agents. The terms "resistant" and "sensitive" lack standardization for corneal infections. Preliminary results suggest that a MIC of approximately 2 to 8 μg/ml separates sensitive from resistant strains for some agents, but further data are needed. Until quantitative test results are adequately correlated to intracorneal drug concentrations, in vitro susceptibility test procedures can only provide a relative guide to antimicrobial resistance patterns.

Disc-Diffusion Procedure. In this procedure a standardized broth subculture is inoculated onto Mueller-Hinton agar. Antibiotic-impregnated discs are then applied, and the plate is incubated aerobically. Subsequently the diameter of the zone of inhibition surrounding each disc is measured. By means of an interpretive table, these measurements are translated into susceptible, intermediate, or resistant categories, although these labels relate to drug levels achievable in serum rather than in the eye. The diameter of the zone of inhibition can also be expressed as an approximate MIC. Care should be taken in correlating the susceptibility test results with the clinical therapeutic response. For example, methicillin-resistant staphylococci, as evaluated with an oxacillin disc at 35°C, should be considered resistant to other beta-lactams despite the disc test results. Diffusion procedures are primarily standardized for testing aerobic or facultatively anaerobic bacteria. Slowly growing microorganisms and obligate anaerobes cannot be adequately tested with the disc-diffusion method.

Broth-Dilution Procedure. The tube-dilution test exposes bacteria to serial dilutions of antimicrobial agents in liquid media. This macroscopic test can also be performed using a microdilution method with wells rather than test tubes. Commercially prepared trays are available in both frozen and dry forms. The MIC is the lowest concentration at which no visible growth occurs.

TABLE 74-11 ANTIBACTERIAL AGENTS BY ROUTE OF ADMINISTRATION FOR INITIAL SELECTIVE THERAPY BASED ON GRAM STAIN FINDINGS*

Gram Stain	Gram-Positive Cocci	Gram-Negative Cocci	Gram-Negative Rods	Gram-Positive Rods
Common organisms				
Aerobic	Micrococcaceae (*S. aureus, S. epidermidis*) Streptococcaceae (*S. pneumoniae, S. pyogenes*)	Neisseriaceae (*N. gonorrhoeae, N. meningitidis*)	Pseudomonadaceae (*P. aeruginosa*) Enterobacteriaceae (*Enterobacter* spp., *Klebsiella* spp., *Proteus* spp., *Serratia* spp., *E. coli*) Azotobacteraceae Neisseriaceae (*Moraxellla* spp.) (*Haemophilus* spp.)	Bacillaceae *Corynebacterium* spp.
Anaerobic	Peptococcaceae		Bacteroidaceae	Propionibacteriaceae (*P. acnes*) Bacillaceae
Topical therapy	Cefazolin 50 mg/ml	Ciprofloxacin 3 mg/ml	Tobramycin or gentamicin 13.6 mg/ml	Cefazolin 50 mg/ml
Subconjunctival therapy†	Cefazolin 100 mg	Penicillin G 500,000 units if sensitive	Tobramycin or gentamicin 20 mg	Cefazolin 100 mg
Intravenous therapy†	Cefazolin 1 gm every 8 hours	Ceftriaxone 1 gm (or spectinomycin 2 gm if penicillin-allergic) every 12 hours	Tobramycin or gentamicin 3–7 mg/kg/day	Cefazolin 1 gm every 8 hours

* Broad-spectrum therapy may also be begun with combined agents (e.g., cefazolin and tobramycin) or a single agent, such as fluoroquinolone (e.g., ciprofloxacin) or an extended-spectrum cephalosporin (e.g., ceftazidime).
† The use of subconjunctival and systemic routes depends on the type and severity of ocular infection. Dosages are for normal healthy adults; readjustments may be necessary for children and patients with renal or hepatic dysfunction.

The MLC can be detected by subculturing the wells that show growth inhibition. The determination of the MLC is hampered by methodologic variables including media composition, incubation time, temperature, growth phase, and other confounding factors.

Correct interpretation of sensitivity tests requires knowledge of bacterial survival tactics.[472] In the Eagle effect, a high concentration of a bactericidal antibiotic such as penicillin G can paradoxically produce less lysis than a lower concentration, apparently because the higher drug level blocks not only cell-wall synthetic enzymes but other bacterial proteins as well, resulting in bacteriostasis. Another phenomenon, persistence, is due to the survival of some bacteria during exposure to a bactericidal agent, presumably because at any time some bacteria are in a nonreplicating state. Tolerance is recognized when the MLC is at least 16 times higher than the MIC.

Antimicrobial susceptibility testing generally evaluates the effect of single agents on bacterial growth although a fixed ratio of two or more agents can be incorporated in the procedure. Checkerboard sensitivity testing can be requested to learn the combined effects of two antibiotics. Using two-dimensional titration, an isobologram is plotted, and the fractional inhibitory concentration (FIC) is calculated by dividing the MIC of the drug combination by the MIC of one agent. These results can be used to predict the effects of drug interactions such as synergy or antagonism.

E test. The E test combines disc-diffusion and broth-dilution principles. MIC determination uses a plastic strip with an antibiotic gradient that covers 15 two-fold dilutions. The strip is applied to a bacterial lawn, and after incubation an elliptical or teardrop-shaped inhibitory zone forms. The MIC is read where the growth edge intersects the strip's logarithmic scale.

THERAPY

The goals of therapy for bacterial keratitis are to eliminate the causative agents, to suppress the inflammatory responses, and to restore normal structure. Clinical recognition, laboratory evaluation, and specific antimicrobial therapy are decisive steps in conserving vision. Appropriate management of bacterial keratitis relies on correct interpretation of laboratory information and knowledge of available medical and surgical options.

Antimicrobial therapy involves choosing one or more appropriate antibacterial agents, selecting the optimal routes and dosage, modifying the initial treatment, and terminating therapy.[30,87,204,485] Adjunctive medical therapy can help control symptoms and may minimize complications. Surgical management is generally reserved for progressive corneal destruction and permanent structural alterations.

Initiation of Antibacterial Therapy

Clinical decision-making involves assessing the possibility of actively replicating organisms in the corneal stroma versus that of a nonmicrobial cause. If in doubt, many prefer to initiate treatment rather than miss an early opportunity to halt an infectious process. Because of the wide variety of microorganisms capable of producing bacterial keratitis, clinical and laboratory evaluations are necessary for optimal management.

Initial Antibacterial Selection. Antimicrobial selection is based on the anticipated likelihood of specific microorganisms and susceptibility profiles. Some clinicians[202] use a strategy based on clinical and laboratory data (Plan A), whereas others[31] recommend an initial empirical approach with broad-spectrum therapy subsequently narrowed and tailored to the bacterial isolates (Plan B). In the former plan, specific therapy with a single agent is initiated according to the interpretation of smears of corneal scrapings. In the latter, broad-spectrum therapy with one or more antibacterial agents is begun without reliance on the initial smears and rapid diagnostic tests; but laboratory evaluation is done to guide subsequent treatment modifications. Each initial treatment approach has potential advantages, depending upon the expertise and familiarity of clinical and laboratory personnel with ophthalmic infections. Empiric therapy without cultures may be common[289] but is not commendable.[331]

Plan A: Initial Specific Antibacterial Therapy. Specific bactericidal therapy can be begun based on the results of the smears of corneal scrapings. The morphology of the organism, its Gram staining characteristics, and a knowledge of the organisms most commonly responsible for bacterial keratitis enable a rational choice of initial antibacterial therapy (Table 74-11). While serious infections at other body sites are often treated with two or more additive or synergistic drugs, the relatively high antibiotic concentrations that are achievable in the cornea from topical administration make it possible to use single agents for bacterial keratitis if chosen appropriately. Scleral infection, such as pseudomonal sclerokeratitis, is usually treated with combined topical and intravenous therapy.

Gram-Positive Cocci. A cephalosporin is an appropriate initial choice when gram-positive cocci are identified on smears of corneal scrapings. A first-generation cephalosporin such as cefazolin or cephapirin is clinically effective. Certain second-generation cephalosporins (e.g., cefamandole) and other extended-spectrum cephalosporins (e.g., ceftazidime and moxalactam) can be effective for many gram-positive microorganisms that cause bacterial keratitis. Bacitracin and vancomycin are useful alternatives but are limited by solubility and toxicity problems. Vancomycin is effective for both staphylococci and streptococci and can be considered for patients with a major penicillin allergy, but it is generally reserved as an alternative agent because of its toxic side effects such as impaired epithelial healing. Neomycin-containing preparations are effective against most staphylococci, but many streptococci are resistant, and a local hypersensitivity reaction to neomycin can occur in susceptible individuals.

Gram-Positive Rods. Gram-positive rods include both short bacilli and branching or filamentous forms. Most of these microorganisms are susceptible to gentamicin, an agent that would be useful if improper staining resulted in misidentification of gram-negative organisms. *Corynebacterium* spp. can sometimes be recognized when gram-positive "Chinese-letter" forms are detected. Diphtheroids are usually susceptible to gentamicin or penicillin G. For gram-positive filaments, penicillin G (benzylpenicillin) would be an appropriate choice.

Gram-Negative Cocci. Because the prevalence of penicillinase-producing *Neisseria gonorrhoeae* (PPNG) is increasing, an alternative to penicillin G is now considered when gram-negative cocci are identified. Ceftriaxone is an appropriate choice and is also effective against gram-negative coccobacilli, such as *Haemophilus* spp., that might be mistaken for gonococci. Ciprofloxacin and chloramphenicol, with or without ampicillin or amoxicillin, are also useful for this group of microorganisms and can provide adequate coverage if gram-positive cocci are misidentified on the initial smears as gram-negative cocci. Because short rods such as *Serratia marcescens* may occasionally be misidentified as gram-negative cocci, some clinicians add an aminoglycoside agent until culture results are available unless clinical features suggesting gonococcal keratoconjunctivitis are present.

Gram-Negative Rods. Tobramycin, gentamicin, and other aminoglycosides are effective for most cases of bacterial keratitis caused by gram-negative rods. Despite the relative in vitro resistance of *Pseudomonas* spp. and other gram-negative rods against aminoglycosides, achievable corneal concentrations with topical tobramycin generally exceed the MIC for these organisms. New beta-lactam agents such as extended-spectrum cephalosporins (e.g., cefoperazone and ceftazidime), ureidopenicillins (e.g., ticarcillin and piperacillin), monobactams (e.g., aztreonam), and carbapenems (e.g., imipenem) are also effective for these bacteria but are generally used in combination with an aminoglycoside rather than alone. *Moraxella* spp. are gram-negative diplobacilli that are inhibited by many antibiotics. Because *Azotobacter* spp. can have a similar appearance, however, an aminoglycoside is an appropriate initial choice when paired rods are seen on stained smears. Gram-negative bacilli that are resistant to aminoglycoside antibiotics are infrequently encountered but include *Alcaligenes denitrificans* (formerly *Achromobacter xylosoxidans*),[126,303] *Capnocytophaga* spp.,[130a] *Eikenella corrodens,*[228] *Flavobacterium* spp.,[50] and *Fusobacterium* spp. Beta-lactam agents (e.g., cephalosporins) are effective for some of these resistant genera, but others have limited antimicrobial susceptibility.

Multiple Bacterial Types. When two or more different types of bacteria are seen on smear, combined therapy with a cephalosporin (e.g., cefazolin or ceftazidime) and an aminoglycoside (e.g., tobramycin) is appropriate.

No Microorganisms. If no microorganisms are seen on the initial smears, the decision must be made whether to begin broad-spectrum therapy or to defer treatment pending further clinical observation. If in doubt about the possibility of actively replicating microorganisms, the clinician must decide whether to initiate antibacterial therapy rather than risk worsening while the patient is followed before culture results are available. Broad-spectrum therapy can be achieved with combined cephalosporin (e.g., cefazolin or ceftazidime) and aminoglycoside (e.g., tobramycin or gentamicin) agents or with selected single (e.g., ciprofloxacin) agents.

Plan B: Initial Broad-Spectrum Antibacterial Therapy. In some patients (such as those with prior antimicrobial therapy), stained smears might not reveal the causative microorganisms[8,277] or can lead to incorrect initial therapy in about 10% of cases.[202] Rather than depending on initial laboratory information that might occasionally be misleading, treatment can begin with either combination or single-agent therapy that should be effective against the major pathogens in the community.

Combination Therapy. Combined therapy with a beta-lactam, such as cefazolin, and an aminoglycoside, such as tobramycin, can effectively treat nearly all common causes of suppurative bacterial keratitis. After culture results are available the less effective agent can be stopped. Fixed-combination preparations, such as neomycin-polymyxin B-gramicidin, were originally developed to be effective against multiple bacteria, but variable efficacy against resistant strains and the possibility of toxic or allergic reactions limit their current use for bacterial keratitis.

Single-Agent Therapy. Ophthalmic fluoroquinolone preparations have excellent in vitro activity against common corneal bacterial pathogens.[92,322] Several topical fluoroquinolones are becoming commercially available that are approved for treating bacterial keratitis. Ciprofloxacin 0.3% solution is clinically effective[248] and adverse reactions are mild, although some treated patients develop reversible drug precipitation or crystallization within the superficial stroma of the ulcer (Fig. 74-21). Ofloxacin 0.3% solution appears as effective as combined cefazolin and tobramycin.[291,309a] Other fluoroquinolones such as norfloxacin[445] and lomefloxacin may also be effective in the treatment of bacterial keratitis. Caution is advised for infections caused by organisms with variable susceptibility to the fluoroquinolones such as streptococci, methicillin-resistant staphylococci, anaerobic cocci, and some resistant strains of *P. aeruginosa.*

Other agents that show promise as effective single-agent therapy include the extended-spectrum cephalosporins such as ceftazidime and carbapenems such as imipenem. Certain animal-derived peptides (e.g., magainins from frogs, cecropins from moths, and defensins from human neutrophils and epithelial cells) show promise. Further developments in ophthalmic antimicrobial therapy are anticipated.

Dosages and Routes of Antibacterial Therapy. *Topical Administration.* The initial treatment of bacterial keratitis typically includes topical administration of antibacterial agents in a safe and effective concentration. Multiple antibiotics are commercially available at concentrations designed for the treatment of ocular surface infections. Some of these agents, such as gentamicin and tobramycin, can be fortified to a higher concentration by adding a more concentrated parenteral formulation to the ophthalmic solution. Concentrations higher than those commercially available are equivalent or superior in curing experimental bacterial keratitis.[236,302,476]

Preparation. Some antibiotics are not marketed as topical preparations because of a short shelf life when dissolved. These agents can be freshly made at an appropriate concentration (Table 74-12) by mixing the powder available for intravenous use in an appropriate solvent. An ideal diluent would achieve optimal pH, osmolarity, colloid oncotic pressure, electrolyte composition, and viscosity. Normal tears and aqueous humor are isotonic to blood plasma, but normal saline is not recommended to dissolve topical antibiotics because it may yield a hyperosmolar solution with the drug concentrations that are often used. Furthermore many antibacterial agents prepared from a parenteral preparation are acidic, and buffered solvents are usually preferred. Topical vancomycin prepared with sterile water, normal saline, or a nonphosphate-buffered artificial tear is more acidic, and thus more irritating, than a preparation reconstituted with a phosphate-buffered vehicle;[127] but its activity is retained longer in a slightly acidic solution.

Potential drug interactions, such as may occur between cephalosporin and aminoglycoside antibiotics, are avoided by not mixing two different agents in the same eyedropper vial. Freshly prepared antibiotics can generally be kept at room temperature for one week or longer without significant loss of activity[48,285,323] or risk of contamination[51] but should be replaced every 5 to 7 days.

Topical Application. Topical antibacterial solutions are administered as frequently as one drop every 15 to 30 minutes around the clock, with a minimum of 5 minutes between different eyedrops. This dosing schedule is significantly more effective than eyedrops given every 1 to 2 hours.[97] A loading dose to rapidly elevate the drug level within the corneal stroma can be administered by giving one drop every minute for 5 minutes, repeating this application schedule 30 to 60 minutes later,[143] and then giving a single drop every 30 to 60 minutes. An appropriate plan has proved to be initially intensive applications followed by gradual tapering of less frequent chemotherapy.[98]

By pinching and pulling the lower eyelid, a small pouch of the lower cul-de-sac is made that can simplify proper delivery. Refrigerating solutions might also help because a cold drop will be noticeable when instilled. Two or more medications should be given at alternating dosing intervals to allow maximal contact and penetration. Because there is a maximal volume that can be retained in the conjunctival cul-de-sac, a single solution drop is given at each adminis-

TABLE 74-12 PREPARATION OF TOPICAL ANTIBACTERIAL AGENTS FOR BACTERIAL KERATITIS*

Antibiotic	Amount in Vial	Dilute With	Withdraw	Add to	Final Volume	Final Concentration
Amikacin	250 mg/ml injectable	0	2 ml	8 ml artificial tears	10	50 mg/ml
Bacitracin	50,000 units powder	5 ml	10 ml	Empty bottle	5 ml	100,000 units/ml
Cefazolin†	500 mg powder	2 ml	2 ml	8 ml artificial tears	10 ml	50 mg/ml
Ceftazidime†	500 mg powder	2 ml	2 ml	8 ml artificial tears	10 ml	50 mg/ml
Clindamycin	150 mg/ml injectable	0	1 ml	9 ml artificial tears	10 ml	15 mg/ml
Colistimethate	150 mg powder	2 ml	1.5 ml	8.5 ml artificial tears	10 ml	10 mg/ml
Gentamicin	40 mg/ml injectable	0	2 ml	5 ml ophthalmic solution (3 mg/ml)	7 ml	13.6 mg/ml
Penicillin G	1 million units powder	10 ml	10 ml	Empty bottle	10 ml	100,000 units/ml
	5 million units powder	3 ml	1 ml	9 ml artificial tears	10 ml	100,000 units/ml
Piperacillin†	2 gm powder	10 ml	0.5 ml	9.5 ml artificial tears	10 ml	10 mg/ml
Polymyxin B	50 mg powder	10 ml	10 ml	Empty bottle	10 ml	5 mg/ml
Tobramycin	40 mg/ml injectable	0	2 ml	5 ml ophthalmic solution (3 mg/ml)	7 ml	13.6 mgml
Vancomycin	500 mg powder	10 ml	10 ml	Empty bottle	10 ml	50 mg/ml

* Guidelines for the preparation of ophthalmic pharmaceuticals should be followed. Solvent selection for small diluent volumes should follow manufacturers' recommendations. The topical antimicrobial solution can then be prepared with an artificial tear containing a preservative and dispensed in a sterile eyedropper bottle, or it can be reconstituted using a preservative-free solution and packaged in unit-dose containers.
† Other agents in the group may be formulated at a similar concentration. Fresh solutions should be prepared every 5 to 7 days.

tration. Because the average tear turnover rate is approximately 16% per minute, about 5 minutes are needed for adequate tear replacement and should be the least interval between instillation of different eyedrops. Frequent administration not only enhances corneal penetration but can rinse inflammatory material from the eye. Systemic absorption occurs[100] but is not clinically important in older children and adults. Outpatient management is feasible if patient compliance with the prescribed regimen is possible.[151] Sleep deprivation and confusion can be partially relieved with nursing comfort measures.[321]

Patient factors that affect antibiotic penetration include the blink rate, tear-film dynamics, and conjunctival vascular inflammation.[391] Excessive tearing can dilute topically administered drugs, and conjunctival inflammation removes drugs from the preocular tear film. Reducing lacrimal outflow can decrease the possibility of systemic absorption and help raise the drug level in the tear film and cornea. Simple eyelid closure and digital pressure on the medial canthus retain instilled drugs by impeding drainage into the nasolacrimal duct. Punctal occlusion with intracanalicular collagen plugs can prolong the retention of a topical antibacterial agent and increase corneal penetration.[142] Penetration of hydrophilic agents into the cornea is enhanced by the presence of an epithelial defect, but corneal debridement is not usually performed for this purpose.

Vehicles for Drug Delivery. Topically applied drugs can be delivered in an aqueous solution, suspension, emulsion, gel, or ointment. Corneal drug penetration is affected by an antibiotic's relative lipid and aqueous solubilities and the presence of preservatives and other surface-active agents in the drug-delivery vehicle. A viscous vehicle might aid corneal penetration, but ointments are generally less preferred than solutions. Ointments prolong corneal contact, sustain the drug level in the tear film, and can effectively treat bacterial keratitis.[481] An ointment, however, reduces the bioavailability of some antibiotics, makes it difficult to alter the antibiotic concentration, and tends to slow the penetration of subsequently administered eyedrops. Ointments can be useful for patients who find it difficult to instill eyedrops, for young children whose tearing washes out antibiotic solutions, and for nocturnal use to supplement daytime treatment.

Microcapsules, drug-impregnated liposomes, and other ways of administering topical drug preparations have potential applications in the management of bacterial keratitis.[246] Antibiotics such as gentamicin have been incorporated into phospholipid vesicles, but technologic limitations such as short shelf life and restricted drug-loading capacity have constrained the use of liposomes.[376] Other vehicles such as the cyclodextrins offer opportunities for delivering poorly soluble agents to the eye.

Soft Contact Lenses. Hydrophilic soft contact lenses can be used as corneal drug-delivery devices. With frequent topical administration of a fortified antibiotic, the presence of a soft contact lens can yield higher corneal drug levels after several hours.[57,278] A high-water-content lens soaked in an antibiotic solution yields high levels of drug over several hours. The release rate depends on the drug's concentration; its molecular weight, solubility, and ion charge, and the makeup of the contact lens. The therapeutic advantage of drug delivery with a soft contact lens in the management of bacterial keratitis has not been determined, but a bandage contact lens does not impair the delivery of topical drugs to the cornea and can act as a barrier to corneal infiltration by tear-film neutrophils.

Collagen Shields. Collagen corneal shields, fabricated from porcine or bovine cornea or sclera and composed predominantly of type 1 collagen, can deliver antibiotics to the eye. Shaped like a soft contact lens, the rehydrated shield conforms to most corneal curvatures, and oxygen permeability is similar to or better than hydrophilic contact lenses. As a result of ultraviolet light-induced collagen cross-linking, available shields are intended to dissolve in 12, 24, and 72 hours. Hydrating the shield in an antibiotic solution provides a means for corneal drug delivery;[134] maximal drug absorption occurs within 10 to 15 minutes of soaking. Water-soluble drugs are trapped within the collagen matrix, and some also bind directly. With a presoaked collagen shield, corneal and aqueous humor drug levels are generally highest within the first few hours after application. Different drugs elute from a shield at different rates depending on molecular weight, solubility, and other factors. An aminoglycoside is rapidly released within 30 minutes; other agents are released over several hours. Pharmacokinetic studies show that collagen shields are superior to soft contact lenses[310] or subconjunctival injection[441] in rapidly achieving high tissue levels.

Experimental studies have shown that a drug-soaked collagen shield can aid in the treatment of bacterial keratitis.[179] The short-term efficacy of a drug-soaked collagen shield is equivalent to an initial loading dose of fortified eyedrops.[14] A drug-soaked collagen shield with topical eyedrops administered at least every 6 hours augments drug levels and speeds eradication of experimental bacterial keratitis compared to either a shield or hourly eyedrops alone.[77] An antibiotic-impregnated shield supplemented with topical therapy is not better than the use of half-hourly fortified antibiotics, however.[294]

A collagen shield can deliver one or more antibacterial agents, but combined drugs must be pharmacologically compatible.[395] Admixed gentamicin and cefazolin, for example, will precipitate and cannot be satisfactorily incorporated together. Corticosteroids and some antibiotics (e.g., gentamicin and ciprofloxacin) aggregate into crystalline precipitates on a collagen shield and can result in mechanical trauma to the corneal epithelium. Because shields are available in a limited choice of base curves and diameters, accidental loss can occur. Accelerated dissolution occurs during early bacterial keratitis, and concomitant topical dosing is recommended. Other potential problems with collagen shields include allergic reactions[44] to the material and toxicity related to drug release. The excessive drug concentration that can be delivered into the aqueous humor risks corneal toxicity in patients who have reduced endothelial density or poor tear clearance.[336] Better knowledge of safe and effective drug soaking solutions and improved drug incorporation into a dissolvable shield are needed for appropriate clinical use.

Other methods that may improve penetration and efficacy of a topical antibiotic have been proposed, including drug inserts, corneal lavage, and iontophoresis:

Reservoirs and Delayed Release Devices. Inserts[43] and other sustained release devices[394] can potentially provide initially high levels of an antimicrobial agent and maintain a constant or gradually tapering drug concentration in the precorneal tear film. A drug-soaked cotton pledget and erodible and nonerodible inserts have been tried but are not currently in use. Presoaked collagen discs yield drug levels in the cornea within 30 minutes, but rapid dissolution limits their therapeutic potential at the present.[255]

Corneal Lavage or Bath. Saline irrigation can rinse excess bacteria and inflammatory debris from the ocular surface. Continuous subpalpebral lavage,[56] an infusing scleral contact lens, and a corneal bath or eyecup all expose the cornea to a constant high antibiotic level. These techniques might rarely be considered for bacterial sclerokeratitis, but the patient must be immobilized. These techniques have been successfully used, but the risk of toxicity and patient discomfort limits their routine or widespread use. Subpalpebral lavage does have a potential role in veterinary ophthalmic practice.

For subpalpebral lavage, flexible tubing is used. The end is heated to form a flared, funnel-like opening. After topical and infiltrative anesthesia in the region of the upper eyelid fold and superior fornix, the nonflared end of the tubing is passed through a large-gauge needle after the hub is removed. The tubing is positioned by inserting the trocar needle through the upper, outer fornix and then removing and discarding it. The tube is anchored with sutures and tape. Continuous or intermittent infusion is maintained with a slow drip or pump system. Saline rather than dextrose solution is used for irrigation.

Subcutaneous pumps can deliver a continuous infusion of fluid to the ocular surface. When implanted, a connecting tube opens into the conjunctival sac. While not practical in clinical ophthalmology, these devices have potential research applications.[134]

A corneal bath can be fashioned with a plastic drape or by molding clay, and specially designed eyecups are available. A diluted antibiotic solution fills the reservoir as the patient remains supine, thus bathing the cornea continuously. The duration of bathing can be reduced by accelerating the diffu-

sion of ionic compounds using the technique of iontophoresis.

Iontophoresis. Iontophoresis can enhance the penetration of polar molecules[186] such as vancomycin,[72] tobramycin,[355] and ciprofloxacin.[180] An eyecup or similar device is filled with medication and placed over the cornea; alternatively a drug-soaked pad is placed over the eye or closed eyelids. The instrument is connected to a direct current source. For cationic drugs, the platinum anode is placed in contact with the antimicrobial solution bathing the cornea and the cathode is held in the hand or attached to another part of the body such as the ear. A current of approximately 1 mA is passed through the solution for several minutes. Transient corneal edema is not uncommon, and permanent corneal endothelial cell loss can occur. The procedure can be repeated later or can be followed with topical dosing of eyedrops.

Subconjunctival Injection. Periocular antibiotic injection achieves therapeutic intracorneal drug levels by leakage of the antimicrobial agent into the preocular tear film and by diffusion of the drug from the injection site to the sclera and peripheral cornea. Because leakage into the tears appears more important, subconjunctival rather than subtenon injection is suggested. The role of diffusion is enhanced by putting the injection as close as possible to the site of infection.[25,309]

Experimental models of bacterial keratitis have shown that subconjunctival antibiotics add little to antibacterial efficacy if an adequate concentration and dosing frequency of the topical agent are used.[32] Subconjunctival antibiotic administration is as effective as topical therapy and could rarely be considered as the sole route of drug delivery if topical administration is not possible or reliable. Subconjunctival injections are usually reserved for severe disease in which bacterial keratitis is progressing with threatened perforation or involvement of the adjacent sclera.

Antibacterial agents used for subconjunctival or subtenon injection are prepared from drugs marketed for intravenous or intrathecal use (Table 74-13). Appropriate concentrations are extrapolated from parenteral dosages and based on pharmacokinetic data. The total volume of each set of one or more injections should generally not exceed one milliliter.

For subconjunctival injection the patient should generally be provided an opportunity to give informed consent. A systemic analgesic or anxiolytic agent is considered. Sedation and physical restraint are provided to children. If one anticipates involuntary eyelid squeezing that could dangerously raise the intraocular pressure to rupture a descemetocele, local eyelid akinesia should be given with an anesthetic injection. The conjunctiva to be injected is topically anesthetized with a swab soaked in an anesthetic solution such as 0.5% proparacaine or 4% lidocaine. A small amount (0.1 to 0.25 ml) of 1% or 2% lidocaine can also be injected subconjunctivally with a small-gauge needle before the antibiotic is injected. A local anesthetic does not affect antimicrobial ac-

TABLE 74-13 PREPARATION OF ANTIBACTERIAL AGENTS FOR SUBCONJUNCTIVAL INJECTION

Antibiotic	Amount in Vial	Diluent Volume	Volume to Inject*	Amount in Injection
Amikacin	1 gm/4 ml	0	0.5 ml	125 mg
Cefazolin	500 mg powder	2.5 ml	0.5 ml	100 mg
Clindamycin	300 mg/2 ml	0	0.25 ml	37.5 mg
Gentamicin	80 mg/ml	0	0.5 ml	20 mg
Penicillin G	1 million units powder	4.6 ml	0.5 ml	500,000 units
Tobramycin	80 mg/2 ml	0	0.5 ml	20 mg
Vancomycin	500 mg	10 ml	0.5 ml	25 mg

* Dosage reduction may be indicated in small children.

tivity.[24] The antibacterial agent is then injected with the same or different syringe in the quadrant nearest the site of corneal infection. The needle's bevel should face toward the globe to reduce the risk of accidental perforation. Two antibiotics should not be mixed in the same syringe and should preferably be given at different injection sites. Afterward an ice pack can provide temporary pain relief. Subconjunctival injections can be repeated every 12 to 24 hours during the first few days of therapy.

Pain and subconjunctival hemorrhage commonly occur after periocular antibiotic injection. Epithelial cytotoxicity,[256] corneal edema and endothelial changes,[372] and mydriasis[16] are occasionally encountered. More serious complications include conjunctival necrosis and scarring. The use of preservative-free preparations minimizes these adverse effects.[326] Subconjunctival injections also carry the risk of accidental perforation and excessive transscleral drug penetration with intraocular toxicity. In neonates and young children subconjunctival injection can lead to high drug levels that could cause systemic side effects such as neuromuscular blockade. Thus, lacking a clear clinical advantage,[29,101] subconjunctival antibiotics are generally reserved for the most serious infections.

Systemic Therapy. Some oral agents can lead to detectable drug levels in the preocular tear film and intraocular fluids but are generally of no additional benefit over topical administration. Some oral antibiotics, such as the macrolides and the quinolones, that are concentrated within polymorphonuclear leukocytes can potentially be delivered by inflammatory cells to the site of corneal infection. Parenteral antibiotic administration produces low levels in tears[488] but can attain therapeutic concentrations in the cornea[192] to enhance the drug levels achieved by topical administration. Although not usually necessary for adequate treatment of bacterial keratitis, intravenous therapy can be considered as an adjunct to topical and periocular treatment if the infectious process involves the sclera, when intraocular spread is likely, and whenever there is a risk of systemic involvement, such as gonococcal keratoconjunctivitis,[439] meningococcal keratoconjunctivitis,[22] or neonatal bacterial keratitis.

Peak and trough serum levels can be monitored. The choice of systemic antibacterial therapy is based upon the responsible microorganisms and the possible adverse effects and drug interactions associated with intravenous drugs.

Adjunctive Therapy. Periodic rinsing of the conjunctival discharge and gentle cleansing of crusted matter and dried medications from the eyelids comfort patients and permit better examination. Patching is generally unnecessary during initial therapy, although a protective shield may be useful in the presence of corneal thinning. Frequent cleaning or exchange of any soft contact lens or collagen shield should be ensured.

Initial medical management generally includes a topical cycloplegic-mydriatic agent, such as scopolamine hydrobromide 0.25% or atropine 1%, to ease the discomfort of ciliary spasm and to minimize the formation of iris synechiae. If posterior synechiae have begun to form, maximal dilatation can be achieved with atropine and phenylephrine hydrochloride.

Intraocular pressure should be monitored. If elevated, nonmiotic antiglaucoma agents such as a topical betablocker and/or an oral carbonic anhydrase inhibitor should be considered.

Control of any factors that predisposed to bacterial keratitis should be undertaken if possible. Although surgical correction of structural abnormalities is generally deferred until adequate control of the infectious process, temporizing measures may sometimes be useful. A temporary tarsorrhaphy can correct lagophthalmos or other causes of corneal exposure. Lacrimal outflow should be assessed to exclude chronic dacryocystitis. Punctal plugs may aid in the control of dry eyes, and selected epilation of abnormal eyelashes can be helpful. Adequate nutrition, including vitamin A supplementation, should be provided to malnourished individuals. While clostridial keratitis is exceedingly rare, tetanus prophylaxis might be considered for farming accidents and similar injuries. Patients with gonococcal keratoconjunctivitis should be evaluated for other sexually transmitted diseases and treated presumptively with oral doxycycline or erythromycin for concomitant chlamydial infection.[439]

The decision for hospitalization is generally made on the need for nursing help in the administration of frequent topical eyedrops. Isolation is not usually necessary, although these patients should probably not come in close contact with those undergoing intraocular surgery. Outpatient management is feasible for most patients. Oral analgesia is usually provided, but pain control may be difficult until ocular inflammation abates.

Modification of Antibacterial Therapy

Modifications of the initial antibacterial therapy are based on the clinical response and laboratory data (Table 74-14). If more than one antibacterial agent was initially chosen to provide broad-spectrum coverage, the less effective drug may be discontinued based on culture results. A change in antibacterial therapy should be considered if progressive corneal suppuration occurs despite intensive therapy. Changes in antibacterial agents can be guided by bacterial identification (Table 74-15), and further modifications are based on susceptibility testing. If more than one bacterial species is identified and specific initial therapy was used, the addition of a second agent can be based on anticipated or reported susceptibility data. For culture-negative cases the decision to continue antibacterial therapy must be made on clinical grounds.

Preliminary culture data aid in selecting optimal agents. Treatment modifications for the common bacterial isolates are discussed in the paragraphs that follow.

Gram-Positive Cocci. Initial antibacterial therapy that includes a cephalosporin, such as cefazolin, or a fluoroquinolone, such as ciprofloxacin, is generally adequate and even optimal for most gram-positive cocci. Because methicillin-resistant staphylococci are increasing in prevalence, vancomycin is a useful alternative to cephalosporins;[145] and teicoplanin may prove to be effective. Many gram-positive cocci are resistant to aminoglycosides like gentamicin,[268] and

some streptococci and enterococci are only marginally sensitive to cefazolin and ciprofloxacin. Alternative agents are selected if clinical improvement does not occur. Except for rare strains,[419] penicillin G remains one of the most effective agents against pneumococci. Enterococci that are resistant to multiple antibiotics are best managed with combination therapy including an aminoglycoside agent such as gentamicin and a second agent such as penicillin, ampicillin, or vancomycin. Beta-lactamase inhibitors such as clavulanic acid and sulbactam are now commercially available in combination with a semisynthetic penicillin and have potential ophthalmic use.

Gram-Negative Rods. An aminoglycoside, such as gentamicin or tobramycin, or a fluoroquinolone, such as ciprofloxacin or ofloxacin, is appropriate for most gram-negative rods. The addition of an extended-spectrum penicillin such as ticarcillin or piperacillin is not usually necessary. For aminoglycoside-resistant *P. aeruginosa,* an extended-spectrum cephalosporin (e.g., ceftazidime or cefoperazone) or a carbapenem (e.g., imipenem) may be effective. Gentamicin-resistant strains may be sensitive to amikacin.[141] Older agents such as the polymyxins, including colistin, may still have a therapeutic role.

Anaerobes. When anaerobic bacteria are isolated a change in antibacterial therapy is not usually indicated. These organisms are sensitive to most of the agents usually used in treating bacterial keratitis. In vitro susceptibility testing is difficult to perform but suggests that effective agents include penicillin G, chloramphenicol, and clindamycin.

Follow-Up Evaluation

During initial therapy the patient should be evaluated daily to determine the severity and pace of infection and to judge the response to treatment. Because of the release of bacterial exotoxins that digest corneal tissue and chemotactic factors that stimulate local inflammation, persistent suppuration, ulceration, and necrosis may occur during the first few days despite initially effective therapy. Signs of clinical improvement are generally noticeable within 2 to 3 days of effective therapy. Polymicrobial infection with two or more types of microorganisms can sometimes account for clinical progression if the initial antibiotic selection does not inhibit all causative organisms. Repeat corneal scrapings or corneal biopsy may be indicated for continued worsening, although reliability is impaired by concomitant therapy. If all cultures are negative a nonbacterial cause should be reconsidered.

The area and density of stromal inflammation, the area and depth of epithelial and stromal ulceration, and the amount of intraocular inflammation should be recorded at each examination. Specific biomicroscopic features that suggest clinical improvement include the following: decreasing size and density of the area of stromal inflammation, decreasing cellular infiltration in the adjacent stroma, decreasing edema with disappearing pseudoguttata at the

TABLE 74-14 MODIFICATION OF TREATMENT PLAN BASED ON LABORATORY INFORMATION

Laboratory Data	Management Action
Single microbial isolate	Initiate therapy if patient not being treated
	or
	Reduce combined treatment to a single agent
≥ 2 microbial isolates	Consider adding alternate or second agent if activity spectrum of initial therapy is uncertain
Susceptibility data	Substitute more effective agent if clinical response not acceptable

TABLE 74-15   POSSIBLE MODIFICATIONS IN ANTIMICROBIAL THERAPY

Organism	Topical	Subconjunctival	Intravenous*
Staphylococcus spp., methicillin-resistant	Vancomycin 50 mg/ml	Vancomycin 25 mg	Vancomycin 1 gm every 12 hours
S. pneumoniae	Penicillin G 100,000 units/ml	Penicillin G 500,000 units	Penicillin G 2-6 million units every 4 hours
S. pyogenes	Penicillin G 100,000 units/ml	Penicillin G 500,000 units	Penicillin G 2-6 million units every 4 hours
Enterococcus spp.	Vancomycin 50 mg/ml + gentamicin 13.6 mg/ml	Vancomycin 25 mg	Vancomycin 1 gm every 12 hours
Anaerobic gram-positive cocci	Penicillin G 100,000 units/ml	Penicillin G 500,000 units	Penicillin G 2-6 million units every 12 hours
Neisseria spp., penicillin-resistant	Erythromycin (or bacitracin) ointment	Ceftriaxone 100 mg	Ceftriaxone 1 gm every 12 hours
Pseudomonas spp.	Tobramycin 13.6 mg/ml	Tobramycin 20 mg	Tobramycin 3-7 mg/kg/day
Pseudomonas spp., aminoglycoside-resistant	Ciprofloxacin or ofloxacin 3 mg/ml (or ceftazidime 50 mg/ml or imipenem 5 mg/ml)	Ceftazidime 100 mg	Ceftazidime 1 gm every 8 hours
Moraxella spp.	Gentamicin 13.6 mg/ml	Gentamicin 20 mg	Gentamicin 50-100 mg every 8 hours
Haemophilus spp., chloramphenicol-resistant	Ciprofloxacin 3 mg/ml	Cefotaxime 100 mg	Cefotaxime 1 gm every 8 hours
Acinetobacter spp.	Gentamicin 13.6 mg/ml	Gentamicin 20 mg	Gentamicin 50-100 mg every 8 hours
Corynebacterium spp.	Cefazolin 50 mg/ml (or gentamicin 13.6 mg/ml or vancomycin 50 mg/ml)	Cefazolin 100 mg (or gentamicin 20 mg)	Cefazolin 1 gm every 8 hours
Bacillus spp.	Clindamycin 15 mg/ml	Clindamycin 37.5 mg	Clindamycin 600 mg every 8 hours
Bacteroides spp.	Penicillin G 100,000 units/ml + clindamycin 15 mg/ml	Clindamycin 37.5 mg	Clindamycin 600 mg every 8 hours
Propionibacterium acnes	Cefazolin 50 mg/ml (or imipenem 50 mg/ml)	Cefazolin 100 mg	Cefazolin 1 gm every 8 hours

Modified after Jones DB. Decision making in the management of microbial keratitis, *Ophthalmology* 88:814, 1981.
* For adult with normal renal function.

borders of the infiltrate, blunting of the margins of the focal infiltrate with a progressively more well-defined perimeter, reduction of the anterior-chamber inflammation with a decrease in size of the hypopyon, and progressive reepithelialization. Careful observation of the microstructural changes at the margins of the zone of suppuration can show whether a patient is improving or worsening. Early signs of improvement include enhanced delineation of the inflammatory perimeter, resolution of endothelial pseudoguttata, and stromal edema adjacent to the ulcer's outer edges. Variations in the rate of improvement depend on the following: responsible bacteria, the initial severity and duration of the infection, the intensity of the inflammatory reaction, the presence of concomitant host factors, the efficacy of the antibacterial therapy, the use of concomitant medications, and compliance with the treatment regimen.

The dosing frequency of topical antibacterial therapy is generally reduced every few days and is often begun by doubling the dosing frequency from every 15 to 30 minutes to every 30 to 60 minutes. Subconjunctival and parenteral therapy, if used, can be discontinued within a few days if scleral or intraocular involvement is not anticipated.

Once the frequency of topical application has been reduced to approximately 4 to 6 times daily, the drug concentration can be lowered. Fortified antibiotics are changed to commercially available solutions or ointments to reduce toxicity related to topical antimicrobial therapy. Epithelial healing usually signals resolution; but because toxicity may slow this process, the endpoint of treatment is not necessarily complete reepithelialization. A typical total duration of antimicrobial therapy is 3 to 4 weeks. Prolonged antibacterial therapy may be required for more severe infections. Recrudescent infection has occurred by microorganisms, such as *P. aeruginosa,* that are capable of surviving within corneal cells during antibacterial treatment.

Antiinflammatory Therapy

Corticosteroids. As antimicrobial agents control the infectious process, a topical corticosteroid may be used to suppress the local inflammatory response. The potential advantages of corticosteroid use include reducing postinflammatory scarring, limiting the damage produced by neutrophils, minimizing corneal neovascularization, and permitting reepithelialization. But corneal opacification and a persistent epithelial defect may occur despite topical corticosteroid use, and whether corticosteroids substantially affect outcome remains to be determined. As a result, the indications for optimal use of a topical corticosteroid in bacterial keratitis have not been established.

Adverse Effects. Potential adverse effects of corticosteroids include secondary glaucoma, cataract formation, inhibition of corneal wound healing, and potentiation of corneal infection. By suppressing the host's inflammatory response, the use of corticosteroids without effective antibacterial therapy can permit uncontrolled bacterial replication. Experimental and clinical evidence suggest that the growth of microorganisms such as *P. aeruginosa* is enhanced when corticosteroids are used alone. With incomplete antibacterial therapy, corticosteroids allow bacterial survival. Clinical reports of patients with *P. aeruginosa* keratitis incriminate corticosteroids as a factor in leading to late recrudescence of infection after discontinuation of antibacterial therapy.[55,157]

Corticosteroids should not be used if the efficacy of antibacterial therapy is uncertain. These situations include lack of a culture isolate, lack of antibacterial susceptibility test results, uncertainty about the bactericidal effects of the topical antibacterial agent, or questions about compliance. While maximal antiinflammatory effects are achieved with early corticosteroid use, corticosteroids are usually deferred until clinical response to antibacterial therapy is determined and initial laboratory information is available.

Beneficial Effects. Potential benefits of corticosteroids are suppression of stromal inflammation and prevention of severe corneal opacification. If adequate bactericidal therapy is administered concomitantly, corticosteroids should not accelerate bacterial growth. Experimental studies have shown that the use of topical corticosteroids with effective bactericidal therapy does not impair eradication of intrastromal bacteria.[20,99,250]

Inflammation disrupts the normally transparent stromal lamellae, and healing results in its partial replacement by different collagen fibers. Corticosteroids can impair collagen formation in the injured cornea, but a significant reduction in postinflammatory corneal scarring following corticosteroid use in treated bacterial keratitis has not been demonstrated. Corticosteroids have little if any direct effect on reepithelialization but can be useful for managing a persistent epithelial defect over inflamed stroma. By reducing persistent inflammation, corticosteroids can minimize stromal thinning and speed reepithelialization.

Lacking guidelines for optimal corticosteroid use, topical corticosteroids remain a controversial treatment option. Experimental studies have generally shown that little is to be gained from corticosteroid use very early in the treatment plan but that a corticosteroid can substantially reduce leukocyte recruitment during effective antibacterial therapy. If

clinical improvement is noted within the first few days after the initiation of antibacterial therapy, then a topical corticosteroid can be added,[12,247] based on the severity of corneal inflammation and the expectation of visually disabling structural changes. A prospective clinical trial showed no detrimental effect of topical dexamethasone when begun after antibacterial therapy,[62] but the topical corticosteroid regimen in this study did not show a significant effect on visual outcome.

Clinical Usage. The choice of an ophthalmic corticosteroid can be based on the base compound, its derivative, its formulation, and its concentration.[249] Clinical studies have not compared the use of different products in the management of bacterial keratitis. Widely used preparations include prednisolone phosphate, prednisolone acetate, dexamethasone phosphate, dexamethasone alcohol, fluorometholone alcohol, and fluorometholone acetate. The highest commercially available concentration is generally chosen when initiating corticosteroid therapy. Combined corticosteroid-antibiotic preparations are not usually appropriate during initial therapy of bacterial keratitis but perhaps have a role in the later phases of treatment. Corticosteroids are deferred until after antibacterial therapy has been implemented, although one exception might be those patients who are already receiving a topical corticosteroid for another indication (e.g., herpetic keratitis) before bacterial keratitis is diagnosed. In these patients the dosing frequency and/or concentration of the corticosteroid that is already being used can be continued at a reduced dosage until control of the bacterial infection is established.

Caveats regarding the use of a topical corticosteroid during bacterial keratitis have been recommended:[410] (1) corticosteroids should not be used if the causative microorganism is uncertain or if effective bactericidal therapy is not being provided, and (2) corticosteroids can be considered after several days of antibacterial therapy for persistent corneal inflammation. A risk-benefit analysis must be weighed for each case. For example, a topical corticosteroid might help a patient with a dense stromal infiltrate impinging on the visual axis that is due to bacteria of known sensitivities, whereas corticosteroid therapy may not be useful for patients with such severe corneal involvement that central corneal opacification appears inevitable.

The frequency and concentration of a topical corticosteroid should be adjusted according to the severity of the corneal inflammatory reaction and subsequently gradually tapered corresponding to antibacterial dosage reduction. Rarely are corticosteroids used more often or longer than the concomitant bactericidal agent. Abrupt discontinuation is avoided to prevent possible rebound inflammation. Whether a topical corticosteroid predisposes to recrudescent infection after medical treatment of bacterial keratitis has not been determined. Local corticosteroid injections and oral agents are not generally used.

Better insight into the mechanisms of bacterial invasion

and of the host response aims to create new ways to affect outcome. New agents under development are nonsteroidal antiinflammatory agents, inhibitors of bacterial and host enzymes, and monoclonal antibodies that block key components of inflammatory pathways.

Other Antiinflammatory Agents. Nonsteroidal antiinflammatory agents have a potential role in the management of bacterial keratitis. Cyclooxygenase inhibitors such as indomethacin, diclofenac, flurbiprofen, and ketorolac[133] do not worsen bacterial keratitis, but some inhibitors of prostaglandin synthesis might exacerbate corneal inflammation by shunting arachidonic acid metabolites into the parallel leukotriene pathway if concomitant effective antibacterial therapy is not used.[150] Some nonsteroidal agents may have small additive antibacterial effect when given with bactericidal therapy.

Phosphodiesterase inhibitors have the potential to reduce the recruitment and degranulation of neutrophils but have not been adequately studied in the management of bacterial keratitis. The development of specific inhibitors of leukocyte migration, such as monoclonal antibodies directed against integrins and other adhesion molecules, may prove helpful as a supplement to corticosteroid therapy. The value of antifibrinolytic agents and other antiangiogenic substances has not been evaluated.

New Strategies for Controlling Molecular Mediators

During bacterial keratitis destructive enzymes are released from bacteria, from leukocytes, and from keratocytes and damaged epithelial cells.[39] Enzymes implicated in corneal ulceration include the serine proteases (e.g., plasmin and tissue plasminogen activator) and several metalloproteases released from keratocytes (e.g., collagenases, gelatinases, stromelysins, and matrilysin) and from leukocytes (e.g., collagenase and elastase). Regulated by α_2-macroglobulin, interleukins, and other cytokines, the calcium-dependent metalloproteases are activated from the proenzyme state by cleavage of a propeptide and incorporate zinc cations at the catalytically active site. Inhibition of these and other mediators of corneal inflammation and destruction may soon be feasible.

Metalloproteinase Inhibitors. Zinc chelators such as sodium edetate (NaEDTA), L-cysteine, N-acetylcysteine, and D-penicillamine are nonspecific metalloprotease chelators[132] but are relatively ineffective in controlling corneal inflammation. Additional Zn^{++} can decrease activity, but the use of zinc sulfate is not clinically useful.

Tetracyclines can bind zinc and inhibit collagenases and other metalloenzymes,[253] but their role in the management of bacterial keratitis is unclear. Beta-lactoms are also able to inhibit metalloproteinases.

Synthetic, metal-chelating peptides[54,405] and congeners of α_2-macroglobulin, such as ovomacroglobulin,[292] are under development that inhibit matrix metalloproteinases and, in combination with corticosteroids, reduce corneal angiogenesis. By blocking endogenous collagenolysis and by inhibiting bacterial metalloproteases such as pseudomonal elastase, these substances offer new possibilities in preventing progressive corneal destruction during bacterial keratitis.[138a,149a] Metalloproteinase gene expression can also be suppressed by agents such as corticosteroids and retinoids. Whether a beneficial effect of metalloproteinase inhibition will be limited to the early stages of infection before excessive inflammatory cells have accumulated and whether a significant effect on preserving corneal structure and function will be possible remain to be determined. Perhaps it will be necessary to use a combination of agents that work on different components of corneal wound healing, such as a metalloprotease inhibitor (e.g., a hydroxamate derivative), a serine protease inhibitor (e.g., aprotinin), an extracellular matrix component (e.g., fibronectin), and a mitogenic growth factor (e.g., epidermal growth factor).[382]

A collagen shield, applied to the corneal surface, can potentially compete with stromal collagen as a substrate for liberated collagenases.[381] The rate of dissolution provides a crude index of disease activity because it degrades more rapidly during early, untreated bacterial keratitis than later. Whether a shield can divert sufficient enzyme from the corneal stroma to a clinically important degree remains to be determined.

Inhibitors of Leukocytic Substances. Sodium citrate can limit the respiratory burst of neutrophils, and colchicine is able to inhibit the extracellular release of lysosomal enzyme. These inhibitors of leukocytic migration or degranulation are not clinically used for bacterial keratitis, however.

Antiphlogistic agents that target the production of toxic oxygen metabolites include antioxidant enzymes (e.g., superoxide dismutase and catalase), hydroxyl radical scavengers (e.g., dimethyl sulfoxide), and iron-chelating agents. As scavengers of free radicals, topical antioxidants suppress corneal inflammation but, by reducing the antimicrobial activity of neutrophils, can enhance bacterial growth.[4a] The clinical role of these inhibitors has not been shown in the management of bacterial keratitis.

Inhibitors of Bacterial Substances. Antiserum is rarely indicated during bacterial keratitis. Because of the seriousness of diphtheria and tetanus (death occurs in about 1 of every 10 people with diphtheria and in 3 of every 10 people with tetanus), patients with suspected *C. diphtheriae* or *C. tetani* keratitis should receive antitoxin. The only other current role of systemic immunotherapy during bacterial keratitis is the use of hyperimmune globulin to prevent septicemia in burn patients with pseudomonal keratitis.

Antibodies against bacterial components have shown some preliminary promising results.[466] The commercial availability of different monoclonal antibodies that bind to lipid A, the reactive portion of endotoxin, suggests that an antilipopolysaccharide immunoglobulin might prove useful in gram-negative bacterial keratitis.

Inhibitors of Inflammatory Mediators. Monoclonal antibodies targeted to soluble and cell-surface glycoproteins such as the selectins, which are involved in leukocyte recruitment, diapedesis, and migration, are currently under development.[430] Topical application of monoclonal antibodies directed at the molecules mediating neutrophil-vascular endothelium interactions might reduce the leukocyte-mediated corneal damage of bacterial keratitis.

Various cytokines such as interferons and colony-stimulating factors are involved in bacterial keratitis. If there were a way to rapidly assess whether certain cytokines were being produced or their genes were being expressed, it might be possible to control their effects. Potential ways to modulate proinflammatory cytokines are reducing their synthesis, inhibiting the converting enzyme that cleaves the procytokine, administering neutralizing antibodies to the cytokine, administering blocking antibodies to their receptors, and flooding the system with receptor antagonists or soluble receptors.

Nonpharmacologic Therapy

Corneal debridement and superficial keratectomy can reduce the bacterial load, but surgical intervention is generally postponed until effective bactericidal therapy has begun. Cryotherapy has a bactericidal effect and may rarely be useful in the management of bacterial sclerokeratitis unresponsive to conventional medical management.[82,113] Topical antimicrobial therapy can be synergistic with corneal freezing. Thermal cauterization has also been used.[210]

Laser pulses applied directly to microbial cultures are bactericidal.[214] Corneal irradiation using the argon,[137] carbon dioxide,[371] or excimer[115] laser has been suggested; but photoablation can cause substantial destruction of host tissues and has limited clinical application at this time.

Techniques to Encourage Reepithelialization

Epithelial ulceration is typically present during the early stages of bacterial keratitis but is not a concern unless the epithelial defect persists beyond the duration of antibacterial therapy. Patching is generally avoided early in the course of treatment for bacterial keratitis but might be considered with a persistent epithelial defect after treatment has been tapered.

Bandage Lens. A continuous-wear soft contact lens or collagen shield can promote epithelial healing by providing structural support and by reducing the erosive actions of eyelid movements on the ocular surface. A therapeutic contact lens or collagen shield is generally preferred to patching because these permit continued, uninterrupted use of topical antibacterial eyedrops.

The use of a contact lens or collagen shield should, however, be carefully assessed in patients with delayed epithelial healing. A drug-soaked soft contact lens or collagen shield can expose the cornea to an excessively high antibiotic level

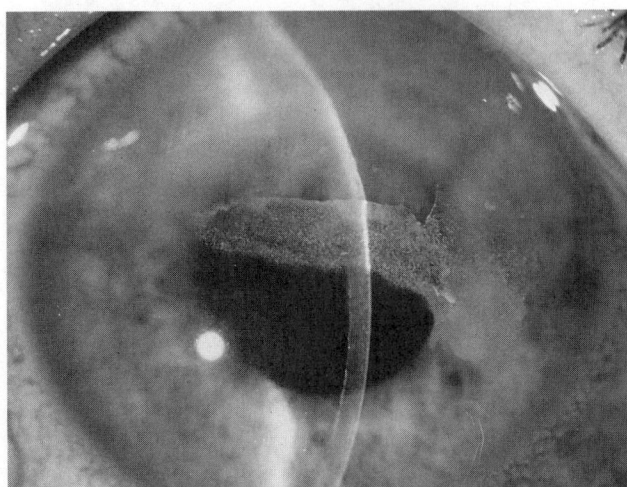

Fig. 74-21. Drug precipitation within superficial cornea during ciprofloxacin therapy.

if the lens or shield is impregnated with a fortified or concentrated eyedrop solution. Also, a soft contact lens or collagen shield permits accumulation of inflammatory and other material that can add to corneal damage. On the other hand, when topical therapy is reduced, a hydrophilic contact lens can help maintain a moist film over an ulcer and minimizes the mechanical irritation of eyelid blinking to promote reepithelialization.

Other Techniques. Epithelial healing can be impaired with persistent stromal inflammation. The judicious use of a topical corticosteroid might aid reepithelialization. Rarely, an elevated island of thickened or inflamed stroma will prevent reepithelialization (Figure 74-22). Superficial keratectomy of tissue above the corneal surface can be therapeutic in these cases.

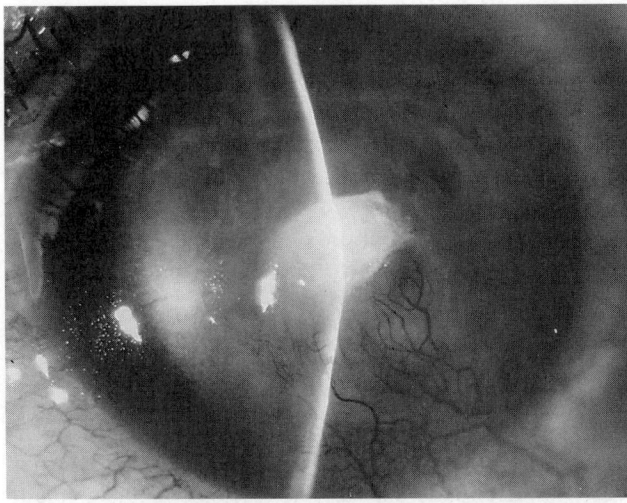

Fig. 74-22. Necrotic stromal outgrowth following treatment of *P. aeruginosa* keratitis, subsequently removed by superficial keratectomy.

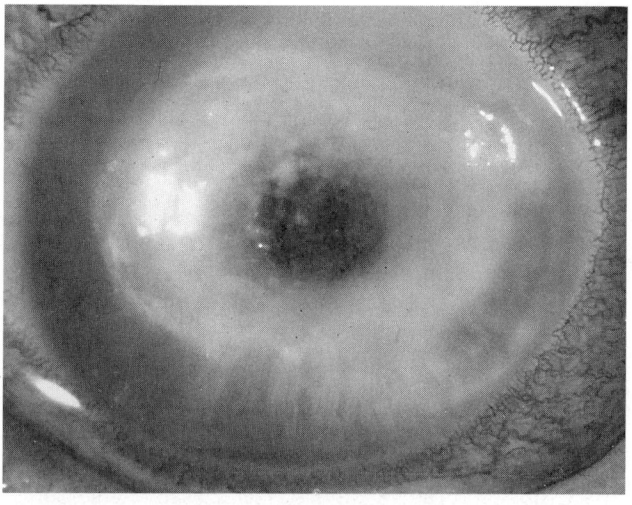

A

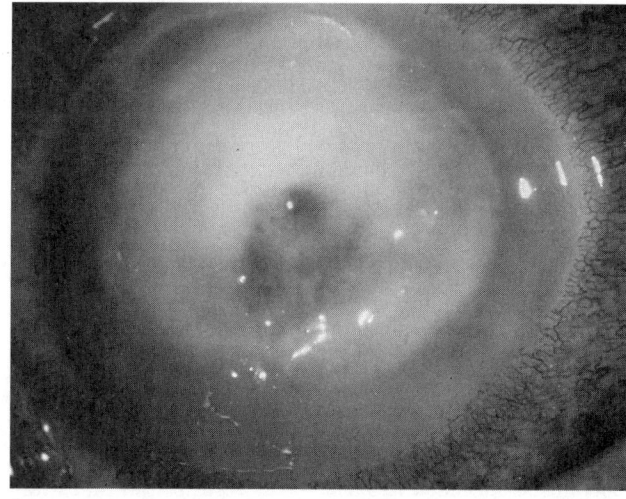

B

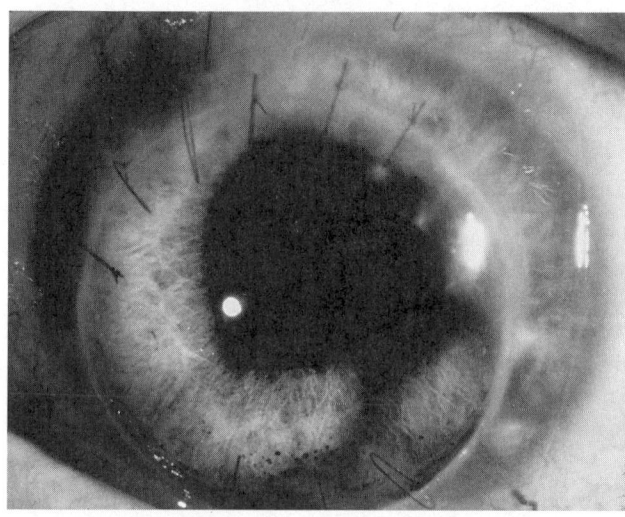

C

Fig. 74-23. Reconstructive keratoplasty following progressive corneal destruction. **A,** Staphylococcal keratitis after corneal trauma. **B,** Progressive corneal thinning with perforation despite 3 weeks of antibacterial therapy. **C,** Tectonic keratoplasty permitted subsequent visual correction.

Various agents, including allantoin, topical fibronectin,[3] and oral tetracycline, have been suggested to speed epithelial healing after bacterial keratitis but are not commonly used.

Surgical Management

Bacterial keratitis is a common cause of corneal perforation.[176] A continuous-wear soft contact lens may help protect an area of stromal ulceration or microperforation from desiccation and the erosive actions of eyelid movements.

Glue. Cyanoacrylate tissue adhesive is useful to provide architectonic reinforcement over an area of corneal thinning or a descemetocele and can seal a small perforation. A bandage soft contact lens is usually applied after the glue has hardened.

Conjunctival Flap. A conjunctival flap can be used for progressive inflammation with corneal thinning[60,193,211] but is an unsatisfactory option for most cases of corneal perforation in bacterial keratitis because of the good chance of an adherent leukoma and secondary glaucoma. Suturing fresh amnion[28] or other mucosal tissue has also been used but is not a recommended alternative.

Keratoplasty. A corneal patch graft can be considered for a small perforation. Dissection should try to get adequate, nonnecrotic borders. Debridement may remove the bulk of bacteria and proteolytic enzymes, but keratectomy risks excising potentially salvageable stroma. Lamellar keratoplasty is generally avoided because residual microorganisms may remain in the deeper cornea.

For necrotic corneal perforations, especially those larger than 2 mm in diameter, penetrating keratoplasty in an inflamed eye (keratoplasty *à chaud*) should be considered.* If possible, surgery is deferred until initial antimicrobial ther-

---

*References 34, 131, 172, 421, 426, 462.

apy has been begun.[226,306] Excisional keratoplasty is considered for progressive stromal inflammation,[86] particularly if limbal or scleral involvement is present.[352] Topical and systemic corticosteroids are sometimes used preoperatively to reduce inflammation. Less than 5% of cases of treated bacterial keratitis require therapeutic keratoplasty to cure the infection,[131] and half of these have concurrent conditions that impair host defenses.[222]

The use of a supportive scleral ring with conjunctival recession or peritomy can be helpful in performing a corneal transplant for bacterial keratitis. A suction or mechanical trephine helps to reduce wound distortion in a perforated eye. Alternatively the surface can be marked with a hand-held trephine, and the incision deepened with a sharp blade.[90] Trephination margins or freehand dissection should encompass the infected zone. Total corneal transplantation may be required to achieve adequate recipient margins.[64,227]

The techniques of reconstructive sclerokeratoplasty[81] and iridoplasty[84] help maintain the anterior-chamber angle. Reforming the anterior chamber before trephination and preparing an accessible sclerotomy site can help prevent unplanned vitreous loss. While corneal perforation can result in an anterior polar cataract, the lens may not need to be extracted because its presence might help minimize extension of suppurative inflammation into the posterior segment. On the other hand, necrotic iris tissue and a ruptured or markedly intumescent lens should be removed. Adequate aqueous flow should be ensured by one or more peripheral iridectomies, lysis of posterior synechiae, and an oversized graft. Interrupted sutures are recommended. The primary goals in these severely diseased eyes are the reestablishment of structural integrity and the elimination of viable microorganisms (Figure 74-23).

The excised corneal button can be cut aseptically in the operating room to submit sections for both histopathologic evaluation and microbiologic assessment. Cultures may also be obtained of aqueous humor or an inflammatory iris membrane if available. Postoperatively, topical antibacterial therapy is generally continued and topical corticosteroids are begun. Intravenous antibiotic administration is considered if endophthalmitis is suspected.

PROGNOSIS

Despite the availability of effective antibiotics that achieve bacteriologic cure, corneal inflammation and structural alteration limit an optimal visual outcome in many cases of bacterial keratitis. Corneal opacification following bacterial keratitis depends upon multiple factors including preexisting corneal conditions, the causative microorganisms,[239] and the extent of involvement. A worse clinical and visual outcome is associated with larger initial infiltrate sizes, especially when caused by *Pseudomonas* spp. Antibacterial and corticosteroid therapy seek to minimize permanent corneal scarring. Whether antibiotic selection or concentration,[411] corticosteroid use, or other treatment factors affect outcome has not yet been determined.

Approximately one third of treated patients subsequently improve to a visual acuity of 20/40 or better, one third have vision between 20/40 and 20/200, and about one third have visual loss of 20/200 or worse. The most common reasons for visual disability are stromal scarring and irregular astigmatism. Corneal infections in both eyes, such as those related to dry-eye syndromes and contact lens wear,[465] can lead to severe visual loss.

Cicatrization frequently leaves a slightly depressed facet that can fill in with a thickened epithelial layer. Calcific

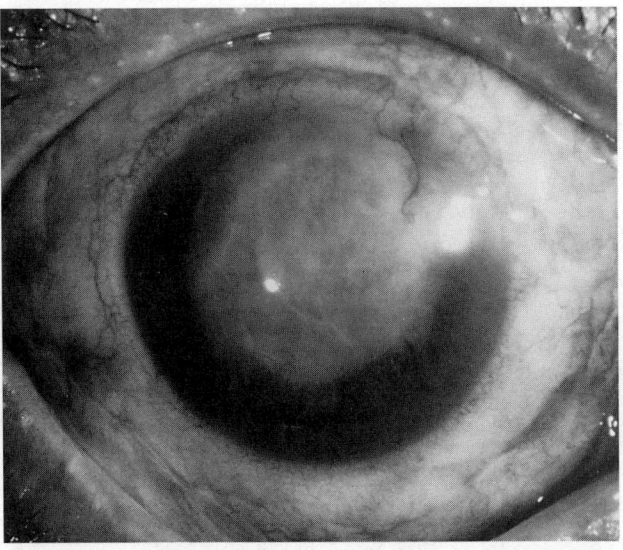

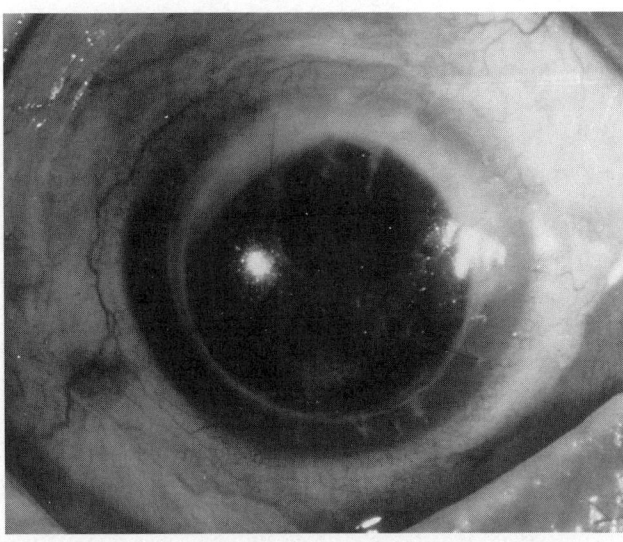

A   B

Fig. 74-24.   Optical keratoplasty for postbacterial corneal opacification. **A,** Residual corneal scar following treatment of *P. aeruginosa* keratitis. **B,** Corneal transplant after suture removal.

deposition and corneal neovascularization occurs with chronic inflammation. Gradual improvement in corneal clarity sometimes occurs after several months, perhaps more often in children.

A contact lens may improve vision in some patients with irregular astigmatism. If residual scarring with impaired vision persists, optical corneal transplantation can be electively considered (Figure 74-24). Of all corneal transplants performed in the United States each year, 0.5% to 1% are in patients with corneal changes occurring because of bacterial keratitis.

Approximately 70% of therapeutic grafts performed for bacterial keratitis remain clear.[131,172,222] Success is better when the graft diameter is 9 mm or less.[222] About half of those with a clear graft recover vision of 20/60 or better. The causes of visual loss include various postinflammatory and postoperative conditions, such as iris synechiae with secondary glaucoma, pupillary membrane, cataract, macular edema, and retinal detachment. Up to one half will develop allograft rejection.

PREVENTION

In many parts of the world bacterial keratitis is a leading cause of corneal blindness. Further advances in the outcome of bacterial keratitis will not come from better antibiotics but from improved methods of drug delivery and from new therapeutic approaches based on an understanding of disease mechanisms. Equally important is the development of preventive strategies that can reduce opportunities predisposing to corneal infection.

Bacterial keratitis can be prevented by recognizing and minimizing potential risk factors. Because the pathogenesis of bacterial keratitis involves the parallel factors of both a suitable portal of entry and the presence of bacteria at the corneal surface, strategies are feasible to reduce or avoid these occurrences.

Any common-sense advice that prevents a corneal epithelial defect can avoid the risk of bacterial keratitis. Practical suggestions are tailored to individual risk factors:

- Protective eyewear is recommended in the primary prevention of industrial and agricultural eye injuries.
- Factors that lead to recurrent or persistent epithelial erosions should be avoided if possible.
- Dry-eye syndromes and causes of corneal exposure ought to be managed properly, particularly in comatose patients.
- Topical anesthetics must not be provided to patients for repeated use.
- No contaminated instruments or materials should be allowed to touch the corneal surface.

Contact lens fitting must ensure a proper fit with adequate lens movement that curtails corneal touch and tear-film stagnation. Keeping the contact lens storage case clean has an important protective benefit in avoiding ulcerative keratitis.[377] Care must be taken to use sterile solutions; homemade saline using tap or distilled water should not be used as a contact lens rinse except before heat disinfection. A daily-wear schedule is recommended for most contact lens patients.[465] Extended-wear lenses should be removed at least every week for cleaning and disinfection. Patients fitted with a therapeutic contact lens must be frequently and carefully followed until reepithelialization has occurred and the lens removed. Recommendations regarding contact lens disinfection and insertion need to be followed scrupulously.

In a similar way, care should be taken to avoid contamination of topical ophthalmic agents and their containers. Microorganisms are frequently introduced inadvertently into ocular medications during use,[378] and this problem is potentially influenced by eyedropper bottle design.[79] Unit-dose containers are available for some commonly used ophthalmic agents.[223] The development of a practical microbial detection kit would enable regular monitoring of contamination of solutions and contact lenses.

The use of prophylactic antibiotics to prevent bacterial keratitis remains controversial. There is no consensus on the use or selection of prophylactic topical antimicrobial agents in herpetic keratitis,[45,469] during contact lens wear,[76] with tear deficiency states,[315] after chemical injuries, following nonpenetrating corneal trauma, or following corneal transplantation.[216] Prolonged delay after exogenous contamination could affect clinical efficacy. Some agents are competitive inhibitors of tear lysozyme and could impair one of the cornea's natural defenses.[392] Microbial keratitis has occurred despite the use of prophylactic antibiotics in these conditions.

Passive[299] and active[174,234] systemic immunization provides partial protection against experimental bacterial keratitis. Human vaccination might be feasible[135] and is actively being assessed in veterinary practice to prevent *Moraxella bovis* keratoconjunctivitis in cattle. Whether people vaccinated against pneumococci, *H. influenzae,* or other bacteria are protected against eye infections by these organisms has not been determined. Topical administration of specific antibodies might have a preventive or therapeutic role.[213] Similarly, lectins that mask corneal surface glycoconjugates show promise in experimental studies,[42] but their prophylactic use is limited by the multiple ways bacteria attach to the cornea.[348] These and other strategies for blocking bacterial adhesion or invasion are under investigation.[341a]

By identifying specific risk factors and designing preventive measures, the risk of corneal infection can potentially be reduced. Better understanding of the pathogenesis of bacterial keratitis will lead to innovative opportunities for prophylaxis and management in the control of this common eye disease.

REFERENCES

1. Abraham EP, Chain E, Fletcher CM et al.: Further observations on penicillin, *Lancet* 2:177-188, 1941.
2. Adair FW, Liauw HL, Geftic SG, Gelzer J: Reduced virulence of *Pseudomonas aeruginosa* grown in the presence of benzalkonium chloride, *J Clin Microbiol* 1:175-179, 1975.
3. Adamova NA, Gorgiladze TU, Artemov AV: Effektivnost' lecheniia iazvennykh porazhenii rogovitsy fibronektinom, *Oftalmol Zh* 4:245-248, 1990.
4. Alfonso EC, Miller D: Detection of ocular infections. In Prior RB, editor: *Clinical applications of the limulus amoebocyte lysate test,* 121-133, Boca Raton, Fla, 1990, CRC Press.
4a. Alió JL, Artola A, Serra A et al.: Effect of topical antioxidant therapy on experimental infectious keratitis, *Cornea* 14:175-179, 1995.
5. Algan M, George JL, Lion C et al.: Abces de cornée à *Pasteurella* consecutif à un traumatisme par griffe de chat, *Bull Soc Ophtalmol Fr* 89:581-583, 1989.
6. Al'Hazzaa SAF, Tabbara KF: Bacterial keratitis after penetrating keratoplasty, *Ophthalmology* 95:1504-1508, 1988.
7. Al-Samarrai AR, Sunba MSN: Bacterial corneal ulcers among Arabs in Kuwait, *Ophthalmic Res* 21:278-284, 1989.
8. Ammous MW, Noor Sunba MS: The nature of ulcerative keratitis in Kuwait (clinical and microbiological study), *APMIS Suppl* 3:104-106, 1988.
9. Anderson EL, Stager D, Levin DL: *Pseudomonas aeruginosa* corneal infections in seriously ill children, *Clin Pediatr* 21:123-124, 1982.
10. Ando E, Ando Y, Inoue M et al.: Inhibition of corneal inflammation by an acylated superoxide dismutase derivative, *Invest Ophthalmol Vis Sci* 31:1963-1967, 1990.
11. Aristimuño B, Nirankari VS, Hemady RK, Rodrigues MM: Spontaneous ulcerative keratitis in immunocompromised patients, *Am J Ophthalmol* 115:202-208, 1993.
12. Aronson SB, Moore TE Jr: Corticosteroid therapy in central stromal keratitis, *Am J Ophthalmol* 67:873-896, 1969.
13. Asbell P, Stenson S: Ulcerative keratitis: survey of thirty years' laboratory experience, *Arch Ophthalmol* 100:77-83, 1982.
14. Assil KK, Zarnegar SR, Fouraker BD, Schanzlin DJ: Efficacy of tobramycin-soaked collagen shields vs tobramycin eyedrop loading dose for sustained treatment of experimental *Pseudomonas aeruginosa*-induced keratitis in rabbits, *Am J Ophthalmol* 113:418-423, 1992.
15. Aswad MI, John T, Barza M et al.: Bacterial adherence to extended wear soft contact lenses, *Ophthalmology* 97:296-302, 1990.
16. Awan KJ: Mydriasis and conjunctival paresthesia from local gentamicin, *Am J Ophthalmol* 99:723-724, 1985.
17. Axenfeld T: *The bacteriology of the eye,* New York, 1908, William Wood (Translated by A MacNab).
18. Babushkin AE, Gimranov RM: Povrezhdenie rogovitsy zhalom pchely, oslozhnennoe prisoedineniem sinegnoinoi i gerpesvirusnoi infektsii, *Vestn Oftalmol* 106(5):65, 1990.
19. Badenoch PR, Coster DJ: Antimicrobial activity of topical anaesthetic preparations, *Br J Ophthalmol* 66:364-367, 1982.
20. Badenoch PR, Hay GJ, McDonald PJ, Coster DJ: A rat model of bacterial keratitis: effect of antibiotics and corticosteroid, *Arch Ophthalmol* 103:718-722, 1985.
21. Barlati S, Marchina E, Quaranta CA et al.: Analysis of fibronectin, plasminogen activators and plasminogen in tear fluid as markers of corneal damage and repair, *Exp Eye Res* 51:1-9, 1990.
22. Barquet N, Gasser I, Domingo P et al.: Primary meningococcal conjunctivitis: report of 21 patients and review, *Rev Infect Dis* 12:838-847, 1990.
23. Barth G: Animal models of bacterial corneal ulcers. In Tabbara KF, Cello RM, editors: *Animal models of ocular diseases,* 129-135, Springfield, Ill, 1984, Charles C Thomas.
24. Barza M, Ernst C, Baum J, Weinstein L: Effect of lidocaine on the antibacterial activity of seven antibiotics, *Arch Ophthalmol* 92:514-515, 1974.
25. Barza M, Kane A, Baum J: Regional differences in ocular concentration of gentamicin after subconjunctival and retrobulbar injection in the rabbit, *Am J Ophthalmol* 83:407-413, 1977.
26. Bates AK, Kirkness CM, Ficker LA et al.: Microbial keratitis after penetrating keratoplasty, *Eye* 4:74-78, 1990.
27. Bates AK, Morris RJ, Stapleton F et al.: 'Sterile' corneal infiltrates in contact lens wearers, *Eye* 3:803-810, 1989.
28. Batmanov IuE, Egorova KS, Kolesnikova LN: Primenemie svezhego amniona v lechenii zabolevanii rogovitsy, *Vestn Oftalmol* 106(5):17-19, 1990.
29. Baum J: Treatment of bacterial ulcers of the cornea in the rabbit: a comparison of administration by eye drops and subconjunctival injections, *Trans Am Ophthalmol Soc* 80:369-390, 1982.
30. Baum J: Therapy for ocular bacterial infection, *Trans Ophthalmol Soc UK* 105:69-77, 1986.
31. Baum JL: Initial therapy of suspected microbial corneal ulcers. I. Broad antibiotic therapy based on prevalence of organisms, *Surv Ophthalmol* 24:97-105, 1979.
32. Baum J, Barza M: Topical vs subconjunctival treatment of bacterial corneal ulcers, *Ophthalmology* 90:162-168, 1983.
33. Baum J, Fedukowicz HB, Jordan A: A survey of *Moraxella* corneal ulcers in a derelict population, *Am J Ophthalmol* 90:476-480, 1980.
34. Behrens-Baumann W: Ergebnisse der Keratoplastik à chaud, *Klin Monatsbl Augenheilkd* 185:25-27, 1984.
35. Belmont JB, Ostler HB, Dawson CR et al.: Noninfectious ring-shaped keratitis associated with *Pseudomonas aeruginosa,* *Am J Ophthalmol* 93:338-341, 1982.
36. Benson WH, Lanier JD: Comparison of techniques for culturing corneal ulcers, *Ophthalmology* 99:800-804, 1992.
37. Berk RS, Montgomery IN, Hazlett LD: Serum antibody and ocular responses to murine corneal infection caused by *Pseudomonas aeruginosa,* *Infect Immun* 56:3076-3080, 1988.
38. Berk RS, Montgomery IN, Hazlett LD, Abel EL: Paternal alcohol consumption: effects on ocular response and serum antibody response to *Pseudomonas aeruginosa* infection in offspring, *Alcohol Clin Exp Res* 13:795-798, 1989.
39. Berman M: Regulation of collagenase: therapeutic considerations, *Trans Ophthalmol Soc UK* 98:397-405, 1978.
40. Berman M, Manseau E, Law M, Aiken D: Ulceration is correlated with degradation of fibrin and fibrinectin at the corneal surface, *Invest Ophthalmol Vis Sci* 24:1358-1366, 1983.
41. Billings FS: Keratitis contagiosa in cattle, *Buffalo M & S J* 28:499-504, 1888-1889.
42. Blaylock WK, Yue BY, Robin JB: The use of concanavalin A to competitively inhibit *Pseudomonas aeruginosa* adherence to rabbit corneal epithelium, *CLAO J* 16:223-227, 1990.
43. Bloomfield SE, Miyata T, Dunn MW et al.: Soluble gentamicin ophthalmic insert as a drug delivery system, *Arch Ophthalmol* 96:885-887, 1978.
44. Boerner CF: Allergic response to a porcine collagen corneal shield, *Arch Ophthalmol* 106:171, 1988.
45. Boisjoly HM, Pavan-Langston D, Kenyon KR, Baker AS: Superinfections in herpes simplex keratitis, *Am J Ophthalmol* 96:354-361, 1983.
46. Bowden FW III, Cohen EJ, Arentsen JJ, Laibson PR: Patterns of lens care practices and lens product contamination in contact lens associated microbial keratitis, *CLAO J* 15:49-54, 1989.
47. Bowden HH, Sutphin JE: Nosocomial *Pseudomonas* keratitis in a critical-care nurse, *Am J Ophthalmol* 101:612-613, 1986.
48. Bowe BE, Snyder JW, Eiferman RA: An in vitro study of the potency and stability of fortified ophthalmic antibiotic preparations, *Am J Ophthalmol* 111:686-689, 1991.
49. Briggs WE: Sub-conjunctival injections in the treatment of eye diseases, *JAMA* 23:407-408, 1894.
50. Bucci FA Jr, Holland EJ: *Flavobacterium meningosepticum* keratitis successfully treated with topical trimethoprim-sulfamethoxazole, *Am J Ophthalmol* 111:116-118, 1991.
51. Bueche MJ et al.: The incidence of contamination in fortified ophthalmic antibiotics, *Cornea* (in press).
52. Buehler PO, Schein OD, Stamler JF et al.: The increased risk of ulcerative keratitis among disposable soft contact lens users, *Arch Ophthalmol* 110:1555-1558, 1992.
52a. Bukanov N, Ravi VN, Miller D et al.: *Pseudomonas aeruginosa* corneal ulcer isolates distinguished using the arbitrarily primed PCR DNA fingerprinting method, *Curr Eye Res* 13:783-790, 1994.
53. Burnette WC, Foos RY: Infectious crystalline keratopathy in a neonatal infant, *Cornea* 9:108-114, 1990.

54. Burns FR, Paterson CA, Gray RD, Wells JT: Inhibition of *Pseudomonas aeruginosa* elastase and *Pseudomonas* keratitis using a thiol-based peptide, *Antimicrob Agents Chemother* 34:2065-2069, 1990.

55. Burns RP: *Pseudomonas aeruginosa* keratitis: mixed infections of the eye, *Am J Ophthalmol* 67:257-262, 1969.

56. Burris TE, Newsom DI, Rowsey JJ: Hessburg subpalpebral antibiotic lavage of *Pseudomonas* corneal and corneoscleral ulcers, *Cornea* 1:347-355, 1982.

57. Busin M, Spitznas M: Sustained gentamicin release by presoaked medicated bandage contact lenses, *Ophthalmology* 95:796-798, 1988.

58. Butrus SI, Klotz SA: Contact lens surface deposits increase the adhesion of *Pseudomonas aeruginosa, Curr Eye Res* 9:717-724, 1990.

59. Butrus SI, Klotz SA, Misra RP: The adherence of *Pseudomonas aeruginosa* to soft contact lenses, *Ophthalmology* 94:1310-1314, 1987.

60. Buxton JN, Fox ML: Conjunctival flaps in the treatment of refractory *Pseudomonas* corneal abscess, *Ann Ophthalmol* 18:315-318, 1986.

61. Callahan MA, Kimura SJ: Slit beam ruler, *Am J Ophthalmol* 81:851-853, 1976.

62. Carmichael TR, Gelfand Y, Welsh NH: Topical steroids in the treatment of central and paracentral corneal ulcers, *Br J Ophthalmol* 74:528-531, 1990.

63. Carmichael TR, Wolpert M, Koornhof HJ: Corneal ulceration at an urban African hospital, *Br J Ophthalmol* 69:920-926, 1985.

63a. Carta F, Pinna A, Zanetti S et al.: Corneal ulcer caused by *Aeromonas* species, *Am J Ophthalmol* 118:530-531, 1994.

64. Cavanagh HD, Jones DB: Complications of penetrating keratoplasty: therapeutic keratoplasty. In *Cornea, refractive surgery and contact lens: transactions of the New Orleans Academy of Ophthalmology,* 251-258, New York, 1987, Raven Press.

65. Cavanagh HD, Leveille AS: Extended-wear contact lenses in patients with corneal grafts and aphakia, *Ophthalmology* 89:643-650, 1982.

66. Cavanaugh TB, Gottsch JD: Infectious keratitis and cyanoacrylate adhesive, *Am J Ophthalmol* 111:466-472, 1991.

67. Chambers WA, Belin MW, Parenti DM, Simon GL: Corneal ulcers in house staff: are risk factors identifiable? *Ann Ophthalmol* 20:172-175, 1988.

68. Chandler JW, Milam DF: Diphtheria corneal ulcers, *Arch Ophthalmol* 96:53-56, 1978.

69. Characklis WG, Marshall KC: *Biofilms,* New York, 1990, Wiley Interscience.

69a. Charteris DG, Batterbury M, Armstrong M, Tullo AB: Suppurative keratitis caused by *Streptococcus pneumoniae* after cataract surgery, *Br J Ophthalmol* 78:847-849, 1994.

70. Chew S-J, Beuerman RW, Assouline M et al.: Early diagnosis of infectious keratitis with in vivo real time confocal microscopy, *CLAO J* 18:197-201, 1992.

71. Chirambo MC, Tielsch JM, Jr West KP et al.: Blindness and visual impairment in southern Malawi, *Bull World Health Organ* 64:567-572, 1986.

72. Choi TB, Lee DA: Transscleral and transcorneal iontophoresis of vancomycin in rabbit eyes, *J Ocul Pharmacol* 4:153-164, 1988.

73. Chumbley LC, Thompson IM: Epidemiology of trachoma in the West Bank and Gaza Strip, *Eye* 2:463-470, 1988.

74. Chusid MJ, Davis SD: Polymorphonuclear leukocyte kinetics in experimentally induced keratitis, *Arch Ophthalmol* 103:270-274, 1985.

75. Chusid MJ, Nelson DB, Meyer LA: The role of the polymorphonuclear leukocyte in the induction of corneal edema, *Invest Ophthalmol Vis Sci* 27:1466-1469, 1986.

76. Clemons CS, Cohen EJ, Arentsen JJ et al.: *Pseudomonas* ulcers following patching of corneal abrasions associated with contact lens wear, *CLAO J* 13:161-164, 1987.

77. Clinch TE, Hobden JA, Hill JM et al.: Collagen shields containing tobramycin for sustained therapy (24 hours) of experimental *Pseudomonas* keratitis, *CLAO J* 18:245-247, 1992.

78. Clinch TE, Palmon FE, Robinson MJ et al.: Microbial keratitis in children, *Am J Ophthalmol* 117:65-71, 1994.

79. Coad CT, Osato MS, Wilhelmus KR: Bacterial contamination of eyedrop dispensers, *Am J Ophthalmol* 98:548-551, 1984.

80. Cobo LM, Coster DJ, Peacock J: *Moraxella* keratitis in a nonalcoholic population, *Br J Ophthalmol* 65:683-686, 1981.

81. Cobo M, Ortiz JR, Sanfran SG: Sclerokeratoplasty with maintenance of the angle, *Am J Ophthalmol* 113:533-537, 1992.

82. Codere F, Brownstein S, Jackson B: *Pseudomonas aeruginosa* scleritis, *Am J Ophthalmol* 91:706-710, 1981.

83. Cohen EJ, Gonzalez C, Leavitt KG et al.: Corneal ulcers associated with contact lenses including experience with disposable lenses, *CLAO J* 17:173-176, 1991.

84. Cohen EJ, Kenyon KR, Dohlman CH: Iridoplasty for prevention of post-keratoplasty angle closure and glaucomas, *Ophthalmic Surg* 13:994-996, 1982.

85. Cohn H, Mondino BJ, Brown SI, Hall GD: Marginal corneal ulcers with acute beta streptococcal conjunctivitis and chronic dacryocystitis, *Am J Ophthalmol* 87:541-543, 1979.

86. Cooper RL, Constable IJ: Draining pus from the cornea, *Aust J Ophthalmol* 11:287-294, 1983.

87. Coster DJ: Management of suppurative keratitis, *Trans Ophthalmol Soc NZ* 34:59-63, 1982.

88. Coster DJ, Bodenoch PR: Host, microbial, and pharmacological factors affecting the outcome of suppurative keratitis, *Br J Ophthalmol* 71:96-101, 1987.

89. Cottingham AJ, Berkeley RG, Nordan LT et al.: *Bacterial corneal ulcers following keratorefractive surgery: a retrospective study of 14,163 procedures,* Ocular Microbiology and Immunology Group meeting, San Francisco, 1986.

90. Cowden JW, Copeland RA Jr, Schneider MS: Large diameter therapeutic penetrating keratoplasties, *Refract Corneal Surg* 5:244-248, 1989.

91. Cruz OA, Sabir SM, Capo H, Alfonso EC: Microbial keratitis in childhood, *Ophthalmology* 100:192-196, 1993.

92. Cutarelli PE, Lass JH, Lazarus HM et al.: Topical fluoroquinolones: antimicrobial activity and in vitro corneal epithelial toxicity, *Curr Eye Res* 10:557-563, 1991.

93. Dart JKG: Predisposing factors in microbial keratitis: the significance of contact lens wear, *Br J Ophthalmol* 72:926-930, 1988.

94. Dart JKG: Disease and risks associated with contact lenses, *Br J Ophthalmol* 77:49-53, 1993.

95. Dart JKG, Seal DV: Pathogenesis and therapy of *Pseudomonas aeruginosa* keratitis, *Eye* 2(suppl):S46-S55, 1988.

96. Dart JKG, Stapleton F, Minassian D: Contact lenses and other risk factors in microbial keratitis, *Lancet* 338:650-653, 1991.

97. Davis SD, Sarff LD, Hyndiuk RA: Antibiotic therapy of experimental *Pseudomonas* keratitis in guinea pigs, *Arch Ophthalmol* 95:1638-1643, 1977.

98. Davis SD, Sarff LD, Hyndiuk RA: Bacteriologic cure of experimental *Pseudomonas* keratitis, *Invest Ophthalmol Vis Sci* 17:916-918, 1978.

99. Davis SD, Sarff LD, Hyndiuk RA: Corticosteroid in experimentally induced *Pseudomonas* keratitis: failure of prednisolone to impair the efficacy of tobramycin and carbenicillin therapy, *Arch Ophthalmol* 96:126-128, 1978.

100. Davis SD, Sarff LD, Hyndiuk RA: Therapeutic effect of topical antibiotic on untreated eye in experimental keratitis, *Can J Ophthalmol* 13:273-276, 1978.

101. Davis SD, Sarff LD, Hyndiuk RA: Comparison of therapeutic routes in experimental *Pseudomonas* keratitis, *Am J Ophthalmol* 87:710-716, 1979.

102. Davison CR, Tuft SJ, Dart JKG: Conjunctival necrosis after administration of topical fortified aminoglycosides, *Am J Ophthalmol* 111:690-693, 1991.

103. DeBroff BM, Donahue SP, Caputo BJ et al.: Clinical characteristics of corneal foreign bodies and their associated culture results, *Cornea* 20:128-130, 1994.

104. DeCarlo JD, Van Horn DL, Hyndiuk RA, Davis SD: Increased susceptibility to infection in experimental xerophthalmia, *Arch Ophthalmol* 99:1614-1617, 1981.

105. Derick RJ, Kelley CG, Gersman M: Contact lens related corneal ulcers at the Ohio State University Hospitals 1983-1987, *CLAO J* 15:268-270, 1989.

106. de Smet MD, Chan CC, Nussenblatt RB, Palestine AG: *Capnocytophaga canimorsus* as the cause of a chronic corneal infection, *Am J Ophthalmol* 109:240-242, 1990.

107. DiBisceglie AM, Carmichael TR: Factors predisposing to central corneal ulceration in a developing population, *S Afr Med J* 71(12):769-770, 1987.

108. Dixon JM, Young CA Jr, Baldone JA et al.: Complications associated with the wearing of contact lenses, *JAMA* 195:901-903, 1966.

109. Dohlman CH, Zucker BB: Long-term treatment with idoxuridine and steroids: a complication in herpetic keratitis, *Arch Ophthalmol* 74:172-174, 1965.

110. Donaldson DD: *Atlas of external diseases of the eye,* vol 3, *Cornea and sclera,* ed 2, St Louis, 1980, Mosby.

111. Donzis PB, Mondino BJ, Weissman BA: *Bacillus* keratitis associated with contaminated contact lens care systems, *Am J Ophthalmol* 105:195-197, 1988.

112. Driebe WT Jr, Stern GA: Microbial keratitis following corneal transplantation, *Cornea* 2:41-45, 1983.

113. Eiferman RA: Cryotherapy of *Pseudomonas* keratitis and scleritis, *Arch Ophthalmol* 97:1637-1639, 1979.

114. Eiferman RA, Flaherty KT, Rivard AK: Persistent corneal defect caused by *Listeria monocytogenes, Am J Ophthalmol* 109:97-98, 1990.

115. Eiferman RA, Forgey DR, Cook YD: Excimer laser ablation of infectious crystalline keratopathy, *Arch Ophthalmol* 110:18, 1992.

116. Eiferman RA, Levartovsky S, Box JD: Anaerobic *Capnocytophaga* corneal ulcer, *Am J Ophthalmol* 105:427, 1988.

117. Eiferman RA, Ogden LL, Snyder J: Anaerobic peptostreptococcal keratitis, *Am J Ophthalmol* 100:335-336, 1985.

118. Eiferman RA, Snyder JW: Antibacterial effect of cyanoacrylate glue, *Arch Ophthalmol* 101:958-960, 1983.

119. Elander TR, Goldberg MA, Salinger CL et al.: Microbial changes in the ocular environment with contact lens wear, *CLAO J* 18:53-55, 1992.

120. Erie JC, Nevitt MP, Hodge DO, Ballard DJ: Incidence of ulcerative keratitis in a defined population from 1950 through 1988, *Arch Ophthalmol* 111:1665-1671, 1993.

121. Fahmy JA, Moller S, Bentzon MW: Bacterial flora of the normal conjunctiva. II. Methods of obtaining cultures, *Acta Ophthalmol* 53:237-253, 1975.

122. Feaster FT, Nisbet RM, Barber JC: *Aeromonas hydrophila* corneal ulcer, *Am J Ophthalmol* 85:114-117, 1978.

123. Fedukowicz HB, Stenson S: *External infections of the eye: bacterial, viral, mycotic with noninfectious and immunologic diseases,* ed 3, 17-81, Norwalk, Conn, 1985, Appleton-Century-Crofts.

124. Feist RM, Sugar J, Tessler H: Radial keratoneuritis in *Pseudomonas* keratitis, *Arch Ophthalmol* 109:774-775, 1991.

125. Feng CM: The causes of blindness by corneal diseases in 3,499 cases, *Chung Hua Yen Ko Tsa Chih* 26:151-153, 1990.

126. Fiscella R, Noth J: *Achromobacter xylosoxidans* corneal ulcer in a therapeutic soft contact lens wearer, *Cornea* 8:267-269, 1989.

127. Fleischer AB, Hoover DL, Khan JA et al.: Topical vancomycin formulation for methicillin-resistant *Staphylococcus epidermidis* blepharoconjunctivitis, *Am J Ophthalmol* 101:283-287, 1986.

128. Fleiszig SMJ, Efron N: Microbial flora in eyes of current and former contact lens wearers, *J Clin Microbiol* 30:1156-1161, 1992.

129. Fleiszig SMJ, Efron N, Pier GB: Extended contact lens wear enhances *Pseudomonas aeruginosa* adherence to human corneal epithelium, *Invest Ophthalmol Vis Sci* 33:2908-2916, 1992.

130. Fong LP, Ormerod LD, Kenyon KR, Foster CS: Microbial keratitis complicating penetrating keratoplasty, *Ophthalmology* 95:1269-1275, 1988.

130a. Font RL, Jay V, Misra RP et al.: *Capnocytophaga* keratitis. A clinicopathologic study of three patients, including electron microscopic observations, *Ophthalmology* 101:1929-1934, 1994.

131. Forster RK: The role of excisional keratoplasty in microbial keratitis. In Cavanagh HD, editor: *The cornea: transactions of the World Congress on the Cornea III,* 529-533, New York, 1988, Raven Press.

132. Francois J: Collagenase and collagenase inhibitors, *Trans Am Ophthalmol Soc* 75:285-315, 1977.

133. Fraser-Smith EB, Matthews TR: Effect of ketorolac on *Pseudomonas aeruginosa* ocular infection in rabbits, *J Ocul Pharmacol* 4:101-109, 1988.

134. Friedberg ML, Pleyer U, Mondino BJ: Device drug delivery to the eye. Collagen shields, iontophoresis, and pumps, *Ophthalmology* 98:725-732, 1991.

135. Friedman MG: Antibodies in human tears during and after infection, *Surv Ophthalmol* 35:151-157, 1990.

136. Friendlaender MH: Corneal biopsy, *Int Ophthalmol Clin* 28:101-102, 1988.

137. Fromer C, L'Esperance F: Argon laser phototherapy of *Pseudomonas* corneal ulcers, *Invest Ophthalmol Vis Sci* 10:1-8, 1971.

138. Fuchs E: (Translated by A Duane) *Text-book of ophthalmology,* ed 2, New York, 1892, D Appleton. (Republished by Classics of Ophthalmology Library, Birmingham, Ala, 1988, Gryphon Editions.)

138a. Galardy RE, Cassabonne ME, Giese C et al.: Low molecular weight inhibitors in corneal ulceration, *Ann NY Acad Sci* 732:315-323, 1994.

139. Garcia-Olivares E, Carreras B, Gallardo JM: Presence of Langerhans cells in the cornea of *Klebsiella* keratoconjunctivitis mice, *Invest Ophthalmol Vis Sci* 29:108-111, 1988.

140. Gasparrini E: Il diplococco di Frankel in patologia oculare: studio sperimentale e clinico, *Ann Ottol* 22:131-134, 1893.

141. Gelender H, Rettich C: Gentamicin-resistant *Pseudomonas aeruginosa* corneal ulcers, *Cornea* 3:21-26, 1984.

141a. Ghabrial R, Climent A, Cevallos VE, Ostler HB: Laboratory results of corneal scrapings in microbial keratitis, *Ann Ophthalmol* 27:40-45, 1995.

142. Gilbert ML, Wilhelmus KR, Osato MS: Intracanalicular collagen implants enhance topical antibiotic bioavailability, *Cornea* 5:167-171, 1986.

143. Glasser DB, Gardner S, Ellis JG, Pettit TH: Loading doses and extended dosing intervals in topical gentamicin therapy, *Am J Ophthalmol* 99:329-332, 1985.

144. Glynn RJ, Schein OD, Seddon JM et al.: The incidence of ulcerative keratitis among aphakic contact lens wearers in New England, *Arch Ophthalmol* 109:104-107, 1991.

145. Goodman DF, Gottsch JD: Methicillin-resistant *Staphylococcus epidermidis* keratitis treated with vancomycin, *Arch Ophthalmol* 106:1570-1571, 1988.

146. Goodman DF, Gottsch JD, Smith PW et al.: Lamellar keratectomy and repeat epikeratoplasty following failed epikeratoplasty: a clinicopathologic report, *Cornea* 8:295-298, 1989.

147. Goosey JD, Mosteller MW, Kaufman HE: Radiating folds in Descemet's membrane as a sign of impending corneal perforation, *Am J Ophthalmol* 98:625-686, 1984.

148. Gradle H: *Bacteria and the germ theory of disease,* Chicago, 1883, WT Keener.

149. Grassus B: *De oculis eorumque egritudinibus et curis,* Ferrara, 1474, Severinus. (Republished by Classics of Ophthalmology Library, Birmingham, Ala, 1985, Gryphon Editions.)

149a. Gray RD, Paterson CA: Application of peptide-based matrix metalloproteinase inhibitors in corneal ulceration, *Ann NY Acad Sci* 732:206-216, 1994.

150. Gritz DC, Lee TY, Kwitko S, McDonnell PJ: Topical anti-inflammatory agents in an animal model of microbial keratitis, *Arch Ophthalmol* 108:1001-1005, 1990.

151. Groden LR, Brinser JH: Outpatient treatment of microbial corneal ulcers, *Arch Ophthalmol* 104:84-86, 1986.

152. Groden LR, Rodnite J, Brinser JH, Genvert GI: Acridine orange and gram stains in infectious keratitis, *Cornea* 9:122-124, 1990.

153. Gross ND, Meyer RF: *Enterobacter cloacae* ulceration in a failed corneal graft: a case report, *Br J Ophthalmol* 69:542-544, 1985.

154. Gudmundsson OG, Ormerod LD, Kenyon KR et al.: Factors influencing predilection and outcome in bacterial keratitis, *Cornea* 8:115-121, 1989.

155. Guillemeau J (Trans by AH): *A worthy treatise of the eyes: contayning the knowledge and cure of one hundreth and thirteen diseases—incident unto them,* London, 1577, R Waldegraue. (Republished by Classics of Ophthalmology Library, Birmingham, Ala, 1989, Gryphon Editions.)

156. Haldimann R, Konig H: Ulcus corneae durch *Mima polymorpha, Ophthalmologica* 161:98-103, 1970.

157. Harbin T: Recurrence of a corneal *Pseudomonas* infection after topical steroid therapy: report of a case, *Am J Ophthalmol* 58:670-674, 1964.

158. Harris DJ Jr, Stulting RD, Waring GO III, Wilson LA: Late bacterial and fungal keratitis after corneal transplantation: spectrum of pathogens, graft survival, and visual prognosis, *Ophthalmology* 95:1450-1457, 1988.

159. Harrison SM: A new diagnostic unit for corneal ulcers, *Ann Ophthalmol* 7:677-684, 1975.

160. Harrison SM: Grading corneal ulcers, *Ann Ophthalmol* 7:537-542, 1975.

161. Hazlett LD, Berk RS, Iglewski BH: Microscopic characterization of ocular damage produced by *Pseudomonas aeruginosa* toxin A, *Infect Immun* 34:1025-1035, 1981.

162. Hazlett LD, Iglewski BH, Berk RS: Experimental *Pseudomonas* exotoxin A mediated ocular damage in mouse pups: microscopic observations, *Ophthalmic Res* 14:401-408, 1982.

163. Hazlett LD, Kreindler FB, Berk RS, Barrett R: Aging alters the phagocytic capability of inflammatory cells induced into cornea, *Curr Eye Res* 9:129-138, 1990.

164. Hazlett LD, Moon MM, Singh A et al.: Analysis of adhesion, piliation, protease production and ocular infectivity of several *P. aeruginosa* strains, *Curr Eye Res* 10:351-362, 1991.

165. Hazlett LD, Moon MM, Strejc M, Berk RS: Evidence for N-acetyl-mannosamine as an ocular receptor for *P. aeruginosa* adherence to scarified cornea, *Invest Ophthalmol Vis Sci* 28:1978-1985, 1987.

166. Hazlett LD, Rosen DD, Berk RS: *Pseudomonas* eye infections in cyclophosphamide-treated mice, *Invest Ophthalmol Vis Sci* 16:649-652, 1977.

167. Hazlett LD, Wells PA, Berk RS: Scanning electron microscopy of the normal and experimentally infected ocular surface, *Scan Electron Microsc* 3:1379-1389, 1984.

168. Heidemann DG, Alfonso E, Forster RK et al.: *Branhamella catarrhalis* keratitis, *Am J Ophthalmol* 103:576-581, 1987.

169. Heidemann DG, Dunn SP, Diskin JA, Aiken TB: *Corynbacterium striatus* keratitis, *Cornea* 10:81-82, 1991.

170. Hemady RK, Griffin N, Aristimuño B: Recurrent corneal infections in a patient with the acquired immunodeficiency syndrome, *Cornea* 12:266-269, 1993.

171. Herbst RW: *Herellea* corneal ulcer associated with the use of soft contact lenses, *Br J Ophthalmol* 56:848-850, 1972.

172. Hill JC: Use of penetrating keratoplasty in acute bacterial keratitis, *Br J Ophthalmol* 70:502-506, 1986.

173. Hilton E, Adams AA, Uliss A et al.: Nosocomial bacterial eye infections in intensive-care units, *Lancet* 1:1318-1320, 1983.

174. Hirao Y, Homma JY: Therapeutic effect of immunization with OEP, protease toxoid and elastase toxoid on corneal ulcers in mice due to *Pseudomonas aeruginosa* infection, *Jpn J Exp Med* 48:41-51, 1978.

175. Hirschberg J: (Translated by FC Blodi). *The history of ophthalmology,* vol 7, 254-256, Bonn, 1976, JP Wayenborgh Verlag.

176. Hirst LW, Smiddy WE, Stark WJ: Corneal perforation: changing methods of treatment, 1960-1980, *Ophthalmology* 89:630-635, 1982.

177. Ho AC, Rapuano CJ: *Pasteurella multocida* keratitis and corneal laceration from a cat scratch, *Ophthalmic Surg* 24:346-348, 1993.

178. Hobden JA, Hill JM, Engel LS, O'Callaghan RJ: Age and therapeutic outcome of experimental *Pseudomonas aeruginosa* keratitis treated with ciprofloxacin, prednisolone, and flurbiprofen, *Antimicrob Agents Chemother* 37:1856-1859, 1993.

178a. Hobden JA, Masinick SA, Barrett RP, Hazlett LD: Aged mice fail to upregulate ICAM-1 after *Pseudomonas aeruginosa* corneal infection, *Invest Ophthalmol Vis Sci* 36:1107-1114, 1995.

179. Hobden JA, Reidy JJ, O'Callaghan RJ et al.: Treatment of experimental *Pseudomonas* keratitis using collagen shields containing tobramycin, *Arch Ophthalmol* 106:1605-1607, 1988.

180. Hobden JA, Reidy JJ, O'Callaghan RJ et al.: Ciprofloxacin iontophoresis for aminoglycoside-resistant pseudomonal keratitis, *Invest Ophthalmol Vis Sci* 31:1940-1944, 1990.

181. Hodges EJ, Friedlaender MH, Lee A, Okumoto M: Effect of minimal antibiotic treatment on bacterial keratitis, *Cornea* 8:188-190, 1989.

182. Holbach LM, Bialasiewicz AA, Boltze HJ: Necrotizing ring ulcer of the cornea caused by exogenous *Listeria monocytogenes* serotype IV b infection, *Am J Ophthalmol* 106:105-106, 1988.

183. Holland S, Alfonso E, Gelender H et al.: Corneal ulcer due to *Listeria monocytogenes, Cornea* 6:144-146, 1987.

184. Howe TR, Iglewski BH: Isolation and characterization of alkaline protease-deficient mutants of *Pseudomonas aeruginosa* in vitro and in a mouse eye model, *Infect Immun* 43:1058-1063, 1984.

185. Howes EL, Cruse VK, Kwok MT: Mononuclear cells in the corneal response to endotoxin, *Invest Ophthalmol Vis Sci* 22:494-501, 1982.

186. Hughes L, Maurice DM: A fresh look at iontophoresis, *Arch Ophthalmol* 102:1825-1829, 1984.

187. Hutton WL, Sexton RR: Atypical *Pseudomonas* corneal ulcers in semicomatose patients, *Am J Ophthalmol* 73:37-39, 1972.

188. Hwang DG, McDonnell PJ: Polymicrobial keratitis resulting from a dental pick injury, *Am J Ophthalmol* 115:252-254, 1993.

189. Hy YH: An analysis of 1,048 cases of corneal disease, *Chung Hua Yen Ko Tsa Chih* 27:19-21, 1991.

190. Hyndiuk RA: Experimental *Pseudomonas* keratitis. I. Sequential electron microscopy. II. Comparative therapy trials, *Trans Am Ophthalmol Soc* 79:541-624, 1981.

191. Iglewski BH, Burns RP, Gipson IK: Pathogenesis of corneal damage from *Pseudomas* exotoxin A, *Invest Ophthalmol Vis Sci* 16:73-76, 1977.

192. Insler MS, Helm CJ, George WJ: Topical vs systemic gentamicin penetration into the human cornea and aqueous humor, *Arch Ophthalmol* 105:922-924, 1987.

193. Insler MS, Pechous B: Conjunctival flaps revisited, *Ophthalmic Surg* 18:455-458, 1987.

194. Janda WM, Hellerman DV, Zeiger B, Brody BB: Isolation of *Klebsiella ozaenae* from a corneal abscess, *Am J Clin Pathol* 83:655-657, 1985.

195. Jensen OL, Gluud BS: Bacterial growth in the conjunctival sac and the local defense of the outer eye, *Acta Ophthalmol* 63 (suppl 173):80-82, 1985.

196. John T: How safe are disposable soft contact lenses? *Am J Ophthalmol* 111:766-768, 1991.

197. Johnson AP, Wool BM, Johnson MK: Adherence of *Staphylococcus aureus* to rabbit corneal epithelial cells, *Arch Ophthalmol* 102:1229-1231, 1984.

198. Johnson MK, Hobden JA, Hagenah M et al.: The role of pneumolysin in ocular infections with *Streptococcus pneumoniae, Curr Eye Res* 9:1107-1114, 1990.

199. Jones DB: Early diagnosis and therapy of bacterial corneal ulcers, *Int Ophthalmol Clin* 13(4):1-28, 1973.

200. Jones DB: A plan for antimicrobial therapy in bacterial keratitis, *Trans Am Acad Ophthalmol Otolaryngol* 79:OP95-OP103, 1975.

201. Jones DB: Pathogenesis of bacterial and fungal keratitis, *Trans Ophthalmol Soc UK* 98:367-371, 1978.

202. Jones DB: Initial therapy of suspected microbial corneal ulcers. II. Specific antibiotic therapy based on corneal smears, *Surv Ophthalmol* 24:97, 105-116, 1979.

203. Jones DB: Strategy for the initial management of suspected microbial keratitis: symposium on medical and surgical diseases of the cornea. In *Transactions of the New Orleans Academy of Ophthalmology,* St Louis, 1980, CV Mosby.

204. Jones DB: Decision making in the management of microbial keratitis, *Ophthalmology* 88:814-820, 1981.

205. Jones DB: Introduction: pathogenesis and therapy of infectious diseases: an overview. In Suran A, Gery I, Nussenblatt RB, editors: *Immunology of the eye: workshop. III. Immunologic aspects of ocular disease: infection, inflammation and allergy, Immunol Abstr,* 1981 (sp suppl):3-19.

206. Jones DB: Polymicrobial keratitis, *Trans Am Ophthalmol Soc* 79:153-167, 1981.

207. Reference deleted in proofs.

208. Jones DB, Robinson NM: Anaerobic ocular infections, *Trans Am Acad Ophthalmol Otolaryngol* 83:309-331, 1977.

209. Kamata R, Matsumoto K, Okamura R et al.: The serratial 56K protease as a major pathogenic factor in serratial keratitis: clinical and experimental study, *Ophthalmology* 92:1452-1459, 1985.

210. Kasparov AA, Oganesiants VA, Riabokon' BV, Gorbovitskaia GE: Mikrodiatermokoaguliatsiia v lechenii gerpeticheskogo keratita, *Vestn Oftalmol* 106(1):37-41, 1990.

211. Katz N, Wadud S, Ayazuddin M: Corneal ulcer disease in Bangladesh, *Ann Ophthalmol* 15:834-836, 1983.

212. Kawaharajo K, Homma JY: Pathogenesis of the mouse keratitis produced with *Pseudomonas aeruginosa, Jpn J Exp Med* 45:515-524, 1975.

213. Kawaharajo K, Homma JY: Synergistic effect of immune gamma-globulin fraction on protection by antibiotic against corneal ulcers in experimental mice infected with *Pseudomonas aeruginosa, Jpn J Exp Med* 46:155-165, 1976.

214. Keates RH, Drago PC, Rothchild EJ: Effect of excimer laser on microbiological organisms, *Ophthalmic Surg* 19:715-718, 1988.

215. Kelly L, Eliason J: *Eikenella corrodens* keratitis: case report, *Br J Ophthalmol* 73:22-24, 1989.

216. Kelly LD, Phan TM, Steinert RF: Evaluation of prophylactic antibiotic use in patients with corneal graft infection, *Invest Ophthalmol Vis Sci* 32:1170, 1991.

217. Kennedy P: *Ophthalmographia: or, a treatise of the eye, in two parts,* London, 1713, B. Lintott. (Republished by Classics of Ophthalmology Library, Birmingham, Ala, 1988, Gryphon Editions.)

218. Kent HD, Cohen EJ, Laibson PR, Arentsen JJ: Microbial keratitis and corneal ulceration associated with therapeutic soft contact lenses, *CLAO J* 16:49-52, 1990.

219. Kenyon KR: Inflammatory mechanisms in corneal ulceration, *Trans Am Ophthalmol Soc* 83:610-663, 1985.

220. Kerr N, Stern GA: Bacterial keratitis associated with vernal keratoconjunctivitis, *Cornea* 11:355-359, 1992.

221. Kiel RJ, Crane LR, Aguilar J et al.: Corneal perforation caused by dysgonic fermenter-2, *JAMA* 257:3269-3270, 1987.

222. Killingsworth DW, Stern GA, Driebe WT et al.: Results of therapeutic penetrating keratoplasty, *Ophthalmology* 100:534-541, 1993.

223. Kimura SJ: Fluorescein paper: a simple means of insuring the use of sterile fluorescein, *Am J Ophthalmol* 34:446-447, 1951.

224. Kincaid MC, Fouraker BD, Schanzlin DJ: Infectious crystalline keratopathy after relaxing incisions, *Am J Ophthalmol* 111:374-375, 1991.

225. Kintner JC, Grossniklaus HE, Lass JH, Jacobs G: Infectious crystalline keratopathy associated with topical anesthetic abuse, *Cornea* 9:77-80, 1990.

226. Kirkness CM, McSteele AD, Rice NS: Penetrating keratoplasty in the management of suppurative keratitis, *Dev Ophthalmol* 18:172-175, 1989.

227. Kirkness CM, Ficker LA, Rice NS, Steele AD: Large corneal grafts can be successful, *Eye* 3:48-55, 1989.

228. Klein B, Couch J, Thompson J: Ocular infections associated with *Eikenella corrodens, Am J Ophthalmol* 109:127-131, 1990.

229. Klotz SA, Au YK, Misra RP: A partial-thickness epithelial defect increases the adherence of *Pseudomonas aeruginosa* to the cornea, *Invest Ophthalmol Vis Sci* 30:1069-1074, 1989.

230. Klotz SA, Butrus SI, Misra RP, Osato MS: The contribution of bacterial surface hydrophobicity to the process of adherence of *Pseudomonas aerugonisa* to hydrophilic contact lenses, *Curr Eye Res* 8:195-202, 1989.

231. Klussmann KG, Viti AJ, Macsai MS: A black and white method for illustration and reproduction of corneal pathology, *Ophthalmology* 99(suppl):124, 1992.

232. Koidou-Tsiligianni A, Alfonso E, Forster RK: Ulcerative keratitis associated with contact lens wear, *Am J Ophthalmol* 108:64-67, 1989.

233. Kreger AS: Pathogenesis of *Pseudomonas aeruginosa* ocular diseases, *Rev Infect Dis* 5(suppl 5):S931-S935, 1983.

234. Kreger AS, Lyerly DM, Hazlett LD, Berk RS: Immunization against experimental *Pseudomonas aeruginosa* and *Serratia marcescens* keratitis: vaccination with lipopolysaccharide endotoxins and proteases, *Invest Ophthalmol Vis Sci* 27:932-939, 1986.

235. Kupferman A, Leibowitz HM: Quantitation of bacterial infection and antibiotic effect in the cornea, *Arch Ophthalmol* 94:1981-1984, 1976.

236. Kupferman A, Leibowitz HM: Topical antibiotic therapy of *Pseudomonas aeruginosa* keratitis, *Arch Ophthalmol* 97:1699-1702, 1979.

237. Lal H, Ahluwalia BK, Khurana AK et al.: Serum and tear immunoglobulins in bacterial, fungal and viral corneal ulcers, *Acta Ophthalmol* 68:71-74, 1990.

237a. Lal H, Khurana AK: Tear immunoglobulins and lysozyme levels in corneal ulcers. In Sullivan DA, editor: *Lacrimal gland, tear film, and dry eye syndromes. Basic science and clinical relevance. Advances in experimental medicine and biology,* vol 350, New York, 1994, Plenum.

238. Lande MA, Birk DE, Nagpal ML, Rader RL: Phagocytic properties of human keratocyte cultures, *Invest Ophthalmol Vis Sci* 20:481-489, 1981.

239. Lass JH, Haaf J, Foster CS, Belcher C: Visual outcome in eight cases of *Serratia marcescens* keratitis, *Am J Ophthalmol* 92:384-390, 1981.

240. Lawin-Brussel CA, Refojo MF, Leong FL et al.: Time course of experimental *Pseudomonas aeruginosa* keratitis in contact lens overwear, *Arch Ophthalmol* 108:1012-1019, 1990.

241. Lawin-Brussel CA, Refojo MF, Leong FL, Kenyon KR: *Pseudomonas* attachment to low-water and high-water, ionic and nonionic new and rabbit-worn soft contact lenses, *Invest Ophthalmol Vis Sci* 32:657-662, 1991.

242. Lawrence W: *A treatise on the diseases of the eye,* 104, 114, London, 1833, J Churchill. (Republished by Classics of Ophthalmology Library, Birmingham, Ala, 1987, Gryphon Editions.)

243. Leahey AB, Avery RL, Gottsch JD et al.: Suture abscesses after penetrating keratoplasty, *Cornea* 12:489-492, 1993.

244. Leber T: *Die Entstehung der Entzündung,* Leipzig, 1891, W Engelmann.

245. Lee P, Green WR: Corneal biopsy: indications, techniques, and a report of a series of 87 cases, *Ophthalmology* 97:718-721, 1990.

246. Lee VHL, Urrea PT, Smith RE, Schanzlin DJ: Ocular drug bioavailability from topically applied liposomes, *Surv Ophthalmol* 29:335-348, 1985.

247. Leibowitz HM: Management of inflammation in the cornea and conjunctiva, *Ophthalmology* 87:753-758, 1980.

248. Leibowitz HM: Clinical evaluation of ciprofloxacin 0.3% ophthalmic solution for treatment of bacterial keratitis, *Am J Ophthalmol* 112:34S-47S, 1991.

249. Leibowitz HM, Kupferman A: Antiinflammatory medications, *Int Ophthalmol Clin* 20(3):117-134, 1980.

250. Leibowitz HM, Kupferman A: Topically administered corticosteroids: effect on antibiotic-treated bacterial keratitis, *Arch Ophthalmol* 98:1287-1290, 1980.

251. Lembach RG, Ringel DM: Factitious bilateral crystalline keratopathy, *Cornea* 9:246-248, 1990.

252. Lemp MA: Is the dry eye contact lens wearer at risk? Yes, *Cornea* 9(suppl 1):S48-50, 1990.

253. Levy JH, Katz HR: Effect of systemic tetracycline on progression of *Pseudomonas aeruginosa* keratitis in the rabbit, *Ann Ophthalmol* 22:179-183, 1990.

254. Li WW, Grayson G, Folkman J, D'Amore PA: Sustained-release endotoxin: a model for inducing corneal neovascularization, *Invest Ophthalmol Vis Sci* 32:2906-2911, 1991.

255. Liang F-Q, Viola RS, del Cerro M, Aquavella JV: Noncross-linked collagen discs and cross-linked collagen shields in the delivery of gentamicin to rabbits eyes, *Invest Ophthalmol Vis Sci* 33:2194-2198, 1992.

256. Libert J, Ketelbant-Balasse PE, van Hoof F et al.: Cellular toxicity of gentamicin, *Am J Ophthalmol* 87:405-411, 1979.

257. Liesegang TJ, Forster RK: Spectrum of microbial keratitis in south Florida, *Am J Ophthalmol* 90:38-47, 1980.

258. Liesegang TJ, Jones DB, Robinson NM: *Azotobacter* keratitis, *Arch Ophthalmol* 99:1587-1590, 1981.

259. Lotti R, Dart JKG: Cataract as a complication of severe microbial keratitis, *Eye* 6:400-403, 1992.

260. Lubniewski AJ, Houchin KW, Holland EJ et al.: Posterior infectious crystalline keratopathy with *Staphylococcus epidermidis, Ophthalmology* 97:1454-1459, 1990.

260a. Luchs JI, d'Aversa G, Udell IJ: Ulcerative keratitis associated with spontaneous corneal erosions, *Invest Ophthalmol Vis Sci* 36(4):540, 1995.

261. Lyerly D, Gray L, Kreger A: Characterization of rabbit corneal damage produced by *Serratia* keratitis and by a *Serratia* protease, *Infect Immun* 33:927-932, 1981.

262. Lyon DB, Newman SA: Secondary bacterial keratitis in herpes zoster ophthalmicus, *Cornea* 6:283-285, 1987.

263. Mackowiak PA: The normal microbial flora, *New Eng J Med* 307:83-93, 1982.

264. MacNab A: *Ulceration of the cornea,* London, 1907, Baillière, Tindall & Cox.

265. MacNab A: The bacteriology of ulceration of the cornea, *Ophthalmoscope* 8:629, 1910.

266. MacRae S, Herman C, Stulting RD et al.: Corneal ulcer and adverse reaction rates in premarket contact lens studies, *Am J Ophthalmol* 111:457-465, 1991.

267. Macsai MS, Hillman DS, Robin JB: *Branhamella* keratitis resistant to penicillin and cephalosporins: case reports, *Arch Ophthalmol* 106:1506-1507, 1988.

268. Mader TH, Maher KL, Stulting RD: Gentamicin resistance in staphylococcal corneal ulcers, *Cornea* 10:408-410, 1991.

269. Mahajan VM: Ulcerative keratitis: an analysis of laboratory data in 674 cases, *J Ocul Ther Surg* 4:138-141, 1985.

270. Mahajan VM, Reddy TN, Agarwal LP: Toxigenic strains of *Staphylococcus epidermidis* and their experimental corneal pathogenicity in rabbits, *Int Ophthalmol* 5:155-161, 1982.

271. Majekodunmi S, Odugbemi T: *Clostridium welchii* corneal ulcer: a case report, *Can J Ophthalmol* 10:290-292, 1975.

272. Mandelbaum S, Waring III GO, Forster RK et al.: Late development of ulcerative keratitis in radial keratotomy scars, *Arch Ophthalmol* 104:1156-1160, 1986.

273. Manthey KF: Erregernachweis bei bakterieller Keratitis mit Immufluoreszenz, *Fortschr Ophthalmol* 79:310-312, 1982.

274. Marioneaux SJ, Cohen EJ, Arentsen JJ, Laibson PR: *Moraxella* keratitis, *Cornea* 10:21-24, 1991.

275. Marmer RH: Radial keratotomy complications, *Ann Ophthalmol* 19:409-411, 1987.

276. Martorina M: Spontaneous corneal perforation with expulsive hemorrhage, *Ann Ophthalmol* 25:324-325, 1993.

277. Maske R, Hill JC, Oliver SP: Management of bacterial corneal ulcers, *Br J Ophthalmol* 70:199-201, 1986.

278. Matoba AY, McCulley JP: The effect of therapeutic soft contact lenses on antibiotic delivery to the cornea, *Ophthalmology* 92:97-99, 1985.

278a. Matoba AY, O'Brien TP, Wilhelmus KR, Jones DB: Infectious crystalline keratopathy due to *Streptococcus pneumoniae:* possible association with serotype, *Ophthalmology* 101:1000-1004, 1994.

279. Matoba AY, Torres J, Wilhelmus KR et al.: Bacterial keratitis after radial keratotomy, *Ophthalmology* 96:1171-1175, 1989.

280. Matsumoto K, Shams NBK, Hanninen LA, Kenyon KR: Cleavage and activation of corneal matrix metalloproteases by *Pseudomonas aeruginosa* proteases, *Invest Ophthalmol Vis Sci* 34:1945-1953, 1993.

281. Matsumoto K, Yamamoto T, Kamata R, Maeda H: Pathogenesis of serratial infection: activation of the Hageman factor–prekallikrein cascade by serratial protease, *J Biochem* 96:739-749, 1984.

282. Matthews TD, Frazer DG, Minassian DC et al.: Risks of keratitis and patterns of use with disposable contact lenses, *Arch Ophthalmol* 110:1559-1562, 1992.

283. Maudgal PC, Missotten L: *Acinetobacter* keratoconjunctivitis clinically resembling keratitis sicca, *Bull Soc Belge Ophtalmol* 182:25-32, 1978.

284. Mayo MS, Schlitzer RL, Ward MA et al.: Association of *Pseudomonas* and *Serratia* corneal ulcers with use of contaminated solutions, *J Clin Microbiol* 25:1398-1400, 1987.

285. McBride HA, Martinez DR, Trang JM et al.: Stability of gentamicin sulfate and tobramycin sulfate in extemporaneously prepared ophthalmic solutions at 8 degrees C, *Am J Hosp Pharm* 48:507-509, 1991.

286. McClellan KA, Bernard PJ, Billson FA: Microbial investigations in keratitis at the Sydney Eye Hospital, *Aust NZ J Ophthalmol* 17:413-416, 1989.

287. McCulloch RR, Torres JG, Wilhelmus KR et al.: Biofilm on contaminated hydrogel contact lenses protects adherent *Pseudomonas* aeruginosa from antibacterial therapy, *Invest Ophthalmol Vis Sci* 29(suppl):228, 1988.

288. McDonnell PJ, Kwitko S, McDonnell JM et al.: Characterization of infectious crystalline keratitis caused by a human isolate of *Streptococcus mitis, Arch Ophthalmol* 109:1147-1151, 1991.

289. McDonnell PJ, Nobe J, Gauderman WJ et al.: Community care of corneal ulcers, *Am J Ophthalmol* 114:531-538, 1992.

290. Millar MR, Inglis T: Influence of lysozyme on aggregation of *Staphylococcus aureus, J Clin Microbiol* 25:1587-1590, 1987.

291. Mitsui Y, Sakuragi S, Tamura O et al.: Effect of ofloxacin ophthalmic solution in the treatment of external bacterial infections of the eye, *Folia Ophthalmol Jpn* 37:1115, 1986.

292. Miyagawa S, Kamata R, Matsumoto K et al.: Inhibitory effects of ovomacroglobulin on bacterial keratitis in rabbits, *Graefes Arch Clin Exp Ophthalmol* 229:281-286, 1991.

293. Mollee T, Kelly P, Tilse M: Isolation of *Kingella kingae* from a corneal ulcer, *J Clin Microbiol* 30:2516-2517, 1992.

294. Mondino BJ: Collagen shields, *Am J Ophthalmol* 112:587-590, 1991.

295. Mondino BJ, Brown SI, Rabin BS: Role of complement in corneal inflammation, *Trans Ophthalmol Soc UK* 98:363-366, 1978.

296. Mondino BJ, Sumner HL: Generation of complement-derived anaphylatoxins in normal human donor corneas, *Invest Ophthalmol Vis Sci* 31:1945-1949, 1990.

297. Mondino BJ, Bath PE, Foos RY et al.: Absent meibomian glands in the ectrodactyly, ectodermal dysplasia, cleft lip-palate syndrome, *Am J Ophthalmol* 97:496-500, 1984.

298. Mondino BJ, Rabin BS, Kessler E et al.: Corneal rings with gram-negative bacteria, *Arch Ophthalmol* 95:2222-2225, 1977.

299. Moon MM, Hazlett LD, Hancock RE et al.: Monoclonal antibodies provide protection against ocular *Pseudomonas aerugonisa* infection, *Invest Ophthalmol Vis Sci* 29:1277-1284, 1988.

300. Musch DC, Sugar A, Meyer RF: Demographic and predisposing factors in corneal ulceration, *Arch Ophthalmol* 101:1545-1548, 1983.

301. Nanda M, Pflugfelder SC, Holland S: Fulminant pseudomonal keratitis and scleritis in human immodeficiency virus-infected patients, *Arch Ophthalmol* 109:503-505, 1991.

302. Nassif KF, Davis SD, Hyndiuk RA et al.: Factors that influence the efficacy of topical gentamicin prophylaxis for experimental *Pseudomonas* keratitis, *Am J Ophthalmol* 94:216, 1982.

303. Newman PE, Hider P, Waring GO III et al.: Corneal ulcer due to *Achromobacter xylosoxidans, Br J Ophthalmol* 68:472-474, 1984.

304. Newton C, Moore MB, Kaufman HE: Corneal biopsy in chronic keratitis, *Arch Ophthalmol* 105:577-578, 1987.

305. Nissenkorn I, Wood TO: Secondary bacterial infections in herpes simplex keratitis, *Ann Ophthalmol* 14:757-759, 1982.

306. Nobe JR, Moura BT, Robin JB, Smith RE: Results of penetrating keratoplasty for the treatment of corneal perforations, *Arch Ophthalmol* 108:939-941, 1990.

307. Noble EM: *A treatise on opthalmy; and those diseases which are induced by inflammations of the eyes: with new methods of cure,* Birmingham, 1800, Swinney & Hawkins. (Republished by Classics of Ophthalmology Library, Birmingham, Ala, 1991, Gryphon Editions.)

308. Norn M: Tear stix tests for leucocyte-esterase, nitrite, haemoglobin, and albumin in normals and in a clinical series, *Acta Ophthalmol* 67:192-198, 1989.

309. Oakley DE, Weeks RD, Ellis PP: Corneal distribution of subconjunctival antibiotics, *Am J Ophthalmol* 81:307-312, 1976.

309a. O'Brien TP et al.: Comparative clinical efficacy of topical ofloxacin vs combined fortified cefazolin and tobramycin in therapy of bacterial keratitis, *Arch Ophthalmol* (in press).

310. O'Brien TP, Sawusch MR, Dick JD, Gottsch JD: Use of collagen corneal shields versus soft contact lenses to enhance penetration of topical tobramycin, *J Cataract Refract Surg* 14:505-507, 1988.

311. O'Brien TP, Wilhelmus KR: Bacterial keratitis in trichothiodystrophy, *Can J Ophthalmol* 30:200, 1995.

312. Olijnyk I, Marchese AL, McDonald JE: The use of disposable cautery to scrape corneal ulcers, *Am J Ophthalmol* 90:110, 1980.

313. Ormerod LD: Causation and management of microbial keratitis in subtropical Africa, *Ophthalmology* 94:1662-1668, 1987.

314. Ormerod LD: Causes and management of bacterial keratitis in the elderly, *Can J Ophthalmol* 24:112-116, 1989.

315. Ormerod LD, Fong LP, Foster CS: Corneal infection in mucosal scarring disorders and Sjögren's syndrome, *Am J Ophthalmol* 105:512-518, 1988.

316. Ormerod LD, Foster CS, Paton BG et al.: Ocular *Capnocytophaga* infection in an edentulous, immunocompetent host, *Cornea* 7:218-222, 1988.

317. Ormerod LD, Gomez DS, Schanzlin DJ et al.: Chronic alcoholism and microbial keratitis, *Br J Ophthalmol* 72:155-159, 1988.

318. Ormerod LD, Hertzmark E, Gomez DS et al.: Epidemiology of microbial keratitis in southern California: a multivariate analysis, *Ophthalmology* 94:1322-1333, 1987.

319. Ormerod LD, Murphree AL, Gomez DS et al.: Microbial keratitis in children, *Ophthalmology* 93:449-455, 1986.

320. Ormerod LD, Ruoff KL, Meisler DM et al.: Infectious crystalline keratopathy: role of nutritionally variant streptococci and other bacterial factors, *Ophthalmology* 98:159-169, 1991.

321. Orticio LP: Confusion and the patient on an intensive topical ocular antibiotic regimen: a case analysis, *J Ophthalmic Nurs Technol* 9:145-151, 1990.

322. Osato MS, Jensen HG, Trousdale MD et al.: The comparative in vitro activity of ofloxacin and selected ophthalmic antimicrobial agents against ocular bacterial isolates, *Am J Ophthalmol* 108:380-386, 1989.

323. Osborn E, Baum JL, Ernst C, Koch P: The stability of ten antibiotics in artificial tear solutions, *Am J Ophthalmol* 82:775-780, 1976.

324. Ostler HB, Okumoto M, Wilkey C: The changing pattern of the etiology of central bacterial corneal (hypopyon) ulcers, *Trans Pac Coast Ophthalmol Soc* 57:235-246, 1976.

325. Pamel GJ, Buckley DJ, Frucht J et al.: *Capnocytophaga* keratitis, *Am J Ophthalmol* 107:193-194, 1989.

326. Pande M, Ghanchi F: The role of preservatives in the conjunctival toxicity of subconjunctival gentamicin injection, *Br J Ophthalmol* 76:235-237, 1992.

327. Panjwani N, Clark B, Cohen M et al.: Differential binding of *P. aeruginosa* and *S. aureus* to corneal epithelium in culture, *Invest Ophthalmol Vis Sci* 31:696-701, 1990.

328. Panjwani N, Zaidi TS, Gigstad JE et al.: Binding of *Pseudomonas aeruginosa* to neutral glycosphingolipids of rabbit corneal epithelium, *Infect Immun* 58:114-118, 1990.

329. Patitsas C, Rockwood EJ, Meisler DM, McMahon JT: Infectious crystalline keratopathy occuring in an eye subsequent to glaucoma filtering surgery with postoperative subconjunctival 5-fluorouracil, *Ophthalmic Surg* 22:412-413, 1991.

330. Paton BG, Ormerod LD, Peppe J, Kenyon KR: Evidence for a feline reservoir for dysgonic fermenter 2 keratitis, *J Clin Microbiol* 26:2439-2440, 1988.

331. Pepose JS, Wilhelmus KR: Divergent approaches to the management of corneal ulcers, *Am J Ophthalmol* 114:630-632, 1992.

332. Perry LD, Brinser JH, Kolodner H: Anaerobic corneal ulcers, *Ophthalmology* 89:636-642, 1982.

333. Petit PJ: Sur une forme particulière d'infection cornéenne à type serpigineaux, *Ann Oculist* 121:166, 1899.

334. Petroutsos G, Guimaraes R, Giraud J, Pouliquen Y: Antibiotics and corneal epithelial wound healing, *Arch Ophthalmol* 101:1775-1778, 1983.

335. Pfister RR, Haddox JL, Yuille-Barr D et al.: Amino acid composition of a neutrophil respiratory burst stimulant: evidence for a protein, noncollagenous source, *Invest Ophthalmol Vis Sci* 32:2112-2118, 1991.

336. Pflugfelder SC, Murchison JF: Corneal toxicity with an antibiotic/steroid-soaked collagen shield, *Arch Ophthalmol* 110:20, 1992.

337. Pharmakakis N, Papadakis E, Gartaganis S et al.: Etude histologique des lesions cornéennes créés par la glycoliproproteine Slime-GLP du *Pseudomonas aeruginosa, Ophtalmologie* 4:72-75, 1990.

338. Philipp W, Göttinger W: T6-positive Langerhans cells in diseased corneas, *Invest Ophthalmol Vis Sci* 32:2492-2497, 1991.

339. Philipp W, Göttinger W: Leukocyte adhesion molecules in diseased corneas, *Invest Ophthalmol Vis Sci* 34:2449-2459, 1993.

340. Poggio EC, Abelson M: Complications and symptoms in disposable extibded wear lenses compared with conventional soft daily wear and soft extended wear lenses, *CLAO J* 19:31-39, 1993.

341. Poggio EC, Glynn RJ, Schein OD et al.: The incidence of ulcerative keratitis among users of daily-wear and extended-wear soft contact lenses, *New Eng J Med* 321:779-783, 1989.

341a. Portolés M, Austin F, Nos-Barberá S et al.: Effect of poloxamer 407 on the adherence of *Pseudomonas aeruginosa* to corneal epithelial cells, *Cornea* 14:56-61, 1995.

342. Pramhus C, Runyan TE, Lindberg RB: Ocular flora in the severely burned patient, *Arch Ophthalmol* 96:1421-1424, 1978.

343. Presley GD, Hale LM: Corneal ulcer due to *Bacterium anitratum, Am J Ophthalmol* 65:571-572, 1968.

344. Preston MJ, Kernack K, Berk RS: Kinetics of serum and ocular antibody responses in susceptible mice that received a secondary corneal infection with *Pseudomonas aeruginosa, Infect Immun* 61:2713-2716, 1993.

345. Rabinovitch J, Cohen EJ, Genvert GI et al.: Seasonal variation in contact lens-associated corneal ulcers, *Can J Ophthalmol* 22:155-156, 1987.

346. Ramphal R, McNiece MT, Polack FM: Adherence of *Pseudomonas aeruginosa* to the injured cornea: a step in the pathogenesis of corneal infections, *Ann Ophthalmol* 13:421-425, 1981.

347. Rashid ER, Waring GO III: Complications of radial and transverse keratotomy, *Surv Ophthalmol* 34:73-106, 1989/1990.

348. Reichert R, Stern GA: Quantitative adherence of bacteria to human corneal epithelial cells, *Arch Ophthalmol* 102:1394, 1984.

349. Reichert RW, Das ND, Zam ZS: Adherence properties of *Pseudomonas* pili to epithelial cells of the human cornea, *Curr Eye Res* 2:289-293, 1982/1983.

350. Reiss GR, Campbell RJ, Bourne WM: Infectious crystalline keratopathy, *Surv Ophthalmol* 31:69-72, 1986/1987.

351. Remeijer L, van Rij G, Mooij CM et al.: Infectious crystalline keratopathy, *Doc Ophthalmol* 67:95-103, 1987.

352. Reynolds MG, Alfonso E: Treatment of infectious scleritis and keratoscleritis, *Am J Ophthalmol* 112:543-547, 1991.

353. Robin JB, Schmidt L, Haimov T et al.: Fluorescein-conjugated lectin visualization of infectious organisms. In Cavanagh HD, editor: *The cornea: transactions of the World Congress on the Cornea III,* 485-489, New York, 1988, Raven Press.

353a. Roman F: The short history of heat cauterisation of the cornea, *Br J Ophthalmol* 79:236, 1995.

354. Romano A: New approach for early, simple, and rapid detection of acute eye infections, *Metab Pediatr Syst Ophthalmol* 11:53-57, 1988.

355. Rootman DS, Hobden JA, Jantzen JA et al.: Iontophoresis of tobramycin for the treatment of experimental *Pseudomonas* keratitis in the rabbit, *Arch Ophthalmol* 106:262-265, 1988.

356. Rosenfeld SI, Mandelbaum S, Corrent GF et al.: Granular epithelial keratopathy as an unusual manifestation of *Pseudomonas* keratitis associated with extended-wear soft contact lenses, *Am J Ophthalmol* 109:17-22, 1990.

357. Rosenwasser GOD, Holland S, Pflugfelder SC et al.: Topical anesthetic abuse, *Ophthalmology* 97:967-972, 1990.

358. Roser W: Ueber Hypopyonkeratitis, *Albrecht von Graefes Arch Ophthalmol* 2(pt 2):151-157, 1856.

359. Rotkis WM: Infections. In Brightbill FS, editor: *Corneal surgery: theory, technique, and tissue,* 322-325, St Louis, 1986, Mosby.

360. Roussel TJ, Osato MS, Wilhelmus KR: *Capnocytophaga* keratitis, *Br J Ophthalmol* 69:187-188, 1985.

361. Rowley W: *A treatise on one hundred and eighteen principal diseases of the eyes and eyelids, etc. in which are communicated several new discoveries relative to the cure of defects in vision: with many original prescriptions* (Translated from von Plenck JJR: *Doctrina de morbis oculorum*), 218, London, 1790, J Wingrove. (Republished by Classics of Ophthalmology Library, Birmingham, Ala, 1988, Gryphon Editions.)

362. Ruben M: Acute eye disease secondary to contact-lens wear: report of a census, *Lancet* 1:138-140, 1976.

363. Rubinfeld RS, Cohen EJ, Arentsen JJ, Laibson PR: Diphtheroids as ocular pathogens, *Am J Ophthalmol* 108:251-254, 1989.

364. Rudner XL, Zheng Z, Berk RS et al.: Corneal epithelial glycoproteins exhibit *Pseudomonas aeruginosa* pilus binding activity, *Invest Ophthalmol Vis Sci* 33:2185-2193, 1992.

365. Saari KM, Parvi V: Occupational eye injuries in Finland, *Acta Ophthalmol* 161(suppl):17-28, 1984.

366. Sachs R, Zagelbaum BM, Hersh PS: Corneal complications associated with the use of crack cocaine, *Ophthalmology* 100:187-191, 1993.

367. Saemisch T: *Das Ulcus corneae serpens und seine Therapie, eine Klinische Studie,* Bonn, 1870, M Cohen & Sohn.

368. Saini JS, Rao GN, Aquavella JV: Post-keratoplasty corneal ulcers and bandage lenses, *Acta Ophthalmol* 66:99-103, 1988.

368a. Sampath R, Ridgway AE, Leatherbarrow B: Bacterial keratitis following excimer laser photorefractive keratectomy: a case report, *Eye* 8:481-482, 1994.

369. Samples JR, Buettner H: Corneal ulcer caused by a biologic insecticide (*Bacillus thuringiensis*), *Am J Ophthalmol* 95:258-260, 1983.

370. Reference deleted in proofs.

371. Sarno EM, Robin JB, Garabet A, Schanzlin DJ: Carbon dioxide laser therapy of *Pseudomonas aeruginosa* keratitis, *Am J Ophthalmol* 97:791-792, 1984.

372. Sasamoto K, Akagi Y, Kodama Y, Itoi M: Corneal endothelial changes caused by ophthalmic drugs, *Cornea* 3:37-41, 1984.

373. Sattler H: Über bacillen Panophthalmitis, *Bericht Versammlung Ophth Gesellsch Stuttgart* 21:201-207, 1891/1892.

374. Saunders JC: *A treatise on some practical points relating to the diseases of the eye,* 77-83, London, 1811, Longman, Hurst, Rees, Orme, & Brown. (Republished by Classics of Ophthalmology Library, Birmingham, Ala, 1986, Gryphon Editions.)

375. Scarpa A: *Practical observations on the principal diseases of the eyes: illustrated with cases,* 297, London, 1806, T Cadell & W Davies. (Republished by Classics of Ophthalmology Library, Birmingham, Ala, 1984, Gryphon Editions.)

376. Schaeffer HE, Krohn DL: Liposomes in topical drug delivery, *Invest Ophthalmol Vis Sci* 22:220-227, 1982.

377. Schein OD, Glynn RJ, Poggio EC et al.: The relative risk of ulcerative keratitis among users of daily-wear and extended-wear soft contact lenses: a case-control study, *New Eng J Med* 321:773-778, 1989.

378. Schein OD, Hibberd PL, Starck T et al.: Microbial contamination of in-use ocular medications, *Arch Ophthalmol* 110:82-85, 1992.

379. Schein OD, Ormerod LD, Barrauquer E et al.: Microbiology of contact lens-related keratitis, *Cornea* 8:281-285, 1989.

380. Schein OD, Wasson PJ, Boruchoff SA, Kenyon KR: Microbial keratitis associated with contaminated ocular medications, *Am J Ophthalmol* 105:361-365, 1988.

381. Schiff WM, Speaker MG, McCormick SA: The collagen shield as a collagenase inhibitor and clinical indicator of collagenase activity on the ocular surface, *CLAO J* 18:59-63, 1992.

382. Schultz GS, Strelow S, Stern GA et al.: Treatment of alkali-injured rabbit corneas with a synthetic inhibitor of matrix metalloproteinases, *Invest Ophthalmol Vis Sci* 33:3325-3331, 1992.

383. Schwab L, Tizazu T: Destructive epidemic *Neisseria gonorrhoeae* keratoconjunctivitis in African adults, *Br J Ophthalmol* 69:525-528, 1985.

384. Scott GI: Traumatic ulcers of the cornea in miners: a survey of the changing picture during the 25 years 1928-1953, *Trans Ophthalmol Soc UK* 74:105-116, 1954.

385. Seal DV: The effect of ageing and disease on tear constituents, *Trans Ophthalmol Soc UK* 104:355-362, 1985.

386. Seal DV, McGill JI, Mackie IA et al.: Bacteriology and tear protein profiles of the dry eye, *Br J Ophthalmol* 70:122-125, 1986.

387. Selinger DS, Selinger RC, Reed WP: Resistance to infection of the external eye: the role of tears, *Surv Ophthalmol* 24:33-38, 1979/1980.

388. Sen DK, Sarin GS: Immunoglobulin concentrations in human tears in ocular diseases, *Br J Ophthalmol* 63:297-300, 1979.

389. Sendele DD, Kenyon KR, Wolf G, Hanninen LA: Epithelial abrasion precipitates stromal ulceration in the vitamin A-deficient rat cornea, *Invest Ophthalmol Vis Sci* 23:64-72, 1982.

390. Shams NB, Sigel MM, Davis RM: Interferon-gamma, *Staphylococcus aureus,* and lipopolysaccharide/silica enhance interleukin-1 beta production by human corneal cells, *Reg Immunol* 2:136-148, 1989.

391. Shell JW: Pharmacokinetics of topically applied ophthalmic drugs, *Surv Ophthalmol* 26:207-218, 1981/1982.

392. Shiono T, Hayasaka S: Aminoglycoside antibiotics and lysosomal enzymes of human tears, *Arch Ophthalmol* 103:1747-1749, 1985.

393. Shivitz IA, Arrowsmith PN: Delayed keratitis after radial keratotomy, *Arch Ophthalmol* 104:1153-1155, 1986.

394. Shofner RS, Kaufman HE, Hill JM: New horizons in drug delivery, *Ophthalmol Clin NA* 2:15-24, 1989.

395. Silbiger J, Stern GA: Evaluation of corneal collagen shields as a drug delivery device for the treatment of experimental *Pseudomonas* keratitis, *Ophthalmology* 99:889-892, 1992.

396. Singh A, Hazlett L, Berk RS: Characterization of pseudomonal adherence to unwounded cornea, *Invest Ophthalmol Vis Sci* 32:2096-2104, 1991.

397. Smith SG, Herman WK, Lindstrom RL, Doughman DJ: A method of collecting culture material from corneal ulcers, *Am J Ophthalmol* 97:105-106, 1984.

398. Smith SG, Lindstrom RL, Nelson JD et al.: Corneal ulcer-infiltrate associated with soft contact lens use following penetrating keratoplasty, *Cornea* 3:131-134, 1984.

399. Smolin G: The role of tears in the prevention of infections, *Int Ophthalmol Clin* 27:25-26, 1987.

400. Smolin G, Tabbara K, Whitcher J: *Infectious diseases of the eye,* 82-84, Baltimore, 1984, Williams & Wilkins.

401. Sobol WM, Torres Gomez J, Osato MS, Wilhelmus KR: Rapid streptococcal antigen detection in experimental keratitis, *Am J Ophthalmol* 107:60-64, 1989.

402. Sokol JL, Masur SK, Asbell PA, Holosin JM: Layer-by-layer desquamation of corneal epithelium and maturation of tear-facing membranes, *Invest Ophthalmol Vis Sci* 31:294-304, 1990.

403. Sokol PA: Surface expression of ferripyochelin-binding protein is required for virulence of *Pseudomas aeruginosa, Infect Immun* 55:2021-2025, 1987.

404. Sommer A: Effects of vitamin A deficiency on the ocular surface, *Ophthalmology* 90:592-600, 1983.

405. Spierer A, Kessler A: The effect of 2-mercaptoacetyl-L-phenylalanyl-L-leucine, a specific inhibitor of *Pseudomonas aeruginosa* elastase, on experimental *Pseudomonas* keratitis in rabbit eyes, *Curr Eye Res* 3:645-650, 1984.

406. Spurr-Michaud SJ, Barza M, Gipson IK: An organ culture system for study of adherence of *Pseudomonas aeruginosa* to normal and wounded corneas, *Invest Ophthalmol Vis Sci* 29:379-386, 1988.

407. Stein RM, Clinch TE, Cohen EJ et al.: Infected vs sterile corneal infiltrates in contact lens wearers, *Am J Ophthalmol* 105:632-636, 1988.

408. Stern GA: *Moraxella* corneal ulcers: poor response to medical treatment, *Ann Ophthalmol* 14:295-298, 1982.

409. Stern GA: *Pseudomonas* keratitis and contact lens wear: the lens/eye is at fault, *Cornea* 9(suppl 1):S36-S38, 1990.

410. Stern GA, Buttross M: Use of corticosteroids in combination with antimicrobial drugs in the treatment of infectious corneal disease, *Ophthalmology* 98:847-853, 1991.

411. Stern GA, Driebe WT: The effect of fortified antibiotic therapy on the visual outcome of severe bacterial corneal ulcers, *Cornea* 1:341-345, 1982.

412. Stern GA, Hodes BL, Stock EL: *Clostridium perfringens* corneal ulcer, *Arch Ophthalmol* 97:661-663, 1979.

413. Stern GA, Lubniewski A, Allen C: The interaction between *Pseudomonas aeruginosa* and the corneal epithelium: an electron microscopic study, *Arch Ophthalmol* 103:1221-1225, 1985.

414. Stern GA, Stock EL: Experimental *Bacteroides fragilis* keratitis, *Arch Ophthalmol* 96:2264-2266, 1978.

415. Stern GA, Zam AS: The pathogenesis of contact lens-associated *Pseudomonas aeruginosa* corneal ulceration. I. The effect of contact lens coatings on adherence of *Pseudomonas aeruginosa* to soft contact lenses, *Cornea* 5:41-45, 1986.

416. Stern GA, Schemmer GB, Farber RD, Gorovoy MS: Effect of topical antibiotic solutions on corneal epithelial wound healing, *Arch Ophthalmol* 101:644-647, 1983.

417. Steuhl K-P, Döring G, Henni A et al.: Relevance of host-derived and bacterial factors in *Pseudomonas aeruginosa* corneal infections, *Invest Ophthalmol Vis Sci* 28:1559-1568, 1987.

418. Stonecipher KG, Jensen HG, Kastl PR et al.: Ocular infections associated with *Comamonas acidovorans, Am J Ophthalmol* 112:46-49, 1991.

419. Sutphin JE, Pflugfelder SP, Wilhelmus KR, Jones DB: Penicillin-resistant *Streptococcus pneumoniae* keratitis, *Am J Ophthalmol* 97:388-389, 1984.

420. Tabbara KF, Tarabay N: *Bacillus licheniformis* corneal ulcer, *Am J Ophthalmol* 87:717-719, 1979.

421. Taylor DM, Stern AL: Reconstructive keratoplasty in the management of conditions leading to corneal destruction, *Ophthalmology* 87:892-904, 1980.

422. Tazawa H: Adherence of *Pseudomonas aeruginosa* to the rabbit corneal epithelium, *Nippon Ganka Gakkai Zasshi* 94:269-276, 1990.

423. Templeton WC, Eiferman RA, Snyder JW et al.: *Serratia* keratitis transmitted by contaminated eyedroppers, *Am J Ophthalmol* 93:723-726, 1982.

424. Tervo T, Salonen EM, Vahen A et al.: Elevation of tear fluid plasmin in corneal disease, *Acta Ophthalmol* 66:393-399, 1988.

425. Theodore FH, Feinstein R: Preparation and maintenance of sterile ophthalmic solutions, *JAMA* 152:1631-1633, 1953.

426. Thiel HJ, Weidle EG: Keratoplasty 'à chaud': results and complications, *Dev Ophthalmol* 11:68-74, 1985.

427. Thygeson P: Acute central (hypopyon) ulcers of the corneal, *Calif Med* 69:18-21, 1948.

428. Thygeson P, Hogan MJ, Kimura SJ: Cortisone and hydrocortisone in ocular infections, *Trans Am Acad Ophthalmol Otolaryngol* 57:64-85, 1953.

429. Ticho BH, Urban RC Jr, Safran MJ, Saggau DD: *Capnocytophaga* keratitis associated with poor dentition and human immunodeficiency virus infection, *Am J Ophthalmol* 109:352-353, 1990.

430. Till GO, Lee S, Mulligan MS et al.: Adhesion molecules in experimental phacoanaphylactic endophthalmitis, *Invest Ophthalmol Vis Sci* 33:3417-3423, 1992.

431. Tjia KF, van Putten JP, Pels E, Zanen HC: The interaction between *Neisseria gonorrhoeae* and the human cornea in organ culture: an electron microscopic study, *Graefes Arch Clin Exp Ophthalmol* 226:341-345, 1988.

432. Tobias JD, Starke JR, Tosi MF: *Shigella* keratitis: a report of two cases and a review of the literature, *Pediatr Infect Dis* 6:79-81, 1987.

433. Torres Gomez J, Robinson NM, Osato MS, Wilhelmus KR: Comparison of acridine orange and gram stains in bacterial keratitis, *Am J Ophthalmol* 106:735-737, 1988.

434. Trinkaus-Randall V, Leibowitz HM, Ryan WJ, Kupferman A: Quantification of stromal destruction in the inflamed cornea, *Invest Ophthalmol Vis Sci* 32:603-609, 1991.

435. Tuberville AW, Wood TO: Corneal ulcers in corneal transplants, *Curr Eye Res* 1:479-485, 1981.

436. Twining SS, Lohr KM, Moulder JE: The immune system in experimental *Pseudomonas* keratitis: model and early effects, *Invest Ophthalmol Vis Sci* 27:507-515, 1986.

437. Twining SS, Kirschner SE, Mahnke LA, Frank DW: Effect of *Pseudomonas aeruginosa* elastase, alkaline protease, and exotoxin A on corneal proteinases and proteins, *Invest Ophthalmol Vis Sci* 34:2699-2712, 1993.

438. Uhthoff W, Axenfeld T: Beiträge zur pathologischen Anatomie und Bakteriologie der eiterigen Keratitis des Menschen, *Albrecht von Graefes Arch Ophthalmol* 42(1):1-130, 1896.

439. Ullman S, Roussel TJ, Forster RK: Gonococcal keratoconjunctivitis, *Surv Ophthalmol* 32:199-208, 1987/1988.

440. Ullman S, Roussel TJ, Culbertson WW et al.: *Neisseria gonorrhoeae* keratoconjunctivitis, *Ophthalmology* 94:525-531, 1987.

441. Unterman SR, Rootman DS, Hill JM et al.: Collagen shield drug delivery: therapeutic concentrations of tobramycin in the rabbit cornea and aqueous humor, *J Cataract Refract Surg* 14:500-504, 1988.

442. Upadhyay MP, Karmacharya PCD, Koirala S et al.: Epidemiologic characteristics, predisposing factors, and etiologic diagnosis of corneal ulceration in Nepal, *Am J Ophthalmol* 111:92-99, 1991.

443. Upadhyay MP, Rai NC, Brandt F et al.: Corneal ulcers in Nepal, *Graefes Arch Clin Exp Ophthalmol* 219:55-59, 1982.

444. Upadhyay MP, Shah DN, Karmacharya PC et al.: Antibiotic prophylaxis for ocular surface trauma: a preliminary report. Asia Pacific Acad of Ophthalmol, Bangladesh, 1993.

445. Vajpayee RB, Gupta SK, Angra SK, Munjal A: Topical norfloxacin therapy in *Pseudomonas* corneal ulceration, *Cornea* 10:268-271, 1991.

446. Valenton MJ, Tan RV: Secondary ocular bacterial infection in hypovitaminosis A xerophthalmia, *Am J Ophthalmol* 80:673-677, 1975.

447. Van Horn DL, Davis SD, Hyndiuk RA, Pederson HJ: Experimental *Pseudomonas* keratitis in the rabbit: bacteriologic, clinical, and microscopic observations, *Invest Ophthalmol Vis Sci* 20:213-221, 1981.

448. van Setten GB, Tervo T, Tarkkanen A: Akute keratitis und die Kontamination von Kontaktlinsenpflegesystemen mit *Bacillus cereus, Klin Monatsbl Augenheilkd* 195:28-31, 1989.

449. Vaughan DG Jr: The contamination of fluorescein solutions: with special reference to *Pseudomonas aeruginosa* (bacillus pyocyanene), *Am J Ophthalmol* 39:55-61, 1955.

450. Vaughn DG Jr: Corneal ulcers, *Surv Ophthalmol* 3:203-215, 1958.

451. Verhagen C, Breebaart AV, Kijlstra A: The effects of complement depletion on corneal inflammation in rats, *Invest Ophthalmol Vis Sci* 33:273-279, 1992.

452. von Arlt FR: (Translated by L Ware). *Clinical studies on diseases of the eye including those of the conjunctiva, cornea, sclerotic, iris and ciliary body,* 135-180, Philadelphia, 1885, P Blakiston, Son & Co, 1885. (Republished by Classics of Ophthalmology Library, Birmingham, Ala, 1987, Gryphon Editions.)

453. Wainwright M, Swan HT: CG Paine and the earliest surviving clinical records of penicillin therapy, *Med Hist* 30:42-56, 1986.

453a. Wakil A, Hassman E, Lam S: Infectious corneal ulcers associated with crack cocaine, *Ann Ophthalmol* 27:96-100, 1995.

454. Wan WL, Farkas GC, May WN et al.: The clinical characteristics and course of adult gonococcal conjunctivitis, *Am J Ophthalmol* 102:575-583, 1986.

455. Wand M, Olive GM Jr, Mangiaracine AB: Corneal perforation and iris prolapse due to *Mima polymorpha, Arch Ophthalmol* 93:239-241, 1975.

456. Wardrop J: *Essays on the morbid anatomy of the human eye,* 5-21, Edinburgh, 1808, G Ramsay. (Republished by Classics of Ophthalmology Library, Birmingham, Ala, 1984, Gryphon Editions.)

457. Ware J: *Remarks on the ophthalmy, psorophthalmy and purulent eye with methods of cure, considerably used: and cases annexed, in proof of their utility,* London, 1780, C Dilly.

458. Waring GO III, Laibson PR: A systematic method of drawing corneal pathologic conditions, *Arch Ophthalmol* 95:1540-1542, 1977.

459. Watt PJ: Pathogenic mechanisms or organisms virulent to the eye, *Trans Ophthalmol Soc UK* 105:26-31, 1986.

460. Webb RM, Duke MA: Bacterial infection of a neurotrophic cornea in an immunocompromised subject, *Cornea* 4:14-18, 1985/1986.

461. Webb RM, Tabbara KF: Indolent bacterial corneal ulcers, *Cornea* 1:337-339, 1982.

462. Weidle EG, Thiel HJ: Keratoplastik à chaud als therapeutische Massnahme bei akuten Hornhautinfektionen, *Klin Monatsbl Augerkeilkd* 184:520-528, 1984.

463. Weisenthal RW, Krachmer JH, Folberg R et al.: Postkeratoplasty crystalline deposits mimicking bacterial infectious crystalline keratopathy, *Am J Ophthalmol* 105:70-74, 1988.

464. Weiss JL, Williams P, Lindstrom RL, Doughman DJ: The use of tissue adhesive in corneal perforations, *Ophthalmology* 90:610-615, 1983.

465. Weissman BA, Mondino BJ: Is daily wear better than extended wear? Arguments in favor of daily wear, *Cornea* 9(suppl 1):S25-S27, 1990.

466. Welsh NH, Rauch AJ, Gaffin SL: Topical immunotherapy for *Pseudomonas* keratitis in rabbits: use of antilipopolysaccharide plasma, *Br J Ophthalmol* 68:828-832, 1984.

467. Whitehouse G, Reid K, Hudson B et al.: Corneal biopsy in microbial keratitis, *Aust N Z J Ophthalmol* 19:193-196, 1991.

468. Wiggins RL: Experimental studies on the eye with polymyxin B, *Am J Ophthalmol* 35(5, pt II):83-100, 1952.

469. Wilhelmus KR: Suppurative corneal ulceration following herpetic keratitis, *Doc Ophthalmol* 53:17-36, 1982.

470. Wilhelmus KR: Bacterial corneal ulcers, *Int Ophthalmol Clin* 24(2):1-16, 1984.

471. Wilhelmus KR: The importance of having lysozyme, *Cornea* 4:69-70, 1985/1986.

472. Wilhelmus KR: Survival of the fittest, *Cornea* 5:67-68, 1986.

473. Wilhelmus KR: Review of clinical experience with microbial keratitis associated with contact lenses, *CLAO J* 13:211-214, 1987.

474. Wilhelmus KR: Bacterial keratitis complicating absolute glaucoma, *Glaucoma* 10:57-59, 1988.

475. Wilhelmus KR: Microbial keratitis associated with contact lens wear. In Kastl PR, editor: *Contact lenses: the CLAO guide to basic science and clinical practice,* vol 3, 41.1-41.19, Dubuque, 1995, Kendall/Hunt.

476. Wilhelmus KR, Gilbert ML, Osato MS: Tobramycin in ophthalmology, *Surv Ophthalmol* 32:111-122, 1987.

477. Wilhelmus KR, Hamburg S: Bacterial keratitis following radial keratotomy, *Cornea* 2:143-146, 1983.

478. Wilhelmus KR, Peacock J, Coster DJ: *Branhamella* keratitis, *Br J Ophthalmol* 64:892-895, 1980.

479. Wilhelmus KR, Peacock J, Coster DJ: The role of the gram stain in the management of suppurative keratitis. In Trevor-Roper PD, editor: *The cornea in health and disease,* 399-402. Sixth Congress of the European Society of Ophthalmology, London, 1981, Royal Society of Medicine.

480. Wilhelmus KR, Robinson NM, Jones DB: *Bacterionema matruchotii* ocular infections, *Am J Ophthalmol* 87:143-147, 1979.

481. Wilhelmus KR, Hyndiuk RA, Caldwell DR et al.: Ciprofloxacin ophthalmic ointment 0.3% in the treatment of bacterial keratitis, *Arch Ophthalmol* 111:1210-1218, 1993.

481a. Wilhelmus KR, Liesegang TJ, Osato MS, Jones DB: *Cumitech 13A: laboratory diagnosis of ocular infections,* Washington, DC, 1994, American Society for Microbiology.

482. Williams G, McClellan K, Billson F: Suppurative keratitis in rural Bangladesh: the value of Gram stain in planning management, *Int Ophthalmol* 15:131-135, 1991.

483. Williams G, Billson F, Husain R et al.: Microbiological diagnosis of suppurative keratitis in Bangladesh, *Br J Ophthalmol* 71:315-321, 1987.

484. Wilson FM: Adverse external ocular effects of topical opthalmic therapy: an epidemiologic, laboratory and clinical study, *Trans Am Ophthalmol Soc* 81:854-965, 1983.

485. Wilson LA: Acute bacterial infection of the eye: bacterial keratitis and endophthalmitis, *Trans Ophthalmol Soc UK* 105:43-60, 1986.

486. Wilson LA, Julian AJ, Ahearn DG: The survival and growth of microorganisms in mascara during use, *Am J Ophthalmol* 79:596-601, 1975.

487. Wilson LA, Sikes RK: *Pseudomonas aeruginosa* corneal infection related to mascara application trauma: Georgia, *MMWR* 39:47-48, 1990.

488. Woo FL, Johnson AP, Insler MS et al.: Gentamicin, tobramycin, amikacin, and netilmicin levels in tears following intravenous administration, *Arch Ophthalmol* 103:216-218, 1985.

489. Woods DE, Sokol PA, Iglewski BH: Modulatory effect of iron on the pathogenesis of *Pseudomas aeruginosa* mouse corneal infections, *Infect Immun* 35:461-464, 1982.

490. Yamaguchi K, Okumoto M, Stern G et al.: Idoxuridine and bacterial corneal infection, *Am J Ophthalmol* 87:202-205, 1979.

491. Zabel RW, Winegarden T, Holland EJ, Doughman DJ: *Acinetobacter* corneal ulcer after penetrating keratoplasty, *Am J Ophthalmol* 107:677-678, 1989.

492. Zaidman GW: *Propionibacterium acnes* keratitis, *Am J Ophthalmol* 113:596-598, 1992.

493. Zaidman GW, Coudron P, Piros J: *Listeria monocytogenes* keratitis, *Am J Ophthalmol* 109:334-339, 1990.

494. Zirm M: Die Bedeutung von Proteinaseinhibitoren in der Tranenflussigkeit, *Klin Monatsbl Augenheilkd* 177:759-767, 1980.

495. Zirm M, Ritzinger I: Der diagnostische und prognostische Wert einer Alpha-1-Antitrypsinbestimmung in der Tramenflussigkeit, *Klin Monatsbl Augenheilkd* 173:221-225, 1978.

75 Nontuberculous Mycobacterial Diseases

TERRENCE P. O'BRIEN, ALICE Y. MATOBA

Shortly after discovery of the tubercule bacillus by Koch in 1882, the existence of mycobacteria other than the causal agents of tuberculosis and leprosy was recognized. Although isolated infrequently from clinical specimens in the past, the relative importance of these other mycobacterial species has progressively increased in recent years. This change is associated with improved microbiologic diagnostic methods and an increased number of patients with abnormal local host defenses or systemic deficits of immunity. Ocular infection, principally keratitis, may be caused by several mycobacteria other than the tubercule bacilli. This chapter examines the classification, epidemiology, clinical features, laboratory diagnosis, and evolving therapies of ocular infections caused by these mycobacteria.

MYCOBACTERIOLOGY

Mycobacterium, the only genus in the family Mycobacteriaceae, contains over 50 species including *M. tuberculosis* and *M. leprae,* the causal agents of tuberculosis and leprosy, respectively. Controversy exists over the aggregate designation of "other" mycobacterial species. Members of the other species have been termed *atypical, anonymous, paratubercule, nontuberculous* bacilli (NTB), and *mycobacteria other than tubercule bacilli* (MOTT). Because they are recognized with increasing frequency, these organisms are no longer anonymous, and they are not atypical, except in their differences from the *M. tuberculosis* and *M. leprae.* For these reasons the terms *nontuberculous mycobacteria* and MOTT have gained increasing favor. As an adjective, however, "nontuberculous" is somewhat inaccurate, because these organisms often do elicit histologic "tubercules" in infected nonocular tissues.

Historically, classification of the nontuberculosis mycobacteria has been based on growth and pigmentation characteristics. Early classification schemes* divided the species

of *Mycobacterium* into four groups based on pigment production, rate of growth, and colony characteristics of the organisms. The four major groups have generally been referred to as photochromogenic, scotochromogenic, nonchromogenic, and rapidly growing mycobacteria. Runyon group I consists of slow-growing photochromogens species that produce carotenoid pigments upon exposure to light. Runyon group II consists of slow-growing scotochromogens that produce a yellow-orange pigment when grown either in light or dark. Runyon group III consists of "nonphotochromogens" that may contain white, tan, or pale yellow pigment. Members of Runyon group IV are designated as rapid growers. The species of other mycobacteria are differentiated on the basis of a variety of morphologic, physiologic, and biochemical characteristics (Table 75-1).

The vast majority of ocular infections that result in clinical disease have been caused by mycobacterial isolates that are rapid growers (group IV), especially *M. fortuitum* or *M. chelonae. M. chelonae* contains two major subspecies: *chelonae* and *abscessus.*

HISTORICAL BACKGROUND

In 1938 an organism isolated from a cold abscess of a Brazilian woman became known as *M. fortuitum.*[8] This acid-fast bacillus was determined to be identical to an organism isolated in 1932 from abscesses in the lymph gland in cows.[42a,72] *M. fortuitum* was later recognized as a potential cause of pulmonary disease.[25] It soon became known that the nontuberculous mycobacteria, formerly conceived as saprophytic organisms, could produce a progressive, potentially fatal disease that is clinically, roentgenographically, and pathologically indistinguishable from lesions produced by *M. tuberculosis.*

EPIDEMIOLOGY

Unlike *M. tuberculosis* and *M. leprae,* other mycobacterial species generally are found free in the natural environment. It is generally assumed that these organisms are con-

---

*Timpe and Runyon, 1954; Runyon, 1959.

TABLE 75-1 DISTINGUISHING LABORATORY CHARACTERISTICS OF MEDICALLY IMPORTANT MYCOBACTERIA

Organism	Optimum Temp (C)	Growth Rate (Days)	Niacin	Nitrate Reduction	Catalase 25	Catalase 68	Tween Hydrolysis	Urease	Arylsulfatase	Growth in 5% NaCl	Iron Uptake
M tuberculosis	37	12-28	+	+	Weak	–	–	+	–	–	–
M. bovis	37	21-40	–	–	Weak	–	–	+	–	–	–
Photochromogens (Runyon group I)											
M. kansasii	37	10-21	–	+	Strong	+	+	+	–	–	–
M. marinum	32	7-14	–	–	Weak	±	+	+	–	–	–
M. simiae	37	7-14	+	–	Strong	+	–	+	–	–	–
Scotochromogens (Runyon group II)											
M. scrofulaceum	37	10-28	–	–	Strong	+	–	+	–	–	–
M. szulgai	37	12-28	–	+	Strong	+	±	+	±	–	–
M. gordonae	37	10-28	–	–	Strong	+	+	–	–	–	–
M. flavescens	37	7-10	–	+	Strong	+	+	+	–	+	–
Nonchromogens (Runyon group III)											
M. avium intracellulare	37	10-21	–	–	Weak	+	–	–	–	–	–
M. xenopi	42	14-28	–	–	Weak	+	–	–	±	–	–
M. ulcerans	32	28-60	–	–	Strong	+	–	–	–	–	–
M. gastri	37	10-21	–	–	Weak	–	+	+	–	–	–
M. terrae	37	10-21	–	+	Strong	+	+	–	–	–	–
M. triviale	37	10-21	–	+	Strong	+	+	–	±	+	–
Rapid growers (Runyon group IV)											
M. fortuitum	37	3-7	–	+	Strong	+	±	+	+	+	+
M. chelonae sp. *abscessus*	37	3-7	–	–	Strong	+	–	+	+	+	–
M. chelonae sp. *chelonae*	37	3-7	–	–	Strong	+	–	+	+	–	–
M. smegmatis	37	3-7	–	+	Strong	±	+	–	–	+	+

(Data from references 54, 63, 74)

tracted from environmental sources and not from other infected humans, as in the case of tuberculosis or leprosy.

Many of the nontuberculous mycobacteria species are ubiquitous and have been found in soil, water, domestic and wild animals, milk, and other food stuffs. Many species have been isolated from a variety of fresh water sources including laboratory and municipal tap water.[10,14,18] Runyon group IV mycobacteria have been documented to multiply readily in commercial distilled water, with persistence of viable stationary-phase populations for over 1 year.[4] *M. fortuitum* and *M. chelonae* are generally more resistant to chemical disinfectants, such as chlorine, than coliforms or other gram-negative bacteria.[4] The widespread presence of Runyon group IV mycobacteria and their relative resistance may account for the identification of several clusters of cases of ocular infections associated with office procedures.[45,51] To prevent office-related outbreaks, recommendations for sterilization of instruments include the use of heat or high-level disinfection with a chemical germicide such as those registered by the Environmental Protection Agency as sterilants and disinfectants.[37]

The frequency of isolation of nontuberculous mycobacteria has increased and the spectrum of human disease has broadened over the last decade.[74] In a recent survey, organisms other than *M. tuberculosis* were found to account for 35% of isolations of potentially pathogenic mycobacteria. In a review of 125 patients with disease caused by rapidly growing mycobacteria, five (4%) had ocular infection, all involving the cornea.[68] *M. chelonae* has been isolated more frequently from ocular infections than *M. fortuitum* in recent years, although they are encountered with equal frequency in nonocular infections.[68]

The vast majority of ocular infections by nontuberculous mycobacteria involve the cornea and are principally caused by the rapid growers *M. fortuitum* and *M. chelonae*. Since the first documented case,[64] *M. fortuitum* has been recognized as an opportunistic pathogen capable of causing intractable keratitis frequently resistant to multiple antibiotics. Although first described in 1953, it was not until 1978 that *M. chelonae* was identified as a causal agent of keratitis.[14] Between 1965 and 1974 virtually all of the reported cases of keratitis secondary to nontuberculous mycobacteria were attributed to *M. fortuitum*.* In more recent years (1978 to 1994) there has been a preponderance of *M. chelonae* isolates that have accounted for the majority of reported corneal infections.† *M. fortuitum* complex is composed of the species *M. fortuitum* and *M. chelonae*, which were not accepted as distinct organisms until 1972.[19,28] As a result some early reports regarding these organisms may have identified the species incorrectly.

Other mycobacterial species also implicated as causes of keratitis include *M. gordonae*,[44] *M. marinum*,[58] and *M. avium-intracellulare*.[27]

CLINICAL FEATURES

A variety of clinical syndromes associated with nontuberculous mycobacteria have been identified (Table 75-2). In tuberculosis, isolation of a single colony of *M. tuberculosis* is always clinically significant. In contrast, the nontuberculous mycobacteria may colonize body surfaces or secretions for prolonged periods without causing disease. Moreover, nontuberculous mycobacteria are ubiquitous in soil, water, and dust and are frequent contaminants of clinical specimens. Thus the differentiation between contamination, colonization, and disease is often difficult.

Nonocular Infections

M. fortuitum complex is a ubiquitous organism that can survive nutritional deprivation and temperature extremes. Most human infections are the result of inoculation during accidental trauma, injection, or surgery. The precise source of surgical contamination has sometimes been indeterminant. Water used to cool a cardioplegia solution was suggested as the source of an outbreak of sternal osteomyelitis following open heart surgery.[29] Contaminated gentian violet used for skin marking was the source of a series of wound infections in plastic surgery.[56] Pulmonary infection with the *M. fortuitum* complex may be acquired hematogenously or by aspiration. Unlike transmission of *M. tuberculosis*, no person-to-person spread has been documented.

Sporadic nontuberculous mycobacteria infections have involved almost every tissue and organ system following cardiothoracic surgery, peritoneal dialysis, hemodialysis, augmentation mammoplasty, and arthroplasty.[68] Infections of the skin and soft tissues with *M. fortuitum* complex have been encountered most frequently. Bronchopulmonary infections usually occur following aspiration in persons with severe underlying diseases or immunosuppression. Other clinical syndromes infrequently encountered include lymphadenitis, suppurative arthritis, osteomyelitis, endocarditis, meningitis, peritonitis, chronic urinary infection, solid pulmonary nodules, bacteremia related to indwelling intravenous catheters, and otitis media.

Keratitis

Clinically, nontuberculous mycobacteria produce relatively slow-progressing keratitis, which may mimic the indolent course of disease caused by other organisms such as fungi, anaerobic bacteria, or herpes simplex virus. Environmental exposure to nontuberculous mycobacteria is the most common route of inoculation, and many patients have a history of antecedent trauma or prior surgery such as penetrating keratoplasty or radial keratotomy. Clinical infection

---

*References 13, 32, 33, 34, 59, 64, 73,75, 77.
†References 7, 13, 21, 27, 30, 38, 39, 40, 41, 43, 44, 45, 50, 51, 58, 69.

TABLE 75-2 CLINICAL SYNDROMES ASSOCIATED WITH NONTUBERCULOUS MYCOBACTERIA

Syndrome	Relatively Common Causes	Less-Frequent Causes
Chronic bronchopulmonary disease (usually adults)	*Mycobacterium avium-intracellulare, M. kansasii*	*M. szulgai, M. xenopi, M. simiae, M. scrofulaceum, M. fortuitum, M. chelone, M. malmoense*
Cervical or other local lymphadenitis (especially children)	*M. avium-intracellulare, M. scrofulaceum*	*M. kansasii, M. fortuitum, M. chelonae*
Skin and soft tissue (swimming pool granuloma)	*M. marinum*	
Sporotrichoid	*M. marinum*	*M. fortuitum, M. chelonae, M. kansasii*
Abscesses, ulcers, sinus tracts	*M. fortuitum, M. chelonae*	*M. haemophilum*
Chronic ulcer	*M. ulcerans*	
Hyperimmune reactions	*M. avium-intracellulare, M. kansasii*	
Skeletal, bone, joint, tendon infection	*M. kansasii, M. avium-intracellulare, M. fortuitum, M. chelonae*	*M. marinum, M. scrofulaceum*
Disseminated infection	*M. avium-intracellulare, M. kansasii*	*M. fortuitum, M. chelonae, M. scrofulaceum*
Genitourinary disease (relatively rare)	*M. avium-intracellulare*	*M. kansasii*

(Data from references 5, 74)

usually develops 2 to 8 weeks after the corneal trauma, but delayed-onset keratitis, occurring as long as 2 years after radial keratotomy, has been reported.[39] Often the patient has been treated with topical corticosteroid prior to the identification of the infection, but it is not clear in many cases whether the infection developed subsequent to or prior to the initiation of corticosteroid therapy. Experimental studies have suggested that *M. fortuitum* keratitis in rabbits is made worse by corticosteroid use.[47]

It is often not possible to differentiate clinically between keratitis caused by nontuberculous mycobacteria and infections attributable to other microorganisms. The typical clinical features include slow evolution and a relative paucity of suppuration (Fig. 75-1), although dense stromal abscesses may form and rarely corneal perforation may occur. Multi-

focal lesions may be visible at presentation (Fig. 75-2). Satellite lesions may also develop as the infection worsens (Fig. 75-3). The presenting corneal lesion has occasionally been linear and described as dendriform with accompanying epithelial ulceration. Nevertheless, differentiation from herpes simplex virus keratitis should be possible; the ability to produce true dendritic epithelial keratitis is unique to certain members of the herpesvirus group. In misdiagnosed cases lack of response to conventional antibacterial or antiviral therapy should raise the possibility of nontuberculous mycobacteria infection. In addition to the more typical features, a broad spectrum of unusual clinical presentations has been reported including ring stromal infiltrate[50] and infectious crystalline keratopathy.[21]

In the earliest stages of disease, the corneal stroma has

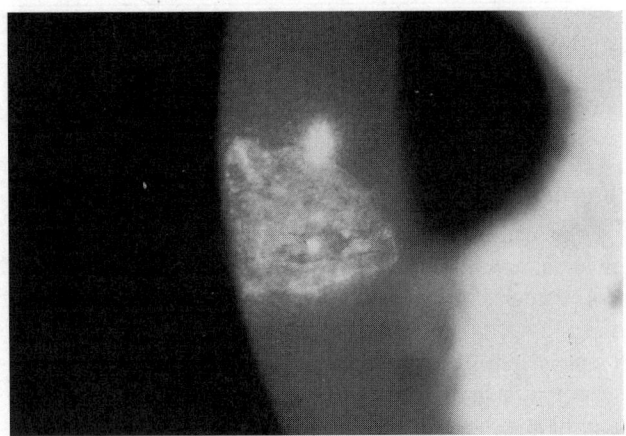

Fig. 75-1. *M. chelonae* keratitis following injury with a corn husk.

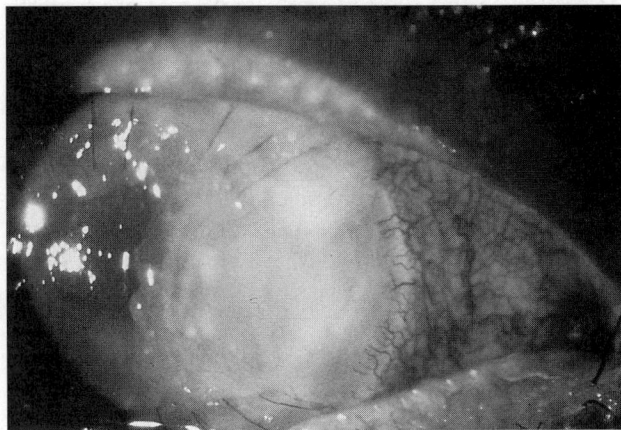

Fig. 75-2. *M. chelonae* keratitis noted 2 months after penetrating keratoplasty. Courtesy of Dan B. Jones, MD.

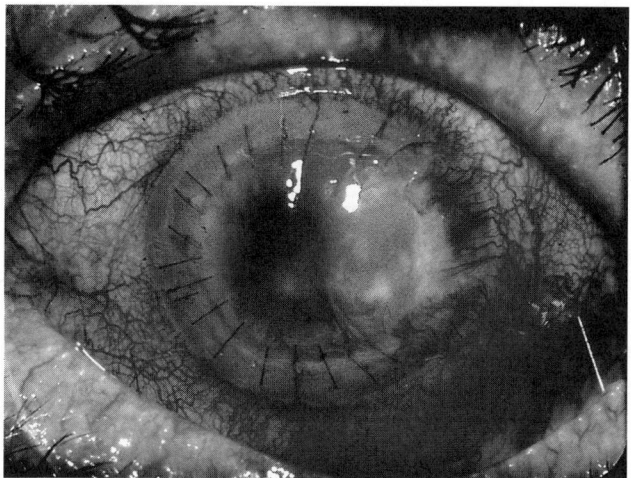

Fig. 75-3. A midstromal "satellite" lesion developed central to the original area of involvement following initial response to topical amikacin therapy. (Figure also in color insert.)

been characterized by thin, radiating lines within the corneal stroma, which give the appearance of "cracked glass."[33] This change lasts for only a few days and may be attributed to separation of the corneal lamellae as organisms spread within the stroma. It may also account for the occasional reports of disease resembling infectious crystalline keratopathy, a disorder that is usually caused by viridans group streptococci.

Extraocular Infections

Noncorneal infections caused by nontuberculous mycobacteria are reported uncommonly. Several cases of extraocular infection, including orbital granuloma,[60] dacryocystitis,[24] and canaliculitis[52] after probing of the nasal lacrimal duct, have been observed. One of the patients had no apparent evidence of systemic disease or compromised immunity. The infections presented as mass lesions associated with variable inflammation; in the case of dacryocystitis, ulceration of the overlying skin developed during the 7 months the patient was lost to follow-up.[24]

Scleritis

A case of scleral abscess caused by *M. chelonae* has been reported following removal of a scleral buckle in an elderly man.[48] Subconjunctival nodules progressed to necrotizing scleral laceration. Although the mycobacteria were not isolated from office solutions, the authors believed that the organisms might have been introduced during removal of the buckle in their office.

Endophthalmitis

Intraocular infection with nontuberculous mycobacteria from both endogenous and exogenous routes has been reported. Endophthalmitis caused by members of Runyon group IV following uncomplicated secondary intraocular lens implantation and cataract extraction has been observed.[53] Infection with the *M. chelonae* subspecies *abscessus* produced multiple spherical white opacities in the anterior vitreous humor, suggestive of fungal infection. In the second infection an organism that was only identified as a pigment-producing member of Runyon group IV produced a nonspecific low-grade uveitis with fibrinous pupillary membrane formation. The one reported case of endogenous *M. chelonae* endophthalmitis[1] occurred in an immunosuppressed 67-year-old man with mycobacteremia in association with osteomyelitis of both calcanei. The unilateral infection evolved rapidly and was characterized by a marked anterior chamber reaction with a small hypopyon and a moderate vitreous humor inflammatory reaction.

Other nontuberculous mycobacterial species have also been implicated as possible causes of uveitis. Sera from a heterogenous group of patients with uveitis were significantly more reactive to nontuberculous mycobacterial antigens than sera from control patients.[71] No patient-disease patterns could be linked with positive reactions; however, nontuberculous mycobacterial species should be considered in the differential diagnosis of chronic low-grade intraocular inflammation, along with other organisms of low virulence including *Propionibacterium acnes*.

PATHOLOGY

Levinson and Harrison[34] described the histopathologic finding of a case of ulcerative keratitis with marked corneal thinning that required therapeutic tectonic keratoplasty. The cellular infiltrate contained equal numbers of neutrophils and mononuclear cells. Special acid-fast stains revealed the presence of acid-fast bacilli. Cultures taken from the edge of the ulcer prior to corneal transplantation revealed *M. fortuitum*. Zimmerman, Turner, and McTigue[77] described the histopathologic features of two cases of *M. fortuitum* keratitis. One case had marked corneal thinning with descemetocele formation followed by perforation. The other infection followed penetrating keratoplasty. In both cases *M. fortuitum* elicited an acute suppurative response rather than a granulomatous reaction. Complete necrosis of the central stroma was observed in the case that ultimately perforated. Microscopic examination of both corneas disclosed areas of extracellular acid-fast bacilli with microabscesses containing intracellular acid-fast organisms.

A variety of detailed pathologic studies have failed to detect grosser microscopic abnormalities that might permit differentiation of one mycobacteria species from another. For example, pulmonary tissues from patients infected with *M. tuberculosis, M. kansasii,* and several of the less commonly encountered species may appear histopathologically identical. Examination of lymph nodes from patients infected with a variety of mycobacteria species has shown a broad spectrum of possible inflammatory responses. Both acute and chronic inflammatory responses have been observed. Acute suppuration, nonnecrotic epithelial tubercules, and caseation have been recorded alone or in combination within the same lymph node. In general, the nontuberculous mycobacteria are somewhat less virulent than *M. tuberculosis* in most laboratory animals. Thus initiation of experimental infection is usually difficult, even using immunosuppressive agents.[47,63]

The poor response of these nontuberculous mycobacteria to conventional antibiotic treatment may result in chronic intractable ulceration with prolonged recruitment of inflammatory cells and their mediators, potentially contributing to stromal destruction.

PATHOGENESIS

The nontuberculous mycobacteria are opportunistic pathogens that produce lesions in areas where local resistance is compromised. Predisposing factors are essential in the pathogenesis of disease by these organisms.[42] There is an apparent direct relationship between nontuberculous mycobacterial pulmonary disease and preexisting injury to the lung, such as emphysema and silicosis.[5,55]

The portal of entry for nontuberculous mycobacteria in disease is not always determined. Nontuberculous mycobacterial organisms are frequently recovered from gastric washings in healthy individuals, suggesting ingestion as a possible route.[2] Among children, the tonsils and adenoids may be a source of infection in a scrofula-like syndrome. The organisms are deposited in the cervical nodes, either by hematogenous or lymphogenous spread.[49] Primary inoculation of nontuberculous mycobacteria through the skin is a well-established route of infection.[36]

Pulmonary infections with *M. fortuitum* complex have been associated with achalasia.[17] Patients with achalasia were found in some way to be specifically susceptible to infection by *M. fortuitum* complex organisms; the infections were apparently due to repeated aspirations of milk followed by invasion of mycobacteria. Experimental studies demonstrated that the presence of a lipoid substance enhanced the virulence of the nontuberculous mycobacteria organisms.[31] These investigations suggested that nontuberculous mycobacteria might be protected from phagocytosis if surrounded by fatty material. A case of mineral oil granuloma of the lung associated with fast-growing nontuberculous mycobacteria has also been reported.[49a] The mineral oil was postulated to increase the virulence of the mycobacteria. Mastitis in cattle has also been observed with fast-growing nontuberculous mycobacteria organisms that is made worse by treatment with drugs solubilized in an oily vehicle.[54]

Because nearly all reported cases of nontuberculous mycobacterial keratitis have followed physical trauma, surgery, or contact lens use, a breakdown in natural host defenses appears to be an important factor in the pathogenesis of disease.

Infection results in multiple foci of disease at various levels within the corneal stroma. The presence of organisms stimulates a mixed acute and chronic inflammatory response.[11,47] The development of granulomatous inflammation appears to play an important part in protecting the cornea against nontuberculous mycobacterial keratitis.[47] Granulomatous inflammation performs a valuable role in preventing the spread of mycobacterial infections and clearing mycobacteria from infected tissue. The suppression of granulomatous inflammation by corticosteroids, which can be long-lasting, may account for the severe and prolonged keratitis seen in patients treated with topical corticosteroids.

LABORATORY INVESTIGATIONS

Ocular infection by nontuberculous mycobacteria may occasionally be suspected by clinical presentation, but the microbiology laboratory is required to confirm the diagnosis and to identify the specific causal agent. Because of their ubiquity in soil, water, and dust, nontuberculous mycobacteria are potentially frequent contaminants of clinical specimens. Thus differentiation between contamination and clinical disease may be problematic. Nontuberculous mycobacteria are sometimes isolated from normal skin and sputum specimens, but their isolation from corneal or intraocular specimens is highly suggestive of infection and should be treated accordingly.

Successful laboratory diagnosis of nontuberculous mycobacterial infection is highly dependent on the vigilance of the clinician. Specific tests must be ordered because these organisms stain poorly by screening dyes, such as Gram stain and acridine orange, and may grow poorly on conventional media. Lectins, which are glycoproteins that can bind specifically to carbohydrate moieties in microbial cell walls, have been used in the fluorescein-conjugated form to visualize many isolates of mycobacteria successfully (Fig. 75-4).[23] Once the presence of the mycobacteria has been identified, a more specific stain such as the Ziehl-Neelsen acid-fast stain can be employed (Fig. 75-5). The state of being acid-fast, a characteristic feature of mycobacteria, is the ability to resist decolorization by acid following staining with carbol fuchsin that is believed to be due to the binding of the dye by mycolic acids present in the cell wall. It is not absolutely specific for mycobacteria. Fungal and bacterial spores, as well as members of the genus *Nocardia,* are also partially acid-fast.

The recommended culture media for the isolation of mycobacteria include Lowenstein-Jensen, Petragnani, Middlebrook 7H10, and Middlebrook 7H11. Although nontuberculous mycobacteria will sometimes proliferate on blood or chocolate agar, media more specific for mycobacteria are necessary for optimal growth. Selected media such as selective 7H11 (Mitchison medium) should be used in addition to the nonselective media. Although members of Runyon group IV are "rapid growers" and may produce positive

Fig. 75-4. Fluorescein-conjugated lectin stain visualizing *M. chelonae* on smear.

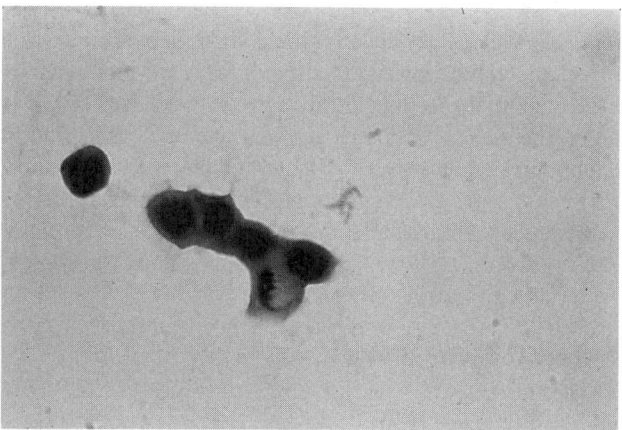

Fig. 75-5. Ziehl-Neelsen acid-fast stain of nontuberculous mycobacteria.

cultures within 7 days, "slow growers" may require several weeks for isolation. In general, antibiotic susceptibility testing requires several weeks for completion, even for the rapid growers. For this reason, tests for susceptibility to antimicrobial agents should be initiated as soon as it is apparent that the organism implicated in disease is likely to grow.

In the past the nontuberculous mycobacterial antigen skin tests have been of limited value.[3,26] Newly formulated nontuberculous mycobacteria antigens available from the Centers for Disease Control and Prevention have been useful in the evaluation of children with lymphadenitis.[9] Their value in the evaluation and management of ocular and periocular infection is not known, however.

THERAPY

The recommended initial therapy for keratitis with acid-fast-stain positive corneal scrapings remains topical administration of amikacin.[62] The current recommended dose of amikacin is 10 to 20 mg/ml, 1 drop every ½ hour as indicated. Slightly higher concentrations and more frequent applications may be used if the clinical response is not adequate.

Concentrations of amikacin as high as 100 mg/ml have been used, without success in some patients.[11] Based on clinical experience and animal studies, prolonged therapy is required, even with organisms believed to be susceptible to a given antibiotic on in vitro testing.

Subconjunctival amikacin (20 mg in 0.5 cc) may be used adjunctively. Systemic amikacin is not routinely used but may be added in selected cases with corneal perforation or extension of infection to involve the sclera.

Other antibiotics reported to be effective against a significant number of isolates of *M. fortuitum* and *M. chelonae* include cefoxitin, ciprofloxacin, doxycycline, erythromycin, imipenem, kanamycin, netilmicin, ofloxacin, and tobramycin. Sulfamethoxazole may sometimes have activity against nontuberculous mycobacteria.

The fluoroquinolones have been shown to be active against the mycobacteria that are most important for causing disease in humans, including some species highly resistant to standard antituberculous drugs. *M. fortuitum* is highly susceptible to the fluoroquinolones, the most active of which have been ciprofloxacin and ofloxacin.* The minimal inhibitory concentrations of ciprofloxacin have varied from 0.01 to 12.5 mg/L. The MICs of ofloxacin have ranged from 0.03 to 1.2 mg/L and no resistant strains have been identified.

In contrast, with the exception of the results reported by Gay, DeYoung, and Roberts[16] and Garcia-Rodriquez and associates[15] for ciprofloxacin, the majority of investigators have found almost all isolates of *M. chelonae* resistant to both ciprofloxacin and ofloxacin.

Experimental animal models[20,46,61] and isolated clinical reports[22] have suggested that topical ciprofloxacin alone or in combination with topical amikacin may be useful in the treatment of nontuberculous mycobacterial keratitis. Experimental studies assessing the in vivo efficacy of newer macrolides, including clarithromycin,[12,35] suggest a potential role in the therapy of *M. fortuitum* keratitis. Nevertheless, limited clinical experience and the reported relative resistance of the *M. chelonae* isolates dictate that caution in patient selection should be exercised in the use of newer fluoroquinolones or macrolides.

Experience with corneal infection by nontuberculous mycobacteria other than *M. fortuitum* or *M. chelonae* is very limited. The ocular isolate of *M. gordonae* was reported to be sensitive to amikacin, as well as to antituberculous medications including ethambutol, rifampin, and streptomycin.[44] The *M. marinum* isolate was sensitive to ethambutol and rifampin, but resistant to isoniazid and streptomycin.[58]

The recognition of corneal infections caused by nontu-

---

*References 15, 16, 57, 66, 67, 76.

berculous mycobacteria other than *M. fortuitum* or *M. chelonae,* as well as the prolonged and unpredictable course of these infections underscore the necessity of obtaining in vitro sensitivity testing for all patients with acid-fast isolates. The therapy of nontuberculous mycobacterial keratitis is complicated, however, by the relatively poor correlation between in vitro susceptibility profiles and clinical response to treatment. Following initial response, the infection may become worse,[38,51] even if the pathogen remains "sensitive" by in vitro susceptibility testing.

Surgical Management

Debridement is a useful adjunctive measure in cases poorly responsive to medical therapy; in one case, debridement alone appeared to cure a superficial corneal infection.[11] Therapeutic penetrating keratoplasty is sometimes indicated and is often successful in arresting the infection in cases in which no improvement occurs despite intensive medical therapy.

Treatment of Noncorneal Infections

One patient with sclerokeratitis caused by *M. chelonae* was treated with debridement and intravenous cefoxitin.[48] Local recurrence was noted at 4 weeks. Topical kanamycin and oral sulfamethoxazole led to resolution. Endophthalmitis attributable to *M. chelonae* has been treated with intravitreal amikacin (250 to 400 micrograms) and a variety of topical and systemic antibiotics, with variable success.[1,53]

No specific recommendations can be made regarding patients with dacryocystitis or orbital granulomata because so few cases are known. One patient with *M. chelonae* dacryocystitis improved following treatment with intravenous amikacin and cefotaxime.[48] The patient with *M. fortuitum* dacryocystitis was lost to follow-up for 7 months. She returned with an ulcerated abscess of the lower eyelid. This lesion was treated with cryotherapy, which was followed by slow healing.[24] The patient with the orbital abscess infected by *M. chelonae* was treated with subtotal excision and oral erythromycin, with good response.[60] In general, systemic therapy, with local excision when appropriate, appears to be the most successful management strategy. Newer macrolides with longer serum half-lives and improved tissue penetration may have a potentially beneficial role.

Corticosteroids

Because of the probable role of corticosteroids in exacerbating mycobacterial infections, avoidance of topical corticosteroid therapy is an important component in the management of these infections. If nontuberculous mycobacterial keratitis is suspected, topical corticosteroid therapy should be discontinued or avoided until the infection can be ruled out.

REFERENCES

1. Ambler JS, Meisler DM, Zakor ZN et al.: Endogenous *Mycobacterium chelonae* endophthalmitis, *Am J Ophthalmol* 108:338-339, 1989.
2. Atwell RJ, Paratt PC: Unclassified mycobacteria in the gastric contents of healthy personnel in patients of a tuberculosis hospital, *Am Rev Resp Dis* 81:888, 1960.
3. Brennan PJ: Structure of the typing antigens of atypical mycobacteria: a brief review of present knowledge, *Rev Infect Dis* 3:905, 1981.
4. Carson LA, Peterson NJ, Favero MS, Aguero SM: Growth characteristics of atypical mycobacteria in water and their comparative resistance to disinfectants, *Appl Environ Microbiol* 36:839-846, 1978.
5. Chapman JS: Atypical mycobacterial infections: pathogenesis, clinical manifestations and treatment, *Med Clin North Am* 51:503, 1967.
6. Dalvisio JR, Pankey GA, Wallace RJ, Jones DB: Clinical usefulness of amikacin and doxycycline in the treatment of infection due to *Mycobacterium fortuitum* and *Mycobacterium chelonei*, *Rev Infect Dis* 3:1068-1074, 1981.
7. Dansby W, Morgan AB, Gilman WN et al.: Epidemiological notes and reports. *Mycobacterium chelonei* infections following eye surgery, *MMWR* 32:591-598, 1983.
8. de Costa P, Cruz Brazi J: Mycobacterium fortuitum um novo bacilo acido-resistente patogenico para o homen, *Acta Med,* 1:297-301, 1938.
9. Del Baccaro MA, Mendelman PM, Nolan C: Diagnostic usefulness of mycobacterial skin test antigens in childhood lymphadenitis, *Pediatr Infect Dis J* 8:210-215, 1989.
10. Dizon D, Milhailescu C, Bae HC: A simple procedure for detection of *Mycobacterium gordonae* in water causing false-positive acid-fast smears, *J Clin Microbiol* 3:211, 1976.
11. Dugel PU, Holland GN, Brown HH et al.: *Mycobacterium chelonei* keratitis, *Am J Ophthalmol* 105:661-669, 1988.
12. Field AJ, Backhoff IK, Dick JD, O'Brien TP: Comparative topical treatment of *Mycobacterium fortuitum* keratitis in rabbits, *Invest Ophthalmol Vis Sci* 34:851, 1993.
13. Gangadharam PR, Lanier JD, Jones DB: Keratitis due to *Mycobacterium chelonei*, *Tubercle* 59:55-60, 1978.
14. Gangadharam PR, Lockhart JA, Awe RJ, Jenkins DE: Mycobacterial contamination through tap water, *Am Rev Respir Dis* 113:894, 1976.
15. Garcia-Rodriguez JA, Garcia-Sanchez JE, Gomez-Garcia AC et al.: In vitro activity of the new quinolones, with special reference to *Mycobacterium, Nocardia,* and *Rhodococcus*, *Rev Infect Dis* 10(suppl 1):S53-S55, 1988.
16. Gay JD, DeYoung DR, Roberts GD: In vitro activities of norfloxacin and ciprofloxacin against *Mycobacterium* tuberculosis, *M. avium* complex, *M. chelonei, M. fortuitum,* and *M. kansasii*, *Antimicrob Agents Chemother* 26:94-96, 1984.
17. Gibson JB: Infection of the lungs by saprophytic mycobacteria in achalasia of the cardia with report of a fatal case showing lipoid pneumonia due to mild, *J Pathol Bacteriol* 65:239, 1953.
18. Goslee S, Wolinsky E: Water as a source of potentially pathogenic mycobacteria, *Am Rev Respir Dis* 113:287-292, 1976.
19. Haas H, Michel J, Sacks T: Identification of *Mycobacterium fortuitum, Mycobacterium abscessus,* and *Mycobacterium borstelense* by polyacrylamide gel electrophoresis of their cell proteins, *Int J Syst Bacteriol* 24:366, 1974.
20. Helm CJ, Holland GN, Lin R et al.: Comparison of topical antibiotics for treating *Mycobacterium fortuitum* keratitis in an animal model, *Am J Ophthalmol* 116:700-707, 1993.
21. Hu FR: Infectious crystalline keratopathy caused by *Mycobacterium fortuitum* and *Pseudomonas aeruginosa*, *Am J Ophthalmol* 109:738-739, 1990.
22. Hwang DG, Biswell R: Ciprofloxacin therapy of *Mycobacterium chelonae* keratitis, *Am J Ophthalmol* 115:114-115, 1993.
23. Jackson M, Chan R, Matoba AY, Robin JB: The use of fluorescein conjugated lectins for visualizing atypical mycobacteria, *Arch Ophthalmol* 107:1206-1209, 1989.
24. Katowitz JA, Kropp TM: *Mycobacterium fortuitum* as a cause for nasolacrimal obstruction and granulomatous eyelid disease, *Ophthalmic Surg* 18:97-99, 1987.
25. Keltz H, Colton R, Lester W: Studies on atypical acid fast organisms obtained from patients with pulmonary tuberculosis, *Am Rev Respir Dis* 103:290, 1957.

26. Kim TC, Arora NS, Aldrich TK et al.: Atypical mycobacterial infections: a clinical study of 92 patients, *South Med J* 74:1304-1308, 1981.

27. Knapp A, Stern GA, Hood CI: *Mycobacterium avium-intracellulare* corneal ulcer, *Cornea* 6:175-180, 1987.

28. Kubica GP, Baess I, Gordon RE et al.: A cooperative numerical analysis of rapidly growing mycobacteria, *J Gen Microbiol* 73:55, 1972.

29. Kuritsky JN, Bullen MG, Broome CV et al.: Sternal wound infections and endocarditis due to organisms of the *Mycobacterium fortuitum* complex, *Ann Intern Med* 98:938-939, 1982.

30. Laflamme MY, Poisson M, Chehade N: *Mycobacterium chelonei* keratitis following penetrating keratoplasty, *Can J Ophthalmol* 22:178-180, 1987.

31. Laporte F: Contributional'etude des bacilles paratuberculeux propriete pathogenes, *Ann Pasteur,* 65:282-325, 1940.

32. Lauring LM, Wergeland FL, Sack GE: Anonymous mycobacterium keratitis, *Am J Ophthalmol* 67:130-133, 1969.

33. Lazar M, Nemet P, Bracha R et al.: *Mycobacterium fortuitum* keratitis, *Am J Ophthalmol* 78:530-532, 1974.

34. Levenson DS, Harrison CH: *Mycobacterium fortuitum* corneal ulcer, *Arch Ophthalmol* 75:189-191, 1966.

35. Lin R, Holland GN, Helm CJ et al.: Comparative efficacy of topical ciprofloxacin for treating *Mycobacterium fortuitum* and *Mycobacterium chelonae* keratitis in an animal model, *Am J Ophthalmol* 117:657-662, 1994.

36. Linell F, Norden A: Mycobacterium balnei: a new acid fast bacillus occurring in swimming pools capable of producing skin lesions in humans, *Acta Tuberc Scand* (suppl 33):1-84, 1954.

37. Lowry PW, Jarvis WR, Oberle AD et al.: *Mycobacterium chelonei* causing otitis media in an ear-nose-throat practice, *N Engl J Med* 319:978-982, 1988.

38. Matoba AY: *Mycobacterium chelonae* keratitis, *Am J Ophthalmol* 103:595-596, 1987.

39. Matoba AY, Torres J, Wilhelmus KR et al.: Bacterial keratitis after radial keratotomy, *Ophthalmology* 96:1171-1175, 1989.

40. McClellan KA, Bernard PJ, Robinson LP et al.: Atypical mycobacterial keratitis, *Aust NZ J Ophthalmol* 17:103-105, 1989.

41. Meisler DM, Friedlander MH, Okumoto M: *Mycobacterium chelonei* keratitis, *Am J Ophthalmol* 94:398-401, 1982.

42. Merck JJ, Soule EH, Alford AG: The histopathology of lesions caused by infection with unclassified acid fast bacteria in man: report of 25 cases, *Am J Clin Pathol* 41:244, 1964.

42a. Minett FC: Avian tuberculosis in cattle in Great Britain, *J Comp Pathol Ther* 45:317, 1932.

43. Mirate DJ, Hull DS, Steel JH Jr et al.: *Mycobacterium chelonei* keratitis: a case report, *Br J Ophthalmol* 67:324-326, 1983.

44. Moore MB, Newton C, Kaufman HE: Chronic keratitis caused by *Mycobacterium gordonae, Am J Ophthalmol* 102:516-521, 1986.

45. Newman PE, Goodman RA, Waring GO III et al.: A cluster of cases of *Mycobacterium chelonei* keratitis associated with outpatient office procedures, *Am J Ophthalmol* 97:344-348, 1984.

46. O'Brien TP, Sawusch MR, Dick JD, Gottsch JD: Comparative topical treatment of atypical mycobacterial keratitis in rabbits, *Invest Ophthalmol Vis Sci* 30:363, 1989.

47. Paschal JF, Holland GN, Sison RF et al.: *Mycobacterium fortuitum* keratitis: clinicopathologic correlates and corticosteroid effects in an animal model, *Cornea* 11:493-499, 1992.

48. Pope Jr J, Sternberg Jr P, McLane NJ et al.: *Mycobacterium chelonae* scleral abscess after removal of a scleral buckle, *Am J Ophthalmol* 107:557-558, 1989.

49. Prissick EH, Masson HM: Cervical lymphadenitis in children caused by chromogenic mycobacteria, *Canad MAJ* 75:798-803, 1956.

49a. Quest JL, Arean Jr VM, Brenner HA: Group IV atypical *Mycobacterium* infection occurring in associated with mineral oil granuloma of lungs, *Am Rev Respir Dis* 95:659, 1967.

50. Richardson P, Crawford GJ, Smith DW et al.: *Mycobacterium chelonei* keratitis, *Aust NZ J Ophthalmol* 17:195-196, 1989.

51. Robin JB, Beatty RF, Dunn S et al.: *Mycobacterium chelonei* keratitis after radial keratotomy, *Am J Ophthalmol* 102:72-79, 1986.

52. Rootman DS, Insler MS, Wolfley DE: Canaliculitis caused by *Mycobacterium chelonae* after lacrimal intubation with silicone tubes, *Can J Ophthalmol* 24:221-222, 1989.

53. Roussel TJ, Stern WH, Goodman DF, Whitcher JP: Postoperative mycobacterial endophthalmitis, *Am J Ophthalmol* 107:403-406, 1989.

54. Runyon EH: Anonymous mycobacteria in pulmonary disease, *Med Clin North Am* 43:273-289, 1959.

55. Runyon EH: Recent developments in mycobacteriosis. In Chapman JS, editor: *Anonymous mycobacteria in human disease,* Springfield, 1960, Charles C Thomas.

56. Safranek TJ, Jarris WR, Carson LA et al.: Mycobacterium chelonae wound infections after plastic surgery employing contaminated gentian violet skin marking solution, *N Engl J Med* 317:197-201, 1987.

57. Saito H, Watanabe T, Tomioka H, Sato K: Susceptibility of various mycobacteria to quinolones, *Rev Infect Dis* 10(suppl 1):52, 1988.

58. Schonherr U, Naumann GOH, Lang GK et al.: Sclerokeratitis caused by *Mycobacterium marinum* 108:607-608, 1989.

59. Sexton RP: *Mycobacterium fortuitum* infection of the cornea. In Polack FM, editor: *Corneal and external diseases of the eye,* Springfield, Illinois, 1976, Charles C Thomas.

60. Smith RE, Salz JJ, Moors R et al.: *Mycobacterium chelonei* and orbital granuloma after tear duct probing, *Am J Ophthalmol* 89:139-141, 1980.

61. Stevens RK, Holland GN, Paschal JF et al.: *Mycobacterium fortuitum* keratitis: a comparison of topical ciprofloxacin and amikacin in an animal model, *Cornea* 11:500-504, 1992.

62. Swenson JM, Wallace RJ Jr, Silcox VA, Thornsberry C: Antimicrobial sensitivity of five subgroups of *Mycobacterium fortuitum* and *Mycobacterium chelonae, Antimicrob Agents Chemother* 28:807-811, 1985.

63. Turner L: Atypical mycobacterial infections in ophthalmology, *Trans Am Ophthalmol Soc* 68:667-729, 1970.

64. Turner L, Stinson I: *Mycobacterium fortuitum* as a cause of corneal ulcer, *Am J Ophthalmol* 60:329-331, 1965.

65. Valero-Guillen PL, Martin-Luengo F, Quintanilla: In vitro activity of some quinone derivatives against *Mycobacterium fortuitum, J Antimicrob Chemother* 15:254-255, 1985.

66. Van Cackenberghe DV: Comparative in-vitro activities of ten fluoroquinolones and fusidic acid against *Mycobacterium* spp., *J Antimicrob Chemother* 26:381-386, 1990.

67. Wallace RJ, Bedsole G, Sumter G et al.: Activities of ciprofloxacin and ofloxacin against rapidly growing mycobacteria with demonstration of acquired resistance following single-drug therapy, *Antimicrob Agents Chemother* 34:65-70, 1990.

68. Wallace RJ, Swenson JM, Silcox VA et al.: Spectrum of disease due to rapidly growing mycobacteria, *Rev Infect Dis* 5:657-679, 1983.

69. Waylard GW, Stacey AR, Marsh RJ: *Mycobacterium chelonei* infection of a corneal graft, *Br J Ophthalmol* 71:690-693, 1987.

70. Wayne LG, Kubica GP: Mycobacteria. In Holt JG, editor: *Bergey's manual of systemic bacteriology,* vol 2, Baltimore, 1986, Williams and Wilkins.

71. Weber JC, Schlaegel TF: Atypical mycobacteria and uveitis, *Am J Ophthalmol* 72:167-170, 1971.

72. Wells AG, Agius E, Smith N: *Mycobacterium fortuitum, Am Rev Tuberc* 72:53-64, 1955.

73. Willis W, Laibson PR: Intractable *Mycobacterium fortuitum* corneal ulcer in man, *Am J Ophthalmol* 71:500-504, 1971.

74. Woods GL, Washington JA II: Mycobacteria other than *Mycobacterium* tuberculosis: review of microbiologic and clinical aspects, *Rev Infect Dis* 9:275-294, 1987.

75. Wunsh SE, Boyle GL, Leopold IH et al.: *Mycobacterium fortuitum* infection of corneal graft, *Arch Ophthalmol* 82:602-607, 1969.

76. Young LS, Berlin OGW, Inderlied CB: Activity of ciprofloxacin and other fluorinated quinolones against mycobacteria, *Am J Med* 82(suppl 4A):23-26, 1987.

77. Zimmerman LE, Turner L, McTigue JW: *Mycobacterium fortuitum* infection of the cornea, *Arch Ophthalmol* 82:596-601, 1969.

76 Nocardial and Actinomycotic Keratitis

ANDREW J.W. HUANG, STEPHEN C. PFLUGFELDER

The bacterial order Actinomycetales comprises three families: Mycobacteriaceae, Actinomycetaceae, and Streptomycetaceae. *Nocardia* and *Actinomyces* are members of the family Actinomycetaceae. Both genera grow as fragile branching filaments that tend to fragment into bacillary and coccoid forms,[22] producing chains of either conidia or arthrospores (Fig. 76-1). *Nocardia* species are aerobic and partially acid-fast, whereas *Actinomyces* species are anaerobic and not acid-fast. With their filamentous growth and mycelia-like colonies, these two actinomycetes have a striking resemblance to fungi.

Confusion may arise in differentiating *Nocardia* species from rapid-growing nontuberculous mycobacteria. Similarities exist between mycobacteria and *Nocardia* species with respect to antigens of the cell wall and bacteriophage susceptibility.[38] *Nocardia* organisms, however, are differentiated from mycobacteria because they are only partially acid-fast and form fragmenting mycelia with true branching. Furthermore, the lipid composition of the cell walls between the two groups also differs.[21] *Nocardia* species and other aerobic pathogenic actinomycetes have a complex cell wall that contains mesodiaminopimelic acid, arabinose, and galactose.[9]

HISTORICAL BACKGROUND

Nocardia and *Actinomyces* organisms are soil organisms, often found in decaying organic matter such as wet hay or straw. Though distributed worldwide, *Nocardia* corneal infections are rarely encountered. The commonly identified species are *N. asteroides, N. brasiliensis, N. otitidis-caviarum, N. farcinica,* and *N. transvaliensis. N. asteroides,* the most common species, was named after Nocard, a French bacteriologist and veterinary pathologist, and for the starlike appearance of the colonies on the agar plate.[9]

EPIDEMIOLOGY

The two most common modes of *Nocardia* infections are (1) inhalation of organisms with suppurative or cavitary pulmonary infection, often simulating tuberculosis, and (2) contamination of skin wounds with soil, causing a localized mycetoma. Pulmonary or generalized *Nocardia* infections have become increasingly prevalent in immunocompromised patients. *Nocardia* organisms may occasionally cause infections in other tissues such as the brain, kidney, and bone. Most intraocular *Nocardia* infections are caused by metastatic spread from pulmonary or other infections,[10,12,19,28,36] although some follow surgical trauma.[28] Endogenous nocardiosis occurs principally in patients with systemic immunosuppression related to antineoplastic therapy or systemic corticosteroids.[24,30]

Nocardial keratitis is usually preceded by minor corneal trauma. Besides keratitis* — conjunctivitis,[27] dacryoadenitis,[1] uveitis,[26] endophthalmitis,[34,36] and contaminated scleral buckles have been reported. Corneal infections of variable severity have been seen more frequently in males, in young adults, and in rural areas. Such preponderances are related to the predisposing roles of minor corneal trauma and soil contact. *Nocardia* organisms represent less than 1% of the corneal isolates from infectious keratitis.

PATHOGENESIS

N. asteroides is a facultative intracellular organism that can persist and grow within macrophages. No exotoxins have been described. *Nocardia* organisms usually do not multiply quickly enough within host tissues to produce a fulminant infection. The nocardial cell wall, composed of a variety of complex lipids, peptides, and polysaccharides, is important in its pathogenicity. Chemical differences in the cell walls of various strains at different stages of growth may explain variations in the pathogenicities of such organisms.[7] Iron seems to be an important factor for the intracellular growth of most *Nocardia* organisms.

The host defense mechanisms against *Nocardia* infections are not completely understood. In general, natural defense is a combination of innate immunity and specific acquired immunity. The exact nature of specific acquired

---

*References 6, 11, 14, 16, 17, 18, 29, 31, 32, 35, 37, 40, 41.

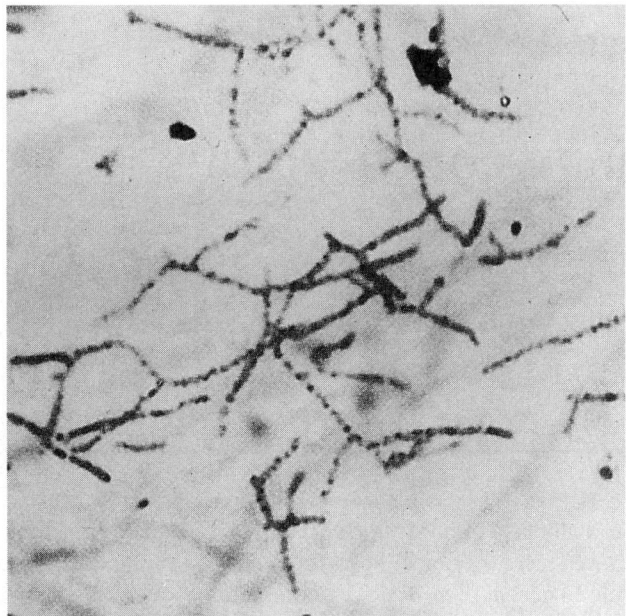

Fig. 76-1. Branching, gram-positive filaments of *Nocardia asteroides* from a corneal scraping.

humoral immunity and cell-mediated immunity contributing to the defense against *Nocardia* infections remains relatively unclear. Both humoral antibodies and delayed hypersensitivity to nocardial antigens have been found in persons with systemic nocardiosis.[3] Studies have also suggested that the resistance to *Nocardia* infections, in contrast to other bacteria such as *Salmonella* organisms, is independent of humoral immunity.[4]

Cell-mediated immunity may play an important role in protection. T-lymphocytes[5] and nonspecifically activated macrophages[15] can inhibit the growth of *N. asteroides*. Furthermore, an animal model of *N. asteroides* keratitis showed that untreated, small corneal lesions eventually healed with vascularization.[29] In infected eyes treated with topical corticosteroids for 3 weeks, large granulomatous lesions with extension into the anterior chamber developed in one third of the steroid-treated rabbits, whereas no intraocular extension was noted in the eyes with keratitis not treated with steroids. The suppression of cell-mediated immunity by corticosteroids is mainly due to macrophage inhibition rather than to T cell suppression. Steroids might have inhibited the macrophages by stabilizing the lysosomal granules and inhibiting the release of lysosomal enzymes, thereby preventing the destruction of phagocytized intracellular *Nocardia* organisms.

CLINICAL FEATURES

Nocardial Keratitis

Nocardial keratitis is characterized by a relatively slow and recalcitrant keratitis. Delay in identification of the causative organism sometimes causes the mistaken topical administration of corticosteroids as adjunctive therapy prior to specific diagnosis. The use of corticosteroids may be a possible predisposing factor compromising the ocular immunity that helps control the infection.

The characteristic morphology of nocardial keratitis is its resemblance to filamentous fungal ulcers. *Nocardia* species should be kept in mind as possible causative organisms in cases (in which a fungal infection is suspected) that do not respond to antifungal therapy. Minimal involvement of the epithelium with nonspecific punctate epitheliopathy is often encountered (Fig. 76-2). The infiltrate is usually located in the midperiphery of the cornea, adjacent to sites of minor corneal trauma or abrasion, with superficial or midstromal involvement. The typical ulcer has a gray, sloughing base and undermined, overhanging necrotic edges. A "brush-fire" border of the infiltrate can at times be observed (Fig. 76-3). Multiple foci of infection or satellite lesions can sometimes be encountered (Figs. 76-3 and 76-4).

Nocardial keratitis is usually refractory to conventional topical antibiotics, resulting in a protracted clinical course and progressive extension of the keratitis. Corneal thinning and a moderate anterior chamber reaction or hypopyon can be observed (Fig. 76-4). The stromal involvement can be grossly granular or nodular in appearance. Eventual resolution leaves superficial stromal scarring and surface irregularities. The differential diagnosis of nocardial keratitis should include *Moraxella* species, nontuberculous mycobacteria, and fungi.

Nocardia species are a somewhat rare cause of primary conjunctivitis[27] that may be either mucopurulent or granulomatous, sometimes associated with the development of sub-

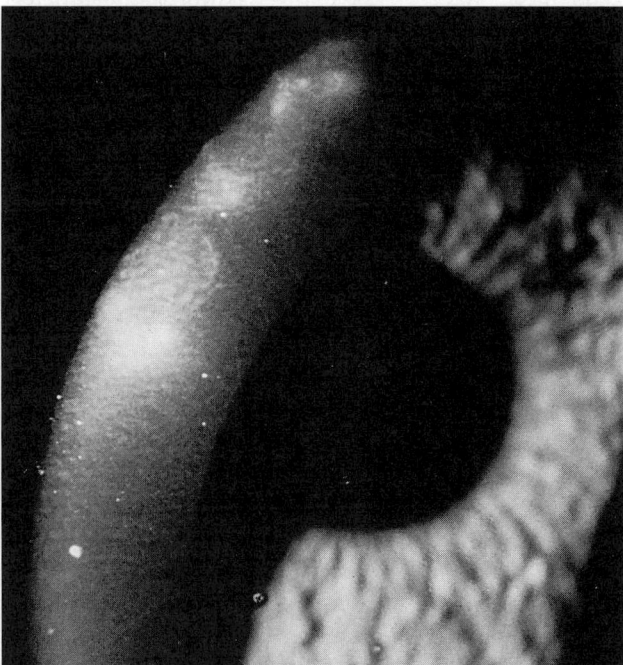

Fig. 76-2. Superficial punctate epitheliopathy and subepithelial infiltrates during early nocardial keratitis.

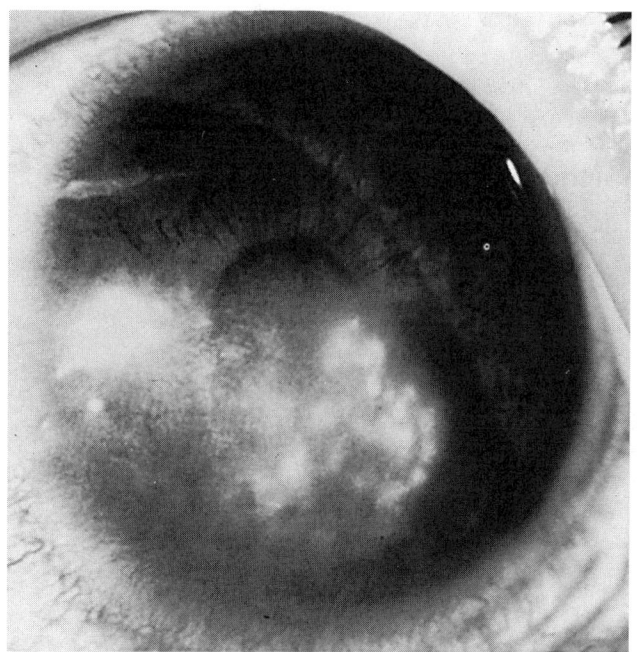

Fig. 76-3. Multifocal, chalky-white infiltrates with minimal inflammation during established nocardial keratitis.

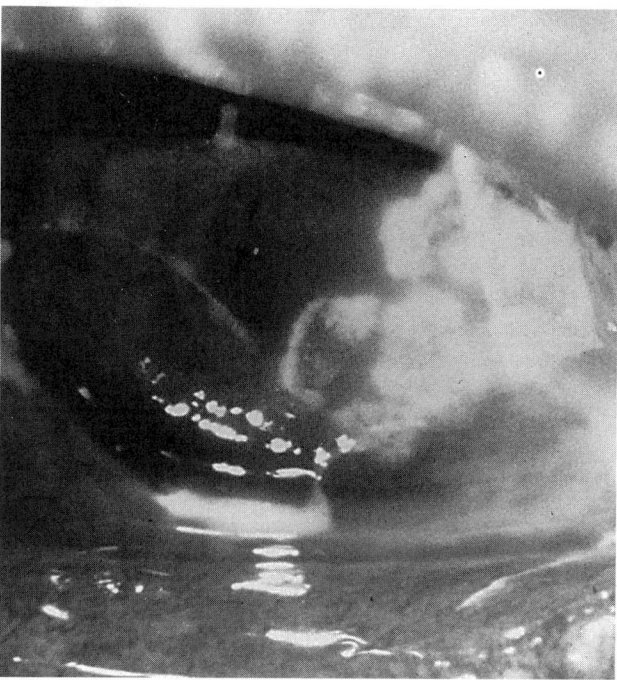

Fig. 76-4. Progressive nocardial keratitis.

conjunctival scar tissue and an interstitial or superficial punctate keratitis. Corneal ulcer may occur from the direct extension from conjunctivitis.

Actinomycotic Keratitis

A primary corneal ulcer attributable to *Actinomyces* species is rare and usually follows corneal trauma. Most reported cases of keratitis are due to *A. israelii*.[33] Actinomycotic keratitis is characterized by a dry ulceration with central necrosis, surrounded by a gutter of demarcation.[8,27] In contrast to nocardial keratitis, iritis and hypopyon usually accompany actinomycotic keratitis. In severe keratitis, descemetocele and perforation may occur.

LABORATORY INVESTIGATIONS

Nocardia organisms are gram-positive, branching pleomorphic rods with intermittent or beaded staining patterns, especially when invading tissues. The organisms stain black with the methenamine silver stain. They are partially acid-fast by the Ziehl-Neelsen technique with acid decolorization.

In early cultures, branching of filaments at right angles is distinctive. In old colonies, these tend to fragment, producing bacillary and coccoid forms more closely resembling bacteria than fungi. The acid-fast characteristics are more obvious in tissue and less evident in culture.

N. asteroides reduces nitrates to nitrites and does not hydrolyze casein, tyrosine, or xanthine.[9] Acid is produced from adonitol, arbutin, dextrin, D-fructose, D-glucose, and occasionally mannose and rhamnose.[9] No acid production is noted from lactose or xylose. Urea, esculin, allantoin, and benzidine are hydrolyzed.

In culture, *Nocardia* organisms are not fastidious but tend to grow slowly. The colonies will grow on most bacterial, fungal, or mycobacterial media that lack antibiotics. Blood and Sabouraud agars are good substrates for pathogenic *Nocardia* organisms that usually grow satisfactorily at temperatures between 35° to 37°C. Growth of *N. asteroides* is facilitated by 10% carbon dioxide. In pure culture, the colonies often grow out after only 48 hours of incubation, but in mixed cultures or in primary isolation from clinical materials, the colonies can take as long as 2 to 4 weeks to appear. The colonies grow well in an aerobic environment, either smooth and moist, waxy and hard, or rough with a velvety surface caused by rudimentary aerial mycelia. They may have a waxy or powdery starlike appearance, and the colonies can be white, tan, buff, or yellow-to-blond in coloration.

Antibiotic susceptibility can be assessed by disc-diffusion and broth-dilution methods. Different *Nocardia* strains vary in antibiotic sensitivity.[7,13,20,23,39] Susceptibility testing varies according to pH and type of agar used in the assay.[17] Thus in vitro susceptibility results may not correlate well with clinical response. Most *Nocardia* isolates are sensitive to sulfonamides such as sulfamethoxazole, trimethoprim-sulfamethoxazole, doxycycline, and amikacin (Table 76-1). Moderate or inconsistent sensitivity occurs to gentamicin, tobramycin, azithromycin, and clarithromycin. Most are resistant to trimethoprim, penicillin and other beta-lactam agents,[13,20] vancomycin, and ciprofloxacin. Many strains produce beta-lactamase.

Actinomyces organisms are usually susceptible to penicillins and cephalosporins.

TABLE 76-1 SENSITIVITY OF CORNEAL ISOLATES OF *NOCARDIA ASTEROIDES* AND *N. BRASILIENSIS*

	MIC$_{50}$*	MIC$_{90}$†	% Sensitive
Trimethoprim-sulfamethoxazole	<.047	>4.0	100%
Doxycycline	<1.5	>4	100%
Amikacin	<.75	>12	100%
Tobramycin	<.75	>48	92%
Gentamicin	<1.5	>16	83%
Imipenem	<2	>32	50%
Ciprofloxacin	>32	>32	25%
Trimethoprim	>32	>32	0
Vancomycin	>256	>256	0
Penicillin	>256	>256	0

*MIC$_{50}$ = Concentration of antibiotic required to inhibit 50% of the isolates.
†MIC$_{90}$ = Concentration of antibiotic required to inhibit 90% of the isolates.

THERAPY

Nocardial Keratitis

Sulfonamides, both systemic and topical, have remained the drug of choice for ocular *Nocardia* infections. Trimethoprim-sulfamethoxazole combinations have also been used successfully in systemic as well as ocular nocardiosis.[2,14,25]

Antibacterial agents. Initial treatment of nocardial keratitis should include topical and systemic trimethoprim-sulfamethoxazole. In the event of refractory or severe keratitis, topical amikacin can be considered with oral doxycycline or minocycline. Newer fluoroquinolones and macrolides show disappointing results against this organism. Because corticosteroids suppress cell-mediated immunity that is pivotal in eradicating the organisms, the use of topical corticosteroids for nocardial keratitis should be limited to the severe cases with extensive intraocular inflammation.

Disease may progress despite appropriate therapy. Diagnostic and excisional biopsies may be considered to facilitate the diagnosis and reduce the extent of corneal involvement.

Successful medical management is feasible. Corneal scarring is often minimal. Nocardial keratitis tends to heal with peripheral corneal vascularization or with vascularized scars. The visual prognosis is usually optimistic.

Surgical management. In the presence of progressive corneal thinning despite prolonged medical therapy, surgical intervention with conjunctival flap or keratoplasty can be considered. Extension beyond the limbus with scleral involvement can sometimes be encountered. Superficial keratectomy and partial-thickness sclerectomy, followed by lamellar corneoscleral patch graft, may effectively eradicate

nocardial keratoscleritis. With deep stromal involvement, penetrating keratoplasty may be required. Judicious use of postoperative antibiotics and corticosteroids may facilitate resolution of corneal and intraocular inflammation.

Actinomycotic Keratitis

The treatment of actinomycotic keratitis used to be excision of necrotic tissue followed by cauterization. Good results have been obtained by subconjunctival penicillin together with systemic iodides. Alternatively, topical sulfacetamide or penicillin can be used.

REFERENCES

1. Archibald RG: Primary nocardiosis of the lacrimal gland, *Lancet* 2:847, 1918.
2. Baikie AG, MacDonald CB, Mundy GR: Systemic nocardiosis treated with trimethoprim and sulphamethoxazole, *Lancet* 2:261, 1970.
3. Beaman BL: Possible mechanisms of nocardial pathogenesis. In Goodfellow M, Brownell GH, Serrano JA, editors: *Biology of the Nocardia* New York, 1976, Academic Press.
4. Beaman BL, Gershwin ME, Ahmed A et al.: Response of CBA/NxDBA2/F$_1$ mice to Nocardia asteroides, *Infect Immun* 35:111-116, 1982.
5. Beaman BL, Gershwin ME, Maslan S: Infectious agents in immunodeficient murine models: pathogenicity of Nocardia asteroides in congenitally athymic (nude) and hereditarily asplenic (Dh/+) mice, *Infect Immun* 20:381-387, 1978.
6. Benedict WL, Iverson HA: Chronic keratoconjunctivitis associated with Nocardia, *Arch Ophthalmol* 32:89-92, 1944.
7. Boiron P, Provost F: In vitro susceptibility testing of Nocardia spp. and its taxonomic implication, *J Antimicrob Chemother* 22:623-629, 1988.
8. Bruce GM, Locatcher-Khorazo D: Actinomyces: recovery of the streptothrix in a case of superficial punctate keratitis, *Arch Ophthalmol* 27:294-298, 1942.
9. Bullock JD: Endogenous ocular nocardiosis: a clinical and experimental study, *Trans Am Ophthalmol Soc* 81:451-531, 1983.
10. Burpee JC, Starke WR: Bilateral metastatic intraocular nocardiosis, *Arch Ophthalmol* 86:666-669, 1971.
11. Climenhaga DB, Tokarewicz AC, Willis NR: Nocardia keratitis, *Can J Ophthalmol* 19:284-286, 1984.
12. Davidson S, Foerster HC: Intraocular nocardial abscess, endogenous, *Trans Am Acad Ophthalmol Otolaryngol* 71:847-850, 1967.
13. Dewsnup DH, Wright DN: In vitro susceptibility of Nocardia asteroides to 25 antimicrobial agents, *Antimicrob Agents Chemother* 25:165-167, 1984.
14. Donnenfeld ED, Cohen EJ, Barza M, Baum J: Treatment of Nocardia keratitis with topical trimethoprim-sulfamethoxazole, *Am J Ophthalmol* 99:601-602, 1985.
15. Filice GA, Beaman BL, Remington JS: Effects of activated macrophages on Nocardia asteroides, *Infect Immun* 27:643-649, 1980.
16. Gingrich WD: Keratomycosis, *JAMA* 179:602-608, 1962.
17. Hirst LW, Harrison KG, Merz WG, Stark WJ: Nocardia asteroides keratitis, *Br J Ophthalmol* 63:449-454, 1979.
18. Hirst LW, Merz WG, Green WR: Nocardia asteroides corneal ulcer, *Am J Ophthalmol* 94:123-124.
19. Jampol IM, Strauch BS, Albert DM: Intraocular nocardiosis, *Am J Ophthalmol* 76:568-573, 1973.
20. Kitzis MD, Gutmann L, Acan JF: In vitro susceptibility of Nocardia asteroides to 21-β-lactam antibiotics, in combination with three β-lactamase inhibitors and its relationship to the β-lactamase content, *J Antimicrob Chemother* 15:23-30, 1985.
21. Lechevalier MP, Horan AC, Lechevalier II: Lipid composition in the classification of Nocardiae and Myobacteria, *J Bacteriol* 105:313-318, 1971.
22. Lennette EH, Spaulding FH, Truant JP: *Manual of clinical microbiology*, ed 3, Washington, DC, 1985, American Society for Microbiology.

23. Lerner PI, Baum GL: Antimicrobial susceptibility of Nocardia species, *Antimicrob Agents Chemother* 4:85-93, 1973.

24. Lissner GS, O'Grady R, Chromokos E: Endogenous intraocular Nocardia asteroides in Hodgkins disease, *Am J Ophthalmol* 86:388-394, 1978.

25. Maderazo EG, Quintiliani R: Treatment of nocardial infection with trimethoprim and sulfamethoxazole, *Am J Med* 57:671-675, 1974.

26. McCarthy JL, Kennedy RJ, Hazard JB: Experimental ocular infection with Nocardia asteroides in the normal rabbits, *Arch Ophthalmol* 62:425-433, 1959.

27. McLean JM: Oculomycosis, *Trans Am Acad Ophthalmol Otolaryngol* 67:149-163, 1963.

28. Meyer SL, Font RL, Shaver RP: Intraocular nocardiosis: report of three cases, *Arch Ophthalmol* 83:536-541, 1970.

29. Newmark E, Polack FM, Ellison AC: Report of a case of Nocardia asteroides keratitis, *Am J Ophthalmol* 72:813-815, 1971.

30. Panijayanond P, Olsson CA, Spivack ML et al.: Intraocular nocardiosis in a renal transplant patient, *Arch Surg* 104:845-847, 1972.

31. Penikett EJK, Rees DL: *Nocardia asteroides* infection, *Am J Ophthalmol* 53:1006-1008, 1962.

32. Ralph RA, Lemp MA, Liss G: Nocardia asteroides keratitis: a case report, *Br J Ophthalmol* 60:104-106, 1976.

33. Roche F: Actynomycose aigue de la cornée, *Bull Soc Ophtalmol Fr* 218-221, 1949.

34. Rogers SJ, Johnson BL: Endogenous Nocardia endophthalmitis: report of a case in a patient treated for lymphocytic lymphoma, *Ann Ophthalmol* 9:1123-1131, 1977.

35. Schardt WM, Unsworth AC, Hayes CV: Corneal ulcer due to Nocardia asteroides, *Am J Ophthalmol* 42:303-305, 1956.

36. Sher NA, Hill CW, Eifrig DE: Bilateral intraocular Nocardia asteroides infection, *Arch Ophthalmol* 95:1415-1418, 1977.

37. Sigtenhorst ML, Gingrich WD: Bacteriologic studies of keratitis, *South Med J* 50:346-350, 1975.

38. Tsukamura M: Relationship between Mycobacterium and Nocardia, *Jap J Microbiol* 14:187-195, 1970.

39. Wallace RJ, Septimus EJ, Musher DM, Martin RR: Disk diffusion susceptibility testing of *Nocardia* species, *J Infect Dis* 135:568-576, 1977.

40. Zimmerman LE: Mycotic keratitis, *Lab Invest* 11:1151-1160, 1962.

41. Zimmerman LE: Keratomycosis, *Surv Ophthalmol* 8:1-25, 1963.

77 Fungal Keratitis

DENIS M. O'DAY

Fungal infections of the cornea were once considered rare and unusual events. In the last two decades, however, there has been a seemingly dramatic increase in the frequency of these infections.[42] Indiscriminate use of antibiotics and corticosteroids has been blamed by some for this phenomenon, but it is more likely that increased clinical awareness and improved diagnostic capabilities have allowed more frequent recognition of this type of infection.

In the past it was not uncommon for a patient to lose an eye as a result of fungal infection. Improved diagnostic techniques and recent advances in therapy have improved the prognosis to the extent that the majority of these infections can now be controlled. Useful vision can be preserved in most cases.

EPIDEMIOLOGY

Keratomycosis is relatively uncommon in the Western world. As a result it has been difficult to accumulate a broad experience with the disease. The literature abounds with single case reports providing insights into the management of difficult or unusual cases, but contributing little to the understanding of the prevalence of particular fungal pathogens or responses to treatment.

Over the years several centers in the United States have collected their experiences with these infections, accumulating numerous cases for analysis.* Ophthalmologists in tropical countries have followed suit.[31,53,91,100] As a result of these efforts, a view of the relative frequency of organisms is beginning to emerge.

The total annual number of cases of fungal keratitis in the United States is approximately 1500. Fungal keratitis is much more common in agrarian, tropical countries.

RISK FACTORS

Fungi are a normal part of the microbial environment. Although the eye is continuously exposed to these microorganisms, the normal external ocular defenses, including the eyelids and tear components, provide adequate protection. Favorable conditions for fungal attachment to corneal epithelial cells (a prerequisite for invasion) are not present in the normal cornea. Fungal infections, in the absence of a precipitating event, are unusual in the human cornea.

The importance of trauma, often trivial and frequently associated with plant material, is well documented in the initiation of fungal infection.[19] In the southern United States and in tropical regions elsewhere in the world, trauma is the most important precipitating cause of keratomycosis. This fact is readily understandable in view of the ubiquitous presence of fungi in these areas (Fig. 77-1). In cooler climates a different spectrum of disease is seen with fungal infection. In these regions mycotic keratitis often occurs in association with dry eye (Fig. 77-2) or in corneas with extensive structural alteration (Fig. 77-3).[61]

It is clear from both individual case reports and published series of cases over the years, that preponderance of a particular fungal genus is likely in a given geographic area. The literature also suggests that many different species and genera of fungi can cause corneal infections. The ability of a given fungus to infect the cornea is probably more related to the condition of the patient or the patient's eye than it is on the specific fungus. The isolates vary by region. In the southern United States septate filamentous fungi, most commonly *Fusarium* or *Aspergillus* species, are more frequent. In the northern states infections caused by *Candida* species are prevalent. Worldwide, *Fusarium* and *Aspergillus* are the most notable fungal pathogens in both frequency and severity.[62]

CLINICAL FEATURES

The onset of a fungal infection of the cornea is almost always insidious. Trauma, usually with vegetable matter, is frequently the precipitating event in an otherwise normal eye. It may be days or even weeks before the infection is

---

*References 8, 14, 21, 42, 45, 46, 48, 57, 84, 110.

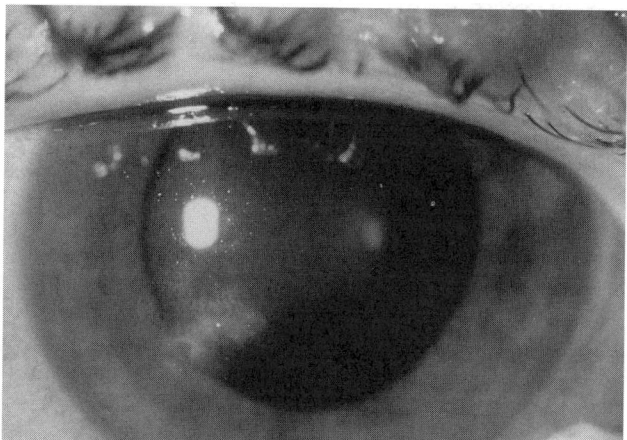

Fig. 77-1. Keratomycosis in early stages 5 days following corneal abrasion. *Acremonium* sp. was isolated.

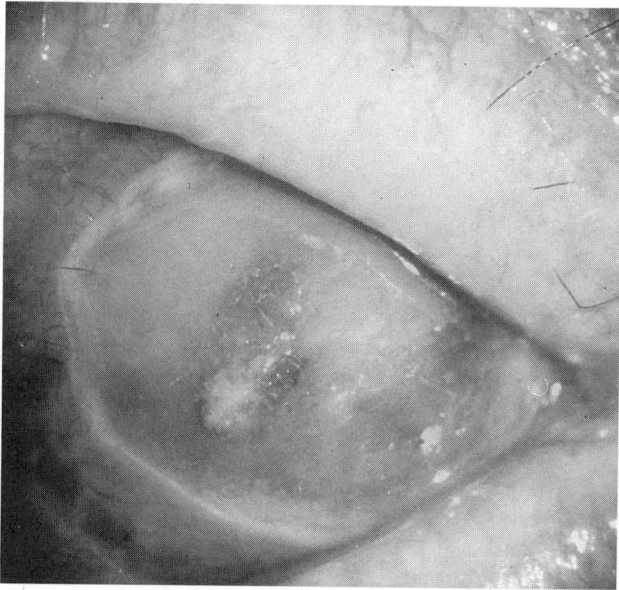

Fig. 77-3. Colonies of *Candida albicans* growing on the corneal surface of a patient with ocular pemphigoid.

recognized, and it is not uncommon for the traumatized epithelium to heal completely before signs of infection supervene. During this latent period the patient may experience little or no discomfort, and the eye may appear to respond to topically applied antibiotics. However, within a highly variable interval, lasting from days to sometimes weeks, the patient becomes aware of discomfort and photophobia, and there may be an accompanying discharge.

During this period a persistent infiltrate at the site of the previous superficial injury is often present. With time, the infiltrate gradually increases in size and density. The epithelium tends to heal over this inflammatory focus, although there may be recurrent episodes of epithelial breakdown. The cornea becomes slightly thickened, and "satellite" lesions may develop peripheral to the focal area of infiltration. If the infiltrate is not overwhelmingly dense, it may be possible, under high magnification, to see actual

fungal filaments coursing through the stroma parallel to the lamellae. In some instances, a partial or complete Wessely ring develops around the central lesions, indicative of antigen-antibody interaction with resultant chemotaxis of polymorphonuclear leukocytes (Fig. 77-4). It is important to remember that findings such as "satellite" lesions and a Wessely ring, though used as strong clinical evidence of fungal infection, may occur in other inflammatory conditions, particularly herpes simplex and acanthamoebic keratitis.

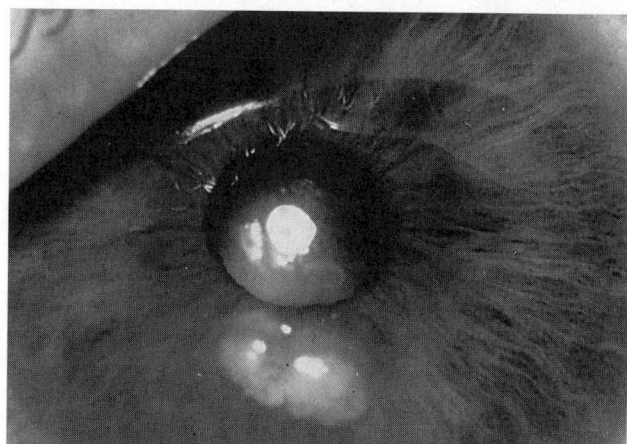

Fig. 77-2. *Candida albicans* keratitis in a patient with dry eyes due to Sjögren syndrome.

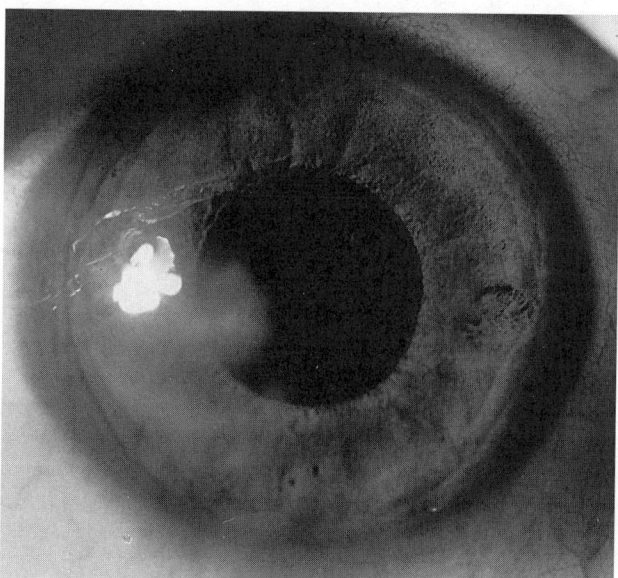

Fig. 77-4. Fungal keratitis with Wessely immune ring partially surrounding the area of active infection.

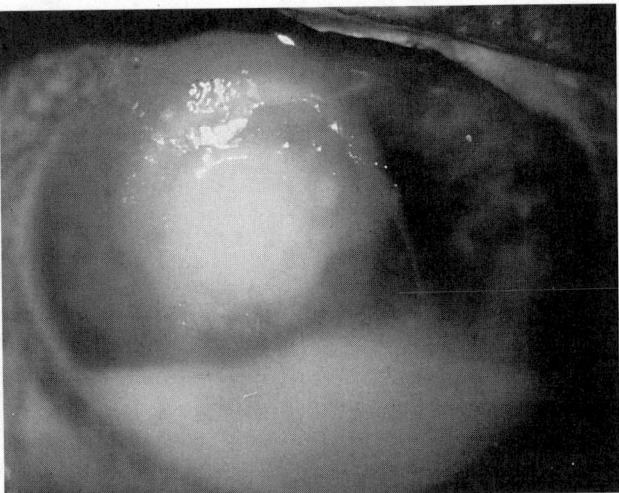

Fig. 77-5. Keratomycosis caused by *Fusarium solani* with hypopyon, partial immune ring, and marked injection.

Untreated, the inflammatory signs gradually progress, causing permanent breakdown of the epithelium, stromal ulceration, and, in some cases, the formation of a descemetocele. Eventually the cornea may perforate. Neovascularization may also occur as a result of the inflammatory stimulus, and ultimately the cornea may be left severely scarred. Associated signs, indicative of the intensity of the developing inflammation, are the presence of ciliary injection and hypopyon (Fig. 77-5). It is not uncommon to see a hypopyon develop in association with corneal infection by a filamentous fungus, even when the lesions appear superficial. Fungi can invade the deep corneal stroma with great rapidity and may gain access to the anterior chamber (Fig. 77-6).[61]

PATHOGENESIS

Fungal corneal pathogens can be divided into three groups. The filamentous fungi are multicellular organisms that produce tubular projections known as hyphae. Hyphae may be septate (Fig. 77-7), having distinct divisions between cellular elements, or nonseptate. Septate filamentous fungi

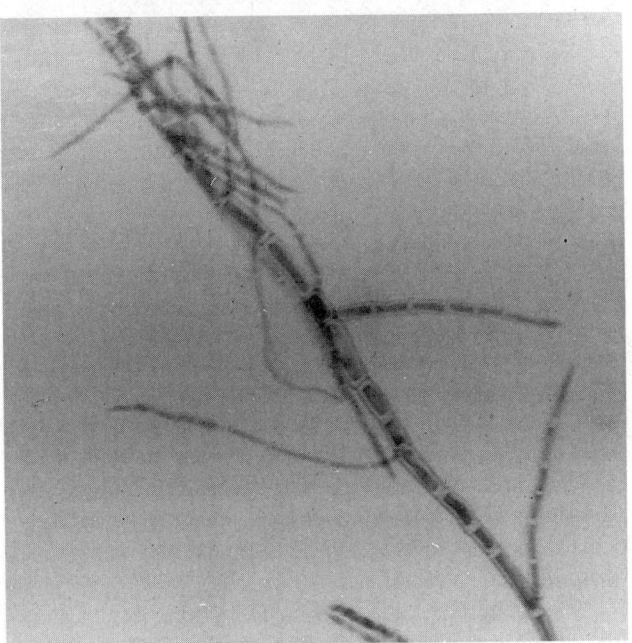

Fig. 77-7. Lactophenol cotton blue stain of fungal hyphae (in vitro); note the cross septations.

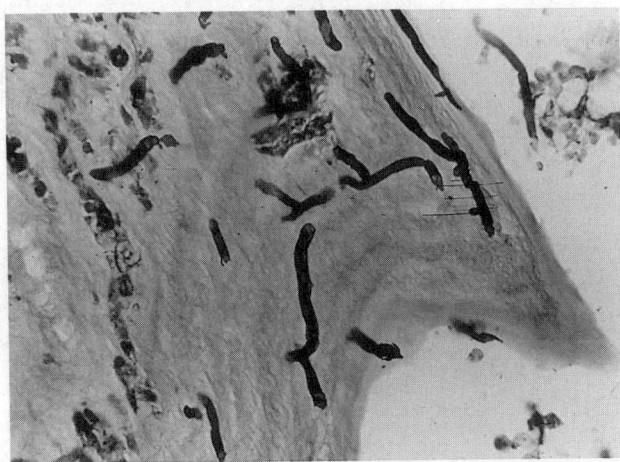

Fig. 77-6. Keratoplasty button showing hyphae at the level of Descemet membrane with invasion of the anterior chamber.

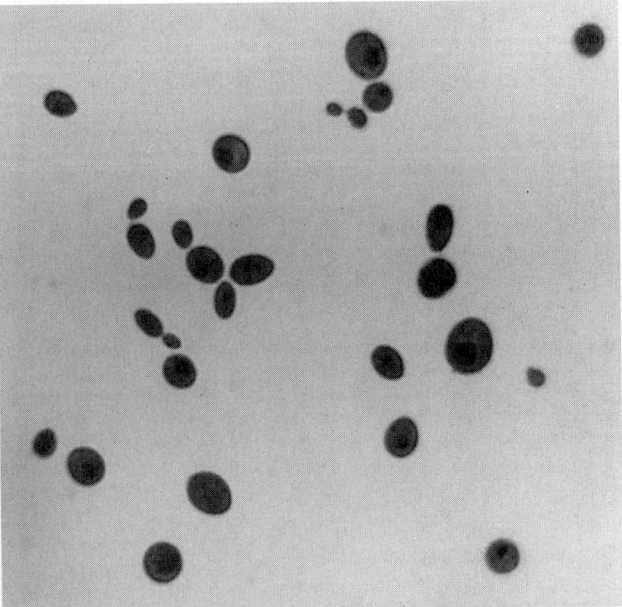

Fig. 77-8. *Candida parapsilosis* in a budding phase of growth in vitro.

are the most important group to cause corneal disease and include *Fusarium* and *Aspergillus* species. The nonseptate filamentous fungi, such as the Zygomycetes, *Rhizopus,* and *Mucor,* are extremely rare as corneal pathogens. Yeasts, making up the second group, are unicellular organisms that reproduce by budding (Fig. 77-8). They may, however, also form hyphae or pseudohyphae. This ability may affect their potential role as pathogenic fungi. *Candida* and *Cryptococcus* species are the yeasts most commonly involved in intraocular infections. Dimorphic fungi can exist in both filamentous and nonfilamentous forms. This third group of fungi, including *Histoplasma,* rarely infects the cornea but is more commonly responsible for hematogenously-spread ocular and orbital diseases. Thus filamentous fungi and yeasts are the most important common corneal pathogens.[62]

LABORATORY INVESTIGATIONS

A major factor in the improved management of fungal infection has been the ability to detect the fungus, thus facilitating the selection of appropriate therapy. A standard, general approach to the management of any suspected keratitis should be followed in every case, because it is impossible on clinical grounds to determine with certainty the infectious cause of the corneal ulcer. In addition, combined infections with bacteria and fungi, or even with multiple fungi, can occur.

Selection of the appropriate media for culture is based on the need to recover the most frequently encountered bacterial and fungal pathogens. Blood agar, Sabouraud dextrose agar, thioglycollate broth, and brain-heart infusion should be routinely employed. When indicated (and this applies particularly to cases in children or instances in which *Haemophilus* infection is suspected), chocolate agar may be substituted for blood agar or used as an additional plate. Fresh culture media should always be used. Media containing inhibitory compounds, such as cycloheximide, should be avoided because they may prevent the recovery of organisms known to be pathogenic in the human cornea that are saprophytes or nonpathogens in other sites.

Techniques for obtaining cultures and inoculating media have been well standardized. The media are listed in the box. Following the application of a topical anesthesia, the epithelium over the lesion, if intact, should be removed. The surface of the lesion and the margins are scraped vigorously with a Kimura spatula or similar instrument. The isolate is then transferred to the culture plate by making a row of "C" marks, reversing the edge of the spatula with each "C", so that all material on the spatula is transferred to the plate. The spatula is then flamed, allowed to cool, and the process is repeated until several rows of "C" streaks have been made on each agar plate. For inoculation into liquid media, the spatula is briefly immersed directly in the culture fluid or wiped onto a cotton swab, which is then inoculated into the medium. Unfortunately, these diagnostic techniques are somewhat cumbersome and present opportunities for contamination by airborne organisms.

Recent studies have demonstrated that direct rubbing of the lesion with either a calcium alginate swab moistened with trypticase soy broth,[3] or a rayon swab moistened with thioglycollate broth[106] may provide a more effective means of recovering isolates in culture from corneal ulcers than the traditional method of scraping with a spatula. Further studies are needed to determine the role of the moistening agent used. There is some concern that this technique may collect tear-film contaminants and could provide additional nutrition to the organisms infecting the cornea.

In vitro susceptibility testing for fungi is available, and clinical decisions can be made on the basis of these tests.[83] The evidence that such studies are of value in selecting therapy in a particular case is still lacking, however. A handful of correlation studies have been performed—all concerned with *Candida* infection and all in animals.[72,73,96] Two studies, the first to involve the eye, have also demonstrated a correlation between in vivo efficacy and in vitro susceptibility for both amphotericin B and natamycin.[73,96] Although these experimental studies suggest that broad correlations can be made, in vitro testing is still very imprecise. Consistency within, let alone between, laboratories is difficult to achieve.[83] Many variables, including inoculum size, media composition, pH, temperature, oxygen tension, and time of reading the endpoint, all influence the values obtained. There is, as yet, no general agreement on how to standardize testing and, until this is achieved, it is doubtful that in vitro testing should be performed for decision-making purposes in particular cases. Ultimately, it remains a most important goal of fungal research.

THERAPY

The morphologic state of fungi in tissue has an important bearing on pharmacologic management. In the cornea both yeasts and filamentous fungi may be present in filamentous forms. The hyphal cell membrane is thus a crucial element to consider in the development of effective antifungal therapy. In addition to its barrier function, the fungal cell membrane modulates electrolyte and solute exchange, and controls the internal homeostasis of the fungal cell. All cell membranes

---

CULTURE MEDIA FOR SUSPECTED FUNGAL KERATITIS

Blood agar
Chocolate agar
Sabouraud dextrose agar without cycloheximide
Brain-heart infusion broth
Thioglycollate broth

contain sterols, but ergosterol is the sterol unique to fungi. In mammalian cell membranes, the principal sterol is cholesterol. Most antifungal agents capitalize on this key difference in plasma membrane constituents to damage the fungal cells while minimizing damage to host mammalian cells.[2]

Effective eradication of fungi is frequently difficult because of the deeply invasive nature of the infectious process. Penetration of the fungus through the cornea into the anterior chamber may occur. Therefore the ideal agent for treating fungal keratitis should exhibit pharmacologic properties that include excellent corneal and intraocular penetration.

Currently available antifungal agents can be divided into three groups: the polyenes, the imidazoles, and the fluorinated pyrimidines (Table 77-1).

Polyenes

The first effective antifungal agents discovered were the polyenes.[28] These compounds share a common molecular structure consisting of a conjugated double-bond system of variable size linked to mycosamine, an amino acid sugar. The various members of this group are classified according to the number of double bonds present. Polyenes bind preferentially to fungal ergosterol, thereby altering membrane permeability and disrupting the fungal cell. Larger polyenes (those with 35 or more carbon atoms), such as nystatin and amphotericin B, and smaller polyenes, such as natamycin, differ in their interaction with fungal cell membrane ergosterol. The larger polyenes, in binding to the cell membrane, are thought to create channels that span the cell membrane and allow electrolyte movement. Polyenes too small to bridge the width of the cell membrane may alter membrane permeability by creating localized disruptions in the membrane.[58]

Amphotericin B (Fungizone, Fungispec, Fungilin, Ampho-Moronal). Amphotericin B, a heptaene polyene (7 double bonds), was the first polyene effective in treating systemic mycoses. Produced by *Streptomyces nodosus,* it was identified in a soil culture from Venezuela in 1956 by Gold, Stout, Pagano, and Donovick.[28] Amphotericin B is insoluble in water and relatively unstable at 37°C. The commercial manufacture of this preparation Fungizone* overcomes these difficulties by dissolving amphotericin B in acid and adding sodium deoxycholate. In vivo, the rapid tissue binding characteristic of amphotericin B limits the actual amount of drug that is bioactive. In vitro, methyl esterification of amphotericin B was attempted to enhance water solubility while maintaining good antifungal activity. Development of amphotericin B methyl ester and similar

---

*E.R. Squibb & Sons, Princeton, NJ.

TABLE 77-1 ANTIFUNGAL AGENTS

Polyenes	Imidazoles	Triazoles	Fluorinated Pyrimidines
Amphotericin B	Miconazole	Fluconazole	Flucytosine
Natamycin	Clotrimazole	Itraconazole	
Nystatin	Ketoconazole	Saperconazole	
	Econazole		

analogues was halted, however, when evidence of severe toxicity emerged.[17]

Route of Administration. Amphotericin B for intravenous use is dispensed in vials containing 50 mg of amphotericin B powder, 41 mg of sodium deoxycholate, and a sodium phosphate buffer. The powder is initially reconstituted to a concentration of 5 mg/ml in 10 ml of sterile water for injection. For topical application, this solution is further diluted with sterile water to concentrations of 0.05% to 0.15%.[110,111] When stored at 36°C, it retains potency for 1 week. Care must be taken to handle the solution in an aseptic manner as the preparation does not contain a bacteriostatic agent.

The efficacy of topical amphotericin B has been studied clinically and experimentally using concentrations ranging from 0.003% to 0.3%.[74] The corneal epithelium appears to be a powerful barrier to corneal penetration of the drug. In experimental animals, intact epithelia prevented the corneal penetration of topical amphotericin B 0.15%, whereas epithelial debridement greatly increased drug penetration into the cornea.[65,66] Topical amphotericin B efficacy in an animal model of keratitis was also greatly enhanced by removal of the epithelial barrier.[69]

Evidence suggests topical amphotericin B can penetrate deep corneal stroma and enter the aqueous. Amphotericin B 0.15% administered topically was present in the cornea and aqueous of rabbit eyes inflamed by the intrastromal injection of clove oil.[66] Although only 7% of the drug was in a bioactive form in the corneal tissue and 5% in the aqueous, this amount appeared adequate for susceptible organisms.[65,72]

Topical amphotericin B has been used to treat mycotic keratitis since 1959, although toxicity has been a troublesome complication. Amphotericin B diluted to a concentration of 0.15% is efficacious and produces far fewer toxic effects than the higher concentrations previously used.[111] Because of residual problems with toxicity, even at this concentration, the concentration has been reduced to 0.05%. Even with this lower concentration the drug continued to show efficacy in another small series of cases.[110]

The efficacy of dilute amphotericin B has also been established in experimental studies.[74] Although the optimal rate of administration is not precisely established, animal experiments suggest that following very rapid administration (every 5 minutes for 1 hour) drug levels within the therapeutic range can rapidly be achieved in the cornea.[66] After this intensive treatment period, a less-frequent rate of administration may maintain adequate drug levels in the cornea.[65,66]

Subconjunctival administration of amphotericin B has been advocated for the treatment of fungal keratitis. The injections, however, are quite painful and poorly tolerated. Ulceration and necrosis of the overlying conjunctival epithelium may occur. In rabbits, subconjunctival injections of amphotericin B produced only trace amounts of the drug in the aqueous model,[76] while inducing severe inflammatory changes in the conjunctiva, sclera, and anterior uvea (Fig. 77-9).

The use of systemic amphotericin B in the treatment of fungal keratitis has not been studied experimentally to a significant extent. In one animal model of chemical keratitis, amphotericin B could not be detected in the aqueous after intravenous administration.[29] Intravenous administration carries a serious risk of systemic effects, including renal toxicity, chills, fever, phlebitis, and anemia.[58]

Efficacy and Spectrum of Activity. In the treatment of systemic mycoses, amphotericin B is often the most efficacious agent against yeasts, particularly *Candida* and *Cryptococcus* spp. It is much less useful in filamentous fungal infections, however. In the eye, the situation is similar. Studies of experimental *Candida albicans* keratitis showed topical amphotericin B, in concentrations of 0.15% or 0.075%, superior in efficacy to 5% natamycin, 1% flucytosine, 1% miconazole, 1% econazole, and 1% ketocona-

zole.[69,75] Although amphotericin B exerts antifungal activity against *Aspergillus,* it appears of limited usefulness against most filamentous fungi.

In addition to its direct fungicidal activity, amphotericin B has modest immunoadjuvant properties. Administration of systemic amphotericin B in a murine model was associated with an increase in the number of antibody-producing cells in the spleen and lymph nodes. Amphotericin B may interact with T-lymphocytes to enhance host resistance to infection.[94] Whether topical amphotericin B also exhibits immunoadjuvant properties is unknown.

Toxicity. The toxic effects of topical amphotericin B appear to be related in part to the effects of the bile salt, sodium deoxycholate, used as a solubilizer. These effects include chemosis, burning, epithelial clouding, and punctate epithelial erosions. In extreme cases the cornea may assume a greenish hue. In the rabbit, topical 1% amphotericin B retarded the healing of epithelial defects. Toxicity of topical amphotericin B can be minimized by using more dilute preparations (0.15% and less).[110,111]

Natamycin (Pimaricin, Pimafucin, Natacyn, Myoprozine, Tennecetin). Natamycin is a tetraene polyene that is the only antifungal commercially available in the United States in a topical ophthalmic form (Natacyn 5%*). The agent, discovered in 1958, is one of the most valuable ocular antifungal agents discovered to date.[97]

Route of Administration. Natacyn, a commercial preparation of natamycin, may be stored at room temperature or refrigerated, but exposure to light or temperature extremes should be avoided. Like other polyenes, it is insoluble in water. The commercial preparation is a 5% suspension that must be shaken well before use. Natamycin often adheres to areas of corneal ulceration, perhaps increasing the duration of drug contact. The drug cannot be administered systemically.

Although the optimal dosing schedule for topical administration is not known, a loading dose approach in which one drop is instilled into the conjunctival sac at half-hour intervals appears appropriate initially. This rate can then be gradually reduced to 1 hourly drop (6 to 8 times daily) after the first 3 to 4 days of administration.

Natamycin has been considered to be poorly absorbed by the cornea. Its demonstrated efficacy in proven extensive fungal keratitis and the results of a recent experimental study suggest, however, that this may not be the case. Large amounts of radiolabeled natamycin can be detected in the cornea after intensive topical administration.[66] Moreover, substantial levels can be detected in the aqueous. What has been thought to be poor corneal penetration may actually be

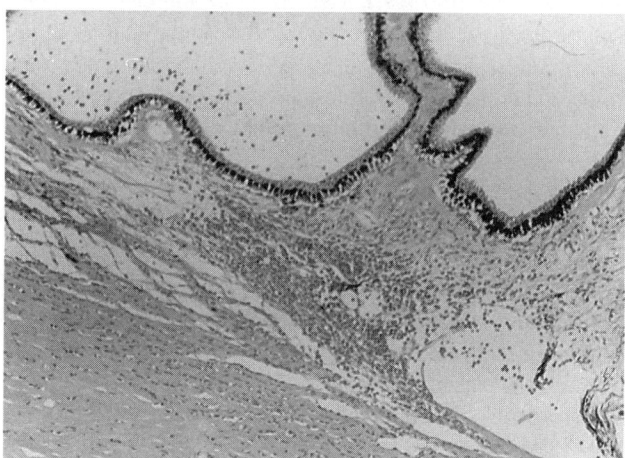

Fig. 77-9. Severe inflammatory changes in the ciliary body of a rabbit eye 24 hours following the injection of 1500 μg of amphotericin B.

---

*Alcon Laboratories, Ft Worth, TX.

poor bioavailability. Because of high tissue binding, only about 2% of total tissue natamycin in the cornea is in a bioavailable state. Fortunately, the relatively high total corneal drug concentration ensures that adequate amounts of bioactive drug are available. As with amphotericin B, the corneal epithelium is a major barrier to corneal penetration. Removal of the epithelium dramatically enhances penetration and efficacy.[66,69]

Efficacy and Spectrum of Activity. Natamycin is effective against many filamentous fungi and has been of particular use in the treatment of *Fusarium* and *Aspergillus* infections, the commonest cause of fungal keratitis around the world.[62] Treatment failures do occur, but numerous series of patients have established the primacy of natamycin in the treatment of fungal infections caused by filamentous fungi.[20,47,60] Yeasts, such as *Candida* species, tend to be less sensitive to treatment with natamycin.

Toxicity. In general, topical natamycin is well tolerated. Corneal toxicity, usually in the form of punctate keratitis, is uncommon, although low-grade inflammation may develop with prolonged use. In an animal model, natamycin did not retard the healing of corneal epithelial defects.[22] The development of conjunctival necrosis following subconjunctival injection precludes its use by this route.

Nystatin (Mycostatin, Moronal, Fungicidin, Mycolog, Candio-Hermal, Diastatin, Nyspes, Nystan, Nystavescent, Polyfungin A). Nystatin was the first polyene antibiotic to be identified.[34] It has been recommended for topical ocular use, but corneal toxicity and poor ocular penetration limit its value. Parenteral administration is not well tolerated.

Imidazoles

In 1965 the antiprotozoal compound thiabendazole, a substituted benzimidazole, was shown to have antifungal activity in vitro. This discovery led to the development of a new class of potent antifungal agents, the imidazoles. Several of these—miconazole, ketoconazole, fluconazole, itraconazole, and clotrimazole—are now commercially available in the United States. In general, imidazoles exhibit fungistatic activities in vitro at low concentrations and fungicidal activity at high concentrations. They appear to have two distinct mechanisms of action.[98] Inhibition of ergosterol synthesis is believed responsible for the fungistatic activity observed at low concentrations.[98] Fungicidal activity observed at higher concentrations appears to be due to direct membrane damage to the fungal cell wall that is unrelated to inhibition of ergosterol synthesis.[2] This fungicidal effect is dependent on the growth phase of the susceptible organism and is observed with clotrimazole and miconazole, but not with ketoconazole. The drug levels required to produce the fungicidal activity, however, are higher than can be reasonably attained and sustained within ocular tissues. From a practical standpoint, the imidazole compounds exhibit fungistatic activity only. In addition, the variable spectrum of activity among the imidazoles may be due in part to a differential affinity for phospholipid components of the fungal cell membrane.[54]

Miconazole (Monistat, Micatin, Gyno-daktarin, Dermonistat). Miconazole, first synthesized in Belgium in 1969, is a phenethyl imidazole.[27] In addition to its antifungal properties, miconazole also exhibits mild activity against gram-positive bacteria.[102]

Route of Administration. The antifungal activity of miconazole appears to result from an alteration in the fungal cell wall that induces permeability changes. It can be administered by subconjunctival, topical, and intravenous routes. In the rabbit, the pharmacokinetics of subconjunctivally administered miconazole are poor.[23] When given intravenously, miconazole can be detected in the aqueous humor. According to case reports, intravenously administered miconazole has been used successfully to treat human corneal fungal infections.[40]

Miconazole can be prepared for topical administration as a 1% drop in polyethylene glycol or as a 2% cream. The commercially available intravenous preparation (Monistat) can be administered topically (10 mg/ml) or by subconjunctival injection (5 to 10 mg). The corneal epithelium appears to be a potent barrier following topical administration, but the drug easily enters the debrided cornea.[23]

Efficacy and Spectrum of Activity. Miconazole has a broad spectrum of activity against yeast and filamentous fungi in vitro, although individual strains may be resistant.

Toxicity. Topical miconazole 1% exhibits minimal toxicity characterized by conjunctival injection and punctate epithelial corneal erosions. In a rabbit model, the rate of healing of epithelial defects was not retarded by administration of 1% miconazole drops.[22] Similarly, subconjunctival miconazole appears to be well tolerated.[23]

Ketoconazole (Nizoral). Ketoconazole inhibits ergosterol synthesis in vivo, thus damaging the fungal cell wall and altering electrolyte concentration. The increased water solubility and enhanced systemic adsorption of ketoconazole are valuable properties of this drug that set it apart from the earlier imidazoles.[99]

Route of Administration. Chu, Foster, Moran, and Giovanoni[9] reported that ketoconazole can produce good drug levels in the cornea when administered topically, subconjunctivally, or orally. More recently, Savani, Perfect, Cobo, and Durack[93] reported high levels in the aqueous, but very low corneal levels 4 hours after an oral dose of 80 mg.

Initial experience with oral and topical ketoconazole in the treatment of human corneal infection has been promising.[39] The most reliable predictor of success is the severity of the infection at initiation of therapy. Most patients with "nonsevere" infections show an "excellent" response, but only one fourth of patients with "severe" ulcers achieved an "excellent" response.[86] Patients with corneal ulcers caused by infection with *Fusarium solani* have been successfully treated with orally administered ketoconazole, 300 mg per day. Using combined therapy of topical and subconjunctival miconazole and oral ketoconazole, healing occurred in a series of 13 of 20 patients with fungal corneal ulcers.[18]

Ketoconazole can be administered as a topical preparation in concentrations ranging from 1% to 5%. The optimal dosing schedule of topical ketoconazole has yet to be determined.

Efficacy and Spectrum of Activity. In vitro, ketoconazole has a wide spectrum of activity. Clinically, the agent appears effective against some species of *Candida, Aspergillus, Fusarium* and *Curvularia,* in particular.[99] In one animal study of a stromal *Aspergillus* infection, however, neither topical nor oral ketoconazole was effective in eradicating the infection, despite moderate sensitivity to the drug in vitro.[52] Further work is needed before the appropriate role of ketoconazole is elucidated fully.

Toxicity. Systemically administered ketoconazole appears to be relatively safe, although hepatotoxicity has been reported, as evidenced by increased liver enzymes. The hepatotoxicity of systemic ketoconazole is usually reversible with cessation of the drug, although recovery may be slow; rarely, death has been reported.[56] Topical preparations of ketoconazole are well tolerated; 1% ketoconazole did not retard the closure of epithelial defects in the rabbit cornea.[22]

Fluconazole (Diflucan). Fluconazole is a member of a new group of agents, the triazoles, derived from the imidazoles. The primary antifungal activity of fluconazole is against yeasts and certain filamentous fungi.[16,51,82,89]

Route of Administration. Fluconazole is water soluble and has excellent absorption when given orally.[55] In contrast to the polyenes and the imidazoles, fluconazole has a low affinity for plasma proteins.[38,93] After oral and intravenous administration, the agent is distributed in body tissues including brain and eye.[24,64] Experimental single-dose studies (20 mg/kg) showed that a once- or twice-a-day administration was sufficient to maintain therapeutic levels in the cornea against most susceptible fungi.[64]

Fluconazole can be used topically as a 0.2% solution in a balanced salt solution with adequate corneal and aqueous levels attainable.[7] Following subconjunctival administration peak corneal concentrations occur soon after injection and drop rapidly in the first 8 hours.[50]

Efficacy and Spectrum of Activity. Fluconazole has good anticandidal activity, and there is some evidence of activity against *Aspergillus* sp. also.[16,51,82,89] Although there are no case series or controlled trials of therapy in patients with this agent for ophthalmic infection, studies with systemic mycoses and isolated case reports of corneal and intraocular infections suggest that fluconazole may be a preferred alternative to amphotericin B for candidal infections and should be considered as adjunctive therapy for infections caused by aspergillic. Experience with experimental infections in rab-

bit corneas has been disappointing, although this agent may have value in endogenous endophthalmitis.[80,107] Fluconazole appears to be the first antifungal agent with potential value as systemic therapy for severe corneal and anterior segment fungal infections.

Itraconazole (Sporanox). Itraconazole, also a member of the triazole group of compounds, has a spectrum of activity similar to that of ketoconazole and fluconazole. There is indirect evidence of better activity against filamentous fungi, particularly *Aspergillus fumigatus.**

Route of Administration. Itraconazole is poorly soluble in water and is highly protein bound, limiting its bioavailability in tissue. Tissue levels are inferior to those achieved with fluconazole on systemic administration. Studies indicate a poor penetration of the cerebrospinal fluid.[93] Paradoxically, itraconazole, despite this seemingly poor pharmacologic profile, has demonstrated efficacy on systemic administration in a number of different experimental infections and in human case studies.† Corneal penetration was reported to be < 0.05 μg/g following systemic administration.[93] Studies with subconjunctival itraconazole indicate a superior pharmacokinetic profile compared to other azole compounds. Subconjunctival injection may be a useful route of therapy.[50]

Itraconazole shows a much higher affinity in vitro for cytochrome P450 than either fluconazole or miconazole.[105] This fact may partially explain observations of clinical efficacy despite lower tissue concentrations.

Efficacy and Spectrum of Activity. Itraconazole has a spectrum of activity similar to that of ketoconazole and fluconazole. Studies of topical therapy have not been reported. A recent report of subconjunctival therapy of experimental aspergillic keratitis showed a therapeutic effect over a 5-day treatment period.[35]

Saperconazole. Saperconazole is an experimental lipophilic triazole that appears to be highly effective against *Aspergillus* sp. as well as *Candida albicans* in vitro.‡

Route of Administration. Like most azole compounds, saperconazole is poorly soluble in water. This problem is being addressed by the concurrent development of hydroxypropyl-β-cyclodextrin as a vehicle to aid in solubilizing lipophilic agents.

Following topical administration in rabbits, excellent corneal penetration was observed in eyes that had been debrided of corneal epithelium; the corneal epithelium was a significant barrier to drug penetration. Ocular uptake was generally poor following oral administration of the drug. Thirty minutes following topical administration, 40% of the drug found in the cornea was biologically active.[67]

---

*References 6, 10, 11-13, 33, 36, 87, 101, 108, 109.
†References 6, 10, 13, 32, 33, 87, 101, 108, 109.
‡References 4, 11, 12, 26, 41, 79, 81, 90, 103, 104.

Efficacy and Spectrum of Activity. Although there are few studies of in vivo therapeutic efficacy,[26,81,104] saperconazole shows promise as a topically applied antifungal agent. **Clotrimazole (Canesten, Lotrimin, Mycosporin).** First synthesized by the Bayer Research Laboratories in Germany in 1967, clotrimazole is a chlorinated trityl imidazole.

Route of Administration. A topical ophthalmic preparation of clotrimazole can be made with 1% clotrimazole in arachis (peanut) oil.[42] Canesten,* a commercial topical preparation, is not available in the United States.[43] A dermatologic cream containing clotrimazole 1% (Lotrimin cream 1%) is tolerated when applied to the eye.[78] Care must be taken, however, not to use the dermatologic lotion that contains harmful alcohols.

Clotrimazole is poorly soluble in water and cannot be given parenterally. It is rapidly absorbed by mouth, however, and satisfactory blood levels can be maintained for a week or two after the initiation of therapy. Unfortunately, clotrimazole induces microsomal enzyme oxidation, so these drug levels cannot be maintained. Hepatotoxicity, nausea, and diarrhea have been reported with systemic administration.[58,61]

Efficacy and Spectrum of Activity. In vitro clotrimazole has broad antifungal activity. In vivo efficacy studies are lacking for this agent.

Toxicity. Topical clotrimazole 1% in arachis oil or as the dermatologic cream has been well tolerated in humans, but punctate keratopathy and ocular irritation have been reported from long-term use.[22,78] The safety and efficacy of subconjunctival and intracameral clotrimazole have not been thoroughly evaluated.

Econazole (Ecostatin, Pevaryl). Econazole, a dichlorimidazole, exhibits a wide spectrum of activity against filamentous fungi in vitro.[77] It appears to be less effective than miconazole against *Candida* species. A topical preparation of econazole 1% can be prepared and appears to be well tolerated.[42] There are no plans to market econazole in the United States at the present time.

Fluorinated Pyrimidines

Flucytosine (5-Fluorocytosine, Alcobon, Ancobon, Ancotil). Flucytosine (5-fluorocytosine) is a fluorinated pyrimidine that was first synthesized in 1957 as an antimetabolite in the treatment of leukemia. The antifungal properties of flucytosine were first described by Grunberg, Titsworth, and Bennett[30] in 1963.

Route of Administration. Flucytosine is transported across the fungal cell membrane by a specific permease elaborated by certain fungi. Once in the cell, the agent is deaminated to fluorouracil, a thymidine analogue that blocks further fungal thymidine synthesis.[15] Because mammalian

cells do not normally metabolize flucytosine, it does not inhibit metabolic processes in mammalian cells. The drug is well absorbed by the gastrointestinal tract. Therapeutic levels can be achieved in adults with the administration of a dosage of 50 to 150 mg/kg/day in divided doses.[15]

Flucytosine is moderately soluble in water. A topical preparation can be made by dissolving the contents of a capsule of flucytosine in artificial tears.[22] The solution should be filtered before use to remove any undissolved material. Flucytosine has been used with success as a 1% solution topically.[88] In an animal model of *Candida albicans* keratitis, 1% flucytosine was ranked in efficacy behind 0.15% and 0.075% amphotericin B and 5% natamycin, but was found more efficacious than 1% miconazole.[75] The efficacy of subconjunctival flucytosine has yet to be established.

Efficacy and Spectrum of Activity. Flucytosine is active against yeasts, including *Candida* and *Cryptococcus*.[61] Some fungal strains lack the specific permease to transport the drug into the cell and are resistant to flucytosine.[85] Resistance can also be induced with prolonged therapy.[37] For this reason, flucytosine should not be administered alone in the treatment of keratomycoses. It can be used as an adjunct in the treatment of yeast keratitis but has been supplanted by the availability of newer azoles.

Toxicity. Flucytosine given orally is well tolerated by patients. Mild gastrointestinal toxicity, including nausea, vomiting, and diarrhea, has been reported. In some cases hepatotoxicity may develop, as evidenced by elevated levels of serum transaminase and alkaline phosphotase. 5-Fluorocytosine in the gastrointestinal tract is metabolized by bacteria to fluorouracil; this metabolic product can produce bone marrow toxicity. Usually these gastrointestinal and liver manifestations can be reversed when the drug is stopped. Because flucytosine is largely excreted by the kidneys, caution should be exercised in patients with renal failure.[61]

Topical flucytosine is well tolerated. In one animal study the 1% solution did not impair epithelial wound healing.[22]

Combination Therapy

The less-than-desirable efficacy of most antifungal agents has spurred attempts at enhancement. Perhaps the most promising possibility involves potentiating antifungal activity through the silmultaneous administration of several antifungal agents. The pharmacology of such combinations is complex, but data from in vitro studies suggest the possible antagonism as well as potentiation of antifungal activity. In addition, certain antibiotics, such as tetracycline and rifampin, seem to enhance the efficacy of other agents. To date most studies have been carried out in vitro because of a lack of a suitable animal model to study their effects precisely.

In animal studies the combination of amphotericin B 0.5% and subconjunctival rifampin was found more effective than amphotericin B alone.[95] Rifampin, an antibacterial agent, given alone is ineffective against fungi. Amphotericin

---

*Bayer Laboratories.

B, by altering the fungal cell wall, may allow rifampin to enter the fungal cell where it inhibits RNA synthesis. There is also evidence of synergy, or at least an additive effect, between amphotericin B and 5-fluorocytosine, but this interaction is quite complex.[1] In addition, the combination of natamycin and ketoconazole was found beneficial in an animal model of *Aspergillus* infection.[51] The concept of combination therapy appears to offer opportunities for increasing the efficacy of existing agents, although detailed studies have yet to be done.

There is also a risk of an antagonistic effect by combining antifungal agents. Antagonism between amphotericin B and the imidazoles has been demonstrated in an experimental model.[5] In vitro studies are contradictory on this point, producing evidence for both potentiating and antagonizing actions. To some degree, this may be the consequence of the experimental design, but it may also reflect the complexity of the interaction between the antifungal agent and the organism. Thus it seems clear from several animal and in vitro studies that a number of factors determine whether a particular combination is antagonistic, without any additive effect, or able to potentiate the antifungal activity. Such factors, as the stage in the life cycle of the organism and the order of administration of the agents and their dosage, appear to be important. Length of treatment may also be a factor. These variables can be manipulated in vitro, but the relevance of such experiments to the clinical situation is unclear.

Corticosteroids

The interaction between corticosteroids and topical antifungal agents is complex. When an experimental corneal fungal infection is treated with corticosteroids alone, the result is a worsening of infection.[25,70,71] The concomitant use of corticosteroids and antifungal agents remains controversial, however. Topical 1% prednisolone acetate adversely influenced the efficacy of 5% natamycin, 1% flucytosine, and 1% miconazole applied topically, but did not adversely affect the efficacy of amphotericin B applied topically in an animal model of candidal keratomycosis.[71] In a rabbit model of *Aspergillus* corneal infection, the simultaneous administration of topical dexamethasone phosphate 0.001% and topical natamycin 5% suppressed inflammation without exacerbating the fungal infectious process.[60]

The introduction of corticosteroids into the management of fungal keratitis should be approached with great caution. Topical antifungal agents are largely fungistatic at best and usually of uncertain efficacy in a given case. Suppressing the host response in this situation runs the risk of tipping the scales in favor of the infective organism.[63,68]

Principles of Treatment

The decision whether to treat a patient with an antifungal agent is influenced heavily by the interpretation of laboratory data. There is rarely justification for empirical treatment with antifungals without corroborating evidence of a fungal cause. Drug toxicity and the necessity for a prolonged treatment period mitigate against the use of these agents empirically. Only in a vision-threatening situation, when the clinical findings are strongly suggestive of fungal infection, is the use of these agents without culture confirmation warranted.

Treatment with an antifungal agent may be initiated on the basis of smear cytology alone, if the findings are clearcut and support the clinical evaluation. In this instance, it is unnecessary to await fungal isolation and identification, which may be delayed for an extended period of time. When the corneal lesion has an appearance consistent with that of a fungal infection but the smear is negative, it is usually appropriate to withhold therapy while awaiting the culture results. Repeated attempts at obtaining an isolate are often unsuccessful in resolving the diagnostic dilemma. Corneal biopsy should be strongly considered if the infection is deeply situated or surface cultures remain negative.

These are differing views regarding the selection of the initial antifungal agent based on the smear cytology. Some investigators advocate topical natamycin 5% as the drug of first choice for superficial keratomycoses, regardless of whether septate hyphae or yeast elements are identified on the smear; additional antifungal agents are added for deep corneal infections. Another therapeutic viewpoint is to choose different initial antifungal agents if the smear reveals budding elements rather than hyphae.

If a smear reveals unequivocal septate hyphal fragments, suggesting that a filamentous fungus is the responsible pathogen, there is general agreement that 5% natamycin is the drug of choice. Initially, the agent is administered hourly for several days. The dosage can then be gradually reduced. If natamycin is unavailable, 0.15% amphotericin B drops can be used.

When yeasts or pseudohyphae are present in the smear, treatment with topical 0.15% amphotericin B is indicated. Animal studies suggest that a loading dose approach, giving the agent every 5 minutes for 1 hour and then hourly, is of benefit. Natamycin 5% is both a more expensive and less efficacious alternative than amphotericin B in the initial treatment of yeast keratomycoses.

Once the organism has been identified by culture, treatment may be modified. Most authors, however, recommend natamycin for filamentous fungus infections regardless of the identification of the organism. Amphotericin B appears to be less efficacious against filamentous fungi and is probably best reserved for those situations in which natamycin is unavailable. Some strains of *Aspergillus, Cladosporium,* and *Penicillium* are sensitive to flucytosine in vitro.[11] Although treatment with topical flucytosine 1% hourly has been suggested, the efficacy of this form of therapy has not been proved. Amphotericin B is indicated for the primary treatment of yeast infections. Occasional strains of *Candida al-*

bicans appear resistant to amphotericin B. For these infections, topical natamycin, topical fluconazole, or topical miconazole appears to be a useful alternative. The same approach should be used for infections with *Candida parapsilosis* if initial therapy with amphotericin B fails.

In contrast to the rapid response seen with effective treatment of bacterial infections in the cornea, fungal keratitis resolves slowly over a period of weeks. As a result it is sometimes difficult to detect small changes in the clinical appearance. In addition, topical antifungal agent toxicity leading to punctate keratitis, chemosis, and conjunctival injection can readily confuse the clinical picture. Recurrent corneal epithelial erosions may also occur as a result of drug toxicity.

Signs of improvement of a fungal corneal ulcer include a lessening of pain, decrease in size of the infiltrate, disappearance of satellite lesions, and rounding out of the feathery margins of the ulcer. Negative scrapings during the treatment are not always an indication of fungal eradication as the fungi may become deep-seated and inaccessible to superficial isolation attempts. Therapy should be maintained for at least 6 weeks.

Surgical Intervention

The preferred management of keratomycosis is pharmacologic. Although there have been reports of the successful use of penetrating keratoplasty in the acute phase of the infection,[49,92] this is not really necessary with the improved armamentarium of more effective antifungal agents. Keratoplasty should be reserved for visual restoration following corneal scarring and for the acute management of corneal perforation. Fortunately, corneal perforation is relatively uncommon in the early stages of keratomycosis unless there has been an accompanying penetrating injury. If corneal perforation occurs in the course of treatment, penetrating keratoplasty is indicated. The use of glue, therapeutic lens, or a collagen lens may provide additional time to continue medical therapy. Once fungi gain intracameral access, the prognosis worsens considerably.

Fungi may gain access to the anterior chamber and intraocular structures by direct spread from the infected cornea, as a result of corneal perforation in the course of the infection or from a penetrating injury. Once intraocular fungi gain intracameral access they become extremely difficult to eradicate (Fig. 77-10). This observation is particularly true of filamentous fungi, such as *Fusarium solani* and *Aspergillus fumigatus*. Fortunately, the majority of fungal infections remain localized to the cornea and show little tendency to invade aggressively.

The onset of intraocular spread is difficult to recognize. Signs may include the apparent worsening of the keratomycosis, especially with deepening spread despite intensive topical therapy. An enlarging hypopyon in the face of therapy is not uncommon. Worsening pain and signs of intraoc-

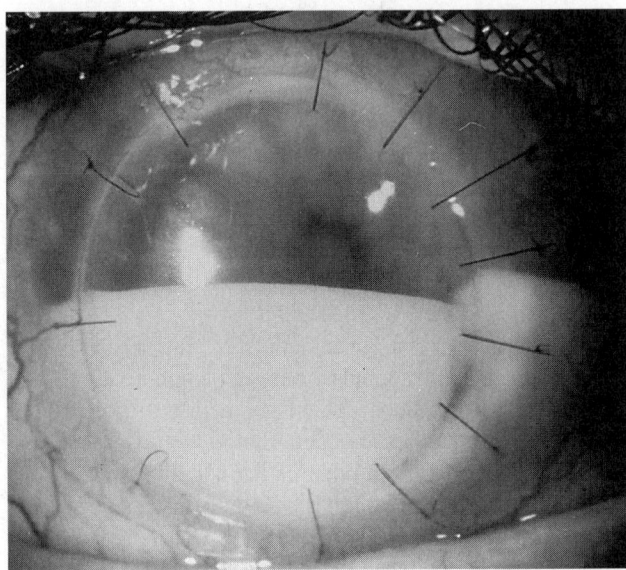

Fig. 77-10. Recrudescent fungal infection following reconstructive keratoplasty.

ular inflammation, including an increase in ciliary flush, a shallowing of the anterior chamber as a result of the development of fungal glaucoma,[44] the development of focal nodular lesions on the surface of the iris, or posterior spread from the endothelium in the region of the corneal lesion, are hallmarks of intraocular invasion.

With intraocular spread, a large therapeutic keratoplasty should be performed in an attempt to excise infected corneal tissue. Lateral spread in the cornea by fungal hyphae often precedes signs of inflammation, so a clear margin should be provided around the lesion if at all possible. The corneal button should be cultured for residual fungi. On removing the corneal disc, the aqueous fluid should be cultured, and any nodules present should be carefully excised and sent for culture. If possible, an intact lens should not be removed. If there is evidence of lenticular invasion, an extracapsular procedure should be performed to preserve the posterior capsule as a barrier to vitreous cavity invasion. Lens material should be sent for culture. After removal of the lens is completed, the entire anterior chamber and the posterior chamber should be irrigated with amphotericin B for several minutes, after which the new corneal button is sutured into place. Therapy with topical antifungal agents should be initiated immediately postoperatively along with systemic antifungal therapy, either with fluconazole or itraconazole.

Corticosteroid therapy should be used with great caution, especially in the initial 2 to 3 weeks following surgery. Corticosteroids have great potential to enhance fungal infections and to mask the signs of the accompanying inflammation. The efficacy of current antifungal agents is limited.

REFERENCES

1. Beggs WH: Mechanisms of synergistic interactions between amphotericin B and flucytosine, *J Antimicrob Chemother* 17:402-404, 1986.

2. Beggs WH, Hughes CE: Exploitation of the direct cell damaging action of antifungal azoles, *Diagn Microbiol Infect Dis* 6:1-3, 1987.

3. Benson WH, Lanier JD: Comparison of techniques for culturing corneal ulcers, *Ophthalmology* 99:800-804, 1992.

4. Borgers M, van de Ven MA, van Cutsem J: Structural degeneration of *Aspergillus fumigatus* after exposure to saperconazole, *J Med Vet Mycol* 27:381-389, 1989.

5. Brajtburg J, Kobayashi D, Medoff G, Kobayashi GS: Antifungal action of amphotericin B in combination with other polyene or imidazole antibiotics, *J Infect Dis* 146:138-146, 1982.

6. Carlson AN, Foulks GN, Perfect JR, Kim JH: Fungal scleritis after cataract surgery: successful outcome using itraconazole, *Cornea* 11:151-154, 1992.

7. Cheng CJ, Yee RW, Ludden TM et al.: Ocular penetration and pharmacokinetics of topical fluconazole, *Invest Ophthalmol Vis Sci Suppl* 32(4):1169, 1991.

8. Chin GN, Hyndiuk RA, Kwasny GP, Schultz RO: Keratomycosis in Wisconsin, *Am J Ophthalmol* 79:121-125, 1975.

9. Chu W, Foster CS, Moran K, Giovanoni R: Intraocular penetration of ketoconazole in rabbits, *Invest Ophthalmol Vis Sci Suppl* 18:133, 1979.

10. Delescluse J, Cauwenbergh G, Degreef H: Itraconazole, a new orally active antifungal, in the treatment of pityriasis versicolor, *Br J Dermatol* 114:701-703, 1986.

11. Denning DW, Hanson LH, Perlman AM, Stevens DA: In vitro susceptibility and synergy studies of *Aspergillus* species to conventional and new agents, *Diagn Microbiol Infect Dis* 15:21-34, 1992.

12. Denning DW, Hanson LH, Stevens DA: In vitro activity of saperconazole (R66 905) compared with amphotericin B and itraconazole against *Aspergillus sp., Eur J Clin Microbiol Infect Dis* 9:693-697, 1990. (Erratum *Eur J Clin Microbiol Infect Dis* 10:49, 1991).

13. Denning DW, Tucker RM, Hanson LH, Stevens DA: Treatment of invasive aspergillosis with itraconazole, *Am J Med* 86:791-800, 1989.

14. Doughman DJ, Leavenworth NM, Campbell RC, Lindstrom RL: Fungal keratitis at the University of Minnesota: 1971-1981, *Trans Am Ophthalmol Soc* 80:235-237, 1982.

15. Drouhet E, Dupont B: Evolution of antifungal agents: past, present, and future, *Rev Infect Dis* 9(suppl 1):S4-S14, 1987.

16. Dupont B, Drouhet E: Fluconazole in the management of oropharyngeal candidosis in a predominately HIV antibody-positive group of patients, *J Med Vet Mycol* 26:67-71, 1988.

17. Ellis WG, Sobel RA, Neilsen SL: Leukoencephalopathy in patients treated with amphotericin B methyl ester, *J Infect Dis* 146:125-137, 1982.

18. Fitzsimmons R, Peters AL, Med M: Miconazole and ketoconazole as a satisfactory first-line treatment for keratomycosis, *Am J Ophthalmol* 101:605-608, 1986.

19. Forster RK: Fungal keratitis and conjunctivitis. Clinical disease. In Smolin G, Thoft RA, editors: *The cornea: scientific foundation and clinical practice,* 228-240, Boston, 1994, Little, Brown.

20. Forster RK, Rebell G: The diagnosis and management of keratomycoses. II. Medical and surgical management, *Arch Ophthalmol* 93:1134-1136, 1975.

21. Foster CS: Miconazole therapy for keratomycosis, *Am J Ophthalmol* 91:622-629, 1981.

22. Foster CS, Lass JH, Moran-Wallace K, Giovanoni R: Ocular toxicity of topical antifungal agents, *Arch Ophthalmol* 99:1081-1084, 1981.

23. Foster CS, Stefanyszyn M: Intraocular penetration of miconazole in rabbits, *Arch Ophthalmol* 97:1703-1706, 1979.

24. Foulds G, Brennan DR, Wajszczuk C et al.: Fluconazole penetration into cerebrospinal fluids in humans, *J Clin Pharmacol* 28:363-366, 1988.

25. Francois J, Risjsselaere M: Corticosteroids and ocular mycoses: Experimental study, *Ann Ophthalmol* 6:207-217, 1974.

26. Fu KP, Isaacson D, Foleno B, LoCoco J: Saperconazole: in vitro and in vivo anticandidal activity, *Chemotherapy* 38:174-178, 1992.

27. Godefroi EG, Heeres J, van Cutsem JH, Janssen PAJ: The preparation and antimycotic properties of derivatives of 1-phenylethylimidazole, *J Med Chem* 12:784-791, 1969.

28. Gold W, Stout HA, Pagano JF, Donovick R: Amphotericin A & B: antifungal antibiotics produced by a streptomycete. I. In vitro studies, *Antibiot Annu* 3:579-586, 1955/1956.

29. Green WR, Bennett JE, Goos RD: Ocular penetration of amphotericin B, *Arch Ophthalmol* 73:769-775, 1965.

30. Grunberg E, Titsworth E, Bennett M: Chemotherapeutic activity of 5-fluorocytosine, *Antimicrob Agents Chemother* 3:566-568, 1963.

31. Gugnani JC, Guypta S, Talwar RS: Role of opportunistic fungi in ocular infections in Nigeria, *Mycopathologia* 65:155-166, 1978.

32. Hay RJ: First international symposium of itraconazole: a summary, *Rev Infect Dis* 9:S1-S2, 1987.

33. Hay RJ, Clayton YM, Moore MK, Midgely G: An evaluation of itraconazole in the management of onychomycosis, *Br J Dermatol* 119:359-366, 1988.

34. Hazen EL, Brown R: Fungicidin, an antibiotic produced by a soil actinomycete, *Proc Soc Exp Biol* 76:93-97, 1951.

35. Head WS, O'Day DM, Robinson RD, Yang R: Effects of preinoculation therapy versus postinoculation therapy with itraconazole in experimental *Aspergillus* keratitis in rabbits, *Invest Ophthalmol Vis Sci Suppl* 34(4):845, 1993.

36. Hector RF, Yee E: Evaluation of Bay R 3783 in rodent models of superficial and systemic candidiasis, meningeal cryptococcosis, and pulmonary aspergillosis, *Antimicrob Agents Chemother* 34:448-454, 1990.

37. Hoeprich PA, Ingraham JL, Klecker E, Winship MJ: Development of resistance to 5-fluorocytosine in *Candida parapsilosis* during therapy, *J Infect Dis* 130:112-118, 1974.

38. Humphrey MJ, Jevons S, Tarbit MH: Pharmacokinetic evaluation of UK-49,858, a metabolically stable triazole antifungal drug, in animals and humans, *Antimicrob Agents Chemother* 28:648-653, 1985.

39. Ishibashi Y: Oral ketoconazole therapy for keratomycosis, *Am J Ophthalmol* 95:342-345, 1983.

40. Ishibashi Y, Matsumoto Y: Intravenous miconazole in the treatment of keratomycosis, *Am J Ophthalmol* 97:646-647, 1984.

41. Jansen T, Borgers M, van de Ven MA et al.: The effects of saperconazole on the morphology of *Candida albicans, Pityrosporum ovale* and *Trichophyton rubrum* in vitro, *J Med Vet Mycol* 29:293-303, 1991.

42. Jones BR: Principles in the management of oculomycosis, *Am J Ophthalmol* 79:719-751, 1975.

43. Jones BR, Clayton YM, Jones DB et al.: The place of Canesten in the management of oculomycoses, *Munch Med Wochenschr* 118:97, 1976.

44. Jones BR, Jones DB, Lim AS et al.: Corneal and intraocular infection due to *Fusarium solani, Trans Ophthalmol Soc UK* 89:757-759, 1970.

45. Jones DB: Strategy for the initial management of suspected microbial keratitis. In New Orleans Academy of Ophthalmology (editor): *Symposium on medical and surgical diseases of the cornea,* 86-119, St Louis, 1980, Mosby.

46. Jones DB: Fungal keratitis. In Duane T, editor: *Clinical ophthalmology,* vol 4, 1-13, Hagerstown, MD, 1985, Harper & Row.

47. Jones DB, Forster RK, Rebell G: *Fusarium solani* keratitis treated with natamycin (pimaricin): eighteen consecutive cases, *Arch Ophthalmol* 88:147-154, 1972.

48. Jones DB, Sexton R, Rebell G: Mycotic keratitis in south Florida: a review of 39 cases, *Trans Ophthalmol Soc UK* 89:781-797, 1969.

49. Killingsworth DW, Stern GA, Driebe WT et al.: Results of therapeutic penetrating keratoplasty, *Ophthalmology* 100:534-541, 1993.

50. Klippenstein K, Robinson RD, O'Day DM et al.: A rapid method for screening potential subconjunctival antifungal agents, *Invest Ophthalmol Vis Sci Suppl* 31(4):451, 1990.

51. Kobayashi GS, Travis SJ, Medoff G: Comparison of fluconazole and amphotericin B in treating histoplasmosis in immunosuppressed mice, *Antimicrob Agents Chemother* 31:2005-2006, 1987.

52. Komadina TG, Wilkes TDI, Shock JP et al.: Treatment of *Aspergillus fumigatus* keratitis in rabbits with oral and topical ketoconazole, *Am J Ophthalmol* 99:476-479, 1985.

53. Koul RL, Pratap VB: Keratomycosis in Luknow, *Br J Ophthalmol* 59:47-51, 1975.

54. Kuroda S, Uno J, Arai T: Target substances of some antifungal agents in the cell membrane, *Antimicrob Agents Chemother* 13:454-459, 1978.

55. Lazar JD, Hilligoss DM: The clinical pharmacology of fluconazole, *Semin Oncol* 17:14-18, 1990.

56. Lewis JH, Zimmerman HJ, Benson GD, Ishak KG: Hepatic injury associated with ketoconazole therapy: analysis of 33 cases, *Gastroenterology* 86:503-513, 1984.

57. Liesegang TJ, Forster RK: Spectrum of microbial keratitis in south Florida, *Am J Ophthalmol* 90:38-47, 1980.

58. Medoff G, Kobayaski GS: Strategies in the treatment of systemic fungal infections, *N Engl J Med* 302:145-155, 1980.

59. Newmark E, Ellison AC, Kaufman HE: Pimaricin therapy of *Cephalosporium* and *Fusarium* keratitis, *Am J Ophthalmol* 69:458-466, 1970.

60. Newmark E, Ellison AC, Kaufman HE: Combined pimaricin and dexamethasone therapy for keratomycosis, *Am J Ophthalmol* 71:718-722, 1971.

61. O'Day DM: Antifungal agents in corneal disorders. In Leibowitz H, editor: *Corneal disorders: clinical diagnosis and management,* Philadelphia, 1984, WB Saunders.

62. O'Day DM: Selection of appropriate antifungal therapy, *Cornea* 6:238-245, 1987.

63. O'Day DM: Corticosteroids: an unresolved debate, *Ophthalmology* 98:845-846, 1991.

64. O'Day DM, Foulds G, Williams TE et al.: Ocular uptake of fluconazole following oral administration, *Arch Ophthalmol* 108:1006-1008, 1990.

65. O'Day DM, Head WS, Robinson RD, Clanton JA: Bioavailability and penetration of topical amphotericin B in the anterior segment of the rabbit eye, *J Ocul Pharmacol* 2:371-378, 1986.

66. O'Day DM, Head WS, Robinson RD, Clanton JA: Corneal penetration of topical amphotericin B and natamycin, *Curr Eye Res* 5:877-882, 1986.

67. O'Day DM, Head WS, Robinson RD et al.: Ocular pharmacokinetics of saperconazole in rabbits. A potential agent against keratomycoses, *Arch Ophthalmol* 110:550-554, 1992. (Erratum *Arch Ophthalmol* 110:1597, 1992).

68. O'Day DM, Moore TE, Aronson SB: Deep fungal corneal abscess—combined corticosteroid therapy, *Arch Ophthalmol* 86:414-419, 1971.

69. O'Day DM, Ray WA, Head WS, Robinson RD: Influence of the corneal epithelium on the efficacy of topical antifungal agents, *Invest Ophthalmol Vis Sci* 25:855-859, 1984.

70. O'Day DM, Ray WA, Head WS et al.: Influence of corticosteroid on experimentally induced keratomycosis, *Arch Ophthalmol* 109:1601-1604, 1991.

71. O'Day DM, Ray WA, Robinson RD, Head WS: Efficacy of antifungal agents in the cornea. II. Influence of corticosteroids, *Invest Ophthalmol Vis Sci* 25:331-335, 1984.

72. O'Day DM, Ray WA, Robinson RD, Head WS: Correlation of *in vitro* and *in vivo* susceptibility of *Candida albicans* to amphotericin B and natamycin, *Invest Ophthalmol Vis Sci* 28:596-598, 1987.

73. O'Day DM, Ray WA, Robinson RD et al.: *In vitro* and *in vivo* susceptibility of *Candida* keratitis to topical polyenes, *Invest Ophthalmol Vis Sci* 28:874-880, 1987.

74. O'Day DM, Ray WA, Robinson RD et al.: Differences in response *in vivo* to amphotericin B among *Candida albicans* strains, *Invest Ophthalmol Vis Sci* 32:1569-1572, 1991.

75. O'Day DM, Robinson RD, Head WS: Efficacy of antifungal agents in the cornea. I. A comparative study, *Invest Ophthalmol Vis Sci* 24:1098-1102, 1983.

76. O'Day DM, Smith R, Stevens JB et al.: Toxicity and pharmacokinetics of subconjunctival amphotericin B: an experimental study, *Cornea* 10:411-417, 1991.

77. Oji EO, Clayton YM: The role of econazole in the management of oculomycosis, *Int Ophthalmol* 4:137-142, 1981.

78. Osato MS, Gilbert ML, Trautwein LM: Ocular toxicity and efficacy of 1% clotrimazole in amoebic keratitis: ocular Microbiology and Immunology Group abstracts, twenty-first annual meeting, New Orleans, Nov 8, 1986.

79. Otčenášek M: Susceptibility of clinical isolates of fungi to saperconazole, *Mycopathologia* 118:179-183, 1992.

80. Park SS, D'Amico DJ, Paton B, Baker AS: Treatment of exogenous *Candida* endophthalmitis in rabbits with oral fluconazole or combination fluconazole and flucytosine, *Invest Ophthalmol Vis Sci Suppl* 34(4):1258, 1993.

81. Patterson TF, George D, Miniter P, Andriole VT: Saperconazole therapy in a rabbit model of invasive aspergillosis, *Antimicrob Agents Chemother* 36:2681-2685, 1992.

82. Perfect JR, Savani DV, Durack DT: Comparison of itraconazole and fluconazole in treatment of cryptococcal meningitis and *Candida* pyelonephritis in rabbits, *Antimicrob Agents Chemother* 29:579-583, 1986.

83. Pfaller MA et al.: Collaborative investigation of variables in susceptible testing of yeasts, *Antimicrob Agents Chemother* 34:1648-1654, 1990.

84. Polack FM, Kaufman HE, Newmark E: Keratomycosis. Medical and surgical treatment, *Arch Ophthalmol* 85:410-416, 1971.

85. Polak A, Scholer HJ: Mode of action of 5-fluorocytosine and mechanisms of resistance, *Chemotherapy* 21:113-130, 1975.

86. Rajasekaran J, Thomas PA, Srinivasan R: Ketoconazole in keratomycosis. *Proceedings of the XXV International Congress of Ophthalmology,* Rome, May 4-10, 1986.

87. Restrepo A, Robledo J, Gomez I et al.: Itraconazole therapy in lymphangitic and cutaneous sporotrichosis, *Arch Dermatol* 122:413-417, 1986.

88. Richards AB, Jones BR, Whitwell J, Clayton YM: Corneal and intraocular infection by *Candida albicans* treated with 5-fluorocytosine, *Trans Ophthalmol Soc UK* 89:867-885, 1969.

89. Richardson K, Brammer KW, Marriott MS, Troke PF: Activity of UK-49,858, a bistriazole derivative against experimental infections with *Candida albicans* and *Trichophyton mentagrophytes, Antimicrob Agents Chemother* 27:832-835, 1985.

90. Robinson N, Penland R, Osato M, Richardson SW: Comparative efficacy of new azole antifungal agents against human ocular isolates, *Invest Ophthalmol Vis Sci Suppl* 31:451, 1990.

91. Sandhu DK, Randhawa IS: Studies on the air-borne fungal spores in Amritsar: their role in keratomycosis, *Mycopathologia* 68:47-52, 1979.

92. Sanitato JJ, Kelley CG, Kaufman HE: Surgical management of peripheral fungal keratitis, *Arch Ophthalmol* 102:1506-1509, 1984.

93. Savani DV, Perfect JR, Cobo LM, Durack DT: Penetration of new azole compounds into the eye and efficacy in experimental *Candida* endophthalmitis, *Antimicrob Agents Chemother* 31:6-10, 1987.

94. Shirley SF: Immunopotentiating effects of amphotericin B, *J Immunol* 123:2878-2889, 1979.

95. Stern GA, Okumoto M, Smolin G: Combined amphotericin B and rifampin treatment of experimental *Candida albicans* keratitis, *Arch Ophthalmol* 97:721-722, 1979.

96. Stiller RL, Bennett JE, Scholer JH et al.: Correlation of *in vitro* susceptibility test results with *in vivo* response: flucytosine therapy in a systemic candidiasis model, *J Infect Dis* 147:1070-1077, 1983.

97. Struyck AP, Hoette I, Drost G et al.: Pimaricin, a new antifungal antibiotic, *Antibiot Annu* 878-879, 1957/1958.

98. Sud IJ, Feingold DS: Mechanisms of action of the antimycotic imidazoles, *J Invest Dermatol* 76:438-441, 1981.

99. Thienpont D, Van Cutsem J, Van Gerven F et al.: Ketoconazole, a new broad spectrum orally active antimycotics, *Experientia* 35:606-609, 1979.

100. Thomas PA, Ravi CMK, Rajasekaran J: Microbial keratitis—a study of 774 cases and review of the literature, *J Madras St Ophthalmol Assoc* 23:13-21, 1986.

101. Van Cutsem J: *In vitro* antifungal spectrum of itraconazole and treatment of systemic mycoses with old and new antimycotic agents, *Chemotherapy* 38(suppl 1):3-11, 1992.

102. Van Cutsem JM, Thienpont D: Miconazole, a broad-spectrum antimycotic with antibacterial activity, *Chemotherapy* 17:392-404, 1972.

103. Van Cutsem J, Van Gerven F, Janssen PAJ: R66-905, a new potent broad-spectrum antifungal triazole with topical, oral and parenteral activity. Program and abstracts of the 10th Congress of the International Society of Human and Animal Mycology, Barcelona, Spain, June 27-July 1, 1988 (abstract).

104. Van Cutsem J, Van Gerven F, Janssen PA: Oral and parenteral therapy with saperconazole (R66 905) of invasive aspergillosis in normal and immunocompromised animals, *Antimicrob Agents Chemother* 33:2063-2068, 1989.

105. Vanden Bossche J, Marichal P, Gorrens J, Coene MC: Biochemical basis for the activity and selectivity of oral antifungal drugs, *Br J Clin Pract Symp Suppl* 71:41-46, 1990.

106. Varga JH, Wolf TC, Jensen HG: Swab cultures of corneal ulcers, *Ophthalmology* 99:1346, 1992.

107. Vives T, Yee RW, Jalcedo K et al.: Topical 0.2% fluconazole in rabbit fungal-induced keratitis, *Invest Ophthalmol Vis Sci Suppl* 33(4):776, 1992.

108. Viviani MA et al.: Experience with itraconazole in cryptococcosis and aspergillosis, *J Infect* 18:151-154, 1989.

109. Viviani MA, Tortorano AM, Malaspina C et al.: Surveillance and treatment of liver transplant recipients for candidiasis and aspergillosis, *Eur J Epidemiol* 8:433-436, 1992.

110. Wood TO, Tuberville AW: Keratomycosis and amphotericin B, *Trans Am Ophthalmol Soc* 83:397-409, 1985.

111. Wood TO, Williford W: Treatment of keratomycosis with amphotericin B 0.15%, *Am J Ophthalmol* 81:847-849, 1976.

78 Acanthamoebic Keratitis

HASSAN ALIZADEH, JERRY Y. NIEDERKORN, JAMES P. McCULLEY

Acanthamoeba species are ubiquitous protozoa that have been isolated from diverse habitats. Acanthamoebic keratitis was first recognized in 1973 and has become an uncommon but important infection.

HISTORICAL BACKGROUND

Free-living amoebae were first described by Rösel Von Rosenhof in 1755.[55] Dujardin[14] found numerous limax amoebae (the term ''limax'' was used for small amoebae with sluggish movement) from water samples collected from the river Seine in France. In a notable paper published by Franchini,[21] small amoebae were also recovered from the surface of ''lettuce'' plants and called ''amoeba lettuce''.[40,69] In 1930 Castellanii[4] reported that limax amoeba contaminating an agar plate consumed bacteria and yeast growing on the medium. This observation led to methods for culturing free-living amoeba. Based on morphology, free-living, limax amoebae were reclassified from the genus *Hartmannella* to a new genus, *Acanthamoeba*[13,73] (Table 78-1).

Acanthamoebic keratitis is a severe, progressive, and potentially blinding infection of the cornea. The first case of acanthamoebic keratitis was reported in 1973 in a 59-year-old cattleman from southern Texas with a history of ocular trauma and exposure to contaminated water.[27] Between 1973 and 1981 only five additional cases were reported. The number of cases increased gradually from 1981 through 1984, with an increased incidence of acanthamoebic keratitis occurring during the late 1980s.[46,63]

EPIDEMIOLOGY

Acanthamoeba species have been isolated from a wide variety of environments, including public water supplies and swimming pools,[37,54] fresh water ponds and lakes,[35,41] hot tubs,[56] bottled mineral water,[53] and soil.[3] Subclinical exposure is probably common in healthy people; parasites have been isolated from the nose and throat of healthy, asymptomatic individuals.[6,74] Serologic surveys have shown that antibodies against *Acanthamoeba* can be found in a high percentage of normal human subjects.[7,12]

Keratitis is the most common human infection caused by *Acanthamoeba*. Various nonocular infections caused by free-living amoebae have been reported, but most of these have been cases of granulomatous meningoencephalitis.[36,40]

Acanthamoebic keratitis has become a growing clinical problem that is closely associated with contact lens wear. Up until 1989 approximately 250 cases of acanthamoebic keratitis had been reported to the Centers for Disease Control and Prevention.[38] Despite the widespread use of contact lenses, the occurrence of this disease is relatively low, suggesting that additional risk factors are involved in the development of corneal infection with *Acanthamoeba*.

RISK FACTORS

There are several important risk factors associated with acanthamoebic keratitis, with the vast majority of patients having at least one of these identifiable factors (i.e., corneal trauma, contaminated water, and contact lenses). Exposure to contaminated water or soil has been found in a small number of patients. Approximately 71% to 85% of patients with acanthamoebic keratitis are contact lens wearers.[45,46,64]

No single type of contact lens has been excluded from association with acanthamoebic keratitis. Daily-wear soft contact lens patients account for approximately 75% of the patients, 14% wore extended wear contact lenses, 6% wore hard contact lenses, and 4% wore rigid gas permeable lenses.[46] In another study Stehr-Green and associates[64] reported that most patients (95%) had at least one risk factor for acanthamoebic keratitis, and of the 85% of patients who wore contact lenses, most wore daily-wear (56%) or extended-wear soft lenses (19%). A few patients (26%) had a history of corneal trauma before developing acanthamoebic keratitis, and 25% of patients had a history of exposure to contaminated water.

Acanthamoeba trophozoites adhere not only to worn lenses, but also to new contact lenses of all types.[26] The contact lens serves as a carrier for *Acanthamoeba*. Isolation of *Acanthamoeba* from commercial bottled water as well as tap water may explain the high incidence of acanthamoebic

TABLE 78-1 CLASSIFICATION OF *ACANTHAMOEBA*

Kingdom:	Protista
Subkingdom:	Protozoa
Phylum:	Sacromastigophora
Subphylum:	Sarcodina
Superclass:	Rhizopoda
Class:	Lobosea
Subclass:	Gymnamoebia
Order:	Amoebida
Suborder:	Acanthopodina
Family:	Acanthamoebida
Genus:	Acanthamoeba
Species:	Isolated from human cornea
	A. castellanii
	A. culbertsoni
	A. polyphaga
	A. hatchetti

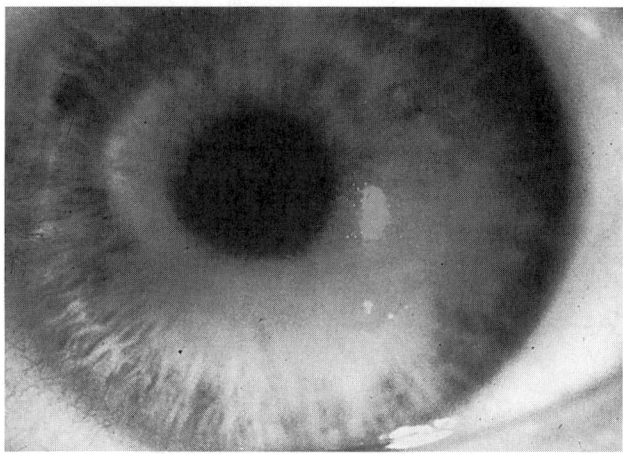

Fig. 78-1. Patchy stromal infiltration caused by *Acanthamoeba* infection.

keratitis in the patients using nonsterile distilled water and salt tablets to store and clean contact lenses. A limited association of acanthamoebic keratitis with contamination from saliva and nonpreserved bottled saline has been observed previously.[46] Any contact lens is a potential carrier of *Acanthamoeba* to the ocular surface after being exposed to a contaminated fluid source.

It is not known whether an epithelial defect is required for adherence and invasion of the cornea by *Acanthamoeba*. A significantly greater number of parasites bound to abraded Chinese hamster corneal buttons than to intact, nonabraded corneas.[71] Moreover, corneal epithelial abrasion is necessary for the establishment of an animal model of contact lens–related acanthamoebic keratitis.[71] Other risk factors that contribute to the development of acanthamoebic keratitis in contact lens wearers may be related to host susceptibility, defects in mucosal immunity, or other subtle defects in host defense mechanisms.

Acanthamoeba can adhere to and penetrate intact human corneal epithelium.[49,70] Acanthamoebic keratitis should be considered as a possibility in any patient who is a contact lens wearer who shows symptoms of corneal inflammation. This is especially true if there are other conditions in the history, such as the use of distilled water and salt tablets to make homemade saline, and excessive pain, relative to the clinical appearance of the cornea.

CLINICAL FEATURES

Patients with acanthamoebic keratitis are typically young, healthy individuals. Males and females are equally affected, and many are contact lens wearers.[43] The most commonly infected contact lens wearers are those who wear daily soft contact lenses. Another frequently found association in the past was the use of nonpreserved saline made from bottled water and salt tablets. These patients typically have no antecedent eye trauma or surgery.

Acanthamoebic keratitis is most frequently unilateral, but bilateral cases have occurred.[22a] One of the most important features of the disease is that patients have severe pain far out of proportion to the clinical signs, at least in the early phases of the infection. The epithelial irregularity and dendriform changes of *Acanthamoeba* infection represent an early stage of disease. The occurrence of patchy anterior stromal infiltrates (Fig. 78-1), crescents, and rings that become more circumscribed and confluent (Fig. 78-2) are later manifestations. *Acanthamoeba* cysts can sometimes be visualized.[5] Some patients have a stage of disease mimicking disciform stromal keratitis, and others develop radial neuritis.[47] The occurrence of lacunar-like changes, satellite lesions, necrotizing inflammation, and stromal abscess formation signal advanced infection. The lack of corneal neovascularization is striking. Two forms of scleral inflam-

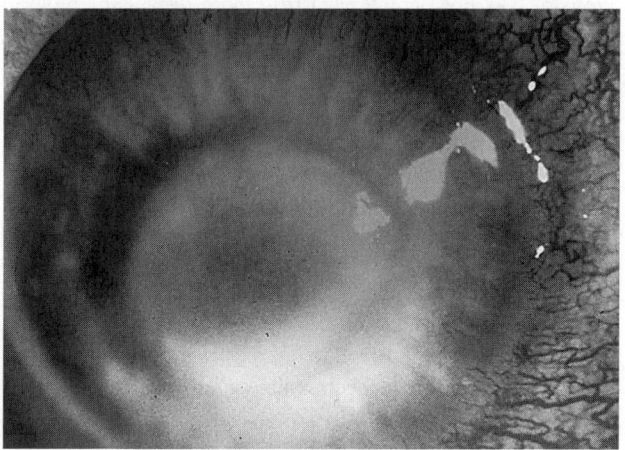

Fig. 78-2. Progressive infection leading to ring infiltrate.

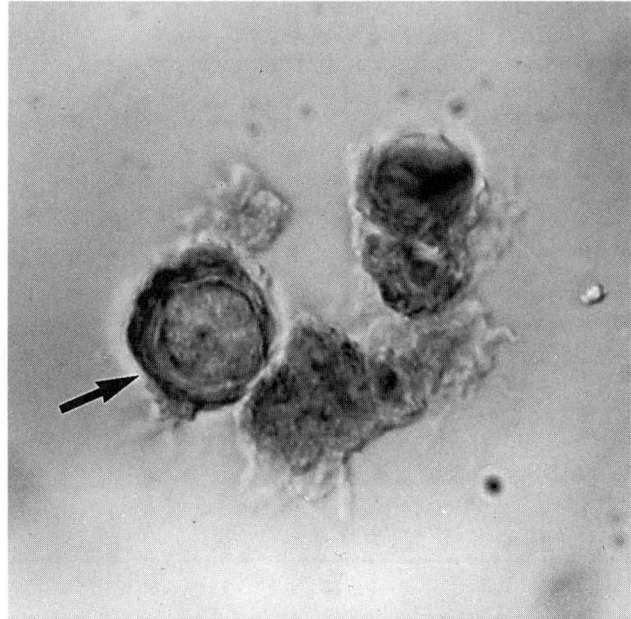

Fig. 78-3. Two stages in the life cycle of *Acanthamoeba:* trophozoites and cyst *(arrow).*

mation occur in acanthamoebic keratitis patients[39]: severe anterior scleritis with a nodular component contiguous to the area of inflamed cornea and posterior scleritis with or without optic neuritis (see box).

The recurrent epithelial breakdown, overlying ring infiltrates, and abscesses lead to the frequent diagnosis of ring abscesses being caused by herpes simplex virus. Stromal involvement prior to the development of a ring abscess varies tremendously. There can be single or multiple anterior stromal infiltrates, a nummular keratitis appearance at one or all levels of the stroma, or the formation of dense single or multiple stromal infiltrates.

The most characteristic form of stromal disease occurs late and is characterized by a ring infiltrate or abscess that can consist of single, multiple, or overlapping rings. The explanation has been elusive because pathologic specimens usually demonstrate few organisms and minimal inflammatory cells. It has been suggested that infiltrating neutrophils were responsible for collagenolysis through the elaboration of various proteases. *Acanthamoeba* elaborate collagenolytic enzymes that not only degrade collagen in vitro, however, but also produce lesions that parallel those characteristically found in human patients diagnosed with acanthamoebic keratitis.[24]

Bacterial, fungal, or viral infections occurring concurrently with acanthamoebic keratitis have been reported previously. It is not known what role these organisms have in the pathogenesis of acanthamoebic keratitis. In a few cases initial corneal cultures showed the occurrence of bacterial infection such as *Staphylococcus epidermidis,*[10] *Staphylococcus aureus,*[10,27] *Streptococcus* species,[29] and *Propionibacterium magnus.*[1]

PATHOGENESIS

Acanthamoeba has two stages in its life cycle, an active trophozoite and a dormant cyst. The size of trophozoites of *Acanthamoeba* varies among species but generally measures 10 to 25 μm in length and is characterized by a single nucleus and spinelike pseudopodia called "acanthapodia." Trophozoites encyst in an unfavorable environment. The cyst is characterized by a wrinkled ectocyst wall measuring approximately 10 to 25 μm in diameter (Fig. 78-3).

The pathogenesis of acanthamoebic keratitis can follow two pathways.[66] The first pathway is restricted to the epithelium without involvement of the stroma and has a good prognosis. The second pathway culminates in the parasites entering the stroma, resulting in extensive necrosis, edema, and infiltration of polymorphonuclear leukocytes.[22]

Adherence and Invasion

The first step in the initiation of amoebic infection is attachment to the epithelial surface. Amoebae bind to the corneal surface and produce epithelial thinning and necrosis. Eventually the parasites enter the stroma, resulting in necrosis, edema, disruption of the stromal lamellae, and an intense polymorphonuclear inflammatory response.[42] *Acanthamoeba* trophozoites produce cytopathic effects on a variety of cultured mammalian cells including human corneal epithelium.[11,31,72] Both pathogenic and nonpathogenic amoebae produce cytopathic effects in cell culture, however.[8,72] Possession of cytolytic machinery does not necessarily convey pathogenicity.

Potential pathways for cell-mediated killing of target cells by *Acanthamoeba* are shown schematically in Fig. 78-4. The cytopathic effect could result from (*A*) phagocytosis, (*B*) spontaneous exocytosis, or (*C*) membrane-initiated exocytosis. A cytolytic, pore-forming protein may be involved in target-cell killing. Target-cell death induced by *Entamoeba histolytica, Naegleria fowleri,* cytolytic T lymphocytes, and complement all involve membrane disruption by a pore-forming protein that is inserted into target-cell membrane.[77,78] For *Acanthamoeba* infection it is not clear whether the target cells have to be damaged before they can

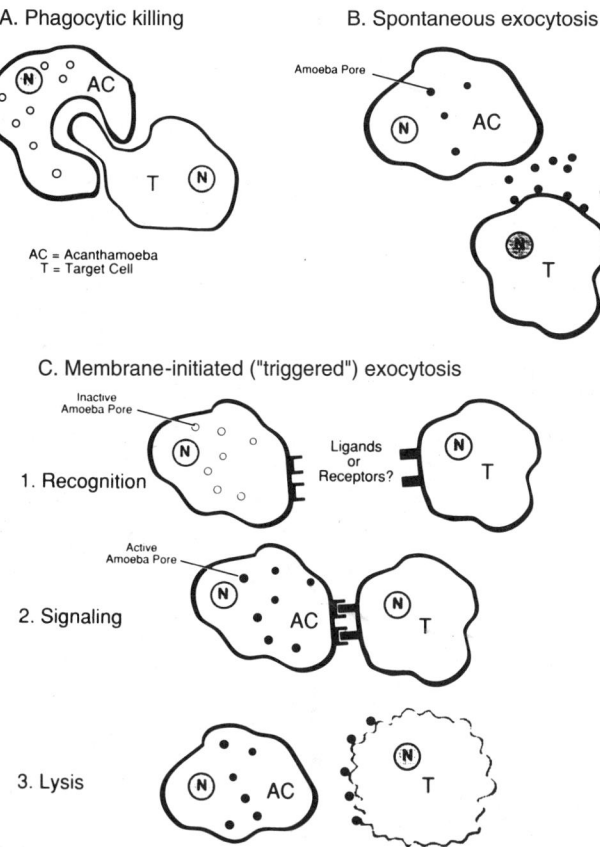

A. Phagocytic killing

B. Spontaneous exocytosis

Amoeba Pore

AC = Acanthamoeba
T = Target Cell

C. Membrane-initiated ("triggered") exocytosis

Inactive
Amoeba Pore

1. Recognition

Ligands
or
Receptors?

Active
Amoeba Pore

2. Signaling

3. Lysis

Fig. 78-4. Potential methods of cell-mediated killing of target cell (T) by *Acanthamoeba* (AC).

be phagocytosed, but amoebae seldom ingest target cells at first contact.[22] Experiments with *E. histolytica* demonstrate that amoebae rapidly and firmly bind to the plasma membranes of target cells and induce marked changes in their permeability of cations. The resulting pores render target cells highly permeable to sodium and calcium ions.[23] The mechanisms of adherence and cytopathogenicity by *Acanthamoeba* remain to be determined.

Once in the corneal stroma, *A. castellanii* secretes a collagenolytic enzyme that produces severe necrosis, edema, inflammation, and ringlike infiltrates.[24] Nonpathogenic soil isolates of *Acanthamoeba* produce similar enzymes yet do not produce corneal disease in vivo. Culture supernatants from an ocular isolate of *A. castellanii* display plasminogen activator, but this activity is not present in cell cultures from a nonpathogenic soil isolate of *A. castellanii*.[72] Thus it is possible that the pathogenesis of acanthamoebic keratitis involves the activation of plasminogen to active plasmin, which, in turn, promotes the parasite's penetration into the corneal epithelium.

Axenic cultures of *A. castellanii* contained a collagenolytic enzyme that digested collagen shields and purified type I collagen in vitro. When selective enzyme inhibitors were used, it was found that parasites produced both collagenase and other proteolytic enzymes. Most of the collagenolytic activity was directly attributable to specific collagenase, however. Intrastromal injection of sterile *Acanthamoeba*-conditioned medium into the corneas of rats produced corneal lesions that clinically and histopathologically mimicked those found in patients diagnosed with acanthamoebic keratitis. Thus soluble parasite-derived factors are capable of producing lesions characteristic of human acanthamoebic keratitis. These findings further suggest that the stromal degradation in acanthamoebic keratitis may be caused in large part by parasite-derived collagenase.[24]

Inflammatory Response

Little information is available on immunologic effector mechanisms or mechanisms of immunopathogenesis in acanthamoebic keratitis. Several studies have demonstrated that antibody and complement are involved in the lysis of *Acanthamoeba* in vitro.[17,19,65,75] The amoebolytic activity of antibody is enhanced by the presence of macrophages and neutrophils.[18,65]

Pathologic investigations of human and animal specimens reveal that severe inflammatory responses occur in acanthamoebic keratitis.[33,42] Macrophages are predominant during the early stage of experimental infection.[33] Because an intact inflammatory response is needed for full expression of clinical acanthamoebic keratitis, animals subjected to severe chronic immunosuppression[20,57] are not valid counterparts to human patients diagnosed with acanthamoebic keratitis. Attempts to produce acanthamoebic keratitis in rats and mice fail to produce convincing evidence that these hosts developed corneal lesions that resembled the human counterpart. Previous models involved injection of parasites with or without bacteria into the cornea rather than induction by contact lenses.[2,31] *Acanthamoeba* species are apparently host specific.[51]

Studies have also evaluated the cellular immune response to *A. castellanii*. In the presence of normal serum, macrophages from naive rats produced minimal lysis of trophozoites in vitro. Macrophages armed with serum from immunized rats, with crude aqueous extract of *A. castellanii* antigens and activated with rat recombinant γ interferon (1,000 units/well), produced 43% cytolysis of parasites in a 6-hour assay. By contrast, macrophages collected from immunized rats and activated with immune serum plus rat recombinant γ interferon lysed almost twice as many parasites (i.e., 70% cytolysis) as macrophages collected from naive rats and similarly activated. Macrophages from both naive rats and rats immunized with *Acanthamoeba* antigens responded chemotactically to parasite antigens.[65]

Animal Models

Binding studies indicate that trophozoites do not bind to the intact corneal epithelium of mice, rats, cotton rats, horses, guinea pigs, cows, chickens, dogs, or rabbits. Parasites adhered, invaded, and produced severe damage to human, pig, and Chinese hamster corneas, however. These in vitro results suggest that the pig and Chinese hamster corneas might serve as animal models for acanthamoebic keratitis.[51]

The prediction that the pig would be susceptible to acanthamoebic keratitis was confirmed through a series of experiments in which parasite-laden hydrophilic soft contact lenses were placed onto the abraded corneas of Yucatan micropigs.[25] Pigs developed corneal infections that clinically and histopathologically mimicked the human counterpart. Three distinct stages of disease became apparent and were categorized as follows: acute, condensed infiltrate, and resolution stages. Importantly, viable parasites were isolated from the lesions and were cultured in vitro. In addition, cysts could be identified deep within the stroma of histologic specimens taken during the resolution stage of infection. The characteristic dense, white, ringlike infiltrates, stromal edema, keratic precipitates, and the chronic nature of the infections were similar to those observed in human acanthamoebic keratitis. Histopathologic examination of infected corneas revealed extensive neutrophilic infiltrates, stromal necrosis, and disorganization of collagen lamellae. Similar lesions were not elicited by sterile contact lenses placed onto abraded corneas. Moreover, the bacterial flora of the diseased eyes did not differ from the normal flora in the pig's eye. Similar results were found in subsequent studies using less expensive domestic pigs.

The Chinese hamster, like the pig, is also susceptible to acanthamoebic keratitis. Parasites bound extensively to miniature contact lenses fashioned from dialysis tubing. The lenses were applied to intact or abraded corneas of Chinese hamsters. Of the various techniques for exposing corneas to viable parasites, only exposure via parasite-laden contact lenses produced corneal infection in a large number of hamsters. Keratitis was characterized by epithelial ulceration, stromal infiltrate, edema, and neovascularization. Corneal epithelial defects promoted parasite binding. None of the hamsters with intact corneal epithelia were infected following exposure to parasite-laden contact lenses, but 66% of the hamsters whose corneal epithelial surfaces were abraded prior to exposure to parasite-laden contact lenses developed severe keratitis. Induction of Langerhans-cell migration into the central corneal epithelium by instillation of sterile latex beads or by the intracorneal injection of interleukin-1 before exposing the corneas to parasite-laden contact lenses resulted in a significant reduction in the incidence and severity of acanthamoebic keratitis.[71]

These experimental results indicate that the pathogenic potential of *Acanthamoeba* is correlated with the parasite's capacity to bind to corneal epithelium, respond chemotactically to corneal endothelial extracts, elaborate plasminogen activators, and produce cytopathic effects on corneal epithelium.[72] Acute inflammation and delayed hypersensitivity are involved in the host response to corneal infection.

LABORATORY INVESTIGATIONS

Confirmatory laboratory tests are important in the diagnosis of acanthamoebic keratitis. This fact is especially important considering the very long treatment that is required for patients with acanthamoebic keratitis. Confocal microscopy may make it possible to visualize organisms in vivo,[75a] but laboratory testing is usually required. A number of diagnostic tests are available.

Corneal scrapings or biopsy should be inoculated into culture media. The use of a confluent lawn of *Escherichia coli* (monoxenic culture) on nonnutrient agar enhances recovery. Enteric gram-negative rods such as *E. coli* and *Enterobacter* species serve as a food source for *Acanthamoeba,* which will eat the bacteria and leave identifiable tracks. The *E. coli* will not fill in these tracks, because the bacteria are plated on nonnutrient agar. Other methods of culturing the organism have been suggested, such as peptone–yeast-extract broth without added bacteria (axenic culture), in mammalian tissue culture, or various types of blood agar.

Tissue specimens, corneal smears, contact lenses, and swabs may be kept in Page saline and then sent to the laboratory. Corneal scraping, contact lenses, and filtered contact lens solution can be cultured on plates containing nonnutrient agar at 35°C for at least 7 days. If cysts are present, however, the material should be cultured for a longer period to excyst to the trophozoite stage.

Microscopy can provide rapid identification. Trophozoites can be identified by the presence of the contractile vacuole, which will disappear and reappear within a few seconds. For a wet-mount preparation, contact lens solution is best centrifuged at slow speed (250 g), and then the sediment is transferred to the slide and covered with a coverslip. The prepared slide can be examined under phase microscopy, and the motile trophozoite can be seen with a large karyosome and contractile vacuole.

If an epithelial or subepithelial abnormality is observed, scraping and biopsy is very useful to identify the parasite. Scraping of the cornea by a sterile scalpel can be performed under local anesthesia by placing a drop of anesthetic on the patient's cornea. The material can be used either for slide preparation or cultured on a nonnutrient agar plate as described previously.

Amoebae in corneal scrapings have been identified by staining with Gram staining (Fig. 78-5), Giemsa-Wright (Hemacolor) staining, and Gomori-Wheatley trichrome staining. Calcofluor white,[59] which stains the wall of cysts but not trophozoites, is an excellent stain but requires access to a fluorescent microscope (Fig. 78-6).

If there are no active epithelial lesions, but there are accessible stromal lesions, a biopsy is recommended. The biopsy specimens can be cultured on a nonnutrient agar plate or stained with hematoxylin and eosin, periodic acid-Schiff, methenamine silver, calcofluor white, or fluorescein-labeled antibodies directed against *Acanthamoeba*. The latter two approaches require access to a fluorescent microscope for

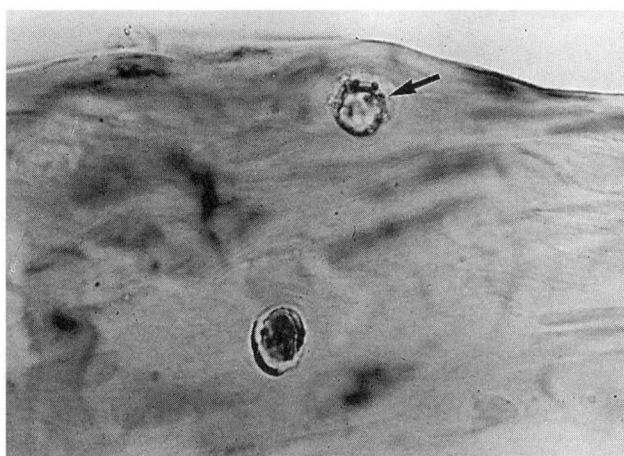

Fig. 78-5. *Acanthamoeba* cyst *(arrow)* in corneal scraping of patient with acanthamoebic keratitis.

effective observation. It is much easier to recognize the characteristic double-walled cysts than trophozoites, which can be confused with other cellular forms.

Keratoplasty specimens can be processed by histology or cultured in nonnutrient agar plates. Tissue should be fixed in formalin and preferably embedded in paraffin. Various histologic stains can be used to identify amoeba. Because lymphocytes and inflammatory cells infiltrate the infected cornea, it is important to identify the amoeba not only by histologic staining but also with immunofluorescent antibody against *Acanthamoeba.* Moreover, electron microscopy of a corneal transplant may be used to identify the parasites. The other method is to culture the parasite from the corneal button; in this case the tissue should be homogenized and then cultured in nonnutrient agar.

Acanthamoeba can be recognized because of its cyst structure and acanthapodia, but species identification is difficult. The Pussard-Pons system uses differences in cyst morphology to classify different species of *Acanthamoeba.*

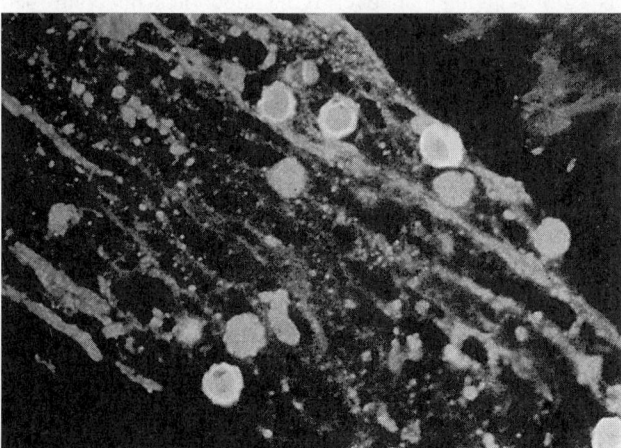

Fig. 78-6. *Acanthamoeba* cysts in corneal biopsy cultured for 10 days in nonnutrient agar to allow trophozoites to encyst.

More recently isoenzyme analysis has been used to classify different strains of *Acanthamoeba.* Restriction enzyme analysis of either mitochondrial DNA or cellular DNA often has not correlated with morphologic characteristics of different species. At present the identification of *Acanthamoeba* is based on morphologic, biologic, and physiologic characteristics.

DIFFERENTIAL DIAGNOSIS

The diagnosis of acanthamoebic keratitis is aided by a high degree of suspicion on the part of the ophthalmologist, as well as several characteristic clinical appearances that may be present. Corneal *Acanthamoeba* infection can mimic a number of other types of corneal disease, including bacterial, viral, or fungal keratitis. It is frequently misdiagnosed as herpes simplex stromal keratitis. Early infection and recurrent epithelial breakdown may produce a dendriform pattern. Cultures taken from these lesions can induce changes on cell-culture plates, because *Acanthamoeba* can destroy individual cells. The severe pain and the annular infiltrate associated with acanthamoebic keratitis may aid clinical differentiation.

THERAPY

Antimicrobial Agents

Acanthamoeba is highly resistant to available chemotherapeutic agents. A combination of antibiotics, antiprotozoal, antifungal, antiparasitic, and antiviral drugs have been tested against *Acanthamoeba.*[44,45,48,76] Ocular application of several drugs have suggested several compounds of potential clinical use (see box), but more than one agent is usually suggested.

Diamidine derivatives include dibrompropamidine

ANTIMICROBIAL AGENTS USED IN THE TREATMENT OF ACANTHAMOEBIC KERATITIS

Aminoglycosides
  Neomycin
  Paromomycin
Diamidines
  Dibrompropamidine
  Hexamidine
  Propamidine
Imidazoles
  Clotrimazole
  Fluconazole
  Itraconazole
  Ketoconazole
  Miconazole
Antiseptic biocides
  Chlorhexidine
  Polyhexamethylene biguanide

0.15% (Brolene ointment), hydroxystilbamidine, hexamidine 0.1% (Desomedine), propamidine isethionate 0.1% (Brolene solution), pentamidine isethionate 0.05% to 0.1% (Pentam 300), and diminazene aceturate. Imidazole derivatives (e.g., miconazole 10 mg/ml, clotrimazole 1%, and metronidazole) and aminoglycoside derivatives (neomycin-polymyxin B-gramicidin and paromomycin) have been successfully used for treatment of acanthamoebic keratitis. Systemic imidazoles (e.g., ketoconazole, fluconazole, or itraconazole) are also recommended.

Topical treatment usually begins with hourly instillations around the clock for approximately 48 hours, and the frequency gradually is decreased to hourly instillation during waking hours. Medications are tapered with the goal of maintaining the patient on topical application 3 to 4 times a day for several months.

Medications are more effective against the trophozoite form as compared to the cyst. It is estimated that the initial therapy kills many of the trophozoites while stimulating other trophozoites to encyst. Therefore with the frequency of maintenance at 3 to 4 times a day, the cysts are apt to excyst, leading to a burst of trophozoite activity and thus causing recrudescence. When this condition occurs it is important to increase the frequency of the medications to reestablish therapeutic control. Agents such as topical clotrimazole,[15] topical polyhexamethylene biguanide (PHMB),[32] or topical chlorhexidine,[23a] can be added to the regimen. PHMB is cysticidal at a low concentration and is not very toxic to the corneal epithelium. The ideal medical therapy of acanthamoebic keratitis is yet to be adequately established, however.

Antiinflammatory Agents

The pain, which is often severe in these patients, can be managed with an oral noncorticosteroidal antiinflammatory agent such as sulindac.[30] Narcotics can usually be avoided. A retrobulbar alcohol block has occasionally been used.

Patients with a misdiagnosis of herpes simplex keratitis should have their antiviral agent discontinued. The corticosteroids should be tapered off as quickly as possible.

The role of corticosteroids in the treatment of acanthamoebic keratitis has not been determined. Corticosteroids can suppress the host immune and inflammatory responses; therefore corticosteroid use may permit the parasite to escape the host defense mechanisms, in turn exacerbating the disease. It is also possible that corticosteroid treatments reduce inflammatory reactions caused by parasites, in turn reducing the severity of the disease. Moreover, the use of topical corticosteroids may also inhibit morphogenesis of the organism in which it can transform back and forth from cyst to trophozoite stages. Therefore it is difficult to conclude whether the use of corticosteroids is beneficial or has adverse effects.

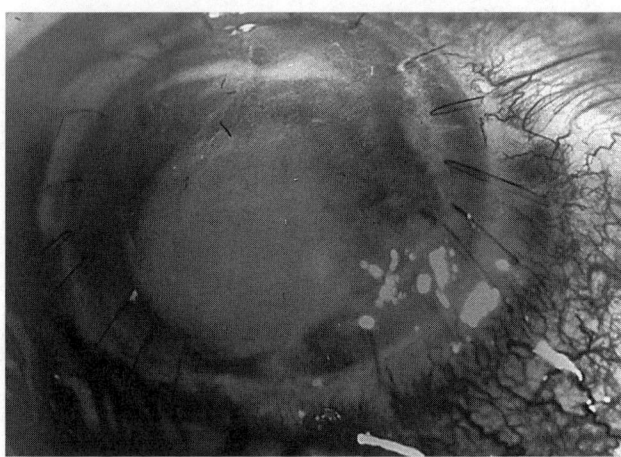

Fig. 78-7. Recurrence of acanthamoebic keratitis in corneal graft.

Surgical Management

Epithelial debridement has been used for management of acanthamoebic keratitis. This procedure may not be successful, however, if the parasites penetrate into the stroma. Surgical debridement can improve the penetration of drugs into the cornea and facilitates the removal of pathogens from the lesion.[1] Debridement is usually effective in the early phases of acanthamoebic keratitis, however, only if it is used with a combination of antiamoebic drugs.[1]

Cryotherapy has been used either with or without penetrating keratoplasty.[1] Effort has been made to use cryotherapy at the time of penetrating keratoplasty to destroy any remaining organisms before transplantation. Trophozoites are killed when subjected to temperatures ranging from -50 to $130°C$, but cysts survive when subjected to similar freezing temperatures. Cryotherapy treatment without corneal transplantation can cause extensive damage to the cornea including opacification, thinning, increased inflammation, necrosis, and vascularization.

Penetrating keratoplasty is deferred until there is a medical cure of the infectious process unless one must do surgery as a globe-saving maneuver. If the infection is not controlled and a penetrating keratoplasty is done, the infection often recurs in the graft (Fig. 78-7) with the greatest devastation in the area of the wound.

PREVENTION

Considering the devastating nature of the disease process and the many problems that ophthalmologists still face with therapy, it is most important to attempt to prevent the disease.

Contact Lens Precautions

Acanthamoebic keratitis occurs predominately in patients who are contact lens wearers. Exposure to contaminated fluids is the major problem. The frequent association of the disease with homemade saline made from distilled water and salt tablets led several companies to withdraw voluntarily from the salt-tablet market. Distilled water and salt tablets should not be used by anyone to make saline. It is unrealistic to expect that a person can use a large container of distilled water over time in making saline without running the risk of significant contamination of the distilled water. Additionally, patients typically keep the large container of distilled water in their kitchen or toilet area, neither of which would be considered a very sterile environment. The use of large containers of intravenous fluids or buffering solutions commonly found in hospitals and laboratories raises the risk for contamination and therefore should not be used for lens care.

Commercial heat sterilization units are effective in killing both *Acanthamoeba* trophozoites and cysts.[36] This method is effective for sterilizing contact lenses, as long as the lens is not contaminated after sterilization and before reinsertion onto the eye. Hydrogen peroxide is effective in killing both trophozoites and cysts if the organism is exposed to the hydrogen peroxide for two hours. Hydrogen peroxide systems that allow one to add the deactivating agent at a certain time after the lens is placed into hydrogen peroxide can be used effectively to kill *Acanthamoeba*, providing that the hydrogen peroxide deactivator is not added before the *Acanthamoeba* have been killed.[58,62] The reagents that are found in the various cold sterilization solutions have been examined previously. There is some variability in time exposure required for those that are effective.[60] Cold sterilization preservatives that are effective require 4 hours of exposure for the *Acanthamoeba* trophozoites to be killed.[61]

Preservatives that have been found to be effective are benzalkonium chloride, thimerosal with ethylenediaminetetraacetic acid (EDTA), chlorhexidine, and polyaminopropyl biguanide at appropriate concentrations. Sorbate, sorbic acid, polyquaternium, thimerosal alone, and EDTA alone are relatively ineffective in killing *Acanthamoeba*.[61]

Immunization

Immunity plays an important role in the pathogenesis of infections by free-living amoebae such as *Naegleria* sp.[9,68] Passively transferred immune serum protects mice against a lethal intranasal inoculation of *N. fowleri*. Protection resides in the IgG fraction of immune serum. Whether a similar situation applies to acanthamoebic keratitis has yet to be determined.

As in other protozoal infections, cytokines play an important role in the immune resistance to acanthamoebic keratitis. For example, γ interferon significantly increases the ability of macrophages to kill *Acanthamoeba* trophozoites in vitro.[65] Although γ interferon also exerts direct antiparasitic effects on plasmodium and toxoplasma, it is not known if a similar condition occurs with *Acanthamoeba*.

The role played by the secretory immune system in protecting against *Acanthamoeba* is unknown. It has been suggested that immunity protects against a wide variety of infections at the mucosal surfaces. Secretory IgA antibodies can prevent binding of bacteria and internalization of viruses at the mucosal surfaces.[14,28] Two independent studies have shown that partial immunity to trachoma in monkeys and guinea pigs is correlated with the appearance of IgA antibodies in their ocular secretions.[50,52] Specific antibody-producing plasma cells can be stimulated in the conjunctiva either by enteric priming with cholera toxin followed by conjunctival challenge or by repeated conjunctival immunization alone.[67] These latter findings suggest that ocular priming together with enteric priming might be sufficient to induce ocular mucosal immunity and therefore may have practical value for inducing protection against acanthamoebic keratitis.[1] Immunization may offer a future means of protection against this serious protozoal infection.

REFERENCES

1. Alizadeh H, He Y, McCulley JP et al.: Successful immunization against *Acanthamoeba* keratitis in a pig model, *Cornea* 14:180-186, 1995.
1a. Auran JD, Starr MB, Jakobiec FA: *Acanthamoeba* keratitis. A review of the literature, *Cornea* 6:2, 1987.
2. Badenoch PR et al.: Pathogenicity of *Acanthamoeba* and *Corynebacterium* in the rat cornea, *Arch Ophthalmol* 108:107-112, 1990.
3. Brown TJ, Cursons RTM, Keys EA: Amoeba from antarctic soil and water, *Appl Environ Microbiol* 44:491, 1982.
4. Castellani A: An amoeba found in cultures of yeast: preliminary note, *J Trop Med Hyg* 33:160, 1930.
5. Cavanagh HD et al.: Clinical and diagnostic use of in vivo confocal microscopy in patients with corneal disease, *Ophthalmology* 100:1444, 1993.
6. Cerva L, Serbus C, Skocil V: Isolation of limax amoeba from the nasal mucosa of man, *Folia Parasitol* 20:97, 1973.
7. Cerva L: *Acanthamoeba culbertsoni* and *Naegleria fowleri*: occurrence of antibodies in man, *J Hyg Epidemiol Microbiol Immunol* 33:99, 1989.
8. Chang SL: Small, free-living amebas: cultivation, quantitation, identification, pathogenesis, and resistance, *Current topics in comparative pathobiology*, 202-254, New York, 1971, Academic Press.
9. Cleary SF, Marciano-Cabral F: Soluble amoebicidal factors mediated cytolysis of *Naegleria fowleri* by activated macrophages, *Cell Immunol* 101:62, 1986.
10. Cohen EJ et al.: Medical and surgical treatment of *Acanthamoeba* keratitis, *Am J Ophthalmol* 103:615-625, 1987.
11. Cursons RTM, Brown TJ: Use of cell cultures as an indicator of pathogenicity of free-living amoebae, *J Clin Pathol* 31:1, 1978.
12. Cursons RTM et al.: Immunity to pathogenic free-living amoeba: role of humoral antibody, *Infect Immun* 29:401, 1980.
13. Douglas M: Notes on the classification of the amoeba found by Castellani in cultures of a yeast-like fungus, *J Trop Med Hyg* 33:258, 1930.
14. Douglas RG et al.: Rhinovirus neutralizing antibody in tears, parotid saliva nasal secretions and serum, *J Immunol* 99:297, 1967.
15. Driebe WT Jr et al.: *Acanthamoeba* keratitis: potential role for topical clotrimazole in combination chemotherapy, *Arch Ophthalmol* 106:1196, 1988.
16. Dujardin F: Historie naturelle des zoophytes infusoires, *Librairie Encyclopédique de Roret*, Paris, 1841.
17. Ferrante A: Free living amoeba: pathogenicity and immunity, *Parasit Immunol* 13:31, 1991.
18. Ferrante A: Immunity to *Acanthamoeba*, *Rev Infect Dis* 13(suppl 5):S403, 1991.
19. Ferrante A, Rowan-Kelly B: Activation of the alternative pathway of complement by *Acanthamoeba culbertsoni*, *Clin Exp Immunol* 54:477, 1983.
20. Font RL et al.: An animal model of *Acanthamoeba* keratitis, *Invest Ophthalmol Vis Sci* 20(suppl):8, 1981.
21. Franchini G: Sur une amibe de la laitue (Latuca Sativa), *Bull Soc Pathol Exot* 15:784, 1922.

22. Garner A: Pathology of acanthamoebic infection. In Cavanagh HD, editor: *The cornea: transactions of the world congress on the cornea III*, 535-539, New York, 1988, Raven Press.

22a. Giovannini A, Tittavelli R, Bertelli E, et al.: Bilateral *Acanthamoeba* keratitis in a gas-permeable contact lens wearer, *Ophthalmologica* 208:321-324, 1994.

23. Gitler C, Calef E, Rosenberg I: Cytopathogenicity of *Entamoeba histolytica*, *Philos Trans R Soc Lond* B307:73, 1984.

23a. Hay J, Kirkness CM, Seal DV, Wright P: Drug resistance and *Acanthamoeba* keratitis: the quest for alternative antiprotozoal chemotherapy, *Eye* 8:555-563, 1994.

24. He YG et al.: In vivo and in vitro collagenolytic activity of *Acanthamoeba castellanii*, *Invest Ophthalmol Vis Sci* 31:2235, 1990.

25. He YG et al.: A pig model of *Acanthamoeba* keratitis: transmission via contaminated contact lenses, *Invest Ophthalmol Vis Sci* 33:126, 1992.

26. John T, Desai D, and Sam D: Adherence of *Acanthamoeba castellanii* cysts and trophozoites to extended wear soft contact lenses, *Rev Infect Dis* 13(suppl 5):S419, 1991.

27. Jones DB, Visvesvara GS, Robinson NM: *Acanthamoeba polyphaga* keratitis and *Acanthamoeba* uveitis associated with fatal meningoencephalitis, *Trans Ophthalmol Soc UK* 95:221, 1975.

28. Kasel JA et al.: Human influenza: aspects of the immune response to vaccination, *Ann Intern Med* 71:369, 1969.

29. Key et al.: Keratitis due to *Acanthamoeba castellanii:* a clinico pathologic case report, *Arch Ophthalmol* 98:475, 1980.

30. Koenig BS et al.: *Acanthamoeba* keratitis associated with gas-permeable contact lens wear, *Am J Ophthalmol* 103:832, 1987.

31. Larkin DFP, Berry M, Easty DL: In vitro corneal pathogenicity of *Acanthamoeba*, *Eye* 5:560, 1991.

32. Larkin DFP, Easty DL: Experimental *Acanthamoeba* keratitis. I. Preliminary findings, *Br J Ophthalmol* 74:421, 1990.

33. Larkin DFP, Easty DL: Experimental *Acanthamoeba* keratitis: immunohistochemical evaluation, *Br J Ophthalmol* 75:421, 1991.

34. Larkin DFP et al.: Treatment of *Acanthamoeba* keratitis with polyhexamethylene biguanide, *Ophthalmology* 99:185, 1992.

35. Lewis EJ, Sawyer TK: *Acanthamoeba tibiashii* n.s.p.: a new species of fresh water Amoebida (Acanthamoebidae), *Trans Am Microbiol Soc* 98:543, 1974.

36. Ludwing HI et al.: Susceptibility of *Acanthamoeba* to soft contact lens disinfection systems, *Invest Ophthalmol Vis Sci* 27:626, 1986.

37. Lyons TB, Kapur R: Limax amoeba in public swimming pools of Albany, Schenectady, and Ransselaer Counties, New York: their concentration, correlations, and significance, *Appl Environ Microbiol* 2:27, 1977.

38. Ma P et al.: *Naegleria* and *Acanthamoeba* infectious: review, *Rev Infect Dis* 12:490, 1990.

39. Mannis MK et al.: *Acanthamoeba* sclerokeratitis: determining diagnostic criteria, *Arch Ophthalmol* 104:1313, 1986.

40. Martinez AJ: Free-living amoeba: pathogenic aspects, a review, *Protozool Abst* 7:293, 1983.

41. Martinez AJ: *Free living amoebas: natural history, prevention, diagnosis, pathology and treatment of disease*, Boca Raton, Fl, 1985, CRC Press.

42. Mathers et al.: Immunopathology and electron microscopy of Acanthamoeba keratitis, *Am J Ophthalmol* 103:626, 1987.

43. McCulley JP: Clinical perspectives of *Acanthamoeba* keratitis, *Ophthalmology (Japan)* 33:727, 1991.

44. Moore MB, McCulley JP: Treatment of *Acanthamoeba* keratitis, *Am J Ophthalmol* 104:310, 1987.

45. Moore MB, McCulley JP: *Acanthamoeba* keratitis associated with contact lenses: six consecutive cases of successful management, *Br J Ophthalmol* 73:271, 1989.

46. Moore MB et al.: *Acanthamoeba* keratitis associated with soft contact lenses, *Am J Ophthalmol* 100:396, 1985.

47. Moore MB et al.: Radial keratoneuritis as a presenting sign in *Acanthamoeba* keratitis, *Ophthalmology* 93:1310, 1986.

48. Moore MB et al.: A growing problem in soft and hard contact lens wearers, *Ophthalmology* 94:1654, 1987.

49. Moore MB et al.: In vitro penetration of human corneal epithelium by *Acanthamoeba castellanii:* a scanning and transmission electron microscopy study, *Cornea* 10:291, 1991.

50. Murray ES et al.: Immunity to chlamydial infections of the eye. I. The role of circulatory and secretory antibodies in resistance to reinfection with guinea pig inclusion conjunctivitis, *J Immunol* 110:1518, 1973.

51. Niederkorn JY et al.: Susceptibility of corneas from various animal species to in vitro binding and invasion by *Acanthamoeba castellanii. Invest Ophthalmol Vis Sci* 33:104, 1992.

52. Peters JH et al.: Development of local and systemic immunity in trachoma of man and animals. In Dayton DH Jr et al., editors: *The secretory immunologic system,* proceedings of conference on the secretory immunologic system, Washington DC, 1969, US Government Printing Office.

53. Rivera F et al.: Bottled mineral water polluted by protozoa in Mexico, *J Protozool* 28:54, 1981.

54. Rivera F et al.: Survey of pathogenic and free-living amoeba inhabiting swimming pool water in Mexico City, *Environ Res* 32:205, 1983.

55. Rösel von Rosenhof AJ: Der kleine Proteus, Der Monat-herausgeg, *Infekten-Belustigungen* 3:622, 1755.

56. Samples JR et al.: *Acanthamoeba* keratitis possibly acquired from a hot tub, *Arch Ophthalmol* 102:707, 1984.

57. Schlaegel TF, Culbertson CG: Experimental Hartmannella optic neuritis and uveitis, *Ann Ophthalmol* 4:103, 1972.

58. Silvany RE, Dougherty JM, McCulley JP: The effect of contact lens preservatives on *Acanthamoeba, Ophthalmology* 98:854, 1991.

59. Silvany RE, Luckenbach MW, Moore MB: The rapid detection of *Acanthamoeba* in paraffin-embedded sections of corneal tissue with calcofluor white, *Arch Ophthalmol* 105:1366, 1987.

60. Silvany RE, Moore MB, McCulley JP: The effect of less than four hour exposures of thimerosal, benzalkonium chloride, and chlorhexidine on *Acanthamoeba castellanii* and *Acanthamoeba polyphaga, Invest Ophthalmol Vis Sci* 30:41, 1989.

61. Silvany RE et al.: The effect of contact lens solutions on two species of *Acanthamoeba Invest Ophthalmol Vis Sci* 29(suppl):253, 1988.

62. Silvany RE et al.: The effect of currently available contact lens disinfection systems on *Acanthamoeba castellanii* and *Acanthamoeba polyphaga, Ophthalmology* 97:286, 1990.

63. Stehr-Green JK, Bailey TM, Visvesvara GS: The epidemiology of *Acanthamoeba* keratitis in the United States, *Am J Ophthalmol* 107:331, 1989.

64. Stehr-Green JK et al.: *Acanthamoeba* keratitis in soft contact lens wearers: a case-control study, *JAMA* 258:57, 1987.

65. Stewart GL et al.: Chemotactic response of macrophages to *Acanthamoeba castellanii* antigen and antibody-dependent macrophage-mediated killing of the parasite, *J Parasitol* 78:849, 1992.

66. Stopak SS et al.: Growth of *Acanthamoeba* on human corneal epithelial cells and keratocytes in vitro, *Invest Ophthalmol Vis Sci* 32:354, 1991.

67. Taylor HR et al.: Secretory immune cellular traffic between the gut and the eye. In O'Connor GR, Chandler JW, editors: *Proceedings of the third international symposium on the immunology and immunopathology of the eye,* 208-211, New York, 1985, Masson Publishing USA.

68. Thong YH et al.: Resistance of mice to *Naegleria fowleri* in experimental amoebic meningoencephalitis transferred by immune serum, *Am J Trop Med Hyg* 27:238, 1978.

69. Ubelaker JE: *Acanthamoeba* spp.: "Opportunistic pathogens," *Trans Am Microsc Soc* 110:289, 1991.

70. Ubelaker JE et al.: In vitro adherence of *Acanthamoeba castellanii* to human corneal epithelium: a scanning and transmission electron microscopy study, *Cornea* 10:299, 1991.

71. van Klink F, Alizadeh H, He Y et al.: The role of contact lenses, trauma, and Langerhans cells in a Chinese hamster model of *Acanthamoeba* keratitis, *Invest Ophthalmol Vis Sci* 34:1937-1944, 1993.

72. van Klink F, Alizadeh H, Stewart GL et al.: Characterization and pathogenic potential of a soil isolate and an ocular isolate of *Acanthamoeba castellanii* in relation to *Acanthamoeba* keratitis, Curr Eye Res 11:1207-1220, 1992.

73. Volkonsky M: *Hartmannella castellanii* Douglas, et classification des hartmannelles, *Arch Zool Exp Gene* 72:317, 1931.

74. Wang SS, Feldman HA: Isolation of Hartmannella species from human throats, *New Eng J Med* 277:1174, 1967.

75. Whitman LY, Marciano-Cabral F: Susceptibility of pathogenic and non-pathogenic Naegleria spp. to complement mediated lysis, *Infect Immun* 55:2442, 1987.

75a. Winchester K, Mathers WD, Sutphin JE, Daley TE: Diagnosis of *Acanthamoeba* keratitis in vivo with confocal microscopy. *Cornea* 14:10-17, 1995.

76. Wright P, Warhurst D, Jones BR: *Acanthamoeba* keratitis successfully treated medically, *Br J Ophthalmol* 69:778, 1985.

77. Yong JDE, Lowrey DM: Biochemical and functional characteristics of a membrane-associated pore-forming protein from the pathogenic amoeboflagellate *Naegeleria fowleri, J Biol Chem* 164:1077, 1989.

78. Young JDE, Liu CC: Multiple mechanisms of lymphocytic mediated killing, *Immunol Today* 9:140, 1988.

79 Microsporidiosis

CAREEN YEN LOWDER, LOUIS A. WILSON

Microsporidia are ubiquitous organisms known to parasitize every major animal group, both vertebrate and invertebrate, including amphibians, fish, insects, reptiles, birds, and rodents. They can cause a variety of human diseases, involving multiple organ systems, in both immunocompetent and immunosuppressed patients. They are an uncommon, but well-documented, cause of keratitis, which has been associated most recently with the acquired immunodeficiency syndrome (AIDS).

PARASITOLOGY

Microsporidia, an order within the phylum Microspora, consists of ubiquitous obligate intracellular spore-forming protozoans. Three phases characterize the life cycle of Microsporidia, and all occur within the infected host cell: (1) infective, (2) proliferative (merogony and schizogony), and (3) sporogony. Sporogony results in the production of spores, which are resistant to environmental and chemical stresses and are the infective form of Microsporidia (Fig. 79-1). Each spore has a thick two-layered cell wall that encloses a coiled polar filament or polar tubule, as well as one or two nuclei, a polaroplast, and a vacuole (Fig. 79-2).

The coiled polar tubule present in all microsporidial spores is the identifying feature of this parasite. The polar tubule is attached to the spore cell wall by an anchoring disc. Infection occurs by direct invasion of host cells and is accomplished by extrusion of the polar tubule, which penetrates the host cell allowing passage of spore contents to the host cell.[7]

Four genera have been implicated in human infections: *Enterocytozoon, Pleistophora, Nosema,* and *Encephalitozoon.* Various ultrastructural features serve to distinguish and classify the microorganisms in the appropriate genus: (1) the number of coils formed by the polar tubule, (2) the size of the spore, (3) the number and configuration of the nuclei in the spore, and (4) the relationship between the parasite and the host cell (whether there is a parasitophorous vacuole, and whether the vacuole is a product of the host cell or the parasite).[4]

Prior to 1992 *Enterocytozoon bieneusi* was the only microsporidian implicated in the malabsorption and chronic diarrhea syndrome in patients with AIDS. *Enterocytozoon* sp. spores are small, measuring approximately 1.0 by 1.5 μm, and are characterized by multinucleated organisms that develop in direct contact with the host cell cytoplasm and are never associated with a vacuole. A new microsporidian species, yet unclassified, has been recovered from small bowel biopsies of patients with AIDS and chronic diarrhea. This new species develops within a septated vacuole of parasitic origin. In contrast to *E. bieneusi,* which are only observed within enterocytes, this new species spreads to different sites within the host, such as kidney, liver, peritoneal cavity, and central nervous system.[21]

In 1985 *Pleistophora* sp. was recovered from the skeletal muscles of a man with progressive muscle weakness.[16] *Pleistophora* sp. spores are slightly larger, measuring approximately 2.8 by 3.4 μm and are characterized by development in clusters of more than eight spores within a parasite-formed parasitophorous vacuole. The polar tubule has about 11 coils. The organism is usually found in the skeletal muscles of fish.

Spores of the genus *Nosema* measure approximately 2.0 by 4.0 μm and contain two abutted nuclei (diplokaryon). The polar tubule has 10 or more coils, and the spores are in direct contact with the cell cytoplasm; there is no pansporoblastic membrane nor a parasitophorous vacuole.

The genus *Encephalitozoon* has small spores measuring approximately 1.0 by 2.0 μm, the polar tubule has five to seven coils, and the organism develops within a parasitophorous vacuole of host origin.

EPIDEMIOLOGY

Only eight cases of human microsporidial infection were reported between 1959 and 1990 in immunocompetent patients or immunocompromised individuals without AIDS.[9] Four of the cases involved the eye.[1,4,11,22] Since 1985 microsporidia have been demonstrated to be the causal agents of enteritis in over 75 patients with AIDS, chronic diarrhea,

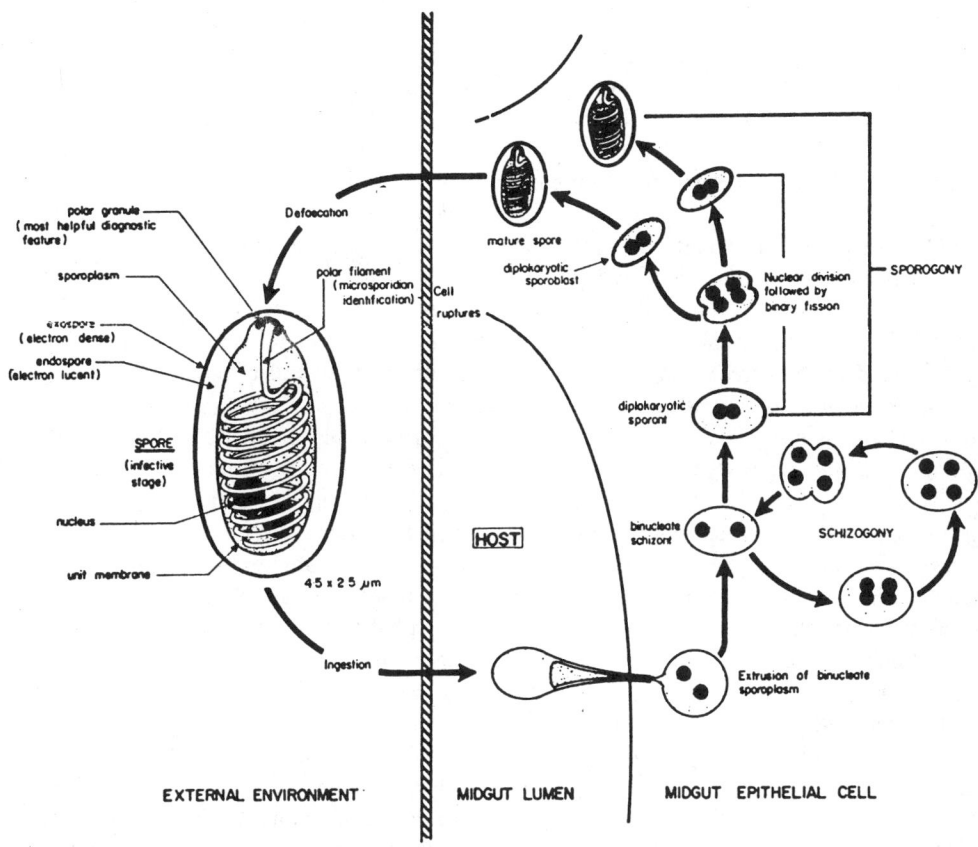

Fig. 79-1. Life-cycle diagram of *Nosema apicalis*. (Reprinted with permission from Tabbara KF, Hyndiuk RA, editors: *Infections of the Eye,* 184, Boston, 1986, Little, Brown.)

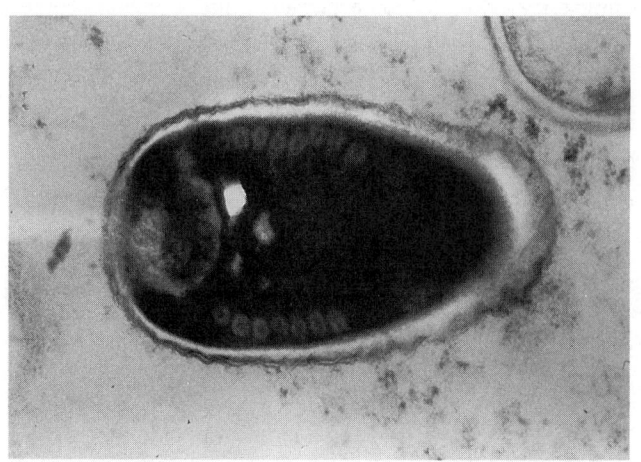

Fig. 79-2. Transmission electron photomicrograph of a microsporidial spore in a conjunctival epithelial cell ($\times$ 99,000). (Reprinted with permission from Diesenhouse MC, Wilson LA, Corrent GF et al.: Treatment of microsporidial keratoconjunctivitis with topical fumagillin, *Am J Ophthalmol* 115:293-298, 1993. Copyright by The Ophthalmic Publishing Company.)

and weight loss.[21,29,33] Since 1990 at least 14 cases of microsporidial keratoconjunctivitis have been reported in patients with AIDS.*

Exposure to farm animals, proximity to the tropics, and trauma are factors postulated in the development of microsporidiosis. Direct inoculation is postulated in ocular dis-

ease. Horizontal transmission may be the most important source of infection in ocular microsporidiosis. Schwartz and associates[24] reported concomitant tracheobronchial, ocular, and urinary tract involvement in a patient with *Encephalitozoon hellem* infection. *E. hellem* was also detected in the urinary sediment of two patients reported by Diesenhouse and associates.[13] Urine to finger to eye transmission may be responsible for horizontal spread in humans.[24,25]

*References 4, 13, 15, 17, 20, 25, 32.

CLINICAL FEATURES

Microsporidia can cause severe, persistent enteritis, especially in immunosuppressed patients; affected individuals develop malabsorption syndromes with chronic diarrhea and weight loss. Disseminated infections can involve the lungs and respiratory tract, kidneys, liver, heart and other muscles, and the central nervous system.

The first case of human microsporidial infection, reported in 1959, was from the genus *Encephalitozoon*.[19] A Japanese boy exposed to farm animals developed headache, convulsions, and recurrent fever. Microsporidia of the genus *Encephalitozoon* were found in the cerebral spinal fluid and urine of this patient. A second report appeared in 1984. A 3-year-old Colombian boy developed seizures and hepatomegaly; *Encephalitozoon cuniculi* was identified in urine specimens.[2]

The first reported case of *Nosema* sp. human infection was in 1973. *Nosema connori* was found widely disseminated in a 4-month-old infant with combined immunodeficiency, who presented with diarrhea, malabsorption, and athymic dysplasia. Organisms were identified in the kidney, adrenal cortex, liver, lungs, myocardium, and arterial walls. Large numbers of organisms were present within infected tissues, but elicited little host inflammatory response except in the diaphragm.[18]

Ocular Disease

There are two clinical presentations of ocular microsporidial infections. A corneal stromal keratitis occurs in immunocompetent patients, and an epithelial keratopathy and conjunctivitis occurs in patients with AIDS. To date, the genus *Nosema* (or reported as *Nosema*-like) has been the only causal agent demonstrated in the corneal stromal keratitis of immunocompetent individuals, and only the genus *Encephalitozoon* has been implicated in the keratoconjunctivitis associated with AIDS.

Immunocompetent Patients. The first case of ocular microsporidial infection was reported in 1973. An 11-year-old boy presented to the Eye Hospital in Colombo, Ceylon with light perception vision in his right eye. The cornea was scarred and vascularized, and the patient reported having been gored by a goat 6 years previously. Penetrating keratoplasty was performed, and histopathology of the corneal button revealed necrotic stroma surrounded by acute inflammatory cells. Refractile oval bodies measuring approximately 3.5 by 1.5 μm were present in the deep stroma immediately above Descemet membrane. Based on the morphologic appearance, the authors called this organism *Nosema cuniculi*.[1] Recently, because the nucleation of the organism was not observed and the genus designation not proved, Canning and Lom[8] transferred this parasite to the genus *Microsporidium* (a genus developed for unclassified organisms) subtype *ceylonensis*.

The second case of ocular infection was reported in 1981.[22] A 26-year-old woman from Botswana, Africa had a 4-month history of a painful left eye when she presented for examination. The eye had no light perception, and the cornea had a central perforated corneal ulcer. The enucleated specimen revealed numerous small, oval organisms measuring 2.5 by 4.5 μm anterior to Descemet membrane. Electron microscopic studies revealed 11 to 13 coils in the polar tubule and organisms that were free in the host cell cytoplasm, but the nuclear characteristics were not studied. The authors classified this organism as *Nosema* sp. Because of the lack of knowledge of the nuclear arrangement of this organism, this parasite was also transferred to the genus *Microsporidium*, subtype *africanum*.[8]

In 1990 Davis and associates[11] reported a case of microsporidial infection of the cornea in a 45-year-old man from South Carolina. The patient was healthy and had no history of prior trauma. He presented with decreased vision in his left eye. The initial examination revealed a midstromal infiltrate associated with stromal edema, a small central area of epithelial irregularity, and iritis. The stromal infiltrate enlarged over the next 11 months (despite treatment with topical corticosteroids and neomycin/bacitracin/polymyxin eye drops), and a penetrating keratoplasty was performed (Fig. 79-3). Histopathologic examination of the corneal specimen revealed large numbers of spores within the stroma and a lack of an inflammatory cellular response[11] (Fig. 79-4). This microsporidial organism was isolated and propagated in vitro.[27] The spores measured 3.7 by 1.0 μm and contained two closely abutted nuclei, identifying the organism as a diplokaryon. Replication occurred in direct contact with the host cell cytoplasm (absence of a parasitophorous vacuole). The polar tubule had five to six coils. These features were different from previously described species of *Nosema*, and the organism was therefore named *Nosema corneum* (Fig. 79-5).

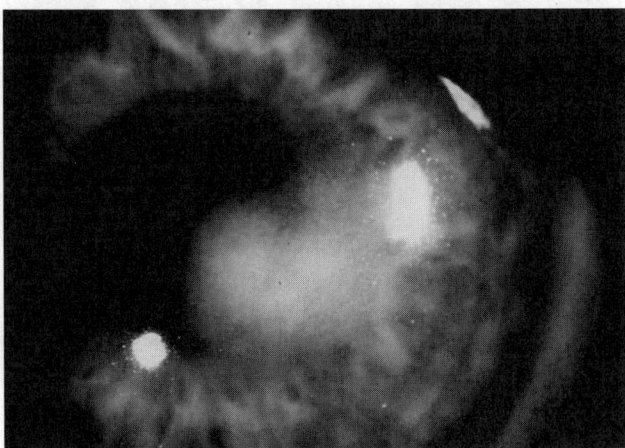

Fig. 79-3. Microsporidial stromal keratitis. (Reprinted with permission from Davis RM, Font RL, Keisler MS, Shadduck DVM: Corneal microsporidiosis: a case report including ultrastructural observations, *Ophthalmology* 97:953-957, 1990.)

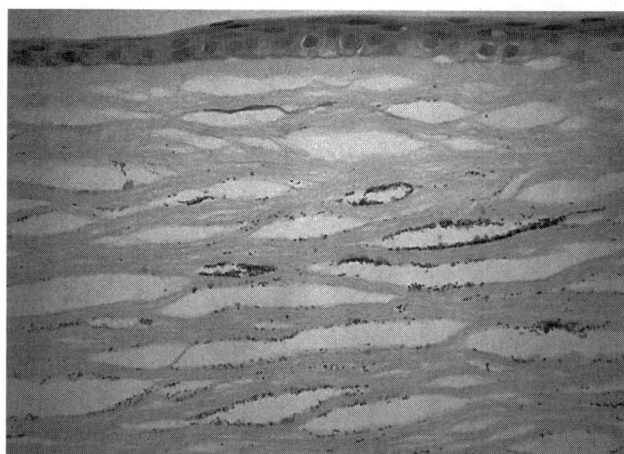

Fig. 79-4. Low power view of anterior corneal stroma. Large numbers of gram-positive spores are located both intracellularly and extracellularly (Brown and Hopps; × 100). (Reprinted with permission from Davis RM, Font RL, Keisler MS, Shadduck DVM: Corneal microsporidiosis: a case report including ultrastructural observations, *Ophthalmology* 97:953-957, 1990.)

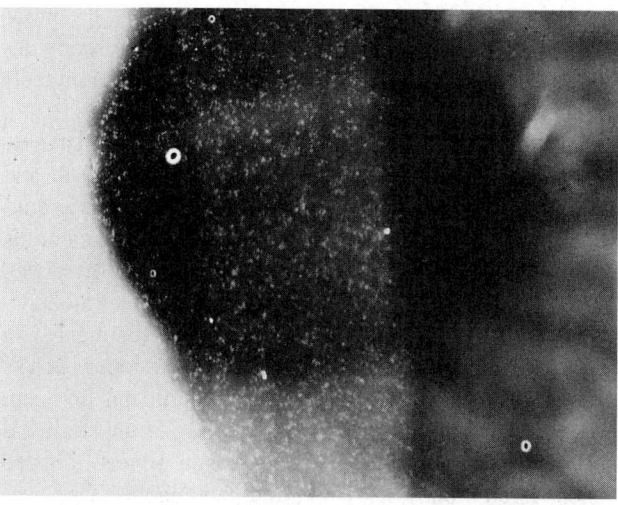

Fig. 79-6. Slit lamp photograph of punctate epithelial keratopathy. (Reprinted with permission from Lowder CY, Meisler DM, McMahon JT et al.: Microsporidia infection of the cornea in an HIV-positive man, *Am J Ophthalmol* 109:242-244, 1990. Copyright by The Ophthalmic Publishing Company.)

The other report of stromal keratitis involved a 39-year-old immunocompetent man from Ohio who presented with blurred vision in his left eye. A corneal foreign body was removed but the corneal ulcer persisted. Examination of the corneal biopsy specimen revealed microsporidial spores measuring 3.0 by 5.0 μm that had 11 to 12 coils of the polar tubule, nuclei in diplokaryon arrangement, and replication within the host cell cytoplasm. All of these features are consistent with the genus *Nosema*, and the subspecies has been named *ocularum*.[4] These results were reported in 1991 by Richard Lembach in the Symposium on Opportunistic Microsporidians from AIDS Isolates.[28]

The stromal keratitis reported in immunocompetent individuals led to a failed graft and loss of the eye in the two early reports. The patient reported by Davis and associates[11] had a penetrating keratoplasty without recurrence of microsporidiosis. The slow progression of stromal keratitis and absence of inflammatory cells may have been secondary to the use of topical corticosteroids.

Immunosuppressed Patients. The first reports of microsporidial keratoconjunctivitis appeared in 1990. Fourteen cases have since been reported in the United States and one in Great Britain. Lowder and associates[17] reported the first case of microsporidial infection of the cornea in an HIV-seropositive man. The patient was a 30-year-old homosexual man with AIDS-related complex and no prior history of opportunistic infections. He had a 3-month history of red eyes associated with crusting that had been unresponsive to topical antibiotics. Visual acuities were 20/25 in each eye. The conjunctiva had a mixed follicular-papillary reaction, and the cornea had a diffuse coarse punctate epithelial keratopathy (Fig. 79-6). Cultures were negative. The corneal epithelium was scraped after the visual acuities decreased to 20/60 with progression of epithelial keratopathy over the next few months. The corneal scrapings were submitted for cultures and histopathologic examination. Cultures of the corneal scrapings were negative. The organisms were poorly visualized in corneal scrapings stained with hematoxylin and eosin; gray granular organisms were present in vacuoles within the cytoplasm of the epithelial cells. Gram-positive oval bodies were found within corneal epithelial cells, and no inflammatory cells were present. A periodic acid Schiff

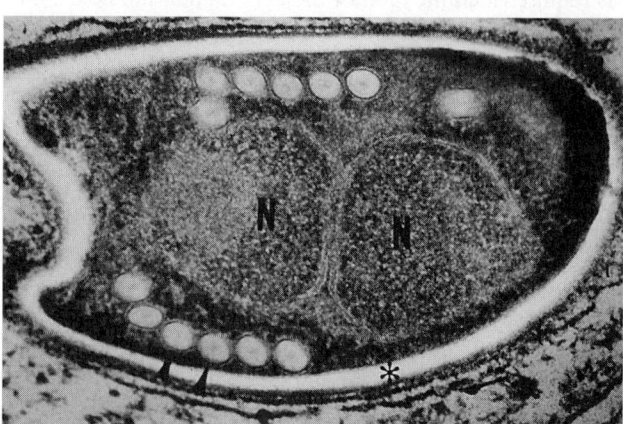

Fig. 79-5. Electron micrograph of a mature spore displaying distinct cell wall and double abutted nuclei (N) and a polar filament with six coils (× 80,000). (Reprinted with permission from Davis RM, Font RL, Keisler MS, Shadduck DVM: Corneal microsporidiosis: a case report including ultrastructural observations, *Ophthalmology* 97:953-957, 1990.)

(PAS) stain-positive body was noted in many of the intracellular inclusions. Transmission electron microscopy revealed spores measuring 1.0 by 2.0 μm and six to eight coils of the polar tubule[17] (Fig. 79-7).

Electron microscopic features of the organism isolated by Lowder and associates[17] were further studied by Cali and associates.[5,6] Although the microorganism had features consistent with *Encephalitozoon cuniculi,* a parasitophorous vacuole could not be identified. The organism has been termed *Encephalitozoon*-like.[5,6] The epithelial keratopathy in this patient continued to progress despite treatment with numerous courses of combination topical antibiotics such as neomycin/polymyxin/bacitracin and the antiparasitic agent propamidine isethionate 0.1%. Progression of the epithelial keratopathy led to increasing symptoms of dryness, blurred vision, foreign body sensation, and photophobia. One year later, examination revealed loss of conjunctival luster, coalescence of the coarse punctate areas of epithelial keratopathy, and corneal vascularization. The epithelial keratopathy appeared to improve when the patient was placed on oral itraconazole for cryptococcal meningitis, but eventually the disease continued its relentless progression.

Three additional cases of microsporidial keratoconjunctivitis from New York were reported by Friedberg and associates[15] in 1990. All had AIDS, with previous episodes of opportunistic infections, such as *Pneumocystis carinii* pneumonia, and/or Kaposi sarcoma. The presenting symptoms in all three cases were similar, consisting of photophobia, blurred vision, and foreign body sensation. Examination of all three cases revealed a superficial corneal epithelial keratopathy characterized by coarse staining and nonstaining epithelial opacities, minimal conjunctival involvement, decreased conjunctival luster, and the presence of a fusiform swelling in the inferior fornix.[15] In contrast to the report by

Lowder and associates,[17] Friedberg and associates[15] recovered microsporidial organisms from an inferior forniceal conjunctival biopsy specimen in one patient and from conjunctival scrapings of the inferior palpebral conjunctiva in a second patient. Diagnosis of the third patient was based on the clinical appearance.

Didier and associates[12] recovered the same organism from cultures of all three patients from New York. Although the organism had the morphologic characteristics of *Encephalitozoon cuniculi,* SDS polyacrylamide gel electrophoresis revealed different protein profiles, and the organism involved in the three infections was named *Encephalitozoon hellem.*[12]

The other reported cases also occurred in patients with AIDS, and the organisms were morphologically of the *Encephalitozoon* genus.[4,20,32] The clinicopathologic features, including immunofluorescent antibody demonstration of microsporidia, were reported for seven additional patients with ocular disease by Schwartz and associates.[25] All patients had markedly decreased levels of CD4+ T-lymphocytes (mean, 26/μl). Light and electron microscopic studies of cornea, conjunctival biopsies, cytologic specimens, and intact globes revealed microsporidia of the genus *Encephalitozoon.* Immunofluorescent antibody techniques were required for species identification of *Encephalitozoon hellem* in all seven patients, since morphologically and ultrastructurally, *E. hellem* is identical to *E. cuniculi.* A total of 11 cases of microsporidia ocular infection in HIV-seropositive patients have been attributed to *E. hellem,* suggesting that human infection by the genus *Encephalitozoon* may be predominantly, if not solely, a result of *E. hellem* infection.

LABORATORY INVESTIGATIONS

Microsporidia are difficult to recover in culture. Diagnosis requires identification of the coiled polar tubule distinctive for this parasite by transmission electron microscopy of biopsy specimens. The organism may be identified with gram-stained scrapings (Fig. 79-8), swabs, or biopsy specimens of the conjunctiva, avoiding the risk of secondary infection associated with corneal scraping. The organism stains gram-positive. The organisms have variable staining characteristics with Gomori methenamine silver, acid-fast, and Giemsa stains. The presence of a PAS-positive body at one end of the oval structure, the mature spore, is diagnostic for microsporidia at the light microscopic level. The organism is poorly visualized on hematoxylin and eosin stained sections. Serologic tests are not reliable.

Although morphologic identification of microsporidia to the genus level can be obtained by histochemical and electron microscopic studies, determination of species can only be made by antibody or biochemical studies. Antiserum to *Encephalitozoon hellem* has been produced by the Division of Parasitic Diseases of the Centers for Disease Control and Prevention, and was used by Schwartz and associates[25] in

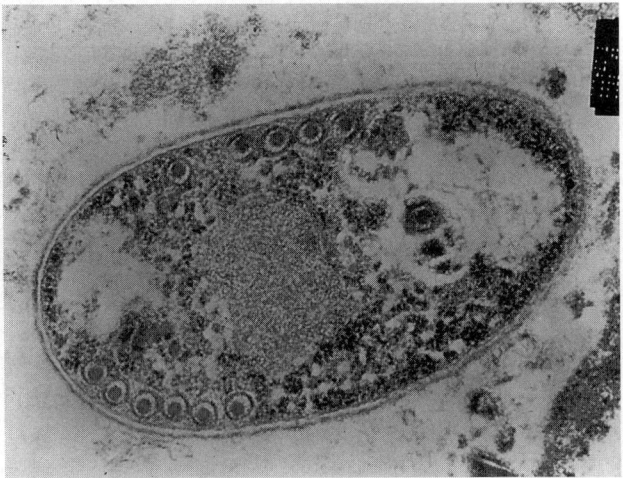

Fig. 79-7. Transmission electron micrograph of a microsporidial spore of *Encephalitozoon* sp. Ultrastructural features include cell wall, coiled filament, polar vacuole, and a single nucleus.

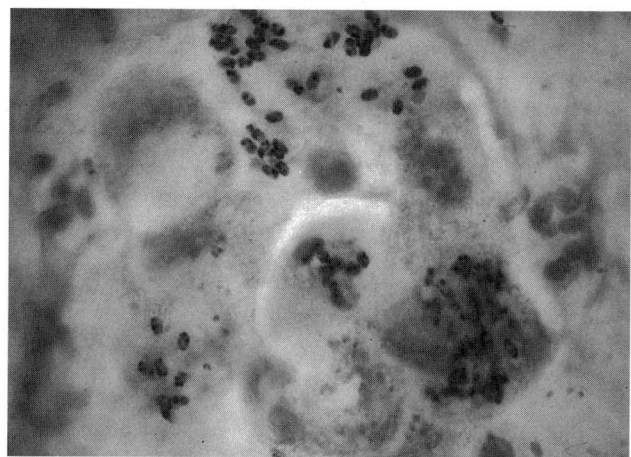

Fig. 79-8.   Gram stain of a smear of a conjunctival scraping. Numerous ovoid gram-positive organisms are within the cytoplasm of conjunctival epithelial cells (×290). (Reprinted with permission from Diesenhouse MC, Wilson LA, Corrent GF et al.: Treatment of microsporidial keratoconjunctivitis with topical fumagillin, *Am J Ophthalmol* 115:293-298, 1993. Copyright by The Ophthalmic Publishing Company.)

the identification of *Encephalitozoon hellem* as the infectious agent.[13,25,30,31] The increasing identification of microsporidia in human infections is most likely secondary to increased awareness of microsporidia as potential opportunistic pathogens.[4,7,12]

THERAPY

The epithelial keratopathy and conjunctivitis caused by microsporidia in patients with AIDS are unresponsive to combination antibiotics. Yee and associates[32] reported resolution of microsporidial keratoconjunctivitis in an AIDS patient who was started on oral itraconazole, 200 mg orally twice a day, for concurrent cryptococcal meningitis. The patient had previously been treated with topical neomycin/polymyxin B sulfate/dexamethasone and topical intravenous preparation of trimethoprim/sulfisoxazole without improvement. After 6 weeks on oral itraconazole, the patient's foreign body sensation and punctate staining decreased, and repeat conjunctival scrapings revealed no organisms.

Trimethoprim had been used with limited success in managing microsporidial diarrhea[10]; but when it was used topically, it had no effect on patients treated by Diesenhouse and associates[13] or Yee and associates.[32] Metronidazole, an antiprotozoal drug previously reported to be useful in managing HIV-positive patients with gastrointestinal microsporidiosis,[14] was equally ineffective when used topically in the treatment of microsporidial keratoconjunctivitis.[13]

Thiabendazole is an anthelmintic benzimidazole with larvacidal activity and some suggestion of activity against protozoan parasites. Nevertheless, a 0.4% suspension applied topically had no effect in the management of at least

one case of microsporidial keratoconjunctivitis.[13] Albendazole, a related benzimidazole, has been reported effective in managing intestinal microsporidiosis caused by *Enterocytozoon bieneusi,* when administered orally[3]; but its topical use for microsporidial keratoconjunctivitis has not been reported.

Propamidine isethionate 0.1% (Brolene) 6 times daily for 3 weeks led to resolution of microsporidial keratoconjunctivitis in the patient reported by Metcalfe and associates.[20] Transmission electron microscopy confirmed the lack of intracellular parasites following treatment with Brolene. Recurrence was documented after Brolene was discontinued. The patient reported by Lowder and associates[17] failed to resolve on either Brolene or itraconazole.

Diesenhouse and associates[13] have reported on the use of fumagillin in the management of *Encephalitozoon hellem* keratoconjunctivitis. They used the water soluble form of the drug fumagillin bicyclohexylammonium salt (Fumadil B). The drug may be obtained from Mid-Continent Agrimarketing (Overland Park, Kansas) and contains approximately 23 mg of fumagillin per gram of dry powder. The topical solution is prepared by adding 60 mg of Fumadil B to 20 ml of sterile saline protected from light and filtered with a 0.22 μm cellulose acetate filter. The final preparation contains 3 mg/ml of Fumadil B or 70 μm/ml of fumagillin. Fumadil B is used commercially to control nosematosis, a microsporidial disease of honey bees caused by *Nosema apis.* Using this preparation, Shadduck[26] observed a significant inhibitory effect by fumagillin on the in vitro multiplication of rabbit and canine isolates of *Encephalitozoon cu-*

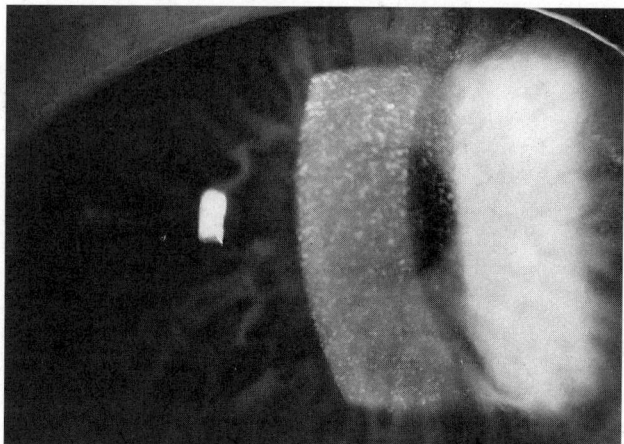

Fig. 79-9.   Coarse white epithelial infiltrates and erosions in a patient with microsporidial epithelial keratopathy prior to treatment with topical fumagillin. (Reprinted with permission from Schwartz DA, Visvesvara GS, Diesenhouse MC et al.: Pathologic features and immunofluorescent antibody demonstration of ocular microsporidiosis *(Encephalitozoon hellem)* in seven patients with acquired immunodeficiency syndrome, *Am J Ophthalmol* 115:285-292, 1993. Copyright by The Ophthalmic Publishing Company.)

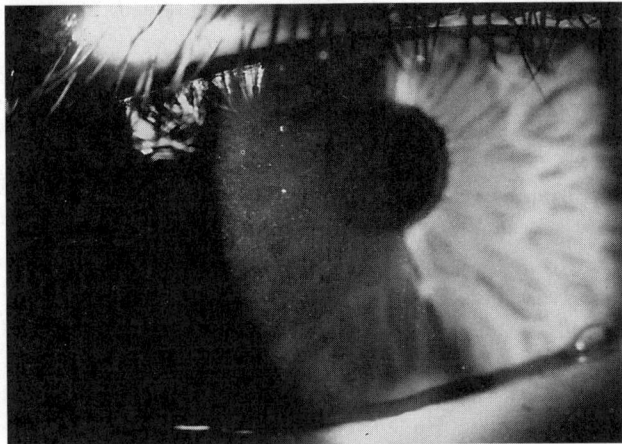

Fig. 79-10. Left cornea after 5 weeks of topical fumagillin (Fumadil B) therapy. Small scattered irregular white intraepithelial opacities persist. (Reprinted with permission from Diesenhouse MC, Wilson LA, Corrent GF et al.: Treatment of microsporidial keratoconjunctivitis with topical fumagillin, *Am J Ophthalmol* 115:293-298, 1993. Copyright by The Ophthalmic Publishing Company.)

niculi. The drug did not entirely eliminate the organism from the previously infected cell cultures, and on discontinuation of the drug, a number of organisms returned to pretreatment levels. Diesenhouse and associates[13] treated their patients with fumagillin hourly for 1 week, with decrease of symptoms as well as conjunctival hyperemia and corneal changes (Figs. 79-9, 79-10). Although scattered intraepithelial opacities were still present, the epithelium was not eroded, nor did it stain with fluorescein. Frequency of instillation was reduced to every 2 hours for 1 week, and the patient was

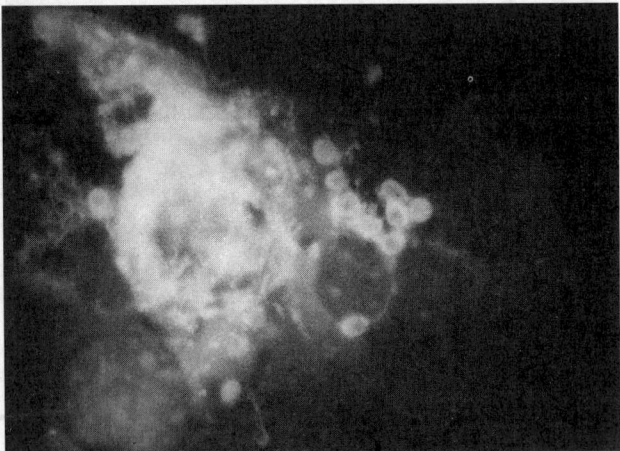

Fig. 79-11. Microsporidial organisms reacted intensely with species-specific antisera using indirect immunofluorescent assay (× 1000). (Reprinted with permission from Diesenhouse MC, Wilson LA, Corrent GF et al.: Treatment of microsporidial keratoconjunctivitis with topical fumagillin, *Am J Ophthalmol* 115:293-298, 1993. Copyright by The Ophthalmic Publishing Company.)

maintained on 1 drop 5 times daily. The patient became asymptomatic but continued to have white intraepithelial opacities. Conjunctival scrapings and immunofluorescent antibody assays continued to be positive during therapy, suggesting persistence of *Encephalitozoon cuniculi* spores during treatment (Fig. 79-11).[13]

SUMMARY

The clinical appearance of ocular microsporidiosis in the immunocompromised individual with AIDS differs markedly from that seen in the immunocompetent host. All of the reported cases in patients with AIDS had a slowly progressive corneal epithelial keratopathy without stromal involvement. Electron microscopic examination of biopsy specimens revealed organisms with the morphologic characteristics of genus *Encephalitozoon*. Reports of successful treatment with fumagillin are promising.[13,23] The stromal keratitis in the immunocompetent individual is associated with a severe inflammatory reaction unless modified by the use of topical corticosteroids. In all cases the organism identified was a member of the genus *Nosema* or was *Nosema*-like. Treatment appears to require the surgical excision of infected necrotic tissue. The distinct clinical appearances may be due to the individual's immunologic status and ability to mount an inflammatory response or to the specific clinical syndromes elicited by two different genera of microsporidia.

REFERENCES

1. Ashton N, Wirasinha PA: Encephalitozoonosis (Nosematosis) of the cornea, *Br J Ophthalmol* 57:669-674, 1973.
2. Bergquist NR, Stintzing G, Smedman L et al.: Diagnosis of encephalitozoonosis in man by serological tests, *BMJ* 288:902, 1984.
3. Blanshard C, Ellis DS, Tovey DG et al.: Treatment of intestinal microsporidiosis with Albendazole in patients with AIDS, *AIDS* 6:311, 1992.
4. Bryan RT, Cali A, Owen RL, Spencer HC: Microsporidia: opportunistic pathogens in patients with AIDS. In Sun T, editor: *Progress in clinical parasitology,* 2:1-26, Philadelphia, 1991, Field and Wood.
5. Cali A, Meisler DM, Lowder CY et al.: Corneal microsporidioses: characterization and identification, *J Protozool* 38:2155-2175, 1991.
6. Cali A, Meisler DM, Lowder CY et al.: Corneal microsporidiosis in a patient with AIDS, *Am J Trop Med Hyg* 44:463-468, 1991.
7. Cali A, Owen R: Microsporidiosis. In Balows A, Hausler WJ, editors: *The laboratory diagnosis of infectious diseases: principles and practice,* vol 1, New York, 1988, Springer-Verlag.
8. Canning EU, Lom J: *The microsporidia of vertebrates,* London, 1986, Academic Press.
9. Center for Disease Control: Microsporidian keratoconjunctivitis in patients with AIDS, *MMWR* 39:188-189, 1990.
10. Current WL, Owen RL: Cryptosporidiosis and Microsporidiosis. In Farthing MJG, Keusch GT, editors: *Enteric infection: mechanisms, manifestations and management,* 223-249, London, 1989, Chapman and Hall Medical.
11. Davis RM, Font RL, Keisler MS, Shadduck DVM: Corneal microsporidiosis: a case report including ultrastructural observations, *Ophthalmology* 97:953-957, 1990.
12. Didier ES, Didier PJ, Friedberg DN et al.: Isolation and characterization of a new human microsporidian, *Encephalitozoon hellem* (n.sp.), keratoconjunctivitis, *J Infect Dis* 163:617, 1991.
13. Diesenhouse MC, Wilson LA, Corrent GF et al.: Treatment of microsporidial keratoconjunctivitis with topical fumagillin, *Am J Ophthalmol* 115:293-298, 1993.

14. Eeftinck Schattenkerk JKM, van Gool T, van Ketel RJ et al.: Clinical significance of small intestinal microsporidiosis in HIV-1 infected individuals, *Lancet* 337:895, 1991.

15. Friedberg DN, Stenson SM, Orenstein JM et al.: Microsporidial keratoconjunctivitis in acquired immunodeficiency syndrome, *Arch Ophthalmol* 108:504-508, 1990.

16. Ledford DK, Overman MD, Gonzalvo A et al.: Microsporidiosis myositis in a patient with acquired immunodeficiency syndrome, *Ann Intern Med* 102:628-630, 1985.

17. Lowder CY, Meisler DM, McMahon JT et al.: Microsporidia infection of the cornea in an HIV-positive man, *Am J Ophthalmol* 109:242-244, 1990.

18. Margileth AM, Strano AJ, Chandra R et al.: Disseminated nosematosis in an immunologically compromised infant, *Arch Pathol* 95:145-150, 1973.

19. Matsubayashi H, Koike T, Mikata T, Hagiwara S: A case of *Encephalitozoon*-like body infection in man, *Arch Pathol* 67:181-187, 1959.

20. Metcalfe TW, Doran RM, Rowlands PL et al.: Microsporidial keratoconjunctivitis in a patient with AIDS, *Br J Ophthalmol* 76:177-178, 1992.

21. Orenstein JM, Tenner M, Cali A, Kotter DP: A microsporidia previously undescribed in humans, infecting enterocytes and macrophages and associated with diarrhea in an acquired immunodeficiency syndrome patient, *Hum Pathol* 23:722-728, 1992.

22. Pinnolis M, Egbert PR, Font RL, Winter FC: Nosematosis of the cornea, *Arch Ophthalmol* 99:1044-1047, 1981.

23. Rosberger D, Serdarevic O: Treatment of Microsporidia keratoconjunctivitis with fumagillin in a patient with AIDS (submitted for publication).

24. Schwartz DA, Bryan RT, Hewan-Lowe KO et al.: Disseminated microsporidiosis *(Encephalitozoon hellem)* and AIDS: autopsy evidence for respiratory acquisition, *Arch Pathol Lab Med* 116:660, 1992.

25. Schwartz DA, Visvesvara GS, Diesenhouse MC et al.: Pathologic features and immunofluorescent antibody demonstration of ocular microsporidiosis *(Encephalitozoon hellen)* in seven patients with acquired immunodeficiency syndrome, *Am J Ophthalmol* 115:285-292, 1993.

26. Shadduck JA: Effect of fumagillin on in vitro multiplication of *Encephalitozoon cuniculi, J Protozool* 27:202, 1980.

27. Shadduck JA, Meccoli RA, Davis R, Font RL: Isolation of a microsporidian from a human patient, *J Infect Dis* 162:773-736, 1990.

28. Symposium on opportunistic microsporidians from AIDS isolates, Bozeman, Montana, July 1, 1991.

29. Terada S, Reddy R, Jeffers LJ et al.: Microsporidian hepatitis in the acquired immunodeficiency syndrome, *Ann Intern Med* 107:61-62, 1987.

30. Visvesvara GS, Leitch GJ, Moura HM et al.: Culture, electron microscopy, and immunoblat studies on a microsporidian parasite isolated from the urine of a patient with AIDS, *J Protozool* 38:105S, 1991.

31. Visvesvara GS, Leitch GJ, Moura HM et al.: Growth characteristics, electron microscopy, and antigenic analysis of the microsporidian isolated from a patient with AIDS, *Am J Trop Med Hyg* 45(suppl):133, 1991.

32. Yee RW, Fermin OT, Martinez J et al.: Resolution of microsporidial epithelial keratopathy in a patient with AIDS, *Ophthalmology* 98:198-201, 1991.

33. Zender HE, Arrigoni E, Eckert J, Kapanci Y: A case of *Encephalitozoon cuniculi* peritonitis in a patient with AIDS, *Am J Clin Pathol* 92:352-356, 1989.

80 Microbial Scleritis

MICHAEL B. RAIZMAN

Infections of the sclera present in many ways and manifest the entire range of severity of inflammation from subclinical to rapidly destructive. In general, scleral infections may be classified into two groups. The first, exogenous infections, is more common and includes posttraumatic and postsurgical infections, as well as extensions from adjacent infections such as keratitis, chorioretinitis, or panophthalmitis. These exogenous infections tend to be acute, suppurative, and destructive. Less common are those cases of scleritis in the second group, endogenous infections. These often present in a way that resembles noninfectious diffuse, nodular, or necrotizing scleritis. Scleritis associated with systemic infections such as syphilis and tuberculosis falls into this category.

EPIDEMIOLOGY

Infections of the sclera are rare. Infection is responsible for scleritis in roughly 4% to 18% of cases of scleritis in a tertiary care setting.[23,40,54] The proportion of infectious cases of scleritis in the general population is almost certainly lower. Scleritis, or inflammation of the sclera, is most often immune-mediated and without an infectious cause.[53,54]

Most cases of infectious scleritis develop from spread of infection to the sclera from adjacent keratitis or severe endophthalmitis. Trauma can lead to infectious scleritis and sclerokeratitis. Reports of infectious scleritis increased following the advent of scleral buckling surgery and with the use of beta-irradiation or mitomycin in conjunction with pterygium excision. Infectious scleritis is found worldwide but especially in those regions where severe bacterial keratitis is prevalent.

RISK FACTORS

Bacteria, viruses, fungi, and parasites are all capable of infecting the sclera (see box). Organisms reach and infect the sclera in a variety of ways (see box).

The most likely route of scleral infection is spread from contiguous ocular structures. Most commonly the sclera is infected by migration of organisms from the adjacent cornea in cases of keratitis.* In a typical scenario, pseudomonal keratitis spreads from the peripheral cornea to the limbal tissues and finally into the sclera if uncontrolled. The predilection for *Pseudomonas* sp. to spread into the sclera probably relates to the virulence of the organism. Why certain patients with pseudomonal keratitis develop extension into the sclera and most others do not is not known, but presumed factors include corticosteroid use, old age, and diabetes mellitus.[13,25,38] Organisms may also spread from the underlying choroid in severe endophthalmitis, usually following surgery or trauma or from localized chorioretinitis.† Infections of the conjunctiva or orbital tissues almost never involve the sclera, but occasionally scleritis will follow orbital cellulitis, dacryocystitis, sinusitis, or severe conjunctivitis.[16,25,26]

Organisms may reach the sclera via the circulation with deposition of septic emboli in or near the sclera. This is the presumed mechanism of infection in cases without antecedent trauma, surgery, or associated corneal infection. Although organisms may directly infect the sclera, many forms of scleral inflammation associated with systemic infections represent an immune response in the absence of scleral organisms. Scleritis may occur in response to foreign antigen or from release of autoantigens in the sclera occurring in association with infection rather than actual invasion of replicating organism, but this mechanism lacks solid clinical or experimental support.

Trauma can introduce organisms directly into the sclera in penetrating injuries. Foreign bodies that lodge in or pass through the sclera may harbor organisms (see chapters 92 and 93).[12] Infectious scleritis after trauma is quite rare; the intraocular tissues are far more susceptible to posttraumatic infection than the sclera.

Scleral buckling materials cause infections rarely and the

---

*References 1, 17, 18, 29, 35, 38, 41.
†References 25, 39, 45, 46, 49, 55, 60.

INFECTIOUS AGENTS ASSOCIATED WITH SCLERITIS

Direct Invasion
  Bacteria
    Pseudomonas aeruginosa
    Pseudomonas fluorescens
    Staphylococcus aureus
    Staphylococcus epidermidis
    Streptococcus pneumoniae
    Streptococcus equinus
    Serratia marcescens
    Corynebacterium spp.
    Proteus spp.
    Moraxella spp.
    Nocardia spp.
    Escherischia coli
    Mycobacterium chelonei
  Fungi
    Aspergillus spp.
    Paecilomyces spp.
    Sporothrix schenckii
    Blastomyces spp.
    Acremonium spp.
  Viruses
    Varicella-zoster
    Herpes simplex
Reactive Inflammation
  Bacteria
    Mycobacterium tuberculosis
    Mycobacterium leprae
    Treponema pallidum
    Borrelia burgdorferi
  Parasites
    Acanthamoeba sp.
    Toxoplasma gondii
    Toxocara canis
    Insect larva

RISK FACTORS FOR INFECTIOUS SCLERITIS

Extension from adjacent structures
  Keratitis
  Choroiditis
  Endophthalmitis
  Conjunctivitis
  Orbital cellulitis
  Dacryocystitis
  Sinusitis
Traumatic, with or without foreign body
Postsurgical
  Scleral buckle
  Pterygium excision, especially with beta irradiation or mitomycin application
  Cataract extraction
  Glaucoma filtration surgery
  Suture abscess
Associated with systemic infections

incidence appears to be decreasing, probably because of better materials, surgical techniques, and antibiotic prophylaxis.* Any buckling material can cause infection—sponge or silicone, explant or implant. The source of infection in such cases is presumed to be organisms introduced at the time of surgery, although a conjunctival fistula can be a path for conjunctival flora and other exogenous microbes. Sutures and other foreign materials may also harbor organisms and lead to infections in the sclera.[53]

Surgical manipulation of the sclera may lead to infectious scleritis, even in the absence of sutures and other foreign materials. Scleritis may develop in a scleral tunnel following cataract extraction in association with endophthalmitis.[3,10,36]

Ischemia and necrosis in the sclera can lead to infection

following beta-irradiation in association with pterygium excision.* Presumably the radiation leads to vascular closure with subsequent scleral necrosis allowing entry of organisms. Such infections have been reported years after surgery and irradiation. Similar cases can develop after mitomycin therapy to prevent recurrence of pterygia following excision.[43]

CLINICAL FEATURES

Two principal forms of infectious scleritis occur: suppurative and nonsuppurative. Suppurative scleritis is associated with spread of adjacent infection or following trauma or surgery. Nonsuppurative scleral inflammation is associated with a systemic infectious disease.

Keratoscleritis

Most cases of infectious scleritis result from severe bacterial infections of the cornea but viral, fungal, and parasitic keratitis may also expand into a keratoscleritis. Gram-negative bacteria, most commonly *Pseudomonas aeruginosa,* can spread from the cornea to the sclera.† Pseudomonal scleritis without keratitis has also been reported.[13] *Staphylococcus aureus,*[26,44] *Streptococcus pneumoniae*[41] (Fig. 80-1), *Mycobacterium chelonei,*[8,41] herpes simplex,[53] varicella-zoster,[50,58] *Aspergillus* sp.,[30] *Acremonium* sp.,[41] and *Acanthamoeba* sp.[29] have also been reported to cause keratoscleritis. Patients who are immunosuppressed, especially those with AIDS, can have fulminant keratoscleritis with poor response to therapy.[35]

Infection of the peripheral cornea that spreads to the limbus will first demonstrate limbal erythema, usually with

---

*References 19, 20, 27, 28, 32, 60.

*References 19, 25, 30, 32, 33, 49.
†References 1, 13, 17, 18, 35, 38.

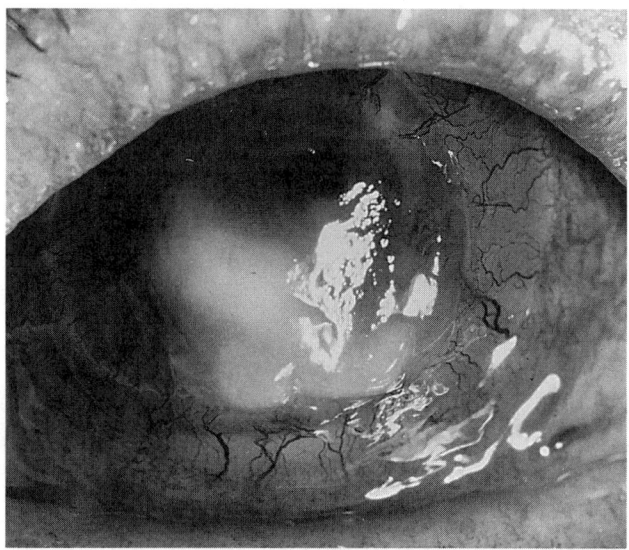

Fig. 80-1. *Streptococcus pneumoniae* infection of the cornea and adjacent inferior sclera with corneal perforation following corneal transplantation.

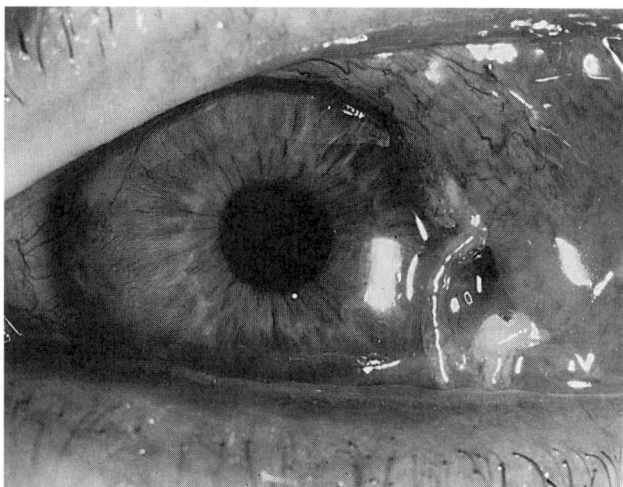

Fig. 80-2. *Staphylococcus aureus* infection of the sclera following conjunctival resection and scleral biopsy in a patient with peripheral ulcerative keratitis caused by Wegener granulomatosis. Note the purulent discharge.

edema and infiltrate. There may be no conjunctival epithelial defect. If inadequately treated the scleral inflammation will spread posteriorly and circumferentially. Pain may increase with infection of the sclera. Scleral involvement in cases of corneal infection decreases the prognosis for control of the infection but can be successfully treated as outlined below.

Panophthalmitis

Scleritis may result from progression of severe endophthalmitis of any cause. Most cases occur after trauma or surgery. Eyes with endophthalmitis are usually intensely hyperemic, so the first sign of scleral infection may be scleral thinning, uveal prolapse, or scleral perforation. Many of these eyes are hypotonous. The prognosis for restoration of vision is dismal. Abscess and necrosis in a scleral tunnel following cataract extraction in two patients were associated with *Staphylococcus aureus* and *Streptococcus equinus* endophthalmitis, respectively;[36] and both patients lost all vision.

Less commonly intraocular infections from endogenous causes may extend into the sclera and present as a scleritis. Such cases of toxoplasmic[45] and toxocaral scleritis[23,39,46] have been reported. Scleral inflammation in these cases may be part of a granulomatous reaction rather than direct invasion.

Scleritis Following Scleral Buckling Surgery

Infection associated with a scleral buckle may present in several ways.* The patient may experience pain and a foreign-body sensation. Signs and symptoms of posterior uveitis may develop. An abscess may be seen in the choroid or retina on ophthalmoscopy. A portion of the buckle may extrude and be evident on external examination. A subcon-

junctival abscess can be seen in some cases. In others a purulent discharge is noted. Additional signs may include subconjunctival hemorrhage, conjunctival granuloma, recurrent retinal detachment, proliferative vitreoretinopathy, and scleral perforation.

Scleral infection from a buckle may develop immediately after surgery or years later. Reported causative organisms include *S. aureus, Pseudomonas* sp., and *Proteus* sp.[19,20,28] In one unusual case noninfectious scleral inflammation took on the appearance of a scleral buckle.[4]

Postpterygium Excision Scleritis

Infections after pterygium excision are exceedingly rare. When infections do occur following this common procedure they are almost always associated with the postoperative use of beta-irradiation* or mitomycin[43] at the excision site. Both of these strategies have been used in attempts to reduce the likelihood of recurrence of the pterygium. Patients have pain, redness, scleral necrosis, and a purulent discharge. Biomicroscopically visible occlusion of the conjunctival and scleral vessels with scleral necrosis is typical. Infection may follow. *S. pneumoniae* is the most common organism in this setting. An analogous streptococcal infection may occur in the setting of chronic scleritis without previous surgery,[2] suggesting that *S. pneumoniae* organisms have a predilection for necrotic sclera.

Other Postsurgical Scleritis

Scleral inflammation at the site of recent or remote surgery should prompt consideration of an infectious process (Fig. 80-2). Infections of the sclera can occur in cataract

---

*References 19, 20, 27, 28, 32, 60.

*References 9, 25, 30, 32, 33, 49.

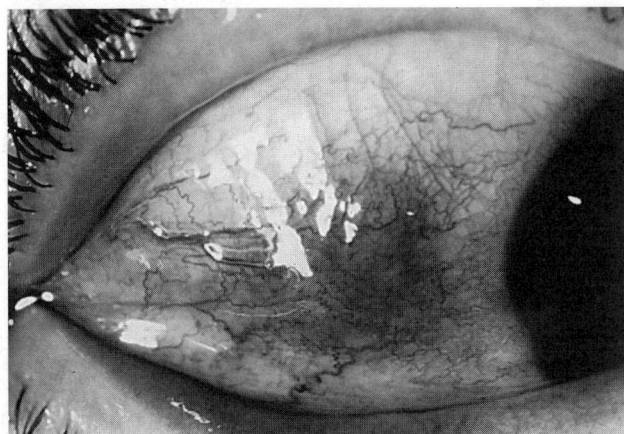

Fig. 80-3. Localized nodular scleritis in a patient with active herpes zoster ophthalmicus.

wounds[3,10,36] and following strabismus[23] and glaucoma filtering surgery.[41] Pain, hyperemia, a purulent discharge, and scleral necrosis are typical signs. Although bacterial infections are most likely in this setting, fungal scleritis[10] has been identified after cataract surgery.

Varicella-Zoster and Herpes Simplex Scleritis

Though not commonly recognized, scleral involvement in varicella-zoster infection can occur and may be associated with stromal keratitis.[50] Patients may have no symptoms or may experience pain, photophobia, and blurry vision. The severity of symptoms probably reflects the degree of corneal involvement. Ocular signs may include diffuse or focal conjunctival and scleral edema and hyperemia, tenderness to palpation, and concurrent corneal infiltrates.

Similar signs and symptoms can follow herpes zoster ophthalmicus with involvement of the sclera[50,53,58,59] (Fig. 80-3). Ischemia with occlusion of the conjunctival and scleral vessels is typical. In one series of 86 patients followed with herpes zoster ophthalmicus, three patients developed scleral inflammation.[58] Scleritis in this setting is usually accompanied by keratitis and uveitis. Chronic inflammation can lead to scleral nodules, thinning, and uveal prolapse.

Herpes simplex virus rarely infects the sclera. If epithelial herpetic disease spreads or involves the limbal conjunctiva primarily, the underlying sclera may become inflamed (Fig. 80-4).

Syphilitic Scleritis

Syphilis can lead to inflammation in any ocular structure. Syphilitic scleritis is rare (less than 5% of cases of scleritis in a referral practice) but has been reported with the secondary, tertiary, and congenital forms of the disease.* Inflammation may be restricted to the episclera or be associated with dif-

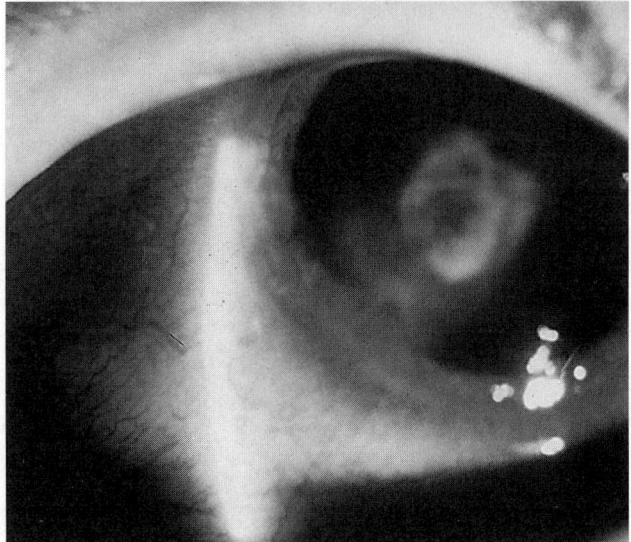

Fig. 80-4. Herpes simplex keratitis with scleritis. After multiple episodes of epithelial and stromal herpes simplex keratitis, this woman developed limbal inflammation extending clockwise from 4 to 8 o'clock. A deeper area of scleral edema with a purple hue was noted at 8 o'clock, consistent with scleritis.

fuse inflammation, including uveitis. Nodular scleritis or diffuse scleritis has been reported. Evidence of prior interstitial keratitis will be found in cases of congenital syphilis. Patients will usually have positive serologic tests for *Treponema pallidum* and may respond to systemic penicillin or other appropriate antibiotics. The role of the spirochete in causing scleritis is uncertain, however. The inflammation may result from a vasculitis rather than direct infection of the sclera. The diagnosis may be hard to prove, but response to antibiotic therapy and the absence of connective-tissue disorders that can cause scleritis strongly suggests syphilis as a cause for scleritis in such cases.

Tuberculous Scleritis

Although the incidence of tuberculosis in the United States is increasing, ocular tuberculosis remains rare.[21] Even more rare is scleral involvement* (Fig. 80-5). Although Verhoeff[52] and others thought that scleritis (and uveitis) was often caused by tuberculosis, of 10,524 patients with tuberculosis examined in a sanitorium between 1940 and 1966, only 14 (0.13%) had evidence of scleritis.[15] Rarely are bacilli found on biopsy of the sclera, suggesting a hypersensitivity reaction rather than direct infection of the sclera. Definitive diagnosis is difficult.

Patients may be asymptomatic or have pain, redness, and discharge. The discharge can be mucopurulent. Diffuse scleritis, ulceration, or scleral nodules may be seen. Uveitis with corneal opacification and vascularization often accompany tuberculous scleritis.

---

*References 14, 25, 56, 57.

*References 5, 15, 21, 23, 25, 34, 51.

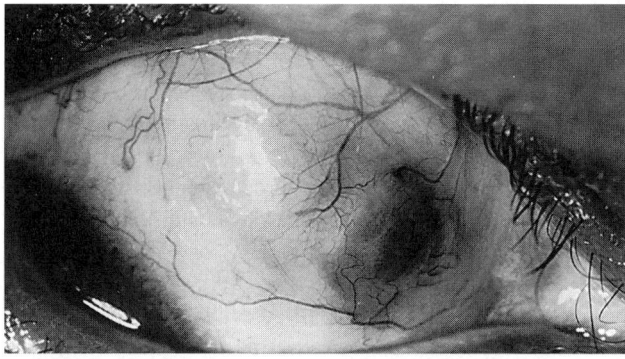

Fig. 80-5. Scleral thinning in a patient with previous anterior scleritis. The scleritis resolved, leaving this appearance following systemic therapy for pulmonary tuberculosis. The scleral biopsy showed nonspecific chronic inflammation; no organisms were found on culture or demonstrated with staining of biopsy sections.

CLINICAL SIGNS OF INFECTIOUS SCLERITIS
Subconjunctival nodule
Subconjunctival abscess
Scleral necrosis
Nodular or diffuse scleritis
Conjunctival or episcleral hyperemia
Mucopurulent discharge
Subconjunctival hemorrhage
Uveitis
Uveal prolapse
Scleral perforation
Conjunctival ulceration

Lepromatous Scleritis

The prevalence of scleritis in patients with Hansen disease is unknown but is probably rare.[6,24,25,51] Lepromas of the conjunctiva and episclera can be the first site of ocular involvement owing to the relatively low temperature on the ocular surface. Lepromas are nodular and may appear gelatinous. They are most common near the limbus, especially in the interpalpebral zone (3 and 9 o'clock). Although these lepromas contain bacilli, hypersensitivity reactions (including immune-complex vasculitis) may be responsible for other lepromatous scleritis. Patients may be asymptomatic or complain of pain, redness, and a foreign-body sensation.

PATHOGENESIS

Regardless of the cause of the infection, destruction of scleral tissue is a combination of proteolytic and other enzymes released from host leukocytes and organisms. Severity depends on the organism and duration of the infection.[25] Some infections cause scleral inflammation by hypersensitivity reactions rather than actual scleral invasion of organisms. In other cases no organisms will be seen on section because the inflammatory response has destroyed them, or the biopsy material was obtained from an area adjacent to active infection.

Necrosis of the sclera during microbial scleritis is commonly seen, with or without abscess. There may be thickening of the adjacent superciliary or superchoroidal space. Acute or chronic inflammatory cells are often abundant. Granulomatous inflammation will be seen in most cases of tuberculosis and herpetic scleritis. In herpes simplex and varicella-zoster virus scleritis, an occlusive vasculitis with areas of ischemic necrosis may be noted. Any other ocular structure may also be inflamed, depending on the cause and extent of the scleritis.

DIFFERENTIAL DIAGNOSIS

The clinical findings in a case of infectious scleritis, including the presentation, natural history, and disease course,

are dependent on the precipitating cause of the infection. The patient's symptoms are nonspecific and often similar to those in infectious keratitis. They may include pain, redness, tenderness to touch, blurred vision, and purulent discharge. The potential clinical signs are myriad (see box). When present, subconjunctival nodules may be yellow or red in color. The overlying conjunctiva may be intact or ulcerated. The appearance may be similar to noninfectious diffuse, nodular, or necrotizing scleritis. In most cases of infectious scleritis, the process is readily apparent, with obvious concurrent keratitis, recent trauma, or previous ocular surgery.

Infection of the sclera in association with systemic infection is less common and can be more difficult to recognize, requiring a careful history, review of systems, physical examination, and laboratory investigation in many cases. Scleritis associated with systemic disease may appear similar to noninfectious scleritis. These cases require an investigation for noninfectious causes of scleritis, most importantly rheumatoid arthritis, Wegener granulomatosis, inflammatory bowel disease, relapsing polychondritis, systemic lupus erythematosus, and polyarteritis nodosa.

LABORATORY INVESTIGATIONS

Most cases of infectious scleritis are associated with other ocular infection, and the diagnosis is established by culturing material from the infected cornea or vitreous. In cases of scleritis where no obvious infection is present, a careful history is required. Previous surgery (especially pterygium excision), trauma, known infectious and collagen-vascular diseases, and risk factors for tuberculosis and syphilis should be determined.

Ocular examination should include careful binocular indirect ophthalmoscopy. A physical examination should also be performed. Laboratory studies may routinely include syphilis serologies (FTA-ABS or MHA-TP), antineutrophil cytoplasmic antibodies (ANCA), and chest x-ray. Other useful tests in selected settings include complete blood count, antinuclear antibodies (if other signs of collagen-vascular disease are present), rheumatoid factor, antiDNA (if other signs of lupus are present), and PPD skin testing with controls. Occasionally, B-scan ultrasonography and CT or MR imaging of the orbits can detect posterior scleritis, mass lesions, or orbital inflammation.

Cultures of obviously infected tissues should always be performed. As with corneal ulcers, Gram and Giemsa stains should be obtained with placement of scrapings on blood, chocolate, and Sabouraud agar. If tuberculosis is a consideration, specimens should be stained for acid-fast bacilli and cultures performed on Löwenstein-Jensen medium. Scleritis with possible acanthamoebic infection requires additional staining of specimens with calcofluor white or specific antibodies and plating on nonnutrient agar overlayed with *E. coli*. Scleral scrapings are usually deferred if corneal material can be obtained.

Biopsy of inflamed sclera should be reserved for cases in which a diagnosis is not determined by the preceding steps and intervention will be altered based on the results. Care should be taken when performing a biopsy on inflamed sclera. This sclera may be thin and could result in uveal prolapse. It is worth having donor sclera available at the time of biopsy. Biopsy material may be cultured as well as fixed, sectioned, and stained for histopathologic examination for infectious organisms. In unusual cases, electron microscopy may be helpful. A number of case reports include rare organisms,* some found only by culture or microscopic evaluation of biopsy material.

THERAPY

Effective treatment of infectious scleritis usually requires culture or pathologic evidence of a causative organism. In some cases of scleritis suspected to arise from tuberculosis, varicella-zoster, herpes simplex, or syphilis, presumptive therapy may be considered. Therapy of tuberculosis scleritis should be with multiple agents, and may include isoniazid, rifampin, pyrazinamide, and ethambutol or streptomycin. Zoster scleritis may respond to topical or systemic corticosteroids; acyclovir appears to be helpful for many forms of ocular inflammation related to zoster infections. Herpes simplex scleritis is usually responsive to topical antiviral agents and can worsen if active infection is treated with corticosteroids. Syphilitic scleritis usually responds to systemic penicillin therapy. Whether penicillin therapy should be intravenous for 7 to 10 days or if intramuscular penicillin is adequate has not been determined. Topical and systemic corticosteroids may be helpful, depending on the degree of ocular inflammation.

Foreign bodies and foreign material such as sutures or scleral buckling components must be removed if associated with infection. Retinal detachment following removal of infected elements is unusual, although necrotic scleral perfo-

ration can occur. Scleral grafts may be required after removal of the buckle.

Medical treatment of scleritis caused by bacteria can be successful. The prognosis is worse with bacterial keratoscleritis. Initial therapy of scleritis follows that for bacterial keratitis, with intensive topical broad-spectrum antibiotics. Topical therapy may be altered based on Gram stain, culture, and sensitivity results. It is common for clinicians to add intravenous antibiotics when infection of the sclera is associated with keratitis. This is a generally accepted clinical practice, though studies have not been done to clarify the added benefit of parenteral therapy. Given the poor outcome in most cases of bacterial keratoscleritis treated with drops alone, more aggressive approaches seem reasonable. Use of a combination of intravenous ceftazidime and an aminoglycoside (tobramycin or gentamicin) in combination with topical fortified antibiotics has been reported to be effective in three patients with pseudomonal scleritis or sclerokeratitis.[22]

A number of series support surgical intervention in cases of keratoscleritis. Cryotherapy appears to be a useful adjunct to topical and parenteral antibiotics, especially in cases of pseudomonal infection.[17,41] Morbidity from cryotherapy is low. Direct treatment of necrotic sclera with the cryoprobe following conjunctival resection may be effective for several reasons. Destruction of the organisms may occur, alterations in the host tissue may enhance the elimination of organisms and the healing process, and penetration of antibiotic through host tissues and the organism may be increased.

Combining surgical debridement of infected tissue with cryotherapy may further improve response to medical therapy. In cases of severe destruction of the cornea or scleral perforation, lamellar or full-thickness scleral and corneal grafting may be helpful and can be successful.[42] Grafting should probably be reserved for cases that do not respond to cryotherapy in combination with topical and parenteral antibiotics, or those cases where perforation of the globe has occurred or is imminent.

PROGNOSIS

The outcome in cases of isolated infectious scleritis is good. Because the primary function of the sclera is tectonic, if adjacent ocular structures are unaffected and perforation does not occur, the visual outcome is usually excellent. The prognosis in cases following surgery and with endophthalmitis depends on the extent of damage to other intraocular structures; these cases have a worse prognosis. Most cases of scleritis extending from infectious keratitis do poorly if treated with medical therapy alone. The prognosis is enhanced in selected cases with the addition of cryotherapy and corneoscleral grafting. In any case with associated corneal disease, vision may be reduced by corneal scarring. Many eyes with infection following pterygium surgery are left with high astigmatism.

---

*References 6-8, 11, 23, 31, 33, 37, 44, 47, 48.

REFERENCES

1. Alfonso E, Kenyon KR, Ormerod LD et al.: *Pseudomonas* corneoscleritis, *Am J Ophthalmol* 103:90-98, 1987.
2. Altman AJ, Cohen EJ, Berger ST, Mondino BJ: Scleritis and *Streptococcus* pneumoniae, *Cornea* 10:341-345, 1991.
3. Berler DK, Alper MG: Scleral abscesses and ectasia caused by *Pseudomonas aeruginosa*, *Ann Ophthalmol* 14:665-667, 1982.
4. Bidwell AE, Jampol LM, O'Grady R: Scleritis resembling a scleral buckle, *Arch Ophthalmol* 111:865, 1993.
5. Bloomfield SE, Mondino B, Gray GF: Scleral tuberculosis, *Arch Ophthalmol* 94:954-956, 1976.
6. Brooks JG Jr, Mills RA, Coster DJ: Nocardial scleritis, *Am J Ophthalmol* 114:371-372, 1992.
7. Brunette I, Stulting RD: *Sporothrix schenckii* scleritis, *Am J Ophthalmol* 114:370-371, 1992.
8. Bullington RH Jr., Lanier JD, Font RL: Nontuberculous mycobacterial keratitis: report of two cases and review of the literature, *Arch Ophthalmol* 110:519-524, 1992.
9. Cameron ME: Preventable complications of pterygium excision with beta-irradiation, *Br J Ophthalmol* 56:52-56, 1972.
10. Carlson AN, Foulks GN, Perfect JR, Kim JH: Fungal scleritis after cataract surgery: successful outcome using itraconazole, *Cornea* 11:151-154, 1992.
11. Caronia R, Liebman J, Speaker M, Ritch R: *Corynebacterium* scleritis, *Am J Ophthalmol* 117:405-406, 1994.
12. Cobo LM: Inflammation of the sclera, *Int Ophthalmol Clin* 23:159, 1982.
13. Codere F, Brownstein S, Jackson WB: *Pseudomonas aeruginosa* scleritis, *Am J Ophthalmol* 91:706-710, 1981.
14. Deodati F, Bec P, Labro JB, Barrioulet Y: Sclérite syphilitique: aspect clinique et angiographique, *Bull Soc Ophtalmol Fr* 71:63-65, 1971.
15. Donahue HC: Ophthalmologic experience in a tuberculosis sanatorium, *Am J Ophthalmol* 64:742-748, 1967.
16. Duke-Elder S, Leigh AG: *Diseases of the outer eye,* vol 7, part 2, 841-852, 1024-1034, London, 1965, Henry Kimpton.
17. Eiferman RA: Cryotherapy of *Pseudomonas* keratitis and scleritis, *Arch Ophthalmol* 97:1637-1639, 1979.
18. Eiferman RA: *Pseudomonas* scleritis, *Am J Ophthalmol* 93:133, 1982.
19. Hagler WS, Jarrett II WH, Smith JA: Infections after retinal detachment surgery, *South Med J* 68:1564, 1975.
20. Hahn YS, Lincoff A, Lincoff H, Kreissig I: Infection after sponge implantation for scleral buckling, *Am J Ophthalmol* 87:180, 1979.
21. Helm CJ, Holland GN: Ocular tuberculosis, *Surv Ophthalmol* 38:229-256, 1993.
22. Helm CJ, Holland GN, Webster RG, et al.: Treatment of *Pseudomonas* scleritis with intravenous ceftazidime and aminoglycosides, *Invest Ophthalmol Vis Sci* 35:1748, 1994.
23. Hemady R, Sainz de la Maza M, Raizman MB, Foster CS: Six cases of scleritis associated with systemic infection, *Am J Ophthalmol* 114:55-62, 1992.
24. Holmes WJ: Leprosy of the eye, *Trans Am Ophthalmol Soc* 55:145, 1957.
25. Jackson WB: Infections of sclera. In Tabbara KF, Hyndiuk RA, editors: *Infections of the eye,* 481, Boston, 1986, Little, Brown.
26. Lebensohn JE: Suppurative conjunctivitis with scleral involvement, *Am J Ophthalmol* 78:856, 1974.
27. Lincoff HA, McLean JM, Nano H: Scleral abscess I: a complication of retinal detachment buckling procedures, *Arch Ophthalmol* 74:641, 1965.
28. Lindsey PS, Pierce H, Welch RB: Removal of scleral buckling elements: causes and complications, *Arch Ophthalmol* 101:570, 1983.
29. Mannis MJ, Tamaru R, Roth AM et al.: *Acanthamoeba* sclerokeratitis: determining diagnostic criteria, *Arch Ophthalmol* 104:1313, 1986.
30. Margo CE, Polack FM, Mood CI: *Aspergillus* panophthalmitis complicating treatment of pterygium, *Cornea* 7:285, 1988.
31. Maskin SL: Infectious scleritis after a diabetic foot ulcer, *Am J Ophthalmol* 115:254-255, 1993.
32. Milauskas AT, Duke JR: Mycotic scleral abscess: report of a case following a scleral buckling operation for retinal detachment, *Am J Ophthalmol* 63:951, 1967.
33. Moriarty AP, Crawford GJ, McAllister IL, Constable IJ: Bilateral streptococcal corneoscleritis complicating beta irradiation induced scleral necrosis, *Br J Ophthalmol* 77:251-252, 1993.
34. Nanda M, Pflugfelder SC, Holland S: *Mycobacterium tuberculosis* scleritis, *Am J Ophthalmol* 108:736-737, 1989.
35. Nanda M, Pflugfelder SC, Holland S: Fulminant pseudomonal keratitis and scleritis in human immunodeficiency virus–infected patients, *Arch Ophthalmol* 109:503-505, 1991.
36. Ormerod LD, Puklin JE, McHenry JG, McDermott ML: Scleral flap necrosis and infectious endophthalmitis after cataract surgery with a scleral tunnel incision, *Ophthalmology* 100:159-163, 1993.
37. Podedworny W, Suie T: Mycotic infection of the sclera, *Am J Ophthalmol* 63:951-953, 1967.
38. Raber IM, Laibson PR, Kurz GH et al.: *Pseudomonas* corneoscleral ulcers, *Am J Ophthalmol* 92:353-362, 1981.
39. Raistrick ER, Dean Hart JCD: Ocular toxocariasis in adults, *Br J Ophthalmol* 60:365, 1976.
40. Rao NA, Marak GE, Hidayat AA: Necrotizing scleritis: a clinico-pathologic study of 41 cases, *Ophthalmology* 92:1542, 1985.
41. Reynolds MG, Alfonso E: Treatment of infectious scleritis and keratoscleritis, *Am J Ophthalmol* 112:543, 1991.
42. Rockwood EJ, Meisler DM: Scleritis. In Abbott RL, editor: *Surgical intervention in corneal and external diseases,* 181-185, Orlando, 1987, Harcourt Brace Jovanovich.
43. Rubinfeld RS, Pfister RR, Stein RM et al.: Serious complications of topical mitomycin-C after pterygium surgery, *Ophthalmology* 99:1647-1654, 1992.
44. Sainz de la Maza M, Hemady RK, Foster CS: Infectious scleritis: report of four cases, *Doc Ophthalmol* 83:33-41, 1993.
45. Schuman JS, Weinberg RS, Ferry AP, Guerry RK: Toxoplasmic scleritis, *Ophthalmology* 95:1399-1403, 1988.
46. Shields JA: Ocular toxocariasis: a review, *Surv Ophthalmol* 28:361, 1984.
47. Stenson S, Brookner A, Rosenthalm S: Bilateral endogenous necrotizing scleritis due to *Aspergillus oryzea*, *Ann Ophthalmol* 14:67-72, 1982.
48. Tabbara KF: Other parasitic infections. In Tabbara KF, Hyndiuk RA, editors: *Infections of the Eye,* 682-688, Boston, 1986, Little, Brown and Company.
49. Tarr KH, Constable IJ: *Pseudomonas* endophthalmitis associated with scleral necrosis, *Br J Ophthalmol* 64:676, 1980.
50. Threlkeld AB, Eliot D, O'Brien TP: Scleritis associated with varicella-zoster disciform stromal keratitis, *Am J Ophthalmol* 113:721-722, 1992.
51. Trucksis M, Baker AS: Mycobacterial diseases: tuberculosis and leprosy. In Albert DM, Jakobiec FA, editors: *Principles and practice of ophthalmology: clinical practice,* 3011-3020, Philadelphia, 1994, WB Saunders.
52. Verhoeff FH: Tuberculous scleritis, a commonly unrecognized form of tuberculosis, *Boston Med Surg J* 156:317-321, 1907.
53. Watson P: Diseases of the sclera and episclera. In Duane TD, Jaeger EA, editors: *Clinical ophthalmology,* 1-39, vol 4, Philadelphia, 1985, Harper & Row.
54. Watson PG, Hayreh SS: Scleritis and episcleritis, *Br J Ophthalmol* 60:163-191, 1976.
55. Weinberg RS: Endogenous bacterial and fungal infections of the retina and choroid. In Tabbara KF, Hyndiuk RA, editors: *Infections of the eye,* 501-503, Boston, 1986, Little, Brown.
56. Whitcup SM, Raizman MB: Spirochetal infections and the eye, In Albert DM, Jakobiec FA, editors: *Principles and practice of ophthalmology: clinical practice,* 3078-3092, Philadelphia, 1994, WB Saunders.
57. Wilhelmus KR, Yokoyama CM: Syphilitic episcleritis and scleritis, *Am J Ophthalmol* 104:595-597, 1987.
58. Womack LW, Liesegang TJ: Complications of herpes zoster ophthalmicus, *Arch Ophthalmol* 101:42-45, 1983.
59. Zaal MJ, Maudgal PC, Rietveld E, Suir EP: Chronic ocular zoster, *Curr Eye Res* 10:125-130, 1991.
60. Zinn KM, Ferry AP: Massive scleral necrosis from a *Pseudomonas* infection following scleral buckling and pars plana vitrectomy surgery, *Mt Sinai J Med* 47:618-621, 1980.

81 Cytomegalovirus Diseases

GARY N. HOLLAND, ADNAN TUFAIL, M. COLIN JORDAN

Cytomegalovirus (CMV) is a ubiquitous member of the herpes group of viruses. Infection with CMV is very common among the general population, but in most cases it does not cause clinically apparent disease. Cytomegalovirus is, however, a well-known cause of serious, even life-threatening, disease in immunosuppressed individuals and in congenitally infected newborns. Cytomegalovirus retinitis has emerged from obscurity in recent years to become an important cause of blindness because of its association with the acquired immunodeficiency syndrome (AIDS); in fact, because of the AIDS epidemic, CMV retinitis is now believed to be the most common single cause of posterior uveitis in many large urban areas of North America.[252] Additional attention was focused on CMV retinitis in the 1980s and 1990s by the introduction of new antiviral drugs having activity against CMV.

VIROLOGY

Cytomegalovirus is an enveloped, linear, double-stranded DNA virus and is a member of the family Herpesviridae and subfamily Betaherpesvirinae. Human CMV has been designated type species human herpesvirus 5 (human cytomegalovirus) by the International Committee on Taxonomy of Viruses.[250] Cytomegalovirus is species-specific; in addition to human CMV, there are well-characterized CMV strains that affect the rat, mouse, monkey, and guinea pig. All CMVs are similar to other herpesviruses in morphology and in their ability to produce latent infections and undergo reactivation.

Morphologically, CMV has a central DNA-containing core surrounded by a capsid composed of 162 capsomeres, each of which is hexagonal in cross section. The capsid is surrounded by a poorly demarcated area, the tegmentum, and an envelope. The genome of CMV is the largest of the herpesvirus group. It is approximately 230,000 base pairs in length and has a molecular weight of 15,106 daltons[121,366] The DNA structure is similar to that of herpes simplex virus; they both contain long and short unique sequences bounded by terminally repetitive segments. The long and short sequences can be orientated in two directions so that four DNA isomers are produced by cells in culture. The genome has a coding capacity for over 80 proteins of average molecular weight.[223] The entire CMV genome has been sequenced[14]; it contains areas that are homologous with human chromosomal DNA,[327] which has led to speculation that CMV may be oncogenic. The genome also contains an area of homology with HLA class I specificities, but the implications of this finding are not known.[15]

The cells in which CMV initially replicates and the sites of persistence have not been clearly defined. Thus the nature of the virus receptor is not known. Cytomegalovirus replicates readily in fibroblasts in vitro, and much of the understanding of the virus is derived from such studies. Other human cell types are only moderately permissive in culture.[214]

A cascade system is involved in controlling the synthesis of proteins from the genome of CMV.[382] The immediate-early or α group of proteins is synthesized first, which allows the transcription of messenger RNA for the second group of proteins, the early or β proteins. Immediate-early proteins are rapidly expressed in the host nucleus after virus absorption and penetration; their presence may be the only evidence of infection in cells in which the virus does not replicate.[264] Early proteins allow DNA replication to proceed by encoding replicative enzymes such as DNA polymerase. The late or γ proteins are the last to be synthesized. Most or all of the immediate-early and early proteins are nonstructural, whereas most of the late proteins are structural for the virus. The cascade system does not apply as rigorously to CMV as to other herpesviruses, as several late structural proteins have been shown to be transcribed and translated before viral DNA synthesis.[248]

Cytomegalovirus may cause abortive infections in some cells and lytic infections in others. In nonpermissive cells the lytic cycle can be blocked at any of the steps between absorption and virion production. The outcome of CMV infection is host cell-dependent and species-specific. Different CMVs vary with respect to the range of host cells in which there is expression of genes for immediate-early proteins (which may have implications for understanding latency and abortive infections) and in which viral DNA replication can occur.[222] Human CMV is the most restricted for both. Simian CMV has the broadest range of host cells in which there can be expression of genes for immediate-early proteins, whereas murine CMV has the broadest range of host cells in which DNA synthesis can occur.

Infectious enveloped virus particles result when nucleocapsids, formed in the nucleus of the host cell, acquire an envelope derived from both the endoplasmic reticulum and the internal nuclear membrane of the cell.[347] The envelope glycoproteins, such as the gB, gC11, and the gH complex, contain antigens that stimulate host immune responses.[245,316]

A number of different human CMV strains can be differentiated by both the size and number of additions to the terminal ends of the long and short components of the genome.[381] The restriction endonuclease profiles of various human CMV strains share many similarities, but no two profiles are identical. Strains grouped by variations in the structure of gB of the viral envelope have been related to survival in bone marrow transplant recipients with CMV disease, but the basis for this relationship is not known.[114]

HISTORICAL BACKGROUND

The history of research into CMV and the diseases it causes has been outlined by Ho.[158] In 1921 Goodpasture and Talbot[131] introduced the term *cytomegalia* to describe the presence of large mononuclear inclusions in various organs in the autopsy of a 6-week-old child. Similar findings in newborns suspected to have syphilis or other congenital infections had been described earlier in the century by other investigators, who thought that the cytomegalic cells were protozoa. Goodpasture and Talbot disagreed with this theory, as did subsequent investigators. In 1925 Von Glahn and Pappenheimer[396] described identical findings for the first time in an adult, and suggested that the inclusions were caused by a virus similar to those of the herpesvirus group. Over the next several years, additional congenital cases were reported in symptomatic newborns, and a viral causation became accepted.

In 1932 Farber and Wolbach[93] showed, in a large autopsy series, that clinically inapparent infection could also occur. In 1950 Wyatt and associates[410] suggested the term *generalized cytomegalic inclusion disease* to describe the lethal infection in newborns and showed that the diagnosis could be made on cytologic examination of the urine.

The viral agent responsible for cytomegalic inclusion disease was first visualized by electron microscopy in 1953 by Minders.[261] In the mid-1950s CMV was finally isolated and grown in tissue culture independently by Smith,[360] by Weller and associates,[403] and by Rowe and associates.[326]

The spectrum of diseases known to be caused by CMV was expanded in 1965, when Klemola and Kaariainen[211] described a CMV-associated infectious mononucleosis-like syndrome in immunocompetent adults. More important in recent years has been the role of CMV as an opportunistic pathogen in immunosuppressed patients. The growing number of bone marrow and solid organ transplantations as well as the increasing use of immunosuppressive drugs were associated with the emergence of pneumonitis, colitis, hepatitis, encephalitis, and other life-threatening diseases caused by CMV.[159] Then in 1981 CMV was recognized as one of the most common opportunistic infections in patients with AIDS.

CMV infection of the eye was first recognized in newborns with cytomegalic inclusion disease. In 1947 Kalfayan[201] reported the presence of cytomegalic cells with nuclear inclusions at the "sclerocorneal junction," in episcleral tissue, and in ciliary body tissue of one infant. As more cases were seen in the 1950s and 1960s, it became obvious that the retina was the primary site of ocular disease in infants with disseminated CMV infection.[83,242,259,358,387]

The first confirmed case of CMV retinitis in an adult was reported by Smith[358] in 1964*; a 61-year-old woman who had been treated with chemotherapy for Hodgkin disease was found to have bilateral retinal necrosis with typical cytomegalic cells in the retina at autopsy. Moeller and associates[265] were able to identify less than 50 reported cases in the English language literature of CMV retinitis in patients with noncongenital CMV disease before the AIDS epidemic.†

In the first published case series of patients with AIDS-related eye disease, Holland and associates[167] reported CMV retinitis to be a complication of the syndrome. An additional single case of AIDS-related CMV retinitis was published at approximately the same time by Friedman and associates.[112] Other early case series confirmed that CMV retinitis was the most common opportunistic infection of the eye in patients with AIDS.[108,209,284,325] The importance of CMV retinitis in the AIDS epidemic is reflected in the fact that fear of blindness is believed to be the leading cause of suicide among patients with AIDS.[54] With the introduction of ganciclovir in 1984, CMV retinitis became a treatable disease.[96]

---

*Some authors have cited a previous report by Foerster[101] as the first case of acquired CMV retinitis. At a 1959 uveitis symposium Foerster described a 59-year-old woman with a history of chronic unilateral uveitis, who was otherwise healthy. The eye was enucleated, and examination revealed retinal necrosis and intranuclear inclusions. Although there was some speculation among symposium participants that CMV infection was the cause of the uveitis, there was no additional evidence to support that diagnosis.

†References 1, 5, 7, 17, 24, 28, 44, 50, 52, 64, 98, 239, 240, 243, 256, 271, 301, 306, 329, 358, 392, 398, 411.

EPIDEMIOLOGY

Cytomegalovirus infects a large proportion of adults throughout the world; rates vary depending on the group being studied, but in many populations it exceeds 50%. The prevalence of seropositivity increases with age;[404] it varies geographically, with higher rates found in developing countries;[216] and it is more prevalent in lower socioeconomic groups.[216] Serologic evidence of CMV infection is present in 40% to 100% of patients with AIDS;[311] in the United States, the rate is lowest among heterosexual patients with AIDS, but is almost universal among HIV-infected homosexual or bisexual men.[77]

Transmission

Transmission of CMV is not completely understood, but appears to require close contact with an individual who is excreting virus in urine, saliva, or other body fluids. Sexual contact is an important mode of transmission in some populations, such as homosexual men. Cytomegalovirus can also be transmitted by transfusion of cellular blood products or transplantation of infected organs.[210] The highest rates of CMV transmission (approximately 95%) occur in liver transplant recipients. Infants can be infected in utero or in the perinatal period through ingestion of infected breast milk or by other exposures.

The risk of CMV transmission to health-care workers has been a subject of controversy, but most evidence suggests that the risk of transmission during patient care activities is small. Congenitally infected infants excrete CMV into nasopharyngeal secretions and urine for many months or years, but health-care workers who have contact with these infants did not have an increased rate of CMV infection when compared to the general population.[85] There has also been no evidence of an increased rate of CMV acquisition among health care workers who have frequent contact with HIV-infected patients, despite the high rate of CMV disease in these patients.[124,218]

Congenital Disease

An estimated 30,000 to 40,000 infants are born with CMV infections in the United States each year.[73,374] The rate of congenital CMV infection is 0.5% to 2.4% of live births, making it the most common intrauterine infection.[2,73,145,253,291] Congenital CMV infection remains subclinical in 90% of cases.[2,73,374]

Infection during pregnancy may occur by sexual or nonsexual routes of transmission[289] and remains asymptomatic in the majority of women.[369,370] Neonatal CMV infection can result from either primary or recurrent maternal infection during pregnancy, but nearly all clinical disease at birth results from primary maternal infection.[2,102] With primary maternal infections, the rate of symptomatic neonatal disease has been reported to be 5% to 15%.[369,370,374] Stagno and Whitley[374] estimate that 40% of mothers with primary infec-

tions transmit CMV to the fetus, but of these infections, only 10% to 15% result in symptomatic disease at birth. Symptomatic disease is also believed to be more frequent when maternal infection occurs earlier in pregnancy.[369] In contrast, neonatal infection resulting from recurrent maternal CMV infection is rarely symptomatic, which suggests that maternal antibodies offer some protection against congenital disease.

The incidence of congenital CMV infection is highest in low socioeconomic groups. The rate of CMV infection among women of childbearing age is inversely related to socioeconomic status, but among CMV-infected women, transplacental transmission of virus is more common in lower socioeconomic groups, for unknown reasons.[370] Infants with congenital infections are more likely to be symptomatic when born to mothers in higher socioeconomic groups, however, because a greater proportion of these pregnant women are susceptible to primary CMV infections.[370]

The risk of congenital CMV infection is reported to be higher in second and third pregnancies because of the increased risk of maternal infection from young children within the household who may have been infected with the virus at school or daycare facilities.[289,369]

There is a 20% to 30% mortality rate among patients with symptomatic cytomegalic inclusion disease.[253,291] Of survivors, approximately 90% will have damage to the central nervous system (CNS) or organs of perception during the first few years of life, with resulting mental retardation, learning disabilities, hearing loss, or seizures.[2,291] Among infants with subclinical disease at birth, 5% to 15% will go on to develop CNS damage later in childhood.*

Cytomegalovirus infection of newborns acquired in the perinatal period from exposure to infected cervical infections, breast milk, or other nongenital sources usually does not result in severe disease or neurologic sequelae. In contrast, CMV infection following blood transfusion from a CMV seropositive donor can result in fatal or severe neonatal disease, as occurs with intrauterine transmission.[413]

Acquired Disease

Infectious mononucleosis-like syndromes are caused by CMV in 6% to 8% of cases.[177,212] Only a very small percentage of immunocompetent patients infected with CMV develop clinical disease, and there are no known risk factors that predict the development of symptomatic disease in this population. The rate of clinical disease is higher with transfusion-associated infections in otherwise healthy individuals; it is approximately 1% per unit of whole blood. Following infection, virus may be shed for 2 to 3 years.

---

*References 73, 145, 289, 291, 369, 370, 374.

Immunosuppressed Patients

In a review of four studies dealing with the development of CMV disease after kidney transplantation, Ho[158] calculated that an average of 83% of individuals (range 78% to 88%) developed symptomatic disease after primary infections, and that an average of 44% (range 20% to 69%) developed symptomatic disease following reactivation of CMV infection.

Homosexual, HIV-infected men who excrete CMV in the semen have an increased rate of CMV disease, and this rate is increased further if more than one strain of CMV is shed in semen.[227]

There is an increasing prevalence of CMV disease among patients with AIDS.[117,176,203,267] In a study of 844 HIV-infected men, Hoover and associates[176] found that CMV disease eventually developed in 44.9% of the individuals who had received prophylaxis against *Pneumocystis carinii* pneumonia, but in only 24.8% of the individuals who did not receive such prophylaxis. These results suggest that the increased survival associated with prophylaxis against other life-threatening infections places patients at risk for CMV disease, because it is a late manifestation of AIDS.

Ocular Disease

CMV retinitis will develop in 5% to 30% of newborns with clinically-apparent congenital CMV infection.* In 1990 a registry of newborns with cytomegalic inclusion disease was established for surveillance purposes; among the first 100 cases, 15% had retinal disease.[73] Fowler and associates[102] found that CMV retinitis was more common among infants born to mothers with primary CMV infection (7 of 112 infants, 6%) than among infants born to mothers with recurrent CMV infection (1 of 54 infants, 2%), although the difference was not statistically significant. Retinal "hyperpigmentation" also has been reported[111,253,371]; this finding may represent foci of healed disease, and therefore, the true prevalence of CMV retinitis may be higher than reported.

Cytomegalovirus retinitis usually develops in infants with disseminated CMV infection that is clinically apparent at birth, but has been reported as the only manifestation of CMV infection.[402] Some investigators have stated that CMV retinitis will not develop if it is not present at birth,[16,371] but, in fact, cases have been reported in which retinal disease developed several weeks after birth.[143] Furthermore, Alford and associates[2] stated that 2% of newborns with subclinical infections may develop late "chorioretinitis," but they provide no details about these cases. Late development of retinal disease in previously uninfected eyes has not been reported as a complication of cytomegalic inclusion disease in other series. Cytomegalovirus retinitis has not been seen in infants with perinatally acquired CMV infection, even

among those who develop symptomatic disease.[371] Maternal antibodies, if present, may offer some protection against disease in these cases.

Cytomegalovirus Retinitis in Patients with AIDS. Cytomegalovirus retinitis is the most common ocular infection in patients with AIDS in the United States.[170,182,283,343] The reported prevalence of AIDS-related CMV retinitis varies from 4% of ambulatory patients (primarily intravenous drug abusers)[325] to 34% of eyes in an autopsy series of male homosexuals.[294] This discrepancy may reflect the fact that CMV retinitis occurs late in the course of AIDS, and that male homosexual patients have a much higher frequency of CMV seropositivity. Most data have been generated from nonrandom series that potentially suffer from a variety of referral biases. In an early autopsy study of all patients with AIDS who died at UCLA, which was performed at a time when it was common to admit all patients to the hospital during the terminal stages of the disease, it was found that 25% of patients had CMV retinitis.[171] Most investigators believe that the true prevalence of CMV retinitis among patients with AIDS has been approximately 15% to 25%. Cytomegalovirus retinitis is uncommon among African patients with AIDS.[208]

CMV retinitis is usually a late manifestation of HIV disease. Although CMV retinitis is an "index disease" for AIDS (meaning that, in the absence of other risk factors, its presence alone is sufficient for making a diagnosis of AIDS),[39] only about 2% of patients with AIDS have CMV retinitis as the first and only manifestation of the syndrome.[353] It is estimated that the risk of developing CMV retinitis as the first manifestation of AIDS is less than 0.5% during the first 7 years after infection with HIV.[353] The reported duration of AIDS before the development of CMV retinitis has varied from medians of 9 to 10 months[146,175] to a mean of 18 months.[296] The range, however, is broad (0 to 45 months).[175] Holland and associates[175] found no evidence that this interval was changing during the first several years of the AIDS epidemic, despite increasing patient survival.

It is now more common to consider rates of CMV retinitis over time and in relationship to immune function, rather than the prevalence of disease for all patients with AIDS. In a prospective study of 132 HIV-infected patients (with CD4+ T-lymphocytes less than 200 per μl) recruited from two ambulatory medical care clinics, Kuppermann and associates[220] found CMV retinitis in 20%. The same authors found that 26 of 87 patients (30%) with CD4+ T-lymphocyte counts less than 50 per μl had CMV retinitis.

There appears to be an increasing prevalence of CMV retinitis among patients with AIDS, which parallels the increased rate of all CMV disease in this population, as discussed previously. It has also been suggested that CMV retinitis is more common in homosexual men with AIDS than in other risk groups, owing to different levels of exposure to CMV.[325,367]

---

*References 65, 73, 102, 111, 253, 291, 371, 402.

Cytomegalovirus retinitis is reported less commonly among HIV-infected children than among HIV-infected adults.[66] Cytomegalovirus retinitis in HIV-infected children generally does not develop for several years after birth, which reflects its association with declining immune function. Although CMV retinitis has been reported in HIV-infected infants,[66,197,230,334] its occurrence at birth is not diagnostic of AIDS, as it may be a manifestation of congenital cytomegalic inclusion disease.

Cytomegalovirus retinitis is more common among patients with AIDS than among other severely immunosuppressed individuals. Before the AIDS epidemic, renal allograft recipients were the most common group to develop CMV retinitis.[86,301] Other groups that may develop CMV retinitis include recipients of heart[204,301,310] or bone marrow transplants[4,49]; and patients with a variety of malignancies, including Hodgkin disease,[265] other lymphomas,[301] leukemia,[206] and solid tumors.[301] The occurrence of CMV retinitis in patients with malignancies is usually associated with the use of immunosuppressive chemotherapy. Cytomegalovirus retinitis has also been associated with the use of systemic corticosteroid therapy.[17]

Reported rates of CMV retinitis among renal transplant recipients have been between 1% and 5%.[5,99,280,306] Infection is most common among patients with prolonged CMV viremia.[98] Possible factors for the higher rate of CMV retinitis among patients with AIDS are discussed in the Pathogenesis section. The current incidence of opportunistic infections in transplant patients may be lower than previously reported because more selective immunosuppressive therapy is now used to prevent allograft rejections. There has been an overall drop in the incidence of CMV infections in cardiac transplant patients during the 2 months after surgery from 15% in patients receiving azathioprine and prednisone to 3% in patients receiving cyclosporine.[200]

RISK FACTORS

Acquired CMV infection usually results from close contact with individuals who are shedding virus. Demographic factors associated with increased rates of virus transmission and congenital disease are presented in the Epidemiology section. Less commonly, infection results from transfusion of blood or transplantation of organs from infected donors.

The primary risk factor for the development of serious clinical CMV disease (other than cytomegalic inclusion disease in newborns) in newly infected or latently infected individuals is immunosuppression.

Ocular Disease

CMV retinitis occurs only in severely immunocompromised patients. There appears to be a relationship between CMV retinitis and CMV viremia in patients with AIDS. Salmon and associates[331] found that CMV viremia at the development of AIDS was predictive of tissue-invasive CMV disease; 14 of 28 patients (50%) with positive CMV blood cultures developed disease, after a mean interval of 7.7 ± 6.3 months, in contrast to only 4 of 43 patients (9.3%) with negative blood cultures after a mean interval of 11.8 ± 3.8 months ($P < 0.001$). Survival and mean CD4+ T-lymphocyte counts were not different between groups. Zurlo and associates[417] also found that CMV viremia and viruria in patients with AIDS were statistically associated with development of tissue-invasive CMV disease, but pointed out that the positive predictive values of CMV viremia (35%) and CMV viruria (28%) for development of disease within 6 months were relatively low. Fiala and associates[98] also suggested a relationship between the duration of CMV viremia and development of CMV retinitis in organ transplant recipients.

CMV Retinitis in Patients with AIDS. The only systemic risk factor that has been clearly associated with development of CMV retinitis in HIV-infected patients is a low CD4+ T-lymphocyte count.[220,296] The infection almost always occurs in patients with counts less than 50 per μl; the mean counts reported for patients with CMV retinitis have been 8 to 15.6 per μl.[220,296]

In a retrospective study of 135 patients, 26 of whom developed CMV retinitis during 27 months of follow-up, Pertel and associates[296] found that the odds ratio for developing CMV retinitis was 4.62 ($P = 0.002$) for patients with baseline CD4+ T-lymphocyte counts of 0 to 50 per μl when compared to those with counts of 101 to 250 per μl. The proportion of patients developing CMV retinitis at 27 months, grouped by baseline CD4+ T-lymphocyte count, is shown in Table 81-1. In the same study the mean duration before development of CMV retinitis in 24 of 26 patients with a CD4+ T-lymphocyte count less than 50 per μl was 13.1 months.

Despite its strong association with low CD4+ T-lymphocyte counts, CMV retinitis has been seen occasionally in patients with counts above 100 per μl.[53,95,160] An association has also been identified between CMV retinitis and low CD8+ T-lymphocyte counts,[236] but it could not be determined from initial studies whether low CD8+ T-lymphocyte counts place a patient at risk independent of CD4+ T-lymphocyte. If so, it might explain the occasional cases of CMV retinitis in patients with high CD4+ T-lymphocyte counts.

As discussed in the Epidemiology section, CMV retinitis may be more common in homosexual patients with AIDS than in other risk groups. As discussed in the Pathogenesis section, the retinal microvasculopathy associated with HIV infection may be associated with the increased prevalence of CMV retinitis in patients with AIDS when compared to other immunosuppressed populations. Cotton-wool spots, the most common clinical manifestation of the microvasculopathy, are more common in patients with the full AIDS illness than in other HIV-infected individuals and are fre-

TABLE 81-1   CUMULATIVE INCIDENCE OF CMV RETINITIS VERSUS
BASELINE CD4+ T-LYMPHOCYTES COUNT

Baseline CD4+ T-Lymphocyte Count (per μl)	Cumulative Percentage Having CMV Retinitis at Specified Intervals After Baseline Examination*		
	9 Months	18 Months	27 Months
0-50	21.9	33.6	41.9
50-100	8.9	26.3	26.3
100-250	0	6.7	14.7

Adapted from Pertel P, Hirschtick R, Phair J et al.: Risk of developing cytomegalovirus retinitis in persons infected
with the human immunodeficiency virus, *J Acquir Immune Defic Syndr* 5:1069-1074, 1992.
*$P = 0.003$, log-rank test.

quently seen in patients prior to the development of CMV retinitis.[170] The presence of isolated cotton-wool spots, however, has never been confirmed as an independent risk factor for development of CMV retinitis.

The identification of risk factors for CMV retinitis in HIV-infected patients makes screening programs for the identification of asymptomatic disease more practical. Kuppermann and associates[220] advocate examining patients with CD4+ T-lymphocyte counts less than 50 per μl every 3 to 4 months. In this prospective study all 14 patients found to have previously undiagnosed CMV retinitis on screening examination reported no symptoms, although several patients actually had visual changes when instructed how to look for them. In contrast, MacGregor and associates[238] found no asymptomatic CMV retinitis among 78 patients with CD4+ T-lymphocyte less than 100 per μl.

Although other investigators have advocated similar screening programs, there have been no data upon which to base the recommended intervals, nor have there been studies to determine whether long-term visual outcomes are affected by screening programs. Others have suggested patient education programs regarding early symptoms of disease as a more practical alternative to widespread screening.[163] This suggestion is based on the assumptions that even asymptomatic patients will develop recognizable symptoms after short intervals, and that the amount of lesion enlargement that might occur before symptoms develop will be small and will not affect response to treatment and final visual outcomes. Furthermore, even if patients are screened, they will develop new lesions throughout the interval between examinations, and it is unlikely that educated patients who develop new lesions in the earlier part of that interval would remain asymptomatic until the next scheduled examination. Therefore, in practical terms, it is likely that most new lesions will actually be identified because of patient symptoms and self-referral, even if screening programs become more widespread. Because it will be impossible to determine how long CMV retinitis remains asymptomatic, rational decisions re-

garding the value of screening or appropriate screening intervals will require a study of outcomes.

It is appropriate to examine selected asymptomatic patients for CMV retinitis if they have additional risk factors for infection, including new or persistent viremia, nonocular CMV infections, and/or sudden declines in immune function.

CLINICAL FEATURES

Clinical disorders caused by CMV infection depend on the immune status of the host and mode of virus transmission. They can be grouped into the following categories: congenital disease, acquired disease in immunocompetent older children and adults, and disease in immunosuppressed individuals. Cytomegalovirus retinitis occurs only in patients with congenital disease or in patients who are immunosuppressed.

Congenital Disease

Cytomegalic inclusion disease in congenitally infected newborns primarily affects the reticuloendothelial system and CNS, and differentiation from congenital toxoplasmosis may be difficult in some cases. Characteristic findings include hepatomegaly (the most common finding at birth), splenomegaly, jaundice, petechiae, and respiratory distress[2,253,402]; but these clinical findings may not be apparent within the first 24 hours of life.[2,253] Congenital heart disease has been reported in association with cytomegalic inclusion disease, but is not common.[253] Cytomegalovirus interstitial pneumonia in otherwise normal neonates occurs occasionally.

Although intelligence may develop normally, mental retardation, varying from mild to severe, is common.[253] Other CNS disorders include deafness, seizures, microcephaly, motor disabilities, and behavioral disorders.[145,253,402] Intracranial calcifications may be seen. Intrauterine growth retardation and prematurity are common sequelae of congenital CMV infection.

Acquired Disease

CMV infection in immunocompetent older children and adults is usually asymptomatic, but patients may develop a syndrome resembling infectious mononucleosis. Patients with this syndrome usually present with nonspecific symptoms of myalgia, malaise, headache, fever, and sore throat. Lymphadenopathy and hepatosplenomegaly may occur. Rarely, CMV infection may result in interstitial pneumonia,[212] hepatitis,[23] Guillain-Barre syndrome,[338] encephalitis,[399] thrombocytopenia,[148] and myocarditis.[399] Children tend to have more respiratory complications than adults.

Immunosuppressed Patients

An infectious mononucleosis-like syndrome, which is indistinguishable from the disease seen in immunocompetent hosts, is the most common clinical presentation of systemic CMV disease among immunosuppressed individuals and is particularly common in solid organ transplant recipients. It may progress to invasive organ disease. The syndrome may occur with both newly acquired and reactivated infections.

Cytomegalovirus is the most common life-threatening opportunistic viral pathogen in patients with AIDS,[188] and in one autopsy series, over half of the patients dying from any AIDS-related complication had CMV infection of at least one organ.[268] As prophylaxis regimens against *P. carinii* pneumonia have become widespread, CMV infection has emerged as the most frequent initial AIDS-related illness.[176]

It is estimated that up to 20% of patients with AIDS will develop CMV related-gastrointestinal disease.[69] Cytomegalovirus esophagitis is a common cause of dysphagia in patients with AIDS. Diagnosis requires endoscopic biopsy showing extensive ulceration with intranuclear inclusions at the ulcer margin; the exclusion of other potential causes; and an appropriate clinical setting of severe immunosuppression.[405] Colitis/ileitis will develop in 10% of patients with AIDS; symptoms are nonspecific and include fever, weight loss, diarrhea, abdominal pain, and occasionally hemorrhage and perforation. As with CMV esophagitis, the diagnosis depends on colonoscopic biopsy with the identification of inclusion bodies and the exclusion of other potential causes.[361] Frequently, multiple pathogens may be present, and it may be difficult to identify the cause of clinical disease. Cytomegalovirus is an infrequent cause of hepatitis and biliary tract disease.[21]

Cytomegalovirus can be detected in culture from a high proportion of lung tissue or bronchial fluids obtained from patients with AIDS; in one study, 43% of specimens were culture-positive.[27] Cultures cannot distinguish between colonization by CMV and tissue-destructive infection, however.[260] Furthermore, the presence of inclusion bodies in the lung does not necessarily implicate CMV as the cause of clinical disease, unless other causes have been excluded.[254] Only 4% of patients with AIDS and pneumonitis have been found to have CMV as the sole pathogen.[272] In contrast,

CMV pneumonitis in immunosuppressed solid organ or bone marrow transplant recipients is common, and isolation of CMV from lung tissue or bronchial fluids is associated with a poor prognosis in bone marrow transplant recipients.[257]

Cytomegalovirus infection of the nervous system in patients with AIDS may cause a number of disorders, including meningoencephalitis, polyradiculomyelitis, and peripheral neuropathy.[63,249,330] The role of CMV in the AIDS dementia complex is uncertain, but it is probable that HIV itself, rather than CMV, is the main causal agent.[274] In patients with AIDS, there is a large variation in the reported rates of CMV infection in the CNS; based on autopsy examinations, rates range from approximately 20% to 60%.[32,298,406] The exact contribution of CMV infection to clinically apparent CNS disease is unknown. Cytomegalovirus meningoencephalitis may also occur in immunosuppressed individuals after solid organ transplantation.[75]

Other disorders attributed to CMV in patients with AIDS have included adrenalitis,[127] thyroiditis,[104] epididymitis,[313] and dermatitis.[389]

Ocular Disease

Ocular CMV infection is primarily a disease of the retina, although there have been isolated reports of infection involving other ocular structures, as described at the end of this subsection. Detailed information about CMV retinitis is derived almost exclusively from patients with AIDS; possible differences in CMV retinitis between patients with AIDS and others at risk are identified in the following discussion.

Cytomegalovirus Retinitis. Terminology used to describe CMV retinitis lesions is listed in the Appendix to this chapter. The diagnosis of CMV retinitis is based on clinical findings. Untreated disease can have a variety of clinical presentations, with variable amounts of retinal whitening or opacification (caused by edema and necrosis), retinal hemorrhage, and vascular sheathing. Two distinct clinical types of CMV retinitis have been described, based on retinal characteristics. The *fulminant/edematous* variant corresponds to the classic appearance of disease, which was recognized before the AIDS epidemic. These lesions tend to have the following characteristics: dense confluent areas of retinal opacification (through which choroidal details cannot be seen) involving both the border and central areas of the lesions; and the absence of clear central atrophic areas (unless the lesions are large, involving 25% or more of the retina) (Fig. 81-1). Other suggestive, but not definitive, characteristics of fulminant/edematous lesions are the following: location along vessels; hemorrhage sufficient to obscure underlying choroidal or retinal detail; and inflammatory vascular sheathing.

The *indolent/granular* variant is defined by the following characteristics: only faint, grainy opacification of the retina (through which choroidal details can be seen); only trace

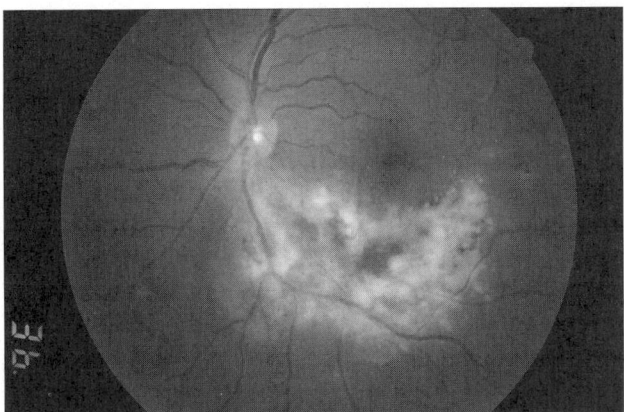

Fig. 81-1. Fulminant/edematous variant of untreated CMV retinitis along the inferotemporal vascular arcade in the left eye of a patient with AIDS. (Figure also in color insert.)

(punctate) or no hemorrhage; and no inflammatory vascular sheathing (Fig. 81-2). Other suggestive, but not definitive, characteristics of indolent/granular lesions are the following: circular or oval shape; location not overlying arterioles or venules; and opacification of the lesion border only, with the presence of a clear atrophic central area.

Both lesion variants have an irregular, dry-appearing, granular border, which is the most characteristic feature of CMV retinitis. There can be a variable number of distinct *satellite* lesions, which are considered to be encompassed within the lesion border (Fig. 81-3). Other clinical features that suggest a diagnosis of CMV retinitis include relatively slow enlargement of lesions and minimal vitreous humor and anterior chamber inflammatory reactions. These two variants seem to exist at the ends of a disease spectrum, and many lesions, which cannot be classified as one clinical type or the other, are considered *indeterminant* in type. It is also

generally impossible to classify early lesions (less than 2 optic disc areas in size) as one clinical type or the other (Fig. 81-4). Clinical type designations are appropriate only for untreated lesions; treated lesions that are not completely inactive will almost always have features similar to the indolent/granular variant of untreated disease.

In occasional patients, severe retinal periphlebitis has been the most prominent feature of AIDS-related CMV retinitis[122,368] (Fig. 81-5). Such patients have foci of CMV retinitis typical of the fulminant/edematous variant somewhere in the fundus, but also have dense inflammatory sheathing of vessels throughout the retina, even remote from the site of infection. In their initial 1982 report Holland and associates[167,170] included retinal vasculitis of unknown cause among the ophthalmic manifestations of AIDS, on the basis of a patient who had severe perivascular sheathing throughout the fundus. The patient also had retinal opacities surrounding the optic disc, and in retrospect, probably had unrecognized CMV retinitis. The appearance of the vascular changes in these patients has been likened to *frosted branch angiitis,* a syndrome initially described in otherwise healthy individuals. (Patients with frosted branch angiitis do not have foci of retinal necrosis, however, and the relation between these disorders, if any, is unknown.) Perivascular inflammatory cells remote from foci of CMV-induced retinal necrosis can be found in many patients,[170] however, and those who appear to have frosted branch angiitis can be thought of as having an extreme form of the fulminant/edematous variant of disease.

The reason for variations in retinal lesion appearance are not known. Henderly and associates[153] suggested that indolent/granular lesions may be more common in the peripheral retina. In a study of 234 patients by other investigators, 66% of eyes with fulminant/edematous lesions had Zone 1 (see Fig. 81-6 for location) involvement, whereas only 36% of

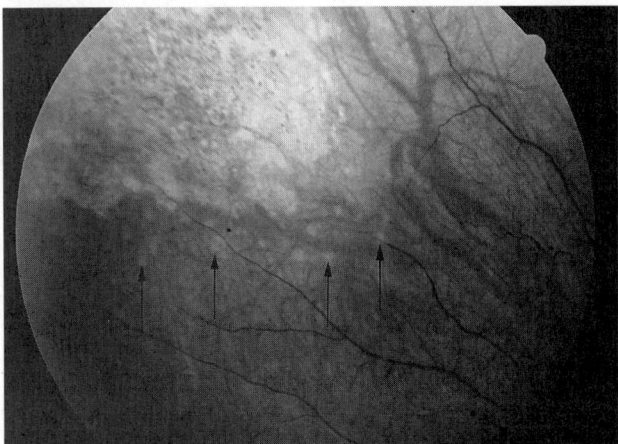

Fig. 81-2. Indolent/granular variant of untreated CMV retinitis in the peripheral retina of a patient with AIDS. Only the posterior border of the oval lesion, which straddles the border of Zones 2 and 3 of the retina, is visible. (Figure also in color insert.)

Fig. 81-3. Untreated CMV retinitis in the superotemporal quadrant of the right eye. There are a number of satellite lesions at the border of between infected and normal retina *(arrows).* (Figure also in color insert.)

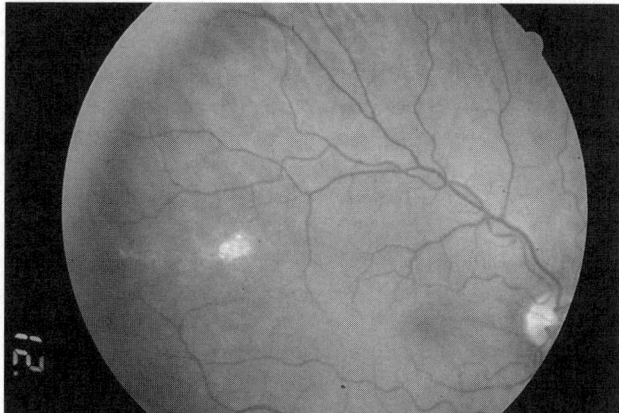

Fig. 81-4. Early CMV retinitis lesion in the right eye of a patient with AIDS. There is fine granularity of the retina adjacent to the solid opacity.

eyes with indolent/granular lesions had Zone 1 involvement.[384] Anatomic factors may therefore influence the character of lesions. The appearance of lesions at diagnosis might also reflect treatments the patient is already receiving. Several investigators have reported at least partial or transient resolution of lesions in patients receiving acyclovir, zidovudine, or both (see Therapy section). Because many HIV-infected patients are receiving these medications for other indications, it is possible that variations in the appearance of lesions reflect the use of these or other drugs.[164] Finally, the severity of a patient's immunosuppression may affect his or her ability to control CMV infection in the absence of any antiviral drugs, and therefore may affect the amount of retinal opacification of untreated lesions.[22]

The variation in lesion appearances was emphasized initially to ensure that even lesions without the classic appear-

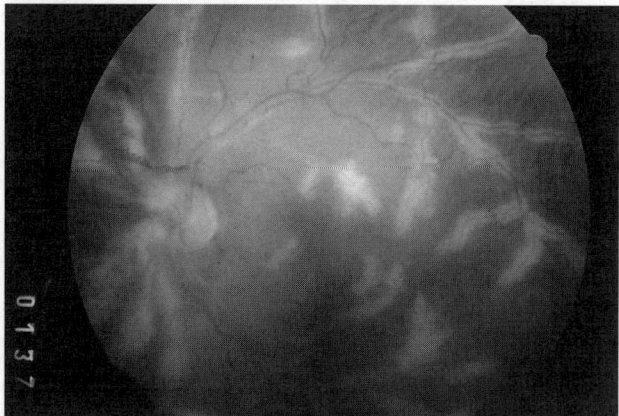

Fig. 81-5. Marked inflammatory vascular sheathing in the left eye of a patient with AIDS and CMV retinitis. The only focus of CMV retinitis is nasal to the optic disc at the left border of the photograph. The vascular involvement in such cases resembles "frosted branch angiitis."

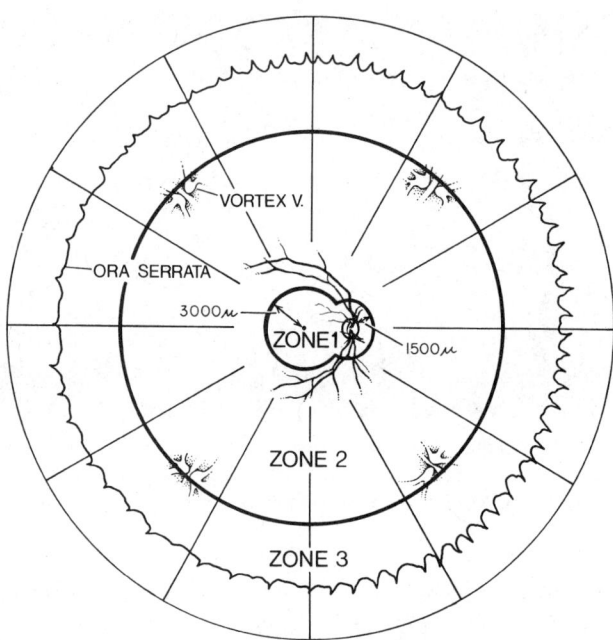

Fig. 81-6. Retinal zones. Reprinted with permission from Holland GN, Buhles WC, Mastre B et al.: A controlled retrospective study of ganciclovir treatment for cytomegalovirus retinopathy: use of a standardized system for the assessment of disease outcome, *Arch Ophthalmol* 107:1759-1766, 1989. Copyright 1989 American Medical Association.

ance of CMV retinitis would be diagnosed accurately. Variations in appearance may have some prognostic implications as well, however. There has been limited evidence that the rate of lesion enlargement in untreated patients is slower for indolent/granular lesions.[173] Slower enlargement of these lesions would explain the atrophic central area; as the lesions spread centrifugally, necrotic debris would be cleared from the oldest sites of disease before lesions became very large.

Patients with Zone 1 lesions may develop serous exudation of fluid into the macula with exudative retinal detachment.[118,172,294] Gangan and associates[118] found lipid exudates and/or exudative retinal detachments in 35 of 214 eyes (16%) with CMV retinitis in Zone 1. The majority of their patients had parapapillary lesions, and they hypothesized that the optic nerve was the source of fluid. Other cases had lesions up to 3000 μm from the fovea without optic disc involvement; in those cases the parafoveal vessels were believed to be the source of fluid.[118] Pepose and associates[294] found exudative retinal detachments at autopsy in 10 of 35 eyes with CMV retinitis. Exudative retinal detachment of the macula is one cause of reversible vision loss in patients with CMV retinitis.[118,172]

The proportion of patients with bilateral CMV retinitis at diagnosis has ranged from approximately 20% to 40% in most reports.[137,153,384] Most patients have only one descrete focus of disease per eye at presentation, and it is very uncommon to present with more than three lesions per eye.

Eyes with CMV retinitis will have mild cellular reactions in the aqueous and vitreous humors. Anterior segment inflammation is never severe enough to cause redness, pain, or synechiae formation between the iris and lens. Small, translucent, spicular keratic precipitates may develop. The vitreous humor never contains enough inflammatory material to obscure view of the retina, although vitreous humor haze may increase over time, especially after many months of disease that is very extensive in area.

Inflammatory signs are more variable in CMV retinitis patients who are immunosuppressed for reasons other than HIV infection,[256] and may increase as patients are taken off immunosuppressive medications.[86] This increase suggests that the lack of a prominent inflammatory reaction in patients with AIDS may reflect the specific immunologic defects associated with HIV infection.

The optic nerve can become infected with CMV* (Fig. 81-7). "Optic neuritis" was reported in 32% of patients in one series; in all cases CMV retinitis was adjacent to the optic disc.[321] Gross and associates[138] distinguished two types of optic nerve involvement: cases in which CMV retinitis extends posteriorly to involve the optic disc margin (termed Type I disease by the authors); and cases of isolated optic nerve and peripapillary CMV infection of the retina (termed Type II). Patients with optic disc swelling associated with parapapillary CMV retinitis can retain good central vision, although dense altitudinal and horizontal visual field defects may occur[138]; in such cases there may be no histologic evidence of CMV infection of the nerve. In contrast, patients with isolated optic disc infection have early afferent pupillary defects and rapid deterioration of vision to no light perception, even with antiviral therapy.[138] The majority of patients with peripapillary CMV retinitis do not develop infection of the optic nerve.[35]

Cytomegalovirus retinitis in newborns is commonly reported to occur in the peripheral retina, but may develop anywhere in the fundus. Retinal hemorrhages and vascular sheathing have been associated findings, as in immunocompromised adults.[387] Infection also may involve the optic nerve,[259,387] and optic atrophy has been a common finding.[73,111,371]

Symptoms. The symptoms of CMV retinitis include blurring of vision, scotomata ("blind spots"), and floaters. The specific symptoms experienced by an individual patient depend on the location of lesions in the eye. Even small foci of disease in the far periphery of the retina can cause floaters, which probably represent changes in the consistency of the vitreous humor induced by the adjacent retinal infection. Lesions that are more posterior in the fundus can cause scotomata, characterized by distortion or absence of images. Scotomata related to CMV retinitis usually have sharp borders.

---

*References 113, 138, 139, 275, 293, 322.

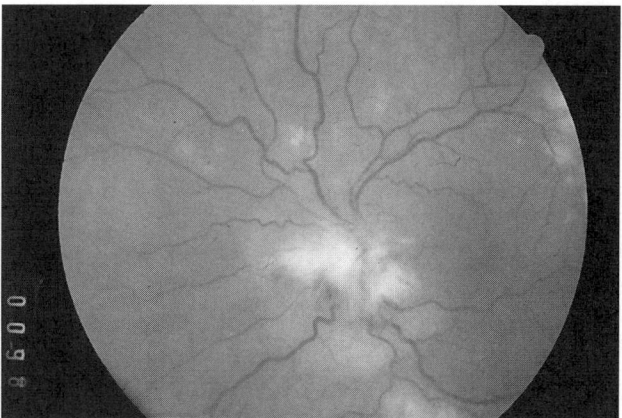

Fig. 81-7. CMV papillitis in the left eye in a patient with AIDS. There is also an exudative retinal detachment surrounding the swollen optic disc.

Lesions near the fovea or optic disc may cause blurring of vision. This blurring, which will be constant for both close and distant objects of regard, should not be confused with the symptoms of presbyopia (the inability to focus clearly on close objects without reading glasses), which normally develop in the early 40s (also a common age for patients with AIDS-related CMV retinitis).

Some patients may complain only of a vague sensation that the quality of vision has changed. In patients with unilateral disease, normal vision in the uninvolved eye can mask symptoms in the eye with CMV retinitis, unless vision is checked in each eye individually by covering one eye and then the other. Occasionally patients will be completely asymptomatic, especially if lesions are in the peripheral retina.

Symptoms of retinal detachment include increased floaters, photopsia ("flashing lights"), new scotomata or sudden enlargement of existing scotomata, the sensation of a curtain over one's vision, or sudden blurring of vision. Small peripheral retinal detachments can be asymptomatic, however.

Natural History of Cytomegalovirus Retinitis. Untreated CMV retinitis in patients with AIDS is a relentlessly progressive disease. Cytomegalovirus retinitis frequently begins adjacent to retinal vessels in the posterior pole, which is consistent with the belief that virus reaches the eye via the bloodstream. Lesions enlarge in an irregular fashion (Fig. 81-8). Also, the rate of border advancement is generally faster in an anterior direction toward the ora serrata than in a posterior direction toward the fovea.[173] Cytomegalovirus retinitis has been considered a "foveal-sparing" disease. In a series of organ transplant patients with CMV retinitis reported by Egbert and associates[86] prior to the AIDS epidemic, only 4 of 21 eyes had macular involvement. Gross and associates[137] found no cases of foveal infection among their patients with AIDS and CMV retinitis. In patients with

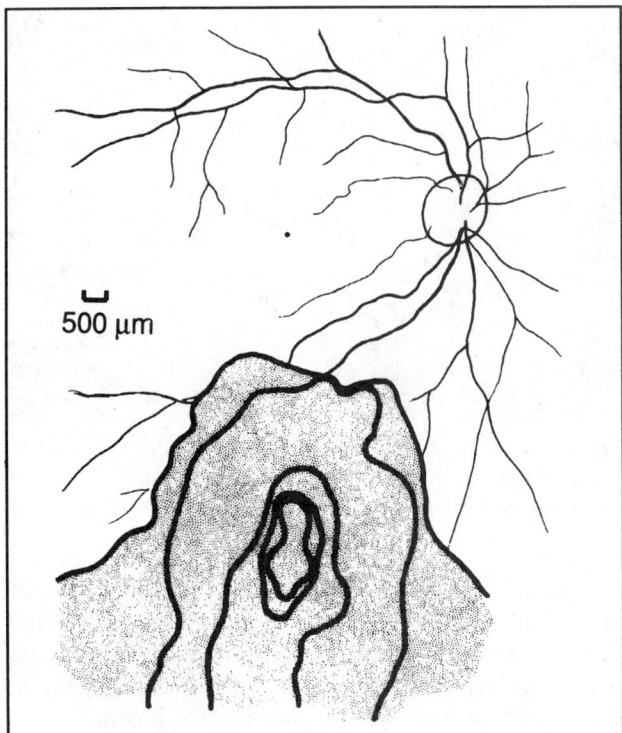

Fig. 81-8. Diagram of the enlargement of an untreated CMV retinitis lesion over time. *Bold lines* within the shaded area indicate borders of the lesion on successive examination dates: *innermost line,* the position of the border at baseline; and other *solid lines,* border position on the following examination days: 7, 21, 34, and 48. Reprinted with permission from Holland GN, Shuler JD: Progression rates of cytomegalovirus retinopathy in ganciclovir-treated and untreated patients, *Arch Ophthalmol* 110:1435-1442, 1992. Copyright 1992 American Medical Association.

AIDS, disease expands toward the fovea at a median rate of approximately 24 μm/day,[173] but posterior movement directly toward the fovea appears to slow as it nears the fovea, and disease moves circumferentially around the fovea (Fig. 81-9). As a consequence, the fovea is generally the last area of the retina to be destroyed. A fairly high rate of foveal involvement in early autopsy series of patients with AIDS[294] may have reflected the fact that progression of CMV retinitis into the macula could not be stopped prior to the introduction of ganciclovir and foscarnet therapy.

In untreated disease the entire retina will be destroyed over a period of approximately 6 months. In most cases the destruction is attributable to enlargement of the initial lesions; new disease foci develop infrequently during the course of disease. Necrotizing CMV infection does not extend beyond the retina.[294] Areas of retinal necrosis are eventually replaced by a thin gliotic membrane, and there can be fine pigmentary mottling throughout the area of scar formation[284] (Fig. 81-10). The lack of darkly pigmented scars, as occurs with healing of some other retinal infections such as

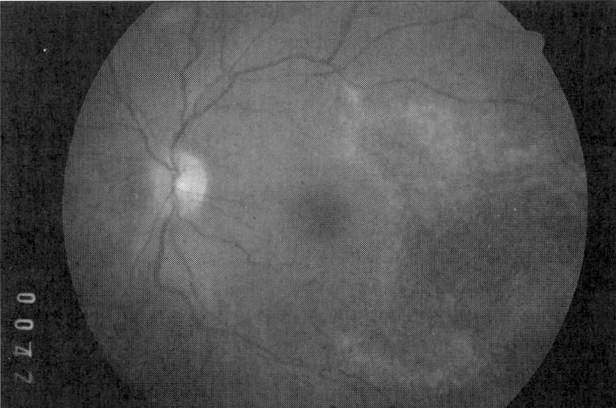

Fig. 81-9. CMV retinitis in the left eye of a patient with AIDS. Despite treatment with ganciclovir, the lesion border has reactivated and is advancing. Posterior advancement slows as it nears the fovea; as a result the advancing border appears to be moving circumferentially around the fovea.

toxoplasmic retinochoroiditis, is presumably caused by total destruction of the retinal pigment epithelium (RPE).

Spontaneous resolution of AIDS-related CMV retinitis in the absence of antiviral therapy has not been reported. A case of "transient spontaneous regression" of CMV retinitis in a patient with AIDS has been described, in which a lesion typical of CMV retinitis lost its opacification over a several week period without specific anti-CMV therapy.[269] The improvement was not permanent, however, and there was no mention of whether or not the patient was receiving antiretroviral therapy, which is believed to alter lesion appearance in some cases (see Therapy section). Furthermore, the diagnosis was not confirmed histopathologically, and the patient had a history of toxoplasmosis and syphilis, both of

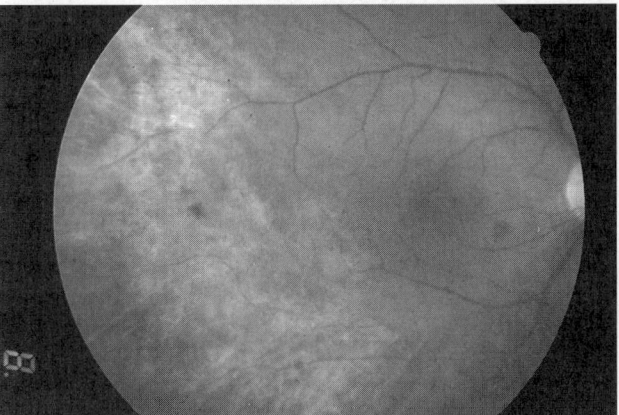

Fig. 81-10. Inactive, temporally located CMV retinitis in a patient with AIDS who is receiving foscarnet therapy. The border of the lesion has no opacity. The central portion of the lesion is characterized by gliosis and mild pigment stippling.

which can cause a severe retinopathy in HIV-infected individuals.

The natural history of CMV retinitis in congenitally infected infants is less well understood. In a study of 12 patients with cytomegalic inclusion disease who were followed for 3 to 12 years after birth, Berenberg and Nankervis[16] reported that 4 of 12 "continued to have retinal involvement." No information was given about the activity of these lesions or changes that occurred during serial examinations. Berenberg and Nankervis may simply have observed scarring from old sites of infection. Based on isolated case reports, lesions apparently can be active for many months, during which time extensive areas of the retina can be destroyed. Lesions eventually become quiescent, leaving areas of atrophy and scarring.[33,143] Pigmentation of the scar may occur, giving the fundus a finely mottled appearance, as in adults.

Other Ocular Lesions. Despite its apparent predilection for retinal tissue, CMV is found occasionally in other ocular tissues. Cytomegalovirus was cultured from the ocular surface of an immunocompetent patient with CMV-associated lymphadenopathy and a mild nonpurulent conjunctivitis.[119] Cytomegalovirus was cultured from a patient with AIDS and conjunctivitis[209]; autopsy examination revealed no virus in the lacrimal gland, and the characteristics of the conjunctivitis were not described. Cytomegalovirus infection was demonstrated histopathologically in a biopsy specimen from a patient with AIDS and an inflamed caruncle.[92] The virus has also been found by electron microscopy in the conjunctiva of an HIV-infected patient without clinical signs of disease related to CMV,[29] and has been isolated from conjunctival swabs of patients undergoing bone marrow transplantation.[168] In one series CMV could be found in tears of 19.5% of children with leukemia,[52] but the site of infection was not determined. Cytomegalovirus infection of keratocytes was found in a failed corneal graft treated with topical cyclosporine 2% and prednisolone acetate 1%.*

It has been suggested by some authors that CMV infection is a cause of decreased tear production in immunocompetent and immunosuppressed patients,[88,209] although there is little evidence to support this hypothesis.

Cytomegalovirus has been cultured from lens material aspirated from an otherwise healthy 3-year-old child with bilateral iridocyclitis and cataracts.[149] A causal relationship was not established.

Branch retinal artery occlusions in an immunocompetent patient with serologic evidence of acute CMV infection has been reported,[71] although the mechanism by which systemic infection by CMV would cause such vascular events is unknown.

Developmental anomalies reported to be associated with cytomegalic inclusion disease include microphthalmus,[157,259] optic nerve hypoplasia, optic nerve colobomata,[157] anophthalmia,[111] and Peter anomaly.[111] Strabismus and nystagmus have been seen in patients with cytomegalic inclusion disease, but a causal relationship has not been established.[371] Cataracts were reported in a stillborn infant with CMV retinitis.[83]

Sundmacher and associates[386] reported a case of disciform-like corneal clouding and increased intraocular pressure that they hypothesized to be the result of CMV corneal endotheliitis and trabeculitis, based on the isolation of CMV from aqueous humor and conjunctiva. Histopathologic confirmation of tissue infection was not obtained, however.

PATHOLOGY

Cytomegalovirus infection occurs in a variety of tissues and cell types, but infection of macrophages and endothelial cells is seen frequently in vivo. A unique histopathologic finding in tissues infected by CMV is the presence of giant (or cytomegalic) cells, which classically have type A intranuclear inclusions[51] (Fig. 81-11). The cytomegalic cells are typically two to four times larger than surrounding cells, with a large round-oval nucleus that is often eccentrically displaced. The eosinophilic nuclear inclusion may be surrounded by a clear halo, giving rise to an "owl's eye" appearance. Basophilic granular inclusions may also be found in the cytoplasm. The origin of the cytomegalic cells is unresolved. Because cytomegalic cells are frequently associated with ductal epithelium, they may be of epithelial origin, even though epithelial cells are not permissive to CMV in vitro.[158]

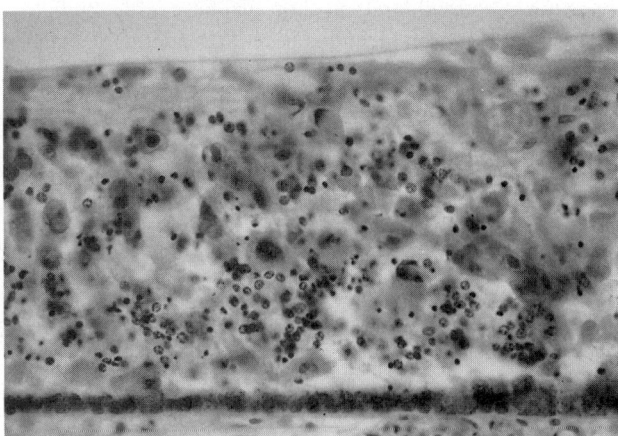

Fig. 81-11. Light micrograph of CMV retinitis demonstrating full thickness retinal necrosis with scattered cytomegalic cells. (Hematoxylin-eosin, original magnification ×110.) Photograph courtesy of Robert Y. Foos MD.

*S.R. Wehrly, MD, unpublished data, presented at the annual meeting of the Ocular Microbiology and Immunology Group, San Francisco, CA, October 1994.

Ocular Disease

A number of publications have described the histopathologic features of CMV retinitis in patients with AIDS* and other immunodeficiency states.[64] Electron microscopic and immunohistochemical studies identify CMV viral particles and antigen in a patchy distribution throughout all layers of the retina and occasionally in contiguous RPE cells.[294] Infection results in retinal necrosis with complete disruption of all retinal layers (Fig. 81-12). Cytomegalic cells can be seen throughout the necrotic retina. There may be a sharp demarcation between normal and necrotic retina, or there may be a transition zone containing isolated cytomegalic cells and partially disrupted retinal elements.

It is uncommon to find CMV in intraocular tissues other than the retina. Cytomegalovirus has been detected rarely in the iris stroma and ciliary body of patients with AIDS.[57,294,388] Viral antigens are rarely identified in choroidal tissue of patients with AIDS and CMV retinitis.[294,323] When present in the choroid, viral antigen has been found in association with vessels and is not always adjacent to areas of CMV retinitis, suggesting that the virus reaches the choroid through independent hematogenous spread, rather than by extension of infection from retina.[294] Uveal tissue inflammation has been seen in congenitally infected infants with CMV retinitis,[259,359,387] but infection of the choroid, iris, and ciliary body occurs rarely, if at all.

Cells with CMV viral inclusions may be seen in the choroidal and retinal vascular lumina.[43,393] In immunosuppressed patients without HIV infection, the spread of disease along vessels has been attributed to infection of vascular endothelial cells, which break free and travel through the retinal circulation.[64] In support of this hypothesis, inclusion bodies have been identified in retinal endothelial cells of organ transplant patients with CMV retinitis. In patients with AIDS and CMV retinitis, endothelial cell inclusions have been reported rarely in choroidal tissue,[10,323] but CMV antigen has not been identified in retinal endothelial cells by immunohistochemical techniques, even in vessels that travel through areas of retinopathy.[170] Thus although endothelial cell infection is seen in a variety of tissues, it may not play an important role in the spread of CMV retinitis in patients with AIDS. It has been hypothesized that virus spreads adjacent to vessels in the anatomic spaces of Virchow.[173]

In most cases CMV infection elicits only a mild cellular inflammatory response in the retina.† It is usually characterized by a sparse infiltrate of mononuclear cells in both patients with AIDS and those immunosuppressed by other mechanisms. Lymphocytes are the predominant cell type. In addition, however, 22% to 50% of patients with AIDS and CMV retinitis have foci of neutrophilic infiltrates in retinal

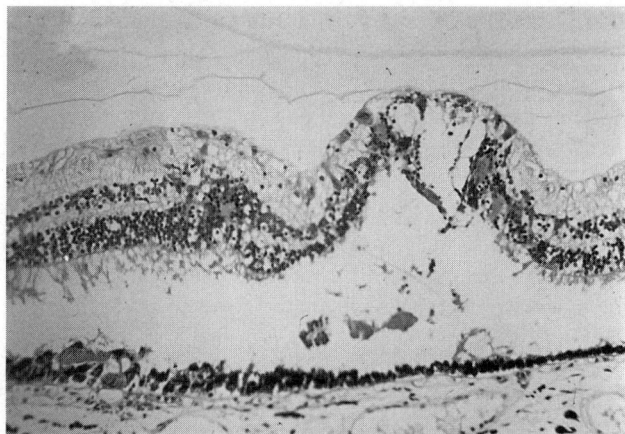

Fig. 81-12. Light micrograph of CMV retinitis demonstrating abrupt transition between the normal architecture of the uninfected retina *(left)* and full thickness necrosis caused by CMV infection. There is also a focus of retinal pigment epithelial infection in the lower left. (Hematoxylin-eosin, original magnification ×27.)

tissue at autopsy.[284,294] This finding is not typical of CMV retinitis in patients without HIV infection. The difference has been attributed to intact granulocyte function and chemotaxis in patients with AIDS, in contrast to infants, organ transplant recipients, and patients with malignancies who can have more severe quantitative or qualitative granulocyte dysfunction.[294] Patients on immunosuppressive drugs can develop marked inflammatory reactions to CMV retinitis when the drug therapy is withdrawn.[86]

Pepose and associates[294] performed an in situ analysis of T-lymphocyte subsets on choroidal tissue of two patients with AIDS and CMV retinitis: there was a reversal of the normal T-helper to T-cytotoxic/suppressor cell ratio, which parallels changes seen in the blood of patients with AIDS; a normal reaction was seen in choroidal tissue of normal controls.

A variety of stimuli (CMV antigen, immune complex deposition, and tissue necrosis) may be responsible for the production of chemotactic factors leading to inflammatory cell infiltration. Immunochemical studies have revealed deposition of IgG, IgA, and, to a lesser extent, IgM and C3c in retinal tissue and within retinal arteriolar walls.[294] Many IgA-bearing plasma cells were present in one case.[170] There is poor correlation between the distribution of tissue-bound immunoglobulins, acute inflammatory cells, and CMV antigens.[294] It is therefore possible that the acute inflammatory reaction present in some eyes may be in response to stimuli other than CMV.

The perivascular inflammatory sheathing that is seen clinically in cases of CMV retinitis is composed of neutrophils, and is consistent with an immune complex-mediated vasculitis; CMV antigen is not identified in the affected vessels[170,294] (Fig. 81-13).

A secondary choroiditis consisting of mononuclear cells

---

*References 10, 170, 195, 196, 276, 284, 294, 342, 343, 346.
†References 10, 55, 139, 155, 195, 276, 393.

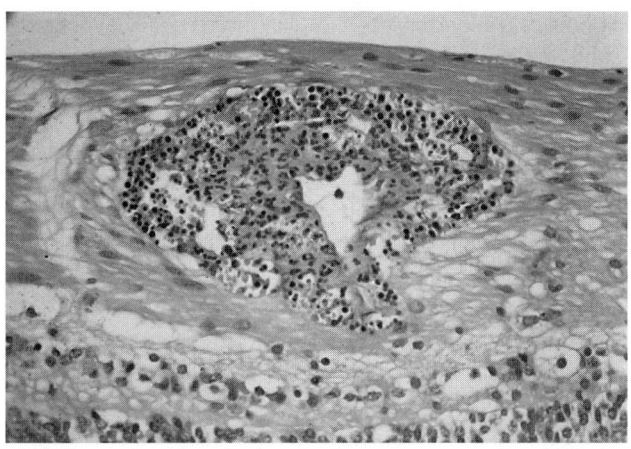

Fig. 81-13. Light micrograph of uninfected superficial retina in an eye with CMV retinitis elsewhere. Wall of inferotemporal retinal vein (which drains the region of CMV retinitis) is markedly thickened with an infiltrate of neutrophils and the lumen is significantly narrowed. (Hematoxylin-eosin, original magnification ×52.) Reprinted with permission from Holland GN, Pepose JS, Pettit TH et al.: Acquired immune deficiency syndrome: ocular manifestations, *Ophthalmology* 90:859-873, 1983.

or neutrophils may occur subjacent to areas of CMV retinitis without identifiable viral antigens in the inflamed choroid.[294] In areas where CMV antigens can be identified in choroid, only a minimal cellular inflammatory reaction is elicited.[294]

The vitreous humor usually remains remarkably free of inflammatory material, despite the presence of virus in the vitreous cavity.[10]

In the acute stage of disease there may be subretinal fluid with exudative retinal detachment.[294] In the later stages of CMV retinitis the necrotic retina thins with formation of multiple retinal holes, which predispose patients to retinal detachment. Eventually the necrotic retinal is replaced by a thin gliotic membrane. At this stage CMV particles cannot be identified in the eye histologically.

COMPLICATIONS

The sequelae of congenital CMV infection and CMV infection in immunocompromised hosts have been discussed in the Clinical Features section. Acquired CMV infection in healthy adults is not believed to have any serious long-term consequences.

CMV infection itself may cause immunosuppression, making patients more susceptible to other opportunistic infections. In HIV-infected individuals, CMV may transactivate HIV, thereby facilitating progression of HIV-induced disease, as discussed in the Pathogenesis section.

Cytomegalovirus Retinitis

CMV may spread from the retina to involve the optic nerve, with severe loss of vision. Branch retinal artery occlusions have been reported in association with optic nerve involvement.[321] Optic disc neovascularization, attributed to nonperfusion of infected retina, has been reported as a rare complication of CMV retinitis.[228] The major complication of CMV retinitis, however, is rhegmatogenous retinal detachment.

Retinal Detachments. Rhegmatogenous retinal detachments occur when fluid gains access to the subretinal space through holes in necrotic retina. Because of retinochoroidal adhesions at the borders of lesions, the configuration of these retinal detachments may lead to the mistaken impression that they are exudative.[28,107,256] Prior to the AIDS epidemic rhegmatogenous retinal detachments were considered a late complication of the disease; they occurred as edema resolved and retinal holes developed in the healing process.[28,256]

The reported prevalence of rhegmatogenous retinal detachments in patients with AIDS and CMV retinitis has ranged from approximately 15% to 35%.[107,137,174,180,321] The reported intervals from diagnosis of CMV retinitis to retinal detachment have ranged from medians of approximately 4 months[179,181] to a mean of approximately 7 months.[109] The risk of retinal detachment increases over time. Jabs and associates[181] estimated a cumulative risk of 50% for retinal detachment at 1 year, and the Studies of the Ocular Complications of AIDS (SOCA) Research Group reported a risk of 28% at 6 months.[384] Freeman and associates[106] found a smaller risk among their patients: 11% at 6 months and 24% at 1 year. Laser retinopexy has not been effective in preventing retinal detachments.[109]

In addition to duration of disease, the rate of retinal detachments is related to a number of disease characteristics, including location of lesions and extent of infection. Several studies have confirmed an increased risk of retinal detachments in patients with infection extending to the ora serrata.[107,181] Lesions in the anterior portion of the retina underlie the vitreous base, where the vitreous body is normally adherent to the retina. Any traction of the vitreous body on infected retina can result in the formation of retinal tears and can facilitate movement of fluid to the subretinal space.

Jabs and associates,[181] who found that patients with CMV retinitis lesions involving more than 50% of the retina at diagnosis had an increased rate of retinal detachment, were not able to establish a relationship between lesion size at baseline and detachment rates for patients with lesions smaller than 50%. In contrast, Freeman and associates[106] compared retinal detachment rates to extent of disease at the time of detachment and found that among patients with less than 50% of the peripheral retina involved, the risk of retinal detachment did in fact grow as the extent of disease increased. Freeman and associates[106] did not find a relationship between detachment rates and increasing extent of disease when more than 50% of the peripheral retina was involved, however.

Multiple studies have suggested that patients with active retinitis are more likely to have retinal detachments,[106,351] although other studies have not found such a relationship.[181] With completely inactive lesions, there may be sufficient chorioretinal scarring to prevent retinal detachment.[351]

When antiviral agents became available for the treatment of CMV retinitis, there was some concern that use of these drugs was associated with increased rates of retinal detachment.[107,174] It has been suggested that antiviral drugs hasten the development of rhegmatogenous retinal detachments by accelerating the healing of lesions, at which time retinal holes are more likely to develop.[174] Freeman and associates[107] also suggested that ganciclovir might magnify the risk of detachment by reducing adhesive scar formation. The increased number of retinal detachments seen after the introduction of anti-CMV therapies may simply reflect the increasing survival of patients that was occurring at the same time; in the early years of the AIDS epidemic many patients simply did not survive long enough to develop rhegmatogenous retinal detachments. In fact, Jabs and associates[181] found that antiviral therapy delayed detachments by unclear mechanisms; they could not attribute this finding to an effect of treatment on lesion size or location. Sidikaro and associates[351] found large differences in the length of time that patients were on antiviral therapy before detachment occurred, suggesting that the direct effect of drug therapy on retinal detachment rates, if any, is probably small.

A majority of patients in several studies have had retinal detachments in both eyes.[219,351] The presence of a retinal detachment in the opposite eye is a risk factor for rhegmatogenous retinal detachment.[106] This observation suggests that patients with bilateral disease have similar extents of disease and location of lesions in each eye, or that host factors may influence the risk of retinal detachment. Irvine[179] has identified one such factor; he noted an increased prevalence of myopia in patients who developed retinal detachments.

The growing use of invasive local therapies for treatment of CMV retinitis, such as intravitreous drug injections or implantation of intraocular devices for sustained release of ganciclovir, may increase the number of retinal detachments or hasten their development by disruption of the vitreous base.

Retinal detachments associated with CMV retinitis are among the most difficult to repair, because of extensive retinal necrosis, multiple-hole formation, and the high prevalence of associated proliferative vitreoretinopathy.[79,107,181,351] Rhegmatogenous retinal detachments in patients with CMV retinitis are usually repaired with silicone oil tamponade after vitrectomy; the procedure has been described in detail in several recent publications.* Studies have documented good anatomic success rates with these procedures. Lim and

---

*References 107, 109, 179, 181, 219, 234, 282, 351.

associates[234] reported a 64% rate of total retinal reattachment at last patient follow-up; in 86% of their patients the macula was reattached at last follow-up. Kuppermann and associates[219] reported a final total retinal reattachment rate of 82% and a final macular reattachment rate of 92%. When detachments recur, they usually involve the inferior retina.[179]

The use of intraocular silicone oil has several side effects that can affect a patient's vision. It alters a patient's refractive status by causing a marked hyperopic shift.[109,162,179] Silicone oil has also been observed to reduce a patient's accommodative amplitudes.[179] There is also a high rate of silicone oil-induced cataract formation.

Early reports documented poor visual acuity[181,351] and progressive decline in vision[79,179,351] after retinal detachment repair. A variety of factors may contribute to poor vision. Sidikaro and associates[351] believed that progression of CMV retinitis was responsible for continued loss of vision in their patients. Dugel and associates[79] attributed vision loss to the high rate of optic atrophy seen in patients after surgery. Optic atrophy may be caused by increased intraocular pressure during and after surgery.[79] Also, patients with AIDS are known to have alterations in blood flow[89]; as a result, there may be poor retinal and/or optic disc perfusion during surgery when fluid infusions elevate intraocular pressure.[79,162] Dugel and associates[79] have argued against silicone oil toxicity as a cause of optic atrophy. Kuppermann and associates[219] do not believe that optic atrophy can be attributed to retinal detachment repairs. They found no difference in the amount of optic atrophy between eyes that underwent surgery and opposite, infected eyes that did not. Instead, they attributed optic atrophy to the extent of retinitis in the affected eye.

Cataracts can contribute to decreased vision, but despite the high rate of cataract formation with the use of silicone oil, cataract was not the factor that limited vision for most patients in several series.[179,219,351]

Whether or not the macula has detached before surgical repair did not influence final vision in one study.[219] Lim and associates[234] found that the best visual outcomes were related to good preoperative visual acuity, early surgical intervention, absence of preoperative optic atrophy, and lack of macular CMV infection.

Visual outcomes have been improving.[109,234] Kuppermann and associates[219] reported a mean best corrected visual acuity of 20/66 (range 20/20 to 20/200) for all patients undergoing retinal detachment repair, achieved at a mean interval of 6.5 weeks after surgery. Mean final visual acuity among their patients was 20/100 (range 20/25 to no light perception) at a mean follow-up interval of 20 weeks. Lim and associates[234] reported that 71% of their patients had visual acuity of 20/200 or better at last follow-up. Factors contributing to the improvement in outcomes probably include patient selection, earlier intervention, improved surgical techniques, and earlier diagnosis and medical treatment of CMV infection.[234]

Despite the fact that final visual results have been modest in many patients, they are much better than the results (hand motion level or worse)[181,351] for patients who do not undergo surgery.

Patients undergoing surgical repair of a retinal detachment should be informed that the use of silicone oil makes visual rehabilitation of repaired eyes difficult, and that best corrected vision may be worse after surgery. In cases in which vision is better in the opposite eye, patients should be informed that good binocular vision after surgery may not be possible, but that the procedure is being performed to preserve some vision in the involved eye, in case vision is eventually lost in the other eye. Several reports have suggested that ultimately, vision in an eye that has undergone retinal detachment repair may be better than in the opposite eye, because of the high rate of bilateral disease and bilateral detachments.[179,219,234]

PATHOGENESIS

CMV disease can result from primary exogenous acquisition of the virus, from congenital infection, or from reactivation of endogenous/latent virus, but the pathogenesis of CMV infection in each setting is yet to be fully elucidated. Life- and sight-threatening CMV diseases in adults occur only in immunosuppressed individuals; prior to the AIDS epidemic, they were seen exclusively in patients with defects in cellular immunity related to disease or immunosuppressive drugs. Isolated case reports of CMV retinitis in immunocompetent adults have not been confirmed by culture or tissue examination.[41,88,101] In one such reported case, retinal lesions were probably cotton-wool spots, not CMV retinitis.[88,192]

Spread of the Virus

Following primary infection, CMV is disseminated by the bloodstream to various organs, with virtually all virus particles cell-associated during this process. Cytomegalovirus can be recovered from peripheral blood granulocytes, which may contain large amounts of viral DNA.[52,98,246,332] Molecular studies have also found the viral genome in monocytes, although they are usually culture negative. In some studies viral RNA is identified only in monocytes,[394] whereas in other studies viral RNA is found in both monocytes and neutrophils.[59,126] Early viral antigens can usually be detected in the nuclei of neutrophils during viremia, which has been termed "CMV antigenemia."[134] An in situ hybridization study found that both mononuclear cells and neutrophils were involved in the dissemination of murine CMV, although infection of mononuclear cells predominated.[11] Although replication within mononuclear cells can be shown, it is unclear whether it contributes substantially to disease pathogenesis. A biphasic viremia has been observed in a murine model; the primary viremia results in murine CMV dissemination to the reticuloendothelial organs, whereas the secondary, more intense, viremia follows virus amplification.[48]

Once clinically apparent CMV disease develops, viremia is virtually always present. Patients with AIDS and visceral organ CMV disease, especially colitis, have twentyfold to twenty-fivefold greater amounts of CMV DNA in their granulocytes than those with only CMV retinitis or CMV viremia without organ involvement.[333] Presumably, this high-grade viremia reflects the greater amount of virus replication and tissue injury that occurs with visceral organ infection when compared to retinal infection. Similar patterns were seen in solid organ transplant recipients with visceral organ CMV disease when compared to those with viremia without organ involvement. In contrast, the amounts of CMV DNA in granulocytes of bone marrow transplant recipients were low (whether or not visceral organ CMV disease was present), possibly reflecting a modulating effect of graft-versus-host disease. Cytomegalovirus DNA, but not infectious virus, has also been detected free in the plasma during viremia.[31,409]

Following initial infection, CMV is disseminated to many organs. It is commonly found in the urine, in secretions from the oropharynx and vagina, and in semen.[47,84,135,290] In animal studies the heart, lungs, spleen, liver, kidneys, adrenals, and bone marrow have been shown to be infected during the first few weeks following exposure. In humans CMV has been detected in a variety of organs including the kidney, spleen, salivary gland, brain, inner ear, lungs, and gastrointestinal tract.[120,135,158] Using immunohistochemical techniques, CMV has been detected in endothelial, epithelial, smooth muscle, and parenchymal cells.[25,273,297]

Organs contain infectious virus for variable lengths of time, depending on the host immune status. If the host is immunocompetent, the infection is usually subclinical, despite diffuse organ involvement. In congenitally infected newborns and immunosuppressed older children and adults, replicating CMV is found in many organs, and there is a prolonged period of virus excretion in urine and saliva.[158]

In the immunosuppressed host retinal infection can occur at the time of primary infection or after reactivation of latent CMV. Whether latent CMV exists in retinal cells remains to be clarified. It is assumed, however, that in patients with chronic infection, virus reaches the eye to cause CMV retinitis by hematogenous spread after reactivation elsewhere in the body. Sludging of blood flow and damage to the retinal microvasculature, which occur commonly in HIV-infected patients, may increase the contact time between CMV-infected leukocytes, which might become trapped in abnormal capillary nets and retinal tissue; this hypothesis is discussed in the subsection Factors Affecting Disease Severity.

Chronic Infection and Latency

CMV has an affinity for the salivary glands, where it produces a persistent infection with shedding of virus into the saliva, which may be a means of virus transmission in a population.[158] Such excretion may occur in normal individuals without CMV disease.[135] Cytomegalovirus may also persist in the body after primary infection in a latent state in which the viral genome is present, but gene expression is either limited or does not occur at all, and infectious virus particles are not produced.[380]

From evidence in human and animal studies, it is probable that all seropositive individuals harbor latent virus that can reactivate.[158] Knowledge about mechanisms and sites of latency is incomplete, but cellular blood elements are one probable site. Information regarding the location of latent CMV is indirect and is based primarily on epidemiologic data, in which CMV is transmitted by blood transfusion and organ transplantation. Seroconversion that occurs after blood transfusion is proportional to the amount of blood transfused.[307] Rates are less than 1% per unit of blood.[135,202,390] The rate of seroconversion decreases with the transfusion of leukocyte-poor blood.[226] The identification of CMV DNA in blood leukocytes (especially mononuclear cells) by PCR techniques also suggest that they are sites of latency, although these results are difficult to interpret because of positive results in some seronegative controls.[38,376] Viral RNA can be detected in T-lymphocytes by in situ hybridization techniques during latency, in the absence of viral antigens or infectious particles.[38,376]

Cytomegalovirus may also persist in a variety of other cell types in different organs. Murine CMV has been shown to persist in salivary glands, prostatic tissue, heart, spleen, and bone marrow.[198,199,408] Murine CMV DNA has been detected by PCR techniques in the kidney, salivary gland, and spleen in latent infection,[48,213] and by in situ DNA hybridization and PCR techniques in the liver, lung, spleen, heart, kidneys, and adrenals. In the spleen, the latent viral DNA has been detected primarily in the stromal or "red pulp" rather than in the lymphoid follicles.[255,305] Similar findings are obtained with immunohistochemical techniques using monoclonal antibodies specific for an immediate-early protein of CMV.[391] Human CMV DNA has been demonstrated in monocytes, endothelium, macrophages, and smooth muscle in arteries of individuals with and without atherosclerotic disease.[154,297,412] It is probable that there is more than one cell type in which CMV latency can occur.

The host's failure to eradicate CMV may be attributable to either ineffective immune response or escape mechanisms on the part of the virus, such as downregulation of cell surface viral molecules.[30] A discrepancy in the sites of local virus production and latency has been observed in a murine model,[13] reflecting the cytocidal nature of active CMV infection, which prevents latency in those tissues in which productive infection occurs.

Immune Response

Host defense to CMV may involve innate nonspecific immune mechanisms, as well as specific humoral and cellular immunity.[354] Because CMV has the ability to persist and remain latent, it is clear that the immune defenses are only partly successful in combating CMV infection. In some cases the immune response may even contribute to pathology.

Mononuclear phagocytes and natural killer (NK) cells appear to be important in early resistance to infection. If mice are depleted of NK cells, there is an increased severity and duration of murine CMV infection.[349] It is not clear whether the same phenomenon is true for man, but in rare patients with a depletion in NK cells, there is an increase in herpetic infections, including CMV infection.[19] Natural killer cells and macrophages also produce interferon-γ (IFN-γ) and IFN-α, which have a variety of antiviral effects. They may influence the development of CD4+ T-lymphocyte cells, enhance NK activity, and increase MHC class I expression on cells.

Immunohistochemical studies of CMV-infected retina from patients with AIDS have revealed the expression of an inducible form of nitric oxide synthetase in glial cells.[70] Host production of toxic nitrogen intermediates is a known antimicrobial mechanism; Dighiero and associates[70] hypothesized that these products may also damage retinal tissue, although they presented no evidence to support that hypothesis.

Humoral Immunity. Humoral immunity is probably not the main defense against CMV, as CMV disease occurs most commonly in patients who have depressed cell-mediated immunity and develops despite the presence of circulating antibodies. Nevertheless, there is evidence that humoral immunity does play some protective role; the presence of maternal antibody appears to protect newborns from the development of symptomatic CMV disease,[370] and immune globulin may be protective against the development of pneumonitis in bone marrow transplant recipients.[407] In studies of rats, administration of hyperimmune serum protected against CMV-related mortality and dissemination.[375] In studies of mice, hyperimmune serum reduced virus reproduction, but not latency.[350]

Antibody is capable of direct binding only to extracellular virus. IgA, which is produced in 90% of primary CMV infections, may protect epithelial surfaces.[232] In immunocompetent patients, both IgG and IgM are produced early in the primary infection; IgG antibodies persist throughout life, whereas IgM antibodies disappear after the first month of a primary infection, although they may reappear during reactivation. Immunosuppressed patients may fail to produce IgM on initial exposure to the virus. Antibodies to a number of specific CMV proteins can be identified,[225] but it has been difficult to identify the importance of reactions against specific proteins because of the complex nature of the polypeptide profile of CMV. Antibody to phosphoprotein p150, a component of the viral matrix, is a useful marker of infection,[224] but may not be detectable early.[320] Other immunogenic proteins are the 28-, 35-, and 52-KDa DNA-binding proteins. The envelope glycoproteins gC11 complex, gB, and gH are also known to be immunogenic,[315] although it is not clear whether they produce protective immunity. Antibody to gB may have some protective effect; it develops concurrently with the initial IgG and IgM response, and its levels increase during secondary infections.[245] Antibody to gH is detected in HIV-seronegative individuals transiently after recent infection; in contrast, HIV-infected individuals may have high sustained levels of antibodies to gH, possibly in response to multiple episodes of CMV reactivation or reinfection.[315,316] Antibody to gH has been decreased in titer or absent in HIV-positive patients with CD4+ T-lymphocyte counts less than 100 per μl and/or with CMV retinitis, whereas levels of antibody to gB were increased.[316] Rasmussen and associates[316] have interpreted this finding possibly to mean that anti-gH antibodies are protective against the development of CMV retinitis, although they did not show that the absence of these antibodies was an independent predictor of disease.

Cell-Mediated Immunity and Cytokines. T-lymphocytes play the most important role in host defenses against CMV. The mechanisms by which T-lymphocytes mediate defense against CMV are multiple, but include cytolysis of infected cells and cytokine production. Cell-mediated immunity to CMV has been studied by tests that look at: (1) the effector arm of the immune response, (2) antigen recognition, and (3) both functions. Tests of lymphocyte blastogenesis have been used most often to study recognition of CMV antigen. Most healthy seropositive individuals have a positive response,[302] indicating the presence of circulating T-lymphocyte memory cells specific for CMV. In contrast, few congenitally or perinatally infected individuals have a positive response.[287] This failure to respond typically recovers by age 3 to 5 years, when viruria stops. Impaired test response in mothers has been shown to be a risk factor for intrauterine transmission of CMV.[378] Solid organ transplant recipients with CMV disease have been shown to have depressed lymphocyte blastogenic responses to CMV.[235,287,302] In children with leukemia an impaired blastogenic response to CMV has been found, which may contribute to prolonged excretion of CMV in the urine.[178] Lymphocyte transformation responses have been shown to increase significantly 1 to 12 months after symptomatic, acquired CMV infection in immunocompetent individuals.[231]

Cytotoxic tests for CMV have been used to examine both recognition and effector functions. Cell-mediated cytotoxicity by CD8+ T-lymphocytes has been strongly implicated in the control of CMV infection.[312] Studies involving bone marrow transplant recipients suggest that a diminished specific CD8+ T-lymphocyte response is associated with a

poor outcome in CMV pneumonitis.[312] Transfer of CMV-specific CD8+ T-lymphocytes may be protective against CMV pneumonitis in bone marrow transplant recipients.[319]

Cytomegalovirus infection is known to alter production of several cytokines. Cytomegalovirus infection of fibroblasts result in the release of IFN-β, which induces upregulation of HLA class I molecule expression, presumably on nearby uninfected cells.[140] This action may facilitate recognition of viral antigens by the immune system. Conversely, other studies of CMV-infected fibroblasts have shown a fall in HLA class I molecule levels in the infected cells themselves.[141] Increased production of IFN-β and tissue necrosis factor (TNF)-α has been shown to occur in human CMV-infected fibroblasts co-cultured with T-lymphocytes that have been activated in vivo.[80] Interferon-γ has been shown to suppress murine CMV viral expression in microglial cells of mice.[344] Elevation of serum interleukin-6 (IL)-6, IL-8, and C-reactive protein occurs in patients with CMV infection.[270,345] In immunosuppressed rats, TNF-α production has been shown to be induced by replicating rat CMV in a variety of cell types.[144] Genes for immediate-early proteins of human CMV have been found to upregulate TNF-α expression, which may account for some of the inflammatory manifestations of CMV infection.[123] Vitreous humor from patients with AIDS and CMV retinitis contains increased levels of IFN-β when compared to eyes from controls without HIV-infection (who were undergoing vitreoretinal surgical procedures for a variety of reasons).[266] Infection of fibroblasts and vascular endothelium by CMV increases the expression of adhesion molecules LFA-3 and ICAM-1[141] and HLA-DR on the cell surfaces.[339,397] The enhanced endothelial HLA-DR expression is probably mediated by IFN-β release.[397]

Cytomegalovirus induces transforming growth factor (TGF)-β1, which downregulates host immune responses and independently can enhance viral replication.[258]

Effect of Cytomegalovirus on Host Immunity

Cytomegalovirus infection is known to have an immunosuppressive effect on the host. Although the exact basis for this effect has yet to be established, the presence of CMV in circulating cells suggests that virus-leukocyte interactions play a key role in this immunosuppression.[394] Other abnormalities include a decrease in NK cells[341] and decreased cytotoxic T-lymphocyte activity.[340] There is also a depression of interferon production by mononuclear cells in recently acquired CMV infection.[231] Infants with cytomegalic inclusion disease have persistent defects in cell mediated immunity, as indicated by decreased in vitro lymphocyte blastogenic response to CMV antigens.[2,370] Animal studies also confirm an immunosuppressive effect of CMV; for example, acute murine CMV infection in mice results in depressed numbers of tissue CD4+ T-lymphocytes.[304]

Factors Affecting Disease Severity

Human CMV strains can be grouped by similarities in amino acid sequence of glycoprotein B of the viral envelope. In a study of bone marrow transplant recipients with CMV disease, survival appeared to be related to the CMV group being excreted.[114] Whether such variations in CMV strains have implications for CMV retinitis is not known.

A variety of factors may be responsible for the difference in frequency of CMV retinitis between HIV-infected patients and those who are immunosuppressed for other reasons; they include the possibility of differences in the nature of immunosuppression among HIV-infected individuals, more severe or prolonged viremia, or transactivation of CMV by HIV in retinal tissue, as discussed in the following subsection. Also, the frequent development of CMV retinitis in patients with AIDS may be related in part to the retinal microvasculopathy associated with HIV infection.[105,128,277,294] Ultrastructural studies of retinal capillaries have demonstrated microaneurysms, narrowing and occlusion of vascular lumina, basal lamina thickening, and swelling of endothelial cells and loss of pericytes with an increased ratio of endothelial cells to pericytes. This microvascular disease may facilitate access of virus to retinal tissue through damaged vessel walls. In an autopsy study, Glasgow and Weisberger[128] have shown that these vascular changes are more severe in eyes with CMV retinitis; they hypothesized that the vascular changes may predispose to development of infection, but they could not rule out the possibility that the more severe vasculopathy is secondary to the CMV retinitis or that it may be an independent reflection of the more advanced state of AIDS in which CMV retinitis develops.

Hematogenous spread of virus to the eye is supported by the finding of CMV-like viral particles within macrophages in the choroidal circulation of an AIDS patient with CMV viremia.[284] Autopsy studies have shown aggregates of lymphocytes in vessels leading to areas of CMV retinitis.[128] Sludging of blood flow through the retinal circulation may also contribute to infection by increasing the contact time between circulating infected cells and retina.[89]

Interactions with Other Infectious Agents

Cytomegalovirus may be a cofactor in the development of AIDS; its immunosuppressive effect may accelerate and facilitate HIV infection. Conversely, CMV infections are facilitated by the immunosuppression of AIDS.[355] Furthermore, transactivation between the two viruses has been shown in vitro.[62,355] Co-infection of cells in culture enhances CMV production.[355] Also, the gene region of CMV that codes for immediate-early proteins augments gene expression governed by the HIV promotor.[62] Cytomegalovirus has also been shown to enhance lysis of HIV-infected T-lymphoblasts.[37] Clinical cohort studies are divided as to whether CMV infection alters the progression of AIDS.[193,400]

HIV can infect retinal cells,[303,356] but there is no evidence that it alone can cause a clinically apparent inflammatory or necrotizing retinopathy. In some cases both HIV and CMV have been found in the same retinal cells at autopsy.[356] Interactions between the two viruses may enhance the activity of CMV in co-infected cells and may be one reason CMV retinitis is more severe in some patients.[355]

CMV has also been found to co-infect retinal cells with human herpes virus-6, although the implications of this finding are unknown.[309]

Animal Models of Ocular Disease

Because human CMV is highly species-specific, the study of human CMV infections in animal models is difficult. Attention has therefore been focused on murine CMV infections in mice as a possible model for the study of human CMV retinitis. Holland and associates[166] showed that murine CMV was capable of causing retinal necrosis in immunosuppressed mice. Other investigators have subsequently studied the role of immune defenses against murine CMV retinitis.[6,11,78] Depletion of CD4+ and/or CD8+ T-lymphocytes is necessary for development of murine CMV retinitis; a study by Atherton and associates[6] suggested that CD8+ T-lymphocytes play a more important role in protection against disease than CD4+ T-lypmphocytes.

There are many differences between murine and human CMV infections of the eye, and extrapolations about disease mechanisms to human CMV retinitis should be made with caution. For example, murine CMV seems to have a propensity for uveal tissue, unlike its human counterpart.[166] Also, susceptibility of murine and human CMV isolates to various antiviral agents is very different, making these models of little use for investigation of new antiviral agents.

To produce an animal model of ocular disease in which human CMV can be grown, DiLoreto and associates[72] inoculated human fetal retinal tissue into the anterior chamber of immunodeficient mice. Subsequent intraocular inoculation of human CMV resulted in a productive infection in the engrafted tissue. This model may be useful for the study of immune defenses and drug therapy.

Recently a rabbit model of disease using human CMV has been reported.[81] Chorioretinal inflammation and destruction was seen, but additional study will be required to determine the extent to which the lesions and the course of disease mimic human retinal infection.

DIFFERENTIAL DIAGNOSIS

The most common disorders confused with CMV retinitis clinically are listed in Table 81-2. They include other infectious retinopathies, retinal vascular lesions, and some forms of intraocular lymphoma. Endogenous bacterial retinitis is a rare disorder in patients with AIDS that also might be confused with CMV retinitis.[61] In patients with AIDS CMV retinitis is much more common than any of the disorders in its differential diagnosis. In patients who are immunosuppressed for other reasons, however, toxoplasmic retinochoroiditis may be as common as CMV retinitis.[87]

The severity of inflammatory reactions in the anterior segment and vitreous humor is an important differentiating feature. Patients with AIDS and CMV retinitis rarely have more than a mild to moderate cellular reaction in the anterior chamber and do not develop signs of severe anterior segment inflammation, such as red and painful eyes or posterior synechiae between the iris and lens. They may develop small, translucent, and grainy keratic precipitates, but they never develop large or mutton-fat keratic precipitates. The vitreous humor is usually very clear, although patients with extensive or prolonged infection may eventually develop varying degrees of vitreous humor haze; it is never severe enough to obscure view of the fundus, however. In contrast, patients with toxoplasmic retinochoroiditis, syphilitic retinitis, fungal retinitis, and the acute retinal necrosis syndrome variant of varicella-zoster virus retinitis can develop severe intraocular inflammatory reactions.

In evaluating patients it should be remembered that CMV retinitis can occur concurrently with other retinal infections, including toxoplasmic retinochoroiditis,[90,116] cryptococcal retinitis,[276] and herpes simplex virus retinitis.[293] Concurrent infections should be considered in any patient with CMV retinitis who has atypical features of disease or incomplete initial response to antiviral therapy.

It has been suggested that in immunocompromised patients, CMV and certain other agents such as *Toxoplasma gondii* or *Pneumocystis carinii* infect tissues concurrently at rates higher than would be predicted from the independent frequencies of each. Possible explanations include further immunosuppression by CMV infection, transport of CMV to tissues by other organisms serving as vectors, or through other symbiotic relationships.[328] In patients with AIDS some eyes with concurrent CMV retinitis and toxoplasmic retinochoroiditis have had the infections in anatomically different parts of the retina[90]; thus, they may simply be coincidental, as a result of the high rate of CMV retinitis.

Noninfectious disorders can also be confused with CMV retinitis. Intraocular lymphoma with retinal involvement can mimic an infectious necrotizing retinopathy.[336,377] Although intraocular lymphoma is closely associated with intracranial lymphoma, ocular disease can become apparent before development of other neurologic symptoms. Large or atypical cotton-wool spots can be mistaken for very early CMV retinitis. Differentiation is best made on the basis of disease course. Cotton-wool spots will not enlarge over 1 to 2 weeks of observation and may begin to fade; in contrast, small CMV retinitis lesions will enlarge slowly and granular borders will become evident. Observation for 1 to 2 weeks of a CMV retinitis lesion that is the size of a cotton-wool spot poses little risk to the patient, unless it is immediately adjacent to the fovea. Branch retinal vein occlusions are

believed to be more common among HIV-infected patients. They are characterized by wedge-shaped areas of intraretinal hemorrhage with retinal edema that can be confused with the fulminant/edematous variant of CMV retinitis; they can be distinguished from CMV retinitis, however, by the lack of a granular border that advances over time.

Other disorders that can have clinical features resembling CMV retinitis include Coats disease[262] and the occlusive retinal vasculopathy of Behçet disease. These diseases are not associated with severe immunosuppression and therefore will be seen in very different clinical settings than CMV retinitis.

LABORATORY INVESTIGATIONS

A variety of laboratory tests are available or in development to assist in the evaluation of CMV disease. Because CMV can exist in tissues without causing disease, the results of diagnostic tests should be interpreted in the context of the clinical findings and with the exclusion of other possible causes for disease.

Virus Cultures

Cytomegalovirus isolated from a variety of clinical specimens, such as blood, urine, saliva, and tissue biopsies, can be grown in cell culture, usually using human fibroblasts. If a sample cannot be inoculated immediately onto the cell culture, it should be placed in a viral transport media. The typical cytopathic effect of CMV in tissue culture consists of round or elongated, enlarged refractile cells.[158] The time to development of this characteristic cytopathic effect ranges from a few days to as long as 6 weeks, but usually occurs in 2 to 3 weeks.

Rapid culture systems have been developed to reduce the time to a positive result. These systems detect immediate-early or early proteins produced by replicating CMV within 8 to 32 hours of cell culture infection, using monoclonal antibodies in a fluorescence assay.[136] Rapid culture systems can also employ shell vial cultures, in which monoclonal antibody to early antigen is added after centrifugation[292]; centrifugation increases the sensitivity of virus detection.[130] Rapid culture techniques may be insensitive to antigenic variation among different CMV strains because they rely on monoclonal antibodies to specific proteins. Although virus isolation is an important diagnostic technique, it does not necessarily confirm tissue-destructive disease.

Antibody Tests

Positive serologic tests indicate that the host has become infected with CMV at sometime in the past, but they do not indicate tissue-destructive disease. Recent CMV infection is indicated by development of anti-CMV IgG antibodies in a previously seronegative individual, or by at least a twofold rise in anti-CMV IgG antibody titer on serial specimens tested in parallel. The presence of anti-CMV IgM antibodies

TABLE 81-2 IMPORTANT DISORDERS IN THE DIFFERENTIAL DIAGNOSIS OF CMV RETINITIS

Disorder	Possible Differentiating Features*
A. Infectious diseases	
1. Varicella-zoster virus retinitis	
a. ARN syndrome variant	• Association with cutaneous zoster (concurrent, recent, or remote) • Occlusive vasculopathy • Marked inflammation in vitreous humor or anterior chamber • Optic neuritis • Scleritis • Rapid progression • Pain
b. PORN syndrome variant	• Multifocality • Rapid progression • Deep homogeneous retinal opacification • Early perifoveal lesions
2. Herpes simplex virus (HSV) retinitis†	• Edematous, homogeneous lesions • Association with HSV encephalitis • May have features of ARN syndrome as above • Rapid progression
3. Syphilitic retinitis	• Granular infiltrates without retinal necrosis (upper figure a) or subretinal plaquoid lesions (lower figure b) • Prominent anterior chamber inflammatory reaction with posterior synechiae and large keratic precipitates • Prominent vitreous humor inflammatory reaction • Cutaneous signs of secondary syphilis • CD4+ T-lymphocyte count may be high

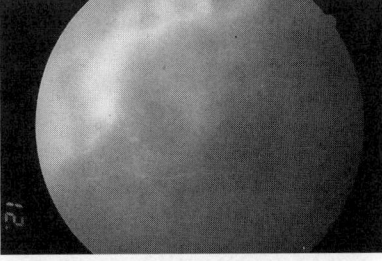

A 1a. ARN syndrome.

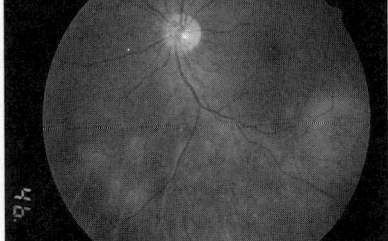

A 1b. PORN syndrome.

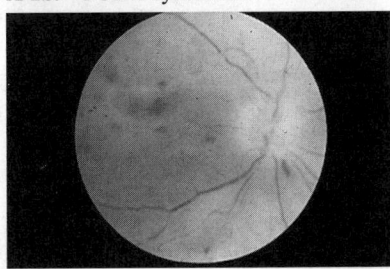

A 2. Herpes simplex virus retinitis.

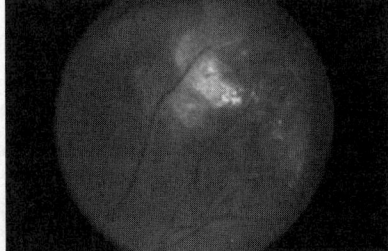

A 3a. Syphilitic retinitis.

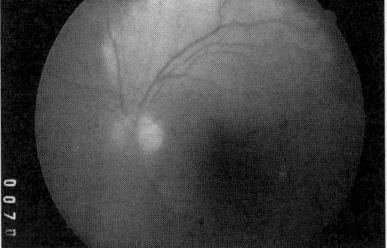

A 3b. Subretinal placoid lesion caused by syphilis.

ARN = acute retinal necrosis
PORN = progressive retinal necrosis

*Features may not be present in each case, but if present, help to rule out CMV retinitis.
†Rare; typical appearance not established, especially in patients with AIDS.
Photographs reprinted with permission as follows: **A 1b,** reprinted with permission from Engstrom RE Jr, Holland GN, Margolis TP et al.: The progressive outer retinal necrosis syndrome: a variant of necrotizing herpetic retinopathy in patients with AIDS, *Ophthalmology* 101:1488-1502, 1994; **A 2,** photograph

Disorder	Possible Differentiating Features*	
4. Toxoplasmic retinochoroiditis	• Thick-appearing lesions • Sharply defined lesion borders • Early perifoveal lesions • Old chorioretinal scars • Red, painful eye • Prominent anterior chamber inflammatory reaction with posterior synechiae and large keratic precipitates • Prominent vitreous humor inflammatory reaction • Focal intracranial ring-enhancing lesions	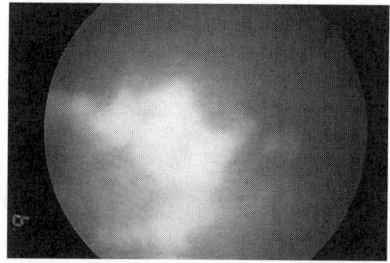 **A 4.** Toxoplasmosic retinochoroiditis.
5. Fungal retinitis	• Multifocality • Prominent anterior chamber inflammatory reaction with posterior synechiae and large keratic precipitates • Prominent vitreous humor inflammatory reaction • Lesions predominantly in posterior pole • CD4+ T-lymphocyte count may be high	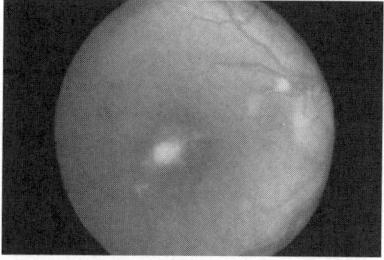 **A 5.** Candidal chorioretinitis.
B. Vascular disorders 1. Cotton-wool spots	• Absence of intraocular inflammatory reactions • Involvement of inner retinal layers only • Predominantly in peripapillary locations • Feathery or ''squiggly'' shape with sharp borders • Lack of progressive enlargement over 1-2 weeks; resolution over 4-6 weeks • Lack of symptoms	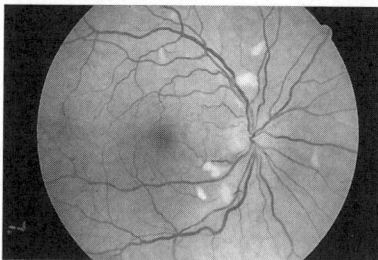 **B 1.** Cotton-wool spots.
2. Retinal vein occlusions	• Extensive intraretinal hemorrhage with mild retinal whitening • Wedge-shaped area of involvement surrounding retinal venule (branch retinal vein occlusion) or involvement of all four retinal quadrants (central retinal vein occlusion, illustrated) • Lack of granular lesion border • Cotton-wool spots at border of hemorrhagic area • Stasis or occlusion on fluorescein angiogram	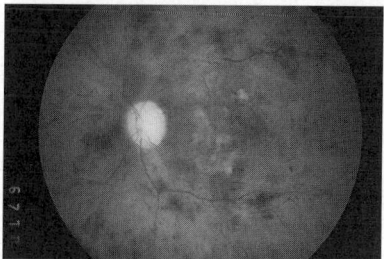 **B 2.** Retinal vein occlusion.
C. Neoplasms 1. Intraocular lymphoma	• Subretinal material with retinal elevations • Prominent vitreous humor cells • Focal intracranial lesion	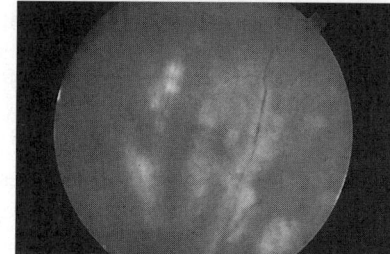 **C 1.** Intraocular lymphoma.

courtesy of JS Pepose, MD PhD. Reprinted with permission from Pepose JA, Kreiger AE, Tomiyasu U et al.: Immunocytologic localization of herpes simplex type 1 viral antigens in herpetic retinitis and encephalitis in adult, *Ophthalmology* 92:160-166, 1985; **A 3a,** reprinted with permission from Holland GN: AIDS: retinal and choroidal infections. In Ryan SJ, Lewis H, editors. *Medical and surgical retina: advances controversies and management,* St Louis, 1994, Mosby-Year Book; **A 3b,** reprinted with permission from Holland GN: AIDS: retinal and choroidal infections. In Ryan SJ, Lewis H, editors. *Medical and surgical retina: advances controversies and management,* St Louis, 1994, Mosby-Year Book; **A 4,** reprinted with permission from Elkins BS, Holland GN, Opremcak EM et al.: Ocular toxoplasmosis misdiagnosed as cytomegalovirus retinopathy in immunocompromised patients, *Ophthalmology* 101:499-507, 1994; **A 5,** photograph courtesy of JP Dunn Jr, MD. Reprinted with permission from Dunn JP: Uveitis in Children. In *Focal points: clinical modules for ophthalmologists,* ed 4, 1995, American Academy of Ophthalmology; **C 1,** reprinted with permission from Schanzer MC, Font RL, O'Malley RE: Primary ocular malignant lymphoma associated with the acquired immune deficiency syndrome, *Ophthalmology* 98:88-91, 1991. (Figures also in color insert.)

suggests, but does not confirm, recent infection; anti-CMV IgM antibodies may persist for many months after infection or can develop during virus reactivation, and tests for IgM antibodies may be falsely positive in the presence of rheumatoid factor.[318] Changes in antibody titers may not occur in immunocompromised individuals.[244] For these reasons, serologic tests have limited utility for diagnosis of CMV disease in patients with AIDS.

The complement fixation test has been a widely used serologic test for CMV infection and has been used in most seroepidemiologic studies, but it lacks sensitivity.[372,373] This test is usually directed against antigens of CMV strain AD169, but does not discriminate between various human strains of CMV.[314] The indirect immunofluorescence antibody test can give false positive results, as CMV infected cells develop Fc receptors that bind IgG antibodies, giving rise to nonspecific staining.[115,207] The anticomplement immunofluorescence test is more sensitive than the complement fixation test, is quick to perform, and does not result in false positives, as with the immunofluorescent antibody test.[314] Other tests that have been used to detect CMV include virus neutralization tests, enzyme-linked immunosorbent assays, radioimmunoassays, latex agglutination tests, and immune adherence hemagglutination tests.

Serologic tests have applications in a variety of situations, including the evaluation of clinical disease in newborns, the evaluation of patients prior to organ transplantation, and the screening of organ donors. Current serologic tests have little utility in the evaluation of CMV retinitis, however, because of the high prevalence of seropositivity in populations at risk for this infection. Cytomegalovirus retinitis has been reported in a patient with AIDS who had no evidence of CMV infection by the complement fixation test on serum.[275]

In cases of presumed CMV retinitis, antibody levels can be determined in aqueous or vitreous humor and compared to serum levels as a test for intraocular antibody production. To control for passive diffusion of anti-CMV serum antibodies into the eye, the ratio of intraocular to serum antibodies must be compared to the ratio of total immunoglobulin or a similar-size molecule that would not be produced locally. Some investigators prefer to use a specific IgG antibody to a common agent that does not cause intraocular disease (such as adenovirus), which will have a similar molecular weight. The comparison of ratios can be expressed mathematically as follows to calculate a value that has come to be called the Witmer or Witmer-Goldmann coefficient: [antibody titer (fluid) × total immunoglobulin (serum)] ÷ [antibody titer (serum) × total immunoglobulin (fluid)]. In calculating the coefficient, the reciprocal of the fractional titer is used in the formula (e.g. for a titer of 1 : 64, the numeral 64 is used). Theoretically, values greater than 1 would indicate local production of antibody, but practical experience has shown that larger values are needed to identify one of the necrotiz-

ing herpetic retinopathies accurately. A possible source of error in determining intraocular antibody production is polyclonal B-lymphocyte activation. No absolute values can be used reliably to diagnose disease in all cases. A more useful application of this technique may be to compare the magnitude of the Witmer-Goldmann coefficient for several pathogens in the differential diagnosis of a lesion; the highest value would indicate the most likely cause. This technique has been used to distinguish between CMV retinitis, varicella-zoster virus retinitis, and toxoplasmic retinochoroiditis in patients with AIDS.[60]

Anterior chamber paracentesis to obtain an aqueous humor specimen for testing can be performed safely as a simple office procedure, but there is a small risk of intraocular infection or damage to the lens or cornea. Vitreous humor sampling is generally reserved for patients who are undergoing retinovitreous surgical procedures, such as a vitrectomy associated with retinal detachment repair. Techniques for determination of antibody titers on the extremely small (generally 0.1 to 0.2 ml) sample sizes obtained from the eye are discussed by Davis and associates.[60]

Histologic Studies

A histologic diagnosis of CMV infection can be based on the presence of large cytomegalic cells with intranuclear inclusions surrounded by an owl's eye halo. Occasionally, granular, basophilic inclusions may be seen in the cytoplasm; the presence of these cytoplasmic inclusions may help to differentiate infection by CMV from infection by other members of the herpes group of viruses.[158] Cytomegalovirus can often be cultured when no histologic changes are evident, however.[363] Also, cytomegalic cells do not develop with abortive or latent infections.

If productive CMV infection is suspected and no cytomegalic cells are present, light microscopy should be supplemented with immunocytochemical techniques using labeled antibodies to detect viral antigens. Immunohistochemical techniques using monoclonal antibodies against CMV will show staining in all layers of the neurosensory retina and RPE.[337]

Nucleic Acid Detection

Detection of the CMV genome in tissue may be made either by in situ hybridization or by PCR techniques. In situ hybridization is a sensitive technique for detection of CMV DNA or RNA in tissue specimens,[273] but has it low sensitivity for detecting DNA in bronchoalveolar lavage samples.[129] Anti-CMV antibodies may not detect a viral antigen in tissues fixed with formalin or in extensively necrotic retina; in those situations, detection of the viral genome may be more useful for diagnosis.[152] In situ hybridization is both sensitive and specific for detection of CMV in the retinal tissue of patients with active CMV retinitis, but it may be less useful in cases of treated CMV retinitis in which virus is not replicating.[152]

The PCR technique has been used to detect both primary and reactivated CMV disease.[18,65] With respect to ocular infections, PCR has been used to detect CMV in aqueous humor, vitreous humor, subretinal fluid, and in formalin-fixed ocular tissue sections.[20,97,103] Although CMV retinitis can usually be diagnosed on clinical appearance alone, there may be a role for PCR techniques on ocular fluids in confirming the diagnosis of atypical lesions. Antiviral treatment may have a confounding effect on PCR technique results, however. Although Fox and associates[103] found no loss of sensitivity in detecting CMV DNA in vitreous- and aqueous-humor samples after treatment with ganciclovir, Gerna and associates[125] identified CMV in 12 of 12 aqueous humor samples (100%) prior to treatment, but in only 4 of 12 aqueous humor samples (33%) after the start of foscarnet therapy. McCann and associates[251] have reported a sensitive and specific diagnostic assay to detect CMV in vitreous humor samples using PCR techniques. They estimated a 95% sensitivity in detecting CMV in patients with untreated, clinically diagnosed CMV retinitis, but a sensitivity of only 48% in diagnosing cases of CMV retinitis treated with systemic ganciclovir or foscarnet. Most important, they had no false positive tests on vitreous humor from patients with a variety of other intraocular disorders.

Polymerase chain reaction techniques are extremely sensitive, and even very small amounts of contaminating DNA may be amplified, resulting in false positive results. Nested PCR techniques may reduce background amplification and increase sensitivity.[263] In one study detection of free CMV DNA in plasma by PCR techniques was predictive of CMV disease in at least some patients with AIDS.*

THERAPY

Early attempts to treat CMV disease met with only limited success; agents included vidarabine, transfer factor, and IFN-α.[40,42,301,329] The AIDS epidemic stimulated the development of several new antiviral drugs with anti-CMV activity. The first to become available were ganciclovir and foscarnet for intravenous administration; the following discussion is based on experience with these drugs, although the concepts of treatment will be applicable to new agents as they become available. In 1995 the following agents were under clinical investigation for possible use in treatment of CMV retinitis: cidofovir, a nucleotide analog that inhibits DNA polymerase[364]; lobucovir, a cyclobutyl derivative of guanine that also acts by inhibition of DNA polymerase,[279] and ISIS-2922, a phosphorothioate oligonucleotide complementary to messenger RNA that encodes regulatory proteins

of the immediate early region 2 of human CMV (an "antisense" drug).[8]

In patients who are iatrogenically immunosuppressed, the most effective treatment for CMV disease is to stop or reduce the dose of the immunosuppressive drugs that are being administered. If that is not possible, treatment with systemic anti-CMV agents should be administered until immunocompetence is restored. Patients with CMV retinitis who are immunosuppressed for reasons other than HIV infection respond better to antiviral therapy than patients with AIDS.[56,285]

Photocoagulation of the retina has not been effective at preventing spread of CMV retinitis.[379]

Monitoring Therapy

It was difficult to interpret and compare early reports regarding the effects of ganciclovir on CMV retinitis because investigators described the disease and its response to therapy with poorly defined terms, and they used a variety of unrelated outcome measures. These problems arose from the fact that there had been no previous experience with treatment of CMV retinitis and very little was known about its natural history. In response to this problem, standardized nomenclature was adopted, and an algorithm for assessment of response to antiviral treatment was developed in anticipation of future clinical trials.[165] Terminology used in the evaluation and management of CMV retinitis is listed in the Appendix to this chapter. The nomenclature and concepts are also applicable to routine patient care.

Because no current therapy is completely effective at preventing spread of CMV retinitis, it is important to document the status of disease at diagnosis and follow patients carefully for signs of change in their disease. At baseline examination, the following parameters are documented: best corrected visual acuity in each eye; the number of descrete lesions in each eye; the location of lesions; and the extent of disease. The location of lesions is identified using a system of zones (Fig. 81-6). The location of lesions has important prognostic implications. Zone 1 lesions, or those in the macular and peripapillary areas, are considered immediately vision-threatening. Zone 3 lesions, because they underlie the vitreous base (a broad area of attachment between the retina and vitreous body), can be associated with vitreoretinal traction, and are more likely to result in retinal detachments. The extent of disease is identified using the following semiquantitative categories: less than 10% of retina involved, 11% to 25% of the retina involved, 26% to 50% of the retina involved, or greater than 50% of retina involved. For reference, the macula (the area encircled by the major temporal vascular arcades) is approximately 5% of the total retinal area.

The goal of treatment for CMV retinitis is to prevent CMV from destroying additional normal retinal tissue. This concept is the basis for the algorithm used to follow the

---

*M. Shinkai, unpublished data presented at the 34th Interscience Conference on Antimicrobial Agents and Chemotherapy, Orlando, Florida, USA, October 1994

course of disease and its response to treatment[165] (Fig. 81-14). It uses three parameters: development of new retinal lesions, enlargement of preexisting lesions, and change in opacification (whiteness) of lesion borders. Progression of disease is defined as the development of new lesions or the enlargement of preexisting lesions. Enlargement of preexisting lesions is most easily identified by the advancement of any segment of a lesion border toward previously uninfected retina. In clinical studies an arbitrary threshold distance of linear advancement from baseline (usually 750 microns) is required before disease is considered to have progressed. The direction of border advancement is also important; posterior advancement of a lesion can threaten the macula or optic disc. Change in border position is determined by its relationship to fundus landmarks, such as retinal vessels, and can be determined most accurately by a comparison of serial retinal photographs. The interval between start of therapy and either enlargement of lesions or development of new lesions ("time to progression") has been used as a measure of treatment efficacy.

The opacity of lesion borders is also monitored because it is believed to reflect viral activity. Change in the opacity of lesions is the most obvious effect of treatment (Fig. 81-15) but is not a reliable surrogate for change in the size of lesions;[165] even minimally opaque lesions can continue to enlarge, with destruction of additional retina. Nevertheless, for lesions that have not enlarged, change in border opacity from the previous examination may help to predict outcomes.[165] Increasing border opacity usually predicts eventual enlargement of lesions (Fig. 81-16). Lesions enlarging on therapy will generally have mildly opaque borders, a condition which has been called "smoldering retinitis."

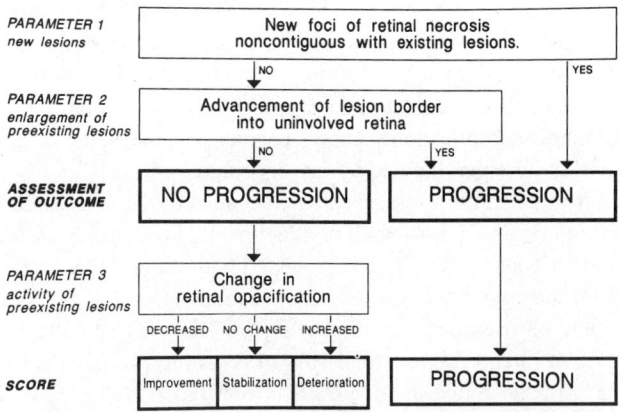

ASSESSMENT OF CMV RETINOPATHY OUTCOME

Fig. 81-14. Algorithm used to evaluate the response of CMV retinitis to antiviral therapy. Reprinted with permission from Holland GN, Buhles WC, Mastre B et al.: A controlled retrospective study of ganciclovir treatment for cytomegalovirus retinopathy: use of a standardized system for the assessment of disease outcome, *Arch Ophthalmol* 107:1759-1766, 1989. Copyright 1989 American Medical Association.

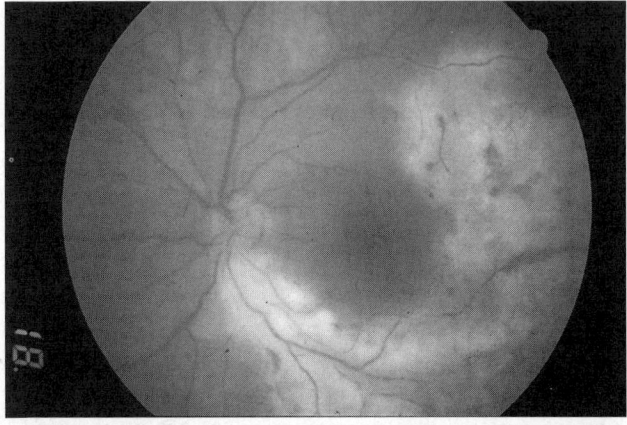

A

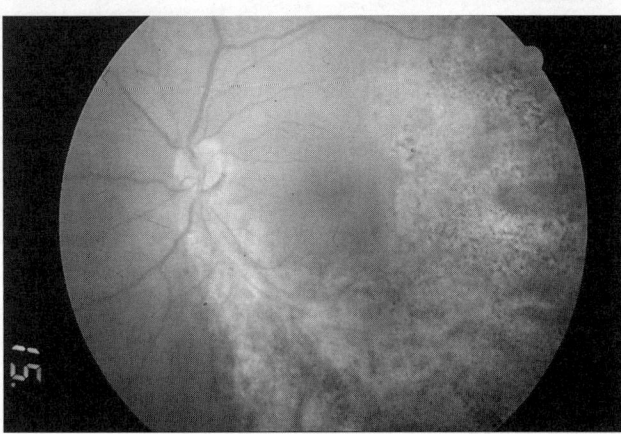

B

Fig. 81-15. **A,** Untreated CMV retinitis in the left eye of a patient with AIDS. **B,** The same eye 2 months later during successful therapy with intravenous ganciclovir; the lesion is inactive and there has been no change in the position of the lesion borders.

Comparison of serial retinal photographs is the best means of identifying the presence of subtle retinal opacities and changing opacification over time. If opaque lesion borders have not advanced, changes in therapy are not warranted; in some cases stable opacity of the border may represent gliosis with calcification or necrotic debris that has not cleared instead of active viral disease.[205] Persistent opacities in the central portion of the lesion do not signify active retinitis (Fig. 81-17).

Perivascular inflammatory sheathing resolves rapidly with the initiation of therapy, but this change is not a reliable measure of eventual treatment efficacy. Recurrence of perivascular inflammatory sheathing is an important sign of disease reactivation.

Other outcome measures, such as retinal detachments or visual acuity, are not considered to be direct measures of treatment efficacy. For example, active lesions in the anterior retina can continue to enlarge with little immediate effect on central vision. Conversely, a small lesion near the fovea can have a profound effect on vision, and even if treatment prevents further enlargement of a parafoveal lesion, vision may deteriorate further because of scarring and retinal traction, retinal detachment, or other changes that occur in the healing process. Preservation of vision is a measure of long-term treatment success, however.

Visual field determinations have been used to monitor patients with CMV retinitis.[9,384] Serial determinations can demonstrate progressive loss of visual field in patients treated for CMV retinitis,[384] but measurement of visual field changes is probably not sufficiently sensitive to identify the early changes associated with disease reactivation and progression. Amsler grids are useful for self-monitoring by motivated patients who have lesions in that portion of Zone 1 that is responsible for the central 20 degrees of vision (corresponding to the approximate area contained by the major temporal vascular arcades). An Amsler grid consists of a pattern of crossing horizontal and vertical lines with a central dot for fixation. Patients hold the printed grid 14 inches away from the eye and look at the central dot; scotomata corresponding to retinal lesions can be identified as blank or gray areas or areas of distortion. Each eye must be tested separately. There will generally be a sharp demarcation of scotoma borders, which allows patients to recognize advancement of a lesion border if it occurs. Amsler grids can also be used to screen for immediately vision-threatening new lesions. For lesions outside of the central 20 degrees of vision, patients can monitor themselves in a similar, albeit less precise, manner by looking at a newspaper page held at a constant distance from the face.

Intravenous Ganciclovir and Foscarnet

Ganciclovir and foscarnet suppress CMV replication, but do not eliminate virus from the eye. Electron microscopic studies of eyes with CMV retinitis that have been treated

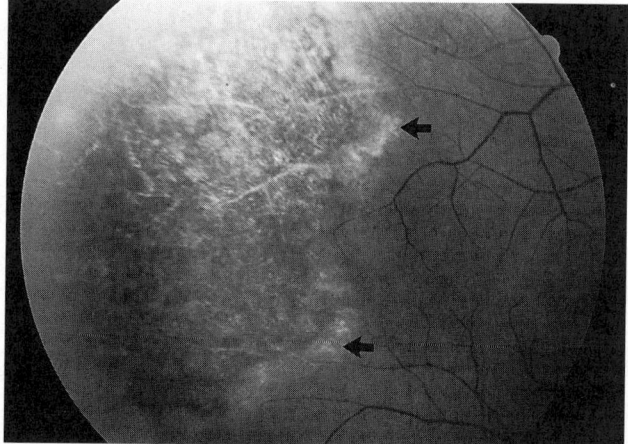

Fig. 81-16. Treated CMV retinitis in the temporal retina of the right eye of a patient with AIDS. There is faint opacity of the lesion borders *(arrows)* indicating reactivation of disease.

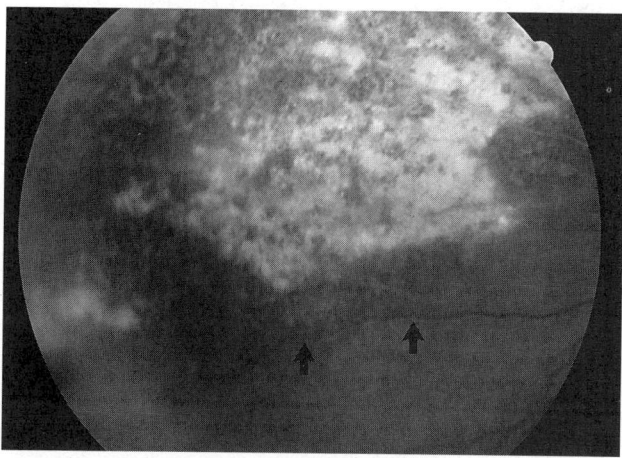

Fig. 81-17. Treated CMV retinitis in the superonasal quadrant of the left eye of a patient with AIDS. The white scarring is in the central area of the lesion and does not indicate disease activity. There is no opacity of the lesion border, which is adjacent to the retinal vessel *(arrows)*.

with ganciclovir show viral particles at the borders of lesions; the appearance of the particles is consistent with ineffective viral replication.[295]

Based on early clinical experience with ganciclovir and foscarnet, a similar treatment regimen has evolved for both drugs.* Patients are given an initial *induction* course of therapy (ganciclovir: 5 mg/kg every 12 hours for 14 days; foscarnet: 60 mg/kg every 8 hours for 14 days) to inhibit viral replication and prevent further enlargement of lesions. This induction therapy is followed by life-long secondary prophylaxis or *maintenance* therapy (USA Food and Drug Administration-approved regimens, ganciclovir: 5 mg/kg daily or 6 mg/kg 5 out of 7 days; foscarnet: 90 to 120 mg/kg daily) to prevent disease reactivation.

Objective Signs of Efficacy. There is no apparent difference in the ability of ganciclovir and foscarnet to control CMV retinitis. The following paragraphs describe the results of a large, prospective, and randomized clinical trial conducted by the SOCA Research Group in which treatment of newly diagnosed CMV retinitis with intravenous ganciclovir and intravenous foscarnet were compared.[383,384] There was no statistical difference between the two drugs in their abilities to control CMV retinitis. The median time to disease progression was approximately 7 weeks for each drug (47 days for the ganciclovir-assigned group; 53 days for the foscarnet-assigned group), and progression was observed in 85% of patients by 120 days of therapy. Disease became harder to control over time; the interval to next progression decreased after each consecutive reactivation of disease. The time to first progression was not predictive of the number of

---

*References 46, 137, 153, 172, 174, 183, 189, 190, 229, 281, 285.

subsequent reactivations. Among patients with unilateral disease at baseline, approximately 17% developed bilateral disease at 6 months.

Baseline factors associated with an increased risk of progression were (1) bilateral disease and (2) a CD4+ T-lymphocyte count less than 14 per μl. Baseline factors not associated with an increased risk of progression were location of lesions, size of lesions, appearance of lesions, the interval from the diagnosis of AIDS to the diagnosis of CMV retinitis, antiretroviral drug use, and Karnofsky score.

There is no role for the use of antiinflammatory drugs, such as corticosteroids, in the management of CMV retinitis. Perivascular inflammatory sheathing in patients with CMV retinitis, even if very severe, resolves with antiviral therapy alone.[368]

Visual Outcomes. Despite continuous maintenance therapy with either intravenous ganciclovir or intravenous foscarnet, patients continued to lose vision, albeit at a slow rate. Central visual acuity in involved eyes declined three lines or more on modified Baily-Lovie charts (a doubling of the visual angle) at a rate of 94 events per 100 person-years. Expressed differently, vision decreased at a rate of 2.5 letters per month (approximately one line on the eye chart every 2 months). Nevertheless, it is now rare for patients with AIDS to die without any vision as a result of CMV retinitis.

Progressive visual field loss also occurred in involved eyes. Baseline visual field scores were determined using kinetic perimetry along 12 meridians, with summation of the degrees of field along each meridian; the median baseline visual field score was 711 degrees. Involved eyes lost 30 degrees from their baseline score per month (an area representing approximately 5% of the total visual field).

The probability that central vision would be worse than 20/40 was 0.34 (i.e. 34% of patients would have that level of vision) at 6 months for involved eyes treated with ganciclovir. The median time to a visual acuity of less than 20/100 for all involved eyes treated with ganciclovir was 346 days. Rates were not significantly different for patients treated with foscarnet.

In patients with bilateral CMV retinitis, the ability to function is determined by vision in the better eye; the SOCA Research Group therefore considered visual outcomes using the better eye for each patient as well. They found that the probability of vision less than 20/40 at 6 months was 0.07 for patients treated with ganciclovir, and 0.12 for patients treated with foscarnet; overall 91% of patients maintained visual acuity better than 20/40 at 6 months in their better eye.

Baseline factors associated with a worse visual outcome included an initial visual acuity less than 20/40 in the involved eye, decreased vision in the involved eye before treatment, fulminant/edematous lesions, and CD4+ T-lymphocyte count less than 14 per μl. Not only was visual acuity worse, but eyes with a baseline visual acuity less than 20/40

had greater *rates* of vision loss during treatment than those with baseline visual acuities greater than 20/40. This observation probably reflects the location of lesions; eyes with visual acuity less than 20/40 are more likely to have lesions adjacent to the fovea or optic disc. With minimal progression, such lesions could cause profound vision loss. Decreased vision could also result from scarring or atrophy of tissues after inactivation of virus, which would not occur with lesions remote from the posterior pole. Treatment is therefore expected to be more effective if initiated before vision loss. A similar observation was made by Holland and Shuler[173] in a retrospective study of patients treated with ganciclovir.

Fulminant/edematous lesions may progress faster than indolent granular lesions,[173] although the SOCA Research Group did not identify a difference in time to first progression between patients with indolent/granular lesions and those with fulminant/edematous lesions. A more likely explanation is that fulminant/edematous lesions are more often located in the posterior retina,[153,384] where they have a greater chance of causing damage to the optic nerve or fovea.

Cytomegalovirus retinitis adjacent to and involving the optic disc has a poor prognosis despite treatment, although improvement of vision with ganciclovir therapy has been reported.[322]

Central vision may improve with initial therapy in patients with Zone 1 lesions who have exudation of fluid into the macula, but who do not have foveal infections.[118,172] Gangan and associates[118] found that vision improved in 22 of 23 such eyes (96%) as fluid resorbed with successful treatment; patients gained 1 to 7 lines of vision on the Snellen eye chart (mean, 2.5 lines).

Survival. The SOCA Research Group did find a statistically significant difference between treatment groups for patient survival. Those who received foscarnet had a median survival approximately 4 months longer than those who received only ganciclovir, as discussed in the Prognosis section. The cause for the differential survival could not be determined. It is possible that survival was prolonged by foscarnet, since it has antiretroviral activity. This hypothesis is supported by the finding that survival is longer in patients on higher maintenance doses of foscarnet.[185] The differential survival might also be attributable, in part, to other factors that were not controlled in the trial. Patients taking ganciclovir were less able to tolerate zidovudine, a drug known to increase patient survival, as ganciclovir and zidovudine both cause bone marrow suppression.[160] Various analyses could not identify differential use of antiretroviral agents as a factor in the survival results, however.

Toxicities and Complications. Ganciclovir and foscarnet maintenance therapy doses are limited by their toxicities. Ganciclovir is a bone marrow suppressant; in early series, up to 38% of patients developed dose-limiting neutropenia.[174] Neutropenia can now be corrected with the concurrent use of the leukocyte growth factors sargramostim [ganulocyte-monocyte colony stimulating factor (GM-CSF)] and filgrastim [granulocyte colony stimulating factor (G-CSF)].[147]

Foscarnet therapy is associated with a greater incidence of side effects that require discontinuation of drug administration than ganciclovir.[383] The major toxicity of foscarnet is renal impairment. Serum creatinine increased to 260 μmol/l or above at a rate of 0.30 per person-year at risk in patients treated by the SOCA Research Group.[383]

Because they have similar abilities to control CMV retinitis, the decision to begin treatment with ganciclovir or foscarnet should be based on nonophthalmic factors, such as patient tolerance and toxicity.

Indwelling catheters can be infected, resulting in sepsis. This complication has been reported to occur at a rate of 2 per 1000 catheter-days.[308,357]

Effects of Other Drugs

There are several case reports in which zidovudine therapy alone appeared to cause inactivation of CMV retinitis.[55,142] Because zidovudine itself has no activity against CMV, the effect is presumably through enhancement of the patient's own immune defenses or by its suppression of HIV, which is known to enhance CMV activity in vitro. The effect of zidovudine treatment on CMV retinitis may not be apparent for several weeks and may be only temporary. In most patients zidovudine does not prevent enlargement of CMV retinitis lesions.

Fay and associates[94] described three patients with apparently inactive CMV retinitis who had not received ganciclovir or foscarnet prior to diagnosis. Two of the three were taking zidovudine, and all had taken acyclovir. One of the patients was not subsequently treated with specific anti-CMV therapy and lesions remained quiescent for 11 weeks. In an uncontrolled study Sha and associates[348] used intravenous acyclovir and oral zidovudine as maintenance therapy for 10 patients with CMV retinitis after ganciclovir induction. When compared to historic controls, time to reactivation and progression was shorter than with ganciclovir or foscarnet maintenance therapy, but was longer than for untreated patients. Acyclovir has poor activity against CMV at levels normally achieved in vivo, but based on these reports, the combination of zidovudine and acyclovir may have some effect on CMV retinitis. In general, however, the use of high-dose oral acyclovir does not appear to influence the rate or severity of CMV disease in patients with AIDS whose CD4+ T-lymphocyte counts are less than 150 per μl.[415]

Long-Term Systemic Therapy

The most difficult problem in the management of CMV retinitis is prevention of disease progression during long-term maintenance therapy. Disease will reactivate and progress in nearly all patients, if they survive long enough. The cause of late disease reactivations is probably multifactorial.

In most cases the first reactivation of CMV retinitis can again be brought under control by administering induction-level doses of the same drug being used for maintenance therapy,[137] which suggests that drug levels achieved with maintenance therapy are simply too low to prevent disease reactivation (Fig. 81-18). An inverse relation between ganciclovir dosage and CMV viremia in patients receiving maintenance therapy has also been shown.[194]

Viruses that are relatively resistant to ganciclovir and/or foscarnet have been isolated from patients undergoing therapy for CMV retinitis.* In some cases there has been a relationship between drug resistance and clinical signs of disease progression,[82,91,100] but such a relationship has not been found in all patients.[76]

The fact that disease reactivation and progression comes at increasingly shorter intervals after multiple reinductions may be due to increasing viral drug resistance but may also reflect further waning of the patient's immune defenses. Gross and associates[137] reported a relationship between progression of disease and low T-lymphocyte counts.

With these possibilities in mind, a number of treatment strategies have been proposed to deal with disease progression. They include the use of increased doses of drug, switching from one drug to another,[186] and use of multiple drug therapy. Continued administration of induction-level ganciclovir is possible in many patients, with the concurrent use of a leukocyte growth factor. Holland and associates[169] showed that among patients receiving foscarnet, the rate with which CMV retinitis spreads may be slower in patients treated with higher drug doses during maintenance therapy. There is in vitro evidence that ganciclovir and foscarnet act synergistically against CMV,[110,241] and combined maintenance therapy using both drugs has been used in some patients.[100,187,401] Although this therapy may be useful for the most refractory of cases, it is probably not practical for routine use.

In some long-term survivors CMV retinitis can no longer be completely controlled, even with aggressive therapy, and there is continued enlargement of lesions. Even if disease activity cannot be completely eliminated with drug therapy, patients probably receive a therapeutic benefit from continued drug administration through the slowing of disease progression.[173]

In some patients lesions can continue to expand slowly and circumferentially throughout the peripheral retina, with little retinal opacification. This phenomenon has been called "smoldering disease" or "creeping scars" by some investigators. This phenomenon can occur even in the early stages of therapy, for unknown reasons.

Local Therapy

Direct placement of ganciclovir or foscarnet into the eye has been studied as an alternative therapy to intravenous

---

*References 76, 82, 91, 100, 186, 385.

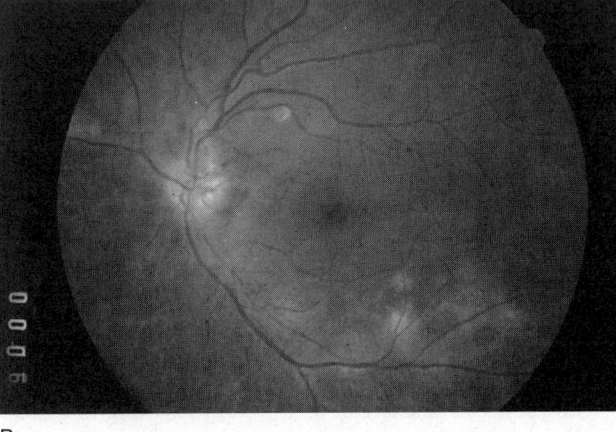

A

B

C

Fig. 81-18. **A,** CMV retinitis in the left eye of a patient with AIDS during intravenous ganciclovir therapy. The wedge-shaped area of disease is inferior to the optic disc, with its temporal border adjacent to the inferonasal vascular arcades. The lesion is inactive. **B,** The same eye, 2 months later, during continuous intravenous ganciclovir maintenance therapy. The temporal border has reactivated. **C,** The same eye, following re-induction therapy with intravenous ganciclovir. The lesion has again become inactive. Reprinted with permission from: Holland, GN: An update on AIDS-related cytomegalovirus retinitis. In *Focal points: clinical modules for ophthalmologists (5),* American Academy of Ophthalmology, 1991.

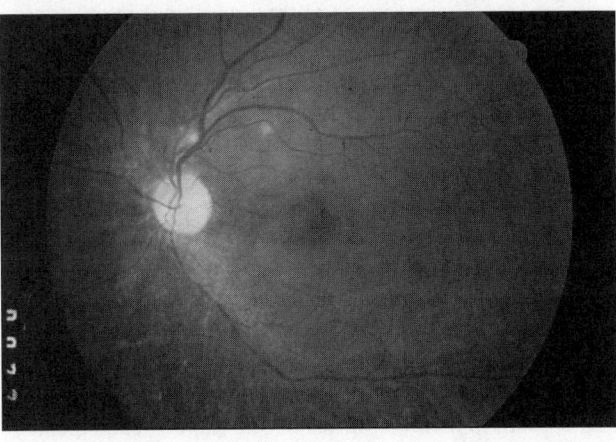

administration of drug. Interest in this local therapy arose initially out of concern about the systemic toxicity of ganciclovir, when alternative therapies were not available. It has also been advocated by some investigators as supplementation to systemic therapy, either following reactivation and enlargement of lesions[395] or to improve the efficacy of intravenous drug at the onset of treatment.[58,416] The desire for convenience and the observation that direct delivery of drug to the eye may actually be more effective than intravenously administered drug for delaying time to progression[247] are the reasons that interest in local therapy continues. Supplementation of local drug levels in patients receiving oral formulations of anti-CMV drugs (which may have low bioavailability) is viewed by many as the most promising future role for local therapy.

Serial intravitreous injections of ganciclovir have been studied by several groups of investigators; the most common regimen has been to inject 200 micrograms of drug 2 or 3 times weekly for 2 to 3 weeks as induction therapy, followed by weekly injections of the same dose, as maintenance therapy. Stabilization or quiescence of disease was observed in the majority of reported eyes.[36,45,150,395] Data is hard to interpret, however, because (1) patients were not studied in ran-

domized clinical trials, and (2) patients included a heterogeneous group, treated with a variety of regimens, for a variety of indications.

Foscarnet has also been delivered by intravitreous injection.[67,68,233] A dose of 1200 micrograms of drug per injection is used; injections have been given every 2 or 3 days for induction therapy followed by weekly injections for maintenance therapy.

The problems associated with once or twice weekly intravitreous injections stimulated interest in an intraocular device for sustained release of ganciclovir, which was introduced in 1992.[362] Martin and associates[247] reported the results of a study in which 26 patients with untreated CMV retinitis in Zones 2 and/or 3 were randomized to receive an intraocular device or to have therapy deferred until there was progression of disease. Median time to disease progression in the group receiving intraocular devices was 226 days compared to 15 days for the deferral group. Many factors can influence study results, and different studies should be compared with caution. Nevertheless, there is a very large difference between the median times to disease progression in the Martin and associates study (226 days) and in the SOCA Research Group study (47 days) for patients receiving intravenous ganciclovir. This difference probably represents a real disparity in the abilities to contain disease of drugs administered by intraocular devices and drugs delivered intravenously at maintenance therapy doses, especially as results were determined by the same fundus photograph reading center.[247,384]

Direct delivery of drugs to the eye offers the advantage of high levels at the site of infection. Ganciclovir levels in the vitreous humor after maintenance intravenous infusion are subtherapeutic for many CMV isolates.[221] Although vitreous humor drug levels are relevant for bacterial or fungal intraocular infection, where organisms invade the vitreous body with abscess formation, they may be less relevant for CMV infection, which is restricted to retinal tissue. Kuppermann and associates[221] have argued that vitreous humor levels reflect retinal levels because of equilibrium, but this fact has not been confirmed. Retinal drug levels are difficult to measure, but high levels presumably can be achieved in tissue from intravenously administered drug, because of breakdown of the blood ocular barrier. Ganciclovir levels in the subretinal space at the time of retinal detachment repair are similar to those measured simultaneously in the plasma.[184]

Intraocular devices offer the additional advantage of drug release at a steady rate, thereby avoiding the fluctuating drug levels associated with intermittent dosing, which might affect efficacy and facilitate emergence of resistant virus strains.

The study by Martin and associates[247] did not address the efficacy of intraocular devices for treatment of progressive disease in patients who have already received intravenously administered drug, and who may have strains of virus resistant to ganciclovir. Earlier studies by Anand and associates,[3] however, suggest that there may be a role for intraocular devices in such salvage therapy.

Although time to disease progression is an important objective measure of a drug's ability to suppress virus activity, it does not necessarily reflect the efficacy of long-term therapy in terms of final visual outcomes. The ability of intraocular devices to prevent enlargement of lesions must be weighed against the risk of new bilateral disease, nonocular CMV disease, and early retinal detachments. In the study by Martin and associates,[247] 50% of patients with unilateral disease who were treated with an intraocular device had developed bilateral disease at 6 months. In contrast, the cumulative risk of bilateral disease in the SOCA Research Group study was only 27% at 6 months in patients receiving intravenous ganciclovir.[384] Once an eye develops CMV retinopathy, it is at risk for retinal detachment, regardless of the success with which it is controlled medically.

Invasive procedures may increase the rate of retinal detachment, but this association is difficult to establish during local treatment of CMV retinitis, as retinal detachment is a well-known complication of necrotizing infectious retinopathies, even if disease is medically controlled. Retinal de-

tachments may develop sooner when eyes are treated with intraocular devices, however. The SOCA Research Group identified the risk of retinal detachment among patients receiving intravenous ganciclovir to be 27% at 6 months[384] ; in another study of 38 patients with retinal detachment who had been treated with systemic therapy, the median time to detachment was 4 months. [181] In the study by Martin and associates,[247] retinal detachment or retinal tear occurred in 18% of eyes, but 5 of 7 retinal detachments occurred sooner than 65 days after implantation of the intraocular device.

The fact that local therapy does not treat nonocular disease has also been viewed as a major disadvantage. All patients with untreated CMV retinopathy have evidence of nonocular tissue-invasive CMV infections at autopsy,[294] although the rate with which these infections cause clinically apparent disease is hard to determine. Nonocular, clinically apparent CMV disease occurred in 8 of 26 patients (31%) with intraocular devices reported by Martin and associates[247]; and in at least one patient, death was attributed to CMV infection. Systemic therapy for CMV retinitis has been shown to decrease the incidence of nonocular CMV infections,[268] but in the absence of clinically apparent nonocular CMV disease, the need to administer systemic anti-CMV therapy has not been well established. Systemic therapy appears to prolong patient survival,[175,185] but it has never been shown that early treatment of nonocular CMV infection is any more beneficial than treating the clinical manifestations of infections when they develop.

Reported complications of local therapy include scleral induration, mild-to-moderate vitreous humor haze, iritis, mild to severe vitreous hemorrhage, and infectious endophthalmitis.[36,45,150,151,247] The incidence of endophthalmitis is not known. Invasion of the vitreous base results in development of localized granulation tissue and vitreous body traction that can lead to retinal detachment, even after a single needle perforation of the pars plana.[217] Milder complications that may not affect final vision have included mild vitreous hemorrhage and astigmatism after implantation of intraocular devices.

There have been no clinical reports suggesting toxicity among patients undergoing local therapy. In a single report, however, Yoshizumi and associates[414] described vacuolization of photoreceptor outer segments with repeated intravitreal injections of 100 micrograms of ganciclovir in a rabbit model.

The limitations of serial intravitreous injections and implantation of intraocular devices has led to the investigation of other techniques for drug delivery. They include the injection of liposome-encapsulated drugs,[74] which would require less frequent administration of drug and yet avoid the large surgical incision associated with implantation of intraocular devices, and transscleral iontophoresis of drug,[335] which would have the benefits of a noninvasive procedure.

Goals of Therapy

With increasing survival and the fact that most patients with CMV retinitis will eventually have progression of disease, it is important to consider the goals of therapy. The definition of progression used for clinical trials has been useful for studying new drugs, but is too rigid to indicate treatment failure in clinical practice. In lesions outside the major vascular arcades, it may be acceptable to observe small amounts of lesion enlargement over a prolonged period of treatment, especially late in the course of infection, in lieu of overly aggressive therapy that may place the patient at risk for systemic or local complications. Some investigators have considered protection of Zone 1 a realistic goal for long-term therapy.

Deferral of Therapy

It has been suggested that treatment of small CMV retinitis lesions in Zones 2 and 3 may be deferred for short periods of time without placing patients at risk of vision loss, but this issue has been a subject of controversy.[164] Faced with the prospect of life-long intravenous drug therapy, there are several reasons why patients and clinicians might prefer to delay the start of therapy. Short periods of deferral will (1) allow patients to be evaluated and prepared for treatment in an unhurried manner, (2) postpone the risk of drug toxicity and sepsis from catheter infections, (3) reduce the risk of adverse drug interactions, and (4) delay the expense and inconvenience of therapy.[163]

Deferral may be acceptable because of several factors in the natural history of CMV retinitis: the slow enlargement of lesions, the infrequency with which new lesions develop, and the rare development of new lesions in the foveal area. Extent of disease at diagnosis is believed to reflect duration of untreated CMV retinitis, but has not been found to be related to visual outcome or response to therapy.[285,384] Based on differences in extent of CMV retinitis at diagnosis, therapy has, in effect, been deferred for many patients before they are first examined. In clinical practice periods of deferral are rarely longer than 2 to 3 weeks; therapy is usually started when posterior advancement of lesion borders is first documented. Deferral of therapy is not appropriate for patients with Zone 1 lesions.

There are equally cogent arguments in favor of immediate treatment. It will further reduce the risk of developing new lesions, and it presumably treats clinically inapparent, nonocular sites of CMV infection that might eventually be life-threatening. As less toxic drug therapies are developed, risk/benefit analyses will undoubtedly favor earlier treatment.

Treatment of Children

Experience with antiviral therapy for CMV disease is more limited in infants and older children than in adults. Ganciclovir is being investigated as a treatment for the clinical manifestations of cytomegalic inclusion disease, including CMV retinitis, in congenitally infected newborns.[161,278,317] The most appropriate dose and the effect of treatment on the long-term sequelae of CMV infection have not yet been determined, however. Also, the required length of treatment for CMV retinitis in this setting is not known. Cytomegalovirus retinitis in HIV-infected children has been treated successfully with ganciclovir[230,324,334] or ganciclovir and foscarnet.[34]

PROGNOSIS

The prognosis for infants with congenital CMV infection depends on the severity of disease in the perinatal period. For infants with symptomatic cytomegalic inclusion disease prior to the availability of anti-CMV drugs, prognosis has been quite poor. Pass and associates[291] found that 10 of 34 symptomatic infants (29%) died, and among 23 survivors, 21 (91%) developed severe CNS disorders in the first few years of life. The majority had microcephaly and intellectual impairment. Signs of old retinitis and/or optic atrophy were present in 5 of 23 (22%); defects of vision were difficult to assess because of mental retardation. The effect of anti-CMV therapy on long-term outcomes for infants with cytomegalic inclusion disease is under study.

An autopsy study of 47 HIV-infected individuals indicated that CMV retinitis is associated with an increased risk of CMV encephalitis; 10 of 24 patients (42%) with CMV retinitis had CMV encephalitis in contrast to only 1 of 23 patients (4%) without CMV retinitis.[35] The relative risk of CMV encephalitis increased from 9.5 to 13 when CMV retinitis was in the peripapillary retina. Evidence from this study suggested that CMV encephalitis occurred later in life than CMV retinitis, however, and that CMV encephalitis develops despite systemic treatment with antiviral drugs.

Vision

Since the introduction of specific anti-CMV therapies, the prognosis for retention of useful vision in patients with CMV retinitis has been excellent. At 6 months after the start of intravenous ganciclovir or foscarnet therapy, at least 88% of patients will retain 20/40 or better central visual acuity in the better eye (see Therapy section).[384] The major threat to vision currently is rhegmatogenous retinal detachments (see Complications section).

Survival

Because CMV retinitis is a marker for the presence of nonocular, tissue-invasive CMV disease,[294] and because CMV is suspected to cause or contribute to the death of many patients with AIDS, the relationship between CMV retinitis and survival has been studied extensively. During the first few years of the AIDS epidemic, CMV retinitis was considered to be a preterminal event, with no patients surviving longer than 6 weeks in one study.[170] Survival of patients with CMV disease has increased since the start of the epidemic.[146,175] This change can be attributed to improved general medical care of patients with AIDS (and especially to improved management of opportunistic infections), to the use of antiretroviral agents, and to the use of prophylaxis against *P. carinii* pneumonia and other opportunistic infections.

Several studies have also suggested that the use of anti-CMV therapy has contributed to increased survival.[175,185,215,300] In a retrospective, nonrandomized study shortly after the introduction of ganciclovir, Holland and associates[175] found a significant difference in survival between patients whose CMV retinitis was not treated (median 2 months) and those receiving ganciclovir (median 7 months, $P < 0.001$). Not only were patients not randomized, the investigators were not able to control for medical factors related to survival (hemoglobin, absolute lymphocyte count);[146] therefore, the influence of ganciclovir could not be confirmed. Harb and associates[146] could not confirm an effect of ganciclovir or foscarnet on survival in another retrospective study.

The SOCA Research Group found a difference in survival between patients with CMV retinitis who were initially treated with ganciclovir (median 8.5 months) and those initially treated with foscarnet (median 12.6 months, $P = 0.007$).[383] These survival statistics for patients receiving foscarnet are supported by another recent, uncontrolled study in which median patient survival was 13.5 months.[300] In that study over 25% of patients survived longer than 2 years.

In the SOCA Research Group study, excess mortality among patients receiving ganciclovir could not be attributed to a differential use of antiretroviral agents, which are known to affect survival. It has been hypothesized that patients receiving foscarnet survived longer because foscarnet also has antiretroviral activity, whereas ganciclovir does not.[383] This hypothesis is supported by a subsequent study of patients with AIDS and CMV retinitis that showed a positive relationship between survival and dosage of foscarnet used for maintenance therapy.[185]

In a 1989 report Jabs and associates[180] found that patients with a "complete" response of lesions to ganciclovir therapy had a longer median survival (5.5 months) than patients with a partial response (3.1 months) or no response (1.0 months). They attributed the differences in survival and response to different levels of immunosuppression.

The duration of anti-CMV therapy has not been shown to be related to survival[146,300]; therefore, short periods of deferral prior to initiation of treatment for CMV retinitis probably do not affect patient mortality. The location of CMV retinitis lesions had no apparent prognostic significance for survival in one study.[175]

For patients whose index diagnosis for AIDS is CMV retinitis, the interval from diagnosis of CMV retinitis to death appears to be longer than for patients whose CMV retinitis develops later, but their overall survival after diagnosis of AIDS is shorter.[175] Although Holland and associates[175] also found a weak inverse correlation between the interval from diagnosis of AIDS to diagnosis of CMV retinitis and the interval from diagnosis of CMV retinitis to death for patients whose CMV retinitis was untreated, no such relationship existed for patients who received ganciclovir. Therefore the interval from diagnosis of AIDS to diagnosis of CMV retinopathy probably has no prognostic significance for survival in the current setting in which all patients are routinely treated.

Jacobson[191] found that the presence or absence of CMV retinitis was not related to survival for patients after a first episode of *P. carinii* pneumonia.

PREVENTION

Shedding of CMV in the saliva of infected children has been implicated in the transmission of CMV in day care centers.[288] Although CMV may be shed from the respiratory system, epidemiologic evidence argues against airborne transmission of virus between immunocompetent children.[288] Because knowledge of the modes of CMV transmission is incomplete, specific recommendations for health care workers and pregnant women have not been produced, despite the fact that some investigators believe that these groups are at increased risk of infection.[286] Simple hygiene measures, such as handwashing, probably play an important role in prevention of CMV transmission.[210]

To prevent CMV infection in high-risk groups, such as organ transplant recipients, premature infants, and patients with AIDS, exposure of seronegative individuals to exogenous sources of CMV, such as blood transfusions from seropositive donors, should be avoided, and organs for transplantation should be obtained from seronegative donors.[159] Other successful preventative measures are the use of leukocyte-poor blood transfusions during bone marrow transplantation[26] and intravenous immune globulin in renal transplant patients.[365] Although IFN-α has a moderate effect in preventing CMV infection in renal transplant recipients, it is not used clinically, because it increases the risk of acute graft rejection.[156] Other studies, however, have provided conflicting data regarding this action of interferon.[237]

"Pre-emptive" ganciclovir therapy reduces the incidence of CMV disease in bone marrow and solid organ transplant recipients who develop positive surveillance cultures. Thus this therapy may improve patient survival.[133,352] The use of true prophylaxis at the time of engraftment is controversial, as toxicity may outweigh benefits.[132]

The only form of active immunization that has been used clinically is a live-attenuated vaccine against the Towne strain of CMV. This vaccine has not been shown to reduce the incidence of CMV disease, but has been shown to reduce the rate of severe disease by 80% to 100% in high-risk seronegative renal transplant recipients with kidneys from seropositive donors.[12,299] The Towne strain of CMV is not isolated from such patients after transplantation. The development of CMV subunit vaccines against antigens such as the glycoproteins gB or gH, IE1 protein, pp 65, and pp 150, may prove more effective for the prevention of infection.

Prophylactic Drug Therapy

In a prospective, randomized, and masked study oral ganciclovir was shown to reduce the proportion of HIV-infected patients with CD4+ T-lymphocyte counts less than 100 who developed CMV retinitis during a 12-month treatment period from 20% to 11% ($P = 0.001$).*

Development of effective primary prophylaxis programs for prevention of CMV retinitis is a top priority. To be practical, these programs will require not only an oral drug, but better knowledge of risk factors for the development of CMV retinitis, so that only those patients at highest risk will be treated.

REFERENCES

1. Aaberg TM, Cesarz TJ, Rytel MW: Correlation of virology and clinical course of cytomegalovirus retinitis, *Am J Ophthalmol* 74:407-417, 1972.
2. Alford CA, Pass RF, Stagno S: Early and late developmental abnormalities associated with congenital cytomegalovirus and toxoplasma infections, *Prog Clin Biol Res* 163B:343-349, 1985.
3. Anand R, Nightingale SD, Fish RH et al.: Control of cytomegalovirus retinitis using sustained release of intraocular ganciclovir, *Arch Ophthalmol* 111:223-227, 1993.
4. Aschan J, Ringden O, Ljungman P et al.: Foscarnet for treatment of cytomegalovirus infections in bone marrow transplant recipients, *Scand J Infect Dis* 24:143-150, 1992.
5. Astle JN, Ellis PP: Ocular complications in renal transplant patients, *Ann Ophthalmol* 6:1269-1274, 1974.
6. Atherton SS, Newell CK, Kanter MY, Cousins SW: T cell depletion increases susceptibility to murine cytomegalovirus retinitis, *Invest Ophthalmol Vis Sci* 33:3353-3360, 1992.
7. Augsburger JJ, Henry RY: Retinal aneurysms in adult cytomegalovirus retinitis, *Am J Ophthalmol* 86:794-797, 1978.
8. Azad RF, Driver VB, Tanaka K et al.: Antiviral activity of a phosphorothioate oligonucleotide complementary to RNA of the human cytomegalovirus major immediate-early region, *Antimicrob Agents Chemother* 37:1945-1954, 1993.
9. Bachman DM, Bruni LM, DiGioia RA et al.: Visual field testing in the management of cytomegalovirus retinitis, *Ophthalmology* 99:1393-1399, 1992.
10. Bachman DM, Rodrigues MM, Chu FC et al.: Culture-proven cytomegalovirus retinitis in a homosexual man with the acquired immunodeficiency syndrome, *Ophthalmology* 89:797-804, 1982.
11. Bale JF, O'Neil ME, Folberg R: Murine cytomegalovirus ocular infection in immunocompetent and cyclophosphamide-treated mice: potentiation of ocular infection by cyclophosphamide, *Invest Ophthalmol Vis Sci* 32:1749-1756, 1991.
12. Balfour HH, Welo PK, Sachs GW: Cytomegalovirus vaccine trial in 400 renal transplant candidates, *Transplant Proc* 17:81-83, 1985.
13. Balthesen M, Dreher L, Lucin P, Reddehase MJ: The establishment of cytomegalovirus latency in organs is not linked to local virus production during primary infection, *J Gen Virol* 75:2329-2336, 1994.
14. Bankier AT, Beck S, Bohni R et al.: The DNA sequence of the human cytomegalovirus genome, *DNA Seq* 2:1-12, 1991.
15. Beck S, Barrell BG: Human cytomegalovirus encodes a glycoprotein homologous to MHC class-I antigens, *Nature* 331:269-272, 1988.
16. Berenberg W, Nankervis G: Long-term follow-up of cytomegalic inclusion disease of infancy, *Pediatrics* 46:403-410, 1970.
17. Berger BB, Weinberg RS, Tessler HH et al.: Bilateral cytomegalovirus panuveitis after high-dose corticosteroid therapy, *Am J Ophthalmol* 88:1020-1025, 1979.
18. Bevan IS, Daw RA, Day PJ et al.: Polymerase chain reaction for detection of human cytomegalovirus infection in a blood donor population, *Br J Haematol* 78:94-99, 1991.
19. Biron CA, Byron KS, Sullivan JL: Severe herpesvirus infections in an adolescent without natural killer cells, *N Engl J Med* 320:1731-1735, 1989.
20. Biswas J, Mayr AJ, Martin WJ, Rao NA: Detection of human cytomegalovirus in ocular tissue by polymerase chain reaction and in situ DNA hybridization, *Graefes Arch Clin Exp Ophthalmol* 231:66-70, 1993.
21. Blanchard C: Treatment of HIV-related cytomegalovirus disease of the gastrointestinal tract with foscarnet, *J Acquir Immune Defic Syndr Hum Retrovirol* 5(suppl 1):25-28, 1992.
22. Bloom JN, Palestine AG: The diagnosis of cytomegalovirus retinitis, *Ann Intern Med* 109:963-969, 1988.
23. Bonkowsky HL, Lee RV, Klatskin G: Acute granulomatous hepatitis: occurrence in cytomegalovirus mononucleosis, *JAMA* 233:1284-1288, 1975.
24. Boone WB, O'Reilly RJ, Pahwa S et al.: Acquired CMV chorioretinitis in severe combined immunodeficiency, *Clin Immunol Immunopathol* 9:129-133, 1978.
25. Borisch B, Jahn G, Scholl BC et al.: Detection of human cytomegalovirus DNA and viral antigens in tissues of different manifestations of CMV infection, *Virchows Arch B Cell Pathol Incl Mol Pathol* 55:93-99, 1988.
26. Bowden RA, Slichter SJ, Sayers MH et al.: Use of leukocyte-depleted platelets and cytomegalovirus-seronegative red blood cells for prevention of primary cytomegalovirus infection after marrow transplant, *Blood* 78:246-250, 1991.
27. Broaddus C, Dake MD, Stulbarg MS et al.: Bronchoalveolar lavage and transbronchial biopsy for the diagnosis of pulmonary infections in the acquired immunodeficiency syndrome, *Ann Intern Med* 102:747-752, 1985.
28. Broughton WL, Cupples HP, Parver LM: Bilateral retinal detachment following cytomegalovirus retinitis, *Arch Ophthalmol* 96:618-619, 1978.
29. Brown HH, Glasgow BJ, Holland GN, Foos RY: Cytomegalovirus infection of the conjunctiva in AIDS, *Am J Ophthalmol* 106:102-104, 1988.
30. Bruggeman CA: Cytomegalovirus and latency: an overview, *Virchows Arch B Cell Pathol Incl Mol Pathol* 64:325-333, 1993.
31. Brytting M, Xu W, Wahren B, Sundqvist VA: Cytomegalovirus DNA detection in sera from patients with active cytomegalovirus infections, *J Clin Microbiol* 30:1937-1941, 1992.
32. Burns DK, Risser RC, White CL: The neuropathology of human immunodeficiency virus infection: the Dallas, Texas experience, *Arch Pathol Lab Med* 115:1112-1124, 1991.
33. Burns RP: Cytomegalic inclusion disease uveitis, *Acta Ophthalmol* 61:376-387, 1959.
34. Butler KM, De Smet MD, Husson RN et al.: Treatment of aggressive cytomegalovirus retinitis with ganciclovir in combination with foscarnet in a child infected with human immunodeficiency virus, *J Pediatr* 120:483-486, 1992.
35. Bylsma SS, Achim CL, Wiley CA et al.: The predictive value of cytomegalovirus retinitis for cytomegalovirus encephalitis in aquired immunodeficiency syndrome, *Arch Ophthalmol* 113:89-95, 1995.
36. Cantrill HL, Henry K, Melroe NH et al.: Treatment of cytomegalovirus retinitis with intravitreal ganciclovir: long-term results, *Ophthalmology* 96:367-374, 1989.
37. Casareale D, Fiala M, Chang CM et al.: Cytomegalovirus enhances lysis of HIV-infected T lymphoblasts, *Int J Cancer* 44:124-130, 1989.

*Stephen A. Spector, MD, unpublished data presented at the 34th Interscience Conference on Antimicrobial Agents and Chemotherapy, Orlando, Florida, USA, October 1994.

38. Cassol SA, Poon MC, Pal R et al.: Primer-mediated enzymatic amplification of cytomegalovirus (CMV) DNA: application to the early diagnosis of CMV infection in marrow transplant recipients, *J Clin Invest* 83:1109-1115, 1989.

39. Centers for Disease Control: Revision of the Centers for Disease Control surveillance case definition for aquired immunodeficiency syndrome, *MMWR* 36(supp):1S-16S, 1987.

40. Ch'ien LT, Cannon NJ, Whitley RJ et al.: Effect of adenine arabinoside on cytomegalovirus infections, *J Infect Dis* 130:32-39, 1974.

41. Chawla HB, Ford MJ, Munro JF et al.: Ocular involvement in cytomegalovirus infection in a previously healthy adult, *BMJ* 2:281-282, 1976.

42. Chou SW: Acquisition of donor strains of cytomegalovirus by renal-transplant recipients, *N Engl J Med* 314:1418-1423, 1986.

43. Christensen L, Beeman HW, Allen A: Cytomegalic inclusion disease, *Arch Ophthalmol* 57:90-99, 1957.

44. Chumbley LC, Robertson DM, Smith TF, Campbell RJ: Adult cytomegalovirus inclusion retino-uveitis, *Am J Ophthalmol* 80:807-816, 1975.

45. Cochereau-Massin I, Lehoang P, Lautier-Frau M et al.: Efficacy and tolerance of intravitreal ganciclovir in cytomegalovirus retinitis in acquired immune deficiency syndrome, *Ophthalmology* 98:1348-1353; discussion 1353-1355, 1991.

46. Collaborative DHPG Treatment Study Group: Treatment of serious cytomegalovirus infections with 9-(1,3-dihydroxy-2-propoxymethyl)guanine in patients with AIDS and other immunodeficiencies, *N Engl J Med* 314:801-805, 1986.

47. Collier AC, Meyers JD, Corey L et al.: Cytomegalovirus infection in homosexual men: relationship to sexual practices, antibody to human immunodeficiency virus, and cell-mediated immunity, *Am J Med* 82:593-601, 1987.

48. Collins TM, Quirk MR, Jordan MC: Biphasic viremia and viral gene expression in leukocytes during acute cytomegalovirus infection of mice, *J Virol* 68:6305-6311, 1994.

49. Coskuncan NM, Jabs DA, Dunn JP et al.: The eye in bone marrow transplantation: VI. Retinal complications, *Arch Ophthalmol* 112:372-379, 1994.

50. Coulson AS, Lucas ZJ, Condy M, Cohn R: Forty-day fever: an epidemic of cytomegalovirus disease in a renal transplant population, *West J Med* 120:1-7, 1974.

51. Cowdry A: The problem of intranuclear inclusions in virus disease, *Arch Pathol* 18:525-542, 1934.

52. Cox F, Meyer D, Hughes WT: Cytomegalovirus in tears from patients with normal eyes and with acute cytomegalovirus chorioretinitis, *Am J Ophthalmol* 80:817-824, 1975.

53. Crowe SM, Carlin JB, Stewart KI et al.: Predictive value of CD4 lymphocyte numbers for the development of opportunistic infections and malignancies in HIV-infected persons, *J Acquir Immune Defic Syndr* 4:770-776, 1991.

54. Culbertson WW: Infections of the retina in AIDS, *Int Ophthalmol Clin* 29:108-118, 1989.

55. D'Amico DJ, Skolnik PR, Kosloff BR et al.: Resolution of cytomegalovirus retinitis with zidovudine therapy: case report, *Arch Ophthalmol* 106:1168-1169, 1988.

56. D'Antonio D, Iacone A, Fioritoni G et al.: Patterns of cytomegalovirus retinitis in immunocompromised patients treated with 9-(2-hydroxy-1-(hydroxymethyl)ethoxymethyl) guanine (ganciclovir), *J Chemother* 3:162-166, 1991.

57. Daicker B: Cytomegalovirus panuveitis with infection of corneotrabecular endothelium in AIDS, *Ophthalmologica* 197:169-175, 1988.

58. Daikos GL, Pulido J, Kathpalia SB, Jackson GG: Intravenous and intraocular ganciclovir for CMV retinitis in patients with AIDS or chemotherapeutic immunosuppression, *Br J Ophthalmol* 72:521-524, 1988.

59. Dankner WM, McCutchan JA, Richman DD et al.: Localization of human cytomegalovirus in peripheral blood leukocytes by in situ hybridization, *J Infect Dis* 161:31-36, 1990.

60. Davis JL, Feuer W, Culbertson WW, Pflugfelder SC: Interpretation of intraocular and serum antibody levels in necrotizing retinitis, *Retina* 15:233-240, 1995.

61. Davis JL, Nussenblatt RB, Bachman DM et al.: Endogenous bacterial retinitis in AIDS, *Am J Ophthalmol* 107:613-623, 1989.

62. Davis MG, Kenney SC, Kamine J et al.: Immediate-early gene region of human cytomegalovirus trans-activates the promoter of human immunodeficiency virus, *Proc Natl Acad Sci USA* 84:8642-8646, 1987.

63. de Gans J, Portegies P, Tiessens G et al.: Therapy for cytomegalovirus polyradiculomyelitis in patients with AIDS: treatment with ganciclovir, *AIDS* 4:421-425, 1990.

64. De Venecia G, Zu Rhein GM, Pratt MV, Kisken W: Cytomegalic inclusion retinitis in an adult, *Arch Ophthalmol* 86:44-57, 1971.

65. Demmler GJ: Infectious Diseases Society of America and Centers for Disease Control, summary of a workshop on surveillance for congenital cytomegalovirus disease, *Rev Infect Dis* 13:315-329, 1991.

66. Dennehy PJ, Warman R, Flynn JT et al.: Ocular manifestations in pediatric patients with acquired immunodeficiency syndrome, *Arch Ophthalmol* 107:978-982, 1989.

67. Diaz-Llopis M, Chipont E, Sanchez S et al.: Intravitreal foscarnet for cytomegalovirus retinitis in a patient with acquired immunodeficiency syndrome, *Am J Ophthalmol* 114:742-747, 1992.

68. Diaz-Llopis M, Espana E, Munoz G et al.: High dose intravitreal foscarnet in the treatment of cytomegalovirus retinitis in AIDS, *Br J Ophthalmol* 78:120-124, 1994.

69. Dieterich DT, Kotler DP, Busch DF et al.: Ganciclovir treatment of cytomegalovirus colitis in AIDS: a randomized, double-blind, placebo-controlled multicenter study, *J Infect Dis* 167:278-282, 1993.

70. Dighiero P, Reux I, Hauw JJ et al.: Expression of inducible nitric oxide synthase in cytomegalovirus-infected glial cells of retinas from AIDS patients, *Neurosci Lett* 166:31-34, 1994.

71. Digre KB, Blodi CF, Bale JF: Cytomegalovirus infection in a healthy adult associated with recurrent branch retinal artery occlusion, *Retina* 7:230-232, 1987.

72. DiLoreto DJ, Epstein LG, Lazar ES et al.: Cytomegalovirus infection of human retinal tissue: an in vivo model, *Lab Invest* 71:141-148, 1994.

73. Dobbins JG, Stewart JA, Demmler GJ: Surveillance of congenital cytomegalovirus disease, 1990-1991: collaborating Registry Group, *MMWR CDC Surveill Summ* 41:35-39, 1992.

74. Dolnak DR, Munguia D, Wiley CA et al.: Lack of retinal toxicity of the anticytomegalovirus drug (S)-1-(3-hydroxy-2-phosphonylmethoxypropyl) cytosine, *Invest Ophthalmol Vis Sci* 33:1557-1563, 1992.

75. Dorfman LJ: Cytomegalovirus encephalitis in adults, *Neurology* 23:136-144, 1973.

76. Drew WL, Miner RC, Busch DF et al.: Prevalence of resistance in patients receiving ganciclovir for serious cytomegalovirus infection, *J Infect Dis* 163:716-719, 1991.

77. Drew WL, Mintz L, Miner RC et al.: Prevalence of cytomegalovirus infection in homosexual men, *J Infect Dis* 143:188-192, 1981.

78. Duan Y, Ji Z, Atherton SS: Dissemination and replication of MCMV after supraciliary inoculation in immunosuppressed BALB/c mice, *Invest Ophthalmol Vis Sci* 35:1124-1131, 1994.

79. Dugel PU, Liggett PE, Lee MB et al.: Repair of retinal detachment caused by cytomegalovirus retinitis in patients with the acquired immunodeficiency syndrome, *Am J Ophthalmol* 112:235-242, 1991.

80. Duncombe AS, Meager A, Prentice HG et al.: Gamma-interferon and tumour necrosis factor production after bone marrow transplantation is augmented by exposure to marrow fibroblasts infected with cytomegalovirus, *Blood* 76:1046-1053, 1990.

81. Dunkel EC, de Freitas D, Scheer DI et al.: A rabbit model for human cytomegalovirus-induced chorioretinal disease, *J Infect Dis* 168:336-344, 1993.

82. Dunn JP, MacCumber MW, Forman MS et al.: Viral sensitivity testing in patients with cytomegalovirus retinitis clinically resistant to foscarnet or ganciclovir, *Am J Ophthalmol* 119:587-596, 1995.

83. Dvorak-Theobald G: Cytomegalic incusion disease, report of a case, *Am J Ophthalmol* 309:950-953, 1959.

84. Dworsky M, Yow M, Stagno S et al.: Cytomegalovirus infection of breast milk and transmission in infancy, *Pediatrics* 72:295-299, 1983.

85. Dworsky ME, Welch K, Cassady G, Stagno S: Occupational risk for primary cytomegalovirus infection among pediatric health-care workers, *N Engl J Med* 309:950-953, 1983.

86. Egbert PR, Pollard RB, Gallagher JG, Merigan TC: Cytomegalovirus retinitis in immunosuppressed hosts: II. Ocular manifestations, *Ann Intern Med* 93:664-670, 1980.

87. Elkins BS, Holland GN, Opremcak EM et al.: Ocular toxoplasmosis misdiagnosed as cytomegalovirus retinopathy in immunocompromised patients, *Ophthalmology* 101:499-507, 1994.

88. England AC, Miller SA, Maki DG: Ocular findings of acute cytomegalovirus infection in an immunologically competent adult, *N Engl J Med* 307:94-95, 1982.

89. Engstrom RE, Holland GN, Hardy WD, Meiselman HJ: Hemorheologic abnormalities in patients with human immunodeficiency virus infection and ophthalmic microvasculopathy, *Am J Ophthalmol* 109:153-161, 1990.

90. Engstrom RE, Holland GN, Nussenblatt RB, Jabs DA: Current practices in the management of ocular toxoplasmosis, *Am J Ophthalmol* 111:601-610, 1991.

91. Erice A, Chou S, Biron KK et al.: Progressive disease due to ganciclovir-resistant cytomegalovirus in immunocompromised patients, *N Engl J Med* 320:289-293, 1989.

92. Espana-Gregori E, Vera-Sempere FJ, Cano-Parra J et al.: Cytomegalovirus infection of the caruncle in the acquired immunodeficiency syndrome, *Am J Ophthalmol* 117:406-407, 1994 (letter).

93. Farber S, Wolbach SG: Intranuclear and cytoplasmic inclusions (''protazoan-like bodies'') in the salivary glands and other organs of infants, *Am J Pathol* 8:123-135, 1932.

94. Fay MT, Freeman WR, Wiley CA et al.: Atypical retinitis in patients with the acquired immunodeficiency syndrome, *Am J Ophthalmol* 105:483-490, 1988.

95. Fekrat S, Dunn JP, Lee D et al.: Cytomegalovirus retinitis in HIV-infected patients with elevated CD4+ counts, *Arch Ophthalmol* 113:18, 1995.

96. Felsenstein D, D'Amico DJ, Hirsch MS et al.: Treatment of cytomegalovirus retinitis with 9-[2-hydroxy-1-(hydroxymethyl)ethoxymethyl]guanine, *Ann Intern Med* 103:377-380, 1985.

97. Fenner TE, Garweg J, Hufert FT et al.: Diagnosis of human cytomegalovirus-induced retinitis in human immunodeficiency virus type 1-infected subjects by using the polymerase chain reaction, *J Clin Microbiol* 29:2621-2622, 1991.

98. Fiala M, Chatterjee SN, Carson S et al.: Cytomegalovirus retinitis secondary to chronic viremia in phagocytic leukocytes, *Am J Ophthalmol* 84:567-573, 1977.

99. Fiala M, Payne JE, Berne TV et al.: Epidemiology of cytomegalovirus infection after transplantation and immunosuppression, *J Infect Dis* 132:421-433, 1975.

100. Flores-Aguilar M, Kuppermann BD, Quiceno JI et al.: Pathophysiology and treatment of clinically resistant cytomegalovirus retinitis, *Ophthalmology* 100:1022-1031, 1993.

101. Foerster HW: Pathology of granulomatous uveitis, *Surv Ophthalmol* 4:283-326, 1959.

102. Fowler KB, Stagno S, Pass RF et al.: The outcome of congenital cytomegalovirus infection in relation to maternal antibody status, *N Engl J Med* 326:663-667, 1992.

103. Fox GM, Crouse CA, Chuang EL et al.: Detection of herpesvirus DNA in vitreous and aqueous specimens by the polymerase chain reaction, *Arch Ophthalmol* 109:266-271, 1991.

104. Frank TS, LiVolsi VA, Connor AM: Cytomegalovirus infection of the thyroid in immunocompromised adults, *Yale J Biol Med* 60:1-8, 1987.

105. Freeman WR, Chen A, Henderly DE et al.: Prevalence and significance of acquired immunodeficiency syndrome-related retinal microvasculopathy, *Am J Ophthalmol* 107:229-235, 1989.

106. Freeman WR, Friedberg DN, Berry C et al.: Risk factors for development of rhegmatogenous retinal detachment in patients with cytomegalovirus retinitis, *Am J Ophthalmol* 116:713-720, 1993.

107. Freeman WR, Henderly DE, Wan WL et al.: Prevalence, pathophysiology, and treatment of rhegmatogenous retinal detachment in treated cytomegalovirus retinitis, *Am J Ophthalmol* 103:527-536, 1987.

108. Freeman WR, Lerner CW, Mines JA et al.: A prospective study of the ophthalmologic findings in the acquired immune deficiency syndrome, *Am J Ophthalmol* 97:133-142, 1984.

109. Freeman WR, Quiceno JI, Crapotta JA et al.: Surgical repair of rhegmatogenous retinal detachment in immunosuppressed patients with cytomegalovirus retinitis, *Ophthalmology* 99:466-474, 1992.

110. Freitas VR, Fraser-Smith EB, Matthews TR: Increased efficacy of ganciclovir in combination with foscarnet against cytomegalovirus and herpes simplex virus type 2 in vitro and in vivo, *Antiviral Res* 12:205-212, 1989.

111. Frenkel LD, Keys MP, Hefferen SJ et al.: Unusual eye abnormalities associated with congenital cytomegalovirus infection, *Pediatrics* 66:763-766, 1980.

112. Friedman AH, Freeman WR, Orellana J et al.: Cytomegalovirus retinitis and immunodeficiency in homosexual males, *Lancet* 1:958, 1982 (letter).

113. Friedman DI: Neuro-ophthalmic manifestations of human immunodeficiency virus infection, *Neurol Clin* 9:55-72, 1991.

114. Fries BC, Chou S, Boeckh M, Torok-Storb B: Frequency distribution of cytomegalovirus envelope glycoprotein genotypes in bone marrow transplant recipients, *J Infect Dis* 169:769-774, 1994.

115. Furukawa T, Hornberger E, Sakuma S, Plotkin SA: Demonstration of immunoglobuliin G receptors induce by human cytomegalovirus, *J Clin Microbiol* 2:332-336, 1975.

116. Gagliuso DJ, Teich SA, Friedman AH, Orellana J: Ocular toxoplasmosis in AIDS patients, *Trans Am Ophthalmol Soc* 88:63-86; discussion 86-88, 1990.

117. Gallant JE, Moore RD, Richman DD et al.: Incidence and natural history of cytomegalovirus disease in patients with advanced human immunodeficiency virus disease treated with zidovudine: the Zidovudine Epidemiology Study Group, *J Infect Dis* 166:1223-1227, 1992.

118. Gangan PA, Besen G, Munguia D, Freeman WR: Macular serous exudation in patients with acquired immunodeficiency syndrome and cytomegalovirus retinitis, *Am J Ophthalmol* 118:212-219, 1994.

119. Garau J, Kabins S, DeNosaquo S et al.: Spontaneous cytomegalovirus mononucleosis with conjunctivitis, *Arch Intern Med* 137:1631-1632, 1977.

120. Gass P, Kiessling M, Schafer P et al.: Detection of human cytomegalovirus DNA in paraffin sections of human brain by polymerase chain reaction and the occurrence of false negative results, *J Neurol Neurosurg Psychiatry* 56:211-214, 1993.

121. Geelen JL, Walig C, Wertheim P, van der Noordaa J: Human cytomegalovirus DNA: I. Molecular weight and infectivity, *J Virol* 26:813-816, 1978.

122. Geier SA, Nasemann J, Klauss V et al.: Frosted branch angiitis associated with cytomegalovirus retinitis, *Am J Ophthalmol* 114:514-516, 1992 (letter, comment).

123. Geist LJ, Monick MM, Stinski MF, Hunninghake GW: The immediate early genes of human cytomegalovirus upregulate tumor necrosis factor-alpha gene expression, *J Clin Invest* 93:474-478, 1994.

124. Gerberding JL, Bryant-LeBlanc CE, Nelson K et al.: Risk of transmitting the human immunodeficiency virus, cytomegalovirus, and hepatitis B virus to health care workers exposed to patients with AIDS and AIDS-related conditions, *J Infect Dis* 156:1-8, 1987.

125. Gerna G, Baldanti F, Sarasini A et al.: Effect of foscarnet induction treatment on quantitation of human cytomegalovirus (HCMV) DNA in peripheral blood polymorphonuclear leukocytes and aqueous humor of AIDS patients with HCMV retinitis: the Italian Foscarnet Study Group, *Antimicrob Agents Chemother* 38:38-44, 1994.

126. Gerna G, Zipeto D, Percivalle E et al.: Human cytomegalovirus infection of the major leukocyte subpopulations and evidence for initial viral replication in polymorphonuclear leukocytes from viremic patients, *J Infect Dis* 166:1236-1244, 1992.

127. Glasgow BJ, Steinsapir KD, Anders K, Layfield LJ: Adrenal pathology in the acquired immune deficiency syndrome, *Am J Clin Pathol* 84:594-597, 1985.

128. Glasgow BJ, Weisberger AK: A quantitative and cartographic study of retinal microvasculopathy in acquired immunodeficiency syndrome, *Am J Ophthalmol* 118:46-56, 1994.

129. Gleaves CA, Myerson D, Bowden RA et al.: Direct detection of cytomegalovirus from the bronchoalveolar lavage samples using a rapid in situ DNA hybridization assay, *J Clin Microbiol* 27:2429-2432, 1989.

130. Gleaves CA, Smith TF, Shuster EA, Pearson GR: Rapid detection of cytomegalovirus in MRC-5 cells inoculated with urine specimens by using low-speed centrifugation and monoclonal antibody to an early antigen, *J Clin Microbiol* 19:917-919, 1984.

131. Goodpasture EM, Talbot FB: Concerning the nature of ''protazoan-like'' cells in certain lesions of infancy. *Am J Dis Child* 21:415-425, 1921.

132. Goodrich JM, Bowden RA, Fisher L et al.: Ganciclovir prophylaxis to prevent cytomegalovirus disease after allogeneic marrow transplant, *Ann Intern Med* 118:173-178, 1993.

133. Goodrich JM, Mori M, Gleaves CA et al.: Early treatment with ganciclovir to prevent cytomegalovirus disease after allogeneic bone marrow transplantation, *N Engl J Med* 325:1601-1607, 1991.

134. Grefte A, van der Giessen M, van Son W, The TH: Circulating cytomegalovirus (CMV)-infected endothelial cells in patients with an active CMV infection, *J Infect Dis* 167:270-277, 1993.

135. Griffiths PD, Grundy JE: The status of CMV as a human pathogen, *Epidemiol Infect* 100:1-15, 1988.

136. Griffiths PD, Panjwani DD, Stirk PR et al.: Rapid diagnosis of cytomegalovirus infection in immunocompromised patients by detection of early antigen fluorescent foci, *Lancet* 2:1242-1245, 1984.

137. Gross JG, Bozzette SA, Mathews WC et al.: Longitudinal study of cytomegalovirus retinitis in acquired immune deficiency syndrome, *Ophthalmology* 97:681-686, 1990.

138. Gross JG, Sadun AA, Wiley CA, Freeman WR: Severe visual loss related to isolated peripapillary retinal and optic nerve head cytomegalovirus infection, *Am J Ophthalmol* 108:691-698, 1989.

139. Grossniklaus HE, Frank KE, Tomsak RL: Cytomegalovirus retinitis and optic neuritis in acquired immune deficiency syndrome: report of a case, *Ophthalmology* 94:1601-1604, 1987.

140. Grundy JE, Ayles HM, McKeating JA et al.: Enhancement of class 1 HLA antigen expression by cytomegalovirus: role in amplification of virus infection, *J Med Virol* 25:483-495, 1988.

141. Grundy JE, Downes KL: Up-regulation of LFA-3 and ICAM-1 on the surface of fibroblasts infected with cytomegalovirus, *Immunology* 78:405-412, 1993.

142. Guyer DR, Jabs DA, Brant AM et al.: Regression of cytomegalovirus retinitis with zidovudine: a clinicopathologic correlation, *Arch Ophthalmol* 107:868-874, 1989.

143. Guyton TB, Ehrlich F, Blanc WA et al.: New observations in generalised cytomegalic-inclusion disease of the newborn: report of a case with chorioretinitis, *N Engl J Med* 257:803-807, 1957.

144. Haagmans BL, van den Eertwegh AJ, Claassen E et al.: Tumour necrosis factor-alpha production during cytomegalovirus infection in immunosuppressed rats, *J Gen Virol* 75:779-787, 1994.

145. Hanshaw JB: Congenital cytomegalovirus infection: a fifteen year perspective, *J Infect Dis* 123:555-561, 1971.

146. Harb GE, Bacchetti P, Jacobson MA: Survival of patients with AIDS and cytomegalovirus disease treated with ganciclovir or foscarnet, *AIDS* 5:959-965, 1991.

147. Hardy WD: Combined ganciclovir and recombinant human granulocyte-macrophage colony-stimulating factor in the treatment of cytomegalovirus retinitis in AIDS patients, *J Acquir Immune Defic Syndr* 4(suppl 1):S22-S28, 1991.

148. Harris AI, Meyer RJ, Brody EA: Cytomegalovirus-induced thrombocytopenia and hemolysis in an adult, *Ann Intern Med* 83:670-671, 1975 (letter).

149. Hart WM, Reed CA, Freedman HL, Burde RM: Cytomegalovirus in juvenile iridocyclitis, *Am J Ophthalmol* 86:329-331, 1978.

150. Heinemann MH: Long-term intravitreal ganciclovir therapy for cytomegalovirus retinopathy, *Arch Ophthalmol* 107:1767-1772, 1989.

151. Heinemann MH: Staphylococcus epidermidis endophthalmitis complicating intravitreal antiviral therapy of cytomegalovirus retinitis: case report, *Arch Ophthalmol* 107:643-644, 1989.

152. Henderly DE, Atalla LR, Freeman WR, Rao NA: Demonstration of cytomegalovirus retinitis by in situ DNA hybridization, *Retina* 8:177-181, 1988.

153. Henderly DE, Freeman WR, Causey DM, Rao NA: Cytomegalovirus retinitis and response to therapy with ganciclovir, *Ophthalmology* 94:425-434, 1987.

154. Hendrix MG, Salimans MM, van Boven CP, Bruggeman CA: High prevalence of latently present cytomegalovirus in arterial walls of patients suffering from grade III atherosclerosis, *Am J Pathol* 136:23-28, 1990.

155. Hennis HL, Scott AA, Apple DJ: Cytomegalovirus retinitis, *Surv Ophthalmol* 34:193-203, 1989.

156. Hirsch MS, Schooley RT, Cosimi AB et al.: Effects of interferon-alpha on cytomegalovirus reactivation syndromes in renal-transplant recipients, *N Engl J Med* 308:1489-1493, 1983.

157. Hittner HM, Desmond MM, Montgomery JR: Optic nerve manifestations of human congenital cytomegalovirus infection, *Am J Ophthalmol* 81:661-665, 1976.

158. Ho M: *Cytomegalovirus: biology and infection,* ed 2, New York, 1991, Plenum.

159. Ho M, Suwansirikul S, Dowling JN et al.: The transplanted kidney as a source of cytomegalovirus infection, *N Engl J Med* 293:1109-1112, 1975.

160. Hochster H, Dieterich D, Bozzette S et al.: Toxicity of combined ganciclovir and zidovudine for cytomegalovirus disease associated with AIDS: an AIDS Clinical Trials Group Study, *Ann Intern Med* 113:111-117, 1990.

161. Hocker JR, Cook LN, Adams G, Rabalais GP: Ganciclovir therapy of congenital cytomegalovirus pneumonia, *Pediatr Infect Dis J* 9:743-745, 1990.

162. Holland GN: The management of retinal detachments in patients with acquired immunodeficiency syndrome, *Arch Ophthalmol* 109:791-793, 1991 (editorial).

163. Holland GN: Acquired immunodeficiency syndrome and ophthalmology: the first decade, *Am J Ophthalmol* 114:86-95, 1992.

164. Holland GN: AIDS: retinal and choroidal infections. In Ryan SJ, Lewis H, editors: *Medical and surgical retina: advances, controversies and management,* St. Louis, 1994, Mosby.

165. Holland GN, Buhles WC, Mastre B et al.: A controlled retrospective study of ganciclovir treatment for cytomegalovirus retinopathy: use of a standardized system for the assessment of disease outcome, *Arch Ophthalmol* 107:1759-1766, 1989.

166. Holland GN, Fang EN, Glasgow BJ et al.: Necrotizing retinopathy after intraocular inoculation of murine cytomegalovirus in immunosuppressed adult mice, *Invest Ophthalmol Vis Sci* 31:2326-2334, 1990.

167. Holland GN, Gottlieb MS, Yee RD et al.: Ocular disorders associated with a new severe acquired cellular immunodeficiency syndrome, *Am J Ophthalmol* 93:393-402, 1982.

168. Holland GN, Levinson RD: Ocular infections associated with the aquired immune deficiency syndrome. In Tasman W, Jaeger EA, editors: *Duane's foundation of clinical ophthalmology,* ed 2, Hargerstown, 1994, Lippincott.

169. Holland GN, Levinson RD, Jacobson MA, AIDS Clinical Trials Group Protocol 915 Team: A dose-related difference in progression rates of cytomegalovirus retinopathy during foscarnet maintenance therapy, *Am J Ophthalmol* 119:576-586, 1995.

170. Holland GN, Pepose JS, Pettit TH et al.: Acquired immune deficiency syndrome: ocular manifestations, *Ophthalmology* 90:859-873, 1983.

171. Holland GN, Pepose JS, Simons KB et al.: Ocular disease in the aquired immune deficiency syndrome: cilincopathological correlations. In Secchi AG, Fregona IA, editors: *Modern trends in immunology and immunopathology of the eye,* Milano, 1989, Masson S.p.A.

172. Holland GN, Sakamoto MJ, Hardy D et al.: Treatment of cytomegalovirus retinopathy in patients with acquired immunodeficiency syndrome: use of the experimental drug 9-[2-hydroxy-1-(hydroxymethyl)ethoxymethyl]guanine, *Arch Ophthalmol* 104:1794-1800, 1986.

173. Holland GN, Shuler JD: Progression rates of cytomegalovirus retinopathy in ganciclovir-treated and untreated patients, *Arch Ophthalmol* 110:1435-1442, 1992.

174. Holland GN, Sidikaro Y, Kreiger AE et al.: Treatment of cytomegalovirus retinopathy with ganciclovir, *Ophthalmology* 94:815-823, 1987.

175. Holland GN, Sison RF, Jatulis DE et al.: Survival of patients with the acquired immune deficiency syndrome after development of cytomegalovirus retinopathy: UCLA CMV Retinopathy Study Group, *Ophthalmology* 97:204-211, 1990.

176. Hoover DR, Saah AJ, Bacellar H et al.: Clinical manifestations of AIDS in the era of pneumocystis prophylaxis: multicenter AIDS Cohort Study, *N Engl J Med* 329:1922-1926, 1993.

177. Horwitz CA, Henle W, Henle G et al.: Heterophil-negative infectious mononucleosis and mononucleosis-like illnesses: laboratory confirmation of 43 cases, *Am J Med* 63:947-957, 1977.

178. Ihara T, Yasuda N, Isaji M et al.: Impaired cell-mediated immunity to cytomegalovirus (CMV) in leukemic children with prolonged CMV viruria, *Leuk Res* 18:485-491, 1994.

179. Irvine AR: Treatment of retinal detachment due to cytomegalovirus retinitis in patients with AIDS, *Trans Am Ophthalmol Soc* 89:349-363; discussion 363-367, 1991.

180. Jabs DA, Enger C, Bartlett JG: Cytomegalovirus retinitis and acquired immunodeficiency syndrome, *Arch Ophthalmol* 107:75-80, 1989.

181. Jabs DA, Enger C, Haller J, de Bustros S: Retinal detachments in patients with cytomegalovirus retinitis, *Arch Ophthalmol* 109:794-799, 1991.

182. Jabs DA, Green WR, Fox R et al.: Ocular manifestations of the acquired immune deficiency syndrome, *Ophthalmology* 96:1092-1099, 1989.

183. Jabs DA, Newman C, de Bustros S, Polk BF: Treatment of cytomegalovirus retinitis with ganciclovir, *Ophthalmology* 94:824-830, 1987.

184. Jabs DA, Wingard JR, de Bustros S et al.: BW B759U for cytomegalovirus retinitis: intraocular drug penetration, *Arch Ophthalmol* 104:1436-1437, 1986.

185. Jacobson MA, Causey D, Polsky B et al.: A dose-ranging study of daily maintenance intravenous foscarnet therapy for cytomegalovirus retinitis in AIDS, *J Infect Dis* 168:444-448, 1993.

186. Jacobson MA, Drew WL, Feinberg J et al.: Foscarnet therapy for ganciclovir-resistant cytomegalovirus retinitis in patients with AIDS, *J Infect Dis* 163:1348-1351, 1991.

187. Jacobson MA, Kramer F, Basiakos Y et al.: Randomised phase 1 trial of two different combination foscarnet and ganciclovir chronic maintenance regimens for AIDS patients with cytomegalovirus retinitis: AIDS clinical trials group protocol 151, *J Infect Dis* 170:189-193, 1994.

188. Jacobson MA, Mills J: Serious cytomegalovirus disease in the acquired immunodeficiency syndrome (AIDS): clinical findings, diagnosis, and treatment, *Ann Intern Med* 108:585-594, 1988.

189. Jacobson MA, O'Donnell JJ, Brodie HR et al.: Randomized prospective trial of ganciclovir maintenance therapy for cytomegalovirus retinitis, *J Med Virol* 25:339-349, 1988.

190. Jacobson MA, O'Donnell JJ, Mills J: Foscarnet treatment of cytomegalovirus retinitis in patients with the acquired immunodeficiency syndrome, *Antimicrob Agents Chemother* 33:736-741, 1989.

191. Jacobson MA, O'Donnell JJ, Porteous D et al.: Retinal and gastrointestinal disease due to cytomegalovirus in patients with the acquired immune deficiency syndrome: prevalence, natural history, and response to ganciclovir therapy, *QJM* 67:473-486, 1988.

192. Jampol LM: Ocular findings of acute cytomegalovirus infection, *N Engl J Med* 307:1584, 1982 (letter).

193. Jason J, Lui KJ, Ragni MV et al.: Risk of developing AIDS in HIV-infected cohorts of hemophilic and homosexual men, *JAMA* 261:725-727, 1989.

194. Jennens ID, Lucas CR, Sandland AM et al.: Cytomegalovirus cultures during maintenance DHPG therapy for cytomegalovirus (CMV) retinitis in acquired immunodeficiency syndrome (AIDS), *J Med Virol* 30:42-44, 1990.

195. Jensen OA, Gerstoft J, Thomsen HK, Marner K: Cytomegalovirus retinitis in the acquired immunodeficiency syndrome (AIDS): light-microscopical, ultrastructural and immunohistochemical examination of a case, *Acta Ophthalmol (Copenh)* 62:1-9, 1984.

196. Jensen OA, Klinken L: Pathology of the brain and the eye in the acquired immune deficiency syndrome (AIDS): a comparison of lesions in consecutive autopsy material, *Ampis* 97:325-333, 1989.

197. Jonckheer T, de Selys A, Pierre C et al.: [Retinitis in an infant infected with HIV] Retinite chez un nourrisson infecte par le VIH, *Arch Fr Pediatr* 47:585-586, 1990.

198. Jordan MC, Mar VL: Spontaneous activation of latent cytomegalovirus from murine spleen explants: role of lymphocytes and macrophages in release and replication of virus, *J Clin Invest* 70:762-768, 1982.

199. Jordan MC, Takagi JL, Stevens JG: Activation of latent murine cytomegalovirus in vivo and in vitro: a pathogenetic role for acute infection, *J Infect Dis* 145:699-705, 1982.

200. Kahan BD: Immunosuppressive therapy with cyclosporine for cardiac transplantation, *Circulation* 75:40-56, 1987.

201. Kalfayan B: Inclusion disease in infancy, *Arch Pathol* 44:467-476, 1947.

202. Kane RC, Rousseau WE, Noble GR et al.: Cytomegalovirus infection in a volunteer blood donor population, *Infect Immun* 11:719-723, 1975.

203. Katz MH, Hessol NA, Buchbinder SP et al.: Temporal trends of opportunistic infections and malignancies in homosexual men with AIDS, *J Infect Dis* 170:198-202, 1994.

204. Keay S, Petersen E, Icenogle T et al.: Ganciclovir treatment of serious cytomegalovirus infection in heart and heart-lung transplant recipients, *Rev Infect Dis* 10(suppl 3):S563-S572, 1988.

205. Keefe KS, Freeman WR, Peterson TJ et al.: Atypical healing of cytomegalovirus retinitis: significance of persistent border opacification, *Ophthalmology* 99:1377-1384, 1992.

206. Keith CG, La Nauze J: Cytomegalovirus retinitis, *Med J Aust* 1:24-26, 1980.

207. Keller R, Peitchel R, Goldman JN, Goldman M: An IgG-Fc receptor induced in cytomegalovirus-infected human fibroblasts, *J Immunol* 116:772-777, 1976.

208. Kestelyn P: Ocular problems in AIDS, *Int Ophthalmol* 14:165-172, 1990.

209. Khadem M, Kalish SB, Goldsmith J et al.: Ophthalmologic findings in acquired immune deficiency syndrome (AIDS), *Arch Ophthalmol* 102:201-206, 1984.

210. Kinney JS, Onorato IM, Stewart JA et al.: Cytomegaloviral infection and disease, *J Infect Dis* 151:772-774, 1985.

211. Klemola E, Kaariainen L: Cytomegalovirus as a possible cause of a disease resembling infectious mononucleosis, *BMJ* 5470:1099-1102, 1965.

212. Klemola E, Stenstrom R, Essen RV: Pneumonia as a clinical manifestation of cytomegalovirus infection in previously healthy adults, *Scand J Infect Dis* 4:7-10, 1972.

213. Klotman ME, Henry SC, Greene RC et al.: Detection of mouse cytomegalovirus nucleic acid in latently infected mice by in vitro enzymatic amplification, *J Infect Dis* 161:220-225, 1990.

214. Knowles WA: In-vitro cultivation of human cytomegalovirus in thyroid epithelial cells, *Arch Virol* 50:119-124, 1976.

215. Kotler DP, Culpepper-Morgan JA, Tierney AR, Klein EB: Treatment of disseminated cytomegalovirus infection with 9-(1,3 dihydroxy-2-propoxymethyl)guanine: evidence of prolonged survival in patients with the acquired immunodeficiency syndrome, *AIDS Res* 2:299-308, 1986.

216. Krech U: Complement-fixing antibodies against cytomegalovirus in different parts of the world, *Bull World Health Organ* 49:103-106, 1973.

217. Kreiger AE, Foos RY, Yoshizumi MO: Intravitreous granulation tissue and retinal detachment following pars plana injection for cytomegalovirus retinopathy, *Graefes Arch Clin Exp Ophthalmol* 230:197-198, 1992.

218. Kuhls TL, Viker S, Parris NB et al.: Occupational risk of HIV, HBV and HSV-2 infections in health care personnel caring for AIDS patients, *Am J Public Health* 77:1306-1309, 1987.

219. Kuppermann BD, Flores-Aguilar M, Quiceno JI et al.: A masked prospective evaluation of outcome parameters for cytomegalovirus-related retinal detachment surgery in patients with acquired immune deficiency syndrome, *Ophthalmology* 101:46-55, 1994.

220. Kuppermann BD, Petty JG, Richman DD et al.: Correlation between CD4+ counts and prevalence of cytomegalovirus retinitis and human immunodeficiency virus-related noninfectious retinal vasculopathy in patients with acquired immunodeficiency syndrome, *Am J Ophthalmol* 115:575-582, 1993.

221. Kuppermann BD, Quiceno JI, Flores-Aguilar M et al.: Intravitreal ganciclovir concentration after intravenous administration in AIDS patients with cytomegalovirus retinitis: implications for therapy, *J Infect Dis* 168:1506-1509, 1993.

222. Lafemina RL, Hayward GS: Differences in cell-type-specific blocks to immediate early gene expression and DNA replication of human, simian and murine cytomegalovirus, *J Gen Virol* 69:355-374, 1988.

223. Landini MP, Michelson S: Human cytomegalovirus proteins, *Prog Med Virol* 35:152-185, 1988.

224. Landini MP, Mirolo G, Coppolecchia P et al.: Serum antibodies to individual cytomegalovirus structural polypeptides in renal transplant recipients during viral infection, *Microbiol Immunol* 30:683-695, 1986.

225. Landini MP, Rossier E, Schmitz H: Antibodies to human cytomegalovirus structural polypeptides during primary infection, *J Virol Methods* 22:309-317, 1988.

226. Lang DJ, Ebert PA, Rodgers BM et al.: Reduction of postperfusion cytomegalovirus-infections following the use of leukocyte depleted blood, *Transfusion* 17:391-395, 1977.

227. Leach CT, Detels R, Hennessey K et al.: A longitudinal study of cytomegalovirus infection in human immunodeficiency virus type 1-seropositive homosexual men: molecular epidemiology and association with disease progression, *J Infect Dis* 170:293-298, 1994.

228. Lee S, Ai E: Disc neovascularization in patients with AIDS and cytomegalovirus retinitis, *Retina* 11:305-308, 1991.

229. Lehoang P, Girard B, Robinet M et al.: Foscarnet in the treatment of cytomegalovirus retinitis in acquired immune deficiency syndrome, *Ophthalmology* 96:865-873; discussion 873-874, 1989.

230. Levin AV, Zeichner S, Duker JS et al.: Cytomegalovirus retinitis in an infant with acquired immunodeficiency syndrome, *Pediatrics* 84:683-687, 1989.

231. Levin MJ, Rinaldo CR, Leary PL et al.: Immune response to herpesvirus antigens in adults with acute cytomegaloviral mononucleosis, *J Infect Dis* 140:851-857, 1979.

232. Levy E, Sarov I: Determination of IgA antibodies to human cytomegalovirus by enzyme-linked immunosorbent assay (ELISA), *J Med Virol* 6:249-257, 1980.

233. Lieberman RM, Orellana J, Melton RC: Efficacy of intravitreal foscarnet in a patient with AIDS, *N Engl J Med* 330:868-869, 1994 (letter).

234. Lim JI, Enger C, Haller JA et al.: Improved visual results after surgical repair of cytomegalovirus-related retinal detachments, *Ophthalmology* 101:264-269, 1994.

235. Linnemann CC, Kauffman CA, First MR et al.: Cellular immune response to cytomegalovirus infection after renal transplantation, *Infect Immun* 22:176-180, 1978.

236. Lowder CY, Butler CP, Dodds EM et al.: CD8+ T lymphocytes and CMV retinitis in patients with AIDS, *Am J Ophthalmol* 120:283-290, 1995.

237. Lui SF, Ali AA, Grundy JE et al.: Double-blind, placebo-controlled trial of human lymphoblastoid interferon prophylaxis of cytomegalovirus infection in renal transplant recipients, *Nephrol Dial Transplant* 7:1230-1237, 1992.

238. MacGregor RR, Pakola SJ, Graziani AL et al.: Evidence of active cytomegalovirus infection in clinically stable HIV-infected individuals with CD4-positive lymphocyte counts below $100/\mu l$ of blood: features and relationship to risk of subsequent CMV retinitis, *J Acquir Immune Defic Syndr Human Retrovirol* 1995 (in press).

239. Madge GE: Cytomegalovirus infection of the eye in a case of renal homotransplantation, *Med Coll Va Q* 8:251-255, 1972.

240. Malek GH, Kisken WA: Problems in diagnosis and treatment in renal transplantation, *Am J Surg* 119:334-336, 1970.

241. Manischewitz JF, Quinnan GV, Lane HC, Wittek AE: Synergistic effect of ganciclovir and foscarnet on cytomegalovirus replication in vitro, *Antimicrob Agents Chemother* 34:373-375, 1990.

242. Manschot WA, Daaman CBF: A case of cytomegalic inclusion disease with ocular involvement, *Ophthalmologica* 143:137-140, 1962.

243. Marmor MF, Egbert PR, Egbert BM, Marmor JB: Optic nerve head involvement with cytomegalovirus in an adult with lymphoma, *Arch Ophthalmol* 96:1252-1254, 1978.

244. Marsano L, Perrillo RP, Flye MW et al.: Comparison of culture and serology for the diagnosis of cytomegalovirus infection in kidney and liver transplant recipients, *J Infect Dis* 161:454-461, 1990.

245. Marshall GS, Stout GG, Knights ME et al.: Ontogeny of glycoprotein gB-specific antibody and neutralizing activity during natural cytomegalovirus infection, *J Med Virol* 43:77-83, 1994.

246. Martin DC, Katzenstein DA, Yu GS, Jordan MC: Cytomegalovirus viremia detected by molecular hybridization and electron microscopy, *Ann Intern Med* 100:222-225, 1984.

247. Martin DF, Parks DJ, Mellow SD et al.: Treatment of cytomegalovirus retinitis with an intraocular sustained-release ganciclovir implant: a randomized controlled clinical trial, *Arch Ophthalmol* 112:1531-1539, 1994.

248. Martinez J, St Jeor SC: Molecular cloning and analysis of three cDNA clones homologous to human cytomegalovirus RNAs present during late infection, *J Virol* 60:531-538, 1986.

249. Masdeu JC, Small CB, Weiss L et al.: Multifocal cytomegalovirus encephalitis in AIDS, *Ann Neurol* 23:97-99, 1988.

250. Matthews RE: Third report of the International Committee on Taxonomy of Viruses. Classification and nomenclature of viruses, *Intervirology* 12:129-296, 1979.

251. McCann JD, Margolis TP, Wong MG et al.: A sensitive and specific polymerase chain reaction based assay for the diagnosis of CMV retinitis, *Am J Ophthalmol* 120:219-226, 1995.

252. McCannel C, Holland GN, Helm CJ et al.: Causes of uveitis in the general practice of ophthalmology, *Am J Ophthalmol* 1995 (in press).

253. McCracken GH, Shinefield HMR, Cobb K et al.: Congenital cytomegalic inclusion disease: a longitudinal study of 20 patients, *Am J Dis Child* 117:522-539, 1969.

254. McKenzie R, Travis WD, Dolan SA et al.: The causes of death in patients with human immunodeficiency virus infection: a clinical and pathologic study with emphasis on the role of pulmonary diseases, *Medicine (Baltimore)* 70:326-343, 1991.

255. Mercer JA, Wiley CA, Spector DH: Pathogenesis of murine cytomegalovirus infection: identification of infected cells in the spleen during acute and latent infections, *J Virol* 62:987-997, 1988.

256. Meredith TA, Aaberg TM, Reeser FH: Rhegmatogenous retinal detachment complicating cytomegalovirus retinitis, *Am J Ophthalmol* 87:793-796, 1979.

257. Meyers JD, Flournoy N, Thomas ED: Nonbacterial pneumonia after allogeneic marrow transplantation: a review of ten years' experience, *Rev Infect Dis* 4:1119-1132, 1982.

258. Michelson S, Alcami J, Kim SJ et al.: Human cytomegalovirus infection induces transcription and secretion of transforming growth factor beta 1, *J Virol* 68:5730-5737, 1994.

259. Miklos G, Orban T: Ophthalmic lesions due to cytomegalic inclusion disease. *Ophthalmologica* 148:98-106, 1964.

260. Millar AB, Patou G, Miller RF et al.: Cytomegalovirus in the lungs of patients with AIDS: respiratory pathogen or passenger? *Am Rev Respir Dis* 141:1474-1477, 1990.

261. Minders WH: Die aetiologie der cytomegalia infantum, *Schweiz Med Wochenschr* 83:1180-1182, 1953.

262. Miralles GD: Cytomegalovirus retinitis: when looks can deceive, *Lancet* 342:51-52, 1993 (letter).

263. Mitchell SM, Fox JD, Tedder RS et al.: Vitreous fluid sampling and viral genome detection for the diagnosis of viral retinitis in patients with AIDS, *J Med Virol* 43:336-340, 1994.

264. Mocarski ES, Stinski MF: Persistence of the cytomegalovirus genome in human cells, *J Virol* 31:761-775, 1979.

265. Moeller MB, Gutman RA, Hamilton JD: Acquired cytomegalovirus retinitis: four new cases and a review of the literature with implications for management, *Am J Nephrol* 2:251-255, 1982.

266. Mondino BJ, Sidikaro Y, Mayer FJ, Sumner HL: Inflammatory mediators in the vitreous humor of AIDS patients with retinitis, *Invest Ophthalmol Vis Sci* 31:798-804, 1990.

267. Montaner JS, Le T, Hogg R et al.: The changing spectrum of AIDS index diseases in Canada, *AIDS* 8:693-696, 1994.

268. Morinelli EN, Dugel PU, Lee M et al.: Opportunistic intraocular infections in AIDS, *Trans Am Ophthalmol Soc* 90:97-108; discussion 108-109, 1992.

269. Muller-Jensen K, Fischer JT, Meyer HJ: Transient spontaneous regression of cytomegalovirus retinitis in AIDS, *Ophthalmologica* 203:154-156, 1991.

270. Murayama T, Kuno K, Jisaki F et al.: Enhancement human cytomegalovirus replication in a human lung fibroblast cell line by interleukin-8, *J Virol* 68:7582-7585, 1994.

271. Murray HW, Knox DL, Green WR, Susel RM: Cytomegalovirus retinitis in adults: a manifestation of disseminated viral infection, *Am J Med* 63:574-584, 1977.

272. Murray JF, Felton CP, Garay SM et al.: Pulmonary complications of the acquired immunodeficiency syndrome: report of a National Heart, Lung, and Blood Institute workshop, *N Engl J Med* 310:1682-1688, 1984.

273. Myerson D, Hackman RC, Nelson JA et al.: Widespread presence of histologically occult cytomegalovirus, *Hum Pathol* 15:430-439, 1984.

274. Navia BA, Jordan BD, Price RW: The AIDS dementia complex: I. Clinical features, *Ann Neurol* 19:517-524, 1986.

275. Neuwirth J, Gutman I, Hofeldt AJ et al.: Cytomegalovirus retinitis in a young homosexual male with acquired immunodeficiency, *Ophthalmology* 89:805-808, 1982.

276. Newman NM, Mandel MR, Gullett J, Fujikawa L: Clinical and histologic findings in opportunistic ocular infections: part of a new syndrome of acquired immunodeficiency, *Arch Ophthalmol* 101:396-401, 1983.

277. Newsome DA, Green WR, Miller ED et al.: Microvascular aspects of acquired immune deficiency syndrome retinopathy, *Am J Ophthalmol* 98:590-601, 1984.

278. Nigro G, Scholz H, Bartmann U: Ganciclovir therapy for symptomatic congenital cytomegalovirus infection in infants: a two-regimen experience, *J Pediatr* 124:318-322, 1994.

279. Norbeck DW, Kern E, Hayashi S et al.: Cyclobut-A and cyclobut-G: broad-spectrum antiviral agents with potential utility for the therapy of AIDS, *J Med Chem* 33:1281-1285, 1990.

280. Oberman AE, Chatterjee SN: Ocular complications in renal transplant recipients, *West J Med* 123:184-187, 1975.

281. Orellana J, Teich SA, Friedman AH et al.: Combined short- and long-term therapy for the treatment of cytomegalovirus retinitis using ganciclovir (BW B759U), *Ophthalmology* 94:831-838, 1987.

282. Orellana J, Teich SA, Lieberman RM et al.: Treatment of retinal detachments in patients with the acquired immune deficiency syndrome, *Ophthalmology* 98:939-943, 1991.

283. Palestine AG, Polis MA, De Smet MD et al.: A randomized, controlled trial of foscarnet in the treatment of cytomegalovirus retinitis in patients with AIDS, *Ann Intern Med* 115:665-673, 1991.

284. Palestine AG, Rodrigues MM, Macher AM et al.: Ophthalmic involvement in acquired immunodeficiency syndrome, *Ophthalmology* 91:1092-1099, 1984.

285. Palestine AG, Stevens GJ, Lane HC et al.: Treatment of cytomegalovirus retinitis with dihydroxy propoxymethyl guanine, *Am J Ophthalmol* 101:95-101, 1986.

286. Pass RF: Epidemiology and transmission of cytomegalovirus, *J Infect Dis* 152:243-248, 1985.

287. Pass RF, Dworsky ME, Whitley RJ et al.: Specific lymphocyte blastogenic responses in children with cytomegalovirus and herpes simplex virus infections acquired early in infancy, *Infect Immun* 34:166-170, 1981.

288. Pass RF, Hutto C, Ricks R, Cloud GA: Increased rate of cytomegalovirus infection among parents of children attending day-care centers, *N Engl J Med* 314:1414-1418, 1986.

289. Pass RF, Little EA, Stagno S et al.: Young children as a probable source of maternal and congenital cytomegalovirus infection, *N Engl J Med* 316:1366-1370, 1987.

290. Pass RF, Stagno S, Dworsky ME et al.: Excretion of cytomegalovirus in mothers: observations after delivery of congenitally infected and normal infants, *J Infect Dis* 146:1-6, 1982.

291. Pass RF, Stagno S, Myers GJ, Alford CA: Outcome of symptomatic congenital cytomegalovirus infection: results of long-term longitudinal follow-up, *Pediatrics* 66:758-762, 1980.

292. Paya CV, Smith TF, Ludwig J, Hermans PE: Rapid shell vial culture and tissue histology compared with serology for the rapid diagnosis of cytomegalovirus infection in liver transplantation, *Mayo Clin Proc* 64:670-675, 1989.

293. Pepose JS, Hilborne LH, Cancilla PA, Foos RY: Concurrent herpes simplex and cytomegalovirus retinitis and encephalitis in the acquired immune deficiency syndrome (AIDS), *Ophthalmology* 91:1669-1677, 1984.

294. Pepose JS, Holland GN, Nestor MS et al.: Acquired immune deficiency syndrome: pathogenic mechanisms of ocular disease, *Ophthalmology* 92:472-484, 1985.

295. Pepose JS, Newman C, Bach MC et al.: Pathologic features of cytomegalovirus retinopathy after treatment with the antiviral agent ganciclovir, *Ophthalmology* 94:414-424, 1987.

296. Pertel P, Hirschtick R, Phair J et al.: Risk of developing cytomegalovirus retinitis in persons infected with the human immunodeficiency virus, *J Acquir Immune Defic Syndr* 5:1069-1074, 1992.

297. Petrie BL, Melnick JL, Adam E et al.: Nucleic acid sequences of cytomegalovirus in cells cultured from human arterial tissue, *J Infect Dis* 155:158-159, 1987 (letter).

298. Pillay D, Lipman MC, Lee CA et al.: A clinico-pathological audit of opportunistic viral infections in HIV-infected patients, *AIDS* 7:969-974, 1993.

299. Plotkin SA, Starr SE, Friedman HM et al.: Effect of Towne live virus vaccine on cytomegalovirus disease after renal transplant: a controlled trial, *Ann Intern Med* 114:525-531, 1991.

300. Polis MA, deSmet MD, Baird BF et al.: Increased survival of a cohort of patients with acquired immunodeficiency syndrome and cytomegalovirus retinitis who received sodium phosphonoformate (foscarnet), *Am J Med* 94:175-180, 1993.

301. Pollard RB, Egbert PR, Gallagher JG, Merigan TC: Cytomegalovirus retinitis in immunosuppressed hosts: I. Natural history and effects of treatment with adenine arabinoside, *Ann Intern Med* 93:655-664, 1980.

302. Pollard RB, Rand KH, Arvin AM, Merigan TC: Cell-mediated immunity of cytomegalovirus infection in normal subjects and cardiac transplant patients, *J Infect Dis* 137:541-549, 1978.

303. Pomerantz RJ, Kuritzkes DR, de la Monte SM et al.: Infection of the retina by human immunodeficiency virus type I, *N Engl J Med* 317:1643-1647, 1987.

304. Pomeroy C, Filice GA, Hitt JA, Jordan MC: Cytomegalovirus-induced reactivation of Toxoplasma gondii pneumonia in mice: lung lymphocyte phenotypes and suppressor function, *J Infect Dis* 166:677-681, 1992.

305. Pomeroy C, Hilleren PJ, Jordan MC: Latent murine cytomegalovirus DNA in splenic stromal cells of mice, *J Virol* 65:3330-3334, 1991.

306. Porter R, Crombie AL, Gardner PS, Uldall RP: Incidence of ocular complications in patients undergoing renal transplantation, *BMJ* 3:133-136, 1972.

307. Prince AM, Szmuness W, Millian SJ, David DS: A serologic study of cytomegalovirus infections associated with blood transfusions, *N Engl J Med* 284:1125-1131, 1971.

308. Pritchard JA, Nelson JM, Burns L et al.: Infections caused by central venous catheters in patients with aquired immune deficiency syndrome, *South Med J* 81:1496-1498, 1988.

309. Qavi HB, Green MT, SeGall GK, Font RL: Demonstration of HIV-1 and HHV-6 in AIDS-associated retinitis, *Curr Eye Res* 8:379-387, 1989.

310. Quinlan MF, Salmon JF: Ophthalmic complications after heart transplantation, *J Heart Lung Transplant* 12:252-255, 1993.

311. Quinn TC, Piot P, McCormick JB et al.: Serologic and immunologic studies in patients with AIDS in North America and Africa: the potential role of infectious agents as cofactors in human immunodeficiency virus infection, *JAMA* 257:2617-2621, 1987.

312. Quinnan GV, Kirmani N, Rook AH et al.: Cytotoxic t cells in cytomegalovirus infection: HLA-restricted T-lymphocyte and non-T-lymphocyte cytotoxic responses correlate with recovery from cytomegalovirus infection in bone-marrow-transplant recipients, *N Engl J Med* 307:7-13, 1982.

313. Randazzo RF, Hulette CM, Gottlieb MS, Rajfer J: Cytomegaloviral epididymitis in a patient with the acquired immune deficiency syndrome, *J Urol* 136:1095-1097, 1986.

314. Rao N, Waruszewski DT, Armstrong JA et al.: Evaluation of anticomplement immunofluorescence test in cytomegalovirus infection, *J Clin Microbiol* 6:633-638, 1977.

315. Rasmussen L, Matkin C, Spaete R et al.: Antibody response to human cytomegalovirus glycoproteins gB and gH after natural infection in humans, *J Infect Dis* 164:835-842, 1991.

316. Rasmussen L, Morris S, Wolitz R et al.: Deficiency in antibody response to human cytomegalovirus glycoprotein gH in human immunodeficiency virus-infected patients at risk for cytomegalovirus retinitis, *J Infect Dis* 170:673-677, 1994.

317. Reigstad H, Bjerknes R, Markestad T, Myrmel H: Ganciclovir therapy of congenital cytomegalovirus disease, *Acta Paediatr* 81:707-708, 1992.

318. Reimer CB, Black CM, Phillips DJ et al.: The specificity of fetal IgM: antibody or anti-antibody? *Ann NY Acad Sci* 23:77-93, 1975.

319. Riddell SR, Watanabe KS, Goodrich JM et al.: Restoration of viral immunity in immunodeficient humans by the adoptive transfer of T cell clones, *Science* 257:238-241, 1992.

320. Ripalti A, Landini MP, Mocarski ES, La Placa M: Identification and preliminary use of recombinant lambda gt11 fusion proteins in human cytomegalovirus diagnosis, *J Gen Virol* 70:1247-1251, 1989.

321. Roarty JD, Fisher EJ, Nussbaum JJ: Long-term visual morbidity of cytomegalovirus retinitis in patients with acquired immune deficiency syndrome, *Ophthalmology* 100:1685-1688, 1993.

322. Robinson MR, Streeten BW, Hampton GR et al.: Treatment of cytomegalovirus optic neuritis with dihydroxy propoxymethyl guanine, *Am J Ophthalmol* 102:533-534, 1986.

323. Rodrigues MM, Palestine A, Nussenblatt R et al.: Unilateral cytomegalovirus retinochoroiditis and bilateral cytoid bodies in a bisexual man with the acquired immunodeficiency syndrome, *Ophthalmology* 90:1577-1582, 1983.

324. Rosecan LR, Stahl-Bayliss CM, Kalman CM, Laskin OL: Antiviral therapy for cytomegalovirus retinitis in AIDS with dihydroxy propoxymethyl guanine, *Am J Ophthalmol* 101:405-418, 1986.

325. Rosenberg PR, Uliss AE, Friedland GH et al.: Acquired immunodeficiency syndrome: ophthalmic manifestations in ambulatory patients, *Ophthalmology* 90:874-878, 1983.

326. Rowe WP, Hartley JW, Waterman S: Cytopathogenic agent resembling human salivary gland virus recovered from tissue cultures of human adenoid, *Proc Soc Exp Biol Med* 92:418-424, 1956.

327. Ruger R, Bornkamm GW, Fleckenstein B: Human cytomegalovirus DNA sequences with homologies to the cellular genome, *J Gen Virol* 65:1351-1364, 1984.

328. Ryning FW, Mills J: *Pneumocystis carinii, Toxoplasma gondii, Cytomegalovirus* and the compromised host, *West J Med* 130:18-34, 1979.

329. Rytel MW, Aaberg TM, Dee TH, Heim LH: Therapy of cytomegalovirus retinitis with transfer factor, *Cell Immunol* 19:8-21, 1975.

330. Said G, Lacroix C, Chemouilli P et al.: Cytomegalovirus neuropathy in acquired immunodeficiency syndrome: a clinical and pathological study, *Ann Neurol* 29:139-146, 1991.

331. Salmon D, Lacassin F, Harzic M et al.: Predictive value of cytomegalovirus viraemia for the occurrence of CMV organ involvement in AIDS, *J Med Virol* 32:160-163, 1990.

332. Saltzman RL, Quirk MR, Jordan MC: Disseminated cytomegalovirus infection: molecular analysis of virus and leukocyte interactions in viremia, *J Clin Invest* 81:75-81, 1988.

333. Saltzman RL, Quirk MR, Jordan MC: High levels of circulating cytomegalovirus DNA reflect visceral organ disease in viremic immunosuppressed patients other than marrow recipients, *J Clin Invest* 90:1832-1838, 1992.

334. Salvador F, Blanco R, Colin A et al.: Cytomegalovirus retinitis in pediatric acquired immunodeficiency syndrome: report of two cases, *J Pediatr Ophthalmol Strabismus* 30:159-162, 1993.

335. Sarraf D, Equi RA, Holland GN et al.: Transscleral iontophoresis of foscarnet, *Am J Ophthalmol* 115:748-754, 1993.

336. Schanzer MC, Font RL, O'Malley RE: Primary ocular malignant lymphoma associated with the acquired immune deficiency syndrome, *Ophthalmology* 98:88-91, 1991.

337. Schmitt-Graff A, Neuen-Jacob E, Rettig B, Sundmacher R: Evidence for cytomegalovirus and human immunodeficiency virus infection of the retina in AIDS, *Virchows Arch A Pathol Anat Histopathol* 416:249-253, 1990.

338. Schmitz H, Enders G: Cytomegalovirus as a frequent cause of Guillain-Barre syndrome, *J Med Virol* 1:21-27, 1977.

339. Scholz M, Hamann A, Blaheta RA et al.: Cytomegalovirus- and interferon-related effects on human endothelial cells: cytomegalovirus infection reduces upregulation of HLA class II antigen expression after treatment with interferon-gamma, *Hum Immunol* 35:230-238, 1992.

340. Schrier RD, Oldstone MB: Recent clinical isolates of cytomegalovirus suppress human cytomegalovirus-specific human leukocyte antigen-restricted cytotoxic T-lymphocyte activity, *J Virol* 59:127-131, 1986.

341. Schrier RD, Rice GP, Oldstone MB: Suppression of natural killer cell activity and T cell proliferation by fresh isolates of human cytomegalovirus, *J Infect Dis* 153:1084-1091, 1986.

342. Schuman JS, Friedman AH: Retinal manifestations of the acquired immune deficiency syndrome (AIDS): cytomegalovirus, candida albicans, cryptococcus, toxoplasmosis and *Pneumocystis carinii, Trans Ophthalmol Soc UK* 103:177-190, 1983.

343. Schuman JS, Orellana J, Friedman AH, Teich SA: Aquired immunodeficiency syndrome (AIDS), *Surv Ophthalmol* 31:384-410, 1987.

344. Schut RL, Gekker G, Hu S et al.: Cytomegalovirus replication in murine microglial cell cultures: suppression of permissive infection by interferon-gamma, *J Infect Dis* 169:1092-1096, 1994.

345. Schwaighofer H, Herold M, Schwarz T et al.: Serum levels of interleukin 6, interleukin 8, and C-reactive protein after human allogeneic bone marrow transplantation, *Transplantation* 58:430-436, 1994.

346. Seregard S: Retinochoroiditis in the acquired immune deficiency syndrome: findings in consecutive post-mortem examinations, *Acta Ophthalmol (Copenh)* 72:223-228, 1994.

347. Severi B, Landini MP, Musiani M: A study of the passage of human cytomegalovirus from the nucleus to the cytoplasm, *Microbiologica* 2:265-273, 1979.

348. Sha BE, Benson CA, Deutsch TA et al.: Suppression of cytomegalovirus retinitis in persons with AIDS with high-dose intravenous acyclovir, *J Infect Dis* 164:777-780, 1991.

349. Shanley JD: In vivo administration of monoclonal antibody to the NK 1.1 antigen of natural killer cells: effect on acute murine cytomegalovirus infection, *J Med Virol* 30:58-60, 1990.

350. Shanley JD, Jordan MC, Stevens JG: Modification by adoptive humoral immunity of murine cytomegalovirus infection, *J Infect Dis* 143:231-237, 1981.

351. Sidikaro Y, Silver L, Holland GN, Kreiger AE: Rhegmatogenous retinal detachments in patients with AIDS and necrotizing retinal infections, *Ophthalmology* 98:129-135, 1991.

352. Singh N, Yu VL, Mieles L et al.: High-dose acyclovir compared with short-course preemptive ganciclovir therapy to prevent cytomegalovirus disease in liver transplant recipients: a randomized trial, *Ann Intern Med* 120:375-381, 1994.

353. Sison RF, Holland GN, MacArthur LJ et al.: Cytomegalovirus retinopathy as the initial manifestation of the acquired immunodeficiency syndrome, *Am J Ophthalmol* 112:243-249, 1991 (published erratum appears in *Am J Ophthalmol* 112(5):618, 1991).

354. Sissons JG: The immunology of cytomegalovirus infection, *J R Coll Physicians Lond* 20:40-44, 1986.

355. Skolnik PR, Kosloff BR, Hirsch MS: Bidirectional interactions between human immunodeficiency virus type 1 and cytomegalovirus, *J Infect Dis* 157:508-514, 1988.

356. Skolnik PR, Pomerantz RJ, de la Monte SM et al.: Dual infection of retina with human immunodeficiency virus type 1 and cytomegalovirus, *Am J Ophthalmol* 107:361-372, 1989.

357. Skoutelis AT, Murphy RL, MacDonell KB et al.: Indwelling central venous catheter infections in patients with aquired immune deficiency syndrome, *J Acquir Immune Defic Syndr* 3:335-342, 1990.

358. Smith ME: Retinal involvement in adult cytomegalic inclusion disease, *Arch Ophthalmol* 72:44-49, 1964.

359. Smith ME, Zimmerman LE, Harley RD: Ocular involvement in congenital cytomegalic inclusion disease, *Arch Ophthalmol* 76:696-699, 1966.

360. Smith MG: Propargation of salivary gland virus of the mouse in tissue cultures. *Proc Soc Exp Biol Med* 86:434-440, 1954.

361. Smith PD, Lane HC, Gill VJ et al.: Intestinal infections in patients with the acquired immunodeficiency syndrome (AIDS): etiology and response to therapy, *Ann Intern Med* 108:328-333, 1988.

362. Smith TF, Holley KE, Keys TF, Macasaet FF: Cytomegalovirus studies of autopsy tissue: I. Virus isolation, *Am J Clin Pathol* 63:854-858, 1975.

363. Smith TJ: Intravitreal sustained-release ganciclovir, *Arch Ophthalmol* 110:255-258, 1992.

364. Snoeck R, Sakuma T, De Clercq E et al.: (S)-1-(3-hydroxy-2-phosphonylmethoxypropyl)cytosine, a potent and selective inhibitor of human cytomegalovirus replication, *Antimicrob Agents Chemother* 32:1839-1844, 1988.

365. Snydman DR, Werner BG, Heinze-Lacey B et al.: Use of cytomegalovirus immune globulin to prevent cytomegalovirus disease in renal-transplant recipients, *N Engl J Med* 317:1049-1054, 1987.

366. Somogyi T, Colimon R, Michelson S: An illustrated guide to the structure of the human cytomegalovirus genome and a review of transcription data, *Prog Med Virol* 33:99-133, 1986.

367. Spaide RF, Podhorzer J, Coleman S et al.: Risk factors for CMV retinitis, *American Academy of Ophthalmology Annual Meeting: Supp to Ophthalmol* 140, 1994 (abstract).

368. Spaide RF, Vitale AT, Toth IR, Oliver JM: Frosted branch angiitis associated with cytomegalovirus retinitis, *Am J Ophthalmol* 113:522-528, 1992.

369. Stagno S, Pass RF, Cloud G et al.: Primary cytomegalovirus infection in pregnancy: incidence, transmission to fetus, and clinical outcome, *JAMA* 256:1904-1908, 1986.

370. Stagno S, Pass RF, Dworsky ME et al.: Congenital cytomegalovirus infection: the relative importance of primary and recurrent maternal infection, *N Engl J Med* 306:945-949, 1982.

371. Stagno S, Reynolds DW, Amos CS et al.: Auditory and visual defects resulting from symptomatic and subclinical congenital cytomegaloviral and toxoplasma infections, *Pediatrics* 59:669-678, 1977.

372. Stagno S, Reynolds DW, Huang E et al.: Congenital cytomegalovirus infection: occurrence in an immune population, *N Engl J Med* 296:1254-1258, 1977.

373. Stagno S, Reynolds DW, Tsaiantos A et al.: Comparative serial viriologic and serologic studies of symptomatic and subclinical congenitally and natally acquired cytomegalovirus infections, *J Infect Dis* 132:568-577, 1975.

374. Stagno S, Whitley RJ: Herpesvirus infections of pregnancy: Part I: Cytomegalovirus and Epstein-Barr virus infections, *N Engl J Med* 313:1270-1274, 1985.

375. Stals FS, Bosman F, van Boven CP, Bruggeman CA: An animal model for therapeutic intervention studies of CMV infection in the immunocompromised host, *Arch Virol* 114:91-107, 1990.

376. Stanier P, Taylor DL, Kitchen AD et al.: Persistence of cytomegalovirus in mononuclear cells in peripheral blood from blood donors, *BMJ* 299:897-898, 1989.

377. Stanton CA, Sloan B III, Slusher MM, Greven CM: Acquired immunodeficiency syndrome-related primary intraocular lymphoma, *Arch Ophthalmol* 110:1614-1617, 1992.

378. Stern H, Hunnington G, Booth J, Moncrieff D: An early marker of fetal infection after primary cytomegalovirus infection in pregnancy, *BMJ* 292:718-720, 1986.

379. Stevens G, Palestine A, Rodrigues MM et al.: Failure of argon laser to halt cytomegalovirus retinitis, *Retina* 6:119-122, 1986.

380. Stevens JG: Human herpesviruses: a consideration of the latent state, *Microbiol Rev* 53:318-332, 1989.

381. Stinski M: Molecular biology of cytomegalovirus repliction. In Ho M, editors: *Cytomegalovirus: biology and infection,* ed 2, New York, 1991, Plenum.

382. Stinski MF, Thomsen DR, Whaten MW: Structure and function of the human cytomegalovirus genome. In Stinski MF, Thomsen DR, Whaten MW, editors: *The human herpesvirus, an interdisciplinary perspective,* New York, 1980, Elsevier.

383. Studies of Ocular Complications of AIDS (SOCA) Research Group in collaboration with the AIDS Clinical Trials Group (ACTG): Mortality in patients with the acquired immunodeficiency syndrome treated with either foscarnet or ganciclovir for cytomegalovirus retinitis, *N Engl J Med* 326:213-220, 1992.

384. Studies of Ocular Complications of AIDS (SOCA) Research Group in collaboration with the AIDS Clinical Trials Group (ACTG): Forscarnet-ganciclovir ctomegalovirus retinitis trial: IV. Visual outcomes, *Ophthalmology* 7:1250-1261, 1994.

385. Sullivan V, Coen DM: Isolation of foscarnet-resistant human cytomegalovirus patterns of resistance and sensitivity to other antiviral drugs, *J Infect Dis* 164:781-784, 1991.

386. Sundmacher R, Neumann-Haefelin D, Mattes A, Cantell K: Connatal monosymptomatic corneal endotheliitis by cytomegalovirus. In Sundmacher R, editors: *Herpetic eye diseases,* Munich, 1981, JF Bergmann Verlag.

387. Tarkkanen A, Merenmies L, Holmstrom T: Ocular involvement in congenital cytomegalic inclusion disease, *J Pediatr Ophthalmol* 9:82-86, 1972.

388. Teich SA, Castle J, Friedman AH et al.: Active cytomegalovirus particles in the eyes of an AIDS patient being treated with 9-[2-hydroxy-1-(hydroxymethyl) ethoxymethyl] guanine (ganciclovir), *Br J Ophthalmol* 72:293-298, 1988.

389. Thiboutot DM, Beckford A, Mart CR et al.: Cytomegalovirus diaper dermatitis, *Arch Dermatol* 127:396-398, 1991.

390. Tolpin MD, Stewart JA, Warren D et al.: Transfusion transmission of cytomegalovirus confirmed by restriction endonuclease analysis, *J Pediatr* 107:953-956, 1985.

391. Toorkey CB, Carrigan DR: Immunohistochemical detection of an immediate early antigen of human cytomegalovirus in normal tissues, *J Infect Dis* 160:741-751, 1989.

392. Toy JL, Knowlden RP: Cytomegalovirus retinitis misdiagnosed as Hodgkin's lymphoma deposits, *BMJ* 2:1398-1399, 1978.

393. Tsukahara I, Ueno I, Kawanishi H: Retinal changes in human cytomegalovirus infection: an electron microscopic study, *Am J Ophthalmol* 62:1153-1160, 1966.

394. Turtinen LW, Saltzman R, Jordan MC, Haase AT: Interactions of human cytomegalovirus with leukocytes in vivo: analysis by in situ hybridization, *Microb Pathog* 3:287-297, 1987.

395. Ussery FM, Gibson SR, Conklin RH et al.: Intravitreal ganciclovir in the treatment of AIDS-associated cytomegalovirus retinitis, *Ophthalmology* 95:640-648, 1988.

396. Von Glahn WC, Pappenheimer AM: Intranuclear inclusions in visceral disease, *Am J Pathol* 1:445-466, 1925.

397. Waldman WJ, Knight DA, VanBuskirk A et al.: Endothelial HLA class II induction mediated by allogeneic T cells activated by cytomegalovirus-infected cultured endothelial cells, *Transplant Proc* 25:1439-1440, 1993.

398. Wallow IH, Arnold W: Electron microscopic demonstration of intraretinal virus particle in cytomegalic inclusion disease, *Ophthalmic Res* 4:211-217, 1972.

399. Waris E, Rasanen O, Kreus KE, Kreus R: Fatal cytomegalovirus disease in a previously healthy adult, *Scand J Infect Dis* 4:61-67, 1972.

400. Webster A, Lee CA, Cook DG et al.: Cytomegalovirus infection and progression towards AIDS in haemophiliacs with human immunodeficiency virus infection, *Lancet* 2:63-66, 1989.

401. Weinberg DV, Murphy R, Naughton K: Combined daily therapy with intravenous ganciclovir and foscarnet for patients with recurrent cytomegalovirus retinitis, *Am J Ophthalmol* 117:776-782, 1994.

402. Weller TH, Hanshaw JB: Virologic and clinical observations on cytomegalic inclusion disease, *N Engl J Med* 266:1233-1244, 1962.

403. Weller TH, McCauley JC, Craig JM: Isolation of intranuclear producing agents from infants with illnesses resembling cytomegalovirus inclusion disease, *Proc Soc Exp Biol Med* 94:4-12, 1957.

404. Wentworth BB, Alexander ER: Seroepidemiology of infectious due to members of the herpesvirus group, *Am J Epidemiol* 94:496-507, 1971.

405. Wilcox CM: Esophageal disease in the acquired immunodeficiency syndrome: etiology, diagnosis, and management, *Am J Med* 92:412-421, 1992.

406. Wiley CA, Nelson JA: Role of human immunodeficiency virus and cytomegalovirus in AIDS encephalitis, *Am J Pathol* 133:73-81, 1988.

407. Winston DJ, Ho WG, Champlin RE: Cytomegalovirus infections after allogeneic bone marrow transplantation, *Rev Infect Dis* 12(suppl 7):S776-S792, 1990.

408. Wise TG, Manischewitz JE, Quinnan GV et al.: Latent cytomegalovirus infection of BALB/c mouse spleens detected by an explant culture technique, *J Gen Virol* 44:551-556, 1979.

409. Wolf DG, Spector SA: Early diagnosis of human cytomegalovirus disease in transplant recipients by DNA amplification in plasma, *Transplantation* 56:330-334, 1993.

410. Wyatt JP, Saxton J, Lee RS: Generalized cytomegalic inclusion disease. *J Pediatr* 36:271-294, 1950.

411. Wyhinny GJ, Apple DJ, Guastella FR, Vygantas CM: Adult cytomegalic inclusion retinitis, *Am J Ophthalmol* 76:773-781, 1973.

412. Yamashiroya HM, Ghosh L, Yang R, Robertson AL: Herpesviridae in the coronary arteries and aorta of young trauma victims, *Am J Pathol* 130:71-79, 1988.

413. Yeager AS, Grumet FC, Hafleigh EB et al.: Prevention of transfusion-acquired cytomegalovirus infections in newborn infants, *J Pediatr* 98:281-287, 1981.

414. Yoshizumi MO, Lee D, Vinci V, Fajardo S: Ocular toxicity of multiple intravitreal DHPG injections, *Graefes Arch Clin Exp Ophthalmol* 228:350-355, 1990.

415. Youle MS, Gazzard BG, Johnson MA et al.: Effects of high-dose oral acyclovir on herpesvirus disease and survival in patients with advanced HIV disease: a double-blind, placebo-controlled study: European-Australian Acyclovir Study Group, *AIDS* 8:641-649, 1994.

416. Young SH, Morlet N, Heery S et al.: High dose intravitreal ganciclovir in the treatment of cytomegalovirus retinitis, *Med J Aust* 157:370-373, 1992.

417. Zurlo JJ, O'Neill D, Polis MA et al.: Lack of clinical utility of cytomegalovirus blood and urine cultures in patients with HIV infection, *Ann Intern Med* 118:12-17, 1993.

Appendix 81-1: Terminology Used in the Evaluation and Management of CMV Retinitis

I. Lesion characteristics
  A. Satellites: Small discrete opacities at the interface between infected and uninfected retina; correspond to early sites of CMV infection.
  B. Lesion border: The interface between infected and uninfected retina, where virus replication occurs, and where activity of disease and response to treatment are assessed. For study purposes, the border is usually considered a strip of retina, 1000 microns wide, that encompasses all satellite lesions.
  C. Lesion types (used only to describe untreated lesions)
    1. Fulminant/edematous lesions: Characterized by dense, confluent areas of retinal opacification in the lesion border through which choroidal details cannot be seen; hemorrhage sufficient to obscure underlying choroidal or retinal detail; absence of a clear central atrophic area, unless the lesion involves more than 25% of the retina. Other characteristics that are suggestive, but not required, include a perivascular location and inflammatory vascular sheathing. Patients with fulminant/edematous lesions who have severe and extensive inflammatory sheathing of retinal vessels in areas remote from foci of infection are sometimes considered to have frosted branch angiitis.
    2. Indolent/granular lesions: Characterized by faint or grainy retinal opacification in all areas of the lesion border, through which choroidal details can be seen; a few punctate or no hemorrhages; and no inflammatory vascular sheathing. Other characteristics suggestive, but not required, include a circular or oval shape and the presence of a clear atrophic central area.
  D. Disease activity
    1. Active lesions: Those lesions with opaque or white borders caused by edema and necrosis, indicating persistent virus production. Persistent opacities in the central portions of lesions may represent gliosis or calcification and are not considered to be signs of active infection.
    2. Inactive lesions (quiescent disease): Those lesions with no opacity of the border.
II. Location of lesions
  A. Retinal zones*
    1. Zone 1: The area extending 3000 microns from the center of the fovea or 1500 microns from the border of the optic disc; CMV retinitis in this area is considered immediately vision-threatening. For reference in calculating distances, the optic disc is commonly assumed to be 1500 microns in diameter.
    2. Zone 2: The area anterior to zone 1 and extending to the anterior border of the ampullae of the vortex veins; generally the farthest area anteriorly that can be photographed easily.
    3. Zone 3: The area anterior to Zone 2, extending to the ora serrata.
    4. Peripheral disease: An inexact term generally used to denote lesions in Zones 2 and 3 only.
III. Evolution of lesions
  A. Border advancement:* Movement of an active lesion border into previously uninfected retina, resulting in enlargement of a lesion. Coalescence of satellite lesions is not considered border advancement. Slow, continued advancement of lesion borders is sometimes referred to as ''smoldering disease.''
  B. Progression:* Enlargement of preexisting lesions (identified on retinal photographs as border advancement) or development of discrete new lesions. Progression is not defined by changes in disease activity.
  C. Changes in disease activity:* Used to describe active lesions when progression has not occurred; based on changes in the density of border opacification, its homogeneity and confluence, and the ability to see underlying choroidal details; used as a predictor of eventual lesion evolution.
    1. Stabilization: No change in border opacification.
    2. Improvement: Any area of decreased border activity without increased activity elsewhere; assumed to signify decreased virus production. Also termed regression.
    3. Deterioration: Any area of increased border activity (including coalescence of satellite lesions), regardless of changes elsewhere; assumed to signify increased virus production. Progression (enlargement of lesions) usually follows deterioration after a short period of time.
    4. Relapse (reactivation): Recurrence of border activity after a period of disease quiescence.

---

*Adapted from: Holland GN, Buhles WC, Mastre B et al.: A controlled retrospective study on ganciclovir treatment for cytomegalovirus retinopathy: use of a standardized system for the assessment of disease outcome, *Arch Ophthalmol* 107:1759-1766, 1989.

82 Varicella-Zoster Virus Diseases: Posterior Segment of the Eye

WILLIAM W. CULBERTSON, RICHARD D. DIX

Varicella-zoster virus (VZV) is an uncommon cause of necrotizing retinitis that occurs both in healthy and immunocompromised patients, with or without other systemic manifestations of VZV infection. Retinitis develops either from reactivation of latent, previously acquired VZV infection or during the course of primary infection. Clinical disease usually conforms to typical patterns of retinitis such as acute retinal necrosis (ARN) syndrome or progressive outer retinal necrosis (PORN) syndrome. Visual consequences may be mild or severe, usually from retinal detachment. Medical and surgical management is only partially effective in preventing vision loss. The pathogenesis of the retinitis is poorly understood; knowledge regarding the site(s) of latency, the factor(s) responsible for VZV reactivation, and the manner by which the virus gains access to the eye remains incomplete.

HISTORICAL BACKGROUND

Before the late 1970s very few cases of presumed VZV retinitis had been published.[26,45,147,255] The retinitis was always reported in association with zoster ophthalmicus, both in healthy and immunocompromised patients. Nonspecific descriptions of the fundus findings in these patients included retinochoroiditis and papillitis.

In 1971 Urayama and associates in Japan reported six cases of what they called *unilateral acute uveitis with retinal periarteritis and detachment.*[294] This disorder, which was later shown to be caused by either VZV or herpes simplex virus (HSV), had been known in Japan as *Kirisawa uveitis,* named in honor of Professor Nagonori Kirisawa in Sendai, Japan. In this beautifully illustrated paper, Urayama and associates emphasized the distinguishing features of VZV retinitis: peripheral retinal necrosis, retinal arteritis, vitritis, and late rhegmatogenous retinal detachment. Additional descriptive papers were reported over the next 10 years in Japan.[16,159,211] Western authors, apparently unaware of the Japanese papers, began reporting similar cases with names such as *vasoocclusive retinitis*[305] or *bilateral acute retinal necrosis* (BARN).* In 1982 Fisher and associates[86] summarized the cases that had been previously reported by the Japanese authors and by Western authors under the inclusive term *acute retinal necrosis.*

Culbertson and associates,[55] in a companion paper to that of Fisher and associates, demonstrated the presence of a member of the herpes virus family on histopathologic and electron microscopic evaluation of a blind eye enucleated during the active phase of ARN syndrome. Two years later VZV was demonstrated to be the specific causal agent for some cases of ARN syndrome.[58] Later studies showed that HSV could also cause an identical clinical picture.[78,110,166,182,183]

The retinitis in these early papers was reported to occur in healthy patients with no other recent systemic evidence of clinical VZV infection. Later it was shown that VZV retinitis occasionally occurred during the course of varicella (chickenpox)[46,155,186,188,189] or following cutaneous zoster (shingles),[27,311,319] and that it could occur in immunocompromised patients.[90,143] PORN syndrome, which is clinically distinct and occurs in patients with advanced AIDS, was first described by Forster and associates[87] in 1989. In 1994 Engstrom and associates[84] published a large series of cases with PORN syndrome and established specific diagnostic criteria for this clinical entity.

Recently Holland and the American Uveitis Society have attempted to define and unify the spectrum of presumed herpetic retinitis under the umbrella designation *necrotizing herpetic retinopathy* (see Acute VZV Retinitis).[128]

EPIDEMIOLOGY

The prevalence of VZV retinitis has been found to be nearly equal in men and women. The age of individuals developing the disease ranges from the newborn period to the ninth decade of life, although the majority of cases de-

---

*References 178, 225, 242, 244, 263, 292, 313.

velop in the fifth to seventh decades of life.[54,66,75] Both healthy and immunocompromised patients are affected. VZV retinitis may occur congenitally,[161,194] during the course of a primary infection associated with chickenpox,[59,189] or as a recurrence of latent, previously acquired infection.[51,53] There has been an observed tendency for VZV retinitis to develop during the fall and spring (unpublished data). The disease has been reported worldwide, but it is uncertain why it was not recognized and reported earlier than the 1970s. A genetic predisposition conferred by HLA subtypes has been reported in both the United States and Japan, as discussed later in this chapter.[130,181]

RISK FACTORS

Early descriptions of ARN syndrome characterized it as occurring in otherwise healthy individuals of all ages.[56,86] Subsequent reports, however, have indicated that other factors may predispose an individual to develop VZV-induced ARN syndrome.

Temporal Association with Outbreaks of Cutaneous Zoster

There are numerous reports of a recent episode of cutaneous zoster (including, but not exclusively zoster ophthalmicus) occurring before the onset of VZV-induced ARN syndrome in patients who are not overtly immunosuppressed.* For example, Browning and associates[27] described seven patients in whom ARN syndrome developed shortly after cutaneous zoster. The length of time between the skin infection and the ocular manifestations ranged from 5 days to 3 months. Only two of the seven cases involved the ophthalmic branch of the trigeminal nerve ipsilateral to the affected eye. In four of the patients the dermatitis was remote from the eye. Primary VZV infection (chickenpox) has also been observed to precede VZV retinitis,† usually within one month before the development of ocular disease. In contrast to typical ARN syndrome, however, cases occurring after recent chickenpox have been found to be less severe[59,186,189] and resemble a mild form of retinitis described by Matsuo and associates.[187] Although chickenpox and cutaneous zoster are common disorders, only rarely does VZV retinitis occur in temporal association with them. Conversely a majority of healthy patients with ARN syndrome only occasionally exhibit a temporal association with outbreaks of cutaneous zoster or chickenpox. No doubt other factors, possibly related to one or more immune irregularities, ultimately contribute to the development of ARN syndrome in this patient population.

In sharp contrast, the onset of VZV retinitis in patients with AIDS is temporally related to recent outbreaks of cutaneous zoster in the majority of cases.[84,87,177] This association is not surprising because VZV is a common opportunistic pathogen in this population; as many as 21% of all AIDS patients report a recent history of cutaneous zoster.[145] Indeed, Engstrom and associates[84] documented a known history of cutaneous zoster in 22 of 33 (67%) patients with AIDS and PORN syndrome. In this series, however, active cutaneous disease at time of diagnosis of VZV retinitis was uncommon, although ocular disease coincident with an eruption of cutaneous zoster has been reported.[177]

Immunogenetics of the Host

Patients with VZV retinitis have been found to have certain HLA antigens more frequently than the general population. HLA antigens are proteins produced by the histocompatibility complex of genes. These proteins have been divided into distinct classes.[268] Class I antigens are expressed on the surface of all nucleated cells and are represented by the HLA-A, -B, and -C antigens. Class II antigens have a more restricted tissue distribution, being expressed primarily on cells of the immune system (e.g., B-lymphocytes, a proportion of activated T-lymphocytes, antigen-presenting cells, and activated macrophages). The region of the major histocompatibility complex, which carries the genes for class II antigens, is known as the HLA-D region. Class I and II antigens were originally described as transplantation antigens involved in the rejection of organ grafts. It is now recognized, however, that their principal biologic function is to govern interactions between cells, particularly those cells comprising the immune system. In particular, class I antigens govern interactions between cytotoxic T-lymphocytes and their target cells, whereas class II antigens restrict the interaction of T-lymphocytes with antigen-presenting cells.[268]

An association between HLA specificities and several forms of uveitis is well established. Strongest associations exist between birdshot choroidopathy with HLA-A29; unilateral anterior uveitis of sudden onset with HLA-B27; and Behçet disease with HLA-B51.[208,210,226] Because VZV retinitis is uncommon, although systemic VZV infection is frequent, a special HLA association has been sought. Holland and associates[130] detected a significantly higher frequency of HLA-DQw7 antigen and phenotype Bw62,DR4 in a group of white caucasian patients with ARN syndrome in the United States, supporting the hypothesis that immunogenetic factors are indeed important in the disease process. Similarly an association between ARN syndrome and several HLA phenotypes has been recognized in Japanese patients; they include HLA-Aw33, B44 and DRw6.[136,295] Of pathogenetic interest is the finding that a higher frequency of HLA-DR9 (50%) is found in Japanese patients who have fulminant ARN syndrome when compared with patients who have milder forms of the disease (0%).[181] Thus the severity of ARN syndrome may be determined by immune response or immune suppression genes.

---

*References 27, 94, 147, 256, 260, 311, 318.
†References 18, 33, 46, 59, 155, 189.

An immunogenetic predisposition for ARN syndrome might involve a variety of mechanisms.[130] Possibilities include an increased susceptibility to infection with members of the herpesvirus family, altered immune responses leading to inadequate control of infection once initiated, or an increased frequency of reactivation of latent virus.

Immune Status of the Host

The likelihood of developing recurrent VZV disease and the severity of the disease increases with age.[132,229] Aging is also associated with a progressive decline in cell-mediated immunity in general[303] and a decline in cellular immunity to VZV in particular.[32,119,196,245] Patients immunosuppressed by human immunodeficiency virus type 1 (HIV-1) infection also exhibit an increased prevalence of recurrent VZV infection.* A strong inverse correlation therefore exists between declining VZV-specific cellular immunity and the incidence of VZV-associated diseases.[251] This relationship raises the distinct possibility that VZV-induced ARN syndrome evolves in a setting of either diminished or impaired cell-mediated immunity to the virus.[1,123,295] Alterations in cytokine profiles, especially those oriented toward a strong CD4+ T-lymphocyte–mediated, delayed type of hypersensitivity response (Th1-type response),[42,124,197,289] might also predispose to disease.

Altamirano and associates[1] recently proposed that immune dysfunction is the underlying reason for development of ARN syndrome. They described an atypical case of VZV-induced ARN syndrome that occurred in an elderly woman who experienced a subacute disease course accompanied by relapses over a 4-year period. Depressed cellular immunity was initially suggested by widespread lumbar cutaneous zoster. Additional studies revealed cutaneous anergy to several common antigens (e.g., tetanus diphtheria, *Streptococcus* sp., tuberculin, and *Candida albicans* antigen) and depressed lymphocyte activity as measured by in vitro antigen and mitogen stimulation assays. In comparison, absolute and relative numbers of B-lymphocytes were found to be increased. The authors concluded that the protracted course of ARN syndrome in this patient was due to long-term dysregulation of immune responses and commented that similar findings were obtained upon examination of seven additional patients with ARN syndrome. Usui has also documented transient cutaneous anergy to tuberculin and VZV antigens during the course of ARN syndrome, with recovery to expected levels three months later.[295] It is therefore possible that VZV retinitis may develop either because of a temporary subclinical decline in immune surveillance in otherwise healthy people or because of more obvious immunodepression, as occurs with aging or AIDS.[205,235]

CLINICAL FEATURES

VZV retinitis occurs uncommonly during the course of a primary, first-time systemic infection, either in association with congenital VZV infection or following chickenpox. Much more frequently, VZV retinitis develops as a reactivated infection in adults who have a history of chickenpox as children. Both healthy and immunocompromised patients may develop VZV retinitis during either primary or recurrent VZV infection. Although necrotizing retinitis is observed in all cases, the clinical presentation may vary in severity.

Congenital VZV Retinitis

Retinopathy, optic nerve atrophy and hypoplasia, microphthalmia, and cataracts have been reported as ocular disorders observed in infants whose mothers contracted varicella* or had cutaneous zoster during pregnancy.[74,150] Other systemic manifestations of congenital VZV infection have included skin scars, retardation, and limb hypoplasia. Up to 38% of children with congenital VZV infection have chorioretinal scars suggestive of intrauterine infection.[67]

The chorioretinal scars typically show chorioretinal atrophy with either central or peripheral pigmentation. The scars may be located in the posterior or the peripheral retina. The appearance of the retinal scar may mimic congenital toxoplasmic retinochoroiditis scars. Serologic studies of both the infant and mother may be required to differentiate these two possibilities. There has been no report to date of active necrotizing retinitis during the neonatal period, and presumably the fetal infection has resolved by the time of delivery or shortly thereafter.

Chickenpox-Associated VZV Retinitis

A mild self-limited form of necrotizing retinitis develops rarely during chickenpox.† Of the eleven reported cases in the literature only three cases occurred in children,[33,46,59] the rest being in adults. All three of the patients reported by Matsuo had mild immunosuppression (i.e., lung disease, prednisone therapy, and pregnancy).[188,189] In approximately 30% of cases the retinitis was bilateral.

Typically, patients develop symptoms of floaters corresponding to vitritis as the chickenpox skin lesions are fading. Mild necrotizing retinitis is observed in the peripheral retina and is usually confined to one quadrant of the retina. Retinal arteriolitis is limited to the vicinity of the retinitis. Retinal detachment and optic neuropathy do not occur, and vision remains good after the retinitis resolves, usually within two or three weeks after onset. Although acyclovir has been used orally or intravenously in these patients, it is unclear whether there is any beneficial effect of treatment, because the retini-

---

*References 31, 133, 145, 151, 250, 260.

*References 37, 67, 91, 162, 193, 194, 234.
†References 18, 33, 46, 59, 155, 186, 188, 189.

tis appears to resolve quickly with or without acyclovir treatment. The disproportionate predilection for involvement of adults versus children probably reflects the tendency for extradermal systemic involvement when adults develop chickenpox.

A single case of choroiditis with an overlying serous retinal detachment in a 29-year-old woman with chickenpox has been reported by Deegan and associates.[63] A similar lesion in a 27-year-old woman has been observed (unpublished data) (Fig. 82-1). In both patients the choroiditis developed as the cutaneous lesions were resolving. The serous detachment and choroidal lesions resolved with full return of vision after intravenous acyclovir treatment.

Acute VZV Retinitis

The disorder first described in 1971 by Uruyama, now known as ARN syndrome, is an acute disorder characterized by primarily peripheral, necrotizing retinitis, retinal arteriolitis, and frequent retinal detachment.[294] It is now known to be caused by both VZV and HSV. These clinical features occur together in the same eye and constitute a characteristic clinical syndrome that has been defined recently by Holland and the American Uveitis Society.[128] The following clinical characteristics should be present if the designation of ARN syndrome is to be used: focal, well-demarcated areas of retinal necrosis located in the peripheral retina (outside of the major temporal vascular arcades); rapid, circumferential progression of necrosis (if antiviral therapy has not been administered); evidence of occlusive vasculopathy; and a prominent inflammatory reaction in the vitreous humor and anterior chamber. Infected patients usually have no obvious predisposing characteristics and they may be either healthy or immunosuppressed. A few may have experienced previous cutaneous zoster either in the ophthalmic or in a nonophthalmic dermatome.

Initial symptoms consist of ocular discomfort (especially

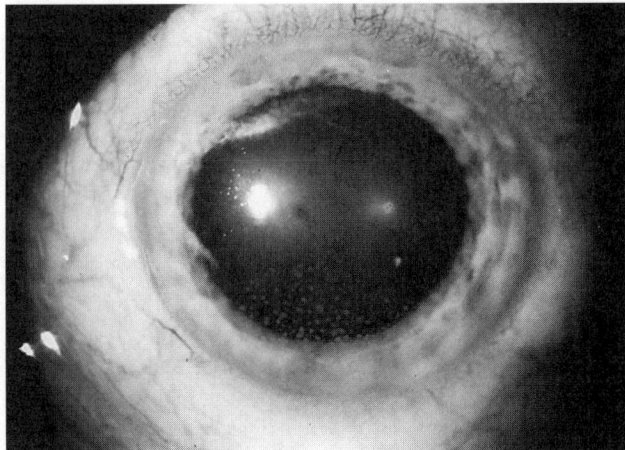

Fig. 82-2. ARN syndrome variant of VZV retinitis with granulomatous anterior uveitis.

on eye movement), photophobia, and floaters. The affected eye becomes red with episcleral injection and an anterior granulomatous iridocyclitis is typically present (Fig. 82-2). Granulomatous keratic precipitates, cells, and proteinaceous flare in the anterior chamber, and elevated intraocular pressure are observed along with an increasing number of cells in the vitreous humor.

The earliest retinitis consists of round or oval deep, yellow-white lesions at the level of the retinal pigment epithelium or deep retina in the postequitorial fundus, typically sparing the macula area. At this time retinal arteriolitis may be seen affecting both posterior and peripheral arterioles (Fig. 82-3). Mild optic disc edema is usually present early in the course of the disease. Over the next 3 to 5 days, patches of yellow-white necrotizing retinitis develop in the peripheral retina, rapidly spreading peripherally and circumferentially over the next 5 to 10 days. The retinitis may remain limited to less than one quadrant of involvement, may in-

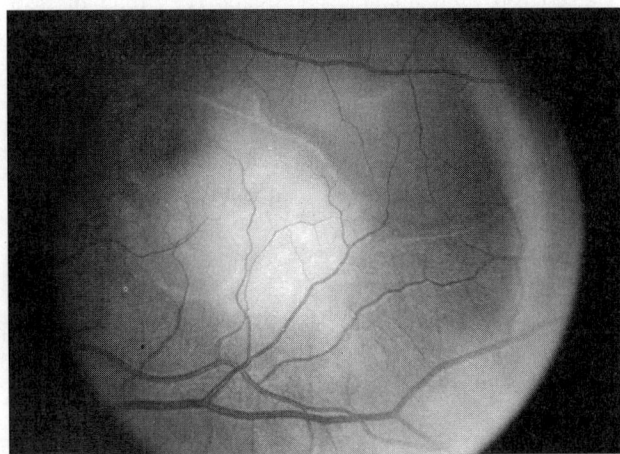

Fig. 82-1. Choroiditis in patient with chickenpox. There is overlying serous retinal detachment.

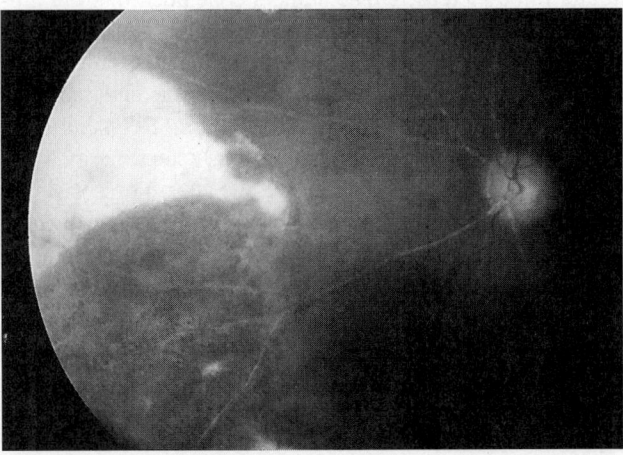

Fig. 82-3. Retinal arteriolitis in patient with ARN syndrome.

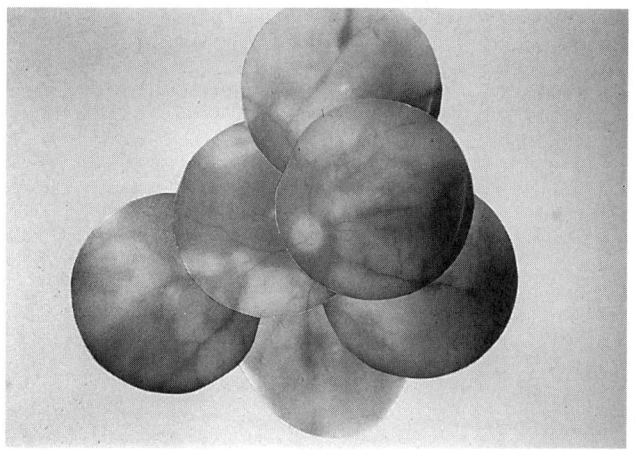

Fig. 82-4. Peripheral necrotizing retinitis in patient with ARN syndrome.

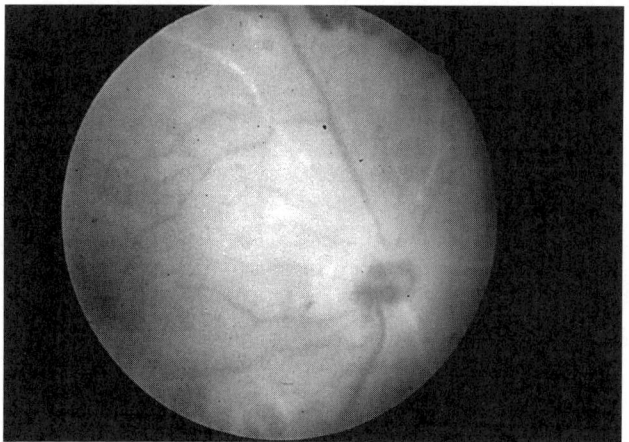

Fig. 82-6. Optic neuropathy in patient with ARN syndrome.

volve multiple peripheral quadrants of the retina, or may become confluent in the periphery (Fig. 82-4). Interestingly, the retinitis almost never extends more posteriorly than the major temporal vascular arcades; the posterior pole is spared from the acute progression of the retinitis. Vitritis increases, sometimes limiting visualization of the fundus in severe cases. An exudative retinal detachment occasionally develops in the inferior periphery. There may be areas of intraretinal hemorrhage. Vitritis gradually increases in severity, and both optic disc edema and retinal arteriolitis increase. Occasionally central retinal artery or central retinal vein occlusions may occur, causing a sudden decrease in vision (Fig. 82-5). Alternatively, optic neuropathy may precipitously reduce central vision. Optic disc swelling is pale in color, and there may be a rapid decrease in central vision or the development of an altitudinal field defect (Fig. 82-6).

Eventually, the retinitis begins to regress from the leading edge, from around venules, and from within the lesion, giving a "Swiss cheese" appearance. Regression is noted

within 5 days in acyclovir-treated patients and by three weeks in untreated patients. Transparent atrophic retina and hard yellow exudates remain behind in the wake of the clearing retinitis. The vitreous debris continues to increase as necrotic retinal debris is sloughed into the vitreous humor.

Fine salt-and-pepper pigmentation develops in the areas of atrophic retina. An adherent retinochoroidal scar does not form because of the full-thickness retinal necrosis. During the phases of activity and regression of the retinitis, good vision may be retained if retinovascular occlusion or optic neuropathy does not occur and if the vitreous haze is not severe. The papillitis gradually resolves, the affected retinal arterioles become attenuated, and the vitritis increases. Retinal detachment occurs in over 75% of severe cases at 4 to 8 weeks after the onset of retinitis.[21]

Both eyes are ultimately affected in 24%[54] to 80%[214] of untreated cases. Both eyes may be affected initially or there may be an interval of 5 to 20 days between involvement of the two eyes; longer intervals ranging from 3 to 26 years have been reported.* Intravenous acyclovir treatment appears to reduce the development of bilateral disease significantly.[21,214] The severity of disease in one eye is not necessarily correlated with the severity in the fellow eye. Recurrence of VZV retinitis in the same eye appears to be more common in patients with AIDS[149] and is rare in healthy patients.[202]

VZV retinitis may occasionally develop shortly before or after cutaneous zoster.[27,311] In cases where disease follows zoster ophthalmicus, the affected eye may be on the opposite side from the involved dermatome. In immunocompromised patients almost all cases of acute VZV retinitis are preceded by one or more episodes of shingles.†

When VZV retinitis occurs in immunocompromised pa-

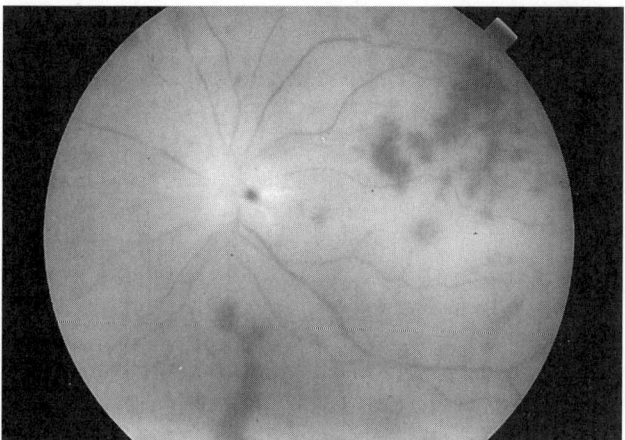

Fig. 82-5. ARN syndrome presenting as central retinal artery occlusion.

*References 86, 171, 179, 185, 285, 288.
†References 26, 36, 38, 92, 94, 120, 221, 256, 260.

tients, it may conform either to the clinical pattern of the ARN syndrome[128] or to the more recently described PORN syndrome.[84,87,177] ARN syndrome may occur in the setting of AIDS,* pharmacologic immunosuppression,[144] lymphoproliferative neoplasm,[92] or congenital immunosuppression.[94,287] In some populations it has been reported to be the second most common cause of retinitis in patients with AIDS, after CMV retinitis,[84] although in other populations it is the third most common cause of retinitis after toxoplasmic retinochoroiditis.[221] When the ARN syndrome variant occurs in patients with AIDS, it is more extensive with a greater tendency to bilaterality (90%), retinal detachment (80%), and poorer final visual acuity (80% less than 20/20) than in the general population.[223a] Although the retinitis ultimately resolves, it is less responsive to antiviral agents and may recur from 2 to 12 weeks later.[149]

Progressive Outer Retinal Necrosis Syndrome

Progressive outer retinal necrosis syndrome, a form of VZV retinitis first described by Forster and associates,[87] is characterized by deep retinal opacification and minimal vitritis occurring in patients with advanced AIDS.[77,84,177] Studies by Margolis and associates[177] and by Engstrom and associates[84] have defined the clinical and histopathologic features of PORN syndrome.

Symptoms of PORN syndrome consist of painless reduction in central vision or constriction of visual fields. There is a minimal, nongranulomatous anterior chamber inflammatory reaction and no vitritis. Multifocal areas of retinitis of various sizes are found in both the posterior pole and in the midretina and peripheral retina (Fig. 82-7). The retinitis progressively spreads outwardly and peripherally, often becoming confluent and involving the entire retina. In PORN syndrome, retinal vasculitis (20%) and optic neuritis (17%) are less commonly observed than in the ARN syndrome variant of VZV retinitis, but PORN syndrome is more often bilateral (71%).[84] The visual prognosis is universally poor because of limited responsiveness to antiviral agents and a high incidence of retinal detachment.

A retrospective review of 38 patients (65 eyes) with PORN syndrome at four academic institutions was summarized by Engstrom and associates.[84] Results revealed anterior segment inflammation in only 23 (38%) of 60 eyes examined and inflammatory cells in the vitreous humor of only 15 (25%) of 61 eyes. Nevertheless, all eyes had multifocal, discrete lesions of the outer retina that progressed to confluence and full-thickness retinal involvement as the lesions enlarged. Whereas 14 (23%) of 62 eyes had predominantly multifocal disease with little or no areas of confluence, 25 (40%) of the eyes had confluent retinal involvement. Retinal vasculopathy, observed in areas within or adjacent to ret-

---

*References 36, 38, 40, 90, 93, 221, 232.

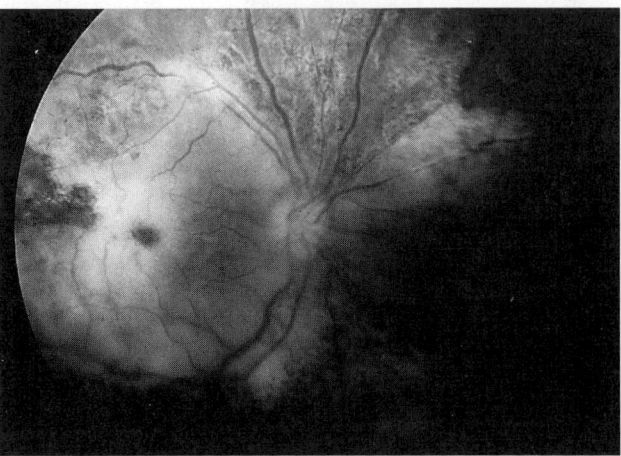

Fig. 82-7.   Deep retinitis posterior to vascular arcades in case of PORN syndrome.

inal necrosis, was found in only 13 (21%) of 61 eyes. Manifestations included vascular sheathing (7 eyes) or vascular occlusion (6 eyes). Similarly, optic nerve abnormalities were noted in only 11 (17%) of 65 eyes; they included optic disc swelling, hyperemia, and optic atrophy. Features that help to distinguish it from AIDS-related CMV retinitis include multifocality, lack of granular borders, lack of extensive retinal hemorrhage, and an extremely rapid spread.[84]

Multifocal Choroiditis

Multifocal choroidal lesions without retinitis have been reported following zoster ophthalmicus.[2,20,142] Yellow, white, round, or oval atrophic choroidal lesions develop, but apparently have no effect on vision and require no treatment.[120,204] The cause is uncertain, but local viral infection of posterior ciliary nerves with surrounding inflammation may be the cause.

PATHOLOGY

Acute Retinal Necrosis Syndrome

The histopathologic features of eyes with VZV retinitis have been described for both the acute[55,58,90,170,184] and resolution[241,243,272,294] stages of the disease. Culbertson and associates[55,58] reported the pathologic findings of two eyes, enucleated during the active phase of the disease. In the anterior segment, chronic iridocyclitis and perivasculitis with inflammatory cells along the anterior surface of the iris and infiltrating the trabecular meshwork and the ciliary body were noted. Posterior segment disease is dominated by widespread full-thickness retinal necrosis and hemorrhagic retinitis, typical of viral retinitis. Inflammatory cells (consisting primarily of lymphocytes) and necrotic retinal debris extend into the overlying vitreous humor. Areas of necrotic retina are often sharply demarcated from adjacent areas of

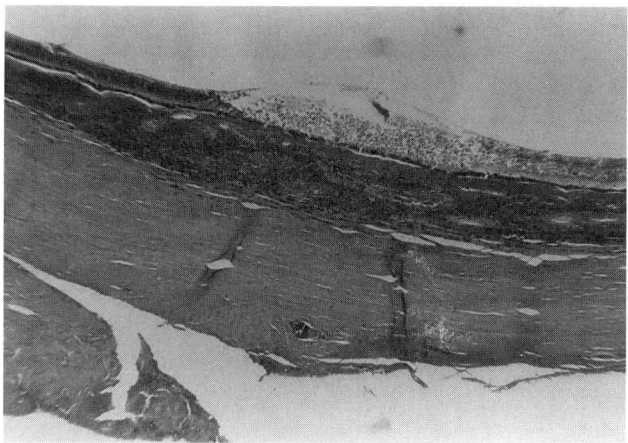

Fig. 82-8. Retinal "vesicle" with necrotic retina. Underlying choroid is thickened with inflammatory cells. (Hematoxylin-eosin; orig. mag 160×.)

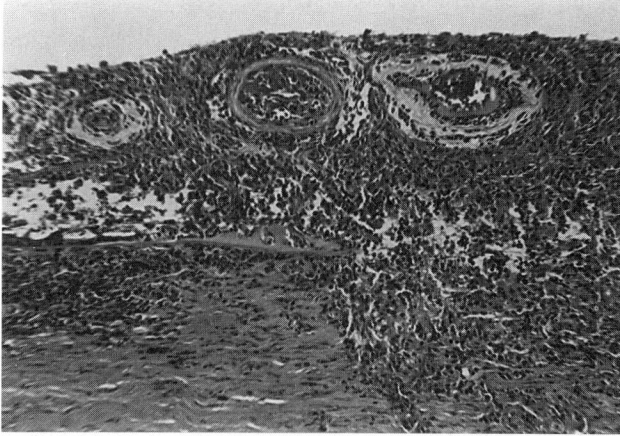

Fig. 82-9. Occluded retinal vessels immediately adjacent to optic disc in case of ARN syndrome.

relatively intact retina that contain cells with eosinophilic intracytoplasmic inclusions, predominantly in the inner nuclear layer (Fig. 82-8). Immunohistochemical staining has revealed VZV-specific antigens localized to peripheral retinal tissue in the transition zone between normal and necrotic retina. Eosinophilic intranuclear inclusion bodies are observed occasionally within retinal pigment epithelium subjacent to focal areas of full-thickness retinal necrosis. VZV antigens have also been detected in scattered retinal pigment epithelial cells, but more extensively in cells in both the inner and outer retina.

Retinal vascular involvement ranges from chronic perivascular inflammation to complete occlusion of the vessel lumen by swollen endothelial cells (Fig. 82-9). Thrombosis and endothelial cell necrosis may also be present in areas of hemorrhagic retinitis, although neither virus inclusions nor virus antigens have been observed in the endothelium of retinal vessels. Beneath areas of necrotic retina a mononuclear cell infiltrate comprised of lymphocytes and predominantly plasma cells may double the thickness of the choroid, and the choriocapillaris appears occluded in these areas. In comparison, the choroidal infiltrate is less intense and the choriocapillaris is better preserved under areas of preserved retina. The optic disc is edematous with a perivascular infiltration of chronic inflammatory cells, and the optic nerve has been found to be largely necrotic, heavily infiltrated with plasma cells, but devoid of virus antigens. In summary, the typical histopathologic features of VZV retinitis during the active phase of disease include a diffuse necrotizing retinitis, occlusive vasculitis, optic neuritis, and papillitis associated with chronic panuveitis characterized by dense plasmalymphocytic infiltration. Electron microscopy has revealed large quantities of typical herpetic virus particles (Fig. 82-10) in all layers of the neuroretina.*

In comparison, Rummelt and associates[241] described the histopathologic features of an eye that was enucleated following resolution of VZV retinitis at 32 months after the clinical onset of bilateral ARN syndrome. Light microscopic examination of this eye revealed a chronic plasmalymphocytic infiltrate in the pars plana of the ciliary body associated with necrosis of the retinal pigment epithelium. Areas of prior full-thickness retinal necrosis were either completely absent or replaced by a glial scar. Remnants of retinal tissue showed marked epiretinal gliosis. The thickened choroid was partly infiltrated by lymphocytes and mononuclear cells bearing eosinophilic intracytoplasmic and intranuclear virus inclusions, but in other areas a marked granulomatous inflammatory reaction was predominant. In addition, cellular thrombi obstructed vessels of the retina and choriocapillaris. VZV antigen expression was noted by immunohistochemical staining only in plasmalymphocytic infiltrates of the

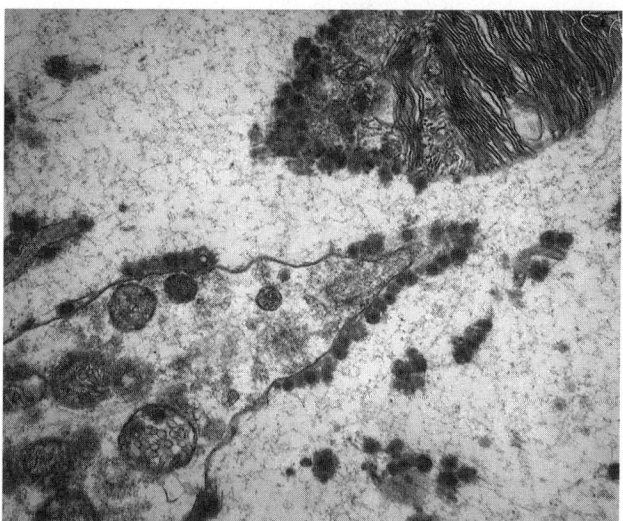

Fig. 82-10. Herpes virus in deep retina in case of ARN syndrome. (mag. 16,000×.)

---

*References 55, 58, 90, 141, 170, 203, 209.

choroid, specifically within inclusion-bearing mononuclear cells. Preserved areas of retina showed a perivascular plasmalymphocytic infiltration of retinal vessels, with some retinal arteries showing a complete occlusion of their lumen due to a fibrinoid necrosis of the vessel walls. The optic nerve was markedly atrophic and showed a chronic inflammatory infiltrate. No VZV antigen expression was detected in preserved retinal remnants, the retinal vascular endothelium, or the optic nerve, however. In summary, the central histopathologic features of VZV retinitis during late stages of the disease include extensive glial scarring and epiretinal gliosis, granulomatous choroiditis, optic neuritis with ischemic optic atrophy, and a perivascular cellular infiltration of the retinal arterioles. Abundant eosinophilic virus inclusion bodies are also present in mononuclear cells found mainly in the peripheral choroid.

Progressive Outer Retinal Necrosis Syndrome

The histopathologic features of PORN syndrome in patients with AIDS have only recently been described. Forster and associates[87] initially examined a retinal biopsy specimen taken from an HIV-1–infected patient with unilateral PORN syndrome suspected to be associated with VZV infection. Light microscopic analysis of this specimen revealed extensive glial tissue containing occasional inflammatory cells, but without evidence of intranuclear or intracytoplasmic virus inclusions. Enucleated eyes taken from two patients with AIDS and PORN syndrome were later examined histopathologically by Margolis and associates.[177] Light microscopic examination of these eyes showed a clinically normal anterior chamber with the exception of a few lymphocytes found in the ciliary muscle of one eye. The retinas, however, showed variable inflammation and necrosis ranging from areas of full-thickness retinal necrosis in one eye to necrosis localized primarily to the outer nuclear layer of the retina in the other eye. In both eyes a variable inflammatory response was observed in the choroid. The choriocapillaris had an intense lymphocytic infiltrate in some areas, whereas the lymphocytic infiltrate involved all layers of the choroid in other areas. In any given region of the fundus, however, the degree of choroidal inflammation was not related to the degree of retinal necrosis. The optic nerves of these eyes also exhibited necrosis and a marked lymphocytic infiltrate. Significantly, herpesvirus particles and VZV-specific antigens were demonstrated in the outer retinal layers of both eyes, although intranuclear or intracytoplasmic virus inclusions were notably absent in cells of the retina, choroid, and optic nerve.

The typical histopathologic features of AIDS-related PORN-syndrome variant of VZV retinitis during the active phase of disease appear to include multifocal full-thickness or outer retinal necrosis associated with minimal intraocular inflammation and hemorrhage, occasional retinal vasculopathy, and occasional optic nerve abnormalities.

COMPLICATIONS

In contrast to other forms of necrotizing retinitis, such as CMV retinitis or toxoplasmic retinochoroiditis, ARN syndrome does not usually cause vision loss as a direct result of virus-induced retinal necrosis of central visual structures, such as the macula or papillomacular bundle. Instead poor vision is a consequence of retinal and choroidal vasculopathy, optic neuritis, and/or retinal detachment.

Vasculopathy

Compromised vascular perfusion of both the retinal and choroidal circulation contributes to the damage caused by VZV retinitis. Fibrinoid necrosis and thrombosis of retinal vessels[55,58] leads to reduced flow or occlusion of the central retinal artery and vein and in branch arterioles and venules.[233] Retinal arteriolitis may be observed clinically with ARN syndrome before extensive retinitis.* Occlusion of the central retinal artery, or less often the central retinal vein, has been reported and may be the presenting sign of ARN syndrome.[51,95,96] Peripheral attenuation or blockage of retinal arterial flow is observed angiographically, most prominently in the areas of retinitis.[86] The choriocapillaris is occluded under areas of retinal necrosis. Large areas of choroidal nonperfusion are observed outside the areas of necrotizing retinitis.[96] Ando and associates[4,5] have demonstrated increased platelet adhesiveness with ARN syndrome, theoretically leading to increased vascular thrombosis. Thus ischemic damage may occur in both the choroid and the inner and outer retina as the result of VZV retinitis.[55,118] Less vasculopathy has been observed in the chickenpox-associated retinitis[55,188] and PORN-syndrome variants of VZV retinitis than in ARN syndrome, although some patients with ARN syndrome may have only minimal vasculopathy on clinical examination.[84]

Optic Neuropathy

Pale, apparently ischemic swelling of the optic disc is a common (approximately 50%) observation in patients with ARN syndrome,[55,58,261,262,294] and is less common (less than 20%) with PORN syndrome.[84,232] A profound decrease in central vision may occur abruptly with visual field changes that are consistent with an ischemic and/or compressive optic neuropathy. Visual acuity may drop to no perception of light, but may return to 20/20 following treatment (unpublished data). Optic nerve vasculitis, intraneural necrosis, and optic nerve edema have all been implicated as the cause of the optic neuropathy. Both echography and neuroimaging of the optic nerve demonstrate intraneural or optic nerve sheath enlargement.[261,262]

---

*References 54, 86, 95, 96, 211, 294.

Retinal Detachment

Retinal detachment is the primary cause of vision loss in patients with VZV retinitis and occurs in 24% to 80%* of affected eyes. The more extensive and severe the retinitis, the greater is the risk of retinal detachment.[190] Typically detachment occurs approximately two months after the onset of retinitis, usually following resolution of the active phase of disease.[23] Large retinal breaks form at the junction of necrotic and unaffected retina, often in several quadrants. The combination of large, multiple retinal breaks and inflammation-induced organization of the vitreous humor leads to the highest frequency of retinal detachment of any ocular disease.[54] Severe vitreous humor organization and proliferative vitreoretinopathy are common late sequelae.[313]

PATHOGENESIS

Molecular Biology

VZV is a relatively large, enveloped, DNA virus that belongs to the family Herpesviridae. Like HSV type 1 and type 2, VZV is an alphaherpesvirus. Members of this herpesvirus subfamily exhibit a relatively short reproductive cycle, rapid spread and efficient destruction of tissue culture cells, and the capacity to establish latent infections primarily, but not exclusively, in sensory ganglia.[236] Thus VZV is a neurotropic herpesvirus, a pathogenetic characteristic that no doubt contributes to its ability to invade the retina and produce an acute necrotizing retinitis.

The genome of VZV is approximately 125,000 base pairs in length (80 to 87 $\times$ 10^6 daltons),[98,236] making it the smallest of the human herpesviruses. The complete DNA sequence has been determined which predicts 70 unique genes that encode for at least 68 unique proteins.[60] Of these proteins, approximately 33 appear to be structural proteins that make up the mature virus particle,[265] with at least five of the proteins being envelope glycoproteins that are involved in eliciting VZV-specific humoral and cell-mediated immune responses.[7] Functions have been assigned to some of the other gene products either by direct analysis or by comparison with analogous sequences of known HSV-1 proteins, but the majority remain undefined.[165] Moreover, the inability to generate high titers of cell-free stocks of VZV, which is normally highly cell-associated, has prevented extensive analysis of VZV gene regulation. Such in vitro studies with high-titer stocks of HSV-1 have facilitated synchronous infection of cell monolayers, thereby allowing identification of distinct classes of HSV-1 genes (i.e., immediate-early, early, and late genes) and their temporal expression during the course of productive infection.[237] Identification of the regulatory factors for each gene class has ultimately provided important insights into the pathogenesis of HSV-1 infections, insights not gained as yet for VZV. Putative immediate-early genes for VZV have nonetheless been identified through sequence homology to analogous HSV-1 genes.[60,265]

Numerous strains of VZV have been recognized by DNA restriction enzyme analysis of clinical isolates from widely varying geographic locations.[117,131,276,309] Epidemiologically related strains show identical "fingerprint" patterns of DNA fragment mobility that remain stable upon virus passage.[283,309] Nonepidemiologically related strains, however, exhibit different DNA fingerprints, and these strains can often be distinguished with just one or two restriction enzymes.[103,117,131,276,309] The fact that clinical isolates of VZV can be fingerprinted by DNA cleavage analysis can be useful in tracing transmission of individual virus strains from one person to the next and in comparing multiple virus isolates recovered from different fluids and tissues of the same person. In this regard multiple VZV strains have been recovered from the same person.[131] Whether VZV strains differ in their tropisms or pathogenicity within the host remains to be determined.

Latency

Viruses are fundamentally intracellular parasites that usurp the energy and protein synthesizing machinery of the cell to manufacture new infectious virus particles. Such productive infections usually result in the death of the cell or at least impairment of the cell's specialized functions. A main feature of the biology of herpesviruses, however, is their unique capacity to establish and maintain latent infections within specialized cells of the host and reactivate later in life to produce episodes of productive infection that may lead to clinical disease. Historically, latency has been defined operationally (i.e., the inability to recover infectious virus from disrupted cells known to harbor the virus genome). Instead the viable, undisrupted cells must be explanted or cocultivated in tissue culture for days to weeks to allow in vitro reactivation of the virus genome which ultimately leads to virus replication and production of infectious virus particles. It is noteworthy that the operational definition of latency originally implied that the virus genome is completely dormant during latent herpesvirus infection.

More recent work has shown that the genome of several neurotropic herpesviruses (both human and nonhuman) is indeed transcriptionally active during latency.[50] For example, HSV-1 expresses large quantities of virus-specific RNA during latency ("latency-associated transcript" or LAT) that maps to the ICP0 region of the genome.[274] Although precise functions have not been assigned to the LAT gene of HSV-1, deletion mutants of HSV-1 lacking the LAT gene are fully capable of establishing latent infections, yet they exhibit reduced efficiency of reactivation in vitro and in animal models.[146,164,258] Thus the LAT gene of HSV-1 is thought to facilitate the process of reactivation rather than play a role in the establishment or maintenance of latency.

---

*References 22, 41, 54, 86, 114, 211, 212.

Nevertheless, the LAT provides a molecular marker for HSV-1 latency, one that supplements the operational definition of herpes virus latency.

Many aspects of VZV latency and reactivation are unique among the neurotropic herpes viruses (reviewed by Croen and Straus[49]), as illustrated by comparison with HSV-1. First, whereas HSV-1 is readily recovered from latently infected sensory ganglia by explantation or cocultivation techniques,[17,273] VZV cannot be reactivated from sensory ganglia using identical techniques,[195,222] although genomic VZV DNA and virus-specific transcripts have been detected by some investigators.* Thus unlike HSV-1, VZV does not appear to replicate well within sensory neurons, suggesting greater difficulty in reactivation and subsequent spread to peripheral sites. This interpretation is consistent with clinical observations regarding recurrent HSV-1 versus recurrent VZV disease. A wide variety of stimuli trigger reactivation of HSV-1, including fever, trauma, ultraviolet light, and hormonal changes. In sharp contrast, however, VZV is not consistently induced to reactivate by any of these stimuli. The absence of a VZV gene equivalent to LAT and ICP0 of HSV-1 may account for its reduced reactivation frequency.[50,60] Second, unlike HSV-1, VZV can become latent in nonneuronal cells of the ganglion, such as satellite cells, endothelial cells, and fibroblast-like cells.[50,167,275] That VZV does not reside within the neuron could explain further the failure of VZV reactivation following exposure to stimuli that typically induces HSV-1 reactivation. Transmission of virus to the neuron following reactivation from satellite cells could also be an inefficient process, perhaps blocked by various components of an immune response. In many ways, therefore, VZV appears to be unique among the neurotropic herpesviruses with regard to latency and reactivation. The overall impact of these unique features on VZV pathogenesis and therapeutic regimens to control VZV disease must await further investigations.

Primary and Recurrent VZV Infection

Two distinct clinical disorders involving the skin are caused by VZV in humans: varicella and zoster.[99,109] Varicella is a primary virus infection that usually occurs as a highly contagious, generalized exanthem in children. Reactivation of latent VZV later in life causes cutaneous zoster, which produces painful vesicular eruptions restricted to one or more adjacent sensory dermatomes. Restriction enzyme analysis has shown no detectable differences between matched virus isolates obtained during distinct episodes of chickenpox and shingles from the same individual.[139,277] Thus both syndromes are caused by the same virus.

The pathogenesis of varicella and zoster in immunocompetent patients is not completely understood. In children

---

*References 104, 105, 135, 173, 174, 299.

VZV infects the mucosa of the upper respiratory tract and oropharynx, which results in an asymptomatic primary viremia. The virus then spreads to cells of the reticuloendothelial system where it replicates. This incubation period is followed by a secondary viremia during which virus replicates within blood mononuclear cells.[106] The secondary viremia is associated with prodromal symptoms (fever, chills, headache, and malaise) that progress to focal cutaneous and mucosal lesions characteristic of the disease. Virus is ultimately cleared from the blood following stimulation of VZV-specific humoral and cell-mediated immune responses during the secondary viremia.[7] Of these, cellular immune responses and possibly interferon-alpha are apparently required to limit VZV infection,[9] because antibody response to VZV does not correlate with the severity of varicella.[108,302]

During primary infection VZV spreads centripetally by neural routes from the skin and mucosal lesions to the corresponding sensory ganglia via the contiguous sensory nerve endings and sensory nerve fibers, although the virus may also seed the ganglia hematogenously. Once in the ganglia, it establishes a latent infection, probably in satellite cells that surround the neurons.[50,167,275] Later in life, reactivated virus may travel centrifugally down the sensory nerves to the skin and produce the clusters of vesicles along the dermatome that are the hallmark of zoster. Of historic note, the standard diagram of the sensory dermatomes of humans usually attributed to the turn-of-the-century work of Head and Campbell originated from a detailed study of zoster.[148]

A decline in immune competence, especially VZV-specific cell-mediated immunity, is common to most patients with segmental zoster. The age-adjusted risk of zoster in the HIV-1-infected population has been found to be 17 times higher when compared with a control homosexual population,[31] although the development of zoster is not predictive of more rapid progression of HIV-1 infection. The frequency of zoster radiculitis in HIV-1-infected individuals appears to range from 2% to 4%.[165,191] The clinical picture of segmental zoster, however, appears to be similar in both immunocompetent and HIV-1-infected individuals: a cutaneous eruption characterized by pain and vesicles on an erythematous base in a pattern reflecting involvement of one or several dermatomes. Any dermatome may be involved, but the pattern is not random and usually reflects the dermatomes in which the rash of varicella was most dense. Thus the trunk is most frequently affected, followed by the face and extremities. The areas supplied by the trigeminal nerve (especially the ophthalmic division) and thoracic ganglia (T3-L2) are most commonly involved, with lesions less commonly found on the extremities. Other cranial nerves may also be involved.

On occasion the immune response prevents the formation of cutaneous lesions, but fails to prevent necrosis and inflammation at the ganglion level. Thus severe ganglionitis, often associated with neuralgia, may occur in the absence of vesicles. It is noteworthy that some degree of cutaneous dissemination may follow segmental zoster, suggesting an associated viremia.[91] Indeed, VZV-specific DNA has been detected in circulating mononuclear cells during zoster.[107] VZV DNA has also been detected by polymerase chain reaction (PCR) analysis of peripheral blood mononuclear cells of the elderly, even in the absence of recent zoster.[68]

Neurologic complications of VZV infection have been recognized clinically in patients with varicella and in those with zoster. VZV is presumed to cause a spectrum of neurologic illnesses, including cranial and peripheral nerve palsies, transverse myelitis, ascending myelitis, encephalitis, leukoencephalopathy, and a contralateral hemiplegia caused by cerebral vasculitis associated with zoster ophthalmicus[44,104] (see Chapter 72).

Animal Models

Our understanding of the pathogenesis of HSV disease has been enhanced greatly by the availability of several useful animal models of disease that closely mimic HSV infection in humans.[69] Unfortunately, few animal models of VZV disease exist to help in the elucidation of questions relating to the pathophysiology of varicella and recurrent zoster in humans. This paucity of animal models probably reflects the relative species-specificity of the virus, which does not replicate well in nonhuman cell lines.

VZV has been found to infect nonhuman primates. Oral or nasal inoculation of the common marmoset with VZV results in a mild pneumonitis, but no other clinical disease.[227] Naturally occurring varicella has also been observed in the gorilla with virus recovered from vesicular lesions.[200] The guinea pig, however, has proved to be the most promising animal for development of clinically relevant in vivo models of VZV infection. Using virus adapted to fetal guinea pig cells in culture, several investigators have demonstrated VZV infection of weanling guinea pigs following inoculation of virus by the intranasal, intratracheal, subcutaneous, intramuscular, or intracranial routes.[180,198,199] Of particular interest to VZV-associated ocular disease is a guinea pig model of corneal infection described by Pavin-Langston and Dunkel[216] (see Chapter 72). Briefly, corneal intrastromal inoculation of guinea pigs with tissue culture–adapted VZV results in acute corneal infection that progresses to a diffuse punctate keratitis with microdendrites that is characteristic of VZV anterior segment disease. Moreover, virus disseminates via neural routes to the trigeminal ganglia, midbrain, cerebellum, and superior cervical ganglia in a high percentage of animals. More recent work by these investigators[64,65,238,318] has succeeded in producing VZV infection of the cornea and trigeminal ganglia in rabbits. This animal model will no doubt be useful in evaluating various systemic and topical therapeutic regimens to manage VZV infection of the eye.[25]

It is noteworthy that the few existing animal models of VZV ocular disease have been oriented toward investigation of anterior segment disease and trigeminal ganglia infection. At the present, however, there exists no specific animal model to study directly the pathophysiology of VZV retinitis.[25] Nevertheless, studies utilizing the "von Szily" animal model for primary HSV-1 retinitis in rabbits[301] and mice[304] indicate that this model (see Chapter 83) shares many features with VZV-induced ARN syndrome, perhaps providing important insights into the pathogenetic events involved during evolution of the disease. The most intriguing similarities between the animal model and ARN syndrome in humans include the development of unilateral HSV-1-induced retinitis and subclinical encephalitis with optic nerve, optic tract, and lateral geniculate ganglia involvement. In the mouse model, inoculation of HSV-1 (KOS strain) into the anterior chamber of one eye of a euthymic BALB/c mouse produces a necrotizing retinitis in the uninoculated contralateral eye within 7 to 10 days of infection.[304] In sharp contrast, the infected eye appears to be protected from fulminant necrosis, although significant retinal damage does indeed occur as determined by abnormal retinal electrophysiology and other findings.[111]

Infectious virus can also be recovered from brain tissue in the absence of detectable clinical encephalitis with peak virus titers found on day 5 to 7 postinfection.[11] Virus spread from the eye to the central nervous system (CNS) appears to occur via parasympathetic fibers of the oculomotor nerve that supply the iris and ciliary body.[11,176,300] Subsequent virus spread within the brain appears to be limited to nuclei of the visual system and the suprachiasmatic area of the hypothalamus, with virus ultimately reaching the contralateral eye from the brain via retrograde axonal transport through the optic nerve.[300] Thus virus spread apparently occurs by neural routes in this animal model rather than by hematogenous ones. One limitation of this animal model of ARN syndrome, however, is its apparent virus strain-specificity; some HSV-1 strains other than KOS,[122,129,134] including a clinical isolate from an ARN syndrome patient,[72] produce not only bilateral retinitis, but also clinical encephalitis and death following unilateral anterior chamber inoculation.

The retinal disease that develops in the contralateral eye of BALB/c mice inoculated intracamerally with HSV-1 (KOS strain) presents with several unique pathophysiologic features. Retinitis begins with the focal expression of virus genes and virus-induced antigens on infected ganglion cells and/or Muller cells of the retina, followed shortly thereafter by infiltration of neutrophils and mononuclear leukocytes into the retina. Clinical examination of mouse eyes at this early stage of retinitis shows findings similar to those associated with human ARN syndrome.[48] Approximately three days after the onset of retinitis, the abrupt appearance of retinal necrosis occurs in association with rapid loss of all retinal architecture. Over time the inflammation subsides, ultimately leaving a fibroproliferative scar to replace the retinal tissue.

In terms of the pathophysiology of retinal disease in the contralateral eye, the relative contributions of virus replication and host cell infection versus the specific immune response to virus antigens have been extremely difficult to ascertain. This difficulty arises from the inherent complexity of the animal model, which involves virus replication at several sites and virus spread over time (days) from the inoculated eye, through the CNS, to the contralateral eye where retinal disease ultimately occurs. Nevertheless, several studies have suggested a role for virus-specific immune responses as mediators of immunopathology during evolution of retinal disease in the contralateral eye.[13,14,19,280,316] On the other hand, a role for virus replication in the development of retinal damage has been suggested by studies in athymic nude mice.[12] These animals develop bilateral retinal necrosis, although some of the histopathologic features of disease in athymic mice suggest a slower and less explosive course than that observed in euthymic animals. The mechanism(s) whereby retinal necrosis develops remains controversial, although immunopathogenic mechanisms, vascular occlusion, and anatomic factors (schisis) have been implicated.[47,71]

In addition to its contribution to retinal injury, the immune system may also regulate the spread of virus from the inoculated eye, into and through the CNS, and into the contralateral eye. Intravenous administration of HSV-1–specific, in vitro–activated, cytotoxic T-lymphocytes before ocular inoculation apparently limits the spread of virus and protects the animals from contralateral retinitis.[137,317] In contrast, a possible protective role for antibody remains unclear. Passive transfer studies using hyperimmune HSV-1 rabbit serum have suggested that neutralizing antibody fails to prevent virus spread and does not influence the development of contralateral retinitis[70]; protection has been achieved in similar passive transfer studies, however, using monoclonal antibodies to individual HSV-1–specific antigens.[10]

Although immune responses may regulate virus spread in this animal model, immune privilege also appears to facilitate virus spread. Following anterior chamber inoculation, BALB/c mice fail to mount a vigorous delayed hypersensitivity response to HSV-1 because of the development of virus-induced anterior chamber associated immune deviation (ACAID)[279] (see Chapter 7). Consequently, complete and effective maturation of cytotoxic T-lymphocytes fails to occur within the inoculated eye due to the absence of T-lymphocyte help. Without localized HSV-1–specific delayed hypersensitivity and cytotoxic T-lymphocyte responses to contain virus infection within the inoculated eye, virus escapes into the brain, replicates, and eventually invades the contralateral retina. A different outcome is observed, however, in mouse strains genetically resistant to

HSV-1–induced ACAID, as occurs in HSV-1 (KOS strain)–infected C57BL/6 mice.[156] In these animals a vigorous delayed hypersensitivity reaction to HSV-1 is associated with reduced virus spread and the absence of contralateral retinitis. Whether ACAID plays a role in the pathogenesis of ARN syndrome in humans remains to be shown. These animal studies presumably have implications for understanding of VZV retinitis as well, because of the marked similarity between ARN syndrome caused by HSV and ARN syndrome caused by VZV.

Pathophysiology of VZV Retinitis

The precise pathogenetic events that lead to VZV retinitis are unknown. Questions remain regarding the origin of virus responsible for retinitis, the route(s) by which virus spreads to the retina to produce disease, and the pathogenesis of retinal tissue destruction. The pathophysiology of the disease is particularly puzzling when one considers that VZV infection is prevalent in the general population,[224] yet the occurrence of VZV-induced ARN syndrome is a relatively rare event in apparently healthy individuals. This paradox might be explained by a rare mutation in the VZV genome that results in a new virus strain with unusual retinovirulent properties. Precedence for this possibility has been provided by the work of Thompson and associates,[290] which demonstrated that changes in a relatively small portion of the HSV-1 genome results in a 10-million fold increase in the neurovirulent properties of the virus in mice. Similarly, Yeung and associates[312] traced the neuroinvasiveness of HSV-1 (i.e., the capacity to replicate in the trigeminal ganglia of mice and spread from the eye to the CNS) to specific nucleotide sequences found within the DNA polymerase gene of the virus. A comparison of the restriction endonuclease patterns of virus isolates from patients with ARN syndrome to those of typical wild-type VZV strains has shown them to be similar, however, with no evidence for mutation.[218] Furthermore, those isolates display similar sensitivities to a panel of antiviral drugs,[218] suggesting that mutations do not exist in either the thymidine kinase or DNA polymerase genes of the virus. If VZV retinitis does not arise from a retinovirulent mutant virus strain, it remains enigmatic why a virus such as VZV that has been recognized for centuries should give rise to a relatively "new" ocular syndrome. Definitive resolution of the mutant virus hypothesis, however, must await complete sequencing of the genome of isolate from a patient with ARN syndrome and its direct comparison with the known DNA sequence of a reference VZV strain.[60]

What is the origin of virus responsible for VZV retinitis? Cutaneous zoster is believed to represent endogenous reactivation of VZV that has been latent in a sensory ganglia since the time of childhood varicella.[132,138,277] It is also possible for a person who has already experienced chickenpox to be superinfected subclinically with a second VZV strain acquired from an exogenous source.[8,101] Thus VZV retinitis could represent either endogenous reactivation or exogenous reinfection by VZV. Of these possibilities, reported cases of VZV-induced ARN syndrome that are temporally related to outbreaks of cutaneous zoster would support virus reactivation from sensory ganglia as the source of virus.* Nevertheless, the observation that varicella can precede the appearance of ARN syndrome[18,33,46,59,155] provides evidence that retinitis may also occur as a consequence of primary VZV infection.

By what route(s) does virus spread to the retina to produce disease? Two possibilities present themselves. Because VZV is a neurotropic virus, the most obvious route to consider is neural. It has been postulated that VZV reactivates from a trigeminal ganglion and spreads via sympathetic or sensory nerves to the posterior segment to initiate retinitis in the ipsilateral eye.[27,55,75,76] Clinical observations do not support this mechanism, however, because only rarely do patients with zoster ophthalmicus develop ipsilateral ARN syndrome.[80,204,308] It has therefore been suggested that upon reactivation from a trigeminal ganglion, virus spreads to the retina of the contralateral eye by retrograde axonal transport via the optic nerve[24,85,166,240] in a fashion similar to that observed in an experimental mouse model of necrotizing herpetic retinopathy using HSV-1, as discussed previously in this chapter.[71,300] Enlargement of the optic nerve sheath has been observed in some patients with ARN syndrome,[166,261,262] and the optic nerve may be necrotic and heavily infiltrated with plasma cells. Nevertheless, virus particles and virus-specific antigens have not been detected in the optic nerve of enucleated eyes.[27] It is possible that the absence of virus particles or antigens in these specimens merely reflects the late point in the course of the disease, when enucleation occurred, and that virus is indeed neurally transported during initial stages of the disease.

Alternatively, it is possible that a transient viremia is responsible for VZV-induced ARN syndrome.[6,27,58] Virus could seed the blood either from endogenous sources (e.g., reactivation of latent virus from sensory ganglia or active cutaneous zoster vesicles) or exogenous sources (e.g., contact with a person shedding virus). Blood-borne dissemination of virus to the eye could account for several key features of the disease noted in some patients; they include (1) the potential bilateral and often multifocal nature of the disease, (2) the temporal involvement of dermatomes that are remote from the eye, and (3) the potential development of ARN syndrome during the course of primary VZV infection (varicella).

What are the pathogenetic events that lead to retinal tissue destruction during the evolution of VZV retinitis? Immunohistochemical staining of the retinal arteriolar walls of

eyes with ARN syndrome has revealed immunoglobulins, fibrinogen, and complement component C3c in a pattern that corresponds with the presence of VZV-specific antigens, suggesting that virus antigen-induced inflammation causes localized breakdown of the blood-retinal barrier.[58] Immune complexes of VZV antigen and immunoglobulin could therefore accumulate in the perivascular area[206] and contribute to the occlusive vasculitis that is a major histopathologic feature of ARN syndrome. This finding is reminiscent of the cerebral angiitis associated with zoster ophthalmicus and delayed contralateral hemiparesis that may be caused by VZV infection of the cerebral vasculature.[126] A generalized platelet hyperaggregation could also predispose to retinal and choriocapillaris occlusion.[5] Breakdown of the blood-retinal barrier due to vasculitis would permit diffusion of inflammatory and immunocompetent cells, inflammatory products, and various cytokines into the vitreous cavity, the latter possibly contributing to proliferative vitreoretinopathy that complicates the disease through stimulation of fibroblasts and retinal pigment epithelium.

The evolution of full-thickness retinal necrosis with ARN syndrome is complex and probably multifactorial.[58] Because VZV-specific antigens have been detected in scattered retinal pigment epithelium and more extensively in cells in both the inner and outer retina,[58] direct virus-induced cytopathic effect no doubt contributes to destruction of the retinal tissue. The brush fire–like expansion of the leading edge of the retinitis is probably due to the fact that VZV is highly cell-associated and spreads from cell to cell during replication. Indeed, it is in the leading edge of infected but not yet necrotic retina that the majority of virus particles are found. Additional factors that contribute to retinal necrosis include virus-stimulated inflammation and virus-induced immune responses involving CD4+ and/or CD8+ T-lymphocytes, inner and outer retinal ischemia due to a combination of retinal arteriolar and choriocapillaris occlusion, and vitreous traction on the necrotic retina.[58] All of these elements contribute to various extents and lead eventually to rhegmatogenous retinal detachment.

DIFFERENTIAL DIAGNOSIS

Varicella-zoster virus retinitis should be differentiated from other disorders that are characterized clinically by large, flat, white retinal lesions including HSV, CMV, toxoplasmic and syphilitic retinitides, large cell lymphoma, and the retinitis of Behçet disease.[54,75,213] Both VZV and HSV can cause ARN syndrome that is identical in presentation.[78,110,166,182,183]

CMV retinitis is a chronic, slowly evolving disease occurring exclusively in immunosuppressed patients. There is little or no discomfort and minimal vitritis and retinal arteriolitis. Retinal lesions are found anywhere in the retina, often in an arcuate pattern. The retinitis slowly expands in a brush fire–like fashion in the retina. Active areas of retinitis

---

*References 27, 46, 80, 92, 94, 144, 147, 204, 215, 256, 257, 260.

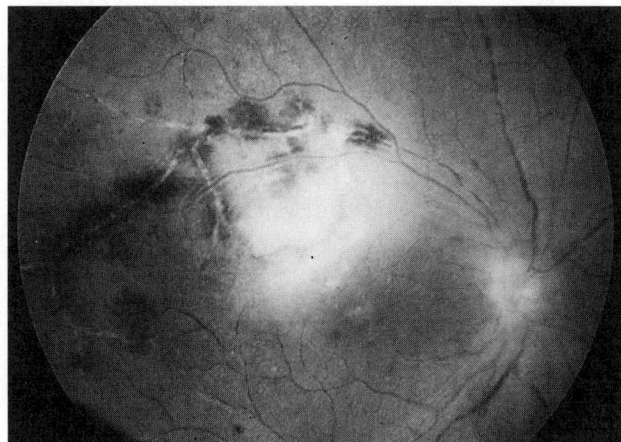

Fig. 82-11. Retinitis in patient with Behçet syndrome simulating ARN syndrome.

border atrophic retina throughout the fundus. CMV retinitis does not spontaneously resolve and instead relentlessly progresses if untreated.

Toxoplasmic retinochoroiditis in otherwise healthy patients is usually characterized by a focal area of retinitis adjacent to an old pigmented chorioretinal scar, with overlying vitritis. Usually the retinitis is more confined or localized than with ARN syndrome, but retinal arteriolitis may be prominent in both diseases. The patient often recalls having had previous episodes of floaters and/or retinitis typical of the recurrent nature of toxoplasmic retinochoroiditis. Multifocal chorioretinal scars may be seen in both eyes.

Syphilis may cause localized or large areas of retinal opacification with vitritis and sometimes a hypopyon. Patients may recall a primary genital chancre or the rash of secondary syphilis. Serology for active syphilis is positive for VDRL and FTA-ABS. The retinal manifestations of Behçet disease have occasionally been confused with ARN syndrome when retinal vasculitis is accompanied by atypically large areas of retinal whitening (Fig. 82-11). Nonocular manifestations, such as oral and genital ulcers, arthritis, and cutaneous lesions, as well as a history of hypopyon uveitis, helps differentiate these two entities.

Large cell lymphoma (reticulum cell sarcoma) may cause vitritis and subretinal areas of well-circumscribed white infiltrates.[209] Retinal arteriolitis is uncommon. Progression is very slow compared to VZV retinitis. Vitreous humor biopsy may be required to confirm the diagnosis.

LABORATORY INVESTIGATIONS

The clinical diagnosis of VZV retinitis is usually based upon a constellation of evolving signs and symptoms. Laboratory investigation and diagnostic tests are oriented toward either detection of the virus or detection of a local, intraocular antibody response to the virus.[217] Rapid identification of VZV as a causal agent of ARN syndrome can have impor-

tant therapeutic consequences and may facilitate early antiviral intervention, thereby influencing the clinical course of the disease.

Detection of Virus

Recovery of infectious virus is the definitive way to confirm a diagnosis of VZV retinitis, as has been done previously.[58,121] Virus can be recovered by inoculation of vitreous humor or retinal tissue onto monolayers of cells, usually fibroblasts of human origin, grown in tissue culture. The appearance of VZV-induced cytopathology often requires a week or more, although centrifugation culture in shell vials may hasten the appearance of cytopathology to within 24 to 48 hours after inoculation.[252] It must be emphasized, however, that VZV is extremely labile (to a greater extent than HSV), and clinical specimens should be inoculated directly onto indicator cell monolayers immediately after collection to avoid false-negative results. When cytopathology appears, confirmation of identity is accomplished immunologically by immunofluorescence assay using VZV-specific monoclonal antibodies. Whether specimens obtained by vitrectomy or endoretinal biopsy are of equal sensitivity in virus recovery is unclear. Virus recovery is most likely when specimens are taken during the acute phase of the disease, rather than using specimens taken from eyes with chronically detached atrophic retinas when the overall amount of virus is reduced.[90] Acyclovir treatment will also reduce the likelihood of infectious virus recovery.

Detection of virus-specific antigens in cells of vitreous humor aspirates has also been used to assist in making a diagnosis of VZV-induced ARN syndrome.[269,270,297] In this procedure, cells collected at time of vitrectomy are pelleted by centrifugation onto glass slides and subjected to immunofluorescence assay. Care must be taken to include appropriate controls to avoid false-positive or false-negative interpretations of immunofluorescence. This approach, however, may have some advantages over virus culture. When the two techniques were compared directly, Soushi and associates[270] found antigen-positive cells in the vitreous humor aspirates of two of four cases of ARN syndrome suspected to be of VZV origin, while cultures of aspirate samples from all four cases remained negative for infectious virus. In addition, identification of virus antigen in vitreous humor by immunofluorescence was accomplished within hours of vitrectomy, whereas several days to weeks were required to isolate virus in culture. Although this procedure may assist in the rapid diagnosis of VZV retinitis, it nonetheless has limitations. The presence of local antibody within the vitreous humor (discussed later in this chapter) may block virus-specific antigens, and small quantities of obtainable vitreous humor aspirate may limit its usefulness.

Advances in biotechnology have allowed for the rapid detection of virus-specific nucleic acid within small-volume samples of intraocular fluids by use of a PCR assay.[81,89] This highly sensitive methodology has been used recently to detect VZV genomic sequences in ocular samples (aqueous humors and vitreous, or subretinal fluid) from patients with clinically diagnosed ARN syndrome.[100,207,298] Of six patients in early stages of ARN syndrome from whom samples of aqueous humor were tested by PCR assay, Usui and associates[298] found that four were positive for the presence of VZV DNA, while the other two were positive for HSV DNA. In comparison, among four patients with ARN syndrome in relatively late stages of disease following treatment with acyclovir from whom samples of vitreous humor was obtained and tested, only one was found to have detectable VZV-specific DNA sequences. Neither CMV nor human herpesvirus 6 (HHV-6) DNA sequences were detected in any sample. Thus the PCR amplification technique appears to be a very useful tool of apparent high sensitivity and high specificity in establishing a causal diagnosis of VZV retinitis in patients in early stages of the disease. It requires only small sample volumes and can be performed in a matter of hours. Nevertheless, at present the assay requires meticulous technical performance and confirmation by probe hybridization to avoid problems of specificity and contamination that could yield false-positive results.[125] Perhaps future biotechnologic advances will simplify and standardize PCR methodology, possibly through the use of biotinylated primers and an immobilized complementary probe coupled with nonisotopic colorimetric development in a standard enzyme immunoassay format.[219,247]

Detection of Local Antibody Synthesis

Diagnosis of a virus infection can be accomplished indirectly through detection and quantitation of an antibody response to the virus. Historically a fourfold increase in serum antibody titer over time has been considered indicative of an active systemic infection, but such an increase does not always occur in ocular disease. Indeed, Pepose and associates[219] identified quantitative changes in antibody titers to VZV in acute and convalescent sera from only two of six patients with clinical signs of ARN syndrome, and these two patients suffered from cutaneous zoster. A review of the literature indicated that a diagnostic increase or decrease in antibodies to VZV (and other herpesviruses) in serial serum samples has been found in only 39% of patients (13 of 33) examined with ARN syndrome.[219] Similar findings have been reported by de Boer and associates.[62]

Antibodies can be detected within ocular fluids, however, during the course of uveitis or retinitis caused by a variety of infectious microorganisms.[15,79,157,158,230] These intraocular antibodies may originate from one of two sources. They may be of systemic (serum) origin due to compromise of the blood-ocular barrier or, alternatively, they may be synthesized locally within the eye by infiltrating B-lymphocytes. The most common method used to differentiate between local versus systemic origination of intraocular antibody involves calculation of the Goldmann-Witmer coefficient,[15,307] which is determined by comparison of the intraocular fluid : serum ratio of the immunoglobulin in question to the intraocular fluid : serum ratio of total immunoglobulin. Theoretically a coefficient above 1.0 indicates a local production of antibodies within the eye.

Application of the Goldmann-Witmer coefficient to paired serum and ocular fluid samples for detection of intraocular VZV antibody synthesis has been found to be of diagnostic value in a number patients with suspected ARN syndrome,* even in early stages of the disease.[62,219] Sensitivity of this method to detect VZV (or HSV) antibody synthesis within the eye was estimated to be 57% (16 of 28 patients) in one study[62] and 86% (12 of 14 patients) in another.[219] It must be emphasized, however, that confirmation of VZV retinitis in these patients was ultimately not obtained through examination of retinal tissues for the presence of virus by histopathologic or immunohistochemical means.

Usui and associates[298] directly compared the diagnostic value of the Goldmann-Whitmer coefficient with that of PCR amplication technology using vitreous humor from a small number of patients with ARN syndrome. One patient who was tested in an extremely early stage of the disease was PCR-positive for HSV DNA, yet failed to exhibit an antibody ratio that would predict a specific virus infection. Conversely, among four acyclovir-treated ARN syndrome patients in relatively late stages of disease, the antibody ratio was found to be predictive of VZV infection in all four patients, although only one was PCR-positive for VZV DNA. These findings suggest that the antibody quotient is often not helpful diagnostically in early stages of disease, but that the PCR assay can be particularly useful at this disease stage. Perhaps detection of intraocular antibody synthesis in combination with PCR technology will enhance further the sensitivity and specificity needed for a rapid and definitive diagnosis of VZV retinitis.

Detection of intrathecal antibody synthesis to VZV and other herpesviruses may also be of diagnostic value in some cases of ARN syndrome. Enlargement of the optic nerve sheath associated with prominent optic disc edema has been observed in some cases.[169,261,262] Lewis and associates,[166] however, documented definitive CNS involvement in a patient with clinical features of ARN syndrome from whom HSV-1 was recovered from vitreous humor. Of significance, this patient had normal neurologic signs and symptoms even though magnetic resonance imaging studies revealed lesions of the lateral geniculate, optic tracts, and chiasm. Magnetic resonance imaging abnormalities were also observed in a patient with ARN syndrome who had had zoster ophthalmicus.[85]

---

*References 15, 32, 39, 62, 140, 161, 172, 219, 231, 281, 295.

These findings prompted el Azazi and associates[82] to postulate that subclinical herpesvirus infection of the CNS accompanies ARN syndrome in some cases, resulting in a virus-induced antibody response within the blood-brain barrier. To explore this possibility, matched cerebrospinal fluid and serum samples taken from three patients with ARN syndrome (who were judged normal by clinical neurologic examination) were analyzed for evidence of local antibody synthesis to VZV or other herpesviruses. Intrathecally synthesized antibody to VZV, HSV-1, or HSV-2 was indeed detected in the cerebrospinal fluid; each patient had antibody to a single, different virus. While suggesting an alternative diagnostic approach for VZV-induced ARN syndrome, this procedure is useful only if virus infection of the brain occurs in a substantial number of patients, and if there is direct correlation between VZV retinitis and subclinical CNS infection. Clearly additional work must be done to explore this very intriguing possibility.

THERAPY

Treatment of VZV retinitis is directed towards suppressing the retinitis in the affected eye, preventing retinitis in the fellow eye, minimizing the effects of vasculopathy and optic neuropathy, and preventing and repairing retinal detachment. A lack of controlled studies has prevented an accurate comparison of the efficacy of various strategies used to achieve these goals.

Antiviral Agents

Antiviral agents have been employed intravenously and intraocularly[190,220] in the treatment of VZV retinitis ever since a virus cause was recognized.[55,58] Acyclovir has been the predominant antiviral agent studied* although other agents including ganciclovir[61,83,175,281] have been used. Isolates of VZV from cases of ARN syndrome appear to have normal sensitivity to acyclovir and other antiviral agents.[218]

Initial evaluation of intravenous acyclovir treatment of severe cases of ARN syndrome by Blumenkranz and associates[21] showed that new lesions were prevented and that regression of existing lesions began within four days of the onset of treatment. Active retinitis had resolved within 33 days of initiation of treatment in all cases, but it is uncertain if this course is significantly different from untreated cases of similar severity. Acyclovir treatment did not positively affect the rate of retinal detachment because 73% of cases had retinal detachment despite treatment. Additional studies by other investigators have not demonstrated that acyclovir treatment of eyes already affected by ARN syndrome has any beneficial effect in prevention of vision loss or retinal detachment.†

---

*References 21, 62, 127, 138, 171, 185, 214, 218, 232, 246, 253, 254, 298.
†References 57, 60, 127, 139, 170, 185, 214, 218, 232, 240, 246, 253, 254, 298.

With PORN syndrome, acyclovir or ganciclovir treatment alone or combined acyclovir/ganciclovir treatment does not appreciably retard the progression of retinitis or improve the visual prognosis.[61,83,175] This lack of effect may indicate the severe immunosuppression of these patients or possibly the development of antiviral resistance of VZV in patients with AIDS. Prophylactic maintenance acyclovir treatment may be added to prevent recurrence of ARN syndrome in immunosuppressed patients.[73,255,278]

Acyclovir treatment apparently decreases significantly the incidence of involvement of the fellow eye in patients with ARN syndrome if it has not yet been affected at the time of initiation of antiviral treatment. In the study of Blumenkranz and associates[21], no new retinal lesions developed in the fellow eye after initiation of antiviral treatment. In a study by Paley and associates[214], only 13% of acyclovir-treated patients developed ARN syndrome in the fellow eye, compared to 70% of untreated patients.

Acyclovir has been administered intraocularly to patients with ARN syndrome usually at the time of vitrectomy by adding acyclovir to the infusion fluid.[190,220] Although intravitreous levels of acyclovir may be theoretically inadequate in patients with ARN syndrome because of poor retinal perfusion, inhibitory levels of acyclovir have been detected in the vitreous humor after intravenous administration.[254,253] It is impossible to determine from the small number of reported cases that were treated intravitreous whether there is any practical clinical advantage of intravitreous administration of acyclovir compared to intravenous administration.

Antiinflammatory Drugs

Corticosteroids have been administered systemically by the oral or intravenous route in an attempt to suppress the inflammatory components of the vasculopathy and optic neuropathy and to decrease vitreous organization.[33,52,53] Although it is the clinical impression of ophthalmologists that intraocular inflammation is decreased and that there is no adverse effect of corticosteroid treatment, the efficacy of this therapy has not yet been confirmed.

Management of Vasculopathy

Vasculopathy has been treated with strategies designed to decrease clotting, including the use of warfarin sodium[56] and aspirin to decrease platelet adhesiveness.[4,5] Corticosteroid treatment probably decreases inflammation in arteries, veins, and in the choriocapillaris.

Some patients appear to have benefited from plasma exchange therapy.[203] Photocoagulation has been effective in treatment of retinal neovascularization.[232]

Management of Optic Neuropathy

Optic neuropathy has been treated with corticosteroids for inflammation and with anticlotting measures to minimize thrombosis of vessels serving the optic nerve, as described previously.[53] Sergott and associates[260] have reported visual benefit from surgical optic nerve sheath decompression in a group of patients who experienced rapidly decreasing vision and who had ultrasonographic or neuroimaging evidence of enlargement of the optic nerve and/or its perineural sheath. It is uncertain if patients with slowly decreasing vision might respond as well.

Management and Prevention of Retinal Detachment

Retinal detachment is the most common cause of vision loss in patients with VZV retinitis, occurring in 24%[86] to 80%[41,271] of affected eyes. Although technical advances have increased the rate of successful reattachment, visual results are still poor. Consequently attempts to prevent retinal detachment have been investigated.[56] Prophylactic delimiting argon laser photocoagulation has been administered posterior to the posterior border of retinitis during the acute phase of retinitis. Studies by Han and associates[113] and Sternberg and associates[271] have shown a low rate of retinal detachment following prophylactic argon laser treatment in groups of patients with relatively mild ARN syndrome. It is not clear, however, that the retinal detachment risk is reduced in eyes with more extensive retinitis. In severe cases dense vitritis often prohibits adequate laser treatment.

For severe cases other investigators have used prophylactic pars plana vitrectomy and endolaser treatment, both with and without scleral buckling, to prevent retinal detachment.* These uncontrolled studies have generally shown a lower-than-expected retinal detachment rate.

Retinal detachment in patients with ARN syndrome is difficult to repair because of the presence of multiple, posteriorly positioned retinal tears in association with intraocular inflammation. Surgical reattachment rates have improved from 22%[41] to 90%[22] or more. Current surgical repair technique utilizes pars plana vitrectomy, endolaser and internal tamponade, with or without lensectomy and scleral buckling.† Numerous reports of successful mechanical reattachment with silicone oil have been published recently.‡

PROGNOSIS

The overall prognosis for final visual acuity with VZV retinitis is primarily dependent on the extent and severity of retinitis. The risk of retinal artery and vein occlusion, optic neuropathy, and retinal detachment appears to be roughly proportional to the number of quadrants of peripheral retina with necrotizing retinitis. Immunosuppressed patients have the worst visual outcome, primarily because of the extensiveness of the retinitis and consequent high incidence of retinal detachment.

---

*References 34, 139, 152, 153, 168, 220, 249, 264, 288, 291, 309.
†References 3, 21-23, 88, 153, 154, 160, 170, 192, 201, 212, 224, 232, 248, 249, 254, 267, 281, 286, 292.
‡References 3, 170, 201, 232, 249, 259, 267, 286.

In an early review of the cases of ARN syndrome reported up to 1984, Culbertson and Blumenkranz[54] found that 76% of affected eyes ultimately saw worse than 20/200. Since these early reports it has become evident that VZV retinitis comprises a spectrum of disease severity. Mild cases with limited peripheral retinitis, arteriolitis, and optic neuropathy commonly have good visual acuity and a low incidence of retinal detachment.[187] In a 1991 study of 22 patients (26 eyes) with ARN syndrome, Matsuo and associates[190] found that best final visual acuity occurred in patients with the fewest quadrants of retinal involvement, the least arteriolitis, and in patients younger than 50 years of age. Early intravenous acyclovir treatment had no correlation with final vision. Usui[295] found that patients who had ARN syndrome caused by VZV had worse vision, more extensive retinitis and retinal arteriolitis and more frequent retinal detachment than patients with ARN syndrome caused by HSV.

In an early study (1984) of retinal detachment surgery in patients with ARN syndrome, Clarkson and associates[41] found that 63% of detached retinas were successfully reattached surgically, and 56% of these eyes saw better than 20/200. A similar study by the same group five years later revealed a 94% reattachment rate using more sophisticated surgical techniques, but only 40% of the eyes successfully reattached saw better than 20/200.[23]

Higher retinal reattachment rates up to 100% have been reported in smaller series with individual cases seeing better than 20/40.[22] Once the retina detaches, however, even if successfully repaired, the general prognosis for vision remains poor.

When VZV retinitis occurs in immunosuppressed patients, the visual prognosis is worse than in healthy patients. Only 20% of patients with AIDS who have ARN syndrome see better than 20/200 in the affected eye.[223a] With PORN syndrome, two thirds (67%) of eyes had no light perception.[83]

PREVENTION

VZV Vaccine

Although treatment of preexisting VZV retinitis can be achieved through antiviral chemotherapy, prophylactic strategies should be considered to prevent the occurrence of retinitis in VZV-infected individuals or to protect the uninvolved fellow eye from future retinal disease in individuals who have already experienced unilateral VZV-induced ARN syndrome. One approach to prevent the occurrence of VZV retinitis is use of a live attenuated vaccine developed originally by Takahashi and associates[282,284] (see Chapter 72). Several questions have been raised about its long-term safety and efficacy, including persistence of immunity, degree of attenuation, risk of secondary spread, possible oncogenicity, and potential for reactivation with development of zoster. To date, however, the vaccine appears to be relatively safe, immunogenic, and protective against severe varicella in healthy children and adults as well as in certain immuno-compromised patients, including children with leuke-mia.[99,315]

Because VZV-induced ARN syndrome can originate from reactivated virus and can be temporally related to episodes of cutaneous zoster (see Risk Factors), the potential for outbreaks of zoster in vaccine recipients is of particular interest to ophthalmologists. Cases of zoster have indeed been observed in both immunocompetent and immunosuppressed vaccine recipients in the United States[98,112,223,306] and in Japan.[116] Thus there is no doubt that the vaccine virus strain (the Oka strain) is capable of causing latent infection and later reactivating to produce cutaneous disease. Fortunately the cases have all been mild, and the dermatome involved often correlates with the site of vaccination. No VZV ocular disease has been noted. Virus isolates generally have been the vaccine strain as determined by restriction endonuclease analysis, but wild-type VZV strains also have been seen.[98,112,116,306] The dermatome involved with wild-type virus, however, does not seem to be related to the vaccination site.[98,112] The incidence of zoster in vaccine recipients has generally been low, approximately 2% over a ten-year period in a study of leukemic vaccine recipients.[102] Thus, zoster in vaccine recipients appears to be no more common, and perhaps less common, than in natural infection.[30,115,163] The potential prophylactic value of the vaccine to prevent reactivation of latent VZV in adults who have already experienced varicella has not yet been investigated.

Despite current data suggesting that the risk-to-benefit ratio of the live attenuated Oka vaccine is favorable, questions remain about its long-term safety and the longevity of immunity. For example, the degree and even the nature of attenuation of the Oka vaccine strain are unknown, although the virus appears to be clinically attenuated.[293] Nevertheless, concerns persist about possible reversion of the virus strain to one that possesses original wild-type virulence and pathogenicity. In addition, waning immunity in adults after childhood vaccination would undoubtedly be associated with increased morbidity and mortality due to renewed susceptibility to natural infection late in life.[99] Finally, because varicella is usually a benign and generally inevitable disease in immunologically normal children and often provides life-long immunity, a proposal for universal VZV vaccination is highly controversial.[28] Whether vaccine recipients would be protected against development of VZV retinitis or show a higher prevalence for VZV ocular disease later in life remains a topic of debate and must await long-term prospective studies of vaccinees.

Immune-Based Prophylaxis

Passive transfer of antibodies is the most widely used and oldest form of immunotherapy. It is therefore not surprising that an area of clinical investigation has focused on the use of VZV hyperimmune globulin to prevent or modify postex-posure disease. Initial attempts at passive immunization employed large doses of standard immune globulin that was found to attenuate, but not prevent, varicella in immunocompetent children if administered within three days of exposure.[239] In comparison, administration of a high-titer VZV immune globulin preparation (VZIG) was found not only to prevent varicella in normal children under similar circumstances,[29] but also to modify disease in immunosuppressed children.[314] Similarly zoster-immune plasma (ZIP), a convalescent VZV plasma preparation, also modifies or prevents varicella in susceptible high-risk children.[97] Recipients of either VZIG or ZIP who ultimately develop clinical disease usually show a mild disease course that is associated with prolonged incubation period. This clinical course is significantly different from that observed in high-risk children with unmodified varicella, which is usually severe and potentially life-threatening.

Guidelines for the use of the VZV immune globulins have been published by the Centers for Disease Control and Prevention.[35] Due to its general unavailability, use of VZIG has been historically restricted to high-risk children who have been exposed to varicella. A new method for preparing VZIG from outdated banked blood[314] has increased its availability, however. Thus passive immunization can now be used more freely and perhaps can be extended to susceptible adults, especially pregnant women. Prophylactic use of VZIG could even prove to be an important adjunct to traditional antiviral chemotherapy for prevention of VZV retinitis in the uninvolved fellow eye of individuals suffering from unilateral ARN syndrome of VZV origin. Clinical trials evaluating the potential efficacy of such combination prophylaxis have not yet been carried out, however.

Antiviral Chemotherapy

Although acyclovir hastens the resolution of unilateral VZV retinitis, at least one third of patients with ARN syndrome ultimately develop bilateral disease. In most instances retinitis develops in the fellow eye within six weeks of the onset of symptoms in the first eye, although in some cases a period of years may elapse. Paley and associates[214] studied the potential protective effect of acyclovir treatment on the fellow eye in a review of 54 patients with unilateral ARN syndrome. Of this group 31 patients were treated with acyclovir (1,500 mg/m^2/day of acyclovir administered intravenously for 7 to 10 days followed by oral maintenance doses of acyclovir for two to four weeks), whereas 23 patients who had not received acyclovir served as controls. Results revealed that the fellow eyes of 27 of 31 (87.1%) acyclovir-treated patients remained disease-free throughout a median follow-up of 12 months. In sharp contrast, only 7 of 23 (30.4%) patients not treated with acyclovir had fellow eyes that remained disease-free throughout a median follow-up of 11 months. Furthermore, two years after initial treatment, the proportion of eyes that remained disease-free was 75.3% for acyclovir-treated patients, compared to 35.1% for the untreated control patients. These results therefore support the assertion that acyclovir treatment has prophylactic value and effectively reduces the risk of future development of retinitis in the fellow eye of patients with unilateral ARN syndrome.

REFERENCES

1. Altamirano D et al.: Acute retinal necrosis: a result of immune dysfunction? Report of a case with subacute evolution and relapses in a patient with impaired cellular immunity, *Ophthalmologica* 208:49-53, 1994.
2. Amano Y et al.: A new fundus finding in patients with zoster ophthalmicus, *Am J Ophthalmol* 102:532-533, 1986.
3. Anand R, Fischer DH: Silicone oil in the management of retinal detachment with acute retinal necrosis. In Freeman HM, Tolentino FI, editors: *Proliferative vitreoretinopathy,* New York, 1989, Springer-Verlag.
4. Ando F et al.: Platelet function in six of Kirisawa's uveitis, *Folia Ophthalmol Jpn* 33:976-982, 1982.
5. Ando F et al.: Platelet function in bilateral acute retinal necrosis, *Am J Ophthalmol* 96:27-32, 1983.
6. Arbeit RD et al.: Infection of human peripheral blood mononuclear cells by varicella-zoster virus, *Intervirology* 18:56-65, 1982.
7. Arvin A: Clinical manifestations of varicella and herpes zoster and the immune response to varicella-zoster virus. In Hyman RW, editor: *Natural history of varicella-zoster virus,* 67-130, Boca Raton, Fla, 1987, CRC Press.
8. Arvin AM et al.: Immunologic evidence of reinfection with varicella-zoster virus, *J Infect Dis* 148(2):200-205, 1983.
9. Arvin AM et al.: Early immune response in healthy and immunocompromised subjects with primary varicella-zoster virus infection, *J Infect Dis* 154:422-429, 1986.
10. Atherton SS: Protection from retinal necrosis by passive transfer of monoclonal antibody specific for herpes simplex virus glycoprotein D, *Curr Eye Res* 11:45-52, 1992.
11. Atherton SS, Streilein JW: Two waves of virus following anterior chamber inoculation with HSV-1, *Invest Ophthalmol Vis Sci* 28:571-579, 1987.
12. Atherton SS et al.: Histopathologic study of herpes virus-induced retinitis in athymic BALB/c mice: evidence for an immunopathologic process, *Curr Eye Res* 8:1179-1192, 1989.
13. Azumi A et al.: Modulation of murine herpes simplex virus type 1 retinitis in the uninoculated eye by CD4 + T lymphocytes, *Invest Ophthalmol Vis Sci* 35:54-63, 1994.
14. Azumi SS et al.: Virus replication and recruitment of CD4 + T-cells to the uninjected eye in murine HSV-1 retinitis, *Invest Ophthalmol Vis Sci* 35(suppl):1333, 1994.
15. Baarsma GX et al.: Analysis of local antibody production in the vitreous humor of patients with severe uveitis, *Am J Ophthalmol* 112:147-150, 1991.
16. Bando K et al.: Six cases of so called "Kirisawa type" uveitis, *Jpn J Ophthalmol* 33:1515-1521, 1979.
17. Baringer JR, Swoveland P: Recovery of herpes simplex virus from human trigeminal ganglions, *N Engl J Med* 288:648-650, 1973.
18. Barondes MJ et al.: Acute retinal necrosis after chickenpox in a healthy adult, *Ann Ophthalmol* 24:335-336, 1992.
19. Berra A et al.: The role of macrophages in the pathogenesis of HSV-1 induced chorioretinitis in BALB/c mice, *Invest Ophthalmol Vis Sci* 35:2990-2998, 1994.
20. Bloom SM, Sandy-McCoy L: Multifocal choroiditis uveitis occurring after herpes zoster ophthalmicus, *Am J Ophthalmol* 108:733-734, 1989.
21. Blumenkranz MS et al.: Treatment of the acute retinal necrosis syndrome with intravenous acyclovir, *Ophthalmology* 93:296-300, 1986.
22. Blumenkranz MS et al.: Vitrectomy for retinal detachment associated with acute retinal necrosis, *Am J Ophthalmol* 106:426-429, 1988.
23. Blumenkranz MS et al.: Visual results and complications after retinal reattachment in the acute retinal necrosis syndrome, *Retina* 9:170-174, 1989.
24. Bosem ME et al.: Optic nerve involvement in viral spread in herpes simplex virus type 1 retinitis, *Invest Ophthalmol Vis Sci* 31:1683-1689, 1990.
25. Brik D et al.: Efficacy of high- and low-dose acyclovir during VZV ocular infection in the rabbit, *Invest Ophthalmol Vis Sci* 33(suppl):788, 1992.
26. Brown RM, Mendis U: Retinal arteritis complicating herpes zoster ophthalmicus, *Br J Ophthalmol* 57:344-346, 1973.
27. Browning DJ et al.: Association of varicella zoster dermatitis with acute retinal necrosis syndrome, *Ophthalmology* 94:602-606, 1987.
28. Brundell PA: Protection against varicella, *Pediatrics* 59:1-2, 1977.
29. Brunell PA et al.: Prevention of varicella by zoster immune globulin, *N Engl J Med* 280:1191-1194, 1969.
30. Brunell PA et al.: Risk of herpes zoster in children with leukemia: varicella vaccine compared with history of chickenpox, *Pediatrics* 77:53-56, 1986.
31. Buchbinder S et al.: Herpes zoster and human immunodeficiency virus infection, *J Infect Dis* 166:1153-1156, 1992.
32. Burke BL et al.: Immune responses to varicella-zoster in the aged, *Arch Intern Med* 142:292-293, 1982.
33. Capone A Jr, Meredith TA: Central visual loss caused by chickenpox retinitis in a 2-year-old child, *Am J Ophthalmol* 113:592-593, 1992.
34. Carney MD et al.: Acute retinal necrosis, *Retina* 6:85-94, 1986.
35. Centers for Disease Control: Varicella-zoster immune globulin for the prevention of chickenpox: recommendations of the Immunizations Practices Advisory Committee, *Ann Intern Med* 100:859-865, 1984.
36. Chambers RB et al.: Varicella-zoster retinitis in human immunodeficiency virus infection, *Arch Ophthalmol* 107:960-961, 1989.
37. Charles NC et al.: Ocular pathology of the congenital varicella syndrome, *Arch Ophthalmol* 95:2034-2037, 1977.
38. Chess J, Marcus DM: Zoster-related bilateral acute retinal necrosis syndrome as presenting signs in AIDS, *Ann Ophthalmol* 20:431-435, 1988.
39. Chung Y et al.: Acute retinal necrosis combined with rising of varicella-zoster antibody titer in the intraocular fluid, *J Formos Med Assoc* 86:662, 1987.
40. Ciancas F. et al.: Acute retinal necrosis syndrome, *Arch Soc Espan Oftalmol* 63:137-144, 1992.
41. Clarkson JG et al.: Retinal detachment following the acute retinal necrosis syndrome, *Ophthalmology* 91:1665-1668, 1984.
42. Clerici M, Shearer GM: The TH1 to TH2 shift is a critical step in the etiology of HIV infection, *Immunol Today* 14:107-111, 1993.
43. Cobo M et al.: Oral acyclovir in the therapy of acute herpes zoster ophthalmicus, *Ophthalmology* 93:763-770, 1986.
44. Cohen B, Dix RD: Cytomegalovirus and other herpesviruses. In Levy RM, Berger J, editors: *AIDS and the nervous system,* ed 2, New York, 1995, Raven Press (in press).
45. Collier M: Two rare ocular manifestations of ophthalmic zoster: retinal periarteritis, *Bull Soc Ophthalmol* pp 737-741, 1959.
46. Copenhaver RM: Chickenpox with retinopathy, *Arch Ophthalmol* 75:199-200, 1966.
47. Cousins SW et al.: Schisis contributes to necrosis in experimental HSV-1 retinitis, *Exp Eye Res* 48:745-760, 1987.
48. Cousins SW et al.: Herpes simplex retinitis in the mouse: clinicopathologic correlations, *Invest Ophthalmol Vis Sci* 30:1485-1494, 1989.
49. Croen KD, Straus SE: Varicella-zoster virus latency, *Annu Rev Microbiol* 45:265-282, 1991.
50. Croen KD et al.: Patterns of gene expression and sites of latency in human nerve ganglia are different for varicella-zoster and herpes simplex viruses, *Proc Natl Acad Sci USA* 85:9773-9777, 1988.
51. Culbertson WW: Infections of the retina in AIDS. In G Smolin and MH Friedlander, editors: *AIDS and ophthalmology. Int Ophthalmol Clinics,* 108-118, Boston, 1989, Little, Brown.
52. Culbertson WW, Atherton SS: Acute retinal necrosis, *Jpn Rev Clin Ophthalmol* 86:2668-2679, 1992.
53. Culbertson WW, Atherton SS: Acute retinal necrosis and similar retinitis syndromes, *Ophthalmology* 33:129-143, 1993.

54. Culbertson WW, Blumenkranz MS: The acute retinal necrosis syndrome. In Blodi FC, editor: *Herpes simplex infections of the eye,* 77-89, New York, 1984, Churchill Livingstone.

55. Culbertson WW et al.: The acute retinal necrosis syndrome. Part 2: Histopathology and etiology, *Ophthalmology* 89:1317-1325, 1982.

56. Culbertson WW et al.: Acute retinal necrosis, *Am J Ophthalmol* 96:683-685, 1983.

57. Culbertson WW et al.: Treatment of the acute retinal necrosis syndrome. In Saari KM, editor: *Uveitis update: proceedings of the first international symposium of uveitis held in Hanasaari, Espoo, Finland on May 16-19, 1984,* 251-255, Amsterdam, 1984, Excerpta Medica.

58. Culbertson WW et al.: Varicella zoster virus is a cause of the acute retinal necrosis syndrome, *Ophthalmology* 93:559-569, 1986.

59. Culbertson WW et al.: Chickenpox-associated acute retinal necrosis syndrome, *Ophthalmology* 98:1641-1646, 1991.

60. Davidson AJ, Scott JE: The complete DNA sequence of varicella-zoster virus, *J Gen Virol* 67:1759-1816, 1986.

61. Reference deleted in page proofs.

62. de Boer JH et al.: Detection of intraocular antibody production to herpesviruses in acute retinal necrosis syndrome, *Am J Ophthalmol* 117:201-210, 1994.

63. Deegan WF III, Duker JS: Unifocal choroiditis in primary varicella zoster (chickenpox), *Arch Ophthalmol* 112:735-736, 1994.

64. de Freitas D et al.: Varicella-zoster virus RNA expression in rabbit corneas and trigeminal ganglia after intranasal and intrastromal inoculation, *Invest Ophthalmol Vis Sci* 31(suppl):312, 1990.

65. de Freitas D et al.: Ocular VZV in the rabbit: clinical disease, virus, and VZV RNA detection, *Invest Ophthalmol Vis Sci* 32(suppl):987, 1991.

66. de la Paz M, Young LHY: Acute retinal necrosis syndrome, *Semin Ophthalmol* 8:61-69, 1993.

67. de Nicola LK, Hanshaw JB: Congenital and neonatal varicella, *J Pediatr* 94:175-176, 1979.

68. Devlin ME et al.: Peripheral blood mononuclear cells of the elderly contain varicella-zoster virus DNA, *J Infect Dis* 165:619-622, 1992.

69. Dix RD, Mills J: Experimental mouse models of herpes simplex virus infection. In Zak O, Sande MA, editors: *Experimental models in antimicrobial chemotherapy,* vol 2, 219-258, New York, 1986, Academic Press.

70. Dix RD et al.: Effect of passively-administered neutralizing antibody on the development of herpes simplex virus type 1 retinitis, *Invest Ophthalmol Vis Sci* 27(suppl):117, 1986.

71. Dix RD et al.: Histopathologic characteristics of two forms of experimental herpes simplex virus retinitis, *Curr Eye Res* 6:47-52, 1987.

72. Dix RD et al.: Bilateral retinal disease following unilateral inoculation of mice with a HSV-1 isolate from a patient with acute retinal necrosis, *Invest Ophthalmol Vis Sci* 31(suppl):314, 1990.

73. Douglas JM et al.: A double-blind study of oral acyclovir for suppression of recurrence of genital herpes simplex virus infection, *N Engl J Med* 310:1551, 1984.

74. Duehr PA: Herpes zoster as a cause of congenital cataract, *Am J Ophthalmol* 39:157-161, 1955.

75. Duker JS, Blumenkranz MS: Diagnosis and management of the acute retinal necrosis (ARN) syndrome, *Surv Ophthalmol* 35:327-343, 1991.

76. Duker JS, Fischer DH: Acute retinal necrosis. In Tasman WS, Jaeger EA, editors: *Duane's clinical ophthalmology,* vol 4, Philadelphia, JB Lippincott.

77. Duker JS, Shakin EP: Rapidly progressive outer retinal necrosis in the acquired immunodeficiency syndrome, *Am J Ophthalmol* 111:255-256, 1991.

78. Duker JS et al.: Rapidly progressive acute retinal necrosis secondary to herpes simplex virus type 1, *Ophthalmology* 97:1638-1643, 1990.

79. Dussaix E et al.: New approaches to the detection of locally produced antiviral antibodies in the aqueous of patients with endogenous uveitis, *Ophthalmologica* 194:145-149, 1987.

80. Edgerton AE: Herpes zoster ophthalmicus: report of cases and review of the literature, *Arch Ophthalmol* 34:40-62, 1945.

81. Eisenstein BI: The polymerase chain reaction: a new method of using molecular genetics for medical diagnosis, *N Engl J Med* 322:178-183.

82. el Azazi M et al.: Intrathecal antibody production against viruses of the herpesvirus family in acute retinal necrosis syndrome, *Am J Ophthalmol* 112:76-82, 1991.

83. Engstrom RE Jr, Holland GN: Chronic herpes zoster virus keratitis associated with the acquired immunodeficiency syndrome, *Am J Ophthalmol* 105:556-559, 1988.

84. Engstrom RE Jr et al.: The progressive outer retinal necrosis syndrome: a variant of necrotizing herpetic retinopathy in patients with AIDS, *Ophthalmology* 101:1488-1502, 1994.

85. Farrell TA et al.: Magnetic resonance imaging in a patient with herpes zoster keratouveitis and contralateral acute retinal necrosis, *Am J Ophthalmol* 112:735-736, 1991.

86. Fisher JP et al.: The acute retinal necrosis syndrome. Part 1. Clinical manifestations, *Ophthalmology* 89:1309-1316, 1982.

87. Forster DJ et al.: Rapidly progressive outer retinal necrosis in the acquired immunodeficiency syndrome, *Am J Ophthalmol* 110:341-348, 1990.

88. Fox GM, Blumenkranz M: Giant retinal pigment epithelial tears in acute retinal necrosis, *Am J Ophthalmol* 116:302-306, 1993.

89. Fox GM et al.: Detection of herpesvirus DNA in vitreous and aqueous specimens by the polymerase chain reaction, *Arch Ophthalmol* 109:266-271, 1991.

90. Freeman WR et al.: Demonstration of herpes group virus in acute retinal necrosis syndrome, *Am J Ophthalmol* 102:701-709, 1986.

91. Frey HM et al.: Congenital varicella: case report of a serologically proved long-term survivor, *Pediatrics* 59:110-112, 1977.

92. Friberg TR, Jost BF: Acute retinal necrosis in an immunosuppressed patient, *Am J Ophthalmol* 98:515-517, 1984.

93. Friedman SM et al.: Varicella-zoster retinitis as the initial manifestation of the acquired immunodeficiency syndrome, *Am J Ophthalmol* 117:536-538, 1994.

94. Gartry DS et al.: Acute retinal necrosis syndrome, *Br J Ophthalmol* 75:292-297, 1991.

95. Gass JDM: Acute herpetic thrombotic retinal angiitis and necrotizing neuroretinitis ("Acute retinal necrosis syndrome"). In *Symposium of medical and surgical diseases of the retina and vitreous: transactions of the New Orleans academy of ophthalmology,* St Louis, 1983, Mosby.

96. Gass JDM: Acute retinal necrosis. In *Stereoscopic atlas of macular diseases,* vol 2, St Louis, 1987, Mosby.

97. Geiser CF et al.: Prophylaxis of varicella in children with neoplastic disease: comparative results with zoster immune plasma and gamma globulin, *Cancer* 35:1027-1030, 1975.

98. Gelb LD: Varicella-zoster virus: molecular biology. In Roizman B, Whitley RJ, Lopez C, editors: *The human herpesviruses,* New York, 1993, Raven Press.

99. Gelb LD: Varicella-zoster virus: clinical aspects. In Roizman B, Whitley RJ, Lopez C, editors: *The human herpesviruses,* New York, 1993, Raven Press.

100. Gerling J et al.: Diagnosis and management of the acute retinal necrosis syndrome, *Ger J Ophthalmol* 1:388-393, 1992.

101. Gershon A et al.: Can varicella-zoster (VZ) virus cause re-infection? Abstract, *Pediatr Res* 17:270A, 1983.

102. Gershon AA et al.: Live attenuated varicella vaccine use in immunocompromised children and adults, *Pediatrics* 78:757-762, 1986.

103. Gharabaghi F et al.: A rapid and simplified micromethod for subtyping varicella zoster virus, *J Med Virol* 31:129-134, 1990.

104. Gilden DH, Vafai A: Varicella zoster. In McKendall RR, editor: *Handbook of clinical neurology,* vol 12, *Viral disease,* Amsterdam, 1989, Elsevier.

105. Gilden DH et al.: Varicella-zoster virus DNA in human sensory ganglia, *Nature* 306:478-480, 1983.

106. Gilden DH et al.: Varicella-zoster virus infection of human mononuclear cells, *Virus Res* 7:117-129, 1987.

107. Gilden DH et al.: Persistence of varicella-zoster virus DNA in blood mononuclear cells of patients with varicella or zoster, *Virus Genes* 2:299-305, 1989.

108. Gold E: Serologic and virus-isolation studies of patients with varicella or herpes-zoster infection, *N Engl J Med* 274:181-185, 1966.

109. Grose C: Varicella-zoster virus: pathogenesis of the human diseases, the virus and viral replication. In Hyman RW, editor: *Natural history of varicella-zoster virus,* 1-66, Boca Raton, Fla, 1987, CRC Press.

110. Grutzmacher RD et al.: Herpes simplex chorioretinitis in a healthy adult, *Am J Ophthalmol* 96:788-796, 1983.

111. Hamasaki DI et al.: Bilateral alterations of the ERG and retinal histology following unilateral HSV-1 inoculation, *Invest Ophthalmol Vis Sci* 29:1242-1254, 1988.

112. Hammerschlag MR et al.: Herpes zoster in an adult recipient of live attenuated varicella vaccine, *J Infect Dis* 160:535-537, 1989.

113. Han DP et al.: Laser photocoagulation in the acute retinal necrosis syndrome, *Arch Ophthalmol* 105:1051-1054, 1987.

114. Hara Y et al.: Clinical features of 31 cases of Kirisawa-type uveitis, *Jpn J Clin Ophthalmol* 44:633-666, 1990.

115. Hardy I et al.: The incidence of zoster after immunization with live attenuated varicella vaccine: a study of children with leukemia, Varicella Vaccine Collaborative Study Group, *N Engl J Med* 325:1545-1550, 1991.

116. Hayakawa Y et al.: Biologic and biophysical markers of a live varicella vaccine strain (Oka): identification of clinical isolates from vaccine recipients, *J Infect Dis* 149:956-963, 1984.

117. Hayakawa Y et al.: Analysis of varicella-zoster virus DNAs of clinical isolates by endonuclease *Hpa*I, *J Gen Virol* 67:1817-1829, 1986.

118. Hayreh SS: So-called acute retinal necrosis syndrome—an acute ocular panvasculitis syndrome, *Dev Ophthalmol* 10:40-77, 1985.

119. Hayward AR, Herberger M: Lymphocyte responses to varicella zoster virus in the elderly, *J Clin Immunol* 7:174-178, 1987.

120. Hedges TR III, Albert DM: The progression of the ocular abnormalities of herpes zoster: histopathologic observations of nine cases, *Ophthalmology* 89:165-176, 1982.

121. Hellinger WC et al.: Varicella-zoster virus retinitis in a patient with AIDS-related complex: case report and brief review of the acute retinal necrosis syndrome, *Clin Infect Dis* 16:208-212, 1993.

122. Hemady R et al.: Herpes simplex virus type-1 strain influence on chorioretinal disease patterns following intracameral inoculation in Igh-1 disparate mice, *Invest Ophthalmol Vis Sci* 30:1750-1757, 1989.

123. Herbort CP et al.: Acute retinal necrosis, a consequence of cellular immune dysfunction, *Fortschr Ophthalmol* 88(Suppl II):394, 1991.

124. Higa K et al.: T-lymphocytes in otherwise healthy patients with herpes zoster and relationships to the duration of acute herpetic pain, *Pain* 51:111-118, 1992.

125. Higuchi R, Kwok S: Avoiding false positive with PCR, *Nature* 339:237-238, 1989; erratum p 490.

126. Hilt DC et al.: Herpes zoster ophthalmicus and delayed contralateral hemiparesis caused by cerebral angiitis: diagnosis and management approaches, *Ann Neurol* 14:543-553, 1983.

127. Hirst LW et al.: Successful management of acute retinal necrosis with intravenous acyclovir, *Ann Ophthalmol* 19:445-448, 1987.

128. Holland GN: Executive committee of the American Uveitis Society. Standard diagnostic criteria for the acute retinal necrosis syndrome, *Am J Ophthalmol* 117:663-667, 1994.

129. Holland GN et al.: A microscopic study of herpes simplex virus retinopathy in mice, *Invest Ophthalmol Vis Sci* 28:1181-1190, 1987.

130. Holland GN et al.: An association between acute retinal necrosis syndrome and HLA-DQw7 and phenotype Bw62,DR4, *Am J Ophthalmol* 108:370-374, 1989.

131. Hondo R et al.: Genome variations among varicella-zoster virus isolates derived from different individuals and from the same individual, *Arch Virol* 93:1-12, 1987.

132. Hope-Simpson RE: The nature of herpes zoster: a long-term study and a new hypothesis, *Proc R Soc Med* 58:9-21, 1965.

133. Hoppenjans WB et al.: Prolonged cutaneous herpes zoster in acquired immunodeficiency syndrome, *Arch Dermatol* 126:1048, 1990.

134. Hurst L et al.: Comparative neuroinvasiveness, neurovirulence, and retinovirulence of two KOS strains of herpes simplex virus type 1, *Invest Ophthalmol Vis Sci* (Suppl)32:801, 1991.

135. Hyman RW et al.: Varicella-zoster virus RNA in human trigeminal ganglia, *Lancet* 2:814-816, 1983.

136. Ichikawa T et al.: HLA antigens of patients with Kirisawa's uveitis and herpetic keratitis, *Atarashii Ganka* 6:107-111, 1989.

137. Igietseme JU et al.: Protection of mice from herpes simplex virus-induced retinitis by in vitro-activated immune cells, *J Virol* 63:4808-4813, 1989.

138. Ilyid JP et al.: Comparison of the DNAs of varicella-zoster viruses isolated from clinical cases of varicella and herpes zoster, *Virology* 82:345-352, 1977.

139. Immonen I et al.: Acute retinal necrosis syndrome treated with vitrectomy and intravenous acyclovir, *Acta Ophthalmol* 67:106-108, 1989.

140. Immura N et al.: Rise of antibody titter for varicella-zoster virus in the aqueous and vitreous in two cases with Kirisawa uveitis, *Jpn J Clin Ophthalmol* 39:101-106, 1985.

141. Inoue H et al.: Virus particles in Kirisawa-Urayama type uveitis, *Jpn J Clin Ophthalmol* 43:307-311, 1989.

142. Iwamoto Y et al.: A case of herpes zoster ophthalmicus with choroidal involvement, *Jpn J Clin Ophthalmol* 40:945-948, 1986.

143. Jabs DA et al.: Presumed varicella-zoster retinitis in immunocompromised patients, *Retina* 7:9-13, 1987.

144. Jampol LM: Acute retinal necrosis (letter), *Am J Ophthalmol* 93:254-255, 1982.

145. Jansen RS et al.: Neurological and neurophysiological manifestations of HIV-1 infection: association with AIDS-related complex but not asymptomatic HIV-1 infection, *Ann Neurol* 26:592-600, 1989.

146. Javier RT et al.: A herpes simplex virus transcript abundant in latently infected neurons is dispensable for establishment of the latent state, *Virology* 166:254-257, 1988.

147. Jensen J: A case of herpes zoster ophthalmicus complicated with neuroretinitis, *Acta Ophthalmol* 26:551-554, 1948.

148. Johnson RT: *Viral infections of the nervous system,* New York, 1982, Raven Press.

149. Johnston WH et al.: Recurrence of presumed varicella-zoster virus retinopathy in patients with acquired immunodeficiency syndrome, *Am J Ophthalmol* 116:42-50, 1993.

150. Jones KL et al.: Offspring of women infected with varicella during pregnancy a prospective study, *Teratology* 49(1):29-32, 1994.

151. Jura E et al.: Varicella-zoster virus infections in children infected with human immunodeficiency virus, *Pediatr Infect Dis J* 8:586-590, 1989.

152. Karsenti G et al.: La retinite necrosante augue: a propos de deux cas, *J Fr Ophthalmol* 8:133-197, 1985.

153. Kawaai G et al.: A case of Kirisawa-type uveitis treated by vitrectomy, *Jpn Clin Ophthalmol* 30:21-25, 1991.

154. Kawamoto M, Kato S: Vitreous surgery for acute retinal necrosis, *Jpn Rev Clin Ophthalmol* 30:39-45, 1991.

155. Kelly SP, Rosenthal AR: Chickenpox chorioretinitis, *Br J Ophthalmol* 74:698-699, 1990.

156. Kielty D et al.: HSV-1 retinitis and delayed hypersensitivity in DBA/2 and C57BL/6 mice, *Invest Ophthalmol Vis Sci* 28:1994-1999, 1987.

157. Kijlstra A: The value of laboratory testing in uveitis, *Eye* 4:732-736, 1990.

158. Kijlstra A et al.: Laboratory tests in uveitis: new developments in the analysis of local antibody production, *Doc Ophthalmol* 75:225-231, 1990.

159. Kometani J, Asayama T: A case of specific uveitis occurring acutely in the right eye, *Folia Ophthalmol Jpn* 29:1397-1401, 1978.

160. Kreiger AE: Management of combined inflammatory and rhegmatogenous retinal detachments (ARN and AIDS). In Ryan SJ, editor: *Retina,* 591-598, St Louis, 1989, Mosby.

161. Kumashiro O et al.: Increased antibody titer for herpes zoster virus in the intraocular fluids in a case of Kirisawa uveitis, *Rinsho Ganka* 41:902-906, 1987.

162. Lambert SR et al.: Ocular manifestations of the congenital varicella syndrome, *Arch Ophthalmol* 107:52-56, 1989.

163. Lawrence R et al.: The risk of zoster after varicella vaccination in children with leukemia, *N Engl J Med* 318:543-548, 1988.

164. Leib DA et al.: A deletion of mutant of latency-associated transcript of herpes simplex virus type 1 reactivates from the latent state with reduced frequency, *J Virol* 63:2893-2900, 1989.

165. Lcvy RM et al.: Neurological manifestations of the acquired immunodeficiency syndrome (AIDS): experience of UCSF and review of the literature, *J Neurosurg* 62:475-495, 1985.

166. Lewis ML et al.: Herpes simplex virus type 1: a cause of the acute retinal necrosis syndrome, *Ophthalmology* 96:875-878, 1989.

167. Liesegang TJ: Biology and molecular aspects of herpes simplex and varicella-zoster virus infections, *Ophthalmology* 99:781-799, 1991.

168. Lightman S: Acute retinal necrosis, *Br J Ophthalmol* 75:449, 1991.

169. Litoff D, Catalona RA: Herpes zoster optic neuritis in human immunodeficiency virus infection, *Arch Ophthalmol* 108:782-783, 1990.

170. Lucke K et al.: Acute retinal necrosis, *Klin Monatsbl Augenheilkd* 193:602-607, 1988.

171. Ludwig IH et al.: The acute retinal necrosis syndrome: possible herpes simplex retinitis, *Ophthalmology* 91:1659-1664, 1984.

172. Luyendijk L et al.: Detection of locally produced antibodies to herpes viruses in the aqueous of patients with acquired immune deficiency syndrome (AIDS) or acute retinal necrosis syndrome (ARN), *Curr Eye Res* 9(Suppl):7-11, 1990.

173. Mahalingam R et al.: Latent varicella-zoster viral DNA in human trigeminal and thoracic ganglia, *N Engl J Med* 323:627-631, 1990.

174. Mahalingam R et al.: Localization of herpes simplex virus and varicella zoster virus DNA in human ganglia, *Ann Neurol* 31:444-448, 1992.

175. Margolies T et al.: Acute retinal necrosis syndrome presenting with papillitis and arcuate neuroretinitis, *Ophthalmology* 95:937-940, 1988.

176. Margolis TP et al.: Selective spread of herpes simplex virus in the central nervous system after ocular infection, *J Virol* 63:4756-4761, 1989.

177. Margolis TP et al.: Varicella-zoster virus retinitis in patients with the acquired immunodeficiency syndrome, *Am J Ophthalmol* 112:119-131, 1991.

178. Martenet AC: Necrose retinienne peripherique et decollement retinien total d'origine vasculaire. *5th Congress de la Societè Européene d'Ophtalmologie,* 180-182, Hamburg, 1976. Stuttgart, F Enke, 1978.

179. Martinez J et al.: Delayed bilateral involvement in the acute retinal necrosis syndrome, *Am J Ophthalmol* 113:103-104, 1992.

180. Matsunaga Y et al.: Experimental infection and immune response of guinea pigs with varicella-zoster virus, *Infect Immunol* 37:407-412, 1982.

181. Matsuo T, Matsuo N: HLA-DR9 associated with the severity of acute retinal necrosis syndrome, *Ophthalmologica* 203:133-137, 1991.

182. Matsuo T et al.: Immune complex containing herpes virus antigen in a patient with acute retinal necrosis, *Am J Ophthalmol* 101:368-371, 1986.

183. Matsuo T et al.: Immunological studies of uveitis: 1. Immune complex containing herpes virus antigens in four patients with acute retinal necrosis syndrome, *Jpn J Ophthalmol* 30:472-479, 1986.

184. Matsuo T et al.: Cytological and immunological study of the aqueous humor in acute retinal necrosis syndrome, *Ophthalmologica* 195:38-44, 1987.

185. Matsuo T et al.: Mild type acute retinal necrosis syndrome involving both eyes at three-year intervals, *Jpn J Ophthalmol* 31:455-460, 1987.

186. Matsuo T et al.: Acute retinal necrosis following chickenpox in pregnant woman, *Jpn J Ophthalmol* 32:70-74, 1988.

187. Matuso T et al.: A proposed mild type of acute retinal necrosis, *Am J Ophthalmol* 105:579-583, 1988.

188. Matsuo T et al.: Acute retinal necrosis as a novel complication of chickenpox in adults, *Br J Ophthalmol* 74:443-444, 1990.

189. Matsuo T et al.: Acute retinal necrosis developing after chickenpox in adults, *Jpn J Clin Ophthalmol* 44:605-607, 1990.

190. Matsuo T et al.: Factors associated with poor visual outcome in acute retinal necrosis, *Br J Ophthalmol* 75:450-454, 1991.

191. McArthur JC: Neurologic manifestations of AIDS, *Medicine* 66:407-437, 1987.

192. McDonald HR et al.: Surgical management of retinal detachment associated with the acute retinal necrosis syndrome, *Br J Ophthalmol* 75:455-458, 1991.

193. McKendry JBJ, Bailey JD: Congenital varicella associated with multiple defects, *Can Med Assoc J* 108:66-68, 1973.

194. Mendivil A et al.: Ocular manifestations of the congenital varicella-zoster syndrome, *Ophthalmologica* 205:191-193, 1992.

195. Meurisse EV: Laboratory studies on the varicella-zoster virus, *J Med Microbiol* 2:317-325, 1969.

196. Miller AE: Selective decline in cellular immune response to varicella-zoster in the elderly, *Neurology* 30:582-587, 1980.

197. Mosmann TR, Coffman RL: Th1 and Th2 cells: different patterns of lymphokine secretion lead to different functional properties, *Ann Rev Immunol* 7:145-173, 1989.

198. Myers MG et al.: Experimental infection of guinea pigs with varicella-zoster virus, *J Infect Dis* 142:414-420, 1980.

199. Myers MG et al.: Varicella-zoster virus infection of strain 2 guinea pigs, *J Infect Dis* 151:106-113, 1985.

200. Myers MG et al.: Varicella in the gorilla, *J Med Virol* 23:317-322, 1987.

201. Nagae Y et al.: Pars plana vitrectomy and silicone tamponade for Kirisawa's uveitis, *Jpn J Clin Ophthalmol* 39:819-822, 1985.

202. Naito T et al.: A case of recurrent acute retinal necrosis, *Jpn Rev Clin Ophthalmol* 30:26-28, 1991.

203. Nakayama T et al.: Clinical investigations of acute retinal necrosis 3: ultrastructure of biopsy specimens and possibility of herpes virus infection, *Folia Ophthalmol Jpn* 35:1029-1036, 1984.

204. Naumann G et al.: Histopathology of herpes zoster ophthalmicus, *Am J Ophthalmol* 656:533-541, 1968.

205. Neumeyer DA, Hirsh MS: Inversion of T cell subsets before herpes zoster infection, *N Engl Med J* 314:1456, 1986.

206. Nielsen H et al.: Circulating immune complexes and complement-fixing antibodies in patients with varicella-zoster infection: relationship to debut of the disease, *Scand J Infect Dis* 12:21-26, 1980.

207. Nishi M et al.: Polymerase chain reaction for the detection of the varicella-zoster genome in ocular samples from patients with acute retinal necrosis, *Am J Ophthalmol* 114:603-609, 1992.

208. Nussenblatt RB et al.: Birdshot retinochoroidopathy associated with HLA-A29 antigen and immune responsiveness to retinal s-antigen, *Am J Ophthalmol* 94:147-158, 1982.

209. Offret H et al.: Retinal lymphoma, retinal necrosis. Identification of retinal viral particles and anti-herpetic antibodies in the vitreous body, *J Fr Ophthalmol* 13:51, 1990.

210. Ohno S et al.: Close association of HLA-Bw51 with Behçet's disease, *Arch Ophthalmol* 100:1455-1458, 1982.

211. Okinami S, Tsukahara I: Acute severe uveitis with retinal vasculitis and retinal detachment, *Ophthalmologica* 179:276-285, 1979.

212. Okinami S et al.: A surgical treatment for acute retinal necrosis, *Jpn Rev Clin Ophthalmol* 30:17-20, 1991.

213. Okuma M et al.: Posterior fundus lesion masqueraded in a case with acute retinal necrosis, *Jpn J Clin Ophthalmol* 43:347-350, 1989.

214. Palay DA et al.: Decrease in the risk of bilateral acute retinal necrosis by acyclovir therapy, *Am J Ophthalmol* 112:250-255, 1991.

215. Partamian LG et al.: Herpes simplex type 1 retinitis in an adult with systemic herpes zoster, *Am J Ophthalmol* 92:215-220, 1981.

216. Pavin-Langston D, Dunkel EC: Ocular varicella-zoster virus infection in the guinea pig, *Arch Ophthalmol* 107:1068-1072, 1989.

217. Pepose JS: Infectious retinitis: diagnostic modalities, *Ophthalmology* 93:570-573, 1986.

218. Pepose JS, Biron K: Antiviral sensitivity of the acute retinal necrosis syndrome virus, *Curr Eye Res* 6:201-205, 1987.

219. Pepose JS et al.: Herpesvirus antibody levels in the etiologic diagnosis of the acute retinal necrosis syndrome, *Am J Ophthalmol* 113:248-256, 1992.

220. Peyman GA et al.: Vitrectomy and intravitreal antiviral drug therapy in acute retinal necrosis syndrome, *Arch Ophthalmol* 102:1619-1621, 1984.

221. Pfaffl W et al.: Acute retinal necrosis and HIV infection, *Fortschr Ophthalmol* 88:705-711, 1991.

222. Plotkin SA et al.: Attempts to recover varicella virus from ganglia (letter), *Ann Neurol* 2:249, 1977.

223. Plotkin SA et al.: Zoster in normal children after varicella vaccine, *J Infect Dis* 159:1000-1001, 1989.

223a. Prado A, Davis JL, Heilskov T: Acute necrotizing viral retinitis in HIV infection and AIDS, *Invest Ophthalmol Vis Sci* 34(suppl):1109, 1993.

224. Preblud SR: Varicella: complications and costs, *Pediatrics* 78:728-735, 1986.

225. Price FW, Schlaegel TF: Bilateral acute retinal necrosis, *Am J Ophthalmol* 89:419-424, 1980.

226. Priem HA et al.: HLA typing in birdshot chorioretinopathy, *Am J Ophthalmol* 105:182-185, 1988.

227. Provost PJ et al.: Successful infection of the common marmoset with human varicella-zoster virus, *J Virol* 61:2951-2955, 1987.

228. Rabinovitch T et al.: Bilateral acute retinal necrosis syndrome, *Am J Ophthalmol* 108:735-736, 1989.

229. Ragozzino MW et al.: Population-based study of herpes zoster and its sequelae, *Medicine* 61:310-316, 1982.

230. Rai T et al.: Antibody quotient value for the diagnosis of herpetic uveitis. In Belfort R Jr, Petrilli AMN, Nussenblatt R, editors: *World uveitis symposium,* 511-520, Brazil, 1989, Roca Ltda.

231. Reese L et al.: Intraocular antibody production suggests herpes zoster in only one cause of acute retinal necrosis (ARN), *Invest Ophthalmol Vis Sci* 27(suppl):12, 1986.

232. Regillo CD et al.: Repair of retinitis-related retinal detachments with silicone oil in patients with acquired immunodeficiency syndrome, *Am J Ophthalmol* 113:21-27, 1992.

233. Regillo CD et al.: Hemodynamic alterations in the acute retinal necrosis syndrome, *Ophthalmology* 100:1171-1176, 1993.

234. Rinvik R: Congenital varicella encephalitis in surviving infant, *Am J Dis Child* 117:231-235, 1969.

235. Rochat C et al.: Immune dysfunction in acute retinal necrosis (ARN) in HIV-negative patients. Presented at Sixth International Symposium on the Immunology and Immunopathology of the Eye, Washington, DC June 22-24, 1994, (abstract).

236. Roizman B: The family herpes viride: a brief introduction. In Roizman B, Whitley RJ, Lopez C, editors: *The human herpesviruses,* 11-68, New York, 1993, Raven Press.

237. Roizman B, Sears AE: Herpes simplex viruses and their replication. In Roizman B, Whitley RJ, Lopez C, editors: *The human herpesviruses,* 1-9, New York, 1993, Raven Press.

238. Rong BL et al.: Accurate quantiation of varicella zoster virus (VZV) genomic DNA in infected rabbit ocular tissue using quantitative competitive PCR (QC-PCR), *Invest Ophthalmol Vis Sci* (Suppl)33:1347, 1992.

239. Ross AH: Modification of chickenpox in family contacts by administration of gamma globulin, *N Engl J Med* 267:369-376, 1962.

240. Rostad SW et al.: Transsynaptic spread of varicella zoster virus through the visual system: a mechanism of viral dissemination in the central nervous system, *Hum Pathol* 20:174-179, 1989.

241. Rummelt V et al.: Detection of varicella zoster virus DNA and viral antigen in the late stage of bilateral acute retinal necrosis syndrome, *Arch Ophthalmol* 110:1132-1136, 1992.

242. Runger-Brandle E et al.: Bilateral acute retinal necrosis (BARN): identification of the presumed infectious agent, *Ophthalmology* 91:1648-1657, 1984.

243. Saari KM: Association of acute retinal necrosis with herpetic infection. In Saari KM, editor: *Uveitis update; proceedings of the first international symposium on uveitis held in Hanasaari, Espoo, Finland on May 16-19, 1984,* 233-249, Amsterdam, 1984, Excerpta Medica.

244. Saari KM et al.: Bilateral acute retinal necrosis, *Am J Ophthalmol* 93:403-411, 1982.

245. Saibara T et al.: Depressed immune functions in the early phase of varicella-zoster virus reactivation, *J Med Virol* 39:242-245, 1993.

246. Sakai J et al.: Comparative efficacy of antiherpes drugs in acute retinal necrosis, *Jpn Rev Clin Ophthalmol* 85:876-881, 1991.

247. Saiki RK et al.: Genetic analysis of amplified DNA immobilized sequence-specific oligonucleotide probes, *Proc Natl Acad Sci USA* 86:6230-6234, 1989.

248. Saiki RK et al.: Comparative efficacy of antiherpes drugs in acute retinal necrosis, *Jpn Rec Clin Ophthalmol* 85:876-881, 1991.

249. Sakuma T et al.: Surgery for acute retinal necrosis: effects and early surgical intervention, *Jpn Rev Clin Ophthalmol* 30:3-7, 1991.

250. Sandor EV et al.: Herpes zoster ophthalmicus in patients at risk for the acquired immune deficiency syndrome (AIDS), *Am J Ophthalmol* 101:153, 1986.

251. Schimpff S et al.: Varicella-zoster infection in patients with cancer, *Ann Intern Med* 76:241-254, 1972.

252. Schirm J et al.: Rapid detection of varicella-zoster virus in clinical specimens using monoclonal antibodies on shell vials and smears, *J Med Virol* 28:1-6, 1989.

253. Schulman JA, Peyman GA: Management of viral retinitis, *Ophthalmol Surg* 19:876-884, 1988.

254. Schulman JA et al.: Parenterally administered acyclovir for viral retinitis associated with AIDS, *Arch Ophthalmol* 102:1750, 1984.

255. Schwab IR: Oral acyclovir in the management of herpes simplex ocular infections, *Ophthalmology* 95:423-429, 1988.

256. Schwartz JN et al.: Necrotizing retinopathy with herpes zoster ophthalmicus, *Arch Pathol Lab Med* 100:386-391, 1976.

257. Schwoerer J et al.: Acute retinal necrosis: a new pathophysiological hypothesis, *Ophthalmologica* 203:172-175.

258. Sedarati R et al.: Herpes simplex virus type 1 latency-associated transcription plays no role in establishment or maintenance of a latent infection in murine sensory neurons, *J Virol* 63:4455-4458, 1989.

259. Seki F et al.: Surgical treatment of Kirisawa-Urayama uveitis, *Jpn Rev Clin Ophthalmol* 30:876-881, 1991.

260. Sellitti TP et al.: Association of herpes zoster ophthalmicus with acquired immunodeficiency syndrome and acute retinal necrosis, *Am J Ophthalmol* 116:297-301, 1993.

261. Sergott RC et al.: Optic nerve involvement in the acute retinal necrosis, *Arch Ophthalmol* 103:1160-1162, 1985.

262. Sergott RD et al.: Acute retinal necrosis neuropathy: clinical profile and surgical therapy, *Arch Ophthalmol* 197:692-696, 1989.

263. Severin M, Neubauer H: Bilateral acute retinal necrosis, *Ophthalmologica* 192:199-203, 1981.

264. Shibata T et al.: Three cases of Kirisawa-type uveitis treated with the encircling procedure of retinal detachment, *Folia Ophthalmol Jpn* 34:2115-2121, 1983.

265. Shiraki K, Hyman RW: The immediate early proteins of varicella-zoster virus, *Virology* 156:423-426, 1987.

266. Shiraki K et al.: Polypeptides of varicella-zoster virus (VZV) and immunological relationship of VZV and herpes simplex virus (HSV), *J Gen Virol* 61:255-269, 1982.

267. Sidikaro Y et al.: Rhegmatogenous retinal detachments in patients with AIDS and necrotizing retinal infections, *Ophthalmology* 98:129-135, 1991.

268. Sissons JGP, Oldstone MBA: Host response to viral infections. In Fields BN, Knipe DM, Chanock RM et al., editors: *Virology,* 265-279, New York, 1985, Raven Press.

269. Soushi S et al.: Positive varicella-zoster virus antigen in the vitreous of a case with acute retinal necrosis syndrome, *Rinsho Ganka* 41:199-202, 1987.

270. Soushi S et al.: Demonstration of varicella-zoster virus antigens in the vitreous aspirates of patients with acute retinal necrosis syndrome, *Ophthalmology* 95:1394-1398, 1988.

271. Sternberg P Jr et al.: Photocoagulation to prevent retinal detachment in acute retinal necrosis, *Ophthalmology* 95:1389-1393, 1988.

272. Sternberg P et al.: Acute retinal necrosis syndrome, *Retina* 2:145-151, 1982.

273. Stevens JG, Cook ML: Latent herpes simplex virus in spinal ganglia of mice, *Science* 173:843-845, 1971.

274. Stevens JG et al.: RNA complimentary to a herpesvirus gene mRNA is prominent in latently infected neurons, *Science* 235:1056-1059, 1987.

275. Straus SE: Clinical and biological differences between recurrent herpes simplex virus and varicella-zoster virus infections, *JAMA* 262:3455-3458, 1989.

276. Straus SE et al.: Genomic differences among varicella-zoster virus isolates, *J Gen Virol* 64:1031-1041, 1983.

277. Straus SE et al.: Endonuclease analysis of viral DNA from varicella and subsequent zoster infections in the same patient, *N Engl J Med* 311:1362-1364, 1984.

278. Straus SE et al.: Suppression of frequently recurring genital herpes. A placebo-controlled double blind trial of oral acyclovir, *N Engl J Med* 310:1545, 1984.

279. Streilein JW et al.: A critical role for ACAID in the distinctive pattern of retinitis that follows anterior chamber inoculation of HSV-1, *Curr Eye Res* 6:127-131, 1987.

280. Streilein JW et al.: Evidence that precursor cytotoxic T cells mediate acute necrosis in HSV-1-infected retinas, *Curr Eye Res* 10:81-86, 1991.

281. Suttorp-Schulten MSA et al.: Aqueous chamber tap and serology in acute retinal necrosis, *Am J Ophthalmol* 108:327-328, 1989.

282. Takahaski M: A vaccine to prevent chickenpox. In Hyman RW, editor: *Natural history of varicella-zoster virus,* 61-67, Boca Raton, Fla, 1987, CRC Press.

283. Takahashi M et al.: Comparative restriction endonuclease analysis of varicella zoster virus clinical isolates, *Med Microbiol Immunol* (Berl) 178:61-67, 1989.

284. Takahaski M et al.: Immunization of the elderly and patients with collagen vascular diseases with live varicella vaccine and use of varicella skin antigen, *J Infect Dis* 166(suppl 1):S58-S62, 1992.

285. Takayama H et al.: Ocular and systemic manifestations of Kirisawa's uveitis, *Jpn J Clin Ophthalmol* 38:369-375, 1984.

286. Tanaka N, Ozawa K: Surgical treatment of acute retinal necrosis syndrome, *Jpn Rev Clin Ophthalmol* 30:13-20, 1991.

287. Tanaka N et al.: Varicella-zoster viral retinitis in an immunodeficient newborn infant, *Jpn J Clin Ophthalmol* 41:759-762, 1987.

288. Tanifugi Y et al.: A case of Kirisawa type uveitis, *Jpn Rev Clin Ophthalmol* 75:225-228, 1981.

289. Terada K et al.: Natural killer cell activity in herpes zoster in children without underlying disease, *Scand J Infect Dis* 25(4):521-524, 1993.

290. Thompson RL et al.: Physical location of a herpes simplex virus type-1 gene function(s) specifically associated with a 10 million-fold increase in HSV neurovirulence, *Virology* 131:180-192, 1983.

291. Tokura T et al.: Surgical outcome in acute retinal necrosis, *Jpn Rev Clin Ophthalmol* 30:34-38, 1991.

292. Topilow HW et al.: Bilateral acute retinal necrosis: clinical and ultrastructural study, *Arch Ophthalmol* 100:1901-1908, 1982.

293. Tsolia M et al.: Live attenuated varicella vaccine: evidence that the virus is attenuated and the importance of skin lesions in transmission of varicella-zoster virus, *J Pediatr* 116:184-189, 1990.

294. Uruyama A et al.: Unilateral acute uveitis with retinal periarteritis and detachment, *Jpn J Clin Ophthalmol* 25:607-629, 1971.

295. Usui M: Clinical differences in the pattern of Kirisawa-Uruyama uveitis induced by different herpes viruses, *Jpn Rev Clin Ophthalmol* 85:868-875, 1991.

296. Usui M et al.: Electron microscopic study and biochemical analysis on the vitreous of uveitis: two cases of Kirisawa's uveitis, *Jpn J Clin Ophthalmol* 38:381-387, 1984.

297. Usui M et al.: The detection of varicella-zoster virus antigen from vitreous humor in 3 cases with Kirisawa-Uruyama type uveitis, *Nippon Ganka Gakkai Zasshi* 92:1398-1405, 1988.

298. Usui M et al.: Polymerase chain reaction for diagnosis of herpetic intraocular inflammation, *Ocular Immunol Inflammation* 1:105-112, 1993.

299. Vafai A et al.: Expression of varicella-zoster virus and herpes simplex virus in normal trigeminal ganglia, *Proc Natl Acad Sci USA* 85:2362-2366, 1988.

300. Vann V, Atherton SS: Neural spread of herpes simplex virus after anterior chamber inoculation, *Invest Ophthalmol Vis Sci* 32:2462-2472, 1991.

301. von Szily A: Experimental endogenous transmission of infection from bulbus to bulbus, *Klin Monatsbl Augenheilkd* 75:593-602, 1924.

302. Weigle KA, Grose C: Molecular dissection of the humoral immune response to individual varicella-zoster viral proteins during chickenpox, quiescence, reinfection, and reactivation, *J Infect Dis* 149:741-749, 1984.

303. Weksler ME: Immune senescence, *Ann Neurol* 35:S35-S37, 1994.

304. Whittum JA et al.: Ocular disease induced in mice by anterior chamber inoculation of herpes simplex virus, *Invest Ophthalmol Vis Sci* 25:1065-1073, 1984.

305. Willerson D et al.: Necrotizing vasoocclusive retinitis, *Am J Ophthalmol* 84:209-219, 1977.

306. Williams DL et al.: Herpes zoster following varicella vaccine in a child with acute lymphocytic leukemia, *J Pediatr* 106:259-261, 1985.

307. Witmer R: Clinical implications of aqueous humor studies in uveitis, *Am J Ophthalmol* 86:39-43, 1978.

308. Womack LW, Liesegang TJ: Complications of herpes zoster ophthalmicus, *Arch Ophthalmol* 101:42-45, 1983.

309. Yamamoto S et al.: Restriction endonuclease analysis of varicella-zoster virus DNAs, *Kurume Med J* 38:45-50, 1991.

310. Yamamoto S et al.: Herpes simplex virus genomes were detected in the aqueous humor in five cases of acute retinal necrosis, *Jpn J Clin Ophthalmol* 46:665-667, 1992.

311. Yeo JH et al.: Acute retinal necrosis syndrome following herpes zoster dermatitis, *Ophthalmology* 93:1418-1422, 1986.

312. Yeung KC et al.: Differences in the capacity of two herpes simplex virus isolates to spread from eye to brain map to 1610 base pairs of DNA found in the gene for DNA polymerase, *Curr Eye Res* 10(Suppl):31-37, 1990.

313. Young NJ, Bird AC: Bilateral acute retinal necrosis, *Br J Ophthalmol* 62:581-590, 1978.

314. Zaia FA et al.: A practical method for preparation of varicella zoster immune globulin, *J Infect Dis* 137:601-604, 1978.

315. Zaia JA et al.: Evaluation of varicella-zoster immune globulin: protection of immunosuppressed children after household exposure to varicella, *J Infect Dis* 147:737-743, 1983.

316. Zaltas MM et al.: Immunohistopathologic findings in herpes simplex virus chorioretinitis in the von Szily model, *Invest Ophthalmol Vis Sci* 33:68-77, 1992.

317. Zhao M et al.: Immune effector cell (IEC)-mediated protection from HSV-1 retinitis occurs in the central nervous system (CNS), *Invest Ophthalmol Vis Sci* (Suppl)35:1682, 1994.

318. Zhu Q et al.: Varicella zoster virus dissemination and detection by PCR after ocular infection in rabbits, *Invest Ophthalmol Vis Sci* (Suppl)34:1680, 1993.

319. Ziehut M et al.: Akute nekrotisdierende retinitis nach varicella-zoster-virus-infektion, *Klin Monatsbl Augenheilkd* 194:52-58, 1989.

83 Herpes Simplex Virus Diseases: Posterior Segment of the Eye

TODD P. MARGOLIS, SALLY S. ATHERTON

Although herpes simplex virus (HSV) is commonly included as a causal agent in the differential diagnosis of infectious retinitis, well-documented cases of HSV retinitis are rare, and relatively few studies have described the clinical and pathologic features of this disease. As a result, the clinical features characterizing human HSV retinitis have been poorly defined, a problem complicated by the variable presentation of this disease which seems to depend on the age and immune status of the infected host. Within the framework of these limitations, this chapter attempts to summarize the clinical and pathologic features of human HSV retinitis.

EPIDEMIOLOGY

Congenital and Neonatal Disease

HSV infection, along with toxoplasmosis, syphilis, rubella, histoplasmosis, and cytomegalovirus (CMV) infection, has been classically described in the differential diagnosis of intrauterine retinal infection, but documented cases of congenital HSV retinitis are rare. Furthermore, many of the cases of HSV retinitis reported as "congenital" were probably acquired during labor and delivery, either as an ascending maternal genital infection associated with ruptured membranes or during passage of the infant through the birth canal. In this review congenital HSV retinitis will be defined as disease transmitted during gestation, before the process of labor and delivery.

Almost without exception, all cases of congenital HSV retinitis are associated with other clinical evidence of intrauterine infection with HSV-1 or HSV-2. Most cases have associated central nervous system (CNS) abnormalities and skin findings, related either to viral teratogenicity or chronic persistent viral infection. In addition, the retinal findings in these infants occur bilaterally, reflecting the systemic nature of the disease. Unlike neonatally acquired HSV infection, congenital HSV infection usually occurs with mothers who give a history of new onset HSV-2 genital disease during pregnancy (usually during the second trimester). Evidence of active genital infection in the mothers of these infants at delivery is extremely rare.

Much more is known about the epidemiology of neonatal HSV infection than of congenital HSV-related disease. In part this fact is due to the greater ease in making a diagnosis, since viral isolates can be easily obtained. In general neonatal HSV infection occurs with an equal prevalence in males and females. It is more commonly observed in lower socioeconomic classes and in association with a first full-term pregnancy.[40] According to Whitley and associates,[71] about 30% of mothers have signs or symptoms of HSV genital infection around the time of delivery, and over 50% of affected infants are born prematurely. Skin involvement is never seen in 20% of infected neonates, so the absence of viral skin lesions does not rule out a diagnosis of neonatal HSV infection. Active ocular infection occurs in 20% to 25% of HSV infected neonates, with about 5% developing HSV retinitis. A much higher prevalence of ocular infection has been observed in neonates with HSV encephalitis. Of these infants, 60% have ocular involvement, and 20% to 25% have active HSV retinitis.[41] Although about 35% of neonatal HSV disease is caused by HSV-1,[10] all reported cases of neonatal HSV retinitis except one[54] have been associated with HSV-2 infection.

Neonatal ocular infection with HSV is a bilateral disease occurring in infants 2 days to 2 weeks of age. Retinal findings, however, may not be apparent until 1 month of age or older. Most cases of neonatal HSV retinitis occur in association with HSV infection of the CNS, but only about 20% have been associated with HSV conjunctivitis, keratitis, or disseminated dermatitis.[41]

Adult Disease

As with neonatal HSV retinitis, most well-documented cases of adult HSV retinitis have been bilateral and have occurred in patients with an associated encephalitis. This disease occurs in otherwise healthy adults with no well-defined risk factors. Based on reported cases in the medical literature, males are twice as likely to have this disease as females, and the average age of onset is 43 years. For all cases in which the virus was isolated and typing was carried out, the causal agent was HSV-1.

Only a handful of well-documented cases of HSV retinitis have been described in adults without a concurrent encephalitis. Based on reported cases, males are twice as likely to have retinitis without a concurrent encephalitis as females, and the average age of onset is 29 years. In all cases in which the virus was isolated and typing was carried out, the causal agent was HSV-1. Nevertheless, in a few cases, serologic evidence suggests HSV-2 may have been the causal agent.[32,34,63a] Despite the absence of clinical signs and symptoms of an encephalitis in these patients, most had bilateral disease.

Immunosuppressed Patients. Well-documented cases of HSV retinitis in immune compromised individuals have been described exclusively in males, ages 41 to 75, with clinical histories significant for malignancy, organ transplantation, or AIDS.[47,50,62] As might be expected, all of these cases occurred in association with a fatal encephalitis. Similar to the other adult forms of HSV retinitis, only HSV-1 has been found in the retinas and brains of these patients.

CLINICAL FEATURES

Congenital and Neonatal Disease

The clinical findings in congenital HSV infection of the retina are variable and probably largely dependent on the size of the viral inoculum and stage of development of the affected fetus. Infections acquired during the first and second trimesters of pregnancy are associated with a variable degree of ocular teratogenesis and/or retinochoroidal scarring, whereas infections acquired late in the third trimester are usually persistent and may be indistinguishable in presentation from neonatal disease.

Most of what has been learned about the ocular manifestations of congenital HSV infection during the first and second trimesters of fetal development has come from case reports in the nonophthalmic literature. In these reports the ocular findings usually received scant attention, and the funduscopic examination revealed either a white atrophic scar or a "classic" salt-and-pepper pigmentary pattern. Associated systemic teratogenic anomalies have typically included congenital heart disease, short digits, soft nails, intrauterine growth retardation, fibrosis and pigmentation of the skin, and abnormalities of the CNS.

In a few case reports descriptions of HSV-related congenital ocular disease have been a little more revealing. Komorous and associates[25] described two patients with presumed congenital HSV infection as suggested by intrauterine growth retardation, microcephaly, encephalitis, and psychomotor retardation. Optic atrophy and healed retinochoroiditis were described in the first patient, who also had bilateral nystagmus, and bilateral white vitreous masses. Retinochoroidal scars associated with microphthalmia, microcornea, and posterior lenticular opacification were described in the second patient.

Hutto and associates[22] described eight cases of longstanding retinochoroiditis in neonates congenitally infected with HSV. These infants suffered CNS abnormalities including microcephaly and atrophy. Mitchell and McCall[39] described a case of transplacentally acquired HSV infection with large areas of well-healed superior retinochoroiditis in a developmentally delayed child. In one of the rare cases described in the ophthalmic literature, Reynolds and associates[55] described the case of an infant with large bilateral white macular scars characterized by atrophic areas with variable border pigmentation, low-lying vitreous cicatricial changes, and traction on the optic disc. There was no evidence of active intraocular inflammation. As might be expected from an infection that took place early during fetal development, this child had a number of systemic manifestations of congenital HSV infection including intrauterine growth retardation, hypopigmented skin lesions, and CNS abnormalities.

In neonates HSV retinitis is typically diagnosed between 10 and 90 days of age. Diagnosis delays can sometimes be attributed to poor views of the posterior pole, as a consequence of decreased corneal clarity. In other well-documented cases, however, the retina initially appears normal, progressing to active disease at a later time. The clinical course of this disease is poorly defined, but according to most descriptions, early disease begins posterior to the equator and is characterized by well-demarcated patches of yellow-white retinal exudate associated with a variable degree of perivasculitis, vitreous humor inflammatory reaction, and superficial and deep retinal hemorrhage. There is often a sharp demarcation of normal and diseased retina. As the inflammatory phase of the disease resolves, optic atrophy and well-defined hypopigmentary and hyperpigmentary changes become the prominent findings. Although most reports simply describe late alterations in the pigmentary pattern of the fundus, Reersted and Hansen[54] described elevated retinochoroidal scarring in the equatorial region of the fundus, and Hagler and associates[19] described a 360° equatorial band of retinal pigment epithelium (RPE) changes associated with attenuation of the vasculature. In cases in which the acute phase of the disease has been extensive and associated with vascular occlusion, late findings may include neovascularization and detachment of the retina.[78]

Two published investigations have made a particular point of studying the ocular findings of children with a history of neonatal HSV infection, and their findings are worth discussing. Tarkkanen and Laatikainen[63] studied five children, 6 to 9 years of age, with histories of neonatal HSV-2 infection. Four of these children had bilateral retinal and/or

RPE atrophy and associated attenuation of the retinal vasculature. Furthermore, three children had exotropia, two had optic atrophy, and two had late inflammatory changes of the vitreous humor. One patient, with a history of neonatal HSV infection without ocular findings, developed bilateral exudative retinitis at age 5, raising the possibility of reactivation of latent virus from intraocular tissue.

In the second study el Azazi and associates[13] examined 32 children, 1 to 15 years after neonatal HSV infection. In this series 16 of the 17 children with neurologic impairment as a consequence of neonatal HSV infection also had ocular abnormalities. In contrast, only three of the 15 neurologically healthy children had late ocular findings. Overall, nine of the 32 children with a history of neonatal HSV infection had retinochoroidal scars, which were largely described as well-defined areas of coarse hypopigmentation and hyperpigmentation located anterior to the equator.

The results of these studies suggest that a much higher percentage of children with neonatal HSV infection have associated retinal involvement (at least 28%, based on late pigmentary changes) than has been reported based on examinations during the neonatal period (4%). Furthermore, the results of these studies suggest a much higher attack rate of retina anterior to the equator than has been suggested by studies carried out during the neonatal period. These differences can probably be attributed to the difficulty in examining the newborn and the delay in appearance of pigmentary disturbances after the acute inflammatory episode. An alternative explanation is that either virus or viral antigen persists in the retina for years, continuing to incite inflammatory changes in the RPE. All in all, it would appear that fulminant retinitis associated with neonatal HSV-2 infection is a rare occurrence, even in children with neurologic or other ocular involvement, but late disturbances of the RPE are common.

Because the ocular findings associated with congenital and neonatal HSV infections can be extremely variable and may be limited to nondistinct pigmentary changes, it is often difficult to distinguish HSV retinitis from other causes of inflammatory retinal disease in the newborn such as CMV infection, syphilis, toxoplasmosis, varicella-zoster virus (VZV) infection, rubella, and toxocariasis. As such, careful attention should be paid to the features of systemic disease in these patients when attempting to make a diagnosis. Laboratory tests, especially virus cultures and virus-specific serum IgM antibody (which does not cross the placental barrier), may be particularly helpful in this regard.

Adult Disease

Many of the well-documented cases of HSV retinitis described in the medical literature have occurred in patients with associated viral encephalitis. In this setting the onset of HSV ocular disease may not be noted for days or even weeks following the clinical onset of encephalitis. HSV retinitis in these patients usually presents as a rapidly progressive bilateral disease characterized by retinal whitening, vasculitis, papilledema, and a variable degree of nerve fiber layer hemorrhage (Fig. 83-1). Exudative or rhegmatogenous retinal detachment is a common complication and may occur early in the course of the disease. Other associated ocular findings have included keratitis (filamentary and dendritic), iritis, and mild vitreous clouding. Bloom and associates[3] have suggested that the combined findings of multiple flame-shaped hemorrhages and massive exudative retinal detachments in a patient with encephalitis should alert the clinician to consider possible HSV infection.

There are at least two clinical cases in which presumed HSV retinitis occurred years after recovery from HSV encephalitis. The first case, described by Sekizawa and associates,[61] was a 30-year-old man who developed HSV retinitis 2.5 years after an episode of HSV encephalitis. The diagnosis of HSV encephalitis was made by typical clinical and radiographic findings as well as an increase in CSF anti-HSV antibody titer, and the diagnosis of HSV retinitis was made by a high intraocular anti-HSV antibody titer in an eye with vitreous humor cells, yellow-white patches of retinal necrosis and perivascular infiltrates, and hemorrhage. In a second, unpublished case, seen at the Francis I. Proctor Foundation in San Francisco, California, an 80-year-old woman developed extensive retinal necrosis 5 years after recovery from an episode of presumed HSV encephalitis. HSV was suspected to be the cause of her encephalitis based on typical clinical and radiologic findings. The diagnosis of HSV retinitis was made by (1) electron microscopic detection of herpesvirus particles in necrotic retina and (2) detection of HSV DNA within the retina and vitreous humor of the infected eye through the use of a polymerase chain reaction (PCR)-based assay system (Fig. 83-2). Neither patient developed recurrent symptomatic CNS disease at the time of their retinal infection. Sekizawa and associates[61] have suggested that this disease might be a consequence of reactivation of HSV from ocular tissue in which a latent infection had been established during the initial viremia or encephalitis.

Although the clinical pattern of HSV retinal disease may vary considerably from person to person (and perhaps from virus strain to virus strain), it is still possible to consider the usual pattern of this disease. Patients will commonly present with blurred vision, as a result of inflammatory debris in the vitreous humor, and (in some cases) ocular pain, indicative of inflammation of the anterior segment of the eye. The inflammatory response in the anterior chamber and vitreous humor may be quite severe, limiting examination of the retina, but where a thorough view is possible, HSV retinitis is characterized by marked retinal edema, exudate, hemorrhage, and vascular occlusion. Disease may start in either the posterior pole, equator, or periphery and is commonly associated with optic disc swelling and late rhegmatogenous retinal detachment. Prognosis is poor, in part because of the

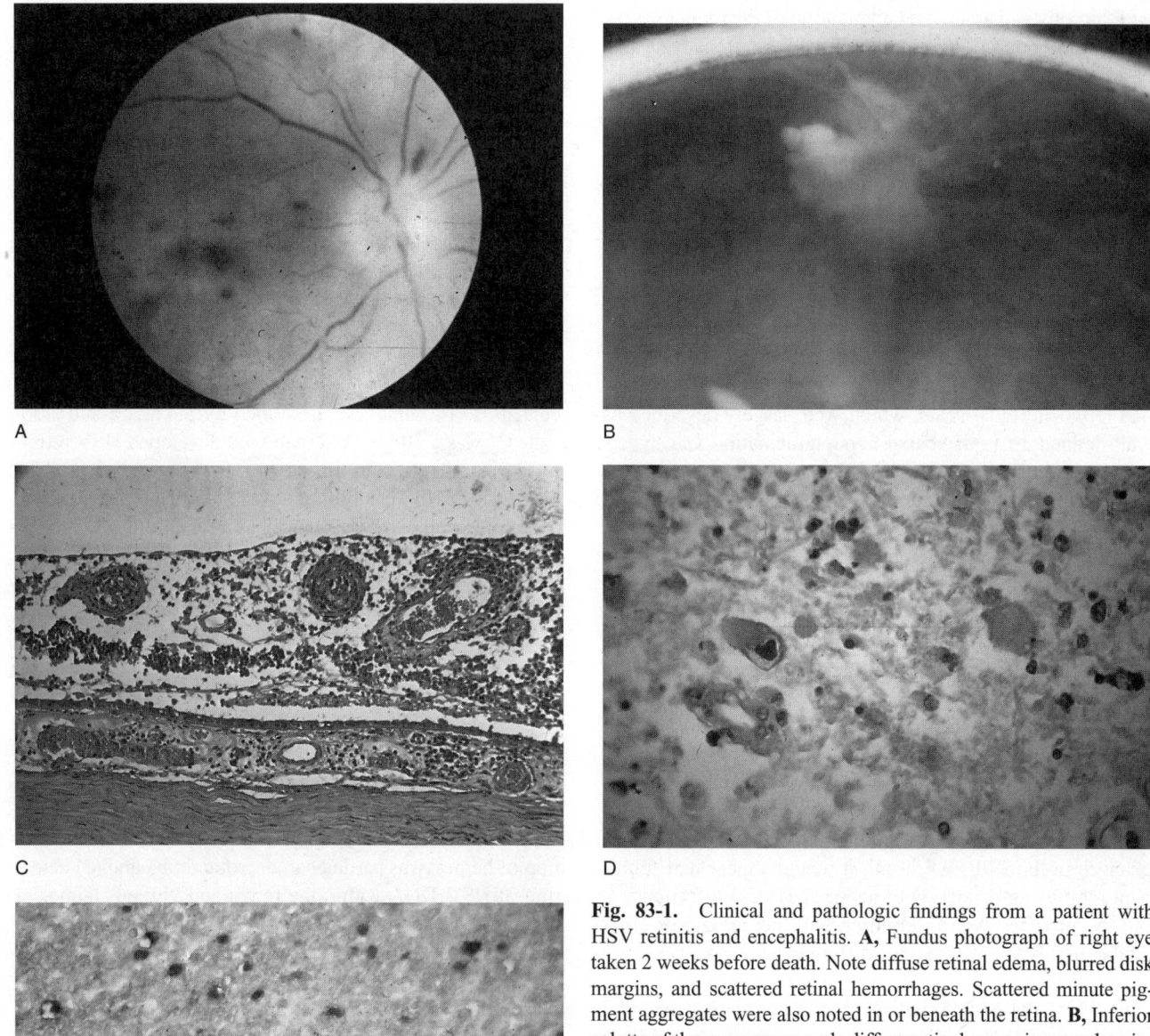

Fig. 83-1. Clinical and pathologic findings from a patient with HSV retinitis and encephalitis. **A,** Fundus photograph of right eye taken 2 weeks before death. Note diffuse retinal edema, blurred disk margins, and scattered retinal hemorrhages. Scattered minute pigment aggregates were also noted in or beneath the retina. **B,** Inferior calotte of the same eye reveals diffuse retinal necrosis, granular pigment epithelium, and vitreous humor haze. **C,** Retinal tissue section stained immunohistochemically for herpes simplex virus antigens. Note occlusion of the arteriolar lumen secondary to mural leukocytic infiltrate as well as dense staining for HSV in the RPE. **D,** Herpes simplex viral antigens as seen with immunohistochemical staining in oligodendroglia in the right optic nerve. **E,** Herpes simplex viral antigens are seen with immunohistochemical staining in cells scattered throughout the left temporal lobe of the brain. (A, B, E reprinted with permission from Pepose JS, Kreiger AE, Tomiyasu U et al.: Immunocytologic localization of herpes simplex type 1 viral antigens in herpetic retinitis and encephalitis in an adult, *Ophthalmology* 92:160-166, 1985.)

rapid and destructive nature of this disease, but also because of delays in diagnosis and treatment.

There are at least five published cases of presumed HSV retinitis in otherwise healthy adults in which the diagnosis was confirmed by culture of HSV from ocular tissues.

Pavan-Langston and Brockhurst[48] described the case of a 34-year-old woman with bilateral panuveitis characterized by choroidal hemorrhage, choroidal and intraretinal exudates, retinal edema, and narrowing (but not occlusion) of the retinal arterioles. An interesting characteristic of this

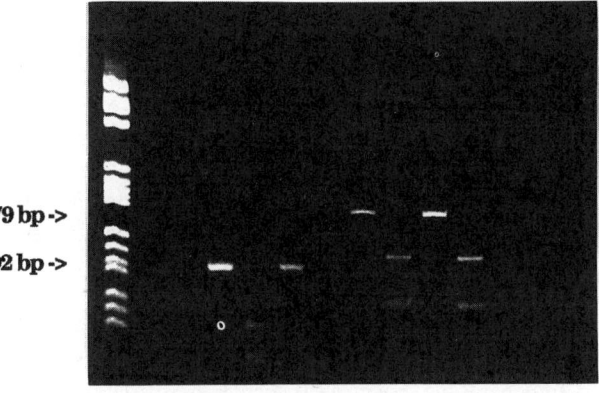

Fig. 83-2. Ethidium bromide stained polyacrylamide gel of PCR amplification products. Two independent primer sets were used to assay for detection of HSV DNA sequences from vitreous humor specimen taken from a patient with a necrotizing retinitis 5 years after an episode of HSV encephalitis. Bands of the appropriate molecular weight were confirmed as amplified HSV DNA by restriction enzyme analysis. Lane 1: molecular weight standards, Lane 2: negative control (buffer), Lane 3: control vitreous humor, Lane 4: purified HSV DNA, Lane 5: Rsa-1 digest of purified HSV DNA, Lane 6: retinal biopsy using first primer set, Lane 7: Rsa-1 digest of retinal biopsy DNA amplified with first primer set, Lane 8: retinal biopsy using second primer set, Lane 9: Rsa-1 digest of retinal biopsy DNA amplified with second primer set, Lane 10: purified HSV DNA; Lane 11: Rsa-1 digest of purified HSV DNA, Lane 12: control vitreous humor, Lane 13: negative control (buffer).

case was the development of discrete yellow plaques at the level of the retinal pigment epithelium. The patient had a facial HSV eruption a few days prior to the onset of the retinal disease, and HSV was cultured from the aqueous humor of one of the involved eyes. More recently, Grutzmacher and associates[18] described the clinical course of a 20-year-old man with bilateral multifocal retinochoroiditis characterized by early fluffy deep retinal edema without hemorrhage or vasculitis. He developed late swelling of the optic disk of one eye but failed to develop retinal detachment. A diagnosis of HSV retinitis was made by positive viral culture of the vitreous humor and the retina of one of the involved eyes.

Acute Retinal Necrosis Syndrome. The remaining three culture-proven cases presented with clinical features characteristic of the acute retinal necrosis (ARN) syndrome, which are distinct from those described previously.[12,21a,28] Each of these three individuals was less than 38 years old, which is consistent with the concept that in younger individuals HSV is more likely than VZV to cause ARN syndrome.[31,45] A second feature that may help to distinguish cases of HSV-associated ARN syndrome is an exudative retinal detachment. As noted by Duker and associates,[12] exudative retinal detachment is a common characteristic of HSV retinitis, but is not commonly associated with ARN syndrome caused by VZV.

ARN syndrome has also been described in a number of cases in which HSV-1 was suspected as the causal agent, but virus was not recovered by culture. Immonen and associates,[23] Sarkies and associates,[58] and Matsuo and associates[37] all diagnosed HSV-1 as the causal agent of ARN syndrome, based on the levels of anti-HSV-1 antibodies in intraocular fluids. Ludwig and associates[31] and Willerson and associates[75] depended on the concomitant appearance of recurrent HSV facial skin lesions, and Matsuo and associates[37] relied on the presence of both antibody titers to HSV and HSV antigen-containing immune complexes in ocular fluids to make the diagnosis. In all of these reports the clinical presentation included the classic features of ARN syndrome: retinal whitening with confluent necrosis, vitritis, and retinal vasculitis.

Immunosuppressed Patients. HSV retinitis has also been reported in immune compromised patients. The ophthalmoscopic findings described for presumed HSV retinitis in this population have been extremely variable and may reflect, in part, the degree of immunosuppression of the host. Partamian and associates[47] described the case of a 72-year-old man with Lennert lymphoma, who developed a white-yellow multifocal retinitis with cloudy overlying vitreous humor and optic nerve involvement, concurrently with culture-proven HSV blepharoconjunctivitis. There was no mention of retinal hemorrhage, vasculitis, or retinal detachment in the description of this case. In contrast, in a case of disseminated HSV infection in a renal allograft recipient, Uninsky and associates[68] described marked vitreous humor haze and multifocal retinal whitening accompanied by retinal hemorrhage, vascular sheathing, and late exudative retinal detachment—a description more consistent with HSV retinitis observed in immunocompetent individuals. Finally, presumed HSV-2 retinitis occurred in a 45-year-old woman receiving systemic corticosteroids following surgical resection of a sphenoid ridge meningioma.[34] The clinical findings in this case fell somewhere between those described by the two other groups; there was retinal whitening and vitritis with vascular sheathing but no hemorrhage or exudative retinal detachment (Fig. 83-3).

HSV might also be responsible for retinitis in some patients with AIDS, either as a sole pathogen or via co-infection with CMV. In a histopathologic study, Pepose and associates[49] reported co-localization of CMV and HSV antigens in the retina of a patient with AIDS and HSV encephalitis. It is important to note that this patient's clinical examination was consistent with typical CMV retinitis. There are two similar, unpublished cases of patients with AIDS and typical CMV retinitis in whom postmortem cultures revealed both CMV and HSV in ocular tissues.* Unlike the case described by Pepose and associates,[49] neither of

---

*Jacob P. Lalezari, MD, University of California, San Francisco, personal communication.

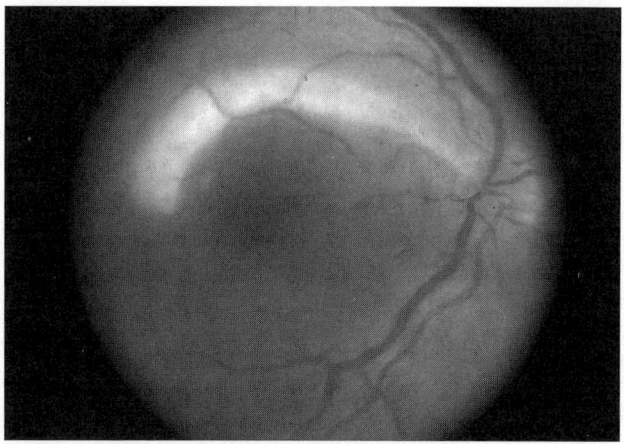

A

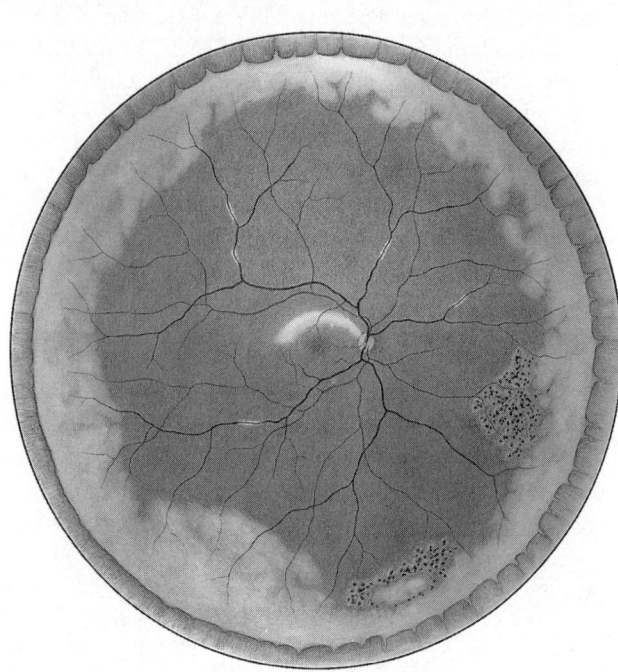

B

Fig. 83-3. **A,** Fundus photograph of a patient with presumed HSV-2 retinitis. Note the unusual pattern of arcuate neuroretinitis early in the course of infection. **B,** Retinal drawing of the same eye 18 days after the initial ophthalmologic evaluation. By this time, a 360° peripheral retinitis as well as a dense vitritis and midperipheral vasculitis had developed. (Reprinted with permission from Margolis T, Irvine AR, Hoyt WF, Hyman R: Acute retinal necrosis syndrome presenting with papillitis and arcuate neuroretinitis, *Ophthalmology,* 95:937-940, 1988.)

these patients had clinical evidence of HSV encephalitis before their death. Thus in all three of these cases, the clinical picture was that of typical CMV retinitis. In contrast, Sidikaro and associates[62] described three cases of possible HSV retinitis in patients with AIDS in which the clinical findings differed considerably from that observed with CMV retinitis. All three cases were characterized by bilateral deep multifocal retinal opacification that rapidly progressed to co-

alescent retinal necrosis and rhegmatogenous retinal detachment. Vascular occlusion and retinal hemorrhages were present, but only late in the course of the disease. For two reasons it is possible these cases of retinitis were not caused by HSV, but by another herpesvirus such as VZV: (1) the clinical findings of these patients appear very similar to those of the progressive outer retinal necrosis syndrome,[13a] and (2) the diagnosis in these cases was not based on positive viral cultures, but on a history of vesicular skin lesions and ultrastructural evidence of herpesvirus family particles in biopsy specimens.

PATHOLOGY

In general the few clinical specimens available for histopathologic study of HSV retinitis have been obtained late in the course of the disease, after extensive retinal necrosis has occurred. As such they provide a narrow temporal window on the pathologic processes at work.

Congenital and Neonatal Disease

There are no reported histopathologic studies of congenital HSV retinitis. In contrast, there are a few published reports in which the pathologic features of neonatal HSV retinitis have been described; the first is a study by Cogan and associates.[8] In this report the investigators studied the eyes of a 4-month-old infant who developed HSV encephalitis and retinitis at 3 weeks of age. Their report, therefore, should be considered a histopathologic description of a late stage of this disease. Not surprisingly, they found extensive bilateral destruction of the retinas, which were reduced to thin glial membranes, and complete loss of all neuronal tissue of the optic nerves. Unexpected findings included a proliferative metaplasia of the RPE, a relative lack of retinal inflammatory cells, and almost complete sparing of the anterior segments and choroids. The rapid course of the disease, its symmetry, and its selective involvement of the neural retina led the authors to conclude that the observed ocular destruction was most likely caused by an immunologic process rather than direct viral infection of the retinas. Similar findings and a comparable conclusion were subsequently reported by Cibis.[5]

The results of two subsequent studies, however, led investigators to substantially different conclusions.[6,77] In both cases studies were carried out on autopsy specimens obtained within 2 weeks of the observed onset of retinal disease. Thus a much earlier point in the course of HSV infection was represented. In addition to the full thickness retinal necrosis, RPE metaplasia, and optic nerve atrophy observed in earlier studies, these tissues displayed a sharp demarcation between involved and uninvolved retina, with substantial inflammatory cell infiltrate of the involved regions of retina and adjacent choroid. Furthermore, by both light and electron microscopy, viral inclusions consistent with HSV were noted within all layers of involved retina, especially in the transition zone between necrotic and healthy retina.

Viral inclusions were only rarely noted in the choroid or retinal vascular endothelium. In all published reports hemorrhage contributed minimally to the overall pathologic picture.

Adult Disease

Most of the tissue used for histopathologic study has come from patients who died from an associated HSV encephalitis. The most comprehensive of these studies involve the work of Minckler and associates,[38] Johnson and associates,[24] and Pepose and associates.[50] Although the pictures described by these investigators are similar in some respects, they differ in many ways as well. In all three studies the anterior segment was spared, but there was acute and chronic inflammation of the retina, RPE, and optic nerve, with both light and electron microscopic evidence (intranuclear Cowdry type A bodies as well as viral capsids approximately 100 nm in diameter) of a direct herpesvirus infection of these tissues. In contrast, the degree of retinal necrosis, vascular occlusion, and hemorrhage, as well as perivascular and choroidal inflammatory infiltration varied widely in these reports. Furthermore, whereas Minckler and associates[38] noted a massive exudative retinal detachment, this finding had not been described by the other investigators.

PATHOGENESIS

The pathogenesis of HSV retinitis in human beings remains obscure. Very few samples of HSV-infected human retinal tissue are available for study, and in most of these cases the specimens only represent one time point (usually the end point) in the course of disease. This situation has made it very difficult to describe the sequence of events leading up to the development of HSV retinitis. Understanding the pathogenesis of HSV retinitis is further complicated by the fact that a documented primary or reactivated infection by HSV at a nonocular site may be separated in time from the onset of HSV ocular disease.

In considering the pathogenesis of HSV retinitis, both virus and host factors are likely to be important. For example, the site of the original infection, the virulence of the virus, and its ability to replicate and spread through host tissues contribute to development of herpetic disease, whereas the age, immunologic status, and innate resistance of the host also influence the outcome of either a primary or reactivated HSV infection.

Animal Models

Much of the information about the pathogenesis of herpesvirus infections has been obtained using animal models, and the results from such studies provide insights into the pathogenesis of HSV infections in human patients. In considering HSV retinitis in particular, one of the underlying questions is how does the virus gain access to the retina? There are at least three routes by which HSV might enter the retina: (1) hematogenous, (2) direct spread from an infected anterior segment of the eye to the posterior segment, and (3) from the CNS to the retina.

The capacity of HSV to replicate in neurons and to spread via axonal transport[9] must be considered in any attempt to describe disease mechanisms caused by these viruses. Although HSV usually enters the nervous system primarily through sensory neurons, studies in experimental animals also indicate that HSV can infect the CNS by retrograde axonal transport of somatic motor neurons.[46,67] HSV has also been shown to spread along autonomic nerves to parasympathetic and sympathetic (especially the superior cervical ganglion) secretomotor neurons.[36,59,64,65] The ability of HSV to spread via neuronal pathways was described by Goodpasture and Teague[16] and Goodpasture[15] and has been confirmed by more recent investigations. In 1982 Anderson and Field[1] demonstrated that intravenous injection of virus does not result in ocular infection. Even in human patients with disseminated HSV infection with concomitant retinitis, cultures of the blood are usually negative for virus.[17] Because of the predilection of HSV for neurons and the apparent inability of the virus to spread in the blood, it is not likely that virus infection of the retina results from hematogenous spread of the virus.

The second route, direct spread of virus from the anterior to the posterior segment of the eye, is also probably not the primary route by which virus gains access to the retina, since patients with HSV anterior uveitis do not appear to be at increased risk of developing HSV retinitis. It is thus likely that the anterior chamber inflammation noted in many cases of HSV retinitis represents either simultaneous infection of both the anterior and posterior segments of the eye or inflammatory "spillover" phenomenon in the anterior segment.

The third route of spread, from the CNS to the optic nerve and from there frequently to the retina, appears to be the most likely route by which HSV gains access to the retina. Support for this contention is derived from both human cases and from studies using animals. The strong association between HSV retinitis and encephalitis provides support for virus spread from the CNS to the eye as the most likely and/or most common cause of HSV retinitis. Because spread of virus cannot be directly followed in human patients, much of the work to determine routes of virus spread has been performed using animal models of CNS and ocular infection. Results from these studies have described several pathways by which HSV might be able to gain access to the retina in human patients. Intracerebral inoculation of HSV (both HSV-1 and HSV-2) as well as other neurotropic viruses (for example, Borna disease virus) is followed by retinitis.[26,27,30,44,53]

Following intracerebral inoculation, the percentage of animals with retinitis varies. In the case of murine models of HSV disease, this percentage depends both on the strain of the mouse and on the virulence of the infecting virus. In studies in which an extremely neurovirulent strain of virus is inoculated intracerebrally, animals with encephalitis may not survive long enough to develop retinitis. In animals that do develop retinitis, spread to the retina has been shown to occur via the optic nerve and its connections within the CNS. One drawback of intracerebral inoculation is that direct inoculation of HSV into the CNS only provides information about the spread of virus from the brain to the eye during and following a primary HSV encephalitis. This model will probably not provide insight into the pathogenesis of human HSV retinitis in which primary HSV inoculation must have occurred at a more peripheral site (and where retinitis may be the consequence of reactivation of latent infection).

Spread of HSV from the anterior segment of an injected eye to the retina of the opposite, uninjected eye was documented in 1924 by von Szily, who reported that injection of HSV into one eye of a rabbit produces retinal necrosis in the noninoculated, contralateral eye.[70] These findings were confirmed recently by other investigators using both rabbits and mice. In 1984 Whittum and associates[72] reported that uniocular anterior chamber inoculation of HSV-1 (KOS strain) into euthymic BALB/c mice results in acute retinitis followed by retinal necrosis in the contralateral eye 8 to 10 days after virus inoculation. In this model the anterior segment of the uninoculated eye exhibits mild iridocyclitis, but virus infection of the anterior segment is not observed. In the injected eye the pattern of involvement is reversed, and there is massive inflammation of the anterior segment.[73] Curiously, although retinal folding and mild-to-moderate vitritis are observed in the posterior segment, the retina of the inoculated eye is not infected with virus and does not become necrotic.[74] Besides sharing some clinical similarities with viral retinopathies observed in human patients, the von Szily model of HSV retinitis has provided additional insight into the pathways by which virus might spread to the retina in human beings following virus infection at a peripheral site.

Several tracing studies in which mice were infected with different strains of HSV-1 via the anterior chamber have described the route by which HSV leaves the injected eye and enters the CNS.[35,52,69] These studies demonstrated that virus spread is limited to synaptically related sites. Initial spread of the virus from the anterior segment of the eye occurs via sensory fibers of the ophthalmic division of the trigeminal nerve and parasympathetic fibers of the oculomotor nerve. The trigeminal route provides a direct pathway for the spread of neuroinvasive strains of HSV-1 to the brainstem nucleus of the spinal trigeminal tract, and from there to other synaptically related CNS nuclei (Fig. 83-4). In contrast, less neuroinvasive strains of HSV-1, such as KOS, rarely spread along this route beyond the primary sensory neurons of the trigeminal ganglion.

In contrast, the parasympathetic route provides a pathway

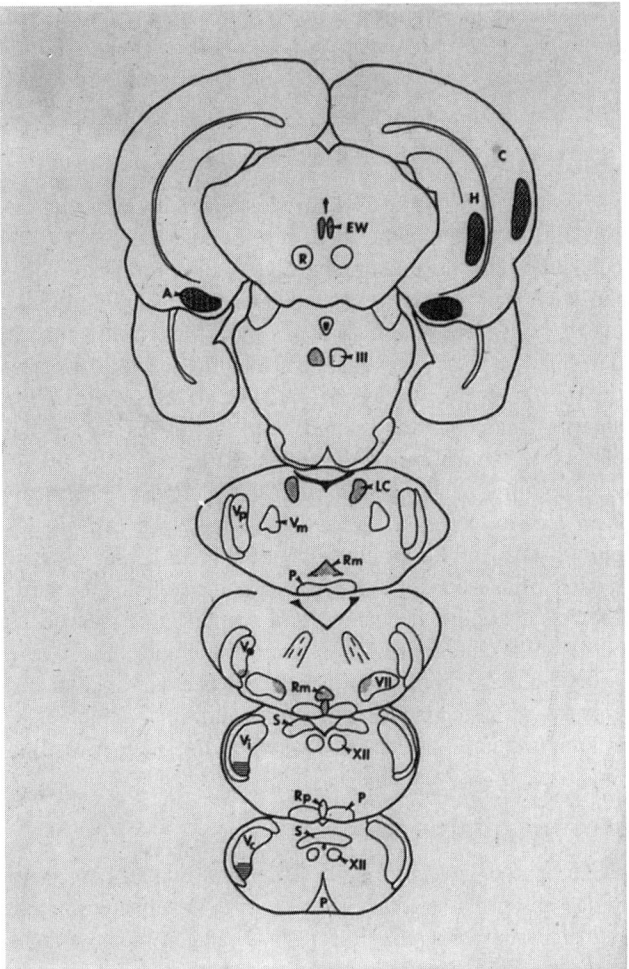

Fig. 83-4. Diagram summarizing the spread of McKrae strain HSV in the CNS of mice after anterior chamber inoculation. Darker shaded regions represent the location of productive viral infection at 4 days postinoculation; lighter shaded areas represent sites where productive viral infection was first found at 5 days postinoculation; and circles represent sites where productive viral infection was first found at 7 days postinoculation. *A,* amygdala complex; *C,* cerebral cortex; *H,* hippocampal formation; *LC,* nucleus locus coeruleus; *S,* nucleus solitarius; *R,* red nucleus, V_c, nucleus caudalis; V_i, nucleus interpolaris; V_o, nucleus orlis; V_m, main sensory nucleus; *Rm,* nucleus raphe magnus; *Rp,* nucleus raphe pallidus; *P,* pyramidal fibers; *III,* oculomotor nucleus; *Vii,* facial nerve nucleus; *Xii,* hypoglossal nucleus.

for the spread of virus to the contralateral eye (Fig. 83-5). In following this route, HSV travels by retrograde axonal transport from the anterior segment of the infected eye to the ipsilateral ciliary ganglion and Edinger-Westphal nucleus. From the ipsilateral Edinger-Westphal nucleus, virus spreads sequentially to the ipsilateral suprachiasmatic nucleus, contralateral optic nerve, and contralateral retina. Two days after HSV first appears in the ipsilateral suprachiasmatic nucleus, it is also found in the contralateral suprachi-

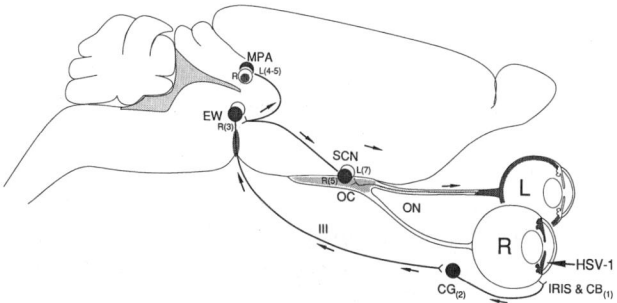

Fig. 83-5. Diagram of the pathway from the anterior segment of one eye to the retina of the contralateral eye. Following anterior chamber inoculation of KOS strain HSV, virus spreads from the anterior segment of the inoculated right eye along parasympathetic motor nerve fibers of the oculomotor nerve to the CNS. The pathway from the inoculated eye *(right)* to the contralateral *(left)* retina is as follows: iris$_R$ → ciliary ganglion (CG)$_R$ → Edinger-Westphal nucleus (EW)$_R$ → suprachiasmatic nucleus (SCN)$_R$ → optic nerve (II)$_L$ → retinal ganglion cells and retina$_L$. Arrows indicate the direction of virus spread and the numbers in parentheses indicate the first day virus is observed at that site. *OC* = optic chiasm, *III* = oculomotor nerve, *MPA* = medial pretectal area. Subscripts: *R* = right (ipsilateral to the site of injection), *L* = left (contralateral to the site of injection).

asmatic nucleus. Curiously, however, sequential spread to the synaptically related ipsilateral optic nerve and retina does not occur. One possible reason why mice infected with relatively avirulent strains of HSV do not develop retinitis in both eyes may be that the host's immune response is mobilized rapidly enough to prevent virus spread from the contralateral suprachiasmatic nucleus (day 7 postinfection), but not rapidly enough to prevent virus spread from the ipsilateral suprachiasmatic nucleus (day 5 postinfection).[2] After anterior chamber inoculation, HSV also spreads by retrograde axonal transport to the sympathetic neurons of the ipsilateral superior cervical ganglion.[33] This route would not be expected to provide access to the visual pathway, however.

In a study of the von Szily model using rabbits,[45a] the contralateral retina became infected after inoculation of HSV into either the anterior chamber or vitreous body of one eye. Selective transection of the ipsilateral retrobulbar optic nerve, without disrupting other neural and vascular connections to that eye, prevented development of contralateral disease in rabbits that received vitreous humor inoculations, but not in those that received anterior chamber inoculations. In contrast, similar selective transection of the contralateral retrobulbar optic nerve prevented development of retinal infection in the contralateral eye, regardless of the site of inoculation in the other eye. These results suggest that HSV can leave the inoculated eye by multiple routes, but that virus reaches the contralateral eye only via the optic nerve.

Knowledge of routes of virus spread from the mouse and rabbit models may provide insight into the mechanism of

HSV retinitis in human beings. By extrapolation from the mouse, the following sequence of events might occur in patients that develop HSV retinitis: (1) infectious HSV, either from a primary infection or reactivation of a latent source (trigeminal, superior cervical, or ciliary ganglion; perhaps even cornea) causes an anterior uveitis; (2) immune mechanisms are incapable of completely restricting virus spread, and the virus travels to the CNS by retrograde axonal transport within the parasympathetic component of the oculomotor nerve; (3) virus spreads along axonal pathways to the suprachiasmatic nuclei and returns to one or both eyes by retrograde axonal transport along the optic nerve; (4) once virus reaches the ganglion cell layer of the retina, virus replication occurs, and the retina is destroyed by both virus- and immune-mediated mechanisms. Alternatively, virus might enter the visual system via brainstem connections with the sensory trigeminal system. This second pathway of spread has yet to be well defined in an animal model.

Immune Response

Because the prevalence of HSV retinitis in humans is extremely low compared to latent trigeminal infection and recurrent anterior segment ocular disease, development of HSV retinitis is most likely caused by failure of the host to contain virus at its usual sites of disease. Although little is known about the mechanisms by which the host restricts spread of HSV in nervous tissue, it is becoming clear that both T-lymphocytes and cytokines (interleukin-1, interferon, and tumor necrosis factor) probably play a critical role in this process.* Furthermore, it is likely that T-lymphocyte subsets contribute differentially to this process. Whereas CD4+ T-lymphocytes probably facilitate production of HSV-1 specific antibody and participate in class II-restricted killing of HSV-infected cells,[11] CD8+ T-lymphocytes probably limit virus spread by class I-restricted cytotoxic killing of infected neurons and glia.

Tissue Destruction

Development of an immune response to HSV, although critical to limiting virus spread, also may contribute to the pathologic changes of HSV-associated disease. In the process of targeted destruction of infected cells, the inflammatory response may destroy adjacent uninfected tissue as well. Although all the usual mechanisms of "innocent bystander" destruction probably contribute to the destruction of cells immediately adjacent to the foci of infection, vascular compromise, as a consequence of an occlusive vasculitis, probably accounts for a substantial amount of the tissue damage that occurs in cases of HSV retinitis.

In an animal study of the pathogenesis of retinal necrosis associated with HSV infection, direct destruction of cells by

---

*References 4, 14, 21, 29, 43, 56, 57, 76.

productive virus infection appeared to play a major role in early retinal changes.[21b] Holland and associates[21b] showed by light and electron microscopy that the earliest events were "collapse" of the photoreceptor layer and disruption of the outer nuclear layer, whereas virus particles were located primarily in the ganglion and inner nuclear layers. Muller cells were consistently infected. The investigators hypothesized that virus reaches the retina via retrograde transport in axons of the optic nerve to produce infection of ganglion cell nuclei, and virus released from ganglion cell nuclei is then taken up by Muller cells. Destruction of Muller cells and their processes, which serve as the supporting neuroglia of the retina, leads to disruption of the outer retinal layers, despite the relative absence of virus particles in that part of the retina. There was little correlation between early retinal destruction and the appearance or anatomic distribution of inflammatory cells, suggesting that inflammation may not play an important role in the earliest events surrounding retinal necrosis. The study did not address the possible role of noncellular immune mechanisms, such as cytokine-induced damage, in the destruction of tissue, however. A heightened inflammatory response followed the development of extensive tissue necrosis.

DIFFERENTIAL DIAGNOSIS

In patients with HSV encephalitis, the cause of an associated retinitis is rarely in question. In contrast, cases of HSV retinitis in which infection is limited to intraocular tissues may be difficult to diagnose on clinical grounds alone. HSV retinitis must be differentiated from retinitis caused by CMV, syphilis, toxoplasmosis, and VZV. In this regard, proper laboratory testing and knowledge of the patient's immune status are critical to making the diagnosis. Both syphilis and toxoplasmosis may be ruled out by serologic testing, and retinal infection with CMV does not occur in an immunocompetent host. Each of these other infectious retinopathies is much more common than HSV retinitis.

LABORATORY INVESTIGATIONS

Tissue culture isolation of HSV is probably the best way to confirm a clinical diagnosis of HSV retinitis. Culture systems are based on the premise that HSV will infect a monolayer of cultured indicator cells, replicate, and produce a characteristic cytopathic effect. Positive cultures are commonly confirmed by immunofluorescence assay, using monoclonal antisera specific for HSV-1 or HSV-2. Positive virus cultures are most likely obtained from retinal biopsy specimens taken at the advancing border of the infected tissue. Virus cultures of the aqueous, vitreous, subretinal fluid, serum, and cerebrospinal fluid are probably equally useful in diagnosing HSV retinitis, but the relative sensitivity of assaying these fluids in cases of HSV retinitis is unknown.

A number of authors of published case reports of presumed HSV retinitis have based their diagnosis, in part, on tissue culture isolation of HSV from temporally related lesions of the skin and cornea. The results of such tests, however, should be interpreted with caution and only used as confirmatory data. This suggestion stems from the work of Nahmias and associates,[42] who studied the association between HSV culture positive skin lesions and temporal lobe brain biopsies in patients with encephalitis and concluded that demonstration of peripheral excretion of HSV is of no diagnostic value in HSV encephalitis. This finding is not surprising, since febrile illness (whatever the cause) is a common trigger for the reactivation of peripheral shedding of HSV. A similar problem exists in trying to interpret the relationship between recurrent peripheral HSV disease and an active retinitis.

Quantitative antibody levels can also contribute to a diagnosis of HSV retinitis. Nevertheless, although serum antibody titers are valuable for determining primary HSV infection (and for excluding a diagnosis of HSV in patients with no serologic evidence of exposure), they may be of limited value in recurrent disease when less than 5% of individuals demonstrate significant changes in anti-HSV serology. As an alternative, investigators are beginning to examine the diagnostic utility of intraocular antibody titers and calculation of the Witmer coefficient in cases of retinitis of presumed viral cause.[51,60] In addition, el Azazi and associates[13] have discussed the diagnostic utility of intrathecal antibody titers in cases of HSV retinitis, and Matsuo and associates[37] reported a case of fulminant retinitis in which the diagnosis of HSV retinitis was based on an ELISA for HSV-1 circulating immune complexes.

Laboratory evaluation can assist in distinguishing HSV retinitis from other nonviral disorders in its differential diagnosis. Furthermore, viral cultures and acute and convalescent antibody titers (serum and ocular) may help to distinguish HSV retinitis from VZV retinitis. In the absence of laboratory tests, it is extremely difficult to differentiate VZV and HSV retinitides because their clinical features are very similar. The clinical features of retinitis caused by syphilis or toxoplasmosis may be largely obscured by an accompanying dense vitritis; laboratory data may help differentiate these infections from HSV retinitis.

With the recent development of molecular biologic techniques for the amplification of unique sequences of DNA, additional tools are becoming available for the diagnosis of ocular infections. In particular, use of PCR techniques may prove extremely valuable in the diagnosis of viral retinitis from small samples of aqueous or vitreous fluid. Clinical studies of the sensitivity and specificity of PCR-based assays need to be carried out before their use in the diagnosis of HSV retinitis becomes widely accepted, however.

The cytologic features of HSV retinitis may have some limited value in confirming a diagnosis of HSV retinitis. Similarly, ultrastructural analysis of involved tissues may be useful in confirming a diagnosis of HSV retinitis but cannot differentiate the causal agent within the herpesvirus family (HSV, VZV, CMV, EBV, and HHV-6 and -7). As such, the limited amount of tissue obtained in the course of a diagnostic retinal biopsy for presumed HSV retinitis might be best put to use for virus cultures, viral DNA amplification by PCR techniques, and immunohistochemical studies for viral antigen. Furthermore, to increase the chance of making a diagnosis through the use of these techniques, biopsy specimens are probably best taken from the leading edge of involved retina.

THERAPY

Antiviral Agents

Systemic antiviral agents have long been the mainstay of therapy for HSV retinitis. Both vidarabine and acyclovir are probably effective, but acyclovir has recently become the drug of choice because of its greater therapeutic index and ease of administration. For neonates the dose of intravenously administered acyclovir is 30 mg/kg/day IV for 10 days to 4 weeks, and for adults it is 5 to 10 mg/kg IV every 8 hours for 7 to 10 days, followed by a prolonged period of oral therapy. Acyclovir is cleared from the circulation by the kidney, and appropriate adjustments in the dosing should be made for patients with renal insufficiency. The major side effect associated with administration of systemic acyclovir is renal toxicity. Acyclovir has also been administered via subconjunctival injection and intravitreous injection (10 to 40 mg/ml), but the role of these routes of administration in the effective therapy of HSV retinitis has yet to be established. Vidarabine is administered as a single intravenous infusion, 15 mg/kg/day, over a 12-hour period. Potential side effects associated with the administration of systemic vidarabine include hepatic toxicity and bone marrow suppression.

Antiinflammatory Agents

The role of corticosteroids in the treatment of HSV retinitis remains controversial. Although it is possible that their use may suppress tissue-damaging inflammation, it may also impair host immunity, thereby inhibiting clearance of the offending viral agent. It may be prudent to institute the use of corticosteroids at least 24 hours after beginning systemic antiviral therapy. In view of the theoretic drawbacks of corticosteroids in the management of HSV retinitis, the use of nonsteroidal antiinflammatory drugs (NSAIDs) that inhibit the cyclooxygenase pathway of arachidonic acid metabolism may prove a more rational approach to the suppression of HSV-related intraocular inflammation. In animal models of bacterial meningitis, the combination of antibiotic and oxindanac, a NSAID, has been of considerable therapeutic advantage over antibiotic alone or a combination of antibiotic and dexamethasone.[66] Similar studies are needed to determine the efficacy of combination therapy with oxindanac,

as well as other antiinflammatory agents, in the treatment of viral retinitis.

Anticoagulation

It has been suggested that anticoagulants, and in particular aspirin, may be of value in the management of HSV retinitis, by virtue of the role these agents may play in reducing the thrombotic component of the occlusive vasculitis that may occur as part of this disease. There is no clinical evidence to support the use of such agents at this time, however. In the event such agents were effective, they would have to be given very early in the course of disease (to prevent thrombosis) and would be of little value later in the disease once vascular occlusion has occurred.

Laser Photocoagulation

Laser photocoagulation of the retina has been advocated to reduce the risk of retinal detachment associated with viral retinitis.[7,20] Nevertheless, very little data are available to support the use of this prophylactic therapy for any form of viral retinitis, and the efficacy of laser photocoagulation has never been studied in well-documented cases of retinitis caused by HSV. Furthermore, given the rarity of HSV retinitis and the variable clinical course it may follow, it is unlikely any well-controlled studies will be carried out to test the effectiveness of this therapy in the near future.

Retinal Detachment Repair

Retinal detachment associated with HSV retinitis may occur early or late in the course of the disease and is usually linked with multiple retinal breaks and vitreous fibrosis. For this reason, retinal detachment is probably best repaired by a combination of advanced vitreoretinal techniques including vitrectomy, epiretinal membrane peeling, endo-laser photocoagulation, fluid gas exchange, and scleral buckle. The successful use of silicone oil in the management of retinal detachment associated with CMV retinitis makes it a likely candidate for the treatment of retinal detachment associated with HSV infection.

PROGNOSIS

In general the prognosis for good visual function following an episode of HSV retinitis of the neonate or adult is poor. Furthermore, many of these patients have severe systemic disease caused by HSV infection, notably, infection of the CNS. As a result, unless the disease is recognized early and treated immediately with high-dose systemic antiviral therapy, the patient's overall prognosis is poor.

REFERENCES

1. Anderson JR, Field HJ: The development of retinitis in mice with non-fatal herpes simplex encephalitis, *Neuropathol Appl Neurobiol* 8:277-287, 1982.

2. Azumi A, Atherton SS: Sparing of the ipsilateral retina following anterior chamber inoculation of HSV-1: requirement for either CD4+ or CD8+ T cells, *Invest Ophthalmol Vis Sci* 35:3251-3259, 1994.

3. Bloom NB, Katz JI, Kaufman HE: Herpes simplex retinitis and encephalitis in an adult, *Arch Ophthalmol* 95:1798-1979, 1977.

4. Chan WL, Javanovic T, Lukic ML: Infiltration of immune T cells in the brain of mice with herpes simplex virus-induced encephalitis, *J Neuroimmunol* 23:195-201, 1989.

5. Cibis GW: Neonatal herpes simplex retinitis, *Graefes Arch Clin Exp Ophthalmol* 196:39-47, 1975.

6. Cibis CW: Herpes simplex retinitis, *Arch Ophthalmol* 96:299-302, 1978.

7. Clarkson JG et al.: Retinal detachment following the acute retinal necrosis syndrome, *Ophthalmology* 91:1665-1668, 1984.

8. Cogan DG et al.: Herpes simplex retinopathy in an infant, *Arch Ophthalmol* 72:641-645, 1964.

9. Cook ML, Stevens JG: Pathogenesis of herpetic neuritis and ganglionitis in mice: evidence of intra-axonal transport of infection, *Infect Immun* 7:272-288, 1973.

10. Corey L et al.: Difference between herpes simplex virus type 1 and type 2 neonatal encephalitis in neurological outcome, *Lancet* January 2:1-4, 1988.

11. Doymaz MZ et al.: MHC II-restricted, CD4+ cytotoxic T lymphocytes specific for herpes simplex virus-1: implications for the development of herpetic stromal keratitis in mice, *Clin Immunol Immunopathol* 61:398-409, 1991.

12. Duker JS et al.: Rapidly progressive acute retinal necrosis secondary to herpes simplex virus, type 1, *Ophthalmology* 97:1638-1643, 1990.

13. el Azazi M, Malm G, Forsgren M: Late ophthalmologic manifestations of neonatal herpes simplex virus infection, *Am J Ophthalmol* 109:1-7, 1990.

13a. Engstrom RE, Holland GN, Margolis TP et al.: The progressive outer retinal necrosis syndrome: a variant of necrotizing herpetic retinopathy in patients with AIDS, *Ophthalmology* 101:1488-1502, 1994.

14. Gebhardt BM, Hill JM: Cellular neuroimmunologic response to ocular herpes simplex virus infection, *J Neuroimmunol* 28:227-236, 1990.

15. Goodpasture EW: Herpetic infection with special reference to involvement of the nervous system, *Medicine* 8:223-243, 1929.

16. Goodpasture EW, Teague O: Transmission of the virus of herpes febrilis along nerves in experimentally infected rabbits, *J Med Res* 44:139-184, 1923.

17. Greer CH: Bilateral necrosing retinitis complicating fatal encephalitis probably due to herpes simplex type 2, *Ophthalmologica* 180:146-150, 1980.

18. Grutzmacher RD et al.: Herpes simplex chorioretinitis in a healthy adult, *Am J Ophthalmol* 96:788-796, 1983.

19. Hagler WS, Walters PV, Nahmias AJ: Ocular involvement in neonatal herpes simplex virus infection, *Arch Ophthalmol* 82:169-176, 1969.

20. Han DP et al.: Laser photocoagulation in the acute retinal necrosis syndrome, *Arch Ophthalmol* 105:1051-1054, 1987.

21. Hartung H-P et al.: Inflammatory mediators in demyelinating disorders of the CNS and PNS, *J Neuroimmunol* 40:197-210, 1992.

21a. Holland GN, The Executive Committee of the American Uveitis Society: Standard diagnostic criteria for the acute retinal necrosis syndrome, *Am J Ophthalmol* 117:663-667, 1994.

21b. Holland GN, Togni BI, Dawson CR, Briones OC: A microscopic study of herpes simplex virus retinopathy in mice, *Invest Ophthalmol Vis Sci* 28:1181-1190, 1987.

22. Hutto C et al.: Intrauterine herpes simplex virus infections, *J Pediatr* 110:97-101, 1987.

23. Immonen I, Laatikainen L, Linnanvuori K: Acute retinal necrosis syndrome treated with vitrectomy and intravenous acyclovir, *Acta Ophthalmologica* 67:106-108, 1989.

24. Johnson BL, Wisotzkey HM: Neuroretinitis associated with herpes simplex encephalitis in an adult, *Am J Ophthalmol* 83:481-489, 1977.

25. Komorous JM et al.: Intrauterine herpes simplex infections, *Arch Dermatol* 113:918-922, 1977.

26. Krey H, Ludmig H, Boschek CB: Multifocal retinopathy in Borna disease virus infected rabbits, *Am J Ophthalmol* 87:157-164, 1979.

27. Krey H, Ludwig H, Gierend M: Borna disease virus-induced retinouveitis treated with immunosuppressive drugs, *Graefes Arch Clin Exp Ophthalmol* 216:111-119, 1981.

28. Lewis ML et al.: Herpes simplex virus type 1: a cause of the acute retinal necrosis syndrome, *Ophthalmology* 96:875-878, 1989.

29. Lindsley MD, Thiemann R, Rodriguez M: Cytotoxic T cells isolated from the central nervous systems of mice infected with Theiler's virus, *J Virol* 65:6612-6620, 1991.

30. Love A, Hill TJ, Maitland NJ: MS strain of type 2 herpes simplex virus produces necrotizing retinitis in mice, *J Neurol Sci* 115:144-152, 1993.

31. Ludwig IH, Zegarra H, Zakov ZN: The acute retinal necrosis syndrome: possible herpes simplex retinitis, *Ophthalmology* 91:1659-1664, 1984.

32. Mahjoub SB et al.: Isolation of a herpes simplex virus type 2 that is retinovirulent in mice, *Curr Eye Res* 8:687-695, 1989.

33. Margolis T et al.: Identifying HSV infected neurons after ocular inoculation, *Curr Eye Res* 6:119-126, 1987.

34. Margolis TP et al.: Selective spread of herpes simplex virus in the central nervous system after ocular inoculation, *J Virol* 63:4756-4761, 1989.

35. Margolis T et al.: Acute retinal necrosis syndrome presenting with papillitis and arcuate neuroretinitis, *Ophthalmology* 95:937-940, 1988.

36. Martin X, Dolivo M: Neuronal and transneuronal tracing in the trigeminal system of the rat using herpes virus suis, *Brain Res* 273:253-276, 1983.

37. Matsuo T et al.: Immune complex containing herpesvirus antigen in a patient with acute retinal necrosis, *Am J Ophthalmol* 101:368-371, 1986.

38. Minckler DS et al.: Herpesvirus hominis encephalitis and retinitis, *Arch Ophthalmol* 94:89-95, 1976.

39. Mitchell JE, McCall FC: Transplacental infection by herpes simplex virus, *Am J Dis Child* 106:121-123, 1963.

40. Nahmias AJ, Hagler WS: Ocular manifestations of herpes simplex in the newborn (neonatal ocular herpes), *Int Ophthalmol Clin* 12:191-213, 1972.

41. Nahmias AJ et al.: Eye infections with herpes simplex viruses in neonates, *Surv Ophthalmol* 21:100-105, 1976.

42. Nahmias AJ et al.: Herpes simplex virus encephalitis: laboratory evaluations and their diagnostic significance, *J Infect Dis* 145:829-836, 1982.

43. Nash AA et al.: Different role for L3T4+ and Lyt2+ T cell subsets in the control of an acute herpes simplex virus infection of the skin and nervous system, *J Gen Virol* 68:825-833, 1987.

44. Norgren RB Jr, Lehman MN: Retrograde transneuronal transport of herpes simplex virus in the retina after injection in the superior colliculus, hypothalamus and optic chiasm, *Brain Res* 479:374-378, 1989.

45. Nussenblatt RB, Palestine AG: Uveitis: fundamentals and clinical practice, St Louis, 1989, Mosby.

45a. Olson RM, Holland GN, Goss SJ et al.: Routes of viral spread in the von Szily model of herpes simplex virus retinopathy, *Curr Eye Res* 6:59-62, 1987.

46. Openshaw H, Ellis W: Herpes simplex virus infection of motor neurons: hypoglossal model, *Infect Immun* 42:409-413, 1983.

47. Partamian LG, Morse PH, Klein HZ: Herpes simplex type 1 retinitis in an adult with systemic herpes zoster, *Am J Ophthalmol* 92:215-220, 1981.

48. Pavan-Langston D, Brockhurst RJ: Herpes simplex panuveitis, *Arch Ophthalmol* 81:783-787, 1969.

49. Pepose JS et al.: Concurrent herpes simplex and cytomegalovirus retinitis and encephalitis in the acquired immune deficiency syndrome (AIDS), *Ophthalmology* 91:1669, 1984.

50. Pepose JS et al.: Immunocytologic localization of herpes simplex type 1 viral antigens in herpetic retinitis and encephalitis in an adult, *Ophthalmology* 92:160-166, 1985.

51. Pepose JS et al.: Herpes virus antibody levels in the etiologic diagnosis of the acute retinal necrosis syndrome, *Am J Ophthalmol* 113:248-256, 1992.

52. Pettit TH et al.: Herpes simplex uveitis: an experimental study with the fluorescein-labeled antibody technique, *Invest Ophthalmol* 4:349-357, 1965.

53. Pfeiffer RL, Dekker CD, Siegel FL: Ocular lesions in mice following intracerebral injection of herpes simplex virus type 1, *Invest Ophthalmol Vis Sci* 24:1070-1080, 1983.

54. Reersted P, Hansen B: Chorioretinitis of the newborn with herpes simplex virus type 1: report of a case, *Acta Ophthalmologica* 57:1096-1100, 1979.

55. Reynolds JD et al.: Congenital herpes simplex retinitis, *Am J Ophthalmol* 102:33-36, 1986.

56. Richt J et al.: Borna disease, a progressive meningoencephalomyelitis as a model for CD4+ T cell-mediated immunopathology in the brain, *J Exp Med* 170:1045-1050, 1989.

57. Richt J et al.: Borna disease virus-induced meningoencephalomyelitis caused by a virus-specific CD4+ T cell-mediated immune reaction, *J Gen Virol* 71:2565-2573, 1990.

58. Sarkies N et al.: Antibodies to herpes simplex virus type I in intraocular fluids of patients with acute retinal necrosis, *Br J Ophthalmol* 70:81-84, 1986.

59. Schimeld C et al.: Spread of herpes simplex virus and distribution of latent infection after intraocular infection of the mouse, *Arch Virol* 85:175-187, 1985.

60. Schwoere J, Othenin-Girard P, Herbort CP: Acute retinal necrosis: a new pathophysiological hypothesis, *Ophthalmologica* 203:172-175, 1991.

61. Sekizawa T et al.: Acute retinitis 2 years after recovery from herpes simplex encephalitis, *Neurology* 41:456, 1991.

62. Sidikaro Y et al.: Rhegmatogenous retinal detachments in patients with AIDS and necrotizing retinal infections, *Ophthalmology* 98:129-135, 1991.

63. Tarkkanen A, Laatikainen L: Late ocular manifestations in neonatal herpes simplex infection, *Br J Ophthalmol* 61:608-616, 1977.

63a. Thompson WS, Culbertson WW, Smiddy WE et al.: Acute retinal necrosis caused by reactivation of herpes simplex virus type 2, *Am J Ophthalmol* 118:205-211, 1994.

64. Tokumaru T, Wilentz J: Iridoplegia and aqueous flare due to acute herpetic keratouveitis, *Can J Ophthalmol* 10:193-200, 1975.

65. Tullo AB et al.: Ocular herpes simplex and the establishment of latent disease, *Trans Ophthalmol Soc UK* 102:15-18, 1982.

66. Tuomanen E: Adjunctive therapy of experimental meningitis: agents other than steroids. In Schonfeld H, Helwig H, editors: Bacterial meningitis, *Antibiot Chemother,* 45:184-191, 1992.

67. Ugolini C: Transneuronal transfer of herpes simplex virus type 1 (HSV-1) from mixed limb nerves to the CNS. I. Sequence of transfer from sensory, motor, and sympathetic nerve fibers to the spinal cord, *J Comp Neurol* 326:527-548, 1992.

68. Uninsky E et al.: Disseminated herpes simplex infection with retinitis in a renal allograft recipient, *Ophthalmology* 90:175, 1983.

69. Vann VR, Atherton SS: Neural spread of herpes simplex virus after anterior chamber inoculation, *Invest Ophthalmol Vis Sci* 32:2462-2472, 1991.

70. von Szily A: Experimentelle endogene infektions übertragung von bulbus zu bulbus, *Klin Monatsbl Augenheilkd* 72:593-602, 1924.

71. Whitley RJ et al.: The natural history of herpes simplex virus infection of mother and newborn, *Pediatrics* 66:489-494, 1980.

72. Whittum JA et al.: Ocular disease induced in mice by anterior chamber inoculation of herpes simplex virus, *Invest Ophthalmol Vis Sci* 25:1065-1073, 1984.

73. Whittum-Hudson J, Farazdaghi M, Prendergast RA: A role for T lymphocytes in preventing experimental herpes simplex virus type 1-induced retinitis, *Invest Ophthalmol Vis Sci* 26:1524-1532, 1985.

74. Whittum-Hudson JA, Pepose JS: Immunologic modulation of virus-induced pathology in a murine model of acute retinal necrosis, *Invest Ophthalmol Vis Sci* 28:1541-1548, 1987.

75. Willerson D, Aaberg TM, Reeser FH: Necrotizing vaso-occlusive retinitis, *Am J Ophthalmol* 84:209-219, 1977.

76. Williamson JSP, Sykes KC, Stohlman SA: Characterization of brain-infiltrating mononuclear cells during infection with mouse hepatitis virus strain JHM, *J Neuroimmunol* 32:199-207, 1991.

77. Yanoff M, Allman M, Fine BS: Congenital herpes simplex virus, type 2, bilateral endophthalmitis, *Trans Am Ophthalmol Soc* LXXV:325-338, 1977.

78. Young GF, Knox DL, Dodge PR: Necrotizing encephalitis and chorioretinitis in a young infant, *Arch Neurol* 13:15-24, 1965.

84 Other Viral Infections of the Retina

E. MITCHEL OPREMCAK

Our ability to diagnose viral infections of the retina has improved greatly over the last decade.[29,86] Advances in vitreoretinal surgery and the development of techniques for chorioretinal/retinal biopsy have provided fresh tissue for study in cases of sight-threatening retinal disease. By employing light and electron microscopy, immunohistochemistry, newer microbial culture techniques, and molecular biologic probes, specific infectious agents have been identified in several disorders.[30,87] Herpes simplex type-1 (HSV-1), herpes simplex type-2 (HSV-2), varicella-zoster, herpes B virus, cytomegalovirus, Epstein-Barr, coxsackievirus B, rubella, Rift Valley Fever virus, influenza A, mumps, measles, and subacute sclerosing panencephalitis viruses have all been shown to be agents of infectious retinitis in man. Other retinal disorders, such as acute posterior multifocal placoid pigment epitheliopathy (APMPPE), acute retinal pigment epitheliitis (ARPE), multiple evanescent white dot syndrome (MEWDS), and Leber idiopathic stellate neuroretinitis often begin with a viral prodrome and may represent manifestations of viral illness as well.[22,32,53,64]

The most important family of viruses capable of infecting the retina are the herpesviruses. Herpes simplex viruses (HSV-1, HSV-2), cytomegalovirus (CMV) and varicella-zoster virus (VZV) are responsible for the vast majority of cases of viral retinitis in the USA. Immunocompromised hosts as well as patients with intact immune systems are susceptible to this family of viruses. For example, the acute retinal necrosis syndrome (ARN/BARN) occurs in healthy adults and is the result of retinal infection with HSV-1, HSV-2 or VZ viruses.[4,10,16,23] In contrast, CMV retinitis affects immunosuppressed patients such as those on chemotherapy, neonates, and patients with AIDS. These syndromes are reviewed separately in other chapters.

The pathogenesis of viral retinitis in man is complex and outside the scope of this chapter. It is important to note that both host and viral factors determine clinical disease course. Viral strain characteristic, virus antigen expression, mutation and variation, cell and tissue tropism, and latent viral infection all govern the development of retinal disease. For example, certain strains of HSV may produce more severe clinical disease (blepharitis, keratitis) than do other less virulent strains,[46] and specific segments of the viral chromosome may govern neuroinvasiveness.[14,108] Viral antigen expression may greatly modify clinical disease course. The absence or alteration of M protein antigen on the measles virus results in a persistent, slow-viral infection of the central nervous system, while inoculation with the wild-type (unaltered M-protein) effects an acute, self-limiting, febrile exanthem.[109] Influenza virus continually makes changes, or "shifts," in its surface antigens. These "new" antigens permit cyclical and widespread "flu" pandemics.[69] The affinity or tropism of a virus for certain tissues also plays a role in viral disease pathogenesis. Several members of the herpesvirus family are inherently neurotropic and therefore infection often involves the brain, nerves and eye. Other viruses (influenza, mumps, measles) have an affinity for epithelium of the respiratory tract and begin their infection in these tissues.[4,10,16,23,69] Finally, latent viral infection and subsequent reactivation may result in recurrent disease such as in CMV and VZV retinitis.[4,10,16,23]

Whereas viral factors play a pivotal role in the pathogenesis of many diseases, host factors (including genetics and the status of the immune system) often determine susceptibility and severity of infection. Certain strains of mice are resistant to HSV-mediated keratitis, retinitis, or encephalitis, while other strains are exceptionally prone to infection.[80,81] As mentioned, the status of the immune system can determine whether a patient is susceptible to infection such as with CMV retinitis.[50,75] In contrast, the rigorous intraocular inflammation observed in ARN/BARN is a result of an intact immune response in healthy subjects directed toward the replicating viral antigens.[4,10,16,23]

This chapter will cover viruses known to be associated with infectious retinitis. Herpes simplex, varicella zoster, and cytomegalovirus/HIV infections will be discussed in separate sections (Table 84-1).

1169

TABLE 84-1 OPHTHALMIC MANIFESTATIONS OF SELECTED VIRAL RETINITIDES

Virus	Vitreous	Vessels	Sensory Retina	RPE	Choroid	Optic Nerve
Herpes B virus	Hemorrhage[95] Scar[95] Vitritis[76]	(—)	Retinal detachment[95] Multifocal necrotizing retinitis[76]	Scar[95]	Chorioretinal scarring[95]	Atrophy[95]
Epstein-Barr virus	Vitritis[11,78,107]	(—)	Macular edema[9,85,89,107,116] Hemorrhage[9,85,116] Multifocal outer retinitis[11] Multifocal choroiditis and panuveitis[78] Chorioretinitis[103]	Scar[60] Pigment changes[11,78,89,103]	Multifocal choroiditis[78] Subretinal neovascular membrane[103]	Edema[9,58,85,89,107]
Coxsackievirus	(—)	(—)	Multifocal chorioretinitis[60]	Scar[60]	(—)	(—)
Rubella						
Acquired	Vitritis[35]	(—)	Grey lesions[92] Exudative RD[63,92]	Exudative RPE detachment[63,92]	(—)	(—)
Congenital	(—)	(—)	Salt and pepper[44,115] Dull foveal reflex[44,115]	SRNVM	(—)	
Rift Valley fever virus	Vitritis[8]	Occlusion[8,28,111]	Macular lesions Exudative RD Hemorrhage Fibrosis[8,28,111]	Scarring	(—)	(—)
Influenza A	(—)	Leakage[54]	Submacular hemorrhage[96] Macular star[54] CME[21] Inner retinitis	(—)	(—)	Edema[21]
Mumps	Vitritis[62]	(—)	White retinitis[62]	Scarring	(—)	Edema[62]
Measles						
Acquired	(—)	Attenuated arterioles[77]	Macular star[26,77] CME[77]	(—)	(—)	Edema[72]
Congenital	(—)	Attenuated[12,61]	Macular star[12,61]	Pigment changes	(—)	(—)
SSPE virus	(—)	(—)	Macular edema White infiltrates Hemorrhage Serous detachment[17,19]	Scarring	Chorioretinitis[19]	Edema[17] Atrophy[19]

HERPES B VIRUS

Virology

Herpes B virus (HV-B), or herpesvirus simiea, is an alphaherpesvirus within the Herpesvirinea family. HV-B is an encapsulated, double-stranded DNA virus (100 nm) with an icosahedral nucleocapsid.[105] Other alphaherpesviruses include herpes simplex type 1 (HSV-1), herpes simplex type 2 (HSV-2) and varicella-zoster virus (VZV).

Epidemiology

Herpes B virus is an endemic virus among macaque monkeys; 30% to 80% of animals are seropositive for HV-B. Transmission to humans occurs through bites or scratches from infected monkeys.[95,105] Human infections have also occurred via puncture wounds from contaminated objects.[76]

Pathogenesis

Herpes B virus gains access to the blood via direct inoculation. Similar to the other alphaherpesviruses, HV-B is neurotropic and inoculation may result in severe encephalo-myelitis and retinitis.[76,95,105] One patient who died from cul-ture-proved HV-B encephalomyelitis was found on autopsy to have a vitritis, panuveitis, optic neuritis and a multifocal necrotizing retinitis.[76] Electron microscopy demonstrated herpesvirus in the retina. Vitreous cultures obtained post mortem were positive for HV-B.

Clinical Features

Herpes B virus causes a rapidly progressive ascending meningitis and encephalitis.[76,105] The infection can be severe and is often fatal despite antiviral therapies. Asymptomatic or latent HV-B infections have not been reported.

Two cases of HV-B encephalomyelitis in monkey handlers have been reported with associated ocular compli-cations and viral retinitis.[76,95] In one case a 29-year-old handler noted sudden loss of vision because of a vitreous hemorrhage.[95] With resolution of the hemorrhage, vitreous organization and widespread chorioretinal scarring were noted throughout the fundus. The patient went on to develop an irreparable retinal detachment. In a second case of fatal HV-B encephalitis, a multifocal, necrotizing retinitis and panuveitis was found on autopsy.[76] These reports suggest that all four alphaherpesviruses appear to be able to infect the retina and cause an ARN/BARN-like syndrome with multifocal, necrotizing retinitis and panuveitis in immuno-competent hosts.[4,10,16,23]

Laboratory Diagnosis

Encephalomyelitis developing in monkey handlers fol-lowing a bite, scratch, or contaminated puncture wound should suggest Herpes B virus infection. In this clinical set-ting the presence of an acute retinal necrosis, vitritis, and subsequent retinal detachment would support a clinical diagnosis of HV-B retinitis. Serologic studies showing a fourfold rise in complement fixation (CF) or enzyme-linked immunosorbent assay (ELISA) antibodies toward HV-B would confirm the diagnosis.[105] Vitreous cultures may isolate HV-B.[76]

Differential Diagnosis

Other viral infections may have a similar fundus appear-ance. Specifically, HSV-1, HSV-2, and VZV can cause an acute, multifocal necrotizing retinitis that would be difficult to distinguish by fundus examination alone.[4,10,16,23] The his-tory of exposure to monkeys is important in establishing the diagnosis. Retinal biopsy may help with the differential diagnosis in severe sight-threatening or medically unrespon-sive cases of suspected viral retinitis.* Other diseases that can affect both the retina and the central nervous system include Lyme disease, rickettsial infections, sarcoidosis, and Behçet disease. These conditions are discussed further in other sections.

---

*References 4, 10, 16, 23, 29, 86.

Treatment and Prognosis

Antiviral agents may play a role in treating HV-B retini-tis. Acyclovir has been shown to be effective in treating the acute retinal necrosis (ARN) syndrome secondary to HSV and VZV when given intravenously at a dose of 1500 mg/ m^2/day.[75] In one fatal case of HV-B encephalitis and retini-tis, the use of both acyclovir and ganciclovir failed to halt the CNS disease. The role of oral corticosteroids is not clear, but there may be a theoretical advantage to using systemic corti-costeroids to minimize the vigorous intraocular inflamma-tion accompanying herpesvirus infections of the retina.[68]

As with other forms of necrotizing retinitis, it appears that HV-B infection can result in retinal breaks and vitreous traction. Vitreoretinal surgical repair may be required in cases of tractional detachment with multiple, posterior reti-nal breaks as observed in viral infection of the retina.[51,82,102]

EPSTEIN-BARR VIRUS

Virology

Epstein-Barr virus (EBV) is a member of the gammaher-pesvirinae genus in the Herpesviridae family.[100] The virus was first identified by Epstein and Barr in 1964 by means of electron microscopy. EBV is a double-stranded DNA virus (100 to 200 nm) with an encapsulated, icosahedral nucleo-capsid.

Epidemiology

Epstein-Barr virus is ubiquitous with as high as 90% of the population demonstrating antibodies to the virus by the third decade of life.[99,100] Asymptomatic shedding of virus in saliva is the primary mode of transmission. The virus can be isolated from the oropharynx in 15% to 25% of all seroposi-tive individuals in the absence of clinical disease. Infectious mononucleosis (IM), or the "kissing disease," peaks during adolescence at ages 14 to 16 in girls and 16 to 18 in boys.[48]

Pathogenesis

Initial viral replication occurs within the oropharyngeal mucosal epithelium. Epstein-Barr virus has surface recep-tors for the C3d marker found on B lymphocytes. This B-cell tropism plays an important role in the pathogenesis of EBV-mediated diseases.[48,99] During an infection, up to 20% of circulating B-cells demonstrate EBV-encoded gene prod-ucts. Once inside the B-cell, EBV may cause B-cell activa-tion or B-cell lysis, or it may establish a latent viral infec-tion. Nonspecific B-cell activation and mononuclear cell proliferation results in a relative lymphocytosis and poly-clonal secretion of immunoglobulin. Heterophil antibodies noted in 50% to 95% of patients with IM are a result of this nonspecific B-cell activation.

Antibodies to several EBV specific antigens develop during the primary infection and are diagnostically help-ful.[99,100] IgM antibodies to the viral capsid antigen (VCA) indicate recent infection. IgG antibodies directed toward this same antigen develop later and persist for life. EBV nuclear antigens (EBNA) can be detected in the nucleus of B-cells within 24 hours of infection and can stimulate anti-EBNA antibody production. These antibodies are detectable within the first 6 to 8 weeks and are lifelong. Antibodies directed toward diffuse and restricted early viral antigens (EA-D and EA-R) occur on 70% of patients with IM, peak at 3 to 4 weeks and become undetectable with resolution of disease. A fourfold rise in IgG and the presence of IgM and EA-D/EA-R antibodies indicate recent infection.

Resolution of the disease occurs with the development of viral neutralizing antibodies that can inactivate extracellular virus.[48,99] As well, an EBV specific, T-cell-mediated immune response controls B-cell proliferation and immunoglobulin production. This cell-mediated immune response appears to be directed at unique lymphocyte-determined membrane antigens (LYDMA) induced on the surface of EBV infected B-cells.

Clinical Features

EBV may produce an acute, recurrent or chronic disorder as a result of a primary, persistent, or latent viral infection.[48,99,100] Infection may be asymptomatic (childhood infections), self-limiting (IM), or resultant in neoplastic disorders. Infectious mononucleosis, nasopharyngeal carcinoma, Burkitt lymphoma, and Sjögren syndrome have all been associated with EBV.* Recently the EBV genome has been detected in Reed-Sternberg cells of Hodgkin disease via in situ DNA hybridization.[74,113]

Ocular involvement with EBV has been reported primarily in patients with infectious mononucleosis. Patients with IM develop sore throat, fever, lymphadenopathy, and hepatosplenomegaly. A follicular conjunctivitis can be noted in 2% to 40% of patients.[31] Stromal keratitis, iritis, episcleritis, optic neuritis, and ophthalmoplegia have been reported during the acute phases of IM.[31,89]

Infectious mononucleosis and EBV have been reported to be associated with several retinal presentations: (1) macular edema, (2) retinal hemorrhages, (3) chorioretinitis, (4) punctate outer retinitis, and (5) a multifocal chorioretinitis and panuveitis (MCP) syndrome.† Karpe and Wising[58] reported severe macular edema and optic neuritis in a 20-year-old patient with IM and loss of central acuity. The macula developed extensive pigmentary changes, but acuity returned to normal. In another report one of three patients with chronic EBV infection developed bilateral macular edema with an associated vitritis, uveitis, and disc edema.[116]

Peil and associates[85] reported a patient with IM who presented with diplopia and intraretinal hemorrhages. Several other authors have reported a similar fundus presenta-

tion. The retinal hemorrhages may be associated with disc and macular edema.[9,11]

Raymond and associates[93] presented a patient with acute IM who developed multiple, gray-white, outer retinal punctate lesions (50 to 75 um). These were located in the midperipheral retina and were associated with a mild vitritis. The macula developed mild pigment epithelial changes.

Nozik and Dorsch[78] described a group of patients with a pseudohistoplasmosis syndrome. Their patients had, in addition to a multifocal choroiditis, a severe panuveitis (MCP) (Fig. 84-1, *A* and *B*). Tiedeman[110] compared EBV serologies of patients with this syndrome with both normal subjects and patients with other forms of uveitis. Patients with MCP had a serologic pattern indicating either recent or chronic EBV infection. In contrast to normal controls and patients with other forms of uveitis, patients with MCP had IgM antibodies against EBV capsid antigens and antibodies to EBV early

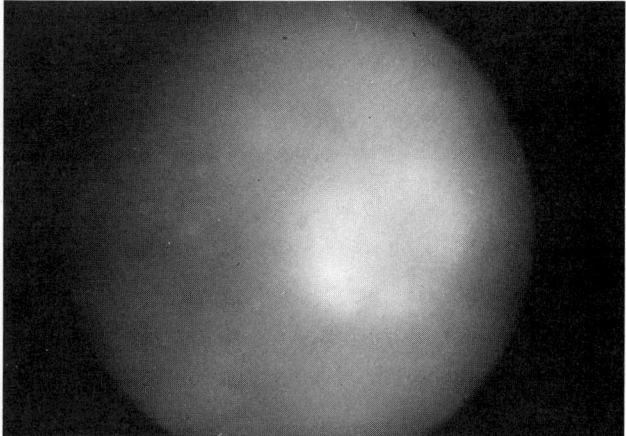

A

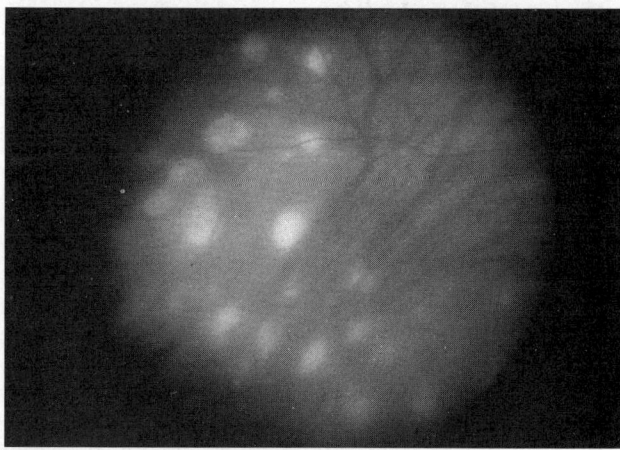

B

Fig. 84-1.   Patient with multifocal choroiditis and panuveitis syndrome. **A,** vitritis and peripapillary pigment changes. **B,** multifocal chorioretinal lesions. History, physical examination, and laboratory testing were negative except for elevated IgM, IgG, and early antigen (EA) titers for Epstein-Barr virus. (Figure **B** also in color insert.)

---

*References 2, 47, 48, 57, 67, 88.
†References 9, 11, 58, 83, 86, 93, 107, 110, 116.

antigens. A role for chronic EBV infection was postulated. Other investigators have not found this strong association.[103] It is interesting to note that MCP and progressive subretinal fibrosis and uveitis syndrome (SFU) may be different stages of the same disease. A chorioretinal biopsy of one patient with SFU showed a predominance of subretinal B-cells.[83] In a series of six patients with SFU followed in the uveitis service at the Ohio State University College of Medicine, EA and IgM antibodies to EBV were found in all six. These two conditions appear to be related and have serologic and histologic findings compatible with EBV infection.

A case report of bilateral retinochoroiditis in a 17-year-old boy with acute IM was reported by Kelly and associates.[60] The patient had a granulomatous iritis, vitritis, and a disc diameter area of discrete retinitis in the macula of both eyes resembling toxoplasmosis. A chorioretinal scar developed following resolution of the active retinitis in 7 days.

Laboratory Diagnosis

Retinal involvement in most cases of IM is uncommon. Fundus lesions developing in the setting of acute IM would support the diagnosis. Serologic testing for heterophile antibodies, IgM antibodies directed against VCA, and antibodies to early viral antigens would help confirm the diagnosis.[99,100]

Differential Diagnosis

The differential diagnosis of retinal edema, retinal hemorrhages, multifocal outer retinitis, and MCP is expansive. Sarcoidosis, tuberculosis, syphilis, toxoplasmosis, histoplasmosis, retinal vascular disorders, and idiopathic retinal white dot syndromes can all present with similar fundus findings. These disorders are discussed in other sections. Characteristic systemic symptoms and serologic studies in IM would serve to distinguish EBV retinitis from these conditions.

Treatment and Prognosis

Retinal involvement in IM is typically mild and self-limiting. Therapy for IM-associated retinitis is chiefly supportive. Retinal edema, intraretinal hemorrhages, and the punctate outer retinal lesions gradually resolve.* One case with more severe retinochoroiditis had loss of central vision because of a macular scar.[60] The prognosis for patients with EBV-associated MCP is more guarded.[78,110] Intraocular inflammation tends to be chronic, and retinal sequelae such as chronic cystoid macular edema and subretinal neovascular membranes are frequent. Systemic corticosteroids and acyclovir may be useful in cases with the sight-threatening complication of chronic intraocular inflammation.

---

*References 9, 11, 58, 85, 93, 107, 110, 116.

COXSACKIEVIRUS

Virology

The coxsackieviruses groups A and B are enteroviruses belonging to the Picornaviridae family.[73] Polioviruses and echoviruses are related to coxsackievirus and are in this same enterovirus subfamily. The virus was first isolated in Coxsackie, New York, by Dalldorf and Sickles in 1948. Coxsackievirus is a small, single-stranded RNA virus (25 to 35 nm) with an unencapsulated, icosahedral nucleocapsid. They are called enteroviruses because of their common isolation from the gastrointestinal tract.

Epidemiology

Man is the only natural host for Coxsackievirus.[73] Epidemics of Coxsackievirus-mediated diseases have been reported in the United States (1963 Coxsackievirus B1, 1972 Coxsackievirus B5). The virus is able to tolerate gastric acids and intestinal enzymes and can survive for long periods of time in untreated sewage.[73] These features play an important role in the epidemiology of enterovirus diseases. Fecal-oral routes of infection are the most common mode of viral transmission. The virus may be spread by respiratory or insect vectors as well. Coxsackieviruses occur more frequently in children and during the summer months.

Pathogenesis

Initial viral replication occurs within the gastrointestinal tract.[73] End-organ infection results from a secondary viremia. The respiratory tract, heart, liver, brain, and gastrointestinal tract are primarily affected in coxsackievirus-mediated disease. Histopathology of infected tissues reveal focal areas of necrosis and cellular infiltration.

Clinical Features

Systemic infections with coxsackieviruses range from subclinical to potentially fatal diseases. Common presentation for coxsackievirus infection includes herpangina, hand-foot-and-mouth disease, pharyngitis, gastroenteritis, aseptic meningitis, encephalitis, myocarditis, hepatitis, and pneumonia.[73]

Coxsackievirus has a unique role in the acute hemorrhagic conjunctivitis syndrome (AHC).[45] Enterovirus 70 has been the dominant agent of AHC since the first epidemics in 1969. AHC is a tropical disease that appears to have evolved from an animal strain of enterovirus. More recently coxsackievirus type A24 has been isolated during epidemics of AHC. These separate strains of enterovirus appear to produce an identical ocular picture characterized by a sudden painful follicular conjunctivitis. Often there is an associated superficial keratitis.

There has been one case report of a bilateral chorioretinitis associated with coxsackievirus B4 infection.[49] An 11-year-old boy developed high fever, fatigue, and abdominal pain. Examination found him to have an aseptic meningitis and hepatitis caused by coxsackievirus B4. He had no ocular complaints. Visual acuity was 20/20. Biomicroscopic and fundus examination found a bilateral chorioretinitis. The white lesions were 0.25 to 1.5 disc diameters in size and located along retinal vessels throughout the midperipheral fundus. The macula and optic nerve were not involved. The lesions resolved spontaneously leaving a chorioretinal scar.

Laboratory Diagnosis

Coxsackievirus retinitis appears to be rare, and ocular involvement may be asymptomatic.[49] The diagnosis would depend upon ophthalmic examination during the course of the systemic viral illness.

Coxsackievirus can be isolated from the conjunctiva, nasopharyngeal secretions, and stool specimens during active disease. Acute and convalescent titers of viral neutralizing antibodies (VNA) have been used extensively during epidemics of coxsackievirus-mediated diseases.[45] A fourfold rise in VNA indicates a recent infection.

Differential Diagnosis

The differential for a multifocal chorioretinitis occurring in children with an acute systemic illness should include Lyme disease and Rocky Mountain spotted fever (RMSF). Serologic testing can help differentiate these conditions, but is not useful during the acute phase. Lyme disease is a tick-borne, spirochetal systemic infection caused by *Borrelia burgdorferi*.[104] This disease occurs during the summer months and can present with fever, malaise, and fatigue. A characteristic annular skin lesion (erythema chronicum migrans) can be found before the onset of central nervous system, cardiac, and joint involvement. Conjunctivitis, iritis, vitritis, and chorioretinitis have been reported in Lyme disease.[1,65] RMSF is another tick-borne disease caused by *Rickettsia rickettsii* that has been associated with chorioretinitis.[91] Fever, malaise, and headache occur with a characteristic skin rash. The skin lesions are small erythematous macules associated with petechial hemorrhages and occur initially on the extremities.

Treatment and Prognosis

Therapy for coxsackievirus infections is primarily supportive. Coxsackievirus retinitis appears to improve spontaneously with resolution of the disease.[49] Visual prognosis appears to be good, and asymptomatic peripheral retinal scars may develop as a sequelae of the disease.

RUBELLA VIRUS

Virology

Rubella virus belongs to the *Rubivirus* genus within the Togaviridae family.[35] The virus is an enveloped, single-stranded RNA virus (50 to 70 nm) with an icosahedral nucleocapsid. In addition to a viral hemagglutinin, the capsule has a viral antigen (V-antigen) and an S-antigen.

Epidemiology

Rubella virus is species-specific with man being the natural host. Rubella (German measles) is endemic and, before widespread vaccination, epidemics occurred in 6- to 9-year cycles.[35] Rubella is spread via droplets expelled from an infected host. The virus is only moderately contagious and typically occurs in children. It is estimated that 10% to 25% of pregnant women may be nonimmune.[92]

Pathogenesis

The virus replicates in the upper respiratory tract epithelium before a more disseminated infection and viremia.[35,92] Viral neutralizing antibodies appear coincident with the rash and may play a role in producing the skin lesions. Rubella may involve the retina in both congenital and acquired forms. Autopsy reports from congenital rubella have shown retinal pigment epithelial degeneration with an occasional phagocytic cell.[63,118] The contiguous choroid and choriocapillaris are uninvolved.

The virus may establish a lifelong, persistent infection.[35] Rubella virus has been isolated from cataracts in children 3 years of age. It has also been cultured from the brain as long as 12 years after congenital infection.

Clinical Features

Rubella can cause both acquired and congenital infections.[92,115] Acquired rubella begins with a mild prodrome consisting of fever, headache, malaise, and conjunctivitis. Lymphadenopathy and splenomegaly may occur.[35,92] The skin rash begins on the trunk and spreads toward the extremities. It follows the initial prodrome by 1 to 3 days and consists of discrete maculopapular lesions. The rash lasts 3 to 5 days (3-day measles). Complications of rubella infection include encephalitis, arthritis, and hemorrhage. Ocular manifestations of acquired rubella include conjunctivitis (70%), superficial keratitis, and iritis.[115] Two cases of acquired rubella retinitis have been reported.[36,44] A bilateral retinitis and associated exudative detachment of the retina were noted, as well as retinal pigment epithelium.[44] The retinal lesions were in the posterior pole and were described as dark gray with atrophy. The optic nerve and retinal vessels were not involved. Fluorescein angiography demonstrated multifocal punctate hyperfluorescent lesions at the level of the choroid. The retinal detachments resolved with oral corticosteroid therapy.

Congenital rubella syndrome was first recognized by Gregg in 1941.[41] This syndrome consists of congenital cataracts, deafness, cardiac malformation, and mild mental retardation.[41,115] The disease is caused by a maternal infection with rubella during the first trimester. Fetal outcome depends on the timing of the transplacental infection. Spontaneous abortion may occur with infections early in the first trimester. Infections in the second or third trimester typically result in normal offspring. Ocular manifestations of congenital rubella include cataract (2% to 15%), glaucoma (10%), iritis and microphthalmia.[71,96,115] Rubella retinitis is perhaps the most common manifestation.[8,74] Fundus examination reveals a widespread fine mottling of the RPE and a diminished foveal light reflex (Fig. 84-2, *A* and *B*). This finding is most prominent within the posterior pole. The optic nerve and retinal vessels are normal. This fundus picture has been called a "salt and pepper fundus" because of the alternating hypopigmented and hyperpigmented changes. Rarely, rubella retinitis may result in disciform macular scar formation.[28] The salt and pepper fundus changes are lifelong.

Laboratory Diagnosis

Acquired rubella retinitis can be diagnosed in the presence of active German measles. Viral culture and the diagnostic fourfold rise in hemagglutination inhibition (HI), complement fixation, or ELISA antibodies confirm the clinical diagnosis.[35] Congenital rubella syndrome can be diagnosed with the history of maternal rubella and the characteristic congenital findings. Viral isolation from the oropharynx and the presence of IgM antibodies in the newborn support the diagnosis.[35,92]

Differential Diagnosis

Bilateral exudative retinal detachments noted in the acquired form of rubella retinitis may also occur in syphilis and VKH syndrome. The skin rash in syphilis typically involves the palms and soles of the feet.[111] Serology can assist in the diagnosis. VKH syndrome can have constitutional symptoms including headache and fatigue.[96] Hearing loss, vitiligo, poliosis and a panuveitis are also noted. The salt and pepper fundus observed in congenital rubella may be similar to luetic retinitis and hereditary retinal degenerations.

Treatment and Prognosis

There is no specific therapy for rubella. Acquired rubella is a self-limiting disease. Acquired rubella retinitis may be treated with oral corticosteroids if severe.[44] Congenital rubella retinitis has a very good visual prognosis. Despite the widespread RPE changes, patients typically enjoy 20/20 to 20/40 acuities with full visual fields. Glaucoma and cataract may be problematic in congenital rubella. Glaucoma therapy is often unsuccessful. Early cataract extraction may be required to prevent severe amblyopia.

RIFT VALLEY FEVER VIRUS

Virology

Rift Valley fever virus (RVFV) is an insect-borne virus in the Bunyaviridae family.[54,101] RVFV is an encapsulated RNA virus (100 nm) with a coiled circular nucleocapsid. The viruses associated with this endemic disease are named after the different regions in Africa from where they originate.

Epidemiology

RVFV is an infectious disease of animals and livestock in eastern portions of Africa and South Africa.[101,112] Goats, cattle, and sheep are the primary host and reservoir for the virus. Mosquitos are thought to be the primary vector for transmission of both between animals and man.

Pathogenesis

The arthropod vector directly inoculates the virus within the bloodstream. The viremia results in the end-organ infection including the retina.

Clinical Features

RVFV causes an acute febrile illness with malaise, chills, myalgias, and headache.[54,112] Incubation time is 2 to 7 days.

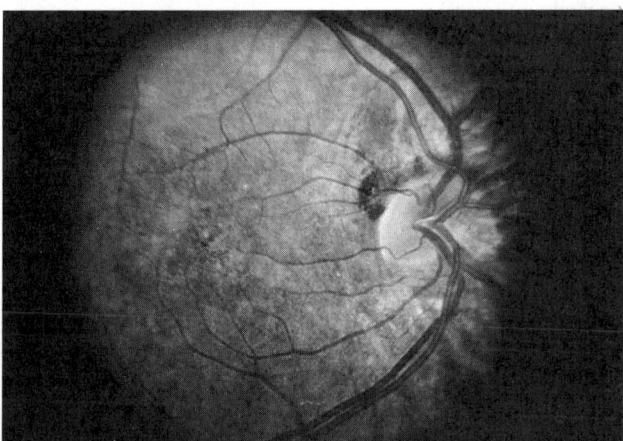

A

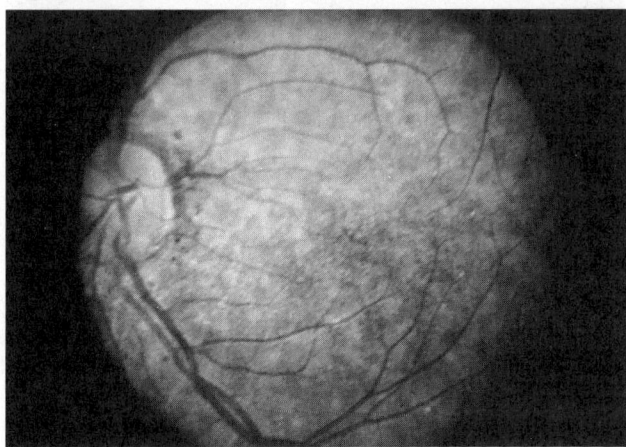

B

Fig. 84-2. Fundus photographs from patient with congenital rubella syndrome. Diffuse "salt and pepper" pigmentary changes can be noted at level of retinal pigment epithelium of both eyes. Notice absent foveal light reflex. Patient had 20/25 visual acuities in both eyes. (Figure **A** also in color insert.)

Gastrointestinal involvement is common later in the disease course. The fever can be high (104°F) and is characteristically relapsing. The disease is usually self-limiting with rapid recovery. In one recent epidemic a 1% mortality rate was noted as a result of encephalitis, hepatitis, and hemorrhagic complications.

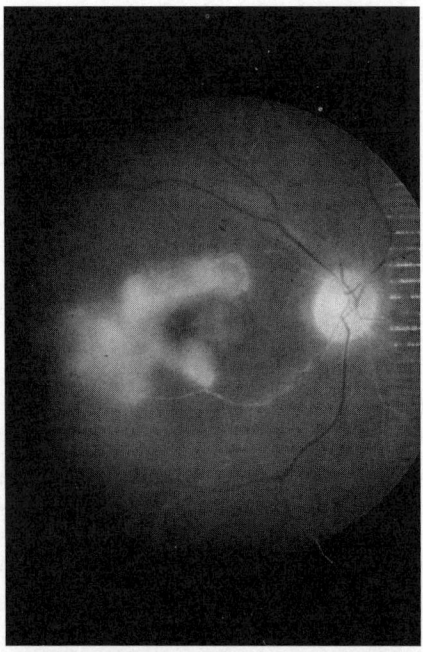

A

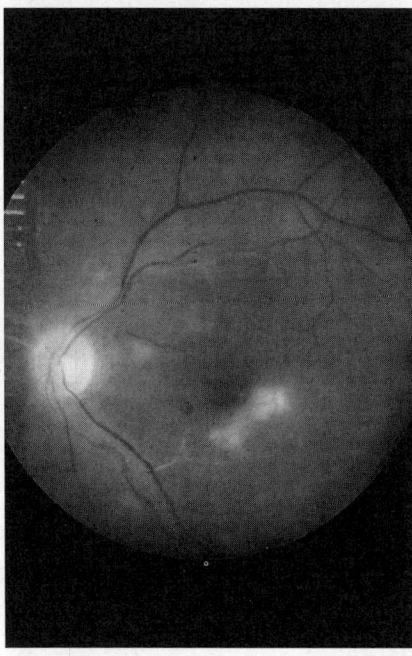

B

Fig. 84-3. Fundus photographs from patient with Rift Valley fever described by Deutman and Klamp. Note hypopigmented area of retinitis in posterior pole and retinal arteriolitis.

Conjunctivitis and uveitis can be found during the acute phases of the disease.[21,101,112] A viral retinitis has been described during several outbreaks of the disease. Typically, patients present with loss of central vision 7 to 21 days following the onset of the fever. Unilateral or bilateral macular, paramacular, and midperipheral retinal exudates and intraretinal hemorrhages are noted on dilated fundus examination. Fluorescein angiography shows retinal vasculitis and vascular occlusion. The retinal lesions resolve over a period of several months (Fig. 84-3).

Laboratory Diagnosis

In endemic areas the diagnosis should be suspected during outbreaks of RVF. The characteristic fundus findings help establish a clinical diagnosis. The virus can be isolated and cultured in mice to confirm the diagnosis.[54] As well, a fourfold rise in CF and HI antibodies toward RVFV can support a recent RVFV infection. Fluorescein angiography may assist in determining the mechanism for the loss of central acuity.

Differential Diagnosis

Lyme disease, rickettsial diseases, and sarcoidosis may present as a febrile systemic illness.[1,65,91,104] History, physical exam, and laboratory testing can help differentiate these disorders as discussed in other chapters.

Treatment and Prognosis

Rift Valley fever is a self-limiting disease and therapy is typically supportive. A small percentage of patients (1%) develop serious complications from the virus including encephalitis, hepatitis, and visceral hemorrhage.[54] RVFV retinitis, if mild and outside the posterior pole, can be observed. In severe sight-threatening cases, corticosteroid therapy could be considered to minimize inflammatory damage. Fifty percent of the patients with severe disease in one series of 80 patients had residual loss of central vision as a result of macular scar formation, epiretinal membrane, ischemic maculopathy, or retinal detachment.[21,101]

INFLUENZA A

Virology

Influenza A virus (IAV) is one type of influenzavirus in the Orthomyxoviridae family.[7] The virus was first isolated in 1933. Influenza A is a single-stranded RNA virus (80 to 120 nm) with an outer lipoprotein envelope and a helical nucleocapsid. Neuraminidase and hemagglutinin are surface glycoproteins within this envelope and are important in viral adherence and entry into cells.

Epidemiology

Epidemics of Influenza A are cyclic (every 2 to 4 years) and occur as a result of major and minor antigenic variations in the surface glycoproteins ("antigenic shifts").[7] These antigenic shifts play an important role in the success of the outbreaks. Epidemics and pandemics of IAV occur typically in the winter months with an overall attack rate of 40%.

Pathogenesis

Influenza A is a pneumotropic virus with affinity to the tracheobronchial epithelial cells. The virus is transmitted by droplets that are exhaled from an infected person.[7] Once in the respiratory tract the virus causes cell lysis and desquamation of the ciliated epithelium.

Clinical Features

Influenza is an acute febrile illness characterized by malaise, headache, and myalgias. The illness lasts 2 to 7 days. Recovery is complete unless secondary bacterial infections occur. Influenza can be serious and may cause cardiopulmonary complications or death in elderly or debilitated patients.

Ocular involvement with influenza includes conjunctivitis, a mild iritis, interstitial keratitis, and dacryoadenitis during the acute illness. Influenza A retinitis has been described by several authors.[61,62,70,90,114] Weinberg and Nerny[114] described a 21-year-old woman with influenza A and bilateral submacular hemorrhages. Examination found her to have 20/20 vision with annular central scotoma. On fundus examination she had a quiet vitreous and normal optic nerve and retinal vessels. Both maculae had small subretinal hemorrhages. The hemorrhages resolved over several weeks and the patient maintained 20/20 vision. A persistent ring-shaped scotoma was noted despite a normal fundus examination two years later.

Kovacs[62] described a 23-year-old man with active influenza A, decreased vision and central scotomas. Dilated fundus examination revealed bilateral macular lipid star formation without hemorrhage. Fluorescein angiography showed retinal capillary leakage in the posterior pole. The fundus lesions and visual acuity return to normal by 6 weeks. Three years later the macula had subtle RPE changes.

More recently Rabon and associates[90] presented a case of serologically proven IAV associated with a bilateral posterior microvasculopathy and secondary macular and disc edema. Vision was reduced to 20/400 bilaterally. Fundus exam demonstrated multifocal white patches in the inner retina. The vitreous was quiet. Fluorescein angiography showed perifoveal capillary leakage and both diffuse and cystoid macular edema. Visual acuities improved over a period of several days, and repeat angiography documented complete resolution of the retinal vascular leakage. Convalescent serum showed a fourfold rise in influenza A titers. Follow-up examination found 20/20 acuities and decreased foveal reflexes bilaterally.

Laboratory Diagnosis

Submacular hemorrhages, macular star formation, and/or retinal capillary microvasculopathy with multifocal inner retinitis occurring in the setting of an influenza epidemic suggest the clinical diagnosis of IAV retinitis. Serologic testing documenting a fourfold rise in IAV titers by ELISA, CF, or HI can help confirm the diagnosis.[7]

Differential Diagnosis

Several disorders can present with submacular hemorrhages. Age-related macular degeneration, ocular histoplasmosis, trauma, and angioid streaks can all result in subretinal neovascular membranes and subretinal hemorrhage in the macula.[12] These disorders do not typically occur with systemic flulike symptoms. As well, spontaneous resolution is rare. Macular lipid stars can occur in measles and mumps virus infections, diabetic retinopathy, hypertension, anterior ischemic optic neuropathy, and Leber idiopathic stellate neuroretinitis.[22]

Treatment

Influenza A retinitis appears to be a self-limiting disorder. All patients had complete resolution of their retinopathy and return of 20/20 vision. One patient had a persistent subjective annular scotoma and another had reduced foveal light reflexes.[90,114] Vaccination for IAV is recommended for those at higher risk for contracting the disease such as health care workers. Others at high risk for complications include the elderly and patients with chronic pulmonary disease, cardiovascular disease, or other debilitating disorders.

MUMPS VIRUS

Virology

Mumps virus (MV) belongs to the Paramyxoviridae family of viruses.[5] The virus is an enveloped RNA virus (85 to 300 nm) with a helical nucleocapsid.

Epidemiology

Man is the only natural host for the mumps virus, although close contact between infected children and their pets has been associated with isolated cases of canine mumps parotitis.[77] Transmission is via direct contact with droplets expelled by an infected host.[5] Most cases of mumps (90%) occur in children. The virus is endemic and can produce epidemics in 2- to 4-year cycles.

Pathogenesis

Mumps virus may start replication directly in the salivary glands or in the epithelial cells of the upper respiratory tract.[5] Secondary viremia disseminates the MV throughout the body. MV can infect the testes, meninges, brain, pancreas, heart, and kidneys.

Clinical Features

Following initial exposure mumps takes 14 to 21 days before disease onset. A viral prodrome consisting of fever, myalgias, headache, and anorexia can occur 1 to 2 days before salivary gland and other organ involvement. Typically the parotid and submandibular glands develop massive swelling and become tender; this condition lasts 1 to 2 weeks.

Ocular involvement with mumps includes dacryoadenitis, conjunctivitis, iritis, optic neuritis, and keratitis.[5] Foster and associates[26] reported a case of unilateral mumps neuroretinitis in a 15-year-old boy. Visual acuity was 20/200 in the involved eye with an afferent pupillary defect. A mild posterior vitritis was noted on biomicroscopy. Fundus examination revealed marked disc edema and hyperemia. A macular star exudate was noted. There were two small white intraretinal lesions noted in the midperipheral retina. Intravenous methylprednisolone was used because of progressive loss of vision. The lesions stabilized and 5 months later vision had improved to 20/40. The two areas of retinitis evolved into a chorioretinal scar.

Laboratory Diagnosis

Mumps have a characteristic clinical picture that is sufficient for diagnosis in most cases. Serologic testing can be performed detecting a fourfold rise in CF antibodies toward S and V mumps antigens, as well as a fourfold rise in antibodies using standard HI neutralization or hemolysis-in-gel assays.[5] IgM antibodies also indicate recent infection.

Differential Diagnosis

Macular lipid stars can be found in influenza A virus and measles virus infections, diabetes, hypertension, anterior ischemic optic neuropathy, and Leber idiopathic stellate neuroretinitis.[22] Sarcoidosis can cause parotid swelling and intraocular inflammation (uveoparotid fever, Heerfordt syndrome). The inflammation is often bilateral with a chronic granulomatous uveitis, vasculitis, and retinitis.[52]

Treatment and Prognosis

Systemic treatment of mumps is supportive with fluids and analgesics. One case of mumps neuroretinitis required IV methylprednisolone therapy because of severe optic nerve and macular involvement.[26] Visual acuity improved to 20/40 with resolution of the acute process. Children over the age of 1 routinely receive a live attenuated mumps vaccination to limit the spread of this virus. A controlled study suggests that hyperimmune gammaglobulin may modify the course of mumps in selected cases.[33]

MEASLES VIRUS

Virology

Measles virus is a morbillivirus in the Paramyxoviridae family.[34] The virus is an enveloped RNA virus (120 to 250 nm) with a coiled helical nucleocapsid core.

Epidemiology

Measles is one of the most common infectious diseases worldwide. Man and monkeys are the only hosts for measles or rubeola virus.[34] The virus is extremely contagious (90% attack rate) and can be spread by either contaminated fomite or direct droplet transmission. Measles is endemic and before widespread immunization occurred in cyclic pandemics of 2 to 3 years.

Pathogenesis

Measles virus replicates in the upper respiratory tract and produces a viremia within the first few days. This first viremia results in infection of the lymphoid tissues. A second, larger viremia occurs resulting in disseminated infection.[34,76] Multinucleated giant cells can be found in the skin lesions, mucous membranes, and the respiratory tract.

Clinical Features

Measles virus (rubeola) can cause both congenital and acquired infections.[34,72] Congenital measles is transmitted via the placenta and can cause fetal demise and serious congenital malformations including deafness and cardiac and skeletal anomalies.

Cataracts have been reported in several cases of congenital measles.[22] Congenital measles retinitis has been observed in two cases.[42,72] Visual acuity was normal. Fundus examination revealed a bilateral fine pigmentary change throughout the retina. Associated retinal edema, macular star formation, and mild arteriolar attenuation were reported in one patient (Fig. 84-4).

Acquired measles presents with a prodrome of persistent cough, conjunctivitis, and fever.[34,106] Koplik spots can be found on the oral mucosa. A pink macular rash appears on the face and trunk and spreads toward the extremities over a period of several days. Complications of measles include encephalitis and myocarditis.[55]

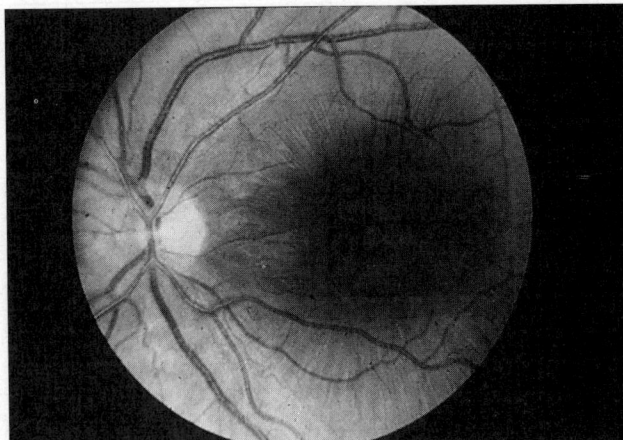

Fig. 84-4. Fundus photograph from patient with measles retinopathy. Macular and disc edema evolved into macular star and subsequent pigmentary changes at level of retinal pigment epithelium. (Figure also in color insert.)

Acquired measles retinitis has been described and characterized as macular edema, neuroretinitis, macular star formation, attenuated arterioles, and disc edema.[6,98] One case of pigmented paravenous dystrophy associated with measles infection was reported.[27] Immunosuppressed patients may develop a more severe clinical course.[43] Fundus examination in one patient on chemotherapy for testicular carcinoma revealed annular depigmented retinal lesions, fine pigmentary changes, and a central serous chorioretinopathy (CSR-like) lesion.

Laboratory Diagnosis

Acquired measles has a characteristic clinical picture. A fourfold rise in HI, CF, or ELISA antibodies confirms the diagnosis.[34] Congenital measles retinopathy may be more difficult to diagnose. A history of maternal measles and the presence of other congenital malformations suggest the diagnosis.

Differential Diagnosis

Other forms of viral retinitis (mumps and influenza A) discussed previously in this chapter may present with retinal edema, macular star formation, and widespread pigmentary changes in the fundus. History, clinical examination, and serologies may assist in differentiating these conditions in atypical presentations. Central serous retinopathy and Leber idiopathic stellate neuroretinitis may also have a similar fundus picture, but may present without the systemic manifestations.

Treatment and Prognosis

The treatment of measles is supportive. No therapy has been described for measles retinitis. Passive immunization in nonimmune pregnant women and debilitated patients may be considered following exposure.

SUBACUTE SCLEROSING PANENCEPHALITIS VIRUS

Virology

Subacute sclerosing panencephalitis (SSPE), or Dawson inclusion body encephalitis, is caused by a variant of the measles virus.[66] SSPE virus is a morbillivirus within the Paramyxoviridae family that differs from the wild-type measles virus by alterations or absence of viral M protein and possibly other envelope components.[13,57,59,84]

Epidemiology

SSPE virus is a slow virus that involves the central nervous system of school-age children (5 to 14 years of age).[66] In rare cases adults have developed SSPE.[17] The frequency of SSPE following measles is 1 to 10 per million cases of measles. Boys are involved more than girls (4:1). Symptoms of SSPE begin 6 to 7 years after the initial measle virus infection. A majority of children who develop SSPE contracted measles at an early age (under 2 years old).

Pathogenesis

In contrast to the acute febrile illness of wild-type measles, SSPE is a persistent slow viral infection of the central nervous system including the cerebrum, cerebellum, spinal cord, and eye. The virus causes a true panencephalitis. On autopsy the brain has inflammatory foci in both the gray and white matter. Intranuclear, eosinophilic inclusion bodies are found in the lesions and contain paramyxovirus on electron microscopy. Immunohistochemical techniques have identified the presence of the measles virus within the brain tissue.[18,19] High titers of measles antibodies are found in the blood and cerebro-spinal fluid (CSF).[15]

In the retina, focal areas of photoreceptor loss and periretinal fibrosis are noted on histopathology.[20,25] Measles virus has also been localized to the retina in the ganglion and inner nuclear layers.

Clinical Features

The incubation time between initial measles infection and onset of neurologic signs is 6 to 7 years. The first stage of the disease begins with behavioral changes and intellectual deterioration. In the second stage progressive neurologic deficits, extrapyramidal signs, and cortical blindness develop. Dementia occurs in the last stage of the disease with death typically within 1 to 3 years of disease onset.[79,97]

Patients with SSPE have ocular findings in 30% to 75% of cases.[40,94] Disc edema, papillitis, and optic atrophy are commonly noted. The most consistent finding is a maculopathy. The contiguous vitreous and choroid are not involved. The retinitis begins as focal macular edema[3,117] (Fig. 84-5, A). This may evolve into a white retinal infiltrate and, in rare cases, may be associated with intraretinal hemorrhage (Fig. 84-5, B). Later in the course of the disease, macular gliosis is noted. Retinal pigmentary changes are often noted on fluorescein angiography. One patient was noted to have serous retinal detachment associated with SSPE.[3] In another series, two patients presented with a focal chorioretinitis.[17]

Laboratory Diagnosis

SSPE should be considered in any school-age child with slowly progressive deterioration in mental function and emotional behavior. The diagnosis requires a high level of clinical suspicion. SSPE retinitis does not necessarily coincide with any specific stage of the disease and may actually precede the onset of CNS symptoms and signs.[37,39] High titers of measles antibody can be found in SSPE and can assist in the diagnosis.[15] Brain biopsy is the most accurate way to confirm the diagnosis.

Differential Diagnosis

Neurologic complaints and macular edema can be found in children with multiple sclerosis–associated intermediate uveitis.[38] Children will present with pars planitis and progressive neurologic signs. MS is not a panencephalitis, and the focal demyelination and neurologic findings would dif-

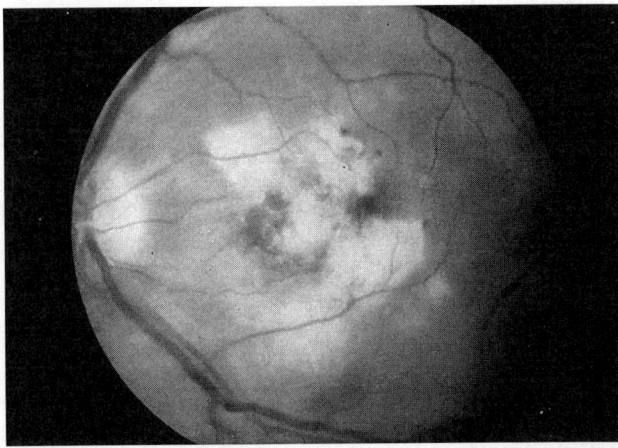

A

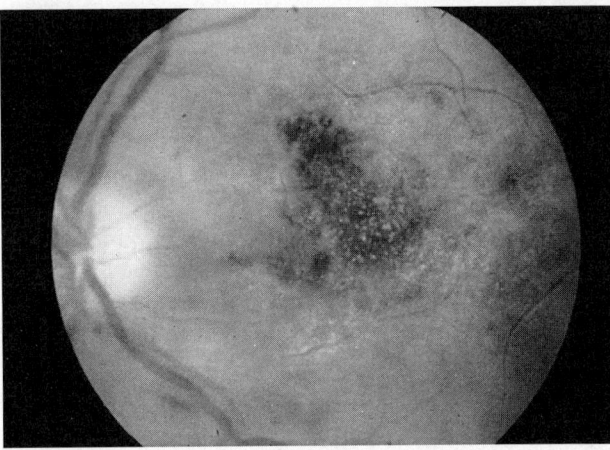

B

Fig. 84-5. From patient with SSPE retinopathy. **A,** Early in course of disease macula may be edematous or have white infiltrate. (Figure **A** also in color insert.) **B,** This may evolve into mild intraretinal hemorrhage.

ferentiate this condition from SSPE. Inflammatory cystoid macular edema would be noted on clinical exam and fluorescein angiography. MRI scan would show focal areas of demyelination.

Treatment and Prognosis

The treatment of SSPE is supportive. Isoprinosine has been shown to delay the neurologic deterioration in SSPE.[24,56] No therapy has been described for SSPE retinitis.

REFERENCES

1. Aaberg TM: The expanding ophthalmologic spectrum of Lyme disease, *Am J Ophthalmol* 107:77-80, 1989.
2. Alspaugh MA, Jensen PC, Rabin H, Tan EM: Lymphocytes transformed by Epstein-Barr virus: induction of nuclear antigens reactive with antibody in rheumatoid arthritis, *J Exp Med* 147:1018-1020, 1978.
3. Andriola M: Maculopathy in subacute sclerosing panencephalitis, *Am J Dis Child* 124:187-189, 1972.
4. Azazi M, Samuelson A, Linde A, Forsgren M: Intrathecal antibody production against viruses of the herpes family in acute retinal necrosis, *Am J Ophthalmol* 112:76-82, 1991.
5. Baum SG, Litman N: Mumps virus. In Mandell GL, Douglas RG, Bennett JE, editors: *Principles and practice of infectious diseases,* ed 3, 1260-1265, New York, 1990, Churchill Livingstone.
6. Bedrossian RH: Neuroretinitis following measles, *J Ped* 46:329-331, 1955.
7. Betts RF, Douglas RG: Influenza virus. In Mandell GL, Douglas RG, Bennett JE, editors: *Principles and practice of infectious diseases,* ed 3, 1306-1325, New York, 1990, Churchill Livingstone.
8. Blankstein SS, Feiman LH: Macular pigmentation following maternal rubella, *Am J Ophthalmol* 35:408-411, 1952.
9. Blaustein A, Caccavo A: Infectious mononucleosis complicated by bilateral papilloretinal edema, *Arch Ophthalmol* 43:853-856, 1950.
10. Blumenkranz MS, Culbertson WW, Clarkson JG, Dix R: Treatment of the acute retinal necrosis syndrome with intravenous acyclovir, *Ophthalmology* 93:296-300, 1986.
11. Boynge TW, Von Hagen KO: Severe optic neuritis in infectious mononucleosis: report of a case, *JAMA* 148:933-935, 1952.
12. Bressler NM, Bressler SB, Fine SL: Age-related macular degeneration, *Surv Ophthalmol* 32:375-413, 1988.
13. Chen TT, Watanabe I, Zeman W: Subacute sclerosing panencephalitis: propagation of measles virus from brain biopsy in tissue culture, *Science* 163:1193-1194, 1967.
14. Chou J, Kern ER, Whitley RJ, Roizman B: Mapping of herpes simplex virus-1 neurovirulence to gamma 34.5, a gene nonessential for growth in culture, *Science* 250:1262-1266, 1990.
15. Connolly JH, Allen I, Hurwitz LJ: Measles-like antibody and antigen in subacute sclerosing panencephalitis, *Lancet* 1:542-544, 1967.
16. Culbertson WW, Blumenkranz MS, Pepose JS et al.: Varicella zoster virus is a cause of the acute retinal necrosis syndrome, *Ophthalmology* 93:559-569, 1986.
17. David P, Maurizio E, Mariotti P, Macchi G: Adult onset of subacute sclerosing panencephalitis: a case report, *Riv Neurol* 60:83-87, 1990.
18. Dawson JR Jr: Cellular inclusions in cerebral lesions of epidemic encephalitis: second report, *Arch Neurol Psychiat* 31:685-700, 1933.
19. Dawson JR Jr: Cellular inclusions in cerebral lesions of lethargic encephalitis, *Am J Pathol* 9:7-15, 1933.
20. Delaey JJ, Hanssens M, Colette P et al.: Subacute sclerosing panencephalitis: fundus changes and histopathologic correlations, *Doc Ophthalmol* 56:11-21, 1983.
21. Deutman AF, Klomp HJ: Rift Valley fever retinitis, *Am J Ophthalmol* 92:38-42, 1981.
22. Dreyer RF, Hopen G, Gass JDM, Smith JL: Leber's idiopathic stellate neuroretinitis, *Arch Ophthalmol* 102:1140-1145, 1984.
23. Duker JS, Nielsen JC, Eagle RC et al.: Rapidly progressive acute retinal necrosis secondary to herpes simplex virus, type 1, *Ophthalmology* 97:1638-1643, 1990.
24. DuRant RH, Dyken PR, Swift AV: The influence of inosoplex treatment on the neurologic disability of patients with subacute sclerosing panencephalitis, *J Pediatr* 101:288-293, 1982.
25. Font RL, Jenis EH, Tuck KD: Measles maculopathy associated with subacute sclerosing panencephalitis: immunofluorescent and immuno-ultrastructural studies, *Arch Pathol Lab Med* 96:168-174, 1973.
26. Foster RE, Lowder CY, Meisler DM et al.: Mumps neuroretinitis in an adolescent, *Am J Ophthalmol* 110:92-93, 1990.
27. Foxman SG, Heckenlively JR, Sinclair SH: Rubeola retinopathy and pigmented paravenous retinochoroidal atrophy, *Am J Ophthalmol* 99:605-606, 1985.
28. Frank KE, Purnell EW: Subretinal neovascularization following rubella retinopathy, *Am J Ophthalmol* 86:462-466, 1978.
29. Freeman WR, Stern WH, Gross JG et al.: Pathologic observations made by retinal biopsy, *Retina* 10:195-204, 1990.
30. Fujikawa LS, Haugen JP: Immunopathology of vitreous and retinochoroidal biopsy in posterior uveitis, *Ophthalmology* 97:1644-1653, 1990.
31. Gardner BP, Margolis TP, Mondino BJ: Conjunctival lymphocytic nodule associated with Epstein-Barr virus, *Am J Ophthalmol* 112:567-571, 1991.
32. Gass JD: Acute posterior multifocal placoid pigment epitheliopathy, *Arch Ophthalmol* 80:177-179, 1968.

33. Gellis SS, McGuiness AC, Peters M: A study of the prevention of mumps orchitis by gammaglobulin, *Am J Med Sci* 210:661-664, 1945.

34. Gershon AA: Measles virus (rubeola). In Mandell GL, Douglas RG, Bennett JE, editors: *Principles and practice of infectious diseases,* ed 3, 1279-1286, New York, 1990, Churchill Livingstone.

35. Gershon AA: Rubella virus (German measles). In Mandell GL, Douglas RG, Bennett JE, editors: *Principles and practice of infectious diseases,* ed 3, 1242-1247, New York, 1990, Churchill Livingstone.

36. Gerstle C, Zinn KM: Rubella-associated retinitis in an adult: report of a case, *Mt Sinai J Med* 43:303-308, 1976.

37. Gilden DH, Rorke LB, Tanaka R: Acute SSPE, *Arch Neurol* 32:644-646, 1975.

38. Giles CL: Peripheral uveitis in patients with multiple sclerosis, *Am J Ophthalmol* 70:17-19, 1970.

39. Gravina RF, Nakanishi AS, Faden A: Subacute sclerosing panencephalitis, *Am J Ophthalmol* 86:106-108, 1978.

40. Green SH, Wirtschafter JD: Ophthalmoscopic findings in subacute sclerosing panencephalitis, *Br J Ophthalmol* 57:780-787, 1932.

41. Gregg NM: Congenital cataract following German measles in the mother, *Trans Ophthalmol Soc Aust* 3:35-46, 1942.

42. Guzinati GC: Suula possibilita de lesion oculari congenita da morbillo e da epatite gridemica, *Bull Ocul* 33:833-841, 1954.

43. Haltia M, Paetau A, Vaheri A et al.: Fatal measles encephalopathy with retinopathy during cytotoxic chemotherapy, *J Neurol Sci* 32:323-330, 1977.

44. Hayashi M, Yoshimura N, Kondo T: Acute rubella retinal pigment epitheliitis in an adult, *Am J Ophthalmol* 93:285-288, 1982.

45. Heirholzer JC, Hatch MH: Acute hemorrhagic conjunctivitis. In Darrell RW, editor: *Viral diseases of the eye,* 165-196, Philadelphia, 1985, Lea & Febiger.

46. Hemady R, Opremcak EM, Zaltas M et al.: Herpes simplex virus type 1 strain influence on chorioretinal disease patterns following intracameral inoculation in Igh-1 disparate mice, *Invest Ophthalmol Vis Sci* 30:1750-1757, 1989.

47. Henle G, Henle W: Epstein-Barr virus-specific IgA serum antibodies as an outstanding feature of nasopharyngeal carcinoma, *Int J Cancer* 17:1-6, 1976.

48. Henle W, Henle G: Epstein-Barr virus and infectious mononucleosis, *New Engl J Med* 288:263-264, 1973.

49. Hirakata K, Oshima T, Azuma N: Chorioretinitis induced by coxsackievirus B4 infection, *Am J Ophthalmol* 109:225-227, 1990.

50. Jabs DA, Enger C, Bartlett JG: Cytomegalovirus retinitis and acquired immunodeficiency syndrome, *Arch Ophthalmol* 107:75-80, 1989.

51. Jabs DA, Enger C, Haller J, de Bustros S: Retinal detachments in patients with cytomegalovirus retinitis, *Arch Ophthalmol* 109:794-799, 1991.

52. Jabs DA, Johns CJ: Ocular involvement in chronic sarcoidosis, *Am J Ophthalmol* 102:297-301, 1986.

53. Jampol LM, Sieving PA, Pugh AS: Multiple evanescent white dot syndrome. I. Clinical findings, *Arch Ophthalmol* 102:671-674, 1984.

54. Johnson KM: California encephalitis and bunyaviral hemorrhagic fevers. In Mandell GL, Douglas RG, Bennett JE, editors: *Principles and practice of infectious diseases,* ed 3, New York, 1990, Churchill Livingstone.

55. Johnson RT, Griffin DE, Hirsch RL et al.: Measles encephalomyelitis: clinical and immunologic studies, *N Engl J Med* 310:137-141, 1984.

56. Jones CE, Dyken PR, Huttenlocher PR: Inosoplex therapy in subacute sclerosing panencephalitis, *Lancet* 1:1034-1036, 1982.

57. Jones JF, Williams M, Schooley RT et al.: Antibodies to Epstein-Barr virus-specific DNase and DNA polymerase in the chronic fatigue syndrome, *Arch Int Med* 148:1957-1960, 1988.

58. Karpe G, Wising P: Retinal changes with acute reduction of vision as initial symptoms of infectious mononucleosis, *Acta Ophthalmol* 26:19-24, 1948.

59. Katz M, Rorke LB, Masland WS: Transmission of an encephalitogenic agent from brains of patients with subacute sclerosing panencephalitis to ferrets: preliminary report, *N Engl J Med* 279:793-796, 1969.

60. Kelly SP, Rosenthal AR, Nicholson KG, Woodward CG: Retinochoroiditis in acute Epstein-Barr virus infection, *Br J Ophthalmol* 73:1002-1003, 1989.

61. Knapp A: Optic neuritis after influenza with changes in the spinal fluid, *Arch Ophthalmol* 45:247-249, 1916.

62. Kovacs B: Alterations of the blood-retina barriers in cases of viral retinitis, *Int Ophthalmol* 8:159-166, 1985.

63. Kresky B, Nauheim JS: Rubella retinitis, *Am J Dis Child* 113:305-310, 1967.

64. Krill AE, Deutman AF: Acute retinal pigment epitheliitis, *Am J Ophthalmol* 74:193-205, 1972.

65. Lang GE, Schonherr U, Naumann GOH: Retinae vasculitis with proliferative retinopathy in a patient with evidence of *Borrelia burgdorferi* infection, *Am J Ophthalmol* 111:243-244, 1991.

66. Lehrich JR: Measles-like virus (subacute sclerosing panencephalitis). In Mandell GL, Douglas RG, Bennett JE, editors: *Principles and practice of infectious diseases,* ed 3, 1286-1289, New York, 1990, Churchill Livingstone.

67. Lenoir GM: Role of the virus, chromosomal translocations and cellular oncogenes in the etiology of Burkitt's lymphoma. In Epstein MW, Achong BG, editors: *The Epstein-Barr virus: recent advances,* 184-207, New York, 1986, John Wiley & Sons.

68. Liesegang TJ: Diagnosis and therapy of herpes zoster ophthalmicus, *Ophthalmology* 98:1216-1229, 1991.

69. Masurel N, Marine WM: Recycling of Asian and Hong Kong influenza virus hemaglutinins in man, *Am J Epidemiol* 97:44-49, 1973.

70. Mathur SP: Macular lesions after influenza, *Br J Ophthalmol* 42:702, 1958.

71. Matoba A: Ocular viral infections, *Pediatr Inf Dis J* 3:358-368, 1984.

72. Metz HS, Harkey ME: Pigmentary retinopathy following maternal measles (morbilli) infection, *Am J Ophthalmol* 66:1107, 1968.

73. Modlin JF: Coxsackieviruses, echoviruses, and newer enteroviruses. In Mandell GL, Douglas RG, Bennett JE, editors: *Principles and practice of infectious diseases,* ed 3, 1367-1383, New York, 1990, Churchill Livingstone.

74. Mueller N, Evens A, Harris NL et al.: Hodgkin's disease and Epstein-Barr virus, *New Engl J Med* 320:689-695, 1989.

75. Murray HW, Knox DL, Green WR, Susel RM: Cytomegalovirus retinitis in adults, *Am J Med* 63:574-584, 1977.

76. Nanda M, Curtin VT, Hilliard JK et al.: Ocular histopathologic findings in a case of human herpes B virus infection, *Arch Ophthalmol* 108:713-716, 1990.

77. Noice F, Bolin FM, Eveleth PF: Incidence of viral parotitis in the domestic dog, *Am J Dis Child* 98:350-352, 1959.

78. Nozik RA, Dorsch W: A new chorioretinopathy associated with anterior uveitis, *Am J Ophthalmol* 76:758-762, 1973.

79. Obenour LC: Subacute sclerosing panencephalitis, *Int Ophthalmol Clin* 12:215-223, 1972.

80. Opremcak EM, Foster CS, Hemady R et al.: Chorioretinal disease patterns in congenic mice following intraocular inoculation with HSV-1, *Invest Ophthalmol Vis Sci* 30:1041-1046, 1989.

81. Opremcak EM, Wells PA, Thompson P et al.: Immunogenetic influence of Igh-1 phenotype on experimental herpes simplex virus type-1 corneal infection, *Invest Ophthalmol Vis Sci* 29:744-748, 1988.

82. Orellana J, Teich SA, Lieberman RM et al.: Treatment of retinal detachments in patients with the acquired immune deficiency syndrome, *Ophthalmology* 98:939-943, 1991.

83. Palestine AG et al.: Histopathology of subretinal fibrosis and uveitis syndrome, *Ophthalmology* 92:838-844, 1985.

84. Payne FE, Baublis JV, Itashi HH: Isolation of measle virus in subacute sclerosing panencephalitis, *N Engl J Med* 281:585-589, 1969.

85. Peil JJ, Thelander HE, Shaw EB: Infectious mononucleosis of the central nervous system with bilateral papilledema, *J Pediatr* 37:661-663, 1950.

86. Pepose JS: Infectious retinitis: diagnostic modalities, *Ophthalmology* 93:570-573, 1986.

87. Peyman GA, Fishman GA, Sanders DR et al.: Biopsy of human scleralchorioretinal tissue, *Invest Ophthalmol Vis Sci* 14:707-710, 1975.

88. Pflugfelder SC, Roussel TJ, Culbertson WW: Primary Sjogrens syndrome after infectious mononucleosis, *JAMA* 257:1049-1051, 1987.

89. Pinnolis M, McCulley JP, Urman JD: Nummular keratitis associated with infectious mononucleosis, *Am J Ophthalmol* 89:791-794, 1980.

90. Rabon RJ, Louis GJ, Zegarra H, Gutman FA: Acute bilateral posterior angiopathy with influenza A viral infection, *Am J Ophthalmol* 103:289-293, 1987.

91. Raoult D, Walker DH: *Rickettsia rickettsii* and other spotted fever group rickettsiae (Rocky Mountain spotted fever and other spotted fevers). In Mandell GL, Douglas RG, Bennett JE, editors: *Principles and practice of infectious diseases,* ed 3, 1465-1471, New York, 1990, Churchill Livingstone.

92. Ray CG: Rubella (''German measles'') and other viral exanthems. In Braunwald E, Isselbacher KJ, Petersdorf RG et al., editors: *Principles and practice of medicine,* ed 11, 684-686, New York, 1987, McGraw-Hill.

93. Raymond LA, Wilson CA, Linnemann CC: Punctate outer retinitis in acute EBV infection, *Am J Ophthalmol* 104:424-425, 1987.

94. Robb RM, Watters GW: Ophthalmic manifestations of subacute sclerosing panencephalitis, *Arch Ophthalmol* 83:426-435, 1970.

95. Roth AM, Purcell: Ocular findings associated with encephalomyelitis caused by herpesvirus simiae, *Am J Ophthalmol* 84:345-348, 1977.

96. Rubsamen PE, Gass JDM: Vogt-Koyanagi-Harada syndrome: clinical course, therapy and long-term visual outcome, *Arch Ophthalmol* 109:682-687, 1991.

97. Salib EA: Subacute sclerosing panencephalitis presenting at the age of 21 as a schizophrenic-like state with bizarre dysmorphic features, *Br J Psychiatry* 152:709-710, 1988.

98. Scheie HG, Morse PH: Rubeola retinopathy, *Arch Ophthalmol* 88:341-344, 1972.

99. Schooley RT: Epstein-Barr virus infections including infectious mononucleosis. In Braunwald E, Isselbacher KJ, Petersdorf RG et al., editors: *Harrison's principles of internal medicine,* ed 11, 699-704, New York, 1987, McGraw-Hill.

100. Schooley RT, Dolin R: Epstein-Barr virus (infectious mononucleosis). In Mandell GL, Douglas RG, Bennett JE, editors: *Principles and practice of infectious diseases,* ed 3, 1172-1185, New York, 1990, Churchill Livingstone.

101. Siam AE, Gharbawi KF, Meegan JM: Ocular complications of Rift Valley fever, *J Egyp Public Health Assoc* 53:185-186, 1978.

102. Sidikaro Y, Silver L, Holland GN, Kreiger AE: Rhegmatogenous retinal detachments in patients with AIDS and necrotizing retinal infections, *Ophthalmology* 98:129-135, 1991.

103. Spaide RF, Sugin S, Yannuzzi LA, DeRosa JT: Epstein-Barr virus antibodies in multifocal choroiditis and panuveitis, *Am J Ophthalmol* 112:410-413, 1991.

104. Steere AC: *Borrelia burgdorferi* (Lyme disease, Lyme borreliosis). In Mandell GL, Douglas RG, Bennett JE, editors: *Principles and practice of infectious diseases,* ed 3, 1819-1827, New York, 1990, Churchill Livingstone.

105. Straus SE: Introduction to herpesviridae. In Mandell GL, Douglas RG, Bennett JE, editors: *Principles and practice of infectious diseases,* ed 3, 1139-1144, New York, 1990, Churchill Livingstone.

106. Suringa DWR, Bank LJ, Ackerman AB: Role of measles virus in skin lesions and Koplik's spots, *N Engl J Med* 283:1139-1144, 1970.

107. Tanner OR: Ocular manifestations of infectious mononucleosis, *Arch Ophthalmol* 51:229-241, 1954.

108. Thompson RL, Devi-Rao GV, Stevens JG, Wagner EK: Rescue of a herpes simplex virus type 1 neurovirulence function with a cloned DNA fragment, *J Virol* 55:504-508, 1985.

109. Thormar H, Mehta PD, Brown HR: Comparison of wild-type and subacute sclerosing panencephalitis strains of measles virus, *J Exp Med* 148:674-691, 1978.

110. Tiedeman JS: Epstein-Barr viral antibodies in multifocal choroiditis and panuveitis, *Am J Ophthalmol* 104:659-663, 1987.

111. Tramont EC: *Treponema pallidum* (syphilis). In Mandell GL, Douglas RG, Bennett JE, editors: *Principles and practice of infectious diseases,* ed 3, 1794-1808, New York, 1990, Churchill Livingstone.

112. Van Velden DJ, Meyer JD, Olivier J et al.: Rift Valley fever affecting humans in South Africa: a clinicopathologic study, *S Afr Med J* 51:867-871, 1977.

113. Weiss LM, Movahed LA, Warnkee RA, Sklar J: Detection of Epstein-Barr viral genomes in Reed-Sternberg cells of Hodgkin's disease, *New Engl J Med* 320:502-506, 1989.

114. Winberg RJ, Nerney JJ: Bilateral submacular hemorrhages with an influenza syndrome, *Ann Ophthalmol* 15:710-712, 1983.

115. Wolf SM: The ocular manifestations of congenital rubella, *J Pediatr Ophthalmol Strabismus* 10:101-141, 1973.

116. Wong KW, D'Amico DJ, Hedges TR et al.: Ocular involvement with chronic Epstein-Barr virus disease, *Arch Ophthalmol* 105:788-790, 1987.

117. Zagami AS, Lethleean AK: Chorioretinitis as a possible very early manifestation of subacute sclerosing panencephalitis, *Aust NZ J Med* 21:350-352, 1991.

118. Zimmerman LE: Histopathologic basis for ocular manifestations of congenital rubella syndrome, *Am J Ophthalmol* 65:837-862, 1968.

85 Toxoplasmosis

GARY N. HOLLAND, G. RICHARD O'CONNOR, RUBENS BELFORT, JR,
JACK S. REMINGTON

Toxoplasma gondii, a protozoan parasite, can cause severe, life-threatening disease, especially in newborns and immunosuppressed patients, and is an important cause of ocular disease in both immunosuppressed and immunocompetent individuals. The organism is widespread in nature, and in many parts of the world, the majority of the population has serologic evidence of infection. *T. gondii* establishes chronic infections in the host, during which encysted organisms persist in tissues without necessarily causing clinical manifestations. The term *toxoplasmosis* refers to clinically apparent disease caused by proliferating organisms.

There is no cure for *T. gondii* infection, but nonocular infections are generally not serious in otherwise healthy adults. In contrast, toxoplasmic retinochoroiditis, which for many years has been considered the most common recognizable cause of posterior uveitis in immunocompetent individuals, can cause severe morbidity. The active phase of retinal disease is self-limited, but it can recur, and the destructive nature of the infection places patients at risk for blindness if tissues critical for vision, such as the optic nerve or macula, are involved. The growing problem of toxoplasmosis in immunosuppressed patients has led to a renewed interest in ocular toxoplasmosis.

PARASITOLOGY

T. gondii is a one-celled, obligate, intracellular protozoan parasite. Its taxonomic classification is listed in the first box. *T. gondii* undergoes a complicated life cycle that includes both sexual and asexual reproduction[81]; it is considered a *coccidian* parasite because it undergoes sexual reproduction in the epithelial cells of the small intestine. Members of the cat family are its only definitive hosts, but hundreds of other species, including mammals, birds, and reptiles, may serve as intermediate hosts.

T. gondii exists in several forms. Oocysts are the products of sexual reproduction and are shed in feces of cats. They are ovoid with a diameter of 10 μm to 12 μm. In nature the oocyst is the hardiest of the various forms of *T. gondii;* in warm, moist soil they can survive for more than a year. They are rendered noninfectious by boiling or dry heat in excess of 66°C. Ingestion of sporulated oocysts can cause infection in either definitive or intermediate hosts.

Tachyzoites (previously known as trophozoites), the obligate intracellular form of the parasite, are able to invade nearly all host tissues. They are crescent-shaped, measuring 7 μm to 8 μm in length by 2.5 μm to 4 μm in diameter (Fig. 85-1). They have a blunt posterior end and a slightly pointed anterior end with an apical complex containing the conoid and other specialized organelles (Fig. 85-2). Tachyzoites move by gliding and flexing. They stain well with Wright and Giesma stains.

Tissue cysts begin to form as early as 6 to 8 days after infection and may persist in a viable state in multiple tissues for the life of the host (Fig. 85-3). They are 10 μm to 100 μm in diameter and are most commonly found in the central nervous system (CNS) and in skeletal and cardiac muscle. The tissue cyst wall contains structural elements contributed by both the parasite and the host; the presence of host materials may in some way prevent stimulation of immunologic reactions against the tissue cyst. The wall, which is composed of complex proteins and polysaccharides, permits passage of water, gases, electrolytes, and amino acids. Organisms within these tissue cysts, which are termed bradyzoites, will continue to replicate slowly by endodyogeny, a special form of cell division described in the following section. A tissue cyst may eventually contain as many as 3000 organisms. They stain well with conventional stains but are well differentiated from surrounding tissues by the use of periodic acid-Schiff stain.

Life Cycle

The reason sexual reproduction, or gametogony, occurs only in cats is not known. It is believed that cats are most commonly infected with *T. gondii* through ingestion of tissue cysts in the flesh of infected birds and rodents, but cats

TAXONOMIC CLASSIFICATION OF *TOXOPLASMA GONDII**

Phylum: Protozoa
Subphylum: Apicomplexa
Class: Sporozoasida
Subclass: Coccidiasina
Order: Eucoccidiorida
Suborder: Eimeriorina
Family: Sarcocystidae
Subfamily: Toxoplasmatinae
Genus: *Toxoplasma*
Species: *gondii* (only one known species)

---

* Adapted from Frenkel JK: Toxoplasmosis: parasite life cycle, pathology, and immunology. In Hammond DM, Long PL, editors: *The coccidia: Eimeria, Isospora, Toxoplasma, and related genera,* Baltimore, 1973, University Park Press.

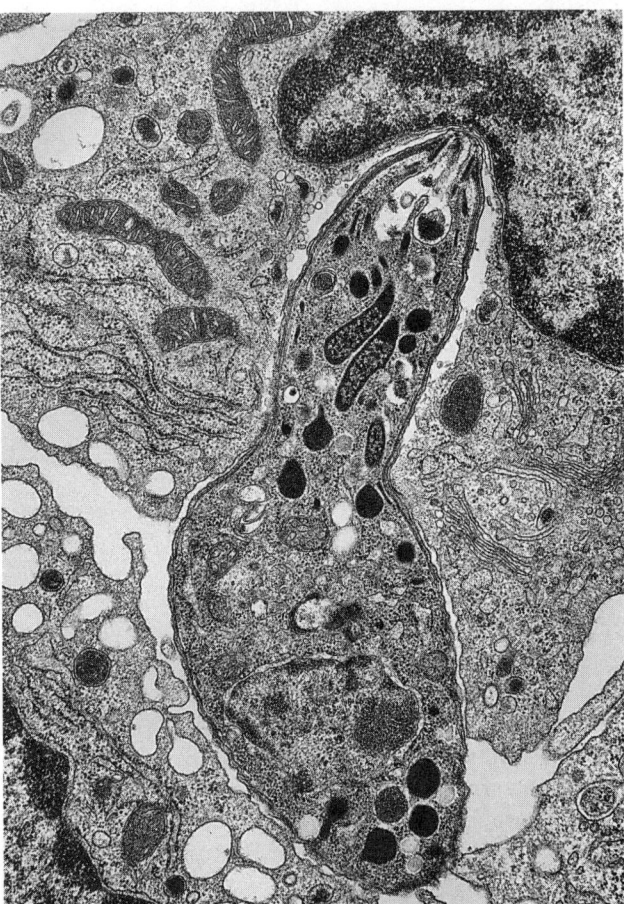

Fig. 85-2. Specimen fixed in the mouse peritoneal cavity 60 seconds after injection of *Toxoplasma gondii,* showing a parasite invading a macrophage. There is disruption and vesiculation of the macrophage plasma membrane around the anterior end of the parasite, although cytoplasmic organelles such as the mitochondria, endoplamsic reticulum, and Golgi complex are well preserved. Correlated studies have shown that the parasites force their entry into host cells treated to inhibit phagocytosis. Micrograph courtesy of Barbara A. Nichols, PhD, San Francisco, CA. Reprinted with permission from Nichols BA, O'Connor GR: Penetration of mouse peritoneal macrophages by the protozoon *Toxoplasma gondii:* new evidence for active invasion and phagocytosis, *Lab Invest* 44:324-335, 1981.

can also become infected through ingestion of sporulated oocysts. In small intestinal epithelial cells of the cat, organisms can develop into sexual forms or gametocytes. During gametogony, male gametocytes (2% to 4% of the total gametocyte population) produce an average of 12 microgametes, which penetrate mature female macrogametes; their union results in an ookinete. The ookinete, or fertilized macrogametocyte, is released by rupture of the host cell and is shed from the intestine of the cat in the form of a noninfectious, unsporulated oocyst. Oocysts are excreted 3 to 24 days after initial infection, depending on the form of *T. gondii* ingested by the cat: 3 to 5 days after ingestion of tissue cysts; 5 to 10 days after ingestion of tachyzoites; and 20 to 24 days after ingestion of oocysts. Millions of oocysts are produced, but they are shed for a period of only 7 to 20 days (average 12 days). Thus individual cats are not a continuing source of infection.

After excretion, sporogony occurs over 2 to 21 days, depending on the ambient temperature. This process results in the formation of an infective oocyst containing two sporocysts, each of which contains four sporozoites. Sporulation does not occur at temperatures of less than 4°C or more than 37°C.[65] As a result of fecal contamination, oocysts are either reingested by cats or are ingested by intermediate hosts. Insects such as cockroaches and flies can serve as vectors for transporting oocysts. It is believed that infection may also be transmitted by inhalation of oocysts, which are then trapped by respiratory secretions and eventually swallowed.[295] After ingestion, sporozoites are liberated from oocysts by diges-

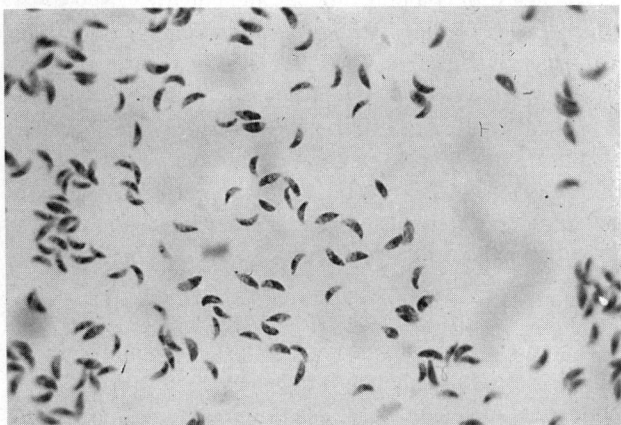

Fig. 85-1. Giemsa-stained smear of an in vitro preparation demonstrating tachyzoite forms of *Toxoplasma gondii.*

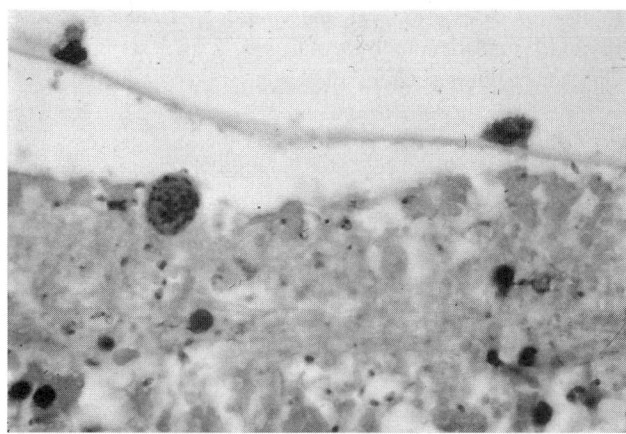

Fig. 85-3. A prominent tissue cyst of *Toxoplasma gondii* in necrotic retina of a patient with AIDS. (Hematoxylin and eosin, original magnification ×160). (Courtesy of Ben J. Glasgow, MD, Los Angeles, CA.)

tive enzymes. Sporozoites invade epithelial cells of the small intestine, where they reproduce rapidly as tachyzoites for several generations by the asexual process of schizogony, in which there is simultaneous cleavage of nuclear and cytoplasmic material. Continued reproduction results in lysis of the host epithelial cells, and tachyzoites are then spread throughout the body in the blood and lymph circulations, where they may invade all cells.

Tachyzoites continue to reproduce by endodyogeny, a specialized form of asexual reproduction in which two daughter cells are produced within the mother parasite and are then released by rupture of the mother cell membrane. This unique form of asexual reproduction occurs only in members of the family Sarcocystidae. With an intact host immune response, replication of tachyzoites eventually ceases, and most organisms are eliminated. Some, however, will form intracellular tissue cysts.

In cats some organisms in the small intestine will develop into gametocytes after several generations of asexual reproduction; thereafter, gametogony can occur in the epithelial cells simultaneously with schizogony. The stimulus for some organisms to become gametocytes is not known.

T. gondii infection can be transmitted by ingestion of tissue cysts when chronically infected animals are eaten by carnivores. Tissue cyst walls are relatively resistant to peptic digestion within the stomach but are susceptible to trypsin digestion in the small intestine, which releases viable organisms. These organisms can tolerate exposure to those same digestive enzymes for several hours. They are thus able to invade the intestinal wall, and the asexual reproductive cycles outline previously are repeated, with dissemination of tachyzoites in the new host. If primary infection occurs during pregnancy, tachyzoites can pass the placenta to infect the developing fetus. *T. gondii* can therefore be perpetuated through carnivorism and congenital transmission without involving the definitive host; nevertheless, cats are felt to play an important role in disease transmission in most areas of the world.

HISTORICAL BACKGROUND

Toxoplasmosis is undoubtedly an ancient disease, but it was not recognized as a specific entity until after the parasite was discovered in the early twentieth century. According to Binazzi,[21] Laveran[160] was probably describing *T. gondii* in a 1900 report of parasites seen in circulating blood cells of the rice bird *(Padda oryzivora)*. Nevertheless, credit is generally given to Nicolle and Manceaux[200,201] for the first description of the organism, which they found in tissues of *Ctenodactylus gundi,* a small North African rodent, in 1908. They named it *Toxoplasma gondii* during the following year; the genus name was derived from the Greek word "toxon" (meaning "arc"), in recognition of the shape of tachyzoites, and the species name was taken from the name of the rodent in which they first recognized it. In 1908 the parasite had also been seen by Splendore[277] in the tissues of a rabbit in Brazil.

The disease toxoplasmosis was possibly described by Darling at the Gorgas Hospital in the Panama Canal Zone in 1908.[35] He reported a case of sarcosporidiosis, based on a muscle biopsy taken from a patient with acute myositis; he was not certain of his diagnosis, however, because of atypical features of the organism he saw in the biopsy specimen. Many years later, Chaves-Carballo[35] re-examined the tissue specimens upon which Darling had made his diagnosis and concluded that the organism was, in fact, most likely *T. gondii.*

A paper by Jankû[130] in 1923 is accepted as the first report of ocular toxoplasmosis.* He found organisms identical to those described by Nicolle and Manceaux in retinal tissue of a baby with microphthalmos, who had died of congenital toxoplasmosis. The child had been given an antemortem diagnosis of typical "coloboma of the macula."

It was not until 1939 that interest finally focused on human toxoplasmosis as a disease of newborns. In that year Wolf, Cowen, and Paige[309] described the isolation of *T. gondii* from the brain and ocular tissues of a child who died of congenital infection. Subsequent study of ocular tissues from that child revealed the presence of *T. gondii* exclusively in the retina, although there was severe inflammation of the subjacent choroid.[151]

Serologic tests for *T. gondii* infection became available in the 1940s. The complement fixation test of Sabin[245] remained positive for only a few months after acute infection, and the neutralizing antibody test of Sabin and Ruchman[247] was difficult to standardize. In 1948, however, introduction

---

*Although Jankû's work was cited by some investigators in the 1950s, details of the original Czech language publication remained largely unknown to the medical community outside of Czechoslovakia, until a German language translation appeared in 1959.[131]

of the Sabin-Feldman dye test[246] made it possible to do large scale epidemiologic studies of toxoplasmosis. It was a sensitive and specific test that detected antibodies against *T. gondii* soon after infection, and it remained positive for the entire lifetime of an infected individual, even without clinically apparent disease. Using this test, it became apparent that there were many asymptomatic carriers of the parasite, among both human beings and domestic animals. It confirmed a worldwide distribution of the infection and helped to establish the fact that *T. gondii* infection could be a cause of an infectious mononucleosis-like disease.[232]

A milestone in the history of ocular toxoplasmosis was the 1952 discovery by Wilder[303] of *T. gondii* in stained sections of eyes that had "intractable chorioretinitis." As a direct result of her observations, it was finally realized that many cases of posterior uveitis in adults that had been attributed to tuberculosis were, in fact, caused by *T. gondii* infection.

Over the next decade, additional clinical and histopathologic studies[115,128,324] characterized ocular toxoplasmosis in newborns and adults more fully, and provided additional proof of disease causation by identification and isolation of the organism from retinal tissue. In 1954 Jacobs and associates[128] were the first to describe the isolation of *T. gondii* from the enucleated eyes of an adult. By the 1960s toxoplasmosis had become accepted as the leading cause of posterior uveitis in the United States and other industrialized countries.

In 1970 the cat was discovered to be the definitive host of *T. gondii* by Frenkel[85] in Kansas and by Hutchison[124] in Scotland. That discovery provided important information for a more detailed understanding of the epidemiology of toxoplasmosis and led to strategies to prevent its transmission, especially to pregnant women.

EPIDEMIOLOGY

In 1972 Kean[145] estimated that 500 million individuals were infected with *T. gondii* worldwide. In the United States serologic evidence of *T. gondii* infection ranges from 3% to 70% of the healthy adult population.[15] The presence of anti-*T. gondii* antibodies in different populations throughout the world varies with social and economic factors, age, and geographic area. Prevalence is highest in tropical areas and is relatively low in hot and arid areas, and in cold regions, such as Iceland.[77,298] At a given latitude, persons at elevations above 5000 feet appear to have lower rates of infection than matched controls at sea level.[209] These variations are attributed to the effect of environmental conditions on oocyte survival. Societies in which there is an increased consumption of raw or undercooked meat and areas affected by poor sanitation have higher rates. In some areas of Central America, the South Pacific, and Western Europe, seropositivity rates exceed 90% by the fourth decade of life.

The majority of acquired *T. gondii* infections in immunocompetent children and adults remain asymptomatic. In 10% to 20% of cases, however, individuals will develop a self-limited lymphadenopathy syndrome,[231] as described in the Clinical Features section.

Transmission

Human beings can be infected by tissue cysts, tachyzoites, or oocysts; ingestion of tissue cysts in undercooked meat is believed to be the most common mode of transmission. The level of infestation varies among species commonly used in meat production; hogs and sheep are more commonly infected than cattle. As many as 25% of pork and lamb samples are found to contain tissue cysts.[64] Oocysts can be ingested with unwashed fruit or vegetables, and tissue cysts can be ingested if hands are not washed after contact with uncooked meat during preparation of meals. Surfaces on which food is prepared can also become contaminated, and be a source of infection.

Inhalation of sporulated oocysts appears to be another mode of transmission. Teutsch and associates[295] described an epidemic of acquired *T. gondii* infection involving 37 individuals who were present at a single riding stable in Atlanta, Georgia, USA. There was no evidence of a common source of oral ingestion among victims of the epidemic, but oocysts were found in dust that covered the floor in an area of the stable frequented by feral cats.

Toxoplasma gondii has been isolated from eggs,[293] and transmission can also occur from ingestion of colostrum or milk containing tachyzoites. Infection after drinking unpasteurized goat milk from a chronically infected animal has been reported.[236,248] O'Connor[206,209] has hypothesized that infection in such cases may occur as a result of transmucosal penetration of tachyzoites through the oral or pharyngeal mucosa, as the acid environment of the stomach should kill *T. gondii* when it is in the tachyzoite form. Nichols and O'Connor[198] have shown that tachyzoites can penetrate mucosa within 15 seconds of contact.

Toxoplasma gondii can be transmitted by transfusion of whole blood or leukocytes[269] and by organ transplantation.[27] Evidence argues against sexual transmission of infection.[209]

Congenital Infection

Transplacental transmission of *T. gondii* to the fetus occurs almost exclusively when infection is acquired by women during pregnancy. Rarely, however, transplacental transmission can occur if an immunocompetent woman acquires infection within the 6 to 8 weeks before conception.[233] Also, chronically infected women who are immunosuppressed may transmit *T. gondii* to the fetus, although such cases appear to be rare.

In the United States, where approximately 70% to 80% of women of childbearing age are at risk for primary infection,[149] the prevalence of acquired toxoplasmosis during pregnancy has been estimated to be 0.2% to 1%.[312]

In most series congenital infection develops in 30% to 50% of infants born to mothers who have serologic evidence of newly-acquired *T. gondii* infection during pregnancy,[56,57,152,164] but the rate of fetal infection is related to the stage of pregnancy during which the mother becomes infected.[6,40,57] Without treatment, it is approximately 10% to 15% during the first trimester, 30% during the second trimester, and 60% during the third trimester.[312] Rates are significantly lower when the mother is treated. The higher rate during the last trimester of pregnancy is possibly caused by the greater vascularity of the placenta at that time. Damage to the fetus, however, is greatest if infection occurs during the first trimester, presumably because of the immaturity of the immune system and the greater impact of injury to organs during the early stages of development.

Estimates of the prevalence of congenital infection have ranged widely: from 1 of 750 to 1 of 8000 live births in the United States and Scandinavia[6,7,149,283,312] to approximately 1 of 300 live births in France.[175]

Maternal immunity protects against fetal transmission; thus women infected before pregnancy are at little or no risk for delivering a child with congenital toxoplasmosis, and women who deliver one child with congenital toxoplasmosis are at little or no risk of having a second infected child.* Reactivation of toxoplasmic retinochoroiditis in an immunocompetent, pregnant women also does not pose a threat to the fetus. There are, however, rare reports of congenital toxoplasmosis in more than one sibling[282] and congenital disease in offspring of women with toxoplasmosis that occurred before pregnancy.[58,91] These exceptional cases have been attributed to immunologic abnormalities or to uterine foci of organisms in the chronic maternal infection. Most cases of toxoplasmosis in multiple siblings, especially when discovered at an older age, probably are attributable to acquired disease in the siblings.[14,166,176]

Disease in Immunosuppressed Patients

Toxoplasma gondii is a common opportunistic pathogen among immunosuppressed patients and is a particularly severe problem in HIV-infected individuals. The prevalence of anti-*T. gondii* antibodies is 15% to 40% among HIV-infected individuals in the United States,[170] but is nearly universal where infection rates are very high in the general population. There may also be an increased risk for primary, acquired *T. gondii* infections among HIV-infected individuals.

Toxoplasmosis is believed to be the most common nonviral infection of the brain in patients with AIDS. Toxoplasmic encephalitis eventually develops in 25% to 50% of patients with antibodies against *T. gondii*.[313,322]

Ocular Disease

Ocular toxoplasmosis has been the most common cause of posterior uveitis in many surveys. Although reported rates vary, it probably accounts for at least 25% of posterior uveitis cases in the United States[110,179,218,314] and over 85% of posterior uveitis cases in southern Brazil.[101]

The prevalence of ocular toxoplasmosis in the United States is not known, but in a frequently cited study, Smith and Ganley[274] found that 5 of 842 individuals (0.6%) in a single small community in Maryland had chorioretinal scars consistent with healed toxoplasmic retinochoroiditis. A similar rate has been found in the state of Alabama.[172] In southern Brazil, an area with a very high rate of *T. gondii* infection, 17.7% of the population was found to have ocular toxoplasmosis.[101]

Toxoplasmic retinochoroiditis is the most common manifestation of congenital *T. gondii* infection; it occurs in 70% to over 90% of all patients with congenital toxoplasmosis.* Eichenwald[69] found that the incidence of retinochoroiditis was related to the type of congenital disease; 94.4% of infants with neurologic disease alone had ocular lesions, whereas only 65.9% of infants with disseminated disease at birth had ocular lesions. Ocular infection may be the only manifestation of congenital toxoplasmosis; 10% of patients have ocular lesions without clear evidence of disease in other organs.[7,73,74]

Approximately 85% of infected infants appear normal at birth, but prospective studies indicate that approximately 85% of those subclinically infected infants, if left untreated, will develop ocular toxoplasmosis.[152,305] In a study of 12 patients with congenital toxoplasmosis, Loewer-Sieger and associates[164] found that 4 had retinochoroidal lesions at age 1. By age 18, 9 of 11 had lesions, 4 of whom had vision loss.

Ocular disease in patients with acquired *T. gondii* infection is believed to be uncommon.[243] In a 1973 publication Perkins[217] reviewed a number of isolated case reports in which acquired ocular toxoplasmosis appeared to be well documented. He estimated that ocular involvement occurred in 2% to 3% of patients with acquired *T. gondii* infection. In the Atlanta epidemic of acquired *T. gondii* infection described previously, only 1 of 37 affected individuals (2.7%) had developed eye disease after 4 years of follow-up.[5] In his 1973 review of ocular toxoplasmosis, Perkins[217] also identified 26 cases of accidental laboratory infection with *T. gondii;* only 2 developed ocular disease, and in both cases the reported lesions were not typical of toxoplasmic retinochoroiditis.

Perkins[217] found that ocular disease was more frequent in patients with acquired toxoplasmosis when the patient also had other CNS involvement; this association may reflect a similar reduction in host defenses in the eye and the brain (for example, neither organ has internal lymphatics). Conversely, an association between ocular disease and infection elsewhere in the CNS may simply reflect the severity of the acquired infection, as suggested by Perkins, rather than a

---

*References 6, 40, 56, 57, 149, 152.

*References 7, 40, 152, 233, 279, 305.

direct relationship between the two sites of disease. It does not appear to reflect a direct extension of infection from one site to the other.

It is commonly believed that the majority of ocular toxoplasmosis cases result from the recurrence of congenital infections. Perkins based this assumption on several observations. Although the prevalence of *T. gondii* infection increases with age, toxoplasmic retinochoroiditis occurs more frequently in the second and third decades than later in life. Also, he found that patients with ocular toxoplasmosis did not have higher titers of anti-*T. gondii* antibodies than individuals in the population without eye disease, as would be expected if ocular involvement occurred at the time of initial infection.

In some areas of the world where seropositivity rates are high, such as Micronesia, ocular toxoplasmosis is rarely seen.[47] This observation has also been used to support the hypothesis that ocular lesions usually result from recurrence of congenital disease. When infection is widespread in a population, first exposure to the organism will usually occur before pregnancy, and congenital transmission will be uncommon. A low rate of ocular disease in populations with high rates of acquired disease in childhood has been used to argue against recurrence of noncongenital disease as a cause of retinal lesions.[209]

The relationship between congenital *T. gondii* infection and ocular disease later in life is being reevaluated. An infrequently reported, but important, subgroup of patients are those in whom toxoplasmic retinochoroiditis is the only manifestation of recently acquired *T. gondii* infection (Fig. 85-4). Perkins[217] assumed that acquired ocular toxoplasmo-

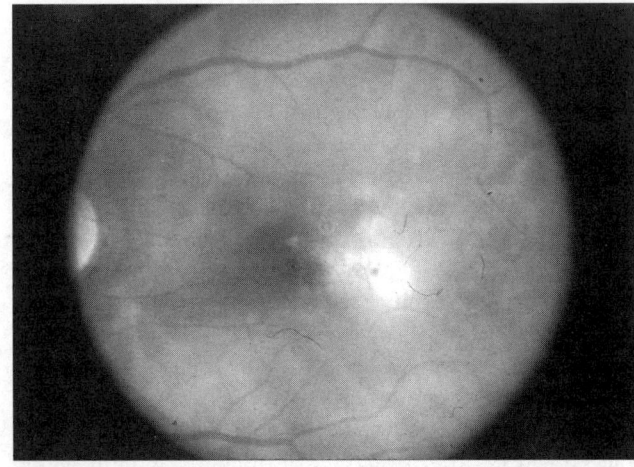

B

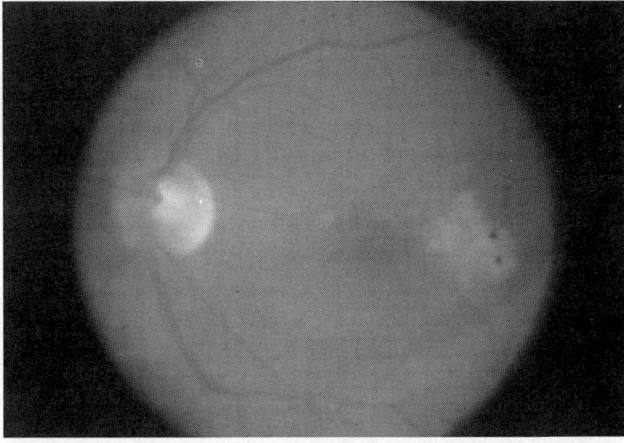

C

Fig. 85-4, cont'd. B, The same fundus photographed approximately 2 years later, following spontaneous reactivation of toxoplasmic retinochoroiditis in the same area. The lesion responded again to medical therapy. **C,** The same fundus photographed 2 years after **B.** The patient has a retinochoroidal scar typical of those seen with ocular toxoplasmosis. (Photographs courtesy of Stephen G. Turner, MD, San Leandro, CA.)

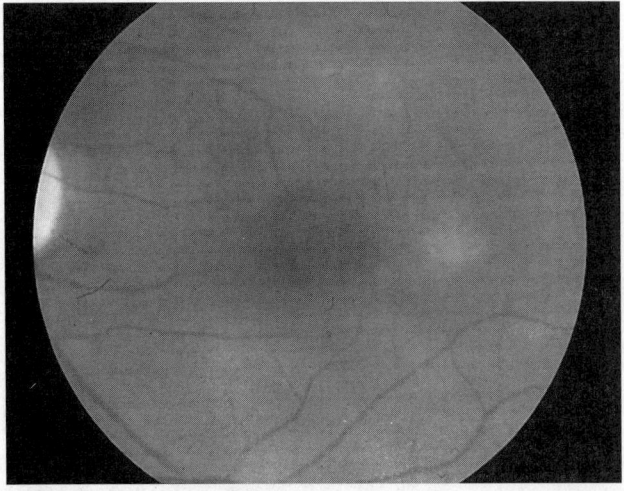

A

Fig. 85-4. A, Left fundus of a 48-year-old woman with a focus of retinitis temporal to the fovea. She had serologic evidence of recently acquired *Toxoplasma gondii* infection but no clinically apparent nonocular disease. The lesion responded to antimicrobial drug therapy and oral corticosteroids.

sis without systemic manifestations of disease should be even less common than ocular disease in patients with symptomatic systemic infections. In a review of published cases of presumed acquired ocular toxoplasmosis without systemic manifestations of disease, he found little evidence to confirm the diagnoses. In contrast, a series of patients whose serologic testing was performed at the Palo Alto Medical Foundation suggests that acquired ocular toxoplasmosis may be more common than heretofore realized.* Such patients have detectable IgM antibodies against *T. gondii* and very high anti-*T. gondii* IgG antibody titers, but do

---

*J.R. Remington, MD, unpublished data.

not have lymphadenopathy or other nonocular clinical disease.

In view of such cases, it may be appropriate to reconsider basic assumptions about the nature of recurrent toxoplasmic retinochoroiditis; it is possible that the retinochoroidal scars from which recurrent disease arises may actually be residua of earlier acquired, but asymptomatic, infections, rather than residua of congenital infections. Initial episodes of acquired toxoplasmic retinochoroiditis might be asymptomatic if lesions are small or located in the peripheral retina. Symptomatic lesions during early childhood might go unrecognized if young individuals do not verbalize their visual changes.

Recent studies from southern Brazil have also challenged traditional concepts about the epidemiology and pathogenesis of ocular disease. In the region of Erechim, a city in the state of Rio Grande do Sul, the prevalence of ocular disease increases with age, and numerous families have been identified in which multiple, nontwin siblings have ocular toxoplasmosis. Congenital toxoplasmosis is uncommon.[101,270] These findings suggest that ocular disease, including recurrent lesions, is related to acquired infection rather than congenital infection. Transmission has been attributed to the common practice of ingesting raw pork during the preparation of sausage in that population.

Several hypotheses have been raised to explain the very high rates of ocular toxoplasmosis among patients with acquired *T. gondii* infection in southern Brazil; they include differences in the age at exposure, duration and intensity of exposure, strain differences, genetic differences in the host population, or co-factors that might affect the course of disease. The relevance of these cases to transmission and pathogenesis of toxoplasmosis in other parts of the world is uncertain.

Disease Recurrence. In a study of 63 patients with recurrent toxoplasmic retinochoroiditis, Friedmann and Knox,[88] found that the age of first symptomatic recurrence ranged between 7 and 57 years. The authors reported that the mean age of first symptomatic recurrence was 25.3 years; review of their published data showed that the median age is younger (between 20 and 24 years) and the 5-year interval in which the greatest number of first episodes occurred was 10 to 14 years. First symptomatic recurrences developed between ages 10 and 35 years in 75% of patients.

Women with a history of ocular toxoplasmosis are believed to have an increased rate of disease recurrence during pregnancy.[208] As stated previously recurrent active disease in immunocompetent women does not pose a threat to the fetus.

Immunosuppressed Patients. Toxoplasmic retinochoroiditis is believed to account for 1% to 3% of retinal infections in patients with AIDS.[37,127] The rate is probably highest among patients in areas of the world with high rates of *T. gondii* infection in the general population, such as France and Brazil. Most descriptions of ocular toxoplasmosis in other immunosuppressed individuals have come from isolated case reports, and prevalence rates are not known.

Ocular toxoplasmosis is much less common in HIV-infected patients than toxoplasmic encephalitis. Frenkel[84] has cited the difference in parasitic load in the eye versus the brain as the probable reason for this difference.

RISK FACTORS

The major risk factor for transmission of *T. gondii* to adults and children is ingestion of undercooked meat; a variety of other modes of transmission are discussed in the Epidemiology section.

Also discussed in the epidemiology section is the fact that congenital infection is related to initial infection of the mother during pregnancy; the risk of transmission to the fetus is highest when maternal infection occurs during the third trimester of pregnancy, but the risk of severe clinical disease is highest if congenital infection occurs during the first trimester.

Immunosuppression is associated with an increased risk of life-threatening toxoplasmosis. Immunosuppression also increases the *severity* of ocular toxoplasmosis when it occurs (see Clinical Features section).

In HIV-infected patients, ocular toxoplasmosis can occur before the development of index diseases diagnostic of AIDS. The risk of life-threatening toxoplasmosis increases when CD4+ T-lymphocyte counts fall below $100/\mu l$.[43] In one study the median CD4+ T-lymphocyte count of patients with AIDS and toxoplasmic encephalitis was $50/\mu l$ (range 0 to $730/\mu l$).[226] Although the median CD4+ T-lymphocyte count specifically associated with toxoplasmic retinochoroiditis is not known, this infection can occur at higher counts than usually associated with cytomegalovirus (CMV) retinitis.[70]

CLINICAL FEATURES

The most common clinical manifestation of acquired *T. gondii* infection is asymptomatic cervical lymphadenopathy. Other commonly involved lymph nodes are those in the suboccipital, supraclavicular, axillary, and inguinal areas. They will generally be nonsuppurative, discrete, of variable firmness, and nontender.[178]

Symptomatic patients may develop sore throat, fever, malaise, night sweats, myalgias, and maculopapular rash.[178] Hepatosplenomegaly may be present, and there may be a few circulating atypical lymphocytes. This disorder resembles infectious mononucleosis, but can be confused with Hodgkin disease or other lymphomas. Symptoms and lymphadenopathy will usually resolve within a few months.

Infection during pregnancy, also usually asymptomatic, can result in a mild systemic illness with lymphadenopathy and skin rash, as in other adults.[6,56,149,312]

Rarely, immunocompetent individuals will develop severe life-threatening disease, with myocarditis, pneumonitis, and/or encephalitis.[15,102]

Congenital Disease

Disseminated infection evident at birth is characterized by jaundice, rash, petechiae caused by thrombocytopenia, encephalitis, fever, anemia, lymphadenopathy, hepatosplenomegaly, pneumonitis, vomiting, and diarrhea. Hydrocephaly or microcephaly, seizures, and other neurologic manifestations may also be apparent in such patients. Markedly elevated CSF protein is a hallmark of congenital toxoplasmosis.[7] Those infants symptomatic at birth will often be left with severe sequelae of infection.

Infants may have congenital infection, yet display no overt clinical signs of disease at birth. Examination of asymptomatic newborns may, however, reveal chorioretinal scars, intracranial calcifications, or other sequelae of infection. Also, infants who appear normal at birth may, after several weeks or months, develop signs and symptoms attributable to CNS infection, including hydrocephalus, intracranial calcifications, psychomotor retardation, deterioration of intellect, deafness, and retinochoroidal lesions.

Longitudinal studies suggest that most infants with subclinical infection at birth will eventually develop signs or symptoms of congenital toxoplasmosis, even months or years later. Wilson and associates[305] found that 11 of 13 infected children who had no signs of disease at birth developed sequelae of infection after a mean follow-up period of 8.3 years. Each had retinochoroidal lesions (mean age at diagnosis, 3.7 years). Five children also developed other neurologic sequelae.

Disease in Immunosuppressed Patients

Toxoplasmosis can be a life-threatening disease in immunosuppressed patients.* Toxoplasmic encephalitis is the most common cause of focal intracranial lesions in patients with AIDS and is the most frequent manifestation of *T. gondii* infection in this population.† The disease usually presents with focal neurologic signs that have a subacute onset. Clinical findings can include mental status changes, seizures, speech abnormalities, weakness, cranial nerve dysfunction, cerebellar signs, meningismus, and neuropsychiatric disorders. Patients will have solitary, or more commonly, multiple contrast-enhancing lesions on computed tomographic (CT) or magnetic resonance imaging (MRI) studies (Fig. 85-5). Less commonly, patients with AIDS will develop diffuse encephalitis.[103] Such patients will have generalized cerebral dysfunction and no focal signs. This form of disease is rapidly fatal.

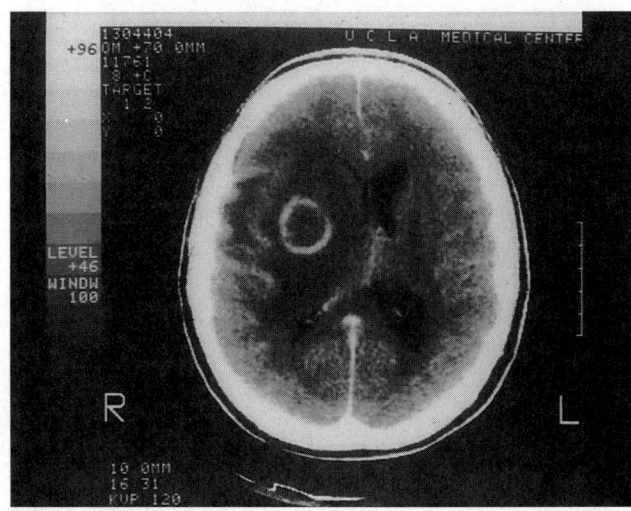

Fig. 85-5. Computed tomographic scan shows a 2-cm contrast-enhanced lesion with surrounding cerebral edema in the right frontoparietal lobe of a patient with AIDS and intercranial toxoplasmosis. (Reprinted with permission from Holland GN, Engstrom RE Jr, Glasgow BJ et al.: Ocular toxoplamosis in patients with the acquired immunodeficiency syndrome, *Am J Ophthalmol* 106:653-667, 1988. Copyright by The Ophthalmic Publishing Company.)

Patients may also develop toxoplasmic myelopathy,[112] which results in motor or sensory dysfunction of the limbs, bladder, and bowels.

The lungs are another site of *T. gondii* infection in patients with AIDS.[31,211,225,253] Toxoplasmic pneumonitis causes a prolonged febrile illness, characterized by cough and dyspnea, that can be confused with *Pneumocystis carinii* pneumonia and pulmonary tuberculosis. Pulmonary disease can lead to acute respiratory failure and hemodynamic abnormalities.[211] Disseminated infection has also been reported to result in septic shock.[167]

Among patients who are immunosuppressed for reasons other than HIV infection, toxoplasmosis has been reported most commonly in organ transplant recipients and those with Hodgkin disease or other lymphomas.[125] Disease most commonly involves the CNS, heart, and lungs. Manifestations are similar to those seen in patients with AIDS, although there may be a higher rate of nonfocal signs in immunosuppressed patients without AIDS who develop toxoplasmic encephalitis.[125]

Ocular Disease

Table 85-1 lists the ocular disorders that may be seen with local or systemic *T. gondii* infections. The retina is the primary site of *T. gondii* infection in the eye. Toxoplasmic retinochoroiditis lesions have the same characteristics, whether they result from congenital or acquired infections. They are usually intensely white, focal lesions with overlying vitreous inflammatory haze. Active lesions that are ac-

---

*References 27, 54, 161, 168-170, 226, 311, 315, 322.
†References 161, 168, 170, 226, 311, 322.

TABLE 85-1 OCULAR DISEASE IN PATIENTS WITH *TOXOPLASMA GONDII* INFECTION

I. Ocular infections
  A. Retina
    1. Recurrent retinochoroiditis*
    2. Acquired retinochoroiditis
  B. Optic nerve
  C. Iris (immunosuppressed patients only)
II. Inflammatory lesions without apparent active ocular infection
  A. Neuroretinitis
  B. Retinal vasculitis (patients with recently acquired systemic toxoplasmosis)
  C. Disorders associated with old, inactive toxoplasmic retinochoroidal scars
    1. Recurrent iridocyclitis
    2. Persistent vitritis

*Recurrent retinochoroiditis is the only lesion seen frequently; others are uncommon.

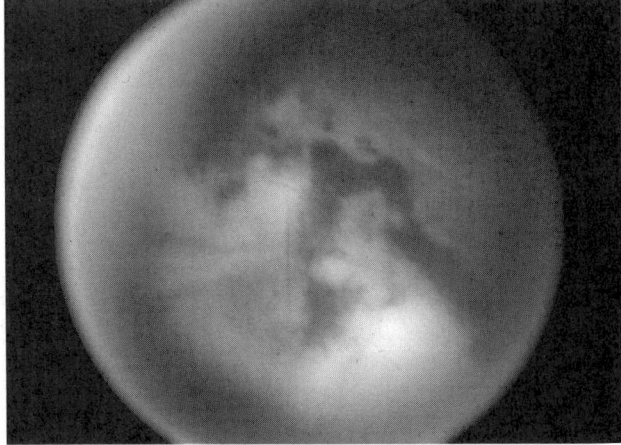

B

Fig. 85-6, cont'd. B, The same eye after resolution of the active retinal infection and vitreous humor inflammatory reaction. There is extensive retinochoroidal scarring.

companied by a severe vitreous inflammatory reaction will have the classic "headlight in the fog" appearance (Fig. 85-6). The choroid is secondarily inflamed, but choroidal lesions do not occur in the absence of retinal infection. There can also be an intense, secondary iridocyclitis.

Recurrent lesions tend to occur at the borders of retinochoroidal scars, which are the remnants of previous disease episodes (Figs. 85-7 to 85-10). Scars are often found in clusters (Fig. 85-7).

Lesions can occur anywhere in the fundus. Among 63 patients examined by Friedmann and Knox,[88] 47 (75%) had active lesions in the posterior pole, whereas 16 (25%) had active lesions in the peripheral retina; this distribution of

lesions may, however, reflect the referral of patients suffering from more serious disease to these investigators. Hogan and associates[114] found that macular lesions were present in only 46% of eyes among all patients with ocular toxoplasmosis who were seen in the Uveitis Survey Clinic of the Francis I. Proctor Foundation in San Francisco, California.

Hogan and associates[114] also found evidence of bilateral infection in 34% of all patients with ocular toxoplasmosis. (Scars can be found in both eyes, but it is unusual to have more than one focus of active infection at any given time in an immunocompetent patient.) Bilateral, macular lesions have been considered one of the hallmarks of congenital disease (Fig. 85-8), whereas acquired infections are gener-

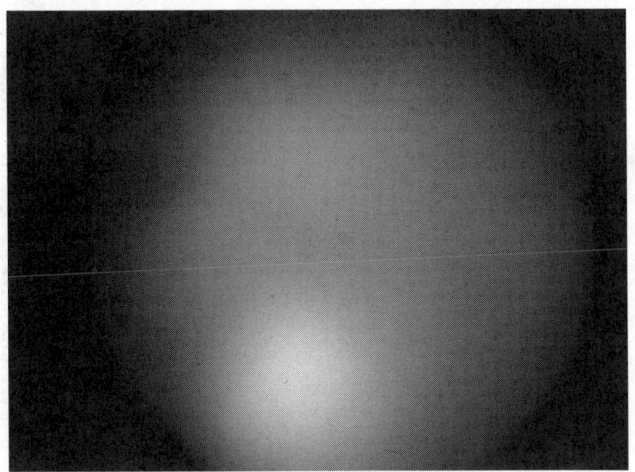

A

Fig. 85-6. A, "Headlight in the fog" appearance of recurrent ocular toxoplamosis in a patient with a severe vitreous humor inflammatory reaction.

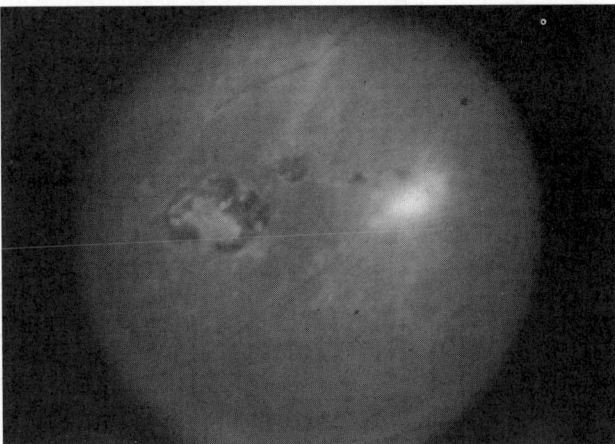

Fig. 85-7. An intensely white focus of recurrent toxoplasmic retinochoroiditis adjacent to a cluster of hyperpigmented retinochoroidal scars associated with past episodes of active disease. There is also patchy inflammatory sheathing of retinal vessels. (Figure also in color insert.)

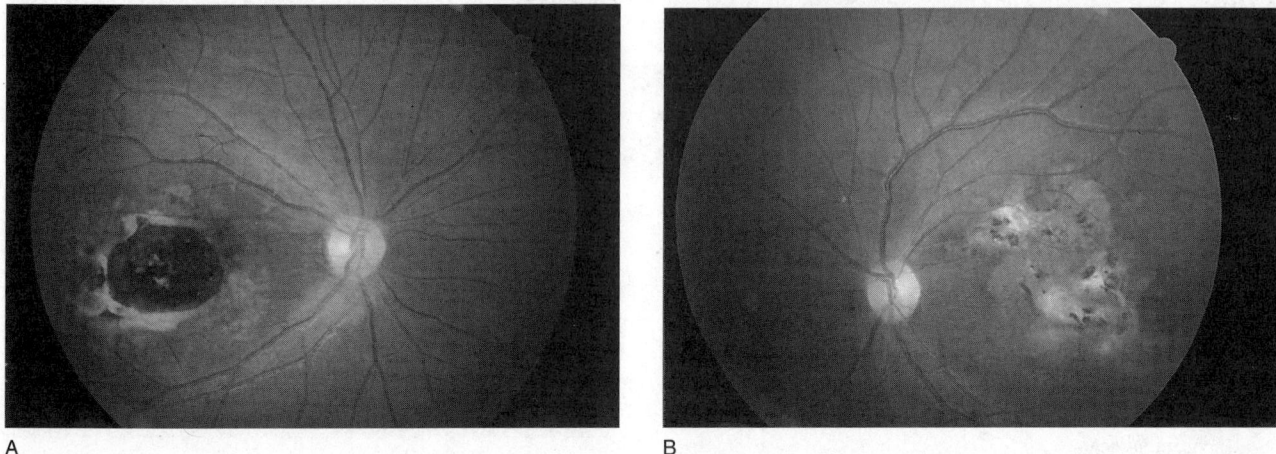

A   B

Fig. 85-8. **A, B,** Bilateral macular retinochoroidal scars in a patient having a history of congenital toxoplasmosis. There is a resolving focus of recurrent disease at the inferior border of the scar in the left eye **(B).**

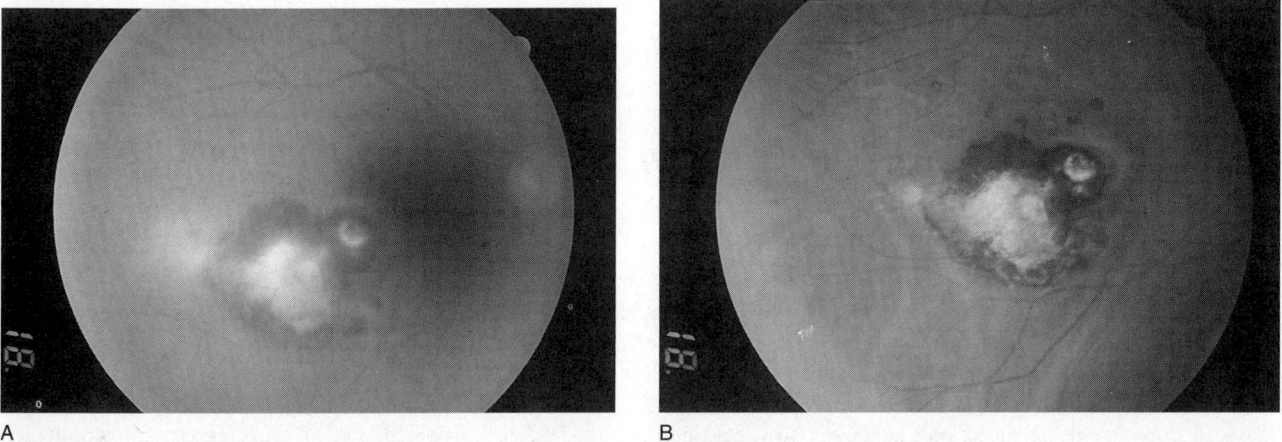

A   B

Fig. 85-9. **A,** The right fundus of a patient with ocular toxoplasmosis. There is a focus of recurrent disease at the temporal (left in photograph) border of the large macular scar. **B,** The same fundus photographed 10 months later. The satellite lesion is inactive and is developing a hyperpigmented border. Vitreous humor inflammatory reaction has cleared.

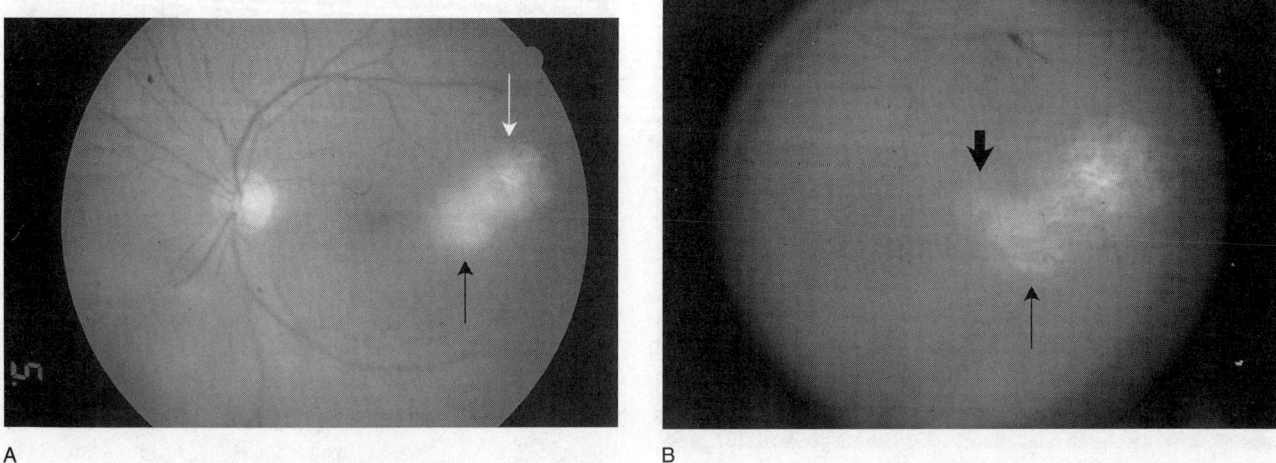

A   B

Fig. 85-10. **A,** The left fundus of a patient with ocular toxoplasmosis. There is a focus of recurrent disease *(black arrow)* at the inferior border of a retinochoroidal scar *(white arrow).* The lesion resolved following treatment with oral therapy consisting of antimicrobial drugs and corticosteroids. **B,** The same fundus 14 months later. The site of the previous recurrence has scarred *(thin arrow),* and there is a new recurrence of disease *(thick arrow)* at the border of that scar and adjacent to the fovea. There is little pigmentation associated with any scars. (Figure also in color insert.)

ally thought to result in unilateral disease. Macular infections and bilateral involvement have been reported in patients with acquired infections, however.[101,114]

The symptoms of recurrent toxoplasmic retinochoriditis include floaters (from vitreous inflammatory debris) and blurring of vision (either from the direct effects of retinal infection, if it occurs in the macula, or from retinal edema). Patients may also develop painful, red eyes from the associated anterior segment inflammatory reaction. Recurrent toxoplasmic retinochoroiditis is not associated with systemic symptoms.

Associated findings and course of disease are considered in the following section in relation to specific patient populations.

Newborns with Congenital Disease. Retinochoroiditis is the most common manifestation of congenital toxoplasmosis, and it will be bilateral in up to 85% of patients.[40,76,183,233] Retinochoroidal lesions are self-limited and may already have healed at birth. In other patients retinal lesions may not develop for months or years after birth, despite well-documented congenital infection.[217]

In a study of 94 children with congenital toxoplasmosis (76 of whom were treated with pyrimethamine and sulfadizine for at least 1 year), Mets and associates[183] found chorioretinal scars in 79% of patients, and bilateral scars in 65%. Peripheral retinal scars were present in 64% of patients, whereas macular scars were present in 58%. Considering the much smaller area of the macula, these results suggest a definite predilection for macular lesions in patients with congenital toxoplasmosis. This predilection may be due to the fact that the posterior pole is vascularized earlier than other portions of the retina, or to the unique vasculature of the fetal macula, which contains end arterioles.

Mets and associates[183] found that 29% of patients with congenital toxoplasmosis had substantial bilateral vision loss (less than 20/40 best corrected vision in the better eye), despite the fact that the majority of their patients were treated throughout the first year of life.

Immunocompetent Patients. In 1969 Friedmann and Knox[88] described three clinical types of retinochoroidal lesions in otherwise healthy patients. *Large destructive lesions* accounted for 56% of their patients. They were generally larger than the area of the optic disc and were the lesions most likely to be associated with complications or decreased vision (Fig. 85-6). *Punctate inner lesions* (27% of their patients) were smaller and associated with less vitreous reaction. *Punctate deep lesions* (17% of their patients) were always located in the macula or peripapillary area and were associated with retinal edema and little or no vitreous inflammatory reaction, presumably because the infected tissue is separated from the vitreous body by uninvolved inner retinal layers (Fig. 85-11). Each lesion type could be associated with old chorioretinal scars. It may not be possible to categorize all cases of toxoplasmic retinochoroiditis into one of these disease types. Punctate inner lesions, for example, may

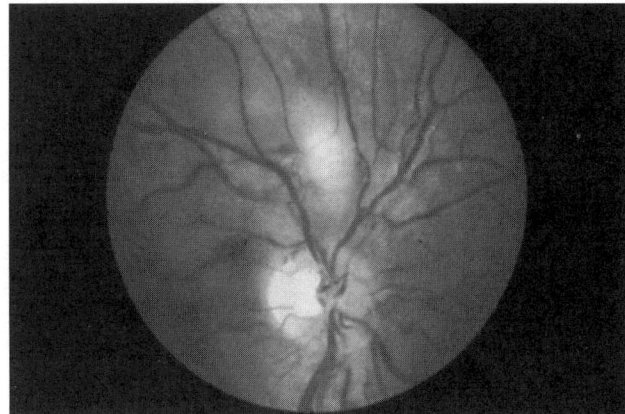

Fig. 85-11. A deep retinal focus of *Toxoplasma gondii* infection superior to the optic nerve head with scattered intraretinal hemorrhages. There is little vitreous humor inflammatory reaction. (Photograph courtesy of David L. Knox, MD, Baltimore, MD.)

simply be earlier or less severe infection than large destructive lesions.

Other investigators have also described *punctate outer retinal toxoplasmosis* as a distinct subset of patients[62,177] (Fig. 85-12). Disease consists of multifocal, gray-white lesions, less than 1000 μm in size, at the level of the deep retina and retinal pigment epithelium. There is little overlying vitreous humor inflammatory reaction. Involvement can be bilateral, and active lesions can recur. Doft and Gass[62] described three patients (two children and a teenager) with these findings, whose lesions resolved spontaneously with the formation of fine granular white dots or small chorioretinal scars. Matthews and Weiter[177] reported an additional five cases, ranging in age from 9 to 41 years. Treatment with antiparasitic agents appeared to be associated with resolution of disease. All of their patients

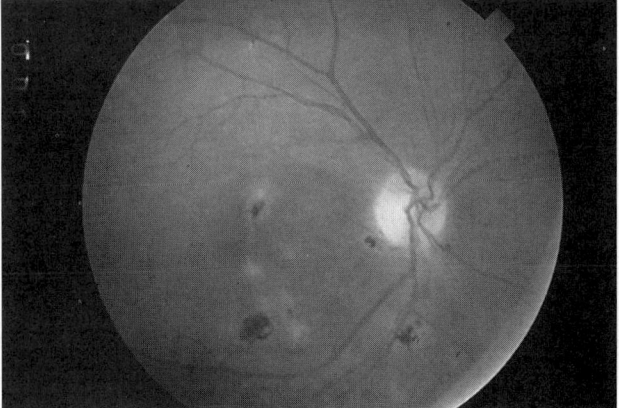

Fig. 85-12. Punctate outer retinal toxoplasmosis in the right eye of a 6-year-old boy. There are multiple, discrete, cream-colored, active lesions inferior to the fovea. Four pigmented scars indicate a history of previous disease. (Photograph courtesy of Fernando Oréfice, MD, Belo Horizonte, Minas Gerais, Brazil.) (Figure also in color insert.)

retained visual acuity of 20/25 or better in the involved eye.

Less commonly, immunocompetent patients can develop a more severe form of disease, characterized by extensive retinal necrosis and panuveitis.[100,114,115,217,222] Inflammation may gradually subside over 9 to 18 months, or the disease can lead to phthisis bulbi.

When *T. gondii* infection involves the optic disc or the retina immediately adjacent to the optic disc, it can result in a papillitis (Fig. 85-13). Such cases are sometimes referred to as Jensen juxtapapillary retinitis. Clinical diagnosis may be difficult, although the character of the lesion and course of disease are similar to toxoplasmic retinochoroiditis elsewhere in the fundus. Such patients may be left with sectoral or nerve fiber bundle visual field defects but can regain good

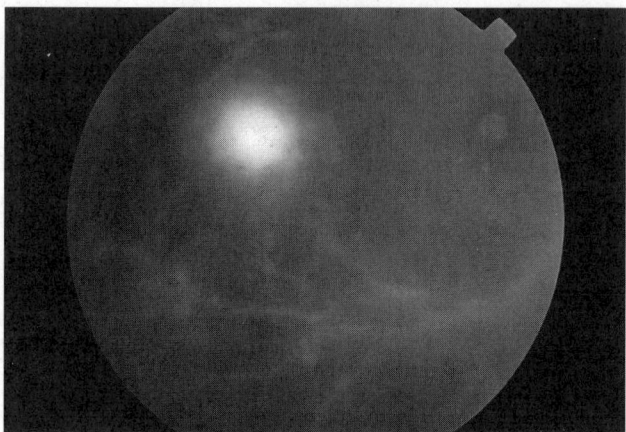

Fig. 85-14. Inflammatory vascular sheathing adjacent to a focus of active toxoplasmic retinochoroiditis. (Photograph courtesy of Cristina Muccioli, MD, Sao Paulo, Brazil.)

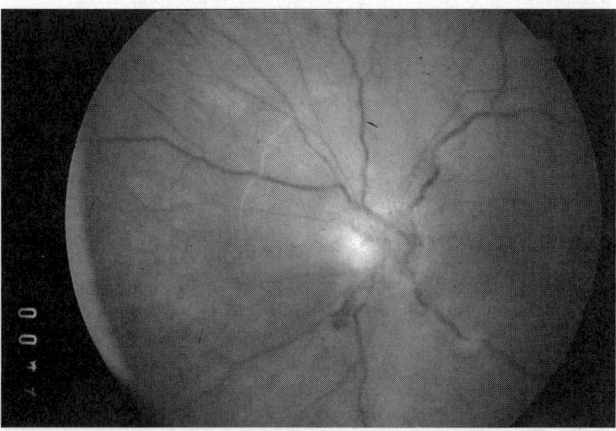

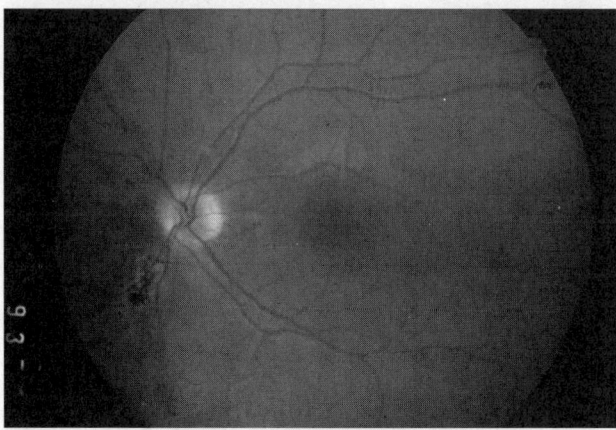

Fig. 85-13. **A,** Left eye of a patient with toxoplasmic papillitis and peripapillary serous retinal detachment. Central visual acuity is 20/60. **B,** The same fundus after treatment using oral antimicrobial agents and corticosteroids and resolution of the papillitis. Central visual acuity has returned to 20/20. The previous papillitis was caused by recurrence of active retinal disease at the border of the small retinochoroidal scar that can be seen inferonasal to the optic disc.

central visual activity after resolution of the inflammatory component of the disease. Patients with macular lesions may also get secondary optic disc swelling.[304]

Signs Associated with Active Disease. Patients with active toxoplasmic retinochoroiditis will occasionally develop inflammatory sheathing of retinal vessels (Fig. 85-14). Vasculitis may develop in response to reactions between circulating antibodies and local *T. gondii* antigens.[204,205,300] Venules are most commonly involved, although both venules and arterioles may be sheathed.[51,205] Affected vessels are usually near the focus of active infections but can also occur in remote areas of the fundus. Patients can develop periarteritis (consisting of diffuse or focal plaquelike, yellow deposits involving major branches of the arteriolar tree[258,308]) that is reminiscent of the changes described by Kyrieleis[154] in patients with presumed ocular tuberculosis. In general, vascular sheathing disappears rapidly with resolution of other inflammatory signs, although the plaquelike lesions in patients with Kyrieleis-type periarteritis may persist.[258]

Several authors have incorrectly cited a report by Jacobs and associates[129] as stating that perivasculitis occurs in 5% of patients with ocular toxoplasmosis. In fact, Jacobs and associates reported that among a group of patients with various forms of uveitis, 5% of those with serologic and skin test evidence of *T. gondii* infection had retinal periphlebitis as their sole form of uveitis. This study was performed before it was generally appreciated that seropositivity is very common in the general population and that necrotizing retinitis is probably the only manifestation of active *T. gondii* infection within the eye of immunocompetent patients. Although the true prevalence of vascular involvement in patients with ocular toxoplasmosis is not known, it is probably much greater than 5%.

Affected vessels are generally not occluded, although Reese and associates[229] described a patient with presumed ocular toxoplasmosis in which extensive retinal necrosis was at least partly attributed to an obliterative retinal vasculitis.

The sclera overlying a focus of toxoplasmic retinochoroiditis can develop a clinically apparent scleritis.[256] Parasites have not been found in scleral tissue of such patients, however.

Course of Disease. In most cases toxoplasmic retinochoroiditis is a self-limited disease. Untreated lesions generally begin to heal after 1 to 2 months, although the time course is variable, and in some cases active disease may persist for months.[114] Rothova and associates[239] found that the most reliable predictor of disease duration was size of lesions; larger lesions took longer to heal. Friedmann and Knox[88] reported that active inflammation can last from 1 week to 2 years. They reported a mean disease duration of 4.2 months, although the median disease duration was less than 3 months; 76 of 127 disease episodes (60%) in their patients lasted less than 3 months. Only 24 of 127 episodes (19%) lasted longer than 6 months. They felt that duration of disease was longer in older patients, but data from their study could not confirm that theory.

As a lesion heals, its borders become more discrete, and it becomes gray-white and less "fuzzy" in appearance as the inflammatory reaction clears. Over several months the borders of lesions may become hyperpigmented. It may also take weeks to months for all vitreous cells and haze to resolve. Large scars will have an atrophic center that is devoid of all retinal and choroidal elements; the underlying sclera gives the lesion its white center.

The frequency of recurrent inflammation attacks varies widely and cannot be predicted (Fig. 85-10). Canamucio and associates[30] found disease recurrence in 16% to 30% of patients treated for toxoplasmic retinochoroiditis. Recurrences developed at 1 week to 28 months after treatment, but the median follow-up period for the whole population was not stated. Rothova and associates[239] found that disease recurred in 49% of patients followed for 3 years. In immunocompetent patients, there will usually be only one recurrent focus of infection at any given episode, even if there are multiple scars in the fundus. Although recurrences usually arise from the borders of preexisting scars, they can also develop in areas remote from scars,[114,183] suggesting that encysted organisms can be present in normal-appearing retina.

Immunosuppressed Patients. Toxoplasmic retinochoroiditis is a serious disorder in HIV-infected patients* and in other immunosuppressed individuals such as cancer patients or organ transplant recipients.† It is generally more severe than in immunocompetent patients, with a broader range of clinical features.

Ocular toxoplasmosis in immunosuppressed patients can be a great diagnostic challenge to ophthalmologists who are

---

*References 20, 37, 70, 75, 90, 185, 221, 255.
†References 113, 116, 199, 214, 215, 272, 319.

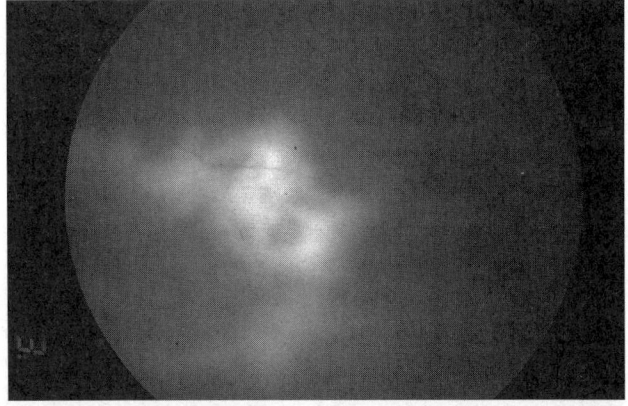

A

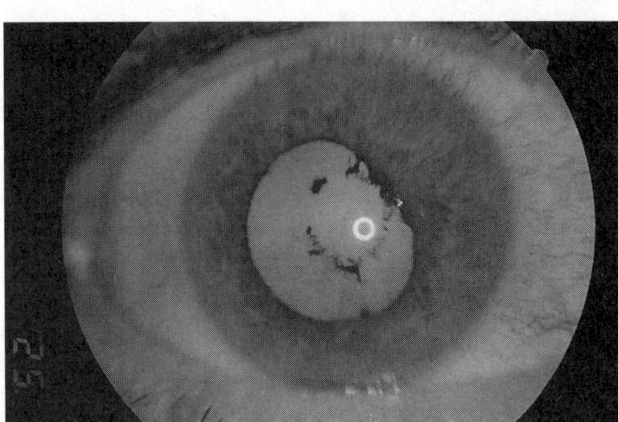

B

Fig. 85-15. **A,** Untreated toxoplasmic retinochoroiditis in the macula of a patient with AIDS. There is densely opaque retinal opacification, and the lesion has relatively sharp borders. There is a marked vitreous humor inflammatory reaction, which prevents a clear view of the fundus. This lesion responded to antimicrobial therapy. (Reprinted with permission from Elkins BS, Holland GN, Opremcak EM et al.: Ocular toxoplasmosis misdiagnosed as cytomegalovirus retinopathy in immunocompromised patients, *Ophthalmology* 101:499-507, 1994.) **B,** Anterior segment of the same eye following initiation of therapy, which included topical prednisolone acetate 1% and scopolamine 1/4%; posterior synechiae between the pupillary margin and anterior lens capsule remain in the superonasal quadrant. There is some residual vascular injection of the conjunctiva.

accustomed to its typical appearance, as described for immunocompetent individuals. In immunosuppressed patients, there can be single lesions, multifocal lesions in one or both eyes, and broad areas of retinal necrosis[116,117] (Figs. 85-15 to 85-19). Small, early lesions may appear to be restricted to the outer or inner retinal layers,[117] but in most reported cases there has been full-thickness retinal necrosis, with the lesions usually being at least several optic disc areas in size.

Although the majority of reported cases in HIV-infected patients have been unilateral,[37,106,117] it is not uncommon to see bilateral cases; 6 of 16 cases (37.5%) reported by Gag-

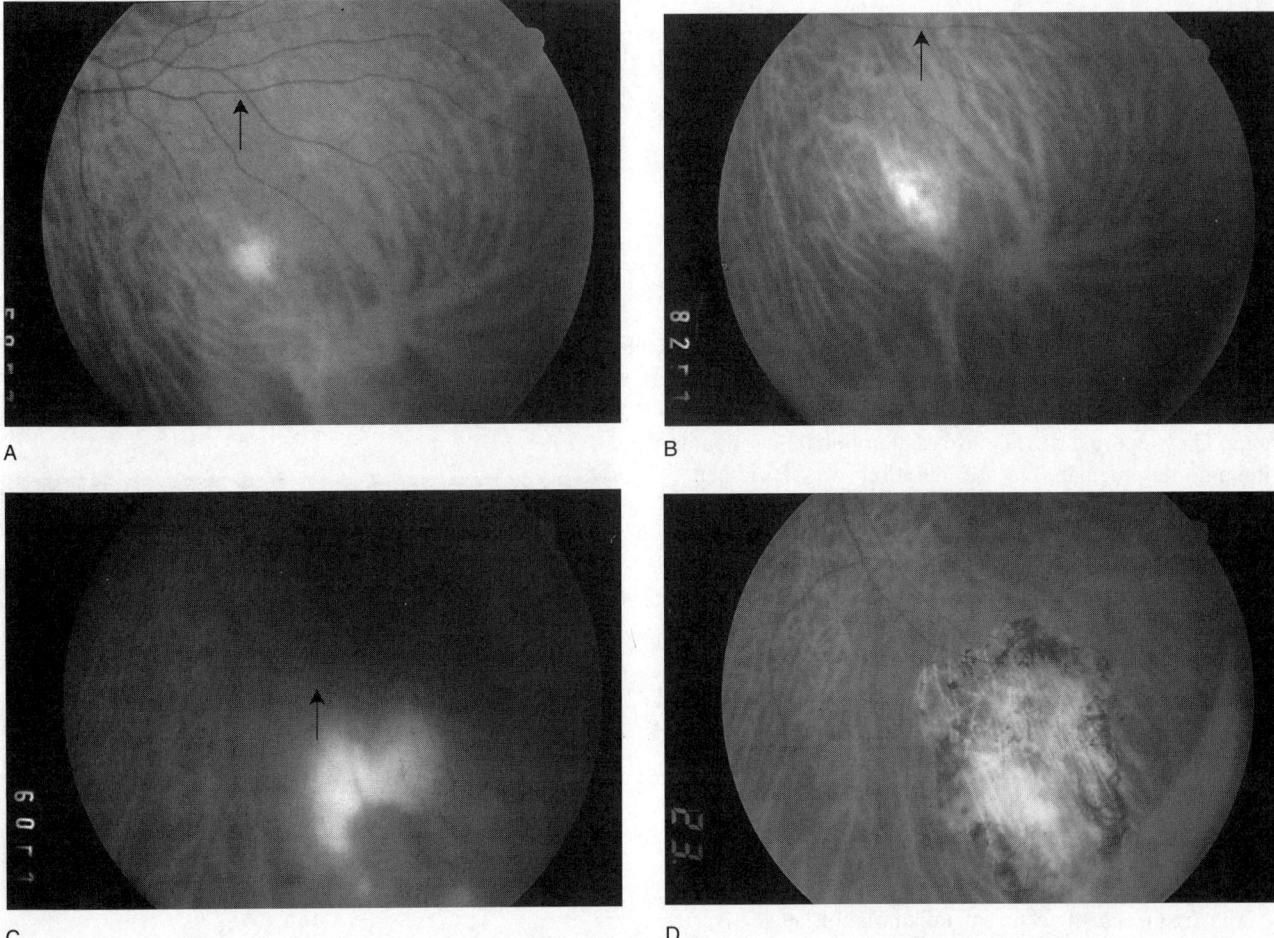

A

B

C

D

Fig. 85-16. **A,** A focus of presumed toxoplasmic retinochoroiditis in the inferotemporal quadrant of the left eye of a patient with AIDS. **B,** The same lesion photographed 1 month later. There has been enlargement of the lesion without antimicrobial therapy. **C,** The same lesion photographed 1 month after **B.** There has been posterior extension of the lesion without antimicrobial therapy. Treatment was begun with pyrimethamine and sulfadiazine at this point. For orientation, *arrows* indicate the same vascular crossing in each photograph. **D,** Four years later, the patient has an inactive retinochoroidal scar. He had been receiving chronic maintenance therapy consisting of oral sulfadiazine. (Fig. 85-16**A** and 85-16**C** reprinted with permission from Holland GN, Engstrom RE Jr, Glasgow BJ et al.: Ocular toxoplamosis in patients with the acquired immunodeficiency syndrome, *Am J Ophthalmol* 106:653-667, 1988. Copyright by The Ophthalmic Publishing Company.)

liuso and associates[90] and 8 of 45 patients (18%) reported by Cochereau-Massin and associates[37] were bilateral.

Although the ability to diagnose toxoplasmic retinochoroiditis in immunosuppressed patients on clinical grounds alone has been questioned,[49] there seem to be several reliable features of *T. gondii* infection that can distinguish toxoplasmic retinochoroiditis from other opportunistic infections.[70] In cases with full-thickness necrosis, the retina appears to have a hard, "indurated" appearance, with sharply demarcated borders. There is usually little retinal hemorrhage within the lesion itself. Even in immunosuppressed patients, there will be an overlying vitreous inflammatory reaction.

There can also be inflammatory vascular sheathing, although the latter sign is not helpful in differentiating ocular toxoplasmosis from other infections, such as CMV retinitis

or syphilitic retinitis. Gagliuso and associates[90] also reported exudative retinal detachments in 2 of their 16 HIV-infected patients with ocular toxoplasmosis.

A prominent inflammatory reaction in the vitreous body and anterior chamber has been described in several reports of HIV-associated ocular toxoplasmosis,[117] whereas other investigators report little associated vitritis or iridocyclitis.[24,90] The difference may be one of interpretation; whereas the degree of secondary inflammation may vary and may be less than might be seen in immunocompetent hosts, inflammatory reactions in the vitreous body exceed those that result from CMV retinitis in patients with AIDS, for example. Anterior segment inflammation in immunosuppressed patients may be so severe that it results in redness, pain, and posterior synechiae (Fig. 85-15).

Lesions will continue to enlarge without treatment, which

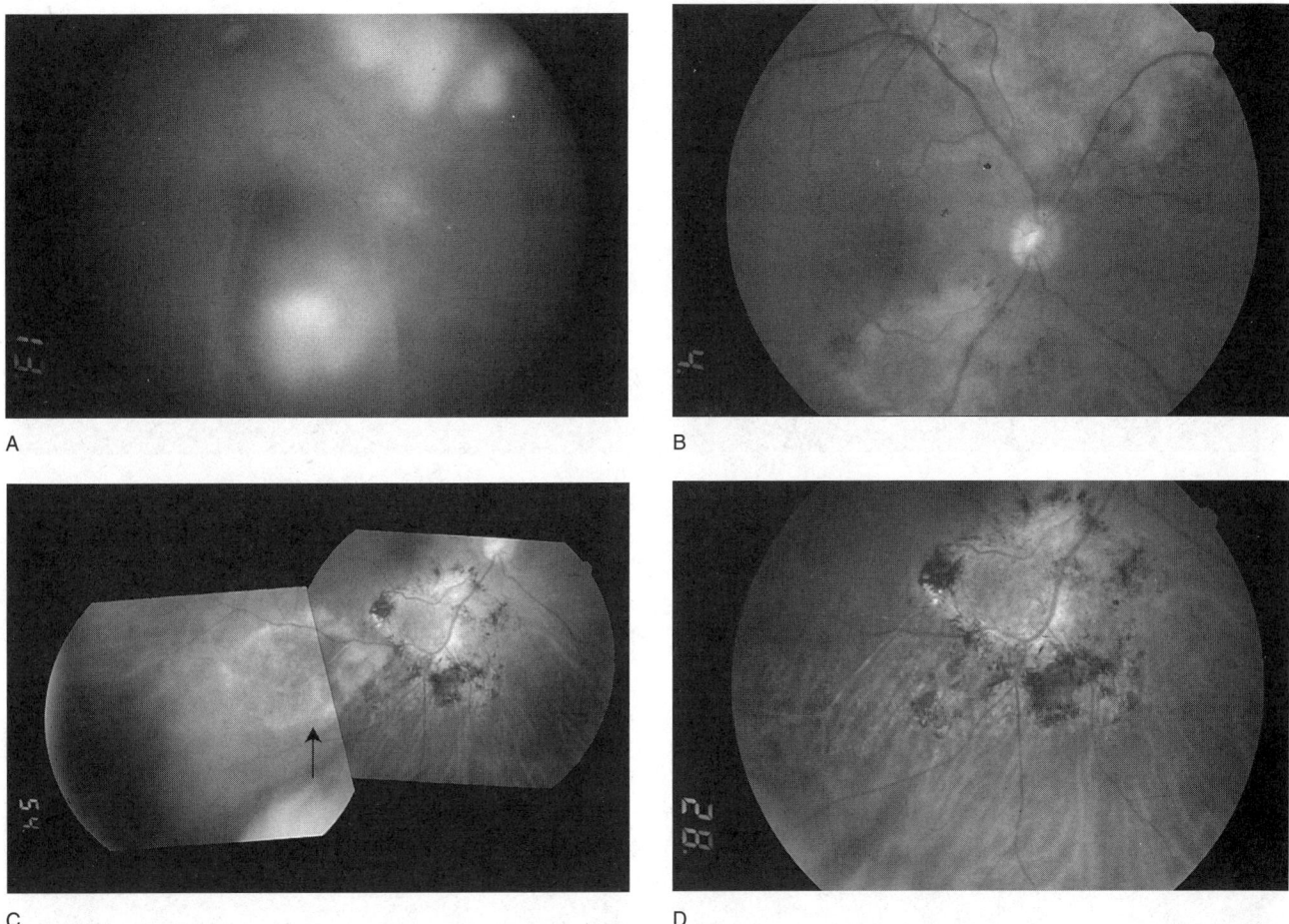

A

B

C

D

Fig. 85-17. **A,** Two peripapillary foci of untreated toxoplasmic retinochoroiditis in a patient with AIDS. There is a marked vitreous humor inflammatory reaction, which prevents a clear view of the fundus. **B,** The same fundus, 5 months later, after treatment with oral pyrimethamine (50 mg daily for 6 weeks). He continued to receive maintenance therapy with oral pyrimethamine (25 mg daily). **C,** Montage of fundus photographs of the same eye, taken 10 months later, shows a new focus of untreated cytomegalovirus (CMV) retinitis *(arrow)* adjacent to the inferotemporal border of the retinochoroidal scar shown in **B.** That scar is inactive and the borders have developed hyperpigmentation. **D,** After 2 months of intravenous ganciclovir therapy, the focus of CMV retinitis appears inactive. This series of photographs illustrates the differences between the active lesions, scars, and vitreous humor inflammatory reactions associated with toxoplasmic retinochoroiditis and CMV retinitis in patients with AIDS. (Reprinted with permission from Elkins BS, Holland GN, Opremcak EM et al.: Ocular toxoplasmosis misdiagnosed as cytomegalovirus retinopathy in immunocompromised patients, *Ophthalmology* 101:499-507, 1994.)

probably explains the fact that most reported patients have had extensive areas of retinal necrosis by the time diagnosis is made (Figs. 85-15 to 85-16). Spontaneous resolution of toxoplasmic retinochoroiditis in HIV-infected patients has not been reported. Progression is generally slow. Rarely, disease can progress to a severe panophthalmitis, and a secondary ''orbitis'' can occur, although *T. gondii* does not extend beyond the intraocular space.[185]

Berger and associates[20] described miliary retinitis as a rare manifestation of ocular toxoplasmosis in a patient with AIDS. Their patient had numerous oval-to-round retinal inflammatory lesions in the posterior pole. They were initially 100 to 500 microns in diameter and slowly enlarged. Lesions did not respond to antiparasitic therapy; diagnosis was made at autopsy.

In most reported cases of ocular toxoplasmosis in immu-nosuppressed patients, there have not been pre-existing scars; none of the 8 cases reported by Holland and associates and only 1 of the 16 cases reported by Gagliuso and associates had such a scar, which suggests the majority of cases are not caused by reactivation of encysted organisms that have persisted in retina from a previously active infection. Instead, ocular disease in immunosuppressed patients may be more commonly caused by newly acquired infection or organisms newly disseminated to the eye from other sites of active disease. Although recurrent toxoplasmosis is a well-known phenomenon in immunosuppressed patients, the number of tissue cysts in nonocular tissue will be much greater than the number in the retina; therefore, the frequency with which organisms disseminate to the eye from nonocular sites of reactivation might be greater than reactivation in the eye itself.

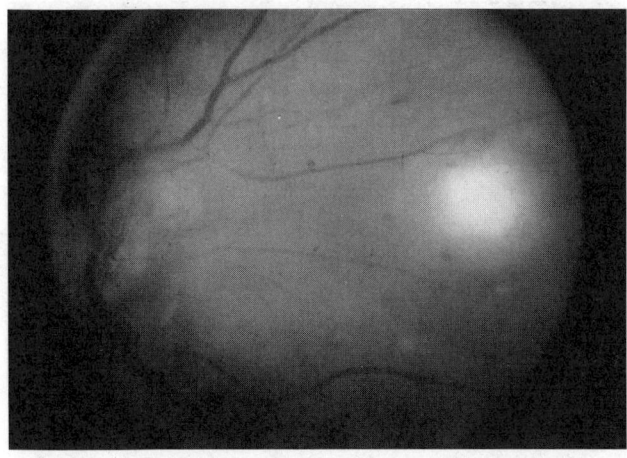

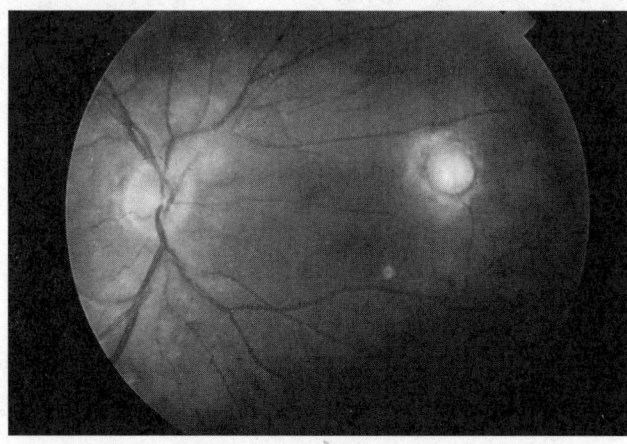

A   B

Fig. 85-18. **A,** The nasal fundus of the right eye of a patient with AIDS and multifocal toxoplasmic retinochoroiditis. There is a prominent lesion in the midperiphery and a less-opaque lesion immediately adjacent to the optic disc. **B,** After 4 months of spiramycin therapy, there has been resolution of active disease with scar formation. (Photographs courtesy of Brian B. Berger, MD, Austin, TX. Reprinted with permission of Holland GN, Engstrom RE Jr, Glasgow BJ et al.: Ocular toxoplamosis in patients with the acquired immunodeficiency syndrome, *Am J Ophthalmol* 106:653-667, 1988. Copyright by The Ophthalmic Publishing Company.)

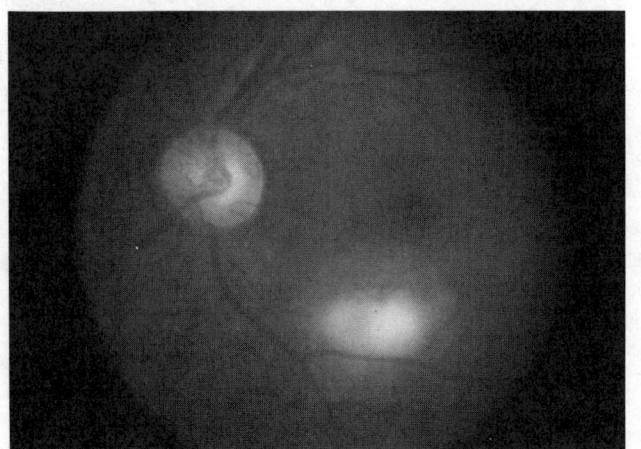

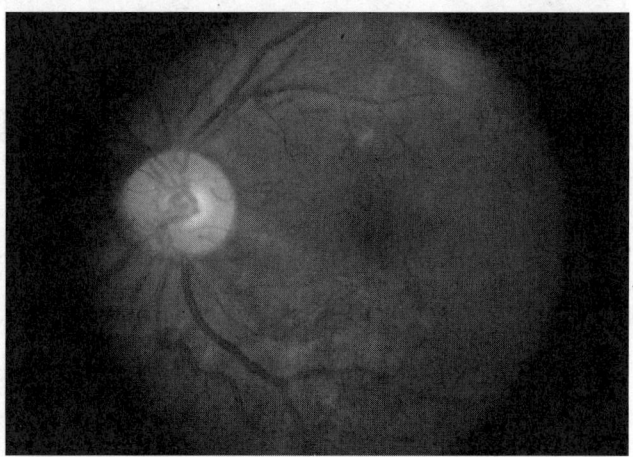

A   B

Fig. 85-19. **A,** A focus of toxoplasmic retinochoroiditis in the inferior macula of the left eye of a patient with AIDS. **B,** Following 2 months of therapy with oral pyrimethamine and sulfadiazine, the lesion has become inactive. Despite retinal damage, the patient did not develop a typical retinochoroidal scar, and blood vessels in the area of infection remain intact. **C,** Late-phase fluorescein angiogram of the same eye highlights the retinal scar, which is characterized by window defects and staining. (Photographs courtesy of Tina M. Chou, MD and James M. Weisz, MD, Los Angeles, CA.)

C

Central nervous system involvement is seen in 29% to 50% of HIV-infected patients with ocular toxoplasmosis.[37,90] Ocular disease may be recognized before any neurologic manifestations of intracranial infection, however.[90,117]

Other Ophthalmic Disorders. Microphthalmos and microcornea are uncommon manifestations of congenital toxoplasmosis.[56,73,74] Nystagmus and strabismus are other manifestations of congenital toxoplasmosis that can either be due to cranial nerve palsies from intracranial disease[220] or to sensory deprivation from extensive retinal infection. Ocular motility disturbances can also occur in adults with acquired infection and toxoplasmic encephalitis.[108,307] Papillitis, papilledema, and optic atrophy are other possible manifestations of toxoplasmic encephalitis.[183,217]

In 1957 Pillat and Thalhammer[222] attributed severe granulomatous iridocyclitis to T. gondii infection of the anterior segment, on the basis of parasite isolation after enucleation of the eye. Other authors[205,217] have questioned their conclusion; Perkins suggested the patient actually had panuveitis, with the iridocyclitis secondary to retinal infection.[217] Other investigators have stated that T. gondii may cause an anterior uveitis on the basis of antibodies found in aqueous humor;[51] nevertheless, it is generally believed that isolated iridocyclitis never occurs as a manifestation of ocular toxoplasmosis in immunocompetent patients. Occasionally, however, patients who have extensive, old, and apparently inactive toxoplasmic retinochoroiditis scars have been found to develop recurrent, transient anterior uveitis and vitritis,[88] possibly on the basis of a reaction to exposed antigens in the retina, but without apparent reactivation and proliferation of parasites.

Infection of the iris with T. gondii has been reported in a patient with AIDS.[230] Iris details could not be seen on clinical exam because of a severe inflammatory reaction, but diagnosis was made histologically at autopsy. In another HIV-infected patient, T. gondii infection of the iris was suspected when iris stromal nodules resolved during medical therapy for toxoplasmic retinochoroiditis.[117]

In the 1960s a variety of intraocular inflammatory disorders, including Coats disease and "geographic choroiditis," were suspected to be caused by T. gondii infection. In his review of reported cases, however, Perkins[217] found little evidence to support such claims. In 1965 Frezzotti and associates[87] isolated T. gondii from an enucleated eye of a patient reported to have uveitis "typical" of Coats disease. A clinical description of the patient's recurrent fundus lesions was not provided in their report, but it is likely that the patient had a severe exudative form of toxoplasmic retinochoroiditis, as described previously. Other cases of Coats disease attributed to T. gondii infection were based on serologic studies only.

Conjunctivitis has been reported in patients with symptomatic, systemic T. gondii infections, although its pathogenesis and relationship to infection has not been well established.[284]

Patients with evidence of recently acquired T. gondii infection, but without evidence of focal intraocular infection, may develop transient retinal vasculitis, vitreous inflammatory reactions, and anterior uveitis.* These findings are reminiscent of those produced in nonhuman primates inoculated with toxoplasmic antigens (see Pathogenesis section) and may therefore represent a noninfectious, immunologic response to disseminated parasites in acquired, systemic T. gondii infections. In 1956 Jacobs and associates[129] reported an infrequent association between serologic and skin test evidence of T. gondii infections and retinal periphlebitis but a causal relationship was not confirmed.[129]

Hausmann and Richard[109] described a patient with serologic evidence of acquired T. gondii infection who developed papillophlebitis, retinal hemorrhages, and subretinal spots in the macula. Fluorescein angiography showed isolated choroidal vascular occlusions. Fundus lesions resolved and decreased vision improved with antimicrobial therapy. Toxoplasma gondii was not histopathologically confirmed to be the cause of the lesions.

Neuroretinitis. There have been several reports of neuroretinitis attributed to T. gondii, in which there was no evidence of active retinal or optic nerve infection.[79,186,237] Cases were characterized by optic nerve edema, papillomacular retinal detachment, splinter hemorrhages, and hard exudates in the macula distributed in a "star" pattern; these findings resemble Leber stellate neuroretinitis, a disease of unknown cause. Patients also have anterior chamber and vitreous body inflammatory cells. Diagnosis was based on evidence of anti-T. gondii antibodies and response to antiparasitic drug therapy. These factors cannot confirm the diagnosis, however, as idiopathic neuroretinitis is a self-limited disease with good visual outcome. Among reported patients with presumed toxoplasmic neuroretinitis, most regained visual acuity of 20/25 or better, although a few had residual optic atrophy and visual field defects.

PATHOLOGY

Toxoplasma gondii is found most commonly in muscle, the heart, and the brain. Active T. gondii infections can stimulate a marked inflammatory response. Macrophages and lymphocytes are the predominant cell type, although plasma cells are frequently seen. Inflammation can be granulomatous or nongranulomatous in nature. Tissue cysts, however, elicit little inflammatory reaction.[68,143,182]

Tissue cysts can form early during a tissue infection; therefore their presence should not be interpreted to mean that the patient has a chronic infection with recurrence of active disease.[241,242]

---

*GN Holland, MD, GR O'Connor, MD, JM Weisz, MD, unpublished data.

Ocular Disease

Ocular toxoplasmosis in immunocompetent patients is characterized histopathologically by foci of coagulative necrosis of the retina with sharply demarcated borders.[227,323] Inflammatory changes, however, can be widespread in the eye, involving the choroid, iris, and trabecular meshwork. Chronic inflammatory cells can also occur in retina remote from the site of infection. Coagulative necrosis of the choroid and adjacent sclera can be seen, although parasites are not found in tissues other than the retina in immunocompetent patients.[323] In a patient with chronic, severe toxoplasmic retinochoroiditis, Rao and Font[227] found a combination of tachyzoites and tissue cysts in affected retina, but the majority of tissue cysts were nonviable and necrotic. They could not identify host elements in the tissue cyst walls.

After resolution of active infection, scarring is characterized by gliosis, obliteration of vessels, and hyperpigmentation at the borders. Calcification can develop.[115]

Tissue cysts can exist in the retina with little disruption of the retinal architecture,[182,199] which helps to explain why recurrences can develop in locations remote from retinochoroidal scars.

Similar histopathologic features have been reported from animal studies of ocular toxoplasmosis. In both mice and rabbits with ocular toxoplasmosis, parasites are most commonly found at the inner retina, in the ganglion cell layer.[182,321] Infection does not spread to tissues other than the retina, although the choroid can become severely inflamed.[182,321] Glial cells are believed to be the most common host cell type for *T. gondii* infections. McMenamin and associates[182] were able to identify probable Muller cell elements in tissue cyst walls in a murine model.

Dutton and associates[68] found that the character of the inflammatory response varied with the severity and duration of disease. An early, low-grade inflammatory response was composed predominantly of macrophages and lymphocytes. As the severity of disease increased, greater numbers of these cells were present, and plasma cells were identified. With severe degrees of inflammation, vasculitis was present. Dutton and associates[68] hypothesized that inflammatory cells contributed to the damage that occurs to outer retinal elements.

Immunosuppressed Individuals. Histopathologic examination of eyes from immunosuppressed patients and toxoplasmic retinochoroiditis reveals both tachyzoites and tissue cysts in areas of retinal necrosis and within retinal pigment epithelial cells[117,199] (Fig. 85-20). The inner retina appears to be the primary site of infection. Holland and associates[117] found the greatest number of parasites to be located in the nerve fiber and ganglion cell layers, frequently adjacent to blood vessels. Fewer organisms were found in outer retinal layers, and they were rare in the photoreceptor layer. Nicholson and associates[199] found *T. gondii* infection to be focused in the inner retina of a patient receiving chronic

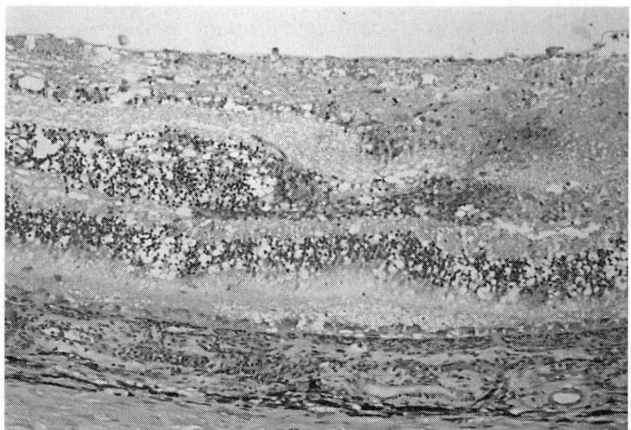

Fig. 85-20. Full thickness retinal necrosis in a patient with AIDS and ocular toxoplasmosis. Numerous tachyzoites were seen in the retina, but there is little inflammatory cell infiltration of the retina. (Hematoxylin and eosin, original magnification × 40.) (Light micrograph courtesy of Ben J. Glasgow, MD, Los Angeles, CA.)

high-dose corticosteroid therapy; in many areas, the outer retina was relatively well preserved. Both necrosis and parasites were located in a paravascular distribution, in proximity to both arterioles and venules.

In immunosuppressed patients, including those with AIDS, parasites can occasionally be found in the choroid and vitreous, and the optic nerve may be infected.[90,106,117,319]

A prominent choroidal inflammatory reaction may be present in immunosuppressed patients with toxoplasmic retinochoroiditis, but there is usually scant inflammatory material in the necrotic retina.[90,117,199]

Based on a review of published cases, the features that appear to distinguish ocular toxoplasmosis in immunosuppressed patients from disease in immunocompetent individuals include a greater number of organisms in retinal lesions, occasional spread of organisms to uveal tissue, and scant inflammatory cells in necrotic retina. A paravascular distribution of organisms appears to be a frequent feature of disease in immunosuppressed patients.

COMPLICATIONS

Toxoplasmic retinochoroiditis can result in permanent, dense scotomata because of retinal necrosis. Central vision will be lost if lesions affect the fovea, maculopapillary bundle, or optic disc. Involvement of the optic disc or the peripapillary retina can also result in optic atrophy. Other reported complications include macular edema and the sequelae of anterior segment inflammation (secondary glaucoma, posterior synechiae, secondary cataracts). Schlaegel and Weber[252] reported mild macular edema in 7 of 60 patients (12%) with ocular toxoplasmosis, but severe cystoid macular edema occurred only rarely.

Vascular complications include subretinal neovascularization[39,78,252,273,304] (Fig. 85-21), retinochoroidal vascular

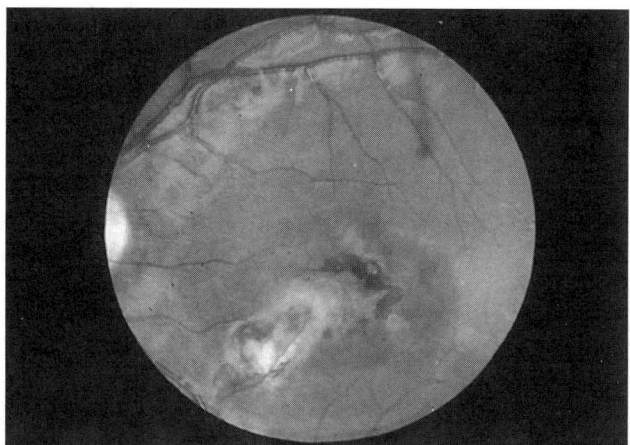

Fig. 85-21. Elevated, parafoveal gray scar with subretinal hemorrhage and serous retinal detachment in a patient with inactive congenital toxoplasmic retinochoroiditis. Fluorescein angiography confirmed the presence of a subretinal neovascular membrane.

anastamoses,[61,146] and obstruction of branch arterioles or venules that pass through areas of infection.[25,92,304] Neovascularization of the retina and the optic disc can occur, resulting in vitreous hemorrhage.[92,99] Subretinal neovascular membranes may be a cause of sudden loss of vision.[78]

Silveira and associates[271] have described pigmentary retinopathy as a complication of recurrent toxoplasmic retinochoroiditis. A group of seven patients (who had had bilateral ocular toxoplasmosis for many years) developed unilateral, sectorial or extensive, diffuse spicular pigmentation of the peripheral retina, resembling retinitis pigmentosa. Electroretinograms could not be recorded from involved eyes, and visual fields were constricted. The pathogenesis of this complication is unknown.

Rhegmatogenous and tractional retinal detachments may occur. Rhegmatogenous retinal detachment is more common in immunosuppressed patients because they are likely to have extensive areas of retinal necrosis in which retinal holes may develop.[117,268]

Serous detachment of the macula is an uncommon finding in patients with posterior segment lesions,[153] and these detachments resolve with medical therapy.

Fuchs Uveitis Syndrome

It has been hypothesized that ocular toxoplasmosis is a cause of Fuchs uveitis syndrome. De Abreu and associates[50] reported that 13 of 23 Brazilian patients (56.5%) with Fuchs uveitis syndrome had anti-*T. gondii* antibodies and retinal lesions consistent with healed toxoplasmic retinochoroiditis. Subsequent investigators have also identified similar scars in 64% to 65% of patients with Fuchs uveitis syndrome in France and West Virginia, USA.[250,257] Development of Fuchs uveitis syndrome has also been documented in a patient with confirmed congenital toxoplasmosis.[155] The rea-

son for this association is not known, but it has been suggested that Fuchs uveitis syndrome may be an autoimmune response to retinal damage from *T. gondii* infection. La Hey and associates[156] confirmed that toxoplasmosis-like scars were more frequent in patients with Fuchs uveitis syndrome than in those with other forms of chronic anterior uveitis, but emphasized that other types of chorioretinal scars were also seen. These investigators could not find an association between Fuchs uveitis syndrome and *T. gondii* infection using serologic testing, immunologic testing, and determination of intraocular antibody production, when an entire population of patients with Fuchs uveitis syndrome was studied. They concluded that *T. gondii* infection was not the sole cause of Fuchs uveitis syndrome, but they could not rule out the possibility that the syndrome might have multiple causes, one of which is ocular toxoplasmosis. A more detailed discussion of this problem is found in Chapter 41.

PATHOGENESIS

T. gondii can reach the eye through the bloodstream as free tachyzoites, but more commonly it is carried in circulating leukocytes, which may be arrested temporarily in terminal capillary loops of the retina. Parasites are then released from the leukocytes following intracellular reproduction and bursting of the cell. Parasitemia is identified commonly in patients with AIDS.[297]

Parasites can be found in the optic nerves of some patients,[117,174] and it has been suggested that *T. gondii* can reach the retina via the optic nerve from intracranial sites of infection.[19] Such transmission would explain the frequent parapapillary location of lesions. Nevertheless, transmission via the optic nerve is not believed to occur in most patients.

Penetration of Host Cells

The fact that *T. gondii* can invade virtually all cells (in contrast to most other intracellular parasites) indicates that the receptors mediating initial attachment are ubiquitous, or that a variety of different receptors can be utilized. Laminin receptors have been implicated; in vitro studies have shown that laminin bound to the surface of tachyzoites attaches to receptors in several cell types, and a variety of laminin receptors have been identified.[89] The major surface protein of *T. gondii*, P30 (SAG-1), also appears to be an important parasite ligand that binds to the host cell in the process of *T. gondii* invasion.[184]

Penetration of host cells is an active process[4,134,198] (Fig. 85-2). After the conoid of the tachyzoite makes contact with the plasmalemma of the host cell membrane, specialized organelles at the anterior end of the parasite (termed rhoptries) protrude through the extended conoid and fuse with the limiting membrane of the parasite.[197] The contents of the rhoptries are then discharged through this membrane. Rhoptries appear to be the source of *penetration enhancing factor*, which alters the host cell membrane.[259] Electron microscopic studies have shown that discontinuities form in the plasmalemma of the host cell prior to penetration,[198] although there has been some controversy as to whether disruption of the plasmalemma occurs during the entry process.[4,138,150]

Once enveloped within the cytoplasm of the host cell, the organism is surrounded by a parasitophorous vacuole that allows *T. gondii* to resist microbicidal activity and normal digestion.[137,267,306] The vacuole forms by invagination of the host cell plasma membrane, which becomes disrupted at the point of entry.[4] Studies by Nichols and associates[197] indicate that a portion of the host cell membrane is incorporated into the vacuole at the time of cell penetration. In macrophages *T. gondii* modifies the vacuole by secretion of membranous vesicles and formation of a reticulate network.[265] This intraphagosomal membrane (IPM) network is composed of major *T. gondii* surface proteins and develops within minutes of entry into the cell.[265] As a part of this process, specialized tubules that are end products of rhoptry secretion can be seen extending to the vacuolar membrane.[197] The IPM network helps to resist normal endocytic processing and digestion of live organisms. The IPM network is also formed during infection of other cell types.[265]

Active entry of tachyzoites into macrophages fails to trigger an oxidative burst with production of toxic oxygen intermediates[266,306] and phagosome acidification.[267] The presence of parasitic components probably contributes to the fact that lysosomes do not fuse with the parasitic vacuole, as they do with other phagosomes.[137] If extracellular tachyzoites are coated with antibody, they can be taken up by host cells through phagocytosis, with entry into the host mediated by Fc receptors. The formation of an IPM network does not occur when killed or antibody-coated parasites are engulfed by macrophages.[137,198] After formation of the phagosome, fusion with lysosomes can occur, and destruction of the parasite ensues.[135] Inhibition by live *T. gondii* of arachidonic acid metabolism within monocyte-derived macrophages may be an important mechanism that prevents phagocytosis of parasites by these cells, as discussed in the next section.[320]

Tissue Cyst Formation

The reason for tissue cyst formation is not understood, but the process may depend on immune mechanisms and/or nutritional and metabolic factors in the host environment. Basic pH and nitric oxide stimulate tissue cyst formation in vitro.[23] Soete and associates[275] found that increased temperature and increased pH induced the expression of bradyzoite-specific antigens and the induction of tissue cysts in vitro, whereas interferon-γ (IFN-γ) did not. These observations suggest that environmental factors can stimulate the formation of tissue cysts without the direct effect of immune defenses. Other studies have shown a role for IFN-γ in tissue cyst formation,[22,136] but its action may be indirect.[275] The presence of IFN-γ appears to slow division of tachyzoites

and prevent the disruption of host cells, thereby allowing formation of intracellular tissue cysts.[136] Another study of stage conversion between tachyzoites and bradyzoites showed that activation of infected, bone marrow-derived murine macrophages by IFN-γ induces expression of bradyzoite-specific antigens. This change appears to be mediated by a direct effect of nitric oxide produced by the macrophages.* It has been hypothesized that humoral immune factors may play a role in the encystment process, as the presence of complement and specific antibody against *T. gondii* in the environment of cultured cells infected with the parasite will also stimulate the formation of tissue cysts in vitro.[262]

Virulence

The severity of toxoplasmosis is dependent on several factors: the size of the parasite inoculum, the strain of *T. gondii,* and the immune status of the host. *T. gondii* isolates vary in many respects: their pathogenicity for mice, their antigenic structure, the immune response they stimulate in animal models, and their behavior in cultures. In an analysis of 28 strains isolated from different host species and from various parts of the world, Sibley and Boothroyd[264] found that virulent strains in mice have an identical genotype, indicating that virulent strains comprise a single clonal lineage. In contrast, nonvirulent strains were polymorphic. The reason for the persistence of this clonality, despite the possibility of a sexual phase that will lead to genetic diversity, is not known. Darde and associates[46a] were able to place 35 isolates into 5 distinct groups based on differences in 6 parasite enzyme systems. The pathogenicity for mice was different for each group. Such differences suggest that strains may also vary in their virulence for human beings.

Different strains of mice appear to have different susceptibility to toxoplasmic encephalitis,[289] suggesting that genetic differences in the host, as well as the parasite, may play a role in severity of disease. This susceptibility to severe disease in mice cannot be attributed to a lack of measurable CD4+ T-lymphocytes, CD8+ T-lymphocytes, tumor necrosis factor-α (TNF-α), IFN-γ, or interleukin-2 (IL-2).[120]

Immune Response

A good deal is known about the immune response to *T. gondii,* owing in part to the availability of animal models of disease. Much of the information about immunologic reactions has been derived from the study of the immune response to *T. gondii* infection in mice.

Parasitic Antigens. Tachyzoites have four major surface membrane proteins with molecular weights of 43, 35, 30,

---

*Uwe Gross and Wolfgang Bohne, unpublished data, presented at the 47th annual meeting of the Society of Protozoologists, Cleveland, Ohio, USA, June 1994

and 22 kiloDaltons (kD); the major surface antigen is p30,[249] although mutant strains devoid of p30 have been described.[139] Immunization with p30 induces CD8+ T-lymphocytes that are cytotoxic for infected macrophages.[148] Both p30 and p22 stimulate antibody production in humans, leading to antibody-dependent complement-mediated lysis of tachyzoites.[140,141] Neither p30 nor p22 is expressed by bradyzoites or sporozoites.

In a study of 40 patients with ocular toxoplasmosis, Nussenblatt and associates[203] found that in vitro lymphocyte proliferative responses were much greater to purified p22 antigen than to p30 antigen, which is generally considered the immunodominant protein. They hypothesized that individuals genetically restricted in their immune response to the p22 antigen (rather than the p30 antigen) might be prone to ocular disease.

Tachyzoites also excrete and secrete antigens (ESA) that elicit both antibody and T-lymphocyte-mediated immune responses.[45,66] Monoclonal antibodies against p30 also inhibit penetration of tachyzoites into host cells.[105]

A variety of other T. gondii proteins are under investigation, some of which appear to induce protective immunity.

Cell-Mediated Immunity. Cell-mediated immunity is the host's major defense against T. gondii infections.[313] A variety of effector cells work together to protect the host against T. gondii; they include T-lymphocytes, macrophages, natural killer (NK) cells, and lymphokine-activated killer (LAK) cells. Within hours after tachyzoites invade tissue in a previously uninfected individual, macrophages can be seen in the tissue, where they become activated by cytokines to kill the parasite. Soon thereafter, lymphocytes, NK cells, monocytes, neutrophils, and eosinophils also enter the areas of infection.

Oral ingestion of T. gondii induces an early T-lymphocyte response in mesenteric lymph nodes.[34] There is a correlation between the strength of this response and survival in murine models of disease.

Resistance to T. gondii depends on both CD4+ and CD8+ T-lymphocytes, but CD8+ T-lymphocytes appear to be the major mediators of protection in some studies.* In mice with toxoplasmic encephalitis, CD8+ T-lymphocytes are the predominant lymphocyte type in the CNS.[120] CD8+ T-lymphocytes act through production of IFN-γ (which activates macrophages) and/or through lysis of cells infected with the parasite.[107,148,286] Toxoplasma gondii infected cell-specific CD8+ cytotoxic T-lymphocytes have been identified in blood from patients with acute toxoplasmosis.[317] CD4+ T-lymphocytes play a regulatory role in both cellular and humoral immune response, and the presence of CD4+ T-lymphocytes is important for adequate response to treatment.[11]

---

*References 10a, 11, 97, 107, 142, 213, 291.

Fusion of T. gondii and host membranes followed by cytoplasmic localization of the parasite appears necessary for MHC class I-restricted antigen presentation for cytotoxic T-lymphocyte reactions.[318] Exogenous antigens can apparently be transferred into this MHC class I-restricted antigen presentation pathway by specialized antigen-presenting cells[278]; bone marrow-derived macrophages appear to be one such cell in murine models of disease.[53]

Resistance to T. gondii is dependent on cytokine-activated macrophages, which act through several effector mechanisms.[9,235,266] Macrophages produce oxygen intermediates that kill T. gondii.[187,194] Oxygen-independent mechanisms include degradation of intracellular tryptophan by expression of indoleamine 2,3-dioxygenase,[190] and production of toxic nitrogen intermediates from L-arginine, by expression of nitric oxide sythetase.[3,94] Although the production of reactive nitrogen intermediates appears to be the major nonoxidative mechanism of intracellular killing of T. gondii by mouse macrophages, its equivalent in humans has not been discovered, as human macrophages have not been shown to produce toxic nitrogen metabolites.

Metabolic products of arachidonic acid via the 5-lipoxygenase pathway (e.g. leukotriene B4, leukotriene C4) also appear to play an important role in killing of T. gondii by phagocytic cells. Nonactivated monocyte-derived macrophages are not cytotoxic to T. gondii. This fact may be explained by the observation that live, but not killed, T. gondii inhibits release of these products by macrophages in vitro. This inhibition is reversed, however, by treating cells with INF-γ.

It has been proposed that microglia, which have phagocytic function and can produce cytokines, may serve the role of macrophages in the CNS.[94] Such a role for cells in the retina has not been studied specifically, however.

Heat shock proteins, which are polypeptides produced by many cell types in response to stress, may play a role in the development of protective immunity against T. gondii. They are expressed in mice infected with strains of T. gondii of low virulence, but not in mice infected with strains of high virulence.[191] Heat shock proteins are recognized by γδ T-lymphocytes, a lymphocyte subset believed to play a role in early immune reactions against infectious agents. Elevated proportions of γδ T-lymphocytes have been found in peripheral blood of patients with acquired toxoplasmosis.[52,251]

Cytokines. Cytokines, particularly IFN-γ and TNF-α, play a critical role in resistance to T. gondii,[18,33,122,288,290] and the kinetics of cytokine production appear to be important in determining the severity of murine toxoplasmosis in different strains of mice.[86] The actions of various cytokines in T. gondii infection have been reviewed by Beamen, Wong, and Remington.[17,18]

Interferon-γ induces macrophage activation.[288,290,292] Interferon-γ is stimulated by P30,[147] and CD4+ T-lymphocytes appear to be its major source. Interferon-γ is also produced by CD8+ T-lymphocytes[95] and NK cells, however.[261] It has also been suggested that IFN-γ may be produced by glial cells,[122] but Hunter and associates[120] suggest that infiltrating cells in the brain are the major source of IFN-γ during toxoplasmic encephalitis.

IFN-γ has been detected in the serum of congenitally infected newborns and of recently infected pregnant women.[228] Among HIV-infected individuals, there is a decreased ability to produce IFN-γ, which is related to the development of opportunistic infections.[188,189]

Tumor necrosis factor-α appears necessary for IFN-γ to activate macrophages to kill T. gondii, and therefore has a modulating role in the immune response against T. gondii.[33,158,159,263] Administration of antibodies against TNF-α causes increased severity of toxoplasmic encephalitis in mice[94] as well as the death of mice infected with an otherwise avirulent strain of T. gondii.[133]

Interleukin-2 appears to be an important mediator of resistance against T. gondii. Administration of IL-2 offers protection to normally susceptible mice.[260] When incubated with peripheral blood, IL-2 induces LAK cells that are cytotoxic to target cells infected with T. gondii, as described in the next section.[260] It does not, however, act through increased macrophage killing of T. gondii.

Interleukin-10 downregulates T. gondii-stimulated IFN-γ production by T-lymphocytes and NK cells and prevents IFN-γ from activating macrophages against T. gondii.[96] Interleukin-6 appears to impair microbicidal activity of macrophages against T. gondii and decreases the ability of IFN-γ to activate macrophages.[16,287]

Other Cellular Defenses. T. gondii may be taken up by phagocytosis and killed by monocytes and neutrophils.

Lymphokine-activated killer cells are cytotoxic for target cells infected with T. gondii.[44,285] They can be induced by IL-2, even in peripheral blood lymphocytes from donors without serologic evidence of T. gondii infection.[285] The induced cells can be either NK or T-lymphocyte phenotypes.

An early defense against T. gondii involves the interaction of macrophages and NK cells. This interaction is an IFN-γ-dependent, but T-lymphocyte-independent, mechanism of immunity. Live or dead T. gondii or T. gondii antigens stimulate macrophages to produce TNF-α and IL-12. These two cytokines act in concert on NK cells to produce IFN-γ, which can then activate macrophages to kill T. gondii. These events occur prior to conventional cellular immunity.[121]

Humoral Immunity. Infection with T. gondii stimulates production of IgG, IgM, IgA, and IgE antibodies. Extracellular tachyzoites coated with antibody and complement will be lysed[254] or killed within phagocytes,[8] but these humoral mechanisms offer no protection against live organisms that are already within cells. Antibodies alone will protect mice only against less virulent strains of T. gondii.[216,313]

Human secretory IgA reduces in vitro infectivity of ta-chyzoites for enterocytes.[171] Anti-p30 monoclonal antibodies reduce the ability of tachyzoites to invade mammalian cells.[105]

Other Protective Mechanisms. T. gondii infection causes release of thromboxane A2 and 13-hydroxy-octadecadienoic acid by platelets.[111] These metabolites may play a role in cytotoxic reactions against T. gondii.

Retinal Lesions

Protection against ocular toxoplasmosis involves many of the same immunologic mechanisms described previously. Treatment of mice with monoclonal antibodies against IFN-γ, TNF-α, or CD4+ and CD8+ T-lymphocytes results in increased severity of ocular lesions, including a heightened inflammatory response and increased numbers of organisms in the retina.[93]

As discussed previously the majority of retinal lesions in patients from the United States and Europe arise at the borders of old retinochoroidal scars, which are typical of those seen in congenital toxoplasmosis. Based on this observation and on epidemiologic evidence, it has been thought that the vast majority of adult cases are recurrent congenital infections in persons without other manifestations of congenital disease.[73,74] It has been shown that live organisms can persist in clinically inactive lesions for many years after birth.[115]

Understanding of the pathogenesis of disease recurrences in the retina is incomplete.[207] Frenkel[83] suggested that recurrences were due to hypersensitivity responses against exposed T. gondii antigens, rather than to proliferation of the parasite. He based this conclusion on experiments with hamsters infected with the related parasite Besnoitia jellisoni, which has a tissue cyst large enough to be seen with a direct ophthalmoscope. He observed spontaneous rupture of tissue cysts, but little invasion of adjacent cells by the released parasites.

More recently, a series of studies at the Francis I. Proctor Foundation using a nonhuman primate model[41] has shed more light on the relative roles of parasitic invasion of retinal cells versus hypersensitivity reactions in the pathogenesis of toxoplasmic retinochoroiditis. Intraocular inoculation of T. gondii results in a focal necrotizing retinochoroiditis with clinical and histopathologic characteristics similar to human disease[41] (Fig. 85-22). In contrast, intraocular inoculation of live T. gondii organisms or T. gondii antigen in previously immunized animals does not produce necrotizing retinochoroiditis.[300] Also, intravenous or intraocular injection of T. gondii antigen in previously infected animals does not produce recurrent necrotizing retinochoroiditis.[195] These animals do, however, develop anterior uveitis, vitreous inflammatory reactions, macular edema, and retinal vasculitis. It is assumed from these results that tissue invasion by live organisms, with subsequent rupture of host cells, plays the major role in the pathogenesis of retinal necrosis in recurrent

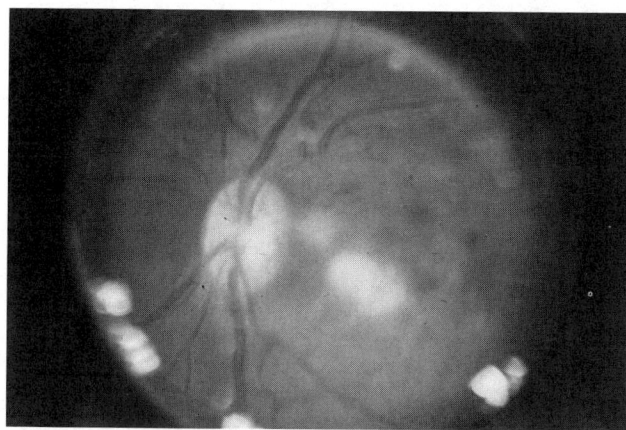

Fig. 85-22. Left fundus of a cynomologus monkey *(Macaca fascicularis)* 10 days after injection of 20,000 *Toxoplasma gondii* organisms into the eye. There is a focus of necrotizing retinitis in the macula, reminiscent of human disease. (Photograph courtesy of William W. Culbertson, MD, Miami, FL; reprinted with permission from Culbertson WW, Tabbara KF, O'Connor GR: Experimental ocular toxoplasmosis in primates, *Arch Ophthalmol* 100:321-323, 1982. Copyright 1982 by The American Medical Association.)

disease, although hypersensitivity reactions are responsible for many of the other clinical signs (such as iritis, retinal vasculitis) that accompany recurrent infections.

Autoimmune reactions may play a role in the pathogenesis of toxoplasmic retinochoroiditis as well.[203,316] Histopathologic study of congenital toxoplasmosis in a murine model revealed selective loss of the photoreceptor layer of the retina,[67] which is similar to the changes seen in experimental uveitis induced by immunization with retinal S-antigen. Nussenblatt and associates[203] found that 40% of patients with ocular toxoplasmosis had lymphocyte proliferative responses to retinal S-antigen. The presence of S-antigen reactivity did not correlate with clinical characteristics or course of disease, however. Reaction to S-antigen was more common in younger patients, suggesting that it does not simply reflect a secondary phenomenon of sensitization to exposed antigens in disease of longer duration. Although antibody responses to retinal antigens have also been reported in patients with ocular toxoplasmosis,[1] this finding could not be confirmed by other investigators.

In immunocompetent hosts, *T. gondii* does not spread to affect ocular tissues other than the retina. The inflammatory reactions that damage the subjacent choroid or anterior segment are attributed to either soluble mediators released from the retinal site of infection or to hypersensitivity reactions to parasitic antigens.

In a study of 38 patients, there was no apparent relationship between HLA types and ocular toxoplasmosis.[203]

Disease Recurrences

The factors that cause reactivation of organisms from retinal tissue cysts are unknown, but may be multiple. Tissue cysts appear to undergo senescent changes with hyalinization of their contents,[227] but it is unknown whether these changes lead to the spontaneous rupture of cyst walls. There is no experimental evidence that trauma precipitates recurrent toxoplasmic retinochoroiditis,[202,210] as previously suspected by some clinicians. It is generally believed that ocular toxoplasmosis recurs with increased frequency during pregnancy,[88,208] which suggests that hormonal factors may also be involved in disease recurrence.

The immune system may play a role in maintaining *T. gondii* in its tissue cyst form. Cytokines are believed to play a role in tissue cyst formation as discussed previously;[22,136] immunosuppression might therefore stimulate stage conversion from bradyzoites to tachyzoites. On the other hand, cellular immunodeficiency may simply permit reactivation of disease by failure to kill organisms that emerge from cysts, without actually initiating cyst breakdown. Studies in vitro have shown that antibodies against *T. gondii* can induce tissue cyst formation,[262] but the significance of this finding for reactivation of tissue cysts in vivo is uncertain. Tissue cysts are formed within cells, where antibody is not active. Humoral immunity therefore may not play an important role in disease recurrence.

Animal models of infection have provided conflicting data regarding the role of immunosuppression as an initiating factor for recurrence of ocular toxoplasmosis. Nozik and O'Connor[202] caused recurrent ocular toxoplasmosis in rabbits using antilymphocyte serum. Although Frenkel[82] described recurrence of ocular toxoplasmosis in hamsters after treatment with irradiation and cortisone, other investigators have not been able to induce such recurrences in other animals. Zimmerman[323] was unable to induce reactivation of encysted organisms with intramuscular cortisone injections in rabbits and guinea pigs. Others have been unable to induce recurrent ocular toxoplasmosis in rabbits after subcutaneous injection of hydrocortisone.[144,202]

Holland and associates[118] were unable to induce disease recurrences in cynomolgus monkeys that had healed toxoplasmic retinochoroidal scars by immunosuppression with total body irradiation. Reinoculation of parasites directly into the eyes of the immunosuppressed monkeys (possibly simulating the release of organisms from a tissue cyst) resulted in the development of second foci of retinal infection.[118] In other studies reinoculation of live parasites into eyes of immunocompetent animals with toxoplasmic retinochoroidal scars did not result in active retinal disease,[210] presumably because specific immunity prevented proliferation of organisms. These results support the hypothesis that immunosuppression does not initiate disease recurrence, but does allow uncontrolled proliferation of organisms if they escape from tissue cysts for other reasons. It is possible, however, that maintenance of *T. gondii* in the tissue cyst form is under the control of cellular immune mechanisms, but does not require the same level of immune function needed to destroy proliferating organisms. Alternatively, it may involve immune mechanisms that are not affected by radiation.

There is little evidence in clinical studies that immunosuppression precipitates recurrence of toxoplasmic retinochoroiditis in patients with inactive scars. It has been noted that patients with AIDS may have retinochoroidal scars without evidence of active disease, despite the presumed presence of encysted organisms at scar borders.[117,196] This observation has not been studied with respect to the severity of immunosuppression, however. Among patients with recurrent toxoplasmic retinochoroiditis, it is very uncommon to see individuals who were receiving immunosuppressive doses of systemic corticosteroids before the onset of the recurrence.

Holland and associates[117] have hypothesized that most cases of ocular toxoplasmosis in immunosuppressed patients are due to acquired disease or to organisms newly disseminated to the eye from nonocular sites of re-activation, as lesions may be multifocal at onset and are seldom associated with pre-existing chorioretinal scars.[117] Re-activation of disease from tissue cysts in normal-appearing retina cannot be ruled out, however.

Interaction with Other Agents

In immunosuppressed patients, *T. gondii* and CMV may infect tissues concurrently at rates higher than would be predicted from the independent frequencies of each.[242] In a mouse model newly acquired murine CMV infection of animals with chronic *T. gondii* infection causes reactivation of *T. gondii* infection with development of pneumonia.[225] Toxoplasmic pneumonia was associated with a murine CMV-induced fall in CD4+ T-lymphocyte count and an influx of CD8+ T-lymphocytes into the lungs. Reactivation of *T. gondii* infection could not be attributed to change in macrophage function.

Concurrent CMV retinitis and toxoplasmic retinochoroiditis have been reported in patients with AIDS.[117] It is unknown whether this association is related to a local change in immune defenses or is simply coincidental because of the high frequency of CMV retinitis.

DIFFERENTIAL DIAGNOSIS

In newborns, toxoplasmosis can be confused with other congenital infections in the "TORCH complex," a group of congenital and perinatally-acquired infectious diseases caused by agents that usually are of low pathogenicity in adults, but can cause severe morbidity in newborns.[192] They include *TO*xoplasmosis, *R*ubella, *C*ytomegalic inclusion disease (caused by CMV), *H*erpes simplex virus infections,

and others, including congenital syphilis. Diagnosis requires serologic tests and/or isolation of pathogens; these conditions cannot be differentiated on clinical grounds alone.

It is unlikely that typical lesions of recurrent toxoplasmic retinochoroiditis, which develop adjacent to retinochoroidal scars, will be confused with other disorders in older children and adults. Serpiginous chorioretinitis is another disorder in which there may be focal inflammation at borders of pre-existing scars, but it is not associated with severe anterior segment inflammation or with multiple peripheral chorioretinal scars, both of which can be present in patients with recurrent ocular toxoplasmosis. Serpiginous chorioretinitis lesions can usually be recognized by the large geographic scarring that occurs in the peripapillary area.

Toxoplasmic papillitis and atypical forms of retinochoroiditis present greater diagnostic challenges. The differential diagnosis of toxoplasmic papillitis includes other infections, such as CMV papillitis in immunosuppressed patients and fungal abscesses in the area of the optic disc; sarcoidosis with optic disc granuloma; various causes of optic neuritis; and anterior ischemic optic neuropathy. The latter disorder will not be associated with a vitreous inflammatory reaction.

If foci of toxoplasmic retinochoroiditis occur near the ora serrata, the inflammatory reaction might be confused with the "snowbanks" seen in the pars planitis syndrome, an idiopathic form of intermediate uveitis (see Chapter 55). It should be relatively easy to differentiate pars planitis syndrome from ocular toxoplasmosis on the basis of its chronic course and bilaterality. Punctate outer retinal toxoplasmosis may be confused with acute posterior multifocal placoid pigment epitheliopathy, punctate inner choroidopathy, or other white dot syndromes (see Chapter 46).

Retinal infections in patients with *acquired* toxoplasmosis may be confused with other disorders. Endogenous spread of fungal or bacterial infection can result in focal retinal lesions, but they can usually be distinguished from toxoplasmic retinochoroiditis by associated nonocular findings or the clinical setting in which they occur. Also, bacterial and fungal infections are more likely to be multifocal, and progress rapidly to endophthalmitis.

Differentiation of toxoplasmic retinochoroiditis from other disorders is most difficult in patients who are immunosuppressed, as lesions (1) can present with a variety of clinical features, (2) are not usually associated with retinal scars, and (3) may result in widespread areas of retinal necrosis that resemble other infections.[117] Toxoplasmosis is most commonly confused with the necrotizing herpetic retinopathies such as CMV retinitis and the acute retinal necrosis syndrome. Elkins and associates[70] described the following clinical features of toxoplasmic retinochoroiditis in immunosuppressed patients that may help to differentiate it from CMV retinitis: densely opaque and thick retinal lesions with smooth borders (as opposed to the dry granular borders of CMV retinitis, Fig. 85-17); prominent vitreous and anterior segment inflammatory reactions, lack of prominent retinal hemorrhage within lesions (although hemorrhage can occur), and solitary central macular lesions (Fig. 85-15). Toxoplasmic retinochoroiditis may also occur at higher CD4+ T-lymphocyte counts than CMV retinitis in HIV-infected individuals.[70]

LABORATORY INVESTIGATIONS

Nonocular *T. gondii* infection produces a variety of nonspecific clinical manifestations, which makes laboratory testing important in the evaluation of patients. Diagnosis can be confirmed by one of the following methods: isolation of *T. gondii* from blood, body fluids, or tissue specimens; histologic demonstration of tachyzoites or tissue cysts in body fluids or tissue specimens; and polymerase chain reaction (PCR) techniques for detection of *T. gondii* DNA in body fluids or tissues.[26,32,173] Isolation techniques involve inoculation of specimens into mice or tissue cultures (the latter being a less sensitive technique). Immunohistochemical staining techniques may help identify tachyzoites and tissue cysts in tissue preparations.

Identification of *T. gondii* in blood or other body fluids generally suggests active infection, whereas isolation from a tissue specimen may simply reflect the presence of tissue cysts in chronic infection.

Characteristic lymph node histology may also establish a diagnosis of recently acquired toxoplasmosis in older children and adults, even if *T. gondii* is not isolated.[63]

Serologic Tests

Serologic tests for demonstration of specific antibodies are used commonly to confirm exposure to *T. gondii* in cases of suspected toxoplasmosis. The presence of anti-*T. gondii* IgG antibodies cannot confirm a diagnosis, however, because (1) such antibodies can persist at high titers for years after an acute infection, and (2) there is a high prevalence of such antibodies in the general population. The presence of antibodies may therefore be unrelated to the clinical disorder being investigated.

In general IgG antibodies appear within 1 to 2 weeks after infection, peak at 1 to 2 months, then fall at variable rates, but they remain detectable for life. IgM antibodies also develop within 1 to 2 weeks after infection. They can persist for up to 1 year at low titers before becoming undetectable. The presence of anti-*T. gondii* IgM antibodies therefore cannot be used as a marker for newly acquired infection, in contrast to common belief. A negative test for IgM antibodies does rule out recently acquired infection, however. IgG antibodies will cross the placenta, but IgM antibodies will not; the presence of IgM antibodies in a newborn therefore indicates congenital infection, whereas IgG antibodies in a newborn may simply indicate passive transfer of maternal antibodies in utero.

Identification of specific anti-*T. gondii* IgA antibodies by immunosorbent assays indicates recent infection and appears to be more sensitive for diagnosis of congenital infection in the fetus and newborn than detection of IgM.[281] IgA antibodies usually disappear by 7 months. Anti-*T. gondii* IgE antibodies are also markers of recent infection, but are detectable for shorter periods than either specific IgM or IgA.[223,310] The titers of IgM, IgA, and IgE antibodies cannot be used to determine how recently the infection was acquired.

Several different serologic tests are available to clinicians; they identify antibodies to different *T. gondii* antigens and have unique patterns of change after infection. The most useful tests are the Sabin-Feldman dye test, the enzyme-linked immunosorbent assay (ELISA), the indirect fluorescent antibody (IFA) test, and the modified direct agglutination test (Table 85-2).

The Sabin-Feldman dye test is the standard reference against which all other serologic tests are compared.[246] It is a neutralization test in which live organisms are exposed to patient serum and complement; the cell membrane of organisms are lysed if specific anti-*T. gondii* IgG antibodies are present in the serum, and the organisms will fail to stain with methylene blue dye. Titers are determined by the dilution at which only 50% of organisms are stained. It is a sensitive and specific test, but is available only through a few reference laboratories because of the need to use live parasites. The titer of antibodies is not correlated with the severity of disease.[10]

The IgG IFA test measures the same antibodies as the dye test and is comparable in sensitivity and specificity, but it is easier, safer, and more economical to perform. In this test a slide preparation of killed tachyzoites is incubated with patient serum; fluorescein-tagged anti-human IgG (or IgM) antibodies are used to identify anti-*T. gondii* antibodies in the test serum that have reacted with the organisms. False positive results can occur in patients with antinuclear antibodies (ANA),[12] and false negative results can occur in patients with low titers of anti-*T. gondii* antibodies. Titers parallel those obtained with the dye test, and high titers can persist for life.

ELISA tests are used widely for detection of anti-*T. gondii* antibodies, but commercially available ELISA tests vary in sensitivity and specificity.

Direct agglutination tests identify the presence of IgG antibodies that bind and agglutinate formalin-preserved whole tachyzoites[59] or antigen-coated latex beads.[299] The technique is not reliable for identifying IgM antibodies. Direct agglutination tests are commercially available in Europe, where they are used for screening pregnant women.

The complement fixation test measures antibodies that appear later than those identified by the dye or IFA tests. They decline earlier, although they also can persist for many years. The test is not routinely available in the United States.

The indirect hemagglutination (IHA) test uses erythro-

TABLE 85-2 COMMON SEROLOGIC TESTS FOR ANTI-*TOXOPLASMA GONDII* ANTIBODIES

Test	Antibodies Identified	Positive Titer[a]	Titer in Chronic Infection[a]	Duration of Positive Test	Causes of False Results
Sabin-Feldman dye test	IgG	1:4[b]	1:4 to >1:2000; stable or slow decrease	Years	
IFA	IgG	1:4	1:8 to 1:2000	Years	False positives ANA
	IgM[c]	1:2 (infants)	<1:20	Weeks to months[d]	False positives ANA, RF
		1:10 (adults)			False negatives high titers of IgG
ELISA	IgG	>6	>6	Years	
	IgM[c,e]	≥2	<2	Months[d]	False positives RF
Direct agglutination	IgG	Varies; rises slowly in acquired infection	Varies	Years	
CF[f]	IgG	1:4	Negative to 1:8	Varies; may persist for years.	
IHA[f]	IgG	1:16; rises very slowly in acquired infection	1:16 to 1:256	Years	

Note: ANA = Antinuclear antibodies.
CF = Complement fixation.
ELISA = Enzyme-linked immunosorbent assay.
IFA = Immunofluorescent antibody.
IHA = Indirect hemagglutination.
RF = Rheumatoid factor.

[a]Titers are representative; values may vary between laboratories.
[b]In patients with strong clinical evidence of toxoplasmic retinochoroiditis, a positive test on undiluted serum may be significant.
[c]Tests for specific anti-*T. gondii* IgA and IgE antibodies may be more reliable for identification of acute and congenital infections.
[d]Occasionally, IgM antibodies can be detected for up to 1 year.
[e]Frequent false positive results preclude routine use of standard IgM-ELISA; double sandwich technique more sensitive and specific.
[f]Antibodies rise later than those identified by dye test or IFA test. CF and IHA tests rarely used in United States.

cytes coated with *T. gondii* antigen, which will agglutinate in the presence of anti-*T. gondii* antibodies in test serum. It also measures antibodies different from those detected in the dye or IFA tests; titers rise later and last longer. It is therefore not a useful screening test for recently acquired infection. False positive tests are more common with the IHA test than with the dye test or IFA test.

IgM antibody can be detected by IFA or ELISA techniques, but false positive results can occur in patients with ANA or rheumatoid factor (RF). Rheumatoid factor can be present in newborns. A double-sandwich IgM ELISA technique avoids these false positive results.[29,193]

The immunosorbent agglutination assay (ISAGA) can be used to detect IgG, IgM, IgA, and IgE. It is a sensitive and specific technique that does not require an enzyme conjugate, and it is read in the same manner as agglutination tests. IgM-ISAGA is more sensitive than IgM-IFA and is not affected by ANA or RF.[234]

Acquired Infections. In a symptomatic, immunocompetent patient, recently acquired disease is *suggested* by dye test or IFA antibody titers greater than 1:1000 and either a positive IgM-IFA titer or a positive IgM-ELISA. Diagnosis cannot be made with certainty, however, because very high stable antibody titers can persist for many years and results can vary between test kits. For a more definitive diagnosis, presumed cases of recently acquired toxoplasmosis should be evaluated by serial testing for both IgG and IgM antibodies at 3-week intervals, and specimens should be tested in parallel. New infection is supported by seroconversion or at least a two-tube rise in titers for either antibody.[28] IgG antibodies detected by the Sabin-Feldman dye or IFA tests will peak at 6 to 8 weeks after infection, then gradually decline over months or years. In many cases antibody titers are already high when patients are first evaluated; in such cases tests for IgM, IgA, and IgE antibodies are useful.

Immunosuppressed Patients. Active disease in immuno-suppressed patients is thought to be caused by reactivation of chronic infections, and therefore serologic testing may not be helpful in differentiating suspected toxoplasmosis from other disorders. Specific IgG antibody titers may be low, and specific IgM, IgA, and IgE may be absent. Confirmation of past exposure may require a panel of multiple tests. Serologic diagnosis of toxoplasmosis in patients with AIDS has been discussed by Wong and associates.[313]

Ocular Disease

Toxoplasmic retinochoroiditis is diagnosed clinically. Parasites are found rarely in intraocular fluids,[104] and invasive diagnostic tests such as retinal biopsy are associated with serious risks that prevent their routine use. Serologic tests should be used only to confirm past exposure to *T. gondii;* it is inappropriate to base a diagnosis of ocular toxoplasmosis on the presence of antibodies alone. Because active retinal lesions are usually foci of recurrent disease, serum IgG titers may be low and IgM may be absent. There have been histologically proven cases of toxoplasmic retinochoroiditis in which serum antibodies could be detected only in undiluted serum.[324] Tests reported to be negative by the laboratory should only be repeated using undiluted serum if there is a high clinical suspicion of infection.[114] The Sabin-Feldman dye test is the only technique that should be used to test undiluted serum, owing to the extremely high rate of false positives that would result with other techniques. A negative test on undiluted serum makes a diagnosis of toxoplasmic retinochoroiditis highly unlikely.

Sensitivity and specificity may vary between different tests and in different clinical situations. Rothova and associates[240] found that an ELISA test for anti-*T. gondii* IgG antibodies was highly sensitive for evaluation of patients with ocular toxoplasmosis. Their results are relevant only for the technique they used, however, and may not be the same for all ELISA test kits. Weiss and associates[301] described three patients with presumed toxoplasmic retinochoroiditis for whom IFA tests were negative, but dye tests were positive; in only one case was an ELISA test positive. In cases of presumed disease in which serologic testing is negative or equivocal, it is appropriate to perform a panel of several tests using a reference laboratory.

There is little experience with the determination of IgA and IgE antibody titers in patients with ocular toxoplasmosis, but IgA antibodies have been found in 86% of adult patients with toxoplasmic retinochoroiditis,[15] and IgE antibodies can be detected in children with toxoplasmic retinochoroiditis.[224]

Serologic testing has not been helpful in the diagnosis of ocular toxoplasmosis in patients with AIDS. Anti-*T. gondii* IgG antibody titers vary widely, and IgM antibodies are uncommon.[117]

In atypical cases of presumed toxoplasmic retinochoroiditis in which the diagnosis is uncertain, antibody levels can also be determined in aqueous or vitreous humor, and compared to serum levels, as a test for intraocular antibody production. To control for passive diffusion of anti-*T. gondii* serum antibodies into the inflamed eye, the ratio of intraocular to serum antibodies must be compared to the ratio of total immunoglobulin or a similar-size molecule that would not be produced locally. Some investigators prefer to use a specific IgG antibody to a common agent that does not cause intraocular disease (such as adenovirus), with a similar molecular weight. The comparison of ratios can be expressed mathematically as follows to calculate a value that has come to be called the Witmer or Witmer-Goldmann coefficient: [Antibody titer (ocular fluid) × total immunoglobulin (serum)] ÷ [Antibody titer (serum) × total immunoglobulin (ocular fluid)]. Titers determined by the dye test, ELISA, and IFA techniques have been used to calculate intraocular antibody production. In calculating the coefficient, the reciprocal of the fractional titer is used in the formula (e.g. for a titer of 1 : 64, the numeral 64 is used). Theoretically, values greater than 1 would indicate local production of antibody, but practical experience has shown that values should be greater than 8 for a diagnosis of toxoplasmic retinochoroiditis.[55]

A possible source of error in determining intraocular antibody production is polyclonal B-lymphocyte activation. No absolute values can be used reliably to diagnose disease in all cases; a more useful application of this technique may be to compare the magnitude of the Witmer-Goldmann coefficient for several pathogens in the differential diagnosis of a lesion; the highest value would indicate the most likely cause. This technique has been used to distinguish between CMV retinitis, varicella-zoster virus retinopathy, and toxoplasmic retinochoroiditis in patients with AIDS.[48]

Determination of intraocular antibody formation is most reliable in cases of recurrent toxoplasmic retinochoroiditis, but may not be positive during the initial stages of reactivation.[55] The coefficient drops to normal levels with resolution of active disease, indicating that a recent antigenic stimulus is necessary for local antibody production. It is not a reliable technique for congenital disease, or in patients who also have recently acquired nonocular disease because of the high level of serum antibodies.[55] The technique is unreliable when the dye test antibody titer is greater than 1 : 1000.

Anterior chamber paracentesis to obtain an aqueous humor specimen for testing can be performed safely as a simple office procedure, but there is a small risk of intraocular infection or damage to the lens or cornea. Vitreous sampling is generally reserved for patients undergoing retinovitreous surgical procedures, such as a vitrectomy associated with retinal detachment repair. Techniques for determination of antibody titers on the extremely small sample sizes obtained from eye (generally 0.1 to 0.2 ml) are discussed by Davis and associates.[48]

Toxoplasma gondii DNA has been identified in ocular tissue sections of patients with presumed toxoplasmic retinochoroiditis by PCR techniques,[20,26] even when typical tissue cysts are not identified on histopathologic examination.[26]

Other Evaluations

Skull x-rays may identify intracranial calcification, which is typical of congenital toxoplasmosis. Immunosuppressed patients suspected of having toxoplasmic encephalitis can be evaluated by CT or MRI studies. Multiple bilateral cerebral lesions will be present on CT scans in 70% to 80% of patients with AIDS and toxoplasmic encephalitis. Lesions are hypodense with enhancement after intravenous contrast.[163] The number of lesions can be underestimated by CT scans; MRI is a more sensitive technique, especially if gadolinium is used for contrast. On MRI scans lesions appear as high signal abnormalities on T2-weighted imaging.[36,132,162]

THERAPY

In most cases *T. gondii* infection is self-limited and asymptomatic. Furthermore, currently available drugs do not eliminate tissue cysts and therefore cannot prevent chronic infection. Treatment is therefore not warranted for the majority of *T. gondii* infections. There are specific situations, however, in which treatment may be extremely important; they include infections in pregnant women, newborns, and immunosuppressed patients. Details regarding the treatment of *T. gondii* infections in these settings are reviewed elsewhere.[15,233,312,313]

It is also generally accepted that treatment is beneficial for ocular infections. Nevertheless, many issues remain unresolved regarding the treatment of ocular toxoplasmosis. This section deals with factors important for making management decisions regarding therapy of ocular infections. Specific details regarding various treatment regimens and the pharmacologic action of the drugs used to treat ocular infections have been reviewed elsewhere.[71,302]

The management of ocular toxoplasmosis in immunocompetent adults is based on the following principles: (1) the active phase of the disease is self-limited; (2) retinal necrosis is due to proliferation of organisms; (3) the immune response to these organisms can also result in additional damage to intraocular tissues; and (4) currently available drugs cannot eliminate tissue cysts and therefore cannot prevent future recurrences. Because the disease is self-limited, many clinicians will not treat small, peripheral retinal lesions that are not immediately vision-threatening, so as to avoid drug-associated side effects (Fig. 85-23).

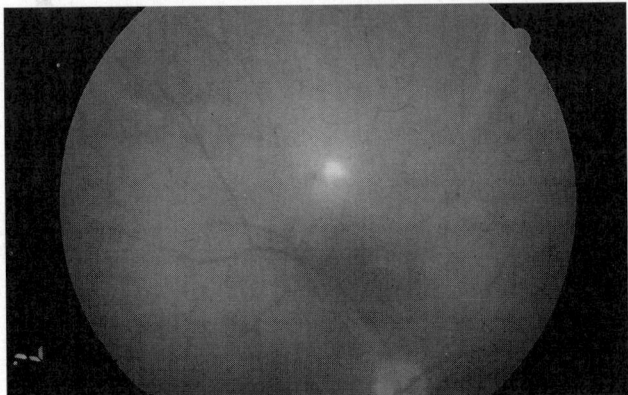

Fig. 85-23. A small focus of recurrent toxoplasmic retinochoroiditis superior to the superotemporal vascular arcades in the right eye of an immunocompetent adult. The vitreous humor inflammatory reaction is mild, and the patient retains central visual acuity of 20/20 in this eye. The lesion resolved spontaneously after several weeks without therapy.

Indications

The goal of medical therapy is to prevent damage to the retina and optic nerve, thereby preventing permanent vision loss. In 1991 Engstrom and associates[71] conducted a survey of all physician members of the American Uveitis Society to determine current practices in the management of ocular toxoplasmosis. Of respondents, only 6% treat all active lesions, regardless of ocular findings. The majority of respondents felt that lesions could be observed without treatment if visual acuity remained 20/20 in the affected eye and lesions were located in the far periphery of the retina. A majority of respondents agreed that the following factors were indications for medical therapy: any decrease in visual acuity, macular or peripapillary lesions, lesions greater than one optic disc diameter in size, lesions associated with a moderate-to-severe vitreous inflammatory reaction, the presence of multiple active lesions, persistence of active disease for greater than 1 month, and any ocular lesions associated with recently acquired infection. Of these factors, lesion size alone was considered least important in management decisions.

Although Matthews and Weiter[177] felt that medical therapy altered the outcome of patients with punctate outer retinal toxoplasmosis, only half of the respondents in the American Uveitis Society survey consider this form of disease a specific indication for treatment. Perhaps this attitude exists because these lesions are not typically associated with vitreous inflammation, and because their natural course appears similar to more typical toxoplasmic retinochorodit is lesions. Other atypical lesions, with a less understood natural course or with signs suggesting a more severe infection (such as multifocal lesions, acquired lesions, and lesions persisting for more than 1 month), are generally considered indications for treatment.

Antimicrobial Agents

In 1953 Eyles and Coleman[72] demonstrated the synergistic action of pyrimethamine and sulfonamides on *T. gondii.* Pyrimethamine interferes with the conversion of folic acid to folinic acid by blocking the enzyme dihydrofolic acid reductase, whereas sulfonamides interfere with the formation of folic acid from para-amino benzoic acid. As a result, errors in nuclear division occur during parasitic replication. Human beings, unlike *T. gondii,* can utilize exogenous folinic acid, which is therefore administered concurrently to prevent bone marrow suppression during treatment. These drugs continue to be the mainstay of treatment for ocular toxoplasmosis. Sulfadiazine, believed the most effective of the sulfonamide agents, has sometimes been difficult to obtain in recent years; as a result, clinicians have used various other sulfonamides for the treatment of ocular toxoplasmosis,[71,212] although an equivalent clinical efficacy has not been confirmed.

The combination of pyrimethamine, sulfadiazine, and corticosteroids, which is considered "classic" therapy for ocular toxoplasmosis (see second box), is the most common drug combination used; it was cited as the treatment of choice by 32% of respondents in the American Uveitis Society survey.[71] When using pyrimethamine for the treatment of toxoplasmosis, patients should be monitored for leukopenia and thrombocytopenia; most clinicians will discontinue therapy for a white blood cell count less than 4,000 cells/μl or a platelet count less than 100,000/μl.[71]

A number of other drugs have also demonstrated in vitro and in vivo efficacy against *T. gondii* and have been used in the treatment of human ocular toxoplasmosis (see third box), but their relative efficacies remains uncertain. They are generally used in multiple drug combinations, both with and without oral corticosteroid therapy.

An additional 27% of American Uveitis Society respondents add clindamycin to the combination of pyrimethamine, sulfadiazine, and corticosteroids ("quadruple therapy") as their treatment of choice, and several use clindamycin as the sole antimicrobial agent in combination with corticosteroids.[71] Clindamycin appears to be concentrated in ocular tissue and can penetrate tissue cyst walls.[294] Although animal experiments showed that clindamycin treatment reduced tissue cyst numbers,[181] there is no clinical evidence to support the concept that clindamycin prevents recurrences.[157]

The AIDS epidemic has stimulated renewed interest in the medical therapy of toxoplasmosis. A goal of ongoing research is to identify drugs, drug combinations, and treatment regimens that will be cysticidal. Atovaquone is a hydroxynaphthoquinone that interferes with pyrimidine synthesis by its effect on the enzyme dihydroorotate dehydrogenase.[13,119,123] The drug acts by a selective and potent inhibition of the mitochondrial electron transport chain in several protozoan parasites. Dihydroorotate dehydrogenase is linked to the mitochondrial electron transport chain by ubiquinone. The drug is believed to be safe and has been well tolerated by patients; the only reported side effect is a transient maculopapular rash. Interest in this compound stems from laboratory studies in mice showing that the drug has both in vitro and in vivo activity against tachyzoites, tissue cyst formation, and bradyzoites found within tissue cysts. Although the drug has been used more commonly for the treatment of *P. carinii* infections and intracranial toxoplasmosis, Lopez and associates[165] have described the successful treatment of ocular toxoplasmosis in a patient with

---

ANTIMICROBIAL DRUGS USED IN THE TREATMENT OF TOXOPLASMOSIS

Dihydrofolate reductase inhibitors
  Pyrimethamine
  Trimethoprim/sulfamethoxazole
Sulfonamides
  Sulfadiazine
  Sulfadiazine/sulfamerazine/sulfamethazine "triple sulfa"
  Sulfisoxazole
Tetracyclines
  Tetracycline
  Minocycline
Other antimicrobial agents
  Clindamycin
  Atovaquone
  Clarithromycin
  Spiramycin

TYPICAL THERAPY FOR OCULAR TOXOPLASMOSIS

Pyrimethamine
  75 mg to 100 mg loading dose given over 24 hours, followed by 25 to 50 mg daily for 4 to 6 weeks depending on clinical response.
Sulfadiazine
  2.0 to 4.0 g loading dose initially, followed by 1.0 g given 4 times daily for 4 to 6 weeks, depending on clinical response.
Prednisone
  40 to 60 mg daily for 2 to 6 weeks depending on clinical response; taper off before discontinuing pyrimethamine/sulfadiazine.
Folinic acid
  5.0 mg tablet or 3.0 mg intravenous preparation given orally, 2 to 3 times weekly during pyrimethamine therapy.

AIDS using atovaquone. Unfortunately, treatment does not prevent the recurrence of toxoplasmic retinochoroiditis.*

Corticosteroids

Corticosteroids are used to decrease problems associated with inflammation, such as macular edema, vitreous inflammatory reaction, and retinal vasculitis. Their use is felt to be especially important for lesions that threaten the macula or optic disc. Because retinal necrosis is believed to be caused by proliferation of *T. gondii,* corticosteroids should not be used without concurrent antimicrobial agents; the suppression of immune defense mechanisms by corticosteroids might lead to fulminant *T. gondii* infection. Corticosteroids alter the immune response and its ability to fight *T. gondii* infection, but they do not completely eliminate the signs of inflammation in the presence of proliferating organisms. Paradoxically, eyes treated with intensive corticosteroid therapy, but without antimicrobial agents, can have heightened signs of inflammation including vascular sheathing, vitreous humor opacification, and marked anterior chamber cells and flare (Fig. 85-24). This profound reaction is presumably in response to the increased proliferation of organisms that occurs in the setting of reduced host defenses, and it can contribute to the loss of an eye from ocular toxoplasmosis.[244] When used with antimicrobial agents, however, corticosteroids have not been shown to worsen the underlying infection.[205]

Initiation of corticosteroid therapy is frequently delayed for 24 to 48 hours to allow adequate blood levels of antimicrobial agents.[71] Whether this delay is clinically necessary is not known.

Periocular injections of corticosteroids should be used with caution, if at all, because of the intense antiinflammatory action of drug administered by this routine. Many investigators have discouraged the use of periocular corticosteroid injections because of experiences in which it has been associated with uncontrollable disease and loss of the eye.[244]

Topical corticosteroids are used to treat the secondary anterior chamber reaction associated with toxoplasmic retinochoroiditis. The frequency of treatment is based on the severity of reaction and the patient's symptoms of redness and discomfort. Topically applied drug has no effect on the retinal infection.

The general approach to medical therapy of most clinicians is to treat patients with a combination of antimicrobial agents and oral corticosteroids until there are definite signs of disease resolution (such as decreased inflammatory reaction and healing of retinal lesions). These signs of improvement usually occur within 4 to 6 weeks. At that time corticosteroids are tapered off. Antimicrobial agents are continued

until the corticosteroids are stopped, then they are discontinued as well. Drug therapy can be stopped before all signs of inflammation have resolved.

Treatment Efficacy

The reported benefits of medical therapy are based primarily on clinical impressions. Response to therapy is difficult to interpret, as there is so much variation in the clinical manifestation of retinal disease, and the disease is usually self-limited, even without treatment.

There have been very few prospective and controlled studies to assess the efficacy of various treatment regimens. In 1956 Perkins and associates[219] found a significant treat-

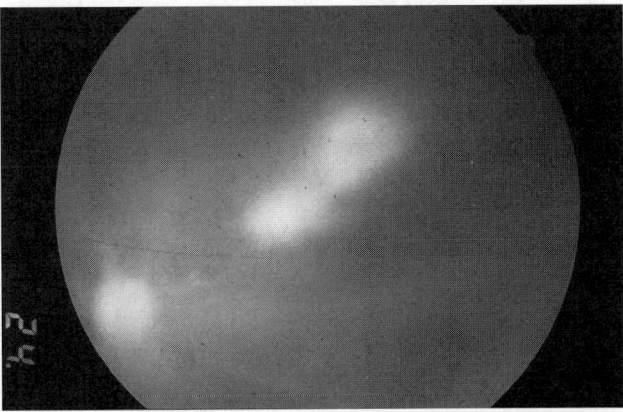

A

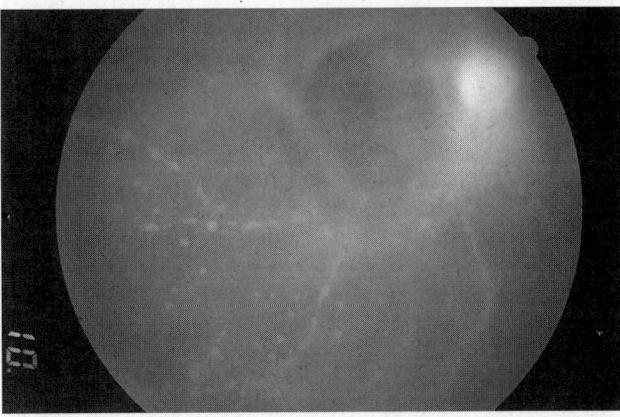

B

Fig. 85-24. **A,** A 39-year-old immunocompetent woman with a history of recurrent ocular toxoplasmosis. Photograph shows an intensely white, active satellite lesion at the inferior border of a retinochoroidal scar. The patient's condition has deteriorated to its current status after treatment with a periocular injection of long-acting corticosteroid. **B,** Macular view of the same eye showing "beading" (inflammatory sheathing) of all retinal vessels. There is a dense vitreous humor inflammatory reaction with membrane formation. Active retinochoroiditis and inflammatory signs resolved slowly over a 6-month period during which the patient was treated with oral pyrimethamine, clindamycin, and folinic acid.

---

*Ruebens Belfort Jr MD PhD, unpublished data.

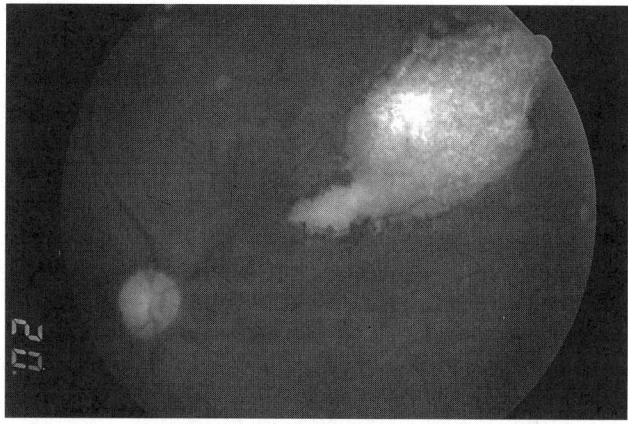

C

Fig. 85-24, cont'd. C, The same fundus, photographed 2 years later. The retinochoroidal scar resulting from the satellite lesion shown in **A** is more excavated (hence, its denser white appearance) than the larger, pre-existing scar; this difference may be due to the more severe disease that resulted from intensive corticosteroid therapy without the use of concurrent antimicrobial agents.

ment benefit with the use of pyrimethamine for selected cases of uveitis. The study was performed before there was a good understanding of the spectrum of disease findings that can be caused by *T. gondii,* and therefore the investigators included 164 cases of active uveitis, regardless of clinical signs. Either pyrimethamine (25 mg daily) or placebo was given to patients. Response to treatment, based on visual acuity, injection, flare, "subjective response," and "objective response," was measured after 4 weeks. Patients also received cortisone (dose unspecified) in some cases; the study was not controlled for this medication, but the investigators did not believe that it influenced the results. A significant difference in outcome was noted between those patients treated with pyrimethamine and those untreated, but only for patients with serologic evidence of *T. gondii* infection. A nonspecific effect of pyrimethamine on uveitis was ruled out by the observation that there was no apparent effect of treatment for serologically negative patients. A benefit of pyrimethamine treatment was not confirmed statistically when only seropositive patients with posterior uveitis were considered, but the investigators made the clinical observation that the "best responses" were seen in cases of circumscribed chorioretinitis.

Acers,[2] in 1964, reported a prospective, randomized study in which therapy using a combination of pyrimethamine (25 mg daily), trisulfapyrimidines (2 g daily), and prednisone (20 mg daily) was compared to corticosteroid therapy alone. After 8 weeks of therapy, they found no difference in the time to disease quiescence, and after 2 years, no difference in recurrence rate (10%). Only 10 patients were treated in each group, however, and therefore the study probably lacked the statistical power to detect differences.

Colin and Harie[38] compared treatment with oral pyrimethamine and sulfadiazine to subconjunctival injections of clindamycin and found no difference in time to healing or recurrence rates, but their study involved only 29 patients.

Rothova and associates[239] compared 3 treatment regimens in a group of 149 patients with toxoplasmic retinochoroiditis. Treated patients received 1 of 3 drug combinations: (1) pyrimethamine (50 mg daily), sulfadiazine (4 g daily), and prednisone; (2) clindamycin (300 mg 4 times daily), sulfadiazine (4 g daily), and prednisone; or (3) trimethoprim/sulfamethoxazole (960 mg twice daily for two weeks, followed by 380 mg twice daily) and prednisone. In each group prednisone (60 mg daily) was given on the third to seventh days, then reduced doses were given on a tapering schedule until discontinued. Treatment was administered to patients in both groups for 4 weeks. A fourth group of patients remained untreated. Although it was a prospective study, the patients were not randomized to one group or another; treatment was based on the institution where patients were treated, and untreated patients were those who had disease in the peripheral retina. A significantly greater proportion of patients receiving pyrimethamine were observed to have a decrease in lesion size during therapy than untreated patients, but there were no other differences between treated and untreated patients in this study. Specifically, none of the treatments affected the duration of activity or recurrence rates. The use of pyrimethamine was associated with a greater incidence of side effects, however.

Adjunctive Therapies

A variety of nonmedical therapies have been used in patients with sight-threatening lesions, in patients intolerant of oral medications, in pregnant patients, and in patients with severe, persistent lesions that did not respond completely to medical therapy. They include laser photocoagulation,[2,238,276,280] cryotherapy,[60] and vitrectomy,[80] but experience with these therapies is limited.[71]

The use of laser photocoagulation and cryotherapy is based on the presumption that these treatments will destroy organisms within lesions (including tissue cysts) and possibly alter antigenic proteins in such a way that they will not stimulate a recurrent immune response. Theoretically they may also help limit the spread of lesions by destroying the surrounding uninfected cells necessary for tachyzoite replication.

Vitrectomy is used most commonly to remove persistent vitreous opacities in otherwise quiet eyes or to relieve retinovitreous traction that may lead to retinal detachment, but it has also been used for severe or persistent vitreous inflammation in patients with active lesions.[80] The goal of vitrectomy in such cases is to remove mediators of inflammation from the eye. Potential complications of vitrectomy include retinal edema, retinal traction, and retinal detachment.

Laser Therapy. The greatest experience to date with non-medical therapies has been with the use of lasers. Xenon arc and argon laser photocoagulation of toxoplasmic retinochoroiditis lesions has been used by several investigators, either in an attempt to prevent disease recurrences or as an alternative to drug therapy in the management of active lesions.[2,238,276,280] It is preferred by some over other tissue-destructive techniques such as cryotherapy because it can be localized to very specific areas of the retina and can be used for lesions in the posterior pole. It cannot be used effectively, however, in eyes with dense vitreous inflammatory reactions or other media opacities. For patients with vitreous opacification, a combination of vitrectomy and argon laser endophotocoagulation has been advocated,[280] although reported experience with such therapy is very limited.

Spalter and associates[276] treated inactive retinochoroidal scars in 24 patients with argon laser photocoagulation as a prophylactic measure. All had had previous recurrences in the treated lesions (range 1 to 8 recurrences, mean 2.6 recurrences), with the interval between recurrences ranging from 4 months to 6 years. The entire area of a lesion was treated with a laser intensity sufficient to create faint blanching of the retina, and a row of treatment spots was placed around the lesion when possible. Recurrences were noted in only two patients; they were two in whom a row of treatment spots could not be administered around the entire lesion because of the proximity to structures critical for vision. The prophylactic advantage of treatment is difficult to assess from this study, however, because the follow-up period (8 to 33 months) was less than the interval between previous recurrences in some cases. In this study no serious side effects occurred with treatment. Some had transient small hemorrhages at the site of treatment that resolved without sequelae, but no patient experienced reactivation of disease attributable to laser therapy, and no retinal tears or detachments developed.

Some investigators,[238] however, have noted potentially serious side effects of laser therapy for toxoplasmic retinochoroiditis, such as epiretinal membrane formation and vitreous hemorrhage. Also, despite apparently adequate therapy, recurrences have been reported.[238] For these reasons, prophylactic treatment of quiescent scars is usually not performed.

Laser therapy is usually reserved for treatment of active disease that has had a prolonged course and appears to be refractory to medical therapy. Ghartey and associates[98] treated five patients with either xenon arc or argon laser photocoagulation in which active lesions did not heal after periods of medical treatment ranging from 1 to 4 months. In one patient media opacities prevented the delivery of adequate energy to the lesions; in the others, disease became quiescent within periods ranging from 3 weeks to 2 months. There was no evidence of disease recurrence in treated lesions for follow-up periods of 9 months to 7 years, despite frequent recurrences before treatment.

Theodossiadis[296] reported the laser treatment of patients with active disease and a history of frequent recurrences. In those cases in which he also treated the scar, patients had no recurrence of disease for 2 to 4 years after treatment. Other investigators have reported marked vitreous reactions after laser therapy for active lesions.[2]

The self-limited nature of ocular toxoplasmosis, its variable course and recurrence rates, as well as the lack of controlled studies make it difficult to interpret the value of adjunctive therapies. In most cases they are reserved for use with medical therapies in the most serious cases, especially those in which frequent recurrences have caused advancement of lesions toward the fovea, or in which prolonged activity has not responded completely to medical therapy. Because tissue cysts can exist in clinically normal-appearing retina, laser therapy cannot be expected to prevent recurrences in all patients.

Laser photocoagulation is also used to treat choroidal neovascularization, when it occurs as a complication of toxoplasmic retinochoroiditis.

Special Clinical Situations

Modification in the treatment of ocular disease may be necessary in specific clinical situations because of differences in disease severity or because of drug toxicity issues.
Pregnant Women. There are two potential reasons to treat women with ocular toxoplasmosis. As in other patients, drug therapy may be administered to treat vision-threatening lesions in the mother. In addition, if ocular lesions are thought to be one manifestation of *acquired* infection, medications may be given with the goal of treating the fetus.

In those cases in which active retinal lesions in the mother are associated with a retinochoroidal scar, the disease can be assumed to be a recurrence of a previous infection. There is no indication that *recurrent* toxoplasmic retinochoroiditis in an immunocompetent, pregnant woman poses a risk to the fetus; the fetus will be at little or no risk because of the protection afforded by preexisting maternal antibodies. In such cases it is desirable to avoid treatment unless the active lesion is in the macula or immediately adjacent to the optic disc.

Pregnant women present a unique therapeutic challenge because conventional medical therapies may be teratogenic. Concern exists about the potential teratogenicity of dihydrofolate reductase inhibitors, although such toxicity has not been convincingly demonstrated in humans.[57] Spiramycin has been recommended as probably having the lowest risk of toxicity for the fetus.[312]

Spiramycin is believed to reduce the rate with which *T. gondii* infection is transmitted from the mother to fetus; treatment is based on the observation that there is a lag between maternal and fetal infection.[312] Spiramycin does not, however, alter the course of disease in fetuses already infected. Spiramycin is not readily available in the United States, although it can be obtained from the U.S. Food and

Drug Administration on a compassionate use basis. If spiramycin is not available, treatment with sulfadiazine has been recommended.[312]

Treatment of congenital *T. gondii* infections in utero is believed to decrease the severity of ophthalmic disease after birth.[42]

Newborns. Toxoplasmic retinochoroiditis lesions have usually healed by birth, and specific treatment for the eyes is not necessary. Active ocular toxoplasmosis in newborns is a manifestation of disseminated disease, and such patients are generally not treated by the ophthalmologist.

Pyrimethamine and sulfonamides are the most commonly used antimicrobial agents for treatment of newborns with congenital toxoplasmosis.* Drug therapy is usually administered continuously for the first year of life.[180,183] Treatment may prevent further progression of ocular lesions[7] and shorten the course of active disease,[69] but it does not prevent late recurrences.[164]

Immunosuppressed Patients. Ocular toxoplasmosis in HIV-infected and other immunosuppressed patients usually responds well to antimicrobial therapy[117] (Figs. 85-16 to 85-19), although lack of response to treatment in severely inflamed eyes of patients with AIDS has been reported.[185]

Response to antimicrobial therapy can be remarkably fast.[90,117] Patients with red, painful eyes and decreased vision from vitritis may notice an improvement in just a few days. Lesions generally heal completely within 4 to 6 weeks. Gagliuso and associates[90] observed that there may be little pigmentary response with healing, in contrast to the hyperpigmented scars frequently seen in immunocompetent patients (Fig. 85-19). The lack of pigmentation may be due to the complete destruction of the retinal pigment epithelium layer, with the severe disease in immunosuppressed patients. In contrast, it may simply reflect the short follow-up of most reported patients with AIDS and ocular toxoplasmosis. Patients with AIDS and toxoplasmic retinochoroiditis who survive many months or years may eventually develop hyperpigmented scar borders (Figs. 85-16 and 85-17).

Because it is a continuously progressive disease, most clinicians will treat all cases of ocular toxoplasmosis in immunosuppressed patients, regardless of the location of lesions or visual acuity at diagnosis.[71] A variety of medications have been used, but many investigators believe that pyrimethamine in combination with at least one other antimicrobial agent is the most effective of the currently available medications.

Pyrimethamine is sometimes avoided, however, for the treatment of patients with AIDS. Pre-existing bone marrow suppression is one reason, and another involves the fact that zidovudine (an antiretroviral agent commonly used to treat HIV infection) has been shown to be antagonistic to pyrimethamine, which may lead to treatment failures if both

agents are used concurrently.[126] There is also a high rate of sulfonamide allergy among HIV-infected patients, which may limit the use of these agents in the treatment of toxoplasmosis.

Corticosteroids are generally not used in combination with antimicrobial agents for treatment of immunosuppressed patients for several reasons: inflammation does not appear to play an important role in tissue destruction; corticosteroids may further impair host defenses; and corticosteroids are generally not necessary for control of vitreous humor and anterior chamber inflammatory reactions. Inflammatory signs resolve rapidly with antimicrobial agents alone.

Disease Recurrences. Without treatment, toxoplasmic retinochoroiditis will probably recur in all patients with AIDS,[117] although there may be a lag of several months before recurrence.[221] Maintenance therapy with lower, sup-

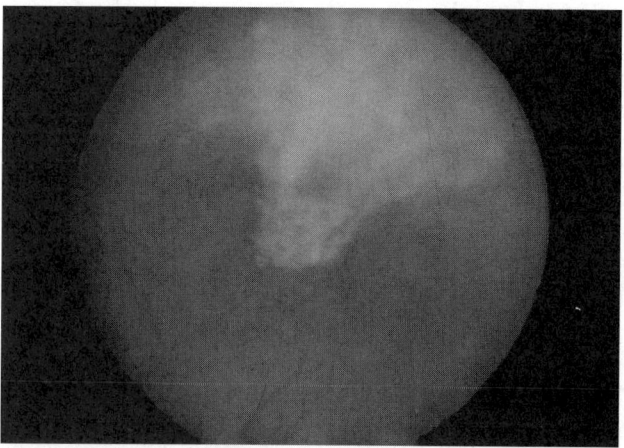

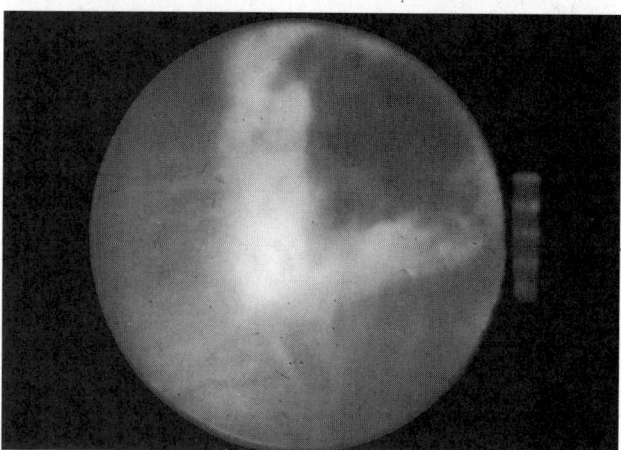

Fig. 85-25. A, Inactive retinochoroidal scar in a patient with AIDS and ocular toxoplasmosis following 1 month of treatment with oral pyrimethamine and sulfadiazine and 5 months of maintenance therapy using oral tetracycline (250 mg 4 times daily). **B,** Recurrent toxoplasmic retinochoroiditis at the borders of the scar (shown in **A**), following discontinuation of tetracycline therapy.

---

*References 7, 40, 56, 57, 69, 71, 149, 152, 164.

pressive doses of antimicrobial agents may prevent the reactivation of disease. A variety of maintenance therapies have been used in an attempt to prevent disease recurrence; they range from continuous, multiple drug therapy to intermittent, single drug therapy. Pyrimethamine has been used, although some clinicians prefer not to use it for chronic therapy because of the disadvantages of this drug cited previously. Uses of single drugs, such as tetracycline, that would not be effective for treatment of active disease have been reported anecdotally to be adequate for maintenance therapy (Fig. 85-25). Clindamycin was the most frequently cited agent for chronic maintenance therapy for immunosuppressed patients in the American Uveitis Society survey.[71]

PROGNOSIS

Toxoplasma gondii infection among immunocompetent adults is generally a benign and self-limited condition. In contrast, congenital toxoplasmosis can result in severe mental and physical impairments, even if the infection is inapparent at birth. Prognosis is poorest for patients symptomatic at birth; the mortality rate is 12%, and only 10% to 15% of surviving infants are left without debilitating sequelae.[69] Toxoplasmosis in immunosuppressed patients is a serious disease with a high mortality, especially when intracranial infection occurs.

Ocular Disease

In otherwise healthy patients with normal baseline visual acuity, the prognosis for retention of vision after episodes of recurrent or acquired toxoplasmic retinochoroiditis is good, because the active disease is self-limited. In a study of 63 patients, Friedmann and Knox[88] reported that in 26 of 58 patients without macular scars (45%), vision eventually dropped to 20/100 or less. An additional 10 patients (17%) had final visual acuities between 20/40 and 20/70. This study may overemphasize the risk of vision loss, however, as almost all patients had been referred to their tertiary care facility. Factors associated with poor visual outcomes included lesions in close proximity to the fovea, large lesions, and disease of long duration. The number of disease recurrences was not related to final visual outcomes.

With early diagnosis and appropriate therapy, the prognosis for retention of vision is also reasonably good for immunosuppressed patients, as the infection can usually be controlled by long-term therapy, using daily administration of one or more antimicrobial drugs.[117]

The factors that lead to severe, progressive disease in some patients, despite the lack of an obvious immunodeficiency state, are not well understood. They may relate to the virulence of different strains of *T. gondii.*

PREVENTION

Current efforts at prevention of toxoplasmosis focus on the interruption of disease transmission to human beings that occurs by ingestion of live tissue cysts or sporulated oocysts. Efforts to prevent disease transmission are especially important for immunosuppressed individuals and seronegative pregnant women. Tissue cysts in meat are destroyed by smoking, curing, and cooking at temperatures in excess of 66°C. Freezing meat at temperatures of $-20°C$ for 24 hours will also kill the tissue cyst form, but many home freezers do not reach that temperature. Fruits and vegetables, which may be contaminated with oocytes, should be washed thoroughly before ingestion. Contact with mucous membranes should be avoided when handling uncooked meat or unwashed vegetables and fruit. Kitchen countertops should be cleaned after working with these items, and hands should be washed. Raw eggs and unpasteurized milk (especially from goats) should not be consumed.

Contamination of closed areas by cat feces should be avoided, as airborne oocysts in dusty environments have been associated with epidemics of acquired toxoplasmosis. To avoid exposure to cat feces, it is commonly recommended that women not clean cat litter pans during pregnancy. Oocytes in cat litter pans can be killed by soaking the pan in nearly boiling water for 5 minutes. If the pan is cleaned daily, oocysts will not have time to sporulate before disposal.

Serologic screening of seronegative pregnant women can be used to reduce the rate of clinically significant congenital toxoplasmosis; appropriate screening techniques have been reviewed by Beaman and associates[15] and by Wong and Remington.[312]

Prevention of *T. gondii* transmission by organ transplantation or transfusion of leukocyte-rich blood products from infected donors is a subject of concern to infectious disease specialists. Prevention strategies have been reviewed by Beaman and associates.[15] It is not the current practice of blood or tissue banks to screen donors routinely for anti-*T. gondii* antibodies.

A goal for prevention of toxoplasmosis has been the development of an effective vaccine against the parasite. The fact that previous maternal infection in immunocompetent women prevents congenital infection suggests that a vaccine could be developed. Immunization of laboratory animals with a multiple antigenic peptide construction derived from p30 (the major surface antigen of *T. gondii*) results in partial protection against a lethal challenge with the parasite,[46] which further supports the possibility that an effective vaccine may eventually be developed. A vaccine for cats would also be useful as a means of interrupting the life cycle of *T. gondii.*

Ocular Disease

If the majority of ocular lesions are the result of disease reactivation, as is currently believed, then prevention of eye disease will ultimately depend on prevention of initial infection. Use of antiparasitic drugs as secondary prophylaxis (maintenance therapy) to prevent reactivation of ocular lesions is not warranted in most patients, as the frequency of recurrent disease is relatively low compared to the proportion of the population that is seropositive, and since many individuals with chorioretinal scars consistent with old toxoplasmic retinochoroiditis do not have a history of disease recurrences. It is apparent, however, that chronic antiparasitic therapy is necessary to prevent recurrences in immunosuppressed patients with recently active retinal lesions.

It has been shown that primary prophylaxis with a number of drug combinations, including trimethoprim-sulfamethoxazole, pyrimethamine-dapsone, and pyrimethamine-sulfadoxine, may decrease the incidence of toxoplasmic encephalitis in patients with AIDS.[313] The effect of primary prophylaxis on the incidence of ocular toxoplasmosis in patients with AIDS is not known, however.*

REFERENCES

1. Abrahams IW, Gregerson DS: Longitudinal study of serum antibody responses to retinal antigens in acute ocular toxoplasmosis, *Am J Ophthalmol* 93:224-231, 1982.
2. Acers TE: Toxoplasmic retinochoroiditis: a double blind therapeutic study, *Arch Ophthalmol* 71:58-63, 1964.
3. Adams LB, Hibbs JB, Taintor RR, Krahenbuhl JL: Microbiostatic effect of murine-activated macrophages for *Toxoplasma gondii:* role for synthesis of inorganic nitrogen oxides from L-arginine, *J Immunol* 144:2725-2729, 1990.
4. Aikawa M, Komata Y, Asai T, Midorikawa O: Transmission and scanning electron microscopy of host cell entry by *Toxoplasma gondii, Am J Pathol* 87:285-296, 1977.
5. Akstein RB, Wilson LA, Teutsch SM: Acquired toxoplasmosis, *Ophthalmology* 89:1299-1302, 1982.
6. Alford CA: Chronic congenital infections of man, *Yale J Biol Med* 55:187-192, 1982.
7. Alford CA, Stagno S, Reynolds DW: Congenital toxoplasmosis: clinical, laboratory, and therapeutic considerations, with special reference to subclinical disease, *Bull NY Acad Med* 50:160-181, 1974.
8. Anderson SE, Bautista SC, Remington JS: Specific antibody-dependent killing of *Toxoplasma gondii* by normal macrophages, *Clin Exp Immunol* 26:375-380, 1976.
9. Anderson SE, Remington JS: Effect of normal and activated human macrophages on *Toxoplasma gondii, J Exp Med* 139:1154-1174, 1974.
10. Anderson SE, Remington JS: The diagnosis of toxoplasmosis, *South Med J* 68:1433-1443, 1975.
10a. Araujo FG: Depletion of L3T4+ (CD4+) T lymphocytes prevents development of resistance to *Toxoplasma gondii* in mice, *Infect Immun* 59:1614-1619, 1991.
11. Araujo FG: Depletion of CD4+ T cells but not inhibition of the protective activity of IFN-gamma prevents cure of toxoplasmosis mediated by drug therapy in mice, *J Immunol* 149:3003-3007, 1992.
12. Araujo FG, Barnett EV, Gentry LO, Remington JS: False-positive anti-*Toxoplasma* fluorescent-antibody tests in patients with antinuclear antibodies, *Appl Microbiol* 22:270-275, 1971.
13. Araujo FG, Huskinson J, Remington JS: Remarkable in vitro and in vivo activities of the hydroxynaphthoquinone 566C80 against tachyzoites and tissue cysts of *Toxoplasma gondii, Antimicrob Agents Chemother* 35:293-299, 1991.
14. Asbell PA, Vermund SH, Hofeldt AJ: Presumed toxoplasmic retinochoroiditis in four siblings, *Am J Ophthalmol* 94:656-663, 1982.
15. Beaman MH, McCabe RE, Remington JS: Toxoplasma gondii. In Mandell GL, Bennett JE, Dolin R, editors: *Principles and practice of infectious diseases,* New York, 1995, Churchill Livingstone.

16. Beaman MH, Remington JS: IL-6 impairs macrophage killing of toxoplasma gondii and IFN gamma function, *Clin Res* 39:176A, 1991 (abstract).
17. Beaman MH, Remington JS: Cytokines and resistance against *Toxoplasma gondii:* evidence from in vivo and in vitro studies. In Sonnenfield G, Czarniecki C, Nancy C et al., editors: *Cytokines and resistance to nonviral pathogenic infections,* 111-119, New York, 1992, Biomedical Press.
18. Beaman MH, Wong SY, Remington JS: Cytokines, *Toxoplasma* and intracellular parasitism, *Immunol Rev* 127:97-117, 1992.
19. Berengo A, Frezzotti R: Active neuro-ophthalmic toxoplasmosis: a clinical study on nineteen patients, *Adv Ophthalmol* 12:265-343, 1962.
20. Berger BB, Egwuagu CE, Freeman WR, Wiley CA: Miliary toxoplasmic retinitis in acquired immunodeficiency syndrome, *Arch Ophthalmol* 111:373-376, 1993.
21. Binazzi M: Historical aspects of cutaneous toxoplasmosis, *Int J Dermatol* 25:401-404, 1986.
22. Bohne W, Heesemann J, Gross U: Induction of bradyzoite-specific *Toxoplasma gondii* antigens in gamma interferon-treated mouse macrophages, *Infect Immun* 61:1141-1145, 1993.
23. Bohne W, Heesemann J, Gross U: Reduced replication of *Toxoplasma gondii* is necessary for induction of bradyzoite-specific antigens: a possible role for nitric oxide in triggering stage conversion, *Infect Immun* 62:1761-1767, 1994.
24. Bottoni F, Gonnella P, Autelitano A, Orzalesi N: Diffuse necrotizing retinochoroiditis in a child with AIDS and toxoplasmic encephalitis, *Graefes Arch Clin Exp Ophthalmol* 228:36-39, 1990.
25. Braunstein RA, Gass DM: Branch artery obstruction caused by acute toxoplasmosis, *Arch Ophthalmol* 98:512-513, 1980.
26. Brezin AP, Egwuagu CE, Burnier MJ et al.: Identification of *Toxoplasma gondii* in paraffin-embedded sections by the polymerase chain reaction, *Am J Ophthalmol* 110:599-604, 1990.
27. Britt RH, Enzmann DR, Remington JS: Intracranial infection in cardiac transplant recipients, *Ann Neurol* 9:107-119, 1981.
28. Brooks RG, McCabe RE, Remington JS: Role of serology in the diagnosis of toxoplasmic lymphadenopathy, *Rev Infect Dis* 9:1055-1062, 1987.
29. Camargo ME, Ferreira AW, Mineo JR et al.: Immunoglobulin G and immunoglobulin M enzyme-linked immunosorbent assays and defined toxoplasmosis serological patterns, *Infect Immun* 21:55-58, 1978.
30. Canamucio CJ, Hallett JW, Leopold IH: Recurrence of treated toxoplasmic uveitis, *Am J Ophthalmol* 55:1035-1039, 1963.
31. Catterall JR, Hofflin JM, Remington JS: Pulmonary toxoplasmosis, *Am Rev Respir Dis* 133:704-705, 1986.
32. Chan CC, Palestine AG, Li Q, Nussenblatt RB: Diagnosis of ocular toxoplasmosis by the use of immunocytology and the polymerase chain reaction, *Am J Ophthalmol* 117:803-805, 1994 (letter).
33. Chang HR, Grau GE, Pechere JC: Role of TNF and IL-1 in infections with *Toxoplasma gondii, Immunology* 69:33-37, 1990.
34. Chardes T, Velge-Roussel F, Mevelec P et al.: Mucosal and systemic cellular immune responses induced by *Toxoplasma gondii* antigens in cyst orally infected mice, *Immunology* 78:421-429, 1993.
35. Chaves-Carballo J: Darling and human sarcosporosis or toxoplasmosis in Panama, *JAMA* 211:1687-1689, 1970.
36. Ciricillo SF, Rosenblum ML: Use of CT and MR imaging to distinguish intracranial lesions and to define the need for biopsy in AIDS patients, *J Neurosurg* 73:720-724, 1990.
37. Cochereau-Massin I, Lehoang P, Lautier-Frau M et al.: Ocular toxoplasmosis in human immunodeficiency virus-infected patients, *Am J Ophthalmol* 114:130-135, 1992.
38. Colin J, Harie JC: Chorioretinites presumees toxoplasmiques: etude comparative des traitements par pyrimethamine et sulfadiazine ou clindamycine, *J Fr Ophtalmol* 12:161-165, 1989.
39. Cotliar AM, Friedman AH: Subretinal neovascularisation in ocular toxoplasmosis, *Br J Ophthalmol* 66:524-529, 1982.
40. Couvreur J, Desmonts G: Congenital and maternal toxoplasmosis: a review of 300 congenital cases, *Dev Med Child Neurol* 4:519-530, 1962.
41. Culbertson WW, Tabbara KF, O'Connor R: Experimental ocular toxoplasmosis in primates, *Arch Ophthalmol* 100:321-323, 1982.

---

*Rajesh C. Rao, MD, Adnan Tufail, FRCOphth, and James M. Weisz, MD, provided valuable assistance in the preparation of this chapter.

42. Daffos F, Forestier F, Capella-Pavlovsky M et al.: Prenatal management of 746 pregnancies at risk for congenital toxoplasmosis, *N Engl J Med* 318:271-275, 1988.

43. Dannemann B, McCutchan JA, Israelski D et al.: Treatment of toxoplasmic encephalitis in patients with AIDS: a randomized trial comparing pyrimethamine plus clindamycin to pyrimethamine plus sulfadiazine: the California Collaborative Treatment Group, *Ann Intern Med* 116:33-43, 1992.

44. Dannemann BR, Morris VA, Araujo FG, Remington JS: Assessment of human natural killer and lymphokine-activated killer cell cytotoxicity against *Toxoplasma gondii* trophozoites and brain cysts, *J Immunol* 143:2684-2691, 1989.

45. Darcy F, Deslee D, Santoro F et al.: Induction of a protective antibody-dependent response against toxoplasmosis by in vitro excreted/secreted antigens from tachyzoites of *Toxoplasma gondii, Parasite Immunol* 10:553-567, 1988.

46. Darcy F, Maes P, Gras-Masse H et al.: Protection of mice and nude rats against toxoplasmosis by a multiple antigenic peptide construction derived from *Toxoplasma gondii* p30 antigen, *J Immunol* 149:3636-3641, 1992.

46a. Darde ML, Bouteille B, Pestre-Alexandre M: Isoenzyme analysis of 35 *Toxoplasma gondii* isolates and the biological and epidemiological implications, *J Parasitol* 78:786-794, 1992.

47. Darrell RW, Kurkland LT, Jacobs L: Chorioretinopathy and toxoplasmosis: an epidemiologic study on a south pacific island, *Arch Ophthalmol* 71:63-68, 1964.

48. Davis JL, Feuer W, Culbertson WW, Pflugfelder SC, Interpretation of intraocular and serum antibody levels in necrotizing retinitis, *Retina,* 1995 (in press).

49. Davis JL, Nussenblatt RB, Bachman DM et al.: Endogenous bacterial retinitis in AIDS, *Am J Ophthalmol* 107:613-623, 1989.

50. de Abreu MT, Belfort RJ, Hirata PS: Fuchs' heterochromic cyclitis and ocular toxoplasmosis, *Am J Ophthalmol* 93:739-744, 1982.

51. de Jong PT: Ocular toxoplasmosis; common and rare symptoms and signs, *Int Ophthalmol* 13:391-397, 1989.

52. De Paoli P, Basaglia G, Gennari D et al.: Phenotypic profile and functional characteristics of human gamma and delta T cells during acute toxoplasmosis, *J Clin Microbiol* 30:729-731, 1992.

53. Denkers EY, Gazzinelli RT, Hieny S et al.: Bone marrow macrophages process exogenous *Toxoplasma gondii* polypeptides for recognition by parasite-specific cytolytic T lymphocytes, *J Immunol* 150:517-526, 1993.

54. Derouin F, Gluckman E, Beauvais B et al.: Toxoplasma infection after human allogeneic bone marrow transplantation: clinical and serological study of 80 patients, *Bone Marrow Transplant* 1:67-73, 1986.

55. Desmonts G: Definitive serological diagnosis of ocular toxoplasmosis, *Arch Ophthalmol* 76:839-851, 1966.

56. Desmonts G, Couvreur J: Toxoplasmosis in pregnancy and its transmission to the fetus, *Bull NY Acad Med* 50:146-159, 1974a.

57. Desmonts G, Couvreur J: Congenital toxoplasmosis: a prospective study of 378 pregnancies, *N Engl J Med* 290:1110-1116, 1974b.

58. Desmonts G, Couvreur J, Thulliez P: Toxoplasmose congenitale: cinq cas de transmission a l'enfant d'une infection maternelle anterieure a la grossesse, *Presse Med* 19:1445-1449, 1990.

59. Desmonts G, Remington JS: Direct agglutination test for diagnosis of *Toxoplasma infection:* method for increasing sensitivity and specificity, *J Clin Microbiol* 11:562-568, 1980.

60. Dobbie JG: Cryotherapy in the management of toxoplasma retinochoroiditis, *Trans Am Acad Ophthalmol Otolaryngol* 72:364-373, 1968.

61. Doft BH: Choroidoretinal vascular anastomosis, *Arch Ophthalmol* 101:1053-1054, 1983.

62. Doft BH, Gass DM: Punctate outer retinal toxoplasmosis, *Arch Ophthalmol* 103:1332-1336, 1985.

63. Dorfman RF, Remington JS: Value of lymph-node biopsy in the diagnosis of acute acquired toxoplasmosis, *N Engl J Med* 289:878-881, 1973.

64. Dubey JP: A review of toxoplasmosis in pigs, *Vet Parasitol* 19:181-223, 1986.

65. Dubey JP, Miller NL, Frenkel JK: The *Toxoplasma gondii* oocyst from cat feces, *J Exp Med* 132:636-662, 1970.

66. Duquesne V, Auriault C, Darcy F et al.: Protection of nude rats against *Toxoplasma* infection by excreted-secreted antigen-specific helper T cells, *Infect Immun* 58:2120-2126, 1990.

67. Dutton GN, Hay J: Toxoplasmic retinochoroiditis—current concepts in pathogenesis, *Trans Ophthalmol Soc UK* 103:503-507, 1983.

68. Dutton GN, McMenamin PG, Hay J, Cameron S: The ultrastructural pathology of congenital murine toxoplasmic retinochoroiditis. Part II: The morphology of the inflammatory changes, *Exp Eye Res* 43:545-560, 1986.

69. Eichenwald HF: A study of congenital toxoplasmosis: with particular emphasis on clinical manifestations, sequellae and therapy. In Siim JC, editors: *Human toxoplasmosis,* Baltimore, 1959, Williams & Wilkins.

70. Elkins BS, Holland GN, Opremcak EM et al.: Ocular toxoplasmosis misdiagnosed as cytomegalovirus retinopathy in immunocompromised patients, *Ophthalmology* 101:499-507, 1994.

71. Engstrom RE, Holland GN, Nussenblatt RB, Jabs DA: Current practices in the management of ocular toxoplasmosis, *Am J Ophthalmol* 111:601-610, 1991.

72. Eyles DE, Coleman N: Synergistic effect of sulphadiazine and daraprim against experimental toxoplasmosis in the mouse, *Antibiot Chemother* 3:483-490, 1953.

73. Fair JR: Congenital toxoplasmosis: chorioretinitis as the only manifestation of the disease, *Am J Ophthalmol* 46:135-254, 1958.

74. Fair JR: Clinical eye findings in congenital toxoplasmosis, *Surv Ophthalmol* 6:923-935, 1961.

75. Falcone PM, Notis C, Merhige K: Toxoplasmic papillitis as the initial manifestation of acquired immunodeficiency syndrome, *Ann Ophthalmol* 25:56-57, 1993.

76. Feldman HA: Congenital toxoplasmosis: a study of one hundred and three cases, *Am J Dis Child* 86:487-489, 1953.

77. Feldman HA, Miller LT: Serological study of ocular toxoplasmosis, *Am J Hyg* 64:320, 1956.

78. Fine SL, Owens SL, Haller JA et al.: Choroidal neovascularization as a late complication of ocular toxoplasmosis, *Am J Ophthalmol* 91:318-322, 1981.

79. Fish RH, Hoskins JC, Kline LB: Toxoplasmosis neuroretinitis, *Ophthalmology* 100:1177-1182, 1993.

80. Fitzgerald CR: Pars plana vitrectomy for vitreous opacity secondary to presumed toxoplasmosis, *Arch Ophthalmol* 98:321-323, 1980.

81. Frenkel JF: Toxoplasmosis: parasite life cycle, pathology, and immunology. In Hammond DM, Long PL, editors: *The Coccidia: eimeria, isospora, toxoplasma, and related genera,* Baltimore, 1973, University Park Press.

82. Frenkel JK: Effect of cortisone, total body irradiation and nitrogen mustard on chronic latent toxoplasmosis, *Am J Pathol* 33:618-619, 1957.

83. Frenkel JK: Pathogenesis of toxoplasmosis with a consideration of cyst rupture in besnoitia infection, *Surv Ophthalmol* 6:799-825, 1961.

84. Frenkel JK: Ocular toxoplasmosis, *JAMA* 272:356, 1994.

85. Frenkel JK, Dubey JP, Miller NL: *Toxoplasma gondii* in cats: fecal stages identified by as coccodian oocysts, *Science* 167:893-896, 1970.

86. Freund YR, Sgarlato G, Jacob CO et al.: Polymorphisms in the tumor necrosis factor alpha (TNF-α) gene correlate with murine resistance to development of toxoplasmic encephalitis and with levels of TNF-α mRNA in infected brain tissue, *J Exp Med* 175:683-688, 1992.

87. Frezzotti R, Berengo A, Guerra R, Cavallini F: Toxoplasmic Coats' retinitis: a parasitologically proved case, *Am J Ophthalmol* 59:1099-1102, 1965.

88. Friedmann CT, Knox DL: Variations in recurrent active toxoplasmic retinochoroiditis, *Arch Ophthalmol* 81:481-493, 1969.

89. Furtado GC, Slowik M, Kleinman HK, Joiner KA: Laminin enhances binding of *Toxoplasma gondii* tachyzoites to J774 murine macrophage cells, *Infect Immun* 60:2337-2342, 1992.

90. Gagliuso DJ, Teich SA, Friedman AH, Orellana J: Ocular toxoplasmosis in AIDS patients, *Trans Am Ophthalmol Soc* 88:63-86; discussion 86-88, 1990.

91. Garcia AG: Congenital toxoplasmosis in two successive sibs, *Arch Dis Child* 43:705-710, 1968.

92. Gaynon MW, Boldrey EE, Strahlman ER, Fine SL: Retinal neovascularization and ocular toxoplasmosis, *Am J Ophthalmol* 98:585-589, 1984.

93. Gazzinelli RT, Brezin A, Li Q et al.: *Toxoplasma gondii:* acquired ocular toxoplasmosis in the murine model, protective role of TNF-α and IFN-γ, *Exp Parasitol* 78:217-229, 1994.

94. Gazzinelli RT, Eltoum I, Wynn TA, Sher A: Acute cerebral toxoplasmosis is induced by in vivo neutralization of TNF-α and correlates with the down-regulated expression of inducible nitric oxide synthase and other markers of macrophage activation, *J Immunol* 151:3672-3681, 1993.

95. Gazzinelli RT, Hakim FT, Hieny S et al.: Synergistic role of CD4+ and CD8+ T lymphocytes in IFN-γ production and protective immunity induced by an attenuated *Toxoplasma gondii* vaccine, *J Immunol* 146:286-292, 1991.

96. Gazzinelli RT, Oswald IP, James SL, Sher A: IL-10 inhibits parasite killing and nitrogen oxide production by IFN-γ-activated macrophages, *J Immunol* 148:1792-1796, 1992.

97. Gazzinelli RT, Xu Y, Hieny S et al.: Simultaneous depletion of CD4+ and CD8+ T lymphocytes is required to reactivate chronic infection with *Toxoplasma gondii, J Immunol* 149:175-180, 1992.

98. Ghartey KN, Brockhurst RJ: Photocoagulation of active toxoplasmic retinochoroiditis, *Am J Ophthalmol* 89:858-864, 1980.

99. Gilbert HD: Unusual presentation of acute ocular toxoplasmosis, *Graefes Arch Clin Exp Ophthalmol* 215:53-58, 1980.

100. Girard P, Kohen D, Chevalier C, Forest A: Necrose retinienne aigue et toxoplasmose oculaire, *Bull Soc Ophtalmol Fr* 84:751-754, 1984.

101. Glasner PD, Silveira C, Kruszon-Moran D et al.: An unusually high prevalence of ocular toxoplasmosis in southern Brazil, *Am J Ophthalmol* 114:136-144, 1992.

102. Grant SC, Klein C: *Toxoplasma gondii* encephalitis in an immunocompetent adult: a case report, *S Afr Med J* 71:585-587, 1987.

103. Gray F, Gherardi R, Wingate E et al.: Diffuse "encephalitic" cerebral toxoplasmosis in AIDS: report of four cases, *J Neurol* 236:273-277, 1989.

104. Greven CM, Teot LA: Cytologic identification of *Toxoplasma gondii* from vitreous fluid, *Arch Ophthalmol* 112:1086-1088, 1994.

105. Grimwood J, Smith JE: *Toxoplasma gondii:* the role of a 30-kDa surface protein in host cell invasion, *Exp Parasitol* 74:106-111, 1992.

106. Grossniklaus HE, Specht CS, Allaire G, Leavitt JA: *Toxoplasma gondii* retinochoroiditis and optic neuritis in acquired immune deficiency syndrome: report of a case, *Ophthalmology* 97:1342-1346, 1990.

107. Hakim FT, Gazzinelli RT, Denkers E et al.: CD8+ T cells from mice vaccinated against *Toxoplasma gondii* are cytotoxic for parasite-infected or antigen-pulsed host cells, *J Immunol* 147:2310-2316, 1991.

108. Hamed LM, Schatz NJ, Galetta SL: Brainstem ocular motility defects and AIDS, *Am J Ophthalmol* 106:437-442, 1988.

109. Hausmann N, Richard G: Acquired ocular toxoplasmosis: a fluorescein angiography study, *Ophthalmology* 98:1647-1651, 1991.

110. Henderly DE, Genstler AJ, Smith RE, Rao NA: Changing patterns of uveitis, *Am J Ophthalmol* 103:131-136, 1987.

111. Henderson WR, Chi EY: Cytotoxic activity of 13-hydroxyoctadecadienoic acid against *Toxoplasma gondii, Parasitology* 105:343-347, 1992.

112. Herskovitz S, Siegel SE, Schneider AT et al.: Spinal cord toxoplasmosis in AIDS, *Neurology* 39:1552-1553, 1989.

113. Hoerni B, Vallat M, Durand M, Pesme D: Ocular toxoplasmosis and Hodgkin's disease: report of two cases, *Arch Ophthalmol* 96:62-63, 1978.

114. Hogan MJ, Kimura SJ, O'Connor GR: Oculat toxoplasmosis, *Arch Ophthalmol* 72:592-600, 1964.

115. Hogan MJ, Zweigart P, Lewis A: Recovery of toxoplasma from a human eye, *Arch Ophthalmol* 60:548-554, 1958.

116. Holland GN: Ocular toxoplasmosis in the immunocompromised host, *Int Ophthalmol* 13:399-402, 1989.

117. Holland GN, Engstrom RE, Glasgow BJ et al.: Ocular toxoplasmosis in patients with the acquired immunodeficiency syndrome, *Am J Ophthalmol* 106:653-667, 1988.

118. Holland GN, O'Connor GR, Diaz RF et al.: Ocular toxoplasmosis in immunosuppressed nonhuman primates, *Invest Ophthalmol Vis Sci* 29:835-842, 1988.

119. Hughes WT, Kennedy W, Shenep JL et al.: Safety and pharmacokinetics of 566C80, a hydroxynaphthoquinone with anti-*Pneumocystis carinii* activity: a phase I study in human immunodeficiency virus (HIV)-infected men, *J Infect Dis* 163:843-848, 1991.

120. Hunter CA, Litton MJ, Remington JS, Abrams JS: Immunocytochemical detection of cytokines in the lymph nodes and brains of mice resistant or susceptible to toxoplasmic encephalitis, *J Infect Dis* 170:939-945, 1994.

121. Hunter CA, Remington JS: Immunopathogenesis of toxoplasmic encephalitis, *J Infect Dis* 170:1057-1067, 1994.

122. Hunter CA, Roberts CW, Alexander J: Kinetics of cytokine mRNA production in the brains of mice with progressive toxoplasmic encephalitis, *Eur J Immunol* 22:2317-2322, 1992.

123. Huskinson-Mark J, Araujo FG, Remington JS: Evaluation of the effect of drugs on the cyst form of *Toxoplasma gondii, J Infect Dis* 164:170-171, 1991.

124. Hutchison WM, Dunachie JF, Work K: The life cycle of the coccidian parasite *Toxoplasma gondii,* in the domestic cat, *Trans R Soc Trop Med Hyg* 89:759-782, 1971.

125. Israelski DM, Remington JS: Toxoplasmosis in the non-AIDS immunocompromised host, *Curr Clin Top Infect Dis* 13:322-356, 1993.

126. Israelski DM, Tom C, Remington JS: Zidovudine antagonizes the action of pyrimethamine in experimental infection with *Toxoplasma gondii, Antimicrob Agents Chemother* 33:30-34, 1989.

127. Jabs DA, Green WR, Fox R et al.: Ocular manifestations of the acquired immune deficiency syndrome, *Ophthalmology* 96:1092-1099, 1989.

128. Jacobs L, Fair JR, Bickerton JH: Adult ocular toxoplasmosis (report of a parisitologically proved case), *Arch Ophthalmol* 52:63, 1954.

129. Jacobs L, Naquin H, Woods AC: A comparison of the toxoplasmin skin tests, the Sabin-Feldman dye tests, and the complement fixation tests for toxoplasmosis in various forms of uveitis, *Bull John Hopkins* 99:1-15, 1956.

130. Jankû J: Pathogensa a pathologica anatomie T. Zv. vrozaneho kolobou zlute skurney oku normal ne velikem a mikrophtalmickem s nalezem parisitu v sitnici, *Cas Lek Cesk* 62:1021-1027, 1923.

131. Jankû J: Die pathogenese und pathologische anatomie des sogenannten angeborenen kloloboms des gelben flecks im normal grossen sowie mikropthalmischen auge mit parasitenbefund in der netzhaut, *Cls Parasit* 6:9-16, 1959.

132. Jarvik JG, Hesselink JR, Kennedy C et al.: Acquired immunodeficiency syndrome: magnetic resonance patterns of brain involvement with pathologic correlation, *Arch Neurol* 45:731-736, 1988.

133. Johnson LL: A protective role for endogenous tumor necrosis factor in *Toxoplasma gondii* infection, *Infect Immun* 60:1979-1983, 1992.

134. Joiner KA, Dubremetz JF: *Toxoplasma gondii:* a protozoan for the nineties, *Infect Immun* 61:1169-1172, 1993.

135. Joiner KA, Fuhrman SA, Miettinen HM et al.: *Toxoplasma gondii:* fusion competence of parasitophorous vacuoles in Fc receptor-transfected fibroblasts, *Science* 249:641-646, 1990.

136. Jones TC, Bienz KA, Erb P: In vitro cultivation of *Toxoplasma gondii* cysts in astrocytes in the presence of gamma interferon, *Infect Immun* 51:147-156, 1986.

137. Jones TC, Hirsch JG: The interaction between *Toxoplasma gondii* and mammalian cells. II. The absence of lysosomal fusion with phagocytic vacuoles containing living parasites, *J Exp Med* 136:1173-1194, 1972.

138. Jones TC, Yeh S, Hirsch JG: The interaction between *Toxoplasma gondii* and mammalian cells. I. Mechanism of entry and intracellular fate of the parasite, *J Exp Med* 136:1157-1172, 1972.

139. Kasper LH: Isolation and characterization of a monoclonal anti-P30 antibody resistant mutant of *Toxoplasma gondii, Parasite Immunol* 9:433-445, 1987.

140. Kasper LH, Crabb JH, Pfefferkorn ER: Isolation and characterization of a monoclonal antibody-resistant antigenic mutant of *Toxoplasma gondii, J Immunol* 129:1694-1699, 1982.

141. Kasper LH, Crabb JH, Pfefferkorn ER: Purification of a major membrane protein of *Toxoplasma gondii* by immunoabsorption with a monoclonal antibody, *J Immunol* 130:2407-2412, 1983.

142. Kasper LH, Khan IA, Ely KH et al.: Antigen-specific (p30) mouse CD8+ T cells are cytotoxic against *Toxoplasma gondii*-infected peritoneal macrophages, *J Immunol* 148:1493-1498, 1992.

143. Kass EH, Andrus SB, Adams RD et al.: Toxoplasmosis in the human adult, *Arch Intern Med* 89:759-782, 1952.

144. Kaufman HE: The effect of corticosteroid on experimental ocular toxoplasmosis, *Am J Ophthalmol* 50:919-926, 1960.

145. Kean BH: Clinical toxoplasmosis—50 years, *Trans R Soc Trop Med Hyg* 66:549-571, 1972.

146. Kennedy JE, Wise GN: Retinochoroidal vascular anastamosis in uveitis, *Am J Ophthalmol* 71:1221-1225, 1971.

147. Khan IA, Eckel ME, Pfefferkorn ER, Kasper LH: Production of gamma interferon by cultured human lymphocytes stimulated by purified membrane protein (P30) from *Toxoplasma gondii, J Infect Dis* 157:979-984, 1988.

148. Khan IA, Smith KA, Kasper LH: Induction of antigen-specific human cytotoxic T cells by *Toxoplasma gondii, J Clin Invest* 85:1879-1886, 1990.

149. Kimball AC, Kean BH, Fuchs F: Congenital toxoplasmosis: a prospective study of 4,048 obstetric patients, *Am J Obstet Gynecol* 111:211-218, 1971.

150. Klainer AS, Krahenbuhl JL, Remington JS: Scanning electron microscopy of *Toxoplasma gondii, J Gen Microbiol* 75:111-118, 1973.

151. Koch FL, Wolf A, Cowen D, Paige BH: Toxoplasmic encephalomyelitis. VII. Significance of ocular lesions in the diagnosis of infantile or congenital toxoplasmosis, *Arch Ophthalmol* 29:1-25, 1943.

152. Koppe JG, Klooterman GJ, de Roever-Bonnet H et al.: Toxoplasmosis and pregnancy, with a long-term follow-up of the children, *Eur J Obstet Gynecol Reprod Biol* 4:101-110, 1974.

153. Kraushar MF, Gluck SB, Pass S: Toxoplasmic retinochoroiditis presenting as serous detachment of the macula, *Ann Ophthalmol* 11:1513-1514, 1979.

154. Kyrieleis W: Uber atypische gerfaesstuberkulose der netzhaut (periareritis "nodosa" tuberculosa), *Arch Augenheilkd* 107:182-190, 1933.

155. La Heij E, Rothova A: Fuchs' heterochromic cyclitis in congenital ocular toxoplasmosis, *Br J Ophthalmol* 75:372-373, 1991.

156. La Hey E, Rothova A, Baarsma S et al.: Fuchs' heterochromic cyclitis is not associated with ocular toxoplasmosis, *Arch Ophthalmol* 110:806-811, 1992.

157. Lakhanpal V, Schocket SS, Nirankari VS: Clindamycin in the treatment of toxoplasmic retinochoroiditis, *Am J Ophthalmol* 95:605-613, 1983.

158. Langermans JA, Van der Hulst ME, Nibbering PH et al.: IFN-γ-induced L-arginine-dependent toxoplasmastatic activity in murine peritoneal macrophages is mediated by endogenous tumor necrosis factor-α, *J Immunol* 148:568-574, 1992.

159. Langermans JA, Van der Hulst ME, Nibbering PH, Van Furth R: Endogenous tumor necrosis factor α is required for enhanced antimicrobial activity against *Toxoplasma gondii* and *Listeria monocytogenes* in recombinant γ interferon-treated mice, *Infect Immun* 60:5107-5112, 1992.

160. Laveran A: Au sujet de l'haematozoaire endoglobulaire de Padda oryzivora, *Compt Rend Soc Biol Paris* 52:19-20, 1900.

161. Levy RM, Bredesen DE, Rosenblum ML: Neurological manifestations of the acquired immunodeficiency syndrome (AIDS): experience at UCSF and review of the literature, *J Neurosurg* 62:475-495, 1985.

162. Levy RM, Mills CM, Posin JP et al.: The efficacy and clinical impact of brain imaging in neurologically symptomatic AIDS patients: a prospective CT/MRI study, *J Acquir Immune Defic Syndr* 3:461-471, 1990.

163. Levy RM, Rosenbloom S, Perrett LV: Neuroradiologic findings in AIDS: a review of 200 cases, *Am J Roentgenol* 147:977-983, 1986.

164. Loewer-Sieger DH, Rothova A, Koppe JG, Kylstra A: Congenital toxoplasmosis, a prospective study based on 1821 pregnant women. In Saari KM, editors: *Uveitis update,* Amsterdam, 1984, Elsevier Science Publishers.

165. Lopez JS, De Smet MD, Masur H et al.: Orally administered 566C80 for treatment of ocular toxoplasmosis in a patient with the acquired immunodeficiency syndrome, *Am J Ophthalmol* 113:331-333, 1992 (letter).

166. Lou P, Kazdan J, Basu PK: Ocular toxoplasmosis in three consecutive siblings, *Arch Ophthalmol* 96:613-614, 1978.

167. Lucet JC, Bailly MP, Bedos JP et al.: Septic shock due to toxoplasmosis in patients infected with the human immunodeficiency virus, *Chest* 104:1054-1058, 1993.

168. Luft BJ, Brooks RG, Conley FK et al.: Toxoplasmic encephalitis in patients with acquired immune deficiency syndrome, *JAMA* 252:913-917, 1984.

169. Luft BJ, Naot Y, Araujo FG et al.: Primary and reactivated toxoplasma infection in patients with cardiac transplants: clinical spectrum and problems in diagnosis in a defined population, *Ann Intern Med* 99:27-31, 1983.

170. Luft BJ, Remington JS: Toxoplamic encephalitis in AIDS, *Clin Infect Dis* 15:211-222, 1992.

171. Mack DG, McLeod R: Human *Toxoplasma gondii*-specific secretory immunoglobulin A reduces *T. gondii* infection of enterocytes in vitro, *J Clin Invest* 90:2585-2592, 1992.

172. Maetz HM, Kleinstein RN, Federico D, Wayne J: Estimated prevalence of ocular toxoplasmosis and toxocariasis in Alabama, *J Infect Dis* 156:414, 1987 (letter).

173. Manners RM, O'Connell S, Guy EC et al.: Use of the polymerase chain reaction in the diagnosis of acquired ocular toxoplasmosis in an immunocompetent adult, *Br J Ophthalmol* 78:583-584, 1994.

174. Manschot WA: Connatal ocular toxoplasmosis, *Arch Ophthalmol* 74:49-54, 1965.

175. Martins MC, Desmonts G, Couvreur J, Ben Rachid MS: Le toxoplasme: la mere et l'enfant, *Arch Fr Pediatr* 22:1183-1190, 1965.

176. Masur H, Jones TC, Lempert JA, Cherubini TD: Outbreak of toxoplasmosis in a family and documentation of acquired retinochoroiditis, *Am J Med* 64:396-402, 1978.

177. Matthews JD, Weiter JJ: Outer retinal toxoplasmosis, *Ophthalmology* 95:941-946, 1988.

178. McCabe RE, Brooks RG, Dorfman RF, Remington JS: Clinical spectrum in 107 cases of toxoplasmic lymphadenopathy, *Rev Infect Dis* 9:754-774, 1987.

179. McCannel C, Holland GN, Helm CJ et al.: Causes of uveitis in the general practice of ophthalmology, *Am J Ophthalmol,* 1995 (in press).

180. McCauley JB, Boyer KM, Patel D et al.: Early and longitudinal evaluations of treated infants and children and untreated historical patients with congenital toxoplasmosis: The Chicago Collaborative Treatment Trial, *Clin Infect Dis* 18:38-72, 1994.

181. McMaster PR, Powers KG, Finerty JF, Lunde MN: The effect of two chlorinated lincomycin analogues against acute toxoplasmosis in mice, *Am J Trop Med Hyg* 22:14-17, 1973.

182. McMenamin PG, Dutton GN, Hay J, Cameron S: The ultrastructural pathology of congenital murine toxoplasmic retinochoroiditis. Part I: The localization and morphology of *Toxoplasma* cysts in the retina, *Exp Eye Res* 43:529-543, 1986.

183. Mets MB, Holfels E, Boyer KM et al.: Congenital toxoplasmosis: the eye manifestations, 1995 (submitted).

184. Mineo JR, Kasper LH: Attachment of *Toxoplasma gondii* to host cells involves major surface protein, SAG-1 (P30), *Exp Parasitol* 79:11-20, 1994.

185. Moorthy RS, Smith RE, Rao NA: Progressive ocular toxoplasmosis in patients with acquired immunodeficiency syndrome, *Am J Ophthalmol* 115:742-747, 1993.

186. Moreno RJ, Weisman J, Waller S: Neuroretinitis: an unusual presentation of ocular toxoplasmosis, *Ann Ophthalmol* 24:68-70, 1992.

187. Murray HW, Cohn ZA: Macrophage oxygen-dependent antimicrobial activity. I. Susceptibility of *Toxoplasma gondii* to oxygen intermediates, *J Exp Med* 150:938-949, 1979.

188. Murray HW, Hillman JK, Rubin BY et al.: Patients at risk for AIDS-related opportunistic infections: clinical manifestations and impaired gamma interferon production, *N Engl J Med* 313:1504-1510, 1985.

189. Murray HW, Rubin BY, Masur H, Roberts RB: Impaired production of lymphokines and immune (γ) interferon in the acquired immunodeficiency syndrome, *N Engl J Med* 310:883-889, 1984.

190. Murray HW, Szuro-Sudol A, Wellner D et al.: Role of tryptophan degradation in respiratory burst-independent antimicrobial activity of gamma interferon-stimulated human macrophages, *Infect Immun* 57:845-849, 1989.

191. Nagasawa H, Oka M, Maeda K et al.: Induction of heat shock protein closely correlates with protection against *Toxoplasma gondii* infection, *Proc Natl Acad Sci USA* 89:3155-3158, 1992.

192. Nahmias AJ, Walls KW, Stewart JA et al.: The TORCH complex-perinatal infection with toxoplasma and rubella, cytomegalo- and herpes simplex viruses, *Pediatr Res* 5:405-406, 1971.

193. Naot Y, Barnett EV, Remington JS: Method for avoiding false-positive results occurring in immunoglobulin M enzyme-linked immunosorbent assays due to presence of both rheumatoid factor and antinuclear antibodies, *J Clin Microbiol* 14:73-78, 1981.

194. Nathan CF, Murray HW, Wiebe ME, Rubin BY: Identification of interferon-γ as the lymphokine that activates human macrophage oxidative metabolism and antimicrobial activity, *J Exp Med* 158:670-689, 1983.

195. Newman PE, Ghosheh R, Tabbara KF et al.: The role of hypersensitivity reactions to toxoplasma antigens in experimental ocular toxoplasmosis in nonhuman primates, *Am J Ophthalmol* 94:159-164, 1982.

196. Newsome DA, Green WR, Miller ED et al.: Microvascular aspects of acquired immune deficiency syndrome retinopathy, *Am J Ophthalmol* 98:590-601, 1984.

197. Nichols BA, Chiappino ML, O'Connor GR: Secretion from the rhoptries of *Toxoplasma gondii* during host-cell invasion, *J Ultrastruct Res* 83:85-98, 1983.

198. Nichols BA, O'Connor GR: Penetration of mouse peritoneal macrophages by the protozoon *Toxoplasma gondii:* new evidence for active invasion and phagocytosis, *Lab Invest* 44:324-335, 1981.

199. Nicholson DH, Wolchok EB: Ocular toxoplasmosis in an adult receiving long-term corticosteroid therapy, *Arch Ophthalmol* 94:248-254, 1976.

200. Nicolle C, Manceaux L: Sur une infection a corps de Leishmen (ou organismes voisins) du gondi, *C R Seances Soc Biol Fil* 147:763-766, 1908.

201. Nicolle C, Manceaux L: Sur une prozaire nouveau du gondi (*Toxoplasma* n.g.), *Arch Inst Pasteur Tunis* 4:97-100, 1909.

202. Nozik RA, O'Connor GR: Studies on experimental ocular toxoplasmosis in the rabbit. II. Attempts to stimulate recurrence by local trauma, epinephrine, and corticosteroids, *Arch Ophthalmol* 84:788-794, 1970.

203. Nussenblatt RB, Mittal KK, Fuhrman S et al.: Lymphocyte proliferative responses of patients with ocular toxoplasmosis to parasite and retinal antigens, *Am J Ophthalmol* 107:632-641, 1989.

204. O'Connor GR: The influence of hypersensitivity on the pathogenesis of ocular toxoplasmosis, *Trans Am Ophthalmol Soc* 68:501-547, 1970.

205. O'Connor GR: Manifestations and management of ocular toxoplasmosis, *Bull N Y Acad Med* 50:192-210, 1974.

206. O'Connor GR: The mucosae as possible sites of entrance for *Toxoplasma gondii.* In O'Connor GR, editors: *Immunologic diseases of the mucous membrane,* New York, 1980, Masson Publishing Group.

207. O'Connor GR: The role of parasite invasion and of hypersensitivity in the pathogenesis of toxoplasmic retinochoroiditis, *Ocular Inflammation Ther* 1:37-46, 1983a.

208. O'Connor GR: Factors related to the initiation and recurrence of uveitis: XL Edward Jackson memorial lecture, *Am J Ophthalmol* 96:577-599, 1983b.

209. O'Connor GR: *Toxoplasma.* In Tasman W, Jaeger EA, editors: *Duane's biomedical foundations of ophthalmology,* Philadelphia, 1987, Harper & Row.

210. O'Connor GR, Nozik RA: Studies on factors influencing the recurrence of ocular toxoplasmosis. In Solanes MP, editors: *Ophthalmology: proceedings of the XXI International Congress,* Amsterdam, 1971, Excerpta Medica.

211. Oksenhendler E, Cadranel J, Sarfati C et al.: *Toxoplasma gondii* pneumonia in patients with the acquired immunodeficiency syndrome, *Am J Med* 88:18N-21N, 1990.

212. Opremcak EM, Scales DK, Sharpe MR: Trimethoprim-sulfamethoxazole therapy for ocular toxoplasmosis, *Ophthalmology* 99:920-925, 1992.

213. Parker SJ, Roberts CW, Alexander J: CD8+ T cells are the major lymphocyte subpopulation involved in the protective immune response to *Toxoplasma gondii* in mice, *Clin Exp Immunol* 84:207-212, 1991.

214. Pass RF, Morris RE, Shaw JF, Diethelm AG: Ocular toxoplasmosis after renal transplantation, *South Med J* 74:1033-1034, 1981.

215. Pauleikhoff D, Messmer E, Beelen DW et al.: Bone-marrow transplantation and toxoplasmic retinochoroiditis, *Graefes Arch Clin Exp Ophthalmol* 225:239-243, 1987.

216. Pavia CS: Protection against experimental toxoplasmosis by adoptive immunotherapy, *J Immunol* 137:2985-2990, 1986.

217. Perkins ES: Ocular toxoplasmosis, *Br J Ophthalmol* 57:1-17, 1973.

218. Perkins ES, Folk J: Uveitis in London and Iowa, *Ophthalmologica* 189:36-40, 1984.

219. Perkins ES, Smith CH, Schofield PB: Treatment of uveitis with pyrimethamine (Daraprim), *Br J Ophthalmol* 40:577-583, 1956.

220. Perry DD, Marritt JC, Greenwood RS et al.: Congenital toxoplasmosis associated with acquired oculomotor nerve (CN III) palsy, *J Pediatr Ophthalmol Strabismus* 19:265-269, 1982.

221. Pillai S, Mahmood MA, Limaye SR: Herpes zoster ophthalmicus, contralateral hemiplegia, and recurrent ocular toxoplasmosis in a patient with acquired immune deficiency syndrome-related complex, *J Neuroophthalmol* 9:229-233; discussion 234-235, 1989.

222. Pillat A, Thalhammer O: Herdformige iridocyclitis als (einige) Manifestation einer ereworbenen Toxoplasmose, atiologisch gesichert durch titerkurve und tierversuch, *Graefes Arch Clin Exp Ophthalmol* 158:403-415, 1957.

223. Pinon JM, Toubas D, Marx C et al.: Detection of specific immunoglobulin E in patients with toxoplasmosis, *J Clin Microbiol* 28:1739-1743, 1990.

224. Poirriez J, Toubas D, Marx-Chemla C et al.: Isotypic characterization of anti-*Toxoplasma gondii* antibodies in 18 cases of congenital toxoplasmic chorioretinitis, *Acta Ophthalmol (Copenh)* 67:164-168, 1989.

225. Pomeroy C, Filice GA: Pulmonary toxoplasmosis: a review, *Clin Infect Dis* 14:863-870, 1992.

226. Porter SB, Sande MA: Toxoplasmosis of the central nervous system in the acquired immunodeficiency syndrome, *N Engl J Med* 327:1643-1648, 1992.

227. Rao NA, Font RL: Toxoplasmic retinochoroiditis: electron-microscopic and immunofluorescence studies of formalin-fixed tissue, *Arch Ophthalmol* 95:273-277, 1977.

228. Raymond J, Poissonnier MH, Thulliez PH et al.: Presence of γ interferon in human acute and congenital toxoplasmosis (published erratum appears in *J Clin Microbiol* 28(12):2853, 1990), *J Clin Microbiol* 28:1434-1437, 1990.

229. Reese LT, Shafer DM, Zweifach P: Acute acquired toxoplasmosis, *Ann Ophthalmol* 13:467-470, 1981.

230. Rehder JR, Burnier MB, Pavesio CE et al.: Acute unilateral toxoplasmic iridocyclitis in an AIDS patient, *Am J Ophthalmol* 106:740-741, 1988.

231. Remington JS: Toxoplasmosis in the adult, *Bull NY Acad Med* 50:211-227, 1974.

232. Remington JS, Barnett CG, Meikel M, Lunde MN: Toxoplasmosis and infectious mononucleosis, *Arch Intern Med* 110:250-259, 1962.

233. Remington JS, Desmonts G: Toxoplasmosis. In Remington JS, Klein JO, editors: *Infectious diseases of the fetus and newborn infant,* ed 4, Philadelphia, 1995, WB Saunders.

234. Remington JS, Eimstad WM, Araujo FG: Detection of immunoglobulin M antibodies with antigen-tagged latex particles in an immunosorbent assay, *J Clin Microbiol* 17:939-941, 1983.

235. Remington JS, Krahenbuhl JL, Mendenhall JW: A role for activated macrophages in resistance to infection with *Toxoplasma, Infect Immun* 6:829-834, 1972.

236. Riemann HP, Meyer ME, Theis JH et al.: Toxoplasmosis in an infant fed unpasteurized goat milk, *J Pediatr* 87:573-576, 1975.

237. Roach ES, Zimmerman CF, Troost BT, Weaver RG: Optic neuritis due to acquired toxoplasmosis, *Pediatr Neurol* 1:114-116, 1985.

238. Rodriguez A: Photocoagulation in toxoplasmic retinochoroiditis, *Am J Ophthalmol* 91(3):417-418, 1981 (letter).

239. Rothova A, Meenken C, Buitenhuis HJ et al.: Therapy for ocular toxoplasmosis, *Am J Ophthalmol* 115:517-523, 1993.

240. Rothova A, van Knapen F, Baarsma GS et al.: Serology in ocular toxoplasmosis, *Br J Ophthalmol* 70:615-622, 1986.

241. Ruskin J, Remington JS: Toxoplasmosis in the compromised host, *Ann Intern Med* 84:193-199, 1976.

242. Ryning FW, Mills J: *Pneumocystis carinii, Toxoplasma gondii, Cytomegalovirus* and the compromised host, *West J Med* 130:18-34, 1979.

243. Saari M, Vuorre I, Neiminen H, Raisanen S: Acquired toxoplasmic chorioretinitis, *Arch Ophthalmol* 94:1485-1488, 1976.

244. Sabates R, Pruett RC, Brockhurst RJ: Fulminant ocular toxoplasmosis, *Am J Ophthalmol* 92:497-503, 1981.

245. Sabin AB: Complement fixation test in toxoplasmosis and persistence of antibody in human beings, *Pediatrics* 4:443-452, 1949.

246. Sabin AB, Feldman HA: Dyes as microchemical indicators of a new immunity phenomenon affecting the protozoon parasite (toxoplasma), *Science* 10:660-663, 1948.

247. Sabin AB, Ruchman I: Characteristics of the toxoplasma neutralising antibody, *Proc Soc Exp Biol Med* 51:1-12, 1942.

248. Sacks JJ, Roberto RR, Brooks NF: Toxoplasmosis infection associated with raw goat's milk, *JAMA* 248:1728-1732, 1982.

249. Santoro F, Charif H, Capron A: The immunodominant epitope of the major membrane tachyzoite protein (P30) of *Toxoplasma gondii*, *Parasite Immunol* 8:631-639, 1986.

250. Saraux H, Laroche L, Lehoang P: Secondary Fuchs's heterochromic cyclitis: a new approach to an old disease, *Ophthalmologica* 190:193-198, 1985.

251. Scalise F, Gerli R, Castellucci G et al.: Lymphocytes bearing the γ δ T-cell receptor in acute toxoplasmosis, *Immunology* 76:668-670, 1992.

252. Schlaegel TF, Weber JC: The macula in ocular toxoplasmosis, *Arch Ophthalmol* 102:697-698, 1984.

253. Schnapp LM, Geaghan SM, Campagna A et al.: *Toxoplasma gondii* pneumonitis in patients infected with the human immunodeficiency virus, *Arch Intern Med* 152:1073-1077, 1992.

254. Schreiber RD, Feldman HA: Identification of the activator system for antibody to *Toxoplasma* as the classical complement pathway, *J Infect Dis* 141:366-369, 1980.

255. Schuman JS, Friedman AH: Retinal manifestations of the acquired immune deficiency syndrome (AIDS): cytomegalovirus, candida albicans, cryptococcus, toxoplasmosis and *Pneumocystis carinii*, *Trans Ophthalmol Soc U K* 103:177-190, 1983.

256. Schuman JS, Weinberg RS, Ferry AP, Guerry RK: Toxoplasmic scleritis, *Ophthalmology* 95:1399-1403, 1988.

257. Schwab IR: The epidemiologic association of Fuchs' heterochromic iridocyclitis and ocular toxoplasmosis, *Am J Ophthalmol* 111:356-362, 1991.

258. Schwartz PL: Segmental retinal periarteritis as a complication of toxoplasmosis, *Ann Ophthalmol* 9:157-162, 1977.

259. Schwartzman JD: Inhibition of a penetration-enhancing factor of *Toxoplasma gondii* by monoclonal antibodies specific for rhoptries, *Infect Immun* 51:760-764, 1986.

260. Sharma SD, Hofflin JM, Remington JS: In vivo recombinant interleukin 2 administration enhances survival against a lethal challenge with *Toxoplasma gondii*, *J Immunol* 135:4160-4163, 1985.

261. Sher A, Oswald IP, Hieny S, Gazzinelli RT: *Toxoplasma gondii* induces a T-independent IFN-γ response in natural killer cells that requires both adherent accessory cells and tumor necrosis factor-α, *J Immunol* 150:3982-3989, 1993.

262. Shimada K, O'Connor GR, Yoneda C: Cyst formation by *Toxoplasma gondii* (RH strain) in vitro: the role of immunologic mechanisms, *Arch Ophthalmol* 92:496-500, 1974.

263. Sibley LD, Adams LB, Fukutomi Y, Krahenbuhl JL: Tumor necrosis factor-α triggers antitoxoplasmal activity of IFN-γ primed macrophages, *J Immunol* 147:2340-2345, 1991.

264. Sibley LD, Boothroyd JC: Virulent strains of *Toxoplasma gondii* comprise a single clonal lineage, *Nature* 359:82-85, 1992.

265. Sibley LD, Krahenbuhl JL, Adams GM, Weidner E: Toxoplasma modifies macrophage phagosomes by secretion of a vesicular network rich in surface proteins, *J Cell Biol* 103:867-874, 1986.

266. Sibley LD, Krahenbuhl JL, Weidner E: Lymphokine activation of J774G8 cells and mouse peritoneal macrophages challenged with *Toxoplasma gondii*, *Infect Immun* 49:760-764, 1985.

267. Sibley LD, Weidner E, Krahenbuhl JL: Phagosome acidification blocked by intracellular *Toxoplasma gondii*, *Nature* 315:416-419, 1985.

268. Sidikaro Y, Silver L, Holland GN, Kreiger AE: Rhegmatogenous retinal detachments in patients with AIDS and necrotizing retinal infections, *Ophthalmology* 98:129-135, 1991.

269. Siegel SE, Lunde MN, Gelderman AH et al.: Transmission of toxoplasmosis by leukocyte transfusion, *Blood* 37:388-394, 1971.

270. Silveira C, Belfort RJ, Burnier MJ, Nussenblatt R: Acquired toxoplasmic infection as the cause of toxoplasmic retinochoroiditis in families, *Am J Ophthalmol* 106:362-364, 1988.

271. Silveira C, Belfort RJ, Nussenblatt R et al.: Unilateral pigmentary retinopathy associated with ocular toxoplasmosis, *Am J Ophthalmol* 107:682-683, 1989.

272. Singer MA, Hagler WS, Grossniklaus HE: *Toxoplasma gondii* retinochoroiditis after liver transplantation, *Retina* 13:40-45, 1993.

273. Skorska I, Soubrane G, Coscas G: Toxoplasmic choroiditis and subretinal neovascularization, *J Fr Ophtalmol* 7:211-218, 1984.

274. Smith RE, Ganley JP: Ophthalmic survey of a community. 1. Abnormalities of the ocular fundus, *Am J Ophthalmol* 74:1126-1130, 1972.

275. Soete M, Camus D, Dubremetz JF: Experimental induction of bradyzoite-specific antigen expression and cyst formation by the RH strain of *Toxoplasma gondii* in vitro, *Exp Parasitol* 78:361-370, 1994.

276. Spalter HF, Campbell CJ, Noyori KS et al.: Prophylactic photocoagulation of recurrent toxoplasmic retinochoroiditis: a preliminary report, *Arch Ophthalmol* 75:21-31, 1966.

277. Splendore A: Un nuovo protazoa parasite de conigli, *Rev Soc Sci San Paulo* 3:109-112, 1908.

278. Staerz UD, Karasuyama H, Garner AM: Cytotoxic T lymphocytes against a soluble protein, *Nature* 329:449-451, 1987.

279. Stagno S, Reynolds DW, Amos CS et al.: Auditory and visual defects resulting from symptomatic and subclinical congenital cytomegaloviral and toxoplasma infections, *Pediatrics* 59:669-678, 1977.

280. Steahly LP: Laser treatment of toxoplasmosis, *Ann Ophthalmol* 21:36-38, 1989.

281. Stepick-Biek P, Thulliez P, Araujo FG, Remington JS: IgA antibodies for diagnosis of acute congenital and acquired toxoplasmosis, *J Infect Dis* 162:270-273, 1990.

282. Stern GA, Romano PE: Congenital ocular toxoplasmosis: possible occurrence in siblings, *Arch Ophthalmol* 96:615-617, 1978.

283. Stray-Pedersen B: A prospective study of acquired toxoplasmosis among 8,043 pregnant women in the Oslo area, *Am J Obstet Gynecol* 136:399-406, 1980.

284. Strom J: Toxoplasmosis due to laboratory infection in two adults, *Acta Med Scan* 139:224-252, 1951.

285. Subauste CS, Dawson L, Remington JS: Human lymphokine-activated killer cells are cytotoxic against cells infected with *Toxoplasma gondii*, *J Exp Med* 176:1511-1519, 1992.

286. Subauste CS, Koniaris AH, Remington JS: Murine CD8+ cytotoxic T lymphocytes lyse *Toxoplasma gondii*-infected cells, *J Immunol* 147:3955-3959, 1991.

287. Subauste CS, Remington JS: Immunity to *Toxoplasma gondii*, *Curr Opin Immunol* 5:532-537, 1993.

288. Suzuki Y, Conley FK, Remington JS: Treatment of toxoplasmic encephalitis in mice with recombinant gamma interferon, *Infect Immun* 58:3050-3055, 1990.

289. Suzuki Y, Joh K, Orellana MA et al.: A gene(s) within the H-2D region determines the development of toxoplasmic encephalitis in mice, *Immunology* 74:732-739, 1991.

290. Suzuki Y, Orellana MA, Schreiber RD, Remington JS: Interferon-γ: the major mediator of resistance against *Toxoplasma gondii*, *Science* 240:516-518, 1988.

291. Suzuki Y, Remington JS: Dual regulation of resistance against *Toxoplasma gondii* infection by Lyt-2+ and Lyt-1+, L3T4+ T cells in mice, *J Immunol* 140:3943-3946, 1988.

292. Suzuki Y, Remington JS: The effect of anti-IFN-γ antibody on the protective effect of Lyt-2+ immune T cells against toxoplasmosis in mice, *J Immunol* 144:1954-1956, 1990.

293. Swartzberg JE, Remington JS: Transmission of *Toxoplasma*, *Am J Dis Child* 129:777-779, 1975.

294. Tabbara KF, O'Connor GR: Ocular tissue absorption of clindamycin phosphate, *Arch Ophthalmol* 93:1180-1185, 1975.

295. Teutsch SM, Juranek DD, Sulzer A et al.: Epidemic toxoplasmosis associated with infected cats, *N Engl J Med* 300:695-699, 1979.

296. Theodossiadis GP, Koutsandrea C, Tzonou A: A comparative study concerning the treatment of active toxoplasmic retinochoroiditis with argon laser and medication (follow-up 2-9 years), *Ophthalmologica* 199:77-83, 1989.

297. Tirard V, Niel G, Rosenheim M et al.: Diagnosis of toxoplasmosis in patients with AIDS by isolation of the parasite from the blood, *N Engl J Med* 324:634, 1991 (letter).

298. Wallace GD: Serologic and epidemiologic observations on three Pacific atolls, *Am J Epidemiol* 90:103, 1969.

299. Walls KW, Remington JS: Evaluation of commercial latex agglutination method for toxoplasmosis, *Diagn Microbiol Infect Dis* 1:265-271, 1983.

300. Webb RM, Tabbara KF, O'Connor GR: Retinal vasculitis in ocular toxoplasmosis in nonhuman primates, *Retina* 4:182-188, 1984.

301. Weiss MJ, Velazquez N, Hofeldt AJ: Serologic tests in the diagnosis of presumed toxoplasmic retinochoroiditis, *Am J Ophthalmol* 109:407-411, 1990.

302. Weisz JM, Holland GN, Rao R et al.: The management of ocular toxoplasmosis, *Surv Ophthalmol,* 1995 (submitted).

303. Wilder HC: Toxoplasma chorioretinitis in adults, *Arch Ophthalmol* 47:425-438, 1952.

304. Willerson DJ, Aaberg TM, Reeser F, Meredith TA: Unusual ocular presentation of acute toxoplasmosis, *Br J Ophthalmol* 61:693-698, 1977.

305. Wilson CB, Remington JS, Stagno S, Reynolds DW: Development of adverse sequelae in children born with subclinical congenital *Toxoplasma* infection, *Pediatrics* 66:767-774, 1980.

306. Wilson CB, Tsai V, Remington JS: Failure to trigger the oxidative metabolic burst by normal macrophages: possible mechanism for survival of intracellular pathogens, *J Exp Med* 151:328-346, 1980.

307. Wilson WB, Sharpe JA, Deck JH: Cerebral blindness and oculomotor nerve palsies in toxoplasmosis, *Am J Ophthalmol* 89:714-718, 1980.

308. Wise GN: Uveitis with secondary retinal arteriosclerosis, *Am J Ophthalmol* 51:797-807, 1961.

309. Wolf A, Cowen D, Paige BH: Human toxoplasmosis: occurrence in infants as an encephalomyelitis; verification by transmission to animals, *Science* 89:226-227, 1939.

310. Wong SY, Hajdu MP, Ramirez R et al.: Role of specific immunoglobulin E in diagnosis of acute toxoplasma infection and toxoplasmosis, *J Clin Microbiol* 31:2952-2959, 1993.

311. Wong SY, Israelski DM, Remington JS: AIDS-associated toxoplasmosis. In Sande MA, Volberding PA, editors: *The medical management of AIDS,* ed 4, Philadelphia, 1994, WB Saunders.

312. Wong SY, Remington JS: Toxoplasmosis in pregnancy, *Clin Infect Dis* 18:853-862, 1994a.

313. Wong SY, Remington JS: Toxoplasmosis in the setting of AIDS. In Broder S, Merigan TC, Bolognesi D, editors: *Textbook of AIDS medicine,* Baltimore, 1994b, Wiliams & Wilkins.

314. Woods AC, Abrahams IW: Uveitis Survey, *Am J Ophthalmol* 51:761-780, 1961.

315. Wreghitt TG, Hakim M, Gray JJ et al.: Toxoplasmosis in heart and heart and lung transplant recipients, *J Clin Pathol* 42:194-199, 1989.

316. Wyler DJ, Blackman HJ, Lunde MN: Cellular hypersensitivity to toxoplasmal and retinal antigens in patients with toxoplasmal retinochoroiditis, *Am J Trop Med Hyg* 29:1181-1186, 1980.

317. Yano A, Aosai F, Ohta M et al.: Antigen presentation by *Toxoplasma gondii*-infected cells to CD4+ proliferative T cells and CD8+ cytotoxic cells, *J Parasitol* 75:411-416, 1989.

318. Yano A, Ohno S, Norose K et al.: Antigen presentation by *Toxoplasma-infected* cells: antigen entry through cell membrane fusion, *Int Arch Allergy Immunol* 98:13-17, 1992.

319. Yeo JH, Jakobiec FA, Iwamoto T et al.: Opportunistic toxoplasmic retinochoroiditis following chemotherapy for systemic lymphoma: a light and electron microscopic study, *Ophthalmology* 90:885-898, 1983.

320. Yong EC, Chi EY, Henderson WR: *Toxoplasma gondii* alters eicosanoid release by human mononuclear phagocytes: role of leukotrienes in interferon gamma-induced antitoxoplasma activity, *J Exp Med* 180:1637-1648, 1994.

321. Yoshizumi MO: Experimental *Toxoplasma* retinitis: a light and electron microscopical study, *Arch Pathol Lab Med* 100:487-490, 1976.

322. Zangerle R, Allerberger F, Pohl P et al.: High risk of developing toxoplasmic encephalitis in AIDS patients seropositive to *Toxoplasma gondii, Med Microbiol Immunol (Berl)* 180:59-66, 1991.

323. Zimmerman LE: Ocular pathology of toxoplasmosis, *Surv Ophthalmol* 6:832-838, 1961.

324. Zscheile FP: Recurrent toxoplasmic retinitis with weakly positive methylene blue dye test, *Arch Ophthalmol* 71:645-648, 1964.

86 Toxocariasis

DAVID W. PARKE II, ROBERT P. SHAVER

Intraocular infection by nematodes of the genus *Toxocara* represents one of the most commonly recognized *parasitic* causes of visual loss in the United States, Canada, and Europe. Generally affecting young children, it may cause a spectrum of ocular disease ranging from asymptomatic posterior segment granulomata to fulminant endophthalmitis and/or total retinal detachment.

HISTORICAL BACKGROUND

Nematodes were first recognized as pathogens in the ocular posterior segment by Wilder[76] in 1950. She reviewed histopathology on 46 children's eyes enucleated because of clinical diagnoses that included retinoblastoma, pseudoglioma, and endophthalmitis. All eyes evidenced a prominent eosinophilic response. In these specimens she noted larvae or nematode larval capsules in 24 cases. At that time *Toxocara* sp. was not appreciated as a cause of human disease.

Although long recognized as an intestinal parasite in dogs and cats, *Toxocara* sp. was first described as a cause of human disease, visceral larval migrans, by Beaver and associates[7] in 1952. They described a group of three patients with eosinophilia and pulmonary, hepatic, neurologic, cardiac, and other symptoms and signs who showed histopathologic evidence of *Toxocara* sp. infection. The term "visceral larval migrans" (VLM) was coined to describe this syndrome and to differentiate it from hookworm-caused cutaneous larval migrans or "creeping eruption". During the 1940s multiple reports had described a condition similar to VLM, and laparotomy had revealed hepatic nodules identified histologically as eosinophilic granulomata.[5,44,49] The link to *Toxocara* sp., however, was not made until Beaver's report.

Nichols subsequently reviewed the specimens reported by Wilder and determined that several represented second-stage *Toxocara* sp. larvae, thus confirming the first specific link of *Toxocara* infection with ocular disease.[47]

Although not characterized completely, the cases initially reported by Wilder indicated a clinical picture of posterior uveitis and retinal detachment producing leukocoria. The clinical spectrum of ocular disease attributed to *Toxocara* sp. infection was expanded over the ensuing two decades by several groups of clinical investigators. Irvine and Irvine[37] in 1959 presented the case of a 4-year-old boy with an inferior retinal detachment, a positive ^{32}P isotope uptake test, and "suspicious cells" on aqueous cytology. Enucleation was performed because of a concern of retinoblastoma, and histologic examination revealed *Toxocara* sp. larval remnants in the midst of a mass of inflammation involving the peripheral retina and vitreous. This report represented the first description of the clinical variant of peripheral "inflammatory granuloma" with coincident vitreous inflammation and traction retinal detachment.

Ashton[1] reported histopathology on four cases, each with a posterior pole whitish retinochoroidal granuloma, that were enucleated because of a suspicion of retinoblastoma. In contradistinction to the cases reported earlier by Wilder and Irvine and Irvine, these eyes showed little posterior segment inflammation or vitreoretinal traction. Again *Toxocara* sp. larvae were present. This observation was augmented the following year, in 1961, by Duguid, who reviewed 28 cases from the Institute of Ophthalmology, London, of ocular infestation with *Toxocara* sp. Thirteen of these cases were proved histologically.[19] In this, the largest series of eyes to date, Duguid made several important observations: (1) All cases were unilateral; (2) the right and left eyes were equally represented; (3) the lack of intraocular calcification is a diagnostic aid in differentiating ocular toxocariasis from retinoblastoma; (4) there are two primary clinical forms: "retinal granuloma" and "chronic endophthalmitis"; and (5) retinal granulomata may remain stable for decades.

Finally, Hogan and associates[35] in 1965 elegantly described the clinical picture and histopathology of peripheral vitreoretinal and retinal changes associated with direct invasion of *Toxocara* sp. in this region of the eye.

EPIDEMIOLOGY

Toxocara canis is a ubiquitous canine parasite, affecting not only dogs, but wolves, foxes, and other canids. (Another *Toxocara* organism, *Toxocara catis,* may be found in domestic cats. That nematode, although commonly recovered from domestic felines, has not been identified histopathologically in human disease).

Although more common in warmer regions, *Toxocara canis* is endemic in all dog populations where it has been sought, regardless of socioeconomic conditions. The precise prevalence in canine populations is not well defined because most studies have used fecal sampling for eggs to assess rates of infection. Older dogs can harbor adult worms that do not shed eggs. Canine infection rates have been found to be higher in strays or where worming of puppies is not customary.* Even well-cared-for dogs and puppies harbor *Toxocara canis* organisms, indicating that the problem is a ubiquitous one.[74]

Toxocara canis eggs are found in soil throughout tropical and temperate climates. The prevalence of eggs in soil is related largely to two factors: climate and the number of dogs in the environment (particularly where strays and poor veterinary services exist). In the United States and western Europe samples taken from parks and other public places have yielded a 10% to 30% contamination rate.[10,34,59] Eggs have even been recovered from soil and dog feces in Montreal. Presumably, snow cover insulates the eggs from freezing even in subzero temperatures.[26]

Human infection with *Toxocara canis* generally presents as a nonspecific mild systemic illness resembling a viral infection or is entirely subclinical. Therefore, the vast majority of cases go clinically unrecognized.[14] Seropositivity varies tremendously, dependent on climate, ambient veterinary care, ages tested, and risk factors (pica and puppy contact). A survey using enzyme-linked immunosorbent assay (ELISA) methodology of adult blood donors in the United Kingdom yielded a 2.8% rate of positive serologies.[18] In a recent study of a rural North Carolina county, Ellis and associates[20] found that 32% of kindergarten children had a positive antibody titer of greater than or equal to 1:16 by ELISA assay, and 23% had a titer of greater than or equal to 1:32. In St. Lucia in the Caribbean, where soil contamination rates were found to be 46%, Thompson and associates[72] found 80% of children had serological evidence of *Toxocara canis* infection by ELISA assay.

The relationship of ocular disease to seropositivity is unclear. Ellis and associates[20] in examining 106 children with positive serologies did not find any evidence of ocular involvement. No controlled large-scale surveillance study for ocular toxocariasis has been performed. Maetz and associates[40] surveyed ophthalmologists and optometrists in Alabama in an attempt to determine disease prevalence. They estimated an attack rate of between 0.1% and 1.1%. The percentage of eyes that were dilated in this study is unknown, however, and examiner diagnostic accuracy was not determined.

RISK FACTORS

Any individual (particularly children) exposed to young (< 4 months of age) puppies, lactating bitches, or to ingestion of contaminated soil is at risk for infection.[61] This risk is enhanced by residence in communities with poor animal control and inadequate deworming of puppies. Veterinarians and animal control officers are at increased risk for seroconversion. Clemett and associates[15] showed a greater than fourfold increase in seropositivity amongst dog breeders in New Zealand and a tenfold increase amongst animal control officers.

CLINICAL FEATURES

It is rare for ocular toxocariasis to coexist with visceral larval migrans (VLM). In a series by Brown,[11] only 5 of 245 cases of ocular toxocariasis reported symptoms of VLM. Active ocular toxocariasis in a patient with active, severe VLM has not been reported. Most reports of VLM where ocular disease is present consist predominantly of a flulike illness. The average age at presentation of ocular disease is also older (7½ yrs) than that for VLM (15 to 30 months).[11]

VLM presentations vary substantially, probably because of factors including patient age, larval load, and distribution of larvae. Most infections are asymptomatic. Three human subjects who received a single dose of 100 to 200 larvae developed a moderate eosinophilia but no subjective complaints.[59] When symptomatic, common complaints and clinical signs include the following: fever, cough and wheeze, malaise, irritability, weight loss, and pruritic eruptions and nodules over trunk and legs.

Laboratory investigations at this stage will generally reveal leukocyte counts of 30,000 to 100,000 per cubic millimeter with 50% to 90% eosinophils. (This eosinophilia may persist months or years and is not indicative only of acute disease). Serum gamma globulins IgG, IgM, and IgE are usually above normal. Anti-A and anti-B titers are also elevated as *Toxocara canis* larval polysaccharide residues stimulate isohemagglutinins.[67] Transient pulmonary infiltrates may be noted on chest x-ray, although severe respiratory distress is rare.

Severe VLM may result in death from myocardial or central nervous system involvement or from an exaggerated immunologic response. Neurologic involvement may include focal or generalized seizures, cerebrospinal fluid eosinophilia, cerebral eosinophilic granulomata, and cerebral larvae.[59]

---

*References 33, 43, 53, 57, 68, 72, 73.

Ocular Toxocariasis

Clinical presentations of ocular toxocariasis may be best differentiated according to the primary tissue or anatomic site of involvement: (1) peripheral retina and vitreous; (2) posterior pole; (3) endophthalmitis; (4) optic nerve; and (5) anterior segment.

Of these presentations, the first two are by far the most common, occurring separately or together. Wilkinson and Welch[78] described peripheral involvement in 44% of eyes with ocular toxocariasis as the most common form of presentation. Hagler and associates[32] reported 100 cases of ocular toxocariasis with posterior disease as the most common presentation. The fourth and fifth presentation types listed above are extraordinarily rare.

Peripheral Retina and Vitreous. It is unclear why the *Toxocara canis* organism has an apparent preference for peripheral fundus involvement. Because most spread is initially hematogenous, this preference may reflect local retinal and/or choroidal vascular microanatomy. The organisms migrate into the retina and incite a massive local inflammatory response, which is appreciated ophthalmoscopically as a local mass of whitish tissue involving retina and peripheral vitreous (Fig. 86-1). Vitreous membranes frequently radiate out from the mass circumferentially around the vitreous and (less commonly) transvitreally. Contraction of the inflammatory membranes may result in the retina becoming "wadded up" into the mass, with localized tractional elevation and formation of characteristic radial retinal falciform folds leading from the peripheral mass to the optic nervehead (Fig. 86-2). As noted by Shields[63] in his excellent review of the subject, some cases of "congenital" folds reported in the literature were due to *Toxocara* canis infection with the peripheral mass unrecognized.

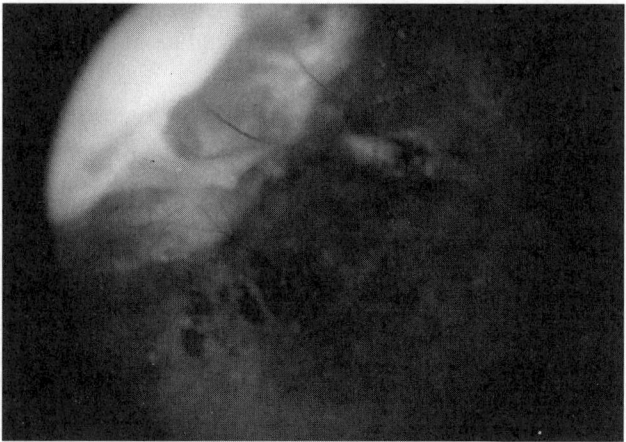

Fig. 86-1. Peripheral inflammatory mass seen following surgical removal of vitreous membranes. Note that retina is drawn up into the mass. Reactive retinal pigment epithelial atrophy and hyperplasia are present just posterior to mass. Residual membranes are noted extending from the mass circumferentially.

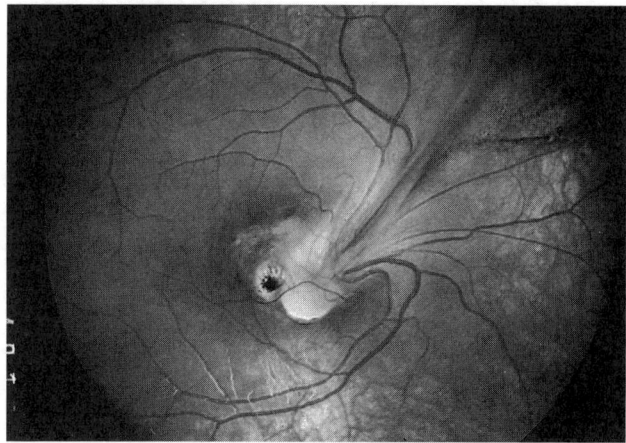

Fig. 86-2. Fundus photograph of superonasal peripheral *Toxocara canis* inflammatory mass causing radial retinal fold. Peripapillary lesion is also present, possibly from second *Toxocara canis* lesion.

Occasionally more than one nidus of inflammation may be apparent, indicating involvement by more than one larva. In some cases with an inferior focus, the circumferential membranes may superficially simulate pars planitis syndrome. The entirely unilateral nature of the disease, presence of a mass, and retinal fold all help in the differential diagnosis, however.

Rarely, epiretinal membranes may form secondarily in the posterior pole, resulting in visual symptoms (Fig. 86-3). Epiretinal membranes in the macular region of a child should prompt a careful search for a peripheral toxocariasis lesion.

Many peripheral lesions, particularly if nasal, are asymptomatic. Symptoms, if present, may be due to vitreous inflammation (in the acute phase of the disease), macular heterotopia from a traction fold, tractional macular detachment, a macular epiretinal membrane, or rhegmatogenous retinal detachment secondary to a traction-induced retinal break (Fig. 86-4).

Posterior Pole. The appearance at presentation of posterior pole lesions is quite heterogeneous. Small children may be unaware of a visual change and may not have disease detected until a visual deprivation strabismus develops, at which time there may be little observable vitreous inflammation and a mature granuloma. If detected early the posterior pole may be only poorly visualized through vitreous cells and only a vague, whitish mass may be noted.

Typically, posterior pole toxocariasis lesions are whitish or greyish-white in color (Fig. 86-5). They may be centered anywhere in the posterior pole, including juxtapapillary and subfoveal locations. Lesion size varies from less than one disc diameter to involvement of the entire macular region. Longstanding masses may have substantial secondary atrophy and hyperplasia of the retinal pigment epithelium. De-

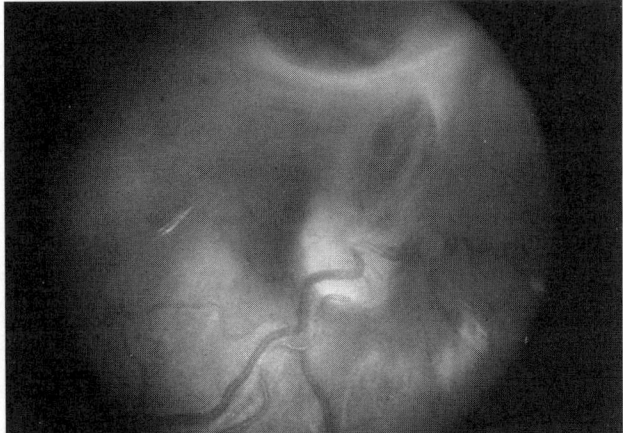

A

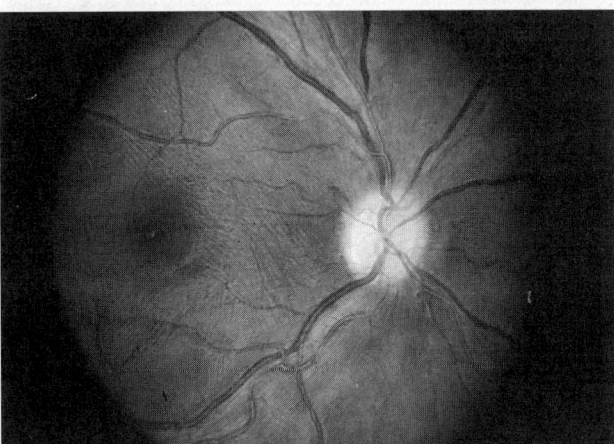

B

Fig. 86-3. **A,** Epiretinal membranes from peripheral lesion causing tractional changes in posterior pole and 20/200 visual acuity. **B,** Postoperative appearance demonstrating relief of tractional changes, absence of macular lesions, and recovery of 20/25 visual acuity.

pending on the anatomic location of the larva there may be minimal vitreous involvement or massive, dense preretinal membrane formation. (In some cases the membrane material arises from the retina itself, resulting in surgical inability to separate the membranes from the retina).[42,66]

Occasionally a dark gray area within the whitish mass may represent the dead larva. Retinochoroidal vascular anastomoses may be visible with vascular invasion of the inflammatory tissue.

Endophthalmitis. Most of the original cases of *Toxocara canis* infection described histopathologically by Wilder presented as endophthalmitis with a whitish vitreitis and retinal detachment.[76] Such eyes were generally enucleated because of suspected bacterial endophthalmitis or retinoblastoma.

Factors causing a massive intraocular inflammatory response, as opposed to a small localized granuloma, are un-

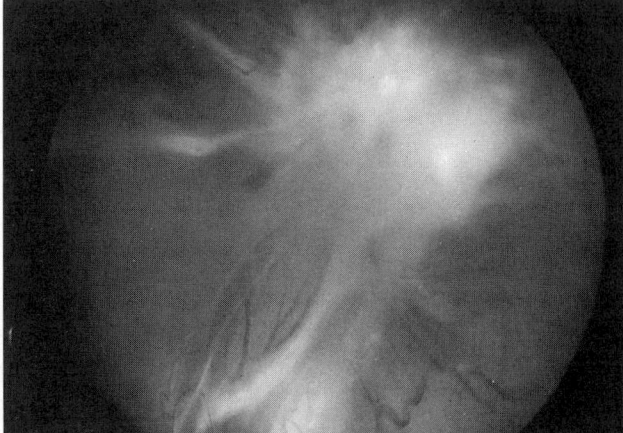

Fig. 86-4. Combined traction/rhegmatogenous retinal detachment in ocular toxocariasis with peripheral inflammatory masses and posterior vitreoretinal membrane formation inducing multiple retinal breaks.

known. The degree of response may be determined by differential host immune response capabilities, organism factors (size or number), or location of the organism within the eye.

When initially seen, such eyes generally are noted to have little or no scleroconjunctivitis or pain. Anterior chamber reaction may range from minimal cellular suspension to a layered hypopyon and fibrin membrane formation. Vitreous cellular reaction may lead to leukocoria and/or to cyclitic membrane development. In its most severe form retinal detachment, neovascular glaucoma, and phthisis bulbi may result.

In many cases, however, the inflammation subsides spontaneously, permitting recognition of a typical posterior pole or peripheral picture of ocular toxocariasis. When the fundus cannot be visualized ophthalmoscopically, B-scan echography may demonstrate a peripheral fundus mass suggesting the diagnosis.

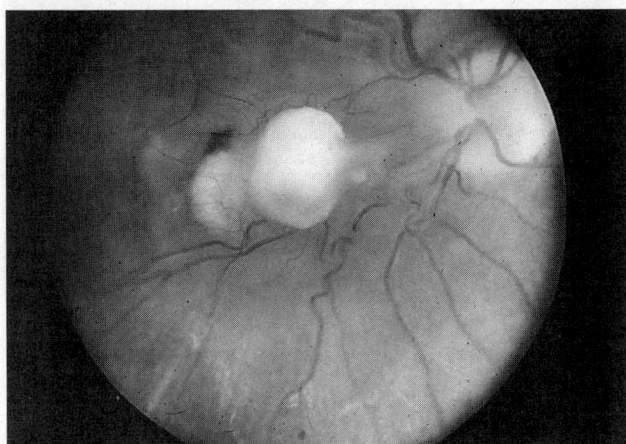

Fig. 86-5. Posterior pole granuloma.

Optic Nerve. A number of reports exist in the literature purporting *Toxocara canis* infection of the optic disc.[9,12,45,50] In fact, some of these cases are only *presumed* toxocariasis cases. It is reasonable, however, to assume that some of these cases do in fact represent *Toxocara canis* infection characterized by optic neuritis, adjacent retinal detachment, and overlying vitreitis.[9] The frequency of this presentation is very low.

Anterior Segment. Several cases of anterior segment *Toxocara canis* infestation have been reported,[4,36] but these cases have not been confirmed histologically. Shields[63] has suggested that anterior segment *Toxocara canis* infestation may result from organisms becoming lodged in end arteries at the corneoscleral limbus. Larvae then migrate into clear cornea and are observed at the slit lamp to be motile. Definitive reports of *Toxocara canis* conjunctivitis are lacking.[2]

Diffuse Chorioretinitis. In addition, diffuse chorioretinitis has been included in the potential spectrum of toxocariasis presentations in prior reviews.[63,77] When Gass and associates[25,23] initially reported patients with what he subsequently called diffuse unilateral subacute neuroretinitis (DUSN), *Toxocara* sp. was mentioned as a possible cause. There are a number of factors suggesting that *Toxocara* sp. is not causally related to DUSN, however. First, there is no confirmatory serology. Second, eyes with DUSN share no clinical similarities with other known cases of ocular toxocariasis. Third, the epidemiologic distributions of DUSN and toxocariasis are not concordant. Finally, the second-stage larva of *Toxocara canis* is smaller than those identified ophthalmoscopically in patients with DUSN.[24] Both *Ancylostoma caninum* and *Baylisascaris procyonis* have been tentatively identified histopathologically in DUSN cases.[22,39] *Toxocara canis* has therefore not been convincingly identified as a cause of diffuse chorioretinitis from meandering subretinal migration of larvae. Sorr[69] reported one case of "meandering ocular toxocariasis" in a sixteen-year-old patient who had a significantly elevated anti-*Toxocara canis* ELISA antibody titer and optic neuritis. Although intriguing, the case remains unconfirmed histologically.

PATHOLOGY

The initial description by Wilder[76] entitled "Nematode Endophthalmitis" published in 1950 was similar to descriptions of nematode infections in other organs. She wrote, "Eosinophilic abscesses sometimes surrounded by epithelioid and giant cells presented a pathologic picture not accounted for by most commonly recognized granulomatous lesions of the eye." Multiple sections of 46 eyes revealed nematode larva or residual hyalin capsules in 24 eyes. It has since been noted that most of these organisms were *Toxocara* sp. larvae.[47] The average width of the *T. canis* second-stage larva is 18 to 21 microns, approximately 2 to 3 times the size of a red blood cell. (Most present-day sectioning is

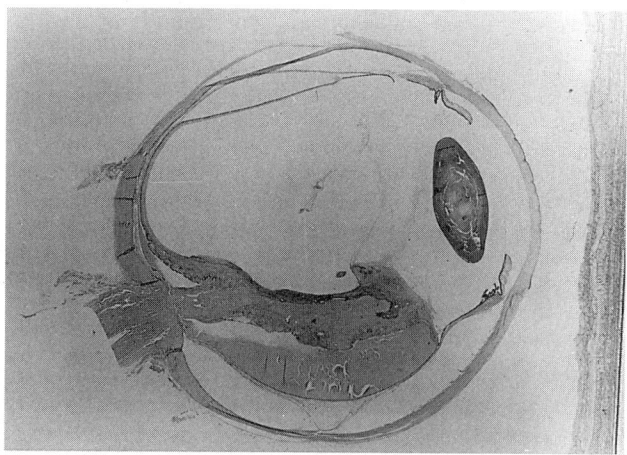

Fig. 86-6. *Toxocara canis* endophthalmitis showing focal eosinophilic abscess with more chronic adjacent granulation tissue response. Traction retinal detachment with subretinal fluid is also present.

at 6 to 8 micron intervals.) On one case Wilder sectioned 2300 cuts before she found the larva.

Because of this time-consuming process, a presumptive diagnosis can be made by the histologic features described by Wilder, even without discovery of the organism or the capsule. Cases enucleated for suspected retinoblastoma or microbial endophthalmitis demonstrate a varying degree of intraocular disorganization, retinal detachment, and vitreous membrane formation (Fig. 86-6). Focal inflammatory masses may be incorporated into retina and overlying vitreous. Underlying retinal pigment epithelium (RPE) is generally involved with atrophy, hyperplasia, and breaks in Bruch membrane (possibly due to transit of the organism).

Inflammatory foci are characterized by granuloma formation with eosinophilic abscesses (Fig. 86-7). Surrounding

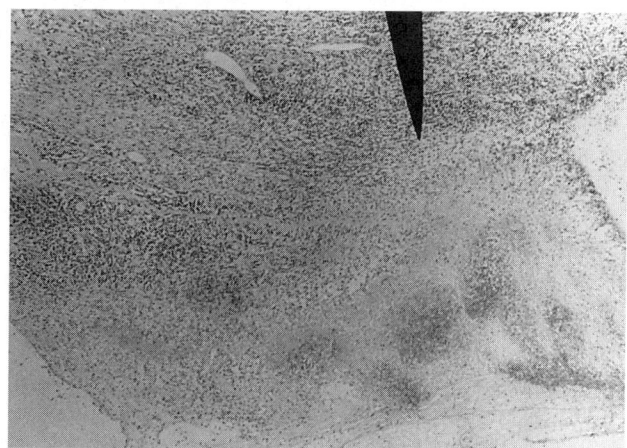

Fig. 86-7. Photomicrograph demonstrating interface between eosinophilic abscess above pointer tip and less eosinophilic granulomatous response below pointer tip.

the eosinophils are epithelioid and giant cells, lymphocytes, plasma cells, and fibroblasts. Cytologic examination of the vitreous and frequently aqueous reveals eosinophilia. Although not absolutely diagnostic of toxocariasis, prominent eosinophilia in a vitreous biopsy specimen should be considered highly indicative of toxocariasis.

COMPLICATIONS

Loss of vision in ocular toxocariasis may be related to direct retinal changes such as macular scar, macular heterotopia, macular traction retinal detachment, epimacular membrane, and rhegmatogenous retinal detachment. It may also be caused by active posterior segment inflammation with severe vitreitis. Loss of vision may also be due to sequelae of inflammation including cyclitic membrane, cataract, and glaucoma. Finally, all vision may be lost because of phthisis resulting from severe intraocular inflammation and/or retinal detachment.

The frequency of severe visual loss in eyes with toxocariasis is unknown because some cases of ocular toxocariasis are asymptomatic or are misdiagnosed. Reported series to date are all retrospective ones, suffering from a bias of recruitment.

PATHOGENESIS

Toxocara canis is a canine roundworm sharing certain characteristics with the feline roundworm Toxocara catis and with the human roundworm Ascaris lumbricoides. The first complete description of the T. canis lifecycle was provided by Sprent in 1958.[71]

Parasite

Adult roundworms grow up to 10 cm in length and excrete about 200,000 eggs each day. The eggs are initially embryonated and further development requires a specific range of temperature and humidity. They can, however, withstand temperatures from − 25°C to 36°C.[29] After a two- to three-week period of development, the ova become infective.[30] They may remain infective for months.

Intermediate Host

Adult dogs may become infected either through ingestion of infective eggs in the soil or through ingestion of larval infected tissue. They may also become infected (or reinfected) by ingestion of larvae or immature adult worms in the vomitus or feces of infected puppies. In the adult dog intestine, first- and second-stage larvae remain within the eggshell.[59] Rupture of the shell discharges third-stage larvae into the intestine. These larvae subsequently can invade the intestinal wall and enter the lymphatics and the bloodstream. Typically this interval is about 24 hours after ingestion.

Larvae may then seed end organs including lung, liver, brain, and eye, producing a VLM-type picture in dogs.[29,70] After migration throughout the body (which may take months) the larvae encyst and become dormant, surviving for many years. Only rarely do larvae complete maturation to fully developed worms.[71] Thus, adult dogs (except lactating bitches) are rarely a source of human infection. Additionally, reinfection (or primary infection) of adult dogs appears to be an uncommon event.

Puppies, however, play a major role in disease transmission. Encysted larvae in pregnant bitches become activated and can migrate transplacentally to infect puppies in utero. The third-stage larval moult occurs before puppy birth. These third-stage larvae migrate to the trachea, moult again, and develop into the adult worm. The adult worms produce eggs that are excreted in puppy feces beginning about four weeks after birth.

Puppies may also be infected by larvae in milk. These larvae are swallowed and complete development in the puppy intestine. Both puppies and the lactating bitch begin to shed ova in their feces by the fourth postparturient week.[59]

Human Infection

Humans are paratenic hosts (like adult dogs). Larval maturation arrests at the second stage after ingestion of infective ova. Eggs are ingested, moult twice to second-stage larvae, and larvae penetrate the intestine and disseminate to tissues. The larvae wander throughout tissues, remaining viable for months. Ocular involvement probably occurs primarily by hematogenous dissemination, although the recovery of organisms from the cornea and larval migration into the vitreous bears witness to the organism's ability to invade tissue.* Humans do not harbor adult worms or excrete eggs. Attempts to recover eggs from human feces are therefore futile.[28,59]

Humans acquire infection either through direct ingestion of eggs in soil (pica) or via contaminated hands or uncooked food. As would be expected, numerous case control studies have identified a relationship between recent exposure to puppies and serologic evidence of Toxocara canis infection.[20,60,61] No similar relationship with toxocariasis has been identified with exposure to cats, kittens, or other animals.

The number of organisms necessary to induce systemic, and particularly ocular, infection remains unknown. Experimental studies in an animal model have indicated that the likelihood of ocular disease increases with an increasing inoculum of organisms. Schantz and associates[60] point out that ocular involvement and severe VLM therefore should logically coexist, which paradoxically they do not.

Ocular toxocariasis and VLM differ with respect to several important characteristics. Ocular toxocariasis and VLM generally do not coexist. Ocular disease occurs in older children than does VLM, and ocular disease generally leads to lower circulating antibody levels than does VLM.[11,60,51,54]

---

*References 4, 6, 11, 13, 48, 52, 58, 70, 75.

Schantz and associates[60] suggest that ocular involvement occurs preferentially in children not previously exposed to *Toxocara canis,* when relatively small numbers of organisms migrate without rapidly eliciting a host response. This hypothesis does not, however, explain the paucity of cases reported in adults, most of whom do not demonstrate an elevated anti-*Toxocara canis* antibody titer.

DIFFERENTIAL DIAGNOSIS

The differential diagnosis of ocular toxocariasis varies with the clinical presentation of the disease. Young children presenting with unilateral severe intraocular inflammation without a recent history of intraocular surgery pose an intriguing differential diagnosis. The initial differential includes the following: traumatic, exogenous infectious endophthalmitis; endogenous bacterial endophthalmitis; severe inflammation such as in the pars planitis syndrome or juvenile rheumatoid arthritis (JRA)—associated uveitis.

Uveitis and Endophthalmitis

Pars planitis syndrome and JRA-associated uveitis can generally be ruled out easily because they are almost always bilateral, albeit asymmetric, conditions (particularly if so severe as to mimic endophthalmitis). Uveitis associated with JRA is restricted to the anterior segment. Patients generally have systemic findings and usually present with signs of chronic ocular inflammation, such as band keratopathy and cataract. JRA patients can also have posterior segment spillover.

Endogenous bacterial endophthalmitis is an important disorder in the differential diagnosis of the endophthalmitic form of toxocariasis. Although endophthalmitis can be an expected complication in patients with septicemia, indwelling catheters, or known sources of septic emboli, such as bacterial endocarditis, metastatic bacterial endophthalmitis can occur in children who appear otherwise well (see chapter 93).

Exogenous infectious endophthalmitis from unrecognized ocular penetration must always be considered. Generally, however, these eyes will be grossly inflamed with substantial pain.

The character of retinal detachments, if present, can aid in differentiating various diseases. Eyes with bullous retinal detachments and toxocariasis are uncommon. Bullous detachment generally implies that a retinal detachment has a rhegmatogenous component. Exudative detachments have not been reported in toxocariasis. Detachments related to *Toxocara* sp. are generally tractional and shallow unless a secondary retinal break occurs. If a bullous or exudative detachment is seen, the differential diagnosis includes the following: retinoblastoma, Coats disease, retinopathy of prematurity, and persistent hyperplastic primary vitreous (PHPV).

Intraocular Neoplasm

Historically, retinoblastoma was the entity most often confused with toxocariasis. Of the 24 eyes examined by Wilder and diagnosed histopathologically as toxocariasis, 20 had been enucleated for a suspected diagnosis of retinoblastoma.[76] Shields and Augsberger[64] reported in 1981 that of 136 children referred to Wills Eye Hospital for retinoblastoma, 26% were found to have toxocariasis, the most common referral misdiagnosis made.

Patients presenting with retinoblastoma are generally younger than those with toxocariasis; they are usually less than age 2 years, whereas most patients with ocular toxocariasis are over age 5 years. As noted earlier, toxocariasis rarely presents acutely with a bullous retinal detachment, as can occur with retinoblastoma, but, if present, the vitreous will generally show vitreitis and careful examination of the peripheral retina will demonstrate the peripheral *Toxocara canis*–associated lesion. Vitreoretinal membranes will be present and the subretinal space is generally clear. In contrast, eyes with endophytic retinoblastoma may demonstrate hazy vitreous, but cellular accumulations will generally be clumps of tumor cells. The lens will be clear (as opposed to eyes with toxocariasis, which may develop cataract). The tumor(s) itself may be visible. If the retinoblastoma is exophytic, the tumor may be seen extending from the retina into the subretinal space.

B-scan echography and/or computerized tomography (CT scanning) may be helpful in demonstrating calcium in cases of retinoblastoma. Serum serologies and (if necessary) aqueous and/or vitreous examination may help to differentiate especially challenging cases. Study of intraocular fluid is generally unnecessary in differentiating retinoblastoma from toxocariasis.

Congenital and Infantile Conditions

Coats disease is generally differentiated easily from cases of toxocariasis that present with retinal detachment. In cases of toxocariasis the detachment is generally tractional, complicated by vitreoretinal membrane formation and vitreous cells. Retinal vasculature is normal in caliber without telangiectases. In Coats disease the detachment is exudative with minimal if any membrane formation and the vitreous is generally clear. The peripheral retinal vasculature demonstrates typical telangiectases. Subretinal exudate (absent in ocular toxocariasis) is prominent.

Patients with retinopathy of prematurity are easily excluded on the basis of disease bilaterality. The peripheral microvascular disease, broad-based nature of the traction, and history of prematurity also help to differentiate the two conditions.

PHPV is a congenital condition and as such is generally diagnosed within the first several weeks or months of life. It is usually associated with microphthalmia, a retrolenticular mass, and a cataract. In more posterior PHPV in which the fundus can be visualized, a hyaloid artery system may be seen along with varying degrees of tractional disorganization of the epipapillary region. Peripheral tractional masses are not present.

Eyes presenting with a peripheral inflammatory mass and retinal traction leading to detachment and falciform folds may be seen in familial exudative vitreoretinopathy (FEVR), retinopathy of prematurity, and occult penetrating ocular injury.

FEVR is an autosomal dominant condition that can present with peripheral vitreoretinal membrane formation and retinal traction, even inducing a falciform foldlike appearance. Such cases can generally be differentiated on the basis of a family history, bilaterality, and associated microvascular changes, however.

Past peripheral retinal penetrating ocular injury, with or without an associated intraocular foreign body, may give rise to a local exuberant membrane formation with vitreoretinal traction. Generally such eyes will not have substantial vitreitis and will have evidence of surrounding retinal pigment epithelial hyperplasia, but such cases generally do not cause macular traction and may be clinically silent. Occasionally the differential diagnosis can be difficult to make in the presence of indeterminate serological tests.

LABORATORY INVESTIGATIONS

Over 95% of patients with VLM will manifest a leukocytosis and hypereosinophilia.[27] In ocular toxocariasis, eosinophilia is generally absent because there is no active, coincident systemic infection. In neither VLM nor ocular toxocariasis can ova or larvae be recovered from stools because the larvae do not come to maturity in the human gastrointestinal tract.

Antibody Testing

Immunodiagnosis has become the prime serologic method for detecting VLM and for confirming the clinical suspicion of ocular toxocariasis. Hemagglutination and complement fixation tests have been described.[21,38] Both have limited sensitivity because they tend to cross-react with other antihelminthic antibodies. Immunofluorescent antibody techniques using larval secretory antigen are highly specific, but lack sensitivity.[30]

ELISA has become the test of choice for evaluating possible cases of toxocariasis. Two Toxocara sp. antigen have been used: the Toxocara sp. embryonated egg (TEE) antigen and the ES antigen derived from Toxocara sp. larvae maintained in long-term culture.[17,18] Initially serum titers of $\geq 1:32$ were felt to be indicative of VLM whereas titers of $\geq 1:8$ were supportive of a diagnosis of ocular toxocariasis, with sensitivity and specificity both greater than 90%.[51,60,65] Many commercial laboratories now report Toxocara sp. ELISA (or EIA) tests in terms of standard deviations (SD) referenced above a normal population. Separate values for IgG, IgM, and IgA can be obtained with any result > 3.0 SD considered positive for systemic infection. (Less than 2.0 SD is interpreted as not detected.)

In interpreting the significance of weakly positive ELISA tests for Toxocara sp. infection, one must bear in mind the epidemiologic data presented earlier. In some geographic locales 10% to 25% of children will show serum antibodies against Toxocara sp.

Vitreous specimens in cases of ocular toxocariasis demonstrate higher ELISA titers than do serum specimens.[8,55] In some cases serum ELISA may be negative with positive aqueous and/or vitreous titers. These titer differentials support the concept of local antibody production.

A negative or weakly positive ELISA performed on serum therefore does not rule out the possibility of ocular toxocariasis, particularly in the face of a compelling clinical picture. Intraocular fluid titers higher than serum titers help confirm the diagnosis, especially if eosinophils are noted on intraocular fluid cytology.

Ocular toxocariasis is foremost a clinical diagnosis. Serum serologic tests are of no clinical utility unless a compatible clinical picture exists. In such situations a markedly positive serum IgM and IgA titers will add weight to the clinical impression of acute inflammation, but markedly positive serum serologies are not commonly found in ocular disease unless it is encountered acutely. A negative or low antibody titer does not rule out the disease. In such circumstances the physician must rely on clinical appearance or on higher intraocular fluid titers. As always, absolute confirmation of ocular toxocariasis requires histopathologic examination.

Radiography

Radiologic imaging techniques may be helpful in cases with opaque media for differentiating retinoblastoma from toxocariasis. CT scanning may detect calcium-containing retinoblastomas. CT scanning is of no benefit in differentiating a toxocariasis lesion from a noncalcified retinoblastoma. MRI studies have demonstrated that toxocariasis lesions are hyperintense in T_1- and proton-weighted MRI scans, as are retinoblastomas. Unlike retinoblastoma, toxocariasis lesions are hyperintense in T_2-weighted MRI scans.[41]

THERAPY

Treatment of ocular toxocariasis depends on three factors: visual potential of the eye, amount of inflammation, and structural macular damage.

The ophthalmologist has the theoretical potential to abate inflammation and repair various types of structural damage. Unfortunately many patients with toxocariasis are diagnosed after the development of irreversible amblyopia or of massive macular photoreceptor and/or retinal pigment epithelial damage. Aggressive surgical intervention to reattach a trac-

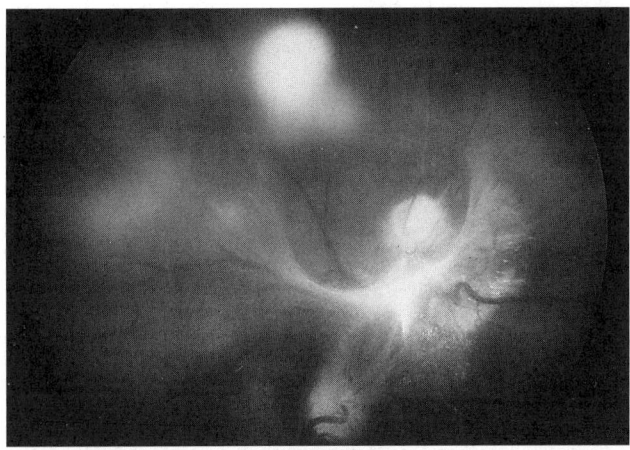

A

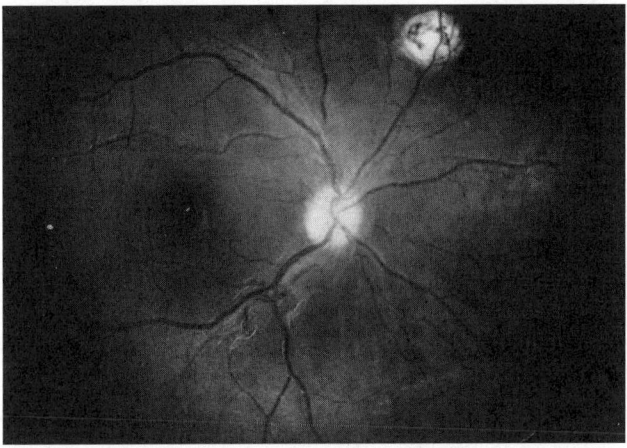

B

Fig. 86-8. **A,** Preoperative appearance of six-year-old with peripheral and midperipheral granulomatous masses and substantial vitreous membrane formation. White lesion superiorly is vitreous microabscess. **B,** Postoperative appearance demonstrating a nidus superonasal to the disc and relief of vitreoretinal traction.

tionally detached macula with all the attendant risks of surgery may not be warranted in such situations.

Systemic or periocular corticosteroids remain the therapeutic mainstay for eyes with active vitreitis. Corticosteroids will help reduce the severity of the vitreitis and decrease the severity and extent of vitreoretinal membranes. Topical corticosteroids are inadequate for the task. Because the usual patient is less than 10 years old, systemic corticosteroids rather than repeated periocular injections are better tolerated. Care must be taken, however, in the peripubescent patient because of effects of systemically administered corticosteroids on the pubertal growth process. Generally corticosteroid therapy is required for weeks to months and a slow drug taper is advisable because of the tendency for rebound inflammation.

The antihelminthic agents thiabendazole and diethylcar-

bamazine have been utilized in small series against VLM and ocular toxocariasis.* Unfortunately no large case control study has compared antihelminthic therapy for VLM or for ocular toxocariasis against observation alone. Most authors feel that although antihelminthic therapy may result in clinical improvement and a decrease in antibody levels, the observed changes may simply represent the disease's natural course.[27,59,63]

Vitrectomy has been employed by a number of different surgeons with some success to (1) remove vitreous cells and membranes (Fig. 86-8), (2) remove epimacular membranes, (3) relieve macular heterotopia and detachment from traction, and (4) repair tractional and tractional rhegmatogenous retinal detachments.[31,32,42,55,66]

PROGNOSIS

Hagler and associates[32] reported that in 17 toxocariasis cases requiring surgery, anatomic reattachment was achieved in 12 cases and vision stabilized or improved in 15 cases. Rodriguez,[55] in a series of 12 eyes, performed surgery for retinal detachment in 8 eyes and for vitreitis and membrane formation in 4 eyes. Five eyes required multiple surgical procedures. Eight eyes experienced an improvement in vision, with six eyes achieving a level of 20/20 to 20/40. Complications of surgery included exacerbation of inflammation, cataract, rhegmatogenous retinal detachment, and cystoid macular edema. Small and associates[66] reported a series of 12 eyes undergoing vitrectomy and membranectomy. All eyes had macular detachment, heterotopia, or distortion preoperatively. Five eyes required reoperation. Ten of 12 eyes were completely reattached, but visual acuity improved in only 7 eyes. Those eyes presenting with good preoperative acuity were the only ones with $\geq$ 20/100 postoperatively. A large fold through the macular region was the preoperative anatomic factor most commonly associated with a poor outcome. Even with membranectomy these folds could not be relieved entirely.

Both Hagler and associates and Small and associates reported late recurrence of detachments in 24% and 42% respectively. These recurrent detachments may be the result of persistent (and occasionally severe) inflammation postoperatively that has been observed to last in some patients for years.[56,66] It has been postulated that this inflammation may be engendered by persistence of antigen in the retina, which has not removed by vitrectomy. Larvae have been demonstrated to remain viable in animal tissue for at least 15 months following inoculation.[75] Several surgeons have been successful in removing the *Toxocara canis* larva. In general the proliferative tissue and retina-encapsulated larvae in the peripheral fundus have been impossible to remove in their entirety without retinectomy.[42]

*References 3, 46, 54, 62, 78, 79.

PREVENTION

Prevention of ocular toxocariasis is theoretically simple. Children (and to a lesser extent adults) should avoid contact with puppy feces from four weeks following their birth until about age four months. Lactating bitches shed infective ova in milk and occasionally in feces for several months following delivery. Piperazine is effective in eradicating adult worms from puppies, and thiabendazole appears effective as well.[16] For maximal effectiveness, puppies and lactating bitches should be treated with antihelminthics first at about two weeks following delivery and then every two weeks until the puppy reaches four months of age. Preliminary data suggest that some antihelminthic agents (such as ivermectin) administered to pregnant bitches during late gestation and early lactation may decrease transmission of organisms to the puppies.[29,59]

Unfortunately direct contact with puppies is only partially effective because ova are found in soil in most communities. Soil contamination is greatest in tropical and subtropical regions and where animal control and veterinary practices are not well developed. Pica therefore remains a major mode of transmission. Children exhibiting this habit should be removed as much as possible from potentially contaminated environments.

REFERENCES

1. Ashton N: Larval granulomatosis of the retina due to *Toxocara*, *Br J Ophthalmol* 44:129-148, 1960.
2. Ashton N, Cook C: Allergic granulomatous nodules of the eyelid and conjunctiva, XXXV Edward Jackson memorial lecture, *Ophthalmology* 86:8-42, 1979.
3. Aur RJA, Pratt CB, Johnson WW: Thiabendazole in visceral larva migrans, *Am J Dis Child* 121:226-229, 1971.
4. Baldone JA, Clark WB, Jung RC: Nematode ophthalmitis: report of two cases, *Am J Ophthalmol* 57:763-766, 1964.
5. Bass MH: Extreme eosinophilia and leukocytosis: unusual clinical syndrome of unknown origin occurring in childhood, *Am J Dis Child* 62:68-80, 1941.
6. Beaver PC: Zoonoses, with particular reference to parasites of veterinary importance. In Soulsby EJL, editor: *Biology of parasites: emphasis on veterinary parasites.* New York, 1966, Academic Press.
7. Beaver PC, Snyder CH, Carrera GM et al.: Chronic eosinophilia due to visceral larval migrans, *Pediatrics* 9:7-19, 1952.
8. Biglan AW, Glickman LT, Lobes Jr LA: Serum and vitreous *Toxocara* antibody in nematode endophthalmitis, *Am J Ophthalmol* 88:898-901, 1979.
9. Bird AC, Smith JL, Curtin VT: Nematode optic neuritis, *Am J Ophthalmol* 69:72-77, 1970.
10. Borg VA, Woodruff AW: Prevalence of infective ova of *Toxocara* species in public places, *Br Med J* 4:470-472, 1973.
11. Brown DH: Ocular *Toxocara canis*. II. Clinical review, *J Pediatr Ophthalmol* 7:182-191, 1970.
12. Brown GC, Tasman WS: Retinal arterial obstruction in association with presumed *Toxocara* neuroretinitis, *Ann Ophthalmol* 13:1385-1387, 1981.
13. Byers B, Kimura SJ: Uveitis after death of a larva in the vitreous cavity, *Am J Ophthalmol* 77:63-66, 1974.
14. Clemett RS, Tuft SJ: Toxocariasis: a neglected entity, *NZ Med J* 517-520, 1983.
15. Clemett RS, Williamson HJE, Hidajat RR et al.: Ocular *Toxocara canis* infections: diagnosis by enzyme immunoassay, *Aust NZ J Ophthalmol* 15:145-150, 1987.
16. Corwin RM, Miller TA: 1978 antihelminthic efficacy of thenium closylate-piperazine phosphate combination tablets against *Toxocara canis* in pups and young dogs, *Am J Vet Res* 39:263-265, 1978.
17. Cypress RH, Karol M, Zidian J et al.: Larva specific antibodies in patients with visceral larva migrans, *J Infect Dis* 135:633-640, 1977.
18. de Savigny DH, Voller A, Woodruff AW: Toxocariasis: serological diagnosis by enzyme immunoassay, *J Clin Pathol* 37:284-288, 1979.
19. Duguid IM: Features of ocular infestation by *Toxocara*, *Br J Ophthalmol* 45:789-796, 1961.
20. Ellis GS, Pakalnis VA, Worley G et al.: *Toxocara canis* infestation: clinical and epidemiological associations with seropositivity in kindergarten children, *Ophthalmology* 93:1032-1037, 1986.
21. Fernando ST: Immunobiological response of the host to *Toxocara canis* (Werner 1782) infection, *Parasitology* 58:547-559, 1968.
22. Gass JDM: *Stereoscopic atlas of macular diseases: diagnosis and treatment,* ed 3, St. Louis, 1987, Mosby.
23. Gass JDM, Lewis RA: Subretinal tracts in ophthalmomyiasis, *Trans Am Acad Ophthalmol Otolaryngol* 81:483-490, 1976.
24. Gass JDM, Olsen KR: Diffuse unilateral subacute neuroretinitis. In Ryan SJ: *Retina,* ed 2, St Louis, 1993, Mosby.
25. Gass JDM, Gilbert WR, Guerry RK et al.: Diffuse unilateral subacute neuroretinitis, *Ophthalmology* 85:521-545, 1978.
26. Ghadirian E, Veins P, Strykowski H et al.: Epidemiology of toxocariasis in the Montreal area, *Can J Public Health* 67:495-498, 1976.
27. Gillespie SH: A review of human toxocariasis, *J Appl Bacteriol* 63:473-479, 1987.
28. Glickman LT, Schantz PM: Epidemiology and pathogenesis of toxocariasis, *Epidemiol Rev* 3:230-250, 1981.
29. Glickman LT, Shofer FS: Zoonotic visceral and ocular larva migrans, *Vet Clin North Am: Small Anim Pract* 17, 1, 1987.
30. Glickman LT, Schantz PM, Dombroske R et al.: Evaluation of serological test for visceral larva migrans, *Am J Trop Med Hyg* 27:492-498, 1978.
31. Grand MG, Roper-Hall G: Pars plana vitrectomy for ocular toxocariasis, *Retina* 1:258-261, 1981.
32. Hagler WH, Pollard ZF, Jarrett WH et al.: Results of surgery for ocular *Toxocara canis*, *Ophthalmology* 88:1081-1086, 1981.
33. Hinman EH, Baker DD: Helmintologic survey of 1315 dogs from New Orleans, with special reference to age resistance, *Am J Trop Med Hyg* 39:101-104, 1936.
34. Hinz E, Baltz I: Intestinal helminths of domestic dogs in the Neckar valley, Federal Republic of Germany, *Int J Zoonosis* 12:211-213, 1985.
35. Hogan MJ, Kimura SJ, Spencer WH: Visceral larval migrans and peripheral retinitis, *J Am Med Assoc* 194:1345-1347, 1965.
36. Irvine AR: Nematodiasis: clinical description and pathology. In Kimura, editor: *Retinal diseases symposium on differential diagnostic problem of posterior uveitis.* Philadelphia, 1966, Lea & Febiger.
37. Irvine WC, Irvine AR Jr: Nematode endophthalmitis: *Toxocara canis*: report of one case, *Am J Ophthalmol* 47:185-191, 1959.
38. Jung RC, Pacheco G: Use of haemagglutination test in visceral larva migrans, *Am J Trop Med Hyg* 9:185-191, 1960.
39. Kazacos KR, Raymond LA, Kazacos EA et al.: The raccoon ascarid: a probable cause of human ocular larval migrans, *Ophthalmology* 92:1735-2744, 1985.
40. Maetz HM, Kleinstein RN, Federico D et al.: Estimated prevalence of ocular toxoplasmosis and toxocariasis in Alabama, *J Infect Dis* 156:414, 1987.
41. Mafee MF, Goldberg MF, Cohen SB et al.: Magnetic resonance imaging versus computed tomography of leukocoric eyes and use of in vitro proton magnetic resonance spectroscopy of retinoblastoma, *Ophthalmology* 96:7, 1989.
42. Maguire AM, Green WR, Michels RG et al.: Recovery of intraocular *Toxocara canis* by pars plana vitrectomy, *Ophthalmology* 97:675-680, 1990.
43. Maplestone PA, Bhaduri NV: The helminth parasites of dogs in Calcutta and their bearing on human parasitology, *Ind J Med Res* 28:595-604, 1940.
44. Milburn C, Ernst K: Eosinophilia-hepatomegaly syndrome of infants and young children, *Pediatrics* 11:358-367, 1953.
45. Molk R: Treatment of toxocaral optic neuritis, *J Clin Neuro Ophthalmol* 2:109-112, 1982.

46. Nelson JD, McConnell TH, Moore DV: Thiabendazole therapy of visceral larva migrans: a case report, *Am J Trop Med Hyg* 15:930-933, 1966.

47. Nichols RL: The etiology of visceral larval migrans. I. Diagnostic morphology of infective second-stage *Toxocara* larvae, *J Parasitol* 42:349-362, 1956.

48. O'Connor PR: Visceral lava migrans of the eye: subretinal tube formation, *Arch Ophthalmol* 88:526-529, 1972.

49. Perlinger JG, Gyorgy P: Chronic eosinophilia: report of a case with necrosis of liver, pulmonary infiltration anemai and ascaris infection, *Am J Dis Child* 73:34-43, 1947.

50. Phillips CI, Mackenzie AD: Toxocaral larval papillitis, *Br Med J* 1:154-155, 1973.

51. Pollard ZF, Jarrett WH, Hagler WS et al.: ELISA for diagnosis of ocular toxocariasis, *Ophthalmology* 86:743-749, 1979.

52. Raistrick ER, Hard JCD: Ocular toxocariasis in adults, *Br J Ophthalmol* 60:365-370, 1976.

53. Read MA, Thompson RCA: Prevalence of *Toxocara canis* and *Toxocara leonina* in dog faeces on the streets of Leeds, *J Helminthol* 50:95-96, 1976.

54. Rey A: Nematode endophthalmitis due to *Toxocara*, *Br J Ophthalmol* 46:616-618, 1962.

55. Rodriguez A: Early pars plana vitrectomy in chronic endophthalmitis of toxocariasis, *Graefes Arch Clin Exp Ophthalmol* 224:218-220, 1986.

56. Rowson NJ: Letters to the editor, *Eye* 7:810, 1993.

57. Rubin LF, Saunders LZ: Intraocular larva migrans in dogs, *Pathol Vet* 2:566-573, 1965.

58. Rubin ML, Kaufman HE, Tierney JP et al.: An intraretinal nematode (a case report), *Trans Am Acad Ophthalmol Otolaryngol* 72:855-866, 1968.

59. Schantz PM, Glickman LT: Current concepts in parasitology: toxocaral visceral larval migrans, *N Engl J Med* 298:436-439, 1978.

60. Schantz PM, Meyer D, Glickman LT: Clinical, serologic and epidemiologic characteristics of ocular otocariasis, *Am J Trop Med Hyg* 28(1):24-28, 1979.

61. Schantz PM, Weis PE, Pollard ZF et al.: Risk factors for toxocaral ocular larva migrans: a case-control study, *Am J Public Health* 70:1269-1272, 1980.

62. Schlaegel TF, Knox DL: Toxocariasis. In Duane TD, editor: *Clinical ophthalmology,* vol 4, Hagerstown, Md, 1976, Harper & Row.

63. Shields JA: Ocular toxocariasis: a review, *Surv Ophthalmol* 28, 5, 1984.

64. Shields JA, Augsburger JJ: Current approaches to the diagnosis and management of retinoblastoma, *Surv Ophthalmol* 15:347-371, 1981.

65. Shields JA, Felberg NT, Federman JF: Discussion of ELISA for diagnosis of ocular toxocariasis, *Ophthalmology* 86:750-752, 1979.

66. Small KW, McCuen BW, deJuan E et al.: Surgical management of retinal traction caused by toxocariasis, *Am J Ophthalmol* 108:10-14, 1989.

67. Smith HV, Kusel JR, Girdwood RWA: The production of human A and B group like substances by in vitro maintained second stage *Toxocara canis* larvae: their presence on the outer larval surfaces and in their excretions/secretions, *Clin Exp Immunol* 54:625-634, 1983.

68. Smith RE, Hagstad H: Vesceral larval migrans: a risk assessment in Baton Rouge, *Int J Zoonoses* 11:189-194, 1984.

69. Sorr EM: Meandering ocular toxocariasis, *Retina* 4:90-96, 1984.

70. Sprent JFA: The life cycles of nematodes in the family *Ascarididea blanchard* 1896, *J Parasitol* 40:608-617, 1954.

71. Sprent JFA: Observations of the development of *Toxocara canis* (Werner 1792) in the dog, *Parasitology* 48:148-209, 1958.

72. Thompson DE, Bundy DAP, Cooper ES et al.: Epidemiological characteristics of *Toxocara canis* zoonotic infection of children in a Caribbean community, *Bull World Health Organ* 64:283-290, 1986.

73. Ugochukwu EI, Ejimadu KN: Studies on the prevalence of gastrointestinal helminths of dogs in Calabar Nigeria, *Int J Zoonoses* 12:214-218, 1985.

74. Vaughn J, Jordan R: Intestinal nematodes in well cared for dogs, *Am J Trop Med Hyg* 9:29-32, 1960.

75. Watzke RC, Oaks JA, Folk JC: *Toxocara canis* infection of the eye: correlation of clinical observations with developing pathology in the primate model, *Arch Ophthalmol* 102:282-291, 1984.

76. Wilder HC: Nematode endophthalmitis, *Trans Am Acad Ophthalmol Otolaryngol* 55:99-109, 1950.

77. Wilkinson CP: Ocular toxocariasis. In Ryan SJ, editor: *Retina,* St Louis, 1993, Mosby.

78. Wilkinson CP, Welch RB: Intraocular *Toxocara, Am J Ophthalmol* 71:921-930, 1971.

79. Wiseman RA, Woodruff AW, Pettitt LE: The treatment of toxocaral infections: some experimental and clinical observations, *Trans R Soc Trop Med Hyg* 65:591-598, 1971.

87 Cysticercosis

ALAN H. FRIEDMAN

Cysticercosis is caused by the encystment of the cestode larva, *Cysticercus cellulosae,* of the tapeworm *Taenia solium.* This parasite causes two types of human disease. Eating undercooked pork containing cysticerci can lead to intestinal taeniasis. Cysticercosis, however, usually results from ingesting eggs from food, water, or other material contaminated with human feces. Larvae that penetrate the intestinal wall can disseminate to the skin, brain, eye, and other tissues.[4]

PARASITOLOGY

The phylum Platyhelminthes (flatworms) contains the class Cestoda that is divided into eight orders. Of these, the order Cyclophyllidea contains the genus *Taenia.* Ocular cysticercosis is due to larvae of the pork tapeworm *T. solium,* although rare cases of *T. saginata* and *T. crassiceps* ocular infection have been encountered. Other cestode infections that have rarely produced ocular or orbital disease are hydatid cysts caused by *Echinococcus* sp. and sparganosis caused by the larvae (spargana) of *Spirometra* sp.

In human tapeworm infection, the adult *T. solium* is found in the upper part of the small intestine and may measure from 4 to 8 meters in length and contain up to 800 to 1000 segments. The head is formed by a rostellum composed of a globular scolex about 1 mm in diameter and containing a double row of hooklets with four suckers. The narrow neck of the tapeworm is 5 cm to 10 cm in length and is connected to the distal segments that each measure 6 by 12 mm and contain 30,000 to 50,000 ova. Segments, called proglottids, pass from the bowel in the feces and may rupture in or outside the stool.

Larvae contain a superficial tegument and a deeper subtegument or parenchyma (Fig. 87-1). The surface of the tegument contains villous processes with cilia that stir up the surrounding fluid. The central core at the base of each microtrix is continuous with syncytial cytoplasm. Metabolites are absorbed at the surface and transported by pinocytotic vesicles. Cytoplasmic processes penetrate the muscle layer into parenchymal cells. The muscle layer contains circular and longitudinal fibers. The parenchyma contains calcareous corpuscles rich in organic substances and inorganic carbonates (Fig. 87-2, *A*) important in neutralizing gastric acids. An osmoregulatory apparatus contains flame cells and an interconnecting systemic of tubules necessary to move water throughout the parasite (Fig. 87-2, *B*). Fluids pass from the flame cell by cilia (Fig. 87-2, *C*) into collecting tubules and toward pores in the tegument.

HISTORICAL BACKGROUND

Milestones in the study of cysticercosis have been reviewed by Duke-Elder.[10a] The first recorded observations of porcine cysticercosis were noted in the Ebers Papyrus (c. 1500 BC) and in the writings of Hippocrates. For centuries it was commonly thought that worms spontaneously generated in the intestinal tract. Von Benenden established the life cycle of the parasite in 1850.

The first clinical observation of cysticercosis of the eye was Soemmering's 1830 report of a cyst in the anterior chamber. The surgical removal of an intracameral cyst was accomplished by Schott soon thereafter. Von Graefe made the first observation of a cysticercus in the vitreous humor in 1854 and was the first to remove an intravitreous cyst. In a report of 90 cases, he found 80 cysts in the posterior segment, 3 in the anterior chamber, 1 in the lens, 5 under the conjunctiva, and 1 in the orbit.

The occurrence of ocular cysticercosis in Europe declined toward the end of the nineteenth century. In Berlin Hirschberg found 70 cases of ocular cysticercosis among 60,000 clinic visits during 1869 to 1885, 3 cases among 78,000 visits during 1886 to 1894, and none among 650,000 patients during 1895 to 1902. This decrease was due in large measure to compulsory meat inspection instituted in Berlin in 1883. Extraintestinal infections with *Taenia solium* larvae are rare in developed countries but still occur in many parts of the world.

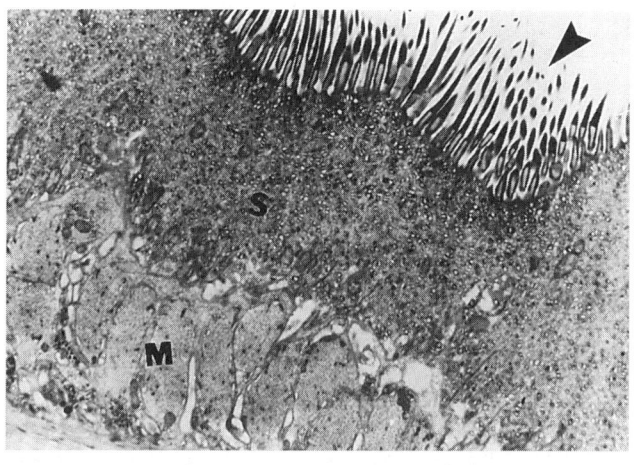

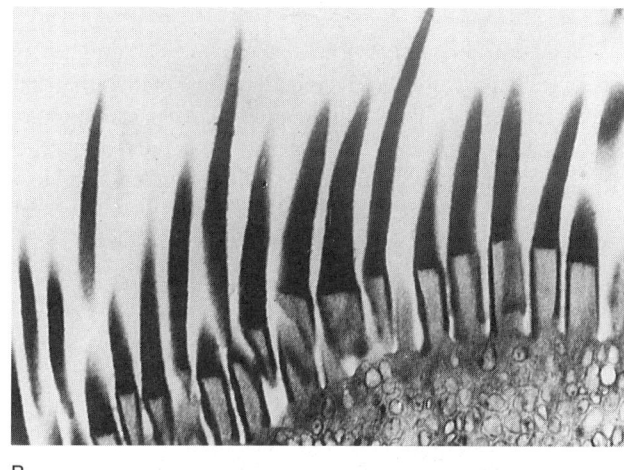

A

B

Fig. 87-1. Electron micrographs of larva of *T. solium.* **A,** Distal syncytial cytoplasm *(S)* with surface microtriches *(arrowhead)* and a contractile muscle layer *(M).* (× 17,000). **B,** Microtriches contain an electron-lucent base separated from a conical tip by a pentalaminate zone. The base has an electron-dense wall and communicates with the distal cytoplasm and its vesicles (× 40,000).

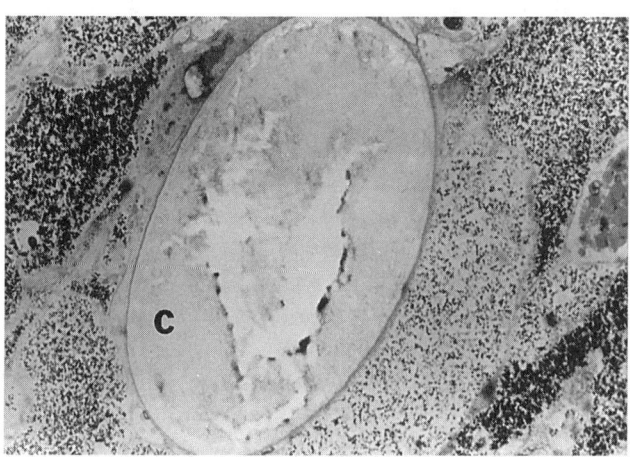

A

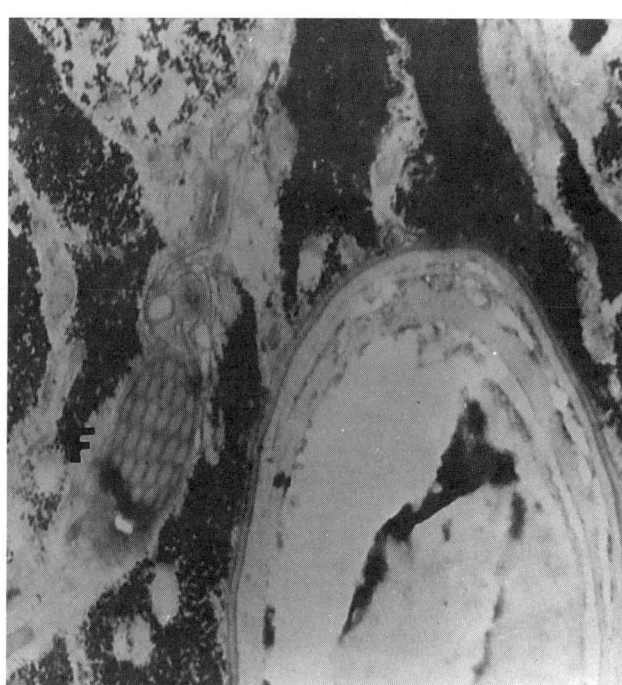

B

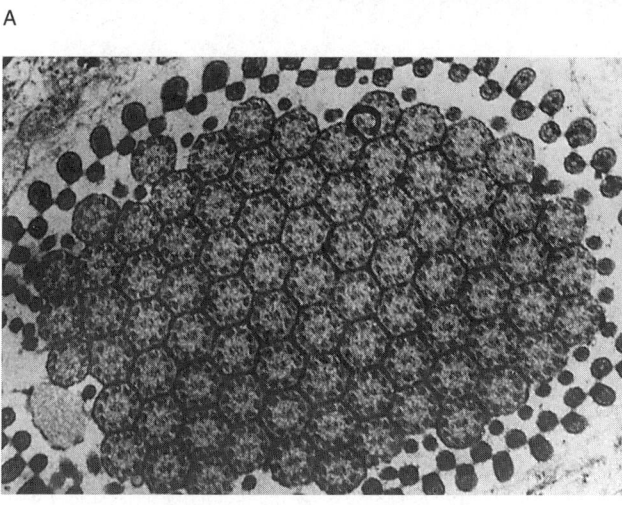

C

Fig. 87-2. Subcellular structure of a cysticercus. **A,** Cells of the parenchyma contain glycogen granules, ribosomes, and calcareous corpuscles *(C).* These vesicles have an electron-dense surface and a granular, electron-lucent core (× 11,000). **B,** Within the parenchyma are osmoregulatory structures and flame cells *(F),* seen here adjacent to a calcareous corpuscle (× 18,000). **C,** Cross section of cilia containing a 9 + 2 structure projecting into the lumen of a collecting tubule (× 30,000).

EPIDEMIOLOGY

Tapeworm infestation occurs worldwide, although it is rare in societies with a high standard of food preparation and among religious cultures that do not eat pork. Cysticercosis, in contrast, occurs in all ethnic groups; it is related more to poverty and poor hygiene than to dietary practices. Most cases of cysticercosis occur in Mexico and other parts of Latin America, India and southern Asia, China, and certain areas of Africa. Neurocysticercosis and ocular cysticercosis seem to be more common in Latin America, whereas skin disease is relatively more common in India.

CLINICAL FEATURES

Disseminated cysticercosis may cause muscle pains, weakness, and fever. Central nervous system involvement may be manifested by meningoencephalitis, seizures, intracranial hypertension with papilledema (Fig. 87-3, *A*), visual field deficits, and mental changes.* Cranial nerve palsies have occurred. A cysticercus involving the optic nerve has been described. Central nervous system lesions are visualized by computed tomography or magnetic resonance imaging (Fig. 87-3, *B*). Cerebral cysts usually measure 1 cm to 4 cm by 0.5 cm to 2 cm. Calcified cysticerci may be seen on radiographs.

Ocular cysticercosis can involve any structure within or around the eye, although the vitreous humor (Fig. 87-4) and retina are most likely to be affected.[7,19,39] Of more than 500 reported cases of ocular cysticercosis, approximately 4% involve the eyelid or orbit, 20% are located subconjunctivally, 8% involve the anterior segment of the eye, and 68% involve the posterior segment.

Eyelid and Orbit

Cysticercosis of the eyelid usually appears as a painless, enlarging nodule that may reach 1 cm to 2 cm in diameter.[13,24,35] Cysticerci within the orbit[22] or lacrimal gland[32] are uncommon. A cysticercus within an extraocular muscle may produce diplopia.[5,10,26,37]

Conjunctiva

Subconjunctival lesions usually appear as somewhat painful, hyperemic epibulbar masses that are sometimes fluctuant.[20,31,33,34]

Anterior Chamber

An intracameral cysticercus is uncommon (only about 20 cases have been reported during the twentieth century). Most are free-floating cysts within the aqueous humor.[14] Others are attached to the iris or to the anterior lens capsule. Minimal inflammation is usually present, although un-

---

*References 2, 8, 15, 21, 23, 25.

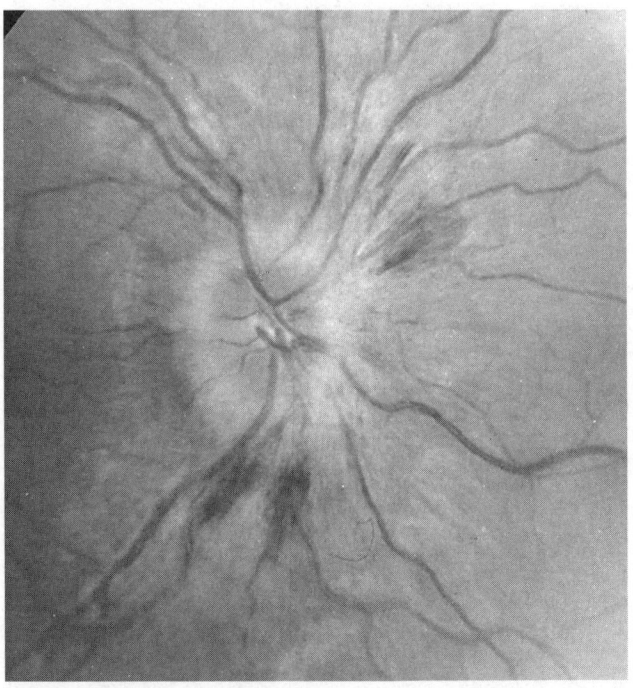

A

B

Fig. 87-3. Neurocysticercosis. **A,** Papilledema in a patient with cerebral cysticercosis. **B,** CT scan showing multiple cystic lesions. (Courtesy of Patricia Cucci, MD).

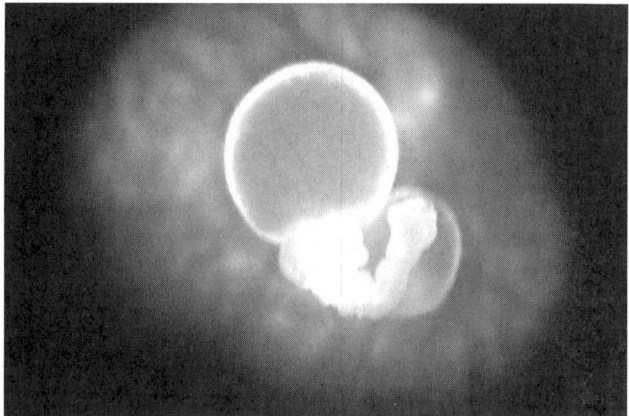

Fig. 87-4. Ocular cysticercosis with larva in the vitreous humor.

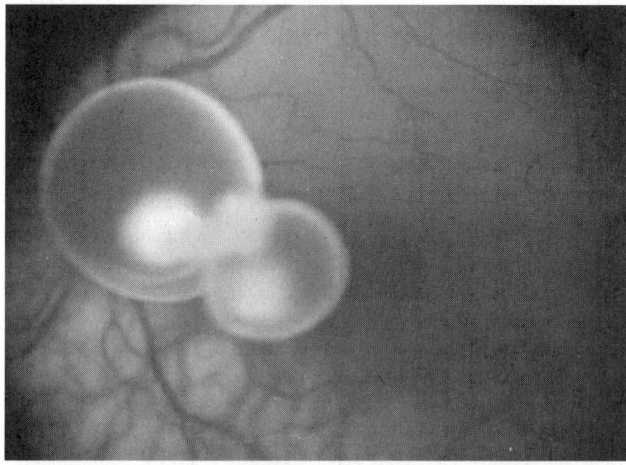

A

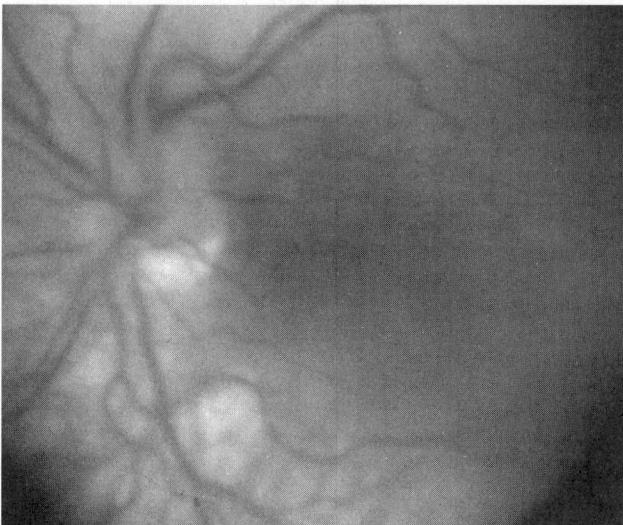

B

Fig. 87-5. Ocular cysticercosis. **A,** Two cysticerci in the vitreous humor, one with an evaginated scolex and the other with an invaginated scolex. **B,** Mild peripapillary choroidal atrophy following pars plana vitrectomy.

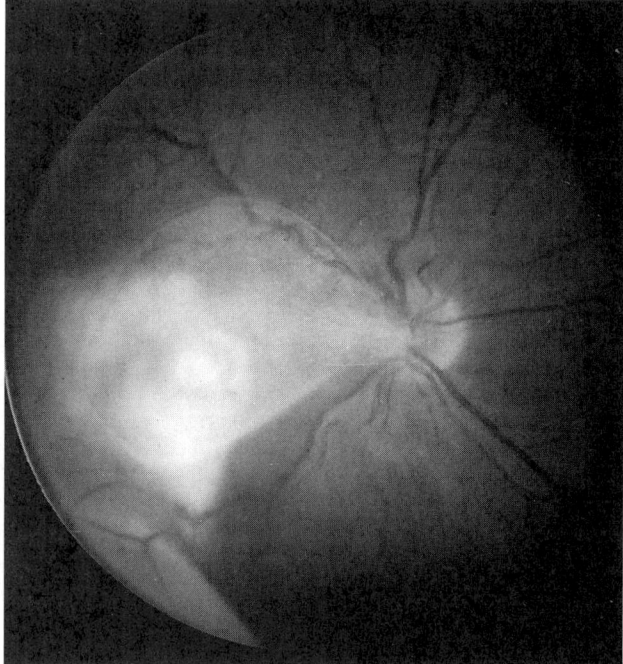

Fig. 87-6. Subretinal cysticercosis with adjacent scarring and an overlying exudative retinal detachment.

treated, degenerated cysts produce a severe iritis. A cysticercus within the lens or cornea is an extremely rare occurrence.

Posterior Segment

A cysticercus of the posterior segment of the eye is usually present in the vitreous humor (Fig. 87-5) or in the subretinal space (Fig. 87-6).[3,16] The parasite is brought to the globe by the posterior ciliary arteries and enters the subretinal space at the posterior pole. Cysticerci may traverse the retina and present in the vitreous humor as a free-floating cyst. The translucent, fluid-filled cyst is approximately 3 to 6 optic disc diameters in size and has a protoscolex that may be invaginated or evaginated. Contraction and undulation of the cyst wall can be accentuated by light. Bilateral multifocal intraocular cysticerci have been described.[38]

Retinal pigment epithelial disturbances, retinal edema, intraretinal hemorrhage, perivascular sheathing, and serous or exudative retinal detachment may be seen. Without removal, a severe exudative choroiditis and vitritis can develop that can lead to disorganization of the globe.

PATHOLOGY

Histopathologic examination of eyelid lesions from patients with cysticercosis shows an inflammatory reaction around the cyst wall. An outermost zone of dense fibrovascular connective tissue surrounds a middle layer of lymphocytes and large histiocytes intermingled with fibroblasts. An inner layer contains neutrophils and eosinophils around the degenerating parasite.

A mild inflammatory reaction accompanies viable intraocular larvae. As the cysticercus degenerates, inflammation within the eye intensifies. Eosinophils, neutrophils, and macrophages surround the dying organism. Enucleated eyes with intraocular cysticercosis have a degenerated, thickened retina detached by a subretinal serous exudate. Cysticerci can be found within the vitreous cavity, in the retina, or in the subretinal space. Degenerated parasites are associated with an intense fibrovascular reaction and sometimes calcification.

PATHOGENESIS

Ova imbibed by the intermediate host (pigs for *T. solium*) develop into larvae (oncospheres and metacestodes) within the pig's intestine. Eggs eaten directly by humans, the definitive host, behave the same as if they were in the intermediate host. Cysticercosis is a parasitic disease usually produced by ingestion of ova of *T. solium* from contaminated food; autoinfection is possible by swallowing one's own infected feces or by reverse peristalsis of intestinal eggs.

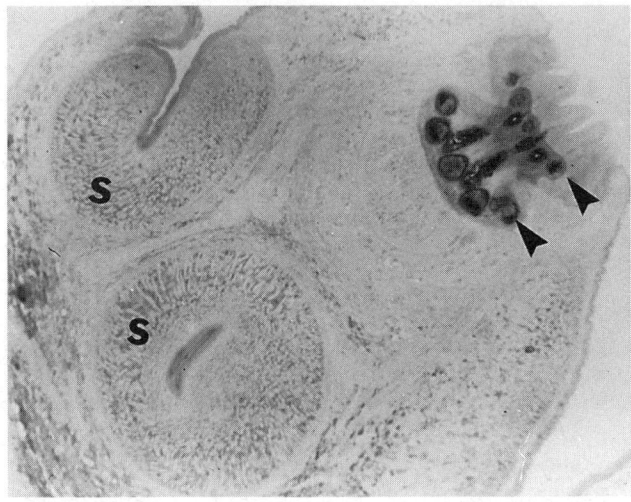

B

Fig. 87-7, cont'd. B, Light micrograph of scolex displaying suckers *(S)* and rostellum with double row of hooklets *(arrowheads)* (toluidine blue, × 150).

Upon emerging from the hatched eggs in the intestine, hexacanth (six-toothed) larvae penetrate the intestinal wall and travel via the lymphatic and vascular systems to subcutaneous tissues, muscles, and the central nervous system. As the larva or oncosphere develops, it becomes a metacestode or cysticercus. At this stage there is complete development of a cystic structure with an inverted scolex and a spiral canal, through which the scolex can evaginate. This process of evagination usually takes place in the small intestine but can also be observed in the eye. When the scolex evaginates it appears with its four cup-shaped suckers and a rostellum containing a double row of hooklets (Fig. 87-7).[11]

Living cysticerci elicit minimal inflammation and persist for years, usually long after any prior intestinal infestation may have occurred. Cysticerci may remain viable in the eye for 2 years or more and for an average of 5 years in the central nervous system.

Host Response

Humoral and cellular immunity to parasitic antigens can be demonstrated during experimental cysticercosis.[6] Immunity appears to play a limited role during disseminated human disease, however. The immune response neither shortens the duration of infection nor reduces susceptibility to reinfection.

DIFFERENTIAL DIAGNOSIS

A cysticercus can be differentiated from a hydatid cyst (produced by *Echinococcus granulosus* or *Echinococcus multilocularis*), a coenurus (produced by *Taenia multiceps*), and ocular sparganosis (produced by *Spirometra mansonoides*) by histopathology of the excised organism. *Echinococcosis multilocularis* produces a multilocular cyst containing a gray gel instead of clear fluid as in a cysticercus.

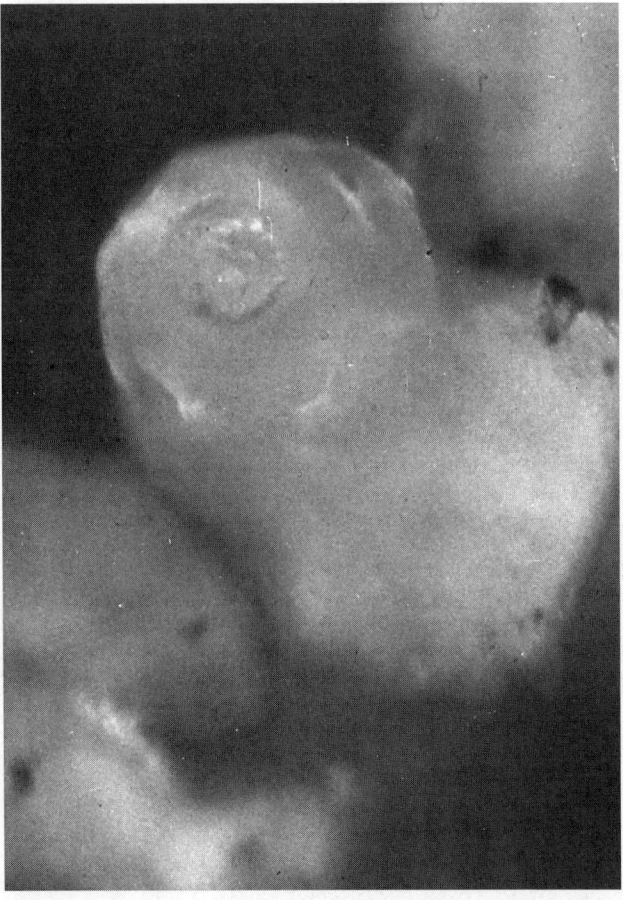

A

Fig. 87-7. Larva of *Taenia solium*. **A,** Scolex on the surface of a cysticercus (× 40).

LABORATORY INVESTIGATIONS

B-scan ultrasonography can confirm the cystic nature of the parasite (Fig. 87-8).[12] Intravenous fluorescein angiography can highlight the secondary fundus changes but will not stain the parasite (Fig. 87-9). Cytology of intraocular cysticercosis can show numerous eosinophils.

An enzyme linked immunosorbent assay (ELISA) test for *T. solium* coproantigens is available to detect previous exposure to the intestinal adult worm if autoinfection is suspected, but this assay is not useful in the diagnosis of ocular cysticercosis.[27] An immunoblot assay for antibody to cysticercal glycoproteins is available at the Centers for Disease Control and Prevention. Antigen detection and nucleic acid probes are under development.

THERAPY

Patients with ocular cysticercosis usually do not harbor adult tapeworms in the intestine. If intestinal taeniasis is suspected, medical treatment consists of a single dose of niclosamide, 2 grams (4 500-mg tablets) chewed one at a time and swallowed with a small amount of water. The dose is titrated for children (1 gram for body weight of 11 to 34 kg, and 1.5 grams for body weight more than 34 kg). Praziquantel is an alternative treatment, used as a single 10 mg/kg dose.

Treatment of intraocular or adnexal cysticercosis is surgical removal of the living organism. Medical treatment can lead to serious ocular inflammation that risks vision loss.[28] Photocoagulation can also release metabolic products or toxins that produce an inflammatory reaction.[29] Intravitreous cysticerci can be removed by pars plana vitrectomy. Subret-

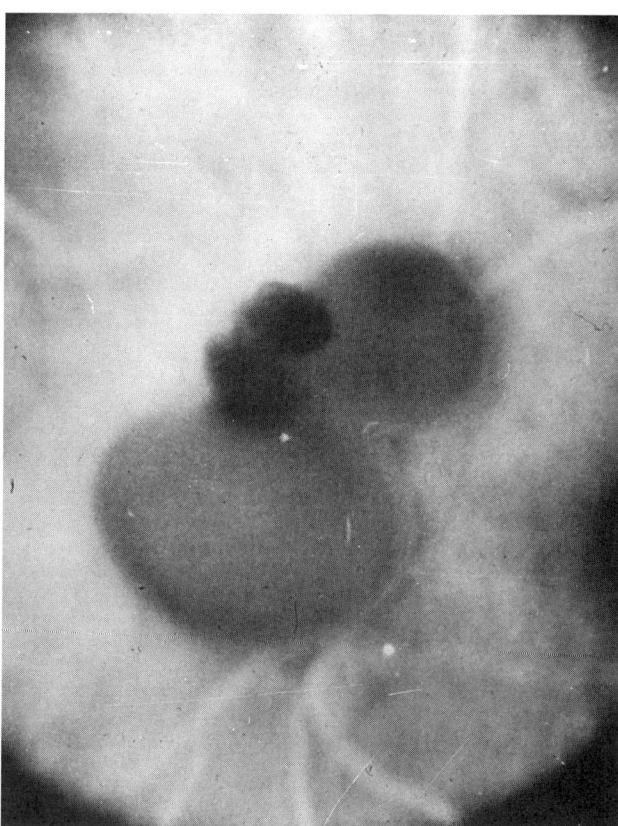

Fig. 87-9. Intravenous fluorescein angiography fails to enhance cysticerci in the vitreous humor.

inal cysticerci can be removed by a transvitreous or a transscleral approach.[1,18,36,40]

An 8-day course of oral albendazole is recommended for parenchymal brain cysticercosis.[9]

PREVENTION

Infection may be prevented by thoroughly cooking pork at a minimal temperature of 56°C (133°F) for at least 5 minutes. Cysticerci in contaminated pork give it a measled appearance. Eating only properly inspected meat is essential. Salting and pickling alone are not effective.

The role of a vaccine in preventing ocular cysticercosis is unknown.[17] Prevention will rely on improvements in hygiene and other international control measures.[30]

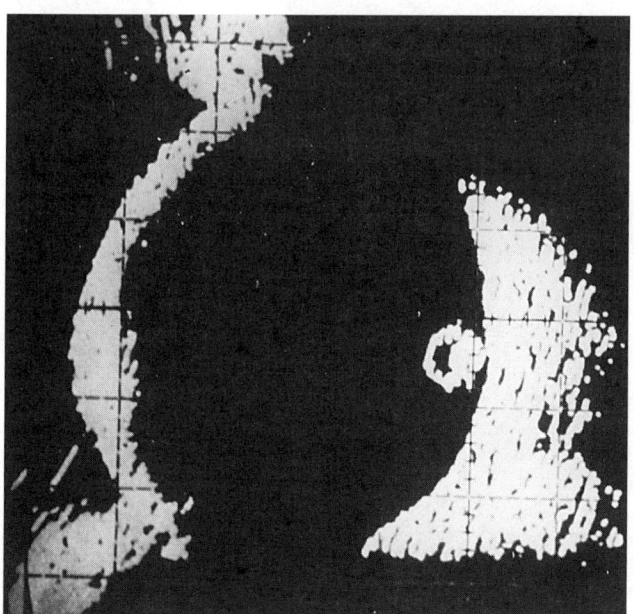

Fig. 87-8. B-scan ultrasound showing a cysticercus in the vitreous cavity adjacent to the optic disc.

REFERENCES

1. Arciniegas A, Gutierrez F: Our experience in the removal of intravitreal and subretinal cysticerci, *Ann Ophthalmol* 20:75-77, 1988.
2. Barry M, Kaldjian LC: Neurocysticercosis, *Semin Neurol* 13:131-143, 1993.
3. Bartholomew RS: Subretinal cysticercosis, *Am J Ophthalmol* 79:670-672, 1975.
4. Botero D, Tanowitz HB, Weiss LM, Wittner M: Taeniasis and cysticercosis, *Infect Dis Clin North Am* 7:683-697, 1993.

5. Brooks AMV, Essex WB, West RH: Cysticercosis of the superior oblique muscle, *Aust J Ophthalmol* 11:119-122, 1983.

6. Cardenas F, Plancarte A, Quiroz H et al.: *Taenia crassiceps:* experimental model of intraocular cysticercosis, *Exp Parasitol* 69:324-329, 1989.

7. Cardenas F, Quiroz H, Plancarte A et al.: *Taenia solium* ocular cysticercosis: findings in 30 cases, *Ann Ophthalmol* 24:25-28, 1992.

8. Case Records of the Massachusetts General Hospital: Case 8-1993, Neurocysticercosis, *New Eng J Med* 328:566-573, 1993.

9. Del Brutto OH, Sotelo J, Roman GC: Therapy for neurocysticercosis: a reappraisal, *Clin Infect Dis* 17:730-735, 1993.

10. DiLoreto DA, Kennedy RA, Neigel JM, Rootman J: Infestation of extraocular muscle by *Cysticercus cellulosae, Br J Ophthalmol* 74:751-752, 1990.

10a. Duke-Elder S: Summary of systemic ophthalmology. In Duke-Elder S, editor: *System of ophthalmology,* vol XV, London, 1976, Henry Kimpton.

11. Friedman AH, Pokorny KS, Suhan J et al.: Electron microscopic observations of intravitreal *Cysticercus cellulosae (Taenia solium), Ophthalmologica* 180:267-273, 1980.

12. Guillory SL, Zinn KM: Intravitreal *Cysticercus cellulosae:* ultrasonographic and fluorescein angiographic features, *Bull NY Acad Med* 56:655-661, 1980.

13. Jampol LM, Caldwell JBH, Albert DM: *Cysticercus cellulosae* in the eyelid, *Arch Ophthalmol* 89:319-320, 1973.

14. Kapoor S, Sood GC, Aurora AL, Sood M: Ocular cysticercosis: report of a free floating cysticercus in the anterior chamber, *Acta Ophthalmol* 55:927-930, 1977.

15. Keane JR: Cysticercosis: unusual neuro-ophthalmologic signs, *J Clin Neuroophthalmol* 13:194-199, 1993.

16. Kruger-Leite E, Jalkh AE, Quiroz H et al.: Intraocular cysticercosis, *Am J Ophthalmol* 99:252-257, 1985.

17. Lightowlers MW, Rickard MD: Vaccination against cestode parasites, *Immunol Cell Biol* 71:443-451, 1993.

18. Luger MH, Stilma JS, Ringens PJ, van Baarlen J: In-toto removal of a subretinal *Cysticercus cellulosae* by pars plana vitrectomy, *Br J Ophthalmol* 75:561-563, 1991.

19. Manschot WA: Intraocular cysticercosis, *Arch Ophthalmol* 80:772-774, 1968.

20. Mehra KS, Nema HV, Nagarajachar J et al.: Conjunctival cysticercosis, *Acta Ophthalmol* 46:980-984, 1968.

21. Mitchell WG, Crawford TP: Intraparenchymal cerebral cysticercosis in children: diagnosis and treatment, *Pediatrics* 82:76-82, 1988.

22. Murthy H, Kumar A, Verma L: Orbital cysticercosis—an ultrasonic diagnosis, *Acta Ophthalmol* 68:612-614, 1990.

23. Nash TE, Neva FA: Recent advances in the diagnosis and treatment of cerebral cysticercosis, *New Eng J Med* 311:1491-1496, 1984.

24. Perry HD, Font RL: Cysticercosis of the eyelid, *Arch Ophthalmol* 96:1255-1257, 1978.

25. Pollard ZF: Cysticercosis: an unusual cause of papilledema, *Ann Ophthalmol* 12:110-112, 1975.

26. Rao VA, Kawatra VK, Ratnakar C: Unusual cause of acquired inflammatory Brown's syndrome, *Can J Ophthalmol* 22:320-323, 1987.

27. Rosas N, Sotelo J, Nieto D: ELISA in the diagnosis of neurocysticercosis, *Arch Neurol* 43:353-356, 1986.

28. Santos R, Chavarria M, Aquirre AE: Failure of medical treatment in two cases of intraocular cysticercosis, *Am J Ophthalmol* 97:249-250, 1984.

29. Santos R, Dalma A, Ortiz E, Sanchez-Bulnes L: Management of subretinal and vitreous cysticercosis: role of photocoagulation and surgery, *Ophthalmology* 86:1501-1507, 1979.

30. Schantz PM, Cruz M, Sarti E, Pawlowski Z: Potential eradicability of taeniasis and cysticercosis, *Bull Pan Am Health Organ* 27:397-403, 1993.

31. Sen DK: *Cysticercus cellulosae* presenting as an epibulbar tumor in an infant, *J Pediatr Ophthalmol Strabismus* 16:251-253, 1979.

32. Sen DK: Acute suppurative dacryoadenitis caused by a *Cysticercus cellulosa, J Pediatr Ophthalmol Strabismus* 19:100-102, 1982.

33. Sen DK, Thomas A: *Cysticercus cellulosae* causing subconjunctival abscess, *Am J Ophthalmol* 68:714-715, 1969.

34. Sen DK, Thomas A: Incidence of subconjunctival cysticercosis, *Acta Ophthalmologica* 47:395-399, 1969.

35. Singh G, Kaur J: Cysticercosis of the eyelid, *Ann Ophthalmol* 14:947-950, 1982.

36. Steinmetz RL, Masket S, Sidikaro Y: The successful removal of a subretinal cysticercus by pars plana vitrectomy, *Retina* 9:276-280, 1989.

37. Stewart CR, Salmon J, Murray AD, Sperryn C: Cysticercosis as a cause of severe medial rectus muscle myositis, *Am J Ophthalmol* 116:501-510, 1993.

38. Topilow HW, Yimoyines DJ, Freeman HM et al.: Bilateral multifocal intraocular cysticercosis, *Ophthalmology* 88:1166-1172, 1981.

39. Welsh NH, Peters AL, Crewe-Brown W et al.: Ocular cysticercosis: a report of 13 cases, *S Afr Med J* 71:719-722, 1987.

40. Zinn KM, Guillory SL, Friedman AH: Removal of intravitreal cysticerci from the surface of the optic nerve head: a pars plana approach, *Arch Ophthalmol* 98:714-718, 1980.

88 Diffuse Unilateral Subacute Neuroretinitis

JANET L. DAVIS, J. DONALD M. GASS

Adult and larval forms of organisms in the class Nematoda have been found in the inner eye. Most of the historic cases involve large (greater than 10 mm) adult worms visible in the anterior chambers of persons from tropical areas with endemic filariasis; they are typically attributed to filarial roundworms (Filarioidea) that inhabit the blood and lymphatic tissues, such as those of the genera *Wuchereria, Loa, Onchocerca,* and *Dracunculus.*[6] Two such cases have been described in the United States.[19,31] Diffuse unilateral subacute neuroretinitis (DUSN) is a more recently described disorder believed to be caused by smaller nematodes.

HISTORICAL BACKGROUND

In 1950 Wilder[35] reported the first cases in which larval forms of nematodal intestinal roundworms (Ascaridoidea: *Ascaris, Toxocara, Ancylostoma, Necator, Strongyloides*) were implicated as a cause of intraocular disease.[35] Forty-six eyes, principally of children from the southeastern United States, enucleated for possible retinoblastoma, were serially sectioned because they contained eosinophilic granulomata of unknown cause. Nematode larvae or hyaline capsules were found in 24 of the cases. The parasites were later determined to be *Toxocara* sp. larvae.[27,28] The formation of a white mass or leukocoria in these cases is presumed to have been the stimulus for enucleation.

Case reports of a clinical syndrome very different from the large worms suspended in intraocular fluid or the small larvae embedded in posterior segment granulomata began to appear in 1952 when a motile, subretinal worm was described and photographed in a living eye by Parsons[30] in Florida. Two other Florida patients were subsequently reported to have living nematodes in the retina that produced a syndrome similar to a macular degeneration or a healed central serous retinopathy; the worms were thought to be *Toxocara canis.*[33]

A live worm was seen in the macula of a North Carolina man in 1966; the fellow eye had lost vision from a macular chorioretinitis of undetermined cause several years previously.[31] Similar subretinal, motile nematodes and pigmentary changes were described in a Kentucky girl and a Michigan man.[32] Raymond and associates[32] suggested that migrating retinal nematodes be included in the differential diagnosis of unilateral pseudoretinitis pigmentosa and unilateral macular degeneration.

A thorough description of a "diffuse unilateral subacute neuroretinitis" in 29 patients was formulated[15] before the connection with the earlier cases of nematodiasis was made. The clinical syndrome had previously been known as "unilateral wipe-out syndrome."[9] A footnote to the original publication on DUSN[15] remarks that two later patients with the same clinical syndrome were observed to have motile, subretinal worms, presumed to be *T. canis,* and the suspicion was raised that all cases of the clinical syndrome might be due to nematode infestation. Since then, efforts have been directed toward identification of the responsible nematodes and to treatment; the clinical description of the syndrome has not been improved.

EPIDEMIOLOGY

DUSN appears to be most common in the southeastern United States and the Caribbean, although a smaller number of cases have been reported from the upper midwestern United States.[11] Two cases have been reported in Brazilian patients[5] and one in a European.[24,26] Increased recognition may ultimately lead to more cases being diagnosed in other parts of the world since nematodes of this type are extremely common. Warm climate may foster the transmission of the parasite because of persistence of the eggs in soil.

DUSN is more prevalent in the young. Of 37 patients, the age at onset of visual symptoms was 5 to 38 years with an average of 14 years.[14] There was a slight male predominance (22 of 37) in this series; the racial distribution was well-matched to the surrounding community (31 white, 6 black).

CLINICAL FEATURES

Recognition of DUSN early in its course is the principal task of the clinician, since treatment may prevent further vision loss but is unlikely to restore vision. Onset is frequently insidious.[15] Because the disorder has been unilateral in all but one case,[15] nearly half of patients in Gass' series[14] had advanced vision loss when they first became symptomatic. Patients who became symptomatic in the early stages of disease typically complained of paracentral or central scotomata,[14] although some noted ocular discomfort,[14] poor night vision,[4] or transient obscurations of vision.[17] Patients are virtually always in good health except for the ocular disorder.[14,15]

Vision in the early stages of disease is good in only a small minority of patients; five out of 36 patients in the largest series to date had vision better than 20/80.[14] Anterior segment inflammation is uncommon, but ciliary flush, keratic precipitates, and a small hypopyon have been reported in one patient.[14] Vitreous humor inflammatory reaction, in contrast, is a fairly constant finding in DUSN.[14] The optic disc may be edematous or exhibit mild pallor in the early stages.[12,14,17] An afferent pupillary defect is the rule.[15]

The most characteristic features of DUSN involve the retina and retinal pigment epithelium. In 14 of 19 patients with early-stage disease, multiple, active-appearing, focal, gray- or yellow-white lesions in the outer retina occurred in clusters, then faded within several days (Figs. 88-1 and 88-2).[14] Successive crops of lesions were observed over 20 months in one patient.[14] Localized serous retinal detachment may accompany the lesions, which are presumed to be responses to toxic metabolic products of the worm. The color of the retinal pigment epithelium undergoes a diffuse change with chronicity, which produces a dull reflex reminiscent of a pseudoretinitis pigmentosa, and focal areas of depigmentation can develop. Retinal arteriolar narrowing, choroidal neovascularization, and cystoid macular edema are less common manifestations of early stage disease.[14]

Less than half of cases reported have had a visible sub-

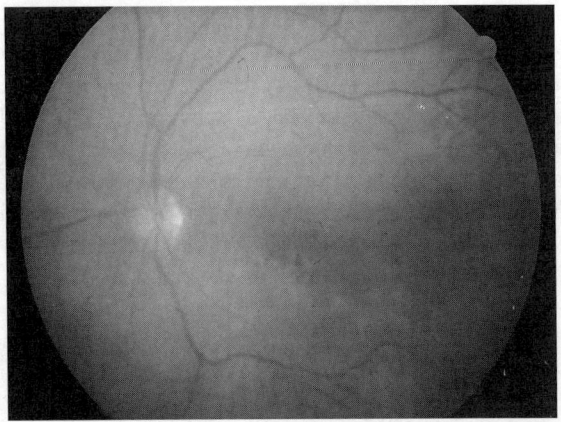

Fig. 88-1. Active, outer retinal, yellow-white lesions in the left eye of a 37-year-old woman with increasing visual complaints for 6 months. Vision was hand motions only with a probable functional overlay. There was very mild optic disc pallor with an afferent pupillary defect and a trace of anterior vitreous cell. (Figure also in color insert.)

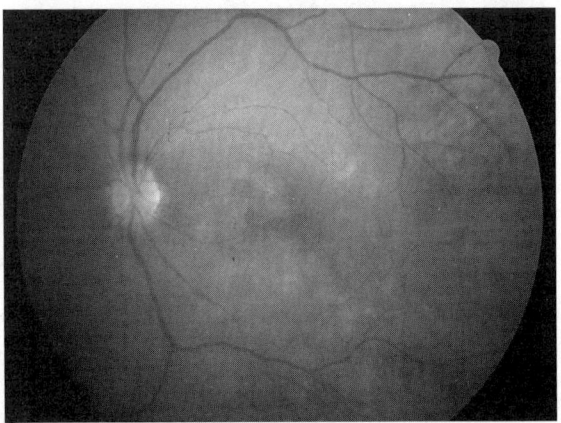

Fig. 88-2. The same eye shown in Fig. 88-1, 12 days later. The active retinal lesions are increased in number and extent and a subretinal worm is visible 2 disc diameters superonasal to the center of the macula at the 11:00 meridian. (Figure also in color insert.)

retinal worm. The subretinal worm is usually observed in early stage disease close to the active retinal lesions before moving, rarely rapidly, to another location. Small worms cannot be seen with indirect ophthalmoscopy using a 20 diopter lens and should be searched for with a contact lens. Motility of the worm is often documented only by change in the configuration of the worm from a coiled circle, to a serpentine, to a figure six or eight over time, although slow coiling and uncoiling movements in the subretinal space have been described.[5] Fundus photography is a great help to document the nematode and is sometimes successful in finding the worm when the clinician fails. Light can irritate the nematode and make it move, which may account for the frequent loss of the worm after an initial sighting. Worms have been detected in eyes for up to 3 years.[11]

Late-stage or inactive disease is accompanied by reduced visual acuity, which is usually 20/400 or less, and large, dense, central scotomata.[4,14,29] Vision can be poor even with minimal optic nerve atrophy and no retinal arteriolar narrowing.[14] The damage to the retina and retinal pigment epithelium is usually widespread, although some quadrants may be asymmetrically affected. Choroidal neovascularization and, in one patient, intraretinal pigment migration, have also been found in late-stage disease.[14]

PATHOLOGY

The histopathology described in one case in the original report of DUSN[15] may not be relevant, since viral inclusions were present. No eosinophilic granulomata, typical for toxocariasis, or traces of parasite were found in that specimen. A subretinal nematode was externalized surgically from a human eye by means of an eye-wall biopsy, with features suggestive of *Ancylostoma caninum,* but a definitive identification could not be made.[10]

PATHOGENESIS

Because the nematodes causing DUSN are probably of the intestinal roundworm type, a fecal-oral route of contamination is likely. Embryonated eggs in contaminated soil or other sources are ingested, penetrate the intestinal wall as motile larvae, and migrate to the subretinal space. The presence in the eye is probably caused by a low frequency, random event in small infestations, since virtually none of the cases described have had systemic disease suggestive of visceral larva migrans. The relative immune privilege of the eye may permit a larva to survive intraocularly, whereas it would be killed by the body's immune defenses in other locations.

Causal Agent

Much speculation has been directed toward the identity of the nematode. Worms of two different sizes have been described,[11] neither of which was thought to be *T. canis,* based on the negative serologic titers in most patients. The smaller worm of 400 to 1000 microns in length is more common in the cases from the southern United States; a larger worm of 1500 to 2000 microns is more common in the northern cases.[11] The smaller worm may actually be *T. canis,* despite earlier doubts. Toxocaral second stage larvae are typically 400 microns in length and rarely grow beyond 450 microns.[27,28] Some DUSN patients do have serum against *T. canis* antibodies[11,29] and it is well known that in some cases of toxocariasis, only intraocular antibodies can be found.[1,7] *Ancylostoma caninum* is another common nematode suggested as a possible cause of DUSN.

Baylisascaris procyonis, an intestinal roundworm of raccoons and skunks, has been proposed for the larger worm. These nematodes potentially meet the size requirements for both the small and large worm since they are 300 microns at hatching and grow to 2000 microns.[22] Three cases of DUSN following contact with raccoons have been reported.[17,24,32] A large percentage of raccoons are infested.[16] *Baylisascaris* sp. larvae are known to produce fatal central nervous system disease in primates and humans[23] and ocular larva migrans in a variety of species.[8,21] Areas of the country in which large numbers of raccoons are infected overlap somewhat with the regions of reported cases of the large nematode DUSN.[20] Because a variety of nematodal species from lower mammals are probably capable of causing DUSN,[2,21] recovery and morphologic identification of a worm from a DUSN eye, if ever achieved, will still not definitively solve the pathogenesis of this disorder.

Other types of parasites may also cause similar disease. Two cases of intraocular infection with *Alaria* sp. (class Trematoda) mesocercariae were recently described that had some clinical features of DUSN, although the infesting larvae were broader than the thin worms typically seen in DUSN.[25]

Animal Models

An experimental model of ascarid endophthalmitis was developed in guinea pigs to investigate the pathologic response leading to vision loss in these cases.[18] Eosinophilic choroiditis, cystic changes in the retinal pigment epithelium, destruction of the photoreceptor outer segments, and outer retinal degeneration were noted distant from focal reactions directed against the intraocular larvae. The choriocapillaris and large choroidal blood vessels were not occluded. Degranulation of eosinophils and mast cells was hypothesized to have released mediators toxic to the photoreceptors and retinal pigment epithelium, thus accounting for the histologic changes.[18]

DIFFERENTIAL DIAGNOSIS

In the early stages of vision loss and vitritis without other visible lesions, retrobulbar neuritis may be suspected. Optic nerve edema may suggest a postviral neuroretinitis. The active outer retinal lesions are most commonly mistaken for acute posterior multifocal placoid pigment epitheliopathy[15] or multiple evanescent white dot syndrome, but virtually any posterior uveitis could be invoked, including multifocal choroiditis and panuveitis syndrome, punctate inner choroidopathy, outer retinal toxoplasmosis, sarcoidosis, birdshot retinochoroidopathy, or Behçet disease.[12] The punched-out chorioretinal scars may also suggest presumed ocular histoplasmosis syndrome.

The late stages with optic atrophy, narrowed retinal vessels, and diffuse pigment epithelial damage may resemble virtually any end-stage process including macular degeneration,[31] atypical retinitis pigmentosa without intraretinal pigment migration,[4,5,15,29,32] or the aftereffects of necrotizing viral retinopathies.

LABORATORY INVESTIGATIONS

Because DUSN is thought to be caused by a random migration of a single larva into the eye, systemic evaluation is expected to be negative, and in virtually all cases, it is. A complete blood count to check for peripheral eosinophilia is probably an adequate screen for visceral larva migrans in patients with negative medical history and examination. A serum antibody for *T. canis* exposure is of interest if obtained with the understanding that it may be negative in cases of confirmed intraocular toxocariasis.[1,7] A test for human serum antibody against *Baylisascaris* sp. is not currently available but would suffer from the same limitations as the *Toxocara* sp. antibody test, since the number of infecting organisms is likely to be small in isolated intraocular disease.[21] Atypical cases may suggest other diagnoses in the differential, which can be excluded by further laboratory testing as appropriate.

Electroretinography is helpful, since most patients will have abnormal electroretinograms (ERG) to a moderate or marked degree, even if tested early in the course of disease.

The B wave is affected more than the A wave, and both rod and cone functions are affected.[14] The ERG is rarely extinguished completely, which offers an important distinction between late-stage DUSN and tapetoretinal degenerations.[4,11,14]

Fluorescein angiography may demonstrate capillary permeability of the optic disc and retinal vessels in the area of active lesions, and cystoid macular edema has been reported.[14] The active deep retinal lesions seen in early disease are hypofluorescent early in the angiogram and become hyperfluorescent in its late stages.[14] Late-stage disease may show a generalized hyperfluorescence related to the alterations in the pigment epithelium and there may be a delay in retinal circulation time.[14]

THERAPY

Corticosteroids have been tried for treatment of DUSN without apparent effect.[11,30] Anthelmintic agents have been ineffective as well.[11] Gass,[13] however, has recently reported successful oral therapy with thiabendazole in four patients with DUSN and moderate-to-severe vitreous humor inflammation.[12] A dose of 22 mg/kg twice daily for 2 to 4 days was used.[13] A beneficial effect of treatment with death of the worm was presumed if an active focus of retinal necrosis developed 1 week after thiabendazole treatment, after which active retinal lesions subsided with formation of a chorioretinal scar, and decreased vitritis and stabilization or improvement in vision occurred. Fading of the lesions could ordinarily be detected within a week after treatment, with a decrease in the intraocular inflammatory reaction by 1 month.[9,13] Thiabendazole treatment is more effective in cases with substantial vitreous humor inflammation, since this inflammatory reaction may help the penetration of the drug into the intraocular tissues.[13]

Ivermectin, an antifilarial agent with broad antiparasitic effects used in veterinary practice, has also been used successfully in four patients with presumed DUSN.[3] It was ineffective in another patient in whom the worm was subsequently found and treated with photocoagulation. This drug, which is used widely for the treatment of onchocerciasis, penetrates the intraocular tissues well and has notably fewer side effects associated with its use than thiabendazole, which commonly produces gastrointestinal and central nervous system symptoms. It is classified as an experimental drug in the United States but is available from the Centers for Disease Control and Prevention. A single dose of 0.15 mg/kg to 0.20 mg/kg in adults is sufficient to cause a marked reduction in intraocular filaria and appears to be larvacidal for the roundworms causing DUSN as well.

Xenon arc or argon laser photocoagulation was used to kill subretinal, motile worms in two patients, one from Kentucky and one from Michigan.[32] Both patients retained vision at their pretreatment level but vision did not improve. Several additional cases have been treated with laser photocoagulation.[4,11,17,34] None of these cases showed a marked increase in intraocular inflammation after destruction of the nematode.

PROGNOSIS

Cases without a visible subretinal nematode may be difficult to diagnose and substantial vision loss may occur. Clinical suspicion should be high in cases of unilateral inflammatory disease, particularly if migratory crops of active outer retinal lesions are seen. If suspicion of DUSN is high and the worm cannot be found, medical treatment with thiabendazole or ivermectin may be effective in halting the disease progression. If the worm can be found, laser photocoagulation is the most direct way of killing the worm. Once the worm is killed or dies, vision appears to stabilize and further degeneration is halted. Modest visual improvement may occur, caused by clearing of the vitreous humor cellular infiltrate or reduction in optic nerve edema after the worm is killed.[3,12,13] The chance of involvement of the second eye is very slight.

REFERENCES

1. Biglan AW, Glickman LT, Lobes LAJ: Serum and vitreous *Toxocara* antibody in nematode endophthalmitis, *Am J Ophthalmol* 88:898-901, 1979.
2. Bowman DD: Diagnostic morphology of four larval ascaridoid nematodes that may cause visceral larva migrans: *Toxascaris leonina, Baylisascaris procyonis, Lagochilascaris sprenti,* and *Hexametra leidyi, J Parasitol* 73:1198-1215, 1987.
3. Callanan D, Davis JL, Cohen SM et al.: The use of ivermectin in diffuse unilateral subacute neuroretinitis, *Ophthalmology* 100(suppl):114, 1993.
4. Carney MD, Combs JL: Diffuse unilateral subacute neuroretinitis, *Br J Ophthalmol* 75:633-635, 1991.
5. Cunha de Souza E, Lustosa da Cunha S, Gass JDM: Diffuse unilateral subacute neuroretinitis in South America, *Arch Ophthalmol* 110:1261-1263, 1992.
6. Duke-Elder S, Perkins ES: Parasitic uveitis. In Duke-Elder S, editor: *System of ophthalmology,* 453-459, vol IX, St Louis, 1966, Mosby.
7. Felberg NT, Shields JA, Federman JL: Antibody to *Toxocara canis* in the aqueous humor, *Arch Ophthalmol* 99:1563-1564, 1981.
8. Fox AS, Kazacos KR, Gould NS et al.: Fatal eosinophilic meningoencephalitis and visceral larva migrans caused by the raccoon ascarid *Baylisascaris procyonis, N Engl J Med* 312:1619-1623, 1985.
9. Gass JDM: *Stereoscopic atlas of macular diseases,* ed 2, St Louis, 1977, Mosby.
10. Gass JDM: *Stereoscopic atlas of macular disease: diagnosis and treatment,* ed 3, St Louis, 1987, Mosby.
11. Gass JDM, Braunstein RA: Further observations concerning the diffuse unilateral subacute neuroretinitis syndrome, *Arch Ophthalmol* 101:1689-1697, 1983.
12. Gass JDM, Callanan DG, Bowman CB: Successful oral therapy for diffuse unilateral subacute neuroretinitis, *Trans Am Ophthalmol Soc* 89:97-112, 1991.
13. Gass JDM, Callanan DG, Bowman CB: Oral therapy in diffuse unilateral subacute neuroretinitis, *Arch Ophthalmol* 110:675-680, 1992.
14. Gass JDM, Gilbert WRJ, Guerry RK, Scelfo R: Diffuse unilateral subacute neuroretinitis, *Ophthalmology* 85:521-545, 1978.
15. Gass JDM, Scelfo R: Diffuse unilateral subacute neuroretinitis, *J R Soc Med* 71:95-111, 1978.
16. Goldberg MA, Ai E, Boyce WM et al.: Diffuse unilateral subacute neuroretinitis: epidemiologic documentation of baylisascaris infestation of the raccoon population of northern California, *Inv Ophthalmol Vis Sci* 33:743, 1992.

17. Goldberg MA, Kazacos KR, Boyce WM et al.: Diffuse unilateral subacute neuroretinitis: morphometric, serologic, and epidemiologic support for *Baylisascaris* as a causative agent, *Ophthalmology* 100:1695-1701, 1993.

18. John T, Barsky HJ, Donnelly JJ, Rockey JH: Retinal pigment epitheliopathy and neuroretinal degeneration in ascarid-infected eyes, *Invest Ophthalmol Vis Sci* 28:1583-1598, 1987.

19. Jones LT, Jordan LW, Sullivan NP: Intraocular nematode worm: report of a case and review of the literature, *Arch Ophthalmol* 20:1006-1012, 1938.

20. Kazacos KR, Boyce WM: *Baylisascaris* larva migrans, *J Am Vet Med Assoc* 195:894-903, 1989.

21. Kazacos KR, Raymond LA, Kazacos EA, Vestre WA: The raccoon ascarid: a probable cause of human ocular larva migrans, *Ophthalmology* 92:1735-1744, 1985.

22. Kazacos KR, Vestre WA, Kazacos EA, Raymond LA: Diffuse unilateral subacute neuroretinitis syndrome: probable cause, *Arch Ophthalmol* 102:967-968, 1984.

23. Kazacos KR, Wirtz WL, Burger PP, Christmas CS: Raccoon ascarid larvae as a cause of fatal central nervous system disease in subhuman primates, *J Am Vet Med Assoc* 179:1089-1094, 1981.

24. Küchle M, Knorr HLJ, Medenblik-Frysch S et al.: Diffuse unilateral subacute neuroretinitis syndrome in a German most likely caused by the raccoon roundworm, *Baylisascaris procyonis, Graefes Arch Clin Exp Ophthalmol* 231:48-51, 1993.

25. McDonald HR, Kazacos KR, Schatz H et al.: Two cases of intraocular infection with Alaria mesocercariae (Trematoda), *Am J Ophthalmol* 117:447-455, 1994. (See correction *Am J Ophthalmol* 118:129, 1994.)

26. Naumann GOH, Knorr HLJ: DUSN occurs in Europe, *Ophthalmology* 101:971-972, 1994.

27. Nichols RL: The etiology of visceral larva migrans. I. Diagnostic morphology of infective second-stage *Toxocara* larva, *J Parasitol* 42:349-362, 1956.

28. Nichols RL: The etiology of visceral larva migrans. II. Comparative larval morphology of *Ascaris lumbricoides, Necator americanus, Strongyloides stercoralis,* and *Ancylostoma caninum, J Parasitol* 42:363-399, 1956.

29. Oppenheim S, Rogell G, Peyser R: Diffuse unilateral subacute neuroretinitis, *Ann Ophthalmol* 17:336-338, 1985.

30. Parsons HE: Nematode chorioretinitis: report of a case, with photographs of a viable worm, *Arch Ophthalmol* 47:799-800, 1952.

31. Price JAJ, Wadsworth JAC: An intra-retinal worm: report of a case of macular retinopathy caused by invasion of the retina by a worm, *Arch Ophthalmol* 83:768-770, 1970.

32. Raymond LA, Gutierrez Y, Strong LE et al.: Living retinal nematode (filarial-like) destroyed with photocoagulation, *Ophthalmology* 85:944-949, 1978.

33. Rubin ML, Kaufman HE, Tierney JP, Lucas HC: An intraretinal nematode (a case report), *Trans Am Acad Ophthalmol Otolaryngol* 72:855-866, 1968.

34. Sivalingam A, Goldberg RE, Augsburger J, Frank P: Diffuse unilateral subacute neuroretinitis, *Arch Ophthalmol* 109:1028, 1991.

35. Wilder HC: Nematode endophthalmitis, *Trans Am Acad Ophthalmol Otolaryngol* 55:99-109, 1950.

89 Brucellosis

KHALID F. TABBARA

Brucellosis is a zoonotic systemic infection caused by the aerobic bacterial genus *Brucella*. In the past the pathogens severely affected meat and milk worldwide. Legislative measures in many countries have now brought brucellosis in humans and animals under control, although it continues to be a health problem in certain regions of the world.

BACTERIOLOGY

There are several species of *Brucella,* and each species has one or more hosts. The principal hosts of *B. melitensis* are sheep, goats, and camels. The principal host of *B. abortus* is cattle, *B. suis* is pigs, *B. canis* is dogs, *B. ovis* is sheep, and *B. neotomae* is rats.[7] The major causes of the disease in humans are *B. melitensis, B. abortus,* and *B. suis.*

Brucella spp. organisms are gram-negative intracellular coccobacilli that have the ability to persist in milk for several days and may remain in cheese for weeks. The organisms have been reported to survive in dust for several weeks. Brucellae are killed when they are heated to 60°C for 10 minutes.

HISTORICAL BACKGROUND

Brucellosis was recognized as a clinical entity in 1860 among British soldiers serving in Malta. In 1887 Sir David Bruce[6] recovered the responsible organism from the spleens of army personnel dying with undulant fever. In 1905 goats on this Mediterranean island were found to harbor these bacteria. Subsequent studies showed that brucellosis affected livestock in many countries.

EPIDEMIOLOGY

Brucellosis occurs worldwide and affects about 500,000 people each year. Pasteurization, cattle immunization, and slaughter of infected animals have reduced the incidence of human brucellosis to less than one case in one million population in many countries. Abattoir workers are at risk for the disease because of their contact with infected cattle or swine. The use of unpasteurized dairy products accounts for cases in developing parts of the world.

Cases of *B. melitensis* infection have been reported in Kuwait and Saudi Arabia,[14] but brucellosis is not limited to certain ethnic groups. Travelers to areas where brucellosis is endemic may acquire the disease, even during a short visit, by consuming contaminated milk or milk products such as cheese. Transboundary transmission of the disease is further promoted by the intercontinental export of contaminated meat, milk products, and animals.

Laboratory workers may acquire the disease during the processing of *Brucella* spp. cultures or by handling infected body fluids.[3,13]

CLINICAL FEATURES

Systemic brucellosis manifests in two stages: acute brucellosis and chronic brucellosis.

The clinical manifestations of acute brucellosis include fever, fatigue, malaise, anorexia, abdominal pain, night sweats, headache, and arthralgia. Children may display weight loss, malaise, arthralgia, hepatosplenomegaly, lymphocytosis, and elevation in liver enzymes.[5,15]

The illness enters the chronic phase if the disease is untreated or the diagnosis is missed. Skeletal and neurologic complications may occur. Patients may develop arthritis of the knees or ankles; sacroiliitis is also common. The disease may be confused with autoimmune rheumatic disorders, particularly when uveitis, another manifestation of chronic brucellosis, is present. Spondylitis, osteomyelitis, and paravertebral abscesses may occur, simulating tuberculosis. Neurologic manifestations include meningitis, encephalitis, and peripheral nerve involvement such as sciatica. Other chronic manifestations include skin rash, bronchopneumonia, pleurisy, endocarditis, orchitis, and placentitis.

Ocular Disorders

The eye may be involved in both the acute and chronic stages of brucellosis, although ocular disease is uncommon. In 100 consecutive patients with systemic brucellosis seen in Saudi Arabia, the prevalence of ocular involvement was

TABLE 89-1 OCULAR MANIFESTATIONS OF BRUCELLOSIS

Active Disease	Complications
Granulomatous iridocyclitis	Posterior synechiae
Nongranulomatous iridocyclitis	Secondary glaucoma
Vitritis	Secondary cataract
Choroiditis	Tractional retinal detachment
Retinitis	
Retinal vasculitis	
Optic neuritis	
Scleritis	
Endophthalmitis	
Papilledema	

found to be 3%. Uveitis is the most common eye manifestation.

The ocular findings are variable. They can be mild or severe, in the latter case often leading to vision loss.[1,2] The disease is usually unilateral: in seven consecutive patients with ocular brucellosis seen in Saudi Arabia, the disease was bilateral in one patient and unilateral in six. The clinical findings of ocular brucellosis are summarized in Table 89-1.

The most frequent ocular finding in both acute and chronic brucellosis is uveitis. Intraocular inflammation may present as anterior uveitis, chorioretinitis, or panuveitis with vitritis.

Anterior uveitis can be granulomatous or nongranulomatous. Mutton-fat keratic precipitates may be found. Unilateral geographic choroiditis may involve the retina and progress into a localized necrotic granuloma. Vitreous humor inflammatory reactions are common. Patients treated with topical corticosteroids display anterior nongranulomatous uveitis. Uveitis caused by brucellosis can be confused with uveitis during tuberculosis and with idiopathic uveitis in a patient with rheumatism.

In the acute phase of the disease, the patient may also develop unilateral endogenous endophthalmitis with hypopyon. In one reported case, blood IgG and IgM for *B. melitensis* were elevated, and *B. melitensis* (biotype 3) was isolated from the vitreous humor.[4]

Papilledema is another finding in acute brucellosis. A case has been reported of a woman who complained to her neurologist of headaches and bilateral papilledema was discovered on examination. Pseudotumor cerebri was diagnosed, but further laboratory work-up revealed evidence of neurobrucellosis and meningeal involvement. This patient recovered completely following antibiotic therapy.*

Other ocular manifestations of acute brucellosis are retinal vasculitis, scleritis (which is usually diffuse but may be nodular), and optic neuritis or perineuritis. Optic nerve in-

*Personal communication with A Al-Kawi, 1993.

volvement may represent an extension of meningeal infection.[1]

In the chronic stage of the disease, anterior or posterior uveitis may occur. Fibrotic vitreous bands may develop, resulting in tractional retinal detachment. Posterior synechiae are common; secondary cataract and glaucoma may also occur.

PATHOGENESIS

In cows, which can be infected for their lifetime, *B. abortus* has a unique predilection for the lymphatics of the uterus; infection of the placenta is common and frequently leads to abortion. Organisms from infected placental tissue cause massive contamination of the grazing environment and may cause infection in humans. Infected cows that deliver successfully and subsequently excrete the organism in their milk. Goats, camels, and sheep infected with *B. melitensis* also yield contaminated milk. Cheese made from contaminated and inadequately pasteurized milk may contain viable *Brucella* spp. organisms.

Brucellosis is transmitted from animals to humans by consumption of raw or inadequately pasteurized milk, contaminated cheese, and infected meat.[17] The disease may also be transmitted to human beings during handling or cutting of infected meat.[9,10] In addition, human beings have also been infected by airborne dissemination of the organism,[12] person-to-person transmission, and by skin contact with an infected cow's placental tissue.[11] The conjunctiva may serve as the portal of entry for *Brucella* spp.

Because of their susceptibility to acidity, brucellae in milk are killed when the milk turns sour; they are also killed by gastric acidity. Consequently, consumption of antacids may increase susceptibility to the organism.[15]

LABORATORY INVESTIGATIONS

Several serologic testing methods for *Brucella* spp. are available. IgM and IgG antibodies are elevated in the acute phase of the disease; these can be detected with an agglutination test, complement fixation, or enzyme linked immunosorbent assay (ELISA). The ELISA test detects antibodies to cell-membrane proteins of pathogenic *Brucella* spp.

The definitive diagnosis is made by isolation of the organism. *Brucella* spp. may be isolated from blood and vitreous humor in patients with endogenous endophthalmitis or severe uveitis with vitreous humor exudates. In one patient with uveitis, the organism was isolated from a paravertebral abscess.[16] Trypticase soy broth is valuable for the recovery of the organism. Castaneda bottles or lysis-centrifugation procedures may enhance recovery. Culture media should be observed for 3 to 6 weeks.

THERAPY

The treatment of choice for brucellosis consists of simultaneous administration of doxycycline (100 mg orally twice daily) and rifampin (300 mg orally twice daily), or a combination of doxycycline and streptomycin.[8] In patients with acute systemic brucellosis, treatment is given for 3 to 4 weeks, but in chronic systemic disease, it should be given for 3 months. Trimethoprim-sulfamethoxazole and aminoglycosides (such as gentamicin, tobramycin, and streptomycin) are also effective. The role of newer agents, such as ciprofloxacin and azithromycin, appears promising.

For ocular brucellosis, additional therapy consisting of subconjunctival injections of tobramycin, 20 mg every other day for a total of 5 doses has been used successfully.

PREVENTION

The control of brucellosis among cattle and swine relies on the identification and slaughter of infected animals. Strain-specific vaccines are available for domesticated livestock.

Limiting endemic infection among cattle, hogs, and other animals is an effective means for preventing human disease. Pasteurization of dairy products, especially milk and cheese, can also reduce the risk of human brucellosis.

REFERENCES

1. Abd Elrazak MM: Brucella optic neuritis, *Arch Int Med* 151:776-778, 1991.
2. Akduman L, Or M, Hasanreisolglu B, Kurtar K: A case of ocular brucellosis: importance of vitreous specimen, *Acta Ophthalmol* 71:130-132, 1993.
3. al-Aska AK, Chagla AH: Laboratory-acquired brucellosis, *J Hosp Infect* 14:69, 1989.
4. al Faran MF: *Brucella melitensis* endogenous endophthalmitis, *Ophthalmologica* 201:19, 1990.
5. Benjamin B, Annobil SH: Childhood brucellosis in southwestern Saudi Arabia: a 5-year experience, *J Trop Pediatr* 38:167-172, 1992.
6. Bruce D: Note on the discovery of microorganism in Malta fever, *Practioner* 39:161, 1887.
7. Christie AB: Brucellosis. In *Infectious disease: epidemiology and clinical practice,* ed 4, 1130, Edinburgh, 1987, Churchill Livingstone.
8. Colmenero Castillo JD, Hernandez Marquez S, Reguera Iglesias JM et al.: Comparative trial of doxycycline plus streptomycin versus doxycycline plus rifampin for the therapy of human brucellosis, *Chemotherapy* 35:146, 1989.
9. Cooper CW: The epidemiology of human brucellosis in a well defined urban population in Saudi Arabia, *J Trop Med Hyg* 94:416-422, 1991.
10. Cooper CW: Risk factors in transmission of brucellosis from animals to humans in Saudi Arabia, *Trans R Soc Trop Med Hyg* 86:206-209, 1992.
11. Grave W, Sturm AW: Brucellosis associated with a beauty parlour, *Lancet* 1:1326, 1983.
12. Kaufman AF, Fox MD, Anderson DC: Airborne spread of brucellosis, *Ann NY Acad Sci* 353:105, 1980.
13. Kiel FW, Khan MY: Brucellosis among hospital employees in Saudi Arabia, *Infect Control Hosp Epidemiol* 14:268, 1993.
14. Madkour MM, Mohamed AE, Talukder MAS, Kudaway AJN: Brucellosis in Saudi Arabia, *Saudi Med J* 6:324, 1985.
15. Steffen R: Antacids: a risk factor in travellers, *Scand J Infect Dis* 9:311, 1977.
16. Tabbara KF, Al Kassimi H: Ocular brucellosis, *Br J Ophthalmol* 74:249, 1990.
17. Young EJ: Human brucellosis, *Rev Infect Dis* 5:821, 1983.

90 Histoplasmosis

DAVID M. BROWN, THOMAS A. WEINGEIST, RONALD E. SMITH

The fungus *Histoplasma capsulatum* has been associated with two distinct ophthalmic disorders: (1) productive *H. capsulatum* infection of ocular tissues, and (2) the presumed ocular histoplasmosis syndrome (POHS), which is believed to be an immunologically-mediated disorder. POHS, which is much more common than productive infection of the eye, will be considered separately at the end of this chapter.

MYCOLOGY

Histoplasma capsulatum is a dimorphic soil fungus existing in mycelial form at 20° to 30°C and in yeast phase at 37°C.[50] *H. capsulatum* is endemic to the central and southeastern United States (particularly the Mississippi and Ohio River valleys) as well as Puerto Rico, and parts of Central America, Asia, Italy, Turkey, Israel, and Australia.[11]

INFECTIOUS HISTOPLASMOSIS

Histoplasma capsulatum infection is usually subclinical or mildly symptomatic, with a flulike reaction. Rarely, however, disseminated infection can be life-threatening. Endogenous or exogenous infections of the eye can result in blindness.

Epidemiology

Infection usually results from incidental exposure to moderate numbers of mycelial fragments in an endemic area. Histoplasmosis, like tuberculosis, primarily infects the lungs. In tuberculosis, the source of infection is an aerosolized droplet of respiratory secretions from a patient infected with *Mycobacterium tuberculosis*. In histoplasmosis the infective mycelial fragments and/or spores enter the lung with dust particles. Unlike tuberculosis, which can be controlled by limiting access to infected patients, exposure to spore-containing soil in endemic areas is nearly unavoidable. Up to 70% of persons living in endemic areas have evidence of previous infection by histoplasmin skin test reactivity.[50] Primary infection can also occur with exposure to highly infectious soil dust in such locations as storm cellars or bat-infested caves.

Clinical Features

In addition to subclinical or mildly symptomatic disease, infection with *H. capsulatum* can result in more severe disorders. Massive exposure to great numbers of fungal elements can produce a violent, acute, febrile disease with a clinical, serologic, and radiologic picture of acute pneumonitis.

The primary lesion in the lung is generally a single focus of bronchopneumonia in incidentally exposed patients, and there will be multiple foci of involvement in those with massive exposure.

Disseminated Histoplasmosis. Disseminated histoplasmosis is a rare disease that occurs in infants with incomplete immune defenses, in immunosuppressed individuals, and (rarely) in normal adults without any known immune defect.[8] The disease is characterized by persistent infection of the monocyte-phagocytic system by *H. capsulatum* organisms throughout the body.

Disseminated histoplasmosis in infants is a debilitating disease presenting with fever (101° to 103°F) and gastrointestinal symptoms. Cough and tachypnea with interstitial pneumonia are seen several weeks later, secondary to heavily parasitized macrophages. The disease is fatal in 5 weeks unless diagnosed and treated aggressively.

Disseminated histoplasmosis in adults is most often seen as one of the life-threatening opportunistic infections associated with acquired immunodeficiency syndrome (AIDS) and other immunocompromised disease states.[71] The disease presents as an acute pneumonitis and fungemia, and can secondarily affect the central nervous system, kidneys, gastrointestinal tract, skin and other distant foci.[70] Histologically, intracellular organisms are found without tissue reaction. Patients with AIDS often have a fulminant course complicated by disseminated intravascular coagulation or acute respiratory distress syndrome.

Ocular Disease. Ocular involvement can include retinitis, optic neuritis, and uveitis.[65] The retinal lesions consist of multiple creamy-white intraretinal and subretinal infiltrates with distinct borders. Some lesions have surrounding retinal hemorrhage, and most are small (⅙ to ¼ optic disc diameter in size). Histopathologically, intracytoplasmic yeast has been demonstrated in the retina, retinal pigment epithelial (RPE) cells, choroidal infiltrates, optic nerve, and uvea.*

Histoplasmic Endophthalmitis. H. capsulatum is a rare cause of severe endophthalmitis both from endogenous dissemination and after intraocular surgery. Patients with systemic disseminated histoplasmosis may develop a panuveitis, vitritis, iritis, or focal retinitis.[69] Cultures demonstrate *H. capsulatum* organisms in the aqueous and vitreous humors, and histology reveals organisms extracellularly in the vitreous humor and both intracellularly and extracellularly in areas of granulomatous inflammation involving the iris, ciliary body, and retina.[18] Exogenous *H. capsulatum* endophthalmitis has also been reported following cataract surgery complicated by vitreous humor incarceration in the wound.[39]

Pathogenesis

H. capsulatum resides and replicates almost exclusively within macrophages after phagocytosis in the lung. Partial or complete encapsulation occurs, and the lesion becomes necrotic in the center. The overwhelming majority of primary foci calcify as they heal. Soon after the pneumonic process starts, regional lymph nodes swell and caseation and calcification occur in the lymphatic chain. The caseated pulmonary lesion and lymph node lesions form the *primary complex* and contain numerous *H. capsulatum* organisms. The majority of these organisms die, but they can be identified for many years in the primary complex because of their chitinous cell walls. Lymphatic and hematogenous dissemination of *H. capsulatum* organisms throughout the body is common in the primary infection, but the dissemination is self-limited and usually benign. The immunologically competent person apparently manages to limit the hematogenous dissemination to circumscribed foci in the spleen and/or liver. The primary infection offers partial protective immunity from subsequent reinfection. Reinfection or reactivation is generally exogenous and occurs only after massive exposure or when an individual's resistance is lowered by disease or extrinsic immunosuppression.

Laboratory Investigations

Diagnosis in the acute illness can be made from positive blood cultures, cultures of mouth ulcers, urine cultures, and tissue biopsies. Liver biopsies are positive in up to 80% of cases.

Therapy

Immunocompetent patients are managed with either amphotericin B or ketoconazole (except in patients with men-

---

*References 9, 18, 24, 31, 49, 51.

ingitis or endocarditis). Treatment of disseminated histoplasmosis in patients with AIDS generally requires high dose amphotericin B (1 to 2.5 grams) followed by either daily ketoconazole (life-long) or long-term intermittent maintenance amphotericin B treatment (weekly).[8]

PRESUMED OCULAR HISTOPLASMOSIS SYNDROME

POHS is a much more common ophthalmic disease than productive *H. capsulatum* infection in the eye, which is rare. POHS has been associated with *H. capsulatum* and is thought to be immunologically mediated in individuals previously exposed to the fungus.

Convincing evidence from epidemiologic studies and animal models continues to support *H. capsulatum* as the causal organism of POHS.[15,54,56] The pathogenesis of POHS lesions and the inciting factors for choroidal neovascular membrane formation are unknown and can only be extrapolated from histopathologic studies of patients with the disease and studies of a nonhuman primate model.

Historical Background

Woods and Whalen[73] first described the entity of presumed ocular histoplasmosis syndrome in 1959. In their review of 295 patients with uveitis, they found that 62 of 186 patients with granulomatous uveitis were positive reactors to the histoplasmin skin test, compared to 16 of 107 patients with nongranulomatous uveitis. Woods and Whalen further subdivided their patients into groups based on histoplasmin reactivity, roentgenographic findings of pulmonary histoplasmosis disease, and reactivity to tuberculin. In a group of nine patients with positive histoplasmin skin reactivity, radiographic evidence of pulmonary calcification, and tuberculin anergy, they noted a unique fundus appearance consisting of peripheral focal spots of chorioretinal atrophy ("histo spots") and central cystic lesions that often progressed into Junius-Kuhnt disciform macular scars. They noted that the peripheral lesions were usually about one-third disc diameter in size, often somewhat yellowish in color, and either depigmented or sparsely pigmented. The central lesions were either in the macula or contiguous with it and were often associated with edema, subretinal exudate, and hemorrhage (Fig. 90-1). None of these patients had anterior uveitis, and the vitreous humor was clear in most patients. Woods and Whalen described another 10 patients with similar findings but with confounding variables such as positive tuberculin skin test or elevated anti-*Toxoplasma gondii* antibody titers. In this combined series 26 of 31 eyes with uveitis secondary to presumed histoplasmosis had both peripheral and central lesions; 4 eyes had only peripheral lesions; and 1 eye had only a central active lesion. Woods and Whalen concluded that it was reasonable to assume a cause-and-effect relationship between benign systemic histoplasmosis and the typical ocular lesions seen in these patients.

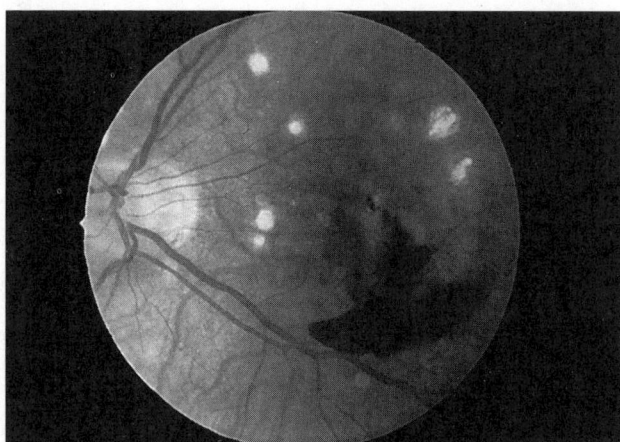

Fig. 90-1. The classic triad of presumed ocular histoplasmosis syndrome is demonstrated with peripapillary atrophy, "punched-out" chorioretinal lesions, and a hemorrhagic choroidal neovascular membrane.

Since 1959 POHS has been well described.* Thousands of patients with the syndrome have been identified and laser photocoagulation treatment regimens for its associated choroidal neovascular membranes have been refined and tested by multicenter national trials. Woods and Whalen's basic supposition that this entity is caused by the organism *H. capsulatum* has never been definitively proved, however. The organism has not been positively identified in POHS lesions despite attempts with microbiology culture techniques, light and electron microscopy, and immunohistochemistry.[36,49,69]

Epidemiology

In 1970 Ellis and Schlaegel[13] polled United States and foreign medical schools regarding their experiences with POHS and compared the results to known histoplasmin skin test sensitivity patterns. They noted a correlation between endemic POHS cases and areas of the United States along the Mississippi and Ohio rivers where the highest prevalence of histoplasmin skin test reactors exists.

In an epidemiologic study of POHS in Walkersville, Maryland, 842 people were examined by indirect ophthalmoscopy, and 22 definite or highly suspected cases of POHS were identified by two separate uveitis experts without access to the histoplasmin skin test results.[59] Positive skin tests were found in 59% of the general population, and all 22 subjects with presumed histoplasmosis were positive reactors. The subjects with histo spots had a larger mean diameter of induration in response to the histoplasmin test (12.4 mm) than those who responded to the test dose; this response suggests a relationship between the ocular lesions and *H.*

---

*References 3, 40, 46, 50, 54, 58, 59, 61.

capsulatum. Among persons with positive skin tests, 4.4% were found to have POHS lesions and only 1 case of disciform macular disease was noted.

Clinical Features

Schlaegel[46] described clinical features of POHS in 190 patients diagnosed by a characteristic clinical picture and a positive histoplasmin skin test. Males represented 63% of the reported cases and the peak age of involvement was between 30 and 40 years. Disease was diagnosed in the first eye in September, October, and November in 42% of patients. Schlaegel characterized histo spots as small, yellow, moderately soft, disseminated lesions that were randomly scattered, usually nonpigmented, atrophic areas measuring 0.1 to 0.5 optic disc diameters in size and involving the RPE and choroid (Fig. 90-2). In the acute stage, a slight yellowish swelling of the choroid and occasionally a slight ground glasslike haze in the overlying retina occur. In the atrophic stage, a slight depression of the RPE and choroid exists, but the lesion is usually not "punched-out." Choroidal vessels are rarely seen through the lesion. The number of chorioretinal scars varies in patients from one to four per eye, although some eyes may have as many as 70 chorioretinal lesions.[61] Peripheral lesions occur in both eyes in approximately two thirds of cases.

Peripapillary choroiditis is seen frequently in POHS and generally appears as a pigmented crescent around the optic disc inside an atrophic depigmented area (Fig. 90-3). Schlaegel[46] found that 70% of patients with macular disease had bilateral "circumpapillary choroiditis," and an additional 15% had peripapillary changes in only one eye. Only 18% to 28% of patients without macular disease (only peripheral lesions) have peripapillary changes, however.[61]

Fountain and Schlaegel[14] described linear streaks at the equator in 26 of 536 patients with POHS, and they termed this finding a "fourth sign" of the syndrome (Fig. 90-4).[14]

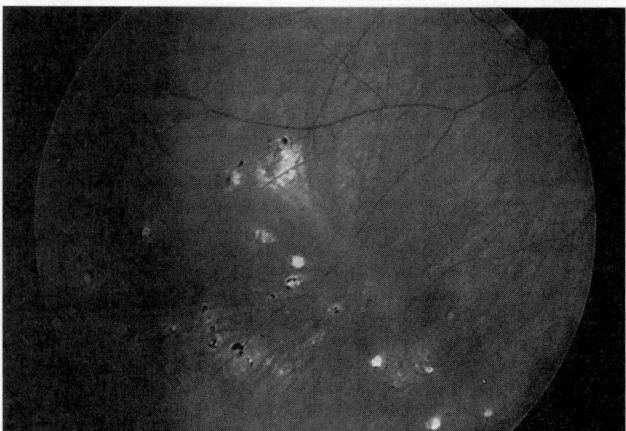

Fig. 90-2. Peripheral "punched-out" lesions typical of POHS (histo spots).

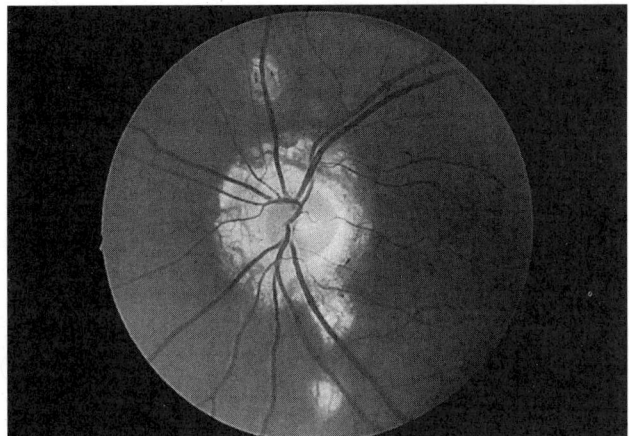

Fig. 90-3. Peripapillary atrophy may be extensive and circumferential or confined primarily to the temporal side of the optic disc.

These streaks, which consist of hypopigmented and hyperpigmented circumlinear peripheral chorioretinal scars (multiple histo spots), have also been seen in the multifocal choroiditis and panuveitis syndrome and in pathologic myopia.[5,64]

The vitreous humor is clear in POHS, with cells rarely seen in either the anterior chamber or vitreous cavity. When vitreous humor cells are seen, other entities, such as multifocal choroiditis with panuveitis syndrome, should be considered.[12]

Seven percent of Schlaegel's patients showed reactivation of a previously noted inactive POHS lesion (noted as a hemorrhagic area adjacent to the histo spot) after histoplasmin skin testing.[46] Because of this increased risk following skin reactivity testing, the histoplasmin skin test is now rarely performed.

Pathology

Several disputed histopathology reports have attempted to identify *H. capsulatum* within ocular tissues as part of POHS.[29,42] Maumenee[35] described the presence of *H. capsulatum* organisms in a disciform scar of an eye believed to harbor a malignant melanoma. This case is disputed by Zimmerman because the organism could only be identified by Gomori methenamine silver and not by routine hematoxylin and eosin stains.[18] Roth[41] published a histopathologic report in which he claimed to demonstrate *H. capsulatum* organisms in disciform macular lesions, peripapillary lesions, and peripheral atrophic scars in both eyes of a patient with POHS. Gass and Zimmerman[17] disputed the findings because some, if not all, of the structures purported to be organisms in the ocular tissue were small calcific bodies and not fungi.

Histopathologic studies of subretinal neovascular membranes removed by subretinal surgery in patients with POHS demonstrate fibrovascular tissue interposed between Bruch membrane and the RPE.[44] Cellular components present in the membranes include RPE cells, vascular endothelium, photoreceptor cells, macrophages, erythrocytes, ghost erythrocytes, myofibroblasts, glial cells, smooth-muscle cells, and lymphocytes. Extracellular constituents include collagen fibrils, fragments of Bruch membrane and choroid, and fibrin. The histopathologic studies are consistent with a nonspecific healing response to a local stimulus or injury. The ultrastructural features found were similar to neovascular membranes in age-related macular degeneration (AMD), except basal laminar deposits are not seen in POHS membranes. Bruch membrane is normal thickness in the POHS membrane specimens, and the lesions are focal in POHS compared to excised AMD membranes, which exhibit diffuse intra-Bruch membrane disease. This presence of normal RPE-Bruch membrane layers probably accounts for the relatively better visual prognosis for removal of membranes in patients with POHS than for patients with AMD.

Complications

The most serious complication of POHS is choroidal neovascularization of the macula. Each year, at least 2000 young and middle-aged adults in the United States have substantial loss of central vision secondary to POHS-related choroidal neovascular lesions.[38] Schlaegel noted that 33% of 100 patients diagnosed with POHS had bilateral choroidal neovascular membranes over 1 to 7 years of follow-up. Several studies have demonstrated the poor visual outcome of macular subretinal neovascular membranes that are not treated (50% to 70% with a final visual acuity of 20/200 or less).[30,38] Nevertheless, 10% to 16% of patients with macular choroidal neovascular membranes (including those with subfoveal membranes) will retain vision of 20/40 or better over long-term follow-up. Factors associated with retaining vision better than 20/40 include the following: age less than 30 years, smaller membrane size, less involvement of the foveal avascular zone, and absence of vision loss from POHS in the other eye.[30,38]

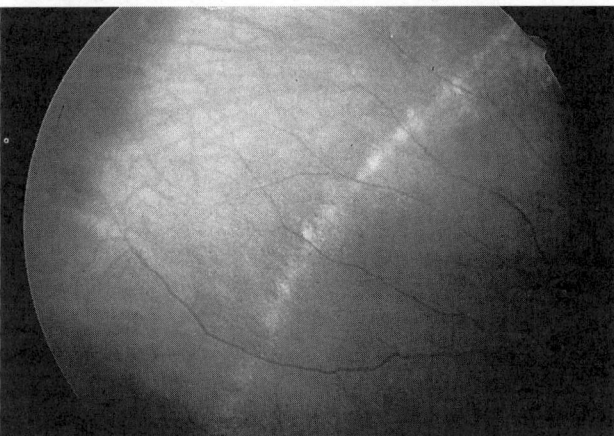

Fig. 90-4. Peripheral linear streak in a patient with POHS.

Choroidal neovascularization generally occurs at sites of antecedent POHS scars in the macula or peripapillary region (Fig. 90-5).

Pathogenesis

HLA-B7 has been reported to be significantly more common in patients with POHS and macular choroidal neovascular membranes (14 of 18 patients)[6,8] than in patients with only peripheral atrophic spots (4 of 15 patients).[36] HLA-DRw2 is associated with disciform macular lesions (21 of 26 patients) and patients with only peripheral lesions (8 of 13 patients).[37] The association of HLA-B7 with disciform macular lesions, but not with peripheral lesions, implies a genetic predisposition in a subset of POHS patients to develop choroidal neovascularization. The presence of HLA-B7 may identify patients at greater risk of developing active posterior pole lesions. Currently, HLA typing is not commonly performed because of its expense and because of the large number of asymptomatic POHS patients.

Lymphocyte infiltrates are present in human POHS lesions.[25,36] The significance of persistent foci of lymphocytes in the choroid is unknown. It is possible that such occult foci of lymphocytes may be the potential site and source for reactivation of the "de novo" lesions that appear to arise from normal retina.[10,28,55] Furthermore, in humans the appearance of "new foci" or continually changing peripheral and central POHS scars may be the result of chronic, low-grade choroiditis. This inflammation may eventually involve the RPE to the extent that it begins to proliferate or lose pigmentation, thereby causing the lesion to become clinically obvious months or even years after initial infection.

Animal Models. Animal models of experimental histoplasmic choroiditis have been developed in rabbits and in monkeys.[62,63,72] Primate models of experimental histoplasmic choroiditis provide some of the most convincing evidence that *H. capsulatum* produces the chorioretinal lesions associated with POHS in humans. The models also increase understanding of the pathophysiology of the disease and appear to explain some of the confusing clinical aspects of human POHS.

The primate model uses stump-tailed monkeys *(Macaca speciosa)* and rhesus monkeys *(Macaca mulatta)* inoculated with 5000 organisms of *H. capsulatum* per pound of monkey directly into the internal carotid artery.[56] An acute choroiditis appears 3 to 4 days after injection. Some early foci are not clinically visible, but fluorescein angiography shows early blocking of fluorescence and late staining in the choroid. Within 5 to 7 days of injection, multiple foci become clinically apparent as discrete, round, poorly circumscribed, yellowish lesions.[62] The severity of the disease varies from a few visible lesions to confluent choroiditis and serous detachment. The histoplasmin skin test becomes positive 2 to 4 weeks after injection. Six weeks after infection, it is no longer possible to demonstrate organisms by histologic techniques or culture. Histopathology of the acute lesions demonstrates mononuclear cell infiltrates of the choroid containing macrophages with phagocytized yeast phase organisms. The vitreous humor, retina, and anterior uveal structures are rarely affected, although damage to Bruch membrane is detectable by transmission electron microscopy.

The resolution stage (when organisms can no longer be identified in lesions) begins 6 weeks postinfection. It is characterized by four distinct clinical patterns evolving from acute experimental histoplasmic choroiditis: (1) atrophic scars (chorioretinal adhesions), (2) RPE window defects, (3) subclinical lesions identified only by fluorescein angiography, and (4) "disappearing" lesions characterized by a "normal" fundus examination and normal fluorescein angiography.

Atrophic Scars. Atrophic scars are focal, circumscribed, round or oval, yellowish-white, have slightly hazy margins, and are less than ½ optic disc diameter in size. Throughout the acute phase, and during a 3-year follow-up period, the hypopigmented portion of these lesions does not change appreciably in size or appearance. Fluorescein angiography typically reveals an early window defect and fluorescence persisting into the late phase. The region immediately surrounding the depigmented foci occasionally develops pigmentary changes, beginning 20 to 40 days after infection, and typically consisting of a halo of increased pigmentation that progresses for up to 1 year. In other cases the surrounding fundus becomes slightly hypopigmented and contains scattered pigment clumps giving a mottled appearance to the region. Light microscopy of the atrophic scars reveals loss of the RPE, occasional migration of RPE into the overlying retina, and focal adherence of the choroid to the retina.[57] The outer photoreceptor segments are absent, with variable disruption of the outer and inner retina and clumping of pigment. A round cell infiltrate consisting of lymphocytes, macrophages, and plasma cells is present in the underlying choroid. Ultrastructural analysis reveals alteration of Bruch membrane within areas of chorioretinal adhesion.

Retinal Pigment Epithelial Window Defects. In some animals the foci of acute choroiditis resolve with no ensuing chorioretinal scar formation, leaving a mottled appearance of the RPE. Fluorescein angiography reveals window defects with some areas of minimal late staining. Histopathologic examination of these lesions also reveals an underlying chronic lymphocytic infiltrate in the choroid and alterations of the RPE, Bruch membrane, and the choriocapillaris.

Subclinical Lesions. In many animals acute lesions resolve with no abnormalities detected by ophthalmoscopy, but some of these subclinical lesions can be detected on fluorescein angiography as areas of faint, late staining. By the end of the first month, these lesions evolve from clinically obvious lesions to subtle hypopigmented areas. Lesions gradually fade and clinically disappear (in some cases) 1 to 4 months after injection. Histopathologic examination

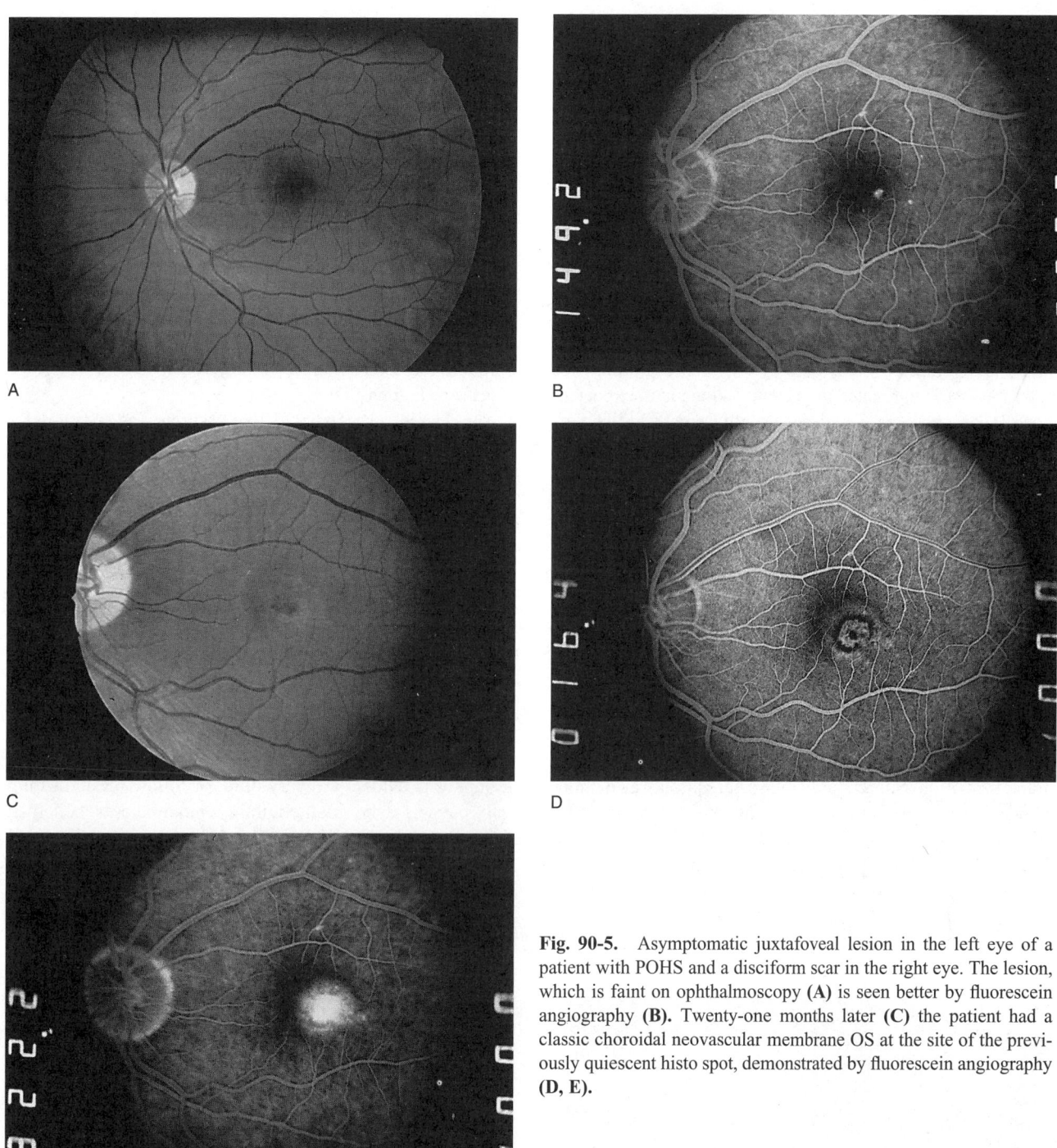

A

B

C

D

E

Fig. 90-5. Asymptomatic juxtafoveal lesion in the left eye of a patient with POHS and a disciform scar in the right eye. The lesion, which is faint on ophthalmoscopy **(A)** is seen better by fluorescein angiography **(B).** Twenty-one months later **(C)** the patient had a classic choroidal neovascular membrane OS at the site of the previously quiescent histo spot, demonstrated by fluorescein angiography **(D, E).**

of these lesions reveals an intact RPE-Bruch membrane-choriocapillaris complex with the presence of focal aggregates of lymphocytes and plasma cells in the choroid.

"Disappearing" Lesions. Some lesions completely disappear by both clinical and fluorescein angiographic examinations. In these cases no abnormalities are detectable on

follow-up examinations. Many acute lesions disappear on follow-up. Of 49 originally infected eyes, an average of 14.9 foci of acute choroiditis per eye were identifiable by clinical exams and angiography 10 to 14 days after infection. Six months after infection, an average of only 5.9 lesions per eye in 32 eyes remained visible by ophthalmoscopy, and 11.2

lesions per eye could be identified by fluorescein angiography. At 1 year, these numbers were reduced to an average of 4.8 and 8.5 lesions per eye by funduscopic exam and fluorescein angiography, respectively. In 18 eyes followed 2 to 3 years, only 3.2 and 6.6 lesions per eye were visible on funduscopic and fluorescein angiographic exams. Histopathologic examination of these ''disappearing lesions'' reveals multiple foci of lymphocytes in the choroid underlying normal retina, RPE, and Bruch membrane (Fig. 90-6). These lymphocytic infiltrates persist for as long as 3 years after apparent infection. Immunopathology studies of these lymphocytes reveal a decrease in the total number of lymphocytes over time, but continued presence of both T-lymphocytes and mature B-lymphocytes.[1] The finding of B-lymphocyte aggregates in chronic lesions is unexpected, since B-lymphocytes would not usually remain in the choroid without an antigenic stimulus. Perhaps this stimulus is the nondegraded chitinous cell wall material of *H. capsulatum* remaining after the acute choroidal disease and/or other sequestered ocular antigens related to acute and chronic damage to Bruch membrane and the RPE complex.

Implications for Human Disease. An important finding in the primate model is the histopathologic absence of organisms 6 weeks following infection.[22] This finding reinforces the clinical impression that amphotericin B has no role in the treatment of later macular disease when replicating organisms are no longer present.

The primate model does not answer the question of inciting factors for reactivation or choroidal neovascular membrane formation. Subretinal neovascularization was demonstrated in only one subhuman primate eye 30 months after injection of *H. capsulatum* organisms.[26] This membrane was found only on routine histopathologic sectioning. It could not be demonstrated by routine fluorescein angiography performed at 11 and 21 days, and 1, 3, 6, 9, 12, 18, 24, and

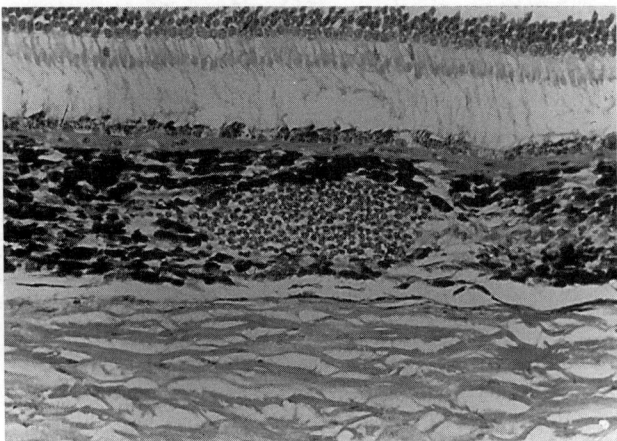

Fig. 90-6. A cluster of lymphocytes in the choroid of a primate eye approximately 1 year after injection of *H. capsulatum* organisms. The eye is otherwise quiet and asymptomatic (hematoxylin and eosin, × 63).

30 months after injection. Histopathologic examination revealed subretinal neovascularization between Bruch membrane and the degenerated retinal inner segments. The vessels were continuous with tight junctional complexes, which probably explains the lack of leakage on fluorescein angiography. The significance of this occult neovascular net is unknown but implies that asymptomatic choroidal neovascular membranes may occur in POHS.

Therapy

Because *H. capsulatum* organisms are not found in the animal model 6 weeks after infection, and no organisms have been identified in human histopathologic specimens, amphotericin B has no place in the treatment of the macular disease in human POHS.

Laser Trials. The National Eye Institute has sponsored a multicenter controlled clinical trial, the Ocular Histoplasmosis Study (OHS), designed to determine whether argon laser photocoagulation is useful in preventing severe visual acuity loss in eyes with choroidal neovascular membranes associated with POHS. The first phase of the study was designed to address choroidal neovascular membranes within 200 to 2500 microns from the geometric center of the foveal avascular zone.[20] Eligible patients were assigned to photocoagulation (n = 124) or to observation only (n = 121). At a median follow-up of 18 months, 34.2% (39 of 114) of untreated eyes versus 9.4% (11 of 117) of treated eyes had lost 6 or more lines of visual acuity from the baseline level. The superiority of argon laser photocoagulation for all subgroups was evident at every point of follow-up, indicating that patients who met eligibility requirements benefited from treatment. Eligibility requirements included visual acuity better than 20/100 and symptoms related to the neovascular membrane (such as decreased acuity, Amsler grid distortion, metamorphopsia, or uniocular diplopia), as well as a choroidal neovascular membrane 200 to 2500 microns from the center of the foveal avascular zone that was evident on fluorescein angiography.

Long-term analysis of 132 patients initially treated by argon laser photocoagulation in the OHS extrafoveal treatment trial revealed 30% of treated eyes had recurrences of choroidal neovascular membranes following laser treatment.[22] Most recurrences were early, with 22% occurring within 6 months; the figure increased only to 28% 2 years after treatment. Of the 40 patients with 1 or more recurrences, 31 had recurrence contiguous to a previously treated area, and 8 patients developed an independent choroidal neovascular membrane. Despite these recurrences, treated patients had improved visual outcome over untreated patients. A loss of 6 or more lines at 3 years after randomization occurred in 48% of patients in the untreated group, compared with only 9% in the treated group (Table 90-1).[21] Recurrences were treated (in 65% of patients) if they remained 200 microns from the center of the foveal avascular zone. Eyes with recurrences had an average visual acuity of

TABLE 90-1 PERCENT OF PATIENTS WITH VISUAL LOSS OF SIX OR MORE LINES AT THREE YEARS AFTER RANDOMIZATION

	OHS Study (extrafoveal)	OHS-Krypton (juxtafoveal)
Treated patients	9%	4.6%
Untreated patients	48%	24.6%

Data from Group MPS: Argon laser photocoagulation for neovascular maculopathy: three-year results from randomized clinical trials, *Arch Ophthalmol* 104:694-701, 1986; and Persistent and recurrent neovascularization after krypton laser photocoagulation for neovascular lesions of ocular histoplasmosis, *Arch Ophthalmol* 107:344-352, 1989.

20/62 at 3 years follow-up. This relatively good visual acuity in treated eyes with recurrent membranes is superior to natural history studies and reinforces the benefit of argon laser photocoagulation. The early recurrences underscore the necessity of close follow-up of patients with clinical, angiographic, and Amsler grid examinations after argon laser photocoagulation.

The Ocular Histoplasmosis Study (Krypton Laser) was a multicenter controlled clinical trial designed to determine whether krypton red laser photocoagulation was of value in "juxtafoveal" POHS choroidal neovascular membranes (1 to 199 microns from the center of the foveal avascular zone) or choroidal neovascular membranes (greater than 200 microns from the center of the foveal avascular zone with hemorrhage or pigment extending within 200 microns of the center of the foveal avascular zone). Patients were assigned to photocoagulation (n = 143) or to observation only (n = 145). One year after randomization, 24.8% (31 of 125) of untreated eyes, in contrast with 6.6% (8 of 121) of treated eyes, had lost 6 or more lines of visual acuity. By 3 years after randomization, the corresponding values were 24.6% (15 of 61) and 4.6% (3 of 64). Persistent choroidal neovascular membranes were observed in 23% of treated patients, with recurrent choroidal neovascular membranes in an additional 8%.[23] No recurrences were seen after 2 years. Data regarding visual loss in these studies are summarized in Table 90-1.

Complications have been reported with laser photocoagulation to choroidal neovascular membranes. Scars from juxtafoveal laser treatment may extend over time to involve the center of the foveal avascular zone.[52] Argon laser photocoagulation scars in patients with POHS were found to expand toward the foveal avascular zone at a rate of 152 microns per year for the first 2 years following laser treatment and 22 microns per year thereafter.[52] After 10 years the average scar was 3.23 times larger than the original treatment area. Macular hole formation attributed to argon laser treatment has also been described in patients with POHS.[34]

The macular photocoagulation treatment trial did not address subfoveal neovascular membranes. Most ophthalmol-ogists do not recommend laser ablation because this treatment always creates a dense central scotoma.

Surgical Treatment. In 1991 Thomas and Kaplan[67] reported two cases of POHS in which subfoveal neovascular membranes were removed successfully with surgery. Both patients noted improved visual acuity (from 20/400 to 20/20 in one and to 20/40 in the other) 3 to 7 months after surgery. In 1992 Thomas and associates[66] and Berger and Kaplan[4] reported the short-term outcome of a series of 20 and 15 patients, respectively. Thomas and associates' study[66] of 20 patients demonstrated improvement in visual acuity (2 Snellen lines or more) in 6 of 20 eyes followed 1 to 8 months after subretinal surgery. Only 4 patients had final visual acuities better than 20/100, and no patients had final visual acuities better than 20/50. Berger and Kaplan[4] reported visual acuity improvement (2 or more Snellen lines) in 8 of 15 cases of POHS. Follow-up ranged from 1 week to 6 months (except 1 patient who was followed for 48 months). Six patients had final visual acuities better than 20/100, with four patients recovering vision to 20/40 or better.

Long-term follow-up studies are indicated to assess the efficacy of subretinal neovascular membrane surgical excision in patients with POHS.

Corticosteroids. Some ophthalmologists advocate the use of systemic or periocular corticosteroids in patients with subfoveal subretinal neovascular membranes. Schlaegel[45,48] has advocated the administration of oral corticosteroids immediately upon symptomatology of macular lesions, with continuation until laser photocoagulation is administered.[27] Olk[38] found no significant difference between visual outcome in an uncontrolled trial of 25 eyes treated with corticosteroids that were compared to 41 untreated eyes. Olk's patients, however, had varying amounts of drug and different routes of corticosteroid administration.

The presence of lymphocyte infiltrates in POHS lesions[25,36] and the persistent foci of lymphocytes in the choroid suggest a role for corticosteroids. The possibility that reactivation of previously inactive histo spots and de novo lesions is secondary to persistent low-grade inflammation is the rationale for use of sub-Tenon corticosteroids in cases not amenable to surgical treatment. Histopathologic studies of treated choroidal neovascular membranes in POHS imply that the neovascular process may be a nonspecific healing response to a specific stimulus.[19,36,44,53] Antiinflammatory agents may modify this mechanism by limiting the inciting stimulus as well as reducing the resulting reparative process. Although no definitive proof exists regarding efficacy, sub-Tenon injection of corticosteroid should be considered if symptomatic macular disease is present and no subretinal neovascular membrane can be detected (or if detected, is not treatable by laser).

In cases that have no demonstrable subretinal neovascular membrane (by fluoroscein angiography), or in which the net is subfoveal or otherwise untreatable by laser, sub-Tenon injection of long-acting corticosteroids and/or administration of systemic corticosteroids should be considered as a therapeutic trial.

Prognosis

Gass and Wilkinson[16] noted an excellent visual prognosis for asymptomatic eyes when there is no ophthalmoscopic or angiographic evidence of focal chorioretinal scars in the macula or paramacular region. When atrophic scars are present in one eye of a patient with a POHS-related neovascular membrane, the rate of neovascular membrane development in the contralateral eye is 20.7% over 30 months. This rate of a choroidal neovascular membrane formation in a second eye, which has been confirmed in further studies to be 8% to 24% over 3 years,[2] justifies periodic exams and Amsler grid testing in patients with macular POHS lesions. It is well documented, however, that de novo subretinal neovascularization can occur in areas without preexisting atrophic scars or pigmentary changes,* so even patients without macular lesions are at risk for subretinal neovascular membranes.

The appropriate management of patients with subfoveal, subretinal neovascularization in the treatment of POHS remains controversial. Seven percent of patients with no treatment may have spontaneous improvement of vision,[4] and many documented cases of excellent visual acuity following spontaneous involution of the subretinal neovascular membranes exist.[7] Youth, involvement of less than 50% of the foveal avascular zone, membrane extent less than 200 microns beyond the center of the foveal avascular zone, and good initial visual acuity are factors that correlate with a good visual outcome.[38]

REFERENCES

1. Anderson A, Clifford W, Palvolgyi I et al.: Immunopathology of chronic experimental histoplasmic choroiditis in the primate, *Invest Ophthalmol Vis Sci* 33:1637-1641, 1992.
2. Argon laser photocoagulation for neovascular maculopathy: three-year results from randomized clinical trials, Macular Photocoagulation Study Group, *Arch Ophthalmol* 104:694-701, 1986.
3. Baskin MA, Jampol LM, Huamonte FU et al.: Macular lesions in blacks with the presumed ocular histoplasmosis syndrome, *Am J Ophthalmol* 89:77-83, 1980.
4. Berger AS, Kaplan HJ: Clinical experience with the surgical removal of subfoveal neovascular membranes—short-term postoperative results, *Ophthalmology* 99:969-975, 1992.
5. Bottoni FG, Deutman AF, Aandekerk AL: Presumed ocular histoplasmosis syndrome and linear streak lesions, *Br J Ophthalmol* 73:528-535, 1989.
6. Braley RE, Meredith TA, Aaberg TM et al.: The prevalence of HLA-B7 in presumed ocular histoplasmosis, *Am J Ophthalmol* 85:859, 1978.
7. Campochiaro PA, Morgan KM, Conway BP et al.: Spontaneous involution of subfoveal neovascularization, *Am J Ophthalmol* 109:668-675, 1990.
8. Cohen PR, Grossman ME, Silvers DN: Disseminated histoplasmosis and human immunodeficiency virus, *Int J Dermatol* 30:614-622, 1991.

9. Craig EL, Suie T: Histoplasma capsulatum in human ocular tissue, *Arch Ophthalmol* 91:285-289, 1974.
10. Davidorf FR: The role of T-lymphocytes in the reactivation of presumed ocular histoplasmosis scars, *Int Ophthalmol Clin* 15:111-124, 1975.
11. Denning DW: Epidemiology and pathogenesis of systemic fungal infections in the immunocompromised host, *J Antimicrob Chemother* 28(suppl B):1-16, 1991.
12. Dreyer RF, Gass DJ: Multifocal choroiditis and panuveitis: a syndrome that mimics ocular histoplasmosis, *Arch Ophthalmol* 102:1776-1784, 1984.
13. Ellis FD, Schlaegel TF: The geographic localization of presumed histoplasmic choroiditis, *Am J Ophthalmol* 75:953-956, 1973.
14. Fountain JA, Schlaegel TF: Linear streaks of the equator in the presumed ocular histoplasmosis syndrome, *Arch Ophthalmol* 99:246-248, 1981.
15. Ganley JP: Epidemiologic characteristics of presumed ocular histoplasmosis, *Acta Ophthalmol Suppl* 119:1-63, 1973.
16. Gass JDM, Wilkinson CP: Follow-up study of presumed ocular histoplasmosis, *Trans Am Acad Ophthalmol Otolaryngol* 75:572-593, 1972.
17. Gass JDM, Zimmerman LE: Histopathologic demonstration of *Histoplasma capsulatum*, *Am J Ophthalmol* 85:725, 1978.
18. Goldstein BG, Buettner H: Histoplasmic endophthalmitis: a clinicopathologic correlation, *Arch Ophthalmol* 101:774-777, 1983.
19. Green WR: Clinicopathologic studies of treated choroidal neovascular membranes: a review and report of two cases, *Retina* 11:328-356, 1991.
20. Group MPS: Argon laser photocoagulation for ocular histoplasmosis: results of a randomized clinical trial, *Arch Ophthalmol* 101:1347-1357, 1983.
21. Group MPS: Argon laser photocoagulation for neovascular maculopathy: three-year results from randomized clinical trials, *Arch Ophthalmol* 104:694-701, 1986.
22. Group MPS: Recurrent choroidal neovascularization after argon laser photocoagulation for neovascular maculopathy, *Arch Ophthalmol* 104:503-512, 1986.
23. Group MPS: Persistent and recurrent neovascularization after krypton laser photocoagulation for neovascular lesions of ocular histoplasmosis, *Arch Ophthalmol* 107:344-352, 1989.
24. Hoefnagels KL, Pijpers PM: Histoplasma capsulatum in a human eye, *Am J Ophthalmol* 63:715-723, 1967.
25. Irvine AR, Spencer WH, Hogan MJ et al.: Presumed chronic ocular histoplasmosis syndrome: a clinical-pathologic case report, *Trans Am Ophthalmol Soc* 94:91, 1976.
26. Jester JV, Smith RE: Subretinal neovascularization after experimental ocular histoplasmosis in a subhuman primate, *Am J Ophthalmol* 100:252-258, 1985.
27. Kaiser RJ, Torsch T, O'Connor PR: Prognostic criteria in macular histoplasmic choroiditis, *Int Ophthalmol Clin* 15:41-49, 1975.
28. Kaplan HJ, Waldrep JC: Immunological basis of presumed ocular histoplasmosis, *Int Ophthalmol Clin* 23:19-31, 1983.
29. Khalil MK: Histopathology of presumed ocular histoplasmosis, *Am J Ophthalmol* 94:369-376, 1982.
30. Kleiner RC, Ratner DM, Enger C et al.: Subfoveal neovascularization in the ocular histoplasmosis syndrome: a natural history study, *Retina* 8:225-229, 1988.
31. Klintworth GK, Hollingsworth AS, Lusman PA et al.: Granulomatous choroiditis in a case of disseminated histoplasmosis: histologic demonstration of *Histoplasma capsulatum* in choroidal lesions, *Arch Ophthalmol* 90:45-48, 1973.
32. Krill AE, Chishti MI, Klien BA et al.: Multifocal inner choroiditis, *Trans Am Acad Ophthalmol Otolaryngol* 73:222-245, 1969.
33. Lewis ML, Van NM, Gass JD: Follow-up study of presumed ocular histoplasmosis syndrome, *Ophthalmology* 87:390-399, 1980.
34. Lim JI, Schachat AP, Conway B: Macular hole formation following laser photocoagulation of choroidal neovascular membranes in a patient with presumed ocular histoplasmosis, *Arch Ophthalmol* 109:1500-1501, 1991 (letter).
35. Maumenee AE: Clinical entities in "uveitis": an approach to the study of intraocular inflammation, *Am J Ophthalmol* 69:1-27, 1970.
36. Meredith TA, Green WR, Key SN et al.: Ocular histoplasmosis: clinicopathologic correlation of 3 cases, *Surv Ophthalmol* 22:189-205, 1977.

---

*References 25, 32, 33, 43, 47, 60, 68.

37. Meredith TA, Smith RE, Duquesnoy RJ: Association of HLA-DRw2 antigen with presumed ocular histoplasmosis, *Am J Ophthalmol* 89:70-76, 1980.

38. Olk RJ, Burgess DB, McCormack PA: Subfoveal and juxtafoveal subretinal neovascularization in the presumed ocular histoplasmosis syndrome, *Ophthalmology* 91:1592-1602, 1984.

39. Pulido JS, Folberg R, Carter KD et al.: Histoplasma capsulatum endophthalmitis after cataract extraction, *Ophthalmology* 97:217-220, 1990.

40. Rivers MB, Pulido JS, Folk JC: Ill-defined choroidal neovascularization within ocular histoplasmosis scars, *Retina* 12:90-95, 1992.

41. Roth AM: *Histoplasma capsulatum* in the presumed ocular histoplasmosis syndrome, *Am J Ophthalmol* 84:293-298, 1977.

42. Ryan SJ: Histopathological correlates of presumed ocular histoplasmosis, *Int Ophthalmol Clin* 15:125-137, 1975.

43. Ryan SJ: De novo subretinal neovascularization in the histoplasmosis syndrome, *Arch Ophthalmol* 94:321-327, 1976.

44. Saxe SJ, Grossniklaus HE, Lopez PF et al.: Ultrastructural features of surgically excised subretinal neovascular membranes in the ocular histoplasmosis syndrome, *Arch Ophthalmol* 111:88-95, 1993.

45. Schlaegel TF Jr: *Ocular histoplasmosis,* New York, 1977, Grune and Straton.

46. Schlaegel TF, Weber JC, Helveston E et al.: Presumed histoplasmic choroiditis, *Am J Ophthalmol* 63:919-925, 1967.

47. Schlaegel TJ: The natural history of histo spots in the disc-macula area, *Int Ophthalmol Clin* 15:19-28, 1975.

48. Schlaegel TJ: Corticosteroids in the treatment of ocular histoplasmosis, *Int Ophthalmol Clin* 23:111-123, 1983.

49. Scholz R, Green WR, Kutys R et al.: Histoplasma capsulatum in the eye, *Ophthalmology* 91:1100-1104, 1984.

50. Schwarz J: *Histoplasmosis,* New York, 1981, Praeger Publishers.

51. Schwarz J, Salfelder K, Viloria JE: Histoplasma capsulatum in vessels of the choroid, *Ann Ophthalmol* 9:633-636, 1977.

52. Shah SS, Schachat AP, Murphy RP et al.: The evolution of argon laser photocoagulation scars in patients with the ocular histoplasmosis syndrome, *Arch Ophthalmol* 106:1533-1536, 1988.

53. Sheffer A, Green WR, Fine SL et al.: Presumed ocular histoplasmosis syndrome: a clinicopathologic correlation of a treated case, *Arch Ophthalmol* 98:335-340, 1980.

54. Smith RE: Studies of the presumed ocular histoplasmosis syndrome, *Trans Ophthalmol Soc UK* 328-334, 1981.

55. Smith RE: Natural history and reactivation studies of experimental ocular histoplasmosis in a primate model, *Trans Am Ophthalmol Soc* 80:695-757, 1982.

56. Smith RE, Dunn S, Jester JV: Natural history of experimental histoplasmic choroiditis in the primate. I. Clinical features, *Invest Ophthalmol Vis Sci* 25:801-809, 1984.

57. Smith RE, Dunn S, Jester JV: Natural history of experimental histoplasmic choroiditis in the primate. II. Histopathologic features, *Invest Ophthalmol Vis Sci* 25:810-819, 1984.

58. Smith RE, Ganley JP: Ophthalmic survey of a community. I. Abnormalities of the ocular fundus, *Am J Ophthalmol* 74:1126-1130, 1972.

59. Smith RE, Ganley JP: Presumed ocular histoplasmosis. I. Histoplasmin skin test sensitivity in cases identified during a community survey, *Arch Ophthalmol* 87:245-250, 1972.

60. Smith RE, Ganley JP: The natural history of non-disciform ocular histoplasmosis, *Can J Ophthalmol* 12:114-120, 1977.

61. Smith RE, Ganley JP, Knox DL: Presumed ocular histoplasmosis. II. Patterns of peripheral and peripapillary scarring in persons with nonmacular disease, *Arch Ophthalmol* 87:251-257, 1972.

62. Smith RE, Macy JI, Parret C et al.: Variations in acute multifocal histoplasmic choroiditis in the primate, *Invest Ophthalmol Vis Sci* 17:1005, 1978.

63. Smith RE, O'Connor GR, Halde CJ et al.: Clinical course in rabbits after experimental induction of ocular histoplasmosis, *Am J Ophthalmol* 76:284-293, 1973.

64. Spaide RF, Yannuzzi LA, Freund KB: Linear streaks in multifocal choroiditis and panuveitis, *Retina* 11:229-231, 1991.

65. Specht CS, Mitchell KT, Bauman AE et al.: Ocular histoplasmosis with retinitis in a patient with acquired immune deficiency syndrome, *Ophthalmology* 98:1356-1359, 1991.

66. Thomas MA, Grand MG, Williams DF et al.: Surgical management of subfoveal choroidal neovascularization, *Ophthalmology* 99:952-968, 1992.

67. Thomas MA, Kaplan HJ: Surgical removal of subfoveal neovascularization in the presumed ocular histoplasmosis syndrome, *Am J Ophthalmol* 111:1-7, 1991.

68. Watzke RC: Presumed histoplasmosis syndrome, *Trans New Orleans Acad Ophthalmol* 31:89-96, 1983.

69. Weingeist TA, Watzke RC: Ocular involvement by histoplasma capsulatum, *Int Ophthalmol Clin* 23:33-47, 1983.

70. Wheat LJ, Batteiger BE, Sathapatayavongs B: Histoplasma capsulatum infections of the central nervous system: a clinical review, *Medicine (Baltimore)* 69:244-260, 1990.

71. Wheat LJ, Connolly SP, Baker RL et al.: Disseminated histoplasmosis in the acquired immune deficiency syndrome: clinical findings, diagnosis and treatment, and review of the literature, *Medicine (Baltimore)* 69:361-374, 1990.

72. Wong VG, Kwon CK, Green WR et al.: Focal choroidopathy in experimental ocular histoplasmosis, *Trans Am Acad Ophthalmol Otolaryngol* 77:OP769-777, 1973.

73. Woods AC, Wahlen HE: The probable role of benign histoplasmosis in the etiology of granulomatous uveitis, *Trans Am Ophthalmol Soc* 57:318-343, 1959.

91 Endogenous Fungal Endophthalmitis

THOMAS H. PETTIT, JOHN E. EDWARDS JR, ERIC P. PURDY, JOHN D. BULLOCK

Fungi constitute a prominent and diverse group among the myriad of microorganisms that coexist with man in both his external and internal environments. Despite their ubiquitous nature, only a limited number of fungi produce infections of the eye, of which only a few cause endogenous fungal endophthalmitis. Nevertheless, the prevalence of endogenous fungal endophthalmitis is increasing due to the growing number of iatrogenically induced infections.

In contrast to exogenous infections, which enter the eye either directly during penetrating trauma or surgery or by extension of infection from adjacent tissues, endogenous infections reach the eye via the bloodstream, usually as part of a disseminated infection. Endogenous intraocular infections are classified by the infectious agent and the area of ocular involvement: choroiditis, retinitis, chorioretinitis, retinochoroiditis, endophthalmitis, or panophthalmitis. Endogenous intraocular fungal infections arise from circulating fungal elements that become lodged in the fine vessels of the retina and uvea, where they initiate a focal choroiditis, retinitis, or cyclitis. When this initial focus of infection extends into the vitreous, producing inflammation and the potential for the fungal infection to involve all of the internal structures of the eye, endogenous fungal endophthalmitis results.

The major causes of endogenous fungal infections in the eye include *Aspergillus* species, *Blastomyces dermatitidis*, *Candida* species, *Coccidioides immitis*, *Cryptococcus neoformans*, *Histoplasma capsulatum*, *Pseudallescheria boydii*, and *Sporothrix schenckii*. Most of these organisms are capable of producing endophthalmitis, but they may produce only a localized infection and present as a focal chorioretinitis or a granuloma in the eye. Coccidioidomycosis and histoplasmosis are not included in this chapter but are presented elsewhere under separate chapter headings (Chapters 103 and 90 respectively).

CANDIDIASIS

Candida species are recognized as the most common causes of endogenous fungal endophthalmitis and are one of the most common of all endogenous infections of the eye.

Candida species are notable as accounting for 7% to 15% of all hospital-acquired infections in the United States.[201] Clinical evidence of endogenous candidal endophthalmitis (ECE) found by examination of the ocular fundus is recognized as an extremely useful and important marker for disseminated candidiasis, a major nosocomial infection affecting an estimated 120,000 patients annually in this country.[47,76,110] The term candidiasis indicates the presence of a parenchymatous infection caused by *Candida* species. The infection may be localized to one organ, but is more likely multifocal or disseminated, involving simultaneously a variety of vital organs such as the kidney, heart, eye, skin, and bone, and in terminal stages, the brain, liver, spleen, and lung.[76] In contrast, the term candidemia denotes merely the presence, confirmable by culture, of *Candida* species in the bloodstream.

Mycology

More than 100 species of *Candida* have been identified, but less than a dozen are clinically important pathogens in man.[201] The *Candida* species producing disease in humans, for the most part, live commensally as part of the normal flora on the mucocutaneous surfaces of man's gastrointestinal (GI), genitourinary (GU), and respiratory systems. These ubiquitous yeasts coexist with man worldwide and can be isolated from the oropharynx and GI tract of up to 50% of healthy asymptomatic individuals.[76] *Candida* species can be recovered frequently from soil, food, and occasionally from other areas in the environment.[201] *Candida* species can be cultured readily on blood agar and Sabouraud glucose media, where they can be identified in 24 to 48 hours as smooth, dome-shaped, creamy white colonies with a pasty appearance. They are readily recognized in cultures and in clinical specimens where they may exist as a budding yeast and/or in a pseudomycelial form, depending on the medium.

Epidemiology

Prior to 1970 endogenous candidal endophthalmitis was rarely recognized, and then usually only at autopsy.[139] In the early 1970s an increasing incidence of endogenous candidal endophthalmitis was noted; this event paralleled an increase in the frequency of candidemia and disseminated candidiasis.[68,143] With the study of this outbreak of candidal infections, the relationship between disseminated candidiasis, endogenous candidal endophthalmitis, and candidemia became clearer.[60,82,83]

Approximately a third of patients with candidemia will develop candidiasis. A 5-year study published by Griffin and associates[82] in 1974 found that of 82 patients with candidemia, 30% had clinical or autopsy evidence of endogenous candidal chorioretinitis or endophthalmitis. In a 1982 report of 38 patients with candidemia, Parke and associates[153] found 11 (29%) who developed candidal chorioretinitis. All patients developing ocular candidal infections in this series had multiple positive blood cultures for Candida species. In a prospective study of hospitalized patients published in 1989, Brooks[33] found chorioretinitis consistent with candidal infection in 28% of patients with candidemia.

Endogenous candidal endophthalmitis is associated with a very high incidence of coexistant disseminated candidiasis. The eye is an important clinical marker for disseminated candidiasis, a life-threatening and treatable systemic fungal infection. In a study of 39 autopsy cases of ECE, Edwards and associates[60] found 77% (30 cases) had evidence of candidal infection in other major organs. Other autopsy and clinical studies have noted from 78% to 88% of patients with candidal chorioretinitis also have tissue-invasive infection of other organs.[82,83,153] The kidney and heart are the most common sites of nonocular infection. Conversely, two autopsy series of patients with disseminated candidiasis found that approximately 80% of cases had candidal lesions in the eye.[82,153] The close parallel between ocular and systemic foci of fungal infection at the time of death is an important observation. Autopsy cases frequently represent advanced disease, however, and therefore, they may not accurately reflect the degree of multiorgan involvement present during the earlier stages of candidemia and candidiasis.

Risk Factors

In ECE, infectious fungal elements reach the eye (via the bloodstream) from (1) fungal colonies on indwelling venous catheter tips, (2) foci of infection remote to the eye, or (3) contaminated injections self-administered by intravenous drug abusers. Intermittent or persistent candidemia leads to disseminated candidiasis in which the eye is the most visible locus of infection available to the physician for monitoring.

The increase in disseminated candidiasis occurring in the early 1970s was predominately a complication of aggressive medical and surgical therapeutic efforts in seriously ill patients. In the late 1970s reports of ECE associated with intravenous drug abuse began to appear. With the expansion of the drug culture during the 1980s, increasing numbers of cases of ECE in drug abusers were reported at a time when

case reports unrelated to drug abuse were declining. Although a 1990 review identified intravenous drug abuse as "the most common [single] predisposing factor in cases of endogenous fungal endophthalmitis,"[31] nosocomial ECE, as a group, still appears to be a more frequent form of disease overall.

Important in the early detection of ECE is an awareness of the clinical setting and predisposing factors leading to candidemia. The most notable factors include broad-spectrum systemic antimicrobial use, indwelling intravenous catheters, parenteral hyperalimentation, recent major surgery (particularly of the GI tract), a prolonged postoperative course of recovery, generalized immunosuppression (associated with malnutrition, debilitating disease, iatrogenic neutropenia, and corticosteroid use), and intravenous drug abuse. Candidemia in newborns and fungal infections of the vagina are other potential risk factors.

The 1973 report by Griffin and associates[83] drew attention to a number of predisposing factors. The paper described six patients who developed endogenous candidal endophthalmitis while hospitalized. All patients had surgery and intravenous catheters, and five of them had bacterial sepsis. Candidemia developed 6 to 58 days after the placement of the intravenous catheters. Candida species were cultured from the intravenous catheter tips, and visual symptoms developed 3 to 15 days after blood cultures confirmed the presence of candidemia. In the same paper 11 of 15 patients with candidal chorioretinitis (studied at autopsy) had a history of sepsis caused by Escherichia coli or Pseudomonas species, and 9 of the 15 had GI tract perforations. Sepsis is probably not a predisposing factor by itself but merely leads to antibiotic use, which is a predisposing factor.

In 1974 Edwards and associates,[60] summarizing 62 previously reported cases and 14 unpublished cases, noted that 88% of the patients had received some type of intravenous infusion. These infusions were via indwelling catheters in 46% of cases. Systemic antibiotics had been received by 84% of the patients, and 63% had had major surgery (with 60% of the procedures on the GI tract). Other debilitating diseases in this same group of patients included malignancies (21%), diabetes mellitus (13%), and alcoholism and liver disease (8%). In these studies patients at greatest risk were those who underwent complicated GI tract surgery and (1) received intravenous hyperalimentation, (2) experienced prolonged antibiotic therapy, and (3) had indwelling intravascular catheters or other devices for complex postoperative care. The prominence of iatrogenic factors in this group of patients is striking. Many of them had complicated GI surgery with a guarded prognosis followed by a stormy postoperative course leading to a long period of recovery or even death.

Drug Abuse. Intravenous drug abusers are at significant risk for developing ECE.[3,74,75,172,197] They tend to be young adults without obvious systemic disease. The source of contamination is not identified in most cases, but undoubtedly relates to nonsterile paraphernalia and drug preparation. Efforts to isolate *Candida* species from pure heroin and from heroin samples confiscated in drug raids have been unsuccessful.[119,197] Diacetyl morphine has a fungicidal effect on *C. albicans*.[119] In 1986 contaminated preserved lemon juice used to dissolve heroin was traced to an outbreak of *C. albicans* endophthalmitis amongst intravenous drug abusers in Glasgow.[173,174]

In the mid-1980s a syndrome comprised of disseminated candidiasis, characteristic skin pustules, deep-seated scalp nodules, endophthalmitis, costochondritis, osteomyelitis, and occasional pleuropulmonary involvement was identified in intravenous heroin abusers.[58a] The localized, small, epidemic-like outbreaks occurring in clusters appeared to be related to the use of Iranian or brown heroin.[119] Blood and urine cultures were negative, although *Candida* species were isolated from lesions of the skin, joints, and costal cartilage.

On initial examination drug abusers with ECE tend to show more vitreous reaction than other risk groups, possibly because of their delay in seeking care. They also may show less evidence of disseminated candidiasis than other risk groups. This observation may relate to their younger age, a pattern of more transient candidemia, and the general lack of other debilitating disease.

Lesions in the eye compatible with ECE are seen in 40% to 60% of the drug abusers with disseminated candidiasis.[119] For intravenous drug abusers, the eye becomes a particularly important organ for monitoring the internal milieu. Any patient with a history of intravenous drug abuse and uveitis should be evaluated for ECE, as well as other fungal and bacterial causes of intraocular infection that can occur with a disseminated infection.

Neonatal Infections. Low birth weight infants and normal birth weight infants undergoing prolonged hospitalization are particularly susceptible to candidal chorioretinitis that may progress to endophthalmitis. Candidal chorioretinitis is the most common intraocular fungal infection in infants.[14,94,151] The factors predisposing to its development resemble those seen in the adult.[14] The presence of *Candida* species in the eye in infants, as in adults, signals evidence of probable disseminated candidiasis.[151]

Infants at risk are usually severely ill, have central venous lines for long periods, and are receiving multiple antibiotics and hyperalimentation; a significant number also have had abdominal surgery.[147,151] Up to 3% of very low birth weight newborns (< 1500 grams) develop systemic candidiasis.[13,14,100]

The increased risk of candidiasis in newborns may reflect immature host defenses, as the capability of the neonatal leukocyte to kill *Candida* species organisms is less than that of adult leukocytes.[209] This reduced leukocyte capacity may lead to a more exuberant inflammatory reaction in infants with candidal endophthalmitis.

Vaginal Infections. Seven cases with ocular lesions clinically consistent with intraocular candidal infections, and presumed to be of endogenous origin, have been reported in women with candidal vaginitis or vaginal colonization.[36,112,137,143,147] Three cases were in postpartum women, whereas the others were unassociated with childbirth. Neither candidemia nor disseminated candidiasis was documented in any of these patients. In one recent case with vaginitis, karyotype analysis found the identical strain of *C. albicans* in cultures from the vitreous and the patient's fingernails.[112]

It is possible that candidemia may occur during delivery, in the early postpartum period, or at other times leading to disseminated infection, but the incidence of ECE related to a vaginal source must be very low, considering how frequently *Candida* species are present in the vagina.

Factors Promoting Fungal Growth. Normally *Candida* species are found only in small numbers on the mucosal surfaces of the human body. There they compete for nutrients and adherence sites with the more numerous bacterial microflora. A variety of factors may promote the proliferation of *Candida* species on mucosal surfaces, allowing them to replace the resident bacterial flora and to alter the natural barriers inhibiting candidal overgrowth and tissue invasion. The most important factor promoting fungal growth in the human body is the prolonged use of broad-spectrum antibiotics that suppress the normal bacterial microflora, allowing *Candida* species to flourish.[59,80,201] Other factors that may promote fungal growth in the body include the following: (1) diabetes mellitus, which increases available glucose (an important *Candida* species nutrient), (2) a low pH, which enhances the transferrin release of iron required by *Candida* species to grow, (3) corticosteroid use, which may increase available glucose and at the same time suppress phagocytic and lymphocytic activity, and (4) ileus associated with abdominal disease and surgery, which may encourage yeast overgrowth. The massive proliferation of *Candida* species in the GI or GU tracts may weaken the mucosal defenses to tissue invasion and allow fungi access to the circulation.[201]

Indwelling venous catheters and other intravascular devices can become foci for fungal adherence and proliferation,[163,201] providing a source for intermittent candidemia, thereby seeding fungi throughout the vascular system.[64,83,91] Abdominal surgery, endoscopy, or other manipulation may produce additional seeding of fungi into the circulation.

Clinical Features

In ECE the patients' general condition may obscure their awareness of early symptoms. Intravenous drug abusers may deny or fail to recognize visual symptoms. Many postoperative and seriously ill patients are too sick to pay attention to the onset of floaters, localized scotomata, subtle changes in vision, photophobia, ciliary injection, or even ocular pain. Early extramacular or peripheral fundus lesions produce little or no visual symptoms. With macular lesions or significant vitreous involvement most patients become symptomatic, unless they are too ill to respond.

In the early studies of ECE, over half the patients had vitreous involvement and multiple fundus lesions when first examined, and two thirds had lesions in both eyes at the time of their initial symptoms.[60,83] The majority of early lesions of ECE originate in the inner choroid as an intense focal inflammatory reaction surrounding a small locus of *Candida* species organisms. A small percentage begin as a localized retinitis. The earliest lesions may be difficult to see with ophthalmoscopy but may show up well on fluorescein angiography, with which they appear as an area of hypofluorescence with late staining. The characteristic appearance of a candidal lesion in the fundus is a creamy-white, round or oval, ⅛ to ¼ disc-diameter in size, circumscribed chorioretinal lesion with overlying vitreous inflammation of varying intensity (Figs. 91-1 and 91-2).

As the infectious focus breaks into the vitreous it enlarges in a globular fashion, with budding extensions. Vitreous extension is accompanied by focal perivascular inflammatory deposits and increasing vitreous haze, with strandlike clusters of inflammatory cells and diffuse cellular infiltration. Lesions are commonly multifocal and located in both eyes. Small focal intraretinal hemorrhages occur fairly frequently, and when they surround small lesions may have the appearance of a Roth spot. Focal retinal necrosis and scarring combined with vitreoretinal membrane formation and contraction are the major causes of permanent vision loss (Fig. 91-3, *A* and *B*). Vitreous inflammation may be so severe that it obscures the view of the fundus and makes clinical diagnosis difficult.

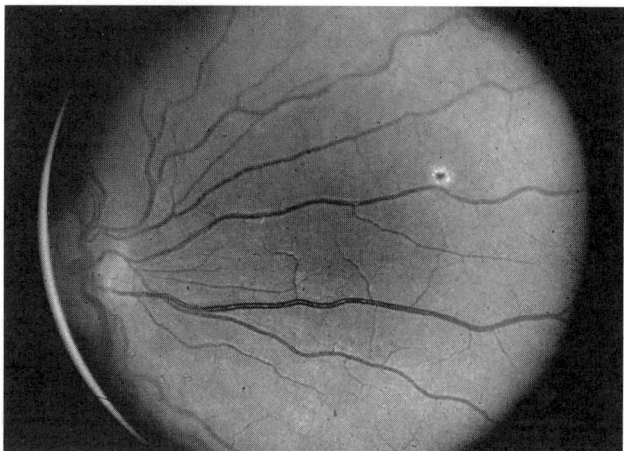

Fig. 91-2. Same lesion as in Fig. 91-1, following treatment with intravenous amphotericin B. Note hypopigmented scar with central pigmentation.

Candidal infections progress at a much slower pace than most bacterial infections and may take days or weeks to produce the damage bacterial infections can cause over a few hours or days. Prompt diagnosis and treatment have a much better chance of salvaging vision in ECE than in bacterial endophthalmitis. Anterior segment inflammation lags behind posterior segment inflammation but mirrors the intensity of the vitreous reaction and may slowly progress from minimal to severe iridocyclitis with synechiae, hypopyon, pupillary block (Fig. 91-4), and even a ciliary body abcess. Vision loss varies depending on the degree of macular, retinovitreal, and anterior segment involvement. Misdiagnosis or ineffective therapy may result in perforation or phthisis.

Pathology

Histologically the chorioretinal lesions of early ECE show an intense localized inflammatory reaction (arising in the choroid) composed of suppurative and granulomatous elements surrounding a small nidus of *Candida* species organisms. From the inner choroid the inflammatory reaction breaks through Bruch membrane into the retina to produce a localized retinal microabscess (Fig. 91-5). In the absence of effective treatment, the infectious nidus along with its surrounding inflammatory response enlarges, ruptures through the internal limiting lamina, and spills into the vitreous. The characteristic budding yeast and pseudohyphae of *Candida* species are seen in small numbers in the choroid, where the process originates, and become more numerous as the process extends into the retina (Fig. 91-6) and avascular vitreous.

The host's immune defenses are better able to confine the infectious process on the vascular margins of the lesion located in the choroid and retina than on the avascular perimeter adjacent to the vitreous. Thus the infectious process ex-

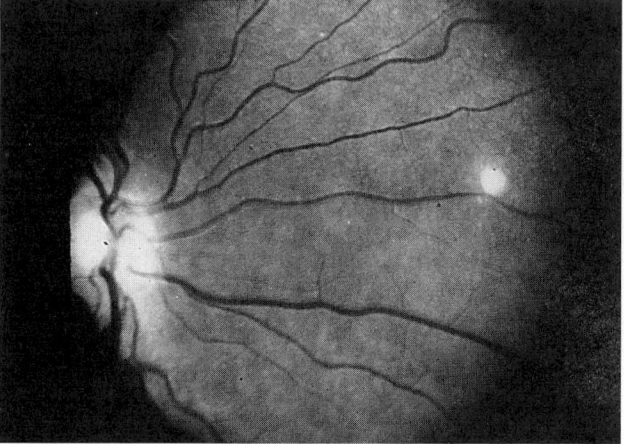

Fig. 91-1. Typical early lesion of candidal chorioretinitis located nasal to the optic disc. Other similar lesions were seen elsewhere in this eye and in the opposite eye. The inflammatory reaction overlying the lesion extends into the vitreous, partially obscuring the adjacent vessel.

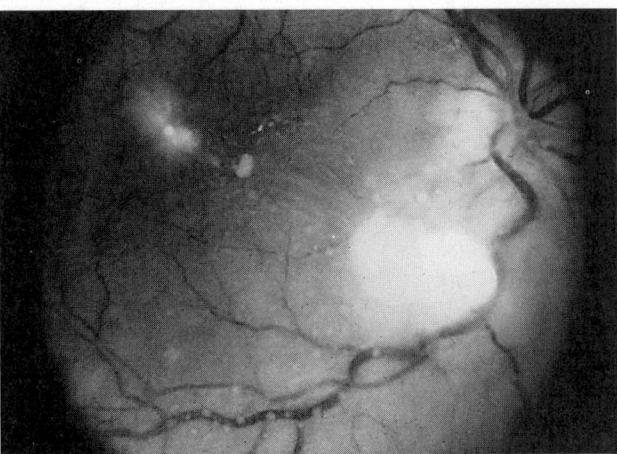

A

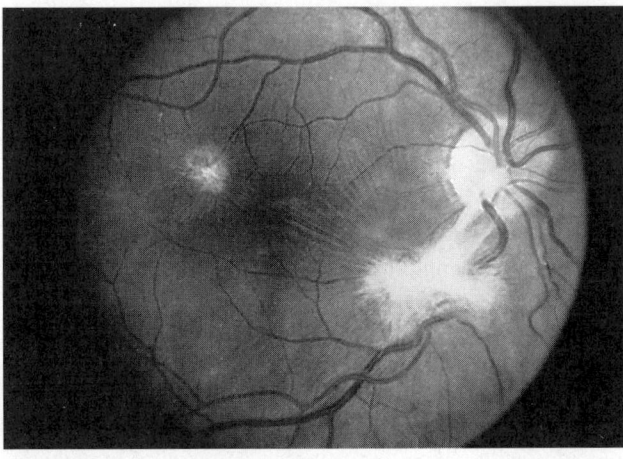

B

Fig. 91-3. Photos of candidal endophthalmitis before and after successful treatment with amphotericin B. This major vitreous involvement developed from multifocal lesions originating in the choroid. In **A** note the globular budding masses of vitreous inflammation and the perivascular inflammatory reaction. In **B** note the extensive vitreous traction with secondary effects on the macula and the retinal vessels. Reprinted with permission from Holland GN: Endogenous fungal infections of the retina and choroid. In Ryan SJ, editor: *Retina,* vol 2, *Medical Retina,* ed 2, 1607-1619, St Louis, 1994, Mosby.

tends toward and into the vitreous. In the vitreous the inflammatory reaction forms a vitreous abscess with a nidus of proliferating *Candida* species surrounded by an intense inflammatory infiltrate composed of numerous neutrophils, lymphocytes, and plasma cells. The more intense host immune response in the vascular tissues of the choroid and retina slows the lateral extension of the infection along the plane of the choroid and retina. In the vitreous leukocytes are scattered in declining numbers as they extend away from the candidal micro-abscess, except where they cluster in increased numbers along vessels or on vitreous strands.

Perivasculitis, papillitis, and localized serous retinal detachments commonly accompany an expanding intravitreous infection. In the late stages of ECE, traction retinal detachments associated with proliferative vitreoretinopathy and cyclitic membranes are found.

Pathogenesis

Predominance of *Candida albicans*. Most of the *Candida* species isolated from endogenous fungal endophthalmitis

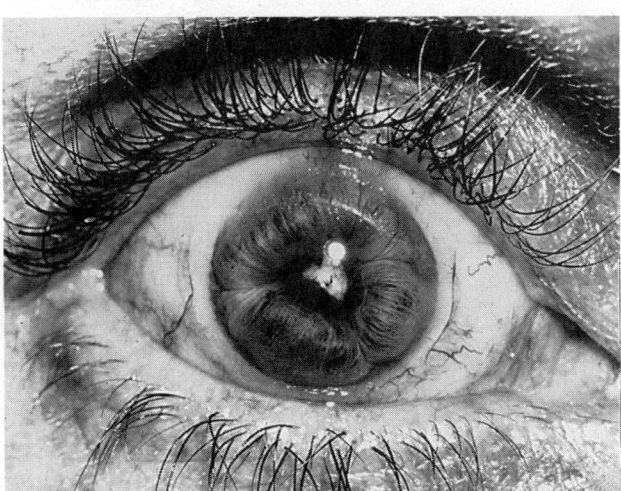

Fig. 91-4. An atrophic eye with pupillary block, a hypermature cataract and a disorganized retina that resulted from failure to diagnose and appropriately treat candidal endophthalmitis. Patient's initial eye symptoms began the day of discharge from the hospital, following prolonged hospitalization for multiple fractures related to a motorcycle accident. Despite the fact that candidemia was noted during hospitalization, candidal endophthalmitis was not suspected until 8 weeks after patient was discharged.

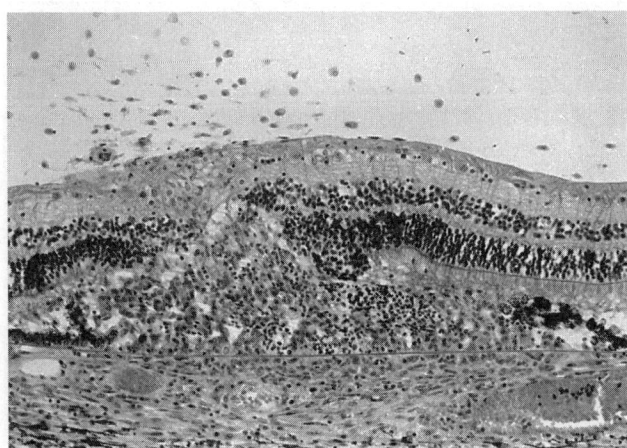

Fig. 91-5. Histopathology of focal candidal chorioretinitis. Note the inflammatory locus is centered in the choroid and retina with inflammatory cells in the overlying vitreous. All retinal layers have been disrupted focally by acute and chronic inflammatory cells. (Hematoxylin-eosin, ×200.) Photograph courtesy of Robert Y. Foos, MD.

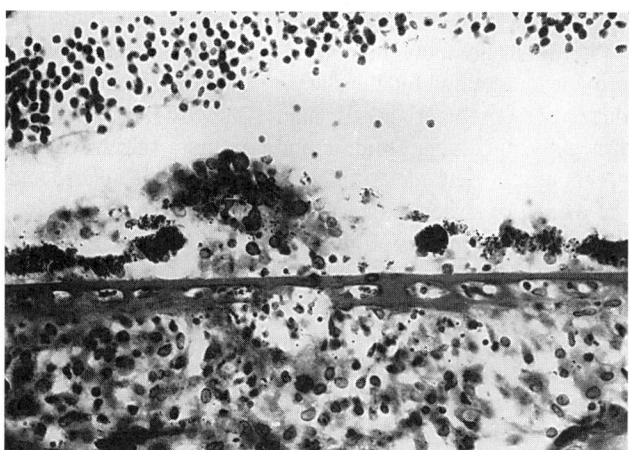

Fig. 91-6. Candida yeast forms in necrotic retina and choroid from an autopsy case of candidal endophthalmitis. Note Bruch membrane and choriocapillaris running horizontally. (Hematoxylin-eosin, ×430.)

are *Candida albicans,* suggesting that this species may be more likely than other *Candida* species to infect the eye. Of 15 autopsy cases reported by Griffin and associates,[83] 12 were *C. albicans,* 2 were *C. tropicalis,* and 1 was *C. parapsilosis.* In a series of 38 patients with candidemia followed by Parke and associates,[153] 11 developed candidal chorioretinitis. Of these, 10 had *C. albicans* isolated from the blood, whereas only 1 had *C. tropicalis* isolated. Of the total of 38 patients with candidemia in Parke's study, 27 had *C. albicans* candidemia.

Two independent laboratory studies of disseminated candidiasis with endophthalmitis produced in a rabbit model suggest a similar tendency for *C. albicans* to involve the eye.[62,101] The reason for this preference for the eye is not understood. It has been observed that *C. albicans* rapidly forms germ tubes in serum, whereas other *Candida* species do not.[147] It is possible that the germ tubes of *C. albicans* lodge in the choriocapillaris more readily than other yeast forms. Disparities in the production of protease and phospholipases have also been suggested as contributing factors to differences in the ocular pathogenicity of various *Candida* species.[147] A recent review[102] of endophthalmitis caused by nonalbican species suggests that *Candida* species other than *C. albicans* are not as likely to infect the choroid and retina. It does not necessarily follow, however, that these nonalbican species are any less capable of producing disseminated candidiasis by seeding organs other than the eye.

Host Factors. Certain host factors may contribute to the development of candidal chorioretinitis in the presence of candidemia. There is a clinical impression that candidal lesions in the fundus are more common in postsurgical patients than in nonsurgical patients with severe neutropenia secondary to certain malignancies and chemotherapy.[147] In the presence of neutropenia the host may be unable to mobi-

lize enough neutrophils to produce visible lesions around fungal foci in the choroid and retina. In a study of hematogenous disseminated candidiasis in an immunosuppressed (nitrogen-mustard-induced neutropenia) model in the rabbit, lesions of candidal chorioretinitis were uncommon and atypical if the animals were severely neutropenic.[92] These observations, though fragmentary, should alert the physician to consider that in patients with severe neutropenia the typical lesions of endogenous candidal endophthalmitis may not develop fully enough to be visible even in the presence of disseminated candidiasis.

Immune Response. The body's immunologic defenses are capable of clearing rather large numbers of candidal organisms entering the bloodstream, but these defenses can be overwhelmed by persistent candidemia. Both humoral and cell-mediated immunity are involved in the body's defenses. Agglutination factors and other components of serum promote clumping of *Candida* species and enhance phagocytosis.[59] Neutrophil-mediated phagocytosis and the complement system are key elements in the defense against *Candida* species. Neutrophils, monocytes, and macrophages are all capable of candidacidal activity. A principal candidacidal mechanism of the neutrophil involves the myeloperoxidase, hydrogen peroxide, and/or superoxide anion systems.[59] An abundant neutrophil infiltrate is a hallmark of candidal lesions.

Differential Diagnosis

In the majority of reported cases the diagnosis of ECE has been clinical and based on the combination of a characteristic clinical setting, compatible fundus lesions, and isolation of *Candida* species from blood, urine, or a nonocular site.[31,60,83,96] Fundus lesions that might be confused with candidal infection include other forms of infectious chorioretinitis, cotton wool spots, leukemic infiltrates, and drusen. Most other fungal infections producing chorioretinitis cannot be differentiated from candidal infections on the basis of clinical appearance alone. The frequent hemorrhagic component of cytomegalovirus (CMV) retinitis and its lack of associated intraocular inflammation as well as the more indolent course of ocular toxoplasmosis help distinguish those infections from candidal chorioretinitis.

Laboratory Investigations

In the presence of a typical lesion in the fundus, a history of *Candida* species cultured from the blood, urine, intravascular catheters, or other body sources days or weeks prior to the onset of symptoms can be very helpful in providing support for a presumptive diagnosis of ECE. Isolation of *Candida* species directly from the inner eye can provide a definitive diagnosis but is not routinely required. The clinical appearance of the ocular lesions may be quite characteristic, and in most cases the risk of a diagnostic vitrectomy can be avoided.

In the case of a diagnostic dilemma or when a suspected

case is not responding to therapy, a vitrectomy provides the best chance of obtaining an isolate and a definitive diagnosis. The inconsistency of diagnostic vitreous taps without vitrectomy make them a poor second choice as they frequently fail to sample the locus of infection.[3,90] Anterior chamber aspiration is not helpful for diagnostic cultures[90] but in the future may prove useful for identifying local synthesis of anticandidal antibodies.[22,132] Unfortunately, even pars plana vitrectomy is not always successful in recovering the causative organism. Although vitrectomy does pose some risks, it offers unique benefits such as the following: (1) the debulking of inflammatory and infectious material from the vitreous, (2) the acquisition of a larger sample for laboratory study, (3) the potential for concentrating the vitreous sample by centrifugation or filtration to give a better yield on culture, and (4) the opportunity for the injection of antifungal agents directly into the vitreous. The laboratory should be alerted when a vitrectomy specimen is anticipated so that appropriate handling and media are available. In the absence of appropriate fungal media, vitreous samples may be innoculated directly into blood culture bottles.[31]

Future development of highly specific immunologic probes to identify candidal antigens or antibodies in small samples of vitreous or aqueous humor may provide a quicker and safer means of definitive diagnosis.

Therapy

With rare exception, antifungal therapy is indicated in cases of ECE.* Such an exception was reported by Dellon and associates[49] in 1975, when removal of a contaminated intravenous catheter alone, without any antifungal therapy, was followed by complete resolution of candidal chorioretinitis. The expected course of untreated intraocular candidal infections is progression to endophthalmitis and severe loss of vision. Early recognition and treatment, however, can lead to recovery of good vision, provided the process has not involved the macula.

Amphotericin B. Systemic amphotericin B, administered intravenously, is currently the drug of choice in the treatment of ECE.[59,147,165] Amphotericin B is a heptaene polyene antibiotic that binds to sterols in the cell membrane of sensitive fungi, producing permeability changes, cell injury, and ultimately cell death. It may be fungistatic or fungicidal depending on fungal sensitivity and the tissue levels of amphotericin B.

In treating early cases of ECE in which the lesions are confined to the choroid and retina, a minimal cumulative dose of at least 200 mg may be adequate to control the infection. If there is significant vitreous involvement or if the lesion is not responding promptly to initial treatment, flucytosine can be added and therapy continued until the total

---

*References 32, 59, 96, 134, 147, 165.

cumulative dose of amphotericin B is between 1000 and 1500 mg. Regrettably, no controlled studies are available to provide guidelines for the duration of therapy or the total dose of amphotericin B and flucytosine required.[59] Currently, treatment duration and total dose of intravenous amphotericin B are determined by the clinical response and the degree of systemic or nonocular involvement.

In an autopsy series reported by Edwards and associates,[60] a subgroup of 7 patients who received 200 mg or more of amphotericin B showed the best rate of healing, whereas 5 of 6 patients in another subgroup who received less than 200 mg still had active candidal lesions in the eye at autopsy. In the same study,[60] only 1 of 7 patients receiving greater than 1000 mg of amphotericin B were found to have active lesions at autopsy.

Early clinical experience with candidal chorioretinitis without vitreous invasion suggested that a total dose of amphotericin B of 1000 mg would provide adequate therapy.[83] With more extensive disease, total dosages averaging 1500 mg up to 3000 mg have been recommended.[76,165] Even with longer treatment and higher levels of total drug delivered, treatment failures occur. Despite its significant systemic toxicity and poor penetration into the eye, intravenous amphotericin B definitely facilitates clearing of ECE and remains the primary antifungal agent in the treatment of ECE.

Prior to commencing treatment with amphotericin B, patients receive a test dose, usually 1 mg of drug in 20 ml of 5% dextrose in water given intravenously over 30 minutes. In the absence of severe side effects, such as hypotension or cardiac arrhythmias, treatment is initiated 1 hour later using 0.7 mg/kg of amphotericin B in 500 ml of 5% dextrose in water by slow intravenous infusion over 2 to 6 hours. The patient is observed carefully for side effects. Usually the patient will tolerate a full 0.7 mg/kg given on the first day. If severe side effects occur, the infusion can be given more slowly or may need to be discontinued prior to the administration of the full dose. Efforts should be made to reach a 0.7 to 1.0 mg/kg/day dosage as quickly as possible, rather than using a previously popular approach of incrementally advancing the dosage by 5 to 10 mg each day. The drug is infused slowly over 4 to 6 hours in 500 ml of 5% dextrose in water.[31,96] Although controversial, rapid rates of infusion over 1 to 2 hours have been advocated. The total cumulative dose of amphotericin B and the length of treatment vary from case to case depending on the therapeutic response and extent of disease. Early signs of a therapeutic response may be recognized after only 7 days; there will be a gradual clearing of vitreous inflammation and a beginning to the resolution of the chorioretinal lesions. Antifungal therapy is continued until the chorioretinal lesions clear or become discrete scars.

Lesions confined to the choroid or with minimal retinal involvement may clear and leave well-demarcated, hypopigmented or lightly pigmented scars without demonstrable functional deficit (Fig. 91-2). Lesions extending through the retina and into the vitreous stimulate glial and fibrovascular proliferation with formation of full-thickness retinal scars, epiretinal membranes, macular pucker, vitreous bands, retinal traction, and retinal detachments (Figs. 91-3A, B). It may be extremely difficult to determine when the infectious element has been cleared. Close observation is required, even after antifungal treatment has been completed.

Eyes successfully cleared of infection may show additional late changes, with gradual development of epiretinal membranes, macular pucker, vitreous traction bands, and retinal detachments. These eyes may benefit from vitrectomy with membrane peeling, sectioning, and removal.[134]

Side Effects. The therapeutic usefulness of amphotericin B is limited by its toxic side effects, which include anaphylaxis (rare), thrombocytopenia, anemia, generalized pain, convulsions, phlebitis, chills, fever, flushing, headache, hypotension, cardiac arrhythmias, and anorexia. Renal toxicity with renal dysfunction and azotemia, which occurs in 80% of patients, is the most significant side effect. Although the renal side effects are usually reversible with cessation of therapy, some reduction in glomerular filtration may persist.

Ophthalmologists should not try to manage antifungal therapy in patients with ECE without enlisting the aid of an internist skilled in infectious diseases. Active monitoring of renal function, the ocular lesions, and the patient's underlying systemic disease is required on an ongoing basis.

Neonates on amphotericin B are particularly susceptible to nephrotoxicity leading to anuria. Thus special caution is advised in neonates, and daily dosages of amphotericin B exceeding 0.5 mg/kg/day are not recommended in the low birth weight infant.[15] Combined use of amphotericin B and flucytosine entails additional risks of renal and hepatic toxicity. Renal and hepatic function should be evaluated at the onset of treatment and monitored in all infants receiving these drugs. When ECE is identified early in infants, medical treatment alone can be successful, and retained vision can be "good" in eyes where the macular area has been spared.[6]

Intravitreous Injections. The systemic toxicity and the limited penetration of intravenously administered amphotericin B into vitreous humor led to the investigation of intravitreous injection of amphotericin B as an adjunct to intravenous therapy for the treatment of ECE.[17,57,186] Despite some controversy concerning the toxicity of intravitreously administered drugs, 5 and 10 ug doses of intravitreous amphotericin B have been used in patients.[17,32,112,115,186] A rabbit model of candidal endophthalmitis using similar doses failed to demonstrate toxicity.[97] Stern and associates[186] used intravitreous injections of 5 ug of amphotericin B without apparent toxicity in the successful treatment of intraocular candidal infection. Because of its retinal toxicity, amphotericin B must be delivered slowly into the central vitreous

body—as far from the retina as possible, for even small amounts close to the retina can produce retinal injury. Animal studies of intravitreous injections of amphotericin B in eyes that have undergone vitrectomy have demonstrated more rapid clearance of amphotericin B and the potential for enhanced retinal toxicity in these eyes.[57] How often and how many times intravitreous injections of amphotericin B may be repeated has not been established.

Because of the frequent association of disseminated candidiasis with ECE, intravitreous amphotericin B is best viewed as an adjunct to intravenous therapy rather than a substitute for it.[96,147] Treatment of intraocular candidal infections with vitrectomy and intravitreous amphotericin B alone (without systemic antifungal agents) has been suggested by some authors, but it is not favored by internists because it fails to address the need for treatment of the frequently associated systemic candidiasis.

Flucytosine. Edwards and associates[59,147] have recommended the use of oral flucytosine in combination with intravenous amphotericin B for treatment of ECE in special circumstances. The use of flucytosine alone is not recommended because of the frequent occurrence of primary and secondary drug resistance.[59,76] Up to 50% of *Candida* species isolates taken from patients prior to treatment are resistant to flucytosine, and the development of resistance during treatment is not uncommon.[61] Combination therapy is indicated in cases in which the macula is threatened or the inflammatory response is extensive and/or rapidly progressive.[147] Flucytosine is administered orally, 50 to 100 mg/kg/day, in divided doses at 6-hour intervals.

A combination of amphotericin B and flucytosine is currently the recommended treatment for candidal meningitis.[147] In a study of 17 patients with candidal meningitis who were placed on this combined therapy, the median time to sterilization of cerebral spinal fluid cultures was 7 days.[147] Fifteen of the seventeen patients in this series were improved or cured.

The antifungal selectivity of flucytosine relates to its unique property of conversion to fluorouracil in fungal cells, but not in the host's cells. Combined therapy seems to be synergistic against *Candida* species. It has been suggested that amphotericin B damages the fungal cell wall, permitting enhanced penetration of flucytosine. This synergism may exist even in cases in which the fungi are resistant to flucytosine alone.[61] Combination therapy has been used successfully in the treatment of intraocular candidal infections in neonates[13,100] and adults. Patients receiving flucytosine require close monitoring of their renal, hematologic, and hepatic status. Flucytosine is absorbed readily by mouth and is excreted by glomerular filtration. Ninety percent of the drug can be recovered unchanged from the urine. In patients with impaired renal function, flucytosine is not excreted at the normal rate and may rise to toxic levels in the blood. Daily monitoring of flucytosine levels is necessary in these cases.

Other Antifungal Drugs. A combination of intravenous amphotericin B and rifampin has been used successfully in the treatment of one patient with ECE, and in vitro synergism using this combination has been documented.[122] Other clinical reports using this combination have not been forthcoming.

The introduction of the azole derivatives miconazole, ketoconazole, itraconazole, and fluconazole stimulated considerable interest in their potential use in the treatment of ECE. The azoles have shown good antifungal activity in vitro. Intraocular penetration studies in the rabbit both with and without inflammation have demonstrated penetration in the following rank order: fluconazole > ketoconazole > itraconazole.[164] In the inflamed rabbit eye, fluconazole levels in the aqueous humor approach 65% of serum levels.[164] The azoles can reduce the number of fungi found in the eye in experimental ECE in rabbits when treatment is initiated within 24 hours of innoculation.[164] If treatment is delayed for 7 days after innoculation, ketoconazole is the only one of these azole derivatives that significantly reduced the fungal counts in the eye.[164]

A study of the long-term treatment of rabbits with experimental disseminated candidiasis and ECE compared fluconazole and amphotericin B.[67] For the first 17 days of treatment, the two groups demonstrated a similar clinical course and initial decline in the intraocular fungal counts. After 24 days of treatment, however, the endophthalmitis had worsened and the fungal colony counts had risen in the fluconazole-treated rabbits, whereas in the amphotericin B group, the fungal colony counts from all organs sampled were below detectable levels. Only in the amphotericin B group was the severity of the eye involvement statistically better than in the saline-treated controls.[67]

Direct comparison of ketoconazole and amphotericin B in an animal model has not been reported.[147] Ketoconazole used as a single agent in the treatment of ECE has been unsuccessful.[165] Others have advised against its use in systemic candidiasis.[76]

Available data suggest that none of the azole derivatives are as effective as amphotericin B. A limited number of cases of ECE treated with fluconazole or ketoconazole combined with intravitreal amphotericin B, some with and some without vitrectomy, have been reported.[17,112,115,194,198] Significant antagonism in the anticandidal effect of amphotericin B and ketoconazole has been reported when these drugs are used in combination both in vitro and in experimental animals.[157a,190] The use of ketoconazole in combination with amphotericin B is not recommended; exposure of *C. albicans* to ketoconazole may result in resistance of the organisms to amphotericin B.[96,157a,163a,190]

The clinical cases reported to date and the available laboratory data have not established the place for the azoles in the treatment of ECE, but more extensive clinical studies are in progress.

Surgical Treatment. Vitrectomy combined with intravitreous amphotericin B has been beneficial in the treatment of selected cases of ECE.* Indications for vitrectomy in ECE include eyes with prominent vitreous involvement and eyes showing progressive disease despite intensive medical therapy. In these cases vitrectomy was useful as a means of debulking the vitreous of inflammatory debris and fungal elements and confirming the presumptive diagnosis of ECE. An added benefit has been the ability to deliver a therapeutic level of amphotericin B intraocularly without systemic toxicity and with limited local toxicity. Vitrectomy also can remove the scaffolding for vitreoretinal traction bands and epiretinal membranes that can contribute to late-developing macular pucker and retinal detachments. In eyes successfully treated for ECE, but with residual vision loss due to late-developing epiretinal membranes and traction bands, pars plana vitrectomy and membranectomy have been successful in improving vision from 20/400 to 20/25 in one eye and to a lesser degree in three others.[134]

A 1990 report with long-term follow-up of infants with ECE and systemic candidiasis advised against the use of vitrectomy and intravitreal injections in infants. Anatomic and visual results were better in those infants treated with systemic antifungals alone.[6]

Prevention

Awareness of the clinical setting and the risk factors associated with ECE has led to preventive management of patients at-risk. Selection of materials for indwelling catheters and other intravascular devices along with standardization of care procedures helps decrease the occurrence of candidemia. The earlier candidemia is detected, the better the chance for elimination of vascular seeding of fungi and prevention of candidal chorioretinitis, ECE, and disseminated candidiasis. The earlier focal candidal chorioretinitis is recognized, the better the prognosis for successful treatment. Early detection could possibly mean the prevention of both candidal endophthalmitis and severe vision loss. Patients at risk for candidemia should be monitored regularly with blood and urine cultures. In the presence of bacteremia, concomitant fungi may not grow in culture.[59] In 45% of patients with candidemia, blood and urine cultures drawn at the same time will grow the same yeast.[64] When blood cultures are positive for *Candida* species, the following procedures should be considered to reduce factors contributing to overgrowth and systemic spread of *Candida* species:

1. Central venous catheters should be removed (or at least changed), as thrombotic material on the tip of the catheter provides a nidus for colonization by yeast; these catheters also should not be placed over a preexisting wire.

---

*References 17, 32, 112, 115, 134, 182, 186.

2. Broad-spectrum or combined antibiotics should be discontinued, and other antibiotics should be targeted and used only as needed.
3. Hyperglycemia should be corrected.
4. Corticosteroids should be reduced or withdrawn if possible.
5. Patients should be reevaluated regularly for evidence of disseminated candidiasis or a change in their general condition and monitored for resolution or persistence of candidemia.
6. The need for antifungal therapy should be evaluated on an ongoing basis. In the past when the preceding steps were taken, the patient was frequently observed without the institution of antifungal therapy. Recently there has been an inclination to treat even transient candidemia in an effort to avoid the potential late complications of candidemia, especially ECE and osteomyelitis, and to avoid underdiagnosis of the widespread dissemination that a single positive blood culture may signify.[76] In the immunosuppressed patient, treatment with amphotericin B in the range of 500 to 1000 mg has been recommended empirically.[76]

The most critical initial step in the prevention and management of ECE and systemic candidiasis is recognition of this important infectious fungal disease complex and the risk factors that will alert the physician to the threat it poses to patients under his care. Colleagues outside of ophthalmology should also be instructed about the usefulness of the ocular fundus examination in recognizing this life-threatening disseminated fungal infection. Because early lesions can be asymptomatic, all patients with candidemia or who are at high risk for candidemia should be warned to report any eye symptoms and should have at least two dilated funduscopic examinations a week apart. The frequency of subsequent examinations depends on a patient's ocular symptoms and general medical condition.

ASPERGILLOSIS

Aspergillus species cause a variety of disease processes, from simple hypersensitivity allergic reactions against airborne or foodborne spores or mycelial fragments to fatal invasive systemic aspergillosis.

Mycology

About 21 of the 900 species and subspecies of *Aspergillus* species cause invasive human disease; of these, only 5 cause endogenous endophthalmitis (*A. flavus, A. fumigatus, A. candidus, A. niger,* and *A. terreus*). *Aspergillus* species is the second most frequent cause of endogenous fungal endophthalmitis, following *Candida* species.[103,145,160]

The genus name *Aspergillus* was first conceived by the Florentine botanist Micheli in 1729, because the conidiophore and conidia of *Aspergillus* species closely resembled the aspergillum, a perforated globe used to sprinkle holy water during religious ceremonies.[140] *Aspergillus* species are ubiquitous fungi, commonly isolated from soil, vegetation, grains, decaying organic matter, air, and human skin and nasopharyngeal mucosa. *A. fumigatus,* the most frequently encountered pathogenic species in humans, is the species most often associated with invasive systemic disease.[145,160]

The microscopic morphology of *Aspergillus* species is variable, depending on the particular species and the medium conditions. In culture, all *Aspergillus* species have characteristic branching septate hyphae with long stalks (conidiophores). *Aspergillus* species grow quickly on Sabouraud agar as flat, white, velvety filamentous colonies, which usually become pigmented within 48 hours because of conidiophore formation. *A. fumigatus* colonies are typically greenish-gray or blue-green.[136,145,160]

Epidemiology

In a recent review of 30 culture-proven cases of endogenous aspergillic endophthalmitis (EAE), patient ages ranged from infancy to 83 years, with a mean age of 39 years. A 2 : 1 male-to-female ratio was noted, and 7 of the 30 cases had bilateral eye involvement. Most of the patients were immunosuppressed or were intravenous drug abusers. Although *A. fumigatus* was the predominant species isolated, 10 patients were infected with *A. flavus,* and 9 of these 10 were intravenous drug abusers.[11] It has been suggested that intravenous drug users are more likely to become infected with *A. flavus.*[56]

Risk Factors

Intravenous drug abuse has been the most frequent predisposing factor among the cases of EAE reported since 1975.[56,117,142,162,207] This patient population is at particular risk for EAE because the ubiquitous organisms are injected directly into the bloodstream from contaminated drugs, needles, or syringes.[56,141,207] Frequent intravenous illicit drug injection also causes suppression of lymphocyte reactivity.[144]

Other predisposing diagnoses resulting in an immunocompromised or debilitated state in reported cases of EAE include the following:

- Organ transplantation with use of corticosteroids and immunosuppressive drugs,[25,148,206]
- Acute myelogenous leukemia under treatment with chemotherapy,[99]
- Chronic lymphocytic leukemia,[103]
- Primary thrombocytosis treated with immunosuppressive agents,[50]
- Polyclonal gammopathy,[133]
- Bronchial carcinoid and iatrogenic Cushing syndrome,[149]

- Intraocular large cell sarcoma,[28]
- Miliary tuberculosis,[72]
- Chronic bronchitis and pneumonia in a child,[118]
- Allergic bronchopulmonary aspergillosis and use of corticosteroids,[26]
- Prematurity in an infant,[152]
- Alcoholism, and
- Goodpasture syndrome.[31]

Endogenous aspergillic endophthalmitis has also been reported in patients with aspergillic endocarditis involving both natural and prosthetic valves.[26,113,199] In a review of aspergillic endocarditis, 3 of 29 patients also had endophthalmitis.[104]

Clinical Features

The broad range of manifestations of noninvasive disease caused by *Aspergillus* species encompasses all types of hypersensitivity reactions. Atopic patients may develop IgE-mediated type I reactions to inhaled *Aspergillus* species allergens, resulting in asthma. Allergic bronchopulmonary aspergillosis (ABPA) is mediated by type I and type III reactions, and is characterized by asthma, eosinophilia, pulmonary infiltrates, mucus plugs, and positive serology. Also, 46% to 83% of patients with ABPA have positive sputum cultures for *Aspergillus* species. Extrinsic allergic alveolitis occurs in nonatopic hosts. It is manifested by fever, dyspnea, cough, myalgias, and leukocytosis several hours after inhalation of *Aspergillus* species antigen.[18,127,128,145]

Various forms of noninvasive aspergillosis are characterized by colonization of open pulmonary cavities, paranasal sinuses, the nasal cavity, ear canals, skin, nails, conjunctiva, or eyelids by *Aspergillus* species. Aspergilloma is a pulmonary fungal mass that arises within a lung cavity; the condition is associated with preexisting pulmonary disease.[18,145]

Invasive Aspergillosis. Invasive aspergillosis may be localized, as in invasive pulmonary aspergillosis, or disseminated, with involvement of multiple sites including the GI tract, liver, kidney, brain, heart, skin, eye, and orbit. Invasive aspergillosis has increased in frequency, primarily in immunocompromised hosts. Patients with leukemia, lymphoma, and other malignancies, those on immunosuppressive medications for organ transplantation, and patients with AIDS now represent the majority of cases with invasive aspergillosis. The hyphae invade blood vessel walls, resulting in thrombosis and infarction. Without prompt treatment, disseminated aspergillosis is nearly always fatal in immunocompromised hosts.[18,113,133,145,210]

Ocular Disease. The first case of EAE was reported by Dimmer[54] in 1913. To date there have been over 40 cases of EAE reported in the literature.* Initial symptoms include blurred vision, eye pain, photophobia, redness, conjunctival chemosis, and periocular swelling.* Typical clinical findings are cells in the anterior chamber and vitreous, keratic precipitates, hypopyon, chorioretinitis, perivasculitis, or retinal hemorrhages.[26,28,56,141,178] EAE may be the presenting feature of disseminated aspergillosis.[50] The chorioretinitis may be characterized by depigmented discrete lesions, Roth spots, or elevated pale yellow, fluffy chorioretinal lesions.[25,85,117] Choroidal and retinal vascular occlusion by fungal hyphae also have been reported.[25,103,133,206,210] In one case reported by Khurana and associates[105] the lens was directly invaded by *Aspergillus* species organisms. The disease may progress, resulting in an anterior chamber inflammatory mass, vitreous opacities, serous or exudative retinal detachment, choroidal or vitreous abscess formation, and intravitreous granulomata.†

Bilateral acute necrotizing aspergillic retinitis, with chorioretinal vascular invasion and positive postmortem vitreous cultures, was reported in a 52-year-old immunocompromised heart transplant recipient. This patient also had disseminated CMV infection; thus, some of the retinal findings may have resulted from CMV retinitis.[25] Weiss and associates[206] also described a case of disseminated and intraocular concomitant infection with *Aspergillus* sp. (endophthalmitis) and CMV (retinitis) in a renal transplant patient.

The case reported by Sihota and associates[178] involved a 15-day-old infant with bilateral EAE who was apparently otherwise healthy. The patient required enucleation of one phthisical eye, but the other eye was successfully treated with amphotericin B alone. This case represents the youngest reported patient with EAE to date.

Aside from endogenous endophthalmitis, other reported cases of ophthalmic involvement by *Aspergillus* species include exogenous endophthalmitis,[35,86,123,126,131] fungal keratitis,[192] orbital abscess,[87] orbital apex syndrome,[180] ischemic posterior optic neuropathy,[203] and optic neuropathy associated with aspergillic ethmoid sinusitis.[46]

Pathogenesis

In an animal model of endogenous fungal endophthalmitis, Aziz and associates[11] inoculated control and immunosuppressed rabbits with a virulent strain of *A. fumigatus*. This organism had been isolated from the postmortem heart and lungs of an immunosuppressed renal transplant recipient who died with respiratory failure and disseminated aspergillosis. All seven of the immunosuppressed rabbits and seven of the eight immunocompetent rabbits developed intraocular infection with *Aspergillus* species (Figs. 91-7 and 91-8). A separate stock laboratory isolate of *A. fumigatus* failed to cause intraocular infection in any rabbits. This failure sug-

---

*References 10, 25, 30, 31, 54, 56, 66, 85, 103, 113, 133, 202.

---

*References 26, 31, 56, 103, 118, 141, 148.
†References 30, 56, 118, 141, 148, 162, 178, 202.

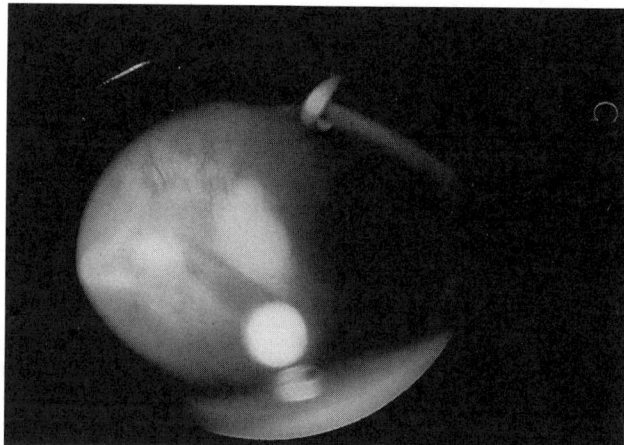

Fig. 91-7. Photograph demonstrating a large intravitreous granuloma appearing as a white "fluff ball" 24 days after injection of A. fumigatus organisms in an immunocompetent rabbit. An adjacent tractional retinal detachment is also present. (Reprinted with permission from Aziz AA, Bullock JD, McGuire TW et al.: *Aspergillus* endophthalmitis: a clinical and experimental study, *Trans Am Ophthalmol Soc* 90:317-346, 1992.)

gests that either the stock culture isolate had a very low virulence or the isolate from the postmortem renal transplant recipient had an unusually high virulence. This variability in virulence may partially explain the wide disparity in disease severity observed with aspergillosis.[11]

The authors noted a lack of vascular occlusion and thrombosis in the histologic analysis of the choroid and retina in the infected animals. They suggested that most of the intraocular injury in EAE may result from the intense inflammation,[11] rather than from vascular occlusion and infarction, as suggested by other investigators.[25,99,133,206]

Differential Diagnosis

The differential diagnosis of EAE includes exogenous aspergillic endophthalmitis, which is usually caused by penetrating injuries involving organic or vegetative material, fungal keratitis with subsequent perforation, or postoperative infection after previous ocular surgery.[35,86,123,126,131] A thorough history should reveal an exogenous source. Fungal endophthalmitis caused by other fungi, particularly *Candida* species, *Cryptococcus* species, and *Pseudallescheria* species, may produce symptoms and clinical findings similar to those of EAE. Fungal cultures or systemic signs of a specific fungal infection may be helpful in differentiating these organisms. Endogenous endophthalmitis secondary to the bacteria *Nocardia asteroides* or *Actinomyces israelii*, may resemble endogenous fungal endophthalmitis as well.[31]

Depending on the degree of severity of the endophthalmitis, the symptoms and findings may be confused with anterior uveitis, pars planitis syndrome, ocular sarcoidosis or tuberculosis, large cell lymphoma, the white-dot syndromes, retinal vasculitis, or acute retinal necrosis syndrome.

Laboratory Investigations

The diagnosis of EAE depends on a high index of suspicion in patients with predisposing factors such as documented systemic infection caused by *Aspergillus* species, immunosuppression, or intravenous drug abuse. If the clinical findings are compatible with EAE, confirmation of the disease often depends on indirect evidence such as the presence of hyphae on biopsies or smears, or positive cultures from nonocular sites including blood, sputum, indwelling catheter tips, bronchoalveolar lavage, or open lung biopsy. Blood cultures are only rarely positive.

Fungal serology (immunodiffusion) has a sensitivity of 80% to 100% for cases of ABPA or aspergilloma, but is not helpful in invasive aspergillosis. Serology, therefore, may be of limited value in the diagnosis of EAE.[18,113,145,210]

Robin and associates[161] have described the use of fluorescein-conjugated lectins to detect and differentiate *Aspergillus* species, *Candida* species, and *Fusarium* species in culture isolates, tissue samples, and fixed histologic specimens.

Although vitreous aspirates may yield positive fungal cultures for *Aspergillus* species, anterior chamber aspirates are of no value. If a vitrectomy is performed, the aspirate should be cultured and examined for hyphae. Histologic examination of tissue specimens reveals septate hyphae with dichotomous branching using Gomori methenamine silver or periodic acid-Schiff stains. Conidiophores are often absent in tissue. *Candida* species have a different histologic appearance, with presence of yeast forms, hyphae with a smaller diameter, and lack of true hyphal branching.[11,31,210]

Two additional tissue stains, calcofluor and ink-potassium hydroxide, have been valuable in identifying *Aspergillus* species, *Candida* species, and *Fusarium* species in ocular

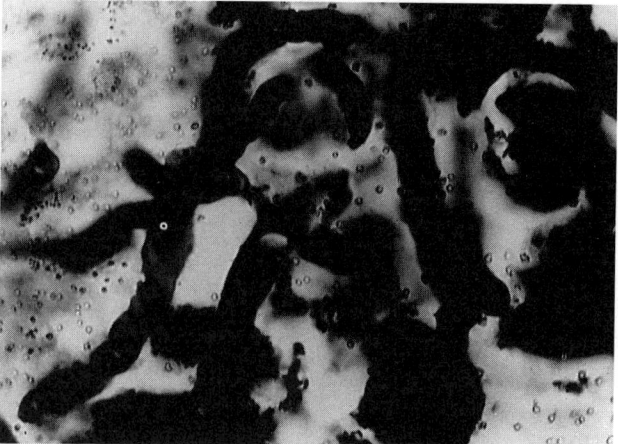

Fig. 91-8. Photomicrograph of the choroid of an immunosuppressed rabbit 4 days after injection of *Aspergillus fumigatus*, demonstrating many septate hyphae that stain with Gomori methenamine silver stain. (×1000.) (Reprinted with permission from Aziz AA, Bullock JD, McGuire TW et al.: *Aspergillus* endophthalmitis: a clinical and experimental study, *Trans Am Ophthalmol Soc* 90:317-346, 1992.)

tissue samples, biopsy specimens, and corneal scrapings. Although the calcofluor method provides more rapid results, the ink-potassium hydroxide method is more sensitive and specific.[8]

Jain and associates[98] investigated the use of electroretinography (ERG) in the early diagnosis of aspergillic endophthalmitis in an animal model. They observed statistically significant increases in b-wave amplitudes 2 to 5 days after injection, before ophthalmoscopic signs of infection were noted. With the onset of clinically apparent infection, b-wave amplitudes fell below baseline preinjection levels, and eventually became unrecordable.

Therapy

Successful management and therapy of EAE depends on early diagnosis, before irreversible intraocular injury has occurred. Treatment includes administration of systemic antifungal agents, and in most cases, surgical intervention, including vitrectomy and instillation of intravitreous amphotericin B.[4,18,85,117,178] Intravenous amphotericin B has been a major component in the treatment of EAE.[18]

Animal studies have suggested there may be some additive therapeutic effect with the concomitant use of amphotericin B and either 5-flucytosine or rifampin, but clinical data have been inadequate to determine the efficacy of these agents in aspergillosis.[18,107]

Ketoconazole, an oral imidazole antifungal agent, is effective against *Aspergillus* species isolates in vitro,[195] but has had limited clinical efficacy in the treatment of invasive aspergillosis or aspergillic keratitis.[111,188] Of the newer, less toxic imidazoles, itraconazole is more effective than fluconazole in the treatment of invasive aspergillosis, but its penetration into the eye is less than that of fluconazole or ketoconazole.[164] Itraconazole may be useful for prophylaxis against aspergillosis in granulocytopenic patients.[188,196] There are no data on the efficacy of these agents in EAE.

Only one case of successful EAE treatment with intravenous amphotericin B alone has been described.[178] Other reported cases of EAE survival with salvage of vision have involved the use of pars plana vitrectomy, with or without intravitreous amphotericin B, along with intravenous amphotericin B.[56,117,141,162,206] Most of these patients also received oral flucytosine.[56,117,141,162] Enucleation may be indicated in cases of overwhelming infection with irreversible loss of vision.[11,50,178]

Prognosis

The prognosis for salvage of useful vision in EAE is poor unless early diagnosis and aggressive treatment with intravenous amphotericin B and possibly vitrectomy with intravitreous amphotericin B are provided. The mortality rate is high for immunocompromised patients with invasive aspergillosis and EAE.[11,25,50,103,202] Survival is much better for intravenous drug users with EAE.[11,117,141]

PSEUDALLESCHERIOSIS

Pseudallescheria boydii is an opportunistic fungus with a low inherent virulence that can produce many of the same disease processes typically associated with *Aspergillus* species.[65,136] Because of this similarity in clinical spectrum and the identical histologic morphology, *Pseudallescheria* species has been referred to as a "great imitator."[159]

Mycology

The mycologic terminology representing this organism has been somewhat confusing. *Pseudallescheria boydii* is the current name for the sexual (perfect) state, and *Scedosporium apiospermum* is the preferred name for the asexual (imperfect) state. Older terms for the sexual state (*Allescheria boydii* and *Petriellidium boydii*) and for the asexual state (*Monosporium apiospermum*) are encountered in the literature as well.[19,65,136]

P. boydii is present worldwide in soil, stagnant and flowing water sources, coastal areas, sewage, manure, and vegetation.[19,136] Potted plants have been identified as a potential source of *P. boydii* and other opportunistic fungi in immunocompromised, hospitalized patients.[191] The thin, septate, branching hyphae of *P. boydii* and *Aspergillus* species in tissue sections are identical. Also, both organisms cause similar pathologic reactions, with vascular invasion, hemorrhage, infarction, and necrosis. Although both fungi grow well on Sabouraud agar, the colony appearance is helpful in distinguishing them. *A. fumigatus* usually produces greenish colonies in culture, whereas *P. boydii* is velvety white and becomes dark gray in appearance. Indeed, definitive fungal cultures are the most reliable method of differentiating *P. boydii* from *Aspergillus* species.[19,136,159]

Clinical Features

P. boydii is the organism responsible for Madura foot (maduromycosis), a localized form of mycetoma. This destructive subcutaneous chronic infection is secondary to traumatic implantation of organisms and can involve bone as well as soft tissue.[19,159] Mycetomata are most often encountered in tropical areas, but have been reported sporadically in the United States and Europe.[189]

Many of the disease manifestations of *P. boydii* are very similar to those caused by *Aspergillus* species. Fungal masses caused by *P. boydii* (pseudallescheromas) in lung cavities, kidney, and brain are analogous to aspergillomas.[167,168] One reported case of mixed allergic bronchopulmonary fungal disease caused by *Aspergillus* species and *P. boydii* underscores the clinical similarity of these two organisms.[116]

P. boydii causes invasive infections including sinusitis, otitis, pulmonary infection, prosthetic and native valve endocarditis, prostatitis, meningitis, brain abscess, arthritis, osteomyelitis, and disseminated disease.* As with aspergillosis, dissemination is more likely in immunocompromised hosts.[193] Disseminated pseudallescheriasis has been reported in patients on immunosuppressive therapy,[193] as well as those with leukemia,[168,177] AIDS,[158] chronic granulomatous disease,[156] Cushing syndrome,[7] and diabetes mellitus.[21,136] Other reported causes of invasive or disseminated pseudallescheriasis include near drowning, penetrating trauma, and intravenous drug abuse.[9,21,136] Iatrogenic cases have also occurred.

McGuire and associates[136] reviewed 17 cases of human ocular infections caused by *P. boydii*. Five of these cases can be considered truly endogenous endophthalmitis caused by *Pseudallescheria* species.[40,124,138,181,187] The other cases included exogenous endophthalmitis following cataract surgery (1 patient), invasive keratitis (7 patients), orbital infection caused by penetrating trauma (2 patients), conjunctival and eyelid mycetoma (1 patient), and maxillary sinusitis with loss of vision (1 patient).[136] One of two cases of endogenous endophthalmitis caused by *Pseudallescheria* species later reported by Pfeifer and associates[155] was not listed in the review by McGuire and Bullock, and represents the sixth documented case.

Eye pain was the most common symptom in five of the six cases, followed by decreased or blurred vision, photophobia, and tearing. Examination findings included visual acuity ranging from 20/200 to no light perception, conjunctival chemosis and injection, anterior chamber cells and flare, hypopyon, retinal depigmentation, chorioretinal abscesses, vitritis, vitreous abscesses, and proptosis.† In one case the fundus lesions were described as intraretinal, fluffy white exudative lesions.[187] All six reported cases had positive vitreous cultures for *P. boydii*.[136,155]

Predisposing factors in the six cases included systemic lupus erythematosis with immunosuppressive therapy,[124] immunosuppression following renal transplantation[40] and cardiac transplantation,[155] progressive pulmonary fibrosis,[155] fungal endocarditis and aortic graft infection,[187] and near drowning caused by aspiration of muddy water during a seizure.[138] The patients' ages ranged from 15 to 52 years, with 4 males and 2 females.[136,155]

Five of the six reported patients with endogenous endophthalmitis caused by *Pseudallescheria* species died of disseminated pseudallescheriasis, their underlying disease, and/or multisystem diseases.[136,155] The single surviving patient recovered after enucleation of the involved eye, but this patient did not have disseminated disease.[124] Three of the five patients who died had also undergone enucleation or evisceration following aggressive treatment with antifungal agents and/or vitrectomy.‡

---

*References 19, 21, 158, 168, 177, 184, 193.
†References 9, 40, 124, 136, 138, 155, 181, 187.
‡References 9, 40, 136, 138, 155, 181, 187.

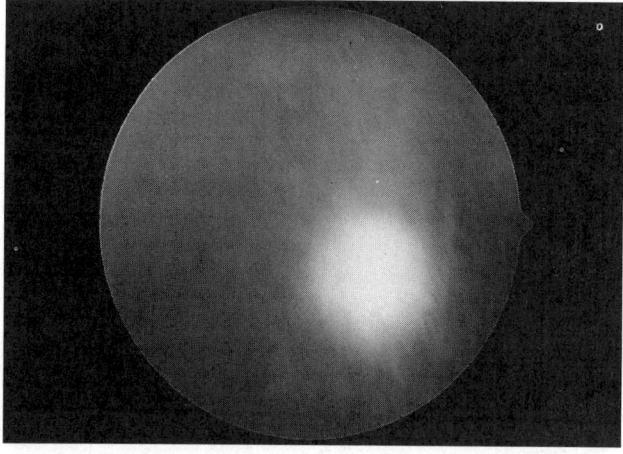

Fig. 91-9. Fundus photograph of an immunosuppressed rabbit, demonstrating white choroidal lesion 6 days after challenge with *Pseudallescheri boydii*. (Reprinted with permission from McGuire TW, Bullock JD, Bullock JD Jr et al.: Fungal endophthalmitis: an experimental study with a review of 17 human ocular cases, *Arch Ophthalmol* 109:1289-1296, 1991. Copyright 1991, The American Medical Association.)

Pathogenesis

In an animal model of endogenous endophthalmitis caused by *Pseudallescheria* species, McGuire and associates[136] produced exogenous and endogenous endophthalmitis caused by *Pseudallescheria* species in immunocompromised and control animals. The animals with endogenous endophthalmitis developed a spectrum of findings including chorioretinal abscesses, hypopyon, lens destruction, and fulminant endophthalmitis with vitreous abscess formation (Figs. 91-9 and 91-10). *P. boydii* was histologically indistinguishable from *Aspergillus fumigatus* in tissue specimens.

Differential Diagnosis

The differential diagnosis for endogenous endophthalmitis caused by *Pseudallescheria* species is similar to that previously discussed for EAE. Although intravenous drug abuse is a significant predisposing factor in EAE, near drowning is a known risk factor for invasive pseudallescheriasis. Immunosuppression is a predisposing factor for both infections. A history of the inciting factors may be helpful in differentiating EAE and endogenous endophthalmitis caused by *Pseudallescheria* species in some cases.

Laboratory Investigations

Definitive diagnosis of endogenous endophthalmitis caused by *Pseudallescheria* species depends on the identification of *P. boydii* in fungal cultures of vitreous obtained either during a diagnostic vitreous biopsy or at the time of pars plana vitrectomy. The presence of septate hyphae, vascular invasion, and abscess formation on histopathology is not diagnostic for endogenous endophthalmitis caused by

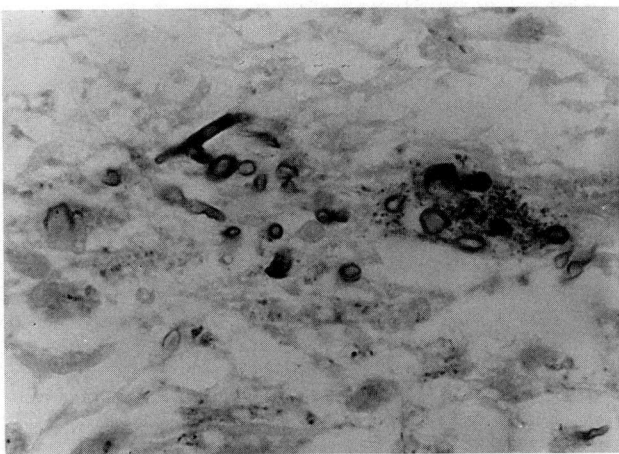

Fig. 91-10. Photomicrograph of choroidal abscess shown in Fig. 91-9, revealing hyphal fragments of *Pseudallescheri boydii.* (Gomori methenamine silver stain ×1000.) (Reprinted with permission from McGuire TW, Bullock JD, Bullock JD Jr et al.: Fungal endophthalmitis: an experimental study with a review of 17 human ocular cases, *Arch Ophthalmol* 109:1289-1296, 1991. Copyright 1991, The American Medical Association.)

Pseudallescheria species, but gives sufficient information to begin antifungal therapy, while awaiting culture results.[19]

Phillips and Weiner[157] successfully utilized monoclonal antibodies with peroxidase immunohistochemical methods on tissue samples from infected patients to differentiate *Aspergillus* species from *P. boydii* and other filamentous fungi.

Therapy

In view of the dismal outcome in reported patients with endogenous endophthalmitis caused by *Pseudallescheria* species, early aggressive treatment with systemic antifungal agents and surgical intervention is warranted. Several treatment failures with intravenous amphotericin B and oral flucytosine for disseminated pseudallescheriasis have been reported.[19,124,155] Likewise, four of the six cases of endogenous endophthalmitis caused by *Pseudallescheria* species initially received intravitreous amphotericin B; one required enucleation, and the other three died.[40,124,155] One patient, who received intravenous amphotericin B followed by intravenous miconazole, subsequently died.[138] The sixth patient died following treatment with intravenous and intravitreous miconazole, which is reported to be the drug of choice for systemic pseudallescheriasis.[136,159,187]

Oral ketoconazole and fluconazole can achieve therapeutic blood levels above minimal inhibitory concentrations, but these antifungal agents have not been studied sufficiently in patients or animal models with endogenous endophthalmitis caused by *Pseudallescheria* species. The three patients with endogenous endophthalmitis caused by

Pseudallescheria species who had received fluconazole during treatment, all died.[136,155] Patients with localized nonocular pseudallescheriasis have been successfully treated with systemic miconazole or ketoconazole.[7,73,124,136]

Surgical treatment with pars plana vitrectomy was performed in three of the six cases with endogenous endophthalmitis caused by *Pseudallescheria* species. The other three patients had only partial or diagnostic vitrectomies. Despite this intervention, two of the three patients who had undergone pars plana vitrectomies required enucleation, and all three subsequently died.[136,155]

Current management recommendations include early treatment with intravenous and intravitreous miconazole, consideration of concomitant treatment with fluconazole, close monitoring of antifungal drug levels and minimal inhibitory concentrations, and prompt surgical intervention, including complete pars plana vitrectomy and timely enucleation, when indicated.[136,155]

CRYPTOCOCCOSIS

Cryptococcosis is a systemic disease caused by *Cryptococcus neoformans,* a round encapsulated fungus with worldwide distribution. The fungus is found in bird droppings, contaminated soil, and (occasionally) on fruits and other vegetation.

Mycology

C. neoformans is a budding, spore-forming yeast that produces smooth, yellow or tan colonies on culture media. Four serotypes (A, B, C, and D) can be identified using immunofluorescence or agglutination. Systemic disease is most often acquired through inhalation of aerosolized organisms.[53]

Risk Factors

Predisposing factors among patients with cryptococcal endophthalmitis included cryptococcal meningitis, AIDS, lymphoma, polyarteritis nodosa and diabetes with long-term use of corticosteroids, chronic active hepatitis with use of prednisone and azathioprine, alcoholism, and uremia. Patients with cryptococcal meningitis can be immunocompetent.[31,93,204] If patients with cryptococcal chorioretinitis are included, additional predisposing factors have been systemic lupus erythematosis, polycythemia rubra vera with use of immunosuppressive agents, renal transplantation and immunosuppression, and exposure to pigeons.[1,31,51] Organ transplant recipients have a 2% to 3% risk of developing cryptococcosis, and patients with AIDS have a 7% to 13% risk.[31,77]

Clinical Features

Systemic features of cryptococcosis vary widely and include meningitis, pneumonia, mucocutaneous lesions, multiple skin lesions, and ocular involvement. Less common manifestations are pyelonephritis, endocarditis, hepatitis, and prostatitis. The patterns of central nervous system (CNS) involvement are meningitis, meningoencephalitis, and cryptococcoma (toruloma).[31,53]

C. neoformans has become an important CNS pathogen in patients immunosuppressed by AIDS or other causes. In such patients it usually causes chronic meningitis, which frequently results in papilledema, optic neuropathy, and chiasmal involvement. Other neuro-ophthalmic manifestations include optic atrophy, cranial nerve palsies, nystagmus, and internuclear ophthalmoplegia. Cryptococcal meningitis is usually fatal without systemic antifungal therapy, and even with treatments the relapse rate is about 50% in patients with AIDS. Fluconazole has been used as a long-term oral maintenance therapy in an attempt to prevent such recurrences.[53,77]

Ocular Disease. Additional reported ophthalmic manifestations of *C. neoformans* infection are choroiditis,[31,37] retinitis,[1] uveitis,[45] inflammatory iris mass,[42] keratitis,[45] conjunctival granuloma,[16] phthisis bulbi,[200] periorbital necrotizing fasciitis,[58] orbital infection,[45,58] exogenous endophthalmitis following penetrating keratoplasty,[23] and endogenous endophthalmitis.* Most patients with intraocular involvement also have cryptococcal meningitis. Extension occurs via a hematogenous or leptomeningeal route.[31,37]

The most common intraocular manifestation is chorioretinitis. Typically, several yellow or white, subretinal, slightly elevated lesions one-fifth to one optic disc diameter in size are observed. Investigators have theorized that intraocular disease usually evolves from choroiditis to chorioretinitis, followed by extension into the vitreous and anterior segment, resulting in uveitis, vitritis, and endophthalmitis.[31,37,45]

Endogenous cryptococcal endophthalmitis was first reported in 1948.[205] Three of the twelve cases of intraocular cryptococcosis reported by Hiles and Font[93] in 1968 had endophthalmitis. The exact number of previously reported cases of true endogenous cryptococcal endophthalmitis is difficult to ascertain, because previous reviews have included cases of choroiditis or retinitis. Brod and associates[31] stated that 17 cases had been reported in an earlier 1975 review, and 15 more cases were presented in their 1990 review. On closer analysis, however, about half of the cited cases are found to be limited to choroiditis or chorioretinitis, without documented clinical findings to support a diagnosis of endophthalmitis. Similarly, in a recent review of 20 cases of "cryptococcal endophthalmitis" only 10 cases could be considered truly endogenous cryptococcal endophthalmitis. The others were limited to chorioiditis or retinitis (eight cases), or were cases of exogenous endophthalmitis (two cases).[51] Using strict criteria for true endogenous cryptococ-

cal endophthalmitis narrows the number of cases reported in the literature to approximately 15.*

Presenting symptoms in patients with endogenous cryptococcal endophthalmitis were blurred or decreased vision, eye pain, photophobia, floaters, and ocular injection. Patients with concomitant cryptococcal meningitis also suffered from headache and nausea. Bilateral eye involvement was present in 6 of the 15 endophthalmitis cases, but the second eye had only chorioretinitis in three of these cases. Ophthalmic findings were variable and included conjunctival injection, anterior chamber cell and flare, mutton fat keratic precipitates, posterior synechiae, yellow or white chorioretinal lesions, retinal perivascular sheathing, subretinal exudate or localized serous retinal detachment, vitreous cells, severe vitreous inflammation with fluffy exudates, preretinal or vitreous abscesses, retinal detachment, and phthisis bulbi.† With fluorescein angiography, the chorioretinal lesions are hypofluorescent early and exhibit diffuse staining late in the study.[95,176]

Four of the fifteen patients with endogenous cryptococcal endophthalmitis died. Of the 11 survivors, 10 patients either underwent enucleation or became blind in at least one involved eye.[31,51,200] One patient had resolution following treatment with flucytosine and intravenous and intravitreous amphotericin B.[150] Three of the six patients with bilateral involvement were reported to have resolution in the less involved eye, but these eyes had chorioretinitis rather than endophthalmitis.[93,95,176] Eight patients developed retinal detachments during their clinical course. Five of these patients underwent enucleation, and the other three had delayed-onset or chronic retinal detachment following an initial improvement on antifungal therapy. Among the cases with true endophthalmitis that had documented visual outcome, the acuity ranged from 5/200 to light perception. Persistent retinal detachment, optic atrophy, and dense cataract limited visual improvement in these patients.‡

Differential Diagnosis

Other diagnostic considerations for cases with clinical features similar to endogenous cryptococcal endophthalmitis are ocular tuberculosis, sarcoidosis, choroidal pneumocystosis, retinochoroiditis caused by *Toxoplasma gondii*, intraocular lymphoma, and endophthalmitis caused by other fungal organisms.[31,51,89] Inaccurate diagnosis has resulted in inappropriate initial therapy in several cases.[31,89,129,166,176]

Laboratory Investigations

The diagnosis of endogenous cryptococcal endophthalmitis is a presumptive one in a patient with the characteristic

---

*References 51, 63, 81, 89, 93, 95, 129, 150, 166, 176, 204, 205.

---

*References 31, 51, 63, 81, 89, 93, 95, 129, 150, 166, 176, 200, 204, 205.
†References 1, 31, 51, 89, 93, 95, 129, 150, 166, 176, 200, 204, 205.
‡References 31, 51, 63, 81, 89, 93, 95, 129, 150, 204.

fundus lesions, vitritis, and documented cryptococcal meningitis or disseminated cryptococcosis. If the causative organism is not known, early diagnostic vitreous humor tap or vitrectomy should be performed for fungal stains (including India ink) and cultures.[51,89,95,129,150] Also, the fluid should be tested for cryptococcal antigen.

Hiss and associates[95] performed fine-needle aspiration of a retinovitreous abscess through the pars plana, and obtained positive smears and cultures for *C. neoformans* from 0.1 ml of fluid.

In several of the reported cases of endogenous cryptococcal endophthalmitis, diagnosis was not made until enucleation or autopsy. Histopathologic examination may reveal *C. neoformans* organisms in the choroid, retina, and vitreous, and a granulomatous choroiditis with noncaseating areas of necrosis. Other findings may include optic nerve invasion, preretinal or vitreous abscess, vitreous inflammatory opacification, retinal detachment, or phthisis bulbi.* In immunocompromised patients, including those with AIDS, there may be little or no inflammatory reaction in tissues at the site of infection or in the ocular fluids.[10a,37,104a,149a,153a]

Cerebrospinal fluid analysis, including cryptococcal antigen testing and fungal culture, is important if signs of chronic meningitis are present.[53,77] Cryptococcal serology and fungal cultures of blood, sputum, or urine are often helpful in patients with disseminated disease.[53]

Therapy

Treatment of endogenous cryptococcal endophthalmitis depends on the disease severity and may require a combination of systemic antifungal agents, intravitreous amphotericin B, and pars plana vitrectomy.[31,204] Combined therapy with oral flucytosine and intravenous amphotericin B has been the recommended treatment of choice for patients with disseminated or meningeal cryptococcosis. Oral fluconazole has been successful in some AIDS patients and others who cannot tolerate the renal toxicity and bone marrow suppression of this combined therapy.[53,77] Intravenous miconazole also has been used for cryptococcal meningitis.[31] Cases of cryptococcal choroiditis or retinitis have been successfully treated with parenteral amphotericin B,[37] fluconazole,[1] or itraconazole.[51]

The early reported cases of endogenous cryptococcal endophthalmitis were treated with enucleation alone, before modern antifungal agents were available.[51,93] Most of the cases since the 1970s have been treated with amphotericin B, and six also received flucytosine. Four patients were given intravitreous amphotericin B (5 to 7 μg), and two of these patients underwent pars plana vitrectomy. Enucleation was not required in the cases treated with intravitreous amphotericin B, but visual outcome was still poor.†

---

*References 31, 37, 51, 95, 200, 204.
†References 31, 51, 89, 95, 129, 150.

If cryptococcal organisms are seen on the India ink stain at the time of diagnostic vitreous humor tap or vitrectomy, intravitreous amphotericin B should be administered immediately, and systemic therapy should be initiated. Early pars plana vitrectomy is recommended if severe vitritis fails to clear or worsens on antifungal therapy. Enucleation can be considered if the outcome is a blind, painful eye.

SPOROTRICHOSIS

Sporotrichosis, caused by the filamentous branching fungus *Sporothrix schenckii,* is classified as a subcutaneous mycosis because it is usually acquired by traumatic implantation through the skin. The first case attributed to *S. schenckii* was reported in 1898, and in the 1940s a large outbreak of nearly 3000 cases occurred in South African gold mines as a result of contaminated timber beams.[125]

Mycology

Sporothrix schenckii is a dimorphic fungus with yeastlike and filamentous mold stages. In enriched culture medium at 37°C and in tissues, the variable yeastlike cells may be round, oval, or cigar-shaped. On Sabouraud agar at 25°C, *S. schenckii* grows as a filamentous white mold that becomes brownish black. Minute spores form on the fine, branching hyphae.[20,125]

Epidemiology

S. schenckii is distributed throughout the world, but it is particularly common in tropical or temperate regions. It is a common saprophyte, found in soil and on plants, thorns, wood, straw, and reeds.[125] Outbreaks of sporotrichosis have involved gardeners, agricultural workers, miners,[20] meat-packers,[52] and sphagnum moss handlers.[55] Sporotrichosis also can be inoculated by insect stings, animal bites,[31] cat scratches,[78] or by handling contaminated fish.[125]

Risk Factors

Disseminated or pulmonary sporotrichosis has been reported (1) in a renal transplant recipient and (2) in several cases with immunosuppression or debilitating conditions including alcoholism, diabetes, use of corticosteroids, multiple myeloma, lymphoma, other malignancies, and AIDS.*

Clinical Features

The most common form of sporotrichosis is a chronic subcutaneous nodular granuloma, usually with spreading lymphatic involvement, following traumatic implantation. Subcutaneous and lymphatic nodules may ulcerate. In 23% of cases, the primary lesion remains "fixed," without lymphatic involvement. The disease usually originates on the extremities or the face, and may persist for years. Mucocu-

---

*References 20, 31, 84, 114, 125, 175.

taneous sporotrichosis also is usually caused by traumatic implantation.[20,125]

Pulmonary sporotrichosis is uncommon and is acquired through inhalation in endemic areas or in an immunocompromised host. Disseminated disease occurs after hematogenous spread from a primary pulmonary or subcutaneous site. Reported manifestations of extracutaneous or disseminated sporotrichosis include fungal arthritis, osteomyelitis, diffuse skin lesions, meningitis, ocular infections, and vocal cord granulomata.[2,20,84,125,170]

Ocular Disease. Most cases of ocular sporotrichosis have an exogenous cause and are acquired through a puncture or scratch injury to the conjunctiva, cornea, or eyelids by a contaminated object. Witherspoon and associates[208] reported a case of exogenous *S. schenckii* endophthalmitis in a 13-year-old boy who was struck in his eye with a stick. They also reviewed previous cases of exogenous and endogenous ocular sporotrichosis, citing older reviews by Gordon[79] in 1947, and Francois and Rysselaere[71] in 1972.

Most cases in the 1947 review were exogenous and involved the eyelids, conjunctiva, cornea, lacrimal excretory system, or orbit.[79,208] In 1909 the first case of endogenous *S. schenckii* endophthalmitis (in a patient with disseminated disease) was reported by DeBeurmann and Gourgerot.[48] Fourteen of the 18 cases of intraocular sporotrichosis reported in the 1972 review were endogenous, resulting from disseminated sporotrichosis. The other four were cases of postoperative exogenous *S. schenckii* endophthalmitis following cataract surgery.[71]

Presenting symptoms in endogenous *S. schenckii* endophthalmitis include decreased vision, pain, and ocular redness. Most cases have signs of anterior segment inflammation including granulomatous or nongranulomatous keratic precipitates, iris nodules, and hypopyon. Later sequelae may include posterior synechiae, glaucoma, cataract, and phthisis bulbi. Posterior segment involvement may be manifested by choroiditis, vitritis, or a fluffy white retinal lesion.*

Most patients with endogenous *S. schenckii* endophthalmitis eventually require enucleation. One problem is the difficulty in culturing the organism from blood, urine, or intraocular fluids. Several cases in the Witherspoon[208] study were not accurately diagnosed until enucleation. In addition, most of the previously reported cases occurred before amphotericin B or modern vitreoretinal surgical techniques were available.

A more recent case of endogenous *S. schenckii* endophthalmitis involved a 30-year-old man with AIDS and disseminated sporotrichosis. He had a granulomatous uveitis that worsened following topical and subconjunctival corticosteroids. An aqueous aspirate was positive for *S. schenckii,* and he received treatment with intravitreous and intravenous amphotericin B. His intraocular inflammation

deteriorated despite negative repeat aqueous and vitreous cultures, and enucleation became necessary.[114]

Pathology

Histopathologic and electron microscopic examination of the eye from the patient with AIDS discussed previously revealed severe inflammatory changes, with granulomatous uveitis, lens opacification, a whitish flocculent material filling the anterior and posterior chambers, and scattered *S. schenckii* organisms with disrupted protoplasm.[114] Cultures of the intraocular fluids were negative. In this patient the inflammatory process worsened despite the apparent fungicidal effectiveness of therapy.[114] Additional histopathologic findings in other patients with endogenous *S. schenckii* endophthalmitis include a granulomatous necrotizing chorioretinitis,[69] organisms throughout many intraocular tissues, and intracellular fungi within inflammatory cells.[31]

Differential Diagnosis

The differential diagnosis of endogenous *S. schenckii* endophthalmitis includes other causes of severe granulomatous intraocular inflammation: ocular tuberculosis, sarcoidosis, and fungal endophthalmitis caused by other organisms.

Laboratory Investigations

Accurate and timely diagnosis is challenging because *S. schenckii* can be very difficult to isolate from blood, urine, or ocular fluids; repeated diagnostic aqueous and vitreous aspiration and culture may be necessary to isolate the organism. If there is another site of infection, such as a cutaneous lesion or fungal arthritis, biopsy or aspiration of that site with culture may be helpful.

Careful examination of Gram, periodic acid-Schiff, or Gomori methenamine silver stains, as well as immunofluorescence histologic studies of a tissue specimen may reveal organisms, even when the cultures are negative.[20,114,125]

Also, specific serologic tests are available to identify antibodies to *S. schenckii* in blood or body fluids.[170,171] Immunodiffusion, ELISA, or Western immunoblot testing can be attempted on aqueous or vitreous fluid as well. Gallium and bone scans have been helpful in localizing areas of involvement in patients with disseminated sporotrichosis.[5]

Therapy

The treatment of sporotrichosis varies with the disease form. Cutaneous disease is treated with a saturated solution of potassium iodide (SSKI),[125] and disseminated or extracutaneous sporotrichosis is usually treated with intravenous amphotericin B.[20] Itraconazole is also very effective against both *S. schenckii* (in vitro) and disseminated sporotrichosis.[12,188] As a result itraconazole is likely to become the drug of choice for both disseminated and nondisseminated forms, as most patients do not accept potassium iodide. Itraconazole, however, is not currently approved by the FDA for sporotrichosis.

---

*References 31, 38, 48, 69, 71, 79, 114, 120, 171, 208.

Although the patient presented by Witherspoon and associates[208] had exogenous *S. schenckii* endophthalmitis, it was the first case to be successfully treated. The patient underwent pars plana lensectomy and vitrectomy, received topical amphotericin B, and had a repeat vitrectomy with injection of intravitreous amphotericin B. It was the first reported case of *S. schenckii* endophthalmitis treated with vitrectomy. His vision improved from light perception to 20/50. All of the 17 previous cases of endogenous and exogenous *S. schenckii* endophthalmitis resulted in enucleation.[208] Aggressive treatment with systemic antifungal agents (amphotericin B and/or itraconazole), pars plana vitrectomy, and intravitreous amphotericin B is therefore advised.

BLASTOMYCOSIS

Blastomycosis is a systemic pyogranulomatous disease caused by the dimorphic fungus *Blastomyces dermatitidis*. It was first described by Gilchrist in Chicago in 1894. The older term *North American blastomycosis* is no longer used, because the infection is now recognized in several continents. Also, the term *South American blastomycosis* has been replaced by *paracoccidioidomycosis,* which is caused by *Paracoccidioides brasiliensis*.[29,41]

Mycology

B. dermatitidis exists as a mycelial form with branching hyphae at room temperatures, and as a yeast form in culture and tissues at 37°C. The mycelial form grows well on Sabouraud agar as a white-to-tan colony. Final identification depends on conversion to the characteristic yeast form at 37°C. The yeast cells (which have a thick cell wall and 8 to 12 nuclei) reproduce by budding.[41]

Epidemiology

Most cases of blastomycosis have been reported in the United States and Canada, with sporadic cases in Central America, South America, and Africa. The organism has been isolated from soil in endemic areas and has infected domestic animals, although direct spread to humans has not been reported. The male to female ratio of patients with blastomycosis is 6 : 1, and many patients have had exposure to soil near waterways.[29,41,109]

Clinical Features

Although blastomycosis is most often acquired through the lungs, many patients initially have few or no symptoms. Active pulmonary disease may present as an acute pneumonitis, a miliary disease, a chronic granulomatous process, or a lung mass. Hematogenous seeding may result in lesions in nearly any organ or tissue in the body, particularly skin, bone, GU tract, liver, spleen, lymph nodes, and mucous membranes. Involvement of the CNS, heart, joints, eye, thyroid, or adrenal gland is uncommon. Multiple skin lesions (which are observed in 40% to 80% of cases) are usually painless, crusted, erythematous nodules or plaques on the face or extremities. Disseminated disease may progress over weeks to years and lead to death.

Few cases have been described in immunocompromised patients.[29,41] Butka and associates[34] reported a renal transplant recipient who developed disseminated blastomycosis following accidental inoculation in the veterinarian's office where she worked.

The pathophysiology of blastomycosis involves a combination of pyogenic and granulomatous inflammatory reactions. *B. dermatitidis* in the yeast form may be seen in tissue sections, using Gomori methenamine silver or periodic acid-Schiff stains.[41]

Ocular Disease. Ophthalmic manifestations of blastomycosis include skin lesions involving the eyelids, lesions on the conjunctiva or cornea, orbital infection, choroiditis, and a few reported cases of endophthalmitis.[31] The first case of endogenous *B. dermatitidis* endophthalmitis was described in 1914 by Churchill and Stober.[43] *B. dermatitidis* was isolated from the vitreous in a patient with disseminated blastomycosis.

Several subsequent cases of intraocular *B. dermatitidis* infection have shown localized involvement of the anterior segment,[169] angle, and ciliary body,[39] as well as single or multiple choroidal lesions.[121,179] Sinskey and Anderson[179] described a patient with miliary blastomycosis who had multiple yellow-white choroidal lesions (0.125 disc diameter) that were identified as choroidal granulomata on postmortem histopathologic examination. A patient reported by Lewis and associates[121] had a single large, yellow, oval, elevated lesion that measured 1 by 1.5 optic disc diameters. Neither of these patients had vitritis, nor should they be considered true cases of endophthalmitis.

In addition to the case reported in 1914, two other patients with endogenous *B. dermatitides* endophthalmitis have been discussed in the literature. Presenting symptoms were nonspecific: pain, blurred vision, and evidence of uveitis. The case described in 1967 by Font and associates[70] presented with findings of anterior uveitis, secondary glaucoma, and no view of the fundus. The eye perforated, became blind and painful, and was enucleated. A correct diagnosis was made only after examination of the enucleated globe. Findings included panophthalmitis and organisms within the choroid, retina, sclera, and optic nerve sheaths.

Bond and associates[27] described a 49-year-old outdoor laborer with sarcoidosis who developed presumed *B. dermatitidis* endophthalmitis and biopsy-proven cutaneous blastomycosis lesions. His ocular examination revealed signs of bilateral anterior uveitis, cells in the vitreous, and bilateral choroidal lesions. There was a large, pale, yellow, elevated choroidal lesion in the right eye, and three smaller, whiter lesions in the left eye. Because of an initial diagnosis of sarcoidosis, the patient was treated with systemic corticosteroids. The vitritis worsened in the right eye. After the correct diagnosis of blastomycosis was made by biopsy and culture of the skin lesions and positive *B. dermatitides* serology, the patient was treated with intravenous amphotericin B. Renal toxicity limited the duration of amphotericin B therapy, and the patient was subsequently treated with intravenous hydroxystilbamidine, intrathecal amphotericin B, then intravenous miconazole. The patient eventually died of disseminated blastomycosis with CNS involvement, and bacterial pneumonia. The vitritis and choroiditis had largely cleared following treatment with IV amphotericin B.[27] Postmortem examination was refused.

Among the three cases of endogenous *B. dermatitidis* endophthalmitis reported since 1967, only the one presented by Bond and associates[27] had definite predisposing factors. The patient had been an outdoor laborer, presumably in contact with *B. dermatitidis* in the environment. Also, he was immunocompromised as the result of a long-standing history of sarcoidosis with pulmonary involvement and treatment with systemic corticosteroids.

Differential Diagnosis

Differential diagnoses to consider in a patient with endogenous *B. dermatitidis* endophthalmitis are ocular sarcoidosis, tuberculosis, endophthalmitis caused by *Cryptococcus* species or other fungi, and posterior scleritis.[27,127]

Laboratory Investigations

Because of the myriad of cutaneous and systemic manifestations of blastomycosis, and because of the variable and nonspecific ocular findings of infection, a high index of suspicion and appropriate diagnostic testing are necessary for correct diagnosis. Fungal cultures and microscopic examination of potassium hydroxide wet mount slide preparations of blood, sputum, prostatic secretions, skin lesions, and aqueous and vitreous aspirates are the most valuable. After initial growth at 30°C, fungal cultures also should be examined following incubation at 37°C, so as to detect the characteristic budding, thick-walled yeast forms.

In the past, serologic tests have been neither specific, nor sensitive enough to be clinically helpful.[29,41] Enzyme immunoassay (EIA) appears to be more sensitive than immunodiffusion or complement fixation, however.[108]

Gomori methenamine silver or periodic acid-Schiff stains allow detection of yeast-form organisms in tissue sections.[29] Margo and associates[130] discussed the use of the natural autofluorescence of *B. dermatitidis* organisms in fixed tissue specimens to identify an unsuspected case of periocular blastomycosis in a patient thought to have squamous cell carcinoma.

Therapy

Previously, the treatment of choice for all clinical forms of blastomycosis was amphotericin B. Although this drug is still advised for patients with CNS involvement or other

life-threatening disease, clinical trials have proved the efficacy of oral ketoconazole at a dosage of 400 mg/day for 6 months.[29,41,188] Intravenous miconazole and oral itraconazole also have achieved therapeutic success in several reported cases.[185] Itraconazole is now considered the drug of choice.

Of the three cases of endogenous *B. dermatitidis* endophthalmitis, two ended in enucleation; in each of these, the diagnosis was made only following enucleation.[43,70] The other patient died of disseminated blastomycosis and bacterial pneumonia, following treatment with several antifungal agents.[27] No cases have been treated with intravitreous antifungal agents or vitrectomy.

As with other cases of fungal endophthalmitis, optimal treatment of endogenous *B. dermatitidis* endophthalmitis demands early diagnosis, assisted by vitreous and aqueous aspiration with fungal cultures, and prompt treatment with systemic antifungal agents. Intravitreous amphotericin B and pars plana vitrectomy are recommended if a clinically important amount of vitreous inflammation is present.

REFERENCES

1. Agarwal A, Gupta A, Sakhuja V et al.: Retinitis following disseminated cryptococcosis in a renal allograft recipient: efficacy of oral fluconazole, *Acta Ophthalmol* 69:402-405, 1991.
2. Agger WA, Seager GM: Granulomas of the vocal cords caused by *Sporothrix schenckii, Laryngoscope* 95:595-596, 1985.
3. Aguilar GL et al.: Candidal endophthalmitis after intravenous drug abuse, *Arch Ophthalmol* 97:96-100, 1979.
4. Aisner J, Wiernik PH, Schimpff SC: Treatment of invasive aspergillosis: relation of early diagnosis and treatment and response, *Ann Int Med* 86:539-543, 1977.
5. Anees A, Ali A, Fordham EW: Abnormal bone and gallium scans in a case of multifocal systemic sporotrichosis, *Clin Nucl Med* 11:663-664, 1986.
6. Annable WL, Kachmer ML, DiMarco M et al.: Long-term follow up of candidal endophthalmitis in the premature infant, *J of Pediatric Ophthalmol and Strabismus* 27:103-106, 1990.
7. Ansari RA, Hindson DA, Stevens DL et al.: *Pseudallescheria boydii* arthritis and osteomyelitis in a patient with Cushing's disease, *South Med J* 80:90-92, 1987.
8. Arffa RC, Avni I, Ishibashi Y et al.: Calcofluor and ink-potassium hydroxide preparations for identifying fungi, *Am J Ophthalmol* 100:719-723, 1985.
9. Armin AR, Reddy VB, Orfei E: Fungal endocarditis caused by *Pseudallescheria (Petriellidium) boydii* in an intravenous drug abuser, *Tex Heart Inst J* 14:321-324, 1987.
10. *Aspergillus* endophthalmitis in intravenous-drug users—Kentucky, *MMWR* 39(3):48-49, 1990.
10a. Avendaõ J, Tanishima T, Kuwabara T: Ocular cryptococcosis, *Am J Ophthalmol* 86:110-113, 1978.
11. Aziz AA, Bullock JD, McGuire TW et al.: *Aspergillus* endophthalmitis: a clinical and experimental study, *Trans Am Ophthalmol Soc* 90:317-346, 1992.
12. Baker JH, Goodpasture HC, Kuhns HR Jr et al.: Fungemia caused by an amphotericin B-resistant isolate of *Sporothrix schencki*: successful treatment with itraconazole, *Arch Pathol Lab Med* 113:1279-1281, 1989.
13. Baley JE, Annable WL, Kliegman RM: Candidal endophthalmitis in the premature infant, *J Pediatr* 98:458-461, 1981.
14. Baley JE, Kliegman RM, Fanaroff AA: Disseminated fungal infections in very low-birth-weight infants: clinical manifestations and epidemiology, *Pediatrics* 73:144-152, 1984.

15. Baley JE, Kliegman RM, Fanaroff AA: Disseminated fungal infections in very low-birth-weight infants: therapeutic toxicity, *Pediatrics* 73:153-157, 1984.

16. Balmes R, Bialasiewicz AA, Busse H: Conjunctival cryptococcosis preceding human immunodeficiency virus seroconversion, *Am J Ophthalmol* 113:719-721, 1992.

17. Barrie T: The place of elective vitrectomy in the management of patients with candidal endophthalmitis, *Graefes' Arch Clin Exp Ophthalmol* 225:107-113, 1987.

18. Bennett JE: *Aspergillus* species. In Mandell GL, Douglas RG Jr, Bennett JE, editors: *Principles and practice of infectious diseases,* ed 2, 1447-1451, New York, 1985, John Wiley & Sons.

19. Bennett JE: Miscellaneous fungi. In Mandell GL, Douglas RG Jr, Bennett JE, editors: *Principles and practice of infectious diseases,* ed 2, 1502-1504, New York, 1985, John Wiley & Sons.

20. Bennett JE: *Sporothrix schenckii.* In Mandell GL, Douglas RG Jr, Bennett JE, editors: *Principles and practice of infectious diseases,* ed 2, 1456-1458, New York, 1985, John Wiley & Sons.

21. Berenguer J, Diaz-Mediavilla J, Urra D et al.: Central nervous system infection caused by *Pseudallescheria boydii:* case report and review, *Rev Infect Dis* 11:890-896, 1989.

22. Bessieres MH, Malecaze F, Linas MD et al.: Local production of specific antibodies in the aqueous humor in experimental candidal endophthalmia in rabbits, *Ann Biol Clin (Paris)* 45:651-656, 1987.

23. Beyt BE Jr, Waltman SR: Cryptococcal endophthalmitis after corneal transplantation, *N Eng J Med* 298:825-826, 1978.

24. Blumenkranz MS, Stevens DA: Therapy of endogenous fungal endophthalmitis: miconazole or amphotericin B for coccidioidal and candidal infection, *Arch Ophthalmol* 98:1216-1220, 1980.

25. Bodoia RD, Kinyoun JL, Qingli L et al.: *Aspergillus* necrotizing retinitis: a clinico-pathologic study and review, *Retina* 9:226-231, 1989.

26. Boldrey EE: Bilateral endogenous *Aspergillus* endophthalmitis, *Retina* 1:171-174, 1981.

27. Bond WI, Sanders CV, Joffe L et al.: Presumed blastomycosis endophthalmitis, *Ann Ophthalmol* 14:1183-1188, 1982.

28. Bosley TM, Kaufman KJ, Folberg R et al.: Disseminated aspergillosis in a patient with ocular reticulum cell sarcoma, *Br J Ophthalmol* 71:526-530, 1987.

29. Bradsher RW: Blastomycosis. In Strickland GT, editor: *Hunter's tropical medicine,* ed 7, 530-533, Philadelphia, 1991, WB Saunders.

30. Brasseur G, Retout A, Charlin JF et al.: Endophthalmitis caused by *Aspergillus* (anatomo-clinical study of a case), *Bull Soc Ophtalmol Fr* 89:305-310, 1989.

31. Brod RD, Clarkson JG, Flynn HW Jr et al.: Endogenous fungal endophthalmitis. In Duane TD, Jaeger EA, editors: *Clinical ophthalmology,* vol 3, Hagerstown, MD, 1990, Harper & Row.

32. Brod RD, Flynn HW Jr, Clarkson JG et al.: Endogenous candidal endophthalmitis, *Ophthalmology* 97:666-674, 1990.

33. Brooks RG: Prospective study of candidal endophthalmitis in hospitalized patients with candidemia, *Arch Intern Med* 149:2226-2228, 1989.

34. Butka BJ, Bennett SR, Johnson AC: Disseminated inoculation blastomycosis in a renal transplant recipient, *Am Rev Respir Dis* 130:1180-1183, 1984.

35. Cameron JA, Antonios SR, Cotter JB et al.: Endophthalmitis from contaminated donor corneas following penetrating keratoplasty, *Arch Ophthalmol* 109:54-59, 1991.

36. Cantrill HL, Rodman WF, Ramsay RC, Knobloch WH: Postpartum candidal endophthalmitis, *JAMA* 234:1163-1165, 1980.

37. Carney MD, Combs JL, Waschler W: Cryptococcal choroiditis, *Retina* 10:27-32, 1990.

38. Cassady JR, Foerster HC: *Sporotrichum schenckii* endophthalmitis, *Arch Ophthalmol* 85:71-75, 1971.

39. Cassady JV: Uveal blastomycosis, *Arch Ophthalmol* 35:84-97, 1946.

40. Caya JG, Farmer SG, Williams GA et al.: Bilateral *Pseudallescheria boydii* endophthalmitis in an immunocompromised patient, *Wis Med J* 87:11-14, 1988.

41. Chapman SW: *Blastomyces dermatitidis.* In Mandell GL, Douglas RG Jr, Bennett JE, editors: *Principles and practice of infectious diseases,* ed 2, 1477-1485, 1985, John Wiley & Sons.

42. Charles NC, Boxrud CA, Small EA: Cryptococcosis of the anterior segment in acquired immune deficiency syndrome, *Ophthalmology* 99:813-816, 1992.

43. Churchill T, Stober AM: A case of systemic blastomycosis, *Arch Intern Med* 13:568-574, 1914.

44. Clinch TE et al.: Infantile endogenous candidal endophthalmitis presenting as a cataract, *Surv Ophthalmol* 34:107-112, 1989.

45. Condon PI, Terry SI, Falconer H: Cryptococcal eye disease, *Doc Ophthalmol* 44:49-56, 1977.

46. Corvisier N, Gray F, Gherardi R et al.: Aspergillosis of ethmoid sinus and optic nerve, with arteritis and rupture of the internal carotid artery, *Surg Neurol* 28:311-315, 1987.

47. Crislip MA, Edwards JE Jr: Candidiasis, *Infect Dis Clin North Am* 3:103-133, 1989.

48. DeBeurmann CL, Gourgerot H: Sporotrichose cachectisante mortelle, *Bull Mem Soc Med Hop Paris* 26:1046, 1909.

49. Dellon AL, Stark WJ, Chretien PB: Spontaneous resolution of endogenous candidal endophthalmitis complicating intravenous hyperalimentation, *Am J Ophthalmol* 79:648-654, 1975.

50. Demicco DD, Reichman RC, Violett EJ et al.: Disseminated aspergillosis presenting with endophthalmitis: a case report and a review of the literature, *Cancer* 53:1995-2001, 1984.

51. Denning DW, Armstrong RW, Fishman M et al.: Endophthalmitis in a patient with disseminated cryptococcosis and AIDS who was treated with itraconazole, *Rev Infect Dis* 13:1126-1130, 1991.

52. Dewan N, Bedi S, O'Donohue WJ Jr: Primary pulmonary sporotrichosis occurring in two meat packers, *Nebr Med J* 71:37-39, 1986.

53. Diamond RD: Cryptococcus neoformans. In Mandell GL, Douglas RG Jr, Bennett JE, editors: *Principles and practice of infectious diseases,* ed 2, 1985, John Wiley & Sons.

54. Dimmer F: Ein Fall von Schimmel pilzerkrankung des Auges, *Klin Monatsbl Augenheilkd* 51:194-198, 1913.

55. Dixon DM, Salkin IF, Duncan RA et al.: Isolation and characterization of *Sporothrix schenckii* from clinical and environmental sources associated with the largest U.S. epidemic of sporotrichosis, *J Clin Microbiol* 29:1106-1113, 1991.

56. Doft BH, Clarkson JG, Rebell G et al.: Endogenous *Aspergillus* endophthalmitis in drug abusers, *Arch Ophthalmol* 98:859-862, 1980.

57. Doft BH, Weiskopf J, Nilsson-Ehle et al.: Amphotericin clearance in vitrectomized versus nonvitrectomized eyes, *Ophthalmology* 92:1601-1605, 1985.

58. Doorenbos-Bot ACC, Hooymans JMM, Blanksma LJ: Periorbital necrotising fasciitis due to *Cryptococcus neoformans* in a healthy young man, *Doc Ophthalmol* 75:315-320, 1990.

58a. Dupont E, Droubet E: Cutaneous, ocular and osteoarticular candidiasis in heroin addicts: new clinical and therapeutic aspects in 38 patients, *J Infect Dis* 152:577-591, 1985.

59. Edwards JE Jr: *Candida* species. In Mandell GL, Douglas RG Jr, Bennett JE, editors: *Principles and practice of infectious diseases,* ed 3, 1943-1958, New York, 1990, Churchill Livingstone.

60. Edwards JE Jr, Foos RY, Montgomerie JZ et al.: Ocular manifestations of candidal septicemia: review of seventy-six cases of hematogenous candidal endophthalmitis, *Medicine* 53:47-75, 1974.

61. Edwards JE Jr, Lehrer RI, Stiehm ER et al.: Severe candidal infections: clinical perspective, immune defense mechanisms, and current concepts of therapy, *Ann Int Med* 89:91-106, 1978.

62. Edwards JE Jr, Montgomerie JZ, Ishida K et al.: Experimental hematogenous endophthalmitis due to *Candida:* species variation in pathogenicity, *J Infect Dis* 135:294-297, 1977.

63. Ehrhorn J, Grosse G, Staib F et al.: Intraokulare cryptococcose, *Klin Monatsbl Augenheilkd* 168:577-583, 1976.

64. Eilard T: Isolation of fungi in blood cultures, *Scand J Infect Dis* 19:145-156, 1987.

65. Elder BL, Roberts GD: Pseudallescheriasis. In Sarosi GA, Davies SF, editors: *Fungal diseases of the lung,* 205-215, New York, 1986, Grune & Stratton.

66. Elliot JH, O'Day DM, Gutow GS et al.: Mycotic endophthalmitis in drug abusers, *Am J Ophthalmol* 88:66-71, 1978.

67. Filler SG, Crislip MA, Mayer CL et al.: Comparison of fluconazole and amphotericin B for treatment of disseminated candidiasis and endophthalmitis in rabbits, *Antimicrob Agent Chemother* 35:288-292, 1991.

68. Fishman LS, Griffin JR, Sapico FL et al.: Hematogenous candidal endophthalmitis: a complication of candidemia, *N Eng J Med* 286:675-681, 1972.

69. Font RL, Jakobiec FA: Granulomatous necrotizing retinochoroiditis caused by *Sporotrichum schenckii:* report of a case including immunofluorescence and electron microscopical studies, *Arch Ophthalmol* 94:1513-1519, 1976.

70. Font RL, Spaulding AG, Green WR: Endogenous mycotic panophthalmitis caused by *Blastomyces dermatitidis:* report of a case and a review of the literature, *Arch Ophthalmol* 77:217-222, 1967.

71. Francois J, Rysselaere M: *Oculomycosis,* 69-81, Springfield, IL, 1972, Charles C Thomas.

72. Friedman AH, Chishti MI, Henkind P: Endogenous ocular aspergillosis, *Ophthalmologica* 168:197-205, 1974.

73. Galgiani JN, Stevens DA, Graybill JR et al.: *Pseudallescheria boydii* infections treated with ketoconazole, *Chest* 86:219-224, 1984.

74. Gallo J, Playfair J, Gregory-Roberts J et al.: Fungal endophthalmitis in narcotic abusers: medical and surgical therapy in 10 patients, *Med J Austr* 142:386-388, 1985.

75. Getnick RA, Rodriguez MM: Endogenous fungal endophthalmitis in a drug addict, *Am J Ophthalmol* 77:680-683, 1974.

76. Gold JWM: Infections due to fungi, *Actinomyces* and *Nocardia.* In Reese GE, Betts RG, editors: *A practical approach to infectious disease,* ed 2, 512-527, Boston, 1991, Little, Brown.

77. Golnik KC, Newman SA, Wispelway B: Cryptococcal optic neuropathy in the acquired immune deficiency syndrome, *J Clin Neuroophthalmol* 11:96-103, 1991.

78. Gonzalez-Cabo JF, de las Heras-Guillamon M, Latre-Cequiel MV et al.: Feline sporotrichosis: a case report, *Mycopathologia* 108:149-154, 1989.

79. Gordon DM: Ocular sporotrichosis, *Arch Ophthalmol* 37:56-72, 1947.

80. Graham E, Chignell AH, Eykyn S: Candidal endophthalmitis: a complication of prolonged intravenous therapy and antibiotic treatment, *J Infect* 13:167-173, 1986.

81. Grieco MH, Freilich DB, Louria DB: Diagnosis of cryptococcal uveitis with hypertonic media, *Am J Ophthalmol* 72:171-174, 1971.

82. Griffin JR, Foos RY, Pettit TH: Relationship between candidal endophthalmitis, candidemia, and disseminated candidiasis, *Concilium Ophthalmologicum,* 22nd, Paris, 1974 Masson.

83. Griffin JR, Pettit TH, Fishman LS, Foos RY: Blood-borne candidal endophthalmitis: a clinical and pathologic study of 21 cases, *Arch Ophthalmol* 89:450-456, 1973.

84. Gullberg RM, Quintanilla A, Levin ML et al.: Sporotrichosis: recurrent cutaneous, articular, and central nervous system infection in a renal transplant recipient, *Rev Infect Dis* 9:369-375, 1987.

85. Halperin LS, Roseman RL: Successful treatment of a subretinal abscess in an intravenous drug abusers, *Arch Ophthalmol* 106:1651-1652, 1988.

86. Hanish SJ, Perlmutter JC, Boucher C et al.: Exogenous aspergillic endophthalmitis, *Ann Ophthalmol* 16:417-419, 1984.

87. Harris GJ, Will BR: Orbital aspergillosis: conservative debridement and local amphotericin irrigation, *Ophthalmic Plast Reconstr Surg* 5:207-211, 1989.

88. Heinemann MH, Bloom AF, Horowitz J: *Candida albicans* endophthalmitis in a patient with AIDS, *Arch Ophthalmol* 105:1172-1173, 1987.

89. Henderly DE, Liggett PE, Rao NA: Cryptococcal chorioretinitis and endophthalmitis, *Retina* 7:75-79, 1987.

90. Henderson DK, Edwards JE Jr, Ishida K et al.: Experimental hematogenous candidal endophthalmitis, diagnostic approaches, *Infect Immun* 23:858-862, 1979.

91. Henderson DK, Edwards JE Jr, Montgomerie JZ: Hematogenous candidal endophthalmitis in patients receiving parenteral hyperalimentation fluids, *J Infect Dis* 143:655-661, 1981.

92. Henderson DK, Hockey LJ, Vukalcic LJ et al.: Effect of immunosuppression on the development of experimental hematogenous candidal endophthalmitis, *Infect Immun* 27:628-631, 1980.

93. Hiles DA, Font RL: Bilateral intraocular cryptococcosis with unilateral spontaneous regression: report of a case and review of the literature, *Am J Ophthalmol* 65:98-108, 1968.

94. Hill HR, Mitchell TG, Matsen JM: Recovery from disseminated candidiasis in a premature neonate, *Pediatrics* 53:748-752, 1974.

95. Hiss PW, Shields JA, Augsburger JJ: Solitary retinovitreal abscess as the initial manifestation of cryptococcosis, *Ophthalmology* 95:162-165, 1988.

96. Holland GN: Endogenous fungal infections of the retina and choroid. In Ryan SJ, editor: *Retina,* vol 2, 629-636, St Louis, 1989, Mosby.

97. Huang K, Peyman G, McGetrick J: Vitrectomy in experimental endophthalmitis. Part I fungal endophthalmitis, *Ophthalmol Surg* 10:84-87, 1979.

98. Jain VK, Dawson WW, Engel HM et al.: Electroretinograms in early fungal endophthalmitis, *Doc Ophthalmol* 69:227-235, 1988.

99. Jampol LM, Dyckman S, Maniates V et al.: Retinal and choroidal infarction from *Aspergillus:* clinical diagnosis and clinicopathologic correlations, *Trans Am Ophthalmol Soc* 86:422-436; discussion 437-440, 1989.

100. Johnson DE, Thompson TR, Green TP et al.: Systemic candidiasis in very low-birth-weight infants (< 1,500 grams), *Pediatrics* 73:138-143, 1984.

101. Jones DB: Chemotherapy of experimental endogenous *Candida albicans* endophthalmitis, *Trans Am Ophthalmol Soc* 76:846-895, 1980.

102. Joshi N, Hamory BH: Endophthalmitis caused by non-*albicans* species of *Candida, Rev Infect Dis* 13:281-287, 1991.

103. Kalina PH, Campbell RJ: *Aspergillus terreus* endophthalmitis in a patient with chronic lymphocytic leukemia, *Arch Ophthalmol* 109:102-103, 1991.

104. Kammer RB, Utz JP: *Aspergillus* species endocarditis: the new face of a not so rare disease, *Am J Med* 56:506, 1974.

104a. Khodadoust AA, Payne JW: Cryptococcal (torular) retinitis: a clinicopathologic case report, *Am J Ophthalmol* 67:745-750, 1969.

105. Khurana AK, Mathur SK, Ahluwalia BK et al.: An unusual case of endogenous *Aspergillus* endophthalmitis, *Acta Ophthalmol Copenh* 67:315-318, 1989.

106. Kinyoun JL: Treatment of candidal endophthalmitis, *Retina* 2:215-222, 1982.

107. Kitahara M, Seth VK, Medoff G et al.: Activity of amphotericin B, 5-fluorocytosine and rifampin against six clinical isolates of *Aspergillus, Antimicrob Agents Chemother* 9:915-919, 1976.

108. Klein BS, Kuritsky JN, Chappell WA et al.: Comparison of the enzyme immunoassay, immunodiffusion, and complement fixation tests in detecting antibody in human serum to the A antigen of *Blastomyces dermatitidis, Am Rev Respir Dis* 133:144-148, 1986.

109. Klein BS, Vergeront JM, DiSalvo AF et al.: Two outbreaks of blastomycosis along rivers in Wisconsin. Isolation of *Blastomyces dermatitidis* from riverbank soil and evidence of its transmission along waterways, *Am Rev Respir Dis* 136:1333-1338, 1987.

110. Klein JJ, Watanakunakorn C: Hospital-acquired fungemia. Its natural course and clinical significance, *Am J Med* 67:51-58, 1979.

111. Komadina TG, Wilkes TD, Shock JP et al.: Treatment of *Aspergillus fumigatus* keratitis in rabbits with oral and topical ketoconazole, *Am J Ophthalmol* 99:476-479, 1985.

112. Kostick DA, Foster RE, Lowder CY et al.: Endogenous endophthalmitis caused by *Candida albicans* in a healthy woman, *Am J Ophthalmol* 113:593-595, 1992.

113. Kotwal MR, Rinchhen CZ: Primary aspergillosis with multisystem dissemination, *Lancet* 1:562, 1981.

114. Kurosawa A, Pollock SC, Collins MP et al.: *Sporothrix schenckii* endophthalmitis in a patient with human immunodeficiency virus infection, *Arch Ophthalmol* 106:376-380, 1988.

115. Laatikainen L, Tuominen M, Dickhoff KV: Treatment of endogenous fungal endophthalmitis with systemic fluconazole with or without vitrectomy, *Am J Ophthalmol* 113:205-207, 1992.

116. Lake FR, Tribe AE, McAleer R et al.: Mixed allergic bronchopulmonary fungal disease due to *Pseudallescheria boydii* and *Aspergillus, Thorax* 45:489-491, 1990.

117. Lance SE, Friberg TR, Kowalski RP: *Aspergillus flavus* endophthalmitis and retinitis in an intravenous drug abuser: a therapeutic success, *Ophthalmology* 95:947-949, 1988.

118. Lederman IR, Madge G: Endogenous intraocular aspergillosis, *Arch Ophthalmol* 76:233-237, 1966.

119. Leen CL, Brettle RP: Fungal infections in drug users, *J Antimicrob Chemother* 28(suppl A):83-96, 1991.

120. Levy JH: Intraocular sporotrichosis: report of a case, *Arch Ophthalmol* 85:574-579, 1971.

121. Lewis H, Aaberg TM, Fary DRB et al.: Latent disseminated blastomycosis with choroidal involvement, *Arch Ophthalmol* 106:527-530, 1988.

122. Lou P, Kazdan J, Bannatyne RM et al.: Successful treatment of candidal endophthalmitis with a synergistic combination of amphotericin B and refampin, *Am J Ophthalmol* 83:12-15, 1977.

123. Lubniewski A, Olk RJ, Grand MG: Ocular dangers in the garden. A new menace-nylon line lawn trimmers, *Ophthalmology* 95:906-910, 1988.

124. Lutwick LI, Galgiani JN, Johnson RH et al.: Visceral fungal infections due to *Petriellidium boydii (Allescheria boydii), Am J Med* 61:632-639, 1976.

125. Mackenzie DWR: Subcutaneous mycoses. In Strickland GT, editor: *Hunter's tropical medicine,* ed 7, 510-515, Philadelphia, 1991, WB Saunders.

126. Mahajan VM: Postoperative ocular infections: an analysis of laboratory data on 750 cases, *Ann Ophthalmol* 16:847-848, 1984.

127. Malo JL, Hawkins R, Pepys J: Studies in chronic allergic bronchopulmonary aspergillosis. I. Clinical and physiological findings, *Thorax* 32:254-261, 1977.

128. Malo JL, Longbottom J, Mitchell J et al.: Studies in chronic allergic bronchopulmonary aspergillosis. III. Immunologic findings, *Thorax* 32:269-274, 1977.

129. Malton ML, Rinkhoff JS, Doft BS et al.: Cryptococcal endophthalmitis and meningitis associated with acute psychosis and exudative retinal detachment, *Am J Ophthalmol* 104:438-439, 1987.

130. Margo CE, Bombardier T: The diagnostic value of fungal autofluorescence, *Surv Ophthalmol* 29:374-376, 1985.

131. Margo CE, Polack FM, Hood CI: *Aspergillus* panophthalmitis complicating treatment of pterygium, *Cornea* 7:285-289, 1988.

132. Mathis A, Malecaze F, Bessieres MH et al.: Immunological analysis of the aqueous humour in candidal endophthalmitis, *Br J Ophthalmol* 72:313-316, 1988.

133. McCormick WF, Schochet SS Jr, Weaver PR et al.: Disseminated aspergillosis, *Aspergillus* endophthalmitis, optic nerve infarction and carotid artery thrombosis, *Arch Pathol* 99:353-359, 1975.

134. McDonald HR, De Bustro S, Sipperley JO: Vitrectomy for epiretinal membranes with candidal chorioretinitis, *Ophthalmology* 97:466-469, 1990.

135. McDonnell PJ, McDonnel JM, Brown RH et al.: Ocular involvement in patients with fungal infections, *Ophthalmology* 92:706-709, 1985.

136. McGuire TW, Bullock JD, Bullock JD Jr et al.: Fungal endophthalmitis: an experimental study with a review of 17 human ocular cases, *Arch Ophthalmol* 109:1289-1296, 1991.

137. McLean JM: Oculomycosis: The XIX Jackson Memorial Lecture, *Am J Ophthalmol* 56:537-549, 1963.

138. Meadow WL, Tipple MA, Rippon JW: Endophthalmitis caused by *Petriellidium boydii, AJDC* 135:378-380, 1981.

139. Miale JB: *Candida albicans* infection confused with tuberculosis, *Arch Pathol* 35:427-437, 1943.

140. Micheli PH: *Nova plantarum genera juxta tournefortii methodum disposita,* Florence, 1729.

141. Michelson JB, Freeman SD, Boydan DG: Aspergillic endophthalmitis in a drug abuser, *Ann Ophthalmol* 14:1051-1054, 1982.

142. Michelson JB, Friedlander MH: Endophthalmitis of drug abuse, *Int Ophthalmol Clin* 27(2):120-126, 1987.

143. Michelson PE, Stark WJ, Reeser F, Green WR: Endogenous candidal endophthalmitis, *Int Ophthalmol Clin* 11(3):125-147, 1971.

144. Mientjes GH, Miedema F, van Ameijden EJ et al.: Frequent injecting impairs lymphocyte reactivity in HIV-positive and HIV-negative drug users, *AIDS* 5(1):35-41, 1991.

145. Mitchell TG: Opportunistic mycoses. In Joklik WK, Willett HP, Amos DB, editors: *Zinsser microbiology,* ed 17, 1417-1420, New York, 1980, Appleton-Century-Crofts.

146. Montgomerie JZ, Edwards JE: Association of infection due to *Candida albicans* with intravenous hyperalimentation, *J Infect Dis* 137:197-201, 1978.

147. Moyer DV, Edwards Jr JE: Candidal endophthalmitis and central nervous system infection. In Bodey GP, editor: *Candidiasis, pathogenesis, diagnosis and treatment,* 331-355, New York, 1993, Raven Press.

148. Naidoff MA, Green WR: Endogenous aspergillic endophthalmitis occurring after kidney transplant, *Am J Ophthalmol* 79:502-509, 1975.

149. Naylor CD, Shkrum MJ, Edmonds MW et al.: Pulmonary aspergillosis and endophthalmitis: complications of Cushing's syndrome, *Can Med Assoc J* 138:719-720, 1988.

149a. Newman NM et al.: Clinical and histologic findings in opportunistic ocular infections: part of a new syndrome of acquired immunodeficiency, *Arch Ophthalmol* 101:396, 1983.

150. O'Dowd GJ, Frable WJ: Cryptococcal endophthalmitis: diagnostic vitreous aspiration cytology, *Am J Clin Pathol* 79:382-385, 1983.

151. Palmer EA: Endogenous candidal endophthalmitis in infants, *Am J Ophthalmol* 89:388-395, 1980.

152. Paradis AJ, Roberts L: Endogenous ocular aspergillosis, *Arch Ophthalmol* 69:765-769, 1963.

153. Parke DW, Jones DB, Gentry LO: Endogenous endophthalmitis among patients with candidemia, *Ophthalmology* 89:789-796, 1982.

153a. Pepose JS, Holland GN, Nestor MS et al.: Acquired immune deficiency syndrome: pathogenic mechanisms of ocular disease, *Ophthalmology* 92:472-484, 1985.

154. Perraut LE Jr, Perraut LE, Bleiman B et al.: Successful treatment of *Candida albicans* with intravitreal amphotericin B, *Arch Ophthalmol* 99:1565-1567, 1981.

155. Pfeifer JD, Grand G, Thomas MA et al.: Endogenous *Pseudallescheria boydii* endophthalmitis: clinicopathologic findings in two cases, *Arch Ophthalmol* 109:1714-1717, 1991.

156. Phillips P, Forbes JC, Speert DP: Disseminated infection with *Pseudallescheria boydii* in a patient with chronic granulomatous disease: response to gamma-interferon plus antifungal chemotherapy, *Pediatr Infect Dis J* 10:536-539, 1991.

157. Phillips P, Weiner MH: Invasive aspergillosis diagnosed by immunohistochemistry with monoclonal and polyclonal reagents, *Hum Pathol* 18:1015-1024, 1987.

157a. Polak A: Combination therapy with antifungal drugs, *Mycoses* 31:45-53, 1988.

158. Raffanti SP, Fyfe B, Carriero S et al.: Native valve endocarditis due to *Pseudallescheria boydii* in a patient with AIDS: case report and review, *Rev Infect Dis* 12:993-996, 1990.

159. Rippon JW: Petriellidiosis: the great imitator, *Clin Microbiol Newsletter* 3:57-58, 1981.

160. Rippon JW: The pathogenic fungi and the pathogenic *Actinomycetes.* In *Medical Mycology,* ed 3, 618-650, Philadelphia, 1988, WB Saunders.

161. Robin JB, Arffa RC, Avni I et al.: Rapid visualization of three common fungi using fluorescein-conjugated lectins, *Invest Ophthalmol Vis Sci* 27:500-506, 1986.

162. Roney P, Barr CC, Chun CH et al.: Endogenous *Aspergillus* endophthalmitis, *Rev Infect Dis* 8:955-958, 1986.

163. Rotresen D, Calderine RA, Edwards JE Jr: Adherence of *Candida* species to host tissues and plastic surfaces, *Rev Infect Dis* 8:73-85, 1986.

163a. Sande MA, Mandell GL: Antimicrobial agents: antifungal and antiviral agents. In Gilman AG, Goodman LS, Rall TW, Murad F, editors: *The pharmacological basis of therapeutics,* ed 7, 1219-1239, New York, 1985, Macmillan.

164. Savani DV et al.: Penetration of new azole compounds into the eye and efficacy in experimental candidal endophthalmitis, *Antimicrob Agent Chemother* 31:6-10, 1987.

165. Schmid S, Martenet AC, Oelz O: Candidal endophthalmitis: clinical presentation, treatment and outcome in 23 patients, *Infection* 19:21-24, 1991.

166. Schulman JA, Leveque C, Coats M et al.: Fatal disseminated cryptococcosis following intraocular involvement, *Br J Ophthalmol* 72:171-175, 1988.

167. Schwartz DA: Organ-specific variation in the morphology of the fungomas (fungus balls) of *Pseudallescheria boydii.* Development within necrotic host tissue, *Arch Pathol Lab Med* 113:476-480, 1989.

168. Schwartz DA, Amenta PS, Finkelstein SD: Cerebral *Pseudallescheria boydii* infection: unique occurrence of fungus ball formation in the brain, *Clin Neurol Neurosurg* 91:79-84, 1989.

169. Schwartz VJ: Intra-ocular blastomycosis, *Arch Ophthalmol* 5:581-590, 1931.

170. Scott EN, Kaufman L, Brown AC et al.: Serologic studies in the diagnosis and management of meningitis due to *Sporothrix schenckii, N Engl J Med* 317:935-940, 1987.
171. Scott EN, Muchmore HG: Immunoblot analysis of antibody responses to *Sporothrix schenckii, J Clin Microbiol* 27:300-304, 1989.
172. Servant JB, Dutton GN, Augsburger JJ et al.: Candidal endophthalmitis in Glaswegian heroin addicts: report of an epidemic, *Trans Ophthalmol Soc UK* 104:297-308, 1985.
173. Shankland GS, Richardson MD: Epidemiology of an outbreak of candidal endophthalmitis in heroin addicts: identification of possible source of infection by biotyping, *J Med Vet Mycol* 26:199-202, 1988.
174. Shankland GS, Richardson MD: Possible role of preserved lemon juice in the epidemiology of candidal endophthalmitis in heroin addicts, *Eur J Clin Microbiol Infect Dis* 8:87-89, 1989.
175. Shaw JC, Levinson W, Montanaro A: Sporotrichosis in the acquired immuno-deficiency syndrome, *J Am Acad Dermatol* 21:1145-1147, 1989.
176. Shields JA, Wright DM, Augsburger JJ et al.: Cryptococcal chorioretinitis, *Am J Ophthalmol* 89:210-218, 1980.
177. Shih L, Lee N: Disseminated petriellidiosis (allescheriasis) in a patient with refractory acute lymphoblastic leukaemia, *J Clin Pathol* 37:78-82, 1984.
178. Sihota R, Agarwal HC, Grover AK et al.: *Aspergillus* endophthalmitis, *Br J Ophthalmol* 71:611-613, 1987.
179. Sinskey RM, Anderson WB: Miliary blastomycosis with metastatic spread to posterior uvea of both eyes, *Arch Ophthalmol* 54:602-604, 1955.
180. Slavin ML: Primary aspergillosis of the orbital apex, *Arch Ophthalmol* 109:1502-1503, 1991.
181. Smith ME: Endogenous *Pseudallescheria boydii* endophthalmitis. Presented at the Verhoeff Society, Houston, April 6-7, 1990.
182. Snip RC, Michels RG: Pars plana vitrectomy in the management of endogenous candidal endophthalmitis, *Am J Ophthalmol* 82:699-704, 1976.
183. Souri EN, Green WR: Intravitreal amphotericin B toxicity, *Am J Ophthalmol* 78:77-86, 1974.
184. Stamm MA, Frable MA: Invasive sinusitis due to *Pseudallescheria boydii* in an immunocompetent host, *South Med J* 85:439-441, 1992.
185. Steck WD: Blastomycosis, *Dermatol Clin* 7:241-250, 1989.
186. Stern GA, Fetkenhour CL, O'Grady RB: Intravitreal amphotericin B treatment of candidal endophthalmitis, *Arch Ophthalmol* 95:89-93, 1977.
187. Stern RM, Zakov ZN, Meisler DM et al.: Endogenous *Pseudallescheria boydii* endophthalmitis: a clinicopathologic report, *Cleve Clin Q* 53:197-203, 1986.
188. Stevens DA: The new generation of antifungal drugs, *Eur J Clin Microbiol Infect Dis* 7:732-735, 1988.
189. Stierstorfer MB, Schwartz BK, McGuire JB et al.: *Pseudallescheria boydii* mycetoma in northern New England, *Int J Dermatol* 27:383-387, 1988.
190. Sud IJ, Feingold DS: Effect of ketoconazole on the fungicidal action of amphotericin B in *Candida albicans, Antimicrob Agents Chemother* 23:185-187, 1983.
191. Summerbell RC, Krajden S, Kane J: Potted plants in hospitals as reservoirs of pathogenic fungi, *Mycopathologia* 106:13-22, 1989.
192. Sundaram BM, Badrinath S, Subramanian S: Studies on mycotic keratitis, *Mycoses* 32:568-572, 1989.
193. Travis LB, Roberts GD, Wilson WR: Clinical significance of *Pseudallescheria boydii:* a review of 10 years' experience, *Mayo Clin Proc* 60:531-537, 1985.
194. Urbak SF, Degn T: Fluconazole in the treatment of *Candida albicans* endophthalmitis, *Acta Ophthalmol* 70:528-529, 1992.
195. VanCutsem J: The antifungal activity of ketoconazole, *Am J Med* 74(1B):9-15, 1983.
196. VanCutsem J: Oral, topical and parenteral antifungal treatment with itraconazole in normal and in immunocompromised animals, *Mycoses* 32(suppl 1):14-34, 1989.
197. Vastine DW, Horsley W, Guth SB et al.: Endogenous candidal endophthalmitis associated with heroin use, *Arch Ophthalmol* 94:1805, 1976.
198. Venditti M, De Bernardis F, Micozzi A et al.: Fluconazole treatment of catheter-related right-sided endocarditis caused by *Candida albicans* and associated with endophthalmitis and folliculitis, *Clin Infect Dis* 14:422-426, 1992.
199. Vishniavsky N, Sagar KB, Markowitz SM: *Aspergillus fumigatus* endocarditis on a normal heart valve, *South Med J* 76:506-508, 1983.
200. Vogiatzis KV, Makley TA, Werling K: Cryptococcosis in a phthisical eye, *Ann Ophthalmol* 13:434-435, 1981.
201. Wade JC: Epidemiology of *Candida* infections. In Bodey GP, editor: *Candidiasis, pathogenesis, diagnosis and treatment,* 85-107, New York, 1993, Raven Press.
202. Walinder PE, Kock E: Endogenous fungus endophthalmitis, *Acta Ophthalmol* 49:263-271, 1971.
203. Weinstein JM, Morris GL, ZuRhein GM et al.: Posterior ischemic optic neuropathy due to *Aspergillus fumigatus, J Clin Neuro Ophthalmol* 9:7-13, 1989.
204. Weis RP, Everett ED, Sprouse R et al.: Endogenous cryptococcal endophthalmitis, *South Med J* 74:482-483, 1981.
205. Weiss C, Perry IH, Shevky MC: Infection of the human eye with *Cryptococcus neoformans (Torula histolytica; Cryptococcus hominis):* a clinical and experimental study with a new diagnostic method, *Arch Ophthalmol* 39:739-751, 1948.
206. Weiss JN, Hutchins RK, Balogh K: Simultaneous *Aspergillus* endophthalmitis and cytomegalovirus retinitis after kidney transplantation, *Retina* 8:193-198, 1988.
207. Wilmarth SS, May DR, Roth AM et al.: *Aspergillus* endophthalmitis in an intravenous drug abuser, *Ann Ophthalmol* 15:470-472, 1983.
208. Witherspoon CD, Kuhn F, Owens D et al.: Endophthalmitis due to *Sporothrix schenckii* after penetrating ocular injury, *Ann Ophthalmol* 22:385-388, 1990.
209. Xanthou M et al.: Phagocytosis and killing ability of *Candida albicans* by blood leucocytes of healthy term and preterm babies, *Arch Dis Child* 50:72-75, 1975.
210. Young RC, Bennett JE, Vogel CL et al.: Aspergillosis. The spectrum of the disease in 98 patients, *Medicine* 49:147-173, 1970.

92 Endogenous Bacterial Endophthalmitis

JOHN P. WHITCHER, ALEXANDER R. IRVINE

Bacterial endophthalmitis is an extremely serious and potentially blinding ocular infection, which is usually associated with recent intraocular surgery. Other presentations of bacterial endophthalmitis occur, however, and a complete classification should include the following: (1) acute postoperative bacterial endophthalmitis, (2) late-onset postoperative endophthalmitis, (3) endophthalmitis secondary to an infected filtering bleb, (4) posttraumatic endophthalmitis, (5) endophthalmitis secondary to contiguous spread, and (6) metastatic or endogenous bacterial endophthalmitis. Advances in recent years in the medical and surgical treatment of the first five types of endophthalmitis in the preceding list have resulted in marked improvement in visual prognosis.[20,27] Treatment of endogenous bacterial endophthalmitis remains controversial, however, and visual results are often disappointing.[36]

HISTORICAL BACKGROUND

Endogenous bacterial endophthalmitis was first recognized as a distinct clinical entity by Virchow[69] in 1856. The first review of world literature was reported by Seginni[22] in 1922. He found 106 cases of laboratory-confirmed metastatic bacterial endophthalmitis, and in 1933 Lumbroso[22] reported 91 additional cases that had occurred in the intervening 10 years. In 1977 Shammas[63] reviewed the literature from 1935 to 1975 and found 102 proven cases of endogenous bacterial endophthalmitis. This report was followed by the most comprehensive appraisal of the subject by Greenwald and associates[36] in 1986, in which another 72 cases were added from the intervening decade, as well as 5 cases of their own. A review of the literature since 1986 reveals that endogenous bacterial endophthalmitis continues to be a persistent problem. There were 66 laboratory-proven cases of endogenous bacterial endophthalmitis in 35 reports from 1987 to the present.* The total of all reported cases of en-

dogenous bacterial endophthalmitis from its recognition as a clinical entity in the middle of the nineteenth century until today is, therefore, less than 500 cases. Despite the relatively small number of patients affected, endogenous bacterial endophthalmitis remains an important problem because of the severity of the infection and the frequently dismal visual outcome.

EPIDEMIOLOGY

The epidemiology of the disease has changed considerably over the years. Until the 1940s *Neisseria meningitidis* accounted for more than 50% of all infections, followed by *Streptococcus pneumoniae* and *Staphylococcus aureus*.[63] After 1945 infection with other bacterial pathogens, especially gram-negative bacilli (*Escherichia* sp., *Pseudomonas* sp., and *Proteus* sp.) began to occur more frequently. By 1986 Greenwald and associates[36] reported that *Bacillus cereus* had become the most frequent cause of endogenous bacterial endophthalmitis. Their findings were confirmed by other reports,[17,40,68] but there was also an increased incidence of infections caused by bacteria of low pathogenicity in immunologically compromised hosts. In the last 5 years an extraordinary variety of bacterial pathogens have been reported as causes of endogenous endophthalmitis. The list includes the following: *Propionibacterium acnes*,[56] *Yersinia pestis*,[9] *Clostridium septicum*,[35] group G streptococci,[5] *Serratia marcescens*,[19] bacille Calmette-Guérin,[49] *Enterobacter agglomerans* (*Erwinia* species),[73] *Aeromonas hydrophila*,[31] *Mycobacterium chelonei*,[3] *Brucella melitensis*,[2] *Salmonella arizonae*,[7] *Listeria monocytogenes*,[39] group C streptococci,[54] *Kingella kingae,* and a number of more common gram-negative organisms. Even though *Bacillus cereus* continues to remain the most common cause of endogenous bacterial endophthalmitis, there have been several series reported in which *Klebsiella pneumoniae* was the most common pathogen isolated.[11,33,47,50,53] These cases have occurred in patients with diabetes and/or with pyogenic liver abscesses, except for one case that occurred after shock wave lithotripsy.

---

*References 2, 3, 5, 7-13, 16, 17, 19, 24, 31-33, 35, 38-40, 43, 45, 47, 49, 50, 53-56, 61, 62, 68, 71, 73.

The decrease in *Neisseria meningitidis* as the most commonly isolated bacterial pathogen was due to the advent of antibiotics in the 1940s and the marked sensitivity of this organism to penicillin. The wide variety of subsequent bacterial pathogens causing endogenous endophthalmitis is understandable given the sporadic occurrence of this rare disease. The emergence of *Bacillus cereus* as the current most frequently isolated organism is surprising. It can be explained, however, by the almost invariable association of intravenous drug use with its occurrence.[36] Almost all organisms that cause endogenous endophthalmitis, with the exception of *Neisseria meningitidis* and *Haemophilus influenzae,* require a host predisposed to infection.

CLINICAL FEATURES

The clinical presentation of endogenous bacterial endophthalmitis can be extremely variable. The usual clinical terms (such as mild, moderate, and severe) are not adequate for describing the complicated differences existing between the various forms of the disease. Greenwald and associates[36] proposed a system of classification dividing metastatic bacterial endophthalmitis into several distinct clinical presentations. In an attempt to quantitate the differences between mild localized infections and cases with overwhelming intraocular sepsis, the classification ranges from focal anterior or posterior infections to diffuse anterior or posterior infections, to panophthalmitis. The clinical findings present in each category of intraocular infections are listed in Table 92-1.

Anterior Focal Infection

Focal anterior bacterial infections usually involve the iris or ciliary body.[44] Lesions in the iris frequently appear as discrete whitish nodules or plaques, 1 to 3 mm in diameter, associated with a moderate-to-marked anterior chamber reaction. When several foci are present there may be an associated hypopyon. There is usually a sluggish pupillary reaction to light. Vitreous details are seen with difficulty because of the severe anterior reaction. With adequate dilation of the pupil, however, the retina can usually be observed with the indirect ophthalmoscope, and it appears to be normal. Intraocular pressure can be normal or elevated.

Posterior Focal Infection

Focal posterior bacterial infections usually involve the retina but may also involve the choroid. Lesions are 1 to 10 disc diameters in size, white or yellowish, and associated with moderate-to-marked cellular reaction with moderate vitreous haze. There is usually only mild external evidence of inflammation, but there may be cells in the aqueous and occasionally a hypopyon. Keratic precipitates are sometimes seen. The intraocular pressure is low or normal, and the pupil reacts sluggishly. If the posterior focus of infection is located near a muscle insertion, there may be underaction of the muscle in that direction.[45] Usually, if the posterior infection is localized, at least some portion of the retina or red reflex can be seen with the indirect ophthalmoscope after dilating the pupil.

Anterior Diffuse Infection

Anterior diffuse endogenous bacterial endophthalmitis is usually characterized by signs of severe anterior segment inflammation: conjunctival injection and chemosis, corneal edema, marked anterior chamber reaction with a fibrin clot and significant hypopyon, and a nonreactive pupil with or without posterior synechia. The vitreous is seen with difficulty because of the severity of the anterior chamber reaction, and no retinal detail is visible. Ultrasonography dem-

TABLE 92-1 CLINICAL CLASSIFICATION OF ENDOGENOUS BACTERIAL ENDOPHTHALMITIS

	Anterior Focal	Posterior Focal	Anterior Diffuse	Posterior Diffuse
Conjunctival reaction	Mild to moderate	Normal or mild	Moderate to marked	Mild to marked
Cornea	Mild-to-moderate haze	Clear with ± precipitate	Moderate-to-marked haze	Clear-to-mild haze
Anterior chamber reaction	Moderate to marked ± hypopyon	Mild to moderate ± hypopyon	Marked to reaction ± hypopyon	Mild to marked ± hypopyon
Iris, pupillary reaction	Microabscess, poor movement ± late synechia	Iris clear, limited with no synechia	Poorly seen, no movement ± synechia	Limited movement ± synechia
Vitreous reaction	Poorly seen ± anterior opacity	Moderate-to-marked cells, moderate haze	Poorly seen ± anterior opacity	Marked cells to opaque
Retina (when seen)	Normal	Discrete lesions	Normal	White retina ± emboli
Tension	Normal to high	Low to normal	Typically high	Variable
Visual prognosis	Excellent	Good	Good	Poor

Modified after Greenwald MJ, Wohl LG, Sell CH: Metastatic bacterial endophthalmitis: a contemporary reappraisal, *Surv Ophthalmol* 31:81-101, 1986.

onstrates a clear vitreous, however, and subsequent examination reveals that the retina is not involved. Typically the intraocular pressure is markedly elevated.

Posterior Diffuse Infection

Posterior diffuse endogenous bacterial endophthalmitis involves the vitreous and retina with such an intense inflammatory reaction that all retinal detail is obscured. In the early course of the disease whitish emboli may be seen scattered in multiple sites in the retinal arteries with associated perivascular hemorrhages. As the infection progresses the retina becomes totally necrotic and the vitreous is filled with inflammatory cells. Vitreous abscess formation and organization frequently occur. The anterior segment remains only moderately involved until late in the disease. A hypopyon may be present and the pupillary reaction is quickly lost as the retina is destroyed. The intraocular pressure is usually low as the disease progresses.

Panophthalmitis

In severe cases of endogenous bacterial endophthalmitis there is involvement of both the anterior and posterior segments of the eye as well as the adjacent extraocular tissues. Signs of panophthalmitis include marked eyelid edema, chemosis of the conjunctiva, proptosis, and limitation of motion. All details of the anterior chamber and iris are lost, and there is usually a prominent hypopyon. The pupil is fixed, and the vitreous and retina cannot be seen. Typically the intraocular pressure is high. Development of a panophthalmitis usually indicates a massive septic embolization of an extremely virulent organism into the intraocular and extraocular blood vessels.

Natural History

Anterior focal bacterial infections may be so mild and so localized that there is hesitancy to use the term endophthalmitis. They can progress rapidly, however, and cause more fulminant infections if they are not treated. A smoldering anterior focal infection may lead to late posterior synechia, iris bombé, and glaucoma. Usually the chance for a good visual outcome is excellent, assuming proper antibiotic treatment. Posterior focal infections are more problematic. Focal areas of infection in the retina and choroid are usually caused by relatively small numbers of organisms that have entered the ocular circulation. As long as the bacteria do not break through the choroidal and retinal tissue into the vitreous, the infection remains localized and there is limitation of the inflammatory response. When the organisms invade the vitreous, the infection very quickly overcomes the inflammatory reaction holding the pathogens in check. As long as the posterior infection remains focal, the chance of visual recovery is good, assuming appropriate antibiotic treatment.

Anterior diffuse endogenous bacterial endophthalmitis is an ocular emergency of the highest order. If the severe generalized anterior infection is not treated immediately, it can quickly spread to involve the entire eye. In the initial stages, however, the retina and vitreous are still uninvolved, and there is an excellent chance for good visual recovery with aggressive appropriate antibiotic therapy. Blindness is usually caused by a delay in treatment.

Posterior diffuse endogenous bacterial endophthalmitis is usually the result of occlusion of the central retinal artery by a septic embolus, followed by seeding of organisms over the entire retina. Ischemia may play a prominent role in the poor visual prognosis. Light perception is usually lost within hours, and the retina is destroyed before therapy can be initiated. Greenwald and associates,[36] in their review of the literature, did not find a single case of posterior diffuse endophthalmitis that recovered useful vision, regardless of management.

Panophthalmitis is also a rapidly developing, disastrous infection that destroys the globe and invades the orbit, producing total necrosis of the retina and all intraocular structures. Every reported case in the literature has resulted in blindness, phthisis, or enucleation.[36] Significantly, some cases of endogenous bacterial endophthalmitis initially confined to the anterior or posterior segment evolved into panophthalmitis when there was a delay in initiation of appropriate antibiotic treatment.[37] Depending on the virulence of the bacterial pathogen, progression of a panophthalmitis may be life threatening.

PATHOLOGY

Pathologic specimens obtained from the enucleated eyes of patients who had suffered metastatic intraocular bacterial infections revealed that in most cases the bacteria are seeded in the small capillaries in the peripheral retina or in blood vessels in the iris or ciliary body. At this point, before the perivascular ocular tissues are invaded, the infection is probably most susceptible to aggressive systemic antibiotic therapy, but delay in initiation of therapy allows the septic emboli to enlarge and produce necrotic foci in the surrounding intraocular structures. The iris and ciliary body microabscesses, which are collections of polymorphonuclear leukocytes (PMNs) around colonies of bacteria, rupture into the aqueous, initially spilling PMNs, and later bacteria, into the anterior chamber. An anterior focal infection quickly becomes diffuse as more PMNs are released and more iris tissue becomes necrotic. In the posterior segment a similar process of bacterial invasion occurs in the perivascular tissue. With multiplication of bacterial organisms, PMNs engulf all areas of the retina in an attempt to wall off the increasing numbers of bacteria. Further retinal necrosis produces breaks in Bruch membrane, and PMNs and bacteria are released into the overlying vitreous. As the vitreous provides a more hospitable environment for growth than the aqueous, the bacteria quickly multiply and are surrounded by a dense inflammatory cellular infiltrate, which results in the formation of a vitreous abscess. At this point a diffuse posterior bacterial endophthalmitis develops, and if the infection is allowed to continue unchecked a panophthalmitis may result involving all the intraocular tissues as well as contiguous extraocular structures.

PATHOGENESIS

Endogenous bacterial endophthalmitis occurs secondary to the hematogenous spread of bacteria to the eye from a site of infection in the body or from contaminated intravenous catheters or needles. Any disease process that produces a septicemia can lead to development of endophthalmitis. Overwhelming bacterial infections, such as meningitis (caused by *Neisseria meningitidis* or *Haemophilus influenzae*) or a severe bacteremic pneumonia (caused by *Streptococcus pneumoniae*), are the most likely disorders to produce the proper conditions, which allow entry of the organisms into the retinal or uveal circulation. Patients of any age may be affected, but often there is a higher incidence in young adults or pediatric patients.[32] Often the site of infection in the body is occult and may require a careful history and physical to detect. Urinary tract infections, endocarditis, septic arthritis, gastrointestinal infections, liver abscesses, and infected skin wounds should be considered if the source of the septicemia is not obvious. Involvement of both eyes occurs in one fourth of all cases. If involvement is unilateral, however, the right eye is affected twice as often as the left, presumably because of more direct blood flow to the right carotid artery.[36] Host factors are of paramount importance in predisposing an individual to metastatic endophthalmitis. A number of commonly associated conditions are listed in the box.

In contrast to exogenous forms of endophthalmitis, the bacteria responsible for the infection in endogenous endophthalmitis are not inoculated directly into the vitreous.

Instead they enter into the uveal or retinal circulation as scattered organisms, or in a bolus, and lodge in the small capillaries. To invade the ocular tissues and produce infection these bacteria must cross the blood-ocular barrier and establish a septic focus. It is likely that only after this focus of infection has been established in close proximity to the blood vessels can large numbers of bacterial organisms break through into the aqueous or vitreous and produce a true endophthalmitis. This natural delay in the clinical evolution of most cases of endogenous bacterial endophthalmitis has important implications for the diagnosis and treatment of the disease at an early stage. First, because the focus of infection usually develops in the retina prior to breaking through into the vitreous, there is a "window of opportunity" for early clinical diagnosis by careful retinal examination. Second, because early development of the focus of infection in the retina must take place in proximity to the retinal blood vessels, treatment with high doses of systemic antibiotics should reach the pathogens in high enough con-

PREDISPOSING HOST FACTORS FOR ENDOGENOUS BACTERIAL ENDOPHTHALMITIS
Chronic alcoholism
Liver abscess/GI infections
Diabetes mellitus
Recent surgery/trauma
Heart abnormalities/endocarditis
Pediatric or newborn infant
Leukemia/lymphoma
Other malignancy
Renal failure
Asplenia
Intravenous drug abuse
Septic arthritis
Infected skin wounds
Urinary tract infections
Pneumonia
Meningitis
Corticosteroid therapy
Acquired immunodeficiency syndrome
General debility/aging

Modified after Greenwald MJ, Wohl LG, Sell CH: Metastatic bacterial endophthalmitis: a contemporary reappraisal, *Surv Ophthalmol* 31:71-101, 1986.

centrations to eliminate them or at least to attenuate the infectious process. If a large septic bolus passes through the central retinal artery and disseminates throughout the retina very rapidly, however, an overwhelming retinal necrosis may occur, allowing the bacteria to quickly invade the vitreous. In such a case, where the initial inoculum is very large, even extremely high doses of appropriate systemic antibiotics will not eliminate the overwhelming numbers of organisms.

Immunologically compromised patients who lack the capacity to mount a normal immune response to these foci of infection are especially susceptible to rapid development of an overwhelming intraocular infectious process. Any defect in the immune system secondary to an underlying condition such as leukemia, lymphoma, hypogammaglobulinemia, or corticosteroid therapy may enhance the rapid development of the infection. In some reports diabetics have been found to be more susceptible to metastatic infection,[16,38,50] and several series have implicated chronic cirrhosis with pyogenic liver abscess and associated debilitation as a major factor predisposing patients to endogenous *Klebsiella pneumoniae* endophthalmitis.[11-13,53] Neonates are also more susceptible to infections, presumably because of their immature immune system.[62] Patients with acquired immunodeficiency syndrome (AIDS) may also develop endogenous bacterial retinitis,[18] but surprisingly few cases have been reported. Low virulence pathogens such as *Staphylococcus epidermidis* have been implicated in several instances.[30] In contrast to other bacterial organisms responsible for metastatic endophthalmitis, *Listeria monocytogenes* appears to be unique in its ability to produce a fulminous infection in otherwise healthy, immunologically competent individuals.[4]

DIFFERENTIAL DIAGNOSIS

Because of the various clinical presentations of endogenous bacterial endophthalmitis, the differential diagnosis includes a diverse list of clinical entities. An anterior focal bacterial infection may easily be confused with any of the disease entities, either infectious or noninfectious, that cause acute anterior uveitis (see box). Individuals who are HLA-B27 positive can develop a severe acute iritis with a hypopyon. A similar clinical picture can be seen with ankylosing spondylitis, Behçet syndrome, and Reiter syndrome. Anterior focal infections may also mimic more

---

DIFFERENTIAL DIAGNOSIS OF ENDOGENOUS BACTERIAL ENDOPHTHALMITIS

Anterior Focal and Diffuse Inflammation
Acute noninfectious uveitis of unknown cause
Behçet syndrome
Reiter syndrome
HLA-B27-associated uveitis
Sarcoidosis
Syphilis
Tuberculosis
Herpes simplex virus-associated anterior uveitis
Zoster ophthalmicus
Fuch uveitis syndrome
Glaucomatocyclitis crisis
Acute angle-closure glaucoma
Posterior Focal and Diffuse Inflammation
Endogenous candidal endophthalmitis
Cryptococcosis
Blastomycosis
Histoplasmosis
Choroidal pneumocystosis
Toxoplasmosis
Toxocariasis
Cytomegalovirus retinitis
Herpes simplex virus retinitis
Varicella-zoster virus retinitis
Epstein-Barr virus infection
Tuberculosis
Syphilis
Sympathetic ophthalmia
Intraocular lymphoma
Leukemia
Metastatic tumors

---

chronic causes of iritis such as sarcoidosis, although the microabscesses present in the iris are usually readily distinguished from the Busacca nodules characteristic of chronic inflammatory conditions. A number of infectious processes such as syphilis, tuberculosis, herpes simplex virus infection, and varicella-zoster virus infection can mimic a focal or diffuse anterior bacterial infection with a marked anterior chamber reaction and/or a hypopyon. Fuchs uveitis syndrome and the acute onset of a glaucomatocyclitic crisis can also be confused with an anterior bacterial infection, as can an attack of acute angle-closure glaucoma. All of these entities should be considered and ruled out by appropriate clinical evaluation or diagnostic studies.

The problem of distinguishing posterior focal or diffuse endogenous bacterial endophthalmitis from other clinical entities becomes much more difficult. Posterior focal infections may be mimicked by a number of disease processes, especially fungal infections. *Candida albicans* is the single most common pathogen causing endogenous fungal endophthalmitis.[14] Those patients at greatest risk are patients on hyperalimentation and hemodialysis. The typical clinical findings are small retinal exudates that grow and extend into the surrounding retina and into the vitreous. Intraretinal hemorrhages with white centers, papillitis, and anterior uveitis with hypopyon are common. Untreated, candidal endophthalmitis progresses to vitreoretinal abscess formation, retinal necrosis, vitreous organization, and retinal detachment.[67] Other fungal organisms that can cause infections mimicking posterior focal bacterial infections with progression to diffuse involvement include *Cryptococcus neoformans*,[41] *Aspergillus* sp.,[48,72] *Blastomyces dermatitidis*,[59] and *Histoplasma capsulatum*.[34]

Opportunistic protozoa may also produce focal posterior lesions in the retina and choroid. In patients with AIDS, *Pneumocystis carinii* causes a characteristic bilateral multifocal choroidopathy.[29] Toxoplasmosis produces a focal retinochoroiditis with typical satellite lesions adjacent to chorioretinal scars, mild-to-moderate overlying vitreous reaction, and anterior uveitis.[42] In contrast, *Toxicara canis* infections can present as full-blown posterior endophthalmitis that can only be diagnosed by vitrectomy[51] or by careful echography.[70]

Viral diseases that can mimic a posterior focal bacterial infection include infections with cytomegalovirus (CMV), herpes simplex virus, and varicella-zoster virus.[60] Cytomegalovirus retinitis is the most common opportunistic ocular infection associated with AIDS; it is characterized by confluent patches of retinal necrosis frequently associated with hemorrhages and perivascular sheathing.[65] CMV retinitis may be the initial manifestation of AIDS in up to 15% of undiagnosed patients.[64] Very early, small foci of disease might be mistaken for a bacterial retinitis before developing the granular border characteristic of CMV retinitis. This infection does not occur in otherwise normal hosts. Acute retinal necrosis (ARN) syndrome, which produces vasculitis, confluent necrotizing retinitis, a moderate-to-severe vitritis, and anterior segment inflammation, may be mistaken for a posterior bacterial infection. The ARN syndrome is caused by the herpes simplex virus or varicella-zoster virus, and infection can lead to late retinal detachment and blindness.[23] Epstein-Barr virus has also been implicated in producing a multifocal choroiditis and panuveitis, but recent serologic evidence is equivocal.[66] Other infectious causes include tuberculosis and syphilis.[52] Appropriate skin tests and serologic evaluation should aid in ruling out these entities as causes of posterior infection.

Noninfectious disorders that should be considered in the differential diagnosis of posterior focal and diffuse endophthalmitis include those entities already listed under anterior focal and diffuse causes in the box on page 1291, as well as sympathetic ophthalmia,[1] diffuse infiltrating retinoblastoma,[6] primary lymphoma (reticulum cell sarcoma),[58] leukemia, and metastatic tumors. Other necrotic tumors such as choroidal melanoma can also occasionally mimic a severe posterior infection.

LABORATORY INVESTIGATIONS

The diagnosis of endogenous bacterial endophthalmitis depends first of all on a high degree of suspicion by the clinician that this rare problem may be responsible for the clinical findings. The varied presentations of a metastatic bacterial infection make a clinical diagnosis even more difficult. In addition to careful documentation of signs of infection in the anterior and posterior segments of the eye, the risk factors predisposing the patient to septicemia and bacterial seeding of the intraocular tissues must be thoroughly investigated (see box on page 1290). At this point, if a diagnosis of endogenous bacterial endophthalmitis is warranted, the clinician is obligated to proceed immediately with the appropriate clinical and laboratory investigations to avert the potentially blinding complications that can result from a missed diagnosis or a delay in the initiation of appropriate therapy (Table 92-2).

Nonocular Specimens and Tests

As an important first step, blood cultures should be obtained on all patients. Three separate cultures should be obtained in the same manner as recommended for any patient who may have a potentially life-threatening septicemia. As the genitourinary tract and kidneys are often implicated as the source of a bacterial infection, urine cultures should be obtained routinely on all patients.[24] Bacterial cultures of other nonocular sites in the body should also be obtained, depending on the systemic symptoms of the patient. Cultures of the throat, for example, may reveal the source of a beta hemolytic streptococcal infection. Sputum cultures in a patient with upper respiratory symptoms might yield a possible culture for pneumococcus.[10] Sputum should also be

TABLE 92-2 DIAGNOSIS OF ENDOGENOUS BACTERIAL ENDOPHTHALMITIS

	Anterior Focal	Posterior Focal	Anterior Diffuse	Posterior Diffuse
Blood cultures	Yes	Yes	Yes	Yes
Urine cultures	Yes	Yes	Yes	Yes
Other cultures	CSF, sputum, infected skin wounds, liver abscesses, intraabdominal abscesses, infected joints, as indicated			
Aqueous aspiration	Yes	No	Yes	No
Vitreous aspiration	No	Yes*	No	Yes

Modified after Greenwald and associates: Metastatic bacterial endophthalmitis: a contemporary reappraisal, *Surv Ophthalmol* 31:81-101, 1986.
* Only after other cultures are negative or if infection is not improving.

examined for acid-fast organisms. Stool cultures are indicated in any patient with gastrointestinal symptoms. Any skin wounds that are clinically infected should be debrided and cultured. Infected joints, which can provide a source for bacteremia, should be aspirated and cultured. Other more occult sites of infection, such as liver abscesses, should be aspirated and cultured, as they are responsible for an increasing number of intraocular bacterial infections.[11,12] Cerebrospinal fluid (CSF) should be cultured in any patient in which meningitis cannot be definitely ruled out (Table 92-2). Even though meningitis has declined from its previous status as the main cause of endogenous bacterial endophthalmitis, it should always be kept in mind as a possible source of infection, and the CSF should be cultured accordingly.

Other deep-seated occult foci should be considered including endocarditis, osteomyelitis, intraabdominal abscesses, and abscesses of the lungs, kidneys, and retroperitoneal space. Greenwald and associates[36] reported that 80% of 65 patients with metastatic bacterial endophthalmitis had positive bacterial cultures from blood and other nonocular sources. The importance of nonocular cultures cannot be overemphasized in diagnosing metastatic ocular infections.

In some cases the source of infection is so obscure that other diagnostic tests must be pursued. Depending on the patient's physical signs and symptoms; conventional x-ray studies, computerized tomography, and nuclear magnetic resonance imaging studies may be diagnostic. Echocardiography, abdominal ultrasonography, and appropriate scanning techniques using radioactive markers may also help to locate the focus of infection. Close collaboration with an infectious disease consultant is extremely helpful in most cases.

Ocular Specimens and Tests

The main diagnostic goal in all cases of endogenous bacterial endophthalmitis is to identify the bacterial pathogen producing the infection. Unlike other forms of endophthalmitis in which the bacteria is already in the aqueous or vitreous at the time of clinical diagnosis, in metastatic endophthalmitis there may be only a small septic focus present in the iris, ciliary body, retina, or choroid at the initial presentation. The recommendation of Forster and associates[28] that the vitreous should always be cultured in preference to the aqueous is based on experience with exogenous endophthalmitis and not with endogenous infections. In cases of anterior focal or diffuse endophthalmitis, aqueous aspiration is indicated to make a diagnosis (Table 92-2). In cases of focal anterior infection an attempt to aspirate the microabscess in the infected area should be made if the abscess is in an accessible location. In most cases of endogenous bacterial endophthalmitis the patient is phakic. Aqueous aspiration is therefore a high-risk procedure because of the danger of inadvertently nicking the lens capsule and producing a cataract. The aspiration should be performed through a stab incision made at the limbus, using a 25-gauge needle on a tuberculin syringe. No more than 0.1 m should be aspirated. Cultures can then be inoculated onto solid media and into liquid media following the recommendations of Forster.[26] Greenwald and associates[36] reported that no untreated case of anterior endophthalmitis in their series had a negative aqueous culture; aqueous cultures were also positive in nine cases of panophthalmitis that they reviewed. Aqueous cultures are positive prior to treatment except when the infection is confined to the posterior segment. They are then of questionable value.

The issue of whether or not a vitreous aspiration and culture should be done depends largely on the site of involvement and the severity of the infectious process. Vitreous cultures are not recommended in cases of anterior focal or diffuse infection (Table 92-2). At the other end of the spectrum, in diffuse posterior bacterial infection involving the vitreous, there is no doubt that a culture of the vitreous aspirate can be of crucial diagnostic importance. Whether or not to do a vitreous culture becomes equivocal in those cases in which a well-localized posterior focal infectious process has not yet broken through the inner layers of the retina to involve the vitreous. In these patients the chance of a positive bacterial culture is small. Even though there is cellular infiltration and haze in the vitreous over the site of the septic focus, viable bacteria are unlikely. In this situation it is advisable to reculture all other suspicious nonocular sites, including the blood, and to perform a vitreous aspirate only if the other cultures continue to be negative and the infection appears to be getting worse clinically. Vitreous aspiration should be performed in the standard fashion, entering the eye through a stab incision inferotemporally 4 mm posterior to the limbus. The aspiration should be performed with a 22-gauge needle on a tuberculin syringe under direct observation. No more than 0.2 to 0.3 ml of liquid vitreous should be aspirated. Preferably the aspirate should be taken from the site of greatest vitreous involvement, although great care must be taken not to create a retinal tear.

Laboratory Techniques

With few exceptions, ocular bacterial pathogens grow readily in standard media. In most cases aqueous and vitreous aspirates are inoculated on separate blood agar, chocolate agar, brain-heart infusion (BHI) liquid broth, and thioglycolate broth. Chocolate agar should be inoculated as well as blood agar because *Haemophilus influenzae* and *Neisseria meningitidis* will only grow on chocolate agar. Thioglycolate and BHI broth have the advantage of allowing the growth of both aerobic and anaerobic organisms. When numbers of bacterial organisms are small, as they frequently are in aspirates from the aqueous and vitreous in cases of endophthalmitis, liquid media is also more sensitive and will support the growth of a very small inoculum of bacteria. The disadvantage in using liquid media is that it is easily contaminated by bacteria in the laboratory or by other nonvirulent pathogens present on the surface of the patient's eye at the time of aspiration. These contaminants can overgrow a liquid medium and lead to false assumptions regarding the true cause of infection. In addition to bacterial cultures on standard media, special media may be used when atypical bacterial pathogens such as *Mycobacterium tuberculosis* are suspected. A small amount of the aspirate should also be inoculated onto several microscopic slides and stained with Gram and Giemsa stain for immediate diagnosis. One or two unstained slides should be held in reserve in the event that unusual stains are needed (such as acid-fast stains) to diagnose atypical bacterial organisms. Recently a new culture method for diagnosing infectious endophthalmitis has been reported in which vitreous aspirates are inoculated directly into blood culture bottles.[46] This relatively simple method may be an acceptable adjunct or alternative to more sophisticated laboratory techniques for culturing vitreous aspirates in infectious endophthalmitis.

THERAPY

Endogenous bacterial endophthalmitis is a medical emergency. As in the management of exogenous endophthalmitis, time is the crucial element in determining whether or not a patient will retain useful vision. Any delay in appropriate aggressive antibiotic therapy can result in a poor visual outcome.

The other important point to keep in mind is that in most cases of endogenous endophthalmitis, intensive systemic treatment is the most effective route for delivering antibiotics to the site of infection. An appreciation of this concept requires that the clinician think of endogenous endophthalmitis as a unique entity within the general classification of endophthalmitis. The therapeutic approach is the same one would use in treating any other generalized systemic infectious disease. The dosages of antibiotics are the same as those recommended for the treatment of meningitis or any other serious life-threatening infection.

Systemic Antibiotics

The most critical element in the treatment of endogenous bacterial endophthalmitis is prompt initiation of intensive intravenous antibiotic administration[36] (Table 92-3). The dosages should be based on serum drug levels. The choice of drug depends on culture and sensitivity results, and systemic treatment should be continued for 2 to 3 weeks or longer, until it is certain that the systemic infection has been eradicated. Because of the varied species of bacteria responsible for infection, the choice of antibiotics prior to obtaining results from culture and sensitivities depends on the most likely source of the infection. In previously healthy children, penicillin G or ampicillin is indicated, especially if there is evidence of meningitis or endocarditis. If *Haemophilus influenzae* is the possible pathogen, systemic chloramphenicol should be added because of its excellent penetration across the blood-ocular barrier and because of its marked effectiveness against this organism. When the intraocular bacterial pathogen is unknown and no focus of systemic infection is evident, a combination of ceftazidime 1.0 gram intravenously every 12 hours and vancomycin 1.0 gram intravenously every 12 hours can be used to cover the entire spectrum of possible organisms. Ceftazidime has excellent penetration into the ocular tissues and is effective against almost all strains of *Pseudomonas* sp. and many other gram-negative organisms. Vancomycin has excellent broad-spectrum coverage against all gram-positive organisms, including almost all strains of penicillinase-producing staphylococci and all strains of streptococci. Ototoxicity and renal toxicity must be monitored. Wang and associates[71] have reported excellent visual results in two cases of metastatic endophthalmitis (caused by *Klebsiella pneumoniae* and *Enterobacter agglomerans*) using high doses of parenteral ceftriaxone (2.0 grams intravenously every 12 hours). Other investigators have recommended a combination of ceftriaxone 1.0 gram intravenously every 12 hours and gentamicin

80 mg intravenously every 8 hours.[25] In any case where *Bacillus cereus* is suspected, a combination of parenteral vancomycin and gentamicin appears to be most effective.[18]

Local Antibiotics

Subconjunctival or sub-Tenon injections of antibiotic are of no value in posterior focal and diffuse endogenous endophthalmitis. They may be of use, however, in both anterior focal and anterior diffuse infections (Table 92-3). An initial subconjunctival injection of 40 mg of tobramycin and 125 mg of cefazolin should be given as soon as treatment is initiated in anterior bacterial infections. Presumably enough antibiotic penetrates into the aqueous to aid in containing the infection while systemic concentrations of the antibiotics are reaching therapeutic levels.

Antibiotic drops are of less value than periocular injections in anterior segment infections and are of no value in posterior bacterial infections. Many clinicians prescribe them because of the severity of the infectious process, but from a theoretical point of view they are optional.

Intravitreal antibiotic injections have revolutionized the treatment of exogenous bacterial endophthalmitis, but in endogenous bacterial infections their usefulness is of questionable value. Certainly they are not indicated in almost all cases of anterior focal and diffuse endophthalmitis because of the good visual results obtained with systemic treatment. In posterior focal infections the question of intravitreal antibiotics becomes more complicated. The majority of cases with posterior focal infections do well with systemic antibiotics alone. Nevertheless, if after 1 to 2 days of maximum systemic antibiotic treatment there is continued clinical deterioration and further retinal necrosis with breakthrough into the vitreous, intravitreal antibiotics should be given. If the bacterial pathogen has not been isolated, broad-spectrum coverage can be obtained by giving 1.0 mg of vancomycin in 0.1 ml and 1.0 mg of ceftazidime in 0.1 ml intravitreally. In the past gentamicin has been the drug of choice for intravitreal injection, but many reports of retinal toxicity have lead to the use of other, less-toxic medications.[15] Cases of posterior diffuse bacterial infections should be treated early with intravitreal antibiotics.

Corticosteroids

Corticosteroids can be administered topically and periocularly in cases of anterior focal and diffuse disease to prevent complications (such as glaucoma or synechiae) of the inflammatory reaction. Topical prednisolone acetate 1.0% can be given hourly for severe anterior chamber reactions with hypopyon, and dexamethasone phosphate (4 mg in 1.0 ml) can be given as a subconjunctival injection daily (if necessary). In severe cases of posterior infection when intravitreal antibiotics are being administered, 0.4 mg of parenteral dexamethasone phosphate without preservatives can be given intravitreally in 0.1 ml. In severe infections in

TABLE 92-3 TREATMENT OF ENDOGENOUS BACTERIAL ENDOPHTHALMITIS

	Anterior Focal	Posterior Focal	Anterior Diffuse	Posterior Diffuse
Intravenous antibiotics	Yes	Yes	Yes	Yes
Periocular antibiotics	Yes	No	Yes	No
Intravitreal antibiotics	No	Yes*	No	Yes
Topical antibiotics	Optional	No	Optional	No

Modified after Greenwald MJ, Wohl LG, Sell CH: Metastatic bacterial endophthalmitis: a contemporary reappraisal, *Surv Ophthalmol* 31:81-101, 1986.
* Only after 1 to 2 days of appropriate systemic antibiotics, if deteriorating.

which retinal necrosis and hemorrhage are continuing, 120 to 140 mg of prednisone can be given orally every day for a short period of time. In addition, it is important to administer mydriatic drops to prevent posterior synechia, and any elevation in intraocular pressure should be treated with topical beta adrenergic blocking agents or with oral carbonic anhydrase inhibitors.

Surgical Management

Advances in the surgical treatment of intraocular infections have resulted in improvement of the visual prognosis in cases of postoperative and traumatic endophthalmitis in recent years,[57] but the surgical management of metastatic endophthalmitis is controversial.[36] Vitrectomy should not be considered in anterior focal or diffuse infections or in posterior focal bacterial infections that are responding to treatment. Vitrectomy may improve the prognosis of posterior diffuse endophthalmitis in which marked vitritis and vitreous abscess are part of the clinical presentation. Garg and associates[32] reported 10 cases of metastatic endophthalmitis, all of which responded poorly to medical management. Seven of the ten patients eventually underwent vitrectomy, and four of the seven developed useful vision of 6/60 or better. Pars plana vitrectomy may, therefore, have a definite role in the management of cases of severe posterior diffuse bacterial endophthalmitis. Vitrectomy should be followed by intraocular antibiotics combining amikacin 0.4 mg or ceftazidime 1.0 mg with vancomycin 1.0 mg.[21]

PROGNOSIS

The visual prognosis in the milder forms of endogenous bacterial endophthalmitis is surprisingly good. Anterior focal bacterial infections have an excellent chance for the recovery of normal vision if they are properly diagnosed and treated in a timely fashion (Table 92-1). Similarly, anterior diffuse endophthalmitis and posterior focal bacterial infections (if treated in an expeditious manner) may be expected to recover useful vision in a relatively high percentage of patients. Unfortunately the visual prognosis for patients with posterior diffuse bacterial endophthalmitis is very guarded. This group of patients may benefit from a combination of intensive parenteral antibiotic treatment and vitrectomy followed by intravitreal antibiotics. Once a patient has progressed to panophthalmitis, the visual outcome is uniformly dismal, despite heroic therapeutic measures.

The key factors affecting visual outcome include (1) the pathogenicity of the organism, (2) the size of the bacterial inoculum, (3) the primary site of embolization in the eye, and (4) the delay in time between clinical diagnosis and initiation of appropriate antibiotic therapy. All of these factors are beyond the control of the clinician, except the urgency with which treatment is begun after the diagnosis has been made. Pathogenic organisms such as *Bacillus cereus* uniformly result in a blind eye or in panophthalmitis, despite the treatment instituted. The size of the bacterial inoculum is often a function of the severity of the underlying systemic disease process or the seriousness of the primary focus of infection. The site of septic embolization is largely by chance, although organisms such as *Haemophilus influenzae* seem to preferentially involve the anterior segment. Improvements in visual outcome depend almost entirely on the speed with which aggressive and appropriate systemic antibiotic treatment is initiated.

PREVENTION

Prevention of endogenous bacterial endophthalmitis does not lie within the scope of the practice of the clinician. Eradication of all systemic bacterial infections would certainly eliminate the majority of cases, but many of these infections are occult and are not manifest until complications like metastatic endophthalmitis have occurred. It is within the scope of the clinician, however, to examine patients who are at risk for developing metastatic bacterial endophthalmitis. Patients who are immunocompromised, whether from AIDS, diabetes mellitus, or chronic alcoholism, and who have signs or symptoms of systemic infection should have a retinal examination if possible. In a series of 180 patients with pyogenic liver abscess, Chiu and associates[12] found the prevalence of metastatic endophthalmitis to be 1.7%, but patients who specifically had *Klebsiella* sp. cultured from their abscess had a prevalence of 5.2%. The authors concluded that a high index of suspicion is critical in making an early diagnosis and preventing blindness in those patients who are at high risk of developing endogenous bacterial endophthalmitis.

Any patient who has at least one of the host factors (see box on page 1290) should be considered at risk for the development of endogenous bacterial endophthalmitis. The importance of metastatic endophthalmitis as the initial manifestation of a generalized septicemia should constantly be kept in mind. Patients at risk should have periodic dilated examinations of their retina, especially if they have any symptoms of ocular inflammation, photophobia, or blurred vision. The eye should be searched for septic foci of infection, and if the clinical diagnosis of endogenous bacterial endophthalmitis is made, early systemic treatment should be started to prevent blindness and to avert the life-threatening complications of sepsis.

REFERENCES

1. Albert DM, Diaz-Rohena R: A historical review of sympathetic ophthalmia and its epidemiology, *Surv Ophthalmol* 34:1-14, 1989.
2. al Farou MF: Brucella melitensis endophthalmitis, *Ophthalmologica* 201:19-22, 1990.
3. Ambler JS et al.: Endogenous Mycobacterium chelonae endophthalmitis, *Am J Ophthalmol* 108:338-339, 1989.
4. Bagnarello AG et al.: Listeria monocytogenes endophthalmitis, *Arch Ophthalmol* 95:1004-1005, 1977.
5. Berkey PB, Rolston K: Group G streptocci as a cause of bacterial endophthalmitis, *Arch Ophthalmol* 106:171-172, 1988.

6. Bhatnagar R, Vine AK: Diffuse infiltrating retinoblastoma, *Ophthalmology* 98:1657-1661, 1991.

7. Caravalho J Jr et al.: Endogenous endophthalmitis due to Salmonella arizonae and Hafnia alvei, *South Med J* 83:325-327, 1990.

8. Carden SM et al.: Kingella kingae endophthalmitis in an infant, *Aust NZ J Ophthalmol* 19:217-220, 1991.

9. Carter DB, Ellis PP: Yersinia pestis endophthalmitis, *Am J Ophthalmol* 103:721-722, 1987.

10. Cheesbrough JS et al.: Metastatic pneumococcal endophthalmitis: report of two cases and review of literature, *J Infect* 20:231-236, 1990.

11. Cheng DL et al.: Septic metastatic lesions of pyogenic liver abscess: their association with Klebsiella pneumoniae bacteremia in diabetic patients, *Arch Int Med* 151:1557-1559, 1991.

12. Chiu CT, Lin DY, Liaw YF: Metastatic septic endophthalmitis in pyogenic liver abscess, *J Clin Gastroenterol* 10:524-527, 1988.

13. Chiu KW, Liaw YF: Endogenous septic endophthalmitis in severe acute hepatitis with septicemia, *J Clin Gastroenterol* 13:694-696, 1991.

14. Clinch TE et al.: Infantile endogenous Candida endophthalmitis presenting as a cataract, *Surv Ophthalmol* 34:107-112, 1989.

15. Conway BP, Campochiaro PA: Macular infarction after endophthalmitis treated with vitrectomy and intravitreal gentamicin, *Arch Ophthalmol* 104:367-371, 1986.

16. Cordido M et al.: Bilateral metastatic endophthalmitis in diabetes, *Acta Ophthalmologica* 69:266-267, 1991.

17. Cowan CL et al.: Endogenous Bacillus cereus panophthalmitis, *Ann Ophthalmol* 19:65-68, 1987.

18. Davis JL et al.: Endogenous bacterial retinitis in AIDS, *Am J Ophthalmol* 107:613-623, 1989.

19. de Courten C, Sancho P, Ben Ezra D: Metastatic Serratia marcescens endophthalmitis, *J Pediatr Ophthalmol Strabismus* 25:45-47, 1988.

20. Diamond JG: Intraocular management of endophthalmitis, a systematic approach, *Arch Ophthalmol* 99:96-99, 1981.

21. Doft BH: The endophthalmitis vitrectomy study, *Arch Ophthalmol* 109:487-488, 1991.

22. Duke-Elder S: Diseases of the uveal tract. In *System of ophthalmology*, vol 9, St Louis, 1966, Mosby.

23. Duker JS, Blumenkranz MS: Diagnosis and management of the acute retinal necrosis (ARN) syndrome, *Surv Ophthalmol* 35:327-343, 1991.

24. Faraawi R, Fong IW: Escherichia coli emphysematous endophthalmitis and pyelonephritis: case report and review of the literature, part 2, *Am J Med* 84 (3):636-639, 1988.

25. Flynn HW et al.: Endophthalmitis therapy: changing antibiotic sensitivity patterns and current therapeutic recommendations, *Arch Ophthalmol* 109:175-176, 1991.

26. Forster RK: Endophthalmitis: diagnostic cultures and visual results, *Arch Ophthalmol* 92:387-392, 1974.

27. Forster RK, Abbott RL, Gelender H: Management of infectious endophthalmitis, *Ophthalmology* 87:313-318, 1980.

28. Forster RK et al.: Further observations on the diagnosis, cause, and treatment of endophthalmitis, *Am J Ophthalmol* 81:52-56, 1976.

29. Foster RE et al.: Presumed Pneumocystis carinii choroiditis: unifocal presentation, regression with intravenous pentamidine, and choroiditis recurrence, *Ophthalmology* 98:1360-1365, 1991.

30. Freeman WR et al.: Retinopathy before the diagnosis of AIDS, *Ann Ophthalmol* 21:468-474, 1989.

31. Frieling et al.: Endogenous Aeromonas hydrophilia endophthalmitis, *Ann Ophthalmol* 21:117-118, 1989.

32. Garg SP, Talwar D, Verma LK: Metastatic endophthalmitis: a reappraisal, *Ann Ophthalmol* 23:74-78, 1991.

33. Glassman RM et al.: Endogenous Klebsiella endophthalmitis: case report, *Mt Sinai J Med* 56:326-329, 1989.

34. Goldstein BG, Buettner KF: Histoplasmic endophthalmitis: a clinicopathologic correlation, *Arch Ophthalmol* 101:774-777, 1983.

35. Green MT et al.: Endogenous Clostridium panophthalmitis, *Ophthalmology* 94:435-438, 1987.

36. Greenwald MJ, Wohl LG, Sell CH: Metastatic bacterial endophthalmitis: a contemporary reappraisal, *Surv Ophthalmol* 31:81-101, 1986.

37. Hatem G, Merritt JC, Cowan CL Jr: Bacillus cereus panophthalmitis after intravenous heroin, *Ann Ophthalmol* 11:431-440, 1979.

38. Havunjian RH, Goldberg RA, Hepler RS: Bacterial endogenous endophthalmitis in a patient with diabetes and renal papillary necrosis, *Am J Ophthalmol* 111:654, 1991.

39. Heidemann DG et al.: Endogenous Listeria monocytogenes endophthalmitis presenting as keratouveitis, *Cornea* 9:179-180, 1990.

40. Hemady R et al.: Bacillus-induced endophthalmitis: new series of 10 cases and review of the literature, *Br J Ophthalmol* 74:26-29, 1990.

41. Hiss PW, Shields JA, Augsburger JJ: Solitary retinovitreal abscess as the initial manifestation of cryptococcosis, *Ophthalmology* 95:162-165, 1988.

42. Holland GN et al.: Ocular toxoplasmosis in patients with the acquired immunodeficiency syndrome, *Am J Ophthalmol* 106:653-667, 1988.

43. Hornblass A et al.: Endogenous orbital cellulitis and endogenous endophthalmitis in subacute bacterial endocarditis, *Am J Ophthalmol* 108:196-197, 1989.

44. Horner WD, Cordes FC: Metastatic abscess of iris and ciliary body, *Am J Ophthalmol* 14:628-633, 1931.

45. Ishibashi Y et al.: Endogenous Nocardia asteroides endophthalmitis in a patient with systemic lupus erythematosus, *Br J Ophthalmol* 74:433-436, 1990.

46. Joondeph BC et al.: A new culture method for infectious endophthalmitis, *Arch Ophthalmol* 107:1334-1337, 1989.

47. Kremer I et al.: Klebsiella metastatic endophthalmitis—a complication of shock wave lithotripsy, *Ophthalmol Surg* 21:206-208, 1990.

48. Lance SE, Friberg TR, Kowalski RP: Aspergillus flavus endophthalmitis and retinitis in an intravenous drug abuser, *Ophthalmology* 95:947-949, 1988.

49. Lester H et al.: Bacillus calmette-guerin (BCG) endophthalmitis, *Retina* 8:182-184, 1988.

50. Liao HR et al.: Endogenous Klebsiella pneumoniae endophthalmitis in diabetic patients, *Can J Ophthalmol* 27:143-147, 1992.

51. Maguire AM et al.: Recovery of intraocular Toxocara canis by pars plana vitrectomy, *Ophthalmology* 97:675-680, 1990.

52. Margo CE, Hamed LM: Ocular syphilis, *Surv Ophthalmol* 37:203-220, 1992.

53. Martinez M et al.: Septic endophthalmitis associated with bacteremia and liver abscess caused by Klebsiella pneumoniae, *Bol Asoc Med P R* 83:845-846, 1991.

54. Moffett DG Jr, Edward DP: Anterior segment necrosis associated with endogenous endophthalmitis secondary to group C Streptococcal septicemia, *Can J Ophthalmol* 26:283-287, 1991.

55. O'Brien CJ, Kyle GM: Metastatic Staphylococcus aureus endophthalmitis: a case report, *Br J Ophthalmol* 72:189-191, 1988.

56. Ormerod LD et al.: Anaerobic bacterial endophthalmitis, *Ophthalmology* 94:799-808, 1987.

57. Peyman GA, Raichand M, Bennett TO: Management of endophthalmitis with pars plana vitrectomy, *Br J Ophthalmol* 64:472-475, 1980.

58. Ridley ME et al.: Retinal manifestations of ocular lymphoma (reticulum cell sarcoma), *Ophthalmology* 99:1153-1161, 1992.

59. Safneck JR, Hogg GR, Napier LB: Endophthalmitis due to Blastomyces dermatitidis, *Ophthalmology* 97:212-216, 1990.

60. Schulman JA, Peyman GA: Management of viral retinitis, *Ophthalmic Surg* 19:876-884, 1988.

61. Schutze GE, Englund JA, Bresee JS: Pseudomonas aeruginosa endogenous endophthalmitis in a neonate, *Pediatr Infect Dis J* 8:893-895, 1989.

62. Sekimoto M et al.: Endogenous Escherichia coli endophthalmitis in a patient with autosomal-dominant polycystic kidney, *Ann Ophthalmol* 23:458-459, 1991.

63. Shammas HF: Endogenous E. coli endophthalmitis, *Surv Ophthalmol* 21:429-435, 1977.

64. Sison RF et al.: Cytomegalovirus retinopathy as the initial manifestation of the acquired immunodeficiency syndrome, *Am J Ophthalmol* 112:243-249, 1991.

65. Skolnik PR et al.: Dual infection of retina with human immunodeficiency virus type 1 and cytomegalovirus, *Am J Ophthalmol* 107:361-372, 1989.

66. Spaide RF et al.: Epstein-Barr virus antibodies in multifocal choroiditis and panuveitis, *Am J Ophthalmol* 112:410-413, 1991.

67. Uliss AE, Walsh JB: Candida endophthalmitis, *Ophthalmology* 90:1378, 1983.
68. Vahey JB, Flynn HW Jr: Results in the management of Bacillus endophthalmitis, *Ophthalmic Surg* 22:681-686, 1991.
69. Virchow R: Uber capillare embolie, *Virchows Arch Pathol Anat* 9:307, 1856.
70. Wan WL et al.: Echographic characteristics of ocular toxoplasmosis, *Ophthalmology* 98:28-32, 1991.
71. Wang FD et al.: Successful treatment of metastatic endophthalmitis. Case reports, *Ophthalmologica* 198:124-128, 1989.
72. Wilmarth SS et al.: Aspergillus endophthalmitis in an intravenous drug user, *Ann Ophthalmol* 15:470-476, 1983.
73. Zeiter et al.: Endogenous endophthalmitis with lenticular abscess caused by Enterobacter agglomerans (Erwinia species), *Ophthalmic Surg* 20:9-12, 1989.

93 Exogenous Endophthalmitis

SID MANDELBAUM, RICHARD K. FORSTER

Endophthalmitis, or inflammation of intraocular tissues, is most frequently caused by microbial organisms. Much less commonly, endophthalmitis results from direct physical or chemical tissue injury or from immunologic or neoplastic processes. In clinical practice the term *endophthalmitis* generally refers to microbial endophthalmitis. Microbial endophthalmitis may be caused by organisms from the external environment entering the eye (usually after ocular surgery or penetrating ocular trauma, and termed *exogenous endophthalmitis*) or as a result of hematogenous spread of organisms to the eye (often termed *endogenous endophthalmitis*). The pathogenesis, clinical setting, clinical features, and to some extent the treatment of endogenous endophthalmitis differ from endophthalmitis caused by exogenously-introduced organisms. This chapter will be devoted to a discussion of exogenous endophthalmitis.

Most cases of exogenous endophthalmitis develop following intraocular surgery. Endophthalmitis may occur after any surgical procedure during which there has been communication between the interior of the eye and the external environment. Because cataract extraction is by far the most common ophthalmic surgical procedure, most cases of postoperative endophthalmitis follow cataract surgery. Endophthalmitis has also developed after seemingly "minor" surgical procedures such as strabismus surgery with inadvertent scleral perforation,[143] anterior chamber paracentesis,[83] repositioning of a lens implant,[52] and posterior capsulotomy performed with a needle.[52,136] These cases serve as reminders that the possibility of exogenously-introduced infection must be considered after any surgical procedure that breaches the integrity of the corneoscleral wall of the eye, no matter how "minor" this breach may seem.

Although most cases of postoperative endophthalmitis become evident shortly after the surgical procedure, some cases may not manifest for months or even years postoperatively. These "late" cases fall into two groups: in the first, organisms enter the eye long after the operation, and endophthalmitis develops rapidly. These patients must have an avenue for the infecting organisms to enter the eye, such as a wound dehiscence or a filtering bleb. The second group (cases with what has been called *chronic endophthalmitis*) comprises patients who manifest the inflammation late, but in whom all evidence indicates that the organisms have actually been present within the eye since the surgical procedure itself. Organisms isolated from this group of patients have been relatively less virulent, such as *Propionibacterium acnes, Staphylococcus epidermidis,* and fungi.

As a result of penetrating eye injuries, particularly destructive organisms may gain access to the eye. Ocular damage resulting from the injury may combine with the infectious process to cause very severe ocular damage.

On the basis of large clinical series, it has been determined that certain organisms predominate in these different categories of exogenous endophthalmitis, resulting in variations in the clinical presentation and prognosis. Awareness of these differences allows for modifications in the therapeutic approach based on the most likely causative organisms.

HISTORICAL BACKGROUND

A seminal study that increased our understanding of the pathophysiology of microbial endophthalmitis was the laboratory investigation reported by Maylath and Leopold[107] in 1955, in which they demonstrated in a rabbit model that the anterior chamber was more capable of resisting exogenously-introduced bacteria than was the posterior chamber. In this model large numbers of organisms introduced into the anterior chamber might not cause endophthalmitis, whereas even a small number of organisms injected into the vitreous cavity would result in progressive ocular infection.

During this era the diagnosis of endophthalmitis was based upon clinical examination and inference of the intraocular infectious agent from conjunctival cultures. Theodore[163] in 1964 emphasized that the intraocular infection could be caused by organisms that were completely different from those isolated from conjunctival cultures and recommended anterior chamber paracentesis for diagnosis of endophthalmitis. Allansmith and associates[7] in 1970 reported culturing the infectious agent from 5 of 14 cases of suspected postoperative endophthalmitis in whom they performed an anterior chamber diagnostic tap. In an experimental rabbit model reported in 1972, Tucker and Forster[166] confirmed the potential value of anterior chamber paracentesis in diagnosis of endophthalmitis.

Recognizing the importance of the vitreous in the infectious process, Forster began diagnostically aspirating the vitreous directly. In 1974 he reported that some eyes with clinical signs of endophthalmitis, but negative aqueous cultures, did grow organisms from vitreous aspirates.[62] In a subsequent larger clinical series in 1976 Forster and associates[66] confirmed that organisms could frequently be grown from the vitreous despite negative aqueous cultures. In a later series reported in 1980 Forster and associates[65] found that of 78 culture-positive eyes, 27 had growth from the vitreous only while the aqueous specimen was culture-negative. Occasional cases have been documented, however, where organisms grew from the aqueous despite a negative vitreous culture.[52,65] Accordingly it has been recommended that both aqueous and vitreous be sampled to provide the highest yield when obtaining cultures in patients with endophthalmitis.[52]

As the number of patients treated in clinical series increased, it was recognized that specific organisms were more likely to cause endophthalmitis in the different clinical categories of presentation: acute postoperative,[52,65] bleb-related,[101] and posttraumatic.[3,26,27] Patients developing low-grade, chronic intraocular inflammation with granulomatous features after cataract extraction were reported in the early to mid 1980s and were thought to have phacoanaphylactic endophthalmitis.[2,9,110,170] In 1986 Meisler and associates[112] reported 6 patients with chronic postoperative endophthalmitis clinically indistinguishable from these cases, but from whose vitreous or aqueous specimens they isolated *Propionibacterium* species, usually *P. acnes*. Although other causative organisms of this syndrome have been subsequently reported, the most frequent isolate remains *Propionibacterium* sp. The recognition that this syndrome is microbial in cause affirms the principle that all cases of endophthalmitis should be assumed to be microbial, with evaluation of extensive cultures (including anaerobic cultures properly maintained for 2 weeks), smears, and histopathologic specimens performed before cases are ascribed to a culture-negative category.

Therapeutically, the concept of intraocular administration of antibiotics (then penicillin) was first recommended by von Sallmann[169] in 1944. As then used, this approach to therapy was not effective clinically, and was abandoned for decades. In the 1970s Peyman and associates[11,40,73,106,131] and Forster and associates[36,58,173] revived interest in intravitreal antibiotic administration, determined nontoxic intravitreal doses of selected antibiotics, and tested them in experimental models. In 1974 both Peyman[132] and Forster[62] reported the successful treatment of several eyes with endophthalmitis with intravitreal antibiotics. Multiple additional reports of successful treatment of patients with endophthalmitis followed,[46,65,66,168] and intravitreal administration of antibiotics rapidly became the accepted standard of care.

Preliminary investigation of the use of vitrectomy in an experimental rabbit model of *Pseudomonas aeruginosa* endophthalmitis by Peyman and associates[131a] in 1975 did not demonstrate better results than other methods of treatment, although histopathology did show removal of abscess products. In 1976 Cottingham and Forster[38] did demonstrate that a combination of vitrectomy and intraocular antibiotics was more effective in sterilizing *Staphylococcus aureus* endophthalmitis in a rabbit model than were antibiotics alone. The combination of vitrectomy and intraocular antibiotics was quickly applied to patients with endophthalmitis,[54,65,66,168] and this approach has been used for varying indications since. The inability to ascertain the optimum role and timing of vitrectomy in patients with endophthalmitis based on existing clinical series has prompted a prospective, randomized, ongoing multicenter trial.[49]

EPIDEMIOLOGY

Improvements in aseptic and in surgical techniques, and increased precision in the diagnosis of endophthalmitis over the past years with the use of cultures of intraocular fluids, make older data on the incidence of this condition less relevant than recently-performed studies. Two recent studies have determined the incidence of postoperative endophthalmitis using different approaches.

Postsurgical Endophthalmitis

Kattan and associates[87] reviewed a series of 30,002 intraocular surgical procedures performed by many different surgeons at one university-affiliated, specialty eye hospital between 1984 and 1989. They determined the following incidences of culture-proved microbial endophthalmitis, making the assumption that any cases of endophthalmitis that developed returned to the same institution for treatment: after extracapsular cataract extraction with or without intraocular lens implantation—0.072% (17 of 23,625 cases); after penetrating keratoplasty—0.11% (2 of 1,783 cases); after glaucoma filtering surgery—0.061% (1 of 1,632 cases); after secondary intraocular lens insertion—0.30% (3 of 988 cases); after pars plana vitrectomy—0.051% (1 of 1974 cases).

Javitt and associates[80] used a national Medicare database to analyze the likelihood of rehospitalization for endophthalmitis within one year of having undergone cataract extraction. They evaluated 338,141 Medicare beneficiaries over age 65 who had undergone cataract extraction in a U.S. hospital in 1984, representing approximately one half of all

Medicare patients who underwent cataract extraction that year. As opposed to Kattan's study, in which extensive clinical information was available for each patient, this study was performed based on discharge coding for each patient's hospitalization with no detailed clinical information available. Javitt determined a risk of rehospitalization for endophthalmitis within one month of initial surgery of 0.085% for extracapsular cataract extraction (ECCE) and 0.11% for intracapsular cataract extraction (ICCE). Including cases rehospitalized within one year of initial surgery increased the incidence to 0.12% for ECCE and 0.17% for ICCE. Javitt did not have the data to allow determination of which of these cases were culture-positive.

Kattan's study may underestimate the true rate of endophthalmitis because some individuals may have sought treatment at another hospital; Javitt's study probably overestimates the rate of microbial endophthalmitis both by including cases admitted as endophthalmitis that were actually a different entity and by including culture-negative cases. The actual incidence of endophthalmitis caused by microbial organisms after cataract extraction as performed in the United States in the mid-1980s is probably bracketed by these two studies.

Far fewer patients undergo keratoplasty than cataract extraction, making determination of the incidence of endophthalmitis after keratoplasty less accurate. In general, somewhat higher incidences have been reported after keratoplasty than after cataract extraction, ranging from 0.11% to 0.77%.* This higher incidence is not surprising, because patients undergoing keratoplasty have not only the risks of the surgical intervention but also the additional potential risk that the donor cornea they receive might be contaminated.

The likelihood of developing endophthalmitis "late" after cataract extraction has not been evaluated; some of these cases were likely included in Javitt's series, which tabulated incidences of rehospitalization up to one year postoperatively. This subgroup of patients is heterogenous, including patients who develop wound problems with secondary infection as well as patients with chronic endophthalmitis that becomes manifest late after surgery.

Posttraumatic Endophthalmitis

As would be expected, the incidence of microbial endophthalmitis developing after ocular trauma appears to be considerably higher than after elective ocular surgery. Typical series have far fewer cases, with widely varying incidences.[13,26,27] The setting in which the trauma occurs appears to affect the likelihood of developing intraocular infection. Boldt and associates[26] analyzed their cases of endophthalmitis developing after ocular trauma over a 10-year period. They found that 30% (24 of 80) of individuals who sustained

---

*References 4, 8, 31, 61, 87, 88, 95.

an injury in a rural setting (farm or other outdoor work) developed endophthalmitis, compared with 11% (23 of 204) of patients whose injury occurred in a nonrural environment. Feist and associates[56] reported six patients who sustained penetrating ocular injuries caused by eating utensils recently in contact with the oral cavity: 67% (4 of 6) developed culture-positive endophthalmitis. The large number of pathogenic bacteria present in the oral cavity apparently make this type of injury particularly likely to result in endophthalmitis.

RISK FACTORS

For endophthalmitis to develop, a sufficiently large number of microorganisms must enter the eye so that they cannot be eliminated by host defenses. Risk factors may be broadly divided into two categories: (1) those factors that increase the likelihood of pathogenic organisms entering the eye and (2) those factors that might make it less likely for the eye to be able to eliminate these organisms before they progress to cause severe intraocular inflammation.

Surgical Contamination

Clusters of cases of endophthalmitis have been traced to contaminated intraocular irrigating solutions[157] and to contaminated intraocular lenses.[70,130] Inadequate sterilization of any fluid, instrument, or prosthetic device used in surgery upon the eye certainly poses a risk factor for the development of endophthalmitis. Sterilization techniques for intraocular lenses have become well standardized, and there have been no infections related to inadequate sterilization of intraocular lenses reported in the United States for more than a decade.

Accumulating evidence indicates that the causative organisms in the majority of cases of postoperative endophthalmitis derive from the patients own periocular microbial flora.[152] Situations in which the quantity or virulence of periocular organisms are increased would, therefore, likely pose an increased risk of microbial endophthalmitis. Patients with blepharitis or with nasolacrimal sac stasis or infection would be among those presumably at greater risk for endophthalmitis after intraocular surgery. A recent case report has suggested that a patient with a functioning Jones tube might be at increased risk of postoperative endophthalmitis by retrograde passage of airway secretions and organisms onto the operative field.[120] Similarly, Morris and associates[119] have emphasized that patients wearing an ocular prosthesis may be at increased risk of postoperative endophthalmitis developing in their contralateral eye because of the pathogens that may be harbored in the prosthetic socket and on the conjunctiva of the operative eye, even without evidence of overt infection.

The operating room and operating room personnel provide other potential sources of contamination. Factors that increase the number of airborne organisms in proximity to the operating field could increase the likelihood of endophthalmitis.[5] It has been suggested that conversation, particularly shouting, within the operating room increases the risk of endophthalmitis by increasing the number of airborne organisms.[145] In one case the source of the infecting organism in a patient who developed endophthalmitis was traced to a member of the operating team with respiratory tract disease.[151]

Postoperative Complications

In the vast majority of cases of endophthalmitis the infecting organism apparently gains access to the interior of the eye at the time of the surgical procedure. In certain settings microorganisms may have access to the eye subsequently. These situations pose specific risks for the development of endophthalmitis. In a review of 83 cases of endophthalmitis Driebe and associates[52] found that 22% of the patients they evaluated had problems with the cataract section, which were thought to contribute directly to the development of the intraocular infection. Wound leaks, wound dehiscence caused by premature suture removal or degradation of absorbable sutures, and vitreous wicks were noted in this group of patients and provided sites for potential entry of organisms into the eye after the surgical procedure itself. While this series had a particularly high incidence of wound complications, it serves to stress the importance of maintaining a closed globe postoperatively to avoid an increased risk of endophthalmitis. The recent advent of "sutureless" cataract surgery has resulted in renewed interest in this issue. There have been several reports of patients developing microbial endophthalmitis after sutureless cataract extraction.[76,118,158] Some of these patients had undergone secondary intraocular manipulations and at least one had developed a filtering bleb. The few cases reported to date provide insufficient information to determine whether the relative risk of microbial endophthalmitis is increased after sutureless surgery. The key factor in preventing subsequent entry of microorganisms is that the cataract section be sealed at the close of the surgical procedure, whether by sutures or by an incision architecture that provides a truly watertight internal corneal seal without sutures. Incision architectures need to be carefully evaluated; any that are prone to a "ball-valve" effect until they heal would pose an increased risk of late infection.

Any suture or device left in the eye may become a risk factor for endophthalmitis subsequently if it becomes exposed to the external environment, thus providing a potential pathway along which organisms may enter the eye. Late development of endophthalmitis has been reported after implantation of a sclerally-sutured posterior chamber lens where the scleral fixation sutures became exposed[75] and after glaucoma surgery with placement of a seton when the seton subsequently became exposed because of erosion of the overlying conjunctiva.[90]

Patients with filtering blebs, either intentionally created for treatment of glaucoma or developing inadvertently after cataract extraction, are uniquely susceptible to the development of endophthalmitis while the bleb is present. Although a few of these patients have ruptured filtering blebs at the time of presentation, the vast majority have intact blebs with presumed trans-conjunctival penetration of the organisms into the eye.[101] Although it has been stated that thin-walled blebs are more at risk for the development of late infection than thicker-walled blebs,[74] firm evidence for this supposition is lacking. It is certainly evident that the generally thicker-walled blebs resulting from trabeculectomy are not immune to late endophthalmitis, as numerous cases have been reported after trabeculectomy.[68,101] The incidence of late onset bleb-related endophthalmitis in patients who underwent trabeculectomy with adjunctive 5-fluorouracil therapy was retrospectively examined in a series of 229 consecutive patients by Wolner and associates,[171] who found a higher incidence of infection when the filter was positioned inferiorly (9.4%, or 9 of 96) compared with when the filter was positioned superiorly (3.0% or 4/133). Only 2 of these 13 eyes had hypopyon and vitreous involvement requiring vitreous cultures, however; the other 11 had inflammation confined to the bleb and anterior segment. It is therefore uncertain whether these represented true intraocular infection.

Certain factors other than bleb location have been suggested as additional risks in patients with filtering blebs. Because of the retrospective nature of the studies, none can be statistically confirmed but should be considered associations that are suspicious as risk factors. A number of patients with blebs have developed endophthalmitis while using contact lenses.[101] It is well recognized that contact lenses and lens solutions are frequently contaminated with microorganisms.[135] The presence of a contaminated lens on the surface of the eye would likely increase the number and variety of organisms that might find their way to the surface of the bleb. Particularly if the contact lens rubs the filtering bleb, it could damage the conjunctival epithelium sufficiently to increase the adherence of organisms to the surface of the bleb, potentially aiding in their subsequent intraocular penetration. Other patients have developed bleb-associated endophthalmitis after episodes of conjunctivitis or recent upper respiratory infections. Contaminated eye drops would certainly also pose a particular risk for patients with filtering blebs.

Intraocular Microorganisms

A recent unexpected finding has been the high incidence of positive cultures of fluid aspirated from the anterior chamber at the conclusion of uncomplicated extracapsular cataract extraction. Two studies have reported that viable bacteria were isolated from anterior chamber aspirates in 29% and 43% of cases at the conclusion of surgery.[47,146]

None of these patients developed endophthalmitis. These studies suggest that the anterior chamber has the ability to clear small inocula of bacteria without developing endophthalmitis. Sometimes, for reasons that are not understood and which may vary from case to case, this clearing mechanism fails and endophthalmitis develops.

Maylath and Leopold[107] in 1955 demonstrated that injection of bacteria into the vitreous of rabbits would result in endophthalmitis, though injection of similar numbers of bacteria into the anterior chamber would not. This finding indicated that the vitreous is better able to support bacterial growth than is the aqueous. More recently, experimental studies in primates have extended this observation by showing that similar bacterial inoculums introduced into the anterior chamber of the eye after cataract extraction were more likely to result in development of endophthalmitis if the posterior capsule was not intact than if it remained intact.[21-23,140] These experimental studies suggest that an intact posterior capsule-zonular system may to some degree function as a barrier, relatively limiting spread of organisms from the anterior chamber to the vitreous, from which the eye appears less capable of eliminating them. Based on these experimental data, it would be expected that intraoperative vitreous loss or development of some "communication" between the anterior chamber and vitreous cavity would pose a risk factor for development of endophthalmitis; clinical data confirm this anticipated increased risk.[52,80,114] In a case-control study recently performed by Menikoff and associates,[114] for example, operative procedures in which a defect in the posterior lens capsule or zonules developed, or during which instrumentation of the vitreous was required, had a nearly fourteenfold increased risk of endophthalmitis compared with procedures in which these did not occur.

Appropriately sterilized intraocular lenses are themselves not contaminated with microorganisms. They may possibly act as vehicles by which organisms may be transported into the eye, however, if organisms present in the conjunctival sac or on the ocular surface come into contact with and adhere to the intraocular lens during the insertion process. Recent experimental data[48,139] indicate that certain bacteria preferentially adhere to polypropylene (Prolene) lens material compared with polymethyl methacrylate (PMMA). An epidemiologic study by Menikoff, Speaker and associates[114] has determined that intraocular lenses containing Prolene haptics represent a significant risk factor for the development of microbial endophthalmitis relative to lenses that are composed entirely of PMMA. If confirmed by other investigators these data would provide an indication for avoiding the use of intraocular lenses containing Prolene.

Host Susceptibility

It is known that patients with compromise of their immune system are particularly at risk for the development of endogenous, blood-borne endophthalmitis.[123] Although specific data are not available for immunocompromised patients undergoing ocular surgery, it is likely that these patients may also be less capable of eliminating organisms exogenously introduced into the eye. It has been determined that diabetes mellitus does pose a risk factor for the development of postoperative endophthalmitis.[87]

CLINICAL FEATURES

The clinical features of a particular case of endophthalmitis will vary depending on the clinical category, the infecting organism, the time that has elapsed since entry of the organism into the eye, and therapy that has been administered. The cardinal sign of endophthalmitis is inflammation greater than expected at that point in the patient's clinical course. Unusual intraocular inflammation after ocular surgery, trauma, or in a patient with a filtering bleb should alert the ophthalmologist to consider the possibility of microbial endophthalmitis.

Acute Postsurgical Endophthalmitis

Postoperative endophthalmitis will usually present from 2 to 7 days after the surgical procedure. Most patients will experience increasing discomfort progressing to pain, sometimes very severe. A subgroup of patients may not experience any pain, despite advanced intraocular inflammation[45]; lack of pain should certainly not exclude this diagnosis from consideration. Visual acuity is typically reduced; patients may not recognize this as abnormal, however, in the immediate postoperative period. Eyelid swelling, conjunctival chemosis, hyperemia and exudate, and corneal edema and infiltration are variably present, again depending on the virulence of the organism and stage of the process. Development of a ring corneal infiltrate is a sign of infection by a virulent organism; these findings have been described in association with infection by gram-negative rods, *Bacillus* species, virulent strains of *Staphylococcus aureus,* and streptococci.[96] There is always anterior chamber reaction with flare and cells and frequently a hypopyon and formation of fibrin strands (Fig. 93-1). If the vitreous cavity can be visualized, vitritis will be present in all but the earliest stages of the inflammatory process. Retinal periphlebitis has been recognized as a relatively early sign of bacterial endophthalmitis, both clinically and in experimental animal models, probably because of increased vascular permeability and leukocyte migration caused by the infecting organisms.[127] Retinal hemorrhages may also be seen.[71]

The time of recognizable onset and speed of progression of signs and symptoms varies considerably. Infections caused by the most virulent bacteria (e.g., *Bacillus* species, gram-negative bacteria, streptococci) may present very shortly after surgery and may have explosive courses. By contrast, infection caused by organisms of lower virulence may not become evident for many days or weeks after surgery. Even in cases of endophthalmitis caused by the same

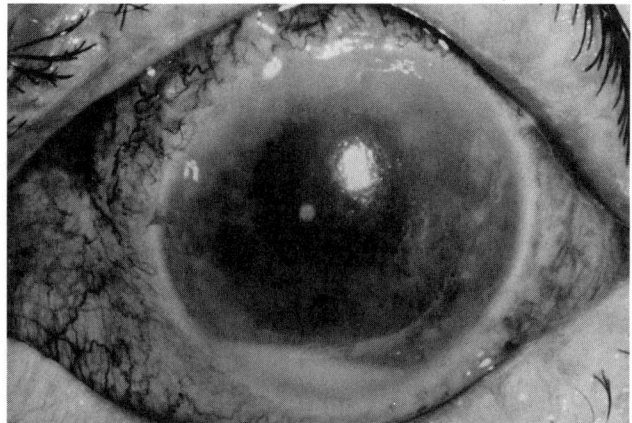

Fig. 93-1. Endophthalmitis after cataract extraction. Note conjunctival injection, corneal haze with blurring of light reflex, and hypopyon with fibrin strand in anterior chamber. Viridans streptococci were isolated from vitreous specimen.

species, the presentation may vary greatly. In a review of 90 cases of endophthalmitis caused by coagulase-negative staphylococci, Ormerod and associates[125] described patterns that ranged from an acute and moderately severe presentation to a milder, more chronic pattern. Twenty-nine percent of their cases were diagnosed within 4 days of surgery and 63% within the first week, but over a third of the patients showed symptoms more than one week after the initiating event.

Delayed-Onset Postsurgical Endophthalmitis

At the end of the spectrum is a group of patients with an unusual, recently recognized form of postoperative endophthalmitis, which may not present for months or, in rare cases, even years after surgery.[111] The term "chronic" has been applied to this category of endophthalmitis because, unless appropriately treated, the inflammation is usually very persistent once it presents. The course of the inflammation tends to be stuttering, with exacerbations and remissions. Initially the inflammation is usually responsive to corticosteroids; with time, increased doses of corticosteroids are often required, but may have less and less effect on the inflammatory process. Various organisms have been isolated from patients with symptoms of chronic endophthalmitis, but the most common has been *Propionibacterium acnes*.[100]

Patients with chronic endophthalmitis generally have both vitritis and iridocyclitis, sometimes severe enough to result in a hypopyon. Granulomatous precipitates on the corneal endothelium and/or on the surfaces of the intraocular lens implant are frequently noted during the clinical course. Most of the reported cases of propionibacterial endophthalmitis have had one or more creamy-white plaques present within the peripheral capsular bag or between the lens implant and the posterior capsule[67,111] (Fig. 93-2). Beaded strands of fibrin have been observed in some eyes.[174]

Exogenous fungal endophthalmitis, a relatively unusual condition, has previously been described as having a latency period of weeks to months after inoculation.[162,164] Whereas the average case of fungal endophthalmitis has a later onset than the typical case of bacterial endophthalmitis, patients with exogenous fungal endophthalmitis may show symptoms within the first week after surgery.[133] Pain is generally, but not invariably, a less prominent feature of fungal as compared with bacterial endophthalmitis. Patients with fungal endophthalmitis tend to develop more localized inflammation, typically in the anterior chamber, in the anterior vitreous, or on the iris surface, frequently at the pupillary margin[133,162,164]; patients can, however, also have the diffuse intraocular inflammation characteristic of bacterial endophthalmitis.[133]

Bleb-Associated Endophthalmitis

Patients with filtering blebs who develop endophthalmitis typically suddenly develop pain, redness, and decreased visual acuity without warning. Once present, intraocular inflammation usually proceeds very rapidly. Only rarely can a predisposing condition other than the presence of the bleb be recognized. In a series of 36 patients with filtering bleb endophthalmitis reviewed retrospectively,[101] five patients recalled symptoms compatible with a recent episode of conjunctivitis, two had relatively recent upper respiratory

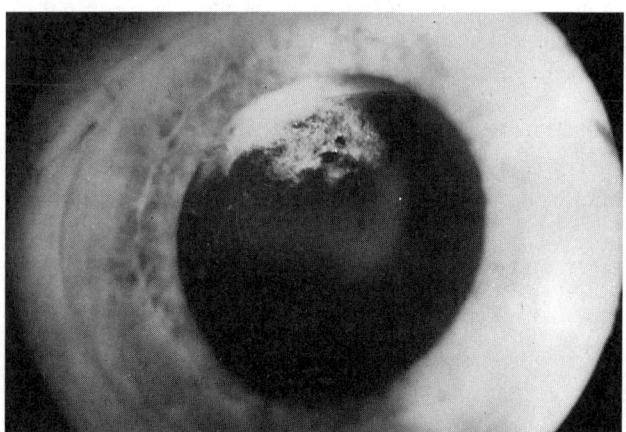

Fig. 93-2. White capsular plaque present between posterior chamber lens implant and posterior capsule in right eye of man who underwent extracapsular cataract extraction and lens implant 16 months previously. Patient had abruptly developed vitritis and iridocyclitis severe enough to reduce visual acuity to hand movements 7 months after surgery. Corticosteroids were used to suppress intraocular inflammation. Peripheral capsular plaque was then recognized, which gradually enlarged over subsequent months.

Pars plana vitrectomy, excision of posterior capsular plaque with intraocular scissors and forceps, and intraocular injection of vancomycin were performed. Cultures of plaque and of vitrectomy specimen grew *Propionibacterium acnes*. Final visual acuity returned to 20/25.

infections, and four had been using contact lenses. The remaining patients recognized nothing unusual before abrupt development of symptoms. Most blebs appeared biomicroscopically intact; only three were ruptured, with two additional blebs being Seidel-positive. Inflammatory cells and debris are usually present within the filtering bleb itself, as well as in the anterior chamber and in the vitreous (Fig. 93-3).

A less severe form of inflammation in patients with filtering blebs has recently been described[28,171] and termed "blebitis" by Brown and associates.[28] During the period of observation inflammation was generally confined to the bleb and anterior chamber, with only a rare patient having vitritis. Many patients had symptoms for several days before seeking attention. Most patients had thin blebs; leakage from the bleb was common before, during, and after the episode. In view of the general lack of evident vitreous involvement, patients were treated with topical and parenteral antibiotics, without intraocular antibiotic injections. Anterior chamber aspiration was performed in several eyes, all of which were culture-negative. All patients improved, with most regaining their previous visual acuities. It was presumed that these patients had intraocular infections because of the sudden onset of the inflammation and the rapid improvement with administration of antibiotics. This presumption may be correct, but the marked difference in clinical course and the substantially better visual outcome compared with previously reported series[68,74,101] suggests that these patients with more limited inflammation were, at the least, infected by less virulent organisms than the patients previously described with postbleb endophthalmitis.

Posttraumatic Endophthalmitis

The signs and symptoms of endophthalmitis developing after ocular trauma may be difficult to separate from those

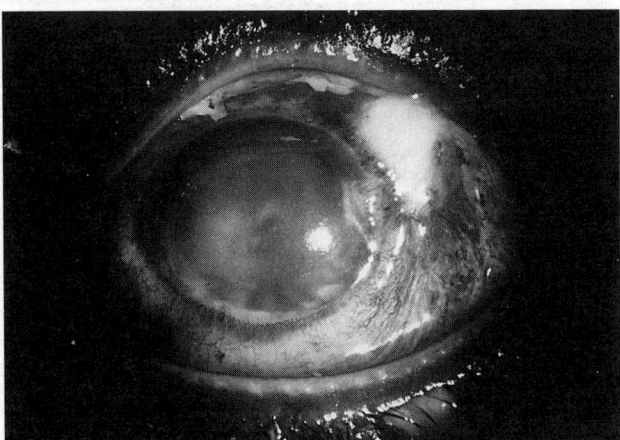

Fig. 93-3. Abrupt development of endophthalmitis in left eye of phakic 28-year-old male approximately 10 years after glaucoma filtering surgery. Note inflammatory material within intact superotemporal filtering bleb and extensive anterior chamber inflammation. Aqueous and vitreous culture grew *Streptococcus pneumoniae.*

caused by the tissue injury resulting from the traumatic event itself. Pain and decreased vision are so frequent after ocular trauma that it often falls upon the ophthalmologist to determine whether the extent of intraocular inflammation is such that a superimposed infection should be considered. The multiple variables involved in ocular trauma and the broad range of inflammation that can result make this decision particularly difficult. The frequency of virulent organisms isolated after trauma, particularly *Bacillus* species,[121] underscore the importance of maintaining a particularly high index of suspicion in this clinical setting, for it is likely that prompt initiation of therapy provides the greatest opportunity to salvage eyes infected by these virulent organisms.[144] Attention to the setting in which the trauma occurred may help in determining which patients are more likely to become infected. For example, in one series of patients with intraocular foreign bodies, 9.2% (33 of 358) of eyes with home- or occupation-related injuries developed endophthalmitis as compared with only 0.8% (1 of 128) of eyes injured in recreation, motor vehicle, or assault settings.[165] Similarly, as previously noted, there was a much higher incidence of endophthalmitis developing after injuries in rural settings than in nonrural locations.[26]

PATHOLOGY

Exogenous endophthalmitis is usually characterized by an acute, suppurative, nongranulomatous intraocular inflammation. Because of the acute nature of the process, the predominant cell is the polymorphonuclear leukocyte. The extent of ocular inflammation is determined by the virulence of the causative organism, the stage of the infectious process, and the effectiveness of any treatment that has been rendered. Cells, inflammatory and necrotic debris, and microorganisms will be present in the anterior chamber and in the vitreous cavity. In advanced cases an abscess may form within the vitreous cavity. Cellular infiltration may involve the cornea, iris, ciliary body, retina, and choroid as well as the anterior chamber and vitreous cavity. Depending on the duration of the process, a secondary chronic nongranulomatous inflammatory infiltrate may develop. In endophthalmitis (as distinguished from panophthalmitis) there is no inflammatory reaction in the sclera.[172]

In a recent histopathologic study of a rabbit model of exogenous endophthalmitis,[63a] various inocula of vancomycin-sensitive *Enterococcus faecalis, Staphylococcus aureus, Staphylococcus epidermidis,* and *Bacillus cereus* were inoculated into the vitreous of aphakic rabbit eyes. Cellular inflammatory reaction was graded semiquantitatively in both noncavitary ocular tissues (cornea, iris, ciliary body, retina, choroid, sclera, and optic nerve) and in the ocular cavities (anterior and posterior chambers, and anterior and posterior vitreous), and was compared to the clinical response. Considering the natural history over 72 hours, the summation average of ocular cavity and noncavitary mean inflammatory scores correlated highly to the clinical response scores. These studies were repeated in eyes treated with vancomycin, with and without vitrectomy. Vancomycin, either with or without vitrectomy, did little to reduce the overall inflammatory response of the four etiologic agents. When vitrectomy was combined with vancomycin injection, by 72 hours there was some reduction in the noncavitary inflammatory response. In the case of *S. epidermidis* in particular, the noncavitary inflammatory response produced little tissue damage, probably accounting for the generally relatively good prognosis for salvaged vision in eyes infected with this organism.

In cases of chronic postoperative endophthalmitis caused by *Propionibacterium acnes,* there are granulomatous features to the intraocular inflammation. Large collections of propionibacterial organisms have been found sequestered adjacent to the lens capsule. A striking pathologic feature of this entity has been the paucity of inflammatory cells surrounding these large collections of organisms.

COMPLICATIONS

Before use of intravitreal antibiotics, exogenous microbial endophthalmitis almost always resulted in loss of vision of the affected eye.[141] Even with current therapy, cases with particularly severe inflammation may develop hypotony and ultimately phthisis bulbi, despite sterilization of the infectious process.

Retinal detachment may develop following treatment for endophthalmitis. In Kattan's series,[87] 10% (3 of 29) of patients developed retinal detachment in the 2 months following treatment for endophthalmitis. In the series reported by Nelsen and associates,[119a] 21% (7 of 33) of patients treated with vitrectomy developed subsequent retinal detachments, compared with 9% (2 of 22) who were treated with vitreous tap and intravitreal antibiotics. The data in Olson's series[124] was consistent with a similar observation: the retinal detachment rate was higher after vitrectomy than after treatment with vitreous tap and intravitreal antibiotics, 14% versus 5%. In neither series, however, was treatment randomized. Eyes with more severe inflammation were treated using vitrectomy, whereas those with milder inflammation at presentation underwent vitreous taps and intravitreal antibiotic injections only. It is therefore difficult to determine the relative roles of disease severity and therapeutic modality in development of retinal detachment after vitrectomy. These series do make it clear that peripheral retinal examination must be carefully and frequently performed to detect retinal breaks in the period after treatment for endophthalmitis.

Macular edema develops not infrequently after endophthalmitis. The incidence and natural history of this complication when occurring after microbial endophthalmitis has not been well defined. There are multiple potential causes for macular edema in these patients, including the intense intraocular inflammation and the surgical and pharmacological intervention required.

A variety of anterior segment conditions may result from an episode of endophthalmitis, including peripheral anterior synechiae (which may be extensive enough to cause secondary glaucoma), posterior synechiae (which may result in a bombé iris configuration), corneal edema, and posterior capsule opacification. These anterior segment complications are amenable to medical and surgical management.

PATHOGENESIS

Among those cases of acute postoperative endophthalmitis suspected of being microbial in recent large series, organisms have been isolated from 73% to 83% of eyes.[52,87,124] About three fourths of the isolated organisms have been gram-positive. Approximately half of the gram-positive isolates have been coagulase-negative staphylococci. Coagulase-negative staphylococci have been found to be the most common isolates from cases of postoperative endophthalmitis in many clinical series.[46,52,124,137] The next most common isolates have been *Staphylococcus aureus* and the streptococci. Sixteen percent of the isolates in one series were gram-negative and 8% were fungal.[52]

The pathogenetic spectrum is quite different in the other clinical categories of endophthalmitis. In a relatively large series of patients who developed late endophthalmitis associated with filtering blebs,[101] for example, none of the cases was caused by *Staphylococcus epidermidis* and only 2 of 30 culture-positive cases were caused by *Staphylococcus aureus.* By far the most common isolate in this group were streptococcal species, accounting for 57% (17 of 30) cases. *Haemophilus influenzae,* an extremely rare cause of endophthalmitis acutely after surgery, was responsible for 23% (7 of 30) of the late postbleb cases. These marked differences in the distribution of organisms are compatible with different mechanisms of infection. Organisms entering the eye during surgery are likely those that reside on the eyelid margins or periocular skin; hence the very high incidence of staphylococci. The bacteria associated with bleb-related endophthalmitis must be capable of penetrating intact conjunctiva overlying filtering blebs in order to enter the eye; thus the high incidence of more virulent organisms with this capability, particularly streptococci.

In patients who sustain penetrating trauma, *Bacillus* species is a particularly frequent pathogen, isolated from as many as 46% of cases in one series.[26] Other frequent pathogens are organisms common in the environment and periocularly, especially *Staphylococcus epidermidis,* streptococci, gram-negative organisms, and fungi.[3,26,27] Because the source of the infecting organism can be so varied, a particularly wide spectrum of organisms has been isolated from patients with posttraumatic endophthalmitis.

The most frequent isolate from eyes with chronic endophthalmitis has been *Propionibacterium acnes.* Other organisms capable of causing this unusual clinical condition include staphylococci (more commonly *S. epidermidis*), anaerobic streptococci, *Actinomyces* species, and a variety of fungi, especially *Candida* species.[100]

DIFFERENTIAL DIAGNOSIS

Any cause of increased postoperative inflammation must be considered in the differential diagnosis of postoperative endophthalmitis. Foreign materials or chemical solutions introduced into the eye intraoperatively may cause a sterile inflammatory response. For example, in the past, clusters of cases of sterile postoperative inflammation have been traced to residual polishing compounds and sterilizing agents on intraocular lenses.[113,153] Retained lens nucleus or cortex, particularly if mixed with vitreous, may result in a marked inflammatory response. Incarceration of iris or vitreous in the wound may cause mild inflammation. Complicated surgical procedures requiring additional operating time, instrumentation, and/or vitreous manipulation are more likely to be followed by greater inflammation postoperatively. Patients who have been receiving chronic miotic therapy, particularly if their irides are very darkly pigmented, and diabetic patients are particularly prone to develop considerable inflammation postoperatively, especially if the procedure required unusual iris manipulation (e.g., creating and then closing a sector iridectomy during cataract extraction). Finally, for reasons that are unclear, some patients not in any of these categories respond to intraocular manipulation with greater-than-expected iridocyclitis.

Marked intraocular inflammation present on the first postoperative visit the morning after surgery may pose a particularly challenging clinical situation. Excessive intraocular inflammation resulting from the surgical procedure itself or the individual patient characteristics described above will usually be most prominent the first day after surgery. Infection, on the other hand, frequently requires an additional 24 to 48 hours of replication time before there are a sufficient number of intraocular organisms to induce significant intraocular inflammation. Because cases of microbial endophthalmitis have developed on the first postoperative day, however, and because such cases are usually caused by virulent organisms, it is not safe for the clinician to assume that severe, early inflammation definitely implies a noninfectious cause. Although intensive topical antiinflammatory therapy and observation may be an appropriate therapeutic choice in a specific case, the observation periods should be measured in hours rather than in days, and the patient should be prepared for surgical intervention if that becomes necessary.

In patients who develop a suspicious increase in intraocular inflammation during the first postoperative week, there are no clinical signs or symptoms that can be used reliably to distinguish inflammation caused by microbial organisms from that which is sterile. The risks of delaying therapy in such patients are usually greater than the risks of culturing and treating an eye that proves to be culture-negative.

Therefore, initiating diagnostic and therapeutic intervention is preferred when treating a patient who develops postoperative inflammation that suggests the possibility of microbial endophthalmitis.

In a patient who develops late signs of endophthalmitis (that is, inflammation developing more than several weeks after surgery), the major diagnostic consideration is whether there is any breach in the corneoscleral wall such as a subtle wound dehiscence, a filtering bleb, or a loose, eroded suture along or through which organisms might have entered the eye. If so, this must be considered as acute endophthalmitis, thus requiring emergency intervention because it may be caused by virulent organisms. If the corneoscleral wall of the eye is intact, the causative organisms must have been introduced into the eye at the time of the surgical procedure (excluding a rare case of coincident, blood-borne metastatic endophthalmitis). In general, this finding implies organisms of lower virulence.

Certain noninfectious entities should be considered in the differential diagnosis of late-onset, chronic endophthalmitis. Epithelial downgrowth can simulate this entity. On careful biomicroscopic examination, the intraocularly shed epithelial cells are generally larger than inflammatory cells and are often accompanied by a glassy epithelial membrane on the iris surface and/or corneal endothelium. Recurrent intraocular hemorrhages (presumably because of erosion of a blood vessel in the iris or ciliary body by an intraocular lens haptic) can likewise simulate intraocular inflammation. Careful examination of the circulating cells and the episodic nature of the hemorrhages will usually allow these to be distinguished. Vitreous incarceration may cause chronic postoperative inflammation, often accompanied by cystoid macular edema.

Inflammation caused by retained cortex or nuclear fragments is generally evident from the history and clinical examination. The lens-related syndrome that has been the most difficult to differentiate from chronic microbial endophthalmitis has been phacoanaphylactic endophthalmitis, also termed phacoantigenic uveitis. This entity is thought to be an immunologic response resulting from an abrogation of tolerance to lens protein.[103] Patients thought to have phacoanaphylactic endophthalmitis after extracapsular cataract extraction and intraocular lens insertion were reported in the early to mid 1980s.[2,9,170] After Meisler and associates[112] reported a group of patients with clinical features indistinguishable from phacoanaphylactic endophthalmitis, but from whose vitreous or aqueous specimens they isolated *Propionibacterium* species, it was recognized that fastidious microbial organisms could cause chronic endophthalmitis. Particularly careful microbiologic and histopathologic examination of these cases since then has usually revealed a causative organism.

In patients with filtering blebs who suddenly develop intraocular inflammation, microbial endophthalmitis should be the primary concern. If there is evidence of vitreous inflammation, or if the status of the vitreous cannot be ascertained, the patient should be treated as if the endophthalmitis is potentially fulminant. If the vitreous is clear and the inflammation remains localized to the bleb and anterior segment only, the process may be "blebitis," described previously. In either case the patient should remain under medical supervision until the cause of the inflammation has been clarified, and therapy appropriate to the condition has been provided.

LABORATORY INVESTIGATIONS

Although initial therapy for presumed microbial endophthalmitis is usually broad-spectrum, determination of the infecting agent is important for modification of subsequent therapy, particularly if the patient's course after initial treatment is not as expected. The vitreous is the intraocular fluid that is most likely to yield the infecting organism, even if the surgical manipulation or injury is confined to the anterior segment and even if the eye is phakic.[69] Multiple clinical cases in which both aqueous and vitreous have been sampled and cultured have documented that the vitreous is often culture-positive despite no growth from the aqueous.[52,65,87] Aqueous should also be cultured, however, as in both experimental animals[21-23] and in occasional clinical cases there has been growth only from the aqueous.[25,52,65]

Specimen Collection

Patients suspected of having microbial endophthalmitis are generally taken to the operating room to obtain samples for culture and to initiate antimicrobial therapy. A retrobulbar block with supplemental sedation will usually provide sufficient anesthesia. Rare patients have such extensive periocular inflammation that adequate anesthesia and akinesia cannot be achieved with a regional block and general anesthesia may be required. A partial-thickness peripheral keratotomy is fashioned with a blade, and a 25- or 27-gauge needle attached to a tuberculin syringe is then inserted through the keratotomy into the anterior chamber. This two-step technique generally allows better control than if the needle were inserted directly through the entire corneal thickness. About 0.1 ml of aqueous is aspirated. This sample should then be inoculated directly onto culture media and onto slides for subsequent staining.

The anterior chamber usually reforms rapidly while the aqueous specimens are being plated. Attention is then directed to obtaining a vitreous sample. Vitreous may be obtained either by aspiration through a needle, by a limited vitreous biopsy using vitrectomy instrumentation, or as part of a vitrectomy performed therapeutically. For vitreous aspirations a pars plana sclerotomy is fashioned 3.5 to 4.0 mm posterior to the limbus. A 22-gauge needle attached to a 3-cc syringe is then passed through the sclerotomy into the anterior vitreous; inserting the needle through the sclerotomy

facilitates its passage into the eye with minimal pressure on the globe. The depth of insertion of the needle into the eye should be carefully monitored to make certain that it extends only approximately halfway across the globe. The reflection of the microscope light from the needle should be observed in the pupillary opening through the microscope before aspirating vitreous. With careful manipulation of the needle a pocket of liquid vitreous will usually be encountered, allowing aspiration of 0.2 to 0.3 ml of liquid vitreous.

If gentle aspiration in several locations does not yield liquid vitreous, a vitreous suction-cutter is used to obtain a vitreous specimen. The sclerotomy is enlarged appropriately to accommodate the instrument. A second sclerotomy is generally required to allow for infusion to keep the globe from collapsing. Occasionally infusion is not required if only a small amount of vitreous is removed with a collection syringe used to provide manual suction for the vitreous cutter. Any portion of the collection tubing or syringes with which the specimen might come into contact must, of course, be sterile to avoid contamination of the specimen.

Culture Processing

Aqueous and vitreous specimens should be separately dripped onto fresh culture plates; ideally the plates should be brought directly to the operating room so that the specimens can be inoculated as soon as they are obtained. The specimen drops should be allowed to dry on the plates before the plates are moved or turned over. Standard culture media include blood agar, chocolate agar maintained in an enriched carbon dioxide environment, and liquid thioglycollate broth (or other anaerobic media), all maintained at 37°C to optimize bacterial growth. Sabouraud agar and blood agar should be inoculated and maintained at 25°C (room temperature) to optimize fungal isolation in cases where fungal cause is a consideration. Drops placed on slides should be subsequently processed with Gram and Giemsa stains. If fungi are a strong consideration, a slide should be reserved for staining with Grocott-Gomori methenamine silver.

If a therapeutic vitrectomy is performed, an initial specimen may be collected before using infusion and should be plated separately for optimum yield. The specimen obtained after the therapeutic vitrectomy will be vitreous diluted with infusion fluid. The culture yield of this material can be increased by passing the entire specimen through a sterile membrane filter to concentrate it. Sterile technique is used to cut the membrane filter into segments, which are directly placed onto appropriate culture plates and may also be placed into liquid media[65] (Fig. 93-4).

Facilities for concentrating a specimen with a membrane filter may not always be available. Joondeph and associates[84] have recommended inoculating blood culture bottles with vitrectomy specimens in these situations. They found the results of this technique to correlate well with results using the membrane filter system just described, although in

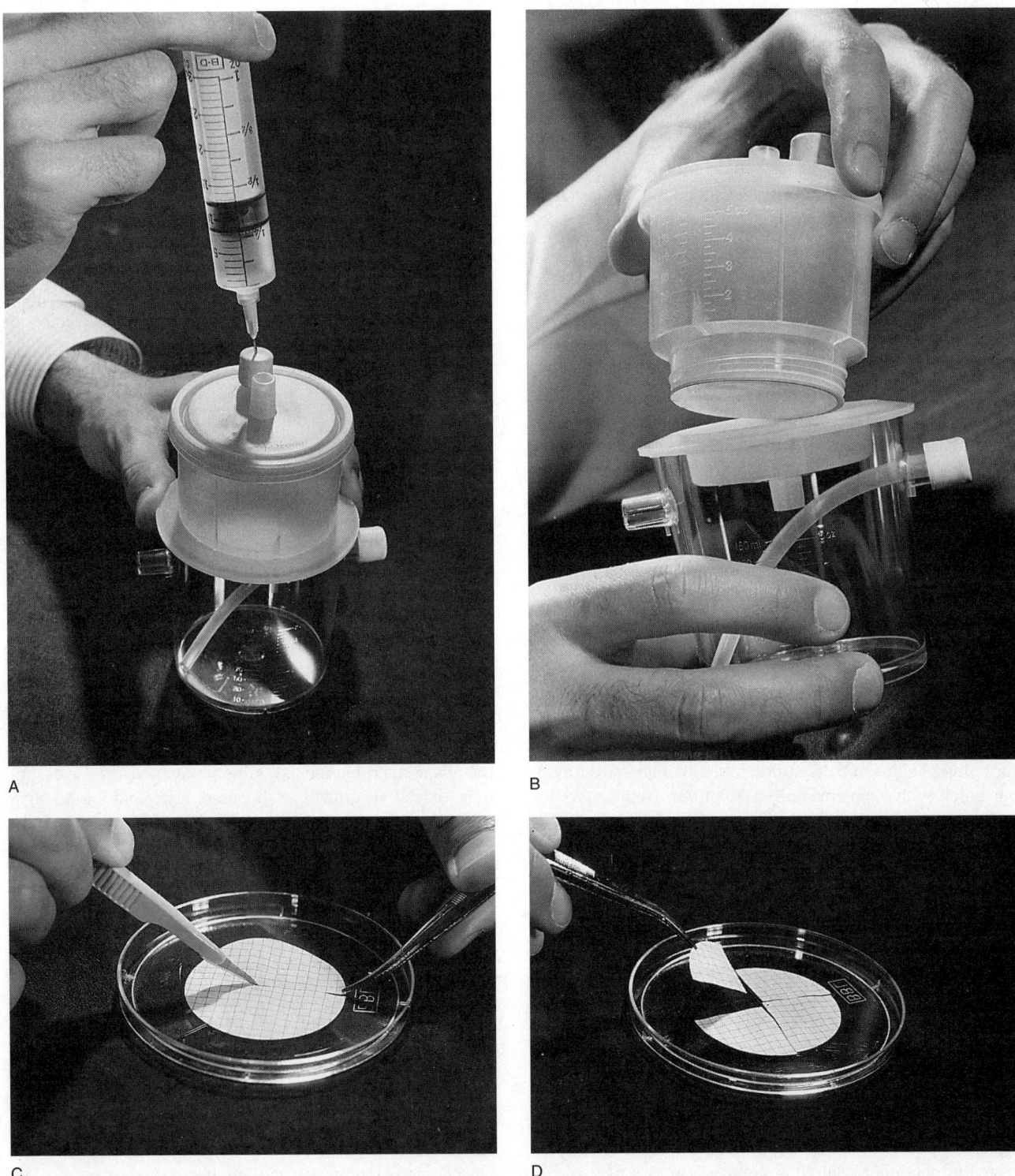

A

B

C

D

Fig. 93-4. Technique for concentrating and culturing vitrectomy specimen. **A,** Vitrectomy fluid, which has been drawn into syringe, is injected into upper chamber of filter system (Falcon 7102, Oxnard, Calif). Rubber cap is sterile. Suction generated by vacuum pump is then applied to lower chamber, drawing specimen through sterile filter located between two chambers. **B,** Upper and lower chambers are separated. **C,** Using sterile technique, filter paper is cut into segments. **D,** Filter paper should be handled only by edges to minimize risk of contamination.

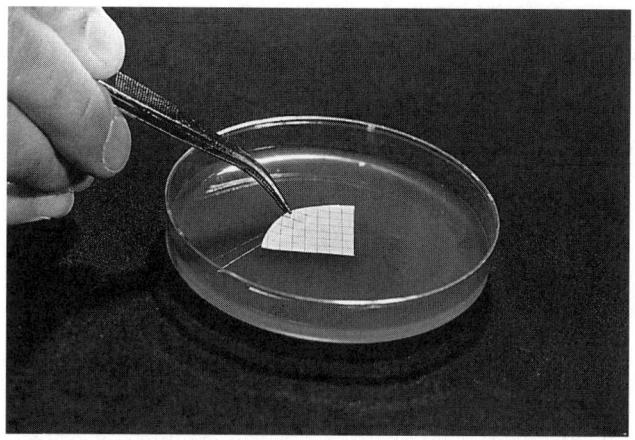

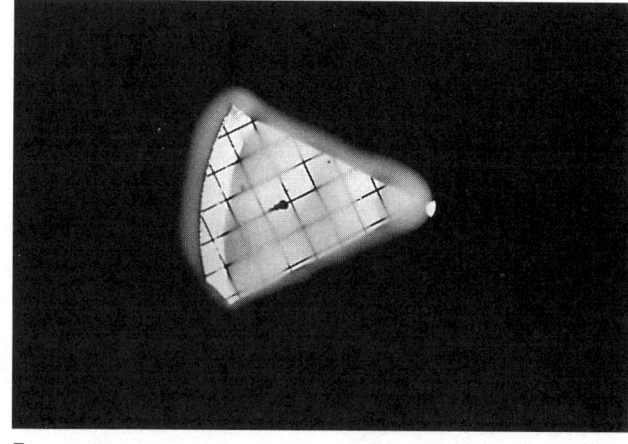

E

F

Fig. 93-4, cont'd. **E,** Each segment of filter paper is placed right side up on agar plate. Alternatively, filter paper may be placed into liquid culture media. **F,** Confluent growth of *Serratia marcescens* on filter paper/agar plate. Drops of vitrectomy specimen that were separately cultured without concentration failed to grow any organisms.

a laboratory comparison the membrane filter system was slightly more sensitive than the blood culture bottles.[84] Direct inoculation of blood culture bottles can be performed immediately in the operating room, minimizes handling of the specimen, thereby potentially reducing the risks of contamination, and is readily performed on nights and weekends when many cases of endophthalmitis are managed and when microbiology staff may not be available. The blood culture bottles were less sensitive for isolating *Haemophilus influenzae* and *Propionibacterium acnes,* however. Also, the identification of organisms isolated from blood culture bottles may require an additional step because the organism must be subcultured for identification and sensitivity testing. Inoculation of blood culture bottles may be a useful adjunct and occasionally a simple alternative to more sophisticated specimen-concentrating techniques, depending on circumstances and available facilities.

In cases of chronic endophthalmitis or in patients in whom there is a strong suspicion of fungal endophthalmitis, a diagnostic vitrectomy directed to the site of maximal inflammatory involvement is preferred to aspiration of liquid vitreous. In both of these circumstances, there is a greater tendency for organisms to be loculated and to be obtained only from the specific involved area. Removal of a small amount of vitreous by a tap is thus likely to be subject to greater sampling error in these cases than in the usual case of bacterial endophthalmitis where the organisms are more diffusely distributed through the vitreous cavity. In patients with chronic endophthalmitis caused by *Propionibacterium acnes* or similar organisms, excision and culture of apparently involved portions of the peripheral posterior capsule will increase the likelihood of isolating the causative organism. In these patients additional anaerobic media should be inoculated and cultures should be maintained for two weeks,

because the organisms may require this period of time to grow.[111]

THERAPY

The goal of therapy in a patient with microbial endophthalmitis is the rapid eradication of the infection, while minimizing the structural and functional ocular damage resulting from the treatment and from the underlying infectious process. Once samples of the aqueous and vitreous have been obtained, the mainstay of therapy has become the injection of antibiotics directly into the vitreous. Antibiotics are also usually administered systemically, periocularly, and topically. Corticosteroids are often used to limit the severe inflammation that accompanies intraocular infection. Vitrectomy is increasingly performed as a component of initial therapy in the management of endophthalmitis, although its precise role is still debated.

Antimicrobial Agents

Through the early 1980s some clinicians continued to advocate treatment of endophthalmitis with periocular and parenteral antibiotics alone, particularly for infection with less virulent organisms.[18,122] Subsequently, however, there has been consensus that direct intravitreal injection is the best approach for most rapidly achieving effective antibiotic concentrations within the vitreous,[19] and this treatment has become the standard of care. This approach represents a logical route for drug delivery to the site most affected by the infectious process, particularly given the difficulties of achieving adequate vitreous drug levels by other routes of administration.[14]

Intravitreal Administration. Antibiotics injected intravitreally diffuse through the vitreous cavity over the next few hours; in one experimental study, diffusion was complete within eight hours of administration.[20] Antibiotics are eliminated from the vitreous cavity either by active excretion across the retina or by diffusion into the anterior chamber and subsequent elimination via aqueous humor outflow channels, depending on the particular antibiotic.[17,86] Antibiotics are more rapidly cleared from the vitreous cavity if the eye is aphakic or has undergone vitrectomy; intraocular inflammation may either increase or decrease the rapidity of clearance depending on the primary route by which the particular antibiotic is eliminated from the vitreous cavity.[20,36,50,57,134]

Along with the capability of rapidly achieving therapeutic vitreous levels, however, direct intravitreal administration also incurs the potential risk of causing visually significant retinal toxicity. Initial determinations of the "safe" doses of intravitreal antibiotics to avoid retinal toxicity were based upon the results of light microscopy and electroretinography in experimental animal eyes.[11,173] More recent studies have used electron microscopic examination of the ultrastructure of the retina to define more precisely antibiotic-associated toxicity. The aminoglycosides were the first class of antibiotics whose effects were examined in this manner.[41,42] The earliest toxic effects recognizable in these ultrastructural studies were the accumulation of lysosomal inclusions within retinal pigment epithelial cells. For gentamicin this early toxicity was noted with doses of 200 μg (0.2 mg); for tobramycin the threshold dose was 500 μg, and for amikacin 750 μg. As higher doses of aminoglycosides were administered, there was a progression of damage ranging from disorganization of photoreceptor outer segments to their disappearance and eventually to full thickness retinal necrosis. Vancomycin and ceftazidime have also been evaluated with relatively similar toxic effects noted, though at different doses.[33,134] The threshold for retinal damage was similar in eyes that had undergone lens extraction or vitrectomy combined with lensectomy, despite differences in the rates of drug clearance from these eyes, suggesting that toxicity was more likely a function of peak drug concentration rather than the duration of exposure.[160]

Number of Injections. Although a single intravitreal antibiotic injection will eradicate the infection in many patients with endophthalmitis, some patients remain culture-positive despite the intravitreal antibiotics.[52,78,156] Frequently these patients are infected by particularly virulent organisms, especially streptococci and gram-negative organisms. At the other extreme some of these patients have endophthalmitis caused by organisms that replicate relatively slowly, such as *P. acnes* or fungi.

Depending on the clinical response of the patient and the virulence of the isolated organism, therefore, repeat intravitreal antibiotic injection may be a consideration at approximately 48 hours after initial antibiotic administration. Oum and associates[126] determined that repeated injections of the combination of vancomycin (1.0 mg) and amikacin

(400 μg) caused progressively greater retinal toxicity; in comparison, there was no toxicity recognized from a single injection of this antibiotic combination. Stern[155] limited the reinjection to only one antibiotic (because the nature of the infecting organism should be known by the time of the reinjection) and reduced the dosage of the subsequent injections, but still found increasing retinal toxicity with repeated intravitreal injections.

Retinal Toxicity. From the clinical standpoint the most devastating antibiotic-related toxicity has been severe macular ischemia and infarction, which has been recognized in a small percentage of patients who have received intravitreal and/or subconjunctival aminoglycosides.[32,37,85,108] The fundus appearance of these patients is similar to patients who have sustained a retinal arterial occlusion, with a cherry red spot within an edematous macula and vascular nonperfusion with abrupt margins evident by examination and by fluorescein angiography. With only rare exceptions, affected patients have lost central vision. In an effort to determine how common this complication was Campochiaro and Conway[32] conducted a retrospective survey and identified 93 such cases. In this series macular infarction occurred after intravitreal administration of not only gentamicin, but also after administration of amikacin (which had been suggested as less likely to cause retinal toxicity).[41] The complication occurred not only in eyes that had undergone vitrectomy but also eyes that had not. Although errors in drug dilution may have occurred in some cases, in many there was near certainty that the medication administered was the recommended dose of 100 to 200 μg of gentamicin or 400 μg of amikacin.[34] Twenty-three of these identified cases of macular infarction occurred in association with prophylactic subconjunctival aminoglycoside administration after uncomplicated anterior segment surgery rather than after treatment for endophthalmitis. In most of these inadvertent intraocular administration of medication was presumed, although in several the injection needle was thought very unlikely to have penetrated the eye. These cases raise significant concerns regarding not only intravitreal but also periocular administration of aminoglycosides, even at the lowest of the doses that have been recommended.

The mechanism of this toxicity is uncertain. Because the medications need to be diluted to achieve the proper dose and concentration, there is potential for error in preparing the antibiotic. Preparation by hospital pharmacists according to standardized, written protocols has been determined to be the method least likely to result in errors in drug dosage.[81] In many of the reported cases, however, antibiotics were prepared in this manner, with high levels of confidence that an amount close to that intended had been administered.[34] Because the macula is the most dependent portion of the eye when the patient is supine, it has been postulated that gravitational effects may contribute to macular toxicity. In some reported cases the zone of nonperfusion was limited to a portion of the macula, as might occur if the patient's head was tilted when the medication was administered intravitreally.[34] Experimental studies in rabbits have also suggested that gravitational effects might be a factor in macular toxicity.[98]

Although gravity may put the most dependent portion of the macula at particular risk after intravitreal injection, it does not explain why the same dosage of medication administered intravitreally may be well tolerated by most patients, yet cause such severe toxic effects in a small number of others. Until the precise mechanism of toxicity is understood, the answer to this question will only be speculative. Individual variability is likely an important factor in this drug toxicity.[138]

Dosage. The specific antibiotics used for intravitreal injection have changed since this approach to therapy was first used and will undoubtedly continue to evolve based on changing susceptibility patterns of the organisms isolated and on accumulating information regarding drug toxicity. To date there is no one drug available with a sufficiently broad spectrum of activity for it to be used as a sole agent. Because the infecting agent is not known at the time intravitreal antibiotics are initially administered and because the causative organism may be either gram-negative or gram-positive, two antibiotics, each with a different spectrum of activity, are generally administered.

Vancomycin, 1.0 mg in 0.1 cc, is the antibiotic currently administered to provide coverage for gram-positive organisms.[134] This drug was substituted for cefazolin, which had been previously used, because of the increasing frequency of staphylococci resistant to methicillin and to the cephalosporins.[44,59,93,149] In patients who develop endophthalmitis after trauma, *Bacillus* species are a frequent cause of a fulminant and particularly destructive intraocular infection.[3,121] Although *Bacillus* species are sensitive to vancomycin in vitro, and endophthalmitis caused by *Bacillus* has been successfully treated with vancomycin, there is somewhat greater clinical experience with clindamycin (1.0 mg in 0.1 cc) in this setting; it can be used in place of vancomycin in posttraumatic endophthalmitis.[121,128,144]

In virtually all recommended therapeutic regimens until recently, an aminoglycoside has been the antibiotic used to provide the coverage required for gram-negative organisms and for the additive effect this class of agents provides against some gram-positive organisms when combined with vancomycin.[134] Because toxic effects had been noted in initial animal studies with gentamicin doses of 200 μg,[173] a threshold toxicity dose that was subsequently confirmed by electron microscopic studies,[41,42] gentamicin doses of 100 μg were recommended. Some clinicians substituted amikacin at doses of 200 to 400 μg, based on animal data indicating it was less toxic to the retina.[41] The reports of macular infarction occurring after aminoglycoside administration (reviewed in this section), even when the medications

were administered at these "conservative" doses, have prompted reconsideration of aminoglycoside use in the treatment of endophthalmitis.[34,51] Ceftazidime, a third-generation cephalosporin that provides excellent gram-negative coverage, has been recently evaluated in the laboratory and found effective for all those gram-negative isolates against which it was tested.[78] An intraocular dose of 2.25 mg of ceftazidime did not produce recognizable retinal toxicity by clinical examination or by light or electron microscopy in a primate model.[33] Early reports of clinical use of ceftazidime in patients with endophthalmitis have been encouraging.[1,97] At this time, however, a small number of patients have been treated with intraocular ceftazidime; additional experience as to its clinical efficacy and reassurance as to its safety needs to be gained before it can receive an unqualified recommendation as a replacement for an aminoglycoside in the treatment of endophthalmitis.

Systemic Administration. The role of systemic antibiotics in the treatment of endophthalmitis is uncertain. It is possible to treat endophthalmitis successfully without the use of systemic antibiotics,[129] and certainly there are potential adverse side effects to their administration, particularly the aminoglycosides. Systemically administered gentamicin is known to penetrate poorly into the vitreous.[142] Systemically administered cefazolin[12] and ciprofloxacin[94] can, however, produce vitreous levels above the minimum inhibitory concentrations for many organisms, even when measured in uninflamed eyes. Vitreous levels of antibiotics administered systemically are likely to be higher in inflamed eyes because of breakdown of the blood-vitreous barrier.[12] Additionally, repeated administration of systemic antibiotics results in accumulation of the antibiotic within the vitreous cavity, thus achieving higher levels than after a single dose.[104] Because vitreous levels of antibiotics injected directly into the vitreous decline with time, this cumulative feature of systemically-administered antibiotics may be especially helpful in maintaining a drug level within the vitreous. In light of these considerations, many clinicians continue to administer systemic antibiotics when treating endophthalmitis. The patient's systemic status should be carefully monitored, with special attention to renal function if intravenous aminoglycosides or vancomycin are used. The national Endophthalmitis Vitrectomy Study (EVS) currently underway is evaluating in a randomized fashion the efficacy of a combination of systemic antibiotics (ceftazidime and amikacin) when administered in conjunction with intravitreal antibiotics.[49]

Local Administration. In addition to intravitreal and systemic administration, antibiotics are also usually administered subconjunctivally and topically. Vitreous levels achieved in humans by subconjunctival antibiotics are extremely low, however.[15,16] It should be recognized that although subconjunctival and topical antibiotics produce high anterior segment levels, they do not achieve therapeutically useful levels of antibiotic within the vitreous cavity.

Corticosteroids

Microbial endophthalmitis generally elicits intense intraocular inflammation, which contributes to the direct destructive effects of the bacteria and bacterial toxins. Corticosteroids administered subconjunctivally and topically are helpful in diminishing the anterior segment inflammatory sequelae of endophthalmitis. Systemic corticosteroids in doses equivalent to 40 to 80 mg of prednisone are also often used to decrease both anterior segment and vitreous inflammation, depending on the severity of the intraocular inflammation and the patient's age and health. It should be recognized that systemic corticosteroids may have life-threatening complications even if used for only several days, particularly in the elderly.

Because the most effective method of antibiotic delivery is into the vitreous, can corticosteroids also be administered intravitreally? Direct intravitreal administration of dexamethasone sodium phosphate was suggested and evaluated in a rabbit model by Graham and Peyman.[72] They determined that 400 μg did not produce any ophthalmoscopic, electroretinographic, or light microscopic abnormalities. In a more recent ultrastructural study transient, reversible staining of rabbit Müller cells was noted at approximately the same dosage of dexamethasone sodium phosphate; doses of 800 μg or higher caused more toxic effects.[92] In an experimental rabbit model of Pseudomonas aeruginosa endophthalmitis, a combination of intravitreal dexamethasone and gentamicin resulted in less inflammation than when gentamicin alone was used in those groups in which therapy was initiated within 5 hours of inoculation.[72] In eyes in which treatment was initiated later the addition of the intraocular corticosteroid was not beneficial in reducing intraocular inflammation. In another experimental rabbit model infected with methicillin-resistant Staphylococcus epidermidis where treatment was initiated 24 hours after inoculation, Smith and associates[148] found both by clinical examination and histopathological evaluation that there was less intense inflammation in eyes treated with intravitreal dexamethasone and vancomycin as compared with eyes treated with vancomycin alone. In other experimental models of S. epidermidis endophthalmitis, the addition of corticosteroids was also beneficial in reducing inflammation[105,115]; in one of the studies the effect of intravitreal corticosteroids was no different from that of systemic corticosteroids, but the antiinflammatory benefit was evident only when vitrectomy was also performed as part of the therapy.[115] Stern,[155] using quantitative microbiologic techniques applied to a rabbit model of Staphylococcus aureus endophthalmitis, determined that concurrent use of intravitreal corticosteroids had neither a positive nor a negative effect on the effectiveness of intravitreal antibiotics. The lack of interference of corticosteroids used in this manner with the microbicidal effects of the intravitreal antibiotics is critical; there would be no benefit to reduction of inflammation if elimination of bacteria were compromised.

Clinical data regarding the effect of intravitreal corticosteroids is more difficult to obtain because of the wide variability in individual cases. Intravitreal dexamethasone sodium phosphate along with appropriate antibiotics has been used in the initial therapy of endophthalmitis caused by virulent bacterial organisms without any evident potentiation of the underlying infectious process.[78] There is general agreement that corticosteroids should be avoided if the clinical picture suggests a fungal etiology.

Vitrectomy

The precise role of vitrectomy in the therapy of endophthalmitis has generated more debate than perhaps any other aspect of management. Experimental animal studies have generally supported the beneficial effects of vitrectomy in this setting. Cottingham and Forster[38] first demonstrated that in a phakic rabbit model of Staphylococcus aureus endophthalmitis, more eyes were sterilized by combining vitrectomy with antibiotics than by antibiotics alone. In subsequent experimental animal studies by other investigators,[77,109,115,161] the benefit provided by vitrectomy has been more rapid clearing of inflammatory material from the eye rather than more effective sterilization of the eye. In a series of elegant experimental studies applying quantitative bacteriologic methods to a rabbit model of S. aureus postoperative endophthalmitis, Stern[155] has recently demonstrated that vitrectomy combined with a single intravitreal injection of vancomycin significantly reduced the bacterial concentration in the vitreous and sterilized a higher percentage of eyes, compared with injection of vancomycin without vitrectomy. His results therefore quantitatively confirmed those obtained by Cottingham and Forster[38] in 1976.

Clinical corroboration of these experimental animal observations has been difficult to obtain. In some clinical series of exogenous endophthalmitis the results have been worse in patients treated with vitrectomy,[24,46,52,124] in others about the same,[65] and in yet others, patients who underwent vitrectomy fared better.[78] It is inappropriate to draw conclusions as to the optimum therapeutic approach from these data, because in none of these studies was vitrectomy a randomized variable applied to a group of patients otherwise comparable in terms of the infecting agents or severity of the inflammatory process. In most but not all reported series, more severely affected eyes underwent vitrectomy, thus biasing the visual outcome results.

The theoretical advantages of vitrectomy in the management of endophthalmitis include direct removal of infecting organisms and their toxins, removal of inflammatory cells and mediators that have been mobilized into the vitreous, possible elimination of sequestered pockets within the vitreous cavity, better fluid circulation within the vitreous allowing for better antibiotic distribution, clearing of vitreous opacity, and removal of membranes that might subsequently cause traction retinal detachment. On the other hand, vitrectomy can be a technically difficult procedure to perform in inflamed eyes. Visualization is frequently suboptimal because of corneal edema and cellular infiltration, as well as anterior chamber inflammation. Vascular engorgement secondary to inflammation may increase the risk of intraocular or postoperative bleeding. The more edematous retina may be more friable and, in combination with suboptimal visualization, predisposes to the development of retinal breaks. In view of these conflicting factors, the generally beneficial effects of vitrectomy in experimental studies, and the difficulty in drawing conclusions from retrospective clinical series, a prospective, randomized, multicenter clinical trial, the Endophthalmitis Vitrectomy Study, has been undertaken in an attempt to define the role of vitrectomy better in the management of postoperative endophthalmitis.[49]

Special Therapeutic Considerations

Complete reviews of the management of endophthalmitis, including specific details of therapy and techniques for proper antibiotic dilution and administration are available.[60,64,91,99] Selected therapeutic considerations that apply to particular categories of exogenous endophthalmitis will be discussed here.

Filtering Blebs. Endophthalmitis developing in patients with filtering blebs is usually caused by virulent organisms.[101] The visual prognosis of these eyes has been very poor when treated with intraocular antibiotics without vitrectomy.[101] Despite the uncertainty regarding the precise role of vitrectomy, the recommendation is to include as complete a vitrectomy as can be safely performed in the initial therapy of patients who have filtering blebs and develop endophthalmitis. This approach, along with appropriate intravitreal antibiotics to cover the streptococcal and *Haemophilus influenzae* organisms most commonly isolated, may offer the best option for salvaging these eyes otherwise usually lost to the consequences of overwhelming inflammation.[101]

Chronic Postoperative Endophthalmitis. A different treatment strategy is required for patients with chronic endophthalmitis than for those with the more common acute postoperative infection.[100] Once it has been ascertained with absolute certainty that the corneoscleral wall is intact, any causative microbial agent can be presumed to have been introduced at the time of surgery, implying an organism of lower virulence. Pars plana vitrectomy represents a reasonable approach in this setting, removing those portions of the capsule that are involved with a capsular plaque. Intraocular scissors and forceps may facilitate removal of these portions of the capsule for culture and histopathologic examination. This procedure is valuable not only diagnostically, but is also likely to be helpful therapeutically by removing sequestered organisms. Intravitreal administration of vancomycin alone (1.0 mg in 0.1 cc) is appropriate in this situation, because this antibiotic is active against the gram-positive bacteria that have been isolated.

Subsequent therapy will depend on the clinical course

and the organism that is ultimately isolated. Repeat intraocular injections, removal of additional portions of capsule not previously recognized as having been involved, and ultimately removal of the entire capsular bag and intraocular lens implant may be necessary to eradicate the underlying infectious process.

Fungal Endophthalmitis. In patients with visible involvement of ocular tissues, results are best if the involved ocular tissues are fully excised and repeated doses of antifungals are administered intraocularly.[133] In patients with diffuse rather than focal involvement, vitrectomy should be performed, also followed by repeated intraocular antifungal administration. Amphotericin B (5 to 10 μg intraocularly) remains the agent to which most isolates are sensitive.[133] If *Paecilomyces lilacinus* is isolated,[117] or if amphotericin B is not effective, intraocular miconazole (25 μg) may be administered. Administration of systemic amphotericin B should be individualized, given its considerable toxicity and the documented ability to eradicate certain cases of fungal endophthalmitis without systemic therapy.[133,159] Oral ketoconazole, which is generally well tolerated, may be useful in those patients infected with sensitive organisms.[133]

PROGNOSIS

As data that includes the results of aqueous and vitreous cultures have been accumulated from various clinical series over the past two decades, it has become apparent that the outcome in cases of exogenous endophthalmitis is primarily related to the virulence of the infecting organism. Results have often been reported based on the category of clinical presentation: for example, acute postoperative,[52,124] chronic postoperative,[67,111] bleb-associated,[101] posttraumatic.[3,26] While this grouping provides clinically useful information, the major differences in outcomes between these groups (with the exception of associated structural ocular injuries resulting from trauma) can be principally accounted for on the basis of differences in the spectrum of infecting organisms associated with these clinical categories. For example, patients with filtering blebs who develop endophthalmitis are almost invariably infected with virulent organisms, usually strep species or hemophilus.[101] The bleb allows these organisms to enter the eye, but the nature of the organism rather than the presence of the bleb is the primary reason why the patient's visual outcome is so poor. There is now a sufficient data base of patients managed using current therapeutic approaches to allow evaluation of outcome based on the infecting organism itself.[24,44,78,102,125]

Bacillus cereus is among the most virulent and destructive of organisms to cause endophthalmitis. Rarely seen as a cause of postoperative endophthalmitis, it is one of the most frequent organisms isolated from eyes that develop endophthalmitis after perforating or penetrating trauma,[26,27,121,144,165] particularly if the injury occurs where soil contamination is likely.[26,121] Only rarely is useful vision salvaged from an eye infected with *B. cereus*.[3,144] Most reported cases have lost all light perception, and many have required evisceration or enucleation.[26,27,121,165,167] The rapidity of progression of the infectious process in bacillus-infected eyes is striking, occurring over hours; the best hope for salvage in these cases seems to be with immediate intervention based on the principles discussed previously.

Pseudomonas aeruginosa, a gram-negative rod, is also a highly virulent organism with poor visual outcome. Of the 12 cases of endophthalmitis caused by this organism reported in a recent series, only 1 recovered 20/400 or better visual acuity.[78] *P. aeruginosa* was also the most common species of the gram-negative organisms reported, accounting for 23% of the 53 cases in the series. The four eyes infected with other *Pseudomonas* species had better outcomes, with all four achieving vision better than 20/400.[78]

The outcome in cases of endophthalmitis caused by other gram-negative organisms in this series was slightly better than that resulting from *Pseudomonas* species. Fifty-seven percent (21 of 37) of these cases achieved 20/400 or better visual acuity. These infections may be difficult to eradicate: of the 19 eyes that underwent culture of samples removed at the time of a retap and reinjection of antibiotic, 14 remained culture-positive. The potential severity of gram-negative endophthalmitis is underscored by the fact that 36% (19 of 53) of the total group either lost all light perception or underwent evisceration or enucleation.[78]

Endophthalmitis caused by streptococci has proved to have a worse visual prognosis than might have been expected. In a recent large series of 48 cases,[102] only 15 eyes (31.3%) achieved 20/400 or better vision. Sixteen of the 48 eyes (33.3%) deteriorated to no light perception or were enucleated. Of the streptococci, β-hemolytic streptococci had the worst visual outcome, with none of the 5 patients from which this organism was isolated achieving even 20/400 acuity. In other series of streptococcal endophthalmitis, visual results have been even worse. In the patients reported by Jones and associates,[82] 2 of 5 (40%) of eyes infected with viridans group streptococci achieved 20/400 or better acuity; of their remaining 13 patients infected with other streptococci, none achieved better than light perception. Similarly, in a group of patients reported by Bohigian and Olk,[25] none of the 13 eyes infected by streptococci retained even 20/400 acuity.

Staphylococci, particularly *S. epidermidis,* is the most common cause of acute postoperative endophthalmitis. Fortunately patients infected by *S. epidermidis* have a relatively good visual prognosis. In one series 78% of these eyes achieved 20/400 or better acuity, with 33% 20/40 or better.[52] In another large series, results were comparable: 68% achieved at least 20/400, with 38% 20/50 or better.[125]

Propionibacterium acnes is the most frequent isolate from eyes with chronic postoperative endophthalmitis.[100] Visual outcome in these cases has generally been good, although multiple interventions may be required to sterilize the eye. In a series of 9 cases reported from one institution, all final visual acuities were 20/400 or better, with 6 patients achieving 20/60 or better.[174]

The visual outcome of exogenous fungal endophthalmitis is variable because of the diversity of organisms that may be causative, the variability in the clinical setting in which the infection may present, and the extent of ocular involvement before institution of therapy. In the largest series, reported by Pflugfelder and associates,[133] 42% of patients (8 of 19) recovered 20/400 or better visual acuity.

These average visual outcomes provide clinically useful information in the management of patients with endophthalmitis. It is important to recognize that variability does exist from case to case, presumably because of differences in the virulence of the particular infecting organism and in host responses. Even infection by *S. epidermidis* can be devastating and can result in complete loss of vision.[24,125] Conversely, isolation of a virulent organism should not preclude vigorous therapy, because some eyes have been salvaged despite infection with *B. cereus* or *P. aeruginosa.*

Not surprisingly, patients with endophthalmitis that is culture-negative have a much better prognosis than do eyes from which organisms are isolated.[25,52,156] In one large series, 94% (15 of 16) of culture-negative cases recovered 20/400 or better acuity, with 44% 20/40 or better.[52] Presumably these culture-negative eyes are either not infected or, if organisms are present intraocularly, they are of relatively low virulence or have already been partially disabled by host defenses.

Patients with posttraumatic endophthalmitis represent a unique situation in that their prognosis may be significantly affected not only by the infectious agent, but also by the precipitating ocular injury. In particular, the presence of retinal breaks or retinal detachment at the time of primary repair carries with it a particularly poor prognosis.[3,26]

In a recent large series of cases of infectious endophthalmitis, echographic findings on initial presentation were correlated to the infecting organism and to the final outcome.[39] Initially echographically clear vitreous was found to correlate with either culture-negative endophthalmitis or with early streptococcal endophthalmitis. Advanced cases of streptococcal endophthalmitis, on the other hand, had the most severe vitreous inflammation and vitreous membranes. A complete posterior vitreous detachment on echography was also found to be a common feature of streptococcal endophthalmitis. Choroidal detachment on initial echography was strongly associated with endophthalmitis caused by gram-negative organisms. The initial echographic findings that were found to correlate with final vision were density of vitreous opacity, presence of vitreous membranes, presence and extent of retinal detachment, and presence of choroidal detachment.

It is likely that the prognosis of patients with endophthalmitis is also affected by the rapidity of institution of therapy.[46,137,168] In some animal models evaluated, the results of either antibiotics alone or vitrectomy combined with antibiotics were better when therapy was instituted earlier.[38,43] Although the logarithmic rate of bacterial multiplication might suggest itself as a likely cause, other considerations may be even more important. Despite maintaining approximately the same concentration of bacteria within the eye in an experimental model, Stern[155] found that intravitreal antibiotics were much more effective at eradicating bacteria from the vitreous cavity when administered ''early'' rather than ''late.'' He suggested that the increasing purulence that developed within the vitreous with time might interfere with the effectiveness of antibiotic administration.

PREVENTION

Despite improvements in visual outcome with contemporary therapy, endophthalmitis is clearly a condition that is best prevented if at all possible. The apparent decline in the incidence of postoperative endophthalmitis over the past decades can probably be ascribed to an increased awareness and understanding of the complication, improved sterile and surgical techniques, and possibly to an improved use of antibiotics. Postoperative endophthalmitis represents the largest clinical category; patients undergoing eye surgery are the group for whom issues regarding prophylaxis are the most relevant both because of the number of patients affected and because control in this setting is greater than in other categories of endophthalmitis.

Preoperative Antimicrobial Prophylaxis

Recent data obtained by Speaker and associates,[152] using techniques of molecular epidemiology, have convincingly confirmed the previously held belief that most cases of postoperative endophthalmitis are caused by the patient's own flora, either from the patient's eyelid, conjunctiva, or nose. Organisms were recovered from the vitreous that were genetically indistinguishable from the patient's periocular flora in 82% of the cases of postoperative endophthalmitis examined (14 of 17). It has long been known that the lids or conjunctiva of most patients are colonized with organisms capable of causing endophthalmitis.[6,53] The presence of these organisms periocularly in so many individuals, and the verification that these same external ocular organisms cause the intraocular infection in most cases, provides a rationale for reduction of the periocular flora before and during intraocular surgery.

Administration of antibiotics topically preoperatively is one approach that has been considered to reduce organisms present on the lids and conjunctiva. A review of the studies performed indicates that topical antibiotics administered for a brief period preoperatively can reduce the numbers of lid and conjunctival bacteria compared with untreated controls.[63] Although evidence suggests that this approach may also reduce the likelihood of intraocular infection, this pre-

sumption cannot be stated definitively based on available studies.[154] If preoperative topical antibiotics are to be utilized, there is little information available to determine the optimum regimen. In earlier studies gentamicin was the most effective of the antibiotics evaluated at reducing the quantity of periocular organisms.[29,30] The aminoglycosides are not, however, particularly effective against the methicillin-resistant staphylococci that are currently a major cause of postoperative endophthalmitis. Trimethoprim sulfate-polymyxin B sulfate drops or a topical fluoroquinolone may be better choices for broad-spectrum coverage. There is no evidence from which to determine the best administration schedule; from a practical point of view, topical antibiotics are usually administered four times a day beginning several days before surgery and continuing on the day of surgery. Inherent in the use of topical antibiotics is the possibility of local toxicity or a hypersensitivity reaction with tearing, conjunctival hyperemia, or lid edema that may be severe enough to require deferral of the planned surgical procedure.

Another approach to reducing periocular flora is the use of topical antiseptic agents applied to the eye just before surgery. Apt and associates[10] showed that when half-strength (5%) povidone-iodine (Betadine) solution was placed in the conjunctival cul-de-sac as part of the preoperative preparation of the eye, the number of colonies and species of bacteria that could be isolated was reduced compared with controls. In a subsequent study the effect of preoperative preparation with 5% povidone-iodine was compared with administration of a topical antibiotic drop (containing polymyxin B sulfate, neomycin sulfate, and gramicidin) used for 3 days preoperatively.[79] A substantial and similar decrease in the number of colonies and species of bacteria isolated was demonstrated in each group. When the two techniques (preoperative topical antibiotics and 5% povidone-iodine presurgical preparation) were used together, there was an additive effect, rendering 83% of the conjunctival cultures negative.

To evaluate the efficacy of preoperative preparation with topical povidone-iodine, Speaker and Menikoff[150] performed a large, controlled, nonrandomized study in their hospital, incorporating 5% povidone-iodine in the preoperative preparation of patients undergoing surgery in one set of operating rooms and comparing the outcomes with those of patients in adjacent operating rooms where silver protein solution was used in the preoperative preparation instead. They found a significantly lower incidence of postoperative endophthalmitis for patients whose preoperative preparation included 5% povidone-iodine (2 of 3489, or 0.06%) compared with those patients for whom silver protein solution had been used (11 of 4594, or 0.24%). These data provide a relevant clinical correlate to the culture results noted previously. No adverse effects to the use of povidone-iodine solution were noted. The povidone-iodine must be a solution rather than a scrub, however, because the latter is toxic to the eye. Additionally, this preparation should be avoided in patients allergic to iodine.

The goal of preoperative antibiotics and antiseptics is to reduce periocular flora before surgery, thereby minimizing the pool of organisms available to enter the eye at surgery; subconjunctival antibiotics, commonly administered at the conclusion of the surgical procedure, are intended to inhibit any organisms that enter the eye intraoperatively from progressing to endophthalmitis. Recent studies indicating that viable bacteria can be isolated from anterior chamber aspirates obtained at the conclusion of surgery in a significant number of eyes[47,146] provide some rationale for this approach. Although there is negligible vitreous penetration from most antibiotics administered subconjunctivally,[15,16] therapeutic levels can be achieved in the anterior chamber, the most likely site for the presence of bacteria immediately after cataract extraction. Animal models in which cataract extraction was followed by intentional inoculation of bacteria into the vitreous cavity have demonstrated a reduction in the incidence of endophthalmitis when subconjunctival antibiotics were administered.[55,147] The evidence for a beneficial effect of subconjunctival injections in reducing endophthalmitis in clinical series, however, is less convincing. Reported studies have been small,[89] some have been performed in third world settings,[35] and they have generally lacked bacteriologic confirmation of the infecting organism in those cases that have developed endophthalmitis.

It is unknown whether perioperative subconjunctival antibiotics actually reduce the incidence of endophthalmitis, but it is clear that administration of these antibiotics certainly does not prevent the development of endophthalmitis in all cases, even by an organism sensitive to those antibiotics. In Driebe's series of postoperative endophthalmitis,[52] the bacteria isolated from aqueous or vitreous cultures were found to be sensitive to the antibiotics that had previously been administered subconjunctivally in 90% of cases. Similarly, in Kattan's epidemiological review,[87] 65% of the patients who developed endophthalmitis after cataract extraction and had received subconjunctival antibiotics were infected by organisms sensitive to those antibiotics.

In addition to uncertainties regarding efficacy, concerns have recently been raised regarding safety of the aminoglycosides, the antibiotics most frequently administered subconjunctivally. Campochiaro and Conway[32] have collected 23 patients who developed macular infarction apparently resulting from subconjunctival aminoglycoside administration for prophylaxis after anterior segment surgery. Although inadvertent penetration of the eye was thought to provide access for toxic antibiotic doses directly into the vitreous, in at least several cases ocular penetration was thought to be unlikely. Substitution of a different antibiotic may not solve this problem, because other antibiotics are also likely to be toxic if injected directly into the eye. If inadvertent ocular penetration occurs in more cases than would be expected after subconjunctival medication administration, perhaps this approach should be reconsidered. At present, it is probable that the majority of ophthalmic surgeons administer subconjunctival antibiotics to most of their patients at the conclusion of surgery, though the efficacy of this approach is uncertain and the potential for sight-threatening toxicity is of great concern.

In view of these uncertainties, some surgeons have chosen to add very low concentrations of antibiotics to the irrigating solutions used during anterior segment surgery as microbial prophylaxis in place of subconjunctival antibiotics. To date information regarding this approach is largely anecdotal. Although it may have potential merit, careful experimental and clinical studies are required before this approach can be recommended. The risk/benefit ratio must be carefully considered; errors in dilution of added antibiotics could have devastating ocular consequences.

In addition to consideration of these generalized prophylactic measures, it is of great importance to examine critically the individual patient preoperatively to determine and treat appropriately any conditions that may increase that patient's risk of endophthalmitis. This requirement particularly applies to patients with conditions that increase periocular flora: for example, blepharitis, lacrimal drainage system disorders, or an ocular prostheses on the contralateral side. Pretreatment and posttreatment cultures and sensitivity studies may be appropriate in selected cases, with recognition of the variability in the results of sequential lid and conjunctival cultures that may occur in any individual.[6]

Within the operating room, the ophthalmologist should be alert to potential sources of contamination. The periocular skin and the eye should be carefully prepared with the method selected. Draping should be performed in such a way that the lid margins are isolated to the extent possible and so that pooling of irrigating solutions in the conjunctival cul-de-sac is minimized. The intraocular lens should be grasped and inserted into the eye so that it does not touch the lid or ocular surface, to minimize the likelihood of organisms coming into contact with and adhering to the lens. Traffic and conversation in the operating room should be limited to that necessary to perform the procedure, thereby minimizing the potential for airborne microbial contaminants.

Antibiotics After Penetrating Ocular Trauma

Given the high likelihood of endophthalmitis developing after penetrating ocular injury, the consideration of prophylactic antibiotics is recommended for all patients who have sustained such trauma, although there is no evidence to indicate that they reduce the incidence of endophthalmitis. Cefazolin sodium, 1.0 gram may be given every 8 hours intravenously. A systemic aminoglycoside has often been recommended as well,[27] although it must be recognized that vitreous penetration of aminoglycosides given systemically is very poor. Ciprofloxacin is an alternate. Parenteral antibiotics are typically administered for 3 to 5 days. Topical antibiotics are frequently used before surgical repair if their administration will not pose additional risk to the globe and if the nature of the injury is such that the topical medication will not enter the eye. Subconjunctival antibiotics are usually administered at the conclusion of surgical repair. A tetanus toxoid booster should be given if required.

In patients who have a retained intraocular foreign body, evidence indicates that endophthalmitis is less likely to develop in eyes in which primary repair is accomplished within 24 hours of the injury, compared with those who undergo later repair.[165] Ideally, foreign bodies removed from the eye should be cultured; determination of whether the foreign body was contaminated can be very helpful depending on the patient's subsequent course. Intravitreal administration of antibiotics should be considered in those cases of contamination of the foreign body with soil or in which the clinical appearance suggests the possibility of early microbial endophthalmitis.

Care of Filtering Blebs

The routine prophylactic use of topical antibiotics is not recommended for patients with filtering blebs. It is highly unlikely that the lid margins and conjunctiva could be maintained free of bacteria over the long term whatever antibiotic regimen were used, and selection of resistant strains would be likely. Strongly recommended, however, is educating patients with filtering blebs, and ophthalmic office personnel, as to the importance of prompt examination should such a patient develop ocular redness or discomfort. If the examination suggests conjunctivitis cultures should be obtained, and appropriate bactericidal antibiotics should be administered frequently. Such patients must be monitored extremely carefully during treatment, searching for the earliest signs of intraocular inflammation; some patients have developed subsequent endophthalmitis despite appropriate topical therapy for conjunctivitis.

REFERENCES

1. Aaberg TM Jr, Flynn HW Jr, Murray TG: Intraocular ceftazidime as an alternative to the aminoglycosides in the treatment of endophthalmitis, *Arch Ophthalmol* 112:18-19, 1994.
2. Abrahams IW: Diagnosis and surgical management of phacoanaphylactic uveitis following extracapsular cataract extraction with intraocular lens implantation, *J Am Intraocul Implant Soc* 11:444-447, 1985.
3. Affeldt JC, Flynn HW Jr, Forster RK et al.: Microbial endophthalmitis resulting from ocular trauma, *Ophthalmology* 94:407-413, 1987.
4. Aiello LP, Javitt JC, Canner JK: National outcomes of penetrating keratoplasty, *Arch Ophthalmol* 111:509-513, 1993.
5. Allen HF, Mangiaracine AB: Bacterial endophthalmitis after cataract extraction: a study of 22 infections in 20,000 operations, *Arch Ophthalmol* 72:454-462, 1964.
6. Allansmith MR, Anderson RP, Butterworth M: The meaning of preoperative cultures in ophthalmology, *Trans Am Acad Ophthalmol Otolaryngol* 73:683-690, 1969.

7. Allansmith MR, Skaggs C, Kimura SJ: Anterior chamber paracentesis: diagnostic value in postoperative endophthalmitis, *Arch Ophthalmol* 84:745-748, 1970.
8. Antonios SR, Cameron JA, Badr IA et al.: Contamination of donor cornea: postpenetrating keratoplasty endophthalmitis, *Cornea* 10:217-220, 1991.
9. Apple DJ, Mamalis N, Steinmetz RL et al.: Phacoanaphylactic endophthalmitis associated with extracapsular cataract extraction and posterior chamber intraocular lens, *Arch Ophthalmol* 102:1528-1532, 1984.
10. Apt L, Isenberg J, Yoshimori R et al.: Chemical preparation of the eye in ophthalmic surgery. III. Effect of povidone-iodine on the conjunctiva, *Arch Ophthalmol* 102:728-729, 1984.
11. Axelrod AJ, Peyman GA: Intravitreal amphotericin B treatment of experimental fungal endophthalmitis, *Am J Ophthalmol* 76:584-588, 1973.
12. Axelrod JL, Klein RM, Bergen RL et al.: Human vitreous levels of selected antistaphylococcal antibiotics, *Am J Ophthalmol* 100:570-575, 1985.
13. Barr CC: Prognostic factors in corneoscleral lacerations, *Arch Ophthalmol* 1010:919-924, 1983.
14. Barza M: Antibacterial agents in the treatment of ocular infections, *Inf Dis Clin North Am* 3:533-555, 1989.
15. Barza M, Doft B, Lynch E: Ocular penetration of ceftriaxone, ceftazidime, and vancomycin after subconjunctival injection in humans, *Arch Ophthalmol* 111:492-494, 1993.
16. Barza M, Kane A, Baum J: Intraocular penetration of gentamicin after subconjunctival and retrobulbar injection, *Ophthalmology* 85:541-547, 1978.
17. Barza M, Kane A, Baum J: Pharmacokinetics of intravitreal carbenicillin, cefazolin and gentamicin in rhesus monkeys, *Invest Ophthalmol Vis Sci* 24:1602-1606, 1983.
18. Baum JL: Antibiotic administration in the treatment of bacterial endophthalmitis. I. Periocular injections, *Surv Ophthalmol* 21:332-339, 1977.
19. Baum J, Peyman GA, Barza M: Intravitreal administration of antibiotic in the treatment of bacterial endophthalmiti. III. Consensus, *Surv Ophthalmol* 26:204-206, 1982.
20. Ben-Nun J, Joyce DA, Cooper RL et al.: Pharmacokinetics of intravitreal injection: assessment of a gentamicin model by ocular dialysis, *Invest Ophthalmol Vis Sci* 30:1055-1061, 1989.
21. Beyer TL, O'Donnell FE, Goncalves V et al.: Role of the posterior capsule in the prevention of post-operative bacterial endophthalmitis: experimental primate studies and clinical implications, *Br J Ophthalmol* 69:841-846, 1985.
22. Beyer TL, Sharma D, Vogler G et al.: Protective barrier effect of the posterior lens capsule in exogenous bacterial endophthalmitis: an experimental pseudophakic primate study, *J Am Intraocul Implant Soc* 9:293-296, 1983.
23. Beyer TL, Vogler G, Sharma D et al.: Protective barrier effect of the posterior lens capsule in exogenous bacterial endophthalmitis: an experimental primate study, *Invest Ophthalmol Vis Sci* 25:108-112, 1984.
24. Bode DD Jr, Gelender H, Forster RK: A retrospective review of endophthalmitis due to coagulase-negative staphylococci, *Br J Ophthalmol* 69:915-919, 1985.
25. Bohigian GM, Olk RJ: Factors associated with a poor visual result in endophthalmitis, *Am J Ophthalmol* 101:332-341, 1986.
26. Boldt HC, Pulido JS, Blodi CF et al.: Rural endophthalmitis, *Ophthalmology* 96:1722-1726, 1989.
27. Brinton GS, Topping TM, Hyndiuk RA et al.: Post-traumatic endophthalmitis, *Arch Ophthalmol* 102:547-550, 1984.
28. Brown RH, Yang LH, Walker SD et al.: Treatment of bleb infection after glaucoma surgery, *Arch Ophthalmol* 112:57-61, 1994.
29. Burns RP, Oden M: Antibiotic prophylaxis in cataract surgery, *Trans Am Ophthalmol Soc* 70:43-57, 1972.
30. Burns RP, Hansen T, Fraunfelder FT et al.: An experimental model for evaluation of human conjunctivitis and topical antibiotic therapy: comparison of gentamicin and neomycin, *Can J Ophthalmol* 3:132-137, 1968.
31. Cameron JA, Antonios SR, Cotter JB et al.: Endophthalmitis from contaminated donor corneas following penetrating keratoplasty, *Arch Ophthalmol* 109:54-59, 1991.

32. Campochiaro PA, Conway BP: Aminoglycoside toxicity: a survey of retinal specialists; implications for ocular use, *Arch Ophthalmol* 109:946-950, 1991.

33. Campochiaro PA, Green WR: Toxicity of intravitreous ceftazidime in primate retina, *Arch Ophthalmol* 110:1625-1629, 1992.

34. Campochiaro PA, Lim JI, Bloome MA et al.: Aminoglycoside toxicity in the treatment of endophthalmitis, *Arch Ophthalmol* 112:48-53, 1994.

35. Christy NE, Lall P: Postoperative endophthalmitis following cataract surgery, *Arch Ophthalmol* 90:361-366, 1973.

36. Cobo LM, Forster RK: The clearance of intravitreal gentamicin, *Am J Ophthalmol* 92:59-62, 1981.

37. Conway BP, Campochiaro PA: Macular infarction after endophthalmitis treated with vitrectomy and intravitreal gentamicin, *Arch Ophthalmol* 104:367-371, 1986.

38. Cottingham AJ Jr, Forster RK: Vitrectomy in endophthalmitis: results of a study using vitrectomy, intraocular antibiotics, or a combination of both, *Arch Ophthalmol* 94:2078-2081, 1976.

39. Dacey MP, Valencia M, Lee MB et al.: Echographic findings in infectious endophthalmitis, *Arch Ophthalmol* 112:1325-1333, 1994.

40. Daily MJ, Peyman GA, Fishman G: Intravitreal injection of methicillin for treatment of endophthalmitis, *Am J Ophthalmol* 76:343-350, 1973.

41. D'Amico DJ, Caspers-Velu L, Libert J et al.: Comparative toxicity of intravitreal aminoglycoside antibiotics, *Am J Ophthalmol* 100:264-275, 1985.

42. D'Amico DJ, Libert L, Kenyon KR et al.: Retinal toxicity of intravitreal gentamicin: an electron microscopic study, *Invest Ophthalmol Vis Sci* 25:564-572, 1984.

43. Davey PG, Barza M, Stuart M: Dose response of experimental pseudomonas endophthalmitis to ciprofloxacin, gentamicin and impenem: evidence for resistance to "late" treatment of infections, *J Infect Dis* 155:518-523, 1987.

44. Davis JL, Koidou-Tsiligianni A, Pflugfelder SC et al.: Coagulase-negative staphylococcal endophthalmitis: increase in antimicrobial resistance, *Ophthalmology* 95:1404-1410, 1988.

45. Deutsch TA, Goldberg MF: Painless endophthalmitis after cataract surgery, *Ophthalmic Surg* 15:837-840, 1984.

46. Diamond JG: Intraocular management of endophthalmitis: a systemic approach, *Arch Ophthalmol* 99:96-99, 1981.

47. Dickey JB, Thompson KD, Jay WM: Anterior chamber aspirate cultures after uncomplicated cataract surgery, *Am J Ophthalmol* 112:278-282, 1991.

48. Dilly PN, Holmes Sellors PJ: Bacterial adhesion to intraocular lenses, *J Cataract Refract Surg* 15:317-320, 1989.

49. Doft BH: The endophthalmitis vitrectomy study, *Arch Ophthalmol* 109:487-489, 1991 (editorial).

50. Doft BH, Weiskopf J, Nilsson-Ehle I et al.: Amphotericin clearance in vitrectomized versus non-vitrectomized eyes, *Ophthalmology* 92:1601-1605, 1985.

51. Donahue SP, Kowalski RP, Eller AW et al.: Empiric treatment of endophthalmitis: are aminoglycosides necessary?, *Arch Ophthalmol* 112:45-47, 1994.

52. Driebe WT Jr, Mandelbaum S, Forster RK et al.: Pseudophakic endophthalmitis: diagnosis and management, *Ophthalmology* 93:442-448, 1986.

53. Dunnington JH, Locatcher-Khorazo D: Value of cultures before operation for cataract, *Arch Ophthalmol* 34:215-219, 1945.

54. Eichenbaum DM, Jaffe NS, Clayman HM et al.: Pars plana vitrectomy as a primary treatment for acute bacterial endophthalmitis, *Am J Ophthalmol* 86:167-171, 1978.

55. Elliot RD, Katz HR: Inhibition of pseudophakic endophthalmitis in a rabbit model, *Ophthalmic Surg* 18:538-541, 1987.

56. Feist RM, Lim JI, Joondeph BC et al.: Penetrating ocular injury from contaminated eating utensils, *Arch Ophthalmol* 109:63-66, 1991.

57. Ficker L, Meredith TA, Gardner S et al.: Cefazolin levels after intravitreal injection: effects of inflammation and surgery, *Invest Ophthalmol Vis Sci* 31:502-505, 1990.

58. Fisher JP, Civiletto SE, Forster RK: Toxicity, efficacy, and clearance of intravitreally injected cefazolin, *Arch Ophthalmol* 100:650-652, 1982.

59. Flynn HW Jr, Pulido JS, Pflugfelder SC et al.: Endophthalmitis therapy: changing antibiotic sensitivity patterns and current therapeutic recommendations, *Arch Ophthalmol* 109:175-176, 1991.

60. Flynn HW Jr, Pflugfelder SC, Culbertson WW et al.: Recognition, treatment, and prevention of endophthalmitis, *Semin Ophthalmol* 4:69-83, 1989.

61. Fong LP, Gladstone D, Casey TA: Corneo-scleral rim cultures: donor contamination: a case of fungal endophthalmitis transmitted by K-sol stored cornea, *Eye* 2:670-676, 1988.

62. Forster RK: Endophthalmitis: diagnostic cultures and visual results, *Arch Ophthalmol* 92:387-392, 1974.

63. Forster RK: Antibiotic and asepsis. In Sears M, Tarkkanen A, editors: *Surgical pharmacology of the eye,* 57-80, New York, 1985, Raven Press.

63a. Forster RK: Experimental postoperative endophthalmitis, *Trans Am Ophthalmol Soc* 90:505-559, 1992.

64. Forster RK: Endophthalmitis. In Tasman W, Jaeger AE, editors: *Duane's clinical ophthalmology,* vol 4, Philadelphia, 1994 rev ed, JB Lippincott.

65. Forster RK, Abbott RL, Gelender H: Management of infectious endophthalmitis, *Ophthalmology* 87:313-319, 1980.

66. Forster RK, Zachary IG, Cottingham AJ Jr et al.: Further observations on the diagnosis, cause, and treatment of endophthalmitis, *Am J Ophthalmol* 81:52-56, 1976.

67. Fox GM, Joondeph BC, Flynn HW Jr et al.: Delayed-onset pseudophakic endophthalmitis, *Am J Ophthalmol* 111:163-173, 1991.

68. Freedman J, Gupta M, Bunke A: Endophthalmitis after trabeculectomy, *Arch Ophthalmol* 96:1017-1018, 1978.

69. Garfinkel RA, Lipkowitz JL: Efficacy of diagnosis of endophthalmitis in the phakic eye, *Invest Ophthalmol Vis Sci* 27(suppl):315, 1986 (abstract).

70. Gerding DN, Poley BJ, Hall WH et al.: Treatment of pseudomonas endophthalmitis associated with prosthetic intraocular lens implantation, *Am J Ophthalmol* 88:902-908, 1979.

71. Godley BF, Folk JC: Retinal hemorrhages as an early sign of acute bacterial endophthalmitis, *Am J Ophthalmol* 116:247-249, 1993.

72. Graham RO, Peyman GA: Intravitreal injection of dexamethasone: treatment of experimentally-induced endophthalmitis, *Arch Ophthalmol* 92:149-154, 1974.

73. Graham RO, Peyman GA, Fishman G: Intravitreal injection of cephaloridine in the treatment of endophthalmitis, *Arch Ophthalmol* 93:56-61, 1975.

74. Hattenhauer JM, Lipisch MP: Late endophthalmitis after filtering surgery, *Am J Ophthalmol* 72:1097-1101, 1971.

75. Heilskov T, Joondeph BC, Olsen KR et al.: Case report: late endophthalmitis after transscleral fixation of a posterior chamber intraocular lens, *Arch Ophthalmol* 107:1427, 1989.

76. Hessburg TP, Maxwell DP, Diamond JG: Endophthalmitis associated with sutureless cataract surgery, *Arch Ophthalmol* 109:1499, 1991.

77. Huang K, Peyman GA, McGetrick J: Vitrectomy in experimental endophthalmitis. I. Fungal infection, *Ophthalmic Surg* 10:84-86, 1979.

78. Irvine WD, Flynn HW Jr, Miller D et al.: Endophthalmitis caused by gram-negative organisms, *Arch Ophthalmol* 110:1450-1454, 1992.

79. Isenberg SJ, Apt L, Yoshimori R et al.: Chemical preparation of the eye in ophthalmic surgery. IV. Comparison of povidone-iodine on the conjunctiva with a prophylactic antibiotic, *Arch Ophthalmol* 103:1340-1342, 1985.

80. Javitt JC, Vitale S, Canner JK et al.: National outcomes of cataract extraction: endophthalmitis following inpatient surgery, *Arch Ophthalmol* 109:1085-1089, 1991.

81. Jeglum EL, Rosenberg SB, Benson WE: Preparation of intravitreal drug doses, *Ophthalmic Surg* 12:355-359, 1981.

82. Jones S, Cohen EJ, Arentsen JJ et al.: Ocular streptococcal infections, *Cornea* 7:295-299, 1988.

83. Joondeph BC, Joondeph HC: Purulent anterior segment endophthalmitis following paracentesis, *Ophthalmic Surg* 17:91-93, 1986.

84. Joondeph BC, Flynn HW Jr, Miller D et al.: A new culture method for infectious endophthalmitis, *Arch Ophthalmol* 107:1334-1337, 1989.

85. Judson PH: Aminoglycoside macular toxicity after subconjunctival injection, *Arch Ophthalmol* 107:1282-1283, 1989.

86. Kane A, Barza M, Baum J: Intravitreal injection of gentamicin in rabbits, *Invest Ophthalmol Vis Sci* 20:593-597, 1981.

87. Kattan HM, Flynn HW Jr, Pflugfelder S et al.: Nosocomial endophthalmitis survey: current incidence of infection after intraocular surgery, *Ophthalmology* 98:227-238, 1991.

88. Kloess PM, Stulting RD, Waring GO et al.: Bacterial and fungal endophthalmitis after penetrating keratoplasty, *Am J Ophthalmol* 115:309-316, 1993.

89. Kolker AE, Freeman MI, Pettit TH: Prophylactic antibiotics and post-operative endophthalmitis, *Am J Ophthalmol* 63:434-439, 1967.

90. Krebs DB, Liebmann JM, Ritch R et al.: Late infectious endophthalmitis from exposed glaucoma setons, *Arch Ophthalmol* 110:174-175, 1992.

91. Kremer PA, Abbott RL: Management of endophthalmitis, *Ophthalmol Clin N Am* 7:39-50, 1994.

92. Kwak HW, D'Amico DJ: Evaluation of the retinal toxicity and pharmacokinetics of dexamethasone after intravitreal injection, *Arch Ophthalmol* 110:259-266, 1992.

93. Lambert SR, Stern WH: Methicillin- and gentamicin-resistant Staphylococcus epidermidis endophthalmitis after intraocular surgery, *Am J Ophthalmol* 99:725-726, 1985.

94. Lesk MR, Ammann H, Marcil G et al.: The penetration of oral ciprofloxacin into the aqueous humor, vitreous, and subretinal fluid of humans, *Am J Ophthalmol* 115:623-628, 1993.

95. Leveille AS, McMullan FD, Cavanagh HD: Endophthalmitis following penetrating keratoplasty, *Ophthalmology* 90:38-39, 1983.

96. Liesgang TJ, Samples JR, Waller RR: Suppurative interstitial ring keratitis due to streptococcus, *Ann Ophthalmol* 16:392-396, 1984.

97. Lim JI, Campochiaro PA: Successful treatment of gram-negative endophthalmitis with intravitreous ceftazidime, *Arch Ophthalmol* 110:1686, 1992.

98. Lim JI, Anderson CT, Hutchinson A et al.: The role of gravity in gentamicin-induced toxic effects in a rabbit model, *Arch Ophthalmol* 112:1363-1367, 1994.

99. Mandelbaum S, Forster RK: Postoperative endophthalmitis, *Int Ophthalmol Clin* 27:95-106, 1987.

100. Mandelbaum S, Meisler DM: Postoperative chronic microbial endophthalmitis, *Int Ophthalmol Clin* 33:71-79, 1993.

101. Mandelbaum S, Forster RK, Gelender H et al.: Late onset endophthalmitis associated with filtering blebs, *Ophthalmology* 92:964-972, 1985.

102. Mao LK, Flynn HW Jr, Miller D et al.: Endophthalmitis caused by streptococcal species, *Arch Ophthalmol* 110:798-801, 1992.

103. Marak GE Jr: Phacoanaphylactic endophthalmitis, *Surv Ophthalmol* 36:325-339, 1992.

104. Martin DF, Ficker LA, Aguilar HA et al.: Vitreous cefazolin levels after intravenous injection: effects of inflammation, repeated antibiotic doses, and surgery, *Arch Ophthalmol* 108:411-414, 1990.

105. Maxwell DP, Brent BD, Diamond JG et al.: Effect of intravitreal dexamethasone on ocular histopathology in a rabbit model of endophthalmitis, *Ophthalmology* 98:1370-1375, 1991.

106. May DR, Ericson ES, Peyman GA et al.: Intraocular injection of gentamicin: Single injection therapy of experimental bacterial endophthalmitis, *Arch Ophthalmol* 91:487-489, 1974.

107. Maylath FR, Leopold JH: Study of experimental ocular infection, *Am J Ophthalmol* 40:86-101, 1955.

108. McDonald HR, Schatz H, Allen AW et al.: Retinal toxicity secondary to intraocular gentamicin injection, *Ophthalmology* 93:871-877, 1986.

109. McGetrick JJ, Peyman GA: Vitrectomy in experimental endophthalmitis. II. Bacterial endophthalmitis, *Ophthalmic Surg* 10:87-92, 1979.

110. McMahon MS, Weiss JS, Riedel KG et al.: Clinically unsuspected phacoanaphylaxis after extracapsular cataract extraction with intraocular lens implantation, *Br J Ophthalmol* 69:836-840, 1985.

111. Meisler DM, Mandelbaum S: Propionibacterium-associated endophthalmitis after extracapsular extraction: review of reported cases, *Ophthalmology* 96:54-61, 1989.

112. Meisler DM, Palestine AG, Vastine DW et al.: Chronic Propionibacterium endophthalmitis after extracapsular cataract extraction and intraocular lens implantation, *Am J Ophthalmol* 102:733-739, 1986.

113. Meltzer DW: Sterile hypopyon following intraocular lens surgery, *Arch Ophthalmol* 98:100-104, 1980.

114. Menikoff JA, Speaker MG, Marmor M et al.: A case-control study of risk factors for post-operative endophthalmitis, *Ophthalmology* 98:1761-1768, 1991.

115. Meredith TA, Aguilar HE, Miller MJ et al.: Comparative treatment of experimental *Staphylococcus epidermidis* endophthalmitis, *Arch Ophthalmol* 108:857-860, 1990.

116. Mieler WF, Ellis MK, Williams D et al.: Retained intraocular foreign bodies and endophthalmitis, *Ophthalmology* 97:1532-1538, 1990.

117. Miller GR, Rebell G, Magoon RC et al.: Intravitreal antimycotic therapy and the care of mycotic endophthalmitis caused by *Paecilomyces lilacinus* contaminated pseudophakos, *Ophthalmic Surg* 9:54-63, 1978.

118. Miller KM, Glasgow BJ: Bacterial endophthalmitis following sutureless cataract surgery, *Arch Ophthalmol* 111:377-379, 1993.

119. Morris R, Camesasca FI, Byrne J et al.: Postoperative endophthalmitis resulting from prosthesis contamination in a monocular patient, *Am J Ophthalmol* 116:346-349, 1993.

119a. Nelsen PT, Marcus DA, Vovino JA: Retinal detachment following endophthalmitis, *Ophthalmology* 92:1112-1117, 1985.

120. Neuhaus RW: Postcataract surgery endophthalmitis in a patient with a functioning Jones tube, *Ophthal Plast Reconstr Surg* 8:208-209, 1992.

121. O'Day DM, Smith RS, Gregg CR: The problem of bacillus species infection with special emphasis on the virulence of *Bacillus cereus*, *Ophthalmology* 88:833-838, 1981.

122. O'Day DM, Jones DB, Patrinely J et al.: *Staphylococcus epidermidis* endophthalmitis: visual outcome following non-invasive therapy, *Ophthalmology* 89:354-360, 1982.

123. Okada AA, Johnson RP, Liles WC et al.: Endogenous bacterial endophthalmitis: report of a ten-year retrospective study, *Ophthalmology* 101:832-838, 1994.

124. Olson JC, Flynn HW Jr, Forster RK et al.: Results in the treatment of postoperative endophthalmitis, *Ophthalmology* 90:692-699, 1983.

125. Ormerod LD, Ho DD, Becker LE et al.: Endophthalmitis caused by the coagulase-negative staphylococci. I. Disease spectrum and outcome, *Ophthalmology* 100:715-723, 1993.

126. Oum BS, D'Amico DJ, Wong KW: Intravitreal antibiotic therapy with vancomycin and aminoglycoside: an experimental study of combination and repetitive injections, *Arch Ophthalmol* 107:1055-1060, 1989.

127. Packer AJ, Weingeist TA, Abrams GW: Retinal periphlebitis as an early sign of bacterial endophthalmitis, *Am J Ophthalmol* 96:66-71, 1983.

128. Paque JT, Peyman GA: Intravitreal clindamycin phosphate in the treatment of vitreous infection, *Ophthalmic Surg* 5:34-39, 1974.

129. Pavan PR, Brinser JH: Exogenous bacterial endophthalmitis treated without systemic antibiotics, *Am J Ophthalmol* 104:121-126, 1987.

130. Pettit TH, Olson RJ, Foos RY et al.: Fungal endophthalmitis following intraocular lens implantation: a surgical epidemic, *Arch Ophthalmol* 98:1025-1039, 1980.

131. Peyman GA, May DR, Ericson ES et al.: Intraocular injection of gentamicin: Toxic effects and clearance, *Arch Ophthalmol* 92:42-47, 1974.

131a. Peyman GA, Paque JT, Maisels HI et al.: Post-operative endophthalmitis: a comparison of methods for treatment and prophylaxis with gentamicin, *Ophthalmic Surg* 6:45-55, 1975.

132. Peyman GA, Vastine DW, Crouch ER et al.: Clinical use of intravitreal antibiotics to treat bacterial endophthalmitis, *Trans Am Acad Ophthalmol Otolaryngol*, 78:862-875, 1974.

133. Pflugfelder SC, Flynn HW Jr, Zwickey TA et al.: Exogenous fungal endophthalmitis, *Ophthalmology* 95:19-30, 1988.

134. Pflugfelder SC, Hernandez E, Fliesler SJ et al.: Intravitreal vancomycin: retinal toxicity, clearance and interaction with gentamicin, *Arch Ophthalmol* 105:831-837, 1987.

135. Pitts RE, Krachmer JH: Evaluation of soft contact lens disinfection in the home environment, *Arch Ophthalmol* 97:470-472, 1979.

136. Prokop BS: Lest we forget—or, every procedure carries risk, *Ophthalmic Surg* 15:221, 1984.

137. Puliafito CA, Baker AS, Haaf J et al.: Infectious endophthalmitis: review of 36 cases, *Ophthalmology* 89:921-929, 1982.

138. Pulido JS, Shires TK, Flynn HW Jr et al.: Intravitreal aminoglycoside toxicity revisited, *Arch Ophthalmol* 110:1683-1684, 1992.

139. Raskin EM, Speaker MG, McCormick SA et al.: Influence of haptic materials on the adherence of staphylococci to intraocular lenses, *Arch Ophthalmol* 111:250-253, 1993.

140. Records RE, Iwen PC: Experimental bacterial endophthalmitis following extracapsular lens extraction, *Exp Eye Res* 49:729-737, 1989.

141. Rowsey JJ, Newsome DL, Sexton DJ et al.: Endophthalmitis: current approaches, *Ophthalmology* 89:1055-1066, 1982.

142. Rubinstein E, Goldfarb J, Keren G et al.: The penetration of gentamicin into the vitreous humor in man, *Invest Ophthalmol Vis Sci* 24:637-639, 1983.

143. Salamon SM, Friberg TR, Luxenberg MN: Endophthalmitis after strabismus surgery, *Am J Ophthalmol* 93:39-41, 1982.

144. Schemmer GB, Driebe WT: Post-traumatic *Bacillus cereus* endophthalmitis, *Arch Ophthalmol* 105:342-344, 1987.

145. Schiff FS: The shouting surgeon as a possible source of endophthalmitis, *Ophthalmic Surg* 21:438-440, 1990.

146. Sherwood DR, Rich WJ, Jacob JS et al.: Bacterial contamination of intraocular and extraocular fluids during extracapsular cataract extraction, *Eye* 3:308-312, 1989.

147. Shockley RK, Fishman P, Aziz M et al.: Subconjunctival administration of ceftazidime in pigmented rabbit eyes, *Arch Ophthalmol* 104:266-268, 1986.

148. Smith MA, D'Aversa G, Sorenson JA et al.: Treatment of experimental methicillin-resistant *Staphylococcus epidermidis* endophthalmitis with intravitreal vancomycin and dexamethasone, *Clin Infect Dis* 17(3), 1993 (Abstract 104).

149. Smith MA, Sorenson JA, Lowy FD et al.: Treatment of experimental methicillin-resistant *Staphylococcus epidermidis* endophthalmitis with intravitreal vancomycin, *Ophthalmology* 93:1328-1335, 1986.

150. Speaker MG, Menikoff JA: Prophylaxis of endophthalmitis with topical povidone-iodine, *Ophthalmology* 98:1769-1775, 1991.

151. Speaker MG, Menikoff JA: Postoperative endophthalmitis: pathogenesis, prophylaxis, and management, *Int Ophthalmol Clin* 33:51-70, 1993.

152. Speaker MG, Milch FA, Shah MK et al.: Role of external bacterial flora in the pathogenesis of acute postoperative endophthalmitis, *Ophthalmology* 98:639-650, 1991.

153. Stark WJ, Rosenblum P, Maumenee AE et al.: Postoperative inflammatory reactions to intraocular lenses sterilized with ethylene-oxide, *Ophthalmology* 87:385-389, 1980.

154. Starr MB, Lally JM: Antimicrobial prophylaxis for ophthalmic surgery, *Surv Ophthalmol* 39:485-501, 1995.

155. Stern GA: Factors affecting the efficacy of antibiotics in the treatment of experimental postoperative endophthalmitis, *Trans Am Ophthalmol Soc* 91:775-844, 1993.

156. Stern GA, Engel HM, Driebe WT: The treatment of postoperative endophthalmitis: results of differing approaches to treatment, *Ophthalmology* 96:62-67, 1989.

157. Stern WH, Tamura E, Jacobs RA et al.: Epidemic post-surgical *Candida parapsilosis* endophthalmitis: clinical findings and management of 15 consecutive cases, *Ophthalmology* 92:1701-1709, 1985.

158. Stonecipher KG, Parmley VC, Jensen H et al.: Infectious endophthalmitis following sutureless cataract surgery, *Arch Ophthalmol* 109:1562-1563, 1991.

159. Stransky TJ: Postoperative endophthalmitis secondary to *Candida parapsilosis:* a case treated by vitrectomy and intravitreous therapy, *Retina* 1:179-185, 1981.

160. Talamo JH, D'Amico DJ, Hanninen LA et al.: The influence of aphakia and vitrectomy on experimental retinal toxicity of aminoglycoside antibiotics, *Am J Ophthalmol* 100:840-847, 1985.

161. Talley AR, D'Amico DJ, Talamo H et al.: The role of vitrectomy in the treatment of post-operative bacterial endophthalmitis, *Arch Ophthalmol* 105:1699-1702, 1987.

162. Theodore FH: Mycotic endophthalmitis after cataract surgery, *Int Ophthalmol Clin* 4:861-881, 1961.

163. Theodore FH: Bacterial endophthalmitis after cataract surgery, *Int Ophthalmol Clin* 4:839-859, 1964.

164. Theodore FH: Etiology and diagnosis of fungal postoperative endophthalmitis, *Ophthalmology* 85:327-340, 1978.

165. Thompson JT, Parver LM, Enger CL et al.: Infectious endophthalmitis after penetrating injuries with retained intraocular foreign bodies, *Ophthalmology* 100:1468-1474, 1993.

166. Tucker DN, Forster RK: Experimental bacterial endophthalmitis, *Arch Ophthalmol* 88:647-649, 1972.

167. Vahey JB, Flynn HW Jr: Results in the management of bacillus endophthalmitis, *Ophthalmic Surg* 22:681-686, 1991.

168. Vastine DW, Peyman GA, Guth SB: Visual prognosis in bacterial endophthalmitis treated with intravitreal antibiotics, *Ophthalmic Surg* 10:76-83, 1979.

169. von Sallmann L, Meyer K: Penetration of penicillin into the eye, *Arch Ophthalmol* 31:1-7, 1944.

170. Wohl LG, Lucier AC, Kline OR Jr et al.: Pseudophakic phacoanaphylactic endophthalmitis, *Ophthalmic Surg* 17:234-237, 1986.

171. Wolner B, Liebmann JM, Sassani JW et al.: Late bleb-related endophthalmitis after trabeculectomy with adjunctive 5-fluorouracil, *Ophthalmology* 98:1053-1060, 1991.

172. Yanoff M, Fine BS: Nongranulomatous inflammation: uveitis, endophthalmitis, panophthalmitis, and sequelae. In Duane TD, Jaeger AE, editors: *Biomedical foundations of ophthalmology,* vol 3, Philadelphia, 1985, Harper & Row.

173. Zachary IG, Forster RK: Experimental intravitreal gentamicin, *Am J Ophthalmol* 82:604-611, 1976.

174. Zambrano W, Flynn HW Jr, Pflugfelder SC et al.: Management options for *Propionibacterium acnes* endophthalmitis, *Ophthalmology* 96:1100-1105, 1989.

94 Orbital Infections

DIANE J. KRAUS, JOHN D. BULLOCK

Orbital infections are infrequent but can provoke rapid and permanent visual loss and can lead to death.

HISTORICAL BACKGROUND

Orbital infection is classically associated with sinusitis, and this relationship was first detailed by Hippocrates (460 to 370 BC).[74] Maitre Jean (1740) and Demarquay (1860) were among the first to describe orbital abscesses.[74] Birch-Hirschfeld (1905)[25] accurately expounded on the clinical nature and importance of the sinuses in the pathogenesis of orbital inflammation. Of the 684 orbital infections he studied, 60% reached the orbit by direct extension from the paranasal sinuses.[25]

ANATOMY

Organisms can reach the orbit by many routes. An infection anterior to the orbital septum, a structure that usually prevents posterior extension of organisms into the orbit, is termed preseptal or periorbital cellulitis. Orbital cellulitis refers to infection behind the orbital septum. Signs of periorbital cellulitis include eyelid redness and swelling and an absence of ocular manifestations, whereas orbital cellulitis typically causes visual loss, pain, proptosis, conjunctival chemosis, ophthalmoplegia and pupillary abnormalities.

Infection can extend from the sinuses, face, nose, eyelids, globe, lacrimal sac, lacrimal gland, teeth, or intracranial structures to involve the orbit. Direct inoculation with organisms occurs by injury to the orbital structures via trauma, especially when it is associated with a fracture, foreign body retention, or orbital or ocular surgery. Metastatic seeding from a distant infection may settle in the orbit and is termed endogenous orbital infection.

Many mechanisms play a role in the development of bacterial, fungal, and parasitic invasion of the orbit. The pathogenesis of orbital infections is best understood in terms of orbital and periorbital anatomy.[51,74,132,255]

Orbital Anatomy

Seven bones contribute to the pyramidal shape of the orbit: the ethmoid, palatine, lacrimal, zygoma, frontal, maxillary, and sphenoid. These bones also form the nasal cavities, paranasal sinuses, and intracranial cavity. The orbit is in intimate contact with these adjacent chambers because these bones are thin and perforated by many neurovascular foramina.

The main foramina of the orbit are the following:

1. The superior orbital fissure, which is between the greater and lesser wings of the sphenoid, contains the first, third, fourth, and sixth cranial nerves, the ophthalmic division of the fifth cranial nerve, sympathetic nerves, and the superior ophthalmic vein.
2. The inferior orbital fissure, between the sphenoid, maxillary and palatine bones, connects the orbit with the temporal fossa and contains the maxillary division of the fifth cranial nerve, the zygomatic nerve, and the inferior ophthalmic vein.
3. The optic canal, which lies within the lesser wing of the sphenoid, transmits the ophthalmic artery, optic nerve, and sympathetic nerves.
4. The anterior and posterior ethmoidal foramina transmit ethmoidal arteries and nerves through the medial orbital wall at the frontoethmoid suture.
5. The zygomaticotemporal and zygomaticofacial foramina contain the zygomatic nerves and vessels, which pass from the lateral orbital wall to the cheek and temporal fossa.
6. The frontosphenoid foramina are located in the frontosphenoid suture and transmit arterial anastomoses between the middle meningeal and lacrimal arteries.
7. The nasolacrimal canal contains the nasolacrimal duct, which empties into the nose beneath the inferior turbinate.

In addition to these foramina, several random bony defects occur in the orbital bones, especially the ethmoid and maxillary. For instance, the lamina papyracea of the medial orbital wall, besides being very thin and perforated by numerous foramina, usually possesses many congenital dehiscences (of Zuckerkandl).[175] These foramina and defects allow for the easy spread of infection from the ethmoid air cells to the medial orbital subperiosteal space. This space is the most common location for a subperiosteal abscess caused by acute sinusitis. The roof of the ethmoid air cells also contains many foramina and dehiscences and may thus allow an ethmoidal infection to reach up into the intracranial cavity to cause meningitis or an epidural, subdural, or frontal lobe abscess. Rarely, bone necrosis from septic processes results in direct extension of infection into the orbit.

Vascular System of the Orbit. The venous system of the orbits, soft tissues (including the lacrimal sac and duct), paranasal sinuses, and intracranial cavity anastomose with one another. Venous extension of infection (septic thrombophlebitis) can occur easily from one compartment to another. Infectious thrombosis may occur and allow clots to travel throughout the system. The main orbital vein, the superior ophthalmic vein, drains into the cavernous sinus; the smaller inferior ophthalmic vein empties into the superior ophthalmic vein and the pterygoid plexus. The primary ethmoid and superior maxillary sinus venous drainage runs through the orbital system.[51,147,175,255] The major facial-orbital anastomoses include the frontal, angular, and anterior facial veins. Because none of the veins through the midface and skull base contain valves, infection can spread easily. The smooth-muscle cells in the connective-tissue septa that surround the orbital venous system do help limit local retrograde phlebitis.[19,20]

The cavernous sinus in the middle cranial fossa is a venous plexus that communicates directly or indirectly with the superior and inferior ophthalmic, central retinal, facial, inferior cerebral, hypophyseal, superficial middle cerebral and middle meningeal veins, the pterygoid plexus, and the sphenoparietal, inferior petrosal, superior petrosal, and opposite cavernous sinuses. The carotid siphon and sympathetic plexus sit within the cavernous sinus. The lateral wall contains the third, fourth, and sixth cranial nerves and the first and second divisions of the fifth cranial nerve. Cavernous sinus thrombosis may result from disease processes of the face, eyes, orbit, sinuses, nasal and oral pharynx, middle ear, and cerebral structures.

No true lymphatic system has been identified in the orbit. If one does exist, some authors feel that it probably contributes to the pathogenesis of orbital infection.[123,175]

Orbital Periosteum. The periorbita, or orbital periosteum, and orbital septum are the main support tissues of the orbit. Orbital periosteum is loosely attached to bone except at sutures, fissures, foramina, and canals (where it fuses with the periosteum on the other side of the bone), at the optic foramen and superior orbital fissure (where it fuses to the dura), at the inferior orbital fissure (where it becomes continuous with pterygopalatine fossa periosteum), and anteriorly (where it adheres to the orbital margins and fuses with the facial periosteum and fascial sheaths to form the arcus marginalis). The orbital septum, an inelastic fibrous tissue layer, originates from the arcus marginalis at the anterior orbital margins and attaches to the levator and tarsal plates. It is the main soft-tissue barrier between the orbit and the eyelids.

Because the periorbita is not a tight barrier between the orbit and sinuses, the orbital subperiosteal space represents a potential space in which an abscess may develop and enlarge rapidly at the onset of infection. The inelastic orbital septum, although thin and incomplete, limits the anterior spread of orbital infection. The orbital bones limit spread in any other direction. Orbital tissue pressure can increase and potentially compromise the globe. Intraorbital abscesses, which are not anatomically confined because orbital fibrous septa are not complete, may also lead to visual loss. They develop more insidiously from tissue necrosis, however, and cause morbidity by tissue destruction rather than by high orbital pressure.

Sinuses. Approximately two thirds of the orbit is surrounded by the paranasal sinuses. The topographic relationship between the orbit and sinuses varies widely because sinus development differs among individuals.[80,255]

The maxillary sinuses and ethmoidal air cells start to develop from the nasal chambers in the second trimester of gestation, are aerated at birth, and reach adult sizes by 12 to 15 years of age. The roof of the antrum may border part or all of the inferior orbital rim and usually extends as far back as the inferior orbital fissure. The ethmoidal air cells sit within the frontal, maxillary, and lacrimal bones between the superior half of the nasal cavity and the orbit. They are adjacent to the medial orbital wall, and occasionally they extend superiorly and laterally to the orbit. The frontal sinuses do not become pneumatized (and are not radiographically evident) until about the sixth year of life.

Adult size of the orbit, which varies from nonexistent to a size that abuts the whole orbital roof back to the optic foramen and middle cranial fossa, is reached at puberty. The frontal sinus, like the ethmoids, usually come in direct contact with the anterior cranial fossa. The orbital wall of the frontal sinus rarely contains dehiscences. Sphenoid sinus development begins around the fourth fetal month. Pneumatization and expansion into the sphenoid, and sometimes into the pterygoid and occipital bones, occurs at about four years of age and continues sporadically until puberty. The anatomical relationships between the sphenoid, posterior ethmoids, cavernous sinus, and orbit are extremely variable. The optic canal is usually superolateral to the sphenoid sinus wall, but the canal may be located within the sinus or abut the opposite sinus.[255] Although visual loss can occur directly from sphenoid sinus pathology, infection of the sphenoid sinus is relatively rare, probably because the ostium is very high in the nasal cavity.[80]

The brain and meninges lie posterior, superior, and lateral to the orbit. Intracranial infectious processes may impinge upon the orbit through the superior or inferior orbital fissures.

BACTERIAL ORBITAL INFECTION

Bacterial orbital infections are usually caused by *Streptococcus pneumoniae,* other streptococci, *Staphylococcus aureus, Haemophilus influenzae,* and/or anaerobes. Extension of infection from the paranasal sinuses, facial soft tissues, and dentition cause most cases of orbital infection. Lacrimal, systemic, intracranial, or intraocular infections can involve the orbit. Trauma, with or without foreign body retention, and systemic factors predispose to orbital cellulitis.

Risk Factors

Sinusitis. Sinusitis remains the most frequent cause of orbital infection even though orbital complications from sinusitis have decreased in the antibiotic era. Inadequate treatment, virulent organisms, delay in diagnosis, and decreased host defenses allow sinus infection to progress and threaten vision and life.

Epidemiology of Sinusitis-Related Orbital Cellulitis. The incidence of orbital complications from sinusitis varies.[79,98,213,218,265] In one large series,[79] only 2% of 6770 patients with sinusitis had ocular or orbital manifestations. The majority of these patients and those from other series[98,213,218] exhibited preseptal infection rather than true orbital complications. Sinusitis was responsible for 56% to 85% of cases of preseptal and orbital cellulitis reported in several series.* In a series of true orbital cellulitis 61% had radiographic evidence of sinusitis.[21] Acute sinusitis and its orbital complications (Fig. 94-1) occur more frequently in children under 18 years of age.† Older individuals tend to develop more severe orbital disease.[218,271] Some series have noted more left- than right-sided orbital involvement,[90,213,219] and others have found males more susceptible than females.[92,98,130,265] Bilateral involvement can occur.[176,213]

Pathogenesis of Sinusitis-Related Orbital Cellulitis. How sinus infection begins is only partially known. The mucosal lining of the nasal and sinus cavities is respiratory mucous membrane. The cilia of the sinus's pseudostratified columnar epithelium continuously remove material out through the sinus ostia into the nose, keeping the sinuses sterile.[181] The two main factors known to contribute to the pathogenesis of sinus infection, ciliary dysfunction and sinus osteal obstruction, allow secretions to pool in the sinuses.[160,181] Bacteria from the oral and nasal cavities can then multiply and penetrate the sinus mucosal lining, initiating suppuration and infection through activation of the humoral and cellular immune systems.[47,160,181] Impaired ciliary action commonly occurs when viruses—especially adenovirus, influenza virus, coronavirus, and rhinoviruses —invade the sinus mucous layer.[47,181] Subsequently, the sinus mucosal lining becomes edematous and inflamed and mucous secretions become thicker. The sinus ostium can then occlude, allowing bacterial infection. Sinusitis occurs more commonly in children in the winter months when they are most likely to develop upper respiratory tract infections. Their sinus ostia are more easily obstructed than adult ostia.[79,80,92,213] Infection further impairs ciliary function and phagocytic activity, reduces oxygen tension and pH, and increases the amount of carbon dioxide present.* The reduced oxygen tension, along with the decrease in the oxidation-reduction potential, allows anaerobic bacteria to proliferate.[47,133,164]

Allergic reactions, which cause mucosal edema, thickened secretions, and polyp formation, can also occlude sinus ostia and cause infectious sinusitis. Other factors predisposing to sinusitis include nasal foreign bodies (especially feeding tubes in hospitalized patients),[149] adenoiditis, tonsillitis, asthma, mucoceles, nasopharyngeal tumors, a deviated septum, and the immotile cilia syndrome.[80] Immunocompromised patients[36] and individuals with impaired resistance caused by diabetes mellitus, sickle cell anemia,[265] juvenile rheumatoid arthritis,[265] and Wegener granulomatosis[273] are susceptible to sinoorbital infections (Fig. 94-2).

Variation in the development among the sinuses is age-related. Maxillary sinusitis is most common in infancy and early childhood (Fig. 94-3). Ethmoiditis is common in later childhood. Frontal sinusitis occurs in adolescence.[91,123] Adults are most prone to frontoethmoiditis.

Sinus infection has easy access to the orbit. The primary modes of extension are through neurovascular foramina, open suture lines (especially the ethmomaxillary and frontoethmoid suture lines), congenital bony defects (especially of the lamina papyracea and maxillary roof), areas of bone necrosis (caused by the interruption of periosteal blood flow by increased intrasinus pressure), and retrograde thrombophlebitis.

Sinusitis causes orbital congestion and chemosis by decreasing orbital venous return. Inflammation anterior and/or posterior to the orbital septum (i.e., preseptal and/or orbital cellulitis) ensues.

An abscess may rapidly occur between the orbital wall and periosteum, especially medially from ethmoiditis. Suppuration in the superior and inferior orbital walls may develop from extension of medial wall infection or from frontal or maxillary sinusitis. Subperiosteal abscesses may break through the lid skin to form a fistula. An orbital abscess (i.e., purulence within the retrobulbar tissues) may develop sec-

---

*References 92, 98, 130, 176, 213, 218, 265.
†References 92, 130, 176, 213, 218, 219, 265, 273.

---

*References 47, 48, 77, 160, 164, 232.

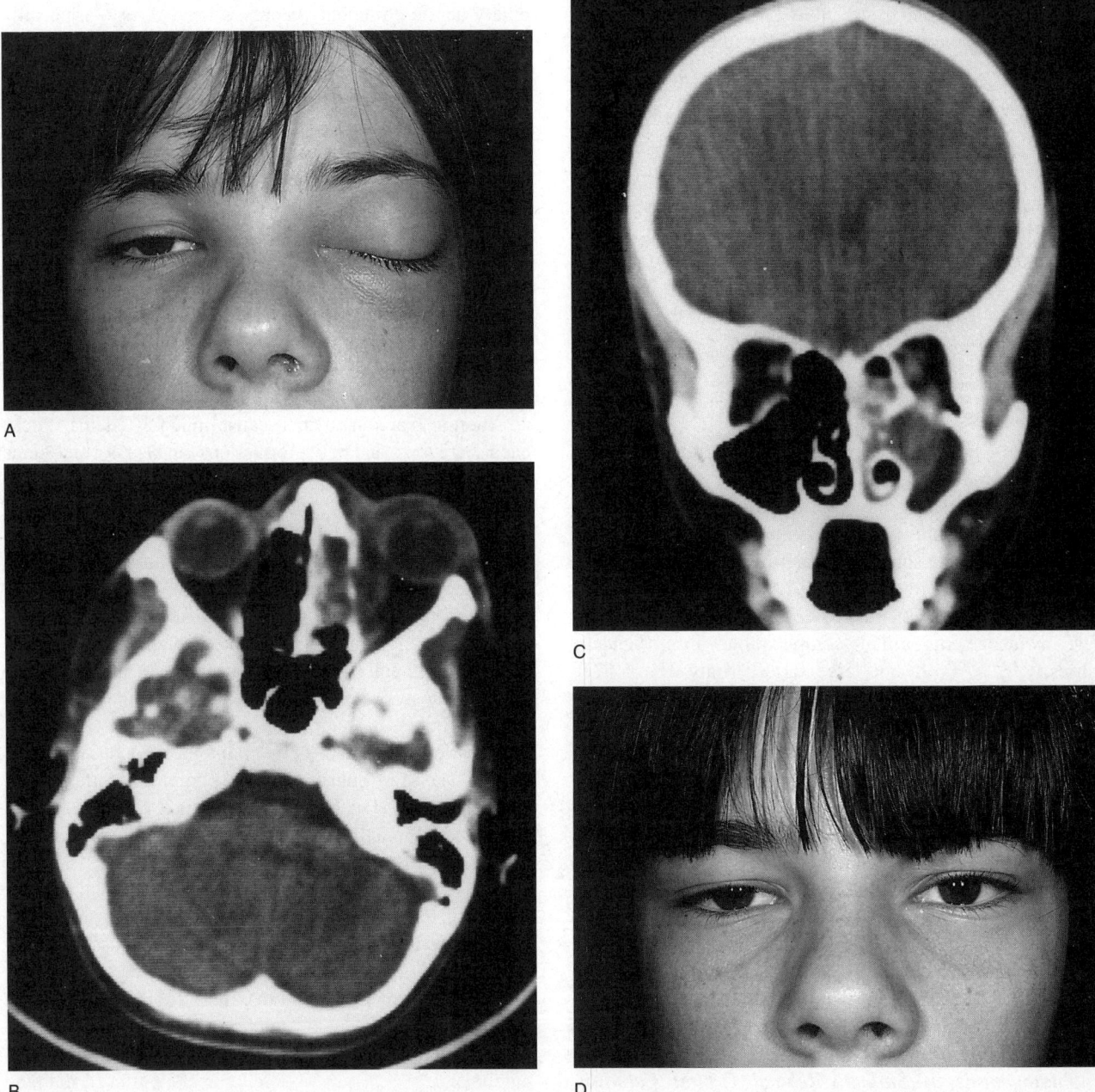

Fig. 94-1. **A,** Left orbital cellulitis and medial subperiosteal abscess in 12-year-old boy, secondary to left pansinusitis. *Staphylococcus epidermidis* and diphtheroids were cultured from nasal swab. Blood cultures were negative. **B,** Axial CT scan localized medial subperiosteal orbital abscess. **C,** Coronal CT scan confirmed involvement of left ethmoidal and maxillary sinuses. **D,** Orbital cellulitis resolved following treatment with cefamandole and cefaclor.

ondary to extension of a subperiosteal abscess or from severe orbital cellulitis with tissue necrosis. A subperiosteal orbital hematoma results when a subperiosteal vessel is ruptured by increased venous pressure from sinoorbital congestion or by direct extension of infection.[53,110]

Visual loss can develop because of corneal damage secondary to proptosis or neurotrophic keratitis, sustained elevation of intraocular pressure, thrombophlebitis of ocular vasculature, central retinal artery occlusion, septic or inflammatory optic neuritis, and panophthalmitis. Occasionally visual loss may occur as one of the first manifestations of sphenoethmoiditis.[237] Intracranial extension of infection, especially to the cavernous sinus, most commonly occurs by retrograde thrombophlebitis.[54,123,243] Other modes include direct spread of infection through the orbital apex, cribiform plate, sphenoid sinus, or frontal sinus.

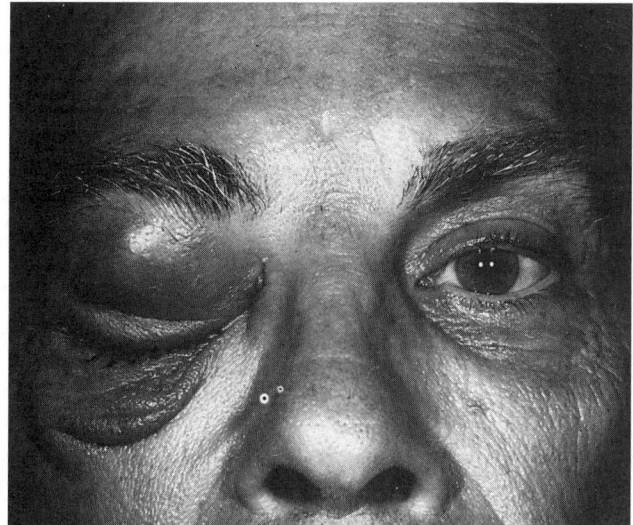

A

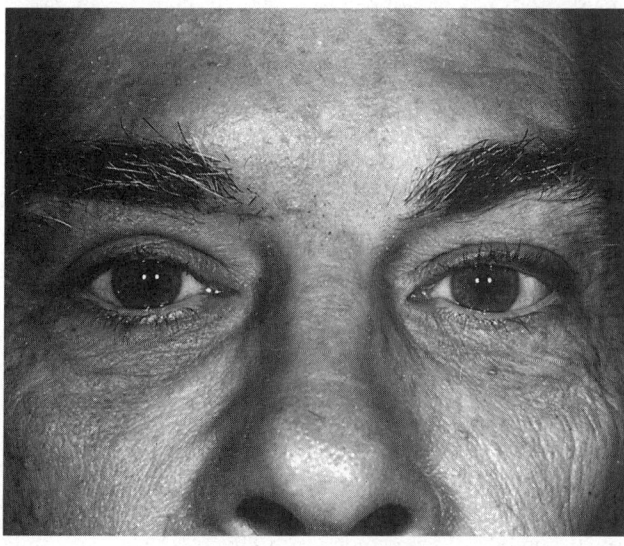

C

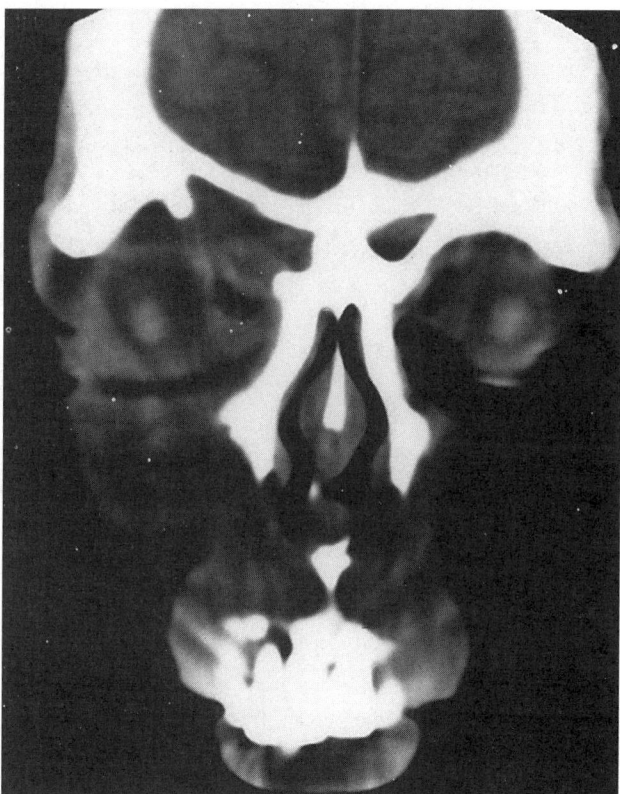

B

Fig. 94-2. **A,** Right pansinusitis secondary to *Propionibacterium acnes* in a 54-year-old HIV-seropositive male. **B,** Coronal CT scan showed right orbital cellulitis, frontal sinusitis, and bony defects in right supranasal orbit. **C,** Three weeks later after treatment with intravenous ceftazidime, metronidazole, and cefuroxime and surgical drainage of right orbit with removal of necrotic bone and drainage of right frontal, ethmoidal, and maxillary sinuses.

Orbital Trauma. Trauma that violates the orbital septum can produce diffuse orbital infection by the direct introduction of bacteria from the skin surface (especially *Staphylococcus* sp.) or on the object causing the trauma. Dog and human bites tend to lead to polymicrobial infections. Blunt and penetrating trauma both can cause hemorrhage, edema, and/or bone fragments that obstruct sinus drainage, creating an environment ideal for bacteria proliferation.[97,107,133,285] Upon orbital wall fracture, sinus infection may spread directly into the orbit.[97,274,285] Patients with penetrating wounds may exhibit signs of infection within 48 to 72 hours or longer, especially if a foreign body was introduced.[82,253] Orbital infections secondary to orbital fractures vary in onset time, and antibiotics given within three hours of the trauma causing the fracture may be effective prophylaxis.[97,107,274]

Orbital Surgery. Orbital infection may follow a variety of ocular, eyelid and orbital procedures including blepharo-plasty,[10] strabismus surgery,[74,129,262,266,278] orbital fracture repair,[134,169,210,274] dacryocystorhinostomy,[134] retinal surgery,[134,210] enucleation with sphere implantation,[210] molteno placement,[138] cataract extraction with intraocular lens implant,[145] and endophthalmitis.[134] Orbital signs of infection from direct spread of the organisms introduced at surgery typically appear within 24 to 72 hours, even with the use of prophylactic local or parenteral antibiotics. After appropriate cultures and the institution of medical treatment, any implanted material must usually be removed.

Contiguous Spread of Infection to the Orbit. Primary infection of the eyelids, preseptal or facial tissues; the globe; the central nervous system; the lacrimal sac or lacrimal gland; and dentition may involve the orbit. Osteomyelitis of the maxillary bone (which usually occurs in newborns)[90,210] and conjunctivitis (primarily caused by *Haemophilus influenzae*)[235] can also spread to the orbit. Infection reaches the

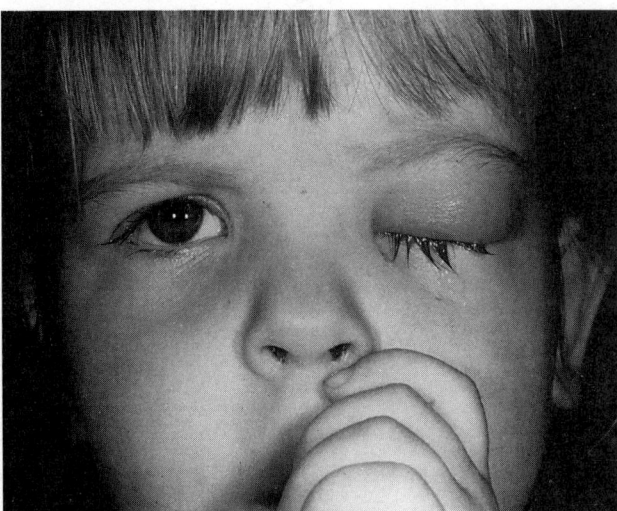

Fig. 94-3. Left orbital cellulitis secondary to *Haemophilus influenzae*. This 19-month-old infant improved rapidly with intravenous ampicillin.

orbit through local tissue planes, from thrombophlebitis, or via involvement of the paranasal sinuses.* Rarely, intracranial infection can erode through the orbital roof or the superior orbital fissure to form a subperiosteal abscess, or affect the cavernous sinus and then the orbital veins.[74,90]

Odontogenic infections gain entrance to the orbit by several pathways, the most common of which is through the paranasal sinuses. As many as 20% of all cases of sinusitis may have a dental origin.[38,146] The apices of maxillary molars and premolars are in close apposition with the floor of the maxillary sinus. Occasionally the apices of these teeth are in direct contact with the mucous membrane of the sinus. During extraction of an abscessed tooth, the floor of the sinus may be fractured, resulting in inoculation of the antrum with purulent material.[38,118] An abscess originating in the maxillary molars may penetrate the buccal cortical plate above the origin of the buccinator muscle and spread to the soft tissues of the cheek.[26,135] Orbital involvement may then ensue, either by direct spread through local tissue planes or by an ascending facial thrombophlebitis.[26,38,135,233] Infections of the maxillary molars may also spread posteriorly into the infratemporal and pterygopalatine fossae.[26,38,94,114,135] Purulent material may then extend along the tuberosity of the maxilla and thus gain access to the orbit through the inferior orbital fissure.[26,38,135] This fissure is usually closed by a strong facia and smooth muscle fibers; an opening is often found at its lateral aspect, however.[281]

Of all the causes of orbital cellulitis from direct spread, odontogenic orbital infections in particular have the poten-

tial to cause the most morbidity and mortality.[9,37,38,186] Sequelae include optic neuritis, optic atrophy causing blindness, cavernous sinus thrombosis, superior orbital fissure syndrome, orbital apex syndrome, meningitis, brain abscess, subdural empyema, and death.[37,38]

Sepsis. Endogenous (pyemic) orbital infection can result from bacteremia. Orbital seeding has been reported to occur in immunocompromised patients with pulmonary infection,[210] urinary tract infection,[210] endocarditis,[124] meningitis,[101] and dental[37,38] infection. Newborns with pulmonary or skin infections are susceptible.[40,119] Endophthalmitis and osteomyelitis may also occur.

Clinical Features

The most common manifestations of acute sinusitis resemble those of an acute upper respiratory tract infection. Sinusitis, however, tends to be more severe and last beyond seven days. Signs include nasal congestion with purulent, malodorous discharge; persistent cough; malaise; anorexia; leukocytosis; headache; and pain over the involved sinus(es). Children may or may not exhibit any of these classic signs. They tend not to experience the dull headache and facial pain that adults develop.[80] Fever is not a consistent finding in adults or children, even if they have orbital involvement.* Infants and young children with sinusitis may not show symptoms until orbital or intracranial infection occurs.[80] For any age group the onset of orbital complications of sinusitis may be rapid and overshadow any nasal or sinus findings.[205,277]

Orbital infections caused by sinusitis were classically categorized according to their anatomic location by Hubert[127] in 1937. He described five subgroups of orbital complications: eyelid edema, orbital cellulitis, orbital abscess, subperiosteal abscess, and cavernous sinus thrombosis.[127] Hubert's classification has been implemented and modified by a number of contemporary authors.† These anatomic classifications remain clinically useful because they help to determine treatment and prognosis, not because they represent an orderly progression of clinical disease. They may occur together and may or may not evolve from one another. For instance, sudden and rapid cavernous sinus or orbital apex infection may result from early spread of sphenoid sinusitis. Abscess formation can occur promptly or insidiously. Factors such as organism virulence, host immune status, and prior treatment add to the variations noted in clinical presentations.

Bacteriology. No signs or symptoms of bacterial orbital cellulitis are specific for any one organism.[153,210,218]

The main sinus pathogens for all age groups repre-

---

*References 8, 38, 107, 134, 210, 254.

---

*References 107, 115, 148, 181, 265, 271.
†References 32, 107, 112, 148, 176, 178, 182, 183, 205, 218, 219, 222, 265, 271, 273, 277.

sent those organisms responsible for orbital cellulitis and abscess, namely, *Streptococcus pneumoniae*, other streptococci, *Staphylococcus aureus* and *Haemophilus influenzae*.* These are the organisms primarily recovered on surgical intervention and thus they only partially reflect the causative bacteria for cases treated medically. Children six months to five years of age are particularly susceptible to *Haemophilus influenzae* infection because they mount a poor humoral antibody response to polysaccharide-encapsulated organisms.[157,210,213,218,235] Immunization with the *Haemophilus influenzae* B vaccine may not affect the incidence of *H. influenzae* sinusitis or cellulitis.[181] *Streptococcus faecalis*,[76] *Streptococcus milleri*,[277] *Pseudomonas aeruginosa*,[272] *Eikenella corrodens*,[117,220] *Branhamella catarrhalis*,[153] *Staphylococcus epidermidis*,[210] diphtheroids,[112,210] *Escherichia coli*,[210] and other gram-negatives have also been reported to cause infection. Anaerobes encountered in sinogenic orbital infection, with or without aerobic infection, include peptostreptococci, *Propionibacterium* sp., *Veillonella* sp., *Bacteroides* sp., *Fusobacterium* sp., and *Eubacterium*.† Adults are more likely to harbor polymicrobial and anaerobic infection, many of which go unnoticed because of prior antibiotic treatment and inadequate anaerobic culture techniques.[33,182,210]

Complications

Inflammatory Edema or Preseptal Cellulitis. Preseptal cellulitis presents with eyelid edema, erythema, warmth, and pain, which are most prominent near the sinus of origin. Chemosis and slight proptosis may occur.[51,218] Extraocular movements and visual acuity remain normal. Abscess formation anterior to the orbital septum is rare.[153]

Subperiosteal Orbital Hematoma. Both frontal and ethmoidal sinusitis have been reported to cause a superior or, more rarely, medial subperiosteal hematoma, sometimes with a subperiosteal abscess.[45,53,110,275] Proptosis with downward displacement of the globe, orbital pain, ophthalmoplegia, and decreased visual acuity occur.

Subperiosteal Abscess. Globe displacement away from the abscess and pain on globe movement toward the abscess are the clinical hallmarks of subperiosteal suppuration. Increasing pain, proptosis, ophthalmoplegia, chemosis, and decreased vision occur as the abscess enlarges. Orbital cellulitis and orbital abscess may be present.

Orbital Cellulitis. Orbital cellulitis is characterized by severe eyelid edema, pain, chemosis and proptosis (usually axial), and partial or complete ophthalmoplegia with pain on globe motion. Ocular signs include visual loss, an afferent pupillary defect, elevated intraocular pressure, optic nerve edema with periphlebitis, and retinal venous congestion. An

orbital apex syndrome, panophthalmitis, or intracranial infection may develop.[150,210,237]

Orbital Abscess. The clinical manifestations of orbital abscess resemble those of orbital cellulitis. Visual loss on a septic or vascular basis, as well as from high intraorbital pressure, is usually profound.

Cavernous Sinus Thrombosis. Symptoms and signs of cavernous sinus thrombosis are local inflammation with chemosis and pain; intraocular pressure elevation; visual loss; dilated pupil or afferent defect; third, fourth, and sixth cranial nerve palsies; corneal hypesthesia from fifth cranial nerve involvement; engorged fundus vasculature with retinal hemorrhage and edema; central retinal artery occlusion; optic nerve edema and perivasculitis; proptosis and third, fourth, and sixth cranial nerve palsies of the contralateral orbit; edema over the mastoid emissary vein; and altered mental status. Reportedly early manifestations include an isolated contralateral oculomotor palsy, meningeal signs, ptosis, diplopia and photophobia.[191,203] Findings that help differentiate cavernous sinus thrombosis from orbital cellulitis include more ophthalmoplegia than proptosis, corneal hypesthesia, bilateral orbital congestion, and ophthalmoplegia and neurologic signs.[134]

Headache, vomiting, fever, altered consciousness, nuchal rigidity, ataxia, and other neurologic signs may occur with central nervous system infection.[80,120,243] Meningitis, cerebritis, and epidural, subdural, and parenchymal abscesses can develop. Sepsis and death may ensue.

Differential Diagnosis

Sinogenic orbital infection must be distinguished from other causes of inflammatory proptosis, namely orbital pseudotumor,[28,134,207,210] myositis,[16] Wegener granulomatosis,[273] thyroid orbitopathy,[134,210,215] orbital hemorrhage,[176] orbital retinoblastoma,[126,230] rhabdomyosarcoma,[134,162,176] leukemia,[103] metastatic carcinoma with necrosis,[134,211] histiocytosis X,[134,176] temporal arteritis,[55] plasma cell tumors,[69,142] and mucoceles or sinus tumors with or without concomitant infection.[80,140] Atypical infection from tuberculosis, syphilis, or pathogenic fungi must be suspected when the clinical scenario suggests it. When clinical findings are nonspecific, radiography and tissue specimens usually allow one to determine the cause of the inflammatory proptosis.

Laboratory Investigations

Aside from careful clinical examination, prompt diagnosis of sinogenic orbital infection requires laboratory investigation and radiologic evaluation. White blood cell counts are usually, but not always, above 10,000/mm³.[107,130,148,271]

Cultures. Nasal, conjunctival, and oropharyngeal cultures do not provide any useful information and may be misleading, whereas cultures of sinus aspirates and surgical speci-

---

*References 33, 107, 108, 133, 134, 190.
†References 51, 53, 110, 123, 130, 218, 238.

mens reliably establish the cause of the inflammation.* Cultures obtained on surgical drainages of abscesses may be sterile from prior treatment.[218,219] Because the main bacteria that cause sinusitis are well known, sinus aspiration is performed only when a patient is unresponsive to traditional treatment, is immunocompromised, or has advanced disease on presentation.[181] When sinus aspiration is necessary, or when surgical intervention is warranted, material should be Gram-stained and inoculated onto blood agar, chocolate agar, Sabouraud agar, and thioglycollate broth. In cases of orbital trauma or surgery, cultures of any wound drainage should be performed. Blood cultures, which are rarely positive in adults,[148,210] tend to be positive in children under four years of age.[218,219,265,271] *Haemophilus influenzae* most commonly causes bacteremia.[157,218,265] Lumbar puncture should be performed if clinical evidence of meningitis exists and CT does not reveal any midline shift.[218,219]

Radiography. Upright Waters, Caldwell, submental vertex, and lateral views of the paranasal sinuses should be obtained when infection is suspected. Common radiographic characteristics of sinusitis include mucosal thickening, complete sinus opacification, and air/fluid levels. Sinus x-rays are difficult to interpret and therefore are of questionable value in very young children.† Schramm and associates[218] found that 40% of healthy children under one year of age had x-ray findings indicative of sinusitis, while only 5% of children aged one to three years had false positive films. After age four, sinus radiographs became reliable. Sinus ultrasonography can also confirm the presence of acute infection.[181,219]

Any individual exhibiting orbital signs of infection should undergo computerized tomography (CT). The development of abscess cavities does not correlate with any specific clinical finding.‡ CT scanning accurately localizes abscesses, demonstrates the full extent of the infection, and monitors disease progression or improvement. Sinus involvement can be documented and again is demonstrated by mucosal thickening, opacification, and air/fluid levels. Bone erosion and osteomyelitis are easily seen. Most commonly infected are the ethmoid sinus, maxillary sinus, and multiple sinuses. Preseptal cellulitis appears as lid and facial edema without proptosis. Orbital cellulitis is appreciated by visualizing intraconal and extraconal obliteration of fat shadows, displacement of the muscle cone and globe with tenting of the posterior globe, or air/fluid levels in an intraconal or extraconal mass. The latter finding denotes an orbital abscess.[96,210,268] Scleral thickening with contrast enhancement denotes globe involvement. Subperiosteal abscesses appear as uniform or heterogeneous, low-density masses with a smooth, convex border on the orbital side.[95,210] When intravenous contrast agents are used, mature abscesses exhibit enhancing walls. Orbital ultrasonography may also help diagnose an orbital abscess.* Apical lesions, however, will be missed by ultrasonography.[134,242] Inflammatory edema or phlegmon and subperiosteal hematoma may resemble subperiosteal abscess on CT.† The use of intravenous contrast, although generally not required, is absolutely essential to delineate suspected intracranial infection.[134,152,252,268] Low narrow axial cuts of the frontal lobes help determine if cerebritis or abscess exists.[134] Coronal sections help further define orbital roof, medial orbital wall, and cavernous sinus anatomy.[7,152] Clinical diagnosis of cavernous sinus thrombosis can be difficult. CT scan findings include enlarged superior orbital vein(s), enlarged extraocular muscle(s), an expanded cavernous sinus with irregular filling defects, and cerebral infarct.[7,68,210,268] In cases of orbital trauma a CT scan can delineate the extent of infection and injury and will help to discern any foreign bodies.[107,134]

Magnetic resonance imaging (MRI) for bacterial orbital infection does not seem to provide any additional information. Its diagnostic use is limited in septic cavernous sinus thrombosis.[68]

Therapy

Medical Treatment. Hospitalization for intravenous antibiotics and for further evaluation and treatment is recommended for patients with orbital infections. Initial therapy should be broad to cover staphylococci, streptococci, *Haemophilus influenzae,* anaerobes, and some gram-negative bacteria, and then tailored to the culture results.

Specific antibiotic regimes change frequently. Still effective is the use of a penicillinase-resistant agent, namely nafcillin or methicillin, or cefazolin, a first-generation cephalosporin, usually with one of the following: (1) chloramphenicol, which covers anaerobes, streptococci and ampicillin-resistant *Haemophilus influenzae*; (2) penicillin G and moxalactam, for broader gram-negative and anaerobic coverage; or (3) piperacillin, again for broader gram-negative and anaerobic coverage.

Cefuroxime, a second-generation cephalosporin, can also be used as a first-line antibiotic because it covers *S. aureus,* pneumococcus, group A streptococci, anaerobes, and *Haemophilus influenzae*. Chloramphenicol, moxalactam, and cefuroxime cross the blood-brain barrier. Cefotaxime, a third-generation cephalosporin, also crosses the blood-brain barrier and is effective against coagulase-positive staphylococci, streptococci, gram-negative bacteria including *Haemophilus influenzae,* and anaerobes. Vancomycin or clindamycin are alternatives if there exists a history of penicillin anaphylaxis.

Nasal decongestants, such as phenylephrine 0.125% or 0.25% for children or oxymetazoline hydrochloride 0.05%

---

*References 78, 148, 176, 218, 219, 240, 265.
†References 176, 218, 219, 231, 240, 263, 271, 273.
‡References 24, 78, 104, 105, 121, 182.

*References 98, 106, 148, 210, 218, 219.
†References 50, 78, 95, 105, 155, 182.

for adults, and heat encourage drainage. Oral decongestants are usually not recommended.[181]

The total duration of parenteral antibiotic treatment depends on clinical response, usually continuing for 10 for 14 days or longer in patients requiring surgery or those with osteomyelitis or intracranial disease. Oral antibiotics should be instituted for 10 to 14 days after hospital discharge. Oral amoxicillin/clavulante potassium or an oral broad-spectrum cephalosporin may be given. Quinolones may be used in adults.[181]

Visual acuity, pupil exam, corneal sensation, degree of proptosis, intraocular pressure, fundus exam, neurologic status, temperature, and white blood cell count must all be assessed frequently, sometimes every two to four hours.

Surgical Management. Surgical intervention should be based not only on CT scan characteristics but on clinical manifestations and disease course. CT demonstration of a subperiosteal abscess does not in itself necessarily indicate the need for surgical drainage.* As long as vision is not threatened a 48-hour trial with intravenous antibiotics and local care is usually warranted.[105,121,212,241] Indications for surgical drainage include failure to defervesce with intravenous antibiotics, visual loss (less than 20/60), increasing proptosis, isolated muscle weakness, and continued fever.[112,134,210,218] Antibiotic infusion into the avascular subperiosteal space may be suboptimal, and any patient with proptosis and limited motility that does not completely resolve should undergo repeat CT scan to rule out an occult subperiosteal abscess. Repeat CT scan should also be obtained upon disease progression or suspected central nervous system involvement. Intracranial abscesses require immediate neurosurgical consultation because drainage by craniotomy is usually necessary. The treatment of cavernous sinus thrombosis consists of high-dose antibiotics and supportive care. Anticoagulant, fibrinolytic and corticosteriod therapy are controversial.[93,205]

The CT location of abscesses and sinus disease determines the surgical approach. The need for sinus drainage may be determined in consultation with an otorhinolaryngologist. Children do not usually require drainage, whereas adults frequently need sinus surgery.[210] Most common is a medial orbital abscess with ethmoiditis, which requires a medial orbital incision between the inner canthus and bridge of the nose, avoiding the trochlea and staying above the medial canthal tendon. The incision is carried through the periosteum, which is then elevated until the abscess drains. An ethmoidectomy may be performed. A small Penrose drain is left in the cavity and placed out through the skin incision or out the nares. Dissection should remain in the subperiosteal space in order to prevent intraconal infection unless an orbital abscess must also be evacuated. Frontal sinusitis with or without a superior orbital abscess can be

drained through this incision but sometimes necessitates a craniotomy. A lateral superior orbital rim incision is frequently required for sufficient exposure and evacuation. Maxillary sinus drainage may be accomplished via an intranasal antrostomy through the inferior meatus.

In cases of orbital cellulitis following trauma, surgical exploration for foreign-body removal is performed through the entry wound after instituting parenteral treatment.[134] Abscess drainage is performed as required. Tetanus immunization is provided.[224]

Prevention

There is no known way to prevent sinusitis.[181] Appropriate, aggressive, and prompt treatment should prevent permanent sequelae and death from complicated sinusitis. Although outcome is generally good, impaired visual acuity is usually not reversible.[51,153] The incidence of permanent visual loss has been reported from about 10% to 33%.[107,176,192,219,242] Schramm and associates' series[218] of 303 patients had a 5% overall complication rate, with one fatality. Gans and associates[92] reported two deaths among 190 cases. Intracranial extension, which occurs in approximately 4% of cases,[134] still carries about a 20% to 40% mortality rate,[33,165] and cavernous sinus thrombosis has nearly an 80% mortality.[71]

ORBITAL TUBERCULOSIS

Myocobacterium tuberculosis is a ubiquitous, aerobic, nonsporulating bacillus that causes a necrotizing granulomatous infection. Tuberculosis has remained a serious worldwide health problem since ancient times.

Epidemiology

In Western countries tuberculosis is most common among nursing-home residents, alcoholics, drug abusers, immigrants, prison inmates, the homeless, and people infected with the human immunodeficiency virus (HIV). Mainly because of the HIV epidemic, the incidence of tuberculosis in the United States has started to increase since 1985.[4] Approximately 1800 tuberculosis-related deaths occur in the United States each year.[234]

Clinical Features

Tuberculous periostitis presents as a chronic, insidious, nontender inflammation, most commonly of the malar bone, and usually in the first or second decade of life. Over months edema and discoloration of the overlying skin can progress to cold abscess, fistula formation, cicatrization, and regional lymphadenitis. Tuberculomas, firm masses of chronic granulomatous inflammation, can occur anywhere in the orbit and at any age. They cause gradual painless proptosis and sclerosis and thus mimic benign and malignant tumors, orbital pseudotumors, and fungal infections. They occasionally involve extraocular muscles and present bilaterally. Tuberculomas may also start in the maxillary or ethmoid sinus,

---

*References 50, 78, 96, 98, 105, 121, 155, 182, 212, 241, 252.

erode into the orbit, and fistulize to the skin. Overt signs of chronic sinusitis accompany this presentation. Epiphora and epistaxis are also common symptoms, as they are with sinus malignancies. Tuberculosis of the lacrimal gland usually presents as a unilateral sclerosing mass, causing gradual painless ptosis, lid edema, and inferior globe displacement with proptosis.

Pathogenesis

In the United States tuberculosis is almost invariably acquired by inhaling organisms exhaled by another human. In the lungs the bacilli elude humoral immune defenses by multiplying inside the alveolar macrophages that phagocytize them. For about two months the organisms silently invade the lungs, lymphatics, and then the blood stream until the activation of cell-mediated immunity results in granulomatous inflammation. The interactions between different sets of T cells and infected macrophages produce interleukins that enhance the effectiveness of macrophages.[139] At this time the majority of the bacilli are killed. If the host's immune mechanisms are not intact overt disease may develop. Usually some bacilli remain dormant until many years after initial infection, when disease reactivation can occur because of altered host immunity or for no known reason.

Approximately 80% of cases of tuberculosis affect the lung.[234] The incidence of orbital tuberculosis is probably much less than 1%. Orbital infection occurs either by hematogenous spread causing a periostitis[6,225] or orbital tuberculoma* or by direct extension from adjacent structures, especially the paranasal sinuses,[131,143,244] lacrimal gland,[17,180,225] or the globe.[72,74]

Laboratory Investigations

Systemic signs and symptoms of tuberculosis may or may not be present. Diagnosis depends on a thorough physical examination to detect systemic tuberculosis, on the results of the tuberculin skin test and, most definitively, on orbital tissue examination revealing caseating granulomas with sclerosis or, rarely, acid-fast bacilli. Tuberculous bacilli from orbital lesions almost never grow from tissue culture. The diagnosis is not easy and sometimes a trial of antituberculosis medicine is warranted. Radiologic findings are nonspecific. Newer diagnostic techniques are being developed.[234]

Therapy

While biopsy is almost always necessary, surgical removal of *all* involved tissue is controversial. Systemic therapy, classically with a combination of isoniazid, rifampin pyrazinamide, and/or ethambutol, is necessary. The exact

regimen is determined by the extent of the disease, the presence of drug-resistant organisms, and any concomitant medical or social problems. Treatment is usually continued for at least nine months. The prognosis for orbital tuberculosis is good: visual loss is rare.

Prevention

Tuberculosis is preventable. The efficacy of the current vaccine for tuberculosis, bacillus Calmette-Guérin (BCG), varies. Newer vaccines are being developed.[139]

ORBITAL SYPHILIS

Syphilis is a sexually transmitted or congenital infection that has been increasing in incidence since the late 1980s.

Epidemiology

Orbital syphilis, first extensively described by MacKenzie in 1840,[74] has never been a common manifestation of treponemal infection. Its incidence is probably much less than 1%.[59] Orbital involvement becomes evident in the late secondary and tertiary stages of acquired or congenital syphilis.

Clinical Features

One case of secondary syphilis causing pain, proptosis, and lacrimal gland inflammation imitating orbital pseudotumor was reported by Spoor and associates.[246] Secondary and tertiary syphilis may cause a diffuse or localized orbital periostitis.

Gumma formation with or without periostitis can occur anywhere in the orbit, including the lacrimal gland and extraocular muscles, in a diffuse or localized pattern or can spread to the orbit from the paranasal sinuses, central nervous system, or surrounding soft tissues.

Signs and symptoms depend on disease location but classically include orbital pain or neuralgia (which may predate all other findings), proptosis, ophthalmoplegia, ptosis, bone sclerosis or absorption, and findings indicative of an orbital apex syndrome.[59,74,210] Visual loss can occur and bilateral orbital involvement is common.

Pathogenesis

The causative bacteria, *Treponema pallidum,* a thin, motile, flagellated spirochete whose only host is man, is transmitted when sexual contact occurs with someone who has the mucocutaneous lesions found in the primary and secondary stages. Pregnant women in any disease stage can transmit syphilis to their fetus.

T. pallidum crosses intact mucous membranes and rapidly invades the lymphatic and circulatory systems. Spirochetemia continues through the development of a chancre at the inoculation site (primary stage) and through the occurrence of multiple systemic manifestations from florid infection (secondary stage) until the host's immune response

---

*References 143, 170, 180, 184, 225, 229.

suppresses spirochete duplication. A so-called latent stage follows, at which time no clinical signs and symptoms are present. Tertiary syphilis represents an insidious inflammatory disease that can affect any organ system. Neurologic, cardiovascular, and gummatous syphilis occur at this stage.

Laboratory Investigations

The diagnosis of syphilis is almost always made by serologic testing. Nontreponemal tests (VDRL and RPR) detect the nonspecific IgM and IgG antibodies formed against a lipoidal antigen. Reactivity varies slightly depending on disease stage. A reactive VDRL in cerebral spinal fluid always indicates acute central nervous system syphilis. Serial titers can be used to determine response to therapy. In patients with tertiary syphilis serum VDRL titers may remain slightly reactive even after adequate therapy. Treponemal tests (FTA-ABS and MHA-TP) specifically determine if antitreponemal antibody is present. Once positive they remain as such. Because the FTA-ABS test is more sensitive than the VDRL and RPR in late syphilis, any patient with suspected ocular or orbital syphilis should undergo both types of tests. The presence of antitreponemal antibodies in the cerebral spinal fluid does not necessarily indicate acute neurosyphilis. Patients with neuroophthalmic and orbital abnormalities and reactive serum FTA-ABS should undergo lumbar puncture to check for reactive cerebral spinal fluid VDRL and lymphocyte pleocytosis characteristic of neurosyphilis.

CT scans of orbital and central nervous system gummata and the radiologic findings of periostitis are nonspecific. Biopsy material, obtained when the diagnosis is questionable, should demonstrate the typical obliterative endarteriolitis present at all disease stages. The microscopic appearance of gummata of tertiary syphilis, as opposed to other granulomatous and mass lesions, shows caseating granulomata with prominent endarteriolitis.

Therapy

Parenteral penicillin G has remained the main treatment of syphilis for over 40 years. Other effective antibiotics include the tetracyclines, erythromycin, and third-generation cephalosporins. The present recommended therapy for any patient with orbital syphilis is similar to that for neurosyphilis, namely intravenous crystalline penicillin G, 2 to 4 million units every four hours for 10 to 14 days followed by benzathine penicillin G, 2 to 4 million units intramuscularly weekly for three weeks.[59,66,67] Even longer therapy by continuous penicillin infusion may be necessary to cure neurosyphilis effectively, especially in patients with concomitant HIV infection.[59,173] Recovery from orbital syphilis, which usually begins in approximately three to six weeks, depends on the degree of damage and the duration of the disease.

ORBITAL ASPERGILLOSIS

Aspergillus species, named by Micheli in 1729 and first described in man by Bennett in 1844,[70] rarely afflicts the orbit. Of the twenty species that definitely cause disease in man, *A. fumigatus, A. flavus, A. niger,* and *A. oryzae* are the most frequent pathogens.[209] The most common disease types in immunocompromised patients are pulmonary followed by sinus, central nervous system, and disseminated aspergillosis.[11,161] Aspergillosis, particularly *A. flavus,* along with mucormycosis cause most of the increasing number of paranasal sinus fungal infections.[217,248] Aspergillosis of the orbit is usually secondary to direct extension from the paranasal sinuses, the maxillary sinus in particular, or more rarely, secondary to hematogenous dissemination.[15,109,171] Primary orbital aspergillosis does occur in both immunocompetent and immunocompromised patients.* Invasion of the sinuses and lungs has also been reported in healthy individuals.[61,100,279,286]

Epidemiology

The incidence of infection with these ubiquitous saprophytes has increased because of the enlarging immunocompromised population who endure most of the morbidity and mortality from fungal disease.[11,109] These organisms presently lag behind only *Candida* species as the most common opportunistic mycotic infection requiring hospitalization.[209] The incidence of candidiasis and aspergillosis has tripled from 1980 to 1990.[208]

Risk Factors

Prolonged hospitalization increases the risk of mycotic infection, especially for patients with renal failure, hematologic malignancies, diabetes, sarcoidosis, tuberculosis, extensive burns, transplanted organs, prosthetic devices, or following multiple surgical procedures.[247] Common sources of fungal spores in hospitals, such as ventilation systems, construction sites, plants or flowers, radiology departments, and operating rooms, may result in inhalation or direct inoculation of a pathogenic quantity of spores.[11] *Aspergillus* sp. can gain access to the body from invasive monitoring devices, hyperalimentation ports, and dialysis or urinary catheters.[247] Intravenous drug users may directly inoculate themselves with contaminated drugs, needles, or syringes.

Although the immune status of the patient is the most important factor determining susceptibility to aspergillosis, individuals with no predisposing disease states do acquire serious fungal infection. Sinusitis in healthy individuals most probably results when the sinus ostium becomes occluded and a hypoxic environment allows fungal proliferation.[217,248] Sinus involvement is divided into four forms: noninvasive, allergic, invasive, and fulminant.[111,217] Factors

---

*References 14, 36, 52, 57, 73, 116, 125, 236, 279.

that contribute to local or noninvasive infection include chronic allergic or bacterial sinusitis, nasal polyposis, septal deviation, hot and humid climate, foreign body, and trauma. The mechanism by which aspergillosis that is contained within the sinus cavity becomes invasive and proceeds, in either a chronic or fulminant manner, to destroy the sinuses and involve the orbit or brain is unknown. Invasive pulmonary aspergillosis[34,188] and disseminated aspergillosis[171] have also been reported in immunocompetent hosts.

The pathogenesis of primary orbital aspergillosis (that is, with no other apparent organ involvement) may involve hematogenous spread from an occult source but remains obscure. The immune status of the affected individual may or may not be intact.

Clinical Features

The clinical manifestations of orbital aspergillosis resemble those found in other types of orbital infections, namely periorbital pain, proptosis, diplopia, decreased visual acuity, conjunctival chemosis, and ophthalmoplegia. The most common form of orbital invasion, from adjacent sinuses, may present insidiously with an enlarging mass causing gradual proptosis and neurologic symptoms over months to years or aggressively causing fever, sinoorbital pain, acute orbital congestion, necrotizing sinusitis, and neurologic signs and symptoms.[217] Because the organism possesses a tendency to invade blood vessels, infection results in thrombosis and infarction of involved tissues. In this regard central retinal artery occlusion or ischemic optic neuropathy may occur.[270] Proptosis and sinus disease are the most common presentations (75%), followed by central nervous system signs and symptoms (32%), decreased vision (28%), pain (23%), and extraocular muscle paresis (9%).[116] The overall mortality in one series was approximately 28%; central nervous system involvement incurred an 80% mortality.[116]

The disseminated form of aspergillosis may involve the orbit in an aggressive, necrotizing fashion, but endogenous endophthalmitis is more common.[172,210] Primary orbital aspergillosis almost always manifests as an orbital apex syndrome with decreased vision, pain, ophthalmoplegia, decreased corneal sensation, and usually, but not always, proptosis.[52,116] Cavernous sinus and central nervous system involvement occurs via extension of infection through the ophthalmic veins and is associated with a high mortality.

Pathogenesis

Aspergillus spores, constantly released into the atmosphere by the asexual reproductive structures known as conidiophores, commonly colonize human respiratory and digestive tracts, but cannot cross intact mucous membranes or skin because they do not possess keratolytic enzymes.[111] Also, phagocytic response prevents inhaled spores from germinating. Rarely, *A. fumigatus* can produce elastase,

phagocytosis inhibitors, and complement inhibitors and thus become more virulent.[156] Exactly how *Aspergillus* sp. become pathogenic remains unclear. A combination of local and systemic conditions are probably necessary. Several types of immunosuppression predispose to locally invasive and disseminated infection, the most important of which is neutropenia.* Instead of using phagocytosis, neutrophils bond to the surface of hyphae to destroy them. When neutrophils become defective, usually secondary to chemotherapy, leukemia, or chronic granulomatous disease, fungi can become invasive. Total granulocyte counts below 500 cells/ mm^3 and prolonged granulocytopenia (greater than two weeks) are definite risk factors.[216,247] Treatment with broad-spectrum antibiotics, which increase the number of spores colonizing the respiratory tract by 100-fold, and corticosteroid use, which inhibits macrophage function, intensify susceptibility. Chemotherapy and irradiation may also promote invasive fungal infection by damaging mucosal barriers.[216,247] Weakened cellular immunity, most commonly from lymphoma or acquired immunodeficiency syndrome (AIDS), is a predisposing factor for invasive aspergillosis, but defective humoral immunity does not seem to be a risk factor.[248]

Differential Diagnosis

Because of the different presentations orbital aspergillosis can imitate many disease states including malignant neoplasm, sinus tumor, mucopyocele, orbital pseudotumor, lethal midline granuloma, tuberculosis, and sarcoidosis. Primary orbital aspergillosis can be mistaken for corticosteroid-responsive optic neuropathy.[236,245]

Mucorales sp., *Pseudallescheria boydii*, *Fusarium* sp., *Curvularia* sp., *Penicillium* sp., *Cladosporium* sp., *Candida* sp., *Coccidioides immitis*, *Rhinosporidium seeberi*, *Sporothrix schenkii*, *Blastomyces dermatitidis*, *Actinomyces*, *Nocardia asteroides*, *Bipolaris* sp., *Histoplasma capsulatum* var. *duboisii*, and *Mycobacterium fortuitum-chelonal* complex may also cause orbital infections.†

Laboratory Investigations

Aspergillosis is notorious for the diagnostic quandary it presents. Polymicrobial infection is often present, and cultures from blood and tissue are usually negative for *Aspergillus*. Diagnosis demands a positive culture from a normally sterile area; a biopsy showing septate hyphae 3 to 6 microns in diameter that branch at an average angle of 45° is suggestive. *Aspergillus* sp. grows on blood or Sabouraud agar and stain with hematoxylin and eosin (if properly fixed), Gomori methenamine-silver, Gridley, and periodic acid-Schiff.

---

*References 11, 36, 161, 216, 247, 248.
†References 36, 167, 172, 179, 187, 209, 210, 250, 260.

Diagnosis almost always requires multiple biopsies, either by fine needle aspiration[1] or from surgical debridement(s). Histologically, a variable degree of granulomatous inflammation, necrotizing vasculitis with infarction, and suppuration are present (Fig. 94-4), depending on the patient's immunologic status and duration of the infection.[111,125,163] Individuals with AIDS develop less of a granulomatous response and more necrosis and suppuration.[261]

Radiologic studies, including plain films, computed tomography, and magnetic resonance imaging, are not specific for mycosis. Serum precipitating antibodies to *Aspergillus* sp. and other new immunologic assays suggest but do not yet definitively confirm infection.[41,42,65,151,209]

Therapy

Surgical debulking, antifungal therapy, improvement of immune status, and prophylaxis together play an important role in the management of invasive orbital aspergillosis. Conservative versus aggressive surgical debridement is controversial, but most investigators agree that surgery remains crucial for accurate diagnosis and effective therapy.* The drug of choice for treatment of all forms of aspergillosis is amphotericin B. The typical systemic dose ranges from 0.5 to 1.5 mg/kg/day intravenously with higher doses, if tolerated, for poor clinical response or severe neutropenia. Central nervous system involvement may require intrathecal infusions.[251] Local irrigation with amphotericin B may improve efficacy of surgical debridement.[141] A nasal spray preparation seems promising for the prophylaxis of invasive aspergillosis.[201]

In vitro studies and case reports indicate that the concomitant use of flucytosine or rifampin with amphotericin B may exert, respectively, an additive or synergistic inhibitory effect on *Aspergillus* sp. in humans[30,198,199,251] and may prevent relapses of invasive aspergillosis in high risk patients.[137,216] This combination therapy allows a reduction of the daily dosage of amphotericin B and therefore results in a reduction of systemic polyene toxicity.[251,264] Fewer side effects, but higher serum levels, can be obtained with the investigational liposomal preparation of amphotericin B.[42,158,251,264,269]

Newer antimycotic agents, in particular the triazoles, fluconazole and itraconazole, achieve excellent in vitro and in vivo activity against *Aspergillus* sp.[64,113,251,256,257] Their efficacy for prophylaxis and cure of invasive aspergillosis in patients with protracted neutropenia is not known.[60,113,193,201,251] Whatever the antifungal therapy, it must be continued well after the resolution of granulocytopenia.[216] Controlled studies correlating dosage to clinical response do not yet exist.[63] Chemoprophylaxis, in addition to traditional prevention by reducing airborne spores with

---

*References 63, 73, 109, 134, 210, 248.

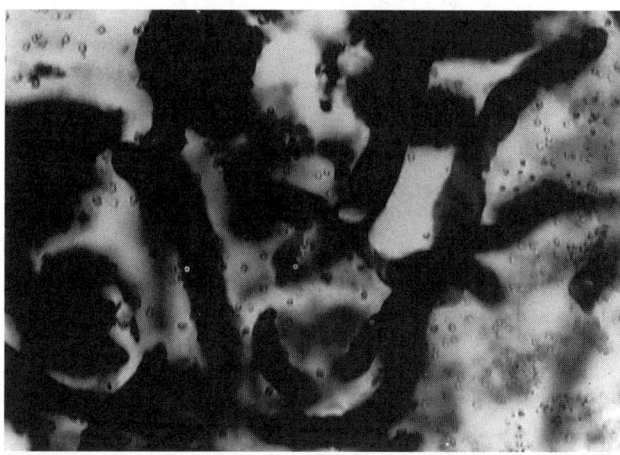

Fig. 94-4. *Aspergillus fumigatus* from orbital biopsy of patient with fungal orbital cellulitis, showing large branching hyphae with occasional septa. (Methenamine silver × 1000.)

special ventilation systems, may be crucial for individuals with leukemia or neutropenia and in bone marrow recipients.[122,201,251]

Early diagnosis and treatment, and restoration of immune defense mechanisms, are the main factors that influence survival in all forms of invasive aspergillar infections. Mortality in patients whose immune status cannot be improved and those with central nervous system involvement approaches 100%, regardless of the treatment mode.[63,125,216] Immunocompromised as well as healthy individuals with orbital cellulitis and/or sinusitis who demonstrate only a marginal response to antibacterials must be suspected of harboring a fungal infection.

Prevention

Methods of prevention including empiric use of antimycotic agents, newer antifungal drugs, and granulocyte transfusions are all under further investigation, especially to decrease mortality in high-risk patients.[63,141,251]

ORBITAL MUCORMYCOSIS

The highly aggressive fungal infection called mucormycosis, first described in humans by Paultauf[194] in 1885, is most commonly caused by three genera from the fungal class Zygomycetes, order Mucorales and family Mucoraceae, namely *Rhizopus, Mucor,* and *Absidia.*

Epidemiology

Mucormycosis may afflict virtually any anatomic site, but usually takes one of five forms: rhino-orbito-cerebral, pulmonary, gastrointestinal, cutaneous and disseminated. Although the rhino-orbito-cerebral type is the most common, the incidence of disseminated mucormycosis continues to rise with the increase in the number of immunocompromised patients.[209] The orbit may be involved by either the rhino-orbito-cerebral route or, more rarely, the disseminated form. This occurs by direct spread from the paranasal sinuses or nasolacrimal duct and/or secondary to hematogenous seeding.[3,22,43,154] Orbital extension from the sinuses occurs in about 67% to 85% of cases.[98,99,189] Direct spread is facilitated by vascular invasion with endothelial injury and growth of hyphae into blood vessel lumens, especially arteries. To date, approximately 208 cases of rhino-orbito-cerebral mucormycosis have been reported since 1970, when effective treatment became available.[282] Over 50% of these patients had diabetes mellitus.[282] Mucormycosis occurs almost exclusively in immunocompromised patients, especially those with diabetes mellitus or renal failure.* Rare reports of infection in apparently healthy individuals do exist.[49,195,204,249,284]

Risk Factors

Any individual with a quantitative or qualitative defect in neutrophil function (especially caused by leukemia and lymphoma),[23,62,206] a chronic granulomatous disease,[189] or chemotherapy,[189] is predisposed to mucormycosis. Because of the use of immunosuppressive agents to prevent rejection, renal transplant patients with or without diabetes are especially prone.[46,136,177] Dialysis patients, particularly those being treated with deferoxamine, are at risk for infection.[1,29,258] Iron represents an important growth factor for Mucorales.[1,13] Serum transferrin binds iron such that it becomes unavailable to pathogens. Deferoxamine provides iron to Mucorales and may also alter granulocyte and lymphocyte function.[258] Deferoxamine has been demonstrated to promote Mucor sp. pathogenicity in vitro[29] and in vivo.[1,29] Mortality is substantially higher in these patients.[282]

Other conditions associated with mucormycosis include dehydration and diarrhea, with or without acidosis;[3,70,174,249] cirrhosis;[46,89,189] hepatic failure;[249] aplastic anemia;[86,189] Fanconi anemia;[202] systemic lupus erythematosus;[189] multiple myeloma;[189] cholesteatoma;[189] polyarteritis nodosa;[189] viral myocarditis;[31,189] extensive malignancies;[189] severe burns;[189] trauma;[35,259] intravenous drug abuse;[58,223] and HIV infection.[58] Treatment with broad-spectrum antibiotics or corticosteroids are only occasionally a risk factor.[18,221] The mechanism by which apparently healthy patients acquire mucormycosis is not currently known.[49,195,204,249,284]

Clinical Features

The clinical manifestations of rhino-orbito-cerebromucormycosis reported after 1970 include fever (44%), nasal ulceration or actual necrosis (38%), periorbital or facial edema (34%), decreased vision (30%), ophthalmoplegia (29%), sinusitis (26%), headache (25%), facial pain (22%), decreased mental status (22%), leukocytosis (19%), nasal

---

*References 27, 36, 39, 83, 102, 189, 197, 249.

discharge (18%), nasal stuffiness (17%), corneal anesthesia (17%), orbital cellulitis (16%), and proptosis (16%).[282] Necrosis of facial skin and bone with typical black eschar formation is usually a late manifestation of mucormycosis.[84] The classic presentation in a susceptible patient is with unilateral severe headache and facial pain, nasal stuffiness with granular or purulent discharge, facial or eyelid edema, fever, and leukocytosis.

As fungi invade orbital blood vessels to cause ischemic necrosis, cranial nerve abnormalities arise. A partial or complete superior orbital fissure syndrome or orbital apex syndrome is characteristic. Visual loss is typically sudden, caused by an apex syndrome, central retinal artery occlusion, or ophthalmic artery occlusion. Proptosis results from venous congestion or from frank cellulitis possibly with orbital abscess.

Infectious spread into the cavernous sinus leads to cavernous sinus thrombosis, the diagnosis of which is made difficult because ophthalmoplegia, proptosis, chemosis, and lid edema may already exist from orbital invasion. Cavernous sinus thrombosis with visual loss is more typical of Mucor sp. infection, whereas thrombosis with normal vision typifies bacterial orbital invasion.[3,128] Mental status changes often develop with orbital mucormycosis. Intracranial extension occurs via orbital vessels, the orbital apex, or the cribiform plate. Brain abscesses pose a frequent problem for drug addicts and AIDS patients.[209]

A high index of suspicion is necessary for diagnosis, even in a susceptible patient. The differential diagnosis is similar to that of orbital aspergillosis. It is controversial whether any radiologic findings exist specific for Murcorales infection. CT nonenhancement of the superior ophthalmic artery and vein may represent a specific sign of orbital mucormycosis.[89,144] CT imaging of sinus infection resembles benign mucosal thickening: air/fluid levels are usually not present.[89] Other common findings include medial rectus thickening, optic nerve enlargement, and increased orbital apex density.[84] Bone destruction is a late finding. MRI findings, although nonspecific, probably demonstrate the extent of disease as well as CT scan.[89] MRI may prove crucial for the detection of early vascular and intracranial invasion.[283]

Pathogenesis

Like Aspergillus sp., the genera of Mucorales are ubiquitous saprophytes abundant in soil, air, most ventilation systems, and almost any body orifice including the nose and pharynx. Inhaled or swallowed spores are prevented from germinating by macrophages.[154] If the phagocytic response fails, however, the hyphae allowed to form from germination can establish infection. They are not as easily destroyed as the spores.[75] The main predisposition to Mucorales infection, a state of metabolic acidosis usually secondary to diabetes mellitus or uremia, alters the phagocytic response by decreasing phagocytosis[44] and decreasing migration and tissue accumulation of polymorphonuclear leukocytes and fibroblasts.[196,228] The immune response to mucormycosis also depends on a dialyzable, humoral anti*Rhizopus* sp. factor.[136] This inhibitory factor could not be found in serum from a patient with diabetic ketoacidosis.[87] Studies using *Rhizopus* sp. have also demonstrated that its growth increases in glucose-rich, acidotic environments because it possesses a ketone reductase system.[3,200] *Rhizopus* also thrives in the presence of unbound iron, whose serum concentration increases because of the decreased iron-binding capacity of transferrin in the face of metabolic acidosis.[13] Any form of metabolic acidosis is a predisposing factor,[70,174,204] but diabetic patients who are neither hyperglycemic nor acidotic are also at risk. The factors responsible for infection in these individuals are not presently known.

Laboratory Investigations

Mucorales grow on most culture media without inhibitors.[154] Tissue identification remains necessary for definitive diagnosis because the organisms are ubiquitous and are common laboratory contaminants.[154,221,249]

Histologic samples, especially in necrotic areas, demonstrate broad, irregular, nonseptate hyphae that branch at right angles. The diameter of some hyphae approximate that of aspergillus species, that is, 5 to 10 microns. Others are 50 microns and should not be confused with small blood vessels, which have a similar size.[221,249] Mucorales stain best with Gomori methenamine-silver (Fig. 94-5), hematoxalin and eosin, and periodic acid-Schiff preparations.[84,221] To find hyphae multiple specimens (fresh, frozen, and fixed) are often necessary.[128]

Therapy

Treatment requires systemic antifungal therapy, surgical debridement, adequate sinus and orbital drainage, and improvement of immune status. Surgical debridement of all necrotic tissue is crucial, often quite mutilating, and usually calls for multiple operations.[2,27,88,185,239] Serial radiologic imaging identifies the extent of disease and response to treatment. Orbital exenteration, which could be life-saving, is usually considered only in an acutely infected orbit with a blind, immobile eye.[3,84,147,154,221]

The antifungal medication of choice for mucormycosis is amphotericin B. Because disease progression is rapid, dosages should reach 0.7 to 1.5 mg/kg/day intravenously as rapidly as possible. A cumulative dose of 2.0 to 4.0 grams is usually necessary.[3,154] Local irrigation with amphotericin B helps improve its efficacy.[147,239] Fewer side effects and possibly higher efficacy has been obtained with liposomal amphotericin B.[85,159,269] Further studies must be performed in order to clarify the role of combination therapy for mucormycosis, consisting of amphotericin B with 5-fluorocytosine, rifampin, tetracycline, fluconazole, itraconazole, or the new allylamine derivatives.[5,214,227,267]

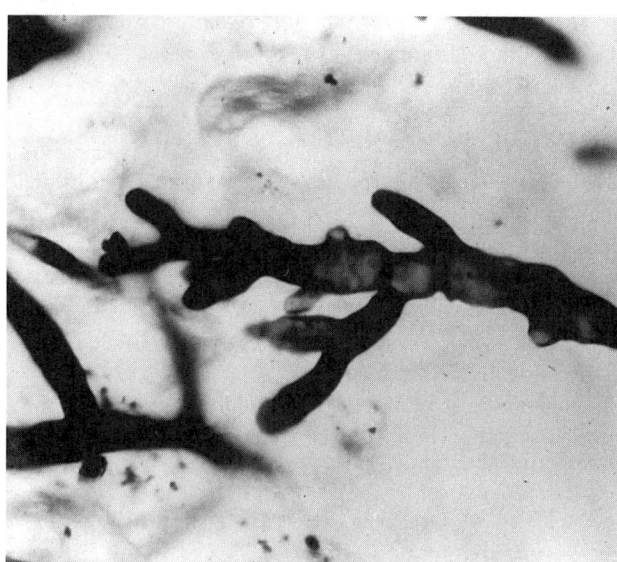

Fig. 94-5. Nasal mucosa of a diabetic patient with orbital phycomycosis caused by *Rhizopus arrhizus*. (Methenamine silver × 400.)

Hyperbaric oxygen treatments possess a fungistatic effect and may also help affected patients by decreasing tissue hypoxia, enhancing oxygen dependent cidal mechanisms, and decreasing tissue acidosis.[56,81] Hyperbaric oxygen improves survival, and some recommend it as part of the initial therapy for mucormycosis.[282]

Prognosis

With advances in diagnosis and treatment, the mortality rate for rhino-orbital-cerebral mucormycosis has decreased from 88%[83,189] to under 30%.[27,189] Survival rates remain higher for diabetics than for patients compromised by other diseases.[89] Five-year survival rates range from 20% to 45% for individuals with intracranial disease.[12,89,189,206] Factors statistically correlated with a poorer prognosis include the following: delayed diagnosis in treatment, hemiparesis or hemiplegia, bilateral sinus involvement, leukemia, renal disease, and deferoxamine treatment.[282]

PARASITIC ORBITAL INFECTION

Even in endemic areas orbital parasitic infestation is relatively uncommon. Hematogenous dissemination of *Echinococcus granulosus* causes a slow-growing hydatid cyst.[226] Orbital hydatid cysts represent up to 1% of all hydatid disease in the Middle East and East Africa.[74,166] Symptoms and signs resemble those of any mass lesion. Cellulitis is rare.[226] CT scanning may show the characteristic thin, calcified cyst wall. Surgical excision with adequate exposure is required to drain the contents, irrigate with alcohol to kill the scoleces, and then excise the cyst wall completely.

Other parasites that may afflict the orbital and periocular tissues include *Dirofilaria tenuis* (periorbital), *Trichinella* sp. (extraocular muscles), *Taenia solium, Schistosoma* sp. (lacrimal gland), *Entamoeba* sp., *Onchocerca* sp., *Coenurus* sp., and *Ascaris* sp.[74,134,210]

ORBITAL MYIASIS

Fly larvae have been reported to infest orbital, periorbital, and ocular structures.[168,276,280] Fly eggs are usually transported by mosquitos and hatch to emit larvae that can burrow into intact skin.[276] The resultant local inflammation with fistula formation can become superinfected with bacteria. Alternatively, larvae can infest neglected wounds, especially in debilitated individuals.[280]

Maggots must be removed manually with ether or turpentine irrigation.[210,280] Any concomitant bacterial infection should also be treated.

REFERENCES

1. Abe F, Inaba H, Katoh T et al.: Effects of iron and desferrioxamine on Rhizopus infection, *Mycopathologia* 110:87-91, 1990.
2. Abedi E, Sismanis A, Choi K et al.: Twenty-five years' experience treating cerebro-rhino-orbital mucormycosis, *Laryngoscope* 94:1060-1062, 1984.
3. Abramson E, Wilson D, Arky RA: Rhinocerebral phycomycosis in association with diabetic ketoacidosis, *Ann Intern Med* 66:735-742, 1967.
4. Abrutyn E: Multi-drug resistant nosocomial TB: newest facet of the HIV epidemic, *Hosp Pract* 27:11, 15-16, 1992.
5. Abruzzo GK, Fromtling RA, Turnbull TA et al.: Effects of bifonazole, fluconazole, itraconazole, and terbinafine on the chemiluminescence response of immune cells, *J Antimicrob Chemother* 20:61-68, 1987.
6. Agrawal PK, Nath J, Jain BS: Orbital involvement in tuberculosis, *Indian J Ophthalmol* 25:12-16, 1977.
7. Ahmadi J, Keane JR, Segall HD et al.: CT observations pertinent to septic cavernous sinus thrombosis, *AJNR* 6:755-758, 1985.
8. Ahrens-Palumbo MJ, Ballen PH: Primary dacryocystitis causing orbital cellulitis, *Ann Ophthalmol* 14:600-601, 1982.
9. Allan BP, Egbert MA, Myall RWT: Orbital abscess of odontogenic origin. Case report and review of the literature, *J Oral Maxillofac Surg* 20:268-270, 1991.
10. Allen MV, Cohen KL, Grimson BS: Orbital cellulitis secondary to dacryocystitis following blepharoplasty, *Ann Ophthalmol* 17:498, 1985.
11. Anaissie E, Bodey GP: Nosocomial fungal infections: old problems and new challenges, *Infect Dis Clin North Am* 3:867-882, 1989.
12. Anaissie EJ, Shikhani AH: Rhinocerebral mucormycosis with internal carotid occlusion: report of two cases and review of the literature, *Laryngoscope* 95:1107-1113, 1985.
13. Artis WM, Fountain JA, Delcher HK et al.: A mechanism of susceptibility to mucormycosis in diabetic ketoacidosis: transferrin and iron availability, *Diabetes* 31:109-114, 1982.
14. Austin P, Dekker A, Kennerdell JS: Orbital aspergillosis: report of a case diagnosed by fine needle aspiration biopsy, *Acta Cytol* 27:166-169, 1983.
15. Axelsson H, Carlsöö B, Weibring J et al.: Aspergillosis of the maxillary sinus, *Acta Otolaryngol* 86:303-308, 1978.
16. Bach MC, Knowland M, Schuyler WBJ: Acute orbital myositis mimicking orbital cellulitis, *Ann Intern Med* 109:243-245, 1988.
17. Baghdassarin SA, Zakharia H, Asdourian KK: Report of a case of bilateral caseous tuberculosis dacryoadenitis, *Am J Ophthalmol* 74:744-746, 1972.
18. Bauer H, Wallace GL Jr, Sheldon WH: The effects of cortisone and chemical inflammation on experimental mucormycosis (*rhizopus oryzae* infection), *Yale J Biol Med* 29:839-395, 1957.
19. Bergen MP: Relationships between the arteries and veins and the connective tissue system in the human orbit. I. The retrobulbar part of the orbit: apical region, *Acta Morphol Neerl Scand* 20:1-17, 1982.
20. Bergen MP: Relationships between the arteries and veins and the connective tissue system in the human orbit. II. The retrobulbar part of the orbit: septal complex region, *Acta Morphol Neerl Scand* 20:17-27, 1982.
21. Bergin DJ, Wright JE: Orbital cellulitis, *Br J Ophthalmol* 70:174-178, 1986.
22. Bergstrom LV, Hemenway WG, Barnhart RA: Rhinocerebral and otologic mucormycosis, *Ann Otol Rhinol Laryngol* 79:70-81, 1970.
23. Bhaduri S, Kurrle E, Vanek E et al.: Mucormycosis in the immunocompromised host, *Infection* 11:170-172, 1983.
24. Bilaniuk LT, Zimmerman RA: Computer-assisted tomography: sinus lesions with orbital involvement, *Head Neck Surg* 2:293-301, 1980.
25. Birch-Hirschfeld A: Zur diagnostik und pathologie der orbitaltumoren, *Berl Versamm Dtsch Ophthalmol Ges* 32:127-135, 1905.
26. Birn H: Spread of dental infections, *Dent Pract Dent Rec* 22:347, 1972.
27. Blitzer A, Lawson W, Meyers BR et al.: Patient survival factors in paranasal sinus mucormycosis, *Laryngoscope* 90:635-648, 1980.
28. Blodi FC: Field Marshall Radetzky's orbital abscess, *Doc Ophthalmol* 71:205-219, 1989.
29. Boelaert JR, Fenves AZ, Coburn JW: Deferoxamine therapy and mucormycosis in dialysis patients: report of an international registry, *Am J Kidney Dis* 18:660-667, 1991.
30. Bradley SF, McGuire NM, Kauffman CA: Sino-orbital and cerebral aspergillosis: cure with medical therapy, *Mykosen* 30:379-385, 1987.
31. Bray WH, Giangiacomo J, Ide CH: Orbital apex syndrome, *Surv Ophthalmol* 32:136-140, 1987.
32. Brook I: Bacteriology of chronic maxillary sinusitis in adults, *Ann Otol Rhinol Laryngol* 98:426-428, 1989.
33. Brook I, Friedman EM, Rodriguez WJ et al.: Complications of sinusitis in children, *Pediatrics* 66:569-572, 1980.
34. Brown E, Freedman S, Arbert R et al.: Invasive pulmonary aspergillosis in an apparently non-immunocompromised host, *Am J Med* 69:624-627, 1980.
35. Bullock JD: Mucormycosis following cataract extraction. In Emery JM, Paton D, editors: *Current concepts in cataract surgery,* 349-355, St Louis, 1976, Mosby.
36. Bullock JD: Orbital infections in the immunocompromised patient, *Ophthal Plast Reconstr Surg* 2:189-196, 1986.
37. Bullock JD, Fleishman JA: Orbital cellulitis following dental extraction. *Trans Am Ophthalmol Soc* 82:111-133, 1984.
38. Bullock JD, Fleishman JA: The spread of odontogenic infections to the orbit: diagnosis and management, *J Oral Maxillofac Surg* 43:749-755, 1985.
39. Bullock JD, Jampol LM, Fezza AJ: Two cases of orbital phycomycosis with recovery, *Am J Ophthalmol* 78:811-815, 1974.
40. Burnard ED: Proptosis as the first sign of orbital sepsis in the newborn, *Br J Ophthalmol* 43:9, 1959.
41. Burnie JP: Antigen detection in invasive aspergillosis, *J Immunol Methods* 143:187-195, 1991.
42. Burnie JP: Developments in the serological diagnosis of opportunistic fungal infections, *J Antimicrob Chemother* 28(suppl A):23-33, 1991.
43. Burns RP: Mucormycosis of the sinuses, orbit and central nervous system, *Trans Pacific Coast Oto-Ophthalmol Soc* 40:83-101, 1959.
44. Bybee JD, Rogers DE: The phagocytic activity of polymorphonuclear leukocytes obtained from patients with diabetes mellitus, *J Lab Clin Med* 64:1-13, 1964.
45. Calcaterra TC, Trapp TK: Unilateral proptosis, *Otolaryngol Clin North Am* 21:53, 1988.
46. Carbone KM, Pennington LR, Gimenez LF et al.: Mucormycosis in renal transplant patients: a report of two cases and review of the literature, *Q J Med* 57:825-831, 1985.
47. Carenfelt C: Pathogenesis of sinus empyema, *Ann Otol Rhinol Laryngol* 88:16-20, 1979.
48. Carenfelt C, Lundberg C: Purulent and non-purulent maxillary sinus secretions with respect to pO_2, pCO_2 and pH, *Acta Otolaryngol* 84:138-144, 1977.
49. Castelli JB, Pallin JL: Lethal rhinocerebral phycomycosis in a healthy adult: a case report and review of the literature, *Otolaryngology* 86:696-703, 1978.
50. Catalano RA, Smoot CN: Subperiosteal orbital masses in children with orbital cellulitis: time for a reevaluation? *J Pediatr Ophthalmol Strabismus* 27:141-142, 1990.

51. Chandler JR, Langenbrunner DJ, Stevens ER: The pathogenesis of orbital complications in acute sinusitis, *Laryngoscope* 80:1414-1428, 1970.

52. Chandra P, Ahluwalia BK, Chugh TD: Primary orbital aspergilloma, *Br J Ophthalmol* 54:693-696, 1970.

53. Choi S, Lawson W, Urken ML: Subperiosteal orbital hematoma: an unusual complication of sinusitis, *Arch Otolaryngol Head Neck Surg* 114:1464, 1988.

54. Clairmont AA, Per-Lee JH: Complications of acute frontal sinusitis, *Am Fam Physician* 11:80-84, 1975.

55. Clark AE, Victor WH: An unusual presentation of temporal arteritis, *Ann Ophthalmol* 19:343-346, 1987.

56. Couch L, Theilen F, Mader JT: Rhinocerebral mucormycosis with cerebral extension successfully treated with adjunctive hyperbaric oxygen therapy, *Arch Otolaryngol Head Neck Surg* 114:791-794, 1988.

57. Crivelli G, Riviera LC: Unilateral blindness from aspergilloma at the right optic foramen: case report, *J Neurosurg* 33:207-211, 1970.

58. Cuadrado LM, Guerrero A, Asenjo JALG et al.: Cerebral mucormycosis in two cases of acquired immunodeficiency syndrome, *Arch Neurol* 45:109-111, 1988.

59. Currie JN, Coppeto JR, Lessell S: Chronic syphilitic meningitis resulting in superior orbital fissure syndrome and posterior fossa gumma: a report of two cases followed for twenty years, *J Clin Neuro-ophthalmol* 8:145-159, 1988.

60. De Beule K, De Doncker P, Cauwenbergh G et al.: The treatment of aspergillosis and aspergilloma with itraconazole, clinical results of an open international study (1982-1987), *Mycoses* 31:476-485, 1988.

61. De Foer C, Fossion E, Vaillant JM: Sinus aspergillosis, *J Craniomaxillofac Surg* 18:33-40, 1990.

62. del Palacio HA, Fereres J, Larregla G et al.: Nosocomial infection by Rhizomucor pusillus in a clinical haematology unit, *J Hosp Infect* 4:45-49, 1983.

63. Denning DW, Stevens DA: Antifungal and surgical treatment of invasive aspergillosis: review of 2121 published cases, *Rev Infect Dis* 12:1147-1201, 1990.

64. Denning DW, Tucker RM, Hanson LH et al.: Treatment of invasive aspergillosis with itraconazole, *Am J Med* 86:791-800, 1989.

65. de Repentigny L: Serological techniques for diagnosis of fungal infection, *Eur J Clin Microbiol Infect Dis* 8:362-375, 1989.

66. Deschenes J, Seamone CD, Baines MG: The ocular manifestations of sexually transmitted diseases, *Can J Ophthalmol* 25:177-185, 1990.

67. Deschenes J, Seamone CD, Baines MG: Acquired ocular syphilis: diagnosis and treatment, *Ann Ophthalmol* 24:134-138, 1992.

68. deSlegte RG, Kaiser MC, van der Baan S et al.: Computed tomographic diagnosis of septic sinus thrombosis and their complications, *Neuroradiology* 30:160-165, 1988.

69. deSmet MD, Rootman J: Orbital manifestations of plasmacytic lymphoproliferations, *Ophthalmology* 94:995-1003, 1987.

70. DeWeese DD, Schleuning AJ II, Robinson LB: Mucormycosis of the nose and paranasal sinuses, *Laryngoscope* 75:1398-1407, 1965.

71. DiNubile MJ: Septic thrombosis of the cavernous sinuses, *Arch Neurol* 45:567-572, 1988.

72. Donahue HC: Ophthalmologic experience in a tuberculosis sanitorium, *Am J Ophthalmol* 64:742-748, 1967.

73. Dortzbach RK, Segrest DR: Orbital aspergillosis, *Ophthalmic Surg* 14:240-244, 1983.

74. Duke-Elder S, MacFaul PA: The ocular adnexa: inflammations of the orbit. In Duke-Elder S, editor: *System of ophthalmology,* vol 13, part 2, 859-933, St Louis, 1974, Mosby.

75. Edwards JE: Zygomycosis. In Hoeprich PD, Jordan MC, Ronald AR, eds: *Infectious diseases: a treatise of infectious processes,* ed 5, Philadelphia, 1994, Lippincott.

76. Elitsur Y, Biedner BZ, Bar-Ziv J: Ethmoiditis, conjunctivitis and orbital cellulitis due to *Enterococcus* infection, *Clin Pediatr* 23:123, 1984.

77. English G: *Sinusitis,* Hagerstown, Md, 1981, Harper & Row.

78. Eustis HS, Armstrong DC, Buncic JR et al.: Staging of orbital cellulitis in children: computerized tomography characteristics and treatment guidelines, *J Pediatr Ophthalmol Strabismus* 23:246-251, 1986.

79. Fearon B, Edmonds B, Bird R: Orbital-facial complications of sinusitis in children, *Laryngoscope* 89:947-953, 1979.

80. Fearon B, McMillin BD: Sinusitis in infants and children. In Blitzer A, Lawson W, Friedman WH, editors: *Surgery of the paranasal sinuses,* ed 2, 421-432, Philadelphia, 1991, WB Saunders.

81. Ferguson BJ, Mitchell TG, Moon R et al.: Adjunctive hyperbaric oxygen for treatment of rhinocerebral mucormycosis, *Rev Infect Dis* 10:551-559, 1988.

82. Ferguson EC: Deep, wooden foreign bodies of the orbit: a report of two cases. *Trans Am Acad Ophthalmol Otolaryngol* 74:778, 1970.

83. Ferry AP: Cerebral mucormycosis (phycomycosis). Ocular findings and review of the literature, *Surv Ophthalmol* 6:1-24, 1961.

84. Ferry AP, Abedi S: Diagnosis and management of rhino-orbitocerebral mucormycosis (phycomycosis): a report of 16 personally observed cases, *Ophthalmology* 90:1096-1104, 1983.

85. Fisher EW, Toma A, Fisher PH et al.: Rhinocerebral mucormycosis: use of liposomal amphotericin B, *J Laryngol Otol* 105:575-577, 1991.

86. Forteza G, Burgeno M, Martorell V et al.: Rhinocerebral mucormycosis, *J Craniomaxillofac Surg* 16:80-84, 1988.

87. Gale GR, Welch AM: Studies of opportunistic fungi. I. Inhibition of Rhizipus oryzae by human serum, *Am J Med Sci* 241:604-612, 1961.

88. Galetta SL, Wulc AE, Goldberg HI et al.: Rhinocerebral mucormycosis: management and survival after carotid occlusion, *Ann Neurol* 28:103-107, 1990.

89. Gamba JL, Woodruff WW, Djang WT, Yeates AE: Craniofacial mucormycosis: assessment with CT, *Radiology* 160:207-212, 1986.

90. Gamble RC: Acute inflammations of the orbit in children, *Arch Ophthalmol* 10:483, 1933.

91. Gamble RC: Orbital abscesses, *Arch Ophthalmol* 18:633-641, 1937.

92. Gans H, Sekula J, Wlodyka J: Treatment of acute orbital complications, *Arch Otolaryngol* 100:329-332, 1974.

93. Geggel HS, Isenberg SJ: Cavernous sinus thrombosis as a cause of unilateral blindness, *Ann Ophthalmol* 14:569, 1982.

94. Gold RS, Sager E: Pansinusitis, orbital cellulitis, and blindness as sequelae of delayed treatment of dental abscess, *J Oral Surg* 32:40, 1974.

95. Gold SC, Arrigg PG, Hedges TR: Computerized tomography in the management of acute orbital cellulitis, *Ophthalmic Surg* 18:753-756, 1987.

96. Goldberg F, Berne AS, Oski FA: Differentiation of orbital cellulitis from preseptal cellulitis by computed tomography, *Pediatrics* 62:1000-1005, 1978.

97. Goldfarb MS, Hoffman DS, Rosenberg S: Orbital cellulitis and orbital fractures, *Ann Ophthalmol* 19:97-99, 1987.

98. Goodwin WJ Jr: Orbital complications of ethmoiditis, *Otolaryngol Clin North Am* 18:139-147, 1985.

99. Green WH, Goldberg HI, Wohl GT: Mucormycosis infection of the craniofacial structures, *AJR* 101:802-806, 1967.

100. Green WR, Font RL, Zimmerman LE: Aspergillosis of the orbit: report of ten cases and review of the literature, *Arch Ophthalmol* 82:302-313, 1969.

101. Greewald MJ, Wohl LG, Sell CH: Metastatic bacterial endophthalmitis: a contemporary reappraisal, *Surv Ophthalmol* 31:81, 1986.

102. Gregory JL, Golden A, Haymaher W: Mucormycosis of the central nervous system: a report of three cases, *Bull John Hopkins Hosp* 73:405-419, 1943.

103. Grossniklaus HE, Wojno TH: Leukemic infiltrate appearing as periorbital cellulitis, *Arch Ophthalmol* 108:484, 1990.

104. Gutowski WM, Mulbury PE, Hengerer AS et al.: The role of CT scans in managing the orbital complications of ethmoiditis, *Int J Pediatr Otorhinolaryngol* 15:117-128, 1988.

105. Handler LC, Davey IC, Hill JC et al.: The acute orbit: differentiation of orbital cellulitis from subperiosteal abscess by computerized tomography, *Neuroradiology* 33:15-18, 1991.

106. Harr DL, Quencer RM, Abrams GW: Computed tomography and ultrasound in evaluation of orbital infection and pseudotumor, *Neuroradiology* 142:395-401, 1982.

107. Harris GJ: Subperiosteal abscess of the orbit, *Arch Ophthalmol* 101:751-757, 1983.

108. Harris GJ: Subperiosteal inflammation of the orbit: a bacteriological analysis of 17 cases, *Arch Ophthalmol* 106:947-952, 1988.

109. Harris GJ, Will BR: Orbital aspergillosis: conservative debridement and local amphotericin irrigation, *Ophthalmic Plast Reconstruct Surg* 5:207-211, 1989.

110. Harris GJ, Kay MC, Nilles JJ: Orbital hematoma secondary to frontal sinusitis, *Ophthalmology* 85:1229-1234, 1978.

111. Hartwick RW, Batsakis JG: Pathology consultation: sinus aspergillosis and allergic fungal sinusitis, *Ann Otol Rhinol Laryngol* 100:427-430, 1991.

112. Hawkins DB, Clark RW: Orbital involvement in acute sinusitis: lessons from 24 childhood patients, *Clin Pediatr* 16:464-471, 1977.

113. Hay RJ: Antifungal therapy and the new azole compounds, *J Antimicrob Chemother* 28(suppl A):35-46, 1991.

114. Haymaker W: Fatal infections of the central nervous system and meninges after tooth extraction with analysis of 28 cases, *Am J Orthod* 31:117, 1945.

115. Haynes RE, Cramblett HG: Acute ethmoiditis: its relationship to orbital cellulitis, *Am J Dis Child* 114:261, 1967.

116. Hedges TR, Leung LE: Parasellar and orbital apex syndrome caused by aspergillosis, *Neurology* 26:117-120, 1976.

117. Hemady R, Zimmerman A, Katzen BW et al.: Orbital cellulitis caused by *Eikenella corrodens*, *Am J Ophthalmol* 114:584-588, 1992.

118. Hempstead BE: Intranasal surgical treatment of chronic maxillary sinusitis, *Arch Otolaryngol* 6:426, 1927.

119. Hepner R, Hagar D: Staphylococcal orbital sepsis in newborn infants, *South Med J* 53:922, 1960.

120. Hirsch JF, Roux FX, Sainte-Rose C et al.: Brain abscess in childhood, *Childs Brain* 10:251-265, 1983.

121. Hirsch M, Lifshitz T: Computerized tomography in the diagnosis and treatment of orbital cellulitis, *Pediatr Radiol* 18:302-305, 1988.

122. Höffken G: Fungal infections during neutropenia: the role of prophylaxis, *Mycoses* 32(suppl 1):88-95, 1989.

123. Hornblass A, Herschorn BJ, Stern K et al.: Orbital abscess, *Surv Ophthalmol* 29:169-178, 1984.

124. Hornblass A, To K, Coden DJ et al.: Endogenous orbital cellulitis and endogenous endophthalmitis in subacute bacterial endocarditis, *Am J Ophthalmol* 108:196-197, 1989.

125. Houle TVJ, Ellis PP: Aspergillosis of the orbit with immunosuppressive therapy, *Surv Ophthalmol* 20:35-42, 1975.

126. Howard GM, Ellsworth RM: Differential diagnosis of retinoblastoma: a statistical survey of 500 children, *Am J Ophthalmol* 60:618-621, 1965.

127. Hubert L: Orbital infections due to nasal sinusitis: a study of 114 cases, *N Y J Med* 37:1559, 1937.

128. Humphry RC, Wright G, Rich WJ et al.: Acute proptosis and blindness in a patient with orbital phycomycosis, *J R Soc Med* 82:304-305, 1989.

129. Ing MR: Infection following strabismus surgery, *Ophthalmic Surg* 22:41, 1991.

130. Jackson K, Baker SR: Clinical implications of orbital cellulitis, *Laryngoscope* 96:568-574, 1986.

131. Jain MR, Chunduwat HS, Batra V: Tuberculosis of the maxillary antrum of the orbit, *Indian J. Ophthalmol* 1:18-20, 1979.

132. Jarrett WH, Gutman FA: Ocular complications of infection in the paranasal sinuses, *Arch Ophthalmol* 81:683, 1969.

133. Jedrzynski MS, Bullock JD, McGuire TW et al.: Anaerobic orbital cellulitis: a clinical and experimental study, *Trans Am Ophthalmol Soc* 89:313-347, 1991.

134. Jones DB, Steinkuller PG: Microbial preseptal and orbital cellulitis. In Duane TB, editor: *Clinical ophthalmology,* vol 4, 1, New York, 1989, Harper & Row.

135. Kaban LB, McGill T: Orbital cellulitis of dental origin: differential diagnosis and the use of the computed tomography as a diagnostic aid, *J Oral Surg* 38:682, 1980.

136. Kaplan AH, Poza-Juncal E, Shapiro R et al.: Cure of mucormycosis in a renal transplant patient receiving cyclosporin with maintenance of immunosuppression, *Am J Nephrol* 8:139-142, 1988.

137. Karp JE, Burch PA, Merz WG: An approach to intensive antileukemia therapy in patients with previous invasive aspergillosis, *Am J Med* 85:203-206, 1988.

138. Karr DJ, Weinberger E, Mills RP: An unusual case of cellulitis associated with a molteno implant in a one-year-old child, *J Pediatr Ophthalmol Strabismus* 27:107, 1990.

139. Kaufman SH: Vaccines against tubuclerosis: the impact of modern biotechnology, *Scand J Infect Dis* (suppl)76:54-59, 1990.

140. Kaufman SJ: Orbital mucopyoceles: two cases and a review, *Surv Ophthalmol* 25:253-262, 1981.

141. Kavanagh KT, Parham DM, Hughes WT et al.: Fungal sinusitis in immunocompromised children with neoplasms, *Ann Otol Rhinol Laryngol* 100:331-336, 1991.

142. Kelly SP, Lloyd IC, Anderson H et al.: Solitary extramedullary plasmacytoma of the maxillary antrum and orbit presenting as acute bacterial orbital cellulitis, *Br J Ophthalmol* 75:438-439, 1991.

143. Khalil M, Lindley S, Matouk E: Tuberculosis of the orbit, *Ophthalmology* 92:624-627, 1985.

144. Kilpatrick C, Tress B, King J: Computed tomography of rhinocerebral mucormycosis, *Neuroradiology* 26:71-73, 1984.

145. Kimbrough BO, Young AB, Modica LA: Orbital cellulitis and cavernous sinus thrombosis after cataract extraction and lens implantation, *Ann Ophthalmol* 24:313-317, 1992.

146. Knight JS, Stacy GC: Antral infection of dental origin with a report of a case via an unusual dental route, *Aust Dent J* 8:483, 1963.

147. Kohn R, Hepler R: Management of limited rhino-orbital mucormycosis without exenteration, *Ophthalmology* 92:1440-1444, 1985.

148. Krohel GB, Krauss HR, Winnick V: Orbital abscess: presentation, diagnosis, therapy and sequalae, *Ophthalmology* 89:492-498, 1982.

149. Kronberg FG, Goodwin WJ Jr: Sinusitis in intensive care unit patients, *Laryngoscope* 95:936-938, 1985.

150. Kronschnabel EF: Orbital apex syndrome due to sinus infection, *Laryngoscope* 84:353, 1974.

151. Kurup VP, Kumar A: Immunodiagnosis of aspergillosis, *Clin Microbiol Rev* 4:439-456, 1991.

152. Langham-Brown JJ, Rhys-Williams S: Computed tomography of acute orbital infection: the importance of coronal sections, *Clin Radiol* 40:471-474, 1989.

153. Lawson W: Orbital complications of sinusitis. In Blitzer A, Lawson W, Friedman WH, editors: *Surgery of the paranasal sinuses,* ed 2, 457-469, 1991, Philadelphia, WB Saunders.

154. Lehrer RI, Howard DH, Sypherd PS et al.: Mucormycosis, *Ann Intern Med* 93(Part 1):93-108, 1980.

155. Lemke BN, Gonnering RS, Weinstein JM: Orbital cellulitis with periosteal elevation, *Ophthal Plast Reconstr Surg* 3:1-7, 1987.

156. Levitz SM: Aspergillosis. Systemic fungal infections: diagnosis and treatment II, *Infect Dis Clin North Am* 3:1-18, 1989.

157. Londer L, Nelson DL: Orbital cellulitis due to *Haemophilus influenzae*, *Arch Ophthalmol* 91:89-91, 1974.

158. Lopez-Berestein G, Bodey GP, Fainstein V et al.: Treatment of systemic fungal infections with liposomal amphotericin B, *Arch Intern Med* 149:2533-2536, 1989.

159. Lopez-Berestein G, Fainstein V, Hopfer R et al.: Liposomal amphotericin B for the treatment of systemic fungal infections in patients with cancer: a preliminary study, *J Infect Dis* 151:704-710, 1985.

160. Lundberg C, Engquist S: Pathogenesis of maxillary sinusitis, *Scand J Infect Dis* 39(suppl):53-55, 1983.

161. Maartens G, Wood MJ: The clinical presentation and diagnosis of invasive fungal infections, *J Antimicrob Chemother* 28(suppl A):13-22, 1991.

162. Macy JI, Mandelbaum SH, Minckler DS: Ocular pathology for clinicians. 8. Orbital cellulitis, *Ophthalmology* 87:1309-1313, 1980.

163. Mahajan VM: Experimental orbital mycosis, *Mycoses* 31:11-16, 1988.

164. Mandell GL, Douglas RG, Bennett JE, editors: *Principles and practice of infectious diseases,* ed 3, New York, 1989, Churchill Livingstone.

165. Maniglia AJ, Goodwin WJ, Arnold JE et al.: Intracranial abscesses secondary to nasal, sinus, and orbital infections in adults and children, *Arch Otolaryngol Head Neck Surg* 115:1424-1429, 1989.

166. Marouf LM, Azar DT, Hemadeh R et al.: Orbital echinococcosis in unilateral exophthalmos, *Orbit* 6:213-216, 1987.

167. Maskin SL, Fetchick RJ, Leone CR et al.: *Bipolaris hawaiiensis*-caused phaeohyphomycotic orbitopathy: a devastating fungal sinusitis in an apparently immunocompetent host, *Ophthalmology* 96:175-179, 1989.

168. Mathur SP, Makhija JM: Invasion of the orbit by maggots, *Br J Ophthalmol* 51:406, 1967.

169. Mauriello JA: Complications of orbital trauma surgery, *Adv Ophthalmic Plast Reconst Surg* 7:99-115, 1988.

170. Maurya OPS, Patel R, Thakur B et al.: Tuberculoma of the orbit: a case report, *Indian J Ophthalmol* 38:191-192, 1990.

171. McCormick WF, Schochet SS, Weaver PR et al.: Disseminated aspergillosis: aspergillus endophthalmitis, optic nerve infarction, and carotid artery thrombosis, *Arch Pathol* 99:353-359, 1975.

172. McGuire TW, Bullock JD, Bullock JD Jr et al.: Fungal endophthalmitis: an experimental study with a review of 17 human ocular cases, *Arch Ophthalmol* 109:1289-1296, 1991.

173. McLeish WM, Pulido JS, Holland F et al.: The ocular manifestations of syphilis in the human immunodeficiency virus type I infected host, *Ophthalmology* 97:196-203, 1990.

174. Miller RD, Steinkuller PG, Naegele D: Nonfatal maxillocerebral mucormycosis with orbital involvement in a dehydrated infant, *Ann Ophthalmol* 12:1065-1068, 1980.

175. Mills RP, Kartush JM: Orbital wall thickness and the spread of infection from the paranasal sinuses, *Clin Otolaryngol* 10:209-216, 1985.

176. Moloney JR, Badham NJ, McRae A: The acute orbit: preseptal (periorbital) cellulitis, subperiosteal abscess, and orbital cellulitis due to sinusitis, *J Laryngol Otol Suppl* 12:1-18, 1987.

177. Morduchowicz G, Shmueli D, Shapira Z et al.: Rhinocerebral mucormycosis in renal transplant recipients: report of three cases and review of the literature, *Rev Infect Dis* 8:441-446, 1986.

178. Morgan PR, Morrison WV: Complications of frontal and ethmoid sinusitis, *Laryngoscope* 90:661-666, 1980.

179. Morriss FH, Spock A: Intracranial aneurysm secondary to mycotic orbital and sinus infection: report of a case implicating *Penicillium* as an opportunistic fungus, *Am J Dis Child* 119:357-362, 1970.

180. Mortada A: Tuberculoma of the orbit and lacrimal gland, *Br J Ophthalmol* 55:565-567, 1971.

181. Neu HC: Infectious diseases of the sinuses. In Blitzer A, Lawson W, Friedman WH, editors: *Surgery of the paranasal sinuses,* ed 2, 161-166, Philadelphia, 1991, WB Saunders.

182. Noel LP, Clarke WN, MacDonald N: Clinical management of orbital cellulitis in children, *Can J Ophthalmol* 25:11-16, 1990.

183. Noel LP, Clarke WN, Peacocke TA: Periorbital and orbital cellulitis in childhood, *Can J Ophthalmol* 16:178-180, 1981.

184. Oakhill A, Shah KJ, Thompson AG et al.: Orbital tuberculosis in childhood, *Br J Ophthalmol* 66:396-397, 1982.

185. Ochi JW, Harris JP, Feldman JI et al.: Rhinocerebral mucormycosis: results of aggressive surgical debridement and amphotericin B, *Laryngoscope* 98:1339-1342, 1988.

186. Ogundiya DA, Keith DA, Mirowski J: Cavernous sinus thrombosis and blindness as complications of an odontogenic infection: report of a case and review of literature, *J Oral Maxillofac Surg* 47:1317-1321, 1989.

187. Olurin O, Lucas AO, Oyediran ABO: Orbital histoplasmosis due to *Histoplasma duboisii, Am J Ophthalmol* 68:14-18, 1969.

188. O'Silva H, Burke JF, Cho SY: Disseminated aspergillosis in a presumably immunocompetent host, *JAMA* 248:1495-1497, 1982.

189. Parfrey NA: Improved diagnosis and prognosis of mucormycosis: a clinicopathologic study of 33 cases, *Medicine* 65:113-123, 1986.

190. Partamian LG, Jay WM, Fritz KJ: Anaerobic orbital cellulitis, *Ann Ophthalmol* 15:123-126, 1983.

191. Pascarelli E, Lemlich A: Diplopia and photophobia as premonitory symptoms in cavernous sinus thrombosis, *Ann Otol* 73:210, 1964.

192. Patt BS, Manning SC: Blindness resulting from orbital complications of sinusitis, *Otolaryngol Head Neck Surg* 104:789-795, 1991.

193. Patterson TF, George D, Miniter P et al.: The role of fluconazole in the early treatment and prophylaxis of experimental invasive aspergillosis, *J Infect Dis* 164:575-580, 1991.

194. Paultauf A: Mycosis mucorina; ein beitraq zur kenntniss der menschlichen fadenpilzerkrankurnen, *Virchows Arch* 102:543-564, 1885.

195. Pennisi AK, Parenti DM, Stevens A et al.: Paranasal sinus mucormycosis in an immunologically competent host, *Am J Otolaryngol* 6:471-473, 1985.

196. Perillie PE, Nolan JP, Finch SC: Studies of the resistance to infection in diabetes mellitus: local exudative cellular response, *J Lab Clin Med* 59:1008, 1962.

197. Pillsbury HC, Fischer ND: Rhinocerebral mucormycosis, *Arch Otolaryngol Head Neck Surg* 103:600-604, 1977.

198. Polak A: Combination therapy with antifungal drugs, *Mycoses* 31(suppl 2):45-53, 1988.

199. Polak A: Combination therapy for systemic mycosis, *Infection* 17:203-209, 1989.

200. Polli C: On the incidence of ketone reductase in microorganisms, *Pathol Microbiol* 28:93, 1965.

201. Powles RL, Milliken S: The prophylaxis of fungal infections, *J Antimicrob Chemother* 28(suppl A):97-103, 1991.

202. Press GA, Weindling SM, Hesselink JR et al.: Rhinocerebral mucormycosis: MR manifestations, *J Comput Assist Tomogr* 12:744-749, 1988.

203. Price CD, Hameroff SB, Richards RD: Cavernous sinus thrombosis and orbital cellulitis, *South Med J* 64:1243, 1971.

204. Quattrocolo G, Pignatta P, Dimanico U et al.: Rhinocerebral mucormycosis and internal carotid artery thrombosis in a previously healthy patient, *Acta Neurol Belg* 90:20-26, 1990.

205. Quick CA, Payne E: Complicated acute sinusitis, *Laryngoscope* 82:1248-1263, 1972.

206. Rangel-Guerra R, Martinez HR, Saenz C: Mucormycosis report of 11 cases, *Arch Neurol* 42:578-581, 1985.

207. Reidy JJ, Giltner J, Apple DJ et al.: Paranasal sinusitis, orbital abscess, and inflammatory tumors of the orbit, *Ophthalmic Surg* 18:363-366, 1987.

208. Richardson MD: Opportunistic and pathogenic fungi, *J Antimicrob Chemother* 28(suppl A):1-11, 1991.

209. Rogers AL, Kennedy MJ: Opportunistic hyaline hyphomycetes. In Hausler WJ Jr, Herrmann KL, Isenberg HD, Shadomy HJ, editors: *Manual of clinical microbiology,* ed 5, 659-673, Washington, DC, 1991, American Society for Microbiology.

210. Rootman J, Robertson W, Lapointe JS: Inflammatory diseases. In Rootman J, editor: *Diseases of the orbit: a multi-disciplinary approach,* Philadelphia, 143-159, 1988, JP Lippincott.

211. Rootman J, Roth AM, Crawford JB et al.: Extensive squamous cell carcinoma of the conjunctiva presenting as orbital cellulitis: the hermit syndrome, *Can J Ophthalmol* 22:40-44, 1987.

212. Rubin SE, Rubin LG, Zito J et al.: Medical management of orbital subperiosteal abscess in children, *J Pediatr Ophthalmol Strabismus* 26:21-27, 1989.

213. Rubinstein JB, Handler SD: Orbital and periorbital cellulitis in children, *Head Neck Surg* 5:15-21, 1982.

214. Ryder NS: Mechanism of action and biochemical selectivity of allylamine antimycotic agents, *Ann NY Acad Sci* 544:208-220, 1988.

215. Sanders MD, Brown P: Acute presentation of thyroid ophthalmopathy, *Trans Ophthalmol Soc UK* 105:720, 1986.

216. Saral R: Candida and aspergillus infections in immunocompromised patients: an overview, *Rev Infect Dis* 13:487-492, 1991.

217. Sarti EJ, Lucente FE: Aspergillosis of the paranasal sinuses, *Ear Nose Throat J* 67:824-831, 1988.

218. Schramm VL, Curtin HV, Kennerdell JS: Evaluation of orbital cellulitis and results of treatment, *Laryngoscope* 92:732-738, 1982.

219. Schramm VL, Myers EN, Kennerdell JS: Orbital complications of acute sinusitis: evaluation, management, and outcome, *Otolaryngol Head Neck Surg* 86:221-230, 1978.

220. Schwartz H, Baskin MA, Ilkiw A et al.: An unusual organism causing orbital cellulitis, *Br J Ophthalmol* 63:710-712, 1979.

221. Schwartz JN, Donnelly EH, Klintworth GK: Ocular and orbital phycomycosis, *Surv Ophthalmol* 22:30-28, 1977.

222. Scott GI: Orbital cellulitis and cavernous sinus thrombosis, *Trans Ophthalmol Soc UK* 80:435-450, 1960.

223. Scully RE, Mark EJ, McNeely WF et al.: Case records of the Massachusetts General Hospital, *New Engl J Med* 323:1823-1833, 1990.

224. Searl SS: Minor trauma, disastrous results, *Surv Ophthalmol* 31:337, 1987.

225. Sen DK: Tuberculosis of the orbit and lacrimal gland: a clinical study of 14 cases, *J Pediatr Ophthalmol Strabismus* 17:232-238, 1980.

226. Sevel D, Sapeika RJ: Hydatid cyst of the orbit, *Surv Ophthalmol* 22:101-105, 1977.

227. Shadomy S, Espinel-Ingroff, Gebhart RJ: In-vitro studies with SF-327, a new orally active allylamine derivative: Sabouraudia: *J Med Vet Mycology* 23:125-132, 1985.

228. Sheldon WH, Bauer H: The development of the acute inflammatory response to experimental cutaneous mucormycosis in normal and diabetic rabbits, *J Exp Med* 110:845-852, 1959.

229. Sheridan PH, Edman JB, Starr SE: Tuberculosis presenting as an orbital mass, *Pediatrics* 67:874-875, 1981.

230. Shields JA, Shields CL, Suvarnamani C et al.: Retinoblastoma manifesting as orbital cellulitis, *Am J Ophthalmol* 112:442-449, 1991.

231. Shopfner CE, Rossi JO: Roentgen evaluation of the paranasal sinuses in children, *Am J Roentgenol Radium Ther Nucl Med* 118:176, 1973.

232. Shurin P: Inflammatory diseases of the nose and paranasal sinuses. In Bluestone D, Stool SE, editors: *Pediatric otolaryngology,* vol 1, Philadelphia, 1983, WB Saunders.

233. Sicher H, DuBrul EL: *Oral anatomy,* ed 7, 498-518, St Louis, 1980, Mosby.

234. Simon HB: Infections due to mycobacteria. In Rubenstein E, Federman DD, editors: *Scientific American medicine,* 1-23, New York, 1993, Scientific American.

235. Simpson GT, McGill TlJ, Healy GB: *Hemophilus influenzae* type B soft tissue infections of the head and neck, *Laryngoscope* 91:17-30, 1981.

236. Slavin ML: Primary aspergillosis of the orbital apex, *Arch Ophthalmol* 109:1502-1503, 1991.

237. Slavin ML, Glaser JS: Acute severe irreversible visual loss with sphenoethmoiditis-'posterior' orbital cellulitis, *Arch Ophthalmol* 105:345-348, 1987.

238. Smith AT, Spencer JT: Orbital complications resulting from lesions of the sinuses, *Ann Otol Rhinol Laryngol* 57:5-27, 1948.

239. Smith JL, Stevens DA: Survival in cerebro-rhino-orbital zygomycosis and cavernous sinus thrombosis with combined therapy, *South Med J* 79:501-504, 1986.

240. Smith TF, O'Day D, Wright PF: Clinical implications of preseptal (periorbital) cellulitis in childhood, *Pediatrics* 62:1006-1009, 1978.

241. Souliere CR, Antoine GA, Martin MP et al.: Selective nonsurgical management of subperiosteal abscess of the orbit: computerized tomography and clinical course as indication for surgical drainage, *Int J Pediatr Otorhinolaryngol* 19:109-119, 1990.

242. Spires JR, Smith RJH: Bacterial infections of the orbital and periorbital soft-tissues in children, *Laryngoscope* 96:763-767, 1986.

243. Spires JR, Smith RJ, Catlin FI: Brain abscesses in the young, *Otolaryngol Head Neck Surg* 93:468-474, 1985.

244. Spoor TC, Harding SA: Orbital tuberculosis, *Am J Ophthalmol* 91:644-647, 1981.

245. Spoor TC, Hartel WC, Harding S et al.: Aspergillosis presenting as a corticosteroid-responsive optic neuropathy, *J Clin Neuro-ophthalmol* 2:103-107, 1982.

246. Spoor TC, Wynn P, Hartel WC et al.: Ocular syphilis: acute and chronic, *J Clin Neuro-ophthalmol* 3:197-203, 1983.

247. Stein DK, Sugar AM: Fungal infections in the immunocompromised host, *Diagn Microbiol Infect Dis* 12:221S-228S, 1989.

248. Stevens MH: Primary fungal infections of the paranasal sinuses, *Am J Otolaryngol* 2:348-357, 1981.

249. Straatsma BR, Zimmerman LE, Gass JDM: Phycomycosis: a clinicopathologic study of fifty-one cases, *Lab Invest* 11(Part 1):963-985, 1962.

250. Streeten BW, Rabuzzi DD, Jones DB: Sporotrichosis of the orbital margin, *Am J Ophthalmol* 77:750-755, 1974.

251. Terrell CL, Hughes CE: Antifungal agents used for deep-seated mycotic infections, *Mayo Clin Proc* 67:69-91, 1992.

252. Towbin R, Han BK, Kaufman RA et al.: Postseptal cellulitis: CT in diagnosis and management, *Head and Neck Radiology* 158:735, 1986.

253. Townsend DJ, Beyer-Machule CK, Fabian RL: Osteomyelitis of the orbit: a case report, *Ophthal Plas Reconstr Surg* 2:15-19, 1986.

254. Ullman S, Pflugfelder SC, Hughes R et al.: *Bacillus cereus* panophthalmitis manifesting as an orbital cellulitis, *Am J Ophthalmol* 103:105-106, 1987.

255. Vail DT: Orbital complications in sinus disease: a review, *Am J Ophthalmol* 1931:202-208.

256. Van Cutsem J: Oral, topical and parenteral antifungal treatment with itraconazole in normal and in immunocompromised animals, *Mycoses* 32(suppl 1):14-34, 1989.

257. Van Cutsem J, Van Gerven F, Janssen PAJ: Oral and parenteral therapy with saperconazole (R 66905) of invasive aspergillosis in normal and immunocompromised animals, *Antimicrob Agents Chemother* 33:2063-2068, 1989.

258. Vandevelde L, Bondewel C, Dubois M et al.: Mucorales and deferoxamin: from saprophytic to pathogenic state, *Acta Otorhinolaryngol Belg* 44:429-433, 1990.

259. Venezio FR, Sexton DJ, Forsythe R et al.: Mucormycosis after open fracture injury, *South Med J* 78:1516-1517, 1985.

260. Vida L, Moel SA: Systemic North American blastomycosis with orbital involvement, *Am J Ophthalmol* 77:240-242, 1974.

261. Vitale AT, Spaide RF, Warren FA et al.: Orbital aspergillosis in an immunocompromised host, *Am J Ophthalmol* 113:725-726, 1992.

262. von Noordan GK: Orbital cellulitis following extraocular muscle surgery, *Am J Ophthalmol* 74:627, 1972.

263. Wald ER, Pang D, Milmoe GJ et al.: Sinusitis and its complications in the pediatric patient, *Pediatr Clin North Am* 28:777-796, 1981.

264. Walsh TJ, Pizzo A: Treatment of systemic fungal infections: recent progress and current problems, *Eur J Clin Microbiol Infect Dis* 7:460-475, 1988.

265. Watters EC, Wallar PH, Hiles DA et al.: Acute orbital cellulitis, *Arch Ophthalmol* 94:785-788, 1976.

266. Weakley BR: Orbital cellulitis complicating strabismus surgery: a case report and review of the literature, *Ann Ophthalmol* 23:454-457, 1991.

267. Webb D: New antifungal agents: clinical and laboratory issues, *Clin Microbiol Newsletter* 13:129-136, 1991.

268. Weber AL: Inflammatory diseases of the paranasal sinuses and mucoceles, *Otolaryngol Clin North Am* 21:421-437, 1988.

269. Weber RS, Lopez-Berestein G: Treatment of invasive aspergillus sinusitis with liposomal-amphotericin B, *Laryngoscope* 97:937-941, 1987.

270. Weinstein JM, Morris GL, ZuRhein GM et al.: Posterior ischemic optic neuropathy due to aspergillus fumigatus, *J Clin Neuro Ophthalmol* 9:7-13, 1989.

271. Weiss A, Friendly D, Eglin K et al.: Bacterial periorbital and orbital cellulitis in childhood, *Ophthalmology* 90:195-203, 1983.

272. Weiss IS: Pseudomonas orbital cellulitis, *Am J Ophthalmol* 87:368-370, 1979.

273. Welsh LW, Welsh JJ: Orbital complications of sinus disease, *Laryngoscope* 84:848-856, 1974.

274. Westfall CT, Shore JW: Isolated fractures of the orbital floor: risk of infection and the role of antibiotic prophylaxis, *Ophthalmic Surg* 22:409, 1991.

275. Wheeler JM: Orbital cyst without epithelial lining, *Arch Ophthalmol* 18:356, 1937.

276. Wilhelmus KR: Myiasis palpebrum, *Am J Ophthalmol* 101:496, 1986.

277. Williams BJ, Harrison HC: Subperiosteal abscesses of the orbit due to sinusitis in childhood, *Aust N Z J Ophthalmol* 19:29-36, 1991.

278. Wilson ME, Paul TO: Orbital cellulitis following strabismus surgery, *Ophthalmic Surg* 18:92, 1987.

279. Wolter JR: Diagnosis and management of orbital aspergillosis, *Ann Ophthalmol* Jan:17-20, 1976.

280. Wood TR, Slight JR: Bilateral orbital myiasis, *Arch Ophthalmol* 84:692, 1970.

281. Wunderer S: Die Ausbreitung der retromaxillaren Abszesse im Lichte neurerer anatomischer Forschung, *Ost Z Stomat* 52:651, 1955.

282. Yohai RA, Bullock JD, Aziz AA et al.: Survival factors in rhino-orbito-cerebral mucormycosis, *Surv Ophthalmol* 39:3-22, 1994.

283. Yousem DM, Galetta SL, Gusnard DA et al.: MR findings in rhinocerebral mucormycosis, *J Comput Assist Tomogr* 13:878-882, 1989.

284. Zak SM, Katz B: Successfully treated spheno-orbital mucormycosis in an otherwise healthy adult, *Ann Ophthalmol* 17:344-348, 1985.

285. Zimmerman RA, Bilaniuk LT: CT of orbital infection and its cerebral complications, *AJR* 134:45, 1980.

286. Zinneman HH: Sino-orbital aspergillosis: report of a case and review of the literature, *Minn Med* Jul:661-664, 1972.

95 Infectious Dacryoadenitis

THOMAS D. FITZSIMMONS, STEVEN E. WILSON, ROBERT H. KENNEDY

The lacrimal gland is a bilobate exocrine gland located in the anterior superotemporal orbit. The orbital lobe is separated from the smaller palpebral lobe by the lateral extension of the levator aponeurosis. Excretory ducts pass through the palpebral lobe and drain tears into the superior conjunctival fornix via 6 to 12 ductules located approximately 5 mm above the superior border of the tarsus. The gland has a rich vascular and nerve supply.

HISTORICAL BACKGROUND

Awareness of the lacrimal gland has existed since at least the time of the ancient Greeks.[24] Schmidt is credited with the introduction of the term dacryoadenitis in 1803, referring to inflammation of the lacrimal gland.[53]

EPIDEMIOLOGY

Dacryoadenitis caused by infection is a rare disease; the medical literature consists primarily of single case reports or small series. The combined experience in two historical reviews provides an incidence rate of approximately one case of dacryoadenitis per 10,000 ophthalmology patients, but infectious dacryoadenitis was not specified and probably occurs much less frequently.[11,53] Males and females appear equally affected, with the possible exception of metastatic gonorrheal dacryoadenitis, in which a 5:1 male-to-female predominance has been reported.[53] Infectious dacryoadenitis has been described in persons as young as 4 years[23,59] and as old as 82 years.[5]

CLINICAL FEATURES

Dacryoadenitis may involve the palpebral and orbital lobes separately or together. The infection may be acute, subacute, or chronic. With the exception of mumps dacryoadenitis, acute infections tend to be unilateral. Chronic infections are more often bilateral.

Acute palpebral dacryoadenitis typically has a sudden onset of pain in the superotemporal orbit. The upper eyelid is red, swollen, and tender, often causing ptosis with an S-shaped lid (Fig. 95-1). Eversion of the upper lid reveals an enlarged, inflamed lacrimal gland (Fig. 95-2). The surrounding conjunctiva is injected and chemotic. A mucopurulent discharge is often present, but suppuration rarely occurs. Infection may be accompanied by mild fever and a general malaise. Preauricular and cervical nodes are often swollen and tender. Motility may be limited in abduction.[11,23,33,66] Vision is not usually affected.

Chronic dacryoadenitis is characterized by gradual, painless enlargement of the lacrimal gland over several months. Ptosis is present and a firm, tender mass can often be palpated. Superficial punctate keratopathy was reported in a patient with tuberculous dacryoadenitis.[44] Tuberculous dacryoadenitis has been reported in the absence of infection involving other organs.[59]

PATHOLOGY

Few histologic examinations of acute infectious dacryoadenitis have been reported.[11,32,39,49,53] Acute infections are characterized by a combined lymphocytic and leukocytic infiltration in the gland, with the connective-tissue elements affected more greatly than the secretory portions. The duct epithelium shows fatty degeneration. Ducts are filled with inflammatory cells that may plug the lumen and cause wide distension. Blood vessels may show thrombi, arteritic changes, or necrosis. Tuberculous dacryoadenitis is characterized by the presence of epitheloid and giant cells with caseous necrosis. Tissue sections from any cause rarely demonstrate microorganisms.

PATHOGENESIS

Many infectious agents have been cited as causes of dacryoadenitis, but all are exceedingly uncommon. Few organisms have actually been cultured or identified histopathologically (see box).

No evidence exists that the lacrimal gland carries a normal flora, although its conjunctival surface does. Organisms can infect the lacrimal gland by four main routes: (1) directly, as in trauma, (2) through nerves, (3) by retrograde passage from the conjunctiva through the ductules, or (4)

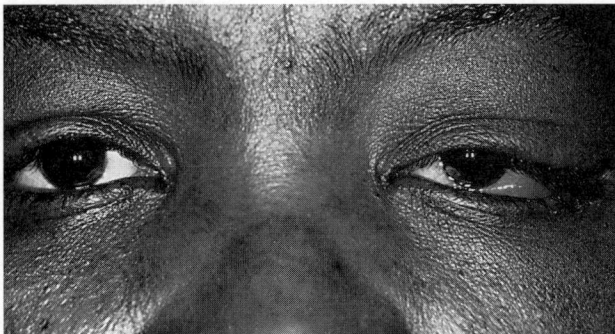

Fig. 95-1. Forty-nine-year-old woman with acute dacryoadenitis. Left upper eyelid is swollen with typical S-shaped appearance and conjunctiva is chemotic.

through blood. Hematogenous spread is probably the most common route of infection.

The lacrimal gland has histologic and physiologic similarities to other exocrine tissues, particularly the parotid gland. Two viruses can affect the lacrimal and parotid glands preferentially: mumps virus and Epstein-Barr virus.

Before the advent of widespread vaccination, the mumps virus may have been the most common cause of infectious dacryoadenitis. An incidence of 20% dacryoadenitis in mumps is widely quoted, but this figure dates from a single epidemic among soldiers in 1903.[54] Different mumps virus strains probably have different propensities for causing lacrimal gland infections. Dacryoadenitis has been described before, during, and after parotid gland swelling.[54] Cases of "lacrimal mumps" have also been reported in the absence of any apparent parotid gland disease.[54]

Epstein-Barr virus (EBV) is a cause of infectious mononucleosis, also called glandular fever, and may play a role in the pathogenesis of Sjögren syndrome. Despite the common occurrence of infectious mononucleosis, symptomatic lacri-

---

ORGANISMS IMPLICATED IN DACRYOADENITIS

Viruses
  Arbovirus[11]
  Epstein-Barr virus*
  Herpes simplex virus[10,19,29,71]
  Human immunodeficiency virus[26,57]
  Influenza virus[11]
  Measles virus[11]
  Mumps virus[11,21,32,54]
  Varicella-zoster virus[4,11,28,46,52]

Bacteria
  Brucella sp.[11]
  Chlamydia trachomatis[11,39,43]
  Corynebacterium diphtheriae[11]
  Haemophilus influenzae (aegyptius)[11]
  Moraxella catarrhalis
  Moraxella lacunata[11]
  Mycobacterium leprae[1,11,25]
  Mycobacterium tuberculosis†
  Neisseria gonorrhoeae[11,53]
  Nocardia sp.[20]
  Salmonella typhi[11]
  Staphylococcus sp.[11,23,28,33]
  Streptococcus sp.[11]
  Streptococcus pneumoniae[11]
  Treponema pallidum[11,23]

Fungi
  Actinomyces sp.[11,20]
  Pseudallescheria boydii[20]
  Cryptococcus sp.[20]
  Histoplasma capsulatum[11,20]

Parasites
  Cysticercus cellulosae (Taenia solium) sp.[60]
  Schistosoma haematobium[27]

---

*References 11, 19, 22, 28, 33, 35, 41, 48-51, 69, 70.
†References 2, 3, 5, 11, 12, 14, 15, 37, 40, 44, 45, 58, 59, 65.

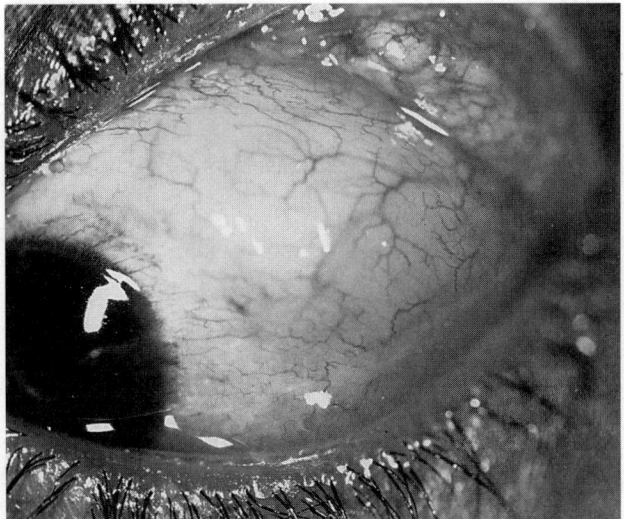

Fig. 95-2. Eversion of upper eyelid reveals a red, swollen, palpebral lobe of the lacrimal gland.

mal gland inflammation has rarely been reported with this infection.[11,28,64] Latent or subclinical EBV infection of the lacrimal gland may provide a stimulus for autoimmune destruction of the gland and resultant dryness of the eye.[16,18] Keratoconjunctivitis sicca has been attributed to EBV infection[22,70], the complement (CD 21)/EBV receptor has been detected in the lacrimal gland[51], and EBV DNA has been detected in some patients with Sjögren syndrome using polymerase chain reaction and DNA probe techniques.[7,17,50,56] Some investigators dispute the finding of increased EBV DNA in patients with Sjögren syndrome.[8,67] Aqueous tear deficiency has been associated with infection by human immunodeficiency virus (HIV).[26,57]

The lacrimal gland has been postulated to be a repository for latent herpes simplex virus. Experimental infection of rabbits with herpes simplex virus has shown that the lacrimal gland is among the first tissues to harbor reproducing virus particles, presumably through retrograde infection.[47] The virus has been cultured from tears of asymptomatic patients and found in lacrimal gland biopsies of patients with herpes simplex corneal disease.[29,30] Still, few cases of dacryoadenitis have been positively linked to the herpes simplex virus, and little further supporting evidence for a major role of the lacrimal gland in herpes simplex virus disease has emerged.

Staphylococcal, streptococcal, and gonococcal infections are the most frequent causes of acute suppurative dacryoadenitis. Tuberculosis is a reported cause of chronic dacryoadenitis. Bacterial infections, however, are very uncommon. Infection of the lacrimal gland by fungi and other organisms is exceedingly rare.

DIFFERENTIAL DIAGNOSIS

The differential diagnosis of dacryoadenitis includes virtually all diseases affecting the superotemporal orbit (see box).* Many of these diseases are more common than infectious dacryoadenitis. The recognition of chronic infectious dacryoadenitis is particularly difficult.

A hordeolum and a lid abscess are usually easily distinguishable from infectious dacryoadenitis by virtue of their restriction to the lid. Orbital cellulitis is characterized by marked impairment of extraocular motility, proptosis, and visual loss. Periostitis is not a common feature of dacryoadenitis, and bone pain suggests other disorders. Pseudotu-

---

DIFFERENTIAL DIAGNOSIS OF INFECTIOUS DACRYOADENITIS

Adenocarcinoma, adenoid cystic carcinoma of the lacrimal gland
Benign mixed tumor of the lacrimal gland
Dermoid, epidermoid cyst
Eosinophilic granuloma
Epithelial inclusion cyst
Foreign body
Hordeolum
Lacrimal duct cyst
Leukemia
Lymphoma
Orbital amyloidosis
Orbital cellulitis
Periostitis
Prolapsed lacrimal gland
Pseudotumor
Radiation injury
Sarcoidosis
Wegener granulomatosis

---

*References 6, 11, 13, 28, 31, 34, 36, 42, 53, 55, 61, 63, 67.

---

mor and other orbital inflammatory syndromes involving the lacrimal gland do not respond to antibiotic therapy but generally respond quickly to systemic corticosteroids.

Sarcoidosis affecting the lacrimal gland is more common than chronic infectious dacryoadenitis. Systemic sarcoidosis may be diagnosed by physical examination, radiologic evidence of typical hilar adenopathy, elevated angiotensin converting enzyme levels, and abnormal gallium scans.

Many lacrimal gland disorders require biopsy to establish the diagnosis and initiate appropriate therapy.

LABORATORY INVESTIGATIONS

Any mucopurulent discharge from the conjunctiva or skin should be cultured. The leukocyte count and erythrocyte sedimentation rate may be elevated in acute disease. Blood cultures are usually negative.

Specific laboratory tests can be considered if a particular disease is suspected, as follows:

- Mumps—complement fixation titers, including S/V ratio
- Epstein-Barr virus—EBV titers, including anti-VCA IgM and IgG antibodies and anti-EBNA antibodies
- AIDS—HIV testing
- Trachoma—Giemsa stain, culture
- Tuberculosis—TB skin test, sputum culture
- Syphilis—nonspecific antibody tests (VDRL, RPR), specific treponemal antibody tests (FTA-ABS, MHA-TP).

Radiography and Ultrasonography

Computerized tomography is often obtained to define the nature and extent of masses in the area of the lacrimal gland. In dacryoadenitis, scans show a large ovoid mass in the lacrimal gland fossa, which may enhance with contrast agents (Fig. 95-3). Bone destruction is not a feature of infectious dacryoadenitis and suggests other diseases such as a lacrimal gland tumor, eosinophilic granuloma or dermoid cyst. Ultrasonography can be useful in detecting low reflectance areas of an abscessed lacrimal gland.[23]

Biopsy

The definitive diagnosis of chronic lacrimal gland disorders requires biopsy. The skin and orbicularis muscle are incised in the upper lid crease or directly over the swollen gland. The orbital septum is opened and the enlarged lacrimal gland is identified. A small piece of lacrimal gland tissue is removed for histology and microbiologic studies. Transconjunctival biopsy of the palpebral lobe of the lacrimal gland may be indicated in some situations but caution is advised to avoid excising ductules of the gland, which may result in a dry eye.

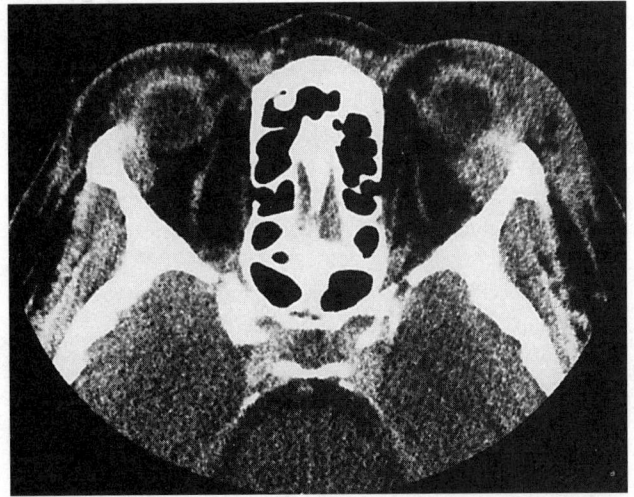

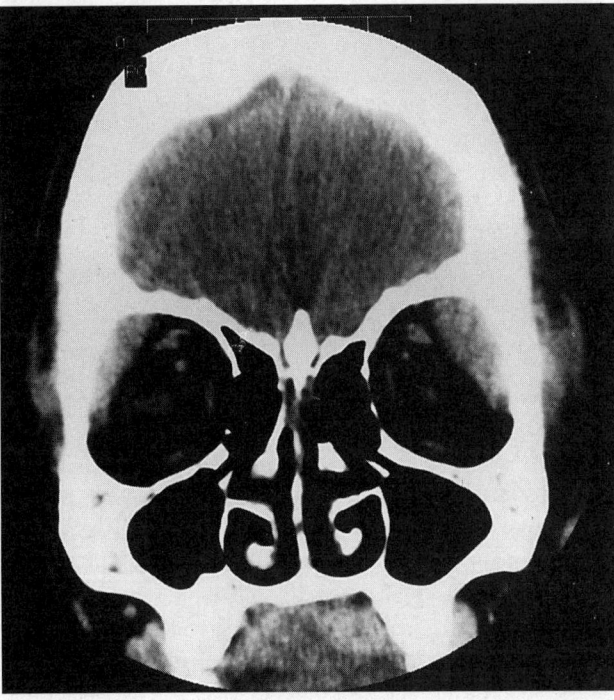

Fig. 95-3. **A,** Axial view orbital CT scan of acute dacryoadenitis shows enlarged lacrimal gland on left side. **B,** Coronal view orbital CT scan posterior to globes shows enlargement of both lacrimal glands, left greater than right.

THERAPY

Initial treatment is usually determined by the severity of presenting symptoms. Mild cases of infectious dacryoadenitis can be treated as variants of conjunctivitis. Conservative management includes vasoconstrictor eyedrops and, if a mucopurulent discharge is present, topical broad-spectrum antibiotic drops. It should be noted that topical treatment alone will not penetrate the lacrimal tissue suffi-

ciently to provide therapeutic drug levels but can treat an inciting or associated conjunctivitis.

Systemic, broad-spectrum antibiotic therapy is often used for dacryoadenitis with cellulitis. Antibiotic therapy can be guided by conjunctival cultures, the diagnosis of concurrent systemic infection, and the patient's response. An abscess of the lacrimal gland should be incised and drained. General supportive measures such as warm compresses to the lids, lavage of the conjunctival sac, and analgesics may provide relief.

Acute infectious dacryoadenitis generally runs a benign course with resolution after several days to weeks. Inappropriately treated systemic infections may result in recurrence of dacryoadenitis.[58]

PROGNOSIS

The prognosis for dacryoadenitis is generally very good, with few sequelae. Lacrimal duct cysts may be the consequence of previous glandular infection.[6] Suppuration can occur, with or without fistula formation. A case of an untreated suppurative dacryoadenitis was reported in which pus tracked posteriorly into the orbit and cavernous sinus, causing a fatal meningitis.[11]

Tear production is usually not affected but may be diminished.[2,41] Subclinical EBV and HIV infections of the lacrimal gland may play a role in the development of a dry eye syndrome. Trachoma can cause a dry eye from conjunctival scarring of the ductules and accessory lacrimal glands, but infection of the nerve supply of the lacrimal gland and actual parenchymal destruction of the lacrimal gland have been suggested as additional mechanisms.[25,43]

Although not a result of lacrimal gland infection, mention is made of the rare syndrome of crocodile tears, also known as the gustolacrimal reflex. This syndrome consists of unilateral lacrimation associated with eating or drinking and occurs most often as a consequence of Bell palsy or facial nerve trauma.[38] The cause is felt to be misdirection of regenerating autonomic nerves to the lacrimal gland.[38] The crocodile tear syndrome has been noted after two infections that involve the facial nerve: herpes zoster oticus[9] and leprosy.[62]

REFERENCES

1. Abraham JC: Prevention and treatment of eye complications in leprosy, *Lepr India* 48(suppl 4):763-769, 1976.
2. Baghdassarian SA, Zakharia H, Asdourian KK: Report of a case of bilateral caseous tuberculous dacryoadenitis, *Am J Ophthalmol* 74:744-746, 1972.
3. Boudet C, Arnaud B, Bullier B: Tuberculose de la glande lacrymale, *Bull Soc Ophtalmol* 103-109, 1971.
4. Bouzas A: Canalicular inflammation in ophthalmic cases of herpes zoster and herpes simplex, *Am J Ophthalmol* 60:713-716, 1965.
5. Chauvaud D et al.: An unusual observation of a case of tuberculous dacryoadenitis, *Arch Ophthalmol* 37:41-46, 1977.
6. Conway ST: Bilateral lacrimal duct cyst, *Ophthalmic Surg* 19:811-813, 1988.
7. Crouse CA et al.: Detection of Epstein-Barr virus genomes in normal human lacrimal glands, *J Clin Microbiol* 28:1026-1032, 1990.
8. Deacon LM et al.: Frequency of EBV DNA detection in Sjögren's syndrome, *Am J Med* 92:453-454, 1992.

9. De la Fuente Arjona L: The crocodile tear syndrome: apropos of a case, *An Otorhinolaringol Ibero Am* 13:185-193, 1986.

10. Docherty JJ, Chopan M: The latent herpes simplex virus, *Bacteriol Rev* 38:337-355, 1974.

11. Duke-Elder S, MacFaul PA: Inflammations of the lacrimal gland (dacryoadenitis). In Duke-Elder S, editor: *System of ophthalmology,* vol 13, *The ocular adnexa,* St. Louis, 1974, CV Mosby.

12. Enculescu A: A tuberculous etiology in Mikulicz's syndrome, *Ophtalmologia* 36:276, 1992.

13. Feldman RB et al.: Solitary eosinophilic granuloma of the lateral orbital wall, *Am J Ophthalmol* 100:318-323, 1985.

14. Filippone C, Muzzi M: Further data on a case of primary tuberculosis of the lacrimal gland, *Atti Accad Fisiocrit Siena* 16:537-542, 1967.

15. Filippone C, Muzzi M: On an infrequent localization of primary tuberculosis of the lacrimal gland, *Atti Accad Fisiocrit Siena* 16:531-536, 1967.

16. Flescher E, Talal N: Do viruses contribute to the development of Sjögren's syndrome?, *Am J Med* 90:283-285, 1991.

17. Fox RI, Pearson G, Vaughan JH: Detection of Epstein-Barr virus–associated antigens and DNA in salivary gland biopsies from patients with Sjögren's syndrome, *J Immunol* 137:3162-3168, 1986.

18. Fox RI et al.: Reactivation of Epstein-Barr virus in Sjögren's syndrome, *Springer Semin Immunopathol* 13:217-231, 1991.

19. Fox RI et al.: Potential role of Epstein-Barr virus in Sjögren's syndrome and rheumatoid arthritis, *J Rheumatol* 19:18-24, 1992.

20. Francois J, Rysselaere M: *Oculomycoses,* Springfield, 1972, Charles C. Thomas.

21. Galpine JF, Walkowski J: A case of mumps with involvement of the lacrimal glands, *Br Med J* 1069-1070, 1952.

22. Gaston JS, Rowe M, Bacon P: Sjögren's syndrome after infection by Epstein-Barr virus, *J Rheumatol* 17:558-561, 1990.

23. Harris GJ, Snyder RW: Lacrimal gland abscess, *Am J Ophthalmol* 104:193-194, 1987.

24. Hirschberg J: *The history of ophthalmology,* vol 1, Bonn, 1982, Wayenborgh.

25. Hodges EJ et al.: Keratoconjunctivitis sicca in leprosy, *Lepr Rev* 58:413-417, 1987.

26. Itescu S, Brancato LJ, Winchester R: A sicca syndrome in HIV infection: association with HLA-DR5 and CD8 lymphocytosis, *Lancet* i:466-468, 1989.

27. Jakobiec FA, Gess L, Zimmerman LE: Granulomatous dacryoadenitis caused by *Schistosoma haematobium, Arch Ophthalmol* 95:278-280, 1977.

28. Jones BR: The clinical features and etiology of dacryoadenitis, *Trans Ophthalmol Soc UK* 75:435-450, 1955.

29. Kaufman HE, Brown DC, Ellison ED: Herpes virus in the lacrimal gland, conjunctiva and cornea of man: a chronic infection, *Am J Ophthalmol* 65:32-35, 1968.

30. Kaufman HE, Brown DC, Ellison ED: Recurrent herpes in the rabbit and man, *Science* 156:1628-1629, 1967.

31. Kennerdell JS, Dresner SC: The nonspecific orbital inflammatory syndromes, *Surv Ophthalmol* 29:93-103, 1984.

32. Krishna N, Lyda W: Acute suppurative dacryoadenitis as a sequel to mumps, *Arch Ophthalmol* 59:350-351, 1958.

33. Krishnasamy M, Chandran S: Acute suppurative dacryoadenitis, *Med J Malaysia* 42(2):137-138, 1987.

34. Leavitt JA, Butrus SI: Wegener's granulomatosis presenting as dacryoadenitis, *Cornea* 10:542-545, 1991.

35. Levine J et al.: Detection of the complement (CD21)/Epstein-Barr virus receptor in human lacrimal gland and ocular surface epithelia, *Reg Immunol* 3:164-170, 1990-91.

36. Levine MR, Buckman G: Primary localized orbital amyloidosis, *Ann Ophthalmol* 18:165-167, 1986.

37. Madhukar K et al.: Tuberculosis of the lacrimal gland, *J Trop Med Hyg* 94:150-151, 1991.

38. McCoy FJ, Goodman RC: The crocodile tear syndrome, *Plast Reconstr Surg* 63:58-62, 1979.

39. Mortada A: Trachomatous acute palpebral dacryoadenitis, *Rev Int Trach* 44(1):15-19, 1967.

40. Mortada A: Tuberculoma of the orbit and lacrimal gland, *Br J Ophthalmol* 55:565-567, 1971.

41. Nesher N, Kleinman Y, Zauberman H: Temporary keratitis sicca secondary to bilateral acute dacryoadenitis, *Harefuah* 110:554-556, 1986.

42. Nowinski T, Flanagan J, Ruchman M: Lacrimal gland enlargement in familial sarcoidosis, *Ophthalmology* 90:909-913, 1983.

43. Nurmamedov NN, Rsaulkuliev Ula: Hypofunction of the lacrimal apparatus of trachomatous origin, *Vestn Oftalmol* 3:76-77, 1975.

44. Offret G, Renard G, Pasticier Dhermy MP: A case of bilateral tuberculosis dacryoadenitis, *Bull Soc Ophtalmol Fr* 74:557-567, 1974.

45. Panda A, Singhal V: Tuberculosis of lacrimal gland, *Indian J Pediatr* 56:531-533, 1989.

46. Paufique L et al.: Zosterian dacryo-adenitis, *Bull Soc Ophtalmol Fr* 65:1116-1118, 1965.

47. Pavan-Langston D, Nesburn AB: The chronology of primary herpes simplex infection of the eye and adnexal glands, *Arch Ophthalmol* 80:258-264, 1968.

48. Pepose JS et al.: Mononuclear cell phenotypes and immunoglobulin gene rearrangements in lacrimal gland biopsies from patients with Sjögren's syndrome, *Ophthalmology* 97:1599-1605, 1990.

49. Pflugfelder SC, Roussell TJ, Culbertson WW: Primary Sjögren's syndrome after infectious mononucleosis, *JAMA* 257:1049-1050, 1987.

50. Pflugfelder SC et al.: Amplification of Epstein-Barr virus genomic sequences in blood cells, lacrimal glands, and tears from primary Sjögren's syndrome patients, *Ophthalmology* 97:976-984, 1990.

51. Pflugfelder SC et al.: Epstein-Barr virus infection and immunologic dysfunction in patients with aqueous tear deficiency, *Ophthalmology* 97:313-323, 1990.

52. Ravault MP et al.: Dacryoadenite zonateuse associée à des lesions cornéennes, *Bull Soc Ophtalmol Fr* 5:511-514, 1967.

53. Richardson JM: Acute metastatic gonorrheal dacryoadenitis, *Arch Ophthalmology* 28:93-133, 1942.

54. Riffenburgh RS: Ocular manifestations of mumps, *Arch Ophthalmol* 66:155-159, 1961.

55. Roy FH: *Ocular differential diagnosis,* Philadelphia, 1993, Lea & Febiger.

56. Saito I et al.: Detection of Epstein-Barr virus DNA by polymerase chain reaction in blood and tissue biopsies from patients with Sjögren's syndrome, *J Exp Med* 169:2191-2198, 1989.

57. Schiødt M et al.: Parotid gland enlargement and xerostomia associated with labial sialoadenitis in HIV-infected patients, *J Autoimmun* 2:415-425, 1989.

58. Segal N et al.: Orbital pseudotumor: chronic tuberculous myositis and dacryoadenitis, *Rev Chir Oncol Radiol ORL Oftalmol Stomatol Ser Oftalmol* 24:69-72, 1980.

59. Sen DK: Tuberculosis of the orbit and lacrimal gland: a clinical study of 14 cases, *J Pediatr Ophthalmol Strabismus* 17:232-238, 1980.

60. Sen DK: Acute suppurative dacryoadenitis caused by a cysticercus cellulosa, *J Pediatr Ophthalmol Strabismus* 19:100-102, 1982.

61. Shields CL et al.: Clinicopathologic review of 142 cases of lacrimal gland lesions, *Ophthalmology* 96:431-435, 1989.

62. Sinha HK, Prakash AP: Syndrome of crocodile tears caused by lepra bacilli, *Lepr India* 50:392-395, 1978.

63. Stephens LC et al.: Acute radiation injury of ocular adnexa, *Arch Ophthalmol* 106:389-391, 1988.

64. Tanner OR: Ocular manifestations of infectious mononucleosis, *Arch Ophthalmol* 51:229-241, 1954.

65. Torok M, Schnitzler A, Krasznai G: Tuberculous dacryoadenitis, *Klin Monatsbl Augenheilkd* 159:223-227, 1971.

66. Ullman S, Sergott R: Abduction deficit secondary to presumed bacterial dacryoadenitis, *Arch Ophthalmol* 104:1127-1128, 1986.

67. Venables PJW et al.: A seroepidemiological study of cytomegalovirus and Epstein-Barr virus in rheumatoid arthritis and sicca syndrome, *Ann Rheum Dis* 44:742-746, 1985.

68. Weinreb RN: Diagnosing sarcoidosis by transconjunctival biopsy of the lacrimal gland, *Am J Ophthalmol* 97:573-576, 1984.

69. Whittingham S, McNeilage J, Mackay IR: Primary Sjögren's syndrome after infectious mononucleosis, *Ann Intern Med* 102:490-493, 1985.

70. Whittingham S, McNeilage LJ, Mackay IR: Epstein-Barr virus as an etiological agent in primary Sjögren's syndrome, *Med Hypotheses* 22:373-386, 1987.

71. Zarrabi: Acute dacryoadenitis with dendritic keratitis, *Bull Soc Fr Ophtalmol* 18:57-58, 1958.

96 Infections of the Lacrimal Drainage System

NICHOLAS T. ILIFF

Infections of the lacrimal excretory system include canaliculitis and acute and chronic dacryocystitis in adults, children, and newborns.

HISTORICAL BACKGROUND

Infection in the area of the lacrimal sac was mentioned in the Code of Hammurabi in the second millennium BC. Inflammation was described as occurring at the nasal canthus with subsequent rupture of the sac and fistulization.[80] The gross manifestation of lacrimal abscess and fistula on the face led to reports from the earliest times suggesting a "rotting of the nasoorbital bones or drainage from the brain."

In the second century AD Galen proposed the caruncle as the cause for blocking tear secretion followed by lacrimal fistulization, and the focus on the caruncle as the cause of the problem continued through the Middle Ages. During the Renaissance Vesalias and Fallopias presented a reasonably accurate description of the lacrimal system.[29]

Early in the 18th century Maître Jean first suggested that tears and secretions (which he felt were secreted by the sac) caused abscess when stasis occurred.[80] It was not until Stahl wrote in 1702 on the pathologic manifestations and described acute, chronic, and ulcerative afflictions of the nasolacrimal canal that the concept of inflammation of the canal was advanced as the basis for the disease.[29] In the late 19th century Peters showed that neonatal dacryocystitis was a result of blockage of the lacrimal ostium.[80]

Development of Lacrimal Surgery

The first treatment of abscess in the lacrimal sac consisted of rubbing the eyes with a mixture of honey, antimonia, and wood powder, described in the Ebers Papyrus in approximately 1150 BC. Pliny the Elder in the first century AD described a treatment with the herb *Aegylopia fatua,* or wild oat. At about the same time Celsus recommended opening the fistula to the bone and cauterizing the bone with a hot iron. Galen in the second century AD also described the use of grapevine ashes, aegylopia juice, vinegar, honey, and carob for the treatment for sac infection.

Probing of the lacrimal fossa and perforation of the lacrimal bone was described by Al-Ghafiqi of Cordoba in the 12th century AD. But it was not until 1710 that irrigation through the puncta, comparable to what is currently done, was introduced by Anel. Pallucci in 1762 used linen thread to provide a stent to maintain patency; in the 19th century ophthalmologists used copper and platinum wires for the same purpose. Dacryocystorhinostomy was described by Toti in 1904 and modified in 1921 by Dupuy-Dutemps and Bouguet. Improved versions of this technique are the basis of modern lacrimal surgery.[80]

ANATOMY

The punctum is a funnel-shaped structure surrounded by a ring of connective tissue that is approximately 0.2 to 0.3 mm in diameter. The upper and lower puncta open on a slight elevation of the posterior margin of the lid corresponding to the junction of the cilia and lacrimal portions of the lids. Inferior to the punctum is the vertical component of the canaliculus which is 2 mm in length and 1 ½ to 2 mm in diameter. The canaliculi lie within the eyelid margin and proceed medially for 8 mm and then join, in most cases, the common canaliculus, 3 to 5 mm in length, which empties into the lacrimal sac at the junction of its upper third and lower two thirds. The common internal punctum may have folds of tissues surrounding it acting as a valve, which may prevent decompression at the lacrimal sac in cases of mucocele or pyocele.

The lacrimal sac rests on the periosteum lining the bony lacrimal fossa and is covered by a firm fascial extension of the periosteum. The frontal process of the maxilla anteriorly and the lacrimal bone posteriorly form the lacrimal fossa. The position of the lacrimal fossa is comparable to the middle meatus of the nose with the upper portion contiguous with the anterior ethmoid air cells. In some cases the ethmoid air cells may extend sufficiently anteriorly and inferiorly to be between the lacrimal fossa and nasal cavity. The fundus of the sac extends superiorly posterior to the medial canthal tendon. It is the relationship with the medial canthal tendon that causes abscesses or fistulas to appear in nearly all cases below the inferior border of the tendon. Swelling above the tendon suggests tumor rather than inflammatory disease.

The nasolacrimal duct is formed by a continuation of the sac inferiorly to where it enters the nose at the inferior meatus. The nasolacrimal canal, through which the nasolacrimal duct passes, is 12 mm in length. The approximate distance from the external naris to the opening of the duct in an adult is 30 to 35 mm. A mucous membrane ridge, the valve of Hasner, is present at the opening of the duct and functions to prevent reflux of air or nasal discharge into the nasolacrimal system. There are folds of mucous membrane that act as valves within the sac, but these probably have little effect on tear flow.

Lacrimal Outflow Obstruction

Infectious processes involving the lacrimal excretory system are influenced by the juxtaposition of the lacrimal sac to the orbit, sinuses, and nose, with resulting multiple possibilities for obstruction of flow and stasis. Infection within the sac is, in most cases, dependent on obstruction of flow. In rare instances infections can be related to a foreign body or to tumor growth within the lacrimal sac. The canaliculus can also develop infection; this condition is less related to obstruction, however. The juxtaposition of the sac to the ethmoid and maxillary sinuses and the orbit leave it prone to external compression or associated inflammation with pathologic processes involving these structures. The necessity for the nasolacrimal duct to drain into the nose leaves it vulnerable to nasal pathology, which could obstruct the opening at the valve of Hasner. Conjunctival and lid disease can adversely impact the function of the punctum and canaliculus with the possibility for secondary infection.

CANALICULITIS

Epidemiology

Approximately 2% of patients with lacrimal disease have canaliculitis.[27] The average age is 54 years (range 14 to 96 years).[82] While one report suggests the inferior canaliculus is more frequently affected than the superior,[27] the study was of a small number of patients and there is no good evidence of preferential site. Elliot[30] reported nine cases, two upper, two both, and five lower in women ranging in age from 10 to 58 years.

Clinical Features

Epiphora is usually the presenting symptom of canaliculitis. Unilateral mucopurulent conjunctivitis, which may be chronic or recurring and which may center around the me-

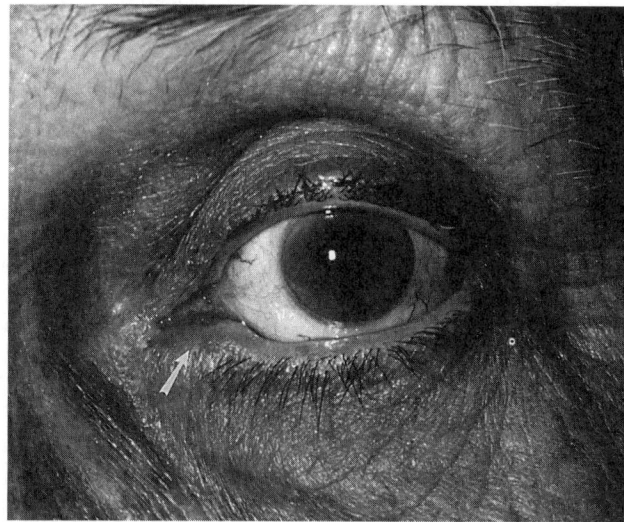

Fig. 96-1.   Left lower canalicutitis. Canalicular area is swollen, tender, and erythematous *(arrow).*

dial canthus, is a frequent finding. These processes may go on for months to years. As the area of the canaliculus swells and becomes erythematous (Fig. 96-1), the inflammation can be mistaken for a chalazion.[14] The punctum may be swollen shut or pouting.

In advanced canaliculitis, canalicular diverticuli can form. The diverticuli can become quite large, as large as the lacrimal sac itself, and spontaneous fistula formation has been reported.[29] Concretions can be expressed by pressing on each side of the canaliculus toward the punctum (Fig. 96-2). The type of concretion depends on the infectious agent.

Throughout the course of the disease it may be possible to irrigate or probe the system. Firm concretions cause a gritty

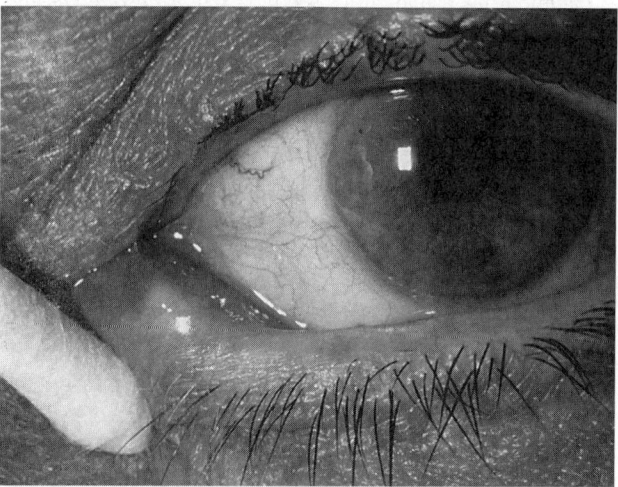

Fig. 96-2.   Canaliculitis. Pressure on canalicular area causes expression of purulent material from this markedly distended canaliculus.

feeling as the probe is passed. The punctum may be blocked with the material filling the canaliculus. Dacryocystograms show an irregularity to the canalicular epithelium and may demonstrate diverticula or filling defects caused by the concretions.[98a]

Pathogenesis

The cause of canaliculitis is not known, nor is it known whether the diverticula that are observed with the disease are part of the cause or a result of the chronic infection. There may be congenital diverticula that provide nidus areas for the beginning of infection and present an anaerobic environment. *Actinomyces* sp. tends to cause suppurative tracts, and diverticula may be a result, rather than a cause, of canaliculitis.[82]

Nonsuppurative canalicular inflammation can occur secondary to periocular infections caused by herpes simplex virus, varicella-zoster virus, or *Chlamydia trachomatis*. Trachomatous canaliculitis results from the spread from the conjunctiva to the canaliculus. Granulomatous reaction occurs in the pericanalicular tissue and mucous membrane with resultant purulent discharge. Ultimately, however, cicatricial contraction leads to sunstantial stricture of the canaliculus. Secondary infection then occurs.[29]

Conjunctival inflammation may sometimes spread into the canaliculus and cause a follicular canaliculitis.[29] While not part of the spectrum of primary suppurative canaliculitis, inflammation and stenosis can obstruct the canaliculus secondary to pericanalicular infection. This condition differs from suppurative canaliculitis, characterized by primary canalicular infection with purulent discharge originating in the canaliculus and evident at the punctum.

Secondary canaliculitis can also occur as a result of spread of infection from either acute or chronic dacryocystitis.[29] Retained foreign bodies have been reported as a cause of canaliculitis. Canaliculitis secondary to *Enterobacter* and *Klebsiella* species can occur from a retained Veirs rod,[9] and *Mycobacterium chelonei* canaliculitis has complicated silicone intubation.[96]

Laboratory Investigations

Actinomyces israelii is a commonly identified cause of canaliculitis. Originally termed *Streptothrix*, this anaerobic gram-positive bacterium was described by Israel in 1878.[23] It is part of the normal flora in the human mouth.

Actinomycetes are bacteria but may be confused with fungi because they tend to be filamentous. They orient in radially arranged branching clumps. Although the microscopic appearance may be that of fungi, actinomycetes lack nuclear membranes, have bacterial cell walls, and undergo genetic recombination typical of bacteria and not fungi.[25]

A. israelii causes suppurative sinus tracts and scarring. An exudate is produced containing granules that have been termed "sulphur granules" (Fig. 96-3). These yellowish,

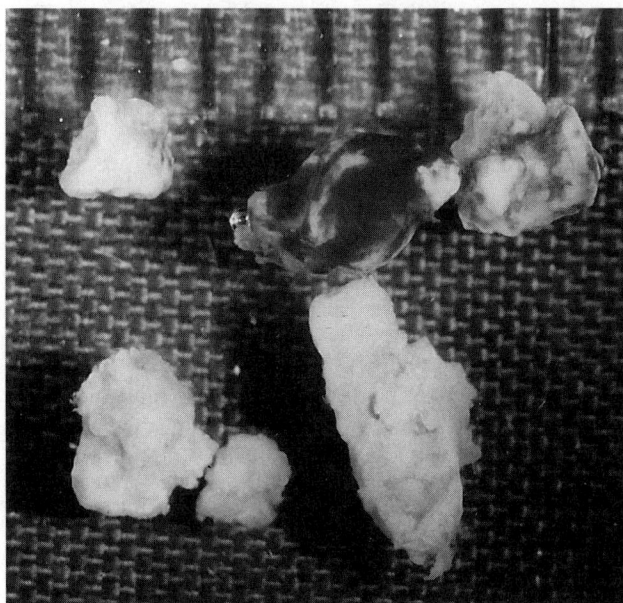

Fig. 96-3. "Sulphur granules" seen with *Actinomyces israelii* and *Propionibacterium propionicum (Arachnia propionica)* canaliculitis.

cheese-like granules have a gritty consistency. When examined with the Gram stain, masses of gram-positive branching filamentous organisms are seen.

A second anaerobic organism implicated as a cause of canalicular infection is *Propionibacterium propionicum*.[17,111a] Originally believed to be a new species in the genus *Actinomyces*, it was reclassified to *Arachnia propionica*[100] and then shown to be related to the propionibacteria. It differs from *A. israelii* in that it produces propionic acid in broth and does not ferment arabinose, cellobiose, salicin, or xylose. It has different surface antigens and contains diaminopimelic acid in its cell wall.[15] The Gram stain appearances of *A. israelii* and *P. propionicum* are similar, and cases of canaliculitis due to the latter organism may have been ascribed to *A. israelii*.[100]

Pine and associates[89] in 1961 examined the normal flora of the human lacrimal system and did not find anaerobic actinomycetes; they did find the anaerobe *Proprionibacterium acnes*, however, suggesting that the lacrimal system contains an anaerobic environment but that the actinomycetes are not normally present. Another anaerobic bacillus, *Fusobacterium nucleatum*, is a gram-negative organism that has been reported to cause suppurative canaliculitis.[112] Although it is present in normal oral flora, it is found in the canaliculi only when there is active canaliculitis.[89] The suggestion is that the most common cause of canaliculitis is infection with normal anaerobic oral flora.

Of the multitude of bacteria and fungi that have been found to cause canaliculitis, some are associated with characteristic clinical findings that may suggest the nature of the organism. The diverticula and concretions commonly seen with *A. israelii* infections can also occur as a result of fusobacterial infections.[112] Rubbery concretions occur in the presence of candidal infections, whereas *Aspergillus niger* causes brown or black debris to accumulate.[82] *Enterobacter cloacae,* a common intestinal organism also found in soil and water, produces a tenacious mucoid material within the canaliculus.[19]

Other reported causes of suppurative canaliculitis include *Eikenella corrodens, Candida* sp., *Aspergillus* sp., *Fusorium* sp., *Streptomyces somaliensis,*[99] *Rhinosporidium seeberi,*[2] *Nocardia asteroides,*[87] *Sporotrichum* sp.,[2] *Cephalosporium* sp.,[2] and *Pityrosporum pachydermatis.*[95]

Gram stains of the exudate and concretions should be done, and Giemsa stain may be helpful in identifying fungi. Anaerobic and fungal cultures similarly may be helpful in some cases, but aerobic cultures are of no value for isolating the most common causes of canaliculitis.

Therapy

Whereas laboratory identification of the causative organism may be helpful in guiding medical therapy, the cornerstone of treatment is surgery. Topical and systemic therapy with antibiotics is ineffective unless there is surgical removal of concretions and debris.[111a]

A probe is inserted in the canaliculus and incision made through the adjacent conjunctiva into the dilated canaliculus. A small curette can be used to remove the debris. The incision need not be closed. Irrigation with an antibacterial preparation at the time of surgery and treatment with oral antibiotics for seven to ten days may be helpful. *A. israelii* is resistant to aminoglycosides (such as neomycin, gentamicin, and tobramycin), but is sensitive to penicillin, erythromycin, tetracycline, and bacitracin.[82] Resolution is usually prompt and recurrences are rare.

Simple curettage through the punctum, without canaliculotomy, has been reported to be curative.[86] However, silicone intubation and repeat curettage are sometimes needed. Silicone intubation is sometimes added to canaliculotomy during the primary procedure.

DACRYOCYSTITIS

Epidemiology

Dacryocystitis is rare in childhood and adolescence.[29] When it occurs in the pediatric age group (excluding neonatal dacryocystitis), suspicion should be heightened to the presence of an underlying disorder, particularly if the process is bilateral. Exanthematous diseases that contribute to chronic inflammation of the lacrimal sac in childhood and adolescence can lead to chronic dacryocystitis. Of a series of acquired (noncongenital) dacryocystitis in patients up to age 15, one half had had chicken pox and one third had had small pox.[22] Rarer disorders such as sinus histiocytosis[61] and mu-

cocutaneous lymph node syndrome (Kawasaki disease)[72] have been reported as predisposing factors in the development of dacryocystitis in children.

Dacryocystitis is predominantly a disease of middle-aged adults. Females are affected four times more often than males.[111] The narrower lumen of the bony nasolacrimal canal in females may be a contributing factor.[29] Females have a narrower nose than males,[29] and hormonal influences have been thought to play a part.[109] The disease is rarer in the black population than in the white population, possibly due to differences in the nasolacrimal canal which is shorter, wider, less sinuous, and has a larger ostium in black people. Reports from the early 20th century suggest white people are more likely affected in tropical than temperate countries.[29] While dacryocystitis is usually sporadic, familial and autosomal-dominant inheritance patterns have been reported.[111]

Pathogenesis

Dacryocystitis can be secondary to pericystic inflammation and infections, gross infections in the nose and sinuses, or conjunctival diseases. In a majority of cases, primary dacryocystitis is secondary to nasolacrimal duct obstruction. The cause of the obstruction may be endogenous, exogenous, or of an unknown cause. Inflammation with secondary constriction of the nasolacrimal duct is a frequent cause for obstruction, but the cause for the inflammation is not clear.

Clinicopathologic studies of the lacrimal sac demonstrated the effects of chronic inflammation in the lacrimal sac.[71] Of patients who had a dacryocystorhinostomy (DCR), 40% had had one or more episodes of dacryocystitis. Chronic inflammatory changes were noted in patients who had been tearing only and in those who had had previous attacks of dacryocystitis. A chronic, low-grade inflammation leads to fibrosis of the lacrimal sac and the common internal punctum. The pseudostratified, ciliated, columnar epithelium of the lacrimal sac undergoes changes of squamous metaplasia, hyperplasia with loss of goblet cells, and ulceration. Most patients have evidence of chronic subepithelial inflammatory cell infiltrates, consisting predominately of lymphocytes and plasma cells. Subepithelial fibrosis is present in most cases. A similar process can occur in the nasolacrimal duct. Chronic inflammation causes secondary fibrosis that, in turn, causes gradual narrowing of the nasolacrimal duct until complete obstruction occurs.[66]

When the lacrimal passages are functioning normally, protection is provided by the flow of tears and the resistance of the mucosa itself to infection. Even severe bacterial infections of the conjunctiva rarely extend down into the sac. Thus stasis within the sac is a prerequisite for the development of infection. Any swelling will lead to blockage because of the confines of the narrow, bony canal. A partially stenosed canal is more sensitive to the effects of inflammation. The numerous folds and valves in the mucous membrane of the sac combine with a submucosa that is vascular, leading, with little insult, to enough swelling to cause a fluid backup.

Risk Factors

Congenital Variations. Congenital variations in the shape and size of the osseous canal impact on the chance of developing dacryocystitis and may explain some familial transmission of the disease. Heinonin in 1920 and Seidenari in 1947 described cases of dacryocystitis associated with narrowing of the osseous canal occurring in patients with a flat nose and narrow face. Whitnall related a narrow osseous canal to an underdeveloped lacrimal bone.[29]

Associated Nasal or Sinus Disease. Nasal disease can be an important cause of lacrimal outflow obstruction. Mechanical obstruction can result from enlargement or flattening of the inferior turbinate, which can nearly obliterate the anterior part of the inferior meatus and may cause a chronic local rhinitis. Septal deviation can compress the inferior turbinate against the lateral nasal wall. Congestive, inflammatory, and hypertrophic conditions of the nasal mucosa can cause obstruction. Atrophic conditions of the nose are also associated with dacryocystitis. Atrophic rhinitis was found in over one third of cases of dacryocystitis.[29] While there is some argument as to the part sinus disease plays in the cause of dacryocystitis, there are many reports that suggest a relationship. Kuhnt, in 1914, reported that 68% of cases of dacryocystitis had sinus disease and an additional 23% had probable sinus disease.[29] Although it is suggested that infections spread by venous or lymphatic pathways to the lacrimal area and in some cases by direct continuity, lacrimal outflow obstruction from nasal mucosal disease related to sinus inflammation is a more likely mechanism.[29]

Nasolacrimal duct obstruction has been associated with nasal allergy.[102] Viral or bacterial pharyngitis and rhinitis can produce sufficient nasal mucosal edema, lymphoid hyperplasia, and exudate to cause obstruction of the nasolacrimal duct and dacryocystitis.[43]

Extrinsic Neoplasia. External compression of the nasolacrimal duct or of the lacrimal sac can cause secondary dacryocystitis. Benign or malignant neoplasia of the adjacent paranasal sinuses or of the nasal cavity can impinge on the outflow channel. Dacryocystitis may be the presenting sign of a paranasal sinus neoplasm.[16] Secondary involvement of the lacrimal drainage system by lesions affecting adjacent structures is more common than primary neoplasia of the system.[8] Invasion or compression has been related to adenoid cystic carcinoma,[76] sebaceous gland carcinoma,[64] and osteoma.[40,107] Nasolacrimal obstruction has occurred secondary to adenoid cystic carcinoma, basal cell carcinoma, esthesioneuroblastoma, intraosseus cavernous hemangioma, leukemia, lymphoma, mucoepidermoid carcinoma, squamous cell carcinoma, and orbital lesions such as rhabdomyosarcoma.[8] Tumors that arise within the maxillary antrum can occlude the nasolacrimal duct, and squamous cell carcinoma is the most common.[24,47,59,78] Sinus histiocytosis can cause lacrimal obstruction by intrinsic involvement of the lacrimal drainage system[28] or by involvement of nasal mucosa adjacent to the nasolacrimal duct ostium.[37,38,61]

Tumors of the Lacrimal Sac. Primary neoplasms of the lacrimal sac are less common as a cause of dacryocystitis than are those involving the system secondarily. A bloodstained discharge from the puncta is strongly suggestive of neoplastic involvement of the sac.[33] The most common lesions are those of an epithelial origin, including papillomas and squamous cell carcinomas.*

Of tumors of the lacrimal sac, 25% are pseudotumors or inflammatory granulomata.[94] Pyogenic granulomata of the sac are reported associated with chronic dacryocystitis and in one study represented 53% of lacrimal sac tumors.[3]

Polyps of the lacrimal sac present a chronic inflammation and suppuration, and pus occasionally emits from the puncta.[33] Human papillomavirus infection of the lacrimal sac has been linked to benign and malignant primary epithelial tumors in the sac.[67] Other tumors intrinsic to the sac include hemangiopericytoma[97] and, rarely, adenoid cystic carcinoma.[65]

Trauma. Iatrogenic trauma to the nasolacrimal duct with secondary dacryocystitis can occur following nasal, sinus, or orbital surgery.[22,36,39,101] Craniofacial procedures can also result in lacrimal obstruction.[8]

Noniatrogenic trauma is a frequent cause of lacrimal drainage obstruction.[45,103,117] Orbital floor fracture repair can result in secondary lacrimal obstruction as a result of impingement of the implanted alloplastic plate on the lacrimal system. The obstruction of the lacrimal system can occur many years after the repair.[73] Midfacial traumas, particularly those associated with fractures of the nose, maxilla, and medial orbit, can easily cause partial or complete obstruction as a result of the shifting of bone fragments.[58,60]

Systemic Disease. Systemic infections have been associated with nasolacrimal duct obstruction and dacryocystitis. Influenza, scarlet fever, diphtheria, syphilis, and chickenpox have been reported to cause dacryocystitis or be dacryocystitis-associated.[29] can involve the lacrimal sac directly and cause acute dacryocystitis.[48] Dacryocystitis can be a complication of Wegener granulomatosis, and dacryocystorhinostomy in these patients can be complicated by necrosis and fistulization at the wound.† Acute dacryocystitis has been reported in association with nasopharyngeal hyperplasia secondary to infectious mononucleosis in a child.[4]

Dacryoliths. Calculi of the lacrimal sac were reported as early as 1922,[42] but the mechanism by which these masses form is still to be elucidated. Several substances have been identified in dacryoliths, including calcium, phosphates, ammonium, and cystine.[70] Calcium, phosphates, and ammo-

---

*References 2, 8, 33, 34, 49, 52, 54, 75, 98, 110.

†Dacryocystectomy is recommended for treatment of dacryocystitis in these patients.[53]

nium are found in the tears but not in large concentrations. In nonmycotic dacryoliths, inflammatory plaques on mucosal tissue provide a nidus for ion aggregation.[70] Dacryoliths may show coagulase-negative staphylococci, urate, phosphate, and fibrin.[63] Urate is derived from the cellular purine degradation, suggesting that dacryolith formation occurs as the result of slow aggregation of cellular debris for an extended period. Finding antikeratin antibodies in a dacryolith supports this theory.[26] Inflammation, with resultant fibrin aggregation, may be due to stagnant infection or irritation by the stone. Medications have been reported to play a part, and adrenochrome dacryoliths have been found.[105]

It has been suggested that fungi play a part in dacryolith formation,[10,32,116] but there are many reports of dacryoliths in which no fungi were found.[50,60,114] Special studies are seldom used to evaluate dacryoliths, and the exact relationship of fungi is unknown.

The reported prevalence of dacryolithiasis in all patients having DCRs is approximately 14%.[50] Patients with a dacryolith tend to be younger (average age 45) than most patients undergoing DCRs (average age 52) and tend to give a longer history (4.8 years) of intermittent epiphora and intermittent epiphora and pain.[50,60] Dacryoliths are more commonly found during dacryocystorhinostomy in patients who had prior dacryocystitis[50] and in younger patients.[60]

Clinical Features

Acute Dacryocystitis. Acute dacryocystitis presents with a painful inflammatory response in the medial canthal area. Pain may radiate into the frontal area or down into the teeth. Swelling may be initially diffuse, localizing at a point under the medial canthal ligament as the process progresses. Erythema of the overlying skin and that of the lower lid and cheek is common. The elevation in the area of the lacrimal sac may be obscured by a diffuse swelling (Fig. 96-4). Point tenderness just below the medial canthal ligament is a con-

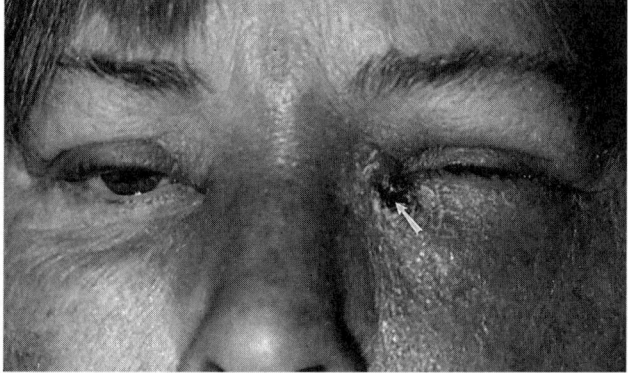

Fig. 96-4. Acute dacryocystitis can be associated with diffuse erythema and swelling, which ultimately led in this patient to perforation and drainage through skin leaving eschar *(arrow)*.

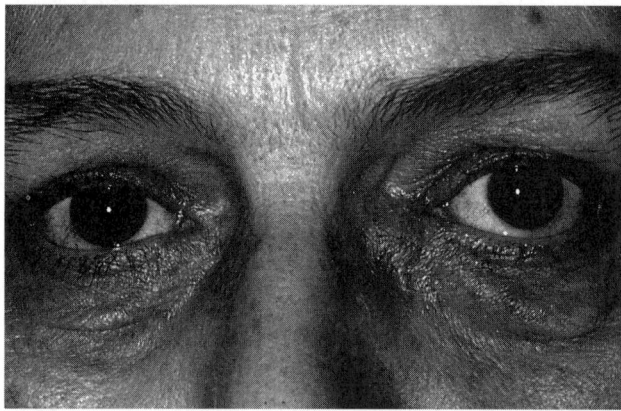

Fig. 96-5. Chronic dacryocystitis associated with swelling and erythema inferior to left medial canthal ligament.

stant finding. Frequently it is not possible to express purulent material from the puncta because swelling closes off the common canaliculus. There may be a progression to spontaneous rupture of the abscess within days. Following perforation through the skin, temporary quieting of the infection occurs, with recurrence of pressure, pain, and inflammation some time after the skin closes. Occasionally a fistula forms allowing chronic drainage.

Chronic Dacryocystitis. Chronic dacryocystitis is associated with epiphora and often conjunctivitis. There is swelling and erythema inferior to the medial canthal ligament (Fig. 96-5). Episodes wax and wane. It may be possible to express mucopurulent material from the puncta by exerting pressure on the lacrimal sac. Occasionally a chronic lacrimal mucocele can become infected and form a distended pyocele. Progression to the clinical picture of acute dacryocystitis can occur.

Laboratory Investigations

Gram-positive cocci are the most common cause of acute dacryocystitis. In 1941 staphylococci, pneumococci, and other streptococci were most prevalent. Other organisms include diphtheroids and coliform bacteria. Recent reports suggest *Staphylococcus aureus* and coagulase-negative staphylococci play a prominent role in dacryocystitis.[18,21,55] At least one half of patients undergoing DCR for chronic dacryocystitis have a positive intraoperative culture,[21] although antibiotic treatment before culture could have affected the spectrum and relative prevalence of pathogens. The finding of staphylococcal species as being most prevalent is supported by the reports of others.* This finding is in contrast to several reports of *Streptococcus pneumoniae* as the most common organism.[29,106,108,111] Recent reports suggest a prevalence of *Streptococcus pneumoniae* from 2% to

---

*References 18, 55, 57, 74, 77, 85.

15%.[6,13,21,55] Up to one third of cases grow two or more organisms.[13,21]

Approximately one fourth to one half of isolates from cases of dacryocystitis are gram-negative organisms,[18,21,55] most commonly *Pseudomonas aeruginosa*[21] and *Escherichia coli.*[55]

Anaerobic bacteria have rarely been reported as a cause of dacryocystitis. *Actinomyces israelii* is frequently associated with canaliculitis, but only a few cases have been reported as a cause of dacryocystitis. When dacryocystitis occurs as the result of *A. israelii,* the course is characterized by periods of quiescence interspersed with acute fistulizing exacerbations.[12] Implicated as predisposing factors for anaerobic growth are the following: (1) obstruction of the lacrimal system combined with further depletion of oxygen by growth of aerobic bacteria in the normally relatively anaerobic lacrimal passages, (2) the presence of foreign bodies, and (3) surgical manipulation. While reports of anaerobic involvement may be limited because careful anaerobic cultures often are not done, Codin and associates[21] found 7% to be culture-positive for anaerobic bacteria, and the majority (66.7%) were *Propionibacterium acnes.*

Fungi have on occasion been implicated as a cause of dacryocystitis. For the most part, single case reports are found in the literature, and the role of fungal organisms and lacrimal sac infections remains unknown. *Candida albicans* is the most commonly identified organism.[20,92,115] *Candida parapsilosis, Candida krusei, Candida parakrusei, Aspergillus* sp., sporotrichosis, trichophytosis, and *Pityrosporum orbiculare* have been reported to cause dacryocystitis.[47] Other fungi reported to cause dacryocystitis are blastomycosis,[108] chromoblastomycosis,[106] rhinosporidiosis,[29] cryptococcosis,[29] cephalosporiosis,[29] and actinomycosis organisms.[29]

Fungal infection has been associated with dacryoliths (Fig. 96-6),[115] but, as has been noted, it is not clear whether the dacryoliths result from the fungal infection or the fungi develop secondary to the dacryolith. Broad-spectrum antibiotics are frequently used empirically in treatment of dacryocystitis and this may have some impact on the prevalence of fungal organisms. The techniques used to determine the presence of fungi undoubtedly also impact on reported prevalence of these organisms. Cultures of dacryoliths sometimes yield aerobes (e.g., *P. aeruginosa* and *S. pneumoniae*), anaerobes (e.g., *Bacteroides* and *Fusarium* species), and fungi (e.g., *Cladosporium* and *Alternaria* species).[10] Special stains sometimes show fungal elements. Others[60,104] have found no infectious agents in the stones.

Organisms rarely reported as causative agents in dacryocystitis include *Chlamydia trachomatis,*[5] *Treponema pallidum,*[106] *Mycobacterium tuberculosis,*[106] and *Mycobacterium fortuitum.*[62] Papillomavirus infection of the lacrimal sac has been linked to primary epithelial tumors in the sac and dacryocystitis.[67]

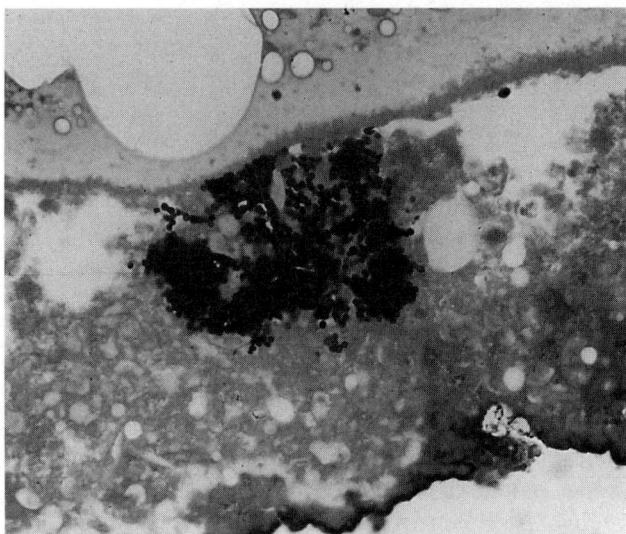

Fig. 96-6. Dacryolith with budding yeast forms of *Candida albicans.*

Complications

Although dacryocystitis rarely is associated with secondary complications, when complications occur they can be substantial. Endophthalmitis following suture removal for penetrating keratoplasty has been reported as being secondary to dacryocystitis.[113] Purgason and Hornblass reported one unfortunate patient who developed *Streptococcus viridans* endophthalmitis following cataract extraction.[92] This organism was isolated from the punctum on that side. A second patient had a corneal ulcer that cultured positive for *Candida albicans* and this organism was cultured from both lacrimal systems. Orbital cellulitis[1] and recurrent facial cellulitis with fistula formation after midfacial trauma[20] have been reported secondary to dacryocystitis.

Therapy

Purulent material that can be expressed from the puncta should be sent for Gram stain, culture, and sensitivity testing. Broad-spectrum antibiotics can be instituted until culture results are available. Most bacterial isolates are susceptible to bacitracin, fluoroquinolones, and aminoglycosides,[55] although methicillin-resistant and gentamicin-resistant staphylococci are occasionally encountered. Sulfonamides are poorly effective.

Moderate to severe cases of acute dacryocystitis may require decompression of the sac by incision and drainage. Acute dacryocystitis treated with even the appropriate antibiotics may progress to spontaneous perforation because penetration of antibiotic agent into the sac is poor. Incision and drainage is a temporizing measure. Its effectiveness may be increased by irrigation of the sac with antibiotic solution and by filling the cavity with antibiotic ointment.[18]

Dacryocystorhinostomy is the definitive treatment and

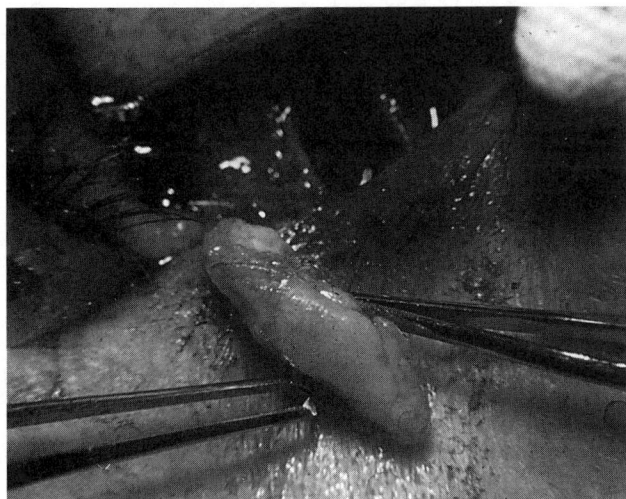

Fig. 96-7. Dacryolith that had formed cast of lacrimal sac is removed at time of dacryocystorhinostomy.

can be done during the acute stages of the disorder (Fig. 96-7). Surgery at the time of acute dacryocystitis can be made considerably more difficult by the attendant hyperemia and induration, which make bleeding a problem and exposure difficult.

NEONATAL DACRYOCYSTITIS

Acute dacryocystitis in the infant causes an acutely distended lacrimal sac, a different picture from the more common one seen with neonatal lacrimal obstruction, which is characterized by epiphora, crusting of the lashes, and regurgitation of mucoid or mucopurulent material when pressure is applied to the lacrimal sac. In neonatal dacryocystitis, there is a rapid evolution of a substantial inflammatory response and progression to perforation and drainage of purulent material through the skin.

Epidemiology

Nasolacrimal duct obstruction at the level of the Hasner valve at birth is relatively common with 6% to 10% of newborn infants having the obstruction.[46,83] Resolution of the obstruction occurs in nearly half by six months of age by massaging and conservative management[91]; 95% resolve by eight months of age with conservative management.[81] There was continued resolution up to 13 months, and by 18 months of age the passage was open in 85% of cases.[88]

Acute neonatal dacryocystitis occurs in about 3% of infants with congenital lacrimal obstruction.[90] It occurs rarely in the first week of life.[11] Most newborn babies and 80% of premature babies have normal tear secretion on the first day of life,[84] and it has been postulated that the sac contents (tears) could get infected during prolonged labor.[93] Bilateral acute dacryocystitis has been reported to occur in a newborn premature infant.[11]

Laboratory Investigations

Gram-positive cocci are responsible for the majority of cases of congenital dacryocystitis in infants as in adults. *Streptococcus pneumoniae* is the most prevalent organism,[7] however, as compared to *Staphylococcus aureus* in the adult. *S. aureus* or *S. epidermidis* are isolated in about one fourth of cases. Other organisms include *Micrococcus* sp., *Pseudomonas aeruginosa*, *Acinetobacter* sp., and diphtheroids. A negative culture is usually due to prior antibiotic therapy or lack of anaerobic culture facilities.

Susceptibility results show the greatest number of isolates are sensitive to erythromycin and cloxacillin sodium, and few are sensitive to gentamicin. The *S. aureus* exhibited 93.3% in vitro sensitivity to cloxacillin sodium with an excellent in vivo response. While *S. epidermidis* has been felt to be normal flora, a number of reports suggest its pathogenicity in certain situations, and it should not be ignored.[56,68,69] *S. epidermidis* was sensitive to cloxacillin sodium in all cases and also sensitive to erythromycin, gentamicin, and chloramphenicol in 80%. The emergence of penicillin-resistant pneumococci[68] suggests the need for broad-spectrum therapy.

The flora of the unilateral dacryocystitis does not correlate with that of the conjunctiva of the contralateral eye or the nasal flora. Conjunctival and nasal flora probably play no role in the causation of congenital dacryocystitis. Bacterial flora and antibiotic sensitivity can change during therapy.[7]

Fungi are isolated in up to one third of cases of congenital dacryocystitis, usually in association with various bacteria. *Candida albicans* is the most prevalent and is the most common fungus of the normal conjunctiva. Fungal flora is probably aided by use of broad-spectrum antibiotics in the presence of mucopurulent material. Fungi isolated probably represent colonization by saprophytic organisms and not necessarily actual fungal dacryocystitis.[41]

Therapy

The hallmark of treatment of congenital dacryocystitis is probing. When dacryocystitis occurs within the first three weeks of life, probing results in rapid resolution.[90] Few newborns will continue to have epiphora and require subsequent probing with silicone intubation. Systemic and topical antibiotics may be used before probing or probing can be done on the day of diagnosis without any prior antibiotic treatment.

A lacrimal sac abscess may occur in the newborn from delayed treatment of nasolacrimal duct obstruction.[31] Incision and drainage are recommended, especially if local and systemic antibiotics do not work.[35] Bacteremia after infant nasolacrimal duct probing has been reported but appears to be an uncommon event.[44,90]

REFERENCES

1. Allen MV, Cohen KL, Grimson DS: Orbital cellulitis secondary to dacryocystitis following blephroplasty, *Ann Ophthalmol* 17:498-499, 1985.
2. Ashton M, Choyce DP, Fison LG: Carcinoma of the lacrimal sac, *Br J Ophthalmol* 35:366-376, 1951.
3. Asiyo MN, Stefani FH: Pyogenic granulomas of the lacrimal sac, *Eye* 6:97-101, 1992.
4. Atkinson PL, Ansons AM, Patterson A: Infectious mononucleosis presenting as bilateral acute dacryocystitis, *Br J Ophthalmol* 74:750, 1990.
5. Bahnasawi SA, Abdalla MI, Gahly AF et al.: Trachomas of the lacrimal sac, *Woll Ophthalmol Soc Egypt* 69:619-627, 1976.
6. Bale RN: Dacryocystitis: bacteriological study and its relation with nasal pathology, *Indian J Ophthalmol* 35:178-182, 1987.
7. Bareja U, Ghose S: Clinicobacteriological correlates of congenital dacryocystitis, *Indian J Ophthalmol* 38:66-69, 1990.
8. Bartley GB: Acquired lacrimal drainage obstruction: an etiologic classification system, case reports, and a review of the literature. III. *Ophthalmol Plast Reconstr Surg* 9:11-26, 1993.
9. Becker BB: Retained Veirs rod and canaliculitis, *Am J Ophthalmol* 111:251-252, 1991.
10. Berlin AJ, Rath R, Rich L: Lacrimal system dacryoliths, *Ophthalmic Surg* 11:435-436, 1980.
11. Berson D, Landau L: Bilateral acute dacryocystitis in a premature infant, *J Pediatr Ophthalmol Strabismus* 15:168-169, 1978.
12. Blanksma LJ, Slijper J: Actinomycotic dacryocystitis, *Ophthalmologica* 176:145-149, 1977.
13. Blicker JA, Buffam FV: Lacrimal sac, conjunctival, and nasal culture results in dacryocystorhinostomy patients, *Ophthalmol Plast Reconstr Surg* 9:43-46, 1993.
13a. Brazier JS, Hall V: *Propionibacterium propionicum* and infections of the lacrimal apparatus, *Clin Infect Dis* 17:892-893, 1993.
14. Brinckerhoff AJ: Actinomyces of the inferior lacrimal canaliculus, *Am J Ophthalmol* 1942, 25:978-981.
15. Brock DW, Georg LK, Brown JM et al.: Actinomycosis caused by *Arachnia propionica, Am J Clin Pathol* 59:66-77, 1973.
16. Bruckmuhler W: Eosinophilic adenoma of the nose and ethmoid bone simulating a malignant tumor, *Laryngol Rhinol Otol* 65:346-347, 1986.
17. Buchanan BB, Pine L: Characterization of a propionic acid producing actinomycete, *Actinomyces propionicus, J Gen Microbiol* 28:305-323, 1962.
18. Cahill KV, Burns JA: Management of acute dacryocystitis in adults, *Ophthalmol Plast Reconstr Surgery* 9:38-42, 1993.
19. Chumbley LC: Canaliculitis caused by *Enterobacter cloacae*: report of a case, *Br J Ophthalmol* 68:364-366, 1984.
20. Codere F, Anderson RL: Bilateral *Candida albicans* dacryocystitis with facial cellulitis, *Can J Ophthalmol* 17:176-177, 1982.
21. Codin DJ, Hornblass A, Haas BD: Clinical bacteriology of dacryocystitis in adults, *Ophthalmol Plast Reconstr Surg* 9:125-131, 1993.
22. Colvard DM, Waller RR, Neault RW, DeSanto LW: Nasolacrimal duct obstruction following transantral-ethmoidal orbital decompression, *Ophthalmic Surg* 10:25-28, 1979.
23. Conant NF, Smith DT, Baker RD et al., editors: *Manual of clinical mycology,* ed 3, 1-37, Philadelphia, 1971, WB Saunders.
24. Conley JJ: Sinus tumors invading the orbit, *Trans Am Acad Ophthalmol Otolaryngol* 70:615-619, 1966.
25. Davis BD, Dulbecco R, Eisen HN et al., editors: *Microbiology,* New York, 1967, Harper & Row.
26. Daxecker F, Philipp W, Muller-Holzner E, Tessadri R: Analysis of a dacryolith, *Ophthalmologica* 195:125-127, 1987.
27. DeMant E, Hurwitz JJ: Canaliculitis: review of 12 cases, *Can J Ophthalmol,* 15:73-75, 1980.
28. Dolman PJ, Harris GJ, Weiland LH: Sinus histiocytosis involving the lacrimal sac and duct: a clinical pathological case, *Arch Ophthalmol* 209:1582-1584, 1991.
29. Duke-Elder S, MacFaul PA: The ocular adnexa: lacrimal, orbital and para-orbital diseases. In Duke-Elder S, editor: *System of ophthalmology,* vol B, part 2, 699-724, St Louis, 1974, Mosby.
30. Elliot AJ: Streptothricosis of the lacrimal canaliculi: report of nine cases, *Am J Ophthalmol* 24:682-686, 1941.
31. Ffooks OO: Dacryocystitis in infancy, *Br J Ophthalmol* 46:422-434, 1962.
32. Fine M, Waring WS: Mycotic obstruction of the nasolacrimal duct *(Candida albicans), Arch Ophthalmol* 38:39-42, 1947.
33. Flanagan JC, Stokes DP: Lacrimal sac tumors, *Ophthalmology* 85:1282-1287, 1978.
34. Flanagan JC, Zolli CL: Lacrimal sac tumors: surgical management. In Lindberg JB, editor: *Lacrimal surgery,* 203-226, New York, 1988, Churchill Livingstone.
35. Flanagan JC, McLachlan DL, Shannon GM: Diseases of the lacrimal apparatus. In Nelson LB, Calhoun JH, Harley RD, editors: *Pediatric ophthalmology,* ed 3, 396-411, Philadelphia, 1991, WB Saunders.
36. Flowers RS, Anderson R: Injury to the lacrimal apparatus during rhinoplasty, *Plast Reconstr Surg* 42:577-581, 1968.
37. Foucar E, Rosai J, Dorfman RF: Sinus histiocytosis with massive lymph adenopathy: ear, nose, and throat manifestations, *Arch Otolaryngol Head Neck Surg* 104:687-693, 1978.
38. Foucar E, Rosai J, Dorfman RF: The ophthalmologic manifestations of sinus histiocytosis with massive lymph adenopathy, *Am J Ophthalmol* 87:354-367, 1979.
39. Freedman HM, Kern EB: Complications of intranasal ethmoidectomy: a review of 1000 consecutive operations, *Laryngoscope* 89:421-432, 1979.
40. Garfin SW: Etiology of dacryocystitis and epiphora, *Arch Ophthalmol* 27:167-188, 1942.
41. Ghose S, Mahajan VM: Fungal flora in congenital dacryocystitis, *Indian J Ophthalmol* 30:189-190, 1990.
42. Gifford SR: Ocular sporotrichosis, *Arch Ophthalmol* 51:54-57, 1922.
43. Goldberg SH, Fedok FG, Botek AA: Acute dacryocystitis secondary exudative rhinitis, *Ophthal Plast Reconstr Surg* 9:51-52, 1993.
44. Gordon RA, Schaeffer A, Sood S: Bacteremia following nasolacrimal duct probing, *Ophthalmology* 97(suppl):149, 1990.
45. Gruss JS, Hurwitz JJ, Nik NA, Kassel EE: The pattern and incidence of nasolacrimal injury and naso-orbital-ethmoid fractures: the role of delayed assessment and dacryocystorhinostomy, *Br J Plast Surg* 38:116-121, 1985.
46. Guerry D, Kendig EL: Congenital impatency of the nasolacrimal duct, *Arch Ophthalmol* 39:193-204, 1948.
47. Hanssens M, Rysselaere M, Domen F: Candida parapsilosis associated with dacryoliths in obstructive dacryocystitis, *Bull Soc Belge Ophtalmol* 201:71-81, 1982.
48. Harris GJ, Williams GA, Clark GP: Sarcoidosis of the lacrimal sac, *Arch Ophthalmol* 99:1198-1201, 1981.
49. Harry J, Ashton N: The pathology of tumours of the lacrimal sac, *Trans Ophthalmol Soc UK* 88:19-34, 1968.
50. Hawes MJ: The dacryolithiasis syndrome, *Ophthalmol Plast Reconstr Surg* 4:87-90, 1988.
51. Helveston EM, Ellis FD: *Pediatric ophthalmology practice,* ed 2, 100, St Louis, 1984, Mosby.
52. Hird RB: Papilloma of the lacrymal sac, *Br J Ophthalmol* 16:416-417, 1932.
53. Holds JB, Anderson RL, Wolin MJ: Dacryochstectomy for the treatment of dacryocystitis patients with Wegener's granulomatosis, *Ophthalmic Surg* 20:443-444, 1989.
54. Hornblass A, Jakobiec FA, Bosniak S, Flanagan J: The diagnosis and management of epithelial tumors of the lacrimal sac, *Ophthalmology* 87:476-489, 1980.
55. Huber-Spitzy V, Steinkogler FJ, Huber E et al.: Acquired dacryocystitis: microbiology and conservative therapy, *Acta Ophthalmologica* 70:745-749, 1992.
56. Hurley R: Epidemic conjunctivitis in the newborn associated with coagulase negative staphylococci, *J Obstet Gynaecol Br Commonw* 73:990-992, 1966.
57. Hurwitz JJ, Rogers KJ: Management of acquired dacryocystitis, *Can J Ophthalmol* 38:233-236, 1983.
58. Iliff NT: The management of lacrimal trauma occurring with midfacial fractures, *Probl Plast Reconstr Surg* 1:420, 1991.
59. Johnson LN, Krohel GB, Yeon EB, Parnes SM: Sinus tumors invading the orbit, *Ophthalmology* 91:209-217, 1984.
60. Jones LT: Tear sac foreign bodies, *Am J Ophthalmol* 60:111-113, 1965.
61. Karcioglu ZA, Allam B, Ansler MS: Ocular involvement in sinus histiocytosis with massive lymphadenopathy, *Br J Ophthalmol* 72:793-795, 1988.

62. Katowitz JA, Kropp TM: *Mycobacterium fortuitum* as a cause for nasolacrimal obstruction and granulomatous eyelid disease, *Ophthalmic Surg* 18:97-99, 1987.

63. Kaye-Wilson LG: Spontaneous passage of a dacryolith, *Br J Ophthalmol* 75:564, 1991.

64. Khan JA, Grove AS Jr, Joseph MP, Goodman M: Sebaceous carcinoma: diuretic use, lacrimal system spread, and surgical margins, *Ophthalmol Plast Reconst Surg* 5:227-234, 1989.

65. Kincaid MC, Meis JM, Lee MW: Adenoid cystic carcinoma of the lacrimal sac, *Ophthalmology* 96:1655-1658, 1989.

66. Linberg JV, McCormick SA: Primary acquired nasolacrimal duct obstruction: a clinicopathologic report and biopsy technique, *Ophthalmology* 93:1055-1063, 1986.

67. Madreperla SA, Green WR, Daniel R, Shah KV: Human papillomavirus in primary epithelial tumors of the lacrimal sac, *Ophthalmology* 100:569-573, 1993.

68. Mahajan VM: Acute bacterial infections of the eye: their aetiology and treatment, *Br J Ophthalmol* 67:191-194, 1983.

69. Mahajan VM, Alexander TA, Jain RK et al.: Role of coagulase negative staphylococci and micrococci in ocular disease, *J Clin Pathol* 33:1169-1173, 1980.

70. Matlzman BA, Favetta JR: Dacryolithiasis, *Ann Ophthalmol* 473-475, 1979.

71. Mauriello JA Jr, Palydowycz S, DeLuca J: Clinicopathologic study of lacrimal sac and nasal mucosa in 44 patients with complete acquired nasolacrimal duct obstruction, *Ophthalmol Plast Reconstr Surg* 8:13-21, 1992.

72. Mauriello JA, Stabile C, Wagner RS: Dacrocystitis following Kawasaki's disease, *Ophthalmol Plast Reconstr Surg* 2:209-211, 1986.

73. Mauriello JA Jr, Fiore PM, Kotch M, Norblass A: Dacryocystitis. a late complication of orbital floor fracture repair with implant, *Ophthalmology* 94:248-250, 1987.

74. McGill J, Goulding NJ, Liakos G et al.: Pathophysiology of bacterial infection in the external eye, *Trans Ophthalmol Soc UK* 102:7-10, 1982.

75. Milder B, Smith ME: Carcinoma of the lacrimal sac, *Am J Ophthalmol* 65:782-784, 1968.

76. Miller CL, Offutt WN, Kielar RA: Adenoid cystic carcinoma of the antrum and epiphora, *Am J Ophthalmol* 83:582-586, 1977.

77. Mindlin AM: Non-surgical treatment of acute dacryocystitis. In Bosinak SL, Smith BC, editors: *Advances in ophthalmic and plastic reconstructive surgery,* New York, 1984, Pergamon Press.

78. Mohan H, Sen DK, Gupta DK: Orbital affection in nasal and paranasal neoplasms, *Acta Ophthalmol* 47:289-294, 1969.

79. Mukherjee PK, Jain PC, Mishra RK: Exanthemata: a causative factor of chronic dacryocystitis in children, *J All-India Ophthalmol Soc* 17:27-30, 1969.

80. Murube-del-Castillo J: A history of dacryology. In Milder B, Weil BA, editors: *The lacrimal system,* 3-8, Norwalk, 1983, Appleton-Century-Crofts.

81. Nelson LB, Calhoun JH, Benduke H: Medical management of congenital nasolacrimal duct obstruction, *Ophthalmology* 92:1187-1190, 1985.

82. Nunery WR, Wilson FM: Suppurative Canaliculitis. In Bosniak SL, Smith BC, editors: *Advances in ophthalmic plastic and reconstructive surgery,* 157-164, New York, 1984, Pergamon Press.

83. Obi S, Yamamoto K: Clinical studies on neonatal dacryocystitis, *J Clin Ophthalmol* 19:391-396, 1965.

84. Patrick RD: Lacrimal secretion in full-term and premature babies, *Trans Ophthalmol Soc UK* 94:283-290, 1974.

85. Pavan-Langston D: Diagnosis and therapy of common eye infections: bacterial, viral, fungal, *Compr Ther* 9:33-42, 1983.

86. Pavilack MA, Frueh BR: Thorough curettage in the treatment of chronic canaliculitis, *Arch Ophthalmol* 110:200-202, 1992.

87. Penikett E, Rees D: *Nocardia asteroides* infection of the nasal lacrimal system, *Am J Ophthalmol* 53:1006, 1962.

88. Peterson RA, Rebb RM: The natural course of congenital obstruction of the nasolacrimal duct, *J Pediatr Ophthalmol Strabismus* 15:246-250, 1978.

89. Pine L, Shearin WA, Gonzales CA: Mycotic flora of the lachrymal duct, *Am J Ophthalmol* 52:619-625, 1961.

90. Pollard Z: Treatment of acute dacryocystitis in neonates, *J Pediatr Ophthalmol Strabismus* 28:341-343, 1991.

91. Pollard ZP: Tear duct obstruction in children, *Clin Pediatr* 18:487-490, 1979.

92. Purgason PA, Hornblass A, Loeffler M: Atypical presentation of fungal dacryocystitis: a report of two cases, *Ophthalmology* 99:1430-1432, 1992.

93. Radnót M, Bolcs S: Acute dacryocystitis in the newborn infant. In Veirs ER, editor: *The lacrimal system,* St Louis, 1971, Mosby.

94. Radnót M, Gall J: Tumoren des tränensackes, *Ophthalmolgica* 151:1-22, 1966.

95. Romano A, Segal E, Blumenthal M: Canaliculitis with isolation of *Pityrosporum pachydermatis,* *Br J Ophthalmol* 62:732-734, 1978.

96. Rootman DS, Insler MS, Wolfley DE: Canaliculitis caused by *Mycobacterium chelonae* after lacrimal intubation with silicone tubes, *Can J Ophthalmol* 24:221, 1989.

97. Roth SI, August CZ, Lissner GS, O'Grady RB: Hemangiopericytoma of the lacrimal sac, *Ophthalmology* 98:925-927, 1991.

98. Ryan SJ, Font RL: Primary epithelial neoplasms of the lacrimal sac, *Am J Ophthalmol* 76:73-88, 1973.

98a. Sathananthan N, Sullivan TJ, Rose GE, Moseley IF: Intubation dacryocystography in patients with a clinical diagnosis of chronic canaliculitis ("streptothrik"), *Br J Radiol* 66:389-393, 1993.

99. Savir J, Henig E, Lehrer N: Exogenous mycotic infections of the eye and adnexa, *Ann Ophthalmol* 10:1013-1018, 1978.

100. Seal DV, McGill G, Flanagan D et al.: Lacrimal canaliculitis due to *Arachnia propionica,* *Br J Ophthalmol* 65:10-13, 1981.

101. Seiff SR, Shore N: Nasolacrimal drainage system obstruction after orbital decompression, *Am J Ophthalmol* 106:204-209, 1988.

102. Senke RF: Pseudolacrimal duct obstruction caused by nasal allergy, *Ophthalmic Surg* 20:63-67, 1989.

103. Smith B: Late bilateral naso-orbital fracture and dacryostenosis, *Trans Am Acad Ophthalmol Otolaryngol* 76:1378-1379, 1972.

104. Smith B, Tenzel RR, Buffam FV et al.: Acute dacryocystic retention, *Arch Ophthalmol* 94:1903-1909, 1976.

105. Spaeth GL: Nasolacrimal duct obstruction caused by topical epinephrine, *Arch Ophthalmol* 77:355-357, 1967.

106. Starr MB: Lacrimal drainage system infections. In Smith BC, Della Rocca RC, Nesi FA et al., editors: *Ophthalmic plastic and reconstructive surgery,* St Louis, 1987, Mosby.

107. Sternberg I, Levine MR: Ethmoidal sinus osteom: a primary cause of nasolacrimal obstruction and dacryocystorhinostomy failure, *Ophthalmic Surg* 15:295-297, 1984.

108. Tabbara KF, Hynduik RA: *Infections of the eye,* Boston, 1986, Little, Brown.

109. Tannenbaum M, McCord CD: The lacrimal drainage system. In Tasman W, Jaeger EA, editors: *Duane's clinical ophthalmology,* Philadelphia, 1991, JB Lippincott.

110. Tennent JN III: Diseases of lids and lacrymal apparatus. I. Carcinoma of the lacrymal sac: report of two cases, *Trans Ophthalmol Soc UK* 53:93-101, 1933.

111. Traquair HM: Chronic dacryocystitis: its causation and treatment, *Arch Ophthalmol* 26:165-180, 1941.

111a. V'ecsei VP, Huber-Spitzy V, Arocker-Mettinger E, Steinkogler FJ: Canaliculitis: difficulties in diagnosis, differential diagnosis and comparison between conservative and surgical treatment, *Ophthalmologica* 208:314-317, 1994.

112. Weinberg RJ, Sartoris MJ, Buerger GF Jr et al.: Fusobacterium in presumed *Actinomyces canaliculitis,* *Am J Ophthalmol* 84:371-374, 1977.

113. Weiss JL, Nelson JD, Lindstrom RL et al.: Bacterial endophthalmitis following penetrating keratoplasty suture removal, *Cornea* 3:278-280, 1984/85.

114. Wilkins RB, Pressly JP: Diagnosis and incidence of lacrimal calculi, *Ophthalmic Surg* 32:787, 1980.

115. Wolter JR, Deitz MR: Candidiasis of the lacrimal sac, *Am J Ophthalmol* 55:153-155, 1963.

116. Wolter JR, Stratford T, Harrell ER: Cast-like fungus obstruction of the nasolacrimal duct, *Arch Ophthalmol* 55:320-322, 1956.

117. Zolli CL, Shannon GN: Dacryocystorhinostomy: a review of 119 cases, *Ophthalmic Surg* 13:905-910, 1982.

97 Measles, Mumps, and Rubella

STEVEN F. LEE, GREGG T. LUEDER

MEASLES

Measles is an acute, highly contagious viral disease. It is characterized by fever, conjunctivitis, coryza, cough, a specific enanthem of the oral mucosa (Koplik spots), and a generalized maculopapular eruption.

Epidemiology

Because measles is a highly contagious, acute infectious disease resulting in lifelong immunity and with no animal reservoir, populations of several hundred thousand are required to provide a sufficient supply of susceptible individuals to sustain the presence of the virus. In less developed nations of the world, over a million children die each year as a result of measles. It is hoped that inclusion of the live attenuated measles vaccine in the World Health Organization's expanded program on immunization will reduce this morbidity and mortality.

The use of the measles vaccine for the past three decades in the United States has made measles a rare disease among American children. The introduction of a required second dose of vaccine has been associated with record low levels of transmission. Complete eradication has not occurred because of lack of vaccination, primary vaccine failure, and importation of measles from other countries.

Before the introduction of the measles vaccine, epidemics occurred at two- to three-year intervals and lasted three to four months.[2] Cases still occur in the United States, most commonly in young children who are not immunized and occasionally in teenagers who were immunized during childhood.[31]

Clinical Features

Systemic Findings. There is a clinically silent incubation period of approximately ten days. During this time lymphopenia may occur. Following the incubation period the prodromal phase begins with a mild fever, conjunctivitis, cough, and coryza. The fever is a result of cellular reaction to viral infection. The temperature gradually increases over a five-day period. A rash appears on the third to fifth day after the onset of symptoms. Two or three days after the start of the rash, the fever abates. The conjunctivitis, cough, and coryza all result from mucous membrane inflammation. The conjunctivitis and coryza usually subside just after the patient becomes afebrile. The cough may persist for one to two weeks.

Koplik spots appear on the oral mucosa two to three days after the onset of symptoms and two to three days before the rash. The lesions are small, irregular bright red spots with a bluish-white speck at each center.[28] After two to three days, the spots coalesce to form a diffuse erythematous background upon which are many minute blue-white elevations. The spots then begin to slough off with a fading of the erythema. By the third day of the rash the mucous membrane returns to a normal appearance.

The rash of measles begins three to five days after the onset of the prodrome. The first maculopapular lesions are seen behind the ear, along the hairline, forehead, and upper part of the neck. The rash then spreads to the face, trunk, and upper extremities. The feet may be involved by the third day. The initial lesions then fade and clear by the fourth day of the rash. The early lesions blanch with pressure. The fading rash has a brownish appearance that does not blanch with pressure.

Ocular Findings. *Conjunctiva.* In the prodromal phase a conjunctivitis may or may not be clinically apparent. At this time the virus is replicating throughout the body, including the subepithelial conjunctival lymphoid tissue. The surrounding tissue reaction causes the conjunctivitis. The palpebral conjunctiva is involved more often than the bulbar conjunctiva. A watery or mucoid discharge is common, whereas purulent discharge usually indicates a secondary bacterial infection. Marked chemosis may be present. Koplik spots of the caruncle and conjunctiva have been reported.[11] In severe cases membranous conjunctivitis may occur on the conjunctiva.[13] The conjunctivitis resolves seven to ten days after the start of the prodrome.

1357

Conjunctival epithelial lesions can be identified with rose bengal or lissamine green. These lesions appear at the time of the prodrome and are not seen after the rash resolves. The number and shape of these lesions vary greatly. They can be singular, multiple, or large and confluent. The lesions are observed on the nasal interpalpebral bulbar conjunctiva more frequently than temporally. They are uncommon on the palpebral conjunctiva.[10]

The individual lesions resolve without treatment within one to two days. Measles antigen has been demonstrated in the epithelial layer of conjunctival biopsies.[10] No subepithelial measles antigens could be demonstrated. The loss of epithelium may be due to a breakdown of intercellular adhesions.

Cornea. The corneal epithelial lesions can be stained with fluorescein, rose bengal, or lissamine green. These lesions are contiguous with the conjunctival lesions. The number and shape of the corneal and conjunctival lesions are similar. Bowman's membrane and stroma are not affected. A superficial punctate keratitis typically occurs first near the limbus and it may spread to involve the central cornea.[9] The peak incidence of corneal lesions occurs the day after the appearance of the rash. The keratitis then rapidly improves with complete resolution within two weeks.

In a prospective evaluation of 248 children with measles, Dekkers[9] found a 76% incidence of keratitis. The duration and the peripheral-to-central progression of the keratitis may be due to the avascularity of the cornea, which increases the time needed for circulating neutralizing antibodies to reach the virus.[9]

Corneal erosions may complicate measles infection within two weeks of the rash. They may occur after the resolution of the initial keratitis. Intercellular adhesions are diminished in areas of measles erosions, and migrating corneal epithelium does not adhere well to the basement membrane.

Postmeasles Blindness. Postmeasles blindness (PMB) may be caused by neurologic or ocular sequelae of measles, including optic neuritis, chorioretinitis, or corneal complications. In developing countries the corneal complications of measles are a notable cause of childhood blindness. Studies in Africa have shown that 14% to 33% of childhood blindness is due to measles.[1,5] Measles blinds approximately 1% of infected African children.[36,37] Corneal ulceration and corneal PMB are indistinguishable. Characteristics of corneal PMB include ulceration, perforation, leukoma, and phthisis bulbi.

The cause of corneal PMB is multifactorial. Foster and Summer[15] studied a large group of Tanzanian children with corneal ulcers and identified four mechanisms by which measles produced this complication. The first was a concomitant herpes simplex virus infection, which was found in 21% of measles-associated ulcers. This association has also been reported by others.[48] The second was the use of folk remedies, which were associated with 17% of the ulcers.

The ingredients in these remedies are not known, but they are believed to include human and animal urine and plant substances. The third mechanism was confluence of measles keratitis. This type of corneal ulcer generally healed without sequelae after treatment with antibiotics and patching.

The most common mechanism in Foster and Sommer's study was concomitant vitamin A deficiency, which accounted for 50% of measles-associated ulceration.[15] The vitamin A deficiency results from a decreased dietary intake and increased demand during the acute illness. The children may also have decreased stores of vitamin A as a result of ongoing malnutrition. In addition, these children with caloric malnutrition may have low levels of retinol binding protein, leading to defective release and transport of vitamin A from the liver to the peripheral tissues. Vitamin A does not appear to play a role in the milder form of keratitis associated with measles. In a study comparing patients with measles with and without keratitis, Reddy and associates[40] found no significant difference in vitamin A levels between the two groups.

Pathogenesis

Measles is a member of the genus *Morbillivirus,* family Paramyxoviridae.[27] The measles virion has a core of linear, single-stranded RNA. The virion is spherical, enveloped, and pleomorphic with a diameter ranging between 100 and 250 nm.[27] The virus is inactivated by heat, cold, ultraviolet light, ether, and trypsin. Humans are the only natural host.

The measles virus is transmitted via the airborne route and contact with infected nasopharyngeal secretions. The virus is present in respiratory secretions from the beginning of the prodromal phase until several days after the rash appears.[25] The measles virus enters the respiratory tract, oropharynx, or conjunctiva by droplet spread. Local replication occurs for the first few days. Further replication occurs when the infection is disseminated throughout the reticuloendothelial system via virus-laden leukocytes. Replication at these secondary reticuloendothelial sites causes a lymphoid hyperplasia and multinucleated giant-cell formation. The secondary viremia is a result of the dissemination of the virus to the remainder of the body. Monocytes and lymphocytes deliver the virus at this stage.[38]

Approximately ten days after the primary infection, the prodromal symptoms and signs are produced by viral replication and the immune response throughout the body. Multinucleated giant cells with eosinophilic cytoplasmic inclusion bodies are present in lymphoid and epithelial tissues. Koplik spots and the skin rash are histopathologically similar, demonstrating multinucleated giant cells, parakeratosis, and dyskeratosis.[45]

Laboratory Investigations and Pathology

The diagnosis of measles is easily done clinically. The cough, conjunctivitis, coryza, distinct rash, and Koplik spots are pathognomonic. The differential diagnosis includes Rocky Mountain spotted fever, scarlet fever, meningococcemia, and varicella.

Laboratory diagnosis of measles is useful when the incidence is low and public health measures will be undertaken. Rapid tests include demonstration of measles virus antigen in nasopharyngeal secretions by fluorescent antibody staining using measles-specific monoclonal antibodies. An alternative approach to rapid diagnosis is the detection of measles-specific IgM antibodies.

Less sensitive and specific laboratory tests are also available. It is possible to isolate the virus in primary human or monkey cell cultures before the appearance of the rash,[25] but this practice is time-consuming and relatively insensitive. During the prodrome and the first three days of the rash, giant cells are present in respiratory secretions, the epithelial surface of the conjunctiva, buccal mucosa, nasal mucosa, and pharynx. These secretions can be rapidly stained with Papanicolaou or Wright stain to identify multinucleated giant cells with eosinophilic inclusions in the nucleus and cytoplasm.

Hemagglutination inhibition by the enzyme-linked immunosorbent assay (ELISA), radioimmunoassay, or passive hemagglutination can determine paired serum antibody concentration. Antibodies appear within the first three days of the rash. Two to four weeks later the titers are at their peak. These antibodies persist for years after infection or immunization. Measles infection is demonstrated by a fourfold or greater increase in antibody titer. By means of the ELISA or radioimmunoassay, the measles virus-specific IgM antibodies can be shown in early serum samples. This approach is very useful for rapid diagnosis with a sensitivity of greater than 90%. Other laboratory findings include leukopenia and electroencephalographic changes.

Therapy

Measles is typically a self-limited disease, and treatment is chiefly supportive. Antimicrobial therapy does not alter an uncomplicated infection. Secondary bacterial infections, however, should be treated with the proper antimicrobial agents.

It is possible to prevent measles infection in exposed patients by treatment with immune globulin. Immune globulin may be used in contacts who are particularly susceptible to infection, such as immunocompromised patients, pregnant women, and infants less than one year of age. The disease may be prevented if the immune globulin is administered within five days of exposure.

The ocular manifestations of measles are treated symptomatically. Conjunctivitis and keratitis are treated with antibiotics to prevent secondary bacterial infections. Vitamin A supplements may be used in those patients who are deficient. Topical antiviral medication is indicated in patients with herpes simplex keratitis.

Subacute Sclerosing Panencephalitis

Subacute sclerosing panencephalitis (SSPE) is a rare, slowly progressive disease that is a late complication of measles. The incidence is approximately 1 per 100,000 cases. There is a mean interval of 6 to 7 years between the measles infection and the onset of symptoms of SSPE. Most children with SSPE have had measles within the first two years of life. SSPE has features of a slowly progressive viral infection. The early clinical signs are declining mental faculties, behavioral changes, and myoclonic seizures. Later signs include progressive neurological deterioration and decerebrate rigidity. The white and gray matter of the brain are involved. Death usually occurs within three years of the onset of SSPE. Laboratory findings in SSPE include a characteristic electroencephalogram, cerebrospinal fluid globulin elevation, high serum measles antibody titer, and a cerebrospinal fluid oligoclonal measles antibody.

There is widespread central nervous system involvement in SSPE and a concomitant high incidence of ocular involvement. The most common ocular findings are macular abnormalities, optic nerve atrophy, and papilledema.[19] Other ocular findings in SSPE include peripheral retinitis, ocular motility disorders, nystagmus, ptosis, and visual disturbances.[19,33,43] Cortical blindness may develop during the course of SSPE without any ocular signs.

The most common ocular manifestation of SSPE is a focal abnormality of the fovea (Fig. 97-1). In Green and Wirtschaffer's study,[19] 57% of patients had macular pigmentary changes and 36% had retinitis in the macular area. Contraction of the internal limiting membrane may be associated with these changes. The severity of the retinitis does not correlate with the progression of SSPE. The inflammation is generally limited to the retina. Histopathologic examination of a macular lesion in one patient revealed swollen

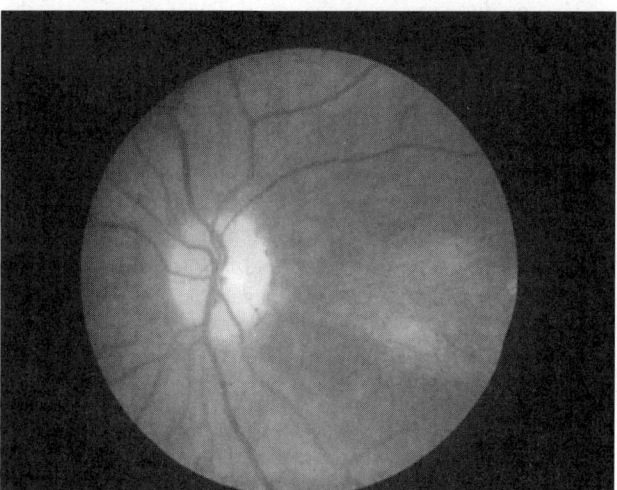

Fig. 97-1. Subacute sclerosing panencephalitis. Macular pigmentary abnormality and temporal pallor of optic nerve head are seen. (Photo courtesy of Morton Smith, MD.)

ganglion cells, nerve fibre layer atrophy, and granular changes in the pigment epithelium of the macula.[33]

Before the appearance of other neurological manifestations of SSPE, opthalmic signs may be detected.[18] SSPE should be included in the differential diagnosis of a patient with unexplained optic nerve atrophy or retinitis. Early treatment of SSPE with inosiplex has been reported to delay the neurologic progression of the disease.[24]

MUMPS

Mumps is an acute contagious viral disease commonly characterized by enlargement of the parotid glands. There is a wide spectrum in the clinical presentation of mumps, including subclinical infection, parotitis, orchitis, meningoencephalitis, and pancreatitis.

Epidemiology

Mumps is mainly a disease of childhood. It usually occurs after the first year of life. This delay is due in part to passive immunity from maternal antibodies acquired by the fetus. These antibodies appear to protect the infant during the first year of life. Studies have shown that maternal complement-fixating and hemagglutination-inhibiting antibodies directed against mumps are present at birth, but they are usually undetectable after eight weeks of age, although they may remain detectable by more sensitive assays such as ELISA. It is postulated that the antibodies are effective but difficult to detect during the first year.[6]

Mumps was an endemic disease in most prevaccine urban areas. There were approximately 190,000 reported cases of mumps in 1967, when the live attenuated virus vaccine became available in the United States. In 1991 the number of reported cases was about 4000.

Pathogenesis

The mumps virus is of the genus *Paramyxovirus* in the family Paramyxoviridae. The mumps virion is enveloped and pleomorphic, ranging in size from 90 to 135 nm. The RNA genome is single-stranded, nonsegmented, and negative-sense. There are two glycoproteins at the virion surface. One induces lipid membrane fusion and the other mediates neuraminidase activity and hemagglutination.

The in vitro cytopathic effects of mumps virus are dependent on the particular host cells and isolates. Henle and associates[22] described a large homogeneous mass of cytoplasm enclosing numerous nuclei in tissue culture of infected human epithelial cells. Other effects include cell pyknosis, spindle formation, and cytoplasmic vacuolization. The growth of mumps virus in cell culture may induce hemagglutination; this property is useful in the detection of the virus in inoculated cell cultures. The infectivity of the virus is lost after four days at room temperature. The virus remains infective for years when stored below 20°C. Inactivation occurs with heat at 55°C for 20 minutes, 0.2% formalin, ether, and ultraviolet irradiation.[29]

Man is the only natural host of mumps virus. Virus droplets spread to the oral or upper respiratory tract mucosal epithelium. Primary viral replication then occurs. During the 18-day incubation period there is a lymphatic spread of the virus and viremia. The virus then localizes in glandular or nervous tissue. The parotid gland is most commonly involved along with other salivary glands. The virus can be isolated from saliva, cerebrospinal fluid, blood, and urine in the acute phase.[52]

Live attenuated and killed mumps viruses have been used for vaccines. The disadvantages of killed virus include short-term immunity, the need for a second dose to induce a more lasting protection, and a state of hypersensitivity. In the hypersensitive state, the patient may have a severe reaction when exposed to live mumps virus. The current mumps vaccine is a live attenuated virus vaccine that achieves a 95% seroconversion rate. The immunity is long lasting after a single vaccination. It is currently recommended that all children, adolescents, and adults be vaccinated. Infants normally receive the vaccine at 12 to 15 months of age.

Standard immune globulin is not effective in preventing mumps. Immune globulin made from convalescent mumps serum is of questionable efficacy. One study showed a decreased incidence of orchitis when patients were given convalescent immune globulin, but another study did not show evidence of prevention of orchitis.[16,41]

Clinical Features

Systemic Findings. After infection with the mumps virus there is an 18-day incubation period. A subclinical infection occurs in 30% to 40% of infected patients. In the remaining patients symptoms are variable. Typically the incubation period ends with fever, headache, anorexia, and malaise. Within two days there is noticeable swelling and pain of the parotid gland. The pain is aggravated by jaw movement. The opening of Stenson's duct is usually red and prominent with a clear discharge. Both parotid glands are involved in approximately 75% to 90% of cases. The parotid gland reaches its maximum size within a few days. The fever and parotid gland swelling resolve within one week. Submaxillary and sublingual gland swelling is infrequent.

Orchitis may follow parotitis. It affects about 25% of males who develop mumps after puberty. The incidence of bilateral orchitis is approximately 2%. Affected patients experience testicular pain, swelling, and tenderness. The symptoms gradually subside after four days. It is common to have some degree of atrophy after orchitis, although impotence and sterility are uncommon.

A common manifestation of mumps is central nervous system (CNS) involvement. Approximately 10% of patients develop symptoms of meningitis. Mumps meningitis usually develops about five days following the onset of parotitis. Less commonly it may precede the parotitis or occur in its absence. The symptoms of mumps meningitis are fever, vomiting, neck stiffness, headache, and lethargy. Asymptomatic CNS involvement is not uncommon. Cerebrospinal fluid pleocytosis was found in 20% of infected patients who lacked meningeal signs or symptoms.[14] Examination of the cerebrospinal fluid shows an increase in protein, normal glucose, and a pleocytosis with a predominance of lymphocytes. The electroencephalogram is usually normal.

Less common manifestations of mumps include pancreatitis, oophoritis, mastitis, thyroiditis, arthritis, and myocarditis.

Ocular Findings. *Lacrimal Gland.* Dacryoadenitis is the most common ocular manifestation of mumps.[49] It usually coincides with the parotitis, but it may precede the parotitis or occur without detectable salivary gland enlargement. The latter condition is known as lacrimal mumps. The dacryoadenitis is usually bilateral and nonsuppurative. Lacrimal gland tenderness, chemosis, lid edema, and hyperemia are present. The lacrimal gland remains swollen for approximately three days, followed by resolution of edema and pain. There are usually no sequelae.[42]

Conjunctiva. The conjunctival changes in mumps may be due to direct infection of the conjunctival secretory glands or hyperemia of the conjunctival blood vessels. Follicular conjunctivitis associated with documented mumps virus isolation has been reported.[34]

Cornea. The keratitis associated with mumps has been reviewed by Riffenburgh.[42] Corneal changes typically are seen five days following the parotitis. Symptoms include photophobia, tearing, rapid visual loss, and little pain. Typically there is unilateral involvement with severe and extensive keratitis. The cornea may appear gray with white interlacing fibrillae.[8] The epithelium is usually intact. An accompanying iritis has been reported.[35] The keratitis resolves spontaneously after two to three weeks without vascularization. Residual small opacities may be seen, but usually they do not affect visual acuity.

Intraocular Pressure. Hypotony associated with mumps keratitis was reported by Slagsvold[44] in a 27-year-old patient. The intraocular pressure dropped to 4 mmHg but returned to normal within two weeks. The hypotony was probably secondary to a mild iritis. Increased intraocular pressure was reported by Polland and Thorburn[39] in a 43-year-old patient whose intraocular pressure rose to 50 mmHg one week after the onset of parotitis. No iritis was present. The pressure normalized in one week with corticosteroids and acetazolamide. The prompt response to corticosteroids suggested that trabeculitis was responsible for the elevated pressure.

Uveitis and Scleritis. Anterior uveitis may be seen within two weeks of the onset of parotitis. It is associated with multiple organ involvement, especially orchitis. The typical symptoms and signs of anterior uveitis are reported. These include a red eye, pain, photophobia, and decreased vision. Physical examination reveals conjunctival injection, anterior chamber cell and flare, and keratic precipitates. The uveitis responds to topical corticosteroids and cycloplegics and typically lasts one to four weeks.[42] Episcleritis and scleritis are rare and are usually noted within two weeks of the onset of clinical mumps.[46] The majority of cases resolve quickly and leave no sequelae.[42]

Neuro-Ophthalmic Complications. Optic neuritis is the second most common ocular complication of mumps.[42] The usual clinical picture is one of papillitis with a hyperemic disc and surrounding retinal edema. Most cases resolve spontaneously without complications, but residual optic atrophy may occur.[42] Cranial nerve palsies may occur, usually as a sequela of meningitis. Opsoclonus-myoclonus associated with acute cerebellar ataxia has been reported.[23]

Laboratory Investigations

The diagnosis of mumps is usually based on the symptoms and clinical finding of parotitis. In atypical cases the diagnosis may be confirmed by culture of the virus from blood, cerebrospinal fluid, urine, or saliva. Serologic diagnosis of mumps can be accomplished using standard complement-fixation, hemagglutinin-inhibition, neutralization, or hemolysis-in-gel assays, as well as the rapid ELISA. A fourfold increase or decrease in mumps antibodies in acute versus convalescent sera would be considered diagnostic. Determination of virus-specific IgM and IgG levels on a single acute phase serum should also provide reasonable sensitivity. Classic serology defined two mumps antigens (the S and the V antigens) with the complement-fixation assay. These antigens are largely composed of the nucleocapsid (NP) and hemagglutinin-neuramidase (HN) viral proteins, respectively. Antibodies to the viral S antigen are present early in the course of the disease, whereas antibodies to the V antigen occur later. The diagnosis of mumps can therefore be confirmed by a fourfold or greater rise in the anti-V titer during convalescence.

Therapy

There is no effective treatment for mumps. Treatment is supportive, with bedrest and analgesia as needed. The keratitis associated with mumps resolves spontaneously and does not require treatment. Patients with iritis may require topical steroids and cycloplegic treatment.

RUBELLA

Rubella was first described in the 1800s as a mild morbilliform rash, occasional fever, and lymphadenopathy. Rubella is primarily a childhood disease and is endemic throughout the world.

Epidemiology

In 1941 Sir Norman Gregg,[20] an ophthalmologist, reported a group of children with cataracts, congenital heart disease, and deafness. He correlated this syndrome with maternal rubella in early pregnancy. This finding was the first recognition of a virus as a teratogenic agent.

The rubella virus was cultivated in tissue culture in 1962,

in turn leading to the development of an effective vaccine. Widespread use of the vaccine was initiated in the United States in 1969. The last major epidemic of rubella in the United States occurred in 1964. In that year an estimated 20,000 infants were born with evidence of the congenital rubella syndrome (CRS). Since the introduction of the vaccine there has been a steady decline of CRS, with only two reported cases in 1985.[7] The live rubella virus vaccine produces an antibody response in greater than 95% of susceptible persons who are older than one year of age.

Clinical Features

Systemic Findings. There is a two- to three-week incubation period after infection before the first symptoms of rubella are noted. There is an initial malaise and generalized lymphadenopathy. Commonly the cervical, postauricular and suboccipital nodes are enlarged and tender. A few days later the rash becomes apparent, although it may be minimal and can easily be overlooked. It begins on the face and spreads rapidly over the trunk. The skin changes begin as maculopapules. They typically become pinpoint on the second day and resolve by the third day. Mild joint tenderness may occur. Very few systemic complications are associated with rubella infection.

The congenital rubella syndrome is characterized by intrauterine growth retardation, cataracts, microcephaly, deafness, congenital heart disease, and mental retardation. Low birth weight for gestational age is common. Petechial and purpuric eruption associated with thrombocytopenia may occur during the first weeks of life.[3] The platelet count usually returns to normal within one month.

Disabling congenital heart disease occurs in 1% of infants with CRS. The most common cardiac lesions are atrial and ventricular septal defects and patent ductus arteriosus with or without pulmonary artery stenosis. Myocardial necrosis has also been reported.[47]

Hearing loss occurs in up to 44% of patients.[26] It is usually bilateral but may be unilateral. Hearing loss can be minimal or severe. It is thought to result from degeneration or maldevelopment of the organ of Corti and the cochlea. Speech defects may occur in patients with severe bilateral hearing loss.

Central nervous system involvement may result in microcephaly and mental retardation. Chronic infection of the brain may occur, and live virus may be found in the cerebrospinal fluid (CSF) up to one year of age.[30] Progressive rubella panencephalitis, resulting in severe neurologic deterioration, has been described.[30] This deterioration is associated with high titers of rubella antibodies in the CSF and serum and live virus isolation from the brain.

Ocular Findings. *Cornea.* The congenital rubella syndrome may be associated with corneal edema, which varies from mild to severe. The corneal edema may result from corneal endotheliopathy or an elevation in intraocular pressure. Ac-

tive virus found in the aqueous humor may cause an endotheliopathy. Dense corneal clouding does not clear as well as milder corneal haze.[50,51] Hydrops has been reported in a seven-day-old infant who died from congenital rubella.[53] Histopathologic examination revealed a large central bulla, a large gap in the Descemet's membrane, and marked stromal hydropic degeneration.

Iris and Ciliary Body. If the rubella virus infects the fetus at the seventh or eighth week of gestation the development of the iris, ciliary body, and anterior chamber angle may be disturbed. The pigment epithelium of the iris and ciliary body can necrose and vacuolize.[53] The iris dilator muscle and stroma can become atrophic. The lack of inflammation in response to the rubella infection at this early stage of development reflects the inability of the fetus to mount an adequate immune response.[53] In contrast, chronic anterior uveitis may be observed postnatally. This persistent nongranulomatous inflammation can cause permanent damage to the anterior angle structures.

Lens. Maternal rubella infection during the first trimester may result in cataract formation. Intracellular virus can dramatically slow the fetal cell replication rate. This decreased rate of replication results in the retention of nuclei in lens fibers (Fig. 97-2). The cataract in rubella is usually dense centrally with a less opaque peripheral cortex and capsule (Fig. 97-3). Forward displacement of the iris may result from an increase in the anterior-posterior diameter of the lens. Less often there is a thinning of the lens. Congenital aphakia secondary to CRS has been described.[21]

Virus persists in the lens for at least one year in a majority of patients. Care should be taken during cataract surgery to minimize exposure to lens material. A severe inflammatory response may occur after surgery.[51] High doses of topical corticosteroids are usually needed to control the inflammatory response. Early surgery and aggressive treatment to

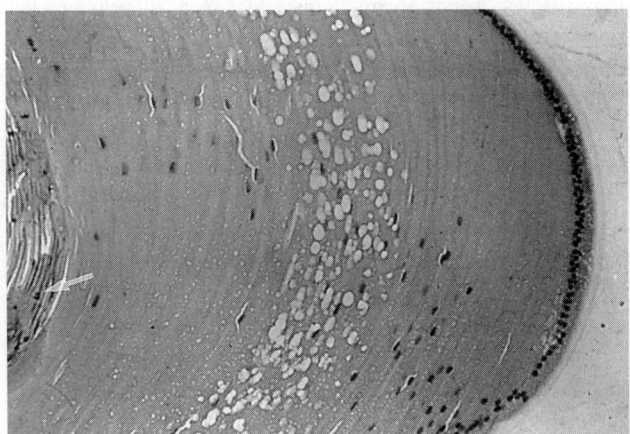

Fig. 97-2. Photomicrograph of lens in congenital rubella syndrome. Note persistence of lens fiber nuclei in the normally acellular nuclear portion of the lens *(arrow)*. (Photo courtesy of G. Frank Judisch, MD.)

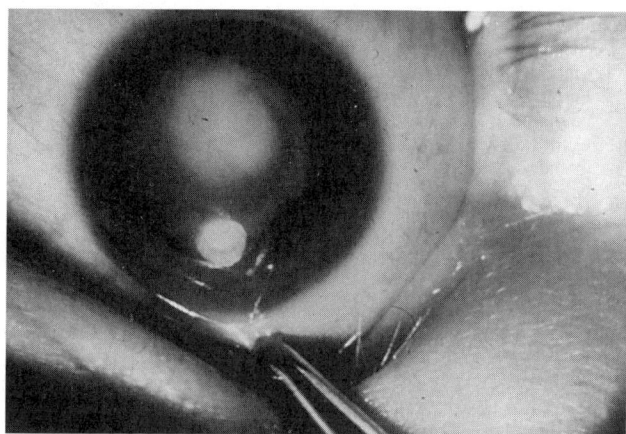

Fig. 97-3. Cataract in congenital rubella syndrome. Note central density with less opaque peripheral lens. (Photo courtesy of G. Frank Judisch, MD.)

prevent amblyopia will maximize the visual outcome. Other rubella-related pathology such as glaucoma, optic neuropathy, and oculomotor disorders may affect the final visual result.

Retina. Retinopathy is the most common ocular manifestation of CRS. It was found in 22% of patients reported by Wolff.[50] There is tremendous variation in the descriptions of rubella retinopathy. The changes may be bone-spiculelike, mottled, finely stippled, or blotchy (Fig. 97-4). The condition may be bilateral, unilateral, central, or peripheral. Rubella retinopathy may be progressive with uneven development of retinal pigment epithelium. A majority of patients will have vision better than 20/60. Histopathologic studies of affected retinas reveal depigmentation of the retinal pigment epithelium without signs of inflammation.[53]

Glaucoma. Approximately 10% of children with congenital rubella will develop glaucoma.[50] Prenatal glaucoma usually results in poor vision. There are several causes of glaucoma in patients with rubella: chronic inflammation, enlarged cataractous lenses causing angle closure, and anatomic abnormalities similar to those seen in primary infantile glaucoma. The diagnosis should be suspected in patients with corneal edema. The glaucoma may not be recognized until after the perinatal period.

Microphthalmos. Microphthalmos and/or microcornea were found in 10% of patients with CRS in Wolff's study.[50] Microphthalmos is often associated with cataract. Most microphthalmic patients have visual acuities less than 20/100. Zimmerman[53] believes that the microphthalmos reflects the growth-slowing effect of the virus on developing tissues.

Pathogenesis

The rubella virus is a member of the Togaviridae family. The virus contains a single-stranded RNA genome surrounded by a lipid envelope or "toga." E1 and E2 glycopeptides make up the envelope glycoprotein. Rubella virus

is inactivated by temperatures above 37°C, a pH above 8.1 or below 6.8, ultraviolet irradiation, ether, and formalin. It is resistant to antibiotics, thimerosal, and 5-iodo-2-deoxyuridine.

Maternal infection and viremia may lead to placental infection followed by fetal viremia. The virus may disseminate to many fetal organs. The most critical factor in the pathogenesis of congenital rubella is the time of infection. Maternal rubella before conception has not been shown to cause intrauterine infection.[12] Before the fourth month of gestation the fetus is more susceptible to chronic infection and damage. Defects from congenital rubella are unlikely when an infection occurs after the 17th week of gestation.

The pathogenesis of rubella embryopathy has not been determined on a cellular level. The main theories are that the virus inhibits cellular multiplication, produces chronic persistent infection during organogenesis, or a combination of both. The fetal immune response to congenital rubella results in production of fetal IgM antibody during the third trimester. This titer peaks at three to six months of age and is markedly diminished by one year of age. Passively acquired maternal IgG is present at birth and is no longer detectable after a few months. By 12 months of age infected infants predominantly produce IgG antibody. Rubella virus is excreted in the nasopharynx and urine in over 80% of newborns with congenital rubella. After 20 months of age, 3% will shed the virus. One patient shed the virus at 29 years of age.[32]

Laboratory Investigations

Patients with rubella typically have a history of malaise and cervical lymph node enlargement before the appearance of the rash. Because of the nonspecific nature of these manifestations the clinical diagnosis of rubella is not considered reliable.

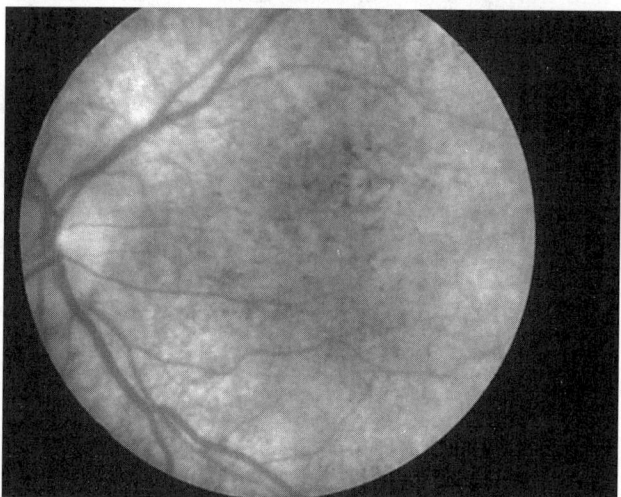

Fig. 97-4. Retinopathy in congenital rubella syndrome. Note granular ("salt and pepper") appearance of retinal pigment epithelium. (Photo courtesy of Morton Smith, MD.)

The laboratory diagnosis of rubella includes virus isolation and serology. Adults and neonates can provide virus samples easily from throat swabs. In congenital rubella the virus can be isolated from lymphocytes, bone marrow, blood, urine, feces, CSF, conjunctiva, and amniotic fluid.[4] Rubella antibody titers can be obtained by latex agglutination, hemagglutination-inhibition, complement-fixation assays, or ELISA.

Maternal rubella infection is diagnosed by a serial rise in maternal rubella IgG antibody titer or by the presence of maternal IgM antibodies to rubella virus. Measurement of IgM is a better approach than serial IgG testing because only a single specimen is required. This test is widely available through state health departments and commercial laboratories.

In the neonate IgG antibodies may be maternal because IgG crosses the placenta. IgM does not cross the placenta and it may be produced by the neonate in response to rubella infection. The presence of IgM antibodies confirms the diagnosis of rubella in neonates.

Therapy

The treatment of rubella is symptomatic. Analgesics and bedrest are mainstays of treatment. Immunoglobulin administration is not recommended to pregnant women who have been exposed to rubella.[17] The corneal manifestations are usually self-limiting, although severe corneal haze may require corneal transplantation. Patients with glaucoma and cataracts secondary to CRS need early surgery and aggressive treatment to prevent amblyopia. The glaucoma associated with CRS is difficult to manage medically and surgically.[51]

REFERENCES

1. Benezra D, Chirombo MC: Incidence and causes of blindness among the under 5 age group in Malawi, *Br J Ophthalmol* 61:154, 1977.
2. Black FL: Measles. In Evans A, editor: *Viral infections of humans: epidemiology and control,* New York, 1989, Plenum Press.
3. Brody JA et al.: Rubella epidemic on St Paul Island in the Pribilofs 1963: epidemiologic, clinical and serological findings, *JAMA* 191:619, 1965.
4. Center for Disease Control: Rubella and congenital rubella: United States, *MMWR* 35:129, 1986.
5. Chirambo MC, Benezra D: Causes of blindness among students in blind school institutions in a developing country, *Br J Ophthalmol* 60:665, 1976.
6. Christie AB: Mumps. In *Infectious diseases: epidemiology and clinical practice,* New York, 1987, Churchill Livingstone.
7. Christie AB: Rubella. In *Infectious diseases: epidemiology and clinical practice,* New York, 1987, Churchill Livingstone.
8. Danielson RW, Long JC: Keratitis due to mumps, *Am J Ophthalmol* 24:655, 1941.
9. Dekkers NWHM: The cornea in measles, *Doc Ophthalmol* 52:1, 1981.
10. Dekkers NWHM: The cornea in measles. In *Viral diseases of the eye,* Philadelphia, 1985, Lea & Febiger.
11. Duke-Elder: Diseases of the outer eye. In *System of ophthalmology,* St Louis, Mo 1965, CV Mosby.
12. Enders G et al.: Outcome of confirmed periconceptional maternal rubella, *Lancet* 1:1445, 1988.
13. Fedukowicz HB: Measles. In *External infections of the eye,* New York, 1978, Appleton-Century-Crofts.
14. Finkelstein H: Meningo-encephalitis in mumps, *JAMA* 3:17, 1938.
15. Foster A, Sommer A: Corneal ulceration, measles, and childhood blindness in Tanzania, *Br J Ophthalmol* 71:331, 1987.
16. Gellis SS et al.: A study of the prevention of mumps orchitis by gamma globulin, *Am J Med Sci* 210:661, 1945.
17. Gibbs RS, Sweet RL: Maternal and fetal infections. In *Maternal fetal medicine principles and practice,* Philadelphia, 1994, Saunders.
18. Gravina RF et al.: Subacute sclerosing panencephalitis, *Am J Ophthalmol* 86:106, 1978.
19. Green SH, Wirtschaffer JD: Ophthalmoscopic findings in subacute sclerosing panencephalitis, *B J Ophthalmol* 57:780, 1973.
20. Gregg NM: Congenital cataract following German measles in the mother, *Trans Ophthalmol Soc Aust* 3:35, 1941.
21. Hartwig NG et al.: The anterior eye segment in virus induced primary congenital aphakia, *Acta Morphol Nederl-Scand* 26:283, 1988/89.
22. Henle G et al.: Cytolytic effects of mumps virus in tissue cultures of epithelial cells, *Proc Soc Exp Biol Med* 87:386, 1954.
23. Ichiba N et al.: Mumps-induced opsoclonus-myoclonus and ataxia, *Pediatr Neurol* 4:224, 1988.
24. Jones CE et al.: Inosiplex therapy in subacute sclerosing panencephalitis, *Lancet* 1:1034, 1982.
25. Katz SL, Enders JF: Measles virus. In Horsfall FL Jr and Tamms I, editors: *Viral and rickettsial infections of man,* Philadelphia, 1965, JB Lippincott.
26. Keir EH: Results of rubella in pregnancy. II. Hearing defects, *Med J Austr* 2:691, 1965.
27. Kingsbury DW et al.: Paramyxoviridae, *Intervirology* 10:137, 1978.
28. Koplik H: The diagnosis of the invasion of measles from a study of the exanthema as it appears on the buccal mucous membrane, *Arch Pediatr* 13:918, 1896.
29. Krugman S et al.: Mumps. In *Infectious diseases of children,* St Louis, 1992, Mosby.
30. Krugman S et al.: Rubella. In *Infectious diseases of children,* St Louis, 1992, Mosby.
31. Markowitz LE et al.: Patterns of transmission in measles outbreaks in the United States 1985-1986, *N Engl J Med* 320:75, 1989.
32. Menser MA et al.: Rubella viremia in a 29-year-old woman with congenital rubella, *Lancet* 2:797, 1971.
33. Meyer E et al.: Subacute sclerosing panencephalitis: clinicopathological study of the eyes, *J Pediatr Ophthalmol Strabismus* 15:19, 1978.
34. Meyer RF et al.: Mumps conjunctivitis, *Am J Ophthalmol* 78:1022, 1974.
35. Mickatavage R, Amdur J: A case report of mumps keratitis, *Arch Ophthalmol* 69:758, 1963.
36. Morley D: Severe measles in the tropics, *Br Med J* 1:297, 1969.
37. Morley DC et al.: Measles in East and Central Africa, *East Afr Med J* 44:497, 1967.
38. Norrby E, Oxman MN: Measles virus. In Fields BN, Knipe DM and associates, editors: *Virology,* New York, 1990, Raven Press.
39. Polland W, Thorburn W: Transient glaucoma as a manifestation of mumps, *Acta Ophthalmol* 54:779, 1976.
40. Reddy V et al.: Relationship between measles, malnutrition, and blindness: a prospective study in Indian children, *Am J Clin Nutr* 44:924, 1986.
41. Reed D et al.: A mumps epidemic on St George Island, Alaska, *JAMA* 199:113, 1967.
42. Riffenburgh RS: Ocular manifestations of mumps, *Am J Ophthalmol* 66:739, 1961.
43. Robb RM, Vatters GV: Ophthalmic manifestations of subacute sclerosing panencephalitis, *Arch Ophthalmol* 83:426, 1970.
44. Slagsvold JE: Acute ocular hypotony as a manifestation of mumps, *Acta Ophthalmol* 58:288, 1980.
45. Suringa DNR et al.: Role of measles virus in skin lesions and Koplik's spots, *N Engl J Med* 283:1139, 1970.
46. Swan JW, Penn RF: Scleritis following mumps, *Am J Ophthalmol* 53:366, 1962.
47. Tondury G, Smith DW: Fetal rubella pathology, *J Pediatr* 58:867, 1966.

48. Ukety TO, Maertens K: Ocular ulcerative herpes following measles in Kinshasa, Zaire, *Curr Eye Res* 10(suppl 1):131, 1991.
49. Villard H: Complications oculaires des oreillons, *Arch Ophthalmol* 44:492, 1927.
50. Wolff SM: The ocular manifestations of congenital rubella: a prospective study of 328 cases of congenital rubella, *J Pediatr Ophthalmol* 10:101, 1973.
51. Wolff SM: Rubella syndrome. In *Viral diseases of the eye.*, Philadelphia, 1985, Lea & Febiger.
52. Wolinsky JS, Waxham MN: Mumps virus. In Fields BN, Knipe DM and associates, editors: *Virology,* New York, 1990, Raven Press.
53. Zimmerman LE: Histopathologic basis for ocular manifestations of congenital rubella syndrome, *Am J Ophthalmol* 65:837, 1958.

98 Human T-Lymphotropic Virus, Type I Associated Disease

MANABU MOCHIZUKI, TOSHIKI WATANABE,
KAZUNARI YAMAGUCHI, KAZUO TAJIMA

Human T-lymphotropic virus type I (HTLV-I) is a human retrovirus that is highly endemic in some regions of the globe and known to be a causative agent of HTLV-I related disorders, such as T-cell malignancies (adult T-cell leukemia and T-cell lymphoma [ATL]),* progressive myelopathy (HTLV-I myelopathy)† and uveitis (HTLV-I uveitis).‡ Retroviruses are single-stranded RNA viruses, encoding for an RNA-dependent DNA polymerase (reverse transcriptase), which translates the viral RNA into a DNA provirus, which in turn is rapidly integrated into the cell genome.[10]

Retroviruses are classified into two subfamilies, that is, oncoviruses and lentiviruses. Oncoviruses are associated with hematologic proliferations and tumors of the connective tissues in many animal species. In humans this subfamily is represented by HTLV-I. Recent studies have found a related virus, HTLV type II (HTLV-II), although the relevance of HTLV-II to human diseases is not proved. The second subfamily of retroviruses, lentiviruses, induce chronic and progressive pulmonary and/or neurologic diseases in a number of animal species. In humans this subfamily is represented by a lentivirus previously known as HTLV-III, which has been shown to be the causative agent of acquired immunodeficiency syndrome (AIDS) and is now named human immunodeficiency virus (HIV-1 and HIV-2).[10]

Retroviruses have existed from ancient times, but the diseases caused by these human retroviruses have been recognized only since the early 1980s. Evidence indicating the significant role of these viruses in human diseases has been forthcoming from clinical and basic research employing epidemiologic, virologic, immunologic, and molecular biologic techniques. These studies have provided important insights into the profound health implications of the human retroviruses. This fact is also true in ophthalmology, where recent reports have shown a variety of ocular manifestations of HTLV-I–related diseases (adult T-cell leukemia and HTLV-I myelopathy) and a pathogenic role of HTLV-I in a specific type of uveitis in asymptomatic carriers of the virus (HTLV-I uveitis).

HISTORICAL BACKGROUND

The discovery of ATL ushered in some dramatic developments in oncology and, unexpectedly, in neurology and ophthalmology. The disease was first internationally recognized in 1977 by Takatsuki and associates.[96,101] HTLV (human T-cell leukemia virus), the pathogen of ATL, was first reported by Gallo's group in 1980.[69] They isolated HTLV from cultured cells taken from one patient with an aggressive variant of mycosis fungoides and from another with Sézary syndrome. Although both patients were said to have cutaneous T-cell lymphoma, they had some unusual features which, in retrospect, link them to the clinical entity now called ATL.

In Japan, Miyoshi and associates[43] established the first cell line MT-1 from an ATL patient, then successfully cocultured ATL cells with umbilical cord blood lymphocytes and obtained the type C retrovirus high-producing cell line MT-2. Hinuma and associates[18] demonstrated that ATL patients have antibodies against presumed viral antigens ATLA (ATL-associated antigens) on MT-1 cells. Subsequently a retrovirus was isolated, characterized, and named ATLV (adult T-cell leukemia virus) by Yoshida and associates.[116] Since it was shown that HTLV and ATLV are, in fact, identical,[105] the term HTLV-I has been commonly used.[81,106]

Immediately after the discovery of ATL and HTLV-I, the acquired immunodeficiency syndrome (AIDS) began to be recognized, and a retrovirus, the human immunodeficiency virus (HIV), was also found to be a causative agent in this disease. The advances made in the worldwide study of AIDS owe much to the knowledge gained during the studies to

---

*References 18, 44, 69, 70, 91, 94, 97, 101, 105, 106.
†References 5, 7, 13, 27, 29, 58, 64-69, 75, 100.
‡References 3, 22, 38, 45-49, 57, 63, 77, 87, 113, 120, 121.

identify the relation between ATL and HTLV-I. For example, almost identical methods for isolation of HTLV-I were used for isolation of HIV.

Following the initial description of ATL and discovery of HTLV-I, the virus was shown to be associated with other human diseases. The most extensively described of these is a chronic neurologic disorder known as tropical spastic paraparesis/HTLV-I–associated myelopathy (TSP/HAM or HTLV-I myelopathy).[37,112] Recent studies by Mochizuki and associates* have demonstrated that the virus is also significantly associated with a specific type of uveitis, which is now considered to be the third clinical entity caused by the virus and called HTLV-I uveitis.

EPIDEMIOLOGY

Geographic Distribution

According to the evidence obtained from the biennial nationwide surveillance of ATL caused by HTLV-I in Japan, the annual incidence of ATL was estimated to be 700 in Japan (Table 98-1).[94] As shown in Fig. 98-1, ATL patients have been observed throughout Japan, mostly in the coastal areas along the Pacific Ocean. More than 50% of ATL cases were distributed in Kyushu, 10% in Hokkaido and Tohoku, and 25% in metropolitan cities, that is, Tokyo, Osaka, and Nagoya. One of the most important epidemiologic features of ATL in Japan is the geographic distribution of the birthplaces of ATL patients. Most of those registered in metropolitan areas had been born and brought up in Kyushu and southern Shikoku, which is the most endemic area of ATL in Japan. The geographic distribution of ATL is consistently related to the distribution of HTLV-I carriers; it is estimated that there are approximately 1.2 million HTLV-I carriers in Japan and those are found mainly among people in the endemic areas of ATL (Fig. 98-2). Corresponding to the geographic distribution of ATL patients, patients with other HTLV-I associated diseases—for example, chronic myelopathy (HTLV-I myelopathy), uveitis without defined causes (HTLV-I uveitis), chronic and/or interstitial bronchitis (HAB)—have been detected in the HTLV-I epidemic areas.

The worldwide geographic and ethnologic distribution of HTLV-I was reviewed in 1992.[90] Outside of Japan, HTLV-I carriers have very rarely been detected in Asian countries. In the Philippines a hunting-gathering people (the Aeta group) even now carry HTLV-I. It was recently reported that several percent of indigenous people in northern Iran and southern India were carriers. In Oceania, HTLV-I carriers were detected among Melanesians in Australia, Papua New Guinea, the Solomon Islands, and Vanuatu. In Africa, carriers of HTLV-I are clustered in the central and western equa-

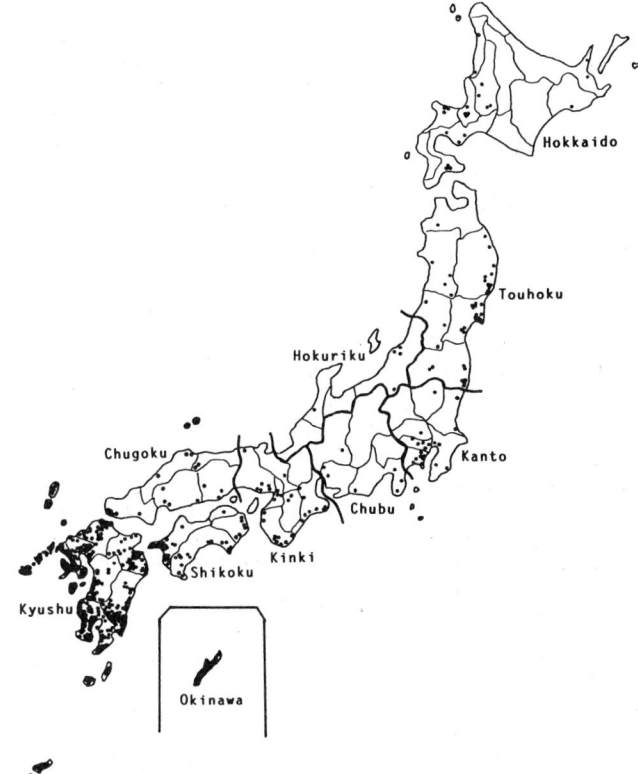

Fig. 98-1. Geographic distribution of 654 patients with ATL in Japan (1986-87). Each dot indicates one patient. (From Tajima K, T- and B-cell malignancy study group: The 4th nationwide study of adult T-cell leukemia/lymphoma (ATL in Japan): estimates of risk of ATL and its geographical and clinical features, *Int J Cancer* 45:237-243, 1990.)

torial countries. In North African and European countries very few carriers of HTLV-I were detected. In America, HTLV-I carriers fall into two groups, Amerindians and African Americans. Among Amerindians in South America, HTLV-I carriers are mainly clustered in Andean groups, but not in groups living along the Amazon and Orinoco rivers.

Age and Sex Distribution

The age of onset of ATL in Japan is over 25 and more than 90% of ATL patients are over 40 years old (Table 98-2).[94] The chronologic increment of the average age of ATL patients is observed, that is, 52 years in 1980 and 59 years in 1988. Sex discrepancy in the average age of ATL patients was not observed though the age mode was younger in males than in females. The age-specific incidence rate of ATL increased steeply with age between 40 and 70 years of age and then decreased in both sexes.

From a cross-sectional seroepidemiologic survey on HTLV-I carriers in Tsushima Island, the rate of HTLV-I carriers among healthy people increased with age and was remarkably higher in females (28.7%) than in males (21.5%) older than 30 years of age (Table 98-3),[95] especially in the

*References 3, 22, 38, 45-49, 57, 63, 77, 87, 113, 120, 121.

TABLE 98-1   NATIONAL SURVEILLANCE OF ADULT T-CELL LEUKEMIA/
LYMPHOMA CAUSED BY HTLV-1 1986-87

District	Population (100,000)	Hospitals (>200 Beds)	Estimated Number Carrier	Estimated Number ATL	Registered Number of ATL Residence	Registered Number of ATL Birth
Hokkaido/Tohoku	154.3 (12.8)	201 (15.7)	108,000	65 (9.3)	58 (8.8)	62 (9.5)
Hokuriku/San-in	69.8 (5.8)	91 (7.1)	24,400	15 (2.0)	12 (1.8)	16 (2.4)
Kanto	366.5 (30.4)	305 (23.9)	128,300	77 (11.0)	70 (10.7)	19 (2.9)
Chubu	164.8 (13.7)	160 (12.5)	57,700	35 (5.0)	29 (4.4)	12 (1.8)
Kinki	60.4 (5.0)	75 (5.9)	21,100	12 (1.7)	12 (1.8)	9 (1.4)
Osaka/Hyougo	135.2 (11.2)	153 (12.0)	141,900	85 (12.2)	77 (11.7)	10 (1.5)
Chugoku/Shikoku	92.9 (7.7)	116 (9.1)	32,500	20 (2.9)	27 (4.1)	17 (2.6)
Kii/South Shikoku	18.7 (1.5)	32 (2.5)	39,300	24 (3.4)	34 (5.2)	52 (8.0)
Kyushu	144.6 (12.0)	154 (12.1)	607,300	364 (52.2)	338 (51.4)	457 (69.9)
Total	1,207.2 (100%)	1,287 (100%)	1,160,500	697 (100%)	657 (100%)	654 (100%)

1: The location of each district in Japan corresponds to that in the map of figure 98-1.
2: The carrier rate of HTLV-I among general population in each district.
3: Annual incidence of ATL in each district was calculated from the incidence rate of 0.6 per 1,000 adult HTLV-I carriers.
4: Three cases were excluded because they were born outside of Japan.
Data source: Tajima K, T- and B-cell malignancy study group: The 4th nationwide study of adult T-cell leukemia/ lymphoma (ATL in Japan): estimates of risk of ATL and its geographical and clinical features, *Int J Cancer* 45:237-243, 1990.

TABLE 98-2   AGE AND SEX DISTRIBUTION OF PATIENTS WITH ADULT
T-CELL LEUKEMIA/LYMPHOMA

Age (Years)	Total Cases	Sex Distribution Male	Sex Distribution Female	Sex Distribution (Ratio)	Proportional Distribution Male	Proportional Distribution Female	Proportional Distribution Total
20-24	2	1	1	(1.00)	0.3	0.3	0.3
25-29	7	5	2	(2.00)	1.7	0.7	1.1
30-34	10	7	3	(2.33)	2.0	1.0	1.5
35-39	39	15	24	(0.63)	4.2	8.1	6.0
40-44	42	20	22	(0.91)	5.6	7.4	6.4
45-49	64	42	22	(1.91)	11.7	7.4	9.8
50-54	83	51	32	(1.59)	14.2	10.8	12.7
55-59	107	60	83	(1.28)	16.8	15.9	16.4
60-64	102	52	50	(1.05)	15.5	16.9	15.6
65-69	82	37	45	(0.82)	10.3	15.3	12.6
70-74	71	44	27	(1.69)	12.3	9.2	10.9
75-79	26	17	9	(1.89)	4.7	3.1	4.0
80-84	12	5	7	(0.71)	1.4	2.4	1.8
85-	6	2	4	(0.50)	0.6	1.4	0.9
Total	653	358	295	(1.21)	100%	100%	100%
40-	595	330 /	265	(1.25)	92.2 /	89.8	91.1

Data source: Tajima K, T- and B-cell malignancy study group: The 4th nationwide study of adult T-cell leukemia/ lymphoma (ATL in Japan): estimates of risk of ATL and its geographical and clinical features, *Int J Cancer* 45:237-243, 1990.

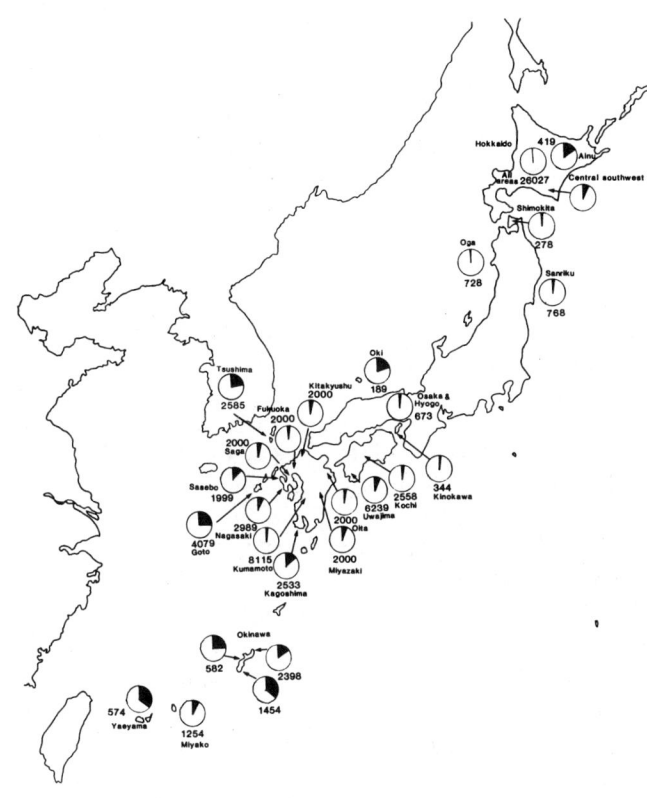

Fig. 98-2. Geographic distribution of HTLV-I carriers in Japan. Shaded part of each circle represents percentage of antibody positives; figures under each circle indicate numbers of subjects tested. (From Tajima K, Hinuma Y: Epidemiology of HTLV-I/II in Japan and the world. In Takatsuki K, Hinuma Y, Yoshida M, editors: *Advances in adult T-cell leukemia and HTLV-I research.* Gann monograph on cancer research, Tokyo, 1992, Japan Scientific Societies Press.)

TABLE 98-3 AGE- AND SEX-SPECIFIC POSITIVE RATE OF ANTI-HTLV-I ANTIBODY AMONG INHABITANTS FROM THE MASS HEALTH SURVEILLANCE AND PATIENTS FROM THE GENERAL HOSPITAL IN TSUSHIMA (1985-87)

Age (Years)	Male			Female		
	Subject	Positives	(%)	Subjects	Positives	(%)
1-4*	349	10	2.9	303	8	2.6
5-9*	316	4	1.3	262	5	1.9
10-14*	198	4	2.0	216	9	4.2
15-19*	81	3	3.7	134	4	3.0
20-24#	—	—	—	667	47	7.0
25-29#	—	—	—	1299	80	6.2
30-34	51	5	9.8	144	23	16.0
35-39	121	25	20.7	256	57	22.3
40-44	179	39	21.8	422	94	22.3
45-49	292	53	18.8	535	119	22.2
50-54	378	79	20.9	713	195	27.3
55-59	420	85	20.2	737	217	29.4
60-64	358	79	22.1	653	190	29.1
65-69	283	60	21.2	481	172	35.8
70-74	220	60	27.3	323	117	36.2
75-79	139	36	25.9	215	77	35.8
80-	68	16	23.5	109	55	50.5
Total	2499	537	21.5	4588	1316	28.7
40-	2327	507	21.8	4188	1236	29.5

* Patients from the general hospital
# Pregnant women
Data source: Tajima K et al.: Ethno-epidemiology of ATL in Japan with special references to the mongoloid dispersal. In Takatsuki K, editor: *Adult T-cell leukemia,* Oxford University Press (in press).

over-40 age group. The incidence of ATL is predominant in males, however, with a 1.2 male-to-female ratio. The rate of HTLV-I carriers was not high among children even in this ATL endemic area.

RISK FACTORS

Transmission Routes of HTLV-I

Distinctive features were observed in the age- and sex-specific distribution of HTLV-I carriers, which showed remarkable discrepancy in HTLV-I carrier rates between two different generation groups, the younger and the older (> 40 years), and between male and female in the older generation (Table 98-3). It is suggested that these findings are associated with the unique transmission routes. From the epidemiologic analysis of family clustering of HTLV-I carriers, the following major transmission routes are suggested[92]: vertical transmission from mother to child, horizontal transmission between husband and wife through sexual contact, and parenteral transmission via blood transfusion.

The most important route is vertical transmission from mother to child. Recent studies have shown that breast feeding poses a risk for HTLV-I transmission from mother to child, particularly from mothers with HTLV-I antigen positive lymphocytes in their breast milk.[30] It has been suggested that HTLV-I infection is caused in part by the transmission through placenta. The detailed mechanism of HTLV-I infection through breast milk and via placenta is not yet clarified, however.

Vertical transmission will have occurred by approximately 1 to 2 years after birth of the child and will remain stable until young adulthood. A prospective 15-year follow-up study showed no change over time from a 3-year-old baby to a 20-year-old young adult.[33] It might be rare for an antibody expression after transmission of HTLV-I to be delayed as long as several decades, and therefore it has been suggested that the seroconversion after vertical transmission of HTLV-I occurs during the first 3 years. The recent study reported that the overall infection rate from carrier mothers to their children (younger than 19 years) was estimated at 10% to 30%.[90,95]

The second important route of natural transmission is horizontal transmission between men and women by sexual contact, both heterosexual primarily from men to women and male homosexual.[6] In terms of the risk of HTLV-I transmission between spouses, the fact that the infected T-cell of the HTLV-I carrier must enter inside the noncarrier's body means that transmission from wife to husband does not easily happen. A study of married couples strongly suggests that HTLV-I is transmitted mainly from husband to wife.[92] The detection of anti-HTLV-I–antibody in semen from carrier males supported the possibility of the one-way transmission of HTLV-I from male to female via semen.[52]

Recently parenteral infection, mostly by blood transfusion, also has become an important transmission route for HTLV-I.[62] It was shown that the average infection rate of HTLV-I by blood transfusion was around 60% to 70% when noncarrier recipients received blood with cell components donated by HTLV-I-carrier donors. In this case dose-response relationship can be seen and fresh blood posed a greater risk of HTLV-I infection than blood stored for one or two weeks before transfusion. Furthermore, no recipients were observed who were infected with HTLV-I after transfusion of cell-free blood components, for example, frozen plasma. Recently the virus has been transmitted among intravenous drug abusers, presumably through the passage of infected blood lymphocytes in shared needles.[34,74]

Risk for HTLV-I–Associated Diseases among Carriers

Adult T-Cell Leukemia/Lymphoma (ATL). As mentioned previously it is estimated that there are approximately 1.2 million HTLV-I carriers in Japan and more than 700 ATL cases occur annually among these carriers.[94] Therefore the incidence of ATL is estimated to reach at least 7000 cases during the next 10 years. Even though a cross-sectional study shows that the positive rate of anti-HTLV antibody is relatively low in children, an effective control strategy for the prevention of HTLV-I infection is required in the ATL endemic areas. Many healthy carriers live in the ATL endemic areas in Japan despite the fact that HTLV-I infection is a main causative agent for ATL manifestation. This fact suggests that HTLV-I infection alone does not necessarily cause the onset of ATL. The annual incidence rate of ATL among HTLV-I carriers older than 40 years is estimated at 0.47 to 1.14 in Kyushu (Table 98-4). The cumulative (life span of 70 years) incidence of ATL among HTLV-I carriers in Japan is estimated at 2.5% (3 to 5% in males and 1 to 2% in females) if competing risks for other diseases are neglected.[90]

HTLV-I Myelopathy. Approximately 1200 patients with HTLV-I myelopathy have been reported in many parts of the world. In Japan a nationwide survey documented more than 700 patients with the disease.[67] The endemic area of HTLV-I myelopathy is consistent with the area where HTLV-I carriers and/or ATL are highly prevalent. Approximately 450 patients with HTLV-I myelopathy have been reported from other countries such as those in the Caribbean basin, South America, and Africa. The disease was also reported among Japanese migrants to Hawaii and Caribbean migrants to the United Kingdom, United States, and France. A strong association of HTLV-I myelopathy with blood transfusion was demonstrated. Familial occurrence has been reported. The incidence of HTLV-I myelopathy among HTLV-I infected persons was estimated at 3.1×10^{-5} cases/year: assuming a lifetime of 75 years, the lifetime incidence is approximately one quarter of 1%. The mean age of onset was 43 years and the male-to-female ratio of occurrence was 1 : 2.9.

TABLE 98-4   ESTIMATED INCIDENCE RATE AMONG 1000 HTLV-I
CARRIERS IN THE ATL ENDEMIC AREAS OF JAPAN

Age (Years)	Tajima (Kyushu) Male & Female	Kondo (Uwajima) Male	Kondo (Uwajima) Female	Tokudome (Saga) Male	Tokudome (Saga) Female
30-	0.23	0.95	0.41	0.00	0.48
40-	0.47	0.83	0.66	1.19	0.63
50-	0.94	2.10	0.33	1.16	0.58
60-	1.14	2.00	0.98	1.20	0.78
>40	0.75	1.50	0.58	1.06	0.61
Cumulative rate in 40-69	24.5	49.3	17.2	35.5	19.7

Data source: Tajima K, Hinuma Y: Epidemiology of HTLV-I/II in Japan and the world. In Takatsuki K, Hinuma Y, Yoshida M, editors: *Advances in adult T-cell leukemia and HTLV-I research:* Gann monograph on cancer research, Tokyo, 1992, Japan Scientific Societies Press.

HTLV-I Uveitis. Because there are no systematic epidemiologic studies of the geographic distribution of HTLV-I uveitis, it is not easy to calculate the annual incidence rate of this disease even in Japan. From the number of patients with HTLV-I uveitis collected by expert clinicians in Japan, the risk for this disease appears to be lower than that of ATL. To assess accurately the risk for HTLV-I uveitis among HTLV-I carriers, however, a more systematic nationwide surveillance is needed.

CLINICAL FEATURES OF HTLV-I UVEITIS

A possible association between HTLV-I infection and uveitis was suggested by many case reports with uveitis in HTLV-I carriers.[32,39,54,59-61] The first set of evidence to indicate the causative implication of HTLV-I in uveitis was reported by Mochizuki and associates,* who showed clinical and laboratory data consisting of seroepidemiology, clinical features, detection of proviral DNA and mRNA of HTLV-I from ocular tissues, and detection of viral particles from T-cell clones derived from the aqueous humor of the patient. The evidence implicating a significant association and pathogenic role of HTLV-I with a specific type of uveitis will be discussed here on the basis of data reported by Mochizuki and associates.

Seroepidemiology

The seroepidemiologic studies were carried out at two hospitals in Kyushu, southwestern Japan: Miyata Eye Hospital at Miyakonojo, located in an HTLV-I endemic area; and Kurume University Hospital at Kurume, located in a less endemic area.[45-48] The subjects of their study were patients with various ocular diseases: patients with uveitis with de-

fined causes (for example, Behçet disease, Vogt-Koyanagi-Harada syndrome, ocular toxoplasmosis, CMV retinitis); patients with uveitis with unknown cause (idiopathic uveitis); patients with nonuveitic ocular diseases such as age-related cataract, retinal detachment, glaucoma, and strabismus at the two hospitals; and some healthy volunteers. Patients with ATL and HTLV-I myelopathy were excluded from their studies.

The seropositivity of HTLV-I in various ocular disorders was examined by the particle agglutination assay and the enzyme-linked immunosorbent assay. Samples positive for HTLV-I by both assays were taken as seropositive and those positive by one of the assays were further analyzed by Western blotting assay. The overall HTLV-I seroprevalence of the tested patients was 23% (157 of 686 patients) in Miyakonojo and 8% (44 of 523 patients) in Kurume.[49] In Miyakonojo the HTLV-I seroprevalence in patients with uveitis with defined cause and that in patients with nonuveitic ocular diseases was 10% (11 of 106 patients) and 19% (75 of 395 patients), respectively. The seroprevalence in both groups increased with the age of the patients (Fig. 98-3).[49] The HTLV-I seroprevalence in the general population in this area (Miyakonojo) was 11.5%[89] and the seroprevalence in the general population is known to increase with age.[93] Therefore the uveitis patients with defined cause and the patients with nonuveitic ocular diseases in the study were considered to reflect the general population in this area. Conversely the seroprevalence of the virus in patients with idiopathic uveitis (38%, 71 of 185 patients) was significantly higher than that in the other two groups (P < 0.01) (Fig. 98-3).[49]

More striking was the age distribution of the HTLV-I seroprevalence in idiopathic uveitis: it was much higher in younger patients (aged 20 through 49 years) with idiopathic uveitis (49%, 37 of 75 patients) than it was in patients with uveitis with defined cause (12%, 6 of 50 patients) or in pa-

---

*References 3, 22, 38, 45-49, 57, 63, 77, 87, 113, 120, 121.

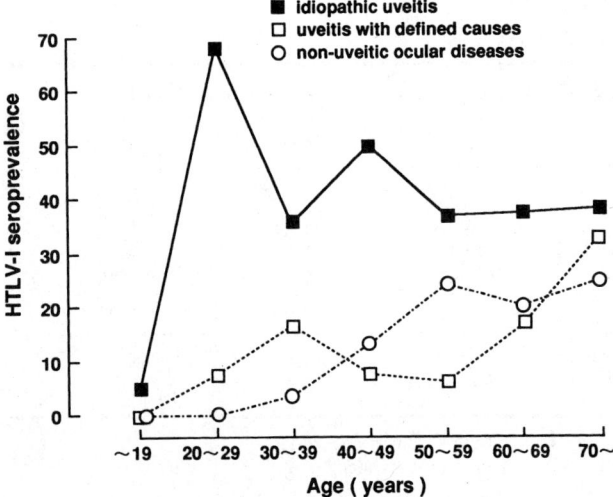

Fig. 98-3. Age distribution of seroprevalence of HTLV-I in HTLV-I endemic area (Miyakonojo). (From Mochizuki M and associates: Human T lymphotropic virus type I uveitis, *Br J Ophthalmol* 78:149-154, 1994.)

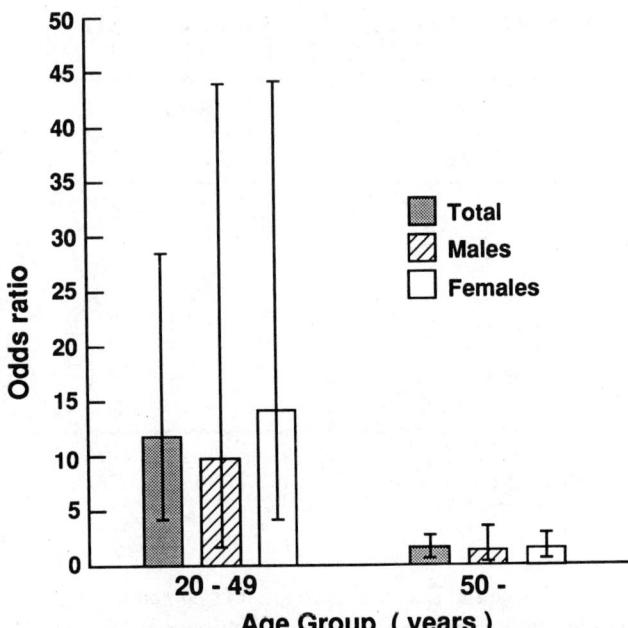

Fig. 98-4. Risk for HTLV-I infection in cases of idiopathic uveitis. (From Mochizuki M et al.: Human T lymphotropic virus type I uveitis, *Br J Ophthalmol* 78:149-154, 1994.)

tients with nonuveitic ocular diseases (6%, 5 of 80 patients) in the same age group.[49] A similar distribution was observed even in the HTLV-I less endemic Kurume. The odds ratio was computed as an estimate of the relative risk of HTLV-I infection in the three groups (Table 98-5). In younger patients (20 to 49 years) the odds ratio of idiopathic uveitis for HTLV-I infection was estimated at 14.6 (95% confidence interval [CI]:5.3 to 40.2) in Miyakonojo and 12.0 (95% CI:1.5 to 95.5) in Kurume. On the other hand, in older patients (≥ 50 years) the odds ratio was much lower: 2.0 (95% CI:1.2 to 3.3) and 1.8 (95% CI:0.7 to 4.4) in Miyakonojo and Kurume, respectively.[49] The odds ratio of uveitis with defined causes for HTLV-I infection in both age groups was very low even in Miyakonojo (Table 98-6). When stratified by sex, it was found in Miyakonojo that the odds ratio of idiopathic uveitis for HTLV-I infection was relatively uniform, estimated at 10.0 (95% CI:2.2 to 45.0) in males and

14.6 (95% CI:4.7 to 45.0) in females in the younger age group. The odds ratio in the older age group was equally low in both sexes: 1.6 (95% CI:0.7 to 3.5) in males and 1.8 (95% CI:1.1 to 3.0) in females (Fig. 98-4).[49]

This epidemiologic finding of a trend for declining odds ratio for HTLV-I with age is important, because the opposite is true for carriers of HTLV-I in the general population. This implies that early exposure to HTLV-I is important, and the uniform odds ratio when stratified by sex suggests that most transmission that is important for uveitogenesis is prenatal. These epidemiologic data indicate that the idiopathic uveitis in asymptomatic carriers of HTLV-I is a distinct clinical entity, like ATL and HTLV-I myelopathy, and it can be named HTLV-I uveitis.

TABLE 98-5 RISK OF HTLV-I INFECTION FOR UVEITIS ACCORDING TO AGE GROUP

| | Miyakonojo | | | | Kurume | | | |
| | 20-49 Years | | ≧ 50 Years | | 20-49 Years | | ≧ 50 Years | |
Disease	+/−[1]	Odds Ratio (95% CI)[2]	+/−	Odds Ratio (95% CI)	+/−	Odds Ratio (95% CI)	+/−	Odds Ratio (95% CI)
Idiopathic uveitis	37/38	14.6 (5.3-40.2)**	33/55	2.0 (1.2-3.3)*	14/41	12.0 (1.5-95.5)*	8/54	1.8 (0.7-4.4)
Uveitis with defined causes	6/44	2.1 (0.6-7.1)	5/42	0.4 (0.2-1.0)	5/68	2.6 (0.3-22.9)	1/35	0.3 (0.0-2.7)
Nonuveitic ocular diseases	5/75	1.0	70/233	1.0	1/35	1.0	14/167	1.0

[1] +/−: HTLV-I seropositive, [2] 95% CI: 95% confidence interval
** P < 0.001, * P < 0.01
From Mochizuki M et al.: Human T lymphotropic virus type I uveitis, *Br J Ophthalmol* 78:149-154, 1994.

TABLE 98-6 RISK OF HUMAN T-CELL LYMPHOTROPIC VIRUS TYPE I
INFECTION FOR INITIAL SYMPTOMS OF IDIOPATHIC UVEITIS

Symptoms	Present antihuman T-cell lymphotropic virus type I antibody		Absent antihuman T-cell lymphotropic virus type I antibody		Odds ratio (95% confidence interval)
	Seropositive patients (*N* = 93)	Seronegative patients (*N* = 222)	Seropositive patients (*N* = 93)	Seronegative patients (*N* = 222)	
Floaters	41	37	52	185	3.94 (2.296-6.769)*
Foggy vision	40	93	53	129	1.05 (0.642-1.708)
Blurring of vision	21	35	72	187	1.56 (0.851-2.855)
Hyperemia of the eye	6	59	87	163	0.19 (0.0790.459)*
Ocular pain	5	34	88	188	0.31 (0.119-0.831)†
Others	9	18	84	204	1.21 (0.524-2.811)

* $P < 0.01$, † $P < 0.05$
From Yoshimura et al.: Clinical and immunological features of human T-cell lymphotropic virus type I uveitis, *Am J Ophthalmol* 116:156-163, 1993.

Although the incidence rate of ATL among 1000 HTLV-I carriers is estimated at 2.0 in males and 0.5 in females, the cumulative risk for ATL in carriers during a 70-year life span is 2.5%, and the lifetime incidence of HTLV-I myelopathy for 75 years is estimated at 0.25%, no such epidemiologic studies on HTLV-I uveitis have been done; this research remains for future investigations. When HTLV-I uveitis is taken as one of the causes of uveitis, the disease is the leading cause in Miyakonojo and the fourth common cause in Kurume (Fig. 98-5).[22]

Clinical Features

The clinical features of 93 patients with idiopathic uveitis who were seropositive for HTLV-I (HTLV-I uveitis) were analyzed.[120] All the patients had no evidence of uveitis with defined cause except for the seropositivity to HTLV-I, even after extensive systemic and ophthalmic examinations and careful determination of the disease history. The onset age of

uveitis distributed from 19 years to 75 years with the mean age of 46 years. The major symptoms at the initial presentation were sudden onset of floaters (44% of the patients), foggy vision (43%), and blurred vision (23%). The inflammation was unilateral (55% of the patients) or bilateral (45%). The ocular signs of the 93 patients consisted of iritis (96%), vitreous opacities (87%), retinal vasculitis (70%), and retinal exudates and hemorrhages (13%). As for the anatomic diagnosis of uveitis according to the criteria of the International Uveitis Study Group,[8] 13 patients (14%) had an anterior uveitis and 56 patients (60%) had an intermediate uveitis in which the vitreous opacities (fine cells and laceworklike membranous opacities) were the most impressive findings and were accompanied by mild iritis and mild retinal vasculitis but no uveoretinal lesions. Two patients (2%) had a posterior uveitis and 22 patients (24%) had a panuveitis. Examples of ophthalmoscopic pictures in HTLV-I uveitis are shown in Fig. 98-6. In summary, HTLV-I uveitis occurs with a sudden onset of floaters, foggy vision, or blurred vision in one eye or both eyes. The uveitis is characterized by moderate or heavy vitreous opacities with mild iritis and mild retinal vasculitis, which can be classified as intermediate uveitis.

These clinical observation simply analyzed the ophthalmic manifestations of uveitis in seropositive patients and had no control group. Yoshimura and associates[120] compared the ophthalmic manifestations of idiopathic uveitis in HTLV-I seropositive patients (HTLV-I uveitis group, *n* = 93) and those in seronegative patients (*n* = 222) as a control group to determine the clinical features of the uveitis associated with HTLV-I. The HTLV-I uveitis group had (1) significantly more female patients, (2) a higher incidence of floaters and lower incidence of hyperemia and ocular pain as initial symptoms (Table 98-6), (3) a higher incidence of vitreous opacities and retinal vasculitis as ocular signs (Table 98-7), and (4) more patients with an intermedi-

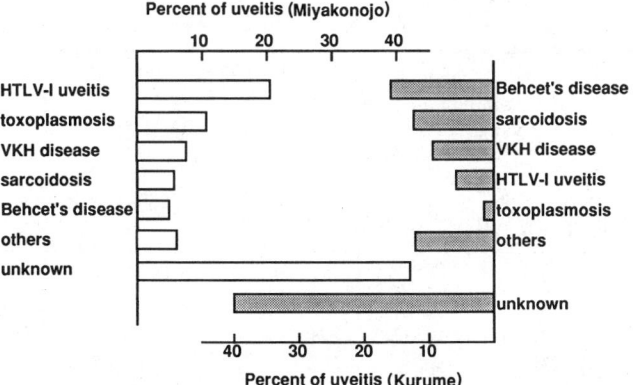

Fig. 98-5. Causes of uveitis in Kurume and Miyakonojo □: patients in Miyakonojo, ■: patients in Kurume. (Data source: Ikeda E et al.: Epidemiological study of uveitis in north Kyushu and south Kyushu, *Jpn J Clin Ophthalmol* 90:11-23, 1993 [in Japanese].)

TABLE 98-7 RISK OF HUMAN T-CELL LYMPHOTROPIC VIRUS TYPE I INFECTION FOR OCULAR FINDINGS OF IOIOPATHIC UVEITIS

Ocular Findings	Present Antihuman T-cell Lymphotropic Virus Type I Antibody		Absent Antihuman T-cell Lymphotropic Virus Type I Antibody		Odds ratio (95% Confidence Interval)
	Seropositive Patients (N = 93)	Seronegative Patients (N = 222)	Seropositive Patients (N = 93)	Seronegative Patients (N = 222)	
(1) Anterior segment					
Cells and flare	89	220	4	2	0.20 (0.036-1.124)
Keratic precipitates					
Fine	69	155	24	67	1.24 (0.720-2.145)
Muttonfat-like	10	41	83	181	0.53 (0.254-1.113)
Iris nodules	25	49	68	173	1.30 (0.743-2.267)
Anterior synechia	9	46	84	176	0.41 (0.192-0.877)†
Posterior synechia	5	46	88	176	0.21 (0.083-0.566)*
(2) Vitreous body					
Vitreous opacities	81	121	12	101	5.63 (2.908-10.915)*
Membranous	52	41	41	181	5.59 (3.291-9.527)*
Fine cells	22	61	71	161	0.82 (0.466-1.434)
Snowball-like	15	24	78	198	1.59 (0.791-3.183)
(3) Ocular fundus					
Retinal vasculitis	65	86	28	136	3.67 (2.185-6.168)*
Chorioretinal exudates	10	40	83	182	0.55 (0.262-1.149)
Retinal hemorrhages	2	23	91	199	0.19 (0.044-0.824)†
Cystoid macular edema	7	12	86	210	1.42 (0.543-3.740)
Hyperemia of optic disc	12	29	81	193	0.99 (0.479-2.028)

* P < 0.01, † P < 0.05

From Yoshimura et al.: Clinical and immunological features of human T-cell lymphotropic virus type I uveitis, *Am J Ophthalmol* 116:156-163, 1993.

ate uveitis and fewer patients with an anterior uveitis (Table 98-8).

Yamaguchi and associates[113] reported an interesting observation in HTLV-I uveitis patients, that is, an association with Graves disease. Sixteen of 93 patients with HTLV-I uveitis (17%) had a previous history of Graves disease. Fifteen patients were female (15/60, 25% of females) and one was male (1/33, 3% of males). Interestingly, uveitis occurred after the onset of Graves disease in all cases. On the other hand, none of 222 seronegative patients with idio-

TABLE 98-8 RISK OF HTLV-I INFECTION AS A CAUSE OF IDIOPATHIC UVEITIS BY ANATOMIC SITE

Anatomical Site (Anatomical Diagnosis)	Present Antihuman T-cell Lymphotropic Virus Type I Antibody		Absent Antihuman T-cell Lymphotropic Virus Type I Antibody		Odds ratio (95% Confidence Interval)
	Seropositive Patients (N = 93)	Seronegative Patients (N = 222)	Seropositive Patients (N = 93)	Seronegative Patients (N = 222)	
Anterior uveitis	13	104	80	118	0.18 (0.097-0.351)*
Intermediate uveitis	56	53	37	169	4.83 (2.877-8.096)*
Posterior uveitis	2	1	91	221	4.86 (0.435-54.233)
Panuveitis	22	64	71	158	0.77 (0.437-1.399)

* P < 0.01

From Yoshimura et al.: Clinical and immunological features of human T-cell lymphotropic virus type I uveitis, *Am J Ophthalmol* 116:156-163, 1993.

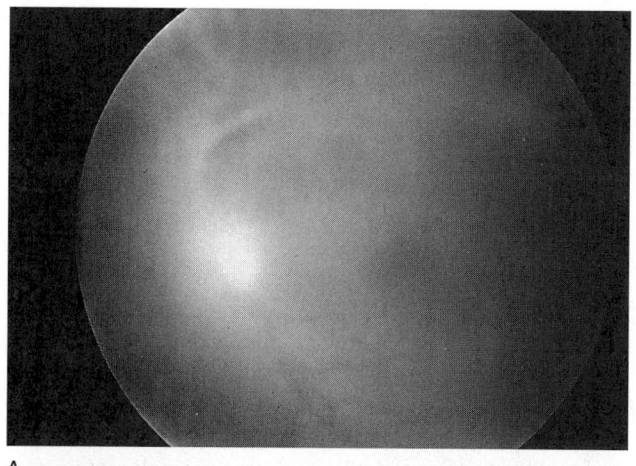

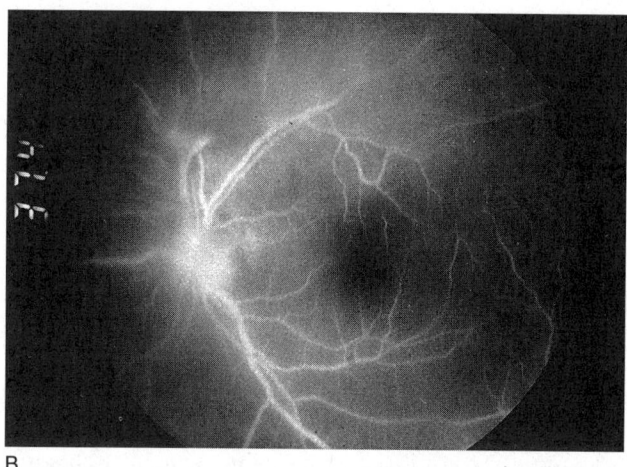

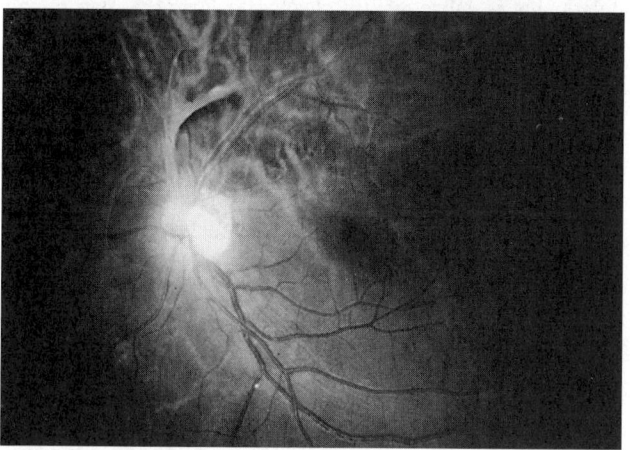

Fig. 98-6. Ocular fundus picture of HTLV-I uveitis (25-year-old man). Patient complained of sudden onset of floaters and blurring vision in left eye. **A,** Fundus picture showing heavy vitreous opacities and retinal vasodilation in left eye at initial presentation (visual acuity: 20/60). **B,** Fluorescein angiography of eye demonstrating dye leakage from retinal blood vessels **C,** Fundus picture of same eye after treatment with topical and systemic corticosteroids showing marked improvement of uveitis (visual acuity: 20/20).

pathic uveitis had a history of Graves disease. Reasons for the correlation between HTLV-I uveitis and Graves disease are not yet known, but this finding suggests that some immune-mediated mechanisms are involved in HTLV-I uveitis.

Another noteworthy observation in the patients with HTLV-I uveitis is the familial clustering of the disease. Araki and associates[3] have found two familial cases: (1) a 62-year-old woman and her 66-year-old sister and (2) a 52-year-old woman and her 26-year-old daughter. All the patients were suffering from uveitis characterized by dense vitreous opacities with mild iritis and mild retinal vasculitis and had negative results of systemic and ophthalmologic examinations except for seropositive response to HTLV-I. None of the patients had ever received a blood transfusion and their husbands were seronegative for HTLV-I, suggesting that the transmission of the virus to the patients was from their mothers, probably via breast-feeding.

Diagnostic Criteria

The diagnosis of HTLV-I uveitis is based on the seropositivity for HTLV-I with no systemic evidence of HTLV-I-

related diseases (ATL and HTLV-I myelopathy) and exclusion of other uveitis entities with defined cause. Therefore all clinical entries of uveitis with defined cause should be excluded by careful determination of the disease history and routine examinations for uveitis, that is, visual acuity, intraocular pressure by applanation tonometry, slit-lamp biomicroscopy, gonioscopy, direct or indirect ophthalmoscopy, and fluorescein angiography. The routine systemic examinations include peripheral blood analysis, blood chemistry, thoracic roentgenogram, tuberculin skin test, serologic test for syphilis, toxoplasmosis and HTLV-I, and angiotensin-converting enzyme. If the serologic test for HTLV-I is positive, careful hematologic and neurologic examinations are needed to differentiate HTLV-I uveitis from two other HTLV-I-related diseases, that is, ATL and HTLV-I myelopathy. A transbronchial lung biopsy, an examination of cerebrospinal fluid, neurologic tests, and analysis of HLA antigens are recommended in case of need. HTLV-I uveitis patients should not have systemic symptoms that are compatible with other types of uveitis, such as Behçet disease (oral aphthous ulcer, skin lesions, genital ulceration), Vogt-

Koyanagi-Harada syndrome (headache, alopecia, dysacusia), ankylosing spondylitis (back pain) and sarcoidosis (skin lesions).

PATHOGENESIS

Molecular Virology

Classification. HTLV-I is one member of the class of retroviruses that include bovine leukemia virus (BLV),[76] simian T-cell leukemia virus (STLV),[107,108] and HTLV-II.[83] These viruses have been taxonomically grouped within the oncovirus subfamily of the Retroviridae and are distinct from the other pathogenic human retrovirus, the AIDS viruses (HIV),[103] which are classified as members of the lentivirus subfamily of retroviruses. Some of the biologic properties and the molecular structure of viruses in the HTLV-I/HTLV-II/BLV group of retroviruses are quite distinct from those of other members of the oncovirus subfamily of retroviruses. Although these are oncogenic and transforming viruses, they do not harbor oncogene sequences derived from the cellular genome,[81] and their replication is regulated by at least two other genes known as tax and rex.[23,88] Thus it may be appropriate to group these viruses into a separate subfamily.

Genetic Structure of HTLV-I. The genetic structure of the HTLV-I is similar to that of other retroviruses, with the major virion proteins encoded 5'-gag-pol-env-3' (Fig. 98-7).[81] In addition to the usual complement of gag, pol, and env genes, however, there is a region at the 3' end of the genome not found in other replication-competent retroviruses. Initially this region was referred to as the pX region because of its unknown function. Two new genes have now been identified within this region, tax gene and rex gene. The tax gene encodes a protein (Tax1) that is responsible for transcriptional activation of the long terminal repeat (LTR).[88] The rex protein (Rex1) is encoded in a partially overlapping region of tax and has been shown to regulate gene expression posttranscriptionally, accumulating the unspliced or singly spliced form of the HTLV-I mRNA.[25]

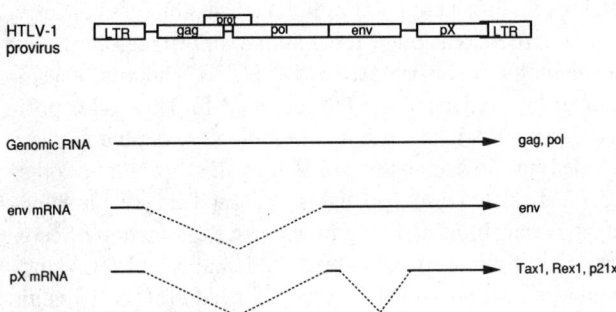

Fig. 98-7. Structure and expression of HTLV-I gene. **A,** Schematic organization of the HTLV-I provirus genome. **B,** Three major species of transcribed mRNA and proteins encoded by them.

Three mRNA species have been identified for HTLV-I (Fig. 98-7). Similar to the other retroviruses the full length RNA, transcribed from the U3-R junction in the 5'LTR and terminating at the R-U5 junction in the 3'LTR, is utilized for synthesis of gag and pol gene products and is also utilized as the genomic RNA packaged into virions. A subgenomic mRNA (env mRNA) where one intron is spliced out encodes the env gene product. A second subgenomic mRNA (pX mRNA) has an additional intron removed and encodes both Tax1 and Rex1.[82] The tax gene methionine initiation codon is the same as that for env and is contained within the second exon of the mRNA. The initiation codon for Rex1 is also located within the second exon but is 59 nucleotides upstream.

The gag region is initially translated as a polyprotein precursor that is subsequently cleaved to form the mature gag polypeptides. There are three of these, comprising 19-kilodalton (kD), 24-kD and 15-kD products (p19, p24 and p15, respectively).[15] By homology to other retroviruses, these three proteins are believed to comprise the matrix, capsid, and nucleocapsid proteins, respectively. Like other retrovirus gag products the p19 is posttranslationally modified and contains myristic acid at the NH2 terminal. At the 3' end, the gag-open reading frame overlaps the 5' end of the reading frame that encodes the protease (Fig. 98-7).[25] In HTLV-I the protease is encoded by a different reading frame that spans the 3' part of the gag region and 5' part of the pol region. Synthesis of the protease as part of the gag polyprotein precursor is likely to be accomplished by ribosomal frameshifting. The protease was shown to be responsible for processing the mature gag products and for generating the mature protease molecule by autocatalysis.

The polymerase region contains the largest open reading frame in the HTLV-I genome, potentially able to encode an 896-amino-acid product. As the 5' end of the pol gene is overlapped by the protease gene, a second ribosomal frameshifting event is necessary to express the pol gene. Based on homology with other retroviruses, the 5' portion of the pol gene is predicted to encode the reverse transcriptase protein, and sequences further downstream are predicted to encode probable integrase and RNAse H functions. HTLV-I reverse transcriptase functions most efficiently using Mg^{2+} rather than Mn^{2+} as the required divalent cation.

The env gene product is a glycosylated polyprotein of 61 to 69 kD. The nonglycosylated precursor is 54 kD. This protein is cleaved into the mature products, the 46-kD surface glycoprotein (gp46) and 21-kD transmembrane (p21).[25]

Two unique nonvirion proteins, Tax1 and Rex1, are translated from pX mRNA (Fig. 98-7). Tax1 is located in the nucleus of the infected cells in the region operationally defined as the nuclear matrix. It is a transacting transcriptional transactivator that increases the rate of transcription initiation from the promotor located in the 5'LTR of the provirus genome. It has been shown that Tax1 is capable of transacti-

TRANSACTIVATION OF CELLULAR GENES BY TAX1
Genes
1. IL-2 (interleukin-2)
2. IL-2Rα (interleukin-2 receptor alpha chain)
3. IL-3 (interleukin-3)
4. IL-4 (interleukin-4)
5. GM-CSF (granulocyte-macrophage colony-stimulating factor)
6. c-fos
7. globin genes
8. TGF β-1 (transforming growth factor beta-1)
9. PTHrP (parathyroid hormone-related protein)
10. EGR-1, -2 (early growth responsive gene-1, -2)

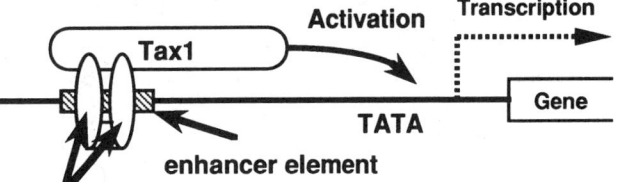

Fig. 98-8. Transcriptional transactivation by HTLV-I Tax 1: schematic illustration of model for mechanism of transactivation of gene expression by Tax 1 in collaboration with cellular transcriptional factors.

vating heterologous promotors in addition to its own LTR. To date various cellular and viral promotors have been shown to be transactivated by Tax1 (box).*

Tax1 does not bind directly to the promotor sequence and acts on the promoters through the interaction with cellular transcriptional factors (Fig. 98-8). The rex gene of HTLV-I encodes proteins of 27 and 21 kD, Rex1 and p21^X, respectively.[31] They share the carboxy-terminal portion. The protein p21^X is synthesized from an internal methionine initiation codon. Rex1 is localized to the nucleus and is phosphorylated. Rex1 has been shown to increase the ratio of the genomic and env mRNA to pX mRNA acting at a posttranscriptional level. Of the three species of the viral mRNA, the pX mRNA is first expressed followed by abundant expression of all the three messages as a result of transactivation by Tax1. In 48 hours the amount of pX mRNA decreases through the effect of Rex1, leaving a prolonged low level of expression of genomic and env mRNA. Nonstructural proteins encoded in the pX region thus control the efficient replication of HTLV-I.[115]

Transactivation Mechanism. The molecular mechanism by which Tax1 transactivates gene expression has been the focus of research. In the transactivation of HTLV-I gene expression, the three repeats of 21bp sequence in the U3 region of LTR was shown to work as the enhancer.[84] Because Tax1 does not bind to DNA directly, some cellular factors bind to the 21bp motif and interact with Tax1, transactivating transcription. Some of these factors with leucine-zipper structure have been cloned by the Southwestern blot technique using the 21bp oligomer as a probe.[122] Their function is now being investigated.

The molecular mechanism of transactivation of cellular genes by Tax1 has also been studied extensively. Tax1 responsive elements were shown to be those of cellular tran-

scription factors characterized previously including NFκB (nuclear factor) element and AP-1 sites.[1,35] They are so diverse that no consensus Tax1 responsive element has been identified, which suggests that a variety of cellular transcriptional factors could cooperate with Tax1. In the absence of growth stimulation, Tax1 transactivates the expression of immediate early genes such as c-fos, EGR-1 and EGR-2, through interaction with p67^{SRF} (serum responsive factor) that bind to an element containing specific nucleodite sequence, CArG box.[12] This mechanism may be one of the main reasons for the abnormal proliferation of the infected cells including nonlymphoid cells.

Transformation of Cells by HTLV-I. HTLV-I will immortalize normal human peripheral blood T cells in vitro, resulting in continuous proliferation in the absence of exogenous IL-2.[44,71] The transformed cells are mostly CD4+ phenotype with surface markers of activated T cells and produce a wide spectrum of cytokines including IL-1, IL-3, IFN-γ, GM-CSF, and PTHrP.[41-42,104,109,114] It was reported that IL-2 independent immortalization of T cells is mediated by Tax1, which is explained by acquisition of IL-2:IL-2R autocrine mechanism through transactivation of these genes. Moreover, fibroblast cell lines were transformed by Tax1 to show anchorage-independent growth and tumor formation in nude mice.[99] For transformation of primary fibroblasts, it was demonstrated that Tax1 needs cooperation with EJ-ras oncogene.[72] These results show a mechanism of cellular transformation other than IL-2:IL-2R autocrine system.

Tropism of HTLV-I Infection. Other than lymphocytes, various types of cells (such as fibroblasts, epithelial cells, and endothelial cells) were shown to be infected with HTLV-I in vitro by cocultivating with x-ray irradiated virus producing cell lines.* Productive infection with HTLV-I has been shown only in a few cells of nonlymphoid origin such as fibrosarcoma cells, kidney epithelial cells, fibroblasts, and endothelial cells.[9,21,119] in vivo target cells are not well characterized, however. CD4+ T-cells have been shown to be the main target cells,[73] while there are evidences for in-

---

*References 2, 11, 24, 41, 42, 79, 109.

*References 9, 18, 19, 21, 24, 50, 119.

fection of B-cells.[36] Infection of HTLV-I is thought to be mediated by a cellular receptor, but the receptor has not yet been identified. A study using hybrid cells and VSV pseudotypes suggested that the infection was encoded by a gene on the chromosome 17.[84]

NATURAL HISTORY

HTLV-I–Associated Diseases

Adult T-Cell Leukemia/Lymphoma (ATL)

Etiology. The causal association of HTLV-I is based on the following observations: (1) the areas of high incidence of ATL correspond closely with those of high prevalence of HTLV-I infection as extensively studied in Japan; (2) HTLV-I immortalizes human CD4 T cells; (3) HTLV-I proviral DNA was demonstrated in ATL neoplastic cells; and (4) all individuals with ATL have antibodies against HTLV-I. HTLV-I is therefore the first retrovirus directly associated with human malignancy.

Clinical Features. The following summarizes current knowledge about ATL:[112]

1. The disease occurs in adults. The age at the onset ranges from the 20s to the 80s, with an average at 58 years. The male-to-female ratio is 1.4 : 1.

2. The predominant physical findings at the onset are peripheral lymph node enlargement (60%), hepatomegaly (26%), splenomegaly (22%), and skin lesions (39%). Hypercalcemia (32%) is frequently associated with ATL. Other symptoms are abdominal pain, diarrhea, pleural effusion, ascites, cough, sputum, and abnormal shadow on chest x-ray films.

3. The white blood cell (WBC) count ranges from normal to 500×10^9/liter. Leukemic cells resemble Sézary cells, having indented or lobulated nuclei. The surface phenotype of ATL cells characterized by monoclonal antibodies is CD3+, CD4+, CD8−, and CD25+, and CD7 is typically absent.[16] Some patients have a mixed phenotype of CD4+/CD8+, and very rarely, CD8 alone. The unusual phenotypes of ATL cells have been reported to be associated with poor prognosis as compared with the cases with the typical cell surface phenotype.

4. The survival time in acute and lymphoma-type ATL ranges from 2 weeks to more than 1 year. Causes of death are pulmonary complications including *Pneumocystis carinii* pneumonia, hypercalcemia,[109] cryptococcal meningitis, disseminated herpes zoster, and disseminated intravascular coagulopathies.

5. All patients were positive for antiHTLV-I antibody and leukemia/lymphoma cells contained monoclonally integrated HTLV-I proviral DNA,[111] although the integration site varied among individuals.

These features and the clinical course, ATL subtype, frequency of hypercalcemia and opportunistic infections, cell morphology, phenotypic profile, and response to treatment appear to be the same for Japanese, Caribbean, and African ATL patients. The only difference is age at onset: the average for the Caribbean and African ATL patients is 43 years (range 19 to 62), whereas that of Japanese patients at diagnosis is older.

Classification and Diagnostic Criteria for Clinical Subtype. Shimoyama and members of the Lymphoma Study Group (1984 to 1987) proposed the following diagnostic criteria for classifying 818 cases of ATL collected in a nationwide survey in Japan into four clinical subtypes: smoldering, chronic, lymphoma, and acute type (Table 98-9).[86]

1. Smoldering type, 5% or more abnormal lymphocytes of T-cell nature in peripheral blood (PB), normal lymphocyte level ($< 4 \times 10^9$/liter), no hypercalcemia, LDH value of up to $1.5 \times$ the normal upper limit, no lymphadenopathy, no involvement of other organs. Skin and pulmonary lesion(s) may be present. In patients with less than 5% abnormal T-lymphocytes in PB, at least one histologically-proven skin or pulmonary lesion should be present.[110]

2. Chronic type, absolute lymphocytosis (4×10^9/liter or more) with T-lymphocytosis more than 3.5×10^9/liter; LDH value up to twice the normal upper limit; no hypercalcemia; no involvement of CNS, bone, or gastrointestinal tract; and neither ascites nor pleural effusion. Lymphadenopathy and involvement of liver, spleen, skin, and lung may be present.

3. Lymphoma type, no lymphocytosis, 1% or less abnormal T-lymphocytes, and histologically-proven lymphadenopathy with or without extranodal lesions.

4. Acute type, remaining ATL patients who have the usual leukemic manifestation and tumor lesions but do not fall into any of the three other types.

Therapy. The results of ATL treatment in the past have been unfavorable. In general, patients with acute and lymphoma-type ATL should be treated with combination chemotherapy such as CHOP, VEPA or COMLA directed toward achieving a cure. Those patients showing hypercalcemia, high LDH levels, and an abnormal increase in white blood cells, however, have a 50% survival time of less than 6 months.[85] Patients often die of severe respiratory infection or hypercalcemia. Analysis of the data of the clinical trials conducted in Japan revealed that three prognostic factors—high LDH levels, highly leukemic state, and poor performance status—were significantly associated with poor response and survival rates of patients with ATL. On the other hand, regardless of treatment, chronic and smoldering-type ATL have a longer course. Aggressive chemotherapy may induce severe respiratory infection. Therefore an independent treatment protocol for chronic and smoldering-type ATL, different from that for acute and lymphoma-type ATL, must be established. In light of the disappointing results from conventional combination chemotherapy, new approaches to the treatment of ATL should be developed.

HTLV-I Myelopathy (Tropical Spastic Paraparesis). The association of tropical spastic paraparesis (TSP) with HTLV-I was first demonstrated in 1985 when a serologic

TABLE 98-9   DIAGNOSTIC CRITERIA FOR CLINICAL SUBTYPE OF ADULT T-CELL LEUKEMIA/LYMPHOMA

	Smouldering	Chronic	Lymphoma	Acute
Anti-HTLV-I antibody	+	+	+	+
Lymphocyte ($\times 10^9$/l)	<4	≥4[a]	<4	*
Abnormal T-lymphocytes	≥5%	+[b]	≤1%	+[b]
Flower cells of T-cell marker	Occasionally	Occasionally	No	+
LDH	≤1.5N	≤2N	*	*
Corrected CA (mmol/l)	<2.74	<2.74	*	*
Histology—proven lymphadenopathy	No	*	+	*
Tumor lesion				
Skin	**	*	*	*
Lung	**	*	*	*
Lymph node	No	*	Yes	*
Liver	No	*	*	*
Spleen	No	*	*	*
CNS	No	No	*	*
Bone	No	No	*	*
Ascites	No	No	*	*
Pleural effusion	No	No	*	*
GI tract	No	No	*	*

N, normal upper limit; GI, gastrointestinal.
* No essential qualification except terms required for other subtype(s), ** No essential qualification if other terms are fulfilled, but histology-prove malignant lesion(s) is required in case abnormal T-lymphocytes are less than 5% in peripheral blood.
[a] Accompanied by T-lymphocytosis (3.5 × 10^9/1 or more).[b] In case abnormal T-lymphocytes are less than 5% in peripheral blood, histology-proved tumor lesion is required.
From Shimoyama M, members of lymphoma study group: Diagnostic criteria and classification of clinical subtypes of adult T-cell leukemia lymphoma, *Br J Hematol* 79:428-439, 1991.

study in Martinique found that 59% of patients with TSP had antibodies to HTLV-I.[13] Other independent work also found an association between HTLV-I and spastic paraparesis (HTLV-I–associated myelopathy).[64] The two diseases are now considered identical. Very recently Hollsberg and Hafler[20] reported a review article on pathogenesis of diseases induced by human lymphotropic virus type I infection and they referred to these two diseases as HTLV-I myelopathy. Here the neurologic diseases are also referred to as HTLV-I myelopathy.

Clinical Features. The clinical and laboratory guidelines for the diagnosis of HTLV-I myelopathy are summarized in box.[68] The main neurologic features of HTLV-I myelopathy consist of the following: spasticity and/or hyperreflexia of lower extremities in 98%, urinary bladder disturbance in 94%, lower extremity muscle weakness in 88%, sensory disturbances in 56%, and cerebellar ataxia in 5%. The incubation period (from infection to onset) is assumed to be months, years, or decades.

Patients with HTLV-I myelopathy have high antibody titers of HTLV-I both in serum and CSF. Abnormal "flowerlike" lymphocytes can be seen in 1% of peripheral lymphocytes. In MRI, high signals of T2-weighted spin echo are observed in the white matter of the brain similar to those found in multiple sclerosis.

Pathology. Autopsies of cases mostly reveal severe involvement of the thoracic spinal cord. Histopathologic studies include mononuclear cell infiltration, marked myelin and axonal destruction, and astrocytic gliosis. Immunocytochemical staining of spinal cords suggests that immune responses in the spinal cord lesions of the patients gradually change along with the duration of illness. CD4, CD8 cells and macrophages were evenly distributed in active-chronic inflammatory lesions. In contrast the predominance of CD8 cells in inactive-chronic inflammatory lesions were noted.

Because the viruses detected from the lymphocytes of ATL and HTLV-I myelopathy are identical,[118] the host factors including HLA may therefore play important roles in the immunogenesis. High immune responsiveness against HTLV-I, such as high levels of HTLV-I antibodies in serum and cerebrospinal fluid (links to specific HLA haplotypes), has been demonstrated, suggesting that host factors are important in determining susceptibility to HTLV-I myelopathy.

Therapy. No specific treatment is known for HAM/TSP. Oral prednisolone showed a transient beneficial effect in some patients with HAM/TSP. Intrathecal hydrocortisone, intravenous methylprednisolone, plasmapheresis, α-interferon, oral azathioprine, and danazol have been tried and also show transient effects.

DIAGNOSTIC GUIDELINES FOR HUMAN T-LYMPHOTROPIC VIRUS TYPE I-ASSOCIATED MYELOPATHY/TROPICAL SPASTIC PARAPARESIS (WHO, 1989)

I. Clinical diagnosis

The florid clinical picture of chronic spastic paraparesis is not always seen when the patient first presents. A single symptom or physical sign may be the only evidence of early HAM/TSP.

A. Age and sex incidence

Mostly sporadic and adult, but sometimes familial; occasionally seen in childhood; females predominant.

B. Onset

Usually insidious but may be sudden.

C. Main neurological manifestations

1. Chronic spastic paraparesis, which usually progresses slowly, sometimes remains static after initial progression.
2. Weakness of the lower limbs, more marked proximally.
3. Bladder disturbance usually an early feature; constipation usually occurs later; impotence or decreased libido is common.
4. Sensory symptoms such as tingling, pins and needles, burning, etc. are more prominent than objective physical signs.
5. Low lumbar pain with radiation to the legs is common.
6. Vibration sense is frequently impaired; proprioception is less often affected.
7. Hyperreflexia of the lower limbs, often with clonus and Babinski sign.
8. Hyperreflexia of upper limbs; positive Hoffmann and Trömner signs frequent; weakness may be absent.
9. Exaggerated jaw jerk in some patients.

D. Less frequent neurological findings Cerebellar signs, optic atrophy, deafness, nystagmus, other cranial nerve deficits, hand tremor, absent or depressed ankle jerk. Convulsions, cognitive impairment, dementia, or impaired consciousness are rare.

E. Other neurological manifestations that may be associated with HAM/TSP Muscular atrophy, fasciculations (rare), polymyositis, peripheral neuropathy, polyradiculopathy, cranial neuropathy, meningtis, encephalopathy.

F. Systemic nonneurological manifestations that may be associated with HAM/TSP Pulmonary alveolitis, uveitis, Sjögren syndrome, arthropathy, vasculitis, ichthyosis, cryoglobulinemia, monoclonal gammopathy, adult T-cell leukemia/lymphoma.

II. Laboratory diagnosis

A. Presence of HTLV-I antibodies or antigens in blood and cerebrospinal fluid (CSF).
B. CSF may show mild lymphocyte plecytosis.
C. Lobulated lymphocyte may be present in blood and/or CSF.
D. Mild to moderate increase of protein may be present in CSF.
E. Viral isolation when possible from blood and/or CSF.

From Osame M et al.: HTLV-I–associated myelopathy (HAM): epidemiology, clinical features, and pathomechanism. In Takatsuki K, Hinuma Y, Yoshida M, editors: *Advances in adult T-cell leukemia and HTLV-I research,* Gann monograph on cancer research, Tokyo, 1992, Japan Scientific Societies Press.

HTLV-I Uveitis. Some proportion of HTLV-I carriers develop a specific type of uveitis and this uveitis is considered to be the third clinical entity associated with HTLV-I infection. The details of seroepidemiology, clinical features, laboratory findings, therapy, and prognosis of the disease will be discussed in a later section.

Other HTLV-I–Associated Diseases. Infection with HTLV-I can indirectly cause many other diseases via the induction of immunodeficiency, such as chronic lung diseases, opportunistic lung infections, cancer of other organs,[4] monoclonal gammopathy,[40] strongyloidiasis,[51] nonspecific dermatomycosis, and HTLV-I associated lymphadenitis[62] (Fig. 98-9). The fact that HTLV-I proviruses are detected as polyclonal integration in most of these patients, especially in HTLV-I myelopathy and strongyloidiasis, indicates that the viruses are widespread among lymphocytes.

Disorders such as arthropathy, polymyositis, and Sjögren syndrome have also been discussed in association with HTLV-I in Japan. Some cases of infective dermatitis with some features of immunodeficiency in Caribbean children have also been linked to HTLV-I.

Ocular Manifestations in HTLV-I–Associated Diseases

The first documentation of the ocular involvement in HTLV-I–infected individuals was reported in 1988 by Vernant and associates,[102] who reported five cases of Sjögren syndrome in patients with tropical spastic paraparesis. In the same year Kabayama and associates[28] reported two patients with ATL who had ocular manifestations: cytomegalovirus retinitis in one case and episcleritis in the other. Since then a number of cases with various ocular manifestations have

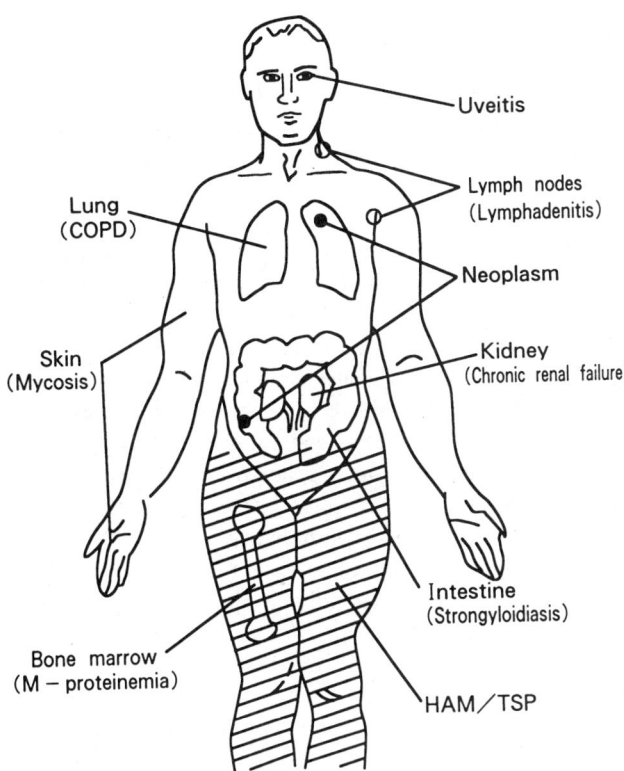

Fig. 98-9. HTLV-I-related diseases. (From Takatsuki K and associates: Adult T-cell leukemia and HTLV-I related diseases. In *Advances in adult T-cell leukemia and HTLV-I research.* Tokyo, 1992, Japan Scientific Societies Press.)

been reported in HTLV-I–infected patients, mainly from HTLV-I endemic areas in Japan.* These ocular manifestations can be classified into three groups based on the HTLV-I–related systemic conditions: (1) opportunistic infections and tumor infiltration in patients with ATL, (2) ocular manifestations characterized by either retinal angiopathy or inflammatory reactions in patients with HTLV-I myelopathy, and (3) uveitis in HTLV-I asymptomatic carriers. The first two categories will be discussed in this section.

Adult T-Cell Leukemia/Lymphoma. Ocular manifestations in patients with ATL are either direct infiltration of malignant cells in ocular tissues or various opportunistic infections in the eye. The most common ocular manifestation in patients with ATL is cytomegalovirus retinitis. Ohba and associates[60] examined 20 patients with ATL; one of the patients had cytomegalovirus retinitis in association with the immunocompromised state of the patient. In Kyushu, an HTLV-I–endemic area in Japan, ATL is one of the most common immunocompromised conditions that can cause cytomegalovirus retinitis.

Another case in Ohba's series had a neoplastic lesion of elevated nontender purplish nodules on the eyelid as a part of generalized lymphoma.[60] Kohno and associates[32] reported

*References 3, 22, 26, 32, 39, 45-49, 53-57, 59-61, 78, 80, 87, 98, 120, 121.

three cases with ATL who developed tumors under the palpebral conjunctiva. Histologic examinations using biopsy tissues disclosed that the tumor was heavily infiltrated by leukemic cells (ATL cells). Fig. 98-10 shows an example of a fundus picture and an echogram of an intraocular lesion in a 76-year-old man with ATL who complained of blurring of vision in his left eye and was referred to the clinic. Cytologic examinations of the cells in the anterior chamber of the patient disclosed the presence of ATL cells in the aqueous humor, suggesting that the intraocular tumor is ATL infiltration.

HTLV-I Myelopathy. As discussed previously HTLV-I myelopathy is a chronic progressive inflammatory disorder in the central nervous system caused by HTLV-I. The ocular manifestations in HTLV-I myelopathy were first examined by Ohba and associates.[60] Previous reports by this group[61,69-71] and many others mainly from Japan[17,26,32,80,98] suggest that some patients with HTLV-I myelopathy may have various ocular manifestations consisting of iritis, vitreous opacities, retinal vasculitis, pigmentary retinal degener-

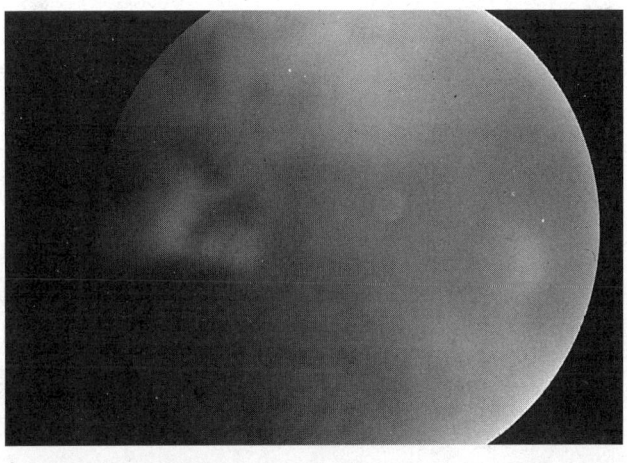

A

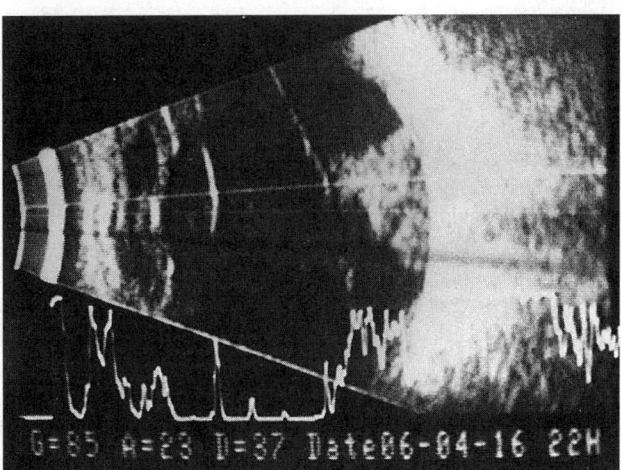

B

Fig. 98-10. Intraocular tumor in a patient with ATL (76-year-old man). **A,** Ocular fundus picture. **B,** Echogram.

ation, retinal microangiopathy (cotton-wool spots and retinal hemorrhages), and Sjögren syndrome. Although many case reports have been published, the incidence of these ocular involvements in HTLV-I myelopathy is not yet clarified. In one of the earlier reports by Ohba and associates,[59] five of 20 patients with HTLV-I myelopathy (25%) had either vascular or inflammatory lesions in the eye, such as granulomatous anterior uveitis, membranous vitreous opacities, and cotton-wool spots in the posterior retina. Another clinical study by Kohno and associates[32] reported that eight of 22 patients with HTLV-I myelopathy (36.4%) had either vitreous opacities or retinal hemorrhages. The number of patients with HTLV-I myelopathy in these studies was too small to estimate the incidence of ocular manifestations in HTLV-I myelopathy, however.

Fig. 98-11 shows the ocular fundus and fluorescein angiography of the left eye in a 55-year-old woman with HTLV-I myelopathy. The patient was referred to the uveitis clinic because of the sudden onset of floaters and blurring of vision in both eyes. As seen in the pictures, she had moderate vitre-

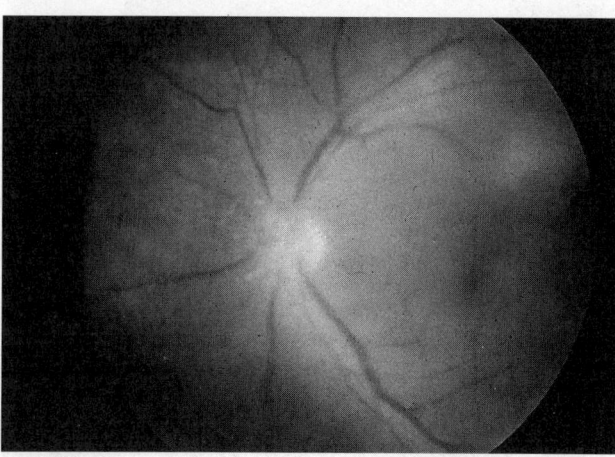

A

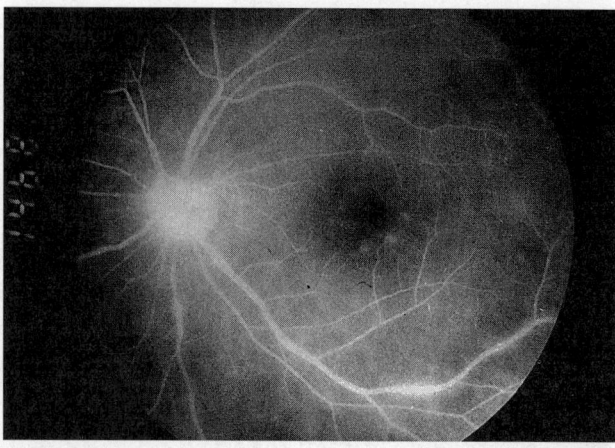

B

Fig. 98-11. Eye with uveitis with HTLV-I myelopathy (55-year-old man). **A,** Ocular fundus picture. **B,** Fluorescein angiography.

ous opacities accompanied by mild iritis. The fluorescein angiography disclosed moderate dye leakage from the retinal blood vessels, indicating the presence of retinal vasculitis. The ocular manifestations improved by therapy with topical and systemic corticosteroid.

DIFFERENTIAL DIAGNOSIS

Similar to sarcoidosis, HTLV-I uveitis may develop granulomatous uveitis with muttonfat-like keratic precipitates, iris nodules, snowball vitreous opacities, and periphlebitis. Therefore the differential diagnosis between the two diseases only by ocular findings is very difficult in some cases. Patients with HTLV-I uveitis, however, have normal chest x-ray findings and normal levels of angiotensin-converting enzyme. In addition, bronchoalveolar lavage (BAL) findings in HTLV-I uveitis differ from those of patients with sarcoidosis. Both diseases show increased total cell counts and T-lymphocytosis in BAL fluid. Patients with sarcoidosis have markedly elevated CD4+-T lymphocytes in BAL fluid, resulting in a high CD4+/CD8+ ratio (6.3 ± 3.8). On the other hand, patients with HTLV-I uveitis show a high proportion of CD8+-T lymphocytes in BAL fluid, resulting in a relatively low CD4+/CD8+ ratio (1.1 ± 0.4).

HTLV-I uveitis may have diffuse retinal vasculitis like Behçet syndrome. Retinal vasculitis in HTLV-I uveitis is usually mild, however, and is rarely accompanied by retinal hemorrhages and retinal exudates. None of the patients with HTLV-I uveitis have hypopyon iridis. However, Behçet syndrome with mild degree of ocular inflammation should be differentiated from HTLV-I uveitis by careful determination of disease history and systemic examinations.

The presenting symptom of VKH disease is sudden onset of bilateral blurring of vision with characteristic systemic symptoms such as headache and disacausia, which are never seen in patients with HTLV-I uveitis. The multifocal serous retinal detachment in the posterior pole of the fundus in VKH disease is not seen in HTLV-I uveitis.

HTLV-I uveitis does not have any types (focal, multifocal, geographic, diffuse) of retinal necrotic lesions and therefore the disease can be differentiated from CMV retinitis, ARN syndrome, toxoplasmosis, and toxocariasis.

Both candidiasis and HTLV-I uveitis may have vitreous opacities that cause floaters as the presenting symptoms. HTLV-I uveitis has no multifocal chorioretinitis manifesting small, round, white, slightly elevated lesions that are the common clinical features of candidiasis, however.

The presenting symptom is usually floaters in both pars planitis and HTLV-I uveitis, and the two diseases may have snowball-like vitreous opacities and cystoid macular edema. HTLV-I uveitis, however, never has the hallmark of pars planitis, snowbanking, which is the grey-white plaque involving the inferior pars plana.

LABORATORY INVESTIGATIONS

The cells floating in the anterior chamber of the eye with HTLV-I uveitis consisted of lymphocytes ($>$95%) with a small proportion of macrophages. No malignant cells were detected in the aqueous humor of the patients. Using these cells in the aqueous humor, the presence of HTLV-I-infected cells at the local site of ocular inflammation was examined by polymerase chain reaction (PCR) (Fig. 98-12).[46,57] HTLV-I proviral DNA was detected in all nine tested samples from the patients by PCR with pol and/or gag primers. Conversely the proviral DNA was not detected in any tested samples from seronegative patients with other types of uveitis. Additionally, the proviral DNA was not detected in two seropositive patients (one with toxoplasmosis and the other with Behçet syndrome) with uveitis from defined causes. These data thus suggest that HTLV-I-infected cells are present at the local site of HTLV-I uveitis. Furthermore, expression of viral mRNA was detected by RT-PCR from the inflammatory cells in the aqueous humor in two of the tested patients with HTLV-I uveitis. These molecular biologic data thus suggest that the HTLV-I-infected cells play a role in the pathophysiology and pathogenesis of the uveitis. A quantitative assay of HTLV-I–infected cells by PCR revealed that the mean (SD) number of HTLV-I–infected cells in the peripheral

TABLE 98-10   PERIPHERAL LYMPHOCYTES' SURFACE PHENOTYPE IN IDIOPATHIC UVEITIS BY HUMAN T-CELL LYMPHOTROPIC VIRUS TYPE I INFECTION

Peripheral Lymphocytes' Surface Phenotype	Antihuman T-cell Lymphotropic Virus Type I Antibody		P Value (Student T Test)
	Seropositive Patients (N = 19)	Seronegative Patients (N = 15)	
CD1	0.3 ± 0.2*	0.2 ± 0.1	
CD2	76.9 ± 15.4	74.5 ± 15.7	
CD3	59.9 ± 13.7	59.8 ± 15.0	
CD4	42.7 ± 11.5	30.9 ± 9.5	<0.01
CD7	49.5 ± 17.5	58.0 ± 10.4	
CD8	25.5 ± 5.2	34.3 ± 10.5	<0.01
CD19	9.0 ± 5.3	9.9 ± 3.7	
CD25	2.5 ± 2.3	1.2 ± 0.8	<0.05
DR	21.9 ± 5.7	24.2 ± 7.9	
CD4/8 ratio	1.7 ± 0.6	1.0 ± 0.4	<0.01

From Yoshimura et al.: Clinical and immunological features of human T-cell lymphotropic virus type I uveitis, *Am J Ophthalmol* 116:156–163, 1993.
* mean ± standard deviation

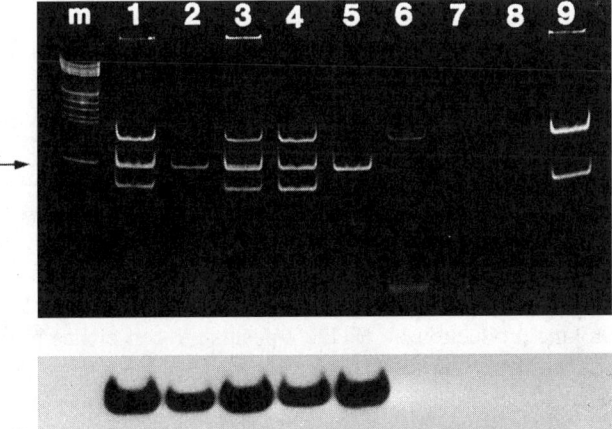

Fig. 98-12. Detection of HTLV-I provirus by polymerase chain reaction with gag primer. One fourth of DNA extracted from infiltrating cells in aqueous humor was subjected to PCR with HTLV-I gag primer. Upper panel shows result of ethidium bromide staining of PCR product by polyacrylamide gel electrophoresis; lower panel is autoradiogram of specific PCR product by filter hybridization with ³²P-labeled internal oligomer probe. m; molecular weight marker, *HaeIII*-digested pBPR322, lane 1; ATL, lanes 2-5; HTLV-I uveitis, lane 6; toxoplasmosis of HTLV-I carrier, lanes 7 and 8; Behçet disease of HTLV-I noncarrier, lane 9; negative control, CEM. (From Mochizuki M et al.: HTLV-I uveitis: a distinct clinical entity caused by HTLV-I, *Jpn J Cancer Res* 83:236-239, 1992.)

blood in patients with HTLV-I uveitis was 3.84% (4.45%) of peripheral mononuclear cells, which was intermediate between the values in asymptomatic carriers [0.54% (1.11%)] and HTLV-I myelopathy patients [11.63% (7.67%)].[63]

The antibody level to HTLV-I in 93 patients with HTLV-I uveitis varied from 1:64 to 1:8192 by particle agglutination assay; this level was similar to that of HTLV-I-asymptomatic carriers but lower than that of HTLV-I myelopathy patients.[48] The antibody to the virus in the aqueous humor was also detected from all tested samples in patients with HTLV-I uveitis.[48] The surface phenotype of peripheral lymphocytes in patients with HTLV-I uveitis was analyzed with a laser flow cytometry using monoclonal antibodies to surface antigens of lymphocytes and compared to those in seronegative patients with idiopathic uveitis: the CD4 fraction was elevated and the CD8 fraction was lowered, thereby elevating the CD4/8 ratio in the HTLV-I uveitis group as compared with the seronegative group (Table 98-10).[120] Furthermore, the CD25 fraction of T lymphocytes, which represents activated T lymphocytes with expression of interleukin 2 receptors on the cell surface, was significantly elevated in patients with HTLV-I uveitis (2.5 ± 5.7% vs. 1.2 ± 0.8%; P < 0.05).[121] The levels of soluble interleukin 2 receptors (sIL2R or sCD25) in the serum were also significantly higher in patients with HTLV-I uveitis than in seronegative healthy controls.[48]

More direct implication of HTLV-I in the pathogenesis of HTLV-I uveitis has been provided by Sagawa, Iho, and Mochizuki[77] using T-cell clones derived from intraocular tissues of HTLV-I uveitis. They established IL-2 dependent T-cell clones (TCC) from the aqueous humor of two patients

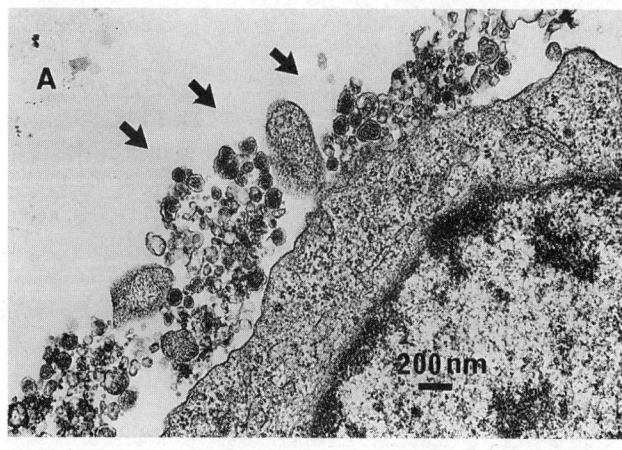

Fig. 98-13. Detection of HTLV-I-associated protein and HTLV-I virus particles on a TCC established from the aqueous humor of a patient with HTLV-I uveitis. **A,** Expression of HTLV-I env gp46 on the cell surface of U16 clone was detected by immunofluorescence method and a confocal laser scanning microscope. **B,** HTLV-I virus particles on U16 clone were detected by electron microscopic analysis. [From Sagawa K et al.: Immunopathological mechanisms of human T cell lymphotropic virus type 1 (HTLV-I) uveitis: detection of HTLV-I-infected T cells in the eye and their constitutive cytokine production, *J Clin Invest* 95:852-858, 1995.]

with HTLV-I uveitis and characterized to better understand the immunopathology of HTLV-I uveitis. Proviral DNA of HTLV-I was identified in 55 out of 94 (59%) or 13 out of 36 (36%) TCC from the ocular fluid or the peripheral blood of these patients, respectively. HTLV-I env and gag proteins were detectable in two HTLV-I provirus-positive TCC (U16 and U25) using the monoclonal antibodies (Fig. 98-13). Furthermore, the electron microscopic observation of the TCC (U16) identified HTLV-I virus particles, the mean diameter of which was 102 nm (Fig. 98-13). These data provided direct evidence of HTLV-I infection in intraocular region of the disease.

Masuoka and associates[38] investigated the clonality of HTLV-I-infected T cells in a patient with HTLV-I uveitis. Eleven TCC were established from the aqueous humor (6 clones) and the peripheral blood (5 clones) of a patient with the disease, and the clonality of the HTLV-I-infected T cells was studied by sequencing the T-cell receptor α gene after the amplification of T-cell receptor α cDNA using an adapter-ligation method and RT-PCR. T-cell receptor use was different for each of 11 TCC, encompassing 8 different HTLV-I-infected TCC (4 from the aqueous humor and 4 from peripheral blood) and 3 HTLV-I negative TCC. The results demonstrated polyclonal use of T-cell receptor α for HTLV-I-infected cells in the ocular lesion and the peripheral blood, suggesting that these T cells are not precursors of the leukemic cells associated with malignant transformation. Instead, they might be randomly infected with HTLV-I in the process of HTLV-I uveitis.

The HTLV-I-infected TCC established by Sagawa and associates[77] produced significant amounts of IL-1α (12,699 pg/ml), IL-2 (61 pg/ml), IL-3 (428 pg/ml), IL-6 (1,336 pg/ml), IL-8 (1,268 pg/ml), IL-10 (28 pg/ml), TNF-α (289 pg/ml), IFN-y (5,095 pg/ml), and GM-CSF (2,886 pg/ml) in the absence of any stimuli. In contrast, HTLV-I negative TCC from the patients did not produce these cytokines. They are potent cytokines capable of inducing immune reactions and inflammation at the tissue level. These data suggest that cytokine production by HTLV-I-positive T-cell clones in the intraocular tissues is at least responsible for uveitis associated with HTLV-I.

These laboratory data thus suggest that the immune-mediated mechanisms, particularly by CD4+ T-cells, play a role in the pathogenesis of HTLV-I uveitis.

THERAPY AND PROGNOSIS IN HTLV-I UVEITIS

HTLV-I uveitis with a mild degree of ocular inflammation can be managed by therapy with topical noncorticosteroidal antiinflammatory drugs and mydriatics. The instillation or the periocular injection of corticosteroids is used when the patients have moderate inflammatory activities in the vitreous cavity. If the vitreous inflammatory activity and the retinal vasculitis is severe, oral corticosteroids (0.5 to 1.0

TABLE 98-11   EFFECT OF TREATMENT ON VISUAL OUTCOME ACCORDING TO HTLV-I SEROREACTIVITY IN IDIOPATHIC UVEITIS

Pre Therapy Visual Acuity	Proportion of Good Visual Acuity ($\geq$ 20/25) After Therapy		P Value (X^2 Test)
	Human T-Cell Lymphotropic Virus Type I Seropositive	Human T-Cell Lymphotropic Virus Type I Seronegative	
20/25 or better	75/76 (99%)	158/177 (89%)	<0.05
20/25 to 20/60	26/29 (90%)	30/56 (54%)	<0.01
20/60 or worse	10/15 (67%)	11/46 (24%)	<0.01
Total	111/120 (92%)	199/279 (71%)	<0.01

From Yoshimura et al.: Clinical and immunological features of human T-cell lymphotropic virus type I uveitis, *Am J Ophthalmol* 116:156-163, 1993.

mg/Kg of predonisolone) is given for one week, then the dosage is decreased gradually. A long-term administration of systemic corticosteroid should be avoided, however, because the long-term prognosis of the disease under immunosuppressive conditions is unknown. The intraocular inflammation is markedly improved in 4 to 6 weeks on the therapies described here, and complete remission will be achieved. The visual prognosis of the disease is good in most cases. The inflammation may reccur in one half of cases; the interval between one inflammatory episode to another varies from a few months to several years.

According to Yoshimura and associates,[120] the visual prognosis of 93 patients with HTLV-I uveitis was good: 76 of 120 eyes (63%) in the 85 patients with long follow-up had good visual acuity (20/25 or better) after therapy with topical and/or systemic corticosteroids, 29 eyes (24%) had fairly good visual acuity (worse than 20/25 but better than 20/60), and 15 eyes (13%) had poor visual acuity (20/60 or worse). When compared to seronegative idiopathic uveitis, HTLV-I uveitis had statistically better visual prognosis than those in the seronegative group (Table 98-11).

At present no information is available whether patients with HTLV-I uveitis may develop HTLV-I myelopathy or even the malignant disorder (ATL) in the future. A long-term follow-up of the patients with HTLV-I uveitis is needed to observe such long-term prognosis. In addition, systemic immunosuppressive drugs including corticosteroids should be given with great caution.

REFERENCES

1. Alexandre C, Verrier B: Four regulatory elements in the human c-fos promoter mediate transactivation by HTLV-I Tax protein, *Oncogene* 6:543-551, 1991.
2. Arai N et al.: Complete nucleotide sequence of the chromosomal gene for human IL-4 and its expression, *J Immunol* 142:274-282, 1989.
3. Araki S et al.: Familial clustering of human T-lymphotopic virus type I uveitis, *Br J Ophthalmol,* 77:747-748, 1993.
4. Asou N et al.: HTLV-I seroprevalence in patients with malignancy, *Cancer* 58:903-907, 1986.
5. Bartholomew C et al.: HTLV-I and tropical spastic paraparesis, *Lancet* ii:99-100, 1986.
6. Bartholomew C et al.: Transmission of HTLV-I and HIV among homosexual men in Trinidad, *JAMA* 257:2604-2608, 1987.
7. Bhagavati S et al.: Detection of human T-cell lymphoma/leukemia virus type I DNA and antigen in spinal fluid and blood of patients with chronic progressive myelopathy, *New Eng J Med* 318:1141-1147, 1988.
8. Bloch-Michel E, Nussenblatt RB: International uveitis study group recommendations for the evaluation of intraocular inflammatory disease, *Am J Ophthalmol* 103:234-235, 1987.
9. Clapham P et al.: Productive infection and cell-free transmission of human T-cell leukemia virus in a nonlymphoid cell line, *Science* 222:1125-1127, 1983.
10. de The G: HTLV-I and chronic progressive encephalomyelopathies: an immunovirololgical perspective. In Roman GC, Osame M, editors: *HTLV-I and the nervous system,* 3-8, New York, 1989, Alan R Liss.
11. Fujii M, Sassone-Corci P, Verma I: c-fos promoter trans-activation by tax1 protein of human T-cell leukemia virus type I, *Proc Natl Acad Sci USA* 85:8526-8530, 1988.
12. Fujii M et al.: Interaction of HTLV-I Tax1 with p67SRF causes the aberrant induction of cellular immediate early genes through CArG boxes, *Genes Dev* 6:2066-2074, 1992.
13. Gessain A et al.: Antibodies to human T-lymphotropic virus type I in patients with tropical spastic paraparesis, *Lancet* ii:407-410, 1985.
14. Hattori S et al.: Identification of envelope glycoprotein encoded by ENV gene of human T-cell leukemia virus, *Jpn J Cancer Res (Gann)* 74:790-793, 1983.
15. Hattori S et al.: Identification of gag and env gene products of human T-cell leukemia virus (HTLV), *Virology* 136:338-346, 1984.
16. Hattori T et al.: Surface phenotype of Japanese ATL cells characterized by monoclonal antibodies, *Blood* 58:645-647, 1981.
17. Hayasaka S et al.: Retinal vasculitis in a mother and her son with human T-lymphotropic virus type I associated myelopathy, *Br J Ophthalmol* 75:566-567, 1991.
18. Hinuma Y et al.: Adult T-cell leukemia: antigen in an ATL cell line and detection of antibodies to the antigen in human sera, *Proc Natl Acad Sci USA* 78:6476-6480, 1981.
19. Ho DD, Rota TR, Hirsch MS: Infection of human endothelial cells by human T-lymphotropic virus type I, *Proc Natl Acad Sci USA* 81:7588-7590, 1984.
20. Hollsberg P, Hafler DA: Pathogenesis of diseases induced by human lymphotropic virus type I infection, *New Eng J Med* 328:1173-1182, 1993.
21. Hoxie JA, Matthews DM, Cines DB: Infection of human endothelial cells by human T-cell leukemia virus type I, *Proc Natl Acad Sci USA* 81:7591-7595, 1984.
22. Ikeda E et al.: Epidemiological study of uveitis in north Kyushu and south Kyushu, *Jpn J Clin Ophthalmol* 90:11-23, 1993 (in Japanese).
23. Inoue J, Yoshida M, Seiki M: Transcriptional (p40x) and posttranscriptional (p27x III) regulators are required for the expression and replication of human T-cell leukemia virus type I genes, *Proc Natl Acad Sci USA* 84:3653-3657, 1987.

24. Inoue J et al.: Induction of interleukin 2 receptor gene expression by p40x encoded by human T-cell leukemia virus type I, *EMBO J* 5:2883-2888, 1986.

25. Inoue J et al.: Nucleotide sequence of the protease coding region in an infectious DNA of simian retrovirus (STLV) of the HTLV-I family, *Virology* 150:187-193, 1986.

26. Ishimoto S et al.: Interferon-a for the treatment of retinal vasculitis associated with human T-lymphotropic virus type I myelopathy (HAM), *Acta Soc Ophthalmol Jpn* 94:769-773, 1990.

27. Jacobson S et al.: Isolation of an HTLV-I-like retrovirus from patient with tropical spastic paraperesis, *Nature* 331:540, 1988.

28. Kabayama Y et al.: Ocular disorders associated with adult T-cell leukemia, *Jpn J Clin Ophthalmol* 42:139-141, 1988 (in Japanese).

29. Kawano F et al.: HTLV-I associated myelopathy/tropical spastic paraparesis with adult T-cell leukemia, *Leukemia* 6:66-67, 1992.

30. Kinoshita K et al.: Demonstration of adult T-cell leukemia virus antigen in milk from three sero-positive mothers, *Jpn J Cancer Res* 75:103-105, 1984.

31. Kiyokawa T et al.: p27x-III and p21x-III proteins encoded by the pX sequence of human T-cell leukemia virus type 1, *Proc Natl Acad Sci USA* 82:8359-8363, 1985.

32. Kohno T, Arita T, Okamoto R: Ocular manifestations in human T-lymphotropic virus type I infection, *Folia Ophthalmol Jpn* 41:2182-2188, 1990.

33. Kusuhara K et al.: Mother-to-child transmission of human T-cell leukemia virus type I (HTLV-I): a fifteen-year follow-up study in Okinawa, Japan, *Int J Cancer* 40:755-757, 1987.

34. Lee H et al.: High rate of HTLV-II infection in seropositive IV drug abusers in New Orleans, *Science* 244:471-475, 1990.

35. Leung K, Nabel GJ: HTLV-I transactivator induces interleukin-2 receptor expression through an NF-kB-like factor, *Nature* 333:776-778, 1988.

36. Longo DL et al.: Isolation of HTLV-transformed B-lymphocyte clone from a patient with HTLV-associated adult T-cell leukemia, *Nature* 310:505-506, 1984.

37. Maeda Y et al.: Prevalence of possible adult T-cell leukemia virus carriers among volunteer blood donors in Japan: a nationwide study, *Int J Cancer* 33:717-720, 1984.

38. Masuoka K et al.: Polyclonal use of T-cell receptor α for human T-cell lymphotropic virus type I-infected T cells, *Invest Ophthalmol Vis Sci* 36:254-258, 1995.

39. Matsuo K et al.: Retinal vasculitis in healthy carriers of HTLV-I, *Folia Ophthalmol Jpn* 41:764-770, 1990 (in Japanese).

40. Matsuzaki H et al.: Monoclonal gammopathies in adult T-cell leukemia, *Cancer* 56:1380-1383, 1985.

41. Miyatake S et al.: Activation of T cell derived lymphokine genes in T cells and fibroblasts: effects of human T cell leukemia virus type I p40x protein and bovine papilloma virus encoded E2 protein, *Nucleic Acid Res* 16:6547-6566, 1988.

42. Miyatake S et al.: T-cell activation signals and human T-cell leukemia virus type I-encoded p40x protein activate the mouse granulocyte-macrophage colony-stimulating factor gene through a common DNA element, *Mol Cell Biol* 8:5581-5587, 1988.

43. Miyoshi I et al.: A novel T-cell line derived from adult T-cell leukemia, *Jpn J Cancer Res (Gann)* 71:155-156, 1980.

44. Miyoshi I et al.: Type C virus particles in a cord T-cell line derived by co-cultivating normal human cord leukocytes and human leukemic T-cells, *Nature* 294:770-771, 1981.

45. Mochizuki M et al.: HTLV-I and uveitis, *Lancet* i:1110, 1992.

46. Mochizuki M et al.: HTLV-I uveitis: a distinct clinical entity caused by HTLV-I, *Jpn J Cancer Res* 83:236-239, 1992.

47. Mochizuki M et al.: Uveitis associated with human T-cell lymphotropic virus type I, *Am J Ophthalmol* 114:123-129, 1992.

48. Mochizuki M et al.: Uveitis associated with human T lymphotropic virus type I: seroepidemiological, clinical, and virological studies, *J Inf Dis* 166:943-944, 1992.

49. Mochizuki M et al.: Human T lymphotropic virus type I uveitis, *Br J Ophthalmol* 78:149-154, 1994.

50. Nagy K et al.: Human T-cell leukemia virus type I: induction of syncytia and inhibition by patients' sera, *Int J Cancer* 32:321-328, 1983.

51. Nakada K et al.: Monoclonal integration of HTLV-I proviral DNA in patients with strongyloidiasis, *Int J Cancer* 40:145-148, 1987.

52. Nakano S et al.: Search for possible routes of vertical and horizontal transmission of adult T-cell leukemia virus, *Jpn J Cancer Res* 75:1044-1045, 1984.

53. Nakao K, Matsumoto M, Ohba N: Seroprevalence of antibodies to HTLV-I in patients with ocular disorders, *Br J Ophthalmol* 75:76-78, 1991.

54. Nakao K, Ohba N, Mastumoto M: Noninfectious anterior uveitis in patients infected with human T-lymphpotropic virus type I, *Jpn J Ophthalmol* 33:472-481, 1989.

55. Nakao K et al.: Cotton-wool spots on the retina in patients infected with human T-lymphotropic virus type I (HTLV-I), *Folia Ophthalmol Jpn* 40:2051-2057, 1989.

56. Nakao K et al.: Pigmentary retinal degeneration in patients with HTLV-I-associated myelopathy, *Jpn J Ophthalmol* 33:383-391, 1989.

57. Nakashima S et al.: Uveitis in human T-lymphotropic virus type I (HTLV-I) carriers. III. A molecular biological study, *Acta Soc Ophthalmol Jpn* 97:741-746, 1993.

58. Nishimoto N et al.: Elevated levels of interleukin-6 in serum and cerebrospinal fluid of HTLV-I associated myelopathy/tropical spastic paraparesis, *J Neurol Sci* 97:183-193, 1990.

59. Ohba N et al.: Ocular disorders in patients infected with human T-lymphotropic virus type I, *J Eye* 5:265-267, 1988 (in Japanese).

60. Ohba N et al.: Ophthalmological complications of HTLV-I infections. In Roma GC, Osame M, editors: *HTLV-I and the nervous system,* New York, 1988, Alan R Liss.

61. Ohba N et al.: Ocular manifestations in patients infected with human T-lymphotropic virus type I, *Jpn J Ophthalmol* 33:1-12, 1989.

62. Ohshima K et al.: HTLV-I associated lymphadenopathy, *Cancer* 69:239-248, 1992.

63. Ono A et al.: Increased number of circulating HTLV-I infected cells in peripheral blood mononuclear cells of HTLV-I uveitis patients: a quantitative polymerase chain reaction study, *Br J Ophthalmol* 79:270-276, 1995.

64. Osame M et al.: HTLV-I associated myelopathy, a new clinical entity, *Lancet* i:1031-1032, 1986.

65. Osame M et al.: Chronic progressive myelopathy associated with elevated antibodies to human T-lymphotropic virus type I and adult T-cell leukemialike cells, *Ann Nuerol* 21:117-122, 1987.

66. Osame M et al.: HTLV-I associated myelopathy (HAM), treatment trials, retrospective survey and clinical and laboratory findings, *Hematol Rev* 3:271-284, 1990.

67. Osame M et al.: Nationwide survey of HTLV-I associated myelopathy in Japan: association with blood transfusion, *Ann Neurol* 28:51-56, 1990.

68. Osame M et al.: HTLV-I-associated myelopathy (HAM): epidemiology, clinical features, and pathomechanism. In Takatsuki K, Hinuma Y, Yoshida M, editors: *Advances in adult T-cell leukemia and HTLV-I research,* Gann monograph on cancer research, 57-68, Tokyo, 1992, Japan Scientific Societies Press.

69. Poiesz BJ et al.: Detection and isolation of type-C retrovirus particles from fresh and cultured lymphocytes of patients with cutaneous T-cell lymphoma, *Pro Natl Acad Sci USA* 77:7415-7419, 1980.

70. Popovic M et al.: The virus of Japanese adult T-cell leukemia is a member of the human T-cell leukemia virus group, *Nature* 300:63-66, 1982.

71. Popovic M et al.: Transformation of human umbilical cord blood T cells by human T-cell leukemia/lymphoma virus, *Proc Natl Acad Sci USA* 80:5402-5406, 1983.

72. Pozzati R, Vogel J, Jay G: The human T-lymphotropic virus type I tax gene can cooperate with the ras oncogene to induce neoplastic transformation of cells, *Mol Cel Biol* 10:413-417, 1990.

73. Richardson JH et al.: In vivo cellular tropism of human T-cell leukemia virus type 1, *J Virol* 64:5682-5685, 1990.

74. Robert-Gurroff M et al.: Prevalence of antibodies to HTLV-I, -II, -III, in intravenous drug abusers from an AIDS endemic region, *JAMA* 255:3133-3137, 1986.

75. Rodgers-Johnson P et al.: HTLV-I and HTLV-III antibodies and tropical spastic paraparesis, *Lancet* ii:1247-1248, 1985.

76. Sagata N et al.: Comparison of the entire genomes of bovine leukemia virus and human T-cell leukemia virus and characterization of their unidentified open reading frames, *EMBO J* 3:3231-3237, 1984.

77. Sagawa et al.: Immunopathological mechanisms of human T cell lymphotropic virus type 1 (HTLV-I) uveitis: detection of HTLV-I-infected T cells in the eye and their constitutive cytokine production, *J Clin Invest* 95:852-858, 1995.

78. Sakai Y et al.: Interferon-α for the treatment of retinal vasculitis associated with human T-lymphotropic virus type I myelopathy (HAM), *Acta Soc Ophthalmol Jpn* 94:769-773, 1990 (in Japanese).

79. Sakamoto KM et al.: HTLV-I and HTLV-II tax trans-activate the human EGR-1 promoter through different cis-acting sequences, *Oncogene* 7:2125-2130, 1992.

80. Sasaki K et al.: Retinal vasculitis in human T-lymphotropic virus type I associated myelopathy, *Br J Ophthalmol* 73:812-815, 1989.

81. Seiki M et al.: Human adult T-cell leukemia virus: complete nucleotide sequence of the provirus genome integrated in leukemic cell DNA, *Proc Natl Acad Sci USA* 80:3618-3622, 1983.

82. Seiki M et al.: Expression of the pX gene of HTLV-I: general splicing mechanism in the HTLV family, *Science* 228:1532-1534, 1985.

83. Shimotohno K et al.: Complete nucleotide sequence of an infectious clone of human T-cell leukemia virus type II: a new open reading frame for the protease gene, *Proc Natl Acad Sci USA* 82:3101-3105, 1985.

84. Shimotohno K et al.: Requirement of multiple copies of a 21-nucleotide sequence in the U3 regions of human T-cell leukemia virus type I and type II long terminal repeats for transacting activating of transcription, *Proc Natl Acad Sci USA* 83:8112-8116, 1986.

85. Shimoyama M et al.: Major prognostic factors of adult patients with advanced T-cell lymphoma/leukemia, *J Clin Oncol* 6:1088-1097, 1988.

86. Shimoyama M, members of lymphoma study group: Diagnostic criteria and classification of clinical subtypes of adult T-cell leukemia/lymphoma, *Br J Hematol* 79:428-439, 1991.

87. Shirao M et al.: Uveitis in human T-lymphotropic virus type I (HTLV-I) carriers. II. A seroepidemiological study, *Acta Soc Ophthalmol Jpn* 97:726-732, 1993.

88. Sodoroski JG, Rosen CA, Haseltine WA: A transcriptional activator protein encoded by the x-lor region of the human T-cell leukemia virus, *Science* 228:1430-1434, 1984.

89. Tachibana N et al.: Anti-human T-cell leukemia virus antibody distribution in Miyazaki Prefecture, *J Jpn Infect Dis* 58:717-722, 1984 (in Japanese).

90. Tajima K, Hinuma Y: Epidemiology of HTLV-I/II in Japan and the world. In Takatsuki K, Hinuma Y, Yoshida M, editors: *Advances in adult T-cell leukemia and HTLV-I research:* Gann monograph on cancer research, 129-149, Tokyo, 1992, Japan Scientific Societies Press.

91. Tajima K et al.: Geographical features and epidemiological approach to endemic T-cell leukemia/lymphoma in Japan, *Jpn J Clin Oncol* 9(suppl 1):495-504, 1979.

92. Tajima K et al.: Epidemiological analysis of the distribution of antibody to adult T-cell leukemia-virus associated antigen (ATLA): possible horizontal transmission of adult T-cell leukemia virus, *Jpn J Cancer Res* 73:893-901, 1982.

93. Tajima K et al.: Epidemiological features of HTLV-I carriers and incidence of ATL in an ATL-endemic island: a report of the community-based cooperative study in Tsushima, Japan, *Int J Cancer* 40:741-746, 1987.

94. Tajima K, T- and B-cell malignancy study group: The 4th nationwide study of adult T-cell leukemia/lymphoma (ATL in Japan): estimates of risk of ATL and its geographical and clinical features, *Int J Cancer* 45:237-243, 1990.

95. Tajima K et al.: Ethno-epidemiology of ATL in Japan with special reference to the mongoloid dispersal. In Takatsuki K, editor: *Adult T-cell leukemia,* Oxford University Press (in press).

96. Takatsuki K et al.: Adult T cell leukemia in Japan. In Seno S, Takaku F, Irino S, editors: *Topics in hematology,* 73-77, New York, 1977, Excerpta Medica.

97. Takatsuki K et al.: Adult T-cell leukemia and HTLV-I related diseases. In *Advances in adult T-cell leukemia and HTLV-I research,* 1-15, Tokyo, 1992, Japan Scientific Societies Press.

98. Tamai K, Shirai S: Uveitis associated with human T-lymphotropic virus type I infection, *Folia Ophthalmol Jpn* 42:44-48, 1991 (in Japanese).

99. Tanaka A et al.: Oncogenic transformation by the tax gene of human T-cell leukemia virus type I in vitro, *Proc Natl Acad Sci USA* 87:1071-1075, 1990.

100. Tsujimoto A et al.: Nucleotide sequence analysis of a provirus derived from HTLV-I associated myelopathy (HAM), *Mol Biol Med* 5:29-42, 1988.

101. Uchiyama T et al.: Adult T-cell leukemia: clinical and hematologic features of 16 cases, *Blood* 50:481-492, 1977.

102. Vernant JC et al.: T-lymphocyte alveolitis, tropical spastic paresis, and Sjögren syndrome, *Lancet* i:177, 1988.

103. Wain-Hobson S et al.: Nucleotide sequence of the AIDS virus, LAV, *Cell* 40:9-17, 1985.

104. Wano Y et al.: Interleukin 1 gene expression in adult T cell leukemia, *J Clin Invest* 80:911-915, 1987.

105. Watanabe T, Seiki M, Yoshida M: ATLV (Japanese isolated) and HTLV (U.S. isolated) are the same strain of retrovirus, *Virology* 133:238-241, 1984.

106. Watanabe T, Seiki M, Yoshida M: HTLV type I (U.S. isolate) and ATLV (Japanese isolate) are the same species of human retrovirus, *Virology* 69:1255-1258, 1984.

107. Watanabe T et al.: Sequence homology of the simian retrovirus genome with human T-cell leukemia virus type I, *Virology* 144:59-65, 1985.

108. Watanabe T et al.: Human T-cell leukemia virus type 1 is a member of the African subtype of simian viruses (STLV), *Virology* 148:385-387, 1986.

109. Watanabe T et al.: Constitutive expression of parathyroid hormone-related protein (PTHrP) gene in HTLV-I carriers and adult T cell leukemia patients which can be transactivated by HTLV-I Tax gene, *J Exp Med* 172:759-765, 1990.

110. Yamaguchi K et al.: A proposal for smoldering adult T-cell leukemia: a clinicopathologic study of 5 cases, *Blood* 62:758-766, 1983.

111. Yamaguchi K et al.: The detection of human T-cell leukemia virus proviral DNA and its application for classification and diagnosis of T-cell malignancy, *Blood* 63:1235-1240, 1984.

112. Yamaguchi K et al.: Pathogenesis of adult T-cell leukemia from clinical pathologic features. In Blattner W, editor: *Human retrovirology: HTLV,* 163-171, New York, 1990, Raven Press.

113. Yamaguchi K et al.: Human T-lymphotropic virus type I uveitis after Graves' disease, *Br J Ophthalmol* 78:163-166, 1994.

114. Yang Y et al.: Human IL-3 (multi-CSF): identification by expression cloning of a novel hematopoietic growth factor related to murine IL-3, *Cell* 47:3-10, 1986.

115. Yoshida M: Expression of the HTLV-I genome and its association with a unique T-cell malignancy, *Biochimica et Biophysica Acta* 907:145-159, 1987.

116. Yoshida M, Miyoshi I, Hinuma Y: Isolation and characterization of retrovirus from cell lines of human adult T cell leukemia and its implication in the disease, *Proc Natl Acad Sci USA* 79:2031-2035, 1982.

117. Yoshida M et al.: Monoclonal integration of human T-cell leukemia provirus in all primary tumors of adult T-cell leukemia suggests causative role of human T-cell leukemia virus in the disease, *Proc Natl Acad Sci USA* 81:2534-2537, 1984.

118. Yoshida M et al.: Viruses detected in HTLV-I associated myelopathy (HAM) and adult T-cell leukemia (ATL) are identical in DNA blotting assay, *Lancet* i:1085-1086, 1987.

119. Yoshikura H et al.: Isolation of HTLV derived from Japanese adult T-cell leukemia patients in human diploid fibroblast strain IMR90 and the biological characters of the infected cells, *Int J Cancer* 33:745-749, 1984.

120. Yoshimura K et al.: Clinical and immunological features of human T-cell lymphotropic virus type I uveitis, *Am J Ophthalmol* 116:156-163, 1993.

121. Yoshimura K et al.: Uveitis in human T-lymphotropic virus type I (HTLV-I) carriers. II. An analysis of clinical features, *Acta Soc Ophthalmol Jpn* 97:733-740, 1993.

122. Yoshimura T, Fujisawa J, Yoshida M: Multiple cDNA clones encoding nuclear proteins that bind to the tax-dependent enhancer of HTLV-I: all contain a leucine zipper structure and basic amino acid domain, *EMBO J* 9:2537-2542, 1990.

99 Cat-Scratch Disease

DAN B. JONES

Cat-scratch disease is a subacute bacterial infection of the skin, soft tissue, and regional lymph nodes that typically follows contact with a cat or kitten. The infection is characterized by an erythematous papule or pustule at the primary inoculation site and regional lymphadenitis. Disseminated complications are rare. Recent evidence supports *Bartonella (Rochalimaea) henselae,* a small gram-negative rod, as the principal cause of cat-scratch disease.

Ocular cat-scratch disease occurs in two principal forms: (1) unilateral conjunctivitis characterized by serous conjunctival discharge, granuloma formation with or without conjunctival ulceration, and preauricular or submandibular lymphadenopathy presumably caused by direct inoculation to the ocular surface; and (2) intraocular inflammation characterized by unilateral or bilateral optic neuritis, retinitis, and vitreitis, presumably caused by disseminated infection from a primary, cutaneous inoculation site. Cat-scratch disease is probably the most common cause of Parinaud oculoglandular syndrome.

HISTORICAL BACKGROUND

In 1889 Parinaud[31] reported three patients with similar features of follicular conjunctivitis, mucofibrinous conjunctival discharge, clear cornea, regional lymphadenopathy, moderate low-grade fever, and a chronic course. Microbiologic or histopathologic studies were not defined. He suspected animals as a source of the condition because one patient was a butcher and another, a child, lived near a slaughter house.[5] In 1898 Gifford[15] termed the condition, "Parinaud's conjunctivitis." The entity was subsequently designated "Parinaud's oculoglandular syndrome" in distinction to "Parinaud's syndrome" of supranuclear paralysis of upgaze described by the same author.

In 1913 Verhoeff[42] identified bacteria in tissue specimens from patients with Parinaud oculoglandular syndrome and classified the organism as leptothrix. Others[43,47] isolated gram-negative, pleomorphic bacteria from patients with Parinaud oculoglandular syndrome and attributed the disease to leptothrix. Several authors noted a history of cat exposure among patients and suspected that the infection was spread by animals.[18,19,48] Later studies established leptothrix to be a saprophyte and not the pathogenic agent of cat-scratch disease or Parinaud oculoglandular syndrome.[7]

In 1950 the first case of cat-scratch disease was reported by Debré and associates[9] in a six-year-old Parisian boy. Infection was confirmed by a positive skin test with antigen provided by Foshay, a microbiologist at the University of Cincinnati.[25] Of note, as early as 1931 Debré described suppurative epitrochlear lymphadenitis in a 10-year-old boy with intimate cat contact and scratches.[25] Foshay also recognized several cases of a similar disease in 1932, prepared an antigen from aspirated pus from lymph nodes, and is credited with giving the entity the name "cat-scratch fever."[19] Multiple case series in France[9,30] and the United States[8] subsequently appeared and established cat-scratch disease as a distinct clinical entity.

Presme and Marchand[5,33] first confirmed cat-scratch disease in Parinaud oculoglandular syndrome in 1950. A six-year-old child developed unilateral conjunctivitis, preauricular lymphadenopathy, and fever following a cat scratch and bite. An intradermal skin test with antigen prepared in Debré's laboratory was positive.[7] Multiple reports of cat-scratch disease conjunctivitis confirmed by the cat-scratch skin test soon followed.

EPIDEMIOLOGY

Cat-scratch disease occurs in immunocompetent individuals of all ages throughout the world and is considered the most common cause of chronic regional lymphadenopathy in children and young adults. Eighty percent of patients are younger than 21 years of age. Fifty-five to sixty percent of cases are males.[20,26] A recent survey suggested that the disease may be more common in whites than blacks.[20] In temperate climates the disease is more common in the months of September through March, although the basis for seasonal variation has not been defined.

A review of three national databases[20] estimated that cat-scratch disease affects approximately 22,000 persons and results in the hospitalization of approximately 2000 persons annually in the United States. Multiple cases among family members occur, generally in families with one or more cats. Veterinarians have a greater risk of exposure to the disease as shown by skin test reactivity.[16,21] Human-to-human transmission of cat-scratch disease has not been documented.

RISK FACTORS

The principal animal vector of cat-scratch disease is the domestic cat or kitten, a role further defined by the elucidation of *B. henselae* in the pathogenesis of the disease. More than 27 million households in the United States have at least one cat.[40] In a series of more than 2000 cases of cat-scratch disease,[26,27] 95% of individuals reported a history of contact with a cat or kitten; 73% had a cat scratch. Four percent had contact with a dog only; 1% had no history of animal contact. In individuals who developed cat-scratch disease following minor injury with a thorn or stick, the majority reported that a cat licked the skin wound.

The route of inoculation in cat-scratch conjunctivitis is presumably hand-to-eye contact from either the cat's mouth, claws, or coat, and possibly by autoinoculation from a primary site elsewhere on the body. Approximately 5% to 10% of reported cases of cat-scratch disease develop as conjunctivitis.[27]

Among cases of cat-scratch disease occurring over a 13-month period in Connecticut, patients were (1) 15 times more likely than cat-owning control subjects to have at least one pet kitten 12 months old or younger, (2) 27 times more likely to have been scratched or bitten by a kitten, and (3) 29 times more likely to have at least 1 kitten with fleas.[49] Among serum samples from patients' cats, 81% were positive for antibodies to *B. henselae* as compared to 38% from control cats.[49] *B. henselae* was identified by culture, polymerase chain reaction, restriction fragment length polymorphism analysis, and DNA sequencing in seven cats among four patients with intimate cat contact and bacillary angiomatosis attributed to *B. henselae*.[23] *B. henselae* was also detected in fleas taken from an infected cat (by both direct culture and polymerase chain reaction) and isolated from 41% of blood samples taken from pet and impounded cats in California.[23] In addition, *B. henselae* was repeatedly isolated over a period of 3 weeks from the blood of a cat shown to have specific antibodies.[35] *B. henselae* antibodies are detectable in 14% to 44% of cats.

The role of other vectors in the transmission of cat-scratch disease to humans is uncertain. The cat flea, *Ctenocephalides felis,* is ubiquitous, has a life cycle spanning more than 1 year, and bites both cats and humans. Arthropod vectors (lice, ticks, and mites) transmit *Bartonella quintana* and most other pathogenic members of the family Rickettsiaceae to humans.[23] *C. felis* also commonly infects dogs and is known as a "dog flea." *B. henselae* is found in fleas, but it is unknown if these ectoparasites transmit the organism to animal hosts.

BACTERIOLOGY

Bartonella are small gram-negative rods of the α-2 subgroup of Proteobacteria assigned to the family Rickettsiacea (Fig. 99-1). The genus *Bartonella* comprises four species: *B. quintana, B. henselae, B. elizabethae,* and *B. vinsonii*. Three have been associated with six principal clinical syndromes in humans (Table 99-1).

Although *B. henselae* and *A. felis* are morphologically similar in tissue by Warthin-Starry staining, the organisms differ in genome size and total guanosine and cytosine content, lack of DNA relatedness on DNA-hybridization studies, and low level of sequence homology 16S ribosomal RNA gene.[1] *A. felis* is only distantly related to the genus *Bartonella* (Fig. 99-1). Although both organisms have been

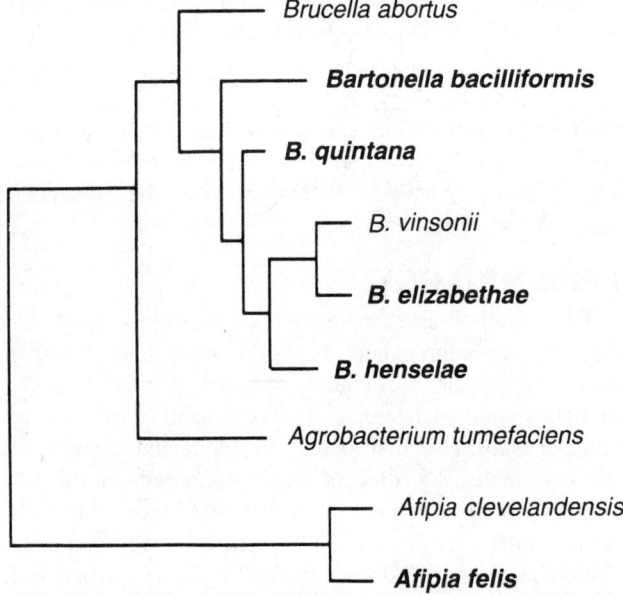

Fig. 99-1. Selected members of the α-2 subgroup of Proteobacteria. (Modified from Adal KA et al.: *N Engl J Med* 330:1509-1515, 1994.)

TABLE 99-1 CLINICAL SYNDROMES ASSOCIATED WITH *BARTONELLA*

Syndrome	Species
Cutaneous bacillary angiomatosis	*B. quintana, B. henselae*
Extracutaneous infection	*B. quintana, B. henselae, B. elizabethae*
Bacillary peliosis of the liver and spleen	*B. quintana, B. henselae*
Fever and relapsing bacteremia	*B. quintana, B. henselae*
Cat-scratch disease (regional lymphadenitis)	*B. henselae*
Trench fever	*B. quintana*
Encephalitis	*B. henselae*
Parinaud oculoglandular syndrome	*B. henselae, B. quintana*

identified as etiologic agents of cat-scratch disease, recent serologic and microbiologic studies provide convincing evidence that *B. henselae* is the principal cause.

CLINICAL FEATURES

Conjunctivitis

In cat-scratch disease conjunctivitis, initial symptoms occur within 3 to 10 days following inoculation, prior to the development of lymphadenopathy and systemic symptoms, and include mild foreign body sensation, lid edema, conjunctival hyperemia, and tearing. Simultaneous ocular and cutaneous inoculation is rare.[44] The conjunctivitis is typically unilateral and may be restricted to diffuse hyperemia and edema of the tarsal and bulbar conjunctiva with prominent follicular hypertrophy. The conjunctival discharge is generally clear and watery; purulent conjunctivitis is rare.[44] Single or multiple, raised or flat, gelatinous, hyperemic granulomatous lesions develop on either the superior or inferior tarsal conjunctiva, fornix, or bulbar conjunctiva (Figs. 99-2, 99-3). The most commonly reported site of granuloma formation is the upper tarsal conjunctiva.[5,44] The lesions may remain solid, densely yellow-white and opaque or become necrotic with ulceration (Fig. 99-4). Corneal involvement is uncommon; but fine and coarse punctate epithelial erosion, small epithelial defects, and small local infiltrates may occur. Concurrent intraocular inflammation is not a feature of ocular surface infection.

Regional lymphadenopathy either develops concurrently with the conjunctival signs or follows within 7 to 14 days. Unilateral preauricular, submandibular, and cervical lymphadenopathy is typical. The nodes are initially firm and tender. The overlying skin may become warm, red, and indurated. Ten to forty percent of lymph nodes become suppurative with formation of a sinus track to the skin sur-

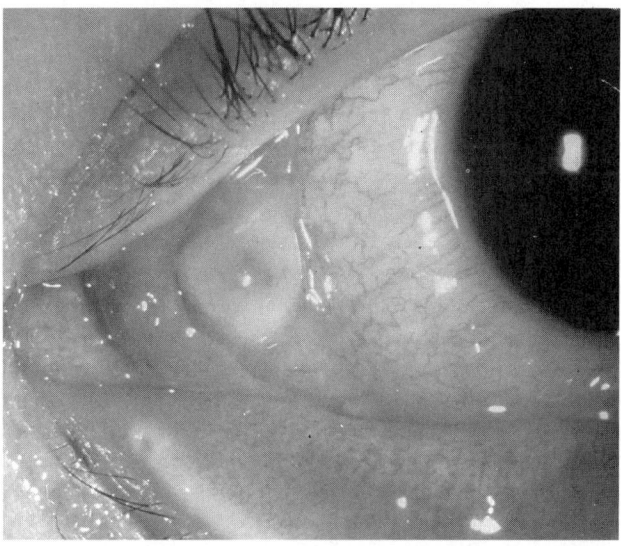

Fig. 99-3. Cat-scratch disease conjunctivitis. Ulcerated granulomatous nodule on the bulbar conjunctiva of an 8-year-old boy. Pleomorphic gram-negative bacilli in biopsy of lesion by Warthin-Starry stain.

face. Disseminated lymphadenopathy is uncommon. Follicular conjunctivitis and granulomatous conjunctival lesions resolve spontaneously. Significant conjunctival scarring does not occur. Serious ocular sequelae have not been reported. Regional lymphadenopathy typically resolves in 4 to 6 weeks but may persist for periods up to 12 months or longer.

Mild systemic symptoms including chills, fever, head-

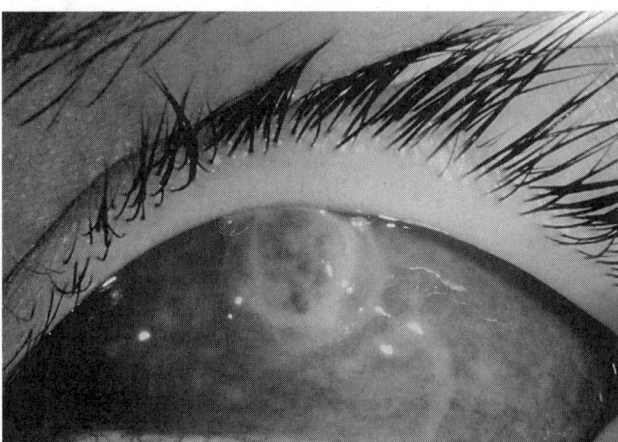

Fig. 99-2. Cat-scratch disease conjunctivitis. Granulomatous nodule on the upper tarsal conjunctiva of an 11-year-old girl. Pleomorphic gram-negative bacilli in biopsy of lesion by Warthin-Starry stain.

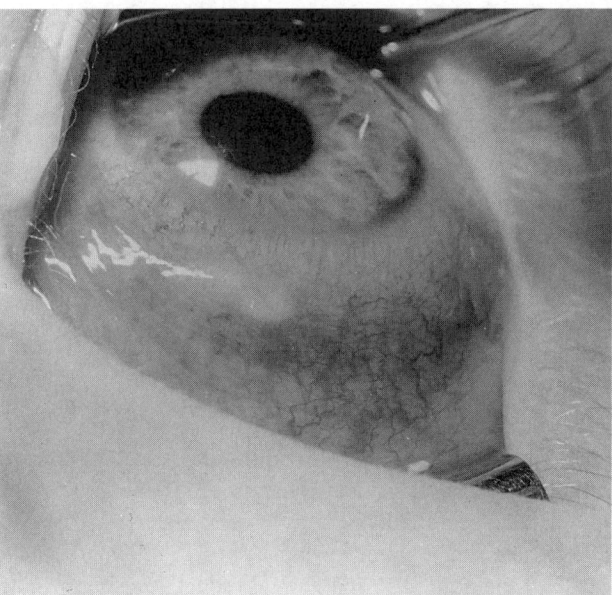

Fig. 99-4. Cat-scratch disease conjunctivitis. Ulcerated nodules on the inferior bulbar conjunctiva of a 22-month-old girl. Pleomorphic gram-negative bacilli in biopsy of lesion by Warthin-Starry stain. (Figure also in color insert.)

ache, anorexia, and malaise occur in approximately 10% to 28% of individuals with all forms of cat-scratch disease.[27] Severe, disseminated complications occur in approximately 2% of individuals and include encephalopathy, encephalitis, radiculopathy, erythema nodosum, thrombocytopenic purpura, osteolytic bone lesions, granulomatous hepatitis and splenitis.

Optic Neuritis

Intraocular inflammation attributable to cat-scratch disease was first described by Sweeney and Drance[39] in 1970. A 39-year-old individual experienced blurred vision in the right eye and weakness of the left hand 10 days following the onset of a pustular lesion on a finger of the left hand. These symptoms were accompanied by regional lymphadenopathy, fever, malaise, and nausea. Visual acuity was 20/400 in the right eye. A central scotoma and slowly reactive pupil were present. Intraocular inflammation was characterized by disc edema, dilated retinal veins, retinal edema, and macular star figure. Histopathologic features of a biopsied lymph node were compatible with cat-scratch disease, and a cat-scratch skin test was positive. Weakness of the left hand was attributed to compressive neuropathy of the median nerve by lymphadenopathy. Vision improved to 20/30 following intravenous ACTH. Others[11,14] subsequently recognized cat-scratch disease as a possible cause of Leber idiopathic stellate neuroretinitis, characterized by unilateral disc edema and macular star figure. In a series of 2006 cases of cat-scratch disease during the period of 1957 to 1993, Margileth and Hadfield[27] identified 30 cases of neuroretinitis.

The neuroretinitis is characterized by unilateral or bilateral decreased vision during the evolution of a primary cutaneous inoculation site and regional lymphadenitis. Neuroretinitis has not been recognized as a complication of cat-scratch disease conjunctivitis or in conjunction with acute encephalopathy.[6] Bilateral neuroretinitis has been reported in a patient with acquired immunodeficiency syndrome[38] and in immunocompetent individuals.[13,17] Initial reduction in visual acuity ranges from 20/25 to light perception. Associated findings include impaired color vision, central scotoma, and afferent pupillary defect. The optic nerve is elevated and edematous with dilated surface capillaries, often accompanied by edema of the nerve fiber layer as well as macular serous detachment and star figure formation (Fig. 99-5). Cells are present in the posterior and anterior vitreous. Peripapillary and diffuse intraretinal hemorrhages occur. White intraretinal infiltrates; yellow-orange subretinal, peripapillary, and perifoveal lesions; focal choroiditis; and necrotizing retinitis have been described.[13,17,27a] Fluorescein angiography typically reveals hyperfluorescence of the optic disc and normal retinal vasculature. The optic nerve edema and retinitis resolve over 4 to 12 months, generally with recovery of good vision in the range of 20/40 or better, without other sequelae.

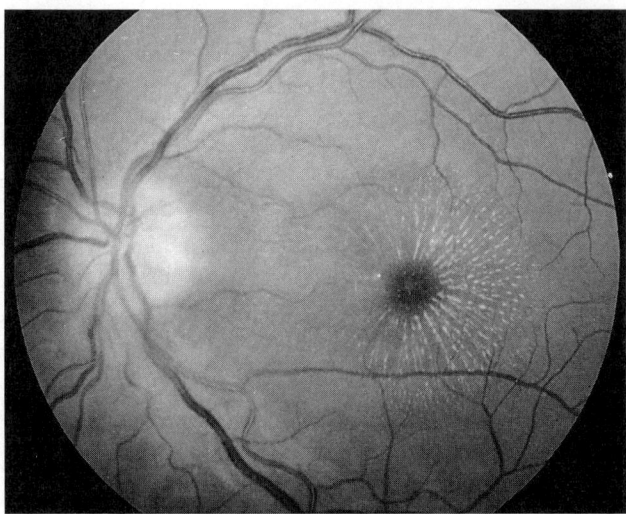

Fig. 99-5. Cat-scratch disease neuroretinitis. Acute loss of vision in a 21-year-old man following 2 weeks of fever, chills, night sweats, arthralgias, and headache. Close contact with a new kitten. Vision of 20/400 left eye and afferent pupillary light reflex. Note segmental disc edema and macular star figure. Acute antibody titer to *Bartonella henselae* of 1:1064. Convalescent titer 8 weeks later of 1:128. (Courtesy of Ralph A. Sawyer, MD.) (Figure also in color insert.)

Detection of organisms in lymph node material from patients with cat-scratch disease neuroretinitis was first reported by Ulrich and associates[41] in 1992. Warthin-Starry silver stain was used to identify typical bacilli in a tender axillary lymph node from a 6-year-old girl. This young patient had developed neuroretinitis 2 weeks following multiple scratches from a litter of kittens. Fish and associates[13] also identified gram-negative bacilli by Warthin-Starry silver staining of a lymph node biopsy in a 22-year-old man with neuroretinitis, 1 month following a cat bite of the left hand. Golnick and associates[17] recently detected *B. henselae* and *B. quintana* antibody titers equal to or greater than 1:256 in four patients with unilateral or bilateral intraocular inflammation characterized by vitreitis, optic disc edema, retinal lesions, and macular star. Each had intimate contact with cats.

DIFFERENTIAL DIAGNOSIS

Parinaud Oculoglandular Syndrome

Parinaud oculoglandular syndrome is granulomatous conjunctivitis, with or without follicle formation or ulceration, and unilateral preauricular or submandibular lymphadenopathy. Other conditions that produce granulomatous, necrotizing, or ulcerative conjunctivitis with regional lymphadenopathy are rare and include tularemia, tuberculosis, sporotrichosis, syphilis, and lymphogranuloma venereum.

Ocular tularemia is caused by hand-to-eye inoculation of *Francisella tularensis,* most commonly among hunters and tradesmen with contact with infected tissue of rabbits or squirrels. Unilateral or bilateral conjunctival involvement develops, characterized by necrotizing, ulcerative conjunctivitis with purulent discharge and suppurative regional lymphadenopathy. Fever and prostration may occur.

Tuberculous conjunctivitis results from a direct inoculation of *Mycobacterium tuberculosis* via infected sputum, blood, or other tissue, often in health-care personnel. Autoinoculation may occur in individuals with pulmonary tuberculosis by hand-to-eye transmission of sputum. Diffuse conjunctival hyperemia and edema precede the development of focal, necrotizing granulomatous lesions on the tarsal or bulbar conjunctiva. Membranous conjunctivitis may develop. Regional lymphadenopathy is common and progresses slowly. Without proper intervention and treatment, necrotizing scleritis and nonsuppurative keratitis may occur.

Ocular sporotrichosis results from direct inoculation from *Sporothrix schenckii*. Single or multiple soft, yellow-white conjunctival lesions develop and ulcerate, accompanied by regional lymphadenopathy. Similar-appearing conjunctival lesions seldom occur. Other fungal infections rarely reported to cause granulomatous conjunctivitis are actinomycosis, blastomycosis, and coccidioidomycosis.

Conjunctival lesions develop via direct inoculation in primary syphilis, characterized by diffuse conjunctival hyperemia within 2 to 4 weeks of inoculation. This hyperemia is followed by focal conjunctival necrosis and ulceration accompanied by mild pain, discharge, lid edema, and regional lymphadenopathy. Lesions in secondary syphilis include diffuse, simple conjunctivitis and nodular granulomatous conjunctivitis and scleritis. Ocular gumma formation in tertiary syphilis is extremely rare.

Lymphogranuloma venereum conjunctival infection is rare and occurs by ocular inoculation of genital secretions infected by serotypes L-1, L-2, and L-3 of *Chlamydia trachomatis*. Granulomatous conjunctivitis, profound lid edema, and preauricular lymphadenopathy develop and progress to conjunctivitis and corneal scarring if untreated.

Epstein-Barr virus occasionally produces nonsuppurative dacryoadenitis accompanied by marked hyperemia and edema of the superior tarsal and bulbar conjunctiva, serous conjunctival discharge, lid edema, and tender preauricular and submandibular lymphadenopathy. Conjunctival ulceration and necrosis are not features.

Optic Neuritis

The development of unilateral or bilateral optic neuritis or neuroretinitis in an individual with a history of cat contact should prompt the consideration of cat-scratch disease. Other similar forms of optic neuritis or retinitis may occasionally be caused by *Treponema pallidum, Toxoplasma gondii,* or *Toxocara canis,* but can usually be distinguished by other features and are not accompanied by a macular star figure.

PATHOLOGY

B. henselae can be identified in tissue and blood by polymerase chain reaction (PCR) coupled with hybridization or DNA sequencing. The PCR-restriction fragment length polymorphism method is relatively rapid and simple to perform and employs analysis of the citrate synthetase gene DNA.[10,24] Le and associates[24] identified *B. henselae* by PCR and oligonucleotide probe in material extracted from a swab of an ulcerated, conjunctival nodule in a man with human immunodeficiency virus who had oculoglandular syndrome.

Although cat-scratch disease conjunctivitis can be confirmed by the identification of small, pleomorphic bacilli in stained sections of conjunctival or regional lymph nodes, the histopathologic features do not distinguish *B. henselae* from *A. felis. Bartonella* species can be detected by Warthin-Starry silver, Steiner silver, and Brown-Hopps tissue stains. Histopathologic features of conjunctival tissue and lymph nodes are similar and are characterized by granulomatous necrosis, mixed cellular infiltrate, and reactive follicular hyperplasia. A central avascular necrotic area surrounded by lymphocytes with giant cells and histocytes is typical (Fig. 99-6). Bacilli may be massed in vessel walls and accompanied by swollen endothelial cells and obliteration of the vessel lumen (Fig. 99-7). Stellate granulomata and caseating necrosis may occur. Bacilli are more likely found in the presence of necrosis and granuloma formation.

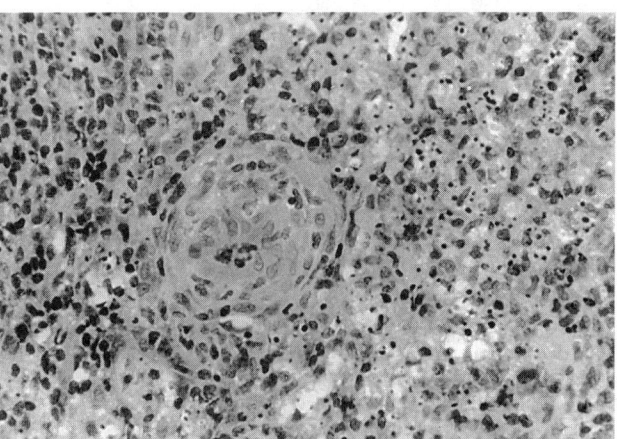

Fig. 99-6. Histopathologic appearance of conjunctival lesion (Fig. 99-4) in cat-scratch disease conjunctivitis. Stromal infiltrate of pleomorphic histocytes, small lymphocytes, and scattered nuclear debris. Occlusion of lumen of the vessel by endothelial cell proliferation. Mononuclear cell infiltrate of vascular wall. (Hematoxylin-eosin stain, 100 ×.)

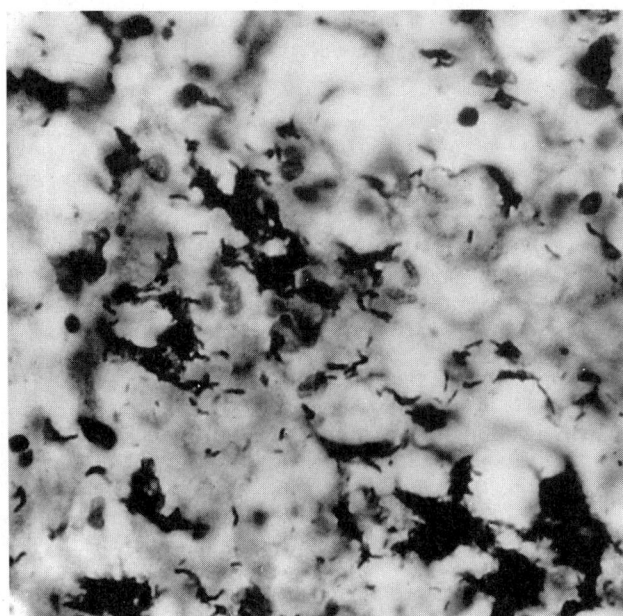

Fig. 99-7. Histopathologic appearance of conjunctival lesion (Fig. 99-4) in cat-scratch disease. Single and clusters of dark staining bacilli within the lesion. (Warthin-Starry stain, 252 ×.)

PATHOGENESIS

The potential role of a bacterium in the pathogenesis of cat-scratch disease remained conjectural until 1983. At this time Wear and associates[45] (at the Armed Forces Institute of Pathology) used the Warthin-Starry silver impregnation stain to identify delicate, pleomorphic gram-negative bacilli in lymph nodes from patients with cat-scratch disease. Similar gram-negative pleomorphic bacilli were subsequently identified in the primary inoculation site of patients with cat-scratch disease[28] and in conjunctival lesions of patients with oculoglandular syndrome.[44]

In 1988 English and associates[12] cultured a gram-negative bacterium morphologically identical to the vegetative and wall-defective forms seen in human tissues from lymph nodes with cat-scratch disease. Some patients also had fourfold or greater rises in antibody titer against the cultured bacterium. This organism was named *Afipia felis*[4] and was presumed to be the causative agent of cat-scratch disease. The genus name was derived from the abbreviation for the Armed Forces Institute of Pathology (AFIP), at which the type strain of the species was initially isolated. *A. felis* is a member of the α-2 subgroup of Proteobacteria (see Fig. 99-1). The organism is 0.2 to 0.5 μm in diameter and 0.2 to 2.5 μm long; pleomorphic when grown in brain-heart infusion broth; catalase-, citrate-, and D-mannitol-negative; possesses a single flagellum; and grows on buffered charcoal-yeast extract agar.

B. henselae was initially implicated as a causative agent of cat-scratch disease by Regnery and associates[36] in 1992. Using indirect fluorescent antibody tests, these researchers detected *B. henselae* antibodies among 88% of patients with cat-scratch disease versus 6% of healthy control individuals. *B. henselae* had initially been characterized by Relman and associates[37] in 1990. These researchers used polymerase chain reaction in tissue from three patients with bacillary angiomatosis and AIDS. The agent was subsequently identified as a new *Rochalimaea* species designated as *R. henselae*.[34,46] Further characterization has resulted in reclassification into the family Bartonellaceae.[4a]

Speculation that bacillary angiomatosis and cat-scratch disease were caused by the same organism was based on (1) the demonstration of similar, pleomorphic gram-negative bacilli in affected tissues by the Warthin-Starry stain, and (2) the development of bacillary angiomatosis following cat-scratch wounds.[22] Perkins and associates[32] subsequently identified rochalimaea-like species by polymerase chain reaction in five preparations of skin test antigens used for diagnosis of cat-scratch disease; each of the antigen preparations was negative for *A. felis* by polymerase chain reaction by random chromosomal DNA primers. *B. henselae* was also identified by polymerase chain reaction coupled with DNA sequence analysis in two additional cat-scratch disease skin test antigen materials.[2] *B. henselae* was subsequently isolated from infected lymph nodes in two immunocompetent patients with intimate contact with cats.[10] In another series[49] 84% of patients with cat-scratch disease had antibody titers (of 1 : 64 or higher) to *B. henselae,* as compared with 33% of samples from cat-owning control subjects. Anderson and associates[3] identified *B. henselae* in 84% of lymph node samples by polymerase chain reaction from patients with cat-scratch disease. Of note, no samples were positive for *B. quintana* or *A. felis.* In addition, 95% of blood samples from the cat-scratch disease cases had immunofluorescent antibody titers (of 1 : 64 or greater) to *B. henselae.*

LABORATORY INVESTIGATIONS

Prior to the development of new laboratory methods, the diagnosis of cat-scratch disease traditionally required the presence of three of four criteria: a history of cat or animal contact, scratch, or primary inoculation lesion; negative studies for other causes of lymphadenopathy; positive skin test with cat-scratch antigen; and characteristic histopathologic features in biopsied material. With the development of new laboratory tests, the diagnostic criteria should be redefined. Ideally these criteria should include identification of *B. henselae* or *A. felis* (1) by culture or nucleic acid hybridization or (2) by the presence of specific antibody.

Direct Identification

B. henselae can be isolated from primary inoculation sites, lymph nodes, and blood. For primary isolation, tissue samples and blood should be directly inoculated onto fresh blood, chocolate, and heart infusion agar and the plates incubated in increased CO_2 at 35°C and held for as long as 6 weeks. The Rickettsiae Laboratory of the National Center for Infectious Diseases of the Centers for Disease Control and Prevention (CDC) recommends commercial rabbit blood agar but has also isolated the organism on sheep blood tryptic soy agar and a defined liquid medium.[47a] *Bartonella* colonies are nonhemolytic, rough and dry, and yellow to gray in color, and typically appear no earlier than 9 days on primary incubation media. The organism can be isolated from blood by a blood culture system. Automated systems may not register positive for growth by CO_2-sensing techniques and should either be subcultured onto solid media or cultured using a lysis-centrifugation system. *A. felis* can be cultured on the same media and under identical conditions used to isolate *B. henselae.*

B. henselae is a pleomorphic, curved gram-negative rod that appears brightly fluorescent by acridine orange stain. The organism is X-factor dependent, and catalase-, oxidase-, and urease-negative. Identification is aided by membrane fatty acid analysis by gas chromatography or by use of a commercial system for identification of fastidious organisms.[1]

Serology

Antibodies to *B. henselae* can be detected in blood by indirect fluorescent antibody testing and by enzyme immunoassay.[1] The CDC Rickettsiae Laboratory currently provides indirect fluorescent antibody testing for *B. henselae* and *B. quintana* to physicians and state health departments. The enzyme immunoassay is more sensitive than the indirect fluorescent antibody test for *B. henselae* and is available from specialty laboratories.[1,22a]

Skin Test

The cat-scratch skin test antigen is prepared from purulent aspirate from a lymph node of a patient with proven cat-scratch disease and is available from multiple sources including the Uniformed Services University of the Health Sciences, Armed Forces Institute of Pathology, and Andrew M. Margileth (University of Virginia Medical Center, Charlottesville, Virginia). The skin test antigen (0.1 ml) is injected intradermally on the flexor surface of the arm. A positive reaction is a 5 mm diameter of induration, read at 48 hours postinoculation.

A positive intradermal skin test reaction requires approximately 4 weeks to develop from the onset of the primary lesion and at least 3 weeks from the onset of lymphadenopathy. The cat-scratch skin test antigen reaction remains positive for many years. The sensitivity of the skin test is 79% to 100% with specificity of 90% to 98% and negative predictive values of 78% to 100%.[26]

Other Tests

Consideration of other causes of oculoglandular syndrome should prompt inclusion of other microbiologic and serologic tests. Excised conjunctival material or aspirate from a lymph node should be inoculated to glucose-cystine-tellurite, Löwenstein-Jensen, and Sabouraud agar media for isolation of *Francisella tularensis, Mycobacterium tuberculosis,* and *Sporothrix schenckii,* respectively. *Chlamydia trachomatis* in lymphogranuloma venereum (LGV) can be detected by direct fluorescent antibody tests (MicroTrak, Syva) from conjunctival swabbing, or by culture onto McCoy cells; the Frei skin test is positive in approximately 50% of patients with LGV. Blood should be obtained for VDRL and MHA-TP testing for syphilis and for specific antibody determinations (to viral capsid antigen and nuclear antigen) for Epstein-Barr viral infection.

THERAPY

The ideal treatment of ocular cat-scratch disease has not been defined. Adequate clinical trials in cat-scratch disease or other infections caused by *Bartonella* species have not been conducted. Dolan and associates[10] performed broth microdilution antimicrobial susceptibility testing on three isolates of *B. henselae.* The organisms were broadly susceptible to a variety of agents including ampicillin (range of ≤ 0.03 to 0.06 μg/ml), cefotaxime (≤ 0.03 to 0.06), ceftriaxone (≤ 0.015), rifampin (≤ 0.03), tetracycline (≤ 0.12), erythromycin (≤ 0.25), azithromycin (≤ 0.03), clarithromycin (≤ 0.3), trimethoprim-sulfamethoxazole (1:19, 0.25 to 1.00), ciprofloxacin (0.5), temafloxacin (0.5), and gentamicin (0.5 to 1.0). *A. felis* is susceptible in vitro to imipenem, ceftriaxone, rifampin, amikacin, and tobramycin.[4,28,29]

For the treatment of *Bartonella* bacillary angiomatosis, bacillary peliosis hepatis, and bacteremic syndrome, oral erythromycin (500 mg 4 times daily) is the current drug of choice.[1] Excellent clinical responses have also been obtained with oral doxycycline. Dolan and associates[10] reported resolution of lymphadenopathy in two immunocompetent patients with cat-scratch disease attributable to *R. henselae* following oral doxycycline with ciprofloxacin and oral cephradine with doxycycline, respectively. Le and associates[24] noted rapid resolution of conjunctival nodularity and regional lymphadenopathy in *B. henselae* infection following oral ciprofloxacin (750 mg twice daily) and rifampin (600 mg daily), after initial failure of topical and oral ciprofloxacin. Among four patients (with intraocular inflammation, vitreitis, optic nerve edema, and retinitis) who had serologic evidence of *Bartonella* infection: two improved following oral ciprofloxacin (500 mg twice daily) and prednisone (40 mg daily initially), and two after oral doxycycline (250 mg four times daily) alone and oral ciprofloxacin (500 mg twice daily), alone.[17] A retrospective study of 202 patients with all forms of cat-scratch disease suggested efficacy of oral rifampin, oral ciprofloxacin, oral trimethoprim-sulfamethoxazole, and intramuscular gentamicin.[25]

The prognosis of ocular cat-scratch disease is excellent. Serious sequelae have not been reported following conjunctivitis. Normal acuity is recovered within one to four weeks after starting antibiotic therapy for *B. henselae* neuroretinitis. Permanent reduction in vision or other ocular complications have not occurred in patients with various forms of intraocular inflammation.

PREVENTION

Cat owners should seek periodic veterinary care to minimize flea infestation and to maintain current rabies and other vaccinations. Contact between infected kittens and cats and humans should be minimized by avoiding rough play with pets and strays. Any cat bite or scratch should be immediately washed and disinfected.

Prevention of cat-scratch disease will require the development of an effective vaccine against *B. henselae* (and possibly *A. felis*) in cats. Other measures seem unlikely, such as (1) control of infection by antibiotic treatments in cats or (2) eradication of the cat flea, *Ctenocephalides felis,* or multiple potential tick vectors.

REFERENCES

1. Adal KA, Cockerell CJ, Petri WA Jr: Cat scratch disease, bacillary angiomatosis, and other infections due to *Rochalimaea, N Engl J Med* 330:1509-1515, 1994.
2. Anderson B, Kelly C, Threlkel R et al.: Detection of *Rochalimaea henselae* in cat-scratch disease skin test antigens, *J Infect Dis* 168:1034-1036, 1993.
3. Anderson B, Sims K, Regnery R et al.: Detection of *Rochalimaea henselae* DNA in specimens from cat scratch disease patients by PCR, *J Clin Microbiol* 32:942-948, 1994.
4. Brenner DJ, Hollis DG, Moss CW et al.: Proposal of *Afipia* gen. nov., with *Afipia felis* sp. nov. (formerly the cat scratch disease bacillus), *Afipia clevelandensis* sp. nov. (formerly the Cleveland Clinic Foundation strain), *Afipia broomeae* sp. nov., and three unnamed genospecies, *J Clin Microbiol* 29:2450-2460, 1991.
4a. Brenner DJ, O'Connor SP, Winkler HH, Steigerwalt AG: Proposals to verify the genera *Bartonella* and *Rochalimaea,* with descriptions of *Bartonella quintana* comb. nov., *Bartonella vinsonii* comb. nov., *Bartonella henselae* comb. nov., and *Bartonella elizabethae* comb. nov., and to remove the family Bartonellacaea from the order Richettsiales, *Int J Syst Bacteriol* 43:777-786, 1993.
5. Carithers HA: Oculoglandular disease of Parinaud: a manifestation of cat-scratch disease, *Am J Dis Child* 132:1195-1200, 1978.
6. Carithers HA and Margileth AM: Cat-scratch disease: acute endephalopathy and other neurologic manifestations, *Am J Dis Child* 145:98-101, 1991.
7. Cassady JV, Culbertson CS: Cat scratch disease and Parinaud's oculolandular syndromes, *Arch Ophthalmol* 50:68-74, 1953.
8. Daniels WP, MacMurray FG: Cat-scratch disease. Report on one hundred sixty cases, *JAMA* 154:1247-1251, 1954.
9. Debré R, Lamy M, Jammett ML et al.: La maladie des griffes de chat, *Bull Mem Soc Med Hôp Paris* 66:76-79, 1950.
10. Dolan MJ, Wong MT, Regenery R et al.: Syndrome of *Rochalimaea henselae* adenitis suggesting cat scratch disease, *Arch Int Med* 118:331-336, 1993.
11. Dreyer RF, Hopen G, Gass DM et al.: Leber's idiopathic stellate neuroretinitis, *Arch Ophthalmol* 102:1140-1145, 1984.
12. English CK, Wear DJ, Margileth AM et al.: Cat-scratch disease. Isolation and culture of the bacterial agent, *JAMA* 259:1347-1352, 1988.
13. Fish RH, Hogan RN, Nightingale SD et al.: Peripapillary angiomatosis associated with cat-scratch neuroretinitis, *Arch Ophthalmol* 110:323, 1992.
14. Gass JDM: Diseases of the optic nerve that may simulate macular disease, *Trans Am Acad Ophthalmol Otolaryngol* 83:763-770, 1977.

15. Gifford H: Five cases of Parinaud's conjunctivitis, *Am J Ophthalmol* 15:193-200, 1898.
16. Gifford H: Skin test reactions to cat scratch disease among veterinarians, *Arch Int Med* 95:828-833, 1955.
17. Golnik KC, Marotto ME, Fanous MM et al.: Ophthalmic manifestations of *Rochalimaea* species, *Am J Ophthalmol* 118:145-151, 1994.
18. Henry M: Oculoglandular conjunctivitis due to leptothrix, *J Ped* 37:535-544, 1950.
19. Henry M: Leptothricosis conjunctivae (Parinaud's conjunctivitis), *Trans Pacific Coast Oto-ophthalmol Soc* 33:173-196, 1952.
20. Jackson LA, Perkins BA, Wenger JD: Cat scratch disease in the United States: an analysis of three national databases, *Am J Public Health* 83:1707-1711, 1993.
21. Kalter SS: A survey of cat scratch disease among veterinarians, *JAMA* 144:1281-1282, 1964.
22. Kemper CA, Lombard CM, Deresinsk SC et al.: Visceral bacillary epithelioid angiomatosis: possible manifestations of disseminated cat scratch disease in immunocompromised host: a report of two cases, *Am J Med* 89:216-222, 1990.
22a. Kessler DF, Cruz OA: Serologic confirmation of *Rochalimaea* in cat-scratch disease, *Ann Ophthalmol* 27:33-35, 1995.
23. Koehler JE, Glaser CA, Tappero JW: *Rochalimaea henselae* infection. A new zoonosis with the domestic cat as reservoir, *JAMA* 271:531-535, 1994.
24. Le HH, Palay DA, Anderson B et al.: Conjunctival swab to diagnose ocular cat scratch disease, *Am J Ophthalmol* 118:249-250, 1994.
25. Margileth AM: Antibiotic therapy for cat-scratch disease: clinical study of therapeutic outcome in 268 patients and a review of the literature, *Pediatr Infect Dis J* 11:474-478, 1992.
26. Margileth AM: Cat scratch disease. In *Advances in pediatric infectious diseases,* vol 8, 1-21, 1993, Mosby.
27. Margileth AM, Hadfield T: Cat scratch disease: etiology, pathogenesis, diagnosis, and management, American Society of Clinical Pathologists Spring 1994 Teleconference Series, April 21, 1994.
28. Margileth AM, Wear DJ, Hadfield TL et al.: Cat-scratch disease. Bacteria in skin at the primary inoculation site, *JAMA* 252:928-931, 1984.
29. Maurin M, Lepochere H, Mallet D et al.: Antibiotic susceptibilities in *Afipia felis* in axenic medium and in cells, *Antimicrob Agents Chemother* 34:1410-1413, 1993.
29a. McCrary B, Cockerham W, Pierce P: Neuroretinitis in cat-scratch disease associated with the macular star, *Pediatr Infect Dis* 13:838-839, 1994.
30. Mollaret P, Reilly J, Bastin R et al.: Sur un adenopathie regionale subaigue et spontanement curable, avec intradermo-reaction et lesions ganglionnaires particulieres, *Bull Mem Soc Med Hôp Paris* 66:424-449, 1950.
31. Parinaud H: Conjunctivite infectieuse paraissant transmisé à l'homme par les animaux, *Bull Soc Ophtalmol Paris* 2:29-31, 1889.
32. Perkins BA, Swaminathan B, Jackson L et al.: Case 22-1992—pathogenesis of cat scratch disease, *N Engl J Med* 327:1599-1600, 1992.
33. Presme P, Marchand E: Sur un nouveau type de conjonctivite infectieuse probablement transmisé par le chat, *J Méd Bordeaux* 127:127-131, 1950.
34. Regnery RL, Anderson BE, Clarridge JE et al.: Characterization of a novel "*Rochalimae* species, *R. henselae* sp. nov., isolated from blood of a febrile, human immunodeficiency virus-positive patient, *J Clin Microbiol* 30:265-274, 1992.
35. Regnery RL, Martin M, Olson J: Naturally occurring "*Rochalimaea henselae*" infection in domestic cat, *Lancet* 340:557-558, 1992.
36. Regnery RL, Olson JG, Perkins BA et al.: Serological response to "*Rochalimaea henselae*" antigen in suspected cat-scratch disease, *Lancet* 339:1443-1445, 1992.
37. Relman DA, Loutit JS, Schmidt TM et al.: The agent of bacillary angiomatosis. An approach to the identification of uncultured pathogens, *N Engl J Med* 323:1573-1580, 1990.
38. Schlossberg D, Morad Y, Krouse TB et al.: Culture-proved disseminated cat-scratch disease in acquired immunodeficiency syndrome, *Arch Intern Med* 149:1437-1439, 1989.
39. Sweeney VP, Drance SM: Optic neuritis and comprehensive neuropathy associated with cat scratch disease, *Can Med Assoc J* 103:1380-1381, 1970.

40. Troutman CM: Cat owners and their use of veterinary services, *J Am Vet Med Assoc* 193:1217-1219, 1988.

41. Ulrich GG, Waecker NJ, Meister SJ et al.: Cat scratch disease associated with neuroretinitis in a 6-year-old girl, *Ophthalmology* 99:246-250, 1992.

42. Verhoeff FJ: Parinaud's conjunctivitis, a mycotic disease due to hitherto undescribed filamentous organism, *Arch Ophthalmol* 42:345-351, 1913.

43. Verhoeff FH, King MJ: Leptotrichosis conjunctivae (Parinaud's conjunctivitis), *Arch Ophthalmol* 9:701-714, 1933.

44. Wear DJ, Malaty RH, Zimmerman LE et al.: Cat scratch disease bacilli in the conjunctiva of patients with Parinaud's oculoglandular syndrome, *Ophthalmology* 92:1282-1287, 1985.

45. Wear DJ, Margileth AM, Hadfield TL et al.: Cat scratch disease: a bacterial infection, *Science* 221:1403-1405, 1983.

46. Welch DF, Pickett DA, Slater LN: *R. henselae* sp. nov., a cause of septicemia, bacillary angiomatosis, and parenchymal bacillary peliosis, *J Clin Microbiol* 30:275-280, 1992.

47. Wherry WB, Ray V: Cultures of a leptothrix from a case of Parinaud's oculoglandular conjunctivitis, *J Infect Dis* 22:554-558, 1918.

47a. Wong MT, Thornton DC, Kennedy RC, Dolan MJ: A chemically defined liquid medium that support primary isolation of *Rochalimaea (Bartonella) henselae* from blood and tissue specimens, *J Clin Microbiol* 33:742-744, 1995.

48. Wright RE: Isolation of Verhoeff's leptothrix in a case of Parinaud's syndrome, *Arch Ophthalmol* 18:233-236, 1937.

49. Zangwill KM, Hamilton DH, Perkins BA et al.: Cat scratch disease in Connecticut. Epidemiology, risk factors, and evaluation of a new diagnostic test, *N Engl J Med* 329:8-13, 1993.

100 Whipple Disease

SANDY T. FELDMAN, WILLIAM R. FREEMAN, LELAND S. RICKMAN

The ocular manifestations of Whipple disease may result from direct infection of the eye or may be secondary to involvement of the central nervous system (see box). Individuals with eye disease may have little or no gastrointestinal or neurologic symptoms. Identification of the organism, *Tropheryma whippelii,* is leading to earlier diagnosis and a better understanding of the pathogenesis of this uncommon disease.

HISTORICAL BACKGROUND

Whipple disease was first described in 1907 in a 36-year-old male physician with migratory polyarthritis, cough, diarrhea with malabsorption, weight loss, and mesenteric lymphadenopathy.[52] Whipple hypothesized the cause was infectious, as rod-shaped organisms were detected in silver-stained sections. He also noted the disease (1) occurred more commonly in whites (99%) and males (86%); (2) was limited to North America, United Kingdom, and Europe; and (3) mimicked lymphoma, collagen-vascular disease, sarcoidosis, and other diseases that present with diarrhea, malabsorption syndrome, pericarditis, and dementia.[10]

The histological criteria for diagnosing Whipple disease were first reported by Black-Schaffer[5] in 1948. The criteria included finding nonlipid containing macrophages throughout the lamina propria of the intestines and colon as well as detecting lipogranulomatous reaction of mesenteric lymph nodes. Black-Schaffer[5] reported positive periodic acid-Schiff (PAS) staining of the macrophages and advocated usage of the name "Whipple's disease" and not "intestinal lipodystrophy" as Whipple had suggested.[10]

The development of electron microscopy aided in the visualization of the organism in the early 1960s.[8,55] The organisms were bacillary shaped, measuring $1.0\ \mu$ by $0.2\ \mu$, with a plasma membrane, capsule external to the membrane, and an inner core of electron-dense material. At the light level, these were identified by PAS, silver, and other special stains as gram-positive bacteria. The mechanism responsible for malabsorption was found to be due to bacterial invasion of the intestinal epithelium and not blockage of the lymphatics. Invasion of many other cell types including the endothe-

lium of lymphatic and capillary vessels, polymorphonuclear leukocytes, plasma cells, lymphocytes, and mast cells was also detected.[11,55] Unlike other bacteria, the Whipple bacillus is located intracellularly and extracellularly.

To date, no one has been able to culture the organism. Nonetheless, molecular biologic techniques has enabled identification of this elusive organism and phylogenetic classification.[37,39]

EPIDEMIOLOGY

Whipple disease is a rare systemic disorder. Dobbins[10] reviewed the literature and reported that there were 617 cases from the early 1900s through 1986. The disease occurs predominantly in Caucasians; only 15 cases have been reported in non-Caucasians.[10] The majority of reported patients are young (average age, 49 years) and male (86%). Approximately 66% of the individuals with Whipple disease have an occupation with soil and/or animal contact. Death caused by Whipple disease occurs in roughly 26% of cases, either because of lack of treatment, relapse, or predisposing factor for other illness.

CLINICAL FEATURES

Although frequently found at autopsy in multiple tissues, clinical evidence of organ dysfunction is predominately reflected by changes in the small bowel, central nervous system, joints (arthralgias and arthritis), and skin (hyperpigmentation). The initial description of a physician with Whipple disease in 1907 included diarrhea with malabsorption and weight loss, migratory polyarthritis, cough, and mesenteric adenopathy.[10,52] The gastrointestinal tract, brain, and heart are often the end organs affected in Whipple disease. The most common findings include weight loss (70% to 100%), malabsorption (93%), hypotension (63% to 83%), lymphadenopathy (52% to 55%), fever (38% to 58%), peripheral edema (18% to 34%), abdominal tenderness (48% to 54%), mesenteric and retroperitoneal lymphadenopathy leading to palpable abdominal masses (18% to 24%), endocarditis (25%), and hyperpigmentation of the skin (25% to 33%).[31]

```
┌─────────────────────────────────────────┐
│       OPHTHALMIC MANIFESTATIONS OF       │
│             WHIPPLE DISEASE              │
├─────────────────────────────────────────┤
│  Ocular Findings                         │
│    Conjunctivitis                        │
│    Keratitis                             │
│    Iridocyclitis                         │
│      Keratitic precipitates              │
│      Iris nodules                        │
│      Vitreitis                           │
│      Secondary glaucoma                   │
│    Choroiditis                           │
│    Retinitis                             │
│    Retinal vasculitis                    │
│      Retinal hemorrhage                  │
│      Vitreous hemorrhage                 │
│      Retinal neovascularization          │
│  Orbital and Neuro-Ophthalmic Findings   │
│    Orbital myositis                      │
│    External ophthalmoplegia              │
│      Ptosis                              │
│    Internal ophthalmoplegia              │
│    Supranuclear ophthalmoplegia          │
│    Nystagmus                             │
│    Papilledema                           │
│      Cecocentral scotoma                 │
│      Optic atrophy                       │
└─────────────────────────────────────────┘
```

A low-grade fever is frequently seen, with occasional temperature spikes over 102°F. Routine laboratory tests (such as the leukocyte count), which are usually elevated with systemic infections, are generally normal but may reveal a leukocytosis or leukopenia.

Intestinal Manifestations

Gastrointestinal manifestations are usually the most prominent symptoms. Clinical illness is most often characterized by the gradual development of diarrhea with evidence of malabsorption (steatorrhea) and weight loss with ill-defined abdominal pain. Routine laboratory tests may reveal a normocytic anemia, evidence of liver synthetic dysfunction (hypoalbuminemia, prolonged prothrombin time), or hypocholesterolemia. Stool studies may reveal increased stool fat excretion; and studies of small intestinal absorptive capacity, such as a decreased D-xylose absorption test. Mesenteric lymphadenopathy is frequently found by imaging studies or at autopsy.

Extraintestinal Manifestations

Migratory arthralgias or a seronegative arthritis of the large joints is quite common and may precede gastrointestinal symptoms by years. Peripheral lymphadenopathy is frequent and occasionally hepatosplenomegaly may be seen.

Central Nervous System. Both parenchymal and meningeal involvement with *T. whippelii* are not uncommon findings; however, clinical findings are less frequent than histopathologic evidence of infection. Dementia, ophthalmoloplegia, and myoclonus are the most frequently reported neurologic signs,[10] and this "classic" triad should suggest Whipple disease.[34] Parenchymal cerebral hemisphere involvement may cause dementia, personality changes, or paresis. Obstructive hydrocephalus and hypothalamic signs (hypersomnia, insomnia, polydipsia, and polyphagia) have also been reported.

Several cases of Whipple disease have been reported with minimal gastrointestinal signs or symptoms; however, histopathologic findings of gastrointestinal infection with *T. whippelii* are usually present.[15,27,29,44,49] There are rare cases reported in which patients with CNS Whipple disease are found not to have gastrointestinal involvement by either premortem or postmortem examinations of the small intestine.[6,14,24,42,53] It is unknown how often CNS Whipple disease actually exists in the absence of gastrointestinal tract infection.

Cardiopulmonary System. Endocarditis, myocarditis, pericarditis, and coronary arteritis have been well described in patients with Whipple disease, although not in a prospective manner. Nonbacterial (marantic) endocarditis causing chronic aortic regurgitation has been well described and was present in Whipple's initial description of the syndrome. Pancarditis or polyserositis (pericarditis, pleuritis, and/or peritonitis) may occur and suggest the presence of a collagen-vascular disease.

Mediastinal adenopathy with or without pleural effusions has been described. Cough is sometimes a prominent complaint. Histopathology may show granulomatous changes, and the disease may mimic sarcoidosis.

Skin. Hyperpigmentation of the skin is seen in approximately 50% of patients and does not reflect adrenal insufficiency.[31] It is suggestive of Whipple disease in the presence of weight loss, diarrhea, and hypotension.

Ocular Manifestations

Involvement of the eye was first reported in 1949.[25] The eye may serve as a primary or secondary target or may be involved as a result of both primary and secondary involvement. The eye findings result from CNS infection in the majority of cases, occur concurrently to CNS infection in a minor percentage of cases, and are intraocular without CNS involvement in only a few cases. There have been many cases of Whipple disease with mainly ocular involvement and minimal gastrointestinal or CNS symptoms.[3,18,27] There is only one case in which ocular findings were detected in the absence of extraocular manifestations.[40] This patient had recurrent and worsening ocular inflammation with two negative duodenal biopsies at the light microscopic level. Her only systemic manifestation was weight loss. Eventually, the diagnosis was made from light microscopy of vitreous

TABLE 100-1 OCULAR FINDINGS OF WHIPPLE DISEASE—WITH OR WITHOUT NEUROLOGIC OR GASTROINTESTINAL MANIFESTATIONS

Author, Year	Number of Patients	Ocular Findings	CNS Disease	GI Disease	Comments
Jones,[25] 1949	1	Optic atrophy	Headache		
Hendrix,[21] 1950	1	Reduced vision	Headaches, radicular pain of lower extremities		
Tracey,[50] 1950	1	Reduced vision			
Paulley,[35] 1952	1	Optic nerve atrophy	Peculiar behavior		
Ritama,[41] 1953	1	Sudden partial loss of vision	"Giddiness, Loss of taste"		
Kruecke, 1962 (Cited by Switz,[48] 1969)	1	Retina	Positive		
Lampert,[28] 1962	1	Nystagmus, gaze palsy			
Enzinger,[13] 1963	1	Reduced vision			PAS-positive deposits at autopsy
Badenoch,[4] 1963	1	Fluctuating gaze palsies, nystagmus, reduced vision, nonreactive pupils	Encephalopathy	Positive premortem	PAS-positive staining with macrophages in CNS at autopsy
Dybkaer,[12] 1965	1	Vitreous hemorrhage			
Smith,[45] 1965	1	Ophthalmoplegia, bilateral ptosis, nystagmus, keratitis	Headaches, myoclonus, confusion		PAS-positive deposits in CNS
Knox,[27] 1968	1	Vitreitis, retinal hemorrhage, papilledema, no iris nodules	Bilateral hearing loss with tinnitus	Positive jejunal biopsy	
Malamud, Harrington (Reviewed in Knox,[27] 1968)	1	Choroiditis, anterior uveitis, retinal vasculitis	Bizarre personality, seizure	"Mild diarrhea"	PAS-positive deposits in brain
Stoupel,[46] 1969	1	Pale optic discs, ophthalmoplegia	Myoclonus	Positive in intestines postmortem	
Switz,[48] 1969	1	Papilledema, retinal hemorrhages, vitreitis	Bilateral hearing deficit, premortem	Positive at autopsy	Postmortem PAS-positivity in optic nerves
Vazquez-Rodriguez,[51] 1972	1	Papilledema			
Henry,[22] 1974	1	Bilateral central scotoma			
Silbert,[44] 1976	1	Ophthalmoplegia	Hypersomnia, memory loss	No symptoms, but positive at autopsy	Postmortem diagnosis
Moorthy,[32] 1977	1	Supranuclear ophthalmoplegia	Positive	Positive biopsy only	Diagnosed by electron microscopy of intestinal biopsy

1400

Reference	No.	Ocular findings	Status	Systemic/biopsy	Comments
Finelli,[15] 1977	3	Uveitis, choroiditis, supranuclear ophthalmoplegia	Positive	Negative jejunal biopsy, positive at autopsy	
Leland,[30] 1978	1	Secondary glaucoma, conjunctival hyperemia, keratitis, anterior uveitis	No symptoms	Positive jejunal biopsy	
Font,[17] 1978	1	Vitreitis, retinitis	Postmortem diagnosis	No symptoms, no biopsy	PAS-positive macrophages in vitreous and retina
Feurle,[14] 1979	2	Nystagmus	Positive	Negative jejunal biopsy	
Johnson,[24] 1980	1	Uveitis, supranuclear ophthalmoplegia	Positive	Negative small bowel biopsy	
Gartner,[18] 1980	1	Ophthalmoplegia, vitreitis	Positive	Negative by history	Extraocular muscle involvement by biopsy
Halperin,[19] 1981	1	Nystagmus	Premortem mass lesion	Negative jejunal biopsy	
Selsky,[43] 1984	1	Bilateral vitreous opacities	None reported	Negative jejunal biopsy	
Avila,[3] 1984	2	Papilledema, retinitis, choroiditis	Negative	Positive by biopsy	
Keinath,[26] 1985	1	Nystagmus			
Adams,[1] 1987	1	Supranuclear ophthalmoplegia	Positive	Negative at autopsy	
Nath,[33] 1987	1	Supranuclear ophthalmoplegia	Premortem		
Fleming,[16] 1988	1	Ophthalmoplegia			AIDS
Hausser-Hauw,[20] 1988	1	Ophthalmoplegia, ptosis, "oculomasticator myorhythmia"	Positive	Positive for symptoms	
Brown,[7] 1990	1	Nystagmus	Positive premortem focal lesion		
Wroe,[54] 1991	1	Papilledema	Positive	Negative jejunal/duodenal biopsy	Intracerebral mass lesion
Disdier,[9] 1991	1	Chemosis, myositis	Negative	Positive duodenal biopsy	
Playford,[36] 1992	1	Retinal vasculitis, reduced vision	No symptoms initially	Positive	Jarisch-Herxheimer reaction
Relman,[39] 1992	1	Uveitis	Negative	Positive duodenal biopsy	
Schrenk,[42a] 1994	1	Panuveitis	No symptoms	Positive jejunal biopsy	
Rickman,[40] 1995	1	Iridocyclitis, corneal endothelial precipitates, vitreitis, iris nodules, retinitis, disc neovascularization	Negative	Positive duodenal biopsy	PAS-positive macrophages in vitreous, PCR analysis of vitreous and duodenum
Knox,[27a] 1995	1	Supranuclear ophthalmoplegia, ocular and facial myoclonus	Positive	Positive	PAS-positive macrophages in eye

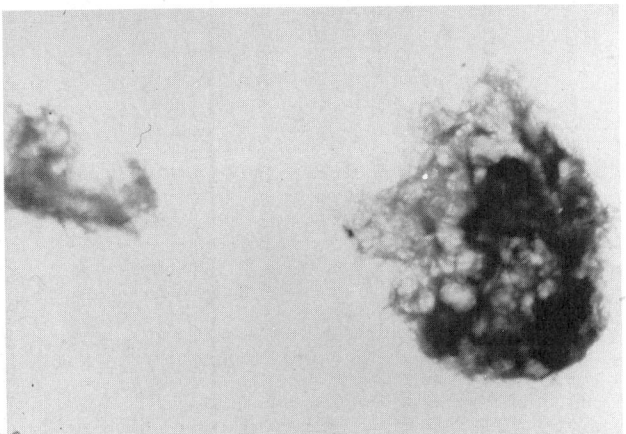

Fig. 100-1. PAS-positive material from a vitreous biopsy.

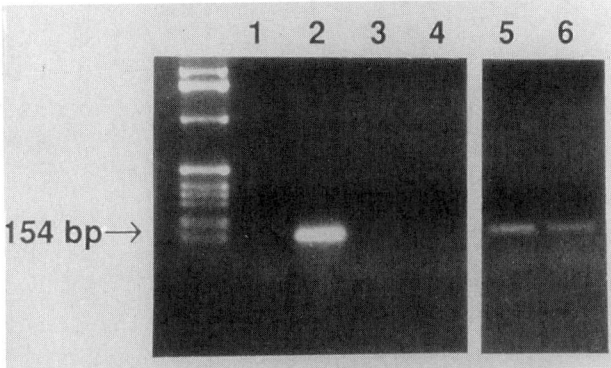

Fig. 100-2. Polymerase chain reaction result confirming *T. whippelii* in the vitreous (lane 5) and duodenum (lane 6) in a patient with chronic uveitis. [Reprinted with permission from Rickman L, Freeman WR, Green WR et al.: Brief report: uveitis caused by *Tropheryma whippelii* (Whipple's bacillus), *N Engl J Med* 332:363-366, 1995.]

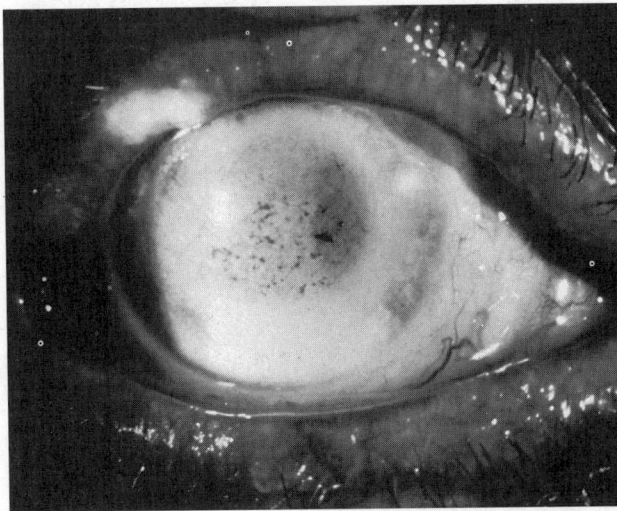

Fig. 100-3. Marked anterior-chamber inflammation with confluent corneal deposits.

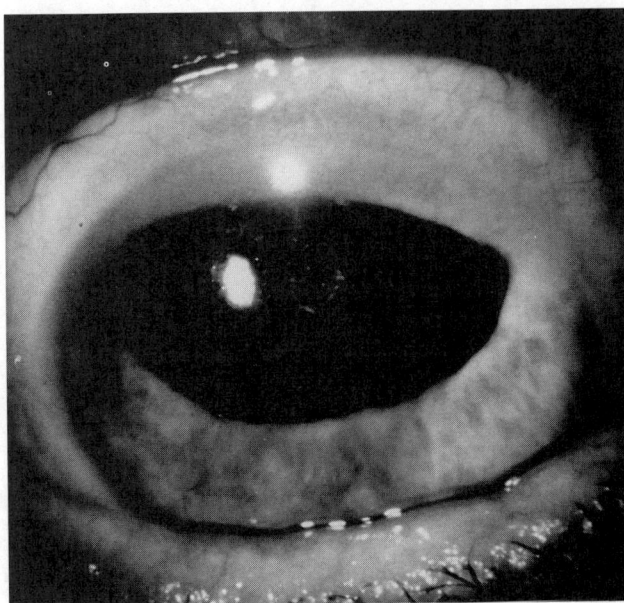

Fig. 100-4. Chronic uveitis with multiple iris nodules caused by Whipple disease.

fluid (Fig. 100-1) and polymerase chain reaction (PCR) analysis of the vitreous and duodenal tissue (Fig. 100-2).[40]

Table 100-1 summarizes the findings in reported cases with eye involvement. The most common ocular manifestations include reduced visual acuity,[1,48] papilledema,[48,51] optic atrophy,[25] uveitis,[15,24,30] choroiditis,[15] retinitis,[17] vitreitis,[27,39,43] vitreous hemorrhages,[43] keratitis,[30,45] ophthalmoplegia,[16,26] external ophthalmoplegia and keratitis,[45] supranuclear ophthalmoplegia,[15,20,23,33] gaze palsies,[4] nystagmus,[4,19,26] bilateral central scotoma,[22] and chemosis.[9] Signs associated with posterior fossa disease such as external ophthalmoplegia,[4,28] gaze palsies,[4,28] and pupillary abnormalities[4,45] have also been described. New findings in Whipple disease include flocculent corneal endothelial precipitates (Fig. 100-3), iris nodules (Fig. 100-4), and retinal neovascularization.

PATHOLOGY

The diagnosis of Whipple disease is usually made by examination of a duodenal biopsy at the light and electron microscopic level. PAS-positive macrophages within the lamina propria of "clubbed," abnormal microvilli are pathognomonic of Whipple disease and result from breakdown of the cell wall of the bacillus. Large lipid deposits are also present throughout the lamina propria. Polymorphonuclear leukocytes, eosinophils, and macrophages, not normally found in the epithelium, are often detected.[2]

Electron microscopic evaluation confirms the light microscopic findings.[11] The microvilli are sparse. The majority of organisms are located not in the lumen, but in the base of the epithelium and in the intercellular spaces, suggesting the epithelial degeneration results from bacterial invasion. The macrophages of the lamina propria show bacteria and their breakdown products. A key feature is the presence of bacteria in an extracellular location.

DIFFERENTIAL DIAGNOSIS

Clinical findings may suggest diffuse involvement of the gastrointestinal tract. Therefore, the differential diagnosis usually includes human immunodeficiency virus and related opportunistic infections such as disseminated *Mycobacterium avium-intracellulare* infection, inflammatory bowel disease, or infiltrative small bowel neoplasms.

Gastrointestinal *Histoplasma capsulatum* or nontuberculous mycobacterial infection may be differentiated from infection caused by *Tropheryma whippelii* by the use of special stains. Not infrequently, the clinical presentation may be a fever of unknown origin, a sarcoidosis-like syndrome, a wasting condition, or a collagen-vascular disease.

LABORATORY INVESTIGATIONS

A major obstacle in Whipple disease is the inability to culture the bacillus and prove it is responsible for the disease. Nonetheless, advances in molecular biology have led to the identification of uncultured bacteria in peptic ulcer disease and in Whipple disease.[38,39,47] Using PCR, a technique that involves amplifying bacterial 16S ribosomal RNA (rRNA) from infected tissue, Relman and associates[39] identified a new organism directly from infected tissue and named this agent, *Tropheryma whippelii.* The 16S rRNA, which is found in all living cells, is helpful in identifying the phylogeny of bacteria, as slow mutations occur over time. Sequence differences help to characterize the organisms in the evolutionary tree. *T. whippelii* belongs to the Actinomycetes family and has a unique sequence not previously identified. Like Actinomycetes, *T. whippelii* is gram-positive and PAS-positive, probably because of its unique cell-wall structure.

Commercial laboratories do not routinely perform PCR to diagnose Whipple disease. This technology, however, is available to investigators; and, in the next decade, PCR is likely to be increasingly used in clinical practice. The use of broad-range bacterial primers with overlapping 16S gene sequences permits identification of organisms such as *T. whippelii* in infected tissues, whereas specific primers are useful for confirming the presence of an organism and thus, diagnosing disease. PCR has been used to identify *T. whippelii* in vitreous fluid from a patient with chronic uveitis without systemic manifestations (Fig. 100-2).[40] In using PCR to diagnose *T. whippelii,* fresh-frozen tissue is better than formalin-fixed tissue.

THERAPY

The natural history of untreated Whipple disease has a uniformly poor prognosis. Relapse after short courses of antibiotics (i.e., less than 1 year) are frequent, and at least 1 year of therapy is recommended. PAS-positive macrophages may persist for years within the lamina propria after several years of adequate therapy; therefore, routine intestinal biopsies are generally not indicated. Close clinical follow-up is indicated for early detection of relapse.

There are no prospective comparative studies of the treatment of Whipple disease. Several choices for antimicrobial therapy are available. Trimethoprim/sulfamethoxazole is generally considered the drug of choice based on clinical experience and the good penetration of the blood-brain barrier. Trimethoprim/sulfamethoxazole is usually given orally after a 10- to 14-day initial course of parenterally administered penicillin and streptomycin. For patients unable to tolerate sulfonamides, parenteral penicillin and streptomycin for 2 weeks followed by oral penicillin for 1 year is generally well tolerated and may treat subclinical CNS disease. Clinical experience with ceftriaxone is limited, although promising. Other alternative agents with clinical efficacy include tetracycline, doxycycline, or (rarely) chloramphenicol. Treatment with all agents is generally given for at least 1 year to prevent relapse.

For patients with malabsorption, supplementation with folate, vitamin K, vitamin B_{12}, and iron may be appropriate.

PROGNOSIS

One retrospective study of 88 patients showed relapse rates, depending on the antibiotic(s) used, of 0% to 43%, with CNS relapses ranging from 0% to 25%.[26] The rate of CNS relapse was highest with either penicillin or tetracycline used as single agents, whereas the overall non-CNS relapse rate was similar with either penicillin, penicillin plus streptomycin, or tetracycline. The lowest CNS relapse rates were found with the use of agents that penetrate noninflamed meninges well (i.e., trimethoprim/sulfamethoxazole) or in patients who received penicillin plus streptomycin (with or without tetracycline).

REFERENCES

1. Adams M, Rhyner PA, Day J et al.: Whipple's disease confined to the central nervous system, *Ann Neurol* 21:104-108, 1987.
2. Austin LL, Dobbins WO III: Intraepithelial leukocytes of the intestinal mucosa in normal man and in Whipple's disease: a light- and electron-microscopic study, *Dig Dis Sci* 27:311-320, 1982.
3. Avila MP, Jalkh AE, Feldman E et al.: Manifestations of Whipple's disease in the posterior segment of the eye, *Arch Ophthalmol* 102:384-390, 1984.
4. Badenoch J, Richards WCD, Oppenheimer DR: Encephalopathy in a case of Whipple's disease, *J Neurol Neurosurg Psychiatry* 26:203-210, 1963.
5. Black-Schaffer B: Tinctoral demonstration of glycoprotein in Whipple's disease, *Proc Soc Exp Biol Med* 72:225-227, 1949.
6. Bleibel JM, Cabane J, Kardouss J et al.: Maladie de Whipple à forme hypothalamique: effect favorable de la rifampicine, *Ann Med Interne* 134:723-727, 1983.
7. Brown AP, Lane JC, Murayama S, Vollmer DG: Whipple's disease presenting with isolated neurological symptoms, *J Neurosurg* 73:623-627, 1990.
8. Cohen AS, Schimmel EM, Holt PR, Isselbacher KJ: Ultrastructural abnormalities in Whipple's disease, *Proc Soc Exp Biol Med* 105:411-414, 1960.

9. Disdier P, Harle JR, Vidal-Morris D et al.: Chemosis associated with Whipple's disease, *Am J Ophthalmol* 112:217-219, 1991.

10. Dobbins WO III: *Whipple's disease,* 242, Springfield, Illinois, 1987, Charles C. Thomas.

11. Dobbins WO III, Ruffin JM: A light and electron microscopic study of bacterial invasion in Whipple's disease, *Am J Pathol* 51:221-242, 1967.

12. Dybkaer R: Diagnosis, pathology and treatment of Whipple's disease, illustrated by two cases, *Dan Med Bull* 12:138-142, 1965.

13. Enzinger FM, Helwig EB: Whipple's disease, a review of the literature and report of fifteen patients, *Virchow's Arch Pathol Anat* 366:238-268, 1963.

14. Feurle GE, Vok B, Waldherr R: Cerebral Whipple's disease with negative jejunal histology, *N Engl J Med* 300:907-908, 1979.

15. Finelli PF, McEntee WJ, Lessel S et al.: Whipple's disease with predominantly neuroophthalmic manifestations, *Ann Neurol* 1:247-252, 1977.

16. Fleming JL, Wiesner RH, Shorter RG: Whipple's disease: clinical, biochemical and histopathologic features and assessment of treatment in 29 patients, *Mayo Clin Proc* 63:539-551, 1988.

17. Font RL, Rao NA, Issarescu S, McEntee WJ: Ocular involvement in Whipple's disease: light and electron microscopic observations, *Arch Ophthalmol* 96:1431-1436, 1978.

18. Gartner J: Whipple's disease of the central nervous system associated with ophthalmopleagia externa and severe asteroid hyalitis: a clinicopathologic study, *Doc Ophthalmol* 49:155-187, 1980.

19. Grossman RI, Davis KR, Halperin J: Cranial computed tomography in Whipple's disease, *J Comput Assist Tomogr* 5:246-248, 1981.

20. Hausser-Hauw C, Roullet E, Robert R, Marteau R: Oculo-facio-skeletal myorhythmia as a cerebral complication of systemic Whipple's disease, *Mov Disord* 3:179-184, 1988.

21. Hendrix JP, Black-Schaeffer B, Withers RW, Handler P: Whipple's intestinal lipodystrophy: report of 4 cases, *Arch Intern Med* 85:91-131, 1950.

22. Henry C, Cuffia C, Soussou A: Un cas de maladie de Whipple se compliquant de scotome central bilateral, *Bull Soc Ophtalmol Fr* 74:1111-1114, 1974.

23. Jankovic J: Whipple's disease of the central nervous system in AIDS, *N Engl J Med* 315:1029-1030, 1986.

24. Johnson L, Diamond I: Cerebral Whipple's disease diagnosis by brain biopsy, *Am J Clin Pathol* 74:486-490, 1980.

25. Jones FA, Paulley JW: Intestinal lipodystrophy (Whipple's disease), *Lancet* 1:214-216, 1949.

26. Keinath RD, Merrell DE, Vlietstra R, Dobbins WO III: Antibiotic treatment and relapse in Whipple's disease: long-term follow-up of 88 patients, *Gastroenterology* 88:1867-1873, 1985.

27. Knox DL, Bayless TM, Yarley JH, Charache P: Whipple's disease presenting with ocular inflammation and minimal intestinal symptoms, *Johns Hopkins Med J* 123:175-182, 1968.

27a. Knox DL, Green WR, Troncoso JC et al.: Cerebral ocular Whipple's disease: a 62-year odyssey from death to diagnosis, *Neurology* 45:617-625, 1995.

28. Lampert P, Tom MI, Cummings JN: Encephalopathy in Whipple's disease—a histochemical study, *Neurology* 12:65-71, 1962.

29. LaPointe LR, LaMarche J, Salloum A, Beaudry R: Meningoependymitis in Whipple's disease, *Can J Neurol Sci* 7:163-167, 1980.

30. Leland TM, Chambers JK: Ocular findings in Whipple's disease, *South Med J* 71:335-338, 1978.

31. Maizel H, Ruffin JM, Dobbins WO III: Whipple's disease: a review of 19 patients from one hospital and a review of the literature since 1950, *Medicine* 49:175-205, 1970.

32. Moorthy S, Nolley G, Hermos JA: Whipple's disease with minimal intestinal involvement, *Gut* 18:152-155, 1977.

33. Nath A, Jankovic J, Pettigrew LC: Movement disorders and AIDS, *Neurology* 37:37-41, 1987.

34. Pallis CA, Lewis PD: Neurology of gastrointestinal disease. In Vinken RJ, Bruyn GW, editors: *Handbook of clinical neurology,* vol 39, 449-468, Amsterdam, North Holland, 1980.

35. Paulley JW: A case of Whipple's disease (intestinal lipodystrophy), *Gastroenterology* 22:128-133, 1952.

36. Playford RJ, Schulenburg E, Herrington CS, Hodgson HJ: Whipple's disease complicated by a retinal Jarisch-Herxheimer reaction: a case report, *Gut* 33:132-134, 1992.

37. Relman DA: PCR-based detection of the uncultured bacillus of Whipple's disease. In Persing DH, Smith TF, Tenover FC, White TJ, editors: *Diagnostic molecular microbiology: principles and applications,* 496-500, Washington, DC, 1993, American Society for Microbiology.

38. Relman DA, Loutit JS, Schmidt TM et al.: The agent of bacillary angiomatosis: an approach to the identification of uncultured pathogens, *N Engl J Med* 323:1573-1580, 1990.

39. Relman DA, Schmidt TM, MacDermott RP, Falkow S: Identification of the uncultured bacillus of Whipple's disease, *N Engl J Med* 327:293-301, 1992.

40. Rickman L, Freeman WR, Green WR et al.: Brief report: uveitis caused by *Tropheryma whippelii* (Whipple's bacillus), *N Engl J Med* 332:363-366, 1995.

41. Ritama V, Haapanen L: Intestinal lipodystrophy (Whipple's disease), *Ann Med Intern Fenn* 42:221-239, 1953.

42. Romanul CA, Radvany J, Rosales RK: Whipple's disease confined to the brain: a case studied clinically and pathologically, *J Neurol Neurosurg Psychiatry* 40:901-909, 1977.

42a. Schrenk M, Metz K, Heiligenhaus A et al.: Augen beteiligung bei Morbus Whipple, *Klin Monatsbl Augenheilkd* 204:538-541, 1994.

43. Selsky E, Knox DL, Maumenee AE, Green WR: Ocular involvement in Whipple's disease, *Retina* 4:103-106, 1984.

44. Silbert SW, Parker E, Horenstein S: Whipple's disease of the central nervous system, *Acta Neuropathol* 36:31-38, 1976.

45. Smith WT, French JM, Gottsman M et al.: Cerebral complications of Whipple's disease, *Brain* 88:137-150, 1965.

46. Stoupel N, Monseu G, Pardoe A et al.: Encephalitis with myoclonus in Whipple's disease, *J Neurol Neurosurg Psychiatry* 32:338-343, 1969.

47. Sung JJ, Chung SC, Ling TK et al.: Antibacterial treatment of gasteric ulcers associated with helicobacter pylori, *N Engl J Med* 332:139-142, 1995.

48. Switz DM, Casey TR, Bogaty GV: Whipple's disease and papilledema, *Arch Intern Med* 123:74-77, 1969.

49. Thompson DG, Ledingham JM, Howard AJ, Brown CL: Meningitis in Whipple's disease, *Br Med J* 2:14-15, 1978.

50. Tracey ML, Brolsma MP: Whipple's disease (lipophagia granulomatosa): report of one case, *Gastroenterology* 15:366-369, 1950.

51. Vazquez Rodriguez JJ, Silva Pozo J, Segura A et al.: Whipplesche krankheit und papilloedem, *Z Gastroenterol* 10:475-482, 1972.

52. Whipple GH: A hitherto undescribed disease characterized anatomically by deposits of fat and fatty acids in the intestinal and mesenteric lymphatic tissues, *Johns Hopkins Hosp Bull* 18:382-391, 1907.

53. Winfield J, Dourmashkin RR, Gumpel JM: Diagnostic difficulties in Whipple's disease, *J R Soc Med* 72:859-863, 1979.

54. Wroe SJ, Pires M, Harding B et al.: Whipple's disease confined to the CNS presenting with multiple intracerebral mass lesions, *J Neurol Neurosurg Psychiatry* 54:989-992, 1991.

55. Yardley JH, Hendrix TR: Combined electron and light microscopy in Whipple's disease, *Bull Johns Hopkins Hosp* 109:80-98, 1961.

101 Tuberculosis

JAMES P. DUNN, CRAIG J. HELM, PAUL T. DAVIDSON

It is important to distinguish between *tuberculous infection* and *tuberculosis (TB)*. Tuberculous infection results from exposure to the obligate aerobic *Mycobacterium tuberculosis* bacillus without clinical, radiographic, or bacteriologic evidence of disease. Patients with tuberculous infection alone are not contagious. Tuberculosis occurs when there is disease involving one or more body organs.

EPIDEMIOLOGY

Worldwide there are approximately 8 million new cases of TB and 3 million deaths from TB each year.[99,116] An estimated 1700 million people (one third of the world's population) have been infected with *Mycobacterium tuberculosis,* but the demographics of infection are related to standard of living; 80% of infected individuals in industrialized countries are 50 years or older, whereas 75% of those in developing countries are less than 50 years old.[116] Less than 5% of TB cases worldwide are associated with human immunodeficiency virus (HIV) infection, with the majority of cases concentrated in subSaharan Africa, but case rates have increased up to 100% in some areas in the last 5 years as a result of dual infection.[116]

Reported TB cases in the United States declined steadily from 84,304 in 1953 (when uniform national reporting of TB was initiated) to 22,253 in 1984, or approximately 5% each year.[49] The annual risk of TB decreased in the same period from 53/100,000 population in 1953 to 9.4/100,000 in 1984, a reduction of 82.3%. Between 1984 and 1992, however, the case rate increased to 10.5/100,000 population, or 26,283 new cases.[53] Using the earlier trend to calculate expected cases, there were 51,700 more cases than expected between 1985 and 1992.[53]

Elimination of (or cutbacks in) public health programs designed to reduce TB have had three predictable consequences.[31] First, there is a resurgence in the disease among those groups whose access to medical care is already limited. Second, there is a growing problem with compliance to TB therapy, thus enhancing the development of multiple drug-resistant TB (MDR-TB). Third, a reduction in TB-related drug research has meant that few new drugs have become available to treat TB, and some older drugs have become unavailable. Multiple drug-resistant TB has therefore become even more difficult to treat. Control programs that failed to maintain a vigorous TB public health policy have seen a dramatic increase in both TB and MDR-TB. It remains to be seen, however, whether these trends will translate into increased numbers of ocular TB.

HIV infection is the single most important reason for the increase in TB in some areas of the United States.[43,46,67] The incidence of TB in patients with the acquired immunodeficiency syndrome (AIDS) is almost 500 times that of the general population.[18] The largest increases in TB have occurred in 25- to 44-year-old men, the group that accounts for nearly 70% of all patients with AIDS through 1990.[45] In a prospective study of tuberculin-positive intravenous drug users followed in a methadone treatment center, the incidence of TB was 7.9% per year among those who were initially HIV-positive, compared to none among those who were HIV-negative.[171] Finally, the prevalence of HIV infection among new TB patients is as high as 50% in New York City and several other urban areas.[31,45,161] A diagnosis of clinical TB in an HIV-infected patient, regardless of site, fulfills the Centers for Disease Control and Prevention criteria for the diagnosis of AIDS.[48]

There may be an astonishingly rapid progression from tuberculous infection to clinical disease in HIV-infected patients. DiPerri and associates[72] reported a nosocomial outbreak of TB among 18 HIV-infected inpatients; 8 patients developed TB, including 7 who developed active disease within 60 days of exposure to the index case. Of particular note was the fact that none of the 4 exposed patients with a previously positive tuberculin skin test developed the disease, suggesting the importance of a functioning immune system in preventing TB. Daley and associates[67] reported the development of active TB within 4 months in 11 (37%) of 30 residents of a housing facility for HIV-infected patients who were exposed to a patient with active disease, while four others (13%) developed newly positive tuberculin skin tests. At least 6 of 28 exposed staff members developed newly positive tuberculin-test reactions, of whom one developed pulmonary TB 6 months after exposure. Dooley and associates[74] reported nosocomial transmission of TB in 8 of 48 exposed patients in a hospital unit for HIV-infected patients. Furthermore the study found a markedly higher prevalence of tuberculous infection among HIV unit and internal medicine ward nurses (55%) than other nurses (19%). Pierce and associates[155] reported skin conversion in 30 (19%) of 158 hospital workers and 11 (17%) of 65 hospice workers exposed to an AIDS patient whose diagnosis of pulmonary TB was obscured by concurrent *Pneumocystis carinii* and *Mycobacterium avium* complex infection, thus delaying proper isolation.

HIV infection alone, however, does not account for the excess cases of TB noted above.[45] Other populations at increased risk include immigrants and refugees,[40,57,108] members of racial and ethnic minorities,[45] homeless individuals in shelters,[44,133,146] prisoners,[29,187] intravenous drug users,[31] and immunosuppressed patients. There may be considerable overlap among these risk groups,[31] which are most likely to suffer from predisposing medical conditions such as poor nutrition, alcoholism, illicit drug use, psychological stress, overcrowding, and limited access to medical care. In areas with large numbers of high-risk individuals, such as central Harlem in New York City, case rates may exceed 300 per 100,000 population.[49]

Extrapulmonary TB formerly comprised about 10% to 15% of all cases of TB[92,97] but is increasing in frequency.[85] One community hospital found that extrapulmonary infections accounted for 37% of all new TB cases in an 11-year period.[196] Certain extrapulmonary sites, such as the lymph nodes, musculoskeletal system, and genitourinary tract, are most frequently affected.[8] The incidence of extrapulmonary TB in the United States rose 20% between 1984 and 1989, compared to a 3% increase in pulmonary TB,[18] in large part due to dual infection with HIV.[21,175,182] Chaisson[54] found at least one extrapulmonary site of disease in 60% of TB patients with AIDS compared to 28% in TB patients without AIDS. In HIV-infected persons, lymphatic and disseminated TB are the most common extrapulmonary presentations.[156]

Ocular Disease

Ocular TB involving any tissue of the eye is uncommon. Dutt and associates[77] reported ophthalmic involvement in only 3 of 402 sites of extrapulmonary TB. Donahue[73] found that 1.4% of more than 10,000 patients in one sanatorium were treated for ocular TB between 1940 and 966. Among the presentations were 14 cases of interstitial keratitis, 23 cases of sclerokeratitis, and 3 corneal ulcers.

The choroid is probably the most commonly infected intraocular structure. Woods[198] estimated that the choroid is involved in about 1% of patients with pulmonary TB. The percentage of patients with uveitis due to TB at one institution declined from 8.6% in 1956 to 1960 to 2.6% from 1961 to 1966 to 0.28% from 1966 to 1970.[168] Tuberculosis accounted for less than 1% of uveitis cases in a more recent study in Los Angeles.[103]

Eyre[84] reported a prevalence of conjunctival TB of 1 in 2500 among patients with ocular complaints, compiled in an area with a high rate of TB. Phlyctenular keratoconjunctivitis occurs in up to 35% of patients in populations with high rates of *M. tuberculosis* infection, such as Alaskan Eskimos.[189] It occurs most commonly in the first and second decades of life, and girls are more commonly affected than boys.[153] In contrast, Donahue[73] found only 6 cases of phlyctenular conjunctivitis in 10,524 patients with TB.

The impact of the AIDS epidemic on rates of ocular TB remains unclear. There are few published reports of ocular TB in HIV-infected patients.[25,64] Shafer and associates[175] reported no cases of ocular TB in 199 consecutive HIV-infected patients with extrapulmonary TB. Small and associates[182] reviewed 132 patients with AIDS and TB in whom the TB was entirely extrapulmonary in 30% and both pulmonary and extrapulmonary in 32% of patients; no ocular involvement was reported. Nevertheless it is reasonable to expect that ocular TB in HIV-infected patients will become more frequent as their life expectancy increases.

CLINICAL FEATURES

The diagnosis of extrapulmonary TB in general may be difficult; only 25% of patients have a history of TB,[179] and approximately 50% of patients have normal chest x-rays[8] and no evidence of pulmonary TB. Three broad clinical categories of extrapulmonary disease have been described.[179] The first is subacute, progressive, life-threatening disease; examples include miliary TB, tuberculous meningitis, and TB of the pericardium and great vessels. Choroidal tubercles are uncommonly found, but are very important diagnostically.[149] Tuberculin skin testing is negative in up to 20% of these patients because of overwhelming disease. Death occurs within a few weeks without treatment.

The second category is TB of serosal surfaces, including pleuritis and peritonitis. The tuberculin test is usually positive, and the prognosis, with or without therapy, is better than in subacute disease.

The third, and most common category of extrapulmonary disease is infection of individual organs. Examples include tuberculous arthritis, osteomyelitis, lymphadenitis, and genitourinary disease. Patients are often afebrile and may have no systemic complaints. Tuberculin skin testing is almost always positive. Local organ dysfunction and destruction follows an indolent course.

Ocular Disease

Tuberculosis may affect any ocular structure. Intraocular or orbital disease occurs as a result of hematogenous dissemination, whereas external disease may occur from either exogenous or endogenous sources. It is important to remember that many descriptions of ocular TB were written before the availability of topical and systemic corticosteroids or antituberculosis drugs and that few reports of ocular TB associated with HIV infection have yet been published.[25,64] The ophthalmologist must therefore be alert to the possibility of ''atypical'' lesions in current practice because of these factors.

Eyelids and Conjunctivae. Tuberculosis of the eyelids may cause bilateral eyelid abscesses[136] or tarsitis, simulating a chalazion.[139]

Tuberculosis of the conjunctiva may result from primary inoculation,[84] by contiguous spread of lupus vulgaris from the face[61] or adjacent sinus disease, or by hematogenous dissemination of pulmonary disease.[198] Redness, lacrimation, mucopurulent discharge, and eyelid swelling may be mild or absent.[13] Primary lesions present as unilateral nodular[198] or ulcerated[55] conjunctivitis associated with regional lymphadenopathy.[14,40] Children are most commonly affected.[198] Secondary lesions resulting from spread of contiguous disease or hematogenous dissemination are more common in older patients, may be bilateral, and may cause regional lymphadenopathy.[15,198] Conjunctival TB is among the causes of Parinaud oculoglandular syndrome.

Phlyctenulosis. Tuberculosis was once the leading cause of phlyctenular keratoconjunctivitis, but is now a much less common cause than *Staphylococcus* sp. The two causes cannot be distinguished accurately on clinical features of the lesion. A phlycten (from the Greek word for blister) is an inflamed nodule of lymphoid tissue near the limbus that results from a delayed-type hypersensitivity to foreign protein. Tuberculous phlyctenular keratoconjunctivitis usually occurs in malnourished, older children, and is more common in girls. Symptoms usually last one to two weeks and consist of tearing, blepharospasm, pain, and photophobia. The severity of these symptoms depends on the site of involvement, with corneal phlyctenulosis being much more severe than conjunctival disease. Recurrence is frequent and may develop in a different site. Conjunctival phlyctenules are usually found adjacent to the limbus, but may occur anywhere on the bulbar conjunctiva. The lesions are small and hyperemic with a central pink-white nodule that becomes gray and soft over several days. Corneal phlyctenules begin at the limbus as an elevated nodule with a trailing sheath of dilated vessels. The central area undergoes necrosis over several weeks. Healing is accompanied by a variety of patterns of scarring.[154] Recurrent lesions may progress centrally, but do not cross the central cornea. De novo corneal lesions are not thought to occur.[7]

Other Corneal Disease. Corneal TB may manifest as either interstitial keratitis,[198] keratoconjunctivitis with stromal infiltration,[4] or an extension of scleral or uveal tract TB.[73,145] It has been suggested that tuberculous interstitial keratitis, in contrast to syphilitic interstitial keratitis, is usually unilateral and more anterior, with more frequent attacks.[198]

Sclera. Although TB was considered a frequent cause of scleritis earlier in the twentieth century,[198] it was considered rare by 1926.[195] Tuberculosis accounted for only one of 130 cases of scleritis in one study.[102] Watson and Hayreh[194] found active TB in one of 217 cases of episcleritis and in four of 301 cases of scleritis. Tuberculous scleritis is characterized by scleral and conjunctival ulceration and is usually not severely painful.[27,73,102,145,165] Focal, necrotizing anterior scleritis is the most common presentation[27,102,145,165] but may be diffuse.[194] Scleral perforation may occur.[28] The margins are usually raised. Adjacent interstitial keratitis may be present if the infection is near the limbus. In one case scleral angiography showed marked nonperfusion.[145] Physical examination may reveal regional preauricular and submandibular lymphadenopathy.[165] Tuberculous scleritis should be suspected when a necrotizing lesion occurs in a patient with a positive chest x-ray or PPD skin test. Scrapings that reveal acid-fast bacilli and a positive culture are confirmatory, but a negative result does not rule out the diagnosis.[198]

Uvea. Tuberculosis has accounted for a progressively smaller percentage of uveitis cases in the United States over the past 50 years.[168] Nevertheless, up to 32% of childhood uveitis in developing countries may be due to TB.[172] Tuberculous uveitis may appear as a chronic granulomatous iridocyclitis,[162,168] peripheral uveitis,[157] disseminated choroiditis, or panuveitis.[3,172] The diagnosis is presumptive if no tissue is available for biopsy and is based on exclusion of other uveitides (such as sarcoidosis, syphilis, toxoplasmosis) by appropriate tests, positive tuberculin skin testing, pulmonary radiographic evidence of TB, and a response to empiric antituberculosis therapy.

The iris[16] and ciliary body[147] may both be sites of hematogenous dissemination of *M. tuberculosis*. Anterior uveal involvement tends to run a protracted course.[147] The associated iridocyclitis is usually granulomatous, characterized by mutton-fat keratic precipitates, extensive posterior synechiae, and secondary glaucoma.[76,162,197] Nongranulomatous iridocyclitis may also occur. Miliary TB may cause seeding of the iris with development of small, grey nodules surrounded by a network of fine blood vessels.[198] Such lesions must be distinguished from sarcoid nodules, which are larger and more pink. In rare cases a conglomerate tubercle of the iris grows rapidly, invades the cornea by direct extension, and causes painful glaucoma or even perforation.[147,158,197]

Because of the extensive choroidal blood supply, choroidal tubercles and tuberculomata (large, solitary masses) are the most common ocular manifestations of disease that result from hematogenous dissemination.[71,147] Choroidal tubercles most commonly occur in miliary TB,[106] but may occur in other forms of the disease, with or without concurrent active pulmonary TB,[34,131,142] and may be the only sign of dissemination.[110,125] Blurred vision may be the only symptom. The tubercles are usually yellow or grey-white, one quarter to two optic disc diameters in size, with somewhat irregular edges. They may become pigmented with time. The lesions are usually unilateral and most frequent in the posterior pole, ranging in number from one[34,93,121] to 60[57] but usually less than five.[131] There may be an overlying sensory retinal detachment[34,110] (Fig. 101-1). A marked anterior uveitis and retinal vasculitis may occur rarely;[25,98,183] in general, however, these reactions are uncommon, perhaps in part because patients with miliary TB are unable to mount an effective immunologic response to infection.[76] Choroidal hemorrhages[178] and subretinal neovascularization[57,98] have been described.

Retina. Retinal involvement in TB is usually a result of extension from choroidal disease. Isolated retinal TB is rare.[162,198] Saini and associates[164] described a retinal mass in a 3-year-old child that was clinically suspicious for retinoblastoma but was histopathologically found to be tuberculous following enucleation. No choroidal disease was found. Periphlebitis, or less commonly periarteritis, is the most common manifestation of retinal TB.[75,162] Perivasculitis may precede[155,168] or develop concurrently with pulmonary TB.[89,162] The perivasculitis may occur without underlying choroidal disease.[151] Tubercles in the central retinal vein may obstruct the lumen of the vessel.[89] Retinal vein occlusion[89] and capillary closure with subsequent neovascularization[157] are potential complications. Failure to find acid-fast bacilli histopathologically does not rule out a tuberculous process.[198] A positive tuberculin test and response to antituberculosis therapy supports the diagnosis. Treatment of tuberculous retinitis using oral corticosteroids may contribute to the development of miliary TB if not given in combination with antituberculosis chemotherapy.[162,176]

An immune mechanism has been proposed in the pathogenesis of retinal periphlebitis in patients with tuberculin hypersensitivity,[80,162] an association sometimes noted in Eales disease.[80,160] This entity is characterized by recurrent retinal and vitreous hemorrhages, most commonly affecting healthy young adult males. The majority of patients present with sudden, painless, unilateral vision loss due to vitreous hemorrhage, usually with involvement of the other eye after several months.[160] Retinal periphlebitis, peripheral vascular sheathing, or retinal capillary nonperfusion, arteriovenous shunts, and retinal neovascularization are among the findings.[81,160] There may be associated neurologic disease.[70] Renie and associates[160] found that 24% of patients had concomitant bilateral sensorineural hearing loss. There is an increased prevalence of tuberculin skin test positivity in these patients, although active pulmonary disease is uncommon.[160] Giant cells, caseation, and acid-fast bacilli are not found histopathologically,[81] and patients usually respond to treatment with systemic corticosteroids[162] but not antituberculosis chemotherapy.[81] Eales disease may, in fact, have multiple causes, and must be distinguished from sarcoidosis, syphilis, Behçet disease, multiple sclerosis, sickle cell disease, and idiopathic retinal vasculitis.

Endophthalmitis. Tuberculous endophthalmitis is a highly destructive process with rapid onset resulting from direct infection of intraocular structures.[69,78,134,137,147] Granulomatous uveitis and painful glaucoma are present. Based on three cases, Ni and associates[147] suggested that children or severely ill adults are usually affected, but endophthalmitis in intravenous drug users[137] or otherwise healthy adults has been reported.[69,78]

Orbit. Tuberculosis involving soft tissue of the orbital space usually occurs as a result of hematogenous dissemination, but may also result from extension of orbital periostitis.[6] Affected patients are usually under 20 years of age, living in highly endemic areas.* The onset is usually insidious, with proptosis or spontaneous fistulization of an orbital abscess as the presenting sign.[6,151,173] The lacrimal gland may be involved.[122,143]

Neuroophthalmic Disease. Meningitis is the most common cause of neuroophthalmic disease in patients with TB.[119] HIV-infected patients are at increased risk of tuberculous

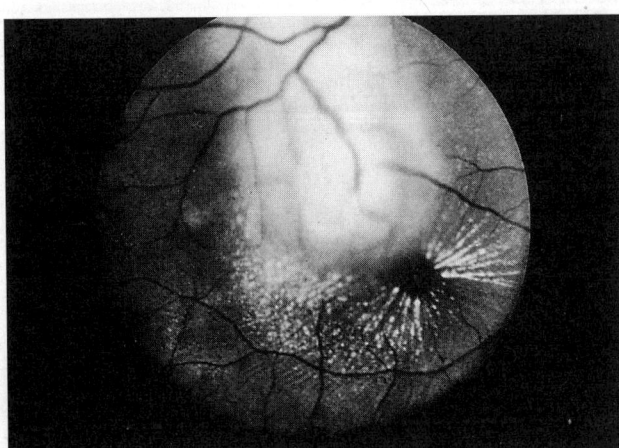

Fig. 101-1. Raised yellowish choroidal tuberculoma with surrounding serous elevation of neurosensory retina, intraretinal exudation, and macular star. (Reprinted with permission from Cangemi FE, Friedman AH, Josephberg R: Tuberculoma of the choroid, *Ophthalmology* 87:252-258, 1980.)

---

*References 6, 17, 113, 127, 132, 166.

meningitis, but the clinical manifestations and outcome do not appear different from those in patients without HIV infection.[21] Sixth and, less frequently, third cranial nerve palsies may occur as a result of increased intracranial pressure; both are associated with high mortality rates.[119] A variety of pupillary abnormalities may occur. Optic nerve involvement may take the form of chiasmatic arachnoiditis, papilledema, or optic neuritis.[119] Tuberculous meningitis is a far more common cause of optic neuritis than is tuberculous retinal periphlebitis.[198] Optic neuropathy may respond to antituberculosis chemotherapy.[125] Progressive necrosis and caseation of nerve tissue lead to optic atrophy.[198]

PATHOLOGY

Histopathologically, phlyctenules are characterized by a dense accumulation of lymphocytes, histiocytes, and plasma cells; neutrophils may be seen in acute stages. There is a notable absence of giant cells, eosinophils, follicles, and acid-fast bacilli.

Choroidal tubercles are similar to tubercles found elsewhere in the body[131] (Fig. 101-2). Granulomata may be caseating or noncaseating. The characteristic epithelioid or giant cells may be absent in disseminated TB,[64] but stains for acid-fast bacilli are positive. In contrast to the histopathology of choroidal tuberculomata, endophthalmitis is marked by caseation necrosis and large amounts of exudation.[125,147]

PATHOGENESIS

In the United States approximately 30% of the close contacts of newly identified patients with pulmonary TB have positive tuberculin skin tests (indicative of *M. tuberculosis* infection), presumably acquired from the index patient.[24] In HIV-negative patients, such new TB infections usually remain inactive; clinically evident TB develops at a rate of

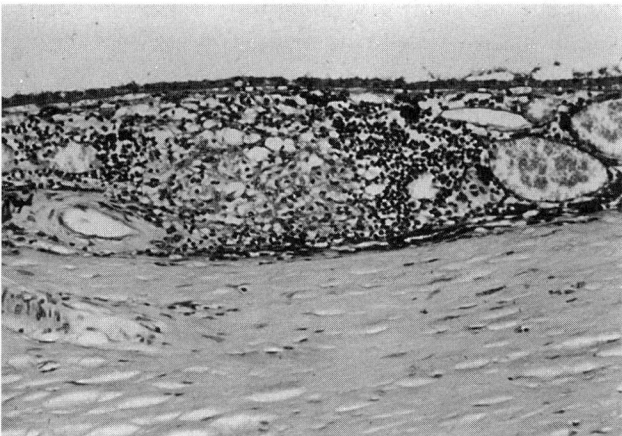

Fig. 101-2. Tuberculous choroidal granuloma. (Hematoxylineosin × 220.) (Courtesy W. Richard Green, MD.)

about 4% per year for the first two years, with a lifetime risk of only 5% to 15%.[92] In contrast, the chance of an HIV-positive, *M. tuberculosis*-infected person developing active disease is about 8% each year.[18]

In at least 90% of patients with active TB in developed countries, clinical illness is the result of reactivation of previous disease; at least 7% of these patients have a history of inadequately treated TB.[36] Newly acquired tuberculous infection in HIV-infected patients may rapidly progress to active disease.[46,67,72,74] Patients with other causes of altered immunity, such as the elderly, diabetics, alcoholics, and those with malignancies, are also at greater risk of reactivation.[12] Exogenous reinfection is an uncommon but potentially important cause of TB, especially in patients whose immunity acquired by previous infection may be incomplete because of stress, malnutrition, and concomitant disease.[146] Patients with TB acquired through reinfection may be more contagious and have more lung cavitation than those patients with reactivated disease.

Primary Infection

With the virtual elimination of bovine TB in the United States, infection with *M. tuberculosis* occurs primarily by inhalation of airborne bacilli. The number of bacilli necessary to establish infection depends on host immunity, the virulence of the bacilli, and genetic resistance of the recipient.[68] Because of their small size (0.2 × 5.0 microns), the bacilli are able to bypass the upper airway defense mechanisms and lodge in pulmonary alveoli. The lower lung fields are most commonly infected, presumably because of gravity and greater ventilation of the lung bases. Alveolar macrophages nonspecifically ingest and either kill or inhibit the bacilli; cell-mediated immunity is not involved at this stage.[68] If not killed, tubercle bacilli multiply slowly within macrophages, but provoke minimal inflammatory reaction in the nonimmune host because they secrete no enzymes or toxins. Lymphatic invasion follows, with spread to regional lymph nodes and eventual hematogenous dissemination. Organs with high blood flow and a high oxygen tension are particularly susceptible to infection; the lung apices are most frequently involved, but any organ may be affected.[179]

After several weeks two specific host defense mechanisms develop, both involving a complex interaction between macrophages and T-lymphocytes.[68,95,111] Delayed-type hypersensitivity causes tubercle formation, in which caseous necrosis surrounds and destroys the nonactivated macrophages harboring growing bacilli. Delayed-type hypersensitivity may be driven by the lymphokine tumor necrosis factor-β and the monokine tumor necrosis factor (TNF)-α, both of which probably contribute to the associated tissue damage.[115,192]

Tubercle bacilli can survive but not multiply within the anoxic and acidic caseous environment. In cell-mediated immunity, macrophages that have ingested tubercle bacilli present mycobacterial antigens to T-lymphocytes, which then secrete lymphokines that activate macrophages (epithelioid cells) specifically to destroy any bacilli that escape areas of caseation. Both CD4+ (helper) T-lymphocytes and CD8+ (suppressor) T-lymphocytes are involved.[110] Cell-mediated immunity is thought to be driven primarily by interferon-γ, but other cytokines may also be important.[95]

Subsequent healing may be inapparent or result in calcification, recognized radiographically in the lower lobe as the Ghon complex. These lesions contain small numbers of inactive but viable mycobacteria. Further exogenous infection is prevented in the immunocompetent host because of the enhanced granuloma formation in alveoli.[179] The tuberculin skin test becomes positive after 6 to 8 weeks as cell-mediated immunity develops.

Over 90% of primarily infected patients remain asymptomatic and can be identified only by conversion of the tuberculin skin test from negative to positive.[179] As a result of incomplete immunity, approximately 5% of infected persons develop progressive primary disease within one to two years after infection. Such disease may manifest in a variety of forms, including miliary TB. An additional 5% of infected individuals develop disease several or many years later.

Reactivation

Failure of either T-lymphocyte or macrophage function may allow dormant bacilli to reactivate. Reactivation (post-primary) TB is most common within a few years of initial infection or following host immune suppression because of factors such as neoplastic disease, malnutrition, aging, or viral illness, including HIV infection. Uncommon associations include gastrectomy and corticosteroid therapy.

Because *M. tuberculosis* is a more virulent organism than those that cause opportunistic infections (e.g., *Pneumocystis carinii*), the development of TB requires less impairment of host defenses and occurs earlier in the course of HIV infection than *P. carinii* pneumonia.[200] Among HIV-infected patients, those with lower total lymphocyte and CD4+ T-lymphocyte counts are more likely to develop TB.[72]

A variety of host defenses against *M. tuberculosis* are impaired in HIV-infected patients, including the effectiveness of alveolar macrophages, antigen-presenting function, clonal proliferation of CD4+ T-lymphocytes, and elaboration of soluble factors such as interferon-γ and interleukin-2.[200] Most cases of TB in patients with AIDS are caused by the reduced ability of the host to produce cell-mediated immunity.[68] The result is poorly formed granulomata,[144] inability to kill the intracytoplasmic mycobacteria, and bloodstream infection.[166] The poor T-lymphocyte immune response among HIV-infected patients accounts for the reduced frequency of cavitary lesions and fibrosis seen on chest x-ray and the increased frequency of miliary infil-

trates and both intrathoracic and extrathoracic lymphadenopathy.[156] Ironically, expression of TNF-α may induce HIV expression in cells of both T-lymphocyte and monocyte lineage, so that immune activation in HIV-1–associated TB may actually accelerate progression to AIDS.[193]

Ocular Disease

Ocular manifestations may be attributed to either infection or noninfectious, immunologic reactions. Immune reactions to tuberculoprotein may cause phlyctenulosis, interstitial keratitis, and possibly retinal vasculitis. Primary infectious ocular TB results from direct inoculation with the organism and is limited almost entirely to corneal and conjunctival disease. The organism may reach subepithelial tissue following trauma[87] or may be carried into the tissue by phagocytes in cases of chronic conjunctivitis with intact epithelium.[30] Both of these mechanisms are extremely rare. Much more common is secondary infectious ocular TB, which results from contiguous spread of infection from adjacent structures such as the nasal sinuses, or hematogenous dissemination from pulmonary infection. As with hematogenous dissemination of other diseases, such as metastatic carcinoma, the choroid is far more commonly involved than the orbit or retina.

The pathophysiology of tuberculous phlyctenular keratoconjunctivitis is unclear, but presumably is due to delayed hypersensitivity to foreign protein.[150] Phlyctenulosis rarely occurs in patients with active pulmonary TB,[73] which may be related to the impairment of cellular immunity in patients with systemic disease.[150] In populations with a high prevalence of TB, phlyctenulosis is common.[189] Furthermore, the incidence of positive tuberculin skin tests is much higher in patients with corneal opacities than in those without.[154] Despite these epidemiologic associations, however, animal models of phlyctenulosis have yielded conflicting results.[101] Gibson[91] noted that instillation of tuberculoprotein in the conjunctival sacs of tuberculous rabbits induced phlyctenule formation, but Thygeson and associates[190] were unable to duplicate these findings. Presumably sensitization occurs as a result of bacteremia from early lung disease, but it has been pointed out that many questions remain unanswered.[7] It is not known what precipitates attacks; why attacks are focal; why phlyctenules form from tuberculoprotein but not most other bacterial proteins; why children, especially girls, are more frequently affected; why there is no associated uveitis; or why some attacks abort themselves, whereas others progress to more central involvement and scarring.

Possible causes of retinal vasculitis in patients with TB include hematogenous dissemination of infection, inflammation from adjacent choroidal lesions, or hypersensitivity reactions.[75] Eales disease in particular may be a clinical entity with multiple causes, because not all patients have positive tuberculin skin tests. Rapid improvement of retinal vasculitis following treatment with antituberculosis chemotherapy[89,162] is consistent with an infectious cause in some cases.

Burgoyne and associates[32] reported a case of tuberculin skin-test-induced uveitis with serous retinal detachments in the absence of TB, suggesting that hypersensitivity to tuberculoprotein may mediate some forms of intraocular inflammation. Elliot[80] suggested that the hemorrhage and exudation in Eales disease result from local reaction in a vessel wall sensitized to tuberculoprotein.

Animal models using live tubercle bacilli injected into the carotid artery or directly into the eye have rarely produced retinal disease, and heat-killed bacilli produce ocular lesions similar to those that occur after the injection of living organisms.[86,148]

DIFFERENTIAL DIAGNOSIS

Tuberculous phlyctenules must be distinguished from staphylococcal phlyctenules, bacterial ulcers, marginal ulcers, inflamed pingueculae, and vernal keratoconjunctivitis. A negative intermediate strength PPD skin test (described later in this chapter) and normal chest x-ray lessen the likelihood of, but do not eliminate, TB as a cause of keratoconjunctivitis.

The differential diagnosis of tuberculous scleritis includes infectious scleritis caused by agents such as varicella-zoster virus or *Aspergillus* sp., syphilis or other bacterial infection,[102] and scleritis associated with systemic vasculitis. In the latter case, the erythrocyte sedimentation rates may be elevated. Biopsy and culture of scleral tissue will also be helpful in selected cases. It is essential to make the correct diagnosis, because treatment with oral or topical corticosteroids may delay the diagnosis and markedly worsen the status of tuberculous scleritis.

The differential diagnosis of tuberculous choroidal tubercles includes syphilis, toxoplasmosis, toxocariasis, histoplasmosis, sarcoidosis, melanoma, metastatic carcinoma, and retinoblastoma. Choroidal tubercles associated with disseminated tuberculosis have been reported in patients with renal allografts[121] and AIDS.[25,64] Such lesions in immunocompromised patients must be distinguished from lymphoma, choroidal pneumocystosis, cryptococcosis, candidal chorioretinitis, and nontuberculous mycobacterial infection.

Tuberculous endophthalmitis may be mistaken for syphilis,[147] retinoblastoma,[134] pseudotumor,[147] or metastatic carcinoma.[69]

LABORATORY INVESTIGATIONS

All patients with suspected TB should undergo skin testing, chest x-ray if the skin test is abnormal or if the patient is symptomatic, and sputum induction for acid-fast smears if the chest x-ray is abnormal. Histologic examination and culture of tissues may be necessary, depending on whether there are signs and symptoms of extrapulmonary disease. A variety of other diagnostic tests may confirm mycobacterial infection. They include liver, lymph node, and bone marrow biopsy, stool for acid-fast smear, and cultures of blood, urine, cerebrospinal fluid, and pleural fluid.

It is essential to consider the possibility of coinfection with HIV when evaluating a patient for TB, because the incidence of atypical presentations and false-negative diagnostic tests increases with the severity of the HIV disease.[18,54,156,188] Chest roentgenography is perhaps the most sensitive test for pulmonary TB. In situations in which the logistic problems of large and rapid turnover make it difficult to have skin tests placed and read consistently (such as prisons), chest x-rays have been recommended as a better screening measure for TB than the PPD skin test.[181] The CDC recommends routine chest x-rays in patients with symptomatic HIV infection for the detection of occult TB,[37] although the usefulness of such testing in patients without respiratory complaints has not been studied.

Radiology

The most common radiographic findings in immunocompetent patients with reactivation disease are infiltrates or cavitation in the apical and/or posterior segment of the upper lobe.[138] Lower lobe infiltrates and pleural effusions are less commonly seen.[191] Cavitation and upper lobe infiltrates are also common in TB patients with early HIV disease and relatively well-preserved immune function. As the HIV infection becomes more severe, the chest x-ray more frequently reveals hilar adenopathy, pleural effusion, or miliary disease, which are features also seen in primary TB in immunocompetent patients. Rarely, the chest x-ray may be normal or show diffuse interstitial infiltrates.[18]

Skin Testing

Skin testing is performed with purified protein derivative (PPD), which is derived from autoclaved and extracted cultures of *M. tuberculosis*. Three strengths are available: 1, 5, and 250 tuberculin units (TU). The intermediate strength (5 TU in 0.1 ml) is most commonly used and is the standard for determining a positive or negative result. The material is injected intradermally on the volar forearm surface and the amount of induration measured in 48 to 72 hours.[159]

Tuberculin hypersensitivity is mediated by T-lymphocytes and is determined in part by the patient's immunologic status.[12,96,128] Designating the result simply as "positive" or "negative" based on the amount of induration is an oversimplification of a complex reaction. The American Thoracic Society and CDC consider reactions of 5 mm or more to be positive in very-high-risk individuals (those with abnormal chest x-rays, recent contacts of patients with infectious TB, and HIV-infected patients), 10 mm or more to be positive in high-risk patients (foreign-born individuals, HIV-negative intravenous drug users, members of low socioeconomic background, and those with medical conditions that increase the risk of TB), and 15 mm or more positive in individuals with none of the risk factors just mentioned.[12] Graham and associates[96] have proposed that induration of 2 mm or greater is a better cutoff for a positive test in HIV-infected patients. There is no specific amount of induration that confirms TB, and a negative test does not exclude the diagnosis.[141]

The specificity of testing increases with larger areas of induration. False-positive tests may occur as a result of atypical mycobacterial infections or previous vaccination with bacille Calmette-Guérin (BCG), whereas false-negative reactions may occur as a result of aging, sarcoidosis, uremia, Hodgkin disease, corticosteroid use, overwhelming tuberculous illness, and viral diseases such as measles, mumps, or HIV disease.[22,104,161] The sensitivity of skin testing declines as co-infection with HIV becomes more severe.[22,141] Anergy occurs in less than 10% of patients with CD4+ T-lymphocyte counts greater than $500/\mu l$, but in approximately 80% of those with counts less than $50/\mu l$.[42] In one study 71% of HIV-infected patients with tuberculosis diagnosed at least 2 years before they developed AIDS had skin tests 10 mm or more in diameter, compared to 33% of patients with AIDS and TB.[161]

A two-step procedure, in which the 5 TU skin test, if negative, is repeated one week later, may reduce the number of false-negative tests in patients with waning sensitivity, such as the elderly, without causing true conversion, a phenomenon known as the "booster effect."[191] Anergy testing with mumps antigen, tetanus toxoid, or *Candida* sp. antigen may help to confirm a truly negative PPD.[96] Anergy to PPD and control skin tests in an HIV-infected patient is a risk factor for progression to AIDS.[22]

Interpretation of tuberculin testing in patients vaccinated with BCG is difficult, although tuberculin sensitivity in such patients declines over time. Individuals with a positive PPD should be managed without regard to a history of BCG vaccination unless it was received within the previous year.[159]

Smears and Cultures

Detection of acid-fast bacilli in a tissue smear has been the traditional means of disease confirmation. Detection of acid-fast bacilli is done with either the Ziehl-Neelsen stain, which stains mycobacteria as red rods or coccobacilli on a blue background, or the auramine O fluorescence stain, which stains mycobacteria as yellow fluorescing rods on a dark background. Between 5×10^3 and 1×10^4 acid-fast bacilli per ml of tissue must be present to be detected by microscopy.[100] Fluorescence testing on sputum specimens is easier and more sensitive than Ziehl-Neelsen staining, but the two tests are comparable on tissue specimens.[112] Both tests have limited specificity, because a positive test does not rule out the presence of mycobacteria other than *M. tuberculosis*.

Culture of *M. tuberculosis* has traditionally involved egg-based media (such as Löwenstein-Jensen) or agar-based media. Agar-based media, such as Middlebrook-Cohn 7H10 agar and 7H11 agar, allow a more rapid recovery of growth (within 2 to 4 weeks) and offer a better opportunity to study colony morphology than egg-based media.[100] Selective 7H11 agar, which contains antibiotics that inhibit the growth of nonmycobacterial contaminants, is helpful as a backup to plain agar. Because some isolates grow on one medium but not another, both egg-based and agar-based media should be used. In addition, Middlebrook 7H12 broth, a liquid medium currently marketed as BACTEC 12B vials,* can provide radiometric detection of growth within 1 to 2 weeks. Even if no growth is detected in BACTEC 12B vials and on agar plates, a culture can be reported as negative only after 8 weeks of unsuccessful incubation of Lowenstein-Jensen slants.[100]

Three successive sputum samples of adequate quality should be obtained for smear and culture in patients suspected of having pulmonary TB.[200] The sensitivity of an acid-fast smear of sputum decreases in patients with more severe HIV infection and in those with miliary TB.[200] One study, however, reported that failure to obtain adequate numbers of sputum for acid-fast smear and mycobacterial culture was the most common cause of delayed diagnosis of TB, rather than atypical manifestations of the disease.[118]

If sputum smears are negative, bronchoscopy may be indicated. Smears of bronchoalveolar-lavage fluid or transbronchial biopsy specimens are particularly useful in the diagnosis or exclusion of nontuberculous diseases such as Kaposi sarcoma or *Pneumocystis carinii* pneumonia.[18]

Acid-fast smears of stool are positive in 40% of patients with TB and HIV infection, but such findings usually do not indicate gastrointestinal disease.[18]

Concurrent infection with *Mycobacterium avium* complex (MAC), which occurs in as many as one third of patients with AIDS,[105] makes the diagnosis of TB more difficult, because MAC infection cannot be differentiated from TB by acid-fast stains and MAC may overgrow culture media.[124] When *M. tuberculosis* and MAC are both present, newer diagnostic methods such as radiometric culture techniques[82] and DNA probes[153] may provide sensitive and rapid diagnosis. The polymerase chain reaction has also been used to make rapid diagnosis of *M. tuberculosis* infection,[62,152] particularly in extrapulmonary disease.[124] The false-positive rate, false-negative rate, reproducibility, and predictive value of these newer tests are not fully understood, however, and therefore their clinical role is not yet defined.[50]

Ocular Disease

The diagnosis of extrapulmonary TB in general may be difficult. Only 25% of patients have a history of TB[179] and

---

*Becton Dickinson Diagnostic Instrument Systems, Cockeysville, MD.

approximately 50% of patients have normal chest x-rays.[8] Blood cultures for *M. tuberculosis* may be useful in diagnosing extrapulmonary disease, particularly in cases of miliary disease.[175] Not surprisingly, there are reports of ocular TB with a negative chest x-ray[125,147] or skin test[69] or both.[19,183]

Duke-Elder and Perkins[76] stated in 1966 that "a positive diagnosis [of ocular TB] can be made in those cases of miliary or proliferative lesions in which there is no evidence of other disease liable to cause a granulomatous uveitis and which exhibit tuberculous disease elsewhere, particularly if specific therapy induces a favourable response." Ocular TB may occur, however, with atypical systemic disease, or in patients with no systemic disease. A high degree of clinical suspicion is therefore the key to diagnosis. Consultation with an infectious disease or pulmonary disease expert is imperative for proper systemic diagnosis and therapy.

According to Woods,[197] the pathologic criteria for diagnosis of ocular TB are the following: (1) formation of a typical tubercle composed of epithelioid and giant cells, (2) presence of caseation necrosis, (Fig. 101-3) (3) identification of tubercle bacillus by acid-fast stain, and (4) correlation with history and general physical examination. Often, however, the acid-fast bacilli cannot be demonstrated in the tissue.

Diagnosis of superficial ocular TB lesions may be made on the characteristic biopsy findings of caseating granulomata with Langhans giant cells and acid-fast bacilli. Biopsy findings may reveal culture-negative, nonspecific granulomatous inflammation, however, which can be mistaken for sarcoidosis.[158] Easily accessible sites include the eyelid,[136] conjunctiva,[15,55,61,180] lacrimal gland,[151] and sclera.[27,145] Clinically suspicious lesions despite equivocal biopsy results should be treated for TB before results of cultures become available, which may take

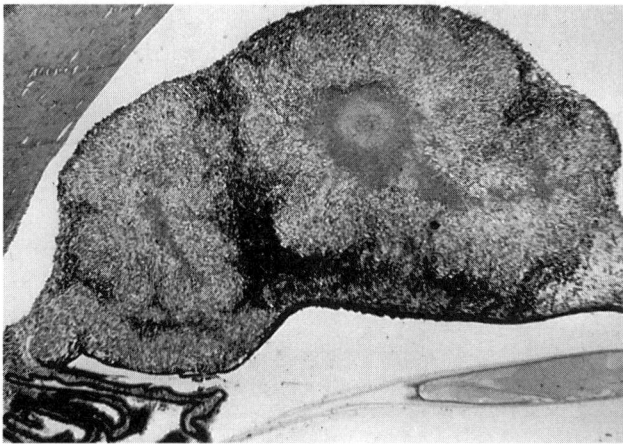

Fig. 101-3. Tuberculous iris mass with caseating granuloma. (Hematoxylin-eosin × 110.) (Courtesy W. Richard Green, MD.)

up to four weeks or longer.[15] It is important to obtain antituberculosis drug sensitivities on any *M. tuberculosis* isolates.

Patients with orbital TB have usually had positive tuberculin skin testing and pulmonary evidence of TB. Orbital radiographs reveal bony erosion.[6,173] The finding of acid-fast bacilli on biopsy is diagnostic, but false-negatives may occur.

Diagnosis of tuberculous choroiditis, retinal vasculitis, or panophthalmitis is more difficult. In most cases the clinician will rely on a combination of epidemiologic factors, evidence of systemic disease, characteristic ocular findings, and possibly a therapeutic treatment trial to make the diagnosis. Helpful clinical diagnostic signs include mutton-fat keratic precipitates, Koeppe nodules, and rapid formation of posterior synechiae.[71,162] Chorioretinal endobiopsy may allow definitive diagnosis of posterior tuberculous uveitis,[19] but is impractical in most cases. Enucleation of one eye may be necessary in some bilateral cases to make the diagnosis.[69,158]

Skin Testing of Patients with Uveitis. Routine tuberculin skin testing in patients with uveitis has been advocated[3] but is rarely helpful, because a positive test is usually incidental. Rosenbaum and Wernick[163] calculated that a patient with uveitis and a positive PPD but no other signs of TB has only a 1% probability of having active TB. There is no proof of the theory that increased intraocular inflammation following tuberculin testing indicates that the ocular lesion is tuberculous.[84] Furthermore there is a risk of tuberculin skin test–induced uveitis in the absence of TB.[32]

Use of Therapeutic Trials for Diagnosis. Abrams, Schlaegel, and associates[2,169] have advocated the isoniazid therapeutic test for diagnosis of suspected tuberculous uveitis. Isoniazid is given in a dose of 300 mg daily for three weeks. If there is dramatic improvement of the inflammatory signs, a presumptive diagnosis is made and a full course of multiple drug antituberculosis therapy is instituted. The value of this test is unsubstantiated. The clinician must distinguish between a therapeutic effect of the INH and a natural fluctuation in the course of chronic uveitis of some other origin. In addition the diagnostic value of therapeutic trials is diminished by the increased prevalence of drug-resistant strains of *M. tuberculosis,* including those causing ocular disease.[114] Furthermore the use of single drugs is not acceptable; even a course of therapy as short as 3 weeks can result in resistance of organisms, although development of resistance is rare, if the infection involves a small number of organisms.

Adjunctive Tests. The fluorescein angiographic and echographic characteristics of choroidal tubercles have been described. Both early hyperflouorescence[34] and early blocking defects[167] have been reported; such differences may reflect the degree to which the retinal pigment epithelium is damaged.[34] Large vessels within the lesion are absent. There is intense late staining. Multiple early blocking defects with late hyperfluorescence were seen in a case of multiple tubercles associated with subretinal neovascular membranes.[56] Goldberg[93] described enlarged retinal vessels overlying a solitary macular tuberculoma without retinochoroidal anastamoses; he suggested that this pattern may help to distinguish tuberculous lesions from other granulomatous processes such as toxoplasmosis, toxocariasis, and syphilis. Following treatment, there is no leakage into surrounding tissue.[107]

Ultrasonography may show low internal reflectivity and high vascularity, simulating a melanoma.[26] Lyon and associates[121] also noted low internal reflectivity on A-scan but found a hypoechoic (solid) mass on B-scan. Jabbour and associates[110] noted variable patterns on A-scan; the B-scan revealed a solid elevated mass with absence of scleral echo, which was felt to be due to absorption by inflammatory cells. Lyon and associates[121] suggested that the combination of fluorescein angiography and ultrasonography is usually sufficient to rule out a choroidal melanoma, but cannot reliably distinguish a tuberculoma from other inflammatory choroidal masses.

Elevated levels of lactate dehydrogenase[63] or soluble antigen fluorescent antibody[140] from aqueous specimens have been reported, but these tests have not achieved widespread use. The radioactive phosphorus test may be positive, so that a choroidal tubercle simulates a melanoma.[26,177] Various serologic tests have been reported to aid in the diagnosis of tuberculous endophthalmitis,[63] uveitis,[140] keratoconjunctivitis,[150] and meningitis,[83] but are not commonly available or of proved benefit.

THERAPY

All hospitalized patients with potentially infectious TB should be placed in respiratory isolation rooms with negative pressure relative to adjacent areas and started on antituberculosis therapy.[38] Adequate air flow is a problem in many older hospitals.[74] The most commonly used drugs to treat TB are isoniazid, rifampin, pyrazinamide (PZA), ethambutol, and streptomycin (Table 101-1). Other accepted drugs included cycloserine, ethionamide, para-aminosalicylic acid (PAS), capreomycin, and kanamycin. Various new drugs have been investigated, including amikacin, the fluoroquinolones, macrolides, and phenazines, but to date none has achieved widespread acceptance.[66] Rifampin is effective against not only actively multiplying organisms but nearly dormant ones. PZA is effective in the acidic internal environment of the macrophage, thus further enhancing therapeutic options. Dosages for currently approved antituberculosis drugs are listed in Table 101-1.

Drug therapy for pulmonary and extrapulmonary TB is usually similar. It must be noted that controlled studies of the treatment for extrapulmonary (including ocular) TB are lacking because of the variety of sites involved, the relatively small number of patients affected, the difficulty in defining an endpoint to treatment, and the difficulty in assessing the relative contribution of surgery and drug therapy in many cases.[97] Treatment of TB in any site, however, must take into account a patient's immune status and the likelihood of resistant organisms.

The use of single-drug therapy for pulmonary TB is associated with a high rate of resistance, as indicated previously.[123,135] Tuberculosis must therefore always be treated with multiple drugs. In immunocompetent patients living in areas where the rate of drug resistance is low, a regimen of isoniazid and rifampin for six months, along with PZA for the first two months, may be sufficient.[51] Most patients with TB, however, should receive empiric treatment with a four-drug regimen consisting of isoniazid, rifampin, pyrazinamide, and either streptomycin or ethambutol.[51,123] If the organism is sensitive to all drugs, the streptomycin or ethambutol can be discontinued. The PZA should be continued for at least the first 2 months. Isoniazid and rifampin should be continued for at least 6 months, including at least 3 months after sputum culture conversion. In patients with HIV infection, meningitis, or disseminated disease, therapy should probably be continued for at least 9 months, including 6 months after sputum culture conversion. Recent recommendations of the American Thoracic Society and the

TABLE 101-1 CURRENT RECOMMENDATIONS FOR INITIAL TREATMENT OF TUBERCULOSIS

| Drug | Daily Dose | | Route | Maximal Daily Dose |
	Children	Adults		
Isoniazid	10–20 mg/kg	5 mg/kg	oral*	300 mg
Rifampin	10–20 mg/kg	10 mg/kg	oral*	600 mg
Pyrazinamide	15–30 mg/kg	15–30 mg/kg	oral	2 gm
Streptomycin	20–40 mg/kg	15 mg/kg†	intramuscular	1 gm†
Ethambutol	15–25 mg/kg	15–25 mg/kg	oral	2.5 gm

From Helm CJ, Holland GN: Ocular Tuberculosis. *Surv Ophthalmol* 38:229–256, 1993.
* Also available in parenteral preparations.
† Streptomycin should be limited to 10 mg/kg (maximum daily dose 750 mg) in persons older than 60 years.

CDC indicate that treatment should be the same whether the patient is HIV-positive or not, however.[11]

Over 95% of immunocompetent patients who complete a full course of therapy are successfully treated.[21] Compliant HIV-infected patients also have a good prognosis,[182] although there are reports of relapse despite sustained treatment.[174]

Compared to self-administered daily therapy, directly observed intermittent therapy for TB in patients with HIV infection is highly effective and associated with better adherence to therapy and survival.[9]

Lack of compliance,[5,31,123,182] drug resistance,[79,92,123] and inadequate primary therapy[123] are the most important factors in the failure of therapy. Brudney and Dobkin[31] found that 159 (89%) of 178 TB patients discharged from a large New York City public hospital were lost to follow-up and failed to complete therapy. Even worse, of the 40 patients who were readmitted for active TB within one year of initial discharge, 35 were again lost to follow-up after discharge. Noncompliance was significantly associated with homelessness, alcoholism, and the use of crack cocaine.

Treatment of Drug-Resistant Infection

Drug resistance may be primary or secondary. The frequency of primary resistance (drug resistance in patients with no prior antituberculosis therapy) was about 8.5% in the United States even before the AIDS epidemic, but was as high as 20% in some locations.[117] Younger patients and those of Asian or Hispanic descent had higher rates. Secondary resistance is particularly common in noncompliant patients and should be suspected in any case of relapse.[92] Because TB is most likely to develop in patients in whom compliance is a problem (drug addicts, alcoholics, the homeless, immigrants with limited access to health care), the emergence of drug resistance is an ongoing concern.[79]

Multiple drug resistant TB has been a devastating consequence of the HIV epidemic and the breakdown of the health-care infrastructure responsible for the treatment of TB.[41,43,51,185] Strains resistant to isoniazid and rifampin, or even all five first-line drugs, have now been reported in at least 15 states.[41] Over 90% of these cases have occurred in patients with advanced HIV disease and over 70% have been fatal.[41] Culture-positive TB cases in the United States in the first quarter of 1991 demonstrated resistance to isoniazid and/or rifampin in 9.5% of cases and MDR-TB was found in 3.5%.[23]

In New York City primary resistance to at least one drug increased from 10% in 1984 to 23% in 1991, while resistance to both isoniazid and rifampin increased from 3% to 7%.[41] When secondary resistance is included, one third of all TB cases in New York City were resistant to at least one drug by 1991.

Treatment for MDR-TB should include at least four but possibly as many as six or seven drugs for 18 to 36 months.[109] The difficulty in obtaining such drugs as streptomycin, PAS, isoniazid, cycloserine, and ethionamide in the United States[47,186] has hampered treatment of MDR-TB. Despite sustained therapy, relapse and mortality rates are high[41] and some investigators have called for mandatory confinement during treatment of the disease.[31]

Ocular Disease

Therapy of ocular TB follows the principles outlined above for extrapulmonary disease. With the exception of tuberculous phlyctenulosis, which usually responds to topical corticosteroids, therapy must be systemic. Adjunctive therapy with topical corticosteroids or topical antibiotics drugs such as isoniazid, streptomycin, or amikacin may be indicated for anterior segment involvement.[101,145] Amikacin, which is structurally similar to kanamycin, has not been widely used in the treatment of TB but is highly active against *M. tuberculosis in vitro*.[11] There is no evidence that ocular TB responds better or faster to treatment than does other extrapulmonary disease.

There is no role for systemic corticosteroid therapy in the treatment of infectious ocular TB. Both early clinical experience and animal models[199] showed that the use of corticosteroids in combination with antituberculosis chemotherapy was associated with a prolonged disease course and a high incidence of recurrence; the drug regimen cited in this 1958 report are considered inadequate currently.

Treatment of ocular TB should be coordinated with knowledgeable specialists. While there has been only one report of ocular TB caused by MDR-TB to date,[114] the possibility that similar cases will eventually occur is a compelling reason to obtain proper cultures from ocular specimens whenever possible. Therapy is potentially toxic[60] or, rarely, even fatal.[51,184] Drug interactions may pose a major problem,[92] especially in HIV-infected patients.[14,182] The ophthalmologist not only evaluates response to treatment, but also can help determine whether toxicity to certain drugs such as ethambutol and isoniazid has developed.*

In addition to treatment of underlying TB, treatment of tuberculous phlyctenulosis consists of topical corticosteroids tapered over one week; cycloplegic agents are also helpful. Systemic corticosteroids are absolutely contraindicated.[197] Conjunctival lesions causing only mild symptoms may respond to topical astrigents. Mucopurulent discharge suggests secondary bacterial infection and should be treated accordingly. Conjunctival lesions heal without scarring, but corneal phlyctenules leave superficial scars of variable severity. Phlyctenular keratoconjunctivitis will heal without treatment but may cause blindness due to corneal scarring.

Treatment of tuberculous interstitial keratitis consists of

---

*References 20, 33, 35, 88, 90, 120, 202.

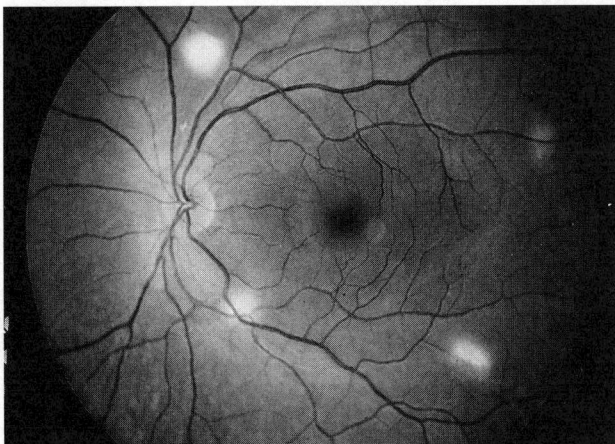

Fig. 101-4. Healed lesions in HIV-positive patient with presumed choroidal TB; note sharp borders and loss of retinal pigment epithelium.

topical corticosteroids and cycloplegics; antituberculosis drugs are indicated for the systemic disease, but have no effect on the ocular disease.[201] Corneal infiltrates associated with phlyctenulosis may also benefit from addition of topical corticosteroids.[4] Resolution of sclerokeratitis is usually achieved with systemic antituberculosis chemotherapy alone.[4,145]

Treatment of tuberculous scleritis consists of oral therapy, which may be supplemented with topical amikacin[145] or streptomycin if the organism is sensitive.[27,165] Resolution may take several months.[27,102] A similar response to antituberculosis chemotherapy is seen with treatment of choroidal tubercles. Treated lesions become larger, paler, and more distinct with time, leaving behind sharply demarcated scars (Fig. 101-4).

PROGNOSIS

There are too few cases of ocular TB to determine its association with mortality. In HIV-infected patients, pulmonary and extrapulmonary TB are associated with a high short-term mortality rate,[182] despite the fact that TB has been considered to occur early in the course of HIV disease. The best hope for treatment lies in prevention of tuberculous infection and in reducing the progression of tuberculous infection to TB.

PREVENTION

It is essential for healthy, exposed individuals to understand the risk of contracting TB. HIV-infected patients with TB may become infectious soon after exposure.[46,67,72,74] Unlike diseases such as *Pneumocystis carinii* pneumonia that are not transmitted to immunocompetent persons, TB (including MDR-TB) is potentially contagious for healthcare workers,[39,74] families, and other close contacts of infected patients.[181] Thorough evaluation of such exposed individu-

als is critical, with prompt institution of preventive treatment for those who develop a positive tuberculin skin test. Healthcare workers potentially exposed to TB should have a PPD skin test upon hiring and every 12 months thereafter, if negative.[38] The need for a high index of suspicion of TB is emphasized by Dooley and associates,[74] who noted that almost half of the patients who developed TB were admitted to regular hospital rooms before their TB was diagnosed.

Drug Prophylaxis

For HIV-infected patients who are exposed to TB, limited data suggest that prophylaxis with isoniazid is effective.[67,170] Tuberculin skin testing is of limited value in this group of patients in determining exposure.[67] Consideration should be given to treating *all* anergic, tuberculin-negative persons whose risk of tuberculous infection is estimated to be greater than 10% after active TB has been excluded.[1,42] Given the potential for rapid progression from infection to disease,[72,74] however, therapy with multiple drugs should be initiated if there is any evidence of active disease based on chest x-ray and the patient's symptoms. The National Institute of Allergy and Infectious Disease has begun a multicenter study to evaluate the effectiveness of a 2-month regimen of rifampin and PZA in preventing TB in PPD-positive, HIV-infected patients.[94]

Vaccination

A point should be made about vaccination with BCG. This vaccine, which has not been widely used in the United States, reduces the risk of the more severe forms of TB in infants and children.[11] The ability of BCG to prevent adult forms of TB remains unproved,[116] although it may reduce the risk of active TB cases and death.[58]

Vaccination has limited potential benefit in developed countries because most TB in these countries develops in patients who have already been infected and who will not benefit from BCG.[11] BCG is recommended in infants and children with negative tuberculin skin tests who are at high risk of intimate and prolonged exposure to patients with infectious pulmonary TB or who are continuously exposed to patients with TB resistant to both isoniazid and rifampin.[11] The vaccine is also recommended for tuberculin-negative infants and children in groups in which the rate of new infection exceeds 1% per year and in whom regular access to health care is limited.[11] Immunosuppressed individuals should not receive BCG. Individuals with a positive PPD should in general be managed without regard to a history of BCG.[59,159]

Strategies

The Advisory Committee for the Elimination of Tuberculosis (ACET) of the Department of Health and Human Services has made recommendations for the goal of reducing TB among populations with particularly high risk of the disease.[49] Such populations include foreign-born persons entering the United States and racial and ethnic minorities born in the United States. Recommendations include (1) community programs to increase awareness of the disease, (2) better training of healthcare providers within at-risk communities, (3) better screening of at-risk populations, (4) increasing the speed and completeness with which confirmed and suspected TB cases are reported to appropriate health departments, and (5) improving the availability and quality of TB healthcare service in at-risk communities. All foreign-born persons applying for permanent entry in the United States should be screened for TB; those with known or suspected active disease should be prevented from entering until treatment has rendered them noninfectious. Those persons with noninfectious TB should be allowed to enter.[40] The ACET has set a goal of eliminating TB from the United States by the year 2010.

Improved drug treatment of TB will require ensuring that old antituberculosis drugs remain available; improving access to available drugs; and expediting the development, testing, and approval of new drugs. Granting orphan-drug status to antituberculosis drugs, approving generic forms of some drugs, and accepting foreign data for approval of new drugs are some of the measures being taken by the Food and Drug Administration.

Failure to treat TB aggressively has had profound economic ramifications. In 1964 the International Union Against Tuberculosis reported that "there are 15 million people with TB in the world and the cost of their treatment would be negligible." Fewer than 10 years ago the CDC estimated that TB could be eradicated in the United States for an annual cost of about $30 million.[130] In 1992 the CDC asked for $540 million just to control the disease. New York City, under court order, has had to build a modern communicable disease prison facility to treat inmates with TB, at a cost of up to $500,000 for each of 42 beds.[181]

Directly observed therapy (DOT), in which visiting healthcare workers directly supervise patients taking their antituberculosis medications at home or in outpatient settings, is a cost-effective means of decreasing spread of the disease and reducing the risk of MDR-TB.[51] The CDC estimates that every dollar spent on observed pill-taking saves $4 in drug and hospital treatments for resistant cases that are prevented. It remains to be seen whether current public health measures, in the face of increasing numbers of HIV-infected patients and limited health care budgets, are up to the task of controlling TB.

REFERENCES

1. Abeles H, Farber SJ, Sarlo J: Tuberculosis in anergic HIV-infected drug users, *JAMA* 269:473-474, 1993 (letter).

2. Abrams J, Schlaegel AB, Schlaegel TF Jr: The role of the isoniazid therapeutic test in tuberculous uveitis, *Am J Ophthalmol* 94:511-515, 1982.

3. Abrams J, Schlaegel TF Jr: The tuberculin skin test in the diagnosis of tuberculous uveitis, *Am J Ophthalmol* 96:295-298, 1983.

4. Aclimandos WA, Kerr-Muir M: Tuberculous keratoconjunctivitis, *Br J Ophthalmol* 76:175-176, 1992.

5. Addington WW: Patient compliance: the most serious remaining problem in the control of tuberculosis in the United States, *Chest* 76:741-743, 1979.

6. Agrawal PK, Nath J, Jain BS: Orbital involvement in tuberculosis, *Indian J Ophthalmol* 76:175-176, 1977.

7. Allansmith MA, Ross RN: Phlyctenular keratoconjunctivitis. In Tasman W, Jaeger EA, editors: *Duane's clinical ophthalmology,* Philadelphia, 1989, JB Lippincott.

8. Alvarez S, McCabe WR: Extrapulmonary tuberculosis revisited: a Baltimore review of experience at Boston City and other hospitals, *Medicine* (Baltimore) 63:25, 1984.

9. Alwood K, Keruly J, Moore-Rice K et al.: Effectiveness of supervised, intermittent therapy for tuberculosis in HIV-invested patients, *AIDS* 8:1103-1108, 1994.

10. American Thoracic Society: Control of tuberculosis in the United States, *Am Rev Respir Dis* 146:1623-1633, 1992.

11. American Thoracic Society: Treatment of tuberculosis and tuberculous infection in adults and children, *Am J Respir Crit Care Med* 149:1359-1374, 1994.

12. American Thoracic Society and Centers for Disease Control: Diagnostic standards and classification of tuberculosis, *Am Rev Respir Dis* 142:725-735, 1990.

13. Anhalt EF, Zavell S, Chang G, Byron HM: Conjunctival tuberculosis, *Am J Ophthalmol* 50:265-269, 1960.

14. Antoniskis D, Easley AC, Espina BM et al.: Combined toxicity of zidovudine and antituberculosis chemotherapy, *Am Rev Respir Dis* 145:430-434, 1992.

15. Archer D, Bird A: Primary tuberculosis of the conjunctiva, *Br J Ophthalmol* 51:679-687, 1967.

16. Asensi F, Otero MC, Perez-Tamarit D et al.: Tuberculous iridocyclitis in a three-year-old girl, *Clin Pediatr* 30:605-606, 1991.

17. Baghdassarian SA, Zakharia H, Adourian KK: Report of a case of bilateral caseous tuberculous dacryoadenitis, *Am J Ophthalmol* 74:744-746, 1972.

18. Barnes PF, Bloch AB, Davidson PT et al.: Tuberculosis in patients with human immunodeficiency virus infection, *N Engl J Med* 324:1644-1650, 1991.

19. Barondes MJ, Sponsel WE, Stevens TS et al.: Tuberculous choroiditis diagnosed by chorioretinal endobiopsy, *Am J Ophthalmol* 112:460-461, 1991.

20. Barron GJ, Tepper L, Iovine G: Ocular toxicity from ethambutol, *Am J Ophthalmol* 77:256-260, 1974.

21. Berenguer J, Moreno S, Laguna F et al.: Tuberculous meningitis in patients infected with the human immunodeficiency virus, *N Engl J Med* 326:668-672, 1992.

22. Blatt SP, Hendrix CW, Butzin CA et al.: Delayed-type hypersensitivity skin testing predicts progression to AIDS in HIV-infected patients, *Ann Intern Med* 119:177-184, 1993.

23. Bloch AB, Cauthen GM, Onorato IM et al.: Nationwide survey of drug-resistant tuberculosis in the United States, *JAMA* 271:665-671, 1994.

24. Bloch AB, Rieder HL, Kelly GD et al.: The epidemiology of tuberculosis in the United States, *Semin Respir Infect* 4:17-170, 1989.

25. Blodi BA, Johnson MW, McLeish WM, Gass JDM: Presumed choroidal tuberculosis in a human immunodeficiency virus infected host, *Am J Ophthalmol* 108:605-607, 1989.

26. Blodi F: Choroidal tuberculoma simulating a melanoma, *Klin Monatsbl Augenheilk* 170:845, 1977.

27. Bloomfield SE, Mondino B, Gray GF: Scleral tuberculosis, *Arch Ophthalmol* 94:954-956, 1976.

28. Bonnet P: Scleritis symptomatic of miliary granulomas in the choroid, *Bull Soc Ophtalmol Fr* 2:144, 1952.

29. Braun MM, Truman BI, Maguire B et al.: Increasing incidence of tuberculosis in a prison inmate population: association with HIV infection, *JAMA* 261:393-397, 1989.

30. Bruckner Z: Etude histologique de la permeabilite de la conjonctive aux bacilles tuberculeus, *Ann Ocul* 166:804-824, 1929.

31. Brudney K, Dobkin J: Resurgent tuberculosis in New York City: human immunodeficiency virus, homelessness, and the decline of tuberculosis control programs, *Am Rev Respir Dis* 144:745-749, 1991.

32. Burgoyne CF, Verstraeten TC, Friberg TR: Tuberculin skin test–induced uveitis in the absence of tuberculosis, *Graefes Arch Clin Exp Ophthalmol* 229:232-236, 1991.

33. Byrd RB, Horn RB, Solomon DA, Griggs A: Toxic effects of isoniazid in tuberculous chemoprophylaxis: role of biochemical monitoring in 1000 patients, *JAMA* 241:1239-1241, 1979.

34. Cangemi FE, Friedman AH, Josephberg R: Tuberculoma of the choroid, *Ophthalmology* 87:252-258, 1980.

35. Carr RE, Henkind P: Ocular manifestations of ethambutol: toxic amblyopia after administration of an experimental antituberculous drug, *Arch Ophthalmol* 67:566-571, 1962.

36. Centers for Disease Control: Patients with recurrent tuberculosis, *MMWR* 30:645, 1981.

37. Centers for Disease Control: Diagnosis and management of mycobacterial infection and disease in persons with human T-lymphotropic virus type-III lymphadenopathy-associated virus infection, *MMWR* 35:448-452, 1986.

38. Centers for Disease Control: Guidelines for preventing the transmission of tuberculosis in health-care settings, with special focus on HIV-related issues, *MMWR* 39(RR-17):1-29, 1990.

39. Centers for Disease Control: Nosocomial transmission of multi drug-resistant tuberculosis to health-care workers and HIV-infected patients in an urban hospital—Florida, *MMWR* 39:718-722, 1990.

40. Centers for Disease Control: Tuberculosis among foreign-born persons entering the United States: recommendations of the advisory committee for elimination of tuberculosis, *MMWR* 39(RR-18):1-21, 1990.

41. Centers for Disease Control: Nosocomial transmission of multi drug-resistant tuberculosis among HIV-infected persons—Florida and New York, 1988-1991, *MMWR* 40:585-591, 1991.

42. Centers for Disease Control: Purified protein derivative (PPD)-tuberculin anergy and HIV-infection: guidelines for anergy testing and management of anergic persons at risk of tuberculosis, *MMWR* 40(RR-5):27-33, 1991.

43. Centers for Disease Control: Transmission of multi drug-resistant tuberculosis from an HIV-positive client in a residential substance-abuse treatment facility—Michigan, *MMWR* 40:129-131, 1991.

44. Centers for Disease Control: Tuberculosis among homeless shelter residents, *MMWR* 40:869-877, 1991.

45. Centers for Disease Control: Tuberculosis morbidity in the United States: final data, 1990, *MMWR* 40(SS-3):23-28, 1991.

46. Centers for Disease Control: Tuberculosis outbreak among persons in a residential facility for HIV-infected persons—San Francisco, *MMWR* 40:649-651, 1991.

47. Centers for Disease Control: Availability of streptomycin and para-aminosalicylic acid—United States, *MMWR* 41:243, 1992.

48. Centers for Disease Control: 1993 revised classification system for HIV infection and expanded surveillance case definition for AIDS among adolescents and adults, *MMWR* 41(RR-17):1-19, 1992.

49. Centers for Disease Control: Prevention and control of tuberculosis in U.S. communities with at-risk minority populations and prevention and control of tuberculosis among homeless persons: recommendations of the advisory council for the elimination of tuberculosis, *MMWR* 41(RR-5):1-23, 1992.

50. Centers for Disease Control: Diagnosis of tuberculosis by nucleic acid amplification methods applied to clinical specimens, *MMWR* 42:686, 1993.

51. Centers for Disease Control: Initial therapy for tuberculosis in the era of multidrug resistance: recommendations of the advisory council for the elimination of tuberculosis, *MMWR* 42(RR-7):1-8, 1993.

52. Centers for Disease Control: Severe isoniazid-associated hepatitis—New York, 1991-1993, *MMWR* 42:545-547, 1993.

53. Centers for Disease Control: Tuberculosis morbidity—United States, 1992, *MMWR* 42:696-704, 1993.

54. Chaisson RE: Tuberculosis in patients with the acquired immunodeficiency syndrome: clinical features, response to therapy, and survival, *Am Rev Respir Dis* 136:570, 1987.

55. Chandler AC, Locatcher-Khorago D: Primary tuberculosis of the conjunctiva, *Arch Ophthalmol* 71:202-205, 1964.

56. Chung YM, Yeh TS, Sheu SJ, Liu JH: Macular subretinal neovascularization in choroidal tuberculosis, *Ann Ophthalmol* 21:225-229, 1989.

57. Ciesielski SD, See JR, Esposito DH, Hunter N: The epidemiology of tuberculosis among North Carolina farm workers, *JAMA* 265:1715-1719, 1991.

58. Colditz GA, Brewer TF, Berkey CS et al.: Efficacy of BCG vaccine in the prevention of tuberculosis: meta-analysis of the published literature, *JAMA* 271:698-702, 1994.

59. Committee on Infectious Diseases: Screening for tuberculosis in infants and children, *Pediatrics* 93:131-134, 1994.

60. Comstock GW, Edwards PQ: The competing risks of tuberculosis and hepatitis for adult tuberculin reactors, *Am Rev Resp Dis* 111:573-577, 1975.

61. Cook CD, Hainsworth M: Tuberculosis of the conjunctiva occurring in association with a neighboring lupus vulgaris lesion, *Br J Ophthalmol* 74:315-316, 1990.

62. Cousins DV, Wilton SD, Francis BR, Gow BL: The use of polymerase chain reaction for rapid diagnosis of tuberculosis, *J Clin Microbiol* 30:255-258, 1992.

63. Croxatto JO, Hulsbus R, Lombardi A: Unsuspected mycobacterial endophthalmitis with increased aqueous lactate dehydrogenase levels in a child, *Ann Ophthalmol* 21:233-237, 1989.

64. Croxatto JO, Mestre C, Puente S, Gonzalez G: Nonreactive tuberculosis in a patient with acquired immune deficiency syndrome, *Am J Ophthalmol* 102:559-660, 1986.

65. Cummings MM: Diagnostic methods in tuberculosis, *Am J Clin Pathol* 21:684-689, 1991.

66. Cynamon MH, Klemens SP: New antimycobacterial agents, *Clin Chest Med* 10:355-364, 1989.

67. Daley CL, Small PM, Schecter GF et al.: An outbreak of tuberculosis with accelerated progression among persons infected with the human immunodeficiency virus: an analysis using restriction-fragment-length polymorphisms, *N Engl J Med* 326:231-235, 1992.

68. Dannenberg AM Jr: Delayed-type hypersensitivity and cell-mediated immunity in the pathogenesis of tuberculosis, *Immunol Today* 12:228, 1991.

69. Darrell RW: Acute tuberculosis panophthalmitis, *Arch Ophthalmol* 78:51-54, 1967.

70. Dastur DK, Singhal BS: Eales' disease with neurological involvement. II. Pathology and pathogenesis, *J Neurol Sci* 27:323-345, 1976.

71. Dinning WJ, Marston S: Cutaneous and ocular tuberculosis: a review, *J R Soc Med* 78:576-581, 1985.

72. Diperri G, Cruciani M, Danzi MC et al.: Nosocomial epidemic of active tuberculosis among HIV-infected patients, *Lancet* 2:1502-1504, 1989.

73. Donahue HC: Ophthalmologic experience in a tuberculosis sanatorium, *Am J Ophthalmol* 64:742-478, 1967.

74. Dooley SW, Villarino ME, Lawrence M et al.: Nosocomial transmission of tuberculosis in a hospital unit for HIV-infected patients, *JAMA* 267:2632-2635, 1992.

75. Duke-Elder S, Dobree JH: *System of ophthalmology: diseases of the retina,* vol. 10, St Louis, 1967, Mosby.

76. Duke-Elder S, Perkins ES: *System of ophthalmology: diseases of the uveal tract,* vol 9, St Louis, 1966, Mosby.

77. Dutt AK, Moers D, Stead WW: Short-course chemotherapy for extra-pulmonary tuberculosis: nine years' experience, *Ann Intern Med* 104:712, 1986.

78. Dvorak-Theobald G: Acute tuberculosis endophthalmitis: report of a case, *Am J Ophthalmol* 45:403, 1958.

79. Edlin BR, Tokars JI, Grieco MH et al.: An outbreak of multi-drug resistant tuberculosis among hospitalized patients with the acquired immunodeficiency syndrome, *N Engl J Med* 326:1514-1521, 1992.

80. Elliot A: Recurrent intraocular hemorrhage in young adults (Eale's disease): a report of thirty-one cases, *Trans Am Ophthalmol Soc* 52:811, 1954.

81. Elliot AJ: 30-year observation of patients with Eales's disease, *Am J Ophthalmol* 80:404-408, 1975.

82. Ellner PD: Rapid detection and identification of pathogenic mycobacteria by combining radiometric and nucleic acid probe methods, *J Clin Microbiol* 26:1349-1352, 1988.

83. Ena J, Crespo MJ, Valls V, de Salamanca RE: Adenosine deaminase activity in cerebrospinal fluid: a useful test for meningeal tuberculosis, even in patients with AIDS, *J Infect Dis* 158:896, 1988 (letter).

84. Eyre JNH: Tuberculosis of the conjunctiva, *Lancet* 1:1319, 1912.

85. Farer LS, Lowell AM, Meador MP: Extrapulmonary tuberculosis in the United States, *Am J Epidemiol* 109:205-217, 1979.

86. Finnoff WC: Changes found in eyes of rabbits following injection of living tubercle bacilli into the common carotid artery, *Am J Ophthalmol* 7:81-89, 1924.

87. Finnoff WC: Ocular tuberculosis, experimental and clinical, *Arch Ophthalmol* 53:1330-1336, 1924.

88. Fledelius HC, Petrera JE, Skjodt K, Trojaborg W: Ocular ethambutol toxicity, *Acta Ophthalmol* 65:251-255, 1987.

89. Fountain JA, Werner RB: Tuberculous retinal vasculitis, *Retina* 4:48-50, 1984.

90. Fraunfelder FT, Meyer SM: Ocular toxicology. In Tasman W, Jaeger EA, editors: *Duane's clinical ophthalmology,* vol 5, 1-24, Philadelphia, 1990, JB Lippincott.

91. Gibson WS: The etiology of phlyctenular conjunctivitis, *Am J Dis Child* 15:81-115, 1918.

92. Glassroth J, Robins G, Snider DE Jr: Tuberculosis in the 1980's, *N Engl J Med* 302:1441-1450, 1980.

93. Goldberg MF: Presumed tuberculous maculopathy, *Retina* 2:47, 1982.

94. Gordin F: Tuberculosis control: back to the future? *JAMA* 267:2649-2650, 1992.

95. Graham NMH, Chaisson RE: Tuberculosis and HIV infection: epidemiology, pathogenesis, and clinical aspects, *Ann Allergy* 71:421-428, 1993.

96. Graham NMH, Nelson KE, Solomon L et al.: Prevalence of tuberculin positivity and skin test anergy in HIV-1–seropositive and –seronegative intravenous drug users, *JAMA* 267:369-373, 1992.

97. Grosset JH: Present status of chemotherapy for tuberculosis, *Rev Inf Dis* 11(S2):S347, 1989.

98. Gur S, Silverstone BZ, Zylberman R, Berson D: Chorioretinitis and extrapulmonary tuberculosis, *Ann Ophthalmol* 19:112-115, 1987.

99. Harries AD: Tuberculosis and human immunodeficiency virus infection in developing countries, *Lancet* 335:387-390, 1990.

100. Heifets LB, Good RC: Current laboratory methods for the diagnosis of tuberculosis. In Bloom BR, editor: *Tuberculosis: pathogenesis, protection, and control,* Washington, DC, 1994, American Society for Microbiology.

101. Helm CJ, Holland GN: Ocular tuberculosis, *Surv Ophthalmol* 38:229-256, 1993.

102. Hemady R, Sainz de la Maza M, Raizman MB, Foster CS: Six cases of scleritis associated with systemic infection, *Am J Ophthalmol* 114:55-62, 1992.

103. Henderly DE, Genstler AJ, Smith RE, Rao NA: Changing patterns of uveitis, *Am J Ophthalmol* 103:131-136, 1987.

104. Holden M, Dubin MR, Diamond PH: Frequency of negative intermediate-strength tuberculin sensitivity in patients with active tuberculosis, *N Engl J Med* 285:1506-1509, 1971.

105. Hoy J, Mijch A, Sandland M et al.: Quadruple drug therapy for *Mycobacterium avium-intracellulare* bacteremia in AIDS patients, *J Infect Dis* 161:801-805, 1990.

106. Illingworth RS, Wright T: Tubercles of the choroid, *BMJ* 2:365, 1948.

107. Inoue S, Ubuka M: A case of choroidal miliary tuberculosis as studied by fluorescence fundus photography, *Jpn J Ophthalmol* 23:256, 1972.

108. Iralu JV, Maguire JH: Pulmonary infections in immigrants and refugees, *Semin Respir Infect* 6:235-246, 1991.

109. Iseman MD: Treatment of multidrug-resistant tuberculosis, *N Engl J Med* 329:784-791, 1994.

110. Jabbour NM, Faris B, Trempe CL: A case of pulmonary tuberculosis presenting with a choroidal tuberculoma, *Ophthalmology* 92:834-837, 1985.

111. Kaufmann SHE: The macrophage in tuberculosis: sinner or saint? The T cell decides, *Pathobiology* 59:153, 1991.

112. Kent PT, Kubica GP: *Public health mycobacteriology: a guide for the level III laboratory,* US Department of Health and Human Services, Public Health Service, Atlanta, Georgia, 1985, Centers for Disease Control.

113. Khalil M, Lindley S, Matouk E: Tuberculosis of the orbit, *Ophthalmology* 92:1624-1627, 1985.

114. Kim JY, Carroll CP, Opremcak EM: Antibiotic-resistant tuberculosis choroiditis, *Am J Ophthalmol* 115:259-260, 1993.

115. Kindler V, Sappino AP, Grau GE et al.: The inducing role of tumor necrosis factor in the development of bactericidal granulomas during BCG infection, *Cell* 56:731-740, 1989.

116. Kochi A: The global tuberculosis situation and the new control strategy of the World Health Organization, *Tubercle* 72:1-6, 1991.

117. Kopanoff DE, Kilburn JO, Glassroth JL et al.: A continuing survey of tuberculosis primary drug resistance in the United States: March 1975 to November 1977: a United States Public Health Service cooperative study, *Am Rev Respir Dis* 118:835-842, 1978.

118. Kramer F, Modilevsky T, Waliany AR et al.: Delayed diagnosis of tuberculosis in patients with human immunodeficiency virus infection, *Am J Med* 89:451-456, 1990.

119. Lamba PA, Bhalla JS, Mullick DN: Ocular manifestations of tubercular meningitis: a clinico-biochemical study, *J Pediatr Ophthalmol Strabismus* 23:123-125, 1986.

120. Leibold JE: Drugs having a toxic effect on the optic nerve, *Int Ophthalmol Clin* 11:137-144, 1971.

121. Lyon CE, Grimson BS, Peiffer RLL, Merritt JC: Clinicopathological correlation of a solitary choroidal tuberculoma, *Ophthalmology* 92:845-850, 1985.

122. Madhukar K, Bhide M, Prasad CE: Tuberculosis of the lacrimal gland, *J Trop Med Hyg* 94:150-151, 1991.

123. Mahmoudi A, Iseman MD: Pitfalls in the care of patients with tuberculosis: common errors and their association with the acquisition of drug resistance, *JAMA* 270:65-68, 1993.

124. Manjunath N, Shankar P, Rajan L et al.: Evaluation of a polymerase chain reaction for the diagnosis of tuberculosis, *Tubercle* 72:21-27, 1991.

125. Mansour AM, Haymond R: Choroidal tuberculomas without evidence of extraocular tuberculosis, *Graefes Arch Clin Exp Ophthalmol* 228:382-385, 1990.

126. Mansour AM: Renal allograft tuberculosis, *Tubercle* 71:147-148, 1990.

127. Maria DL, Mundala SH: Sub-periosteal tuberculoma of the left lateral wall of orbit, *Indian J Ophthalmol* 29:47-49, 1981.

128. Markowitz N, Hansen NI, Wilcosky TC et al.: Tuberculin and anergy testing in HIV-seropositive and HIV-seronegative persons, *Ann Intern Med* 119:185-193, 1993.

129. Marwick C: Do worldwide outbreaks mean tuberculosis again becomes "captain of all these men of death?", *JAMA* 267:1174-1175, 1992.

130. Marwick C: Resurgence of tuberculosis prompts US search for effective drugs, expanded research effort, *JAMA* 269:191-192, 1993.

131. Massaro D, Katz S, Sachs M: Choroidal tubercles: a clue to hematogenous tuberculosis, *Ann Intern Med* 231-241, 1964.

132. Maurya OPS, Patel V, Thakur V, Singh TR: Tuberculoma of the orbit: a case report, *Indian J Ophthalmol* 38:191-192, 1990.

133. McAdam JM, Brickner PW, Scharer LL et al.: The spectrum of tuberculosis in a New York City men's shelter clinic (1982-1988), *Chest* 97:798-805, 1990.

134. McMoli TE, Mordi VPN, Grange A, Abiose A: Tuberculous panophthalmitis, *J Pediatr Ophthalmol Strabismus* 15:383-385, 1978.

135. Medical Research Council Investigation: Streptomycin treatment of pulmonary tuberculosis, *BMJ* 2:769-782, 1948.

136. Mehta DK, Sanhikamal, Ashok P: Bilateral tubercular lid abscess: a case report, *Indian J Ophthalmol* 37:98, 1989.

137. Menezo JL, Martinez-Costa R, Marin F et al.: Tuberculous panophthalmitis associated with drug abuse, *Int Ophthalmol* 10:235-240, 1987.

138. Miller W: Tuberculosis in the adult, *Postgrad Radiol* 1:147-167, 1981.

139. Mohan K, Prasad P, Banerjee AK, Dhir SP: Tubercular tarsitis, *Indian J Ophthalmol* 33:115-116, 1985.

140. Mohan M, Garg SP, Kumar H et al.: SAFA test as an aid to the diagnosis of ocular tuberculosis, *Indian J Ophthalmol* 38:57-60, 1990.

141. Moreno S, Baraia-Etxaburu J, Bouza E et al.: Risk for developing tuberculosis among anergic patients infected with HIV, *Ann Intern Med* 119:194-198, 1993.

142. Morse ML, Karr DJ, Mendelman PM: Ocular tuberculosis in a five-month-old, *Pediatr Inf Dis J* 7:514-516, 1988.

143. Mortada A: Tuberculoma of the orbit and lacrimal gland, *Br J Ophthalmol* 55:565-567, 1971.

144. Nambuya A, Sewankambo N, Mugerwa J et al.: Tuberculosis lymphadenitis associated with human immunodeficiency virus (HIV) in Uganda, *J Clin Pathol* 41:93-96, 1988.

145. Nanda M, Pflugfelder SC, Holland S: Mycobacterium tuberculosis scleritis, *Am J Ophthalmol* 108:736-737, 1989.

146. Nardell E, McInnis B, Thomas B, Weidhaas S: Exogenous reinfection with tuberculosis in a shelter for the homeless, *N Engl J Med* 315:1570-1575, 1986.

147. Ni C, Papale JJ, Robinson NL et al.: Uveal tuberculosis, *Int Ophthalmol Clin* 22(3):103-124, 1982.

148. Ohmart WA: Experimental tuberculosis of the eye, *Am J Ophthalmol* 16:773-778, 1933.

149. Olazabal F: Choroidal tubercles: a neglected sign, *JAMA* 200:374, 1967.

150. Ostler HB, Lanier JD: Phlyctenular keratoconjunctivitis with special reference to the staphylococcal type, *Trans Pacific Coast Oto-Ophthalmol Soc* 55:237, 1974.

151. Panda A, Singhal V: Tuberculosis of lacrimal gland, *Indian J Pediatr* 56:531-533, 1989.

152. Peneau A, Moinard D, Berard I et al.: Detection of mycobacteria using the polymerase chain reaction, *Eur J Clin Microbiol Infect Dis* 11:270-271, 1992.

153. Peterson EM, Lu R, Floyd C et al.: Direct identification of *mycobacterium tuberculosis, Mycobacterium avium* and *Mycobacterium intracellulare* from amplified primary cultures in BACTEC media using DNA probes, *J Clin Microbiol* 27:1543-1547, 1989.

154. Philip RN, Comstock GW, Shelton JH: Phlyctenular keratoconjunctivitis among Eskimos in southwestern Alaska, *Am Rev Respir Dis* 91:171, 1965.

155. Pierce JR Jr, Sims SL, Holman GH: Transmission of tuberculosis to hospital workers by a patient with AIDS, *Chest* 101:581-582, 1992.

156. Pitchenik AE, Fertel D: Tuberculosis and nontuberculous mycobacterial disease, *Med Clin North Am* 76:121-171, 1992.

157. Psilas K, Aspiotis M, Petroutsos G et al.: Anti-tuberculosis therapy in the treatment of peripheral uveitis, *Ann Ophthalmol* 23:254-258, 1991.

158. Regillo CD, Shields CL, Shields JA et al.: Ocular tuberculosis, *JAMA* 266:1490, 1991.

159. Reichman LB: Tuberculin skin testing, *Chest* 76:764-770, 1979.

160. Renie WA, Murphy RP, Anderson KC et al.: The evaluation of patients with Eales' disease, *Retina* 3:243-248, 1983.

161. Rieder HL, Cauthen M, Bloch AB et al.: Tuberculosis and acquired immunodeficiency syndrome—Florida, *Arch Int Med* 149:1268-1273, 1989.

162. Rosen PH, Spalton DJ, Graham EM: Intraocular tuberculosis, *Eye* 4:486-492, 1990.

163. Rosenbaum JT, Wernick R: The utility of routine screening of patients with uveitis for systemic lupus erythematosus or tuberculosis: a bayesian analysis, *Arch Ophthalmol* 108:1291-1293, 1990.

164. Saini JS, Mukherjee AK, Nadkarni: Primary tuberculosis of the retina, *Br J Ophthalmol* 70:533-535, 1986.

165. Saini JS, Sharma A, Pillai P: Scleral tuberculosis, *Trop Geogr Med* 40:350-352, 1988.

166. Saltzman BR, Motyl MR, Friedland GH et al.: *Mycobacterium tuberculosis* bacteremia in the acquired immunodeficiency syndrome, *JAMA* 256:390-391, 1986.

167. Santoni G, Fiore C, Lupidi G, Galuppo L: Choroidal miliary tuberculosis: fluoroangiographic study, *Ophthalmologica* 184:6, 1982.

168. Schlaegel TF Jr, O'Connor GR: Metastatic nonsuppurative uveitis, *Int Ophthalmol Clin* 17:87-108, 1977.

169. Schlaegel TF Jr, O'Connor GR: Tuberculosis and syphilis, *Arch Ophthalmol* 99:2206-2207, 1981.

170. Selwyn P: Multi drug-resistant tuberculosis in HIV disease and AIDS, *AIDS Clin Care* 4:45, 1992.

171. Selwyn PA, Hartel D, Lewis VA et al.: A prospective study of the risk of tuberculosis among intravenous drug users with human immunodeficiency infection, *N Engl J Med* 320:545-550, 1989.

172. Sen DK: Endogenous uveitis in Indian children: analysis of 94 cases, *J Pediatr Ophthalmol* 14:25-32, 1977.

173. Sen DK: Tuberculosis of the orbit and lacrimal gland: a clinical study of 14 cases, *J Pediatr Ophthalmol Strabismus* 17:232-238, 1980.

174. Shafer RW, Jones WD: Relapse of tuberculosis in a patient with the acquired immunodeficiency syndrome despite 12 months of antituberculosis therapy and continuation of isoniazid, *Tubercle* 272:149-151, 1991.

175. Shafer RW, Kim DS, Weiss JP, Quale JM: Extrapulmonary tuberculosis in patients with human immunodeficiency virus infection, *Medicine* 70:384-397, 1991.

176. Shah SM, Howard RS, Sarkies NJC, Graham EM: Tuberculosis presenting as retinal vasculitis, *J R Soc Med* 54:10, 1988.

177. Shammas HF, Burton TC, Weingeist TA: False-positive results with the radioactive phosphorus test, *Arch Ophthalmol* 95:2190, 1977.

178. Shiono T, Abe S, Horiuchi T: A case of miliary tuberculosis with disseminated choroidal hemorrhages, *Br J Ophthalmol* 74:317-319, 1990.

179. Simon HB: Mycobacteria. In Rubenstein E, Federman DD, editors: *Scientific American medicine,* New York, 1984, Scientific American.

180. Singh I, Chaudhary U, Arora B: Tuberculoma of the conjunctiva, *J Indian Med Assoc* 87:265-266, 1989.

181. Skolnick AA: Correction facility TB rates soar: some jails bring back chest roentgenograms, *JAMA* 268:3175-3176, 1992.

182. Small PM, Schecter GF, Goodman PC et al.: Treatment of tuberculosis in patients with advanced human immunodeficiency virus infection, *N Engl J Med* 324:289-294, 1991.

183. Smith RE: Tuberculoma of the choroid, *Ophthalmology* 87:257-258, 1980 (discussion).

184. Snider DE Jr, Caras GJ: Isoniazid-associated hepatitis deaths: a review of available information, *Am Rev Respir Dis* 145:494-497, 1992.

185. Snider DE Jr, Cauthen GM, Farer LS et al.: Drug-resistant tuberculosis, *Am Rev Respir Dis* 144:732, 1991 (letter).

186. Snider DE Jr, Roper WL: The new tuberculosis, *N Engl J Med* 326:703-705, 1992.

187. Stead WW: Undetected tuberculosis in prison: source of infection for community at large, *JAMA* 240:2544-2547, 1978.

188. Theuer CP, Hopewell PC, Elias D et al.: Human immunodeficiency virus infection in tuberculosis patients, *J Infect Dis* 162:8-12, 1990.

189. Thygeson P: Observations on nontuberculous phlyctenular keratoconjunctivitis, *Trans Am Acad Ophthalmol Otolaryngol* 58:128-132, 1954.

190. Thygeson P, Diaz-Bonnet V, Okumoto M: Phlyctenulosis: attempts to produce an experimental model with BCG, *Invest Ophthalmol* 1:262-266, 1962.

191. Van den Brande P, Vijgen J, Demedts M: Clinical spectrum of pulmonary tuberculosis in older patients: comparison with younger patients, *J Gerontol* 46:M204-209, 1991.

192. Wallis RS, Paranjape R, Phillips M: Identification by two-dimensional gel electrophoresis of a 58-kilodalton tumor necrosis factor-inducing protein of *Mycobacterium tuberculosis, Infect Immun* 61:627-632, 1993.

193. Wallis RS, Vjecha M, Amir-Tahmasseb M et al.: Influence of tuberculosis on human immunodeficiency virus (HIV-1): enhanced cytokine expression and elevated B$_2$-microglobulin in HIV-1 associated tuberculosis, *J Infect Dis* 167:43-48, 1993.

194. Watson PG, Hayreh SS: Scleritis and episcleritis, *Br J Ophthalmol* 60:163-191, 1976.

195. Weeks JE: Tuberculosis of the eye, *Am J Ophthalmol* 9:243-246, 1926.

196. Weir MR, Thornton GF: Extrapulmonary tuberculosis: experience of a community hospital and review of the literature, *Am J Med* 79:467-478, 1985.

197. Woods AC: *Endogenous inflammation of the uveal tract,* 340-350, Baltimore, 1961, Williams and Wilkins.

198. Woods AC: Ocular tuberculosis. In Sorsby A, editor: *Modern ophthalmology,* 105-140, Philadelphia, 1972, JB Lippincott.

199. Woods AC, Wood R, Senterfit LB: Studies in experimental ocular tuberculosis, *Arch Ophthalmol* 59:559-578, 1958.

200. Yamaguchi E, Reichman LB: Pulmonary tuberculosis in the HIV-positive patient, *Inf Dis Clin North Am* 5:623-633, 1991.

201. Yee RW, Hyndiuk RA: Interstitial keratitis. In Tabbara KF, Hyndiuk RA, editors: *Infections of the eye,* 605-606, Boston, 1986, Little, Brown and Co.

202. Yonekura Y, Mori T, Kondo N: Optic nerve complications of ethambutol, *Folia Ophthalmol Jpn* 20:545-549, 1969.

102 Hansen Disease

NAUSHAD HUSSEIN, H. BRUCE OSTLER

Hansen disease—better known as leprosy—is one of the oldest clinically described diseases of human beings.[7] Throughout history the term *leprosy* has provoked fear and an aura of horror, resulting in an intolerable social stigma toward affected individuals.

MYCOBACTERIOLOGY

M. leprae belongs to the order Actinomycetales and family Mycobacteriaceae.[46a] The organism is a gram-positive, strongly acid-fast bacillus. It is an obligate intercellular parasite primarily of macrophages and Schwann cells and is the only mycobacterium that infects peripheral nerves. Its long generation time (12 to 13 days) as compared to *M. tuberculosis* (generation time 20 hours) and *Escherichia coli* (generation time 20 minutes), is unique and consistent with the disease's chronicity. Clinical observations in patients and experimental models of leprosy confirm that *M. leprae* grows best at lower temperatures.

Study of the metabolic pathways of *M. leprae* has revealed several interesting findings such as: (1) the organism has a unique ability among mycobacteria to oxidize some diphenons (e.g., D-dihydroxyphenylalanine [dopa]) that are present in melanin,[32] (2) mycobacteria are generally insensitive to bacterial folate synthetase inhibitors (e.g., dapsone), but the folate synthetase of *M. leprae* has high affinity for dapsone, and (3) bacteria are usually protected from free radicals by enzyme systems such as superoxide dismutase, peroxidase, and catalase, but *M. leprae* has low levels of peroxidase and no catalase.

HISTORICAL BACKGROUND

Leprosy originated in tropical and subtropical Africa and southern Asia over 2500 years ago. Leprosy was often confused with many other chronic and debilitating skin diseases. As the disease was better delineated, a heredity theory became popular to explain the social clustering that often occurred. With the development of the microscope, the germ theory gained favor for many diseases. In 1873 Hansen (1841-1912) discovered the rod-shaped leprosy bacillus. *Mycobacterium leprae* was the first bacterium identified as a cause of human disease. Attempts to grow it on artificial media or tissue cultures have been unsuccessful.

EPIDEMIOLOGY

Leprosy is endemic in parts of Africa, Asia, and Central and South America. It is a major public health problem in most populated areas of the developing world, where the estimated prevalence of leprosy is approximately one case per 1000 population. Current figures from the World Health Organization identify 5.5 million patients with an incidence of about 1 million new patients yearly. Worldwide, approximately 15 million patients have Hansen disease.

The disease occurs in clusters and in families, probably because of shared environment, genetics, and contact. A history of prolonged exposure to the disease is common in new cases. Attack rates in families of untreated lepromatous patients range from 5% to 10%. Up to one half of children with a leprotic parent develop one or more lesions that may heal spontaneously.

Man is the major reservoir and host of *M. leprae*. The upper respiratory tract, nasal mucus, and skin lesions of untreated multibacillary patients are principal sources for transmission of organisms. Overcrowding, poverty, and poor hygiene are risk factors for expression of the disease. Leprosy is only mildly infectious and provokes a slow granulomatous response. The host's immune status determines most manifestations of the disease. Early diagnosis and multidrug treatment rapidly render most patients noncontagious.

Ocular complications occur in 10% to 90% of patients and probably occur more frequently during leprosy than in any other systemic infectious diseases. Eye disease is partly determined by the patient's immune response,[31] ethnicity, and genetic make-up, the type and duration of infection, and the treatment received. The form of ocular inflammation also varies by geography. Corneal disease is common in

Africa and India, whereas iridocyclitis is common in Southeast Asia.*

Approximately 5% to 10% of patients with ocular leprosy are blinded by the disease. A million or more leprosy patients have substantial vision loss from leprosy. Blindness from leprosy is often compounded with other disabilities and deformities that result in social ostracism, economic loss, and family and psychological problems that cannot be adequately quantified.

CLINICAL FEATURES

The disease process begins with bacillary infiltration of predisposed cool and dopa-rich nerve and pigmented tissues (e.g., skin, nasal mucosa, the eye, and ocular adnexa), followed by an inflammatory response leading to functional loss and eventual atrophy and deformity of the involved structures.

Disease Classification

Leprosy patients show a range of clinical and histopathologic findings with the two extremes being (1) lepromatous leprosy (disseminated infection with minimal cell mediated immunity) and (2) tuberculoid leprosy (limited infection with marked cell mediated immunity). The Madrid classification advanced in 1953 divided leprosy into three forms: tuberculoid, lepromatous, and indeterminate. The Ridley and Jopling classification advanced in 1962 and 1966 and later modified has the following six classes: indeterminate (I), tuberculoid (TT), borderline tuberculoid (BT), borderline (BB), borderline lepromatous (BL), and lepromatous (LL).[35,36]

Leprosy patients are also classified into paucibacillary and multibacillary types according to skin smears. Paucibacillary patients have negative skin smears for acid-fast bacilli and would encompass I, TT, and BT of the Ridley-Jopling classification. Multibacillary patients have positive skin smears and are classified as BB, BL, or LL. This grouping is used to define the World Health Organization (WHO) recommendations for type and duration of treatment.

Indeterminate Leprosy. In indeterminate leprosy (I) there are one or only a few hypopigmented, erythematous skin macules, the outer edges of which are not indurated. There is often some slight sensory loss, but the peripheral nerves are not thickened or tender. Histologically there is a scanty lymphocytic-histiocytic infiltration around the skin appendages, peripheral nerves, and blood vessels.

Lepromatous Leprosy. Lepromatous leprosy (LL) patients have multiple diffuse, doughy skin lesions with sensory nerve changes that occur late in the disease. These lesions produce a "leonine facies" and are associated with numerous acid-fast bacilli, macrophages, and histiocytes in tissue

---

*References 1, 3, 4, 12, 20, 27, 28, 44, 46, 47.

biopsy. The histologic findings are evidence of defective cell-mediated immunity in this form.

Borderline Leprosy. Borderline leprosy (BB) has characteristics of both tuberculoid and lepromatous forms of disease. Skin and peripheral nerve involvement are variable and show a variety of both forms clinically and histologically. BB is unstable and usually progresses towards the lepromatous end because of progressive loss of cell-mediated immunity. Occasionally it progresses towards the tuberculoid end as a result of increased cell-mediated immunity.

Reactional States

Acute reactional (inflammatory) states may cause deformities from nerve and soft tissue inflammation and destruction. The reactional states are reversal (type I lepra reactions) and erythema nodosum leprosum (ENL) (type II lepra reactions).

Type I Reaction. The reversal reaction represents a delayed hypersensitivity reaction and is directed towards bacillary antigens. The surrounding tissue is damaged as a result of the reaction. This reaction usually occurs in the borderline and unstable states of leprosy and usually after initiation of treatment; it rarely occurs without treatment. A reversal reaction usually arises from an abrupt increase in cell-mediated immunity, and there is a shift of the disease towards the tuberculoid end (called "upgrading reaction"). It is clinically characterized as fever, edema, hyperemia, infiltration of skin lesions, and severe peripheral neuritis. In borderline disease, it is responsible for loss of nerve function and deformity. A downgrading reaction indicates development of decreased immunity. In this form of reversal reaction, borderline leprosy drifts toward the lepromatous pole. It generally occurs in the absence of treatment.

Type II Reaction. Erythema nodosum leprosum is an immune-complex reaction. It occurs in lepromatous or borderline lepromatous patients as a result of immune complex deposition in skin. Erythema nodosum is characterized by painful erythematous nodules or plaques on the face, arms, and thighs. Fever, malaise, arthritis, orchitis, iridocyclitis, lymphadenopathy, and proteinuria may all occur. The reaction is triggered by a transient imbalance in the patient's immunoregulatory mechanisms. There is an increase in the CD4 : CD8 (T helper/suppressor) ratio resulting in release of bacillary antigens from macrophages, which sets the stage for antibody and antigen to combine, fix complement, and attract neutrophils.

The Lucio phenomenon, which occurs in a few lepromatous patients from Mexico and Central America, is probably a variant of erythema nodosum. It represents an acute allergic vasculitis from immune-complex formation and deposition within the vascular walls caused by release of antigens from infected endothelial cells. The Lucio phenomenon results in infarction of the overlying skin.[23]

Ocular Disease

In 1873 Hansen stated: "There is no disease which so frequently gives rise to disorders of the eye as leprosy does." Certainly the ocular adnexa and the anterior segment of the eye offer an ideal site for *M. leprae* to proliferate. The cooler temperatures, the presence of a rich neurovascular network, and the possibility of ocular immunologic compartmentalization may all be incriminated as contributing to ocular complications during leprosy.

Ocular Adnexa. Lateral thinning of the eyebrows and their subsequent total loss is a common manifestation of leprosy. Superciliary madarosis occurs most commonly in tuberculoid disease but may also be seen in lepromatous types. The thinning begins temporally in the cooler region of the brow and progresses nasally. Lash loss is also common and involves the lower eyelid first. The brow loss may be total and permanent.

Seventh cranial nerve paralysis results in lagophthalmos, lower eyelid ectropion, occasionally upper eyelid entropion, and poor lacrimal drainage (Fig. 102-1). All leprosy patients regardless of their clinical disease are at risk of developing lagophthalmos. Paucibacillary patients and those in a reversal reaction sometimes develop paralytic lagophthalmos early and suddenly. Multibacillary patients develop paresis later in the disease and often also develop anesthesia of the cornea and conjunctiva because of fifth cranial nerve involvement. The fifth and seventh cranial nerve involvement leads to exposure keratitis, dry eyes, dermalization of the conjunctiva and cornea, trichiasis, and susceptibility to trauma resulting in corneal scarring and blindness. (Endemic trachoma in a leprosy population compounds the clinical picture leading to upper eyelid entropion and trichiasis with severe corneal scarring.[38])

Eyelid nodules and placoid lesions may develop in paucibacillary disease, reversal reactions, and erythema nodosum leprosum. There is a positive relationship between type I reversal reaction, lesions on the face, and subsequent lagophthalmos, which may help identify those patients that are most at risk for developing corneal blindness from exposure keratitis.[14,18]

Acute and chronic dacryoadenitis, arising from cellular infiltration and inflammation of the lacrimal gland, may occur in lepromatous leprosy. In tuberculoid disease, denervation of the gland results in keratoconjunctivitis sicca.[13] Severe intranasal infiltration and mucous membrane scarring may lead to nasolacrimal duct obstruction and subsequent dacryocystitis in lepromatous leprosy patients.

Cornea. Exposure conjunctivitis and keratoconjunctivitis often occur in patients with longstanding disease. Corneal hypesthesia may be found in all forms of the disease and may lead to an inadequate blink reflex, which (coupled with lagophthalmos, ectropion, and dry eyes) results in a typical inferior exposure keratoconjunctivitis. This finding should serve as an early warning sign of inadequate protection and an increased risk for bacterial corneal infection.[17,21]

The cornea is susceptible to invasion through the corneal nerves and the surrounding vessels. Early in the disease process, *M. leprae* probably enters the cornea by way of the rich network of limbal ciliary nerves that run radially through the anterior two-thirds of the stroma terminating at the Bowman layer. Hematogenous spread to the cornea occurs later by way of the blood vessels of a corneal pannus.

Intraneural spread in the cornea and the resulting infiltrates are pathognomonic of leprosy and may be the first clinical findings of the disease. They appear as enlarged, edematous, sometimes beaded corneal nerves suggesting a string of pearls. The nerve changes represent transient recurrent granulomatous reactions that may regress spontaneously. Following treatment the lesions sometimes calcify and persist.

Avascular keratitis is characterized by the development of chalky white punctate subepithelial opacities that are first seen in the superior temporal corneal quadrants near the limbus. They are usually found in an asymptomatic, noninflamed eye. Histologically, the lesions represent miliary lepromas and consist of macrophages packed with *M. leprae.* The lesions gradually become confluent and less demarcated, causing the surrounding cornea to be hazy. Later there is destruction of the Bowman layer and superficial vascularization producing the classical lepromatous pannus.

Corneal lepromas appear as large white or yellowish nodules at the limbus (Fig. 102-2). They represent large granulomata and are relatively infrequent except in Japan and South America. They occasionally encroach on the visual axis.

Interstitial keratitis begins in the superior temporal quadrant and may represent a more severe form of avascular keratitis that progresses to necrosis and later vascular inva-

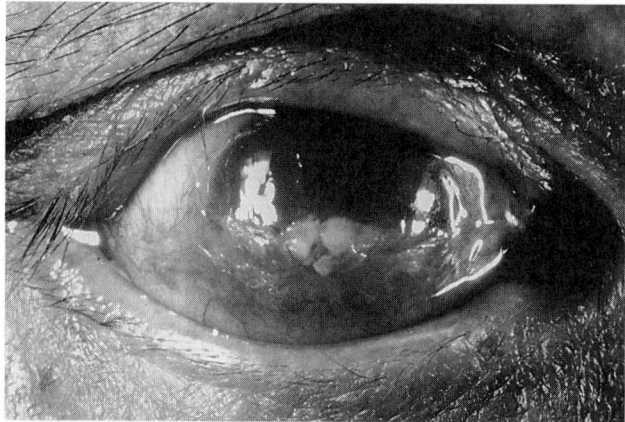

Fig. 102-1. Exposure keratopathy from facial nerve paresis with lagophthalmos caused by Hansen disease.

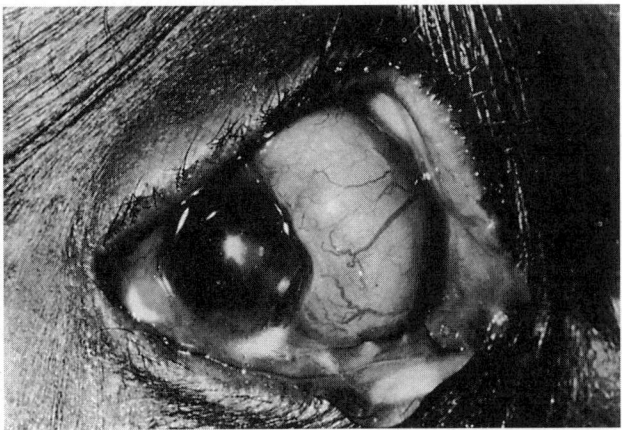

Fig. 102-2. Limbal leproma.

sion (Fig. 102-3). Sometimes it develops as a discoid lesion in the midstroma of the superior cornea without vessels. In the late stages it may progress to involve the visual axis resulting in visual loss.

Sclera. Episcleritis and scleritis occur from direct bacillary invasion or may be immune-mediated, resulting from immune-complex deposition during erythema nodosum reactions. Diffuse and nodular episcleritis is common and is usually found in the cooler interpalipebral fissure area. Scleritis is less common. It presents with excruciating pain and tenderness and is a threat to vision. If the inflammation is protracted or recurrent, it may cause scleral necrosis, ectasia, and a staphyloma.

Anterior Uvea. Because the anterior uvea is heavily pigmented and contains many blood vessels and nerves, it is often severely involved by *M. leprae* in multibacillary disease. Uveitis in leprosy is common and may threaten vision.

There are two distinct clinical forms of uveitis in leprosy patients. One form develops abruptly and is a fulminant granulomatous iridocyclitis that occurs in systemic ery-

thema nodosum reactions. It is often associated with posterior synechiae, peripheral anterior synechiae, increased intraocular pressure, and hypopyon.

The other form is a chronic, low-grade, insidious type of uveitis that may be seen in lepromatous leprosy. It is a major cause of blindness in leprosy and is characterized by minimal ciliary flush, a few anterior chamber cells, and mild to moderate flare. It often progresses to iris atrophy and causes pupillary miosis because of local sympathetic autonomic neuropathy. The small nonreactive pinpoint pupil occurs from early and extensive involvement of the dilator muscle of the iris with relative sparing of the sphincter muscle.[8] When associated with corneal or lens opacities, the pinpoint pupil results in marked reversible vision loss.

Iris pearls, appearing as chalky white particles in the superficial connective tissue of the iris, at the pupillary margin, or in the inferior chamber angle, sometimes are found early in the disease. They represent noninflammatory microlepromas and are pathognomonic for ocular leprosy (Fig. 102-4). Similar lesions have also been observed in the peripheral retina and are possibly carried there by the aqueous humor.[41] Secondary ocular changes arise from sensory, motor, and autonomic nerve involvement in all forms of leprosy. Late in the disease process, atrophy of soft tissues of the adnexa, atrophy of the dilator muscle for the iris, and atrophy of the ciliary body are found.

The ciliary body may represent the site of bacillary activity in early leprosy. Several signs suggest ciliary body dysfunction early in the disease. Premature presbyopia in lepromatous leprosy is common and is probably caused by a parasympathetic neuropathy affecting accommodation.[40]

Intraocular Pressure. Low intraocular pressures with a large fluctuation in pressure during postural changes has been observed early in the disease without other evidence of ocular involvement.[15,22,24] Decreased intraocular pressure can also be found in household contacts of leprosy patients

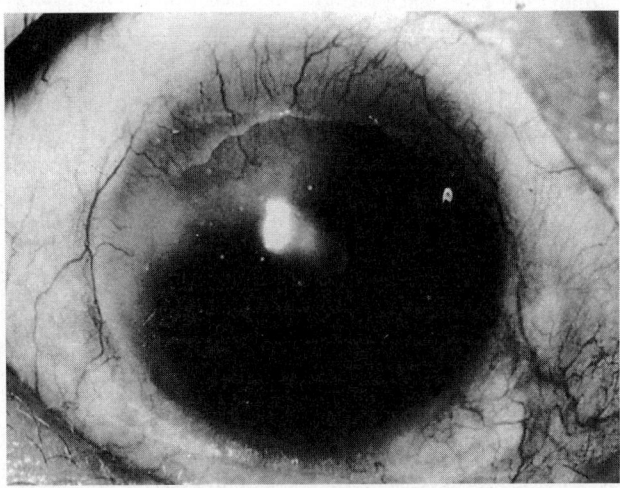

Fig. 102-3. Lepromatous corneal pannus.

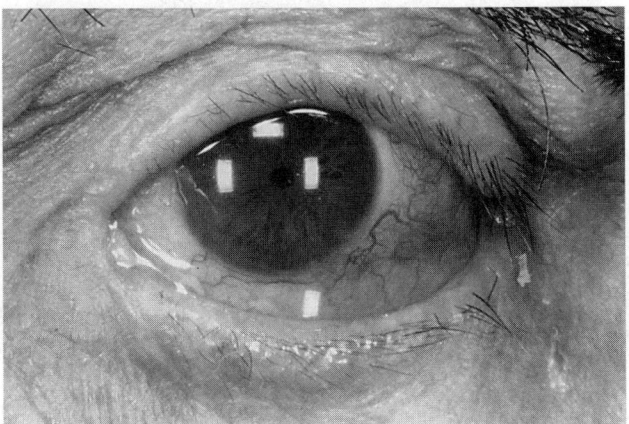

Fig. 102-4. Chronic iridocyclitis with iris pearls in a patient with Hansen disease.

compared to endemic controls.[16] All of these findings suggest early autonomic neuropathy in Hansen disease, although attempts to detect early anterior uveal involvement by measuring pupillary reactions to light and to pharmacologic agents has been equivocal.

Glaucoma and irreversible blindness may arise from anterior and/or posterior synechiae, insult to the aqueous outflow channels, and pupillary occlusion and/or seclusion with iris bombé formation. All patients with leprosy, therefore, should be periodically followed for glaucoma even after they are discharged from therapy.[45]

Lens. Cataracts develop earlier in life in leprosy patients as compared with others because of early ciliary body involvement, loss of intraocular pressure homeostasis, compromised aqueous humor physiology, and lingering uveitis. Cataracts are known to contribute substantially to blindness in leprosy patients. Unfortunately, because of the stigma attached to the disease, many patients are unable to obtain care for this reversible cause of blindness.[33]

PATHOLOGY

Specimens of ocular tissues submitted at postmortem or during intraocular surgical intervention have helped in understanding ocular lepromatous disease.* The primary ocular changes are caused from direct immunologic reactions to *M. leprae* and their antigens in lepromatous patients. In such cases histopathologic specimens show numerous organisms in the conjunctiva, cornea, iris, and ciliary body. These tissues are infiltrated by macrophages, lymphocytes, and plasma cells. Acid-fast bacilli are found inside macrophages, endothelial cells, nerve bundles, pigment epithelium, and smooth muscle cells. Miliary lepromas (macrophages laden with bacilli) are seen around corneal nerves and in iris pearls.

PATHOGENESIS

Limited knowledge of its biochemistry and metabolic processes has restricted attempts to cultivate *M. leprae* in vitro. The development of animal models has contributed greatly to study of the organism and the infection. The mouse footpad infection in normal mice, the development of a T-lymphocyte deficient mouse model, and the discovery of the natural susceptibility of the armadillo and the mangabey monkey have been most helpful.

Host Response

The varied and protracted clinical manifestations of leprosy arise from the immunologic responses of the host against the virtually nontoxic *M. leprae*. Glycolipids are important surface antigens of mycobacteria, and a phenolic glycolipid-I unique to *M. leprae* has been identified. It has

---

*References 2, 19, 25, 26, 34, 39, 43, 48.

an immunodominant trisaccharide segment and serves as a valuable chemical marker for *M. leprae* in infected tissue.

Most HLA studies have been equivocal, but the reported association of HLA-DR2 and tuberculoid leprosy is intriguing. This possibly suggests that the HLA complex determines the granulomatous response and thus the tendency to develop tuberculoid leprosy.[42]

Cell-Mediated Immunity. Following exposure to *M. leprae,* the host's immune response determines the infection's outcome. Cellular immunity is normally responsible for limited bacterial multiplication and is, therefore, essential for protective immunity and resistance against leprosy. Often the cell-mediated immunity indices and humoral immunity indices show an inverse relationship in leprosy. In tuberculoid leprosy there is strong cell-mediated immunity and little humoral immune response, whereas the reverse is true for lepromatous leprosy.

The mechanism of cellular immunodeficiency that allows for uncontrolled proliferation of *M. leprae* in lepromatous leprosy is poorly understood. Studies indicate that there is a decrease in the total number of T-lymphocytes in lepromatous lesions, and the ratio of CD4:CD8 (T helper/suppressor) cells is also low as compared to tuberculoid lesions.[30] Two distinct morphological patterns of lymphocyte distribution have also been identified in both tuberculoid and lepromatous granulomas. In lepromatous leprosy patients, there is profound and specific deficiency of cell-mediated immunity to *M. leprae,* which persists even after prolonged chemotherapy, suggesting that it may also be responsible for the high risk of relapse in these patients. Current evidence at the cellular level suggests that *M. leprae* is present in reactive T-lymphocytes of lepromatous leprosy patients. There is insufficient production and/or availability of interleukin-2 which results in failure of proliferative T-lymphocyte responses and macrophage activation upon exposure to *M. leprae.*

Several theories have been proposed for the development of leprosy. One theory proposes that leprosy patients have a hereditary cellular immunodeficiency that causes them to be unable to mount an effective resistance to infection.[11] The other theory suggests that at an early stage a few replicating organisms gain access to peripheral nerves where they are hidden from recognition by the immune surveillance system. Later, as they multiply, immune tolerance develops, producing a cellular immunodeficiency state. Lepromatous patients may be a heterogeneous group in which different mechanisms are responsible for the development of the specific defect of cellular immunodeficiency.

Humoral Immunity. The role of humoral immune reactions in patients with leprosy is not clear. All leprosy patients respond to antigen by antibody formation. The amount of antibody produced against *M. leprae* may be related to the bacillary load of the patient. Patients with lepromatous disease have hypergamma-globulinemia and an exaggerated antibody response to unrelated immugens such as *Candida albicans* and typhoid H antigen. The serologic profiles of leprosy patients reveal many autoantibodies such as antinuclear, antithyroid, and antisperm antibodies. Lupus cells, rheumatoid factor, and mixed cryoglobulins may also be present. A biologically false-positive test for syphilis is common in lepromatous disease caused by common antigens shared by *M. leprae* and *Treponema pallidum.*

DIFFERENTIAL DIAGNOSIS

Leprosy mimics many neurologic and dermotologic diseases. The presence of a chronic skin or neurologic disorder should raise the possibility of leprosy, especially when there are associated signs of depigmentation and hypesthesia.

Diseases that sometimes mimic leprosy are tinea versicolor, cutaneous mycoses, syphilis, yaws and pinta, tuberculosis, leishmaniasis, onchocerciasis, psoriasis, scleroderma, lichen planus, seborrheic dermatitis, pityriasis alba, sarcoidosis, systemic lupus erythematosus, granuloma annulare, necrobiosis lipoidica, mycosis fungoides, and some of the reticuloses.

LABORATORY INVESTIGATIONS

The diagnosis of leprosy requires a high index of suspicion of the disease. Diagnostic tools are limited, and all cases should be confirmed by histologic means (i.e., biopsy or slit-skin smears). With few exceptions, the clinical diagnosis of leprosy requires at least two of the following three cardinal signs of the disease:

1. Characteristic skin lesions
2. Sensory loss of individual skin lesions or an area of skin supplied by an involved peripheral nerve
3. Enlarged peripheral nerves at a susceptible site.

An adequate history together with examination of the skin in good light and a complete external eye examination are essential to establish the presence of ocular leprosy. Iris pearls and beaded corneal nerves are probably pathognomonic of the disease. Other ocular findings (madarosis, facial nerve palsy with lagophthalmos, recurrent episcleritis or scleritis, and uveitis) are highly suggestive of leprosy in patients with skin and nerve lesions who have lived in an endemic area of the world.

The fifth and seventh cranial nerve functions are established by observation of the frequency of spontaneous complete eyelid blinking, the position and function of the eyelids, tear function, and corneal sensation. The status of the cornea, the irides, pupils, lens opacities, and intraocular pressure must be documented. Patients found to have high risk factors and possible sight-threatening lesions should be given high priority for patient education and management of individual problems.

It is essential to classify leprosy patients properly into multibacillary or paucibacillary types for the correct drug regimen and successful therapy. Skin biopsies in such cases are helpful. In early lesions of indeterminant leprosy, acid-fast bacilli may be found only in a nerve bundle, the subepidermal zone, or arrector pili muscles. Leprosy may cause secondary amyloid deposition in the liver, spleen, kidneys, and adrenal glands in advanced disease.

The lepromin test, although not a diagnostic test for leprosy, is useful for classifying patients once the diagnosis is made. It was described by Mitsuda in 1919 and involves the intradermal injection of a standardized, autoclaved, emulsified preparation of lepromatous tissue. The Fernandez reaction from the lepromin test occurs after 24 to 48 hours, whereas the Mitsuda reaction occurs after 3 to 4 weeks. The reactions are similar to that of a tuberculin test: $0 =$ no reaction; $+/- =$ induration less than 3 mm; $1 + =$ nodular reaction of 3 to 5 mm; and $3 + =$ a nodular reaction of 10 or more mm or a reaction that leads to ulceration regardless of size. Patients with tuberculoid or borderline tuberculoid leprosy have a positive test; patients with lepromatous or borderline lepromatous leprosy have a negative test. Borderline leprosy cases have variable results. A positive Fernandez reaction indicates the amount of existing delayed hypersensitivity to *M. leprae*. A positive Mitsuda reaction indicates the ability for the patient to generate a cell-mediated immune response to the immunizing dose of *M. leprae* that is given with the injection.

THERAPY

Chaulomoogra oil and Promin (glucosulfone) were the first drugs that appeared to have some effect against leprosy. In the early 1940s dapsone was found to be effective and was then widely used for several decades, but prolonged treatment was often necessary, which resulted in noncompliance. In 1960 there was evidence of beginning emergence of secondary sulphone resistance. In 1977 primary dapsone resistance was documented. In 1982 the World Health Organization recommended multidrug therapy for all patients with leprosy to prevent drug resistance and to gain more rapid cures.

Primary drugs that are now used include dapsone, rifampin, clofazimine, and ethionamide (prothionamide). Secondary drugs are thiacetazone, thiambutosine, other long-acting sulphonamides, and some aminoglycosides.

Dapsone and other sulphones are competitive inhibitors with paraaminobenzoic acid for the enzyme dihydropteroate synthetase and thereby block the synthesis of dihydrofolic acid. Dapsone is readily absorbed when taken orally, has a half-life of 28 hours, and is bacteriostatic at doses of 100 mg or more daily. The drug is excreted in the bile and kidneys. Side effects include headaches, various skin rashes, gastrointestinal complaints, psychosis, fever, nephrotic syndrome, and the DDS syndrome (hemolytic anemia, agranulocytosis, hepatitis, peripheral neuropathies, methemoglobinemia, and hypoalbuminuria). No teratogenesis has been demonstrated even when the drug is administered during pregnancy.

Rifampin acts by inhibiting DNA-dependent RNA polymerases of microorganisms and therefore interferes with bacterial DNA synthesis. It is readily absorbed on an empty stomach when taken orally and has a half-life of about 3 hours. It is bactericidal for intracellular and extracellular organisms. Excretion occurs by way of the gastrointestinal tract. Side effects include anorexia, nausea, and vomiting, a flulike syndrome (chills, fever, headaches, and muscle and bone pain), thrombocytopenia, fatigue, drowsiness, headache, pruritis, various skin eruptions, and a reddish discoloration of all body fluids. Teratogenesis has been demonstrated in animals.

Clofazimine is a riminophenezine dye whose mode of action is unknown. It has some antiinflammatory activity and is useful both for treating the infection and for treating reactional states. It is lipophilic and therefore is deposited in fatty tissues and cells of the reticuloendothelial system. It is well-absorbed when taken orally and has a half-life of over 70 days. Side effects are limited primarily to gastrointestinal cramps, epigastric pain, diarrhea, nausea, vomiting, weight loss, decreased sweating and tearing, and a reddish-purple discoloration of exposed skin and mucous membranes including the conjunctiva, cornea, and lepromatous skin lesions.[10] The discoloration disappears some months after the drug is stopped. One serious side effect is that of partial or complete bowel obstruction that is dose-related.

Several multidrug regimens have been suggested. Current recommendations are dapsone and rifampin for paucibacillary cases and the addition of clofazimine for multibacillary cases.

Patients with paucibacillary disease should receive the following:

1. Dapsone (50 mg) daily (unsupervised) and
2. Rifampin (10 mg/kg or as much as 600 mg) monthly (supervised) for a minimum of 6 months. These patients should then be observed for a minimum of 3 years.

Patients with multibacillary disease should receive the following:

1. Dapsone (50 mg) daily (unsupervised)
2. Rifampin (10 mg/kg or as much as 600 mg) monthly (supervised) and
3. Clofazimine (1 to 4 mg/kg) daily (supervised at least once monthly) until slit-skin smears are negative.

Drugs that are useful for reactional states are analgesics (e.g., aspirin), corticosteroids, thalidomide, and clofazimine. For mild reactions consisting of pain, fever, and arthralgia, analgesics are helpful. For skin ulceration and neuritis, corticosteroids are given early and at a dosage sufficient to control the reaction. Antileprosy drugs should always be continued during the reactional state. Leprosy patients

TABLE 102-1 MANAGEMENT OF OCULAR COMPLICATIONS OF LEPROSY

• Madarosis	Island of neurovascular pedical graft from the scalp
• Upper eyelid entropion	Blepharoplasty with correction of lid inversion
• Lower eyelid ectropion	Tarsal strip (Kuhnt-Szymanowski) procedure
• Trichiasis	Cryoablation of abnormal eyelashes
• Dacryocystitis	Systemic antibiotics with dacryocystorhinostomy or dacryocystectomy
• Lagophthalmos with exposure*	Acute: Immediate treatment with prednisone, thalidomide, or clofazamine Chronic: Eyelid exercises using maximum effort with artificial lubricants Tarsorrhaphy or temporalis fasciomuscle transfer
• Limbal lepromas	Systemic antileprosy therapy
• Episcleritis and scleritis	Topical or systemic antiinflammatory agents
• Corneal hypesthesia	Patient education with regular surveillance Eye protection with sunglasses and lubricants
• Acute iridocyclitis	Treatment of systemic erythema nodosum if present Topical corticosteroids and mydriatic/cycloplegic agents Intraocular pressure monitoring
• Chronic iridocyclitis	Topical mydriatic agents Topical corticosteroids if anterior chamber reaction is severe Antileprosy therapy
• Cataract	Cataract extraction without or with intraocular lens implantation depending on the presence or absence of uveitis
• Glaucoma	Standard management for open-angle, angle-closure, or complicated glaucoma with synechia

* With loss of corneal sensation, symptoms of exposure keratitis are lost, and the patient must be educated to rely on signs of increased red eyes and decrease in vision. More follow-up examinations are warranted, and aggressive management of lagophthalmos should be instituted at this stage. Potentially sight-threatening lesions are lagophthalmos, corneal anesthesia, exposure keratopathy, hypotony, acute or chronic iritis, and scleritis.

should also be encouraged to avoid stress and have proper rest because physical and emotional stress can precipitate a reactive episode.

For type I lepra reactions corticosteroids are the treatment of choice. Prednisone (60 to 80 mg) is given daily for severe reactions. If improvement does not occur within 24 to 48 hours, the dosage is increased by 20 to 40 mg daily until a response is seen. Sometimes if the prednisone is given in divided doses, there is a better response. Prednisone should be continued until the skin changes, neuritic pain, and nerve function resolve. It is then tapered carefully and slowly to avoid recurrence of a reaction. The necessity to educate patients about the need to seek help with the first sign of reaction cannot be overemphasized. Clofazamine may also be useful in conjunction with prednisone, but its effectiveness is controversial.

The management of type II lepra reactions (erythema nodosum) is similar in many respects to that of type I reactions, although the reactions tend to be prolonged and may require many months of therapy. It is therefore advisable to use alternate-day therapy with prednisone or clofazimine. Clofazimine (300 mg) daily or every other day can sometimes be used alone if the patient can tolerate the dosage without marked gastrointestinal problems; later the dose can be lowered to 100 mg daily.

Thalidomide, if it can be used, is the drug of choice for erythema nodosum leprosum.[29] It must not be used in women of childbearing age because of its known teratogenicity; otherwise its only side effect is drowsiness, which can be avoided if the drug is given at bedtime. The initial dosage is 100 mg 3 to 4 times daily. Once symptoms are controlled, the drug can be tapered and discontinued after 4 to 6 weeks, then restarted as necessary for recurrent reactions.

The management of ocular complications in leprosy is summarized in Table 102-1. Early recognition of potentially sight-threatening lesions is essential and can prevent blindness.

PROGNOSIS

Most complications of leprosy occur from reactional states with resultant damage to major nerve trunks. All reactional states must be diagnosed early and treated effectively. Patients must be educated to the absolute need to be seen and treated when a reactional state occurs. Primary care workers and ophthalmologists must be aware of the potential sight-threatening lesions and methods of treatment so that patients can be identified and educated to seek care early.

Blinding complications of ocular leprosy usually occur from reversal reactions, erythema nodosum leprosum reactions, or proliferation of M. leprae with secondary tissue inflammation and atrophy. Reversal reactions may occur in borderline (BB) patients at any time during the disease but usually begin soon after treatment is started. The peripheral neuropathy often involves the facial nerve leading to motor and sensory loss with resulting lagophthalmos, exposure keratitis, and scarring of the lower half of the cornea. Trigeminal nerve involvement may also occur in reversal reactions. Sensory neuropathy with corneal anesthesia also occurs from involvement of the long ciliary nerves in scleritis and from invasion of nerve endings in lepromatous disease.

Erythema nodosum leprosum reactions occur in lepromatous forms of leprosy. In many instances they are local, involving the eye without causing systemic signs of ENL. Acute iritis, sclerouveitis, and scleritis may lead to acute blindness and must be treated promptly.

Patients with longstanding and poorly treated multibacillary disease often develop less immediate blindness as a result of keratoconjunctivitis sicca, the development of limbal lepromas, a chronic low-grade iridocyclitis, and cataract.

PREVENTION

A vaccine against M. leprae is being tested, and full development and testing will take at least 10 more years. The vaccine may induce immunity in noninfected patients and induce a high level of immunity in leprosy patients, thus reducing the number of patients developing the highly infectious multibacillary disease and reducing the possibility of relapses of patients who have already been treated.

Leprosy control programs need to be established for early detection, diagnosis, patient classification, and proper treatment in all areas of the world where leprosy is endemic. This process requires continuous training and retraining of medical and paramedical staff involved in the diagnosis and treatment of leprosy, the continuous care of leprosy patients, and an improved standard of living and improved hygiene.

Many blinding complications of Hansen disease are preventable. Potentially sight-threatening lesions must be identified and managed early. Also, ocular disease may occur during or after treatment, and therefore patients must be followed even after completing drug therapy.[9] Ocular disease is often diagnosed by anterior segment and ocular adnexal changes that can be seen on a screening eye examination. Leprosy can serve as a model where blinding complications can be prevented by patient education and medical teamwork.[5,6]

REFERENCES

1. Adala HS et al.: Ocular leprosy in Kenya, East Afr Med J 65:593-601, 1988.
2. Brandt F, Zhou HM: Severity of leprosy eye lesion in armadillos infected with Mycobacterium leprae, Lepr Rev 61:188-192, 1990.
3. Choyce DP: Diagnosis and management of ocular leprosy, Br J Ophthalmol 53:217-223, 1969.
4. Cochrane RG: Leprosy in Korea, Lepr Rev 27:19-28, 1956.
5. Courtright P, Johnson GJ: Prevention of blindness in leprosy, London, 1988, International Centre for Eye Health.
6. Courtright P et al.: Training for primary eye care in leprosy, Bull World Health Organ 68:347-351, 1990.
7. Duke-Elder S: System of ophthalmology, vol 8, 802-844, St Louis, 1965, Mosby.
8. ffytche TJ: Role of iris changes as a cause of blindness in lepromatous leprosy, Br J Ophthalmol 65:231-239, 1981.
9. ffytche TJ: Residual sight-threatening lesion in leprosy patients completing multidrug theraphy and sulphone monotheraphy, Lepr Rev 62:35-43, 1991.
10. Font R et al.: Polychromatic corneal and conjunctival crystals secondary to clofazimine therapy in a leper, Ophthalmology 96:311-315, 1989.

11. Godal T et al.: Evidence that the mechanism of immunological tolerance ('central failure') is operative in the lack of host resistance in lepromatous leprosy, *Scand J Immunol* 1:311-321, 1972.

12. Harrell JD: Ocular leprosy in the Canal Zone, *Int J Lepr* 45:56-60, 1977.

13. Hodges EJ et al.: Keratoconjunctivitis sicca in leprosy, *Lepr Rev* 58:413-417, 1987.

14. Hogeweg M et al.: The significance of facial patches and type I reaction for the development of facial nerve damage in leprosy: a retrospective study among 1226 paucibacillary leprosy patients, *Lepr Rev* 62:143-149, 1991.

15. Hussein N et al.: Low intraocular pressure and postural change in intraocular pressure in Hansen's disease, *Am J Ophthalmol* 108:80-84, 1989.

16. Hussein N et al.: Intraocular pressure decrease in household contacts of patients with Hansen's disease and endemic control subjects, *Am J Ophthalmol* 114:479-483, 1992.

17. Karacorlu MA et al.: Corneal sensitivity and correlations between decreased sensitivity and anterior segment pathology in ocular leprosy, *Br J Ophthalmol* 75:117-119, 1991.

18. Kiran KU et al.: Treatment of recent facial nerve damage with lagophthalmos, using a semistandardized steroid regimen, *Lepr Rev* 62:150-154, 1991.

19. Kirchheimer WF, Storrs EE: Attempts to establish the armadillo (*Dasypus novemcinctus* Linn.) as a model for the study of leprosy. I. Report of lepromatoid leprosy in an experimentally infected armadillo, *Int J Lepr* 39:693-702, 1971.

20. Lamba PA, Rohatgi J: Leprotic keratopathy in India, *Indian J Lepr* 62:186-192, 1990.

21. Lamba PA et al.: Factors influencing corneal involvement in leprosy, *Int J Lepr Other Mycobact Dis* 55:667-671, 1987.

22. Lamba PA et al.: Evidence of sub-clinical uveal involvement in leprosy, *Indian J Ophthalmol* 34:319-323, 1986.

23. Latapi F, Zamora AC: The 'spotted' leprosy of Lucio: an introduction to its clinical histological study, *Int J Lepr* 16:421-429, 1948.

24. Lewallen S et al.: Intraocular pressure and iris denervation of Hansen's disease, *Int J Lepr Other Mycobact Dis* 58:39-43, 1990.

25. Malaty R et al.: Histopathological changes in the eyes of mangabey monkeys with lepromatous leprosy, *Int J Lepr Other Mycobact Dis* 56:443-448, 1988.

26. Malaty R ct al.: Ocular leprosy in nine-banded armadillos following intrastromal inoculation, *Int J Lepr Other Mycobact Dis* 58:554-559, 1990.

27. Malla OK, Brandt F, Anten JGF: Ocular findings in leprosy patients in an institution in Nepal (Khokana), *Br J Ophthalmol* 65:226-230, 1981.

28. McLaren DS, Shaw MJ, Dulley KR: Eye disease in leprosy patients: a study in central Tanganyika, *Int J Lepr* 29:20-28, 1961.

29. Moncada B et al.: Thalidomide: effect on T cell subsets as a possible mechanism of action, *Int J Lepr Other Mycobact Dis* 53:201-205, 1985.

30. Ostler HB: The immunology of Hansen's disease, *Int Ophthalmol Clin* 25:117-131, 1985.

31. Ostler HB: Hansen's disease, *Int Ophthalmol Clin* 30(1):42-45, 1990.

32. Prabhakaran K: Oxidation of 3,4-diphydroxyphenylalanine (DOPA) by *Mycobacterium leprae, Int J Lepr* 35:42-51, 1967.

33. Rao VA et al.: Cataract extraction in leprosy patients, *Lepr Rev* 59:67-70, 1988.

34. Rees RJW: Enchanced susceptibility of thymectomised and irradiated mice to infection with *Mycobacterium leprae, Nature* 211:657-658, 1966.

35. Ridley DS, Jopling WH: A classification of leprosy for research purposes, *Lepr Rev* 33:119-128, 1962.

36. Ridley DS, Jopling WH: A classification of leprosy according to immunity: a five-group system, *Int J Lepr* 34:255-274, 1966.

37. Reference deleted in proofs.

38. Schwab IR et al.: Leprosy in a trachomatous population, *Arch Ophthalmol* 102:240-244, 1984.

39. Shepard CC: The experimental disease that follows the injection of human leprosy bacilli into footpads of mice, *J Exp Med* 112:445-454, 1960.

40. Slem G: Clinical studies of ocular leprosy, *Am J Ophthalmol* 77:431-434, 1971.

41. Somerset EJ, Sen NR: Leprotic lesions of the fundus oculi, *Br J Ophthalmol* 40:167-172, 1956.

42. Stoner GL et al.: Studies on the detection of cell-mediated immunity in lepromatous leprosy using HLA-D−identical siblings, *Scand J Immunol* 15:33-48, 1988.

43. Storrs EE: The nine-banded armadillo: a model for leprosy and other biomedical research, *Int J Lepr* 39:703-714, 1971.

44. Ticho U, Sira IB: Ocular leprosy in Malawi: clinical and therapeutic survey of 8325 leprosy patients, *Br J Ophthalmol* 54:107-112, 1970.

45. Walton RC et al.: Glaucoma in Hansen's disease, *Br J Ophthalmol* 75:270-272, 1991.

46. Wangspa S, Limpaphayom P: Ocular leprosy in Thailand, *Trans Asia Pacific Acad Ophthalmol* 5:153-161, 1976.

46a. Wayne LG, Kubica GP: Mycobacteriaceae. In Holt JG, editor: *Bergey's manual of systematic bacteriology,* vol 2, Baltimore, 1986, Williams and Wilkins.

47. Weerekoon L: Ocular leprosy in Ceylon, *Br J Ophthalmol* 53:457-464, 1969.

48. Zhou HM et al.: Unusual histological lesions in the eye of a leprosy patient, *Int J Lepr Other Mycobact Dis* 55:507-509, 1987.

103 Coccidioidomycosis

ROBERT Y. FOOS, KAMAL A. ZAKKA

Coccidioidomycosis is an infectious disease caused by the dimorphic fungus *Coccidioides immitis*. The disease is endemic in the southwestern and far western United States, in Mexico, and in several South American countries. It is prevalent in California's San Joaquin valley, where it is still known as *San Joaquin fever* or *valley fever*. Most patients experience a subclinical infection. Those that become symptomatic suffer from an acute self-limiting respiratory tract infection, from a chronic pulmonary infection, or occasionally from a chronic disseminated disease involving the skin, bones, and other viscera including the central nervous system.[14,25] Although the ocular adnexa may be affected as part of a disseminated infection, the eye *per se* is very rarely involved.[1,3,9,17,24]

HISTORICAL BACKGROUND

Historical information concerning coccidioidomycosis has been detailed in an excellent textbook by Stevens.[25] The condition was initially recognized (and misdiagnosed as mycosis fungoides caused by a protozoa) in 1892 in Argentina, but the bulk of the subsequent investigative work has been carried out in California and (more recently) in Arizona.[14,25]

Coccidioidal uveitis was reported initially in a clinical study by Levitt in 1948; the patient had a primary pulmonary infection and subsequently developed clinically detectable signs of inflammation of the retina and vitreous humor.[18] Since then there have been 15 cases of coccidioidal uveitis in which pathologic verification has been obtained; 12 have been published and 3 have been presented at annual meetings of ophthalmic pathology societies (Table 103-1).*

EPIDEMIOLOGY

Infection with *C. immitis* occurs sporadically and without regard for age, sex, or race within the endemic areas (lower Sonoran Desert life zone). The portal of entry is the respiratory tract and the infectious agent is an arthroconidia spread by dust, which in turn relates to climatic conditions and to wind activity. Limited exposure (one to a few arthroconidia and only a few hours) can lead to infection; even fomites (fruit, cotton, landfill) from the endemic area can cause disease in people living in nonendemic regions. Except for extremely unusual circumstances, contagion from man to man or from animal to man does not occur. Lifelong immunity (which is associated with skin test reactivity) virtually always follows infection. Rapid population growth, tourism, the AIDS epidemic, and unfavorable weather conditions have led to a significant rise in reported cases in recent years.[7]

Considerably less is known about the epidemiology of coccidioidal uveitis. A retrospective study by Rodenbiker and associates[24] in an endemic area suggests (1) intraocular lesions are associated with benign pulmonary disease as well as with more severe disseminated coccidioidomycosis, and (2) the prevalence of chorioretinal lesions is more common than isolated case reports suggest.

RISK FACTORS

The general population is susceptible to coccidioidomycosis, as the major risk factor is exposure to the arthroconidia of the mycelial phase of *C. immitis*. Exposure is in turn modified by such subfactors as climate and other conditions that favor pulmonary inoculation of organisms (vocation or avocation). Risk factors for severe pulmonary disease or extrapulmonary dissemination include ethnicity (greater in Filipinos, blacks, Hispanics, native Americans, Asians) and intercurrent disease (notably conditions that result in immunosuppression). Women who contract the disease when gravid, especially later in the pregnancy, are at a significantly greater risk to develop severe or disseminated disease. In contrast, the disease in nonpregnant adult white females is most likely to be complicated by erythema nodosum and least likely to undergo dissemination.[25]

---

*References 2, 4-6, 9, 15, 19, 20, 22, 26, 28.

TABLE 103-1 CASES OF COCCIDIOIDAL UVEITIS WITH HISTOPATHOLOGIC VERIFICATION

Case Number	Author Date	Chronic Pulmonary	Extrapulmonary	Uveitis, Anterior vs Posterior	Serology
1	Brown[5] 1958	+	+	A	+
2	Pettit[22] 1967	−	−	A	+
3	Boyden[4] 1970	−	+	P	not recorded
4	Olivaria*[20] 1971	−	+	P	+
5	Bell[2] 1972	+	not recorded	A	not recorded
6	Chandler[6] 1972	−	+	P	not recorded
7	Zakka[28] 1977	−	+	P	+
8	Cutler[9] 1978	+	−	A	+
9	Glasgow[15] 1987	−	+	P	+
10	Ellis† 1989	+	+	P	+
11	Fishman‡ 1990	−	−	P	−
12	Foos§ 1993	−	−	A	−
13	Stone[26] 1993	+	−	A	+
14	Moorthy[19] (case 2) 1995	+	−	A	not recorded
15	Moorthy[19] (case 3) 1995	−	−	A	+

* This case was published separately by Rainin and Little.[23]
† Presented at Hogan Society (Denver, CO, October 1989)
‡ Presented at Hogan Society (Palo Alto, CA, October 1990)
§ Presented at Verhoeff Society (Coral Gables, FL, April 1993) and published by Moorthy (case one).[19]

CLINICAL FEATURES

Systemic coccidioidomycosis becomes manifest clinically in one of four ways: (1) as an asymptomatic subclinical infection, (2) as an acute self-limited pulmonary "flulike" disease (primary pulmonary), (3) as a chronic pulmonary disease (persistent pulmonary), or (4) as a disseminated condition with involvement of the lung or (one to many) other organs.[14,25] Extrapulmonary lesions most commonly are found in the skin, joints, bones, or the meninges. Cutaneous complications of the disease are common and may be seen clinically as:

- Hypersensitivity reactions, including erythema multiforme and erythema nodosum
- Toxic reactions (erythema)
- Disseminated cutaneous infection
- Primary chancriform cutaneous lesions (very rare).

Ocular coccidioidomycosis usually involves the ocular adnexa, with the eyelids and conjunctiva (phlyctenular conjunctivitis) as the most common sites.[27] Coccidioidal uveitis is rare; it can occur in association with any of the four major systemic subsets, or in the absence of clinically detectable systemic disease (Figs. 103-1 and 103-2). The data illustrated in Table 103-1 for the 15 pathologically verified cases of uveitis can be summarized as follows: 8 of 15 involved only the anterior segment; 7 of 15 involved only the posterior segment (none significantly involved both the anterior and posterior segments); 8 of 14 had associated systemic, extrapulmonary, lesions; and 6 of 14 had no lesions (information regarding extrapulmonary lesions is not available for one reported case). Of the eight cases with anterior segment involvement, seven were isolated (there were no other detectable extrapulmonary lesions); five of the seven patients with isolated lesions had appropriate serologic examinations

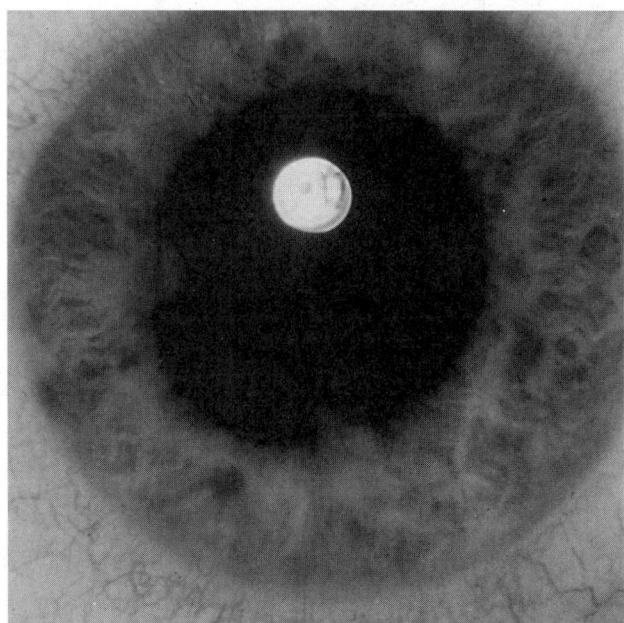

Fig. 103-1. Case 2, anterior uveitis (see Table 103-1). Clinical appearance of the anterior segment 3 months after the patient contracted "idiopathic" iritis (the patient had no other clinical stigmata nor laboratory evidence of coccidioidomycosis). The iris has gray translucent tiny nodules within its stroma, on its surface, and at the six and nine o'clock pupillary margin.

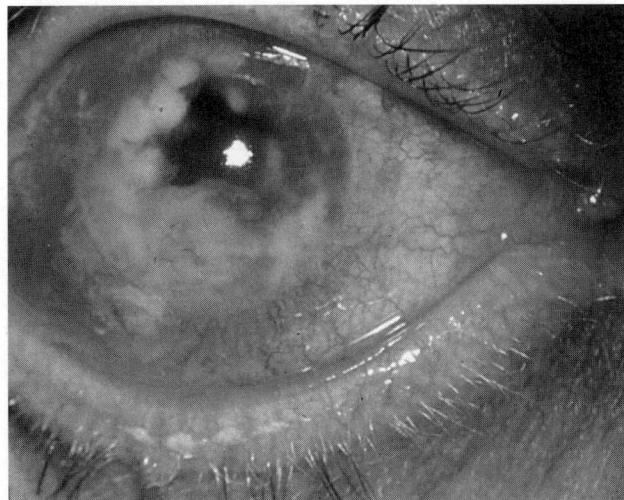

Fig. 103-2. Case 2, anterior uveitis. Clinical appearance of the anterior segment 8 months after onset of iritis. The anterior chamber is now virtually filled with a white nodular exudate that obscures the iris and most of the pupil. A white plaque is noted at the seven o'clock limbus. The conjunctiva is hyperemic and there is a prominent ciliary flush.

for coccidioidomycosis; and one of the four was serologically negative. These data emphasize the following points:

1. Although coccidioidal uveitis is rare (even in endemic areas) this diagnosis must always be considered when confronted with a case of idiopathic uveitis.
2. Systemic lesions may not be present in cases of coccidioidal uveitis to support ophthalmologic observations, especially with anterior segment infections.
3. Serologic evidence of coccidioidal infection also may be lacking, even in the presence of active localized disease.

Culture evidence of infection can be delayed, and biopsy of intraocular lesions can be the most efficient method of making a diagnosis of coccidioidal endophthalmitis, which in turn facilitates earlier treatment.

PATHOLOGY

The tissue reaction to *C. immitis* is typical of most fungal infections; the initial response is acute inflammation (often suppurative), which is usually followed by granulomatous lesions (occasionally including caseous necrosis). The gross appearance of lesions is not distinctive. The diagnosis, however, can be established with the microscopic identification of typical endosporulating spherules in wet-mount preparations, fine needle aspirations, or in tissue sections. Routine hematoxylin and eosin stains demonstrate most spherules readily; Grocott methenamine silver stain or periodic acid-Schiff preparations can also be useful (notably in the identi-

fication of isolated immature endospores) (Fig. 103-3). Granulomatous inflammation is usually diffuse, but can be tuberculoid. Late stages are characterized by fibrosis and occasionally by mineralization.

The pathologic features of coccidioidal uveitis are in concert with those described for systemic lesions. By the time pathologic assistance is obtained, a mixed picture of acute suppurative, nonspecific chronic, and granulomatous inflammation is usually evident. As mentioned in the Clinical Features section, intraocular disease occurs as either an anterior (Figs. 103-3 and 103-4) or a posterior uveitis (Figs. 103-5, 103-6, 103-7); a case in which both the anterior and posterior segments were extensively involved has not been reported. Lesions of the posterior segment are discrete, in-

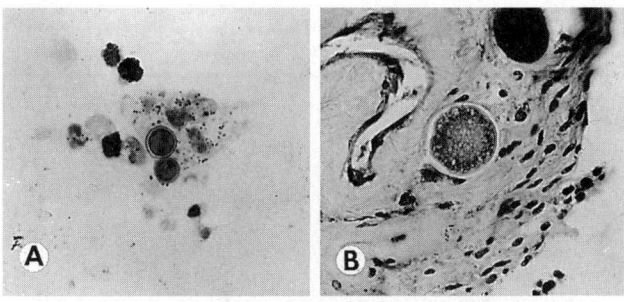

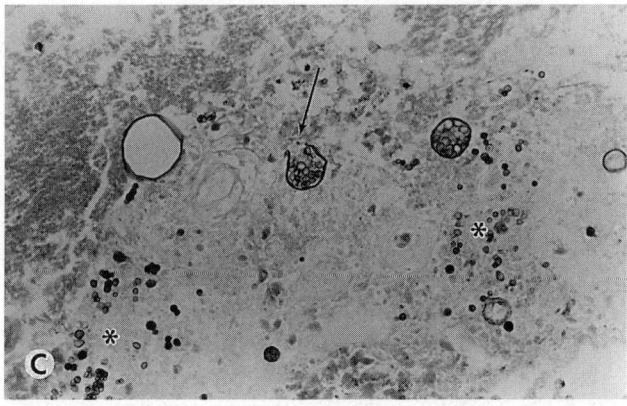

Fig. 103-3. Case 12, anterior uveitis (see Table 103-1). **A,** Washings from an anterior chamber tap show a clump of pigmented debris containing three immature coccidioidal spherules (only the centermost spherule is in sharp focus). (Papanicolaou stain, × 540.) **B,** Biopsy of iris (performed immediately after the anterior chamber tap) showing a mature spherule centrally and a few chronic inflammatory cells along the right-hand margin. (Hematoxylin-eosin, × 540.) **C,** Washings from the vitrectomy/lensectomy procedure performed the day following the anterior chamber tap and iris biopsy. Silver-stained microsection of the paraffin-embedded centrifuged specimen shows all stages of the endospore-spherule cycle of *C. immitis* in animal tissue. The size of the immature endospores *(asterisks)* overlaps that of other fungi (notably *Cryptococcus* sp. and *Histoplasma* sp.). *Arrow* indicates a mature spherule spewing out immature endospores through a point rupture of its wall; spherule on the right contains endospores; the one on the left is empty. (Grocott methenamine silver, × 540.)

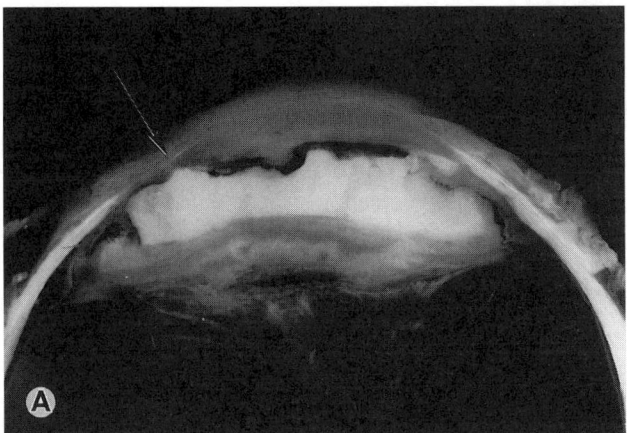

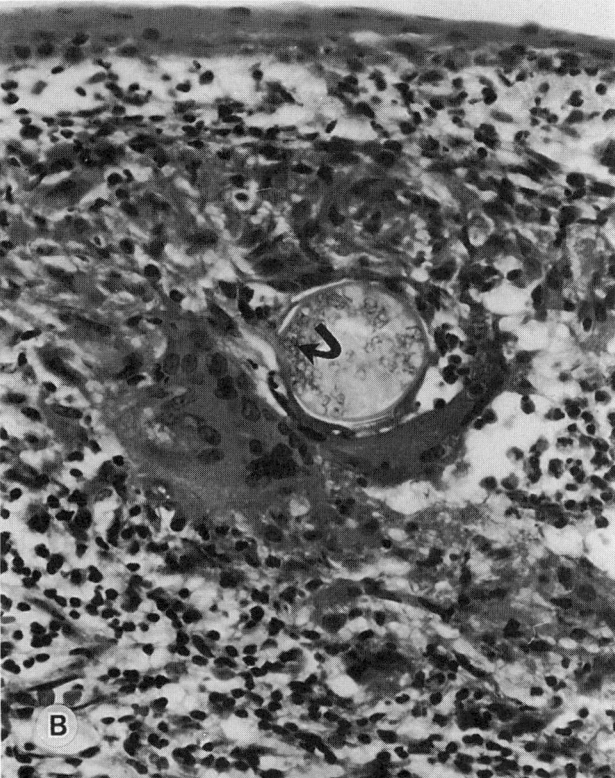

Fig. 103-4. Case 12, anterior uveitis. **A,** Gross appearance of the cut surface of the anterior segment of the enucleated left eye. The anterior and posterior chambers are filled with white semi-solid exudate, which streams into the anterior vitreous humor. At the nasal limbus (the entry site of a prior anterior chamber tap) the inflammatory exudate burrows into the overlying conjunctival stroma *(arrow).* ×5.2 **B,** Subepithelial inflammatory mass at the nasal limbus. There is a mixture of acute *(right of center),* chronic *(left lower corner),* and granulomatous *(center)* inflammation; the latter shows a large multinucleate giant cell containing a mature coccidioidal spherule, which has begun to release its endospores through a point rupture in its wall *(arrow).* (Hematoxylin-eosin, ×540.)

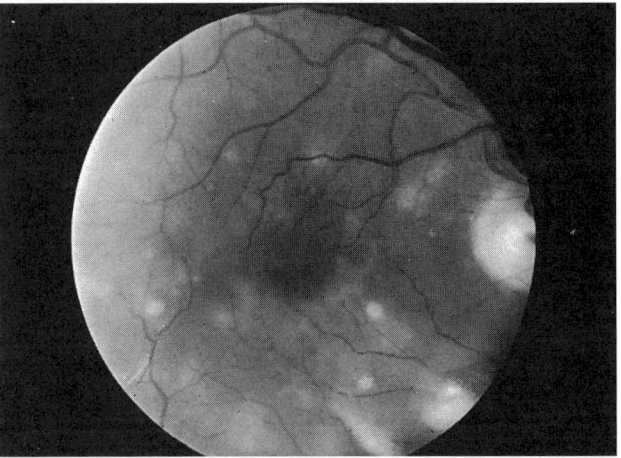

Fig. 103-5. Case 4, posterior uveitis (see Table 103-1). Clinical appearance of the macular region of the right eye (3 months after onset of what became widely disseminated coccidioidomycosis) showing scattered white focal lesions deep to the retina. Photograph courtesy of Dr. E.A. Rainin.

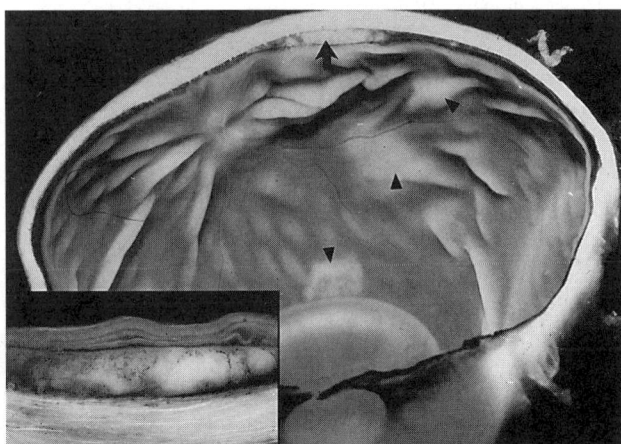

Fig. 103-6. Case 7, posterior uveitis (see Table 103-1). Gross appearance of large patchy choroidal lesions *(arrowheads)* in the large calotte of the left eye in a patient who died of disseminated coccidioidomycosis. *Arrow* shows a choroidal lesion on the cut surface. ×6.7 Inset illustrates the choroidal inflammatory lesion at higher magnification; the choroid is thickened (×2) with a nodular whitish mass. The overlying retina shows only slight edema of the outer plexiform layer (×26).

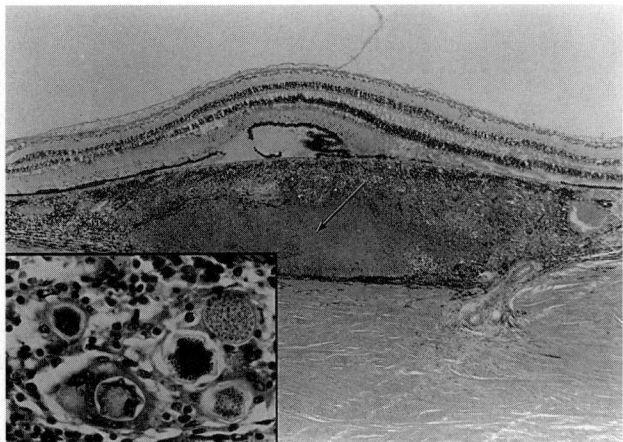

Fig. 103-7. Case 7, posterior uveitis. Microscopic appearance of the submacular choroidal inflammatory mass. Main figure shows caseous necrosis centrally *(arrow),* surrounded by a zone of granulomatous inflammation and chronic inflammation. There is serous detachment of both the pigment epithelium and the retina overlying the inflammation; the retinal inner limiting lamina is artefactually detached. (Hematoxylin-eosin, × 63.) Inset illustrates a cluster of mature and maturing spherules; two are enclosed within multinucleate giant cells. (Hematoxylin-eosin, × 540.)

volving either the choroid (or the retina) and sparing the adjacent retina (or choroid) respectively.[15,28] Additionally, discrete lesions of the posterior retina tend to spare the inlaying vitreous humor, representing a clear distinction from the lesions of *Candida* species that readily spread in a centripetal fashion (from the choroid to the retina and finally to the vitreous humor).[10]

COMPLICATIONS

As the bulk of patients are either asymptomatic or suffer only a mild self-limiting respiratory infection, complications of coccidioidomycosis are very uncommon. When seen, the spectrum of complications varies from persistent cavitary disease of the lung to death from untreated coccidioidal meningitis. This picture has been favorably influenced by the development of suitable drugs, such as amphotericin B and (more recently) the azole class of drugs, but therapeutic failures and rare late relapses continue.

The complications of coccidioidal uveitis follow a similar pattern. Clinically silent chorioretinal scars follow disseminated disease;[3,16,24] such residua are only vision-threatening when they occur in the macula (or more importantly in the fovea).[1,17] Similar scars would be expected to occur in the anterior segment, but this finding has not been reported to date. The pathologist usually sees the therapeutic failures: enucleated eyes in which both systemic and localized treatment has been unable to prevent progression of the disease or its vision-destructive sequelae. Surgically enucleated eyes are virtually always preceded by anterior uveitis, and autopsy enucleated specimens by posterior disease.

PATHOGENESIS

Within the milieu of body fluids and tissue, the inhaled arthroconidia (the end product of the saprobic phase) transform into round cells to initiate repeated endospore-spherule cycles in the body of the host (the parasitic phase). The host response at this stage is complement activation and the resulting acute inflammation (predominantly neutrophilic polymorphonuclear leukocytes). Neutrophils show no significant deterrence to the endospore-spherule cycle, which provides a repetitive stimulus for complement activation, suppuration, and progressive tissue destruction. In time this picture changes to chronic inflammation (and fibrosis), with the appearance of B-lymphocytes and their mature progeny, plasma cells. As the endospores mature into spherules, T-lymphocytes and histiocytes interact to produce a granulomatous response (usually diffuse or zonal, not tuberculoid). The antigen that stimulates the granulomatous inflammation is thought to be some substance in the wall of the spherule. *C. immitis* in tissue does not produce toxins, nor does it have a predilection for vessels that would lead to tissue infarction.[14]

The same microbial-immunologic mechanisms prevail in the ocular uveal tissue; the initial stimulus for coccidioidal uveitis is endospores disseminated through the bloodstream (as no lymphatics are present in the eye).

DIFFERENTIAL DIAGNOSIS

The acute self-limiting respiratory infection can mimic a wide variety of microbial diseases, and skin testing and/or seroconversion must be relied on to establish the diagnosis of coccidioidomycosis. The chronic pulmonary form of the disease can lead either to sharply circumscribed radiodense lesions that resemble carcinoma or to cavities that must be differentiated from those complicating tuberculosis. Disseminated coccidioidomycosis can also clinically imitate a wide spectrum of infectious or even neoplastic lesions. Immunosuppressed patients present additional problems, as they are subject to many opportunistic infections. Thus the diagnosis of disseminated lesions can test the skill of experts and requires a high index of suspicion, laboratory evidence (such as skin testing, serology, or the culture of exudates), or the recognition of the characteristic endosporulating sporangia in body fluids or tissue.

The clinical signs and symptoms of coccidioidal uveitis are equally nonspecific. Of four pathologically verified cases, the ocular lesions were either overlooked (in two cases[15,28]) or undiagnosed for an inordinate length of time (in the others[22]*). To confound the differential diagnosis further, two of the cases (both anterior segment lesions) were isolated; that is, there was no other evidence of extrapulmonary dissemination.[22]* On the basis of limited experience

---

*One case presented by Robert Y. Foos, MD at the Verhoeff Society (Coral Gables, FL, April 1993) and later published by Moorthy and associates.[19] (See case number 12 in Table 103-1.)

with posterior segment cases, it appears that *C. immitis* lesions are much less prone to extend to adjacent tissues (from the choroid to the adjacent retina or vice versa) than other fungal infections. Also unlike other fungal lesions (notably those caused by *Candida* species[10]), the infection rarely extends to the inlaying vitreous humor.

LABORATORY INVESTIGATIONS

Characterization and quantification of anticoccidioidal serum antibodies are the mainstay of the laboratory investigation of *C. immitis* infections. Antibodies to two antigens are measured: a tube precipitin-reacting seroprotein (TP, an IgM), and a complement fixing antibody (CF, an IgG). TP appears initially after an infection and disappears first. CF appears later and persists; CF titers occur in proportion to the extent of the disease (for example, positive readings in dilutions greater than sixteenfold are associated with extrapulmonary dissemination). Simplified tests (using immunodiffusion) for both TP and CF have been introduced (IDTP and IDCF). These tests serve only for qualitative evaluation; the traditional tests for anti-TP and anti-CF antibodies are still used for quantitative information. Rising titers indicate a worsening prognosis and falling titers show improvement. Cross-reactivity in histoplasmosis and cutaneous blastomycosis can occur.

A clinical coccidioidin skin test is also used; it becomes positive 1 week after infection and persists for life (although immunosuppressed patients may become negative). Again, cross-reactions may occur with histoplasmosis and blastomycosis.

THERAPY

Amphotericin B remains the drug of choice for the treatment of chronic pulmonary and disseminated coccidioidomycosis. This drug acts on the cell wall of the organism; the concentrations attainable in tissue are only fungistatic.[13] Amphotericin B must be delivered intravenously in very dilute solutions (typically 0.1 mg/mL). Also, because of its irritative effect on vessel walls and its systemic toxicity (notably nephritic and erythropoietic), the drug must be given slowly to tolerance (often with ameliorative adjunctive therapy), with careful monitoring over a protracted period of time. Apparently because of its molecular size, the drug penetrates poorly into body fluids, which is the rationale for intrathecal treatment of coccidioidal meningitis and intracameral therapy of iridocyclitis and endophthalmitis.

Because of the toxicity and limited efficacy of amphotericin B in many cases, other drugs have been used to treat coccidioidomycosis. The oral azoles (ketoconazole, fluconazole, and itraconazole) are reasonably well tolerated and have some efficacy when used in combination with—or following treatment with—amphotericin B.[8,11] Adjunctive immunotherapy, such as Lawrence transfer factor, appears beneficial in some patients (notably those with immunosuppression).[25]

Coccidioidal uveitis is usually treated in concert with the pulmonary or systemic lesions. When ocular infections are isolated or become vision threatening, however, more aggressive therapeutic strategies may become necessary; these strategies may include procedures such as intracameral injection of antifungal drugs in conjunction with vitrectomy and lensectomy procedures. A typical intracameral injection of amphotericin B (into either the anterior chamber or vitreous cavity) would consist of 0.1 mL containing 5 mcg of drug. Liposomal binding of amphotericin B has been shown experimentally to offer controlled slow release of the drug, and the introduction of this technique may prove useful in overcoming the local toxicity that accompanies intraocular injections.

PROGNOSIS

For most patients infected with *C. immitis* the prognosis is excellent, but for those with severe pulmonary lesions or with disseminated disease, it can often be guarded or poor. Patients at high risk for chronic progressive lesions must often undergo protracted treatment programs (sometimes for years or life) to control infections.

Patients with anterior uveitis have a uniformly poor prognosis; there are no reported cases in which useful vision was preserved following treatment. In contrast, the prognosis with lesions of the posterior segment is good, as shown by the number of patients (with or without treatment) who harbor asymptomatic chorioretinal scars following systemic coccidioidomycosis.[3,16,24]

PREVENTION

Except perhaps for those patients at high risk who reside in endemic areas, measures designed to protect individuals from infection with *C. immitis* are impractical. Although vaccination (using formaldehyde inactivated spherules) has shown some success in decreasing the severity of the disease in experimental animals, clinical studies thus far have been disappointing.[21] Until a safe and efficacious vaccine becomes available, prevention is mainly directed at controlling dust by various means (planting grass as a ground cover, wetting the soil, or oiling roads). Other methods for protecting high risk patients include avoiding endemic areas, wearing masks, and sleeping in air-conditioned houses. With the exception of obviously high-risk patients, there is no solid evidence that treatment of acute pulmonary infections with *C. immitis* prevents the development of chronic progressive pulmonary lesions or of disseminated disease.[14]

REFERENCES

1. Alexander PB, Coodley EL: Disseminated coccidioidomycosis with intraocular involvement, *Am J Ophthalmol* 64:283-289, 1967.
2. Bell R, Font RL: Granulomatous anterior uveitis caused by *Coccidioides immitis*, *Am J Ophthalmol* 74:93-98, 1972.
3. Blumenkranz MS, Stevens DA: Endogenous coccidioidal endophthalmitis, *Ophthalmology* 87:974-984, 1980.
4. Boyden BS, Yee DS: Bilateral coccidioidal choroiditis: a clinicopathological case report, *Trans Am Acad Ophthalmol Otolaryngol* 75:1006-1010, 1971.

5. Brown WC, Kellenberger RE, Hudson KE: Granulomatous uveitis, *Am J Ophthalmol* 45:102-104, 1958.

6. Chandler JW, Kalina RE, Milam DF: Coccidioidal choroiditis following renal transplantation, *Am J Ophthalmol* 74:1080-1085, 1972.

7. Coccidioidomycosis; United States 1991-1992, *MMWR* 42:21-24, 1993.

8. Como JA, Dismukes WE: Oral azole drugs as systemic antifungal therapy, *New Engl J Med* 330:263-272, 1994.

9. Cutler JE, Binder PS, Paul TO, Beamis JF: Metastatic coccidioidal endophthalmitis, *Arch Ophthalmol* 96:689-691, 1978.

10. Edwards JE, Foos RY, Montgomerie JZ, Guze LB: Ocular manifestations of candida septicemia: review of 76 cases of hematogenous Candida endophthalmitis, *Medicine* 53:47-75, 1974.

11. Evans TG, Mayer J, Cohen S et al.: Fluconazole failure in the treatment of invasive mycoses, *J Infect Dis* 164:1232-1235, 1991.

12. Reference deleted in proofs.

13. Foos RY, Zakka KA: Coccidioidomycosis. In Fraunfelder FT, Roy FH, editors: *Current ocular therapy,* 49, Philadelphia, 1980, WB Saunders.

14. Galgiani JN: Coccidioidomycosis, *West J Med* 159:153-171, 1993.

15. Glasgow BJ, Brown HH, Foos RY: Miliary retinitis in coccidioidomycosis, *Am J Ophthalmol* 104:24-27, 1987.

16. Green WR, Bennett JE: Coccidioidomycosis; report of a case with clinical evidence of ocular involvement, *Arch Ophthalmol* 77:337-340, 1967.

17. Lamer L, Paquin F, Lorange G et al.: Macular coccidioidomycosis, *Can J Ophthalmol* 17:121-123, 1982.

18. Levitt JM: Ocular manifestations in coccidioidomycosis, *Am J Ophthalmol* 31:1626-1628, 1948.

19. Moorthy RS, Rao NA, Sidikaro Y, Foos RY: Coccidioidal iridocyclitis, *Ophthalmol* 101:1923-1928, 1994.

20. Olivaria R, Fajardo LE: Ophthalmic coccidioidomycosis; case report and review, *Arch Pathol* 92:191-195, 1971.

21. Pappagianis D, Valley Fever Vaccine Study Group: Evaluation of the killed *Coccidioides immitis* spherule vaccine in humans, *Am Rev Respir Dis* 148:656-660, 1993.

22. Pettit TH, Learn RN, Foos RY: Intraocular coccidioidomycosis, *Arch Ophthalmol* 77:655-661, 1967.

23. Rainin EA, Little HL: Ocular coccidioidomycosis: a clinico-pathologic case report, *Trans Am Acad Ophthalmol Otolaryngol* 76:645-651, 1972.

24. Rodenbiker HT, Ganley JP, Galgiani JN, Axline SG: Prevalence of chorioretinal scars associated with coccidioidomycosis, *Arch Ophthalmol* 99:71-75, 1981.

25. Stevens DA, editor: *Coccidioidomycosis: a text,* New York, 1980, Plenum Medical.

26. Stone JL, Kalina RE: Ocular coccidioidomycosis, *Am J Ophthalmol* 116:249-250, 1993.

27. Wood TR: Ocular coccidioidomycosis: report of a case presenting as Parinauds oculoglandular syndrome, *Am J Ophthalmol* 64:587-590, 1967.

28. Zakka K, Foos RY, Brown WJ: Intraocular coccidioidomycosis, *Surv Ophthalmol* 22:313-321, 1978.

104 Syphilis

KIRK R. WILHELMUS, SHEILA A. LUKEHART

Syphilis is a systemic infection caused by the spirochete *Treponema pallidum,* and the eye is an important focal point. Ocular inflammatory and degenerative changes occur throughout the stages of acquired and congenital syphilis. Viewing syphilis from an ophthalmic perspective gives unique insights into this protean disease.

HISTORICAL BACKGROUND

The fear and folklore of syphilis has fascinated people over centuries. The history of syphilitic eye disease is interwoven with human behavior and public health.[194]

Pre-Columbian Era

The origin of human infection by *T. pallidum* is unknown. Writings from China more than four thousand years ago describe an ulcerative condition that "spread itself throughout the entire volume of blood" resulting in a skin rash and mouth ulcers for which mercury was used. In the New World, paleopathologic investigations have identified skeletal evidence of syphilitic-like disease in prehistoric animals and native humans of pre-Columbian North America.[4] These findings support the theory that a treponemal disease spread from ancient Asia to America and was endemic among the American Indians. The sailors and aboriginal captives who returned with Columbus and subsequent convoys to Spain and Italy may have then taken the "great pox" to Europe.[134]

Preantibiotic Era

Clinical descriptions by Venetian doctors serving at the 1495 battle of the mercenary army in Italy described soldiers with a pustular eruption, some of whom lost their eyesight. Within a few years the great pox had spread throughout Europe and then to the Far East. The pustular skin rash and the rapid development of periostitis and gummas suggest syphilis took a more virulent course during the Renaissance than is usually seen today. Treatment was prolonged and frequently ineffective, although cures were claimed using mercury.

Eye involvement was recognized as one of the many debilitating components of this apparently new disease. "Cold ophthalmia" was often linked to venereal disease. In 1575 Paré noted that syphilitics would sometimes ". . . lose an eye, and often both, or large portions of their eyelids, and even after they were cured the patients remained hideous to behold, on account of their scarred eyes. . . ."

Syphilis remained one of the presumed major causes of uveitis as the signs of intraocular inflammation were detailed in the early 19th century. The ocular complications of neurosyphilis, such as diplopia and visual loss, were first clearly recognized by Ricord in the mid-1800s. Monographs devoted to the ocular findings of venereal diseases[23,67,74,91,181] helped to distinguish the various manifestations of syphilitic eye disease. By the late 19th century at least one half of all cases of iritis, most cases of childhood stromal keratitis, and many forms of ophthalmoplegia were attributed to syphilis. Syphilis was so common that an ophthalmic specialist such as Hutchinson judged that he had seen nearly one million cases![110]

At the beginning of the 20th century syphilis was one of the leading causes of morbidity and mortality.[17] At the turn of the century 5% to 20% of the population of Europe and the United States had syphilis. Neurosyphilis accounted for one fifth of hospitalized mental patients and 10% to 15% of individuals in schools for the blind. It was considered a disease of "bad blood," and its medical and social importance led to the Oslo[28] and Tuskegee[145] studies on untreated syphilis.

Antibiotic Era

Despite its public-health significance, in 1900 the cause of syphilis was unknown; there was no diagnostic test; and no treatment other than mercury had been found. But the groundwork begun 20 years earlier when material was first inoculated into the anterior chamber of rabbit eyes led to the emergence of new knowledge. Between 1900 and 1910 Schaudinn and Hoffman identified *Treponema pallidum* as the cause of venereal syphilis, the Wassermann test was introduced for serologic diagnosis, and Ehrlich showed that arsphenamine was effective for the treatment of syphilis.

These major advances helped, but syphilis remained a major medical disease and an important social stigma. The various ocular manifestations of syphilis could be compiled and classified[75] but not effectively cured. Palliative treat-

TABLE 104-1 SYPHILIS AS A CAUSE OF UVEITIS

	Report Year (Author)	% Due to Syphilis
Prepenicillin era	1853 (von Arlt)	17%
	1905 (Campbell)	70%
	1910 (Igersheimer)	37%
	1911 (Butler)	22%
	1913 (Lang)	6%
	1914 (Goulden)	9%
	1921 (Clapp)	82%
	1923 (Irons)	6%
	1925 (Newton)	13%
	1925 (Elschnig)	20%
	1925 (Weiss)	55%
	1925 (Bruns)	70%
	1930 (Gilbert)	17%
	1931 (Gifford)	17%
	1932 (O'Leary)	6%
	1937 (Copps)	8%
	1941 (Guyton)	16%
	1944 (Woods)	17%
Penicillin era		
Adults	1954 (Woods)	7%
	1956 (Jacobs)	4%
	1958 (Schlaegel)	3%
	1960 (Woods)	2%
	1961 (Woods)	5%
	1961 (Perkins)	1%
	1964 (Lugossi)	0.5%
	1966 (Haut)	1%
	1975 (Saari)	0%
	1976 (Freedman)	1%
	1977 (Ayanru)	0%
	1977 (Cernea)	0.5%
	1980 (Schlaegel)	1%
	1980 (Friedman)	1%
	1988 (Noor Sunba)	5%
Children	1954 (Kimura)	1%
	1958 (Cross)	0%
	1961 (Witmer)	0%
	1964 (Cagianut)	5%
	1964 (Sachsenweger)	2%
	1966 (Bech)	0%
	1966 (Cupak)	0%
	1967 (Braun-Villon)	1%
	1968 (Witmer)	1%
	1969 (Schlaegel)	0%
	1976 (Sen)	1%

ment was sought, and Wagner von Jauregg was awarded the Nobel Prize in 1927 for his work on malariotherapy for neurosyphilis. But it was the demonstration of the efficacy of penicillin against early syphilis in 1943 that heralded renewed optimism about eradicating this disease. By 1954, as a result of widespread treatment and contact-tracing, the World Health Organization estimated that venereal syphilis had fallen to a recent worldwide low of 20 million cases.

In ophthalmology, cases of ocular syphilis were identified for treatment,[85] and animal models of syphilitic eye disease were pursued.[11] Many of the symptoms of syphilis, including its eye manifestations, were so similar to other disease processes that Osler called syphilis the "great imitator."[128] Because of this diagnostic uncertainty, several historic figures were reputed to have had syphilitic eye disease,[5,51] but sorting out who actually did so is difficult. For example, Joyce's chronic iritis was long suspected to be caused by congenital syphilis[58] but probably was not.[99] While in retrospect it may have been formerly overdiagnosed, syphilis as a cause of uveitis and other eye disorders has decreased markedly in the penicillin era (Table 104-1).

Yet syphilis persists and has recently increased in the United States (Fig. 104-1)[25] and throughout the world. The spectrum of syphilitic eye disease continues to expand as the acquired immunodeficiency syndrome (AIDS) affects the clinical picture. Continued advances in medical technology help in confirmation, but, unlike many other infectious diseases, diagnosis is largely based on clinical and serologic findings rather than culture isolation. Recommendations from the 16th century, formulated as the great pox was spreading throughout Europe, are still relevant: "You must gather all the signes in your minde, and comparing them together, attayne to that which is principall, and according to that humor dispose your cure."[1]

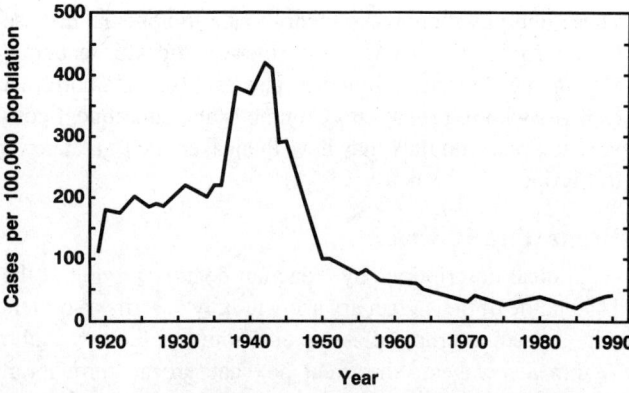

Fig. 104-1. Reported cases of syphilis of all stages by year, United States (Centers for Disease Control and Prevention). Because of poor reporting practices, prevalence of syphilis in early part of twentieth century may be much higher than illustrated. Current actual number of cases may be more than double reported data.

EPIDEMIOLOGY AND RISK FACTORS

The prevalence of syphilis varies widely around the world. Currently, early syphilis affects fewer than 50 people per 100,000 in the United States and western Europe but 200 to 500 cases per 100,000 in parts of Africa and Latin America.[14]

In the United States and other industrialized countries a marked reduction in primary and secondary syphilis was brought about by screening programs and the availability of antimicrobial therapy. An increased rate of reported syphilis in the United States during the late 1970s and early 1980s was linked to a disproportionate number of cases in homosexual and bisexual men. Since the mid-1980s heterosexual transmission, particularly in the medically underserved, has accounted for a further increase in acquired and congenital syphilis.[146] Poverty and illicit drug use, with the exchange of sex for money and drugs like crack cocaine, affect the epidemiology of syphilis and other sexually transmitted diseases. Syphilis is currently the third most frequently reported communicable disease in the United States. The year 2000 objective for the United States is 10 cases of primary or secondary syphilis per 100,000 population (Fig. 104-2).

A prospective ophthalmologic evaluation of large numbers of patients with syphilis has not been undertaken, but an important minority of patients with syphilis have ocular or neuroophthalmic manifestations. Of patients with untreated syphilis, approximately 5% develop uveitis[57,112,194] and 1% progress to optic atrophy.[28,145] Overall, 0.5% of patients with untreated late syphilis develop severe visual disability. Conversely, of patients with various eye diseases, serologic evidence of prior or current syphilis is common in urban centers.[170,175] Syphilis is identified as the cause of ocular disease in approximately 0.1% of patients evaluated in a general ophthalmology clinic[63] and in 2.5% of patients in a referral practice.[180]

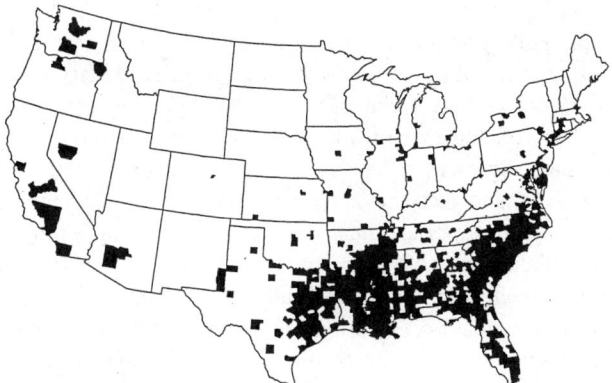

Fig. 104-2. U.S. counties with more than 10 cases of primary or secondary syphilis per 100,000 population (1991, Centers for Disease Control and Prevention).

SYSTEMIC DISEASE

Several mammals are susceptible to experimental spirochetal infections, but syphilis is spread naturally only between humans. Following exposure, syphilis can progress through a sequence of local and systemic manifestations (Fig. 104-3). In acquired syphilis the primary stage of a local skin lesion evolves to a secondary stage of bacteremia with disseminated mucocutaneous lesions and occasional involvement of the eye and central nervous system. A latent stage of subclinical infection is followed in approximately one third of untreated individuals by a tertiary stage with inflammatory and degenerative changes of multiple organs and the central nervous system. Following transplacental infection of the unborn child, congenital syphilis is similarly classified into early and late stages.

Acquired Syphilis

Syphilis is ordinarily contracted by sexual intercourse. Approximately one third of susceptible heterosexual contacts of an infected individual will acquire syphilis. An unusual means of transmission is direct contact with an infected mucocutaneous lesion. When syphilis was more common and syphilitic pharyngitis was treated by cauterization, physicians were liable to develop an eyelid or conjunctival chancre from contaminated sputum.[50] Similar methods of acquiring primary ocular syphilis have been suggested,[21] such as the bizarre epidemic caused by a syphilitic Russian charlatan who removed ocular foreign bodies with her tongue and thereby transmitted the infection.

Formerly transfusion of fresh, unscreened blood was a possible risk factor, but transplantation of tissues and organs and nonmedical tattooing[197] now pose very low risks. Syphilis has not been transmitted by corneal transplantation.[137] *T. pallidum* can probably not survive under the conditions of modern eye-bank storage, and eye banks exclude donors with active syphilis.

Primary Syphilis. The inoculum size and the host's immune status determine the severity and rate of development of the primary lesion. A chancre usually appears 2 to 6 weeks after exposure. This localized skin infection arises in parallel with dissemination of the treponemal organisms by the lymphatic system and bloodstream. A chancre is usually single, painless, nonsuppurative (unless secondarily infected), and hard. Extragenital chancres have occurred on diverse skin and mucous membrane sites. Regional lymphadenopathy is palpable as one or more slightly enlarged lymph nodes (formerly called buboes) that are painless and minimally indurated.

The chancre heals by a localized hypersensitivity-like reaction within 3 to 6 weeks but can persist longer in patients with an altered immune system. Bacterial clearance is thought to be mediated by infiltrating macrophages following development of opsonic antibody.

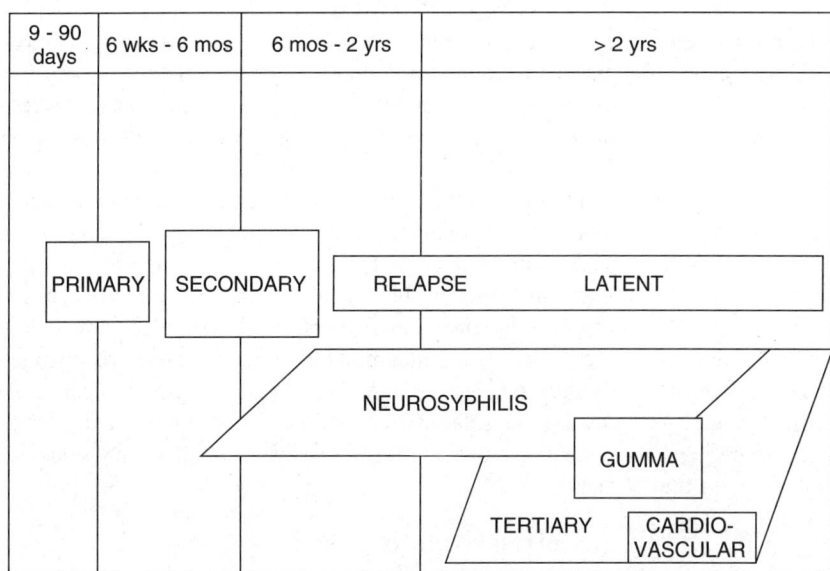

9 - 90 days	6 wks - 6 mos	6 mos - 2 yrs	> 2 yrs

Fig. 104-3. Natural course of syphilis is divided into several clinical stages.

Secondary Syphilis. Despite an effective local immune process, treponemes disseminate and multiply during the several weeks after the primary stage. Signs of secondary syphilis are identified in nearly all untreated patients and appear about 6 weeks after the appearance of the primary chancre, sometimes before the initial lesion has healed. Secondary syphilis typically begins with fever, malaise, headache, sore throat, arthralgia, and nontender generalized lymphadenopathy. Alopecia, liver abnormalities, and kidney involvement are infrequent.

The most commonly recognized clinical sign is a painless, maculopapular skin rash.[26] Usually beginning on the trunk and proximal extremities (Fig. 104-4), syphilids can appear over the entire body, frequently on the palms and soles. Papulosquamous, pustular, and nodular skin lesions resemble psoriasis or acne. Annular lesions may be seen on the face. HIV-infected patients may develop ulceronodular lesions (lues maligna). The skin rash disappears in about 3 weeks but can leave hyperpigmented or hypopigmented spots on the palms, soles, and neck along with brittle nails.

Enlarged or coalescent papules, called condylomata lata, may appear in moist areas such as the groin or perineum. Involvement of hair follicles may cause temporary, patchy (moth-eaten) loss of the head hair, including the eyelashes and eyebrows. Mucous patches are painless, shallow ulcerations of the oral cavity and genitourinary tract, most commonly affecting the buccal mucosa, tongue, tonsils, and urethra. Corresponding lesions of the eye are unusual but can present as papillary conjunctivitis, a conjunctival erosion, or a conjunctival or episcleral nodule.

Anterior uveitis is the most common eye finding of secondary syphilis. Symptomatic uveitis occurred in about 5% of syphilitic patients who went without treatment in the preantibiotic era,[57,114,199] and clinically silent uveitis was reportedly present in many more.[204] Anterior uveitis is still the most likely ocular manifestation of secondary syphilis[69] but is less frequent.[26] The pathogenesis of uveitis appears related to both infectious and immunogenic components. Spirochetemia can seed multiple organs such as the liver, and these invasive bacteria have been identified in aqueous humor aspirates by microscopy during intraocular inflammation in humans[9] and by isolation in experimental neurosyphilis in the rabbit.[104] Circulating immune complexes that occur during secondary syphilis may be involved in the pathogenesis of glomerulonephritis and possibly some forms of ocular inflammation such as uveitis and scleritis.

The central nervous system is affected in up to 40% of individuals during secondary syphilis as determined by cerebrospinal fluid analysis of patients with or without neuro-

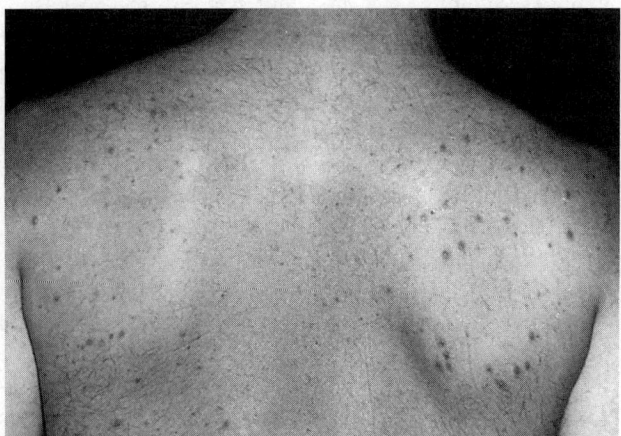

Fig. 104-4. Maculopapular skin rash of secondary syphilis in patient with chorioretinitis. (Reprinted courtesy of Gass JDM, Braunstein RA, Chenoweth RG: Acute syphilic posterior placoid chorioretinitis, *Ophthalmology* 97:1288-1297, 1990.)

logic signs.[98] Acute meningitis occurs in 1% to 2% of patients. Optic neuritis, optic perineuritis, or cranial nerve palsy may be the presenting feature of neurosyphilis.

With or without treatment, the signs of early syphilis gradually resolve. During the next two years, up to 25% of untreated patients develop a relapse of secondary syphilis, frequently presenting with mucous membrane lesions but sometimes only as ocular inflammation. Relapsing syphilis rarely recurs after 4 years unless reinfection intervenes.

Latent Syphilis. Latent syphilis has no overt clinical manifestations, although ocular stigmata of prior syphilitic eye disease (such as corneal ghost vessels or iris synechiae) may be present. The immune response is effective in clearing the billions of organisms present in the primary and secondary lesions and in maintaining the quiescence of the latent stage. While treponemal serologic tests are uniformly positive and cell-mediated immunity can be demonstrated during latent syphilis, infection may be quietly progressing.

The early latent syphilis stage includes the first year following infection, during the time that secondary relapses most likely occur. Relapsing secondary syphilis occurs in about 25% of untreated cases of early latent syphilis. The late latent syphilis stage is defined as the subsequent period that may persist indefinitely or evolve after many decades to the complications of late syphilis. Protective immunity develops in humans during the late latent stage, but reinfection is possible after treatment for early syphilis.

Tertiary Syphilis. In the preantibiotic era one third of persons with untreated syphilis developed a clinical sign of the obliterative endarteritis of late or tertiary syphilis: cardiovascular complications in 10%, gummatous disease in 15%, and neurosyphilis in 8% of all syphilitic people. Since the use of penicillin for early syphilis, the symptomatic manifestations of late syphilis are substantially less common.

Eye signs are noted in approximately 10% of patients with late syphilis, and ocular syphilis can be the sole presenting feature of late syphilis. Anterior uveitis is the most common ocular finding,[39] occurring in approximately 2.5% to 5% of patients with symptomatic late syphilis. Scleritis, retinal vasculitis, and other forms of ocular or periocular inflammation can occur, possibly as a result of granulomatous vasculitis. Gummas have been reported in the uveal tract, eyelid, lacrimal structures, orbit, optic nerve, and chiasm.

Cardiovascular syphilis is due to obliterative endarteritis of the vasa vasorum of the aorta that results in aortitis, aortic aneurysm, and aortic valvular insufficiency. A similar vasculitic process may lead to temporal arteritis.[171] Gummatous syphilis was formerly the most common late complication of syphilis but is now rarely seen. Gummas are necrotic, granulomatous-like lesions produced by focal obliterative endarteritis that can involve the skin, mucous membranes, bones, lungs, liver, and brain. Neurosyphilis is the most frequently recognized feature of late syphilis currently encountered.

Neurosyphilis. Neurosyphilis is commonly considered to be a late manifestation of syphilis, but treponemal invasion of the central nervous system frequently occurs within the initial weeks or months of infection. In many cases of early syphilis central nervous system involvement is asymptomatic, and most patients apparently clear their neurologic infection within two years. Subsequent progression to symptomatic neurosyphilis is uncommon unless no or inadequate therapy has been given or HIV infection coexists.

Symptomatic involvement of the central nervous system encompasses a spectrum of neurologic syndromes:[113] acute and chronic meningitis, gummatous neurosyphilis, meningovascular neurosyphilis with cerebrovascular occlusions, and parenchymatous neurosyphilis. Parenchymatous neurosyphilis encompasses a spectrum of symptoms: frontal lobe degeneration causes general paresis, degeneration of the posterior columns of the spinal cord produces tabes dorsalis, and chronic inflammation of the optic nerve sheaths leads to optic atrophy (Fig. 104-5). Neuroophthalmic signs, particularly pupillary abnormalities, may be a component of any form of neurosyphilis. Necrotizing, infective encephalitis ("quaternary neurosyphilis") and fatal infection ("malignant syphilis") have been described in case reports of immunocompromised states such as AIDS.

Meningitis. Syphilitic meningitis usually occurs within the first year after the onset of acquired syphilis, sometimes presenting during the skin rash of secondary syphilis. Persistent headaches in secondary syphilis probably represent meningeal involvement. Syphilitic meningitis may be acute, subacute, or chronic. Acute meningitis used to be an unusual occurrence but is now identified in some HIV-infected patients with syphilis. Approximately one third of patients with acute syphilitic meningitis have increased intracranial pressure with papilledema. Photophobia is a common feature of acute syphilitic meningitis, and optic neuritis may be the principal clinical finding of early neurosyphilis. Cranial nerve palsies (III, VI, VII, and VIII) are a complication of chronic basilar meningitis. Spinal cord involvement from meningomyelitis is a rare occurrence.

Meningovascular Neurosyphilis. Meningovascular neurosyphilis usually occurs approximately 5 years after infection[71] but may arise during early syphilis in immunocompromised patients. Small-vessel endarteritis may lead to vascular occlusion and cause a stroke syndrome or seizure disorder. The most common neuroophthalmologic manifestation of meningovascular syphilis is a visual field defect caused by occlusive vasculitis affecting the visual pathways of the central nervous system. Hemianopia or quadrantanopia can result from cerebral infarction in the distribution of the middle cerebral artery and is frequently associated with hemiplegia and seizures. Hemianopic visual field defects can also occur with occlusion of the posterior cerebral artery as part of the thalamic syndrome. Posterior inferior cerebellar artery occlusion results in the lateral medullary plate

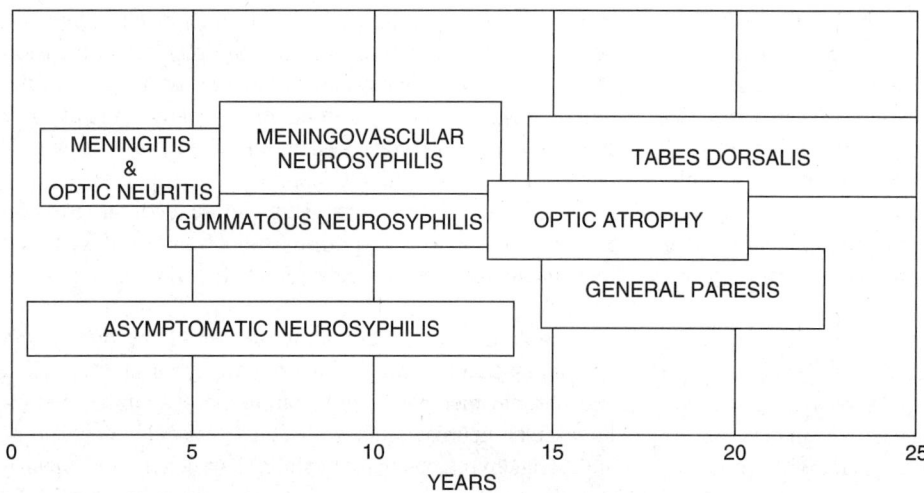

Fig. 104-5. Clinical forms of neurosyphilis. (Modified from Merritt HH, Adams RD, Solomon HC: *Neurosyphilis,* New York, 1946, Oxford University Press.)

syndrome with ipsilateral Horner syndrome and vestibular nystagmus. Internuclear ophthalmoplegia[62] and other brainstem syndromes may develop from obliterative endarteritis of the vertebrobasilar system. Occlusion of the retinal and optic nerve vasculature can also occur. While antimicrobial therapy curbs the progression of meningovascular inflammation, residual sequelae from ischemic damage often persist.

Parenchymatous Neurosyphilis. Parenchymatous neurosyphilis occurs years after infection as the result of postinflammatory neuronal degeneration. Atrophy of the cerebral cortex, posterior columns, optic nerves, and periaqueductal tissue produces neuropsychiatric changes (general paresis), tabes dorsalis, optic atrophy, and pupillary abnormalities, respectively.

General paresis causes memory loss, personality changes with depression or delusions, and seizures. Neurologic findings include sluggishly reacting pupils that later show light-near dissociation and become miotic. Other features of advanced general paresis are a lack of facial expression, tremors of the tongue or facial muscles, and slurred speech. Neuroimaging may show cortical atrophy and multiple small areas resembling infarctions or demyelinating disease. Cortical blindness has been reported as a complication of untreated late syphilis. Progressive disease results in schizophrenia, dementia, and paralysis.

Tabes dorsalis is a late neurosyphilitic syndrome with dysfunction of the dorsal roots and posterior columns of the spinal cord. Symptoms and signs include lightning pains of the legs, acute abdominal pain, diminished deep tendon reflexes, sensory ataxia, and autonomic dysfunction with poor bladder control and impotence. Progressive loss of sensation leads to Charcot joints.

Optic atrophy may accompany other features of parenchymatous degeneration but is often the only obvious clinical sign of late neurosyphilis. Cranial nerve palsies and pupillary changes can occur.

The pathogenesis of the Argyll Robertson pupil is uncertain but is probably due to degeneration in the rostral midbrain (Fig. 104-6). Complete interruption of the internuncial neurons between the pretectal nuclei and the parasympathetic Edinger-Westphal nuclei results in an absent light reaction with a normal near response. Miosis is probably due to interruption of the supranuclear inhibitory neurons from the reticular activating system. Neurologic pupillary changes must be distinguished from iris atrophy and synechiae brought about by syphilitic uveitis.

Congenital Syphilis

Transplacental transmission of *T. pallidum* may occur throughout pregnancy, but harm to the developing child occurs principally after the fourth month when the fetal immune system is developed. Fetal infection is very likely if the mother has early syphilis during pregnancy but also occurs in about one third of infants whose mothers have latent syphilis. Maternal serologic screening is required during pregnancy throughout the United States. Testing should target high-risk mothers during their first and third trimesters and at delivery. Transmission by the infected birth canal during delivery is unusual but has caused chancres on the baby's skin (including the eyelids) that appear soon after

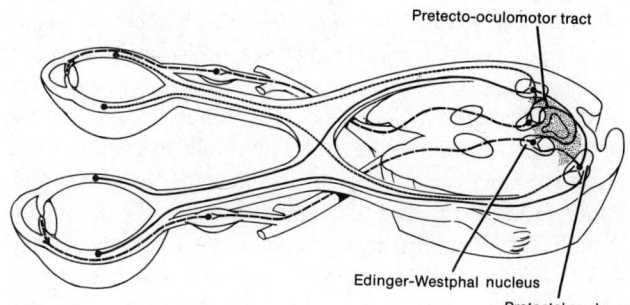

Fig. 104-6. Neuroanatomy of pathways involved in the Argyll Robertson pupil.

birth.[119] Nearly one half of infected fetuses die before or soon after birth; some have developmental ocular abnormalities such as microphthalmia.

Congenital syphilis can be divided into early and late stages that roughly correspond to the secondary and tertiary stages of acquired syphilis. Early congenital syphilis presents before 2 years of age, and late congenital syphilis occurs thereafter.

Early Congenital Syphilis. Early congenital syphilis presents mainly as mucocutaneous lesions and osteochondritis (Table 104-2) that appear about 3 weeks after birth. The maculopapular skin rash usually involves the buttocks, thighs, palms, and soles. Widespread dissemination results in hepatosplenomegaly, anemia, thrombocytopenia, pneumonia, and immune-complex glomerulonephritis. Infectious foci can lead to the residual stigmata of congenital syphilis. For example, condyloma lata along the supraorbital ridges and around the mouth can produce radial fissures (rhagades).

TABLE 104-2   CLINICAL FINDINGS OF CONGENITAL SYPHILIS*

Early Congenital Syphilis	Incidence
Osteochondritis, epiphysitis, periostitis	30-90%
Snuffles	30-90%
Hepatomegaly and/or jaundice	30-90%
Generalized lymphadenopathy	30-50%
Low birth weight or failure to thrive	20%
Mucocutaneous lesions, especially buttocks and thighs	15-60%
Pneumonia	15%
Splenomegaly	10-15%
Anemia and/or thrombocytopenia	10-15%
Pancreatitis	5-10%
Meningoencephalitis	5-60%
Nephrosis	1-5%
Testicular mass	1%
Chorioretinitis and/or iridocyclitis	1%

Late Congenital Syphilis	Incidence
Frontal bossing	70-90%
Short maxillae	70-90%
High palatal arch	70-90%
Hutchinson triad	75%
Notched incisors	60-70%
Stromal keratitis or scarring	5-10%
Deafness	1-5%
Saddle nose	60-75%
Mulberry molars	60-75%
Clavicular sclerosis	30-50%
Prognathous chin	20-30%
Rhagades	1-5%
Scaphoid scapulae	1%

* Compiled from multiple references.

Rhinitis (snuffles) with osteitis of the nasal bones can lead to the saddle-nose deformity and hypertelorism. Periostitis can involve multiple long bones[140] and produce rheumatologic changes such as swelling of the sternoclavicular joint (Higouménaki sign).

Ocular lesions of early congenital syphilis are analogous to those found in acquired secondary syphilis. Mucous patches can appear on the conjunctiva. Uveitis, particularly chorioretinitis, is the principal ocular complication of early congenital syphilis, occurring in approximately 5% of untreated cases. Iridocyclitis can result in secondary cataract or glaucoma. Multifocal chorioretinitis and, less commonly, retinal vasculitis that occur during infancy can be subclinical and can result in a "salt-and-pepper" pattern of pigmentary mottling. Optic neuritis and interstitial keratitis have been reported in early congenital syphilis but usually arise later. Treponemes have been seen by darkfield and fluorescent microscopy from aqueous humor aspirates,[157,166] in the choroid and retina,[122] and in the inflamed corneal stroma of neonates with early congenital syphilis.

Without treatment a latent period ensues. As a result of osteochondritis and perichondritis, bony structural changes arise. The stigmata of congenital syphilis include frontal bossing, supraorbital thickening, sloping skull, short maxilla, arched palate, prominent mandible, sternoclavicular thickening, flared scapula, and sabre shin. Dental abnormalities of the permanent teeth include peg-shaped upper central incisors (Hutchinson teeth) and defective first molars (mulberry or Moon molars). Permanent bony and dental stigmata may be the principal clinical clues of congenital syphilis.[46]

Late Congenital Syphilis. Nonulcerative stromal keratitis is the most common inflammatory sign of untreated late congenital syphilis, appearing in 20% to 50% of cases, more commonly in girls than boys. Maternal therapy before the second trimester or treatment of the infant before the age of 3 months can prevent corneal involvement.[133] After the onset of syphilitic interstitial keratitis, systemic or topical penicillin administration alone has no direct beneficial effect on its course.

Usually occurring between the ages of 5 to 20 years, the pathogenesis of interstitial keratitis is unclear. Experimental stromal keratitis has not been adequately reproduced by intracorneal injection, although corneal edema with iritis has been noted following intracameral or intracranial inoculation.[166] One postulated mechanism is that keratitis results from an immunologic reaction to treponemal antigens deposited in the cornea, although treponemal invasion of clinically normal cornea has not been adequately documented. Because the cornea contains multiple phospholipids, including cardiolipin and phosphatidylcholine,[152] a cross-reacting autoimmune phenomenon is another possible explanation.

Other signs of late congenital syphilis include bilateral knee effusions (Clutton joints) and deafness. Hearing loss in late congenital syphilis is usually stepwise, affecting the high tones first, and tends to begin in one ear before the other. Other symptoms of otosyphilis are vertigo and, rarely, oscillopsia.[106] Electrocochleography of syphilitic labyrinthitis resembles Ménière disease.

Unlike acquired syphilis, cardiovascular complications are very unusual in late congenital syphilis. Similarly, gummatous syphilis is not a common feature of congenital syphilis, although gummas of the nasal septum, palate, and throat have rarely occurred.

The eye and brain manifestations of late congenital neurosyphilis are diverse but infrequent. One fourth of untreated children with congenital syphilis have asymptomatic central nervous system infection that resolves without sequelae. Of the 1% to 3% of untreated cases that develop late-onset anterior uveitis, neurosyphilis should be suspected. Optic neuritis, optic atrophy, cranial nerve palsies, and pupillary abnormalities indicate symptomatic neurosyphilis. Hydrocephalus and other neurologic consequences were once relatively common, but lifelong central nervous system dysfunction following congenital syphilis is now rare.

Syphilis and HIV Infection

Individuals infected with the human immunodeficiency virus (HIV-1) are likely to have serologic evidence of prior syphilis.[102] Risk factors of these two sexually transmitted diseases are similar, and syphilis might increase the risk of transmitting or acquiring HIV from a genital chancre.

HIV infection alters the natural history of syphilis.[70,117,118] HIV-infected patients with syphilis have higher numbers of treponemal bacteria and a higher incidence of disseminated lesions and relapses. Early neurosyphilis and syphilitic eye disease are not unique to people with AIDS, but these complications occur more frequently with HIV infection.[81] Approximately 1% of people with HIV infection have syphilis. Many are latent, but syphilitic uveitis has been diagnosed in up to 0.5% of a series of HIV-infected patients. About 3% of those coinfected with both HIV and *T. pallidum* have symptomatic neurosyphilis that usually presents with a cranial nerve palsy.

Current serologic tests are generally adequate for diagnosing syphilis and for determining efficacy of treatment, but atypical values are sometimes encountered. In some patients with syphilis and early HIV infection, nontreponemal tests may be positive at titers higher than usually expected, and after penicillin therapy a high titer may decline more slowly than usual. Rare instances of impaired antibody production to cardiolipin or treponemal antigens have been reported in established HIV infection, usually in patients with a low CD4 T-lymphocyte level. Seronegative syphilis is an unusual diagnostic dilemma except in patients with advanced immune dysfunction.[59,117]

Posterior uveitis,* retinitis,[79,111,177] optic neuritis,[24,111,202]

---

*References 7, 8, 16, 73, 86, 93, 130, 136, 144.

and optic perineuritis[198] are the most common ocular findings of syphilis in HIV-infected patients. Papilledema[10] and cranial nerve palsies result from acute syphilitic meningitis. Neurosyphilis is almost always present in an HIV-infected patient with syphilitic eye disease and should be suspected in individuals with HIV infection who present with intraocular inflammation, a stroke syndrome, or a seizure disorder. Cerebrospinal fluid examination is necessary, even though interpretation may be difficult because of changes produced by HIV and opportunistic infections. Neuroimaging can reveal changes of meningovascular neurosyphilis (e.g., ischemic infarction) or gummatous disease (e.g., a convexity mass).

Recommended penicillin dosages do not assure a cure. HIV infection seems to impair the treatment response of concurrent ocular syphilis and to increase the likelihood of relapse and early neurosyphilis.[77] Symptomatic neurosyphilis and uveitis have occurred in HIV-infected patients following penicillin treatment. HIV-infected patients with syphilis should be aggressively treated and followed with sequential serologic tests and cerebrospinal fluid examinations. After treatment of syphilitic eye disease, approximately 10% of these patients remain visually impaired in one or both affected eyes.[195]

CLINICAL FEATURES

Clinical signs of syphilis are occasionally manifested in the eye. In the midnineteenth century Hutchinson noted that "syphilitic ophthalmitis . . . may involve any one or all of the different structures of the eyeball."[82] Estimated to cause approximately 1% of certain eye conditions (such as uveitis and optic neuritis), syphilis should still be suspected in any case of unexplained ocular inflammatory disease.[38,121,195] The multiple inflammatory and degenerative changes of the eye[103] can be categorized anatomically according to the clinical stages of acquired or congenital syphilis (Table 104-3).

Orbit and Lacrimal System

Primary Syphilis. Conjunctival inoculation can lead to lacrimal sac infection, but dacryocystitis during primary acquired syphilis is very rare. A lacrimal sac mass produces epiphora and submandibular lymphadenopathy.

Secondary Syphilis. Periostitis and osteitis, characterized by nocturnal pain that increases with heat, can affect one or more orbital walls, rarely bilaterally. Orbital periostitis tends to involve the supraorbital rim and the orbital roof in the region of the supraorbital fissure and can lead to painful, hyperplastic, osteophytic nodules or exostoses. Initial symptoms include tenderness, neuralgia, and pain on movement of the globe. Orbital myositis can occur independently. Erosion into the paranasal sinuses with bony remodeling of the nasal wall may produce chronic dacryocystitis. Mild unilateral or bilateral dacryoadenitis has occurred.

TABLE 104-3 OCULAR FEATURES OF ACQUIRED AND CONGENITAL
SYPHILIS

	Early Syphilis	Late Syphilis	Residual Sequelae
Eyelid	Chancre Eyelid rash Madarosis	Eyelid gumma Tarsitis	Tylosis Poliosis Eyebrow alopecia Rhagades

Conjunctiva	Chancre
	Papillary conjunctivitis
	Conjunctival nodule or
	  erosion
		Granulomatous conjunctivitis	Conjunctival vascular
			  changes

Orbit	Orbital periostitis
	Dacryoadenitis
	Orbital inflammation
	  with proptosis
	Osteophytic nodule
		Gummatous orbital osteitis or periosti-
		  tis (including orbital apex and supe-
		  rior orbital fissure syndromes)
		Gummatous dacryoadenitis
			Orbital deformity
			Lacrimal drainage obstruc-
			  tion
			Dacryocystitis
			Cavernous sinus thrombosis

Cornea	Stromal keratitis	Stromal keratitis	Vascularized corneal scar
			Endothelial and Descemet
			  membrane irregularities
			Salzmann nodular degenera-
			  tion
			Open-angle glaucoma

Sclera	Episcleritis Scleritis	Scleritis	Scleral translucency
Lens			Lens subluxation
Iris & Ciliary Body	Iridocyclitis Iris roseolae or papules	Iris atrophy Granulomatous nodules Ciliary body gumma	Open-angle glaucoma Peripheral anterior synechiae Iridoschisis

Choroid & Retina	Choroiditis
	Chorioretinitis
	Retinitis
	Retinal vasculitis
	Exudative retinal detach-
	  ment
		Choroiditis
		Chorioretinitis
		Retinitis
		Retinal vasculitis
		Exudative retinal detachment
			Chorioretinal atrophy and
			  pigmentation
			Epiretinal gliosis
			Vascular narrowing
			Vascular occlusion
			Choroidal neovascular mem-
			  brane
			Retinal neovascularization
			Macular degeneration
			Neovascular glaucoma

Optic Nerve	Optic neuritis or neuroret- initis Papilledema Optic perineuritis	Optic neuritis or neuroretinitis Papilledema Optic perineuritis Optic nerve gumma Optic atrophy	Optic atrophy
Central Nervous System			
Pupil	Light-near dissociation Miosis Horner syndrome	Light-near dissociation Miosis Horner syndrome Tonic pupils	Variable
Cranial nerves	Cranial nerve palsies (III, IV, VI, VII)	Cranial nerve palsies (III, IV, VI, VII) Trigeminal neuralgia Supranuclear palsies Oculogyric crisis Vestibular nystagmus Periodic alternating nystagmus	Variable
Visual pathways	Visual field defects	Visual field defects Cortical blindness	Variable

Tertiary Syphilis. Gummatous orbital inflammation leading to proptosis resembles orbital pseudotumor.[176] Hyperplastic periostitis can produce nodules along the orbital rim. Inflammation can extend into the extraocular muscles or surround the cranial nerves, such as the abducens nerve and the superior branch of the oculomotor nerve. A superior orbital fissure syndrome[35] or orbital apex syndrome may cause noninflammatory disc edema or can coexist with optic neuritis. Multiple gummas of one or both orbits can produce exophthalmos, ptosis, and extraocular muscle palsies.

Unilateral and bilateral dacryadenitis, which is usually painless, and Mikulicz syndrome have been noted rarely. Syphilitic dacryoadenitis is also caused by erosion of an orbital gumma into the lacrimal gland.

Syphilitic periostitis of the nasal orbital wall can involve the lacrimal drainage system. A gumma of the lacrimal sac resembles acute dacryocystitis but lacks a purulent discharge or abscess. Chronic gummatous dacryocystitis can produce a draining fistula from the enlarging mass.

Early and Late Congenital Syphilis. Orbital periostitis occurring during early congenital syphilis can lead to permanent deformities such as hypertelorism and a flattened nasal bridge. Nasolacrimal duct stenosis can lead to chronic dacryocystitis. Painless dacryoadenitis due to late congenital syphilis presents as a palpable mass in the lacrimal gland.

Eyelids

Primary Syphilis. Chancres of the eyelids with periorbital edema have been reported, presumably due to direct inoculation from contaminated fingers or fomites. Usually appearing as a single lesion of the lower eyelid margin or medial canthus, an eyelid chancre begins as an erythematous papule that enlarges, ulcerates, and resolves over one month. Painless preauricular and submandibular lymphadenopathy are typically present. Conjunctivitis and epithelial keratitis often accompany an eyelid chancre. Superior pannus or infiltrative stromal keratitis can ensue. Residual eyelid notching with focal madarosis may be the only sequelae.

Secondary Syphilis. The eyelid skin can be affected during the maculopapular rash of secondary syphilis,[76,163] sometimes appearing as annular lesions. Pustular or ulcerative marginal blepharitis is unusual but can lead to eyelid scarring and madarosis. Eyelid vitiligo and patchy or generalized alopecia of the eyelashes and eyebrows may be signs of prior infectious dermatitis. Hair regeneration may or may not occur.

Tertiary Syphilis. A subcutaneous gumma of the upper eyelid can occur, resembling an indurated chalazion. Usually a single lesion, multiple or bilateral gummas have been observed. Progressive enlargement of the granulomatous reaction can involve the eyelid margin. Without treatment, necrotic ulceration can erode the tarsus and cause eyelid deformities. Syphilitic tarsitis involves the upper, and less often the lower, eyelid and produces a thickened, fibrotic scar that can obliterate the lacrimal ducts to cause a dry eye.

Early Congenital Syphilis. A chancre of the upper (or, less likely, the lower) eyelid or eyelid margin can occur in a neonate from passage through an infected birth canal. Because congenital syphilis implies transplacental infection, a chancre on an infant's head is properly classified as acquired syphilis. The papular skin rash of early congenital syphilis can involve the eyelids, sometimes producing eyelash loss and clefts at the lateral canthus.

Late Congenital Syphilis. Cicatricial ectropion and other eyelid deformities can develop as a late complication of congenital syphilis.[36] Crow's-feet furrows make affected children appear prematurely old. An eyelid gumma can occur that can produce eyelid and tarsal scarring.

Conjunctiva

Primary Syphilis. A conjunctival chancre can rarely be the initial manifestation of primary syphilis. This lesion tends to occur on the lower bulbar conjunctiva but has been found on the tarsal conjunctiva, caruncle, and limbus. Beginning as a conjunctival nodule or papule, progressive induration produces a pseudomembrane and resembles an oculoglandular syndrome. Marked eyelid edema is usually present with nonsuppurative regional lymphadenopathy.

Secondary Syphilis. The skin rash of secondary syphilis is sometimes associated with papillary conjunctivitis, varying from mild to marked. Mucous patches of the conjunctiva can appear as pale nodules resembling phlyctenules of the bulbar conjunctiva, palpebral conjunctiva, or caruncle and teem with spirochetes. Preauricular lymphadenopathy is common. A superior corneal pannus can occur. Conjunctival mucous patches tend to leave permanent scars that can distort the eyelid margin or cause a dry eye syndrome.

Tertiary Syphilis. Granulomatous conjunctivitis, with or without other features of Parinaud oculoglandular syndrome, can be one of the manifestations of gummatous disease.[173] Either the bulbar or palpebral conjunctiva can be affected, and a limbal gumma has been reported. Nodular or diffuse tarsitis can lead to permanent scarring with deformity of the eyelid margin.

Early Congenital Syphilis. Mucous patches may affect the conjunctiva or caruncle. These lesions begin as an eroded exudate with surrounding hyperemia.

Cornea

Primary Syphilis. The cornea is rarely involved in primary syphilis. A conjunctival or eyelid chancre can initiate stromal inflammation and vascularization with nongranulomatous iritis.

Secondary Syphilis. Marginal corneal infiltrates that may be single or multiple can occur during secondary syphilis, particularly when mucous patches of the conjunctiva are present. Sclerosing keratitis can accompany syphilitic scleritis.

Tertiary Syphilis. Stromal keratitis is commonly linked with untreated congenital syphilis but can also occur during acquired disease (Fig. 104-7). Compared to congenital

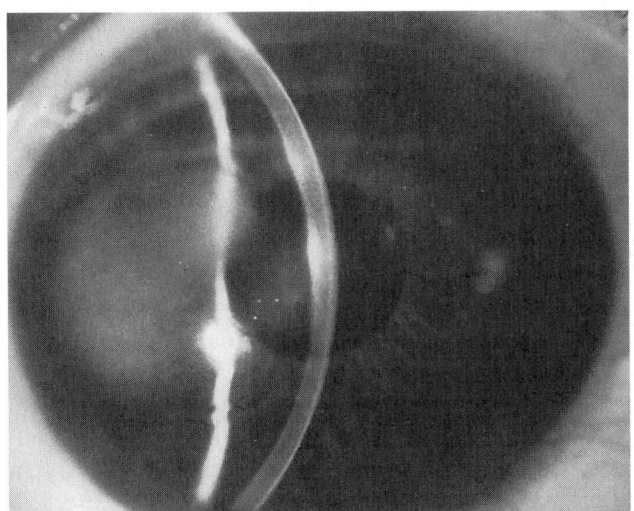

Fig. 104-7. Deep stromal keratitis due to acquired syphilis. No improvement occurred with topical corticosteroids for one month, but gradual resolution followed intramuscular penicillin treatment for syphilis (reactive FTA-ABS).

syphilis in which bilateral interstitial keratitis is typical, the corneal changes of acquired syphilis are usually unilateral. Syphilitic keratitis begins with lymphocytic infiltration of any stromal layer and an associated anterior uveitis. Deep focal stromal keratitis is typical but many variations occur, including marginal ulcerative keratitis,[105] multifocal infiltrates, and deep necrotizing inflammation. Suppurative inflammation of the deep cornea may be a type of gumma. Prolonged corneal inflammation can lead to stromal neovascularization; but, unlike congenital syphilis, stromal keratitis during acquired syphilis results in fewer vessels and is more responsive to penicillin treatment.[18]

Late Congenital Syphilis. Stromal keratitis may occur at any time from birth to middle age but generally begins between the ages of 5 to 20 years. Approximately 40% of surviving cases of untreated congenital syphilis are said to develop corneal involvement. Girls are affected slightly more often than boys. Trauma and other infections sometimes trigger the onset of syphilitic stromal keratitis.

In the 19th century Hutchinson[74] attributed most cases of nonulcerative stromal keratitis to congenital syphilis. Other ophthalmologists described syphilitic keratitis under the headings of "scrofulous corneitis" and parenchymatous keratitis, but Hutchinson's term of interstitial keratitis (IK) has persisted. While applicable to all causes of stromal keratitis, IK usually implies syphilitic corneal disease.[126,174] Other original expressions of Hutchinson's such as "ground-glass cornea," "salmon-colored patch," and "plum-colored eye" vividly depict syphilitic stromal keratitis.[110]

Interstitial keratitis begins with lymphocytic infiltration in the deep stromal layers appearing as a diffuse, ground-glass haziness. Initial findings are deep stromal infiltrates, often in the superior cornea, with pseudoguttata and keratitic

precipitates. Syphilitic stromal keratitis tends to begin at the superior limbus but can begin centrally or remain localized to any quadrant.

Over one to two weeks, punctate opacities coalesce, and deep peripheral inflammation advances centrally and anteriorly. Confluent infiltrates of the deep cornea can produce inflammatory stromal edema resembling disciform keratitis, but patchy infiltrates within a diffuse stromal inflammatory reaction are more typical. Variations include sectoral, peripheral, and multifocal infiltrates. Other atypical forms comprise punctate infiltrates of the posterior cornea (keratitis punctata profunda), deep stromal inflammation in a linear distribution (keratitis linearis migrans), and ringlike stromal keratitis (keratitis centralis annularis). Deep suppurative inflammation (keratitis pustuliformis profunda) and marginal ulcerative keratitis are less common presenting features. Most patients have an associated anterior uveitis.

Superficial and deep stromal neovascularization begins at the limbus and extends radially into the cornea. Stromal inflammation overlying deep corneal blood vessels produces a dull red color called a salmon patch. Focal limbal vascular injection has been described as an epaulet.

Bilateral involvement, sometimes separated by several weeks or months, occurs in about 80% of cases of interstitial keratitis due to congenital syphilis. Without treatment corneal inflammation can persist for several weeks or months before spontaneously subsiding. As an adjunct to systemic penicillin, topical corticosteroid therapy shortens the course of syphilitic keratitis.[139] Resolution usually starts peripherally.

Residual changes of prior IK include stromal opacification and alterations of the Descemet membrane (such as glasleitern, refractive scrolls in a web-like pattern) and endothelium (Fig. 104-8). Stromal ghost vessels persist indefi-

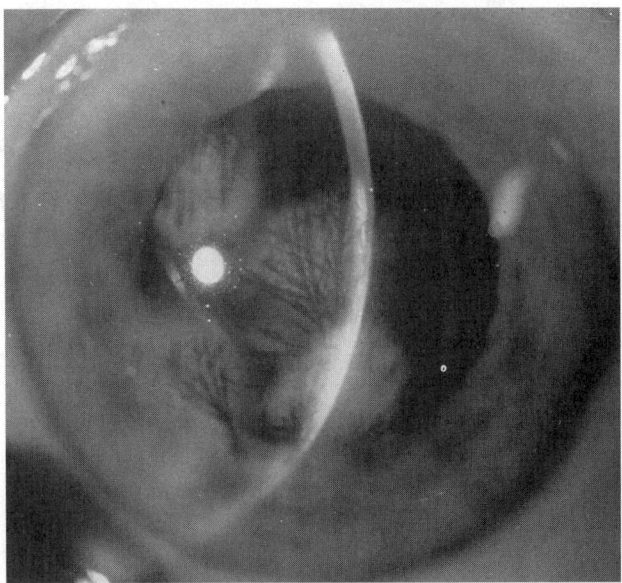

Fig. 104-8. Residual corneal scarring and stromal ghost vessels from prior stromal keratitis due to late congenital syphilis.

nitely but can enlarge or progress in the 5% to 10% of untreated cases that recur. Most cases of postsyphilitic keratopathy are identified as residual vascularized opacification.[92] Histopathologic changes include a posterior collagenous layer, multilaminar retrocorneal ridges or webs, and breaks, scrolls, or striae of the Descemet membrane.[80,143,156,189] Corneal thinning and ectasia, sometimes mimicking keratoglobus, are occasionally encountered. Salzmann nodular degeneration and secondary amyloid accumulation have been reported.[68] Endothelial guttata may gradually progress to bullous keratopathy later in life.

The Hutchinson triad of stromal scarring and vascularization, reduced hearing, and malformed teeth is highly indicative of congenital syphilis. Other stigmata of congenital syphilis, including chorioretinal scars, are frequent. Approximately 15% to 20% of individuals with prior syphilitic stromal keratouveitis are at risk of developing open-angle glaucoma many years later.

Nearly three fourths of patients with interstitial keratitis recover adequate vision. Up to 10% of untreated cases will recur, sometimes decades later. These recurrent episodes of stromal keratitis are usually unilateral and tend to be milder than the first.

Sclera

Secondary Syphilis. Episcleritis with limbal chemosis can occur with no other distinguishing features. Diffuse or nodular scleritis during secondary syphilis (Fig. 104-9) is frequently accompanied by anterior uveitis.[20]

Tertiary Syphilis. Scleritis is an uncommon presentation of late syphilis but may be its only clinical manifestation. Typically presenting as nodular scleritis, any form of scleral inflammation can occur.[65,196] Scleritis must be distinguished from the ciliary flush associated with uveitis. Transscleral

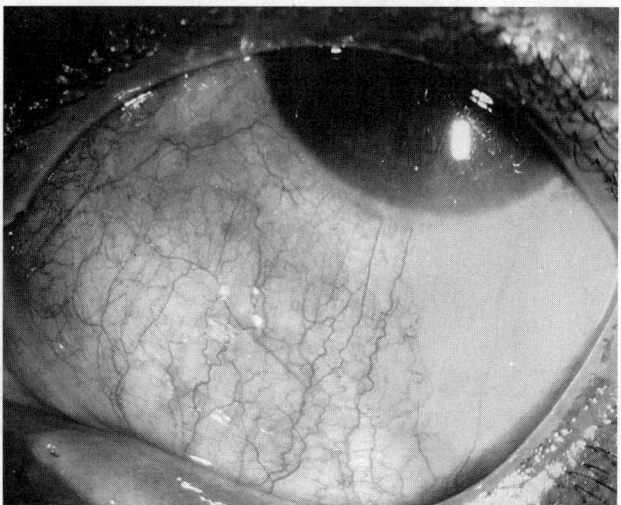

Fig. 104-9. Scleritis as the presenting sign of late syphilis (reactive FTA-ABS and RPR 1:256).

extension of a ciliary body gumma is a rare condition that causes scleral inflammation and dissolution.

Late Congenital Syphilis. Limbal episcleritis may present in the quadrant of active corneal inflammation and neovascularization during acute interstitial keratitis. Scleritis may occur many years later.[196]

Lens

Secondary Syphilis. Anterior uveitis can lead to posterior synechiae and pigment deposition on the lens. Lenticular subluxation has occurred after syphilitic uveitis.[138]

Tertiary Syphilis. Dislocation of the crystalline lens was formerly linked with syphilis, but this association appears tenuous.[147] Similarly, syphilis is not a risk factor for adult-onset cataracts.[161] Finding a positive serologic test for syphilis in patients who have a subluxated lens or who are scheduled for cataract surgery probably reflects demographic rather than causative factors.

Early Congenital Syphilis. Congenital cataract may occur secondary to syphilitic uveitis.[31] Dislocation of a partially resorbed cataractous lens can present as congenital aphakia.

Late Congenital Syphilis. Interstitial keratitis with uveitis can produce a secondary cataract, typically beginning as a brown discoloration of the posterior aspect of the embryonic lens nucleus.

Uvea

Secondary Syphilis. Syphilis as a cause of uveitis has gradually declined in frequency during the 20th century (Table 104-1). Before the discovery of penicillin uveitis was frequently attributed to syphilis, but since 1960 only about 1% of uveitis cases are associated with syphilis.[66]

Syphilitic uveitis cannot necessarily be distinguished from other causes based on the ocular examination alone.[159,172] Physical examination can sometimes show other signs of secondary syphilis such as the skin rash.[101] Iridocyclitis may be the principal clinical sign of relapsing secondary syphilis.[101,141] Patients with persistent uveitis not responding to corticosteroid or immunosuppressive therapy should be evaluated for syphilis.[88,120,149,164]

Anterior uveitis during secondary syphilis typically begins as an acute, unilateral iritis or iridocyclitis. The contralateral eye becomes involved in up to one half of affected patients. The severity of anterior uveitis varies from a subclinical or mild nongranulomatous iritis[205] to severe granulomatous iridocyclitis (Fig. 104-10) with hyphema, hypopyon, vitreitis, and cystoid macular edema. A transient iritis may be a feature of a Jarisch-Herxheimer reaction. Corresponding to the infectious mucocutaneous lesions, transient iris roseolae are engorged vascular tufts of the middle third of the iris that can progress to iris papules.[162] These may evolve to vascularized nodules (Fig. 104-11) that can resolve completely or, less often, lead to sectoral iris atrophy. A syphilitic nodule can rarely present as a fleshy

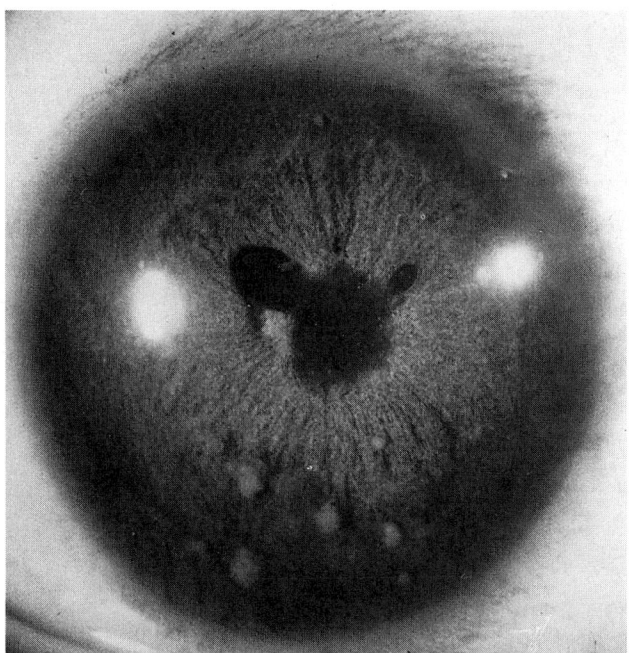

Fig. 104-10. Bilateral granulomatous anterior uveitis with iris nodules during secondary syphilis. (Reprinted with permission from Margo CE, Hamed LM: Ocular syphilis, *Surv Ophthalmol* 37:203-220, 1992.)

mass in the anterior-chamber angle with severe iridocyclitis.[108,160]

Posterior uveitis occurring during secondary syphilis can appear as diffuse or localized choroiditis or chorioretinitis,[62a,100] most often affecting the posterior pole[34] and juxtapapillary area.[42] A focal posterior plaque of chorioretinitis (Fig. 104-12)[34,53] frequently has vitreous cells[9] and a shallow serous retinal detachment[128a] (Figure 104-13). This circumscribed, polymorphous lesion can linger for several weeks and lead to pigmentary changes with retinal and optic nerve atrophy. Multifocal yellow-gray choroidal infiltrates can also occur, may cause areas of localized retinal edema with overlying vitreous cells,[149] and can become confluent. Fluorescein angiography of syphilitic chorioretinitis typically shows early diffuse or leopard-spot hypofluorescence of the involved area with late staining at the level of the retinal pigment epithelium. Subretinal neovascularization is an unusual complication.[200] About one half of all cases of syphilitic posterior uveitis are bilateral, and most are recognized in HIV-infected individuals. Following therapy, mottled depigmentation of the involved retinal pigment epithelium remains.

Progressive posterior uveitis can lead to disc edema, vitreitis, retinal vasculitis,[12] uveal effusion, and exudative retinal detachment.[37] Residual changes of resolved syphilitic chorioretinitis include hyperpigmented stippling of the retinal pigment epithelium, focal or scattered chorioretinal hypopigmented scars, pigment clumping at the borders of cho-

roidal atrophic areas, and pigment migration along retinal blood vessels.

Tertiary Syphilis. Late syphilis may present with anterior or posterior uveitis. Approximately one half of these patients have other signs of disease. One fourth have central nervous system involvement that is frequently asymptomatic. The severity of anterior uveitis during late syphilis varies from mild iritis to severe, chronic iridocyclitis with cystoid macular edema. Gummas of the uveal tract can present as small, miliary granulomas or as a solitary mass. Granulomatous nodules may appear at the pupillary border (Koeppe nodule) or on the peripheral iris (Busacca nodule). A ciliary body

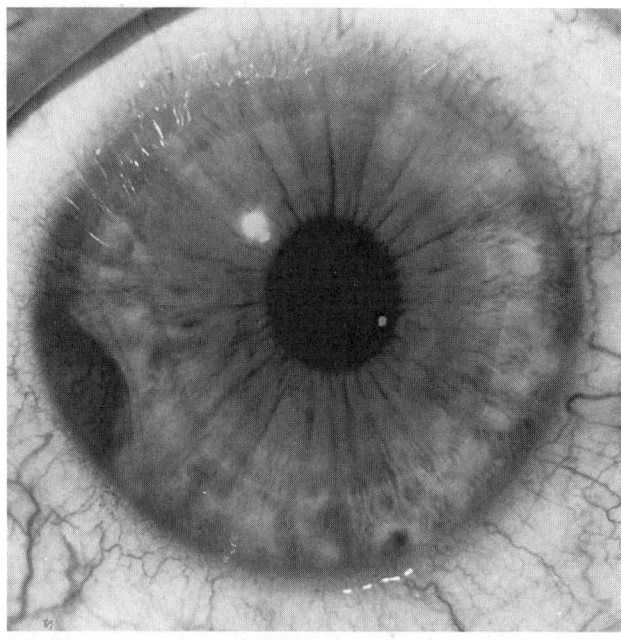

A

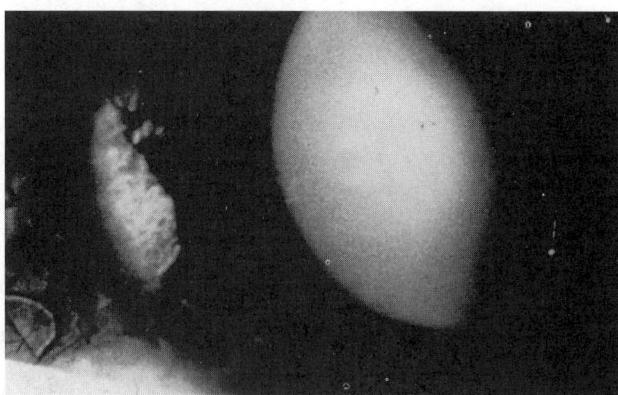

B

Fig. 104-11. Syphilitic iritis. **A,** Vascularized papule at ciliary border of 9 o'clock iris during secondary syphilis. **B,** Anterior-segment fluorescein angiogram confirms lesion's vascularity. (Reprinted courtesy of McCarron MJ, Albert DM: Iridocyclitis and iris mass associated with secondary syphilis, *Ophthalmology* 91:1264-1268, 1984.)

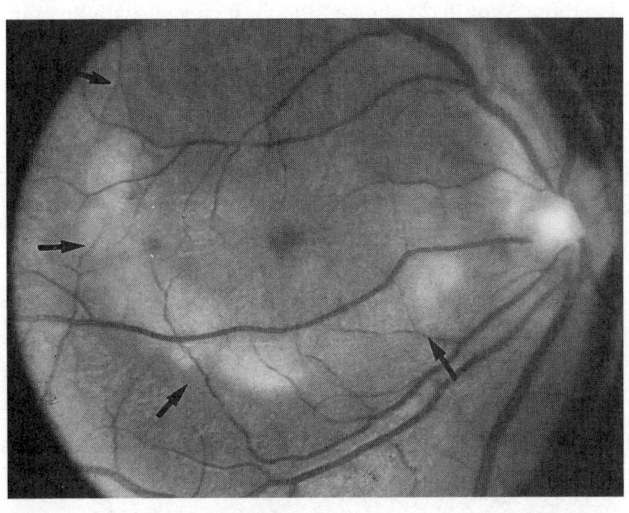

A

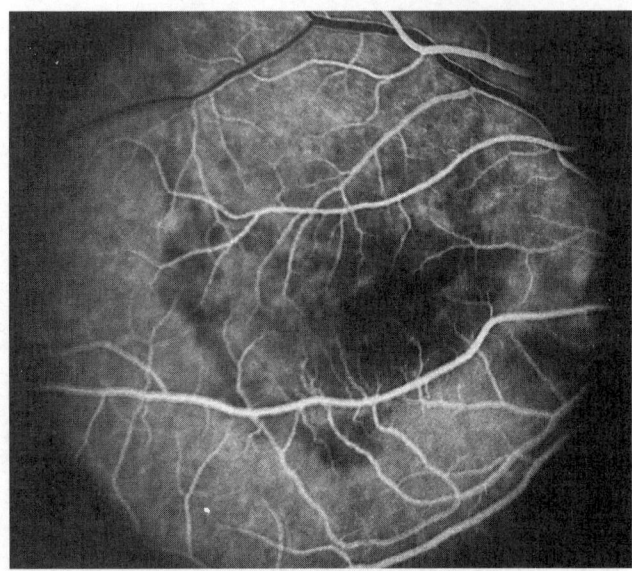

B

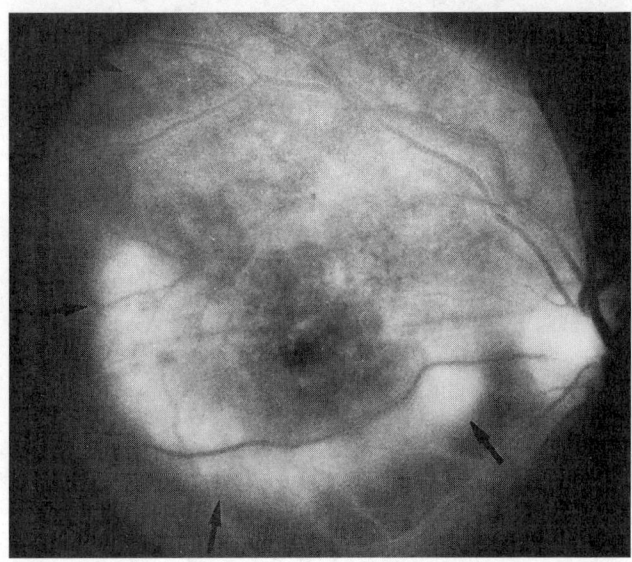

C

Fig. 104-12. Acute syphilitic posterior placoid chorioretinitis. **A,** Localized central chorioretinitis during secondary syphilis. **B,** Early-phase fluorescein angiogram shows mottled hypofluorescence. **C,** Late-phase angiogram shows hyperfluorescence at the level of the retinal pigment epithelium. (Reprinted courtesy of Gass JDM, Braunstein RA, Chenoweth RG: Acute syphilitic posterior placoid chorioretinitis, *Ophthalmology* 97:1288-1297, 1990.)

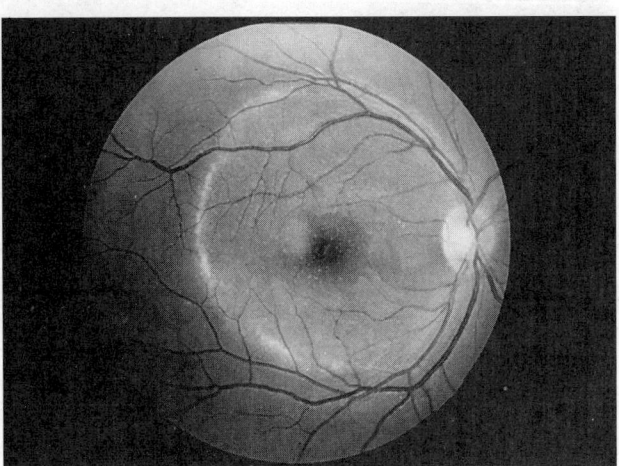

Fig. 104-13. Posterior syphilitic chorioretinitis with serous retinal detachment. (Reprinted with permission from Cunha de Souza E et al.: Unusual central chorioretinitis as the first manifestation of early secondary syphilis, *Am J Ophthalmol* 105:271-276, 1988.)

gumma can present as a reddish-brown tumor in the anterior-chamber angle that can rarely erode through the sclera.

Chorioretinitis may be focal or multifocal.[45] Posterior uveitis can lead to breaks in the Bruch membrane that predispose to subretinal neovascular membrane formation.[61] A gumma of the ciliary body or optic nerve can extend into the choroid and retina, but a gumma of the choroid is very rare.

Early Congenital Syphilis. Acute iritis is the most common eye manifestation of early congenital syphilis and may appear at about 6 months of age in untreated infants. Secondary cataract or glaucoma may follow severe or prolonged iridocyclitis. Posterior uveitis due to congenital syphilis usually begins as multifocal inflammation of the choriocapillaris that is subclinical. Postinflammatory changes consist of diffusely scattered foci of chorioretinal atrophy, patchy proliferation of the retinal pigment epithelium, and narrowed retinal blood vessels. Hypopigmented and hyperpigmented (salt-and-pepper) spots can be diffuse or limited to the periphery, to one quadrant, or to the posterior pole. Visual impairment can result from epiretinal gliosis and optic atrophy.

Late Congenital Syphilis. Anterior uveitis frequently accompanies interstitial keratitis. Iridoschisis has been found in association with corneal changes of prior interstitial keratitis.[49,131] Recurrent iridocyclitis in the adult is an uncommon complication of congenital syphilis. Residual signs of congenital syphilis include multifocal, hypopigmented chorioretinal scars that show window defects on fluorescein angiography (Fig. 104-14). Perivascular sheathing and secondary optic atrophy may be present.

Intraocular Pressure

Hypotony can be a transient feature of syphilitic iridocyclitis or stromal keratouveitis. The intraocular pressure usually returns to normal as the intraocular inflammation subsides.

Glaucoma can be a secondary complication of anterior uveitis or can arise insidiously many years later. Approximately one fourth of patients with syphilitic interstitial keratitis develop secondary glaucoma,[167] usually 15 to 30 years later.[185] Two principal forms of nonuveitic glaucoma are recognized: one resembling primary open-angle glaucoma and another presenting more acutely, usually with a narrow angle.[55]

Chronic open-angle glaucoma can occur from microstructural sclerosis of the trabecular meshwork or from hypertrophy of the Descemet membrane and endothelialization of the anterior-chamber angle. Corticosteroid-induced glaucoma can be a complication of prolonged corticosteroid use in the management of syphilitic stromal keratitis or iritis. Neovascular glaucoma is a rare occurrence but can result from ischemic retinopathy associated with severe syphilitic neuroretinitis.

Acute or chronic narrow-angle glaucoma has occurred

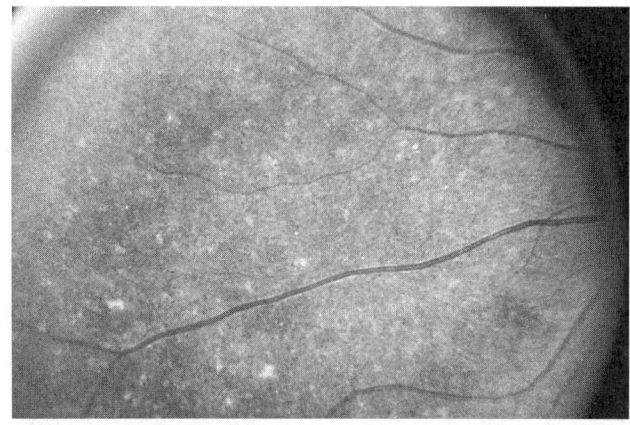

A

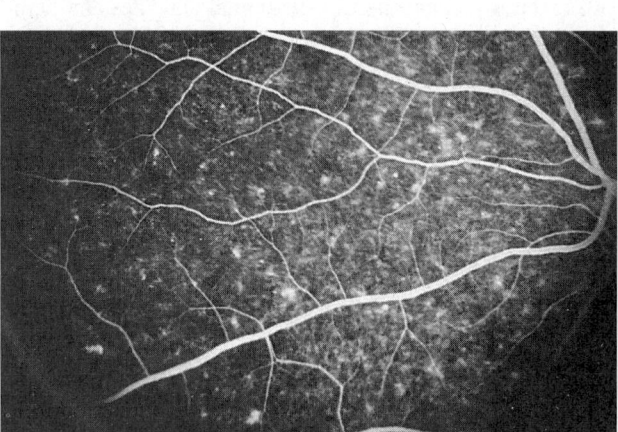

B

Fig. 104-14. Multifocal chorioretinal scars following congenital syphilis. **A,** Scattered hypopigmented spots. **B,** Fluorescein angiogram demonstrates atrophic areas of retinal pigment epithelium.

from postinflammatory iris synechiae, intraepithelial iris cysts,[94] and a congenitally small anterior segment.

Retina

Secondary Syphilis. Posterior uveitis is frequently associated with overlying retinal involvement, and retinochoroiditis can be associated with syphilitic meningitis.[9] Secondary atrophic and pigmentary changes have been termed pseudoretinitis pigmentosa[32,64,165,188] and ''pseudohistoplasmosis.''[40] With extensive inflammation periretinal fibrosis may produce tractional bands between the disc and areas of chorioretinal atrophy. Chorioretinitis can also cause breaks in the Bruch membrane that predispose to a subretinal neovascular membrane[61] and disciform maculopathy.[151]

Syphilitic neuroretinitis presents as papillitis with venous engorgement and peripapillary flame-shaped hemorrhages, periarteriolar sheathing, thickened retina, and stellate macular exudates.[111] Residual changes include optic atrophy and pigmentary mottling around the disc and in the macula.

Necrotizing retinitis may occur,[112,155] frequently associated with panuveitis and retinal vasculitis. Retinitis may be more extensive and bilateral in patients with AIDS (Fig. 104-15). Progressive changes can lead to coalescent patches of yellow-white retinitis resembling acute retinal necrosis.[112] Macrophages predominate in this granulomatous reaction.[13,52] Retinal neovascularization with vitreous hemorrhage has been described as a late complication.

Retinal vasculitis can occur during secondary syphilis,[115] and approximately 5% of all cases of retinal vasculitis are due to syphilis.[125] Associated inflammation includes anterior uveitis, sometimes with granulomatous keratitic precipitates, and vitreous cells over retinal blood vessels and the optic disc.[142] Fluorescein angiography typically shows mural staining with excessive vascular leakage (Fig. 104-16), features that account for the retinal exudates and hemorrhages. Later vascular sheathing and atrophy appear. Occlusive vasculitis with thrombosis can cause acute visual loss.[168] Ischemic retinopathy and diffuse chorioretinitis can lead to retinal neovascularization,[184] glial membranes, and cystoid macular edema.

Tertiary Syphilis. Retinal inflammation may be due to intraocular extension of choroiditis or to peripapillary extension of optic neuritis[3] during meningovascular neurosyphilis. Retinal vasculitis, whether periarteritis[33] or periphlebitis,[60,96] may be associated with chorioretinitis or can be the principal finding.[115] Perivasculitis can lead to narrowed retinal vessels and branch or central retinal vascular occlusion.[2,61,72,132,178] Intraretinal hemorrhages and vitreous hemorrhage occasionally occur.

Congenital Syphilis. Retinal vasculitis can be the major manifestation of congenital syphilis and may precede the clinical onset of neurosyphilis.

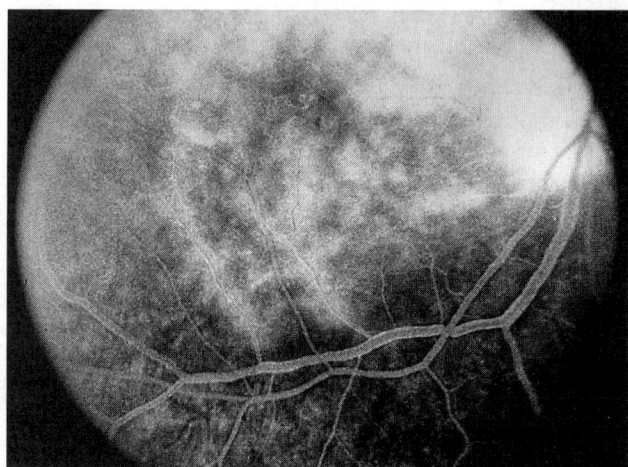

Fig. 104-16. Fluorescein angiogram demonstrates unilateral retinal periphlebitis during acquired syphilis. (Reprinted with permission from Lobes LA Jr, Folk JC: Syphilitic phlebitis simulating branch vein occlusion, *Ann Ophthalmol* 13:825-827, 1981.)

Optic Nerve

Secondary Syphilis. Acute syphilitic meningitis can lead to communicating hydrocephalus with increased intracranial pressure and papilledema.[15,40a] Acute optic nerve swelling can also occur during a Jarisch-Herxheimer reaction.[179] Inflammatory optic disc edema may be due to optic neuritis or optic perineuritis (Table 104-4).

Optic neuritis is more likely to occur during secondary[29] and relapsing[84] syphilis than during tertiary syphilis. Syphilitic optic neuritis generally has no distinctive features.[191] Typical symptoms are reduced vision with a visual field defect such as blindspot enlargement, a central or cecocentral scotoma, or a nerve fiber bundle defect. Papillitis is typically surrounded by gray thickened retina, intraretinal exudates, and perivascular sheathing. Half of affected patients have visible extension into the peripapillary retina.[3] This neuroretinitis is characterized by perivascular lymphocytic inflammation and cellular infiltration into the inner retinal layers.[187] A macular star figure is unusual.[44] Anterior uveitis may also be present[6] and can be the presenting feature.[88] The contralateral eye may be involved concurrently or develop optic neuritis several months later. Retrobulbar neuritis may present with minimal signs of inflammatory disc edema.[202,203] During syphilitic optic neuritis, the electroretinogram is typically normal with a normal implicit time but may have reduced a- and b-wave amplitudes. Syphilitic neuroretinitis is frequently accompanied by abnormal cerebrospinal fluid changes. Treatment for neurosyphilis is indicated.[48]

Optic perineuritis (Fig. 104-17) is a form of syphilitic leptomeningitis, distinguished by inflammatory disc edema with normal intracranial pressure, normal vision, and normal pupils.[150,183] Blindspot enlargement[107] and related visual

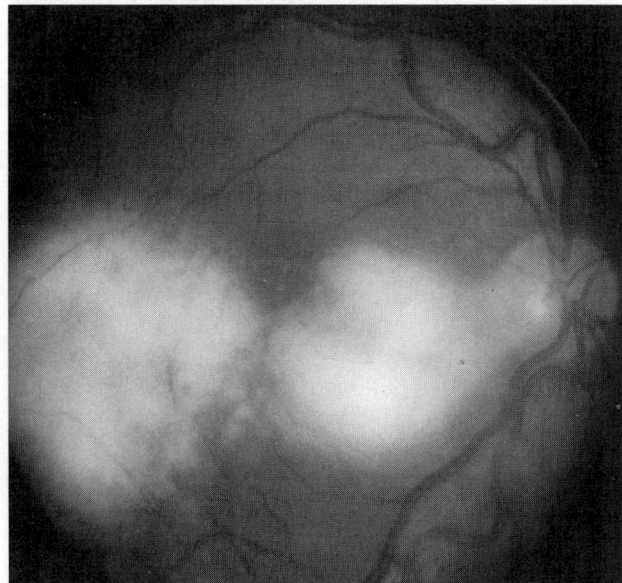

Fig. 104-15. Necrotizing syphilitic retinitis in patient with HIV infection.

TABLE 104-4 CLINICAL DIFFERENTIATION OF VARIOUS CAUSES OF OPTIC DISC EDEMA DURING NEUROSYPHILIS

Condition	Pain	Vision	Visual Field	Pupil	Vitreous Cells	Intracranial Pressure
Papilledema	−	↓	Enlarged blindspot	↓ light reactivity	None	Elevated
Optic neuritis	+	↓	Cecocentral scotoma	↓ light reactivity	Present	Usually normal
Optic perineuritis	+	Normal	Enlarged blindspot	Normal	None	Normal
Optic nerve gumma	±	↓	Cecocentral scotoma	↓ light reactivity	Present	Usually normal
Juxtapapillary choroiditis	±	↓	Cecocentral scotoma	Variable	Present	Normal

field defects may be the presenting features. Anterior uveitis occasionally accompanies optic perineuritis.[95]

Tertiary Syphilis. The optic nerve can be affected during late syphilis in the following ways: optic or retrobulbar neuritis, optic perineuritis, optic nerve gumma, papilledema, and optic atrophy.

Optic neuritis and neuroretinitis occur in approximately 3% of patients with symptomatic meningovascular neurosyphilis and may present without other features of meningitis. Optic perineuritis has also occurred during meningovascular neurosyphilis in association with basilar meningitis. A gumma of the optic nervehead can occur that can subsequently lead to disc neovascularization. Gummas can also arise anywhere along the intraorbital, intracanalicular, or intracranial segments of the optic nerve[169] as well as at the chiasm. Papilledema has been described in late neurosyphilis from chronic intracranial hypertension.[186]

Secondary optic atrophy can ensue from all forms of inflammatory optic nerve disease. The presentation of residual optic atrophy in one eye and optic neuritis in the other can resemble the Foster Kennedy syndrome.[158] Ischemic optic neuropathy can be related to syphilitic vascular disease.[154]

During parenchymatous neurosyphilis, lymphocytic inflammation of the optic nerve sheaths leads to fibrous thickening and adhesions. Subsequent neuronal degeneration begins peripherally and gradually extends toward the center of the optic nerve causing visual field constriction. This progressive optic atrophy usually begins unilaterally but without treatment will almost always involve the other eye. Optic atrophy occurs in 5% of patients with symptomatic parenchymatous neurosyphilis.[71] Optic atrophy is sometimes the presenting feature of tabes dorsalis[19] but may be the sole manifestation of late neurosyphilis.[116] Without adequate therapy, progressive visual loss may lead to blindness over the subsequent decade.[153] Advanced optic atrophy appears as a sharply defined, pale optic disc with an atrophic cup and narrowed retinal arterioles (Fig. 104-18). Although their infectious and inflammatory processes overlap somewhat, electrophysiologic testing can help to distinguish parenchymatous optic atrophy from postneuritic optic atrophy.[83] The visual evoked potential in parenchymatous optic atrophy usually shows an abnormal latency interval.[30]

Early Congenital Syphilis. Optic neuritis is an uncommon presentation of congenital syphilis. Optic atrophy can follow syphilitic chorioretinitis.

Fig. 104-17. Optic perineuritis during secondary syphilis. Evaluation showed normal visual acuity, normal visual evoked potentials, and normal cerebrospinal fluid opening pressure. (Reprinted with permission from Toshniwal P: Optic perineuritis with secondary syphilis, *J Clin Neuro-ophthalmol* 7:6-10, 1987.)

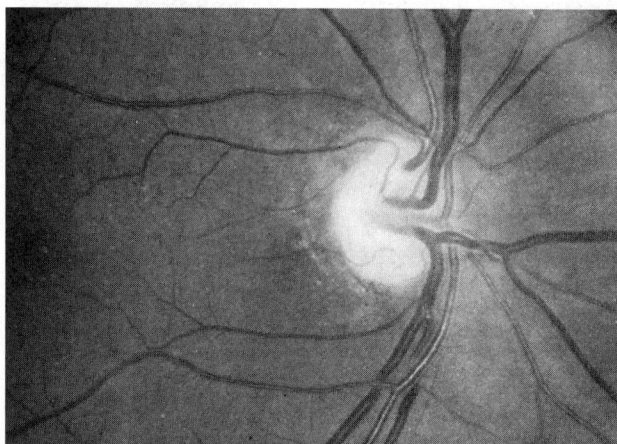

Fig. 104-18. Optic atrophy with hypovascularity of optic nervehead in patient with tabes dorsalis.

Late Congenital Syphilis. Optic atrophy can be a manifestation of degenerative neurosyphilis following congenital infection.

Central Nervous System

Secondary Syphilis. Besides the optic nerve, other cranial nerves may be involved in acute syphilitic meningitis. Third, fourth, and sixth cranial nerve palsies are a complication of basilar meningitis and may persist after other neurologic signs have resolved. Ophthalmologic features of seventh and eighth cranial nerve involvement include ptosis and vestibular nystagmus, respectively. Brainstem involvement can be manifest by a supranuclear gaze palsy.[129] Visual field abnormalities may be due to syphilitic eye disease and to neurosyphilis: a ring scotoma may be caused by syphilitic choroiditis, altitudinal and arcuate defects can result from retinal involvement, and optic neuritis can produce a central or cecocentral scotoma. Irregular bitemporal, or rarely binasal, hemianopia can occur from syphilitic basilar meningitis that affects the optic chiasm. Syphilitic chiasmatic arachnoiditis causes hemianopic and altitudinal visual field defects,[127] can lead to partial or complete visual loss of one or both eyes, and can affect the pituitary gland.

Tertiary Syphilis. One or more cranial nerves may be involved in both the meningovascular and parenchymatous forms of late neurosyphilis.[56]

Cranial nerve palsies during meningovascular neurosyphilis are caused by subacute meningitis and occlusive vasculitis (Fig. 104-19). The oculomotor nerve is the most commonly affected,[148] but trochlear, abducens, facial, and vestibuloauditory nerve palsies also occur. Cranial nerves can be affected by syphilitic vascular changes such as an aneurysm or subdural hematoma. Nuclear or supranuclear palsies can result from brain stem infarction. Single or com-

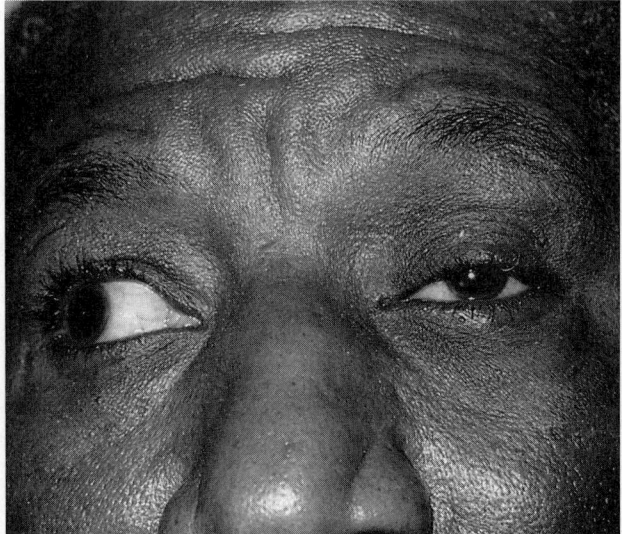

Fig. 104-19. Third nerve palsy due to meningovascular neurosyphilis.

bined cranial nerve palsies can be the presenting feature of gummatous neurosyphilis. Cranial nerves can also be affected by syphilitic periostitis of the supraorbital fissure. Chronic syphilitic meningitis and syphilitic osteitis of the petrous bone can affect the sensory fibers of the trigeminal nerve and might result in neurotrophic keratopathy. Visual field abnormalities can occur from cerebral infarction. Complete or partial homonymous hemianopia or quadrantanopia can result from infarction of the middle cerebral artery as a result of syphilitic arteritis.

Cranial nerve palsies are uncommon during late parenchymatous neurosyphilis although supranuclear palsies and oculogyric crisis have rarely occurred. Subclinical alterations in smooth pursuit and saccadic movements are sometimes detectable. Ptosis can be due to sympathetic or mesencephalic involvement that, with the compensatory brow wrinkling, produces the characteristic tabetic facies. The paresthesias of tabes dorsalis may infrequently be manifest as trigeminal neuralgia. Vestibular nystagmus and periodic alternating nystagmus have been reported.

In the late 19th century Argyll Robertson reported a series of patients with usable vision and small pupils that showed no constriction to light stimulation but normal reactivity to near testing.[97] Other features subsequently noted are normal redilatation following near testing and normal accommodation. Pupillary light-near dissociation is found in approximately 10% of patients with meningovascular neurosyphilis and in most individuals with parenchymatous neurosyphilis. Initially an incomplete picture of normally sized pupils with a sluggish light response is seen.[109] The complete Argyll Robertson pupil is less than 3 mm in diameter with total absence of the light response and a normal near response. Contrary to Argyll Robertson's descriptions, the pupil should dilate satisfactorily to atropine and other mydriatics unless there has been iris atrophy. In parallel with intracranial disease, concomitant syphilitic iritis can cause chronically miotic and irregularly shaped pupils. If treated early in the course of disease, pupillary light-near dissociation can sometimes return to normal.[90]

Other pupillary abnormalities can also appear during neurosyphilis. A lesion near the constrictor nucleus can produce both light and near unresponsiveness. Fixed dilated pupils have occurred with external ophthalmoplegia in late neurosyphilis. Miosis is a component of Horner syndrome that can result from secondary syphilitic meningomyelitis, osteitis, or cardiovascular syphilis. Neurosyphilis may also present as Raeder syndrome.[190] Oculomotor cranial nerve paresis can involve the pupil and has infrequently contributed to paralysis or spasm of accommodation or convergence. Bilateral tonic pupils rarely have been linked with neurosyphilis.[47,201] Chronic iritis can cause pupillary immobility from segmental iris atrophy.

Early and Late Congenital Syphilis. Optic neuritis or a cranial nerve palsy can be the presenting feature of syphilitic meningitis in affected infants. Neuroophthalmic sequelae such as optic atrophy and oculomotor paresis are infrequently encountered. Bilateral total ophthalmoplegia has been reported. Various pupillary changes have been described. The pupils related to late congenital neurosyphilis usually show light-near dissociation but tend to be dilated and fixed rather than miotic.

PATHOGENESIS

Many cultivable treponemes are found in the human oropharynx and gastrointestinal tract, and some are associated with periodontal disease. Human treponemal infections are venereal syphilis, endemic syphilis (bejel), yaws, and pinta (Table 104-5). The term "syphilis" originated from a Renaissance poem relating the story of Syphilis, a shepherd punished by God with a venereal disease. Lues venerea (literally a plague influenced by Venus, the ancient Roman goddess of sensual love) is a 17th century term that is now shortened to lues and used as a euphemistic obfuscation for syphilis.

Etiology

Syphilis is caused by the spirochete *Treponema pallidum* subspecies *pallidum,* named "pale thread" because of its faint microscopic appearance. The organisms are 10 to 13 μm long and 0.15 μm in diameter, just below light microscopic resolution. Treponemes are temperature-sensitive, microaerophilic helical bacteria that are enclosed by a cytoplasmic membrane, a peptidoglycan cell wall, and an outer envelope. At each end 3 endoflagella lie in the periplasmic space between the inner and outer membranes. A single, circular chromosome with 900 kilobase pairs codes for metabolic and structural proteins, including various polypeptide and lipoprotein antigens. Treponemes divide transversely by binary fission and have been genetically stable over the past several decades. The generation time for *T. pallidum* is estimated to be approximately 30 hours during early infection.

Host Response

The pathogenesis of syphilis is complex and poorly understood. *T. pallidum* enters the host by penetrating intact mucosa between endothelial tight junctions or by entering through a small skin abrasion. Within hours, organisms invade local tissues and disseminate via the blood and lymphatic circulation. The host responds with a dramatic local infiltration of mononuclear cells, comprising specifically sensitized T lymphocytes, macrophages, and variable numbers of plasma cells. This inflammatory response is thought to be the principal cause of the primary lesion because *T. pallidum* is not intrinsically cytotoxic and does not elaborate toxins. The chancre ulcerates as the result of obliterative endarteritis of small blood vessels.

Systemic and local antibodies are produced against several treponemal lipid, protein, and lipoprotein antigens. Opsonic antibodies, in concert with the activation of macrophages by treponemal components and/or lymphokines, eradicate nearly all of the local bacteria except for a small subpopulation resistant to opsonophagocytosis that persists at the local site.

Organisms that disseminated during the early days of infection multiply despite the increasing systemic humoral and cellular responses. As the antigenic mass of treponemes at various sites increases, mononuclear inflammation is again triggered, and the disseminated lesions of the secondary stage appear. The lipoprotein and endoflagellar antigens of *T. pallidum* induce the production of various inflammatory mediators, including interleukin-1 and tumor necrosis factor. Local bacterial clearance occurs as during primary syphilis, probably by similar mechanisms.

Late syphilitic lesions develop in a small proportion of

TABLE 104-5 CLASSIFICATION OF SPIROCHETES AFFECTING HUMANS

Order	Family	Genus	Species	Disease
Spirochaetales	Spirochaetaceae	*Treponema*	*T. pallidum* subspecies *pallidum*	Venereal syphilis
			T. pallidum subspecies *endemicum*	Endemic syphilis (Bejel)
			T. pallidum subspecies *pertenue*	Yaws
			T. carateum	Pinta
			T. denticola	Oral commensal
			T. vincentii	Oral commensal
			T. scoliodontum	Oral commensal
			T. refringens	Genital commensal
			T. minutum	Genital commensal
			T. phagedenis	Genital commensal
		Borrelia	*B. recurrentis*	Louse-borne relapsing fever
			Multiple species	Tick-borne relapsing fever
			B. burgdorferi	Lyme borreliosis
		Brachyspira	*B. aalborgii*	Intestinal commensal
	Leptospiraceae	*Leptospira*	*L. interrogans*	Leptospirosis

chronically infected patients. The events that trigger another cycle of disease reactivation are unknown but appear to involve local inflammatory responses to viable organisms. Although treponemes are rarely seen in tertiary lesions, the rapid clinical improvement that follows penicillin therapy provides strong evidence for a bacterial, rather than an autoimmune, cause.

How *T. pallidum* manages to persist in the body despite high titers of circulating antibodies and an intact cellular immune response is not known. Several hypotheses have been raised, including evasion of the host response by an intracellular location, the existence of an immunologically inert outer membrane, and an inappropriate early down-regulation of the host's immune response through prostaglandins and other mediators. Whatever the mechanism, low numbers of slowly dividing treponemes apparently fail to trigger an inflammatory reaction and thereby survive in an immunocompetent person. The stimulus for local inflammation appears to be dependent upon the local antigenic mass (approximately 10 million *T. pallidum* per gram of tissue).

Efforts to unravel the complex host-parasite relationships in syphilis are hampered by the inability to culture *T. pallidum* and the lack of an adequate animal model with well-defined immunologic markers. Improved understanding of the protective antigens of *T. pallidum* and the mechanisms of immunity during syphilis may eventually lead to a successful vaccine.

LABORATORY INVESTIGATIONS

The diagnosis of syphilis is based upon the clinical presentation and serologic testing. Several methods are available for the identification of *T. pallidum* in active syphilis, but direct demonstration of *T. pallidum* is not possible during latent or late syphilis and in almost all forms of ocular syphilis. Reliance on serologic testing of serum and cerebrospinal fluid is necessary.

Demonstration of *T. pallidum*

T. pallidum is a poorly staining bacterium that is so thin as to be invisible with regular light microscopy. Special enhancement techniques, such as darkfield microscopy, silver staining, and immunofluorescence, are needed to enable direct microscopic observation of organisms in material from infectious sites during primary and secondary syphilis.

Careful handling of any potentially infective specimen with disposable gloves is mandatory. After examination slides should be placed directly into a disinfectant solution. If exposure of the collector's mucous membranes, including the ocular surface, accidentally occurs, then saline rinsing and penicillin prophylaxis (as for recent sexual partners) are indicated.

Except for the rare occurrence of an eyelid chancre, direct tests for demonstrating *T. pallidum* are rarely used in clinical ophthalmic practice. Spiral forms resembling *T. pallidum*

have been found in the aqueous humor of patients with syphilis, but the presence and identity of these organisms have been questioned.[54] Enzyme immunoassays could potentially be used to test for intraocular antibody production against *T. pallidum,* and DNA probes might be applied to ocular biopsies.

Darkfield Microscopy. Darkfield and phase-contrast microscopic techniques can identify treponemes from infective specimens. An early lesion is cleaned and debrided to expose the subsurface translucent exudate. A glass slide is touched to this material and examined immediately. Darkfield microscopy uses obliquely applied light from a darkfield condenser that demonstrates treponemes as regularly coiled, white threads against a black background (Fig. 104-20). Motile organisms rotate like a corkscrew and flex along their length.

Silver Staining. Histopathologic processing of skin and mucous membrane specimens during early syphilis typically shows obliterative endarteritis manifested by mononuclear and plasma cell inflammation, a perivascular granulomatous reaction, and fibroblastic proliferative thickening of small blood vessels with endothelial swelling. Silver staining of biopsy material by the Dieterle, Levaditi, Steiner, or other technique can reveal spirochetes.[173] Special care is needed to avoid misinterpreting tissue artifacts as treponemes.

Fluorescent Microscopy. Material collected on a slide is fixed in cold acetone. Fixed smears are tested within 2 weeks because the immunoreactivity of *T. pallidum* may deteriorate over prolonged storage. Polyclonal and monoclonal antibodies are available at reference and research laboratories for direct and indirect immunofluorescent microscopy.

Culture. Viable *T. pallidum* can be maintained in specialized tissue culture for a few days, but sustained in vitro cultivation is not possible. Propagation by intratesticular inoculation in rabbits is not feasible in clinical practice. To perform a rabbit-infectivity test, the clinical specimen is in-

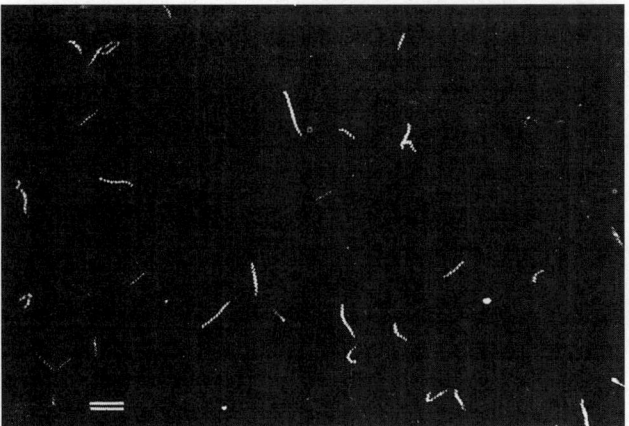

Fig. 104-20. Darkfield microscopy of *T. pallidum* (original magnification, 160×; bar = 10 μ).

oculated into seronegative animals that are maintained on antibiotic-free food and followed for orchitis and seroconversion.

Antigen and DNA Detection Methods. Enzyme immunoassays and DNA probes for *T. pallidum* detection are under development and evaluation. Testing based on the polymerase chain reaction can detect small amounts of *T. pallidum* DNA and might have a role in the diagnosis of infection of the eye or central nervous system.[22,123,192]

Serology

In 1906 Wassermann and associates developed a complement-fixation test for detecting antibodies in patients with syphilis. Later developments using infected liver or uninfected heart extract showed that the antigen was not *T. pallidum* components but rather a phospholipid of mammalian mitochondrial membranes. These findings formed the basis for current serologic assays that are referred to as nontreponemal tests. Subsequently methods using *T. pallidum* antigens were developed and are referred to as treponemal tests. Treponemal tests incorporate an absorption/dilution step to remove cross-reacting antibodies to nonpathogenic treponemes.

Both a nontreponemal test and a treponemal test are used in tandem in the evaluation of any form of syphilis, including suspected syphilitic eye disease (see box). A nontreponemal test is used for screening and quantitation of antibody titer, and a treponemal test is used for diagnostic confirmation of active or prior syphilis. Disease activity usually cor-

relates with antibody titers of nontreponemal tests but not of treponemal tests. Except for about 20% of patients treated during primary syphilis, a reactive treponemal test usually remains reactive for a lifetime.

HIV antibody testing is advised for all patients with syphilis. Retesting is considered 3 months after treatment for early syphilis.

Nontreponemal Tests. During syphilis, antilipoidal antibodies such as anticardiolipin are produced in response to the membrane lipids of *T. pallidum,* modified host lipids, or both. While the immunoglobulin class of antilipoidal antibodies varies with the stage of infection, the nontreponemal tests detect both IgG and IgM.

The Venereal Disease Research Laboratory (VDRL) test was developed in 1946 at the U.S. Centers for Disease Control to detect antilipoidal antibodies (formerly referred to as Wassermann antibodies or reagin). To perform the VDRL slide test, serum or cerebrospinal fluid is added to a mixture of 0.03% cardiolipin, 0.9% cholesterol, and 0.21% lecithin. The presence of antibody produces microscopic flocculation or clumping. In the quantitative VDRL test, serum or cerebrospinal fluid is serially diluted to determine the greatest dilution that is reactive. This dilution indicates the VDRL antibody titer.

The rapid plasma reagin (RPR) card test is a modification of the VDRL test that uses a 0.25% charcoal suspension. The cardiolipin-reagin lattice traps carbon particles to form macroscopically visible black aggregates. Because of rapidity and ease, the RPR test has supplanted the VDRL test in the United States for serum testing, but the VDRL test remains the only approved test for testing cerebrospinal fluid. Related tests include the automated reagin test and the reagin screen test. The same testing method should be used to follow individual patients. RPR titers tend to be slightly higher than corresponding VDRL titers.

Clinical Use. Anticardiolipin antibodies are detectable about one month after the initial infection, persist throughout secondary syphilis, and disappear from the bloodstream in about 25% of untreated individuals during late latent syphilis, tertiary syphilis, or neurosyphilis. In the rare case where secondary syphilis is clinically suspected but the nontreponemal test is nonreactive, a prozone phenomenon due to excess antibody could be responsible, and additional dilutions should be requested. Even without treatment the titer of a nontreponemal test declines slowly over time.

Following therapy repeat quantitative nontreponemal tests should be performed at 3, 6, and 12 months. More frequent testing should be performed for HIV-infected patients with serologic follow-up at 1, 2, 3, 6, 9, and 12 months after treatment.

A fourfold reduction in antibody titer (a change of at least two dilutions) of the same nontreponemal test is needed to demonstrate improvement. With adequate treatment for first-episode early syphilis, the titer declines fourfold by 3 to

---

SEROLOGIC TESTS FOR SYPHILIS

Nontreponemal Tests
  VDRL slide test
  Unheated serum reagin (USR) test
  RPR card test
  Toluidine red unheated serum test (TRUST)
  VISUWELL Reagin ELISA
Treponemal Tests
  FTA-ABS test
  FTA-ABS double-staining test (for incident light microscopy)
  MHA-TP test
  Captia syphilis G test
  Captia syphilis M test (for neonatal congenital syphilis)
  Olympus PK-TP test (for bloodbanking)
  ELISA IgG antitreponemal test (under development)
  Western immunoblot for IgG or IgM antitreponemal antibodies (under development)

Adapted from Larsen SA, Steiner BM, Rudolph AH: Laboratory diagnosis and interpretation of tests for syphilis, *Clin Microbiol Rev* 8:1-21, 1995.

6 months and often becomes nonreactive. Following treatment for late latent or tertiary syphilis, titers may decline more slowly. Approximately one half of patients will remain reactive in low titer, even though adequately treated. All patients with prior syphilis will have a slower decline in titer, regardless of stage. Titer changes of one serial dilution often occur and are not meaningful; only a fourfold or greater increase or decrease in titer is significant, although HIV-infected patients sometimes have fluctuating titers. Lack of expected reduction in the quantitative VDRL titer or an increase in titer suggests treatment failure or reinfection.

False-Positive Interpretation. A reactive VDRL or RPR test can infrequently be due to a biologic false-positive reaction by cross-reactive lipoidal antibodies. Of those with a reactive nontreponemal test, the biologic false-positivity rate is less than 2% in young adults. This rate may be greater in HIV-infected patients and is reported as high as 10% in a geriatric population. Common causes of transient (<6 months) biologic false-positive reactions are recent viral illness, immunization, intravenous drug use, and pregnancy. Approximately 75% of patients with chronic biologic false-positive VDRL tests show a positive lupus-anticoagulant or anticardiolipin test result. Conditions associated with phospholipid antibodies include connective-tissue disorders such as systemic lupus erythematosus and Sjögren syndrome, Behçet disease, Lyme disease, and HIV infection. Ocular features of anticardiolipin syndromes, especially systemic lupus erythematosus, can mimic syphilitic eye disease (such as retinal vasculitis[87] and optic neuritis) and have occurred in HIV-infected and other patients.

Other causes of chronic biologic false-positive reactions include advanced age, hypergammaglobulinemia (such as during leprosy, malaria, and myeloma), and intravenous drug use. Differentiation of a true-positive reaction from a biologic false-positive reaction is accomplished by use of a confirmatory treponemal test.

Treponemal Tests. Treponemal tests include the indirect fluorescent treponemal antibody absorbed (FTA-ABS) test and the microhemagglutination–*Treponema pallidum* (MHA-TP) test. These methods detect both IgG and IgM immunoglobulins to antigenic components of *T. pallidum*.

In the FTA-ABS test, heat-inactivated serum is diluted 1:5 with an absorbing diluent containing culture-filtrate components of *Treponema phagedenis* biotype Reiter to remove cross-reactive antibodies to commensal treponemes. The specimen is then applied onto slide-fixed, lyophilized *T. pallidum* (Nicols strain), and fluoresceinated antihuman immunoglobulin is added for detection by fluorescent microscopy. Intravenous fluorescein does not have an adverse effect on fluorescent treponemal antibody testing.[78] The FTA-ABS double-staining (DS) test incorporates fluorescein-labeled and rhodamine-labeled stains that facilitate use of new fluorescent microscopes with incident illumination.

In the MHA-TP test, serum is diluted 1:80 with absor-

bent and added to a microtiter plate containing lyophilized, formalinized sheep erythrocytes coated with *T. pallidum* fragments. A related assay, the *T. pallidum* hemagglutination (TPHA) test, is commonly used in Europe. A reactive pattern in these tests shows a smooth carpet of agglutinated erythrocytes. The interpretation of each of these specific tests is subjectively qualitative and is usually reported as reactive, borderline, or nonreactive.

Several enzyme-linked immunosorbent assays for anti-*T. pallidum* antibodies are currently being evaluated. Other developments include modifications that distinguish specific immunoglobulin classes (IgG and IgM) that might help to determine infection activity and treatment status.

Clinical Use. Specific tests remain reactive in 98% to 100% of untreated patients with secondary, latent, or late syphilis (Fig. 104-21) despite natural declines in VDRL titer. Most adequately treated patients, except for those treated during first-episode primary syphilis, will also remain reactive by a confirmatory test. Thus a reactive treponemal test indicates either current or prior syphilis and does not determine disease activity or need for treatment.

False-Positive Interpretation. Because of antigenic cross-reactivity, specific serologic tests for syphilis may be positive during other spirochetal infections such as nonvenereal treponematoses (bejel, yaws, and pinta) and Lyme borreliosis.[204] The nontreponemal tests will be reactive in patients with nonvenereal treponematoses but not in Lyme disease.

Cerebrospinal Fluid Testing

Laboratory investigation of neurosyphilis entails examination of cerebrospinal fluid obtained by lumbar puncture. No single test can make the diagnosis of neurosyphilis in all patients. Cerebrospinal fluid leukocytosis (>5 WBC/μL), protein changes, and presence of antibody detected by the VDRL test (RPR is not performed on cerebrospinal fluid) are the most useful laboratory tests. The most common ab-

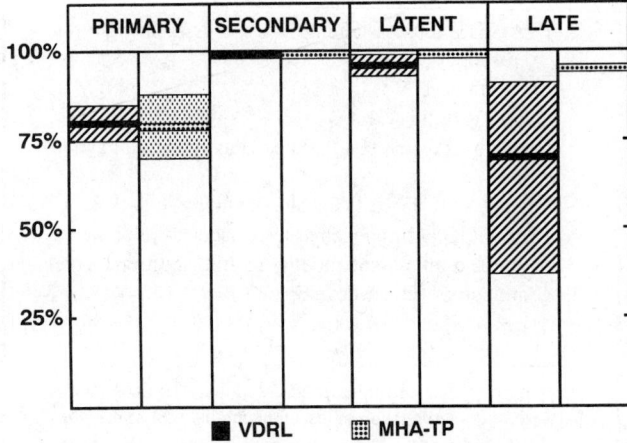

Fig. 104-21. Sensitivity of serologic tests in untreated syphilis.

normalities are mild mononuclear pleocytosis (10 to 400 cells/μL) and elevated protein (0.46 to 2.0 g/L).

Reactivity of the VDRL test in cerebrospinal fluid is a specific but relatively insensitive measure of neurosyphilis. A nonreactive VDRL test on cerebrospinal fluid does not rule out neurosyphilis. Treponemal tests of the cerebrospinal fluid are not generally performed; a reactive FTA-ABS or similar test is inconclusive because antitreponemal IgG antibodies can pass the intact blood-brain barrier, although the test is highly sensitive. Tests to detect antitreponemal IgM antibodies and diagnostic assays for identifying treponemal antigens and *T. pallidum* DNA in the cerebrospinal fluid are under development.

After successful treatment cerebrospinal fluid abnormalities gradually resolve. Inflammatory cells disappear first, then the protein concentration returns to normal, and subsequently the VDRL test becomes negative. Following treatment for neurosyphilis, repeat lumbar punctures should be performed at six-month intervals until the cerebrospinal fluid cell count is normal. Retreatment is considered if the cerebrospinal fluid is not normal by 2 years.

Ophthalmic Indications for Laboratory Evaluation

Serologic Testing. When ocular syphilis or neurosyphilis is clinically suspected, a treponemal test should be obtained.[31,124] A nonreactive treponemal test effectively excludes ocular or neuroophthalmic syphilis. For patients with a reactive treponemal test, a quantitative nontreponemal test, such as the VDRL or RPR test, provides a measure of disease activity and a baseline for subsequent comparison.

Common reasons for requesting serologic testing in ophthalmic practice are the following:

- Anterior or posterior uveitis, especially if not adequately responding to corticosteroid therapy
- Stromal keratitis, especially if herpes simplex eye disease has not been documented
- Scleritis, especially in a young or otherwise healthy patient
- Optic neuritis or progressive optic atrophy
- Pupillary abnormalities, especially light-near dissociation
- Unexplained intraocular inflammation in an HIV-infected individual.

Cerebrospinal Fluid Testing. Laboratory confirmation of neurosyphilis requires cerebrospinal fluid testing. The risk-benefit ratio of performing cerebrospinal fluid analysis during the course of syphilitic eye disease has not been assessed. Lumbar puncture is recommended for patients with syphilitic inflammation of the posterior segment of the eye (1) when there are signs of neurosyphilis such as cranial nerve palsies or pupillary changes and (2) when ocular inflammation occurs in an HIV-infected individual who has

had syphilis, even if previously treated. Cerebrospinal fluid testing of individuals with inactive ocular syphilis, such as residual corneal scarring and inactive uveitis, is based on evidence of prior adequate therapy. Although many individuals with ocular syphilis are treated as for neurosyphilis, cerebrospinal fluid analysis is generally advisable in order to assess intracranial disease activity and to provide a measure for future reference.

Indications for cerebrospinal fluid testing include the following:

- Intraocular inflammation
- Pupillary light-near dissociation
- Optic neuropathy, cranial nerve palsy, or other signs of neuroophthalmic dysfunction
- HIV infection
- Treatment failure, especially if titers increase fourfold
- Serum nontreponemal titer ≥ 1 : 32 for late syphilis.

THERAPY

The principal goals of treatment are to eliminate infectious spirochetes and to prevent or halt the progressive immune and structural responses that contribute to late complications. Because the metabolism and replication rate of *T. pallidum* may slow gradually from early to late syphilis, the dosage of antimicrobial agents that cures early syphilis may not eradicate organisms in late disease. Treatment recommendations (Table 104-6) are based on experimental and clinical observations.

Systemic Treatment

Penicillin remains the treatment of choice for syphilis.[70] The appropriate preparation and length of treatment depend on the stage of syphilis.

A minimal serum level of 0.03 units/ml (0.018 μg/ml) is treponemicidal. This effect is achievable by parenteral penicillin G benzathine, which can maintain treponemicidal serum levels for 7 to 10 days and can cure early syphilis. This form of penicillin, however, fails to cross the blood-brain barrier and does not consistently provide measurable levels in the cerebrospinal fluid and, possibly, in the intraocular fluids. The minimal level of penicillin in cerebrospinal or intraocular fluids that is needed to cure neurosyphilis or syphilitic eye disease has not been determined. Because of decreased drug penetration into these sites, higher doses for more prolonged periods are required for involvement of the central nervous system or the eye.

The efficacy of alternate antibiotics for late syphilis is uncertain, and inadequate therapy may predispose to relapse. Penicillin desensitization is recommended for penicillin-allergic patients who are pregnant or who have neurosyphilis. Penicillin allergy skin testing, by epicutaneous pricks or in-

TABLE 104-6 RECOMMENDED TREATMENT FOR SYPHILIS

Stage	Treatment	Alternative
Primary, secondary, or early (< 1 year) latent syphilis	Penicillin G benzathine 2.4 million units IM (for children: 50,000 units/kg IM, up to adult dose)	Doxycycline 100 mg PO bid for 14 days
Late (> 1 year) latent or tertiary syphilis, with normal CSF	Penicillin G benzathine 2.4 million units IM weekly for 3 successive weeks (for children: 50,000 units/kg IM weekly for 3 weeks, up to adult dose)	Doxycycline 100 mg PO bid for 28 days
Neurosyphilis (symptomatic or asymptomatic)	Penicillin G sodium 2-4 million units every 4 hours IV for 10-14 days[2] *or* Penicillin G procaine 2.4 million units/day IM plus probenecid 500 mg PO qid, both for 10-14 days[2]	None[3]
Any stage of syphilis in an HIV-infected patient	CSF exam is strongly encouraged. If abnormal CSF, treat as for neurosyphilis. If normal CSF, treat according to stage, with diligent follow-up.	Some authorities recommend penicillin G benzathine 2.4 million units IM weekly for 3 successive weeks, or amoxicillin 2 gm PO tid with probenecid 500 mg PO qid for 2-3 weeks, for HIV-infected patients with any stage of syphilis. No controlled studies have been conducted to determine efficacy of these regimens.
Congenital syphilis (infants)	Pencillin G sodium 50,000 units/kg every 8-12 hours IV for 10-14 days *or* Penicillin G procaine 50,000 units/kg/day IM for 10-14 days *or (if follow-up cannot be assured)* Penicillin G benzathine 50,000 units/kg IM in a single dose	None[3]
Pregnancy	Penicillin treatment according to stage, with monthly serologic testing	None[3]
Recent sexual contacts	Penicillin G benzathine 2.4 million units IM	Doxycycline 100 mg PO bid for 14 days
Syphilitic stromal keratitis or anterior uveitis	Pencillin treatment according to stage *and* Topical corticosteroid every 2-4 hours (± topical cycloplegic); taper until resolution of anterior-segment inflammation	None[3]
Syphilitic scleritis, posterior uveitis, or optic neuritis	Penicillin treatment for neurosyphilis *and* Oral prednisone 1 mg/kg PO with gradual taper	None[3]

[1]Ceftriaxone and amoxicillin have activity against *T. pallidum,* but appropriate doses, duration, and clinical efficacy of these agents have not been determined in controlled studies for any stage of syphilis.
[2]Some authorities recommend benzathine penicillin G 2.4 million units IM weekly for 3 successive weeks to follow IV or IM neurosyphilis therapy. Others recommend IV or IM therapy for 21 to 28 days instead of 10 to 14 days.
[3]No alternative to a penicillin is recommended. If penicillin hypersensitivity is confirmed by skin testing, the patient should be desensitized and treated with the recommended course of penicillin. Erythromycin is no longer recommended as alternative therapy.
For further information, refer to Centers for Disease Control and Prevention: 1993 sexually transmitted diseases treatment guidelines, *Morbid Mortal Week Rep* 42:27-46, 1993.

tradermal injections, and oral desensitization can usually be accomplished within a few hours. Doxycycline or tetracycline has been used for penicillin-allergic patients. Some macrolides (e.g., clarithromycin) and cephalosporins (e.g., ceftriaxone) are possible alternatives in tetracycline-intolerant individuals.

In patients without a normal immune response, recommended penicillin dosages may not be adequate. Although few prospective studies have been conducted, patients with HIV infection may require prolonged therapy for syphilis beyond standard dosages and are liable to relapses.[54a,117]

Asymptomatic neurosyphilis must be considered in any

patient with inadequately treated syphilis of more than one year's duration. The need for lumbar puncture should be based on the risks and benefits of diagnosing neurosyphilis.[193] HIV-infected patients with any stage of syphilis should have examination of cerebrospinal fluid and/or receive treatment for neurosyphilis.

When initiating penicillin therapy, patients should be carefully monitored for a Jarisch-Herxheimer reaction, a hypersensitivity response to treponemal antigens. In addition to multiple systemic effects, this reaction may exacerbate ocular inflammation, such as the optic neuritis of acquired syphilis, or precipitate acute neurological signs and pupillary changes. A systemic corticosteroid such as prednisone or dexamethasone is not used during uncomplicated syphilis but is suggested for controlling sight-threatening ocular inflammation.

The management of congenital syphilis depends upon the maternal status, the clinical stage, and the likelihood of neurosyphilis (Fig. 104-22). Alternative antibacterial agents are not used because newborns do not exhibit penicillin sensitivity. Careful evaluation during treatment is necessary because worsening of chorioretinitis and stromal keratitis can occur, presumably as a component of a Jarisch-Herxheimer reaction.

Follow-Up

Clinical evaluation and serologic testing determine treatment efficacy. An appropriate therapeutic response entails the following:

* Reexaminations until ocular inflammation resolves
* Follow-up serum nontreponemal tests that significantly decline in titer and become nonreactive (or stable at a low titer)
* Follow-up lumbar puncture until the cerebrospinal fluid becomes normal.

Serial, quantitative RPR or VDRL serum testing must be done to ensure an adequate therapeutic response. Retesting is recommended at 3, 6, and 12 months after treatment. Failure of the same high-titered nontreponemal test to decrease at least fourfold within a year indicates possible treatment failure or reinfection. Persons who have had prolonged or repeated infection before treatment or a high pretreatment titer are less likely to become seronegative subsequently following therapy. Most will retain a persistently reactive treponemal test.

Any abnormality of the cerebrospinal fluid should be considered suggestive of neurosyphilis. Posttreatment lumbar puncture should be done at six-month intervals until the cell count and protein level are normal and the VDRL titer is significantly lower or nonreactive.

Similar guidelines are used to assess adequacy of penicillin therapy in HIV-infected patients, but the roles of repeat serum and cerebrospinal fluid testing in these patients remain to be better determined.

General medical evaluation is necessary to screen for other sexually transmitted diseases in persons with syphilis. The detection of ocular syphilis should alert one to screen for other sexually transmitted diseases, some of which may or may not have ocular manifestations. The regional health department should be notified,[27] and contact-tracing considered. Recent sexual partners should be presumptively treated with single-dose intramuscular benzathine penicillin.

Ophthalmic Management

Viable treponemes might be able to survive within the eye despite prolonged antimicrobial therapy. Because penicillin penetrates poorly into the eye, sustained high dosages

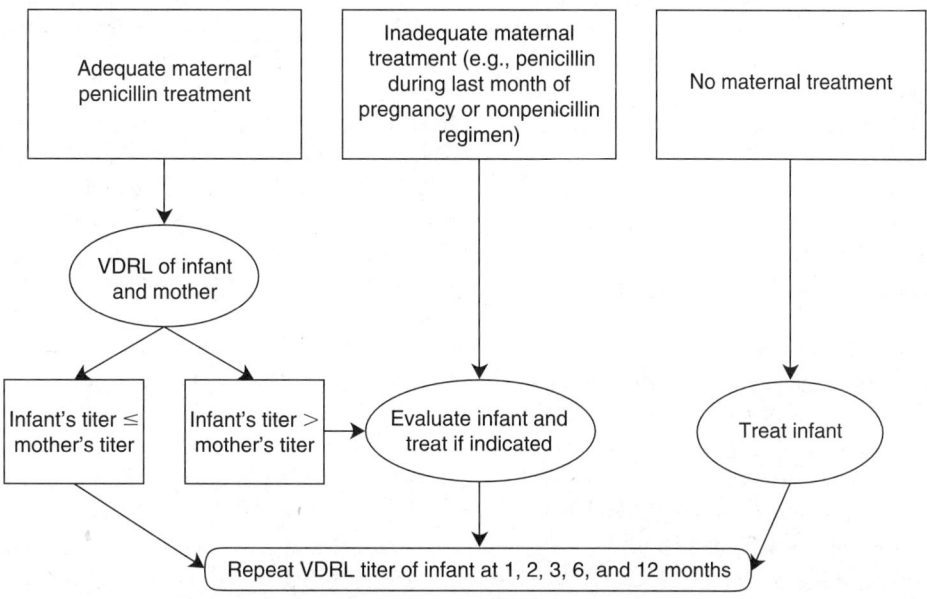

Fig. 104-22. Management of infants born to mothers with syphilis.

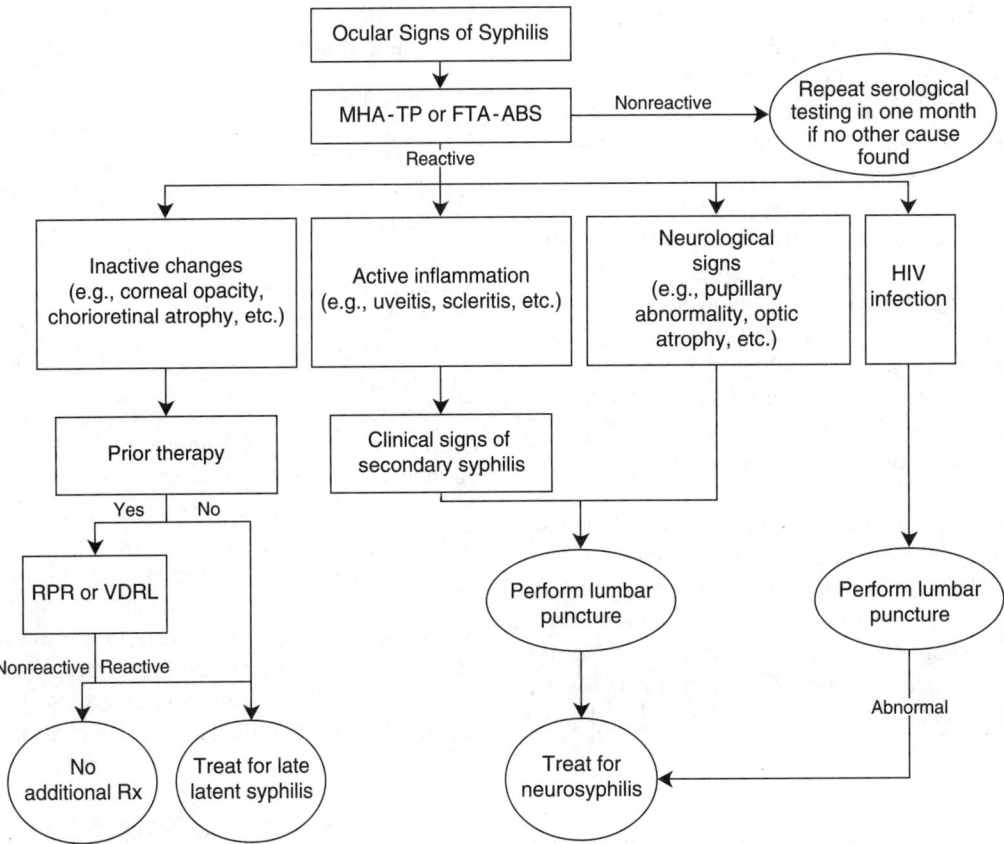

Fig. 104-23. Management of syphilitic eye disease. Quantitative serum RPR or VDRL testing is obtained at time of treatment for future comparisons to evaluate treatment efficacy. Examination of cerebrospinal fluid should be considered to detect asymptomatic neurosyphilis.

are needed.[41] Optimal therapy of syphilitic uveitis and other forms of syphilitic eye disease has not been completely determined.

Therapeutic decision-making for the treatment of syphilitic eye disease is based on prior treatment history, ocular and other signs of syphilis, and serologic testing (Fig. 104-23). Patients with active syphilis who have intraocular inflammation are treated as for neurosyphilis. The role of oral probenecid for enhancing penicillin levels has not been adequately assessed for ocular syphilis but might be a useful adjunct. The efficacy of alternate antibacterial agents such as tetracyclines and fluoroquinolones for the treatment of syphilitic eye disease in penicillin-allergic patients is uncertain, and penicillin desensitization is recommended for these individuals. Topical antibiotics are not needed for syphilitic eye disease.

Adjunctive corticosteroid therapy may be useful for some forms of ocular inflammation during syphilis. A topical corticosteroid can minimize corneal scarring and vascularization during stromal keratitis and can reduce the opportunity for postinflammatory sequelae of anterior uveitis but must sometimes be used for a prolonged period to limit recrudescences. An oral corticosteroid may be helpful for scleritis, posterior uveitis, and optic neuritis and for control of a Jarisch-Herxheimer reaction. Retrobulbar corticosteroid injection may speed resolution of syphilitic optic neuritis.[182] Corticosteroid therapy should never be used alone for ocular syphilis; antibiotic therapy is essential.

Penetrating keratoplasty, with or without cataract extraction, can be performed for residual corneal opacification.[89,135] Corneal opacification from syphilitic interstitial keratitis accounts for approximately 1% of all corneal transplants performed in the United States.[43] Postoperative complications such as glaucoma and allograft rejection may limit a successful outcome.

Permanent visual loss from ocular syphilis has been associated with postinflammatory changes of the posterior segment of the eye, such as retinal ischemia, optic atrophy, macular pigmentary atrophy, and epiretinal membrane. With perceptive clinical recognition, timely serologic testing, and appropriate medical management the blinding complications of syphilitic eye disease are preventable.

REFERENCES

1. Almenar J: De morbo gallica, 1502. In *A prooved practice for all young chirurgians,* London, 1588, Thomas Orwyn (Translated by W Clowes).
2. Appen RE, Wray SH, Cogan DG: Central retinal artery occlusion, *Am J Ophthalmol* 79:374-381, 1975.

3. Arruga J, Valentines J, Mauri F et al.: Neuroretinitis in acquired syphilis, *Ophthalmology* 92:262-270, 1985.
4. Baker BJ, Armelagos GJ: The origin and antiquity of syphilis: paleopathological diagnosis and interpretation, *Curr Anthropol* 29:703-720, 1988.
5. Barnes AC: Diagnosis in retrospect: Mary Tudor, *Obstet Gynecol* 1:585-590, 1953.
6. Barthelmess-Mosler S, Volcker HE: Iritis und Opticus-Meningitis. Erst symptome einer Lues latens, *Klin Monatsbl Augenheilkd* 190:196-198, 1987.
7. Beauvais DA, Michelson JB, Seybold ME et al.: Retroviruses and their play-pals, *Surv Ophthalmol* 34:59-64, 1989.
8. Becerra LI, Ksiazek SM, Savino PJ et al.: Syphilitic uveitis in human immunodeficiency virus–infected and noninfected patients, *Ophthalmology* 96:1727-1730, 1989.
9. Belin MW, Baltch AL, Hay PB: Secondary syphilitic uveitis, *Am J Ophthalmol* 92:210-214, 1981.
10. Berry CD, Hooton TM, Collier AC et al.: Neurologic relapse after benzathine penicillin therapy for secondary syphilis in a patient with HIV infection, *N Engl J Med* 316:1587-1589, 1987.
11. Bertarelli E: Ueber die Transmission der Syphilis auf das Kuninchen, *Zbl Bakt* I Abt 43:167-173, 238-245, 1907.
12. Bialasiewicz AA, Dommer S: Disseminierte Chorioiditis, Papillitis und Vaskulitis retinae als Leitbefund bei Lues II-III, *Klin Monatsbl Augenheilkd* 198:37-43, 1991.
13. Blodi FC, Hervouet F: Syphilitic chorioretinitis: a histologic study, *Arch Ophthalmol* 79:294-296, 1968.
14. Blount JH, Holmes KK: Epidemiology of syphilis and the nonvenereal treponematoses. In Johnson RC, editor: *The biology of parasitic spirochetes*, 157-176, New York, 1976, Academic Press.
15. Bodechtel G, Lund OE: Stauungspapille bei Lues, *Klin Monatsbl Augenheilkd* 175:829-831, 1979.
16. Bouisse V, Cochereau-Massin I, Jobin D et al.: Uvéite syphilitique et infection par le virus de l'immunodéficience humaine, *J Fr Ophtalmol* 14:605-609, 1991.
17. Brandt AM: *No magic bullet: a social history of venereal disease in the United States since 1880*, New York, 1987, Oxford University Press.
18. Brooks AM, Weiner JM, Roberston IF: Interstitial keratitis in untreated latent (late) syphilis, *Aust N Z J Ophthalmol* 14:127-132, 1986.
19. Bruetsch WL: *Syphilitic optic atrophy*, Springfield, Ill, 1953, Charles C Thomas.
20. Buck C: Papulo-ulceroses Syphilid - Lues maligna: ein kasuistischer Beitrag zur klinischen Symptomatik, *Hautarzt* 25:351-353, 1974.
21. Bulkley LD: Unusual methods of acquiring syphilis, with reports of cases, *JAMA* 12:174-176, 1889.
22. Burstain JM, Grimprel E, Lukehart SA et al.: Sensitive detection of *Treponema pallidum* by using the polymerase chain reaction, *J Clin Microbiol* 29:62-69, 1991.
23. Camerarius A, Breyer JF: *De Ophthalmia Venerea*, Tübingen, 1734.
24. Carter JB, Hamill RJ, Matoba AY: Bilateral syphilitic optic neuritis in a patient with a positive test for HIV, *Arch Ophthalmol* 105:1485-1486, 1987.
25. Centers for Disease Control: Primary and secondary syphilis: United States, 1981-1990, *MMWR* 40:314-315, 321-323, 1991.
26. Chapel TA: The signs and symptoms of secondary syphilis, *Sex Transm Dis* 7:161-164, 1980.
27. Chorba TL, Berkelman RL, Safford SK et al.: Mandatory reporting of infectious diseases by clinicians, *JAMA* 262:3018-3026, 1989.
28. Clark EG, Danbolt N: The Oslo study of the natural course of untreated syphilis: an epidemiologic investigation based upon a re-study of the Boeck-Bruusgaard material, *Med Clin North Am* 48:613-623, 1964.
29. Colombati S, Borri P, Tosti G et al.: Two cases of papillitis in patients with early syphilis, *Bull Soc Belge Ophtalmol* 220:69-73, 1986.
30. Conrad B, Benecke R, Musers H et al.: Visual evoked potentials in neurosyphilis, *J Neurol Neurosurg Psychiatry* 46:23-27, 1983.
31. Contreras F, Pereda J: Congenital syphilis of the eye with lens involvement, *Arch Ophthalmol* 96:1052-1053, 1978.
32. Cristiani R: Retinopati a pigmentosa a settore secondaria a leu acquisita, *Ann Ottal* 93:1099-1108, 1967.
33. Crouch ER Jr, Goldberg MF: Retinal periarteritis secondary to syphilis, *Arch Ophthalmol* 93:384-387, 1975.
34. Cunha de Souza E, Jalkh AE, Trempe CL et al.: Unusual central chorioretinitis as the first manifestation of early secondary syphilis, *Am J Ophthalmol* 105:271-276, 1988.
35. Currie JN, Coppeto JR, Lessell S: Chronic syphilitic meningitis resulting in superior orbital fissure syndrome and posterior fossa gumma: a report of two cases followed for 20 years, *J Clin Neuro Ophthalmol* 8:145-155, 1988.
36. Delcourt B, De Laey JP, Dernouchamps JP et al.: Un cas de séquelles oculaires et orbito-faciales de syphilis congénitale, *Bull Soc Belge Ophtalmol* 184:99-107, 1979.
37. DeLuise VP, Clark SW III, Smith JL: Syphilitic retinal detachment and uveal effusion, *Am J Ophthalmol* 94:757-761, 1982.
38. Deschenes J, Seamone C, Baines M: The ocular manifestations of sexually transmitted diseases, *Can J Ophthalmol* 25:177-185, 1990.
39. Deschenes J, Seamone CD, Baines MG: Acquired ocular syphilis: diagnosis and treatment, *Ann Ophthalmol* 24:134-138, 1992.
40. Deutsch TA, Tessler HH: Inflammatory pseudohistoplasmosis, *Ann Ophthalmol* 17:461-465, 1985.
40a. Dobos GJ, Wiek J, Kohler J et al.: Einseitige Erblindung bei Neurolues, *Wien Klin Wochenschr* 105:437-439, 1993.
41. Dunlop EM: Survival of treponemes after treatment: comments, clinical conclusions, and recommendations, *Genitourin Med* 61:293-301, 1985.
42. Eide N, Skjeldal O: Juxtapapillary chorioretinitis in neurosyphilis, *Acta Ophthalmol* 62:351-358, 1984.
43. *Eye banking statistics,* Washington, DC, 1994, Eye Bank Association of America.
44. Fewell AG: Unilateral neuroretinitis of syphilitic origin with a stellate figure at the macula, *Arch Ophthalmol* 8:615-616, 1932.
45. Fiala W, Schipper I, Klern R: Ein Fall von luischer Uveitis unter dem Bild des Morbus Harada, *Klin Monatsbl Augenheilkd* 190:53-55, 1987.
46. Fiumara NJ, Lessell S: The stigmata of late congenital syphilis: an analysis of 100 patients, *Sex Transm Dis* 10:126-129, 1983.
47. Fletcher WA, Sharpe JA: Tonic pupils in neurosyphilis, *Neurology* 36:188-192, 1986.
48. Folk JC, Weingeist TA, Corbett JJ et al.: Syphilitic neuroretinitis, *Am J Ophthalmol* 95:480-486, 1983.
49. Foss AJ, Hykin PG, Benjamin L: Interstitial keratitis and iridoschisis in congenital syphilis, *J Clin Neuro-ophthalmol* 12:167-170, 1992.
50. Fournier A: *Prophylaxie de la syphilis,* 238-243, Paris, 1903, J Rueff.
51. Fuchs J: Freidrich Nietzches Augenleiden, *Muench Med Wochenschr* 120:631-634, 1978.
52. Fujikawa LS, Haugen JP: Immunopathology of vitreous and retinochoroidal biopsy in posterior uveitis, *Ophthalmology* 97:1644-1653, 1990.
53. Gass JDM, Braunstein RA, Chenoweth RG: Acute syphilitic posterior placoid chorioretinitis, *Ophthalmology* 97:1288-1297, 1990.
54. Golden B, Thompson HS: Implications of spiral forms in the eye, *Surv Ophthalmol* 14:179-183, 1969.
54a. Gordon SM, Eaton ME, George R, et al.: The response of symptomatic neurosyphilis to high-dose intravenous penicillin G in patients with human immunodeficiency virus infection, *N Engl J Med* 331:1469-1473, 1994.
55. Grant WM: Late glaucoma after interstitial keratitis, *Am J Ophthalmol* 79:87-91, 1975.
56. Greene BM, Miller NR, Bynum TE: Failure of penicillin G benzathine in the treatment of neurosyphilis, *Arch Intern Med* 140:1117-1118, 1980.
57. Groenouw A. In Graefe A, Saemisch T, editors: *Handbuch der gesamten Augenkeilkunde,* vol 11, 737-862, Leipzig, 1904, W Engelmann.
58. Hall V, Waisbren BA: Syphilis as a major theme of James Joyce's *Ulysses, Arch Intern Med* 140:963-965, 1980.
59. Halperin LS: Neuroretinitis due to seronegative syphilis associated with human immunodeficiency virus, *J Clin Neuro-ophthalmol* 12:171-172, 1992.
60. Halperin LS, Berger AS, Grand MG: Syphilitic disc edema and periphlebitis, *Retina* 10:223-225, 1990.

61. Halperin LS, Lewis H, Blumenkranz MS et al.: Choroidal neovascular membrane and other chorioretinal complications of acquired syphilis, *Am J Ophthalmol* 108:554-562, 1989.

62. Hamed LM, Schatz NJ, Galetta SL: Brainstem ocular motility defects and AIDS, *Am J Ophthalmol* 106:437-442, 1988.

62a. Harada T, Sakamoto R, Nagata A, Majima Y: Uvéite syphilitique, *J Fr Ophtalmol* 17:394-398, 1994.

63. Harden AF, Wright DJM: Clinical aspects of treponemal eye disease: a report of 21 cases, *Proc R Soc Med* 67:817-819, 1974.

64. Heckenlively J: Secondary retinitis pigmentosa, *Doc Ophthalmol Proc* 13:245-248, 1977.

65. Hemady R, Sainz de la Maza M, Raizman MB et al.: Six cases of scleritis associated with systemic infection, *Am J Ophthalmol* 114:55-62, 1992.

66. Henderly DE, Genstler AJ, Smith RE et al.: Changing patterns of uveitis, *Am J Ophthalmol* 103:131-136, 1987.

67. Hewson T: *Observations on the history and the treatment of the ophthalmia accompanying the secondary forms of lues venerea,* London, 1824, Longman, Harst, Rees, Orme, Brown, & Green.

68. Hill JC, Maske R, Bowen RM: Secondary localized amyloidosis of the cornea associated with tertiary syphilis, *Cornea* 9:98-101, 1990.

69. Hira SK, Patel JS, Bhat SG et al.: Clinical manifestations of secondary syphilis, *Int J Dermatol* 26:103-107, 1987.

70. Hook EW III, Marra CM: Acquired syphilis in adults, *N Engl J Med* 326:1060-1069, 1992.

71. Hooshmand H, Escobar MR, Kopf SW: Neurosyphilis, a study of 241 patients, *JAMA* 219:726-729, 1972.

72. Huismans H: Angiopathia retinae syphilitica bei Lues latens seropositiva, *Klin Monatsbl Augenheilkd* 184:48-50, 1984.

73. Hungerbühler U, Kulstrunk M, Osusky R: Uveitis luetica bei einem AIDS-patienten, *Schweiz Med Wochenschr* 118:1762-1766, 1988.

74. Hutchinson J: *A clinical memoir on certain diseases of the eye and ear, consequent on inherited syphilis,* London, 1863, John Churchill. (Republished as Gryphon edition, Birmingham, Ala, 1984, Classics of Ophthalmology Library.)

75. Igersheimer J: *Syphilis und Auge,* Berlin, 1918, Julius Springer.

76. Jeyakumar W, Chithra A, Shanmugasundararaj A: Primary syphilis of the eyelid: case report, *Genitourin Med* 65:192-193, 1989.

77. Johns DR, Tierney M, Felsenstein D: Alteration in the natural history of neurosyphilis by concurrent infection with the human immunodeficiency virus, *N Engl J Med* 316:1569-1572, 1987.

78. Jost BF, Olk RJ, Spurrier MH et al.: Effect of intravenous fluorescein on fluorescent treponemal antibody testing, *Am J Ophthalmol* 102:278-279, 1986.

79. Joyce PW, Haye KR, Ellis ME: Syphilitic retinitis in a homosexual man with concurrent HIV infection: case report, *Genitourin Med* 65:244-247, 1989.

80. Kanai A, Kaufman HE: The retrocorneal ridge in syphilitic and herpetic interstitial keratitis: an electron-microscopic study, *Ann Ophthalmol* 14:120-124, 1982.

81. Katz DA, Berger JR: Neurosyphilis in acquired immunodeficiency syndrome, *Arch Neurol* 46:895-898, 1989.

82. Kelly EC: Sir Jonathan Hutchinson, *Med Classics* 5(3):107-245, 1940.

83. Kerty E, Eide N, Skjeldal O: Visual evoked response in syphilitic optic atrophy: a case report, *Acta Ophthalmol* 64:553-556, 1986.

84. Khamaganova AV, Guseikhanova AG: Izolirovannoe porazhenie zritel'nykh i slukhovykh nervov u bol'noi vtorichnym retsidivnym sifiolisom, *Vestn Dermatol Venerol* (1):74-75, 1988.

85. Klaude JV, Robertson HF: The Wills Hospital clinic for the treatment of ocular syphilis, *Am J Ophthalmol* 13:285-294, 1930.

86. Kleiner RC, Najarian L, Levenson J et al.: AIDS complicated by syphilis can mimic uveitis and Crohn's disease, *Arch Ophthalmol* 105:1486-1487, 1987.

87. Klok AM, Geertzen R, Rothova A et al.: Anticardiolipin antibodies in uveitis, *Curr Eye Res* 11(suppl):209-213, 1992.

88. Kranias G, Schneider D, Raymond LA: A case of syphilitic uveitis, *Am J Ophthalmol* 91:261-263, 1981.

89. Lagoutte F, Dupuy P: L'association kératite interstitielle/cataracte sénile, ses particularities clinics et chirurgicales: à propos de 10 cas, *Bull Soc Ophtalmol Fr* 82:723-724, 1982.

90. Lanigan-O'Keeffe FM: Return to normal of Argyll-Robertson pupils after treatment, *BMJ* 2:1191-1192, 1977.

91. Lawrence W: *A treatise on the venereal diseases of the eye,* London, 1830, John Wilson.

92. Lee ME, Lindquist TD: Syphilitic interstitial keratitis, *JAMA* 262:2921, 1989.

93. Levy JH, Liss RA, Maguire AM: Neurosyphilis and ocular syphilis in patients with concurrent human immunodeficiency virus infection, *Retina* 9:175-180, 1989.

94. Lichter PR, Shaffer RN: Interstitial keratitis and glaucoma, *Am J Ophthalmol* 68:241-248, 1969.

95. Lim SH, Heng LK, Puvanendran K: Secondary syphilis presenting with optic perineuritis and uveitis, *Ann Acad Med Singapore* 19:413-415, 1990.

96. Lobes LA Jr, Folk JC: Syphilitic phlebitis simulating branch vein occlusion, *Ann Ophthalmol* 13:825-827, 1981.

97. Loewenfeld IE: The Argyll Robertson pupil, 1869-1969: a critical survey of the literature, *Surv Ophthalmol* 14:199-299, 1969.

98. Lukehart SA, Hook EW III, Baker-Zander SA et al.: Invasion of the central nervous system by *Treponema pallidum:* implications for diagnosis and treatment, *Ann Intern Med* 109:855-862, 1988.

99. Lyons JB: *Thrust syphilis down to hell and other rejoyceana: studies in the border-lands of literature and medicine,* Dublin, 1988, Glendale Press.

100. MacFaul PA, Catterall RD: Acute choroido-retinitis in secondary syphilis: presence of spiral organisms in the aqueous humour, *Br J Vener Dis* 47:159-161, 1971.

101. Mancel E, Huet-Ernould F, Hugues P et al.: Uvéites syphilitiques, *Bull Soc Ophtalmol Fr* 90:199-204, 1990.

102. Mansour AM: Neuro-ophthalmic findings in acquired immunodeficiency syndrome, *J Clin Neuro-ophthalmol* 10:167-174, 1990.

103. Margo CE, Hamed LM: Ocular syphilis, *Surv Ophthalmol* 37:203-220, 1992.

104. Marra C, Baker-Zander SA, Hook III EW et al.: An experimental model of early central nervous system syphilis, *J Infect Dis* 163:825-829, 1991.

105. Martinez JA, Sutphin JE: Syphilitic interstitial keratitis masquerading as staphylococcal marginal keratitis, *Am J Ophthalmol* 107:431-433, 1989.

106. Maw AR: Bobbing oscillopsia, *Ann Otol Rhinol Laryngol* 80:233-239, 1971.

107. McBurney J, Rosenberg ML: Unilateral syphilitic optic perineuritis presenting as the big blind spot syndrome, *J Clin Neuro-ophthalmol* 7:167-169, 1987.

108. McCarron MJ, Albert DM: Iridocyclitis and iris mass associated with secondary syphilis, *Ophthalmology* 91:1264-1268, 1984.

109. McCrary III JA: The pupil in syphilis. In Smith JL, editor: *Neuro-ophthalmology,* vol 6, 164-182, St Louis, 1972, Mosby.

110. McKusick VA: The clinical observations of Jonathan Hutchinson, *Am J Syphil Gonor Vener Dis* 36:101-126, 1952.

111. McLeish WM, Pulido JS, Holland S et al.: The ocular manifestations of syphilis in the human immunodeficiency virus type 1-infected host, *Ophthalmology* 97:196-203, 1990.

112. Mendelsohn AD, Jampol LM: Syphilitic retinitis: a cause of necrotizing retinitis, *Retina* 4:221-224, 1984.

113. Merritt HH, Adams RD, Solomon HC: *Neurosyphilis,* New York, 1946, Oxford University Press.

114. Moore JE: Syphilitic iritis: a study of 249 patients, *Am J Ophthalmol* 14:110-126, 1931.

115. Morgan CM, Webb RM, O'Connor GR: Atypical syphilitic chorioretinitis and vasculitis, *Retina* 4:225-231, 1984.

116. Moriwaka F, Tashiro K, Matsuura T et al.: Three cases of syphilitic optic atrophy: its clinical features and significance, *No To Shinkei* 39:375-379, 1987.

117. Musher DM, Baughn RE: Neurosyphilis in HIV-infected persons, *N Engl J Med* 331:1516-1517, 1994.

118. Musher DM, Hamill RJ, Baughn RE: Effect of human immunodeficiency virus (HIV) infection on the course of syphilis and on the response to treatment, *Ann Intern Med* 113:872-881, 1990.

119. Nabarro DN: *Congenital syphilis,* Baltimore, 1954, Williams & Wilkins.

120. Neetens A, Smets RM: Ocular complications of neuro-syphilis, *Bull Soc Belge Ophtalmol* 213:83-86, 1986.

121. Neetens A, Smets RM: Ocular lues: a disease wearing many masks, *Bull Soc Belge Ophtalmol* 218:145-152, 1986.

122. Nicol WG, Rios-Montenegro EN, Smith JL: Congenital ocular syphilis, *Am J Ophthalmol* 68:467-471, 1969.
123. Noordhoek GT, Wolters EC, de Jonge ME et al.: Detection by polymerase chain reaction of *Treponema pallidum* DNA in cerebrospinal fluid from neurosyphilis patients before and after antibiotic treatment, *J Clin Microbiol* 29:1976-1984, 1991.
124. O'Connor GR: An interesting case history, *Proctor Bull* 2:1, 1979.
125. O'Day J, Shilling JS, ffytche TJ: Retinal vasculitis, *Trans Ophthalmol Soc U K* 99:163-166, 1979.
126. Oksala A: Studies on interstitial keratitis associated with congenital syphilis occurring in Finland, *Acta Ophthalmol* 30(suppl 38):1-109, 1952.
127. Oliver M, Beller AJ, Behar A: Chiasmal arachnoiditis as a manifeston of generalized arachnoiditis in systemic vascular disease: clinico-pathological report of two cases, *Br J Ophthalmol* 52:227-235, 1968.
128. Osler W: The campaign against syphilis, *Lancet* 1:787-792, 1917.
128a. Ouano DP, Brucker AJ, Saran BR: Macular pseudohypopyon from secondary syphilis, *Am J Ophthalmol* 119:372-374, 1995.
129. Page NGR, Lean JS, Sanders MD: Vertical supranuclear gaze palsy with secondary syphilis, *J Neurol Neurosurg Psychiatry* 45:86-88, 1982.
130. Passo MS, Rosenbaum JT: Ocular syphilis in patients with human immunodeficiency virus infection, *Am J Ophthalmol* 106:1-6, 1988.
131. Pearson PA, Amrien JM, Baldwin LB et al.: Iridoschisis associated with syphilitic interstitial keratitis, *Am J Ophthalmol* 107:88-90, 1989.
132. Primo S: Central retinal vein occlusion in a young patient with sero-positive syphilis, *J Am Optom Assoc* 61:896-902, 1990.
133. Putkonen T: Does early treatment prevent dental changes in congenital syphilis? *Acta Derm Venereol* 43:240-249, 1963.
134. Quétel C: *History of syphilis,* Baltimore, 1990, Johns Hopkins University Press.
135. Rabb MF, Fine M: Penetrating keratoplasty in interstitial keratitis, *Am J Ophthalmol* 67:907-917, 1969.
136. Radolf JD, Kaplan RP: Unusual manifestations of secondary syphilis and abnormal humoral immune response to *Treponema pallidum* antigens in a homosexual man with asymptomatic human immunodeficiency virus infection, *J Am Acad Dermatol* 18:423-428, 1988.
137. Randolph ME: An experimental study of the possibility of transmitting syphilis by a corneal graft, *Am J Ophthalmol* 35:352-357, 1952.
138. Rapkin JS, Bogorad DD: Bilateral dislocation of the crystalline lens in a patient with presumed syphilitic uveitis, *Henry Ford Hosp Med J* 34:207-210, 1986.
139. Rasmussen DH: The treatment of syphilis, *Surv Ophthalmol* 14:184-197, 1969.
140. Rasool MN, Govender S: The skeletal manifestations of congenital syphilis: a review of 197 cases, *J Bone Joint Surg* 71:752-755, 1989.
141. Ratier C, Zenatti C, Bousquet A et al.: Sur un cas d'uvéite syphilitique révélant une syphilis secondaire, *Bull Soc Ophtalmol Fr* 86:15-18, 1986.
142. Regan CD, Foster CS: Retinal vascular diseases: clinical presentation and diagnosis, *Int Ophthalmol Clin* 26(2):25-53, 1986.
143. Renard G, Dhermy P, Pouliquen Y: Dystrophies endothelio-descemetiques secondaires: etude histologique et ultrastructurale, *J Fr Ophtalmol* 4:721-739, 1981.
144. Richards BW, Hessburg TJ, Nussbaum JN: Recurrent syphilitic uveitis, *N Engl J Med* 320:62, 1989.
145. Rockwell DH, Yobs AR, Moore Jr MB: The Tuskegee study of untreated syphilis: the 30th year of observation, *Arch Intern Med* 114:792-798, 1964.
146. Rolfs RT, Nakashima AK: Epidemiology of primary and secondary syphilis in the United States, 1981 through 1989, *JAMA* 264:1432-1437, 1990.
147. Rosenbaum LJ, Podos SM: Traumatic ectopia lentis: some relationships to syphilis and glaucoma, *Am J Ophthalmol* 64:1095-1098, 1967.
148. Rosenhall ULF, Lowhagen G-B, Roupe G: Oculomotor dysfunction in patients with syphilis, *Genitourin Med* 63:83-86, 1987.
149. Ross WH, Sutton HF: Acquired syphilitic uveitis, *Arch Ophthalmol* 98:496-498, 1980.
150. Rush JA, Ryan EJ: Syphilitic optic perineuritis, *Am J Ophthalmol* 91:404-406, 1981.
151. Saari M: Disciform detachment of the macula. III. Secondary to inflammatory diseases, *Acta Ophthalmol* 56:510-517, 1978.
152. Sachedina S, Greiner JV, Glonek T: Membrane phospholipids of the ocular tunica fibrosa, *Invest Ophthalmol Vis Sci* 32:625-632, 1991.
153. Sacks JG, Osher RH, Elconin H: Progressive visual loss in syphilitic optic atrophy, *J Clin Neuro-ophthalmol* 3:5-8, 1983.
154. Sanders MD: Ischaemic papillopathy, *Trans Ophthalmol Soc UK* 91:369-386, 1971.
155. Savir H, Kurz O: Fluorescein angiography in syphilitic retinal vasculitis, *Ann Ophthalmol* 8:713-716, 1976.
156. Scattergood KD, Green WR, Hirst LW: Scrolls of Descemet's membrane in healed syphilitic interstitial keratitis, *Ophthalmology* 90:1518-1523, 1983.
157. Schaffer DB: Eye findings in intrauterine infections, *Clin Perinatol* 8:415-443, 1981.
158. Schatz NJ, Smith JL: Non-tumor causes of the Foster Kennedy syndrome, *J Neurosurg* 27:37-44, 1967.
159. Schlaegel TF Jr, Kao SF: A review (1970-1980) of 28 presumptive cases of syphilitic uveitis, *Am J Ophthalmol* 93:412-414, 1982.
160. Schulman JA, Peyman GA: Syphilitic gummatous iridocyclitis, *Ann Ophthalmol* 21:333-336, 1989.
161. Schwab IR, Armstrong MA, Friedman GD et al.: Cataract extraction: risk factors in a health maintenance organization population under 60 years of age, *Arch Ophthalmol* 106:1062-1065, 1988.
162. Schwartz LL, O'Connor GR: Secondary syphilis with iris papules, *Am J Ophthalmol* 90:380-384, 1980.
163. Sharma VK, Chander RAM, Kumar B et al.: Condylomata lata of the eyelids, *Genitourin Med* 65:124-125, 1989.
164. Shin DH, Kass MA, Kolker AE et al.: Positive FTA-ABS tests in subjects with corticosteroid-induced uveitis, *Am J Ophthalmol* 82:259-260, 1976.
165. Skalka HW: Asymmetric retinitis pigmentosa, luetic retinopathy and the question of unilateral retinitis pigmentosa, *Acta Ophthalmol* 57:351-357, 1979.
166. Smith JL: *Spirochetes in late seronegative syphilis, penicillin notwithstanding,* 137-155, Springfield, Ill, 1969, Charles C Thomas.
167. Smith JL: Testing for congenital syphilis in interstitial keratitis, *Am J Ophthalmol* 72:816-820, 1971.
168. Smith JL: Acute blindness in early syphilis, *Arch Ophthalmol* 90:256-258, 1973.
169. Smith JL, Byrne SF, Cambron CR: Syphiloma/gumma of the optic nerve and human immunodeficiency virus seropositivity, *J Clin Neuro-ophthalmol* 10:175-184, 1990.
170. Smith JL, Crumpton BC, Hummer J: The Bascom Palmer Eye Institute Lyme/syphilis survey, *J Clin Neuro-ophthalmol* 10:255-260, 1990.
171. Smith JL, Israel CW, Harner RE: Syphilitic temporal arteritis, *Arch Ophthalmol* 78:284-288, 1967.
172. Snyers B, Coche F: Uvéite syphilitique: à propos de deux cas, *Bull Soc Belge Ophtalmol* 239:79-86, 1990.
173. Spektor FE, Eagle RC Jr, Nichols CW: Granulomatous conjunctivitis secondary to *Treponema pallidum, Ophthalmology* 88:863-865, 1981.
174. Spicer WTH: Parenchymatous keratitis: intersitital keratitis: uveitis anterior, *Br J Ophthalmol* 8(Suppl 1):1-63, 1924.
175. Spoor TC, Ramocki JM, Nesi FA et al.: Ocular syphilis 1986: prevalence of FTA-ABS reactivity and cerebrospinal fluid findings, *J Clin Neuro-ophthalmol* 7:191-195, 1987.
176. Spoor TC, Wynn P, Hartel WC et al.: Ocular syphilis: acute and chronic, *J Clin Neuro-ophthalmol* 3:197-203, 1983.
177. Stoumbos VD, Klein ML: Syphilitic retinitis in a patient with acquired immunodeficiency syndrome-related complex, *Am J Ophthalmol* 103:103-104, 1987.
178. Susac JO, Hardman JM, Selhorst JB: Microangiopathy of the brain and retina, *Neurology* 29:313-316, 1979.
179. Tait IA: Uveitis due to secondary syphilis, *Br J Vener Dis* 59:397-401, 1983.
180. Tamesis RR, Foster CS: Ocular syphilis, *Ophthalmology* 97:1281-1287, 1990.
181. Terrien F: *Syphilis de l'oeil et de ses annexes,* Paris, 1905, G. Steinheil.
182. Tomsak RL, Lystad LD, Katirji MB et al.: Rapid response of syphilitic optic neuritis to posterior sub-tenon's steroid injection, *J Clin Neuro-ophthalmol* 12:6-7, 1992.
183. Toshniwal P: Optic perineuritis with secondary syphilis, *J Clin Neuro-ophthalmol* 7:6-10, 1987.

184. Touboul JP, LeHoang P, Fontaine M et al.: Uvéites au cours de la syphilis acquise, *J Fr Ophtalmol* 8:321-331, 1985.

185. Tsukahara S: Secondary glaucoma due to inactive congenital syphilitic interstitial keratitis, *Ophthalmologica* 174:188-194, 1977.

186. Van Effenterre G, Haut J, Robineau E et al.: Manifestations ophtalmologiques de la syphilis: a propos de cinq cas, *Bull Soc Ophtalmol Fr* 81:21-25, 1981.

187. Veldman E, Bos PJ: Neuroretinintis in secondary syphilis, *Doc Ophthalmol* 64:23-29, 1986.

188. Volpi U: Pseudo-retinopatia pigmentosa da lue acquisita, *Ann Ottal* 92:408-414, 1966.

189. Waring GO, Font RL, Rodrigues MM et al.: Alterations of Descemet's membrane in interstitial keratitis, *Am J Ophthalmol* 81:773-785, 1976.

190. Watanabe K, Tanahashi N, Nara M: Neurosyphilis presenting with Raeder's syndrome, *Ann Neurol* 25:418, 1989.

191. Weinstein JM, Lexow SS, Ho P et al.: Acute syphilitic optic neuritis, *Arch Ophthalmol* 99:1392-1395, 1981.

192. Wicher K, Noordhoek GT, Abbruscato F et al.: Detection of *Treponema pallidum* in early syphilis by DNA amplification, *J Clin Microbiol* 30:497-500, 1992.

193. Wiesel J, Rose DN, Silver AL et al.: Lumbar puncture in asymptomatic late syphilis: an analysis of the benefits and risks, *Arch Intern Med* 145:465-468, 1985.

194. Wilhelmus KR: The history of ocular syphilis. In Bialasiewicz AA, Schaal KP, editors: *Infectious diseases of the eye,* 494-499, Buren, The Netherlands, 1994, Eolus Press.

195. Wilhelmus KR: Syphilis and the eye. In Bialasiewicz AA, Schaal KP, editors: *Infectious diseases of the eye,* 499-511, Buren, The Netherlands, 1994, Eolus Press.

196. Wilhelmus KR, Yokoyama CM: Syphilitic episcleritis and scleritis, *Am J Ophthalmol* 104:595-597, 1987.

197. Wilkes TD: The complications of dermal tattooing, *Ophthalmic Plast Reconstr Surg* 2:1-6, 1986.

198. Winward KE, Hamed LM, Glaser JS. The spectrum of optic nerve disease in human immunodeficiency virus infection, *Am J Ophthalmol* 107:373-380, 1989.

199. Woods AC: Syphilis of the eye, *Am J Syphil Gonor Vener Dis* 27:133-186, 1943.

200. Yagasaki T, Akiyama K, Nomura H et al.: Two cases of acquired syphilis with acute central chorioretinitis as initial manifestation, *Jpn J Ophthalmol* 36:301-309, 1992.

201. Yasaki S, Ohshima J, Yonekura J et al.: A case of early syphilis presenting general paresis-like symptoms and bilateral tonic pupils, *Rinsho Shinkeigaku* 32:994-999, 1992.

202. Zaidman GW: Neurosyphilis and retrobulbar neuritis in a patients with AIDS, *Ann Ophthalmol* 18:260-261, 1986.

203. Zambrano W, Perez GM, Smith JL: Acute syphilitic blindness in AIDS, *J Clin Neuro-ophthalmol* 7:1-5, 1987.

204. Zierhut M, Kreissig I, Pickert A: Panuveitis with positive serological tests for syphilis and Lyme disease, *J Clin Neuro-ophthalmol* 9:71-75, 1989.

205. Zwink FB, Dunlop EM: Clinically silent anterior uveitis in secondary syphilis, *Trans Ophthalmol Soc UK* 96:148-150, 1976.

105 Endemic Syphilis (Bejel)

KHALID F. TABBARA

There are three major genera of the order Spirochaetales: (1) *Treponema*, (2) *Borrelia*, and (3) *Leptospira*. The pathogenic forms of *Treponema* include *Treponema pallidum*, the causative agent of syphilis; *Treponema pallidum endemicum*, the causative agent of bejel; *Treponema pertenue*, the causative agent of yaws; *Treponema carateum*, the causative agent of pinta; and *Treponema paraluis-cuniculi*, the causative agent of rabbit syphilis. Other *Treponema* are nonpathogenic and form a part of the normal oral flora, including *Treponema macrodentium* and *Treponema vincentii*.

Treponema makes up a group of interrelated organisms that are separated by differences in the types of disorders they produce. The infections caused by *Treponema* are known as treponematoses. Treponematoses fall into four major groups: (1) venereal syphilis, (2) bejel, (3) yaws, and (4) pinta.

HISTORICAL BACKGROUND

It is speculated that treponemal species have their origin in tree-living monkeys of tropical Africa. Inhabitants of dry hot regions of North Africa developed a nonvenereal form of syphilis (bejel), transmitted by bodily contact among adults. Man then served as the main host reservoir for this infection for thousands of years and carried treponemes to the Americas, where they produce yaws or pinta in their new home.

EPIDEMIOLOGY

Bejel occurs in parts of East Africa, the Near East, and Southeast Asia. The disease has also been reported in Bosnia-Herzegovina. Prior to mass treatment under the supervision of the WHO, patients with nonvenereal syphilis made up as much as 5% of the population in endemic areas. Active infection is much less common but still not eradicated.[3] The prevalence of the disease has been decreasing in many parts of the world.[1,4]

The current patchy distribution of the disease is predominantly related to inadequate health services and to an increase in atypical and subclinical forms of the disease. Many clinicians are not familiar with this entity. Furthermore, the disease cannot be differentiated from venereal syphilis on serologic grounds. All available serologic assays for syphilis would be positive in patients with nonvenereal syphilis.

CLINICAL FEATURES

Patients with bejel may develop primary mucocutaneous lesions around the mouth in early childhood. Secondary bejel may occur with skin rash. Osteomyelitis and gumma-like lesions may occur in the tibia in the tertiary stages of the disease. Late manifestations include saddlenose and other facial deformities.[2] Cardiovascular and congenital lesions have not been reported with bejel.

The most frequently encountered ocular lesions consist of anterior uveitis, choroiditis, and chorioretinitis.[5,6] The uveitis may be granulomatous or nongranulomatous. The box summarizes the ocular findings among patients with endemic syphilis (bejel). The majority of patients with bejel have asymptomatic disease.

PATHOGENESIS

As with venereal syphilis, man is the only reservoir of the infection. The onset of the disease is in early childhood, and the infection is usually transmitted via nonvenereal routes: intimate skin contact, kissing, and the use of common fomites or drinking vessels.[1] Familial transmission is common, but congenital transmission has not been reported. The disease is common among nomads but rare in urban communities.[1]

LABORATORY INVESTIGATIONS

All serologic tests for syphilis are positive in patients with bejel, including nonspecific tests (VDRL, and so on) and specific tests (FTA-ABS and MHA-TP). Bejel cannot be differentiated from venereal syphilis on serologic

---

OCULAR MANIFESTATIONS OF ENDEMIC SYPHILIS (BEJEL)

Active Inflammation
  Iridocyclitis
  Choroiditis
  Chorioretinitis
Residual Changes
  Iris atrophy
  Cataract
  Vitreous opacities
  Patchy choroidal atrophy
  Attenuated retinal arterioles
  Optic atrophy

---

grounds. Scrapings may be obtained from skin lesions, and spirochetes may be seen in smears by dark-field microscopy.

THERAPY

The treatment of choice is systemic penicillin therapy consisting of 2.4 million units of benzathine penicillin intramascularly once a week for 3 weeks. Topical mydriatics and prednisolone acetate 1% eye drops may be used for patients with active anterior uveitis. Intraocular inflammation does not respond to systemic penicillin alone.

PREVENTION

Bejel is a preventable and curable cause of uveitis. Early diagnosis and prompt treatment with penicillin may prevent the irreversible damage to the ocular structures. It is not known if bejel affords protection against venereal syphilis.

REFERENCES

1. Csonka GW, Pace JL: Endemic nonvenereal syphilis (bejel) in Saudi Arabia, *Rev Infect Dis* 7(suppl 2):S260-S265, 1985.
2. Erdelyi RL, Molla AA: Burned-out endemic syphilis (bejel): facial deformities and defects in Saudi Arabia, *Plast Reconstr Surg* 74:589-602, 1984.
3. Meheus A, Antal GM: The endemic treponematoses: not yet eradicated, *World Health Stat Q* 45:228-237, 1992.
4. Pace JL: Treponematosis in Saudi Arabia, *Saudi Med J* 4:211-220, 1983.
5. Tabbara KF: Endemic syphilis (bejel), *Int Ophthalmol* 14:379-381, 1990.
6. Tabbara KF, Al Kaff AS, Fadel T: Ocular manifestations of bejel, *Ophthalmology* 96:1087-1091, 1989.

106 Lyme Borreliosis

JOHN R. WITTPENN, PATRICK A. SIBONY, RAYMOND J. DATTWYLER

Lyme disease is a worldwide tick-borne borreliosis with endemic foci distributed throughout North America, Europe, and Northern Asia. Within the United States Lyme disease has become the leading tick-borne infectious disease, and the known range of the tick vector has continued to expand since the disease was first identified (Fig. 106-1).

HISTORICAL BACKGROUND

Erythema chronicum migrans was first noted in 1909 when Afzelius described a skin rash following a tick bite by the sheep tick *Ixodes ricinus,* which was ringlike and migrated by expanding its peripheral borders with central clearing.[4] The term erythema chronicum migrans was coined in 1913 by Lipschütz when he described similar lesions on one patient that lasted as long as 7 months.[55] In 1922 Garin and Bujadoux[38] described a painful radiculoneuritis with a lymphocytic meningitis following a skin rash at the site of a bite by the hedgehog tick *(Ixodes hexagonus).* In the 1940s the triad of painful radiculoneuritis, chronic lymphocytic meningitis, and cranial nerve palsy associated with antecedent tick bites was called Bannwarth syndrome.[7] In 1955 Binder and associates[16] demonstrated the infectious nature of erythema chronicum migrans by placing biopsy specimens (from a lesion) beneath the skin of their own forearms and producing similar skin lesions. They further demonstrated the infectious nature of the lesions by treating themselves with penicillin, resulting in immediate clearing of the lesions.

The description and subsequent identification of the disease in the United States began in the early 1970s when two women living near Lyme, Connecticut, drew attention to the large number of cases of childhood arthritis in the area. The occurrence of severe headaches, skin rashes, and neurologic symptoms along with the recurring arthritic complaints caused them to suspect that the physicians' diagnosis of juvenile rheumatoid arthritis was incorrect. At the request of the Connecticut State Health Department, Steere and associates[91] studied these cases. They documented a geographic cluster of cases of oligoarthritis with seasonal onset that was often preceded by a characteristic skin rash called erythema chonicum migrans (ECM). The condition was labeled Lyme arthritis, and subsequent studies showed that penicillin and tetracycline treatments shortened the duration of the ECM and prevented or treated the Lyme arthritis. These observations suggested an infectious cause.[90]

The causative agent of Lyme disease was identified in 1982 by Burgdorfer,[21] who identified the spirochete associated with Lyme arthritis in the midgut of *Ixodes* ticks collected on Shelter Island, New York. These ticks produced skin rash in rabbits. Subsequent studies by Steere and associates[88] in 1983 revealed serologically identical spirochetes cultured from the blood, skin lesions, cerebrospinal fluid, and *Ixodes* ticks obtained from patients with Lyme disease. Thus the spirochete, *Borrelia burgdorferi,* was conclusively identified as the causitive agent of Lyme disease.

SYSTEMIC DISEASE

Lyme disease is a progressive disease comprised of three stages: stage 1, or early infection, involves the characteristic skin rash and is often associated with constitutional symptoms; stage 2, or disseminated infection, consists of cardiac or neurologic complications; and stage 3, or late infection, involves rheumatologic and central nervous system complications.[83]

This systematic staging of the disease does not parallel the clinical course of many patients, as victims may experience signs or symptoms consistent with any stage of the disease without having experienced a prior stage. For example, only 60% of patients with Lyme disease may recall having a skin rash.[84] Therefore the disease is now more typically divided into early (stage 1) and late (stage 2 or stage 3) manifestations.

Early Infection

Stage 1 or early infection is characterized by the one pathognomonic sign of Lyme disease, the skin rash, ery-

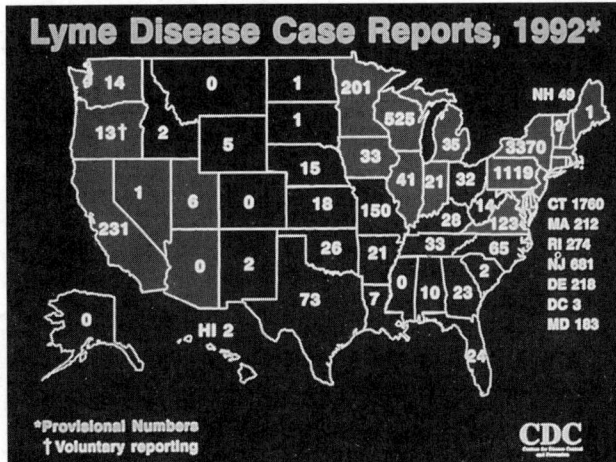

Fig. 106-1. Distribution of reported Lyme cases in 1992 within the United States. (Courtesy of D. Dennis MD, Centers for Disease Control and Prevention.)

thema chronicum migrans (now called erythema migrans). Erythema migrans typically begins several days to weeks after a tick bite as a red macule or papule and expands over a period of days to weeks into a large roundish lesion that may have partial central clearing. Often the expanding skin rash is accompanied by intermittent constitutional symptoms such as fatigue, fever, headache, mild stiff neck, arthralgias, or myalgias. The patient may not recall or have even noticed a tick bite at the site of the rash. The rash will ultimately clear and the constitutional symptoms resolve even without treatment. The documented presence of an erythema migrans rash firmly establishes a diagnosis of Lyme disease. A rash that appears immediately after a tick bite represents a hypersensitivity reaction and is not considered an erythema migrans rash.

Late Manifestations

Late manifestations of Lyme disease primarily involve the musculoskeletal system, the central nervous system, or the cardiac system. Ocular involvement is generally a rare late manifestation of the infection. The cardiac complications of Lyme disease (which occur in approximately 10% of untreated patients) consist of the acute onset of a transient second- or third-degree atrial ventricular conduction defect that generally resolves in days to weeks and is sometimes associated with myocarditis.[85]

The neurologic complications are more protean and found in 10% to 15% of untreated patients. These neurologic complications can include some or all of the following conditions: lymphocytic meningitis, cranial neuritis, radicular neuropathy, or (rarely) encephalomyolitis. The most common cranial neuritis is a facial palsy (Bell palsy) that may present as a bilateral facial palsy. The facial palsy generally resolves in a few weeks (even if untreated), as do the other neurologic manifestations. They may, however, recur or progress to late central nervous system involvement.

The late central nervous system problems are not well described, but include chronic fatigue, neuropsychiatric impairment, chronic encephalitis, and a relapsing encephalomyolitis that can resemble multiple sclerosis.

Musculoskeletal manifestations consist primarily of Lyme arthritis, an oligoarthropathy typically affecting the large joints, particularly the knee, shoulder, elbow, temporal mandibular joint, ankle, wrist, or hip. The attacks may be migratory and are episodic, lasting weeks to months, with asymptomatic intervals between attacks. An occasional patient may develop a chronic arthritis in one or a few joints, but generally there is complete resolution of the inflammation within the affected joint.

CLINICAL FEATURES

The ophthalmic manifestations of Lyme disease have received widespread interest over the past several years, paralleling the increasing frequency and spread of the disease.[1,78] A variety of ophthalmic conditions have been described in patients in each stage of Lyme disease.[49a]

Despite these multiple descriptions, however, the extent and character of the eye findings in Lyme disease have yet to be clearly defined. There are too many uncertainties in establishing a causal relationship between the ocular condition and the infection by the *Borrelia burgdorferi* spirochete. In some of the reported cases the occurrence of ocular findings may be coincidental and unrelated to the presence of Lyme disease. In other cases strict etiologic criteria have not been applied in making a diagnosis of Lyme disease, further complicating attempts to determine any causal relationship between Lyme disease and the ocular condition. These cases often rely only on positive Lyme serology to establish the diagnosis, without acknowledging the well-known limitations of serologic testing.[1,8,22] For example, many of the reported cases have been observed in endemic areas with significant rates of positive serology (5% to 15% or more) among otherwise asymptomatic individuals.[31,32,42,92] The high background rate of seropositivity limits the usefulness of a positive Lyme titer when evaluating the cause of an ophthalmic condition. Seropositivity does not differentiate between past exposure or active ongoing infection. Moreover, the differences in sensitivity and specificity of various serologic assays, interlaboratory variability, and the absence of antibody formation early in the disease add to the difficulties in interpreting the significance of positive Lyme serologies.[57,59,60,80,82]

Ocular Surface

Acute Conjunctivitis. Lyme disease can affect the ocular surface during erythema migrans.[84] Approximately 10% of patients develop conjunctivitis within several days after the onset of the skin rash, sometimes manifested as photophobia or periorbital edema. Acute conjunctivitis is usually mild and short-lived; therefore it often does not require treatment.

Chronic Conjunctivitis. Chronic conjunctivitis and episcleritis are rare manifestations of Lyme disease. One case report described a patient with bilateral chronic follicular conjunctivitis, followed by corneal involvement and episcleritis attributed (based on immunofluorescent antibodies) to late Lyme disease.[36] Another report concerned a patient with a history of migratory arthritis, lethargy, and a skin rash who, 2 years later, developed systemic symptoms with stromal keratitis.[106] Six months after antibacterial and corticosteroid treatment, episcleritis occurred. Whether Lyme disease caused ocular inflammation in these patients is difficult to determine.

Exposure. Exposure keratoconjunctivitis or corneal ulceration may develop as a complication of facial paralysis, a well-established manifestation of Lyme disease.[23,67,72] The duration of the cranial neuropathy is short, and the weakness often begins improving within a few weeks.[67]

Cornea

There have been several reported cases of stromal keratitis occurring as a late manifestation of Lyme disease.* Patients present months to years following the onset of the disease with a painless, progressive blurring of vision and photophobia. The keratitis is characterized by focal infiltrates in a nebular pattern with indistinct borders. The infiltrates are located in the subepithelial layer and throughout the corneal stroma. Occasionally, the keratitis is associated with corneal edema or fine keratic precipitates. Diffuse stromal keratitis has been linked to Lyme disease based on serologic testing, but a direct cause is uncertain.[37]

Lyme keratitis responds to topical corticosteroids but may recur if the corticosteroids are discontinued abruptly. The keratitis does not respond to the use of systemic antibiotics alone and has resulted in some permanent scarring with corneal edema and neovascularization, when left untreated.[51]

One case of Lyme keratitis has been reported in conjunction with Lyme meningitis.[53] In this case the subepithelial corneal infiltrates resolved completely after treatment with intravenous ceftriaxone.

These limited case reports suggest that stromal keratitis is an ocular manifestation of late-stage Lyme disease. The judicious use of topical corticosteroids is indicated in the treatment of Lyme keratitis, especially those cases in which the lesions involve the visual axis.[105a]

The pathogenesis of Lyme keratitis is not known. Most authors[9,51,65] postulate either reactivation of a previous infection, recurrence of an infection secondary to inadequate treatment, or a hypersensitivity response to *B. burgdorferi* antigens. The prompt resolution of corneal inflammation to topical corticosteroids and the lack of response to systemic antibiotics, in most cases, would seem to support immune-mediated mechanisms.

---

*References 9, 13, 14, 36, 43a, 51, 53, 65, 105.

Uvea

Patients with Lyme disease can develop a variety of intraocular inflammations including iridocyclitis, vitreitis, choroiditis, and panuveitis. The inflammation may be secondary to an immune reaction or to direct infection of the intraocular tissues by spirochetes. Experimental studies have demonstrated hematogenous spread of spirochetes into the vitreous following intraperitoneal inoculations.[33]

Panuveitis. There has been only one reported case in which a spirochete, presumably *B. burgdorferi,* was recovered from a human eye.[50,86] In this case the uveitis, which was unusually severe, developed in the early stage of Lyme disease unlike the more common milder presentations seen in the late stage. The case involved a 45-year-old woman from an endemic area, who developed constitutional symptoms and erythema migrans, which responded to systemic cefazolin and oral tetracycline. Two weeks later, following a bee sting, she developed acute iritis that progressed to panuveitis and phthisis, despite the use of topical, subconjunctival, and systemic corticosteroids, as well as systemic antibiotics. Examination of a vitrectomy specimen showed marked necrosis, many neutrophils, and lymphocytes; and Dieterle stains revealed an occasional ''spirochete'' that was ''morphologically compatible'' with *B. burgdorferi.*

Anterior Uveitis. The remaining cases of uveitis described in the literature all occurred in the late stage of the disease. Iridocyclitis with vitreitis is the most common manifestation of intraocular inflammation from Lyme disease.[101] Concomitant findings include keratic precipitates, posterior synechiae, iris nodules, and vitreous snowbanking. Mild pleocytosis of the cerebrospinal fluid can occur along with intraocular inflammation. Occasionally, the uveitis may be associated with optic disc edema secondary to vitreitis.[19] The disc edema is not associated with an optic neuropathy or intracranial hypertension.

Anterior uveitis may, in some cases, be associated with Lyme keratitis.[36,65,105] This anterior uveitis produces fine, white keratic precipitates on the corneal endothelium and generally is not associated with synechiae formation. In at least one case, cells could not be seen floating through the anterior chamber, although there were endothelial deposits present.[65]

Two reports have examined the prevalence of positive Lyme serology among uveitis patients and reached different conclusions.[74,75] One Japanese study examined uveitis patients from an endemic area for Lyme disease.[45] Among the ''unclassified'' uveitis patients, 48% were serologically positive for Lyme disease versus a 5% serologically positive rate for all individuals from the area. Therefore the authors concluded that Lyme disease is a cause of idiopathic or ''unclassified'' uveitis, at least in patients from endemic areas. The second study examined uveitis patients from a nonendemic area.[74] Four patients had positive serologies, but all the Western blots were negative. Therefore this study concluded that a positive serologic test for Lyme disease in uveitis patients is likely to represent a false-positive result.

Posterior Uveitis. There have been several cases of Lyme borelliosis affecting the posterior pole. For example, a 32-year-old woman with constitutional symptoms had iridocyclitis, mild vitreitis, cystoid macular edema, and exudative retinal detachments.[15] These findings, in association with lymphocytic pleocytosis, initially led to the diagnosis of Vogt-Koyanagi-Harada syndrome. Lyme serologies, however, were elevated (IgG 1 : 640, IgM 1 : 40), and the patient improved with oral doxycycline.

Similarly, another patient, exposed to multiple tick bites, developed a rash with fever, headaches, myalgias, and arthralgias.[103] Lumbar puncture showed CSF pleocytosis, and Lyme serologies were positive. After completing a one-month course of oral tetracycline and prednisone, he developed mild vitreitis with exudative retinal detachments and shallow choroidal detachments. He slowly improved with repeated courses of topical corticosteroids, tetracycline, and periocular corticosteroids.

Anecdotal evidence suggests that the uveitis responds to systemic antibiotic treatment,* but many of these patients were treated simultaneously with topical or systemic prednisone. One patient with a 10-year history of pars planitis had received multiple courses of ocular and systemic corticosteroids without improvement.[20] When a reevaluation of the patient revealed a positive Lyme serology, the patient was treated with IV ceftriaxone with complete resolution of all findings.

There have been reports, however, of the uveitis worsening with initiation of antibiotic treatment. For example, one patient with uveitis, a CSF pleocytosis, and positive Lyme serologies was placed on IV antibiotics.[66] Two days following the onset of treatment, he developed an anterior uveitis that subsequently resolved. Kuiper and associates[52] described a 39-year-old woman with a history of tick bites, erythema migrans, bilateral sixth nerve palsies, and CSF pleocytosis. The clinical picture resolved without treatment, but 1 month later she developed bilateral vitreous clouding. She underwent a vitrectomy in the right eye with improvement, but the clouding persisted in the left eye. One year later she developed migratory arthralgias, and a clinical diagnosis of Lyme was made despite a negative serology. She was treated with IV ceftriaxone, which initially produced an increase in clouding of the vitreous on the left, but later produced subsequent clearing and restoration of vision to 20/20 with no further recurrences of any systemic symptoms. This apparent worsening with treatment has led some authors to suggest a mechanism similar to the Herxheimer reaction seen in the treatment of syphilis.[52,58] At least one author recommends the concurrent administration of corticosteroids with the antibiotic treatment for patients with ocular or central nervous system borreliosis.[58]

Tonjes[96] and Bodine[18] each described patients with acute multifocal placoid pigment epitheliopathy (AMPPE), CSF pleocytosis, and positive Lyme serologies that improved on IV antibiotics. Subsequently Wolf and associates[102] tested 18 consecutive AMPPE patients from an endemic area for Lyme disease by serology; all were negative. Therefore the association reported by Tonjes and Bodine may be coincidental.

Retinal Vasculitis. There has been a single report of a retinal vasculitis with mild vitreitis and branch retinal artery occlusion that was attributed to Lyme disease and treated with IV penicillin, but more likely this case represented a case of syphilis.[54] Secondary retinal pigmentary changes have been noted.[49]

Optic Nerve

Papilledema. The most common and unequivocal manifestation of Lyme disease involving the optic nerve is papilledema, defined as optic disc swelling secondary to intracranial hypertension from Lyme meningitis.[47,53,70,73] It is most commonly observed in children with stage 2 disease who suffer from headache, vomiting, or listlessness, and occasionally complain of a horizontal binocular diplopia. On examination, these children are found to have normal visual acuity, enlargement of the blind spot, optic disc swelling (Fig. 106-2) and, in some cases, signs of a sixth nerve palsy. Lumbar puncture reveals an elevated opening pressure and CSF pleocytosis. These patients generally have very positive Lyme titers. They uniformly do well with complete resolution of the papilledema and meningitis following treatment with IV ceftriaxone.

The term pseudotumor cerebri has mistakenly been used to describe these cases. Because these patients almost

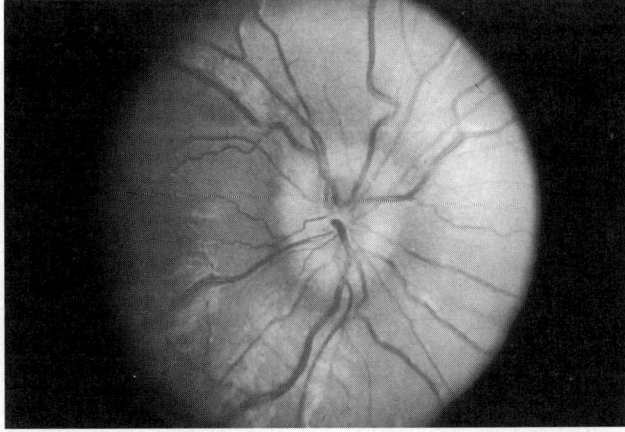

Fig. 106-2. Papilledema in a 7-year-old boy with headache, transient visual obscurations, sixth nerve palsy, meningitis, and a positive Lyme ELISA of 0.655 (0.093 negative cutoff).

---

*References 15, 19, 52, 96, 100, 101, 103.

always had CSF pleocytosis, it would be more correct to attribute the papilledema to meningitis. Occasionally, a spinal tap performed early in the presentation of the disease failed to detect CSF pleocytosis or elevated protein, thereby simulating pseudotumor cerebri. As was shown in one case, however, subsequent taps will show abnormal fluid.[70] Therefore in those patients with optic disc swelling, intracranial hypertension, positive Lyme titers, and a normal CSF, a repeat lumbar puncture might reveal a pleocytosis, thereby confirming a diagnosis of Lyme meningitis.

Optic Perineuritis. Some patients have transient visual obscurations, a nonspecific symptom associated with optic disc edema. One study showed that only two of five patients with transient visual loss experienced swelling of the optic disc, whereas three other patients had optic disc edema without visual changes, and only one of eight patients had intracranial hypertension.[73] Based on this report and others,[104] it has been surmised that patients with normal intracranial pressures and optic disc edema have optic perineuritis, an infiltrating inflammation along the optic nerve sheath that simulates papilledema.[46] Because there were few details concerning the neurovisual status of these patients (e.g., acuity, visual fields, pupillary findings, disc photographs, color vision, etc), it is difficult to assess the significance or reasons for transient visual obscurations without disc edema, or disc edema without intracranial hypertension. Furthermore, without radiographic confirmation of optic nerve sheath thickening or enhancement, it would be difficult, on the basis of these reports alone, to conclude that Lyme disease causes an optic perineuritis. It is, however, a well-established form of luetic optic neuropathy, which might yet be shown to occur in Lyme disease.

Optic Atrophy. An optic neuropathy can develop in the late stages of Lyme disease in association with meningoencephalitis.[53] The first case involved a 59-year-old man with a history of endemic exposure, facial paresis, sixth nerve palsy, and a Lyme titer of 1 : 6400! Despite multiple courses of treatment, symptoms persisted. Five years after the initial presentation, the patient developed a rapidly progressive vision loss to 20/400, an afferent pupillary defect, and bilateral pallor of the optic discs. MRI showed multiple white matter lesions, and CSF was positive for oligoclonal bands, but myelin basic protein was normal. The second case involved a 39-year-old woman with a history of erythema migrans, facial palsy, radiculoneuritis, spastic hemiparesis, a positive T cell response to *B. burgdorferi,* and a Lyme titer (IgG) of 1 : 400. Initial exam showed normal acuities, dyschromatopsia, a mild central scotoma OS, pallor of the optic disc OS, and bilateral sixth nerve palsies. MRI showed multiple areas of demyelination in the brainstem and cortex. Despite treatment with IV ceftriaxone, 5 months later she developed an acute optic neuropathy in the right eye. Syphilis serologies were presumably negative, although the results were not reported in either case.

Several series describing the clinical features of Lyme meningoencephalitis have included some patients with optic neuropathies.[2,41,46,67,98] It would appear that optic neuropathy is an element of Lyme disease with central nervous system involvement, although the specific features have yet to be fully described.

Optic Neuritis. Whether isolated optic neuritis (defined as a rapid decline in vision associated with pain) with objective signs of optic neuropathy, followed by improvement can be a manifestation of Lyme disease is less clear. Unfortunately, most cases of "Lyme optic neuritis" are difficult to distinguish from the demyelinating form of optic neuritis commonly seen in patients or in children with antecedent viral syndromes. For example, in the series reported by Lesser[53] there was one patient with retrobulbar optic neuritis and another patient with neuroretinitis (papillitis associated with stellate macular exudates). Both patients had mild elevation of their Lyme titers and both improved with antibiotic treatment. Similarly, Wu[104] described a 7-year-old boy who developed an annular rash from an insect bite followed by a generalized maculopapular rash and fevers. Several weeks later he was diagnosed with an aseptic meningitis and "papilledema." The presence, however, of a normal intracranial pressure, diminished acuity, cecocentral scotomas, and macular exudates more accurately identified this case as an optic neuritis or neuroretinitis. Immunofluorescent antibody to Lyme was 1 : 256, and the patient improved on IV penicillin. Except for the Lyme titer, this patient's course was entirely consistent with a postviral optic neuritis commonly seen in childhood. Winterkorn,[99] in a review, also briefly described a case of neuroretinitis and positive Lyme titer in which the diagnosis remained unresolved.

Typical features of optic neuritis associated with Lyme disease are onset of vision loss, painful eye movements, and objective signs of optic neuropathy. Most cases have borderline positive Lyme titers, and improvement can occur without specific treatment for Lyme disease.

The most cogent case made for an isolated optic neuritis as a manifestation of Lyme disease was by Jacobson,[48] who had 20 consecutive patients with isolated optic neuritis undergo a battery of serologic tests for Lyme (IFA, ELISA for IgG, IgM, Western immunoblots). Patients with positive titers underwent CSF analysis. Four of the twenty patients (20%) had positive Lyme serologies. In each case the clinical presentation was typical for optic neuritis. Two of the four cases showed a rise in titer for IgM, the presence of specific antibody reactions to *Borrelia* antigens on immunoblot, unusually high cell counts in the CSF, an absence of oligoclonal bands, and an elevation in the Lyme antibody index. These observations led the author to conclude that these two cases were probably related to Lyme disease. The author cautions, however, that all of the patients came from a hyperendemic region with a reported asymptomatic seropositivity rate as high as 15% to 20%,[31,32] identical to the rate observed among his patients with optic neuritis. It is possible that seropositivity in these patients was the result of prior asymptomatic seroconversion.

Ischemic Optic Neuropathy. There are scattered reports of individuals with nonarteritic anterior ischemic optic neuropathy (AION), positive Lyme serologies, and nonspecific constitutional symptoms attributed to Lyme disease.[40,77] An ischemic presentation would be consistent with histopathologic changes reported in Lyme disease. Duray and Steere[34] reported vascular damage, including hypercellular vascular occlusion, following infection with the *B. burgdorferi* spirochete. Nevertheless, the case for Lyme disease causing a nonarteritic ischemic optic neuropathy (AION) remains unconvincing. For example, one report described a 65-year-old man with myalgias and a "strongly positive" Lyme titer, who developed a sudden and persistant vision loss with disc edema.[40] Unfortunately, the details concerning the eye exam and Lyme serologies, as well as the absence of other features specific to Lyme, make it difficult to evaluate the cause of vision loss in this case. In another case a 53-year-old patient with steroid-responsive myalgias, cutaneous hypersensitivity, fevers, paresthesias, and an elevated erythrocyte sedimentation rate (ESR) developed a possible ischemic optic neuropathy associated with a mildly elevated Lyme titer (1:256).[77] Because vasculitis could not be entirely excluded, the cause of the optic neuropathy remained unclear. Finally, another report described a 71-year-old man with classic AION caused by biopsy-proven giant-cell arteritis.[68] The authors claim to have observed a spirochete within a giant cell. The Lyme titer in this patient was not significant at 1:64. Histopathologic diagnosis of *B. burgdorferi* can be difficult, if not misleading.

Jacobson[46] reported seeing several patients with typical nonarteritic anterior ischemic optic neuropathy and positive Lyme titers, but no other clinical features suggestive of Lyme disease within an endemic area. The cerebrospinal fluid in these patients was normal. No treatment was given for Lyme disease. Subsequent follow-up showed no systemic sequelae of Lyme in these patients. Two similar cases confirmed Jacobson's observations (personal observations). Thus the case for Lyme disease as a cause of nonarteritic anterior ischemic optic neuropathy remains very tenuous at best.

Orbit

There has been one report of an orbital myositis attributed to a presumed case of Lyme disease.[81] The case involved a 5-year-old girl who developed a suggestive rash followed by Bell palsy with CSF pleocytosis. The rash and pleocytosis resolved without treatment. Four months later she developed arthritis involving the knee followed by a painful ophthalmoplegia. CT scan of the orbit showed evidence of orbital myositis, which responded to steroid therapy. Serologies were not reported, nor was she apparently treated with antibiotics for Lyme disease. Thus the cause of the orbital myositis in this case remained uncertain, although Lyme disease has been documented to invade skeletal muscles.[6]

Neuro-Ophthalmic Manifestations

Pupillary Abnormalities. There have been a few isolated reports of pupillary abnormalities associated with Lyme disease.[39,53,72] One patient, with a positive history for a tick bite and erythema migrans, subsequently contracted headache, fever, myalgia, malaise, and a stiff neck. Shortly after oral tetracycline, a preganglionic Horner syndrome developed on the patient's left side, which resolved after 10 days of IV ceftriaxone.[39] Another neurologic complication involving the pupils is an Argyll Robertson pupil.[72] Finally, one patient with Lyme meningitis and associated Lyme keratitis developed one pupil that reacted in a "tonic fashion."[53]

Cranial Nerve Palsy. Neurologic complications occur in approximately 10% of patients with late manifestations of Lyme disease, and half of these cases have cranial neuropathies.[72] The development of cranial neuropathies is commonly associated with CSF pleocytosis (93%).[71] Facial paralysis is the single most common cranial neuropathy in Lyme disease.[67,72] Approximately 13% of the cranial neuropathies involve the ocular motor nerves (III, IV, and VI).[71] Nerve VI (unilateral or bilateral) is most commonly involved (9% of cranial neuropathies)* followed by the nerve III (3%)[2,3,76,79,94] and nerve IV (1%).[101]

Sixth nerve palsies often represent a false localizing sign, as many of these patients have intracranial hypertension, meningitis, and papilledema.[46,53,70] Abducens palsies can also develop as a consequence of meningitis alone, without intracranial hypertension.[41,53,76] In either case sixth nerve palsies are frequently associated with other cranial neuropathies, especially the seventh nerve.[3,53,67,76] Whereas most cases presumably affect the peripheral fibers of the sixth nerve, sixth nerve palsies in patients with Lyme encephalitis probably includes some patients with pontine lesions affecting the fascicular portion of the nerve. Such cases may be difficult to distinguish from multiple sclerosis.

PATHOGENESIS

The primary reservoir of the *Borrelia burgdorferi* spirochete is the bloodstream of small rodents such as the white-footed mouse. Humans are incidental hosts for the spirochete and do not contribute to its maintenance in nature. Spirochetes are spread from rodent to rodent or from rodent to humans through the *Ixodes* tick.

The tick passes through three stages in its life cycle, the larva, nymph, and adult stage. During each stage the tick feeds once on an obligate blood meal, at which time it may either acquire the spirochete or pass it on to the host (if it has

---

*References 3, 17, 63, 67, 76, 79, 93, 94.

already acquired the spirochete during a previous blood meal).

The tick eggs are laid in the early spring and hatch approximately 1 month later. The resulting larvae feed anytime from July through September (generally on small rodents) at which time they may acquire the spirochete. They drop off their host and survive the fall and winter in a resting state until molting into nymphs during the second spring. The nymphs feed during the spring and summer. If the nymphs have already been infected during their prior blood meal, they may pass the spirochete on to their host.

Alternatively, they may become infected during this meal. Following this second blood meal, the nymphs molt into adults. In the fall the adults feed and mate, primarily on deer or other large animals such as sheep, racoons, or hedgehogs. The adult ticks survive the winter then drop off in the spring to lay eggs and die.

In New England and the upper Midwest the spirochete is spread through the tick *Ixodes dammini*. In the Pacific Northwest, the spirochete is spread through the *Ixodes pacificus*.

Deer, especially the white-tailed deer, and other large and medium-size animals (such as racoons) serve primarily as a mating ground for the adult ticks and provide the blood meal required for tick egg production. Deer are a host for the spirochete, but are thought to be an incompetant reservoir for the *Borrelia burgdorferi* spirochete.[95]

Humans usually acquire the spirochete from a bite by an infected nymph, although bites by infected larvae or adult ticks can result in the disease. Because nymphs have their primary blood meal in the late spring or early summer, there is a peak seasonal incidence of the disease at these times.

DIFFERENTIAL DIAGNOSIS

Despite the remaining uncertainties regarding the clinical manifestations of ocular Lyme disease, it is clear that there is a considerable overlap with the ophthalmic manifestations of syphilis. This seems especially true in cases of patients with optic neuropathies, keratitis, uveitis, and ocular motor nerve palsies. As all spirochetes share common antigens, serologic tests may cross-react. Depending on the method, Lyme titers may be positive in approximately 20% to 60% of patients with syphilis[61,75]; and 20% of patients with Lyme disease may have a weakly positive FTA-ABS (usually < 1 : 10).[44] Among patients with Lyme, the RPR and MHA-TP are usually negative.[44] A positive Lyme titer with a negative VDRL does not completely rule out syphilis, however, as nearly 30% of patients with primary, latent, or late syphilis will also have a negative VDRL and positive FTA.

Some of the published cases purporting to describe the ophthalmic manifestations of Lyme disease have omitted serologic testing for syphilis (or at least failed to mention the results),[53] and where these studies were performed the results suggest syphilis is at least a plausible alternative, if not the actual cause.[35,54,100,106] Caution must be used in diagnosing Lyme disease in patients from nonendemic regions. For example, one report described a 39-year-old Oklahoman woman with a skin lesion on her breast, diffuse pains, myelopathy, bilateral sixth nerve palsies, and lymphocytic pleocytosis.[35] This patient suffered from what clinically resembled an optic neuritis with mildly elevated Lyme titer (1 : 128) with a negative VDRL, but the FTA and MHA-TP were positive. Similar concerns can be raised in other cases with bilateral optic atrophy,[100] ischemic optic neuropathy[100] and uveitis.[106] Demonstration of specific antibodies to Lyme-specific surface antigens (31kD, 34kD) by Western blot may be the only practical means to distinguish the two diseases when serologies are both positive.[10] Unfortunately, although these antigen studies are highly specific, sensitivity is low and the test is not always helpful.

Distinguishing some of the ophthalmic manifestations of Lyme disease from multiple sclerosis can be even more difficult. If isolated optic neuritis occurs in Lyme disease, it appears clinically indistinguishable from the ordinary form of demyelinating optic neuritis, except for the elevated Lyme titer. The absence of any other findings suggestive of Lyme disease, such as erythema migrans (EM) or facial palsies, in these cases is noteworthy. Moreover, the presence of other neurologic findings, such as CSF pleocytosis or white matter lesions on MRI, may not permit a clear distinction between Lyme and MS. Finally, optic neuritis frequently resolves spontaneously. Thus response to antibiotics is by no means a reliable criterion for establishing the diagnosis of Lyme optic neuritis. Although the demonstration of intrathecal production of Lyme antibodies may help, the possibility must be considered that such associations are merely coincidental; and in some cases treatment will be initiated even when the diagnosis remains uncertain.

Finally, other diseases that may mimic the ocular manifestations of Lyme include viral and postviral syndromes, sarcoidosis, Behçet, Vogt-Koyanagi-Harada, lymphoma, vasculitis, Guillain-Barré, varicella-zoster virus, and others. Consider, for example, one patient with a 5-year history of progressive optic atrophy in one eye and positive Lyme titer. A CT scan performed 5 years earlier was said to be normal, but repeat MRI scan revealed an ipsilateral sphenoid wing meningioma compressing the optic nerve. Patients with ocular conditions possibly related to Lyme disease need to be carefully and fully evaluated to rule out other possible causes.

LABORATORY INVESTIGATIONS

Most bacterial diseases are defined by direct observation or culture of the pathogen. Lyme borreliosis is not readily definable in this manner, and indirect methods are generally used. Recognition by the physician of erythema migrans, the classic skin lesion of *Borrelia burgdorferi* infection, is for all practical purposes diagnostic.[5,11] Unfortunately, this characteristic skin lesion is only recognized in about two thirds of patients, and then only early in the course of the illness.[5,11]

In the absence of a skin rash, the diagnosis of Lyme disease is dependent on the demonstration of an antibody response to *B. burgdorferi* in an appropriate clinical setting.[27,69] Yet, the mere demonstration of an antibody response against *B. burgdorferi* is not diagnostic. Objectively measurable clinical signs must be documented.[27,69] Although vague or nonspecific symptoms such as fatigue, myalgias, or arthralgias may be associated with Lyme disease, they are common to many other illnesses and are not helpful in establishing a diagnosis. Even in instances of objective abnormalities, great care should be taken before a cause-and-effect relationship is assumed between *B. burgdorferi* and a specific sign.

Serologic assays to detect antibodies against *B. burgdorferi* are readily available to the physician. One of two different methods is typically employed: indirect immunofluorescence assay (IFA) or enzyme-linked immunosorbent assay (ELISA). In either case whole *B. burgdorferi* preparations are generally used as the antigen source.[27] The IFA uses fixed *B. burgdorferi* as the antigen substrate and most ELISA's use sonicated spirochetes (with a few using partial purified crude fractions). There is no standardization of these assays, and there are wide differences between laboratories as to how tests are performed, reported, and interpreted. The normal values, sensitivity and specificity, are not comparable between laboratories, even those using the same test kit. Every laboratory must establish its own criteria for anti-*B. burgdorferi* antibody assays, so interlaboratory test results are not directly comparable.

Current assays in which whole *B. burgdorferi* preparations are the antigen source have a high rate of false positives and a poor predictive value when used as screening tests. *B. burgdorferi* expresses a number of common bacterial antigens that are highly cross-reactive with similar antigens expressed by other bacteria.[43,97] Most individuals have detectable antibody against one or more of these antigens. In addition, the 41-kD flagellar-associated antigen of *B. burgdorferi* is highly cross-reactive with similar flagellar antigens expressed by other spirochetes,[24] including *Treponema denticola,* a common cause of periodontal disease. False-positive rates of 2% to 5% are common in these assays because of the high background level of cross-reactive antibodies. Thus because of this cross-reactivity, the presence of antibodies against *B. burgdorferi* does not necessarily mean that a person is actively infected.

Serology results are adjuncts to the diagnosis. To complicate matters further, there are rare instances in which individuals will have serologies within the normal range and yet have active disease.[29,79a] Inadequate antibiotics given early in the course of infection can produce a situation in which an individual fails to maintain a significant antibody response. Therefore if an individual has objective abnormalities clinically compatible with Lyme borreliosis, the diagnosis of *B. burgdorferi* infection should be pursued, even if the peripheral antibody titer is below diagnostic levels. Specimens positive or equivocal by IFA or ELISA should be tested by a Western immunoblot. A second convalescent-phase serum sample may also need to be obtained.

A lumbar puncture and examination of the cerebrospinal fluid should be carried out in all individuals suspected of having central nervous system (CNS) disease. Uncommonly, individuals with negative peripheral serologies will have local antibody production against *B. burgdorferi* in the cerebrospinal fluid.

THERAPY

Presently, there is no consensus on the optimal therapy of Lyme disease. Few randomized, prospective studies on the treatment of *B. burgdorferi* infection have been published, and those have low numbers of patients.[26,89] It is unclear how success or failure should be defined in studies on the treatment of this disease because of the poor state of diagnostic tests. Various authors have handled persistent symptoms differently. Some have assumed that they represent continued infection, whereas others have assumed that they are related to other mechanisms. Whether persistent symptoms are due to continued infection, permanent tissue damage, or some undefined immune mechanism remains to be determined. It is clear that further studies are necessary to define the optimal treatment of this disease. It is also clear, however, that beta lactams and tetracyclines are effective against *B. burgdorferi,* and that the disease is for the most part treated with a high degree of success.[26,89] Some physicians have advocated prolonged therapy, but there has been no evidence presented from controlled prospective studies that would support this practice.

Management of Early Infection

The efficacy of various tetracyclines and penicillins is good in patients with uncomplicated local infection. Studies on the treatment of erythema migrans, however, must be interpreted carefully. *B. burgdorferi* can spread hematogenously early in the course of infection, but this has not always been taken into account. Steere and asssociates[89] randomized between erythromycin, tetracycline, and penicillin for the treatment of patients. The failure rate in their study was 45% to 55%. The majority of patients in that trial who failed had ''minor'' disease manifestations such as headache, fatigue, arthralgias, and transient facial palsies. Only a minority of patients had ''major'' complications, meningo-encephalitis, carditis, or persistent arthritis. Although the categorization of major or minor was arbitrary, and it is now obvious that they both represent persistent infection, tetracycline was declared the drug of choice for the treatment of patients with erythema migrans because none of the 38 patients treated with tetracycline in that study developed a major complication.

More recently, Nadelman and associates[64] published a masked study comparing doxycycline to cefuroxime in the treatment of patients with EM. Patients in that study were considered treatment failures if they had both clinical evidence of persistent disease within 1 year after the initiation of therapy and a positive serology to *B. burgdorferi*. Using that criteria, approximately 10% of patients in each group were failures. If all patients with signs or symptoms (regardless of the serologic status) were considered failures, a different conclusion is obtained. Approximately 30% failed cefuroxime.

Although the optimal treatment of erythema migrans remains to be fully delineated, both amoxicillin and the semisynthetic tetracyclines (doxycycline and minocycline) have an established position in the therapy of patients.[69] In a small randomized trial comparing amoxicillin plus probenecid to doxycycline for the treatment of EM, both drugs were effective and no patient required additional therapy.[28]

Recently, in a large multicenter trial comparing azithromycin to amoxicillin, amoxicillin was significantly more effective than azithromycin in completely resolving the acute manifestations of erythema migrans and in preventing relapse within 6 months after infection.[56] Only 4% (4 of 106) of patients treated with amoxicillin relapsed compared to 18% (20 of 111) treated with azithromycin. The conclusion that azithromycin is not as effective as amoxicillin is in contrast to a small, open trial study that showed comparability between amoxicillin and azithromycin.[62] The differences in size and design (open versus double blind) of these studies may account for the differences between these studies.

A long-term, prospective, double-blind study is needed to directly compare the efficacy of doxycycline and amoxicillin for the treatment of early Lyme disease and the prevention of its long-term sequelae. At present, either amoxicillin (500 mg 3 times a day for 21 days) or doxycycline (100 mg twice a day for 21 days) should be used for the treatment of patients with early *B. burgdorferi* infection. In any case, where there is suspicion of CNS involvement, a lumbar puncture should be performed to rule out active CNS infection, because the latter should be treated with parenteral antibiotics.

Management of Nervous System Disease

Penicillin and ceftriaxone are the most commonly used antimicrobials for the treatment of serious *B. burgdorferi* infection.[69] Acute CNS infection is very responsive to high-dose penicillin therapy in most instances.[69] There are, however, several reports in which acute CNS infection has progressed despite penicillin therapy.[30] Meningopolyradiculitis (Bannwarth syndrome) is somewhat less responsive. Therapy usually halts the progression of meningopolyradiculitis, although, as many as 50% of patients continue to have severe neurologic signs after treatment. Similarly, about 50% or more of patients with Lyme arthritis fail to respond to intravenous penicillin therapy.[87]

Management of Late Complications

Ceftriaxone has been shown superior to penicillin in the treatment of late Lyme borreliosis.[25,26] These studies, however, were small, and larger long-term studies are required to determine the precise role ceftriaxone and other third-generation cephalosporins should play in the treatment of *B. burgdorferi* infection. Currently, patients with disseminated infection, CNS infection, arthritis, cardiac involvement, or compromise of any organ system caused by *B. burgdorferi*, should be treated with 14 to 28 days of ceftriaxone (2 grams once a day). Changes in the preceding recommendations for the treatment of *B. burgdorferi* infection await the completion of further studies.

REFERENCES

1. Aaberg TM: The expanding ophthalmologic spectrum of Lyme disease, *Am J Ophthalmol* 107:77-80, 1989.
2. Ackermann R, Rehse-Kupper B, Gollmer E, Schmidt R: Chronic neurologic manifestations of erythema migrans borreliosis, *Ann NY Acad Sci* 539:16-23, 1988.
3. Ackermann R, Horstrup P, Schmidt R: Tick borne meningopolyneuritis (Garin-Bujadoux, Bannwarth), *Yale J Biol Med* 57:485-490, 1984.
4. Afzelius A: Verhandlungen der Dermatologischen Gesellschaft zu Stockholm, *Arch Dermatol Syph* 101:404, 1910.
5. Asbrink E, Olsson I: Clinical manifestations of erythema chronicum migrans Afzelius in 161 patients: a comparison with Lyme disease, *Acta Derm Venereol* 65:43-52, 1985.
6. Atlas E, Novak SN, Duray PH, Steere AC: Lyme myositis: muscle invasion by *Borrelia burgdorferi*, *Ann Intern Med* 109:245, 1988.
7. Bannworth A: Chronische lymphocytare meningitis, entzunddliche polyneuritis und "rheumtismus," *Arch Psychiatr Nervenki* 113:284, 1941.
8. Barbour AG: Laboratory aspects of Lyme borreliosis, *Clin Microbiol Rev* 1:399-414, 1988.
9. Baum J, Barza M, Weinstein P et al.: Bilateral keratitis as a manifestation of Lyme disease, *Am J Ophthalmol* 105:75-77, 1988.
10. Benach JL, Coleman JL, Golightly MG: A murine IgM monoclonal antibody binds an antigenic determinant in outer surface protein A, an immunodominant basic protein of the Lyme disease spirochete, *J Immunol* 140:265-272, 1988.
11. Berger BW: Dermatologic manifestations of Lyme disease, *Rev Infect Dis* 1989.
12. Berger BW, Kaplan MH, Rothenberg IR, Barbour AG: Isolation and characterization of the Lyme disease spirochete from the skin of patients with erythema chronicum migrans, *J Am Acad Dermatol* 13(3):444-449, 1985.
13. Bertuch AW, Rocco E, Schwartz EG: Eye findings in Lyme disease, *Conn Med* 51:151-152, 1987.
14. Bertuch AW, Rocco E, Schwartz EG: Lyme disease: ocular manifestations, *Ann Ophthalmol* 20:376-378, 1988.
15. Bialasiewicz AA, Ruprecht KW, Naumann GOH, Blenk H: Bilateral diffuse choroiditis and exudative retinal detachments with evidence of Lyme disease, *Am J Ophthalmol* 105:419-420, 1988.
16. Binder E, Doepfmer R, Hornstein O: Experimentelle ubertragung des erythema chronicum migrans von mensch zu mensch, *Hautarzt* 6:494, 1955.
17. Blaumhackl U, Kristoferitsch W, Sluga E, Stanek G: Neurological manifestations of *Borrelia burgdorferi* infections: the enlarging clinical spectrum, *Zbl Bakt Hyg A* 263:334-336, 1986.
18. Bodine SR, Marino J, Camisa TJ, Salvate AJ: Multifocal choroiditis with evidence of Lyme disease, *Ann Ophthalmol* 24:169-173, 1992.
19. Boutros A, Rahn E, Nauheim: Iritis and papillitis as a primary presentation of Lyme disease, *Ann Ophthalmol* 22:24-25, 1990.
20. Breeveld J, Rothova A, Kuiper H: Intermediate uveitis and Lyme borreliosis, *Br J Ophthalmol* 76:181-182, 1992.
21. Burgdorfer W, Barbour AG, Hayes SG: Lyme disease—a tick-borne spirochete? *Science* 216:1317, 1982.

22. Centers for Disease Control: Lyme disease—Connecticut, *MMWR* 37:1, 1988.

23. Clark JR, Carlson RD, Sasaki CT et al.: Facial paralysis in Lyme disease, *Laryngoscope* 95:1341-1344, 1985.

24. Collins C, Peltz G: Immunoreactive epitopes on an expressed recombinant flagellar protein of *Borrelia burgdorferi, Infect Immun* 59:514-520, 1991.

25. Dattwyler RJ, Halperin JJ, Pass H, Luft BJ: Ceftriaxone as effective therapy in refractory Lyme disease, *J Infect Dis* 155:1322-1325, 1988.

26. Dattwyler RJ, Halperin JJ, Volkman DJ, Luft BJ: Treatment of late Lyme boreliosis—randomized comparison of ceftriaxone and penicillin, *Lancet* 2:1191-1194, 1988.

27. Dattwyler RJ, Luft BL: Immunodiagnosis of Lyme borreliosis, *Rheum Dis Clin North Am* 15:727-734, 1989.

28. Dattwyler RJ, Volkman DJ, Conaty SM et al.: Treatment of early Lyme borreliosis, a randomized trial comparing amoxicillin plus probenecid to doxycycline in patients with erythema migrans, *Lancet* 336:1404-1407, 1990.

29. Dattwyler RJ, Volkman DJ, Luft BJ et al.: Seronegative Lyme disease: dissociation of specific T and B lymphocyte responses to *Borrelia burgdorferi, N Engl J Med* 319:1441-1447, 1988.

30. Diringer MN, Halperin JJ, Dattwyler RJ: Lyme menigoencephalitis: report of a severe, penicillin resistant case, *Arthritis Rheum* 30:705-706, 1987.

31. Dlesk A, Broste SK, Marx JL et al.: Lyme serologies by indirect fluorescent antibody assay and enzyme-linked immunosorbent assay in normal residents from an endemic area, *Arthritis Rheum* 31(suppl):98, 1988.

32. Dlesk A, Broste SK, McCarty PA, Mitchell PD: Prevalence of Lyme seropositivity by indirect immunofluorescent antibody assay in normal adult individuals from an endemic area, *Arthritis Rheum* 31(suppl):98, 1988.

33. Duray PH, Johnson RC: The histopathology of experimentally infected hamsters with the Lyme disease spirochete, *Borrelia burgdorferi, Proc Soc Exp Biol Med* 181:263-269, 1986.

34. Duray PH, Steere AC: Clinical pathologic correlations of Lyme disease by stage, *Ann NY Acad Sci* 539:65-79, 1988.

35. Farris BK, Webb RM: Lyme disease and optic neuritis, *J Clin Neuro-ophthalmol* 8:73-78, 1988.

36. Flach AJ, Lavoie PE: Episcleritis, conjunctivitis, and keratitis as ocular manifestations of Lyme disease, *Ophthalmology* 97:973-975, 1990.

37. Fox GM, Heilskov T, Smith JL: Cogan's syndrome and seroreactivity to Lyme Borreliosis, *J Clin Neuro-ophthalmol* 10:83-87, 1990.

38. Garin C, Bujadoux C: Paralysie par les tiques, *J Méd Lyon* 71:765, 1922.

39. Glauser TA, Brennan PJ, Galetta SL: Reversible Horner's syndrome and Lyme disease, *J Clin Neuro-ophthalmol* 9:225-228, 1989.

40. Gustafson R, Svenungsson B, Unosson-Hallnas K: Optic neuropathy in *Borrelia* infection, *J Infect* 17:187-188, 1988.

41. Halperin JJ, Volkmann DJ, Wu P: Central nervous system abnormalities in Lyme neuroborreliosis, *Neurology* 41:1571-1582, 1991.

42. Hanrahan JP, Benach JL, Coleman JL et al.: Incidence and cumulative frequency of endemic Lyme disease in a community, *J Infect Dis* 150:489-496, 1984.

43. Hansen K, Bangsborg JM, Fjordvang H et al.: Immunochemical characterization of and isolation of the gene for a *Borrelia burgdorferi* immunodominant 60-kilodalton antigen common to a wide range of bacteria, *Infect Immun* 56:2047-2053, 1988.

43a. Hoang-Xuan T, Manuel C, Abirached G: Kératite dans la maladie de Lyme, *J Fr Ophtalmol* 17:513-521, 1994.

44. Hunter EF, Russell H, Farshy CE et al.: Evaluation of sera from patients with Lyme disease in FTA-Ab test for syphillis, *Sex Transm Dis* 13:232-236, 1986.

45. Isogai E, Isogai H, Kotake S et al.: Detection of antibodies against *Borrelia burgdorferi* in patients with uveitis, *Am J Ophthalmol* 112:23-30, 1991.

46. Jacobson DM: Neuro-ophthalmic aspects of Lyme disease, *Ophthalmol Clin North Am* 4:463-478, 1991.

47. Jacobson DM, Frens DB: Pseudotumor cerebri syndrome associated with Lyme disease, *Am J Ophthalmol* 107:81-82, 1989.

48. Jacobson DN, Marx JJ, Dlesk A: Frequency and clinical significance of Lyme seropositivity in patients with isolated optic neuritis, *Neurology* 41:706-711, 1991.

49. Karma A, Pirttila TA, Viljanen MK et al.: Secondary retinitis pigmentosa and cerebral demyelination in Lyme borreliosis, *Br J Ophthalmol* 77:120-122, 1993.

49a. Karma A, Seppala I, Mikkila H et al: Diagnosis and clinical characteristics of ocular Lyme borreliosis, *Am J Ophthalmol* 119:127-135, 1995.

50. Kauffmann DJH, Wormser GP: Ocular Lyme disease: case report and review of the literature, *Br J Ophthalmol* 74:325-327, 1990.

51. Kornmehl EW, Lesser RL, Jaros P et al.: Bilateral keratitis in Lyme disease, *Ophthalmology* 96:1194-1197, 1989.

52. Kuiper H, Kaelman JH, Hager MJ: Vitreous clouding associated with Lyme borreliosis, *Am J Ophthalmol* 108:453-454, 1989.

53. Lesser RL, Kornmehl EW, Pachner AR et al.: Neuro-ophthalmic manifestations of Lyme disease, *Ophthalmology* 97:699-706, 1990.

54. Lightman DA, Brod RD: Branch retinal artery occlusion associated with Lyme disease, *Arch Ophthalmol* 109:1198-1199, 1991.

55. Lipschütz B: Ueber eine seltene Erythemform (Erythema chronicum migrancs), *Arch Derm Syph* 118:349, 1913.

56. Reference deleted in proofs.

57. Luger SW, Krauss E: Serologic tests for Lyme disease. Interlaboratory variability, *Arch Intern Med* 150:761-763, 1990.

58. MacDonald AB: Lyme disease: a neuro-ophthalmologic view, *J Clin Neuro-ophthalmol* 7:185-190, 1987.

59. MacDonald AB: Ambiguous serologies in active Lyme borreliosis, *J Clin Neuro-ophthalmol* 8:79, 1988.

60. Magnarelli LA: Quality of Lyme disease tests, *JAMA* 262:3414-3415, 1989.

61. Magnarelli LA, Anderson JF, Johnson RC: Cross-reactivity in serologic tests for Lyme disease and other spirochetal infections, *J Infect Dis* 156:183-188, 1987.

62. Massarotti EM, Luger SW, Rahn DW et al.: Treatment of Lyme disease, *Am J Med* 92:396-403, 1992.

63. Millner M, Schimek MG, Spoork D et al.: Lyme borreliosis in children: a controlled clinical study based on ELISA values, *Eur J Pediatr* 148:527-530, 1989.

64. Nadelman RB, Luger SW, Frank E et al.: Comparison of cefuroxime axetil and doxycycline in the treatment of early Lyme disease, *Ann Intern Med* 117:273-280, 1992.

65. Orlin SE, Lauffer JL: Lyme disease keratitis, *Am J Ophthalmol* 107:678-680, 1989.

66. Oteo JA, Martinez de Artola V, Maravi E, Eiros JM: Lyme disease and uveitis, *Ann Intern Med* 112:883, 1990.

67. Pachner AR, Steere AC: The triad of neurologic manifestations of Lyme disease: meningitis, cranial neuritis, and radiculoneuritis, *Neurology* 35:47-53, 1985.

68. Pizzarello LD, MacDonald AB, Semlear R et al.: Temporal arteritis associated with *Borrelia* infection, *J Clin Neuro-ophthalmol* 9:3-6, 1989.

69. Rahn DW, Malawista SW: Lyme disease: recommendations for diagnosis and treatment, *Ann Intern Med* 114:472-481, 1991.

70. Raucher HS, Kaufman DM, Goldfarb J et al.: Pseudotumor cerebri and Lyme disease: a new association, *J Pediatr* 107:931-933, 1985.

71. Reik L: *Lyme disease and the nervous system,* 57, 59, New York, 1991, Thieme Medical.

72. Reik L, Burgdorfer W, Donaldson JO: Neurologic abnormalities in Lyme disease without erythema chronicum migrans, *Am J Med* 81:73-78, 1986.

73. Reik L, Steere AC, Bartenhagen NH et al.: Neurologic abnormalities of Lyme disease, *Medicine* 58:281-294, 1979.

74. Rosenbaum JT, Rahn DW: Prevalence of Lyme disease among patients with uveitis, *Am J Ophthalmol* 112:462-463, 1991.

75. Russell H, Sampson JS, Schmidt GP et al.: Enzyme-linked immunosorbent assay and indirect immunofluorescence assay for Lyme disease, *J Infect Dis* 149:465-470, 1984.

76. Ryberg B: Bannwarths syndrome (lymphocytic meningoradiculitis) in Sweden, *Yale J Biol Med* 57:499-503, 1984.

77. Schechter SL: Lyme disease associated with optic neuropathy, *Am J Med* 81:143-145, 1986.

78. Schmid GP: The global distribution of Lyme disease, *Rev Infect Dis* 7:41-50, 1985.

79. Schmutzhard E, Pohl P, Stanek G: Involvement of *Borrelia burgdorferi* in cranial nerve affection, *Zbl Bakt Hyg A* 263:333-338, 1986.

79a. Schubert HD, Greenebaum E, Neu HC: Cytologically proven seronegative Lyme chorioditis and vitritis, *Retina* 14:39-42, 1994.

80. Schwartz BS, Goldstein MD, Ribeiro JMC et al.: Antibody testing in Lyme disease: a comparison of results in four laboratories, *JAMA* 262:3431-3434, 1989.

81. Seidenberg KB, Leib ML: Orbital myositis with Lyme disease, *Am J Ophthalmol* 109:13-16, 1990.

82. Smith JL, Parsons TM, Paris-Hamelin AJ, Porschen RK: The prevalence of Lyme disease in a nonendemic area, *J Clin Neuro-ophthalmol* 9:148-155, 1989.

83. Steere AC: Lyme disease, *N Engl J Med* 321:586-596, 1989.

84. Steere AC, Bartenhagen NH, Craft JE et al.: The early clinical manifestations of Lyme disease, *Ann Intern Med* 99:76-82, 1983.

85. Steere A, Batsford WP, Weinberg M et al.: Lyme carditis: cardiac abnormalities of Lyme disease, *Ann Intern Med* 93:8-16, 1980.

86. Steere AC, Duray PH, Kauffmann DJH, Wormser GP: Unilateral blindness caused by infection with the Lyme disease spirochete, *Borrelia burgdorferi, Ann Intern Med* 103:382-384, 1985.

87. Steere AC, Green J, Schoen RT et al.: Successful parenteral penicillin therapy of established Lyme disease, *N Engl J Med* 312:869-873, 1985.

88. Steere AC, Grodzicki RL, Hornblatt AM: The spirochetal etiology of Lyme disease, *N Engl J Med* 308:733-740, 1983.

89. Steere A, Hutchinson GJ, Rahn DW et al.: Treatment of the early manifestations of Lyme disease, *Ann Intern Med* 99:22-27, 1983.

90. Steere AC, Malawista SE, Newman JH et al.: Antibiotic therapy in Lyme disease, *Ann Intern Med* 93:1-8, 1980.

91. Steere AC, Malawista SE, Syndam DR et al.: Lyme arthritis: an epidemic of oligoarthritis in children and adults in three Connecticut communities, *Arthritis Rheum* 20:7-17, 1977.

92. Steere AC, Taylor E, Wilson ML et al.: Longitudinal assessment of the clinical and epidemiologic features of Lyme disease in a defined population, *J Infect Dis* 154:295-300, 1986.

93. Stiernstedt G, Gustafsson R, Karlson M et al.: Clinical manifestations and diagnosis of neuroborreliosis, *Ann NY Acad Sci* 539:46-55, 1988.

94. Stiernstedt G, Skoldenberg B, Garde A et al.: Clinical manifestations of *Borrelia* infections of the nervous system, *Zbl Bakt Hyg A* 263:289-296, 1986.

95. Telford SR: Incompetence of deer as reservoirs of the Lyme disease spirochete, *Am J Trop Med Hyg* 39:105, 1988.

96. Tonjes W, Mielke U, Schmidt HJ et al.: Akute multifokale plakoide pigment epitheliopathie mit entzundlichem liquor befund. Sonderform einer Borreliose? *Dtsch Med Wochenschr* 114:793-795, 1989.

97. Wallich R, Helmis C, Schable V et al.: Evaluation of the genetic divergence among *Borrelia burgdorferi* isolates by use of Osp A, Fla, Hsp60 and Hsp70 gene probes, *Infect Immun* 60:4856-4866, 1992.

98. Weder B, Wiedesheim P, Matter L: Chronic progressive neurological involvement in *Borrelia burgdorferi* infection, *J Neurol* 234:40-43, 1987.

99. Winterkorn JMS: Lyme disease: neurologic and ophthalmic manifestations, *Surv Ophthalmol* 35:191-204, 1990.

100. Winward KE, Smith JL: Ocular disease in Caribbean patients with serologic evidence of Lyme borreliosis, *J Clin Neuro-ophthalmol* 9:65-70, 1989.

101. Winward KE, Smith JL, Culbertson WW, Paris-Hamelin A: Ocular Lyme borreliosis, *Am J Ophthalmol* 108:651-657, 1989.

102. Wolf MD, Folk JC, Nelson JA, Peeples ME: Acute posterior multifocal placoid pigment epitheliopathy and Lyme disease, *Arch Ophthalmol* 110:750, 1992.

103. Wong T: The onset of bilateral uveitis in an elderly man with fever, headache, and rash, *Ophthalmic Surg* 20:154-155, 1989.

104. Wu G, Lincoff H, Ellsworth RM, Haik BG: Optic disc edema and Lyme disease, *Ann Ophthalmol* 18:252-255, 1986.

105. Zaidman GW: Episcleritis and symblepharon associated with Lyme keratitis, *Am J Ophthalmol* 109:487-488, 1990.

105a. Zaidman GW, Wormser GP: Lyme keratitis, *Ophthalmol Clin N Am* 7:597-604, 1994.

106. Zierhut M, Kreissig I, Pickert A: Panuveitis with positive serological tests for syphilis and Lyme disease, *J Clin Neuro-ophthalmol* 9:71-75, 1989.

107 Onchocerciasis

HUGH R. TAYLOR, THOMAS B. NUTMAN

Onchocerciasis is the disease caused by the filarial parasite *Onchocerca volvulus*. It is often called "river blindness" because it occurs in endemic foci along rivers and streams that surround the breeding sites of biting blackflies. These insects transmit the infection from one human to another.

Onchocerciasis is characterized by the presence of relatively few adult worms, macrofilariae, enclosed in nodules and millions of tiny worms, microfilariae, that migrate throughout the body. Blindness is the main disability caused by onchocerciasis, and it relates to the intensity of infection, determined by the duration and intensity of exposure to infected flies.

In 1987 the World Health Organization (WHO) estimated that onchocerciasis, which occurs in 34 countries, affected at least 18 million people (Table 107-1).[168] Over 85 million people were at risk, and at least one third of a million blinded (vision of less than 10/200). The figure for those blinded or visually impaired is acknowledged to be an underestimate, and it has been suggested 2 million people might have visual impairment caused by onchocerciasis.[141]

In hyperendemic areas almost every person will be infected and half of the population will be blinded by onchocerciasis before they die (Fig. 107-1). Once blind, they have a life expectancy of only one third that of the sighted, and most die within 10 years.[118]

HISTORICAL BACKGROUND

Onchocerciasis was first reported in 1875 by British Naval Surgeon John O'Neill.[106] He noted the skin changes among those living along the West Coast of Africa. These changes included papules and vesicles, and the intense itching common in onchocerciasis is still locally called "craw-craw". He took skin snips, examined them under a microscope, and described the presence of mobile microfilariae that emerged.

The characteristic nodules were described in 1893 by Leuckart who also named the parasite *Onchocerca volvulus*,[123] but he did not link the nodules to the skin changes.

The associated ocular involvement was first described by the Guatemalan ophthalmologist Rudolo Robles[124] in 1919. Onchocerciasis is still commonly called Robles disease in Latin America. He also described the acute inflammatory changes of the anterior segment and the acute and chronic skin changes (erisipela de la costa). He recommended the excision of the nodules as a cure.[29]

Pacheco-Luna,[109] who worked with Robles, provided a more detailed description of the forms of keratitis and anterior uveitis. The first description of intraocular microfilariae was made in 1931 by the Mexican ophthalmologist Juan Luis Torroella.[149] The Belgian general physician Jean Hisette in his pioneering studies in the Belgium Congo (Zaire) described in detail the anterior-segment changes that included extensive histopathology and the widespread presence of intraocular microfilariae.[66] He also described the destructive chorioretinal changes that, in the French literature, are often named after him.

Harold Ridley,[123] a British ophthalmologist serving with the British Army in the northern Gold Coast (Ghana), probably gave the most comprehensive description of the ocular manifestations of onchocerciasis. His detailed clinical descriptions of onchochorioretinitis led to the use of the term "Ridley fundus" for onchocercal chorioretinitis.

Since that time many workers have made major contributions to understanding *O. volvulus* and the disease it causes. Prominent among these is the British physician Brian Duke, who changed the study of onchocerciasis into a science, especially the assessment of the effects of treatment. Others who have made outstanding contributions have been the epidemiologic team of John Anderson and Harold Fuglsang, and the French entomologist René Le Berre whose work provided the basis for the successful vector control carried out by the Onchocerciasis Control Program. The most recent advance in the combat against onchocerciasis is ivermectin. This development was in large part due to the work of Mohamed Aziz, a physician from Bangladesh, and Bruce Greene, an American infectious disease physician.

TABLE 107-1 THE DISTRIBUTION OF ONCHOCERCIASIS ESTIMATED NUMBER OF PERSONS AT RISK, INFECTED, AND BLIND (<3/60)

Region	At Risk	Infected	Blind
Africa			
Angola, Benin, Burkina, Faso, Burundi, Cameroon, Central African Republic, Chad, Congo, Côte d'lvoire, Equatorial Guinea, Ethiopia, Gabon, Ghana, Guinea, Guinea Bissau, Liberia, Malawi, Mali, Niger, Nigeria, Senegal, Sierra Leone, Tanzania, Togo, Uganda, Zaire	78,272,500	17,120,500	326,600
Eastern Mediterranean			
Sudan, Yemen	2,060,000	540,000	8,400
Americas			
Brazil, Columbia, Ecuador, Guatemala, Mexico, Venezuela	5,251,280	97,200	1,400
Total	85,583,780	17,757,700	336,400

EPIDEMIOLOGY

Geographic Distribution

Onchocerciasis is endemic across equatorial Africa and in circumscribed areas of Central and South America. Over 90% of those infected live in subSaharan Africa (Fig. 107-2). Geographic foci of infection are often clearly defined and their distribution and size are related to the presence of blackflies.[168] Regional geographic differences in onchocerciasis occur,[9,43] and these are explained by variations in transmission and in the parasite-vector complex, although host factors may also be involved (Table 107-2).

In West Africa there are differences between savanna and forest areas.[35,36,122] In forest areas, despite high rates of transmission and a high prevalence of infection, there is usually less advanced ocular disease and blindness. This finding suggests that the parasites in the forest areas may be both less invasive of the eye or less pathogenic.

Reports from forest and savanna areas in Sierra Leone show a different result.[95,96] Higher rates of ocular involvement occurred in forest areas, although the rates found in the savanna in Sierra Leone were lower than those reported by the OCP.[122]

Some have fallen into the trap of referring to onchocerciasis in the savanna areas as "blinding" onchocerciasis, and that in the forest areas as "nonblinding". This terminology is misleading because, although astounding rates of blindness may be found in some small savanna villages with up to 30% of the village being blind,[5] rates of bilateral blindness of 2% to 5% are not uncommon in forest areas.[96,102] The vast majority of this blindness in these areas is due to onchocerciasis, and these rates are many times greater than those found in nononchocerciasis endemic areas.[164]

These geographic variations have been attributed to many factors including whether a certain blackfly bites around the ankles or the head. It now appears certain that there are a number of different "strains" of *O. volvulus,* each of which is associated with, and transmitted by, a particular species of *Simulium* sp. The species of blackfly also varies from region to region. Recently it has become possible to separate forest and savanna parasites clearly by means of DNA probes.[50] Over the next few years further characteristics of these regional strains of *O. volvulus* are likely to be defined, and further regional or subregional strains need to be identified.

Data based on polymerase chain reaction amplification permits initial sequence analyses of the evolutionary history of *O. volvulus.*[170] These analyses show that although the African savanna and forest strains are quite distinct, the African savanna and the American parasites are very similar. This finding would confirm the long-held belief that onchocerciasis was introduced to Latin America by infected Africans brought to Latin America as slaves[29] and that the fortuitous presence of surrogate blackfly vectors could establish new foci of transmission.

Endemic Environment

O. volvulus is transmitted by the biting blackfly. The blackfly larvae require well-oxygenated water to mature, and eggs are laid in fast-flowing water.[141] Because of seasonal variations in volume and rate of flow, a particular stretch of river may be either a permanent breeding site or a temporary breeding site with breeding occuring only at certain times of the year. Blackflies usually do not travel more than one or two kilometers from their breeding sites, although at times they may be carried hundreds of kilometers by monsoonal winds.[168] Female blackflies require a blood meal to initiate ovulation, and it is during this meal that they may receive or transmit onchocercal parasites.

The geographic distribution of onchocerciasis is characterized by local foci of disease. Foci may vary in intensity but are always located in the vicinity of rivers or streams that form the breeding sites of the blackflies. Foci may be localized to a single breeding site and its adjacent village or they may extend for hundreds of miles and involve whole river complexes.

In general, in the African savanna there are usually a few, clearly defined breeding sites in large rivers. In forest areas,

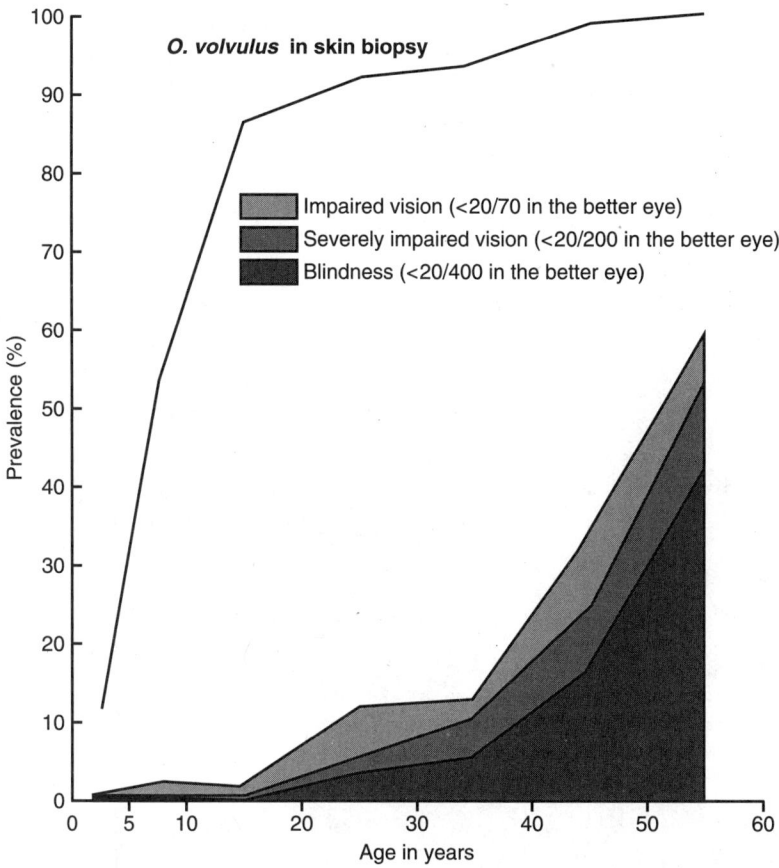

Fig. 107-1. Age-specific prevalence of infection and visual impairment in area of northern Ghana, hyperendemic for onchocerciasis. (With permission World Health Organization Expert Committee Report. Technical Report Series No. 752. Epidemiology of Onchocerciasis. *WHO,* Geneva, 1987.)

smaller and more continuous breeding sites occur along many rivers. In Central America there are many tiny trickles and streams, each supporting a breeding site.

Intensity of Infection

One measure of the risk of infection is the annual transmission potential (ATP), which is the calculated number of infective larvae transmitted to a person who is continuously exposed to blackflies for one year.[168] In the worst areas the ATP may be 90,000 infective larvae per person per year. An ATP of greater than 1500 is associated with a high prevalence of blindness, and values over 2500 are often associated with the subsequent desertion of the involved villages by the populace.[168]

TABLE 107-2 COMPARISON OF GENERAL CHARACTERISTICS OF ONCHOCERCIASIS IN SAVANNA AND RAIN FOREST AREAS OF WEST AFRICA AND CENTRAL AMERICA

	West Africa		Central America
Characteristics	**Rain Forest**	**Savanna**	
Skin counts	Moderate	Very high	Low to moderate
Nodules	More common, usually below waist	Less common, usually below waist	Less common, usually waist
Annual transmission potential	High	Moderate	Low
Prevalence	Very High	High	Low
Blindness	Less common (1% to 2%)	Common (5% to 10%)	Uncommon (Less than 1%)
Major cause of blindness	Chorioretinitis	Sclerosing keratitis	Anterior uveitis
Physiologenic relationship	Distant	Similar	Similar

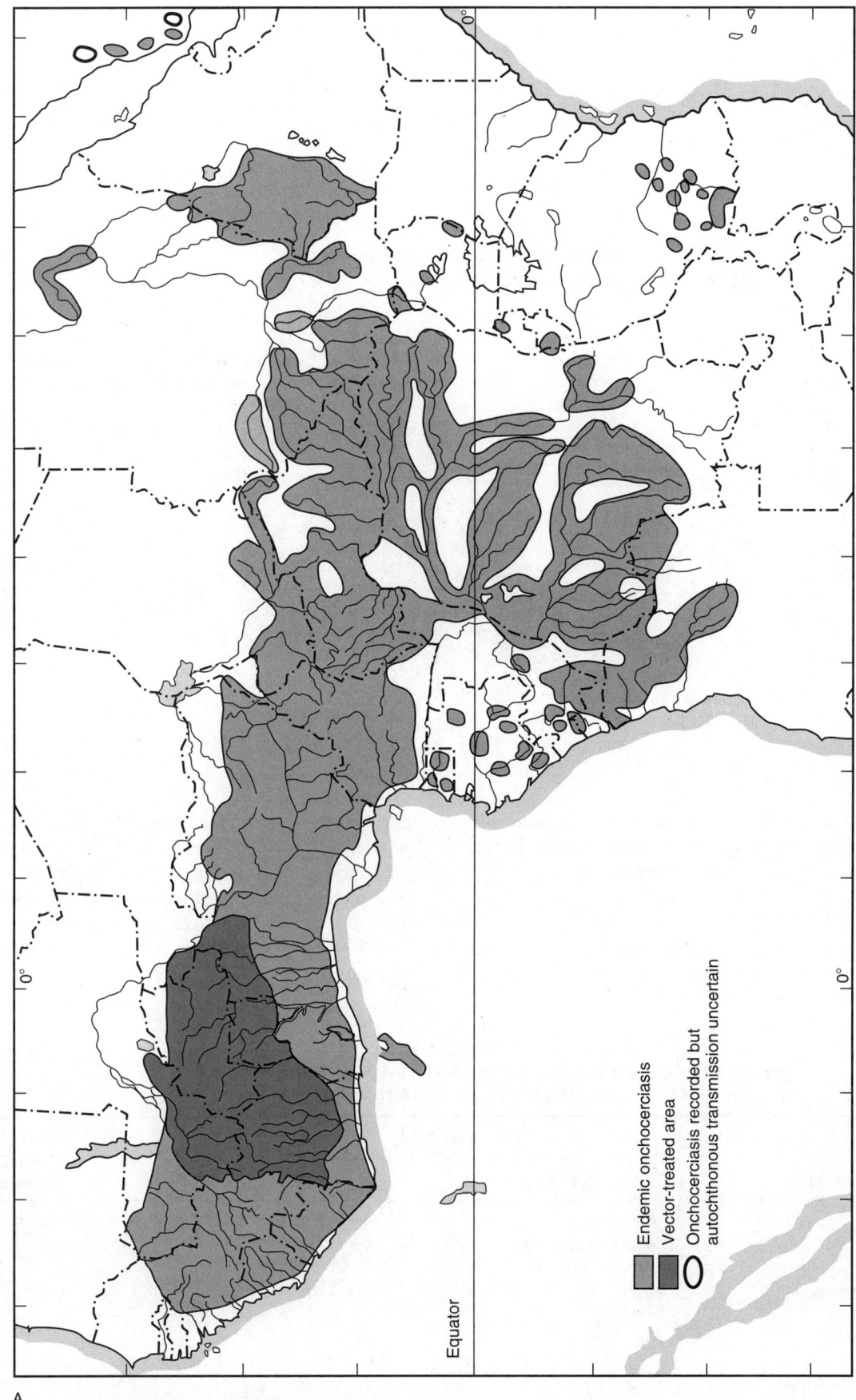

Fig. 107-2. Geographic distribution of onchocerciasis. **A,** in Africa and the Arabian Peninsula.

Endemic onchocerciasis

Vector-treated area

Onchocerciasis recorded but
autochthonous transmission uncertain

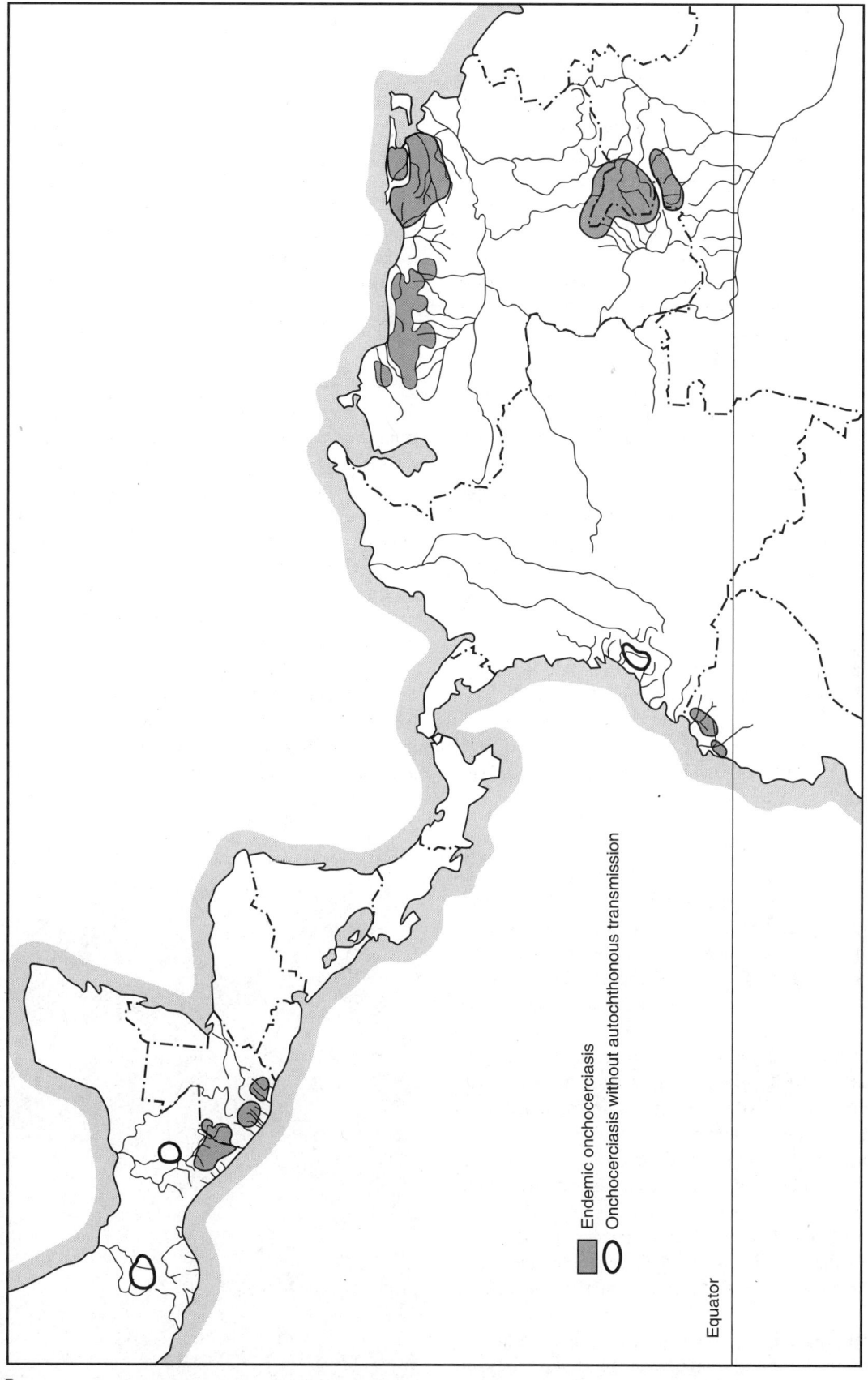

B

Fig. 107-2, cont'd. **B,** in Latin America. (With permission World Health Organization Expert Committee Report. Technical Report Series No. 597. Epidemiology of Onchocerciasis. *WHO,* Geneva, 1987.)

In hyperendemic areas in West Africa most persons are infected with *O. volvulus* during the first years of life (Fig. 107-1). The intensity of infection, measured as the number of microfilariae per milligram of skin snip, increases with host age. Men are often more heavily infected than women, usually because of different occupational exposures. About one third of persons over the age of 15 years will have microfilariae in the anterior chamber of their eyes. Intraocular microfilariae are more common in those who have high skin-snip counts. In the worst affected areas in the African savanna 10% of the population and half of those over the age of 40 will be blind.[168] Severe eye lesions and blindness are more common in heavily infected persons and in areas where more people are infected. The intensity of infection in a person is the cumulative result of many years of exposure.[141]

Although the terms hyperendemic, mesoendemic, and hypoendemic are frequently used in reference to onchocerciasis, there are no clear-cut definitions that have been universally adopted. Frequently a prevalence of greater than 60% is used to define hyperendemicity and a prevalence of less than 20% implies hypoendemicity.

Data from the savanna of West Africa show that there often is a mosaic of endemicity related to the distance a village is from a breeding site. The terms "first-line", "second-line", and "third-line" are used to stratify those villages closest to the breeding sites from those further away.[167] The levels of infection and severity of disease and blindness generally correlate with these classifications.

Socioeconomic Impact

Blindness is the major disability of onchocerciasis and is the factor that makes it such a major public-health problem.[168] It usually affects otherwise healthy adults at their prime of life when they have major responsibility for supporting their families. The loss of these breadwinners in families and villages is devastating among these subsistence farmers and often leads to the abandonment of whole villages in endemic areas. This action is particularly damaging as this land is usually along rivers and often is the only fertile, arable land available. Villages with blindness rates in excess of 5% are not sustainable.[168]

There is a threefold to fourfold increase in mortality associated with blindness.[118] Once persons are blinded by onchocerciasis, life expectancy is reduced by at least 13 years. This increased mortality is due to the impact of blindness on the status of the individuals and their economic and nutritional dependence rather than direct effect of the disease itself.

In central West Africa onchocerciasis has led to a pattern of migration from the fertile hyperendemic river valleys to the barren ridges. After several generations the community moves back to the rivers until the level of endemicity builds up to intolerable levels. Then they once again abandon the

rivers and return to the hills. This cycle may take many generations and possibly has gone on for centuries.[104]

Few studies have looked at the economic cost of onchocerciasis. It is so high that even the expensive Onchocerciasis Control Program was regarded as being cost-effective. Although some argument exists as to how to calculate the precise benefit of the program, it has been compared with measles vaccination in terms of productive years of healthy life added.[52,119,168]

CLINICAL FEATURES

Skin Changes

The skin changes in onchocerciasis cover a broad spectrum from early pruritus and rash through reactive onchodermatitis to the gross and disfiguring late changes (Table 107-3).

The actual bite of the blackfly is usually unnoticed, although a painful weal develops quickly and resolves in two or three days. Some people develop a hypersensitivity to the fly saliva, and they may have a severe reaction around each fly bite.

Pruritus is the most common early manifestation of onchocerciasis.[141] It heralds the onset of onchocerciasis after a latent interval of 6 months to 2 years following initial infection. This period is the time it takes for the first microfilariae to form, migrate into the skin, and die. Itching and scratching may be mild and intermittent or severe and unremitting and can occur anywhere on the body. Scratching can lead to excoriation and secondary infection.[32] A maculopapular rash may develop (Fig. 107-3). Dead microfilariae are found in

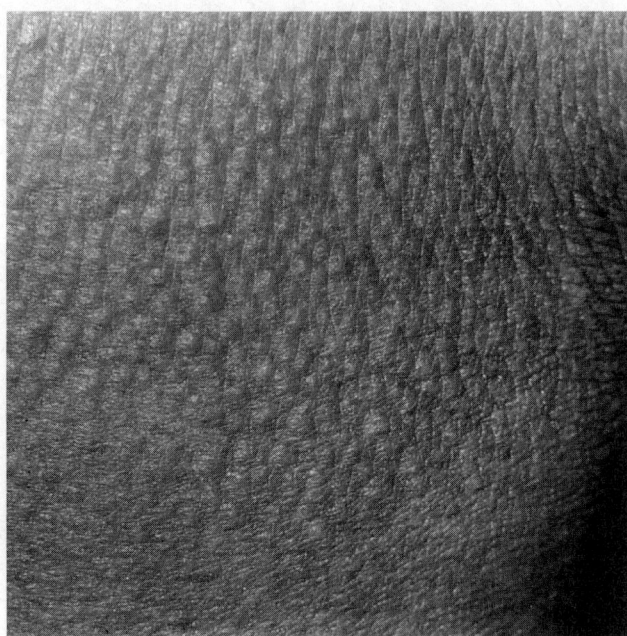

Fig. 107-3. Maculopapular rash typical of onchocerciasis in Mexican male.

TABLE 107-3   CLINICAL FEATURES OF ONCHOCERCIASIS

	Acute	Chronic (reversible)	Chronic (irreversible)
Skin	Pruritis Maculopapular rash Pustular rash	Pruritis Maculopapular rash Onchodermatitis Sowda	Subcutaneous nodules Depigmentation Leopard skin Lichenification
Lymphatic	Lymphadenitis	Lymphadenitis	Shotty lymph nodes
Conjunctiva	Limbitis	Conjunctival injection	—
Cornea	Punctate keratitis	Intracorneal microfilariae	Sclerosing keratitis
Anterior uveitis	Acute uveitis	Intracorneal microfilariae Chronic uveitis	Iris and retropupillary fibrosis (pear-shaped pupil) Inferior posterior Anterior synechia Secondary glaucoma Secondary cataract
Retina/Choroid	Hemorrhage Cotton⁻ wool spots Retinal vasculitis RPE	Intraretinal microfilariae Window defects Other intraretinal deposits	RPE atrophy and pigment clumping Outer retinal atrophy Inner choroidal atrophy Subretinal fibrosis Consecutive optic atrophy Vitreous changes

the papule, which may become vesicular or even pustular. Pruritus may be the sole manifestation of the disease, especially in lightly infected persons, and is often very troublesome in expatriates who are infected as adults.

The earliest pathological changes in the skin are mild and are often limited to a perivasculitis.[32] In more heavily infected persons microfilariae can be found, especially at the epidermal-dermal junction. Live microfilariae are usually not surrounded by inflammatory cells, but dead and disintegrating microfilariae form the center of focal inflammatory infiltrates comprised predominantly of degenerating eosinophils.[31]

Over several years more severe disease leads to alterations in skin pigmentation. Small focal areas of increased pigmentation may develop as may areas of either focal or widespread depigmentation. After many years a particularly characteristic change occurs on the shins, leopard skin (Fig. 107-4). Here there are focal areas of hyperpigmentation surrounding the remaining hair follicles with white hypopigmented skin in between. The simple identification of people with leopard skin has been used to assess the prevalence of onchocerciasis.[49,144]

Severe reactive skin changes (termed onchodermatitis) also occur, especially during the earlier stages of infection. These include thickening of the skin with lichenification and scaling, crusted papules, and deeper erosions with surrounding inflammation and hyperemia. These skin changes can be very disabling. Histologically there is hyperkeratosis, acanthosis, and parakeratosis, with an increase in inflammation and fibrosis. Dermal collagen is disrupted by deposition of increasing amounts of eosinophilic major basic protein and

mucin ground substance and by fibrous scar tissue.[32] With more advanced fibrosis and inflammation, microfilariae become less common in the superficial dermis and are found mainly in the deeper layers. Ultimately the dermis becomes fibrotic and is covered by a thinned and atrophic epithelium. This condition is often referred to clinically as lizard skin. With atrophy of the dermal collagen the skin tends to hang in folds causing "hanging groin" in the inguinal region and leonine facies.

A more severe, localized form of reactive onchodermatitis, seen especially in Yemen, is known by its Arabic name, "sowda", or black-limb.[141] Histologically there is an extensive infiltrate of plasma cells in the skin.[32] Considerable edema and fibrosis occur. Inguinal lymph nodes are enlarged with hyperplasia of germinal centers and some fibrosis. Only occasionally microfilariae are seen in the deep dermis or in skin snips. Patients with onchodermatitis have a high cellular immune response to onchocercal antigens, which is suppressed if their disease becomes generalized.[91]

Nodules

Adult worms are almost always encapsulated in nodules, although at times they may be found free in fascial planes. Most nodules lie in subcutaneous tissue or fascial planes and usually they are firmly fixed to the underlying periosteum or joint capsules (Fig. 107-5).

Nodules are firm, round masses with little or no mobility. Most nodules are found around the pelvis, but they may also occur around the head and shoulders. Nodules also occur on the thorax and in the limbs, where they are often fixed to the skin. Occasionally nodules are found in deeper structures.[32]

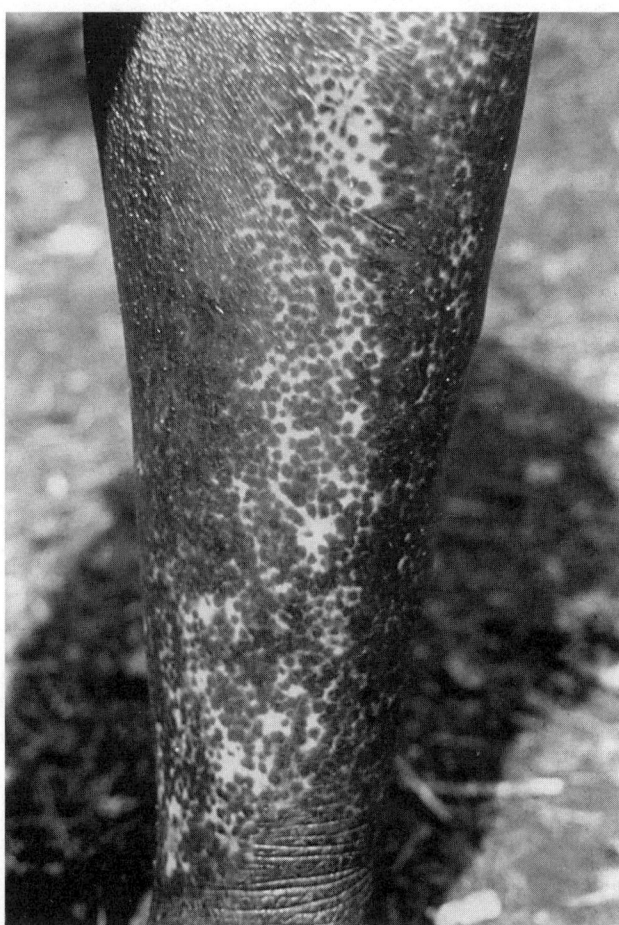

Fig. 107-4. Characteristic leopard skin pigmentary changes in shin of Liberian male. Remaining pigment clusters around residual hair follicles.

New nodules tend to develop around older nodules. Although an individual nodule will usually be 0.25 cm to 1 cm in diameter and contain two or three females and one or two males, large matted conglomerations of nodules can form. Nodules are usually painless and, by themselves, cause little trouble.

Histologically the nodules contain dense scar tissue that surrounds and encases the adult worms. The adults are coiled up like a ball of string.[141] Most of the length of the female is taken up by the long, paired uteri that are normally packed with developing embryonic forms and immature microfilariae. Degenerative females often become calcified. Nodules may show an inflammatory infiltrate of varying intensity and occasionally areas of necrosis and liquefaction. Adult worms may be freed from nodules by collagenase digestion followed by careful dissection (Fig. 107-3). They can then be studied intact.[45]

Lymphatic Involvement

The draining lymph nodes of areas with onchocercal dermatitis become firm and discrete. They are not painful or tender. Although firm lymph nodes may be seen in hanging groin, chronic lymphatic obstruction and lymphedema (common in lymphatic filariasis) are not features of onchocerciasis. Histologically the lymph nodes show capsular fibrosis, atrophic follicles, and dilation of the subcapsular sinusoids and lymphatics. Microfilariae or their remains may be seen in the chronic granulomatous inflammatory infiltrate.[32]

Following treatment with a microfilaricidal drug, a transient reactive lymphadenopathy is quite common. In this case there may be lymphangiitis and enlargement and tenderness of the regional lymph nodes, especially in the axilla and groin. These symptoms may be associated with local lymphedema and a transient peau d'orange change in the skin. A different picture is seen in sowdah, which is characterized by a marked reactive follicular hyperplasia.

Ocular Changes

Microfilariae migrate widely throughout the body. They can enter the eye by invading along scleral vessels and nerves and from the bloodstream. Most, however, probably

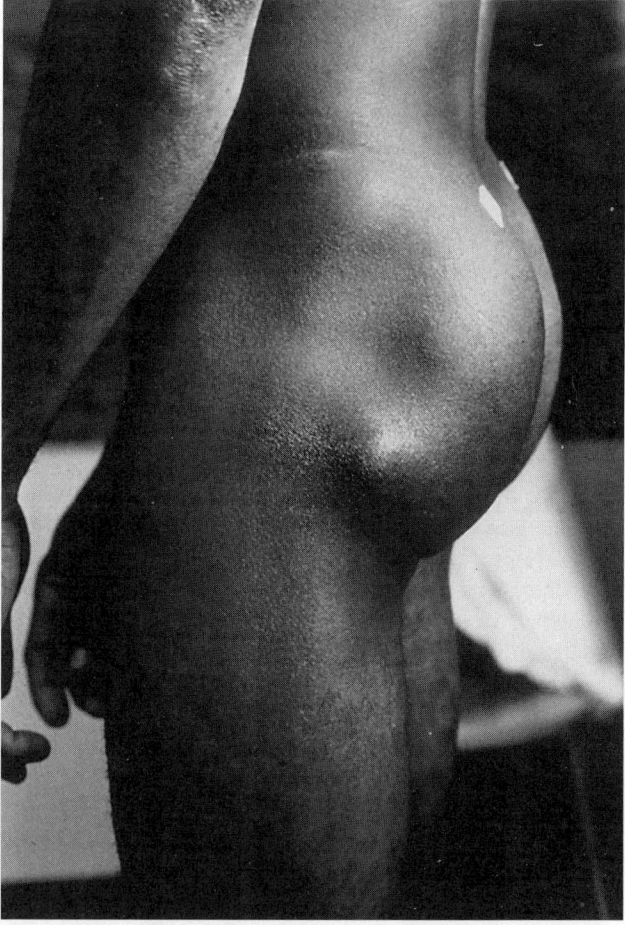

A

Fig. 107-5. Onchocercal nodules. **A,** Cluster of nodules around hips of young Liberian male.

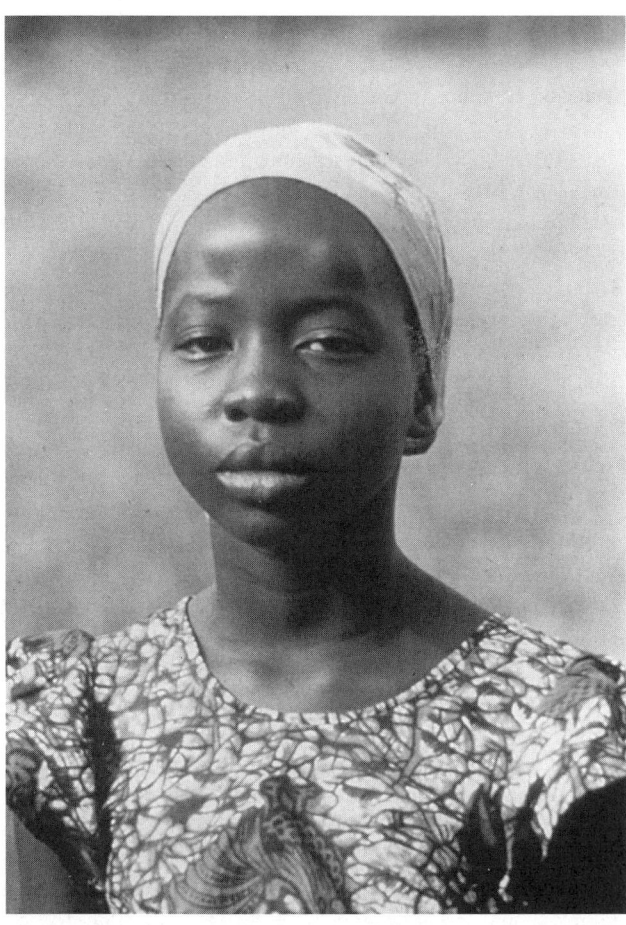

B

Fig. 107-5, cont'd. **B,** Head nodule in Liberian woman. (Photo courtesy H.S. Newland.)

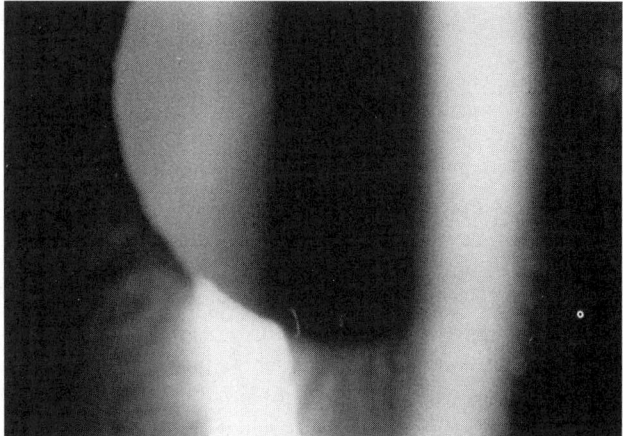

Fig. 107-6. Single microfilaria swimming free in anterior chamber. Microfilaria is just above pupil margin at 6 o'clock position.

appear as small, highly refractile objects with a greenish tinge.[100]

Keratitis. An inflammatory infiltrate surrounds dead microfilariae in the cornea. It appears as an ill-defined punctate, fluffy, or snowflake opacity, about 0.5 mm in diameter in the superficial stroma. These opacities are focal collections of lymphocytes and eosinophils with local edema.[55] Punc-

enter the eye by direct invasion from the surrounding bulbar conjunctiva.[24] The presence of intraocular microfilariae is the earliest sign of ocular involvement (Table 107-3). Microfilariae in the anterior chamber can be seen easily with a slit lamp, especially if the patient sits with the head down for 2 to 5 minutes (Fig. 107-6). This position allows microfilariae in the anterior chamber to fall to the center of the cornea where they can be seen when the patient sits up. The microfilariae are small, wriggling white "worms". They often can be followed as they circulate in convection currents in the aqueous humor.

Live microfilariae in the cornea are more difficult to find because they are immobile, transparent, and coiled.[141] Dead microfilariae are easier to see because they are opaque and straight (Fig. 107-7). Microfilariae are best seen with high magnification (25×) and retroillumination produced by an oblique beam reflected from the iris. Microfilarial numbers are higher in the peripheral cornea, especially in temporal and nasal quadrants. Microfilariae can be found in the retina, anterior vitreous, and at times, attached to the lens capsule or to the Descemet membrane. Intraretinal microfilariae are best seen during contact lens examination of the fundus and

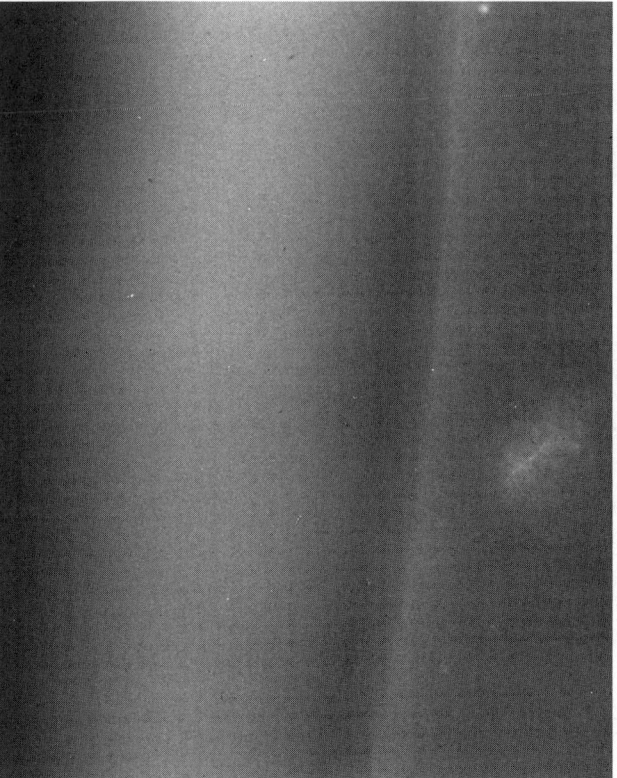

Fig. 107-7. Dead microfilaria, which has become straight and opaque, in cornea. Small fluffy or punctate opacity is forming around it.

tate keratitis is most commonly seen days to weeks after treatment with a microfilicidal drug (especially diethylcarbamazine) when many microfilariae die at one time. Dead microfilariae can sometimes be recognized in the center of these opacities. These opacities clear without visible sequelae.

At times epiphora and limbitis may be seen, especially after diethylcarbamazine treatment.[67] Acute globular limbitis is not common in persons not receiving chemotherapy and may be associated with an increased level of cell-mediated immunity.[53] The small (0.05 mm), pale yellow globules at the limbus are eosinophilic granulomata that are believed to form around dead microfilariae. Other conjunctival lesions have been reported but are not common.[130]

In more advanced disease corneal changes begin at the limbus, initially in the interpalpebral fissure and inferiorly. An increased limbal translucency, or haze, is the earliest change. These changes progress until ultimately the whole cornea is opaque and vascularized in established sclerosing keratitis (Fig. 107-8). The corneal opacity is a fibrovascular pannus and inflammatory infiltrate, composed mainly of lymphocytes and eosinophils, at the level of the Bowman membrane.[55] It advances in an arc that is most marked at each side and below. The remaining areas of clear cornea usually show heavy infiltration of microfilariae. Ultimately the entire cornea becomes opaque. Sclerosing keratitis has been reproduced in an animal model in which various purified antigens are injected into the corneal stroma of systemically immunized guinea pigs.[54]

Anterior Uveitis. The presence and severity of anterior uveitis is variable. A mild nongranulomatous uveitis occurs commonly when there are microfilariae in the anterior chamber or the cornea.[141] An eye may be heavily infiltrated with several hundred microfilariae in either the cornea or the anterior chamber, however, and have no reaction. In other cases a severe anterior uveitis may develop, leading to inferior-posterior synechiae with a characteristic pear-shaped deformity of the pupil and retropupillary fibrosis. Chronic granulomatous anterior uveitis also causes a loss of the iris pigment frill and a pumice-stone appearance of the iris. Extensive synechiae will cause seclusion and occlusion of the pupil, secondary cataract, or secondary glaucoma. Mild uveitis has been related to the microfilarial invasion of the iris, whereas more severe granulomatous uveitis is due to invasion of the ciliary body.[55]

Chorioretinitis. Extensive chorioretinal changes may occur in onchocerciasis. Although the pathogenesis is unclear, some overall perspective is beginning to form from an integration of clinical and experimental observations. There is a spectrum of clinical features that ranges from intraretinal deposits to retinal pigment changes and then to widespread chorioretinal atrophy with loss of all retinal layers (Table 107-3). These changes occur predominantly in the posterior pole, although macular function is often preserved until quite late in the disease.

Clinically and histologically the predominant early changes seem to involve the RPE. There is a dispersion of pigment granules from the RPE. This leads not only to patchy areas of depigmentation that have a granular appearance but also to the presence of fine light brown intraretinal pigment and darker, deeper pigment changes (Fig. 107-9). Later lacunae or holes appear in the residual layer of depigmented RPE. These areas expand and become confluent until in the final stages the RPE has almost entirely disappeared (Fig. 107-10).

Concomitant with these changes is the loss of photoreceptors and outer layers of the retina, leading to consecutive loss of the inner neuroretina, loss of ganglion cells, and subsequent loss of nerve fibers. This condition in turn leads to

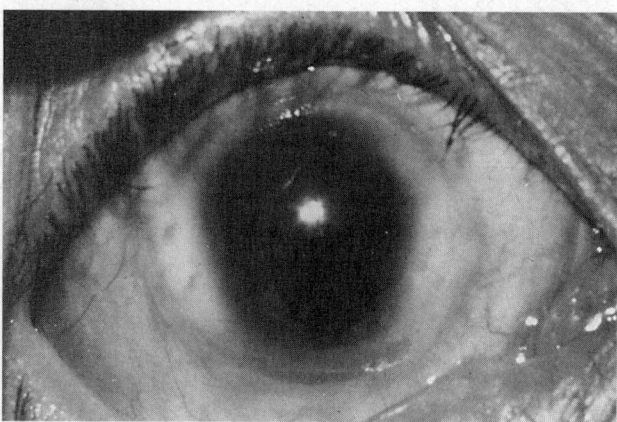

Fig. 107-8. Sclerosing keratitis usually begins at nasal and temporal peripheral cornea and progresses slowly centrally. This Guatemalan man also has pear-shaped distortion of the pupil, which is characteristic of previous onchocercal uveitis. (With permission, Taylor HR: Onchocerciasis. In Tasman W, Jaeger EA, editors: *Duane's clinical ophthalmology*, Philadelphia, 1992, JB Lippincott.) (Figure also in color insert.)

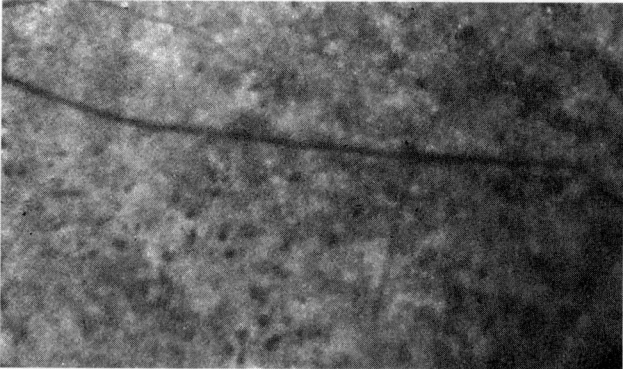

Fig. 107-9. Intraretinal pigment migration and clumping following early changes to retinal pigment epithelium. These changes are usually widespread in posterior pole.

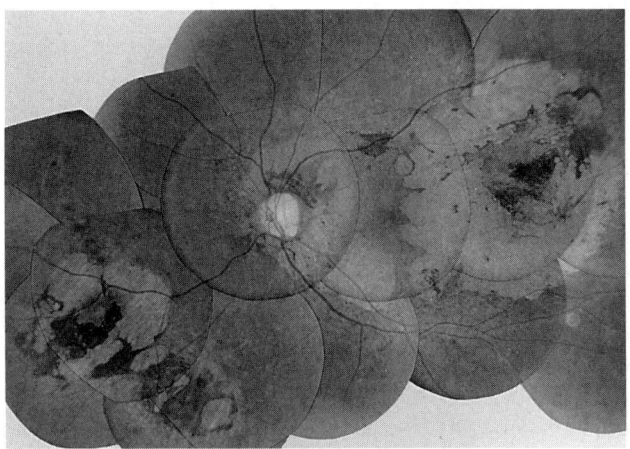

Fig. 107-10.   Montage of fundus of Ghanian male showing severe widespread destruction of retina and choroid. Typically there is temporal and nasal involvement and relative sparing of macula until late in course of disease. (Figure also in color insert.)

optic atrophy. In parallel is progressive inflammation and the loss of the choriocapillaris. Subretinal fibrosis may also occur. These changes appear to progress as a chronic, indolent, low-grade, progressive inflammation. The clinical appearance of the fundus can be quite varied depending on the predominant feature at any given time and the stage of evolution of the disease. Longitudinal studies have shown these changes to be surprisingly dynamic and progressive.[131]

Intraretinal microfilariae may be seen as highly reflective metallic structures in the retina. They often have a white or greenish sheen and are often related to retinal blood vessels. They may be directly observed to move and will change their location from day to day. They are best seen with contact lens examination of the eye.[100]

Intraretinal deposits of two types occur, shiny deposits and white deposits. In a West African forest area shiny deposits occured in about 10% of adults. They were fixed and unchanging.[102,131] White deposits occur twice as often and disappeared or reappeared over a period of months. The cause of these changes is unknown, but they may relate to dead or dying microfilaria in a way comparable to punctate opacities in the cornea.

Intraretinal pigmentation may be seen in over half of those with onchocerciasis.[102] Its distribution varies over time. It becomes more marked with more severe disease, but then disappears as the retina atrophies in advanced chorioretinitis.

Retinal pigment epithelial atrophy is seen initially as a diffuse granularity with translucency on fluorescein angiopathy. Geographic areas of atrophy tend to develop in areas with diffuse changes. The edges of a geographic atrophic area may expand at up to 200 μm per year so that in three years a patch of 1 mm diameter could form.[131] One third of those in a forest area had these changes.[102]

Active retinitis is less common and may occur in about 5% of infected adults. The hemorrhages and cotton-wool spots clear without sequelae as does the vasculitis. Rarely there may be severe retinal vasculitis with active fulminant disease.[141] Subretinal fibrosis is less common and is seen in about 1% of patients.

Not only may optic atrophy occur consecutively to retinal atrophy, but it may occur after optic neuritis, either directly related to the disease itself or precipitated by chemotherapy as part of the generalized Mazzotti reaction.[141,168] The frequency of optic atrophy varies with prevalence and previous treatment with suramin or diethylcarbamazine, but is often between 1% and 5%.

Vitreoretinal abnormalities also occur. They include epiretinal membranes, posterior vitreous detachment, and macular holes.

PATHOGENESIS

Parasitology

Parasite. The parasite *O. volvulus* is one of the filarial nematodes. It is the only onchocercal species to infect man. Other onchocercal species infect cattle, horses, and other large mammals. The filarial nematodes also include *Wuchereria bancrofti* and *Brugia malayi,* both of which produce lymphatic filariasis and elephantitis, and *Loa loa,* the cause of loiasis.

The adult female *O. volvulus* is a white threadlike worm, 50 to 100 cm long and only 0.3 mm across (Fig. 107-11). Adult males have a similar appearance but are thinner and much shorter, being only about 2.5 to 5 cm long. Adult female worms have an average life span of 9 to 10 years but may live up to 15 years. During their lifetime each releases millions of microfilariae. A microfilaria is about 300 μm long and 5 to 10 μm in diameter (Fig. 107-12). A microfilaria will die after 6 to 30 months if it is not taken up by a blackfly.

Vector. Onchocerciasis is transmitted by biting blackflies. Although the species of blackfly vary in different geographic areas, they are all members of the family *Simuliidae.* In the African savanna the main species are grouped as *Simulium damnosum,* a complex of several closely related subspecies.[168] In rain forest areas of Africa *S. yahense* and *S. sanctipauli* are the important vectors. *S. onchraceum* is the main species in Guatemala and Mexico, and *S. metallicum* is found in South America.

Life Cycle. The female blackfly acquires microfilariae when she bites an infected person (Fig. 107-13). The microfilariae pass to the fly's stomach. They then penetrate the gut wall and migrate to the flight muscles. The microfilariae undergo several molts to become third-stage infective larvae. These "L3" larvae migrate to the fly's proboscis to be transferred during the next blood meal. A female fly infected during her first blood meal will be infected during her second meal, but

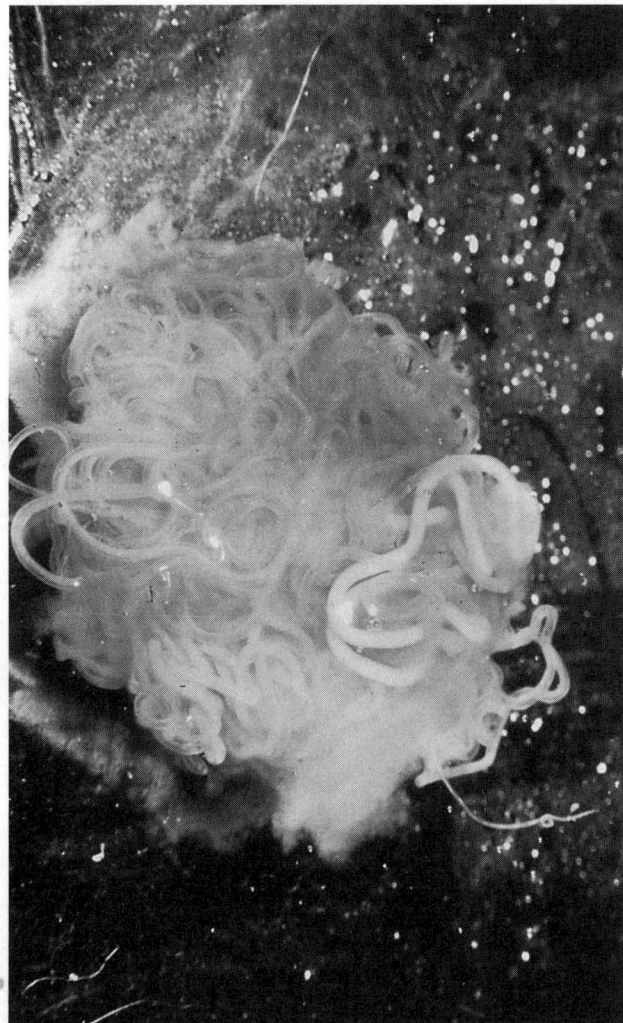

Fig. 107-11. Adult worms of *O. volvulus* can be freed from excised nodules by collagenase digestion, which removes host tissue. This nodule contains two adult females, which are much longer and thicker than the single male worm seen at the edge of the nodule at the upper right. (With permission Taylor HR: Onchocerciasis. In Tasman W, Jaeger EA, editors: *Duane's clinical ophthalmology,* Philadelphia, 1992, JB Lippincott.)

it usually takes until the third blood meal for the L3 larvae to develop and for the fly to become infectious. Most flies die after their third reproductive cycle.

Two to six L3 larvae are transmitted by an infected fly. The infective larvae actively move through the breach in the skin caused by the fly bite and then migrate through the subcutaneous tissues. They rapidly molt within a day or so to become fourth-stage larvae (L4) and four to six weeks later molt for the last time to become immature adult males or female worms. Over a period of about 12 months they develop into mature adult worms.

Most adult worms are encapsulated by host fibrous tissue to form the characteristic nodules (onchocercomata). The adults reproduce sexually and release new microfilariae which migrate through the nodule wall and then spread throughout the body, particularly the skin and the eye.

Microfilariae taken up by another blackfly will continue the cycle as the remaining microfilariae die in the host. The inflammatory reaction initiated by the dead or dying microfilariae is responsible for much of the disease seen in onchocerciasis.

Parasite Factors and Disease. The pathogenesis of disease manifestations in onchocerciasis is largely unknown although punctate, multifocal stromal keratitis has been shown to present an inflammatory focus surrounding dead or dying microfilariae.[57] Because of their vast numbers and wide distribution throughout the body, as well as the clinical correlation between microfilariae and complications,[43] microfilariae are thought to cause many of the disease manifestations. The finding in various tissues of perivascular deposits of immune complexes as well as increased levels of circulating immune complexes[62] also suggests a role for these complexes in the pathogenesis of some lesions.

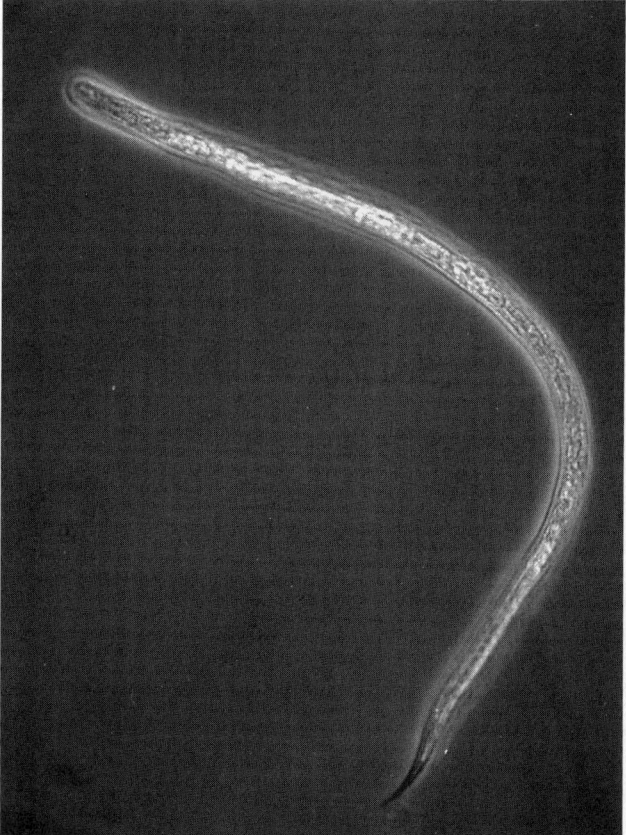

Fig. 107-12. Microfilaria of *O. volvulus* seen by phase-contrast microscopy. Rounded phallic end is clearly distinguished from pointed cortal end. This microfilaria is straightening as it dies. (With permission Taylor HR: Onchocerciasis. In Tasman W, Jaeger EA, editors: *Duane's clinical ophthalmology,* Philadelphia, 1992, JB Lippincott.)

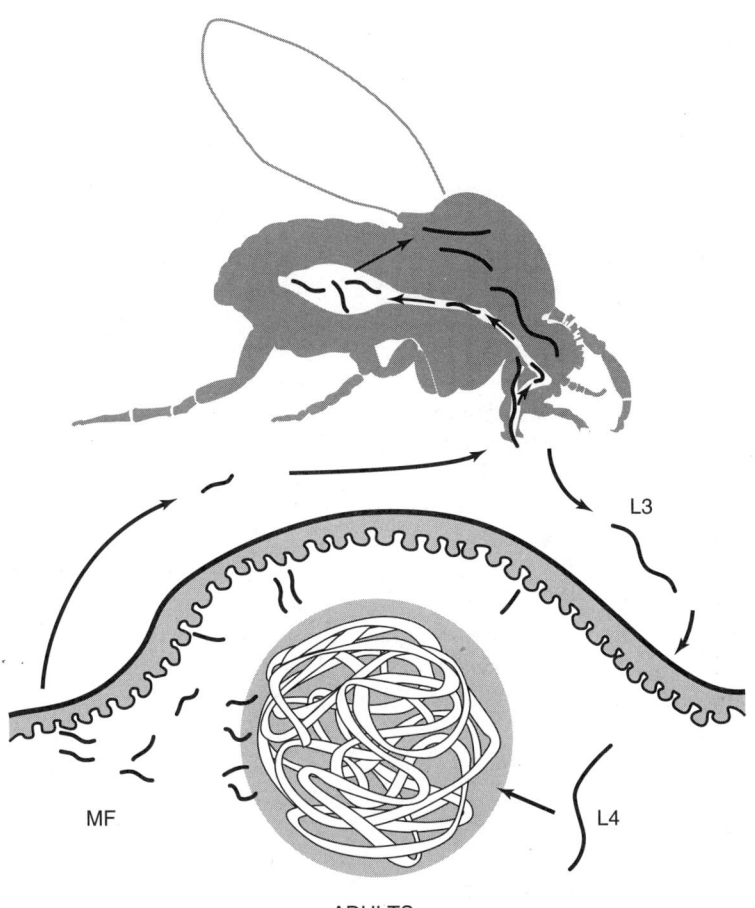

Fig. 107-13. A schematic representation of the life cycle of *Onchocerca volvulus.* Infective larvae (L3) pass from an infected fly to humans. They eventually develop into adult worms, which are found in nodules and release millions of microfilariae (Mf). Microfilariae are taken up by another blackfly and after several molts develop into new infective larvae.

Local Immunosuppression. *Onchocerca* parasites, like other filarial worms, have evolved a number of strategies to avoid the host response. Because parasite-specific T-cell responses are low in patent, generalized onchocerciasis* but antibody responses remain intact, a specific T-cell anergy has been proposed.[72]

Of a more general nature are other mechanisms that play significant roles in down-modulating local immune effector responses. (1) Like other filariae[93] the surfaces of onchocercal parasites are probably associated with human protein that may disguise them from the host immune system. (2) Secretion of immunodominant molecules such as the hapten phosophorylcholine may act both as a local immunosuppressant[75,94] and as a molecule that diverts the attention of the host immune system.[16] (3) The parasites have both secreted and surface-associated proteases[74] that could alter the immune response locally, for example by degrading antibody molecules.[139] (4) They can utilize endogenous and exogenous arachidonic acid to produce and release prostanoids (PGE_2 and prostacyclin) that may inhibit T-cell prolifera-

tion.[80,81] (5) Most helminth parasites including *O. volvulus* and other filarial nematodes have both a physical barrier to the outside world (an extracellular cuticle)[16,92] and surface or secreted antioxidants[65] that might counteract the effects of host granulocytes and macrophages.

Nodules. Over months to years adult worms become encased in a rim of host tissue forming the characteristic nodules known as onchocercomata.[32] The nodule comprises three components: an outer capsular rim, an inflammatory cellular infiltrate, and the enclosed adult worm.[43,57] The rim is comprised of hyalinized and vascularized fibrous tissues, and the adult worm is surrounded by a thick layer of fibrinoid material. Surrounding this fibrin lake is a chronic inflammatory infiltrate usually containing granulocytes, plasma cells, lymphocytes, histiocytes, fibrin, and Russell bodies. Nodules also contain microfilariae outside the adult female; some degenerate, others are phagocytosed by small multinucleate cells, but most pass unharmed to the dermis.

There is an intimate relationship between the cuticle of the adult worm and the capillaries of the host. There is evidence of capillary proliferation around the worms with vessels arborizing into capillary beds that form a sleeve around the adult worm that is contiguous with the central fibrin

*References 53, 58, 70, 71, 88, 136, 138, 156.

lake.[56] Thus the worm has found a niche that is protected from the host immune response but allows for its own nutritional needs.

Microfilariae. Microfilariae can be found in all layers of the skin but are most numerous in the upper dermis. Live microfilariae cause little or no host reaction.[32] However, microfilariae have a finite lifespan so there is natural attrition of these life-cycle stages. Natural microfilarial death is usually associated with eosinophils or eosinophilic granular protein surrounding the cuticle.[69] With disintegration of the parasite comes the migration of neutrophils and macrophages. How the microfilariae evade killing by the host immune system is not known.

The chronic stages of onchocercal skin disease likely results from microfilarial death. Hyperkeratosis, focal parakeratosis, and acanthosis are seen with more advanced changes in the dermis, including lymphatic dilation, tortuosity of dermal vessels, and an increase in extracellular matrix protein.[30,31] Dermal fibroblasts increase in number, presumably leading to the increased fibrosis in the skin. Degeneration of dermal collagen is associated with the loss of elasticity.

Killing of Microfilariae. Information about microfilarial killing in vivo has come from studies of microfilarial death following treatment with microfilaricidal agents such as diethylcarbamazine and ivermectin. Soon after the administration of a microfilaricide the microfilariae undergo a series of morphologic changes and eosinophils and eosinophilic material surround the microfilariae. This material has been shown to be deposits of the highly proinflammatory eosinophilic granular proteins that are toxic to the parasite.[3,69] The microfilariae disintegrate over a period of weeks. These changes occur predominantly in the upper dermis and the epidermal-dermal junction. Clinically microfilarial death causes papules, edema, and urticaria that is probably related to both the eosinophilic infiltrates and mast-cell degranulation.[3]

Host Immune Responses

Humoral Response. Humoral immune responses induced by onchocercal infection include those that are parasite-specific and those that are polyclonal or nonspecific. Hypergammaglobulinemia (IgG and IgM) is common[32] and results from polyclonal B-cell activation either by chronic *O. volvulus* infection or by chronic antigenic stimuli from other concurrent helminthic or protozoal infections. Furthermore, polyclonal IgE elevation is found in the majority of patients.[107] In onchocerciasis, IgE levels are highly elevated and exceed those found in almost any other helminth condition and approach the extreme elevations found in the tropical pulmonary eosinophilia syndrome.[108]

More important are the parasite-specific antibody responses that onchocercal infection engenders. Using a variety of immunological techniques (including immunofluo-

rescence, complement fixation, and enzyme immunoassays employing soluble or detergent extracts as the target antigens) the presence of anti*O. volvulus* antibody (of each isotype) is a constant finding in individuals with onchocerciasis.[157] Because in most studies the onset of infection is not known and there are few studies in children, little data are available that define the evolution of a given antibody response. However, in a cross-sectional, age-related study of children under the age 15 years in a hyperendemic region, antibody (IgG, IgM or IgE) against antigens derived from the adult parasite appeared by age 5 and peaked by age 10.[68,157] These antibody responses correlated with the presence of skin microfilariae. A subset of these children were followed longitudinally; in approximately 10% there was conversion from microfiliaria-negative to positive, a change that was preceded by seroconversion (either IgG or IgE) in all but one.[157]

Although it has been difficult to define the evolution of the immune response after infection in human onchocerciasis, studies in a chimpanzee model of infection have provided insight into the dynamics following infection. Within one month following infection, antigens of developing larvae elicit both humoral and cell-mediated responses against crude *O. volvulus* antigen,[134,135,136] This process is manifested by IgG responses to particular antigens (as assessed by immunoblotting) and by a lymphocyte blastogenic response to soluble worm antigen. There is a parallel rise in IgE directed against parasite antigen.

A definitive role has not been established for antibody in the human immune response against infection with *O. volvulus*. In vitro sera from chronically infected individuals can promote granulocyte adherence to microfilariae and infective larvae[19,78,162]; destruction of microfilariae has also been demonstrated in vitro.[60] The strong promotion of attachment of granulocytes (and in particular eosinophils) to microfilariae in vitro has been correlated with the presence of corneal punctate opacities.[53] This finding suggests that antibodies may be responsible for some inflammatory manifestations of disease in the eye and in the skin. Eosinophils in the skin degranulate around microfilariae and release of eosinophil granule proteins. Eosinophils appear to be a major effector cell of antibody-dependent killing of microfilariae, and local (and perhaps even distant) tissue damage may result from repeated eosinophil degranulation.

Immediate hypersensitivity responses and IgE responses are particularly important in onchocerciasis. The majority of individuals with *O. volvulus* infection have elevated polyclonal serum IgE levels, but only 10% of the increase is directed against parasite antigens.[158] The significance of high-level IgE antibodies is unclear, although IgE antibodies may contribute to the acute inflammatory complications of *O. volvulus* infection, including the ocular lesions.[40] The parallel increase in IgG blocking antibodies may serve to modulate IgE mediated responses.[108]

Immune complexes are found in the serum of individuals infected with *O. volvulus*. Although the functional significance of circulating immune complexes in onchocerciasis is unclear, it is possible that deposition of these immune complexes leads to inflammation and tissue damage in some infected individuals.[60,114] Some correlations have been found between parasite antigen containing circulating immune responses and complications from *O. volvulus* infection.[133]

Cell-Mediated Immune Responses. A hallmark of the cellular response after *O. volvulus* infection is a diminished reactivity both by skin testing and by in vitro lymphocyte activation assays to onchocercal antigens. While the majority of the data suggest that this antigen-specific defect in lymphocyte activation does not extend to nonfilarial antigens, there is evidence of decreased reactivity to tuberculin and tetanus skin testing[70,71,127] and an increased prevalence of leptomatous leprosy in people with onchocerciasis compared with appropriate controls.[120] Further, delayed hypersensitivity reactions and in vitro lymphocyte blastogenesis to streptococcal antigens are reduced in onchocerciasis.[53,58] The dimunition in antigen-specific lymphocyte reactivity is more prominent in individuals with large numbers of skin microfilariae and little cutaneous reaction in contrast to those with highly reactive skin disease and few demonstrable skin microfilariae. One study found that lymphocyte reactivity to parasite antigen in infected young individuals was greater than that in older infected individuals, suggesting that there is an acquired modulation of specific cellular responses.[88,89] In experimentally infected chimpanzees there was a loss of onchocercal antigen-specific cellular reactivity before patency (i.e., the appearance of detectable skin microfilariae), suggesting that the parasite-specific T-cell responses are actively down-regulated as the parasite infection gains a hold on the host.[62] The mechanism by which the cellular reactivity to onchocercal antigens is dampened or modulated is not yet known. Although there is some evidence that exogenous IL-2 restored reactivity to parasite antigen in 45% of infected persons with a specific cellular defect,[53] other studies in onchocerciasis and related filarial diseases have not verified this hypothesis. Intriguing is the concept that, rather than a specific cellular defect, there is a shift away from cells capable of producing IL-2 and interferon gamma and toward an expansion of antigen-reactive cells capable of eliciting IL-4, IL-5, and other cross-regulatory cytokines such as IL-10, TGF-β, IL-12, or PAF.[73]

Pathogenesis of Chorioretinitis. The pathogenesis of the chorioretinal changes is still unclear. Bryant[22] originally suggested that the adult worms may secrete a toxin that affects the fundus and the optic nerve. Ridley[123] postulated that dead microfilariae caused the occlusion of choroidal vessels that lead to retinal atrophy. Rodger[125] believed these chorioretinal changes were due to vitamin A deficiency, although his own clinical trial did not support this hypothesis.

Choyce[29] affirmed that they were all genetic. Others have pointed out the inflammatory component.[55,101]

The intravitreal injection of microfilariae of *O. volvulus* into the vitreous cavity of monkeys produces clinical and histopathologic changes similar to those seen in man.[132] Chorioretinal changes could be induced by either dead or live microfilariae, although they were more marked with live microfilariae. The severity of the changes did not clearly correlate with the cellular or humoral immune response to microfilaria.[40,132] Antiretinal antibodies were not seen.

Some component or exacerbation of chorioretinitis has been attributed to autoimmunity. Some correlations with disease have been reported with circulating immune complexes[60] or antiretinal antibodies,[26,155] although others have found that the presence of antiS-antigen and anti-IRBP antibodies was not specific for onchocerciasis.[153,154] More recently, a 22 kDa antigen has been found in *O. volvulus* that cross-reacts with a 44 kDa component of retinal pigment epithelium (RPE) cells.[20] This antigen has been cloned and expressed in bacteria.

It seems likely that the RPE cells are damaged, either directly or indirectly, by the presence of intraretinal microfilariae. This damage unmasks or exposes epitopes in the RPE and that cross-reacting autoantibodies may then play a role in the continuation or exacerbation of disease. On their own, autoimmune mechanisms do not fully explain the disease process. Animals immunized with *O. volvulus* or various antigen preparations do not spontaneously develop chorioretinitis. The mere presence of microfilariae also does not adequately explain the disease because chorioretinitis is not well correlated to microfilarial densities, unlike the skin and anterior ocular changes.[102] Also unlike the skin and anterior ocular changes, chorioretinitis may continue to progress after the elimination of microfilariae by ivermectin treatment.

Autoimmunity/Cross-Reacting Antigens. Autoimmune reactions have been considered to underlie some of the pathology seen in filarial infections, most notably chorioretinitis in onchocerciasis. With the cloning and sequencing of many human and parasite genes and gene products have come the findings, based on sequence analysis, that there are structural similarities between cloned filarial antigens and molecules that have been implicated in human autoimmune diseases. For example, calreticulin (antibodies to which are found in septemic lupus erythematosus)[126] and possibly the RO/SS-A autoantigen (antibodies to which are found in Sjögren syndrome and lupus)[90] have partial (64%) structural identity with the onchocercal antigen RAL-1, a 42 kDa antigen expressed in infective larvae and adults.[151] Further, patients with onchocerciasis appear to have antibodies that cross-react with the autoantigens, suggesting that autoimmunity may play a role in the pathological responses in onchocerciasis.

Dynamics of the Immune Response Following Treatment

It is thought that the pathological manifestations of onchocerciasis are secondary to the host immune. The modulation of potentially deleterious parasite-specific immune responses may explain why not all those infected develop severe disease. Antibody production is spared for the most part, but cellular responses are impaired in most individuals with generalized onchocerciasis. Because of enhanced posttreatment immunological responsiveness to onchocercal antigens after chemotherapy with diethylcarbamazine, the effect of ivermectin on the host's immunologic responsiveness has important implications, particularly because repeated treatment with ivermectin is anticipated for endemic areas.

Eosinophil Response. Infection with *O. volvulus* causes a peripheral blood eosinophil response, and generally people with onchocerciasis have increased levels of circulating eosinophils. With microfilicidal treatment there is a rapid "mobilization" or migration of microfilariae from the dermis and other organs into the lymphatics, blood, other body fluids, and into the epidermis.[32] Although microfilariae entering the blood may be cleared by the liver or kidney, most microfilariae are destroyed in dermal and epidermal microabscesses, in subcutaneous onchocercal nodules, and in regional lymph nodes.

Within hours of treatment a profound blood eosinopenia occurs concomitant with the accumulation of eosinophils in the skin around damaged microfilariae. Subsequently, eosinophils degranulate and deposit their proinflammatory granular proteins in the dermis and epidermis, causing further inflammation and microfilarial death. The death of the parasites and the rapid movement of blood eosinophils to the skin and other tissues provide a stimulus for bone-marrow production of new eosinophils. By 5 to 7 days after the initiation of treatment there is a marked posttreatment rise in peripheral blood eosinophil levels, levels characteristically above pretreatment levels.[79] Within weeks the levels return to or fall below pretreatment levels. Community-based treatment with ivermectin that interrupts transmission and reduces an individual's microfilarial load by 90 to 100% also reduces the eosinophil levels by 50 to 75%. This finding suggests that the presence of microfilariae is the major stimulus for the eosinophil response seen in onchocerciasis.[91,138]

B-Cell Responses. Although polyclonal IgG and IgE may be elevated in patients with onchocerciasis, immunoglobulin levels may change within weeks of microfilarial therapy.[77,99,137] Changes in quantities of antigen-specific antibodies within the first two weeks following diethylcarbamazine therapy have been documented for the IgG isotype, but not for IgE. Qualitative analyses of these antigen-specific responses (immunoblotting) for both IgG and IgE show enhanced antibody recognition of certain onchocercal antigens. These antigens are presumably released from dying microfilariae.[77]

Long-term assessments of antibody responses have only recently become possible with repeated ivermectin therapy. Repeated ivermectin therapy is associated with decreases in both polyclonal and parasite-specific levels of IgE and IgG (all subclasses).[138] Because antibodies mediate the cellular killing of microfilariae, particularly during treatment, and because high levels of parasite-specific antibodies correlate with circulating immune complexes, possibly causing systemic and ocular complications, these reductions in antibody levels following repeated ivermectin treatment are of great potential importance.

T-Cell Responses. Although parasite-specific, T cell–mediated hyporesponsiveness is a hallmark of onchocerciasis, hyporesponsiveness to nonparasitic antigens has been controversial. There have been many studies of delayed-type hypersensitivity skin testing (using a variety of antigens) that have uniformly demonstrated that patients with active onchocerciasis respond less well to recall antigens administered intradermally than do appropriate control individuals. When in vitro assays of T-cell reactivity are used, the data are more variable. Few studies have addressed changes in cellular responses after treatment of onchocerciasis. Treatment with diethylcarbamazine reversed the antigen-specific defect in T-cell responses in a small group of patients. Cutaneous responses to parasite and nonparasite recall antigens improved following either single or repeated doses of ivermectin as did in vitro assays of cellular proliferation.[89,136,138] This increase in cellular reactivity was not sustained at two years, however, suggesting that during the period of maximal microfilarial death and antigen release there is a stimulus to antigen-driven responses that diminishes after the period of acute immune activation.

LABORATORY INVESTIGATIONS

A definitive diagnosis in an individual can be made by the demonstration of the parasite, either macrofilariae from an excised nodule or microfilariae in small skin snips, in the eye, or rarely in other body fluids such as blood, cerebrospinal fluid, sputum, or urine.[141] A presumptive diagnosis can be made in the presence of typical nodules, skin changes, or ocular features.

Demonstration of Parasites

Skin Snips. Skin-snip testing is a very simple procedure. Small pieces of skin are removed, incubated in a fluid medium, and examined under a microscope for emergent microfilariae (Fig. 107-4). The microfilariae of *O. volvulus* are distinctive and usually are vigorously writhing. In Central and West Africa they may have to be distinguished from the skin-dwelling microfilariae of *Dipetalonema streptocerca* that are shorter (230 to 250 μm), thinner (3 to 5 μm), and have bluntly rounded ends.[23] Microfilariae of *O. volvulus* are longer (300 to 350 μm) and thicker (5 to 9 μm) and have an elongated head and a long, finely pointed tail.

A satisfactory skin snip can be obtained by lifting the skin with the tip of a needle and excising a small saucer-shaped disk of epidermis and superficial dermis with a razor. A better result is achieved by using a scleral punch, which is quick, painless, and bloodless. Microfilariae will emerge from snips incubated for a short time in water, but more prolonged incubation requires a more physiologic incubation solution. Tissue-culture media are commonly used, and snips are incubated in disposable microtiter plates at either room temperature or 37°C. When flat-bottomed microtiter plates are used the snip can be conveniently examined with an inverted microscope.

In an infected person the number of microfilariae that emerge will depend, in part, on the size of the biopsy. Quantitative snips should be weighed and the microfilarial count expressed as the count per milligram of skin. For averaging counts, the geometric mean should be used.[11] The time allowed for microfilariae to emerge is important. One third of the microfilariae will emerge from a snip in the first 15 minutes, and 95% will have emerged in two to three hours. Greater precision is achieved by using either a 24-hour incubation or collagenase digestion of the skin.[128]

In Africa a pair of skin snips for microfilarial counts are usually taken from over each iliac crest. In Central America they are usually taken from each deltoid or scapular region. Two skin snips may not detect microfilariae in patients who are lightly infected; more (usually six snips) are taken from the calf, buttock, and shoulder of each side of the body.[147] Outer canthal skin snips have been suggested as a general indicator of potential ocular involvement but probably reflect higher total counts rather than a particular local ocular risk.

To reduce the risk of transmission of viral hepatitis and the human immunodeficiency virus, the instruments used to collect skin snips require adequate sterilization, usually in glutaraldehyde. Appropriate precautions for handling body fluids must be followed.

Nodule Excision. The clinical detection of a typical nodule is good presumptive evidence of onchocerciasis.[141] Nodules need to be differentiated from lipomas, sebaceous cysts, ganglia, and lymph nodes. A definitive diagnosis can be made if adult worms can be identified in an excised nodule. In West Africa 5% to 10% of the community will have typical nodules and yet have negative skin snips.

Rapid Assessment of Community Endemicity. As the community-based distribution of ivermectin becomes more widely used there has been the need for simple and rapid assessment of the level of endemicity at a community level.[144] Skin snips are less favored because of the time involved, their cost, and the potential for the transmission of viral infections. Because they are invasive, skin snips are not welcomed by most community members. Rates of blindness or of readily detectable leopard skin have been advocated,[49] but because of the relatively low prevalence of these features

(1 to 10%) a large sample size is needed to establish the rate with acceptable precision.

On a community basis the frequency of readily detectable nodules is about half the prevalence of skin snip positivity. Nodule rates are usually fairly stable after 20 years of age. Nodule rates and prevalence of infection are often higher in men, who are also usually more amenable to examination and palpation than women. The examination of a randomly selected sample of 30 men has been advocated as a simple rapid assessment method for use at a community level.[144] Once 3 infected men have been detected (i.e., nodule prevalence is at least 10%), there is a high likelihood that the prevalence of infection is greater than 20%.

Immunological and Molecular Approaches to Diagnosis

Antibody Detection. Attempts to develop sensitive and specific immunoassays to detect *O. volvulus* infection have only recently met with success. The major problem had been cross-reactivity with other nononchocercal filarial species of humans that often coexist with *O. volvulus* in many areas. A low-molecular-weight fraction of crude *O. volvulus* was identified and shown to have less cross-reactivity and thus increased specificity. An enzyme-linked immunosorbent assay (ELISA) using this antigen showed good sensitivity.[68] A recombinant antigen termed Ov-16,[82,83] analogous to one of the antigens in this low-molecular-weight fraction, was cloned, overexpressed, and purified. When Ov-16 was used as the basis for a diagnostic ELISA, the sensitivity and specificity approached 95% and was also able to identify infection in the prepatent period. Concurrently several other potentially diagnostic antigens have been made in recombinant form.[18,84,86,87] An ELISA screen that combines Ov-16, Ov-7, Ov-11, and Ov-33 identifies all infected patients without loss of onchocercal specificity.[18a] These antigens are currently being formatted for use in the field.

Despite the high degree of sensitivity and specificity that immunoassays provide, antibody positivity can be found in individuals who appear free of infection (skin-snip and nodule negative). Thus assays to distinguish between amicrofiladermic-infected individuals and those truly free of infection also have been sought either by detection of parasite antigen circulating in the blood, by detection in the urine, or by identification of onchocercal-specific DNA in the skin, blood, or urine.

Antigen Detection. Direct detection of parasite antigen in tissues or body fluids would have great value in accurately assessing infection status. Several monoclonal and polyclonal antibody-based techniques have been developed for detection of onchocercal antigens, but they have suffered from interference with host antibody and have poor sensitivity and specificity.[64] Even an assay for a recently identified and characterized 23 kDa antigen complexed to antibody suffers from a sensitivity of only 75%.[27]

DNA Probes. The identification of an ~150 base pair, tandemly repeated, noncoding DNA sequence present at about 4000 copies per haploid genome allowed for the development of probes for the species-specific identification of *O. volvulus* in the blackfly vector and also in isolates from human nodules.[50,51,97] Priming the polymerase chain reaction (PCR) with *O. volvulus*–specific primers allows for increased sensitivity (without loss of sensitivity) and the easy identification of small numbers of microfilariae from skin and from infected flies.[98] For diagnostic purposes this PCR-based method has been used successfully to identify onchocercal DNA in skin snips from 100% of skin-snip positive patients (microfilariae range 1 to 210) and also in a few individuals from a hyperendemic area who had consistently negative skin snips.[171] This method has also been used successfully to identify onchocercal DNA in the serum of amicrofilardermic expatriates.* If this method's success continues when applied to larger numbers of patients, it seems likely to replace immunoassays for the definitive diagnosis of onchocerciasis.

THERAPY

The ideal drug to treat onchocerciasis would be an effective macrofilaricide that was safe, did not exacerbate the disease, and could be given as a single oral dose on a mass scale.[141] At present such a drug does not exist despite ongoing research. A drug that comes close to these criteria is ivermectin, which is highly effective, very safe, and is taken as an oral dose. Ivermectin is a microfilaricide, however, and has ill-defined effects on adult worms. Although it rapidly and safely removes microfilariae and hence the stimulus for disease, it does not eliminate the adult worms or cure the infection. Therefore it must be given at repeated intervals until the adult worms eventually die.

The previous mainstay of chemotherapy for onchocerciasis was diethylcarbamazine (DEC). This microfilaricide produced severe side-effects, such as the Mazzotti reaction, and had little or no long-term benefit.[140] It should be no longer used.

Suramin is an effective macrofilaricide that also kills microfilariae. It is inherently toxic and is given by weekly intravenous injections.[44,168] It must be administered under careful supervision because it can produce severe reactions and even death.

Amocarzine is a newly developed macrofilaricidal drug that is effective when given orally.[115] A three-day course kills most adult worms. Neurologic and hepatic side effects and a small therapeutic window appear to limit its usefulness.

Ivermectin has rendered obsolete the two drugs that were previously used: DEC and suramin. Before the introduction of ivermectin, DEC or suramin treatment had been recommended only for those people with the worst disease and the highest risk of developing blindness because of the high incidence of severe reactions seen with these drugs.[140] In comparison ivermectin treatment has such a low rate of adverse reactions that it is widely used in community-based treatment, and the indication for treatment is now that a person lives in an endemic area.

Individual Treatment

Ivermectin is a semisynthetic macrocyclic lactone derived from fermentation of a fungus. It has proved useful in veterinary medicine because it is effective against a wide range of animal parasites.[25] Its pharmacologic effect is as a modulator of GABA-mediated neurotransmitter effects, probably acting through a glutamate-gated chloride channel.[10] Its development revolutionized the treatment of onchocerciasis.

Ivermectin was first tested against onchocerciasis in 1982.[12] Subsequent controlled clinical trials showed that a single dose of ivermectin (200 μg/kg) reduced microfilariae counts as effectively as a one-week course of DEC.[61] The reactions following ivermectin were milder and less frequent than those following DEC.[61,145]

Treatment with DEC produces a severe toxic reaction (the Mazzotti reaction) related to the killing of microfilariae. The occurrence of this reaction severely limits the usefulness of DEC.[141,164] The Mazzotti reaction includes pruritis, a papular or pustular rash, fever, arthralgia, and headache but may at times lead to severe respiratory, renal, and neurologic symptoms and even death. Severe ocular changes also occur with DEC, including photophobia, punctate keratitis, limbitis, severe anterior uveitis, an increase in intraocular microfilariae, acute retinitis, retinal pigment epithelial changes, retinal vasculitis, and optic neuritis.

Further studies indicated that the optimal dose of ivermectin is 150 μg/kg.[142] This dose is usually repeated on an annual basis. Treatment can be given every 6 months to eliminate microfilariae rapidly; but, after two years of treatment, there is no apparent difference between treatment every 6 months or every 12 months as the microfilariae counts continue to fall.[63] A marked effect on skin microfilarial counts persists for 2 years after a single use.

A mild clinical reaction occurs in 10% to 15% of people receiving their initial treatment with ivermectin, with a somewhat more severe reaction seen in 1% to 5%.[28,110,111,159,160] The reactions decrease in frequency and severity with each retreatment. European expatriates complain of skin reactions, especially pruritis, more commonly than those born in endemic areas.[21,37] These reactions are usually mild, however, and settle with aspirin and antihistamines.

The effect of ivermectin on adult worms is less clear-cut.[8,46,47,48] Studies on adult worms have been hampered by

---

*Meredith, unpublished.

the variability of worm burdens, the need for large numbers, and their inherent difficulties. Most studies have shown a sizable reduction in the number of live adult male worms and fewer inseminated female worms after ivermectin treatment. It seems likely that ivermectin kills at least some of the adult male worms.

Ivermectin has two apparent effects on female worms. First, their reproductive capacity is reduced. In the short term this effect is associated with the effects of killing intrauterine microfilariae.[8,46] The paired uteri become packed and clogged with degenerating necrotic debris. It may take 3 to 9 months for this debris to be cleared before normal embryogenesis can resume. In addition, with repeated treatment fewer females produce microfilariae so ivermectin seems to have both a short-term (up to one year) effect of stopping embryogenesis and also a long-term sterilizing effect. Second, repeated doses of ivermectin kill some of the female worms.[47] Although most studies find fewer viable females after ivermectin treatment, the reduction is usually not statistically significant. Further long-term work on larger numbers of worms is needed to clarify the dose response of this effect.

These combined effects on both male and female adult worms explain the prolonged and sustained reduction of microfilarial counts after ivermectin treatment. In contrast, DEC kills microfilariae but does not affect the adults.[7] After DEC treatment, microfilarial counts return to pretreatment levels within one year.

After treatment with ivermectin there is a marked reduction in the uptake of microfilariae by flies, in turn leading to a reduction in transmission.[33] With community-based treatment the transmission potential may be reduced by at least 75%.[34,121,150] A single round of community-based treatment reduces transmission enough to cause a 45% reduction in the incidence of new infection in uninfected children.[148] The impact of ivermectin on transmission should increase with each round of treatment as microfilarial levels are progressively reduced.

Community Distribution

Because of the numbers of people involved and the safety and efficacy of ivermectin, the drug is often distributed by community-based programs rather than on an individual basis. The indication for treatment has evolved to include all those who live in a known endemic area. Pregnant women, lactating mothers of children less than one week old, children weighing less than 15 kg, and those with other intercurrent illnesses are excluded. Treatment is given on a weight-adjusted basis (Table 107-4), although recently a simplified treatment regime based on height has been recommended (Table 107-5).[143] Ivermectin treatment should be repeated once a year for at least 10 years.

Treatment is usually given by community health workers who monitor and treat any adverse reactions occurring

TABLE 107-4 DOSAGE SCHEDULE FOR IVERMECTIN (BASED ON WEIGHT)[166]

Weight	Dosage	Dose Range
15-25 kg	3 mg (½ tablet)	120-176 μg/kg
26-44 kg	6 mg (1 tablet)	136-230 μg/kg
45-64 kg	9 mg (1½ tablets)	141-200 μg/kg
65-85 kg	12 mg (2 tablets)	143-185 μg/kg

within the first 36 hours.[166] Treatment has been shown to be well accepted, well tolerated, safe, and effective.[109,110,111,116,159] It greatly reduces the acute and reversible skin and anterior segment changes and halts the progression of chronic irreversible changes.[112,160] Its effects on the posterior segment have been less well defined with some studies showing ongoing progression,[131] although a recent large-scale study has shown that ivermectin treatment at least halves the risk of developing optic nerve disease.[1] Because of its broad spectrum, ivermectin treatment also has a marked, short-term effect on intestinal parasite loads.[111,161]

By the end of 1992 over 7 million doses of ivermectin had been distributed. The drug is supplied free by its manufacturer, Merck and Company, for the treatment of all patients with onchocerciasis.[152] This unprecedented donation is coordinated for WHO by the Mectizan Expert Committee, which is based at the Carter Presidential Center, Atlanta, Georgia. Funds are still required for the costs of distributing this drug to those who "live beyond the end of the road". Many new initiatives have been taken, including the establishment of the Houston-based River Blindness Foundation, a new foundation whose sole objective is to support the distribution of ivermectin.[14]

Nodulectomy

It is theoretically possible to treat onchocerciasis by the surgical removal of all nodules containing the adult worms. This practice, however, is usually not feasible. Fewer than two thirds of the nodules can be palpated and identified for surgical removal, leaving at least one third of the adult worms undetected. A nodulectomy campaign has been conducted in Guatemala and Mexico for over 50 years but onchocerciasis remains endemic in both these countries.[168] It is

TABLE 107-5 SIMPLIFIED DOSAGE SCHEDULE FOR IVERMECTIN (BASED ON HEIGHT)[143]

Height	Weight	Dosage	Dose Range
95-124 cm	10-30 kg	3 mg (½ tablet)	100-300 μg/kg
125-149 cm	19-63 kg	6 mg (1 tablet)	95-316 μg/kg
≥150 cm	36-95 kg	9 mg (1½ tablets)	95-250 μg/kg

difficult to assess the full impact of these nodulectomy campaigns, but a prospective study in West Africa showed systematic nodulectomy had no lasting effect.[6] There is no evidence that the removal of head nodules, if present, has any impact on the evolution of ocular changes.

PREVENTION

Onchocerciasis should be a straightforward disease to prevent. There is but a single host (mankind) and a single vector (the blackfly). The elimination of host-vector contact would abolish transmission and stop the disease. Alternatively, drugs that kill the adult worm would eliminate the infection and the disease, and drugs that kill microfilariae would remove the stimulus for the disease and stop the disease process. The practical realization of these approaches has been difficult.

Vector Control

Blackflies, especially the larval stage, can be killed by a number of insecticides or larvicides. Onchocerciasis was eliminated from Kenya in the 1950s by the treatment of blackfly breeding sites with DDT. The ecologic consequences of such treatment were later realized. Since then more biodegradable and ecologically appropriate larvicides have become available; these include temephos ("Abate") and *Bacillus thuringiensis* (Bt 14).[76,168]

The most comprehensive and successful vector-control program has been the Onchocerciasis Control Program (OCP). The OCP was initiated in 1974 by the World Health Organization in the Volta River basin of West Africa[168] and now involves 11 countries and 50,000 kilometers of rivers. It aimed to eradicate onchocerciasis as a public health problem by the elimination of blackflies. Systematic spraying of breeding sites was carried out every 7 to 14 days. Seasonal rains alter the distribution of breeding sites and the need for spraying, however. Despite this and other logistic problems, the spraying program has been highly successful in interrupting transmission of infection in this particular area of West Africa.[38] After 15 years of control, 20 million people have been protected against infection and 7 million children born into what have become onchocerciasis-free areas.[117] In some areas spraying has now stopped and blackflies have been allowed to return.[76] Ongoing surveillance is needed to ensure that transmission does not become reestablished.

Vector control has two major limitations. First, it must be continued for a very long time. Adult female worms can live for 15 years, and vector control must be continued for at least that long. Transmission would restart if blackflies returned while microfilariae were still present in the skin of persons infected before the start of vector control.

The second problem is that treated sites can be reinvaded by blackflies from other areas. Although most migration of flies is fairly local, usually along a valley, blackflies can be carried hundreds of miles by monsoonal winds. Repeated local treatment may greatly reduce transmission and the nuisance of biting flies, but it will not eliminate transmission except in areas with isolated breeding sites.[12,105] Even for local treatment every breeding site must be treated, a task that is almost impossible in the African forest and in Latin American endemic areas.

Vector control is not universally applicable. Its main use is in areas of high endemicity where the socioeconomic impact of onchocerciasis is profound and where the breeding sites are relatively few, easily identifiable, and accessible.

Prevention of Fly Bites

The only certain way to prevent onchocerciasis is to avoid being bitten by infected blackflies. Only one to ten in 1000 blackfly bites is likely to be infective, and serious disease usually does not develop unless a person has been infected many times.[141] Known breeding sites should be avoided at the time of maximal fly activity, often early morning and early evening. Protective clothing should be worn and insect repellents should be used.

Even these simple protective measures are often unrealistic or unobtainable, however, to most of the population in endemic areas. Other measures include resiting of homes or villages away from breeding sites and the clearance of rocks and vegetation to smooth the flow of water and remove breeding sites.

Antiinfective Prophylaxis

At present there are no known prophylactic agents or prophylactic drugs effective against the infective larvae. Ivermectin has only a limited action on infective larvae.[146]

Vaccine Development

Strong protective immunity against *O. volvulus* is not an obvious feature. Individuals cured of onchocerciasis can become reinfected following reexposure.[42] The repeated challenge of chimpanzees with living infective larvae or irradiated L3 does not give acquired resistance.[116] Epidemiologic, clinical, and preliminary experimental data from animal studies suggest that some acquired resistance to *O. volvulus* can occur, however.[165]

Epidemiologic data on age-related microfilarial densities suggest that in hyperendemic regions, microfilarial levels plateau in the third decade of life, suggesting that resistance to reinfection occurs despite ongoing infection (concomitant immunity). Studies using radiation-attenuated larvae in animals capable of sustaining natural infection with *Dipetalonema viteae*,[84] *Litomosoides carinii*,[169] *Dirofilaria immitis*,[163] among others, show some degree of protection. More recently there has been a trend towards protection studies using short-term infections with defined life-cycle stages.[2,4] Sensitization of mice to *Onchocerca lienalis* induces resistance to *O. volvulus* microfilariae.[15] Immunization with radiation-attenuated L3 can induce partial protection shown by killing L3 in subcutaneous micropore chamber implants.[103]

More compelling has been the identification of populations in hyperendemic regions of the world who, despite lifelong exposure, appear to be resistant to infection with *O. volvulus.*[156] When immunologic correlates of this immunity have been sought, it has been found that these "putatively immune" individuals produce much more IL-2 to parasite antigen than infected controls.[156] Sera from these and similar populations preferentially recognize certain larval stage antigens.[103] Additionally, isotypic analysis of antibody responses showed that a group of ~20 kDa glycoproteins were specifically recognized by IgG3 of putatively immune individuals and not by those who were infected.[17]

The identification of possible vaccine targets focuses on sera from animals immunized with infective larvae and sera from putatively immune individuals. These sera are differentially screened against antigen preparations on immunoblots or cDNA and/or genomic expression libraries of *O. volvulus* and related parasites. The development of an effective vaccine would open up new ways for controlling human onchocerciasis.

REFERENCES

1. Abiose A et al.: Reduction in incidence of optic nerve disease with annual ivermectin to control onchocerciasis, *Lancet* 341:130-134, 1993.
2. Abraham D et al.: Active and passive immunization of mice against larval *Dirofilaria immitis, J Parasitol* 74:275-282, 1988.
3. Ackerman SJ et al.: Eosinophil degranulation: an immunologic determinant in the pathogenesis of the Mazzotti reaction in human onchocerciasis, *J Immunol* 144:3961-3969, 1990.
4. Abraham D et al.: Identification of surrogate rodent hosts for larval *Onchocerca lienalis* and induction of protective immunity in a model system, *J Parasitol* 78:446-453, 1992.
5. Akogun OB: Eye lesions, blindness and visual impairment in the Taraba river valley, Nigeria, and their relation to onchocercal microfilariae in the skin, *Acta Tropica* 51:143-149, 1992.
6. Albiez EJ: Effects of a single complete nodulectomy on nodule burden and microfilarial density two years later, *Trop Med Parasitol* 36:17-20, 1985.
7. Albiez EJ et al.: Effects of high doses of diethylcarbamazine on adult *Onchocerca volvulus* examined by the collagenase technique and by histology, *Trop Med Parasitol* 39:87-92, 1988.
8. Albiez EJ et al.: Histological examination of onchocercomata after therapy with ivermectin, *Trop Med Parasitol* 39:93-99, 1988.
9. Anderson J et al.: Studies on onchocerciasis in the United Cameroon Republic. III. A four-year follow-up of 6 rain-forest and 6 Sudan-savanna villages, *Trans R Soc Trop Med Hyg* 70:362-373, 1976.
10. Arena JP et al.: Ivermectin-sensitive chloride currents induced by Caenorhabditis elegans RNA in Xenopus oocytes, *Mol Pharmacol* 40:368-374, 1991.
11. Auer CL, Taylor HR, Greene BM: The statistical analysis of microfilarial skin snip counts: stabilization of the variance of microfilarial counts, *Trop Med Parasitol* 35:199-201, 1984.
12. Aziz MA et al.: Efficacy and tolerance of ivermectin in human onchocerciasis, *Lancet* 11:171-173, 1982.
13. Baker RHA, Abdelnur OM: Localized onchocerciasis vector control in the Bahr el Ghazal region of south-western Sudan. II. Control, *Trop Med Parasitol* 36:135-142, 1986.
14. Baldwin WR, Duke BOL: River blindness, *Lancet* 339:1178, 1992.
15. Bianco AE et al.: Immunity to *Onchocerca volvulus* microfilariae in mice and the induction of cross-protection with O. lienalis, *Trop Med Parasitol* 42:188-190, 1991.
16. Blaxter M et al.: Nematode surface coats: actively evading immunity, *Parasitol Today* 8:243-247, 1992.
17. Boyer AE et al.: Guatemalan human onchocerciasis. II. Evidence for IgG3 involvement in acquired immunity to *Onchocerca volvulus* and identification of possible immune-associated antigens, *J Immunol* 146:4001-4010, 1991.

18. Bradley JE et al.: cDNA clone of *Onchocerca volvulus* low molecular weight antigens provide immunologically specific diagnostic probes, *Mol Biochem Parasitol* 46:219-227, 1991.
18a. Bradley JE, Trenholme R, Gillespie AJ et al.: A sensitive serodiagnostic test for onchocerciasis using a cocktail of recombinant antigens, *Am J Trop Med Hyg* 48:198-204, 1993.
19. Brattig NW et al.: Eosinophil-larval-interaction in onchocerciasis: heterogeneity of in vitro adherence of eosinophils to infective third and fourth stage larvae and microfilariae of *Onchocerca volvulus, Parasite Immunol* 13:13-22, 1991.
20. Braun G et al.: Immunological crossreactivity between a cloned antigen of *Onchocerca volvulus* and a component of the retinal pigment epithelium, *J Exp Med* 174:169-177, 1991.
21. Bryan RT, Stokes SL, Spencer HC: Expatriates treated with ivermectin, *Lancet* 337:304, 1991.
22. Bryant J: Endemic retino-choroiditis in the Anglo-Egyptian and its possible relationship to *Onchocerca volvulus, Trans R Soc Trop Med Hyg* 28:523-532, 1935.
23. Buck AA: *Onchocerciasis: symptomatology, pathology, diagnosis,* World Health Organization, Geneva, 1974.
24. Budden FH: Route of entry of *Onchocerca volvulus* microfilariae into the eye, *Trans R Soc Trop Med Hyg* 70:265-266, 1976 (letter).
25. Campbell WC et al.: Ivermectin: a potent new antiparasitic agent, *Science* 221:823-828, 1983.
26. Chan C et al.: Immunopathology of ocular onchocerciasis. II. Antiretinal autoantibodies in serum and ocular fluids, *Ophthalmology* 94:439-443, 1987.
27. Chandrashekar R et al.: Circulating immune complex–associated parasite antigens in human onchocerciasis, *J Infect Dis* 162:1159-1164, 1990.
28. Chijioke CP, Okonkwo PO: Adverse events following mass ivermectin therapy for onchocerciasis, *Trans R Soc Trop Med Hyg* 86:284-286, 1992.
29. Choyce DP: Ocular onchocerciasis in Central America, Africa and British Isles, *Trans R Soc Trop Med Hyg* 58:11-36, 1964.
30. Connor DH, Palmieri JR: Blackfly bites, onchocerciasis and leopard skin, *Trans R Soc Trop Med Hyg* 79:415-417, 1985.
31. Connor DH et al.: Onchocerciasis: onchocercal dermatitis, lymphadenitis and elephantitis in the Ubangi territory, *Hum Pathol* 1:553-579, 1970.
32. Connor DH ct al.: Onchocerciasis. In Strickland G, editor: *Hunter's Tropical Medicine,* ed 6, Philadelphia, 1984, WB Saunders.
33. Cupp EW et al.: The effects of ivermectin on transmission of *Onchocerca volvulus, Science* 231:740-742, 1986.
34. Cupp EW et al.: The effect of multiple ivermectin treatments on infection of *Simulium ochraceum* with *Onchocerca volvulus, Am J Trop Med Hyg* 40:501-506, 1989.
35. Dadzie KY et al.: Ocular onchocerciasis and intensity of infection in the community. II. West African rainforest foci of the vector *Simulium yahense, Trop Med Parasitol* 40:348-354, 1989.
36. Dadzie KY et al.: Ocular onchocerciasis and intensity of infection in the community. III. West African rainforest foci of the vector *Simulium sanctipauli, Trop Med Parasitol* 41:376-382, 1990.
37. Davidson RN, Godrey-Faussett P, Bryceson ADM: Adverse reactions in expatriates treated with ivermectin, *Lancet* 336:1005, 1990.
38. De Sole G, Remme J: Onchocerciasis infection in children born during 14 years of *Simulium* control in West Africa, *Trans R Soc Trop Med Hyg* 85:385-390, 1991.
39. De Sole G et al.: Adverse reactions after large-scale treatment of onchocerciasis with ivermectin: combined results from eight community trials, *Bull World Health Organ* 67:707-719, 1989.
40. Donnelly JJ et al.: Onchocerciasis: experimental models of ocular disease, *Rev Infect Dis* 7:820-825, 1985.
41. Donnelly JJ et al.: Experimental ocular onchocerciasis in cynomolgus monkeys: III. Roles of IgG and IgE autoantibody and cell-mediated immunity in the chorioretinitis elicited by intravitreal *Onchocerca lienalis* microfilariae, *Trop Med Parasitol* 39:111, 1988.
42. Duke BOL: Reinfections with Onchocerca volvulus in cured patients exposed to continuing transmission, *Bull World Health Organ* 39:307-309, 1968.
43. Duke BOL: Geographical aspects of onchocerciasis, *Ann Soc Belge Med Trop* 61:179-186, 1981.

44. Duke BOL: Suramin and the time it takes to kill *Onchocerca volvulus*, *Trop Med Parasitol* 42:346-350, 1991.

45. Duke BOL, Zea-Flores G, Muñoz B: The embryogenesis of *Onchocerca volvulus* over the first year after a single dose of ivermectin, *Trop Med Parasitol* 42:175-180, 1991.

46. Duke BOL et al.: Effects of multiple monthly doses of ivermectin on adult *Onchocerca volvulus*, *Am J Trop Med Hyg* 43:657-664(90-142), 1990.

47. Duke BOL et al.: Viability of adult *Onchocerca volvulus* after six two-weekly doses of ivermectin, *Bull World Health Organ* 69:163-168, 1991.

48. Duke BOL et al.: Effects of three-month doses of ivermectin on adult *Onchocerca volvulus*, *Am J Trop Med Hyg* 46:189-194, 1992.

49. Edungbola LA et al.: "Leopard skin" as a rapid diagnostic index for estimating the endemicity of African onchocerciasis, *Int J Epidemiol* 16:590-594, 1987.

50. Erttmann KD et al.: A DNA sequence specific for forest form *Onchocerca volvulus*, *Nature* 327:415-417, 1987.

51. Erttmann KD et al.: Isolation and characterization of form specific DNA sequences of *O. volvulus*, *Acta Leiden* 59:253-260, 1990.

52. Evans TG, Murray CJL: A critical re-examination of the economics of blindness prevention under the onchocerciasis control programme, *Soc Sci Med* 25:241-249, 1987.

53. Gallin M et al.: Cell-mediated responses in human infection with *Onchocerca volvulus*, *J Immunol* 140:1999-2007, 1988.

54. Gallin MY et al.: Experimental interstitial keratitis induced by *Onchocerca volvulus* antigens, *Arch Ophthalmol* 106:1447-1452, 1988.

55. Garner A: Pathology of ocular onchocerciasis: human and experimental, *Trans R Soc Trop Med Hyg* 70:374-377, 1976.

56. George GH, Palmieri JR, Connor DH: The onchocercal nodule: interrelationship of adult worms and blood vessels, *Am J Trop Med Hyg* 34:1144-1148, 1985.

57. Gibson DW, Duke BOL, Connor DH: Onchocerciasis: a review of clinical, pathological and chemotherapeutic aspects, and vector control program, *Prog Clin Parasitol* 1:57-103, 1989.

58. Greene BM, Fanning MM, Ellner JJ: Non-specific suppression of antigen-induced lymphocyte blastogenesis in *Onchocerca volvulus* infection in man, *Clin Exp Immunol* 52:259-265, 1983.

59. Greene BM, Taylor HR, Aikawa M: Cellular killing of microfilariae of *Onchocerca volvulus*: eosinophil and neutrophil-mediated immune serum-dependent destruction, *J Immunol* 1276:1611-1618, 1981.

60. Greene BM et al.: Ocular and systemic complications of diethylcarbamazine therapy for onchocerciasis: association with circulating immune complexes, *J Infect Dis* 147:890-897, 1983.

61. Greene BM et al.: Comparison of ivermectin and diethylcarbamazine in the treatment of onchocerciasis, *N Engl J Med* 313:133-138, 1985.

62. Greene BM et al.: Humoral and cellular immune responses to *Onchocerca volvulus* infection in humans, *Rev Infect Dis* 7:789-795, 1985.

63. Greene BM et al.: Comparison of 6-, 12-, and 24-monthly dosing with ivermectin for treatment of onchocerciasis, *J Infect Dis* 163:376-380, 1991.

64. Hamilton RG: Application of immunoassay methods in the serodiagnosis of human filariasis, *Rev Infect Dis* 7:837-843, 1985.

65. Henkle KJ et al.: Characterization and molecular cloning of a Cu/Zn superoxide dismutase from the human parasite *Onchocerca volvulus*, *Infect Immun* 59:2063-2069, 1991.

66. Hissette J: Memoire Sur L'*Onchocerca volvulus* "Leuckart" et ses manifestations oculaires au Congo Belge, *Ann Soc Belge Med Trop* 12:433-509, 1932.

67. Jones BR, Anderson J, Fuglsang H: Effects of various concentrations of diethylcarbamazine citrate applied as eye drops in ocular onchocerciasis, and the possibilities of improved therapy from continuous non-pulsed delivery, *Br J Ophthalmol* 62:428-439, 1978.

68. Karam M, Weiss N: Seroepidemiological investigations of onchocerciasis in a hyperendemic area of West Africa, *Am Trop Med Hyg* 34:907-917, 1985.

69. Kephart GM et al.: Deposition of eosinophil granule major basic protein onto microfilariae of *Onchocerca volvulus* in the skin of patients treated with diethylcarbamazine, *Lab Invest* 50:51-61, 1984.

70. Kilian HD, Nielsen G: Cell-mediated and humoral immune responses to BCG and rubella vaccinations and to recall antigens in onchocerciasis patients, *Trop Med Parasitol* 40:445-453, 1989.

71. Kilian HD, Nielsen G: Cell-mediated and humoral immune response to tetanus vaccinations in onchocerciasis patients, *Trop Med Parasitol* 40:285-291, 1989.

72. King CL, Nutman TB: Regulation of the immune response of lymphatic filariasis and onchocerciasis, *Immunol Today* 12:1991.

73. King CL, Nutman TB: Biologic role of helper T-cell subsets in helminth infections, *Chem Immunol* 54:136-165, 1992.

74. Lackey A et al.: Extracellular proteases of *Onchocerca*, *Exp Parasitol* 68:176-185, 1989.

75. Lal RB et al.: Phosphocholine-containing antigens of *Brugia malayi* non-specifically suppress lymphocyte function, *Am J Trop Med Hyg* 42:56-64, 1990.

76. Le Berre R et al.: The WHO onchocerciasis control programme: retrospect and prospects, *Philos Trans R Soc Lond B* 328:721-729, 1990.

77. Lee SJ et al.: Changes in antibody profile after treatment of human onchocerciasis, *J Infect Dis* 162:529-533, 1990.

78. Leke RG et al.: Immunity to *Onchocerca volvulus*: serum-mediated leucocyte adherence to infective larvae in vitro, *Trop Med Parasitol* 40:39-41, 1989.

79. Limaye AP et al.: Interleukin-5 and the post-treatment eosinophilia in patients with onchocerciasis, *J Clin Invest* 88:1418-1421, 1991.

80. Liu LX, Weller PF: Arachidonic acid metabolism in filarial parasites, *Exp Parasitol* 71:496-501, 1990.

81. Liu LX, Serhand CN, Weller PF: Formation of cyclo-oxygenase-derived eicosanoids by a parasitic intravascular nemotode, *Adv Prostaglandin Thromboxane Leukot Res* 1991.

82. Lobos E et al.: Identification of an *Onchocerca volvulus* cDNA encoding a low-molecular-weight antigen uniquely recognized by onchocerciasis patient sera, *Mol Biochem Parasitol* 39:135-145, 1990.

83. Lobos E et al.: An immunogenic *Onchocerca volvulus* antigen: a specific and early marker of infection, *Science* 251:1603-1605, 1991.

84. Lucius R, Ruppel A, Diesfeld HJ: *Dipetalonema viteae*: resistance in *Meriones unguiculatus* with multiple infections of stage-3 larvae, *Exp Parasitol* 62:237-246, 1986.

85. Lucius R et al.: Molecular cloning of an immunodominant antigen of *Onchocerca volvulus*, *J Exp Med* 168:1199-1204, 1988.

86. Lustigman S et al.: *Onchocerca volvulus*: biochemical and morphological characteristics of the surface of third- and fourth-stage larvae, *Exp Parasitol* 71:489-495, 1990.

87. Lustigman S et al.: Identification and characterization of an *Onchocerca volvulus* cDNA clone encoding a microfilarial surface-associated antigen, *Mol Biochem Parasitol* 50:79-93, 1992.

88. Luty AJ et al.: Immunological studies on onchocerciasis in Sierra Leone. 1. Pretreatment baseline data, *Trop Med Parasitol* 41:371-375, 1990.

89. Luty AJ et al.: Immunological studies on onchocerciasis in Sierra Leone. 2. Cell-mediated immune responses after repeated treatment with ivermectin, *Trop Med Parasitol* 43:54-58, 1992.

90. Lux FA et al.: Serological cross-reactivity between a human Ro/SS-A autoantigen (calreticulin) and the lambda Ral-1 antigen of *Onchocercal volvulus*, *J Clin Invest* 89:1945-1951, 1992.

91. Mackenzie CD et al.: Variations in host responses and the pathogenesis of human onchocerciasis, *Rev Infect Dis* 7:802-808, 1985.

92. Maizels R, Selkirk M: Immunology of nematode antigens. In Englund PS, Sher A, editors: *The biology of parasitism: a molecular and immunological approach*, New York, 1988, Adam R Liss.

93. Maizels RM et al.: Human serum albumin is a major component of the surface of microfilariae of *Wuchereria bancrofti*, *Parasite Immunol* 6:185-190, 1984.

94. Maizels RM et al.: Antibody responses to human lymphatic filarial parasites, *Ciba Found Symp* 127:189-202, 1987.

95. McMahon JE et al.: Epidemiological studies of onchocerciasis in forest villages of Sierra Leone, *Trop Med Parasit* 39(suppl 3):251-259, 1988.

96. McMahon JE et al.: Onchocerciasis in Sierra Leone 2: a comparison of forest and savanna villages, *Trans Roy Soc Trop Med Hyg* 82:595-600, 1988.

97. Meredith SE et al.: Cloning and characterization of an *Onchocerca volvulus* specific DNA sequence, *Mol Biochem Parasitol* 36:1-20, 1989.

98. Meredith SE et al.: *Onchocerca volvulus*: application of the polymerase chain reaction to identification and strain differentiation of the parasite, *Exp Parasitol* 73:335-344, 1991.

99. Merino F, Brand A: Immunological studies on onchocercosis patients, *Trop Med Parasitol* 28:229-234, 1977.

100. Murphy RP, Taylor HR, Greene BM: Chorioretinal damage in onchocerciasis, *Am J Ophthalmol* 98:519-521, 1984.

101. Neumann E, Gunders AE: The posterior segment lesion of ocular onchocerciasis: histological aspects, *Isr J Med Sci* 8:8-9, 1971.

102. Newland HS et al.: Ocular manifestations of onchocerciasis in a rain forest area of West Africa, *Br J Ophthalmol* 75:163-169, 1991.

103. Nutman TB et al.: Immunity to onchocerciasis: recognition of larval antigens by humans putatively immune to *Onchocerca volvulus* infection, *J Infect Dis* 163:1128-1133, 1991.

104. Nwoke BEB: The socio-economic aspects of human onchocerciasis in Africa: present appraisal, *J Hyg Epidem Microbiol Immun* 1:37-44, 1990.

105. Ogata K: A trial of onchocerciasis vector control in Guatemala, *Proc XV, joint conference on parasitic diseases,* US-Japan Co-operative Program in Parasitic Diseases, Japan, 1980.

106. O'Neill J: On the presence of a filaria in "craw-craw", *Lancet* 264-267, 1875.

107. Ottesen EA: Immunological aspects of lymphatic filariasis and onchocerciasis in man, *Trans R Soc Trop Med Hyg* 78:9-18, 1984.

108. Ottesen EA: Immediate hypersensitivity responses in the immunopathogenesis of human onchocerciasis, *Rev Infect Dis* 7:796-801, 1985.

109. Pacheco-Luna R: Disturbance of vision in patients harboring certain filarial tumors, *Am J Ophthalmol* 1:122-125, 1918.

110. Pacqué MC et al.: Community-based treatment of onchocerciasis with ivermectin: acceptability and early adverse reactions, *Bull World Health Organ* 67:721-730, 1989.

111. Pacqué MC et al.: Pregnancy outcome after inadvertent ivermectin treatment during community-based distribution, *Lancet* 336:1486-1489, 1990.

112. Pacqué MC et al.: Community-based treatment of onchocerciasis with ivermectin: safety, efficacy and acceptability of yearly treatment, *J Infect Dis* 163:381-385, 1991.

113. Pacqué M et al.: Improvement in severe onchocercal skin disease after a single dose of ivermectin, *Am J Med* 90:590-594, 1991.

114. Paganelli R, Ngu JL, Levinsky RJ: Circulating immune complexes in onchocerciasis, *Clin Exp Immunol* 39:570-575, 1980.

115. Poltera AA et al.: Onchocercacidal effects of amocarzine (CGP 6140) in Latin America, *Lancet* 337:583-584, 1991.

116. Prince AM et al.: Onchocerca volvulus: immunization of chimpanzees with x-irradiated third-stage (L3) larvae, *Exp Parasitol* 74:239-250, 1992.

117. Prod'hon J, Boussinesq M, Fobi G et al.: Lutte contre l'onchocercose par ivermectine: résultats d'une campagne de masse au Nord-Cameroun, *Bulletin de l'Organization mondiale de la Santé* 69:443-450, 1991.

118. Prost A: The burden of blindness in adult males in the savanna villages of West Africa exposed to onchocerciasis, *Trans R Soc Trop Med Hyg* 80:525-527, 1986.

119. Prost A, Prescott N: Cost effectiveness of blindness prevention by the onchocerciasis control programme in Upper Volta, *Bull World Health Organ* 62:795-802, 1984.

120. Prost A, Nebout M, Rougemont A: Leptomatous leprosy and onchocerciasis, *Br Med J* 1:589-590, 1979.

121. Remme J et al.: A community trial of ivermectin in the onchocerciasis focus of Asubende, Ghana. I. Effect on the microfilarial reservoir and the transmission of *Onchocerca Volvulus, Trop Med Parasitol* 40:367-374, 1989.

122. Remme J et al.: Ocular onchocerciasis and intensity of infection in the community. I. West African savanna, *Trop Med Parasitol* 40:340-347, 1989.

123. Ridley H: Ocular onchocerciasis including an investigation in the Gold Coast, *Br J Ophthalmol* Suppl 10:22-23, 1945.

124. Robles R: Onchocercose humaine au Guatémala produisant la cécité et "l'érysipèle du littoral" (Erisipela de la costa), *Bull Soc Path Exot* 12:442-460, 1919.

125. Rodger FC: Posterior degenerative lesion of onchocerciasis, *Br J Ophthalmol* 42:21, 1958.

126. Rokeach LA et al.: Characterization of the autoantigen calreticulin, *J Immunol* 147:3031-3039, 1991.

127. Rougemont A et al.: Tuberculin skin tests and BCG vaccination in hyperendemic areas of onchocerciasis, *Lancet* 1:309, 1977.

128. Schulz-Key H: A simple technique to assess the total number of *Onchocerca volvulus* microfilariae in skin snips, *Trop Med Parasitol* 29:51-54, 1978.

129. Schulz-Key H, Albiez EJ, Buttner DW: Isolation of living adult *Onchocerca volvulus* from nodules, *Trop Med Parasitol* 28:428-430, 1977.

130. Semba RD, Day SH, Spencer WH: Conjunctival nodules associated with onchocerciasis, *Arch Ophthalmol* 103:823-824, 1985.

131. Semba RD et al.: Longitudinal study of lesions of the posterior segment in onchocerciasis, *Ophthalmology* 97:1334-1341, 1990.

132. Semba RD et al.: Experimental ocular onchocerciasis in cynomolgus monkeys: IV. Chorioretinitis elicited by *Onchocerca volvulus* microfilariae, *Invest Ophthalmol Vis Sci* 32:1499-1507, 1991.

133. Sisley BM et al.: Associations between clinical disease, circulating antibodies and C1q-binding immune complexes in human onchocerciasis, *Parasite Immunol* 9:447-463, 1987.

134. Soboslay PT et al.: Experimental onchocerciasis in chimpanzees: cell-mediated immune responses, and production of effects of IL-1 and IL-2 with *Onchocerca volvulus* infection, *J Immunol* 147:346-353, 1991.

135. Soboslay PT et al.: Experimental onchocerciasis in chimpanzees: antibody response and antigen recognition after primary infection with *Onchocerca volvulus, Exp Parasitol* 74:367-380, 1992.

136. Soboslay PT et al.: Ivermectin-facilitated immunity in onchocerciasis: reversal of lymphocytopenia, cellular anergy and deficient cytokine production after single treatment, *Clin Exp Immunol* 89:407-413, 1992.

137. Spry CJ: Alterations in blood eosinophil morphology, binding capacity for complexed IgG and kinetics in patients with tropical (filarial) eosinophilia, *Parasite Immunol* 3:1-22, 1981.

138. Steel C et al.: Immunologic responses to repeated ivermectin treatment in patients with onchocerciasis, *J Infect Dis* 164:581-587, 1991.

139. Tamashiro WK, Rao M, Scott AL: Proteolytic cleavage of IgG and other protein substrates by *Dirofilaria immitis* microfilarial enzymes, *J Parasitol* 73:154-194, 1987.

140. Taylor HR: Recent developments in the treatment of onchocerciasis, *Bull World Health Organ* 62:509-515, 1984.

141. Taylor HR: Onchocerciasis. In Tasman W, Jaeger EA editors: *Duane's clinical ophthalmology,* Philadelphia 1992, JB Lippincott.

142. Taylor HR, Greene BM: The status of ivermectin in the treatment of human onchocerciasis, *Am J Trop Med Hyg* 41:460-466, 1989.

143. Taylor HR, Duke BOL, Gonzales C: Simplified dose schedule of ivermectin, *Lancet* 341:50-51, 1993.

144. Taylor HR, Duke BOL, Muñoz B: The selection of communities for treatment of onchocerciasis with ivermectin, *Trop Med* 43:267-270, 1992.

145. Taylor HR et al.: Comparison of the treatment of ocular onchocerciasis with ivermectin and diethylcarbamazine, *Arch Ophthalmol* 104:863-870, 1986.

146. Taylor HR et al.: Ivermectin prophylaxis against experimental *Onchocerca volvulus* infection in chimpanzees, *Am J Trop Med Hyg* 39:86-90, 1988.

147. Taylor HR, et al.: Reliability of skin snips in the diagnosis of onchocerciasis, *Am J Trop Med Hyg* 41:467-471, 1989.

148. Taylor HR et al.: Impact of mass treatment of onchocerciasis with ivermectin on the transmission of infection, *Science* 250:116-118, 1990.

149. Torroella JL: Nota sobre la observación de microfilarias de *Onchocerca* in vivo en el ojo humano, *Anal Soc Méx Oftal Oto-Rino-Lar* 9:87-88, 1931.

150. Trpis M et al.: Effects of mass treatment of a human population with ivermectin on transmission of *Onchocerca volvulus* by *Simulium yahense* in Liberia, West Africa, *Am J Trop Med Hyg* 42:148-156, 1990.

151. Unnasch TR et al.: Isolation and characterization of expression cDNA clones encoding antigens of *Onchocerca volvulus* infective larvae, *J Clin Invest* 82:262-269, 1988.

152. Vagelos RP: Are prescription drug prices high? *Science* 252:1080-1084, 1991.

153. Van der Lelij A et al.: Cell-mediated immunity against human retinal extract, S-Antigen and interphotoreceptor retinoid binding protein in onchocercal chorioretinopathy, *Invest Ophthalmol Vis Sci* 31:2031-2036, 1990.

154. Van der Lelij A et al.: Humoral autoimmune response against S-antigen and IRBP in ocular onchocerciasis, *Invest Ophthalmol Vis Sci* 31:1374-1380, 1990.

155. Vingtain P et al.: Longitudinal study of microfilarial infestation and humoral immune response to filarial and retinal antigens in onchocerciasis patients treated with ivermectin, *Ophthalmic Res* 20:951-958, 1988.

156. Ward DJ et al.: Onchocerciasis and immunity in humans: enhanced T cell responsiveness to parasite antigen in putatively immune individuals, *J Infect Dis* 157:536-543, 1988.

157. Weiss N, Karam M: Humoral immune responses in human onchocerciasis: detection of serum antibodies in early infections, *Ciba Found Symp* 127:180-188, 1987.

158. Weiss N, Speiser F, Hussain R: IgE antibodies in human onchocerciasis: application of a newly developed radioallergosorbent test (RAST), *Acta Trop* (Basel) 38:353-362, 1981.

159. Whitworth JAG et al.: Community-based treatment with ivermectin, *Lancet* 2:97-98, 1988.

160. Whitworth JAG et al.: A field study of the effect of ivermectin on intestinal helminths in man, *Trans R Soc Trop Med Hyg* 85:232-234, 1991.

161. Whitworth JAG et al.: A community trial of ivermectin for onchocerciasis in Sierra Leone: clinical and parasitological responses to four doses given at six-monthly intervals, *Trans R Soc Trop Med Hyg* 86:277-280, 1992.

162. Williams JF et al.: Cell adherence to microfilariae of *Onchocerca volvulus*: a comparative study, *Ciba Found Symp* 126:146-163, 1987.

163. Wong MM, Guest MF, Lavoipierre MJ: *Dirofilaria immitis*: fate and immunogenicity of irradiated infective stage larvae in beagles, *Exp Parasitol* 35:465-474, 1974.

164. World Health Organization: Data on blindness throughout the world, *WHO Chron* 33:275-283, 1979.

165. World Health Organization: Protective immunity and vaccination in onchocerciasis and lymphatic filariasis: report of the 13th SWG on filariasis, *WHO Document TDR/FIL/SWG 87.3,* 1987.

166. World Health Organization: Strategies for ivermectin distribution through primary health care systems, *WHO/PBL/91.24,* Geneva, 1991.

167. World Health Organization Expert Committee: *Epidemiology of onchocerciasis: technical report series 597,* WHO, Geneva, 1976.

168. World Health Organization Expert Committee: *Epidemiology of onchocerciasis: technical report series 752,* WHO, Geneva, 1987.

169. Zahner H, Wegerhof PH: Immunity to Litomosoides carinii in Mastromys natalensis. II. Effects of chemotherapeutically abbreviated and postpatent primary infections on challenges with various stages of the parasite, *Z Parasitenkd* 72:789-804, 1986.

170. Zimmerman PA et al.: *Onchocerca volvulus* DNA probe classification correlates with epidemiologic patterns of blindness, *J Infect Dis* 165:964-968, 1992.

171. Zimmerman PA, Guderian RH, Aruajo E et al.: Polymerase chain reaction based diagnosis of *Onchocerca volvulus* infection: improved detection of patients with onchocerciasis, *J Infect Dis* 169:686-689, 1994.

108 Ophthalmomyiasis

BEN J. GLASGOW

Ophthalmomyiasis is the invasion of ocular tissues by fly larvae (maggots). Ocular involvement occurs in about 5% of all cases of myiasis.[21] Although much general information has accumulated about myiasis,[6,32,40,66,76] this chapter will focus exclusively on the fly larvae that infect the human eye and its adnexa.

Ophthalmomyiasis may be categorized as ophthalmomyiasis externa, if maggots are confined to the external surface of the eye, or ophthalmomyiasis interna, if maggots invade the eye. Ophthalmomyiasis interna may also be subcategorized as anterior or posterior depending on the ocular segment involved. Maggots that invade the orbit usually coinfect the sinuses and produce a serious and distinctive clinical pattern of disease. For the purposes of this chapter, orbital infestation will be considered as a separate category from ophthalmomyiasis interna or externa. Classification of ophthalmomyiasis is based on taxonomy—the family, genus, and species of fly producing the infection. It is important to consider this classification because some families of flies have unique characteristics that lead to prevailing patterns of clinical disease.

PARASITOLOGY

Classification

The fly is classified as a member of the phylum Arthropoda, subphylum Mandibulata, class Insecta, subclass Endopterygota, order Diptera. There are over 85,000 species of flies in the order Diptera.[48]

The major families of flies that cause ophthalmomyiasis are shown in Table 108-1. The flies that most commonly produce ophthalmomyiasis in the United States are *Oestrus ovis* and *Cuterebra* sp.

Life Cycles

The varied life cycles of the flies have implications regarding the predisposing conditions and severity of ophthalmomyiasis. Flies may have obligatory or facultative life cycles. Obligate larvae feed on and require a host to complete their development (Table 108-1). The natural host varies according to the type of fly (e.g., the sheep is the host for *Oestrus ovis;* the cow is the host for *Hypoderma bovis*). Facultative flies such as *Calliphora* sp. live on organic decaying matter.[46,90] They deposit their ova or larvae in rotting organic debris. Ophthalmomyiasis from facultative flies is often associated with conditions of poor hygiene.

The fly life cycle determines the extent of clinical disease. A botfly whose life cycle entails entry into and migration through the tissues of a natural host is more likely to cause ophthalmomyiasis interna in humans than one that normally does not penetrate host tissues. For example, *Hypoderma bovis* normally penetrates the skin of the natural host, migrates long distances, and invades the eye. In contrast, *Gastrophilus* sp. larvae infest the alimentary tract of horses but do not infiltrate other tissues. As the *Gastrophilus* sp. organisms are unable to invade and migrate through tissues, they usually produce only ophthalmomyiasis externa.

Special adaptations for larval deposition of certain flies may be important in determining clinical disease. For example, three species of screwworms, *Cochliomyia hominivorax, Chrysomyia bezziana,* and *Wohlfahrtia magnifica,* cause overwhelming tissue destruction.[5,112] Simultaneous infestation by many maggots is characteristic of these species,[109] in part because these flies alight directly on their targets, depositing a larger number of larvae. In addition, the larvae produce toxins that prevent healing of the initial wound. Other flies are attracted to the same site, with the end result a severe infestation that destroys tissue.

Oestrus ovis. The adults of *Oestrus ovis* are beelike flies whose natural host is the sheep.[82,83,101] *Oestrus ovis* normally deposits first-instar (immature) larvae in the nostrils of sheep. The adults hover over their target and eject a spray of larvae into the flock of sheep.[54] The larvae attach themselves to the mucous membrane of the nose and penetrate the sinuses. The maggots develop into second- and third-instar larvae in the sinuses. When mature, the larvae fall from the

TABLE 108-1 THE MAJOR FLIES RESPONSIBLE FOR OPHTHALMOMYIASIS

Family	Genus and Species	Natural Host*	Number of Documented Cases
Oestridae	*Oestrus ovis*	sheep	~ 100
	Oedemagena tarandi	reindeer	8
	Gedoelstia sp.	antelope	1
	Rhinoestrus purpureus	horse, zebra	1
Cuterebridae	*Cuterebra* sp.	rodent, rabbit	8
	Dermatobia hominis	bird, cow, dog	5
Hypodermatidae	*Hypoderma bovis*	cow	14
Calliphoridae	*Calliphora* sp.	decaying material	1
	Cochliomyia hominivorax	cow, sheep, goat	3
	Chrysomyia sp.	cow, sheep, goat	3
Sarcophagidae	*Wohlfahrtia* sp.	cow, sheep, hog	1
Gasterophilidae	*Gastrophilus* sp.	horse	2

* Obligatory parasites are associated with animal hosts.

nose to the ground and pupate. Adult flies emerge from the pupae after 3 to 6 weeks and may live up to 1 month. Ophthalmomyiasis caused by *Oestrus ovis* is observed in areas in which sheep raising is prominent. The inaccurate aerial projection of larvae by the adult fly on the wing presumably results in the infection of the human eye.[25] Some authors have claimed that human infection is more common if fewer sheep are present in an endemic area.[48] *Oestrus ovis* larvae usually produce ophthalmomyiasis externa, but on rare occasions they may penetrate the anterior chamber, vitreous humor, or subretinal space.[86]

Hypoderma bovis. Females deposit eggs on the hair of cattle legs. Two to three days later, the larvae penetrate the skin and migrate to visceral organs. After 7 to 8 months they molt in the subcutaneous area on the cow's back. A few weeks later the third-stage instar larvae emerges, drops to the soil, and pupates. Ophthalmomyiasis occurs after the larvae have entered the skin and migrated to the eye. There are a number of lines of evidence supporting the notion that *Hypoderma bovis* grows in the human host for several months before invading the eye: (1) *Hypoderma bovis* infections of the eye are associated with a prolonged history of symptoms such as conjunctival irritation; (2) *Hypoderma bovis* infestations often lead to severe ophthalmomyiasis interna and are associated with such ocular complications as retinal detachment; (3) larvae recovered from eye infestations measure up to 8 mm in length,[96] or are identified as second-stage instar larvae.[9,30,33]

Other Flies. *Oedemagena tarandi* (the reindeer warble fly) has a life cycle similar to that of *Hypoderma bovis*. Each of the 3 larval stages lasts about 3 months; thereafter the organism exits the skin.[106] As with *Hypoderma bovis*, *Oedemagena tarandi* larvae migrate long distances. These flies frequently produce ophthalmomyiasis interna.

Cuterebra sp. (rodent botfly) larvae enter the skin of rodents and rabbits through natural openings and migrate to subcutaneous locations to form warblelike tumors. They may parasitize many unnatural hosts, including man, to produce both internal and external ophthalmomyiasis.[42]

Gastrophilus sp. (horse botfly) larva passes most of its natural life cycle in the horse intestine. The large brown adult flies attach their eggs along the hairs of the horse. The larvae are licked off by the horse and pass from the mouth to the stomach. They attach to the stomach wall while growing and eventually pass from the anus to the ground where they pupate. Humans may become infected after grooming horses.[75] *Gastrophilus* sp. larvae do not naturally invade tissue. Hence, the horse botfly larvae usually cause only external ophthalmomyiasis in humans.[74]

The larvae of screwworms may penetrate tissue and elaborate a collagenase that prevents healing. In natural conditions, the wound rarely heals and secondary ovipositions occur because flies are attracted by the odoriferous suppurating lesion.[59] *Cochliomyia hominivorax* locate their host by olfactory and visual stimuli and deposit several hundred eggs on decaying organic matter.[55] In some cases eggs or larvae may be deposited on the eye by contact with the patient's hand. *Wohlfahrtia* sp. and *Chrysomyia bezziana* have life cycles similar to *Cochliomyia* sp., except they deposit larvae rather than eggs. *Chrysomyia bezziana* larvae use sharp mouth hooks and intersegmental spines to penetrate deeply into tissue and anchor themselves.[97] The larvae molt to the second instar in 12 to 18 hours, transform to the third instar after about 60 hours, and remain in tissue 3 to 4 days. They emerge from the host wound and pupate in about 5 to 10 days. Human infection may occur in the orbit and the multiple maggots may cause intense tissue destruction.

The life cycle of *Dermatobia hominis* is noteworthy because a secondary vector such as a tick, fly, or mosquito may also transmit the disease. The female usually lays eggs on the ventral surface of mosquitoes. The eggs are held by a water-insoluble, quick-drying, cementlike substance. The eggs are released by the heat of a warm-blooded animal. The eggs liberate larvae, one of which penetrates the skin or conjunctiva either directly or through the bite of the vector. An inflammatory nodule develops. The organism creates a hole in the skin (respiratory pore) to obtain oxygen.[113] The larvae molt through 3 instars over the next 4 to 18 weeks. They eventually drop to the ground where they actively bury themselves in the soil for 4 to 11 weeks of pupation. The adult flies mate within 1 day and live for only about 1 week. Knowledge of the requirement for a respiratory pore in the life cycle of *Dermatobia hominis* is helpful in attempted removal of the larvae. Occlusion of the pore with ointment may force the organism to emerge to the surface for oxygen, where it can be removed.

Migration of Larvae. Larvae are quite motile. In ophthalmomyiasis interna, vortex veins and long posterior ciliary vessels may act as conduits for larvae; tracks have been observed to overlie these structures.[68] Larvae migrate vigorously, even between the vitreous humor and the anterior chamber.[78] Larvae may leave the eye spontaneously, as retinal tracks may be found without trace of the organism.[39,42,105]

HISTORICAL BACKGROUND

One of the first cases of ophthalmomyiasis was reported in Austria in 1900.[61] *Hypoderma bovis* was identified. During the attempted removal of maggots, the child died from what was termed chloroform narcosis. Most of the cases reported prior to 1933 were described in children, and more than half were identified as *Hypoderma* sp.[31] These cases were generally associated with poor visual outcomes.[26,52,60,85]

In 1933 DeBoe reported a landmark case in which a maggot was observed to traverse the optic nerve into the vitreous chamber.[26] This case is unique because the portal of entry was directly observed.

Ironically, maggots of the Calliphoridae family have been used to debride necrotic wounds, especially in cases of intractable osteomyelitis.[13,17,56]

EPIDEMIOLOGY

Usually myiasis is found in temperate climates. The known geographic distribution of ophthalmomyiasis is dependent on the regional population of flies, the availability of hosts, and the extent to which scientists report the disease. Hence, the geographic depictions in Figs. 108-1 and 108-2 are incomplete, because in some endemic areas active scientists report every case, whereas in other endemic areas, cases are never reported. Despite this shortcoming, the maps demonstrate a surprisingly unique geographic distribution of each form of ophthalmomyiasis.

As sheep are natural hosts for *Oestrus ovis,* the fly is found in geographic locations where herds are seen (Fig. 108-1). *Oestrus ovis* is the most common cause of ophthalmomyiasis.[1-4] It has a worldwide distribution* and is most commonly found in the Middle East,[47,80] Australia,[16,36,72] Africa,[49,54,92,99,117] South America, and North America[14,22,84,100] (Fig. 108-1). Santa Catalina island, off the coast of southern California, is an endemic area for wild sheep and for *Oestrus ovis.*[11,50,53,91] *Rhinoestrus purpurus* is a related member of the Oestridae family and produces ophthalmomyiasis in northern Iran.[81]

Cuterebra sp. is most common in North America, especially on the east coast (Fig. 108-2). Cases of ophthalmomyiasis have been reported in Alabama,[20,27] Maryland,[28] New York,[80] North Carolina,[23] Pennsylvania,[94] and recently in the western United States[42] (Fig. 108-2).

Hypoderma sp. has caused ophthalmomyiasis in Georgia, Iowa, and Maryland (Fig. 108-2).[30,78,87]

Ophthalmomyiasis caused by *Cochliomyia hominivorax* has been described in Texas and Georgia (Fig. 108-2).[19,46] Conjunctival infestation has been attributed to *Cochliomyia hominivorax* in Jamaica.[89]

Dermatobia hominis is found in tropical regions of Central and South America (Fig. 108-1).[21,98,113] No case of ophthalmomyiasis caused by *Dermatobia hominis* has been well documented in the United States. As the fly requires a vector, it is found in regions where mosquitoes are endemic.

Ophthalmomyiasis from the reindeer fly *(Oedemagena tarandi)* is essentially confined to Scandinavia (Fig. 108-1).

There are other rare causes of ophthalmomyiasis such as *Siphunculina funicola* (eye fly).[12] The fly is identified as part of Chloropidae, genus *Siphunculina.* The eye fly produces myiasis in Indonesia, India, Ceylon, and Java.[12]

RISK FACTORS

Location is an obvious risk factor because flies are concentrated in endemic areas (see preceding Epidemiology section). For obligate larvae, the risk factors are also determined by human exposure to the adult flies and the corresponding natural host. Hence, avocation and vocation are important. Shepherds are at greatest risk for *Oestrus ovis;* hikers on Santa Catalina island are also at risk for *Oestrus ovis;* and horse groomers are at risk for *Gastrophilus* sp. infection.

For facultative larvae, the predisposing environmental conditions are important. The presence of rotting organic material provides a source of food for the larvae. Patients with necrotizing wounds in a setting of inadequate hygiene are susceptible to infestation by maggots.[10]

---

*References 37, 51, 63, 64, 65, 71, 79, 88, 104.

World Distribution of Ophthalmomyiasis

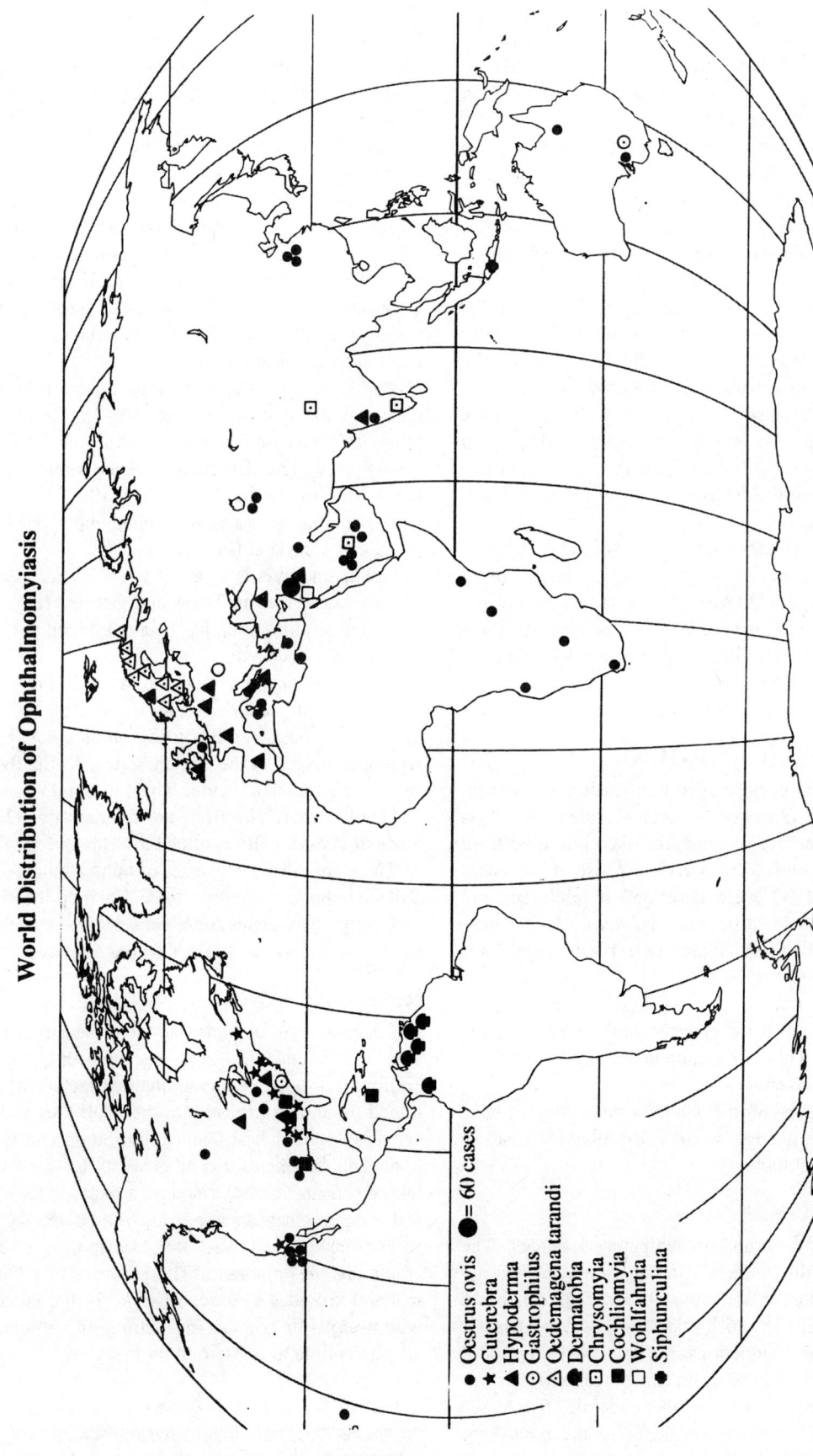

Legend:
- Oestrus ovis ● = 60 cases
- ★ Cuterebra
- ▲ Hypoderma
- ⊙ Gastrophilus
- △ Oedemagena tarandi
- ● Dermatobia
- ▣ Chrysomyia
- ■ Cochliomyia
- ▢ Wohlfahrtia
- ⬟ Siphunculina

Fig. 108-1 Worldwide distribution of the major forms of ophthalmomyiasis. Only reported cases with definite criteria for classification are represented. Very rare species are not shown. (Map adapted and reprinted with permission of Willow Spring Press.)

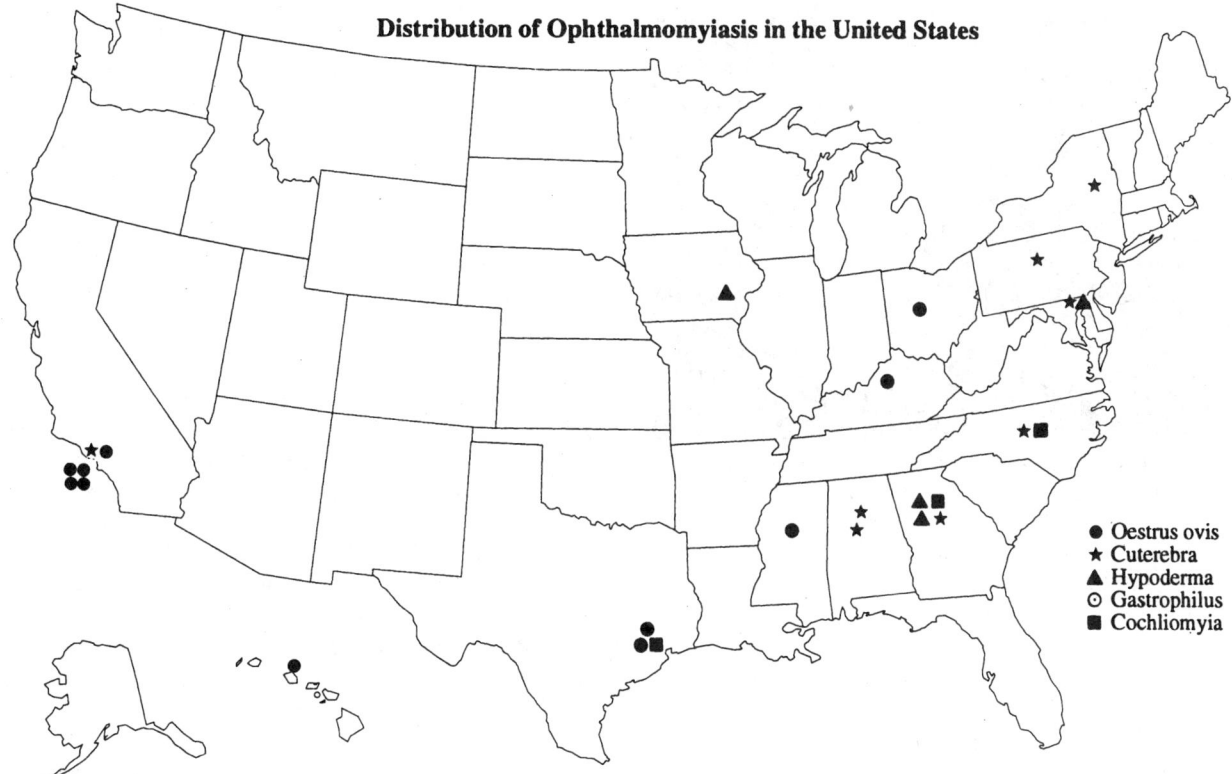

Fig. 108-2   Distribution of ophthalmomyiasis in the United States. Cases shown according to the state in which illness was contracted or reported. (Map adapted and reprinted with permission of Willow Spring Press.)

CLINICAL FEATURES

Ophthalmomyiasis has been documented in human beings age 2 to 88 years of age. The median age is about 25 years. Ophthalmomyiasis is usually unilateral, but bilateral cases have been reported.[68] In some cases bilateral macular disease was presumed to be caused by fly larvae, although maggots were not recovered or pathologically identified.[111] It is uncertain whether these infestations were caused by a single maggot that traversed to the opposite orbit or by multiple maggots.

The clinical features of ophthalmomyiasis are determined by the tissue invaded by the parasite. In ophthalmomyiasis externa, maggots infiltrate the conjunctiva and cornea.[62,80] Larvae may cause conjunctivitis, conjunctival hemorrhage, corneal abrasion, iritis, and subluxation of the lens.[68,106] Direct infiltration of the lens has been reported by an unidentified fly larvae. In this case, the exoskeleton of this organism incited neither inflammation nor cataract after 32 years.[106]

Ophthalmomyiasis interna posterior may cause diminished visual acuity, pain, photophobia, crisscrossing lines (Fig. 108-3),[35,44,103] perception of a copper wire image,[23] vitreous hemorrhage, and tractional retinal detachment.[30]

Myiasis of the orbit is often associated with nose and sinus involvement. Severe tissue destruction is the rule. *Hypoderma* sp. has been reported to cause legal blindness by overwhelming orbital infection caused by multiple maggots. Ocular invasion in these cases was not defined.[70] The most common invaders are *Hypoderma bovis* and *Dermatobia noxialis* or *hominis*.[33] The flies of *Wohlfahrtia magnifica*, *Callitroga marcellaria*, and *Calliphora vomitoria*, however, are capable of penetrating skin and mucous membranes to deposit their eggs directly in these locations. Death may occur in very severe cases.[5,114,115]

Oestrus ovis almost always involves the external part of the eye. All but two of the cases reported have been confined to conjunctiva, fornix, and cornea.[86] One case involved the iris and the second case resulted in posterior disease. The mode of presentation is usually related to a foreign body sensation and the associated inflammatory response produced by the larvae. There are often small conjunctival hemorrhages produced by the claws and spines of the organism. Examination of the conjunctiva usually shows moderate follicular hypertrophy. Visual acuity is often reduced from 20/25 (6/7.5) to 20/100 (6/30) but returns completely in a few days. The diagnosis is predicated on identifying the larva. First-instar larvae are small, less than 1 mm in diameter. The diagnosis requires a careful search; double eversion of the eyelid is often necessary to find maggots in the fornices. Rarely, the inflammatory reaction may be intense and masquerade as bacterial cellulitis.[47] Associated endophthal-

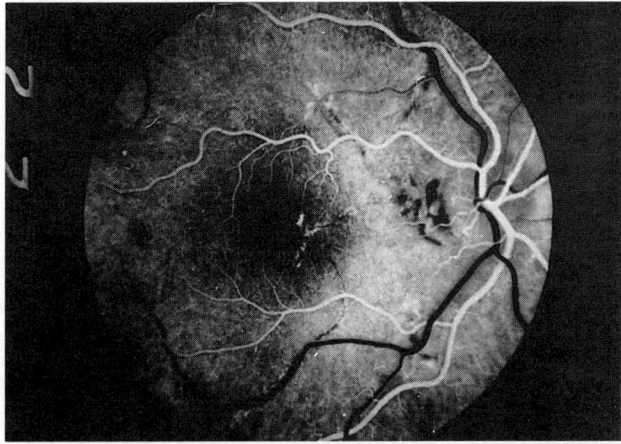

Fig. 108-3 Fluorescein angiogram in arterial-venous phase from the patient shown in Fig. 108-4 shows crisscrossed tracks typical of ophthalmomyiasis interna posterior. (Published with permission from Glasgow BJ, Maggiano JM: *Cuterebra* ophthalmomyiasis, *Am J Ophthalmol* 119:512-513, 1995. Copyright 1995, The Ophthalmic Publishing Company.)

mitis has been reported in a case of *Oestrus ovis* that resulted in blindness.[86] Rarely, *Oestrus ovis* may invade the orbit.[29]

Cuterebrae sp. infestations may present with ophthalmomyiasis externa, ophthalmomyiasis interna, or both (Figs. 108-3 and 108-4). Only eight cases of ophthalmomyiasis caused by *Cuterebrae* sp. have been reported. Four of these cases demonstrated intraocular involvement. Three other cases were confined to the eyelid, and in one case the maggot invaded the corneal stroma.[94] In the cases of ophthalmomyiasis interna posterior, the vision was mildly to severely reduced but improved slightly after treat-

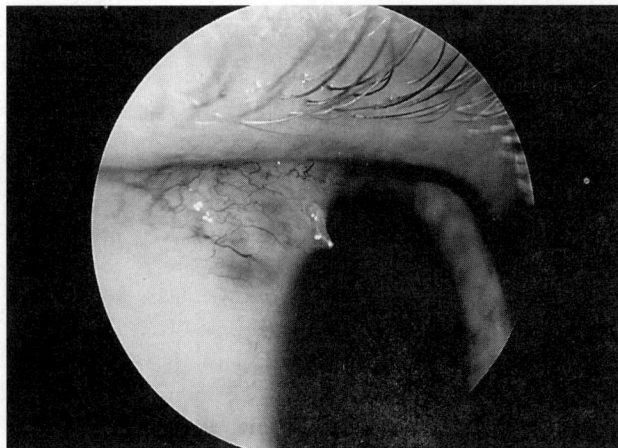

Fig. 108-4 Clinical photograph demonstrates a fly larva in the conjunctiva that proved to be *Cuterebra* sp. (Published with permission from Glasgow BJ, Maggiano JM: *Cuterebra* ophthalmomyiasis, *Am J Ophthalmol* 119:512-513, 1995. Copyright 1995, The Ophthalmic Publishing Company. Photograph courtesy of John Maggiano, MD.)

ment.[23,27,42] An afferent pupillary defect was noted in one case.[23]

Hypoderma bovis is also known as the cattle botfly. *Hypoderma* sp. infection more frequently manifests as ophthalmomyiasis interna; only one case in this survey was solely external. Vision is often severely reduced, and eyes are frequently lost.[45,110] Children are commonly afflicted. *Hypoderma bovis* may reside in the peridural arachnoid space in their natural host, and maggots have been known to infect the human brain.[58]

PATHOLOGY

It is evident from the previous discussion that the type of fly is a clue to the origin, host, severity of involvement, sites of disease, prognosis, and possible prevention of the disease. It is therefore important that suspected fly larvae specimens be examined and classified. In cases of quiescent ophthalmomyiasis interna posterior, in which removal may not be indicated, every effort should be made to classify the maggot with ophthalmic instruments. Larvae that produce external ophthalmomyiasis can often be removed with forceps. Maggots, however, are equipped with intersegmental spines and mouth claws that cling to tissue. Several techniques are available to facilitate removal (see Therapy section). Identification of the maggot may be accomplished with a light microscope. Scanning electron microscopy has been very useful and has been recommended by several authors.[23] Despite these recommendations, the morphologic features of the posterior spiracles and individual spines are within the range of magnification provided by a compound light microscope.[42] The specimen may be fixed in formalin (after appropriate culture), rinsed in buffer, and examined under a dissecting microscope.[42] If the magnification is not sufficient or only a part of the organism is present, the specimen may be cleared in graded glycerol solutions and examined under an elevated coverslip on a glass slide (Fig. 108-5). The organism is placed in a chamber created by 3 to 4

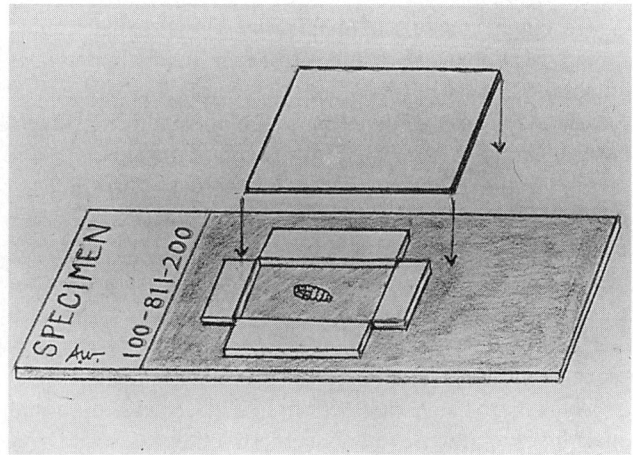

Fig. 108-5 Diagram illustrates method to examine larvae under an elevated coverslip.

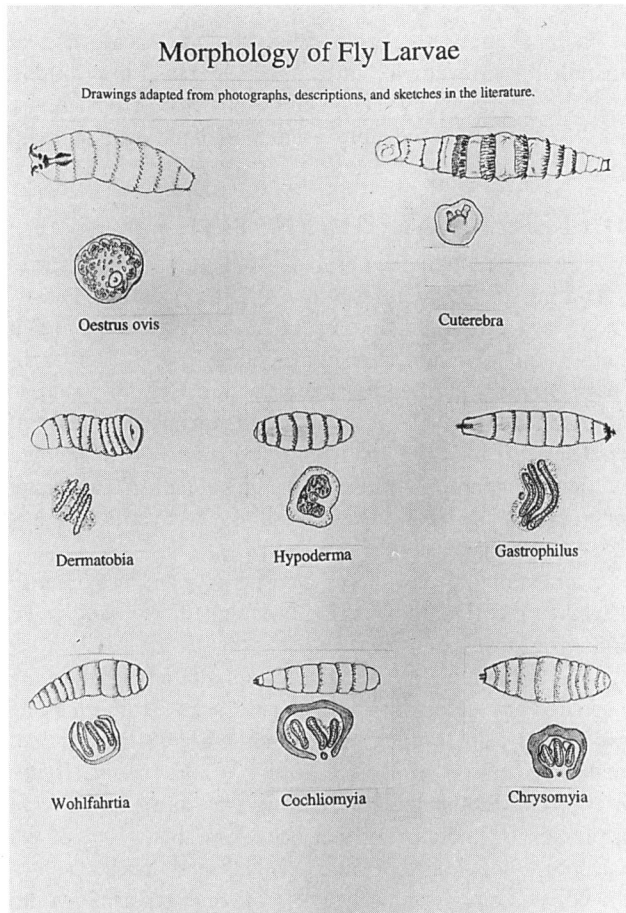

Fig. 108-6 Diagram shows side and posterior views of the common fly larvae that produce ophthalmomyiasis.

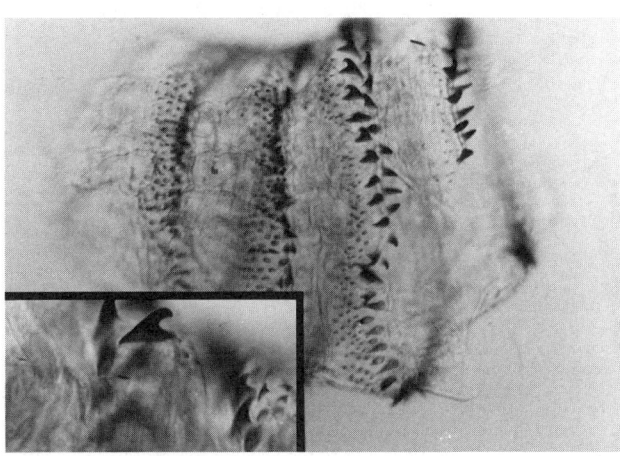

Fig. 108-8 Photomicrograph of *Cuterebra* sp. demonstrating characteristic hooked spines displayed in rows. Specimen was cleared in glycerol and photographed with a compound microscope. (Published with permission from Glasgow BJ, Maggiano JM: *Cuterebra* ophthalmomyiasis, *Am J Ophthalmol* 119:512-513, 1995. Copyright 1995, The Ophthalmic Publishing Company.)

layers of cut cover glass glued to a glass slide. This technique will prevent accidentally crushing the maggot. Photographic documentation is simple with this technique; most pathologists have access to and are familiar with a photomicroscope.

The classification of larvae is accomplished by examination of size, segmentation, anterior and posterior spiracles, mouth hooks, and spines (Fig. 108-6). *Oestrus ovis* shows characteristic oral hooks (Fig. 108-7). In some cases the spines of the thorax are often characteristic and can be used

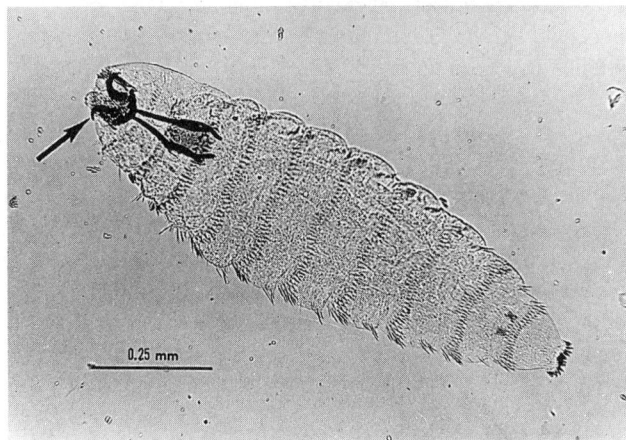

Fig. 108-7 Photomicrograph of *Oestrus ovis* demonstrates large dark oral hooks and a segmented thorax. (Reprinted with the permission of the *Western Journal of Medicine,* Brown, Hitchcock, and Foos: Larval conjunctivitis in California caused by *Oestrus ovis,* 1969, Oct., 111:272-274.)

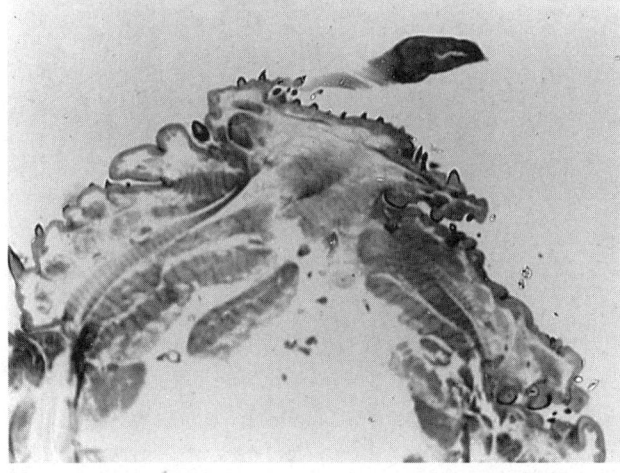

Fig. 108-9 Photomicrograph of a one micron epon embedded section of the *Cuterebra* sp. larva from Figs. 108-3, 108-4, and 108-8 shows developed insect striated muscle and spines. Toluidine blue, original magnification ×40.

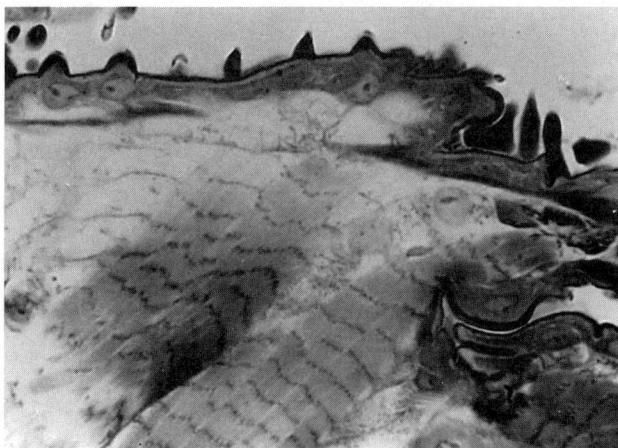

Fig. 108-10 Photomicrograph of the larva from Figs. 108-3, 108-4, 108-8, and 108-9 show a dense cuticle contiguous with spines. Toluidine blue, original magnification ×100.

to identify some maggots (Fig. 108-8). The screwworms contain rows of spines around the anterior edge of each body segment and a body shape that tapers toward the head. This structure resembles a screw.[67]

Three-dimensional visualization of the morphologic structure of the maggot is critical for diagnosis. Histologic sectioning of the organisms is neither necessary nor particularly helpful for identification. Sections show features common to all larvae: well-developed body wall muscle necessary for their accordion-like motility (Fig. 108-9) and a dense cuticle from which the spines emanate (Fig. 108-10 and Fig. 108-11).

In cases undergoing vitrectomy, numerous eosinophils, lymphocytes, plasma cells, and epithelioid cells have been observed.[87]

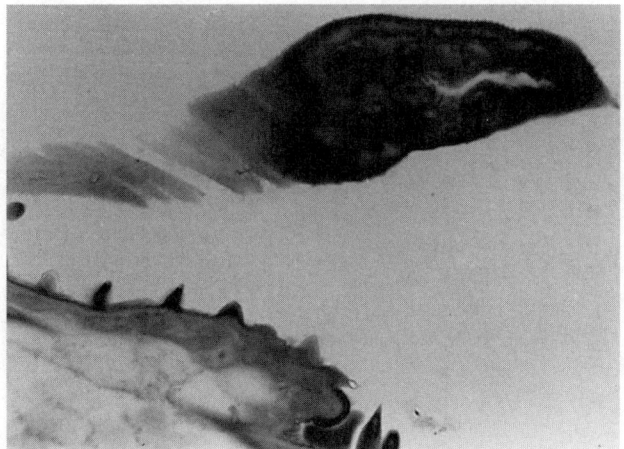

Fig. 108-11 Higher magnification of the larvae in Fig. 108-10 shows the large and small spines. Toluidine blue, original magnification ×400.

COMPLICATIONS

Complications may occur either from the disease or from treatment. For example, vitrectomy may result in proliferative vitreoretinopathy. Death from extensive orbital myiasis has been reported during attempted removal of maggots.[114]

DIFFERENTIAL DIAGNOSIS

The differential diagnosis of ophthalmomyiasis varies according to the manifestations of the disease. Ophthalmomyiasis externa shares clinical features caused by foreign bodies, including irritation, swelling, and erythema. Ophthalmomyiasis is often associated with a local or systemic allergic reaction.[70] Because there is frequently no history of contact with an insect, the local response may be dismissed without an appropriate search for the parasite. Maggots are photophobic, so the fornices should not be overlooked during examination.

Ophthalmomyiasis interna anterior may produce anterior chamber inflammation, cataract, subluxed lens, and/or an inflamed focal iris lesion.

The characteristic findings of ophthalmomyiasis interna posterior are the crisscrossed retinal tracks. Tracks may be produced by other organisms including trematodes,[72,102] nematodes, such as *Toxocara canis*,[43,95] and (rarely) *Histoplasma capsulatum* infection.[68] Linear tracks are also seen in a pigment epitheliopathy that occurs in about 10% of the Chamorro population of Guam. This disease has been associated with amyotrophic lateral sclerosis/Parkinsonism-dementia complex of Guam. Although ophthalmomyiasis was initially suspected, larvae have never been retrieved from the eyes of these patients.[15]

LABORATORY INVESTIGATIONS

Larvae may be cultured for contaminating bacteria by allowing them to crawl over a blood agar plate. In this way, larvae are left intact for classification. Some carry *Streptococcus* sp. group G and may cause cellulitis.[18] *Pseudomonas* sp. has also been cultured.[59]

Geimsa-stained smears of a conjunctival scraping reveal numerous eosinophils.[50] Peripheral eosinophilia has been reported with ophthalmomyiasis, but reports are confounded by the possible presence of other systemic parasites.[108] In other cases associated with eosinophilia, linear tracks were never proved to be caused by a maggot.[30] In addition, in cases of prolonged infection by *Oedemagena tarandi*, eosinophilia was never detected in the course of the disease.[106] Eosinophilia is therefore not a reliable sign of ophthalmomyiasis.

THERAPY

Removal of the larvae (mechanical debridement) remains the mainstay of treatment for ophthalmomyiasis externa. Some clinicians have used .25% physostigmine ophthalmic solution with a combination of antibiotics and corticosteroids. Larvae move rapidly and are difficult to remove. The fact that larvae avoid light and move away from the slit beam of the biomicroscope further complicates their removal.[50] Maggots may be immobilized by the injection of lidocaine in the skin[77] or the topical application of lidocaine and cocaine on the conjunctival surface.[74,109,113]

In the early part of the century, rhino-orbital infections from screwworms were treated with solutions and mixtures of ether, chloroform, turpentine, boracic acid, potassium permanganate, and carbolic acid.[69] Success with these methods has been reported, but use of these substances must be weighed against their toxicity.[114]

Intraocular infestations have required iridectomy, vitrectomy, and retinotomy to remove the maggots. Vitrectomy has been successful in the preservation of vision.[23,87,107] Retinal breaks should be sealed by cryotherapy or laser photocoagulation to prevent rhegmatogenous or tractional retinal detachment.

Argon photocoagulation has been used to destroy subretinal maggots.[34,35] After retrobulbar anesthesia, 10 burns directly on the organism at 400 mW for .1 sec, 200 μm spot size, were successful in killing the larvae. The lack of intraocular inflammation following this treatment was attributed to the intense protein denaturation caused by photocoagulation.[34]

Most authors believe that intraocular dead larvae do not usually incite a significant inflammatory reaction and may be left alone.[57,116] This notion is supported by cases in which dead larvae have been present in the eye for many years without inflammation.[73] An exceptional case with mild iridocyclitis associated with deceased larvae has been documented and successfully managed with corticosteroids and cycloplegics.[75]

PROGNOSIS

The prognosis for patients with ophthalmomyiasis is dependent on the type of larva and the site of infection. *Oestrus ovis* infections are usually external and self-limited. Full recovery of vision is expected. Ophthalmomyiasis interna posterior from *Cuterebrae* sp. and *Hypoderma* sp. may produce severe vision loss if their course includes the macula. Orbital myiasis from screwworms is usually severe and often associated with loss of an eye.[114] Human deaths have been reported from the treatment of overwhelming infestation of the orbit and sinuses.[29]

PREVENTION

Prevention of ophthalmomyiasis is aimed at control of flies. *Gastrophilus* sp. may be controlled by spraying malathion (.12%) on the natural host where larvae are seen.[42] Animals infected with *Dermatobia* sp. and *Hypodermis* sp. have been sprayed with 4% coumaphos. *Oestrus ovis* may be controlled by spraying dichlorvos or fenthion directly into the nostrils of sheep.[41]

Release of sterile males has been effective in controlling facultative flies such as *Cochliomyia hominivorax*.*,[93]

REFERENCES

1. Al-Dabagh M, Al-Mufti N, Shafiq M et al.: A second record from Iraq of human myiasis caused by larvae of the sheep botfly *Oestrus ovis* (L.), *Ann Trop Med Parasitol* 74:73-77, 1980.
2. Anderson WB: Ophthalmomyiasis, *Am J Ophthalmol* 18:699-705, 1935.
3. Archangelsky WN, Braunstein NE: Pathologic anatomy of internal ocular myiasis, *Klin Monatsbl Augenheilkd* 87:340-350, 1931.
4. Avizonis MP: Un cas d'ophthalmomyiasis interna migrans, *Bull Soc Fr Ophtalmol* 48:152-156, 1935.
5. Baruch E, Godel V, Lazar M et al.: Severe external ophthalmomyiasis due to larvae of *Wohlfahrtia* sp., *Isr J Med Sci* 18:815-816, 1982.
6. Beaver PC: *Clinical parasitology,* ed 9, 680-695, Philadelphia, 1984, Lea & Febiger.
7. Better O: Ophthalmomyiasis in the Negev, *Harefuah* 57:7, 1959.
8. Bisley GG: A case of intraocular myiasis in man due to the first stage larva of the oestrid fly *Gedoelstia* spp., *East Afr Med J* 49:768-771, 1972.
9. Blake J: Eye injuries in agriculture, *J Ir Med Assoc* 64:420-423, 1971.
10. Bosniak SL, Schiller JD: Ophthalmomyiasis in an eyelid reconstruction, *Am J Ophthalmol* 109:101-102, 1990.
11. Brown HS Jr., Hitchcock JC Jr, Foos RY: Larval conjunctivitis in California caused by *Oestrus ovis*, *Calif Med* 111:272-274, 1969.
12. Brownstein S, Bernardo AI, Suprapto et al.: Neurofibromatosis with the eye fly *Siphunculina funicola* in an eyelid tumor, *Can J Ophthalmol* 11:261-266, 1976.
13. Bunkis J, Gherini S, Walton RL: Maggot therapy revisited, *West J Med* 142:554-556, 1985.
14. Cameron JA, Shoukrey NM, Al-Garni AA: Conjunctival ophthalmomyiasis caused by the sheep nasal botfly *(Oestrus ovis)*, *Am J Ophthalmol* 112:331-334, 1991.
15. Campbell RJ, Steele JC, Cox TA et al.: Pathologic findings in the retinal pigment epitheliopathy associated with the amyotrophic lateral sclerosis/Parkinsonism-dementia complex of Guam, *Ophthalmology* 100:37-42, 1993.
16. Cher I: External ophthalmomyiasis in Australia, *Med J Aust* 12:335, 1968.
17. Chernin E: Surgical maggots, *South Med J* 79:1143-1145, 1986.
18. Chodosh J, Clarridge J: Ophthalmomyiasis: a review with special reference to *Cochliomyia hominivorax*, *Clin Infect Dis* 14:444-449, 1992.
19. Chodosh J, Clarridge JE, Matoba A: Nosocomial conjunctival ophthalmomyiasis with *Cochliomyia macellaria*, *Am J Ophthalmol* 111:520-521, 1991.
20. Cogen MS, Hays SJ, Dixon JM: Cutaneous myiasis of the eyelid due to *Cuterebra larva*, *JAMA* 258:1795-1796, 1987.
21. Cordero-Moreno R: Etiologic factors in tropical eye diseases, *Am J Ophthalmol* 75:349-364, 1973.
22. Corrin R, Scholten T, Earle J: Ocular myiasis: mobile conjunctival foreign body, *Can Med Assoc J* 132:1291-1292, 1985.
23. Custis PH, Pakalnis VA, Klintworth GK et al.: Posterior internal ophthalmomyiasis: identification of a surgically removed *Cuterebra larva* by scanning electron microscopy, *Ophthalmology* 90:1583-1590, 1983.
24. Dar MS, Amer MB, Dar FK et al.: Ophthalmomyiasis caused by the sheep nasal bot, *Oestrus ovis* (Oestridae) larvae, in the Benghazi area of Eastern Libya, *Trans R Soc Trop Med Hyg* 74:303-306, 1980.

*Acknowledgments—The author is grateful to artist Amy E. Wang and Carol Y. Takami, M.D., for their contributions to this chapter.

25. de Vries LAM, van Bijsterveld OP: Ophthalmooestriasis conjunctivae, *Ophthalmologica* 192:193-197, 1986.

26. DeBoe MP: Dipterous larva passing from the optic nerve into the vitreous chamber, *Arch Ophthalmol* 10:824-825, 1933.

27. Dixon JM, Winkler CH, Nelson JH: Ophthalmomyiasis internal caused by *Cuterebra larva*, *Trans Am Ophthalmol Soc* 67:110-115, 1969.

28. Doxanas MT, Walcher JR, Ludwig RA: Ophthalmomyiasis externa: a case report, *Md Med J* 41:989-991, 1992.

29. Duke-Elder S, editor: *System of ophthalmology*, vol 13, pt 2, 931-932, St Louis, 1974, Mosby.

30. Edwards KM, Meredith TA, Hagler WS et al.: Ophthalmomyiasis interna causing visual loss, *Am J Ophthalmol* 97:605-610, 1984.

31. Eickemeyer KA: Zur Ophthalmomyiasis interna, *Klin Monatsbl Augenheilkd* 130:95-102, 1957.

32. Elgart ML: Flies and myiasis, *Dermatol Clin* 8:237-244, 1990.

33. Fernandez LMG: La Hypodermiasis bovina como parasitos human en españa, *Rev Iber Parasitol* 6:225-238, 1946.

34. Fitzgerald CR, Rubin ML: Intraocular parasite destroyed by photocoagulation, *Arch Ophthalmol* 91:162-164, 1974.

35. Forman AR, Cruess AF, Benson WE: Ophthalmomyiasis treated by argon-laser photocoagulation, *Retina* 4:163-165, 1984.

36. Freney LC, Fox HC: External ophthalmomyiasis caused by *Oestrus ovis* in Queensland, *Med J Aust* 1:310-311, 1974.

37. Gabrielides A, Guiart J: La myose oculaire à *Oestrus ovis* à Constantinople, *Bull Acad Natl Med* 87:253-255, 1922.

38. Garzozi H, Lang Y, Barkay S: External ophthalmomyiasis caused by *Oestrus ovis*, *Isr J Med Sci* 25:162-163, 1989.

39. Gass JD, Lewis RA: Subretinal tracks in ophthalmomyiasis, *Trans Am Acad Ophthalmol Otolaryngol* 81:483-490, 1976.

40. Georgi JR: *Parsitology for veterinarians,* ed 3, Philadelphia, 1980, WB Saunders.

41. Gjotterberg M, Ingemansson SO: Intraocular infestation by the reindeer warble fly larva: an unusual indication for acute vitrectomy, *Br J Ophthalmol* 72:420-423, 1988.

42. Glasgow BJ, Maggiano JM: *Cuterebra* ophthalmomyiasis, *Am J Ophthalmol* 119:512-13, 1995.

43. Goldberg MA, Kazacos KR, Boyce WM et al.: Diffuse unilateral subacute neuroretinitis: morphometric, serologic, and epidemiologic support for Baylisascaris as a causative agent, *Ophthalmology* 100:1695-1701, 1993.

44. Guadalupi U, Pampiglione S: Miasi oculare interna posteriore, *Boll Oculist* 37:17-31, 1958.

45. Haarr M: Ophthalmomyiasis interna posterior, *Acta Ophthalmol (Copenh)* 23:135-141, 1945.

46. Harrison BA, Pearson WG: A case of aural myiasis caused by *Cochliomyia macellaria* (Fabricius), *Mil Med* 133:484-485, 1968.

47. Harvey JT: Sheep botfly: ophthalmomyiasis externa, *Can J Ophthalmol* 21:92-95, 1986.

48. Harwood RF: *Entomology in human and animal health,* ed 7, 296-318, New York, 1979, Macmillan Publishing.

49. Healey MC, Collins RK, Hawkins JA: Ophthalmooestriasis externa, *South Med J* 73:1387-1389, 1980.

50. Hennessy DJ, Sherrill JW, Binder PS: External ophthalmomyiasis caused by *Estrus ovis*, *Am J Ophthalmol* 84:802-805, 1977.

51. Herms WB: Ophthalmomyiasis in man due to *Cephalomyia (Oestrus) ovis* (L.), *J Parasitol* 12:54-56, 1925.

52. Hess C: Severe purulent chorioretinitis with destruction of the retina due to cause not known up to the present time, *Arch Augenh* 74:227-229, 1913.

53. Heyde RRS, Seiff SR, Mucia J: Ophthalmomyiasis externa in California, *West J Med* 144:80-81, 1986.

54. Hoffman BL, Goldsmid JM: Ophthalmomyiasis caused by *Oestrus ovis* L. (Diptera: Oestridae) in Rhodesia, *S Afr Med J* 10:644-645, 1970.

55. Holt GG, Adams TS, Sundet WD: Attraction and ovipositional response of screwworms, *Cochliomyia hominivorax* (Diptera: Calliphoridae) to simulated bovine wounds, *J Med Entomol* 16:248-253, 1979.

56. Horn KL, Cobb AH Jr, Gates GA: Maggot therapy for subacute mastoiditis, *Arch Otolaryngol Head Neck Surg* 102:377-379, 1976.

57. Hunt EW Jr: Unusual case of ophthalmomyiasis interna posterior, *Am J Ophthalmol* 70:978-980, 1970.

58. Kalelioglu M, Aktürk G, Aktürk F et al.: Intracerebral myiasis from *Hypoderma bovis* larva in a child, *J Neurosurg* 71:929-931, 1989.

59. Kersten RC, Shoukrey NM, Tabbara KF: Orbital myiasis, *Ophthalmology* 93:1228-1232, 1986.

60. Kiel E: Über die Erkrankung des Auges durch Fliegenlarven, *Klin Monatsbl Augenheilkd* 124:194-200, 1954.

61. Krautner K: Eine dipterenlarvae in der vorderen Augenkammer, *Atschr Augenh* 4:269-277, 1900.

62. Laborde RP, Kaufman HE, Beyer WB: Intracorneal ophthalmomyiasis, *Arch Ophthalmol* 106:880-881, 1988.

63. Larrouse F: La myiase oculaire a *Oestrus ovis* L. dans la region parisienne, *Bull Soc Pathol Exot* 14:595-601, 1921.

64. Liu YC, Kao CM, Ts'ui M: Conjunctival myiasis due to *Oestrus ovis*: report of three cases, *Chin Med J* 83:190-193, 1964.

65. Loewen U: Ocular myiasis, *Klin Monatsbl Augenheilkd* 169:119-122, 1976.

66. Lukin LG: Human cutaneous myiasis in Brisbane: a prospective study, *Med J Aust* 150:237-240, 1989.

67. Mangan RL, Welch JB: Classification of screwworms (Diptera: Calliphoridae) by larval spine morphology, *J Med Entomol* 27;295-301, 1990.

68. Mason GI: Bilateral ophthalmomyiasis interna, *Am J Ophthalmol* 91:65-70, 1981.

69. Mathur SP, Makhija JM: Invasion of the orbit by maggots, *Br J Ophthalmol* 51:406-407, 1967.

70. Mazzeo V, Ercolani D, Trombetti D et al.: External ophthalmomyiasis: report of four cases, *Int Ophthalmol* 11;73-76, 1987.

71. McDermott S, Schafer MD: Ophthalmomyiasis due to *Oestrus ovis* in South Australia, *Med J Aust* 1:129-130, 1983.

72. McDonald HR, Kazacos KR, Schatz H et al.: Two cases of intraocular infection with Alaria mesocercaria (Trematoda), *Am J Ophthalmol* 117:447-455, 1994.

73. McLane NJ, Howard LJ: Ophthalmomyiasis interna lentis, *South Med J* 83:963-965, 1990.

74. Medownick M, Finkelstein E, Lazarus M et al.: Human external ophthalmomyiasis caused by the horse botfly larva (*Gasterophilus* spp.), *Aust NZ J Ophthalmol* 13:387-390, 1985.

75. Newman PE, Beaver PC, Kozarsky PE et al.: Fly larva adherent to corneal endothelium, *Am J Ophthalmol* 102:211-216, 1986.

76. Norris KR: Myiasis in humans, *Med J Aust* 150:235-237, 1989.

77. Nunzi E, Rongioletti F, Rebora A: Removal of *Dermatobia hominis* larvae (letter), *Arch Dermatol* 122:140, 1986.

78. O'Brien CS, Allen JH: Ophthalmomyiasis interna anterior: report of *Hypoderma* larva in anterior chamber, *Am J Ophthalmol* 22:996-998, 1939.

79. Omar MS, Das AB, Osman NI: External ophthalmomyiasis due to the sheep nostril botfly larva *Oestrus ovis* in Saudi Arabia, *Ann Trop Med Parasitol* 82:221-223, 1988.

80. Perry HD, Donnenfeld ED, Font RL: Intracorneal ophthalmomyiasis, *Am J Ophthalmol* 109:741-742, 1990.

81. Pinkerton AW: Conjunctival myiasis, *JAMA* 215:797, 1971.

82. Pittenger BN: Ocular nyiasis caused by *Oestrus ovis*, *Arch Ophthalmol* 60:1107-1108, 1958.

83. Portchinsky JA: *Oestrus ovis* (L.), its life-history, habits, *Rev Appl Ent Ser B* 1:134-137, 1913.

84. Priour DJ: Ocular myiasis in a Texas sheep shearer, *Tex Med* 76:52-53, 1980.

85. Purtscher A: Entfernung einer lebenden larve von *Hypoderma bovis* aus dem Glaskörper, *Ztschr Augenh* 57:601-605, 1925.

86. Rakusin W: Ocular myiasis interna caused by the sheep nasal bot fly, (*Oestrus ovis*, L.), *S Afr Med J* 44:1155-1157, 1970.

87. Rapoza PA, Michels RG, Semeraro RJ et al.: Vitrectomy for excision of intraocular larva (*Hypoderma* species), *Retina* 6:99-104, 1986.

88. Ratnakar S, Lakshminarayan CA, Ramachandraiah U: Ocular myiasis due to Oestridae, *Indian J Ophthalmol* 22:25-26, 1974.

89. Rawlins SC: Human myiasis in Jamaica, *Trans R Soc Trop Med Hyg* 82:771-772, 1988.

90. Reames MK, Christensen C, Luce EA: The use of maggots in wound debridement, *Ann Plast Surg* 21:388-391, 1988.

91. Reingold WJ, Robin JB, Leipa D et al.: *Oestrus ovis* ophthalmomyiasis externa, *Am J Ophthalmol* 97:7-10, 1984.

92. Richard NF: Ophthalmomyiasis (eye worms): a case report, *J Indiana State Med Assoc* 65:916-917, 1972.

93. Richardson RH, Ellison JR, Averhoff WW: Autocidal control of screwworms in North America, *Science* 215:361-370, 1982.

94. Rodrigues MM, Weiss CB, Muncy DW: Ophthalmomyiasis of the eyelid caused by *Cuterebra* larva, *Am J Ophthalmol* 78:1024-1026, 1974.

95. Rubin ML, Kaufman HE, Tierney JP: An intraretinal nematode, *Trans Am Acad Ophthalmol Otolaryngol* 72:855-866, 1968.

96. Sachs W, Feldman-Muhsam B: A case of intra-ocular myiasis due to *Hypoderma bovis, Isr J Med Sci* 2:778-780, 1966.

97. Sadanand AV: Ocular myiasis due to *Chrysomyia bezziana, J Indian Med Assoc* 59(1):17-18, 1972.

98. Savino DF, Margo CE, McCoy ED et al.: Dermal myiasis of the eyelid, *Ophthalmology* 93:1225-1227, 1986.

99. Schrire L: Conjunctival myiasis due to *Oestrus ovis* L., *S Afr Med J* 42:765-766, 1968.

100. Scott HG: Human myiasis in North America, *Fla Entomol* 47:255-260, 1964.

101. Servicve M: *A guide to medical entomology,* Chapters 12, 13, 28, Hong Kong, 1980, Macmillan Press.

102. Shea M, Maberley AL, Walters J et al.: Intraretinal larval trematode, *Trans Am Acad Ophthalmol Otolaryngol* 77:OP-784-OP-791, 1973.

103. Slusher MM, Holland WD, Weaver RG et al.: Ophthalmomyiasis interna posterior: subretinal tracks and intraocular larvae, *Arch Ophthalmol* 97:885-887, 1979.

104. Smith R: Ophthalmomyiasis in England, *Br J Ophthalmol* 35:242-243, 1950.

105. Steahly LP, Peterson CA: Ophthalmomyiasis, *Ann Ophthalmol* 14:137-139, 1982.

106. Syrdalen P, Nitter T, Mehl R: Ophthalmomyiasis interna posterior: report of case caused by the reindeer warble fly larva and review of previous reported cases, *Br J Ophthalmol* 66:589-593, 1982.

107. Syrdalen P, Stenkula S: Ophthalmomyiasis interna posterior, *Graefes Arch Clin Exp Ophthalmol* 225:103-106, 1987.

108. Tinne JE: The invisible worm, *Lancet* 2:1360, 1970.

109. Verma L, Pakrasi S, Kumar A et al.: External ophthalmomyiasis associated with herpes zoster ophthalmicus, *Can J Ophthalmol* 25:42-43, 1990.

110. Veselý L: K symptomatologii vnútornych oftalmomyiáz, *Cesk Oftalmol* 8:308-313, 1952.

111. Vine AK, Schatz H: Bilateral posterior internal ophthalmomyiasis, *Ann Ophthalmol* 13:1041-1043, 1981.

112. Weizenblatt S: Ophthalmomyiasis externa; larval conjunctivitis in socket, *AMA, Arch Ophthalmol* 50:79-80, 1953.

113. Wilhelmus KR: Myiasis palpebrarum, *Am J Ophthalmol* 101:496-498, 1986.

114. Wood TR, Slight JR: Bilateral orbital myiasis, *Arch Ophthalmol* 84:692-693, 1970.

115. Wright RE: Myiasis with chronic degeneration of cornea, *Am J Ophthalmol* 10:411-412, 1927.

116. Ziemianski MC, Lee KY, Sabates FN: Ophthalmomyiasis interna, *Arch Ophthalmol* 98:1588-1589, 1980.

117. Zumpt F: Ophthalmomyiasis in man, with special reference to the situation in Southern Africa, *S Afr Med J* 37:425-428, 1963.

Index

Page numbers in italics indicate illustrations; *t* indicates tables.